Principles and Practice of
SLEEP MEDICINE

Principles and Practice of
SLEEP MEDICINE

fourth edition

Meir H. Kryger, MD, FRCPC

Professor of Medicine, University of Manitoba
  Faculty of Medicine
Director, Sleep Disorders Center
St. Boniface General Hospital
Winnipeg, Manitoba, Canada

Thomas Roth, PhD

Professor, Department of Psychiatry,
Wayne State University School of Medicine,
Detroit, Michigan
Clinical Professor, Department of Psychiatry
University of Michigan Medical School,
Ann Arbor, Michigan
Division Head, Sleep Disorders and
  Research Center, Henry Ford Hospital
Detroit, Michigan

William C. Dement, MD, PhD

Lowell W. and Josephine Q. Berry Professor of
  Psychiatry and Behavioral Sciences, and
  Director, Sleep Disorders and Research Center
Stanford University School of Medicine
Palo Alto, California

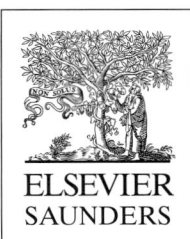

ELSEVIER
SAUNDERS

ELSEVIER
SAUNDERS

The Curtis Center
170 S Independence Mall W 300 E
Philadelphia, PA 19106

Library of Congress Cataloging-in-Publication Data

Principles and practice of sleep medicine / [edited by] Meir H. Kryger, Thomas Roth, William C. Dement.-- 4th ed.
    p. ; cm.
  Includes bibliographical references and index.
  ISBN-13: 978-0-7216-0797-9   ISBN-10: 0-7216-0797-7
    1. Sleep disorders. 2. Sleep. I. Kryger, Meir H. II. Roth, T. (Tom) III. Dement, William C.
  [DNLM: 1. Sleep Disorders. 2. Sleep--physiology. WM 188 P957 2005]
RC547.P75 2005
616.8'498--dc22   2004051416

Acquisitions Editor: Dolores Meloni
Developmental Editor: Marla Sussman
Project Manager: Joan Nikelsky
Design Coordinator: Ellen Zanolle

ISBN-13: 978-0-7216-0797-9
ISBN-10: 0-7216-0797-7

Printed in the United States of America

Last digit is the print number: 9 8 7 6 5 4 3 2

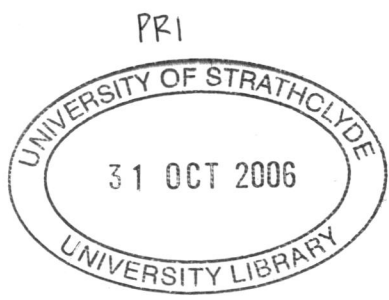

This book is dedicated to our children:

Shelley, Michael, and Steven

Daniel, Adam, Jonathan, and Andrea

Elizabeth, Catherine, and Nicholas

But the tigers come at night,
With their voices soft as thunder,
As they tear your hope apart,
As they turn your dream to shame.

Blessings on him who first invented sleep.—It covers a man all over, thoughts and all, like a cloak.—It is meat for the hungry, drink for the thirsty, heat for the cold, and cold for the hot.—It makes the shepherd equal to the monarch, and the fool to the wise.—There is but one evil in it, and that is that it resembles death, since between a dead man and a sleeping man there is but little difference.

From DON QUIXOTE
by Saavedra M. de Cervantes

"To sleep! To forget!" he said to himself with the serene confidence of a healthy man that if he is tired and sleepy, he will go to sleep at once. And the same instant his head did begin to feel drowsy and he began to drop off into forgetfulness. The waves of the sea of unconsciousness had begun to meet over his head, when all at once—it was as though a violent shock of electricity had passed over him. He started so that he leapt up on the springs of the sofa, and leaning on his arms got in a panic on to his knees. His eyes were wide open as though he had never been asleep. The heaviness in his head and the weariness in his limbs that he had felt a minute before had suddenly gone.

From ANNA KARENINA, Part IV, Chapter XVIII
By Leo Tolstoy

Contributors

Peter Achermann, PhD
Senior Research Associate, Institute of Pharmacology and Toxicology, University of Zurich, Zurich, Switzerland
Sleep Homeostasis and Models of Sleep Regulation

Richard P. Allen, PhD
Assistant Professor, Department of Psychology and Brain Sciences, and Research Associate, Department of Neurology, School of Medicine, Johns Hopkins University, Baltimore, Maryland
Restless Legs Syndrome and Periodic Limb Movements during Sleep

Sonia Ancoli-Israel, PhD
Professor of Psychiatry, University of California, San Diego, School of Medicine; Director, Sleep Disorders Clinic, Department of Psychiatry, Veterans Affairs San Diego Health Care System, San Diego, California
Sleep and Fatigue in Cancer Patients; Actigraphy

Josephine Arendt, BSc, PhD, FRCPath
Professor of Endocrinology (Emeritus), University of Surrey School of Biomedical and Molecular Sciences; Centre for Chronobiology, Neuroendocrinology Section, Guildford, United Kingdom
Sleep Disruption in Jet Lag and Other Circadian Rhythm–Related Disorders

Roseanne Armitage, BSc, MA, PhD
Professor of Psychiatry, University of Michigan Medical School; Director, Sleep and Chronophysiology Laboratory, Ann Arbor, Michigan
The Menstrual Cycle and Circadian Rhythms

Charles W. Atwood, Jr., MD
Assistant Professor of Medicine, University of Pittsburgh School of Medicine; Director, Sleep Disorders Program, VA Pittsburgh Healthcare System; Associate Director, UPMC Sleep Medicine Center, Pittsburgh, Pennsylvania
Medical Therapy for Obstructive Sleep Apnea-Hypopnea Syndrome

Fiona C. Baker, PhD
Post-Doctoral Researcher, Department of Psychology, University of California at Los Angeles, Los Angeles, California; Brain Function Research Unit, School of Physiology, University of the Witwatersrand, Johannesburg, South Africa
The Menstrual Cycle and Circadian Rhythms

Claudio Bassetti, MD
Professor of Neurology, University of Zurich School of Medicine; Vice-Chairman, Department of Neurology, University Hospital Zurich, Zurich, Switzerland
Idiopathic Hypersomnia; Sleep and Stroke

Ali Bassiri, MD
Clinical Instructor, Division of Pulmonary and Critical Care Medicine, Stanford University School of Medicine, Stanford, California; Sleep and Pulmonary Medicine Consultant, Stanford University Medical Center, San Jose, California
Clinical Features and Evaluation of Obstructive Sleep Apnea-Hypopnea Syndrome and the Upper Airway Resistance Syndrome

Maurice D. Baynard, MS
Predoctoral Fellow in Sleep and Chronobiology, Department of Psychiatry, Unit for Experimental Psychiatry, University of Pennsylvania School of Medicine, Philadelphia, Pennsylvania
Chronic Sleep Deprivation

Brock A. Beamer, MD
Assistant Professor of Medicine, Division of Geriatric Medicine and Gerontology, Johns Hopkins University School of Medicine; Medical Staff, Johns Hopkins Bayview Medical Center, Baltimore, Maryland
Sleep Apnea and Metabolic Dysfunction

Ruth M. Benca, MD, PhD
Professor, Department of Psychiatry, University of Wisconsin–Madison School of Medicine, Madison, Wisconsin
Mood Disorders; Sleep and Eating Disorders

Kathleen L. Benson, PhD (*retired*)
Barnstable, Massachusetts;
Formerly, Associate Clinical Professor, Department of Psychiatry and Behavioral Sciences, Stanford University School of Medicine, Stanford, California; Director, Sleep Disorders Program, Veterans Administration Palo Alto Healthcare System, Palo Alto, California
Schizophrenia

Donald L. Bliwise, PhD
Professor of Neurology, Emory University School of Medicine; Director, Program in Sleep, Aging and Chronobiology, Wesley Woods Geriatric Hospital, Atlanta, Georgia
Normal Aging

Bradley F. Boeve, MD
Associate Professor of Neurology, Mayo College of Medicine; Consultant, Department of Neurology and Mayo Sleep Disorders Center, Mayo Clinic, Rochester, Minnesota
Alzheimer's Disease and Other Dementias

Michael H. Bonnet, PhD
Professor, Department of Neurology, Wright State
University School of Medicine; Director, Sleep Laboratory,
Dayton Department of Veterans Affairs Medical Center,
Dayton, Ohio
Acute Sleep Deprivation

Alexander A. Borbély, MD
Professor of Pharmacology, Institute of Pharmacology and
Toxicology, University of Zurich, Zurich,
Switzerland
Sleep Homeostasis and Models of Sleep Regulation

Orfeu M. Buxton, PhD
Instructor in Medicine, Harvard Medical School; Associate
Neuroscientist, Division of Sleep Medicine, Department
of Medicine, Brigham and Women's Hospital, Boston,
Massachusetts
The Human Circadian Timing System and Sleep-Wake Regulation

Daniel J. Buysse, MD
Professor of Psychiatry, University of Pittsburgh
School of Medicine; Director, Clinical Neuroscience
Research Center, and Medical Director, Sleep and
Chronobiology Program, UPMC Presbyterian/Western
Psychiatric Institute and Clinic, Pittsburgh,
Pennsylvania
Clinical Pharmacology of Other Drugs Used as Hypnotics

Christian Cajochen, PhD
Professor (SNF), University of Basel Faculty of Medicine;
Psychiatric University Clinic, Basel, Switzerland
Melatonin in the Regulation of Sleep and Circadian Rhythms

Mary A. Carskadon, PhD
Professor, Psychiatry and Human Behavior, Brown University
Medical School; Director of Sleep and Chronobiology
Research, Bradley Hospital Sleep Research Laboratory,
Providence, Rhode Island
*Normal Human Sleep: An Overview; Daytime Sleepiness
and Alertness; Monitoring and Staging Human Sleep; Evaluating
Sleepiness*

Rosalind Cartwright, PhD
Professor, Rush University Medical College; Affiliated
Scientist, Rush University Medical Center,
Chicago, Illinois
Dreaming as a Mood Regulation System

Michael H. Chase, PhD
Professor Emeritus, Department of Physiology,
University of California at Los Angeles; President/Senior
Researcher, WebSciences International, Los Angeles,
California
Control of Motoneurons during Sleep

Chien Lin Chen, MD
Lecturer, Department of Medicine, Tzu Chi University
School of Medicine; Director, Gastrointestinal Motility
Laboratory, and Attending Physician, Division of
Gastroenterology and Hepatology, Tzu Chi General
Hospital, Hualien, Taiwan
Gastrointestinal Monitoring Techniques

Ronald D. Chervin, MD, MS
Associate Professor, Department of Neurology,
University of Michigan Medical School; Director, Sleep
Disorders Center, University Hospital, Ann Arbor,
Michigan
Use of Clinical Tools and Tests in Sleep Medicine

Camellia P. Clark, MD
Assistant Adjunct Professor of Psychiatry, University of
California, San Diego, School of Medicine La Jolla,
California; Associate Physician, Veterans Medical Research
Foundation, San Diego, California
Medication and Substance Abuse

Michel A. Cramer Bornemann, MD
Staff Physician, Department of Neurology, Department of
Pulmonary & Critical Medicine, Minnesota Regional
Sleep Disorders Center, Hennepin County Medical Center,
Minneapolis, Minnesota; Clinical Scholar Instructor,
Department of Neurology, University of Minnesota School
of Medicine
NREM Sleep–Arousal Parasomnias

Antonio Culebras, MD
Professor, Department of Neurology, Upstate Medical
University, State University of New York at Syracuse;
Consultant, The Sleep Center, Community General
Hospital, Syracuse, New York
Other Neurological Disorders

Charles Andrew Czeisler, PhD, MD
Frank Baldino Jr., PhD, Professor of Sleep Medicine,
Harvard Medical School; Chief, Division of Sleep
Medicine, Department of Medicine,
Brigham and Women's Hospital, Boston,
Massachusetts
*The Human Circadian Timing System and Sleep-Wake
Regulation; Melatonin in the Regulation of Sleep and
Circadian Rhythms*

O'Neill F. D'Cruz, MD
Professor, Departments of Neurology and Pediatrics,
University of North Carolina at Chapel Hill School of
Medicine, Chapel Hill, North Carolina
Cardinal Manifestations of Sleep Disorders

William C. Dement, MD, PhD
Lowell W. and Josephine Q. Berry Professor of
Psychiatry and Behavioral Sciences, and Director,
Sleep Disorders and Research Center, Stanford
University School of Medicine, Palo Alto,
California
*History of Sleep Physiology and Medicine; Normal Human Sleep:
An Overview; Daytime Sleepiness and Alertness; Sleep Medicine,
Public Policy, and Public Health*

Derk-Jan Dijk, PhD
Professor of Sleep and Physiology
Director, Surrey Sleep Research Centre
University of Surrey, Guildford, UK
*Interaction of Sleep Homeostasis and Circadian Rhythmicity:
Dependent or Independent Systems?*

David F. Dinges, PhD
Professor of Psychology, Department of Psychiatry, University of Pennsylvania School of Medicine; Chief, Division of Sleep and Chronobiology, Department of Psychiatry, and Associate Director, Center for Sleep and Respiratory Neurobiology, Philadelphia, Pennsylvania
Chronic Sleep Deprivation; Circadian Rhythms in Sleepiness, Alertness, and Performance; Sleep Medicine, Public Policy, and Public Health

G. William Domhoff, PhD
Research Professor in Psychology, Department of Psychology, University of California, Santa Cruz, California
The Content of Dreams: Methodologic and Theoretical Implications

Neil J. Douglas, MD, DSc, FRCP, FRCPE
Professor of Respiratory and Sleep Medicine, University of Edinburgh; Respiratory Medicine, Royal Infirmary, Edinburgh, United Kingdom
Respiratory Physiology: Control of Ventilation; Asthma and Chronic Obstructive Pulmonary Disease

Sean P. A. Drummond, PhD
Assistant Professor of Psychiatry, University of California, San Diego, School of Medicine, La Jolla; VA San Diego Healthcare System, San Diego, California
Medication and Substance Abuse

Christine Dugovic, PhD
Research Associate Professor, Northwestern University; Center for Sleep and Circadian Biology, Evanston, Illinois
Master Circadian Clock, Master Circadian Rhythm

Jack D. Edinger, PhD
Clinical Professor, Department of Psychiatry and Behavioral Sciences, Duke University School of Medicine; Senior Psychologist, VA Medical Center, Durham, North Carolina
Overview of Insomnia: Definitions, Epidemiology, Differential Diagnosis, and Assessment

Luigi Ferini-Strambi, MD
Associate Professor of Psychology of Sleep and Assistant Professor of Neurology, University Vita-Salute San Raffaele; Director, Sleep Disorders Center, Department of Neurology, San Raffaele Institute, Milan, Italy
Restless Legs Syndrome and Periodic Limb Movements during Sleep

Kathleen A. Ferguson, BSc, MD, FRCP
Associate Professor of Medicine, University of Western Ontario Faculty of Medicine; London Health Sciences Centre, London, Ontario, Canada
Oral Appliances for Sleep-Disordered Breathing

Paul Franken, PhD
Senior Research Scientist, Department of Biological Sciences, Stanford University, Stanford, California
Interaction of Sleep Homeostasis and Circadian Rhythmicity: Dependent or Independent Systems?

Karl A. Franklin, MD, PhD
Associate Professor, Department of Public Health and Clinical Medicine, Umeå University Faculty of Medicine; Consultant Physician, Department of Respiratory Medicine, University Hospital, Umeå, Sweden
Coronary Artery Disease and Obstructive Sleep Apnea

Carlo Franzini, MD
Professor of Human Physiology, Dipartimento di Fisiologia Umana e Generale, University of Bologna Faculty of Medicine, Bologna, Italy
Cardiovascular Physiology: The Peripheral Circulation

Scott Fromherz, MD
Fellow in Sleep Medicine, Stanford Sleep Disorders Clinic, Stanford, California
Narcolepsy: Diagnosis and Management

Charles F. P. George, MD, FRCPC, FCCP, DABSM
Professor of Medicine and Chair, Division of Respirology, University of Western Ontario Faculty of Medicine; Medical Director, Sleep Medicine Clinic and Laboratory, London Health Sciences Centre, London, Ontario, Canada
Neuromuscular Disease; Cognition and Performance in Patients with Obstructive Sleep Apnea

J. Christian Gillin, MD (*deceased*)
Formerly at University of California, San Diego, School of Medicine and VA San Diego Healthcare System, San Diego, California
Medication and Substance Abuse

Paul B. Glovinsky, PhD
Adjunct Professor, Doctoral Program in Experimental Cognition, City University of New York, New York, NY; Clinical Director, Capital Region Sleep/Wake Disorders Center, Albany, New York
Assessment Techniques for Insomnia

Joshua J. Gooley, BA
Program in Neuroscience, Division of Sleep Medicine, Harvard Medical School; Department of Neurology, Beth Israel Deaconess Medical Center, Boston, Massachusetts
Anatomy of the Mammalian Circadian System

Ronald Grunstein, MB, BS, MD, PhD, FRACP
Associate Professor, Department of Medicine, University of Sydney Faculty of Medicine; Head, Sleep Research Group, Woolcock Institute of Medical Research; Head, Centre for Respiratory Failure and Sleep Disorders, Royal Prince Alfred Hospital, Sydney, New South Wales, Australia
Continuous Positive Airway Pressure Treatment for Obstructive Sleep Apnea–Hypopnea Syndrome; Endocrine Disorders

Christian Guilleminault, MD, BiolD
Professor, Sleep Medicine Program, Stanford University School of Medicine; Stanford University Sleep Disorders Clinic, Stanford, California
Narcolepsy: Diagnosis and Management; Idiopathic Hypersomnia; Neuromuscular Disease; Clinical Features and Evaluation of Obstructive Sleep Apnea-Hypopnea Syndrome and the Upper Airway Resistance Syndrome; Surgical Management of Sleep-Disordered Breathing

Ronald M. Harper, PhD
Professor of Neurobiology, Department of Neurology, David Geffen School of Medicine at UCLA, Los Angeles, California
Cardiovascular Physiology: Central and Autonomic Regulation

Jan Hedner, MD, PhD
Professor of Sleep Medicine, Sahlgrenska University Faculty of Medicine; Pulmonary Medicine, Sahlgrenska University Hospital, Göteborg, Sweden
Coronary Artery Disease and Obstructive Sleep Apnea

H. Craig Heller, PhD
Professor, Department of Biological Sciences, Stanford University, Stanford, California
Temperature, Thermoregulation, and Sleep

John H. Herman, PhD
Professor, Department of Psychiatry, University of Texas Southwestern Medical Center at Dallas; Director, Sleep Disorders Center for Children, Children's Medical Center at Dallas, Dallas, Texas
Chronobiologic Monitoring Techniques

Max Hirshkowitz, PhD
Associate Professor, Department of Psychiatry and Department of Medicine, Baylor College of Medicine; Director, Sleep Disorders and Research Center, Michael E. DeBakey Veterans Affairs Medical Center; Clinical Director, Methodist Hospital Diagnostic Sleep Laboratory, VAMC Sleep Center, Houston, Texas
Monitoring Techniques for Evaluating Suspected Sleep-Disordered Breathing; Assessment of Sleep-Related Erections; Evaluating Sleepiness

J. Allan Hobson, MD
Professor of Psychiatry, Harvard Medical School, Boston; Massachusetts Mental Health Center, Boston, Massachusetts
Cardiovascular Physiology: Central and Autonomic Regulation

Victor Hoffstein, MD, PhD
Professor of Medicine, University of Toronto Faculty of Medicine; Staff Respirologist, St. Michael's Hospital, Toronto, Ontario, Canada
Snoring and Upper Airway Resistance

Christer Hublin, MD, PhD
Associate Professor (Docent), Department of Neurology, University of Helsinki School of Medicine; Senior Researcher, Finnish Institute of Occupational Health, Helsinki, Finland
Epidemiology of Sleep Disorders

Shahrokh Javaheri, MD
Professor Emeritus, University of Cincinnati Medical School, Cincinnati, Ohio; Medical Director, Sleepcare Diagnostics, Inc., Mason, OH
Sleep and Cardiovascular Disease: Present and Future; Cardiovascular Effects of Sleep-Related Breathing Disorders; Systemic and Pulmonary Hypertension in Obstructive Sleep Apnea; Heart Failure

Barbara E. Jones, PhD
Professor, Department of Neurology and Neurosurgery, McGill University Faculty of Medicine; Montreal Neurological Institute, Montreal, Quebec, Canada
Basic Mechanisms of Sleep-Wake States

Mark E. Josephson, MD
Herman C. Dana Professor of Medicine, Harvard Medical School; Chief, Cardiovascular Division, and Director, Harvard-Thorndike Electrophysiology Institute and Arrhythmia Service, Beth Israel Deaconess Medical Center, Boston, Massachusetts
Cardiac Arrythmogenesis during Sleep: Mechanisms, Diagnosis, and Therapy

Takafumi Kato, DDS, PhD
Assistant Professor, Institute for Oral Science, Division of Maxillofacial Biology, Matsumoto Dental University, Shiojiri, Nagano, Japan
Sleep Bruxism

Sat Bir Singh Khalsa, PhD
Instructor in Medicine, Harvard Medical School; Associate Neuroscientist, Sleep Disorders Program, Brigham and Women's Hospital, Boston, Massachusetts
The Human Circadian Timing System and Sleep-Wake Regulation

Jean Krieger, MD, PhD
Professor, University Louis Pasteur Faculty of Medicine; Department Head, Service d'Explorations Fonctionnelles du Système Nerveux et de Pathologie du Sommeil, Clinique Neurologique, University of Strasburg Hospitals, Strasburg, France
Respiratory Physiology: Breathing in Normal Subjects

James M. Krueger, PhD
Professor, Department of Veterinary and Comparative Anatomy, Pharmacology and Physiology, Washington State University College of Veterinary Medicine, Pullman, Washington
Host Defense

Meir H. Kryger, MD, FRCPC
Professor of Medicine, University of Manitoba Faculty of Medicine; Director, Sleep Disorders Center, St. Boniface General Hospital, Winnipeg, Manitoba, Canada
Management of Obstructive Sleep Apnea-Hypopnea Syndrome: Overview; Restrictive Lung Disorders; Monitoring Techniques for Evaluating Suspected Sleep-Disordered Breathing

Leszek Kubin, PhD
Research Professor of Physiology, Department of Animal Biology, University of Pennsylvania School of Veterinary Medicine, Philadelphia, Pennsylvania
Respiratory Physiology: Central Neural Control

Samuel T. Kuna, MD
Associate Professor of Medicine, University of Pennsylvania; Chief, Pulmonary, Critical Care and Sleep Section, Philadelphia Veterans Affairs Medical Center, Philadelphia, Pennsylvania
Anatomy and Physiology of Upper Airway Obstruction

Aaron D. Laposky, PhD
Research Assistant Professor, Department of
Neurobiology and Physiology, Northwestern University;
Center for Sleep and Circadian Biology, Evanston,
Illinois
Master Circadian Clock, Master Circadian Rhythm

Gilles J. Lavigne, DMD, MSc, PhD, FRCD
Professor, University of Montreal Faculty of Medicine and
Dentistry; Researcher and Clinician, Hôpital du
Sacré-Coeur de Montréal, Montreal, Quebec,
Canada
Sleep Bruxism; Pain and Sleep

Kathryn A. Lee, PhD, RN
Professor of Nursing, Department of Family Health Care
Nursing; James and Marjorie Livingston Endowed Chair
in Nursing; and Director, Perinatal Nursing Clinical
Specialist Program, University of California, San
Francisco, School of Nursing, San Francisco,
California
Pregnancy and the Postpartum Period

Patrick Leger, MD
Fédération des Pathologies du Sommeil et Institut de
Myologie, Hôpital Pitié Salpêtrière, Paris, France
Noninvasive Ventilation for Chronic Respiratory Failure

Kenneth L. Lichstein, PhD
Professor and Chair, Department of Psychology,
University of Alabama, Tuscaloosa, Alabama
Psychological and Behavioral Treatments for Secondary Insomnias

Alan A. Lowe, DMD, PhD, FRCD(C), FCDS(BC)
Professor and Chair, Division of Orthodontics, University
of British Columbia Faculty of Dentistry, Vancouver,
British Columbia, Canada
Oral Appliances for Sleep-Disordered Breathing

James G. MacFarlane, BSc, PhD
Assistant Professor of Psychiatry, University of Toronto
Faculty of Medicine; Lab Director, Centre for Sleep and
Chronobiology, Toronto, Ontario Canada
Fibromyalgia and Chronic Fatigue Syndromes

Mark W. Mahowald, MD
Professor, Department of Neurology, University of
Minnesota Medical School; Director, Minnesota Regional
Sleep Disorders Center, Hennepin County Medical Center,
Minneapolis, Minnesota
*Epilepsy, Sleep, and Sleep Disorders; NREM Sleep–Arousal
Parasomnias; REM Sleep Parasomnias; Other Parasomnias;
Violent Parasomnias: Forensic Medicine Issues*

Jeannine A. Majde, PhD
Adjunct Professor, Department of Veterinary and
Comparative Anatomy, Pharmacology and Physiology,
Washington State University College of Veterinary
Medicine, Pullman, Washington
Host Defense

Beth A. Malow, MD, MS
Associate Professor, Department of Neurology, Vanderbilt
University School of Medicine; Medical Director,
Vanderbilt Sleep Disorders Laboratory, Nashville,
Tennessee
*Approach to the Patient with Disordered Sleep; Neurologic
Monitoring Techniques*

Christiane Manzini
Research Assistant, University of Montreal Faculty of
Medicine and Dentistry; Center for the Study of Sleep
and Biological Rhythms, Hôpital du Sacré-Coeur de
Montréal, Montreal, Quebec, Canada
Sleep Bruxism

Christina S. McCrae, PhD
Assistant Professor, Center for Gerontological
Studies/Department of Psychology, University of Florida,
Gainesville, Florida
Psychological and Behavioral Treatments for Secondary Insomnias

Dennis McGinty, PhD
Adjunct Professor, Department of Psychology,
UCLA, Los Angeles; Chief of Neurophysiology Research,
Veterans Administration Greater Los Angeles Healthcare
System, Los Angeles, California
Sleep-Promoting Mechanisms in Mammals

Diana McMillan, RN, PhD
Assistant Professor, University of Manitoba Faculty of
Nursing, Winnipeg, Manitoba, Canada
Pain and Sleep

Melanie K. Means, PhD
Staff Psychologist, VA Medical Center, Research Associate,
Department of Psychiatry and Behavioral Sciences,
Duke University Medical Center, Durham,
North Carolina
*Overview of Insomnia: Definitions, Epidemiology, Differential
Diagnosis, and Assessment*

Thomas A. Mellman, MD
Professor and Vice Chair for Research, Department of
Psychiatry, Howard University, Washington, DC
*Dreams and Nightmares in Posttraumatic Stress Disorder;
Anxiety Disorders*

Wallace B. Mendelson, MD
Professor of Psychiatry and Clinical Pharmacology,
University of Chicago, Chicago, Illinois
*Hypnotic Medications: Mechanisms of Action and
Pharmacologic Effects*

Emmanuel Mignot, MD, PhD
Professor of Psychiatry and Behavioral Sciences,
Stanford University School of Medicine; Investigator,
Howard Hughes Medical Institute; Director, Stanford
Center for Narcolepsy, Palo Alto, California
*Wake-Promoting Medications: Basic Mechanisms and
Pharmacology; Narcolepsy: Pharmacology, Pathophysiology,
and Genetics*

Ralph Mistlberger, PhD
Professor, Department of Psychology, Simon Fraser University, Burnaby, British Columbia, Canada
Circadian Rhythms in Mammals: Formal Properties and Environmental Influences

Merrill M. Mitler, MA, PhD
Program Director, National Institute of Neurological Disorders and Stroke, National Institutes of Health, Bethesda, Maryland
Wake-Promoting Medications: Efficacy and Adverse Effects; Evaluating Sleepiness

Murray A. Mittleman, MD, DrPH
Associate Professor of Medicine, Harvard Medical School; Associate Professor of Epidemiology, Harvard School of Public Health, Harvard University; Director, Cardiovascular Epidemiology, Beth Israel Deaconess Medical Center, Boston, Massachusetts
Sleep-Related Cardiac Risk

Karen E. Moe, PhD
Research Associate Professor, Departmernt of Psychiatry and Behavioral Sciences, University of Washington School of Medicine, Seattle, Washington
Menopause

Harvey Moldofsky, MD, Dipl Psych, FRCP(C)
Professor Emeritus, University of Toronto Faculty of Medicine; President and Medical Director, Sleep Disorders Clinic, Centre for Sleep and Chronobiology, Toronto, Ontario, Canada
Fibromyalgia and Chronic Fatigue Syndromes

Timothy H. Monk, PhD, DSc
Professor of Psychiatry, University of Pittsburgh School of Medicine; Director, Human Chronobiology Research Program, Western Psychiatric Institute and Clinic, Pittsburgh, Pennsylvania
Shift Work: Basic Principles

Jacques Montplaisir, MD, PhD, CRCPc
Department of Psychiatry, University of Montreal Faculty of Medicine and Dentistry; Director, Center for the Study of Sleep and Biological Rhythms, Hôpital du Sacré-Coeur de Montréal, Montreal, Quebec, Canada
Restless Legs Syndrome and Periodic Limb Movements during Sleep; Alzheimer's Disease and Other Dementias

Polly Moore, PhD, RPsgT
Visiting Instructor, Psychology Department, University of San Diego; Research Associate, Scripps Clinic Sleep Center, La Jolla, California
Medication and Substance Abuse

Francisco R. Morales, MD
Chairman, Department of Physiology, University of Montevideo Faculty of Medicine, Montevideo, Uruguay; Researcher, Websciences International, Los Angeles, California
Control of Motoneurons during Sleep

Charles M. Morin, PhD
Professor of Psychology, Laval University School of Psychology; Centre d'Etude des Troubles du Sommeil, Centre de Recherche Université Laval/Robert-Giffard, Sainte-Foy, Québec, Canada
Psychological and Behavioral Treatments for Primary Insomnia

Douglas E. Moul, MD, MPH
Assistant Professor of Psychiatry, Department of Psychiatry, University of Pittsburgh School of Medicine; Sleep and Chronobiology Center, Western Psychiatric Institute and Clinic, Pittsburgh, Pennsylvania
Clinical Pharmacology of Other Drugs Used as Hypnotics

Sidney D. Nau, PhD
Research Scientist, Sleep Research Project, Department of Psychology, University of Alabama, Tuscaloosa, Alabama
Psychological and Behavioral Treatments for Secondary Insomnias

Tore A. Nielsen, PhD
Assistant Professor, Department of Psychiatry, University of Montreal Faculty of Medicine and Dentistry; Research Professor, Sleep Study Center, Hôpital du Sacré-Cœur de Montréal, Montreal, Quebec, Canada
Chronobiology of Dreaming; Nightmares and Other Common Dream Disturbances; Disturbed Dreaming in Medical Conditions

Seiji Nishino, MD, PhD
Associate Professor, Department of Psychiatry and Behavioral Sciences, Stanford University School of Medicine, and Associate Director, Center for Narcolepsy, Stanford, California
Wake-Promoting Medications: Basic Mechanisms and Pharmacology

Mary B. O'Malley, MD, PhD
Clinical Instructor, Department of Psychiatry, New York University School of Medicine, New York, New York; Program Director, Sleep Medicine Fellowship, Sleep Disorders Center, Norwalk Hospital, Norwalk, Connecticut
Wake-Promoting Medications: Efficacy and Adverse Effects

John Orem, PhD
Murray Professor of Physiology, Texas Tech University School of Medicine, Lubbock, Texas
Respiratory Physiology: Central Neural Control

William C. Orr, PhD
Clinical Professor of Medicine, Oklahoma University School of Medicine; President and CEO, Lynn Health Science Institute, Oklahoma City, Oklahoma
Gastrointestinal Physiology; Gastrointestinal Disorders; Gastrointestinal Monitoring Techniques

Edward F. Pace-Schott, MS, MA, LMHC
Instructor, Department of Psychiatry, Harvard Medical School; Center for Sleep and Cognition, Beth Israel Deaconess Medical Center, Boston, Massachusetts
The Neurobiology of Dreaming

Pier Luigi Parmeggiani, MD
Emeritus Professor of Physiology, Department of Human and General Physiology, University of Bologna Faculty of Medicine, Bologna, Italy
Physiologic Regulation in Sleep

Barbara L. Parry, MD
Professor of Psychiatry, University of California, San Diego, School of Medicine; Director, Women's Mood Disorders Clinic, La Jolla, California
The Menstrual Cycle and Circadian Rhythms

Markku Partinen, MD, PhD
Associate Professor (Docent), Department of Neurology, University of Helsinki Faculty of Medicine; Chief Physician and Director, Skogby Sleep Clinic, Rinnekoti Research Center, Espoo, Finland
Epidemiology of Sleep Disorders

Yüksel Peker, MD, PhD
Consultant Internist and Pulmonologist, Sleep Unit, Department of Internal Medicine, Skaraborg County Hospital, Lidköping, Sweden
Coronary Artery Disease and Obstructive Sleep Apnea

Rafael Pelayo, MD
Assistant Professor, Department of Psychiatry and Behavioral Science, Stanford University School of Medicine; Stanford Sleep Disorders Clinic, Stanford, California
Idiopathic Hypersomnia

Michael L. Perlis, PhD
Associate Professor, Department of Psychiatry, University of Rochester; Faculty, Neurosciences Program; Director, Sleep and Neurophysiology Research Laboratory, and Director, University of Rochester Behavioral Sleep Medicine Service, Rochester, New York
Etiology and Pathophysiology of Insomnia

Dominique Petit, PhD
Research Assistant, Department of Psychiatry, University of Montreal Faculty of Medicine; Senior Research Assistant, Center for the Study of Sleep and Biological Rhythms, Hôpital du Sacré-Coeur de Montréal, Montreal, Quebec, Canada
Alzheimer's Disease and Other Dementias

Barbara Phillips, MD, MSPH
Professor of Medicine, University of Kentucky College of Medicine; University of Kentucky Hospital, Samaritan Medical Center, Lexington, Kentucky
Management of Obstructive Sleep Apnea-Hypopnea Syndrome: Overview

Wilfred R. Pigeon, PhD
Senior Instructor, Department of Psychiatry, University of Rochester School of Medicine and Dentistry; Research Fellow, University of Rochester Sleep Research and Neurophysiology Laboratory, Rochester, New York
Dreams and Nightmares in Posttraumatic Stress Disorder; Etiology and Pathophysiology of Insomnia

Lawrence H. Pinto, PhD
Professor of Neurobiology, Department of Neurobiology and Physiology, and Associate Director, Center for Functional Genomics, Northwestern University, Evanston, Illinois
Molecular Genetic Basis for Mammalian Circadian Rhythms

Nelson B. Powell, DDS, MD
Adjunct Clinical Professor of Surgery, Department of Otolaryngology–Head and Neck Surgery, and Adjunct Clinical Professor of Sleep Disorders Medicine, Department of Psychiatry and Behavioral Sciences, Stanford University School of Medicine; Stanford University Sleep and Research Center, Stanford, California
Surgical Management of Sleep-Disordered Breathing

Naresh M. Punjabi, MD, PhD
Assistant Professor of Medicine and Epidemiology, Johns Hopkins University School of Medicine; Medical Staff, Division of Pulmonary and Critical Care Medicine, Johns Hopkins Asthma and Allergy Center, Johns Hopkins Hospital, Baltimore, Maryland
Sleep Apnea and Metabolic Dysfunction

Allan Rechtschaffen, PhD
Professor Emeritus, Department of Psychiatry and Department of Psychology, University of Chicago, Chicago, Illinois
Monitoring and Staging Human Sleep

Susan Redline, MD, MPH
Professor of Pediatrics, Medicine, Epidemiology and Biostatistics, Case Western Reserve University School of Medicine; Chief, Division of Clinical Epidemiology, Rainbow Babies and Children's Hospital, Cleveland, Ohio
Genetics of Obstructive Sleep Apnea

Kathryn J. Reid, PhD
Research Assistant Professor, Center for Sleep and Circadian Biology, Northwestern University, Evanston, Illinois
Circadian Disorders of the Sleep-Wake Cycle

John E. Remmers, MD
Professor of Internal Medicine and of Physiology and Biophysics, University of Calgary Faculty of Medicine; Physician, Foothills Hospital, Calgary, Alberta, Canada
Anatomy and Physiology of Upper Airway Obstruction

Robert W. Riley, DDS, MD
Adjunct Clinical Professor of Surgery, Department of Otolaryngology Head and Neck Surgery, and Adjunct Clinical Associate Professor of Sleep Disorders Medicine, Department of Psychiatry and Behavioral Science, Stanford University School of Medicine; Stanford University Sleep and Research Center, Stanford, California
Surgical Management of Sleep-Disordered Breathing

Dominique Robert, MD
Professor of Medicine, University Claude Bernard Faculty of Medicine; Chief, Department of Emergency and Intensive Care Medicine, Hospices Civils de Lyon, Hôpital Edouard Herriot, Lyon, France
Noninvasive Ventilation for Chronic Respiratory Failure

Timothy Roehrs, PhD
Professor, Department of Psychiatry and Behavioral Neuroscience, Wayne State University School of Medicine; Director of Research, Sleep Disorders and Research Center, Henry Ford Hospital, Detroit, Michigan
Daytime Sleepiness and Alertness; Pharmacologic Treatment of Primary Insomnia

Naomi L. Rogers, PhD
Senior Research Fellow, Woolcock Institute of Medical Research, University of Sydney, Sydney, New South Wales, Australia
Chronic Sleep Deprivation

Mark R. Rosekind, PhD
President and Chief Scientist, Alertness Solutions, Cupertino, California
Managing Work Schedules: An Alertness and Safety Perspective

Alan M. Rosenwasser, PhD
Professor of Psychology, University of Maine, Orono, Maine
Physiology of the Mammalian Circadian System

Thomas Roth, PhD
Professor, Department of Psychiatry, Wayne State University School of Medicine, Detroit; Clinical Professor, Department of Psychiatry, University of Michigan Medical School, Ann Arbor; Division Head, Sleep Disorders and Research Center, Henry Ford Hospital, Detroit, Michigan
Daytime Sleepiness and Alertness; Pharmacologic Treatment of Primary Insomnia

Benjamin Rusak, PhD
University Research Professor and Director of Research, Department of Psychiatry, and Professor of Psychology and Pharmacology, Dalhousie University Faculty of Medicine; Director, Chronobiology and Sleep Program, Capital District Health Authority, QEII Health Sciences Centre, Halifax, Nova Scotia, Canada
Circadian Rhythms in Mammals: Formal Properties and Environmental Influences

Mark H. Sanders, MD
Professor of Medicine and Anesthesiology, Director of Research, Pulmonary Sleep Disorders Program, Division of Pulmonary, Allergy and Critical Care Medicine, University of Pittsburgh School of Medicine, Pittsburgh; Montefiore University Hospital, Pittsburgh, Pennsylvania
Medical Therapy for Obstructive Sleep Apnea-Hypopnea Syndrome

Clifford B. Saper, MD, PhD
James Jackson Putnam Professor of Neurology and Neurosciences and Chairman, Department of Neurology, Harvard Medical School; Chairman, Department of Neurology, Beth Israel Deaconess Medical Center, Boston, Massachusetts
Anatomy of the Mammalian Circadian System

Frank A. Scheer, PhD
Research Fellow, Division of Sleep Medicine, Department of Medicine, Harvard Medical School and Brigham and Women's Hospital, Boston, Massachusetts
Melatonin in the Regulation of Sleep and Circadian Rhythms

Carlos H. Schenk, MD
Associate Professor of Psychiatry, University of Minnesota Medical School; Senior Staff Psychiatrist, Minnesota Regional Sleep Disorders Center, Hennepin County Medical Center, Minneapolis, Minnesota
REM Sleep Parasomnias; Violent Parasomnias: Forensic Medicine Issues; Sleep and Eating Disorders

Markus H. Schmidt, MD, PhD
Adjunct Assistant Professor, Department of Neuroscience, The Ohio State University College of Medicine and Public Health, Columbus; Director of Research, Ohio Sleep Medicine and Neuroscience Institute, Dublin, Ohio
Neural Mechanisms of Sleep-Related Penile Erections

Richard J. Schwab, MD
Associate Professor of Medicine, University of Pennsylvania School of Medicine; Co-Medical Director, Penn Sleep Center, Hospital of the University of Pennsylvania, Philadelphia, Pennsylvania
Anatomy and Physiology of Upper Airway Obstruction

Paula K. Schweitzer, PhD
Associate Director, Sleep Medicine and Research Center, Chesterfield, Missouri
Clinical Pharmacology of Other Drugs Used as Hypnotics; Drugs That Disturb Sleep and Wakefulness

Margaret N. Shouse, PhD
Professor IV, Department of Neurobiology, UCLA School of Medicine; Chief, Sleep Disturbance Research, VA Greater Los Angeles Healthcare System, Los Angeles, California
Epilepsy, Sleep, and Sleep Disorders

Jerome M. Siegel, PhD
Professor of Psychiatry and Biobehavioral Sciences, David Geffen School of Medicine at UCLA, Los Angeles; Chief, Neurobiology Research, VA Greater Los Angeles Healthcare System-Sepulveda, North Hills, California
Mammalian Sleep; REM Sleep

Debra J. Skene, BPharm, MSc, PhD
Professor of Neuroendocrinology, University of Surrey School of Biomedical and Molecular Sciences; Centre for Chronobiology, Neuroendocrinology Section, Guildford, United Kingdom
Sleep Disruption in Jet Lag and Other Circadian Rhythm–Related Disorders

Michael T. Smith, PhD
Assistant Professor, Johns Hopkins University School of
Medicine; Clinical Psychologist, Behavioral Medicine
Research Laboratory and Clinic, Johns Hopkins Hospital,
Baltimore, Maryland
Etiology and Pathophysiology of Insomnia

Virend K. Somers, MD, D Phil
Professor of Medicine, Mayo Medical School; Mayo
Clinic, Rochester, Minnesota
Cardiovascular Effects of Sleep-Related Breathing Disorders

Arthur J. Spielman, PhD
Professor, Department of Psychology, The City College
of the City University of New York; Adjunct Clinical
Professor of Psychology in Neuroscience, Weill Medical
College, Cornell University; Associate Director, Center for
Sleep Medicine, New York Presbyterian Hospital; Associate
Director, Center for Sleep Disorders Medicine and Research,
New York Methodist Hospital, New York, New York
Assessment Techniques for Insomnia

Murray B. Stein, MD, MPH, FRCPC
Professor of Psychiatry and Director, Anxiety and
Traumatic Stress Disorders Research and Education
Program, University of California, San Diego, School of
Medicine; Chief, Anxiety and Traumatic Stress Disorders
Programs, VA San Diego Healthcare System, La Jolla,
California
Anxiety Disorders

Mircea Steriade, MD, DSc
Professor of Neuroscience, Laval University Faculty of
Medicine; Department of Anatomy and Physiology,
Quebec, Canada
*Brain Electrical Activity and Sensory Processing during Waking and
Sleep States*

Robert Stickgold, PhD
Assistant Professor of Psychiatry, Harvard Medical School;
Beth Israel-Deaconess Medical Center, Boston Massachusetts
Introduction to Dreams and Their Pathology; Why We Dream

Barbara Stone, BSc, PhD
Principal Consultant, QinetiQ Centre for Human
Sciences, Farnborough, United Kingdom
*Sleep Disruption in Jet Lag and Other Circadian Rhythm–Related
Disorders*

Kristen C. Stone, BA
Clinical Psychology Graduate Student, University of
Memphis, Memphis, Tennessee
Psychological and Behavioral Treatments for Secondary Insomnias

Patrick J. Strollo, Jr., MD
Associate Professor of Medicine, Division of Pulmonary,
Allergy and Critical Care Medicine, Department of
Medicine, University of Pittsburgh School of Medicine;
Medical Director, UPMC Sleep Medicine Center,
Pittsburgh, Pennsylvania
Medical Therapy for Obstructive Sleep Apnea-Hypopnea Syndrome

Ronald Szymusiak, PhD
Adjunct Professor, Department of Medicine, David Geffen
School of Medicine at UCLA, Los Angeles; Research
Scientist, VA Greater Los Angeles Healthcare System,
Los Angeles, California
Sleep-Promoting Mechanisms in Mammals

Jiuan Su Terman, PhD
Research Scientist, New York State Psychiatric Institute,
New York, New York
Light Therapy

Michael Terman, PhD
Professor of Clinical Psychology in Psychiatry, Columbia
University College of Physicians and Surgeons; Director,
Clinical Chronobiology, New York State Psychiatric
Institute, New York, New York
Light Therapy

Michael J. Thorpy, MD
Associate Professor of Neurology, Albert Einstein College
of Medicine of Yeshiva University, Bronx; Director,
Sleep-Wake Disorders Center, Montefiore Medical Center,
Scarsdale, New York
Classification of Sleep Disorders

Irene Tobler, PhD
Professor, Institute of Pharmacology and Toxicology,
University of Zurich, Zurich, Switzerland
Phylogeny of Sleep Regulation; Mammalian Sleep

Claudia Trenkwalder, MD
Professor of Neurology, University of Göttingen School of
Medicine, Göttingen; Medical Director, Paracelsus Elena
Klinik, Special Hospital for Parkinson Disease and
Movement Disorders, Kassel, Germany
Parkinsonism

Fred W. Turek, PhD
Professor, Department of Neurobiology and Physiology,
Northwestern University, and Director, Center for Sleep
and Circadian Biology, Evanston, Illinois
*Master Circadian Clock, Master Circadian Rhythm; Physiology of the
Mammalian Circadian System; Molecular Genetic Basis for
Mammalian Circadian Rhythms; Melatonin in the Regulation of Sleep
and Circadian Rhythms; Introduction: Disorders of Chronobiology*

Eve Van Cauter, PhD
Professor, Department of Medicine, University of Chicago
Pritzker School of Medicine, Chicago, Illinois
Endocrine Physiology

Hans P. A. Van Dongen, MS, PhD
Research Associate Professor of Sleep and Chronobiology
in Psychiatry, University of Pennsylvania School of
Medicine, Philadelphia, Pennsylvania
Circadian Rhythms in Sleepiness, Alertness, and Performance

Bradley V. Vaughn, MD
Associate Professor of Neurology, Department of
Neurology, University of North Carolina at Chapel Hill
School of Medicine, Chapel Hill, North Carolina
Cardinal Manifestations of Sleep Disorders

Richard L. Verrier, PhD
Associate Professor of Medicine, Harvard Medical School; Beth Israel Deaconess Medical Center, Boston, Massachusetts
Cardiovascular Physiology: Central and Autonomic Regulation; Sleep-Related Cardiac Risk; Cardiac Arrythmogenesis during Sleep: Mechanisms, Diagnosis, and Therapy

Martha Hotz Vitaterna, PhD
Research Assistant Professor, Center for Functional Genomics, Northwestern University Center for Functional Genomics, Evanston, Illinois
Molecular Genetic Basis for Mammalian Circadian Rhythms

James K. Walsh, PhD
Adjunct Professor, Department of Psychology, and Clinical Professor, Department of Psychiatry, School of Medicine, Saint Louis University; Executive Director and Senior Scientist, Sleep Medicine and Research Center, St. John's Mercy and St. Luke's Hospitals, Chesterfield, Missouri
Sleep Medicine, Public Policy, and Public Health; Pharmacologic Treatment of Primary Insomnia

Arthur S. Walters, MD
Professor, Department of Neuroscience, Seton Hall University School of Graduate Medical Education, South Orange; Clinical Professor of Neurology, UMDNJ–Robert Wood Johnson Medical School, New Brunswick; New Jersey Neuroscience Institute at JFK Medical Center, Edison, New Jersey
Restless Legs Syndrome and Periodic Limb Movements during Sleep

J. Catesby Ware, PhD
Professor, Departments of Internal Medicine and Psychiatry and Behavioral Sciences, and Chief, Division of Sleep Medicine, Eastern Virginia Medical School; Director, Sleep Disorders Center, Sentara Norfolk General Hospital, Norfolk; Sentara Bayside Hospital, Virginia Beach, Virgina
Assessment of Sleep-Related Erections

Terri E. Weaver, PhD, RN, CS, FAAN
Associate Professor, University of Pennsylvania School of Nursing, Philadelphia, Pennsylvania
Cognition and Performance in Patients with Obstructive Sleep Apnea

John V. Weil, MD
Professor of Medicine (Cardiology), University of Colorado School of Medicine; CVP Research Lab, Denver, Colorado
Respiratory Physiology: Sleep at High Altitudes

David P. White, MD
Gerald E. McGinnis Associate Professor of Medicine, Harvard Medical School; Director, Sleep Disorders Program, Brigham and Women's Hospital, Boston, Massachusetts
Central Sleep Apnea

Amy R. Wolfson, PhD
Associate Professor of Psychology, Department of Psychology, College of the Holy Cross, Worcester, Massachusetts
Pregnancy and the Postpartum Period

Chien-Ming Yang, PhD
Assistant Professor, Department of Psychology, National Chengchi University, Taipei, Taiwan
Assessment Techniques for Insomnia

Terry Young, MS, PhD
Professor of Epidemiology, Department of Population Health Sciences, University of Wisconsin–Madison School of Medicine, Madison, Wisconsin
Systemic and Pulmonary Hypertension in Obstructive Sleep Apnea

Antonio Zadra, PhD
Associate Professor, Department of Psychology, University of Montreal; Dream and Nightmare Laboratory, Hôpital Sacré-Coeur de Montréal, Montreal, Quebec, Canada
Nightmares and Other Common Dream Disturbances

Vincent P. Zarcone, Jr., MD
Emeritus Professor of Psychiatry and Behavioral Science, Stanford University School of Medicine, Stanford; Staff, Sleep Disorders Clinic, Los Altos, California
Schizophrenia

Phyllis C. Zee, MD, PhD
Professor of Neurology and of Neurobiology and Physiology, Northwestern University Feinberg School of Medicine; Director, Sleep Disorders Center, Northwestern Memorial Hospital, Chicago, Illinois
Circadian Disorders of the Sleep-Wake Cycle

Harold Zepelin, PhD
Professor, Clinical Medicine and Psychiatry, Medical College of Ohio, Toledo, Ohio
Mammalian Sleep

Marco Zucconi, MD
Associate Professor of Neurology, Vita-Salute San Raffaele University School of Medicine; Vice-Chief, Sleep Disorders Center, San Raffaele Scientific Institute and Hospital, Milan, Italy
Pain and Sleep

Foreword

There is a time for many words, and there is also a time for sleep.

Homer, The Odyssey

It has been just over 15 years since the publication of the first edition of *Principles and Practice of Sleep Medicine*. That release was noteworthy in that it represented the first comprehensive reference text for the field of sleep medicine – at about half the length of the current edition. Our understanding of the basic mechanisms of sleep and circadian rhythms was immature, and in the clinical arena, important therapeutic interventions such as sleep restriction and nasal continuous positive airway pressure (CPAP) were still relatively new. At the time, there were about 350 certified sleep medicine professionals and 123 accredited sleep centers. The American Board of Sleep Medicine was not yet in existence. Attendance at the Associated Professional Sleep Societies meeting numbered about 700.

Now, as we welcome the arrival of the fourth edition of *Principles and Practice of Sleep Medicine*, it is worth reflecting on the explosive growth that has occurred in our field since that initial 1989 publication. Knowledge of the neurobiological control of sleep-wake and other sleep-related physiology has increased exponentially and, with this, ever-greater opportunities for new, effective diagnostic and treatment strategies emerge. We have seen our field expand to include over 2600 board-certified sleep medicine physicians and 766 accredited programs, while APSS attendance has grown to 5000. Most remarkably, the publication of this edition coincides with the formal recognition of sleep medicine as a medical subspecialty by the Accreditation Council on Graduate Medical Education and the American Board of Medical Specialties. At about the same time, the second edition of the *International Classification of Sleep Disorders* will be released, marking the new strides that have been made in our understanding and classification of sleep disorders.

All of this is by way of pointing out that the field has truly arrived. Our trek from a handful of researchers occupying labs in Chicago, Palo Alto, New York, Lyon, and Bologna to a robust, well-recognized group of health care professionals has been surprisingly brief—a testimony to the remarkable energy, dedication, and foresight of the pioneers on whose shoulders we stand. Despite these successes, however, it remains clear that much more work lies ahead of us than lies behind. Seminal research, such as the identification of the role of hypocretin neurons in sleep-wake control and their dysfunction in narcolepsy, awaits translation into improvements in diagnosis and treatment. More effective therapies, and dissemination strategies for these therapies, must be developed for a host of disorders, particularly insomnia and sleep apnea.

At the heart of all of these challenges lies education. If we are to be successful in continuing the unprecedented development of sleep medicine, we must find the means to expand education about sleep and sleep disorders—from elementary and high schools, through colleges, medical schools, and residencies,

and into the realm of practicing physicians. Such efforts ultimately depend on a reliable, current, and accessible fund of knowledge. *Principles and Practice of Sleep Medicine* has played that central role for students of sleep medicine for almost 2 decades and will doubtless continue to fulfill that function for years to come. Like many great medical reference texts, it has helped to define our field as a specialty of medicine. All of us who have relied so heavily on this text for so many years owe a particular debt of gratitude to Drs. Kryger, Roth, and Dement for their untiring contributions to the growth of sleep medicine.

Michael J. Sateia, MD
President, American Academy of Sleep Medicine
Professor of Psychiatry, Dartmouth Medical School
Lebanon, New Hampshire
Michael.J.Sateia@Dartmouth.edu

On behalf of the National Sleep Foundation, I want to express gratitude for the opportunity to contribute to the foreword to this edition of *Principles and Practice of Sleep Medicine*, and to congratulate Drs. Kryger, Roth, and Dement for compiling this impressive textbook.

In the early 1980s, in a cafeteria on the NIH campus, Bill Dement asked me, "Do you think the body of knowledge in sleep medicine is substantial enough to warrant its own textbook?" After a brief discussion, we agreed that the answer was affirmative. Bill advised me of Meir Kryger's plan to publish a comprehensive medical textbook of the sleep field, *Principles and Practice of Sleep Medicine*, the first edition of which appeared in 1989. Now, over 15 years later, the latest version of the book provides convincing documentation of the exponential expansion in knowledge and the academic vitality of sleep science and sleep medicine.

Principles and Practice of Sleep Medicine serves as an invaluable resource for the sleep medicine practitioner, as well as for clinicians of other specialties, researchers, and students. The data and wisdom within these pages have undoubtedly benefited millions of patients and will continue to do so. Ultimately, however, the knowledge that constitutes a biomedical discipline should be shared, to provide maximum benefit to society. Widespread knowledge dissemination is necessary to increase recognition of sleep disorders, to enhance access to quality care, to prevent sleep-related accidents and injuries, to provide guidance for legislators and regulators, and to save lives. With this in mind, the American Sleep Disorders Association (now the American Academy of Sleep Medicine) established the National Sleep Foundation (NSF) in 1990 as a nonprofit organization dedicated to improving public health and safety by achieving understanding of sleep and sleep disorders. NSF strives to fulfill this mission through public awareness efforts, targeted education programs, support of sleep-related research, and advocacy activities directed toward government agencies, industry, health organizations, academic institutions, and other components of our society.

Our national public health agenda has recently been summarized by United States Surgeon General Richard Carmona, as emphasizing the areas of prevention, preparedness, health disparities, and health literacy.[1] Certainly sleep disorders, sleep deprivation, and chronobiology are components of each of those public health areas, but perhaps most important is our society's relative illiteracy about sleep. In fact, in recognizing the discrepancy between scientific knowledge and its impact on societal practices, Dr. Carmona stated that "sleep disorders probably represent health literacy in our society at its worst." Many of NSF's programs, and the actions of dedicated persons and other organizations, attempt to increase sleep literacy, and some progress is being made. However, for the vast body of knowledge on sleep medicine contained in the pages of *Principles and Practice of Sleep Medicine* to truly affect the health and safety of humankind, an equally tremendous effort is needed to translate science into behavior, practice, and policy. NSF will continue the effort and hopes to work collaboratively with health care professionals and advocates to reduce sleep illiteracy.

James K. Walsh, PhD
Chairman of the Board of Directors
National Sleep Foundation
Washington, DC
walsjk@stlo.smhs.com

I am pleased to have the opportunity to help introduce this fourth edition of the well-established, comprehensive, and highly respected *Principles and Practice of Sleep Medicine*. Sleep physiology and sleep medicine represented a new frontier of knowledge and expertise when the first edition of this book was published in 1989 and were still in their infancy when the second edition was published in 1994. Indeed, the National Center on Sleep Disorders Research (NCSDR) had just been established by the National Institutes of Health (NIH) Revitalization Act of 1993 and was not yet operational.

The legislation further provided for development of a National Sleep Disorders Research Plan. The first Plan, released in 1996, was broad and multidisciplinary and sought to improve health, safety, and productivity by promoting basic, clinical, and applied research on sleep and sleep disorders. The Plan called for developing and strengthening multidisciplinary sleep research to address knowledge gaps, applying new techniques and technologies, and gaining a better understanding of daytime sleepiness and its adverse consequences.

The 2003 National Sleep Disorders Research Plan summarized the new knowledge acquired since the 1996 Plan and concluded with a prioritized listing of recommendations for future research to address gaps in knowledge (http://www.nhlbi.nih.gov/health/prof/sleep/res_plan/index.html). These gaps included the functions of sleep, optimum treatments for sleep disorders, and the nature of human physiology during wakefulness and individual stages of sleep. Both research plans highlighted the current knowledge gaps requiring attention in order to continue improving sleep literacy, to

better understand the health consequences of sleep deprivation and untreated sleep disorders, and to more effectively treat sleep disorder and hence improve health and quality of life. The evolving and expanding content of successive editions of *Principles and Practice of Sleep Medicine* constitutes living proof that dramatic achievements from basic and clinical sleep research have indeed advanced the frontiers of knowledge of sleep neurobiology and sleep disorders.

The third edition of *Principles and Practice of Sleep Medicine*, published in 2000, thus illustrated the increasing scope and interdisciplinary nature of the field since 1994. As a still-maturing research and clinical discipline, however, sleep medicine has again changed greatly since 2000. At NIH, for example, funding for sleep-related research has increased each year and reached $197.1 million in fiscal year 2003—a 170% increase since 1996. This new edition of *Principles and Practice of Sleep Medicine* represents a comprehensive summary of the new frontiers of knowledge achieved since the 2000 edition with regard to normal and abnormal sleep, chronobiology, pharmacology, psychobiology and dreaming, an expanding array of sleep disorders, and the health consequences of untreated sleep disorders. Exemplifying the still-maturing interdisciplinary scope of sleep medicine, this fourth edition includes updated and expanded content for all sections and includes new content for topic areas including neurological and other disorders, endocrine disorders, and women's health.

In summary, one should refer to the 2003 National Sleep Disorders Research Plan for a state-of-the-art summary of present knowledge gaps and prioritized recommendations for future research in sleep and sleep disorders. One should refer to *Principles and Practice of Sleep Medicine*, 4th edition, however, for a comprehensive summary of what we know today about sleep neurobiology and sleep medicine and what we can do today to improve sleep health and quality of life.

Carl E. Hunt, MD
Director, National Center on Sleep Disorders Research
National Heart, Lung, and Blood Institute, NNIH
Bethesda, Maryland
huntc@nhlbi.nih.gov

The release of the fourth edition of *Principles and Practice of Sleep Medicine* is cause not only to applaud this current revision of what has become the benchmark of all texts in the field of sleep, but also to celebrate the recent advances that have been made in sleep research. The study of sleep was still seen as a fringe movement on the edges of mainstream science when a small group of pioneering sleep researchers began meeting together in the early 1960s as the Association for the Psychophysiological Study of Sleep (the original APSS), later to adopt the name Sleep Research Society. Undaunted in their pursuit of a greater understanding of why and how we sleep, these founders of the modern study of sleep established for us a solid foundation of rigorous investigation, sound science, and boundless curiosity. The movement quickly gained momentum, and since that time it has not only achieved a remarkable level of acceptance in both the medical community and the general public but is now its own subspecialty. Among the early pioneers were Drs. Kryger, Roth, and Dement.

This process of maturation and growth has been ultimately dependent upon the vision and foresight of leaders

---

[1]Remarks of Richard H. Carmona, MD, MPH, FACS, United States Surgeon General, at The National Sleep Conference "Frontiers of Knowledge in Sleep & Sleep Disorders: Opportunities for Improving Health and Quality of Life," March 29, 2004, National Institutes of Health, Bethesda, MD.

in the field who have anticipated the challenges and hurdles ahead. It was Dement and his Co-Editor-in-Chief, Dr. Christian Guilleminault,[1] who in the inaugural issue of the journal *SLEEP* wrote, "The message is clear that we are about to witness a dramatic increase in the demand for clinical service and teaching in the area of basic sleep mechanisms and sleep disorders." After recognizing the impending need for more students, scientists, and clinicians to become educated in both the basics and the intricacies of sleep science, the editors of this text chose not to wait for something to be done. Instead, they boldly took upon themselves the challenge of crafting a textbook to fill this void. The result of their efforts was the monumental and historic release of the first edition of *Principles* in 1989.

Now, with the revision of this fourth edition, the editors have continued their commitment to provide the field with the most comprehensive, accurate, and current scientific and clinical data from around the world. They are to be commended for the text's emphasis on the broad body of sleep research, including the presentation of new insights into chronobiology, the relationship between sleep and cardiovascular disorders, the hormonal changes that affect women's health and sleep, and sleep in chronic illness, such as cancer. Every diagnosis and treatment of a sleep disorder is made upon the bedrock of proven research. Much more than simply furthering the study of sleep for the sake of science, this research is used as a basis for improving the health and quality of life of those suffering from disorders of sleep and daytime alertness. This edition will further the editors' goal, stated in the Preface to the first edition, of preventing patients with sleep problems from falling "through the cracks" of the health care system.

While many of the layers of mystery surrounding the nature of sleep have been slowly peeled back through the deliberate process of scientific research, more layers of understanding remain to be unfolded. This text should also serve as motivation for all students of sleep and sleep scientists to strive with even greater purpose to fill in the many gaps of knowledge that remain. As new discoveries and advances are made by future generations of scientists, it will be in part the work of Drs. Kryger, Roth, and Dement, and all the authors that contributed to these volumes, that will be recognized as one of the cornerstones of their achievements.

Sonia Ancoli-Israel, PhD
President, Sleep Research Society
Professor of Psychiatry
University of California San Diego
San Diego, California
sancoliisrael@ucsd.edu

---

[1]Dement W, Guilleminault C. Editorial. *SLEEP* 1978;1:1-2.

Preface to the First Edition

Medical disorders related to sleep are obviously not new. Yet the discipline of sleep disorders medicine is in its infancy. There is a large body of knowledge on which to base the discipline of sleep disorders medicine. We hope that this textbook will play a role in the evolution of this field.

Douglas Hofstadter reviewed how ideas and concepts evolve and are trasmitted.[1] In 1965, Roger Sperry[2] wrote the following: "Ideas cause ideas and help evolve new ideas. They interact with each other and with other mental forces in the same brain, in neighbouring brains, and thanks to global communication, in far distant, foreign brains. And they also interact with the external surroundings to produce *in toto* a burstwise advance in evolution that is far beyond anything to hit the evolutionary scene yet, including the emergence of the living cell." Jacques Monod[3] wrote the following in *Chance and Necessity:* "For a biologist it is tempting to draw a parallel between the evolution of ideas and that of the biosphere. For while the abstract kingdom stands at a yet greater distance above the biosphere than the latter does above the non-living universe, ideas have retained some of the properties of organisms. Like them they tend to perpetuate their structure and to breed; they too can fuse, recombine, segregate their content; indeed they too can evolve, and in this evolution selection must surely play an important role." Hofstadter has called this universe of ideas the ideosphere analogous to the biosphere. The ideosphere's counterpart to the biosphere gene has been called meme by Richard Dawkins.[4] He wrote "just as genes propagate themselves in a gene pool by leaping from body to body via sperm or eggs, so memes propagate themselves in the meme pool by leaping from brain to brain.... If a scientist hears or reads about a good idea, he passes it on to his colleagues and students. He mentions it in his articles and his lectures. If the idea catches on it can be said to propagate itself spreading from brain to brain … memes should be regarded as living structures, not just metaphorically but technically."

Thus, this textbook represents an attempt to summarize the body of science and ideas that up to now has been transmitted verbally, in articles, and in a few more specialized books. The memes in this volume are drawn from a variety of disciplines, including psychology, psychiatry, neurology, pharmacology, internal medicine, pediatrics, and the basic biological sciences. That a field evolves from multidisciplinary roots certainly has precedents in medicine. The field of infectious diseases has its roots in microbiology, and its practitioners are expected to know relevant aspects of internal medicine, surgery, gynecology, and pediatrics. Similarly, oncology has its roots in surgery, hematology, and internal medicine, and its practitioners today must also know virology and molecular biology. Patients with sleep problems in the past have "fallen through the cracks." It is not uncommon to see a patient with classic narcolepsy who has seen 5 to 10 specialists before the diagnosis is finally made. There is a clinical need for physicians to know about sleep and its disorders.

Much of the research in the sleep field has been conducted in animals; thus, a review of sleep mechanisms and the basic sciences relating to sleep must include a certain amount of data obtained in experimental animals. Wherever possible, the focus will be on data obtained from humans. In many cases, these are simply not available.

The book is divided into two parts: The first surveys normal sleep, and the second deals with disorders of sleep. Part I reviews sleep in normal humans, sleep in other species, the anatomy and physiology and pharmacology of sleep mechanisms, chronobiology, and the behavior of various organ systems during sleep. It was felt by the editors that an important aspect of the book should be the basic sciences of sleep. The reason for this focus is that the vast majority of medical schools simply do not teach anything about sleep in their curricula, in either the basic sciences years or the clinical years. Thus, the individual interested in clinical sleep disorders will usually not have the basic science grounding that is necessary for the comprehensive understanding of any clinical field.

The editors also decided that sleep in other species would have to be reviewed in some detail for several reasons. First, much of the research in sleep has been done in animals, and we have learned much about human sleep from such studies. Second, sleep researchers who are likely to do pharmacological or neurophysiological research are likely to use experimental animals. Thus, we thought it was necessary to include a detailed overview of nonhuman sleep.

The second part of the book focuses on the clinical problems most commonly seen by a clinician interested in sleep disorders. No matter what a clinician's primary subspecialty, if he or she is interested in sleep disorders, patients who may have pulmonary problems, psychiatric problems, or neurological problems will be referred. Thus, this section of the book is written by individuals in many medical subspecialties and is aimed at pulmonologists, neurologists, psychiatrists, otolaryngologists, and pediatricians. Some degree of duplication is inevitable in this type of volume. The editors decided that each chapter should be as self-contained as possible, without forcing the reader to go elsewhere in the book from within a chapter.

No field in medicine is static. We are continuously learning to understand new function and dysfunction. The aim of this textbook is to transmit the body of information pertaining to sleep disorders medicine to students, scientists, and clincians concerned with sleep.

Meir H. Kryger, Winnipeg

Thomas Roth, Detroit

William C. Dement, Stanford

1. Hofstadter DR: Chapter 3. *In* Metamagical Themas: Questing for the Essence of Mind and Pattern. Toronto, Bantam Books, 1986.
2. Sperry R: Mind, brain, and humanist values. *In* Platt JR (ed): New Views of the Nature of Man. Chicago, The University of Chicago Press, 1965.
3. Monod J: Chance and Necessity. New York, Vintage Books, 1972.
4. Dawkins R: The Selfish Gene. Oxford, England, Oxford University Press, 1976, p 206.

Preface to the Fourth Edition

There have been dramatic changes in sleep medicine in the past decade. These changes are not simply related to an explosion in the amount of research in sleep disorders but also reflect the fact that sleep has become an issue of public health and personal health, and the names of some sleep disorders have entered the lexicon of everyday conversation. A decade ago, sleep apnea was, in the public's mind, an esoteric medical problem—not any more. Almost everyone knows someone who is being treated for this condition. The public is learning about the dangers of sleep deprivation just as it learned about drunken driving a generation ago.

As new research emerged, the challenge facing the editors was how to organize this new information and present it so that the reader could appreciate both the science and the clinical applications of the science. As *Principles and Practices of Sleep Medicine* enters its fourth edition, users of previous versions will hardly recognize the book. Many changes have been made to make the book more useful. In the previous edition, we experimented by including abstracts at the beginning of the chapters in the first part of the book. Our readers reponded positively and requested that abstracts appear in front of all of the chapters; this has been done. We also asked all of the authors to include at the end of their chapters a "clinical pearl" section in which clinical highlights from the chapter are presented in a few sentences to serve as an important take-home message from the chapter. The illustrations have been redone using color to enhance the graphics; perhaps less noticeable will be that the number of references for most chapters have been reduced, as authors were asked to focus mainly on key references. The role of a book as the only source of references has diminished since most people obtained access to the Internet. Thus, although there are more chapters, the size remains close to that of the previous edition, because there are more pages of text and illustrations and fewer pages of references. Let us know what you think of the changes.

Although the overall organization is the same, with the first part of the book covering the scientific basis of sleep medicine and the second part covering clinical issues, this edition reflects growth in the field. Of the 17 sections in the book, 10 have new section editors. Two new sections have been added: one on women's health and the other on cardiovascular disease.

Knowledge in both of those areas has increased substantially in the past several years.

There are 15 more chapters than in the previous edition, and almost twice as many chapters as in the first edition published just over 15 years ago. Fifty of the chapters deal with new topics or have new authors. Thus, there are many new contributors to the book as well as many new chapters, and some content has been deleted as no longer clinically relevant to the practice of sleep medicine. A textbook is a living structure that grows. It is our intent to respond to clinical needs, new basic science, and clinical research, to meet the needs of our readers and our patients. It is almost exactly 20 years since the editors started to work on the first edition of the book. We are as excited about this edition as we were about the first.

In Memoriam

Two former section editors who were dear to the hearts of many in the sleep medicine community have died. They both played a critical role the development of the first three editions of the book; they will be sorely missed by their friends and colleagues. Dr. Michael Aldrich of the University of Michigan, a neurologist, was a wonderful teacher and a mentor to many. Dr. Chris Gillin of the University of California in San Diego, a psychiatrist, was one of the true giants in the field of sleep and psychiatric disease. Both will be greatly missed by their colleagues and students. They will never be forgotten, because their contributions—of which there were many—are part of the fabric of sleep medicine.

Meir H. Kryger
kryger@sleep.umanitoba.ca
Winnipeg, Manitoba

Thomas Roth
troth1@hfhs.org
Detroit, Michigan

William C. Dement
dement@stanford.edu
Stanford, California

Acknowledgments

It takes several hundred people working together to produce a book the size of *Principles and Practice of Sleep Medicine*. We would like to thank individually all persons who worked on this book, but we cannot, because for many, their important contributions are made "behind the scenes." Included are typists, research assistants, copy editors, illustrators, book designers, proofreaders, and the people involved in the physical production of the book, including its ultimate printing. We want to thank the hundreds of you who have helped put this book together.

We also thank the extraordinary people at Elsevier. We started work on the first edition of *Principles and Practice of Sleep Medicine* about 20 years ago. Individual publishing firms and the publishing industry overall have undergone great changes. The publisher of this book has rotated through about five changes in ownership; for a while, the company was owned by a television network. Throughout these changes, the editorial staff with whom we worked maintained a focused, long-term vision to produce the best textbook possible in the field of sleep medicine. We wish to thank the editorial team over the years that has maintained this vision. These people included Bill Lamsback, Judy Fletcher, Richard Zorab, Cathy Carroll, Todd Hummell, and Dolores Meloni.

Very special thanks must go to Marla Sussman, developmental editor, who received and processed all the chapters and who had the perfect combination of patience, attention to detail, and flexibility, all the while keeping a careful eye on the timetable. Marla had to deal with the diversity of authors and the huge diversity of electronic file formats in order to get the book into production. It was a pleasure working with her.

Joan Nikelsky, project manager, did a splendid job in guiding the transformation of the computerized content of 125 separate chapters through the processes of copyediting, proofreading, production of illustrations, and tracking galley and page proofs. Ellen Zanolle coordinated the beautiful design. All of this labor resulted in the book you now hold in your hands.

The section editors were fantastic. They each chose the authors for their respective sections and were involved in editing the chapters and integrating the content of the chapters into their sections. This was a very difficult task. Many authors produced an absolutely perfect chapter in their first submitted draft. Some chapters had to go through up to 10 revisions until the section editor was satisfied that the chapter could be as good as possible. Two beloved teachers who were also section editors died during the development of the book. Beth Malow took over the section edited by Michael Aldrich. Ruth Benca took responsibility for the section that had been edited by Chris Gillin. A special thanks must go to them for taking over sections under difficult circumstances.

Abbreviations

ACC: anterior cingulate cortex
ACh: acetylcholine
AD-ACL: Activation-Deactivation Adjective Check List
ADHD: attention-deficit/hyperactivity disorder
AHI: apnea-hypopnea index
AMPA: α-amino-3-hydroxy-5-methylisoxazole-4-propionic acid
AMS: acute mountain sickness
ANS: autonomic nervous system
ASPT: advanced sleep phase type
AW: active wakefulness
BA: Brodman area
BAC: blood alcohol content
BF: basal forebrain
BNST: bed nucleus of the stria terminalis
BzRA: benzodiazepine receptor agonist
CAPS: cyclic alternating pattern sequence(s)
CBT: cognitive behavior therapy
CNS: central nervous system
COMT: catechol-*O*-methyltransferase
COPD: chronic obstructive pulmonary disease
CPAP: continuous positive airway pressure
CRP: C-reactive protein
CSN: cold-sensitive neuron
CYP: cytochrome P-450
DA: dopamine
DAT: dopamine transporter
DD: constant dark
DLMO: dim-light melatonin onset
DLPFC: dorsolateral prefrontal cortex
DMD: Duchenne's muscular dystrophy
DSM-IV: *Diagnostic and Statistical Manual of Mental Disorders*, 4th Edition
DSPS: delayed sleep phase syndrome
DSPT: delayed sleep phase type
DTs: delirium tremens
DU: duodenal ulcer
ECG: electrocardiogram/electrocardiographic
EDS: excessive daytime sleepiness
EEG: electroencephalogram, electroencephalographic
EMG: electromyogram
ENS: enteric nervous system
EOG: electrooculogram
EPS: extrapyramidal side effect(s)
EPSP: excitatory postsynaptic potential
ERP: event-related potential
ESS: Epworth Sleepiness Scale
^{18}FDG: 2-deoxy-2-[^{18}F]fluoro-D-glucose
F-DOPA: 6-[^{18}F]fluoro-L-dopa
FEV$_1$: forced expiratory volume in 1 second
fMRI: functional magnetic resonance imaging
FRC: functional residual capacity
GABA: gamma-aminobutyric acid
GAD: generalized anxiety disorder
GAHMS: genioglossus advancement, hyoid myotomy, and suspension

GCD: global cessation of dreaming
GER: gastroesophageal reflux
GHB: gamma-hydroxybutyrate
GHRH: growth hormone–releasing hormone
5-HIAA: 5-hydroxyindole acetic acid
5-HT: 5-hydroxytryptamine (serotonin)
HAPE: high-altitude pulmonary edema
Hcrt: hypocretin
HDI: hypnotic-dependent insomnia
HRV: heart rate variability
HVA: homovanillic acid
ICD: International Classification of Diseases
ICD-9-CM: International Classification of Diseases, 9th Revision, Clinical Modification
ICSD-2: International Classification of Sleep Disorders, Revised
ICV: intracerebroventricular
IGL: intergeniculate leaflet
IL: interleukin
ILD: interstitial lung disease
IPSP: inhibitory postsynaptic potential
kd: kilodalton
KSS: Karolinska Sleepiness Scale
LAUP: laser-assisted uvulopalatoplasty
LD: light–dark
L-dopa: L-dihydroxyphenylalanine, levodopa
LG: lateral geniculate
LL: constant light
LOC: left outer canthus
LPA (or LPOA): lateral preoptic area
LSAT: lowest oxyhemoglobin saturation
LTIH: long-term intermittent hypoxia
MAO: monoamine oxidase
MAOI: monoamine oxidase inhibitor
MDA: methylenedioxyamphetamine
MDMA: methylenedioxymethamphetamine ("ecstasy")
MDP-LD: muramyl dipeptide *N*-actyl-muramyl-L-alanyl-D-isoglutamine
MEG: magnetoencephalography
MI: myocardial infarction
MMC: migrating motor complex
MMO: maxillary and mandibular osteotomy
MnPN: median preoptic nucleus
MNSA: muscle nerve sympathetic vasomotor activity
MPA (or MPOA): medial preoptic area
MPA: medroxyprogesterone acetate
MRA: mandibular repositioning appliance
MSLT: Multiple Sleep Latency Test
MWT: Maintenance of Wakefulness Test
NCSDR: National Center on Sleep Disorders Research
NE: norepinephrine
NET: norepinephrine transporter
NIPPV: nasal intermittent positive-pressure ventilation
NK: natural killer [cell]
NMDA: *N*-methyl-D-aspartate

NO: nitric oxide
NPPV: noninvasive positive-pressure ventilation
NPT: nocturnal penile tumescence
NREM: non–rapid eye movement, non-REM
OCD: obsessive-compulsive disorder
OFC: orbitofrontal cortex
6-OHDA: 6-hydroxydopamine
OHS: obesity–hypoventilation syndrome
OSA: obstructive sleep apnea
OSAHS: obstructive sleep apnea–hypopnea syndrome
OSAS: obstructive sleep apnea syndrome
PCOS: polycystic ovary syndrome
PEEP: positive end-expiratory pressure
PET: positron emission tomography
PGO: ponto-geniculo-occipital [spike]
PIA: pontine inhibitory area
PLMS: periodic limb movements during sleep
    (or PLM)
PMDD: premenstrual dysphoric disorder
POA: preoptic area
POMS: Profile of Mood States
PRC: phase–response curve
PSG: polysomnography, polysomnographic
PTSD: posttraumatic stress disorder
PVN: paraventricular nucleus
PVT: psychomotor vigilance task
QW: quiet wakefulness
RBD: REM sleep behavior disorder
RDI: respiratory disturbance index
REM: rapid eye movement
RFA: radiofrequency ablation
RHT: retinohypothalamic tract
R_{in}: membrane input resistance
RIP: respiratory inductive plethysmography
RLS: restless legs syndrome
RMMA: rhythmic masticatory motor activity
ROC: right outer canthus

ROS: reactive oxygen species (sing. and pl.)
SCN: suprachiasmatic nucleus
SCT: sleep compression therapy
SDB: sleep-disordered breathing
SEMs: small eye movements
SIDS: sudden infant death syndrome
SIT: suggested immobilization test
SND: synucleinopathic disorders
SOREM: sleep-onset REM
SOREMP: sleep-onset REM period
SP: sleep paralysis
SPM: statistical parametric mapping
SRE: sleep-related erection
SRED: sleep-related eating disorder
SRT: sleep restriction therapy
SSEP: somatosensory evoked potential
SSS: Stanford Sleepiness Scale
SSRI: selective serotonin reuptake inhibitor
SWA: slow wave activity
SWS: slow wave sleep
T_a: ambient temperature
TCA: tricyclic antidepressant
THH: terrifying hypnagogic hallucination
TLR: Toll-like receptor
TMJ: temporomandibular joint
TNF: tumor necrosis factor
TRD: tongue-retaining device
UARS: upper airway resistance syndrome
UNS: Ullanlinna Narcolepsy Scale
UPF: uvulopalatal flap
UPPP: uvulopalatopharyngoplasty
VIP: vasoactive intestinal peptide
VLPO: ventrolateral POA (preoptic area)
VMAT2: vascular monoamine transporter-2
VTA: ventral tegmental area
WASO: wake after sleep onset
WSN: warm-sensitive neuron

Contents

Normal Sleep and Its Variations
Timothy Roehrs

1

History of Sleep Physiology and Medicine
William C. Dement

ABSTRACT

There has been great scientific interest in sleep for well over a century, with the discoveries of the electrical activity of the brain, the arousal systems, the circadian system, and rapid eye movement sleep. In spite of these discoveries, the field of sleep medicine has existed for only about 4 decades. The evolution of the field required clinical research, development of clinical services, and changes in society and public policy that recognized the impact of sleep disorders on society. The field is still evolving as new disorders are being discovered, new treatments are being delivered, and basic science is helping us understand the complexity of sleep and its disorders.

Interest in sleep and dreams has existed since the dawn of history. Perhaps only love and human conflict have received more attention from poets and writers. Some of the world's greatest thinkers, such as Aristotle, Hippocrates, Freud, and Pavlov, have attempted to explain the physiologic and psychological bases of sleep and dreaming. However, it is not the purpose of this chapter to present a scholarly review across the ages about prehistoric, biblical, and Elizabethan thoughts and concerns regarding sleep or the history of man's enthrallment with dreams and nightmares. This has been reviewed by others.[1] What is emphasized here for the benefit of the student and the practitioner is the evolution of the key concepts that define and differentiate sleep research and sleep medicine, crucial discoveries and developments in the formative years of the field, and those principles and practices that have stood the test of time.

SLEEP AS A PASSIVE STATE

"Sleep is the intermediate state between wakefulness and death; wakefulness being regarded as the active state of all the animal and intellectual functions, and death as that of their total suspension."[2]

The foregoing is the first sentence of *The Philosophy of Sleep,* a book by Robert MacNish, a member of the faculty of physicians and surgeons of Glasgow; the first American edition was published in 1834 and the Scottish edition somewhat earlier. This sentence exemplifies the overarching historical dichotomy of sleep research and sleep medicine—sleep as a passive process versus sleep as an active process. Until the discovery of rapid eye movements and the duality of sleep, sleep was universally regarded as an inactive state of the brain; with one or two exceptions, most thinkers regarded sleep as the inevitable result of reduced sensory input with the consequent diminishment of brain activity and the occurrence of sleep. Waking up and being awake were considered a reversal of this process, mainly as a result of bombardment of the brain by stimulation from the environment. No real distinction was seen between sleep and other states of quiescence such as coma, stupor, intoxication, hypnosis, anesthesia, and hibernation.

The passive to active historical dichotomy is also given great weight by the modern investigator J. Allan Hobson.[3] In the first sentence of his book *Sleep,* published in 1989, he stated that "more has been learned about sleep in the past 60 years than in the preceding 6,000." He went on, "In this short period of time, researchers have discovered that sleep is a dynamic behavior. Not simply the absence of waking, sleep is a special activity of the brain, controlled by elaborate and precise mechanisms."

Dreams and dreaming were regarded as transient, fleeting interruptions of this quiescent state. Because dreams seem to occur spontaneously and sometimes in response to environmental stimulation (e.g., the well-known alarm clock dreams), the notion of a stimulus that produces the dream was generalized by postulating internal stimulation from the digestive tract or some other internal source. Some anthropologists have suggested that notions of spirituality and the soul arose from primitive peoples' need to explain how their essence could leave the body temporarily at night in a dream and permanently at death.

In addition to the mere reduction of stimulation, a host of less popular theories were espoused to account for the onset of sleep. Vascular theories were proposed from the notion that the blood left the brain to accumulate in the digestive tract, and from the opposite idea—that sleep was due to pressure on the brain by blood. Around the end of the 19th century, various versions of a "hypnotoxin" theory were formulated in which fatigue products (toxins and the like) were accumulated during the day, finally causing sleep, during which they were gradually eliminated. It had, of course, been observed since biblical times that alcohol would induce a sleeplike state. More recently, these observations included other compounds such as opium. Finally, it was noted that caffeine had the power to prevent sleep.

The hypnotoxin theory reached its zenith in 1907 when Legendre and Pieron,[4] the French physiologists, did experiments showing that blood serum from sleep-deprived dogs could induce sleep in dogs that were not sleep deprived. The notion of a toxin's causing the brain to sleep has gradually given way to the notion that there are a number of endogenous "sleep factors" that actively induce sleep by specific mechanisms.

In the 1920s, the University of Chicago physiologist Nathaniel Kleitman carried out a series of sleep deprivation studies and made the simple but brilliant observation that individuals who stayed up all night were generally less sleepy and impaired the next morning than in the middle of their sleepless night. Kleitman argued that this observation was incompatible with the notion of a continual buildup of a hypnotoxin in the brain or blood. In addition, he felt that humans were about as impaired as they would get, that is, very impaired, after about 60 hours of wakefulness, and that longer periods of sleep deprivation would produce little additional change. In the 1939 (first) edition of his comprehensive landmark monograph *Sleep and Wakefulness*, Kleitman[5] summed up by saying, "It is perhaps not sleep that needs to be explained, but wakefulness, and indeed, there may be different kinds of wakefulness at different stages of phylogenetic and ontogenetic development. In spite of sleep being frequently designated as an instinct, or global reaction, an actively initiated process, by excitation or inhibition of cortical or subcortical structures, there is not a single fact about sleep that cannot be equally well interpreted as a let down of the waking activity."

THE ELECTRICAL ACTIVITY OF THE BRAIN

As the 20th century got under way, Camillo Golgi and Santiago Ramón y Cajal had demonstrated that the nervous system was not a mass of fused cells sharing a common cytoplasm but rather a highly intricate network of discrete cells that had the key property of signaling to one another. Luigi Galvani had discovered that the nerve cells of animals produce electricity, and Emil duBois-Reymond and Hermann von Helmholtz found that nerve cells use their electrical capabilities for signaling information to one another. The Scottish physiologist Richard Caton in 1875 demonstrated electrical rhythms in the brains of animals. The centennial of his discovery was commemorated at the 15th annual meeting of the Association for the Psychophysiological Study of Sleep convening at the site of the discovery, Edinburgh, Scotland.

However, it was not until the German psychiatrist Hans Berger[6] recorded electrical activity of the human brain beginning in 1928 and clearly demonstrated differences in these rhythms when subjects were awake or asleep that a real scientific interest commenced. Berger correctly inferred that the signals he recorded, which he called "electroencephalograms," were of brain origin. For the first time, the presence of sleep could be conclusively established without disturbing the sleeper, and, more important, sleep could be continuously and quantitatively measured without disturbing the sleeper.

All the major elements of sleep brain wave patterns were described by Harvey, Hobart, Davis, and others[7-9] at Harvard University in a series of extraordinary papers published in 1937, 1938, and 1939. Blake, Gerard, and Kleitman[10,11] added to this from their studies at the University of Chicago. On the human electroencephalogram (EEG), sleep was characterized by high-amplitude slow waves and spindles, whereas wakefulness was characterized by low-amplitude waves and alpha rhythm. The image of the sleeping brain completely "turned off" gave way to the image of the sleeping brain engaged in slow, synchronized, "idling" neuronal activity. Although it was not widely recognized at the time, these studies were some of the most critical turning points in sleep research. Indeed, Hobson[3] dated the turning point of sleep research to 1928, when Berger began his work on the human EEG. Used today in much the same way as they were in the 1930s, brain wave recordings have been extraordinarily important to sleep research and sleep medicine.

The 1930s also saw one series of investigations that seemed to establish conclusively both the passive theory of sleep and the notion that it occurred in response to reduction of stimulation and activity. These were the investigations of Frederick Bremer,[12,13] reported in 1935 and 1936. These investigations were made possible by the aforementioned development of electroencephalography. Bremer studied brain wave patterns in two cat preparations. One, which Bremer called *encéphale isolé,* was made by a section in the lower part of the medulla. The other, *cerveau isolé,* was made by cutting the midbrain just behind the origin of the oculomotor nerves. The first preparation permitted the study of cortical electrical rhythms under the influence of olfactory, visual, auditory, vestibular, and musculocutaneous impulses; in the second preparation, the field was narrowed almost entirely to the influence of olfactory and visual impulses.

In the first preparation, the brain continued to present manifestations of wakeful activity alternating with phases of sleep as indicated by the EEG. In the second preparation, however, the EEG assumed a definite deep sleep character and remained in this condition. In addition, the eyeballs immediately turned downward with a progressive miosis. Bremer concluded that in sleep there occurs a functional (reversible, of course) deafferentation of the cerebral cortex. The *cerveau isolé* preparation results in a suppression of the incessant influx of nerve impulses, particularly cutaneous and proprioceptive, which are essential for the maintenance of the waking state of the telencephalon. Apparently, olfactory and visual impulses are insufficient to keep the cortex awake. It is probably misleading to assert that physiologists assumed the brain was completely turned off, whatever this metaphor might have meant, because blood flow and, presumably, metabolism continued. However, Bremer and others certainly favored the concept of sleep as a reduction of activity—idling, slow, synchronized, "resting" neuronal activity.

THE ASCENDING RETICULAR SYSTEM

After World War II, insulated, implantable electrodes were developed, and sleep research on animals began in earnest.

In 1949, one of the most important and influential studies dealing with sleep and wakefulness was published: Moruzzi and Magoun's classic paper "Brain Stem Reticular Formation and Activation of the EEG."[14] These authors concluded that "transitions from sleep to wakefulness or from the less extreme states of relaxation and drowsiness to alertness and attention are all characterized by an apparent breaking up of the synchronization of discharge of the elements of the cerebral cortex, an alteration marked in the EEG by the replacement of high voltage, slow waves with low voltage fast activity" (p. 455).

High-frequency electrical stimulation through electrodes implanted in the brainstem reticular formation produced EEG activation and behavioral arousal. Thus, EEG activation, wakefulness, and consciousness were at one end of the continuum; sleep, EEG synchronization, and lack of consciousness were at the other end. This view, as can be seen, is hardly different from the statement by MacNish quoted at the beginning of this chapter.

The demonstration by Starzl and coworkers[15] that sensory collaterals discharge into the reticular formation suggested that a mechanism was present by which sensory stimulation could be transduced into prolonged activation of the brain and sustained wakefulness. By attributing an amplifying and maintaining role to the brainstem core and the conceptual ascending reticular activating system, it was possible to account for the fact that wakefulness outlasts, or is occasionally maintained in the absence of, sensory stimulation.

Chronic lesions in the brainstem reticular formation produced persisting slow waves in the EEG, and immobility. The usual animal for this research was the cat because excellent stereotaxic coordinates had become available in this model.[16] These findings appeared to confirm and extend Bremer's observations. The theory of the reticular activating system was an anatomically based passive theory of sleep or an active theory of wakefulness. Figure 1–1 is from the published proceedings of a symposium entitled *Brain Mechanisms and Consciousness* published in 1954 and probably the first genuine neuroscience bestseller.[17] Horace Magoun had extended his studies to the monkey, and the illustration represents the full flowering of the ascending reticular activating system theory.

EARLY OBSERVATIONS OF SLEEP PATHOLOGY

Insomnia has been described since the dawn of history and attributed to many causes, including a recognition of the association between emotional disturbance and sleep disturbance. Scholars and historians have a duty to bestow credit accurately. However, many discoveries lie fallow for want of a contextual soil in which they may be properly understood and in which they may extend the understanding of more general phenomena. Important early observations were those of von Economo on "sleeping sickness" and of Pavlov, who observed dogs falling asleep during conditioned reflex experiments.

Two early observations about sleep research and sleep medicine stand out. The first is the description in 1880 of narcolepsy by Jean Baptiste Edouard Gélineau (1859–1906), who derived the name narcolepsy from the Greek words *narkosis* (a benumbing) and *lepsis* (to overtake). He was the first to clearly describe the collection of components that constitute the syndrome, although the term *cataplexy* for the emotionally induced muscle weakness was subsequently coined in 1916 by Richard Henneberg.

What might be called the leading sleep disorder of the 20th century, obstructive sleep apnea syndrome, was described in 1836, not by a clinician but by the novelist Charles Dickens. In a series of papers entitled the "Posthumous Papers of the Pickwick Club," Dickens described Joe, a boy who was obese and always excessively sleepy. Joe, a loud snorer, was called Young Dropsy, possibly as a result of having right-sided heart failure. Meir Kryger[18] and Peretz Lavie[19,20] published scholarly accounts of many early references to snoring and conditions that were most certainly manifestations of sleep apnea syndrome. Professor Pierre Passouant[21] provided an account of the life of Gélineau and his landmark description of the narcolepsy syndrome.

SIGMUND FREUD AND THE INTERPRETATION OF DREAMS

By far the most widespread interest in sleep by health professionals was engendered by the theories of Sigmund Freud, specifically about dreams. Of course, the interest was really in dreaming, with sleep as the necessary concomitant. Freud developed psychoanalysis, the technique of dream interpretation, as part of his therapeutic approach to emotional and mental problems. As the concept of the ascending reticular activating system dominated behavioral neurophysiology, so the psychoanalytic theories about dreams dominated the psychological side of the coin. Dreams were thought to be the guardians of sleep and to occur in response to a disturbance in order to obviate waking up, as exemplified in the classic alarm clock dream. Freud's concept that dreaming discharged instinctual energy led directly to the notion of dreaming as a safety valve of the mind. At the time of the discovery of rapid eye movements during sleep (circa 1952), academic psychiatry was dominated by psychoanalysts, and medical students all over America were interpreting one another's dreams.

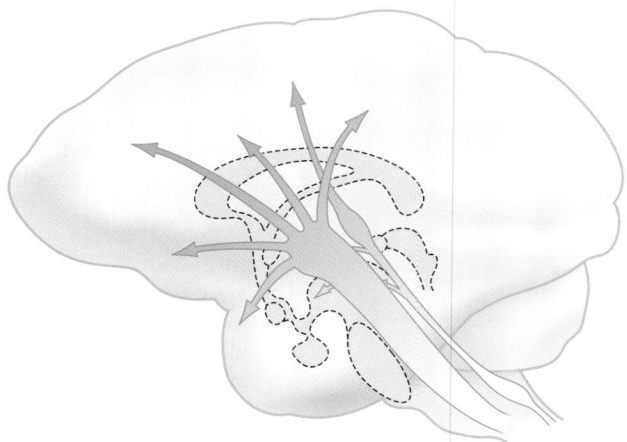

Figure 1–1. Lateral view of the monkey's brain, showing the ascending reticular activating system in the brainstem receiving collaterals from direct afferent paths and projecting primarily to the associational areas of the hemisphere. (Redrawn from Magoun HW: The ascending reticular system and wakefulness. In Adrian ED, Bremer F, Jasper HH [eds]: Brain Mechanisms and Consciousness. A Symposium Organized by the Council for International Organizations of Medical Sciences, 1954. Courtesy of Charles C Thomas, Publisher, Springfield, Ill.)

From the vantage point of today's world, the dream deprivation studies of the early 1960s, engendered and reified by the belief in psychoanalysis, may be regarded by some as a digression from the mainstream of sleep medicine. On the other hand, because the medical–psychiatric establishment had begun to take dreams seriously, it was also ready to support sleep research fairly generously under the guise of dream research.

CHRONOBIOLOGY

Most, but not all, sleep specialists share the opinion that what has been called chronobiology or the study of biologic rhythms is a legitimate part of sleep research and sleep medicine. The 24-hour rhythms in the activities of plants and animals have been recognized for centuries. These biologic 24-hour rhythms were quite reasonably assumed to be a direct consequence of the periodic environmental fluctuation of light and darkness. However, in 1729, Jean Jacques d'Ortous de Mairan described a heliotrope plant that opened its leaves during the day even after de Mairan had moved the plant so that sunlight could not reach it. The plant opened its leaves during the day and folded them for the entire night even though the environment was constant. This was the first demonstration of the persistence of circadian rhythms in the absence of environmental time cues. Figure 1–2,

which represents de Mairan's original experiment, is reproduced from *The Clocks That Time Us* by Moore-Ede and colleagues.[22]

Chronobiology and sleep research developed separately. The following three factors appear to have contributed to this:

1. The long-term studies commonly used in biologic rhythm research precluded continuous recording of brain wave activity. Certainly, in the early days, the latter was far too difficult and not really necessary. The measurement of wheel-running activity was a convenient and widely used method for demonstrating circadian rhythmicity.
2. The favorite animal of sleep research from the 1930s through the 1970s was the cat, and neither cats nor dogs demonstrate clearly defined circadian activity rhythms.
3. The separation between chronobiology and sleep research was further maintained by the tendency for chronobiologists to know very little about sleep, and for sleep researchers to remain ignorant of such biological clock mysteries as phase response curves, entrainment, and internal desynchronization.

THE DISCOVERY OF REM SLEEP

The discovery or identification of the discrete organismic state known as rapid eye movement (REM) sleep should be distinguished from the discovery that rapid eye movements occur during sleep. The historical threads of the discovery of rapid eye movements can be identified. Nathaniel Kleitman (Fig. 1–3), a professor of physiology at the University of Chicago, had long been interested in cycles of activity and

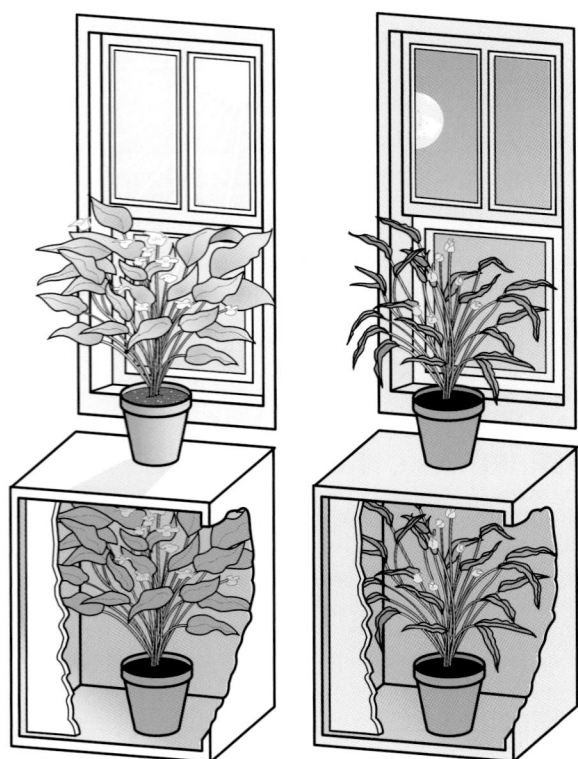

Figure 1–2. Representation of de Mairan's original experiment. When exposed to sunlight during the day *(upper left)*, the leaves of the plant were open; during the night *(upper right)*, the leaves were folded. De Mairan showed that sunlight was not necessary for these leaf movements by placing the plant in total darkness. Even under these constant conditions, the leaves opened during the day *(lower left)* and folded during the night *(lower right)*. (Redrawn from Moore-Ede MC, Sulzman FM, Fuller CA: The Clocks That Time Us: Physiology of the Circadian Timing System. Cambridge, Mass, Harvard University Press, 1982, p 7.)

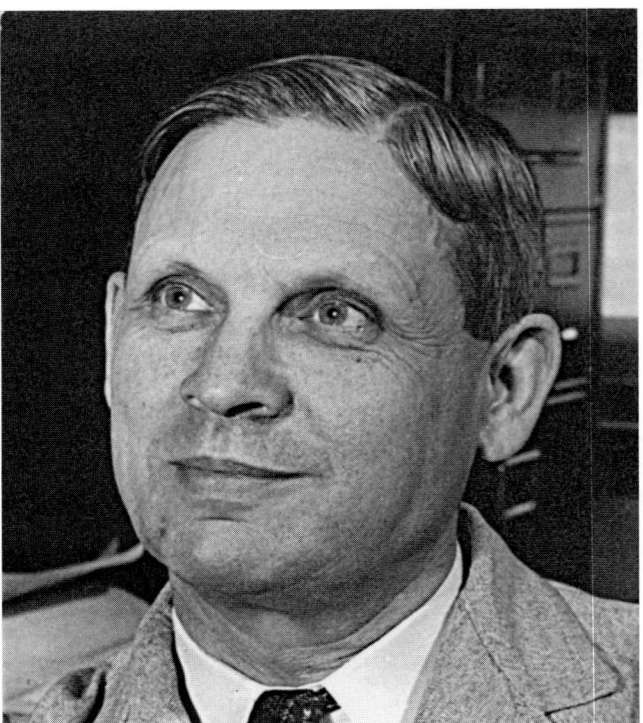

Figure 1–3. Nathaniel Kleitman (circa 1938), Professor of Physiology, University of Chicago, School of Medicine.

inactivity in infants and in the possibility that this cycle ensured that an infant would have an opportunity to respond to hunger. He postulated that the times infants awakened to nurse on a self-demand schedule would be integral multiples of a basic rest–activity cycle. The second thread was Kleitman's interest in eye motility as a possible measure of "depth" of sleep. The reasoning for this was that eye movements had a much greater cortical representation than did almost any other observable motor activity, and that slow, rolling, or pendular eye movements had been described at the onset of sleep with a gradual slowing and disappearance as sleep "deepened."[23]

In 1951, Kleitman assigned the task of observing eye movement to a graduate student in physiology named Eugene Aserinsky. Watching the closed eyes of sleeping infants was tedious, and Aserinsky soon found that it was easier to designate successive 5-minute epochs as "periods of motility" if he observed any movement at all, usually a writhing or twitching of the eyelids, versus "periods of no motility."

After describing an apparent rhythm in eye motility, Kleitman and Aserinsky decided to look for a similar phenomenon in adults. Again, watching the eyes during the day was tedious, and at night was even worse. Casting about, they came upon the method of electrooculography and decided (correctly) that this would be a good way to measure eye motility continuously and would relieve the human observer of the tedium of direct observations. Sometimes in the course of recording electrooculograms (EOGs) during sleep, they saw bursts of electrical potential changes that were quite different from the slow movements at sleep onset.

When they were observing infants, Aserinsky and Kleitman had not differentiated between slow and rapid movements. However, on the EOG, the difference between the slow eye movements at sleep onset and the newly discovered rapid motility was obvious. Initially, there was a great deal of concern that these potentials were electrical artifacts. With their presence on the EOG as a signal, however, it was possible to watch the subject's eyes simultaneously, and when this was done, the distinct movement of the eyes beneath the closed lids was extremely easy to see.

At this point, Aserinsky and Kleitman made two assumptions:

1. These eye movements represented a "lightening" of sleep.
2. Because they were associated with irregular respiration and accelerated heart rate, they might represent dreaming.

The basic sleep cycle was not identified at this time, primarily because the EOG and other physiologic measures, notably the EEG, were not recorded continuously but rather by sampling a few minutes of each hour or half-hour. The sampling strategy was done to conserve paper (there was no research grant) and because there was not a clear reason to record continuously. Also, the schedule made it possible to nap between sampling episodes.

Aserinsky and Kleitman initiated a small series of awakenings, both when rapid eye movements were present and when rapid eye movements were not present, for the purpose of eliciting dream recall. They did not apply sophisticated methods of dream content analysis, but the descriptions of dream content from the two conditions were generally quite different, which made it possible to conclude that rapid eye movements were associated with dreaming. This was, indeed, a breakthrough in sleep research.[24,25]

The occurrence of the eye movements was quite compatible with the contemporary dream theories that dreams occurred when sleep lightened in order to prevent or delay awakening. In other words, dreaming could still be regarded as the "guardian" of sleep. However, it could no longer be assumed that dreams were fleeting and evanescent.

ALL-NIGHT SLEEP RECORDINGS AND THE BASIC SLEEP CYCLE

The seminal Aserinsky and Kleitman paper was published in 1953. It attracted little attention, and no publications on the subject appeared from any other laboratory until 1959. Staying up at night to study sleep remained an undesirable occupation by anyone's standards. In the early 1950s, most previous research on the EEG patterns of sleep, like most approaches to sleep physiology generally, had either equated short periods of sleep with all sleep or relied on intermittent time sampling during the night. The notion of obtaining continuous records throughout typical nights of sleep would have seemed highly extravagant.

However, motivated by the desire to expand and quantify the description of rapid eye movements, Dement and Kleitman[26] did just this over a total of 126 nights with 33 subjects and, by means of a simplified categorization of EEG patterns, scored the paper recordings in their entirety. When they examined these 126 records, they found that there was a predictable sequence of patterns over the course of the night, such as had been hinted at by Aserinsky's study but entirely overlooked in all previous EEG studies of sleep. Although this sequence of regular variations has now been observed tens of thousands of times in hundreds of laboratories, the original description remains essentially unchanged.

The usual sequence was that after the onset of sleep, the EEG progressed fairly rapidly to stage 4, which persisted for varying amounts of time, generally about 30 minutes, and then a lightening took place. Whereas the progression from wakefulness to stage 4 at the beginning of the cycle was almost invariable through a continuum of change, the lightening was usually abrupt and coincident with a body movement or series of body movements. After the termination of stage 4, there was generally a short period of stage 2 or 3 which gave way to stage 1 and rapid eye movements. When the first eye movement period ended, the EEG again progressed through a continuum of change to stage 3 or 4, which persisted for a time and then lightened, often abruptly, with body movement to stage 2, which again gave way to stage 1 and the second rapid eye movement period (see p. 679 of Dement and Kleitman[26]).

Dement and Kleitman found that this cyclical variation of EEG patterns occurred repeatedly throughout the night at intervals of 90 to 100 minutes from the end of one eye movement period to the end of the next. The regular occurrences of REM periods and dreaming strongly suggested that dreams did not occur in response to chance disturbances.

At the time of these observations, sleep was still considered to be a single state. Dement and Kleitman characterized the EEG during REM periods as "emergent stage 1" as opposed to "descending stage 1" at the onset of sleep. The percentage of the total sleep time occupied by REM sleep was between 20% and 25%, and the periods of REM sleep tended to be shorter in the early cycles of the night. Variations in this picture of all-night sleep have been seen over and over in normal humans of both sexes, in widely varying environments and cultures, and, to all intents and purposes, across the life span.

REM SLEEP IN ANIMALS

The developing knowledge of the nature of sleep with rapid eye movements was in direct opposition to the ascending reticular activating system theory and constituted a paradigmatic crisis. The following observations were crucial:

Arousal thresholds in humans were much higher during periods of REM sleep that had a low-amplitude, relatively fast (stage 1) EEG pattern than during similar "light sleep" periods at the onset of sleep.

Rapid eye movements during sleep were discovered in cats; the concomitant brain wave patterns (low-amplitude, fast) were indistinguishable from active wakefulness.

By discarding the sampling approach and recording continuously, a basic 90-minute cycle of sleep without rapid eye movements, alternating with sleep *with* rapid eye movements, was discovered. The all-night sleep patterns had regular, lawful, predictable patterns of occurrence. Continuous recording that revealed a consistent EEG pattern during an entire period of sleep within which bursts of REM occurred, additionally established these as periods of vivid dreaming.

Observations of motor activity in both humans and animals revealed the unique occurrence of an active suppression of spinal motor activity.

Thus, sleep consists not of one state but rather of two distinct organismic states, as different from one another as both are from wakefulness. It had to be conceded that sleep could no longer be thought of as a time of brain inactivity and EEG slowing. By 1960, this fundamental change in our thinking about the nature of sleep was well established; it exists as fact that has not changed in any way since that time.

The discovery of rapid eye movements during sleep in humans, plus the all-night sleep recordings that revealed the regular recurrence of lengthy periods during which rapid eye movements occurred and during which brain wave patterns resembled light sleep, prepared the way for the discovery of REM sleep in cats, in spite of the extremely powerful bias that an "activated" EEG could not be associated with sleep. In the first study of cats, maintaining the insulation and, therefore, the integrity of implanted electrodes had not yet been solved, so an alternative, small pins in the scalp, was used. With this approach, the waking EEG was totally obscured by the electromyogram from the large temporal muscles of the cat. However, when the cat fell asleep, slow waves could be seen, and the transition to REM sleep was clearly observed because muscle potentials were completely suppressed. The cat's rapid eye movements and also the twitching of the whiskers and paws could be directly observed.

It is very difficult today, in 2004, to understand and appreciate the exceedingly controversial nature of these findings. The following note from a more personal account[27] illustrates both the power and the danger of scientific dogma. "I wrote them [the findings] up, but the paper was nearly impossible to publish because it was completely contradictory to the totally dominant neurophysiological theory of the time. The assertion by me that an activated EEG could be associated

with unambiguous sleep was considered to be absurd. As it turned out, previous investigators had observed an activated EEG during sleep in cats[28,29] but simply could not believe it and ascribed it to arousing influences during sleep. A colleague who was assisting me was sufficiently skeptical that he preferred I publish the paper as sole author. After four or five rejections, to my everlasting gratitude, Editor-in-Chief Herbert Jasper accepted the paper without revision for publication in *Electroencephalography and Clinical Neurophysiology*" (see p. 23 of Dement[30]).

It is notable, however, that the significance of the absence of muscle potentials during the REM periods in cats was not appreciated. It remained for Michel Jouvet, working in Lyon, France, to insist on the importance of electromyographic suppression in his early papers,[31,32] the first of which was published in 1959. Hodes and Dement began to study the "H" reflex in humans in 1960, finding complete suppression of reflexes during REM sleep,[33] and Octavio Pompeiano and others in Pisa, Italy, worked out the basic mechanisms of REM atonia in the cat.[34]

THE DUALITY OF SLEEP

Even though the basic non–rapid eye movement (NREM)-REM sleep cycle was well established, the realization that REM sleep was qualitatively different from the remainder of sleep took years to evolve. Jouvet[35] and his colleagues performed an elegant series of investigations on the brainstem mechanisms of sleep that forced the inescapable conclusion that sleep consists of two fundamentally different organismic states. Among his many early contributions were clarification of the role of pontine brainstem systems as the primary anatomic site for REM sleep mechanisms and the clear demonstration that electromyographic activity and muscle tonus are completely suppressed during REM periods and only during REM periods. These investigations began in 1958 and were carried out during 1959 and 1960.

It is now an established fact that atonia is a fundamental characteristic of REM sleep and that it is mediated by an active and highly specialized neuronal system. The pioneering microelectrode studies of Edward Evarts[36] in cats and monkeys, and observations on cerebral blood flow in the cat by Reivich and Kety[37] provided convincing evidence that the brain during REM sleep is very active. Certain areas of the brain appear to be more active in REM sleep than in wakefulness. By now, the notion of sleep as a passive process was totally demolished, although for many years there was a lingering attitude that NREM sleep was essentially inactive and quiet. By 1960, it was possible to define REM sleep as a completely separate organismic state characterized by cerebral activation, active motor inhibition, and, of course, an association with dreaming. The fundamental duality of sleep was an established fact.

PREMONITIONS OF SLEEP MEDICINE

Sleep research, which emphasized all-night sleep recordings, burgeoned in the 1960s and was the legitimate precursor of sleep medicine and particularly of its core clinical test, polysomnography. Much of the research at this time emphasized studies of dreaming and REM sleep and had its roots in a psychoanalytic approach to mental illness, which strongly implicated dreaming in the psychotic process. After sufficient numbers of all-night sleep recordings had been carried out in humans to demonstrate a highly characteristic "normal" sleep architecture, investigators noted a significantly short-ened REM latency in association with endogenous depression.[38] This phenomenon has been intensively investigated ever since. Other important precursors of sleep medicine were the following:

1. Discovery of sleep-onset REM periods in patients with narcolepsy
2. Interest in sleep, epilepsy, and abnormal movement—primarily in France
3. Introduction of benzodiazepines and the use of sleep laboratory studies in defining hypnotic efficacy

SLEEP-ONSET REM PERIODS AND CATAPLEXY

In 1959, a patient with narcolepsy came to the Mount Sinai Hospital in New York City to see Dr. Charles Fisher. At Fisher's suggestion, a sleep recording was begun. Within seconds after he fell asleep, the patient was showing the dramatic, charac-teristic rapid eye movements of REM sleep, as well as saw-tooth waves on the EEG. The first paper documenting sleep-onset REM periods in a single patient was published in 1960 by Gerald Vogel.[39] In a collaborative study between the University of Chicago and the Mount Sinai Hospital, nine patients were studied, and the important sleep-onset REM periods at night were described in a 1963 paper.[40] Subsequent research showed that sleepy patients who did not have cata-plexy did not have sleep-onset REM periods (SOREMPs), and those with cataplexy always had SOREMPs.[41] It was clear that the best explanation for cataplexy was the normal motor inhibitory mechanisms of REM sleep occurring in a preco-cious or abnormal way.

THE NARCOLEPSY CLINIC: A FALSE START

In January 1963, after moving to Stanford University, Dement was eager to test the hypothesis of an association between cataplexy and SOREMPs. However, not a single narcoleptic patient could be identified. A final attempt was made by placing a "want ad," a few words about an inch high, in a daily newspaper, the *San Francisco Chronicle*. More than 100 people responded! About 50 of these patients were bona fide narcoleptics having both sleepiness and cataplexy.

The response to the ad was a noteworthy event in the development of sleep disorders medicine. With one or two exceptions, none of the narcoleptics had ever been diagnosed correctly. A responsibility for their clinical management had to be assumed for their participation in the research. The late Dr. Stephen Mitchell, who had completed his neurology training and was entering a psychiatry residency at Stanford University, joined Dement in creating a narcolepsy clinic in 1964, and they were soon managing well over 100 patients. Mostly, this involved seeing the patients at regular intervals and adjusting their medication. Nonetheless, the seeds of the typical sleep disorders clinic were sowed because at least one daytime polygraphic sleep recording was performed on all patients to look for the presence of SOREMPs, and patients

were questioned exhaustively about their sleep. If possible, an all-night sleep recording was carried out. Unfortunately, most of the patients were unable to pay cash to cover their bills, and insurance companies declared that the recordings of narcoleptic patients were experimental. Because the clinic was unable to generate sufficient income, it was discontinued and most of the patients were referred back to local physicians with instructions about treatment.

EUROPEAN INTEREST

In Europe, a genuine clinical interest in sleep problems had arisen, and it achieved its clearest expression in a 1963 symposium held in Paris, organized by Professor H. Fischgold, and published as *La Sommeil de Nuit Normal et Pathologique* in 1965.[42] The primary clinical emphasis in this symposium was the documentation of sleep-related epileptic seizures and a number of related studies on sleepwalking and night terrors. Investigators from France, Italy, Belgium, Germany, and the Netherlands took part.

BENZODIAZEPINES AND HYPNOTIC EFFICACY STUDIES

Benzodiazepines were introduced in 1960 with the marketing of chlordiazepoxide (Librium). This compound offered a significant advance in terms of safety over barbiturates for the purpose of tranquilizing and sedating. It was quickly followed by diazepam (Valium) and the first benzodiazepine introduced specifically as a hypnotic, flurazepam (Dalmane). Although a number of studies had been done on the effects of drugs on sleep, usually to answer theoretical questions, the first use of the sleep laboratory to evaluate sleeping pills was the 1965 study by Oswald and Priest.[43] An important series of studies establishing the role of the sleep laboratory in the evaluation of hypnotic efficacy was carried out by Anthony Kales and his colleagues at the University of California, Los Angeles.[44] The group also carried out studies of patients with hypothyroidism, asthma, Parkinson's disease, and somnambulism.[45-48]

THE DISCOVERY OF SLEEP APNEA

One of the most important events in the history of sleep disorders medicine occurred in Europe. Sleep apnea was dis-covered independently by Gastaut, Tassinari, and Duron[49] in France and by Jung and Kuhlo in Germany.[50] Both these groups reported their findings in 1965. As noted earlier, scholars have found references to this phenomenon in many places, but this was the first clear-cut recognition and description that had a direct causal continuity to sleep disorders medicine as we know it today. Peretz Lavie has detailed the historical contri-butions made by scientists and clinicians around the world in helping to describe and understand this disorder.[20]

These important findings were widely ignored in America. What should have been an almost inevitable discovery by either the otolaryngologic surgery community or the pulmonary medicine community did not occur because there was no tradition in either specialty for observing breathing carefully during sleep. The well-known and frequently cited study of Burwell and colleagues[51]—although impressive in a literary sense in its evoking of the somnolent boy, Joe, from the "Posthumous Papers of the Pickwick Club"—erred badly in evaluating their somnolent obese patients *only* during waking and attributing the cause of the somnolence to hypercapnia.

The popularity of this paper further reduced the likelihood of discovery of sleep apnea by the pulmonary community. To this day, there is no evidence that hypercapnia causes true somnolence, although, of course, high levels of PCO_2 are associated with impaired cerebral function. Nonetheless, the term *pickwickian* became an instant success as a neologism and may have played a role in stimulating interest in this syndrome by the European neurologists who were also interested in sleep.

A small group of French neurologists who specialized in clinical neurophysiology and electroencephalography were in the vanguard of sleep research. One of the collaborators in the French discovery of sleep apnea, C. Alberto Tassinari, joined the Italian neurologist Elio Lugaresi in Bologna in 1970. These clinical investigators along with Giorgio Coccagna and a host of others over the years performed a crucial series of clinical sleep investigations and, indeed, provided a complete description of the sleep apnea syndrome, including the first observations of the occurrence of sleep apnea in nonobese patients, an account of the cardiovascular correlates, and a clear identification of the importance of snoring and hypersomnolence as diagnostic indicators. These studies are recounted in Lugaresi's book, *Hypersomnia with Periodic Apneas*.[52]

ITALIAN SYMPOSIA

In 1967, Henri Gastaut and Elio Lugaresi (Fig. 1–4) organized a symposium, published as *The Abnormalities of Sleep in Man*,[53] which encompassed issues across a full range of pathologic sleep in humans. This meeting took place in Bologna, Italy, and the papers presented covered many of what are now major topics in the sleep medicine field: insomnia, sleep apnea, narcolepsy, and periodic leg movements during sleep. It was an epic meeting from the point of view of the clinical investigation of sleep; the only major issues not represented were clear concepts of clinical practice models and clear visions of the high population prevalence of sleep disorders.

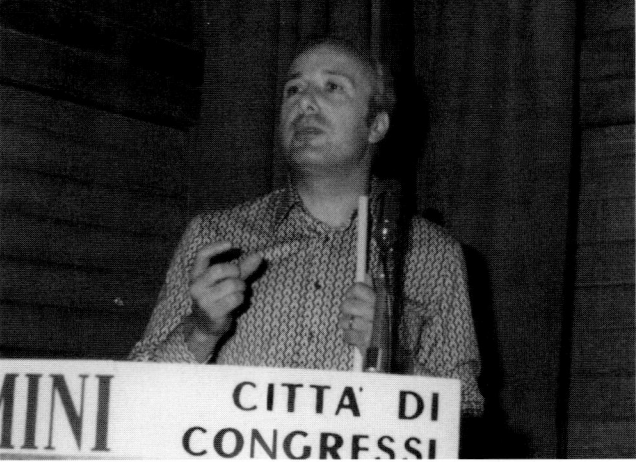

Figure 1–4. Elio Lugaresi, Professor of Neurology, University of Bologna, at the 1972 Rimini symposium.

However, the event that may have finally triggered a serious international interest in sleep apnea syndromes was organized by Lugaresi in 1972 and took place in Rimini, a small resort on the Adriatic coast.[54]

BIRTH PANGS

In spite of all the clinical research, the concept of all-night sleep recordings as a clinical diagnostic test did not emerge unambiguously. It is worth considering the reasons for this failure, partly because they continue to operate today, in altered forms, as impediments to the expansion of the field, and partly to understand the field's long overdue development.

The first important reason was the unprecedented nature of an all-night diagnostic test, particularly if it was conducted on outpatients. The cost of all-night polygraphic recording, in terms of its basic expense, was high enough without adding the cost of hospitalization, which would have legitimized a patient's spending the night in a testing facility, however. To sleep in an outpatient clinic for a diagnostic test was a totally unprecedented, time-intensive, and labor-intensive enterprise and completely in conflict with the image of going to the chemistry laboratory to give a blood sample, breathe into a pulmonary function apparatus, undergo a radiographic examination, and so forth.

A second important barrier was the reluctance of nonhospital clinical professionals to work at night. Although medical house staff are very familiar with night work, they do not generally enjoy it; furthermore, clinicians could not work 24-hour days, first seeing patients and ordering tests, and then conducting the tests themselves.

Finally, only a small number of people understood that complaints of daytime sleepiness and nocturnal sleep disturbance represented anything of clinical significance. Even narcolepsy, which was by the early 1970s fully characterized as an interesting and disabling clinical syndrome requiring sleep recordings for diagnosis, was not recognized in the larger medical community and had too low a prevalence to warrant creating a medical subspecialty. A study carried out in 1972 documented a mean of 15 years from onset of the characteristic symptoms of excessive daytime sleepiness and cataplexy to recognition by a clinician, and the study showed that a mean of 5.5 different physicians were consulted throughout that long interval.[55]

THE EVOLUTION OF SLEEP MEDICINE CLINICAL PRACTICE

The practice of sleep medicine developed in many centers in the 1970s, often as a function of the original research interests of the center. The sleep disorders clinic at Stanford University is in many ways a microcosm of how sleep medicine evolved throughout the world. Patients complaining of insomnia were enrolled in hypnotic efficacy studies, which brought the Stanford group into contact with many insomnia patients and demolished the notion that the majority of such patients had psychiatric problems. An early question was, How reliable are the descriptions of their sleep by these patients? The classic all-night sleep recording gave an answer and yielded a great deal of information. Throughout the second half of the 1960s, as a part of their research, the Stanford group continued to manage patients with narcolepsy. As the group's reputation for expertise in narcolepsy grew, it began to receive referrals for evaluation from physicians all over the United States. Although sleep apnea had not yet been identified (and treated) as a frequent cause of severe daytime sleepiness, it was clear that a number of patients referred with the presumptive diagnosis of narcolepsy certainly did not possess narcolepsy's two cardinal signs, SOREMPs and cataplexy. True pickwickians were an infrequent referral at this time.

In January 1972, Christian Guilleminault, a French neurologist and psychiatrist, joined the Stanford group. He had extensive knowledge of and experience with the European studies of sleep apnea. Until his arrival, the Stanford group had not routinely used respiratory and cardiac sensors in their all-night sleep studies. Starting in 1972, these measurements became a routine part of the all-night diagnostic test, which was named polysomnography in 1974 by Dr. Jerome Holland, a member of the group. Publicity about narcolepsy and excessive sleepiness resulted in a small flow of referrals to the Stanford sleep clinic, usually with the presumptive diagnosis of narcolepsy. During the first year or two, the goal for the practice was to see at least five new patients per week. To foster financial viability, the group did as much as possible, within ethical limits, to publicize its services. Accordingly, there was also a sprinkling of patients, often self-referred, with chronic insomnia. The diagnosis of obstructive sleep apnea in patients with profound excessive daytime sleepiness was nearly always completely unambiguous.

During 1972, the search for sleep abnormality in patients with sleep-related complaints continued; an attempt was made as well to conceptualize the pathophysiologic process both as an entity and as the cause of the presenting symptom. With this approach, a number of phenomena seen during sleep were rapidly linked to the fundamental sleep-related presenting complaints. Toward the end of 1972, the basic concepts and formats of sleep disorders medicine were sculpted to the extent that it was possible to offer a daylong course through Stanford University's Division of Postgraduate Medicine with the title "The Diagnosis and Treatment of Sleep Disorders." The topics covered were normal sleep architecture; the diagnosis and treatment of insomnia with drug-dependent insomnia, pseudoinsomnia, central sleep apnea, and periodic leg movement as diagnostic entities; and the diagnosis and treatment of excessive daytime sleepiness or hypersomnia, with narcolepsy, NREM narcolepsy, and obstructive sleep apnea as diagnostic entities.

The disability and cardiovascular complications of severe sleep apnea were alarming, but at that time, the treatment options were limited to weight loss and chronic tracheostomy. The dramatic results of chronic tracheostomy in ameliorating the symptoms and complications of obstructive sleep apnea had been reported by Lugaresi and coworkers[56] in 1970. However, the notion of using such a treatment was strongly resisted at the time by the medical community, both at Stanford University sleep clinic and elsewhere. Among the first patients who were referred for investigation of their severe somnolence and who eventually had tracheostomy was a 10-year-old boy. The challenges that were met to secure the proper management of this patient can be seen in this account by Christian Guilleminault (personal communication, 1990).

In addition to medical skepticism, a major obstacle to the practice of sleep disorders medicine was the retroactive denial of payment by insurance companies, primarily the largest one in the United States. A 3-year period of educational efforts

directed toward third-party carriers finally culminated in the recognition of polysomnography as a reimbursable diagnostic test in 1975. Another issue was that outpatient clinics that offered overnight testing in polysomnographic testing bedrooms needed to obtain state licensure in order to avoid the licensing requirements of hospitals. This, too, was finally accomplished in 1974.

CASE HISTORY

Raymond M. was a 10½-year-old boy referred to the pediatrics clinic in 1971 for evaluation of unexplained hypertension, which had developed progressively over the preceding 6 months. There was a positive family history of high blood pressure, but never so early in life. Raymond was hospitalized and had determination of renin, angiotensin, and aldosterone, renal function studies including contrast radiographs, and extensive cardiac evaluation. All results had been normal except that his blood pressure oscillated between 140-170/90-100. It was noticed that he was somnolent during the daytime and Dr. S. suggested that I see him for this "unrelated" symptom.

I reviewed Raymond's history with his mother. Raymond had been abnormally sleepy "all his life." However, during the past 2 to 3 years, his schoolteachers were complaining that he would fall asleep in class and was at times a "behavioral problem"—not paying attention, hyperactive, aggressive. His mother confirmed that he had been a very loud snorer since he was very young, at least since age 2, perhaps before.

Physical examination revealed an obese boy with a short neck and a very narrow airway. I recommended a sleep evaluation which was accepted. An esophageal balloon and measurement of end tidal CO_2 was added to the usual array. His esophageal pressure reached 80 to 120 cm H_2O, he had values of 6% end tidal CO_2 at end of apnea, apneic events lasted between 25 and 65 sec, and the apnea index was 55. His Sao_2 [oxygen saturation, arterial] was frequently below 60%.

I called the pediatric resident and informed him that the sleep problem was serious. I also suggested that the sleep problem might be the cause of the as yet unexplained hypertension. The resident could not make sense of my information and passed it to the attending physician. I was finally asked to present my findings at the pediatric case conference, which was led by Dr. S. I came with the recordings, showed the results, and explained why I believed that there was a relationship between the hypertension and the sleep problem. There were a lot of questions. They simply could not believe it. I was asked what treatment I would recommend, and I suggested a tracheostomy. I was asked how many patients had this treatment in the United States, and how many children had ever been treated with tracheostomy. When I had to answer "zero" to both questions, the audience was somewhat shocked. It was decided that such an approach was doubtful at best, and completely unacceptable in a child. However, they did concede that if no improvement was achieved by medical management, Raymond would be reinvestigated, including sleep studies.

This was spring 1972. In the fall, he was, if anything, worse in spite of vigorous medical treatment. At the end of 1972, Raymond finally had his tracheostomy. His blood pressure went down to 90/60 within 10 days, and he was no longer sleepy. During the 5 years we were able to follow Raymond, he remained normotensive and alert, but I had to fight continuously to prevent outside doctors from closing his tracheostomy. I don't know what happened to him since.

CLINICAL SIGNIFICANCE OF EXCESSIVE DAYTIME SLEEPINESS

Christian Guilleminault, in a series of studies, had clearly shown that excessive daytime sleepiness was a major presenting complaint and a pathologic phenomenon unto itself.[57] However, it was recognized that methods to quantify this symptom and the condition in order to show improvement with treatment were not adequate. The Stanford Sleepiness Scale, developed by Hoddes and colleagues,[58] did not give reliable results. The problem was not a crisis, however, because patients with severe apnea and overwhelming daytime sleepiness improved dramatically after tracheostomy, and the reduction in daytime sleepiness was unambiguous. Nonetheless, documenting the pharmacologic treatment of narcolepsy and the objective improvement of sleepiness in patients with less severe sleep apnea continued to be a problem.

The apparent lack of interest in daytime sleepiness by individuals who were devoting their careers to the investigation of sleep has always been puzzling. There is no question but that the current active investigation of this phenomenon is the result of the early interest of sleep disorders specialists. The early neglect of sleepiness is all the more difficult to understand because it is now widely recognized that sleepiness and the tendency to fall asleep during the performance of hazardous tasks is one of the most important problems in our society. A number of reasons have been put forward. One is that sleepiness and drowsiness are negative qualities. A second is that the societal failure to confront the issue was fostered by language ambiguities in identifying sleepiness. A third is that the early sleep laboratory studies focused almost exclusively on REM sleep and nighttime operations with little concern for the daytime except for psychopathology. Finally, the focus with regard to sleep deprivation was on performance from the perspective of human factors rather than on sleepiness as representing a homeostatic response to sleep reduction.

An early attempt to develop an objective measure of sleepiness was that of Yoss and coworkers,[59] who observed pupil diameter directly by video monitoring and described changes in sleep deprivation and narcolepsy. Subsequently designated pupillometry, this technique has not been widely accepted. Dr. Mary Carskadon deserves most of the credit for the development of the latter-day standard approach to the measurement of sleepiness called the Multiple Sleep Latency Test (MSLT). She noted that subjective ratings of sleepiness made before a sleep recording not infrequently predicted the sleep latency. In the spring of 1976, she undertook to establish sleep latency as an objective measurement of the state of sleepiness–alertness by measuring sleep tendency before, during, and after 2 days of total sleep deprivation.[60] The protocol designed for this study has become the standard protocol for the MSLT. The choices of a 20-minute duration of a single test and a 2-hour interval between tests were essentially arbitrary and dictated by the practical demands of that study. This test was then formally applied to the evaluation of sleepiness in patients with narcolepsy[61] and, later, in patients with obstructive sleep apnea syndrome (OSAS).[62]

Carskadon and her colleagues then undertook a monumental study of sleepiness in children by following them longitudinally across the 2nd decade of life, which is also the decade of highest risk for the development of narcolepsy. Using the new MSLT measure, she found that 10-year-old children were completely alert in the daytime, but by the time they reached sexual maturity, they were no longer fully alert with the same amount of sleep at night. Results of this remarkable decade of work and other studies are summarized in an important review.[63]

Early MSLT research established the following important advances in thinking:

1. Daytime sleepiness and nighttime sleep are an interactive continuum, and the adequacy of nighttime sleep absolutely cannot be understood without a complementary measurement of the level of daytime sleepiness or its antonym, alertness.
2. Excessive sleepiness, also known as impaired alertness, was sleep medicine's most important symptom.

RECENT HISTORY

As the decade of the 1970s drew to a close, the consolidation and formalization of the practice of sleep disorders medicine was largely completed. What is now the American Academy of Sleep Medicine was formed and provided a home for professionals interested in sleep and, particularly, the diagnosis and treatment of sleep disorders. This organization began as the Association of Sleep Disorders Centers with five members in 1975. The organization then was responsible for the initiation of the scientific journal *Sleep,* and it fostered the setting of standards through center accreditation and an examination for practitioners by which they were designated Accredited Clinical Polysomnographers.

The first international symposium on narcolepsy took place in the French Languedoc in summer 1975, immediately after the Second International Congress of the Association for the Physiological Study of Sleep in Edinburgh. The former meeting, in addition to being scientifically productive, had landmark significance because it produced the first consensus definition of a specific sleep disorder,[64] drafted, revised, and unanimously endorsed by 65 narcoleptologists of international reputation. The first sleep disorders patient volunteer organization, the American Narcolepsy Association, was also formed in 1975. The *ASDC/APSS Diagnostic Classification of Sleep and Arousal Disorders* was published in fall 1979 after 3 years of extraordinary effort by a small group of dedicated individuals who composed the "nosology" committee chaired by Howard Roffwarg.[65]

Before the 1980s, the only effective treatment for severe OSAS was chronic tracheostomy. This highly effective but personally undesirable approach was replaced by two new procedures—one surgical,[66] the other mechanical.[67] The first was uvulopalatopharyngoplasty, which is giving way to more complex and effective approaches. The second is the widely used and highly effective continuous positive nasal airway pressure technique introduced by the Australian pulmonologist Colin Sullivan. The combination of the high prevalence of OSAS and effective treatments fueled a strong expansion of centers and individuals offering the diagnosis and treatment of sleep disorders to patients. The decade of the 1980s was capped by the publication of sleep medicine's first textbook, *Principles and Practice of Sleep Medicine.*[68] For many years there was only one medical journal devoted to sleep; by 2004 there were seven: *Sleep, Journal of Sleep Research, Sleep and Biological Rhythms, Sleep & Breathing, Sleep Medicine, Sleep Medicine Reviews,* and *Sleep Research Online.* Articles about sleep are now routinely published in the major pulmonary, neurology, and psychiatric journals.

The 1990s saw an acceleration in the acceptance of sleep medicine throughout the world.[69] In spite of this, adequate sleep medicine services are still not readily available everywhere.[70] In the United States, the National Center on Sleep Disorders Research (NCSDR) was established by statute as part of the National Heart, Lung, and Blood Institute of the National Institutes of Health.[71,72] The mandate of NCSDR is to support research, promote educational activities, and coordinate sleep-related activities throughout various branches of the U.S. government. This initiative led to the development of large research projects dealing with various aspects of sleep disorders and the establishment of awards to develop educational materials at all levels of training.

The 1990s also saw the establishment of the National Sleep Foundation[73] as well as other organizations for patients. This foundation points out to the public the dangers of sleepiness, and sponsors the annual National Sleep Awareness Week. As the Internet increases exponentially in size, so do the sleep resources on the Internet, for physicians, patients, and the public. People today know a great deal more about sleep and its disorders than the average person did at the end of the 1980s.

THE CHALLENGE OF THE FUTURE

Chapter 53 of this volume deals with public policy and public health issues. From today's vantage, the greatest challenge for the future is the cost-effective expansion of sleep medicine so that its benefits will be readily available. The major barrier to this availability is the failure of sleep research and sleep medicine to effectively penetrate the educational system at any level. As a consequence, the majority of individuals remain unaware of important facts of sleep and wakefulness, fundamentals of biologic rhythms, and sleep disorders, and particularly of the symptoms that suggest a serious pathologic process. The management of sleep deprivation and its serious consequences in the workplace, particularly in those industries that depend on sustained operations, needs increased attention.

Finally, the education and training of all health professionals, including nurses, has far to go. Take heart! These problems are grand opportunities. Sleep medicine has come into its own. It has made concern for health a truly 24-hours-a-day enterprise, and it has energized a new effort to reveal the secrets of the healthy and unhealthy sleeping brain.

Clinical Pearl

Recent advances in sleep science, sleep medicine, public policy, and communications will foster an educated public that will know a great deal about sleep and its disorders. Clinicians should expect that their patients may have already learned about their sleep disorders from the information sources that are readily available.

REFERENCES

1. Thorpy M: History of sleep and man. In Thorpy M, Yager J (eds): The Encyclopedia of Sleep and Sleep Disorders. New York, Facts on File, 1991.
2. MacNish R: The Philosophy of Sleep. New York, D Appleton, 1834.
3. Hobson J: Sleep. New York, Scientific American Library, 1989.
4. Legendre R, Pieron H: Le probleme des facteurs du sommeil: Resultats d'injections vasculaires et intracerebrales de liquides insomniques. C R Soc Biol 1910;68:1077-1079.
5. Kleitman N: Sleep and Wakefulness. Chicago, University of Chicago Press, 1939.
6. Berger H: Ueber das Elektroenkephalogramm des Menschen. J Psychol Neurol 1930;40:160-179.
7. Davis H, Davis PA, Loomis AL, et al: Changes in human brain potentials during the onset of sleep. Science 1937;86:448-450.
8. Davis H, Davis PA, Loomis AL, et al: Human brain potentials during the onset of sleep. J Neurophysiol 1938;1:24-38.
9. Harvey EN, Loomis AL, Hobart GA: Cerebral states during sleep as studied by human brain potentials. Science 1937;85:443-444.
10. Blake H, Gerard RW: Brain potentials during sleep. Am J Physiol 1937;119:692-703.
11. Blake H, Gerard RW, Kleitman N: Factors influencing brain potentials during sleep. J Neurophysiol 1939;2:48-60.
12. Bremer F: Cerveau "isole" et physiologie du sommeil. C R Soc Biol 1935;118:1235-1241.
13. Bremer F: Cerveau. Nouvelles recherches sur le mecanisme du sommeil. C R Soc Biol 1936;122:460-464.
14. Moruzzi G, Magoun H: Brain stem reticular formation and activation of the EEG. Electroencephalogr Clin Neurophysiol 1949;1:455-473.
15. Starzl TE, Taylor CW, Magoun HW: Collateral afferent excitation of reticular formation of brain stem. J Neurophysiol 1951;14:479.
16. Jasper H, Ajmone-Marsan C: A Stereotaxic Atlas of the Diencephalon of the Cat. Ottawa, Ontario, Canada, The National Research Council of Canada, 1954.
17. Magoun HW: The ascending reticular system and wakefulness. In Adrian ED, Bremer F, Jasper HH (eds): Brain Mechanisms and Consciousness: A Symposium Organized by the Council for International Organizations of Medical Sciences. Springfield, Ill, Charles C Thomas, 1954.
18. Kryger MH: Sleep apnea: From the needles of Dionysius to continuous positive airway pressure. Arch Intern Med 1983;143:2301-2308.
19. Lavie P: Nothing new under the moon: Historical accounts of sleep apnea syndrome. Arch Intern Med 1986;144:2025-2028.
20. Lavie P: Restless Nights: Understanding Snoring and Sleep Apnea. New Haven, Conn, Yale University Press, 2003.
21. Passouant P: Doctor Gélineau (1828-1906): Narcolepsy centennial. Sleep 1981;3:241-246.
22. Moore-Ede M, Sulzman F, Fuller C: The Clocks That Time Us: Physiology of the Circadian Timing System. Cambridge, Mass, Harvard University Press, 1982.
23. Toni G de: I movimenti pendolari dei bulbi oculari dei bambini durante il sonno fisiologico, ed in alcuni stati morbosi. Pediatria 1933;41:489-498.
24. Aserinsky E, Kleitman N: Regularly occurring periods of eye motility, and concomitant phenomena, during sleep. Science 1953;118:273-274.
25. Aserinsky E, Kleitman N: Two types of ocular motility occurring in sleep. J Appl Physiol 1955;8:11-18.
26. Dement W, Kleitman N: Cyclic variations in EEG during sleep and their relation to eye movements, body motility, and dreaming. Electroencephalogr Clin Neurophysiol 1957;9:673-690.
27. Dement W: A personal history of sleep disorders medicine. J Clin Neurophysiol 1990;1:17-47.
28. Derbyshire AJ, Rempel B, Forbes A, et al: The effects of anesthetics on action potentials in the cerebral cortex of the cat. Am J Physiol 1936;116:577-596.

29. Hess R, Koella WP, Akert K: Cortical and subcortical recordings in natural and artificially induced sleep in cats. Electroencephalogr Clin Neurophysiol 1953;5:75-90.

30. Dement W: The occurrence of low voltage, fast electroencephalogram patterns during behavioral sleep in the cat. Electroencephalogr Clin Neurophysiol 1958;10:291-296.

31. Jouvet M, Michel F, Courjon J: Sur un stade d'activite electrique cerebrale rapide au cours du sommeil physiologique. C R Soc Biol 1959;153:1024-1028.

32. Jouvet M, Mounier D: Effects des lesions de la formation reticulaire pontique sur le sommeil du chat. C R Soc Biol 1960;154: 2301-2305.

33. Hodes R, Dement W: Depression of electrically induced reflexes ("H-reflexes") in man during low voltage EEG "sleep." Electroencephalogr Clin Neurophysiol 1964;17:617-629.

34. Pompeiano O: Mechanisms responsible for spinal inhibition during desynchronized sleep: Experimental study. In Guilleminault C, Dement WC, Passouant P (eds): Advances in Sleep Research, vol 3: Narcolepsy. New York, Spectrum, 1976, pp 411-449.

35. Jouvet M: Recherches sur les structures nerveuses et les mecanismes responsales des differentes phases du sommeil physiologique. Arch Ital Biol 1962;100:125-206.

36. Evarts E: Effects of sleep and waking on spontaneous and evoked discharge of single units in visual cortex. Fed Proc 1960;4(suppl):828-837.

37. Reivich M, Kety S: Blood flow and metabolism in the sleeping brain. In Plum F (ed): Brain Dysfunction in Metabolic Disorders. New York, Raven Press, 1968, pp 125-140.

38. Kupfer D, Foster F: Interval between onset of sleep and rapid eye movement sleep as an indicator of depression. Lancet 1972; 2:684-686.

39. Vogel G: Studies in psychophysiology of dreams, III: The dream of narcolepsy. Arch Gen Psychiatry 1960;3:421-428.

40. Rechtschaffen A, Wolpert E, Dement W, et al: Nocturnal sleep of narcoleptics. Electroencephalogr Clin Neurophysiol 1963;15: 599-609.

41. Dement W, Rechtschaffen A, Gulevich G: The nature of the narcoleptic sleep attack. Neurology 1966;16:18-33.

42. Fischgold H (ed): La Sommeil de Nuit Normal et Pathologique: Etudes Electroencephalographiques. Paris, France, Masson et Cie, 1965.

43. Oswald I, Priest R: Five weeks to escape the sleeping pill habit. Br Med J 1965;2:1093-1095.

44. Kales A, Malmstrom EJ, Scharf MB, et al: Psychophysiological and biochemical changes following use and withdrawal of hypnotics. In Kales A (ed): Sleep: Physiology and Pathology. Philadelphia, JB Lippincott, 1969, pp 331-343.

45. Kales A, Beall GN, Bajor GF, et al: Sleep studies in asthmatic adults: Relationship of attacks to sleep stage and time of night. J Allergy 1968;41:164-173.

46. Kales A, Heuser G, Jacobson A, et al: All night sleep studies in hypothyroid patients, before and after treatment. J Clin Endocrinol Metab 1967;27:1593-1599.

47. Kales A, Ansel RD, Markham CH, et al: Sleep in patients with Parkinson's disease and normal subjects prior to and following levodopa administration. Clin Pharmacol Ther 1971;12:397-406.

48. Kales A, Jacobson A, Paulson NJ, et al: Somnambulism: psychophysiological correlates, I: All-night EEG studies. Arch Gen Psychiatry 1966;14:586-594.

49. Gastaut H, Tassinari C, Duron B: Etude polygraphique des manifestations episodiques (hypniques et respiratoires) du syndrome de Pickwick. Rev Neurol 1965;112:568-579.

50. Jung R, Kuhlo W: Neurophysiological studies of abnormal night sleep and the pickwickian syndrome. Prog Brain Res 1965;18:140-159.

51. Burwell CS, Robin ED, Whaley RD, et al: Extreme obesity associated with alveolar hypoventilation: A pickwickian syndrome. Am J Med 1956;21:811-818.

52. Lugaresi E, Coccagna G, Mantovani M: Hypersomnia with Periodic Apneas. New York, Spectrum, 1978.

53. Gastaut H, Lugaresi E, Berti-Ceroni G, et al (eds): The Abnormalities of Sleep in Man. Bologna, Italy, Aulo Gaggi Editore, 1968.

54. Gastaut H, Lugaresi E, Berti-Ceroni G, et al: Pathophysiological, clinical, and nosographic considerations regarding hypersomnia with periodic breathing. Bull Physiopathol Resp 1972;8: 1249-1256.

55. Dement W, Guilleminault C, Zarcone V, et al: The narcolepsy syndrome. In Conn H, Conn R (eds): Current Diagnosis, vol 2. Philadelphia, WB Saunders, 1974, pp 917-921.

56. Lugaresi E, Coccagna G, Mantovani M, et al: Effects de la trachéotomie dans les hypersomnies avec respiration periodique. Rev Neurol 1970;123:267-268.

57. Guilleminault C, Dement W: 235 cases of excessive daytime sleepiness: Diagnosis and tentative classification. J Neurol Sci 1977;31:13-27.

58. Hoddes E, Zarcone V, Smythe H, et al: Quantification of sleepiness: A new approach. Psychophysiology 1973;10:431-436.

59. Yoss R, Moyer N, Hollenhorst R: Pupil size and spontaneous pupillary waves associated with alertness, drowsiness, and sleep. Neurology 1970;20:545-554.

60. Carskadon M, Dement W: Effects of total sleep loss on sleep tendency. Percept Mot Skills 1979;48:495-506.

61. Richardson G, Carskadon M, Flagg W, et al: Excessive daytime sleepiness in man: Multiple sleep latency measurements in narcoleptic and control subjects. Electroencephalogr Clin Neurophysiol 1978;45:621-627.

62. Dement W, Carskadon M, Richardson G: Excessive daytime sleepiness in the sleep apnea syndromes. In Guilleminault C, Dement S (eds): Sleep Apnea Syndromes. New York, Alan R Liss, 1978, pp 23-46.

63. Carskadon M, Dement W: Daytime sleepiness: Quantification of a behavioral state. Neurosci Biobehav Rev 1987;11:307-317.

64. Guilleminault C, Dement W, Passouant P (eds): Narcolepsy. New York, Spectrum, 1976.

65. Sleep Disorders Classification Committee. Diagnostic classification of sleep and arousal disorders, 1st ed. Association of Sleep Disorders Centers and the Association for the Psychophysiological Study of Sleep. Sleep 1979;2:1-137.

66. Fujita S, Conway W, Zorick F, et al: Surgical correction of anatomic abnormalities in obstructive sleep apnea syndrome: Uvulopalatopharyngoplasty. Otolaryngol Head Neck Surg 1981; 89:923-934.

67. Sullivan CE, Issa FG, Berthon-Jones M, et al: Reversal of obstructive sleep apnea by continuous positive airway pressure applied through the nares. Lancet 1981;1:862-865.

68. Kryger M, Roth T, Dement WC: Principles and Practice of Sleep Medicine. Philadelphia, WB Saunders, 1989.

69. International directory of sleep researchers and clinicians. Available at http://www.websciences.org/directory/. Accessed January 2005.

70. Flemons WW, Douglas NJ, Kuna ST, et al: Access to diagnosis and treatment of patients with suspected sleep apnea. Am J Respir Crit Care Med 2004;169:668-672.

71. Lefant C, Kiley JP: Sleep research: Celebration and opportunity. Sleep 1998;21:665-669.

72. National Heart, Lung, and Blood Institute. Sleep Disorders Information. Available at http://www.nhlbi.nih.gov/about/ncsdr/. Accessed January 2005.

73. National Sleep Foundation. Available at http://www.sleepfoundation.org. Accessed January 2005.

2

Normal Human Sleep: An Overview

Mary A. Carskadon
William C. Dement

ABSTRACT

Normal human sleep comprises two states—non–rapid eye movement (NREM) and REM sleep—that alternate cyclically across a sleep episode. State characteristics are well defined: NREM sleep includes a variably synchronous cortical electroencephalogram (EEG; including sleep spindles, K-complexes, and slow waves) associated with low muscle tones and minimal psychological activity; the REM sleep EEG is desynchronized, muscles are atonic, and dreaming is typical. A nightly pattern of sleep in mature humans sleeping on a regular schedule includes several reliable characteristics: Sleep begins in NREM and progresses through deeper NREM stages (stages 2, 3, and 4) before the first episode of REM sleep approximately 80 to 100 minutes later. Thereafter, NREM sleep and REM sleep cycle with a period of approximately 90 minutes. NREM stages 3 and 4 concentrate in the early NREM cycles, and REM sleep episodes lengthen across the night.

Age-related changes are also predictable: Newborns enter REM sleep (called *active sleep*) before NREM (called *quiet sleep*) and have a shorter sleep cycle (approximately 50 minutes); sleep stages emerge as the brain matures during the first year. At birth, active sleep is approximately 50% of total sleep and declines over the first 2 years to approximately 20% to 25%. Slow wave sleep (stages 3 and 4) decreases across adolescence by 40% from preteen years and continues to decline into old age, particularly in men and less so in women. REM sleep as a percentage of total sleep is approximately 20% to 25% across childhood, adolescence, adulthood, and into old age except in dementia. Other factors predictably alter sleep, such as previous sleep–wake history, phase of the circadian timing system, ambient temperature, drugs, and sleep disorders.

A clear appreciation of the normal characteristics of sleep provides a strong background and template for understanding clinical conditions in which "normal" characteristics are altered, and for interpreting certain consequences of sleep disorders. In this chapter, the normal young adult sleep pattern is described as our working baseline pattern. Normative changes due to aging and other factors are described with that background in mind. Several major sleep disorders are highlighted by their differences from the normative pattern.

SLEEP DEFINITIONS

According to a simple behavioral definition, *sleep* is a reversible behavioral state of perceptual disengagement from and unresponsiveness to the environment. It is also true that sleep is a complex amalgam of physiologic and behavioral processes. Sleep is typically (but not necessarily) accompanied by postural recumbence, behavioral quiescence, closed eyes, and all the other indicators one commonly associates with sleeping. In the unusual circumstance, other behaviors can occur during sleep. These behaviors may include sleepwalking, sleeptalking, tooth grinding, and other physical activities. Anomalies involving sleep processes also include intrusions of sleep—sleep itself, dream imagery, or muscle weakness—into wakefulness.

Within sleep, two separate states have been defined on the basis of a constellation of physiologic parameters. These two states, non–rapid eye movement (NREM) and REM, exist in virtually all mammals and birds and are as distinct from one another as each is from wakefulness.

NREM (pronounced "non-REM") sleep is conventionally subdivided into four stages defined along one measurement axis, the electroencephalogram (EEG). The EEG pattern in NREM sleep is commonly described as synchronous, with such characteristic waveforms as sleep spindles, K-complexes, and high-voltage slow waves (Fig. 2–1). The four NREM stages (stages 1, 2, 3, and 4) roughly parallel a depth of sleep continuum, with arousal thresholds generally lowest in stage 1 and highest in stage 4 sleep. NREM sleep is usually associated

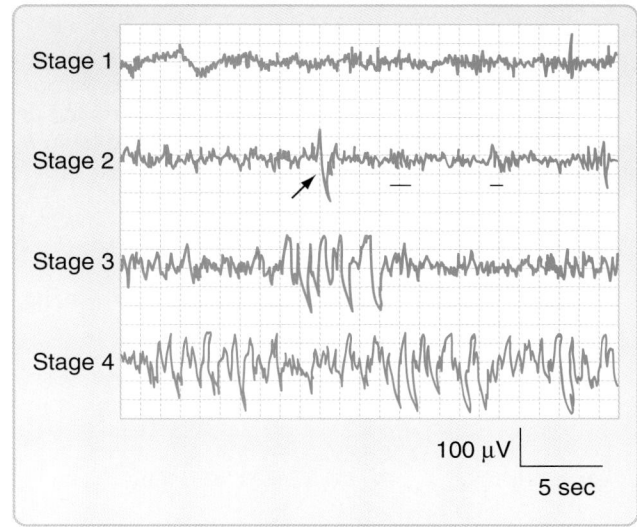

Stage 1

Stage 2

Stage 3

Stage 4

100 μV

5 sec

Figure 2–1. The stages of non–rapid eye movement sleep. The four electroencephalogram tracings depicted here are from a 19-year-old female volunteer. Each tracing was recorded from a referential lead (C3/A2) recorded on a Grass Instruments Co. Model 7D polygraph with a paper speed of 10 mm/second, time constant of 0.3 second, and ½-amplitude high-frequency setting of 30 Hz. On the second tracing, the *arrow* indicates a K-complex, and the *underlining* shows two sleep spindles.

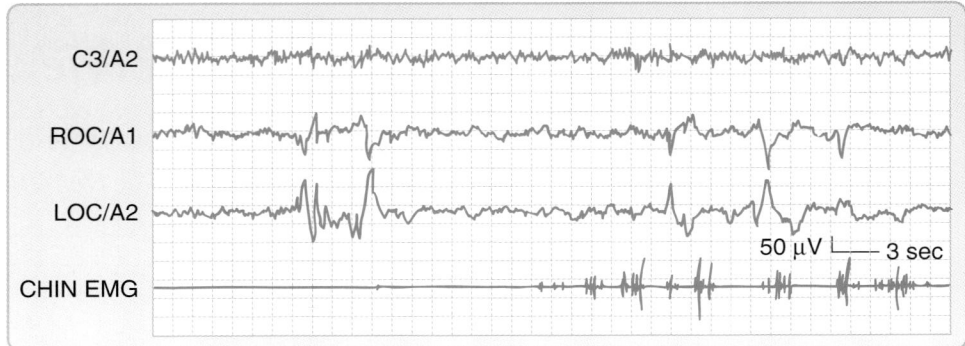

Figure 2–2. Phasic events in human rapid eye movement (REM) sleep. On the left side is a burst of several rapid eye movements (out-of-phase deflections in right outer canthus [ROC]/A1 and left outer canthus [LOC]/A2). On the right side, there are additional rapid eye movements as well as twitches on the electromyographic (EMG) lead. The interval between eye movement bursts and twitches illustrates tonic REM sleep.

with minimal or fragmentary mental activity. A shorthand definition of *NREM sleep* is a relatively inactive yet actively regulating brain in a movable body.

REM sleep, by contrast, is defined by EEG activation, muscle atonia, and episodic bursts of rapid eye movements. REM sleep usually is not divided into stages, although tonic and phasic types of REM sleep are often distinguished for certain research purposes. The tonic versus phasic distinction is based on short-lived events such as eye movements that tend to occur in clusters separated by episodes of relative quiescence. In cats, REM sleep phasic activity is epitomized by bursts of ponto-geniculo-occipital (PGO) waves, which are accompanied peripherally by rapid eye movements, twitching of distal muscles, middle ear muscle activity, and other phasic events that correspond to the phasic event markers easily measurable in human beings. As described in Chapter 116, PGO waves are not usually detectable in human beings. Thus, the most commonly used marker of REM sleep phasic activity in human beings is, of course, the bursts of rapid eye movements (Fig. 2–2); muscle twitches and cardiorespiratory irregularities often accompany the REM bursts. The mental activity of human REM sleep is associated with dreaming, based on vivid dream recall reported after approximately 80% of arousals from this state of sleep.[1] Inhibition of spinal motoneurons by brainstem mechanisms mediates suppression of postural motor tonus in REM sleep. A shorthand definition of *REM sleep*, therefore, is a highly activated brain in a paralyzed body.

SLEEP ONSET

The onset of sleep under normal circumstances in normal adult humans is through NREM sleep. This fundamental principle of normal human sleep reflects a highly reliable finding and is important in considering normal versus pathologic sleep. For example, the abnormal entry into sleep through REM sleep can be a diagnostic sign in adult patients with narcolepsy.

Definition of Sleep Onset

The precise definition of the onset of sleep has been a topic of debate, primarily because there is no single measure that is 100% clear-cut 100% of the time. For example, a change in EEG pattern is not always associated with an individual's perception of sleep; yet even when individuals may report that they are still awake, clear behavioral changes can indicate the presence of sleep. To begin a consideration of this issue, let us examine the three basic polysomnographic measures of sleep and how they change with sleep onset. The electrode placements are described in Chapter 116.

Electromyogram

The electromyogram (EMG) may show a gradual diminution of muscle tonus as sleep approaches, but rarely does a discrete EMG change pinpoint sleep onset. Furthermore, the waking level of the EMG, particularly if the individual is relaxed, can be entirely indistinguishable from that of unequivocal sleep (Fig. 2–3).

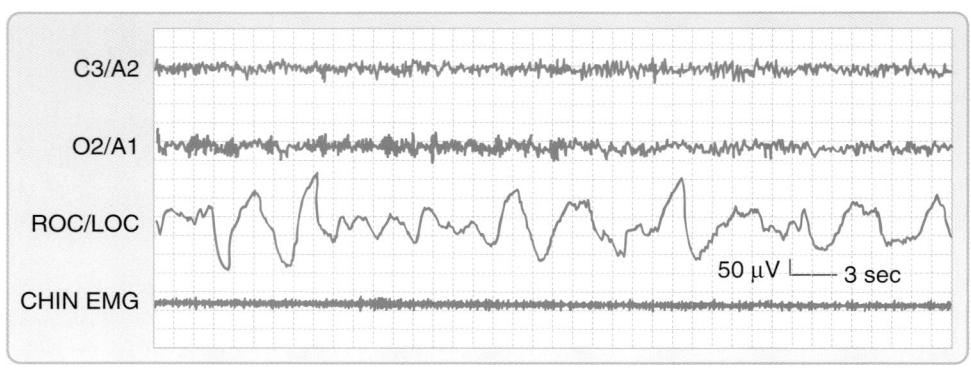

Figure 2–3. The transition from wakefulness to stage 1 sleep. The most marked change is visible on the two electroencephalographic (EEG) channels (C3/A2 and O2/A1), where a clear pattern of rhythmic alpha activity (8 cps) changes to a relatively low-voltage, mixed-frequency pattern at about the middle of the figure. The level of electromyographic (EMG) activity does not change markedly. Slow eye movements (right outer canthus [ROC]/left outer canthus [LOC]) are present throughout this episode, preceding the EEG change by at least 20 seconds. In general, the change in EEG patterns to stage 1 as illustrated here is accepted as the onset of sleep.

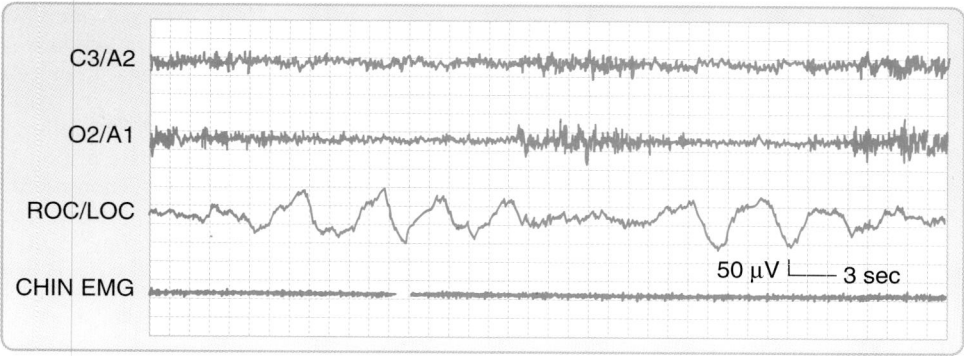

Figure 2–4. A common wake-to-sleep transition pattern. Note that the electroencephalographic pattern changes from wake (rhythmic alpha) to stage 1 (relatively low-voltage, mixed-frequency) sleep twice during this attempt to fall asleep. *EMG,* electromyogram; *LOC,* left outer canthus; *ROC,* right outer canthus.

Electrooculogram

As sleep approaches, the electrooculogram (EOG) shows slow, often asynchronous eye movements (see Fig. 2–3) that usually disappear within several minutes of the EEG changes described next. Occasionally, the onset of these slow eye movements coincides with a person's perceived sleep onset; more often, individuals report that they are awake.

Electroencephalogram

In the simplest circumstance (see Fig. 2–3), the EEG changes from a pattern of clear rhythmic alpha (8 to 13 cycles per second [cps]) activity, particularly in the occipital region, to a relatively low-voltage, mixed-frequency pattern (stage 1 sleep). This EEG change usually occurs seconds to minutes after the start of slow eye movements. With regard to introspection, the onset of a stage 1 EEG pattern may or may not coincide with perceived sleep onset. For this reason, a number of investigators require the presence of specific EEG patterns—the K-complex or sleep spindle (i.e., stage 2 sleep)—to acknowledge sleep onset. Even these stage 2 patterns, however, are not unequivocally associated with perceived sleep.[2] A further complication is that sleep onset frequently does not occur all at once; instead, there may be a wavering of vigilance before "unequivocal" sleep ensues (Fig. 2–4). Thus, it is difficult to accept a single variable as marking sleep onset. As Davis and colleagues[3] wrote many years ago (p. 35):

Is "falling asleep" a unitary event? Our observations suggest that it is not. Different functions, such as sensory awareness, memory, self-consciousness, continuity of logical thought, latency of response to a stimulus, and alterations in the pattern of brain

potentials all go in parallel in a general way, but there are exceptions to every rule.

Nevertheless, a reasonable consensus exists that the EEG change to stage 1, usually heralded or accompanied by slow eye movements, identifies the transition to sleep, provided that another EEG sleep pattern does not intervene. One may not always be able to pinpoint this transition to the millisecond, but it is usually possible to determine the change reliably within several seconds.

Behavioral Concomitants of Sleep Onset

Given the changes in the EEG that accompany the onset of sleep, what are the behavioral correlates of the wake-to-sleep transition? The following material reviews a few common behavioral concomitants of sleep onset. Keep in mind that "different functions may be depressed in different sequence and to different degrees in different subjects and on different occasions" (p. 35).[3]

Simple Behavioral Task

In the first example, volunteers were asked to tap two switches alternately at a steady pace. As shown in Figure 2–5, this simple behavior continues after the onset of slow eye movements and may persist for several seconds after the EEG changes to a stage 1 sleep pattern.[4] The behavior then ceases, usually to recur only after the EEG reverts to a waking pattern. This is an example of what one may think of as the simplest kind of "automatic" behavior pattern. Because such simple behavior may persist past sleep onset and as one passes in and out of

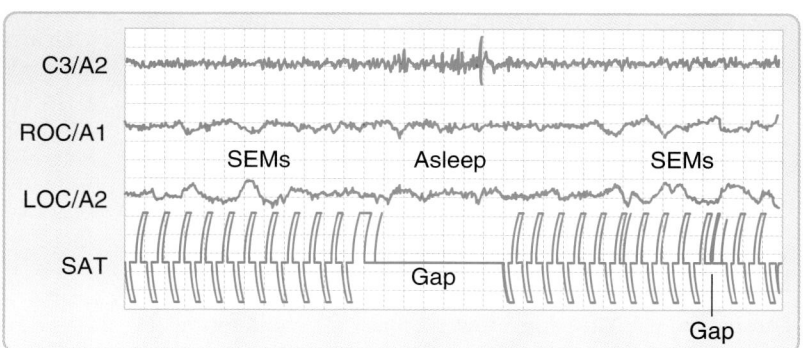

Figure 2–5. Failure to perform a simple behavioral task at the onset of sleep. The volunteer had been deprived of sleep overnight and was required to tap two switches alternately, shown as pen deflections of opposite polarity on the channel labeled SAT. When the electroencephalographic (EEG; C3/A2) pattern changes to stage 1 sleep, the behavior stops, returning when the EEG pattern reverts to wakefulness. LOC, left outer canthus; ROC, right outer canthus; SEMs, slow eye movements. (From Carskadon MA, Dement WC: Effects of total sleep loss on sleep tendency. Percept Mot Skills 1979;48:495-506. © Perceptual and Motor Skills, 1979.)

sleep, it may explain how impaired, drowsy drivers are able to continue down the highway.

Visual Response

A second example of behavioral change at sleep onset derives from an experiment in which a bright light is placed in front of the subject's eyes, and the individual is asked to respond when a light flash is seen by pressing a sensitive microswitch taped to the hand.[5] When the EEG pattern is stage 1 or stage 2 sleep, the response is absent more than 85% of the time. When volunteers are queried afterward, they report that they did not see the light flash, not that they saw the flash but the response was inhibited. This is one example of the perceptual disengagement from the environment that accompanies sleep onset.

Auditory Response

In another domain, the response to sleep onset is examined with a series of tones played over earphones to a subject who is instructed to respond each time a tone is heard. One study of this phenomenon showed that reaction times became longer in proximity to the onset of stage 1 sleep, and responses were absent coincident with a change in EEG to unequivocal sleep.[6] For responses in both visual and auditory modalities, the return of the response after its sleep-related disappearance typically requires the resumption of a waking EEG pattern.

Olfactory Response

When sleeping humans are tasked to respond when they smell something, the response depends in part on sleep state and in part on the particular odorant. In contrast to visual responses, one study showed that responses to graded strengths of peppermint (strong trigeminal stimulant usually perceived as pleasant) and pyridine (strong trigeminal stimulant usually perceived as extremely unpleasant) were well maintained during initial stage 1 sleep.[7] As with other modalities, the response in other sleep stages was significantly poorer: Peppermint simply was not consciously smelled in stages 2 and 4 NREM sleep or in REM sleep; pyridine was never smelled in stage 4 sleep, and only occasionally in stage 2 NREM and in REM sleep.[7] On the other hand, a tone successfully aroused the young adult participants in every stage. One conclusion of this report was that the olfactory system of humans is not a good sentinel system during sleep.

Response to Meaningful Stimuli

One should not infer from the preceding studies that the mind becomes an impenetrable barrier to sensory input at the onset of sleep. Indeed, one of the earliest modern studies of arousability during sleep showed that sleeping human beings were differentially responsive to auditory stimuli of graded intensity.[8] Another way of illustrating sensory sensitivity is shown in experiments that have assessed discriminant responses during sleep to meaningful versus nonmeaningful stimuli, with meaning supplied in a number of ways and response usually measured as evoked K-complexes or arousal. The following are examples.

1. A person tends to have a lower arousal threshold for his or her own name versus someone else's name.[9] In light sleep, for example, one's own name spoken softly will produce an arousal; a similarly applied nonmeaningful stimulus will not. Similarly, a sleeping mother is more likely to hear her own baby's cry than the cry of an unrelated infant.

2. Williams and colleagues[10] showed that the likelihood of an appropriate response during sleep was improved when an otherwise nonmeaningful stimulus was made meaningful by linking the absence of response to punishment (a loud siren, flashing light, and the threat of an electric shock).

From these examples and others, it seems clear that sensory processing at some level does continue after the onset of sleep. Indeed, one recent study has shown with functional magnetic resonance imaging that regional brain activation occurs in response to stimuli during sleep and that different brain regions (middle temporal gyrus and bilateral orbitofrontal cortex) are activated in response to meaningful (person's own name) versus nonmeaningful (beep) stimuli.[11]

Hypnic Myoclonia

What other behaviors accompany the onset of sleep? If you awaken and query someone shortly after the stage 1 sleep EEG pattern appears, the individual usually reports the mental experience as one of losing a direct train of thought and of experiencing vague and fragmentary imagery, usually visual.[12] Another fairly common sleep onset experience is hypnic myoclonia, which is experienced as a general or localized muscle contraction very often associated with rather vivid visual imagery. Hypnic myoclonias are not pathologic events, although they tend to occur more frequently in association with stress or with unusual or irregular sleep schedules.

The precise nature of hypnic myoclonias is not clearly understood. According to one hypothesis, the onset of sleep in these instances is marked by a dissociation of REM sleep components, wherein a breakthrough of the imagery component of REM sleep (hypnagogic hallucination) occurs in the absence of the REM motor inhibitory component. A response by the individual to the image, therefore, results in a movement or jerk. The increased frequency of these events in association with irregular sleep schedules is consistent with the increased probability of REM sleep occurring at the wake-to-sleep transition under such conditions (see later). Although the usual transition in adult human beings is to NREM sleep, the REM portal into sleep, which is the norm in infancy, may become partially opened under unusual circumstances.

Memory Near Sleep Onset

What happens to memory at the onset of sleep? The transition from wake to sleep tends to produce a memory impairment. One view is that it is as if sleep may close the gate between short-term and long-term memory stores. This phenomenon is best described by the following experiment.[13] During a presleep testing session, word pairs were presented to volunteers over a loudspeaker at 1-minute intervals. The subjects were then awakened either 30 seconds or 10 minutes after the onset of sleep (defined as EEG stage 1) and asked to recall those words presented before sleep onset. As illustrated in Figure 2–6, the 30-second condition was associated with a consistent level of recall from the entire 10 minutes before sleep onset. (Primacy and recency effects are apparent, although not large.) In the 10-minute condition, however, recall paralleled

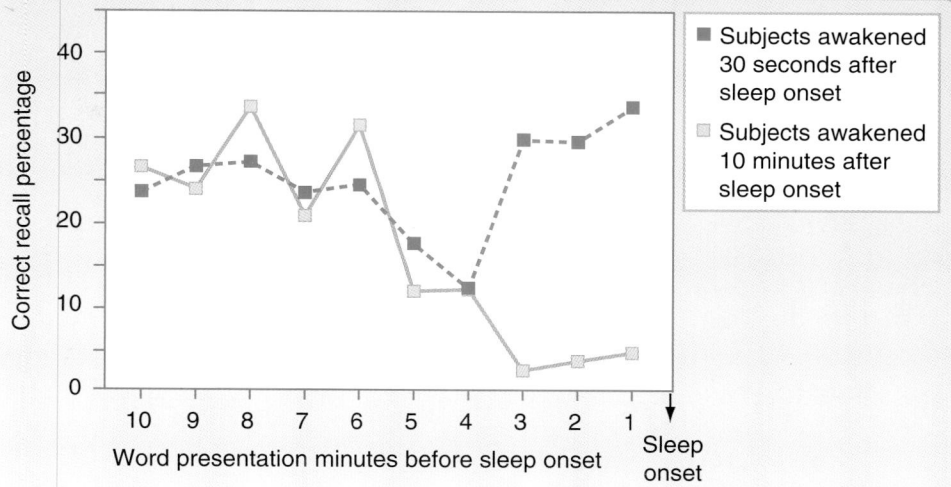

Figure 2–6. Memory is impaired by sleep, as shown by the study results illustrated in this graph. See text for explanation.

that in the 30-second group for only the 10 to 4 minutes before sleep onset and then fell abruptly from that point until sleep onset.

In the 30-second condition, therefore, both longer-term (4 to 10 minutes) and shorter-term (0 to 3 minutes) memory stores remained accessible. In the 10-minute condition, by contrast, words that were in longer-term stores (4 to 10 minutes) before sleep onset were accessible, whereas words that were still in shorter-term stores (0 to 3 minutes) at sleep onset were no longer accessible, that is, had not been consolidated into longer-term memory stores. One conclusion of this experiment is that sleep inactivates the transfer of storage from short- to long-term memory. Another interpretation is that encoding of the material before sleep onset is of insufficient strength to allow recall. The precise moment at which this deficit occurs is not known and may be a continuing process, perhaps reflecting anterograde amnesia. Nevertheless, one may infer that if sleep persists for approximately 10 minutes, memory is lost for the few minutes before sleep. The following experiences represent a few familiar examples of this phenomenon:

1. Inability to grasp the instant of sleep onset in your memory.
2. Forgetting a telephone call that had come in the middle of the night.
3. Forgetting the news you were told when awakened in the night.
4. Not remembering the ringing of your alarm clock.
5. Experiencing morning amnesia for coherent "sleeptalking."
6. Having fleeting dream recall.

Patients with syndromes of excessive sleepiness may experience similar memory problems in the daytime if sleep becomes intrusive.

Learning and Sleep

In contrast to this immediate sleep-related "forgetting," the relevance for sleep to human learning—particularly for consolidation of perceptual and motor learning—is of growing interest.[14,15] The importance of this association has also generated some debate and skepticism.[16] Nevertheless, a spate of recent research is awakening renewed interest in the

topic, and mechanistic studies explaining the roles of REM and NREM sleep more precisely are under examination (see Chapter 47).

PROGRESSION OF SLEEP ACROSS THE NIGHT

Pattern of Sleep in a Normal Young Adult

The simplest description of sleep begins with the ideal case, the normal young adult (Fig. 2–7). In general, no consistent male versus female distinctions have been found in the normal pattern of sleep in young adults. In briefest summary, the normal human adult enters sleep through NREM sleep, REM sleep does not occur until 80 minutes or longer thereafter, and NREM sleep and REM sleep alternate through the night, with an approximately 90-minute cycle (see Chapter 116 for a full description of sleep stages).

First Sleep Cycle

The first cycle of sleep in the normal young adult begins with stage 1 sleep, which usually persists for only a few (1 to 7) minutes at the onset of sleep. Sleep is easily discontinued during stage 1 by, for example, softly calling a person's name, touching the person lightly, quietly closing a door, and so forth. Thus, stage 1 sleep is associated with a low arousal threshold. In addition to its role in the initial wake-to-sleep transition, stage 1 sleep occurs as a transitional stage throughout the night. A common sign of severely disrupted sleep is an increase in the amount and percentage of stage 1 sleep.

Stage 2 NREM sleep, signaled by sleep spindles or K-complexes in the EEG (see Fig. 2–1), follows this brief episode of stage 1 sleep and continues for approximately 10 to 25 minutes. In stage 2 sleep, a more intense stimulus is required to produce arousal. The same stimulus that produced arousal from stage 1 sleep often results in an evoked K-complex but no awakening in stage 2 sleep.

As stage 2 sleep progresses, there is a gradual appearance of high-voltage slow wave activity in the EEG. Eventually, this

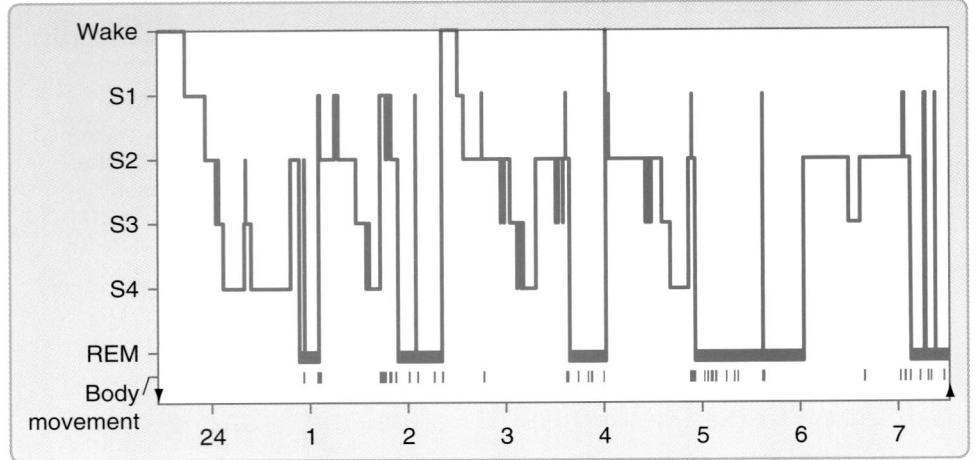

Figure 2–7. The progression of sleep stages across a single night in a normal young adult volunteer is illustrated in this sleep histogram. The text describes the "ideal" or "average" pattern. This histogram was drawn on the basis of a continuous overnight recording of electroencephalogram, electrooculogram, and electromyogram in a normal 19-year-old man. The record was assessed in 30-second epochs for the various sleep stages. REM, rapid eye movement.

activity meets the criteria[17] for stage 3 NREM sleep, that is, high-voltage (at least 75 µV) slow-wave (2 cps) activity accounting for more than 20% but less than 50% of the EEG activity. Stage 3 sleep usually lasts only a few minutes in the first cycle and is transitional to stage 4 as more and more high-voltage slow wave activity occurs. Stage 4 NREM sleep—identified when the high-voltage slow wave activity comprises more than 50% of the record—usually lasts approximately 20 to 40 minutes in the first cycle. An incrementally larger stimulus is usually required to produce an arousal from stage 3 or 4 sleep than from stage 1 or 2 sleep. (Investigators often refer to the combined stages 3 plus 4 sleep as slow wave sleep [SWS], delta sleep, or deep sleep.)

A series of body movements usually signals an "ascent" to lighter NREM sleep stages. There may be a brief (1- or 2-minute) episode of stage 3 sleep, followed by perhaps 5 to 10 minutes of stage 2 sleep interrupted by body movements preceding the initial REM episode. REM sleep in the first cycle of the night is usually short-lived (1 to 5 minutes). The arousal threshold in this REM episode is variable, as is true for REM sleep throughout the night. Theories to explain the variable arousal threshold of REM sleep have suggested that at times, the individual's selective attention to internal stimuli precludes a response, or that the arousal stimulus is incorporated into the ongoing dream story rather than producing an awakening. Certain early experiments examining arousal thresholds in cats found highest thresholds in REM sleep, which was then termed *deep sleep* in this species. Although this terminology is still often used in publications about sleep in animals, it should not be confused with human NREM stages 3 plus 4 sleep, which is also often called *deep sleep*. One should also note that SWS is sometimes used (as is synchronized sleep) as a synonym for all of NREM sleep in other species and is thus distinct from SWS (stages 3 plus 4 NREM) in human beings.

NREM–REM Cycle

NREM sleep and REM sleep continue to alternate through the night in cyclical fashion. REM sleep episodes usually become longer across the night. Stages 3 and 4 sleep occupy less time in the second cycle and may disappear altogether from later cycles, as stage 2 sleep expands to occupy the NREM portion

of the cycle. The average length of the first NREM–REM sleep cycle is approximately 70 to 100 minutes; the average length of the second and later cycles is approximately 90 to 120 minutes. Across the night, the average period of the NREM–REM cycle is approximately 90 to 110 minutes.

Distribution of Sleep Stages across the Night

In the young adult, SWS dominates the NREM portion of the sleep cycle toward the beginning of the night (the first one third); REM sleep episodes are longest in the last one third of the night. Brief episodes of wakefulness tend to intrude later in the night, usually near REM sleep transitions, and usually do not last long enough to be remembered in the morning. The preferential distribution of REM sleep toward the latter portion of the night in normal human adults is thought to be linked to a circadian oscillator and can be gauged by the oscillation of body temperature.[18,19] The preferential distribution of SWS toward the beginning of a sleep episode is not thought to be mediated by circadian processes but is linked to the initiation of sleep, the length of prior wakefulness, and the time course of sleep per se.[20] Thus, these aspects of the normal sleep pattern highlight features of the two-process model of sleep as elaborated on in Chapter 33.

Length of Sleep

The length of nocturnal sleep depends on a great number of factors—of which volitional control is among the most significant in human beings—and it is thus difficult to characterize a "normal" pattern. Most young adults report sleeping approximately 7.5 hours a night on weekday nights and slightly longer, 8.5 hours, on weekend nights. The variability of these figures from person to person and from night to night, however, is quite high. Sleep length also depends on genetic determinants,[21] and one may think of the volitional determinants (staying up late, waking by alarm, and so on) superimposed on the background of a genetic sleep need. The length of sleep is also determined by processes associated with circadian rhythms. Thus, *when* one sleeps helps to determine *how long* one sleeps. In addition, as sleep is extended, the amount of REM sleep increases because REM sleep depends on the persistence of sleep into the peak circadian time in order to occur.

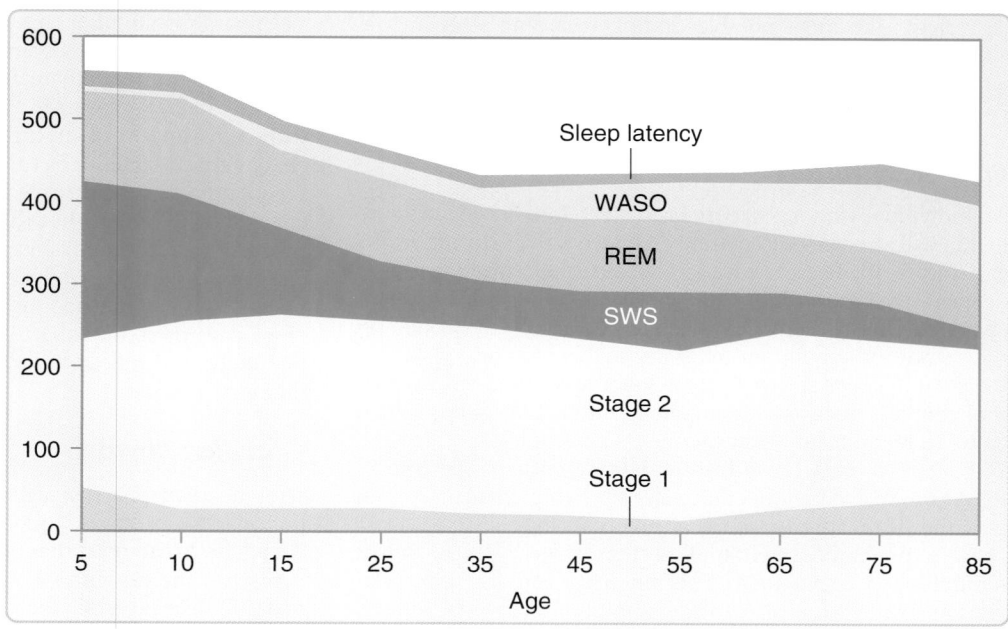

Figure 2–8. Changes in sleep with age. Time (in minutes) for sleep latency and wake time after sleep onset (WASO) and for rapid eye movement (REM) sleep and NREM sleep stages 1, 2, and slow wave sleep (SWS). Summary values are given for ages 5 to 85 years. (Ohayon M, Carskadon MA, Guilleminault C, et al: Meta-analysis of quantitative sleep parameters from childhood to old age in healthy individuals: Developing normative sleep values across the human lifespan. Sleep 2004;27:1255-1273.)

Generalizations about Sleep in the Normal Young Adult

A number of general statements can be made regarding sleep in the normal young adult who is living on a conventional sleep–wake schedule and who is without sleep complaints:

1. Sleep is entered through NREM sleep.
2. NREM sleep and REM sleep alternate with a period near 90 minutes.
3. SWS predominates in the first third of the night and is linked to the initiation of sleep.
4. REM sleep predominates in the last third of the night and is linked to the circadian rhythm of body temperature.
5. Wakefulness in sleep usually accounts for less than 5% of the night.
6. Stage 1 sleep generally constitutes approximately 2% to 5% of sleep.
7. Stage 2 sleep generally constitutes approximately 45% to 55% of sleep.
8. Stage 3 sleep generally constitutes approximately 3% to 8% of sleep.
9. Stage 4 sleep generally constitutes approximately 10% to 15% of sleep.
10. NREM sleep, therefore, is usually 75% to 80% of sleep.
11. REM sleep is usually 20% to 25% of sleep, occurring in four to six discrete episodes.

Factors Modifying Sleep Stage Distribution

Age

The strongest and most consistent factor affecting the pattern of sleep stages across the night is age (Fig. 2–8). The most marked age-related differences in sleep from the patterns described earlier are found in newborn infants. For the first year of life, the transition from wake to sleep is often accomplished through REM sleep (called *active sleep* in newborns).

The cyclical alternation of NREM–REM sleep is present from birth but has a period of approximately 50 to 60 minutes in the newborn compared with approximately 90 minutes in the adult. Infants also only gradually acquire a consolidated nocturnal sleep cycle, and the fully developed EEG patterns of the NREM sleep stages are not present at birth but emerge over the first 2 to 6 months of life. When brain structure and function achieve a level that can support high-voltage slow wave EEG activity, NREM stages 3 and 4 sleep become prominent.

SWS is maximal in young children and decreases markedly with age. The SWS of young children is both qualitatively and quantitatively different from that of older adults. For example, it is nearly impossible to wake youngsters in the SWS of the night's first sleep cycle. In one study,[22] a 123-dB tone failed to produce any sign of arousal in a group of children whose mean age was 10 years. A similar, although less profound qualitative difference distinguishes SWS occurring in the first and later cycles of the night in a given individual. The quantitative change in SWS may best be seen across adolescence, when SWS decreases by nearly 40% during the second decade, even when length of nocturnal sleep remains constant.[23] Feinberg[24] hypothesized that the age-related decline in nocturnal SWS may parallel loss of cortical synaptic density. By age 60 years, SWS may no longer be present, particularly in men. Women appear to maintain SWS later into life than men.

REM sleep as a percentage of total sleep is maintained well into healthy old age; the absolute amount of REM sleep at night has been correlated with intellectual functioning[25] and declines markedly in the case of organic brain dysfunctions of the elderly.[26]

Arousals during sleep increase markedly with age. Extended wake episodes of which the individual is aware and can report, as well as brief and probably unremembered arousals both increase with aging.[27] The latter type of transient arousals may occur with no known correlate but are frequently associated with occult sleep disturbances, such as periodic limb movements during sleep (PLMS) and sleep-related respiratory irregularities, which also become more prevalent in later life.[28,29]

Perhaps the most notable finding regarding sleep in the elderly is the profound increase in interindividual variability,[30] which thus precludes generalizations such as those made for young adults.

Prior Sleep History

An individual who has experienced sleep loss on one or more nights will show a sleep pattern that favors SWS during recovery (Fig. 2–9). Recovery sleep is also usually prolonged and deeper—that is, having a higher arousal threshold throughout—than basal sleep. REM sleep tends to show a rebound on the second or subsequent recovery nights after an episode of sleep loss. Therefore, with total sleep loss, SWS tends to be preferentially recovered compared with REM sleep, which tends to recover only after the recuperation of SWS.

Cases in which an individual is differentially deprived of REM or SWS, either operationally by being awakened each time the sleep pattern occurs, or pharmacologically (see later), show a preferential rebound of that stage of sleep when natural sleep is resumed. This phenomenon has particular relevance in a clinical setting, in which abrupt withdrawal from a therapeutic regimen may result in misleading diagnostic findings (e.g., sleep-onset REM periods [SOREMPs] as a result of a REM sleep rebound) or could conceivably exacerbate a sleep disorder (e.g., if sleep apneas tend to occur preferentially or with greater intensity in the rebounding stage of sleep).

Chronic restriction of nocturnal sleep, an irregular sleep schedule, or frequent disturbance of nocturnal sleep can result in a peculiar distribution of sleep states, most frequently characterized by premature REM sleep, that is, SOREMPs. Such episodes can be associated with hypnagogic hallucinations,

sleep paralysis, or an increased incidence of hypnic myoclonia in individuals with no organic sleep disorder.

Although not strictly related to prior sleep history, the first night of a laboratory sleep evaluation is commonly associated with a disruption of the normal distribution of sleep states, characterized chiefly by a delayed onset of REM sleep.[31] Frequently, this delay takes the form of missing the first REM episode of the night. In other words, the NREM sleep stages progress in a normal fashion, but the first cycle ends with an episode of stage 1 or a brief arousal instead of the expected brief REM sleep episode. In addition, REM sleep episodes are often disrupted, and the total amount of REM sleep on the first night in the sleep laboratory is also usually reduced from the normal value.

Circadian Rhythms

The circadian phase at which sleep occurs affects the distribution of sleep stages. REM sleep, in particular, occurs with a circadian distribution that peaks in the morning hours coincident with the trough of body temperature.[18,19] Thus, if sleep onset is delayed until the peak REM phase of the circadian rhythm—that is, the early morning—REM sleep tends to predominate and may even occur at the onset of sleep. This reversal of the normal sleep-onset pattern is commonly seen in a normal person who acutely undergoes a phase shift, either as a result of a work shift change or a change resulting from jet travel across a number of time zones. Studies of individuals sleeping in environments free of all cues to time have shown that the timing of sleep onset and the length of sleep occur as a function of circadian phase.[32,33] Under these conditions, sleep distribution with reference to the circadian body temperature phase position shows that sleep onset is

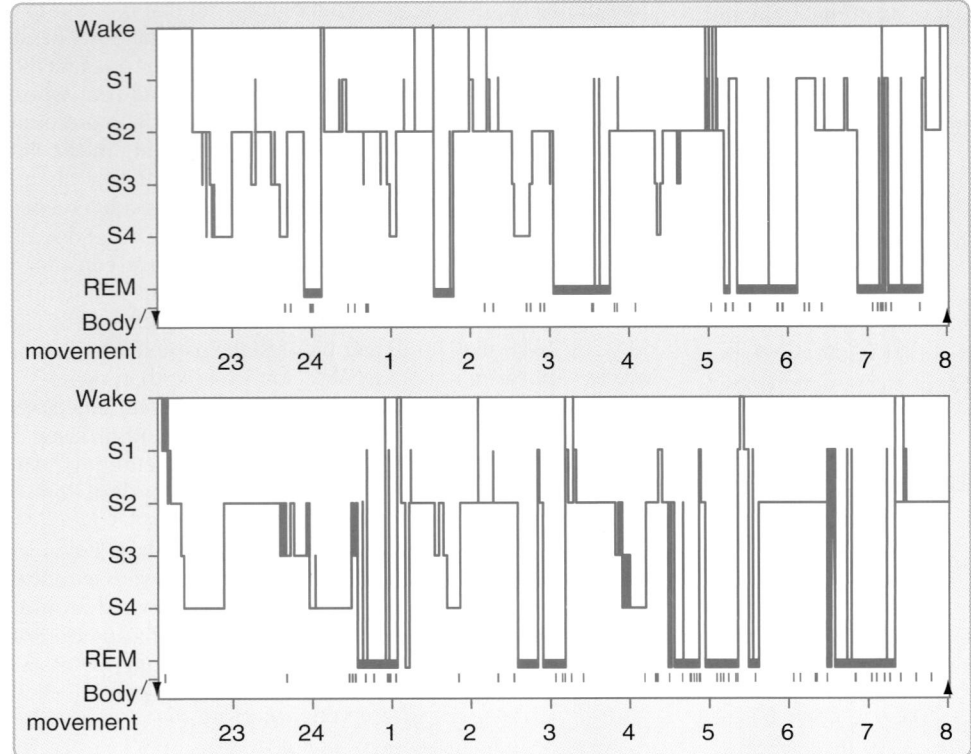

Figure 2–9. The upper histogram shows the baseline sleep pattern of a normal 14-year-old female volunteer. The lower histogram illustrates the sleep pattern in this volunteer for the first recovery night after 38 hours without sleep. Note that the amount of stage 4 sleep on the lower graph is greater than on baseline, and the first rapid eye movement (REM) sleep episode is markedly delayed.

likeliest to occur on the falling limb of the temperature cycle. A secondary peak of sleep onsets, corresponding to afternoon napping, also occurs; the offset of sleep occurs most often on the rising limb of the circadian body temperature curve.[34]

Temperature

Extremes of temperature in the sleeping environment tend to disrupt sleep. REM sleep is commonly more sensitive to temperature-related disruption than is NREM sleep. Accumulated evidence from human beings and other species suggests that mammals have only minimal ability to thermoregulate during REM sleep; in other words, the control of body temperature is virtually poikilothermic in REM sleep.[35] This inability to thermoregulate in REM sleep probably affects the response to temperature extremes and suggests that such conditions are less of a problem early during a night than late, when REM sleep tends to predominate. It should be clear, as well, that sweating or shivering during sleep in response to ambient temperature extremes occurs in NREM sleep and ceases in REM sleep.

Drug Ingestion

The distribution of sleep states and stages is affected by many common drugs, including those typically prescribed in the treatment of sleep disorders as well as those not specifically related to the pharmacotherapy of sleep disorders and those used socially or recreationally. It is unknown whether changes in sleep stage distribution have any relevance to health, illness, or psychological well-being; however, particularly in the context of specific sleep disorders that differentially affect one sleep stage or another, such distinctions may be relevant to diagnosis or treatment. A number of generalizations regarding the effects of certain of the more frequently used compounds on sleep stage distribution follow:

1. Benzodiazepines tend to suppress SWS and have no consistent effect on REM sleep.
2. Tricyclic antidepressants, monoamine oxidase inhibitors, and certain selective serotonin reuptake inhibitors tend to suppress REM sleep. An increased level of motor activity during sleep occurs with certain of these compounds, leading to a pattern of REM sleep without motor inhibition or an increased incidence of PLMS. Fluoxetine is also associated with rapid eye movements across all sleep stages ("Prozac eyes").
3. Withdrawal from drugs that selectively suppress a stage of sleep tends to be associated with a rebound of that sleep stage. Thus, acute withdrawal from a benzodiazepine compound is likely to produce an increase of SWS; acute withdrawal from a tricyclic antidepressant or monoamine oxidase inhibitor is likely to produce an increase of REM sleep. In the latter case, this REM rebound could result in abnormal SOREMPs in the absence of an organic sleep disorder, perhaps leading to a false-positive diagnosis of narcolepsy.
4. Acute presleep alcohol intake produces an increase in SWS and REM sleep suppression early in the night, which is often followed by REM sleep rebound in the latter portion of the night as the alcohol is metabolized.
5. Acute effects of marijuana (tetrahydrocannabinol [THC]) include minimal sleep disruption, characterized by a slight reduction of REM sleep. Chronic ingestion of THC produces a long-term suppression of SWS.[36]

Pathology

Sleep disorders, as well as other nonsleep problems, have an impact on the structure and distribution of sleep. As suggested before, these distinctions appear to be more important in diagnosis and in the consideration of treatments than for any implications about general health or illness resulting from specific sleep stage alterations. Listed are a number of common sleep stage anomalies commonly associated with sleep disorders:

1. *Narcolepsy* is characterized by an abnormally short delay to REM sleep, marked by SOREMPs. This abnormal sleep-onset pattern occurs with some consistency, but not exclusively; that is, NREM sleep onset can also occur. Thus, the preferred diagnostic test consists of several opportunities to fall asleep across a day (see Chapter 120). If REM sleep occurs abnormally on two or more such opportunities, narcolepsy is extremely probable. The occurrence of this abnormal sleep pattern in narcolepsy is thought to be responsible for the rather unusual symptoms of this disorder. In other words, dissociation of components of REM sleep into the waking state results in hypnagogic hallucinations, sleep paralysis, and, most dramatically, cataplexy. Other conditions in which a short REM sleep latency may occur include infancy, in which sleep-onset REM sleep is normal; sleep reversal or jet lag; acute withdrawal from REM-suppressant compounds; chronic restriction or disruption of sleep; and endogenous depression, in which a shortened latency to REM sleep is thought to be a biologic marker of this psychiatric entity.[37] Recent reports have indicated a relatively high prevalence of REM sleep onsets in young adults[38] and in adolescents with early rise times.[39] In the latter, the REM sleep onsets on morning (8:30 and 10:30 AM) naps were related to a delayed circadian phase as indicated by later onset of melatonin secretion.
2. *Sleep apnea syndromes* may be associated with suppression of SWS or REM sleep, secondary to the sleep-related breathing problem. Suppression of SWS occurs most commonly in children with sleep apnea; REM suppression is more common in adults with sleep apnea syndromes. Successful treatment of this sleep disorder, as with nocturnal continuous positive airway pressure, can produce large rebounds of SWS or REM sleep (Fig. 2–10).
3. *Fragmentation of sleep and increased frequency of arousals* occur in association with a number of sleep disorders as well as with medical disorders involving physical pain or discomfort. PLMS, sleep apnea syndromes, chronic fibrositis, and so forth may be associated with tens to hundreds of arousals each night. Brief arousals are prominent in such conditions as allergic rhinitis,[40,41] juvenile rheumatoid arthritis,[42] and Parkinson's disease.[43] In upper airway resistance syndrome,[44] EEG arousals are important markers because the respiratory signs of this syndrome are less obvious than in frank obstructive sleep apnea syndrome, and only subtle indicators may be available.[45] In specific situations, autonomic changes, such as transient changes of blood pressure,[46] may signify arousals; Lofaso and colleagues[47] indicated that autonomic changes are highly correlated with the extent of EEG arousals. Less well studied is the possibility that sleep fragmentation may be associated with subcortical events not visible in the cortical EEG signal. These disorders also often involve an increase in the absolute amount of and the proportion of stage 1 sleep.

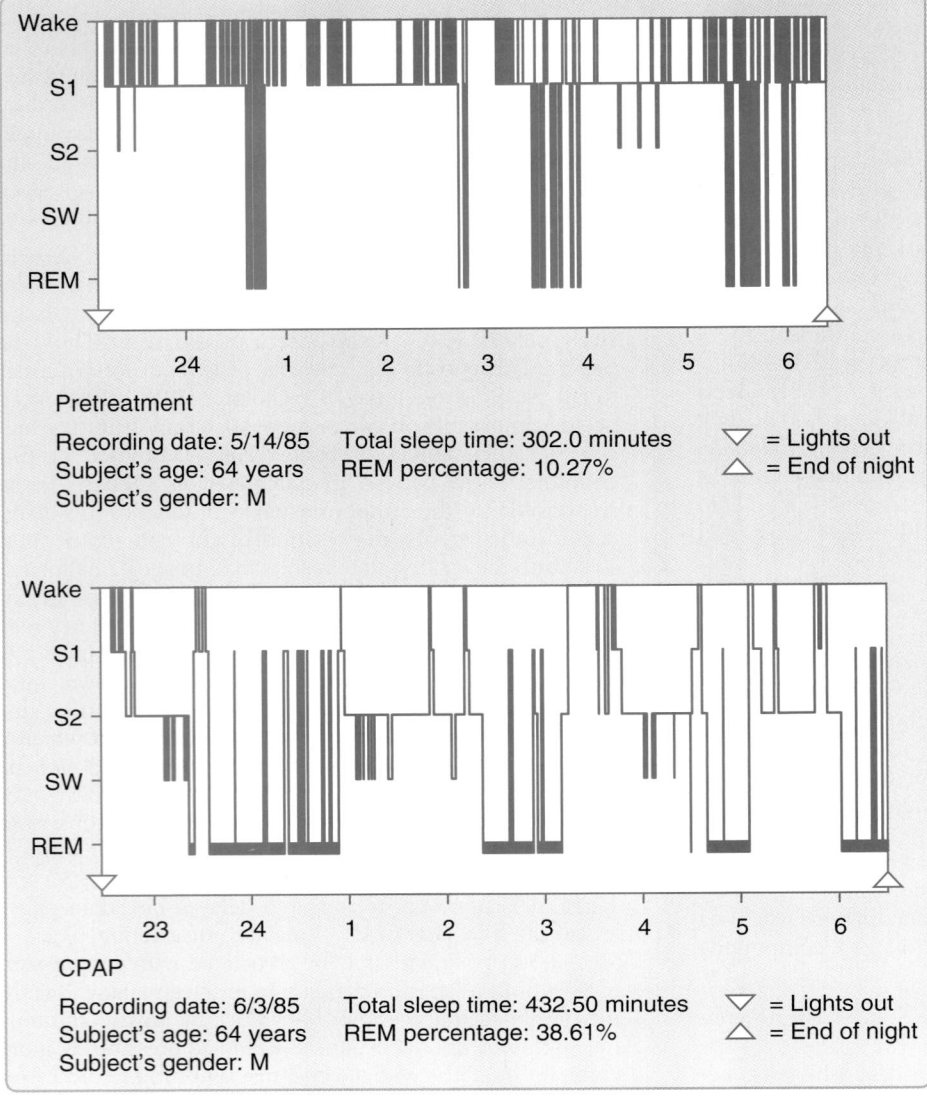

Figure 2–10. These sleep histograms depict the sleep of a 64-year-old male patient with obstructive sleep apnea syndrome. The upper graph shows the sleep pattern before treatment. Note the absence of slow wave (SW; stage 3 or 4) sleep, the preponderance of stage 1 (S1), and the very frequent disruptions. The lower graph shows the sleep pattern in this patient during the second night of treatment with continuous positive airway pressure (CPAP). Note that sleep is much deeper (more SW) and more consolidated, and rapid eye movement (REM) sleep in particular is abnormally increased. The pretreatment REM percentage of sleep was only 10%, versus nearly 40% with treatment. (Data supplied by G. Nino-Murcia, Stanford University Sleep Disorders Center, Stanford, California.)

Pretreatment

Recording date: 5/14/85
Subject's age: 64 years
Subject's gender: M

Total sleep time: 302.0 minutes
REM percentage: 10.27%

▽ = Lights out
△ = End of night

CPAP

Recording date: 6/3/85
Subject's age: 64 years
Subject's gender: M

Total sleep time: 432.50 minutes
REM percentage: 38.61%

▽ = Lights out
△ = End of night

Clinical Pearls

- The clinician should expect to see less SWS (stages 3 and 4) in older individuals, particularly men.
- The clinician may find himself or colleagues denying mid-night communications (nighttime calls) because of memory deficits that occur for events proximal to sleep onset. This phenomenon may also account for memory deficits in excessively sleepy patients.
- Many medications (even if not prescribed for sleep) can affect sleep stages, and their use or discontinuation alters sleep. Thus, REM-suppressant medications, for example, may result in a rebound of REM sleep on discontinuation.
- Certain patients may have sleep complaints (insomnia, hypersomnia) that result from attempts to sleep at a circadian phase that is not in synch.
- Patients who wake with events early in the night may have a disorder affecting NREM sleep; patients who wake with events late in the night may have a disorder affecting REM sleep.

Acknowledgments

The authors thank Joan Mancuso for preparing the figures.

References

1. Dement W, Kleitman N: The relation of eye movements during sleep to dream activity: An objective method for the study of dreaming. J Exp Psychol 1957;53:339-346.
2. Agnew HW, Webb WB: Measurement of sleep onset by EEG criteria. Am J EEG Technol 1972;12:127-134.
3. Davis H, Davis PA, Loomis AL, et al: Human brain potentials during the onset of sleep. J Neurophysiol 1938;1:24-38.
4. Carskadon MA, Dement WC: Effects of total sleep loss on sleep tendency. Percept Mot Skills 1979;48:495-506.
5. Guilleminault C, Phillips R, Dement WC: A syndrome of hypersomnia with automatic behavior. Electroencephalogr Clin Neurophysiol 1975;38:403-413.
6. Ogilvie RD, Wilkinson RT: The detection of sleep onset: Behavioral and physiological convergence. Psychophysiology 1984;21:510-520.
7. Carskadon MA, Herz R: Minimal olfactory perception during sleep: Why odor alarms will not work for humans. Sleep 2004;27:402-405.

8. Williams HL, Hammack JT, Daly RL, et al: Responses to auditory stimulation, sleep loss and the EEG stages of sleep. Electroencephalogr Clin Neurophysiol 1964;16:269-279.

9. Oswald I, Taylor AM, Treisman M: Discriminative responses to stimulation during human sleep. Brain 1960;83:440-453.

10. Williams HL, Morlock HC, Morlock JV: Instrumental behavior during sleep. Psychophysiology 1966;2:208-216.

11. Portas CM, Krakow K, Allen P, et al: Auditory processing across the sleep-wake cycle: Simultaneous EEG and fMRI monitoring in humans. Neuron 2000;28:991-999.

12. Foulkes D: The Psychology of Sleep. New York, Charles Scribner's Sons, 1966.

13. Wyatt JK, Bootzin RR, Anthony J, et al: Does sleep onset produce retrograde amnesia? Sleep Res 1992;21:113.

14. Maquet P: The role of sleep in learning and memory. Science 2001;294:1048-1052.

15. Stickgold R, Hobson JA, Fosse R, et al: Sleep, learning and dreams: Off-line memory reprocessing. Science 2001;294:1052-1057.

16. Siegel J: The REM sleep-memory consolidation hypothesis. Science 2001;294:1058-1063.

17. Rechtschaffen A, Kales A (eds): A Manual of Standardized Terminology, Techniques and Scoring System for Sleep Stages of Human Subjects. Los Angeles, UCLA Brain Information Service/Brain Research Institute, 1968.

18. Czeisler CA, Zimmerman JC, Ronda JM, et al: Timing of REM sleep is coupled to the circadian rhythm of body temperature in man. Sleep 1980;2:329-346.

19. Zulley J: Distribution of REM sleep in entrained 24 hour and free-running sleep-wake cycles. Sleep 1980;2:377-389.

20. Weitzman ED, Czeisler CA, Zimmerman JC, et al: Timing of REM and stages 3 + 4 sleep during temporal isolation in man. Sleep 1980;2:391-407.

21. Karacan I, Moore CA: Genetics and human sleep. Psychiatr Ann 1979;9:11-23.

22. Busby K, Pivik RT: Failure of high intensity auditory stimuli to affect behavioral arousal in children during the first sleep cycle. Pediatr Res 1983;17:802-805.

23. Carskadon MA, Dement WC: Sleepiness in the normal adolescent. In Guilleminault C (ed): Sleep and Its Disorders in Children. New York, Raven Press, 1987, pp 53-66.

24. Feinberg I: Schizophrenia: Caused by a fault in programmed synaptic elimination during adolescence? J Psychiatr Res 1983;17:319-334.

25. Prinz P: Sleep patterns in the healthy aged: Relationship with intellectual function. J Gerontol 1977;32:179-186.

26. Prinz PN, Peskind ER, Vitaliano PP, et al: Changes in the sleep and waking EEGs of nondemented and demented elderly subjects. J Am Geriatr Soc 1982;30:86-93.

27. Carskadon MA, Brown ED, Dement WC: Sleep fragmentation in the elderly: Relationship to daytime sleep tendency. Neurobiol Aging 1982;3:321-327.

28. Ancoli-Israel S, Kripke DF, Mason W, et al: Sleep apnea and nocturnal myoclonus in a senior population. Sleep 1981;4:349-358.

29. Carskadon MA, Dement WC: Respiration during sleep in the aging human. J Gerontol 1981;36:420-423.

30. Williams RL, Karacan I, Hursch CJ: EEG of Human Sleep: Clinical Applications. New York, John Wiley & Sons, 1974.

31. Agnew HW, Webb WB, Williams RL: The first-night effect: An EEG study of sleep. Psychophysiology 1966;2:263-266.

32. Czeisler CA, Weitzman ED, Moore-Ede MC, et al: Human sleep: Its duration and organization depend on its circadian phase. Science 1980;210:1264-1267.

33. Zulley J, Wever R, Aschoff J: The dependence of onset and duration of sleep on the circadian rhythm of rectal temperature. Pflugers Arch 1981;391:314-318.

34. Strogatz SH: The Mathematical Structure of the Human Sleep-Wake Cycle. New York, Springer-Verlag, 1986.

35. Parmeggiani PL: Temperature regulation during sleep: A study in homeostasis. In Orem J, Barnes CD (eds): Physiology in Sleep. New York, Academic Press, 1980, pp 98-143.

36. Freemon FR: The effect of chronically administered delta-9-tetrahydrocannabinol upon the polygraphically monitored sleep of normal volunteers. Drug Alcohol Depend 1982;10:345-353.

37. Kupfer DJ: REM latency: A psychobiologic marker for primary depressive disease. Biol Psychiatry 1976;11:159-174.

38. Bishop C, Rosenthal L, Helmus T, et al: The frequency of multiple sleep onset REM periods among subjects with no excessive daytime sleepiness. Sleep 1996;19:727-730.

39. Carskadon MA, Wolfson AR, Acebo C, et al: Adolescent sleep patterns, circadian timing, and sleepiness at a transition to early school days. Sleep 1998;21:871-881.

40. Lavie P, Gertner R, Zomer J, et al: Breathing disorders in sleep associated with "microarousals" in patients with allergic rhinitis. Acta Otolaryngol 1981;92:529-533.

41. Craig TJ, Teets S, Lehman EB, et al: Nasal congestion secondary to allergic rhinitis as a cause of sleep disturbance and daytime fatigue and the response to topical nasal corticosteroids. J Allergy Clin Immunol 1998;101:633-637.

42. Zamir G, Press J, Tal A, et al: Sleep fragmentation in children with juvenile rheumatoid arthritis. J Rheumatol 1998;25:1191-1197.

43. Stocchi F, Barbato L, Nordera G, et al: Sleep disorders in Parkinson's disease. J Neurol 1998;245(Suppl 1):S15-S18.

44. Guilleminault C, Stoohs R, Clerk A, et al: From obstructive sleep apnea syndrome to upper airway resistance syndrome—consistency of daytime sleepiness. Sleep 1992;15(6 Suppl):S13-S16.

45. Hosselet JJ, Norman RG, Ayappa I, et al: Detection of flow limitation with a nasal cannula/pressure transducer system. Am J Respir Crit Care Med 1998;157:1461-1467.

46. Pitson DJ, Stradling JR: Autonomic markers of arousal during sleep in patients undergoing investigation for obstructive sleep apnoea, their relationship to EEG arousals, respiratory events and subjective sleepiness. J Sleep Res 1998;7:53-59.

47. Lofaso F, Goldenberg F, Dortho MP, et al: Arterial blood pressure response to transient arousals from NREM sleep in nonapneic snorers with sleep fragmentation. Chest 1998;113:985-991.

3

Normal Aging

Donald L. Bliwise

ABSTRACT

Sleep patterns change substantially and continuously with age across adulthood. Altered sleep architecture, such as an increased percentage of time spent in stage 1 and a decreased percentage spent in stage 3/4, is a hallmark of aging, although the changes may be more pronounced in men. The percentage of time spent in rapid eye movement (REM) sleep demonstrates a small (2% to 3%) decrease from middle to old age, and sleep efficiency lowers with age as well, declining from approximately 86% at about age 45 to about 79% in those older than 70. Brief arousals are common in aging and occur at rates of about 15 per hour in elderly individuals without sleep-disordered breathing (SDB) to over twice this in individuals with appreciable SDB. Neurohumoral correlates of changes in architecture include declining growth hormone (correlated with the decreased time spent in stage 3/4), elevated evening cortisol (correlated with the decrease in REM sleep), and increased interleukin-6 (correlated with the increased amount of wake after sleep onset). Inability to phase-shift readily, the occurrence of daytime napping, and lark-like tendencies all characterize the sleep–wake rhythms of older adults. Inability to sustain long bouts of waking and uninterrupted sleep may reflect a fundamental age-dependent change in the homeostatic regulation of sleep. Napping results from multiple factors in old age, ranging from clinical or subclinical disease to functional declines in the sleep homeostasis.

Insomnia is common in people older than 65 years, with about 30% complaining of sleep maintenance problems and about half that number complaining of prolonged sleep latency. Despite having more stage 3/4 sleep, older women are more likely to have sleep complaints and use hypnotics than older men. The presence of medical or psychiatric illness plays an important role in the poor sleep of older people. Both restless legs syndrome and periodic limb movements in sleep increase with aging, although many elderly persons demonstrate substantial numbers of the latter without obvious clinical correlation, which implies that the movements may be an incidental finding. SDB is a very prevalent condition in older adults: as many as 44% of individuals older than 65 demonstrate an apnea/hypopnea index greater than 20 events per hour. Some evidence suggests that SDB in older adults represents an age-dependent condition, and that the clinical significance is different from that of SDB in middle-aged populations. However, some risk factors for SDB in old age may be identical to those in middle age, and the strength of associations between SDB and certain outcomes may not diminish in older adults.

As the populations of industrialized societies age, defining how sleep is affected by age assumes greater importance. In the United States, the average current life expectancy of 77 years means that 80% of residents now live to be at least 65; the fastest-growing segment of the population is composed of those who are 85 and older. These huge numbers force sleep specialists to confront the question, What is *normal?* Investigators often use the term to connote a variety of meanings. In sleep disorders, confusion occurs because the term is used descriptively, to indicate representativeness, as well as clinically, to indicate absence of disease.

Aging is also subject to semantic confusion. Chronologic age has been shown repeatedly to only approximate physiologic age. The decline in slow wave sleep, for example, may occur at a chronologic age far earlier than most age-dependent declines in other biologic functions. Some researchers in gerontology have noted that distance from death may be a far better approximation of the aging process, but too few longitudinal sleep studies exist to yield these types of findings.

In addition to the issue of physiologic age, subjective age must be considered. Because the practice of sleep disorders medicine in geriatrics relies heavily on self-reports of sleep disturbance, subjective appraisal of the older person's symptoms must be considered. Whether an older person views 75% sleep efficiency as insomnia or merely accepts this as a normal part of aging may depend largely on that individual's perspective on growing old. It has been reported that older people are more likely to perceive themselves as having sleep problems when they have difficulty falling asleep rather than difficulty staying asleep, even though the latter continues to be a more commonly reported symptom.[1] In addition, some have suggested that self-reports of sleep, when compared with polysomnographic measurements, are inherently less accurate and valid in older than in younger persons, although evidence for this age difference in other studies is decidedly mixed and varies according to the variables under consideration, including the subject's sex.

Finally, normal aging must be viewed in counterpoint to pathologic aging.[2] Although the prevalence of dementing illnesses is high late in life, determination of the number of normal elderly persons who may be in incipient stages of dementia has seldom been addressed. Additionally, recognition of mental impairments in the more limited domains of memory, executive function, language, attention, and visuospatial ability characterized as being of lesser severity has led to the use of an intermediate diagnostic category entitled mild cognitive impairment (MCI).[3] Few sleep studies of normal aging rely on extensive diagnostic work to eliminate individuals in the earliest stages of mental impairment, and polysomnographic studies in patients with well-defined mild cognitive impairment have yet to be performed.

The point here is not to dismiss all that is known about sleep patterns in normal aging as inadequate but rather to point out the complexities of defining normal aging. Normal aging can never be defined without some arbitrary criteria. Throughout this chapter, aging will be referred to across several species, encompassing what in humans may be considered both "middle-aged" (approximately 40 to 65) and "elderly" (over 65 years). We recognize fully the otherwise arbitrary nature of these verbal and numeric descriptors of processes that are most assuredly gradual and continuous, and that vary widely across individuals. It is also important to recognize that the age-dependent alterations in sleep may simply be secondary manifestations of senescence.

SLEEP ARCHITECTURE

Although age-dependent alterations in sleep architecture have been described for many years, only recently have carefully collected, rigorously scored and analyzed data on large, heterogeneous elderly populations allowed a detailed appreciation of how comorbidities, demographics, and SDB may impact on observed values.[4] Previously, normative sleep architecture data were derived from relatively small samples of selected populations (typically 50 to 100 persons) deemed otherwise "healthy" or "normal," but few of these studies accounted for sleep pathologies (such as SDB) in establishing norms (for compilation of earlier studies, see Bliwise[5]). Recent publication of sleep architecture data from the Sleep Heart Health Study (SHHS)[4] can be considered broadly generalizable to geriatric populations, at least within the limitations of selective survivorship and other aspects of the sampling framework (e.g., single-night, digitally acquired, unattended monitoring) for this major epidemiologic study.

Table 3–1 provides sleep architecture values for 2685 SHHS participants aged 37 to 92; individuals using psychotropics and those having high alcohol intake, restless legs syndrome symptoms, and systemic pain conditions were excluded. About a third of these participants were hypertensive, and about 10% had a history of cardiovascular disease or chronic pulmonary disease. Although age effects are apparent in some measures, gender occupied a far more dramatic role in sleep architecture, in some cases showing considerable divergence between women and men. Most notable in this regard is the

percentage of time spent in stage 3/4, which shows enormous sex differences at every age and, in fact, shows no appreciable decline with aging in women, relative to men, the latter demonstrating a marked cross-sectional decline with aging, as well as huge individual differences in every age group. The extent of these individual differences is emphasized by the fact that even within men, coefficients of variation (i.e., the ratio of variance to mean) in time spent in stage 3/4 far exceeded those for all other sleep variables in both men and women.

Although sex differences in slow wave sleep have been noted previously (see Bliwise[6] for a review), the fact that the age-dependent decline may be confined to men suggests a more limited utility of this biomarker of aging for women. Time spent in stage 1 showed a similar gender-related effect, with increases in this sleep stage usually considered to represent a feature of fragmented, transitional sleep, confined to men only. In contrast, time spent in REM sleep shows a modest decline with age, but the effect was detected in both men and women. Sleep efficiency also declined with age, with mean values of 85.7 (standard deviation [SD] = ±8.3), 83.3 (SD = ±8.9), 80.6 (SD = ±11.7), and 79.2 (SD = ±10.1), in the groups aged 37 to 54, 55 to 60, 61 to 70, and over 70 years, respectively, but without differential effects of gender.

One component of the so-called microarchitectural features of sleep is the number of brief arousals during sleep, and this continues to attract considerable interest as a metric, with particular relevance for the older population. Failure to maintain continuous sleep has, as its basic science counterpart, short bout lengths, a feature highly characteristic of aged sleep in many mammalian species.[5] In elderly persons without SDB, arousal indices from 18 to 27 events per hour have been reported.[7] Among the predominantly elderly subjects (mean age, 61) in the SHHS, the mean (±SD) arousal index showed significant, although relatively small, increases with age, ranging from 16.0 (±8.2) for the 37 to 54 group, to 18.4 (±10.0) for the 55 to 61 group, to 20.3 (±10.5) for the 62 to 70 group, to 21.0 (±11.6) for those older than 70.[4] Other phasic events of non–rapid eye movement (NREM) sleep, such as K-complex and spindle density (the latter thought to reflect, at least partially, the corticothalamic functional integrity of

Table 3–1. Sleep Architecture as a Function of Age

	Percentage of Time Spent in Stage Mean (95% Confidence Interval)							
	Stage 1		Stage 2		Stage 3/4		REM Sleep	
Age	Men	Women	Men	Women	Men	Women	Men	Women
37-54	5.8 (5.2-6.5)	4.6 (4.1-5.3)	61.4 (60.0-62.8)	58.5 (57.1-60.0)	11.2 (9.9-12.6)	14.2 (12.7-15.9)	19.5 (18.8-20.2)	20.9 (20.0-21.8)
55-60	6.3 (5.6-7.0)	5.0 (4.4-5.7)	64.5 (63.2-65.9)	56.2 (54.5-57.8)	8.2 (7.1-9.5)	17.0 (15.2-18.9)	19.1 (18.4-19.8)	20.2 (19.3-21.1)
61-70	7.1 (6.4-7.9)	5.0 (4.4-5.7)	65.2 (63.9-66.5)	57.3 (55.7-58.9)	6.7 (5.7-7.7)	16.7 (14.8-18.6)	18.4 (17.8-19.1)	19.3 (18.4-20.2)
>70	7.6 (6.8-8.5)	4.9 (4.3-5.6)	66.5 (65.1-67.8)	57.1 (55.6-58.7)	5.5 (4.5-6.5)	17.2 (15.5-19.1)	17.8 (17.1-18.5)	18.8 (18.0-19.6)

REM, rapid eye movement.

From Redline S, Kirchner HL, Quan SF, et al: The effects of age, sex, ethnicity, and sleep-disordered breathing on sleep architecture. Arch Intern Med 2004;164:406-418.

Table 3-2. Brief Arousal Index in Elderly Subjects as a Function of Sleep-Disordered Breathing

	Arousal Index Brief Arousals per Hour of Sleep (±SD)	
RDI	**Men**	**Women**
≤5	16.7 (7.7)	14.7 (7.1)
>5 to ≤15	20.5 (8.7)	17.9 (7.8)
>15 to ≤30	25.2 (10.3)	23.2 (10.4)
>30*	39.4 (14.7)	29.7 (13.6)

*Estimated weighted values.

RDI, respiratory disturbance index (apneas plus hypopneas per hour of sleep), a measure of sleep-disordered breathing; SD, standard deviation.

From Redline S, Kirchner HL, Quan SF, et al: The effects of age, sex, ethnicity, and sleep-disordered breathing on sleep architecture. Arch Intern Med 2004;164:406-418.

gamma-aminobutyric acid–ergic [GABAergic] systems), also decrease with age.[8] Although the number of brief arousals, like other metrics of sleep quality, shows a male predominance, the influences of neither age nor gender are as pronounced as the effects of breathing events (Table 3–2). In fact, when accounting for the presence of brief arousals in older adults, the respiratory disturbance index predicts 10-fold more variance than age and fivefold more variance than sex. Higher respiratory disturbance index levels were also associated with slightly lower time spent in REM sleep in both men and

women and with lower amounts of time in stage 3/4 in men. The latter result is consistent with the hypothesis that at least some SDB in both elderly men and elderly women may reflect ventilatory control instability, and that slow wave sleep may be protective (see "Sleep-Disordered Breathing," later).

Insofar as comorbidities are concerned, SHHS sleep architecture data show convergence with epidemiologic data. Selected medical comorbidities (a positive history of cardiovascular disease, hypertension, and stroke) were associated with disturbed sleep architecture, as was smoking, although, curiously, these results were not seen with chronic obstructive pulmonary disease. Consistent with results suggesting that reduced sleep amounts or quality may predispose for metabolic syndrome in old age, diabetic patients had less time spent in stage 3/4, lower sleep efficiencies, and higher numbers of brief arousals and time spent in stage 1. In most cases, however, these effects appeared less salient (i.e., predicted less variance) for sleep architecture than demographic variables such as sex, and to a lesser extent, age, and in some cases, ethnicity,[4] except for the arousal index, where the Respiratory Disturbance Index was by far the single most powerful predictor.

The sex differences in slow wave sleep reported by the SHHS notwithstanding, several aspects of these data must be viewed in the context of prior literature on age-dependent changes in architecture. When period-amplitude analyses are performed, the major change in slow wave sleep ascribed to aging has been a decline in delta wave amplitude rather than wavelength (Fig. 3–1) (see Bliwise[6] for a review). When scored visually using a 75-µV threshold, typical figures for the amount of time spent in stage 3/4 sleep by older adults have often fallen in the 5% to 10% range. The figures reported by the SHHS, particularly for women, are somewhat higher than these conventionally accepted figures. Whether these values represent a more precise rendering of delta activity within

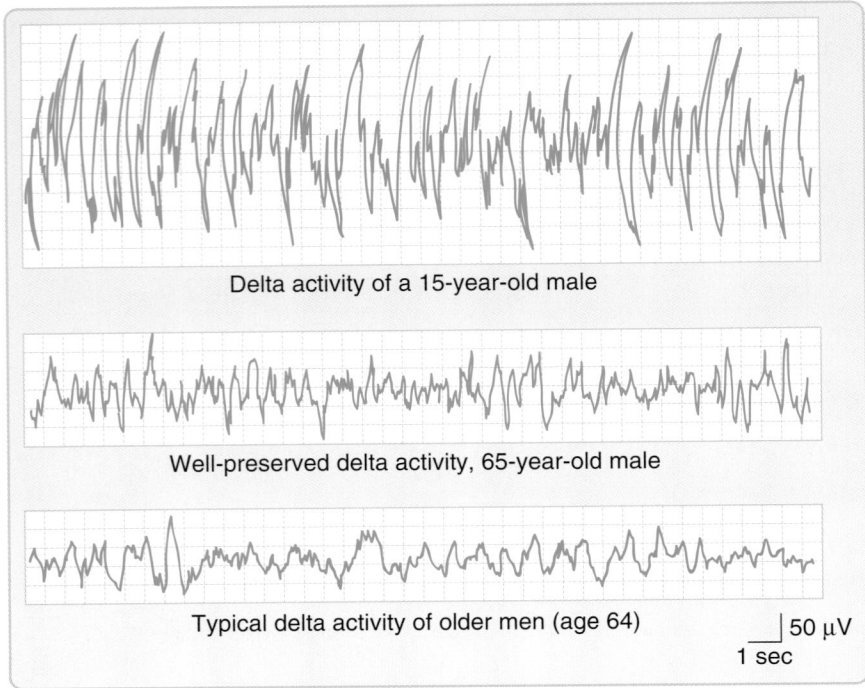

Delta activity of a 15-year-old male

Well-preserved delta activity, 65-year-old male

Typical delta activity of older men (age 64)

50 µV
1 sec

Figure 3–1. Age differences in delta activity. The *top tracing* shows typically abundant high-amplitude delta in an adolescent. The *middle tracing* shows particularly well-preserved delta in an older man. Note the marked decrease in amplitude relative to the adolescent. The *bottom tracing* is a more typical example of delta activity in an older man. Note the number of waves failing to meet the 75-µV amplitude criterion. (From Zepelin H: Normal age related change in sleep. In Chase MH, Weitzman ED [eds]: Sleep Disorders: Basic and Clinical Research. New York, Spectrum, 1983, pp 431-445.)

sleep, perhaps engendered by the visual analyses of electroen- cephalographic waveforms on digital display, or by the simul- taneous availability of precise calibration of the 75-μV criterion for delta waves stipulated by the Rechtschaffen and Kales guidelines,[8a] is unclear. Nonetheless, the strictly con- trolled and exquisitely refined visual analyses conducted by the SHHS represent a standard of polysomnographic technol- ogy aspired to by the field of sleep medicine, and these newly published metrics may well replace existing data and supplant our current understanding of how sleep architecture measures should be benchmarked. Although some laboratories may continue to modify amplitude thresholds for scoring of stage 3/4 sleep, it remains unclear what the functional or operational consequences of such a renormalization would offer, particularly in view of the aforementioned newly acquired reference values. Eventually, presentation of quantified delta activity (using fast Fourier transform or zero-crossing techniques) may come to replace such conventional measures, and some attempts in this regard have been offered.[9]

Age differences in the duration of NREM sleep before the first REM period of the night (REM sleep latency) have been shown in some studies of normal persons and depressed patients (Fig. 3–2). In all likelihood, these findings may reflect changes in the proportion of the first NREM period occupied by slow wave sleep. Some meta-analyses have demonstrated that standardized differences between normal and depressed subjects (e.g., lower sleep efficiencies in the latter) are exag- gerated by age. In normal subjects, the density of eye move- ments in REM sleep is reduced with aging.[10]

PUTATIVE MECHANISMS TO ACCOUNT FOR ALTERED SLEEP ARCHITECTURE IN AGING

Despite the presence of the relatively sophisticated, descriptive data characterizing age dependence in sleep architecture, current understanding of the mechanisms underlying these alterations remains rudimentary at best. Relevant data can be classified into two broad domains: (1) neuroendocrine and other humorally mediated influences, and (2) effects of various neurotransmitters and neuromodulators.

Aging is accompanied by a neuroendocrine cascade involving a decline in the somatotropic, gonadotropic, and hypothalamic- pituitary-adrenal (HPA) axes (see Chapter 32 for a description of age-dependent changes in melatonin and their potential role in the poor sleep quality of older adults). Declines in sleep quality, including but not limited to the decrease in time

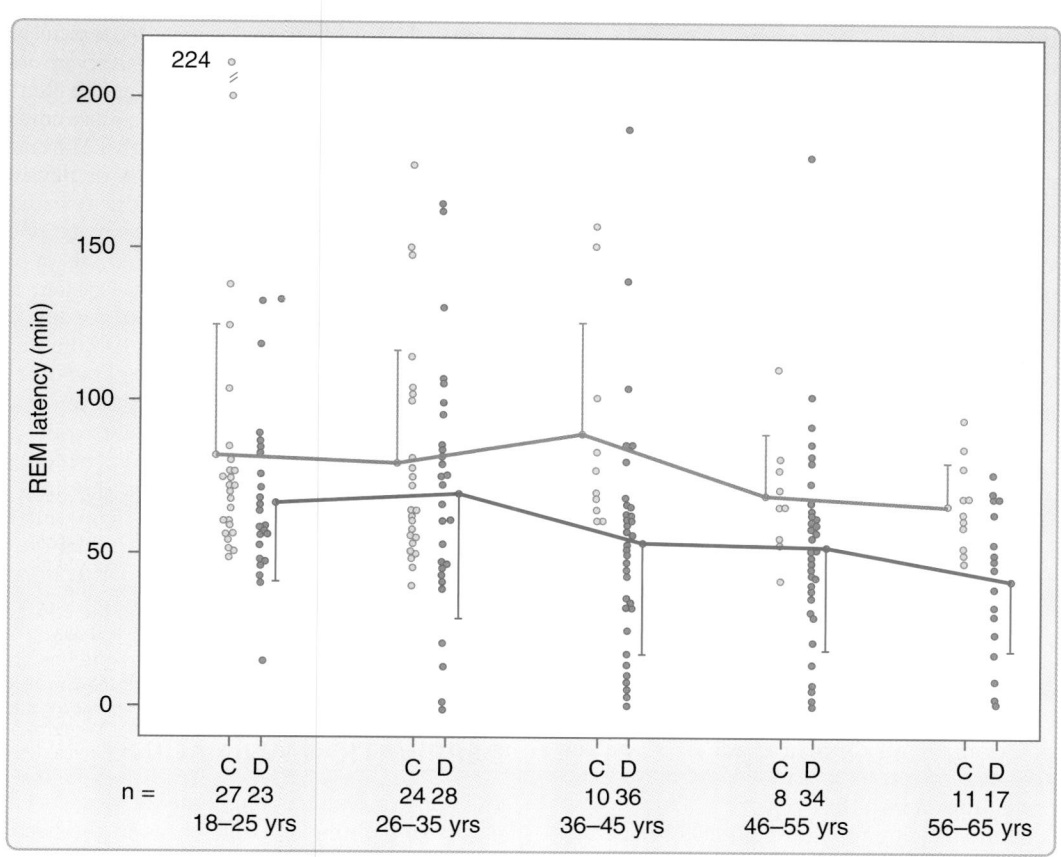

Figure 3–2. Mean, standard deviation, and individual values for REM sleep latency as a function of age in control subjects (C) *(open circles)* and depressed (D) *(closed circles)* patients. REM sleep latency is defined in this study as the time from the first epoch of stage 2 sleep to the first epoch of REM sleep. (From Reiman D, Laver C, Hohagen F, et al: Long term evolution of sleep in depression. In Smirne S, Franceschi M, Ferini-Strambi L [eds]: Sleep and Aging: Proceedings of the Second Milano International Symposium on Sleep, Milano, October 12-14, 1989. Milan, Italy, Masson, 1991, pp 195-204.)

spent in stage 3/4 sleep in men, may partially reflect changes in the somatotropic axis, typically measured by declines in plasma levels of growth hormone during sleep. Age-dependent declines in growth hormone have been noted cross-sectionally to be most pronounced for men aged 16 to 43, with lower apparent rates of decline seen from 44 to 83 years.[11] Insulin-like growth factor 1, a liver-produced polypeptide thought to regulate the anabolic effects of growth hormone, has been shown to correlate with delta activity in elderly men.[12] Because of known interactions between androgens and the somatotropic axis, many of these changes may be secondary to changes in gonadotropins, which, in women, may fundamentally reflect menopause (see Chapter 110).

Activation of the HPA axis, typically indexed by endogenous cortisol levels, has long been associated with aging and is thought to represent a major component of allostatic load, the cumulative lifetime effects of repetitive burden of all forms of stress for the organism.[13] Although the mean 24-hour level of cortisol usually increases with aging, this effect now appears to be conferred largely by the elevation of the evening nadir value, rather than by an exaggeration of the typical morning elevation.[11] The rise in evening level (approximately 20 nmol/L per decade) was most pronounced in subjects over 43 years of age and was related to lower levels of REM sleep. To some extent, the apparent age-dependent decline in percentage time spent in REM sleep could be accounted for by these cortisol elevations. These relationships were noted specifically in men, although there may be reason to think they may occur in women as well,[14] and at least one recent study including both elderly men and women reported a similar effect.[15] In addition to such findings of spontaneous cortisol secretion, direct stimulation of the HPA axis by infusion of corticotropin-releasing hormone was shown to induce more sleep-related arousal in middle-aged men than in younger men.[16]

Mean 24-hour levels of selected proinflammatory cytokines known to be elevated in response to sleep loss, such as interleukin (IL)-6, were shown to be elevated in elderly poor sleepers relative to younger poor sleepers,[15] although another inflammatory marker, tumor necrosis factor-alpha, did not show such elevations. Time-linked associations between elevations in plasma levels of cortisol and IL-6 were also apparent. Within elderly subjects, higher evening IL-6 levels were incrementally related to higher levels of time awake, such that an increase of 1 pg/mL IL-6 was associated with an increased wake time after sleep onset of about 20 minutes. REM sleep was unrelated to IL-6 levels.

When taken together, these cross-sectional data suggest that specific components of sleep architecture with marked age-dependence (stage 3/4, REM sleep, and wake after sleep onset) may have specific humoral correlates (growth hormone, cortisol, and IL-6) indicative of a hyperaroused internal milieu predisposing to insomnia. Given the known interdependence among such measures, future longitudinal data are essential to understand which components of this cascade occur initially and whether these markers precede or follow the polysomnographic changes that they appear to track.

The complex nature of aging processes has also been examined in relation to sleep in several animal models. Dietary restriction, long known to retard aging processes, perhaps by reducing oxidative stress, has recently been examined in relation to sleep in rats. Neither young nor old rats, however, demonstrated appreciable changes in sleep architecture under

a hypocaloric diet.[17] Compromised immunity, also characteristic of aging, was shown to interact with sleep as a function of age. A microbial challenge (lipopolysaccharide) induced slow wave sleep in younger but not in middle-aged rats, whereas reduction in REM sleep was seen in both age groups.[18]

The hypocretin/orexin system, a neuropeptide synthesized by hypothalamic neurons but having diffuse projections to centers crucial for sleep regulation, including the locus coeruleus, the ventral tegmental area, and the tuberomammillary nucleus, is a likely candidate system to undergo deterioration with aging. Studies related to this issue are just beginning to emerge. In humans, cerebrospinal fluid hypocretin-1 showed no age dependence,[19,20] but in the mouse, analyses of mRNA for specific hypocretin receptor subtypes showed lower levels in selected brain regions in older animals. Specifically, mRNA expression for the hypocretin-2 receptor was lower in hippocampus, thalamus, and medulla in the oldest animals (24 months) relative to the youngest (3 months), with some changes in selected regions (e.g., thalamus) as early as 12 months.[21] Changes in the hypocretin-1 receptor, which could be hypothesized to hold more significance for disordered sleep in humans,[20] showed less compelling age differences. Curiously, one report examining whole-brain hypocretin in mice of various ages found a nonsignificant tendency for increased levels of hypocretin-1 receptor with advancing age, a finding that could suggest enhanced, rather than deficient, arousal.[22] Thus, although potentially a viable candidate as a basis for age-dependent changes in sleep, future studies examining the role of the hypocretin/orexin system in aging are required to determine whether this system is relevant for attribution of the sleep alterations observed with aging.

Other regional neurobiologic substrates that might be relevant for aging changes in sleep, such as brainstem serotonin, have not shown age differences when examined in postmortem human tissue by immunohistochemical methods.[23] When analyzed for c-Fos immunoreactivity, cells in the ventral lateral preoptic area of young and old rats, a region predominantly controlled by the GABAergic system and considered critical for sleep generation showed no differences in metabolic activation.[24] However, during 12 hours of sleep deprivation, c-Fos activity throughout the hypothalamus showed induction of this transcription factor in young but not old animals.[25] Basal forebrain studies of adenosine suggested that, although older rats had higher adenosine levels than younger rats in both light and dark periods (findings that would be compatible with more abundant sleep across the 24-hour day), older animals showed a substantial downregulation of the adenosine A1 receptor subtype when microdialyzed, suggesting that changes at the receptor level, either by lower number or by decreased binding affinity, may occur with aging.[26]

EXPERIMENTALLY INDUCED SLEEP DEPRIVATION AND AGING

The construct of age alterations in sleep need and the complexity of defining age differences in the need for sleep have been discussed elsewhere.[6] Recovery effects subsequent to sleep deprivation represent one, but not the only, means of operationalizing sleep need, and such effects can be examined in both humans (Fig. 3–3) and animals with age as an independent variable.

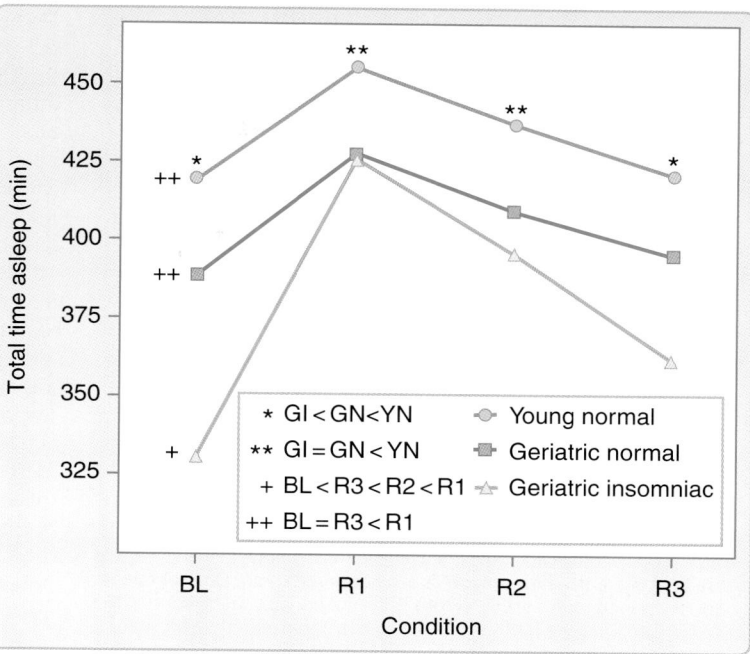

Figure 3–3. Changes in total sleep time after 64 hours of sleep deprivation, as a function of age. BL, baseline; GI, geriatric insomniacs; GN, geriatric normals; R1-R3, recovery nights 1-3; YN, young normals. Significant group differences are indicated by *asterisks,* and significant study night differences by *plus (+) signs.* Note that the effects of sleep deprivation in young and elderly subjects are similar, but age differences in absolute sleep amounts remain. (From Bonnet MH, Rosa RR: Sleep and performance in young adults and older normals and insomniacs during acute sleep loss and recovery. Biol Psychol 1987;25:153-172.)

Relative to young and middle-aged rats, old (24-month) rats undergoing 48 hours of continuous sleep deprivation showed reduced rebound of total sleep time and REM sleep, although high-amplitude, slow wave sleep rebound (analogous to stage 3/4 sleep rebound in humans), did not differentiate older animals from younger animals.[27] Number of sleep bouts, which might be expected to show a decrease during recovery sleep subsequent to deprivation, changed only slightly in older animals relative to younger animals. Even after 12 hours of sleep deprivation, older rats showed a diminished proportional increase in total sleep time relative to younger animals,[24] but the latter study also demonstrated that younger and older animals showed similarly proportional increases in high amplitude slow wave sleep. Strain of animals could not account for these differences across studies.

One approach to examining homeostatic pressure in human sleep in different age groups has been to examine the slow wave activity (analyzed both spectrally and with period–amplitude analysis) during 2-hour daytime naps following various periods of intervening wakefulness (i.e., 2, 5, 8, and 11 hours after morning awakening). Although elderly subjects showed less overall total sleep and lower delta wave activity than younger subjects regardless of time after awakening and both age groups showed increases in sleep as time after awakening increased, the rates of delta activity accumulation as a function of the preceding waking period were equally proportional in young and older subjects.[28] "If homeostatic drive means the absolute amount of delta produced per hour of waking, then drive is obviously diminished in older adults. If, however, homeostatic drive means the proportion of one's delta that increases per hour of waking, homeostatic drive is remarkably similar in young and elderly" (see p. 197 in Feinberg and Campbell[28]).

A related but somewhat different study of 25-hour sleep deprivation employing young and middle-aged subjects, which initiated recovery sleep in the daytime hours (to maximize a potential phase misalignment and allow better appreciation of homeostatic drive), found that middle-aged subjects showed a less steep exponential decline of cumulative slow wave sleep (and spectral measurements of delta power) during recovery.[29] Sleep efficiency during recovery sleep was also lower in the middle-aged subjects. Perhaps of equal importance was the fact that during the prolonged waking period, theta power (suggestive of drowsiness) increased at proportionally identical rates in both young and middle-aged subjects.[30] The juxtaposition of these sets of data (i.e., similar buildups of homeostatic pressure during wake yet inability to show recovery sleep pressure of similar magnitude) suggest that, at least by the time of middle age, homeostatic regulation of sleep and wakefulness undergoes substantial weakening. Curiously, those few studies that have examined the effects of sleep loss on daytime performance measures have shown that elderly subjects appear less influenced by such experimental sleep deprivation,[6] suggesting that the impact of such dysregulation of sleep–wake processes may be of less functional consequence, at least in normal aging.

CIRCADIAN RHYTHMS IN AGING

Age-dependent changes in circadian rhythms have been described in many mammalian species.[31] Data have shown that rest–activity rhythms (and, in some cases, electrophysiologically recorded sleep–wake) become more dispersed around the 24-hour day, and that the free-running period (tau) may shorten with aging, although species or strain differences may impact on these effects to some degree.[31] Such observations, typically made in rodents, have often engendered speculation as to similar tendencies occurring in elderly human subjects living under entrained conditions. Thus, for example, age-dependent impairment in phase shifting (e.g., elderly individuals have more difficulty adapting to shift work), the apparent

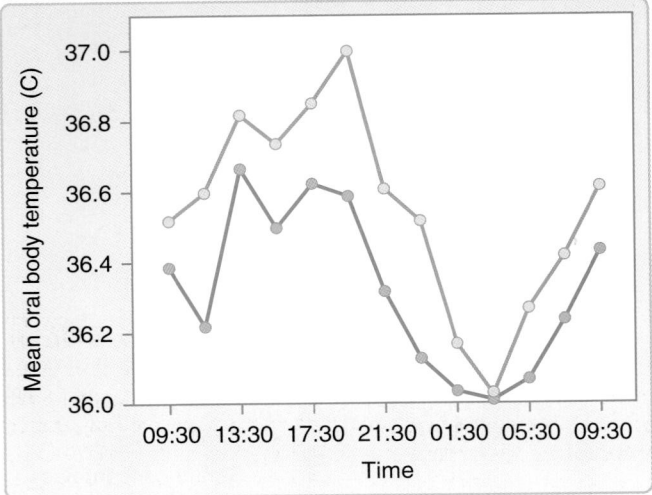

Figure 3–4. Oral temperatures in young *(open circles)* and old *(dark circles)* subjects, showing apparent decreased amplitude and earlier phase in body temperature cycle as a function of aging. Data obtained under entrained conditions. (From Richardson GS, Carskadon MA, Orav EJ: Circadian variation of sleep tendency in elderly and young adult subjects. Sleep 1982;5[suppl 2]:S82-S94.)

flattening of the diurnal sleep–wake rhythm amplitude (e.g., increased daytime napping of older persons), and the apparent "phase-advance" of the sleep–wake cycle (e.g., elderly humans are typically more larklike than owl-like) all suggest phenomenologic parallels between these changes in rodents and humans[32] (Fig. 3–4).

Mechanistically, the aforementioned changes could represent consequences of altered clock function per se, and/or they could also reflect changes in either the inputs to or the outputs from the clock. Regarding the former possibility, rodent studies have confirmed functional age-related change in the suprachiasmatic nucleus, both in glucose utilization and in c-Fos expression. Additionally, fetal transplants of suprachiasmatic nucleus tissue to older animals restored not only rhythm amplitude but also period length. Given evidence of conservation of key molecular components in the biological clock across mammals, it is not surprising that some of the aforementioned changes (e.g., earlier bedtimes and wakeup times) attributed to aging represent endogenous functions of the clock itself. Indeed, a genetic basis for familial advanced sleep phase syndrome has been linked to a mutation in a region homologous to the period gene seen in *Drosophila*.[33]

Examination of aging effects in the context of loss of significant visual input to the circadian timing system represents one attempt to examine the impact of input to the biological clock. A longitudinal study of six completely blind subjects studied over intervals of 10 to 14 years employed the dim light melatonin onset procedure as a marker of circadian phase and found a lengthening, rather than a shortening, of the estimated free-running period. This implied that the apparent phase advance of the sleep–wake cycle seen in older human subjects was caused by factors other than shortening of the endogenous, free-running period.[34] A comparison of the free-running periods of (sighted) young and elderly subjects subjected to a prolonged (approximately 1-month) 28-hour forced desynchrony protocol[35]

showed a virtually identical estimated intrinsic period of 24.18 hours.

The ability to phase shift and entrain to light in elderly humans might be expected to be relatively impaired because of challenges to the visual system that occur as a part of aging (e.g., cataracts, macular degeneration). Indeed, elderly individuals with visual impairment were 30% to 60% more likely to have impaired nighttime sleep than visually unimpaired elderly subjects.[36] A recent study examined the ability of a nonphotic stimulus (i.e., evening exercise) to phase shift melatonin onset in young and elderly humans and found comparable phase delays subsequent to exercise in both groups, thus arguing for the importance of entraining factors other than bright light in shifting rhythms successfully in older adults.[37]

Most current human chronobiology studies attempting to describe age-dependent alterations in the propensity and timing of sleep have focused on elucidating elements downstream from, but interactive with, the circadian system, such as the homeostatic regulation of sleep. Studies using the 28-hour forced desynchrony protocol have shown that, during the assigned (9.33 hour) sleep period, elderly subjects awakened more frequently than younger subjects, regardless of circadian phase, but that the duration of awakenings was virtually identical in young and old subjects.[38] The largest differences in the frequency of awakenings between young and older subjects were detected early, rather than late, in the sleep period, a finding that appears incompatible with the broadly defined "phase-advanced" hypothesis of sleep in older adults, where differences in sleep consolidation should be most pronounced late in the sleep period (i.e., early morning awakening) and would be expected to be minimal just after sleep onset (i.e., early evening sleepiness). Also of note in this study were analyses of sleep structure immediately prior to awakenings from consolidated periods of sleep. With circadian phase controlled, older subjects were far less likely to awaken from stage 1 and far more likely to awaken from stage 2 than were young subjects, suggesting that awakenings in the older subjects were more likely to represent abrupt transitions from NREM sleep than gradual lightening of sleep.[38] These findings can be interpreted as an indication of a reduced homeostatic pressure for continuous bouts of sleep independent of circadian phase in the sleep of older subjects.

Recent studies using the constant routine, a protocol that controls for posture, activity, food intake, light exposure, and sleep itself by having subjects remain in bed in constant low illumination while being deprived of sleep and eating small meals every hour, has allowed elucidation of endogenous phase markers of the circadian system such as melatonin,[39] in this case sampled hourly. As is typical of many studies in entrained conditions, prior to entry into the protocol, elderly subjects demonstrated habitually earlier bedtimes and wake-up times than younger subjects by 66 to 83 minutes and an earlier melatonin rise of nearly 50 minutes. However, the difference between the measures of sleep timing and melatonin rise varied by age of subject; in relationship to their customary bedtimes and wakeup times, elderly individuals' melatonin rises and falls occurred later, rather than earlier, when referenced to their typical sleep period. These data implied that the earlier bedtimes and wakeup times demonstrated by older subjects could not reflect changes in the circadian timing system. Rather, these data suggest a weakening of homeostatic processes in the regulation of sleep and waking, such that maintaining alertness throughout the waking day is challenged by failure to consolidate wakefulness, just as in the 28-hour forced desynchrony, older subjects are less able to consolidate sleep.

INSOMNIA AND ASSOCIATED RISK FACTORS IN OLD AGE

Prevalence, Incidence, and Medical Risk Factors

The prevalence of insomnia in older adults varies across studies, but a range of between 19.0% and 38.4% is typically suggested. In one of the largest surveys of an American population (the Established Populations for Epidemiologic Studies of the Elderly [EPESE], with more than 9000 participants), 29% of the population older than 65 had difficulty maintaining sleep.[40] Relative to sleep maintenance, sleep latency is less likely to be problematic for the elderly population, with prevalence figures on the order of 10% to 19% typically seen,[40] although one study[41] reported a relatively high prevalence of sleep latency problems (36.7%) in a largely rural, older adult population. In nearly all studies, elderly women have a greater probability of sleep complaints (for a review, see Bliwise et al.[42]) and sedative/hypnotic use (for a review, see Carrier and Bliwise[43]) than elderly men. Elderly black individuals generally report fewer sleep complaints than the elderly white population,[44] although a more recent survey in Pennsylvania reported an opposite effect.[45] Figures for regular use of sedatives/hypnotics in elderly populations range from as low as 5% per year to as high as 16% over 4.5 years, 29% over 8 years, 34% over 1 year, and 62% over 3 years.[43]

Much evidence suggests that medical diseases and chronic illness play an important role in much of the poor sleep seen in old age. In fact, when a sufficient number of other causes of poor sleep are taken into account, chronologic age may explain little of the observed prevalence in older adults. A huge array of often co-occurring medical conditions impact and disrupt sleep of elderly populations including *chronic pain conditions,* such as arthritis, hip fracture, fibromyalgia, headache, and back pain; *cardiovascular diseases,* as manifested by hypertension, myocardial infarct, stroke, congestive heart failure, and angina; *respiratory conditions,* such as asthma and bronchitis; and *other systemic diseases,* such as diabetes, gastroesophageal reflux, and duodenal ulcer (for a review, see Carrier and Bliwise[43]). When elderly individuals with such comorbidities are carefully screened, the resulting insomnia prevalence may be only 1% to 3%.[46] Additionally, limitations in mobility, visual impairment, lack of regular exercise, alcohol use, and smoking all contribute to declining sleep quality. Nocturia (nightly awakenings to void) often appear to be associated with poor sleep as well[47] and more recently with SDB.[48] In women, some evidence suggests that menopause may also be associated with declining sleep quality (see Chapter 110).

Several longitudinal studies examining the incidence (i.e., the development of new cases) of insomnia over periods of up to 10 years have been reported. The single best predictor of insomnia continuing longer than 10 years was insomnia at a previous time, although cardiovascular and pulmonary comorbidities conferred risk as well in the population older than 65.[49]

Reported remissions were less likely in older subjects than younger.[50] The EPESE data indicated a yearly incidence of insomnia complaints in the older population of about 5%, with a spontaneous remission rate of about 50% over 3 years.[51] In these data, incident insomnia was related to heart disease, stroke, hip fracture, and new-onset depression. A later report also suggested a risk in dementia.[52] Spontaneous remission of insomnia was related to the resolution of depression, physical illness, and physical disability affecting activities of daily living.[51] Another longitudinal study indicated that higher levels of physical activity were protective for incident insomnia over an 8-year follow-up.[53] Longitudinal analyses of several different birth cohorts over intervals of 24 years have confirmed increased incidence of sleep complaints with aging without obvious secular (cohort) effects, although evidence of historical trends for deceased sedative/hypnotic use and sleep durations were noted.[54]

Psychological and Psychosocial Factors

Despite the importance of the factors intrinsic to sleep in the widespread poor sleep experienced by elderly people, the role of psychological issues must not be dismissed. Loss of a spouse, a yearly occurrence for 1.6% of elderly men and 3.0% of elderly women in the American population, is a particularly devastating condition associated with depression in many older adults. Polysomnographic studies of such geriatric populations who do not have a history of previous depression have shown some of the same findings as in geriatric patients with major depressive disorders. Specifically, such patients demonstrated similar low sleep efficiencies (about 73%). On the other hand, bereaved patients with adjustment reactions (subsyndromally depressed) showed polysomnographic characteristics that did not differ or differed only minimally from elderly controls. Factors salient for geriatric populations, such as retirement, holocaust trauma, and fear of death in sleep, can disrupt sleep, as can anxiety and depression, and there is only mixed evidence that the associations between psychopathology and disturbed sleep, so well demonstrated in younger patients, are in any way abated in older patients.[6]

Treatment Considerations

The overwhelming message from the aforementioned literature regarding the huge number of potential comorbidities disrupting sleep in older adults is that effective insomnia treatment implies that management should focus on primary medical disease and carefully consider the possibility that psychiatric disorder may have preceded the sleep complaint. In practice, of course, the sleep medicine specialist can be asked to offer management apart from such considerations. The following issues should be considered in older adults.

The prevalence of prescription hypnotic medication use in the elderly population is substantial and many elderly people continue to use medications for sleep even when their sleep continues to be disturbed. In one recent study, although both medical and psychological burden predicted hypnotic drug use in older adults, persistent use in older adults over a period of 6 years was far more related to depression than medical disease.[55] Analysis of prescription hypnotic use in 1982 in a study population of 1.1 million Americans[56] showed that higher all-cause mortality and specific-cause mortality were associated with regular use of such medication. In subjects older than 70, these risks were conferred by nightly use, whereas in younger subjects, the risks were apparent at both nightly and more moderate levels of consumption. Whether such risks continue to operate currently, with the widespread use of predominantly GABA–site-specific agonists as hypnotics is unknown, but at very least, these results suggest that nonpharmacologic alternatives or adjunctive treatments for late-life insomnia should always be considered.

Finally, although the poor sleep of old age may have many causes, the possibility exists that poor sleep, if untreated, may lead to adverse outcomes. For example, not only does poor sleep reduce quality of life in older subjects, but several epidemiologic studies examining subjective total sleep times have shown that lower sleep durations, but not necessarily self-reported "insomnia," were associated with higher rates of all-cause mortality.[57] These findings were independent of age. Other studies examining the natural history of insomnia complaints[40] and estimated sleep durations[58] did not support these results. Nonetheless, poor sleep may predispose for psychiatric morbidity; longitudinal studies have noted that poor sleep confers a risk for incident depression in older subjects.[59]

RESTLESS LEGS SYNDROME AND PERIODIC LIMB MOVEMENTS DURING SLEEP

One specific cause of insomnia in older adults is restless legs syndrome (RLS) (see Chapter 70). This condition, characterized by an urge to move the legs, which is usually accompanied by sensations of discomfort, aggravation of symptoms by rest and during the evening or nocturnal hours, and temporary relief of symptoms by movement, is common in elderly populations. A telephone survey in Kentucky noted an average prevalence of 10% in individuals between 30 and 79, and 19% for those of ages 80 and older.[60] However, a primary care survey in rural Idaho noted a peak prevalence of about 30% in 50- to 59-year-olds that declined to about 15% at age 80 and older.[61] Several studies have also reported sex differences, with risks elevated by 50% to 100% in women.[61,62]

Periodic limb movements during sleep (PLMS) are stereotypic, repetitive, nonepileptiform movements of the legs, usually consisting of dorsiflexion of the ankle, but occasionally limited to the great toe or incorporating flexion at the level of knee or hip. They often, but not invariably, occur in conjunction with RLS. Age-dependent increases in the occurrence of PLMS have been noted cross-sectionally in clinical case series without a drop in the oldest groups (e.g., those older than 80 years).[63] Curiously, longitudinal follow-up of elderly subjects did not show increases consistently, perhaps because of inherent variability in PLMS.[64] About 45% of a randomly selected, independently living population over 65 years of age met an arbitrary criterion for the presence of such movements,[63] which makes PLMS at least as common a "pathology" as SDB. Over 5 recording nights, the mean number of PLMS per movement per hour of sleep was 34.5 in a sample of older persons with insomnia; 86% of subjects had a mean movement index of greater than five events per hour of sleep.[65] The prevalence of PLMS in older adults is approximately double that of RLS. Unlike RLS, there may be a male predominance.[63,66]

The discrepancy between the relative prevalence of PLMS and RLS and the failure of a number of studies to show associations between the presence of PLMS and sleep-related symptoms in the absence of full-blown RLS[65] suggests that in many cases, PLMS in older adults may be an incidental finding.[6] At least one recent study including some elderly subjects, however, reported an association between difficulty falling asleep and the presence of PLMS that appeared independent of the presence of RLS symptoms,[66] but a detailed analysis of sleep microarchitecture in relation to PLMS claimed no association with poor subjective sleep quality.[67] Although not specifically investigated in an elderly population, the presence of PLMS in the absence of RLS symptoms may be associated with fewer brief arousals during sleep.[68] In elderly, relative to younger, subjects, PLMS were associated with a reduction in cyclic tachycardia or bradycardia accompanying the movements.[69]

A number of mechanisms may underlie PLMS in old age (for a review, see Bliwise[6]). Current data concerning the pathophysiologic basis of PLMS accompanying RLS have focused largely on iron transport and storage deficiencies, phenomena not uncommon in the elderly population.[70] Elderly RLS patients with serum ferritin levels of less than 45 mg/mL showed subjective improvement following use of ferrous sulfate,[70] although their total iron levels were no different. Because iron represents a key component of production of dopamine, it may play a role in presence of PLMS in some elderly subjects. Several studies of RLS patients in their 50s and 60s with PLMS showed reduced binding for the D2 receptor throughout striatal regions, as assessed with both single photon emission computed tomography[71] and positron emission tomography,[72] and magnetic resonance imaging studies of RLS patients in their 60s have suggested lower levels of brain iron.[73] Whether these results are relevant for elderly individuals with PLMS but without RLS symptoms remains uncertain.

SLEEP-DISORDERED BREATHING

Information relevant to SDB in older adults has expanded substantially in the last 5 years with publications from several major epidemiologic cohorts (the SHHS, the Wisconsin Sleep Cohort Study [WSCS], the Central Pennsylvania Study [CPS], the Honolulu-Asian Study [HAS], and the Cleveland Family Study [CFS]), some of which include sizeable proportions of aged individuals. Within the limitations of the age ranges of these cohorts and their respective sampling strategies, methodologies, and recording approaches, these studies have generated substantial insights into the risk factors and potential outcomes associated with SDB. These studies are all observational. Several randomized treatment trials for SDB are underway or have been completed, but few of these have focused exclusively on geriatric populations.

The previously proposed heuristic model for SDB (Fig. 3–5) posits that the condition represents both an age-related phenomenon (with a specific vulnerability confined to middle age) and an age-dependent phenomenon (with a prevalence that steadily increases throughout the human life course).[6] The articulation and differentiation of these two presumably separate, but chronologically overlapping, conditions continues to be a major focus of researchers. Practically, if the health consequences of SDB in elderly populations are diminished, the necessity to treat the enormous numbers of elderly individuals

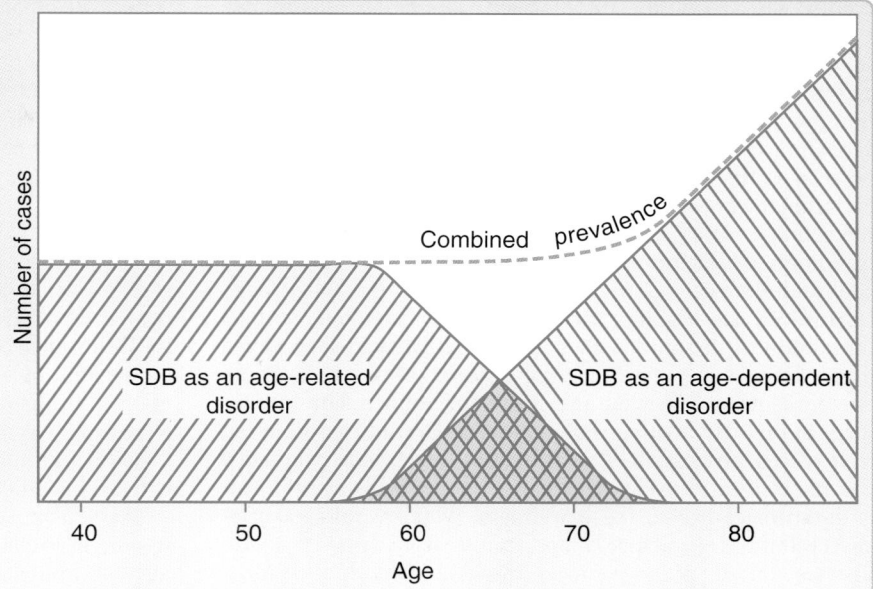

Figure 3–5. Heuristic model suggesting that sleep disordered breathing (SDB) is both an age-related and an age-dependent condition with potential overlap of distributions in the 60- to 70-year-old age range. Cross-sectionally, note that the number of cases observed may remain high and increase with age, despite a presumed decrease in age-related SDB.

with the condition is reduced. One approach to determining the validity of such a model is to examine risk factors to determine whether their constellation is similar in individuals of different ages. The same process can be applied to putative outcomes as well.

Prevalence and Incidence

The earliest study of cross-sectional prevalence of SDB in a community-dwelling, independently living population (in San Diego) over the age of 65 estimated a 44% prevalence of an apnea-hypopnea index (AHI) of at least 20 events per hour.[74] In the SHHS (mean age, 63.5), the prevalence of an AHI of greater than 15 events per hour was somewhat lower, at 18%, probably reflecting the use of full polysomnography in deriving those estimates.[75] Comparable lower prevalence estimates using full polysomnography were also obtained in the CPS, where estimates of 13.3% and 7.2% for 65- to 100-year-old men (AHI greater than 20) and women (AHI greater than 15), respectively, were obtained.[76,77] Cross-sectional analyses of effects of chronologic age in those older than 70 were possible in the SHHS because of the very large number of individuals in this age range (N = 1780). These data suggested a plateau effect above this age.

Far less is known about the incidence of SDB in elderly populations. A report from the San Diego cohort suggested no increment in AHI over an 18-year period unless a concomitant increase in body weight had also occurred.[78] In the younger WSCS cohort, a similar relationship between increased AHI and body weight was also noted over an 8-year period,[79] and the group as a whole appeared to show a small increase in SDB. The most detailed analyses of longitudinal change in AHI appeared in the CFS and demonstrated that, across a wide age range, AHI increased by 30% to 40% over a 5-year follow-up. However, the extent of the change in AHI was dependent on age, sex, and body mass index (BMI). A 60-year-old man, for example, with a BMI of 30 might expect to gain an AHI of 3.6 events per hour over 5 years, whereas a woman

with a similar age and BMI might show a much lower rate of increase (e.g., 1.6 events per hour over 5 years).[80] At a BMI of 22, incidence rates at age 60 were slightly lower, at 2.2 and 1.3 for men and women, respectively. In general, steeper rates of incidence were associated with higher baseline BMI, being male, and an older baseline age. The latter (increased likelihood of incident SDB with advancing years) was consistent with an age-dependent model for SDB in older age groups (see Fig. 3–5).

Risk Factors

Age dependence implies that SDB risk factors might be best considered markers of physiologic or biologic age.[81] In this sense, chronologic age may serve only as a proxy for other risk factors that themselves are age dependent. As a corollary to Figure 3–5, risk factors should operate differently in middle-aged and elderly individuals with SDB. Evidence on this has been mixed. In earlier studies with smaller numbers of individuals and less representative sampling, risk factors such as the BMI appeared to predict SDB equally well in older and in younger populations,[5] despite the fact that few obese individuals survive into old age. In the SHHS, however, several markers of obesity that were significant cross-sectional predictors of SDB in middle-aged populations (neck circumference and waist-to-hip ratio), were no longer significant predictors by ages 70 and 80, respectively.[75] BMI continued to be correlated with SDB even in those older than 80, although the magnitude of the effect was clearly diminished. Early studies also noted a continued male predominance in SDB into old age,[5] and in the SHHS, a male predominance persisted and was undiminished by age.[75] However, in both the WSCS[82] and the CPS,[77] postmenopausal women had rates of SDB that appeared somewhat closer to those of men of similar age. In the CFS, analysis of 5-year incidence rates suggested that by age 50, the male predominance had largely disappeared.[83]

The prevailing view for several decades was that most SDB in older adults consisted of central (i.e., diaphragmatic) events, whereas in the middle-aged population, obstructive events predominated. Considerable evidence has accrued that suggests that obstructive events occur commonly across all age groups.[5] Indeed, specific alterations in upper airway function predisposing to collapse during sleep may operate in old age. Upper airway compliance increases with age[84] and could be related to the overall declines of muscular strength and endurance seen with aging both in the skeletal muscles and in the genioglossus,[85] although some evidence disputes the role of tongue protrusion as a factor in SDB in old age.[86] Elderly edentulous patients appear at particular risk for SDB, perhaps because of an inability to maintain an adequate vertical dimension in the oral cavity.[87] To the extent that sleep apnea may involve changes in structure or function of upper airway afferents in middle-aged patients,[88] age-dependent impairment in oral vibratory sensation and two-point discrimination have also been described in older adults.[89] In older animals, the pharyngeal muscles appear to have a worse profile for endurance relative to the diaphragm, which would enhance susceptibility to collapse,[90] and a shift from type IIa to IIb fibers occurred in the genioglossus in 24-month-old rats, a finding interpreted as conferring susceptibility to fatigue.[91] These and other putatively age-dependent risk factors, shown in Figure 3–6, imply that mechanisms underlying SDB in old age (e.g., the mechanisms affecting airway closure during sleep) may share more similarities with, than differences from, those in middle-aged patients.

At least some unique features predisposing the older person to SDB must be acknowledged. Sleep–wake instability is thought to promote periodic breathing and could predispose older adults to SDB.[92] In the SHHS, the association between reduced stage 3/4 and elevated stage 1 (see "Sleep Architecture," earlier) and higher levels of the respiratory disturbance index[4] can thus be seen not simply as consequences of higher rates of SDB but also as permissive for it. Given the potential importance of state instability in the SDB of the older population, some novel attempts to model the variance in interbreath intervals and frequency and breath-by-breath amplitudes have been undertaken.[93] Apneic event duration has been reported to increase in relation to age.[94]

The APOE4 genotype, a risk factor for Alzheimer's disease, has been shown to be a risk factor for SDB in the middle-aged WSCS cohort[95] but not in the elderly HAS cohort,[96] a difference thought to reflect age dependence. A recent analysis of a subset of the SHHS participants confirmed that the effect of the genotype was more pronounced in individuals younger than 65 rather than older, perhaps reflecting a survivorship phenomenon.[97] The significance of the association between SDB and the APOE4 genotype for the development of dementia in late life has been reviewed elsewhere.[98]

Outcomes

Potential outcomes relevant to SDB in old age include mortality, cardiovascular and neurobehavioral morbidities, and those related to other potential end-organ damage (see Fig. 3–6). In the absence of large-scale, prospective, randomized clinical trials, definitive associations between SDB and adverse outcomes in older adults remain uncertain. (See Bliwise[6] for a discussion of mortality as an outcome of untreated SDB in old age.) The focus in the following paragraphs will be cardiovascular and neurobehavioral morbidities.

Previous studies have suggested an ambiguous picture as to whether relationships between cardiovascular disease and SDB are mitigated in older adults.[6] Data from the SHHS have only partially clarified this situation. For example, when excluding individuals with prevalent cardiovascular disease, associations between SDB (as measured by quartiles of AHI) and various morbidities (including hypertension, diabetes, and lipids) were clearly weaker in the population older than 65 than in the population younger than 65, at least in men.[99] In women, however, the effect was not mitigated by age.[99] Moreover, separate analyses that included individuals with prevalent hypertension and that used multiple measures of SDB (e.g., both AHI *and* cumulative oxygen saturation) demonstrated that the strength of the relationship between hypertension and SDB was *increased* over the age of 65, relative to under 65, depending on the measure used.[100] In yet another report examining associations between multiple measures of SDB and more broadly defined cardiovascular disease (including coronary heart disease, congestive heart failure, and stroke), relationships with SDB, although reduced to some extent by age, were still age independent.[101]

The most obvious neurobehavioral outcome associated with SDB is daytime sleepiness. Although subject to considerable debate about its measurement,[102] an ample body of literature suggests that relationships between SDB and sleepiness are not confined to middle-aged individuals.[6] Perhaps more

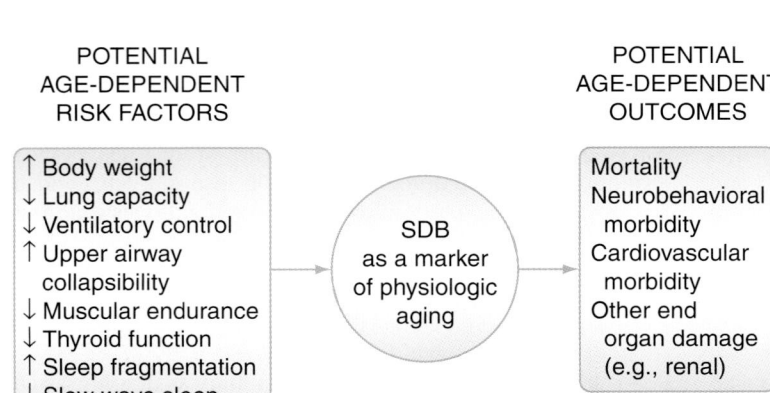

POTENTIAL
AGE-DEPENDENT
RISK FACTORS

↑ Body weight
↓ Lung capacity
↓ Ventilatory control
↑ Upper airway
  collapsibility
↓ Muscular endurance
↓ Thyroid function
↑ Sleep fragmentation
↓ Slow wave sleep

SDB
as a marker
of physiologic
aging

POTENTIAL
AGE-DEPENDENT
OUTCOMES

Mortality
Neurobehavioral
  morbidity
Cardiovascular
  morbidity
Other end
  organ damage
  (e.g., renal)

Figure 3–6. Sleep disordered breathing (SDB) in older adults as an age-dependent condition. Other potentially associated, age-dependent risk factors and outcomes are shown.

provocative is the suggestion that mental impairments, perhaps resembling dementia or, at very least, mild cognitive impairment, may be related to SDB,[103] and considerable research across both middle-aged and elderly subjects has shown such effects.[98] Among newly collected data using brief neuropsychological tests, neither a subset of the SHHS participants[104] nor the survivors from the HAS[105] demonstrated cross-sectional relationships between SDB and poorer mental performances, although in the latter study sleepiness was related to poorer test performances in demented patients. Longitudinal data from the San Diego study, however, showed a relationship between declining mental status test scores and the development of SDB.[106]

Thus, to summarize recent, ongoing data analyses from the major epidemiologic studies of SDB, results are far from conclusive, although some support can be garnered for an age-dependent model of SDB (see Fig. 3–5). Nearly all of the published morbidity data in older adults are cross-sectional and may be subject to various types of selection, period, cohort, and, most assuredly, survivor effects. To expand on the latter point, when examined cross-sectionally, elderly individuals in the SHHS, for example, may show weaker associations between SDB and morbidities because those individuals participating were healthier and survived into old age. Ultimately, the answer to whether SDB in old age is harmful to health will require longitudinal data, which, although still subject to biases, will provide answers less influenced by selective survival.

THE CONUNDRUM OF NAPPING AND SLEEPINESS IN OLD AGE

A time-honored question, asked by professionals and the lay public as well, involves the significance of napping in old age. From the layman's perspective, the questions are "Is it normal to nap?" and "Are naps good for my health?" The sleep specialist may ask fundamentally similar, though more diagnostically inclined, questions such as "What is the probability that daytime naps in a 75-year-old are indicative of SDB?" "Does excessive sleepiness during the day in an older person portend dementia?" and "To what extent does daytime napping adversely affect sleep at night?" These are highly relevant questions for the sleep medicine specialist, made even more difficult by factors related to cultural issues associated with napping, the difficulties in relying on self-reports to derive estimates of the physiologic tendency of sleep during the daytime hours, and the fact that, overarching all other issues, sleeping during the daytime hours in old age is almost assuredly a complex and multiply determined phenomenon.

Studies bearing on the issue of age-dependent, intentional or unintentional napping and sleepiness fall into numerous domains. In human work, data relevant to this topic can be gleaned from epidemiologic, population-based work, various experimental chronobiologic paradigms, studies of human performance, and behavioral intervention studies for geriatric insomnia. Basic science studies include descriptive work from a variety of mammalian species studied at different ages, as well as studies attempting to demonstrate the mechanisms underlying such age-dependent changes. Although convergence among these widely varying methodologies and approaches would help to clarify the fundamental questions posed in the preceding paragraph, there is unfortunately still an incomplete picture. In humans, even the measurement of daytime sleepiness remains a topic of considerable debate.[102]

Sleepiness during the day is not an inevitable component of aging. Studies of *successful aging* (defined as absence of sleep disorders, psychiatric disorders, and medical disease) have shown that elderly people, even well into their 80s, may incur no deficits in daytime alertness on the multiple sleep latency test. On the other hand, subjective reports of absence of daytime sleepiness must be interpreted with suspicion. This is amply illustrated by the June 1997 Gallup Poll, Sleepiness in America, which demonstrated that, despite showing lower Epworth Sleepiness Scale scores relative to younger people, older people were far more likely to use both over-the-counter and prescription medications to maintain daytime alertness and were more likely to hold the belief that it is normal to feel sleepy during the day.[107]

Data demonstrating the complexity and the potential importance of sleepiness in the older population come from several epidemiologic studies. In a cross-sectional analysis of 4500 elderly individuals in the Cardiovascular Health Study, sleepiness (as assessed with the Epworth Sleepiness Scale) was associated with a greater number of nighttime awakenings, nocturnal symptoms of sleep apnea, depression, the presence of congestive heart failure, the use of digitalis and diuretics, limitations in mobility, and the absence of sedative and hypnotic use in both men and women.[108] Additionally, black people tended to be sleepier than white people. Within men only, there was some suggestion that sleepiness was also predicted by lower cognitive function (but not altered brain structure assessed by magnetic resonance imaging) and certain measures of central obesity, whereas in women, a different set of predictors, such as reduced daily exercise and nasal congestion, were more important. These data imply that a host of specific variables consistent with intrinsic lightening of sleep (nighttime awakenings), specific sleep pathologies (symptoms of sleep apnea, nasal congestion), medical disease burden (congestive heart failure), dampening of circadian rhythmicity (bed rest and physical incapacity), psychological issues (depression), and genetics (race, sex) may all contribute to the final common outcome of sleepiness in older adults. A recent case-control study demonstrated that sleepiness in older subjects was associated with functional impairment across a wide spectrum of domains.[109] These data imply that sleepiness in older adults deserves careful evaluation with full consideration of multiple etiologies.

Apart from the prior cross-sectional observations, a number of longitudinal studies suggest that daytime sleepiness or daytime napping portends adverse consequences. Outcomes reported include depression,[110] mortality,[111-113] stroke,[58] myocardial infarct,[58,114] and dementia.[115] The length of follow-up in these studies ranges from 1 to 10 years, and, although convincing, they are not without at least some conflicting evidence. No relationship between daytime sleepiness and mortality occurred in the Canadian Study of Health and Aging.[116] Others have made distinctions between napping and daytime rest without sleeping, with the latter considered to be potentially protective for adverse events.[111] The rationale for napping as protective in old age is to increase the likelihood of a sleep-related fall in blood pressure,[117] an explanation that would appear specious if SDB underlies the phenomenon of sleepiness in the first place and blood pressure does not drop for that reason. Nonetheless, when taken as a whole, the brunt of evidence suggests that napping and sleepiness in old age are unlikely to be indicators of health.

The foregoing epidemiologic evidence notwithstanding, however, it is also possible to view sleepiness in old age in terms far less pathophysiologic. For example, given the studies describing age-dependent changes in sleep regulation in normal human and mammalian sleep (described elsewhere in this chapter), the tendency for older humans to nap during the day could be just as easily viewed as fundamental evidence of altered sleep regulation. As has been described here, many studies of aging in animals have demonstrated waning of the homeostatic drive for sleep, with older animals showing short sleep bouts during their subjective days. In humans, this has been encountered in both studies of challenge, such as sleep deprivation, and in chronobiologic protocols that seek to parse out effects of circadian versus homeostatic regulation. The loss of deep sleep (particularly in men) and the occurrence of brief arousals during sleep serve as indicators of a potentially decreased drive for sleep, which has, as its daytime counterpart, the inability to maintain wakefulness. Beneficial effects of daytime naps on performance in older adults have been demonstrated,[118] and although avoidance of daytime napping is a standard approach to sleep hygiene, studies have shown that daytime naps do adversely affect nocturnal sleep in old age.[119] Sleepiness should always be investigated thoroughly in the older person, but its ultimate meaning and significance may continue to be elusive and determined by multiple factors.

Clinical Pearl

Daytime sleepiness in an elderly person should never be assumed to have a single cause. Best available evidence suggests that overlapping factors, such as nocturnal sleep fragmentation, weakening of homeostatic drive for waking and sleep, altered chronobiology, incipient dementia, and sleep-disordered breathing can all be involved. Although overt pathology may be indicated, the fundamental reorganization of sleep and wakefulness throughout the 24-hour day may also be characteristic of the normal aging process across many mammalian species.

REFERENCES

1. Middelkoop HAM, Smilde-van den Doel DA, Neven AK, et al: Subjective sleep characteristics of 1,485 males and females aged 50-93: Effects of sex and age, and factors related to self-evaluated quality of sleep. J Gerontol A Biol Sci Med Sci 1996;51: M108-M115.
2. Bliwise DL: Sleep disorders in Alzheimer's disease and other dementias. Clin Cornerstone 2004;6:S16-S28.
3. Petersen RC, Doody R, Kurz A, et al: Current concepts in mild cognitive impairment. Arch Neurol 2001;58:1985-1992.
4. Redline S, Kirchner HL, Quan SF, et al: The effects of age, sex, ethnicity, and sleep-disordered breathing on sleep architecture. Arch Intern Med 2004;164:406-418.
5. Bliwise DL: Sleep in normal aging and dementia. Sleep 1993; 16:40-81.
6. Bliwise DL: Normal aging. In Kryger MH, Roth T, Dement WC (eds): Principles and Practice of Sleep Medicine, 3rd ed. Philadelphia, Saunders, 2000, pp 26-42.
7. Boselli M, Parrino L, Smerieri A, et al: Effect of age on EEG arousals in normal sleep. Sleep 1998;21:351-357.
8. Crowley K, Trinder J, Kim Y, et al: The effects of normal aging on sleep spindle and K-complex production. Clin Neurophysiol 2002;113:1615-1622.
8a. Rechtschaffen A, Kales A (eds): A Manual of Standardized Terminology, Techniques and Scoring System for Sleep Stages of Human Subjects. Los Angeles, UCLA Brain Information Service/Brain Research Institute, 1968.
9. Tan X, Campbell IG, Feinberg I: Internight reliability and benchmark values for computer analyses of non-rapid eye movement (NREM) and REM EEG in normal young adult and elderly subjects. Clin Neurophysiol 2001;112:1540-1552.
10. Darchia N, Campbell IG, Feinberg I: Rapid eye movement density is reduced in the normal elderly. Sleep 2003;26:973-977.
11. Van Cauter E, Leproult R, Plat L: Age-related changes in slow wave sleep and REM sleep and relationship with growth hormone and cortisol levels in healthy men. JAMA 2000;284:861-868.
12. Prinz PN, Moe KE, Dulberg EM, et al: Higher plasma IGF-1 levels are associated with increased delta sleep in healthy older men. J Gerontol A Biol Sci Med Sci 1995;50A:M222-M226.
13. Seeman TE, McEwen BS, Rowe JW, et al: Allostatic load as a marker of cumulative biological risk: MacArthur studies of successful aging. Proc Natl Acad Sci U S A 2001;98:4770-4775.
14. Blackman MR: Age-related alterations in sleep quality and neuroendocrine function: Interrelationships and implications. JAMA 2000;284:879-881.
15. Vgontzas AN, Zoumakis M, Bixler EO, et al: Impaired nighttime sleep in healthy old versus young adults is associated with elevated plasma interleukin-6 and cortisol levels: Physiologic and therapeutic implications. J Clin Endocrinol Metab 2003;88: 2087-2095.
16. Vgontzas AN, Bixler EO, Wittman AM, et al: Middle-aged men show higher sensitivity of sleep to the arousing effects of corticotropin-releasing hormone than young men: Clinical implications. J Clin Endocrinol Metab 2001;86:1489-1495.
17. Salin-Pascual RJ, Upadhyay U, Shiromani PJ: Effects of hypocaloric diet on sleep in young and old rats. Neurobiol Aging 2002;23:771-776.
18. Schiffelholz T, Lancel M: Sleep changes induced by lipopolysaccharide in the rat are influenced by age. Am J Physiol Regul Integr Comp Physiol 2001;280:R398-R403.
19. Kanbayashi T, Yano T, Ishiguro H, et al: Hypocretin-1 (orexin-A) levels in human lumbar CSF in different age groups: Infants to elderly persons. Sleep 2002;25:337-339.
20. Mignot E, Lammers GJ, Ripley B, et al: The role of cerebrospinal fluid hypocretin measurement in the diagnosis of narcolepsy and other hypersomnias. Arch Neurol 2002;59:1553-1562.
21. Terao A, Apte-Deshpande A, Morairty S, et al: Age-related decline in hypocretin (orexin) receptor 2 messenger RNA levels in the mouse brain. Neurosci Lett 2002;332:190-194.
22. Lin L, Wisor J, Shiba T, et al: Measurement of hypocretin/orexin content in the mouse brain using an enzyme immunoassay: The effect of circadian time, age and genetic background. Peptides 2002;23:2203-2211.
23. Kloppel S, Kovacs GG, Voigtlander T, et al: Serotonergic nuclei of the raphe are not affected in human ageing. Neuroreport 2001;12:669-671.
24. Shiromani PJ, Lu J, Wagner D, et al: Compensatory sleep response to 12h wakefulness in young and old rats. Am J Physiol Regulatory Integrative Comp Physiol 2000;278:R125-R133.
25. Basheer R, Shiromani PJ: Effects of prolonged wakefulness on c-*fos* and AP1 activity in young and old rats. Brain Res Mol Brain Res 2001;89:153-157.
26. Murillo-Rodriguez E, Blanco-Centurion C, Gerashchenko D, et al: The diurnal rhythm of adenosine levels in the basal forebrain of young and old rats. Neuroscience 2004;123:361-370.
27. Mendelson WB, Bergmann BM: Age-dependent changes in recovery sleep after 48 hours of sleep deprivation in rats. Neurobiol Aging 2000;21:689-693.
28. Feinberg I, Campbell IG: Kinetics of non-rapid eye movement delta production across sleep and waking in young and elderly normal subjects: Theoretical implications. Sleep 2003;26: 192-200.
29. Gaudreau H, Morettini J, Lavoie HB, et al: Effects of a 25-h sleep deprivation on daytime sleep in the middle-aged. Neurobiol Aging 2001;22:461-468.

30. Drapeau C, Carrier J: Fluctuation of waking electroencephalogram and subjective alertness during a 25-hour sleep-deprivation episode in young and middle-aged subjects. Sleep 2004;27:55-60.

31. Brock MA: Chronobiology and aging. J Am Geriatr Soc 1991;39:74-91.

32. Bliwise DL: Sleep and circadian rhythm disorders in aging and dementia. In Turek F, Zee P (eds): Regulation of Sleep and Circadian Rhythms. New York, Marcel Dekker, 1999, pp 487-525.

33. Toh KL, Jones CR, He Y, et al: An hPer2 phosphorylation site mutation in familial advanced sleep phase syndrome. Science 2001;291:1040-1043.

34. Kendall AR, Lewy AJ, Sack RL: Effects of aging on the intrinsic circadian period of totally blind humans. J Biol Rhythms 2001;16:87-95.

35. Czeisler CA, Duffy JF, Shanahan TL, et al: Stability, precision, and near-24-hour period of the human circadian pacemaker. Science 1999;284:2177-2181.

36. Asplund R: Sleep, health and visual impairment in the elderly. Arch Gerontol Geriatr 2000;30:7-15.

37. Baehr EK, Eastman CI, Revelle W, et al: Circadian phase-shifting effects of nocturnal exercise in older compared with young adults. Am J Physiol Regul Integr Comp Physiol 2003; 284:R1542-R1550.

38. Dijk DJ, Duffy JF, Czeisler CA: Age related increase in awakenings: Impaired consolidation of nonREM sleep at all circadian phases. Sleep 2001;24:565-577.

39. Duffy JF, Zeitzer JM, Rimmer DW: Peak of circadian melatonin rhythm occurs later within the sleep of older subjects. Am J Physiol Endocrinol Metab 2002;282:E297-E303.

40. Foley DJ, Monjan AA, Brown SL, et al: Sleep complaints among elderly persons: An epidemiologic study of three communities. Sleep 1995;18:425-432.

41. Ganguli M, Reynolds CF, Gilby JE: Prevalence and persistence of sleep complaints in a rural older community sample: The MoVIES project. J Am Geriatr Soc 1996;44:778-784.

42. Bliwise DL, King AC, Harris RB, et al: Prevalence of self-reported poor sleep in a healthy population aged 50-65. Soc Sci Med 1992;34:49-55.

43. Carrier J, Bliwise DL: Sleep and circadian rhythms in normal aging. In Billiard M (ed): Le Sommeil Normal et Pathologique. Hingham, Mass, Kluwer, 2003, pp 297-332.

44. Blazer DG, Hays JC, Foley DJ: Sleep complaints in older adults: A racial comparison. J Gerontol A Biol Sci Med Sci 1995;50: M280-M284.

45. Bixler EO, Vgontzas AN, Lin HM, et al: Insomnia in central Pennsylvania. J Psychosom Res 2002;53:589-592.

46. Vitiello MV, Moe KE, Prinz PN: Sleep complaints cosegregate with illness in older adults: Clinical research informed by and informing epidemiological studies of sleep. J Psychosom Res 2002;53:555-559.

47. Asplund R: Nocturia in relation to sleep, somatic diseases and medical treatment in the elderly. BJU Int 2002;90:533-536.

48. Endeshaw YW, Johnson TM, Kutner MH, et al: Sleep-disordered breathing and nocturia among older adults. J Am Geriatr Soc 2004;52:957-960.

49. Klink ME, Quan SF, Kaltenborn WT, et al: Risk factors associated with complaints of insomnia in a general adult population. Arch Intern Med 1992;152:1634-1637.

50. Dodge R, Cline MG, Quan SF: The natural history of insomnia and its relationship to respiratory symptoms. Arch Intern Med 1995;155:1797-1800.

51. Foley DJ, Monjan A, Simonsick EM, et al: Incidence and remission of insomnia among elderly adults: An epidemiologic study of 6,800 persons over three years. Sleep 1999;22(Suppl 2): S366-S372.

52. Cricco M, Simonsick EM, Foley DJ: The impact of insomnia on cognitive functioning in older adults. J Am Geriatr Soc 2001;49:1185-1189.

53. Morgan K: Daytime activity and risk factors for late-life insomnia. J Sleep Res 2003;12:231-238.

54. Bjorkelund C, Bengtsson C, Lissner L, et al: Women's sleep: Longitudinal changes and secular trends in a 24-year perspective. Results of the population study of women in Gothenburg, Sweden. Sleep 2002;25:894-896.

55. Dealberto MJ, Seeman T, McAvay GJ, et al: Factors related to current and subsequent psychotropic drug use in an elderly cohort. J Clin Epidemiol 1997;50:357-364.

56. Kripke DF, Klauber MR, Wingard DL, et al: Mortality hazard associated with prescription hypnotics. Biol Psychiatry 1998;43:687-693.

57. Kripke DF, Garfinkel L, Wingard DL, et al: Mortality associated with sleep duration and insomnia. Arch Gen Psychiatry 2002;59:131-136.

58. Qureshi AI, Giles WH, Croft JB, et al: Habitual sleep patterns and risk for stroke and coronary heart disease: A 10-year follow-up from NHANES I. Neurology 1997;48:904-911.

59. Livingston G, Blizard B, Mann A: Does sleep disturbance predict depression in elderly people? A study in inner London. Br J Gen Pract 1993;43:445-448.

60. Phillips B, Young T, Finn L, et al: Epidemiology of restless legs symptoms in adults. Arch Intern Med 2000;160:2137-2141.

61. Nichols DA, Allen RP, Grauke JH, et al: Restless legs syndrome symptoms in primary care: A prevalence study. Arch Intern Med 2003;163:2323-2329.

62. Berger K, Luedemann J, Trenkwalder C, et al: Sex and the risk of restless legs syndrome in the general population. Arch Intern Med 2004;164:196-202.

63. Ancoli-Israel S, Kripke DF, Klauber MR, et al: Periodic limb movements in sleep in community-dwelling elderly. Sleep 1991;14:496-500.

64. Gehrman P, Stepnowsky C, Cohen-Zion M, et al: Long-term follow-up of periodic limb movements in sleep in older adults. Sleep 2002;25:340-343.

65. Youngstedt SD, Kripke DF, Klauber MR, et al: Periodic leg movements during sleep and sleep disturbances in elders. J Gerontol A Biol Sci Med Sci 1998;53:M391-M394.

66. Morrish E, King MA, Pilsworth SN, et al: Periodic limb movement in a community population detected by a new actigraphy technique. Sleep Med 2002;3:489-495.

67. Karadeniz D, Ondze B, Besset A, et al: Are periodic leg movements during sleep (PLMS) responsible for sleep disruption in insomnia patients? Eur J Neurol 2000;7:331-336.

68. Eisensehr I, Ehrenberg BL, Noachtar S: Different sleep characteristics in restless legs syndrome and periodic limb movement disorder. Sleep Med 2003;4:147-152.

69. Gosselin N, Lanfranchi P, Michaud M, et al: Age and gender effects on heart rate activation associated with periodic leg movements in patients with restless legs syndrome. Clin Neurophysiol 2003;114:2188-2195.

70. O'Keeffe ST, Gavin K, Lavan JN: Iron status and restless legs syndrome in the elderly. Age Ageing 1994;23:200-203.

71. Michaud M, Soucy JP, Chabli A, et al: SPECT imaging of striatal pre- and postsynaptic dopaminergic status in restless legs syndrome with periodic leg movements in sleep. J Neurol 2002;249:164-170.

72. Turjanski N, Lees AJ, Brooks DJ: Striatal dopaminergic function in restless legs syndrome: 18F-dopa and 11C-raclopride PET studies. Neurology 1999;52:932-937.

73. Allen RP, Barker PB, Wehrl F, et al: MRI measurement of brain iron in patients with restless legs syndrome. Neurology 2001;56:263-265.

74. Ancoli-Israel S, Coy T: Are breathing disturbances in elderly equivalent to sleep apnea syndrome? Sleep 1994;17:77-83.

75. Young T, Shahar E, Nieto FJ, et al: Predictors of sleep-disordered breathing in community-dwelling adults. Arch Intern Med 2002;162:893-900.

76. Bixler EO, Vgontzas AN, Ten Have T, et al: Effects of age on sleep apnea in men: I. Prevalence and severity. Am J Respir Crit Care Med 1998;157:144-148.

77. Bixler EO, Vgontzas AN, Lin HM, et al: Prevalence of sleep-disordered breathing in women: Effects of gender. Am J Respir Crit Care Med 2001;163:608-613.

78. Ancoli-Israel S, Gehrman P, Kripke DF, et al: Long-term follow-up of sleep disordered breathing in older adults. Sleep Med 2001; 2:511-516.

79. Peppard PE, Young T, Palta M: Longitudinal study of moderate weight change and sleep-disordered breathing. JAMA 2000; 284:3015-3021.

80. Redline S, Schluchter MD, Larkin EK, et al: Predictors of longitudinal change in sleep-disordered breathing in a nonclinic population. Sleep 2003;26:703-709.

81. Bliwise DL: Chronologic age, physiologic age and mortality in sleep apnea. Sleep 1996;19:275-276.

82. Young T, Finn L, Austin D, et al: Menopausal status and sleep-disordered breathing in the Wisconsin Sleep Cohort Study. Am J Respir Crit Care Med 2003;167:1181-1185.

83. Tishler PV, Larkin EK, Schluchter MD, et al: Incidence of sleep-disordered breathing in an urban adult population: The relative importance of risk factors in the development of sleep disordered breathing. JAMA 2003;289:2230-2237.

84. Martin SE, Mathur R, Marshall I, et al: The effect of age, sex, obesity and posture on upper airway size. Eur Respir J 1997; 10:2087-2090.

85. Crow HC, Ship JA: Tongue strength and endurance in different aged individuals. J Gerontol Biol Sci Med Sci 1996;51A: M247-M250.

86. Mortimore IL, Bennett SP, Douglas NJ: Tongue protrusion strength and fatiguability: Relationship to apnoea/hypopnoea index and age. J Sleep Res 2000;9:389-393.

87. Endeshaw Y, Katz S, Ouslander J, Bliwise DL: Association of denture use with sleep-disordered breathing among older adults. J Public Health Dent 2004;64:181-183.

88. Guilleminault C, Li K, Chen NH, et al: Two-point palatal discrimination in patients with upper airway resistance syndrome, obstructive sleep apnea syndrome, and normal control subjects. Chest 2002;122:866-870.

89. Calhoun KH, Gibson B, Hartley L, et al: Oral sensation and aging. In Kuna ST, Suratt PM, Remmers JE (eds): Sleep and Respiration in Aging Adults. New York: Elsevier Science, 1991, pp 215-228.

90. Van Lunteren E, Vafaie H, Salomone RJ: Comparative effects of aging on pharyngeal and diaphragm muscles. Respir Physiol 1995;99:113-125.

91. Oliven A, Carmi N, Coleman R, et al: Age-related changes in upper airway muscles morphological and oxidative properties. Exp Gerontol 2001;36:1673-1686.

92. Pack AI, Silage DA, Millman RP, et al: Spectral analysis of ventilation in elderly subjects awake and asleep. J Appl Physiol 1988;64:1257-1267.

93. Carlson BW, Neelon VJ: Evaluation of variables to characterize respiratory periodicity during sleep in older adults. Biol Res Nurs 2002;3:176-188.

94. Ware C, McBrayer RH, Scott JA: Influence of sex and age on duration and frequency of sleep apnea events. Sleep 2000;23:165-170.

95. Kadotani H, Kadotani T, Young T, et al: Association between apolipoprotein E ε4 and sleep-disordered breathing in adults. JAMA 2001;285:2888-2890.

96. Foley DJ, Masaki K, White L, et al: Relationship between apolipoprotein E ε4 and sleep-disordered breathing at different ages. JAMA 2001;286:1447-1448.

97. Gottlieb DJ, DeStefano AL, Foley DJ, et al: APOE ε4 is associated with obstructive sleep apnea/hypopnea: The Sleep Heart Health Study. Neurology 2004;63:664-668.

98. Bliwise DL: Sleep apnea, APOE4 and Alzheimer's disease 20 years and counting. J Psychosom Res 2002;53:539-546.

99. Newman AB, Nieto FJ, Guidry U, et al: Relation of sleep-disordered breathing to cardiovascular disease risk factors. Am J Epidemiol 2001;154:50-59.

100. Nieto FJ, Young TB, Lind BK, et al: Association of sleep-disordered breathing, sleep apnea, and hypertension in a large community-based study. JAMA 2000;283:1829-1836.

101. Shahar E, Whitney CW, Redline S, et al: Sleep-disordered breathing and cardiovascular disease: Cross sectional results of the Sleep Heart Health Study. Am J Respir Crit Care Med 2001;163:19-25.

102. Bliwise DL: Is the measurement of sleepiness the holy grail of sleep medicine? Am J Respir Crit Care Med 2001;163: 1517-1519.

103. Beebe DW, Gozal D: Obstructive sleep apnea and the prefrontal cortex: Towards a comprehensive model linking nocturnal upper airway obstruction to daytime cognitive and behavioral deficits. J Sleep Res 2002;11:1-16.

104. Boland LL, Shahar E, Iber C, et al: Measures of cognitive function in persons with varying degrees of sleep-disordered breathing: The Sleep Heart Health Study. J Sleep Res 2002;11:265-272.

105. Foley DJ, Masaki K, White L, et al: Sleep-disordered breathing and cognitive impairment in elderly Japanese-American men. Sleep 2003;26:596-599.

106. Cohen-Zion M, Stepnowsky C, Marler M, et al: Changes in cognitive function associated with sleep disordered breathing in older people. J Am Geriatr Soc 2001;49:1622-1627.

107. Gallup Organization: Sleepiness in America. Princeton, NJ, Gallup Organization, June 1997.

108. Whitney CW, Enright PL, Newman AB, et al: Correlates of daytime sleepiness in 4578 elderly persons: The Cardiovascular Health Study. Sleep 1998;21:27-36.

109. Gooneratne NS, Weaver TE, Cater JR, et al: Functional outcomes of excessive daytime sleepiness in older adults. J Am Geriatr Soc 2003;51:642-649.

110. Ford DE, Kamerow DB: Epidemiologic study of sleep disturbances and psychiatric disorders. JAMA 1989;262:1479-1484.

111. Bursztyn M, Ginsberg G, Stessman J: The siesta and mortality in the elderly: Effect of rest without sleep and daytime sleep duration. Sleep 2002;25:187-191.

112. Newman AB, Spiekerman CF, Enright P, et al: Daytime sleepiness predicts mortality and cardiovascular disease in older adults: The Cardiovascular Health Study Research Group. J Am Geriatr Soc 2000;48:115-123.

113. Hays JC, Blazer DG, Foley DJ: Risk of napping: Excessive daytime sleepiness and mortality in an older community population. J Am Geriatr Soc 1996;44:693-698.

114. Campos H, Siles X: Siesta and the risk of coronary heart disease: results from a population-based, case-control study in Costa Rica. Int J Epidemiol 2000;29:429-437.

115. Foley D, Monjan A, Masaki K, et al: Daytime sleepiness is associated with 3-year incident dementia and cognitive decline in older Japanese-American men. J Am Geriatr Soc 2001;49:1628-1632.

116. Rockwood K, Davis HS, Merry HR, et al: Sleep disturbances and mortality: Results from the Canadian Study of Health and Aging. J Am Geriatr Soc 2001;49:639-641.

117. Bursztyn M, Ginsberg G, Hammerman-Rozenberg R, et al: The siesta in the elderly: Risk factor for mortality? Arch Intern Med 1999;159:1582-1586.

118. Monk TH, Buysse DJ, Carrier J, et al: Effects of afternoon "siesta" naps on sleep, alertness, performance and circadian rhythms in the elderly. Sleep 2001;24:680-687.

119. Aber R, Webb WB: Effects of a limited nap on night sleep in older subjects. Psychol Aging 1986;1:300-302.

4

Daytime Sleepiness and Alertness

Timothy Roehrs
Mary A. Carskadon
William C. Dement
Thomas Roth

ABSTRACT

Sleepiness is a problem reported by 10% to 25% of the population, depending on the definition of sleepiness used and the population sampled. It occurs more frequently in young adults and in older adults. Sleepiness is a state of physiologic need, and its intensity is evidenced by how rapidly sleep onset occurs, how easily sleep is disrupted, and how long sleep endures. Validated self-rated scales and physiologic measures are available to assess the presence and degree of sleepiness. The chronicity and irreversibility of sleepiness is indicative of its clinical and pathologic significance. Sleepiness is caused by reduced sleep time, as often seen in otherwise healthy adults; by fragmented and disrupted sleep, as found in patients with primary sleep disorders; by administration of sedating drugs and discontinuation of alerting drugs; and by various neurologic disorders. Sleepiness has a normal circadian rhythm, and it is increased in circadian rhythm misalignments such as those occurring in shift work or jet lag. Excessive and persistent sleepiness is life-threatening, but when its presence is recognized and its etiology identified, it can be successfully treated or at least minimized.

Scientific and clinical attention to sleepiness arose from the recognition of excessive daytime sleepiness (EDS) as a symptom associated with serious life-threatening medical conditions. In the late 1960s, this symptom—which earlier had been ignored, attributed to lifestyle excesses, viewed as a sign of laziness and malingering, or, at best, seen as a sign of narcolepsy—began to be seriously studied by scientist-clinicians. Methods to detect and quantify sleepiness were developed. The result has been a growing scientific literature on the nature of sleepiness and its determinants in clinical populations, in selected populations of healthy volunteers, and in the general population.

This chapter will review information regarding the prevalence of sleepiness in the population. The various methods used to measure sleepiness in the population and in the laboratory will be described and guidelines regarding clinical assessment of sleepiness will be offered. The nature and neurobiologic substrates of sleepiness will be discussed and the known determinants of sleepiness will be described. Finally, the clinical and public health significance of persistent complaints of sleepiness will be discussed.

EPIDEMIOLOGY OF SLEEPINESS

Prevalence estimates of sleepiness in the population vary widely, depending on the definition of sleepiness used and the type of population sampled. Surveys and questionnaires have queried about the experience of a mood or feeling state of sleepiness, fatigue, or tiredness; about falling asleep unintentionally; and about struggling to stay awake and fighting sleep onset. New developments in the epidemiology of sleepiness have included standardized sleepiness scales and physiologic assessments of sleepiness that measure the behavior of falling asleep, the estimated likelihood of its occurrence, and the speed of its actual occurrence. Although another important recent focus has been on sleepiness in children and adolescents, this chapter will address only sleepiness in adults.

Sleepiness in Limited Populations or Populations of Convenience

In surveys of relatively small, selected populations, 0.3% to 36% of respondents reported excessive sleepiness. Surveys with reported excessive sleepiness rates of less than 3% are generally from earlier studies that focused on hypersomnia.[1,2] In later studies, in which rates of 4% to 9% were reported, more specific questions about excessive sleepiness during the day[3] or relative to one's peers[4] were asked. In some surveys, postprandial (or midday) sleepiness was distinguished from sleepiness at other times of the day, a distinction discussed later in regard to the circadian correlates of sleepiness.[5] Somewhat higher rates are reported in other selected populations using sleepiness scales. For example, the Epworth Sleepiness Scale (ESS), a scale that requires the respondent to estimate the likelihood of falling asleep in different situations, was completed by 740 day workers in eight industrial plants in Israel, and 23% of the respondents had ESS scores indicative of excessive sleepiness (i.e., scores greater than 10).[6]

Prevalence rates for sleepiness of 15% and greater have also been found for specific age groups, such as young adults and older adults.[7,8] These survey results are consistent with smaller laboratory studies using a physiologic measure of sleepiness, the Multiple Sleep Latency Test (MSLT), which is described later. Young adults were sleepier, on average, than a comparison group of middle-aged adults; in fact, about 20% of the young adults had mean daily sleep latencies of less than 5 minutes, a level of sleepiness considered pathologic.[9]

Healthy older adults were also found to be physiologically sleepier than middle-aged adults.[10] In surveys of the work force engaged in shift or night work, complaints of excessive sleepiness during waking hours are more frequent than among day workers,[11] and continuous ambulatory electroencephalographic (EEG) field monitoring has confirmed the sleepiness.[12]

Sleepiness in Representative Populations

Representative survey studies of national populations have been done. In a study of a representative sample of the Finnish population, 11% of women and 7% of men reported daytime sleepiness almost every day.[13] In another survey, representative of a large geographic area in Sweden, 12% of respondents thought their sleep was insufficient.[14] In that survey, insufficient sleep, and not its consequent daytime sleepiness, was the focus of the questions. Two recent studies representative of the U.S. population used the MSLT to assess sleepiness. Given the necessary time commitment required of participants in MSLT studies, the representative integrity of study results is critically dependent on the recruitment response rate. From a large southeastern Michigan random sample (N = 1648) representative of the U.S. population, a subsample (n = 259) with a 68% response rate was recruited to undergo a nocturnal polysomnogram and MSLT the following day. The prevalence of excessive sleepiness, defined as an MSLT average sleep latency of less than 6 minutes, was 13%.[15]

In another probability sample of 6947 Wisconsin state employees, a subsample (n = 632), collected with a 52% response rate, slept at home and then completed an MSLT in the laboratory the next day. Twenty-five percent had an average sleep latency of less than 5 minutes.[16] These two studies also used the ESS to assess sleepiness; in the Michigan study, 20% had ESS scores greater than 10, and in the Wisconsin study, 25% had scores greater than 11. The higher prevalence in the Wisconsin study, despite the more stringent definition of sleepiness (MSLT of 5 versus 6 minutes, and ESS of 11 versus 10), could be attributed to an age difference in the samples (51 versus 42 years on average) or the previous night's sleep time and circumstances (habitual at home, on average 7.1 hours versus standard laboratory 8.5 hours). In Figure 4–1, the distribution of sleepiness, defined as the average sleep latency on the MSLT, is illustrated for a representative sample of the Michigan population. The average sleep latency (MSLT) of various clinical samples and after experimental sleep-time manipulations is provided for comparisons.

Risk Factors for Sleepiness

The risk factors for sleepiness identified in the various surveys include hours of daily sleep, employment status, marital status, snoring, and depression. Among 26- to 35-year-old members of a large health maintenance organization in Michigan, respondents reported 6.7 hours of sleep on weekdays and 7.4 hours on weekend days, on average.[17] The hours of sleep were inversely related to daytime sleepiness scores on the

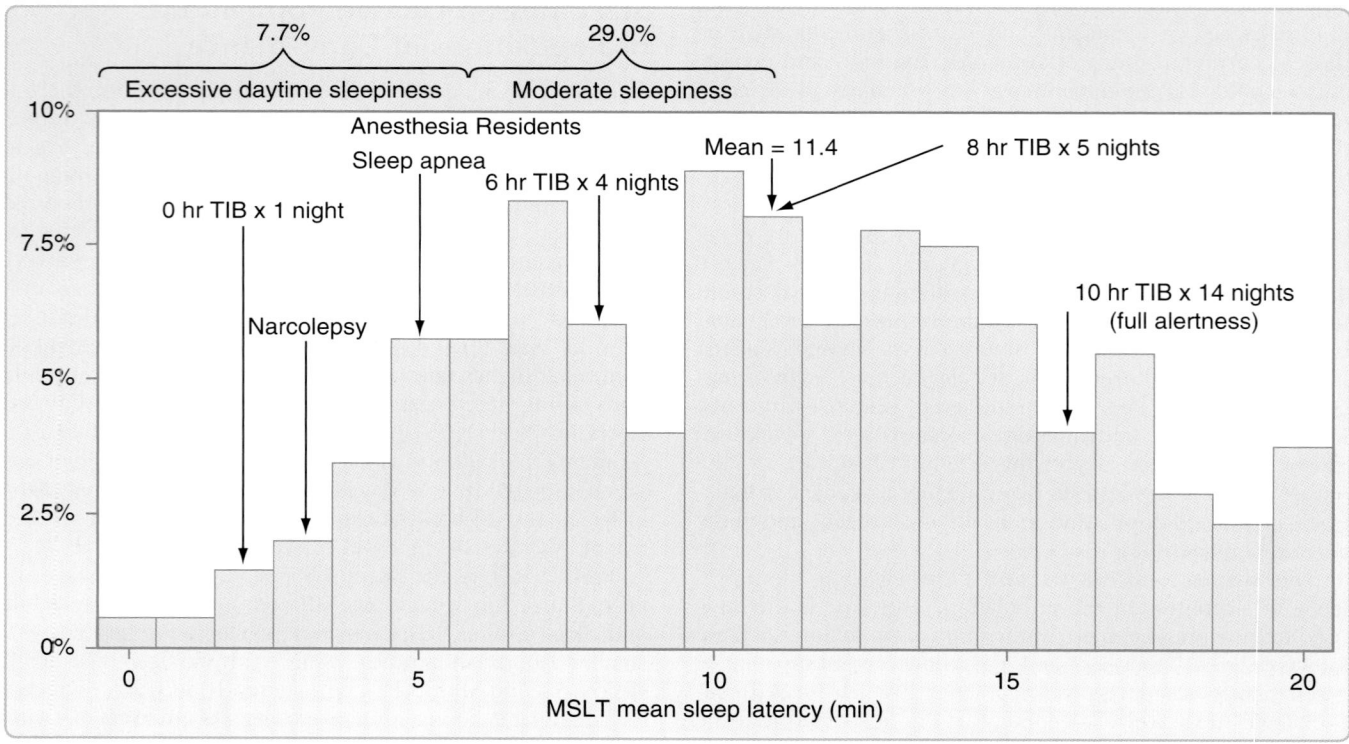

Figure 4–1. The distribution of mean daily sleep latency (minutes) on the multiple sleep latency test (MSLT) in a subsample (n = 259) recruited (68% response rate) from a large southeastern Michigan random sample (N = 1648) representative of the U.S. population. The population mean is 11.4 minutes. This is compared with means reported for various patient groups[60,70,71] and with the means found in healthy individuals after various bedtime manipulations.[23,62] TIB, time in bed.

Sleep–Wake Activity Inventory (SWAI). Both of these variables were related to employment and marital status, with full employment and being single predictive of less sleep time and more sleepiness. Self-reported snoring and depression, as measured by a structured diagnostic interview, were also associated with increased sleepiness. In the Finnish study cited earlier, sleepiness was associated with moderate to severe depression and with snoring more than three times per week.[13]

NATURE OF SLEEPINESS

Physiologic Need State

Sleepiness, according to a consensus among sleep researchers and clinicians, is a basic physiologic need state.[18] It may be likened to hunger or thirst, which are physiologic need states basic to the survival of the individual organism. The presence and intensity of this state can be inferred by how readily sleep onset occurs, how easily sleep is disrupted, and how long sleep endures. Deprivation or restriction of sleep increases sleepiness, and as hunger or thirst is reversible by eating or drinking, sleep reverses sleepiness. In the organism's daily homeostatic economy, severe deprivation states do not normally occur and hence are not routinely responsible for regulating eating or drinking; other factors (e.g., taste, smell, time of day, social factors, biologic variables) modulate these behaviors before severe deprivation states develop. Similarly, routine consumption of sleep is not purely homeostatic but is greatly influenced by social (job, family, friends) and environmental (noise, light, bed) factors.

The subjective experience of sleepiness and its behavioral indicators (yawning, eye rubbing, nodding) can be reduced under conditions of high motivation, excitement, exercise, and competing needs (e.g., hunger, thirst); that is, physiologic sleepiness may not necessarily be manifest. The expression of mild to moderate sleepiness can be masked by any number of factors that are alerting, including motivation, environment, posture, activity, light, and food intake. Studies have shown that average sleep latency on the MSLT is increased by 6 minutes when sitting on as opposed to lying in bed and also by 6 minutes when immediately preceded by a 5-minute walk.[19,20] However, when physiologic sleepiness is most severe and persistent, the ability to reduce its impact on overt behavior wanes. The likelihood of sleep onset increases and the intrusion of microsleeps into ongoing behavior occurs. On the other hand, a physiologically alert (*sleepiness* and *alertness* are used here as antonyms) person does not experience sleepiness or appear sleepy even in the most soporific situations. Heavy meals, warm rooms, boring lectures, and the monotony of long-distance automobile driving unmask physiologic sleepiness when it is present, but they do not cause it.

Within a conventional 24-hour sleep-and-wake schedule, maximum sleepiness ordinarily occurs in the middle of the night when the individual is sleeping, and consequently this sleepiness typically is not experienced or remembered. When forced to be awake in the middle of the night, one experiences loss of energy, fatigue, weariness, difficulty concentrating, and memory lapses. When significant physiologic sleepiness (as a result of reduced sleep quantity or quality) intrudes on one's usual waking activities during the day, similar symptoms are experienced.

Adaptation to the chronic experience of sleepiness probably occurs. Clinicians have reported anecdotally that successfully treated patients frequently comment that they had forgotten the experience of complete alertness. Reduced sensitivity to chronic sleepiness is a probable explanation for the disparities between subjective assessments, even when done with validated scales and the MSLT.[10,21] Typically, it is the most sleepy individuals who show the greatest disparity in subjective versus objective assessments.[10,21] These individuals deny sleepiness despite significant objective indicators of sleepiness. On the other hand, after a 1-night acute sleep restriction, basally alert individuals (ESS mean, 5.6; standard error of the mean, 0.3) were quite accurate in estimating their sleepiness as reflected by the increases in EEG theta activity during a simulated driving task.[22] Studies have also shown that compensation occurs for the cognitive and behavioral effects of experimental sleep restriction and increased sleepiness, particularly when the sleep loss is mild and accumulates at a slow rate.[23] The absence of a readily apparent behavioral deficiency probably also contributes to the subjective–objective disparity seen in chronically sleepy individuals.

The specific nature of this physiologic need state is unclear. Whether sleepiness is unidimensional, varying only in severity, or multidimensional, varying as to etiology or chronicity, has been discussed.[24] If it is unidimensional, whether or not sleepiness and alertness are at opposite poles of the dimension is also an issue. Earlier, it was noted that sleepiness and alertness are being used as antonyms, which suggests a unipolar state. However, it is possible that sleepiness varies from presence to absence and is distinct from alertness. It was noted that sleepiness may be multidimensional, and among the different types of sleepiness cited are rapid eye movement (REM) versus non–rapid eye movement (NREM) sleep, and core versus optional sleepiness.[24] A complete discussion of the heuristic value and of evidence to support these distinctions is beyond the scope of this chapter. Nonetheless, these theoretical perspectives may be colored by different measures, experimental demands, populations studied, and subject or patient motivations (e.g., sensitivity to and capacity to counteract sleepiness).

Neural Substrates of Sleepiness

The substrates of sleepiness have yet to be determined. It is assumed that sleepiness is a central nervous system (CNS) phenomenon with identifiable neural mechanisms and neurochemical correlates. Various electrophysiologic events suggestive of incipient sleep processes appear in behaviorally awake organisms undergoing sleep deprivation. In sleep-deprived animals, ventral hippocampal spike activity, which normally is a characteristic of NREM sleep, increases during behavioral wakefulness and in the absence of the usual cortical EEG changes indicative of sleep.[25] Humans deprived of sleep, or whose sleep is restricted, show identifiable microsleep episodes (brief intrusions of indications of sleep on an EEG) and increased amounts of alpha and theta activity while behaviorally awake.[26] The evidence suggests that these electrophysiologic events are indicants of sleepiness.

A limited number of neuroimaging studies, both structural and functional, have suggested specific brain systems that may be involved in sleepiness. Sleep deprivation in young healthy volunteers reduced regional cerebral glucose metabolism, as assessed by positron emission tomography, in thalamic, basal ganglia, and limbic regions of the brain.[27] Functional magnetic resonance imaging (MRI) after administration of chlorpheniramine (a sedating antihistamine) showed increased frontal and temporal activation when compared with administration of placebo.[28] Because functional MRI is conducted while the subject is performing cognitive tasks, the authors interpreted the increased brain activation as resulting from the increased mental effort, due to sleepiness, required to perform the task. Two groups of patients with severe or slight hypersomnia associated with paramedian thalamic stroke on an MRI showed lesions involving dorsomedial and centromedial thalamic nuclei—bilateral lesions in the severe group and unilateral in the slight group.[29] As yet, these imaging data are not conclusive. They do suggest that it may be possible to identify brain regions and functions that vary with sleepiness. However, the nature of the alteration may depend on the behavioral load imposed on the sleepy subject as well as on the cause of the sleepiness.

The neurochemistry of sleepiness–alertness involves critical and complex issues that have not yet been fully untangled (see Chapters 10, 11, and 31 for a complete discussion). First, a basic issue is whether sleepiness–alertness has a specific neurochemistry that is uniquely different from that associated with the sleep process per se. Second, it is not clear whether sleepiness and alertness are controlled by separate neurochemicals or by a single substance or system. Third, the relation of the neurochemistry of sleepiness–alertness to circadian mechanisms has not yet been determined. Given the number of questions, it should be of no surprise that these are areas of active research.

Neurophysiologic studies of sleep and wake mechanisms have implicated histamine, serotonin, the catecholamines, and acetylcholine in the control of sleep and wake, and these neurotransmitters may also play some role in sleepiness–alertness.[30] Other studies have explored a variety of sleep-inducing substances (e.g., peptides and endocrines) as possible sleep regulators, and any of these substances may prove to be a correlate of sleepiness–alertness.[31] A recently discovered peptide, hypocretin/orexin, has received much attention for its role in the pathophysiology of narcolepsy.[32] It is considered to be a major wake-promoting hypothalamic neuropeptide, and a hypocretin/orexin deficiency has been found in human narcolepsy. However, its role in the homeostatic control of sleep and sleepiness has yet to be determined. It is discussed in greater detail in Chapters 11 and 36.

Pharmacologic studies provide other interesting hypotheses regarding the neurochemistry of sleepiness–alertness. For example, the benzodiazepines induce sleepiness and facilitate gamma-aminobutyric acid (GABA) function at the $GABA_A$ receptor complex, thus implicating this important and diffuse inhibitory neurotransmitter.[33] Another example involves histamine, which is now considered to be a CNS neurotransmitter and is thought to have CNS-arousing activity.[34] Antihistamines that penetrate the CNS produce sleepiness.[35] A recent functional neuroimaging study of histamine H_1 receptors in human brain found that the degree of sleepiness associated with cetirizine (20 mg) was correlated to the degree of H_1 receptor occupancy.[36]

Stimulant drugs suggest several other transmitters and neuromodulators. The mechanism of action of one class of drugs producing psychomotor stimulation and arousal, the amphetamines, is blockade of catecholamine uptake.[37] Another class of stimulants, the methylxanthines, which include caffeine and theophylline, are adenosine receptor antagonists. Adenosine, although not a transmitter in the classic sense, is thought to modulate transmitter activity.[38] It has inhibitory activity in the CNS, inhibiting the two major excitatory neurotransmitters acetylcholine and glutamate. There is growing evidence that adenosine may be a critical, and possibly the key, neurochemical in the homeostatic regulation of sleep.[39] On the other hand, some contradictory evidence limits making definitive conclusions. The space here is too limited to discuss all the evidence in detail. In conclusion, although it is widely held that sleepiness is a physiologic state, its physiologic substrates are as yet not fully defined.

ASSESSMENT OF SLEEPINESS

Quantifying Sleepiness

Behavioral signs of sleepiness include yawning, ptosis, reduced activity, lapses in attention, and head nodding. An individual's subjective report of sleepiness level can also be elicited. As noted earlier, a number of factors such as motivation, stimulation, and competing needs can reduce the behavioral manifestation of sleepiness. Thus, behavioral and subjective indicators often underestimate physiologic sleepiness.

Assessment problems were evident early in research on the daytime consequences of sleep loss. Sleep loss compromises daytime functions; virtually everyone experiences dysphoria and reduced performance efficiency when not sleeping adequately. But a majority of the tasks used to assess the effects of sleep loss are insensitive.[40] In general, only long and monotonous tasks are reliably sensitive to changes in the quantity and quality of nocturnal sleep. An exception is a 10-minute visual vigilance task, completed repeatedly across the day, during which lapses (i.e., response times of 500 msec or longer) and declines in the best response times are increasingly observed as sleep is lost, either during total deprivation or cumulatively over nights of restricted bedtimes.[41]

In various measures of mood, including factor analytic scales, visual analogue scales, and scales for specific aspects of mood, subjects have shown increased fatigue or sleepiness with sleep loss. Among the various subjective measures of sleepiness, the Stanford Sleepiness Scale is the best validated.[42] Yet clinicians have found that chronically sleepy patients may rate themselves alert on this scale even while they are falling asleep behaviorally.[43] All of these scales are state measures that query individuals about how they feel at the present moment.

Another perspective is to view sleepiness behaviorally, as in the likelihood of falling asleep, and thus ask individuals to rate that likelihood in different social circumstances and over longer periods. Two such behavioral rating scales, the ESS and the SWAI, have quite acceptable psychometric properties.[44,45] The ESS has been validated in clinical populations and the SWAI in both clinical and experimental settings. Both ask about falling asleep in settings in which patients typically report falling asleep (e.g., while driving, at church, in social conversation). The time frame over which ratings are to be made is 2 to 4 weeks.

The standard physiologic measure of sleepiness, the MSLT, similarly conceptualizes sleepiness as the tendency to fall asleep by measuring the speed of falling asleep. The MSLT has gained wide acceptance within the field of sleep and sleep disorders as the standard method of quantifying sleepiness.[46] Using standard polysomnographic techniques, this test measures, on repeated opportunities at 2-hour intervals throughout the day, the time it takes to fall asleep while lying in a quiet, dark bedroom. The MSLT is based on the assumption, as outlined earlier, that sleepiness is a physiologic need state that leads to an increased tendency to fall asleep. The reliability and validity of this measure have been documented in a variety of experimental and clinical situations.[47] Motivation does not seem to reduce the impact of sleep loss as measured by the MSLT (as opposed to tests of performance). After total sleep deprivation, subjects can compensate for impaired performance, but they cannot stay awake long while in bed in a darkened room, even if they are instructed to do so.[48]

An alternative to the MSLT, suggested by some clinical investigators, is the Maintenance of Wakefulness Test (MWT). This test requires that subjects lie in bed or sit in a chair in a darkened room and try to remain awake.[49] Like the MSLT, the measure of the ability to remain awake is the latency to sleep onset. The test has not been standardized: there are 20-minute and 40-minute versions, and the subject is variously sitting upright in a chair, lying in bed, or semirecumbent in bed. The reliability of the MWT has not been established either. One study reported sensitivity to the therapeutic effects of continuous positive airway pressure (CPAP) in patients with sleep apnea,[50] and several studies reported sensitivity to the therapeutic effects of stimulants in narcolepsy.[51] A recent study attempted to tease apart the critical factors being measured by the MWT and concluded that, unlike the MSLT, which measures level of sleepiness, the MWT measures the combined effects of level of sleepiness and the degree of arousal as defined by heart rate.[18]

The rationale for the MWT is that, clinically, the critical issue for patients is how long wakefulness can be maintained. A basic assumption underlying this rationale, however, may not be valid: it assumes that a set of circumstances can be evaluated in the laboratory that will reflect an individual's probability of staying awake in the real world. Such a circumstance is not likely because environment, motivation, circadian phase, and any competing drive states all affect an individual's tendency to remain awake. Stated simply, an individual crossing a congested intersection at midday is more likely to stay awake than an individual driving on an isolated highway in the middle of the night. The MSLT, on the other hand, addresses the question of the individual's risk of falling asleep by establishing a setting to maximize the likelihood of sleep onset: all factors competing with falling asleep are removed from the test situation. Thus, the MSLT identifies sleep tendency or clinically identifies maximum risk for the patient. Clearly, the actual risk will vary from individual to individual, from hour to hour, and from environment to environment.

Relationship of Sleepiness to Behavioral Functioning

Given that the MSLT is a valid and reliable measure of sleepiness, the question arises as to how this measure relates to an individual's capacity to function. Direct correlations of the MSLT with other measures of performance under normal conditions have not been too robust.[52] Several studies have found, however, that when sleepiness is at maximum levels, correlations with performance are high. For example, MSLT scores after sleep deprivation,[53] after administration of sedating antihistamines,[54] and after benzodiazepine administration[55] correlate with measures of performance and even prove to be the most sensitive measure.[55] A recent study relating performance lapses on a vigilance task to the cumulative effects of sleep restriction found a function comparable to that of the MSLT under a similar cumulative sleep restriction (Fig. 4–2).[56] The reason many studies have found weak correlations between performance and MSLT at normal or moderate levels of sleepiness is that laboratory performance and MSLT are differentially affected by variables such as age, education, and motivation.

For the most part, the literature relating sleepiness and behavioral functioning has focused on psychomotor and attention behaviors, with the major outcomes being response slowing and attentional lapses. These impairments can be attributed to slowed processing of information and microsleeps—that is, intrusion of sleep-preparatory and sleep-onset behaviors. Recent research has focused on other behavioral domains not as clearly associated with sleep-mediated behaviors, including decision making and pain sensation. Several studies have shown that increased sleepiness is associated with poor risk-taking decisions.[57,58] Sleep loss and its associated sleepiness have also been shown to increase pain sensitivity.[59]

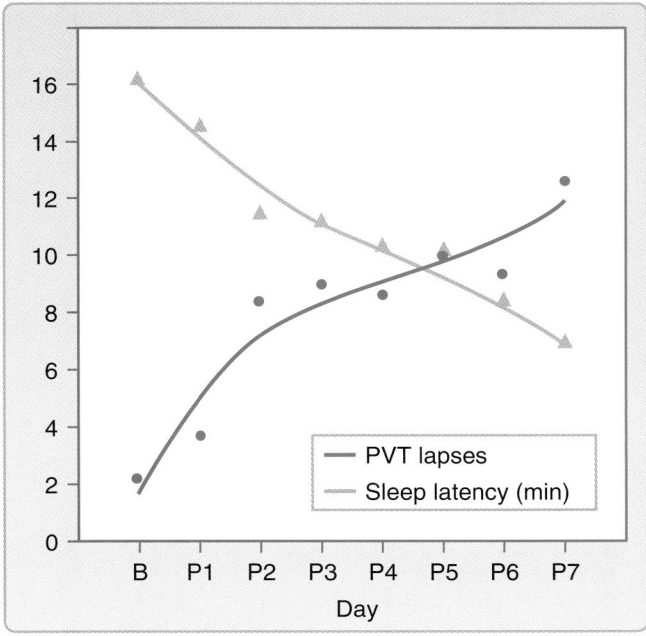

Figure 4–2. Similar functions relating mean daily sleep latency on the multiple sleep latency test (MSLT) and mean daily lapses on the visual psychomotor vigilance test (PVT) to the cumulative effects of sleep restriction (about 5 hours of bedtime nightly) across 7 consecutive nights (P1 to P7). (Redrawn from Dinges DF, Pack F, Williams K, et al: Cumulative sleepiness, mood disturbance, and psychomotor vigilance performance decrements during a week of sleep restricted to 4-5 hours per night. Sleep 1997;20:275.)

Clinical Assessment of Sleepiness

Assessing the clinical significance of a patient's complaint of excessive sleepiness can be complex for an inexperienced clinician. The assessment depends on two important factors: chronicity and reversibility. Chronicity can be explained simply. Although a healthy individual may be acutely sleepy, the patient's sleepiness is persistent and unremitting. As to reversibility, unlike in the healthy person, increased sleep time may not completely or consistently ameliorate a patient's sleepiness. Patients with excessive sleepiness may not complain of sleepiness per se but rather of its consequences: loss of energy, fatigue, lethargy, weariness, lack of initiative, memory lapses, or difficulty concentrating.

To clarify the patient complaint, it is important to focus on soporific situations in which physiologic sleepiness is more likely to be manifest, as discussed earlier. Such situations include watching television, reading, riding in a car, listening to a lecture, or sitting in a warm room. Table 4–1 presents the commonly reported sleep-inducing situations for a large sample of patients with sleep apnea syndrome. After clarifying the complaint, the patient should be asked about the entire day: morning, midday, and evening. As discussed later, most adults experience sleepiness over the midday. However, patients experience sleepiness at other times of the day as well, and often throughout the day. Whenever possible, objective documentation of sleepiness and its severity should be sought. As indicated earlier, the standard and accepted method to document sleepiness objectively is the MSLT.

Guidelines for interpreting the results of the MSLT are available[46] (see Fig. 4–1). A number of case series of patients with disorders of excessive sleepiness have now been published with accompanying MSLT data for each diagnostic classification.[60] These data provide the clinician with guidelines for evaluating the clinical significance of a given patient's MSLT results. Although these data cannot be considered norms, a scheme for ranking MSLT scores to indicate degree of pathology has been suggested.[60] An average daily MSLT score of 5 minutes or fewer suggests pathologic sleepiness, a score of more than 5 minutes but fewer than 10 minutes is considered a diagnostic gray area, and a score of more than 10 minutes is considered to be in the normal range (see Fig. 4–1 for MSLT results in the general population). The MSLT results, however, must also be evaluated with respect to the conditions under which the testing was conducted. Standards have been published for administering the MSLT, which must be followed to obtain a valid, interpretable result.[46]

Determinants of Sleepiness

Quantity of Sleep

The degree of daytime sleepiness is directly related to the amount of nocturnal sleep. (The performance effects of acute and chronic sleep deprivation are discussed in Chapters 5 and 6.) Partial or total sleep deprivation in healthy subjects is followed by increased daytime sleepiness the following day.[47] Therefore, modest nightly sleep restrictions over successive nights accumulate to progressively increase daytime sleepiness and performance lapses[61] (see Fig. 4–1). On the other hand, increased sleep time in healthy young adults, by extending bedtime beyond the usual 7 to 8 hours per night, produces an increase in alertness (i.e., a reduction in sleepiness).[62] Furthermore, the pharmacologic extension of sleep time by an average of 1 hour in older adults produces an increase in mean sleep latency on the MSLT (i.e., increased alertness).[63]

Reduced sleep time explains the excessive sleepiness of several patient and nonpatient groups. For example, a subgroup of sleep clinic patients has been identified whose excessive daytime sleepiness can be attributed to chronic insufficient sleep.[64] These patients show objectively documented excessive sleepiness, have "normal" nocturnal sleep with unusually high sleep efficiency (time asleep per time in bed), and report about 2 hours more sleep on each weekend day than each weekday. Regularizing bedtime and increasing time in bed produces a resolution of their symptoms and normalized MSLT results.[65] The increased sleepiness of healthy young adults also can be attributed to insufficient nocturnal sleep. When the sleepiest 25% of a sample of young adults is given extended time in bed (10 hours) for as long as 5 to 14 consecutive nights, their sleepiness is reduced to a level resembling that of the general population.[64]

Individual differences in tolerability to sleep loss have been reported.[66] These differences can be attributed to a number of possible factors. A difference in the basal level of sleepiness at the start of a sleep time manipulation is quite possible given the range of sleepiness in the general population (see Fig. 4–1). There also may be differences in the sensitivity and responsivity of the sleep homeostat—that is, how large a sleep deficit the system can tolerate and how robustly the sleep homeostat produces sleep when detecting deficiency. Finally, genetic differences in sleep need, the set point around which the sleep homeostat regulates daily sleep time, have long been hypothesized. These are all fertile areas for research.

Quality of Sleep

Daytime sleepiness also relates to the quality and the continuity of a previous night's sleep. Sleep in patients with a number of sleep disorders is punctuated by frequent, brief arousals of 3 to 15 seconds' duration. These arousals are characterized by bursts of EEG speeding or alpha activity and, occasionally, transient increases in skeletal muscle tone. Standard scoring rules for transient EEG arousals have been developed.[67] A transient arousal is illustrated in Figure 4–3. These arousals typically do not result in awakening by either Rechtschaffen and Kales sleep staging criteria or behavioral indicators, and the arousals recur in some conditions as often

Table 4–1.	Sleep-Inducing Situations for Patients with Apnea*	
Situation	**Percentage of Patients**
Watching television	91
Reading	85
Riding in a car	71
Attending church	57
Visiting friends and relatives	54
Driving	50
Working	43
Waiting for a red light	32

*N = 384 patients.

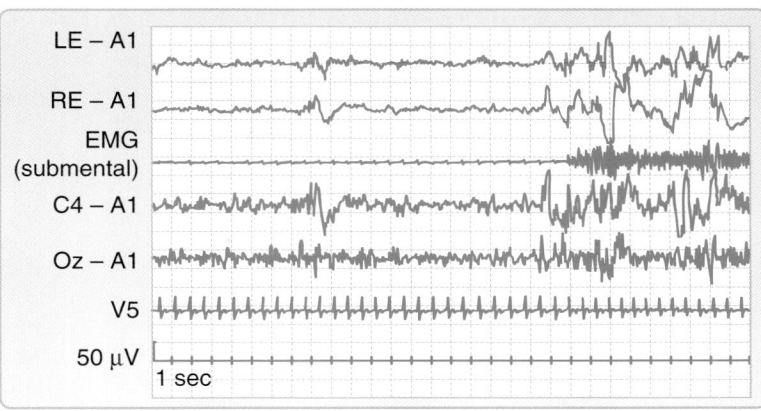

Figure 4–3. A transient arousal (on *right side* of figure) fragmenting sleep. The preexistence of sleep is evident by the K-complex at second 9 of the epoch preceding the arousal. LE-A1, Left electrooculogram referenced to A1; RE-A1, right electrooculogram referenced to A1; EMG, electromyogram from submental muscle; C4-A1, electroencephalogram referenced to A1 from C4 placement; Oz-A1, electroencephalogram referenced to A1 from Oz placement; V5, electrocardiogram from V5 placement. (Redrawn from American Sleep Disorders Association: EEG arousals: Scoring rules and examples. Sleep 1992;15:173-184.)

as one to four times per minute. The arousing stimulus differs in the various disorders and can be identified in some cases (apneas, leg movements, pain) but not in others. Regardless of etiology, the arousals generally do not result in shortened sleep but rather in fragmented or discontinuous sleep, and this fragmentation produces daytime sleepiness.[68]

Correlational evidence suggests a relationship between sleep fragmentation and daytime sleepiness. Fragmentation, as indexed by number of brief EEG arousals, number of shifts from other sleep stages to stage 1 sleep or wake, and the percentage of stage 1 sleep, correlates with EDS in various patient groups.[69] Treatment studies also link sleep fragmentation and excessive sleepiness. Patients with sleep apnea syndrome who are successfully treated by surgery (i.e., the number of apneas is reduced) show a reduced frequency of arousals from sleep as well as a reduced level of sleepiness, whereas those who do not benefit from the surgery (i.e., apneas remain) show no decrease in arousals or sleepiness, despite improved sleeping oxygenation.[70] Similarly, CPAP, by providing a pneumatic airway splint, reduces breathing disturbances and consequent arousals from sleep and reverses EDS.[71] The reversal of daytime sleepiness after CPAP treatment of sleep apnea syndrome is presented in Figure 4–4.

Experimental fragmentation of the sleep of healthy subjects has been produced by inducing arousals with an auditory stimulus. Several studies have shown that subjects awakened at various intervals during the night demonstrate performance decrements and increased sleepiness on the following day.[72] Studies have also fragmented sleep without awakening subjects by terminating the stimulus when there is an EEG sign of arousal rather than when there is a behavioral response. Increased daytime sleepiness (shortened latencies on the MSLT) resulted from nocturnal sleep fragmentation in one study,[73] and in a second study, the recuperative effects (measured as increased latencies on the MSLT) of a nap following sleep deprivation were compromised by fragmenting the sleep during the nap.[74]

One nonclinical population in whom sleep fragmentation is an important determinant of excessive sleepiness is older adults. Many studies have now shown that even older adults without sleep complaints show an increased number of apneas and periodic leg movements during sleep.[75] As noted earlier, older adults as a group are sleepier than other groups.[10] Furthermore, it has been demonstrated that older

adults with the highest frequency of arousal during sleep have the greatest daytime sleepiness.[76]

Circadian Rhythms

A biphasic pattern of objective sleep tendency was observed when healthy young adult and older adult subjects were tested every 2 hours over a complete 24-hour day.[77] During the sleep period (11:30 PM to 8 AM) the latency testing was accomplished by awakening subjects for 15 minutes and then allowing them to return to sleep. Two troughs of alertness—one during the nocturnal hours (about 2 to 6 AM) and another during the daytime hours (about 2 to 6 PM)—were observed. Figure 4–5 shows the biphasic pattern of sleepiness–alertness.

Other research protocols have yielded similar results. In constant routine studies, where external environmental stimulation is minimized and subjects remain awake, superimposed on the expected increase in self-rated fatigue resulting

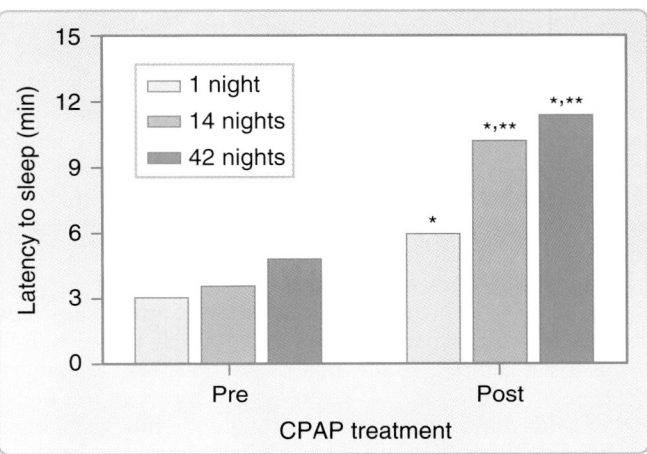

Figure 4–4. Mean daily sleep latency on the multiple sleep latency test (MSLT) in patients with obstructive sleep apnea syndrome before (pre) and after (post) 1, 14, and 42 nights of continuous positive airway pressure (CPAP) treatment. *, $P < .05$; **, $P < .01$. (Redrawn from Lamphere J, Roehrs T, Wittig R, et al: Recovery of alertness after CPAP in apnea. Chest 1989;96:1364-1367.)

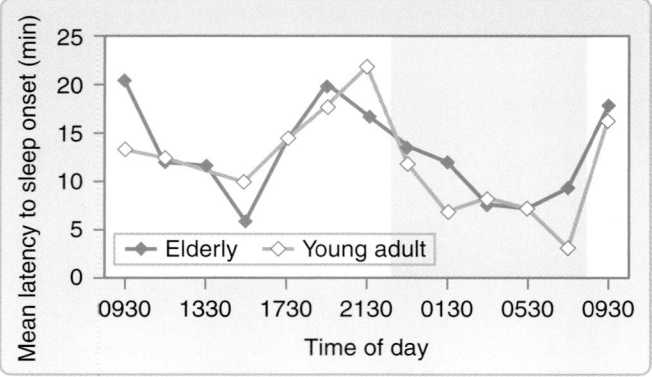

Figure 4–5. Latency to sleep at 4-hour intervals across the 24-hour day. Testing during the daytime followed standard multiple sleep latency test (MSLT) procedures. During the night, from 11:30 PM to 8:00 AM *(shaded area)*, subjects were awakened every 2 hours for 15 minutes, and latency of return to sleep was measured. Elderly subjects (*n* = 10) were 60 to 83 years old; young subjects (*n* = 8) were 19 to 23 years old. (Redrawn from Carskadon MA, Dement WC: Daytime sleepiness: Quantification of a behavioral state. Neurosci Biobehav Rev 1987;111:307-317, Copyright 1987, Elsevier Science.)

from the deprivation of sleep is a biphasic circadian rhythmicity of self-rated fatigue similar to that seen for sleep latency.[78] In another constant routine study in which EEG was continuously monitored, a biphasic pattern of "unintentional sleep" was observed.[79] In studies with sleep scheduled at unusual times, the duration of sleep periods has been used as an index of the level of sleepiness. A pronounced circadian variation in sleep duration is found, with the termination of sleep periods closely related to the biphasic sleep latency function in the studies cited earlier.[80] If individuals are permitted to nap when they are placed in time-free environments, this biphasic pattern becomes quite apparent in the form of a mid-cycle nap.[81]

This circadian rhythm in sleepiness is part of a circadian system in which many biologic processes vary rhythmically over 24 hours. The sleepiness rhythm parallels the circadian variation in body temperature, with shortened latencies occurring in conjunction with temperature troughs.[77] But these two functions, sleep latency and body temperature, are not mirror images of each other; the midday body temperature decline is relatively small compared with that of sleep latency. Further, under free-running conditions, the two functions become dissociated.[82] However, no other biologic rhythm is as closely associated with the circadian rhythm of sleepiness as is body temperature.

Earlier, it was noted that shift workers are unusually sleepy, and jet travelers experience sleepiness acutely in a new time zone. The sleepiness in these two conditions results from the placement of sleep and wakefulness at times that are out of phase with the existing circadian rhythms. Thus, not only is daytime sleep shortened and fragmented but also wakefulness occurs at the peak of sleepiness or the trough of alertness. Several studies have shown that pharmacologic extension and consolidation of out-of-phase sleep can improve daytime sleepiness.[83] Yet, the basal circadian rhythm of sleepiness remains although the overall level of sleepiness has been reduced.

In other words, the synchronization of circadian rhythms to the new sleep–wake schedule is not hastened.

Central Nervous System Drugs

SEDATING DRUG EFFECTS

CNS depressant drugs, as expected, increase sleepiness. Most of these drugs act as agonists at the $GABA_A$ receptor complex. The benzodiazepine hypnotics hasten sleep onset at bedtime and shorten the latency to return to sleep after an awakening during the night (which is their therapeutic purpose), as demonstrated by a number of objective studies.[84] Long-acting benzodiazepines continue to shorten sleep latency on the MSLT the day after bedtime administration.[85] Barbiturates also reduce sleep latency at night, and during the following day they continue to produce sedation as measured by performance testing.[86] The common use of barbiturate hypnotics was discontinued before the development of the MSLT, and, consequently, no studies have used the MSLT to assess their daytime sedating effects. Finally, ethanol administered during the daytime (9 AM) reduces sleep latency in a dose-related manner as measured by the MSLT.[87]

Second-generation antiepileptic drugs, including gabapentin, tiagabine, vigabatrin, pregabalin, and others, enhance GABA activity through various mechanisms that directly or indirectly involve the $GABA_A$ receptor.[88] The sedating effects of these drugs have not been thoroughly documented, but some evidence indicates they do have sedative activity. $GABA_B$ receptor agonists are being investigated as treatments for drug addictions, and the preclinical animal research suggests these drugs may have sedative activity as well.[89]

Antagonists acting at the histamine H_1 receptor also have sedating effects. One of the most commonly reported side effects associated with the use of H_1 antihistamines is daytime sleepiness. Several double-blind, placebo-controlled studies have shown that certain H_1 antihistamines, such as diphenhydramine, increase sleepiness using sleep latency as the objective measure of sleepiness, whereas others, such as terfenadine or loratadine, do not.[90] The difference between these compounds relates to their differential CNS penetration and binding. Other H_1 antihistamines (e.g., tazifylline) are thought to have a greater peripheral compared with central H_1 affinity, and, consequently, effects on daytime sleep latency are found only at relatively high doses.[91]

Antihypertensives, particularly beta adrenoreceptor blockers, are also reported to produce sedation during the daytime.[92] These CNS effects are thought to be related to the differential liposolubility of the various compounds. However, we are unaware of any studies that directly measure the daytime sleepiness produced by beta-blockers; the information is derived from reports of side effects. As noted earlier, it is important to differentiate sleepiness from tiredness or fatigue. Patients may be describing tiredness or fatigue resulting from the drugs' peripheral effects (e.g., lowered cardiac output and blood pressure), not sleepiness, a presumed central effect.

Sedative effects of dopaminergic agonists used in treating Parkinson's disease have been reported as adverse events in clinical trials and in case reports as "sleep attacks" while driving.[93] It is now clear these sleep attacks are not attacks per se but are the expression of excessive sleepiness. Although the dose-related sedative effect of these drugs has been established, the mechanism by which the sedative effects occur is unknown. The dopaminergic agonists are also known to disrupt and fragment sleep.[94] Thus, the excessive sleepiness may be secondary to disturbed sleep, or to a combination of disturbed sleep and direct sedative effects.

ALERTING DRUG EFFECTS

Stimulant drugs reduce sleepiness and increase alertness. The drugs in this group differ in their mechanisms of action. Amphetamine, methylphenidate, and pemoline block dopamine reuptake, and to a lesser extent they enhance the release of norepinephrine, dopamine, and serotonin. The mechanism of modafinil is not established; some evidence suggests that it has a mechanism distinct from the classic stimulants. Amphetamine, methylphenidate, pemoline, and modafinil are used to treat the EDS associated with narcolepsy, and some have been studied as medications to maintain alertness and vigilance in healthy subjects under conditions of sustained sleep loss (e.g., military operations). Studies of patients with narcolepsy using MSLT or MWT have shown improved alertness with amphetamine, methylphenidate, modafinil, and pemoline.[95] There is dispute as to the extent to which the excessive sleepiness of narcoleptics is reversed and about the comparative efficacy of the various drugs. In healthy persons restricted or deprived of sleep, both amphetamine and methylphenidate increase alertness on the MSLT and improve psychomotor performance.[96,97] Caffeine is an adenosine receptor antagonist. In doses equivalent to one to three cups of coffee, caffeine reduced daytime sleepiness on the MSLT in normal subjects after 5 hours of sleep the previous night.[98]

INFLUENCE OF BASAL SLEEPINESS

The preexisting level of sleepiness–alertness interacts with a drug to influence the drug's behavioral effect. In other words, a drug's effect differs when sleepiness is at its maximum compared with its minimum. As noted previously, the basal level of daytime sleepiness can be altered by restricting or extending time in bed[58]; this in turn alters the usual effects of a stimulating versus a sedating drug. A study showed comparable levels of sleepiness–alertness during the day following 5 hours in bed and morning (9 AM) caffeine consumption, compared with 11 hours in bed and morning (9 AM) ethanol ingestion.[98] Follow-up studies explored the dose relationships of ethanol's interaction with basal sleepiness.[99] Dose-related differences in daytime sleepiness after ethanol and 8 hours of sleep were diminished after even 1 night of 5 hours of sleep, although the measured levels of ethanol in the breath were consistent day to day. In other words, sleepiness enhanced the sedative effects of ethanol. In contrast, caffeine and methylphenidate produced a similar increase in alertness, regardless of the basal level of sleepiness. Clinically, these findings imply, for example, that a sleepy driver with minimal blood ethanol levels may be as dangerous as an alert driver who is legally intoxicated.[99]

The basal state of sleepiness also influences drug-seeking behavior. The likelihood that a healthy person without a drug abuse history will self-administer methylphenidate is greatly enhanced after 4 hours of sleep the previous night compared with after 8 hours of sleep. Although not experimentally demonstrated as yet, self-administration of caffeine also is probably influenced by basal state of sleepiness. The high volume of caffeine use probably relates to the high rate of self-medication for sleepiness resulting from chronic insufficient sleep in the population.

Central Nervous System Pathologies

Pathology of the CNS is another determinant of daytime sleepiness. The previously noted hypocretin/orexin deficiency is thought to cause excessive sleepiness in patients with narcolepsy.[100] Another sleep disorder associated with excessive sleepiness and caused by an unknown CNS pathology is idiopathic CNS hypersomnolence.[101] As yet, hypocretin/orexin deficiency has not been shown in this disorder. These two conditions are described in detail in Chapters 64 and 66.

Excessive sleepiness is reported in other neurologic diseases. A study in patients with myotonic dystrophy, type 1, reported excessive sleepiness on the MSLT and reduced cerebrospinal fluid levels of hypocretin/orexin.[102] Sleep attacks have been reported in Parkinson's disease, and assessment with the MSLT suggests they are the expression of excessive daytime sleepiness.[103] What remains unresolved in the excessive sleepiness of Parkinson's disease is the relative contribution of the disease itself, the fragmentation of sleep due to periodic leg movement or apnea, and the dopaminergic drugs used in treating the disease. The previously cited study[103] found no differences in sleepiness as a function of prescribed drug or sleep fragmentation, although further assessment in larger unselected samples is necessary to confirm this finding.

CLINICAL AND PUBLIC HEALTH SIGNIFICANCE OF SLEEPINESS

Although the patients at sleep disorders centers are not representative of the general population, they do provide some indications regarding the clinical significance of sleepiness. Their sleep–wake histories directly indicate the serious impact excessive sleepiness has on their lives.[104] Nearly half the patients with excessive sleepiness report automobile accidents; half report occupational accidents, some life-threatening; and many have lost jobs because of their sleepiness. In addition, sleepiness is considerably disruptive of family life.[105] An elevated automobile accident rate (i.e., sevenfold) among patients with excessive sleepiness has been verified through driving records obtained from motor vehicle agencies.[106]

Population-based information regarding traffic and industrial accidents also suggests a link between sleepiness and life-threatening events. The highest rate of automobile accidents occurs in the early morning hours, which is notable because the fewest automobiles are on the road during these hours. Also during these early morning hours, the greatest degree of sleepiness is experienced.[107] Long-haul truck drivers have accidents most frequently (even corrected for hours driving before the accident) during the early morning hours, again when sleepiness reaches its zenith.[108]

Workers on the graveyard shift were identified as a particularly sleepy subpopulation. In 24-hour ambulatory EEGs of sleep and wakefulness, workers (20% in one study) were found to actually fall asleep during the night shift.[14] Not surprisingly, the poorest job performance consistently occurs during the night shift, and the highest rate of industrial accidents is usually found among workers on this shift. Medical residents are another particularly sleepy subpopulation. In surveys, those reporting 5 or fewer hours of sleep per night were more likely to make medical errors and report serious accidents, and they were twice as likely to be named in medical malpractice suits.[109] In a survey of medical house staff, 49% reported falling asleep while driving and 90% of the episodes occurred after being on call, compared with 13% fall-asleep episodes reported by the medical faculty, and 20 of the 70 house staff were involved in automobile accidents compared with 11 of the 85 faculty.[110]

Cognitive function is also impaired by sleepiness. In children, excessive sleepiness has been associated with learning disabilities,[7] and adults with various disorders of excessive sleepiness also have cognitive and memory problems.[111] The memory deficiencies are not specific to a certain sleep disorder but rather to the sleepiness associated with the disorder. When treated adequately, sleepiness is rectified and the memory and cognitive deficits similarly improve.[112] Results of sleep deprivation studies in healthy patients support the relationship between sleepiness and memory deficiency. Even modest reductions of sleep time are associated with cognitive deficiencies.[113]

Sleepiness also depresses arousability to physiologic challenges: 24-hour sleep deprivation decreases upper airway dilator muscle activity[114] and decreases ventilatory responses to hypercapnia and hypoxia.[115] In a canine model of sleep apnea, periodic disruption of sleep with acoustic stimuli (i.e., sleep fragmentation, in contrast to sleep deprivation) resulted in lengthened response times to airway occlusion, greater oxygen desaturation, increases in inspiratory pressures, and surges in blood pressure.[116] Depressed physiologic responsivity due to sleepiness is clinically significant for patients with sleep apnea and other breathing disorders, as they are all exacerbated by sleepiness. The emerging data on sleepiness and pain threshold, cited earlier, are also clinically significant in the management of both acute and chronic pain conditions.

Finally, life expectancy data directly link excessive sleep (not specifically sleepiness) and mortality. A 1976 study found that men and women who reported sleeping more than 10 hours a day were about 1.8 times more likely to die prematurely than those sleeping between 7 and 8 hours daily.[117] This survey, however, associated hypersomnia and increased mortality and not necessarily EDS, for which the relationship is currently unknown.

Clinical Pearl

Sleepiness, when most excessive and persistent, is a signal to the individual to stop operating—it is dangerous and life-threatening to continue without sleep. And to the clinician, that signal warns that there may be some underlying pathology that can be successfully treated, or, at the very least, its vital, life-threatening impact can be minimized.

REFERENCES

1. Bixler ED, Kales JD, Soldatos CR, et al: Prevalence of sleep disorders in the Los Angeles metropolitan area. Am J Psychiatry 1979;136:1257-1262.
2. Ford DE, Kamerow DB: Epidemiologic study of sleep disturbances and psychiatric disorders. JAMA 1989;262:1479-1484.
3. Billard M, Alperovitch A, Perot C, et al: Excessive daytime somnolence in young men: Prevalence and contributing factors. Sleep 1987;10:297-305.
4. Partinen M: Sleeping habits and sleep disorders of Finnish men before, during, and after military service. Ann Med Milit Fenn 1982;57(Suppl):96.
5. Martikainen K, Hasan J, Uropen H, et al: Daytime sleepiness: A risk factor in community life. Acta Neurol Scand 1992;86:337-341.
6. Melamed S, Oksenberg A: Excessive sleepiness and risk of occupational injuries in non-shift daytime workers. Sleep 2001;25:315-322.
7. Carskadon MA: Patterns of sleep and sleepiness in adolescents. Pediatrician 1990;17:5-12.
8. Asplund R: Daytime sleepiness and napping amongst the elderly in relation to somatic health and medical treatment. J Intern Med 1996;239:261-267.
9. Levine B, Roehrs T, Zorick F, et al: Daytime sleepiness in young adults. Sleep 1988;11:39-46.
10. Dement WC, Carskadon MA: An essay on sleepiness. In Baldy-Mouliner M (ed): Actualités en Medecine Experimentale. Montpellier, France, Euromed, 1981, pp 47-71.
11. Akerstedt T, Frober JE: Shift work and health-interdisciplinary aspects. In Rentos PGR, Shepard RD (eds): Shift Work and Health: A Symposium. Washington, DC, NIOSH, 1976, pp 179-197.
12. Torsvall L, Akerstedt T, Gillander K, et al: Sleep on the night shift: 24h EEG monitoring of spontaneous sleep/wake behavior. Psychophysiology 1989;26:352-358.
13. Hublin C, Kaprio J, Partinen M, et al: Daytime sleepiness in an adult Finnish population. J Intern Med 1996;239:417-423.
14. Broman JE, Lundh LG, Hetta J: Insufficient sleep in the general population. Neurophysiol Clin 1996;26:30-39.
15. Drake CL, Roehrs T, Richardson G, et al: Epidemiology and morbidity of excessive daytime sleepiness. Sleep 2002;25:A91.
16. Punjabi NM, Bandeen-Roche K, Young T: Predictors of objective sleep tendency in the general population. Sleep 2003;26:678-683.
17. Breslau N, Roth T, Rosenthal L, et al: Daytime sleepiness: An epidemiological study of young adults. Am J Public Health 1997;87:1649-1653.
18. Carskadon MA, Dement WC: The multiple sleep latency test: What does it measure? Sleep 1982;5:S67-S72.
19. Bonnet MH, Arand DL: Arousal components which differentiate the MWT from the MSLT. Sleep 2001;24:441-447.
20. Bonnet MH, Arand DL: Sleepiness as measured by the MSLT varies as a function of preceding activity. Sleep 1998;21:477-484.
21. Richardson G, Drake CL, Roehrs T, et al: Habitual sleep time predicts accuracy of self-reported alertness (abstract). Sleep 2002;25:A145.
22. Horne JA, Baulk SD: Awareness of sleepiness when driving. Psychophysiology 2003;41:161-165.
23. Drake C, Roehrs T, Burduvali E, et al: Effects of rapid versus slow accumulation of eight hours of sleep loss. Psychophysiology 2001;38:979-987.
24. Pivik RT: The several qualities of sleepiness: Psychophysiological considerations. In Monk T (ed): Sleep, Sleepiness and Performance. New York, John Wiley & Sons, 1991, pp 3-37.
25. Friedman L, Bergmann BM, Rechtschaffen A: Effects of sleep deprivation on sleepiness, sleep intensity, and subsequent sleep in the rat. Sleep 1979;1:369-391.
26. Strijkstra AM, Beersma DGM, Drayer B, et al: Subjective sleepiness correlates negatively with global alpha (8-12 Hz) and positively with central frontal theta (4-8 Hz) frequencies in the human resting awake electroencephalogram. Neurosci Lett 2003;340:17-20.
27. Wu JC, Gillin JC, Buchsbaum MS, et al: The effect of sleep deprivation on cerebral glucose metabolic rate in normal humans assessed with positron emission tomography. Sleep 1991;14:155-162.

28. Starbuck VN, Kay GG, Platenberg RC: Functional magnetic resonance imaging shows evidence of daytime sleepiness following evening dosing with chlorpheniramine. J Allergy Clin Immunol 1998;101:408.
29. Lovblad KO, Bassetti C, Mathis J, et al: MRI of paramedian thalamic stroke with sleep disturbance. Neuroradiology 1997;39:693-698.
30. Monnier M, Gaillard JM: Biochemical regulation of sleep. Experientia 1980;36:21-24.
31. Inoue S: Sleep substances: Their roles and evolution. In Inoue S, Borbely AA (eds): Endogenous Sleep Substances and Sleep Regulation. Tokyo, Japan Scientific Societies Press, 1985, pp 3-12.
32. Mignot E: A commentary on the neurobiology of the hypocretin/orexin system. Neuropsychopharmacology 2001;25:S5-S13.
33. Gallager DW: Benzodiazepines and gamma-aminobutyric acid. Sleep 1982;5:S3-S11.
34. Pollard H, Schwartz JC: Histamine neuronal pathways and their functions. Trends Neurosci 1987;10:86-89.
35. Roehrs T, Zwyghuizen-Doorenbos A, Roth T: Sedative effects and plasma concentrations following single doses of triazolam, diphenhydramine, ethanol and placebo. Sleep 1993;16:301-305.
36. Tashiro M, Mochizuki H, Iwabuchi K, et al: Roles of histamine in regulation of arousal and cognition: Functional neuroimaging of histamine H1 receptors in human brain. Life Sci 2002;72:409-414.
37. Chiarello RJ, Cole JO: The use of psychostimulants in general psychiatry. Arch Gen Psychiatry 1987;44:286-295.
38. Dunwiddie TV: The physiological role of adenosine in the central nervous system. Int Rev Neurobiol 1985;27:63-139.
39. Porkka-Heiskanen T, Alanko L, Kalinchuk A, et al: Adenosine and sleep. Sleep Med Rev 2002;6:321-332.
40. Webb WB: Sleep deprivation: Total, partial and selective. In Chase MH (ed): The Sleeping Brain. Los Angeles, BIS/BRS, 1972, pp 323-362.
41. Dinges DF, Orne MT, Whithouse WG, et al: Temporal placement of a nap for alertness: Contributions of circadian phase and prior wakefulness. Sleep 1987;10:313-329.
42. Hoddes E, Zarcone VP, Smythe H: Quantification of sleepiness: A new approach. Psychophysiology 1973;10:431-436.
43. Dement WC, Carskadon MA, Richardson G: Excessive daytime sleepiness in the sleep apnea syndrome. In Guilleminault C, Dement WC (eds): Sleep Apnea Syndromes. New York, Alan R Liss, 1978, pp 23-46.
44. Johns MW: Sleepiness in different situations measured by the Epworth Sleepiness Scale. Sleep 1994;17:703-710.
45. Rosenthal L: The sleep-wake activity inventory: A self report measure of daytime sleepiness. Biol Psychiatry 1993;34:810-820.
46. Carskadon MA, Dement WC, Mitler MM, et al: Guidelines for the multiple sleep latency test (MSLT): A standard measure of sleepiness. Sleep 1986;9:519-524.
47. Carskadon MA, Dement WC: Nocturnal determinants of daytime sleepiness. Sleep 1982;5:S73-S81.
48. Hartse KM, Roth T, Zorick FJ: Daytime sleepiness and daytime wakefulness: The effect of instruction. Sleep 1982;5:S107-S118.
49. Mitler MM, Gujavarty KS, Browman CP: Maintenance of wakefulness test: A polysomnographic technique for evaluating treatment efficacy in patients with excessive somnolence. Electroencephalogr Clin Neurophysiol 1982;53:658-661.
50. Sangal RB, Thomas L, Mitler MM: Disorders of excessive sleepiness: Treatment improves ability to stay awake, but does not reduce sleepiness. Chest 1992;102:699-703.
51. Mitler MM, Hajdukovic R: Relative efficacy of drugs for the treatment of sleepiness in narcolepsy. Sleep 1991;14:218-220.
52. Carskadon MA, Harvey K, Dement WC: Acute restriction of nocturnal sleep in children. Percept Mot Skills 1981;53:103-112.
53. Carskadon MA, Dement WC: Effects of total sleep loss on sleep tendency. Percept Mot Skills 1977;48:495-506.
54. Nicholson AN, Stone BM: Impaired performance and the tendency to sleep. Eur J Clin Pharmacol 1986;30:27-32.
55. Roehrs T, Kribbs N, Zorick F, et al: Hypnotic residual effects of benzodiazepines with repeated administration. Sleep 1986;9:309-316.
56. Dinges DF, Pack F, Williams K, et al: Cumulative sleepiness, mood disturbance, and psychomotor vigilance performance decrements during a week of sleep restricted to 4-5 hours per night. Sleep 1997;20:267-277.
57. Harrison Y, Horne JA: The impact of sleep deprivation on decision making: A review. J Exp Psychol Appl 2000;6:236-249.
58. Roehrs T, Greenwald M, Roth T: Risk-taking behavior: Effects of ethanol, caffeine, and basal sleepiness. Sleep 2004;27:887-893.
59. Roehrs TA, Blaisdell B, Greenwald M, et al: Pain threshold and sleep loss. Sleep 2003;26:A196.
60. Van den Hoed J, Kraemer H, Guilleminault C, et al: Disorders of excessive somnolence: Polygraphic and clinical data for 100 patients. Sleep 1981;4:23-37.
61. Carskadon MA, Dement WC: Cumulative effects of sleep restriction on daytime sleepiness. Psychophysiology 1981;18:107-113.
62. Roehrs T, Shore E, Papineau K, et al: A two-week sleep extension in sleepy normals. Sleep 1996;19:576-582.
63. Roehrs T, Zorick F, Wittig R, et al: Efficacy of a reduced triazolam dose in elderly insomniacs. Neurobiol Aging 1985;6:293-296.
64. Roehrs T, Zorick F, Sicklesteel J, et al: Excessive daytime sleepiness associated with insufficient sleep. Sleep 1983;6:319-325.
65. Manber R, Bootzin RR, Acebo C, et al: The effects of regularizing sleep-wake schedules on daytime sleepiness. Sleep 1996;19:432-441.
66. Guilleminault C, Powell NB, Martinez S, et al: Preliminary observations on the effects of sleep time in a sleep restriction paradigm. Sleep Med 2003;4:177-184.
67. The Atlas Task Force: EEG arousals: Scoring rules and examples. Sleep 1992;15:173-184.
68. Stepanski E: The effect of sleep fragmentation on daytime function. Sleep 2002;25:268-276.
69. Stepanski E, Lamphere J, Badia P, et al: Sleep fragmentation and daytime sleepiness. Sleep 1984;7:18-26.
70. Zorick F, Roehrs T, Conway W, et al: Effects of uvulopalatopharyngoplasty on the daytime sleepiness associated with sleep apnea syndrome. Bull Eur Physiopathol Respir 1983;19:600-603.
71. Lamphere J, Roehrs T, Wittig R, et al: Recovery of alertness after CPAP in apnea. Chest 1989;96:1364-1367.
72. Bonnet MH: Performance and sleepiness as a function of the frequency and placement of sleep disruption. Psychophysiology 1986;23:263-271.
73. Stepanski E, Lamphere J, Roehrs T, et al: Experimental sleep fragmentation in normal subjects. Int J Neurosci 1987;33:207-214.
74. Levine B, Roehrs T, Stepanski E, et al: Fragmenting sleep diminishes its recuperative value. Sleep 1987;10:590-599.
75. Ancoli-Israel S, Kripke D, Mason W, et al: Sleep apnea and nocturnal myoclonus in a senior population. Sleep 1981;4:349-358.
76. Carskadon MA, Brown E, Dement WC: Sleep fragmentation in the elderly: Relationship to daytime sleep tendency. Neurobiol Aging 1982;3:321-327.
77. Richardson GS, Carskadon MA, Orav EJ, et al: Circadian variation of sleep tendency in elderly and young adult subjects. Sleep 1982;5:S82-S94.
78. Monk TH: Circadian aspects of subjective sleepiness: A behavioral messenger? In Monk TH (ed): Sleep, Sleepiness and Performance. New York, John Wiley & Sons, 1991, pp 39-63.
79. Carskadon MA, Dement WC: Multiple sleep latency tests during the constant routine. Sleep 1992;15:393-399.

80. Strogatz SH, Kronauer RE, Czeisler CA: Circadian pacemaker interferes with sleep onset at specific times each day: Role in insomnia. Am J Physiol 1987;253:R172-R178.

81. Zulley J, Campbell SS: Napping behavior during "spontaneous internal desynchronization": Sleep remains in synchrony with body temperature. Hum Neurobiol 1985;4:123-126.

82. Jacklet JW: The neurobiology of circadian rhythm generators. Trends Neurosci 1985;8:69-73.

83. Seidel WF, Roth T, Roehrs T, et al: Treatment of a 12-hour shift of sleep schedule with benzodiazepines. Science 1984;22:1262-1264.

84. Roth T, Zorick F, Wittig R, et al: Pharmacological and medical considerations in hypnotic use. Sleep 1982;5:S46-S52.

85. Roth T, Roehrs T: Determinants of residual effects of hypnotics. Accid Anal Prev 1985;17:291-296.

86. Roth T, Zorick F, Sicklesteel J, Stepanski E: Effects of benzodiazepines on sleep and wakefulness. Br J Clin Pharmacol 1981; 11:31S-35S.

87. Zwyghuizen-Doorenbos A, Roehrs T, Lamphere J, et al: Increased daytime sleepiness enhances ethanol's sedative effects. Neuropsychopharmacology 1988;1:279-286.

88. Ashton H, Young AH: GABA-ergic drugs: Exit stage left, enter stage right. J Psychopharmacol 2003;17:174-178.

89. Cousins MS, Roberts DCS, de Wit H: GABA$_B$ receptor agonists for the treatment of drug addiction: A review of recent findings. Drug Alcohol Depend 2002;65:209-220.

90. Roehrs T, Tietz E, Zorick F, et al: Daytime sleepiness and antihistamines. Sleep 1984;7:137-141.

91. Nicholson AN, Stone BM: Antihistamines: Impaired performance and the tendency to sleep. Eur J Clin Pharmacol 1986;30: 27-32.

92. Conway J, Greenwood DT, Middlemiss DN: Central nervous actions of beta-adrenoreceptor antagonists. Clin Sci Mol Med 1978;54:119-124.

93. Olanow CW, Schapira AHV, Roth T: Waking up to sleep episodes in Parkinson's disease. Mov Disord 2000;15:212-215.

94. Clarenbach P: Parkinson's disease and sleep. J Neurol 2000;247:IV20-IV23.

95. Mitler MM, Shafor R, Hajdukovich R, et al: Treatment of narcolepsy: Objective studies on methylphenidate, pemoline and protriptyline. Sleep 1986;9:260-264.

96. Newhouse PA, Belenky G, Thomas M, et al: The effects of d-amphetamine on arousal, cognition, and mood after prolonged total sleep deprivation. Neuropsychopharmacology 1989;2:153-163.

97. Bishop C, Roehrs T, Rosenthal L, et al: Alerting effects of methylphenidate under basal and sleep-deprived conditions. Exp Clin Psychopharmacol 1997;4:344-352.

98. Lumley M, Roehrs T, Asker D, et al: Ethanol and caffeine effects on daytime sleepiness/alertness. Sleep 1987;10:306-312.

99. Roehrs T, Beare D, Zorick F, et al: Sleepiness and ethanol effects on simulated driving. Alcohol Clin Exp Res 1994;18: 154-158.

100. Kilduff TS, Bowersox SS, Kaitin KI, et al: Muscarinic cholinergic receptors and the canine model of narcolepsy. Sleep 1986;9:102-106.

101. American Sleep Disorders Association: International Classification of Sleep Disorders. Lawrence, Kan, Allen Press, 1990.

102. Martinez-Rodriguez JE, Lin L, Iranzo A, et al: Decreased hypocretin-1 (orexin-A) levels in the cerebrospinal fluid of patients with myotonic dystrophy and excessive daytime sleepiness. Sleep 2003;26:287-290.

103. Roth T, Rye DB, Borchert LD, et al: Assessment of sleepiness and unintended sleep in Parkinson's disease patients taking dopamine agonists. Sleep Med 2003;4:275-280.

104. Guilleminault C, Carskadon M: Relationship between sleep disorders and daytime complaints. In Koeller WP, Oevin PW (eds): Sleep 1976. Basel, Karger, 1977, pp 95-100.

105. Broughton R, Ghanem Q, Hishikawa Y, et al: Life effects of narcolepsy in 180 patients from North America, Asia and Europe compared to matched controls. J Can Sci Neurol 1981;8:299-304.

106. Findley LJ, Unverzagt ME, Suratt PM: Automobile accidents involving patients with obstructive apnea. Am Rev Respir Dis 1988;138:337-340.

107. Mitler MM, Carskadon MA, Czeisler CA, et al: Catastrophes, sleep, and public policy: Consensus report. Sleep 1988;11: 100-109.

108. Mackie RR, Miller JC: Effects of hours of service, regularity of schedules, and cargo loading on truck and bus driver fatigue. Washington, DC, U.S. Government Printing Office, 1978, Technical Report 1765-F DOT-HS-5-01142.

109. Baldwin DC, Daugherty SR: Sleep deprivation and fatigue in residency training: Results of a national survey of first- and second-year residents. Sleep 2004;27:217-223.

110. Marcus CL, Loughlin GM: Effect of sleep deprivation on driving safety in housestaff. Sleep 1996;19:763-766.

111. Roehrs TA, Merrion M, Pedrosi B, et al: Neuropsychological function in obstructive sleep apnea syndrome (OSAS) compared to chronic obstructive pulmonary disease (COPD). Sleep 1995;18:382-388.

112. Aguirre M, Broughton RJ, Stuss D: Does memory impairment exist in narcolepsy-cataplexy? J Clin Exp Neuropsychol 1985;7:14-24.

113. Blagrove M, Alexander C, Horne JA: The effects of chronic sleep reduction on the performance of cognitive tasks sensitive to sleep deprivation. Appl Cogn Psychol 1994;9:21-40.

114. Leiter JC, Knuth SL, Barlett D: The effect of sleep deprivation on activity of the genioglossus muscle. Am Rev Respir Dis 1985;132:1242-1245.

115. White DP, Douglas NJ, Pickett CK, et al: Sleep deprivation and control of ventilation. Am Rev Respir Dis 1983;128: 984-986.

116. Brooks D, Horner RL, Kimoff RJ, et al: Effect of obstructive sleep apnea versus sleep fragmentation on responses to airway occlusion. Am J Respir Crit Care Med 1997;155:1609-1617.

117. Kripke DF, Simons NR, Garfinkel L, et al: Short and long sleep and sleeping pills: Is increased mortality associated? Arch Gen Psychiatry 1979;36:103-116.

5

Acute Sleep Deprivation

Michael H. Bonnet

ABSTRACT

Sleep deprivation is an extremely common event in modern society. Sleep loss is accompanied by significant and readily apparent alterations in mood, alertness, and performance. This chapter reviews the behavioral effects of sleep deprivation, including sleep and circadian influences and also arousal system influences, which encompass activity, light, noise, posture, motivation, and drugs. Although the effects of sleep loss are broad, several measures, such as longer tests with little feedback that include external pacing and a memory or vigilance component, seem most sensitive to loss of sleep. Consistent changes in alertness and performance after sleep loss have been reported for many years, but recent work showing similar changes after alcohol ingestion provides a better means of comparatively describing the effects of sleep loss. A number of relatively mild physiologic changes accompany total sleep deprivation in humans. Some changes, such as shift on the electroencephalogram toward rhythms found in deactivation or sleep, are expected. Others, such as alteration in immune function, may hold keys to the function of sleep. Animal sleep deprivation studies have suggested that sleep is centrally important for survival, with especially strong implications for thermoregulation, energy balance, and immune function. Significant controversy remains concerning the loss of specific stages of sleep. Whereas some investigators feel that rapid eye movement (REM) sleep is involved in memory, others feel that much evidence does not support such a global statement. A number of recent studies have shown that high-frequency periodic sleep fragmentation produces nonrestorative sleep that results in sleepiness that is similar in many dimensions to sleepiness after total sleep deprivation. Recovery sleep after sleep loss or sleep fragmentation shows a characteristic pattern of elevated slow wave sleep with elevated sensory thresholds followed by elevated REM sleep.

PERSPECTIVE

Sleep deprivation is both extremely common and critically relevant in our society. As a clinical entity, sleep deprivation is recognized by the diagnosis of insufficient sleep syndrome (International Classification of Diseases [ICD] 307.49-4). As an experimental methodology, sleep deprivation serves as a major tool in understanding the function of sleep. A broad range of physiologic responses and behavioral abilities have been examined after varying periods without sleep, and many lawful relationships have been described. These relationships and the theory they represent are important in their own right, but the findings also serve as an extensive guide to symptoms associated with insufficient sleep. Furthermore, methods developed to lessen the impact of sleep deprivation

also serve as possible clinical treatments for disorders related to insufficient sleep or excessive sleepiness.

This chapter will review behavioral, physiologic, and theoretical implications of acute sleep deprivation. Chronic partial sleep deprivation will be examined in Chapter 6. Two meta-analyses of subtopics of sleep deprivation have been published.[1,2] Both indicated that sleep deprivation has a significant impact on psychomotor performance. One meta-analysis of 27 studies concluded that longer periods of sleep loss had greater impact on performance and that decrements in speed of performance were greater than decreases in accuracy.[1] The other analysis (of 19 studies) concluded that mood measures were more sensitive than cognitive tasks, which were more sensitive than motor tasks[2] during sleep loss.

Studies of sleep deprivation can suffer from some common methodologic problems that should be considered in interpreting them. The most important control issue is that one cannot perform a blinded study. Both experimenter and subject motivation can have a large impact on results, particularly in the behavioral and subjective domains. Motivation effects are frequently apparent near the end of studies (where performance improvement is sometimes found) and also may account for the difficulty in showing decrements early in periods of sleep loss. Animal studies are less susceptible to subject expectation effects, but they may contain additional elements of stress, which may interact with sleep loss and therefore may not be directly comparable with stress control conditions.[3] In addition, almost all sleep loss experiments involve more than simple loss of sleep. Maintenance of wakefulness usually includes upright posture, light, movement, cognition, and all the underlying physiologic processes implied by these activities. The experimental setting itself is usually far from routine. There are studies that have attempted to control some of these factors during sleep loss, but it is probably impossible to control all of these variables in a single experiment.

Over a thousand studies of sleep deprivation have been published during the past 10 years, and the resulting knowledge database has been remarkably consistent. However, new techniques and increasingly sensitive tests continue to add both theoretical and practical understanding of the impact of sleep loss. This review will include discussions of total sleep deprivation, selective sleep stage deprivation, sleep fragmentation, and recovery from sleep deprivation.

TOTAL SLEEP DEPRIVATION

The first published studies of total sleep loss date to 1894 for puppies[4] and to 1896 for humans.[5] The puppy study indicated that prolonged sleep loss in animals could be fatal, an idea dismissed until recent animal studies. The human study included a range of physiologic and behavioral measurements and remains a model study. The areas emphasized in these early studies—behavioral effects, physiologic effects, and animal findings—form the sections of this review.

Behavioral Effects

The clearest effect of sleep loss is sleepiness, and this can be inferred from subjective report, the multiple sleep latency test (MSLT), change on the electroencephalogram (EEG), or simply looking at the face of the participant. The variables that determine the impact of sleep loss have been divided into four categories: sleep and circadian influences, arousal system influences, subject characteristics, and test characteristics. An outline of categories and variables that has grown from the cogent summary by Johnson[6] can be found in Box 5–1.

Sleep and Circadian Influences

Sleep deprivation, like nutritional status, is a relative concept. How an individual responds to sleep loss depends on the prior sleep amount and distribution. Performance during a period of sleep loss is also directly dependent on the length of time awake and the circadian time. Experiments usually try to control these factors by requiring a "normal" night of sleep before initiation of a sleep loss episode. Data from multiple regression analyses of behavioral and EEG data during 64 hours of sleep loss[7,8] suggest that time awake accounts for 25% to 30% of the variance in alertness and that circadian time accounts for about 6% of the variance. When prophylactic naps of varying length were interjected early in a period of sleep loss, it was found that the prophylactic nap sleep accounted for about 5% of the variance in alertness during the sleep deprivation period. In terms of reducing the effect of sleep loss, the overall effect of increasing the prophylactic nap period was linear for additional sleep amounts ranging up to 8 hours. Figure 5–1 displays the effects of time awake and the circadian rhythm on objective alertness as measured by the MSLT and the ability to complete correct symbol substitutions over 64 hours of sleep loss.

Arousal Influences

Environmental and emotional surroundings can have a large impact on the course of a period of sleep loss. In early stages of sleep deprivation, several intervening variables can easily reverse all measurable sleep loss decrements. These influences, which include activity, bright light, noise, temperature, posture, stress, and drugs, have received increased attention in recent years.

ACTIVITY

In one study,[9] a 5-minute walk immediately preceding MSLT evaluations had a large impact (about 6 minutes) on MSLT values. The arousal associated with the walk completely masked the impact of a 50% reduction of nocturnal sleep (about a 2-minute impact on MSLT). It has been shown that a period of exercise immediately before performing tasks provided transient reversal of some psychomotor[10] and subjective[11] decrements secondary to sleep loss. However, more ambitious studies comparing high activity and low activity continuing over 40- to 64-hour periods of sleep deprivation have shown no beneficial effects of exercise on overall performance[12,13] and no differential effects of the exercise on recovery sleep after sleep loss in humans.[13,14] These different results are probably a result of the fact that arousing stimuli act only for a discrete period of time that may be less than 30 minutes[9] and their effects are decreased by increasing sleep loss.[15] There may also be a tradeoff between production of arousal and production of physical fatigue.

BRIGHT LIGHT

It is known that bright light can shift circadian rhythms. Some controversy exists concerning whether bright light can also act as a source of stimulation during sleep loss to help to maintain alertness. Two of five studies found that periods of bright light immediately before sleep onset significantly increased sleep latencies.[16,17] Other studies have found improved night-shift performance under bright light conditions.[18,19] However, the contention has been made that bright light administration in the late evening may simply inhibit melatonin, which promotes sleep, or produce a phase shift to give the appearance of improved performance rather than being intrinsically stimulating.[20]

NOISE

Noise has complex and occasionally negative effects on the performance of well-rested individuals, but small beneficial effects of noise have been reported in several sleep deprivation paradigms.[21,22] It is generally assumed that noise increases arousal level, and, although this may not be beneficial in normal wakefulness, it usually helps during sleep loss.

Box 5–1 **Determinants of the Impact of Sleep Loss**

Sleep and Circadian Influences
Prior sleep amount and distribution
Length of time awake
Circadian time

Arousal Influences
Activity
Bright light
Noise
Temperature
Posture
Drugs
Interest
Motivation
History of exposure to sleep loss

Subject Characteristics
Age
Personality and psychopathology

Test Characteristics and Types
Length of test
Knowledge of results
Test pacing
Proficiency level
Difficulty or complexity of test
Short-term memory requirement
Subjective (versus objective) measures
Electroencephalographic measures (as in the multiple sleep latency test)

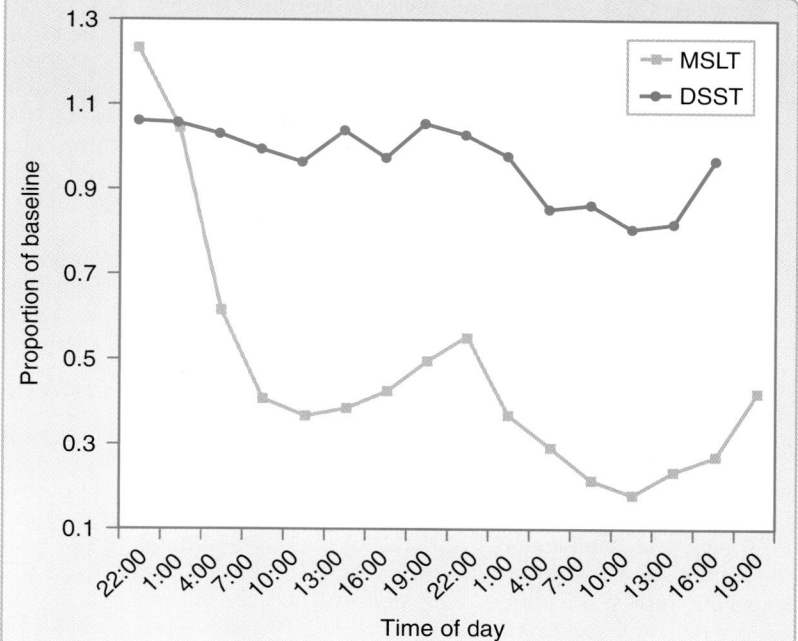

Figure 5–1. Latency to stage 2 sleep *(boxes)* and number of correctly completed symbol substitutions in repeated 5-minute test sessions *(dots)* over a period of 64 hours of sleep deprivation, both expressed as a proportion of baseline values. DSST, digit symbol substitution test; MSLT, multiple sleep latency test. (Data from Bonnet MH, Gomez S, Wirth O, et al: The use of caffeine versus prophylactic naps in sustained performance. Sleep 1995;18:97-104.)

TEMPERATURE

Although temperature variation is commonly used as an acute stimulus to maintain alertness, there is very little research on the effects of ambient temperature interacting with sleep loss. One study has shown that heat (92° F) was effective in increasing performance during the initial minutes of a vigilance task during sleep deprivation.[23] A recent study[24] showed a nonsignificant decrease in subjectively rated sleepiness for about 15 minutes after a car air conditioner was turned on during simulated driving.

POSTURE

One study has shown a significant 6.6-minute increase in sleep latency when subjects were asked to fall asleep in the sitting position (at a 60-degree angle) as opposed to lying down.[25] Such differences in alertness could be accounted for by increasing sympathetic nervous system activity, which occurs with these changes in posture.[26] Greater differences are associated with standing as compared to sitting.[15]

DRUGS

Many drugs have been studied in conjunction with sleep loss. Most studies have examined stimulants, including amphetamine, caffeine, methylphenidate, pemoline, modafinil, nicotine, and cocaine. Amphetamine typically does not improve performance in individuals who have had normal sleep quotas, but positive effects on mood, performance, and alertness have been found after sleep deprivation.[27,28] Newhouse and coworkers[27] administered amphetamine at three doses after 48 hours of sleep loss and reported a classic dose–response curve. A 5-mg dose had little effect, but a 10-mg dose improved performance on a serial mathematics test almost to baseline levels from 1.5 to 2.5 hours after administration. Return to placebo levels occurred 4.5 hours after administration.

After a 20-mg dose, improved performance was maintained for at least 10.5 hours on the mathematics test and alertness on the MSLT was increased for 7 hours. In another study,[29] amphetamine, 20 mg, was administered at three points during 64 hours of sleep loss. Amphetamine (as well as modafinil, 300 mg) reliably increased core temperature over a 4-hour period, improved subjective alertness for 10 or more hours, and improved psychomotor performance over a 6- to 8-hour period.

There are several studies of caffeine use during sleep loss. Three hundred milligrams of caffeine ingested at 23:00 significantly increased alertness as measured by MSLT for 7.5 hours[30] and improved performance for 6 hours.[31] Repeated use of caffeine in 150- to 300-mg doses was effective in maintaining alertness and performance above placebo levels during 48 hours of sleep loss in one study and 44 hours in another.[32,33] In another study,[34] a single 600-mg dose of caffeine significantly increased alertness as measured by MSLT for about 5 hours, although the improvement associated with a single 300-mg dose was not significant. Compared with caffeine, 20 mg of amphetamine showed greater improvement of MSLT values for about 7 hours. The beneficial effect of caffeine 300 mg during periods of sleep loss was approximately equivalent to that seen after a 3- to 4-hour prophylactic nap before the sleep loss period.[30,33] The combination of a 4-hour prophylactic nap followed by 200 mg of caffeine at 01:30 and 07:30 resulted in significantly improved performance (remaining at baseline levels) compared with the nap alone for 24 hours.[35] The combination of naps and caffeine appeared additive[35] and was also superior to the provision of 4 hours of nocturnal naps.[36] The combination of 200 mg of caffeine administered at 22:00 and 02:00 and exposure to 2500-lux bright light had no impact above the effect of caffeine alone on the Maintenance of Wakefulness Test but did provide significant benefit above caffeine alone on a vigilance task at three time points.[32]

Pemoline (37.5 mg per dose twice a day) and methylphenidate (10 mg per dose four times a day) have been examined in one 64-hour sleep loss study.[37] Pemoline improved performance on a tapping task during the first night of sleep loss, whereas methylphenidate was ineffective in increasing performance or alertness above baseline levels. In another study,[38] sleepiness, as measured by MSLT, was reduced by methylphenidate 10 mg twice a day after 1 night of sleep deprivation, and performance on reaction time and vigilance tasks was improved.

Modafinil 200 mg three times a day was shown effective in maintaining MSLT values above placebo levels through 60 hours of sleep loss.[39] Modafinil 300 mg was shown to be equivalent to 20 mg of amphetamine in providing increased body temperature, alertness, and psychomotor performance compared with placebo over 64 hours of sleep deprivation.[29] Modafinil doses of 200 and 400 mg have been shown as effective as caffeine for 12 hours following 40 hours of sleep loss on reaction time performance.[40] An across-study comparison of the impact of modafinil (200 mg three times a day), caffeine (400 mg), and amphetamine (10 and 20 mg) on the MSLT during the second night of total sleep loss[33,39,41] showed that all agents improved alertness compared with placebo groups (which had very low MSLT values, between 12% and 30% of baseline). About 3 hours after medication administration, MSLT was about 54% of baseline after modafinil, 70% of baseline after caffeine, 47% of baseline after amphetamine 10 mg, and 67% of baseline after amphetamine 20 mg administration. About 6 hours after administration, MSLT values had declined to about 40% of baseline following modafinil, 27% of baseline following caffeine, 23% of baseline following amphetamine 10 mg, and 41% of baseline following amphetamine 20 mg.

Nicotine, infused intravenously at doses of 0.25, 0.37, and 0.5 mg after 48 hours of wakefulness, had no significant impact on MSLT or psychomotor performance.[41] Cocaine (96 mg), like amphetamine, did not improve performance in subjects before sleep loss. However, cocaine significantly improved reaction time performance and alertness, as measured by the Profile of Mood States, after 24 and 48 hours of sleep loss.[42]

Recent studies of alcohol have reported decreased alertness. In one study,[43] subjects were tested on MSLT and simulated driving after 0.6 g/kg alcohol or placebo, after normal sleep or 4 hours of sleep. There was a significant main effect for both alcohol and sleep loss, and MSLT latencies were respectively 10.7, 6.3, 6.1, and 4.7 minutes after placebo (normal sleep), placebo (4 hours of sleep), ethanol (normal sleep), and ethanol (4 hours of sleep). Similar results were found in the driving simulator. In addition, three simulator "crashes" occurred, all in the reduced sleep with ethanol condition.

One difficulty in assessing the magnitude of performance effects associated with sleep loss is the lack of a clear standard of pathology for most measures. The fact that society has established very specific rules for blood alcohol content (BAC) with respect to driving has led to the use of impairment associated with blood alcohol level as a standard reference for sleep deprivation as well. Three studies of alcohol use in direct comparison with sleep deprivation have shown similar results on different tasks. In one,[44] response speed on the Mackworth task was reduced by approximately half a second by 03:45 (i.e., after sleep loss) and to a similar extent by a BAC of 0.1%. In another study,[45] hand–eye coordination (in a visual tracking task) declined in a linear fashion during sleep loss and with increasing BAC such that performance was equivalent at

03:00 to a BAC of 0.05%, and equivalent at 08:00 (after a full night of sleep loss) to a BAC of 0.1%. In a third study,[46] performance was measured in a driving simulator after alcohol use or sleep deprivation. After a night of sleep deprivation (at 07:30), subjects averaged one off-road incident (i.e., driving the vehicle off the road) every 5 minutes. This same level of off-road driving was reached with a BAC of 0.08%. These studies suggest that changes in response speed, visual tracking, and driving commonly found during the first night of total sleep deprivation are equivalent to changes associated with legal intoxication. The availability of such a metric shows that performance changes associated with small amounts of sleep loss can have large consequences.

INTEREST

The propensity of individuals to seek all-night poker games or video games attests to the ability of an interesting task to allow individuals to maintain baseline levels of performance for as long as 50 hours of sleep loss.[47] Components of "interest" have not been empirically quantified, but any variable producing increases in arousal could be included.

MOTIVATION

More work has looked at the effect of motivation than interest level during sleep loss, because the same task can usually be examined under low motivation and high motivation conditions. For example, in one study, monetary rewards for "hits" on a vigilance task and "fines" for false alarms[48] resulted in performance being maintained at baseline levels for the first 36 hours of sleep loss in the high incentive group. Performance began to decline during the following 24 hours but remained significantly better than in the "no incentive" group. However, the incentive was ineffective in maintaining performance at a higher level during the third day of sleep loss. Knowledge of results—for example, the publication of daily test results for everyone to see—was sufficient to remove the effects of 1 night of sleep loss.[49] In another variation, simply the knowledge that a prolonged episode of sleep deprivation was going to end in a few hours was sufficient incentive for performance to improve by 30% in a group of soldiers.[50] Clearly, the effects of motivation can be very significant. However, sleep loss effects themselves are probably based on more than motivational effects, as witnessed by the decline in performance on irrelevant tasks such as the completion of crossword puzzles, which had been provided to subjects as a time filler between required performance tasks.[51]

REPEATED PERIODS OF SLEEP LOSS

Two studies of repeated episodes of sleep loss have agreed that the magnitude of performance loss increases as a function of the number of exposures to sleep loss.[49,52] Increasingly poor performance may be secondary to decreased motivation or to familiarity with the sleep deprivation paradigm (resulting in decreased arousal).

Subject Characteristics

The impact of sleep loss on a given individual depends on characteristics that each participant brings to the sleep loss situation. For example, age and personality represent differences in physiologic or psychological function that may interact with the sleep loss event.

AGE

Age appears to play a relatively minor role in the response of humans to loss of sleep. Tests of performance and alertness in older subjects undergoing sleep loss reveal a decrease in performance and alertness similar to that seen in younger individuals. If anything, older subjects had a smaller decrease in psychomotor performance ability at nocturnal times during sleep loss[53,54] than young adults. It has been frequently shown that older individuals perform more poorly than young adults on a broad range of tasks, but this relationship may not be maintained for periods of nocturnal performance or performance during sleep loss. These findings may be explained by the decrease in amplitude of the circadian body-temperature curve in older individuals.[53] The same flattened curve that results in lower temperatures and decreased performance during the day also produces elevated temperatures, as compared with young adults, during the night. These elevated temperatures may improve performance at night as they reduce ability to maintain sleep.

PERSONALITY AND PSYCHOPATHOLOGY

Mood changes, including increased sleepiness, fatigue, irritability, difficulty in concentrating, and disorientation, are commonly reported during periods of sleep loss. Perceptual distortions and hallucinations, primarily of a visual nature, occur in up to 80% of normal individuals, depending on work load, visual demands, and length of deprivation.[55] Such misperceptions are normally quite easy to differentiate from the primarily auditory hallucinations of a schizophrenic patient, but normal individuals undergoing sleep loss may express paranoid thoughts. Two percent of 350 individuals sleep deprived for 112 hours experienced temporary states resembling acute paranoid schizophrenia.[56] Some predisposition toward psychotic behavior existed in individuals who experienced significant paranoia during sleep loss, and the paranoid behavior tended to become more pronounced during the night, with partial recovery during the day and disappearance after recovery sleep. In a review of the area, Johnson concludes, "Each subject's response to sleep loss will depend on his age, physical condition, the stability of his mental health, expectations of those around him, and the support he receives" (from p. 208 of Johnson[57]).

In view of the commonly reported effects of sleep deprivation, it seems quite unusual that one would seek to treat depression by sleep deprivation. However, sleep deprivation has been used as a successful treatment for depression in 40% to 60% of cases for over 30 years.[58] The relationship between sleep and depression is reviewed at more length in Chapter 112. However, one theory proposes that sleep deprivation is more effective in depressed patients with high levels of activation or high central noradrenergic activity because it limits the effects of chronic hyperarousal.[59] As a result, patients felt tired but also had improved mood and energy.

The apparent differential response of depressed patients to sleep deprivation emphasizes that there may be other individual differences in response to sleep deprivation. Studies of highly inbred mouse strains (to study specific gene variation in relation to sleep parameters) have produced mice that characteristically have longer and shorter sleep durations both before and after sleep deprivation.[60] Consistent individual differences in alertness and performance during sleep deprivation have also been found in humans.[61] However, relatively little is known about the relationship of the differential response to sleep deprivation and sleep need in humans (see Bonnet[62] for review). It is equally likely that differential alertness or performance ability during sleep deprivation is dependent on ability to maintain arousal rather than sleep system requirements.[63,64]

Test Characteristics and Types

The measured response to sleep deprivation is critically dependent on the characteristics of the test used. Several specific test characteristics common to sensitive psychomotor tests have been identified.[6] Other measures, such as mood scales and the MSLT, are discussed for comparison.

LENGTH OF TEST

Individuals undergoing sleep loss can usually rally momentarily to perform at their non–sleep-deprived levels, but their ability to maintain that performance decreases as the length of the task increases. For example, subjects attempted significantly fewer addition problems than baseline after 10 minutes of testing after 1 night of sleep loss but reached the same criterion after 6 minutes of testing after the second night of sleep loss. It took 50 minutes of testing to show a significant decrease in percentage of correct problems after 1 night of sleep loss and 10 minutes of testing to reach that criterion after the second night.[65] The common wisdom in sleep loss studies is that performance tests need to be as long as possible and that it is very difficult to show reliable differences during short-term sleep loss from almost any test that is shorter than 10 minutes in duration. Momentary arousal, even as minor as a notification that 5 minutes remained on a task, was sufficient to reverse 75% of the decrement accumulated over 30 minutes of testing.[66]

KNOWLEDGE OF RESULTS

Immediate performance feedback, possibly acting through motivation, has been shown to improve performance during sleep deprivation.[49,66] Simply not giving knowledge of results to subjects with normal sleep doubled their number of very long responses ("gaps") on a serial reaction time test. One night of total sleep loss increased the number of gaps by 9.3 times the baseline level, but provision of immediate knowledge of results decreased the number of gaps to 2.3 times the baseline level. The 2.3 times baseline level was approximately the number of gaps seen after normal sleep when knowledge of results was not given.[49]

TEST PACING

Self-paced tasks are usually more resistant to the effects of sleep loss than tasks that are timed or in which items are presented by the experimenter. In a self-paced task, one can concentrate long enough to complete items correctly and not be penalized for lapses in attention that occur between items. When tasks are externally paced, errors occur when items are presented during lapses in attention.

PROFICIENCY LEVEL

Sleep loss is likely to affect newly learned skills more than well-known activities, as long as arousal level remains constant. For example, in a study of the effects of sleep loss on doctors in training, significant performance decrements were found in first-year surgical residents but not in those in their second to fifth year.[67]

DIFFICULTY OR COMPLEXITY

Performance on simple tasks, such as monitoring a light on a control panel (on/off), declines less than performance on more complex tasks, such as mental subtraction,[68] during sleep loss. Task difficulty can also be adjusted by increasing the speed at which the work must be performed. When 2 seconds were allowed to complete mental arithmetic problems, no significant performance decline was found after 2 nights of sleep loss, but when the rate of presentation was increased to 1.25 seconds, a significant performance decline was found.[69]

SHORT-TERM MEMORY

Impairment of immediate recall for elements placed in short-term memory is a classic finding in sleep deprivation studies.[70] Because subjects are usually required to write down each item as presented, the observed decrements, which can usually be seen after 1 night of sleep loss, do not result from impaired sensory registration of items. Observed decrements may result from a decreased ability to encode,[71] from an increasing inability to rehearse old items (owing to lapses) while the items are being presented, or from a combination of memory effects with reduced ability to respond.

SUBJECTIVE (VERSUS OBJECTIVE) MEASURES

Measures of mood such as sleepiness, fatigue, and ability to think or concentrate are inversely correlated with performance and body temperature during sleep loss.[72] Mood changes are some of the earliest noted indicators of sleep loss. As such, a 1-minute mood scale may be as sensitive to sleep loss as a longer word memory test but less sensitive than a 50-minute vigilance test.[6]

EEG MEASURES

Clear changes on an EEG are seen during sleep loss (see "Neurologic Changes," later). The MSLT was developed as an objective measure of sleepiness. It was validated, in part, by being shown to be sensitive to several types of partial and total sleep loss.[73,74] That the MSLT is more sensitive than the psychomotor tasks can be seen in Figure 5–1, which displays performance changes on the number of symbol substitutions correctly completed in 5-minute test periods and MSLT data.[33]

SUMMARY

Tasks most affected by sleep loss tend to be long, monotonous, without feedback, externally paced, newly learned, and have a memory component. One example of a task containing many of these elements is driving, which was discussed earlier in reference to the effects of alcohol. Since 1994, more than 20 studies have examined the impact of reduced sleep on various measures of driving ability or safety. One study,[75] for example, found that 49% of medical residents who worked on call and averaged 2.7 hours of sleep reported falling asleep at the wheel (90% of the episodes were after being on call). The residents also had 67% more citations for moving violations and 82% more car accidents than the control group.[75]

Physiologic Effects of Sleep Deprivation

Physiologic changes that occur during sleep loss can be categorized into neurologic (including EEG changes), autonomic, and biochemical changes. Physiologic and biochemical effects of sleep deprivation were extensively reviewed by Horne[76] and earlier by Kleitman.[77]

NEUROLOGIC CHANGES

Although it is easy to identify a sleep-deprived individual by appearance and to demonstrate obvious behavioral changes, measurable neurologic changes during sleep loss are relatively minor and quickly reversible. In extended sleep loss studies (205 or more hours), mild nystagmus, hand tremor, intermittent slurring of speech, and ptosis have been noted.[78] Sluggish corneal reflexes, hyperactive gag reflex, hyperactive deep tendon reflexes, and increased sensitivity to pain were reported[79] after deprivation that is more extensive. All of these changes immediately reversed after recovery sleep.

Sleep loss is consistently accompanied by characteristic EEG changes that have been recently reviewed.[80] In careful studies, subjects have been required to stand or be involved in tasks in an attempt to stabilize arousal level. Several studies have reported a generally linear decrease in alpha during sleep loss. In one study, subjects were unable to sustain alpha activity for longer than 10 seconds after 24 hours of sleep loss, and this ability continued to decline to 4 to 6 seconds after 72 hours and 1 to 3 seconds after 120 hours of sleep loss.[81] After 115 hours of sleep loss, eye closure failed to produce alpha activity.[82] In another study, in which individuals were recorded standing with their eyes closed, the percentage of time spent with an alpha pattern in the EEG decreased from 65% in the early deprivation period to about 30% after 100 hours of sleep loss.[83] Delta and theta patterns in the waking EEG were increased from 17% and 12% to 38% and 26% of the time, respectively.[83] No change in beta activity was found in one study,[83] but an increase was found at a central derivation in a second.[84] Performance errors during sleep loss were usually accompanied by a slowing of the EEG[85] that was labeled a "microsleep." However, during sleep loss, a subject may produce delta waves while speaking and clearly awake.[86]

More recently, global decreases in brain activity correlated with increasing sleep loss have been found using positron emission tomography. Larger decreases were found in prefrontal, parietal, and thalamic areas.[87] Functional magnetic resonance imaging has shown increased activity in prefrontal cortex and parietal lobes after sleep loss[88] when measured while subjects performed a verbal learning task. These results have been interpreted as representing increased effort after sleep loss.

Although the neurologic changes associated with significant sleep loss are relatively minor in normal young adults, sleep loss has repeatedly been shown to be a highly activating stress in individuals suffering seizure disorders. Using a period of sleep loss as a "challenge" to elicit abnormal EEG events is currently a standard neurologic test.[89]

AUTONOMIC CHANGES

In humans, autonomic changes, even during prolonged periods of sleep loss, are relatively minor. Individual studies have reported either increases or decreases in systolic blood pressure, diastolic blood pressure, finger pulse volume, heart rate, respiration rate, and tonic and phasic skin conductance. However, the majority of 10 to 15 studies have reported no change in these variables during sleep loss in humans.[76,90,91] Studies that are more recent have suggested that sleep loss does result in about a 20% reduction in response to hypoxia and hypercapnia.[92,93] However, these modifications suggest a transient set point change rather than system failure. Sleep deprivation has been associated with small decreases in the forced expiratory volume in 1 second and the forced vital capacity of the lungs in patients with pulmonary disease.[94] Two studies, one in healthy infants[95] and one in adults,[96] have shown more apneic events and longer apneic events after sleep loss. Brooks and colleagues[97] have shown that apneas become longer as a function of the sleep fragmentation produced by the apneas (as opposed to the respiratory pathology).

Several human studies have found a small (0.3° C to 0.4° C) overall decrease in body temperature during sleep loss.[5,98] Changes in thermoregulation, usually a more vigorous defense against cold, have been found in several human studies,[99] recently reviewed.[100]

Effects of sleep loss on the ability to perform exercise are subtle. Animal studies have consistently shown that sleep deprivation decreases spontaneous activity by up to 40%,[101] but most human studies have focused on maximal exercise ability, where large differences as a function of sleep loss are more difficult to demonstrate. For example, one well-performed study[102] reported a 7% decrease in the maximum volume of oxygen consumed by the body each minute during 64 hours of sleep loss. This change was not associated with heart rate, respiratory exchange ratio, or blood lactate, which remained unchanged. However, there was a decrease in minute ventilation and hemodilution.[103] Recovery from exercise may be slowed by sleep loss.[104] Studies are evenly divided between claims that the amplitude of the circadian rhythm of temperature is increased, decreased, or unchanged during sleep loss.[76]

A well-performed study has shown no sleep deprivation–related changes in whole body metabolism at normal temperatures and in a cold stress situation.[91] These findings in humans are of particular import because a series of elegant studies in rats has shown that after a week of sleep loss, metabolic levels are greatly increased, increased food consumption is accompanied by significant weight loss, and significant difficulty with thermoregulation is apparent (see "Animal Studies," later). Several studies have examined aspects of brain metabolism in animals during short periods of sleep deprivation. Direct measures of brain metabolic rate were not different after a short period of sleep deprivation,[105] although several related enzymes did differ. Another study indicated that some of the noted differences could have been related to stress rather than to sleep deprivation.[106]

BIOCHEMICAL CHANGES

Several studies (10 or more for some variables) have examined various biochemical changes in humans during sleep loss. There is generally no significant change in cortisol,[107] adrenaline and related compounds, catecholamine output,[91,108] hematocrit,[90] plasma glucose,[90] creatinine,[91,109] or magnesium[91] during sleep loss. One study imposed an additional cold stress during sleep loss and still failed to find a physiologic component caused by sleep loss beyond that caused by cold.[91]

Results from analyses of blood components largely parallel the results found in urine components. None of the adrenal or sex hormones (including cortisol, adrenaline, noradrenaline, luteinizing hormone, follicle-stimulating hormone, variants of testosterone, and progesterone) rise during sleep deprivation in humans.[107,110] Some of these hormones actually decreased somewhat during sleep loss, perhaps secondary to sleepiness and decreased physiologic activation. Thyroid activity, as indexed by thyrotropin, thyroxine, and triiodothyronine, was increased, probably secondary to the increased energy requirements of continuous wakefulness.[111] Studies appear about equally divided between those showing an increase in melatonin and those showing no change in melatonin during sleep deprivation.[112,113] Most studies have concluded that there is no significant change in hematocrit levels,[91] erythrocyte count,[114] or plasma glucose during total sleep deprivation in humans.[90] As would be expected, hormones such as noradrenaline, prolactin,[115] and growth hormone, which are dependent on sleep for their circadian rhythmicity or appearance, lose their periodic pattern of excretion during sleep loss (see Spiegel et al.[116] and Parker et al.[117] for excellent reviews). Several studies have reported rebounds in growth hormone during recovery sleep after sleep loss or slow wave sleep (SWS) deprivation.[112,118]

IMMUNE FUNCTION

A number of human studies have examined various aspects of immune function after varying periods of partial or total sleep loss. This work has been recently reviewed[119] and is also discussed in Chapter 21. Several studies have found decreases in natural killer (NK) cell numbers after short periods of sleep deprivation,[120,121] but NK cell activity appears to increase as total sleep loss becomes longer.[120] Some studies have shown increases in interleukin (IL)-1[120,122] and IL-6[123] during total sleep loss. One study that did not find increases in IL-6[124] may have failed because samples were taken only once per day compared with once per hour.[125] In general, immune function studies are difficult to compare because parameters measured, time and number of blood draws, and degree of sleep deprivation vary across studies.

At a more macroscopic level, one study reported the development of respiratory illness or asthma in three subjects after a 64-hour sleep deprivation protocol,[126] but another reported no incidence of illness after a similar protocol.[120] In longer studies involving strenuous exercise and other factors along with sleep loss, increased infection rates are reported about 50% of the time.[127]

One animal study has suggested that mice that had been immunized against a respiratory influenza virus responded to that virus as if they had never been immunized only when exposed after sleep loss.[128] However, in another study,[129] total sleep loss actually slowed the progression of a viral infection in mice. An extensive study of sleep loss in rats (7 to 49 days) was unable to show significant changes in spleen cell numbers, mitogen responses, or in vivo or in vitro splenic antibody-secreting cell responses[130] (see "Animal Studies," later).

GENE EXPRESSION

A recent review of gene expression during wakefulness and extended wakefulness has described a number of changes that occur under these conditions.[131] A number of genes expressed during wakefulness to regulate mitochondrial activity and glucose transport probably reflect increased energy use. However, as sleep deprivation progresses, one gene, for the enzyme arylsulfotransferase (AST), showed stronger induction as a function of length of sleep deprivation. AST induction could reflect a homeostatic response to continuing central noradrenergic activity during sleep loss.[131]

SUMMARY

A large number of studies have reported autonomic, biochemical, and immune function variables during sleep loss. Many of the older studies were based on single observation points before and after sleep loss. Many studies suffer from poor activity controls (i.e., use of activity to maintain wakefulness may produce or mask changes in underlying variables of interest). More recent studies have been able to make use of sampling as often as once per hour and have begun to consider circadian and activity effects. For example, Born and coworkers[132] found that NK cell numbers increased during the night when subjects remained awake (compared with a sleep control) but then decreased on the following afternoon, with the result that numbers averaged across the entire study were about the same in sleep loss and baseline conditions. This means that a study could find an increase, a decrease, or the same number of NK cells based on the time of sampling. Similarly, it has been found that IL-6 was decreased during a night of sleep deprivation compared with the sleep control but increased compared with the control during the next day, so that numbers averaged across the entire study were, again, about the same.[125]

Animal Studies

Modern animal sleep deprivation studies differ from human studies in enough important aspects that they need to be treated separately. Many techniques have been developed to maintain wakefulness in animals,[133] and most of them capitalize on the fact that when an animal falls asleep, muscles relax and the animal takes up more floor space than when sitting or standing awake. Recent extensive reviews in this area are available.[3,134]

Totally sleep-deprived rats developed a characteristic appearance that includes disheveled and clumped fur, skin lesions on tail and paws, and weight loss. The weight loss occurred despite large increases in food intake and with indications that energy expenditure had increased to more than double baseline values. The sleep-deprived rats all died (or were sacrificed at imminent death) within 11 to 22 days of deprivation. In studies that examined rapid eye movement (REM) sleep[135] and SWS[136] deprivation in the same methodologic paradigm, rats developed the same symptoms seen after total sleep loss and died in 16 to 54 days (REM sleep deprivation) or 23 to 66 days (SWS deprivation).

In sleep-deprived rats, body temperature declined as much as 2° C during the second half of the deprivation period.[137] Activity increased 23% from baseline levels, whereas energy expenditure doubled, and this finding was not based on reduced efficiency of energy utilization. Heart rate increased,[135] plasma norepinephrine increased, and plasma thyroxine decreased.[137] Increased energy expenditure could not be explained by increased wakefulness alone or by water exposure. It was concluded that the increased energy expenditure was produced in an attempt to maintain body temperature despite excessive heat loss during deprivation.

One explanation for the sleep loss effects advanced by Everson[138] is that prolonged sleep deprivation impairs host defense against otherwise common bacteria. In an initial study,[139] Everson found bacteria in the blood of five of six rats at the point that sleep deprivation led to a rapid drop in body temperature. However, in a follow-up study, Bergmann and colleagues,[140] while finding bacteremia in 3 of 11 rats early in sleep deprivation, found no evidence of increased life span or bacteremia in 6 rats treated with an antibiotic cocktail during sleep deprivation. This seems to imply that although there may be some breakdown of tissue barriers to microbes late in sleep deprivation in rats, this breakdown is not the cause of many of the common effects and is not the universal cause of death.

More recently, Rechtschaffen and Bergmann[134] suggested three thermoregulatory effects that may be most important in understanding the rat sleep loss data.

1. Rats have been shown to have an increase in temperature set point, associated with loss of non-REM sleep, that causes them to prefer very warm environments and may drive the large increases in energy expenditure.
2. An experiment designed to manipulate temperature set point by administering phentolamine to block vasoconstriction showed that when sleep-deprived rats were tested in cool temperatures, they were unable to recover as they could prior to phentolamine administration.[141]
3. It was noted in several studies that the normal drop in temperature seen at sleep onset disappeared over the course of sleep deprivation in the rats. Late in deprivation, temperature *increased* at sleep onset,[100] and several days of recovery sleep were needed before the normal drops returned.

It is probable that a combination of factors, including hypothermia, stress, energy expenditure, failure of host defense, and malnutrition, accumulate during sleep deprivation to account for eventual death. Rechtschaffen is pessimistic about finding the function of sleep based on these data,[134] but it is likely that sleep serves many functions. Each of these areas—thermoregulation, energy balance, and host defense/immune function—could be seen as an important function of sleep.

SUMMARY

A great deal is known about general physiologic, psychomotor, subjective, and EEG effects of total sleep loss for periods of up to about 11 days in humans. Characteristic circadian decreases in alertness and performance accumulating over time are well documented. Physiologic changes are relatively minor. Total sleep loss in rats appears to be different from total sleep loss in humans. Although eating is usually increased in humans during sleep deprivation,[142] changes in heart rate, weight, metabolism, or most biochemical measures have not been reported. Minor decreases in body temperature are frequently noted in human studies, but the animal studies may report increased body temperature early in deprivation and decreased temperature only after long periods of sleep loss.

A review of the animal studies[143] suggested that human and animal studies are not directly comparable because (1) daily sleep quotients differ, (2) sleep–wake cycle times (the "pressure" to sleep) differ, (3) basal energy expenditure rates differ, (4) life spans differ, (5) surface areas differ, and

(6) survival times during other stresses such as starvation differ. Examination of human versus rat values on each of these parameters indicates that humans should tolerate sleep loss more easily than rats. For example, using basal oxygen consumption as a predictor of energy use, humans should be able to tolerate 2 to 7 months of total sleep deprivation before death. It is also likely that all six of these factors help insulate humans against the effects of sleep loss to some extent as compared with rats. If the combined effects of daily sleep quotients, sleep–wake cycle times, and basal energy expenditure differences are considered, humans might be able to tolerate 2 to 10 years of total sleep loss.

Animal experiments have tried to control for stress by using yoked controls in the deprivation experiments. However, the animal studies cannot determine whether the interaction of profound sleep loss with stress is responsible for the reported effects. Differences between human and rat responses to sleep loss may be moot, because sleep loss of the magnitude apparently required for system failure is unlikely in humans, and the rat studies indicate that animals even near the brink of death appear to recover completely if allowed to sleep.

SELECTIVE SLEEP DEPRIVATION

Selective sleep deprivation experiments attempt to eliminate one or more stages of sleep while having minimal impact on other sleep stages and total sleep time. Studies of selective deprivation were originally intended as a means of determining the functional significance of REM sleep or SWS and typically involved the placement of experimental awakenings or arousals at the onset of the forbidden stage of sleep for one or more nights. A large number of selective deprivation studies were performed in the years after the discovery of REM sleep to test psychoanalytic theories of dreams and pressure to dream. Early experiments[144,145] determined that selective deprivation of REM sleep accomplished by the awakening technique resulted in increasingly frequent attempts by subjects to enter REM sleep. For example, in one study, 17 awakenings were required on the first night, 42 awakenings were required on the fourth night, and 68 awakenings were required on the seventh night to maintain REM sleep deprivation.[145] Large increases in REM sleep amount were also noted when nondisturbed recovery sleep was allowed. Although the EEG effects were large and easily replicated, the impact of REM sleep deprivation on psychological function or performance has been much more difficult to determine.[146]

The following theories attempt to describe the function of REM sleep (see also Chapter 47):

1. The drive facilitation hypothesis[146]
2. The activation synthesis hypothesis[147]
3. The catecholamine restoration hypothesis[148]
4. The cortical homeostasis hypothesis[149]
5. The information-processing hypothesis (see later)
6. The neural growth promotion hypothesis[150]
7. The oculomotor hypothesis[151]
8. The protein synthesis hypothesis
9. The sentinel hypothesis[146]

In recent years, the most frequently studied view of REM sleep function has been the proposal that the activated brain associated with REM sleep is involved in memory consolidation, synthesis of new or adaptive information, or arrangement of information into an internal association framework. Six reviews have been published since 2000. Of interest, four of the reviews concluded that REM sleep, or at least sleep, is significantly involved with memory,[152-155] whereas two reviews concluded that there was little evidence to support a role for REM sleep in human memory.[156,157]

A number of animal studies have shown that REM sleep increases after learning and that REM sleep deprivation after a learning task results in decreased retention (see Peigneux et al.[155] for review). Unfortunately, the results from human REM sleep deprivation studies have not been as supportive as the results of the animal studies, and this suggests that some of the animal results may have been secondary to stress or another intervening variable.[156] Although the human studies have not provided strong support for a role of REM sleep in declarative memory (rote memory or language memory),[154] recent human studies[153,158] found improvement in perceptual performance occurred 8 to 10 hours after a training session only when REM sleep was allowed in the interim. These results have led to the hypothesis that perceptual learning, rather than retention of memorized material, is related to REM sleep.[154] However, such results do not explain why subjects whose REM sleep has been eliminated by the use of monoamine oxidase inhibitors or brainstem injury have no measurable memory deficits.[156]

In contrast to the large number of studies of selective REM sleep deprivation, there are few studies of selective SWS deprivation. Early studies determined that when stage 4 sleep was selectively deprived in humans by an arousal procedure, subjects made increasing efforts to enter the stage and had stage 4 rebounds when sleep was not disturbed.[145,159] In a study specifically comparing the effects of stage 4 and REM sleep deprivation,[145] subjects required five to seven times as many arousals to deprive them of stage 4 sleep than to deprive them of REM sleep during each night of selective sleep deprivation. Recovery nights following stage 4 sleep deprivation were similar to recovery nights following total sleep loss— stage 4 increased only on the first recovery night, and REM sleep, which had not been deprived, increased on recovery nights 2 and 3. In contrast, after REM sleep deprivation, REM sleep was increased throughout 3 recovery nights but there was no increase of stage 4 sleep on any recovery night.

Daytime performance after selective stage 4 and REM deprivation conditions in humans has been tested, but decrements were not found after as many as 7 nights of either stage 4 or REM sleep deprivation.[145,160] It was concluded in these studies that the major predictor of performance during these sleep loss paradigms was the total amount of time spent asleep, regardless of sleep stage parameters.[161]

SLEEP FRAGMENTATION

Sleep is a time-based cumulative process that can be impeded by several types of deprivation and also by systematic disturbance. A number of studies have shown that very brief periodic arousals from sleep reduce the restorative power of sleep. Three extensive reviews of sleep fragmentation have been published recently.[162-164] Two of the reviews specifically compared findings in sleep fragmentation paradigms with findings from sleep deprivation studies.[162,163]

Experimental Sleep Fragmentation

Many studies have examined the relationship between various schedules of sleep fragmentation and residual sleepiness on the following day. Data from eight studies are plotted in Figure 5–2. There is a strong relationship ($r = .775$, $P < .01$) between rate of fragmentation (plotted as minutes of sleep allowed between disturbances) and decrease in sleep latency as measured by MSLT.[162] As expected, increased sleepiness after sleep fragmentation was also associated with decreased psychomotor performance on a broad range of tasks[164] and degraded mood.[163]

In many early studies of sleep fragmentation, total sleep time was reduced and significant changes in sleep parameters, including large reductions in SWS and REM, were found. Thus it became important to differentiate whether the sleep fragmentation effects were related to the periodic disturbance or to partial sleep deprivation or selective sleep stage deprivation. To address this issue, some studies have been carefully designed to produce brief EEG arousals, or even "nonvisible" EEG sleep disturbance, so that there are few[165] or no changes[166] in standard sleep EEG parameters despite the periodic sleep fragmentation. Despite preservation of normal EEG sleep amounts, participants in these studies were still significantly sleepier on the day after sleep fragmentation. In another approach, fragmentation rates, consolidated sleep periods, and SWS amounts were experimentally varied in participants in an attempt to tease out sleep stage effects from fragmentation effects,[167,168] with similar conclusions—residual sleepiness was more related to the sleep fragmentation than to sleep stage parameters.

Another group of studies has directly compared the impact of relatively high rates of sleep fragmentation (usually disturbance every 1 to 2 minutes) with the effect of total sleep deprivation within the same study. In one study, profiles of cortisol and adrenocorticotropic hormone were similar during total sleep deprivation and sleep fragmentation.[169] In two other studies,[167,170] MSLT was decreased to similar low values after both total sleep deprivation and high-frequency sleep fragmentation. In one study,[167] performance loss was the same on a vigilance test after sleep fragmentation and total sleep deprivation but less on addition problems completed and simple reaction time after sleep fragmentation. In another study,[171] a significant increase in apnea/hypopnea index was found after both sleep fragmentation and sleep deprivation, and this increase was actually greater after sleep fragmentation.

These findings of similar impact on hormones, respiratory parameters, psychomotor performance, and objective sleepiness after similar periods of sleep deprivation and sleep fragmentation indicate that there is much in common between the high-frequency sleep fragmentation and total sleep deprivation. Clearly, the restorative function of sleep is severely impaired by high rates of sleep fragmentation. However, as indicated by Figure 5–2, the impact of periodic sleep fragmentation decreases rapidly as the interval between arousals increases, and this has been hypothesized to imply that normal restoration during sleep requires periods of consolidated sleep of 10 to 20 minutes.[172]

More recent studies have examined a broad range of physiologic indices as possible measures of sleep fragmentation.[163] A number of respiratory, cardiac, and alternative EEG measures have been examined, with the general conclusion that most of these physiologic measures, including traditional arousals, are moderately correlated with daytime sleepiness. However, much empirical work needs to be done to determine the extent to which these new measures are simply correlates of EEG arousals rather than new measures of sleep continuity. For example, some investigators posit that K-complexes are associated with arousal because they are reliably accompanied by a small increase in heart rate. Empirically, however, K-complexes have an average frequency of more than one per minute,[173] and one study,[174] using intense tones every 22 seconds for 30 consecutive nights to drive K-complex production, found no changes in sleep latency, recovery sleep, or daytime mood or performance. Such data imply that the "arousal" associated with a periodic small increase in heart rate is not sufficient to reduce the restorative power of sleep. A physiologic event more specific than the EEG arousal remains to be identified.

Sleep Disorders and Fragmentation

The earliest study of sleep fragmentation in dogs documented impaired arousal responses to hypercapnia and hypoxia during sleep.[175] Further studies following dogs with experimentally produced apnea or sleep fragmentation for periods of more than 4 months showed that both the sleep fragmentation procedure and the experimentally produced apnea produced increased time to arousal as well as greater oxygen desaturation, greater peak inspiratory pressure, and greater surges in blood pressure in response to airway occlusion. It was concluded that the sleep fragmentation alone was responsible for the sleepiness symptoms associated with sleep apnea,

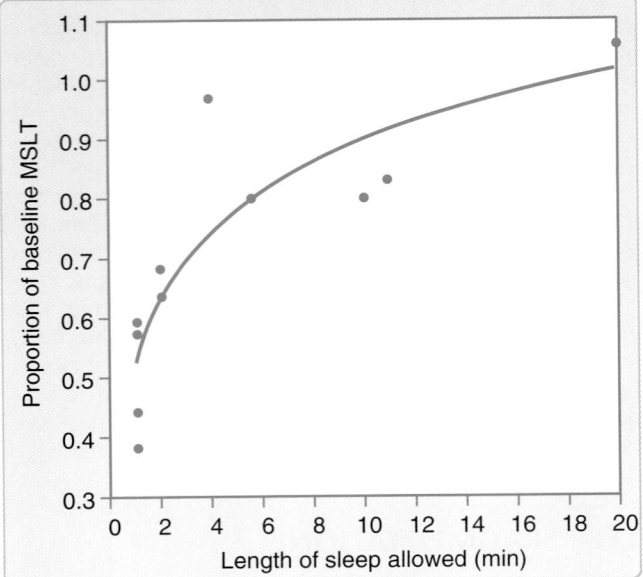

Figure 5–2. Proportion of baseline multiple sleep latency test (MSLT) value (i.e., sleep latency after fragmentation nights divided by sleep latency after baseline) in eight (two separate fragmentation conditions were identified in three studies) sleep fragmentation studies, plotted as a function of the amount of sleep time allowed until disturbance (e.g., "2" means that subjects were aroused briefly after every 2 minutes of sleep). (Adapted from Bonnet MH, Arand DL: Clinical effects of sleep fragmentation versus sleep deprivation. Sleep Med Rev 2003;7:297-310.)

and "the changes in the acute responses to airway occlusion resulting from OSA [obstructive sleep apnea] are primarily the result of the associated sleep fragmentation" (from p. 1609 of Brooks et al.[97]).

Other clinical studies have documented that the number of brief arousals is significantly correlated with the magnitude of daytime sleepiness in groups of patients.[176,177] Traditional sleep stage rebounds (see "Recovery Sleep," next) are seen when the pathology is corrected. After effective treatment of sleep apnea and the corresponding decrease in frequency of arousals during sleep, alertness is improved as measured by either MSLT or reduction in traffic accidents.[178] There are many other instances of sleep fragmentation as a component of medical illnesses (such as fibrositis, intensive care unit syndrome, chronic movement disorders, and chronic pain disorders) and of life requirements (infant care, medical residents). Some of these impositions may not produce the critical number of arousals required for significant decrements in the apnea patients and sleep fragmentation studies. However, most of these situations are a combination of chronic partial sleep loss and chronic sleep fragmentation. The combination of these factors will clearly have greater impact than either factor in isolation.

RECOVERY SLEEP

Sleep is all that is required to reverse the effects of sleep deprivation in almost all circumstances. The EEG characteristics of recovery sleep depend on the amount of prior wakefulness and the circadian time. These effects have been successfully modeled (see Chapter 33).

Performance Effects

Several efforts have been made to assess recovery of performance after sleep deprivation. It is commonly reported that recovery from periods of sleep loss of up to 10 days and nights is rapid and can occur within 1 to 3 nights. Several studies have reported recovery of performance after a single (usually 8-hour) night of sleep after anywhere from 40 to 110 hours of continuous wakefulness.[12,13] Taken together, these experiments suggest that an equal amount of sleep is not required to recover from sleep lost. However, sleep deprivation itself was the main concern of these studies and, therefore, recovery was given minimal attention.

A few studies have specifically examined the rate of performance recovery during sleep in young adults, healthy older subjects, and insomniac patients after 40- and 64-hour sleep loss periods.[53] In such studies, participants were awakened from stage 2 sleep for 20-minute test batteries approximately every 2 hours during baseline and recovery nights. Therefore, it was possible to follow the time course of return to baseline performance during recovery sleep in the three groups. In the young adults, reaction time returned to levels not significantly lower than baseline after 4 hours of recovery sleep following 40 hours of sleep loss. However, reaction time remained significantly slower than baseline in young adults throughout the first night of recovery sleep (including the postsleep morning test) after 64 hours of sleep loss. In contrast, reaction times in both older normal-sleeper and insomniac groups were significantly slower than baseline at 05:30 but had returned to baseline levels by 08:00 following the first recovery night after 64 hours of sleep loss. The young adults not

only recovered more slowly from sleep loss on the initial recovery night but also had some decrease in their reaction times that extended into the second recovery night. This result is consistent with data presented by Carskadon and Dement,[179] who found that older subjects had daytime MSLT values at baseline levels after sleep loss and a single night of recovery sleep, whereas shorter-than-normal latencies continued in young adults.

EEG Effects

A large number of studies have reported consistent effects on sleep EEG when totally sleep-deprived individuals are finally allowed to sleep. If undisturbed, young adults typically sleep only 12 to 15 hours, even after 264 hours of sleep loss.[180] If sleep times are held to 8 hours on recovery nights, effects on sleep stages may be seen for 2 or more nights.

The effects of 40 and 64 hours of sleep loss on recovery sleep stages during the initial recovery night are summarized in Table 5–1 for young adult normal sleepers[14,73,181-183]; young adult short sleepers[184]; young adult long sleepers[184]; 60- to 80-year-old normal sleepers[179,185,186]; 60- to 70-year-old patients with chronic insomnia[185,187]; and 60- to 80-year-old depressed and demented patients.[188,189] The table presents percentage change from baseline data, with an indication of study-to-study variability where the number of studies allowed computation. The table is presented as a summary device so that (1) EEG effects of sleep deprivation can be predicted (roughly by multiplying population baseline values by figures presented in the table), and (2) the potential differential effects of sleep deprivation on EEG recovery sleep as a function of group can be more clearly seen. The results of these several studies indicate that recovery sleep EEG changes that occur as a function of sleep deprivation are remarkably consistent across studies and across several experimental groups including men, women, older subjects, and older insomniac patients. Significant deviations from population recovery values are seen primarily in REM latency changes in depressed and demented patients and in some less-robust differences found in small groups of long and short sleepers. These latter findings might be related to differential sleep stage distributions secondary to long or short sleep times.

On the first recovery night after total sleep loss, there is a large increase in SWS over baseline amounts.[90,187] As would be expected, wake time and stage 1 sleep are usually reduced. Stage 2 and REM sleep may both be decreased on the first recovery night after 64 hours of sleep loss,[53,73] at least in young adults, as a function of increased SWS. In older normal sleepers and insomniac patients, there is less absolute increase in SWS than in young adults on the first recovery night, although the percentage increase in SWS may be as great. Because of less SWS rebound, there may be no change (geriatric normal sleepers) or even an increase in stage 2.[53,189] Recovery sleep stage changes were generally similar regardless of age (see Table 5–1), except that older normal sleepers had a decrease in REM latency during recovery sleep[179,185,189] rather than the increased REM latency common in young adults. It was found that REM latency in the older population was positively correlated with baseline SWS amounts,[185,189] and that sleep-onset REM periods occurred in about 20% of those carefully screened normal sleepers.[185,189] These REM changes were interpreted as being the result of decreased

Table 5–1. Effects* of Sleep Loss on Stages of Recovery Sleep

	Sleep Loss: 40 hr						Sleep Loss: 64 hr	
	Young Adults (SD)	Older Adults (SD)	Depressed	Demented	Short Sleepers	Long Sleepers	Older Normal	Older Insomniacs
Sleep latency	0.38 (0.09)	—	0.22	0.14	—	—	—	—
Wake time	0.44 (0.19)	0.51 (0.11)	—	—	0.13	0.48	—	—
Stage 1	0.42 (0.12)	0.59 (0.14)	0.61	0.68	0.98	0.60	0.56	0.52
Stage 2	0.87 (0.10)	0.95 (0.07)	1.06	1.08	1.38	0.99	1.07	1.20
Stage 3	0.98	1.32 (0.25)	1.14	1.16	—	—	2.36	3.00
Stage 4	2.40	2.06 (0.45)	1.35	1.12	—	—	7.00	5.25
SWS stage	1.53 (0.11)	1.56 (0.23)	1.23	1.15	1.37	1.52	2.56	3.30
REM sleep stage	0.89 (0.13)	1.04 (0.09)	0.84	0.78	1.26	1.03	0.26	0.92
REM sleep latency	1.01 (0.20)	0.77 (0.20)	2.2	2.0	1.13	1.26	0.35	0.96

*The values presented in this table are the mean percentage of baseline levels of the indicated sleep stages for the indicated groups during the first sleep recovery night. Where sufficient studies were available, the standard deviation (SD) around the mean percentage is also given. For example, on their recovery night after one night of sleep loss, young adults have a sleep latency that is 38 ± 9% of their baseline sleep latency. (See text for the references used for each group.)

REM, rapid eye movement; SWS, slow wave sleep.

pressure for SWS in older humans. The REM latency findings did not apply to older depressed or demented individuals. REM rebound effects appear to be related to the amount of lost SWS, so that REM rebound is more likely on an early recovery night when there is less SWS loss as a function either of a shorter period of sleep loss or of age.

On the second recovery night after total sleep loss, SWS amounts approached normal values, and an increase in REM sleep was found in young adults.[73,190] Total sleep time was still elevated. By the third recovery night, all sleep EEG values approached baseline. In situations where REM rebounds on the first sleep recovery night, sleep EEG values may normalize by the second recovery night. Possible exceptions to these general rules include older insomniac patients who have increased total sleep for at least 3 nights after 64 hours of sleep loss,[53] and individuals who have had significant selective REM deprivation.

Relationship between EEG and Psychomotor Performance Recovery Effects

The earliest systematic evaluations of sleep in humans posited that the recuperative value of sleep was directly related to its depth. The consistent data show that recovery sleep after sleep loss seems to result in return to baseline performance levels after much less sleep than had originally been lost. The parallel increase in SWS during recovery leads directly to the speculation that SWS is somehow implicated in the sleep recovery process. Unfortunately, studies designed to test this hypothesis directly by experimentally varying the amount of SWS during the recovery sleep period or during a sleep fragmentation period have not implicated any sleep stages as central in the recovery process. When either SWS or REM was selectively deprived during the initial recovery night after sleep loss, no difference was found between those groups and a group that was allowed a nondisturbed night of recovery sleep.[191] A study of the relationship between systematic sleep

fragmentation and the distribution of SWS came to the same conclusion.[168] However, both studies were not designed to look for the more subtle effects that might have occurred within the initial recovery night.[191]

Horne[142] postulated that only part of a normal night of sleep is essential ("core" sleep), and that the remaining sleep exists primarily as a buffer. In one sense, core sleep could be approximately reduced to SWS and REM. In another sense, core could refer to a period of sleep with high sensory thresholds to reduce the probability of fragmentation by arousals or awakenings. Alternatively, if the restoration that occurs during sleep is viewed as an exponential process instead of as a linear process, rapid changes would occur in the initial hours of sleep and increasingly small increments would occur as sleep continues past 6 or 7 hours.[192] These final small changes may not be easy to measure in typical sleep deprivation studies involving only a few subjects and as a result may give the appearance that the last hour or two of sleep is less essential.

CONCLUSIONS

The physiologic and behavioral effects of sleep loss in humans are consistent and well defined. Unfortunately, several of the consistent findings in human studies do not agree with the findings of the animal studies, and the hope that sleep deprivation would serve as the tool to define the function of sleep has not been realized. It is generally agreed that there is a physiologic imperative to sleep in humans and other mammals and that the drive to sleep can be as strong as the drive to breathe. Future work should (1) address in more detail the microstructure of the sleep process and its relationship to sleep restoration, (2) reconcile response differences among species, (3) examine differences in response to sleep deprivation in normal and depressed humans, (4) explore the interaction between the sleep system and the arousal system, and (5) ensure that our understanding of the lawful relationship between sleep loss, alertness, and behavior be disseminated for use by government and industry.

Clinical Pearl

The impact of sleep deprivation on performance and physiology has been examined in thousands of studies for over a hundred years. These findings might not seem directly relevant in a clinical sense, but it should be remembered that the clinical diagnosis of insufficient sleep syndrome is based on sleep deprivation. Sleepiness symptoms secondary to sleep apnea and periodic limb movements (sleep fragmentation) also evolve from sleep deprivation.

Acknowledgments

The research that underlies this chapter is supported by the Medical Research Service of the Dayton Department of Veterans Affairs Medical Center and Wright State University, Dayton, Ohio. Literature searches were supported by the Sleep-Wake Disorders Research Institute, Dayton, Ohio.

REFERENCES

1. Koslowsky M, Babkoff H: Meta-analysis of the relationship between total sleep deprivation and performance. Chronobiol Int 1992;9:132-136.
2. Pilcher JJ, Huffcutt AI: Effects of sleep deprivation on performance: A meta-analysis. Sleep 1996;19:318-326.
3. Cirelli C, Tononi G: Total sleep deprivation. In Kushida CA (ed): Sleep Deprivation: Basic Science, Physiology, and Behavior. Vol 192: Lung Biology in Health and Disease. New York, Marcel Dekker, 2005, pp 63-80.
4. Manaceine M: Quelques observations experimentales sur l'influence de l'insomnie absolue. Arch Ital Biol 1894;21:322-325.
5. Patrick GTW, Gilbert JA: On the effect of loss of sleep. Psychol Rev 1896;3:469-483.
6. Johnson LC: Sleep deprivation and performance. In Webb WB (ed): Biological Rhythms, Sleep, and Performance. New York, John Wiley & Sons, 1982, pp 111-142.
7. Rosa RR, Bonnet MH: Predicting nighttime alertness following prophylactic naps. Sleep Res 1991;20:417.
8. Mikulincer M, Babkoff H, Caspy T, et al: The effects of 72 hours of sleep loss on psychological variables. Br J Psychol 1989;80:145-162.
9. Bonnet MH, Arand DL: Sleepiness as measured by the MSLT varies as a function of preceding activity. Sleep 1998;21:477-483.
10. Wilkinson RT: Sleep deprivation. In Edholm OG, Bacharach A (eds): The Physiology of Human Survival. New York, Academic Press, 1965, pp 399-430.
11. Leproult R, Van Reeth O, Byrne MM, et al: Sleepiness, performance, and neuroendocrine function during sleep deprivation: Effects of exposure to bright light or exercise. J Biol Rhythms 1997;12:245-258.
12. Lubin A, Hord DJ, Tracy ML, et al: Effects of exercise, bedrest and napping on performance decrement during 40 hours. Psychophysiol 1976;13:334-339.
13. Webb WB, Agnew HWJ: Effects on performance of high and low energy-expenditure during sleep deprivation. Percept Mot Skills 1973;37:511-514.
14. Moses J, Lubin A, Naitoh P, et al: Exercise and sleep loss: Effects on recovery sleep. Psychophysiology 1977;14:414-416.
15. Bonnet MH, Arand DL: Level of arousal and the ability to maintain wakefulness. J Sleep Res 1999;8:247-254.
16. Dijk D-J, Cajochen C, Borbely A: Effect of a single 3-hour exposure to bright light on core body temperature and sleep in humans. Neurosci Lett 1991;121:59-62.
17. Komada Y, Tanaka H, Yamamoto Y, et al: Effects of bright light pre-exposure on sleep onset process. Psychiatry Clin Neurosci 2000;54:365-366.
18. Campbell SS, Dawson D: Enhancement of nighttime alertness and performance with bright ambient light. Physiol Behav 1990; 48:317-320.
19. Dawson D, Encel N, Lushington K: Improving adaptation to simulated night shift: Timed exposure to bright light versus daytime melatonin administration. Sleep 1995;18:11-21.
20. Murphy P, Myers B, Badia P, et al: The effects of bright light on daytime sleep latencies. Sleep Res 1991;20:465.
21. Wilkinson RT: Interaction of noise with knowledge of results and sleep deprivation. J Exp Psychol 1963;66:332-337.
22. Tassi P, Nicolas A, Seegmuller C, et al: Interaction of the alerting effect of noise with partial sleep deprivation and circadian rhythmicity of vigilance. Percept Mot Skills 1993;77:1239-1248.
23. Poulton EC, Edwards RS, Colquhoun WP: The interaction of the loss of a night's sleep with mild heat: Task variables. Ergonomics 1974;17:59-73.
24. Reyner LA, Horne JA: Evaluation of "in-car" countermeasures to sleepiness: Cold air and radio. Sleep 1998;21:46-50.
25. Bonnet MH, Arand DL: Arousal components in the measurement of sleepiness and wakefulness. Sleep 2001;24:441-450.
26. Lindqvist A, Jalonen J, Parviainen P, et al: Effect of posture on spontaneous and thermally stimulated cardiovascular oscillations. Cardiovasc Res 1990;24:373-380.
27. Newhouse PA, Belenky G, Thomas M, et al: The effects of D-amphetamine on arousal, cognition, and mood after prolonged total sleep deprivation. Neuropsychopharmacology 1989;2: 153-164.
28. Caldwell JA, Caldwell JL: An in-flight investigation of the efficacy of dextroamphetamine for sustaining helicopter pilot performance. Aviat Space Environ Med 1997;68:1073-1080.
29. Pigeau R, Naitoh P, Buguet A, et al: Modafinil, D-amphetamine and placebo during 64 hours of sustained mental work: I. Effects on mood, fatigue, cognitive performance and body temperature. J Sleep Res 1995;4:212-228.
30. Walsh JK, Muehlbach MJ, Humm TM, et al: Effect of caffeine on physiological sleep tendency and ability to sustain wakefulness at night. Psychopharmacology 1990;101:271-273.
31. Borland RG, Rogers AS, Nicholson AN, et al: Performance overnight in shiftworkers operating a day-night schedule. Aviat Space Environ Med 1986;57:241-249.
32. Wright KP, Badia P, Myers BL, et al: Combination of bright light and caffeine as a countermeasure for impaired alertness and performance during extended sleep deprivation. J Sleep Res 1997;6:26-35.
33. Bonnet MH, Gomez S, Wirth O, et al: The use of caffeine versus prophylactic naps in sustained performance. Sleep 1995;18: 97-104.
34. Penetar D, McCann U, Thorne D, et al: Caffeine reversal of sleep deprivation effects on alertness and mood. Psychopharmacology 1993;112:359-365.
35. Bonnet MH, Arand DL: The use of prophylactic naps and caffeine to maintain performance during a continuous operation. Ergonomics 1994;37:1009-1020.
36. Bonnet MH, Arand DL: The impact of naps and caffeine on extended nocturnal performance. Physiol Behav 1994;56:103-109.
37. Babkoff H, Kelly TL, Matteson LT, et al: Pemoline and methylphenidate: Interaction with mood, sleepiness, and cognitive performance during 64 hours of sleep deprivation. Mil Psychol 1992;4:235-265.
38. Bishop C, Roehrs T, Rosenthal L, et al: Alerting effects of methylphenidate under basal and sleep-deprived conditions. Exp Clin Psychopharmacol 1997;5:344-352.
39. Lagarde D, Batejat D, Van Beers P, et al: Interest of modafinil, a new psychostimulant, during a sixty-hour sleep deprivation experiment. Fundam Clin Pharmacol 1995;9:271-279.
40. Wesensten J, Belenky G, Kautz MA, et al: Maintaining alertness and performance during sleep deprivation: Modafinil versus caffeine. Psychopharmacology 2002;159:238-247.
41. Newhouse PA, Penetar DM, Fertig JB, et al: Stimulant drug effects on performance and behavior after prolonged sleep deprivation: A comparison of amphetamine, nicotine, and deprenyl. Mil Psychol 1992;4:207-233.

42. Fischman MW, Schuster CR: Cocaine effects in sleep-deprived humans. Psychopharmacology 1980;72:1-8.

43. Roehrs T, Beare D, Zorick F, et al: Sleepiness and ethanol effects on simulated driving. Alcohol Clin Exp Res 1994;18:154-158.

44. Williamson AM, Feyer AM: Moderate sleep deprivation produces impairments in cognitive and motor performance equivalent to legally prescribed levels of alcohol intoxication. Occup Environ Med 2000;57:649-655.

45. Dawson D, Reid K: Fatigue, alcohol and performance impairment (Letter). Nature 1997;388:235.

46. Arnedt JT, Wilde GJ, Munt PW, et al: How do prolonged wakefulness and alcohol compare in the decrements they produce on a simulated driving task? Accid Anal Prev 2001;33:337-344.

47. Wilkinson RT: Effects of up to 60 hours' sleep deprivation on different types of work. Ergonomics 1964;7:175-186.

48. Horne JA, Pettitt AN: High incentive effects on vigilance performance during 72 hours of total sleep deprivation. Acta Psychol 1985;58:123-139.

49. Wilkinson RT: Interaction of lack of sleep with knowledge of results, repeated testing, and individual differences. J Exp Psychol 1961;62:263-271.

50. Haslam DR: The incentive effect and sleep deprivation. Sleep 1983;6:362-368.

51. Bonnet MH, Webb WB: The effect of repetition of relevant and irrelevant tasks over day and night work periods. Ergonomics 1978;21:999-1005.

52. Webb WB, Levy CM: Effects of spaced and repeated total sleep deprivation. Ergonomics 1984;27:45-58.

53. Bonnet MH, Rosa RR: Sleep and performance in young adults and older insomniacs and normals during acute sleep loss and recovery. Biol Psychol 1987;25:153-172.

54. Webb WB: A further analysis of age and sleep deprivation effects. Psychophysiology 1985;22:156-161.

55. Mullaney DJ, Kripke DF, Fleck PA, et al: Sleep loss and nap effects on sustained continuous performance. Psychophysiology 1983;20:643-651.

56. Tyler DB: Psychological changes during experimental sleep deprivation. Dis Nerv Syst 1955;16:293-299.

57. Johnson LC: Physiological and psychological changes following total sleep deprivation. In Kales A (ed): Sleep Physiology and Pathology. Philadelphia, JB Lippincott, 1969, pp 206-220.

58. Giedke H, Schwarzler F: Therapeutic use of sleep deprivation in depression. Sleep Med Rev 2002;6:361-377.

59. Wirz-Justice A, Van den Hoofdakker RH: Sleep deprivation in depression: What do we know, where do we go? Biol Psychiatry 1999;46:445-453.

60. Franken P, Malafosse A, Mehdi T: Genetic determinants of sleep regulation in inbred mice. Sleep 1999;22:155-169.

61. Leproult R, Colecchia EF, Berardi AM, et al: Individual differences in subjective and objective alertness during sleep deprivation are stable and unrelated. Am J Physiol Regul Integr Comp Physiol 2003;284:R280-R290.

62. Bonnet MH: Sleep length. In Kushida CA (ed): Sleep Deprivation: Clinical Issues, Pharmacology, and Sleep Loss Effects. Vol 193: Lung Biology in Health and Disease. New York, Marcel Dekker, 2005, pp 503-514.

63. Bonnet MH, Arand DL: Activity, arousal, and the MSLT in patients with insomnia. Sleep 2000;23:205-212.

64. De Valck E, Cluydts R: Sleepiness as a state-trait phenomenon, comprising both a sleep drive and a wake drive. Med Hypotheses 2003;60:509-512.

65. Donnell JM: Performance decrement as a function of total sleep loss and task duration. Percept Mot Skills 1969;29:711-714.

66. Steyvers FJJM, Gaillard AWK: The effects of sleep deprivation and incentives on human performance. Psychol Res 1993;55:64-70.

67. Light AI, Sun JH, McCool C, et al: The effects of acute sleep deprivation on level of resident training. Curr Surg 1989;46:29-30.

68. Alluisi EA, Coates GD, Morgan BBJ: Effects of temporal stressors on vigilance and information processing. In Mackie RR (ed): Vigilance: Theory, Operational Performance, and Physiological Correlates. New York, Plenum Press, 1977, pp 361-421.

69. Williams HL, Lubin A: Speeded addition and sleep loss. J Exp Psychol 1967;73:313-317.

70. Williams HL, Gieseking CF, Lubin A: Some effects of sleep loss on memory. Percept Mot Skills 1966;23:1287-1293.

71. Nilsson LG, Backman L, Karlsson T: Priming and cued recall in elderly, alcohol intoxicated and sleep deprived subjects: A case of functionally similar memory deficits. Psychol Med 1989;19:423-433.

72. Akerstedt T, Froberg JE, Friberg Y, et al: Melatonin excretion, body temperature and subjective arousal during 64 hours of sleep deprivation. Psychoneuroendocrinology 1979;4:219-225.

73. Carskadon MA, Dement WC: Effects of total sleep loss on sleep tendency. Percept Mot Skills 1979;48:495-506.

74. Carskadon MA, Dement WC: Cumulative effects of sleep restriction on daytime sleepiness. Psychophysiology 1981;18:107-113.

75. Marcus CL, Loughlin GM: Effect of sleep deprivation on driving safety in housestaff. Sleep 1996;19:763-766.

76. Horne JA: A review of the biological effects of total sleep deprivation in man. Biol Psychol 1978;7:55-102.

77. Kleitman N: Sleep and Wakefulness, 2nd ed. Chicago, University of Chicago Press, 1963.

78. Kollar EJ, Namerow N, Pasnau RO, et al: Neurological findings during prolonged sleep deprivation. Neurology 1968;18:836-840.

79. Ross JJ: Neurological findings after prolonged sleep deprivation. Arch Neurol 1965;12:399-403.

80. Finelli LA: Sleep deprivation: Cortical and EEG changes. In Kushida CA (ed): Sleep Deprivation: Basic Science, Physiology, and Behavior. Vol 192: Lung Biology in Health and Disease. New York, Marcel Dekker, 2005, pp 223-264.

81. Rodin EA, Luby ED, Gottleib JS: The EEG during prolonged experimental sleep deprivation. Electroencephalogr Clin Neurophysiol 1962;14:544-551.

82. Naitoh P, Kales A, Kollar EJ, et al: Electroencephalographic activity after prolonged sleep loss. Electroencephalogr Clin Neurophysiol 1969;27:2-11.

83. Naitoh P, Pasnau RO, Kollar EJ: Psychophysiological changes after prolonged deprivation of sleep. Biol Psychiatry 1971;3:309-320.

84. Lorenzo I, Ramos J, Arce C, et al: Effect of total sleep deprivation on reaction time and waking EEG activity in man. Sleep 1995;18:346-354.

85. Williams HL, Granda AM, Jones RC, et al: EEG frequency and finger pulse volume as predictors of reaction time during sleep loss. Electroencephalogr Clin Neurophysiol 1962;14:64-70.

86. Blake H, Gerard RW, Kleitman N: Factors influencing brain potentials during sleep. J Neurophysiol 1939;2:48-60.

87. Thomas M, Sing H, Belenky G, et al: Neural basis of alertness and cognitive performance impairments during sleepiness: I. Effects of 24 h of sleep deprivation on waking human regional brain activity. J Sleep Res 2000;9:335-352.

88. Drummond SP, Gillin JC, Brown GG: Increased cerebral response during a divided attention task following sleep deprivation. J Sleep Res 2001;10:85-92.

89. Pratt KL, Matteson RH, Weckers NJ, et al: EEG activation of epileptics following sleep deprivation. Electroencephalogr Clin Neurophysiol 1968;24:11-15.

90. Kollar EJ, Slater GG, Palmer JO, et al: Stress in subjects undergoing sleep deprivation. Psychosom Med 1966;28:101-113.

91. Fiorica V, Higgins EA, Iampietro PF, et al: Physiological responses of men during sleep deprivation. J Appl Physiol 1968;24:167-176.

92. Schiffman PL, Trontell MC, Mazar MF, et al: Sleep deprivation decreases ventilatory response to CO_2 but not load compensation. Chest 1983;84:695-698.

93. White DP, Douglas NJ, Pickett CK, et al: Sleep deprivation and the control of ventilation. Am Rev Respir Dis 1983;128:984-986.

94. Phillips BA, Cooper KR, Burke TV: The effect of sleep loss on breathing in chronic obstructive pulmonary disease. Chest 1987;91:29-32.

95. Canet E, Gaultier C, D'Allest AM, et al: Effects of sleep deprivation on respiratory events during sleep in healthy infants. J Appl Physiol 1989;66:1158-1163.

96. Persson HE, Svanborg E: Sleep deprivation worsens obstructive sleep apnea: Comparison between diurnal and nocturnal polysomnography. Chest 1996;109:645-650.

97. Brooks D, Horner RL, Kimoff RJ, et al: Effect of obstructive sleep apnea versus sleep fragmentation on responses to airway occlusion. Am J Respir Crit Care Med 1997;155:1609-1617.

98. Minors D, Waterhouse J, Akerstedt T, et al: Effect of sleep loss on core temperature when movement is controlled. Ergonomics 1999;42:647-656.

99. Landis CA, Savage MV, Lentz MJ, et al: Sleep deprivation alters body temperature dynamics to mild cooling and heating not sweating threshold in women. Sleep 1998;21:101-108.

100. Shaw PJ: Thermoregulatory changes. In Kushida CA (ed): Sleep Deprivation: Basic Science, Physiology, and Behavior. Vol 192: Lung Biology in Health and Disease. New York, Marcel Dekker, 2005, pp 319-338.

101. Tobler I, Sigg H: Long-term motor activity recording of dogs and the effect of sleep deprivation. Experientia 1986;42:987-991.

102. Plyley MJ, Shephard RJ, Davis GM, et al: Sleep deprivation and cardiorespiratory function: Influence of intermittent submaximal exercise. Eur J Appl Physiol 1987;56:338-344.

103. Goodman JM, Plyley MJ, Hart LE, et al: Moderate exercise and hemodilution during sleep deprivation. Aviat Space Environ Med 1990;61:139-144.

104. McMurray RG, Brown CF: The effect of sleep loss on high intensity exercise and recovery. Aviat Space Environ Med 1984;55:1031-1035.

105. Van Den Noort S, Brine K: Effect of sleep on brain labile phosphates and metabolic rate. Am J Physiol 1970;218:1434-1439.

106. Mendelson W, Guthrie RD, Guynn R, et al: Rapid eye movement (REM) sleep deprivation, stress and intermediary metabolism. J Neurochem 1974;22:1157-1159.

107. Akerstedt T, Palmblad J, de la Torre B, et al: Adrenocortical and gonadal steroids during sleep deprivation. Sleep 1980;3:23-30.

108. Froberg JE: Twenty-four-hour patterns in human performance, subjective and physiological variables and differences between morning and evening active subjects. Biol Psychol 1977;5:119-134.

109. Kant GJ, Genser SG, Thorne DR, et al: Effects of 72 hour sleep deprivation on urinary cortisol and indices of metabolism. Sleep 1984;7:142-146.

110. Palmblad J, Akerstedt T, Froberg J, et al: Thyroid and adrenomedullary reactions during sleep deprivation. Acta Endocrinol (Copenh) 1979;90:233-239.

111. Gary KA, Winokur A, Douglas SD, et al: Total sleep deprivation and the thyroid axis: Effects of sleep and waking activity. Aviat Space Environ Med 1996;67:513-519.

112. von Treuer K, Norman TR, Armstrong SM: Overnight human plasma melatonin, cortisol, prolactin, TSH, under conditions of normal sleep, sleep deprivation, and sleep recovery. J Pineal Res 1996;20:7-14.

113. Goh VH, Tong TY, Lim C, et al: Effects of one night of sleep deprivation on hormone profiles and performance efficiency. Mil Med 2001;166:427-431.

114. Frank G, Halberg F, Harner R, et al: Circadian periodicity, adrenal corticosteroids, and the EEG of normal man. J Psychiatr Res 1966;4:73-86.

115. Beck U: Hormonal secretion during sleep in man: Modification of growth hormone and prolactin secretion by interruption and selective deprivation of sleep. Int J Neurol 1981;15:17-29.

116. Spiegel K, Leproult R, Van Cauter E: Metabolic and endocrine changes associated with sleep deprivation. In Kushida CA (ed): Sleep Deprivation: Basic Science, Physiology, and Behavior. Vol 192: Lung Biology in Health and Disease. New York, Marcel Dekker, 2005, pp 293-318.

117. Parker DC, Rossman LG, Kripke DF, et al: Endocrine rhythms across sleep-wake cycles in normal young men under basal conditions. In Orem J, Barnes CD (eds): Physiology in Sleep. New York, Academic Press, 1980, pp 146-180.

118. Sassin JF, Parker DC, Johnson LC, et al: Effects of slow wave sleep deprivation on human growth hormone release in sleep: Preliminary study. Life Sci 1969;8:1299-1307.

119. Motivala SJ, Irwin M: Sleep deprivation and immunity. In Kushida CA (ed): Sleep Deprivation: Basic Science, Physiology, and Behavior. Vol 192: Lung Biology in Health and Disease. New York, Marcel Dekker, 2005, pp 359-386.

120. Dinges DF, Douglas SD, Zaugg L, et al: Leukocytosis and natural killer cell function parallel neurobehavioral fatigue induced by 64 hours of sleep deprivation. J Clin Invest 1994; 93:1930-1939.

121. Heisser P, Dickhaus B, Schreiber W, et al: White blood cells and cortisol after sleep deprivation and recovery sleep in humans. Eur Arch Psychiatry Clin Neurosci 2000;250:16-23.

122. Moldofsky H, Lue FA, Davidson JR, et al: Effects of sleep deprivation on human immune functions. FASEB J 1989;3:1972-1977.

123. Shearer WT, Reuben JM, Mullington JM, et al: Soluble TNF-alpha receptor 1 and IL-6 plasma levels in humans subjected to the sleep deprivation model of spaceflight. J Allergy Clin Immunol 2001;107:165-170.

124. Dinges DF, Douglas SD, Hamarman S, et al: Sleep deprivation and human immune function. Adv Neuroimmunol 1995;5:97-110.

125. Vgontzas AN, Papanicolaou DA, Bixler EO, et al: Circadian interleukin-6 secretion and quantity and depth of sleep. J Clin Endocrinol Metab 1999;84:2603-2607.

126. Moldofsky H: Central nervous system and peripheral immune functions and the sleep-wake system. J Psychiatr Neurosci 1994;19:368-374.

127. Boyum A, Wiik P, Gustavsson E, et al: The effect of strenuous exercise, calorie deficiency and sleep deprivation on white blood cells, plasma immunoglobulins and cytokines. Scand J Immunol 1996;43:228-235.

128. Brown R, Pang G, Husband AJ, et al: Suppression of immunity to influenza virus infection in the respiratory tract following sleep disturbance. Reg Immunol 1989;2:321-325.

129. Renegar KB, Crouse D, Floyd RA, et al: Progression of influenza viral infection through the murine respiratory tract: The protective role of sleep deprivation. Sleep 2000;23:859-863.

130. Benca RM, Kushida CA, Everson CA, et al: Sleep deprivation in the rat: VII. Immune function. Sleep 1989;12:47-52.

131. Cirelli C: Functional genomic of sleep and circadian rhythm invited review: How sleep deprivation affects gene expression in the brain—A review of recent findings. J Appl Physiol 2002;92:394-400.

132. Born J, Lange T, Hansen K, et al: Effects of sleep and circadian rhythm on human circulating immune cells. J Immunol 1997; 158:4454-4464.

133. Landis CA: Partial and sleep state selective deprivation. In Kushida CA (ed): Sleep Deprivation: Basic Science, Physiology, and Behavior. Vol 192: Lung Biology in Health and Disease. New York, Marcel Dekker, 2005, pp 81-102.

134. Rechtschaffen A, Bergmann BM: Sleep deprivation in the rat: An update of the 1989 paper. Sleep 2002;25:18-24.

135. Kushida CA, Bergmann BM, Rechtschaffen A: Sleep deprivation in the rat: IV. Paradoxical sleep deprivation. Sleep 1989;12:22-30.

136. Gilliland MA, Bergmann BM, Rechtschaffen A: Sleep deprivation in the rat: VIII. High EEG amplitude sleep deprivation. Sleep 1989;12:53-59.

137. Bergmann BM, Everson CA, Kushida CA, et al: Sleep deprivation in the rat: V. Energy use and mediation. Sleep 1989;12:31-41.

138. Everson CA: Functional consequences of sustained sleep deprivation in the rat. Behav Brain Res 1995;69:43-54.

139. Everson CA: Sustained sleep deprivation impairs host defense. Am J Physiol 1993;265:R1148-R1154.

140. Bergmann BM, Gilliland MA, Feng PF, et al: Are physiological effects of sleep deprivation in the rat mediated by bacterial invasion? Sleep 1996;19:554-562.

141. Obermeyer WH, Bergmann BM, Rechtschaffen A: The effect of sleep deprivation on the thermoregulatory response of rats to phentolamine. Sleep Res 1993;22:340.

142. Horne J: Why We Sleep. New York, Oxford University Press, 1987, pp 1-319.

143. Rechtschaffen A, Bergmann BM, Everson CA, et al: Sleep deprivation in the rat: X. Integration and discussion of the findings. Sleep 1989;12:68-87.

144. Dement WC, Fisher C: Experimental interference with the sleep cycle. Can Psychiatr Assoc J 1963;8:400-405.

145. Agnew HW Jr, Webb WB, Williams RL: Comparison of stage four and 1-REM sleep deprivation. Percept Mot Skills 1967;24:851-858.

146. Pearlman CA: Sleep structure variation and performance. In Webb WB (ed): Biological Rhythms, Sleep, and Performance. New York, John Wiley & Sons, 1982, pp 143-173.

147. Hobson JA, McCarley RW: The brain as a dream state generator: An activation-synthesis hypothesis of the dream process. Am J Psychiatry 1977;134:1335-1348.

148. Stern WC, Morgane PJ: Theoretical view of REM sleep function: Maintenance of catecholamine systems in the central nervous system. Behav Biol 1974;11:1-32.

149. Ephron HS, Carrington P: Rapid eye movement sleep and cortical homeostasis. Psychol Rev 1966;73:500-526.

150. Roffwarg HP, Muzio J, Dement WC: Ontogenetic development of the human sleep-dream cycle. Science 1966;152:604-619.

151. Berger RJ: Oculomotor control: A possible function for REM sleep. Psychol Rev 1969;76:144-164.

152. Maquet P: The role of sleep in learning and memory. Science 2001;294:1048-1052.

153. Stickgold R, Hobson JA, Fosse R, et al: Sleep, learning, and dreams: Off-line memory reprocessing. Science 2001;294:1052-1057.

154. Smith C: Sleep states and memory processes in humans: Procedural versus declarative memory systems. Sleep Med Rev 2001;5:491-506.

155. Peigneux P, Laureys S, Delbeuck X, et al: Sleeping brain, learning brain: The role of sleep for memory systems. Neuroreport 2001;12:A111-A124.

156. Siegel JM: The REM sleep-memory consolidation hypothesis. Science 2001;294:1058-1063.

157. Vertes RP, Eastman KE: The case against memory consolidation in REM sleep. Behav Brain Sci 2000;23:867-876.

158. Karni A, Tanne D, Rubenstein BS, et al: Dependence on REM sleep of overnight improvement of a perceptual skill. Science 1994;265:679-682.

159. Agnew HW, Webb WB, Williams RL: The effects of stage four sleep deprivation. Electroencephalogr Clin Neurophysiol 1964;17:68-70.

160. Johnson LC, Naitoh P, Moses JM, et al: Interaction of REM deprivation and stage 4 deprivation with total sleep loss: Experiment 2. Psychophysiology 1974;11:147-159.

161. Johnson LC: Are stages of sleep related to waking behavior? Am Sci 1973;61:326-338.

162. Bonnet MH, Arand DL: Clinical effects of sleep fragmentation versus sleep deprivation. Sleep Med Rev 2003;7:297-310.

163. Bonnet MH: Sleep fragmentation. In Kushida CA (ed): Sleep Deprivation: Basic Science, Physiology, and Behavior. Vol 192: Lung Biology in Health and Disease. New York, Marcel Dekker, 2005, pp 103-120.

164. Stepanski E: The effect of sleep fragmentation on daytime function. Sleep 2002;25:268-276.

165. Martin SE, Wraith PK, Deary IJ, et al: The effect of nonvisible sleep fragmentation on daytime function. Am J Respir Crit Care Med 1997;155:1596-1601.

166. Stepanski E, Lamphere J, Roehrs T, et al: Experimental sleep fragmentation in normal subjects. Int J Neurosci 1987;33:207-214.

167. Bonnet MH: Performance and sleepiness as a function of frequency and placement of sleep disruption. Psychophysiology 1986;23:263-271.

168. Bonnet MH: Performance and sleepiness following moderate sleep disruption and slow wave sleep deprivation. Physiol Behav 1986;37:915-918.

169. Spath-Schwalbe E, Gofferje M, Kern W, et al: Sleep disruption alters nocturnal ACTH and cortisol secretory patterns. Biol Psychiatry 1991;29:575-584.

170. Levine B, Roehrs T, Stepanski E, et al: Fragmenting sleep diminishes its recuperative value. Sleep 1987;10:590-599.

171. Series F, Roy N, Marc I: Effects of sleep deprivation and sleep fragmentation on upper airway collapsibility in normal subjects. Am J Respir Crit Care Med 1994;150:481-485.

172. Bonnet MH: Infrequent periodic sleep disruption: Effects on sleep, performance and mood. Physiol Behav 1989;45:1049-1055.

173. Johnson LC, Karpan WE: Autonomic correlates of the spontaneous K-complex. Psychophysiology 1968;4:444-452.

174. Townsend RE, Johnson LC, Muzet A: Effects of long term exposure to tone pulse noise on human sleep. Psychophysiology 1973;10:369-375.

175. Phillipson EA, Bowes G, Sullivan CE, et al: The influence of sleep fragmentation on arousal and ventilatory responses to respiratory stimuli. Sleep 1980;3:281-288.

176. Carskadon MA, Brown ED, Dement WC: Sleep fragmentation in the elderly: Relationship to daytime sleep tendency. Neurobiol Aging 1982;3:321-327.

177. Stepanski E, Lamphere J, Badia P, et al: Sleep fragmentation and daytime sleepiness. Sleep 1984;7:18-26.

178. Cassel W, Ploch T, Becker C, et al: Risk of traffic accidents in patients with sleep-disordered breathing: Reduction with nasal CPAP. Eur Respir J 1996;9:2606-2611.

179. Carskadon MA, Dement WC: Sleep loss in elderly volunteers. Sleep 1985;8:207-221.

180. Johnson LC, Slye ES, Dement WC: Electroencephalographic and autonomic activity during and after prolonged sleep deprivation. Psychosom Med 1965;27:415-423.

181. Bonnet MH: The effect of varying prophylactic naps on performance, alertness and mood throughout a 52-hour continuous operation. Sleep 1991;14:307-315.

182. Borbely AA, Baumann F, Brandeis D, et al: Sleep deprivation: Effect on sleep stages and EEG power density in man. Electroencephalogr Clin Neurophysiol 1981;51:483-495.

183. Nakazawa Y, Kotorii M, Ohshima M, et al: Changes in sleep pattern after sleep deprivation. Folia Psychiatr Neurol Jpn 1978;32:85-93.

184. Benoit O, Foret J, Bouard G, et al: Habitual sleep length and patterns of recovery sleep after 24 hour and 36 hour sleep deprivation. Electroencephalogr Clin Neurophysiol 1980;50:477-485.

185. Bonnet MH: Effect of 64 hours of sleep deprivation upon sleep in geriatric normals and insomniacs. Neurobiol Aging 1986;7:89-96.

186. Reynolds CF 3rd, Kupfer DJ, Hoch CC, et al: Sleep deprivation in healthy elderly men and women: Effects on mood and on sleep during recovery. Sleep 1986;9:492-501.

187. Bonnet MH, Arand DL: Sleep loss in aging. Clin Geriatr Med 1989;5:405-420.

188. Reynolds CF 3rd, Kupfer DJ, Hoch CC, et al: Sleep deprivation effects in older endogenous depressed patients. Psychiatry Res 1987;21:95-109.

189. Reynolds CF 3rd, Kupfer DJ, Hoch CC, et al: Sleep deprivation as a probe in the elderly. Arch Gen Psychiatry 1987;44:982-990.

190. Kales A, Tan T, Kollar EJ, et al: Sleep patterns following 205 hours of sleep deprivation. Psychosom Med 1970;32:189-200.

191. Lubin A, Moses JM, Johnson LC, et al: The recuperative effects of REM sleep and stage 4 sleep on human performance after complete sleep loss: Experiment I. Psychophysiology 1974;11:133-146.

192. Jewett ME, Dijk D, Kronauer RE, et al: Dose-response relationship between sleep duration and human psychomotor vigilance and subjective alertness. Sleep 1999;22:171-180.

6

Chronic Sleep Deprivation

David F. Dinges
Naomi L. Rogers
Maurice D. Baynard

ABSTRACT

Chronic sleep restriction is common in today's around-the-clock society, and it results from a wide range of factors, including medical conditions, sleep disorders, shift work, work demands, and social and domestic responsibilities. In contrast, relatively few studies have examined the neurobehavioral and physiologic consequences of chronic sleep restriction in a careful, controlled way. Many early studies provided conflicting reports of the effects on neurobehavioral functions of chronically reducing sleep duration. More recent controlled, dose–response experiments have found that chronic sleep restriction to less than 7 hours per night resulted in cognitive deficits that became progressively worse over time. Subjective assessments of sleepiness and mood were less severely affected. Only limited data are available on the physiologic effects of chronic sleep loss and its consequences for health. The mechanisms underlying the neurobehavioral and physiologic alterations during chronic sleep restriction remain largely unknown. Several theories have been advanced to explain the relationship between chronic sleep restriction and waking functions, but none completely account for the effects or offer a neurobiologic basis for the effects. A better understanding of both the effects of chronic sleep restriction and the mechanisms underlying these effects will be necessary to reduce the risks associated with the long-term accumulation of sleep debt, as well as to advance theories of sleep function.

Chronic sleep restriction occurs frequently and results from a number of factors, including medical conditions (e.g., pain), sleep disorders, work demands (including extended work hours and shift work), and social and domestic responsibilities.[1] Adverse effects on neurobehavioral functioning accumulate as the magnitude of sleep loss escalates, and the result is an increased risk of on-the-job errors, injuries, traffic accidents, personal conflicts, health complaints, and drug use.[2-5]

Chronic sleep restriction, or partial sleep deprivation, has been defined as "preventing subjects from obtaining their usual amount of sleep within a 24-hour period" (on p. 221 of Webb[6]). To determine the effects of chronic sleep loss on a range of neurobehavioral and physiologic variables, a variety of paradigms have been used, including controlled, restricted time in bed for sleep opportunities in both continuous[7] and distributed schedules,[7] gradual reductions in sleep duration over time,[8] selective deprivation of specific sleep stages,[9,10] and situations where the time in bed is individualized, such that it is reduced to a percentage of the individual's habitual time in bed.[11] These studies have ranged from 24 hours[12] to 8 months[8] in length.

The majority of experimental reports and chapter reviews published from the 1970s to the early 1990s concluded that chronic sleep restriction in the range commonly experienced by the general population (i.e., less than 7 hours per night but greater than 4 hours per night) resulted in increased subjective sleepiness but had little or no effect on cognitive performance capabilities. Consequently, there was a widely held belief that individuals could "adapt" to chronic reductions in sleep duration, down to 4 to 5 hours per day. Most of these early reports were limited, however, by a lack of experimental control over a considerable number of critical variables, including sleep actually obtained at night and during the day (e.g., naps) and the use of stimulants (caffeine, nicotine). Most of these early studies also used small sample sizes, failed to include a control group, lacked physiologic measures of sleep and waking, focused on only a few assays of performance or used performance assessments contaminated by practice effects, had infrequent assessment times within and between days, and failed to test quantitatively for cumulative neurobehavioral changes relative to the cumulative sleep debts experienced by the subjects.[11] Controlled experiments that have corrected for these methodologic weaknesses have found markedly different results from those earlier studies. This chapter reviews the cognitive and neurobehavioral consequences of chronic sleep restriction in healthy individuals and the theoretical explanations for these effects.

INCIDENCE OF CHRONIC SLEEP RESTRICTION

The duration of sleep needed to prevent daytime sleepiness, elevated sleep propensity, and cognitive deficits has been a long-standing controversy central to whether chronic sleep restriction may compromise health and behavioral functions. Self-reported sleep durations are frequently less than 8 hours per night. For example, it was recently reported that approximately 20% of more than 1.1 million Americans indicated that they slept 6.5 hours or less each night.[13] Furthermore, in a recent poll of 1000 American adults by the National Sleep Foundation, 15% of subjects (aged 18 to 84 years) reported sleeping less than 6 hours on weekdays and 10% reported sleeping less than 6 hours on weekends over the past year.[14] Scientific perspectives on the duration of sleep that defines chronic sleep restriction have come from a number of theories.

THEORETICAL PERSPECTIVES ON CHRONIC SLEEP RESTRICTION

Basal Sleep Need and Sleep Debt

The amount of sleep habitually obtained by an individual is determined by a variety of factors. Epidemiologic and experimental studies point to a high between-subjects variance in sleep duration, influenced by environmental, genetic, and societal factors. Although not clearly defined in the literature, the concept of basal sleep need has been described as habitual sleep duration in the absence of preexisting sleep debt.[15] Sleep debt has been defined as the fundamental duration of sleep below which waking deficits begin to accumulate.[16] Given these definitions, the basal need for sleep appears to be between 7 and 8 hours per day in healthy adult humans. This number was based on at least one study in which prior sleep debt was completely eliminated through repeated nights of long-duration sleep that stabilized at 8.17 hours.[17] More recently, a large-scale dose–response experiment on chronic sleep restriction statistically estimated daily sleep need to average 8.16 hours per night to avoid detrimental effects on waking functions.[18]

Core Sleep and Optional Sleep Hypothesis

In the 1980s, it was proposed that a normal nocturnal sleep period was composed of two types of sleep relative to functional adaptation: core and optional sleep.[19,20] The initial duration of sleep in the sleep period was referred to as core, or "obligatory," sleep, which was posited to "repair the effects of waking wear and tear on the cerebrum" (on p. 57 of Horne[20]). Initially, the duration of required core sleep was defined as 4 to 5 hours of sleep per night, depending on the duration of the sleep restriction.[20] The duration of core sleep has subsequently been redefined as 6 hours of (good quality, uninterrupted) sleep for most adults.[16] Additional sleep obtained beyond the period of core sleep was considered to be optional, or luxury, sleep, which "fills the tedious hours of darkness until sunrise" (on p. 57 of Horne[20]). This core versus optional theory of sleep need is often presented as analogous to the concept of appetite: hunger drives one to eat until satiated, but additional food can still be consumed beyond what the body requires.[21] It is unknown whether the so-called optional sleep serves any function.

According to the core sleep theory, only the core portion of sleep—which is dominated by slow wave sleep (SWS) and slow wave activity on an electroencephalogram (EEG)—is required to maintain adequate levels of daytime alertness and cognitive functioning.[20] The optional sleep does not contribute to this recovery or maintenance of neurobehavioral capability. This theory was strengthened by results from a mathematical model of sleep and waking functions (the three-process model) that predicted that waking neurobehavioral functions were primarily restored during SWS,[22,23] which makes up only a portion of total sleep time. However, if only the core portion of sleep is required, it would be reasonable to predict that there would be no waking neurobehavioral consequences of chronically restricting sleep to 6 hours per night, and that cognitive deficits would be evident only when sleep durations were reduced below this amount. In contrast to this prediction, however, are findings from a recent study that examined the effects of sleep chronically restricted to 4, 6, or 8 hours of time in bed per night.[18] Cognitive performance measures were relatively stable across 14 days of restriction when 8 hours time in bed was allowed for sleep. However, when time in bed for sleep was reduced to 6 or 4 hours per night, significant cumulative (dose-dependent) decreases in cognitive performance functions and increases in sleepiness were observed.[18]

Adaptation to Sleep Restriction

One hypothesis regarding the effects of sleep restriction on neurobehavioral functioning is that subjects may be acutely affected after the initial restriction of sleep length and may then be able to adapt to the reduced sleep amount, with waking neurocognitive functions unaffected further or returned to baseline levels. Although several studies have suggested that this is the case when sleep duration is restricted to approximately 4 to 6 hours per night for up to 8 months,[8,12,24-26] there is also evidence indicating that subjects show adaptation in subjective reports of sleepiness more than in objective cognitive performance parameters.[18]

One factor thought to be important in adaptation to chronic sleep restriction is the abruptness of the sleep curtailment. Although lacking important controls, reports have appeared that suggest that gradual restriction of sleep duration was more easily tolerated than abrupt curtailment.[27,28] One study examined the relationship between rate of accumulation of sleep loss, to a total of 8 hours, and neurobehavioral performance levels.[29] After 1 night of total sleep deprivation (i.e., a rapid accumulation of 8 hours of sleep loss), neurobehavioral capabilities were significantly reduced. When the accumulation of sleep loss was slower, achieved by chronically restricting sleep to 4 hours per night for 2 nights or 6 hours per night for 4 nights, neurobehavioral performance deficits were evident, but they were of a smaller magnitude than those following the night of total sleep loss. A greater degree of neurobehavioral impairment was evident in those subjects restricted to 4 hours for 2 nights than in those subjects allowed 6 hours per night, leading to the conclusion that during the slowest accumulation of 8 hours of sleep debt (i.e., 6 hours per night for 4 nights), there was evidence of a compensatory adaptive mechanism.

It has also been demonstrated recently that neurocognitive deficits from total sleep loss accumulate more rapidly than those resulting from chronic partial sleep loss.[18] There was evidence that adaptation to restricted sleep schedules was more evident in most subjective measures of sleepiness and alertness but less evident in cognitive performance measures. Despite significant decreases in cognitive functioning across 14 days of sleep restriction to 4 or 6 hours per night, compared with 8 hours per night,[18] there were no systematic sleep-dose–dependent changes over days in waking EEG measures of alpha and theta frequencies.[16] Consequently, different neurobehavioral outcomes showed markedly different responses to chronic sleep restriction, with neurocognitive functions showing the least adaptation, subjective sleepiness measures showing more adaptation, and waking EEG measures as well as non–rapid eye movement (non-REM), SWS measures showing the most adaptation.[16,18]

Two-Process Model

Although the relationship between sleep physiology (architecture) and waking neurobehavioral capabilities, especially in the face of chronic sleep restriction, has yet to be fully elucidated, a number of biomathematical models of sleep–wake regulation have been developed that make predictions about recovery in response to various sleep durations. The basis of almost all current biomathematical models of sleep–wake regulation[30] is the two-process model of sleep regulation.[31,32] This model proposes that two primary components regulate sleep: (1) a homeostatic process that builds up exponentially during wakefulness and declines exponentially during sleep (as measured by slow wave energy or delta power in the non-REM sleep EEG), and (2) a circadian process, with near–24-hour periodicity.

Since its inception, the two-process model has gained widespread acceptance for its explanation of the timing and structure of sleep. Its use has extended to predictions of waking alertness and neurobehavioral functions in response to different sleep–wake scenarios.[23,33,34] This extension of the two-process model was based on observations that as sleep pressure accumulated with increasing time awake, so did waking neurobehavioral or neurocognitive impairment; and as sleep pressure dissipated with time asleep, performance capability improved during the following period of wakefulness. In addition, forced-desynchrony experiments revealed that the sleep homeostatic and circadian processes interacted to create periods of stable wakefulness and consolidated sleep during normal 24-hour days.[35] Hence, it was postulated that waking cognitive function (alertness variable A) could be mathematically modeled as the difference between the quantitative state for the homeostatic process (S) and the quantitative state for the circadian process (C), and thus $A = S - C$. Accordingly, predictions for changes in the neurobehavioral recovery afforded by sleep of varying durations could be made on the basis of sleep–wake times and circadian phase estimates, using the quantitative version of the two-process model.

Recently, the validity of the various biomathematical models based on the two-process model, and their ability to predict actual experimental results of the neurobehavioral effects of chronic sleep restriction were evaluated in a blind test.[36] Because all current models are based on the same underlying principles as the two-process model, all yielded comparable predictions for neurobehavioral functioning in scenarios involving total sleep deprivation or chronic partial sleep restriction. All models could accurately predict waking neurobehavioral responses to total sleep deprivation. However, they all failed to adequately predict sleepiness and cognitive performance responses during chronic sleep restriction.[18,36] Hence, it appears that the extension of the two-process model to prediction of waking alertness[33] does not account for the results of chronic sleep restriction.

Wake Extension Hypothesis

A key feature of the sleep debt and core versus optional sleep hypotheses is the importance placed on cumulative sleep time lost, rather than cumulative wake time cost, in producing the effects of chronic sleep restriction (although the two-process model of sleep regulation describes alterations in the strength of the homeostatic drive for sleep as a function of prior wakefulness). Recently, it was posited that it is the accumulation of wakefulness via its neurobiologic consequences that determines the magnitude and nature of neurobehavioral deficits resulting from chronic sleep restriction.[18] This wake extension hypothesis was proposed to reconcile the results of neurocognitive performance responses to chronic sleep restriction with those from total sleep deprivation.

In a sleep dose–response experiment involving 0, 4, 6, or 8 hours of time in bed each night, it was observed that the accumulation of cognitive performance deficits across days was near-linear for all conditions, but the rate of deterioration was inversely related to the duration of sleep time, with the no-sleep condition producing the fastest rate of deterioration, consistent with the adaptation hypothesis.[18] By the end of the 14-day chronic partial sleep restriction period, the level of cognitive impairments recorded in subjects in the 4-hour sleep restriction condition was equivalent to the level of impairment seen after 1 to 2 nights without any sleep (Fig. 6–1). To understand the relationship between the different sleep loss conditions and the equivalence in performance impairment observed, the amount of cumulative sleep loss for subjects in each condition was calculated.[18] The degree of sleep loss was greater in subjects allowed 4 hours of sleep each night for 14 nights (i.e., losing approximately 55 hours of sleep) than in subjects who remained awake for 88 hours (i.e., losing approximately 25 hours of sleep) (Fig. 6–2A), suggesting that impairments in waking performance should have been much worse in the 4-hour condition. However, this was not the case (see Fig. 6–1).

To reconcile this paradox, wake extension time was defined as the difference between the duration of each continuous wake period and the duration of habitual wake time. Accordingly, cumulative wake time extension was calculated as the sum of all consecutive hours of wakefulness extending beyond the habitual duration of wakefulness that each subject was accustomed to at home. In the 4-hour, 6-hour, and 8-hour sleep restriction conditions, this yielded the same results as for cumulative sleep loss, because the definitions of cumulative wake extension and cumulative sleep loss were arithmetically equivalent. However, for the 0-hour total sleep deprivation condition, each day without sleep added 24 hours to the cumulative wake extension. Thus, over 3 days with 0 hours of sleep, cumulative wake extension was equal to 72 hours for each subject (see Fig. 6–2B), whereas cumulative sleep loss was only 23 hours (see Fig. 6–2A). These results illustrate that cumulative sleep loss and cumulative wake extension are different constructs that can have different quantitative values, depending on the manner in which sleep loss occurs. More importantly, they suggest that sleep debt is perhaps best understood as resulting in additional wakefulness beyond an average of approximately 16 hours a day, which has a neurobiologic cost that accumulates over time.[18]

EFFECTS OF CHRONIC SLEEP RESTRICTION

The effects of sleep loss may be quantified in a number of different ways, using a wide range of physiologic, neurocognitive, behavioral, and subjective tools. Many early studies examining the effects of chronic sleep restriction on cognitive performance were conducted outside a controlled laboratory setting, with little or no control over potentially contaminating factors,

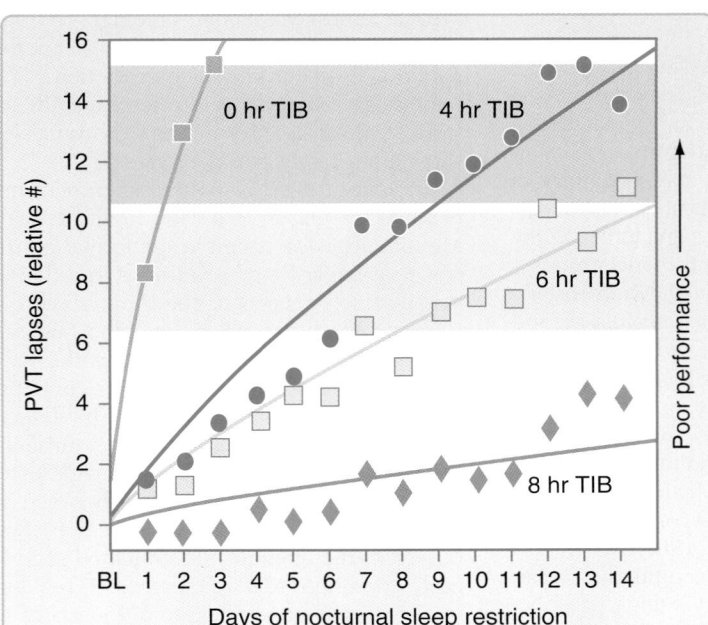

Differences among
conditions
P = .036

Curvature (SEM)
θ = 0.78 (0.04)

Effect sizes
4 hr vs. 8 hr: 1.45
6 hr vs. 8 hr: 0.71
4 hr vs. 6 hr: 0.43

Figure 6–1. Psychomotor vigilance task (PVT) performance lapses under varying doses of daily sleep. Displayed are group averages for subjects in the 8-hour *(diamond)*, 6-hour *(light blue square)*, and 4-hour *(circle)* chronic sleep period time in bed (TIB) across 14 days, and in the 0-hour *(filled square)* sleep condition across 3 days. Subjects were tested every 2 hours each day; data points represent the daily average (07:30 to 23:30) expressed relative to baseline (BL). The curves through the data points represent statistical nonlinear model–based best-fitting profiles of the response to sleep deprivation for subjects in each of the four experimental conditions. The mean ± SE. ranges of neurobehavioral functions for 1 and 2 days of 0 hours of sleep (total sleep deprivation) are shown as *light* and *dark* bands, respectively, allowing comparison of the 3-day total sleep deprivation condition and the 14-day chronic sleep restriction conditions. (Redrawn from Van Dongen HPA, Maislin G, Mullington JM, et al: The cumulative cost of additional wakefulness: Dose-response effects on neurobehavioral functions and sleep physiology from chronic sleep restriction and total sleep deprivation. Sleep 2003;26:117-126.)

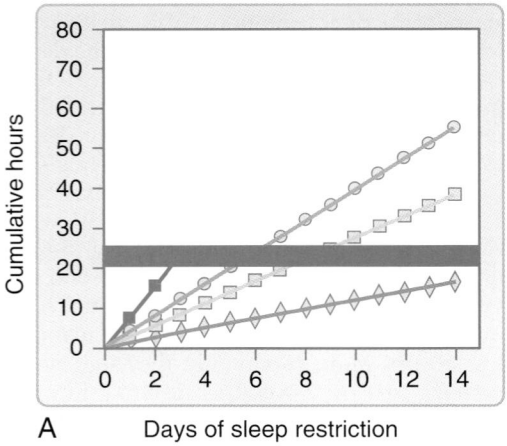

A Days of sleep restriction

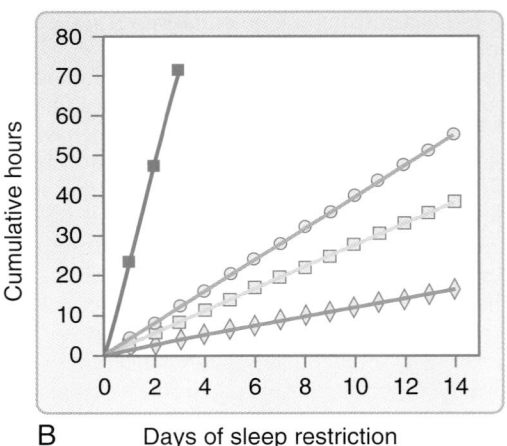

B Days of sleep restriction

Figure 6–2. Cumulative buildup of sleep loss and wake time extension across days of sleep restriction and total sleep loss. **A,** Cumulative sleep loss relative to habitual sleep duration—that is, all hours of sleep habitually obtained (as measured at home during the 5 days prior to the experiment) but not received in the experiment owing to sleep restriction. **B,** Cumulative wake extension relative to habitual wake duration—that is, all consecutive hours of wakefulness in excess of the habitual duration of a wakefulness period. Daily means are shown for subjects in the 8-hour *(diamond)*, 6-hour *(light blue square)*, 4-hour *(circle)*, and 0-hour *(dark blue square)* sleep period conditions. **A** also shows the range (dark blue band) of cumulative sleep loss (relative to habitual sleep duration) after 3 days in the 0-hour sleep condition, which was 23.1 ± 2.6 hours (mean ± SD). This was significantly less than the cumulative sleep loss after 14 days in the 4-hour sleep period condition (t_{20} = 10.58, P < .001). (Redrawn from Van Dongen HPA, Maislin G, Mullington JM, et al: The cumulative cost of additional wakefulness: Dose-response effects on neurobehavioral functions and sleep physiology from chronic sleep restriction and total sleep deprivation. Sleep 2003;26:117-126.)

such as the level of napping, extension of sleep periods, diet, stimulant use (e.g., caffeine, nicotine), activity, or exposure to zeitgebers (environmental time cues). The majority of these studies concluded that there were few or no detrimental effects on waking neurobehavioral capabilities, or subjective effects of the sleep restriction. For example, restriction of nocturnal sleep periods to between approximately 4 and 6 hours per night for up to 8 months produced no significant effects on a range of cognitive outcomes, including vigilance performance,[12,24,25] psychomotor performance,[8] logical reasoning,[37] addition, or working memory.[12] In addition, few effects on subjective assessments of sleepiness[25] or mood were reported.[12]

Later studies, however, with greater experimental control and conducted inside a controlled laboratory setting have demonstrated significant impairment of cognitive functioning and changes in measures of sleep propensity, subjective assessments of sleepiness and mood, and risk of motor vehicle crashes.

Sleep Propensity

With the development and validation of sleep latency measures as sensitive indices of sleep propensity,[38] the effects of chronic sleep restriction could be evaluated physiologically. The daytime Multiple Sleep Latency Test (MSLT)[38] has been shown to systematically vary linearly after 1 night of sleep restricted to between 1 and 5 hours of time in bed.[38] In a seminal experiment, it was reported that progressive decreases in daytime sleep latency occurred (i.e., increases in sleep propensity) across 7 days of sleep restricted to 5 hours per night in healthy young adults,[40] a finding confirmed in a later study using the psychomotor vigilance task (PVT) as a measure of daytime behavioral alertness.[11]

Dose–response effects of chronic sleep restriction on daytime MSLT values have recently been reported in a major sleep study in commercial truck drivers.[26] A significant increase in sleep propensity across 7 days of sleep restricted to either 3 or 5 hours per night was observed, with no increase in sleep propensity found when sleep was restricted to 7 or 9 hours per night.[26] Similarly, sleep propensity (as measured by the maintenance of wakefulness test[41]) during 7 days of sleep restriction to 4 hours per night was reported to increase, especially in subjects whose sleep was restricted by advancing sleep offset.[42] Finally, in an epidemiologic study of predictors of objective sleep tendency in the general population,[43] a dose–response relationship was found between self-reported nighttime sleep duration and objective sleep tendency as measured by MSLT. Persons reporting more than 7.5 hours of sleep had significantly less probability of falling asleep on the MSLT than those reporting between 6.75 and 7.5 hours per night (27% risk of falling asleep), and than those reporting sleep durations less than 6.75 hours per night (73% risk of falling asleep).[43] All of these studies suggest that chronic curtailment of nocturnal sleep increases daytime sleep propensity.

Cognitive Effects

Only a small number of investigators have studied the waking cognitive effects of chronic sleep restriction (e.g., for 7 days) in a controlled, laboratory setting to ensure that subjects obtain only the sleep durations they were assigned, and that they use no stimulants (e.g., caffeine, nicotine) or other techniques to reduce sleepiness. One early study examined the effects of reducing habitual sleep time by 40% for 5 nights.[39] Decreases in performance on a vigilance and simple reaction time performance task were observed across the protocol with sleep restriction. Interestingly, however, there was no effect of sleep restriction on a choice reaction time task, suggesting that not all measures of performance are equally sensitive to chronic sleep restriction. This could result from any of a number of aspects of the tests' psychometric properties (e.g., learning curves) or from their neurobiologic substrates—negative findings provide no insight into the reason for lack of sensitivity.

More recently, two large-scale experimental studies were published that describe dose-related effects of chronic sleep restriction on neurobehavioral performance measures.[18,26] In one study, truck drivers were randomized to 7 nights of 3, 5, 7, or 9 hours of time in bed for sleep per night.[26] Cognitive performance was assessed using the psychomotor vigilance task (PVT). Subjects in the 3- and 5-hour time-in-bed groups experienced a decrease in performance across days of the sleep restriction protocol, with increases in the mean reaction time, in the number of lapses, and in the time for the fastest reaction on the PVT.[26] In the subjects allowed 7 hours of time in bed per night, a significant decrease in mean response speed was also evident, although no effect on lapses was evident. Performance in the group allowed 9 hours of time in bed was stable across the 7 days. As in an earlier report examining cognitive performance effects of 7 nights of sleep restricted to 5 hours per night,[11] there appeared to be an adaptation of subjects to the new sleep schedule, in that cognitive deficits did not appear to continue to accumulate beyond approximately 5 to 6 days of sleep restriction, although neither study evaluated this question statistically.

In an equally large experiment,[18] young adults had their sleep duration restricted to 4, 6, or 8 hours of time in bed per night for 14 nights, and daytime deficits in cognitive functions were observed for lapses on the PVT, for a memory task, and for a cognitive throughput task. These performance deficits accumulated across the experimental protocol in those subjects allowed less than 8 hours of sleep per night.[18] Data from this study demonstrate that sleep restriction–induced deficits continued to accumulate beyond 7 nights of restriction used in other experiments,[11,26,40,44] with performance deficits still increasing at day 14 of the restricted sleep schedule. To quantify the magnitude of cognitive deficits experienced with 14 days of restricted sleep, the findings from the 4, 6, or 8 hours of time in bed dose–response study were compared with cognitive effects of nearly 4 days of total sleep deprivation.[18] This comparison revealed that both 4 and 6 hours of time in bed for sleep per night for 14 nights produced cognitive decrements equivalent to what occur when individuals remain awake for 24 to 48 hours.[18] Other recent studies have reported preliminary findings of chronic sleep restriction on cognitive performance that are complementary to these reports.[45,46]

It appears that the neurocognitive effects of restricting nocturnal sleep to 6 or 4 hours per night on a chronic basis are fundamentally the same as when sleep is chronically restricted but placed diurnally.[47] The primary difference between the nocturnally[18] and diurnally[47] placed restricted sleep periods is that the magnitude of neurobehavioral impairment is significantly greater with daytime sleep compared with nighttime sleep, reflecting a combined influence of the homeostatic and circadian systems.

All these studies suggest that when time in bed for sleep is chronically restricted to less than 7 hours per night in healthy adults, cumulative deficits in a variety of cognitive performance functions become evident. These deficits can accumulate to levels of impairment equivalent to those observed after 1 or even 2 nights of total sleep deprivation.

Subjective Sleepiness and Mood

Although some earlier studies of chronic sleep restriction reported few effects on subjective sleepiness, most subsequent studies have found effects. However, in contrast to reports of continuing accumulation of cognitive deficits associated with chronic sleep restriction, subjective assessments of sleepiness and alertness demonstrate near-saturating functions across periods of sleep restriction. The sensitivity of the Stanford Sleepiness Scale (SSS) to sleep restriction across 5 nights has been demonstrated experimentally, with elevations in subjective sleepiness recorded across the protocol using this scale.[48] It was found, however, that the subjective ratings of sleepiness did not predict the degree of performance impairment induced by the sleep restriction protocol, and they tended to underestimate the degree of neurobehavioral dysfunction induced by the sleep loss. Subsequent studies have demonstrated this to be a common phenomenon.

An additional study reported an immediate increase in subjective sleepiness, using the SSS, when sleep periods were reduced to 5 hours per night.[40] This increase reached a plateau after 4 days of the restricted sleep schedule, however. In the same study, subjective sleepiness was also assessed using a visual analogue scale. This scale showed an increase in sleepiness after 2 nights of restricted sleep, but like the SSS, a plateau after 4 nights of sleep restriction. In a further sleep restriction experiment using a similar experimental paradigm, similar effects on subjective sleepiness, with an immediate increase in SSS scores and Profile of Mood States fatigue scores, which preceded the decrease in neurocognitive functioning by about 1 day, were reported.[11] Consistent with earlier reports, two recent sleep dose–response experiments[18,26] revealed only limited effects of chronic sleep restriction on measures of subjective sleepiness and mood states. Subjective sleepiness and fatigue were elevated in subjects allocated 4 or 6 hours of sleep per night, but the rate of accumulation across restriction days was less than the rate of accumulation of cognitive deficits, and there were initial increases in subjective sleepiness at the beginning of the sleep restriction protocol, with only small increases on subsequent days. Consequently, it appears that subjective assessment of sleepiness during periods of chronic sleep restriction shows an immediate elevation, but this response reaches a plateau after a few days and does not demonstrate the cumulative increases that are evident in cognitive performance measures.

Reports of increased mood disturbance and negative mood states,[11,28] greater effort to perform, and decreased motivation[46] have also been observed during chronic sleep restriction, although like sleepiness reports, these effects are neither large nor ubiquitous. Few studies have examined the incidence of self-reported symptoms during sleep restriction protocols. During a gradual induction of sleep restriction across 6 to 8 months, subjects reported an increased incidence of blurry vision, eye dryness, itching, and aching, and increased hunger.[8] More recently, an increased incidence of headache in subjects restricted to 4 hours of time in bed per night compared with subjects allowed 8 hours was reported.[49]

Driving Performance

One real-world implication of decreased cognitive functioning associated with chronic sleep restriction is decreased driving ability and increased risk of motor vehicle crashes. Few studies, however, have examined the influence of chronic sleep restriction on these parameters. The majority of studies conducted have been anecdotal and have investigated only the effects of short-term sleep restriction on driving ability and crash risk.[50,51] There does appear to be an association, however. A recent epidemiologic study found an increased incidence of sleep-related crashes in drivers reporting less than 7 hours of sleep per night on average.[52] Additional contributing factors to these sleep- or sleepiness-related crashes included poor sleep quality, dissatisfaction with sleep duration (i.e., undersleeping), daytime sleepiness, previous instances of driving drowsy, and time driving and time of day (driving late at night). Studies have also examined the effects of sleep restriction on performance on a driving simulator. Following 1 night of restricted sleep (5 hours), a decrease in performance on a driving simulator, with a concurrent increase in subjectively reported sleepiness, was found.[53] In addition, during chronic sleep restriction in a controlled laboratory, with sleep durations reduced to between 4 and 6 hours per 24 hours, placed either nocturnally or diurnally, significant increases in the rate of accidents on a driving simulator occurred with decreased sleep durations, independent of the timing of the sleep period.[54] A similar finding was reported following 2 nights of restricted sleep.[55]

PHYSIOLOGIC EFFECTS

In addition to the neurobehavioral effects of chronic sleep restriction that have been extensively studied, there is increasing evidence of physiologic and health-related consequences of chronic sleep restriction. In addition to the sleep propensity measures reviewed earlier, different physiologic measures have been employed during sleep restriction studies in an attempt to quantify sleepiness and obtain physiologic correlates of sleepiness and sleep loss. Alterations in other physiologic parameters, such as endocrine and immune activity, have also been recognized and have implications for health status and risk.

Several anecdotal and longitudinal studies have reported an increased incidence and risk of medical disorders and health dysfunction related to shift work schedules, which have been attributed to both circadian disruption and chronic sleep disturbance (for a review, see Rogers and Dinges[56]). Further links between sleep disturbance and health effects have been reported in studies examining insomniac patients and patients with other sleep and medical disorders that disturb sleep.[1] In addition, an elevated mortality risk in those individuals who reported sleeping less than 6.5 hours per night has been recently reported.[13] One provocative discovery from this study was the finding that individuals sleeping more than 7.4 hours per night were also at an elevated risk of mortality. This finding is similar to that reported from the Nurses' Health Study,[57] where subjects reporting greater than 9 hours of sleep per night on average were at a higher risk for coronary events compared with those sleeping 8 hours per night. In addition, an increased risk of coronary events in women obtaining 7 hours of sleep or less per night was observed.[57]

Polysomnography, Waking EEG, and Electrooculogram Effects

Changes in various sleep physiology variables in response to sleep restriction have been reported,[18,58] including alterations in REM sleep and non-REM EEG slow wave energy. These changes have been hypothesized to reflect both increased homeostatic pressure for sleep and the recovery potential of sleep. After acute periods of both total and partial sleep deprivation, a rebound increase in slow wave sleep (SWS) (or deep sleep) has been reported during the first sleep period after the deprivation.[40,59-62] Subsequent studies examining sleep architecture during chronic periods of sleep restriction have demonstrated a consistent conservation of SWS at the expense of other non-REM and REM sleep stages.[18,26,42,58] In addition, elevations in slow wave activity (SWA), derived from spectral analysis of the sleep EEG in the range of 0.5 to 4.5 Hz, during non-REM sleep have also been reported during and after chronic sleep restriction.[18,58] Furthermore, because of the conservation of the amount of SWS and SWA during restricted sleep protocols, independent of sleep duration (e.g., 8 hours of time in bed or 4 hours of time in bed), it has been proposed that, with regard to behavioral and physiologic outcomes, these phenomena provide the recovery aspects of sleep. However, it is also clear that non-REM SWA does not show increases at the levels found after total sleep deprivation or after chronic sleep restriction, even though cognitive performance can be comparably impaired.[18] Consequently, although SWS and non-REM SWA may be conserved in chronic sleep restriction (to 4 to 7 hours per night), they do not appear to reflect the severity of daytime cognitive deficits or to protect against these deficits, raising serious doubts about SWS and non-REM SWA being the only aspects of sleep critical to waking functions.[18]

In addition to examining the EEG during sleep, several researchers have examined changes in the waking EEG as sleep debt and homeostatic pressure for sleep accumulate. Significant increases in power densities in the delta range (3.75 to 4.5 Hz) and decreases in the alpha range (9.25 to 10 Hz) have been reported in subjects exposed to 4 hours of sleep restriction for 4 nights.[58] In contrast, no effect on waking alpha power (8 to 12 Hz) across days of restriction was evident in subjects restricted to 4 or 6 hours of time in bed for sleep per night for 14 nights.[16] An increase in theta power (4 to 8 Hz) across days of the sleep restriction protocol was evident; however, there was no significant difference in theta power changes between restriction conditions.

One further area that has been proposed as a physiologic correlate of increased sleepiness is oculomotor activity. Eye movements and eye closures have been studied during sleep loss protocols, under the premise that changes in the number and rate of movements and eyelid closures are a reflection of increased sleep propensity and precursors of the eventual onset of sleep. It has been demonstrated experimentally that slow eyelid closures during performance are associated with vigilance lapses and are sensitive indices of sleep deprivation,[63] and slow eyelid closures have been found to be a sign of drowsiness while driving.[64,65] Chronic sleep restriction has been reported to lead to a decrease in saccadic velocity in subjects allowed only 3 hours or 5 hours of time in bed for sleep over 7 nights, and to an increase in the latency to pupil constriction.[66] These changes in oculomotor activity were positively correlated with sleep latency, subjective sleepiness measures, and accidents on a simulated driving task.[66]

Endocrine and Metabolic Effects

A number of studies have examined the effects of sleep loss on a range of neuroendocrine variables. Total sleep deprivation reductions in circulating levels of growth hormone,[67,68] leptin,[69] thyroid axis hormones,[70,71] and cortisol,[72,73] with no effect on melatonin,[74] have been reported. In addition, 1 night of sleep restriction has been associated with changes in levels of catecholamines (adrenaline and noradrenaline),[75] thyroid axis hormones (thyroid-stimulating hormone, thyroxine, triiodothyronine), cortisol,[76-79] prolactin, luteinizing hormone, and estradiol, with no effect on growth hormone or follicle-stimulating hormone levels.[80]

A number of recent studies have focused on endocrine and metabolic consequences of chronic sleep restriction. Comparison of sleep restriction (4 hours per night for 6 nights) with sleep extension (12 hours per night for 6 nights) revealed an elevation in evening cortisol, increased sympathetic activation, decreased thyrotropin activity, and decreased glucose tolerance in the restricted versus extended sleep condition.[81] Similarly, an elevation in evening cortisol levels and an advance in the timing of the morning peak in cortisol, so that the relationship between sleep termination and cortisol acrophase was maintained, were found after 10 nights of sleep restricted to 4.2 hours of time in bed for sleep each night compared with baseline measures and a control group allowed 8.2 hours of time in bed for sleep for 10 nights.[82] In the same protocol, significant delays in melatonin onset[83] and in the timing of the peak in growth hormone, equivalent to the delay in sleep onset induced to achieve the restricted sleep period, were found, with no effect on growth hormone levels during the sleep period.[84] Similarly, changes in the timing of the growth hormone secretory profile associated with sleep restriction to 4 hours per night for 6 nights, with a bimodal secretory pattern evolving, have also been reported.[85] In addition, a decrease in leptin levels following sleep restriction to 4 hours per night for either 6 nights or 2 nights, relative to when subjects were allowed 12 hours of sleep per night for the same duration, has been observed.[86] The authors concluded that sleep restriction produced alterations in leptin levels, which in turn altered signaling of hunger and appetite, which may promote increased weight gain and obesity. A decrease in serum leptin was also observed in subjects restricted to 4 hours per night for 7 nights, independent of whether their sleep was restricted via delaying sleep onset or advancing sleep offset.[42]

Immune and Inflammatory Effects

Although it has long been recognized that a relationship between sleep and the immune system exists, the majority of studies examining sleep loss and immune function have concentrated on total sleep deprivation or 1 night of sleep restriction. Changes in natural killer cell activity,[87,88] lymphokine-activated killer cell activity,[88] interleukin-6,[77,89] and soluble tumor necrosis factor-alpha receptor 1[89] have all been reported with total and partial sleep deprivation.

Two recent studies have examined the relationship between chronic sleep duration and antibody production. In one study, it was reported that antibody titers were decreased—by more than 50%—10 days after vaccination for influenza in subjects who were vaccinated immediately after 6 nights of sleep restricted to 4 hours per night, compared with those who were vaccinated after habitual sleep duration.[90] By 3 to 4 weeks after the vaccination, there was no difference in antibody level between the two subject groups. Hence, being in a state of sleep debt appeared to alter the acute immune response to vaccination, decreasing the viability of the vaccine in the short term. In the other study, attenuation in the febrile response to an endotoxin (*Escherichia coli*) challenge in subjects undergoing chronic sleep restriction to 4 hours of time in bed per night for 10 nights, relative to subjects allowed 8 hours of time in bed, was observed.[91]

Cardiovascular Effects

An increase in cardiovascular events and cardiovascular morbidity associated with reduced sleep durations has been highlighted in a number of epidemiologic studies[13,57,92-95] and in a case-control study examining insufficient sleep due to work demands.[96] In the Nurses' Health Study,[57] there was evidence of increased risk of coronary events in women obtaining 7 hours of sleep or less per night compared with those averaging 8 hours per night. In another epidemiologic study, a twofold to threefold increase in risk of cardiovascular events in subjects with an average sleep duration of 5 hours or less per night, or chronically having less than 5 hours of sleep per night at least twice per week, was reported.[96] Similar findings have also been observed in studies examining cardiovascular health in shift workers, who typically experience chronic reductions in sleep duration in addition to circadian disruption.[97-100]

The mechanism underlying the link between chronic sleep restriction and increased cardiovascular risk is unknown, but one potential mechanism may be via activation of inflammatory processes during sleep loss. C-reactive protein (CRP) is an inflammatory marker that is modulated by sleep loss, and it is predictive of increased risk for cardiovascular disease. In a recent report, increased CRP levels were found in obstructive sleep apnea patients, who commonly experience reduced sleep durations because of sleep fragmentation and hypoxia.[101] Furthermore, an increase in CRP levels has been reported following both total and partial sleep deprivation protocols in healthy subjects.[102] It remains to be determined how chronic sleep restriction activates mechanisms involved in cardiovascular morbidity and mortality.

> ### Clinical Pearl
> *The physician should be aware of the pandemic of chronic sleep restriction that accompanies sleep disorders, certain work schedules, and modern lifestyles, and of the adverse effects of chronic sleep restriction on daytime sleep propensity, cognitive functions, driving safety, mood, and physiologic conditions.*

Acknowledgments

The substantive evaluation on which this chapter was based was supported by National Institutes of Health grants NR04281 and RR00040, and by National Aeronautics and Space Administration Cooperative Agreement NCC 9-58 with the National Space Biomedical Research Institute.

REFERENCES

1. Bonnet MH, Arand DL: Clinical effects of sleep fragmentation versus sleep deprivation. Sleep Med Rev 2003;7:297-310.
2. Bell RB, Davison M, Sefcik D: A first survey: Measuring burnout in emergency medicine physician assistants. J Am Acad Phys Assist 2002;15:40-52.
3. Costa G: The problem: Shiftwork. Chronobiol Int 1997;14: 89-98.
4. Davis S, Mirick DK, Stevens RG: Night shift work, light at night, and risk of breast cancer. J Natl Cancer Inst 2001;93: 1557-1562.
5. Dinges DF: An overview of sleepiness and accidents. J Sleep Res 1995;4:4-14.
6. Webb WB: Partial and differential sleep deprivation. In Kales AA (ed): Sleep: Physiology and Pathology—A Symposium. Philadelphia, JB Lippincott, 1969, pp 221-231.
7. Hartley LR: A comparison of continuous and distributed and reduced sleep schedules. Q J Exp Psychol 1974;26:8-14.
8. Friedmann J, Globus G, Huntley A, et al: Performance and mood during and after gradual sleep reduction. Psychophysiology 1977;14:245-250.
9. Walsh JK, Hartman PG, Schweitzer PK: Slow-wave sleep deprivation and waking function. J Sleep Res 1994;3:16-25.
10. Ferrara M, De Gennaro L, Bertini M: The effects of slow-wave sleep (SWS) deprivation and time of night on behavioral performance upon awakening. Physiol Behav 1999;68:55-61.
11. Dinges DF, Pack F, Williams K, et al: Cumulative sleepiness, mood disturbance, and psychomotor vigilance performance decrements during a week of sleep restricted to 4-5 hours per night. Sleep 1997;20:267-277.
12. Webb WB, Agnew HW Jr: The effects of a chronic limitation of sleep length. Psychophysiology 1974;11:265-274.
13. Kripke DF, Garfinkel L, Wingard DL, et al: Mortality associated with sleep duration and insomnia. Arch Gen Psychiatry 2002;59:131-136.
14. National Sleep Foundation: Sleep in America Poll 2002. Washington, DC, National Sleep Foundation, 2002.
15. Dement WC, Vaughan C: The Promise of Sleep. New York, Dell, 1999.
16. Van Dongen HPA, Rogers NL, Dinges DF: Understanding sleep debt: Theoretical and empirical issues. Sleep Biol Rhythms 2003;1:4-12.
17. Wehr TA, Moul DE, Barbato G, et al: Conservation of photoperiod-responsive mechanisms in humans. Am J Physiol 1993;265: R846-R857.
18. Van Dongen HPA, Maislin G, Mullington JM, et al: The cumulative cost of additional wakefulness: Dose-response effects on neurobehavioral functions and sleep physiology from chronic sleep restriction and total sleep deprivation. Sleep 2003;26: 117-126.
19. Horne JA: Sleep function, with particular reference to sleep deprivation. Ann Clin Res 1985;17:199-208.
20. Horne JA: Why We Sleep: The Functions of Sleep in Humans and Other Mammals. Oxford, Oxford University Press, 1988.
21. Bonnet MH: Sleep deprivation. In Kryger MH, Roth T, Dement WC (eds): Principles and Practices of Sleep Medicine. Philadelphia, WB Saunders, 1994, pp 50-67.
22. Folkard S, Akerstedt T: A three-process model of the regulation of alertness-sleepiness. In Broughton RJ, Ogilvie RD (eds): Sleep, Arousal and Performance. Boston, Birkhauser, 1992, pp 11-26.
23. Akerstedt T, Folkard S: The three-process model of alertness and its extension to performance, sleep latency, and sleep length. Chronobiol Int 1997;14:115-123.
24. Lubin A: Performance under sleep loss and fatigue. In Kety SS, Evarts EV, Williams HL (eds): Sleep and Altered States of Consciousness. New York, Williams & Wilkins, 1967, pp 507-513.

25. Horne JA, Pettitt AN: High incentive effects on vigilance performance during 72 hours of total sleep deprivation. Acta Psychol (Amst) 1985;58:123-139.

26. Belenky G, Wesensten NJ, Thorne DR, et al: Patterns of performance degradation and restoration during sleep restriction and subsequent recovery: A sleep dose-response study. J Sleep Res 2003;12:1-12.

27. Horne JA, Wilkinson S: Chronic sleep reduction: Daytime vigilance performance and EEG measures of sleepiness, with particular reference to "practice" effects. Psychophysiology 1985;22:69-78.

28. Johnson LC, MacLeod WL: Sleep and awake behavior during gradual sleep reduction. Percept Mot Skills 1973;36:87-97.

29. Drake CL, Roehrs TA, Burduvali E, et al: Effects of rapid versus slow accumulation of eight hours of sleep loss. Psychophysiology 2001;38:979-987.

30. Mallis MM, Mejdal S, Nguyen TT, Dinges DF: Summary of the key features of seven biomathematical models of human fatigue and performance. Aviat Space Environ Med 2004; 75(Suppl 3):A4-A14.

31. Daan S, Beersma DGM, Borbély AA: Timing of human sleep: Recovery process gated by a circadian pacemaker. Am J Physiol 1984;246:R161-R178.

32. Borbély AA: A two process model of sleep regulation. Hum Neurobiol 1982;1:195-204.

33. Borbély AA, Achermann P: Sleep homeostasis and models of sleep regulation. J Biol Rhythms 1999;14:557-568.

34. Jewett ME, Kronauer RE: Interactive mathematical models of subjective alertness and cognitive throughput in humans. J Biol Rhythms 1999;14:588-597.

35. Dijk DJ, Czeisler CA: Paradoxical timing of the circadian rhythm of sleep propensity serves to consolidate sleep and wakefulness in humans. Neurosci Lett 1994;166:63-68.

36. Van Dongen HPA: Comparison of mathematical model predictions to experimental data of fatigue and performance. Aviat Space Environ Med 2004;75(Suppl 3):A15-A36.

37. Blagrove M, Alexander C, Horne JA: The effects of chronic sleep reduction on the performance of cognitive tasks sensitive to sleep deprivation. Appl Cogn Psychol 1995;9:21-40.

38. Carskadon MA, Dement WC: The multiple sleep latency test: What does it measure? Sleep 1982;5:S67-S72.

39. Herscovitch J, Broughton R: Performance deficits following short-term partial sleep deprivation and subsequent recovery oversleeping. Can J Psychol 1981;35:309-322.

40. Carskadon MA, Dement WC: Cumulative effects of sleep restriction on daytime sleepiness. Psychophysiology 1981;18: 107-113.

41. Mitler MM, Gujavarly KS, Browman CP: Maintenance of wakefulness test: A polysomnographic technique for evaluating treatment in patients. Electroencephalogr Clin Neurophysiol 1982; 53:658-661.

42. Guilleminault C, Powell NB, Martinez S, et al: Preliminary observations on the effects of sleep time in a sleep restriction paradigm. Sleep Med 2003;4:177-184.

43. Punjabi NM, Bandeen-Roche K, Young T: Predictors of objective sleep tendency in the general population. Sleep 2003;26: 678-683.

44. Devoto A, Lucidi F, Violani C, et al: Effects of different sleep reductions on daytime sleepiness. Sleep 1999;22:336-343.

45. Milner CE, Osip SL, Moore JE, et al: Physiological sleepiness and performance during continuous sleep restriction. Sleep 2003;26:A179.

46. Ewing SB, Balachandran DD, LeBeau L, et al: Subjective and objective indices of sleep loss: Effects of chronic partial sleep restriction. Sleep 2002;25:A448.

47. Rogers NL, Van Dongen HPA, Powell I, et al: Neurobehavioural functioning during chronic sleep restriction at an adverse circadian phase. Sleep 2002;25:A126-A127.

48. Herscovitch J, Broughton R: Sensitivity of the Stanford Sleepiness Scale to the effects of cumulative partial sleep deprivation and recovery oversleeping. Sleep 1981;4:83-91.

49. Haack M, Broussard J, Repp A, et al: Increased headache frequency during chronic sleep restriction in healthy human subjects. Sleep 2003;26:A206-A207.

50. Philip P, Ghorayeb I, Stoohs R, et al: Determinants of sleepiness in automobile drivers. J Psychosom Res 1996;41:279-288.

51. Philip P, Taillard J, Guilleminault C, et al: Long distance driving and self-induced sleep deprivation among automobile drivers. Sleep 1999;22:475-480.

52. Stutts JC, Wilkins JW, Osberg JS, et al: Driver risk factors for sleep-related crashes. Accid Anal Prev 2003;35:321-331.

53. Horne JA, Baulk SD: Awareness of sleepiness when driving. Psychophysiology 2004;41:161-165.

54. Dorrian J, Dinges DF, Rider RL, et al: Simulated driving performance during chronic partial sleep deprivation. Sleep 2003;26:A182-A183.

55. Rupp TL, Arnedt JT, Carskadon MA: Effects of sleep restriction on performance of a combined driving simulation/cognitive task. Sleep 2003;26:A193-A194.

56. Rogers NL, Dinges DF: Shiftwork, circadian disruption and consequences. Econ Neurosci 2001;6:58-64.

57. Ayas NT, White DP, Manson JE, et al: A prospective study of sleep duration and coronary heart disease in women. Arch Intern Med 2003;163:205-209.

58. Brunner DP, Dijk DJ, Borbély AA: Repeated partial sleep deprivation progressively changes in EEG during sleep and wakefulness. Sleep 1993;16:100-113.

59. Berger RJ, Oswald I: Effects of sleep deprivation on behaviour, subsequent sleep, and dreaming. J Ment Sci 1962;108:457-465.

60. Dement W, Greenberg S: Changes in total amount of stage four sleep as a function of partial sleep deprivation. Electroencephalogr Clin Neurophysiol 1966;20:523-526.

61. Webb WB, Agnew HW Jr: Sleep: Effects of a restricted regime. Science 1965;150:1745-1747.

62. Williams HL, Hammack JT, Daly RL, et al: Responses to auditory stimulation, sleep loss and the EEG stages of sleep. Electroencephalogr Clin Neurophysiol 1964;16:269-279.

63. Price NJ, Maislin G, Powell JW, et al: Unobtrusive detection of drowsiness-induced PVT lapses using infrared retinal reflectance of slow eyelid closures. Sleep 2003;26:A177-A178.

64. Wierwille WW, Ellsworth LA, Wreggit SS, et al: Research on vehicle-based driver status/performance monitoring: Development, validating, and refinement of algorithms for detection of driver drowsiness. National Traffic Safety Administration Final Report, DOT HS 808 247, 1994.

65. Wierwille WW, Ellsworth LA: Evaluation of driver drowsiness by trained raters. Accid Anal Prev 1994;26:571-581.

66. Russo M, Thomas M, Thorne D, et al: Oculomotor impairment during chronic partial sleep deprivation. Clin Neurophysiol 2003;114:723-736.

67. Radomski MW, Hart LE, Goodman JM, et al: Aerobic fitness and hormonal responses to prolonged sleep deprivation and sustained mental work. Aviat Space Environ Med 1992;63:101-106.

68. Seifritz E, Hemmeter U, Trachsel L, et al: Effects of flumazenil on recovery sleep and hormonal secretion after sleep deprivation in male controls. Psychopharmacology 1995;120:449-456.

69. Mullington JM, Chan JL, Van Dongen HP, et al: Sleep loss reduces diurnal rhythm amplitude of leptin in healthy men. J Neuroendocrinol 2003;15:851-854.

70. Allan JS, Czeisler CA: Persistence of the circadian thyrotropin rhythm under constant conditions and after light-induced shifts of circadian phase. J Clin Endocrinol Metab 1994;79: 508-512.

71. Gary KA, Winokur A, Douglas SD, et al: Total sleep deprivation and the thyroid axis: Effects of sleep and waking activity. Aviat Space Environ Med 1996;67:513-519.

72. Weitzman ED, Zimmerman JC, Czeisler CA, et al: Cortisol secretion is inhibited during sleep in normal man. J Clin Endocrinol Metab 1983;56:352-358.

73. Akerstedt T, Palmblad J, de la Torre B, et al: Adrenocortical and gonadal steroids during sleep deprivation. Sleep 1980;3: 23-30.

74. Morris M, Lack L, Barrett J: The effect of sleep/wake state on nocturnal melatonin excretion. J Pineal Res 1990;9:133-138.

75. Irwin M, Thompson J, Miller C, et al: Effects of sleep and sleep deprivation on catecholamine and interleukin-2 levels in humans: Clinical implications. J Clin Endocrinol Metab 1999; 84:1979-1985.

76. Saletu B, Dietzel M, Lesch OM, et al: Effect of biologically active light and partial sleep deprivation on sleep, awakening and circadian rhythms in normals. Eur Neurol 1986;25:82-92.

77. Redwine L, Hauger RL, Gillin JC, et al: Effects of sleep and sleep deprivation on interleukin-6, growth hormone, cortisol, and melatonin levels in humans. J Clin Endocrinol Metab 2000;85: 3597-3603.

78. Leproult R, Copinschi G, Buxton O, et al: Sleep loss results in an elevation of cortisol levels the next evening. Sleep 1997; 20:865-870.

79. Touitou Y, Benoit O, Foret J, et al: Effects of a two-hour early awakening and of bright light exposure on plasma patterns of cortisol, melatonin, prolactin and testosterone in man. Acta Endocrinol 1992;126:201-205.

80. Baumgartner A, Dietzel M, Saletu B, et al: Influence of partial sleep deprivation on the secretion of thyrotropin, thyroid hormones, growth hormone, prolactin, luteinizing hormone, follicle stimulating hormone, and estradiol in healthy young women. Psychiatry Res 1993;48:153-178.

81. Spiegel K, Leproult R, Van Cauter E: Impact of sleep debt on metabolic and endocrine function. Lancet 1999;354: 1435-1439.

82. Rogers NL, Price NJ, Mullington JM, et al: Plasma cortisol changes following chronic sleep restriction. Sleep 2000;23: A70-A71.

83. Ecker AJ, Schaechter J, Price NJ, et al: Changes in plasma melatonin secretion following chronic sleep restriction. Sleep 2000;23:A184-A185.

84. Orthmann J, Rogers NL, Price NJ, et al: Changes in plasma growth hormone levels following chronic sleep restriction. Sleep 2001;24:A248-A249.

85. Spiegel K, Leproult R, Colecchia EF, et al: Adaptation of the 24-h growth hormone profile to a state of sleep debt. Am J Physiol Regul Integr Comp Physiol 2000;279:R874-R883.

86. Spiegel K, Leproult R, Tasali E, et al: Sleep curtailment results in decreased leptin levels and increased hunger and appetite. Sleep 2003;26:A174.

87. Irwin M, Mascovich A, Gillin JC, et al: Partial sleep deprivation reduces natural killer cell activity in humans. Psychosom Med 1994;56:493-498.

88. Irwin M, McClintick J, Costlow C, et al: Partial night sleep deprivation reduces natural killer and cellular immune responses in humans. FASEB J 1996;10:643-653.

89. Shearer WT, Reuben JM, Mullington JM, et al: Soluble TNF-alpha receptor 1 and IL-6 plasma levels in humans subjected to the sleep deprivation model of spaceflight. J Allergy Clin Immunol 2001;107:165-170.

90. Spiegel K, Sheridan JF, Van Cauter E: Effect of sleep deprivation on response to immunization. JAMA 2002;288:1471-1472.

91. Balachandran DD, Ewing SB, Murray BJ, et al: Human host response during chronic partial sleep deprivation. Sleep 2002;25:A106-A107.

92. Appels A, de Vos Y, van Diest R, et al: Are sleep complaints predictive of future myocardial infarction? Act Nerv Super (Praha) 1987;29:147-151.

93. Eaker ED, Pinsky J, Castelli WP: Myocardial infarction and coronary death among women: Psychosocial predictors from a 20-year follow-up of women in the Framingham Study. Am J Epidemiol 1992;135:854-864.

94. Newman AB, Spiekerman CF, Enright P, et al: Daytime sleepiness predicts mortality and cardiovascular disease in older adults. The Cardiovascular Health Study Research Group [Comment]. J Am Geriatr Soc 2000;48:115-123.

95. Schwartz SW, Cornoni-Huntley J, Cole SR, et al: Are sleep complaints an independent risk factor for myocardial infarction? Ann Epidemiol 1998;8:384-392.

96. Liu Y, Tanaka H, The Fukuoka Heart Study Group: Overtime work, insufficient sleep, and risk of non-fatal acute myocardial infarction in Japanese men. Occup Environ Med 2002;59: 447-451.

97. Tenkanen L, Sjoblom T, Harma M: Joint effect of shift work and adverse life-style factors on the risk of coronary heart disease. Scand J Work Environ Health 1998;24:351-357.

98. Knutsson A, Akerstedt T, Jonsson BG, et al: Increased risk of ischaemic heart disease in shift workers. Lancet 1986;2:89-92.

99. Knutsson A, Hallquist J, Reuterwall C, et al: Shiftwork and myocardial infarction: A case-control study. Occup Environ Med 1999;56:46-50.

100. Koller M: Health risks related to shift work. Int Arch Occup Environ Health 1983;53:59-75.

101. Shamsuzzaman AS, Winnicki M, Lanfranchi P, et al: Elevated C-reactive protein in patients with obstructive sleep apnea. Circulation 2002;105:2462-2464.

102. Meier-Ewert HK, Ridker PM, Rifai N, et al: Effect of sleep loss on C-reactive protein, an inflammatory marker of cardiovascular risk. J Am Coll Cardiol 2004;43:678-683.

7

Phylogeny of Sleep Regulation

Irene Tobler

ABSTRACT

Tracing the evolution of sleep to its origins is an important approach that could provide clues to its functions. Until recently, comparative studies of sleep at different levels of evolution centered on the presence of sleep and its stages in the higher vertebrates (e.g., mammals and birds), and few studies investigated whether sleep or sleeplike states are present also in the lower vertebrates, such as reptiles, amphibians and fish. The limitations were set by the narrow electrophysiologic definition of the vigilance states and their behavioral correlates in mammals that were then applied to nonmammalian species.

Sleep in mammals is finely regulated. A constant daily quota of sleep is maintained through a balance between sleep duration and intensity, a phenomenon that led to the use of the term *sleep homeostasis*. Slow wave activity (SWA; defined as EEG waves in the frequencies between 0.5 and 4 Hz, also referred to as delta activity) in non–rapid eye movement (NREM) sleep is the measure that has found acceptance as an index of sleep intensity. However, other measures, including sleep continuity, arousal threshold, motor activity, and heart rate, can also serve as indicators to document compensatory mechanisms after sleep deprivation. The comparative data addressing the occurrence of these regulatory mechanisms in evolution indicate that a *need* for sleep has evolved that is manifested by its increase as waking is prolonged and by its dissipation when sleep occurs. Therefore, sleep must have an adaptive value that surpasses the constraints of the ubiquitous circadian rest–activity rhythm.

Species belonging to the lower vertebrates (reptiles and fish) and invertebrates (e.g., scorpions, cockroaches, bees, and *Drosophila*) do not meet the electrophysiologic criteria for the definition of sleep, but they do compensate for the loss of sleep. These evolutionarily simpler animals are useful for investigating basic mechanisms of compensatory activity at the molecular and genetic level and thereby provide clues to the functions of sleep.

It is remarkable that the function of sleep is still unknown, although it is generally accepted that sleep leads to some form of recuperation. Making use of the diversity of animals in the investigation of sleep or sleeplike behavior is likely to yield insights into its origins and functional significance. In particular, animals representing different stages of evolution could reveal at which stage sleep evolved and became a necessity for survival. Recent studies in fruit flies show that sleep, with the complexity described for mammalian species, is not a phenomenon unique to the most highly evolved vertebrates— the homeothermic mammals and birds—but is present in simpler manifestations also in arthropods. Its existence in yet lower vertebrates still needs to be clarified. The use of *Drosophila* as a model organism to investigate the molecular regulation of the vigilance states should lead to the identification of the genes regulating sleep in more evolved species.

After sleep deprivation (SD) in mammals, there is typically a compensatory rebound in several variables. This widely occurring phenomenon led to the proposal that the homeostatic aspect of sleep regulation is an essential property of sleep that should be included in a broader definition of sleep.[1] This property sets it apart from the chronobiologic definition of *rest*, with the important consequence that a relatively constant quota of sleep can be fulfilled by the interaction between sleep duration and intensity. This flexibility is especially important when animals are faced with situations in which the opportunity to sleep is limited.

SLEEP REGULATION IN MAMMALS

The Origins and Definition of Sleep Homeostasis

Early studies on sleep were aimed at establishing the presence of NREM and REM sleep in a particular species and determining the amount of each of these states. The implementation of spectral analysis or other methods of signal analysis led to the recognition that there is a continuous process underlying the NREM-REM sleep cycle that is reflected in the time course of SWA in NREM sleep. In mammals, sleep is under homeostatic control. The principle of homeostasis in physiology was defined by W.B. Cannon in 1939 as "the coordinated physiologic processes which maintain most of the steady states in the organism." The term *sleep homeostasis* was coined in 1980 by Borbély,[2] who posited that sleep strives to maintain a constant level by variation of its duration and intensity. A vast amount of data both in humans and rodents shows that homeostatic mechanisms counteract the deviations of sleep from an average reference level. When waking is prolonged, sleep duration, or more importantly, SWA as seen on an EEG during NREM sleep, is enhanced. In contrast, when sleep (in human subjects) is prolonged, or when the subjects are allowed to take a nap during the day, SWA in the subsequent night reaches a predictably lower level compared with a night after a normal wakefulness period. In animals, it is difficult to prolong sleep experimentally. Therefore, it is not known whether animals can "produce" excess sleep. Studies comparing sleep in the laboratory as opposed to sleep in the wild are needed to establish whether the amount of sleep generally reported for animals bred and raised in the laboratory represents "excess" sleep.

The two-process model of sleep regulation postulates that a process S rises during waking and declines during sleep, and that it interacts with process C, which reflects the output of the endogenous circadian pacemaker. SWA best reflects the prior history of sleep and waking and thus is an ideal quantitative marker of the dynamics of the homeostatic process S in humans (see Chapter 33). The time course of the homeostatic variable S was derived from the EEG SWA. The quantitative model accounted for the timing of human sleep,[3] and the interaction of S and C allowed a prediction of the time course of daytime vigilance. In animals, SWA is modulated by the alternation of polyphasic sleep and waking bouts lasting from 4 seconds up to several hours (depending on the minimum criterion to define a sleep epoch). SWA turned out to be the best candidate for a physiologic marker of sleep homeostasis in humans. Is this also true for animals? Strictly speaking, homeostasis is established only when a relationship between the degree of rebound and previous waking duration is established. SWA increases as a function of the duration of the sleep deprivation (Figs. 7–1, 7–2 and 7–3). This has been shown for humans (see Chapter 33), squirrel monkeys, rats, Syrian hamsters, Djungarian hamsters, cats, ground squirrels, and several mouse strains.[4-12] The studies in inbred laboratory mice[13] paved the way for investigations into the mechanisms underlying sleep homeostasis at the genetic level.[5,6,13]

Attempts at simulating SWA in rodents on the basis of the original two-process model of sleep regulation showed that its tenets can be used to predict experimental results in animals. The original formulation was based on an extensive data set derived from experiments in the laboratory rat.[2] Process C was not incorporated. Franken et al.[14] simulated SWA on the basis of the two-process model in rats. The correspondence between the SWA data and the simulations of SWA were optimized when a correction for the SWA-reducing effect of light[15] was incorporated. Light exposure can affect both C and S.[15-17] Attempts to simulate SWA in several strains of mice should help to understand the different dynamics underlying the buildup of sleep pressure and SWA dissipation in different strains.[5,6] It remains to be examined whether sleep homeostasis as conceptualized in the two-process model may be a more general property of mammalian sleep.

Sleep Duration and Intensity of Sleep

The hallmarks of sleep regulation in mammals are sleep duration, sleep consolidation (i.e., brief awakenings and/or duration of consolidated NREM sleep and REM sleep epochs), and EEG "delta power" in NREM sleep, which is synonymous with SWA. A balance between sleep duration and sleep intensity maintains a constant daily quota of sleep. Two factors contribute to this balance—the circadian rest–activity rhythm and the environment—and an increase of total sleep time must occur within the constraints imposed by both. For most animals, it would be maladaptive to engage in long periods of sleep (or wakefulness) during the wrong circadian phase. Generally, compensation for a sleep deficit occurs by relatively small increases of total sleep duration. After periods of extended waking (in the range of 3 to 24 hours), NREM and REM sleep are little increased. Instead, the most striking feature manifested early during recovery sleep is the remarkable increase of slow waves in the NREM sleep EEG; this was first demonstrated in the rabbit[18] and then extensively documented in the rat[19,20] and, more recently, in several species of mice.[5,6,21] The magnitude of the increase in sleep time and/or

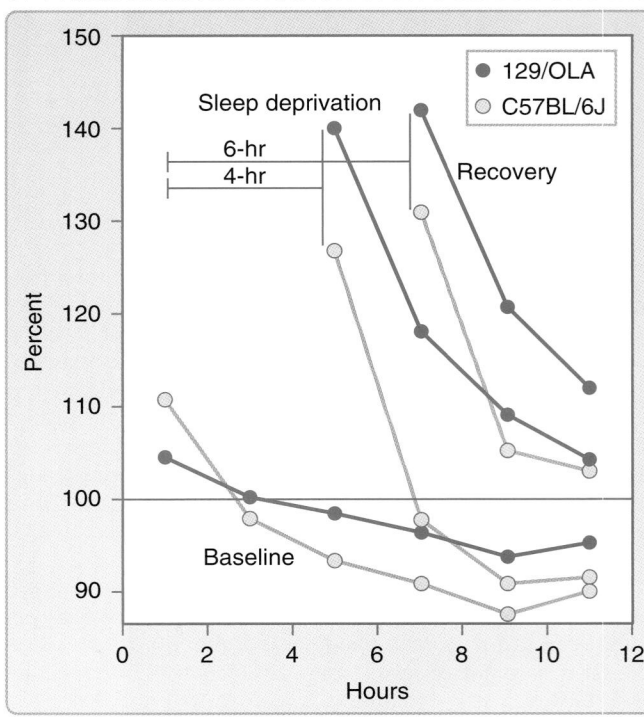

SLOW WAVE ACTIVITY AS A FUNCTION OF PRIOR WAKING DURATION IN TWO MOUSE STRAINS

Figure 7–1. Effect of 4-hour and 6-hour sleep deprivation (SD) by "gentle handling" on slow wave activity (SWA) (electroencephalographic power density, 0.75 to 4.0 Hz) in non–rapid eye movement (NREM) sleep in two inbred mouse strains (129/OLA, n = 7 to 9; and C57BL/6J, n = 7 to 11). Mean hourly values are expressed as percentage of the 12-hour baseline light period value. SWA exhibits a steeper decline in the course of the light period in C57 than in 129/OLA. In both strains, the typical initial significant increase of SWA was observed after 4 hours of SD when compared with the corresponding interval during baseline conditions. After 4 hours of SD, the SWA increase was lower than after 6 hours of SD, and the effect of the 6-hour SD lasted longer than that of the 4-hour SD. The effect after 6 hours of SD persisted during the subsequent dark phase. Total sleep time and REM sleep were increased in the remaining hours of the light period after 6 hours in both strains and after 4 hours in C57 only. The results demonstrate (1) large strain differences in the response to SD, and (2) a clear relationship between the increase in SWA and previous waking duration despite the strain differences. (Modified from Huber R, Deboer T, Tobler I: Effects of sleep deprivation on sleep and sleep EEG in three mouse strains: Empirical data and simulations. Brain Res 2000;857:8-19.)

of SWA in NREM sleep depends on the species, the duration of the deprivation, the efficacy of the deprivation, and the circadian time point at which the deprivation is ended.

It has become generally accepted that SWA reflects NREM sleep intensity.[19,20] Many studies have provided experimental evidence that the arousal threshold is consistently higher during NREM sleep with high amounts of slow waves, compared with more shallow NREM sleep with fewer slow waves.[22-24]

It is still unclear whether it is the waking state per se (i.e., the absence of sleep) or specific aspects of the waking state that are responsible for the increase in SWA. Some early studies addressed this question by using forced locomotion to achieve SD in rats and then comparing rotation rates of the sleep

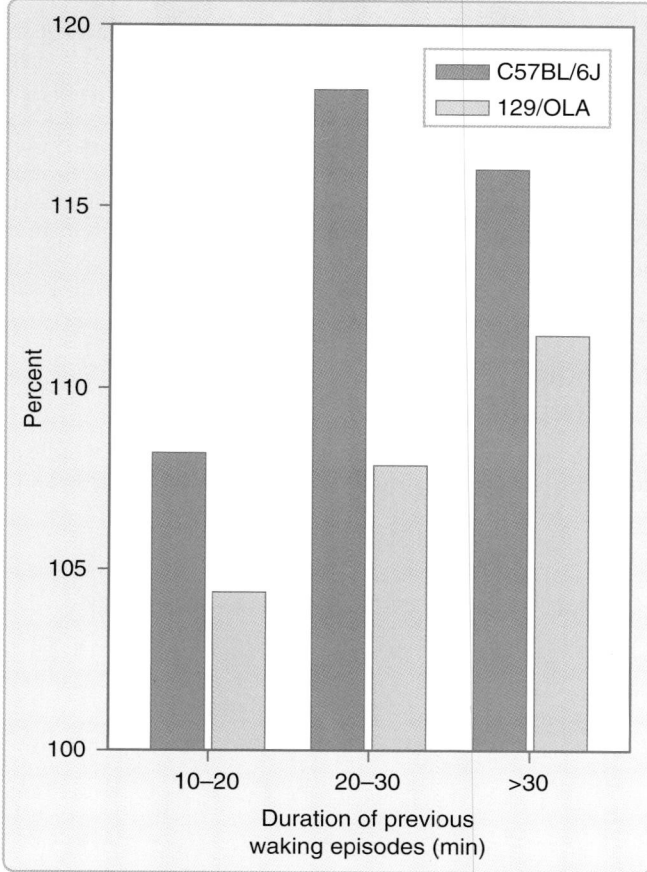

SLOW WAVE ACTIVITY
AFTER SPONTANEOUS WAKING

Figure 7–2. Slow wave activity (SWA) (electroencephalographic power density, 0.75 to 4.0 Hz) in non–rapid eye movement (NREM) sleep after spontaneous waking in the 12-hour baseline light period for two inbred mouse strains, C57BL/6J ($n = 11$) and 129/OLA ($n = 9$). The waking episodes were subdivided into three categories according to their duration (10 to 20, 20 to 30, and longer than 30 minutes). The SWA increase in the 10-minute NREM sleep interval immediately following the waking episode is expressed relative to SWA in NREM sleep in the corresponding 2-hour baseline interval. Even after the short waking interval, both strains show an SWA increase above baseline, and it increases progressively as a function of the duration of the waking episode. (Modified from Huber R, Deboer T, Tobler I: Effects of sleep deprivation on sleep and sleep EEG in three mouse strains: Empirical data and simulations. Brain Res 2000;857:8-19.)

deprivation cylinder,[19,20] and another used the effect of voluntary running activity.[25] No major effect on the magnitude of increase of slow waves in NREM sleep was found. Later SD experiments performed by forced locomotion or by subjecting animals (rat[26] and Syrian hamster[27]) to "gentle handling" showed similar changes of sleep during recovery. The gentle handling procedure consists primarily of keeping the animal active by introducing objects such as tissue and cardboard rolls, by tapping on the cage, and when necessary by tilting the cage. Great care is taken to avoid subjecting the animals to the stress of being touched, and to avoid interference with spontaneous feeding and drinking bouts. When the aim of the SD is

to increase sensory stimulation, further objects such as plastic toys with holes and pieces of wood are introduced (see, e.g., Vyazovskiy et al.[28,29]). A major stress effect on SWA in NREM sleep appears unlikely because the forced locomotion procedure did not entail a significant increase in the level of plasma corticosterone,[30] and the expression patterns of genes were similar after spontaneous wakefulness lasting 3 hours and after 3 hours of enforced SD.[31] The finding that in mice and ground squirrels, SWA in NREM sleep also increased after spontaneous, undisturbed bouts of waking, the magnitude of the increase depending on the duration of the previous waking bout[5,7] (see Fig. 7–2), supports the argument that an increase of EEG slow waves that follows a wakefulness interval is not a stress effect. Thus also the increase in SWA after a period of induced wakefulness is not necessarily a consequence of stress involved in the deprivation procedure. Nevertheless, stressful waking experiences have been shown to lead to an increase of SWA in rats exposed to a social conflict.[32]

The possibility that a global increase in metabolic rate during wakefulness is a critical variable leading to an increase in SWA is improbable because the changes in SWA induced by SD performed both in a warm environment and at room temperature were similar, even though brain temperature was higher in the warm deprivation condition.[33] Metabolic changes at a local level may nevertheless underlie topographic differences in SWA (see "Sleep Regulation: Unihemispheric Sleep and Regional Aspects of Sleep," later).

It is probable that the compensation of sleep after sleep loss may have an adaptive function, unless we postulate that sleep does not have a major function. Under natural conditions, animals need to be vigilant, forage for food, reproduce, and avoid long, continuous bouts of sleep. It is evident that compensating for sleep loss by balancing sleep duration and sleep intensity, depending on the timing and the situation, has added flexibility to sleep.

Daily Time Course of Slow Wave Activity

Because the initial level of EEG SWA in NREM sleep is determined by the prior sleep and waking history, an animal that exhibits a large circadian amplitude of sleep, resulting in predominance of wakefulness in one half of the day, should exhibit high initial SWA values when sleep is prominent. A progressive decline of SWA should result as the need for sleep dissipates. This relationship is evident in nocturnal rodents (e.g., the rat, hamster, and inbred mouse strains), in which SWA is high at light onset. Consistently, in the diurnal chipmunk[34] and in humans, whose main sleep period is at night, the highest SWA values are at the beginning of the dark period. The global progressive SWA decline, which occurs despite the intermittent waking bouts that are typical for most mammals, reveals the presence of a stable, continuous process underlying the sleep–wake pattern. In the rabbit, guinea pig, cat, and blind mole rat, species that exhibit only a small preference for sleep in the light period, the decline of SWA is minor or absent.[35-38] This relationship between the sleep–wake pattern and SWA was also evident in experiments in the rat and Djungarian hamster when the photoperiod was changed. The total amount of sleep was the same in both photoperiods, but sleep was redistributed according to the new light-to-dark ratio.

The time course of SWA followed the new sleep–wake pattern as predicted.[16,17,39] Using a quantitative simulation of NREM sleep homeostasis in the rat and two mouse strains, the biphasic time course of SWA during baseline conditions, during the initial increase after SD, and during the subsequent prolonged negative rebound was reproduced (see Chapter 33, Fig. 33–5).[5,6,14]

Large differences occur in the magnitude of the daily SWA and in SD-induced changes between different mammals and even within mouse strains. Simulations show that the rate of the increase of SWA pressure (process S) in the rat and mouse, reflected by the time constants of its increase, is faster than in human beings (see Chapter 33, Fig. 33–5).[5,6,14] The remarkable difference in the increase of SWA after 4 hours of SD between two relatively small rodents, the Djungarian hamster and inbred mice[40-42] (Fig. 7–3, and see Fig. 7–1) may reflect different levels of process S in these species during baseline conditions. Such an interpretation is supported by the different magnitudes of the SWA response to SD in human long and short sleepers.[43]

Is REM Sleep Homeostatically Regulated?

Both total SD and "selective" REM SD[44-46] elicit a subsequent compensatory increase in the amount of REM sleep in many species including the cat, dog, rat, mouse, and cow. Although the evolutionary origin of REM sleep was a topic of early studies, the REM sleep rebound after SD has never been addressed from an evolutionary perspective. In addition, there is as yet little indication that REM sleep may also have an intensity dimension. Some data in the rat[26,47] and rabbit[35] show an enhancement of theta activity during REM sleep after 24 hours of SD, as well as a progressive decrease in the course of recovery sleep; these factors indicate that theta activity may reflect REM sleep intensity.

Circadian Versus Homeostatic Aspects of Sleep Regulation

Several lines of evidence from animal experiments indicate that the homeostatic (process S) and circadian (process C)

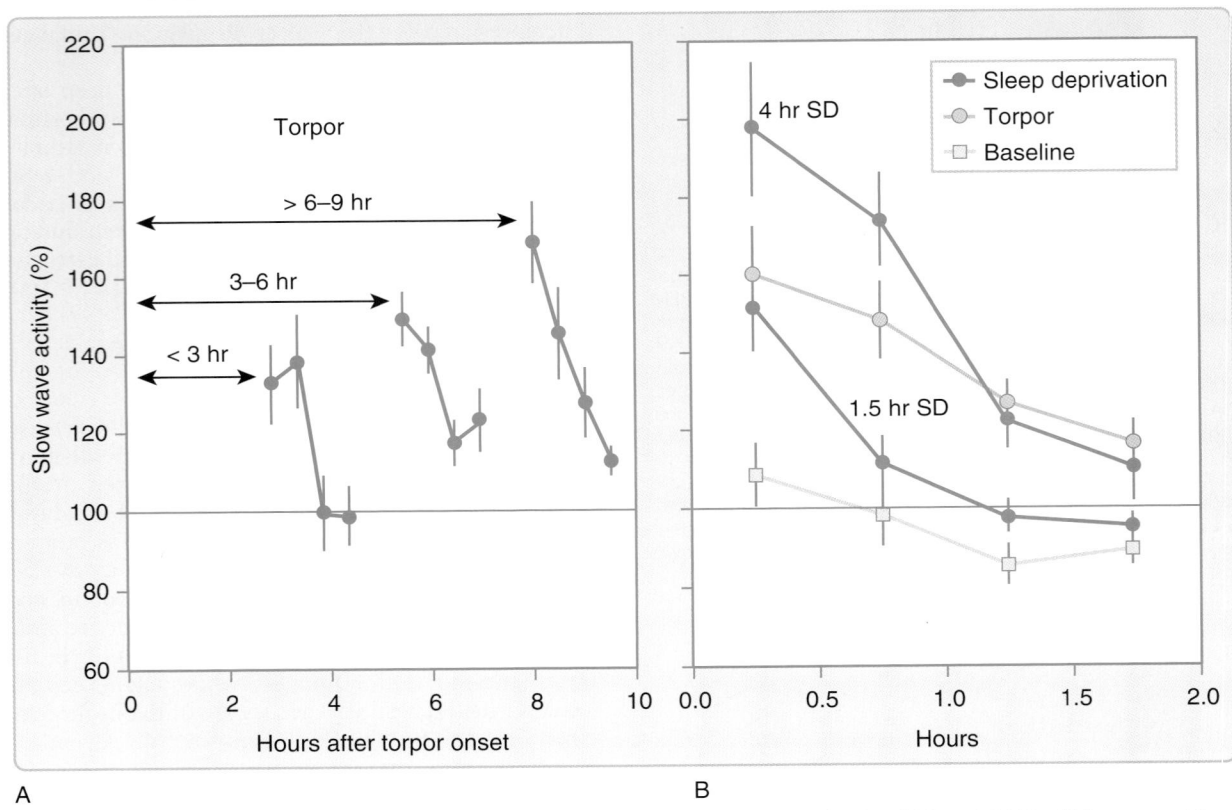

A   **B**

Figure 7–3. Time course of slow wave activity (SWA) (mean electroencephalographic power density, 0.75 to 4.0 Hz) within non–rapid eye movement (NREM) sleep during sleep after torpor episodes of three different durations (less than 3 hours, 3 to 6 hours, and 6 to 9 hours) (**A**) and during baseline, during recovery from 4-hour sleep deprivation (SD), and after torpor (**B**) (mean torpor duration = 4.8 ± 0.3 hours SEM) in the Djungarian hamster, *Phodopus sungorus*. **A,** Mean 30-minute values (*n* = 6, 15, and 7, for less than 3 hours, 3 to 6 hours, and 6 to 9 hours, respectively) for the first 2.5 to 3 hours of recovery after end of torpor. SWA is expressed relative to the 24-hour value of the baseline day without torpor. A linear correlation between torpor bout duration and increase in SWA was significant (*n* = 28, *r* = 0.42, *P* < .05). **B,** Time course of SWA after torpor and after 1.5-hour and 4-hour SD. Mean 30-minute values (*n* = 8, 8, and 7 for 4-hour SD, 6-hour SD, and torpor, respectively). All recordings were performed in a short photoperiod, light–dark (LD) = 8:16, at 16° C to 18° C. (Modified from Deboer T, Tobler I: Sleep regulation in the Djungarian hamster: Comparison of the dynamics leading to the slow-wave activity increase after sleep deprivation and daily torpor. Sleep 2003;26:567-572; and Deboer T, Tobler I: Slow waves in the sleep electroencephalogram after daily torpor are homeostatically regulated. Neuroreport 2000;11:881-885.)

facets of sleep regulation (see Chapter 33) are mediated by separate processes. Seminal experiments in the rat established that an intact circadian rhythm is not a necessary condition for sleep homeostasis. The circadian facet of sleep regulation can be disrupted by lesions of the suprachiasmatic nuclei. Rats made arrhythmic in this manner were subjected to 24-hour SD to test their ability to compensate for sleep loss.[48-50] Both SWA in NREM sleep and the amount of REM sleep increased. These results showed that homeostatic response to SD persists when circadian rhythmicity is abolished (Fig. 7–4A). A similar finding was revealed in arrhythmic flies subjected to SD (see Fig. 7–4B). SD affected neither the phase nor the period of the free-running rest–activity rhythm of intact rats,[51,52] but it led to rapid resetting of the circadian clock in the Syrian hamster.[53] Also, vigilance states can affect the circadian process. Simultaneous recordings of sleep stages and neuronal activity in the suprachiasmatic nucleus of the rat demonstrated a feedback from sleep to the circadian pacemaker.[54]

INCREASE OF SWA AFTER SLEEP DEPRIVATION IN THE RAT

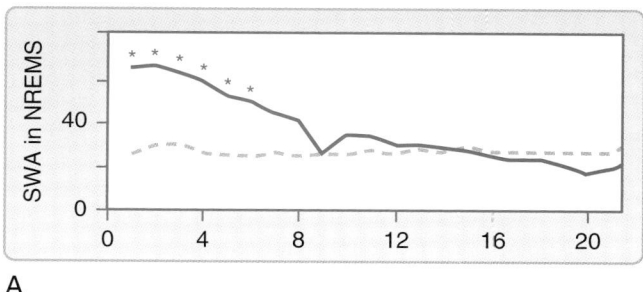

A

INCREASE OF REST IN AN ARRHYTHMIC *DROSOPHILA* MUTANT

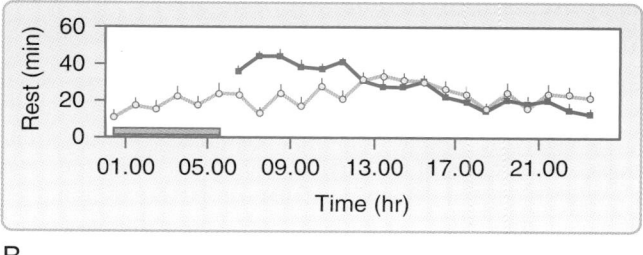

B

Figure 7–4. Independence of the homeostatic aspect of sleep regulation from the circadian component in the rat and the fruit fly *Drosophila*. **A,** Increase of slow wave activity (SWA) in non–rapid eye movement sleep (NREMS) in the rat after bilateral lesion of the nucleus suprachiasmaticus. Mean 3-hour values of sliding averages of 1-hour intervals for the baseline day preceding the 24-hour sleep deprivation (*dashed light blue line*) and the recovery light period (*n* = 5) (*dark blue curve*). (Modified from Tobler I, Borbély AA, Groos G: The effect of sleep deprivation on sleep in rats with suprachiasmatic lesions. Neurosci Lett 1983;42:49-54.) **B,** Increase in duration of rest (minutes) in an arrhythmic per[01] fly mutant recorded in constant darkness. *Blue bar,* 6 hours of deprivation of rest; *light circles,* amount of rest during baseline; *dark squares,* amount of rest during recovery. (From Greenspan RJ, Tononi G, Cirelli C, Shaw JS: Sleep and the fruit-fly. Trends Neurosci 2001;24:142-145.)

Several conflict experiments in animal models examined the relationship between the two processes. In the rat, the conflict was induced by ending a 24-hour SD period either at the onset or in the middle of the dark period, which is the circadian period in which waking predominates.[19,55] SWA showed a rebound in two stages: an immediate increase followed by waking, and then a second, delayed increase at light onset. Because most animals are largely polyphasic, short periods of SD (e.g., 6 hours in rats or mice) can theoretically still elicit considerable increases in sleep duration within the circadian constraint. The magnitude depends on whether recovery is allowed within the light or the dark period. Thus, it is not that an upper threshold in the amount of sleep is reached, as has been often argued. Instead, in the rat, just 3 hours of SD leads to a small but significant increase in SWA with no change in NREM sleep. NREM sleep (and, with a few hours' delay, also REM sleep) was increased only after at least 6 hours of enforced waking.[9,33] When the duration of SD was restricted to 6 hours, once at the beginning of the light period and once at the beginning of the dark period, resulting in a major difference in the amount of sleep loss, there was a difference in the time course and amount of increase in NREM sleep and SWA both in rats and mice (I. Tobler, unpublished findings). When the relationship between NREM sleep and SWA was analyzed by computing slow wave energy (i.e., integrated SWA in NREM sleep), the compensation was identical under both SD conditions (Fig. 7–5).

Even in cats, which show only a minor circadian sleep–wake modulation,[10,37] the effect of a 4-hour SD, performed at two different phases of the light–dark cycle, depended on the phase at which recovery was allowed.[10] The role of the circadian process becomes evident when recovery from SD begins in the circadian phase of predominant waking. The increase in total sleep time was larger than when recovery occurred during the phase where sleep is predominant.

The enhancement of SWA in NREM sleep is less dependent on circadian factors.[55] A series of experiments was performed in squirrel monkeys that were sleep deprived in constant light for 0 to 1.5 circadian cycles. SD was initiated at the beginning of the subjective day and thus ended at different times of the circadian cycle.[4] The authors concluded that in squirrel monkeys, the homeostatic component is weaker than circadian factors in determining the amount of sleep and sleep intensity. However, data obtained in human subjects undergoing a forced desynchrony protocol showed that SWA is subject to only little circadian modulation (see Chapter 33). Results obtained in studies of species that do not have a natural, distinct preference for sleep in a particular circadian phase, such as the guinea pig, rabbits, and some strains of mice,[35,56,57] support the notion that sleep homeostasis is largely independent of circadian rhythm. In guinea pigs after a 6-hour SD, SWA was enhanced during recovery to a similar extent, independent of whether SD occurred in the light or dark period.[58]

The identification of genes underlying circadian rhythms in mice, humans, and *Drosophila* has resulted in renewed interest in the potential interaction between circadian and homeostatic aspects of sleep regulation. Sleep regulation has been investigated in mice in which circadian genes have been knocked out (see review in Franken and Tafti[59]). Studies using mouse mutants with deletions in circadian genes confirmed the presence of sleep homeostasis despite the absence of a circadian

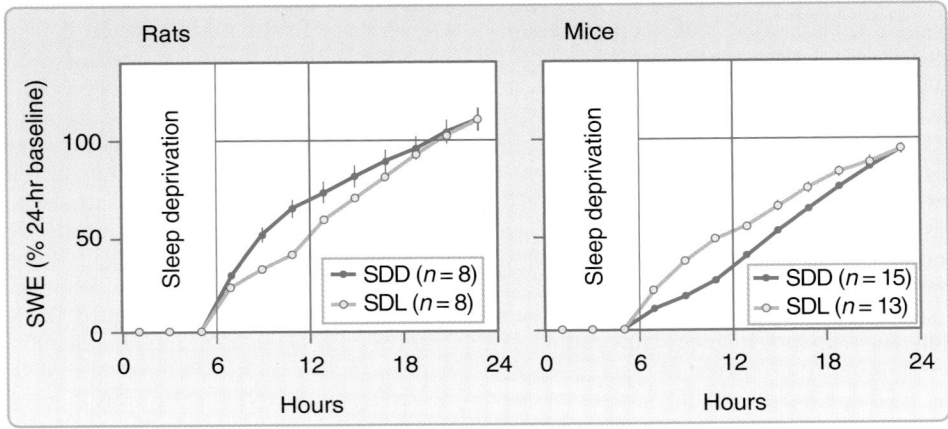

Figure 7–5. Time course of slow wave energy (SWE) (cumulative electroencephalographic power density, 0.75 to 4.0 Hz in non–rapid eye movement [NREM] sleep) for the 18-hour recovery interval after 6-hour sleep deprivation (SD) that began either at light onset (SDL) or dark onset (SDD). Curves connect 2-hour cumulative values of mean SWE (male Sprague-Dawley rats: SDL, $n = 8$; SDD, $n = 8$; male B1 mice [I/LnJ x C57BL/6]: SDL, $n = 13$; SDD, $n = 15$), expressed relative to mean SWE in NREM sleep in the 24-hour baseline. After 6-hour SD performed either at the beginning of the 12-hour light period (SDL) or at the beginning of the 12-hour dark period (SDD) in the rat ($n = 8$) and B1 mice ($n = 13$ to 15), there is a significant increase of NREM sleep as well as of slow wave activity in NREM sleep. The magnitude of the effect and its time course depend on the timing of the SD. The differences in time course become evident when SWE is computed. However, it is notable that in both species, SWE reaches identical values toward the end of the recovery period of both treatments. (Vyazovskiy V, Tobler I, unpublished data.)

rhythm.[60-63] For some mutants, it was claimed that the homeostatic response to SD was weak.[59] There are claims that specific circadian genes may affect sleep homeostasis, but more evidence is needed. Caution is warranted in the interpretation of the effects of SD, because sleep can be changed in duration as well as in intensity. Moreover, the efficacy of the SD procedure used may differ between mouse strains. Simulations based on the two-process model, which accounts for the changes in duration of NREM sleep as well as in its intensity, should reveal whether the differences between strains may be a consequence of different dynamics of the homeostatic process. Thus, it is possible that mouse strains have different time constants for the increase in process S (see Chapter 33).[6]

Special Features

Herbivores: Cows and Horses

In mammals, computation of correlations between body size and amount of sleep indicates that this constitutional variable affects the need for sleep (see Chapter 8). The herbivores, which include species with large body and brain weights, could serve as models to clarify whether sleep regulation is also affected. Many herbivores are ruminants, and this aspect of nutrition may have an impact on the amount of sleep and its regulation that is worth investigating. The effects of prolonging wakefulness were investigated in three ungulate species.

Recumbency was prevented in cows for 14 to 22 hours per day for 2 to 4 weeks, thereby leading primarily to REM sleep deprivation (although NREM sleep and drowsiness were also reduced).[64] During recovery, a rebound occurred in both NREM sleep and REM sleep. A donkey sleep deprived for 48 hours showed an increase in sleep time during recovery.[65]

In ponies, recorded in a stall and outdoors, and subjected to visual and auditory sensory deprivation during the 4-day period in the stall, the amount of NREM sleep increased progressively at the cost of drowsiness, and REM sleep was unchanged. On exposure to the more disturbed conditions outdoors, there was a threefold increase of REM sleep during the first 2 days. This finding was interpreted as a consequence of the relative increase in environmental stimuli.[66,67] These studies indicate that at least some aspects of sleep are regulated also in large herbivores. It is still unknown whether NREM sleep has an intensity component in these animals.

Sleep Regulation: Unihemispheric Sleep and Regional Aspects of Sleep

One of the most interesting specializations of sleep was developed by aquatic mammals belonging to the orders Cetacea, Pinnipedia, and Sirenia. Some species of each of these orders engage in episodes of unihemispheric "deep" sleep (i.e., with a predominance of delta waves) that can last from minutes to several hours, while the other hemisphere exhibits an EEG resembling waking (see, e.g., Oleksenko et al.[68]). It has been mentioned that the invasive recordings with implanted electrodes and the restriction of the animals' movement by the recording cables could have influenced these findings. However, Ridgway[69] recently confirmed his initial findings describing the presence of unihemispheric sleep by behavior (eye closure) and with an EEG in a single bottle-nosed dolphin recorded by telemetry in a small pool. This specialization provided a unique opportunity to investigate whether sleep regulation occurs simultaneously in both brain hemispheres. Keeping six bottle-nosed dolphins awake for 35 to 72 hours resulted in an increase in delta sleep in three of them, and in an early study, it had resulted in a more regular alternation of deep sleep between the brain hemispheres during recovery.[68]

These findings showed that slow waves in NREM sleep represent sleep intensity also in dolphins. The question then was, Is it feasible to sleep deprive a single brain hemisphere, and does this elicit unilateral compensation? SD of one hemisphere attained by disturbing dolphins only when the EEG of one hemisphere was synchronized, while the animals remained undisturbed when slow waves were manifest in the other hemisphere, resulted in a larger compensation of delta sleep during recovery in the deprived hemisphere in seven of the nine deprivations.[68] These data show that sleep does not necessarily encompass the entire brain. It follows that sleep may be a local phenomenon. In humans and rodents, topographic EEG differences between and within hemispheres support this notion (see, e.g., Vyazovskiy et al.[28]). It is possible that the regional differences reflect use-dependent aspects. Sleep may enable recuperation of those regions that were most active during waking. Recent experiments in the rat and in humans[29,29a] are consistent with this notion. The asymmetry in EEG power between the hemispheres during normal sleep in the rat was enhanced during recovery from 6 hours of SD, and stimulation of the whiskers on one side led to a larger increase of EEG power during sleep over the barrel field of the hemisphere contralateral to stimulation compared with the nonstimulated side.[29]

Sleep and Hibernation

Hibernation and daily torpor, both characterized by decreases in metabolism and body and brain temperature that are similar but larger in magnitude than the decreases observed during sleep, can be used as models to understand sleep. Hibernation and daily torpor are specializations that most effectively reduce energy requirements in endothermic animals. During hibernation, body temperature is lowered to approximately 5° C or less for several months,[70] with short (less than 24-hour) euthermic interruptions.[71,72] In daily torpor, temperature is lowered to approximately 15° C to 20° C for several hours during the circadian rest period.[73]

It is puzzling that animals arouse regularly from hibernation despite the high energetic costs of the arousals.[72] It is now well established for several species that the animals arouse from hibernation and, paradoxically, go to sleep. SWA is high at the initiation of the sleep episode and subsequently decreases, exhibiting dynamics that are comparable to those that occur after SD. In three species of ground squirrels, the initial values of SWA during euthermia were higher after long hibernation bouts than after short ones—again, a typical feature for recovery from SD.[71,74,75] Thus hibernation, especially at low temperatures, and daily torpor seem to be incompatible with restorative processes that are expected to occur during sleep.[71,75]

The relationship between the torpid state, subsequent arousal, and SD was extensively investigated in the Djungarian hamster (*Phodopus sungorus sungorus*), in which days with torpor alternating with days at euthermic levels can be compared in the same individuals (for a review, see Deboer and Tobler[42]). As in the hibernating ground squirrels, during euthermia, the initial value of SWA in NREM sleep was high and was followed by a progressive decline closely resembling the pattern during recovery from SD (see Fig. 7–3). Similarly, as after SD, the initial level of SWA was higher after long torpor bouts than after short bouts[76] (see Fig. 7–3), and a

better fit between the duration of torpor or SD and the initial SWA values was attained by a saturating exponential function than by a linear function.[77] The kinetics of the increase in sleep pressure during torpor was 2.75 times slower than after SD in the same species[42] (see Fig. 7–3), supporting the hypothesis that during hypothermia, the hamsters incur a sleep deficit that is recovered by returning to euthermia. It remains to be clarified whether the return to euthermia is triggered by a homeostatic need to recover.

Other Measures for Sleep Regulation

Sleep is apparently regulated relative to an internal reference level. Usually, EEG spectral parameters, especially SWA during NREM sleep, serve as indicators of these regulatory processes in mammals. The compensatory increase of SWA and several other EEG variables after prolonged wakefulness has been abundantly described not only for humans and rodents but also for many other mammals, including two nonhuman primates (the rhesus monkey, *Macaca mulatta*, and squirrel monkey)[4,78,79] and two carnivores, the cat[10-12,37,80] and the dog.[81] However, other variables, such as sleep state continuity as well as the number of epochs with little or no motor activity, also change as a function of the duration of previous wakefulness.

Sleep continuity, defined by the frequency of short wake episodes ("brief awakenings") in the rat, was enhanced after 24-hour SD.[82] The frequency of wake episodes shorter than 32 seconds was reduced, leading to a consolidation of sleep during recovery. In further similar experiments in the rat and other rodents (guinea pigs and laboratory mice), the reduction in the number of brief awakenings correlated with the increase of SWA.[13,26,36,82] The inverse relationship indicates that brief awakenings may represent a behavioral correlate of sleep intensity.[26] The decrease of brief awakenings under sleep pressure may contribute to the reduced variability of the NREM-REM sleep cycle in the rat[82] and bottle-nosed dolphin,[68] and in the cat[84] to the shortening of the sleep cycle and increase in its regularity, and the duration of the single-cell activity discharge cycle in brainstem dorsal raphe nucleus.[84]

During recovery from SD, motor activity during sleep is reduced in humans[85] and in several other mammals. In dogs subjected to SD, motor activity assessed continuously using a portable activity monitor attached to the collar was reduced by 40% during recovery.[86] Similarly, in the rat, motor activity was reduced to 84% of baseline when recovery from 24 hours of SD coincided with dark onset.[19] There are indications that the amount of consecutive rest episodes as a marker for sleep intensity may also be useful to quantify sleep regulation in inbred mouse strains (Tobler, unpublished data). Motor activity is a measure that can be recorded easily and that allows aspects of sleep regulation to be investigated when invasive EEG interventions are not possible, or when sleep cannot be defined by electrophysiologic criteria (see "Sleep Regulation in Invertebrates," later).

SLEEP REGULATION IN NONMAMMALIAN VERTEBRATES

Birds

Sleep in birds (reviewed by Amlaner and Baal[87]) resembles in many ways sleep in mammals, although the limited number of species investigated relative to the large diversity of birds does not allow generalization. The similarity between sleep in birds and in mammals applies especially to the uncontested presence of the two stages NREM sleep and REM sleep, although the duration of REM sleep epochs in birds seems to be relatively short. Whether birds show a homeostatic regulation of sleep that is comparable to that in mammals is important because specific aspects of sleep regulation may be related to homeothermy. It would be important to clarify whether birds have the capacity to increase NREM sleep intensity by enhancing SWA, despite the different anatomy of the bird brain, or if SD affects sleep continuity. A few studies have shown that three vigilance states can be distinguished in birds by spectral analysis of the EEG. In birds, the differences between the sleep stages seem to be much smaller than in mammals,[88] in which NREM sleep power density values in the low-frequency range (0.25 to 6.0 Hz) exceed those of REM sleep and waking by approximately one order of magnitude. In pigeons, SWA in NREM sleep was not affected by SD.[88] It is still an open question whether SWA in birds reflects sleep intensity. The studies are hampered by a lack of knowledge about how long the deprivation should last to obtain a clear effect, and the possibility that birds may have other means to compensate for sleep loss. Moreover, brain anatomy in birds and mammals shows major differences that could be expected to lead to different EEG patterns.

Despite the uncertainty whether sleep in birds has the intensity component seen in mammalian sleep, several other variables were affected by 24-hour SD. Sleep duration, the amount of REM sleep, and electrooculographic activity in waking and in NREM sleep were increased during recovery.[89] In Barbary doves, frequency of eye blinking was a behavioral variable that decreased substantially after 3- to 36-hour SD (achieved by exposing the animals to a ferret on a leash).[90] Moreover, the level of vigilance estimated by the blinking frequency depended on the length of the SD. These findings indicate a need to compensate for sleep loss. There is a tradeoff between the benefits of frequent eye blinking (e.g., optimizing predator detection by increasing vigilance) and sleep with few interruptions.[88,90] The results imply that the birds benefited from sleep with closed eyes, and that those benefits were reduced during SD.

Renewed interest was generated by two studies. EEG recordings in pigeons and mallard ducks showed short epochs of EEG asymmetry during sleep that may resemble unihemispheric sleep in dolphins, despite their short duration. In the birds, these epochs were much shorter and were correlated with unilateral eye-closure. This is in contrast to dolphins, which fail to show such a relationship. Birds that were more exposed to the laboratory surroundings had higher amounts of eye opening and unilateral sleep than when the same birds were in the more protected space between other cages.[91,92] This experimental procedure indicated that the lateralization of behavior is optional and may enhance survival, as it allows one hemisphere to intermittently scan the environment while the other remains in a sleeping state. The occurrence of such episodes may be the clue to "sleeping on the wing," which was recently experimentally determined in frigate birds wearing altimeters,[93] and was postulated years ago on the basis of behavioral observations of swifts. The frigate birds were in constant motion day and night. Alternatively, birds may sleep while they are gliding.

Reptiles

The sleep EEG in reptiles differs in many ways from that in mammals. In particular, the vigilance state–related changes in EEG patterns are different. It is therefore interesting that certain elements in their EEG did respond to SD. Considerable diversity in the appearance of high-voltage slow waves (sharp waves and spikes) superimposed on the waking and sleeping EEG was found, suggesting that this type of EEG activity may be a precursor or a correlate of the slow waves associated with sleep in mammals.[94] In the early 1970s, Flanigan[95] performed a unique set of SD experiments in reptiles belonging to the orders Crocodilia (*Caiman sclerops*), Chelonia (box turtle [*Terrapene carolina*] and red-footed tortoise [*Geochelone carbonaria*]), and Squamata (iguanid lizards, green iguana [*Iguana iguana*], and spiny-tailed lizard, also called black lizard [*Ctenosaura pectinata*]). Depending on the species, the animals were subjected to 24 or 48 hours of stimulation by stroking, handling, or gently tugging the animal's leash when it showed signs of behavioral sleep. The increasing amount of interventions necessary to keep the turtles awake and the loss of muscle tone in the iguanas toward the last hours of SD were clear signs of increasing sleepiness indicating an accumulating need for sleep. During recovery, several variables showed a compensatory rebound: The latency to behavioral sleep decreased, the duration and overall amount of behavioral sleep increased, and EEG spikes were markedly enhanced. The arousal threshold, measured by the response to electrical stimulation of eye potentials or heart rate, was higher during recovery. It seems that reptilian EEG spikes and sharp waves may reflect sleep intensity, and their increase after prolonged wakefulness, like slow waves in mammals, suggests that they may have a functional similarity.

Amphibians and Fish

No experiments have been published investigating compensatory mechanisms after SD in amphibians. In fish, two early studies subjected carp and perch to SD, using behavioral measures to assess its effects.[96] Activation of carp for up to 96 hours by continuous illumination induced decreased latency to sleep behavior during the reinstatement of the dark period,[97] and in perch, the activation induced by exposure to 6 and 12 hours of light during the habitual rest period (i.e., the dark period) resulted in an increase of resting behavior during recovery.[96] The effect depended on the length of the light exposure, confirming the notion that homeostatic mechanisms may also be involved in the regulation of rest in fish. Larvae of the zebrafish *Danio rerio* have recently been shown to exhibit behavioral sleep and rest rebound after rest deprivation.[98] The availability of the genetic map in this lower vertebrate clearly renders it a further candidate to be used for tackling the genetics of sleep regulation at the level of simpler vertebrates.

SLEEP REGULATION IN INVERTEBRATES

Simpler models are better suited to dissect the essence of sleep than mammals and birds, which exhibit the most complex sleep phenotype. Once it was established that sleep in mammals is homeostatically regulated and that variables other than the EEG can be used to define sleep and to demonstrate compensation after prolonged waking, the way was paved to investigate whether arthropods meet the behavioral criteria for sleep.[95,99,100] The criteria have been met, and indeed, arthropods do show a compensatory response after prolongation of the normal waking period. The initial evidence came from two species of cockroaches and the scorpion, the oldest living arthropod (marine scorpions can be traced back to the Silurian period of about 400 million years ago). These studies have been complemented recently by a major effort using the fruit fly, *Drosophila melanogaster*, to dissect the genetics of sleep and sleep regulation.[101-103,105,105a]

Cockroaches (*Leucophea maderae*,[107] *Blaberus giganteus*,[106] and *Periplaneta australasiae*) (K. Sly and R. Brown, unpublished data) were prevented from resting for 3 hours at the end of the daily rest period (it was predicted that a compensatory increase of rest would best be manifested at the time of habitual activity). Rest exhibited a rebound after the deprivation, whereas the control experiment, in which the insects were simply removed from their home cages for 3 hours, elicited a smaller and shorter-lasting decrease of activity and

an increase of immobile, rest episodes. The data provided the first evidence for compensatory mechanisms in invertebrates.[107] In a more refined approach, behavior was scored as "activity" or "rest," but rest was subdivided on the basis of the position of the head, abdomen, and antennae in order to clarify whether substates reflected different thresholds of arousal. In one of the nine behavioral states, characterized by a horizontal body axis with the antennae touching the substrate, the arousal threshold was significantly higher than in all other states. After disturbing the cockroaches for an entire 12-hour dark period, it was this behavioral state that showed a tendency to be increased in duration and frequency after the rest deprivation; however, locomotion was also increased.[106]

Other arthropods, scorpions of the three species *Heterometrus longimanus, Heterometrus spinnifer,* and *Pandinus imperator,* also show a clear daily rhythm of rest and activity, and on the basis of the reaction to a vibration stimulus, an intermediate alert state and a rest state could be defined. Deprivation of rest for 12 hours elicited an initial rise of activity and a significant increase in the resting state (Fig. 7–6).[104]

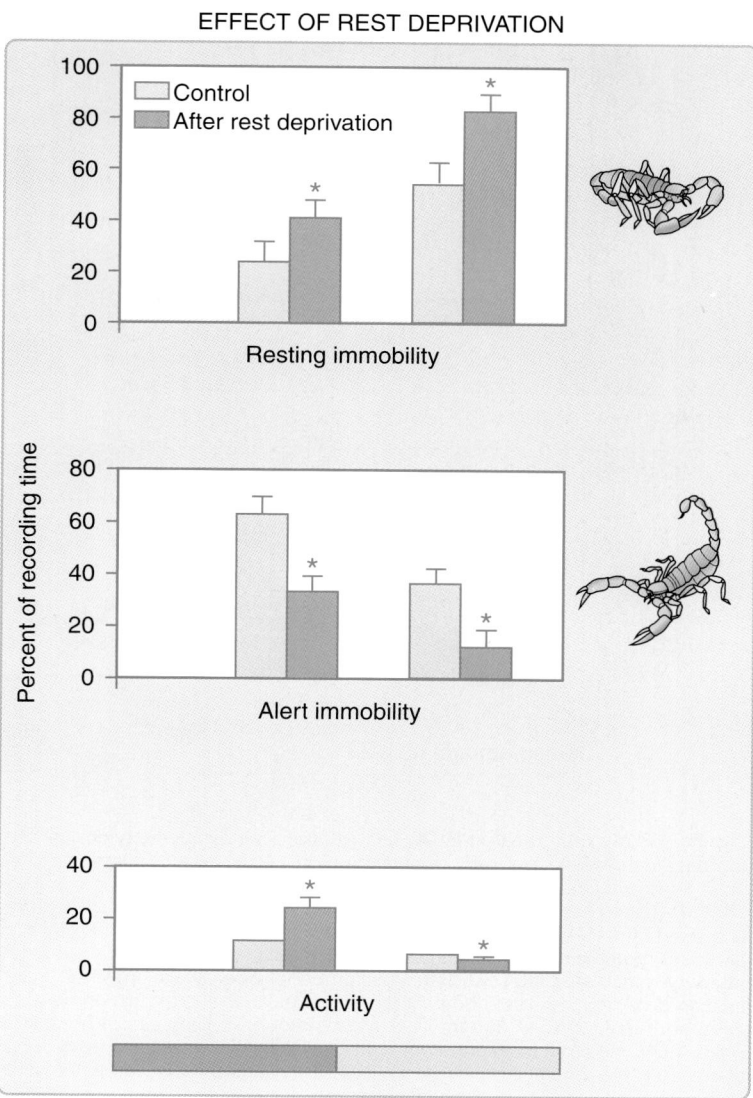

Figure 7–6. Effect of 12-hour rest deprivation on three vigilance states in the scorpion. Mean values ± SEM (*n* = 7) for the 12-hour intervals of the control day and after rest deprivation. *P < .05, Wilcoxon matched pairs signed rank test; differences between control and recovery. Light–dark conditions are indicated by the *dark blue and light blue bar* at the bottom of the figure. (Modified from Tobler I, Stalder J: Rest in the scorpion—a sleep like state? J Comp Physiol [A] 1988;163:227-235.)

The fruit fly *Drosophila* (with its manifold mutants) exhibits a circadian rest–activity rhythm and has significantly contributed to our knowledge. Recently, it was claimed that in the fly, rest is not mere inactivity but fulfills the behavioral criteria for sleep.[103,105] Correlates of sleep and waking were established: the rest–activity pattern was quantified and the arousal thresholds to several types of stimuli were investigated. Further studies have unequivocally established that fruit flies exhibit sleep.[105a] Preventing the flies from attaining rest for different periods of time elicited corresponding increases of rest during recovery (Fig. 7–7A) that were associated with increased sleep continuity and arousal thresholds (see Fig. 7–7B). Thus, both of the factors that contribute to sleep homeostasis in mammals, duration and intensity, have been firmly established for the fruit fly. Moreover, electrical field potentials in the fly brain showed that brain electrical activity in *Drosophila* is reliably correlated with activity state.[108] The definition of sleep and sleep homeostasis in *Drosophila* has led to the screening of thousands of fly mutants (see Fig. 7–7C) and dissecting the genetic components of sleep.

Among lower invertebrates, preliminary experiments in the cuttlefish (*Sepia pharaonis*) showed that they display not only most elements of behavioral sleep but also a rest rebound after 12 hours' prevention of quiescence.[108a]

GENETICS OF SLEEP REGULATION

The availability of tools to study behavior genetics has led to the use of two model systems, the mouse and the fruit fly, to elucidate the genetics of sleep and sleep homeostasis. The sleep comparisons of inbred mouse strains and their backcrosses initiated by Valatx in the mid-1970s were refined and complemented by quantitative trait loci analysis (for a review, see Franken and Tafti[59]). A major gene is postulated to account for the differences between mouse strains in the increase of delta power in NREM sleep after SD. A significant locus was localized to chromosome 3 and named Dps1 (for delta power sleep). The sequencing of the *Drosophila* genome has led to the use of fruit flies as simpler models to investigate sleep. Several hundred fly mutants, including lines derived from

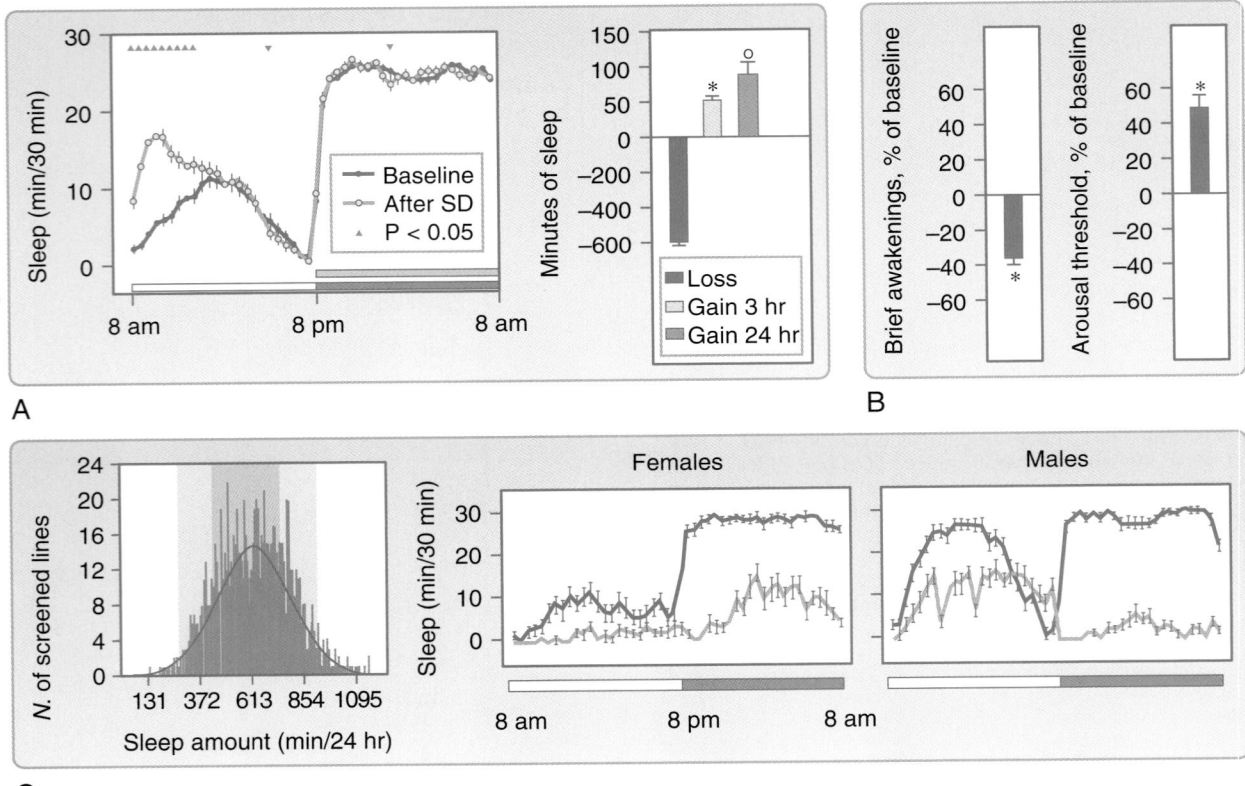

Figure 7–7. Sleep in the fruit fly. **A,** *Left: Filled circles* indicate the typical pattern of sleep in a population of about 100 female wild-type flies during baseline. Flies sleep mostly during the night. *Open circles* indicate sleep amount and distribution after 12 hours of sleep deprivation (SD). Time and duration of SD are indicated by the *light blue bar* on the x-axis. The increase in sleep duration occurs mainly during the first 6 hours after SD (paired *t* tests). Flies were maintained in a 12:12 light–dark cycle (light on at 8 AM). *Right:* Amount of sleep lost (during SD) and of sleep recovered (after SD) for the experiments shown at left. Sleep duration is significantly increased during the first 3 hours after SD. *P < .05; O, P < .1, Duncan's multiple range test. In flies, as in mammals, the amount of sleep recovered after SD represents only a fraction of the sleep lost. **B,** Sleep intensity is increased after SD. *Left:* The number of brief awakenings is reduced during the first 3 hours after SD. *Right:* The arousal threshold is increased during the first 6 hours after SD. Values refer to the experiment shown in **A.** *P < .05, Duncan's multiple range test. **C,** *Left:* Daily amount of sleep in 1547 mutant lines. Mean amount of sleep per 24 hours is 616 ± 169 (mean ± SD; minimum, 131; maximum, 1155). *Shaded areas* show one *(dark blue)* and two *(light blue)* standard deviations from the mean. Only very few mutant lines sleep less than 2 standard deviations from the mean (short sleepers). *Right:* Daily amount of sleep in female and male flies of a short-sleeper line *(light blue lines)*. For comparison, the *dark blue line* in each panel represents the daily amount of sleep in wild-type flies. (From Cirelli C, Huber R, Tononi G. Unpublished data.)

single females collected in the wild, are being screened for short and long sleepers and for flies that lack a homeostatic response to the loss of sleep (reviewed by Cirelli[101]). Already, indications are that there is large variability in sleep homeostasis in flies. *Drosophila* mutants lacking an enzyme involved in the catabolism of monoamines, dopamine acetyl-transferase, as well as the loss-of-circadian-function fly, cyc01, showed enhanced rest rebound after SD, whereas male flies with a null mutation for cycle (BMAL1) showed no rebound or very little rebound (reviewed in Greenspan et al.[109] and Hendricks et al.[110]). Homeostasis was apparently impaired in flies mutant for the clock gene *timeless*, but this result was based on the lack of a rebound after only 6 hours of SD.[103] Longer periods of SD should reveal whether a compensatory response can be induced in these mutants. Many genes in *Drosophila* have a homologous counterpart in mice and humans. These genetic links mean that flies and mice can be used as models, which will eventually lead to greater understanding of sleep in humans.

OUTLOOK

Compensation for the loss of sleep has been found in many mammals. Similar phenomena were described in birds, reptiles, fish, and some invertebrates. Most notably, *Drosophila* exhibits homeostatic compensation of rest after rest deprivation, leading to its use as a model to investigate the underlying mechanisms at the genetic level. In natural environments, there are many disturbances that may prevent animals from obtaining their normal quota of sleep. A large variety of animals have developed mechanisms to compensate for the loss of sleep within the constraints of the circadian rest–activity rhythm by intensifying sleep. This is a powerful indication that there is a benefit to sleep that is reduced during SD and is indispensable.

Rest behavior may be a state from which sleep evolved. A more detailed characterization of rest in different classes of animals is helping to clarify the origin of sleep and to identify the unique properties of sleep in comparison to rest. Sleep, as it is defined in mammals and birds, has many properties that can be identified in lower vertebrates and invertebrates. An important common feature is that sleep is not merely a function of the circadian rest–activity rhythm but is determined by additional regulatory mechanisms. Sleep deprivation in vertebrates and invertebrates elicits compensatory responses. This regulatory property of sleep, which can be considered the essence of sleep, can be used to examine rest in a broad range of animals that, because of the absence of electrophysiologic criteria, are not considered to manifest sleep. The effects of rest deprivation in invertebrates are, in some aspects, analogous to the compensation of sleep after SD in mammals. Elementary properties of sleep may be found that will allow the investigation of the underlying mechanisms in less complex organisms.

It is unknown which genes are essential to control and regulate sleep and sleep homeostasis. The development of gene technology[111] has led, in mice, to the identification of several circadian clock genes and the localization of genomic regions involved in sleep.[59] In rats, gene technology has permitted the recognition of changes in gene expression across the sleep–waking cycle (for reviews, see Cirelli and colleagues[112-114]). Although these technologies allow the application of genetics

to complex systems such as those encountered in mammals, the finding that *Drosophila* exhibits most criteria used to define sleep provides an interesting parallel avenue to clarify the involvement of genes in sleep regulation.

> *Clinical Pearl*
>
> *Hibernation and daily torpor, which are the most effective ways to reduce energy requirements, result in reduction of body temperature and other physiological changes that protect organs that have a high metabolic rate. Lessons learnt from understanding hibernation may lead to new treatments to protect the brain in patients with stroke and traumatic brain injury.*

Acknowledgments

This work was supported by the Swiss National Science Foundation and the Human Frontiers Science Frontier Program. The author thanks Dr. P. Achermann and Dr. A. Borbély for their comments.

REFERENCES

1. Tobler I: Evolution of the sleep process: A phylogenetic approach. Exp Brain Res 1984(Suppl 8):207-226.
2. Borbély AA: Sleep: Circadian rhythm versus recovery process. In Koukkou M, Lehmann D, Angst J (eds): Functional States of the Brain: Their Determinants. Amsterdam, Elsevier, 1980, pp 151-161.
3. Daan S, Beersma DGM, Borbély AA: Timing of human sleep: Recovery process gated by a circadian pacemaker. Am J Physiol 1984;246:R161-R178.
4. Klerman EB, Boulos Z, Edgar DM, et al: Circadian and homeostatic influences on sleep in the squirrel monkey: Sleep after sleep deprivation. Sleep 1999;22:45-59.
5. Huber R, Deboer T, Tobler I: Effects of sleep deprivation on sleep and sleep EEG in three mouse strains: Empirical data and simulations. Brain Res 2000;857:8-19.
6. Franken P, Chollet D, Tafti M: The homeostatic regulation of sleep need is under genetic control. J Neurosci 2001;21:2610-2621.
7. Larkin JE, Heller HC: The disappearing slow wave activity of hibernators. Sleep Res Online 1998;1:96-101.
8. Tobler I, Borbély AA: Sleep EEG in the rat as a function of prior waking. Electroencephalogr Clin Neurophysiol 1986;64:74-76.
9. Tobler I, Borbély AA: The effect of 3-h and 6-h sleep deprivation on sleep and EEG spectra of the rat. Behav Brain Res 1990;36:73-78.
10. Lancel M, van Riezen H, Glatt A: Effects of circadian phase and duration of sleep deprivation on sleep and EEG power spectra in the cat. Brain Res 1991;548:206-214.
11. Lucas EA: Effects of five to seven days of sleep deprivation produced by electrical stimulation of the midbrain reticular formation. Exp Neurol 1975;49:554-568.
12. Ursin R: Differential effect of sleep deprivation on the two slow wave sleep stages in the cat. Acta Physiol Scand 1971;83:352-361.
13. Tobler I, Gaus SE, Deboer T, et al: Altered circadian activity rhythms and sleep in mice devoid of prion protein. Nature 1996;380:639-642.
14. Franken P, Tobler I, Borbély AA: Sleep homeostasis in the rat: Simulation of the time course of EEG slow-wave activity [published erratum appears in Neurosci Lett 1991;132:279]. Neurosci Lett 1991;130:141-144.

15. Tobler I, Franken P, Alföldi P, et al: Room light impairs sleep in the albino rat. Behav Brain Res 1994;63:205-211.

16. Franken P, Tobler I, Borbély AA: Varying photoperiod in the laboratory rat: Profound effect on 24-h sleep pattern but no effect on sleep homeostasis. Am J Physiol 1995;269:R691-R701.

17. Deboer T, Tobler I: Vigilance state episodes and cortical temperature in the Djungarian hamster: The influence of photoperiod and ambient temperature. Pflugers Arch 1997;433:230-237.

18. Pappenheimer JR, Koski G, Fencl V, et al: Extraction of sleep-promoting factor S from cerebrospinal fluid and from brains of sleep-deprived animals. J Neurophysiol 1975;38:1299-1311.

19. Borbély AA, Neuhaus HU: Sleep-deprivation: Effects on sleep and EEG in the rat. J Comp Physiol [A] 1979;133:71-87.

20. Friedman L, Bergmann BM, Rechtschaffen A: Effects of sleep deprivation on sleepiness, sleep intensity, and subsequent sleep in the rat. Sleep 1979;1:369-391.

21. Franken P, Malafosse A, Tafti M: Genetic variation in EEG activity during sleep in inbred mice. Am J Physiol 1998;275:R1127-R1137.

22. Grahnstedt S, Ursin R: Awakening thresholds for electrical brain stimulation in five sleep-waking stages in the cat. Electroencephalogr Clin Neurophysiol 1980;48:222-229.

23. Frederickson CJ, Rechtschaffen A: Effects of sleep deprivation on awakening thresholds and sensory evoked potentials in the rat. Sleep 1978;1:69-82.

24. Neckelmann D, Ursin R: Sleep stages and EEG power spectrum in relation to acoustical stimulus arousal threshold in the rat. Sleep 1993;16:467-477.

25. Hanagasioglu M, Borbély AA: Effect of voluntary locomotor activity on sleep in the rat. Behav Brain Res 1982;4:359-368.

26. Franken P, Dijk DJ, Tobler I, et al: Sleep deprivation in rats: Effects on EEG power spectra, vigilance states, and cortical temperature. Am J Physiol 1991;261:R198-R208.

27. Tobler I, Jaggi K: Sleep and EEG spectra in the Syrian hamster (*Mesocricetus auratus*) under baseline conditions and following sleep deprivation. J Comp Physiol [A] 1987;161:449-459.

28. Vyazovskiy VV, Borbély AA, Tobler I: Interhemispheric sleep EEG asymmetry in the rat is enhanced by sleep deprivation. J Neurophysiol 2002;88:2280-2286.

29. Vyazovskiy V, Borbély AA, Tobler I: Unilateral vibrissae stimulation during waking induces interhemispheric EEG asymmetry during subsequent sleep in the rat. J Sleep Res 2000;9:367-371.

29a. Huber R, Ghilardi MF, Massimini M, Tononi G: Local sleep and learning. Nature 2004;430:78-81.

30. Tobler I, Murison R, Ursin R, et al: The effect of sleep deprivation and recovery sleep on plasma corticosterone in the rat. Neurosci Lett 1983;35:297-300.

31. Cirelli C, Tononi G: Differences in brain gene expression between sleep and waking as revealed by mRNA differential display and cDNA microarray technology. J Sleep Res 1999;8(Suppl 1):44-52.

32. Meerlo P, de Bruin EA, Strijkstra AM, Daan S: A social conflict increases EEG slow-wave activity during subsequent sleep. Physiol Behav 2001;73:331-335.

33. Tobler I, Franken P, Gao B, et al: Sleep deprivation in the rat at different ambient temperatures: Effect on sleep, EEG spectra and brain temperature. Arch Ital Biol 1994;132:39-52.

34. Dijk DJ, Daan S: Sleep EEG spectral analysis in a diurnal rodent: *Eutamias sibiricus*. J Comp Physiol [A] 1989;165:205-215.

35. Tobler I, Franken P, Scherschlicht R: Sleep and EEG spectra in the rabbit under baseline conditions and following sleep deprivation. Physiol Behav 1990;48:121-129.

36. Tobler I, Franken P, Jaggi K: Vigilance states, EEG spectra, and cortical temperature in the guinea pig. Am J Physiol 1993;264:R1125-R1132.

37. Tobler I, Scherschlicht R: Sleep and EEG slow-wave activity in the domestic cat: Effect of sleep deprivation. Behav Brain Res 1990;37:109-118.

38. Tobler I, Herrmann M, Cooper HM, et al: Rest-activity rhythm of the blind mole rat *Spalax ehrenbergi* under different lighting conditions. Behav Brain Res 1998;96:173-183.

39. Palchykova S, Deboer T, Tobler I: Seasonal aspects of sleep in the Djungarian hamster. BMC Neurosci 2003;4:9.

40. Deboer T, Franken P, Tobler I: Sleep and cortical temperature in the Djungarian hamster under baseline conditions and after sleep deprivation. J Comp Physiol [A] 1994;174:145-155.

41. Tobler I, Deboer T, Fischer M: Sleep and sleep regulation in normal and prion protein-deficient mice. J Neurosci 1997;17:1869-1879.

42. Deboer T, Tobler I: Sleep regulation in the Djungarian hamster: Comparison of the dynamics leading to the slow-wave activity increase after sleep deprivation and daily torpor. Sleep 2003;26:1-6.

43. Aeschbach D, Cajochen C, Landolt HP, et al: Homeostatic sleep regulation in habitual short sleepers and long sleepers. Am J Physiol 1996;270:R41-R53.

44. Jouvet D, Vimont P, Delorme F, et al: Etude de la privation sélective de la phase paradoxale de sommeil chez le Chat. C R Seances Soc Biol Fil 1964;4:756-759.

45. Siegel J, Gordon TP: Paradoxical sleep: Deprivation in the cat. Science 1965;148:978-980.

46. Jouvet M: Paradoxical sleep mechanisms. Sleep 1994;17:S77-S83.

47. Borbély AA, Tobler I, Hanagasioglu M: Effect of sleep deprivation on sleep and EEG power spectra in the rat. Behav Brain Res 1984;14:171-182.

48. Mistlberger RE, Bergmann BM, Waldenar W, et al: Recovery sleep following sleep deprivation in intact and suprachiasmatic nuclei-lesioned rats. Sleep 1983;6:217-233.

49. Tobler I, Borbély AA, Groos G: The effect of sleep deprivation on sleep in rats with suprachiasmatic lesions. Neurosci Lett 1983;42:49-54.

50. Trachsel L, Edgar DM, Seidel WF, et al: Sleep homeostasis in suprachiasmatic nuclei-lesioned rats: Effects of sleep deprivation and triazolam administration. Brain Res 1992;589:253-261.

51. Beersma DGM, Daan S, Dijk DJ: Sleep intensity and timing: A model for their circadian control. In Carpenter GA (ed): Some Mathematical Questions in Biology: Circadian Rhythms. Lectures on Mathematics in the Life Sciences, vol 19. Providence, RI, American Mathematical Society, 1987, pp 39-62.

52. Borbély AA: Sleep regulation: Circadian rhythm and homeostasis. Curr Top Neuroendocrinol 1982;1:83-103.

53. Antle MC, Mistlberger RE: Circadian clock resetting by sleep deprivation without exercise in the Syrian hamster. J Neurosci 2000;20:9326-9332.

54. Deboer T, Vansteensel MJ, Détári L, Meijer JH: Sleep states alter activity of suprachiasmatic nucleus neurons. Nat Neurosci 2003;10:1086-1090.

55. Trachsel L, Tobler I, Borbély AA: Sleep regulation in rats: Effects of sleep deprivation, light, and circadian phase. Am J Physiol 1986;251:R1037-R1044.

56. Pellet J, Béraud G: Organisation nychthémérale de la veille et du sommeil chez le cobaye (*Cavia porcellus*): Comparaisons interspécifiques avec le rat et le chat. Physiol Behav 1967;2:131-137.

57. Franken P, Malafosse A, Tafti M: Genetic determinants of sleep regulation in inbred mice. Sleep 1999;22:155-169.

58. Tobler I, Franken P: Sleep homeostasis in the guinea pig: Similar response to sleep deprivation in the light and dark period. Neurosci Lett 1993;164:105-108.

59. Franken P, Tafti M: Genetics of sleep and sleep disorders. Front Biosci 2003;8:e381-e397.

60. Naylor E, Bergmann BM, Krauski K, et al: The circadian *clock* mutation alters sleep homeostasis in the mouse. J Neurosci 2000;20:8138-8143.

61. Franken P, Lopez-Molina L, Marcacci L, et al: The transcription factor DBP affects circadian sleep consolidation and rhythmic EEG activity. J Neurosci 2000;20:617-625.

62. Wisor JP, O'Hara BF, Terao A, et al: A role for cryptochromes in sleep regulation. BMC Neurosci 2002;3:20.

63. Dudley CA, Erbel-Sieler C, Estill SJ, et al: Altered patterns of sleep and behavioral adaptability in NPAS2-deficient mice. Science 2003;301:379-383.

64. Ruckebusch Y: Sleep deprivation in cattle. Brain Res 1974;78: 495-499.

65. Ruckebusch Y: Un problème controversé: La perte de vigilance chez le cheval et la vache au cours du sommeil. Cah Med Vet 1970;39:210-225.

66. Ruckebusch Y: The hypnogram as an index of adaptation of farm animals to changes in their environment. Appl Anim Ethol 1975;2:3-18.

67. Dallaire A, Ruckebusch Y: Sleep patterns in the pony with observations on partial perceptual deprivation. Physiol Behav 1974;12: 789-796.

68. Oleksenko AI, Mukhametov LM, Polyakova IG, et al: Unihemispheric sleep deprivation in bottlenose dolphins. J Sleep Res 1992;1:40-44.

69. Ridgway SH: Asymmetry and symmetry in brain waves from dolphin left and right hemispheres: Some observations after anesthesia, during quiescent hanging behavior, and during visual obstruction. Brain Behav Evol 2002;60:265-274.

70. Barnes BM: Freeze avoidance in a mammal: Body temperatures below 0° C in an arctic hibernator. Science 1989;244: 1593-1595.

71. Daan S, Barnes BM, Strijkstra AM: Warming up for sleep? Ground squirrels sleep during arousal from hibernation. Neurosci Lett 1991;128:265-268.

72. Wang LCH: Energetic and field aspects of mammalian torpor: The Richardson's ground squirrel. In Wang LCH, Hudson JW (eds): Strategies in the Cold. New York, Academic Press, 1978, pp 109-145.

73. Heldmaier G, Steinlechner S: Seasonal pattern and energetics of short daily torpor in the Djungarian hamster, *Phodopus sungorus*. Oecologia 1981;48:265-270.

74. Strijkstra AM, Daan S: Sleep during arousal episodes as a function of prior torpor duration in hibernating European ground squirrels. J Sleep Res 1997;6:36-43.

75. Trachsel L, Edgar DM, Heller HC: Are ground squirrels sleep deprived during hibernation? Am J Physiol 1991;260: R1123-R1129.

76. Deboer T, Tobler I: Sleep EEG after daily torpor in the Djungarian hamster: Similarity to the effects of sleep deprivation. Neurosci Lett 1994;166:35-38.

77. Deboer T, Tobler I: Natural hypothermia and sleep deprivation: Common effects on recovery sleep in the Djungarian hamster. Am J Physiol 1996;271:R1364-R1371.

78. Berger RJ, Meier GW: The effects of selective deprivation of states of sleep in the developing monkey. Psychophysiology 1966; 2:354-371.

79. Pegram GV, Reite ML, Stephens LM, et al: Prolonged sleep deprivation in the monkey: Effects on sleep patterns, brain temperature, and performance. In Primate Electrophysiology, Particularly Related to Sleep. Holloman Air Force Base, NM, 6571st Aeromedical Research Laboratory, 1969, pp 51-53. Report ARL-TR-69-5.

80. Kiyono S, Kawamoto T, Sakakura H, et al: Effects of sleep deprivation upon the paradoxical phase of sleep in cats. Electroencephalogr Clin Neurophysiol 1965;19:34-40.

81. Takahashi Y, Ebihara S, Nakamura Y, et al: Temporal distributions of delta wave sleep and REM sleep during recovery sleep after 12-hour forced wakefulness in dogs: Similarity to human sleep. Neurosci Lett 1978;10:329-334.

82. Trachsel L, Tobler I, Achermann P, et al: Sleep continuity and the REM-nonREM cycle in the rat under baseline conditions and after sleep deprivation. Physiol Behav 1991;49:575-580.

83. Trachsel L, Tobler I, Borbély AA: Electroencephalogram analysis of non-rapid eye movement sleep in rats. Am J Physiol 1988;255:R27-R37.

84. Lydic R, McCarley RW, Hobson JA: Forced activity alters sleep cycle periodicity and dorsal raphe discharge rhythm. Am J Physiol 1984;247:R135-R145.

85. Naitoh P, Muzet A, Johnson LC, et al: Body movements during sleep after sleep loss. Psychophysiology 1973;10: 363-368.

86. Tobler I, Sigg H: Long-term motor activity recording of dogs and the effect of sleep deprivation. Experientia 1986;42: 987-991.

87. Amlaner CJ Jr, Baal NJ: Avian sleep. In Kryger MH, Roth T, Dement WC (eds): Principles and Practice of Sleep Medicine. Philadelphia, WB Saunders, 1994, pp 81-94.

88. Lendrem DW: Sleeping and vigilance in birds. In Koella WP (ed): Sleep, 1982. Basel, Karger, 1983, pp 134-138.

89. Tobler I, Borbély AA: Sleep and EEG spectra in the pigeon (*Columba livia*) under baseline conditions and after sleep deprivation. J Comp Physiol [A] 1988;163:729-738.

90. Lendrem DW: Sleeping and vigilance in birds: II. An experimental study of the Barbary dove (*Streptopelia risoria*). Anim Behav 1984;32:243-248.

91. Rattenborg NC, Lima SL, Amlaner CJ: Half-awake to the risk of predation. Nature 1999;397:397-398.

92. Rattenborg NC, Amlaner CJ, Lima SL: Unilateral eye closure and interhemispheric EEG asymmetry during sleep in the pigeon (*Columba livia*). Brain Behav Evol 2001;58: 323-332.

93. Weimerskirch H, Chastel O, Barbraud C, et al: Frigate birds ride high on thermals. Nature 2003;421:333-334.

94. Hartse KM, Rechtschaffen A: The effect of amphetamine, Nembutal, alpha-methyl-tyrosine, and parachlorophenylalanine on the sleep-related spike activity of the tortoise, *Geochelone carbonaria*, and on the cat ventral hippocampus spike. Brain Behav Evol 1982;21:199-222.

95. Flanigan WFJ: Sleep and wakefulness in Iguanid lizards, *Ctenosaura pectinata* and *Iguana iguana*. Brain Behav Evol 1973;8:401-436.

96. Tobler I, Borbély AA: Effect of rest deprivation on motor activity of fish. J Comp Physiol [A] 1985;157:817-822.

97. Shapiro CM, Hepburn HR: Sleep in a schooling fish, *Tilapia mossambica*. Physiol Behav 1976;16:613-615.

98. Zhdanova IV, Wang SY, Leclair OJ, et al: Melatonin promotes sleep-like state in zebrafish. Brain Res 2001;903:263-268.

99. Piéron H: Le problème physiologique du sommeil. Paris, Masson, 1913.

100. Kaiser W, Steiner-Kaiser J: Neuronal correlates of sleep, wakefulness and arousal in a diurnal insect. Nature 1983;301: 707-709.

101. Cirelli C: Searching for sleep mutants of *Drosophila melanogaster*. Bioessays 2003;25:940-949.

102. Shaw P: Awakening to the behavioral analysis of sleep in *Drosophila*. J Biol Rhythms 2003;18:4-11.

103. Hendricks JC, Finn SM, Panckeri KA, et al: Rest in *Drosophila* is a sleep-like state. Neuron 2000;25:129-138.

104. Tobler I, Stalder J: Rest in the scorpion—a sleep-like state? J Comp Physiol [A] 1988;163:227-235.

105. Shaw PJ, Cirelli C, Greenspan RJ, et al: Correlates of sleep and waking in *Drosophila melanogaster*. Science 2000;287:1834-1837.

105a. Huber R, Hill SL, Holladay C, Biesiadecki M, Tononi G, Cirelli C: Sleep homeostasis in *Drosophila melanogaster*. Sleep 2004;27:628-639.

106. Tobler I, Neuner-Jehle M: 24-h variation of vigilance in the cockroach *Blaberus giganteus*. J Sleep Res 1992;1:231-239.

107. Tobler I: Effect of forced locomotion on the rest–activity cycle of the cockroach. Behav Brain Res 1983;8:351-360.

108. Nitz DA, van Swinderen B, Tononi G, et al: Electrophysiological correlates of rest and activity in *Drosophila melanogaster*. Curr Biol 2002;12:1934-1940.

108a. Duntley SP, Uhles M, Feren S: Sleep in the cuttlefish *Sephia pharaonis*. Sleep 2002;25:A159.

109. Greenspan RJ, Tononi G, Cirelli C, et al: Sleep and the fruit fly. Trends Neurosci 2001;24:142-145.
110. Hendricks JC, Lu S, Kume K, et al: Gender dimorphism in the role of *cycle* (BMAL1) in rest, rest regulation, and longevity in *Drosophila melanogaster*. J Biol Rhythms 2003;18: 12-25.
111. Schibler U, Tafti M: Molecular approaches towards the isolation of sleep-related genes. J Sleep Res 1999;8(Suppl 1):1-10.
112. Cirelli C, Tononi G: Differential expression of plasticity-related genes in waking and sleep and their regulation by the noradrenergic system. J Neurosci 2000;20:9187-9194.
113. Cirelli C, Tononi G: Gene expression in the brain across the sleep-waking cycle. Brain Res 2000;885:303-321.
114. Cirelli C, Gutierrez CM, Tononi G: Extensive and divergent effects of sleep and wakefulness on brain gene expression. Neuron 2004;41:35-43.

8

Mammalian Sleep

Harold Zepelin

Jerome M. Siegel

Irene Tobler

ABSTRACT

Knowledge about sleep comes primarily from research on mammalian species, whose daily sleep quotas range from 4 to 19 hours, with rapid eye movement (REM) sleep occupying 10% to 50% of this time. Findings of REM sleep or elements of it in monotremes have filled a gap in its evolutionary history. To some, this suggests that REM was inherited from reptiles, although the absence of REM in living reptiles casts doubt on this view.

The function of sleep remains controversial.[1] On one hand, restorative theories hold that brain processes during sleep sustain waking behavior (e.g., visual function, learning). On the other hand, the negative correlation of sleep quotas with body size across species suggests that sleep is a state of enforced rest most urgent in species with low energy reserves. Because most of the variance in sleep quotas remains unaccounted for statistically, supplementary theories are in order.

There are strikingly strong correlations of REM sleep quotas with degree of maturity at birth—that is, altricial species, born with a low percentage of adult brain weight after a short gestation period, have higher REM sleep quotas, whereas precocial species have lower quotas. Given other fetal characteristics of altricial species (e.g., lapse of thermoregulation), REM sleep may be a carryover from fetal life.

Most studies on sleep have been performed in mammals. Human beings, cats, rats, and, more recently, many mouse strains have been the most frequent subjects of sleep research, but about 100 other species have also been studied. There are at least two published reports about the daily sleep of mammalian species for each one pertaining to other classes.[2] This not only makes for mammal-centeredness in thinking about sleep but also affords the opportunity for extensive interspecies comparisons that can shed light on the purpose of sleep, which is still without adequate explanation. This chapter considers relevant theories in the light of available findings.

Despite their relative abundance, the mammalian data represent less than 3% of roughly 4260 extant species.

The belief that some mammals do not sleep (e.g., prey species, because of a need for constant vigilance; shrews, because of the need for incessant foraging) has been superseded by systematic observations. Some species, in some circumstances, may be able to postpone sleep for long periods, or sleep may simply be difficult to recognize, as in the ever-swimming, blind Indus dolphin, whose sleep occurs in periods measured in seconds as it contends with strong river currents.[3]

SLEEP CRITERIA

Sleep can usually be identified by sustained quiescence in a species-specific posture accompanied by reduced responsiveness to external stimuli, but a definition of mammalian sleep requires several additional criteria, such as quick reversibility to the wakeful condition and characteristic changes in the electroencephalogram (EEG). Quick reversibility distinguishes sleep from coma and hypothermic states (e.g., hibernation). With only minor exceptions, EEG changes reliably confirm sleep-related change in behavior and brain activity. Another fundamental property of sleep, derived from comparative studies in many species, is its homeostatic regulation. See Chapter 7.

These definitional criteria exhibit notable interspecies variation. Quiescence does not necessarily mean immobility; for example, some cetaceans reportedly swim while sleeping.[4] In terrestrial mammals, lateral and sternoabdominal recumbency with eyes closed are the postures most commonly associated with sleep, but there are striking variations (Figs. 8–1 and 8–2). The horse, elephant, and giraffe, for example, sleep some while standing. Some species (e.g., cattle) sleep while they are ruminating, and many mammals can sleep with eyes semiopen. Choice of sleeping site is another element of species-specific sleep behavior and varies with mode of life and social organization. Burrows, caves, and trees are common sites because of the safety they afford, but some species (e.g., the zebra) sleep in the open and seem to rely on the presence of vigilant conspecifics for protection.[5-8] Ritualistic presleep activity is characteristic of some species, ranging from the circling of a chosen spot (seen in dogs and foxes) to the construction of a nest each evening by chimpanzees.

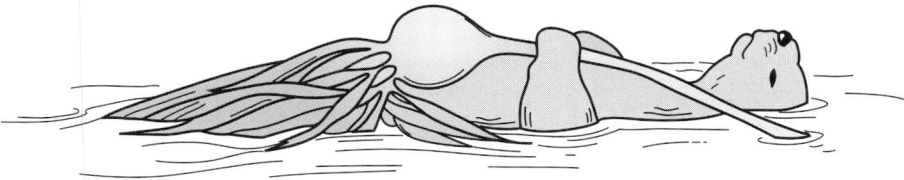

Figure 8–1. Sea otter sleeping "moored" to a float of algae. (From Bourliere F: The Natural History of Mammals, 3rd ed. New York, Alfred A Knopf, 1967, p 68.)

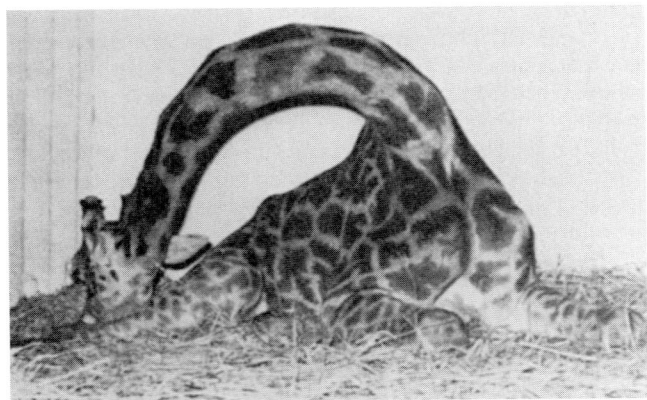

Figure 8–2. Giraffe in a zoo, presumably in paradoxical sleep. (From Immelman K, Gebbing H: Schlaf bei Giraffiden. Z Tierpsychol 1962;19:84-92.)

These preparatory behaviors justify the description of sleep as appetitive, instinctive behavior.

The timing of daily sleep varies with the species and in each case is complementary to the activity pattern, which may be diurnal, nocturnal, crepuscular, or arrhythmic. Sleep tends to be concentrated in a single period each day in adult humans and the great apes, although the latter and people in many cultures take a midday nap. In most mammals, however, sleep is polyphasic, with sleep episodes interrupted by periods of wakefulness. Species also vary in the degree of responsiveness to external stimuli during sleep, some awakening more readily than others.[9,10]

Sleep onset in mammals is associated with a slowing of EEG activity, a rising of EEG amplitude, and a decrease in muscle activity, followed in most species by the appearance of spindling activity, and in all cases culminating in sustained slow activity at relatively high amplitude. Spindling and slow waves are the hallmarks of mammalian quiet or non–rapid eye movement (NREM) sleep (the term *NREM sleep* is used synonymously with slow wave sleep [SWS] in nonhuman mammals).[11,12] The characterization and quantitative analysis of sleep spindles in nonhuman mammals and their significance has received little attention. It is known that spindles are not merely a transition element in the EEG but that they occur also throughout NREM sleep. In some species, however, the distinction between wakefulness and sleep is not always clear-cut. Especially in carnivores, ungulates, and insectivores, there are frequent or protracted periods when spindles or slow EEG components appear sporadically against background behavioral activity that may not be clearly different from that of wakefulness. This characterizes the state commonly described as drowsiness, also referred to as "light sleep" or "spindle sleep." The transition from wakefulness to sleep depends on the derivation—in an occipital derivation, it is abrupt, whereas in the frontal derivation, it is gradual and can be subdivided into "light" and "deep" sleep.[13] It should be noted that spindles in mammals are most apparent in frontal regions, but this does not mean that sleep there is more superficial.

Spindling activity varies from species to species; it occurs over a wide range of amplitudes and at a variety of frequencies (e.g., 11 waves per second in dogs, 6 to 7 Hz in the sloth, 8 to 11 Hz in the opossum, 10 to 16 Hz in rats, 10 to 13 Hz in mice, and 12 to 16 Hz in primates). Slow wave activity (SWA; 0.5 to 4 Hz) differs in its peak frequency depending on species—that is, it is more concentrated at lower frequencies in some species (human beings, rats) than in others (most mice). The considerable differences in amplitude between species are difficult to interpret because technical aspects of the recordings confound them. Although the changes in the EEG spectrum within NREM sleep, especially in SWA, are known to be continuous, NREM sleep is sometimes subdivided into "light" and "deep" sleep, on the basis of the amount of delta wave activity. In most primates, distinct features of the EEG have led to the definition of two stages in NREM sleep.

Another fundamental characteristic of mammalian sleep is its homeostatic self-regulation, which keeps the amount and depth of sleep in equilibrium with prior wakefulness. Sleep loss creates a debt that is repaid, in part, by some lengthening of subsequent sleep and, in addition, by the intensification of SWA, as indicated by its increased amplitude and density[14] (see Chapters 7 and 33).

Mammalian sleep, as is well known, also includes paradoxical sleep (PS), or REM sleep, which is distinguished by desynchronized, low-amplitude EEG activity in association with eye movements, twitching of the extremities, and postural atonia. Eye movements vary in prominence and may even be absent, as in the mole. Detectability of atonia also varies. Rhythmic theta activity (4 to 8 Hz) originating in the hippocampus is a reliable indicator of PS and can be recorded in some animals with implanted epidural electrodes over the parietal or occipital cortex. Theta activity is less evident in frontal recordings. Many studies in mammals benefit from both recording sites by combining frontoparietal electrodes. Other striking features of PS are ponto-geniculo-occipital (PGO) spikes, cardiorespiratory irregularity, and largely inhibited thermoregulatory responsiveness.[15] In all species, PS, defined by several of its behavioral components, is at its height in early life, either in the fetus or in the neonate. It is initially the predominant state—for example, occupying 90% of the kitten's first 10 days of life and perhaps even more time in the infant rat.[16] By virtue of this pattern, PS has been considered ontogenetically primitive sleep, especially because PS time is reduced as electrophysiologic signs of quiet sleep and wakefulness emerge with maturation. However, recent studies investigating the development of EEG patterns in newborn rat pups have questioned this notion. The alternative view is that the vigilance state typical for newborns is a manifestation of the immature nervous system, which becomes progressively more organized and evolves simultaneously both into the typical EEG and behavioral manifestations of PS and into NREM sleep.[17]

The alternation of quiet sleep with periods of REM sleep constitutes the sleep cycle, also known as the NREM-REM (or REM-NREM) cycle, which can be considered the basic organizational unit of mammalian sleep (Fig. 8–3). Duration of the cycle varies widely from species to species, as do daily sleep quotas and the percentage of sleep time occupied by REM sleep. The cyclic organization of sleep is a characteristic shared by mammals and birds, which also share the behavioral and to some extent the EEG criteria of sleep. Notably, birds have a smaller difference in the EEG spectrum between wakefulness and NREM sleep than mammals. It is still an open question whether the bird brain that lacks the structures

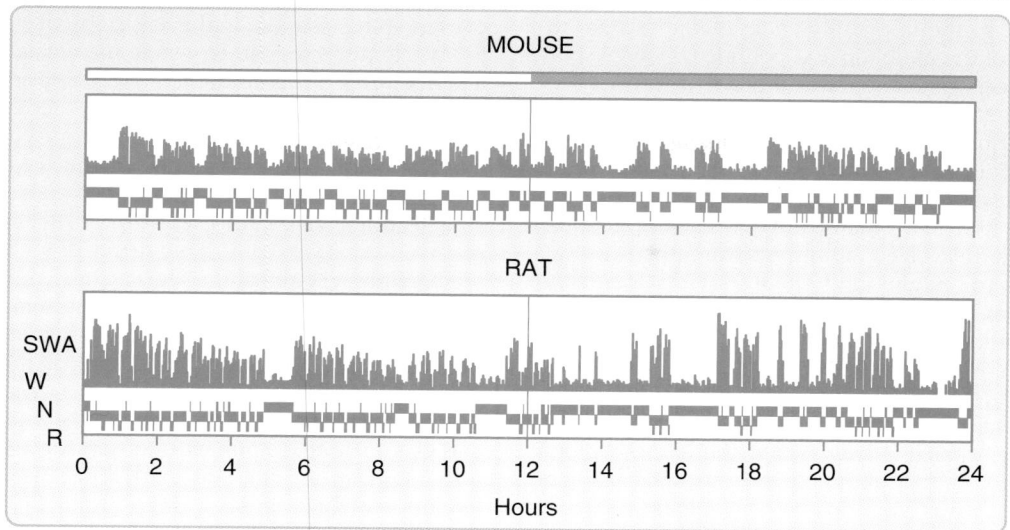

Figure 8–3. Twenty-four-hour distribution of non–rapid eye movement (NREM) sleep (N), REM sleep (R), wakefulness (W), and slow wave activity (SWA—i.e., "delta" power) in a C57BL/6 mouse and a Sprague-Dawley rat recorded in a 12-hour light, 12-hour dark cycle. Note the polyphasic sleep–wakefulness pattern (typical for all nonhuman primates) and the short NREM-REM sleep cycles of 12 to 15 minutes that are typical for small rodents.

responsible for generating slow waves has the capacity to respond to sleep pressure by increasing NREM sleep intensity. Because relatively little is known about avian sleep physiology, other unsuspected differences from mammalian sleep may exist. On the basis of current knowledge, however, what chiefly distinguishes avian from mammalian sleep is the much lower percentage of REM sleep in birds (about 5% of sleep time, on the average, as opposed to 15% to 30% in mammals), the occurrence of REM sleep in clusters, the much briefer REM periods (often less than 10 seconds), and the correspondingly short sleep cycles. It should be noted, however, that there is an immense diversity of bird species, of which few have been recorded.

EVOLUTIONARY HISTORY

The essential similarity of sleep in birds and mammals may well be a clue to the history and function of sleep.[18] The sleep cycle first appears in evolutionary history in association with *endothermy,* which is the maintenance of a high, constant body temperature by metabolic means, as found only in birds and mammals, enabling them to occupy nocturnal niches and survive in cold climates. The alternation between REM and NREM states has yet to be explained, but it is possible that the cycle evolved independently (in parallel) in birds and in mammals, or in their immediate forebears (mammal-like reptiles) (Fig. 8–4). Research on living reptiles has not produced convincing evidence of REM sleep or of sleep organization that might suggest a cycle. Although some studies of reptiles have claimed to see evidence for eye movements and EEG changes during quiescent periods, it remains unclear whether these phenomena were simply transient awakenings or REM sleep.[19] Brain structure and sensorimotor organization in reptiles differ greatly from those in birds and mammals, so it is difficult to draw conclusions about reptilian sleep based on simply observing the electrical activity from screw electrodes positioned on the skull, as can be done in mammals.

However, studies of mammals have localized the neurons driving and responding to REM sleep processes to the brainstem, and these neuronal groups appear to be present in reptiles (see Chapter 10). This can be taken advantage of by recording from these neurons during active and quiescent

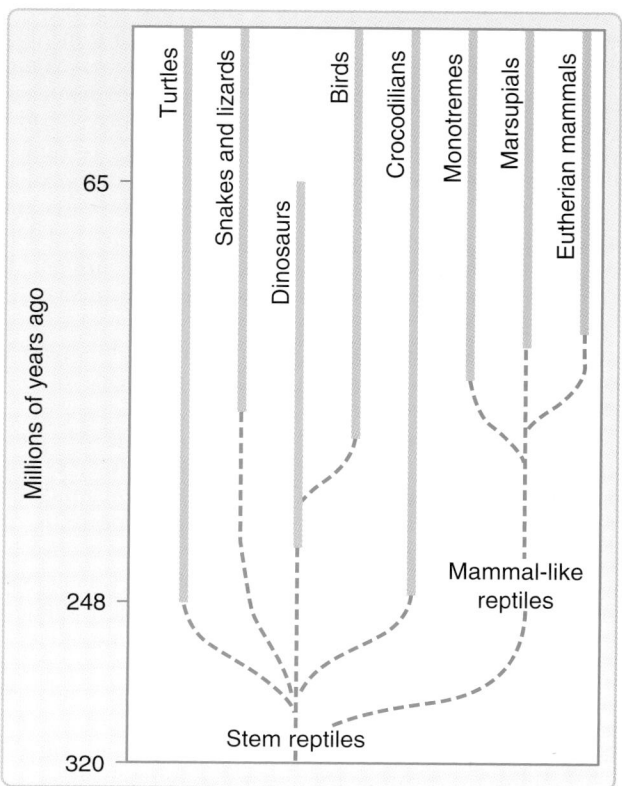

Figure 8–4. Temporal relationships and lines of descent for birds, mammals, and reptiles. *Solid lines* indicate availability of fossil record; *dotted lines* indicate still-uncertain relationships.

states in reptiles. In the first study using this approach, the neuronal activity of the midbrain and pontine regions responsible for REM sleep generation was studied in the turtle.[20] This study found no evidence of cyclicity in neuronal activity during extended quiescent periods and hence no evidence of REM sleep. It would be extremely valuable to confirm these results in other reptilian species. Pending such evidence, these data suggest that REM sleep may not have existed in reptilian species but may have evolved rapidly with endothermy.

A striking finding of the study in turtles was that most brainstem neuronal activity in the observed portions of the midbrain and pontine reticular formation decreased to minimal levels, often completely ceasing, within seconds after movement. In contrast, most brainstem cells in the same brain regions of mammals show tonic activity even during quiet waking. This tonic waking activity presumably allows for more rapid response to sensory inputs. One can speculate that tonic waking activity is accompanied by the need for the inactivity–activity cycle that accompanies mammalian sleep.

Belief that the emergence of PS was relatively recent was encouraged by its reported absence (although quiet sleep was present) in the Australian short-nosed echidna,[21] one of the three surviving monotremes (egg-laying mammals) that diverged early from the main paths of mammalian evolution (see Fig. 8–4). It may seem that some characteristic of the echidna (mode of reproduction, fossorial adaptation, or low body temperature) obviates the need for PS and explains its absence, but this is not the case. The presence of PS in birds shows that it is not related to viviparity. PS is clearly present in other fossorial mammals (e.g., the mole and blind mole rat) and in species with very low body temperature (e.g., the sloth).

Need for qualification of the belief that PS is absent in the echidna is indicated, however, by a finding that, at some times when the echidna's EEG indicates quiet sleep, there are bursts of neuronal activity in its brainstem similar to activity characteristic of REM sleep in therian mammals.[22] This is said to indicate that REM and NREM sleep did not evolve sequentially but as a differentiation of a primitive state that held the seeds of both sleep states. Furthermore, there is now unequivocal evidence of REM sleep in another of the three surviving monotremes, the platypus, occupying 6 to 8 hours per day (more than in any other mammal) and accompanied by eye movements, atonia, twitching, and an elevated response threshold, as generally found in mammalian PS, although with EEG voltage that may be at a level characteristic of quiet sleep in eutherian mammals.[23,24]

Complicating speculation about the history of PS are reports of its absence in the bottle-nosed dolphin and the common porpoise, which cannot be considered primitive mammals[25,26] (see Chapter 10). Most NREM sleep in these species is unihemispheric, consisting of synchronized, slow activity in one cerebral hemisphere and desynchronized activity characteristic of wakefulness in the other. There is no bilateral high-amplitude (delta) sleep. This sleep organization seems necessary to guarantee respiratory function.[27] It has been suggested that PS is also absent on this account, although it is present in the northern fur seal[28] and the manatee,[29] both of which also have unihemispheric sleep. Other reports make it advisable to reserve judgment regarding the absence of PS in any cetaceans. Its possible presence is suggested by a report of quiescent hanging behavior accompanied by twitching in captive beluga whales.[30,31] Penile erections have been reported in the absence of overt sexual behavior in the bottle-nosed dolphin.[32] However, as myoclonus is seen in terrestrial mammals in NREM sleep[32] and nocturnal erections are not always linked to REM sleep in terrestrial mammals,[33] it is unclear whether these observations indicate REM sleep in cetaceans. Unequivocal REM sleep, as identified by EEG and electromyographic (EMG) recording and evidence of elevated arousal thresholds, has not been demonstrated in any cetacean. Even if the twitches that have been observed are eventually demonstrated to be signs of REM sleep, a mystery remains. The maximal number of twitches seen in cetaceans during relatively quiescent periods is of the order of 10 to 20 per day, clustered in two or three short time periods.[31] In terrestrial mammals such as the rat, visual scoring of twitches as has been done in cetaceans registers thousands of twitches each day, most in REM sleep (J. M. Siegel and O. I. Lyamin, unpublished observations). Therefore, even if the twitches in cetaceans mark a REM sleep–like state, the amount of REM sleep in cetaceans would be the lowest among the mammals. Further investigations of cetacean sleep aimed at addressing the question of the amount and nature of REM sleep–like phenomena might provide fundamental insights into the evolution and function of REM sleep.

COMPARATIVE THEORIES

The emerging evolutionary perspective has undermined the previously dominant influence of commonsensical restorative theory, which holds that sleep is for relief of bodily or cerebral deficits caused by waking activity. Restorative theory cannot readily explain the dramatic interspecies variation in daily mammalian sleep quotas (Table 8–1). (For a comprehensive compilation, see *Principles and Practice of Sleep Medicine*, first edition, pp. 39-41. See also Zepelin and Rechtschaffen,[34] Meddis,[35] and Elgar et al.[36,37]).

Inspired by this variation, comparative theories have been advanced as alternatives. Guided by an assumption that sleep varies with complexity of the brain, some of these assert that sleep has cerebral functions. PS has attracted interest in this respect because of its cerebral activation. For example, taking note of instinctive behaviors (e.g., rage) released during PS in cats whose postural atonia is surgically abolished, Jouvet[38] suggested that PS evolved for daily reprogramming of innate behaviors to preserve them in species that rely chiefly on learning. This view is attractive as an explanation for the absence of PS in reptiles and its meagerness in birds, which rely heavily on instinctive behaviors. On the other hand, if the theory is correct, PS quotas should be greatest in mammals with the most learning ability (e.g., primates), but as can be judged by the data in Table 8–1, this is not the case.

In what can be called the eraser theory of REM sleep, Crick and Mitchison have treated its reported absence in the echidna as evidence that it amounts to a mechanism for *reverse learning,* in which stimulation of the forebrain weakens the synaptic strength of undesirable "parasitic modes" of neuronal activity, thus fine-tuning the brain's operation.[39] The echidna, it is said, gets by without REM sleep because its surprisingly large neocortex makes reverse learning unnecessary. If true, an inverse relationship between size of neocortex and REM sleep quotas is to be expected in other species, but supportive data are lacking.[40] Human total sleep time, REM sleep, and percent of sleep time spent in REM sleep are not unusual. Other mammals have much higher or lower amounts of each state.

Table 8–1.	Daily Sleep Quotas in a Sample of Mammalian Species	
Species	Total Daily Sleep Time* (hr)	Daily REM Time (hr)
Echidna	8.5	?
Platypus	14.0	7.0
Opossum	18.0	5.0
Koala	14.5	?
Mole	8.5	2.0
Bat	19.0	3.0
Baboon	9.5	1.0
Humans	8.0	2.0
Armadillo	17.0	3.0
Rabbit	8.0	1.0
Rat	13.0	2.5
Hamster	14.0	3.0
Dolphin	10.0	?
Seal	6.0	1.5
Guinea Pig	9.5	1.0
Cat	12.5	3.0
Ferret	14.5	6.0
Horse	3.0	0.5
Elephant	4.0	?
Giraffe	4.5	0.5

Values are rounded to the half hour and exclude drowsiness. Some values are averages for two or more members of the same genus.

*Total daily sleep time includes daily REM time.

REM, rapid eye movement; ?, reported absence of REM sleep or uncertainty.

This poses a problem for sleep-learning or "information processing" theories of sleep function.[41]

ENERGY CONSERVATION

A major alternative to restorative theory is the view that mammalian sleep is for energy conservation, as suggested by its association with endothermy. Two versions of this view are frequently mistaken to be the same. One of these, advocated by Berger[42] and coworkers, holds that sleep is for reduction of energy expenditure below the level attainable by rest alone. Interdependence of quiet sleep and endothermy is inferred from their concurrent maturation in mammalian infancy and the uninterrupted operation of thermoregulatory processes during quiet sleep at a reduced temperature level.[42,43] The reduced capacity for thermoregulation during PS (see Chapter 24) is considered evidence that PS is a vestige of a reptilian state of ectothermic inactivity. The notion that quiet sleep, torpor, and hibernation are related dormant states with a common purpose, mainly energy conservation, is not upheld by recent data (see Chapter 7). The upsurge and intensification of SWA directly following bouts of torpor or hibernation suggest compensation for loss of sleep during the hypothermic bouts.[44-46] The metabolic expense of heating the body toward euthermia in the periodic interruptions of hibernation is close to the energy saving that results from the immobilization and lower temperature during hibernation.

Above all is the question of whether reduction of metabolic rate is sufficient as the raison d'être for sleep. At most, sleep could effect a metabolic saving of about 15%,[47] and the savings would largely depend on the animal's nutrition[48] and its capacity to remain in quiet wakefulness. There are some species with high sleep quotas and low metabolic rates, a condition traceable to energy-deficient diets.[48] An outstanding example is the endangered koala (see Table 8–1), whose diet consists of rare types of eucalyptus leaves with low nutritional value.[49] Other examples are edentates (e.g., the sloth) and armadillos. Such species cannot afford high activity levels. Their extended sleep seems necessary to ease metabolic pressure and is consistent with a role for sleep in energy conservation. In humans, the overnight saving is more likely to be only 5% to 11%, taking into account the effects of body movement and arousals.[50-52] An argument against the view that sleep is for energy conservation enforced by rest is the reported continuous movement of dolphins while asleep.[3] This is considered evidence of some sleep function other than enforced rest.

Correlational Findings

The second version of energy conservation theory considers the reduction of metabolic rate during sleep to be of minor importance. The principal contribution of sleep (with no qualification regarding PS) is held to be the enforcement of rest so as to set a limit on activity and energy expenditure. This view emerged from Zepelin and Rechtschaffen's[34] comparative study of sleep parameters, potential life span, and other constitutional variables in 53 mammalian species. The study assessed a long-standing belief that species with high daily sleep quotas have relatively long potential life spans because they benefit from lowered metabolism during sleep. The contrary proved to be the case: long-sleeping species are typically short-lived. They also tend to be small in size and high in basal or resting metabolic rate per unit of body weight. There was an impressive correlation (0.63) between sleep quotas and metabolic rate.[53] Together with knowledge that the metabolic cost of physical activity varies inversely with body size[54] and that daily food requirements relative to body size are disproportionately high in small mammals,[55] the finding on metabolic rate led to the conclusion that sleep sets a limit on energy expenditure to the extent necessary to balance a species' energy budget.

Table 8–2 summarizes relevant correlations found in updated analyses of EEG and behavioral sleep data for 85 taxa (species or genera), with missing data for some taxa in each analysis. Despite recent revisions in the sleep data (Asian elephant,[56] giraffe[57]), added data for newly studied species (koala,[58] ferret[59]), and some adjustments and expansion of the data for constitutional variables, the results are quite similar to previous findings. Previous and present correlations of body weight, brain weight, and encephalization quotient with total daily sleep time and cycle length are virtually identical. Consistency was somewhat less for correlations of metabolic rate and the correlations of PS measures. Correlations of quiet sleep time differed most from previous findings. This was because the present analyses made no adjustment of sleep quotas for drowsiness.

Analyses of partial correlations found, as in previous research, that brain weight and cycle length were positively correlated independently of body weight ($r = .64$; $P < .001$), but body weight and cycle length did not correlate independently, thus leaving brain weight alone as a likely determinant

Table 8–2.   Correlations between Sleep Parameters and Constitutional Variables

Constitutional Variables	Total Daily Sleep Time (hr)	Quiet Sleep Time (hr)	Paradoxical Sleep Time (hr)	Paradoxical Sleep (%)	Cycle Length
Body weight	−.53*	−.53*	−.45*	−.12	.83*
	(85)	(65)	(65)	(65)	(33)
Brain weight	−.55*	−.48*	−.52*	−.25	.89*
	(71)	(56)	(54)	(56)	(32)
Metabolic rate	33†	.30‡	.13	−.09	−.82*
	(65)	(51)	(50)	(50)	(29)
Encephalization quotient	−.17	−.10	−.20†	−.30‡	.52†
	(69)	(55)	(53)	(55)	(32)

Common logarithmic transformations were used for the constitutional variables. Log (1 + X) transformations were used for paradoxical sleep values. Number of cases per coefficient is in parentheses.

*$P < .001$
†$P < .01$
‡$P < .05$

of cycle length. Brain weight and body weight both failed to correlate with sleep time independently of each other, as was found in a previous set of analyses.[60] It therefore seems best to consider the correlations of sleep time with brain weight and body weight, without distinction between them, as consequences of *body size*. Multiple regression analysis showed that brain weight and body weight together (i.e., body size) could account for 31% of the variance in sleep time.

Findings similar to those discussed earlier were obtained by Elgar et al.[36,37] in a study based solely on electrographic sleep data for 69 species, with family as the unit of analysis. Agreement between the two sets of findings is important because the choice of families as the taxonomic level for analysis guards against possible inflation of sample size owing to similarities between species with shared phylogenetic backgrounds.

The correlation findings underwrite the view that sleep occurs to enforce rest and keep energy expenditure at an affordable level. There may be less pressure for sleep in large species because of their greater energy reserves. The proportion of fat to body mass increases with size, ranging from less than 5% in the smallest mammals up to 25% to 30% in species weighing 1000 kg.[55] As body size increases, the ratio of surface to body mass decreases and thickness of fur increases. Large mammals consequently have lower *thermal conductance* (flow of heat to the environment) and wider thermoneutral zones. This lessens requirements for active heat production to maintain body temperature. Lindstedt and Boyce,[60] as illustrated by Figure 8–5, have shown that *fasting endurance* (survival time) at thermoneutrality is a function of body size, and the size advantage is accentuated in the cold. Even at thermoneutrality, as the figure shows, survival time is short for small species. Many are frequently only hours away from death by starvation. They may require more sleep to avoid exhaustion of energy reserves. Also consistent with an energy conservation role are the relatively high sleep quotas that all mammals have early in the maturational period, when energy must be channeled into growth.

This version of energy conservation theory befits the requirements of endothermy, which is not only for thermoregulation alone but also for the increased aerobic capacity required for sustained running, climbing, and other vigorous activities. A mammal's basal energy requirement is at least five times that of an ectotherm similar in size and body temperature.[61] This theory is also in accord with findings on prolonged sleep deprivation in rats. With ultimately fatal consequences, the rats suffered from increased metabolism, as shown by weight loss in spite of increased food intake, along with reduced body temperature in spite of increased metabolic rate. Prolonged deprivation of REM sleep alone has similar effects.[62-64] These findings indicate

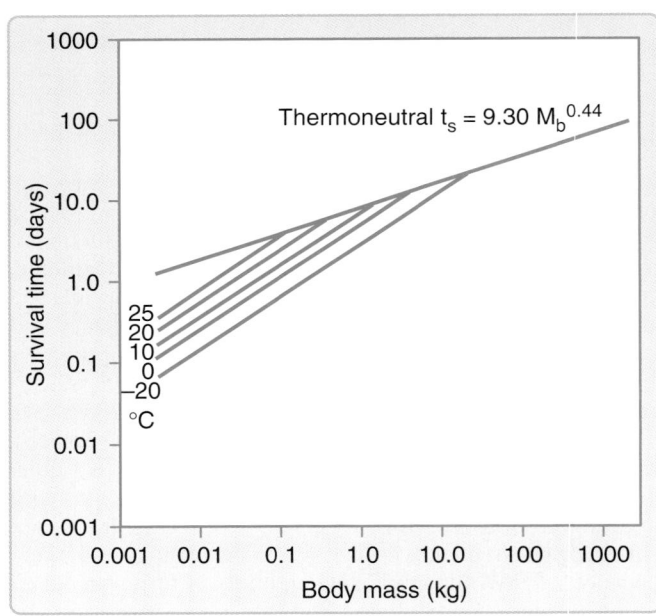

Figure 8–5. Fasting endurance (or survival time) as a function of body size for mammals. The *top line* represents survival time at thermoneutral ambient temperature, where $t_s = 9.30\ M_b^{0.44}$. *Steeper lines* represent survival times at elevated metabolism induced by cold. (From Lindstedt SL, Boyce MS: Seasonality, fasting endurance, and body size in mammals. Am Nat 1985;125:873-878. The University of Chicago Press. All rights reserved.)

an indispensable role for sleep in energy regulation, as suggested by the relationships of sleep quotas and constitutional variables. The convergence here of experimental and correlational findings is theoretically promising.

Immobilization Theory

Because correlational findings in support of energy conservation theory fall short of explaining even half of the variance in sleep quotas, the way is open for other viewpoints. Restorative theories having failed to explain species differences, behavioral theories have come to the fore, expanding the concept of sleep as a state of enforced rest. It is suggested, for example, that large mammals sleep relatively little because they require extra time for foraging.[65] A related view is that the function of sleep amounts to *adaptive nonresponding*,[35,65] meaning that it prevents activity (e.g., foraging) when it would be dangerous or inefficient, and it blocks harmful reactions that might occur in an animal merely resting but aware of ongoing events. Meddis[35] (p. 54) elaborated, "The benefits of sleep depend upon the species. For some the conservation of energy is most valuable, for others, the protection from predation... for others, the timing element." In effect, however, such theory is untestable, for there will always be some need that sleep can be said to meet. Filling spare time can be considered a function of sleep. But how much spare time does a species have? With circular reasoning, it is argued that time in sleep is a measure of spare time (Fig. 8–6).

ECOLOGIC INFLUENCES: THE ALTRICIAL–PRECOCIAL DIMENSION

It is often assumed that species differences in sleep reflect environmental influences, but this is not readily apparent. Probably the clearest case of an ecologically determined characteristic is the unihemispheric sleep found in some marine mammals. Drowsiness in some species seems to have an ecologic basis. Its prominence in ungulates (e.g., the horse) may be a compromise between sleep and alertness to predatory threat. On the other hand, there is no simple explanation for the prominent drowsiness of carnivores (e.g., the cat), which seems like purposeless fraying of sleep.

Predation is the ecologic variable that has attracted most interest. Because of the scarcity of data on the extent to which individual species are subject to predation or have suffered from it in their evolutionary past, judgments of its influence are open to question. Findings by Allison and Cicchetti,[65] however, raised the possibility that PS quotas are reduced by predatory threat because the elevation of sensory thresholds during PS puts prey at a disadvantage.

Relatively neglected in ecologic theorizing about sleep is the role of species differences in reproductive strategies and life histories. Adaptation to the environment occurs not only through fine-tuning of physical and behavioral characteristics but also through changes in the number of offspring and the timing of their maturation. Interspecies variation in sleep may be secondary to such adaptations. Commanding attention in this respect is the variation of REM sleep with maturational variables, as illustrated in Figures 8–7 and 8–8.

In *precocial species*, that is, those born fairly mature (e.g., the guinea pig, sheep), the REM sleep percentage at birth is low and near the adult level. In *altricial species*, that is, those born immature (e.g., the rat, the cat), the REM sleep percentage is initially high and remains relatively high even after maturation.[16] Also indicative of influence by maturational timing is the inverse correlation of REM quotas with gestation time.[34,36]

Previous findings of correlation between daily REM sleep time and degree of maturity at birth were confirmed with expanded data for up to 65 viviparous species or genera (echidna and platypus excluded). For eutherian mammals,

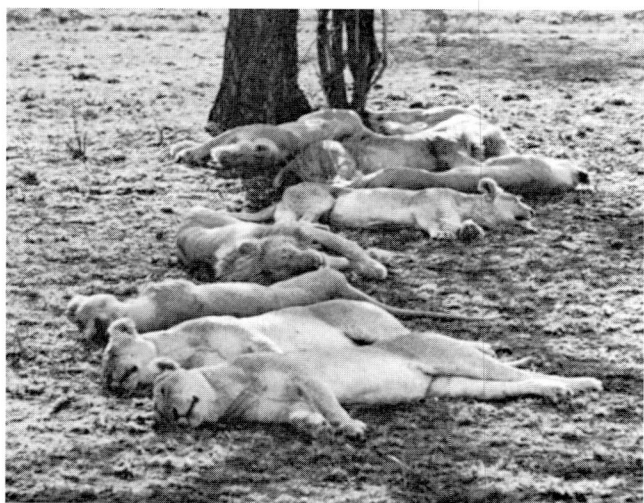

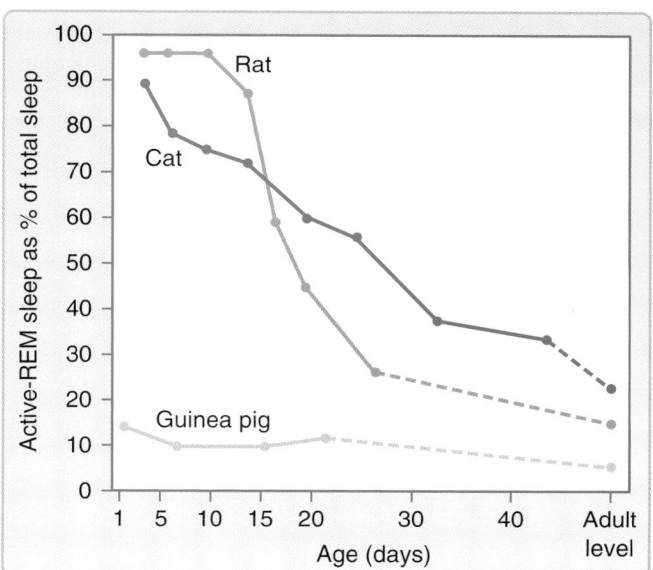

Figure 8–7. Maturational changes in rapid eye movement (REM) sleep as a percentage of total sleep time in two altricial species (rat and cat) and a precocial species (guinea pig). (Reprinted from Jouvet-Mounier D, Astic L, Lacote D: Ontogenesis of the states of sleep in rat, cat, and guinea pig during the first postnatal month. Dev Psychobiol 1970;2:216-239, by permission. Copyright 1970, John Wiley & Sons.)

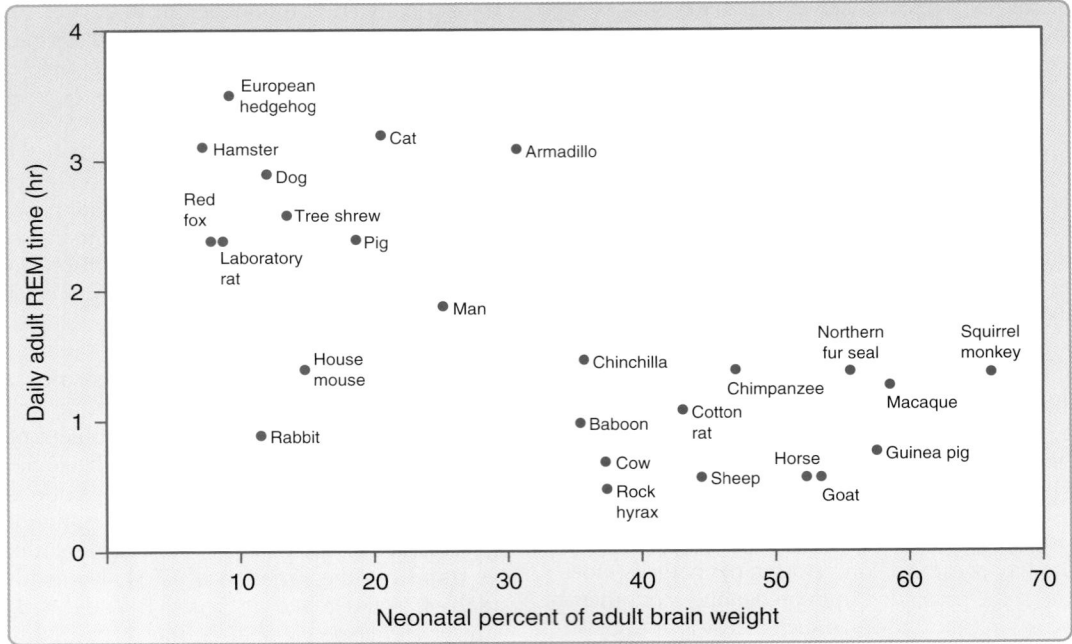

Figure 8–8. Daily rapid eye movement (REM) sleep time in adult mammals as a function of neonatal maturity, represented by the percentage of adult brain weight in neonates of the same species.

the four-point altricial–precocial (A-P) ratings were assigned previously by an expert mammalogist without knowledge of the sleep data (Table 8–3). For this analysis, the author gave marsupials a rating of 1 based on the criteria of the scale. The results, shown in Table 8–4, were independent of body weight and brain weight and differed from previous findings chiefly in terms of a significant correlation in the present research between the PS percentage and the gestation period. It is noteworthy that in the four marsupial species, the two with the shortest gestation periods had PS quotas and percentages radically higher than the others—the highest in the entire sample. The recent findings in the platypus strengthen these correlations, as these animals are highly immature at birth

and they have the highest amount of REM sleep time of any animal yet studied. The absence or minimal presence of PS in cetaceans is understandable on the basis of their extreme precociality.

These analyses also found a correlation of .49 (P < .001) between daily quotas of PS and quiet sleep. In the 49 species with complete data, this correlation with body weight and

Table 8–3.	Altricial–Precocial Scale for Neonates of Viviparous Species
Scale Value	Description
1	Eyes closed; naked; rolls; sometimes can cling (1.5: fur shows)
2	Eyes barely closed or just open; furred; crawls well (2.5: eyes open; can cling)
3	Eyes open; furred; can stand
4	Eyes open; furred; can walk and follow or swim

Intermediate scale values (e.g., 2.8) were assigned to some species.

Adapted from Eisenberg JF. The Mammalian Radiations. Chicago, Ill: University of Chicago Press; 1981. Copyright 1981 by The University of Chicago. All rights reserved.

Table 8–4.	Correlations of Paradoxical Sleep Parameters with Measures of Neonatal Maturity and Reproductive Variables	
Measures of Neonatal Maturity and Reproductive Variables	Paradoxical Sleep Time (hr)	Paradoxical Sleep (%)
Altricial–precocial rating	−.66* (65)	−.45† (64)
Neonatal brain weight (%)	−.61* (27)	−.55† (27)
Gestation period	.63* (60)	−.39† (59)
Litter size	.51* (63)	.41† (62)

To minimize skewness, common logarithmic transformations were used for gestation period and litter size. Log (1 + X) transformations were used for paradoxical sleep values. Number of cases per coefficient is in parentheses.

*P < .001

†P < .01

brain weight partialed out was .28 ($P < .05$). These results are consistent with the view that PS provides endogenous stimulation to the brain to promote recovery from sleep.[66]

The striking relationships between REM quotas and neonatal characteristics give no clear indication of the maturational events that are responsible. If one adopts Parmeggiani's[67] view that REM physiology is under rhombencephalic regulation (as opposed to the hypothalamic regulation in the rest of sleep), then maturation of the hypothalamus may be the critical factor. Given the expression of fetal characteristics (lapse of thermoregulation, respiratory irregularity, and twitching) in REM sleep during maturity, REM sleep could be considered a carryover from fetal life. The difference between mammals and birds in the representation of REM may well be explained by unidentified differences between them in maturational timing.

The association of REM with altriciality takes on added significance with the realization that reptiles are strictly precocial and that altriciality evolved in birds and mammals in conjunction with endothermy. Evolutionary theorists agree that the metabolic cost of endothermy favored altriciality, which meant the birth of exothermic rather than endothermic young. One view is that altriciality reduced the energy requirements for maturation by placing reliance on parental body heat for temperature regulation in the young, allowing their food to be channeled primarily into growth.[68] Another view is that altriciality mainly allowed greater flexibility in meeting energy requirements by shortening gestation and incubation periods, putting off much of the expense of propagation until after birth, thus splitting the expense between parents, both of whom could then forage for the young.[69] Precociality in some mammals evolved as a later adaptation.

Rather than outright inheritance from reptiles, as the finding of REM sleep in the platypus has suggested to some writers, REM sleep seems to be part of the evolution of endothermy, which distinguishes mammals from reptiles. It is simultaneously part of the transition from the strict precociality of reptiles. The limited indications of REM sleep features in the echidna are evidence of this transitional origin as opposed to straightforward inheritance from reptilian forebears.

SUMMARY

Evolutionary history suggests that mammalian sleep developed in association with endothermy, paralleling a similar development of sleep in birds. Consistent with this impression are several clusters of correlated variables that must also be taken into account in theorizing about the function of sleep. One is the correlation of daily mammalian sleep quotas with body weight and weight-specific metabolic rate, indicating greater requirements of sleep in species with low energy reserves. Another is the correlation of REM sleep parameters with A-P status, gestation time, and litter size, indicating the influence of maturational timetables on the prominence of REM sleep and suggesting that it is a byproduct of altriciality and endothermy. Less clearly related to endothermy is the positive correlation of the NREM-REM cycle length with brain weight, a relationship that is also apparent in the increase of cycle length with maturation in mammals. On the basis of an old comparative study that showed a high correlation of mammalian brain weight with cortical acetylcholine content and cholinesterase activity,[70] it could be speculated that cholinergic mechanisms known to influence cycle length are probably its operative link with brain weight.[71]

> **Clinical Pearl**
>
> *Although many sleep parameters differ between species, human sleep does not appear to be qualitatively unique. This factor makes animal models suitable for the investigation of many aspects of sleep pharmacology and pathology.*

Acknowledgment

Thanks to Cathleen S. Zepelin for artwork and assistance with data analysis.

References

1. Rechtschaffen A: Current perspectives on the function of sleep. Perspect Biol Med 1998;41:359-390.
2. Campbell SS, Tobler I: Animal sleep: A review of sleep duration across phylogeny. Neurosci Biobehav Rev 1984;8:269-300.
3. Pilleri G: The blind Indus dolphin, *Platanista indi.* Endeavour 1979;3:48-56.
4. Lyamin OI, Mukhametov LM, Siegel JM: Relationship between sleep and eye state in Cetaceans and Pinnipeds. Arch Ital Biol 2004;142:557-568.
5. Bourliere F: The Natural History of Mammals, 3rd ed. New York, Alfred A Knopf, 1967.
6. Hediger H: Comparative observations on sleep. Proc R Soc Med 1969;62:1-4.
7. Hediger H: The biology of natural sleep in animals. Experientia 1980;36:13-16.
8. Moss C: Portraits in the Wild. Boston, Houghton Mifflin, 1975.
9. Van Twyver H: Sleep patterns in five rodent species. Physiol Behav 1969;4:901-905.
10. Zepelin H: Sleep in the jaguar and the tapir: A prey-predator contrast. Psychophysiology 1970;7:306.
11. Rechtschaffen A, Kales A: A Manual for Standardized Terminology, Techniques, and Scoring System for Sleep Stages of Human Subjects. Washington, DC, Public Health Service, US Government Printing Office, 1968.
12. Ursin R: The two stages of slow wave sleep in the cat and their relation to REM sleep. Brain Res 1968;11:347-356.
13. Huber R, Deboer T, Tobler I: Sleep deprivation in prion protein deficient mice and control mice: Genotype dependent regional rebound. Neuroreport 2002;13:1-4.
14. Borbély AA, Tobler I: Homeostatic and circadian principles in sleep regulation in the rat. In McGinty DJ (ed): Brain Mechanisms of Sleep. New York, Raven Press, 1985, pp 35-44.
15. McGinty DJ, Siegel JM: Sleep states. In Satinoff E, Teitelbaum P (eds): Motivation. (Handbook of Behavioral Neurobiology, vol 6.) New York, Plenum Press, 1983, pp 105-181.
16. Jouvet-Mounier D, Astic L, Lacote D: Ontogenesis of the states of sleep in rat, cat, and guinea pig during the first postnatal month. Dev Psychobiol 1968;2:216-239.
17. Frank MG, Heller C: The ontogeny of mammalian sleep: A reappraisal of alternative hypotheses. J Sleep Res 2003;12:25-34.
18. Allison T, Van Twyver H: The evolution of sleep. Nat Hist 1970;79:56-65.
19. Siegel JM: The evolution of REM sleep. In Lydic R, Baghdoyan HA (eds): Handbook of Behavioral State Control. Boca Raton, Fla, CRC Press, 1999, pp 87-100.
20. Eiland MM, Lyamin OI, Siegel JM: State-related discharge of neurons in the brainstem of freely moving box turtles, *Terrapene carolina major.* Arch Ital Biol 2001;139:23-36.
21. Allison T, Van Twyver H, Goff WR: Electrophysiological studies of the echidna, *Tachyglossus aculeatus:* I. Waking and sleep. Arch Ital Biol 1972;110:145-184.
22. Siegel JM, Manger PR, Nienhuis R, et al: The echidna *Tachyglossus aculeatus* combines REM and non-REM aspects in a single sleep state. J Neurosci 1996;16:3500-3506.

23. Siegel JM: Monotremes and the evolution of REM sleep. Sleep Res Soc Bull 1997;4:31-32.

24. Siegel JM, Manger PR, Nienhuis R, et al: Sleep in the platypus. Neuroscience 1999;91:391-400.

25. Mukhametov LM, Supin AY: EEG study of different behavioral states in free-moving dolphin, *Tursiops truncatus* [in Russian]. Zh Vyssh Nerv Deiat 1975;25:396-401.

26. Mukhametov LM, Poliakova IG: EEG investigation of sleep in porpoises, *Phocoena phocoena* [in Russian]. Zh Vyssh Nerv Deiat 1981;3:333-339.

27. Mukhametov LM, Supin AY, Poliakova IG: Interhemispheric asymmetry of the electroencephalographic sleep patterns in dolphins. Brain Res 1977;124:581-584.

28. Mukhametov LM, Liamin OI, Poliakova IG: Sleep and wakefulness in *Callorhinus ursinus* [in Russian]. Zh Vyssh Nerv Deiat 1984;34:465-471.

29. Mukhametov LM, Lyamin OL, Chetyrbok IS: Sleep and wakefulness in an Amazonian manatee. In Horne JA (ed): Sleep 1990: Proceedings of the Tenth European Congress on Sleep Research, Strasbourg, France, 1990, May 20-25. Bochum, Germany, Pontenagel Press, 1990, pp 119-122.

30. Lyamin OI, Mukhametov LM, Siegel JM, et al: Unihemispheric slow wave sleep and the state of the eyes in a white whale. Behav Brain Res 2002;129:125-129.

31. Lyamin OI, Shpak OV, Nazarenko EA, Mukhametov LM: Muscle jerks during behavioral sleep in a beluga whale (*Delphinapterus leucas L*). Physiol Behav 2002;76:265-270.

32. Coleman RM, Pollak CP, Weitzman ED: Periodic movements in sleep nocturnal myoclonus: Relation to sleep disorders. Ann Neurol 1980;8:416-421.

33. Affanni JM, Cervino CO, Marcos HJ: Absence of penile erections during paradoxical sleep: Peculiar penile events during wakefulness and slow wave sleep in the armadillo. J Sleep Res 2001;10:219-228.

34. Zepelin H, Rechtschaffen A: Mammalian sleep, longevity, and energy metabolism. Brain Behav Evol 1974;10:425-470.

35. Meddis R: The Sleep Instinct. London, Routledge and Kegan Paul, 1977, p 54.

36. Elgar MA, Pagel MD, Harvey PH, et al: Sleep in mammals. Anim Behav 1988;36:1407-1419.

37. Elgar MA, Pagel MD, Harvey PH, et al: Sources of variation in mammalian sleep. Anim Behav 1990;40:991-994.

38. Jouvet M: The function of dreaming: A neurophysiologist's point of view. In Gazzaniga MS, Blakemore C (eds): Handbook of Psychobiology. New York, Academic Press, 1975, pp 499-527.

39. Crick F, Mitchison G: The function of dream sleep. Nature 1983;304:111-114.

40. Zepelin H: Encephalization and species differences in REM sleep: A test of the Crick-Mitchison theory. Sleep Res 1985;14:85.

41. Siegel JM: The REM sleep-memory consolidation hypothesis. Science 2001;294:1058-1063.

42. Berger RJ: Bioenergetic functions of sleep and activity rhythms and their possible relevance to aging. Fed Proc 1975;34:97-102.

43. Glotzbach SF, Heller HC: Central nervous regulation of body temperature during sleep. Science 1976;194:537-539.

44. Walker JM, Berger RJ: Sleep as an adaptation for energy conservation functionally related to hibernation and shallow torpor. Prog Brain Res 1980;53:255-278.

45. Deboer T, Tobler I: Sleep EEG after daily torpor in the Djungarian hamster: Similarity to the effects of sleep deprivation. Neurosci Lett 1994;166:35-38.

46. Trachsel L, Edgar DM, Heller HC: Are ground squirrels sleep-deprived during hibernation? Am J Physiol 1991;260:R1123-R1129.

47. Shapiro CM, Goll CC, Cohen GR, et al: Heat production during sleep. J Appl Physiol 1984;56:671-677.

48. McNab BK: The influence of food habits on the energetics of eutherian mammals. Ecol Monogr 1986;56:1-19.

49. Lee A, Martin R: Life in the slow lane. Nat Hist 1990;8:34-42.

50. Ravussin E, Lillioja S, Anderson TE, et al: Determinants of 24-hour energy expenditure in man: Methods and results using a respiratory chamber. J Clin Invest 1986;78:1568-1578.

51. Garby L, Kurzer MS, Lammert O, et al: Energy expenditure during sleep in men and women: Evaporative and sensible heat losses. Hum Nutr Clin Nutr 1987;41:225-233.

52. Goldberg GR, Prentice AM, Davies HL, et al: Overnight and basal metabolic rates in men and women. Eur J Clin Nutr 1988;42:137-144.

53. Zepelin H: Mammalian sleep, metabolic rate, and body size. Sleep Res 1986;15:62.

54. Schmidt-Nielsen K: Locomotion: Energy cost of swimming, flying, and running. Science 1972;177:222-228.

55. Calder WA III: Size, Function, and Life History. Cambridge, Mass, Harvard University Press, 1984.

56. Tobler I: Behavioral sleep in the Asian elephant in captivity. Sleep 1992;15:1-12.

57. Tobler I, Schwierin B: Behavioural sleep in the giraffe (*Giraffa camelopardalis*) in a zoological garden. J Sleep Res 1996;5:21-32.

58. Nagy KA, Martin RW: Field metabolic rate, water flux, food consumption, and time budget of koalas, *Phascolarctos cinereus*, in Victoria. Aust J Zool 1985;33:655-665.

59. Marks GA, Shaffery JP: A preliminary study of sleep in the ferret, *Mustela putorius furo*: A carnivore with an extremely high proportion of REM sleep. Sleep 1996;19:83-93.

60. Lindstedt SL, Boyce MS: Seasonality, fasting endurance, and body size in mammals. Am Nat 1985;125:873-878.

61. Bennett AF, Ruben JA: Endothermy and activity in vertebrates. Science 1979;206:649-654.

62. Rechtschaffen A, Gilliland MA, Bergmann BM, et al: Physiological correlates of prolonged sleep deprivation in rats. Science 1983;221:182-184.

63. Rechtschaffen A, Bergmann BM, Everson CA, et al: Sleep deprivation in the rat: X. Integration and discussion of the findings. Sleep 1989;12:68-87.

64. Rechtschaffen A, Bergmann BM: Sleep deprivation in the rat by the disk-over-eater method. Behav Brain Res 1995;69:55-63.

65. Allison T, Cicchetti DV: Sleep in mammals: Ecological and constitutional correlates. Science 1976;194:732-734.

66. Vertes RP: A life-sustaining function for REM sleep: A theory. Neurosci Biobehav Rev 1986;10:371-376.

67. Parmeggiani PL: Regulation of physiological functions during sleep in mammals. Experientia 1982;38:1405-1408.

68. Hopson JA: Endothermy, small size, and the origin of mammalian reproduction. Am Nat 1973;107:446-452.

69. Case TJ: Endothermy and parental care in the terrestrial vertebrates. Am Nat 1978;112:861-874.

70. Tower DB, Elliott KAC: Activity of acetylcholine system in cerebral cortex of various unanesthetized mammals. Am J Physiol 1952;168:747-759.

71. Sitaram N, Moore AM, Gillin JC: Experimental acceleration and slowing of REM sleep ultradian rhythm by cholinergic agonist and antagonist. Nature 1978;274:490-492.

Brain Electrical Activity and Sensory Processing during Waking and Sleep States

Mircea Steriade

ABSTRACT

Different types of brain rhythms characterize wakefulness, non–rapid eye movement (NREM) or slow wave sleep (SWS), and rapid eye movement (REM) sleep. Cortical and thalamic neurons display changes in intrinsic and synaptic excitability during shifts between these states of vigilance.

Two main points should be emphasized with regard to brain rhythms. First, the newly discovered slow sleep oscillation (0.5 to 1 Hz), first disclosed in intracellular recordings from cortical and thalamic neurons in animal experiments, and also described with extracellular and intracellular recordings during natural SWS in animals and with EEG and electromyographic recordings during human sleep, has the virtue of entraining other SWS oscillations (spindles and delta waves) in complex wave sequences. This is due to the synchronous firing of cortical neurons whose discharges trigger thalamic circuits. Thus, the neocortex and thalamus constitute a unified oscillatory machine. The best example is the fact that the K-complexes, a major grapho-element of NREM sleep, have the same pattern and rhythmicity as the slow cortical oscillation, and they are followed by a short sequence of spindle waves because thalamic neuronal circuits are set into action. Second, the activation of brain electrical activity during waking and REM sleep is associated with short-scale synchronization of fast (20 to 50 Hz) waves over the cerebral cortex as well as in corticothalamic neuronal loops. Thus, the notion of desynchronization becomes obsolete and should be replaced with the term *EEG activation*.

The first relay station where blockade of synaptic transmission is observed during the period of falling asleep is the thalamus. Synaptic transmission in thalamocortical systems is enhanced during both waking and REM sleep, compared with NREM sleep. During wakefulness, inhibitory periods are shorter than during NREM sleep, but very effective. This provides a mechanism for selection of relevant input signals, as required during an adaptive state.

The states of wakefulness and sleep are characterized by a set of three cardinal physiologic correlates: brain wave activity (electroencephalogram [EEG]), eye movements, and muscle tone. This chapter addresses (1) the morphologic substrates and cellular bases of spontaneous EEG rhythms; and (2) the responses elicited by sensory inputs, and how these responses change during the two basic cerebral conditions of resting and active behavioral states of vigilance.

In the initial sections of this chapter, the basic mechanisms underlying high-amplitude and widely synchronized EEG oscillations during slow wave sleep (SWS) and the neuronal substrates of EEG changes when the state of the brain shifts from SWS to brain arousal are discussed. Work has revealed a series of intrinsic electrophysiologic properties of neurons that have an important role in the patterning of various EEG oscillations.[1] However, the synchronous activation of a neuronal ensemble (or network) requires a mechanism for coordination of the individual oscillations. The determining role of neuronal networks involved in the genesis of SWS oscillations and in their disruption on arousal, as well as the neuronal mechanisms underlying fast rhythms during brain-active states, are discussed in the first part of this chapter. Emphasis is placed on the concept that the cerebral cortex and the thalamus constitute a unified system that generates the coalescence of different brain rhythms into complex wave sequences, which include not only various low-frequency oscillations, but also fast rhythms.

In the second part of the chapter, the dependency of sensory synaptic transmission on the behavioral state of vigilance is analyzed. Data indicate that blockade of afferent information at sleep onset takes place in the thalamus. The enhanced excitability of thalamic and cortical neurons on awakening and during rapid eye movement (REM) sleep is due to brainstem and forebrain modulatory systems. Fine inhibitory sculpturing produces input selection and output tuning.

PRELIMINARY DEFINITIONS

The state of SWS or non-REM (NREM) sleep is easily distinguishable from both wakefulness and REM sleep by high-amplitude and synchronous EEG rhythms. Desynchronization during waking and REM sleep means the disruption of high-amplitude and synchronous EEG waves, and the replacement of low-frequency oscillations by fast rhythms with lower amplitude.[2] However, the spontaneously occurring fast rhythms (20 to 50 Hz, called beta and gamma) during brain-active states are synchronized over restricted distances in the cortex[3] as well as among cortical areas and related thalamic nuclei.[4,5] Therefore, it is better to use the term *activation*[2] than *desynchronization* to designate the electrical activity during waking and REM sleep. The paradox that a similar EEG activity characterizes two states of vigilance that are commonly regarded as extreme poles of the sleep–waking cycle suggests that, with regard to brain cellular activities, waking and REM sleep are closer than is usually believed, and both are opposed to NREM sleep, which is characterized by widely synchronized activities. Indeed, data discussed in this chapter indicate that thalamic and cortical neurons similarly display an increased excitability during both waking and REM sleep. This brain state is called *activation*, a term used at the cellular level and implying a readiness of neuronal networks of the cerebrum to receive afferent information and ensure quick responses. As such, the notion of activation refers to the response readiness of brain neurons either to stimuli from the outside world (as in waking) or to internal drives (as in REM sleep), regardless of whether an overt motor response is generated. Hence, both waking and REM sleep are regarded as brain-activated states, in spite of illogical thought and largely suppressed motor output in REM sleep.

Activation was initially viewed as a globally energizing system of the brain, originating in the brainstem reticular formation.[2,6] Because both processes of excitation and sculpturing inhibition are present in complex integrative tasks of the alert state, one should include inhibition in the process of activation.[7] It was then expected that with an increased level of activation on awakening, both excitatory and inhibitory components of brain responses would increase. Instead, a series of experiments during the 1960s and 1970s reported results suggesting that the increased excitability of thalamic neurons on arousal is due to a global blockade of inhibitory effects acting on them. This embarrassing conclusion was derived from the earlier Zeitgeist that viewed the thalamic reticular nucleus as the only source of thalamic inhibition, as well as from the lack of evidence, during that time, of a significant proportion of inhibitory elements intrinsic to each thalamic nucleus. Since 1980, it has become clear that 20% to 30% of neurons in all major thalamic nuclei of cats and primates operate on a local basis and use gamma-aminobutyric acid (GABA), a potent inhibitory synaptic transmitter.[8] In the section on processing of sensory information, the evidence is further discussed that activation processes in thalamocortical systems involve a direct excitation from the brainstem reticular core, associated with the blockade of long-lasting and cyclic inhibitory potentials that are involved in EEG synchronizing patterns, but also accompanied by preservation and even enhancement of shorter-lasting inhibitory influences, which result in an increased receptive field specificity and orientation selectivity.

CELLULAR BASES OF SYNCHRONOUS OSCILLATIONS AND ACTIVATION PATTERNS IN THALAMOCORTICAL SYSTEMS

Low-Frequency Oscillations in Corticothalamic Networks during NREM Sleep

Three types of oscillations characterize the state of resting sleep: spindle (7 to 14 Hz), delta (1 to 4 Hz), and slow oscillations (<1 Hz).[9] Each of these rhythms originates through intrinsic neuronal properties and network operations in the thalamus and neocortex, even after isolation of these structures (Fig. 9–1). However, in an intact brain, there are no pure

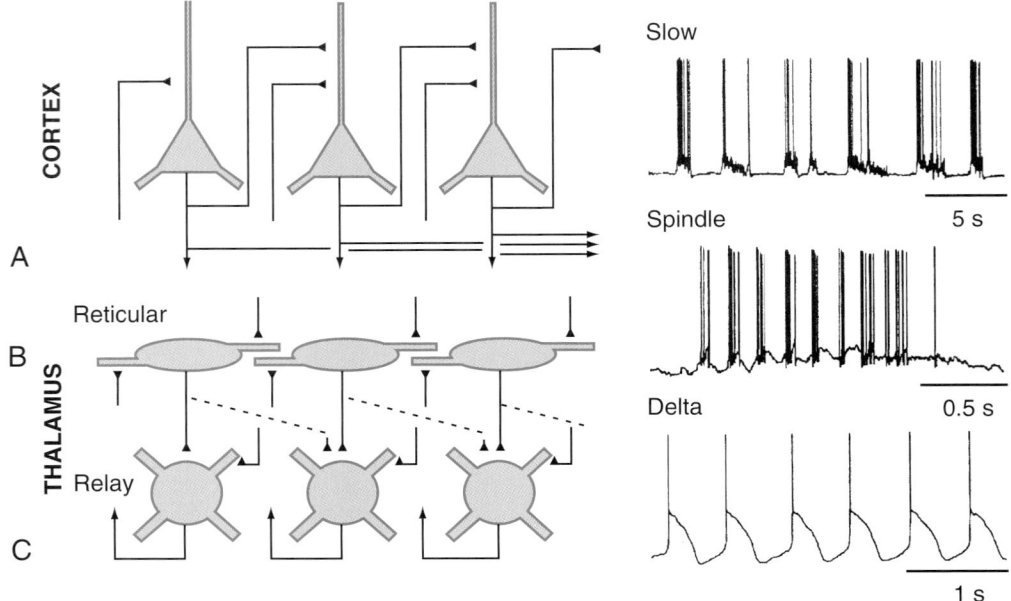

Figure 9–1. For legend see opposite page.

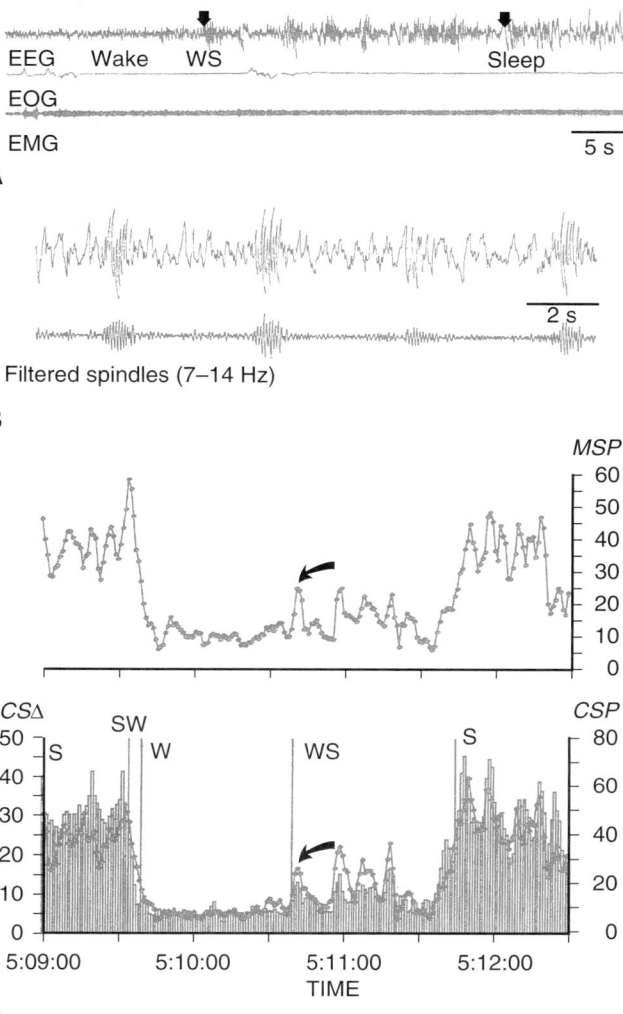

B

Figure 9–2. Electrographic criteria of wake–sleep states and characteristics of spindle rhythmicity. **A,** Behaving cat with chronically implanted electrodes. An electroencephalogram (EEG) from the anterior part (pericruciate areas) of the neocortical surface, an electrooculogram (EOG), and an electromyogram (EMG) of the neck muscles are shown. Spindle oscillations appear during the transitional period between waking and sleep (WS). **B,** Thalamic spindles in a *cerveau isolé* cat with an intercollicular transection. Top trace shows the field electrical activity recorded by means of a microelectrode in the rostral intralaminar (central lateral) nucleus; bottom trace shows spindle waves (filtered from 7 to 14 Hz) from the same period. Note that sequences of spindle waves recur periodically with a slow rhythm. **C,** Normalized amplitudes (ordinates) of simultaneously recorded focal spindle waves in the reticular thalamic nucleus (MSP, *top line-circle trace*), cortical spindle waves (CSP, *bottom line-circle trace*), and cortical slow waves (CSΔ, bottom bar graph) in a behaving cat. Spindles are filtered 7 to 14 Hz; slow waves are filtered 0.5 to 4 Hz. Abscissa indicates real time (hours, minutes, seconds). S, EEG-synchronized sleep; W, waking; SW and WS, transitional periods from S to W and from W to S, respectively. Note desynchronization with decreased wave amplitudes on awakening (SW and W); rhythmic sequences of spindles (recurring with a period of approximately 8 to 10 seconds) in both thalamic and cortical recordings beginning with drowsiness (WS); and increased amplitudes of both spindles and slow waves beginning with S. (Modified from Steriade M, Domich L, Oakson G: Reticularis thalami neurons revisited: activity changes during shifts in states of vigilance. J Neurosci 1986;6:68-81; and Paré D, Steriade M, Deschênes M, et al: Physiological properties of anterior thalamic nuclei, a group devoid of inputs from the reticular thalamic nucleus. J Neurophysiol 1987;57:1669-1685, with permission.)

rhythms because thalamus and neocortex are interconnected, and the recently described cortical slow oscillation has the virtue of grouping different sleep rhythms into complex wave sequences.[10,11] For didactic purposes, I describe each of the three major sleep oscillations separately.

Spindle Oscillation

Spindles appear during early stages of NREM sleep (Fig. 9–2). Spindles are waxing and waning waves at 7 to 14 Hz, grouped in sequences that last 1 to 2 seconds and that recur periodically with a slow rhythm of 0.1 to 0.3 Hz (Fig. 9–2). Both these

rhythms (7 to 14 Hz and 0.1 to 0.3 Hz) should be considered in defining spindle activity. Spindles are generated in the thalamus, but the cerebral cortex plays a major role in their synchronization and virtually simultaneous appearance over widespread thalamic and cortical areas.[12]

The rostral pole of GABAergic thalamic reticular nuclear complex can generate spindle rhythmicity even after disconnection from dorsal thalamic nuclei and cerebral cortex[13] owing to connections among thalamic reticular neurons. The crucial role played by the thalamic reticular nucleus in the generation of sleep spindles was also demonstrated by abolition of spindling in target thalamocortical systems after

Figure 9–1. A, Building blocks of corticothalamic networks and different types of sleep oscillations generated by excitatory glutamatergic neocortical neurons. **B,** Inhibitory gamma-aminobutyric acid (GABA) reticular thalamic neurons. **C,** Excitatory glutamatergic thalamocortical or relay neurons. The direction of axons is indicated by arrows. Short- and long-scale intracortical pathways are illustrated. Divergent axons of thalamic reticular neurons are shown as broken lines. Note the different time calibrations in intracellular traces showing the cortical slow oscillation (~0.3 Hz), the spindles in thalamic reticular neurons (~7 Hz), and the intrinsic, clocklike delta rhythm of thalamocortical neurons (~1.5 Hz). These oscillations might be generated at each of these levels, even after disconnection from afferent inputs. However, in the intact brain, these structures interact and their rhythms are combined in complex wave sequences. (From Steriade M, Contreras D, Amzica F: Synchronized sleep oscillations and their paroxysmal developments. Trends Neurosci 1994;17:199-209, with permission.)

disconnection from the reticular nucleus.[14] Spindles result from repetitive spike bursts in GABAergic reticular cells that produce rhythmic inhibitory postsynaptic potentials (IPSPs) in thalamocortical neurons, leading to postinhibitory rebound spike bursts that are transferred to cortex and produce excitatory postsynaptic potentials (EPSPs) in cortical cells, occasionally leading to action potentials (Fig. 9–3).

Because thalamocortical neurons spend much of their sleep time during spindle-related IPSPs, there is a powerful inhibition of incoming messages in their route to the cerebral cortex. Recording field potentials evoked by stimulation of prethalamic axons (a method that permits the monitoring of the presynaptic deflection, reflecting the magnitude of the afferent volley, together with the synaptically relayed, thalamically generated waves) revealed that the thalamus is the first station where afferent signals are completely blocked from the very onset of sleep (Fig. 9–4). This obliteration of synaptic

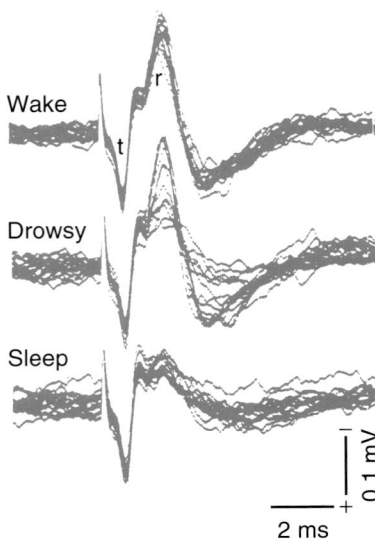

Figure 9–4. Blockade of synaptic transmission in the thalamus at sleep onset in a behaving cat. Field potentials evoked in the ventrolateral thalamic nucleus by stimulation of the cerebellothalamic pathway are shown. The evoked response consists of a presynaptic (tract, t) component and a monosynaptically relayed (r) wave. Note the progressively diminished amplitude of the r wave during drowsiness, up to its complete obliteration during electroencephalogram-synchronized sleep, in spite of lack of changes in the afferent volley monitored by the t component. (M. Steriade, unpublished data, 1988.)

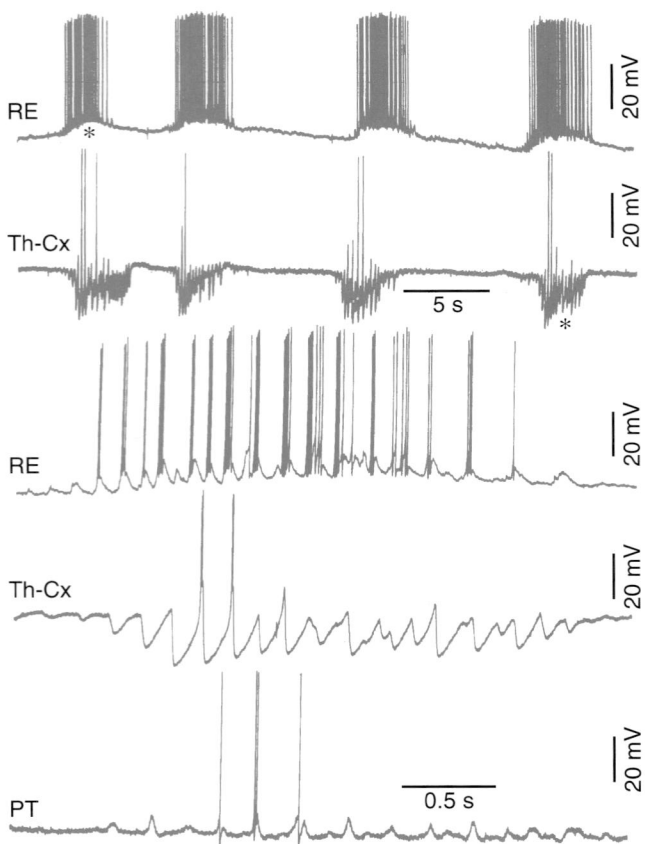

Figure 9–3. Cellular bases of spindling in thalamocortical systems. Intracellular aspects of spindle oscillations in reticular thalamic (RE), thalamocortical (Th-Cx; from the ventrolateral nucleus), and pyramidal tract (PT; from the precruciate gyrus) neurons of a cat under barbiturate anesthesia are shown. The spindle sequences marked by *asterisks* in the top traces of RE and Th-Cx neurons are depicted below at higher speed. Note that spindle oscillations and rhythmic spike bursts develop on a slowly growing and decaying depolarization in the RE neuron; on the contrary, rhythmic hyperpolarizations, occasionally interrupted by low-threshold spikes, underlie spindles in the Th-Cx cell. (Adapted from Steriade M, Deschênes M: Intrathalamic and brainstem-thalamic networks involved in resting and alert states. In Bentivoglio M, Spreafico R [eds]: Thalamic Mechanisms. Amsterdam, Elsevier, 1988, pp 37-62, with permission.)

transmission in the thalamus leads to the deafferentation of the cerebral cortex, a prerequisite for the process of falling asleep. More recently, intracellular recordings from thalamic and cortical neurons have shown that, because of their hyperpolarization during sleep, thalamocortical cells do not transfer to cortex signals from the prethalamic relay station, whereas the internal (corticocortical and corticothalamic) dialogue of the brain may be maintained during sleep.[15]

Although the thalamic gate is closed during NREM sleep, because of obliteration of synaptic transmission, especially during spindle oscillations,[15-17] neurons in the cerebral cortex are quite active during this sleep state,[18] and spindles or their experimental model, augmenting responses, produce enhanced synaptic responsiveness of neocortical neurons.[19,20] This potentiation of cortical responsiveness, which is generated by rhythmic thalamocortical volleys in the frequency range of spindles, represents synaptic plasticity, a mechanism through which memory traces, acquired during wakefulness, are consolidated during NREM sleep. Our data[16,19-21] demonstrate progressively increased neuronal responsiveness during and after spindles or augmenting responses that mimic spindles (Fig. 9–5A) as well as self-sustained activity, like "memory" events, after repeated rhythmic volleys within the frequency range of spindles in corticothalamic networks (Fig. 9–5B). These experimental data are supported by human studies showing the overnight improvement of discrimination skills by early stages of sleep with spindles and increased density of sleep spindles after training on a declarative learning task.[22,23]

The potentiation of cortical neurons' responsiveness is so high during and after augmenting responses or natural spindles that it may take an epileptiform pattern.[20,21] It is known that electrographic and clinical seizures with spike–wave or

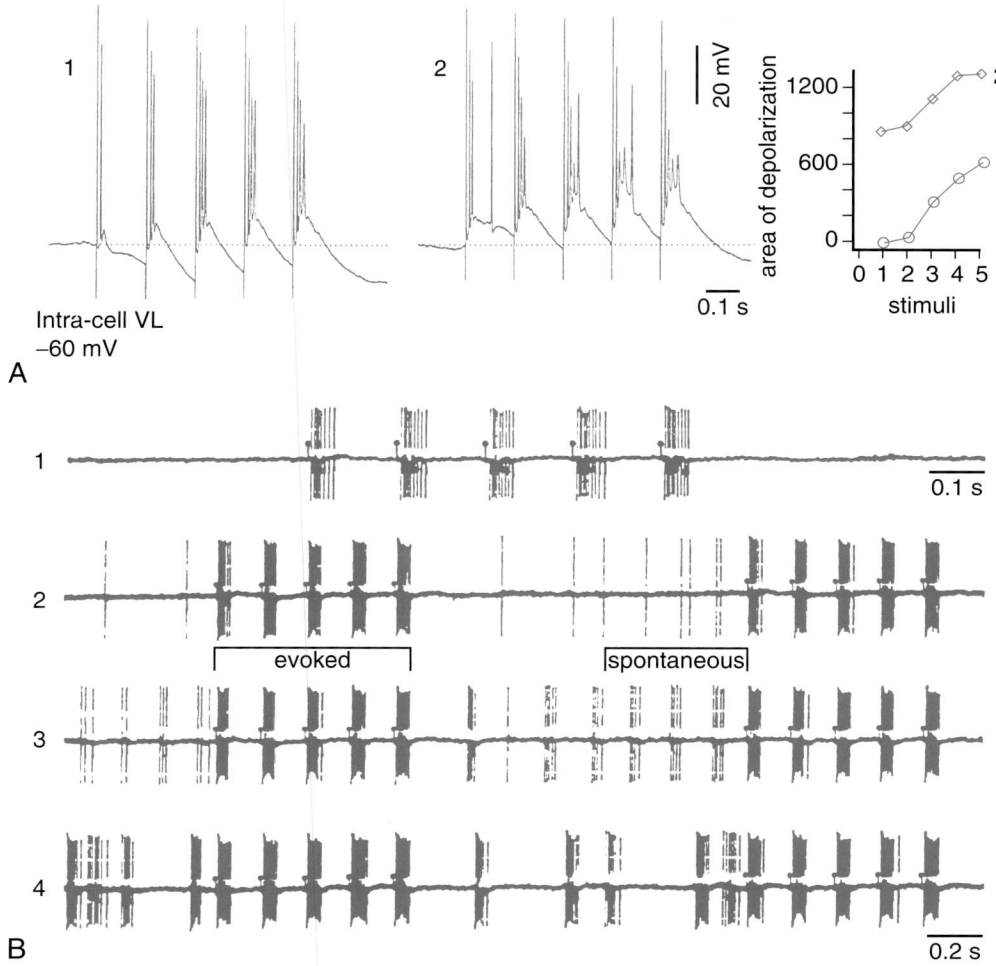

Figure 9–5. Short-term plasticity during and after intrathalamic and corticothalamic augmenting responses. **A,** Cat under ketamine-xylazine anesthesia, with left hemidecortication and callosal cut. Intracellular recordings from thalamocortical ventrolateral (VL) neuron are shown. Pulse trains consisting of five stimuli at 10 Hz were applied to the thalamic VL nucleus every 2 seconds. The type of augmenting illustrated here is high threshold, occurring at a depolarized level. In this case, the responses to a five-shock train consisted of an early antidromic spike, followed by orthodromic spikes displaying progressive augmentation and spike inactivation. Responses to two pulse trains (1 and 2) are illustrated (1 and 2 were separated by 14 seconds). With repetition of pulse trains, inhibitory postsynaptic potentials elicited by preceding stimuli in the train were progressively reduced until their complete obliteration, and spike bursts contained more action potentials with spike inactivation. The graph depicts the increased area of depolarization from the first to the fifth responses in each pulse train as well as from pulse train 1 to pulse-train 2. **B,** Brainstem-transected cat. Cortically evoked spike bursts in thalamic VL neuron (1) are shown. Motor cortex stimulation was applied with pulse trains at 10 Hz delivered every 1.3 seconds. In 1, the pattern of cortically evoked responses at the onset of rhythmic pulse trains (faster speed than in 2 to 4) is presented. In 2 to 4, responses at later stages of stimulation are shown. Stimuli are marked by *dots*. In 2 to 4, stimuli and evoked spike bursts are aligned. Note progressive appearance of spontaneous spike bursts resembling the evoked ones, as a form of "memory" in the corticothalamic circuit. (Modified from Steriade M, Timofeev I: Short-term plasticity during intrathalamic augmenting responses in decorticated cats. J Neurosci 1997;17:3778-3795; and Steriade M: Alertness, quiet sleep, dreaming. In Peters A, Jones EG [eds]: Cerebral Cortex, vol 9. New York, Plenum, 1991, 279-357, with permission.)

polyspike–wave complexes preferentially occur during the NREM sleep state. After protracted stimulation of thalamus or cortex, with rhythmic pulse trains at 10 Hz (within the frequency range of spindles in the cat), simultaneous intracellular recordings from related cortical and thalamic neurons showed an enhanced responsiveness of the cortical neuron, followed by paroxysmal activity; the changes in responsiveness of cortical neurons, which led to self-sustained oscillations of the paroxysmal type, were already initiated during rhythmic stimulation with pulse trains at 10 Hz[21] (Fig. 9–6). Such changes consist of the appearance of "spontaneous"

depolarizing events, occurring between pulse trains and having the same frequency as that used in these pulse trains (see asterisk in the expanded panel at bottom right in Fig. 9–6). That such transformations, from normal (sleep-like) to pathologic (epileptic-like) states, occur in the neocortex in the absence of the thalamus was demonstrated in animals with ipsilateral thalamectomy.[11] The behavioral significance of development from neuronal plasticity, which is beneficial for normal mnemonic functions, to paroxysmal states, in those instances in which repetitive stimuli are prolonged beyond a certain limit, is not yet clearly understood.

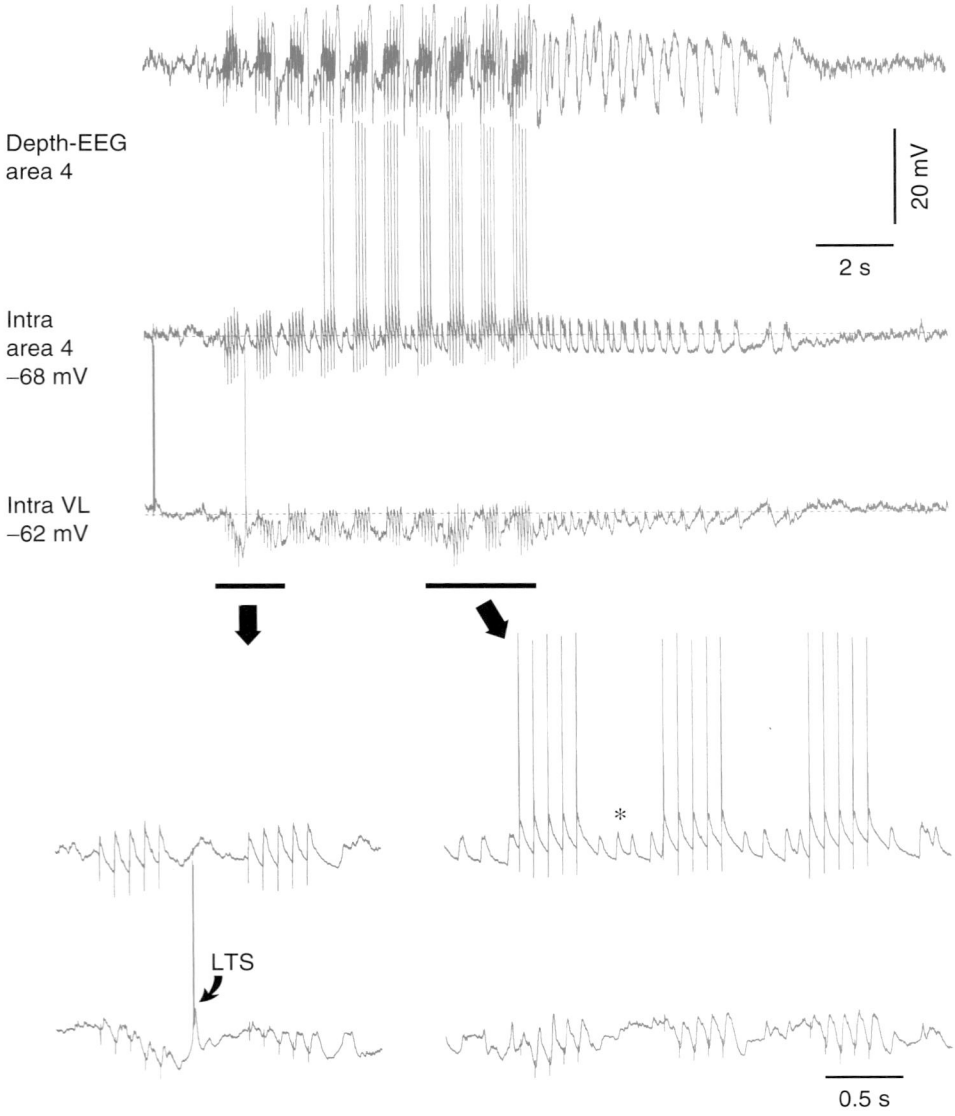

Depth-EEG
area 4

20 mV

2 s

Intra
area 4
–68 mV

Intra VL
–62 mV

LTS

*

0.5 s

Figure 9–6. Plastic changes in cortical responsiveness, leading to self-sustained paroxysmal oscillation, simultaneous with decreased augmenting responses in thalamocortical (TC) neuron in a cat under ketamine-xylazine anesthesia. Dual intracellular recordings from TC neuron in ventrolateral (VL) nucleus and cortical area 4 neuron, together with depth-electroencephalogram (EEG) from area 4 are shown. Stimulation was applied to cortex and consisted of pulse trains at 10 Hz, repeated every second. Two parts, at the beginning and end of stimulation (marked by *horizontal bars* and *arrows*), are expanded at the bottom. Note that although augmenting responses in TC neuron diminished from the second pulse train, cortical augmenting responses were progressively enhanced and, after finishing the stimulation period, a self-sustained oscillation at ~2 Hz ensued, lasting for ~8 seconds. Also note, in cortical neuronal recording, depolarizing events with a similar frequency (10 Hz) to that used in pulse trains, occurring between pulse trains (*asterisk* in bottom right panel). LTS, low-threshold spike. (Unpublished experiments by M. Steriade, I. Timofeev, and F. Grenier.)

Delta Oscillation

The delta oscillation appears during later sleep stages (Fig. 9–2) and has two components. The cortical one survives complete thalamectomy[11,24] and the spectral content in the delta band (1 to 4 Hz) results, at least partially, from the shape and duration of the K-complex.[25] Cortical delta rhythmicity is distinct from the more recently discovered slow oscillation (see later; Fig. 9–7B, C). The other, stereotyped, clocklike component is generated in the thalamus and results from the hyperpolarization-activated interplay between two intrinsic currents of thalamocortical (relay) neurons (see bottom right trace in Fig. 9–1). Although this rhythm is also seen in thalamic slices, after blockage of synaptic transmission[26,27] its appearance at the level of local field potentials and cortical EEG is possible because corticothalamic volleys synchronize thalamocortical cells through the action of inhibitory thalamic reticular neurons[28] that fulfill two requirements: They set the membrane potential of relay cells at the required level of hyperpolarization for the generation of delta oscillation, and they have

projections distributed to the dorsal thalamus which synchronize various relay cells.

Because delta oscillations appear at a more hyperpolarized level of membrane potential in thalamocortical neurons than do spindles,[28] the two sleep oscillations are incompatible in single cells. These intracellular data from anesthetized preparations are supported by results obtained in naturally sleeping animals, showing that thalamic spindles are maximal at sleep onset and decrease thereafter, whereas thalamic delta waves increase gradually during resting sleep. Thus, with increasing hyperpolarization of thalamocortical cells during resting sleep, because of the progressively diminished firing rates of cholinergic and other types of brainstem–thalamic activating neurons,[29] the incidence and amplitude of spindles are largely diminished during deep sleep stages. On the other hand, the reappearance of spindles toward the end of resting sleep[30] is attributable to a relative depolarization of thalamocortical cells, due to the increased firing rates of brainstem–thalamic reticular neurons that display precursor increased rates of spontaneous firing 30 to 60 seconds before the onset of REM sleep.[31]

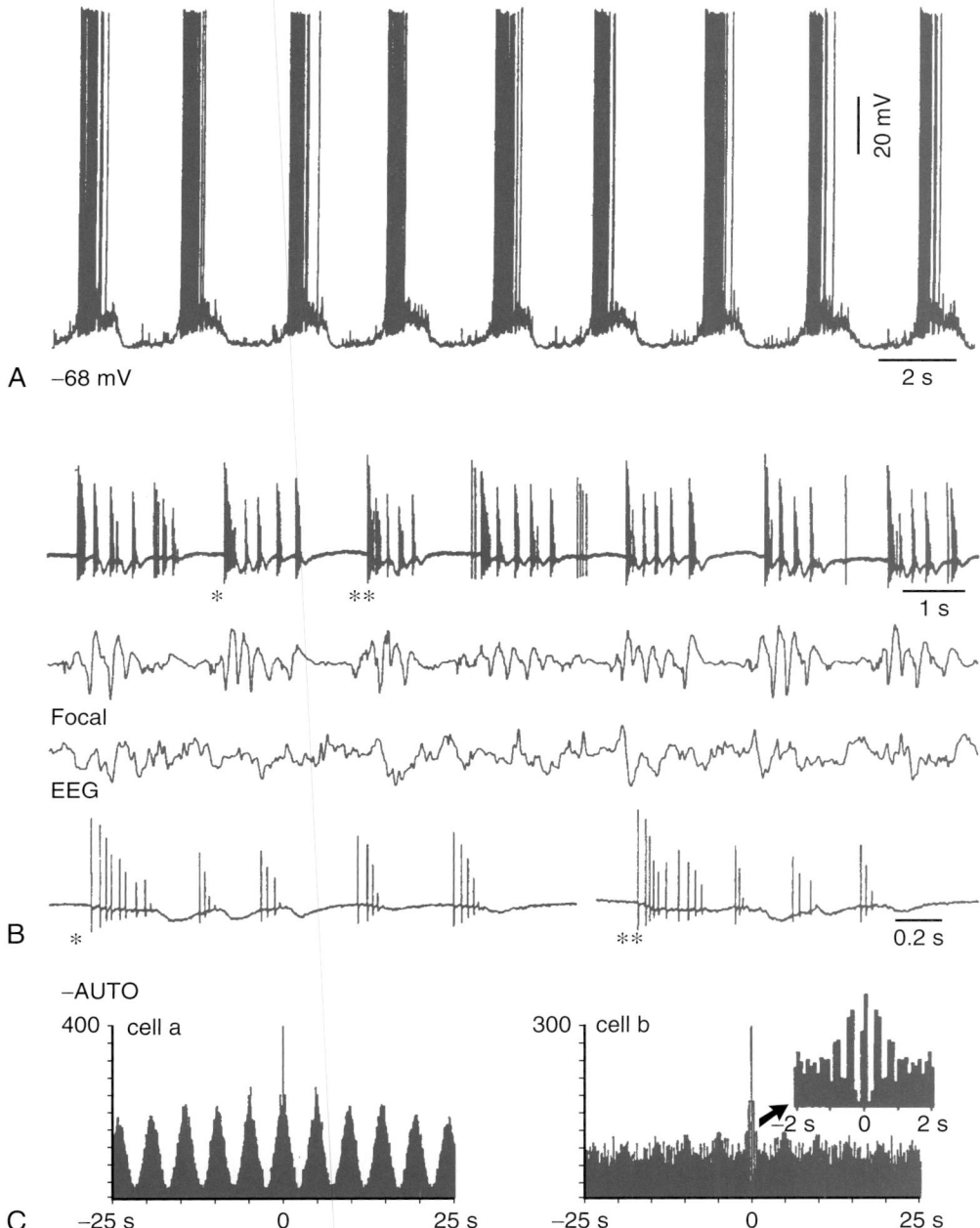

Figure 9–7. The slow sleep oscillation and the delta oscillations are distinct activities, as shown in these intracellular recordings in acutely prepared cats under urethane anesthesia. **A,** Intracellular recording of cortical motor area 4 neuron shows slow oscillation at ~0.35 Hz. **B,** Extra(juxta)cellular recording of bursting neuron from cortical association area 7, together with focal slow waves (through the same microelectrode) and electroencephalogram (EEG). Parts indicated by one or two *asterisks* are expanded at the bottom of the panel. Note sequences of delta waves (3 to 4 Hz) grouped by slow oscillation (~0.4 Hz). **C,** Autocorrelograms of two cells (a and b) recorded from cortical area 4 showing the slow oscillation (~0.2 Hz) and delta rhythmicity (~2.5 Hz, inset in cell b). (Modified from Steriade M, Nuñez A, Amzica F: Intracellular analysis of relations between the slow [<1 Hz] neocortical oscillation and other sleep rhythms of the electroencephalogram. J Neurosci 1993;13:3266-3283; and unpublished data.)

Slow Oscillation

The slow oscillation has a frequency peak at 0.7 to 0.8 Hz in cats under ketamine-xylazine anesthesia[32] as well as during natural sleep of cats[3,5,18,30] and humans.[25,33] The cortical nature of the slow oscillation was demonstrated by its survival in the cerebral cortex after thalamectomy,[11] its absence in the thalamus of decorticated animals,[34] and the disruption of its long-range synchronization after disconnection of intracortical synaptic linkages.[35]

Intracellular analyses of the slow oscillation showed that cortical neurons throughout layers II to VI (many of them with physiologically identified thalamic or callosal inputs or projections) displayed a spontaneous oscillation consisting of prolonged depolarizing and hyperpolarizing components[10] (Fig. 9–7A).

All major cellular classes in the cerebral cortex, as identified by electrophysiologic characteristics and intracellular staining, display the slow oscillation: regularly spiking and intrinsically bursting cells, as well as local-circuit–inhibitory basket cells.[18,32] Both long-axoned and short-axoned cells exhibit similar relations with the EEG components of the slow oscillation: During the depth-positive EEG wave, cortical neurons are hyperpolarized, whereas during the sharp depth-negative EEG deflection, cortical neurons are depolarized. The long-lasting depolarization of the slow oscillation consists of EPSPs, fast prepotentials, and fast IPSPs reflecting the action of synaptically coupled GABAergic local-circuit cortical cells. Data also indicated that the depolarizing component is made up of N-methyl-D-aspartate (NMDA)-mediated as well as non–NMDA-mediated synaptic excitatory events and a voltage-dependent persistent sodium current, $I_{Na(p)}$.[10] The long-lasting hyperpolarization, interrupting the depolarizing envelopes, is a combination of an $I_{K(Ca)}$ and disfacilitation in the corticothalamic network. The disfacilitation mechanism is supported by measurements of the membrane input resistance (R_{in}) showing that R_{in} is highest during the long-lasting hyperpolarizing component of the slow oscillation.[36] The disfacilitation during the hyperpolarization probably occurs because of the progressive $[Ca^{2+}]_{out}$ depletion during the depolarizing phase of the slow oscillation.[37] Dual intracellular recordings in vivo revealed that the overt synchronization of EEG patterns is associated with the simultaneous hyperpolarizations in cortical neurons.[32,35]

Recently, intracellular recordings in chronically implanted, naturally awake and sleeping animals showed that the pattern of the slow oscillation, first described under anesthesia, is similar during natural NREM sleep (SWS).[18] The changes in membrane potential and firing patterns of a regular-spiking neuron (which represents the majority of neocortical neurons) and a fast-spiking neuron (which is most likely a local GABAergic neuron) throughout the sleep–waking cycle are illustrated in Figure 9–8. In the case of the regular-spiking

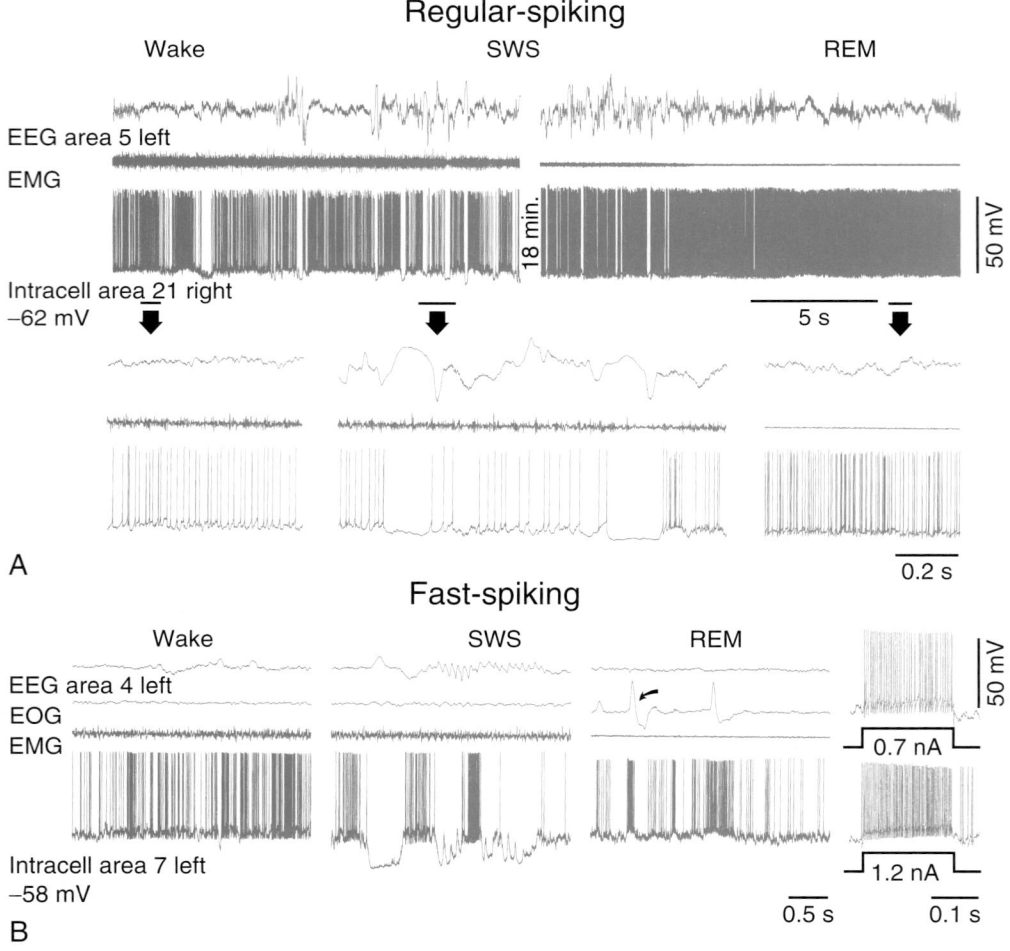

Figure 9–8. Changes in membrane potential and firing patterns during natural wake and sleep states. Intracellular recordings in chronically implanted cat. **A,** Regular-spiking (RS) neuron from association suprasylvian area 21 was recorded together with electromyogram (EMG) and electroencephalogram (EEG) from area 5 during transition from waking to slow wave sleep (SWS) and, further, to rapid eye movement (REM) sleep (nondepicted period of 18 minutes during SWS). Periods in all three tracings marked by *horizontal bars* are expanded at bottom of panel (*arrows*). Note tonic firing during both waking and REM sleep, and cyclic hyperpolarizations associated with depth-positive EEG field potentials during SWS. **B,** Activity of fast-spiking (FS) neuron (see at right responses to depolarizing current pulses) during waking, SWS, and REM sleep. Recording was obtained with KCl-filled pipette. Tonic firing during waking and REM sleep was interrupted during SWS by long periods of hyperpolarizations and spindles, corresponding to EEG depth-positive waves and spindles. (Modified from Steriade M, Timofeev I, Grenier F: Natural waking and sleep states: A view from inside neocortical neurons. J Neurophysiol 2001;85:1969-1985, with permission.)

neuron (Fig. 9–8A), SWS lasted for almost 20 minutes. During this state, neuronal activity was characterized by prolonged, cyclic hyperpolarizations that were associated with depth-positive field EEG potentials, whereas the neuron discharged tonically in both waking and REM sleep. The fast-spiking neuron (Fig. 9–8B) exhibited similar properties, namely tonic discharges during wakefulness, cyclic and prolonged hyperpolarizations during SWS, and again tonic but irregular firing during REM sleep.

The neuronal synchronization implicates both cortical and thalamic neurons. The depolarizing component of the cortically generated slow oscillation is transmitted to thalamic reticular neurons, at which level it triggers rhythmic spike bursts and, consequently, is reflected in thalamocortical cells as rhythmic IPSPs leading to rebound spike bursts.[32,34] This is the mechanism underlying the brief sequence of EEG spindles that follows every cycle of the slow oscillation (Figs. 9–9A and 9–10, CAT). Distinct from the prolonged, waxing-and-waning pattern of spindle oscillations in the decorticated animals or in those under barbiturate anesthesia when cortical neurons display reduced spontaneous activities, the spindles triggered by the corticothalamic volley of the slow oscillation under ketamine-xylazine anesthesia are much shorter. This is because the synchronous excitation of corticothalamic neurons during the slow oscillation entrains, right from the start, a great population of neurons implicated in the genesis of spindles within a thalamic territory, thus explaining the absence of an initial waxing process.

Thus, although the systematization of sleep rhythms into three categories (spindles, delta, slow) may be useful for didactic purposes, in brain-intact animals and humans *the sleep oscillations are not seen in isolation but are grouped by the cortically generated slow oscillation*. The coalescence of the slow and spindle oscillations is especially visible during light sleep.[17,30] However, spindling is not the only sleep rhythm that is modulated and grouped by the cortical slow oscillation. The intrinsically generated delta rhythm of thalamocortical cells is influenced by the slow oscillation because the rhythmic depolarizing corticothalamic drives excite thalamic reticular neurons; these in turn hyperpolarize thalamocortical cells and thus favor the interplay between their intrinsic currents I_h and I_t, leading to generation of clocklike delta potentials that are fed back to cortex and sculpt the slow oscillation[38] (Fig. 9–9B). As to the other component of delta waves, which is generated intracortically after thalamectomy (see earlier), the frequency band of 1 to 4 Hz in the power spectrum during late stages of resting sleep results, at least partially, from the shape of the depth-negative (depolarizing) component of the slow oscillation (0.3 to 0.4 second), which represents the K-complex.[25] Typical delta waves, at a frequency of 2 to 4 Hz, generated by both regular-spiking and intrinsically bursting cortical neurons, are grouped in sequences recurring with the slow rhythm.[11] And, in human sleep EEG, sequential mean amplitudes of delta waves show their periodic recurrence with the rhythm of slow oscillation[10,25] (Fig. 9–10, HUMAN). That delta and slow oscillation represent two distinct phenomena in human sleep EEG was recently demonstrated by showing differences in the dynamics between the slow and delta oscillations; the latter declines in activity from the first to the second non-REM sleep episode, whereas the former does not.[33]

Because the slow oscillation was first described intracellularly under different anesthetics, the similarity between these

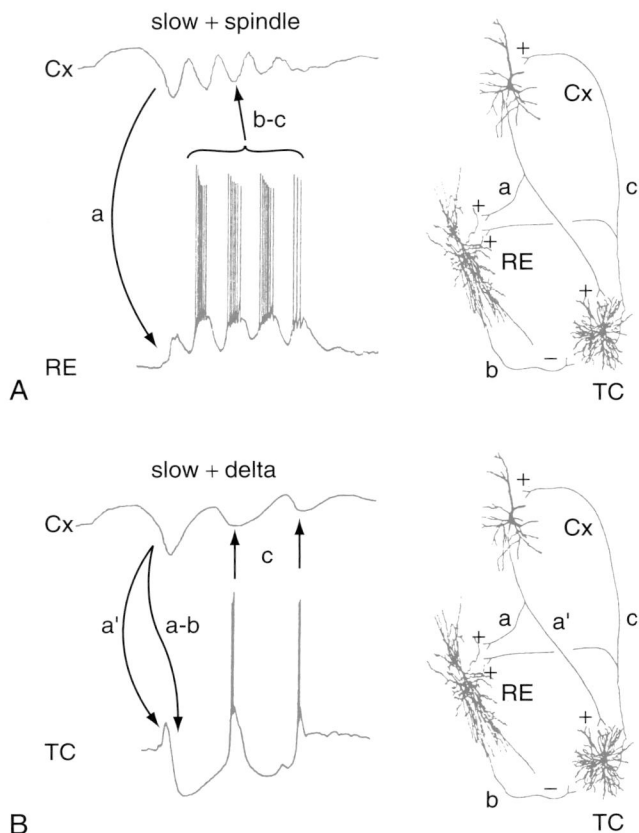

Figure 9–9. Coalescence of the cortical slow oscillation with other slow wave sleep (SWS) rhythms generated in the thalamus. In the left column, two traces represent field potentials from the depth of association cortical area 5 and intracellular recording from thalamic reticular neuron (top and bottom traces, respectively); below, traces represent field potentials from the depth of cortical area 5 and intracellular recording from thalamocortical ventrolateral neuron. In the right column, circuits involved in the generation of the respective SWS pattern are shown. The synaptic projections are indicated with small letters, corresponding to the arrows at left, which indicate the time sequence of the events. **A,** Combination of slow oscillation with a spindle sequence. The depolarizing phase of the field slow oscillation (depth-negative, downward deflection, also called K-complex) in the cortex (Cx) travels through the corticothalamic pathway (a) and triggers in the thalamic reticular nucleus (RE) a spindle sequence that is transferred to thalamocortical cells (TC) of the dorsal thalamus (b) and thereafter back to the cortex (c), where it shapes the tail of the slow oscillatory cycle. **B,** Modulation of slow oscillation by a sequence of clocklike delta waves originating in the thalamus by interplay between two inward currents (I_H and I_T) of thalamocortical neurons. The synchronous activity of cortical neurons during the slow oscillation (depth-negative peak of cortical field potential) travels along the corticothalamic pathway (a') eliciting an excitatory postsynaptic potential, curtailed by an inhibitory postsynaptic potential produced along the cortico-RE (a) and RE-TC (b) projections. The hyperpolarization of the thalamocortical cell generates a sequence of low-threshold potentials crowned by high-frequency spike bursts at delta frequency that may reach the cortex through the thalamocortical link (c). (Modified from Steriade M, Contreras D, Curró Dossi R, Nuñez A: The slow [<1 Hz] oscillation in reticular thalamic and thalamocortical neurons: Scenario of sleep rhythm generation in interacting thalamic and neocortical networks. J Neurosci 1993;13:3284-3299; Steriade M, McCormick DA, Sejnowski TJ: Thalamocortical oscillations in the sleeping and aroused brain. Science 1993;262:679-685; Contreras D, Steriade M: Spindle oscillation in cats: the role of corticothalamic feedback in a thalamically generated rhythm. J Physiol [Lond] 1996;490:159-179; and Amzica F, Steriade M: The functional significance of K-complexes. Sleep Med Rev 2002;6:139-149, with permission.)

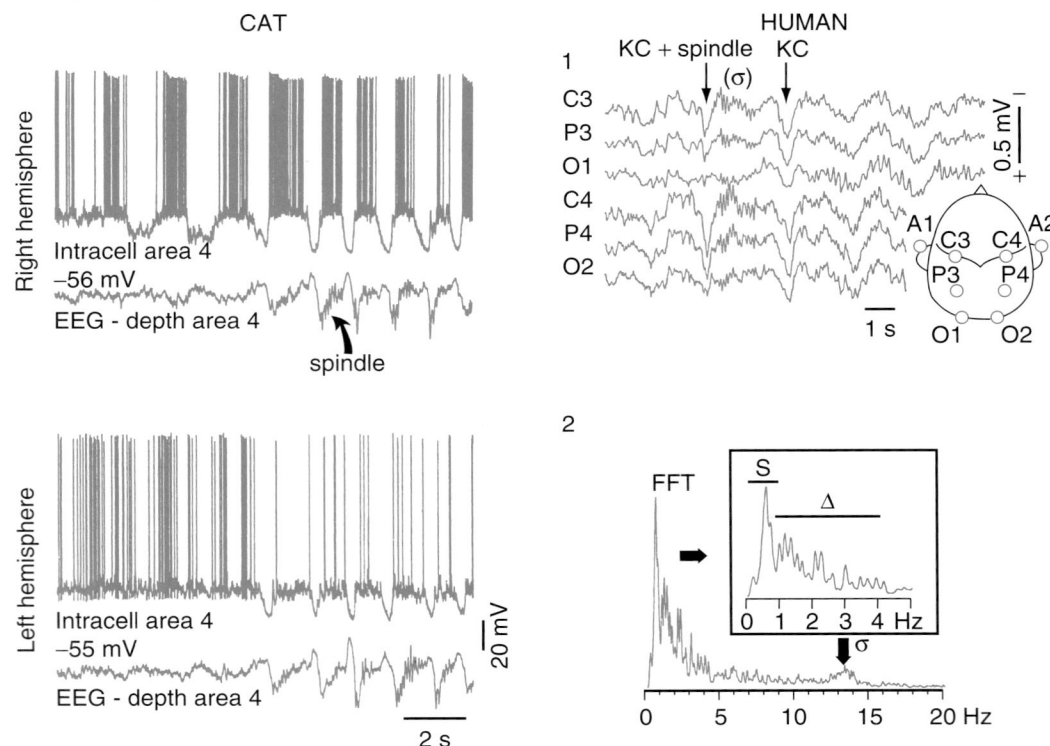

Figure 9–10. The cortical slow oscillation groups thalamically generated spindles. CAT, Dual simultaneous intracellular recordings from right and left cortical area 4. Note spindle during the depolarizing envelope of the slow oscillation and synchronization of electroencephalogram (EEG) when both neurons synchronously display prolonged hyperpolarizations. HUMAN, the K-complex (KC) in natural sleep. **1,** Scalp monopolar recordings with respect to the contralateral ear are shown (see small inset figure). Traces show a short episode from stage 3 non–rapid eye movement sleep. The two *arrows* point to two K-complexes, consisting of a surface-positive wave, followed (or not) by a sequence of spindle (sigma [σ]) waves. Note the synchrony of K-complexes in all recorded sites. **2,** Frequency decomposition of the electrical activity from C3 lead (see **1**) into three frequency bands: slow oscillation (S, 0 to 1 Hz), delta waves (Δ, 1 to 4 Hz) and spindles (σ, 12 to 15 Hz). FFT, fast Fourier transform. (Modified from Steriade M, Contreras D, Amzica F: Synchronized sleep oscillations and their paroxysmal developments. Trends Neurosci 1994;17:199-208; and Amzica F, Steriade M: The K-complex: Its slow [<1 Hz] rhythmicity and relation to delta waves. Neurology 1997;49:952-959, with permission.)

cellular patterns and those observed during natural sleep was validated in extracellular recordings from chronically implanted, unanesthetized animals. Under these conditions, the depth-positive waves are accompanied by silenced firing (because of the cells' hyperpolarizations), whereas depth-negative sharp deflections are associated with brisk firing.[3]

Independent experiments from several laboratories[10,25,33,39-41] have demonstrated the presence of the slow oscillation in human sleep. In our study,[25] during stage 2, scalp recordings showed a prevalent peak (0.8 Hz) within the frequency range of the slow oscillation as well as a minor mode around 15 Hz reflecting spindle waves (Fig. 9–10, HUMAN). The power spectrum revealed a major peak around 1 Hz that became evident from stage 2 and continued throughout resting sleep. These data invite human sleep researchers to consider the two types of oscillatory activities below 4 Hz (delta, 1 to 4 Hz; slow, <1 Hz) and, accordingly, to analyze their results by taking into account the distinctness of these two oscillations.[33]

The slow oscillation groups not only other sleep oscillations (spindles and delta) but fast oscillations (beta/gamma) that are conventionally associated with waking and REM sleep. Indeed, the fast rhythms (20 to 50 Hz) appear on the depolarizing phase of the slow oscillation because these rapid oscillations are voltage (depolarization) dependent. Our concept that different (both low- and high-frequency) brain rhythms are grouped within complex wave sequences by the cortically generated slow oscillation[38,42,43] is supported by human EEG studies showing the grouping of spindles and beta rhythms by the slow oscillation during NREM sleep.[40]

Brainstem–Thalamic Circuits Involved in Brain Activation and Fast Oscillations (20 to 50 Hz) during Waking and REM Sleep

That the brainstem reticular formation has a role in the blockade of low-frequency EEG rhythms is known from early experiments showing that periodic spindle sequences appear on the EEG after transections at the collicular level,[44] and that low-frequency waves are readily erased by high-frequency electrical stimulation of the upper brainstem reticular core.[2] The role of brainstem monoaminergic aggregates, particularly the locus coeruleus, in the tonic EEG desynchronization that characterizes waking and REM sleep can be discounted because bilateral lesions of the locus coeruleus, with a consequent 85% to 95% depletion of cortical norepinephrine, result in control values of EEG activation immediately after recovery from surgery.[45] The firing features of both locus coeruleus and dorsal raphe are opposite in waking and REM sleep, with virtual neuronal silence during the latter state,[29] which is in clear contrast to the similar EEG patterns during these two behavioral states.

Because the replacement of synchronized EEG waves during sleep by EEG activation during natural states of arousal or REM sleep is associated with facilitation of synaptic transmission through major relay thalamic nuclei, these potentiating effects awaited the clarification of the underlying pathways. Moreover, because acetylcholine (ACh) blockers antagonize some components of brainstem–thalamic influences, the morphologic search for these projections should be combined with the immunohistochemical identification of their cholinergic nature. Evidence of such projections to the thalamus after injections of retrograde tracers within the limits of distinct thalamic nuclei is now available for all sensory, motor, associational, reticular, limbic, and intralaminar thalamic nuclei in the cat,[46-48] as well as for associational nuclei in the monkey.[48] All major sensory (visual, auditory, and somesthetic) thalamic nuclei and the ventrolateral nucleus, which is specifically related to the motor cortex, receive fewer than 10% of their brainstem reticular afferents from noncholinergic neurons located in the rostral midbrain reticular formation; they receive 85% to 95% of their brainstem reticular innervation from a region at the midbrain–pontine junction, where two cholinergic nuclear groups are maximally developed. Of the total number of neurons that were retrogradely labeled in these two cholinergic brainstem (pedunculopontine or peribrachial, and laterodorsal tegmental) nuclei after tracer injections in various thalamic nuclei, 70% to 85% were also identified as cholinergic by concurrent visualization of choline acetyltransferase immunoreactivity. Three to eight times more brainstem reticular cells were found to project toward associational thalamic nuclei, and to those nuclear groups that have widespread cortical projections. The more important brainstem projections to the associational and diffusely projecting thalamic nuclei are accounted for by massive projections from noncholinergic brainstem neurons whose synaptic transmitters (peptides, glutamate) remain to be identified.

At their targets, the brainstem–thalamic projections underlie two distinct effects, which represent the main components of activation processes in thalamocortical systems: (1) a direct excitation of thalamocortical neurons; and (2) an inhibition of thalamic reticular neurons, thus disinhibiting thalamocortical neurons and blocking spindle oscillations.

Stimulation of the rostral brainstem reticular formation elicits monosynaptic excitation of thalamocortical neurons (see Steriade and Llinás[1] for a review). Earlier studies conducted on preparations under barbiturate anesthesia have concluded that midbrain reticular stimulation indirectly enhances the synaptic transmission of thalamocortical cells, through a process of disinhibition. It is now established that very small doses (2 mg/kg) of barbiturate block the direct excitatory effect of either brainstem reticular stimulation[49] or ACh application[50] on thalamocortical neurons. In fact, intracellular recordings in unanesthetized animals show that midbrain reticular stimulation in the region of the cholinergic peribrachial nucleus directly depolarizes thalamocortical neurons.[51] The early depolarization is nicotinic in nature, and it starts at latencies compatible with monosynaptic excitation, whereas the late-depolarizing component has a long latency and a very long duration.[49] The prolonged depolarizing response of thalamocortical cells to brainstem cholinergic stimulation is associated with an EEG activation reaction having a similar time course (Fig. 9–11A) and is accompanied by an increase in neuronal excitability[49] (Fig. 9–11B). The association between a prolonged depolarization and an increase in excitability provides the necessary mechanism for the shift from the sleepy state of the closed brain to the activated state characterized by tonic firing and enhanced synaptic responsiveness. The long-lasting depolarization is blocked by scopolamine, a muscarinic antagonist.[49] In those cases in which scopolamine does not succeed in completely blocking the prolonged depolarizing response, other transmitters are probably involved. Peptides (among them substance P) are colocalized in some cholinergic brainstem reticular neurons.

In addition to direct excitation of thalamocortical neurons, brainstem reticular stimulation blocks the spindle-related, rhythmic hyperpolarizing episodes in those neurons.[52] This is due to the blockade of spindle oscillations at the site of their genesis, the reticular thalamic nucleus.[13,14] The effect of stimulating the brainstem peribrachial cholinergic nucleus on intracellularly recorded reticular thalamic neurons is a dual one and consists of two direct and opposed components: a short depolarization and a long-lasting hyperpolarization.[52] The hyperpolarization prevents the occurrence of spindle oscillations and effectively blocks ongoing spindle sequences that normally develop in thalamic reticular cells on a depolarizing envelope. The blockade of spindles by hyperpolarization of reticular thalamic neurons is a muscarinic effect because it is blocked by atropine. This hyperpolarization is associated with a marked conductance increase, probably to K ions.[53] In contrast, the early depolarization is not affected by cholinergic antagonists, and after the blockade of the hyperpolarizing component by atropine, it lasts for 200 msec.

The powerful hyperpolarization elicited by brainstem cholinergic fibers acts on the generalized thalamic inhibition produced by GABAergic thalamic reticular neurons but is quite different from the action exerted by the same system on the other class of thalamic GABAergic neurons, namely, the short-axoned cells intrinsic to each nucleus in the dorsal thalamus. Indirect evidence, discussed in the next section, shows that local inhibitory processes related to discriminatory tasks and attributable to short-axoned interneurons are, in fact, enhanced during natural arousal, brainstem reticular stimulation, or ACh application.

The dampening effect of the brainstem reticular cholinergic system on spindle genesis is consistent with data relating the activity of thalamically projecting midbrain reticular neurons to the appearance of EEG spindles at sleep onset (reviewed in references 1, 29, and 43). Midbrain reticular neurons with antidromically identified projections to the intralaminar thalamus significantly decrease their firing rates during the transitional wake-to-sleep period and reliably slow or completely arrest their discharges approximately 1 second before the onset of spindle sequences in repeated transitions from EEG-desynchronized to EEG-synchronized epochs. The withdrawal of tonic brainstem reticular discharges is probably an effective factor for spindle genesis at two thalamic targets: It creates the hyperpolarization by disfacilitation in thalamocortical neurons; and it removes the source of muscarinic hyperpolarization at the level of thalamic reticular neurons, the spindle pacemaker.

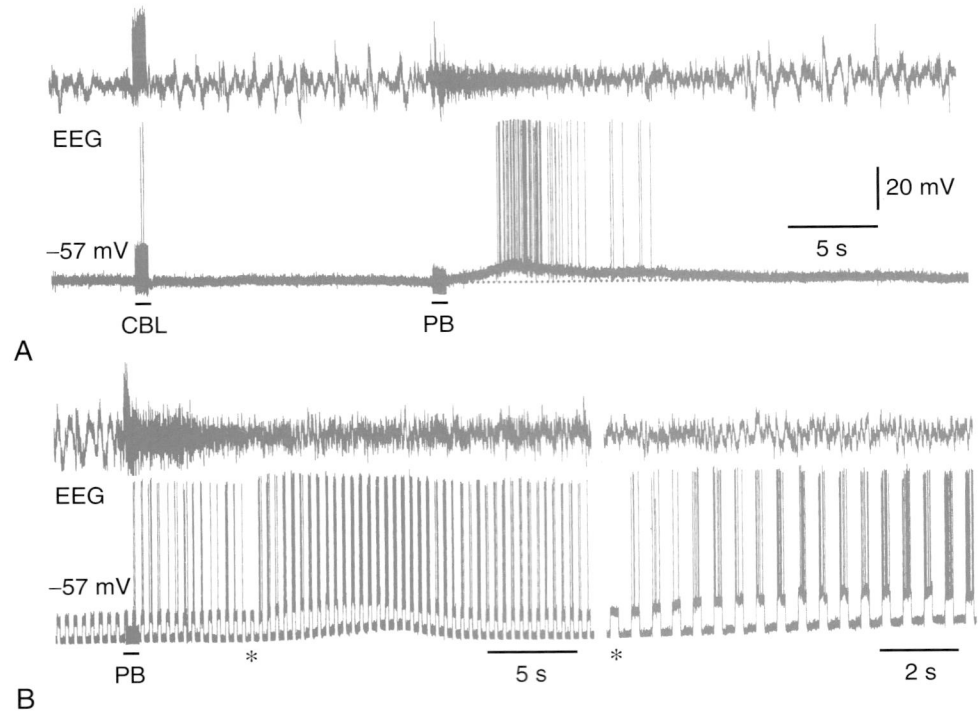

Figure 9–11. Stimulation of the mesopontine cholinergic peribrachial (PB) area induces long-lasting depolarization associated with increased input resistance in the thalamocortical ventrolateral cell. These cellular events are accompanied by desynchronization of ipsilateral electroencephalogram (EEG). **A,** Comparison between the effects of stimulating the contralateral deep cerebellar nuclei (CBL) and ipsilateral PB area to determine whether the effects of PB stimulation are due to activation of PB perikarya or to passing cerebellothalamic axons (for both CBL and PB, stimulation was 1-second pulse train at 30 Hz). Note the similar time course of membrane depolarization and EEG desynchronization in response to PB stimulation. **B,** Membrane conductance tested by injecting depolarizing current pulses. Note the increase in pulse amplitude riding on a 4-mV depolarization. The part indicated by the *asterisk* on the left is depicted at higher speed on the right. (From Curró Dossi R, Paré D, Steriade M: Short-lasting nicotinic and long-lasting muscarinic depolarizing responses of thalamocortical neurons to stimulation of mesopontine cholinergic nuclei. J Neurophysiol 1991;65:393-406, with permission.)

The tonic activating role of the upper brainstem reticular neurons in EEG activation during waking is synergistic with the role played by thalamically projecting medullary reticular neurons in EEG activation during REM sleep.[54] This additional source of EEG activation is required because the destruction of the midbrain reticular formation was found to be much more efficient in impairing EEG activation during waking than during REM sleep. Bulbar reticular neurons (antidromically identified as projecting to thalamic nuclei that, in turn, send axons to widespread cortical areas) significantly increase their firing rates approximately 30 to 60 seconds before the first sign of EEG activation during transition from EEG-synchronized to REM sleep.[54]

The mechanism of cholinergic activation of the cerebral cortex is under investigation. The cortical ACh output increases after brainstem reticular stimulation and during both EEG-activated states of arousal and REM sleep (reviewed in Krnjevic[55]). As discussed earlier, the brainstem reticular cholinergic system plays a decisive role in activation processes in the thalamus, but thalamocortical neurons use aspartate or glutamate as synaptic transmitters, not ACh. There is now evidence of direct projections from the upper brainstem reticular core to cholinergic nuclei of the basal forebrain,[56,57] which are known to have widespread cortical projections. These data indicate that in addition to the noncholinergic thalamocortical activation, the cholinergic activation of the

cerebral cortex is produced by basal forebrain neurons driven by brainstem reticular neurons. Another circuit involves the projection from cholinergic and noncholinergic (GABAergic) basal forebrain neurons located in the substantia innominata and diagonal band nuclei toward a few thalamic nuclear groups, most importantly to the rostral pole of the reticular thalamic complex.[58] The indirect influence of brainstem reticular systems on the synchronizing spindle pacemaker, the reticular thalamic neurons, an influence mediated by basal forebrain neurons, remains to be fully explored.

As mentioned earlier, the reason we call the EEG pattern during waking and REM sleep *activated* and avoid the term *desynchronized* is the occurrence of spontaneous fast (20 to 50 Hz) oscillations that, far from being desynchronized, are coherent within intracortical, intrathalamic, and corticothalamic neuronal networks[3,5] (Fig. 9–12). Fast gamma oscillations are often distinguished from beta oscillations at lower frequencies; however, fast oscillations can double their frequencies during periods as short as 0.5 to 1 second, with an increase in the cell's depolarization.[3] The interest in fast brain oscillations was aroused by claims about their significance in focused attention and in phenomena of binding different features of an object into a global percept.[59] Spatially localized, coherent fast oscillations are present in the background electrical activity, without necessarily requiring optimal sensory stimuli, during all states of vigilance, including NREM sleep as well as deep

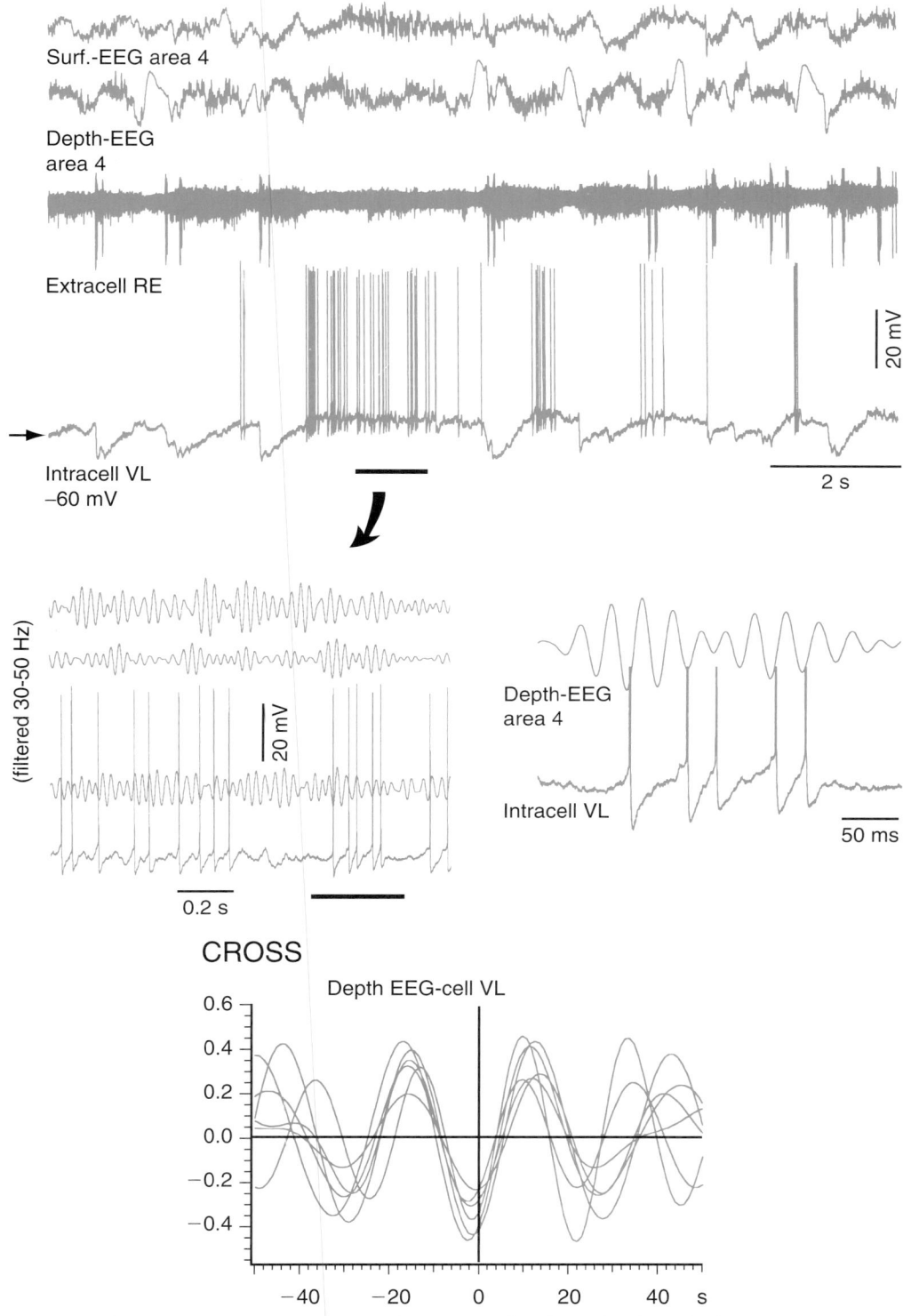

Figure 9–12. Brief episodes of tonic activation are accompanied by sustained and correlated fast rhythms (40 Hz) in cortex and intracellularly recorded thalamocortical (TC) cell. Recordings were obtained in a cat under ketamine and xylazine anesthesia. *Top left*, Four traces represent simultaneous recording of surface- and depth-electroencephalogram (EEG) from precruciate area 4, intracellular activity of TC neuron from the ventrolateral (VL) nucleus, and extracellular discharges of rostrolateral thalamic reticular (RE) neuron. EEG, VL, and RE cells display a slow oscillation (0.7 to 0.8 Hz) consisting of long-lasting, depth-positive EEG waves, leading to sharp depth-negative EEG potentials, related to the initiation of biphasic, long-lasting inhibitory postsynaptic potentials in VL cell. The period from activated epoch is expanded below (*arrow*), with filtered (30- to 50-Hz) activities from surface- and depth-EEG as well as from local field potentials from RE nucleus (picked up by the same microelectrode that served for recording of unitary discharges), and with intracellular activity of VL neuron. Part marked by *horizontal bar* is further expanded at right to show close temporal relations, at ~40 Hz, between the action potentials in VL neuron and depth-negative waves in cortical EEG. CROSS (cross-correlation) is taken from a period of activity without action potentials in VL cell and shows clear-cut relation, with opposition of phase, between depth-EEG and intracellularly recorded VL neuron. (Modified from Steriade M, Contreras D, Amzica F, et al: Synchronization of fast [30-40 Hz] spontaneous oscillations in intrathalamic and thalamocortical networks. J Neurosci 1996;16: 2788-2808, with permission.)

anesthesia, when consciousness is suspended.[3,5] The fast oscillations depend on the depolarization of thalamic and cortical neurons,[3,5] which occurs transiently (but predictably) during the depolarizing phase of the slow sleep oscillation and continuously during behavioral states with tonically increased brain excitability (i.e., waking and REM sleep). Far from being exclusively generated in the cerebral cortex, the fast oscillations also occur in thalamic neurons and are synchronized in corticothalamic networks[60] (Fig. 9–12).

PROCESSING OF SENSORY INFORMATION

Briefly, the synaptic transmission of sensory information through the thalamus and the cerebral cortex is enhanced during the states of waking and REM sleep, compared with EEG-synchronized sleep. The obliteration of synaptic transmission occurs in the thalamus at the first EEG signs of drowsiness, before overt behavioral manifestations of sleep, and despite the unchanged magnitude of the incoming volley (Fig. 9–4). During wakefulness, enhanced synaptic excitability of thalamocortical systems is accompanied by an increased efficacy of the inhibitory sculpturing of afferent information.

Enhanced Excitability

One of the best (and the simplest) methods for investigating state-dependent changes in information processes of thalamic nuclei and cortical areas is the use of field (mass) potentials evoked by stimulation of afferent pathways. This method has the advantages of monitoring the earliest and most rapid deflection that reflects the activity in the presynaptic axons and of ascertaining whether the fluctuations in synaptically evoked components of the thalamic or cortical response depend on parallel modifications in the incoming volley (Fig. 9–4). In detailed analyses on animals, stimuli applied to central pathways (prethalamic fibers, in the case of thalamic responses) are highly artificial and abnormally synchronous. Nonetheless, such central stimuli have the advantage of avoiding unknown alterations at multiple intercalated synapses when peripheral stimulation is used. For an evaluation of this quite old method of centrally evoked field potentials and its use in long-term processes of plasticity, short-term changes during wake and sleep states, and experiments on selective attention and motor set, the reader may consult the monograph by Evarts et al.[61]

Diffuse Brain Activation in Arousal and REM Sleep

The amplitude of the monosynaptically evoked wave of the thalamic and cortical field response is greatly increased both during EEG-activated behavioral states (waking and REM sleep) in chronic experiments and on brainstem reticular stimulation in acutely prepared animals. These changes are observed in all sensory and motor thalamocortical systems. The synaptically relayed component progressively diminishes in amplitude from the very onset of EEG synchronization during drowsiness and is completely obliterated during EEG-synchronized sleep, in spite of the unchanged amplitude of the presynaptic component (Fig. 9–4). *This finding indicates that the thalamus is the first relay station where afferent information is blocked at sleep onset.* Indeed, the excitability of somatosensory cuneothalamic brainstem

neurons does not change from waking to EEG-synchronized sleep.[62] The blockade of synaptic transmission through the thalamus prevents the cerebral cortex from elaborating a response and is a necessary deafferentation prelude to falling asleep.

Besides a parallel increase in spontaneous and evoked discharges during EEG-desynchronized states, another picture emerged when a reduction in spontaneous discharges of cortical neurons on awakening was observed in conjunction with an enhanced probability of their response to afferent stimulation. Thus, most visual cortex neurons reduce their background firing on arousal while simultaneously increasing their responses to optimally oriented moving slits of light.[63] Even when both spontaneous and sensory-evoked discharges are reduced during waking, the ratio of evoked to spontaneous activity becomes higher, which thus indicates a higher signal-to-noise ratio.[64]

These results are explained in the light of data on the action of various modulatory systems. The locus coeruleus acts as an enabling device by suppressing weak inputs and enhancing strong inputs, thus increasing the efficiency of feature extraction from sensory information and switching emphasis from one set of inputs to another.[65] The underlying mechanism of the effects induced by stimulating the locus coeruleus or by iontophoretic application of norepinephrine is a hyperpolarization that accounts for the depressed spontaneous discharges, associated with an increase in input resistance that explains the increased responsiveness to incoming volleys.[66] The association between membrane hyperpolarization and the blockade of afterspike hyperpolarization is a decisive factor in preventing neuronal activation to weak stimuli while enhancing responses to stimuli that overcome inhibition.

Selective Attention

The effects of general arousal can be dissociated from those related to selective attention and initiation of movements. In the experiments conducted by Mountcastle and colleagues,[67] the monkey is in three types of behavioral conditions: a no-trial state, that is, a quiescent state of waking with no involvement in behavioral tasks; a trial state, that is, a condition of attentive fixation on a target when the animal is engaged in a dimming detection task; and an intertrial state, which alternates with the trial state. Although the low degree of responsiveness of parietal cortex visual cells in the intertrial state is virtually equal to that in the no-trial state, the same light-sensitive neurons display a significantly increased excitability during the task mode (Fig. 9–13). The conclusion is that the enhanced responsiveness does not merely occur with changes in general arousal but is more specifically related to the directed attention to the target light. Other studies on the somatosensory cortex of behaving primates have also shown that the response of single neurons increases when the monkey "attends" to the part of the body that is to receive the stimulus.[68] These results are in keeping with data from scalp recordings in human beings, discussed later.

In human beings, sensory information processing can be studied by recording from intact scalp electrical signals as small as 0.1 μV, which are resolved by using computer averaging techniques. A warning stimulus elicits a slow negative potential shift termed *contingent negative variation*, and is followed by an imperative stimulus that evokes an

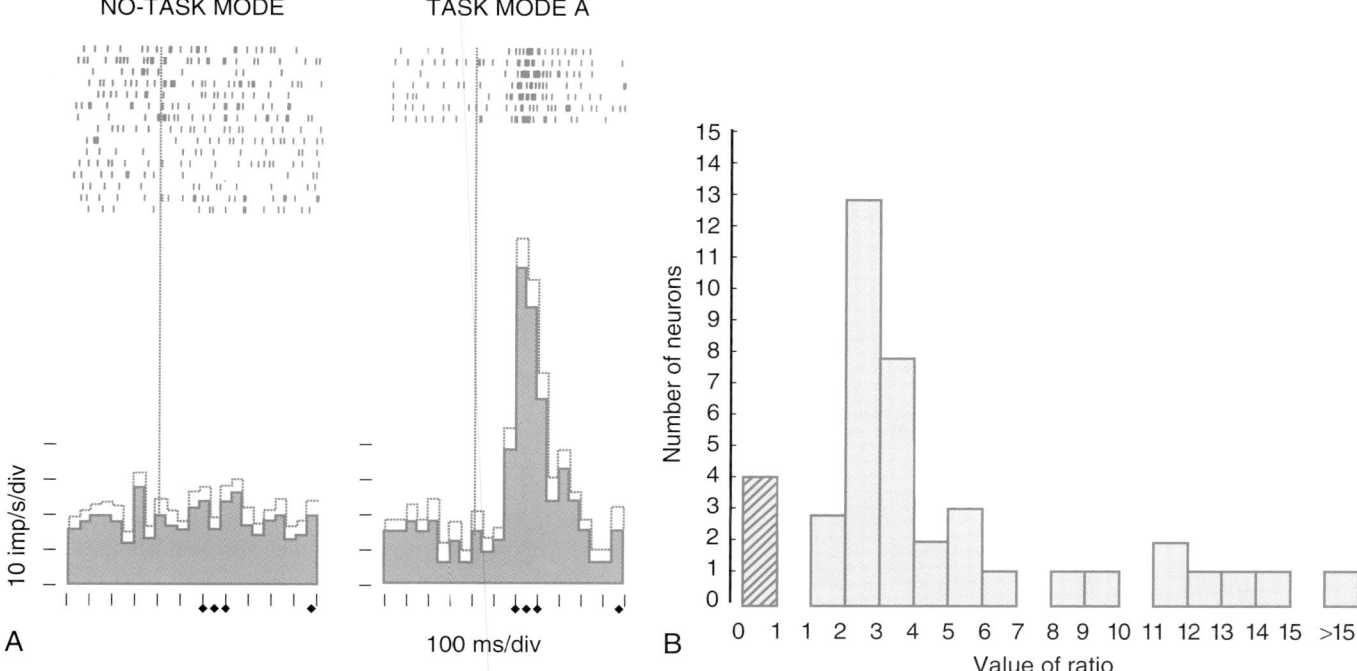

Figure 9–13. Facilitation of the monkey's parietal visual neurons by attentive fixation. **A,** Comparison of responses of parietal light-sensitive neurons to visual stimuli in no-task and task modes (absence of responses during no-task mode compared with strong responses in task mode). Summing histograms: standard error of mean calculated for each bin of the histograms; value shown by *dotted line.* Corresponding bin pairs within the histograms tested for significant differences (*t* test; bin pairs marked with *diamonds* differed at *P* <.05. Overall responses in no-task and task states were compared in the following way. The rate of impulse discharges in the prestimulus period was subtracted from that in the poststimulus period for each trial, and populations of remainders were tested for significant differences (*P* <.05 required) and used to form a facilitation ratio for each neuron. **B,** Ratios for neurons with significant differences plotted in **A**. Facilitation ratio is that of the net increment in response evoked by a light stimulus in a state of interested fixation over that evoked by a physically identical and retinotopically similar stimulus delivered in no-task or intertrial states. Fifty-one neurons showed ratios greater than 1:1 and, of these, the difference was significant at *P* <.05 (*t* test) for 38; values are plotted in histogram. The ratio was fractional for four neurons indicated to the left; for them, the response was significantly greater in the no-task state than during interested fixation. (Adapted from Mountcastle VB, Andersen RA, Motter BO: The influence of attentive fixation upon the excitability of the light-sensitive neurons of the posterior parietal cortex. J Neurosci 1981;1:1218-1235, with permission.)

event-related potential. The scalp-recorded event-related potential consists of a series of components designated by their polarities and peak latencies. In the somatosensory system, all event-related potential components up to and including P14 (a positive wave with 14-msec peak latency) are generated below the thalamus. The first cortical component is the negative wave N20 followed by at least five intracortical components with longer latencies.[69] Although the early components reflecting transmission up to and through the thalamus are unchanged under attentional manipulations, the amplitudes of the P40, N60, and especially P100 and P300 components are increased when the subject is instructed to attend to an infrequent somesthetic stimulus (e.g., to the left thumb) designated as target and to press a button as quickly as possible (with the right index finger) for each such target[70] (Fig. 9–14). Desmedt and colleagues propose that P100 might index the identification of input signals and that P300 reflects the nonspecific postdecision closure. Similarly, the earliest component of the visual cortical response is little affected by psychological variables, whereas subsequent rhythmic waves (which probably reflect intracortical information processing) are selectively enhanced during attention.[71,72]

Circuits Underlying Phasic Events in Alertness and REM Sleep

There are at least two neuronal circuits that are probably involved in phasic processes induced by external sensory stimuli during arousal and in phasic events triggered by brain-stored information during REM sleep.

One of these circuits comprises the GABAergic neurons of the substantia nigra pars reticulata (SNr) and their follower elements in the superior colliculus, peribrachial zone of the upper brainstem reticular formation, and various thalamic nuclei. Novel sensory stimuli that trigger orienting reactions are accompanied by a decrease in the discharge rate of SNr neurons,[73] with a consequent release from tonic inhibition and increased firing in their superior collicular targets, eventually leading (through collicular projections to pontine oculomotor nuclei) to eye movement saccades toward the signal. The decrease in firing rates of GABAergic SNr neurons on sensory stimuli is interpreted as resulting from direct inhibitory inputs arising in GABAergic caudate neurons, which receive projections from some fields in the upper brainstem reticular core, medial and intralaminar thalamic nuclei,

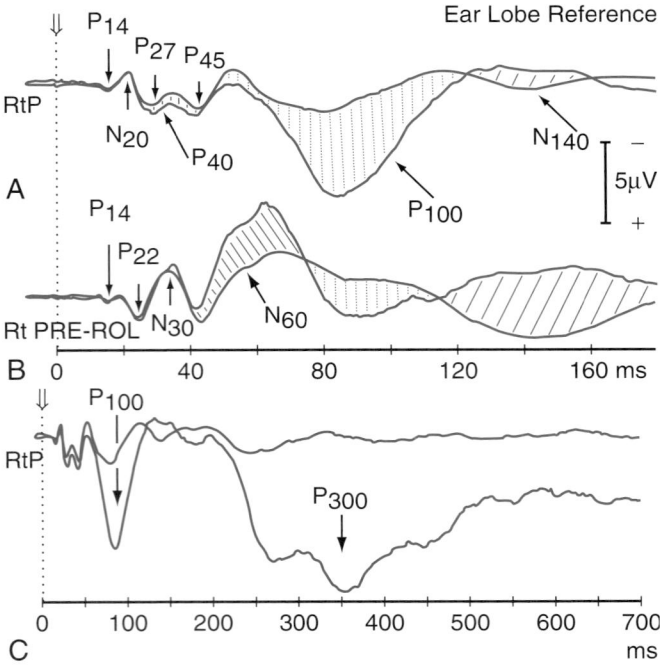

Lt Finger I - P=0.15 - Target - N=645
- P=1.00 - Control no-task

Figure 9–14. Cognitive components in the somatosensory evoked potential (SSEP) of a human to electrical stimuli delivered to the left thumb. The thicker SSEP traces are averaged in runs when the thumb stimuli are infrequent ($P = .15$) targets to which the subject has to respond by pressing a microswitch with the right index finger. Thicker traces were obtained by asking the computer to redraw three times the same trace with an appropriate vertical shift. These SSEPs are superimposed on control SSEPs averaged in other runs of the same experiment when identical thumb stimuli are delivered alone ($P = 1$) at the same intervals and not mixed with any other stimuli. **A,** Right parietal (R + P) scalp derivation. **B,** Right prerolandic (R + PRE-ROL) scalp derivation. **C,** Same trace as **A** displayed on a slower time base. Yoked ear lobes served as reference. The *vertical dotted line* on the left side indicates the time of delivery of the thumb stimulus. The *small arrows* identify standard early SSEP components, namely, the P14 far field, the parietal N20-P27-P45, and the prerolandic P22-N30. Cognitive components identified through divergence of the superimposed traces are indicated by the following symbols: P40 (*vertical lines*), N60 (*oblique lines*), P100 (*vertical rows of dots*), N140 (*widely spaced oblique lines*). Vertical calibration: 5 μV. Horizontal calibration in milliseconds. Negativity of the active scalp electrode registers upward in all traces. (From Desmedt JE, Huy NT, Bourguet M: The cognitive P40, N60 and P100 components of somatosensory evoked potentials and the earliest electrical signs of sensory processing in man. Electroencephalogr Clin Neurophysiol. 1983;56:272-282, with permission.)

and widespread cortical areas.[74] All these structures are the sites of profuse collateralization of sensory pathways. In addition, reciprocal projections link the pars reticulata and pars compacta of the substantia nigra with the cholinergic peribrachial (or pedunculopontine) nucleus of the midbrain–pontine junction.

Therefore, an alerting stimulus would have access to two distinct systems. The first one is the SNr-colliculo-pontine circuit responsible for the phasic shift of gaze involved in the orienting behavior. The relative hyperpolarization of premotor pontine reticular neurons during the alert state[75] is a favorable

condition that underlies their Ca^{2+}-dependent low-threshold spike and superimposed spike bursts, which are operational in driving oculomotor neurons. The second system consists of the brainstem peribrachial and thalamic targets of the SNr that are disinhibited during the periods of silenced firing in the SNr on sensory stimulation. The direct disinhibition of thalamic neurons with widespread cortical projections and depolarizing actions on the superficial cortical layer (such as the cells in the ventromedial thalamic nucleus),[76] together with the secondary brainstem–thalamic activation, is crucial in the EEG activating reaction induced by an alerting stimulus.

Other intra-brainstem and brainstem–thalamic circuits generate the ponto-geniculo-occipital (PGO) waves that are the physiologic correlate of the internal activation of the brain during REM sleep, "the stuff that dreams are made of." PGO waves are sharp field potentials, usually recorded in the visual thalamic (lateral geniculate, or LG) nucleus, where they appear in clusters of up to six waves, closely related to the time occurrence and the direction of eye movement saccades. For example, rightward eye movements are correlated with predominantly right LG waves.[77] Although the original term indicated their presence in the visual pathway, PGO waves largely transcend this sensory system and are disseminated in many thalamic nuclei and in the corresponding cortical areas outside the visual cortex. This widespread distribution of PGO waves is explained by the generalized thalamic projections of PGO generators, the cholinergic neurons of the peribrachial and laterodorsal tegmental nuclei located at the junction of the midbrain and pontine reticular formation. Indeed, peribrachial and some laterodorsal tegmental neurons with antidromically identified projections to thalamic nuclei reliably discharge spike bursts preceding the PGO waves.[29,78-80] PGO waves can also be triggered by stimulating the upper brainstem core when the animal is in REM sleep, which thus suggests a selective gate opening of internal sensory activation during this behavioral state.

How are PGO waves generated? The input sources of the peribrachial, laterodorsal tegmental, and adjacent areas in the upper brainstem reticular formation are in the spinal cord, bulbopontine reticular core, posterior and anterior hypothalamic areas, and cerebral cortex, to mention only some of them. It is likely that initiation of impulses in the PGO generators can be triggered by any of the aforementioned inputs through a mechanism that should conceivably lead to a postinhibitory rebound excitation, because high-frequency spike bursts are the signature of PGO-on peribrachial neurons. The peribrachial neurons can then be regarded as the final link in the brainstem–thalamic path that generates PGO waves in thalamocortical systems. Because these phenomena occur in REM sleep when the brain is disconnected from peripheral sensory gates and because the content of oneiric behavior may relate to past experience, hypothalamic and forebrain structures (which are hypothesized to store some of the emotionally charged information) may be most effective in driving the PGO brainstem neuronal generators.

Sculpturing Inhibition

During waking, the increased response readiness of thalamocortical and corticofugal neurons is accompanied by fine inhibitory sculpturing, which provides input selection and output tuning, the necessary requirements for an adaptive state. The general conclusion based on data discussed in this section is that the inhibitory processes in thalamocortical and corticofugal cells are more effective but much shorter in duration during wakefulness, compared with EEG-synchronized sleep. By inference, the progenitors of short-duration inhibitory events involved in discriminatory tasks would be potentiated during the waking state.

In the thalamus, there are two GABAergic cell types: the reticular neurons, which are leading elements of oscillatory activity during EEG-synchronized sleep, and the short-axoned neurons, which are hypothesized to generate local (intraglomerular) inhibitory processes, which would be effective in input selection during the waking state. Only the reticular neurons were directly investigated during sleep and arousal, brainstem reticular stimulation, and ACh application, both in vivo and in vitro. As yet, there is no study on state-related alterations in the activity of formally identified inhibitory local-circuit thalamic neurons. To complicate the matter, axonal terminals of thalamic reticular neurons contact local-circuit thalamic neurons.[81,82] The functional significance of this finding is the inhibition exerted by one GABAergic cell type on the other, with resulting disinhibition of GABAergic local-circuit cells after disconnection from the thalamic reticular nucleus.[14,83] The consequences of this complex circuit on the target thalamocortical neurons at various levels of vigilance remain unknown. The tremendous variety of local-circuit cortical neurons also remains unexplored with regard to their inhibitory actions across the sleep–waking cycle.

In what follows, the experimental evidence for changes in the inhibitory processes of thalamocortical and corticofugal neurons during states of vigilance is discussed, and state-dependent changes in the activity of inhibitory elements are inferred. The earlier idea of a general disinhibition on arousal evolved and was replaced by the concept of a differential action exerted by brainstem modulatory systems, consisting of the blockade of generalized cyclic inhibition (which underlies spindle genesis) and the preservation or even enhancement of local inhibition involved in discriminatory processes.[1,42] The first type of brainstem-induced cholinergic inhibition that is operational in the blockade of spindles at their site of genesis, the thalamic reticular nucleus, was discussed previously in the section on cellular bases of synchronous oscillations and activation in thalamocortical systems. Data on enhanced inhibitory actions related to input specificity are summarized in the following.

However efficiently midbrain reticular stimulation in acute experiments and natural arousal in behaving animals block cyclic, long-lasting inhibitions in thalamocortical and cortical neurons, neither of these conditions eliminates the early, shorter-lasting inhibitory phase.[84] This result was obtained with both extracellular and intracellular recordings (see details in Steriade[42,43]) and can be related to the improvement of receptive field specificity and orientation selectivity of visual thalamic neurons on arousal.[63] The effect of brainstem reticular stimulation or natural arousal is mainly cholinergic in nature. Indeed, whereas the ACh effect on thalamic reticular neurons is inhibitory and effective in blocking generalized inhibition, the same transmitter induces an improvement in receptive field function.[85,86] This result suggests an ACh-induced potentiation of inhibitory local-circuit thalamic neurons.[87]

The results for inhibitory processes in corticofugal neurons are basically similar to those reported for thalamocortical neurons. Prolonged and cyclic inhibitory periods during behavioral EEG-synchronized sleep develop into significantly shorter but efficient periods of inhibition during wakefulness. The preservation of an initial, short-lasting (20 to 30 msec) inhibitory phase on arousal was reported for both spontaneous and evoked activities of corticospinal neurons.[84]

These data on the facilitatory effects of brainstem reticular stimulation and natural arousal on short-range specific inhibition are congruent with those on the iontophoretic application of ACh to cortical neurons. The increased discrimination applies to receptive field specificity as well as to orientation and direction selectivity.

The common conclusion of these studies on thalamic and cortical inhibitory processes related to discrimination functions is that, during waking, deep but short inhibition provides a mechanism subserving an accurate discrimination of incoming messages, a fine control of performance, and a faithful following of rapidly recurring activity.

Clinical Pearl

A series of studies on EEG sleep rhythms in human subjects[25,33,39] have corroborated data using intracellular recordings from animal experiments in which the newly discovered slow cortical oscillation (0.5 to 1 Hz)[10,11] was differentiated from the classic delta waves (1 to 4 Hz). Moreover, the obsolete notion of different NREM sleep (spindles, delta, slow) and waking (beta and gamma) oscillations considered in isolation has now been replaced by the postulate of coalescing low- as well as high-frequency rhythms under the slow oscillation,[9,30,43] a concept that again has been supported by recent studies in humans.[40] These congruent data should encourage clinical EEG investigators to reanalyze brain rhythms in the light of data arising from intracellular studies in animal experiments.

Acknowledgments

This work was supported by grants from the Canadian Institutes of Health Research, the National Sciences and Engineering Research Council of Canada, the Human Frontier Science Program, and the U.S. National Institutes of Health.

REFERENCES

1. Steriade M, Llinás R: The functional states of the thalamus and the associated neuronal interplay. Physiol Rev 1988;68: 649-742.
2. Moruzzi G, Magoun HW: Brain stem reticular formation and activation of the EEG. Electroencephalogr Clin Neurophysiol 1949;1:455-473.
3. Steriade M, Amzica F, Contreras D: Synchronization of fast (30-40 Hz) spontaneous cortical rhythms during brain activation. J Neurosci 1996;16:392-417.
4. Llinás R., Ribary U: Coherent 40-Hz oscillation characterizes dream state in humans. Proc Natl Acad Sci U S A 1993;90: 2078-2081.
5. Steriade M, Contreras D, Amzica F, Timofeev I: Synchronization of fast (30-40 Hz) spontaneous oscillations in intrathalamic and thalamocortical networks. J Neurosci 1996;16:2788-2808.
6. Moruzzi G: The sleep-waking cycle. Ergebn Physiol 1972;64:1-165.
7. Jasper HH: Recent advances in our understanding of the ascending activities of the reticular system. In Jasper HH, Proctor LD, Knighton RS, et al (eds): Reticular Formation of the Brain. Boston, Little, Brown, 1958, pp 319-331.

8. Jones EG: Thalamus. New York, Plenum Press, 1985.

9. Steriade M: Cellular substrates of brain rhythms. In Niedermeyer E, Lopes da Silva F (eds): Electroencephalography: Basic Principles, Clinical Applications and Related Fields, 4th ed. Baltimore, Williams & Wilkins, 1999, pp 28-75.

10. Steriade M, Nuñez A, Amzica F: A novel slow (<1 Hz) oscillation of neocortical neurons in vivo: Depolarizing and hyperpolarizing components. J Neurosci 1993;13:3252-3265.

11. Steriade M, Nuñez A, Amzica F: Intracellular analysis of relations between the slow (<1 Hz) neocortical oscillation and other sleep rhythms of the electroencephalogram. J Neurosci 1993;13:3266-3283.

12. Contreras D, Destexhe A, Sejnowski TJ, Steriade M: Control of spatiotemporal coherence of a thalamic oscillation by corticothalamic feedback. Science 1996;274:771-774.

13. Steriade M, Domich L, Oakson G, Deschênes M: The deafferented reticularis thalami nucleus generates spindle rhythmicity. J Neurophysiol 1987;57:260-273.

14. Steriade M, Deschênes M, Domich L, Mulle C: Abolition of spindle oscillations in thalamic neurons disconnected from nucleus reticularis thalami. J Neurophysiol 1985;54:1473-1497.

15. Timofeev I, Contreras D, Steriade M: Synaptic responsiveness of cortical and thalamic neurones during various phases of slow sleep oscillation in cat. J Physiol (Lond) 1996;494: 265-278.

16. Steriade M: Alertness, quiet sleep, dreaming. In Peters A, Jones EG (eds): Cerebral Cortex, vol 9: Normal and Altered States of Function. New York, Plenum, 1991, pp 279-357.

17. Steriade M: The corticothalamic system in sleep. Front Biosci 2003;8:878-899.

18. Steriade M, Timofeev I, Grenier F: Natural waking and sleep states: a view from inside neocortical neurons. J Neurophysiol 2001;85:1969-1985.

19. Steriade M, Timofeev I, Grenier F, Dürmüller N: Role of thalamic and cortical neurons in augmenting responses: Dual intracellular recordings in vivo. J Neurosci 1998;18:6425-6443.

20. Timofeev I, Grenier F, Bazhenov M, et al: Short- and medium-term plasticity associated with augmenting responses in cortical slabs and spindles in intact cortex of cats in vivo. J Physiol (Lond) 2002;542:583-598.

21. Steriade M, Timofeev I: Neuronal plasticity in thalamocortical networks during sleep and waking oscillations. Neuron 2003; 37:563-576.

22. Stickgold R, James L, Hobson JA: Visual discrimination learning requires sleep after training. Nat Neurosci 2000;3:1237-1238.

23. Gais S, Mölle M, Helms K, Born J: Learning-dependent increases in sleep density. J Neurosci 2002;22:6830-6834.

24. Villablanca J: Role of the thalamus in sleep control: Sleep-wake-fulness studies in chronic diencephalic and athalamic cats. In Petre-Quadens O, Schlag J (eds): Basic Sleep Mechanisms. New York, Academic Press, 1974, pp 51-81.

25. Amzica F, Steriade M: The K-complex: Its slow (<1 Hz) rhythmicity and relation to delta waves. Neurology 1997;49:952-959.

26. Leresche N, Jassik-Gerschenfeld D, Haby M, et al: Pacemaker-like and other types of spontaneous membrane potential oscillations of thalamocortical cells. Neurosci Lett 1990;113:72-77.

27. McCormick DA, Pape HC: Properties of a hyperpolarization-activated cation current and its role in rhythmic oscillation in thalamic relay neurones. J Physiol (Lond) 1990;431:291-318.

28. Steriade M, Curró Dossi R, Nuñez A: Network modulation of a slow intrinsic oscillation of cat thalamocortical neurons implicated in sleep delta waves: Cortical potentiation and brainstem cholinergic suppression. J Neurosci 1991;11:3200-3217.

29. Steriade M, McCarley RW: Brainstem Control of Wakefulness and Sleep. New York, Plenum, 1990.

30. Steriade M, Amzica F: Coalescence of sleep rhythms and their chronology in corticothalamic networks. Sleep Res Online 1998;1:1-10.

31. Steriade M, Datta S, Paré D, et al: Neuronal activities in brainstem cholinergic nuclei related to tonic activation processes in thalamocortical systems. J Neurosci 1990;10:2541-2559.

32. Contreras D, Steriade M: Cellular basis of EEG slow rhythms: A study of dynamic corticothalamic relationships. J Neurosci 1995;15:604-622.

33. Achermann P, Borbély AA: Low-frequency (<1 Hz) oscillations in the human sleep EEG. Neuroscience 1997;81:213-222.

34. Timofeev I, Steriade M: Low-frequency rhythms in the thalamus of intact-cortex and decorticated cats. J Neurophysiol 1996; 76:4152-4168.

35. Amzica F, Steriade M: Disconnection of intracortical synaptic linkages disrupts synchronization of a slow oscillation. J Neurosci 1995;15:4658-4677.

36. Contreras D, Timofeev I, Steriade M: Mechanisms of long-lasting hyperpolarizations underlying slow sleep oscillations in cat corticothalamic networks. J Physiol (Lond) 1996;494:251-264.

37. Massimini M, Amzica F: Extracellular calcium fluctuations and intracellular potentials in the cortex during the slow sleep oscillation. J Neurophysiol 2001;85:1346-1350.

38. Steriade M, Contreras D, Curró Dossi R, Nuñez A: The slow (<1 Hz) oscillation in reticular thalamic and thalamocortical neurons: Scenario of sleep rhythm generation in interacting thalamic and neocortical networks. J Neurosci 1993;13: 3284-3299.

39. Simon NR, Mandshanden I, Lopes da Silva FH: A MEG study of sleep. Brain Res 2000;860:64-76.

40. Mölle M, Marshall L, Gais S, Born J: Grouping of spindle activity during slow oscillations in human non-REM sleep. J Neurosci 2002;22:10941-10947.

41. Massimini M, Rosanova M, Mariotti M: EEG slow (~1 Hz) waves are associated with nonstationarity of thalamo-cortical sensory processing in the sleeping human. J Neurophysiol 2003;89: 1205-1213.

42. Steriade M: The Intact and Sliced Brain. Cambridge, Mass, MIT Press, 2001.

43. Steriade M: Neuronal Substrates of Sleep and Epilepsy. Cambridge, United Kingdom, Cambridge University Press, 2003.

44. Bremer F: Cerveau "isolé" et physiologie du sommeil. C R Soc Biol (Paris) 1935;118:1235-1241.

45. Jones BE, Harper ST, Halaris AE: Effects of locus coeruleus lesions upon cerebral monoamine content, sleep-wakefulness states and the response to amphetamine in the cat. Brain Res 1977;124: 473-496.

46. Paré D, Smith Y, Parent A, Steriade M: Projections of brainstem core cholinergic and non-cholinergic neurons of cat to intralaminar and reticular thalamic nuclei. Neuroscience 1988;25: 69-86, 1988.

47. Smith Y, Paré D, Deschênes M, et al: Cholinergic and non-cholinergic projections from the upper brainstem core to the visual thalamus in the cat. Exp Brain Res 1988;70:166-180.

48. Steriade, M, Paré D, Parent A, Smith Y: Projections of cholinergic and non-cholinergic neurons of the brainstem core to relay and associational thalamic nuclei in the cat and macaque monkey. Neuroscience 1988;25:47-67.

49. Curró Dossi R, Paré D, Steriade M: Short-lasting nicotinic and long-lasting muscarinic depolarizing responses of thalamocortical neurons to stimulation of mesopontine cholinergic nuclei. J Neurophysiol 1991;65:393-406.

50. Eysel UT, Pape HC, Van Schayck R: Excitatory and differential disinhibitory actions of acetylcholine in the lateral geniculate nucleus of the cat. J Physiol (Lond) 1986;370:233-254.

51. Steriade M, Deschênes M: Intrathalamic and brainstem-thalamic networks involved in resting and alert states. In Bentivoglio M, Spreafico R (eds): Cellular Thalamic Mechanisms. Amsterdam, Elsevier, 1988, pp 51-76.

52. Hu B, Steriade M, Deschênes M: The effects of brainstem peribrachial stimulation on reticular thalamic neurons: The blockage of spindle waves. Neuroscience 1989;31:1-12.

53. McCormick DA, Prince DA: Acetylcholine induces burst firing in thalamic reticular neurones by activating a K+ conductance. Nature 1986;319:147-165.

54. Steriade M, Sakai K, Jouvet M: Bulbothalamic neurons related to thalamocortical activation processes during paradoxical sleep. Exp Brain Res 1984;54:463-475.

55. Krnjevic K: Chemical nature of synaptic transmission in vertebrates. Physiol Rev 1974;54:418-540.

56. Jones BE, Beaudet A: Retrograde labeling of neurons in the brain stem following injections of (^{3}H)choline into the forebrain of the rat. Exp Brain Res 1987;65:437-448.

57. Woolf NJ, Butcher LL: Cholinergic systems in the rat brain: III. Projections from the pontomesencephalic tegmentum to the thalamus, tectum, basal ganglia and basal forebrain. Brain Res Bull 1986;16:603-637, 1986.

58. Steriade M, Parent A, Paré D, Smith Y: Cholinergic and non-cholinergic neurons of cat basal forebrain project to reticular and mediodorsal thalamic nuclei. Brain Res 1987;408: 372-376.

59. Singer W: Synchronization of cortical activity and its putative role in information processing and learning. Annu Rev Physiol 1993;55:349-374.

60. Steriade M: Synchronized activities of coupled oscillators in the cerebral cortex and thalamus at different levels of vigilance. Cereb Cortex 1997;7:583-604.

61. Evarts EV, Shinoda Y, Wise SP: Neurophysiological Approaches to Higher Brain Functions. New York, Wiley, 1984.

62. Carli G, Diete-Spiff K, Pompeiano O: Presynaptic and post-synaptic inhibition of transmission of somatic afferent volleys through the cuneate nucleus during sleep. Arch Ital Biol 1967; 105:52-82.

63. Livingstone MS, Hubel DH: Effects of sleep and arousal on the processing of visual information in the cat. Nature 1981;291: 554-561.

64. Evarts EV: Photically evoked responses in visual cortex units during sleep and waking. J Neurophysiol 1963;26:229-248.

65. Foote SL, Bloom FE, Aston-Jones G: Nucleus locus coeruleus: New evidence of anatomical and physiological specificity. Physiol Rev 1983;63:844-914.

66. Madison DV, Nicoll RA: Actions of noradrenaline recorded intracellularly in rat hippocampal CA1 pyramidal neurones, in vitro. J Physiol (Lond) 1986;72:221-244.

67. Mountcastle VB, Andersen RA, Motter BC: The influence of attentive fixation upon the excitability of the light-sensitive neurons of the posterior parietal cortex. J Neurosci 1981;1:1218-1235.

68. Hyvärinen J, Poranen A, Jokinen Y: Influence of attentive behavior on neuronal responses to vibration in primary somatosensory cortex of the monkey. J Neurophysiol 1980;43:870-882.

69. Desmedt JE, Bourguet M: Color imaging of parietal and frontal somatosensory potential fields evoked by stimulation of median or posterior tibial nerve in man. Electroencephalogr Clin Neurophysiol 1985;62:1-17.

70. Desmedt JE, Huy NT, Bourguet M: The cognitive P40, N60 and P100 components of somatosensory evoked potentials and the earliest electrical signs of sensory processing in man. Electroencephalogr Clin Neurophysiol 1983;56:272-282.

71. Jung R: Neuronal integration in the visual cortex and its significance for visual information. In Rosenblith WA (ed): Sensory Communication. New York, Wiley, 1961, pp 627-674.

72. MacKay DM, Jeffreys DA: Visually evoked potentials and visual perception in man. In Jung R (ed): Handbook of Sensory Physiology, vol VII/3/B. Berlin, Springer, 1973, pp 647-678.

73. Hikosaka O, Wurtz RH: Visual and oculomotor function of monkey substantia nigra pars reticulata: IV. Relation of substantia nigra to superior colliculus. J Neurophysiol 1983;49:1285-1301.

74. Graybiel AM, Ragsdale CW: Fiber connections of the basal ganglia. In Cuenod M, Kreutzberg GW, Bloom FR (eds): Development and Chemical Specificity of Neurons. Amsterdam, Elsevier, 1979, pp 239-283.

75. Ito K, McCarley RW: Alterations in membrane potential and excitability of cat medial pontine reticular formation neurons during changes in naturally occurring sleep-wake states. Brain Res 1984;292:169-175.

76. Glenn LL, Hada J, Roy JP, et al: Anterograde tracer and field potential analysis of the neocortical layer I projection from nucleus ventralis medialis of the thalamus in cat. Neuroscience 1982;7:1861-1877.

77. Nelson JP, McCarley RW, Hobson JA: REM sleep burst neurons, PGO waves, and eye movement information. J Neurophysiol 1983;50:784-797.

78. Hobson JA, Steriade M: Neuronal basis of behavioral state control. In Mountcastle V, Bloom FE (eds): Handbook of Physiology, section 1, vol IV. Bethesda, Md, American Physiological Society, 1986, pp 701-823.

79. Sakai K: Anatomical and physiological basis of paradoxical sleep. In McGinty DA, Morrison A, Drucker-Colin R, Parmeggiani PL (eds): Brain Mechanisms of Sleep. New York, Raven Press, 1985, pp 111-137.

80. Steriade M, Paré D, Datta S, et al: Different cellular types in mesopontine cholinergic nuclei related to ponto-geniculo-occipital waves. J Neurosci 1990;10:2560-2579.

81. Liu XB, Warren RA, Jones EG: Synaptic distribution of afferents from reticular nucleus in ventroposterior nucleus of cat thalamus. J Comp Neurol 1995;352:187-202.

82. Steriade M, Jones EG, McCormick DA: Thalamus, vol 1: Organisation and Function. Oxford, Elsevier, 1997.

83. Steriade M, Domich L, Oakson, G: Reticularis thalamic neurons revisited: Activity changes during shifts in states of vigilance. J Neurosci 1986;6:68-81.

84. Steriade M, Deschênes M: Inhibitory processes and interneuronal apparatus in motor cortex during sleep and waking: II. Recurrent and afferent inhibition of pyramidal tract neurons. J Neurophysiol 1974;37:1093-1113.

85. Sillito AM, Kemp JA: Cholinergic modulation of the functional organization of the cat visual cortex. Brain Res 1983;289:143-155.

86. Sillito AM, Kemp JA, Berardi N: The cholinergic influence on the function of the cat dorsal lateral geniculate nucleus (dLGN). Brain Res 1983;280:299-307.

87. Curró Dossi R, Paré D, Steriade M: Various types of inhibitory postsynaptic potentials in anterior thalamic cells are differentially altered by stimulation of laterodorsal tegmental cholinergic nucleus. Neuroscience 1992;47:279-289.

10

REM Sleep

Jerome M. Siegel

ABSTRACT

Rapid eye movement (REM) sleep was first identified by its most obvious behavior: rapid eye movements during sleep. In most adult mammals, the electroencephalogram (EEG) of the neocortex is low in voltage during REM sleep. The hippocampus has regular high-voltage theta waves throughout REM sleep.

The key brain structure for generating REM sleep is the brainstem, particularly the pons and adjacent portions of the midbrain. These areas and the hypothalamus contain cells that are maximally active in REM sleep, called REM-on cells, and cells that are minimally active in REM sleep, called REM-off cells. Subgroups of REM-on cells use the transmitters gamma-aminobutyric acid (GABA), acetylcholine, glutamate, or glycine. Subgroups of REM-off cells use the transmitters norepinephrine, epinephrine, serotonin, and histamine. It is likely that interactions between REM-on and REM-off cells control the key phenomena of REM sleep.

Destruction of the entire area of midbrain and pons responsible for REM sleep generation can prevent the occurrence of this state. Damage to portions of the brainstem can cause abnormalities in certain aspects of REM sleep. Of particular interest are manipulations that affect the regulation of muscle tone in REM sleep. Lesions in the pons and medulla cause REM sleep to occur without the normal loss of muscle tone. In REM sleep without atonia, animals exhibit locomotor activity, appear to attack imaginary objects, and execute other motor programs during a state that otherwise resembles REM sleep. This syndrome may have some commonalties with the REM sleep behavior disorder seen in humans. Stimulation of portions of the REM sleep–controlling area of the pons can produce a loss of muscle tone in antigravity and respiratory musculature.

Hypocretin neurons, located in the hypothalamus, contribute to the regulation of the activity of norepinephrine, serotonin, histamine, and acetylcholine cell groups and have potent effects on arousal and motor control. Most cases of narcolepsy are caused by a loss of hypocretin neurons.

OVERVIEW

In this chapter I discuss the defining characteristics of rapid eye movement (REM) sleep, including its physiology and neurochemistry. I review how the amounts of REM sleep differ across the animal kingdom. I consider the advantages and disadvantages of the techniques used to investigate the mechanisms generating REM sleep, and discuss the conclusions of these investigations. I examine the mechanisms responsible for the suppression of muscle tone during REM sleep and the pathologic effects of the disruption of these mechanisms. I discuss narcolepsy and its link to mechanisms involved in REM sleep control and especially to the peptide hypocretin. Finally, I speculate about the functions of REM sleep.

WHAT IS REM SLEEP?

REM sleep was discovered by Aserinsky and Kleitman in 1953.[1] They found that it was characterized by the periodic recurrence of rapid eye movements, linked to a dramatic reduction in the amplitude of the electroencephalogram (EEG). They found that the EEG of REM sleep closely resembled the EEG of alert waking and reported that subjects awakened from REM sleep reported vivid dreams. Dement identified a similar state of low-voltage EEG with eye movements in cats.[2] Jouvet then repeated this observation, finding in addition a loss of muscle tone (atonia) in REM sleep and using the name *paradoxical sleep* to refer to this state. The "paradox" was that the EEG resembled that of waking, whereas behaviorally the animal remained asleep and unresponsive.[3] Subsequent authors have described this state as "activated" sleep, or "dream" sleep. Recent work in humans has shown that some mental activity can be present in non-REM sleep but has supported the original finding linking our most vivid dreams to the REM sleep state.[1]

Most early work was done in cats, and it is in the cat that most of the "classic" signs of REM sleep and their generating mechanisms were discovered. Figure 10–1, top, shows the principal electrical signs of REM sleep. These include the reduction in EEG amplitude, particularly in the amplitude of its lower-frequency components. REM sleep is also characterized by a suppression of muscle tone (atonia), visible in the electromyogram (EMG). Erections tend to occur in men and clitoral enlargement in women. Thermoregulation largely ceases, and animal body temperatures drift toward environmental temperatures, as in reptiles.[4] Pupils constrict, reflecting a parasympathetic dominance in the control of the iris. These changes that are present throughout the REM sleep period have been termed its *tonic* features.

Also visible are large electrical potentials that can be most easily recorded in the lateral geniculate nucleus.[5] These potentials originate in the pons, appear after a few milliseconds in the lateral geniculate nucleus, and can be observed with further delay in the occipital cortex, leading to the name *ponto-geniculo-occipital* (PGO) spikes. They occur as large-amplitude, isolated potentials appearing 30 or more seconds before the onset of REM sleep, as defined by EEG and EMG criteria. After REM sleep begins, they arrive in bursts of 3 to 10 waves usually correlated with rapid eye movements. PGO-linked potentials can also be recorded in the motor nuclei of the extraocular muscles, where they trigger the rapid eye movements of REM sleep. They are present, in addition, in thalamic nuclei other than the geniculate and in neocortical regions other than the occipital cortex. In humans, rapid eye

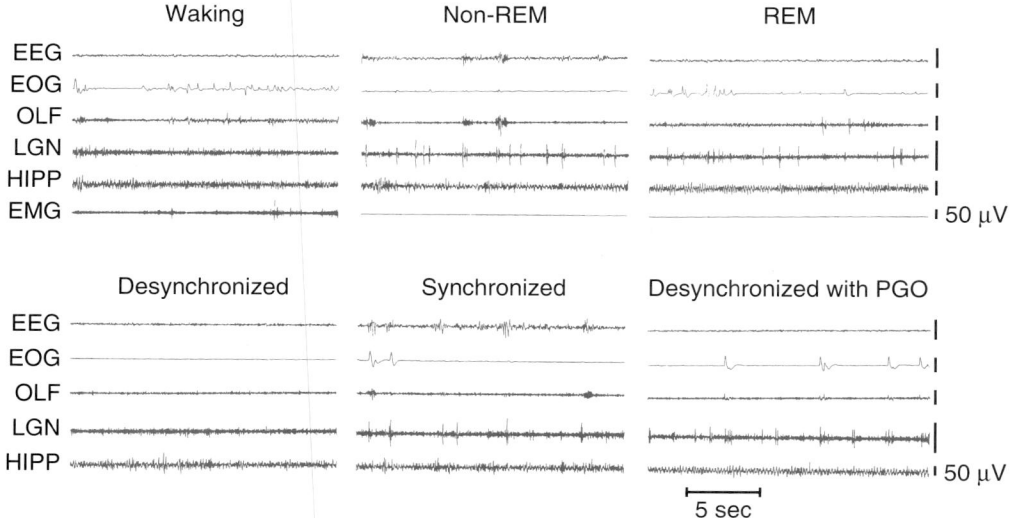

Figure 10–1. *Top,* Polygraph tracings of states seen in the intact cat. *Bottom,* States seen in the forebrain 4 days after transection at the pontomedullary junction. EEG, sensorimotor electroencephalogram; EOG, electrooculogram; OLF, olfactory bulb; LGN, lateral geniculate nucleus; HIPP, hippocampus; EMG, dorsal neck electromyogram. (From Siegel JM, Nienhuis R, Tomaszewski KS: REM sleep signs rostral to chronic transections at the pontomedullary junction. Neurosci Lett 1984;45:241-246, with permission.)

movements are loosely correlated with contractions of the muscles of the middle ear of the sort that accompany speech generation and that are part of the protective response to loud noise.[6] Other muscles also contract during periods of rapid eye movement, briefly breaking through the tonic muscle atonia of REM sleep. There are periods of marked irregularity in respiratory and heart rates during REM sleep, in contrast to non-REM sleep, during which respiration and heart rate are highly regular. There does not appear to be any single pacemaker for all of this irregular activity. Rather, the signals producing twitches of the peripheral or middle ear muscles may lead or follow PGO spikes and rapid eye movements. Bursts of brainstem neuronal activity may likewise lead or follow the activity of any particular recorded muscle.[7-9] These changes that occur episodically in REM sleep have been called its *phasic* features.

As we will see later, certain manipulations of the brainstem can eliminate only the phasic events of REM sleep, whereas others can cause the phasic events to occur in waking; yet other manipulations can affect tonic components. These tonic and phasic features are also expressed to varying extents in different species, and not all of these features are present in all species that have been observed to have REM sleep.

THE DISTRIBUTION OF REM SLEEP IN THE ANIMAL KINGDOM

The identification of REM sleep in the cat indicated that it was not necessarily a correlate of some uniquely human mental state. It soon became apparent that REM sleep was widespread, perhaps even universal in mammals and birds[10] (see Chapter 8). However, a few important exceptions have been identified. Early work investigated the sleep of an egg-laying monotreme mammal, the echidna, an anteater found only in Australia. A thorough study of the echidna EEG by Allison and coworkers showed that this animal did not have any periods of sleep with a low-voltage cortical EEG.[11] This led to the hypothesis that primitive mammals did not have

REM sleep, which must therefore have evolved after the divergence of the monotremes from the placental and marsupial mammalian lines. We reexamined this question, looking at brainstem neuronal activity in addition to the EEG for signs of REM sleep. Although we confirmed Allison and colleagues' observation of no low-voltage EEG during sleep, we found that brainstem neurons exhibited the phasic pattern of activation characteristic of REM sleep while the EEG voltage was elevated.[12] A similar conclusion was reached by Nicol et al.[13]

We then went on to examine the only other available monotreme species, the platypus. We found that most of the sleep time in this animal was also characterized by a high-voltage EEG, as in non-REM sleep. However, dramatic phasic motor activity was visible almost continuously throughout sleep in the platypus. (A video of this activity can be seen at our web site [http://www.npi.ucla.edu/sleepresearch] and at the PPSM web site). The platypus has more REM sleep, approximately 8 hours per day, than any other any other animal.[14] An altered distribution of monoaminergic and particularly cholinergic cells in the brainstems and forebrains of monotreme mammals may be the anatomic substrate of this unusual REM sleep pattern.[15-17] Other animals with high amounts of REM sleep are the ferret, armadillo, and possum (see Chapter 8).

Marine mammals also have unusual sleep patterns that may provide an insight into the evolution and function of REM sleep. Dolphins and other cetaceans have slow waves in only one hemisphere at a time, never showing the bilateral slow waves characteristic of non-REM sleep in terrestrial mammals.[18] This EEG pattern is often present while they swim, avoid obstacles, and appear generally responsive to the environment. If they are disturbed whenever slow waves appear on one side of the brain, they display a rebound of slow waves in that hemisphere when they are subsequently left undisturbed, that is, they have a unihemispheric slow wave sleep (SWS or non-REM sleep) rebound.[19] It is unclear whether dolphins or other cetaceans have REM sleep. One approach to detecting REM sleep in these mammals is to look for signs of phasic events during rest states, although determining which phasic events might correspond to REM sleep twitches and which might be the cetacean equivalent of myoclonic jerks occurring in non-REM sleep is a difficult task. What is already clear is that very few such jerks occur, on the order of 10 to 100 per day, compared with approximately 3000 in the rat. If these events are the correlates of REM sleep in the dolphin, then these animals have some of the smallest amounts of REM sleep observed in any mammalian species, perhaps less than 15 minutes/day.

The fur seal also has an unusual sleep pattern. When quiescent in the water, it assumes an asymmetrical posture, paddling with one flipper while the contralateral flipper remains immobile. The EEG of the hemisphere contralateral to the immobile flipper shows slow waves. Very little REM sleep is seen while the seal is in the water, although REM sleep is apparent on land, when bilateral cortical EEG sleep is seen.[20] Despite the suppression of REM sleep in the water, there is no rebound of REM sleep beyond baseline levels when the seal returns to land.

The average daily amount of REM sleep for a given species appears to be strongly related to how immature it is at birth[21] (see Chapter 8). Animals that are born in a helpless state, as is the case with the platypus, ferret, possum, and armadillo, have high amounts of REM sleep at birth, suggesting that REM sleep may have some role in the development of the brain and body. However, although amounts of REM sleep decrease with age, these animals also have higher amounts of REM sleep as adults, for reasons that remain unclear. In contrast, animals that are born relatively mature, such as the dolphin, which must swim and defend itself from birth, and grazing animals such as the horse or cattle (see Chapter 8), have very little REM sleep either at birth or later in life. Humans fall in the middle, with moderate amounts of REM sleep corresponding to their intermediate level of immaturity at birth.

Birds have REM sleep, although in much smaller amounts than mammals, with REM sleep episodes often lasting only a few seconds.[10] Because birds and mammals diverged from a common reptilian ancestor, we examined sleep in the turtle, using the same neuronal recording technique we had used to detect REM sleep in the echidna. We found no evidence for phasic neuronal activity during sleep.[22] Together, these results suggest a link between REM sleep and homeothermy, but the nature of the link remains unclear.

REM GENERATION MECHANISMS

Technical Considerations: Lesions

More has been learned about brain function and sleep control from brain damage caused by stroke, injury, or infection in patients and by experimentally induced brain lesions in animals, than by any other technique. However, some basic principles need to be borne in mind when interpreting such data.

Brain lesions can result from ischemia, pressure, trauma, and degenerative or metabolic changes. In animals, experimental lesions are most commonly induced by aspiration, transection of the neuraxis, electrolysis, local heating by radiofrequency currents, or by the injection of cytotoxins. The latter include substances such as N-methyl-D-aspartate (NMDA) and kainate that cause cell death by excitotoxicity as well as targeted cytotoxins such as saporin coupled to particular ligands, which kill only cells containing receptors for that ligand. Cytotoxic techniques have the considerable

advantage of sparing axons passing through the region of damage, so that deficits are attributable to the loss of local neurons, rather than axons of passage.

If damage to a particular region causes the loss of a sleep state, one cannot conclude that this is where a "center" for the state resides. Lesion effects are usually maximal immediately after the lesion is created. Swelling and circulatory disruption make the functional loss larger than will be apparent from standard postmortem histologic techniques. The loss of one brain region can also disrupt functions that are organized elsewhere. For example, spinal shock is a well known phenomenon in which severing the spinal cord's connection to more rostral brain regions causes a loss of functions known to be mediated by circuits intrinsic to the spinal cord.

On the other hand, with the passage of time, this sort of denervation-induced shock dissipates. In addition, adaptive changes occur that allow other regions to take over lost functions. This is mediated by sprouting of new connections to compensate for the loss. A striking phenomenon seen after placement of lesions aimed at identifying the brain regions responsible for REM and non-REM sleep is that even massive lesions often produce only a transient disruption of sleep.

A particularly useful approach to the understanding of REM sleep generation has been the transection technique. In this approach, the neuraxis is severed at the spinomedullary junction, at various brainstem levels, or at various forebrain levels by passing a knife across the coronal plane of the neuraxis. Regions rostral to the cut may be left in situ or may be removed. One might expect that such a manipulation would completely prevent sleep phenomena from appearing on either side of this cut, as in the phenomenon of spinal shock. However, to a surprising extent this is not the case. As I review later, REM sleep reappears within hours after some of these lesions. When both parts of the brain remain, signs usually appear on only one side of the cut. This kind of positive evidence is much more easily interpreted than loss of function, because one can with certainty state that the removed regions are not essential for the signs of REM sleep that survive.

Technical Considerations: Stimulation

Sites identified by lesion or anatomic data can be stimulated to identify their roles in sleep control. Older studies used electrical stimulation and were successful in identifying the basal forebrain as a sleep-inducing region (see Chapter 13) and the medial medulla as a region mediating the suppression of muscle tone.[23] Electrical stimulation is an obviously aphysiologic technique, involving the forced depolarization of neuronal membranes by ion flow at a frequency set by the stimulation device, rather than by the patterned afferent impulses that normally control neuronal discharge. For this reason, it has largely been supplanted by administration of neurotransmitter agonists, either by direct microinjection or by diffusion from a microdialysis membrane that is placed in the target area and perfused with high concentrations of agonists. One cannot, however, assume that responses produced by such agonist administration demonstrate a normal role for the applied ligand. For example, many transmitter agonists and antagonists have been administered to the pontine regions thought to trigger REM sleep. In some cases this administration has increased REM sleep. But we can conclude from this only that cells in the region of infusion have receptors for the ligand and have connections to REM sleep–generating mechanisms. Under normal conditions these receptors may not have a role in triggering the state. Only by showing that the administration duplicates the normal pattern of release of the ligand in this area, and that blockade of the activated receptors prevents REM sleep, can a reasonable suspicion be raised that a part of the normal REM sleep control pathway has been identified. Because it is far easier to inject a substance than to collect and quantify physiologically released ligands, there have been many studies implying that various substances are critical for REM sleep control based solely on microinjection. These results must be interpreted with caution.

Technical Considerations: Recording

Observation of the normal pattern of neurotransmitter release and neuronal activity can help determine the neurochemical correlates of sleep states. The natural release of ligands can be most easily determined by placing a tubular dialysis membrane 1 to 5 mm in length in the area of interest and circulating artificial cerebrospinal fluid through it. Neurotransmitters released outside the membrane diffuse through the membrane and can be collected. Each sample is collected at intervals typically ranging from 2 to 10 minutes. The collected dialysates can be analyzed by chromatography, radioimmunoassay, or other means.

Recording the activity of single neurons in vivo can provide a powerful insight into the precise time course of neuronal discharge. Unit activity can be combined with other techniques to make it even more useful. For example, electrical stimulation of potential target areas can be used to identify antidromically the axonal projections of the recorded cell. Intracellular labeling of neurons with dyes, with subsequent immunolabeling of their transmitter, can be used to determine the neurotransmitter phenotype of the recorded cell. Combined dialysis and unit recording or iontophoresis of neurotransmitter from multiple-barrel recording and stimulating micropipettes can be used to determine the transmitter response of the recorded cell, although one cannot easily determine if the effects seen are the direct result of responses in the recorded cell or are mediated by an adjacent responsive cell projecting to the recorded cell. Such distinctions can be made in in vitro studies by blocking synaptic transmission or physically dissociating studied cells, but in this case their role in sleep may not be easily determined.

Although the role of a neuron in fast, synaptically mediated events can be traced by inspection of neuronal discharge and comparison of that discharge with the timing of motor or sensory events, such an approach may be misleading when applied to the analysis of sleep generation. The sleep cycle consists of a gradual coordinated change in EEG, EMG, and other phenomena over a period of seconds to minutes, as waking turns into non-REM sleep and then as non-REM sleep is transformed into REM sleep. Neuronal activity can traverse the human brain in as little as 5 msec. Despite this mismatch of time courses, the "tonic latency," a measure of how long before REM sleep onset activity in a recorded cell changes, has been computed. Neurons purported to show a significant change in activity many seconds or even minutes before REM sleep onset have been reported. However, such a measure is of little utility because at the neuronal level, the activity of key cell groups can best be seen as curvilinear over the sleep cycle,

rather than changing abruptly in the way that activity follows discrete sensory stimulation. A major determinant of the tonic latency, computed as defined previously, is the level of "noise" or variability in the cell's discharge, which affects the difficulty of detecting a significant underlying change in rate. It is therefore not surprising that cell groups designated as "executive neurons" for REM sleep control on the basis of their tonic latencies were later found to have no essential role in the generation of REM sleep.[24] The more appropriate comparison of the unit activity cycle to state control is to compare two different cell types to see what the phase relation is. This kind of study is difficult, involving the simultaneous long-term recording of multiple cells, and is rarely performed. Even in this case, a phase lead does not by itself prove that the "lead" neuron is driving activity seen in the "following" neuron.

Technical Considerations: Summary

Clearly there is no perfect technique for determining the neuronal substrates of sleep states. Nevertheless, there are certain common pitfalls that must be kept in mind in interpreting experimental manipulations designed to analyze sleep states. The next sections explore the major findings derived from lesion, stimulation, and recording studies of REM sleep control mechanisms.

Transection Studies

Sherrington discovered that animals in which the forebrain is removed after transecting the neuraxis in the coronal plane at the rostral border of the superior colliculus, showed tonic excitation of the antigravity muscles or extensors (Fig. 10–2, level A). This decerebrate rigidity was visible as soon as anesthesia was discontinued. Bard and Macht first reported that animals with decerebrate rigidity would show periodic limb relaxation.[25] We now know that Bard and Macht were observing the periodic muscle atonia of REM sleep.

After the discovery of REM sleep in the cat,[2] Jouvet found that this state of EEG desynchrony was normally accompanied by muscle atonia.[3] Jouvet then examined the decerebrate cat preparation used by Sherrington and Bard, now adding measures of muscle tone, eye movement, and EEG. One might have expected that the "dream state" originated in the forebrain, but Jouvet found something quite different. When he recorded in the forebrain after separating the forebrain from the brainstem at the midbrain level (Fig. 10–2, levels A or B), he found no clear evidence of REM sleep. In the first few days after transection, the EEG in the forebrain was always high voltage, but when low-voltage activity appeared, the PGO spikes that help identify REM sleep in the intact animal were absent from the thalamic structures, particularly the lateral geniculate, where they can be most easily recorded. Thus, it appeared that the isolated forebrain had SWS states and possibly waking, but no clear evidence of REM sleep.

In contrast, the midbrain and brainstem behind the cut showed clear evidence of REM sleep. Muscle atonia appeared with a regular periodicity and duration, similar to that of the intact cat's REM sleep periods. This atonia was accompanied by PGO spikes with a similar morphology to those seen in the intact animal. The pupils were highly constricted during atonic periods, as in REM sleep in the intact cat.

An interesting feature of REM sleep in the decerebrate animal is that its frequency and duration varied with the

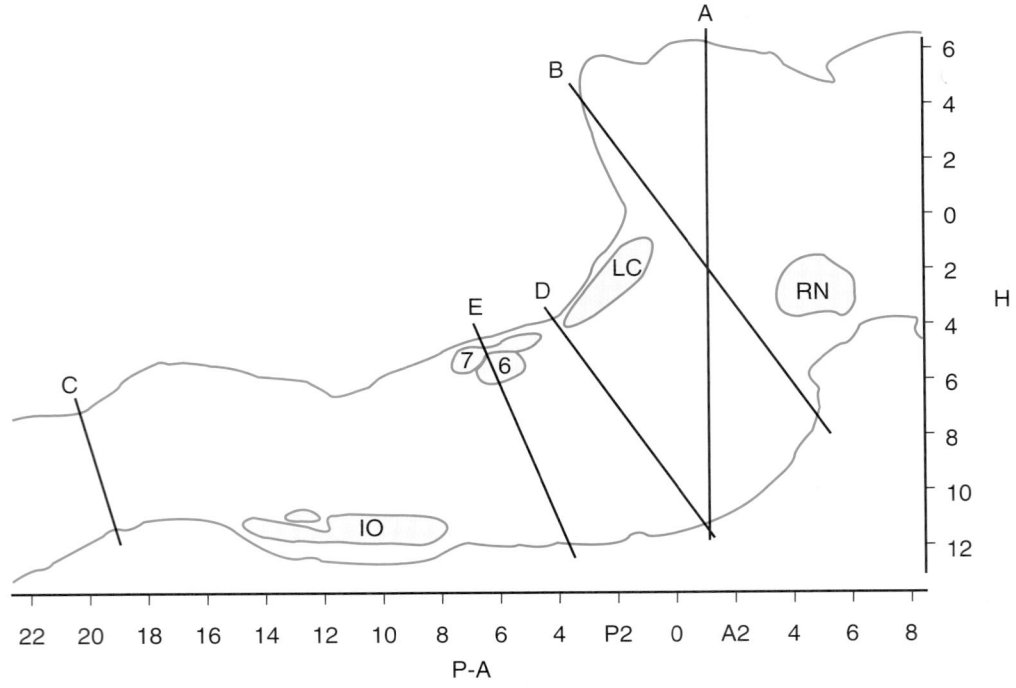

Figure 10–2. Outline of a sagittal section of the brainstem of the cat drawn from level L = 1.6 of the Berman atlas, indicating the level of key brainstem transection studies. A and B, midbrain-pontine junction; D, caudal pons; E, ponto-medullary junction; C, spino-medullary junction; RN, red nucleus; LC, locus coeruleus; 6, abducens nucleus; 7, genu of the facial nerve; IO, inferior olive. H (horizontal) and P-A (posterior-anterior) scales are drawn from the atlas. (From Siegel JM: Pontomedullary interactions in the generation of REM sleep. In McGinty DJ, Drucker-Colin R, Morrison A, Parmeggiani PL [eds]: Brain Mechanisms of Sleep. New York, Raven Press, 1985, pp 157-174, with permission.)

temperature of the animal. In the decerebrate animal, the fore-brain thermoregulatory mechanisms are disconnected from their brainstem effectors. Shivering and panting do not occur at the relatively small temperature shifts that trigger them in the intact animal. For this reason, if the body temperature is not maintained by external heating or cooling, it tends to drift toward room temperature. Arnulf et al.[26] found that if body temperature was maintained at a normal level, little or no REM sleep appeared. But if temperature was allowed to fall, REM sleep amounts increased to levels well above those seen in the intact animal. This suggests that REM sleep facilitatory mechanisms are on balance less impaired by reduced temperature than are REM sleep inhibitory mechanisms. Another way of looking at this phenomenon is that brainstem mechanisms are set to respond to low temperatures by triggering REM sleep, perhaps to stimulate the brainstem, and that high brainstem temperatures inhibit REM sleep. In the absence of forebrain control, major increases in REM sleep can be seen with temperature shifts that do not normally occur in the intact animal. However, a more sensitive mechanism may be operative in the intact animal.

A further localization of the REM sleep control mechanisms can be achieved by examining the sleep of humans or animals in which the brainstem–spinal cord connection has been severed (Fig. 10–2, level C). In this case, normal REM sleep in all its manifestations, except for spinally mediated atonia, is present.[27] Thus, we can conclude that the region between the caudal medulla and rostral midbrain is sufficient to generate REM sleep.

A further localization of REM sleep–generating mechanisms can be achieved by separating the caudal pons from the

medulla (Fig. 10–2, level D or E). In such animals no atonia is present. Furthermore, neuronal activity in the medulla does not resemble that seen across the REM–non-REM sleep cycle, with neuronal discharge very regular for periods of many hours, in contrast to the highly periodic rate modulation that is linked to the phasic events of REM sleep in the intact animal[28] (Fig. 10–3). This demonstrates that the medulla and spinal cord together are not sufficient to generate this aspect of REM sleep.

In contrast, the regions rostral to the cut show aspects of REM sleep[29] (Fig. 10–1, bottom; Fig. 10–4). In these regions we can see the progression from isolated to grouped PGO spikes and the accompanying reduction in PGO spike amplitude that occurs in the pre-REM sleep period and the REM sleep periods in the intact animal. We also see increased forebrain unit activity, with unit spike bursts in conjunction with PGO spikes, just as in REM sleep.[30]

To summarize, this work shows that when pontine regions are connected to the medulla, atonia, the rapid eye movements of REM sleep, and the associated unit activity patterns occur, whereas the medulla and spinal cord together, disconnected from the pons, are not sufficient to generate these local aspects of REM sleep. When the pons is connected to the forebrain, forebrain aspects of REM sleep are seen, but the forebrain without attached pons does not generate these aspects of REM sleep. Further confirmation of the importance of the pons and caudal midbrain comes from the studies of Matsuzaki.[31] They found that when two cuts were placed, one at the junction of the midbrain and pons and the other at the junction of the pons and medulla, one could see periods of PGO spikes in the isolated pons, but no signs of REM sleep in structures rostral or caudal to the pontine island.

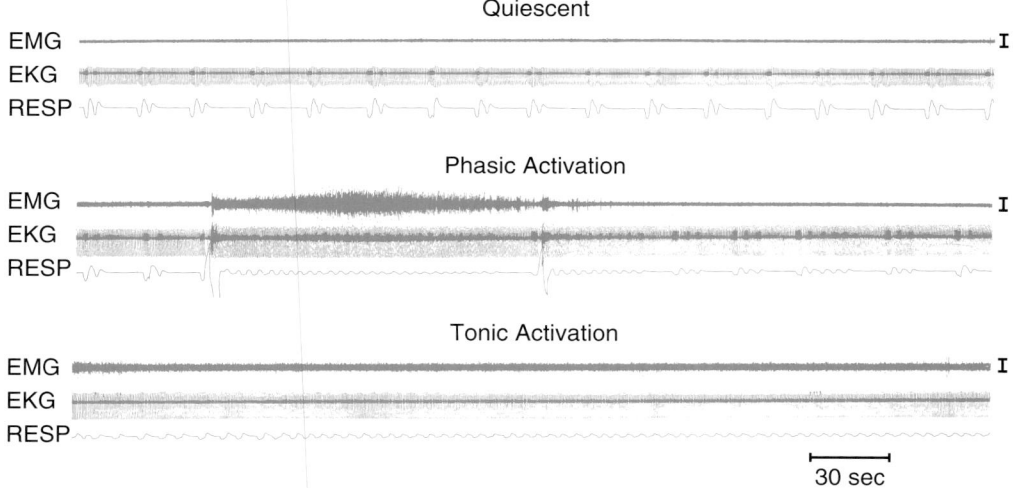

Figure 10–3. States seen in the chronic medullary cat. Note the absence of periods of atonia. EKG, electrocardiogram; EMG, electromyogram; RESP, thoracic strain gauge. Calibration, 50 μV. (From Siegel JM, Tomaszewski KS, Nienhuis R: Behavioral states in the chronic medullary and mid-pontine cat. Electroencephalogr Clin Neurophysiol 1986;63:274-288, with permission.)

These transection studies demonstrate, by positive evidence, that the pons is sufficient to generate the pontine signs of REM sleep, that is, the periodic pattern of PGO spikes and irregular neuronal activity that characterize REM sleep. One can fairly characterize the pons as the crucial region for the generation of REM sleep.

However, it is also clear that the pons alone does not generate REM sleep. Atonia requires the activation of motor inhibitory systems in the medulla. In the intact animal, forebrain mechanisms interact with pontine mechanisms to regulate the amplitude and periodicity of PGO spikes.[32] Extrapolating to human dream imagery, one can hypothesize

that because the structure of REM sleep results from an interaction of forebrain and brainstem mechanisms, the dream itself is not just passively driven from the brainstem, but rather represents the result of a dynamic interaction between forebrain and brainstem structures.

Lesion Studies

The transection studies point to a relatively small portion of the brainstem, the pons and caudal midbrain, as critical for REM sleep generation. Further specification of the critical regions can be achieved by destroying portions of the pons in

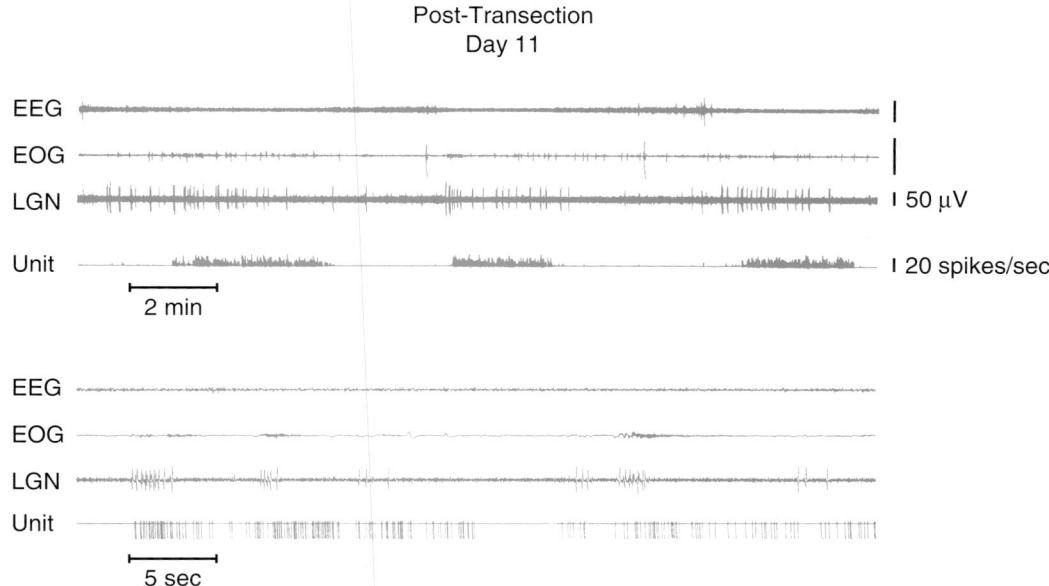

Figure 10–4. Midbrain unit: electroencephalographic (EEG), electrooculographic (EOG), and lateral geniculate nucleus (LGN) activity rostral to chronic transections at the pontomedullary junction. In the upper portion of the figure, the unit channel displays the output of an integrating digital counter resetting at 1-second intervals. In the lower portion, one pulse is produced for each spike by a window discriminator. The figure shows that bursts of PGOs are correlated with increased neuronal ("unit") activity. PGO, ponto-geniculo-occipital. (From Siegel JM: Pontomedullary interactions in the generation of REM sleep. In McGinty DJ, Drucker-Colin R, Morrison A, Parmeggiani PL [eds]: Brain Mechanisms of Sleep. New York, Raven Press, 1985, pp 157-174, with permission.)

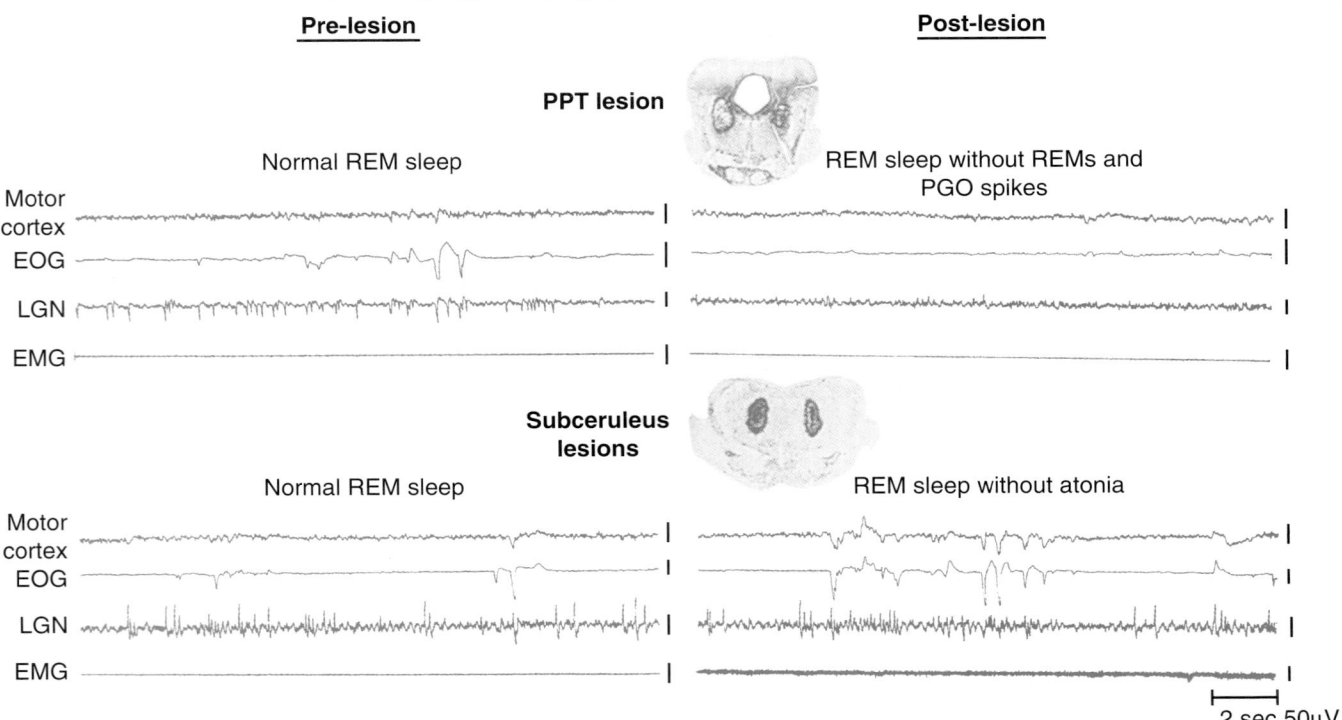

Figure 10–5. Twenty-second polygraph tracings of REM sleep before and after lesions, together with a coronal section through the center of the pontine lesions. Electroencephalographic voltage reduction of REM sleep (recorded from motor cortex) was present after both lesions. *Top,* Radiofrequency lesions of the pedunculopontine region diminished ponto-geniculo-occipital (PGO) spikes and eye movement bursts during REM sleep. *Bottom,* Lesions in the region ventral to the locus coeruleus produced REM sleep without atonia without any diminution of PGO spike or REM frequency. (Reprinted from Shouse MN, Siegel JM: Pontine regulation of REM sleep components in cats: Integrity of the pedunculopontine tegmentum [PPT] is important for phasic events but unnecessary for atonia during REM sleep. Brain Research, vol 571, 50-63, Copyright 1992, with permission from Elsevier Science.)

an otherwise intact animal and seeing which areas are necessary and which are unnecessary for REM sleep generation. An early, exhaustive study by Carli and Zanchetti[33] and other subsequent studies emphasized that lesions of the locus coeruleus[34] and the dorsal raphe[35] nuclei did not block REM sleep. Carli and Zanchetti concluded that lesions that destroyed the region ventral to the locus coeruleus, called the nucleus reticularis pontis oralis or the subcoeruleus region, eliminated or produced a massive decrease in the amount of REM sleep. In their studies, Carli and Zanchetti used the electrolytic lesion technique, in which a current is passed depositing metal that kills cells and axons of passage. As cytotoxic techniques that allowed poisoning of cell bodies without the mechanical damage to the brain substance and axons of passage came into use, these initial conclusions were confirmed and refined. It was shown that neurons in medial regions, including the giant cell region, were not important in REM sleep control because near-total destruction of these cells was followed by normal amounts of REM sleep as soon as anesthesia dissipated.[36] However, lesions of the subcoeruleus and adjacent regions produced with cytotoxins did cause a prolonged loss of REM sleep. According to one study, the extent of this loss was proportional to the percentage of cholinergic cells lost in subcoeruleus and adjacent regions of the brainstem.[37]

Although large lesions may eliminate all aspects of REM sleep, small, bilaterally symmetrical lesions in the pons can eliminate specific aspects of REM sleep. Lesions of lateral pontine structures allow muscle atonia during REM sleep. However, PGO spikes and the associated rapid eye movements are absent when lesions include the region surrounding the superior cerebellar peduncle[38] (Fig. 10–5, top). This points to the role of this lateral region in the generation of PGO waves and the associated phasic activity of REM sleep.

Lesions confined to portions of the subcoeruleus regions identified as critical for REM sleep by Carli and Zanchetti, or to the medial medulla,[39] result in a very unusual syndrome. After non-REM sleep, these animals enter REM sleep as indicated by lack of responsiveness to the environment, PGO spikes, EEG desynchrony, and pupil constriction. However, they lack the muscle atonia that normally characterizes this state[40] (Fig. 10–5, bottom). During "REM sleep without atonia," these animals appear to act out their dreams, attacking objects that are not visible, exhibiting unusual affective behaviors and ataxic locomotion. When "awakened," normal waking behavior resumes. The critical region, termed the *pontine inhibitory area* (PIA), appears to be responsible for the normal coupling of atonia to REM sleep.

Stimulation Studies

The first study showing that stimulation could elicit REM sleep was carried out by George et al.[41] They found that application of the acetylcholine agonist carbachol could elicit REM sleep, but only when it was applied to specific regions of the pons ventral to the locus coeruleus. An impressive proof that a unique REM sleep generation mechanism was being activated was the long duration of the elicited REM sleep periods. Later studies showed that, depending on the exact site, either REM sleep or just atonia could be triggered by such stimulation.[42,43] When stimulation was applied to the lateral regions whose lesion blocked PGO waves, continuous PGO spikes were generated even though the animal was not always behaviorally asleep. More recent studies have found that other chemicals can also trigger atonia or REM sleep when applied to pontine regions. However, the potency of cholinergic agonists in triggering REM sleep remains unique among the tested neurotransmitters.

Neuronal Activity

The transection, lesion, and stimulation studies all point to the same regions of the pons in the control of the state of REM sleep as a whole, and smaller subregions in the control of its individual components. The pons contains a complex variety of cells differing in their neurotransmitter, receptors, and axonal projections. Unit recording techniques allow an analysis of the interplay between these cell groups and their targets to refine further the dissection of REM sleep mechanisms.

Most cells in the *medial* brainstem reticular formation are maximally active in waking, greatly reduce discharge rate in non-REM sleep, and increase discharge rate back to waking levels in REM sleep.[7,8,44-46] Discharge is most regular in non-REM sleep and is relatively irregular in both waking and REM sleep. The similarity of the waking and REM sleep discharge pattern suggests a similar role of these cells in both states. Indeed, most of these cells have been shown to be active in waking in relation to specific lateralized movements of the head and neck, with other cell types linked to equally specific movement of the tongue, face, or limbs. The twitches that are normally visible in facial and limb musculature during REM sleep and the phenomenon of REM sleep without atonia suggest that these cells command motor movement that is blocked by the muscle tone suppression of REM sleep. Lesions of these cells have little or no effect on REM sleep duration or periodicity, but do dramatically prevent movements of the head and neck.[47]

Monoamine-containing cells have a very different discharge profile. Most, if not all noradrenergic[48,49] and serotonergic[50] cells of the midbrain and pontine brainstem and histaminergic[51] cells of the posterior hypothalamus are continuously active during waking, decrease their activity during non-REM sleep, and further reduce or cease activity during REM sleep (Fig. 10–6). As was pointed out earlier, these cell groups are not critical for REM sleep generation, but it is likely that they modulate REM sleep parameters. As is discussed later, the cessation of activity in these cells may be important in the function of REM sleep. The cessation of discharge in monoaminergic cells during REM sleep has been linked to release of GABA onto these cells,[52-55] presumably by REM sleep–active GABAergic brainstem neurons.[56] Administration of a GABA agonist to the raphe cell group increases REM sleep duration,[53] demonstrating a modulatory role for this cell group in REM sleep control.

In contrast to norepinephrine, serotonin, and histamine cell groups, most dopaminergic neurons do not appear to alter their discharge rate across the sleep cycle.[57,58]

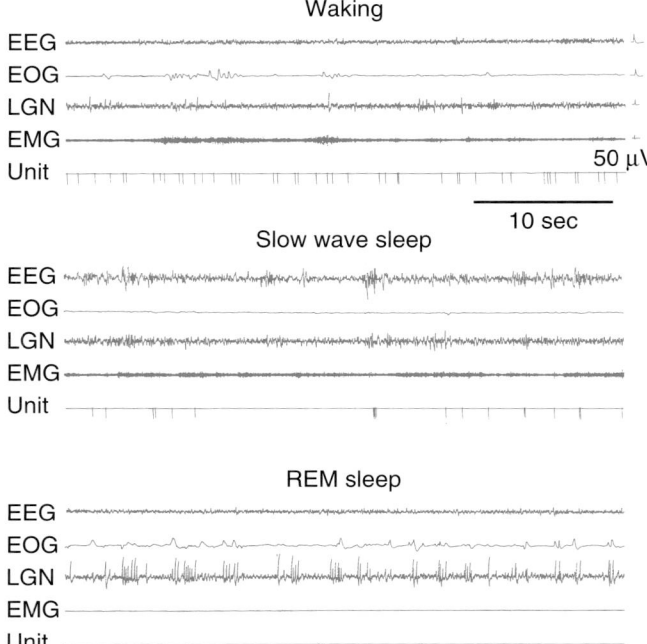

Figure 10–6. Activity of an "REM sleep-off" cell recorded in the locus coeruleus. (From Siegel JM: REM sleep control mechanisms: Evidence from lesion and unit recording studies. In Mayes A [ed]: Sleep Mechanisms and Functions. New York, Van Nostrand Reinhold, 1983, with permission.)

Cholinergic cell groups have an important role in REM sleep control. As was pointed out previously, microinjection of cholinergic agonists into the pons triggers long REM sleep periods. Microdialysis studies show that pontine acetylcholine release is greatly increased during REM sleep compared with either non-REM sleep or waking.[59] Recordings of neuronal activity in the cholinergic cell population demonstrate the substrates of this release. Certain cholinergic cells are maximally active in REM sleep (REM-on cells). Others are active in both waking and REM sleep, as is the case with most reticular cells.[60] Presumably the REM-on cholinergic cells project to the acetylcholine-responsive region in the subcoeruleus area.[61] Other cholinergic cells in lateral pontine regions discharge in bursts before each ipsilateral PGO wave.[62,63] These cells may therefore participate in the triggering of these waves. We know from other studies that PGO waves are tonically inhibited in waking by serotonin input.[64,65] Therefore, it is likely that certain groups of cholinergic cells receive direct or perhaps indirect serotonergic inhibition in waking and that the decrease of this inhibition in non-REM sleep and REM sleep facilitates PGO wave and REM sleep generation.

CONTROL OF MUSCLE TONE

The normal suppression of muscle tone during sleep in general and REM sleep in particular and the failure of the muscle tone suppression system in certain disorders are both of immense clinical importance. During REM sleep, central motor systems are highly active, whereas motoneurons are hyperpolarized (see Chapter 12). The suppression of tone in the tongue and laryngeal muscles is a major contributing factor in sleep apnea (see Chapter 82).

The normal role of the REM sleep atonia system is most dramatically apparent in REM sleep without atonia in animals and in the REM sleep behavior disorder (RBD) in humans (see Chapter 75). However, despite the similarity of RBD to REM sleep without atonia, humans with RBD do not usually have lesions in the areas implicated in feline REM sleep without atonia. One clue to the locus of damage in humans is the progression of RBD to Parkinson's disease in a high percentage of patients. The link between Parkinson's and degenerative changes in the ventral midbrain suggests that the locus for RBD may also be in this region. We have found that lesions in ventral midbrain can release motor activity during REM sleep,[66] consistent with this hypothesis.

Recent work has identified the mechanisms operating at the motoneuronal level to produce muscle tone suppression in REM sleep. Early work using intracellular recording and microiontophoresis had shown that motoneuron hyperpolarization during REM sleep was accompanied by the release of glycine onto motoneurons (see Chapter 12). In recent work it has been shown that both GABA and glycine are released onto motoneurons during atonia.[67] This release occurs in ventral horn motoneurons as well as in hypoglossal motoneurons. In related work it has been shown that norepinephrine and serotonin release onto motoneurons is decreased during atonia.[68] Because these monoamines are known to excite motoneurons and GABA and glycine are known to inhibit them, we can see the coordinated activity of these cell groups as combining disfacilitation and inhibition to produce motoneuron hyperpolarization and hence atonia in REM sleep.

The inhibitory and facilitatory systems are strongly and reciprocally linked. Electrical stimulation of the PIA produces muscle tone suppression. Even though this region is within a few millimeters of the noradrenergic locus coeruleus, stimulation in the PIA that suppresses muscle tone always causes a *cessation* of activity in the noradrenergic neurons of the locus coeruleus[69] and other facilitatory cell groups.[69] Cells that are maximally active in REM sleep (REM-on cells) are present in the PIA and also in the region of the medial medulla that receives PIA projections (Fig. 10–7).

The release of GABA and glycine during REM sleep atonia is most likely mediated by a pathway from the PIA to the medial medulla.[70,71] The pontine region triggering this release not only is sensitive to acetylcholine, but responds to glutamate[72,73] (Fig. 10–8). The medullary region with descending projections to motoneurons can be subdivided into a rostral portion responding to glutamate and a caudal portion responding to acetylcholine.[74,75] The medullary interaction with pontine structures is critical for muscle tone suppression because inactivation of pontine regions greatly reduces the suppressive effects of medullary stimulation on muscle tone.[76,77] This ascending pathway from medulla to pons may mediate the inhibition of the locus coeruleus during atonia and may also help recruit other active inhibitory mechanisms. Thus, damage anywhere in the medial pontomedullary region can block muscle atonia by interrupting ascending and descending portions of the pontomedullary inhibitory system.[78]

Recent work suggests that inhibition of motor output is accompanied by a neurochemically similar inhibition of sensory relays during REM sleep.[79] Such sensory inhibition may be important in preserving sleep in the face of sensory activation produced by twitches breaking through the motor inhibition of REM sleep.

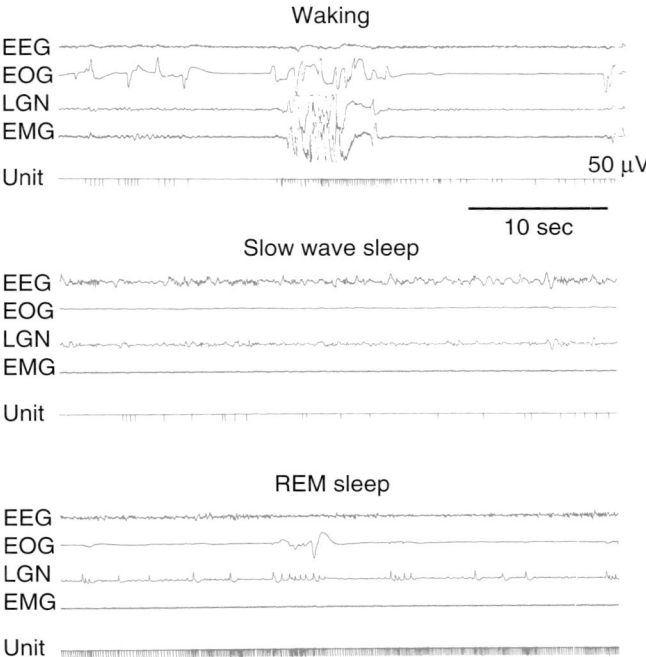

Figure 10–7. Activity of medullary "REM sleep-on" cell. Note the tonic activity during REM sleep. In waking, activity is usually absent even during vigorous movement. However, some activity is seen during movements involving head lowering and postural relaxation. (From Siegel JM, Wheeler RL, McGinty DJ: Activity of medullary reticular formation neurons in the unrestrained cat during waking and sleep. Brain Res 1979;179:49-60, with permission.)

Figure 10–9 illustrates some of the anatomic and neurochemical substrates of the brainstem generation of REM sleep.

NARCOLEPSY

Narcolepsy has long been characterized as a disease of the REM sleep mechanism. Narcoleptics often have REM sleep within 5 minutes of sleep onset, in contrast to normal individuals, who rarely show such "sleep-onset REM sleep." Most narcoleptics experience cataplexy, a sudden loss of muscle tone with the same reflex suppression that is seen in REM sleep. High-amplitude theta activity in the hippocampus, characteristic of REM sleep, is also present in cataplexy.[80] Further evidence for links between narcolepsy and REM sleep comes from studies of neuronal activity during cataplexy. Many of the same cell populations in the pons and medulla that are tonically active only during REM sleep in normal individuals, become active during cataplexy in narcoleptics.[9,81] Likewise, cells in the locus coeruleus, which cease discharge only in REM sleep in normal animals, invariably cease discharge in cataplexy.[82]

However, just as cataplexy differs behaviorally from REM sleep in its maintenance of consciousness, not all neuronal aspects of REM sleep are present during cataplexy. As was explained previously, in the normal animal, noradrenergic, serotonergic, and histaminergic cells are all tonically active in waking, reduce discharge in non-REM sleep, and cease discharge in REM sleep. However, unlike noradrenergic cells, serotonergic cells do not cease discharge during cataplexy,[80,83]

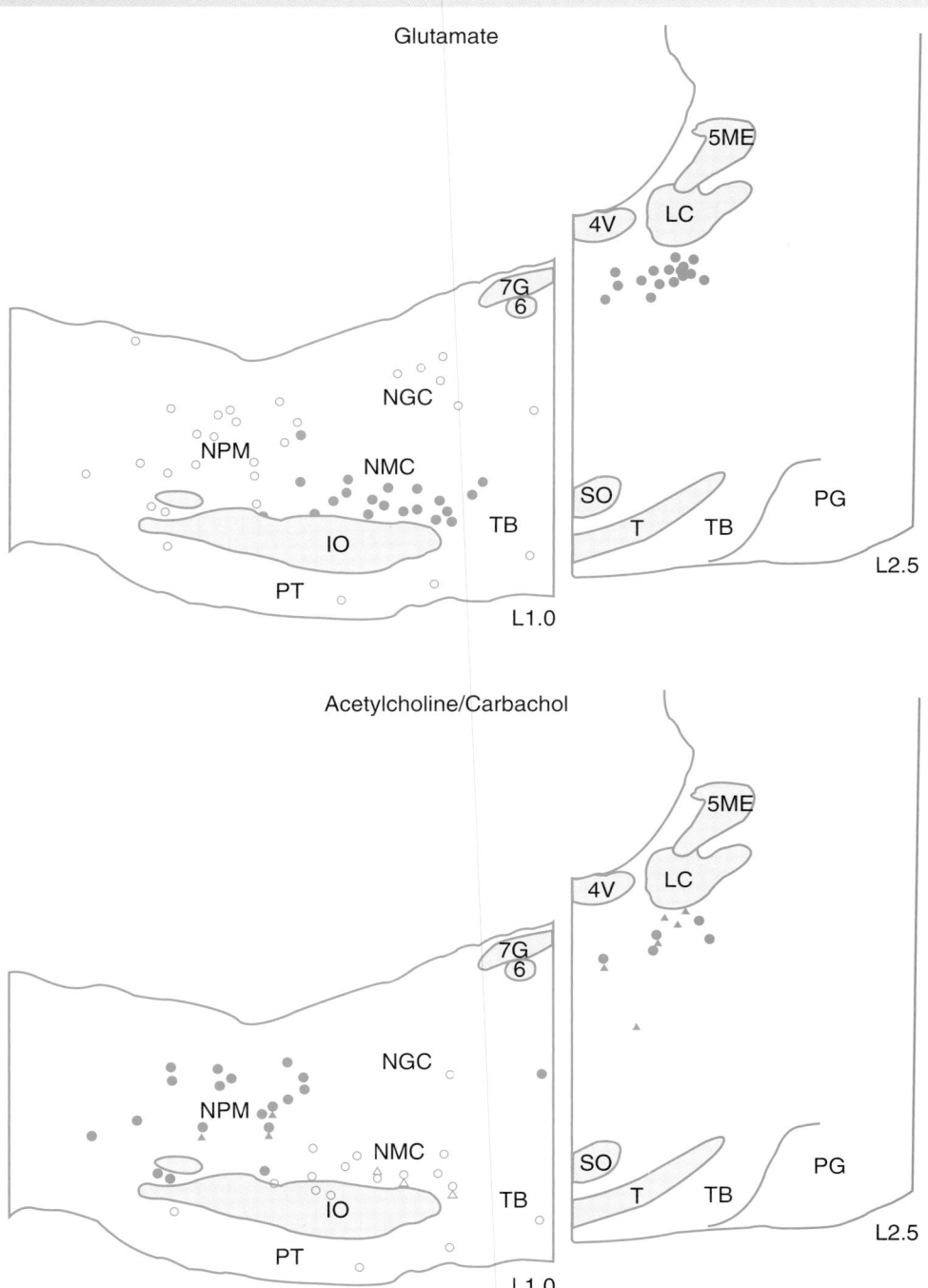

Glutamate

Acetylcholine/Carbachol

Figure 10–8. Sagittal map of pontomedullary inhibitory areas. Electrical stimulation produced atonia at all the points mapped. All electrically defined inhibitory sites were microinjected with glutamate or cholinergic agonists. *Filled symbols* represent points at which microinjections decreased muscle tone (to less than 30% of baseline values or to complete atonia). *Open circles* indicate points at which injections increased or produced no change in baseline values. Glutamate injections are shown at the top, acetylcholine (ACh) and carbachol (Carb) injections at the bottom. At the bottom, *circles* and *triangles* represent ACh and Carb injections, respectively. 4V, fourth ventricle; 5ME, mesencephalic trigeminal tract; 6, abducens nucleus; 7G, genu of the facial nerve; IO, inferior olivary nucleus; LC, locus coeruleus nucleus; NGC, nucleus gigantocellularis; NMC, nucleus magnocellularis; NPM, nucleus paramedianus; PG, pontine gray; PT, pyramidal tract; SO, superior olivary nucleus; T, nucleus of the trapezoid body; TB, trapezoid body. (From Lai YY, Siegel JM: Medullary regions mediating atonia. J Neurosci 1988;8: 4790-4796, with permission.)

only reducing discharge to quiet waking levels. Histaminergic cells actually increase discharge in cataplexy relative to quiet waking levels.[80] These findings allow us to identify some of the cellular substrates of cataplexy. Medullary inhibition and noradrenergic disfacilitation are linked to cataplexy's loss of muscle tone. In contrast, the maintained activity of histamine neurons is a likely substrate for the maintenance of consciousness during cataplexy that distinguishes cataplexy from REM sleep. Thus, the study of neuronal activity in the narcoleptic animal provides an insight into both narcolepsy and the normal role of these cell groups across the sleep cycle.

In 2001, it was discovered that most human narcolepsy was caused by a loss of hypothalamic cells containing the peptide hypocretin (Hcrt, also called orexin).[84,85] It was found that administration of the peptide to genetically narcoleptic dogs reversed symptoms of the disorder,[86] suggesting that similar treatment could be uniquely effective for human narcolepsy.

In further work in normal animals, it was determined that Hcrt was released maximally during motor activity,[87] leading to the hypothesis that release of Hcrt facilitates motor activity during emotionally charged activities of the sort that trigger cataplexy in narcoleptics.[88,89] Even normal individuals

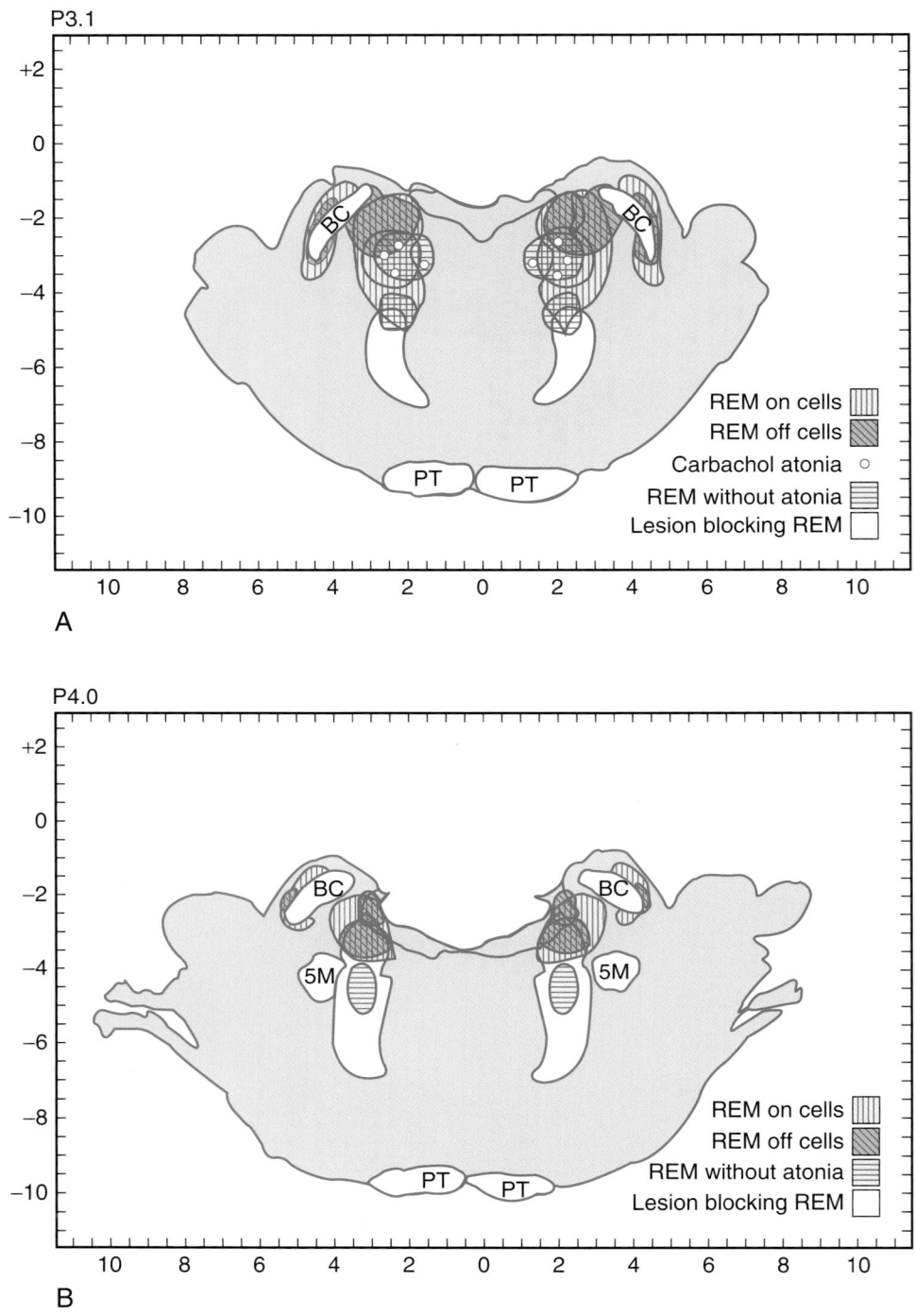

Figure 10–9. A, B, Anatomic relation of "REM sleep-on" and "REM sleep-off" cells, carbachol-induced atonia sites, lesions blocking atonia but not preventing REM sleep, and lesions completely blocking REM sleep. BC, brachium conjuctivum; PT, pyramidal tract; 5M, motor nucleus of the trigeminal nerve. Units are stereotaxic coordinates in mm. (From Siegel JM, Rogawski MA: A function for REM sleep: Regulation of noradrenergic receptor sensitivity. Brain Res 1988;13: 213-233, with permission.)

experience weakness at these times, seen in the "doubling over" that often accompanies laughter or the weakness that can result from sudden-onset, strong emotions. In the absence of the Hcrt-mediated motor facilitation, muscle tone is lost at these times. Hcrt cells also send ascending projections to cortical and basal forebrain regions. In the absence of Hcrt-mediated

facilitation of forebrain arousal centers, waking periods are truncated, resulting in the sleepiness of narcolepsy.[88]

Hcrt appears to act largely by modulating the release of amino acid neurotransmitters.[90] Systemic injection of Hcrt causes a release of glutamate in certain Hcrt-innervated regions, producing a potent postsynaptic excitation.[91,92] In other regions it

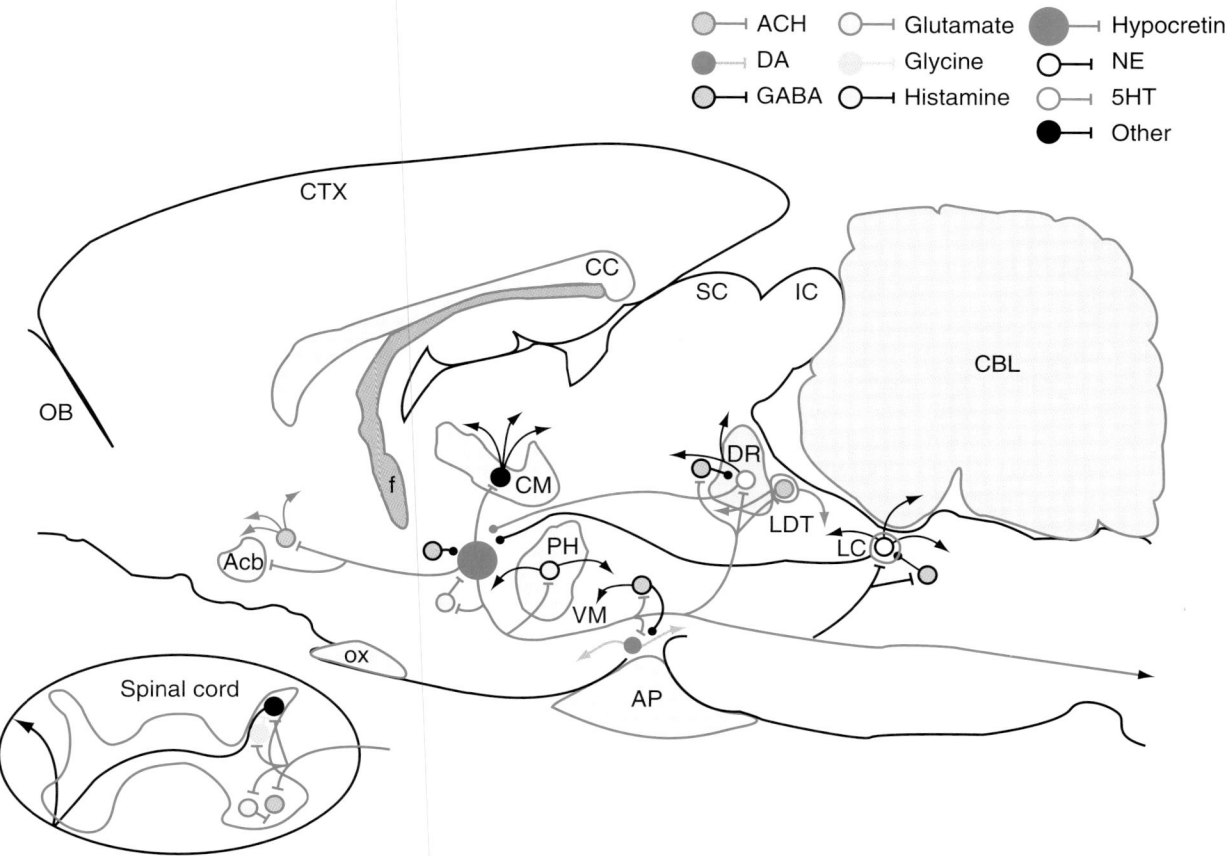

Figure 10–10. Major identified synaptic interactions of hypocretin (Hcrt) neurons. Lines terminated by *perpendicular lines* denote excitation; *circular terminations* indicate inhibition. Arrows indicate direction of projections. CC, corpus callosum; CTX, cortex; 5HT, serotonin; Acb, nucleus accumbens; ACH, acetylcholine; AP, anterior pituitary; CBL, cerebellum; CM, centromedian nucleus of the thalamus; DA, dopamine; DR, dorsal raphe; f, fornix; IC, inferior colliculus; LC, locus coeruleus; LDT, laterodorsal tegmental and pedunculopontine; NE, norepinephrine; OB, olfactory bulb; ox, optic chiasm; PH, posterior hypothalamus; SC, superior colliculus; VM, ventral midbrain. (From color figure in Siegel JM, Ann Rev Psych 2004;55:125-148, with permission.)

facilitates GABA release, producing postsynaptic inhibition.[87,93] The loss of these competing inhibitory and facilitatory influences in narcolepsy appears to leave brain motor regulatory and arousal systems less stable than the tightly regulated balance that can be maintained in the presence of Hcrt (Fig. 10–10). According to this hypothesis, this loss of stability is the underlying cause of narcolepsy, with the result being inappropriate loss of muscle tone in waking and inappropriate increases of muscle tone during sleep, resulting in a striking *increased* incidence of REM behavior disorders in narcoleptics (see Chapter 75). In the same manner, although a principal symptom of narcolepsy is intrusions of sleep into the waking period, narcoleptics sleep poorly at night with frequent awakenings.[94-96] In other words, narcoleptics are not simply weaker and sleepier than normal individuals. Rather, their muscle tone and sleep–waking state regulation is less stable than that in normal subjects as a result of the loss of Hcrt function.

THE FUNCTION OF REM SLEEP

Great progress has been made in localizing the mechanisms that generate REM sleep. As described previously, we know many of the key neurotransmitters and neurons involved. The recent discovery of the role of Hcrt in narcolepsy serves as a reminder that there may still be key cell groups that need to be identified before we can gain fundamental insights into the generation mechanism and functions of REM sleep. Yet despite this caveat, we already understand a substantial amount about what goes on in the brain during REM sleep.

However, the mystery exposed by the discovery of REM sleep remains. We do not know the biologic need that initiates REM sleep. We do not know the source or the REM sleep "debt" that accumulates during REM sleep deprivation.[97]

What is clear is that increased brain activity in REM sleep consumes considerable amounts of metabolic energy. The intense activity shown by most brain neurons, similar to or even more intense than that seen during waking, extracts a price in terms of energy consumption and "wear and tear" on the brain. It is unlikely that such a state would have produced a darwinian advantage and remained so ubiquitous among mammals if it did not have benefits compensating for its obvious costs. But what might these benefits be?

One idea that has gained a great deal of publicity recently is that REM sleep has an important role in memory consolidation. However, the evidence for this is poor. A recent review[98] concludes that a major role for sleep in memory consolidation is unproven and unlikely. Although early animal work suggested that REM sleep deprivation interfered with learning, subsequent studies showed that it was the stress of the REM sleep deprivation procedure rather than the REM sleep loss itself that was critical. A leading proponent of a sleep and memory consolidation relationship has recently concluded that sleep has no role in the consolidation of declarative memory,[99] which would exclude a role for sleep in rote memory, language memory, and conceptual memory, leaving only the possibility of a role in procedural memory, the sort of memory required for learning to ride a bicycle or play a musical instrument. However, studies supporting a role for sleep in the consolidation of human procedural learning have made contradictory claims about similar learning tasks, with some concluding that REM but not non-REM sleep is important, others stating just the reverse, yet others claiming that both sleep states are essential.[98] Millions of humans have taken monoamine oxidase inhibitors or tricyclic antidepressants, often for 10 to 20 years. These drugs profoundly depress or in many cases completely eliminate all detectable aspects of REM sleep. However, there is not a single report of memory deficits attributable to such treatment. Likewise, well-studied individuals with permanent loss of REM sleep resulting from pontine damage show normal learning abilities; the best-studied such individual completed law school after his injury and was last reported to be the puzzle editor of his city newspaper.[100]

Another idea that has been repeatedly suggested is that REM sleep serves to stimulate the brain.[26,101,102] According to this theory, the inactivity of non-REM sleep causes metabolic processes to slow down to an extent that the animal would be unable to respond to a predator or capture prey if one became available. This would leave mammals functioning like reptiles, with slow response after periods of inactivity. This hypothesis explains the appearance of REM sleep after non-REM sleep under most conditions. It also explains the well-documented increased proportion of sleep time in REM sleep as morning approaches in humans. Humans are more alert when aroused from REM sleep than non-REM sleep, consistent with this idea. The very low amounts or absence of REM sleep in dolphins, whose brainstem is continuously active and which never have bilateral EEG synchrony, can be explained by this hypothesis. If one hemisphere is always active, there is no need for the periodic stimulation of REM sleep to maintain the ability to respond rapidly. However, the brain stimulation hypothesis of REM sleep function does not explain why waking does not substitute for REM sleep in terrestrial mammals. REM sleep–deprived individuals have an REM sleep rebound even if they are kept in an active waking state for extended periods.

One phenomenon that may explain REM sleep rebound is the cessation of activity of histamine, norepinephrine, and serotonin neurons during REM sleep. This cessation does not occur during waking and therefore waking would not be expected to substitute for this aspect of REM sleep.[103] Thus, REM sleep rebound may be due to an accumulation of a need to inactivate these aminergic cell groups. Several cellular processes might benefit from the cessation of activity in aminergic cells. Synthesis of these monoamines and their receptors might be facilitated during this period of reduced release. The receptors for these substances might be resensitized in the absence of their agonist. The metabolic pathways involved in the reuptake and inactivation of these transmitters might also

benefit from periods of inactivity. Some, but not all studies have supported this hypothesis.[104-108]

Investigation at the cellular level may lead to an "inside out" explanation of REM sleep function, deriving a functional explanation from a better understanding of the neuronal basis of REM sleep control.

Further relevant literature can be found at http://www.npi.ucla.edu/sleepresearch.

Clinical Pearl

The loss of hypocretin (orexin) neurons is responsible for most human narcolepsy. It is thought that this cell loss may be the result of an immune system attack on these neurons, but convincing evidence for this is lacking. Administration of hypocretin is a promising future avenue for the treatment of narcolepsy. Because the hypocretin system has potent effects on arousal systems, including the norepinephrine, serotonin, acetylcholine, and histamine systems, manipulation of the hypocretin system with agonists and antagonists is likely to be important in further pharmacotherapies for narcolepsy, insomnia, and other sleep disorders.

REFERENCES

1. Aserinsky E, Kleitman N: Regularly occurring periods of eye motility, and concomitant phenomena, during sleep. Science 1953;118:273-274.
2. Dement WC: The occurrence of low voltage, fast, electroencephalogram patterns during behavioral sleep in the cat. Electroencephalogr Clin Neurophysiol 1958;10:291-296.
3. Jouvet M: Recherches sur les structures nerveuses et les mechanismes responsables des differentes phases du sommeil physiologique. Arch Ital Biol 1962;100:125-206.
4. Parmeggiani PL, Zamboni G, Cianci T, Calasso M: Absence of thermoregulatory vasomotor responses during fast wave sleep in cats. Electroencephalogr Clin Neurophysiol 1977;42:372-380.
5. Morrison AR, Bowker RM: The biological significance of PGO spikes in the sleeping cat. Acta Neurobiol Exp 1975;35:821-840.
6. De Gennaro L, Ferrara M: Sleep deprivation and phasic activity of REM sleep: Independence of middle-ear muscle activity from rapid eye movements. Sleep 2000;23:81-85.
7. Siegel JM, Tomaszewski KS: Behavioral organization of reticular formation: Studies in the unrestrained cat: I. Cells related to axial, limb, eye, and other movements. J Neurophysiol 1983;50:696-716.
8. Siegel JM, Tomaszewski KS, Wheeler RL: Behavioral organization of reticular formation: Studies in the unrestrained cat: II. Cells related to facial movements. J Neurophysiol 1983;50:717-723.
9. Siegel JM, Nienhuis R, Fahringer HM, et al: Activity of medial mesopontine units during cataplexy and sleep-waking states in the narcoleptic dog. J Neurosci 1992;12:1640-1646.
10. Amlaner CJ, Ball NJ: Avian sleep. In Kryger MH, Roth T, Dement WC (eds): Principles and Practice of Sleep Medicine. Philadelphia, WB Saunders, 1994, pp 81-94.
11. Allison T, Van Twyver H, Goff WR: Electrophysiological studies of the echidna, *Tachyglossus aculeatus*: I. Waking and sleep. Arch Ital Biol 1972;110:145-184.
12. Siegel JM, Manger P, Nienhuis R, et al: The echidna *Tachyglossus aculeatus* combines REM and nonREM aspects in a single sleep state: Implications for the evolution of sleep. J Neurosci 1996;16:3500-3506.

13. Nicol SC, Andersen NA, Phillips NH, Berger RJ: The echidna manifests typical characteristics of rapid eye movement sleep. Neurosci Lett 2000;283:49-52.

14. Siegel JM, Manger PR, Nienhuis R, et al: Sleep in the platypus. Neuroscience 1999;91:391-400.

15. Manger PR, Fahringer HM, Pettigrew JD, Siegel JM: The distribution and morphological characteristics of catecholaminergic cells in the brain of monotremes as revealed by tyrosine hydroxylase immunohistochemistry. Brain Behav Evol 2003;60:298-314.

16. Manger PR, Fahringer HM, Pettigrew JD, Siegel JM: The distribution and morphological characteristics of serotonergic cells in the brain of monotremes. Brain Behav Evol 2003;60:315-332.

17. Manger PR, Fahringer HM, Pettigrew JD, Siegel JM: The distribution and morphological characteristics of cholinergic cells in the brain of monotremes as revealed by ChAT immunohistochemistry. Brain Behav Evol 2003;60:275-297.

18. Lyamin OI, Mukhametov LM, Siegel JM, et al: Unihemispheric slow wave sleep and the state of the eyes in a white whale. Behav Brain Res 2002;129:125-129.

19. Oleksenko AI, Mukhametov LM, Polykova IG, et al: Unihemispheric sleep deprivation in bottlenose dolphins. J Sleep Res 1992;1:40-44.

20. Mukhametov LM, Lyamin OI, Polyakova IG: Interhemispheric asynchrony of the sleep EEG in northern fur seals. Experientia 1985;41(8):1034-1035.

21. Siegel JM: The evolution of REM sleep. In Lydic R, Baghdoyan HA (eds): Handbook of Behavioral State Control. Boca Raton, Fla, CRC Press, 1999, pp 87-100.

22. Eiland MM, Lyamin OI, Siegel JM: State-related discharge of neurons in the brainstem of freely moving box turtles, *Terrapene carolina major*. Arch Ital Biol 2001;139:23-36.

23. Magoun HW: Bulbar inhibition and facilitation of motor activity. Science 1944;100:549-550.

24. Siegel JM, McGinty DJ: Pontine reticular formation neurons and motor activity. Science 1978;199:207-208.

25. Bard P, Macht MB: The behavior of chronically decerebrate cats. In Wolstenholme GEW, O'Conner CMO (eds): Neurological Basis of Behavior. London, Churchill, 1958, pp 55-75.

26. Arnulf I, Sastre JP, Buda C, Jouvet M: Hyperoxia increases paradoxical sleep rhythm in the pontine cat. Brain Res 1998;807:160-166.

27. Adey WR, Bors E, Porter RW: EEG sleep patterns after high cervical lesions in man. Arch Neurol 1968;19:377-383.

28. Siegel JM, Tomaszewski KS, Nienhuis R: Behavioral states in the chronic medullary and mid-pontine cat. Electroencephalogr Clin Neurophysiol 1986;63:274-288.

29. Siegel JM, Nienhuis R, Tomaszewski KS: REM sleep signs rostral to chronic transections at the pontomedullary junction. Neurosci Lett 1984;45:241-246.

30. Siegel JM: Pontomedullary interactions in the generation of REM sleep. In McGinty DJ, Drucker-Colin R, Morrison A, Parmeggiani PL (eds): Brain Mechanisms of Sleep. New York, Raven Press, 1985, pp 157-174.

31. Matsuzaki M: Differential effects of sodium butyrate and physostigmine upon the activities of para-sleep in acute brain stem preparations. Brain Res 1969;13:247-265.

32. Gadea-Ciria M: Tele-encephalic versus cerebellar control upon ponto-geniculo-occipital waves during paradoxical sleep in the cat. Experientia 1976;32:889-890.

33. Carli G, Zanchetti A: A study of pontine lesions suppressing deep sleep in the cat. Arch Ital Biol 1965;103:725-750.

34. Jones BE, Harper ST, Halaris AE: Effects of locus coeruleus lesions upon cerebral monoamine content, sleep wakefulness states and the response to amphetamine in the cat. Brain Res 1977;124:473-496.

35. Juvancz P: The effect of raphe lesion on sleep in the rat. Brain Res 1980;194:371-376.

36. Sastre JP, Sakai K, Jouvet M: Are the gigantocellular tegmental field neurons responsible for paradoxical sleep? Brain Res 1981;229:147-161.

37. Webster HH, Jones BE: Neurotoxic lesions of the dorsolateral pontomesencephalic tegmentum-cholinergic cell area in the cat: II. Effects upon sleep-waking states. Brain Res 1988;458:285-302.

38. Shouse MN, Siegel JM: Pontine regulation of REM sleep components in cats: Integrity of the pedunculopontine tegmentum (PPT) is important for phasic events but unnecessary for atonia during REM sleep. Brain Res 1992;571:50-63.

39. Schenkel E, Siegel JM: REM sleep without atonia after lesions of the medial medulla. Neurosci Lett 1989;98:159-165.

40. Hendricks JC, Morrison AR, Mann GL: Different behaviors during paradoxical sleep without atonia depend on pontine lesion site. Brain Res 1982;239:81-105.

41. George R, Haslett WL, Jenden DJ: A cholinergic mechanism in the brainstem reticular formation: Induction of paradoxical sleep. Int J Neuropharmacol 1964;3:541-552.

42. Vanni-Mercier G, Sakai K, Lin JS, Jouvet M: Mapping of cholinoceptive brainstem structures responsible for the generation of paradoxical sleep in the cat. Arch Ital Biol 1989;127:133-164.

43. Katayama Y, DeWitt DS, Becker DP, Hayes RL: Behavioral evidence for cholinoceptive pontine inhibitory area: Descending control of spinal motor output and sensory input. Brain Res 1984;296:241-262.

44. Siegel JM, McGinty DJ, Breedlove SM: Sleep and waking activity of pontine gigantocellular field neurons. Exp Neurol 1977;56:553-573.

45. Siegel JM: Behavioral functions of the reticular formation. Brain Res Rev 1979;1:69-105.

46. Siegel JM, Wheeler RL, McGinty DJ: Activity of medullary reticular formation neurons in the unrestrained cat during waking and sleep. Brain Res 1979;179:49-60.

47. Suzuki SS, Siegel JM, Wu MF: Role of pontomedullary reticular formation neurons in horizontal head movements: An ibotenic acid lesion study in the cat. Brain Res 1989;484:78-93.

48. Hobson JA, McCarley RW, Wyzinski PW: Sleep cycle oscillation: Reciprocal discharge by two brainstem neuronal groups. Science 1975;189:55-58.

49. Fenik V, Marchenko V, Janssen P, et al: A5 cells are silenced when REM sleep-like signs are elicited by pontine carbachol. J Appl Physiol 2002;93:1448-1456.

50. McGinty DJ, Harper RM: Dorsal raphe neurons: Depression of firing during sleep in the cat. Brain Res 1976;101:569-575.

51. Steininger TL, Alam MN, Gong H, et al: Sleep-waking discharge of neurons in the posterior lateral hypothalamus of the albino rat. Brain Res 1999;840:138-147.

52. Nitz D, Siegel JM: GABA release in the posterior hypothalamus of the cat as a function of sleep/wake state. Am J Physiol 1996;40:R1707-R1712.

53. Nitz D, Siegel JM: GABA release in the dorsal raphe nucleus: role in the control of REM sleep. Am J Physiol 1997;273:R451-R455.

54. Nitz D, Siegel JM: GABA release in the cat locus coeruleus as a function of the sleep/wake state. Neuroscience 1997;78:795-801.

55. Gervasoni D, Darracq L, Fort P, et al: Electrophysiological evidence that noradrenergic neurons of the rat locus coeruleus are tonically inhibited by GABA during sleep. Eur J Neurosci 1998;10:964-970.

56. Maloney K, Mainville L, Jones B: Differential c-Fos expression in cholinergic, monoaminergic, and GABAergic cell groups of the pontomesencephalic tegmentum after paradoxical sleep deprivation and recovery. J Neurosci 1999;19:3057-3072.

57. Miller JD, Farber J, Gatz P, et al: Activity of mesencephalic dopamine and non-dopamine neurons across stages of sleep and waking in the rat. Brain Res 1983;273:133-141.

58. Shouse MN, Staba RJ, Saquib SF, Farber PR: Monoamines and sleep: Microdialysis findings in pons and amygdala. Brain Res 2000;860:181-189.

59. Kodama T, Takahashi T, Honda Y: Enhancement of acetylcholine release during paradoxical sleep in the dorsal tegmental field of the cat brain stem. Neurosci Lett 1990;114:277-282.

60. Steriade M, Datta S, Pare D, et al: Neuronal activities in brain-stem cholinergic nuclei related to tonic activation processes in thalamocortical systems. J Neurosci 1990;10:2541-2559.

61. Greene RW, Gerber U, McCarley RW: Cholinergic activation of medial pontine reticular formation neurons in vitro. Brain Res 1989;476:154-159.

62. Datta S, Siwek DF: Single cell activity patterns of pedunculo-pontine tegmentum neurons across the sleep-wake cycle in the freely moving rats. J Neurosci Res 2002;70:611-621.

63. Steriade M, Pare D, Datta S, et al: Different cellular types in mesopontine cholinergic nuclei related to ponto-geniculo-occipital waves. J Neurosci 1990;10:2560-2579.

64. Ruch-Monachon MA, Jaffre M, Haefely W: Drugs and PGO waves in the lateral geniculate body of the curarized cat: IV. The effects of acetylcholine, GABA and benzodiazepines on PGO wave activity. Arch Int Pharmacodyn Ther 1976;219: 308-325.

65. Wu MF, Siegel JM: Facilitation of the acoustic startle reflex by ponto-geniculo-occipital waves: Effects of PCPA. Brain Res 1990;532:237-241.

66. Lai YY, Shalita T, Hajnik T, et al: Neurotoxic N-methyl-D-aspartate lesion of the ventral midbrain and mesopontine junction alters sleep-wake organization. Neuroscience 1999;90:469-483.

67. Kodama T, Lai YY, Siegel JM: Changes in inhibitory amino acid release linked to pontine-induced atonia: An in vivo microdialysis study. J Neurosci 2003;23:1548-1554.

68. Lai YY, Kodama T, Siegel JM: Changes in monoamine release in the ventral horn and hypoglossal nucleus linked to pontine inhibition of muscle tone: an in vivo microdialysis study. J Neurosci 2001;21:7384-7391.

69. Mileykovskiy BY, Kiyashchenko LI, Siegel JM: Cessation of activity in red nucleus neurons during stimulation of the medial medulla in decerebrate rats. J Physiol (Lond) 2002;545:997-1006.

70. Lai YY, Clements JR, Wu XY, et al: Brainstem projections to the ventromedial medulla in cat: retrograde transport horseradish peroxidase and immunohistochemical studies. J Comp Neurol 1999;408:419-436.

71. Lai YY, Clements J, Siegel J: Glutamatergic and cholinergic projections to the pontine inhibitory area identified with horse-radish peroxidase retrograde transport and immunohisto-chemistry. J Comp Neurol 1993;336:321-330.

72. Lai YY, Siegel JM: Muscle tone suppression and stepping produced by stimulation of midbrain and rostral pontine reticular formation. J Neurosci 1990;10:2727-2738.

73. Lai YY, Siegel JM: Ponto-medullary glutamate receptors mediating locomotion and muscle tone suppression. J Neurosci 1991;11: 2931-2937.

74. Lai YY, Siegel JM: Medullary regions mediating atonia. J Neurosci 1988;8:4790-4796.

75. Kodama T, Lai YY, Siegel JM: Enhancement of acetyl-choline release during REM sleep in the caudomedial medulla as measured by in vivo microdialysis. Brain Res 1992;580: 348-350.

76. Kohyama J, Lai YY, Siegel JM: Inactivation of the pons blocks medullary-induced muscle tone suppression in the decerebrate cat. Sleep 1998;21:695-699.

77. Siegel JM, Nienhuis R, Tomaszewski KS: Rostral brainstem contributes to medullary inhibition of muscle tone. Brain Res 1983;268:344-348.

78. Kohyama J, Lai YY, Siegel JM: Reticulospinal systems mediate atonia with short and long latencies. J Neurophysiol 1998;80: 1839-1851.

79. Taepavarapruk N, Taepavarapruk P, John J, et al: State-dependent release of glycine in Clarke's column of the upper lumbar spinal cord. Sleep 2003;26:A11-A12.

80. John J, Wu M-F, Boehmer LN, Siegel JM: Cataplexy-active neurons in the posterior hypothalamic-histaminergic region: Implications for the role of histamine in sleep and waking behavior. Neuron 2004;42:619-634.

81. Siegel JM, Nienhuis R, Fahringer H, et al: Neuronal activity in narcolepsy: Identification of cataplexy related cells in the medial medulla. Science 1991;262:1315-1318.

82. Wu MF, Gulyani S, Yao E, et al: Locus coeruleus neurons: Cessation of activity during cataplexy. Neuroscience 1999;91: 1389-1399.

83. Wu MF, John J, Boehmer LN, et al: Activity of dorsal raphe cells across the sleep-waking cycle and during cataplexy in narcoleptic dogs. J Physiol (Lond) 2003;554:202-215.

84. Peyron C, Faraco J, Rogers W, et al: A mutation in a case of early onset narcolepsy and a generalized absence of hypocretin peptides in human narcoleptic brains. Nat Med 2000;6: 991-997.

85. Thannickal TC, Moore RY, Nienhuis R, et al: Reduced number of hypocretin neurons in human narcolepsy. Neuron 2000;27: 469-474.

86. John J, Wu MF, Siegel JM: Systemic administration of hypo-cretin-1 reduces cataplexy and normalizes sleep and waking durations in narcoleptic dogs. Sleep Res Online 2000;3:23-28.

87. Kiyashchenko LI, Mileykovskiy BY, Maidment N, et al: Release of hypocretin (orexin) during waking and sleep states. J Neurosci 2002;22:5282-5286.

88. Siegel JM: Hypocretin (orexin): Role in normal behavior and neuropathology. Annu Rev Psychol 2004;55:125-148.

89. Gulyani S, Wu M-F, Nienhuis R, et al: Cataplexy-related neurons in the amygdala of the narcoleptic dog. Neuroscience 2002;112:355-365.

90. van den Pol AN, Gao XB, Obrietan K, et al: Presynaptic and postsynaptic actions and modulation of neuroendocrine neurons by a new hypothalamic peptide, hypocretin/orexin. J Neurosci 1998;18:7962-7971.

91. John J, Wu M-F, Kodama T, Siegel JM: Intravenously adminis-tered hypocretin-1 alters brain amino acid release: An in vivo microdialysis study in rats. J Physiol (Lond) 2003;548:557-562.

92. Peever JH, Lai YY, Siegel JM: Excitatory effects of hypocretin-1 (orexin-A) in the trigeminal motor nucleus are reversed by NMDA antagonism. J Neurophysiol 2003;89:2591-2600.

93. Liu RJ, van den Pol AN, Aghajanian GK: Hypocretins (orexins) regulate serotonin neurons in the dorsal raphe nucleus by excitatory direct and inhibitory indirect actions. J Neurosci 2002;22:9453-9464.

94. Siegel JM: Narcolepsy: A key role for hypocretins (orexins). Cell 1999;98:409-412.

95. Guilleminault C, Anognos A: Narcolepsy. In Kryger MH, Roth T, Dement WC (eds): Principles and Practice of Sleep Medicine, 3rd ed. Philadelphia, WB Saunders, 2000, pp 676-686.

96. Siegel JM: Narcolepsy. Sci Am 2000;282:76-81.

97. Siegel JM: Why we sleep. Sci Am 2003;289:92-97.

98. Siegel JM: The REM sleep-memory consolidation hypothesis. Science 2001;294:1058-1063.

99. Smith C: Sleep states and memory processes in humans: Procedural versus declarative memory systems. Sleep Med Rev 2001;5:491-506.

100. Lavie P, Pratt H, Scharf B, et al: Localized pontine lesion: nearly total absence of REM sleep. Neurology 1984;34:118-120.

101. Ephron HS, Carrington P: Rapid eye movement sleep and cortical homeostasis. Psychol Rev 1966;73:500-526.

102. Wehr TA: A brain-warming function for REM sleep. Neurosci Biobehav Rev 1992;16:379-397.

103. Mallick BN, Siegel JM, Fahringer H: Changes in pontine unit activity with REM sleep deprivation. Brain Res 1989;515:94-98.

104. Tsai L, Bergman B, Perry B, Rechtschaffen A: Effects of chronic total sleep deprivation on central noradrenergic receptors in rat brain. Brain Res 1993;602:221-227.

105. Hipolide DC, Tufik S, Raymond R, Nobrega JN: Heterogeneous effects of rapid eye movement sleep deprivation on binding to alpha- and beta-adrenergic receptor subtypes in rat brain. Neuroscience 1998;86:977-987.

106. Hipolide DC, Wilson AA, Barlow K, et al: Effects of paradoxical sleep deprivation on serotonin transporter (SERT) binding. Sleep 2003;26:A176.

107. Troncone LRP, Braz S, Benedito MAC, Tufik S: REM sleep deprivation induces a decrease in norepinephrine-stimulated 3H-cyclic AMP accumulation in slices from rat brain. Pharmacol Biochem Behav 1986;25:223-225.

108. Siegel JM, Rogawski MA: A function for REM sleep: Regulation of noradrenergic receptor sensitivity. Brain Res Rev 1988;13: 213-233.

11

Basic Mechanisms of Sleep–Wake States

Barbara E. Jones

ABSTRACT

A state of wakefulness is maintained by neurons in the brainstem reticular formation, which in turn excite neurons in the nonspecific thalamocortical projection system along a dorsal pathway and in the posterior hypothalamus and basal forebrain along a ventral pathway. The thalamocortical, hypothalamocortical, and basalocortical projections serve to activate the cerebral cortex in turn in a long-lasting and widespread manner, stimulating fast activity on the electroencephalogram (EEG). The major population of neurons comprising the ascending reticular activating system use glutamate as a neurotransmitter. Other contributing pontomesencephalic tegmental neurons use acetylcholine. In addition, locus coeruleus neurons containing norepinephrine project diffusely from the brainstem to the entire forebrain, including the cerebral cortex, and thereby serve to stimulate and maintain cortical activation. Similarly, posterior hypothalamic neurons containing histamine and others containing orexin (hypocretin) project diffusely to the forebrain and cortex. Whereas the thalamocortical projection system uses glutamate as a neurotransmitter, the basalocortical system primarily uses acetylcholine. In addition to the smaller neurotransmitter molecules, neurons in these activating systems also contain and often colocalize peptides, including substance P, vasoactive intestinal peptide, and neurotensin, that serve to enhance or prolong their excitatory actions.

For sleep, a shift from sympathetic to parasympathetic regulation occurs, and activating systems are dampened. Neurons in the solitary tract nuclei and in the anterior hypothalamus and preoptic area, constituting parasympathetic control centers, are particularly important in these processes. Serotonergic raphe neurons may also facilitate the onset of sleep. Inhibition of activating systems is effected by particular gamma-aminobutyric acid–ergic (GABAergic) neurons, which are selectively active during slow wave sleep. Dampening the brainstem, hypothalamic, and basal forebrain activating systems leads to disfacilitation and hyperpolarization of thalamocortical systems, which consequently shift their mode of operation from fast, tonic discharge to slow, bursting discharge, reflected as spindles and slow wave activity on the EEG. Certain peptides, such as somatostatin and cortistatin, are colocalized with GABA in particular neurons and may enhance and prolong the inhibition of the activating systems in the initiation and maintenance of slow wave sleep.

Since the 1930s, the basic mechanisms of sleep–wake states have been studied by an interdisciplinary approach to elucidate the neurophysiologic, neuroanatomic, and neurochemical substrates. Through this search, what was initially considered to be a unitary process of sleep emerged as a dual process comprising two distinct states, slow wave sleep and paradoxical or rapid eye movement (REM) sleep. Although normally dependent on the prior occurrence of slow wave sleep, paradoxical sleep is generated by different neural systems than slow wave sleep. In the following historical consideration of basic mechanisms, the term *sleep* refers in a general manner to total sleep when discussing research before 1960 and more specifically to slow wave sleep when reviewing more contemporary research. In the treatment of recent research on the basic mechanisms of sleep–wake states, this chapter deals with the particular mechanisms of slow wave sleep, whereas other chapters focus on the specific mechanisms of paradoxical sleep. The chapter is organized in a historical progression with parallel subdivisions according to the different techniques and approaches applied at different periods.

NEURONAL SYSTEMS IMPLICATED IN SLEEP–WAKE STATE GENERATION

The Activating System

Identification of an Activating System in the Brainstem

In the early 1900s, many physiologists, including, notably, Kleitman, believed that wakefulness and consciousness were maintained by ongoing sensory input to the brain.[1] Bremer showed that in the *cerveau isolé,* or cerebrum isolated from the spinal cord and brainstem by a transection at the mesodiencephalic junction, waking signs were absent and sleep signs predominant, as marked by slow waves on the cerebral cortex and miosis of the pupils.[2] The absence of waking parameters was interpreted at the time as being due to the interruption of sensory inputs from the body and head to the forebrain. In the 1940s, Moruzzi and Magoun questioned this interpretation and suggested instead that it was not interruption of the sensory input to the cerebrum that eliminated wakefulness but interruption of input from the brainstem's netlike core of neurons, the reticular formation. Indeed, they showed that electrical stimulation of the reticular formation, and not of the sensory pathways, produced long-lasting and widespread cortical activation marked by the replacement of cortical slow waves with fast activity[3] (Fig. 11–1). Second, they showed that lesions of the reticular formation, but not of the sensory pathways, produced a loss of cortical activation that was replaced by cortical slow waves and behavioral immobility indicative of coma.[4] Lesions with the most marked and enduring effect were located in the oral pontine and midbrain reticular formation and the posterior hypothalamus and subthalamus,

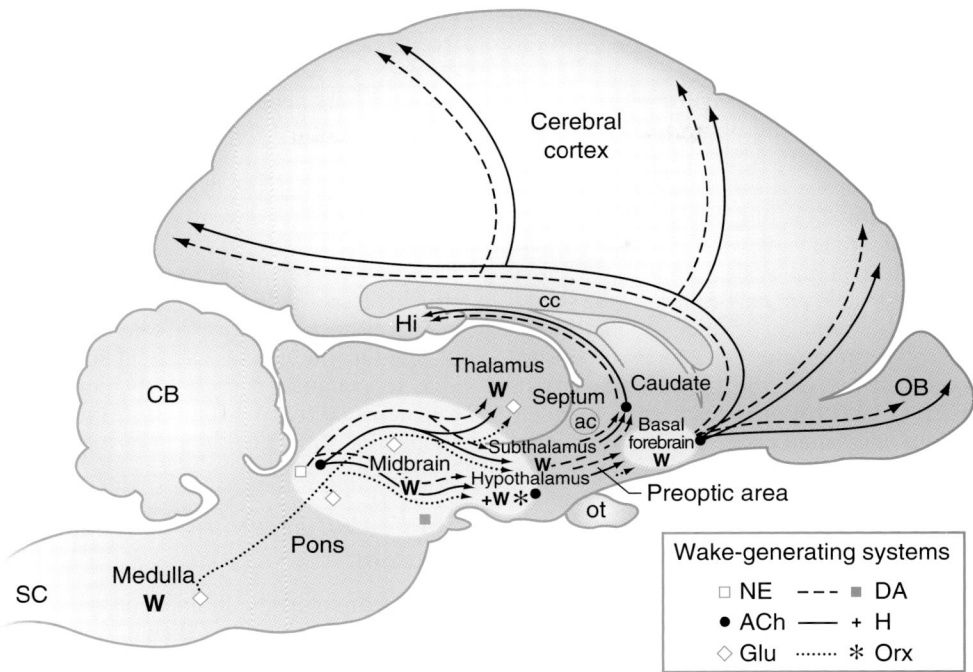

Figure 11–1. Neural systems generating wakefulness. This schematic depiction of a lateral, sagittal section of the cat brain represents neuronal systems implicated in the generation and maintenance of wakefulness. Outlined areas represent the region in the brainstem (oral pontine and midbrain reticular formation) and caudal diencephalon (posterior hypothalamus, subthalamus, and ventral thalamus) and in the basal forebrain where large lesions are associated with a decrease or loss of cortical activation and behavioral activity indicative of wakefulness. Whereas lesions of the central midbrain tegmentum primarily affect cortical activation, lesions of the ventral midbrain tegmentum predominantly alter behavioral arousal. Points marked with "W" (waking) indicate regions where high-frequency electrical stimulation produces cortical activation and arousal, as well as where neurons manifest a higher rate of spontaneous activity during wakefulness than during slow wave sleep (including the medullary, oral pontine, and midbrain reticular formation; the midline and intralaminar thalamic nuclei; the subthalamus and posterior hypothalamus; and the basal forebrain). *Diamond-shaped symbols* represent the neurons of the reticular formation, and *dotted lines* indicate their major ascending projections into the forebrain, which proceed along two major routes. The dorsal route terminates in the nonspecific thalamic nuclei, which in turn project in a widespread manner to the cerebral cortex (not shown). The ventral route passes through and terminates in the subthalamus and posterior hypothalamus and continues into the basal forebrain and septum, where neurons in turn project in a widespread manner to the cerebral cortex and hippocampus. *Squares* represent catecholaminergic neurons of the locus coeruleus (dorsal pons), which contain norepinephrine, and of the substantia nigra and ventral tegmental area (ventral midbrain), which contain dopamine. The noradrenergic neurons are mainly implicated in processes of cortical activation and project (*dashed lines*) directly and diffusely to the cerebral cortex, as well as to the subcortical way stations. The dopaminergic neurons are predominantly implicated in processes of behavioral arousal and responsiveness and project (not shown) heavily into the basal ganglia (including caudate) and frontal cortex. *Solid circles* represent acetylcholine-containing neurons of the brainstem reticular formation (including the laterodorsal and pedunculopontine tegmental nuclei in the dorsal pons and midbrain) and basal forebrain (substantia innominata, diagonal band nuclei, and septum). The brainstem cholinergic neurons project (*solid lines*) to subcortical way stations, including, most importantly, the thalamus, where they excite the nonspecific thalamocortical projection system. The cholinergic basal forebrain neurons project (*solid lines*) in a widespread manner to the cerebral cortex and hippocampus to stimulate cortical activation directly. Contributing in an important manner to the brainstem arousal systems are neurons in the posterior hypothalamus containing histamine and orexin, which project (not shown) diffusely through the brain and directly to the cerebral cortex (not shown). Glutamate-synthesizing neurons (*diamonds*) comprise the projection neurons of the reticular formation, thalamus, and cerebral cortex and are thus critical at all levels in processes of cortical activation and wakefulness. Multiple peptides (not shown), such as substance P, corticotropin-releasing factor, thyrotropin-releasing factor, vasoactive intestinal polypeptide, and neurotensin, may stimulate wakefulness or cortical activation and are often colocalized with one of the other primary neurotransmitters, such as acetylcholine or glutamate. The neuronal systems implicated in the maintenance of wakefulness may be involved in primary processes of sensory transmission and attention, motor response and activity, and orthosympathetic and neuroendocrine (particularly adrenocorticotropic hormone and thyrotropin) responses and regulation, by which they may also enhance and prolong vigilance and arousal. ac, anterior commissure; Ach, acetylcholine; CB, cerebellum; cc, corpus callosum; DA, dopamine; Glu, glutamate; H, histamine; Hi, hippocampus; NE, norepinephrine; OB, olfactory bulb; ot, optic tract; Orx, orexin; SC, spinal cord.

where ascending pathways reach into the forebrain[4,5] (Fig. 11–1). Electrophysiologic and neuroanatomic studies showed that the neurons of the reticular formation receive collateral input from visceral, somatic, and special sensory systems and project in turn by a dorsal pathway to the thalamus and a ventral pathway to the basal forebrain. From thalamus and basal forebrain, impulses are in turn relayed to the cerebral cortex in a widespread manner[5-7] (Fig. 11–1). This system was called the *ascending reticular activating system* and

deemed to be necessary and sufficient for tonic maintenance of cortical activation and behavioral arousal of wakefulness.

In the 1800s, clinical cases of somnolence or coma were found to be due to lesions of the midbrain and posterior diencephalon.[8,9] Based on cases of "encephalitis lethargica" in the early 1900s, von Economo proposed that a "sleep-regulating center" was present in the midbrain and diencephalon and was composed of antagonistic waking and sleeping parts.[10] On the basis of the location of lesions in cases characterized by somnolence, he posited that the waking part was localized in the rostral midbrain tegmentum and caudal diencephalon. Since those observations, many clinical cases of somnolence, stupor, and coma resulting in a loss of consciousness have been reported with lesions in the oral pontine and midbrain tegmentum or posterior hypothalamus and subthalamus.[11,12]

With smaller and more localized lesions in the midbrain and caudal diencephalon, dissociation between the cortical activation and behavioral arousal of wakefulness was subsequently noted in both experimental animal and human cases of somnolence and coma. In animals, lesions of the central midbrain tegmentum were found to produce a deficiency in cortical activation without preventing behavioral responsiveness to sensory stimulation.[13] On the other hand, lesions of the ventral tegmentum and hypothalamus were found to produce a state of behavioral quiescence and unresponsiveness without a loss of cortical activation or alerting. Similar clinical symptoms had previously been noted in humans and were referred to as "akinesia" and "akinetic mutism."[11] It thus appeared that two parallel systems controlled cortical activation and behavioral arousal.

Activating Systems in the Forebrain

Investigation in the 1960s and 1970s indicated that in the chronic course, the brainstem reticular formation was not absolutely necessary for wakefulness because cortical activation could eventually recover given sufficient time after lesions or transections through the brainstem.[14,15] In fact, when lesions were effected gradually in stages, the same total lesions of the midbrain reticular formation that produced long-lasting coma when performed in one operation, were followed by total recovery.[16] This recovery could be explained by a certain amount of regeneration and plasticity that are now known to occur in the central nervous system. However, the recovery could also be interpreted as due to activity of other activating systems located in the forebrain. Indeed, based on recovery of electroencephalographic fast activity in the chronic *cerveau isolé* cat, it was concluded that cortical activation can be independently generated by the forebrain.[15]

Electrophysiologic and lesion studies showed that the activating influence of the reticular formation is transmitted to the cerebral cortex by a dorsal relay through the thalamus and a ventral, extrathalamic relay through the basal forebrain.[5] In the thalamus, electrical stimulation of the midline and intralaminar nuclei, which form the nonspecific thalamocortical projection system, could produce fast activity across the entire cerebral cortex[5] (Fig. 11–1). Ablation of the thalamus in animals led to a loss of cortical activation, which did however recover.[17] Cortical fast activity could still be elicited after thalamic lesions by stimulation of the midbrain reticular formation, indicating that the extrathalamic route and relay to the cortex could be sufficient.[5] Identified by neuroanatomic techniques in the 1970s,[18] this relay to the cortex originates from neurons located in the posterior hypothalamus and basal forebrain (substantia innominata or nucleus basalis of Meynert), which project in a widespread manner to the entire cortical mantle. Electrical stimulation through these regions could produce widespread cortical activation[5] (Fig. 11–1). The posterior hypothalamus was also thought to be important as a waking center because of its regulation of the sympathetic division of the autonomic nervous system.[19,20]

Lesions destroying nerve cell bodies and not nerve fibers of the posterior hypothalamus by neurotoxins have been shown to decrease wakefulness,[21] confirming the importance of hypothalamic neurons and not just fibers ascending from the brainstem for this state. Lesions of cells in the basal forebrain, which project to the cortex, have also been found to be associated with a loss of cortical activation of wakefulness[22,23] (Fig. 11–1). Thus, the essential activating system had to be enlarged to include, in addition to the reticular formation, the posterior hypothalamus–subthalamus and basal forebrain, which receive ascending input from the reticular formation and project in turn to the cerebral cortex.[24] These forebrain systems in the ventral extrathalamic relay also appear to be able to maintain cortical activation of the forebrain in the long-term absence of input from the brainstem reticular formation and thus function independently as activating systems.

Single-Unit Recording of Wake-Active Neurons

Most neurons in the brain were found to discharge at higher rates during wakefulness than during slow wave sleep.[25] In the midbrain reticular formation, most cells were found to have a high rate of tonic discharge in association with cortical fast activity during waking and to decrease their rate of discharge before the onset of cortical slow wave activity and slow wave sleep[26] (Fig. 11–1). These reticular neurons excite in turn neurons of the nonspecific thalamocortical projection system. The thalamic neurons also manifest a high rate of tonic discharge with cortical activation and wakefulness. Through their widespread projections to the cortex, they activate cortical neurons, which fire at high sustained rates with fast cortical activity. Neurons lying in the ventral, extrathalamic pathway in the posterior hypothalamus and basal forebrain have also been found to have a higher rate of firing during wakefulness than during slow wave sleep[27,28] (Fig. 11–1).

Sleep-Generating Systems

Identification of a Sleep-Generating System in the Brainstem

In the 1940s and 1950s, many physiologists believed that sleep was the result of fatigue and decrease in activity of the reticular activating system, thus representing a passive deactivation of the forebrain.[14] However, transections through particular levels of the brain resulted in diminished sleep. Transections of the brainstem behind the oral pontine tegmentum resulted in a total insomnia,[29] indicating that important sleep-generating structures were located in the lower brainstem with the capacity to antagonize the ascending reticular activating system in the upper brainstem.

In clinical cases, slow wave sleep was reported to be diminished or absent with lesions in the lower pons or medulla.[30] These cases show a predominance of alpha activity on the electroencephalogram (EEG), typical of waking, even though behavioral alertness and responsiveness are lacking in what has been referred to as an "alpha coma."

Low-frequency electrical stimulation of the medullary reticular formation, particularly the dorsal medullary reticular formation and the solitary tract nucleus, produced cortical slow wave–activity awake animals[31] (Fig. 11–2). Conversely, lesions

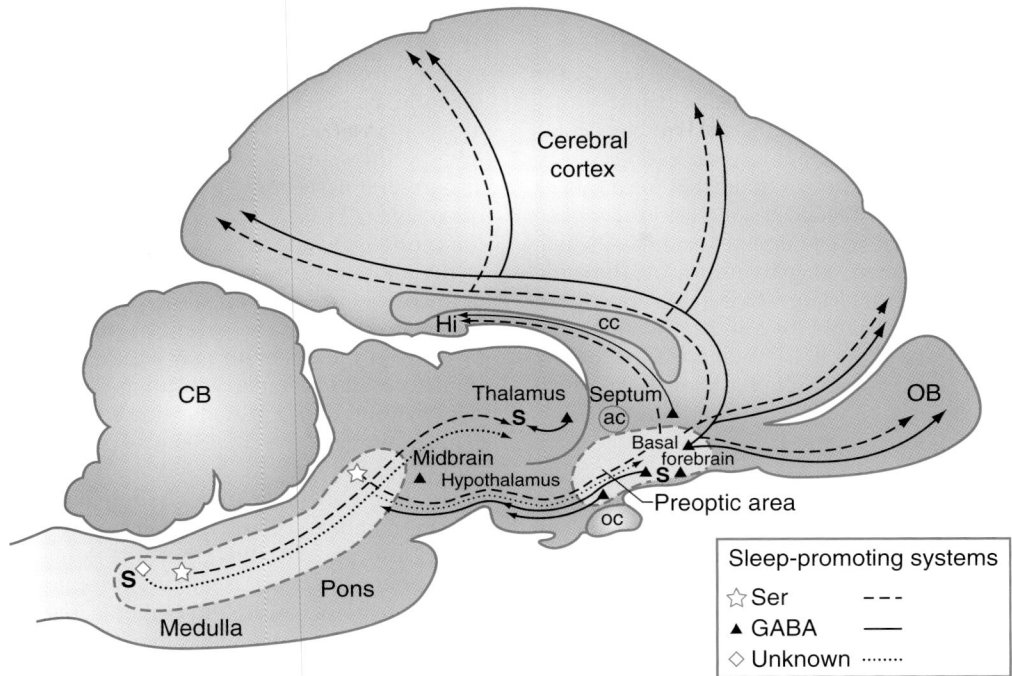

Figure 11–2. Neural systems promoting slow wave sleep. This schematic depiction of a paramedian, sagittal section of the cat brain represents neuronal systems implicated in the facilitation, generation, and maintenance of slow wave sleep. Outlined areas represent the regions in the brainstem (raphe and solitary tract nuclei) and forebrain (anterior hypothalamus, preoptic area, and basal forebrain) where large lesions are associated with a chronic decrease or loss of slow wave sleep. Points marked with "S" (slow wave sleep) indicate regions where low-frequency electrical stimulation produces cortical synchrony and behavioral sleep, as well as where particular neurons manifest a higher rate of spontaneous activity (or typical burst-pause pattern of activity) during slow wave sleep compared with waking (including the solitary tract nucleus, nonspecific thalamic nuclei, anterior hypothalamus-preoptic area, and basal forebrain). *Diamond-shaped symbols* represent neurons of the solitary tract nucleus (of unknown neurotransmitter content) implicated in slow wave sleep regulation, which project (*dotted lines*) forward into the visceral-limbic forebrain. *Stars* represent serotonin-containing neurons of the brainstem raphe nuclei, which may facilitate the onset of slow wave sleep and which project forward into the rostral tegmentum, thalamus, subthalamus, hypothalamus, and basal forebrain and also from the midbrain directly to the cerebral cortex and hippocampus. *Triangles* represent gamma-aminobutyric acid (GABA)–synthesizing neurons located in multiple regions. In the reticular formation, local GABAergic neurons may inhibit surrounding neurons of the ascending reticular activating system. Of the GABAergic neurons in the anterior hypothalamus-preoptic area and basal forebrain-septum, some may also inhibit nearby cholinergic activating neurons, some project (*solid lines*) caudally to the posterior hypothalamus and brainstem to inhibit neurons of the arousal system, and some (*solid lines*) project to the cerebral cortex and hippocampus to dampen cortical activation directly (see Fig. 11–1). GABAergic neurons are also located in the thalamic reticular nucleus, where they play an important role in generating spindles and slow waves of slow wave sleep. Not shown are other neuronal systems or factors implicated in slow wave sleep, including adenosine. Multiple peptides, such as the opiates, somatostatin or cortistatin, and growth hormone–releasing factor, may be involved in slow wave sleep generation and are often colocalized with one of the other primary neurotransmitters, particularly GABA. The neuronal systems implicated in the maintenance of slow wave sleep may be involved in primary processes of sensory inhibition and analgesia, behavioral inhibition, and parasympathetic and neuroendocrine (notably growth hormone) responses and regulation, by which they may also facilitate the onset and maintenance of slow wave sleep. ac, anterior commissure; CB, cerebellum; cc, corpus callosum; Hi, hippocampus; OB, olfactory bulb; oc, optic chiasm; Ser, serotonin.

of these structures produced fast activity in the EEG of sleeping animals.[32] Collectively, these results indicated the presence of neurons in the dorsal medullary reticular formation and the nucleus of the solitary tract that could generate sleep. Their action was hypothesized to be exerted by inhibition of the rostrally located neurons of the ascending reticular activating system, although a direct synchronogenic influence on forebrain systems was also considered possible.

The solitary tract nucleus receives afferent fibers from the glossopharyngeal and vagus (9th and 10th cranial) nerves, which carry afferent input from baroreceptors and chemoreceptors of the thoracic and abdominal viscera. Efferent projections from the solitary tract nucleus and dorsal medullary reticular formation ascend to the level of the rostral pons and midbrain, where many terminate in the parabrachial nuclei.[33] The parabrachial nuclei project rostrally to the thalamus, hypothalamus, preoptic area, amygdala, and orbitofrontal cortex, regions commonly belonging to the visceral-limbic forebrain. The solitary tract nucleus also projects forward although lightly to all of these forebrain structures, except the cortex[34] (Fig. 11–2). From these neuroanatomic data, it appeared that the action of the solitary tract nucleus may not be uniquely through inhibition of the reticular activating system, but also through action on limbic forebrain structures that had also been implicated in sleep generation.

Sleep-Generating Systems in the Forebrain

From the original studies of Bremer with the *cerveau isolé* preparation,[2] it had been known that synchronogenic structures could also be located in the forebrain because cortical slow wave activity occurs continuously in this preparation in absence of brainstem influences. In acute experimental studies applying electrical stimulation, slow cortical activity could be driven or recruited by low-frequency stimulation of the midline thalamus.[35] In chronic preparations, thalamic stimulation was shown to induce natural sleep, as defined by behavioral as well as electroencephalographic criteria (Fig 11–2), findings that led to the conclusion that the thalamus is the "head ganglion of sleep."[36] Such a conclusion has been supported by clinical cases of "fatal familial insomnia," which are associated with selective degeneration of thalamic nuclei.[37] However, experimental lesion studies in animals have shown that although the thalamus may be necessary for the production of cortical spindles, it is not necessary for the generation of cortical slow waves and behavioral sleep, which persist after its complete ablation.[17]

In the early 1900s, von Economo had noted that in some cases of "encephalitis lethargica," insomnia was the prominent symptom, and in such cases the lesions were centered in the anterior hypothalamus.[10] He thus posited that a sleep center was located in the anterior hypothalamus, which would be in opposition to, as well as normally in balance with, the waking center in the posterior hypothalamus. The existence of a sleep facilitatory region in the anterior hypothalamus and preoptic area was subsequently confirmed by lesion studies in animals.[20] It was also demonstrated that electrical stimulation of this area could elicit behavioral suppression and autonomic changes that normally accompany sleep.[19] Electrical stimulation of the basal forebrain and preoptic area was shown to lead to drowsiness followed by natural behavioral and electroencephalographic sleep[38] (Fig. 11–2). Conversely, large lesions of these areas led to an elimination or decrease in sleep and a disruption of the sleep cycle[39] (Fig. 11–2). The anterior hypothalamus, preoptic area, and basal forebrain were thus clearly shown to be important, together with the lower brainstem, for the generation of sleep.

However, it was subsequently shown that these structures were not sufficient for slow wave sleep and that the cerebral cortex and basal ganglia could also contribute to sleep onset and maintenance.[40] Animals without neocortex and striatum (thus called diencephalic cats), but with sleep-inducing structures of both the lower brainstem and the anterior diencephalon intact, did not show a normal sleep cycle but instead a large decrease in slow wave sleep. Although some damage to basal forebrain structures may have occurred in these preparations to explain the decrease in sleep, the results nonetheless suggested that the cerebral cortex and basal ganglia may also have a role in sleep induction or maintenance, perhaps by influence on the activating system of the caudal diencephalon and rostral brainstem. Electrical stimulation of the orbitofrontal cortex and caudate had been shown to produce cortical synchrony and behavioral sleep.[41] Bilateral lesions of the frontal cortex resulted in a permanent moderate reduction of sleep, whereas lesions of the caudate nuclei led to a temporary decrease in sleep.[42] Other lesion studies indicated that the orbitofrontal cortex is particularly important in the generation of slow wave activity and behavioral sleep.[43] Evidence thus suggested that neurons in the orbitofrontal cortex, together with those in basal forebrain, preoptic area, and anterior hypothalamus constitute a forebrain sleep-inducing system.

From neuroanatomic and neurophysiologic studies, several principles were to emerge concerning the links of forebrain sleep-inducing systems with the limbic system and the interaction of this larger system with the brainstem activating system. From early neuroanatomic studies, neurons in the preoptic area and anterior hypothalamus were known to be interconnected with limbic forebrain structures, including, notably, the septum, amygdala, and orbitofrontal cortex, and also to send descending projections to the medial limbic midbrain region[44] (Fig. 11–2). This descending projection went to the central gray and raphe nuclei but also terminated laterally in the midbrain reticular formation.[44,45] Electrical stimulation of the basal forebrain was shown to disrupt ongoing activity in midbrain reticular neurons, showing that sleep-generating neurons in the forebrain may act by antagonizing neurons of the ascending reticular activating system.[46] Connections of the forebrain limbic regions with lower brainstem autonomic centers are also present. Neurons in the anterior hypothalamus project directly to the solitary tract nucleus and adjacent region in the medulla, also sending fibers through, as well as to, the parabrachial nuclei in the pons.[47] The orbitofrontal cortex also projects directly to the solitary tract nucleus, in addition to supplying an important input to the preoptic area, anterior hypothalamus, and parabrachial nuclei.[48] These forebrain and lower brainstem structures form by their interconnections a system that plays an important role in autonomic regulation in addition to having the capacity to influence sleep. The importance of visceral regulatory mechanisms to sleep regulation was originally proposed years ago by Hess and Nauta, who both emphasized the anatomic overlap between centers involved in regulation of the autonomic nervous system and those involved in the sleep–wake cycle.[19] An overlap exists between sleep and parasympathetic centers in the anterior hypothalamus–preoptic area, where stimulation elicits both behavioral and electroencephalographic signs of sleep and in parallel evokes a decrease in blood pressure and heart rate and causes pupillary miosis. Caudally, an overlap exists between waking and orthosympathetic centers in the posterior hypothalamus and midbrain reticular formation, where stimulation elicits behavioral arousal and cortical activation and in parallel stimulates an increase in blood pressure and heart rate and causes pupillary mydriasis.

Single-Unit Recording of Sleep-Active Neurons

Neurons that increase their rate of firing during slow wave sleep are in the minority in the brain and particularly in the brainstem.[25,49] In the region of the solitary tract nucleus, however, a number of neurons have been found to be more active during slow wave sleep than during waking[50] (Fig. 11–2). Such sleep-related cells are invariably intermingled with cells in the same area that show a higher rate of spontaneous activity during wakefulness.

Neurons that increase their overall rate of discharge during slow wave sleep compared with waking were found in the anterior hypothalamus and preoptic area, as well as in the amygdala[49] (Fig. 11–2). Most recently, sleep-active neurons have been found to be concentrated in the ventrolateral preoptic area, where they were first located by their expression of c-Fos, as an indication of neural activity, in association with sleep recovery.[51,52] Sleep-active neurons were also found distributed among wake-active cells in the basal forebrain (including the substantia innominata and diagonal band nuclei; Fig. 11–2).[27]

It originally came as a surprise to the early physiologists to find that neurons in the cerebral cortex are very active during slow wave sleep, given that they discharge in periodic bursts of spikes.[53] However, because of long pauses between the bursts, this pattern of discharge is actually associated with a decrease in average spike rate during slow wave sleep relative to waking, thus allowing a relative rest for the cortical neurons during slow wave sleep. The bursting activity occurs first in association with spindles that are generated in the thalamus by neurons of the thalamic reticular nucleus.[54] As shown by Steriade and colleagues, the thalamic reticular neurons have intrinsic properties that allow them to burst at the frequency of thalamocortical sleep spindles (~12 to 14 Hz) and to pace the thalamocortical projection neurons that they innervate. Through intrinsic properties of the thalamic relay neurons and of cortical projection neurons, other slow oscillations (0.1 to 4 Hz), including delta waves, that characterize slow wave sleep activity are also carried through the thalamocorticothalamic network.[55] This slow activity is also transmitted from the cortex in corticofugal projections to striatum, basal forebrain, brainstem, and spinal cord, as well as to the thalamus, to play the important role in enforcing slow wave sleep through the central nervous system that was originally evident in lesion studies.[43]

CHEMICALS IMPLICATED IN SLEEP–WAKE STATES

In the early 1900s, Pieron demonstrated that transfer of cerebrospinal fluid (CSF) from sleep-deprived animals to undeprived animals caused the undeprived animals to sleep, indicating that a chemical factor accumulated in the brain during waking to generate sleep.[56] Later, in the 1950s and 1960s, it was discovered that the chemicals serving as neurotransmitters in the peripheral nervous system were present in the brain and that drugs acting on these chemicals had profound effects on sleep–wake states. After localization of these neurotransmitters by histochemical techniques, Jouvet proposed that sleep and waking may be generated by specific neurotransmitters contained in specific neuronal systems.[57] Monoamines and acetylcholine were found in neurons in the brainstem that have widespread projections through the brain, suggesting that these neurons were important components of sleep–wake regulating systems. Other small amino acid neurotransmitters and large peptide neuroactive substances are also found in widely projecting systems as well as locally projecting neurons. These varied chemicals have been found to be released at short, medium, or long distances from their targets and to have fast, medium, or long duration actions on their targets. Thus, chemicals of different molecular size may function as neurotransmitters, neuromodulators, or neurohormones to participate collectively in the generation of the sleep–wake cycle.

Chemicals Implicated in Waking

Neurotransmitters or Neuromodulators and Wakefulness

Catecholamines

These chemicals were first shown to be involved in arousal and wakefulness in the 1950s and 1960s.[57] Reserpine, which depletes monoamines, produced a state of inactivity and tranquilization that could be reversed by administration of the catecholamine precursor L-dihydroxyphenylalanine (L-dopa). The precursor administered alone also stimulated a strong and long-lasting arousal and cortical activation. Amphetamine, which was shown to act by releasing the catecholamines, dopamine and norepinephrine, produces an intense behavioral arousal and prolonged vigilance associated with cortical activation. Another stimulant, cocaine, was found to act by blocking reuptake and thus inactivation of catecholamines. Drugs that prevent the enzymatic catabolism of catecholamines by monoamine oxidase cause an intense and prolonged arousal. Similarly, those that inhibit catechol-O-methyltransferase, another catabolic enzyme, stimulate and prolong behavioral arousal and cortical activation alone and to heightened levels when combined with L-dopa.[58] Conversely, wakefulness is decreased after inhibition of catecholamine synthesis by blocking either tyrosine hydroxylase or dopamine-beta-hydroxylase.

Catecholamine perikarya located in the brainstem in regions of the oral pontine and mesencephalic tegmentum are important for the maintenance of wakefulness[59] (Fig. 11–1). The dopamine- and norepinephrine-containing neurons have distinctly different distributions and projections, suggesting different functional roles. Dopamine-containing neurons are localized in the substantia nigra and ventral tegmental area in the midbrain (Fig. 11–1) and are also scattered through the posterior hypothalamus and subthalamus. The dopaminergic neurons of the substantia nigra project forward through the lateral hypothalamus into the neostriatum, to which they provide a dense innervation.[60] Together with those of the ventral tegmental area, these dopaminergic neurons also innervate the basal forebrain, nucleus accumbens, septum, amygdala, and frontal cortex. By these efferent projections, the midbrain dopaminergic neurons may modulate activity in motor and limbic systems. The norepinephrine-containing neurons are found in the pontine tegmentum (Fig. 11–1) and medullary reticular formation.[61] The largest cluster of noradrenergic neurons, giving rise to ascending projections, is in the locus coeruleus nucleus in the dorsolateral pontine tegmentum. Noradrenergic neurons of the locus coeruleus project in a diffuse manner to the entire forebrain, along pathways and terminal areas that overlap to a certain extent with those of the reticular formation but that most uniquely also include all areas of the cerebral cortex[62] (Fig 11–1). Other noradrenergic or adrenergic neurons are scattered through the ventrolateral pontine and medullary reticular formation. Collectively, the noradrenergic and adrenergic brainstem neurons provide innervation to the entire forebrain, brainstem, and spinal cord and thus can directly modulate activity throughout the central nervous system, including the cerebral cortex.

Lesions of the dopamine-containing perikarya in the ventral tegmental area and substantia nigra in the cat produced a state of behavioral unresponsiveness and immobility or akinesia[57,63] (Fig. 11–1). With lesions limited to the ventral midbrain tegmentum, this behaviorally comatose state was not necessarily associated with a decrease in cortical activation of wakefulness. On the other hand, lesions of the central midbrain tegmentum, where the ascending noradrenergic fibers pass, produced a severe decrease in cortical activation of wakefulness (Fig. 11-1). In these animals, behavioral responses to stimulation could be elicited along with cortical activation; however, behavioral somnolence associated with moderately slow electroencephalographic activity was in evidence most of the time when the animals were not stimulated. In summary, dopaminergic neurons of the substantia nigra and ventral tegmental area, which project to the striatum and frontal cortex, play an important role in behavioral arousal, whereas noradrenergic neurons of the locus coeruleus and brainstem, which project diffusely to the forebrain, including the cortex, play an integral role in cortical activation.

Clinical studies provide evidence for the involvement of these chemicals in conditions of akinesia and coma. Cases of akinesia and akinetic mutism often involve lesions of the ventral midbrain tegmentum or ventral posterior hypothalamus, where dopaminergic perikarya and pathways are respectively located.[11] Similarly, advanced cases of parkinsonism associated with severe akinesia involve extensive degeneration of dopaminergic neurons in the midbrain and depletion of dopamine in the striatum.[64] Such akinesia can be improved by treatment with L-dopa. Comas marked by a loss of cortical activation occur with lesions of the mesencephalic reticular formation, through which the ascending noradrenergic pathways course.[65] Improvement of comatose states due to cerebral lesions has also been reported after administration of the catecholamine precursor L-dopa.[66]

Spontaneous recovery from destruction of catecholaminergic neurons has been documented in animals. The recovery of motor function, however, after substantia nigra lesions was shown to depend on intact dopaminergic neurons, which are capable of compensation, plasticity, and regeneration.[67] In such cases, functional recovery can occur if more than 5% of the dopaminergic nigrostriatal projection is left intact by the lesion. With such plasticity, severe long-term deficits may be rare and difficult to detect. Indeed, selective lesions of catecholaminergic neurons produced with 6-hydroxydopamine were found to have small to minimal, transient effects on spontaneous motor activity and cortical activation of wakefulness.[68] Moreover, localized lesions of the noradrenergic locus coeruleus neurons in the oral pontine tegmentum did not produce the loss of wakefulness or cortical activation of the same severity as that associated with midbrain lesions of ascending pathways.[69] On the other hand, reversible cooling of the locus coeruleus has been found to produce sleep in a waking animal, and electrical stimulation has been found to produce arousal in a sleeping animal.[70] These results indicate that collectively, catecholaminergic neurons normally enhance and prolong wakefulness, but may not be essential for behavioral arousal and cortical activation because they represent components of larger and thus redundant neuronal systems.

Single-unit recording and neurotransmitter release studies have substantiated the role of catecholaminergic neurons in arousal processes (Fig. 11–1). Presumed dopaminergic neurons in the substantia nigra and ventral tegmental area have a low basal rate of discharge that is similar across sleep–wake states, although they do increase their discharge and tend to fire in bursts of action potentials in association with significant sensory stimulation, purposive movement, or behavioral arousal.[71] Presumed noradrenergic locus coeruleus neurons are most active during attentive, highly aroused, or stressful waking situations and otherwise show a regular, slow rate of spontaneous activity during quiet waking.[25,72-74] They progressively decrease their rate of discharge during slow wave sleep and virtually cease firing during paradoxical sleep.

Release of dopamine and norepinephrine is greatest during the waking state and, moreover, greatest in association with behavioral arousal.[75,76]

Catecholamines do not act on ionotropic receptors, which open ion channels directly, but instead on metabotropic receptors, which act indirectly on ion channels through second messenger pathways, and are thus more typical of neuromodulators with long-lasting indirect actions than classic neurotransmitters with rapid direct actions. In the thalamus and cortex, stimulation of adrenergic receptors results in a depolarization and excitation of the projection neurons and a switch from the burst discharge mode underlying slow wave sleep to a tonic discharge mode underlying waking.[77] The drug modafinil, which enhances and prolongs wakefulness in humans and animals without eliciting the behavioral excitation associated with amphetamine, was found to act on postsynaptic adrenergic receptors without stimulating catecholamine release like amphetamine.[78,79] These pharmacologic results further substantiate the notion that norepinephrine and adrenergic receptors appear to be particularly important in stimulating and maintaining activating processes in thalamocortical systems, whereas dopaminergic systems are potent in stimulating behavioral arousal. Through widespread or diffuse projections and slow modulatory actions on other systems, catecholamine-containing neurons may collectively stimulate, enhance, or prolong a waking, attentive, and aroused state.

ACETYLCHOLINE

This chemical was known to be important for vigilance and cortical activation during waking from pharmacologic evidence in the 1950s and 1960s.[57,80] Atropine or belladonna, which acts by blocking muscarinic cholinergic receptors, decreases vigilance. This deficit was shown in animals to be due to the appearance of cortical slow wave activity on the cerebral cortex that persisted even during spontaneous movement in what was thus described as the dissociation of EEG and behavior. Conversely, neostigmine, which inhibits the catabolic enzyme acetylcholinesterase and thus prolongs the postsynaptic action of acetylcholine, enhances vigilance in association with prolonged cortical activation. The cholinergic agonists, muscarine and nicotine, enhance or prolong vigilance and cortical fast activity. Acetylcholine thus appears to play an important role in cortical activation, independent of waking behavior, and thus potentially during both waking and paradoxical sleep.[81,82]

Two major groups of cholinergic neurons give rise to forebrain and cortical projections[81,83] (Fig. 11–1). One is located in the oral pontine-caudal mesencephalic reticular formation (in the laterodorsal and pedunculopontine tegmental nuclei) and gives rise to projections into the forebrain, particularly to the midline and intralaminar thalamic nuclei, but also to a lesser degree to the lateral hypothalamus and basal forebrain. Another is made up of cholinergic neurons located in the basal forebrain (nucleus basalis, substantia innominata, nuclei of the diagonal band, and septum), which project in a widespread manner to the entire cortical mantle. The latter cells appear to serve as the ventral, extrathalamic relay from the brainstem reticular formation to the cerebral cortex.

Although the pontomesencephalic cholinergic neurons serve as a component of the ascending reticular activating system, their destruction does not eliminate cortical activation of waking, but eliminates paradoxical sleep.[81] Lesions of the cholinergic neurons of the basal forebrain produce alterations in cortical activity that are similar to those seen after atropine administration, that is, slowing of cortical activity and loss of vigilance[22,23] (Fig. 11–1). Such lesions also alter slow wave sleep.[39,84] The latter effects could be due to destruction of codistributed sleep-active cells, which probably do not contain acetylcholine. Pharmacologic inhibition or inactivation of the cholinergic cells by local microinjections of chemical agents clearly diminishes the high-frequency (30 to 60 Hz gamma) cortical activity that characterizes cortical activation as evident in aroused, attentive awake states and in paradoxical sleep.[85] These results confirm that the cholinergic neurons of the basal forebrain are very important for cortical activation.

Alzheimer's disease, which is associated with a loss of cholinergic innervation of the cerebral cortex and degeneration of cholinergic neurons of the basal forebrain, is characterized by a diffuse slowing of cortical activity.[86,87] In later stages of the disease, sleep is also greatly perturbed, marked by a loss of spindles and slow waves as well as a decrease in REM sleep (see Chapter 71). Such general disruption of the EEG and sleep cycle probably reflects the diffuse degeneration and neurofibrillary changes of multiple cell populations through the brainstem and basal forebrain as well as cortex.[88,89]

Presumed cholinergic pontomesencephalic neurons discharge at higher rates during waking than during slow wave sleep (and often at an even higher rate during paradoxical sleep), as reflected by increased release of acetylcholine from the thalamus[90,91] (Fig. 11–1). Cholinergic basal forebrain neurons are also most active during waking (and paradoxical sleep) compared with slow wave sleep, as reflected by high levels of acetylcholine release from the cortex[85,92] (Fig. 11–1).

Acetylcholine acts on muscarinic and nicotinic receptors in the central nervous system. Muscarinic receptors are metabotropic, associated through second messenger systems with slow and prolonged postsynaptic actions that are predominantly excitatory, although also in some cases inhibitory. Nicotinic receptors are ionotropic, directly linked to ion channels that permit fast postsynaptic excitatory actions. The excitation of pyramidal cells by acetylcholine results in a shift in their mode of firing from a burst discharge associated with cortical slow waves to a tonic discharge associated with cortical fast activity.[77] Cholinergic brainstem and basal forebrain neurons may thus exert a tonic facilitatory influence on transmission and activity in both the thalamus and cortex to promote thalamocortical transmission and fast cortical activity during wakefulness and paradoxical sleep.

Histamine

This chemical has long been assumed to play a role in waking given the well-known sedative effects of the early antihistaminergic drugs[93] (see Chapter 37). Histamine administered directly into the cerebral ventricles has an arousing effect.[94] Histamine-containing neurons are located in the tuberomammillary nuclei and surrounding area of the posterior hypothalamus,[95] where lesions had been shown to be associated with coma or a decrease in wakefulness (Fig. 11–1). Like locus coeruleus neurons, histaminergic neurons give rise to diffuse projections through the brain, including the entire cerebral cortex. Neurotoxic lesions, selective to cell bodies and sparing fibers of passage, of the posterior hypothalamus have been shown to produce a decrease in wakefulness and increase in both slow wave sleep and paradoxical sleep.[21] Putative histaminergic

neurons have also been shown to be most active in association with the cortical activation of wakefulness and turn off during paradoxical sleep.[96] Histamine acts on metabotropic receptors, which are generally excitatory and produce a depolarization and resulting tonic discharge in thalamic and cortical projection neurons, as typically associated with waking, fast cortical activity.[77] Like norepinephrine, histamine would thus promote cortical activation during wakefulness.

Glutamate

The major excitatory neurotransmitter in the brain, glutamate plays a fundamental role in neural activity of the waking brain.[81] Glutamate agonists produce seizures. Some glutamate receptor antagonists (e.g., ketamine) are used as sedatives or anesthetics.[97] Glutamate is found in high concentrations in the large neurons of the brainstem reticular formation and likely serves as the primary neurotransmitter of the ascending reticular activating system[24] (Fig. 11–1). It is also contained in the projection neurons of the thalamus and cerebral cortex.[98] Glutamate is released from the cerebral cortex in greatest quantities in association with cortical activation of spontaneous wakefulness or that evoked by stimulation of the midbrain reticular formation.[99] Glutamate acts on different postsynaptic receptors, including both ionotropic (kainate, α-amino-3-hydroxy-5-methylisoxazole-4-propionic acid [AMPA], and N-methyl-D-aspartate [NMDA]) and metabotropic (trans-aminocyclopentane-1,3-dicarboxylic acid [t-ACPD]) receptors that are generally excitatory but are associated with different durations of excitation and induced patterns of discharge. Stimulation of the different receptors is commonly associated with increased discharge of thalamic and cortical neurons.[77] However, stimulation of NMDA receptors can induce a burst discharge that has been implicated in the burst discharge of pyramidal cells during slow wave sleep.[100] Thus, glutamate, contained in the reticular formation neurons of the brainstem activating system and in most of the projection neurons in the forebrain, is critical for cortical activation and a waking, responsive state. In addition, particular glutamate receptors may also be activated during slow wave sleep in association with a burst mode of discharge.

Cerebrospinal Fluid–Borne Factors, Peptides, and Wakefulness

Wake-promoting factors are suspected of being present in the CSF because wakefulness and activity have been produced in recipient animals after extraction of CSF from waking host animals.[101,102] It has long been suspected that such factors would be peptides, although other chemicals, such as the catecholamines, have been shown to accumulate in the CSF and to vary according to a circadian rhythm.

Peptides have been tested for wake- or sleep-promoting effects by intraventricular administration. This route of administration may or may not mimic physiologic routes of action or reach physiologic sites of action for these factors. Peptides are often colocalized with other smaller molecule neurotransmitters, although they may be differentially released from the same nerve terminals as a function of different levels of neuronal activity. Neuroactive peptides act on metabotropic receptors to produce relatively long-duration presynaptic or postsynaptic effects, some of which serve only to modulate the effects of other neurotransmitters or neuromodulators.

Several peptides, when introduced into the CSF or directly into the brain, enhance cortical activation, waking, and, in some cases, paradoxical sleep. These include *substance P, vasoactive intestinal peptide* (VIP), and *neurotensin*.[103,104] These different peptides are contained in neurons distributed in different regions through the brainstem and forebrain and are thought to act on neurons at a distance from their release sites. In many cases, they may act on or together with catecholaminergic or cholinergic neurons in the brainstem or forebrain. Peptides that stimulate release of pituitary hormones are also contained in neurons that project to other regions of the brain and may thus influence waking and arousal, including *corticotropin-releasing factor* and *thyrotropin-releasing factor*. After intraventricular administration, corticotropin-releasing factor stimulates behavioral arousal associated with prolonged cortical activation.[105] These releasing factors may thus act centrally to alter state and behavior in a manner synergistic with the peripheral effects of their targeted hormones.

Orexin or *hypocretin* was recently discovered as the peptide that is deficient in narcolepsy and would thus play an important role in maintaining waking.[106,107] The neurons that contain orexin are located in the posterior hypothalamus in the region where classic lesions were shown to be associated with decreases in waking or induction of coma, and more recent neurotoxic lesions were associated with increases in slow wave sleep and paradoxical sleep[21] (Fig. 11–1). They give rise to diffuse projections to the brain and spinal cord and can excite neurons in thalamocortical and basalocortical systems as well as other hypothalamic and brainstem arousal systems to stimulate cortical activation and behavioral arousal.[108-112] Orexin neurons could correspond to wake-active and REM sleep–off cells that have been recorded in the perifornical region of the posterior hypothalamus.[113] Given their degeneration in narcolepsy,[114] orexinergic neurons are considered to play a critical role in maintaining waking and preventing sleep, including paradoxical sleep. They may form an important component of the orthosympathetic system of the posterior hypothalamus because they may also stimulate energy metabolism[115] through activation of the sympathetic and hypothalamic-pituitary-adrenal axis, as would be important in association with waking activity.

Wake-Promoting Blood-Borne Factors

Epinephrine, which is normally released in the blood by the adrenal medulla, was shown by intravenous administration in early pharmacologic studies to produce cortical activation in a sleeping animal preparation.[57] Results of multiple studies also suggested that peripherally circulating norepinephrine released by sympathetic discharge could act centrally through the reticular activating system to produce cortical activation and wakefulness. It was only later learned that epinephrine and norepinephrine do not cross the blood–brain barrier. However, epinephrine and other blood-borne substances could act on the specialized circumventricular organs that lie outside the blood–brain barrier and in regions thought to be important in the sleep–wake cycle and in autonomic and neuroendocrine regulation, such as the area postrema in the medulla and the median eminence and organum vasculosum in the hypothalamus.

Histamine, which is produced in peripheral tissues, was shown to produce an arousing effect in rabbits when administered intravenously.[94] Furthermore, higher concentrations of histamine have been measured in the blood of aroused versus sleeping rabbits, which suggests its participation as a neurohumoral factor in the regulation of wakefulness and arousal. Like epinephrine, it must have its effect through regions of the brain that are outside the blood–brain barrier.

The action of peripheral chemical factors, which may also include pituitary hormones such as *corticotropin* and *thyrotropin,* may permit the reinforcement or alteration of centrally generated states. In addition, steroid hormones, such as the glucocorticoids secreted by the adrenal cortex, readily enter the brain and act directly through specific receptors on multiple neurons, by which they may also enhance arousal. Plasma *cortisol* has a very marked circadian rhythm, as measured in humans, reaching a nadir during slow wave sleep in the night and then increasing in the early morning hours before sunrise and awakening, likely reflecting a hormonal preparatory mechanism for the waking state.[116]

Chemicals Implicated in Slow Wave Sleep

Neurotransmitters or Neuromodulators and Slow Wave Sleep

SEROTONIN

Serotonin (5-hydroxytryptamine [5-HT]) appeared in early pharmacologic studies to play a role in sleep–wake states opposite to that of catecholamines because the tranquilization produced by depletion of monoamines with reserpine was not reversed by subsequent administration of the immediate serotonin precursor (5-hydroxytryptophan), as it was by the immediate catecholamine precursor (L-dopa).[57] Monoamine oxidase inhibitors, which primarily block serotonin catabolism, were shown to enhance and prolong slow wave sleep. Conversely, inhibition of serotonin synthesis by blocking tryptophan hydroxylase led to insomnia, which could be reversed by administration of small amounts of the immediate serotonin precursor.

Serotonergic neurons are located in nuclei on the midline or "raphe" through the medulla, pons, and midbrain of the brainstem,[59] suggesting they could comprise part of the brainstem slow wave sleep system[57] (Fig. 11–2). Serotonin raphe neurons provide a diffuse innervation to the brain and spinal cord, the rostrally located (dorsal and central superior) raphe nuclei projecting mainly forward into the forebrain (including the thalamus, hypothalamus, basal forebrain, and all cortical areas), and the caudally located (magnus, pallidus, and obscurus) nuclei projecting mainly caudally into the spinal cord.[117]

Total lesions of the raphe serotonin nuclei produced a total insomnia in the cat[57] (Fig. 11–2). Partial lesions involving the medullary, pontine, or midbrain raphe nuclei were associated with variable decreases in sleep, with the amount of sleep being proportional to the percentage of serotonin remaining in the brain. These results suggested that serotonin raphe neurons constitute an integral component of a brainstem sleep-generating system that lies in the midline midbrain, pontine, and medullary raphe nuclei, as well as in the dorsolateral medullary region of the solitary tract nucleus (see earlier).

Clinical cases of insomnia have been found to be associated with lesions located in the region of the caudal midbrain and pontine tegmentum and particularly involving the midline raphe nuclei at these levels.[30,65,118] In one case of extreme insomnia (or "agrypnie" in a patient with *chorée fibrillarie de Morvan*), administration of the immediate serotonin precursor was found to restore natural slow wave sleep.[119]

Recovery from the insomnia produced by raphe lesions has since been found to occur in animals, particularly after lesions produced by serotonin-selective neurotoxins.[120] Similarly, recovery from the insomnia produced by pharmacologic depletion of serotonin was demonstrated in prolonged chronic studies. It thus appeared that serotonin was not necessary for slow wave sleep.

Further demonstrating the lack of a critical role of serotonergic neurons in the maintenance of sleep, single-unit recordings subsequently revealed that presumed serotonergic raphe neurons actually decreased their rate of firing with the onset and for the duration of slow wave sleep and ceased firing in paradoxical sleep.[121] These single-unit data were supported by results from biochemical studies of serotonin release, which was found to be lower during slow wave sleep and also paradoxical sleep than during wakefulness.[122] On the basis of these results, it was concluded that serotonergic neurons did not play an essential role in sleep maintenance.

Yet, given the overwhelming evidence indicating that serotonin could normally facilitate sleep onset, it appeared that serotonergic neurons must exert an influence during waking that could facilitate sleep onset. Experiments applying electrical stimulation to raphe nuclei had in fact shown that although sleep is not produced by such stimulation, behavioral inhibition and sensory modulation or analgesia are produced.[123,124] Serotonin could thus act by attenuating other systems that normally stimulate cortical activation and arousal. In this regard, serotonin has been shown to have an inhibitory action on cholinergic neurons in both the pontomesencephalic tegmentum and basal forebrain.[125,126] Microinjections of serotonin into the basal forebrain lead to decreases in cortical high-frequency (gamma) electroencephalographic activity, suggesting that serotonin may attenuate cortical activation and be associated with either a quiet waking state or initiation of slow wave sleep.[127] It has also been hypothesized that serotonin neurons may be responsible for the synthesis and accumulation of sleep factors during waking in neurons of the anterior hypothalamus.[128] In summary, serotonin may prepare the brain and organism for slow wave sleep during waking by attenuating activating systems and possibly stimulating accumulation of other sleep factors.

Serotonin acts on multiple receptors, which include second messenger–linked receptors but also ionotropic receptors, and which thus range from long acting to fast acting with inhibitory as well as excitatory effects on different postsynaptic cells. The pharmacologic effects of selective serotonin receptor agonists or antagonists on electroencephalographic activity and sleep have not been clearly interpretable, as is perhaps not surprising given the variety of receptors on diverse projection neurons as well as interneuronal cell populations. It is significant, nonetheless, that the ionotropic excitatory postsynaptic receptor (5-HT$_3$) is found mainly on gamma-aminobutyric acid–ergic (GABAergic) interneurons in the cortex and forebrain[129] and that the major inhibitory postsynaptic receptor (5-HT$_{1A}$) is found on many projection neurons and notably on the cholinergic basal forebrain neurons that are hyperpolarized and inhibited by serotonin through this receptor.[126] In summary, serotonin may thus act through concerted activation of multiple different receptors on different cell types to attenuate cortical activation and thus facilitate the initiation of slow wave sleep.

ADENOSINE

This nucleoside has long been thought to play a role in slow wave sleep because caffeine (methylxanthine), which acts as a stimulant, blocks adenosine receptors.[130] It has been shown that adenosine analogues can increase slow wave sleep and cortical slow wave activity and that this increase can be prevented by administration of caffeine.[131]

Adenosine is found in high concentrations in particular neurons from which it may be released as a neurotransmitter,[132] but is also present in the extracellular space as a degradation product of adenosine triphosphate (ATP), which is packaged and released by many synaptic vesicles, including those containing acetylcholine. Adenosine is also transported out of cells when production of adenosine monophosphate is increased during the formation of ATP from two molecules of adenosine diphosphate, as occurs as a consequence of energy demand.[133] Although extracellular concentrations of adenosine in the brain are higher during waking than during slow wave sleep, these concentrations appear to increase progressively with prolonged waking and to decrease progressively with subsequent sleep, such as to suggest a cumulative extracellular increase in what could be a fatigue-like and sleep-inducing factor in the brain.[134,135]

Adenosine acts as a neuromodulator through second messenger–linked postsynaptic receptors to inhibit neuronal discharge, and also through other receptors to block neurotransmitter release from nerve terminals. It thus suppresses transmission at excitatory synapses in the brain and periphery. It inhibits cholinergic neurons in the brainstem and basal forebrain.[136] In the thalamus and cortex, adenosine hyperpolarizes projection neurons and can facilitate the burst discharge that underlies the slow wave activity of slow wave sleep.[137] Adenosine could thus function in the brain, as it has been shown to do in the body, as a factor that accumulates with continuous activity and acts to protect cells from damage that could result from excess activity.[133] In the brain, its action could be associated with the specialized burst discharge in thalamocortical circuits that underlies slow wave sleep.[138]

GAMMA-AMINOBUTYRIC ACID

GABA, an amino acid which is the major inhibitory neurotransmitter in the brain, has long been thought to have a role in sleep. Many sedative and hypnotic agents, as well as anesthetics, act by enhancing the postsynaptic action of GABA through binding to GABA receptors[139] (see Chapter 36). In clinical cases of so-called idiopathic recurring stupor, an endogenous benzodiazepine-like factor (endozepine) was identified in the CSF and found to be present in elevated levels in association with stuporous episodes that could be reversed with a benzodiazepine antagonist.[140]

GABA-synthesizing neurons (containing the synthetic enzyme glutamic acid decarboxylase) are distributed through the brainstem and forebrain and comprise both interneurons and projection neurons[141] (Fig. 11–2). In the brainstem reticular formation, relatively small GABAergic neurons are intermingled with larger glutamatergic projection neurons and would thus appear to have the capacity through local projections to inhibit the glutamatergic neurons of the ascending reticular activating system.[24] The neurons of the thalamic reticular nucleus that generate thalamocortical spindles contain GABA and simultaneously inhibit while pacing thalamocortical relay neurons by inhibitory postsynaptic potentials.[142] This inhibition of the thalamus, the afferent gateway to the cerebral cortex, is fundamental to slow wave sleep and the loss of consciousness that accompanies it.[143] GABAergic neurons are distributed through the anterior hypothalamus–preoptic area and basal forebrain and some give rise to descending projections to the posterior hypothalamus, where they can inhibit neurons of the activating system.[144,145] A particular cluster of GABAergic neurons that were found to be active (as evidenced by c-Fos expression) during sleep project on histaminergic neurons in the posterior hypothalamus.[52,146] GABA release in the posterior hypothalamus has been found to be significantly higher during slow wave sleep than during waking or paradoxical sleep.[147] There are also GABAergic neurons in the subthalamus, hypothalamus, and basal forebrain that give rise to long ascending projections to the cortex[148,149] (Fig. 11–2). Some of these GABAergic neurons may correspond to long-projecting sleep-active cells recorded in these regions.[85,150] The release of GABA from the cortex was highest in association with cortical slow waves of natural sleep.[99] GABAergic interneurons and projection neurons, however, are certainly active during waking in all regions of the brain and can also be important in pacing fast activity as well as slow activity in the cortex. It would thus be most likely that particular GABAergic cells may be active during sleep or that particular GABAergic receptors may be activated during sleep. Moreover, larger amounts of GABA could be released with the bursting mode of discharge by GABAergic reticularis and other neurons to reach more receptors on more neurons in the thalamus and other regions during slow wave sleep.

GABA acts on two types of receptors, $GABA_A$, which is linked directly to the (chloride) ion channel (and is modulated by benzodiazepines and pentobarbital), and $GABA_B$, which acts through second messenger systems to modulate different (potassium and calcium) ion channels. Although both receptors are generally associated with inhibition, the action of the $GABA_A$ is very rapid, whereas that of the $GABA_B$ is slow and prolonged and includes attenuation of neurotransmitter release as well as neuronal spiking. In the thalamocortical system, $GABA_A$ and $GABA_B$ receptors participate in the hyperpolarization associated with spindling and slow waves.[151,152] $GABA_A$ agonists can enhance spindling and slow wave activity along with sleep in humans.[153] The enhancement of slow wave activity and sleep produced by gamma-hydroxybutyrate in humans may well be mediated through $GABA_B$ receptors.[154,155] In summary, GABAergic transmission is fundamentally involved in the induction and maintenance of slow wave sleep, first by inhibition of activating systems and second by initiating, pacing, and sustaining the thalamocortical burst discharge that underlies spindling and slow wave activity. This involvement must entail, however, selective activity of particular GABAergic neurons or distinct patterns of discharge of GABAergic neurons and resulting selective or prolonged activation of particular GABAergic receptors located on those neurons that serve to maintain waking and consciousness.

Cerebrospinal Fluid–Borne Factors, Peptides, and Slow Wave Sleep

Sleep-inducing factors have been shown to be present in the CSF or brain in multiple animal experiments.[101,102,128] CSF or brain extract removed from a sleep-deprived animal or from an animal in the sleep-intense part of the cycle promotes sleep when it is injected into the ventricles of another animal, even during the awake, active period of the day. Identification of the sleep-promoting factors, however, has proven to be difficult and remains controversial.

Peptides, which are synthesized, stored, and released from neurons of the central nervous system, can act as sleep-promoting factors in particular neuronal systems or throughout the brain by diffusion through the CSF. Attempted isolation of factors from the CSF has not yet yielded any one substance or peptide, although many candidates have been proposed and tested as sleep factors, with ambiguous results. Testing of known peptides by intraventricular administration has revealed several (discussed in the following) that have an effect on sleep. *Opiate* peptides have long been suspected of influencing sleep–wake states, in view of the sensory anesthesia, behavioral stupor, and associated electroencephalographic synchrony produced by the synthetic opiate analogue morphine.[156] Administered by intraventricular route, opiate peptides also produce anesthesia, akinesia, and electroencephalographic hypersynchrony,[157] but they do not appear to induce or increase physiologic slow wave sleep.[158] This negative effect may simply be due to the fact that opiate peptides normally act within specific neuronal circuits and not by release and diffusion through the CSF. The endogenous opiate peptides, including enkephalin, endorphin, and dynorphin, have all been shown to have a role in sensory modulation and analgesia[159] that could be important in the onset and maintenance of sleep. These peptides could thus be involved in attenuation of systems that normally stimulate arousal and waking. *Enkephalin* is contained in neurons that are widely distributed through the brain, including the cerebral cortex, and in neurons within regions involved in slow wave sleep, including the solitary tract nucleus, the preoptic area, and the raphe, where it is colocalized with serotonin.[160] Enkephalin-containing fibers innervate the locus coeruleus noradrenergic neurons; opiates inhibit these neurons and produce a decrease in waking and enhancement of natural slow wave sleep when delivered locally.[161] Derived from proopiomelanocortin, *beta-endorphin* is contained in neurons located in the arcuate region of the hypothalamus that give rise to widespread projections that are particularly dense in the periventricular regions of the hypothalamus and preoptic area.[162] Other beta-endorphin cells are located in the nucleus of the solitary tract.

Somatostatin, administered intraventricularly, produces analgesia, akinesia, and a depression of electroencephalographic activity.[157] Although distributed in multiple systems in the brain, somatostatin-containing neurons are located in the solitary tract nucleus and raphe nuclei.[163] Furthermore, somatostatin is colocalized with GABA in certain neuronal systems, including, notably, neurons of the thalamic reticular nucleus and a proportion of cortical interneurons.[163] Like GABA, somatostatin has been found to have primarily inhibitory effects on central neurons.[164] Like other peptides, it acts on second messenger–linked receptors that are inhibitory to neuronal discharge and also to neurotransmitter release from nerve terminals. *Cortistatin*, which is structurally similar to somatostatin and found in the cerebral cortex, was also found to suppress neuronal activity and to antagonize the effects of acetylcholine on cortical neurons. In addition, this peptide was found to induce cortical slow waves.[165] Because peptides are often colocalized with other smaller neurotransmitters, and somatostatin and cortistatin appear to be commonly colocalized with GABA,[166] it is possible that they may be coreleased with the smaller inhibitory neurotransmitter. Moreover, peptides may be released particularly in association with the bursting discharge of neurons,[167] which would occur in the thalamocortical system during slow wave sleep, where and when somatostatin or cortistatin could be coreleased with GABA and thus further sustain conditions for slow wave activity. *Galanin* is another peptide that is colocalized with other neurotransmitters and notably GABA in the ventrolateral preoptic area in putative sleep-promoting neurons.[146]

Growth hormone–releasing factor, which is produced by neurons in the hypothalamus[168] and stimulates the release of growth hormone by the pituitary, also appears to have slow wave sleep–inducing properties by acting on neurons in the anterior hypothalamus-preoptic area.[105] Its release would accordingly facilitate slow wave sleep at the same time that it would stimulate the surge in growth hormone release from the pituitary that occurs during slow wave sleep in the early part of the night in humans. It should be noted that in these specific systems in the hypothalamus, somatostatin acts to suppress growth hormone release and can also thereby decrease slow wave sleep.[169]

Other substances, including serotonin, that are not peptides and have sleep-inducing effects are found in the CSF. *Prostaglandin D2*, which is synthesized in brain (predominantly by glia) with a circadian fluctuation that is parallel to the sleep–wake cycle, has been shown to induce sleep in animals when it is administered in small amounts into the third ventricle.[170] Cytokines, most particularly *interleukins*, that are now known to be synthesized in the brain (predominantly by glia) also produce sleep and enhance slow wave activity when injected into the ventricles.[171] A brain lipid or *fatty acid amide* was isolated from CSF of sleep-deprived cats that induced physiologic sleep when injected into the ventricles of rats.[172,173] This substance, called *oleamide*, is similar to the anandamides, which are endocannibinoid compounds, and may act through cannibinoid receptors. Oleamide may also act on GABA$_A$ receptors. It thus appears that in addition to neuropeptides that are released by specific neurons, other substances, which may be synthesized by glia as well as neurons and released by nonexocytotic mechanisms from these cells, may participate in facilitating slow wave sleep. Whether such substances accumulate in the CSF and thereby diffuse through the entire brain to exert their effects, remains to be established.

Blood-Borne Factors and Slow Wave Sleep

Presumably produced by platelets, *serotonin* in the blood could act in specialized regions of the brain located outside the blood–brain barrier to facilitate the onset of sleep. This possibility is suggested by the finding that local application of serotonin in the area postrema produced slow wave sleep.[174]

Insulin has been shown to have marked slow wave sleep–inducing effects when it is administered intravenously in animals.[175] It is suggested that the accumulation of insulin during the active, hyperphagic waking periods would lead to the subsequent induction of sleep. Insulin receptors have been found in the brain in circumventricular organs located

outside the blood–brain barrier and in nearby nuclei, notably in the basal hypothalamus and solitary tract, paravagal region.[176] Because the intraventricular administration of insulin has also been shown to induce sleep, it is suggested that its sleep-inducing action would be directly on the brain.

Cholecystokinin is a hormone that is released in the gut after food ingestion and suppresses further food intake. This so-called satiety hormone also promotes rest and may induce slow wave sleep.[177] Another gut hormone, *bombesin*, also released after food ingestion, increases slow wave sleep when it is administered peripherally.[178] These peripheral hormones that are in part responsible for postprandial satiety may thus also contribute to postprandial induction of rest and sleep, either by indirect action through vagal afferents to the solitary tract nucleus or by direct action on circumventricular organs located outside the blood–brain barrier.

Muramyl peptides also originate in the gut from intestinal bacteria and have been shown to have sleep-inducing properties.[177] Like other bacteria and viruses, they also stimulate synthesis and release of cytokines, particularly *interleukins*, that promote slow wave sleep.[171] Thus, sleep may be facilitated through hormones and other peptides that are released from the gut or from the immune system in response to exogenous substances.

Delta sleep-inducing peptide was identified in the blood of rabbits during slow wave sleep produced by low-frequency thalamic stimulation.[179] It was shown to induce sleep when injected into the blood or CSF of recipient rabbits. Although conflicting reports regarding the sleep-inducing effects of delta sleep-inducing peptide in various species have appeared, confirmation of an increase in slow wave sleep has been obtained in mice after intraperitoneal administration of delta sleep-inducing peptide, an increase comparable with that obtained after intraperitoneal administration of sleep-promoting substance isolated from brain tissue.[180] Whether a similar peripheral and central peptide exists, where the peripheral substances are produced, and how they reach relevant receptors in the brain remain to be elucidated.

It would thus appear that as in the regulation of waking, blood-borne substances can have an influence on the central sleep-generating systems, in part through the circumventricular organs by which they all have access to the brain. Included in these factors would accordingly also be certain pituitary hormones, such as *growth hormone* and *prolactin*, which are released maximally during slow wave sleep and may also influence sleep.[177]

CONCLUSIONS

Neurophysiologic and Neuroanatomic Results

The neuronal systems that govern the cyclic alternation between waking and sleep are contained in the isodendritic core of the brain that extends from the medulla through the brainstem and hypothalamus up into the basal forebrain. No structure in this core is uniquely or monolithically involved in the control of one state. Instead, different neurons in the same structure or field of cells are important for sleep versus waking. Despite such an intermingling of sleep-active and wake-active neurons, a differential concentration of such cells may exist in different regions. Thus, it appears that neurons mainly involved in maintaining activation are concentrated in the oral pontine and midbrain central tegmentum and posterior hypothalamus, whereas cells that exert an important sleep-promoting influence are concentrated in the midline brainstem and dorsolateral medullary reticular formation and the anterior hypothalamus-preoptic area, with possible intermingling of the two in the basal forebrain. Just as cells with different activity profiles and primary functional involvements are codistributed in such fields, cells with different projections, including ascending versus descending, are intermingled in the same fields and may thus respectively modulate forebrain and spinal activities during the sleep–wake cycle.

Neurochemical Results

Just as cells with different activities and projections are interdigitated in the reticular core, so cells containing different neuroactive chemicals are intermingled through the same regions. It is thus possible that the specificity of action derives from the neurotransmitter released as well as from the activity and projections of the neurons. Although such a behavioral specificity may not apply to the small amino acid neurotransmitters that are contained and act in multiple local-circuit neurons, it may apply to the amine (more appropriately called) neuromodulators, including catecholamines, acetylcholine, histamine, and serotonin, which are contained in restricted neuronal aggregates located in the reticular core and have widespread projections to the forebrain and spinal cord. Such systems may simultaneously bias or modify the mode of activity of entire populations of neurons in the central nervous system. Moreover, molecules of larger peptides may also function as neuromodulators or even neurohormones that may be responsible for even longer-lasting alterations in neuronal function that would underlie the sleep–wake states and cycle. However, to date, no single chemical neurotransmitter, neuromodulator, or neurohormone has been identified that is necessary or sufficient for the generation and maintenance of sleep or waking. Instead, multiple factors and systems are involved in the onset and maintenance of these states.

Overview of Sleep–Wake Mechanisms

Wakefulness is initiated and reinforced by particular visceral, somatic, and special sensory input, which is transmitted fairly directly to special cortical areas but also, and more important for wakefulness, through collaterals to the brainstem reticular formation, extending from the medulla to the midbrain, in which visceral, somatic, auditory, vestibular, and visual sensory collaterals proliferate. This system overlaps extensively with systems in the brainstem and caudal hypothalamus that regulate the sympathetic nervous system. Activation is transmitted into the forebrain and cortex through the nonspecific thalamocortical projection system and through the subthalamus, hypothalamus, and basal forebrain, where cortically projecting cells are also located. Olfactory sensory input may also influence activation by collateral transmission through the basal forebrain neurons. In this isodendritic core, particular neurons that are distributed through the brainstem, hypothalamus, and basal forebrain are activated more or less during waking, depending on sensory input from internal and external milieus; however, they appear to remain tonically active at some level during this state, irrespective of sensory input,

according to an autochthonous rhythm. This activating system is essential for the maintenance of wakefulness and cortical activation indicative of that state. In this system of cells are located catecholaminergic and cholinergic neurons that are tonically active during wakefulness and that, through particularly long and widespread forebrain projections, may modulate the activity of the subcortical and cortical neurons and circuits to facilitate tonic fast discharge in thalamocortical systems. Histamine-containing neurons and orexin-containing neurons located in the posterior hypothalamus also contribute through long projections to this modulation. The predominant neurotransmitter of neurons of the reticular activating system, as well as thalamic and cortical projection neurons, is glutamate, the excitatory amino acid that is essential for activity in these systems. Certain neuropeptides contained in neurons with relatively long and widespread projections and also colocalized with smaller neurotransmitters, such as substance P, vasoactive intestinal peptide, neurotensin, corticotropin-releasing hormone, and thyrotropin-releasing hormone, may enhance and prolong such actions to promote activation. Certain factors carried in the blood, including epinephrine, histamine, and certain peptides, can serve to reinforce the central state of arousal.

Aided by a decrease in certain types of sensory input and facilitated by an increase in other types of somatic and visceral sensory input, such as warmth and satiation, sleep-inducing neurons become active and promote cortical slow wave activity by dampening the cyclic activity of reticular activating neurons and directly modulating activity in the forebrain. Sleep-inducing neurons are concentrated in the lower brainstem reticular formation and solitary tract nucleus and in the rostral hypothalamus, preoptic area, and basal forebrain, extensively overlapping with autonomic, particularly parasympathetic, regulatory systems. Cortical slow wave activity evolves from a change in the pattern of discharge of cortical and thalamic neurons from tonic and fast to bursting at a slow rate with intervening pauses. Serotonin-containing neurons of the raphe may be important in dampening certain sensory input and attenuating cortical activation in the initiation of slow wave sleep. Adenosine may be a factor that accumulates during waking and could promote slow-bursting discharge in thalamocortical systems. Critical for spindling and slow waves is the activity of GABAergic neurons located in the thalamic reticular nucleus. GABAergic neurons in many other regions, including the reticular formation, hypothalamus, and basal forebrain, also may be important for inhibiting neurons involved in cortical activation. GABAergic neurons located in the hypothalamus and basal forebrain that project to the cortex may be important for initiating and maintaining slow wave activity. Multiple neuropeptide-containing neurons are located in the brainstem and hypothalamic-basal forebrain regions and may, through release of peptide onto other neurons or into the CSF, alter activity and transmission through the forebrain. The peptides somatostatin and cortistatin are colocalized with GABA in neurons in the thalamus and cortex. The sleep-promoting substances of the CSF remain to be identified; however, several known substances, including the opiates, cortistatin, and oleamide, have been shown to have certain sleep-inducing properties when introduced into the CSF. Peripheral factors, such as serotonin, insulin, gut hormones, cytokines, and sleep peptides, may also influence the sleep–wake cycle and facilitate sleep.

In summary, many of the chemical and neuronal substrates of the sleep–wake states have been identified and characterized according to their activity and transmission. Many other chemical neuroactive substances await discovery and, as components of multifarious systems, hold promise to play important roles in the generation of waking and sleep.

Clinical Pearl

Sleep and wakefulness are controlled by diverse neuronal systems containing diverse chemicals in the brain. Thus, lesions can result in either somnolence or insomnia depending on their location. Loss of wakefulness, marked by loss of cortical activation or behavioral arousal, can occur with lesions in the oral pontine and midbrain tegmentum, involving the glutamatergic neurons of the reticular formation, noradrenergic locus coeruleus neurons, cholinergic pontomesencephalic tegmental neurons, or dopaminergic ventral tegmental neurons; lesions in the posterior hypothalamus, involving histaminergic or orexinergic neurons; or lesions in the basal forebrain, involving cholinergic basalis neurons. Loss of natural sleep can occur with lesions located in the lower brainstem or preoptic area in the forebrain, involving particularly GABAergic neurons.

Acknowledgments

The author thanks members of the laboratory, including Lynda Mainville for technical assistance and Elida Arriza for help with illustrations. The author's research has been funded by the Canadian Institutes of Health Research (CIHR) and U.S. National Institutes of Health (NIH).

References

1. Kleitman N: Sleep and Wakefulness. Chicago, University of Chicago Press, 1939.
2. Bremer F: Cerveau 'isole' et physiologie du sommeil. C R Soc Biol (Paris) 1929;102:1235.
3. Moruzzi G, Magoun HW: Brain stem reticular formation and activation of the EEG. Electroencephalogr Clin Neurophysiol 1949;1:455.
4. Lindsley DB, Schreiner LH, Knowles WB, et al: Behavioral and EEG changes following chronic brain stem lesions. Electroencephalogr Clin Neurophysiol 1950;2:483.
5. Starzl TE, Taylor CW, Magoun HW: Ascending conduction in reticular activating system, with special reference to the diencephalon. J Neurophysiol 1951;14:461.
6. Nauta WJH, Kuypers HGJM: Some ascending pathways in the brain stem reticular formation. In: Jasper HH, Proctor LD, Knighton RS, et al (eds): Reticular Formation of the Brain. Boston, Little, Brown, 1958, p 3.
7. Scheibel ME, Scheibel AB: Structural substrates for integrative patterns in the brain stem reticular core. In: Jasper HH, Proctor LD, Knighton RS, et al (eds): Reticular Formation of the Brain. Boston, Little, Brown, 1958, p 31.
8. Gayet M: Affection encephalique (encephalite diffuse probable). Arch Physiol Norm Pathol 1875;2:341.
9. Mauthner L: Zur Pathologie und Physiologie des Schlafes nebst Bermerkungen ueber die "Nona." Wien Klin Wochenschr 1890; 40:961.
10. von Economo C: Encephalitis Lethargica: Its Sequelae and Treatment. London, Oxford University Press, 1931.
11. Plum F, Posner JB: The Diagnosis of Stupor and Coma. Philadelphia, Davis, 1980.
12. Parvizi J, Damasio AR: Neuroanatomical correlates of brainstem coma. Brain 2003;126:1524.
13. Feldman SM, Waller HJ: Dissociation of electrocortical activation and behavioural arousal. Nature 1962;196:1320.
14. Moruzzi G: The sleep-waking cycle. Ergebn Physiol 1972;64:1.
15. Villablanca J: The electrocorticogram in the chronic *cerveau isole* cat. Electroencephalogr Clin Neurophysiol 1965;19:576.
16. Adametz JH: Rate of recovery of functioning in cats with rostral reticular lesions. J Neurosurg 1959;16:85.
17. Villablanca J, Salinas-Zeballos ME: Sleep-wakefulness, EEG and behavioral studies of chronic cats without the thalamus: The 'athalamic' cat. Arch Ital Biol 1972;110:383.
18. Kievit J, Kuypers HGJM: Basal forebrain and hypothalamic connections to frontal and parietal cortex in the rhesus monkey. Science 1975;187:660.
19. Hess WR: The Functional Organization of the Diencephalon. New York, Grune & Stratton, 1957.
20. Nauta WJH: Hypothalamic regulation of sleep in rats: An experimental study. J Neurophysiol 1946;9:285.
21. Sallanon M, Sakai K, Buda C, et al: Increase of paradoxical sleep induced by microinjections of ibotenic acid into the ventrolateral part of the posterior hypothalamus in the cat. Arch Ital Biol 1988;126:87.
22. Stewart DJ, MacFabe DF, Vanderwolf CH: Cholinergic activation of the electrocorticogram: Role of the substantia innominata and effects of atropine and quinuclidinyl benzilate. Brain Res 1984; 322:219.
23. LoConte G, Casamenti F, Bigi V, et al: Effect of magnocellular forebrain nuclei lesions on acetylcholine output from the cerebral cortex, electrocorticogram and behaviour. Arch Ital Biol 1982;120:176.
24. Jones BE: Reticular formation: Cytoarchitecture, transmitters and projections. In Paxinos G (ed): The Rat Nervous System, 2nd ed. Sydney, Academic Press Australia, 1995, p 155.
25. Steriade M, Hobson JA: Neuronal activity during the sleep-waking cycle. Prog Neurobiol 1976;6:155.
26. Steriade M: Mechanisms underlying cortical activation: Neuronal organization and properties of the midbrain reticular core and intralaminar thalamic nuclei. In Pompeiano O, Ajmone Marsan C (eds): Brain Mechanisms and Perceptual Awareness. New York, Raven Press, 1981, p 327.
27. Szymusiak R, McGinty D: Sleep-related neuronal discharge in the basal forebrain of cats. Brain Res 1986;370:82.
28. Sakai K, El Mansari M, Lin J-S, et al: The posterior hypothalamus in the regulation of wakefulness and paradoxical sleep. In Mancia M, Marini G (eds): The Diencephalon and Sleep. New York, Raven Press, 1990 p 171.
29. Batini C, Moruzzi G, Palestini M, et al: Effects of complete pontine transections of the sleep-wakefulness rhythm: The midpontine pretrigeminal preparation. Arch Ital Biol 1959;97:1.
30. Markand ON, Dyken ML: Sleep abnormalities in patients with brain stem lesions. Neurology 1976;26:769.
31. Magnes J, Moruzzi G, Pompeiano O: Synchronization of the EEG produced by low-frequency electrical stimulation of the region of the solitary tract. Arch Ital Biol 1961;99:33.
32. Bonvallet M, Dell P, Hiebel G: Tonus sympathique et activite electrique corticale. Electroencephalogr Clin Neurophysiol 1954;6:119.
33. Norgren R: Projections from the nucleus of the solitary tract in the rat. Neuroscience 1978;3:207.
34. Ricardo JA, Koh ET: Anatomical evidence of direct projections from the nucleus of the solitary tract to the hypothalamus, amygdala, and other forebrain structures in the rat. Brain Res 1978;153:1.
35. Morison RS, Dempsey EW: A study of thalamo-cortical relations. Am J Physiol 1942;135:281.
36. Akert K, Koella WP, Hess RJ: Sleep produced by electrical stimulation of the thalamus. Am J Physiol 1952;168:260.

37. Lugaresi E, Medori R, Montagna P, et al: Fatal familial insomnia and dysautonomia with selective degeneration of thalamic nuclei. N Engl J Med 1986;315:997.

38. Sterman MB, Clemente CD: Forebrain inhibitory mechanisms: Sleep patterns induced by basal forebrain stimulation in the behaving cat. Exp Neurol 1962;6:103.

39. McGinty DJ, Sterman MB: Sleep suppression after basal forebrain lesions in the cat. Science 1968;160:1253.

40. Villablanca J, Marcus R: Sleep-wakefulness, EEG and behavioral studies of chronic cats without neocortex and striatum: The 'diencephalic' cat. Arch Ital Biol 1972;110:348.

41. Penaloza-Rojas JH, Elterman M, Olmos N: Sleep induced by cortical stimulation. Exp Neurol 1964;10:140.

42. Villablanca JR, Marcus RJ, Olmstead CE: Effects of caudate nuclei or frontal cortex ablations in cats: II. Sleep-wakefulness, EEG, and motor activity. Exp Neurol 1976;53:31.

43. Jouvet M: Recherches sur les structures nerveuses et les mécanismes responsables des differentes phases du sommeil physiologique. Arch Ital Biol 1962;100:125.

44. Nauta WJ, Haymaker W: Hypothalamic nuclei and fiber connections. In Haymaker W, Andersoon E, Nauta WJH (eds): The Hypothalamus. Springfield, Ill, Charles C Thomas, 1969, p 136.

45. Swanson LW: An autoradiographic study of the efferent connections of the preoptic region in the rat. J Comp Neurol 1976; 167:227.

46. Lineberry CG, Siegel J: EEG synchronization, behavioral inhibition, and mesencephalic unit effects produced by stimulation of orbital cortex, basal forebrain and caudate nucleus. Brain Res 1971;34:143.

47. Ricardo JA: Hypothalamic pathways involved in metabolic regulatory functions, as identified by track-tracing methods. Adv Metab Disord 1983;10:1.

48. van der Kooy D, Koda LY, McGinty JF, et al: The organization of projections from the cortex, amygdala, and hypothalamus to the nucleus of the solitary tract in rat. J Comp Neurol 1984;224:1.

49. McGinty DJ, Harper RM, Fairbanks MK: Neuronal unit activity and the control of sleep states. Adv Sleep Res 1974;1:173.

50. Eguchi K, Satoh T: Characterization of the neurons in the region of solitary tract nucleus during sleep. Physiol Behav 1980;24:99.

51. Szymusiak R, Alam N, Steininger TL, et al: Sleep-waking discharge patterns of ventrolateral preoptic/anterior hypothalamic neurons in rats. Brain Res 1998;803:178.

52. Sherin JE, Shiromani PJ, McCarley RW, et al: Activation of ventrolateral preoptic neurons during sleep. Science 1996;271:216.

53. Evarts EV: Temporal patterns of discharge of pyramidal tract neurons during sleep and waking in the monkey. J Neurophysiol 1964;27:152.

54. Steriade M, Llinas RR: The functional states of the thalamus and the associated neuronal interplay. Physiol Rev 1988;68:649.

55. Steriade M, Contreras D, Amzica F: Synchronized sleep oscillations and their paroxysmal developments. Trends Neurosci 1994;17:199.

56. Pieron H: Le Probleme Physiologique du Sommeil. Paris, Masson, 1913.

57. Jouvet M: The role of monoamines and acetylcholine-containing neurons in the regulation of the sleep-waking cycle. Ergebn Physiol 1972;64:165.

58. Jones BE: The respective involvement of noradrenaline and its deaminated metabolites in waking and paradoxical sleep: A neuropharmacological model. Brain Res 1972;39:121.

59. Dahlstrom A, Fuxe K: Evidence for the existence of monoamine-containing neurons in the central nervous system: I. Demonstration of monoamines in the cell bodies of brain stem neurons. Acta Physiol Scand Suppl 1964;232:1.

60. Bjorklund A, Lindvall O: Dopamine-containing systems in the CNS. In Bjorklund A, Hokfelt T (eds): Handbook of Chemical Neuroanatomy, vol 2. Classical Transmitters in the CNS, part I. Amsterdam, Elsevier, 1984, p 55.

61. Hokfelt T, Martensson R, Bjorklund A, et al: Distributional maps of tyrosine-hydroxylase-immunoreactive neurons in the rat brain. In Bjorklund A, Hokfelt T (eds): Handbook of Chemical Neuroanatomy, vol 2. Classical Transmitters in the CNS, part I. Amsterdam, Elsevier, 1984, p 277.

62. Jones BE, Yang T-Z: The efferent projections from the reticular formation and the locus coeruleus studied by anterograde and retrograde axonal transport in the rat. J Comp Neurol 1985;242:56.

63. Jones BE, Bobillier P, Pin C, et al: The effect of lesions of catecholamine-containing neurons upon monoamine content of the brain and EEG and behavioral waking in the cat. Brain Res 1973;58:157.

64. Bernheimer H, Birkmayer W, Hornykiewicz O, et al: Brain dopamine and the syndromes of Parkinson and Huntington. J Neurol Sci 1973;20:415.

65. Schott B, Michel D, Mouret J, et al: Monoamines et regulation de la vigilance: II. Syndromes lesionnels du systeme nerveux central. Rev Neurol 1972;127:157.

66. Di Rocco C, Maira G, Meglio M, et al: L-DOPA treatment of comatose states due to cerebral lesions. J Neurosurg Sci 1974;18:169.

67. Stricker EM, Zigmond MJ: Recovery of function following damage to central catecholamine-containing neurons: A neurochemical model for the lateral hypothalamic syndrome. Prog Psychobiol Physiol Psychol 1975;6:121.

68. Laguzzi R, Petitjean F, Pujol JF, et al: Effets de l'injection intraventriculaire de 6-hydroxydopamine: II. Sur le cycle veille-sommeils du chat. Brain Res 1972;48:295.

69. Jones BE, Harper ST, Halaris AE: Effects of locus coeruleus lesions upon cerebral monoamine content, sleep-wakefulness states and the response to amphetamine. Brain Res 1977;124:473.

70. Cespuglio R, Gomez ME, Faradji H, et al: Alterations in the sleep-waking cycle induced by cooling of the locus coeruleus area. Electroencephalogr Clin Neurophysiol 1982;54:570.

71. Ljungberg T, Apicella P, Schultz W: Responses of monkey dopamine neurons during learning of behavioral reactions. J Neurophysiol 1992;67:145.

72. Hobson JA, McCarley RW, Wyzinski PW: Sleep cycle oscillation: Reciprocal discharge by two brainstem neuronal groups. Science 1975;189:55.

73. Jacobs BL: Single unit activity of locus coeruleus neurons in behaving animals. Prog Neurobiol 1986;27:183.

74. Aston-Jones G, Bloom FE: Activity of norepinephrine-containing locus coeruleus neurons in behaving rats anticipates fluctuations in the sleep-waking cycle. J Neurosci 1981;1:876.

75. Trulson ME: Simultaneous recording of substantia nigra neurons and voltametric release of dopamine in the caudate of behaving cats. Brain Res Bull 1985;15:221.

76. Kalen P, Rosegren E, Lindvall O, et al: Hippocampal noradrenaline and serotonin release over 24 hours as measured by the dialysis technique in freely moving rats: Correlation to behavioural activity state, effect of handling and tail-pinch. Eur J Neurosci 1989;1:181.

77. McCormick DA: Neurotransmitter actions in the thalamus and cerebral cortex and their role in neuromodulation of thalamocortical activity. Prog Neurobiol 1992;39:337.

78. Broughton RJ, Fleming JA, George CF, et al: Randomized, double-blind, placebo-controlled crossover trial of modafinil in the treatment of excessive daytime sleepiness in narcolepsy. Neurology 1997;49:444.

79. Lin JS, Roussel B, Akaoka H, et al: Role of catecholamines in the modafinil and amphetamine induced wakefulness: A comparative pharmacological study in the cat. Brain Res 1992;591:319.

80. Domino EF, Yamamoto K, Dren AT: Role of cholinergic mechanisms in states of wakefulness and sleep. Prog Brain Res 1968; 28:113.

81. Jones BE: Arousal systems. Front Biosci 2003;8:S438.

82. Jones BE: The organization of central cholinergic systems and their functional importance in sleep-waking states. Prog Brain Res 1993;98:61.

83. Mesulam M-M, Mufson EJ, Levey AI, et al: Atlas of cholinergic neurons in the forebrain and upper brainstem of the macaque based on monoclonal choline acetyltransferase immunohistochemistry and acetylcholinesterase histochemistry. Neuroscience 1984;12:669.

84. Szymusiak R, McGinty D: Sleep suppression following kainic acid-induced lesions of the basal forebrain. Exp Neurol 1986;94:598.

85. Jones BE: Activity, modulation and role of basal forebrain cholinergic neurons innervating the cerebral cortex. Prog Brain Res 2004;145:157.

86. Prinz PN, Peskind ER, Vitaliano PP, et al: Changes in the sleep and waking EEGs of nondemented and demented elderly subjects. J Am Geriatr Soc 1982;30:86.

87. Frolich L: The cholinergic pathology in Alzheimer's disease: Discrepancies between clinical experience and pathophysiological findings. J Neural Transm 2002;109:1003.

88. Hirano A, Zimmerman HM: Alzheimer's neurofibrillary changes. Arch Neurol 1962;7:227.

89. Ishii T: Distribution of Alzheimer's neurofibrillary changes in the brain stem and hypothalamus of senile dementia. Acta Neuropathol 1966;6:181.

90. El Mansari M, Sakai M, Jouvet M: Unitary characteristics of presumptive cholinergic tegmental neurons during the sleep-waking cycle in freely moving cats. Exp Brain Res 1989;76:519.

91. Williams JA, Comisarow J, Day J, et al: State-dependent release of acetylcholine in rat thalamus measured by *in vivo* microdialysis. J Neurosci 1994;14:5236.

92. Marrosu F, Portas C, Mascia S, et al: Microdialysis measurement of cortical and hippocampal acetylcholine release during sleep-wake cycle in freely moving cats. Brain Res 1995; 671:329.

93. Lin JS, Sakai K, Jouvet M: Evidence for histaminergic arousal mechanisms in the hypothalamus of cats. Neuropharmacology 1988;27:111.

94. Monnier M, Sauer R, Hatt AM: The activating effect of histamine on the central nervous system. Int Rev Neurobiol 1970;12:265.

95. Steinbusch HWM, Mulder AH: Immunohistochemical localization of histamine in neurons and mast cells in the rat brain. In Bjorklund A, Hokfelt T, Kuhar MJ (eds): Handbook of Chemical Neuroanatomy, vol 3. Classical Transmitters in the CNS, part II. Amsterdam, Elsevier, 1984, p 126.

96. Vanni-Mercier G, Sakai K, Jouvet M: Neurones spécifiques de l'eveil dans l'hypothalamus posterieur. C R Acad Sci Paris 1984;298:195.

97. Mayer ML, Westbrook GL: The physiology of excitatory amino acids in the vertebrate central nervous system. Prog Neurobiol 1987;28:197.

98. Ottersen OP, Storm-Mathisen J: Neurons containing or accumulating transmitter amino acids. In Bjorklund A, Hokfelt T, Kuhar MJ (eds): Handbook of Chemical Neuroanatomy, vol 3. Classical Transmitters and Transmitter Receptors in the CNS, part II. Amsterdam, Elsevier, 1984, p 141.

99. Jasper HH, Khan RT, Elliott KAC: Amino acids released from the cerebral cortex in relation to its state of activation. Science 1965;147:1448.

100. Armstrong-James M, Fox K: Evidence for a specific role for cortical NMDA receptors in slow wave sleep. Brain Res 1988;451:189.

101. Ursin R: Endogenous sleep factors. Exp Brain Res 1984; (Suppl 8):118.

102. Fencl V, Koski G, Pappenheimer JR: Factors in cerebrospinal fluid from goats that affect sleep and activity in rats. J Physiol (Lond) 1971;216:565.

103. Riou F, Cespuglio R, Jouvet M: Endogenous peptides and sleep in the rat: I. Peptides decreasing paradoxical sleep. Neuropeptides 1982;2:243.

104. Cape EG, Manns ID, Alonso A, et al: Neurotensin-induced bursting of cholinergic basal forebrain neurons promotes gamma and theta cortical activity together with waking and paradoxical sleep. J Neurosci 2000;20:8452.

105. Ehlers C, Reed TK, Henriksen SJ: Effects of corticotropin-releasing factor and growth hormone-releasing factor on sleep and activity in rats. Neuroendocrinology 1986;42:467.

106. Lin L, Faraco J, Li R, et al: The sleep disorder canine narcolepsy is caused by a mutation in the hypocretin (orexin) receptor 2 gene. Cell 1999;98:365.

107. Chemelli RM, Willie JT, Sinton CM, et al: Narcolepsy in orexin knockout mice: Molecular genetics of sleep regulation. Cell 1999;98:437.

108. Peyron C, Tighe DK, van den Pol AN, et al: Neurons containing hypocretin (orexin) project to multiple neuronal systems. J Neurosci 1998;18:9996.

109. Bourgin P, Huitron-Resendiz S, Spier AD, et al: Hypocretin-1 modulates rapid eye movement sleep through activation of locus coeruleus neurons. J Neurosci 2000;20:7760.

110. Bayer L, Eggermann E, Saint-Mleux B, et al: Selective action of orexin (hypocretin) on nonspecific thalamocortical projection neurons. J Neurosci 2002;22:7835.

111. Eriksson KS, Sergeeva O, Brown RE, et al: Orexin/hypocretin excites the histaminergic neurons of the tuberomammillary nucleus. J Neurosci 2001;21:9273.

112. Eggermann E, Serafin M, Bayer L, et al: Orexins/hypocretins excite basal forebrain cholinergic neurones. Neuroscience 2001;108:177.

113. Alam MN, Gong H, Alam T, et al: Sleep-waking discharge patterns of neurons recorded in the rat perifornical lateral hypothalamic area. J Physiol (Lond) 2002;538:619.

114. Thannickal TC, Moore RY, Nienhuis R, et al: Reduced number of hypocretin neurons in human narcolepsy. Neuron 2000;27:469.

115. Hara J, Beuckmann CT, Nambu T, et al: Genetic ablation of orexin neurons in mice results in narcolepsy, hypophagia, and obesity. Neuron 2001;30:345.

116. Weitzman ED, Zimmerman JC, Czeiler CA, et al: Cortisol secretion is inhibited during sleep in normal men. J Clin Endocrinol Metab 1983;56:352.

117. Steinbusch HWM: Serotonin-immunoreactive neurons and their projections in the CNS. In Bjorklund A, Hokfelt T, Kuhar MJ (eds): Handbook of Chemical Neuroanatomy, vol 3. Classical Transmitters in the CNS, Part II. Amsterdam, Elsevier, 1984, p 68.

118. Freemon FR, Salinas-Garcia RF, Ward JW: Sleep patterns in a patient with a brain stem infarction involving the raphe nucleus. Electroencephalogr Clin Neurophysiol 1974;36:657.

119. Fischer-Perroudon C, Mouret J, Jouvet M: Sur un cas d'agrypnie (4 mois sans sommeil) au cours d'une maladie de Morvan: Effet favorable du 5-hydroxytryptophane. Electroencephalogr Clin Neurophysiol 1974;36:1.

120. Froment J-L, Petitjean F, Bertrand N, et al: Effets de l'injection intracérébrale de 5,6-hydroxytryptamine sur les monoamines cérébrales et les états de sommeil du chat. Brain Res 1974;67:405.

121. McGinty D, Harper RM: Dorsal raphe neurons: Depression of firing during sleep in cats. Brain Res 1976;101:569.

122. Puizillout JJ, Gaudin-Chazal G, Daszuta A, et al: Release of endogenous serotonin from 'encephale isole' cats. J Physiol (Paris) 1979;75:531.

123. Fields HL, Basbaum AI: Brain stem control of spinal pain transmission neurons. Annu Rev Physiol 1978;40:193.

124. Jacobs BL: Electrophysiological and behavioral effects of electrical stimulation of the raphe nuclei in cats. Physiol Behav 1973;11:489.

125. Luebke JI, Greene RW, Semba K, et al: Serotonin hyperpolarizes cholinergic low-threshold burst neurons in the rat laterodorsal tegmental nucleus *in vitro*. Proc Natl Acad Sci U S A 1992; 89:743.

126. Khateb A, Fort P, Alonso A, et al: Pharmacological and immuno-histochemical evidence for a serotonergic input to cholinergic nucleus basalis neurons. Eur J Neurosci 1993;5:541.

127. Cape EG, Jones BE: Differential modulation of high frequency gamma electroencephalogram activity and sleep-wake state by noradrenaline and serotonin microinjections into the region of cholinergic basalis neurons. J Neurosci 1998;18:2653.

128. Jouvet M: Neuromediateurs et facteurs hypnogenes. Rev Neurol (Paris) 1984;140:389.

129. Morales M, Bloom FE: The 5-HT$_3$ receptor is present in different subpopulations of GABAergic neurons in the rat telencephalon. J Neurosci 1997;17:3157.

130. Radulovacki M, Virus RM, Djuricic-Nedelson M, et al: Adenosine and adenosine analogs: Effects on sleep in rats. In McGinty DJ, Morrison A, Drucker-Colin R, et al (eds): Brain Mechanisms of Sleep. New York, Raven Press, 1985, p 235.

131. Benington JH, Kodali SK, Heller HC: Stimulation of A$_1$ adenosine receptors mimics the electroencephalographic effects of sleep deprivation. Brain Res 1995;692:79.

132. Braas KM, Newby AC, Wilson VS, et al: Adenosine-containing neurons in the brain localized by immunocytochemistry. J Neurosci 1986;6:1952.

133. Newby AC: Adenosine and the concept of 'retaliatory metabolites.' Trends Biol Sci 1984;9:42.

134. Porkka-Heiskanen T, Strecker RE, Thakkar M, et al: Adenosine: A mediator of the sleep-inducing effects of prolonged wakefulness. Science 1997;276:1265.

135. Huston JP, Haas HL, Boix F, et al: Extracellular adenosine levels in neostriatum and hippocampus during rest and activity periods of rats. Neuroscience 1996;73:99.

136. Rainnie DG, Grunze HCR, McCarley RW, et al: Adenosine inhibition of mesopontine cholinergic neurons: Implications for EEG arousal. Science 1994;263:689.

137. Pape H-C: Adenosine promotes burst activity in guinea-pig geniculocortical neurones through two different ionic mechanisms. J Physiol (Lond) 1992;447:729.

138. Benington JH, Heller HC: Restoration of brain energy metabolism as the function of sleep. Prog Neurobiol 1995;45:347.

139. Mendelson WB: GABA-benzodiazepine receptor-chloride ionophore complex: Implications for the pharmacology of sleep. In Wauquier A, Monti JM, Gaillard JM, et al (eds): Sleep: Neurotransmitters and Neuromodulators. New York, Raven Press, 1985, p 229.

140. Rothstein JD, Guidotti A, Tinuper P, et al: Endogenous benzodiazepine receptor ligands in idiopathic recurring stupor. Lancet 1992;340:1002.

141. Mugnaini E, Oertel WH: An atlas of the distribution of GABAergic neurons and terminals. In Bjorklund A, Hokfelt T (eds): Handbook of Chemical Neuroanatomy, vol 4. GABA and Neuropeptides in the CNS, part I. Amsterdam, Elsevier, 1985, p 436.

142. Steriade M, Deschenes M: The thalamus as a neuronal oscillator. Brain Res Rev 1984;8:1.

143. Hofle N, Paus T, Reutens D, et al: Regional cerebral blood flow changes as a function of delta and spindle activity during slow wave sleep in humans. J Neurosci 1997;17:4800.

144. Gritti I, Mainville L, Jones BE: Codistribution of GABA- with acetylcholine-synthesizing neurons in the basal forebrain of the rat. J Comp Neurol 1993;329:438.

145. Gritti I, Mainville L, Jones BE: Projections of GABAergic and cholinergic basal forebrain and GABAergic preoptic-anterior hypothalamic neurons to the posterior lateral hypothalamus of the rat. J Comp Neurol 1994;339:251.

146. Sherin JE, Elmquist JK, Torrealba F, et al: Innervation of histaminergic tuberomammillary neurons by GABAergic and galaninergic neurons in the ventrolateral preoptic nucleus of the rat. J Neurosci 1998;18:4705.

147. Nitz D, Siegel JM: GABA release in posterior hypothalamus across sleep-wake cycle. Am J Physiol 1996;271:R1707.

148. Vincent SR, Hokfelt T, Skirboll LR, et al: Hypothalamic gamma-aminobutyric acid neurons project to the neocortex. Science 1983;220:1309.

149. Gritti I, Mainville L, Mancia M, et al: GABAergic and other non-cholinergic basal forebrain neurons project together with cholinergic neurons to meso- and iso-cortex in the rat. J Comp Neurol 1997;383:163.

150. Szymusiak R, McGinty D: Sleep-waking discharge of basal forebrain projection neurons in cats. Brain Res Bull 1989;22:423.

151. Crunelli V, Leresche N: A role for GABA$_B$ receptors in excitation and inhibition of thalamocortical cells. Trends Neurosci 1991;14:16.

152. Krosigk Mv, Bal T, McCormick DA: Cellular mechanisms of a synchronized oscillation in the thalamus. Science 1993;261:361.

153. Faulhaber J, Steiger A, Lancel M: The GABA$_A$ agonist THIP produces slow wave sleep and reduces spindling activity in NREM sleep in humans. Psychopharmacology 1997;130:285.

154. Lapierre O, Montplaisir J, Lamarre M, et al: The effect of gamma-hydroxybutyrate on nocturnal and diurnal sleep of normal subjects: Further considerations on REM sleep-triggering mechanisms. Sleep 1990;13:24.

155. Williams SR, Turner JP, Crunelli V: Gamma-hydroxybutyrate promotes oscillatory activity of rat and cat thalamocortical neurons by a tonic GABA$_B$ receptor-mediated hyperpolarization. Neuroscience 1995;66:135.

156. Bronzino JD, Kelly ML, Cordova C, et al: Amplitude and spectral quantification of the effects of morphine. Electroencephalogr Clin Neurophysiol 1982;53:14.

157. Havlicek V, Friesen HG: Comparison of behavioral effects of somatostatin and beta-endorphin in animals. In Collu R, Ducharme JR, Barbeau A, et al (eds): Central Nervous System Effects of Hypothalamic Hormones and Other Peptides. New York, Raven Press, 1979, p 381.

158. Riou F, Cespuglio R, Jouvet M: Endogenous peptides and sleep in the rat: II. Peptides without significant effect on the sleep-waking cycle. Neuropeptides 1982;2:255.

159. Basbaum AI, Fields HL: Endogenous pain control systems: Brainstem spinal pathways and endorphin circuitry. Annu Rev Neurosci 1984;7:309.

160. Petrusz P, Merchenthaler I, Maderdrut JL: Distribution of enkephalin-containing neurons in the central nervous system. In Bjorklund A, Hokfelt T (eds): Handbook of Chemical Neuroanatomy, vol 4. GABA and Neuropeptides in the CNS, part I. Amsterdam, Elsevier, 1985, p 273.

161. Garzon M, Tejero S, Beneitez AM, et al: Opiate microinjections in the locus coeruleus area of the cat enhance slow wave sleep. Neuropeptides 1995;29:229.

162. Khachaturian H, Lewis ME, Tsou K, et al: β-Endorphin, A-MSH, ACTH, and related peptides. In Bjorklund A, Hokfelt T (eds): Handbook of Chemical Neuroanatomy, vol 4. GABA and Neuropeptides in the CNS, part I. Amsterdam, Elsevier, 1985, p 216.

163. Johansson O, Hokfelt T, Elde RP: Immunohistochemical distribution of somatostatin-like immunoreactivity in the central nervous system of the adult rat. Neuroscience 1984; 13:265.

164. Brown M, Vale W: Central nervous system effects of hypothalamic peptides. Endocrinology 1975;96:1333.

165. de Lecea L, Criado JR, Prospero-Garcia O, et al: A cortical neuropeptide with neuronal depressant and sleep-modulating properties. Nature 1996;381:242.

166. de Lecea L, del Rio JA, Criado JR, et al: Cortistatin is expressed in a distinct subset of cortical interneurons. J Neurosci 1997;17:5868.

167. Hokfelt T: Neuropeptides in perspective: the last ten years. Neuron 1991;7:867.

168. Sawchenko PE, Swanson LW, Rivier J, et al: The distribution of growth hormone-releasing factor (GRF) immunoreactivity in the central nervous system of the rat: An immunohistochemical study using antisera directed against rat hypothalamic GRF. J Comp Neurol 1985;237:100.

169. Beranek L, Obal F, Taishi P, et al: Changes in rat sleep after single and repeated injections of the long-acting somatostatin analog octreotide. Am J Physiol 1997;273:R1484.

170. Ueno R, Honda K, Inoue S, et al: Prostaglandin D2, a cerebral sleep-inducing substance in rats. Proc Natl Acad Sci U S A 1983;80:1735.

171. Krueger JM, Obal FJ, Fang J, et al: The role of cytokines in physiological sleep regulation. Ann NY Acad Sci 2001;933:211.

172. Cravatt BF, Prospero-Garcia O, Siuzdak G, et al: Chemical characterization of a family of brain lipids that induce sleep. Science 1995;268:1506.

173. Lerner RA, Siuzdak G, Prospero-Garcia O, et al: Cerebrodiene: A brain lipid isolated from sleep-deprived cats. Proc Natl Acad Sci U S A 1994;91:9505.

174. Bronzino JD, Morgane PJ, Stern WC: EEG synchronization following application of serotonin to area postrema. Am J Physiol 1972;223:376.

175. Danguir J, Nicolaidis S: Feeding, metabolism and sleep: Peripheral and central mechanisms. In McGinty DJ, Morrison A, Drucker-Colin R, et al (eds): Brain Mechanisms of Sleep. New York, Raven Press, 1985, p 322.

176. van Houten M, Posner BI, Kopriwa BM, et al: Insulin-binding sites in the rat brain: In vivo localization. Endocrinology 1979;105:666.

177. Kapas L, Obal F Jr, Krueger JM: Humoral regulation of sleep. Int Rev Neurobiol 1993;35:131.

178. de Saint Hilaire-Kafi A, Gibbs J, Nicolaidis S: Satiety and sleep: The effects of bombesin. Brain Res 1989;478:152.

179. Monnier M, Dudler L, Gachter R, et al: Delta sleep-inducing peptide (DSIP): EEG and motor activity in rabbits following intravenous administration. Neurosci Lett 1977;6:9.

180. Nagasaki H, Kitahama K, Valatx J-L, et al: Sleep-promoting effect of the sleep-promoting substance (SPS) and delta sleep-inducing peptide (DSIP) in the mouse. Brain Res 1980;192:276.

12

Control of Motoneurons during Sleep

Michael H. Chase

Francisco R. Morales

ABSTRACT

During non–rapid eye movement (NREM) quiet sleep, there is a slight decrease in somatic muscle activity compared with that during wakefulness. During REM sleep, there is a dramatic reduction in ongoing muscle activity to the extent that even background muscle tone is abolished. This occurs because the motoneurons that innervate muscle fibers are actively inhibited. The inhibitory neurotransmitter is glycine.

During active (REM) sleep, however, there also are brief periods of muscle contraction (the "twitches and jerks"), which usually take place during periods of rapid eye movements. These contractions occur due to excitatory processes (postsynaptic potentials) that impinge on motoneurons. Interestingly, even during these periods of excitatory potentials, motoneurons continue to be inhibited by glycine. Thus, throughout REM sleep, there is tonic inhibition of motoneurons, as well as phasically occurring brief periods of motoneuron excitation. Long-duration episodes of REM sleep can be readily induced by the pontine administration of either carbachol or a gamma-aminobutyric acid antagonist, such as bicuculline. The effective site is the nucleus pontis oralis, which is also responsible for initiating motor atonia during REM sleep.

There are various sleep disorders that involve abnormal patterns of motor inhibition, excitation, or both; these include cataplexy, restless leg syndrome, REM sleep behavior disorder, and sleep apnea, among others. These disorders occur in part, or in whole, because of the abnormal expression of the mechanisms, described previously, that control muscle activity during REM sleep.

In human beings, the passage from wakefulness to sleep is accompanied by a decrease in the degree of contraction of muscle fibers—that is, there is a decrease in muscle tone.[1,2] One of the first investigators to describe this reduction in muscle tone was Pakhomov,[3] who used a complex hydrodynamic system of tubes to measure the tonus of the flexors of the fingers. Atonia, or the complete lack of tone of somatic muscles, was subsequently found to occur in human beings during the state of active (i.e., rapid eye movement [REM]) sleep.[1] In 1959, Jouvet and coworkers[4] observed atonia of the neck muscles of the cat during active sleep. In human beings and cats, as well as in many other species,[1,5] there is a decrease in muscle tone during quiet (i.e., non–rapid eye movement [NREM]) sleep and atonia during active sleep. In this chapter, we describe the neural mechanisms that produce hypotonia during quiet sleep and atonia during active sleep.

In the somatic motor system, the alpha motoneuron is defined unambiguously: It is any nerve cell with an axon terminating on skeletal muscle fibers. The significance of motoneurons resides in the fact that they are the principal access of the nervous system to skeletal muscles. Sherrington stressed this point by referring to motoneurons as the final common pathway.[6]

The axon of a motoneuron gives off several terminals, each one innervating a muscle fiber. The motoneuron and the muscle fibers it supplies form a *motor unit*. It is truly a functional unit because all of the muscle fibers supplied by a single motoneuron contract simultaneously.

Command signals, which take the form of trains of action potentials, travel from the initial segment of the motor axon, where they originate, along the motor axon to muscle fibers. Most, but not all, muscles are constantly active when we are awake, especially when we maintain a posture or perform a movement. Their *tone* is due to the asynchronous, sustained firing of motoneurons.

All conscious or reflex commands to initiate or suppress movements are eventually directed to motoneurons. (Unless otherwise specified, all references to motoneurons are to alpha, rather than to gamma, motoneurons.) Activation of motoneurons leads to muscle contraction, and inhibition of motoneurons results in muscle atonia.

It is thought that motoneurons generate action potentials, which they use to initiate muscle contraction by changing the permeability of their cell membrane so ions can diffuse down preestablished electrochemical gradients. The suppression of motoneuron activity is achieved by a change in membrane permeability to certain ions (e.g., Cl^- and K^+). Instead of determining permeability changes themselves, their electrical consequences are directly measured with an intracellularly located recording microelectrode.

Before 1978,[7] all intracellular studies of motoneurons in all animals used acute techniques that required immobilization of the animal and, in most cases, artificial respiration and either anesthesia, decerebration, or spinal transection. However, it is necessary to study neuronal processes during naturally occurring behavioral states because the activity of sensory, motor, and integrative systems is differentially modulated during these states, especially during the background behaviors of sleep and wakefulness.[8] Moreover, certain phenomena are present during only one state of sleep or wakefulness and are nonexistent in the other states.[9]

Consequently, to examine the modulation of membrane potential and synaptic activity during the behaviors of sleep and wakefulness, we developed experimental techniques for intracellular recording from antidromically identified motoneurons that are located in the brainstem and lumbar spinal cord. The preparation is the intact, unanesthetized, undrugged, normally respiring cat; the techniques that are used are illustrated in Figures 12–1 and 12–2. These techniques have also

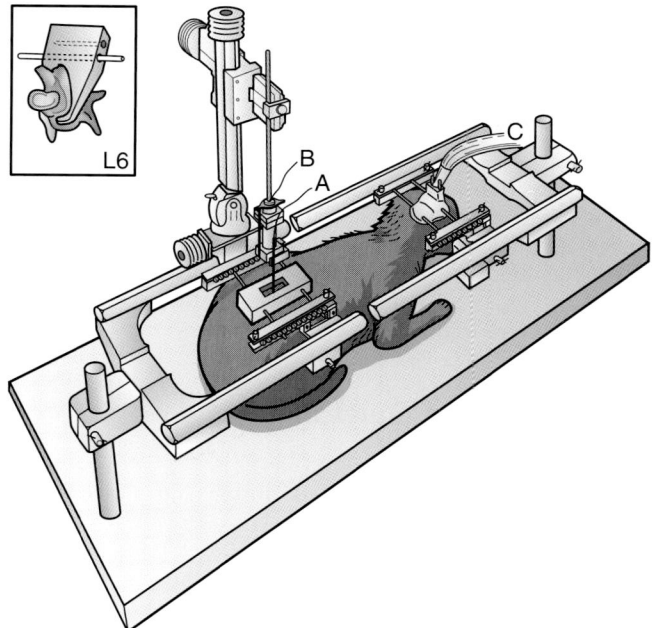

Figure 12–1. Diagram of the chronic cat preparation used to record intracellularly from spinal cord motoneurons. The intracellular electrode carrier is shown with a micropipette (A) being lowered by a microdrive (B) through a hole in the dorsal lamina of L5 to record from cells in the ventral horn (L7–S1 motonuclei). C is a cable connecting permanently placed electrodes with stimulating and recording equipment. *Inset* depicts one of the clamp-and-bar configurations used to immobilize the vertebral column. (From Physiology and Behavior, vol 27, Morales FR, Chase MH, Intracellular recording from spinal cord motoneurons in the chronic cat, 355-362, Copyright 1981, with permission from Elsevier Science.)

been used for intracellular recording from brainstem reticular neurons.[10]

Because the immediate premotor neural circuitry and neurotransmitters that control motoneurons bear the ultimate responsibility for the control of motor tone, this chapter is limited to a discussion of the specific factors that excite and inhibit motoneurons during sleep and wakefulness. At the end of this chapter, the suprasegmental sites and mechanisms that in turn control these controllers are briefly discussed. Unless otherwise specified, the work presented in this chapter represents data obtained from brainstem and spinal cord motoneurons that were reviewed in references 9 and 11 through 14.

BASIC PATTERNS OF MUSCLE ACTIVITY DURING SLEEP

There is a gradual decline in muscle tone (i.e., *hypotonia*) during quiet sleep compared with that during wakefulness. During active sleep, there is a strikingly potent tonic suppression of muscle activity, which often culminates in the complete loss of muscle tone, or *atonia*. In addition, a number of specific patterns of somatomotor suppression occur in the state of active sleep, such as at the onset of active sleep, during REM periods, and during NREM periods. Some of these patterns of suppression operate in conjunction with the concurrent excitation of motoneurons, whose discharge results in myoclonic twitches and jerks.

The two basic mechanisms that may be responsible for the suppression of muscle tone during active sleep are postsynaptic inhibition and disfacilitation (i.e., a reduction in the discharge of tonically active presynaptic excitatory neurons). The two mechanisms may operate continuously, be superimposed on each other at certain times, or act individually for restricted periods. Because measurements of disfacilitation are only indirect in intracellular recording from motoneurons, and to

Figure 12–2. Sagittal sections of the brainstem showing the relationship between various brainstem structures and the intracellular micropipette in the motor V nucleus **(A)**. The recording and stimulating electrodes are drawn approximately to scale. *Inset* **(B)** shows the anatomic and electrophysiologic relationship between the mesencephalic V nucleus and the motor V nucleus. 7N, facial nerve; BC, brachium conjunctivum; FTC, central tegmental field; FTG, gigantocellular tegmental field; FTL, lateral tegmental field; IC, inferior colliculus; INP, nucleus interpositus; PG, pontine gray; RN, red nucleus; SC, superior colliculus. (Reprinted with permission from Chase MH, Chandler SH, Nakamura Y: Intracellular determination of membrane potential of trigeminal motoneurons during sleep and wakefulness. J Neurophysiol 1980; 44:349-358.)

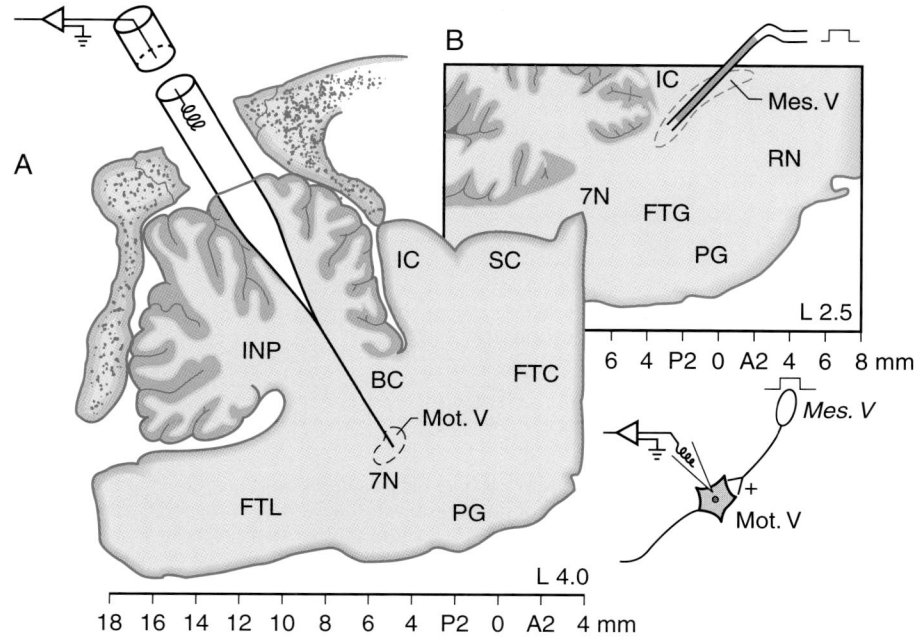

keep our focus centered on the final common executor, the motoneuron, we directed our attention to an exploration of the extent to which postsynaptic inhibition during active sleep could account for muscle atonia and postsynaptic excitation for myoclonic activity. These processes were explored through examination of the state dependence of motoneuron membrane properties and the action potentials and synaptic activity of brainstem and spinal cord motoneurons in the chronic, unanesthetized, undrugged cat during spontaneously occurring episodes of sleep and wakefulness.

Modulation of the Resting Membrane Potential of Motoneurons during Sleep

In the resting state, the membrane potential of a motoneuron is determined by the unequal concentration of ions inside and outside the cell and the differential permeability of its membrane to diverse ions, principally K^+, Na^+, and Cl^-. Experimentally, an initial membrane potential is recorded when the cell is first penetrated with an intracellularly directed microelectrode. A final determination of the resting membrane potential is obtained by taking, as a reference, the voltage recorded by the microelectrode when it is immediately withdrawn from the cell and is located juxtacellularly. In general, when a neuron is hyperpolarized, it is relatively less excitable; when it depolarizes, it is more excitable.

Transitions between Wakefulness and Quiet Sleep

When cats are awake and resting quietly (i.e., drowsy), passage into quiet sleep is accompanied by either a slight hyperpolarization or no discernible change in the level of the membrane potential of the motoneuron. When the animal is alert or actively moving or when the tonic electromyographic activity is

at a high level, the subsequent transition to quiet sleep is accompanied by an increase in the level of membrane polarization–hyperpolarization. However, in most cases, the membrane potential level remains relatively constant because quiet wakefulness or drowsiness usually is the forerunner of quiet sleep.

The transition from quiet sleep to aroused wakefulness is accompanied by membrane depolarization (Fig. 12–3). The degree of depolarization is usually correlated with the level of arousal, as indicated in the initial 15-second period of wakefulness in Figure 12–3 and the subsequent 15-second epoch in which there occurred an increase in neck muscle activity and membrane depolarization.

Transition from Quiet Sleep to Active Sleep

Motoneurons are hyperpolarized during active sleep compared with quiet sleep (Fig. 12–4). The degree of hyperpolarization varies from 2 to 10 mV; its development parallels the various ways in which active sleep emerges from quiet sleep. For example, although the onset of active sleep is demarcated by electroencephalographic desynchronization and a reduction in muscle tone, these indices are not always present at the same time, and either may precede the other as the animal enters the active sleep state. Moreover, electroencephalographic desynchronization and electromyographic suppression (Fig. 12–4, 3- to 4-minute time marks) often are correlated with each other and with membrane hyperpolarization, whereas at other times, hyperpolarization continues to develop beyond the period of the initial onset of electromyographic suppression (Fig. 12–4, 26- to 27-minute time marks). When the muscle units innervated by the recorded motoneurons are monitored, a perfect correlation is observed between the discharge of a motoneuron and the action potentials of individual muscle fibers (Fig. 12–5).

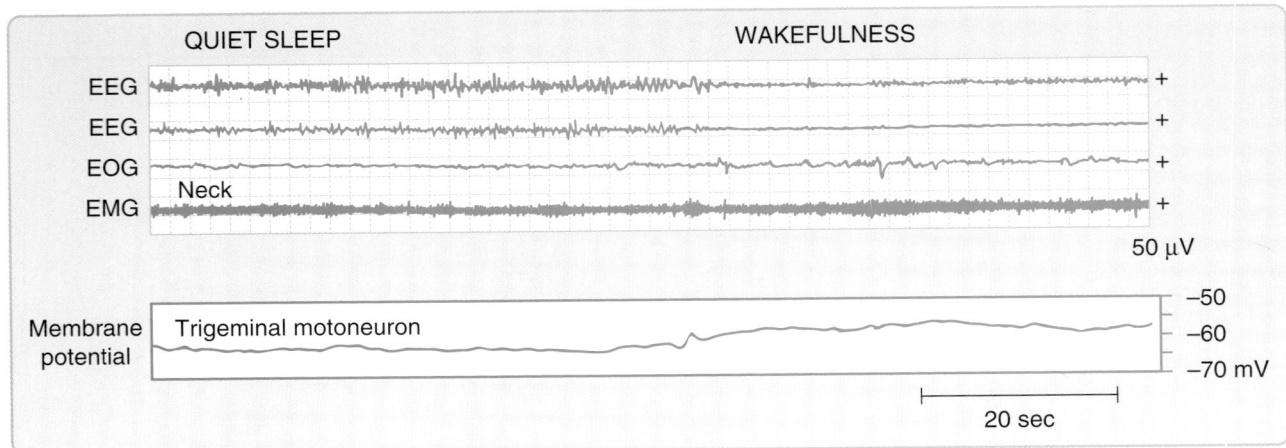

Figure 12–3. Intracellular recording from a trigeminal jaw-closer motoneuron: change in membrane potential during quiet sleep compared with wakefulness. When an extended period of quiet sleep was followed by sustained wakefulness, membrane depolarization occurred. The degree of depolarization was positively correlated with the level of arousal and muscular activity, as portrayed in the middle of the figure when a brief increase in neck electromyographic activity was correlated with a time-locked decrease in membrane polarization. Membrane potential band pass on polygraphic record: direct current to 0.1 Hz. Other polygraphic traces are the same as in Figure 12–4: EEG trace, marginal cortex. EEG, electroencephalogram; EMG, electromyogram; EOG, electrooculogram. (Reprinted with permission from Chase MH, Chandler SH, Nakamura Y: Intracellular determination of membrane potential of trigeminal motoneurons during sleep and wakefulness. J Neurophysiol 1980;44:349-358.)

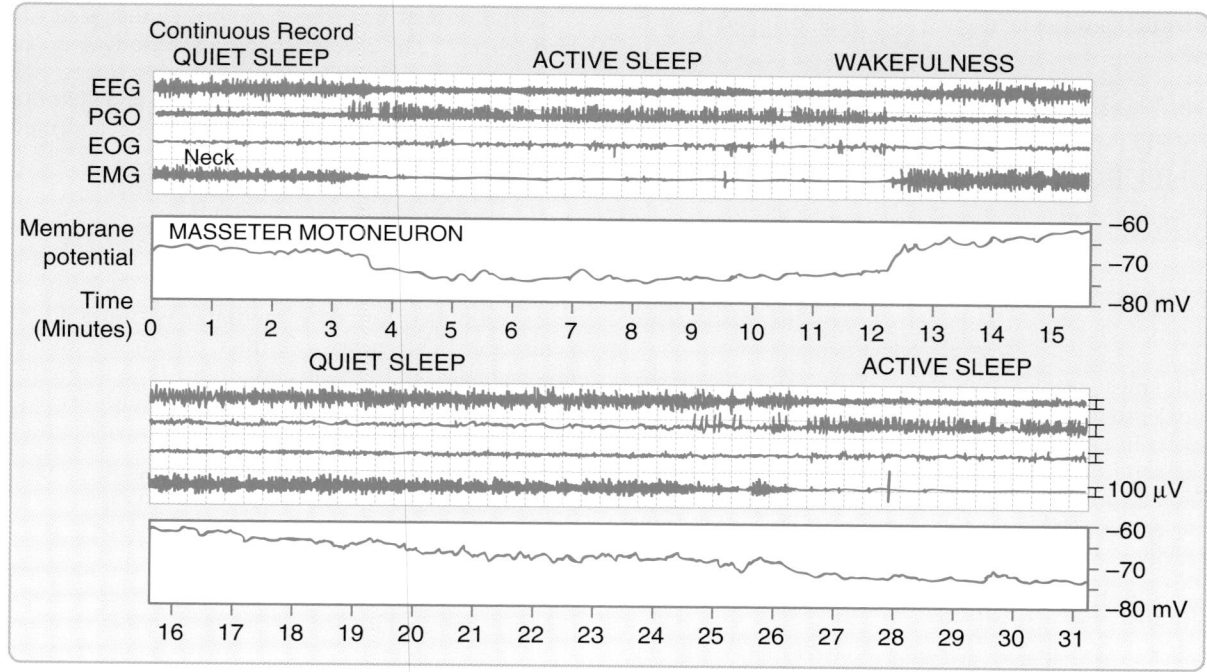

Figure 12–4. Intracellular recording from a trigeminal jaw-closer motoneuron: correlation of membrane potential and state changes. The membrane potential hyperpolarized rather abruptly at 3.5 min in conjunction with the decrease in neck muscle tone and transition from quiet to active sleep. At 12.5 min, the membrane depolarized and the animal awakened. After the animal passed into quiet sleep again, a brief, aborted episode of active sleep occurred at 25.5 min that was accompanied by a phasic period of hyperpolarization. A minute later, the animal once again entered active sleep, and the membrane potential hyperpolarized. EEG trace, marginal cortex, membrane potential band pass on polygraphic record, direct current to 0.1 Hz. EEG, electroencephalogram; EMG, electromyogram; EOG, electrooculogram; PGO, ponto-geniculo-occipital potential. (Reprinted with permission from Chase MH, Chandler SH, Nakamura Y: Intracellular determination of membrane potential of trigeminal motoneurons during sleep and wakefulness. J Neurophysiol 1980;44:349-358.)

Transition from Active Sleep to Wakefulness

When cats awake from active sleep, the membrane potential rapidly depolarizes (Fig. 12–4, 12- to 13-minute and 25- to 26-minute time marks). The degree of depolarization is equal to or exceeds the level maintained during the preceding episode of quiet sleep.

In summary, these data demonstrate that the membrane potential is strongly hyperpolarized during active sleep compared with quiet sleep and wakefulness and, in contrast, that it is only slightly hyperpolarized or remains at the

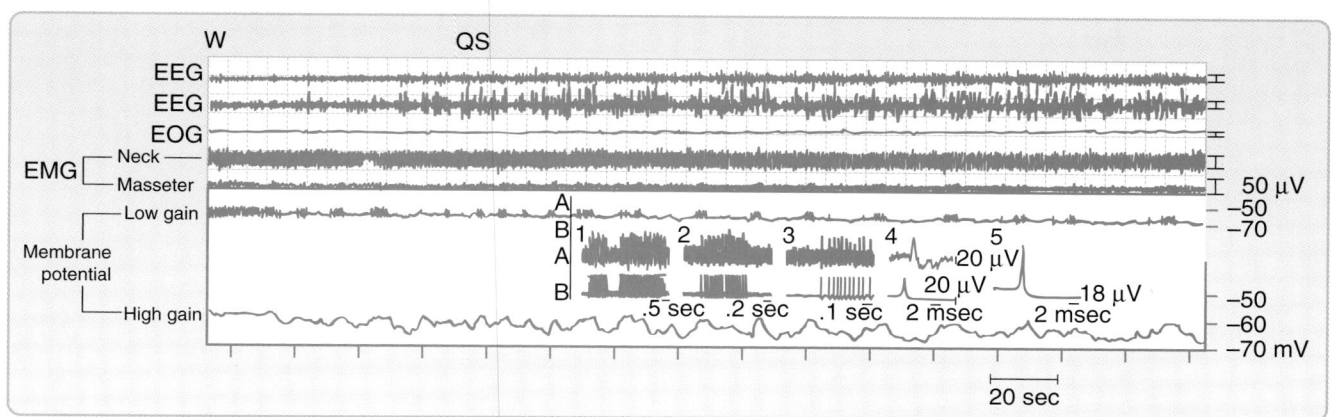

Figure 12–5. Intracellular recording from a masseter motoneuron. This illustrates the gradual increase in membrane potential and decrease in spike occurrence as the animal changed its behavioral state from wakefulness to quiet sleep. An oscilloscopic picture of the activity of an individual masseter motor unit is shown in the *inset*, which portrays the time-locked relationship between an action potential of a masseter muscle unit and each motoneuron spike potential at increasingly faster time bases (A and B, 1-4). In 5, the motoneuron spike is presented at higher gain (spike amplitude, 40 mV). Membrane potential band pass on polygraphic record: low gain, direct current (DC) to 35 Hz; high gain, DC to 0.5 Hz. Top EEG trace, frontal cortex; bottom EEG trace, marginal cortex. EEG, electroencephalogram; EMG, electromyogram; EOG, electrooculogram. (Reprinted with permission from Chase MH, Chandler SH, Nakamura Y: Intracellular determination of membrane potential of trigeminal motoneurons during sleep and wakefulness. J Neurophysiol 1980;44:349-358.)

same potential level when quiet sleep is compared with wakefulness.

ACTION POTENTIAL, RHEOBASE, AND INPUT RESISTANCE OF MOTONEURONS DURING SLEEP

Action Potential

Under natural conditions, motoneurons generate action potentials as the result of a summation of currents generated at synapses on their soma or dendrites. All synaptic currents are integrated in the region of the initial segment of the axon, which is the most excitable portion of the motoneuron. If the voltage drop produced by electrical currents is above a certain threshold level, an action potential is triggered—first in the initial segment and second in the soma. Consequently, motoneuron action potentials exhibit two basic components— the initial segment (IS) and soma-dendritic (SD) spikes—that reflect activity in these two regions of the cell.[15]

Spontaneous Action Potentials

Changes in behavioral state are reflected by variations in the frequency of action potential activity. This finding is evident in masseter motoneurons, which normally present a high level of tonic activity during wakefulness; the sustained discharge of wakefulness first decreases during quiet sleep and then is replaced by brief bursts of spikes (Fig. 12–5).

As the animal changes state from quiet sleep to active sleep, there is an accompanying cessation of spontaneous spike activity (Fig. 12–6). During active sleep, isolated or short bursts of spike potentials are occasionally observed in conjunction with facial twitches and rapid eye movements.

Induced Antidromic Action Potentials

The interval between the IS and SD spikes, which is referred to as the IS-SD delay, is lengthened when the animal enters active sleep, which indicates that motoneuron excitability is depressed during this state. During bursts of rapid eye movements, the IS-SD delay is further prolonged, and there are phasic changes in the peak amplitude of the antidromic spike. These variations in IS and SD spikes are indirect evidence of an increase in conductance of the soma membrane, which is the basis for postsynaptic inhibition.[16,17]

Rheobase

The rheobase is operationally defined as the minimal electrical current that is necessary to elicit an action potential when current is injected into a cell. In considering the effectiveness of an intracellularly applied current pulse in inducing an action potential, attention must be paid not only to the strength of the current but to the time during which it is allowed to flow through the cell. By choosing different voltages as well as pulse durations, a strength–duration curve can be developed that relates these two factors insofar as the

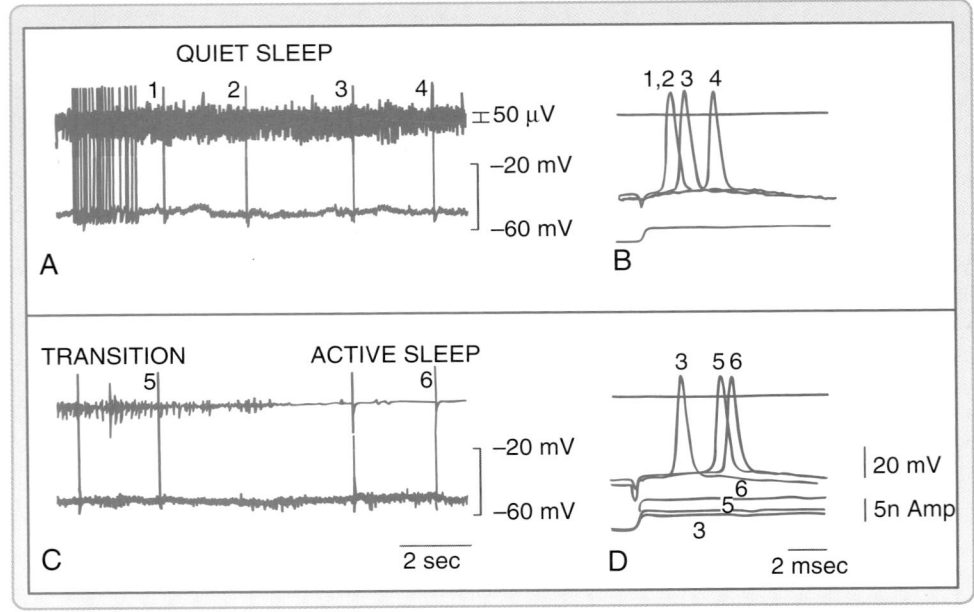

Figure 12–6. Spike generation by intrasomatic stimulation. **A,** After the spontaneous burst of spike activity in the initial portion of the record had receded, four consecutive threshold determinations were performed during quiet sleep using currents of 4 nA with a duration of 20 msec. **B,** Note that membrane potential fluctuations present during quiet sleep were accompanied by changes only in the latency of the direct spikes. **C, D,** An increase in threshold is shown that commenced in the transition period (5) after quiet sleep and was most pronounced during active sleep (6). In **D,** the increase is shown for spikes obtained during quiet sleep (3), the transition period (5), and active sleep (6). During active sleep, a threshold increase of 100% was observed. Note that both the overshoot and the absolute amplitude of the direct spike were smaller during active sleep than during quiet sleep. These reductions in spike size began during the transition period. The lower traces in **B** and **D** reflect the intrasomatic depolarizing current. The heavy line crossing the spike tips represents zero voltage obtained when the electrode was withdrawn from the motoneuron. Upper traces in **A** and **C** are the electromyographic recordings. (Reprinted with permission from Morales FR, Chase MH: Postsynaptic control of lumbar motoneuron excitability during active sleep in the chronic cat. Brain Res 1981;225:279-295.)

effective level of stimulation is concerned, thereby providing an index of the intrinsic excitability of the neuron.

Rheobasic currents during quiet sleep are comparable with those during wakefulness, whereas they are 80% greater in active sleep than in quiet sleep. An example of the increase in rheobasic current during active sleep compared with that during quiet sleep is given in Figure 12–6. These data indicate a dramatic decrease in cellular excitability during active sleep. Although an elevated rheobase is always accompanied by hyperpolarization, hyperpolarization alone cannot completely account for the increase in rheobase currents. An analysis of the data from rheobasic determinations and input resistance indicates that current flow is "shunted" by an increase in membrane conductance during active sleep; moreover, both hyperpolarization and increased conductance appear to contribute to the observed increase in rheobasic current.

Input Resistance

The manner in which a neuron responds to injected subthreshold or synaptic currents is related to its input resistance. This basic electrotonic characteristic of motoneurons depends, in turn, principally on the specific resistivity of the cell membrane, as well as on its area and the geometric characteristics of the dendritic tree.[15]

There is no dramatic difference in motoneuron input resistance when quiet sleep is compared with wakefulness. During active sleep, there is a striking (44%) decrease in input resistance. During active sleep, when rapid eye movements occur, there are frequent phasic decreases in the voltage drop produced by the same current, which indicates a continuously fluctuating motoneuron input resistance.

INDUCED ORTHODROMIC EXCITATORY POSTSYNAPTIC POTENTIALS DURING SLEEP

The amplitude of the Ia monosynaptic excitatory postsynaptic potential (EPSP) is smaller during active sleep than during quiet sleep (Fig. 12–7). The fact that in active sleep there is a decrease in excitability and an increase in membrane conductance, together with motoneuron hyperpolarization, clearly indicates that the EPSP amplitude is depressed by a mechanism of postsynaptic inhibition.[18,19] Phasic periods of additional suppression of EPSP amplitude are present during intense bursts of rapid eye movements in active sleep (Fig. 12–7). These periods are usually accompanied by further hyperpolarization of the postsynaptic membrane and a greater increase in motoneuron conductance. It is evident that phasic enhancements of postsynaptic inhibitory processes act to decrease the size of EPSPs during REM periods.

In summary, the data emerging from analyses of the action potential, rheobase, input resistance, and Ia monosynaptic EPSPs of motoneurons indicate that postsynaptic inhibition is the principal, and probably sufficient, mechanism responsible for atonia of the somatic musculature during active sleep.

SYNAPTIC POTENTIALS RESPONSIBLE FOR POSTSYNAPTIC INHIBITION DURING ACTIVE SLEEP

The preceding section describes the data that indicate motoneurons are subjected to postsynaptic inhibition during

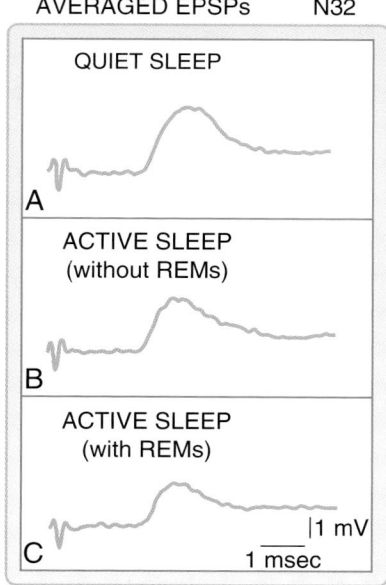

Figure 12–7. Averaged excitatory postsynaptic potential (EPSP) activity (n = 32) during quiet sleep **(A)**, active sleep without rapid eye movements (REMs) **(B)**, and active sleep with REMs **(C)**. Note the decrease in amplitude when active sleep without REMs is compared with quiet sleep, and a further decrease during active sleep with REMs. The averaged peak amplitude decreased 19% during active sleep without REMs and 37% during active sleep with REMs. Peripheral nerve (common peroneal) stimulation: 0.5 V, 0.3 msec. (Reprinted with permission from Morales FR, Chase MH: Postsynaptic control of lumbar motoneuron excitability during active sleep in the chronic cat. Brain Res 1981;225:279-295.)

active sleep. Because the synapse is the point of contact and the site of communication for postsynaptic inhibition, a study of synaptic transmission is central to an understanding of motor control during sleep. In an effort further to elucidate the bases for motoneuron inhibition during active sleep, we analyzed the spontaneous inhibitory postsynaptic potential (IPSP) activity in high-gain intracellular recordings obtained from motoneurons during active sleep, as well as during quiet sleep and wakefulness.

Comparison of Spontaneous Inhibitory Postsynaptic Potentials during Sleep and Wakefulness

During wakefulness and quiet sleep, intracellular records of motoneurons reveal relatively few spontaneous IPSPs. However, during active sleep, a great increase occurs in the number of spontaneous IPSPs (Fig. 12–8A and B). Even more manifest is the development of large-amplitude active sleep–specific IPSPs that are *unique* to this state. The amplitude and time course of these active sleep–specific IPSPs differentiate them from the smaller potentials impinging on the same motoneurons during quiet sleep as well as during active sleep. These large-amplitude active sleep–specific IPSPs are more readily reversed by the iontophoretic injection of chloride ions than are the smaller potentials, a finding that indicates that the responsible synapses are situated closer to the soma region; therefore, they are strategically located to facilitate the suppression of motoneuron activity.

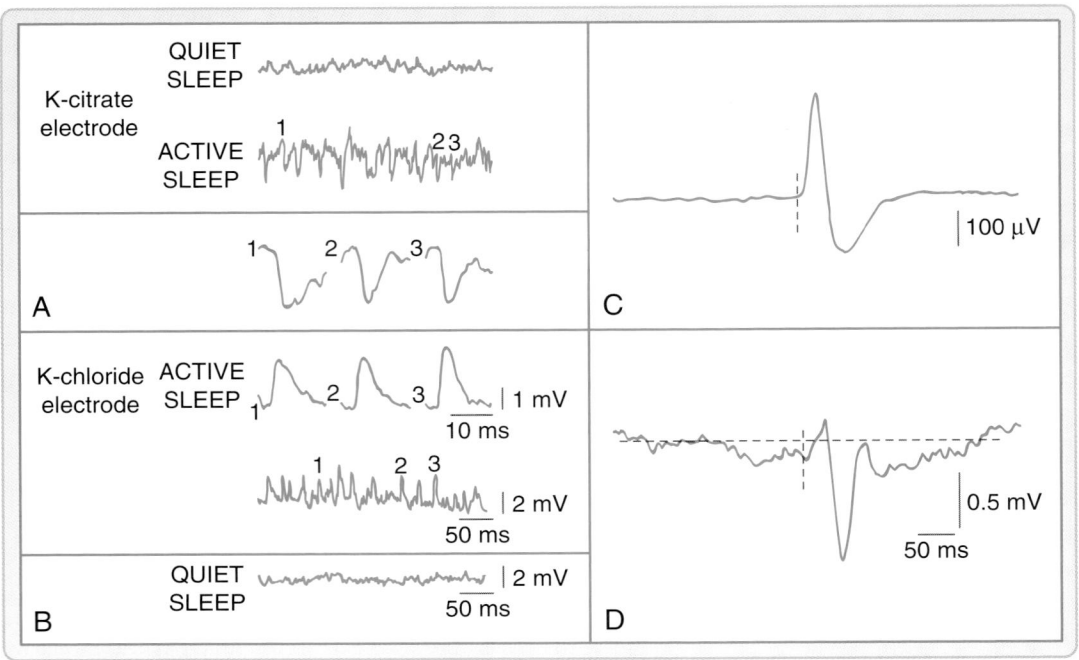

Figure 12–8. A, B, Representative recordings from two different motoneurons during quiet sleep and active sleep using microelectrodes filled with two different electrolyte solutions. **A,** K-citrate electrode. During active sleep, hyperpolarizing potentials were easily distinguishable. Potentials labeled 1 to 3 are shown in an expanded format. Their 10% to 90% amplitude rise times, measured from the digitized record, were 1.4, 1.6, and 1 msec, respectively. **B,** K-chloride electrode. Recordings were maintained for 6 min during quiet sleep without any retention current. A hyperpolarizing current of 10 nA was passed for 45 sec during quiet sleep approximately 1 min before the animal entered into active sleep. The quiet sleep recording of the membrane potential was obtained after current injection had ceased. The active sleep record of the membrane potential revealed the advent of high-frequency depolarizing potentials. In **B,** 1 to 3 are potentials shown in greater detail; their 10% to 90% rise times were 0.95, 1.05, and 1 msec, respectively. Depolarizing potentials like these were never observed during recording with K-citrate electrodes; they are interpreted as being reversed inhibitory potentials. Calibration signals are identical for the two cells. Both records are from sciatic motoneurons. Antidromic action potentials: **A,** 72 mV; **B,** 75 mV. (Reprinted with permission from Morales FR, Chase MH: Repetitive synaptic potentials responsible for inhibition of spinal cord motoneurons during active sleep. Exp Neurol 1982;78:471-476.) **C, D,** Changes in motoneuron membrane potential in conjunction with ipsilateral primary ponto-geniculo-occipital (PGO) waves. **C** and **D** are averages of 50 PGO waves and the corresponding motoneuron membrane potential. In this example, the changes in motoneuron membrane potential that were present in conjunction with PGO waves were the PGO inhibitory postsynaptic potential (PGO-IPSP), the pre-PGO hyperpolarization, and a succession of IPSPs that followed the PGO-IPSP (see text). The *vertical dotted line* marks the foot of the PGO wave, and the *horizontal dotted line* in **D** marks the baseline of the motoneuron membrane potential. (Reprinted with permission from López-Rodríguez F, Chase MH, et al: PGO-related potentials in lumbar motoneurons during active sleep. J Neurophysiol 1992;68:109-116.)

Because the atonia of active sleep is generalized to flexor and extensor muscles,[2] it was expected that every motoneuron innervating hindlimb muscles would show a significant increase in inhibitory activity during active sleep. We therefore compared the IPSP rate within recordings obtained from the same motoneuron (either flexor or extensor) during consecutive behavioral states. This comparison was accomplished by an analysis of the interpotential intervals of IPSPs during quiet sleep, the initial period of active sleep, and the NREM periods of active sleep. The interpotential intervals were significantly shorter during both the initial period of active sleep and the NREM periods of the same active sleep episode than during the preceding quiet sleep episode. It appears as if all motoneurons within pools whose neurons project to flexors as well as extensors receive an increase in inhibitory synaptic input during active sleep.

The occurrence of small-amplitude IPSPs during wakefulness and quiet sleep, albeit of relatively low frequency, was an unpredicted finding, of which the functional significance is unknown. These potentials may reflect the inhibitory control of motoneuron activity that is required to maintain limb position and postural adjustments, and thus they may not be related primarily to motor inhibition vis-à-vis sleep physiology. On the other hand, the increase in IPSP frequency observed in all motoneurons during active sleep was found to be the result not only of the appearance of large-amplitude active sleep–specific IPSPs but of an increase in the number of small-amplitude IPSPs. Therefore, it is possible that the inhibitory system that generates the small IPSPs of active sleep, which undoubtedly contribute to motoneuron inhibition during this state, also functions, albeit to a much lesser degree, during wakefulness and quiet sleep.

It is clear, however, that there is a unique set of inhibitory synapses that generate the active sleep–specific IPSPs. In turn, this observation implies the existence of a unique group of inhibitory interneurons that are responsible for the generation of the active sleep–specific IPSPs driven to discharge, selectively, during active sleep. New evidence gathered with the use of immunohistochemical techniques (see later) supports the hypothesis that rather than being short-axoned cells located in the spinal cord, active sleep inhibitory interneurons are mainly situated in the brainstem and that their long projecting axons end directly on spinal motoneurons.[20] For brainstem motoneurons, the inhibitory interneurons that generate active

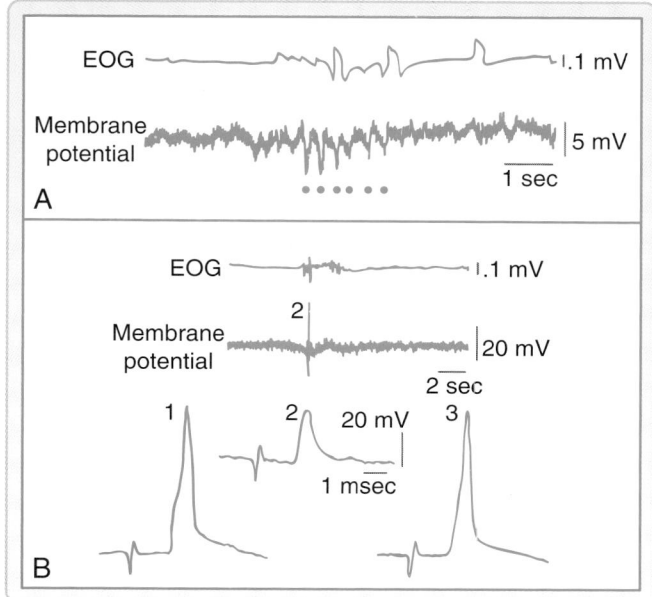

Figure 12–9. Summated hyperpolarizing membrane potential events **(A)** and blockade of antidromic action potential **(B)** during active sleep accompanied by periods of rapid eye movements. **A,** Hyperpolarizing events arise (the most evident indicated by *dots*) that are composed of repetitively occurring inhibitory synaptic potentials. **B,** An antidromic spike was induced immediately before (1) and after (3) a burst of rapid eye movements. When the antidromic action potential coincided with the period of hyperpolarizing potentials, the soma-dendritic spike was blocked and only the initial segment spike was present (2). Data are unfiltered; records were obtained from a peroneal motoneuron in **A** (resting membrane potential: –65 mV) and from a tibial motoneuron in **B** (resting membrane potential: –72 mV). EOG, electrooculogram. (Reprinted with permission from Chase MH, Morales FR: Phasic changes in motoneuron membrane potential during REM periods of active sleep. Neurosci Lett 1982;34:177-182.)

sleep–specific IPSPs are, without doubt, located in the brainstem. Regardless of the location of the interneurons that give rise to the active sleep–specific IPSPs, we suggest that these IPSPs represent the final synaptic expression of a supraspinal inhibitory system that is responsible for promoting the suppression of motoneuron activity and the development of atonia during active sleep.

In association with periods of rapid eye movements during active sleep, phasic enhancement of the postsynaptic inhibition occurs that is directed to motoneurons.[13,21] In addition, in relation to ponto-geniculo-occipital (PGO) activity, there are inhibitory potentials that arise in the membrane potential of both spinal cord and trigeminal motoneurons; these inhibitory changes are reflected in the appearance of a complex pattern of motoneuron hyperpolarization that is centered around PGO waves (Fig. 12–8D). It is clear that a postsynaptic inhibitory process that suppresses motoneuron excitability tonically during active sleep also entails episodes of phasic enhancement during REM periods and PGO waves that further suppress the excitability of motoneurons during active sleep.

EXCITATORY CONTROL OF MOTONEURONS DURING ACTIVE SLEEP

Postsynaptic inhibition is one of the principal synaptic processes affecting motoneurons during the REM periods of active sleep. In fact, all of the inhibitory phenomena that are described in the previous sections are not only present but enhanced during REM periods, including the frequency and amplitude of the active sleep–specific IPSPs (Fig. 12–9). How, then, could there be twitches and jerks of the eyes and limbs during REM periods? The answer is simple because most REM periods are accompanied not only by increased motoneuron inhibition but by strikingly potent motor excitatory drives (Figs. 12–10 and 12–11).

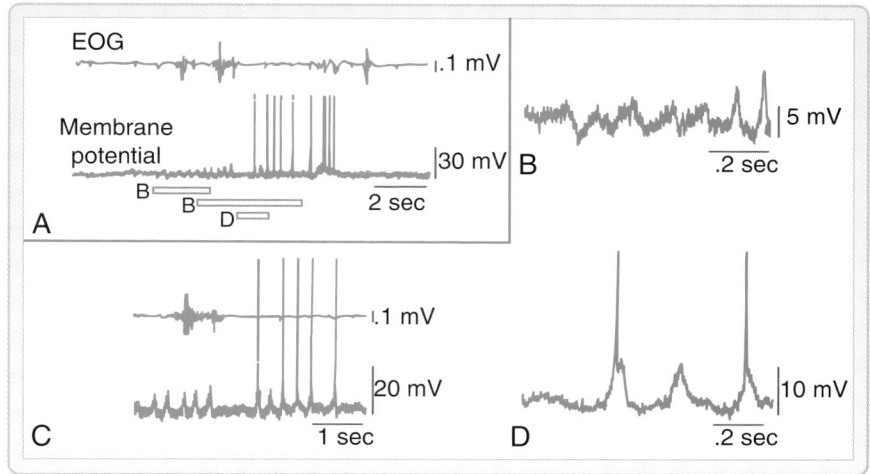

Figure 12–10. A, Summated depolarizing potentials and spike activity in conjunction with active sleep periods of rapid eye movements. EOG, electrooculogram. **B,** During the first burst of eye movements, phasic hyperpolarizing events arose. **C,** In conjunction with the second burst of eye movements, there was a series of rhythmic depolarizing shifts. Action potentials occurred during the third episode of eye movements; they were also present during the interval between the second and third bursts of ocular activity. The recordings over the bars in **A** are presented at a faster sweep speed and greater magnification in **B, C,** and **D.** In **D,** note that spikes arise from the first and third depolarizing shifts, whereas the second does not reach threshold. The action potentials in **C** and **D** are truncated owing to the high gain of the records. Data are unfiltered; records were obtained from a tibial motoneuron (resting membrane potential: –70 mV). (Reprinted with permission from Chase MH, Morales FR. Phasic changes in motoneuron membrane potential during REM periods of active sleep. Neurosci Lett 1982;34:177-182.)

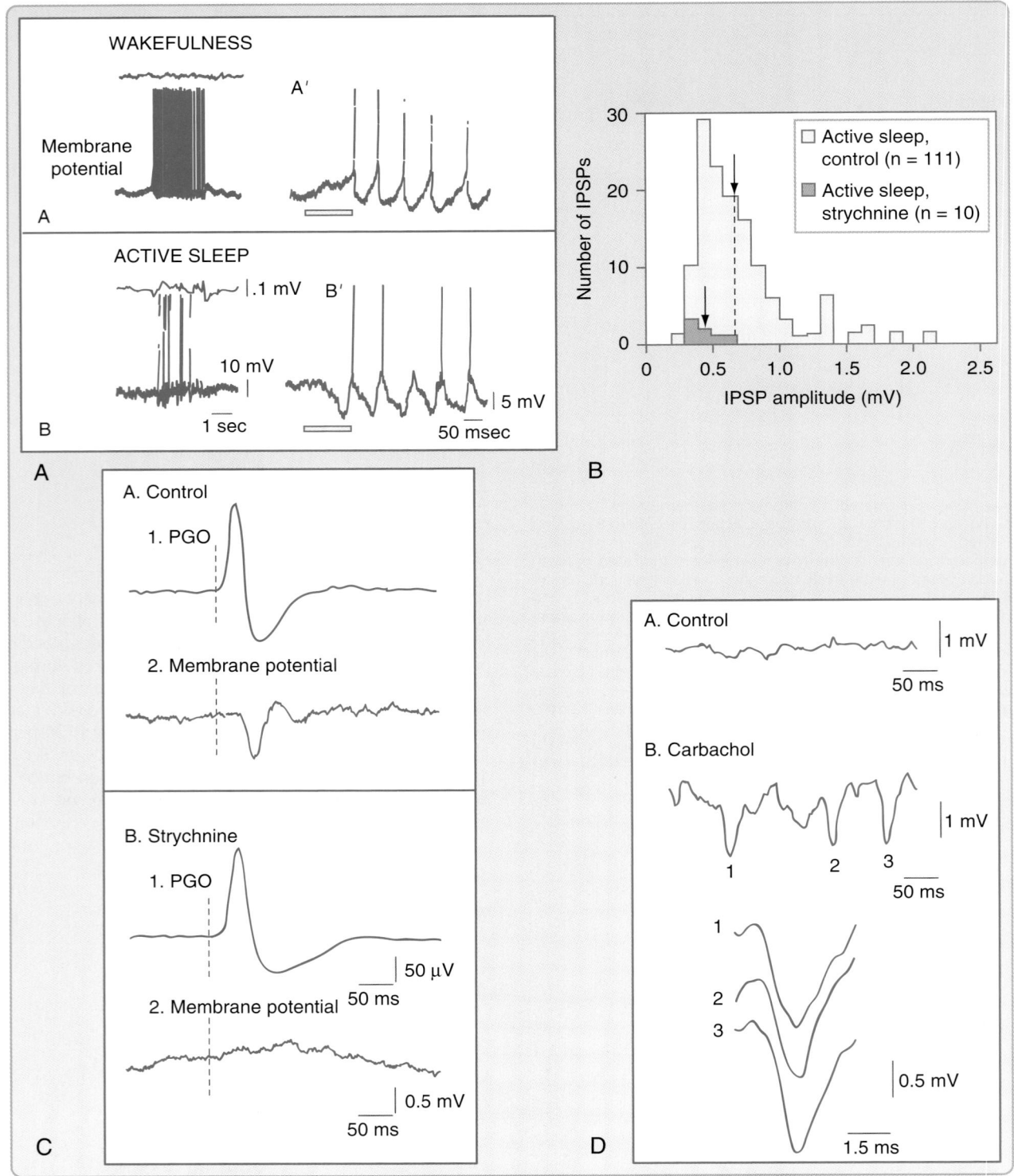

Figure 12–11. A, Action potential generation during wakefulness (A) and a rapid eye movement (REM) period of active sleep (B). Gradual membrane depolarization (*bar* in A′) preceded the development of action potentials during wakefulness, whereas a strong hyperpolarizing drive was evident during a comparable period of active sleep (*bar* in B′). This difference was also observed before the subsequent generation of each action potential during this REM episode. Action potentials in A′ and B′ are truncated owing to the high gain of the recording. Resting membrane potentials are –58 mV in A and –63 mV in B. Data are unfiltered; records were obtained from a single tibial motoneuron. (Reprinted with permission from Chase MH, Morales FR. Phasic changes in motoneuron membrane potential during REM periods of active sleep. Neurosci Lett 1982;34:177-182.) **B,** Distribution of the amplitudes of spontaneous inhibitory postsynaptic potentials (IPSPs) recorded during active sleep from the same lumbar motoneuron before (*light blue histogram*) and after the microiontophoretic ejection of strychnine (*dark blue histogram*). *Arrows* indicate the median value of each IPSP population. Note that before strychnine, 50% of the potentials were larger in amplitude than the largest potential that was detected after the microiontophoretic ejection of strychnine (10 mM, 250 nA, 2.75 min). (Reprinted with permission from Chase MH, Soja PJ, Morales FR: Evidence that glycine mediates the postsynaptic potentials that inhibit lumbar motoneurons during the atonia of active sleep. J Neurosci 1989;9:743-751.) *(Continued)*

The excitatory drives that impinge on motoneurons during REM periods of active sleep are reflected in depolarizing and spike potentials. This pattern of activity is illustrated in Figure 12–10A. During the second cluster of eye movements in this REM episode, there are depolarizing shifts in potential (Fig. 12–10B to D); subthreshold depolarizing potentials and action potentials are also present. These patterns of activation probably reflect descending excitatory activity emanating from supraspinal systems.[2,22]

In contrast to the gradual depolarization that precedes neuronal discharge during wakefulness (Fig. 12–11A, part A), in most instances during active sleep, there is an initial hyperpolarization that is followed immediately by a depolarization shift and action potential generation (Fig. 12–11A, part B). These depolarization shifts in membrane potential appear to be the result of cumulative EPSP activity rather than a reflection of a process of disinhibition, for the following reasons. First, examination of high-gain, high-speed records reveals that each depolarization consists of the summation of wavelets whose form is comparable to that of previously described EPSPs.[23] Second, the depolarizing potentials remain, even though inhibitory processes are reversed by the intracellular injection of chloride ions.

From time to time, for reasons that remain unknown, during the REM periods of active sleep excitatory drives overpower inhibitory drives, motoneurons discharge, and the muscle fibers that they innervate contract. It appears as if, at these times, there is an increase in excitatory drives that is actually accompanied by an increase in inhibitory drives; momentarily, the excitatory drives predominate and motoneurons discharge (Figs. 12–10 and 12–11A). When motoneurons do discharge during the REM periods of active sleep, their activity, as well as the resultant contraction of the muscles that they innervate, is unlike that occurring during any other state. Movements are abrupt, twitchy, and jerky, and without apparent purpose.

The coactivation of excitatory and inhibitory synaptic drives appears, from a functional perspective, to be paradoxical. However, some rationality may be ascribed to each of these processes when they are examined individually. For example, the inhibitory input that is present during active sleep may reflect a need to suppress contraction of the somatic musculature to protect the organism at a time when it is blind and unconscious. Although we do not understand the function of the REM periods of active sleep (and perhaps the rapid eye movements themselves are only an easily observable indicator of a more basic process), we do know that during these periods, most populations of cortical and subcortical cells discharge at rates that often exceed those that occur during wakefulness.[8]

In fact, the activity of practically all motor pathways, including those whose discharge results in movements during wakefulness, is greatly enhanced in an apparently random manner during active sleep (compared with quiet sleep) and, even more strikingly, during the REM periods of active sleep.[8,22,24] It is possible that episodes of motoneuron spike potentials that result in myoclonic activity during REM periods have no specific functional significance but may simply reflect the status of a highly activated nervous system whose motor facilitatory pathways are discharging at extremely high rates. It is also possible that myoclonic activity represents brief episodes of an otherwise integrated behavior that is suppressed by the presence of motor inhibition. Evidently, there is a need during all REM periods for a compensatory increase in motor inhibition to prevent movements (integrated or random) that would otherwise ensue during the activation of motor facilitatory systems.

NEUROTRANSMITTERS MEDIATING THE INHIBITORY SYNAPTIC CONTROL OF MOTONEURONS DURING ACTIVE SLEEP

This section focuses on an investigation of the neurotransmitters that mediate the unique inhibitory potentials that are responsible, at least in part, for the postsynaptic inhibition of motoneurons during active sleep.

In previous studies that were performed on acutely anesthetized or decerebrate cats, microiontophoretic experiments have convincingly demonstrated that strychnine antagonizes the postsynaptic inhibitory actions of alpha- and beta-amino acids, such as glycine and beta-alanine. Indeed, it is generally accepted that glycine is the major inhibitory transmitter at the level of the spinal cord.[25-27] Studies conducted in acute preparations have also indicated that picrotoxin and bicuculline are effective antagonists for the postsynaptic inhibitory actions of gamma-amino acids (e.g., gamma-aminobutyric acid [GABA]).[26,28-30]

In studies,[31,32] the neurotransmitter antagonists strychnine, picrotoxin, and bicuculline were microiontophoretically administered adjacent to the cell body of spinal cord motoneurons while intracellular records were obtained during naturally occurring episodes of sleep and wakefulness.

In these studies, it was determined that the active sleep–specific IPSPs were either diminished in amplitude or abolished after the microiontophoretic application of strychnine (Fig. 12–11B). This finding suggests, on the basis of the

Figure 12–11. cont'd **C,** Averaged ponto-geniculo-occipital (PGO) waves and the membrane potential in lumbar motoneurons recorded in two different cats before (control; A) and after strychnine injection (B). The *vertical bars* are positioned at the foot of the averaged PGO waves. After the injection of strychnine, the PGO-related IPSP was no longer present; instead, a long depolarizing potential occurred (see text for details). (Reprinted with permission from López-Rodríguez F, Morales FR, Soja PJ, et al: Suppression of the PGO-related lumbar motoneuron IPSP by strychnine. Brain Res 1990;535:331-334.) **D,** High-gain intracellular recordings obtained from a single hindlimb motoneuron during precarbachol control conditions (A) and 26 min after carbachol microinjection into the pontine reticular formation (B). After carbachol microinjection, hyperpolarizing potentials were easily distinguishable. Potentials labeled 1 to 3 are shown in an expanded format. These recordings were obtained by using a KCl-filled microelectrode. A 5-nA depolarizing current was injected to displace the membrane potential away from the equilibrium potential; this procedure facilitated the observation of these potentials and also avoided shifting the equilibrium potential to a depolarized value by the retention of chloride ions. The waveforms of these potentials were remarkably similar to those that appear exclusively during active sleep in intact animals under natural conditions (compare, for example, the potentials illustrated in this figure with those of Fig. 2A in Morales and associates).[61] (Reprinted with permission from Morales FR, Engelhardt JK, Soja PJ, et al: Motoneuron properties during motor inhibition produced by microinjection of carbachol into the pontine reticular formation of the decerebrate cat. J Neurophysiol 1987;57:1118-1129.)

documented actions of strychnine, that the neurotransmitter mediating this IPSP activity is glycine or a glycinergic substance. Neither picrotoxin nor bicuculline, when released microiontophoretically near the somas of individual motoneurons, was effective in suppressing the large-amplitude IPSPs of active sleep. Thus, glycine, but not GABA, appears to be the principal postsynaptic inhibitory neurotransmitter responsible for muscle atonia during active sleep. By applying strychnine juxtacellularly through microiontophoresis, we determined that the PGO-related IPSPs are mediated by glycinergic synapses (Fig. 12–11C). We have postulated that the same inhibitory neurons that tonically inhibit motoneurons during active sleep are phasically activated during PGO waves and provide for the phasic enhancement of postsynaptic inhibition that occurs during the phasic events of active sleep. By blocking the PGO-related IPSPs with strychnine, we unmasked a depolarizing potential, which underscores the complexity of motor control that takes place during active sleep, especially during the phasic events of this state.

In a new series of pharmacologic experiments, we applied antagonists of excitatory amino acids juxtacellularly. The broad-spectrum antagonist kynurenic acid completely abolished the phasic depolarizing events that occur during the REM periods of active sleep. The N-methyl-D-aspartate (NMDA) blocker argipressin did not affect these events; therefore, we conclude that the excitatory motor events during REM are mediated by pathways that use an amino acid such as glutamate as their neurotransmitter and that their action is mediated by non-NMDA receptors.[33,34]

PHARMACOLOGIC MODELS OF ACTIVE SLEEP

Since the work of George and colleagues,[35] it has been known that the injection of cholinergic drugs into the brainstem may induce a state that closely resembles active sleep (see, for example, Baghdoyan et al.[36]).

In the decerebrate cat, we demonstrated that carbachol induces a complete abolition of somatomotor rigidity. The mechanisms of this cholinergically induced motor suppression appear to be the same as those that are activated during active sleep (e.g., Fig. 12–11D). The acute decerebrate animal, in which motor suppression is induced by injecting cholinergic substances into the pons, has been used by us and other researchers to explore the synaptic network responsible for the atonia of active sleep and to study the mechanisms of motor suppression of respiratory muscles.[37-40]

Carbachol effects may also be observed in the α-chloralose–anesthetized cat. This preparation is being used intensively to study networks of neurons, the activity of which underlies the physiologic components of active sleep.[41,42] In this preparation, we obtained evidence that makes it very unlikely that Ib inhibitory spinal cord neurons, which are glycinergic inhibitory interneurons, are responsible for the inhibition of motoneurons during active sleep.[43] Previously, we rejected the possibility that Renshaw cells inhibit motoneurons during active sleep (paradoxically, Renshaw cells are themselves inhibited during active sleep).[38] The work of Takakusaki and associates[40] suggests that Ia inhibitory interneurons also do not participate in this process. It is known that entire populations of spinal inhibitory interneurons are not responsible for

the characteristic atonia of active sleep that affects spinal cord musculature.

We have described GABAergic inhibitory processes in the pontine reticular formation that play a key role in the generation and maintenance of wakefulness as well as being involved in the control of active sleep.[44-46] These data emanated from studies in chronic cats in which prolonged periods of wakefulness occur after the injection of GABA as well as GABA$_A$ or GABA$_B$ receptor agonists into the nucleus pontis oralis[47] (Fig. 12–12). The injection of the corresponding antagonists in awake animals results in the rapid induction of REM sleep, and in many cases there was no intercalated episode of quiet (NREM) sleep.[47] We conclude that pontine GABAergic processes are critically involved in the generation and maintenance of wakefulness, and that they also participate in the control of active (REM) sleep and its accompanying patterns of motor inhibition.

SUPRASEGMENTAL CONTROL OF MOTONEURON INHIBITION DURING ACTIVE SLEEP

The existence of active sleep–specific IPSPs reflects the activity of supraspinal centers that, directly or indirectly, activate inhibitory interneurons, which, in turn, discharge selectively during active sleep. We know that some of the neuronal elements that control motor inhibition during active sleep are situated caudal to the anterior border of the mesencephalon because a midbrain transection does not eliminate intermittent periods of motor suppression and correlated epiphenomena during this state (see Chapter 10). On the other hand, after a transection caudal to the medulla, facial muscles continue to be subjected to inhibition during active sleep, whereas limb and trunk musculature is unaffected by changes in the animal's state. Thus, a critical neuronal population responsible for somatomotor inhibition during active sleep must be located within the confines of the lower brainstem. These inhibitory interneurons are the last link in a suprasegmental inhibitory system that controls somatomotor outflow in a state-dependent manner.

Recent evidence appears to corroborate an early postulate by Chase,[48] wherein neurons in the nucleus pontis oralis excite, during active sleep, neurons of the inhibitory region of Magoun and Rhines,[49] which in turn promote the motor inhibition of active sleep. Interestingly, new evidence is emanating from the use of immunocytochemical techniques rather than from the use of classic electrophysiologic procedures. The first immunohistochemical technique used the detection of the nuclear protein c-Fos, which is synthesized during certain patterns of neuronal activity. Immunodetection was performed in brainstem slices of cats that had been sacrificed immediately after 2 hours of continuous active sleep induced by the pontine administration of carbachol.[50] In the ventral region of the medial medullary reticular formation, medial to the facial motor nucleus and lateral to the inferior olive, active sleep–carbachol cats exhibited, bilaterally, a great number of Fos-labeled cells.[50] The region occupied by these cells corresponded, as postulated, to the inhibitory region of Magoun and Rhines.[49] The second immunocytochemical technique consisted of the retrograde labeling of interneurons by using the subunit B of cholera toxin, which was injected into the

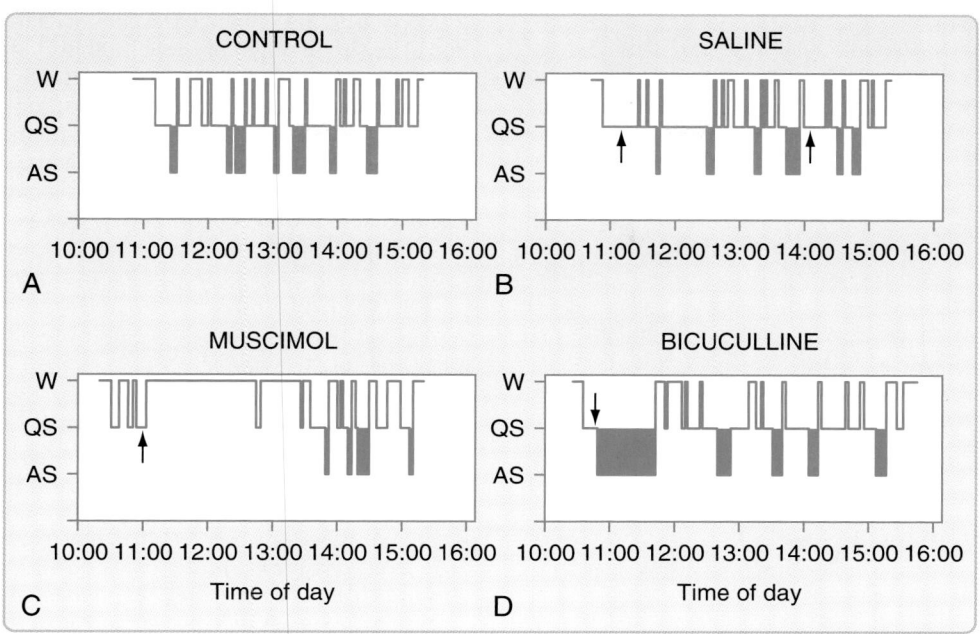

Figure 12–12. Hypnograms obtained under control conditions (**A**) and after the injection of saline (**B**), muscimol (**C**), and bicuculline (**D**) into the nucleus pontis oralis in a representative cat. The temporal distribution of behavioral states during a session with two injections of saline (*vertical arrows* in **B**) were similar to those observed during control sessions. Note that the injection of muscimol (*vertical arrow* in **C**), which was made during a quiet sleep episode, immediately induced wakefulness and blocked the subsequent occurrence of quiet sleep and active sleep for 106 and 141 min, respectively. In contrast, an injection of bicuculline (*vertical arrow* in **D**) induced a short-latency, long-duration episode of active sleep. W, wakefulness; QS, quiet sleep; AS, active sleep. (Modified with permission from Xi M-C, Morales FR, Chase MH: Induction of wakefulness and inhibition of active [REM] sleep by GABAergic processes in the nucleus pontis oralis. Arch Ital Biol 2001;139:25-145.)

trigeminal motor pool.[51] This technique permitted the identification, among all neurons that were activated during active sleep–carbachol, of interneurons that directly innervate the motor nuclei. The most salient result of the combined use of these techniques was the discovery of a subset of neurons in the ventral medulla that were activated during active sleep–carbachol that innervate antigravitatory motor nuclei[52] (Fig. 12–13). These neurons, which we believe are inhibitory premotor neurons that are responsible for the atonia of REM sleep, contain glycine, which produces the postsynaptic inhibition of motoneurons.[52]

The nucleus pontis oralis controls motor activity during REM sleep as well as during wakefulness, as illustrated by the phenomenon of reticular response-reversal, wherein this nucleus is responsible for promoting motor excitation during wakefulness and a diametrically opposite drive, motor inhibition, during REM sleep.[53] Reticular response-reversal is achieved during wakefulness (and NREM/quiet sleep) by the excitation of motoneurons in conjunction with the GABAergic blockade of an inhibitory neuronal pathway from the nucleus pontis oralis to the nucleus reticularis gigantocellularis.[11] During REM sleep, this pathway becomes functional, resulting in the activation of inhibitory glycinergic premotor neurons in the nucleus reticularis gigantocellularis; the activation of these neurons results in the postsynaptic inhibition of motoneurons during REM sleep.[10,11,48,52,54-58,62,63]

The numerous papers that have been published dealing with the role of hypocretin-containing neurons have posited an almost unlimited number of functions, ranging from sleep and wakefulness to reproduction and nociception. In an effort to determine the role of this system in normal and pathologic

processes, we examined the behaviors that were associated with the activation of these neurons.[64,65] Accordingly, we analyzed the c-Fos expression of hypocretinergic neurons in cats and guinea pigs during (1) quiet wakefulness (i.e., in animals awake but at rest and not moving); (2) NREM sleep; and (3) REM sleep; as well as in (4) aroused animals that are exploring their environment. The largest amount of c-Fos expression occurred in aroused animals during exploratory motor behavior, whereas there was practically no expression of c-Fos during NREM sleep and—which is especially important—there was no significant expression during wakefulness when the animals were alert, but not moving. Surprisingly, a larger number of c-Fos–expressing hypocretinergic neurons were observed during REM sleep than during quiet wakefulness.

Thus, it is clear that the hypocretinergic system participates in the control of motor activity during wakefulness in conjunction with movements during specific behaviors as well as during REM sleep, when, through the activation of nucleus pontis oralis and ventral medullary neurons, it enhances motor inhibition. These dual state-dependent actions of the hypocretinergic system reflect the patterns of motor control exerted in conjunction with the phenomenon of reticular response-reversal—that is, hypocretin-containing neurons act at various levels of the neuraxis to support the facilitation of motor activity during wakefulness, whereas their discharge during REM sleep leads to the inhibition of motor activity.[59,60] Because hypocretinergic neurons are located exclusively in areas of the hypothalamus that mediate emotional or motivational behaviors, we propose that the hypocretinergic system is responsible primarily for facilitating motor activities (and secondarily for activating associated motor support systems)

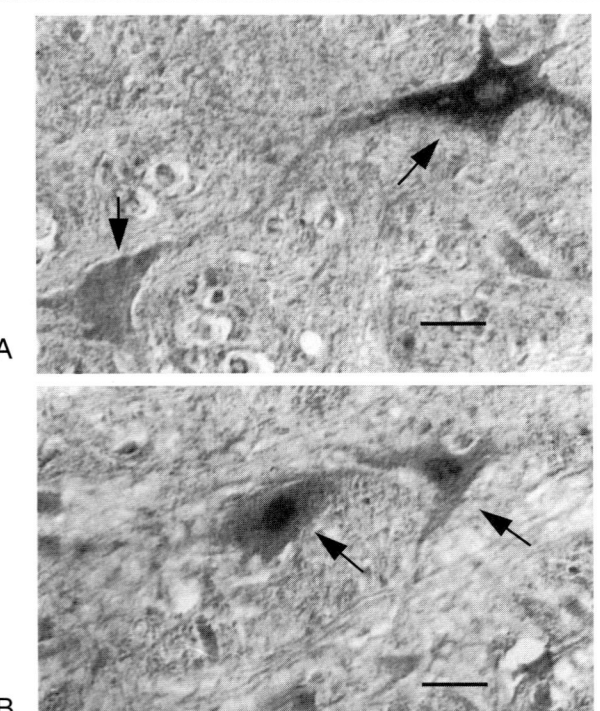

Figure 12–13. Glycine-like immunoreactive neurons in the ventromedial medullary reticular formation of an experimental cat that was injected with cholera toxin B subunit (CTb) in the trigeminal motor nucleus. **A,** This histologic section was processed for both glycine and CTb immunostaining. Two neurons in the magnocellular reticular formation that stained positive to an antibody raised against glycine-conjugated protein may be observed in this photomicrograph. The cell indicated by the *arrow* on the left exhibits glycine-like immuno-reactivity but does not contain CTb. Instead, the cell indicated by the *arrow* on the right exhibits both glycine-like immunoreactivity and CTb retrogradely transported from the motor V deposit. **B,** This histologic section was processed for both glycine and c-Fos immunostaining. Neurons illustrated in **B** (*arrows*), positive to the glycine antibody, express c-Fos during carbachol-induced REM sleep. Scale bars, 15 μm. (Reprinted with permission from Morales FR, Sampogna S, Yamuy J, et al: c-fos expression in brainstem premotor interneurons during cholinergically induced active sleep in the cat. J Neurosci 1999;19: 9508-9518.)

REM periods, by enhanced excitation and enhanced inhibition. The site of origin of these inhibitory drives encompasses the ventromedial medulla. It has also been suggested that this and adjacent regions may, in turn, be activated by more rostrally located nuclei, such as the pontine nucleus pontis oralis. Resolution of the mechanisms of action of the supramedullary control of premotor neurons constitutes a major goal of future experiments.

> *Clinical Pearl*
>
> *To develop the most efficacious treatment for any sleep disorder, the first step is to clarify the genesis of the primary pathologic process. A critical analysis of the literature reveals that a deficiency in hypocretin in humans occurs in conjunction with cataplexy. On the other hand, there are normal levels of hypocretin in individuals who are not cataplectic but experience some or even all of the other symptoms of narcolepsy. Because over a third of naroleptic patients are not cataplectic, it is inaccurate to link a deficiency in hypocretin to narcolepsy. Accordingly, to understand the basis for narcolepsy, studies of hypocretin are irrelevant or misleading; on the other hand, to understand and develop efficacious treatments for cataplexy, they are indispensable. The significant role that hypocretin plays in promoting motor activity is indicated by the increased levels of hypocretin in patients with REM sleep behavior disorder (who exhibit a state-dependent increase in motor activity) as well as by the decreased levels of hypocretin in individuals with cataplexy (who exhibit a state-dependent decrease in motor activity).*

that are necessary for the expression of these emotional and motivationally oriented behaviors.

CONCLUSIONS

In summary, postsynaptic inhibition is a principal process that is responsible not only for the atonia of the somatic musculature during active sleep but for the phasic episodes of decreased motoneuron excitability that accompany bursts of rapid eye movements during this state. These postsynaptic processes depend on the presence of active sleep–specific IPSPs, which are mediated by glycine. The phasic excitation of motoneurons during REM periods is due to EPSPs, which, when present, encounter a motoneuron already subjected to enhanced postsynaptic inhibition.

From the perspective of motoneurons, active sleep can be characterized as a state abundant in the availability of strikingly potent patterns of postsynaptic inhibition and, during

REFERENCES

1. Kleitman N: Sleep and Wakefulness. Chicago, University of Chicago Press, 1963.
2. Pompeiano O: The neurophysiological mechanisms of the postural and motor events during desynchronized sleep. Res Publ Assoc Nerv Ment Dis 1967;45:351-423.
3. Pakhomov AN: A new method of measuring and recording muscle tonus, and its application to the study of the physiology of sleep in man. Fiziol Zh SSSR 1947;33:245-254.
4. Jouvet M, Michel F, Courjon J: Sur en stade d'activité électrique cerébrale rapide au cours du sommeil physiologique. C R Soc Biol (Paris) 1959;153:1024-1028.
5. Chase MH (ed): The Sleeping Brain. Perspectives in the Brain Sciences, vol 1. Los Angeles, Brain Information Service/Brain Research Institute, UCLA, 1972.
6. Sherrington CS: The Integrative Action of the Nervous System. New Haven, Conn, Yale University Press, 1906.
7. Nakamura Y, Goldberg LJ, Chandler SH, et al: Intracellular analysis of trigeminal motoneuron activity during sleep in the cat. Science 1978;199:204-207.
8. Steriade M, Hobson JA: Neuronal activity during the sleep-waking cycle. Prog Neurobiol 1976;6:155-376.
9. Chase MH: The motor functions of the reticular formation are multifaceted and state-determined. In Hobson JM, Brazier MAB (eds): Reticular Formation Revisited. New York, Raven Press, 1980, pp 449-472.
10. Chase MH, Enomoto S, Murakami T, et al: Intracellular potential of medullary reticular neurons during sleep and wakefulness. Exp Neurol 1981;71:226-233.
11. Chase MH: Synaptic mechanisms and circuitry involved in motoneuron control during sleep. Int Rev Neurobiol 1983;24: 213-258.

12. Chase MH, Morales FR: Phasic changes in motoneuron membrane potential during REM periods of active sleep. Neurosci Lett 1982;34:177-182.

13. Chase MH, Morales FR: Subthreshold excitatory activity and motoneuron discharge during REM periods of active sleep. Science 1983;221:1195-1198.

14. Morales FR, Boxer P, Chase MH: Behavioral state-specific inhibitory postsynaptic potentials impinge on cat lumbar motoneurons during active sleep. Exp Neurol 1988;100:583-595.

15. Burke RE, Rudomin P: Spinal neurons and synapses. In Kandel ER (ed): Handbook of Physiology: The Nervous System. Bethesda, Md, American Physiological Society, 1977, pp 877-944.

16. Brock LG, Coombs JS, Eccles JC: Intracellular recording from antidromically activated motoneurons. J Physiol (Lond) 1953;122:429-461.

17. Llinas R, Terzuolo CA: Mechanisms of supraspinal actions upon spinal cord activities: Reticular inhibitory mechanisms on alpha-extensor motoneurons. J Neurophysiol 1964;287:579-591.

18. Cook WA Jr, Cangiano A: Presynaptic and postsynaptic inhibition of spinal motoneurons. J Neurophysiol 1972;35:389-403.

19. Curtis DR, Eccles JC: The time courses of excitatory and inhibitory synaptic actions. J Physiol (Lond) 1959;145:529-546.

20. Holstege JC: The ventro-medial medullary projections to spinal motoneurons: ultrastructure, transmitters and functional aspects. Prog Brain Res 1996;107:159-181.

21. Chase MH, Morales FR: Postsynaptic mechanisms responsible for motor inhibition during active sleep. In Chase MH, Weitzman E (eds): Sleep Disorders: Basic and Clinical Research. New York, Spectrum, 1983, pp 71-94.

22. Marchiafava PL, Pompeiano O: Pyramidal influences on spinal cord during desynchronized sleep. Arch Ital Biol 1964;102:500-529.

23. Burke RE: Composite nature of the monosynaptic excitatory postsynaptic potential. J Neurophysiol 1967;30:1114-1137.

24. Evarts EV: Temporal patterns of discharge of pyramidal tract neurons during sleep and waking in the monkey. J Neurophysiol 1964;27:152-171.

25. Curtis DR, Johnston GAR: Amino acid transmitters in the mammalian central nervous system. Ergebn Physiol 1974;69:97-188.

26. Davidoff RA, Hackmann JE: GABA presynaptic actions. In Rogawski MA, Barker JL (eds): Neurotransmitter Action in the Vertebrate Nervous System. New York, Plenum Press, 1985, pp 3-32.

27. Young AB, McDonald RL: Glycine as a spinal neurotransmitter. In Davidoff RA (ed): Handbook of the Spinal Cord, vol 1: Pharmacology. New York, Marcel Dekker, 1983, pp 1-43.

28. Curtis DR, Hosli L, Johnston GAR, et al: The hyperpolarization of spinal motoneurons by glycine and related amino acids. Exp Brain Res 1968;5:235-258.

29. Krnjevic K, Puil E, Werman R: Bicuculline, benzyl penicillin and inhibitory amino acids in the spinal cord of the cat. Can J Physiol Pharmacol 1976;55:670-680.

30. Nistri A: Spinal cord pharmacology of GABA and chemically related amino acids. In Davidoff RA (ed): Handbook of the Spinal Cord, vol 1: Pharmacology. New York, Marcel Dekker, 1983, pp 45-104.

31. Chase MH, Soja PJ, Finch DM: Pharmacological evidence of postsynaptic factors involved in the suppression of the masseteric reflex during active sleep. Sleep Res 1986;15:3.

32. Soja PJ, Morales FR, Chase MH: Effect of picrotoxin and bicuculline on the waveform characteristics of spontaneous IPSPs involved in motoneuron inhibition during active sleep. Soc Neurosci Abstr 1986;12:154.

33. Soja PJ, López-Rodríguez F, Morales FR, et al: A non-NMDA excitatory amino acid mediates subthreshold synaptic activity influencing cat lumbar motoneurons during quiet and active sleep. Physiologist 1988;31:A26.

34. Soja PJ, López-Rodríguez F, Morales FR, et al: Depolarizing synaptic events influencing cat lumbar motoneurons during rapid eye movement episodes of active sleep are blocked by kynurenic acid. Soc Neurosci Abstr 1988;14:941.

35. George R, Haslett WL, Jenden DJ: A cholinergic mechanism in the brainstem reticular formation: Induction of paradoxical sleep. Int J Neuropharmacol 1964;3:541-552.

36. Baghdoyan HA, Lydic R, Callaway CW, et al: The carbachol-induced enhancement of desynchronized sleep signs is dose-dependent and antagonized by centrally administered atropine. Neuropsychopharmacology 1989;2:67-79.

37. Kubin L, Kimura H, Tojima H, et al: Suppression of hypoglossal motoneurons during the carbachol-induced atonia of REM sleep is not caused by fast synaptic inhibition. Brain Res 1993;611:300-312.

38. Morales FR, Engelhardt JK, Pereda AE, et al: Renshaw cells are inactive during motor inhibition elicited by the pontine microinjection of carbachol. Neurosci Lett 1988;86:289-295.

39. Morales FR, Engelhardt JK, Soja PJ, et al: Motoneuron properties during motor inhibition produced by microinjection of carbachol into the pontine reticular formation of the decerebrate cat. J Neurophysiol 1987;57:1118-1129.

40. Takakusaki K, Ohta Y, Mori S: Single medullary reticulospinal neurons exert postsynaptic inhibitory effects via inhibitory interneurons upon alpha-motoneurons innervating cat hindlimb muscle. Exp Brain Res 1989;74:11-23.

41. López-Rodrguez F, Kohlmeier K, Morales FR, et al: Muscle atonia can be generated by carbachol in cats anesthetized with α-chloralose. Brain Res 1995;699:201-207.

42. Xi M-C, Liu R-H, Yamuy J, et al: Electrophysiological properties of lumbar motoneurons in the α-chloralose-anesthetized cat during carbachol-induced motor inhibition. J Neurophysiol 1997;78:129-136.

43. Xi M-C, Yamuy J, Liu R-H, et al: Dorsal spinocerebellar tract neurons are not subjected to postsynaptic inhibition during carbachol-induced motor inhibition. J Neurophysiol 1997;78:137-144.

44. Xi M-C, Morales FR, Chase MH: GABAergic synaptic transmission in the nucleus pontis oralis: A mechanism controlling the generation of active sleep. Soc Neurosci Abstr 1997;23:1066.

45. Xi M-C, Morales FR, Chase MH: GABAergic but not glycinergic pontine reticular mechanisms are involved in the control of active sleep and wakefulness. Sleep 1998;21:32.

46. Xi M-C, Morales FR, Chase MH: Evidence that wakefulness and REM sleep are controlled by a GABAergic pontine mechanism. J Neurophysiol 1999;82:2015-2019.

47. Xi M-C, Morales FR, Chase MH: Induction of wakefulness and inhibition of active (REM) sleep by GABAergic processes in the nucleus pontis oralis. Arch Ital Biol 2001;139:125-145.

48. Chase MH: A model of central neural processes controlling motor behavior during active sleep and wakefulness. In Desiraju T (ed): Mechanisms in Transmission for Signals for Conscious Behavior. Amsterdam, Elsevier, 1976, pp 99-121.

49. Magoun HW, Rhines R: An inhibitory mechanism in the bulbar reticular formation. J Neurophysiol 1946;9:165-171.

50. Yamuy J, Mancillas JR, Morales FR, et al: C-fos expression in the pons and medulla of the cat during carbachol-induced active sleep. J Neurosci 1993;13:2703-2718.

51. Morales FR, Sampogna, S, Yamuy J, et al: Premotor trigeminal interneurons activated during carbachol-induced active sleep. Soc Neurosci Abstr 1996;22:690.

52. Morales FR, Sampogna S, Yamuy J, et al: c-fos expression in brainstem premotor interneurons during cholinergically induced active sleep in the cat. J Neurosci 1999;19:9508-9518.

53. Chase MH, Babb M: Masseteric reflex response to reticular stimulation reverses during active sleep compared with wakefulness or quiet sleep. Brain Res 1973;59:421-426.

54. Chase MH: State-dependent reversal of a brainstem reflex in *Felix domesticus*. In Ferrendelli JA (ed): Society for Neuroscience Symposia, vol 3: Aspects of Behavioral Neurobiology. Bethesda, Md, Society for Neuroscience 1978, pp 33-65.

55. Chandler SH, Chase MH, Nakamura Y: Intracellular analysis of synaptic mechanisms controlling trigeminal motoneuron activity during sleep and wakefulness. J Neurophysiol 1980;44:359-371.

56. Chandler SH, Nakamura Y, Chase MH: Intracellular analysis of synaptic potentials induced in trigeminal jaw-closer motoneurons by pontomesencephalic reticular stimulation during sleep and wakefulness. J Neurophysiol 1980;44:372-382.

57. Chase MH, Enomoto S, Hiraba K, et al: Role of medullary reticular neurons in the inhibition of trigeminal motoneurons during active sleep. Exp Neurol 1984;84:364-373.

58. Sakai K, Yasuda M, Tomooka K, et al: Activation mechanism and reaction process of the compliment system-the classical pathway [in Japanese]. Nippon Rinsho 1979;37:943-955.

59. Yamuy J, Xi M-C, Fung SJ, et al: Hypocretinergic modulation of the reticular control of lumbar motoneurons during carbachol-induced atonia. Sleep 2003;26:A27-A28.

60. Fung SJ, Yamuy J, Xi M-C, et al: State-dependent control of lumbar motoneurons by the lateral hypothalamus. Sleep 2003;26:A22-A23.

61. Morales FR, Chase MH: Repetitive synaptic potentials responsible for inhibition of spinal cord motoneurons during active sleep. Exp Neurol 1982;78:471-476.

62. Fung SJ, Yamuy J, Xi M-C, et al: Changes in electrophysiological properties of cat hypoglossal motoneurons during carbachol-induced motor inhibition. Brain Res 2000;885:262-272.

63. Yamuy J, Fung SJ, Xi M-C, et al: Hypoglossal motoneurons are postsynaptically inhibited during carbachol-induced rapid eye movement sleep. Neuroscience 1999;94:11-15.

64. Torterolo P, Yamuy J, Sampogna S, et al: Hypothalamic neurons that contain hypocretin (orexin) express c-fos during active wakefulness and carbachol-induced active sleep. Sleep Research Online 2001;4:25-32.

65. Torterolo P, Yamuy J, Sampogna S, et al: Hypocretinergic neurons are primarily involved in activation of the somatomotor system. Sleep 2003;26:25-28.

13

Sleep-Promoting Mechanisms in Mammals

Dennis McGinty
Ronald Szymusiak

ABSTRACT

This chapter summarizes the study of brain mechanisms underlying the occurrence of non–rapid eye movement (NREM) sleep in mammals from early studies of human neuropathology through current attempts to discover the neurochemical basis of NREM sleep homeostasis. Lesions of multiple levels of the brain, including sites in the medulla, mesencephalon, preoptic area (POA) of the hypothalamus, thalamus, and entire neocortex, all markedly reduce the amount of NREM sleep, suggesting that this state requires the activity of functional inhibitory processes at all levels of the brain. Groups of neurons in the POA exhibit increased activity during NREM and REM sleep and respond to physiologic signals such as warming that increase sleep. Circadian signals from the mammalian "clock" in the hypothalamic suprachiasmatic nucleus are also integrated in this brain region. POA sleep-active neurons send inhibitory projections to the diffusely projecting arousal systems of the lateral and posterior hypothalamus and midbrain, including the histaminergic, orexinergic, serotonergic, and noradrenergic systems. By inhibition of these arousal systems, electroencephalographic synchronization can be initiated, and motor activity suppressed. Several putative neurochemical "sleep factors," including adenosine, interleukin-1 and other cytokines, prostaglandin D_2, growth hormone–releasing hormone, and nitric oxide, promote sleep through actions in or adjacent to the POA. Although each of these sleep factors has the capacity to control sleep, our understanding of their roles in normal sleep homeostasis and the neurochemical processes mediating their actions is incomplete.

In this chapter we explore which groups of neurons and neurochemical processes combine to generate the phenomenology of sleep, including patterns of brain activity and peripheral physiology associated with sleep, interactions between non–rapid eye movement (NREM) and REM sleep, temporal properties of states, homeostatic regulation, and circadian distribution. Historically, sleep-promoting or hypnogenic mechanisms were identified on the basis of the effects of brain lesions, specifically, the observation of insomnia following lesions. Recently, putative hypnogenic mechanisms have been identified on the basis of neurochemical processes, that is, the demonstration that activation of a particular neurochemical pathway promotes sleep. We summarize data obtained using both of these approaches.

There is evidence for the existence of sleep promoting mechanisms at all levels of the neuraxis, including both forebrain and brainstem. These will be reviewed first, followed by a summary of more recent findings. One recent focus has been on putative sleep-promoting neurons of the preoptic area (POA) of the hypothalamus and on the interactions of the POA with arousal-promoting neuronal groups localized in the pontine and midbrain reticular formation, posterior (PH) and lateral hypothalamus (LH), and the basal forebrain (BF). This model is supported by data derived from a wide variety of methods, including lesions, neuronal unit recording, local chemical, electrical, and thermal stimulation, anatomic tract tracing, and responses to physiologic manipulations of sleep. We suggest how a POA sleep-promoting mechanism might be related to more widespread sleep-regulatory processes.

DIVERSE BRAIN REGIONS MODULATING NREM SLEEP

Figure 13–1 provides an overview to orient the reader to the neuronal systems and pathways to be discussed in the following review. See Moruzzi[1] for a thoughtful and detailed review of the older work in this area.

The Isolated Forebrain

Early studies examined the physiology of the chronically maintained isolated forebrain or chronic *cerveau isolé* preparation in dogs and cats.[2-4] Animals with complete transverse transections of the brainstem at the level of the midbrain or rostral pons can be maintained and observed for many weeks, with careful nursing. Acutely, after complete midbrain transections, the forebrain exhibited continuous electroencephalographic (EEG) synchronization with slow waves and spindles, but after 1 to 2 weeks, periods of spontaneous EEG activation were seen, which became progressively more sustained. Onset of EEG activation after a sustained synchronized state could be sudden, whereas reonset of synchrony was gradual, much like normal sleep–wake–sleep transitions. During periods of progressive development of full synchronization, olfactory stimuli (a sensory system directly connected to the forebrain) could produce arousal, but such stimuli were ineffective during sustained synchrony. Both rostral and caudal (low) midbrain transections were evaluated. After "low" transections, which preserved the third nerve above the transection, pupillary dilation accompanied EEG activation. If brainstem transections were made still lower, at the midpontine level, an activated forebrain state became predominant immediately after the transection, but with some residual episodes of EEG synchronization.[5] In this midpontine pretrigeminal preparation, the forebrain exhibited evidence of conditioning, and other signs of an integrated waking state.[6] In summary, much evidence suggests that the upper brainstem and forebrain can generate both waking and sleep states.

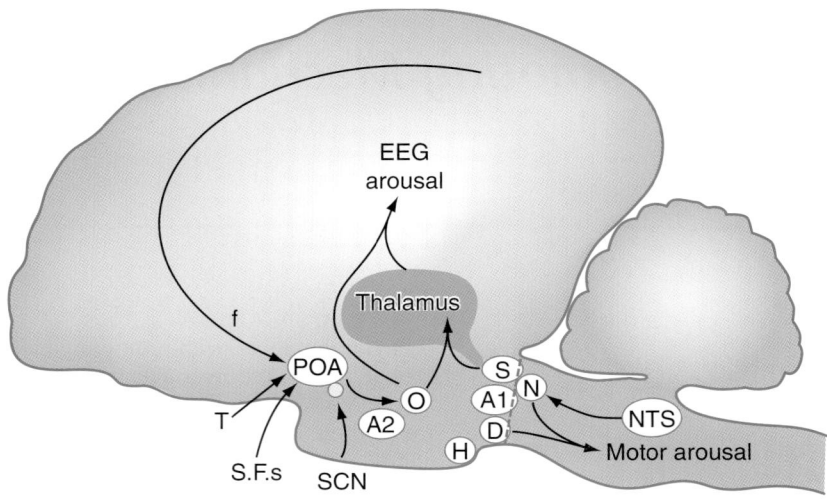

Figure 13–1. Sagittal view of a generic mammalian brain providing an overview of the sleep–wake control networks to be described in the text. The upper brainstem, posterior and lateral hypothalamus, and basal forebrain contain several clusters of neuronal phenotypes with arousal-inducing properties. These clusters include neurons expressing serotonin (S), norepinephrine (N), acetylcholine (A) in both pontomesencephalic and basal forebrain clusters (A1 and A2), dopamine (D), histamine (H), and orexin/hypocretin (O). All of these groups facilitate electroencephalographic (EEG) arousal (waking and rapid eye movement sleep) or motor-behavioral arousal (waking). The arousal systems facilitate forebrain EEG activation both through the thalamus and the basal forebrain and through direct projections to neocortex. Arousal systems also facilitate motor-behavioral arousal through descending pathways. (See Chapter 11 for an extensive discussion of arousal systems.) The arousal-generating neuronal groups are inhibited by sleep-inducing neuronal groups in both the preoptic area of the hypothalamus (POA) and in the region of the nucleus tractus solitarius (NTS) of the medulla. The POA sleep-inducing region is modulated by the circadian clock in the suprachiasmatic nucleus (SCN), by the actions of several neurochemical sleep factors (S.F.s), and by brain and body temperature (T). The thalamus and neocortex also facilitate sleep, possibly through "feedback" (f) to the POA. The *dashed line* indicates a type of brainstem transection that was used in early studies of the neural control of sleep (see text). The exact level of such transections ranged from "high" at the upper midbrain level to "low" at the midpontine level.

After 5 to 9 days of recovery from surgery, the chronic *cerveau isolé* rat preparation exhibited a circadian pattern of EEG activation and synchronization.[7] In this preparation, POA lesions were followed by a continuously activated electroencephalogram, abolishing the circadian facilitation of synchronization. Thus, the POA must play a central role in generating the synchronized state of the *cerveau isolé*.

Diencephalon

Chronic "diencephalic cats," in which neocortex and striatum had been removed except for the piriform cortex, ventral hippocampus, and BF, exhibited three states, behavioral waking with persistent locomotion and orientation to auditory stimuli, a "quiet sleep"–like or NREM-like state with typical cat sleeping postures, and an REM-like state including antigravity muscle atonia, rapid eye movements, muscle twitches, and pontine EEG spikes.[8] Cats even displayed typical motor events after behavioral arousal such as stretching. EEG patterns recorded in the thalamus showed increased amplitude in conjunction with the NREM sleep–like state, although true spindles and slow waves were absent in the chronic state. The thalamic electroencephalogram exhibited desynchronization during the REM-like state.

The chronic diencephalic preparation exhibited greatly reduced amounts of the drowsy state and NREM sleep in the chronic state, usually 25% of that in intact animals. The REM-like state was reduced by more than 90%. This study showed that, at least in the cat, the neocortex and striatum are not required for the behavioral expression of any behaviorally defined sleep–wake state, but are involved in the balance of excitatory and inhibitory processes that affect the regulation of sleep amounts. An NREM-like state occurs in the absence of sleep spindles and slow waves.

Thalamus

The thalamus plays a critical role in regulating cortical EEG patterns during waking and sleep (see Chapter 9). Portions of the thalamus also appear to have hypnogenic functions, although it is unclear which thalamic nuclei are most importantly involved in sleep promotion. Low-frequency stimulation of the midline thalamus produced EEG synchrony and behavioral sleep in cats.[9] However, large lesions of the midline thalamic nuclei in cats did not substantially alter amounts of sleep and waking.[10] Cats subjected to complete thalamectomy (athalamic cats) continue to exhibit episodes of EEG and behavioral sleep and waking, although there is an absence of spindles in the NREM sleep electroencephalogram.[11] Athalamic cats exhibit chronic insomnia, with reductions in both NREM and REM sleep.

A role of the anterior and dorsomedial thalamic nuclei in sleep regulation is suggested by anatomic findings in the very rare human hereditary neurodegenerative (prion) disease, fatal familial insomnia. This disease is characterized by progressive autonomic hyperactivation, motor disturbances, loss of sleep spindles, and severe NREM sleep insomnia, typically beginning after approximately 40 years of age.[12]

Neuropathologic findings reveal severe cell loss and gliosis in the anterior medial thalamus, including the dorsomedial nucleus. Nonthalamic sites of neuronal loss include the inferior olives, neocortex, and cerebellum. Bilateral lesions of the dorsomedial thalamic nucleus in cats cause significant reductions in NREM sleep, with less pronounced decrements in REM sleep.[13] Collectively, these findings suggest an important role for anterior thalamic-limbic cortical circuitry in sleep–wake regulation. However, patients with paramedian thalamic stroke, with magnetic resonance imaging–verified damage to the dorsomedial and centromedial nuclei, present with either severe hypersomnolence or increased daytime sleepiness, not insomnia.[14]

Brainstem

Rudimentary behavioral waking, an NREM-like sleep, and an REM-like sleep can also be generated by the lower brainstem.[15] After recovery from the acute effects of the complete midbrain transections, the motor behavior of the cats could be characterized as having three states, including "waking," identified by crouching, sitting, attempts to walk, dilated pupils, and head orientation to noises. Two sleeplike states were observed. In the first, cats would lie down in a random position, pupils would exhibit reduced but variable miosis, and eyes would exhibit slow and nonconjugate movements. Animals could be aroused by auditory or other stimuli. If this "variable miosis stage" was not disturbed, cats would enter another stage, characterized by complete pupillary miosis, loss of neck muscle tone, and rapid eye movements. This state would be sustained for 20 seconds to 25 minutes. Compared with the variable miosis stage, more intense stimulation was required to produce "arousal" from the extreme miosis state. The latter state closely corresponds to the REM-like state described in decerebrate cats,[16] which led to the search for brainstem REM circuitry. Clearly, the variable miosis state could be identified as an NREM sleep–like state that normally precedes REM sleep. However, the electroencephalogram recorded in the brainstem was not changed across states. If these cats were maintained for approximately 30 days, the variable miosis state occupied approximately 55% of the time and the extreme miosis stage approximately 9% of the time, roughly approximating the amount of NREM and REM sleep in intact cats.

Additional older studies supported the hypothesis that the lower brainstem is responsible for sleep-facilitating processes. Low-frequency electrical stimulation of the dorsal medullary reticular formation in the nucleus of the solitary track produced neocortical EEG synchronization.[17] Lesions[18] or cooling[19] of this site were followed by EEG activation. A sleep-promoting action originating in the lower brainstem was also suggested by the predominance of EEG activation above complete brainstem transections at the midpontine level,[5] as summarized previously. These findings all support a hypothesis that structures below the midpontine level normally inhibit arousal or promote sleep.

Lesions encompassing the ventral pontomesencephalic reticular formation and adjacent ventral structures produced severe, sustained sleep reductions.[20] Both NREM and REM sleep were reduced by approximately 50% 1 month after the lesions. These lesions destroyed 80% of the dopamine-containing neurons in this region. These neurons provide the dopaminergic innervation of the forebrain. However, it has not been determined if dopaminergic neuronal loss underlies the sleep deficit in these animals because other neuronal groups were also damaged.

In summary, widespread structures in the mammalian nervous system, from the neocortex to the lower brainstem, have the capacity to facilitate both sleeplike and waking-like states and to modulate the amounts of sleep.

THE PREOPTIC HYPOTHALAMUS

Preoptic Area and Basal Forebrain Anatomy

Critical forebrain hypnogenic mechanisms are localized in the POA of the hypothalamus and the adjacent BF. The POA extends rostrally to the lamina terminalis and caudally to the anterior hypothalamic nuclei at the level of the optic chiasm. Ventrally, the POA extends to the base of the brain, with the anterior commissure marking the dorsal border. The lateral edge of the optic chiasm approximates the boundary between the medial and lateral POA. More laterally, in the absence of distinct boundaries, the POA merges with the magnocellular BF, a region that contains the corticopetal cholinergic projection system, as well as noncholinergic ascending and descending projection neurons, including a prominent collection of magnocellular gamma-aminobutyric acid–ergic (GABAergic) neurons. Many neuropeptides, hormone-releasing factors, and neurotransmitters are found in the medial POA. In addition to sleep regulation, cells in the POA are critically involved in body temperature control, body fluid balance, cardiovascular regulation, neuroendocrine control, and reproductive physiology and behavior.

A Preoptic Area Sleep-Promoting System

The existence of a POA sleep-promoting area was first proposed more than 70 years ago on the basis of observations that patients with encephalitis and severe insomnia before death were found post mortem to have inflammatory lesions in this area.[21] Other patients with hypersomnia before death had lesions in the vicinity of the PH. These observations suggested the concept of opposing hypothalamic sleep-promoting and wake-promoting systems. In rats, symmetrical bilateral transections of the POA were followed by complete sleeplessness, and symmetrical bilateral transections of the PH were followed by continuous sleep.[22] However, wakefulness could be induced by sensory stimulation, so this resembled normal sleep. Rats with both POA and PH transections exhibited continuous sleep, as did those with PH transections alone. This was interpreted as showing that the POA normally inhibited the PH wake-promoting region.

The existence of a sleep-promoting mechanism in the POA has been confirmed by a variety of methods. Experimental lesions of this area result in insomnia. Bilateral lesions of the POA with diameters of approximately 1 to 2 mm in rats[23] and cats[24] induce partial sleep loss, sometimes followed by partial recovery. Larger, bilateral 3- to 5-mm lesions that extend into the adjacent BF, or transections, induce total or near-total insomnia and sometimes lead to death.[22,25,26] Current evidence suggests that both the location and the size of the lesion in this region determine the magnitude of the sleep deficit. Lesions with diameters under 1 mm produce small sleep deficits.

A recent study suggested that the insomnia produced by POA lesions is due to destruction of galanin-containing neurons in the ventrolateral POA (VLPO). This nucleus was originally identified as containing neurons that exhibit c-*fos* gene expression during sleep (see later). After excitotoxic lesions that were centered on the rat VLPO, but which in every instance produced extensive damage medial, lateral, and dorsal to this nucleus, the degree of sleep loss was positively correlated with loss of neurons in the VLPO. This was interpreted as indicating that loss of VLPO neurons was the critical factor in determining sleep loss. This interpretation is difficult to reconcile with the ability of lesions of the medial POA[27] and the dorsolateral POA[28] that spare the VLPO also to yield severe, persistent insomnia. Cell loss in the VLPO may have been correlated with another, unmeasured variable, such as total lesion volume, which could have been the causative factor mediating severity of sleep loss. To date, there are no published demonstrations that small, specific lesions that target a particular POA subnucleus can yield significant sleep disruption. The concept of a distributed sleep-promoting system is supported by unit recording and c-Fos studies, summarized later.

Several studies have used cell-selective neurotoxins to generate POA lesions,[27,29] showing that loss of local neurons rather than fibers of passage is sufficient to produce experimental insomnia. After POA lesions that resulted in partial sleep loss, implantation of healthy fetal POA tissue into the lesion site prompted the recovery of normal sleep amounts.[30] This finding supports the hypothesis that the hypnogenic process originates in POA neuronal tissue. POA lesions result in transient abnormalities in feeding, body weight, and thermoregulation, but insomnia long outlasts these deficits.[27] Thus, lesion-induced insomnia is not secondary to these other deficits.

After discrete POA lesions that result in partial sleep loss, residual sleep is characterized by reduced delta EEG activity,[31] or low amounts of "deeper" sleep, as defined by EEG slow wave activity.[29] Delta activity in NREM sleep can be increased by POA warming (see later). Because occurrence of delta activity is recognized as a marker of enhanced sleep drive, this finding suggests that POA output contributes to the regulation of sleep drive.

All POA lesions were found to suppress REM as well as NREM sleep. This suggests that NREM and REM sleep are coupled, or that POA mechanisms facilitate REM as well as NREM sleep. In cats with sustained insomnia after POA lesions, administration of a low dose of the anesthetic, pentobarbital, was followed by increased REM sleep, although the identical treatment inhibited REM sleep in intact animals.[32] This study showed that REM sleep–generating mechanisms are not directly disturbed by POA lesions, but that the lesions must result in a process that inhibits or disfacilitates brainstem REM sleep–generating mechanisms.

Electrical stimulation of the ventral POA can induce EEG synchronization and behavioral sleep.[33] This finding led to a prediction that the POA would contain sleep-active neurons. Such findings have been made in cats, rabbits, rats, and kangaroo rats (reviewed in McGinty and Szymusiak[34]). In all studies, sleep-active neurons constituted a minority of the neurons recorded, ranging rather consistently from 21% to 34% in nine studies. Additional work focused on the neuronal activity in specific POA nuclei and relating sleep-active neuronal activity to temperature is discussed further later.

c-Fos Mapping

The further identification of sleep-active neurons was advanced by the application of the c-Fos immunostaining method to this problem.[35] Rapid expression of the protooncogene, c-*fos*, has been identified as a marker of neuronal activation in many brain sites.[36] The presence of c-Fos protein in the nucleus can be readily measured within 30 minutes of neuronal activation with immunostaining methods.

A discrete cluster of neurons exhibiting c-Fos immunoreactivity was found in the VLPO after sustained sleep, but there was little labeling after waking.[35] The VLPO region containing c-Fos immunoreactivity was lateral to the optic chiasm, extending caudally from behind the organum vasculosum of the lamina terminalis to near the emergence of the supraoptic nucleus and extending dorsally from the base of the brain into the lateral preoptic area without a distinct border. The VLPO was also identified as having strong anatomic connections to the histamine-containing arousal-related neuronal group in the tuberomammillary nucleus of the PH. Additional projections of the VLPO include the midbrain dorsal raphe nucleus and the locus coeruleus in the pons.[37,38] VLPO projection neurons contain the inhibitory neuromodulator galanin, which is highly colocalized with the inhibitory neurotransmitter, GABA, in this nucleus.[37,39] VLPO neurons that express c-Fos immunoreactivity after sleep have been shown to express galanin messenger RNA (mRNA)[40] or glutamic acid decarboxylase, the synthetic enzyme for GABA.[41] Collectively, these findings suggest that activation of galaninergic/GABAergic VLPO neurons during sleep could function to inhibit multiple monoaminergic arousal systems in the PH, midbrain, and pons.

We applied the c-Fos immunostaining method to learn more about the anatomic distribution and numbers of POA sleep-active neurons.[42] We examined the distribution of c-Fos–immunoreactive neurons during sleep and waking at a neutral ambient temperature (T_a), 22° C, and a mildly warm T_a compatible with sleep in the rat, 31.5° C. At the neutral T_a, we confirmed the existence of a segregated group of c-Fos–immunoreactive neurons in the VLPO and identified an additional group in the rostral and caudal median preoptic nucleus (MnPN). The MnPN is a midline cell group that widens to form a "cap" around the rostral end of the third ventricle and extends ventrally to the organum vasculosum of the lamina terminalis. Examples of c-Fos immunostaining and the correlations between c-Fos counts and sleep amounts are shown in Figure 13–2. We found in the rostral MnPN that the number of sleep-related c-Fos–immunoreactive neurons was increased during exposure to 31.5° C compared with 22° C. In the VLPO area, the number of c-Fos–immunoreactive neurons was reduced in the heat-sleep condition compared with control-sleep. Most of the MnPN neurons that immunostain for c-Fos protein after sleep also stain for glutamic acid decarboxylase.[41] Like the VLPO, the MnPN projects to both the dorsal raphe nucleus and the locus coeruleus.[43,44] The MnPN also projects to the perifornical lateral hypothalamic area, the location of cell bodies of the hypocretin/orexin arousal system.[44,45]

We used neuronal recording techniques in the rat VLPO and MnPN during sleep and wakefulness to confirm that sleep-related c-Fos immunoreactivity was associated with the presence of neurons with sleep-related discharge patterns, and to examine sequential changes in discharge within sleep episodes.[46,47]

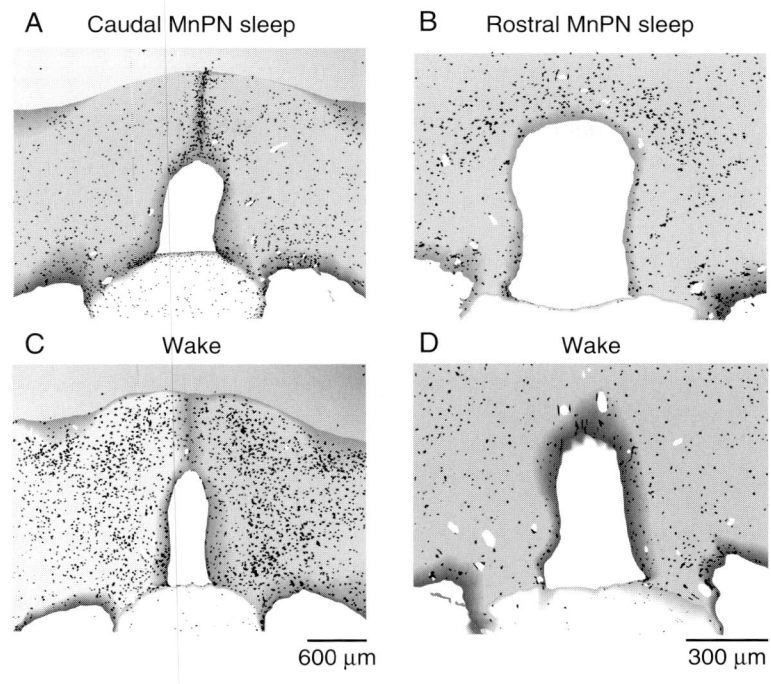

A   Caudal MnPN sleep

B   Rostral MnPN sleep

C   Wake

D   Wake

600 μm

300 μm

ROSTRAL MnPN c-FOS COUNT
vs SLEEP PERCENTAGE

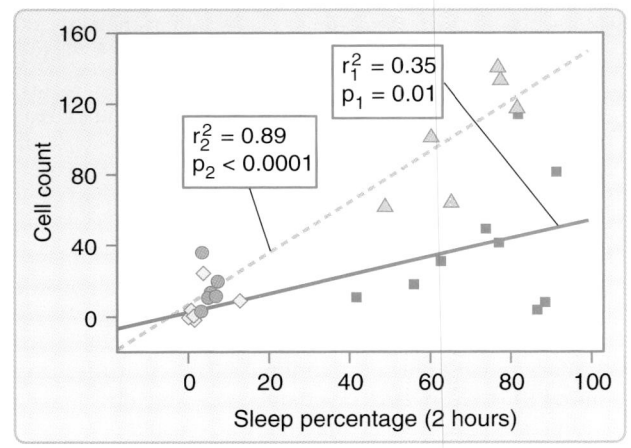

$r_1^2 = 0.35$
$p_1 = 0.01$

$r_2^2 = 0.89$
$p_2 < 0.0001$

CAUDAL MnPN c-FOS COUNT
vs SLEEP PERCENTAGE

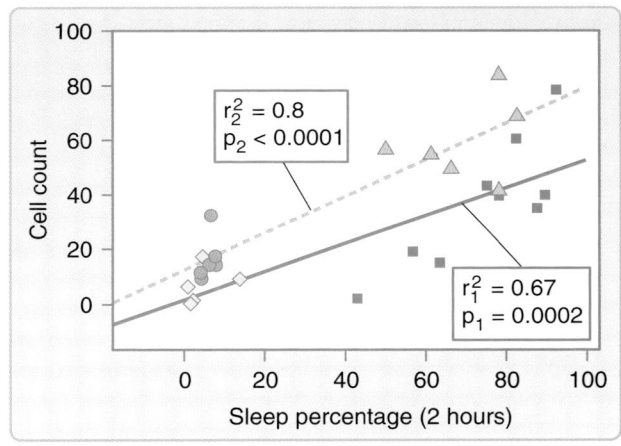

$r_2^2 = 0.8$
$p_2 < 0.0001$

$r_1^2 = 0.67$
$p_1 = 0.0002$

■ Control sleep (CS)
◇ Control wake (CW)

△ Heat sleep (HS)
● Heat wake (HW)

—— Control sleep vs control wake
----- Heat sleep vs heat wake

VLPO c-FOS COUNT vs SLEEP PERCENTAGE

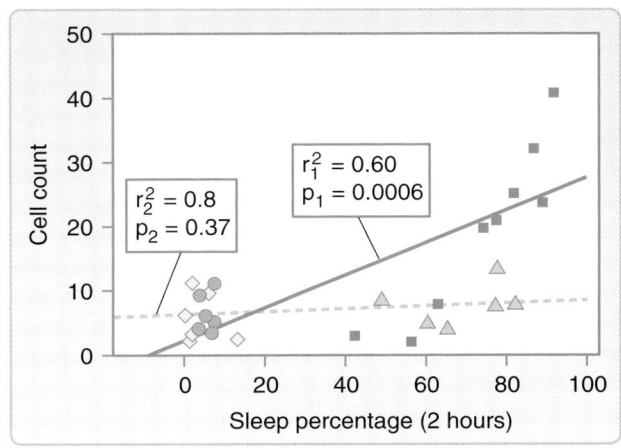

$r_2^2 = 0.8$
$p_2 = 0.37$

$r_1^2 = 0.60$
$p_1 = 0.0006$

Figure 13–2. For legend see next page.

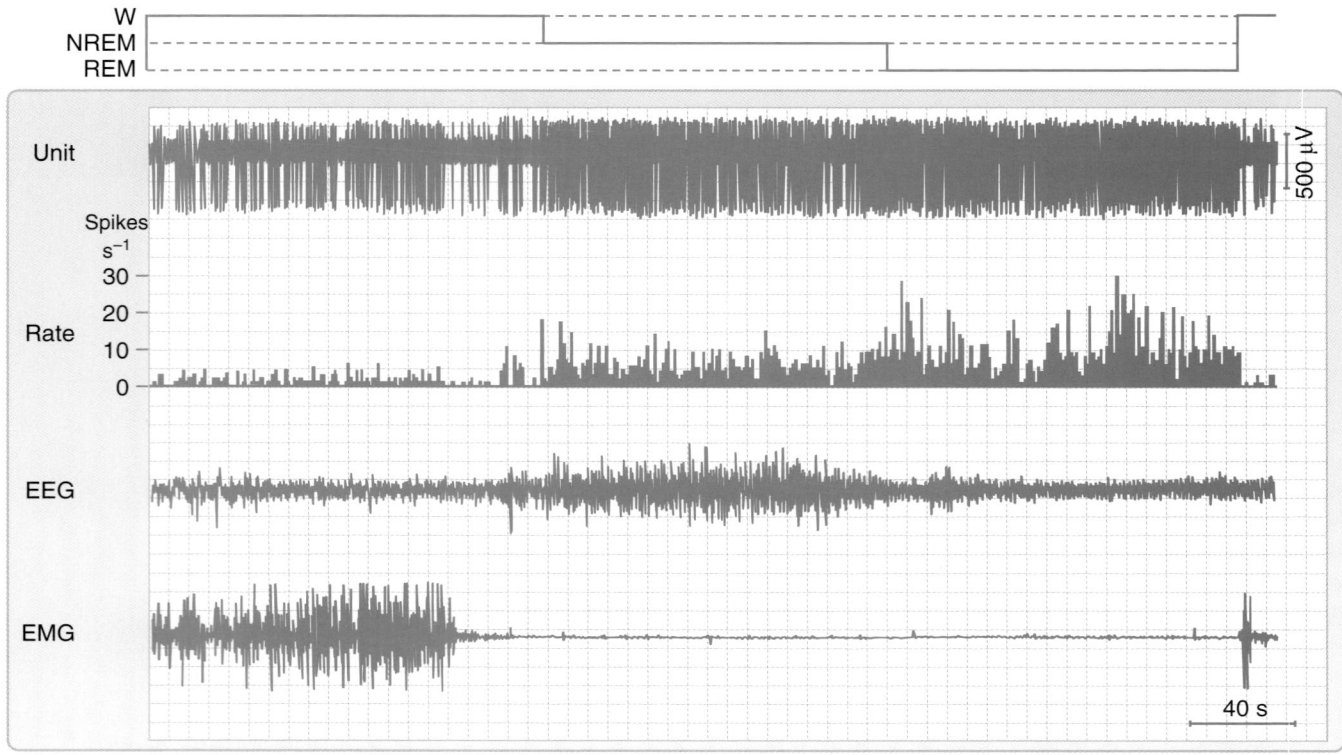

Figure 13–3. Example of a sleep-active neuron in the median preoptic nucleus (MnPN). Shown is a continuous recording of discharge of an MnPN neuron during a wake–non–rapid eye movement (NREM) sleep–REM sleep cycle (*top*). Discharge rate increased at the onset of sleep, which is indicated by the increased amplitude of the electroencephalogram (EEG). Discharge rate increased further in association with REM sleep (*right*). Such sleep-active neurons were the majority of neurons encountered in the MnPN and ventrolateral preoptic area. The presence of sleep-active neurons provides one critical piece of evidence for the importance of a brain region in the facilitation of sleep. EMG, electromyogram. (Reprinted with permission from Suntsova N, Szymusiak R, Alam M, et al: Sleep-waking discharge patterns of median preoptic nucleus neurons in rats. J Physiol [Lond] 2002;543:665-677.)

Approximately 50% of neurons recorded in the VLPO region exhibited sleep-related discharge patterns.[46] Most VLPO neurons were activated during both NREM and REM sleep compared with waking. Most VLPO neurons also exhibited an increase in activity during the immediate transition periods between waking and sleep onset and displayed a progressive increase in discharge rate from light to deep NREM sleep. In response to 12 to 16 hours of sleep deprivation, VLPO neurons exhibited increased activation during sleep, but rates during waking remained the same as in rats that were not sleep deprived.

In a sample of MnPN neurons, 76% exhibited the highest discharge rate during NREM sleep or REM sleep.[47] The largest population (58% of the sample) exhibited elevated discharge rates during both NREM and REM sleep compared with waking, similar to VLPO neurons (Fig. 13–3). Most MnPN cells showed a gradual increase in their firing rates before sleep onset, elevated discharge rates during NREM sleep, and a small, but significant additional increase in discharge rate during REM sleep. Peak discharge rates were observed early in NREM sleep episodes that followed sustained episodes of waking.

The MnPN and VLPO sleep-active neuronal sites were identified because they did not show c-Fos immunoreactivity after waking. Other sites in the POA also exhibited sleep-related c-Fos immunoreactivity, but the same sites showed many c-Fos–immunostained cells after waking. At this time we cannot tell if the cells expressing c-Fos after sleep in these

Figure 13–2. Cont'd. *Upper:* Examples of c-Fos immunostaining of preoptic area (POA) neuronal nuclei, identified by dark spots after either sustained spontaneous sleep or waking. c-Fos immunostaining is a marker of neuronal activation, and provides a method for mapping the localization of sleep-active neurons in the brain. After sleep, increased staining was seen in the midline or around the top of the third ventricle compared with the waking samples. These sites correspond to the caudal and rostral median preoptic nucleus (MnPN). Similar results were seen in the ventrolateral POA (VLPO). In other POA sites, c-Fos immunostaining was seen after both waking and sleep. *Lower:* Regression functions and correlations relating c-Fos counts and sleep amounts before sacrifice among individual animals. In all sites, high correlations were found between sleep amounts and c-Fos counts at a normal ambient temperature. Groups of animals were studied in both normal and warm ambient temperatures. In a warm ambient temperature, c-Fos counts after sleep and correlations between counts and sleep amounts were increased in MnPN sites, but were suppressed in VLPO. (Reprinted with permission from Gong H, Szymusiak R, King J, et al: Sleep-related c-Fos expression in the preoptic hypothalamus: Effects of ambient warming. Am J Physiol 2000;279:R2079-R2088.)

widespread POA areas correspond to sleep-active neurons, or if they are activated by some other process that is present during both sleep and waking. Electrophysiologic studies found sleep-active neurons diffusely in the POA, and lesions that did not include the VLPO or MnPN suppressed sleep (see earlier). This suggests that much of the diffuse sleep-related c-Fos immunoreactivity in POA also labels sleep-active neurons.

THE SLEEP–WAKE SWITCH MODEL

As reviewed previously, sleep-active neurons in the POA are GABAergic and distribute descending projections to arousal-related neuronal groups in the midbrain, PH, and LH. GABA release is increased during NREM sleep and further increased in REM sleep in the PH,[48] and in the dorsal raphe nucleus[49] and locus coeruleus,[50] all sites containing arousal-related neurons.

As is reviewed later, activation of POA warm-sensitive neurons (WSNs) during sleep may be one mechanism underlying inhibition of arousal systems. Local stimulation of POA WSNs inhibits arousal-related neurons in the PH, dorsal raphe nucleus, and locus coeruleus. Reversible inactivation or lesions of the PH counteract the insomnia that follows POA lesions, suggesting that the sleep-inducing output of the POA is directed at PH neurons with wake-promoting functions.[51] Sleep-active neurons in the VLPO and MnPN exhibit discharge rate change profiles across the wake–NREM sleep–REM sleep cycle that are reciprocal to those of wake-promoting neurons of the PH histaminergic, dorsal raphe nucleus serotonergic, and locus coeruleus noradrenergic groups, and to unidentified neurons in the orexinergic neuronal field of the LH (Fig. 13–4). These findings support a hypothesis that the POA sleep-promoting neurons inhibit multiple arousal systems.

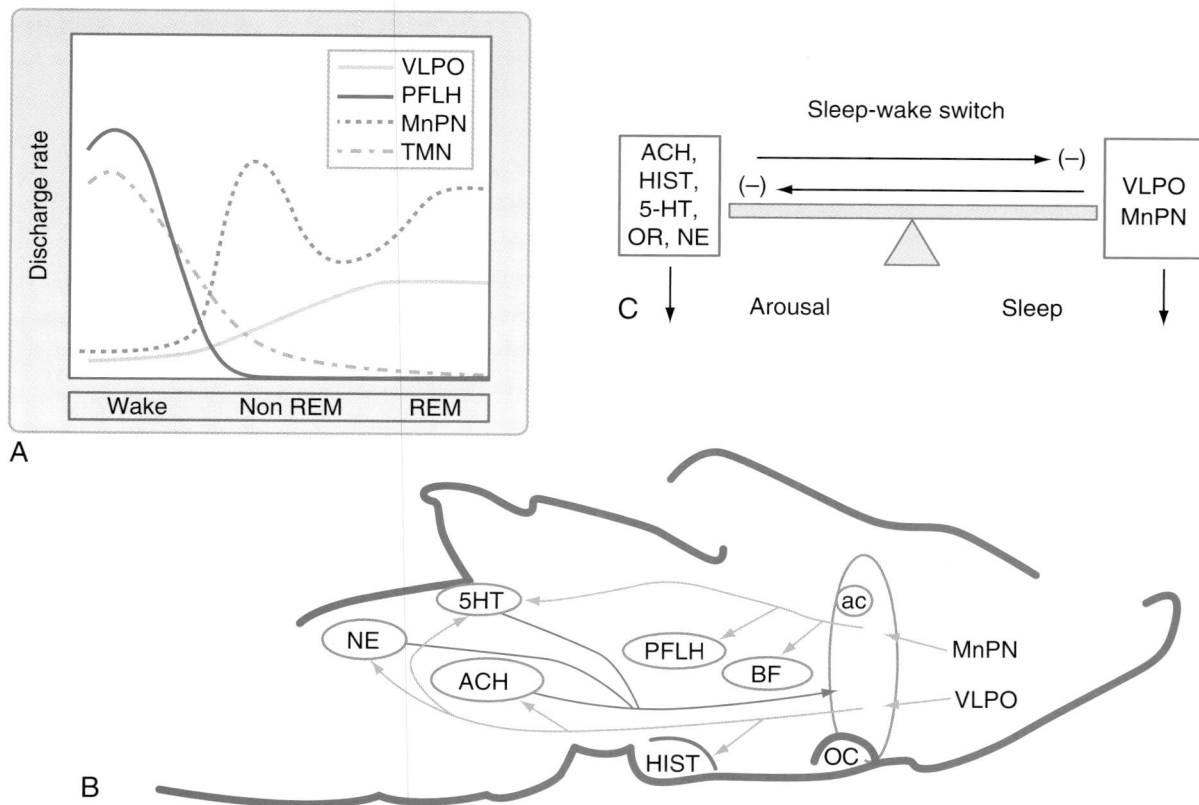

Figure 13–4. Interactions of the preoptic area (POA) sleep-promoting neuronal system with arousal systems that can account for the orchestration of the sleep process. **A,** The neuronal discharge rates across the wake–non–rapid eye movement (NREM) sleep–REM sleep cycle of sleep-active neurons from the ventrolateral POA (VLPO) and median preoptic nucleus (MnPN) and of arousal-related (wake-active) neurons in the perifornical lateral hypothalamus (PFLH) and tuberomammillary nucleus (TMN). These neuronal groups have generally reciprocal discharge patterns, although MnPN and VLPO neurons have peak activity at different times during NREM sleep episodes. The wake-active, NREM sleep–diminished, REM sleep–off discharge pattern shown for TMN and a subgroup of PFLH neurons is also characteristic of putative serotoninergic neurons of the dorsal raphe nucleus and putative noradrenergic neurons (NE) of the locus coeruleus. **B,** Sagittal section of the diencephalon and upper brainstem of the rat showing anatomic interconnections of MnPN and VLPO neurons with arousal-related neuronal groups. The MnPN and VLPO distribute projections to sites of arousal-related activity, including the (1) basal forebrain (BF); (2) PFLH, which includes orexin-containing neurons; (3) histamine (HIST)-containing neurons of the tuberomammillary nucleus; (4) pontomesencephalic acetylcholine(ACH)-containing neurons; (5) pontomesencephalic serotonin (5HT)-containing neurons; and (6) norepinephrine (NE)-containing neurons of the pons in the locus coeruleus. 5HT, NE, and ACH arousal-related neurons provide inhibitory "feedback" to sleep-active neurons. The arousal-related neuronal groups also have widespread additional ascending and descending projections that control state-related functions throughout the brain. **C,** The sleep–wake switch or "flip-flop" model characterized by mutually inhibitory sleep-promoting and arousal-promoting neuronal groups, depicted as a seesaw that can promote stable sleep or waking states. Activity of either sleep-promoting or arousal-promoting neurons inhibits the neurons generating the opposing state. This network provides a mechanism for the global control of brain activity in the sleep–wake cycle. oc, optic chiasm; ac, anterior commissure. (Modified with permission from McGinty D, Szymusiak R: Hypothalamic regulation of sleep and arousal. Front Biosci 2003;8:1074-1083.)

GABAergic neurons in the VLPO region are inhibited by acetylcholine, serotonin, and norepinephrine, transmitters of the arousal systems.[52] MnPN neurons are inhibited by norepinephrine.[53] Thus, arousal and sleep-promoting systems are thought to be mutually inhibitory, suggesting a sleep–wake switch or "flip-flop" model[34,54] (Fig. 13–4). Activation of arousal systems would inhibit sleep-active neurons, thereby removing inhibition from arousal systems, facilitating stable episodes of waking. On the other hand, activation of sleep-promoting neurons would inhibit arousal-related neurons, remove inhibition from sleep-promoting neurons, and thus reinforce consolidated sleep episodes. This model provides a mechanism for the stabilization of both sleep and waking states. Abnormalities in one or more of the components of this system would result in unstable sleep–wake cycles, a typical feature of sleep disorders in which insomnia is an element, and in narcolepsy.

THE ORCHESTRATION OF SLEEP BY THE PREOPTIC AREA

The POA system has anatomic and physiologic properties that provide a basis for the orchestration of the primary components of the sleep process. The POA sleep-promoting system can control EEG patterns through two pathways, direct projections from POA to thalamus,[55] and inhibitory actions on monoaminergic and orexinergic systems,[45] which also project to the thalamus. Activity of monoaminergic and orexinergic neurons facilitates thalamic depolarization through inhibition of potassium channels.[56,57] Thus, inhibition of monoaminergic and orexinergic neurons facilitates hyperpolarization of thalamic neurons, permitting the activation of voltage-dependent membrane currents underlying spindles and slow waves (see Chapter 8). The PH and LH areas facilitate both motor and autonomic activation, under GABAergic control.[58] Sleep-related GABAergic inhibition of the PH and LH provides a basis for sleep-related deactivation of autonomic and motor functions. The POA might facilitate REM sleep episodes by partially suppressing activity of serotonergic and noradrenergic neurons in association with NREM sleep. We speculate that this suppression triggers the activation of brainstem REM sleep–generating neuronal circuitry.[59]

The suprachiasmatic nucleus (SCN) of the POA generates the signals that bring about the circadian patterns of sleep–waking.[60] The anatomic pathways by which the circadian clock in the SCN controls POA sleep-promoting neurons are the focus of recent studies. Lesions of a primary SCN projection target, the subparaventricular zone, eliminate circadian rhythms of sleep–waking.[61] Circadian patterns of sleep–waking are also suppressed by third ventricular infusion of transforming growth factor-α, which is hypothesized to convey the circadian signal from the SCN to the subparaventricular zone.[62] The subparaventricular zone projects indirectly to the VLPO, MnPN, and other POA regions through the dorsomedial hypothalamic nucleus as well as directly to the MnPN.[63,64] Indirect pathways from SCN to VLPO and MnPN through the medial POA were also identified. In diurnal animals, SCN output could inhibit sleep-promoting neurons during the light phase, or facilitate sleep-promoting neurons in the dark phase.

Hierarchical Control Model

In summary, a central role for the POA in the orchestration of sleep is supported by a variety of findings, including the occurrence of insomnia in association with POA neuropathologic processes in humans. On the other hand, as reviewed previously, sleeplike behavior may be generated by an isolated lower brainstem, and sleep is facilitated by the midbrain, thalamus, and neocortex. To rationalize these diverse findings, it is useful to consider a hierarchical control concept, like that applied previously to thermoregulation.[65] In this conceptualization, a fundamental behavior such as rest–activity or sleep–waking is organized at all levels of the neuraxis, just as rest–activity cycles are found in all orders of animals. The POA may act as a master control, integrating sleep-promoting circuitry with sleep homeostatic processes, other behavioral and hormonal regulatory systems, and circadian signals. The limbic system and neocortex are likely sources of additional controls, related to more complex behavioral contingencies, including learned processes such as the location and safety of nesting sites, instinctive behaviors, and sensory stimuli. These controls may be conveyed to the hypothalamus through projections from the neocortex and limbic system.

THE PREOPTIC AREA, THERMOREGULATION, AND CONTROL OF SLEEP

The POA is recognized as a thermoregulatory control site on the basis of the effects of local warming and cooling, lesions, local chemical stimulations studies, and neuronal unit recording studies. For example, local POA warming, using a chronically implanted water-perfused "thermode," induced heat loss responses such as panting.[66] Local POA warming was also shown to trigger NREM sleep or EEG slow wave activity in cats, rabbits, and rats (reviewed in McGinty and Szymusiak[34]). NREM sleep could be tonically increased for several hours with sustained POA warming in kangaroo rats.[67] Local POA warming also increased EEG delta activity in sustained NREM sleep.[68] Enhanced EEG slow wave activity during POA warming was not due to changes in sleep continuity, but was like that induced after sleep deprivation. Because delta EEG activity in sustained sleep is considered to be a measure of sleep drive, this finding supports a hypothesis that sleep drive is modulated by POA thermosensitive neurons. On the other hand, mild POA cooling suppressed both NREM and REM sleep for 3 hours at circadian time 3 to 6, when rats normally sleep almost continuously.[69]

In vivo and in vitro studies have confirmed that the POA contains populations of WSNs and cold-sensitive neurons (CSNs) that are identified by changes in neuronal discharge in response to locally applied mild thermal stimuli.[70] WSNs and CSNs constitute 20% to 25% of neurons in these areas in vivo. We found that most WSNs are sleep active, that is, they exhibit increased discharge during NREM sleep compared with waking, and most CSNs are wake active.[71,72] Increases in WSN discharge and decreases in CSN discharge were found to anticipate EEG changes at sleep onset by several seconds.

As summarized earlier, POA neurons send afferents to putative arousal systems. Local POA warming suppressed the discharge of arousal-related neurons, including PH neurons,[73] midbrain raphe (putatively serotoninergic) neurons,[74] LH neurons in the orexinergic field,[75] and BF arousal-related neurons in the cholinergic field,[76] even when arousal level during warming was carefully controlled (Fig. 13–5). These studies

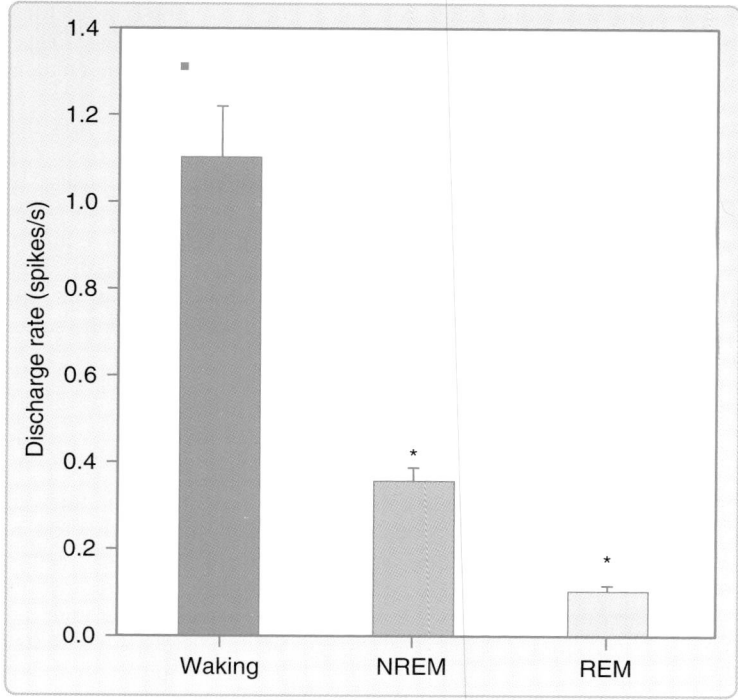

A

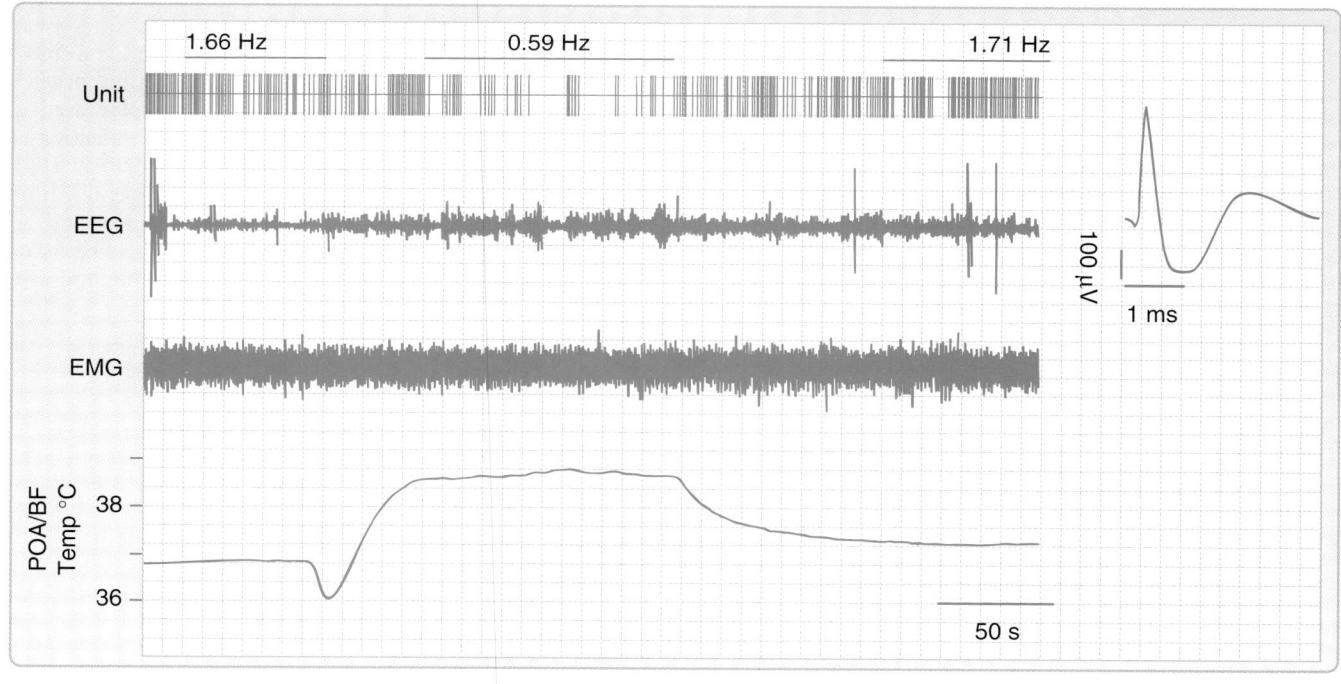

B

Figure 13–5. Effects of activation of preoptic area (POA) warm-sensitive neurons by local warming on discharge of a putative serotoninergic neuron of the dorsal raphe nucleus (DRN) in the rat. **A,** Pattern of activity of DRN neurons across the sleep–wake cycle. Putative DRN serotoninergic neurons exhibit reduced discharge during non–rapid eye movement (NREM) sleep compared with waking, and very low discharge in REM sleep. The identification of this pattern of discharge as representing serotoninergic neurons is supported by several types of indirect evidence. **B,** Effects of POA warming on the discharge of a putative serotoninergic "REM-off" neuron during waking. A POA warming pulse was applied for approximately 100 seconds (see bottom trace). During POA warming, the discharge was reduced by 64%, to a typical NREM sleep rate (from 1.66 to 0.59 Hz on Unit tracing). A waking state was maintained during warming, as shown by electroencephalographic (EEG) and electromyographic (EMG) recordings. Increased discharge of POA warm-sensitive neurons during spontaneous NREM sleep is thought to contribute to the concurrent reduction of DRN discharge. The central role of temperature-sensitive neurons in sleep control provides a mechanistic basis for the coupling of sleep and the circadian temperature rhythm (see text). (Reprinted with permission from Guzman-Marin R, Alam MN, Szymusiak R, et al: Discharge modulation of rat dorsal raphe neurons during sleep and waking: Effects of preoptic/basal forebrain warming. Brain Res 2000;875:23-34.)

show that inhibitory regulation of arousal-related neurons originates in POA WSNs, providing a mechanism for behavioral suppression and EEG synchronization. Although direct evidence is lacking, we can hypothesize that a subset of POA WSNs are GABAergic and have projections to diverse arousal systems.

In summary, activation of POA WSNs suppresses discharge of arousal-promoting neuronal groups, facilitates sleep onset, increases NREM sleep in sustained sleep, and increases delta activity in sleep. WSN neuronal activation occurs before and during spontaneous sleep. Suppression of WSN activation by local POA cooling prevents NREM sleep onset. Thus, it may be hypothesized that NREM sleep is coupled to processes that are regulated by POA WSNs.

The Sleep–Wake Cycle and Thermoregulation

Several types of evidence support the hypothesis that sleep onset is coupled to thermoregulatory processes. Depending on ambient conditions, sleep onset evokes heat loss effector processes such as cutaneous vasodilation and sweating.[77] In humans, sleep onset occurs shortly after a discrete increase in vasodilation of the hands and feet.[78] Vasodilation of these skin surfaces increases heat loss. If "lights-out" is scheduled, sleep latency is shorter if vasodilation has occurred earlier. Sleep in humans and animals is modulated by ambient temperature. Mild to moderate ambient temperature elevation increases coincident sleep as well as subsequent sleep (reviewed in McGinty and Szymusiak[34]). An increase in heat production by selective activation of brown adipose tissue using a beta$_3$-adrenoreceptor agonist increased coincident NREM sleep.[79] Augmentation of sleep by ambient warming in kangaroo rats was prevented by coincident local POA cooling.[67] Because POA cooling would prevent activation of WSNs, this finding suggests that POA WSN activation mediates the sleep augmentation induced by ambient warming.

A circadian temperature cycle is well documented. In humans, sleep normally occurs on the descending phase of the temperature rhythm, but sleep onset evokes a further decrease in temperature, even during continuous bed rest.[80] Self-selected human bedtimes occur at the time of the maximum rate of decline of core body temperature.[81] The association of sleep onset and the circadian temperature rhythm could represent two independent outputs of the circadian oscillator. However, under certain experimental conditions, including short sleep–wake cycles,[82] internal desynchronization,[83] and forced desynchronization,[80] the interactions of the temperature rhythm and sleep propensity can be studied and partially isolated from effects of prior waking. Although sleep may occur at any circadian phase, sleep propensity is greatly increased on the late descending phase of the circadian temperature rhythm and is highest when temperature is low. Awakenings tend to occur as temperature increases, even if sleep time is short. This can be interpreted to mean that low body temperatures directly facilitate sleep or that a mechanism that lowers body temperature also promotes sleep. The latter interpretation is consistent with the evidence, summarized previously, that activation of WSNs promotes sleep. There have been attempts to show that the critical variable is not temperature itself but a correlated variable such as melatonin secretion. Although this is an evolving area of research, some evidence indicates that melatonin is a weak hypnogen at circadian times associated with normal sleep in humans,[84]

and melatonin is released during the active phase in nocturnal animals. At this time, most evidence suggests that sleep is directly coupled to a mechanism that generates the circadian temperature rhythm.

It is unlikely that sleep-related cooling serves a simple thermoregulatory role. Small animals, because of their large surface-to-mass ratio, can readily lose heat when awake, but they sleep much more than large animals.[85] Thus, sleep-associated thermoregulatory processes are likely to serve another function, perhaps related to the higher mass-specific metabolic rate of small animals. In small animals, sleep may help conserve energy through lowered metabolic rate and reduced heat loss (see Chapter 8).

SLEEP-PROMOTING NEUROCHEMICAL AGENTS

Conceptions of sleep control based on neuronal circuitry, like those outlined previously, are deficient in that they do not provide explanations for quantitative features of sleep or sleep homeostasis. In addition, a complete conception should account for biologic variations in sleep such as the high daily sleep quotas in low–body-weight mammalian species and low quotas in very large species, high sleep quotas in infants, slight loss of sleep in aging, sleep facilitation after body heating, and increased sleep propensity during acute infection. To examine these problems, several investigators have examined biochemical mechanisms of sleep control.

Microinjection of a variety of neurochemical substances either directly into the POA or into the adjacent third or lateral ventricles increases NREM sleep. A partial list includes adenosine agonists, prostaglandin D$_2$ (PGD$_2$), proinflammatory cytokines and related molecules including interleukin-1 (IL-1), tumor necrosis factor-α (TNF-α), and muramyl dipeptide; other peptides such as delta sleep–inducing peptide, corticostatin, and growth hormone–releasing hormone (GHRH); as well as oxidized glutathione, desacetyl-α-melanocyte–stimulating hormone (an adrenocorticotropic hormone derivative found in brain), insulin, oleamide, and the benzodiazepine, triazolam (reviewed in McGinty and Szymusiak[34] and Obal and Krueger[86]).

Using the microinjection method, the medial POA was found to be an effective site for the sleep-enhancing effects of GHRH,[87] triazolam,[88] PGD$_2$,[89] and, in one study, adenosine agonists.[90] The adjacent magnocellular BF was an effective site for adenosine agonists in other studies.[91,92] The subarachnoid space under the rostral POA was found to be the most effective hypnogenic site for PGD$_2$.[93] After medial POA lesions, the sleep-enhancing effect of PGD$_2$ administered in the third ventricle was diminished.[94] The specific neuronal phenotypes that are the targets of these injected substances are not clearly established. However, it is logical to hypothesize that the POA sleep-regulating neurons suggested by lesion and other studies are the targets of these neurochemical factors. This hypnogenic neuronal population might be the final common path for several mediators of NREM sleep. We briefly summarize several of these conceptions. See Obal and Kreuger[86] for a detailed and complete review of this field.

Adenosine

Adenosine is recognized as an inhibitory neuromodulator in the central nervous system whose role in sleep is suggested by the potent arousal-producing effects of caffeine, an antagonist of adenosine A_1 receptors. Adenosine and its analogues were found to promote sleep after systemic injection, intraventricular administration, and intra-POA microinjection.[95,96] Recent work has focused on effects of adenosine administration by microdialysis, particularly in the fields of cholinergic neurons in the BF and brainstem in cats,[91,92] or in other brainstem sites in rats.[97] Administration of adenosine or its transport inhibitor increased either NREM or REM sleep, or both, in these sites. In BF, and to a small extent in neocortex, adenosine recovered through microdialysis was found to be increased during sustained waking in cats.[91] No accumulation was found in thalamus, POA, or brainstem sites. An earlier study found increased adenosine release in the hippocampus during the dark (active) phase of the light–dark cycle in rats.[98] Application in the BF of an antisense oligonucleotide to the adenosine A_1 receptor mRNA, which blocks synthesis of receptor protein, slightly reduced spontaneous sleep, but strongly reduced rebound after sleep deprivation.[99] Adenosine A_1 agonists delivered by microdialysis adjacent to BF neurons inhibited wake-active neurons during both waking and sleep.[100] A current hypothesis is that the effects of adenosine on sleep–waking are mediated by BF cholinergic neurons through A_1 receptors.[91] The proposed BF cholinergic neuronal site of action is problematic because destruction of these neurons has little effect on sleep.[101] However, adenosine could act at multiple sites. Adenosine A_{2A} receptors are also present in restricted brain regions. Adenosine A_2 receptor agonists are effective in inducing sleep in dorsal BF sites, in the shell of the nucleus accumbens[102] as well as in the subarachnoid space (see later).

Brain adenosine levels rise when adenosine triphosphate production is reduced; under these conditions, inhibition of neuronal activity is neuroprotective.[103] It has been proposed that increased adenosine is a signal of reduced brain energy reserves that develop during waking, and that sleep is induced as an energy restorative state.[104] With respect to the brain energy restorative concept, some, but not all studies, show reduced cerebral glycogen, an energy supply substrate, after sleep deprivation.[105,106] There is no functional evidence that brain energy supply is compromised after sleep deprivation. This is a critical gap in the theory. Of course, adenosine could be a sleep-promoting signal based on functions other than energy supply limitation.

Proinflammatory Cytokines

Several proinflammatory cytokines have sleep-promoting properties. We summarize work on a well-studied and prototypic molecule, IL-1. IL-1 (usually IL-1β) increases sleep, particularly NREM sleep, when administered intravenously, intraperitoneally, or into the lateral ventricles.[86] Basic findings have been confirmed in rabbits, mice, rats, cats, and monkeys. REM sleep is usually inhibited by IL-1. Much additional evidence supports a hypothesis that IL-1 modulates spontaneous sleep. Intraventricular administration of IL-1 antibodies reduces spontaneous sleep and blocks sleep rebound after sleep deprivation.[107] The administration of the soluble IL-1 receptor antagonist, IL-1ra, which blocks actions of IL-1, also reduces baseline sleep.[107] IL-1 mRNA is increased in the brain during the light phase, when rat sleep is maximal.[108] Sleep deprivation also increases IL-1 mRNA in the brain.[109,110] On the basis of these studies and others, it has been hypothesized

that IL-1 plays a role in spontaneous sleep. Increased sleep associated with peripheral infection may also be mediated by responses to circulating IL-1, either through vagal afferents or through induction of central IL-1 or other hypnogenic signals.[111] Preliminary findings show that POA sleep-active neurons are activated by local application of IL-1, and wake-active neurons are inhibited.[112] Application of IL-1 in other brain sites also promotes sleep.[113]

IL-1 fulfills many criteria for a sleep-promoting signal. Limitations in this conception include lack of evidence connecting IL-1 production to a specific restorative process. It has been suggested that sleep is generated by multiple factors, and IL-1, as one factor, does not have to fulfill all criteria.

Prostaglandin D$_2$

Administration of PGD$_2$ by intraventricular infusion[114] or by microinjection into the POA[89] increases sleep, but the most potent site for administration is the subarachnoid space under the POA and BF.[93] Sleep induced by PGD$_2$ administration is indistinguishable from normal sleep on the basis of EEG analysis. The synthetic enzyme, lipocalin-PGD synthase, is enriched diffusely in arachnoid membrane and choroid plexus,[115] but the receptor, the D-type prostanoid receptor is more localized in the leptomeninges under the BF, just anterior to the POA and also adjacent to the tuberomammillary nucleus, the site of the main collection of histamine-containing neurons.[116] Selective inhibition of lipocalin-PGD synthase with selenium chloride greatly reduced spontaneous sleep, and "knockout" mice lacking the D-type prostanoid receptor were no longer responsive to PGD$_2$. Knockout mice for lipocalin-PGD synthase had normal baseline sleep, but, in contrast to controls, had no rebound increase in NREM sleep after sleep deprivation.[117] The PGD$_2$ concentration was elevated in cerebrospinal fluid during NREM sleep compared with waking and was higher in the light phase in the rat, when sleep amounts are high. Sleep deprivation increased PGD$_2$ contents of the cerebrospinal fluid.[118] On this basis, it was proposed that PGD$_2$ plays a central role in sleep homeostasis. The hypnogenic action of PGD$_2$ is hypothesized to be mediated by adenosine release acting on an adenosine A_2 receptor.[119] Administration of A_2 receptor antagonists blocked the effects of PGD$_2$, and A_2 receptor agonists administered in the subarachnoid space also promoted sleep. Administration of PGD$_2$ in the subarachnoid space was found to induce c-Fos in the VLPO,[120] but this study is difficult to interpret because animals were allowed to sleep, so the increased c-Fos could have resulted from sleep rather than from direct effects of PGD$_2$. However, PGD$_2$ increased discharge of sleep-active neurons in the lateral POA.[121] A functional basis for the role of PGD$_2$ in sleep homeostasis or its primary localization in the meninges has not been identified.

Growth Hormone–Releasing Hormone

GHRH is known primarily for its role in stimulating the release of growth hormone (GH). GH release in association with the initial episodes of sleep has been shown in humans and in rats (see, e.g., Mitsugi and Kimura[122]). GHRH is a peptide with a restricted localization in neurons in the hypothalamic arcuate nucleus and in the adjacent ventromedial and periventricular nuclei. The latter neurons are thought to be the source of projections to the POA and BF. GHRH promotes NREM sleep after intraventricular (rats, rabbits), intravenous and intranasal (humans), or intraperitoneal (mice) administration, or direct microinjection into the POA (reviewed in Obal and Krueger[86]). Blockade of GHRH by administration of a competitive antagonist or by immunoneutralization is followed by reduced sleep and reduced rebound sleep after short-term sleep deprivation.[123,124] Microinjection of a GHRH antagonist into the POA also reduces NREM sleep.[87] Mutant mice with GHRH signaling abnormalities have reduced NREM sleep.[125] GHRH mRNA levels are highest during the first part of the light period, when sleep amounts are highest.[126] GHRH stimulates cultured GABAergic hypothalamic neurons; these may constitute the GHRH target in the sleep-promoting circuit.[127] It has been suggested that GHRH may elicit sleep onset in conjunction with release of GH as a coordinated process for augmenting protein synthesis and protecting proteins from degradation during the fasting associated with sleep. As in the case of IL-1, GHRH is proposed to be one element of a multiple-element sleep-promoting system.[86]

Sleep as "Detoxification" of Glutamatergic Overstimulation or Reactive Oxygen Species

Oxidized glutathione (GSSR) was identified as one of four sleep-promoting substances in brain tissue extracted from sleep-deprived rats.[78] Infusion of GSSR or its reduced form (GSH) into the lateral ventricle of rats during the dark phase was found to increase both NREM and REM sleep.[128] The sleep-enhancing effects of GSSR and GSH could be based on their functions as inhibitory regulators of glutamatergic transmission. Glutamatergic stimulation, in excess, has known neurotoxic functions mediated by N-methyl-D-aspartate (NMDA) receptors. Administration of an NMDA receptor antagonist induces a delayed increase NREM sleep in rats.[129] Thus, GSSR and GSH could function to protect the brain against excess glutamatergic stimulation and potential neurotoxicity, inducing sleep through NMDA receptor blockade.

Reactive oxygen species (ROS) include superoxide anion (O_2^-), hydrogen peroxide (H_2O_2), hydroxyl radical (OH^-), nitric oxide (NO), and peroxynitrite ($OONO^-$). ROS are generated during oxidation reactions or reactions between O_2^- and H_2O_2 or NO. NO is generated through the action of three isoforms of nitric oxide synthase (NOS) that are found in a variety of cell types. These molecules have important signaling and immune functions (e.g., NO is an important vasodilator), but, in excess, may damage cell structure. ROS are normally reduced by constitutive antioxidants such as GSSR, GSH, and different forms of superoxide dismutase (SOD). GSH was reduced in the hypothalamus of rats after 96 hours of sleep deprivation using the platform-over-water method.[130] Five to 11 days of deprivation using the disk-over-water sleep deprivation method reduced Cu/Zn SOD (cytosolic SOD) as well as glutathione peroxidase in hippocampus and brainstem.[131] These studies suggest that, by reducing antioxidant availability, sleep deprivation can increase the risk of oxidative damage, and that sleep is protective against actions of ROS. The possibility that sleep deprivation could cause neuronal damage was suggested by a finding that supraoptic nucleus neurons exhibited signs of subcellular damage after sleep deprivation.[132]

Another study found no evidence of neuronal apoptosis after sleep deprivation, but the latter method may be less sensitive. Supraoptic nucleus neurons may be sensitive to sleep deprivation because of their high rate of protein synthesis.[132]

ROS may play a role in the pathologic processes associated with patients with obstructive sleep apnea (OSA). Patients with OSA exhibit signs of increased oxidative stress, including increased O_2^- production by neutrophils, monocytes, and granulocytes (reviewed in Lavie[133]). Patients also exhibit elevated levels of proteins, such as vascular endothelial growth factor, that are normally induced by ROS.[134] These changes were reversed by continuous positive airway pressure treatment. On the basis of these and several additional findings, it has been proposed that the increased cardiovascular disease in patients with OSA results from oxidative damage to vascular walls.[133] Oxidative stress is a primary theory of both vascular disease and neurodegenerative disease.

The oxidative stress model, however, is incomplete. What are the signaling molecules that increase as a function of sustained wakefulness and promote sleep? Antioxidant enzymes were found to decrease during sleep deprivation and may not directly induce sleep. Do increased levels of ROS molecules directly activate sleep-promoting neurons? One possible signal is NO production, which can be a response to glutamatergic stimulation,[135] cytokines and inflammation, as well as to oxidative stress.[136] Activity of one NO synthetic enzyme, cytosolic NOS, is increased during the dark phase in rats, most strongly in the hypothalamus.[137] There is evidence that NO production is reduced during sleep.[138] Intraventricular or intravenous administration of an NOS inhibitor strongly reduced sleep in rabbits and rats and suppressed the NREM sleep response to sleep deprivation.[139-141] Administration of NO donors increased sleep.[142] NO inhibits oxidative phosphorylation and may stimulate the production of adenosine.[135] NO production could, therefore, be a mediator of several sleep factors.

Adenosine, ROS, glutamate, and NO have brief lives in the synaptic space, no more than a few seconds. If these molecules regulate sleep, they must have sustained release, or they may regulate the gene expression to generate sustained downstream effects. These mechanisms are the subject of current investigations.

SUMMARY

There has been rapid progress in the elucidation of the neural circuitry underlying the facilitation of sleep and the orchestration of NREM sleep. At the center of this circuitry is the POA of the hypothalamus, confirming a 70-year-old hypothesis. POA sleep-promoting circuitry has reciprocal inhibitory connections with several arousal-promoting systems. This model suggests that a delicate balance between the activities of sleep-promoting and arousal-promoting neuronal groups determines state. The circadian clock originating in the SCN has close connections with sleep-promoting neurons to generate the daily rhythm of sleep–waking. Both sleep-promoting and arousal-promoting neuronal groups are modulated by a host of processes, including sensory, autonomic, endocrine, metabolic, and behavioral influences. This conception may shed light on the acute sensitivity of sleep to a wide range of centrally acting drugs and behavioral manipulations. At the same time, the long-term regulation of sleep is relatively stable.

Long-term sleep homeostasis may reflect the actions of several neurochemical processes that express "sleep factors." Some of these sleep factors, including adenosine, PGD_2, IL-1, and GHRH, were found to act directly on POA or adjacent BF neuronal targets. Sleep factors have been linked to distinct functional models of sleep homeostasis, including brain energy supply (adenosine), control of protein synthesis (GHRH), brain cell group "use" or temperature elevation (IL-1), or protection against oxidative or glutamatergic stress (NO, antioxidant enzymes). All of these factors may be involved in sleep homeostasis, but the relative importance of each factor for daily sleep is not established.

Clinical Pearl

In experimental animals, sleep is reduced by a wide variety of localized brain lesions. This may account for the association of insomnia with a variety of neuropathologic processes.

Acknowledgments

Supported by PHS grants MH 47480, MH 04708, MH 61354, MH 63323, and HL 60296, and the Veterans Administration. The authors thank Fiona Baker for helpful comments on the manuscript and Darya Stewart for preparing the figures.

REFERENCES

1. Moruzzi G: The sleep-waking cycle. Ergebn Physiol 1972;64: 1-165.
2. Batsel HL: Electroencephalographic synchronization and desynchronization in the chronic "cerveau isole" of the dog. J Neurophysiol 1960;12:421-430.
3. Batsel HL: Spontaneous desynchronization in the chronic cat "cerveau isole." Arch Ital Biol 1964;102:547-566.
4. Villablanca J: Electroencephalogram in the permanently isolated forebrain of the cat. Science 1962;138:44-46.
5. Batini C, Moruzzi G, Palestini M, et al: Persistent patterns of wakefulness in the pretrigeminal midpontine preparation. Science 1958;128:30-32.
6. Zernicki B: Pretrigeminal cat. Brain Res 1968;9:1-14.
7. Nakata K, Kawamura H: ECoG sleep-waking rhythms and bodily activity in the cerveau isole rat. Physiol Behav 1986;36: 1167-1172.
8. Villablanca J, Marcus R: Sleep-wakefulness, EEG, and behavioral studies of chronic cats without neocortex and striatum: The "diencephalic" cat. Arch Ital Biol 1972;110:348-382.
9. Hess W: The diencephalic sleep centre. In Adrian E, Bremer F, Jasper H (eds): Brain Mechanisms and Consciousness. Oxford, Blackwell, 1954, pp 117-136.
10. Angeleri P, Marchesi GF, Quattrini A: Effects of chronic thalamic lesions on the electrical activity of the neocortex and on sleep. Arch Ital Biol 1969;107:633-667.
11. Villablanca J, Salinas-Zeballos ME: Sleep-wakefulness, EEG and behavioral studies of chronic cats without the thalamus-the "athalamic cat." Arch Ital Biol 1972;110:383-411.
12. Montagna P, Gambetti P, Cortelli P, Lugaresi E: Familial and sporadic fatal insomnia. Lancet Neurol 2003;2:167-176.
13. Marini G, Gritti I, Mancia M: Ibotenic acid lesions of the thalamic medialis dorsalis nucleus in the cat: Effects on the sleep-waking cycle. Neurosci Lett 1988;89:259-264.
14. Lovblad KO, Massetti C, Mathis J, Schroth G: MRI of paramedian thalamic stroke with sleep disturbance. Neuroradiology 1997;39:693-698.
15. Villablanca J: Behavioral and polygraphic study of "sleep" and "wakefulness" in chronic decerebrate cats. Electroencephalogr Clin Neurophysiol 1966;21:562-577.
16. Jouvet M: Neurophysiology of the states of sleep. Physiol Rev 1967;47:117-177.
17. Magnes J, Moruzzi G, Pomeiano O: Synchronization of the EEG produced by low-frequency electrical stimulation of the region of the solitary tract. Arch Ital Biol 1961;99:33-67.
18. Bonvallet M, Allen MB Jr: Prolonged spontaneous and evoked reticular activation following discrete bulbar lesions. Electroencephalogr Clin Neurophysiol 1963;15:969-988.
19. Berlucchi G, Maffei LMG, Stratta P: EEG and behavioral effects elicited by cooling of medulla and pons. Arch Ital Biol 1964; 102:372-392.
20. Lai LL, Shalita T, Hajnik T, et al: Neurotoxic N-methyl-D-aspartate lesion of the ventral midbrain and mesopontine junction alters sleep-wake organization. Neuroscience 1999;90:469-483.
21. von Economo C: Sleep as a problem of localization. J Nerv Ment Dis 1930;71:249-259.
22. Nauta WJH: Hypothalamic regulation of sleep in rats: An experimental study. J Neurophysiol 1946;9:285-316.
23. Asala SA, Okano Y, Honda K, Inoue S: Effects of medial preoptic lesions on sleep and wakefulness in unrestrained rats. Neurosci Lett 1990;114:300-304.
24. Szymusiak R, Danowski J, McGinty D: Exposure to heat restores sleep in cats with preoptic/anterior hypothalamic cell loss. Brain Res 1991;541:134-138.
25. McGinty DJ, Sterman MB: Sleep suppression after basal forebrain lesions in the cat. Science 1968;160:1253-1255.
26. Sallanon M, Sakai K, Denoyer M, Jouvet M: Long lasting insomnia induced by preoptic neuron lesions and its transient reversal by muscimol injection into the posterior hypothalamus. J Neurosci 1989;32:669-683.
27. John J, Kumar V: Effect of NMDA lesion of the medial preoptic neurons on sleep and other functions. Sleep 1998;21:587-598.
28. Schmidt M, Valatx J-L, Sakai K, et al: Role of the lateral preoptic area in sleep-related erectile mechanisms and sleep generation in the rat. J Neurosci 2000;20:6640-6647.
29. Szymusiak R, McGinty D: Sleep suppression following kainic acid-induced lesions of the basal forebrain. Exp Neurol 1986; 94:598-614.
30. John J, Kumar V, Gopinath G: Recovery of sleep after fetal preoptic transplantation in the medial preoptic area-lesioned rats. Sleep 1998;21:601-606.
31. Lu J, Greco M, Shiromani P, Saper C: Effect of lesions of the ventrolateral preoptic nucleus in NREM and REM sleep. J Neurosci 2000;20:3830-3842.
32. Lucas EA, Rogers J, Sterman MB: Effect of amphetamine and pentobarbital on sleep-wake patterns of cats with basal forebrain lesions. Psychopharmacology 1980;68:179-184.
33. Sterman MB, Clemente CD: Forebrain inhibitory mechanisms: Sleep patterns induced by basal forebrain stimulation in the behaving cat. Exp Neurol 1962;6:103-117.
34. McGinty D, Szymusiak R: Brain structures and mechanisms involved in the generation of NREM sleep: Focus on the preoptic hypothalamus. Sleep Med Rev 2001;5:323-342.
35. Sherin JE, Shiromani PJ, McCarley RW, Saper CB: Activation of ventrolateral preoptic neurons during sleep. Science 1996; 271: 216-219.
36. Morgan J, Curran T: Stimulus-transcription coupling in the nervous system: Involvement of the inducible proto-oncogenes fos and jun. Annu Rev Neurosci 1991;14:421-451.
37. Sherin JE, Elmquist JK, Torrealba F, Saper CB: Innervation of histaminergic tuberomammillary neurons by GABAergic and galaninergic neurons in the ventrolateral preoptic nucleus of the rat. J Neurosci 1998;18:4705-4721.
38. Steininger T, Gong H, McGinty D, Szymusiak R: Subregional organization of preoptic area/anterior hypothalamic projections

to arousal-related monoaminergic cell groups. J Comp Neurol 2001;429:638-653.

39. Sherin JE, Shiromani PJ, McCarley RW, Saper CB: Activation of ventrolateral preoptic neurons during sleep. Science 1996;271:216-219.

40. Lu J, Bjorkum AA, Xu MGSE, et al: Selective activation of the extended ventrolateral preoptic nucleus during rapid eye movement sleep. J Neurosci 2002;22:4568-4576.

41. Gong H, McGinty D, Guzman-Marin R, et al: Activation of c-fos in GABAergic neurones in the preoptic area during sleep and in response to sleep deprivation. J Physiol 2004;556(Pt 3):935-946.

42. Gong H, Szymusiak R, King J, et al: Sleep-related c-Fos expression in the preoptic hypothalamus: Effects of ambient warming. Am J Physiol 2000;279:R2079-R2088.

43. Zandetto-Smith A, Johnson A: Chemical topography of efferent projections from the median preoptic nucleus to the pontine monoaminergic cell groups in the rat. Neurosci Lett 1995;199:215-219.

44. Gong H, McGinty D, Szymusiak R: Projections from the median preoptic nucleus to hypocretin and forebrain cholinergic systems in rats (abstract). Sleep 2002;25:A155.

45. Thompson RH, Swanson LW: Structural characterization of a hypothalamic visceromotor pattern generator network. Brain Res Rev 2003;41:153-202.

46. Szymusiak R, Alam N, Steininger T, McGinty D: Sleep-waking discharge patterns of ventrolateral preoptic/anterior hypothalamic neurons in rats. Brain Res 1998;803:178-188.

47. Suntsova N, Szymusiak R, Alam M, et al: Sleep-waking discharge patterns of median preoptic nucleus neurons in rats. J Physiol [Lond] 2002;543:665-677.

48. Nitz D, Siegel JM: GABA release in posterior hypothalamus across sleep-wake cycle. Am J Physiol 1996;271:R1707-R1712.

49. Nitz D, Siegel J: GABA release in the dorsal raphe nucleus: Role in the control of REM sleep. Am J Physiol 1997;273:R451-R455.

50. Nitz D, Siegel JM: GABA release in the locus coeruleus as a function of sleep/wake state. Neuroscience 1997;78:795-801.

51. Sallanon M, Denoyer M, Kitahama K, et al: Long-lasting insomnia induced by preoptic neuron lesions and its transient reversal by muscimol injection into the posterior hypothalamus in the cat. Neuroscience 1989;32:669-683.

52. Gallopin T, Fort P, Eggermann E, et al: Identification of sleep-promoting neurons in vitro. Nature 2000;404:992-995.

53. Bai D, Renaud LP: Median preoptic nucleus neurons: An in vitro patch-clamp analysis of their intrinsic properties and noradrenergic receptors in the rat. Neuroscience 1998;83:905-916.

54. Saper CB, Chou TC, Scammel TE: The sleep switch: hypothalamic control of sleep and wakefulness. Trends Neurosci 2001;24:726-731.

55. Gritti I, Mariotti M, Mancia M: Gabaergic and cholinergic basal forebrain and preoptic-anterior hypothalamic projections to the mediodorsal nucleus of the thalamus of the cat. Neuroscience 1998;85:149-178.

56. McCormick DA, Bal T: Sleep and arousal: thalamocortical mechanisms. Annu Rev Neurosci 1997;20:185-215.

57. Bayer L, Eggermann E, Saint-Mleux B, et al: Selective action of orexin (hypocretin) on nonspecific thalamocortical projection neurons. J Neurosci 2002;22:7835-7839.

58. Waldrop TG, Bauer RM, Iwamoto GA: Microinjections of GABA antagonists into the posterior hypothalamus elicits locomotor movements and cardiorespiratory activation. Brain Res 1988;444:84-94.

59. Suntsova N, Guzman-Marin R, Shouse M, et al: The preoptic sleep-promoting system and absence epilepsy. Soc Neurosci Abstr 2003;33:211.17.

60. Ibuka N, Inouye ST, Kawamura H: Analysis of sleep-wakefulness rhythms in male rats after suprachiasmatic nucleus lesions and ocular enucleation. Brain Res 1977;122:33-47.

61. Lu J, Zhang YH, Chou TC, et al: Contrasting effects of ibotenate lesions of the paraventricular nucleus and subparaventricular zone on sleep-wake cycle and temperature regulation. J Neurosci 2001;21:4864-4874.

62. Kramer A, Yang F-C, Snodgrass P, et al: Regulation of daily locomotor activity and sleep by hypothalamic EGF receptor signaling. Science 2001;294:2511-2515.

63. Deurveilher S, Semba K: Indirect projections from the suprachiasmatic nucleus to the median preoptic nucleus in rat. Brain Res 2003;987:100-106.

64. Deurveilher S, Burns J, Semba K: Indirect projections from the suprachiasmatic nucleus to the ventrolateral preoptic nucleus: A dual tract tracing study in the rat. Eur J Neurosci 2002;16:1195-1213.

65. Satinoff E: Neural organization and evolution of thermal regulation in mammals. Science 1978;201:16-22.

66. Boulant JA: Hypothalamic mechanisms in thermoregulation. Fed Proc 1981;40:2843-2850.

67. Sakaguchi S, Glotzbach SF, Heller HC: Influence of hypothalamic and ambient temperatures on sleep in kangaroo rats. Am J Physiol 1979;237:R80-R88.

68. McGinty D, Siegel J: Brain neuronal unit discharge in freely moving animals: Methods and application in the study of sleep mechanisms. In Morrison A, Epstein A (eds): Progress in Psychobiology and Physiological Psychology, Vol 15. New York, Academic Press, 1992, 85-139.

69. McGinty D, Thomson D, Szymusiak R, Morairty S: Suppression of sleep by local preoptic/anterior hypothalamic cooling. Sleep Res 1996;25:18.

70. Boulant JA, Dean JB: Temperature receptors in the central nervous system. Annu Rev Physiol 1986;48:639-654.

71. Alam MN, McGinty D, Szymusiak R: Neuronal discharge of preoptic/anterior hypothalamic thermosensitive neurons: Relation to NREM sleep. Am J Physiol 1995;269:R1240-R1249.

72. Alam MN, McGinty D, Szymusiak R: Thermosensitive neurons of the diagonal band in rats: Relation to wakefulness and non-rapid eye movement sleep. Brain Res 1997;752:81-89.

73. Krilowicz BL, Szymusiak R, McGinty D: Regulation of posterior lateral hypothalamic arousal related neuronal discharge by preoptic anterior hypothalamic warming. Brain Res 1994;668:30-38.

74. Guzman-Marin R, Alam MN, Szymusiak R, et al: Discharge modulation of rat dorsal raphe neurons during sleep and waking: Effects of preoptic/basal forebrain warming. Brain Res 2000;875:23-34.

75. Methiparra M, Alam MN, Szymusiak R, McGinty D: Preoptic area warming inhibits wake-active neurons in the perifornical lateral hypothalamus. Brain Res 2003;960:165-173.

76. Alam MN, Szymusiak R, McGinty D: Local preoptic/anterior hypothalamic warming alters spontaneous and evoked neuronal activity in the magno-cellular basal forebrain. Brain Res 1995;696:221-230.

77. Heller HC, Glotzbach S, Grahn D, Radeke C: Sleep-dependent changes in the thermoregulatory system. In Lydic R, Biebuyck J (eds): Clinical Physiology of Sleep. Washington, DC, American Physiological Society, 1988, pp 145-158.

78. Inoue S, Honda K, Komoda Y: Sleep as neuronal detoxification and restitution. Behav Brain Res 1995;69:91-95.

79. Dewasmes G, Loos N, Delanaud S, et al: Activation of brown adipose tissue thermogenesis increases slow wave sleep in rat. Neurosci Lett 2003;339:207-210.

80. Dijk DJ, Czeisler CA: Contribution of the circadian pacemaker and the sleep homeostat to sleep propensity, sleep structure, electroencephalic slow waves, and sleep spindle activity in humans. J Neurosci 1995;15:3526-3538.

81. Campbell S, Broughton R: Rapid decline in body temperature before sleep: Fluffing the physiological pillow. Chronobiol Int 1994;11:126-131.

82. Lavie P: Ultradian rhythms: Gates of sleep and wakefulness. In Schulz H, Lavie P (eds): Ultradian Rhythms in Physiology and Behavior. New York, Springer-Verlag, 1985, pp 148-164.

83. Czeisler CA, Weitzman ED, Moore-Ede MC, Zimmerman JC: Human sleep: Its duration and organization depend on its circadian phase. Science 1980;210:1264-1267.

84. Kripke D, Elliot J, Youngstedt S, Smith J: Melatonin: Marvel or marker? Ann Med 1998;30:81-87.

85. Glotzbach SF, Heller HC: Temperature regulation. In Kryger MH, Roth T, Dement WC (eds): Principles and Practice of Sleep Medicine, 2nd ed. Philadelphia, WB Saunders, 1994, pp 260-276.

86. Obal F Jr, Krueger JM: Biochemical regulation of non-rapid-eye-movement sleep. Front Biosci 2003;8:520-550.

87. Zhang J, Obal F Jr, Zheng T, et al: Intrapreoptic microinjection of GHRH or its antagonist alters sleep in rats. J Neurosci 1999; 19:2187-2194.

88. Mendelson WB, Martin JV, Perlis M, Wagner R: Enhancement of sleep by microinjection of triazolam into the medial preoptic area. Neuropsychopharmacology 1989;2:61-66.

89. Ueno R, Ishikawa Y, Nakayama T, Hayaishi O: Prostaglandin D2 induces sleep when microinjected into the preoptic area of conscious rats. Biochem Biophys Res Commun 1982;109:576-582.

90. Radulovacki M, Virus RM, Djuricic-Nedelson M, Green R: Adenosine analogs and sleep in rats. J Pharmacol Exp Ther 1984;228:268-274.

91. Porkka-Heiskanen T, Strecker RE, Thakkar M, et al: Adenosine: A mediator of the sleep-inducing effects of prolonged wakefulness. Science 1997;276:1265-1268.

92. Portas CM, Thakkar M, Rainnie DG, et al: Role of adenosine in behavioral state modulation: A microdialysis study in the freely moving cat. Neuroscience 1997;79:225-235.

93. Matsumura H, Nakajima T, Osaka T, et al: Prostaglandin D2-sensitive, sleep-promoting zone defined in the ventral surface of the rostral basal forebrain. Proc Natl Acad Sci U S A 1994;91:11998-12002.

94. Morairty S, Thomson D, Szymusiak R, et al: The somnogenic effects of prostaglandin D2 infusion in rats with preoptic/anterior hypothalamic lesions. Sleep Res 1996;25:18.

95. Benington JH, Kodali SK, Heller HC: Stimulation of A1 adenosine receptors mimics the electroencephalographic effects of sleep deprivation. Brain Res 1995;692:79-85.

96. Ticho SR, Radulovacki M: Role of adenosine in sleep and temperature regulation in the preoptic area of rats. Pharmacol Biochem Behav 1991;40:33-40.

97. Marks GA, Birabil CG: Enhancement of rapid eye movement sleep in the rat by cholinergic and adenosinergic agonists infused into the pontine reticular formation. Neuroscience 1998;86:29-37.

98. Huston JP, Haas HL, Boix F, et al: Extracellular adenosine levels in neostriatum and hippocampus during rest and activity periods of rats. Neuroscience 1996;73:99-107.

99. Thakkar MM, Winston S, McCarley RM: A1 receptor and adenosinergic homeostatic of sleep-wakefulness: Effects of antisense to the A1 receptor in the basal forebrain. J Neurosci 2003;23:4278-4287.

100. Alam MN, Szymusiak R, Gong H, et al: Adenosinergic modulation of rat basal forebrain neurons during sleep and waking: Neuronal recording with microdialysis. J Physiol (Lond) 1999;521.3:679-690.

101. Bassant MH, Apartis E, Jazat-Poindessous FR, et al: Selective immunolesion of the basal forebrain cholinergic neurons: Effects on hippocampal activity during sleep and wakefulness in the rat. Neurodegeneration 1995;4:61-70.

102. Satoh S, Matsumura H, Koike N, et al: Region-dependent difference in the sleep-promoting potency of an adenosine A2A receptor agonist. Eur J Neurosci 1999;11:1587-1597.

103. Porkka-Heiskanen T, Alanko L, Kalinchuk A, Stenberg D: Adenosine and sleep. Sleep Med Rev 2002;6:321-332.

104. Benington JH, Heller HC: Restoration of brain energy metabolism as the function of sleep. Prog Neurobiol 1995;45:347-360.

105. Franken P, Gip P, Hagiwara G, Heller HC: Changes in brain glycogen after sleep deprivation vary with genotype. Am J Physiol 2003;285:R413-R419.

106. Kong J, Shepel N, Holden CP, et al: Brain glycogen decreases with increased periods of wakefulness: Implications for homeostatic drive for sleep. J Neurosci 2002;22:5581-5587.

107. Opp M, Krueger JM: Interleukin 1-receptor antagonist blocks interleukin 1-induced sleep and fever. Am J Physiol 1991;260:R453-R457.

108. Taishi P, Bredow S, Guha-Thakurta N, Krueger JM: Diurnal variations of interleukin-1 beta mRNA and beta-actin in rat brain. J Neuroimmunol 1997;75:69-74.

109. Opp M, Krueger JM: Interleukin-1 is involved in responses to sleep deprivation in the rabbit. Brain Res 1994;639:57-65.

110. Mackiewicz M, Sollars PJ, Ogilvie MD, Pack AI: Modulation of IL-1b gene expression in rhe rat CNS during sleep deprivation. Neuroreport 1996;7:529-533.

111. Hansen MK, Krueger JM: Subdiaphragmatic vagotomy blocks the sleep and fever-promoting effects of interleukin-1 beta. Am J Physiol 1997;273:R1246-R1253.

112. Alam MN, McGinty D, Imeri L, et al: Effects of interleukin-1 beta on sleep- and wake-active preoptic anterior hypothalamic neurons in unrestrained rats (abstract). Sleep 2001;24:A59.

113. Terao A, Matsumura H, Saito M: Interleukin-1 induces slow wave sleep at the prostaglandin D2-sensitive zone in the rat brain. J Neurosci 1998;18:6599-6607.

114. Inoue S, Honda K, Komoda Y, et al: Differential sleep-promoting effects of five sleep substances nocturnally infused in unrestrained rats. Proc Natl Acad Sci U S A 1984;81:6240-6244.

115. Urade Y, Hayaishi O: Prostaglandin D2 and sleep regulation. Biochim Biophys Acta 1999;1436:606-615.

116. Matsumura H, Takahata R, Hayaishi O: Inhibition of sleep in rats by inorganic selenium compounds, inhibitors of prostaglandin D synthase. Proc Natl Acad Sci U S A 1991;88:9046-9050.

117. Hayaishi O, Urade Y: Prostaglandin D2 in sleep-wake regulation: Recent progress and perspectives. Neuroscientist 2002;8:12-15.

118. Ram A, Pandey HP, Matsumura H, et al: CSF levels of prostaglandins, especially the level of prostaglandin D2, are correlated with increasing propensity towards sleep in rats. Brain Res 1997;751:81-89.

119. Satoh S, Matsumura H, Suzuki F, Hayaishi O: Promotion of sleep mediated by the A2 receptor and possible involvement of this receptor in the sleep induced by prostaglandin D2 in rats. Proc Natl Acad Sci U S A 1996;93:5980-5984.

120. Scammell T, Gerashchenko D, Urade Y, et al: Activation of ventrolateral preoptic neurons by the somnogen prostaglandin D2. Proc Natl Acad Sci U S A 1998;95:7754-7759.

121. Koyama Y, Hayaishi O: Modulation by prostaglandins of activity of sleep-related neurons in the preoptic/anterior hypothalamic areas of rats. Brain Res Bull 1994;33:367-372.

122. Mitsugi N, Kimura F: Simultaneous determination of blood levels of corticosterone and growth hormone in the male rat: Relation to the sleep-wakefulness cycle. Neuroendocrinology 1985;41:125-130.

123. Obal F Jr, Payne L, Kapas L, et al: Inhibition of growth hormone-releasing factor suppresses both sleep and growth hormone secretion in the rat. Brain Res 1991;557:149-153.

124. Obal F Jr, Payne L, Opp M, et al: Growth hormone releasing hormone antibodies suppress sleep and prevent enhancement of sleep after sleep deprivation. Am J Physiol 1992;32:R1078-R1085.

125. Obal F Jr, Fang J, Taishi P, et al: Deficiency of growth hormone-releasing hormone signaling is associated with sleep alterations in the dwarf rat. J Neurosci 2001;2912-2918.

126. Bredow S, Taishi PO, Obal F Jr, et al: Hypothalamic growth hormone-releasing hormone mRNA varies across the day in rats. Neuroreport 1996;7:2501-2505.

127. De A, Churchill L, Obal F Jr, et al: GHRH and IL1 beta increase cytoplasmic Ca2+ levels in cultured hypothalamic GABAergic neurons. Brain Res 2002;949:209-212.

128. Honda Y, Komoda Y, Inoue S: Oxidized glutathione regulates physiological sleep in unrestrained rats. Brain Res 1994;636: 253-258.

129. Campbell IG, Feinberg I: Noncompetitive NMDA channel blockade during waking intensely stimulates NREM delta. J Pharmacol Exp Ther 1996;276:737-742.

130. D'Almeida V, Lobo LL, Hipolide DC, et al: Sleep deprivation induces brain region-specific decreases in glutathione levels. Neuroreport 1998;9:2853-2856.

131. Ramanathan L, Gulyani S, Nienhuis R, Siegel JM: Sleep deprivation decreases superoxide dismutase activity in rat hippocampus and brainstem. Neuroreport 2002;13:1387-1390.

132. Eiland MM, Ramanathan LGS, Gilliland M, et al: Increases in amino-cupric-silver staining of the supraoptic nucleus after sleep deprivation. Brain Res 2002;945:1-8.

133. Lavie L: Obstructive sleep apnoea syndrome: An oxidative stress disorder. Sleep Med Rev 2003;7:35-51.

134. Imagawa S, Yamaguchi Y, Higuchi M: Levels of vascular endothelial growth factor are elevated in patients with obstructive sleep apnea-hypopnea syndrome. Blood 2001;98: 1255-1257.

135. Rosenberg PA, Li Y, Ye M, Zhang Y: Nitric oxide-stimulated increase in extracellular adenosine accumulation in rat forebrain neurons in culture is associated with ATP hydrolysis and inhibition of adenosine kinase activity. J Neurosci 2000; 20:6294-6301.

136. Olivenza R, Mora MA, Lizasoain L, et al: Chronic stress induces the expression of inducible nitric oxide synthase in rat brain cortex. J Neurochem 2000;74:785-791.

137. Ayers NA, Kapas L, Krueger JM: Circadian variation of nitric oxide synthase activity and cytosolic protein levels in rat brain. Brain Res 1996;707:127-130.

138. Burlet S, Cespuglio R: Voltammetric detection of nitric oxide (NO) in the rat brain: its variations throughout the sleep-wake cycle. Neurosci Lett 1997;226:131-135.

139. Ribeiro AC, Gilligan JG, Kapas L: Systemic injection of a nitric oxide synthase inhibitor suppresses sleep responses to sleep deprivation in rats. Am J Physiol 2000;278:R1048-R1056.

140. Kapas L, Fang J, Krueger JM: Inhibition of nitric oxide synthesis inhibits rat sleep. Brain Res 1994;664:189-196.

141. Kapas L, Shibata M, Kimura M, Krueger JM: Inhibition of nitric oxide synthesis suppresses sleep in rabbits. Am J Physiol 1994; 266:R151-R157.

142. Kapas L, Krueger JM: Nitric oxide donors SIN-1 and SNAP promote nonrapid-eye-movement sleep in rats. Brain Res Bull 1996;41:293-298.

Physiology in Sleep

John Orem

Physiologic Regulation in Sleep

Pier Luigi Parmeggiani

ABSTRACT

Physiologic regulation depends on the ultradian wake–sleep cycle. This dependency is the result of functional dominance of phylogenetically different structures of the encephalon in different behavioral states.

The functional similarity of physiologic events during non–rapid eye movement (NREM) sleep in different species and the variety and variability of such events during rapid eye movement (REM) sleep within and between species define the characteristic differences between these states of sleep. Intrinsic nervous processes specific to the state of REM sleep may cause somatic and autonomic variability without relationship to mental content or homeostatic control.

The basic somatic features of NREM sleep are the assumption of a thermoregulatory posture and a decrease in antigravity muscle activity. The basic somatic features of REM sleep are muscle atonia, rapid eye movements, and myoclonic twitches. The basic autonomic feature of NREM sleep is the functional prevalence of parasympathetic influences associated with quiescence of sympathetic activity. The basic autonomic feature of REM sleep is the great variability in sympathetic activity associated with phasic changes in tonic parasympathetic discharge.

In all species, the somatic and visceral phenomena of NREM sleep are indicative of closed-loop operations, automatically maintaining homeostasis at a lower level of energy expenditure compared with quiet wakefulness (QW). In contrast, the somatic and visceral phenomena of REM sleep are characterized in all species by the greatest variability as a result of open-loop operations of central origin impairing the homeostasis of physiologic functions (poikilostasis).

The knowledge of behavioral state–dependent differences in physiologic regulation is fundamental to sleep medicine. For example, the existence of sleep apnea and periodic leg movements in sleep is evidence that physiology must differ in sleep and wakefulness. In this chapter, I address principles of physiologic regulation in sleep so that clinicians and their patients might better understand sleep disorders.

The ultradian wake–sleep cycle consists of the single sequence of at least three behavioral states, which may be called quiet wakefulness (QW), non–rapid eye movement (NREM) sleep, and rapid eye movement (REM) sleep.

Consideration of further subdivisions of sleep behavior and the multifarious behavioral states of active wakefulness (AW) would be outside the scope of this chapter.

In the context of this chapter, the term *physiologic regulation* refers to the nervous control mechanisms of the entire somatic and visceral activity, which is defined here as the "behavior" of the organism. A powerful conceptual tool to facilitate understanding of physiologic regulation is *homeostasis*,[1] which can be experimentally tested across the behavioral continuum by studying stimulus–response relationships in physiologic functions at different levels of integration. Mechanistically, physiologic homeostasis is effected by feedforward and feedback operations that predictively and reactively[2] minimize the influences of internal and external disturbances on the organism. This means that it is necessary to verify whether effector activity maintains (*homeostasis*) or impairs (*poikilostasis*) the stability— within what is conventionally called a normal range—of the fundamental variables of the interstitial and cellular compartments (e.g., temperature, pH, water volume, electrolytes, osmolality, nutrients, oxygen, carbon dioxide) that underlie cellular survival.

However, the homeostasis of such variables is the eventual result of continuous adjustments of "instrumental" variables (e.g., heart rate, stroke volume, cardiac output, vascular resistance, blood pressure, ventilation, muscle force) that are directly affected by the activity of somatic and visceral effectors. It is worth stressing that studies on single variables provide no sound basis for any inference of the behavioral principles of physiologic regulation. As Hess[3] pointed out, "It is essential that the data are interrelated and woven into a theoretical fabric" (p. 4). In this respect, the intensive study of the bioelectrical and behavioral (somatic and visceral) aspects of sleep has shown that the principle of homeostatic regulation of physiologic functions does not apply to all behavioral states.

HOMEOSTASIS VERSUS POIKILOSTASIS OF PHYSIOLOGIC FUNCTIONS IN SLEEP

The demonstration, in terms of reactive homeostasis,[2] that different behavioral states of the ultradian sleep cycle are characterized by either homeostasis (NREM sleep) or poikilostasis (REM sleep) of physiologic functions is based on the criterion

185

of short-latency stimulus–response relationships. This basic functional dichotomy applies to the nervous control of body temperature and of circulatory and respiratory functions. In contrast, gastrointestinal, endocrine, and renal functions do not fit this criterion. For example, many aspects of secretory and gastrointestinal activity are not constrained within the temporal boundaries of single sleep states and appear, at most, to be modulated by changes in the autonomic nervous system outflow during sleep.[4] On the other hand, there are changes in endocrine secretion that are specific to a single sleep state.[5] However, such changes are the result of ultradian or circadian modulation rather than of a homeostatic response to exogenous or endogenous disturbances in terms of reactive homeostasis. On this basis, a survey of experimental results concerning only temperature, cardiovascular, and breathing regulation is presented in this section. The reader interested in further details is referred to the updated Chapters 22 and 23 dealing specifically with these subjects.

SOMATIC BEHAVIOR

Physiologic regulation in wakefulness may involve motor responses that compensate for or avoid internal or external disturbances. For example, the organism can seek shade as a thermoregulatory response (behavioral thermoregulation), and the patient with obstructive sleep apnea may dilate the airway in wakefulness as a compensatory response. In the transition from QW to NREM sleep, the somatic repertory in animals displays the appetitive features of an instinct that consists of the search for a safe and thermally comfortable ecologic niche and the preparation of the body (e.g., grooming) for the natural sleep posture. Subsequently, in NREM sleep, motor behavior is generally more limited, although somnambulism may occur in humans. In general, there is cessation of goal-directed and compensatory motor activity and assumption of a thermoregulatory posture with decreased antigravity muscle activity.[6] Variations in arousal level can lead to periodic leg movements and changes in posture. During REM sleep,[7] muscle atonia, myoclonic twitches, and rapid eye movements are clear signs of a substantial change in motor innervation compared with NREM sleep. The purpose of such fragmented motor activation in REM sleep is not known, but it may be important for development of the nervous system. For example, respiratory movements occur in utero in REM sleep. These movements are not yet necessary for gas exchange, which occurs in the placenta, but they may be the result of a state-specific process that is preparing the organism for existence in the atmosphere after birth.

THERMOREGULATORY FUNCTION

In mammals, homeothermy is controlled by preoptic–hypothalamic integrative mechanisms that drive subordinate brainstem and spinal somatic and visceral mechanisms that elicit thermoregulatory effector responses.

The thermoregulatory responses to ambient thermal loads are present during NREM sleep and absent or depressed during REM sleep. For example, the cat's posture clearly varies in relation to ambient temperature during NREM sleep, whereas the drop in postural muscle tone during REM sleep is unrelated to ambient temperature.[6] Moreover, notwithstanding a positive (warm) thermal load, tachypnea in the cat[8]

and heat-exchange vasodilation in the cat,[9] rabbit,[10] and rat[11] disappear and sweating in humans[12-14] decreases during the episode of REM sleep. Likewise, under a negative (cold) thermal load, shivering in the cat[8] and armadillo,[15-17] heat-exchanger vasoconstriction in the cat,[9] rabbit,[10] and rat,[11] and piloerection in the cat[18] are suppressed during the REM episode. Moreover, the cold-defense function of brown fat is altered in rats.[19]

Thermoregulatory responses elicited by positive and negative thermal loads applied directly to the thermosensitive preoptic–hypothalamic region depend on the behavioral state. In the cat, warming elicits tachypnea[20,21] and heat-exchange vasodilation[9] during NREM sleep, but it has no such effects during REM sleep. Likewise, in the kangaroo rat[22] and marmot,[23] cooling increases oxygen consumption and metabolic heat production during NREM sleep, whereas it is ineffective during REM sleep. A crucial proof of the behavioral state–dependent changes in the function of the preoptic–hypothalamic thermostat has been provided by experiments of direct thermal stimulation of preoptic–hypothalamic thermosensitive neurons across behavioral states in the cat[24-27] and kangaroo rat.[28] The change in thermosensitivity of the majority of such neurons parallels that in thermoregulatory responsiveness to central thermal loads during NREM and REM sleep. Moreover, an indirect proof of this is the disappearance of shivering during REM sleep in a cold ambience in cats with pontine lesions that produce REM sleep without muscle atonia.[18] The result shows that the pontine inhibitory mechanisms eliciting muscle atonia in the normal animal do not underlie the suppression of this thermoregulatory response in REM sleep.

In conclusion, experimental evidence shows that during NREM sleep, thermoregulatory mechanisms are operative as they are in QW, despite some state-dependent differences in the threshold and gain of effector responses to thermal loads.[12,22,29] The other difference with respect to QW is that in NREM sleep, body and hypothalamic temperatures are down-regulated together with energy expenditure.[30-32]

The events during REM sleep are not simply the result of state-dependent changes in the threshold and gain of the different thermoregulatory responses. From the quantitative point of view, REM sleep is characterized by effector activity that not only is functionally inconsistent with the aim of temperature regulation but also lacks any proportional relationship with the intensity of the thermal stimulus. The result is that the temperature of the body changes according to its thermal inertia, as one would expect in a poikilothermic organism.[32,33]

CIRCULATORY FUNCTION

NREM sleep is characterized by a down-regulation of cardiovascular activity of variable intensity depending on the species and its previous level in QW. A decrease in arterial blood pressure occurs in the cat[34] but is lacking in the rabbit[35] and is found less consistently in the rat.[36,37] Of the cardiac variables influencing cardiac output, namely, heart rate and stroke volume, the first is moderately decreased,[34,38] whereas the latter is practically unchanged in cats.[34] There is a significant decrease in heart rate in rats,[37] but the decrease is not statistically significant in rabbits.[35] In humans, a tonic decrease in arterial blood pressure is observed,[39-43] although it has varying intensity in different individuals.[44] Baroreceptor reflex sensitivity is increased in humans.[45] With respect to the vascular conductance, a slight increase occurs in the skin and the mesenteric, iliac, and renal beds in the cat[34] and in the skin of the rabbit[10] and humans.[46,47] On the whole, the cardiovascular changes in NREM sleep are consistent with the changes in respiration and thermoregulation in a condition of postural and motor quiescence.

Different phenomena characterize REM sleep in both animals and humans. According to some, arterial blood pressure falls markedly in cats as a result of a pronounced bradycardia associated with a practically unchanged stroke volume and an increase in total vascular conductance; the increase in vascular conductance in the skin and in the mesenteric and renal beds prevails over the decrease in conductance of the hindlimb muscle vasculature.[34,48] However, according to others,[49] a slight fall in arterial blood pressure was not consistently detected in cats. In addition, another study[50] showed that the bradycardia and hypotension observed in cats during REM sleep may be a long-lasting effect from surgical preparation of the animal for the experiment. Thereafter, heart rate and arterial blood pressure are higher in REM sleep than in NREM sleep. This cardiovascular condition appears to depend on forebrain influences.[51] In the rabbit,[35,52] rat,[36,37] and humans,[39,40,42,43] arterial blood pressure increases from NREM to REM sleep, but the rise is not always related to consistent changes in the primary variables, (i.e., heart rate and vascular conductance).[39,41,53] In the rabbit, renal and fat vascular conductances appear to be decreased during REM sleep.[35] The poor correlation between regional and systemic variables shows that the central integration of cardiovascular functions is altered in REM sleep. As a result, the regional distribution of blood flow is remarkably modified in comparison with NREM sleep.[54]

The variability of heart rate and arterial blood pressure is an important feature of REM sleep in the cat,[55,56] the rat,[36,37] the rabbit,[52] and humans.[39,40,42] It is in general loosely associated with bursts of rapid eye movements, myoclonic twitches, and, probably more often, breathing irregularities. However, such variability is not only the direct result of central changes in the regulation of the autonomic outflow[57]; these changes also activate indirectly a number of feedback loops by affecting the peripherally controlled variables.[38] Therefore, the interaction between the central variability of visceral control during REM sleep and the central effects of activated reflexes are main factors in the generation of the instability of cardiovascular regulation in REM sleep. The importance of such an interaction is also shown by studies in anesthetized[58] and awake[59] cats showing that the central generator underlying the rhythmicity of synchronized cardiac sympathetic nerve activity is subject to reflex modulation by baroreceptor inputs.

In cats, arterial blood pressure during REM sleep is buffered by sinoaortic reflexes.[49,56] After sinoaortic denervation, arterial blood pressure is mildly increased during wakefulness, and it decreases to slightly more than the level that occurs in normal animals during NREM sleep, but it decreases sharply during REM sleep. This decrease in some REM episodes may produce brain ischemia as revealed by the flattening of the electroencephalogram, motor convulsions, and arousal.[56] The marked drop in arterial blood pressure after sinoaortic denervation depends on the greater vasodilation in the splanchnic vascular bed and the reversal of vasoconstriction to vasodilation in the hindlimb muscles.[34,60] Selective removal of either baroreceptor or chemoreceptor afferents showed that the arterial hypotension of REM sleep is buffered in the cat primarily by chemoreceptor reflexes because baroreceptor reflexes are depressed in this species.[34,61,62] In the rat, arterial blood pressure increases during REM sleep, whereas in sinoaortic-denervated rats, hypotension, as occurs in the cat, is observed.[36] However, the role of baroreceptors in REM sleep is still problematic due to long-lasting effects from the surgical preparation of animals for the experiment.[50] Also, the results of baroreceptor studies in humans suggest caution in this respect, because reflex sensitivity may either increase[40] or decrease[45] in REM sleep. Nevertheless, when the results are taken together, it appears likely that circulation in different species is affected by similar central influences in REM sleep, although the eventual pattern of change in cardiovascular variables also depends on species-specific differences in the operation of feedback loops[63] and autoregulation.[64]

With respect to the control of brain integrative centers on brainstem cardiovascular regulation,[65-68] thermoregulatory vasomotion elicited by direct thermal stimulation of the preoptic–hypothalamic region during NREM sleep is suppressed during REM sleep in cats[9] in accord with the reduced responsiveness of preoptic–hypothalamic thermosensitive neurons.[25-28] Moreover, a depression in telencephalic (amygdala, orbital frontal cortex) control over cardiovascular activity has been observed in cats during REM sleep.[69]

VENTILATORY FUNCTION

Conspicuous changes occur in the regulation of breathing across the behavioral states of sleep.[70,71] The transition from wakefulness to NREM sleep is characterized by the inactivation of the "wakefulness" (telencephalic) control mechanism and the release of the automatic control mechanism.[72-75] This transition (stages 1 and 2 of NREM sleep in humans) is characterized by breathing instability[43,76-78] and the appearance of respiratory and circulatory periodic phenomena.[76,79,80] Regular breathing sets in with deep NREM sleep (stages 3 and 4 in humans), when breathing is driven by the automatic control mechanism. The rate decreases and the tidal volume increases slightly; however, ventilation decreases in both humans[79,81] and animals[74,75] according to the metabolic rate. A concomitant increase in alveolar CO_2 partial pressure in humans[79] and animals[71,75] and in arterial CO_2 partial pressure in humans[81,82] and cats[83] associated with a decrease in alveolar and arterial O_2 partial pressure in humans[84] and cats[83] has been observed. Airway resistance is increased.[84,85] These changes in respiratory variables are in agreement with a state of rest at low energy expenditure. Although the operation of the automatic control mechanism appears to be downregulated, it maintains compensatory physiologic responses. Respiratory chemosensitivity to CO_2 is only moderately reduced,[79,81,84,86,87] whereas the hypoxic response is unaffected in humans[88] and in dogs.[89] Moreover, pulmonary inflation and deflation reflexes are active during NREM sleep in both human infants[90] and animals.[71,75,91] The responses to a mechanical respiratory load (airway occlusion, inspiration from a rigid container) are also nearly identical to those observed during wakefulness,[92] thus showing that proprioceptive reflexes of the intercostal muscles are normal during NREM sleep.

The phenomena of REM sleep point to a profound alteration in the activity of the automatic control mechanism of respiration. In fact, the respiratory rhythm in humans and animals is very irregular,[43,76,93,94] with the average frequency being increased or decreased with respect to the rate attained during NREM sleep in eupnea or polypnea, respectively.[29,70] The respiratory activity of the intercostal muscles is diminished in cats and lambs[29,95,96]; in human infants, this depression may even produce paradoxical chest collapse during inspiration.[97] However, ventilation increases in humans[79,90,98,99] and dogs,[100] mostly in temporal relationship to myoclonic twitches.[74] During REM sleep, alveolar ventilation may also be variable as shown by either a decrease[71,75,79] or no change[83,99-101] in alveolar CO_2 partial pressure. It is important to stress that such disturbances are of central origin, as they persist after vagotomy,[71,75,101] sectioning of the spinal cord at T_{1-2},[102,103] afferent denervation of the mid-thoracic chest wall,[75] denervation of the carotid and aortic chemoreceptors and baroreceptors,[83] hypercapnia,[100] and hypoxia.[89] Upper airway resistance increases in humans and cats[85,104,105] and respiratory load compensation is irregular and weak in humans[106-108] and lambs[95] during REM sleep. The alteration of the automatic control mechanism of respiration REM sleep is also shown by other phenomena. In dogs and human infants, respiratory responses to hypercapnia are depressed,[100,109] whereas those to hypoxia are unchanged.[89,98] Pulmonary deflation and inflation reflexes persist in the opossum, although they are more variable than during NREM sleep.[91] In contrast, the inflation reflex is almost abolished during REM sleep in dogs[71,75] and human infants.[90]

Depressed preoptic–hypothalamic influence on respiration during REM sleep as compared with NREM sleep was shown by means of either thermal[20,21] or electrical[110] direct stimulation of this diencephalic region. Moreover, a depression in telencephalic (amygdala, orbital frontal cortex) control on respiration was shown in cats during REM sleep.[111]

CONCLUSIONS

A basic difference between NREM sleep and REM sleep is the functional similarity of the former in different species and the functional variety and variability of the latter within and between species.

In NREM sleep, the changes in visceral regulation are consistent with somatic quiescence, as are the functional prevalence of the parasympathetic over the sympathetic activity, the lowering of metabolic heat production (decrease in muscle tone and in heart and breathing rates), and body temperature (vasodilation of heat exchangers, sweating). Moreover, somatic and visceral regulatory responses to endogenous and exogenous disturbances may be activated during NREM sleep to maintain homeostasis. In conclusion, the stereotypic phenomena of NREM sleep across mammalian species appear to be the coherent result of a common phylogenetic trend to develop a pattern of integrated automatic regulation minimizing energy expenditure. Mechanistically, the regulation of physiologic functions during this stage of sleep is led essentially by diencephalic structures, as shown particularly by the persistence of normal homeothermic regulation.

Concerning REM sleep, it is difficult to establish a rational foundation of the observed functional phenomena in terms of a centrally integrated regulation. Their physiologic aim escapes a teleologic explanation in behavioral terms. Remarkably, cause–effect relationships existing between variables during QW and NREM sleep are suppressed during REM sleep, yet the loss of the specific effects of stimuli during REM sleep is not associated with a loss of their nonspecific arousing influences. The arousal effect, however, requires a much higher stimulus intensity compared with that which normally elicits the specific regulatory response. Thus, REM sleep is characterized by the disintegration of a homeostatic physiologic equilibrium bringing about effector responses of great instability that are primarily of central origin but secondarily complicated by local autoregulation or altered reflex activity, or both. Mechanistically, the leading neural structures in REM sleep are rhombencephalic, as shown by the occurrence of REM sleep phenomena in brainstem preparations.[7,112] However, the physiologic variability appears to depend not only on autochthonous activities of the brainstem but also on changes in the functional relationship between the brainstem and the forebrain.[57] The concept of release, as first proposed by Hughlings Jackson in 1884, appears to apply, for example, to the alteration of functions such as temperature, cardiovascular, and breathing regulation during REM sleep in normal animals. In general, it may be assumed that a critical integrative instability would develop during REM sleep as a result of the impaired homeostatic function at high integration levels. Mechanistically, this instability may be considered to result from a loss of the balance between descending excitatory and inhibitory influences of diencephalic (hypothalamic) and telencephalic structures during REM sleep. In contrast, in QW and NREM sleep, such influences would keep the activity of brainstem and spinal somatic and visceral reflex centers within the range imposed by set point–dependent integrative operations underlying the maintenance of homeostasis.

The impairment of homeostatic control in REM sleep is more dramatic and evident in a function, such as temperature regulation in furry animals, that depends on effector mechanisms strictly subordinated to regulatory structures of the diencephalon (preoptic–hypothalamic region). In functions characterized by more widely distributed control mechanisms, such as circulation and respiration, the features of functional impairment are rather more complex as a result of the persistence of more or less efficient reflex regulation or peripheral autoregulation. Nevertheless, it is evident that functional changes in REM sleep depend essentially on the suppression of a highly integrated homeostatic regulation that is operative in NREM sleep. In comparison with REM sleep, volitional and instinctive drives during AW may also impose a load on or interfere with homeostatic mechanisms at central and/or effector levels to overwhelm their regulatory power. However, such homeostatic mechanisms are still operative and capable of reestablishing the functional equilibrium that so well characterizes QW and NREM sleep. In all species, the somatic and visceral phenomena of NREM sleep are indicative of closed-loop operations, automatically maintaining homeostasis at a lower level of energy expenditure compared with QW. The operative principle is, however, unchanged, which implies a coherent utilization of the parasympathetic and sympathetic divisions of the autonomic nervous system for homeostatic regulation. In contrast, the somatic and visceral activity of REM sleep is characterized in all species by the greatest variability in somatic and autonomic outflow as a result of nonhomeostatic (open-loop) operations. The differences in state-dependent physiologic regulation disclosed with the help of the criterion of homeostasis emphasize the critical role of diencephalic structures in the generation of the somatic and visceral phenomena of the ultradian wake–sleep cycle.

Clinical Pearl

Compensatory responses such as those that occur in obstructive sleep apnea require the phylogenetically advanced functions of wakefulness and are lost in sleep. Automatic reflexive control of somatic and autonomic functions allows homeostatic behavior in NREM sleep without awareness, whereas the open-loop operations of REM sleep elicit physiologic disturbances and can impede reactions to these disturbances.

Acknowledgments

The author is indebted to Dr. John Orem for helpful advice and to Dr. Christine A. Jones for editing the English.

References

1. Cannon WB: Organization for physiological homeostasis. Physiol Rev 1929;9:399-431.
2. Moore-Ede MC: Physiology of the circadian timing system: Predictive versus reactive homeostasis. Am J Physiol 1986;250:R737-R752.
3. Hess WR: Sleep as a phenomenon of the integral organism. In Akert K, Bally C, Schadé JP (eds): Sleep Mechanisms: Progress in Brain Research, vol 18. New York, Elsevier, 1965, pp 3-8.
4. Orr WC: Gastrointestinal physiology. In Kryger MH, Roth T, Dement WC (eds): Principles and Practice of Sleep Medicine, 3rd ed. Philadelphia, Saunders, 2000, pp 279-288.
5. Van Cauter E: Endocrine physiology. In Kryger MH, Roth T, Dement WC (eds): Principles and Practice of Sleep Medicine, 3rd ed. Philadelphia, Saunders, 2000, pp 266-278.
6. Parmeggiani PL, Rabini C: Sleep and environmental temperature. Arch Ital Biol 1970;108:369-387.
7. Jouvet M: Recherches sur les structures nerveuses et les mécanismes responsables des différentes phases du sommeil physiologique. Arch Ital Biol 1962;100:125-206.
8. Parmeggiani PL, Rabini C: Shivering and panting during sleep. Brain Res 1967;6:789-791.
9. Parmeggiani PL, Zamboni G, Cianci T, et al: Absence of thermoregulatory vasomotor responses during fast wave sleep in cats. Electroencephalogr Clin Neurophysiol 1977;42:372-380.
10. Franzini C, Cianci T, Lenzi P, et al: Neural control of vasomotion in rabbit ear is impaired during desynchronized sleep. Am J Physiol 1982;243:R142-R146.
11. Alföldi P, Rubicsek G, Cserni G, et al: Brain and core temperatures and peripheral vasomotion during sleep and wakefulness at various ambient temperatures in the rat. Pflugers Arch 1990;417:336-341.
12. Sagot JC, Amoros C, Candas V, et al: Sweating responses and body temperatures during nocturnal sleep in humans. Am J Physiol 1987;252:R462-R470.
13. Shapiro CM, Moore AT, Mitchell D, et al: How well does man thermoregulate during sleep? Experientia 1974;30:1279-1281.
14. Henane R, Buguet A, Roussel B, et al: Variations in evaporation and body temperature during sleep in man. J Appl Physiol 1977;42:50-55.
15. Prudom AE, Klemm WR: Electrographic correlates of sleep behavior in a primitive mammal, the armadillo Dasypus novemcinctus. Physiol Behav 1973;10:275-282.
16. Van Twyver H, Allison T: Sleep in the armadillo Dasypus novemcinctus at moderate and low ambient temperatures. Brain Behav Evol 1974;9:107-120.
17. Affanni JM, Lisogorsky E, Scaravilli AM: Sleep in the giant South American armadillo Priodontes giganteus (Edentata, Mammalia). Experientia 1972;28:1046-1047.
18. Hendricks JC: Absence of shivering in the cat during paradoxical sleep without atonia. Exp Neurol 1982;75:700-710.
19. Calasso M, Zantedeschi E, Parmeggiani PL: Cold-defense function of brown adipose tissue during sleep. Am J Physiol 1993;265:R1060-R1064.
20. Parmeggiani PL, Franzini C, Lenzi P: Respiratory frequency as a function of preoptic temperature during sleep. Brain Res 1976;111:253-260.
21. Parmeggiani PL, Franzini C, Lenzi P, et al: Threshold of respiratory responses to preoptic heating during sleep in freely moving cats. Brain Res 1973;52:189-201.
22. Glotzbach SF, Heller HC: Central nervous regulation of body temperature during sleep. Science 1976;194:537-539.
23. Florant GL, Turner BM, Heller HC: Temperature regulation during wakefulness, sleep, and hibernation in marmots. Am J Physiol 1978;235:R82-R88.
24. Alam MN, McGinty D, Szymusiak R: Neuronal discharge of preoptic/anterior hypothalamic thermosensitive neurons: Relation to NREM sleep. Am J Physiol 1995;269:R1240-R1249.
25. Alam MN, McGinty D, Szymusiak R: Preoptic/anterior hypothalamic neurons: Thermosensitivity in rapid eye movement sleep. Am J Physiol 1995;269:R1250-R1257.
26. Parmeggiani PL, Azzaroni A, Cevolani D, et al: Responses of anterior hypothalamic-preoptic neurons to direct thermal stimulation during wakefulness and sleep. Brain Res 1983;269:382-385.
27. Parmeggiani PL, Cevolani D, Azzaroni A, et al: Thermosensitivity of anterior hypothalamic-preoptic neurons during the waking-sleeping cycle: A study in brain functional states. Brain Res 1987;415:79-89.
28. Glotzbach SF, Heller HC: Changes in the thermal characteristics of hypothalamic neurons during sleep and wakefulness. Brain Res 1984;309:17-26.
29. Parmeggiani PL, Sabattini L: Electromyographic aspects of postural, respiratory and thermoregulatory mechanisms in sleeping cats. Electroencephalogr Clin Neurophysiol 1972;33:1-13.
30. Brebbia DR, Altshuler KZ: Oxygen consumption rate and electroencephalographic stage of sleep. Science 1965;150:1621-1622.
31. Parmeggiani PL, Agnati LF, Zamboni G, Cianci T: Hypothalamic temperature during the sleep cycle at different ambient temperatures. Electroencephalogr Clin Neurophysiol 1975;38:589-596.
32. Parmeggiani PL, Franzini C, Lenzi P, et al: Inguinal subcutaneous temperature changes in cats sleeping at different environmental temperatures. Brain Res 1971;33:397-404.
33. Walker JM, Walker LE, Harris DV, et al: Cessation of thermoregulation during REM sleep in the pocket mouse. Am J Physiol 1983;244:R114-R118.
34. Mancia G, Zanchetti A: Cardiovascular regulation during sleep. In Orem J, Barnes CD (eds): Physiology in Sleep: Research Topics in Physiology, vol 3. New York, Academic Press, 1980, pp 1-55.
35. Lenzi P, Cianci T, Guidalotti PL, et al: Brain circulation during sleep and its relation to extracerebral hemodynamics. Brain Res 1987;415:14-20.
36. Junqueira LF Jr, Krieger EM: Blood pressure and sleep in the rat in normotension and in neurogenic hypertension. J Physiol 1976;259:725-735.
37. Lacombe J, Nosjean A, Meunier JM, et al: Computer analysis of cardiovascular changes during sleep-wake cycle in Sprague-Dawley rats. Am J Physiol 1988;254:H217-H222.
38. Baust W, Bohnert B: The regulation of heart rate during sleep. Exp Brain Res 1969;7:169-180.

39. Coccagna G, Mantovani M, Lugaresi E: Arterial pressure changes during spontaneous sleep in man. Electroencephalogr Clin Neurophysiol 1971;31:277-281.

40. Jones JV, Sleight P, Smyth HS: Haemodynamic changes during sleep in man. In Ganten D, Pfaff D (eds): Sleep: Current Topics in Endocrinology. New York, Academic Press, 1982, pp 213-272.

41. Khatri IM, Freis ED: Hemodynamic changes during sleep. J Appl Physiol 1967;22:867-873.

42. Scharf SM: Influence of sleep state and breathing on cardiovascular function. In Saunders NA, Sullivan CE (eds): Sleep and Breathing, vol 21. New York, Dekker, 1984, pp 221-239.

43. Snyder F, Hobson JA, Morrison DF, et al: Changes in respiration, heart rate, and systolic blood pressure in human sleep. J Appl Physiol 1964;19:417-422.

44. Mancia G: Autonomic modulation of the cardiovascular system during sleep. N Engl J Med 1993;328:347-349.

45. Conway J, Boon N, Jones JV, et al: Involvement of the baroreceptor reflexes in the changes in blood pressure with sleep and mental arousal. Hypertension 1983;5:746-748.

46. Noll G, Elam M, Kunimoto M, et al: Skin sympathetic nerve activity and effector function during sleep in humans. Acta Physiol Scand 1994;151:319-329.

47. Sindrup JH, Kastrup J, Madsen PL, et al: Nocturnal variations in human lower leg subcutaneous blood flow related to sleep stages. J Appl Physiol 1992;73:1246-1252.

48. Baccelli G, Albertini R, Mancia G, et al: Central and reflex regulation of sympathetic vasoconstrictor activity of limb muscle during desynchronized sleep in the cat. Circ Res 1974;35:625-635.

49. Iwamura Y, Uchino Y, Ozawa S, et al: Spontaneous and reflex discharge of a sympathetic nerve during "para-sleep" in decerebrate cat. Brain Res 1969;16:359-367.

50. Sei H, Sakai K, Kanamori N, et al: Long-term variations of arterial blood pressure during sleep in freely moving cats. Physiol Behav 1994;55:673-679.

51. Kanamori N, Sakai K, Sei H, et al: Effects of decerebration on blood pressure during paradoxical sleep in cats. Brain Res Bull 1995;378:545-549.

52. Dufour R, Court L: Le débit cérébral sanguin au cours du sommeil paradoxal du lapin. Arch Ital Biol 1977;115:57-76.

53. Miki K, Kato M, Kajii S: Relationship between renal sympathetic nerve activity and arterial pressure during REM sleep in rats. Am J Physiol 2003;284:R467-R473.

54. Cianci T, Zoccoli G, Lenzi P, et al: Loss of integrative control of peripheral circulation during desynchronized sleep. Am J Physiol 1991;261:R373-R377.

55. Gassel MM, Ghelarducci B, Marchiafava PL, et al: Phasic changes in blood pressure and heart rate during the rapid eye movement episodes of desynchronized sleep in unrestrained cats. Arch Ital Biol 1964;102:530-544.

56. Guazzi M, Zanchetti A: Blood pressure and heart rate during natural sleep of the cat and their regulation by carotid sinus and aortic reflexes. Arch Ital Biol 1965;103:789-817.

57. Parmeggiani PL: The autonomic nervous system in sleep. In Kryger MH, Roth T, Dement WC (eds): Principles and Practice of Sleep Medicine, 2nd ed. Philadelphia, Saunders, 1994, pp 194-203.

58. Gebber GL, Barman SM, Kocsis B: Coherence of medullary unit activity and sympathetic nerve discharge. Am J Physiol 1990;259:R561-R571.

59. Ninomiya I, Akiyama T, Nishiura N: Mechanism of cardiac-related synchronized cardiac sympathetic nerve activity in awake cats. Am J Physiol 1990;259:R499-R506.

60. Baccelli G, Albertini R, Mancia G, et al: Control of regional circulation by the sino-aortic reflexes during desynchronized sleep in the cat. Cardiovasc Res 1978;12:523-528.

61. Guazzi M, Baccelli G, Zanchetti A: Reflex chemoceptive regulation of arterial pressure during natural sleep in the cat. Am J Physiol 1968;214:969-978.

62. Knuepfer MM, Stumpf H, Stock G: Baroreceptor sensitivity during desynchronized sleep. Exp Neurol 1986;92:323-334.

63. Gilmore JP, Tomomatsu E: Comparison of carotid sinus baroreceptors in dogs, cats, monkeys, and rabbits. Am J Physiol 1984;247:R52-R56.

64. Cowley AW Jr, Hinojosa-Laborde C, Barber BJ, et al: Short-term autoregulation of systemic blood flow and cardiac output. News Physiol Sci 1989;4:219-225.

65. Behbehani MM, Da Costa G: Properties of a projection pathway from the medial preoptic nucleus to the midbrain periaqueductal gray of the rat and its role in the regulation of cardiovascular function. Brain Res 1996;740:141-150.

66. Hirasawa M, Nishihara M, Takahashi M: The rostral ventrolateral medulla mediates suppression of the circulatory system by the ventromedial nucleus of the hypothalamus. Brain Res 1996;724:186-190.

67. Hosoya Y, Sugiura Y, Okado N, et al: Descending input from the hypothalamic paraventricular nucleus to sympathetic preganglionic neurons in the rat. Exp Brain Res 1991;85:10-20.

68. Kanouse K, Yanase-Fujiwara M, Hosono T: Hypothalamic network for thermoregulatory vasomotor control. Am J Physiol 1994;267:R283-R288.

69. Frysinger RC, Marks JD, Trelease RB, et al: Sleep states attenuate the pressor response to central amygdala stimulation. Exp Neurol 1984;83:604-617.

70. Parmeggiani PL: Integrative aspects of hypothalamic influences on respiratory brainstem mechanisms during wakefulness and sleep. In Von Euler C, Lagerkrantz H (eds): Central Nervous Control Mechanisms in Breathing. New York, Pergamon Press, 1979, pp 53-68.

71. Phillipson EA, Bowes G: Control of breathing during sleep. In Cherniack NS, Widdicombe JG (eds): Handbook of Physiology: Section III. The Respiratory System. Bethesda, Md, American Physiological Society, 1986, pp 642-689.

72. Fink BR: Influence of cerebral activity in wakefulness on regulation of breathing. J Appl Physiol 1961;16:15-20.

73. Orem J: Neuronal mechanisms of respiration in REM sleep. Sleep 1980;3:251-267.

74. Orem J, Netick A, Dement WC: Breathing during sleep and wakefulness in the cat. Respir Physiol 1977;30:265-289.

75. Phillipson EA: Regulation of breathing during sleep. Am Rev Respir Dis 1977;115(Suppl):217-224.

76. Duron B: La fonction respiratoire pendant le sommeil physiologique. Bull Physiopathol Respir (Nancy) 1972;8:1031-1057.

77. Gillam PMS: Patterns of respiration in human beings at rest and during sleep. Bull Physiopathol Respir (Nancy) 1972;8:1059-1070.

78. Trinder J, Whitworth F, Kay A, et al: Respiratory instability during sleep onset. J Appl Physiol 1992;73:2462-2469.

79. Bülow K: Respiration and wakefulness in man. Acta Physiol Scand 1963;59(Suppl 209):1-110.

80. Lugaresi E, Coccagna G, Mantovani M, et al: Some periodic phenomena arising during drowsiness and sleep in man. Electroencephalogr Clin Neurophysiol 1972;32:701-705.

81. Birchfield RI, Sieker HO, Heyman A: Alterations in respiratory function during natural sleep. J Lab Clin Med 1959;54:216-222.

82. Birchfield RI, Sieker HO, Heyman A: Alterations in blood gases during natural sleep and narcolepsy. Neurology 1958;8:107-112.

83. Guazzi M, Freis ED: Sinoaortic reflexes and arterial pH, P_{O_2} and P_{CO_2} in wakefulness and sleep. Am J Physiol 1969;217:1623-1627.

84. Robin ED, Whaley RD, Crump GH, et al: Alveolar gas tension, pulmonary ventilation and blood pH during physiological sleep in normal subjects. J Clin Invest 1958;37:981-989.

85. Orem J, Netick A, Dement WC: Increased upper airway resistance to breathing during sleep in the cat. Electroencephalogr Clin Neurophysiol 1977;43:14-22.

86. Bellville JW, Howland WS, Seed JC, et al: The effect of sleep on the respiratory response to carbon dioxide. Anesthesiology 1959;20:628-634.

87. Reed DJ, Kellogg RH: Changes in respiratory response to CO_2 during natural sleep at sea level and at altitude. J Appl Physiol 1958;13:325-330.

88. Reed DJ, Kellogg RH: Effect of sleep on hypoxic stimulation of breathing at sea level and altitude. J Appl Physiol 1960;15:1130-1134.

89. Phillipson EA, Sullivan CE, Read DJC, et al: Ventilatory and waking responses to hypoxia in sleeping dogs. J Appl Physiol 1978;44:512-520.

90. Finer NN, Abroms IF, Taeusch HW Jr: Ventilation and sleep state in the new born infants. J Pediatr 1976;89:100-108.

91. Farber JP, Marlow TA: Pulmonary reflexes and breathing pattern during sleep in the opossum. Respir Physiol 1976;27:73-86.

92. Phillipson EA, Kozar LF, Murphy E: Respiratory load compensation in awake and sleeping dogs. J Appl Physiol 1976;40:895-902.

93. Orem J: Respiratory neurons and sleep. In Kryger MH, Roth T, Dement WC (eds): Principles and Practice of Sleep Medicine, 2nd ed. Philadelphia, Saunders, 1994, pp 177-193.

94. Phillipson EA: Respiratory adaptations in sleep. Annu Rev Physiol 1978;40:133-156.

95. Henderson-Smart DJ, Read DJC: Depression of intercostal and abdominal muscle activity and vulnerability to asphyxia during active sleep in the newborn. In Guilleminault C, Dement WC (eds): Sleep Apnea Syndromes. Kroc Foundation Series. New York, Alan R Liss, 1978, pp 93-117.

96. Duron B: Activité électrique spontanée des muscles intercostaux et de diaphragme chez l'animal chronique. J Physiol (Paris) 1969;61(Suppl 2):282-283.

97. Tusiewicz K, Moldofsky H, Bryan AC: Mechanics of the rib cage and diaphragm during sleep. J Appl Physiol 1977;43:600-602.

98. Bolton DPG, Herman S: Ventilation and sleep state in the newborn. J Physiol 1974;240:67-77.

99. Hathorn MKS: The rate and depth of breathing in new-born infants in different sleep states. J Physiol 1974;243:101-113.

100. Phillipson EA, Kozar LF, Rebuck AS, et al: Ventilatory and waking responses to CO_2 in sleeping dogs. Am Rev Respir Dis 1977;115:251-259.

101. Remmers JE, Bartlett D Jr, Putnam MD: Changes in the respiratory cycle associated with sleep. Respir Physiol 1976;28:227-238.

102. Puizillout JJ, Ternaux JP, Foutz AS, et al: Les stades de sommeil chez la préparation "encéphale isolé": 1. Déclenchement des pointes ponto-géniculo-occipitales et du sommeil phasique à ondes lentes—Role des noyaux du raphé. Electroencephalogr Clin Neurophysiol 1974;37:561-576.

103. Thach BT, Abroms IF, Frantz ID, et al: REM sleep breathing pattern without intercostal muscle influence. Fed Proc 1977;36:445.

104. Henke KG, Dempsey JA, Badr MS, et al: Effect of sleep-induced increases in upper airway resistance on respiratory muscle activity. J Appl Physiol 1991;70:158-168.

105. Wiegand L, Zwillich CW, Wiegand D, et al: Changes in upper airway muscle activation and ventilation during phasic REM sleep in normal men. J Appl Physiol 1991;71:488-497.

106. Frantz ID, Adler SM, Abroms IF, et al: Respiratory responses to airway occlusion in infants: Sleep state and maturation. J Appl Physiol 1976;41:634-638.

107. Henke KG, Badr MS, Skatrud JB, et al: Load compensation and respiratory muscle function during sleep. J Appl Physiol 1992;72:1221-1234.

108. Knill R, Andrews W. Bryan AC, et al: Respiratory load compensation in infants. J Appl Physiol 1976;40:357-361.

109. Bryan HM, Hagan R, Gulston G, et al: CO_2 response and sleep state in infants. Clin Res 1976;24:A689.

110. Parmeggiani PL, Calasso M, Cianci T: Respiratory effects of preoptic-anterior hypothalamic electrical stimulation during sleep in cats. Sleep 1981;4:71-82.

111. Marks JD, Frysinger RC, Harper RM: State-dependent respiratory depression elicited by stimulation of the orbital frontal cortex. Exp Neurol 1987;95:714-729.

112. Futuro-Neto HA, Coote JH: Changes in sympathetic activity to heart and blood vessels during desynchronized sleep. Brain Res 1982;252:259-268.

Cardiovascular Physiology: Central and Autonomic Regulation

Richard L. Verrier

Ronald M. Harper

J. Allan Hobson

ABSTRACT

Because of the close neurohumoral coupling between central structures and cardiorespiratory function, there is a dynamic fluctuation in heart rhythm, arterial blood pressure, coronary artery blood flow, and ventilation. Non–rapid eye movement (NREM) sleep is associated with relative autonomic stability and functional coordination between respiration, pumping action of the heart, and maintenance of arterial blood pressure. During rapid eye movement (REM) sleep, surges in cardiac-bound sympathetic and parasympathetic activity provoke accelerations and pauses in heart rhythm. These occur in association with alterations in ponto-geniculo-occipital activity and theta rhythm that are signs of phasic central nervous system activation in REM. Whereas perturbations in autonomic nervous system activity are well tolerated in normal individuals, those with heart disease may be at risk during REM sleep. The stress on the system has the potential for triggering life-threatening arrhythmias and myocardial infarction. During NREM sleep in the severely compromised heart, there is a potential for hypotension, which can in turn impair blood flow through stenotic coronary vessels. In both states, the coexistence of coronary disease and apnea is associated with heightened risk because of the challenge of dual control of the respiratory and cardiovascular systems.

During a typical night's sleep, a broad spectrum of autonomic patterns unfolds that provides both respite and stress to the cardiovascular system. These effects are the consequences of carefully orchestrated changes in central nervous system (CNS) physiology as the brain periodically reexcites during rapid eye movement (REM) sleep from the relative tranquility of non–rapid eye movement (NREM) sleep.

The main goal of this chapter is to provide insights into the central and peripheral nervous system mechanisms that regulate cardiovascular function during sleep. Particular attention is focused on cardiac electrical stability and coronary artery blood flow because these factors can trigger life-threatening cardiac arrhythmias and myocardial infarction in individuals with heart disease. Attention is also directed toward the central mechanisms underlying the high sympathetic tone found in conditions associated with sleep disordered breathing, including obstructive sleep apnea (OSA) and heart failure, and with cardiovascular function in infants, particularly because perturbations in the regulation of this system during

the nocturnal period may be an important factor in the sudden infant death syndrome (SIDS). The importance of these issues to public health is underscored by the annual toll of nocturnal, sleep-related cardiac events, which account for an estimated 20% of myocardial infarctions (or 250,000) and 15% of sudden cardiac deaths (or 38,000) in the United States.[1] For detailed report and discussion of clinical findings, see Chapters 96-98.

SLEEP-STATE CONTROL OF CARDIOVASCULAR FUNCTION

NREM sleep, the initial stage, is characterized by a period of relative autonomic stability, with vagal nerve dominance and heightened baroreceptor gain. During NREM sleep, a near sinusoidal modulation of heart rate variation occurs due to a coupling with respiratory activity and cardiorespiratory centers in the brain and results in what is termed *normal respiratory sinus arrhythmia* (Fig. 15–1). During inspiration, heart rate accelerates briefly to accommodate increased venous return, resulting in increased cardiac output, whereas during expiration, a progressive slowing in rate ensues. This normal sinus variability in heart rate, particularly during NREM sleep, is generally indicative of cardiac health, whereas the absence of intrinsic variability has been associated with cardiac pathology and advancing age.[2]

The reflexive cardiovascular changes during breathing manifested as cyclical heart rate variation also have a converse relationship, as transient elevation of arterial blood pressure results in a slowing, cessation, or diminution of breathing efforts. This effect is enhanced during sleep,[3] when even small reductions in arterial blood pressure increase respiratory rates.[4,5] These breathing pauses and increased rates apparently serve as compensatory mechanisms to normalize arterial blood pressure. Absence of these normal breathing pauses and diminished breathing variation, as well as reductions in respiration-induced heart rate variation, are characteristic of infants who later succumb to SIDS[6] and may hint at a failure of compensatory mechanisms underlying the syndrome. Reduced heart rate variability is also typical of infants afflicted with congenital central hypoventilation syndrome, a condition in which the drive to breathe is lost during sleep.[7] Obstructive sleep apnea in children is accompanied by exaggerated heart rate variation.[8] Thus, the common denominator of cardiac risk associated with depressed heart rate variability appears to be loss of normal vagal nerve function.

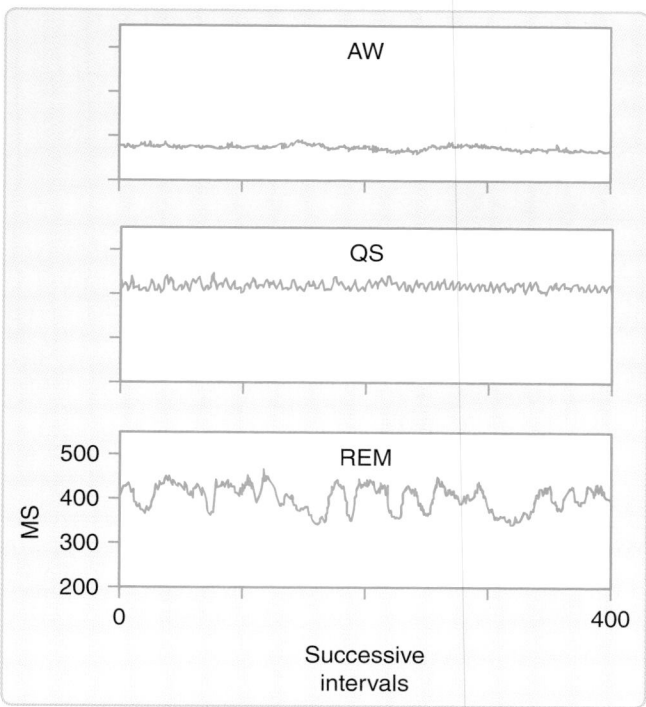

Figure 15-1. The x-axis represents successive heartbeats and the intervals between heartbeats from a healthy 4-month-old infant during quiet sleep (QS), rapid eye movement (REM) sleep, and wakefulness (AW). The y-axis represents time (in milliseconds [MS]) between those heartbeats. Note rapid modulation of intervals during quiet sleep contributed by respiratory variation. Note also lower frequency modulation during REM sleep, and epochs of sustained rapid rate during wakefulness.

Sympathetic nerve activity appears to be relatively stable during NREM sleep, and its cardiovascular input is reduced by more than half from wakefulness to stage 4 of NREM sleep.[9] In general, the autonomic stability of NREM sleep, with hypotension, bradycardia, and reductions in cardiac output and systemic vascular resistance, provide a relatively salutary neurohumoral background during which the heart has an opportunity for metabolic restoration.[10] The bradycardias appear to be caused mainly by an increase in vagal nerve activity, whereas the hypotension is primarily attributable to a reduction in sympathetic vasomotor tone.[11] During transitions from NREM to REM sleep, bursts of vagal nerve activity may result in pauses in heart rhythm and frank asystole.[12]

REM sleep is initiated at 90-minute intervals and, in subserving brain neurochemical functions and behavioral adaptations, can disrupt cardiorespiratory homeostasis.[13] The brain's increased excitability during REM sleep can result in major surges in cardiac sympathetic nerve activity to the coronary vessels. Baroreceptor gain is reduced. Heart rate fluctuates strikingly, with marked episodes of tachycardia and bradycardia.[14,15] Cardiac efferent vagus nerve tone is generally suppressed during REM sleep,[10] and breathing patterns are highly irregular and can lead to oxygen reduction, particularly in patients with pulmonary or cardiac disease.[13] The neurons activating the principal diaphragmatic respiratory muscles normally escape the generalized inhibition,[16] although accessory and upper airway muscles diminish activity.[17] This loss of activity is especially marked in infant thoracic and abdominal

muscles during REM sleep.[18] During sleep apnea, there may be cessation of central respiratory activity or peripheral obstruction several hundred times each night, with the potential for dire consequences for cardiorespiratory activity.

CARDIORESPIRATORY INTERACTIONS

Central Mechanisms

The integration of cardiorespiratory function during sleep is achieved at several levels in the neuraxis. Several pontine and suprapontine, as well as cerebellar, mechanisms have the capability of altering cardiorespiratory patterns during both sleep and wakefulness. The importance of the pontine structures in REM sleep activation has been documented by positron emission tomography imaging studies of REM sleep dreaming, which demonstrate preferential activation of the limbic and paralimbic regions of the forebrain in REM sleep compared with waking or with NREM sleep.[19-21] The orbital frontal cortex, portions of the hippocampal formation, and hypothalamic structures are frequently included among forebrain structures participating in cardiorespiratory patterning, as well as affective behavior. The central nucleus of the amygdala is strategically positioned to regulate cardiac and respiratory functions of affective behavior, because it projects extensively to the parabrachial pons and the nucleus of the solitary tract, the dorsal motor nucleus, and the periaqueductal gray region, all areas exerting significant influences on cardiac action. Portions of the amygdala, hippocampal formation, and frontal and insular cortices all participate in mediating the transient arterial blood pressure elevation elicited by cold pressor challenges or Valsalva maneuvers, as indicated by functional magnetic resonance.[22]

The insular cortex deserves special attention over other cortical areas that express regulatory action on cardiovascular control during sleep and waking states. Both animal and human studies show that the area modulates both sympathetic and parasympathetic action, with sympathetic outflow principally controlled by the right insula, and parasympathetic action by the left[23] (although both sides apparently interact).[24] Of interest for the sleep field are the marked deficits found in the insula in conditions with sleep disordered breathing and high sympathetic tone—namely, heart failure and obstructive sleep apnea. Heart failure patients exhibit severe insular gray matter loss, preferentially on the right side[25] (Fig. 15-2A), and impaired functional magnetic resonance signal responses to cold pressor challenges and to Valsalva maneuvers, in addition to an inability to mount appropriate heart rate responses.[26,27] Patients with OSA also show aberrant heart rate and insular responses to cold pressor and Valsalva challenges, with both amplitude and timing of the neural responses affected in the breathing task.[28,29] Lateralized insular responses are also relevant to epilepsy, because a propensity exists for some types of seizure discharge to occur during sleep states. Seizure discharge can exert profound influences on arterial blood pressure and heart rate,[30] and a unilateral seizure focus could trigger unique autonomic responses. The influence of cortical structures on subcortical sites carries significant import for cardiorespiratory control.

Of all neural structures that can exert control over cardiovascular and respiratory activity in both sleep and waking states, the cerebellum is particularly significant. Although not

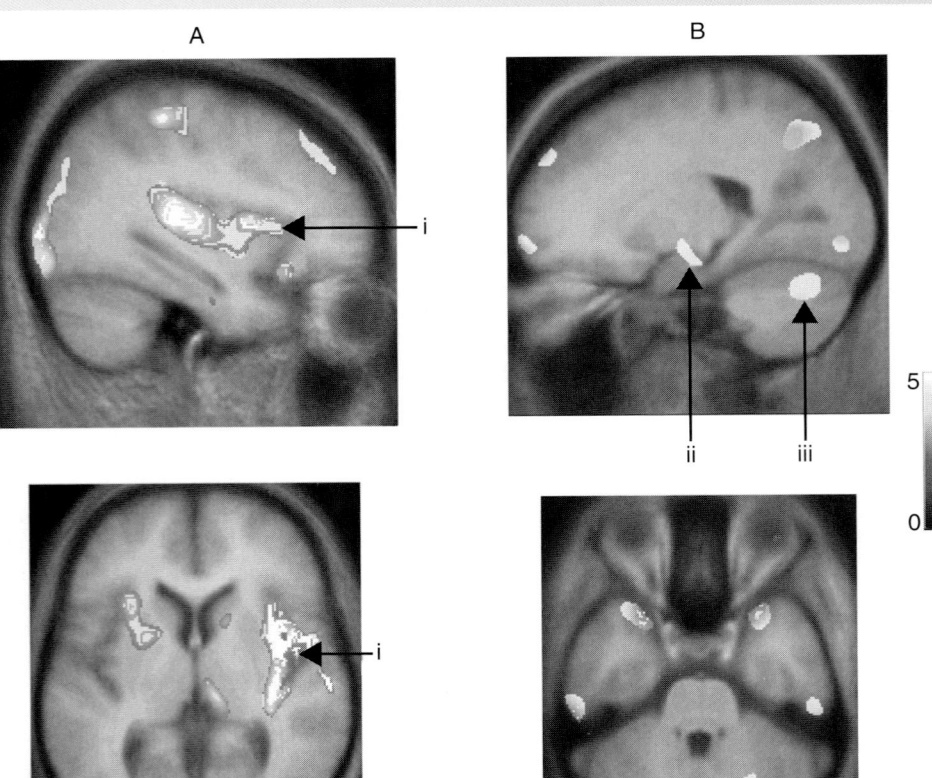

A

B

Figure 15–2. Areas of gray matter loss *(arrows)* within the insula (i) of heart failure patients (*n* = 9) (**A**), and in the hippocampal region (ii) and cerebellum (iii) of OSA patients (*n* = 21) (**B**). Gray matter loss was calculated from structural magnetic resonance imaging scans relative to controls. The 0 to 5 scale represents *t* values; all light areas are significant (*p* < 0.05). (**A,** From Woo MA, Macey PM, Fonarow GC, et al: Regional brain gray matter loss in heart failure. J Appl Physiol 2003;95:677-684; **B,** from Macey PM, Henderson LA, Macey KE, et al: Brain morphology associated with obstructive sleep apnea. Am J Resp Crit Care Med 2002;166: 1382-1387.)

classically considered to be a component of either breathing or cardiac control, a role for the cerebellum has been known for over half a century.[31] A portion of this role is mediated through vestibular/cerebellar mechanisms in regulating blood pressure.[32] Vestibular mechanisms modify arterial blood pressure responses to rapid postural changes, a process familiar to hypotensive individuals who suffer syncope on rising rapidly from the horizontal position. Lesions of the cerebellar fastigial nucleus can result in ineffective compensatory responses to hypotension,[33] with ensuing death. Cerebellar damage, with significant gray matter loss in the cerebellar cortex and deep nuclei, occurs in heart failure cases[25] (see Fig. 15–2B) and in OSA,[34] and may contribute to aberrant state–related cardiovascular control in these syndromes. The contributions of abnormal cerebellar development or cerebellar insults to cardiorespiratory disturbances have long been known.[35-37]

Cardiorespiratory Homeostasis

An important consideration in preserving circulatory homeostasis during sleep is the coordination of control over two systems: the respiratory, essential for oxygen exchange, and the cardiovascular, for blood transport. The difficult balancing act of regulating two motor systems, one that supplies somatic musculature (i.e., diaphragmatic, intercostal, abdominal, and upper airway musculature) and the other involving regulation of autonomic pathways (to the heart and vasculature), is a

formidable task during sleep. This challenge is particularly daunting in individuals who have diseased respiratory or cardiovascular systems, particularly in the form of apnea or heart failure, or in infants, whose developing control systems may become compromised. Activity of the respiratory neurons varies greatly between sleep states, as does the regularity of heart rhythm. Tachycardia, polypnea, sweating, and dramatic elevations in arterial blood pressure secondary to intense autonomic activity occur primarily during REM sleep.

Maintenance of perfusion of vital organs through appropriate arterial blood pressure control is essential for cardiorespiratory homeostasis. Respiratory mechanisms are recruited to support cardiovascular action by assisting venous return and by reflexly altering cardiac rate. REM sleep induces a near paralysis of accessory respiratory muscles and diminishes descending forebrain influences on brainstem control regions.[38,39] Those reorganizations of control during REM sleep have the potential to interfere substantially with compensatory breathing mechanisms that assist arterial blood pressure management, and to remove protective forebrain influences on hypotension or hypertension. The significant interaction between breathing and arterial blood pressure is evident in normalization of blood pressure by continuous positive airway pressure in patients with apnea-induced hypertension.[40]

The control of arterial blood pressure during sleep is of particular interest to those examining potential mechanisms of failure in SIDS. Several reports indicate that the final sequence in SIDS may be the result of failure in cardiac rhythm.[41] Specifically, bradycardia and hypotension, rather than an initial breathing cessation, characterize the final event.[42,43] There may be antecedent tachycardia for up to 3 days. The terminal events in SIDS are similar to the two stages of shock, namely, an initial sympathoexcitation followed by a sudden, centrally triggered sympathoinhibition and bradycardia, leading to a life-threatening fall in arterial blood pressure. Some monitored SIDS cases show a near total loss of arterial blood pressure within a minute of onset of the fatal event. Apparently, the inadequate compensatory mechanisms displayed prior to the fatal event by infants at risk for SIDS fail to provide sufficient support. Because SIDS deaths occur largely during sleep, some interaction of state and compensatory mechanisms is suspected. The prone sleeping position contributes to an enhanced risk for SIDS, which possibly derives from the vestibular and cerebellar contributions to arterial blood pressure control[32] described earlier. Because vestibular mechanisms assist mediation of arterial blood pressure to postural changes, static stimuli, such as those from the prone (as opposed to the supine) position, can directly modify cardiovascular responses to blood pressure challenges.[44-47] Sleep effects on vestibular systems must be considered in examination of arterial blood pressure control mechanisms.

SLEEP STATE–DEPENDENT CHANGES IN HEART RHYTHM

Recent evidence indicates that the pronounced changes in heart rate occurring during REM sleep and transitions between sleep states are attributable to distinct mechanisms associated with specific brain sites rather than representing a continuum of autonomic change.

Heart Rate Surges

Several investigators have reported REM-induced increases in heart rate in experimental animals.[11,14,48-51] Accelerations consisting of an abrupt, although transitory, 35% to 37% increase in rate that are concentrated during phasic REM were observed in canines (Fig. 15–3). These marked heart rate surges are accompanied by a rise in mean arterial blood pressure and are followed by a rate deceleration that is apparently baroreceptor mediated. Because the sequence is completely abolished by interruption of sympathetic neural input to the heart,[48-50] the acceleration does not appear to be dependent on withdrawal of parasympathetic nerve activity.[14,50]

REM sleep state–dependent heart rate surges have also been observed in felines. The rate accelerations are linked to CNS activation as reflected in a concomitant increase in hippocampal

Figure 15–3. Effects of non–rapid eye movement (NREM) sleep (slow wave sleep), rapid eye movement (REM) sleep, and quiet wakefulness on heart rate, phasic and mean arterial blood pressure, phasic and mean left circumflex coronary flow, electroencephalogram (EEG), and electrooculogram (EOG) in the dog. Sleep spindles are evident during NREM sleep, eye movements during REM sleep, and gross eye movements on awakening. Surges in heart rate and coronary flow occur during REM sleep. (From Kirby DA, Verrier RL: Differential effects of sleep stage on coronary hemodynamic function. Am J Physiol 1989;256:H1378-1383.)

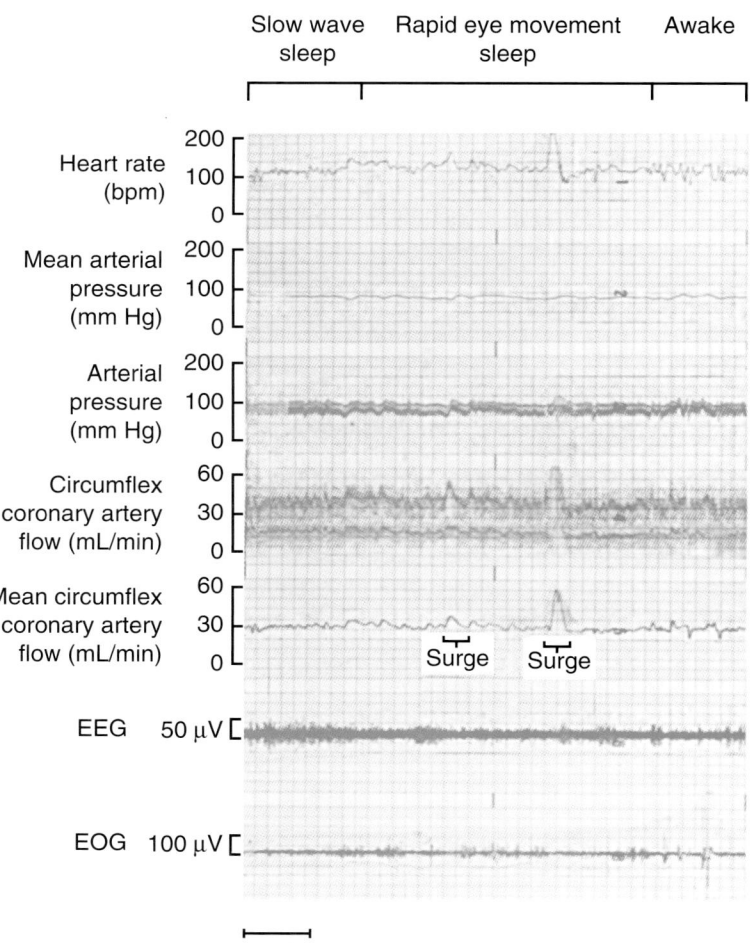

theta frequency, ponto-geniculo-occipital (PGO) activity, and eye movements.[51] In cats, the appearance of theta waves is characteristic of arousal, orienting activity, alertness, and REM sleep.[51-55] The surges are abolished by cardioselective beta-adrenergic blockade with atenolol, suggesting, as in canines, that the peripheral effect is attributable to bursting of cardiac sympathetic efferent fiber activity, which directly affects heart rate. The main difference in rate responses between the two species is that in dogs, the rate acceleration is accompanied within seconds by a baroreflex-mediated deceleration. The precise basis for these differences in the pattern of heart rate responses is unclear, but a plausible explanation is that the canine studies were performed in beagles, a strain that is bred for intense physical activity, which is a factor known to augment baroreceptor responsiveness.

Heart Rhythm Pauses

A complementary finding to centrally mediated heart rate surges is the observation in cats of an abrupt deceleration in heart rhythm that occurs predominantly during tonic REM sleep and is not associated with any preceding or subsequent change in heart rate or arterial blood pressure (Fig. 15–4).[56] The involvement of the vagus nerve appears to be directly initiated by central influences, as there is no antecedent or subsequent change in resting heart rate or arterial blood pressure. The primary involvement of CNS activation is demonstrated by the consistent, antecedent, abrupt cessation of PGO activity and the concomitant interruption of hippocampal theta rhythm. In normal human volunteers, Taylor and colleagues[57] observed heart rate decelerations during REM sleep that preceded eye movement bursts by 3 seconds; they suggested that the phenomenon reflects an orienting response at the onset of dreaming. How these changes in CNS activity lead to the tonic REM sleep–induced increase in vagus nerve tone to suppress sinus node activity remains unknown. Notwithstanding extensive studies of the physiologic and anatomic bases for PGO activity, little is known about its conductivity and functional relationship to heart rhythm control during sleep.

The most likely basis for the abrupt deceleration in heart rate during tonic REM sleep is a change in the centrally induced pattern of autonomic activity to the heart. This could be the result of a decrease in sympathetic nerve activity or of an enhancement of vagus nerve tone, or both in combination. In felines, cardioselective beta$_1$-adrenergic blockade with atenolol did not affect the incidence or magnitude of decelerations, but muscarinic blockade with glycopyrrolate completely abolished the phenomenon. These observations suggest that the tonic REM sleep–induced decelerations are primarily mediated by cardiac vagus nerve efferent fiber activity. It is well known that enhanced vagal activity can abruptly and markedly affect the sinus node firing rate.[58] Because beta-adrenergic blockade exerted no effect on the frequency or magnitude of decelerations, it does not appear that withdrawal of cardiac sympathetic tone is an important factor in the observed rate changes. Respiratory interplay is not an essential component of the deceleration, as the phenomenon often occurs in the absence of a temporal association with inspiratory effort.

This primary heart rate pause phenomenon appears to be distinct from baroreceptor-mediated reductions in heart rate that almost invariably follow accelerations in rate and elevation of arterial blood pressure (Fig. 15–5).[12] This second group of heart rhythm pauses was observed in canines and occurs mainly during the transition from slow wave sleep to desynchronized sleep and more frequently during phasic than tonic REM sleep. They persist for 1 to 8 seconds and are followed by dramatic increases in coronary blood flow averaging 30% and ranging up to 84%, which are independent of metabolic activity of the heart as reflected in the heart rate–blood pressure product. An intense burst of vagus nerve activity appears to produce the phenomenon, because the pauses develop against a background of marked respiratory sinus

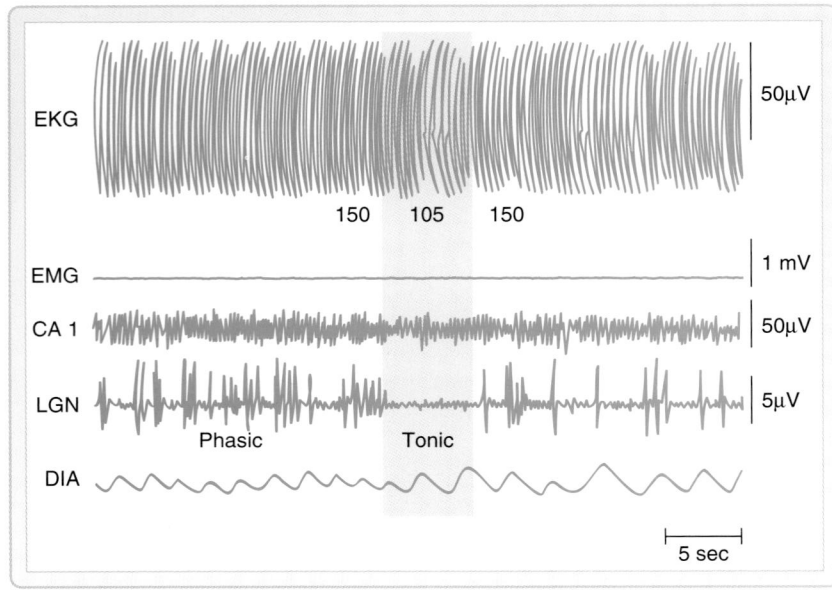

Figure 15–4. Representative polygraphic recording of a primary heart rate deceleration during tonic rapid eye movement (REM) sleep. During this deceleration, heart rate decreased from 150 to 105 bpm, or 30%. The deceleration occurred during a period devoid of ponto-geniculo-occipital (PGO) spikes in the lateral geniculate nucleus (LGN) or theta rhythm in the hippocampal (CA 1) leads. The abrupt decreases in amplitude of hippocampal theta waves (CA 1), PGO waves (LGN), and respiratory rate (DIA) are typical of transitions from phasic to tonic REM. EKG, electrocardiogram; EMG, electromyogram. (From Verrier RL, Lau RT, Wallooppillai U, et al: Primary vagally mediated decelerations in heart rate during tonic rapid eye movement sleep in cats. Am J Physiol 1998;43:R1136-1141.)

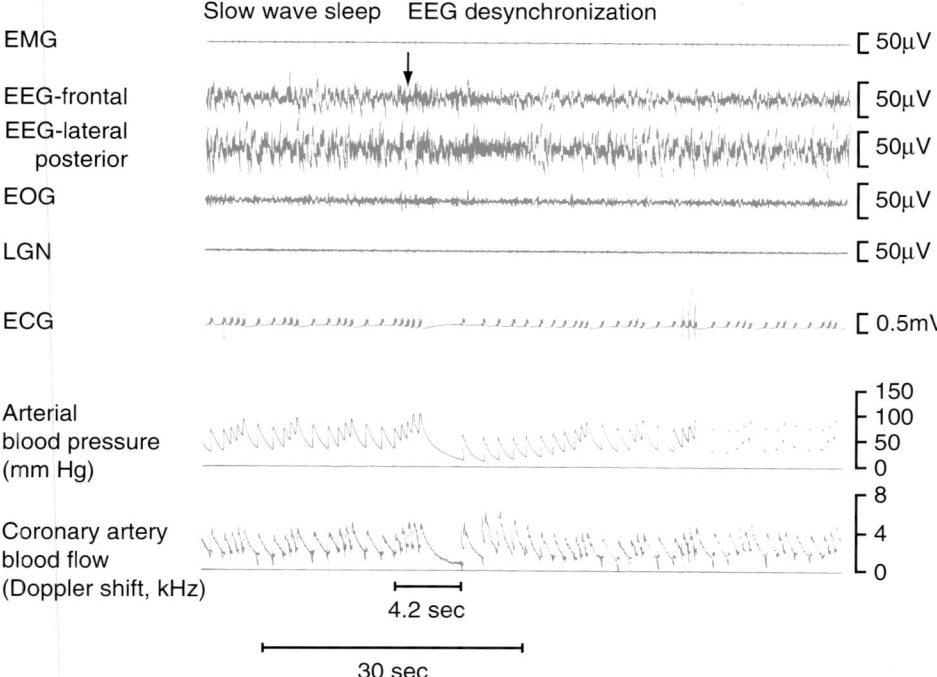

Post-asystole CBF surge during interruption of SWS by EEG desynchronization

Figure 15–5. Coronary blood flow (CBF) surge during deep non–rapid eye movement (NREM) sleep interrupted by electroencephalographic (EEG) desynchronization. This response pattern is common and appears to represent a brief, low-grade arousal. The 4.2-second pause in heart rhythm was followed by a brief increase of 46% in average peak CBF and a decrease of 49% in the heart rate–systolic blood pressure product. ECG, electrocardiogram; EEG, electroencephalogram; EMG, electromyogram; EOG, electrooculogram; LGN, lateral geniculate nucleus field potential recordings; SWS, slow wave sleep. (From Dickerson LW, Huang AH, Nearing BD, et al: Primary coronary vasodilation associated with pauses in heart rhythm during sleep. Am J Physiol 1993;264:R186-196.)

arrhythmia with varying degrees of heart block (with nonconducted P waves) and with low heart rate. Moreover, they could be emulated by electrical stimulation of the vagus nerve. Guilleminault and colleagues[59] documented similar pauses in healthy young adults.

CORONARY ARTERY BLOOD FLOW REGULATION DURING SLEEP

Striking changes in coronary blood flow occur during REM and sleep-state transitions.[12,48-50,60] Vatner and coworkers[60] studied the effects of the sleep–wake cycle on coronary artery function in baboons. During the nocturnal period, when the animals were judged to be asleep by behavioral indicators, coronary blood flow increased sporadically by as much as 100%. The periodic oscillations in blood flow were not associated with alterations in heart rate or arterial blood pressure and occurred while the animals remained motionless with eyes closed. Because the baboons were not instrumented for electroencephalographic recordings, no information was obtained regarding sleep stage, nor was the mechanism for the coronary blood flow surge defined.

Concomitant with the heart rate surges of REM sleep that are observed in canines[48-50] as described earlier were remarkable, episodic surges in coronary blood flow with corresponding decreases in coronary vascular resistance. These phenomena occurred predominantly during periods of REM sleep marked by intense phasic activity as defined by the frequency of eye movements.[50] There were no significant changes in mean arterial blood pressure. Heart rate was elevated during the coronary

flow surges, suggesting an increase in cardiac metabolic activity as the basis for the coronary vasodilation. In fact, the close coupling between rate–pressure product, an index of metabolic demand, and the magnitude of the flow surges indicates that the surges do not constitute a state of myocardial hyperperfusion. These surges in coronary blood flow appear to result from enhanced adrenergic discharge, because they were abolished by bilateral stellectomy, and not from nonspecific effects of somatic activity or respiratory fluctuations.

During severe coronary artery stenosis (with baseline flow reduced by 60%), phasic decreases in coronary arterial blood flow, rather than increases, were observed during REM sleep coincident with these heart rate surges (Fig. 15–6).[49] An increase in adrenergic discharge could lead to a coronary blood flow decrement by at least two possible mechanisms. The first is by stimulation of alpha-adrenergic receptors on the coronary vascular smooth muscle. Such an effect, however, could be only transitory, as alpha-adrenergic stimulation results in brief (10 to 15 seconds) coronary constriction even during sympathetic nerve stimulation in anesthetized animals[61] or during intense arousal associated with aversive behavioral conditioning.[62] The second possible mechanism is mechanical: a decrease in diastolic coronary perfusion time caused by the surges in heart rate. In support of this explanation, we found a strong correlation ($r^2 = 0.96$) between the magnitude of the increase in heart rate and the decrease in coronary blood flow.[49] The link between REM-induced changes in heart rate and the occurrence of myocardial ischemia in patients with advanced coronary artery disease is consistent with the clinical experience of Nowlin and coworkers.[63]

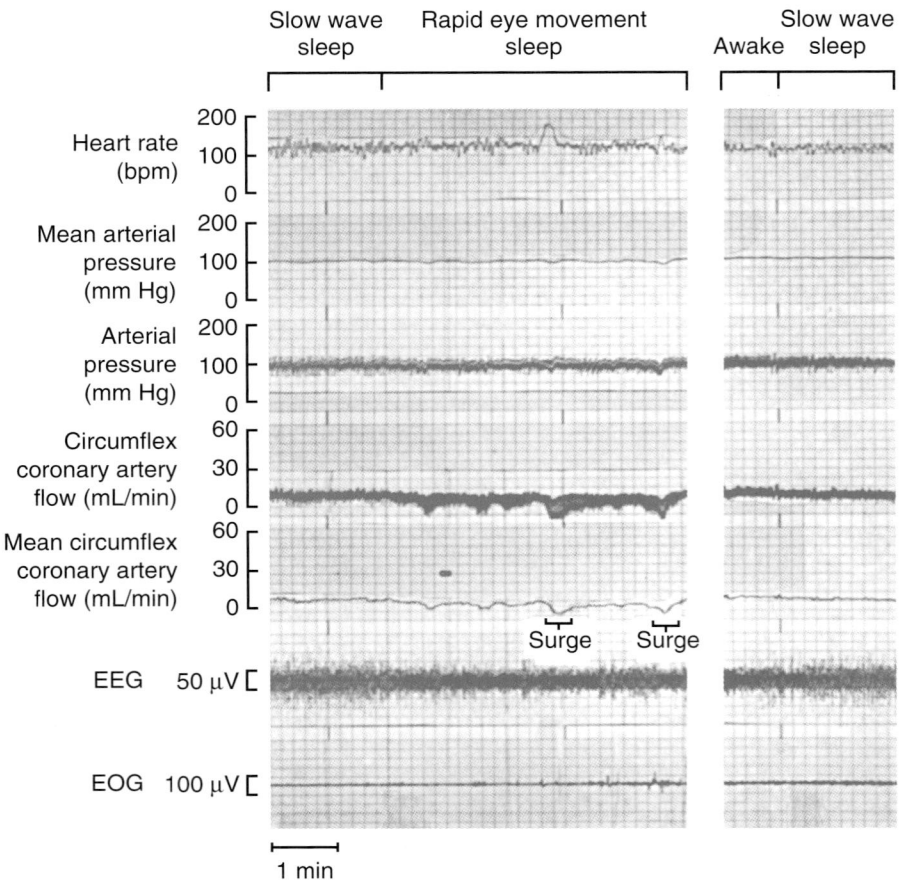

Figure 15–6. Effects of sleep stage on heart rate, mean and phasic arterial blood pressure, and mean and phasic left circumflex coronary artery blood flow in a typical dog during coronary artery stenosis. Note phasic decreases in coronary flow occurring during heart rate surges while the dog is in rapid eye movement (REM) sleep. EEG, electroencephalogram; EOG, electrooculogram. During REM sleep, the EEG reveals a characteristic lower amplitude, higher frequency pattern than in slow wave sleep. The EOG tracing indicates the presence of eye movements during REM but not slow wave sleep. (Reprinted from Kirby DA, Verrier RL: Differential effects of sleep stage on coronary hemodynamic function during stenosis. Physiol Behav 1989;45:1017-1020, with permission.)

IMPACT OF SLEEP ON ARRHYTHMOGENESIS

Central Nervous System Sites Influencing Cardiac Electrical Stability

Extensive investigation of CNS-induced cardiac arrhythmias has provided evidence that triggering of arrhythmias by the CNS is not only the consequence of intense activation of the autonomic nervous system but is also a function of the specific neural pattern elicited. For example, the influence of the vagus nerve on ventricular electrical properties is contingent on the level of sympathetic tone, a phenomenon referred to as accentuated antagonism. The underlying mechanism is that acetylcholine, released by vagal activation, exerts its opposing effects by presynaptic inhibition of norepinephrine release from sympathetic nerve endings and through an antagonism of second messenger formation at the cardiac receptor level.[64] Thus, the balance in cardiac input from either limb of the autonomic nervous system and their interactions must be considered. Another important concept is that triggering of arrhythmias by CNS activity may also depend on several intermediary mechanisms. These include direct effects of neurotransmitters on the myocardium and its specialized conducting system and changes in myocardial perfusion due to alterations in coronary vasomotor tone, enhanced platelet aggregability, or both. The net influence on the heart thus depends on a complex interplay between the specific neural pattern elicited and the underlying cardiac pathology.

Over 80 years ago, Levy[65] demonstrated that ventricular tachyarrhythmias can be elicited in normal animals by stimulating specific areas in the brain. This finding was subsequently confirmed in several species. Hockman and colleagues,[66] using stereotactic techniques, demonstrated that cerebral stimulation and hypothalamic activation evoked a spectrum of ventricular arrhythmias. Stimulation of the posterior hypothalamus causes a 10-fold increase in the incidence of ventricular fibrillation elicited by experimental occlusion of the coronary artery.[67] This enhanced vulnerability was linked to increased sympathetic nerve activity, because beta-adrenergic receptor blockade, but not vagotomy, prevented it. These findings are consistent with clinical reports that cerebrovascular disease (particularly intracranial hemorrhage) can elicit significant cardiac repolarization abnormalities and life-threatening arrhythmias.[68,69] Cryogenic blockade of the thalamic gating mechanism or its output from the frontal cortex to the brainstem[70] and of the amygdala[71] delayed or prevented the occurrence of ventricular fibrillation during stress in pigs.

Ventricular arrhythmias also ensue immediately on cessation of diencephalic or hypothalamic stimulation, but these require intact vagi and stellate ganglia.[72,73] The likely electrophysiologic basis for such post-CNS stimulation arrhythmias is the loss of rate-overdrive suppression of ectopic activity. This phenomenon occurs when the vagus nerve regains its activity after cessation of centrally induced adrenergic stimulation. Accordingly, the enhanced automaticity induced by adrenergic stimulation of ventricular pacemakers is exposed when vagus nerve tone is restored and slows the sinus rate.[73] Although these arrhythmias may be dramatic in appearance (including ventricular tachycardia), they rarely degenerate into ventricular fibrillation.[74] This proarrhythmic effect of dual autonomic activation has been erroneously interpreted as profibrillatory.

The antiarrhythmic influence of beta-adrenergic receptor blockade may result in part from blockade of central beta-adrenergic receptors. Parker and coworkers[75] determined that intracerebroventricular administration of subsystemic doses of *l*-propranolol (but not *d*-propranolol) significantly reduced the incidence of ventricular fibrillation during combined left anterior descending coronary artery occlusion and behavioral stress in the pig. Surprisingly, intravenous administration of even a relatively high dose of *l*-propranolol was ineffectual. The latter result may relate in part to a species dependence because, unlike canines, pigs do not show a suppression of ischemia-induced arrhythmias in response to beta-blockade.[76] It was proposed that the centrally mediated protective effect of beta-blockade is the result of a decrease in sympathetic nerve activity and in plasma norepinephrine concentration.[75,77,78] Importantly, whereas central actions of beta-adrenergic receptor blockers may play an important role in reducing susceptibility to ventricular fibrillation during acute myocardial ischemia, they are unlikely to constitute the sole mechanism, as beta-blockers prevent the profibrillatory effect of direct stimulation of peripheral sympathetic structures such as the stellate ganglia.[79] It is noteworthy that the three beta-blockers that have long-term effects on mortality of cardiac patients (propranolol, metoprolol, and carvedilol) are all lipophilic[80] and therefore cross the blood–brain barrier readily and affect sleep structure, with significant perturbations of sleep continuity.[81]

Autonomic Factors in Arrhythmogenesis during Sleep

NREM sleep is generally salutary with respect to ventricular arrhythmogenesis, as indicated both by extensive studies of neurocardiac interactions and by clinical experience. Activation of the vagus nerve reduces heart rate, increases cardiac electrical stability, and reduces rate–pressure product, an indicator of cardiac metabolic activity, to improve the supply–demand relationship in stenotic coronary artery segments. However, in the setting of severe coronary disease or acute myocardial infarction, hypotension during NREM can lead to myocardial ischemia because of inadequate coronary perfusion pressure and thereby provoke arrhythmias and myocardial infarction.[10,82] The abrupt increases in vagus nerve tone that can occur during periods of REM or sleep-state transitions can result in significant pauses in heart rhythm, bradyarrhythmias, and, potentially, triggered activity, a mechanism of the lethal cardiac arrhythmia torsades de pointes. Patients with the long QT syndrome who have the type 3 phenotype are more prone to experience torsades de pointes at night rather than during stress or exercise.[44] Tonic control of the vagus nerves over the caliber of the epicardial coronary vessels[83] could be an important factor in dynamic regulation of coronary resistance as a function of the sleep–wake cycle.

An important question is whether tonic vagus nerve activity exerts a protective or a deleterious influence on myocardial perfusion and arrhythmogenesis in individuals with atherosclerotic disease. In these patients, nocturnal surges in vagus nerve activity could precipitate myocardial ischemia and arrhythmias as a result of coronary vasoconstriction rather than dilation in atherosclerotic segments, because of impaired release of endothelium-derived relaxing factor.[84]

Because of the attendant surges in sympathetic nerve activity and in heart rate, REM sleep has the potential for triggering ventricular arrhythmias.[85,86] The striking variability of heart rate and breathing pattern can have a significant impact on cardiovascular functioning, as is evident in the development of ischemia and arrhythmias in patients whose myocardium is compromised. Indeed, the only clinical studies in which sleep staging has been employed have identified REM as the state in which arrhythmias occurred.[10,87,88] The increase in sympathetic nerve activity that occurs at the onset of REM sleep[9] provides a potent stimulus for ventricular tachyarrhythmias because of the arrhythmogenic influence of neurally released catecholamines. Sympathetic nerve activation by stimulation of central[65-67,72,73] or peripheral adrenergic structures,[79,89] infusion of catecholamines,[90] or imposition of behavioral stress[91] can increase cardiac vulnerability in the normal and ischemic heart. These profibrillatory influences are substantially blunted by beta-adrenergic receptor blockade.[91] A wide variety of supraventricular arrhythmias can also be induced by autonomic activation.[74]

Enhanced sympathetic nerve activity increases cardiac vulnerability in the normal and in the ischemic heart by complex mechanisms. The major indirect effects include an impaired oxygen supply–demand ratio resulting from increased cardiac metabolic activity and coronary vasoconstriction, particularly in vessels with injured endothelium and in the context of altered preload and afterload. The direct profibrillatory effects on cardiac electrophysiologic function are attributable to derangements in impulse formation or conduction, or both.[74] Increased levels of catecholamines activate beta-adrenergic receptors, which in turn alter adenylate cyclase activity and intracellular calcium flux. These actions are probably mediated by the cyclic nucleotide and protein kinase regulatory cascade, which can alter spatial heterogeneity of calcium transients and consequently increase dispersion of repolarization. The net influence is an increase in susceptibility to ventricular fibrillation.[62,92] Conversely, reduction of cardiac sympathetic drive by stellectomy has proved to be antifibrillatory.

Notwithstanding the evidence that autonomic factors have the potential for significantly altering susceptibility to arrhythmias, the observation that the heart rate surges of REM sleep are conducive to myocardial ischemia, and the epidemiologic data in humans on the extent of sleep-induced cardiac events,[1] there is a paucity of information regarding the effects of myocardial infarction on the cardiovascular system during sleep. Ventricular ectopic activity, but not ventricular fibrillation, has been documented during NREM sleep in pigs after myocardial infarction.[93] This pattern may be attributable to slowing of heart rate and increased vagus nerve activity during NREM sleep, conditions that can inhibit the normal overdrive suppression of ventricular rhythms by sinoatrial node pacemaker activity and result in firing of latent ventricular pacemakers and triggered activity. Snisarenko[94] found significant elevations in heart rate in both the acute (4 to 10 days) and subacute (3 to 12 months) periods following myocardial infarction in a feline model. In the acute period, these effects were accompanied by increased wakefulness, decreased heart rate variability, and severely disordered sleep. In the intervening weeks, sleep quality recovered fully until, in the subacute period, beta-blockade with propranolol led to renewed, pronounced disturbances in sleep structure, with increased wakefulness, reduction in REM sleep, and prolongation of stages 1 and 2 of NREM sleep. He attributed these results to reflex activation of adrenergic, noradrenergic, and dopaminergic nerves in several brain structures after coronary artery ligation.[95]

SUMMARY

Sleep states exert a major impact on cardiorespiratory function. This is a direct consequence of the significant variations in brain states that occur in the normal cycling between NREM and REM sleep. Dynamic fluctuations in CNS variables influence heart rhythm, arterial blood pressure, coronary artery blood flow, and ventilation. Whereas REM-induced surges in sympathetic and parasympathetic nerve activity with accompanying significant surges and pauses in heart rhythm are well tolerated in normal people, patients with heart disease may be at heightened risk for life-threatening arrhythmias and myocardial ischemia and infarction.[63,86] During NREM sleep, in the severely compromised heart, a potential for hypotension exists that can impair blood flow through stenotic coronary vessels to trigger myocardial ischemia or infarction.[10] Damage to central brain areas that regulate autonomic activity and coordinate upper airway and diaphragmatic action can lead to enhanced sympathetic outflow, increasing risk in heart failure and contributing to hypertension in obstructive sleep apnea. Coordination of cardiorespiratory control is especially pivotal in infancy, when developmental immaturity can compromise function and pose special risks. Throughout sleep, the coexistence of coronary disease and apnea is associated with heightened risk of cardiovascular events[96] resulting from the challenge of dual control of the respiratory and cardiovascular systems.

Clinical Pearl

REM sleep is characterized by surges in sympathetic and vagus nerve activity, which are well tolerated in normal individuals but which may result in cardiac arrhythmias, myocardial ischemia, and myocardial infarction in those with heart disease. During NREM sleep, systemic blood pressure may fall, potentially reducing flow through stenotic coronary vessels, which may precipitate cardiac ischemia or infarction. In essence, sleep constitutes an autonomic stress test for the heart, and nighttime monitoring of cardiorespiratory function is of considerable diagnostic value.[97]

Acknowledgments
This work was supported by National Institutes of Health grants P01ES09825 from the National Institute of Environmental Health and MH13923 from the National Institute of Mental Health, and HD22695, HL22418, and HL60296 from the National Institute of Child Health and Human Development and the National Heart, Lung, and Blood Institute, Bethesda, Maryland. Additional support was provided by the Mind-Body Network of the John D. and Catherine T. MacArthur Foundation. The authors thank Sandra S. Verrier for her editorial contributions.

References

1. Lavery CE, Mittleman MA, Cohen MC, et al: Nonuniform nighttime distribution of acute cardiac events: A possible effect of sleep states. Circulation 1997;96:3321-3327.
2. Task Force of the European Society of Cardiology and the North American Society of Pacing and Electrophysiology: Heart rate variability: Standards of measurement, physiological interpretation and clinical use. Circulation 1996;93:1043-1065.
3. Trelease RB, Sieck GC, Marks JD, et al: Respiratory inhibition induced by transient hypertension during sleep. Exp Neurol 1985;90:173-186.
4. Ohtake PJ, Jennings DB: Ventilation is stimulated by small reductions in arterial pressure in the awake dog. J Appl Physiol 1992;73:1549-1557.
5. Harper RM, Gozal D, Forster HV, et al: Imaging of ventral medullary surface activity during blood pressure challenges in awake and anesthetized goats. Am J Physiol 1996;39:R182-191.
6. Schechtman VL, Harper RM, Wilson AJ, et al: Sleep apnea in infants who succumb to the sudden infant death syndrome. Pediatrics 1991;87:841-846.
7. Woo MS, Woo MA, Gozal D, et al: Heart rate variability in congenital central hypoventilation syndrome. Pediatr Res 1992;31:291-296.
8. Aljadeff G, Gozal D, Schechtman VL, et al: Heart rate variability in children with obstructive sleep apnea. Sleep 1997;20:151-157.
9. Somers VK, Dyken ME, Mark AL, et al: Sympathetic nerve activity during sleep in normal subjects. N Engl J Med 1993;328:303-307.
10. Mancia G: Autonomic modulation of the cardiovascular system during sleep. N Engl J Med 1993;328:347-349.
11. Baccelli G, Guazzi M, Mancia G, et al: Neural and non-neural mechanisms influencing circulation during sleep. Nature 1969;223:184-185.
12. Dickerson LW, Huang AH, Nearing BD, et al: Primary coronary vasodilation associated with pauses in heart rhythm during sleep. Am J Physiol 1993;264:R186-196.
13. Harper RM, Frysinger RC, Zhang J, et al: Cardiac and respiratory interactions maintaining homeostasis during sleep. In: Lydic R, Biebuyck JF (eds): Clinical Physiology of Sleep. Bethesda, Md, American Physiological Society, 1988.
14. Gassel MM, Ghelarducci B, Marchiafava PL, et al: Phasic changes in blood pressure and heart rate during the rapid eye movement episodes of desynchronized sleep in unrestrained cats. Arch Ital Biol 1964;102:530-544.
15. Snyder F, Hobson JA, Morrison DF, et al: Changes in respiration, heart rate, and systolic blood pressure in human sleep. J Appl Physiol 1964;19:417-422.
16. Lydic R, Baghdoyan HA: Microdialysis of cat pons reveals enhanced acetylcholine release during state-dependent respiratory depression. Am J Physiol 1991;261:R766-770.
17. Sauerland EK, Harper RM: The human tongue during sleep: Electromyographic activity of the genioglossus muscle. Exp Neurol 1976;51:160-170.
18. Henderson-Smart DJ, Read DJC: Reduced lung volume during behavioral active sleep in the newborn. J Appl Physiol 1979;46:1081-1085.
19. Maquet P, Peters J, Aerts J, et al: Functional neuroanatomy of human rapid-eye-movement sleep and dreaming. Nature 1996;383:163-166.

20. Braun AR, Balkin TJ, Wesenten NJ, et al: Regional cerebral blood flow throughout the sleep-wake cycle: An H2(15)O PET study. Brain 1997;120:1173-1197.

21. Nofzinger EA, Mintun MA, Wiseman M, et al: Forebrain activation in REM sleep: An FDG PET study. Brain Res 1997;770: 192-201.

22. Harper RM, Bandler R, Spriggs D, et al: Lateralized and widespread brain activation during transient blood pressure elevation revealed by magnetic resonance imaging. J Comp Neurol 2000;417:195-204.

23. Oppenheimer SM, Gelb A, Girvin JP, et al: Cardiovascular effects of human insular cortex stimulation. Neurology 1992;42: 1727-1732.

24. Zhang Z, Oppenheimer SM: Characterization, distribution and lateralization of baroreceptor-related neurons in the rat insular cortex. Brain Res 1997;760:243-250.

25. Woo MA, Macey PM, Fonarow GC, et al: Regional brain gray matter loss in heart failure. J Appl Physiol 2003;95:677-684.

26. Harper RM, Woo MA, Macey PM, et al: Diminished cerebellar and hippocampal responses to a cold pressor challenge in heart failure patients revealed by functional magnetic resonance imaging (Abstract). Soc Neurosci Abstr 2002;17:A858.

27. Harper RM, Woo MA, Macey PM, et al: Heart failure patients show deficient heart rate and altered neural fMRI responses to Valsalva maneuvers (Abstract). Soc Neurosci Abstr 2003; 12:A768.

28. Henderson LA, Woo MA, Macey PM, et al: Neural responses during Valsalva maneuvers in obstructive sleep apnea syndrome. J Appl Physiol 2003;94:1063-1074.

29. Harper RM, Macey PM, Henderson LA, et al: FMRI responses to cold pressor challenges in control and obstructive sleep apnea subjects. J Appl Physiol 2003;94:1583-1595.

30. Frysinger RC, Harper RM, Hackel RJ: State-dependent cardiac and respiratory changes associated with complex partial epilepsy. In Engel J Jr, Ojemann GA, Lüders HO (eds): Fundamental Mechanisms of Human Brain Function. New York, Raven Press, 1987, pp 219-226.

31. Moruzzi G: Paleocerebellar inhibition of vasomotor and respiratory carotid sinus reflexes. J Neurophysiol 1940;3:20-32.

32. Yates BJ: Vestibular influences on the autonomic nervous system. Ann N Y Acad Sci 1996:781:458-473.

33. Lutherer LO, Lutherer BC, Dormer KJ, et al: Bilateral lesions of the fastigial nucleus prevent the recovery of blood pressure following hypotension induced by hemorrhage or administration of endotoxin. Brain Res 1983;269:251-257.

34. Macey PM, Henderson LA, Macey KE, et al: Brain morphology associated with obstructive sleep apnea. Am J Resp Crit Care Med 2002;166:1382-1387.

35. Martin R, Roessmann U, Fanaroff A: Massive intracerebellar hemorrhage in low-birth-weight infants. J Pediatr 1976;89: 290-293.

36. Elisevich K, Redekop G: The fastigial pressor response. J Neurosurg 1991;74:147-151.

37. Waters KA, Forbes P, Morielli A, et al: Sleep-disordered breathing in children with myelomeningocele. J Pediatr 1998;132: 672-681.

38. Parmegianni PL, Franzini C, Lenzi P: Respiratory frequency as a function of preoptic temperature during sleep. Brain Res 1976;111:253-260.

39. Frysinger RC, Marks JD, Trelease RB, et al: Sleep states attenuate the pressor response to central amygdala stimulation. Exp Neurol 1984;83:604-617.

40. Somers VK, Dyken ME, Clary MP, et al: Sympathetic neural mechanisms in obstructive sleep apnea. J Clin Invest 1995; 96:1897-1904.

41. Schwartz PJ, Stramba-Badiale M, Segantini A, et al: Prolongation of the QT interval and the sudden infant death syndrome. N Engl J Med 1998;338:1709-1714.

42. Meny RG, Carroll JL, Carbone MT, et al: Cardiorespiratory recordings from infants dying suddenly and unexpectedly at home. Pediatrics 1994;93:43-49.

43. Harper RM, Bandler R: Finding the failure mechanism in the sudden infant death syndrome. Nat Med 1998;4:157-158.

44. Sahni R, Schulze KF, Kashyap S, et al: Body position, sleep states, and cardiorespiratory activity in developing low birth weight infants. Early Hum Dev 1999;54:197-206.

45. Sahni R, Schulze KF, Kashyap S, et al: Postural differences in cardiac dynamics during quiet and active sleep in low birthweight infants. Acta Paediatr 1999;88:1396-1401.

46. Galland BC, Taylor BJ, Bolton DP, et al: Vasoconstriction following spontaneous sighs and head-up tilts in infants sleeping prone and supine. Early Hum Dev 2000;58:119-132.

47. Galland BC, Hayman RM, Taylor BJ, et al: Factors affecting heart rate variability and heart rate responses to tilting in infants aged 1 and 3 months. Pediatr Res 2000;48:360-368.

48. Kirby DA, Verrier RL: Differential effects of sleep stage on coronary hemodynamic function. Am J Physiol 1989;256: H1378-1383.

49. Kirby DA, Verrier RL: Differential effects of sleep stage on coronary hemodynamic function during stenosis. Physiol Behav 1989;45:1017-1020.

50. Dickerson LW, Huang AH, Thurnher MM, et al: Relationship between coronary hemodynamic changes and the phasic events of rapid eye movement sleep. Sleep 1993;16:550-557.

51. Rowe K, Moreno R, Lau RT, et al: Heart rate surges during REM sleep are associated with theta rhythm and PGO activity in the cat. Am J Physiol 1999;277:R843-R849.

52. Sakai K, Sano K, Iwahara S: Eye movements and hippocampal theta activity in cats. Electroencephalogr Clin Neurophysiol 1973;34:547-549.

53. Kemp IR, Kaada BR: The relation of hippocampal theta activity to arousal, attentive behaviour and somato-motor movements in unrestrained cats. Brain Res 1975;95:323-342.

54. Lerma J, Garcia-Austt E: Hippocampal theta rhythm during paradoxical sleep: Effects of afferent stimuli and phase relationships with phasic events. Electroencephalogr Clin Neurophysiol 1985;60:46-54.

55. Sei H, Morita Y: Acceleration of EEG theta wave precedes the phasic surge of arterial pressure during REM sleep in the rat. Neuroreport 1996;7:3059-3062.

56. Verrier RL, Lau RT, Wallooppillai U, et al: Primary vagally mediated decelerations in heart rate during tonic rapid eye movement sleep in cats. Am J Physiol 1998;43:R1136-1141.

57. Taylor WB, Moldofsky H, Furedy JJ: Heart rate deceleration in REM sleep: An orienting reaction interpretation. Psychophysiology 1985;22:110-115.

58. Pappano AJ: Modulation of the heartbeat by the vagus nerve. In: Zipes DP, Jalife J (eds): Cardiac Electrophysiology: From Cell to Bedside. Philadelphia, WB Saunders, 1995, pp 411-422.

59. Guilleminault CP, Pool P, Motta J, et al: Sinus arrest during REM sleep in young adults. N Engl J Med 1984;311:1006-1010.

60. Vatner SF, Franklin D, Higgins CB, et al: Coronary dynamics in unrestrained conscious baboons. Am J Physiol 1971;221: 1396-1401.

61. Feigl EO. Coronary physiology. Physiol Rev 1983;63:1-205.

62. Billman GE, Randall DC: Mechanisms mediating the coronary vascular response to behavioral stress in the dog. Circ Res 1981;48:214-223.

63. Nowlin JB, Troyer WG Jr, Collins WS, et al: The association of nocturnal angina pectoris with dreaming. Ann Intern Med 1965;63:1040-1046.

64. Verrier RL, Antzelevitch C: Autonomic aspects of arrhythmogenesis: The enduring and the new. Curr Opin Cardiol 2004; 19:2-11.

65. Levy AG: The exciting causes of ventricular fibrillation in animals under chloroform anesthesia. Heart 1912;4:319-378.

66. Hockman CH, Mauck HP, Hoff EC: ECG changes resulting from cerebral stimulation: II. A spectrum of ventricular arrhythmias of sympathetic origin. Am Heart J 1966;71:695-700.

67. Verrier RL, Calvert A, Lown B: Effect of posterior hypothalamic stimulation on the ventricular fibrillation threshold. Am J Physiol 1975;228:923-927.

68. Cropp GJ, Manning GW: Electrocardiographic changes simulating myocardial ischemia and infarction associated with spontaneous intracranial hemorrhage. Circulation 1960;22:25-38.

69. Hugenholtz PG: Electrocardiographic abnormalities in cerebral disorders: Report of six cases and review of the literature. Am Heart J 1962;63:451-461.

70. Skinner JE, Reed JC: Blockade of frontocortical-brain stem pathway prevents ventricular fibrillation of ischemic heart. Am J Physiol 1981;240:H156-163.

71. Carpeggiani C, Landisman C, Montaron M-F, et al: Cryoblockade in limbic brain (amygdala) prevents or delays ventricular fibrillation after coronary artery occlusion in psychologically stressed pigs. Circ Res 1992;70:600-606.

72. Korteweg GCJ, Boeles JTF, Ten Cate J: Influence of stimulation of some subcortical areas on electrocardiogram. J Neurophysiol 1957;20:100-107.

73. Manning JW, Cotten M de V: Mechanism of cardiac arrhythmias induced by diencephalic stimulation. Am J Physiol 1962;203:1120-1124.

74. Janse MJ, Wit AL: Electrophysiological mechanisms of ventricular arrhythmias resulting from myocardial ischemia and infarction. Physiol Rev 1989;69:1049-1169.

75. Parker GW, Michael LH, Hartley CJ, et al: Central beta-adrenergic mechanisms may modulate ischemic ventricular fibrillation in pigs. Circ Res 1990;66:259-270.

76. Benfey BG, Elfellah MS, Ogilvie RI, et al: Antiarrhythmic effects of prazosin and propranolol during coronary artery occlusion and reperfusion in dogs and pigs. Br J Pharmacol 1984;82:717-725.

77. Lewis PJ, Haeusler G: Reduction in sympathetic nervous activity as a mechanism for the hypotensive action of propranolol. Nature 1975;256:440.

78. Privitera PJ, Webb JG, Walle T: Effect of centrally administered propranolol on plasma renin activity, plasma norepinephrine, and arterial pressure. Eur J Pharmacol 1979;54:51-60.

79. Schwartz PJ, Vanoli E, Zaza A, et al: The effect of antiarrhythmic drugs on life-threatening arrhythmias induced by the interaction between acute myocardial ischemia and sympathetic hyperactivity. Am Heart J 1985;109:937-948.

80. Hjalmarson A, Olsson G: Myocardial infarction: Effects of beta-blockade. Circulation 1991;84(Suppl 6):VI-101-107.

81. Kostis JB, Rosen RC: Central nervous system effects of beta-adrenergic blocking drugs: The role of ancillary properties. Circulation 1987;75:204-212.

82. Broughton R, Baron R: Sleep patterns in the intensive care unit and on the ward after acute myocardial infarction. Electroencephalogr Clin Neurophysiol 1978;45:348-360.

83. Kovach JA, Gottdiener JS, Verrier RL: Vagal modulation of epicardial coronary artery size in dogs. A two-dimensional intravascular ultrasound study. Circulation 1995;92:2291-2298.

84. Ludmer PL, Selwyn AP, Shook TL, et al: Paradoxical vasoconstriction induced by acetylcholine in atherosclerotic arteries. N Engl J Med 1986;315:1046-1051.

85. Lown B, Verrier RL: Neural activity and ventricular fibrillation. N Engl J Med 1976;294:1165-1170.

86. Andrews TC, Fenton T, Toyosaki N, et al: Subsets of ambulatory myocardial ischemia based on heart rate activity: Circadian distribution and response to anti-ischemic medication. Circulation 1993;88:92-100.

87. Smith R, Johnson L, Rothfeld D, et al: Sleep and cardiac arrhythmias. Arch Intern Med 1972;130:751-753.

88. Rosenblatt G, Hartman E, Zwilling GR: Cardiac irritability during sleep and dreaming. J Psychosom 1973;17:129-134.

89. Verrier RL, Thompson PL, Lown B: Ventricular vulnerability during sympathetic stimulation: Role of heart rate and blood pressure. Cardiovasc Res 1974;8:602-610.

90. Han J, Moe GK: Nonuniform recovery of excitability in ventricular muscle. Circ Res 1964;14:44-60.

91. Kovach JA, Nearing BD, Verrier RL: An angerlike behavioral state potentiates myocardial ischemia-induced T-wave alternans in canines. J Am Coll Cardiol 2001;37:1719-1725.

92. Levy MN: Role of calcium in arrhythmogenesis. Circulation 1989;80(6Suppl):IV:23-30.

93. Skinner JE, Mohr DN, Kellaway P: Sleep-stage regulation of ventricular arrhythmias in the unanesthetized pig. Circ Res 1975;37:342-349.

94. Snisarenko AA: Cardiac rhythm in cats during physiological sleep in experimental myocardial infarction and beta-adrenergic receptor blockade. Cor Vasa 1986;38:306-314.

95. Sole MJ, Hussain MN, Lixfeld W: Activation of brain catecholaminergic neurons by cardiac vagal afferents during acute myocardial ischemia in the rat. Circ Res 1980;47:166-172.

96. Hung J, Whitford EG, Parsons RW, et al: Association of sleep apnoea with myocardial infarction in men. Lancet 1990;336:261-264.

97. Verrier RL, Muller JE, Hobson JA: Sleep, dreams, and sudden death: The case for sleep as an autonomic stress test for the heart. Cardiovasc Res 1996;31:181–211.

Cardiovascular Physiology: The Peripheral Circulation

Carlo Franzini

ABSTRACT

The regulation of physiologic systems changes with state—wakefulness, non–rapid eye movement (NREM) sleep, and rapid eye movement (REM) sleep. This has been demonstrated in studies of thermoregulation and respiration, and it also applies to circulation. The sleep process primarily involves the brain, and changes in cerebral activity are the primary events of sleep. Changes in circulation are modest during NREM sleep but substantial during REM sleep. When the activity of the brain increases in REM sleep, cerebral blood flow also increases. Therefore, during REM sleep, there is flow–metabolism coupling. In contrast, changes in other peripheral beds respond to a sum of central (sympathovagal balance) and peripheral (local activity) changes that are sleep dependent and may conflict with the functional logic of the organs (thermoregulatory, excretory, absorptive). Therefore, whereas cerebral circulation during REM sleep shares the regulatory mechanisms of other brain-activated states, the disrupted integrated control of the remaining peripheral beds is unique to REM sleep. This disruption has no effect under physiologic conditions but may represent a risk factor in pathophysiologic conditions when the control of peripheral resistances is an indispensable adaptive mechanism (e.g., in chronic heart failure).

SLEEP-DEPENDENT CHANGES IN CEREBRAL CIRCULATION

The brain circulation during sleep has been the focus of many studies,[1-4] with the assumption that its understanding might shed light on the elusive issue of sleep function. A review of the literature[5] before 1990 listed more than 80 papers employing many different techniques. The main conclusions were the following:

1. Cerebral blood flow (CBF) mostly decreases during non–rapid eye movement (NREM) sleep, becoming lower than it was during wakefulness, and rises again markedly in rapid eye movement (REM) sleep.
2. Synaptic activity, metabolism, and CBF are related in sleep and in wakefulness.
3. CBF fluctuations result from changes in vascular resistance, but the mechanism was not known.
4. CBF fluctuations are mainly independent of systemic hemodynamic changes, particularly the redistribution of blood flow (BF) in other peripheral beds.

Regional Cerebral Blood Flow Changes during Sleep

More recently, positron emission tomography (PET) and Doppler flowmetry studies have shed light on the spatial and temporal dimension of CBF changes during sleep (see Maquet[6] and Zoccoli et al.[7]).

Maquet et al.[8] found an increased regional BF during REM sleep in the pontine tegmentum, dorsal mesencephalon, thalamic nuclei, amygdala, anterior cingulate, and entorhinal cortex. They interpreted these focal activations as bearing on different aspects of REM sleep neurophysiology and psychophysiology—that is, the centrencephalic (brainstem, thalamus, basal forebrain) origin of the state, its participation in emotional memory consolidation, and its autonomic phenomenology. This accounts for the partial overlap of brain structures (brainstem, anterior cingulate, prefrontal cortex) activated in REM sleep and in states of autonomic cardiovascular arousal during wakefulness.[9] A companion study from the same group examined the functional neuroanatomy of human slow wave sleep.[10] A significant negative correlation was found between the occurrence of NREM sleep and regional CBF in central core structures (pons, mesencephalon, thalamus). These results were recently confirmed, and a further distinction was made between early deactivation (light sleep: pons and thalamus) and late deactivation (deep sleep: encompassing also midbrain and neocortex) with respect to wakefulness levels.[11] A negative correlation has been also reported[12] between sigma (spindle) and delta activity and regional flow in the brainstem reticular formation, cerebellum, and thalamus, whereas at cortical level, both positive and negative correlations of CBF with delta activity were demonstrated. Principal component analysis also indicates decreased thalamic perfusion in NREM sleep.[13] These studies extend to humans the evidence of a reduced metabolic cost of synchronizing modes of operation in the thalamocortical circuitry, which was first shown by measurements of brain glucose uptake in other species (see Franzini[5]); the central role of the thalamus in the genesis of cortical synchronous activity is well established[14] and is confirmed by studies on sleep pathology (e.g., fatal familial insomnia).[15]

The brainstem-thalamo-cortical circuits responsible for the synchronization–desynchronization pattern, however, operate not only in sleep but also in other functional conditions (e.g., under anesthesia). When different anesthetic agents are utilized, a common pattern of reduced 18-fluorodeoxyglucose utilization results in the same anatomic structures (midbrain reticular formation, thalamus, basal forebrain), suggesting that different anesthetics must affect the same anatomic targets to exert their action.[16] The hypothesis is further supported by a study with an anesthetic of a different class (intravenous, as opposed to inhalational); this study reported "an EEG pattern very similar to stage IV sleep" and "a significant covariation between the thalamic and midbrain blood flow changes, suggesting a close functional relationship between the two structures."[17] These structures therefore represent the "common final path" for the synchronization–desynchronization pattern both in sleep and in anesthesia. Accordingly, CBF is rapidly restored in the centrencephalic brainstem–thalamic regions during the process of awakening.[18]

Braun et al.[19] measured CBF during wakefulness before and after sleep, and during NREM and REM sleep. Regional CBF in centrencephalic regions decreased during NREM sleep and increased during REM sleep; at a cortical level, heteromodal frontoparietal association cortices were deactivated during both NREM and REM sleep. This deactivation "may be a defining characteristic of sleep itself"[19] that involves the highest integrative processes of the brain (p.1173); its uniformity across sleep states might relate, in very general terms, to the fact that important features of sleep mental activity are shared by both NREM and REM sleep.[20] On the other hand, deactivation of the primary sensory cortex has been reported in NREM sleep[21] (visual and auditive) and in REM sleep[8] (parietal).

The reported BF changes in central core structures agree in essence with those found in other studies[8,10,12,13]; in contrast, greater variability across studies is apparent in cortical CBF data. Although a stereotypic circulatory and metabolic pattern links specific brain structures (brainstem, thalamus) during the sleep cycle, differences in cortical activation or deactivation often ascribed to differences in the species studied or methods used might well result from interindividual or even intraindividual variability intrinsic to the single sleep cycle. In addition, Braun et al.[19] reported significantly lower CBF values during postsleep wakefulness than during presleep wakefulness; the effect was more pronounced in cortical and limbic structures. The sleep process might thus reset the circulatory and metabolic activity of the brain to a lower level, in accordance with a "restorative" function of sleep (see later).

Cerebral blood perfusion during sleep may change not only quantitatively but also qualitatively. On the basis of local brain temperature changes, Azzaroni and Parmeggiani[22,23] suggested a carotid–vertebral shift in the quotas of CBF during REM sleep.

Spinal cord BF[24,25] also increases in REM sleep. The similar trends of BF changes in brain and spinal cord indicate that the sleep process involves a modulation of the activity in the entire central nervous system. Direct data on spinal cord metabolism during sleep are still lacking.

Maquet et al.,[26] in an attempt to tackle the question of REM sleep function, found that in subjects trained in a probabilistic serial reaction time, brain regions activated during wakefulness (among them striate and extrastriate, motor, premotor and supplementary motor cortices, cerebellum) were also more active during REM sleep, with respect to untrained subjects. This metabolic difference affects neural circuits made selectively operative during wakefulness. The authors correctly point out, however, that their experiments still cannot "identify the specific role of sleep periods in memory trace processing" (p. 833).

Time Course of Cerebral Blood Flow Changes during Sleep

Continuous recording of CBF changes during sleep with flow probes was instrumental in addressing the following issues: (1) the relationship between tonic and phasic cerebral perfusion changes during sleep, (2) the temporal sequence of CBF and sleep-state modifications, and (3) the CBF time course during the night, and the comparison between presleep and postsleep wakefulness levels.

1. In lambs, REM sleep is accompanied by a tonic increase in CBF and by superimposed phasic BF transient changes.[27,28] The analysis of the temporal relationship between cerebral perfusion pressure and CBF changes indicates that a fall in vascular resistance is the primary event that both underlies the tonic CBF increment and initiates the phasic CBF surges associated with transient blood pressure (BP) increases.
2. In rats, laser Doppler probes connected to an optical fiber were stereotaxically implanted in the hippocampus[29,30] and basal forebrain,[31] and relative increments in BF were recorded in the transition from NREM to REM sleep. However, the issue of the temporal relationship between circulatory and sleep-state changes remains unsolved: an early,[31] simultaneous,[30] or late[29] CBF change has been described with respect to the onset of the REM sleep episode. Regional, nonstereotypic differences in brain activation and BF rise with respect to the global state change might explain the different latencies reported.
3. In human adults,[32-34] CBF fluctuates from NREM to REM sleep within the same cycle, but decreases tonically throughout the night, and there are lower values in postsleep wakefulness compared to presleep wakefulness (Fig. 16–1); this corresponds to results obtained with PET[19] and reinforces the hypothesis of a restorative sleep function.

Regulation of Cerebral Circulation during the Sleep–Wake Cycle

The regulation of cerebral circulation aims on the one hand to finely match BF to the metabolic needs of brain activity at a regional level (i.e., flow–metabolism coupling), and, on the other hand, to protect the brain from systemic challenges (PaO_2, $PaCO_2$, pH changes [chemical regulation]; BP fluctuations [autoregulation]).

Flow–Metabolism Coupling

Blood flow, O_2 consumption, and glucose uptake undergo similar changes in the brain in different conditions of active wakefulness (sensory stimulation, selective attention) quiet wakefulness, and sleep (NREM and REM sleep) (see Lenzi et al.[35]).

In fetal lambs[36,37] during low-voltage fast activity (REM sleep equivalent), both O_2 and glucose consumption increase, but cerebral glucose uptake exceeds O_2 uptake. The increased glucose/O_2 quotient indicates a modest but significant anaerobic component in brain metabolism; this might be common to brain-activated states (see Lenzi et al.[35]) and not specific to REM sleep. Madsen,[38] however, calculated that when CBF values during REM sleep are corrected for $PaCO_2$ changes, the cerebral metabolic rate for O_2 remains coupled to CBF and the cerebral metabolic rate for glucose, suggesting an aerobic glucose utilization. The occurrence of anaerobic glycolysis

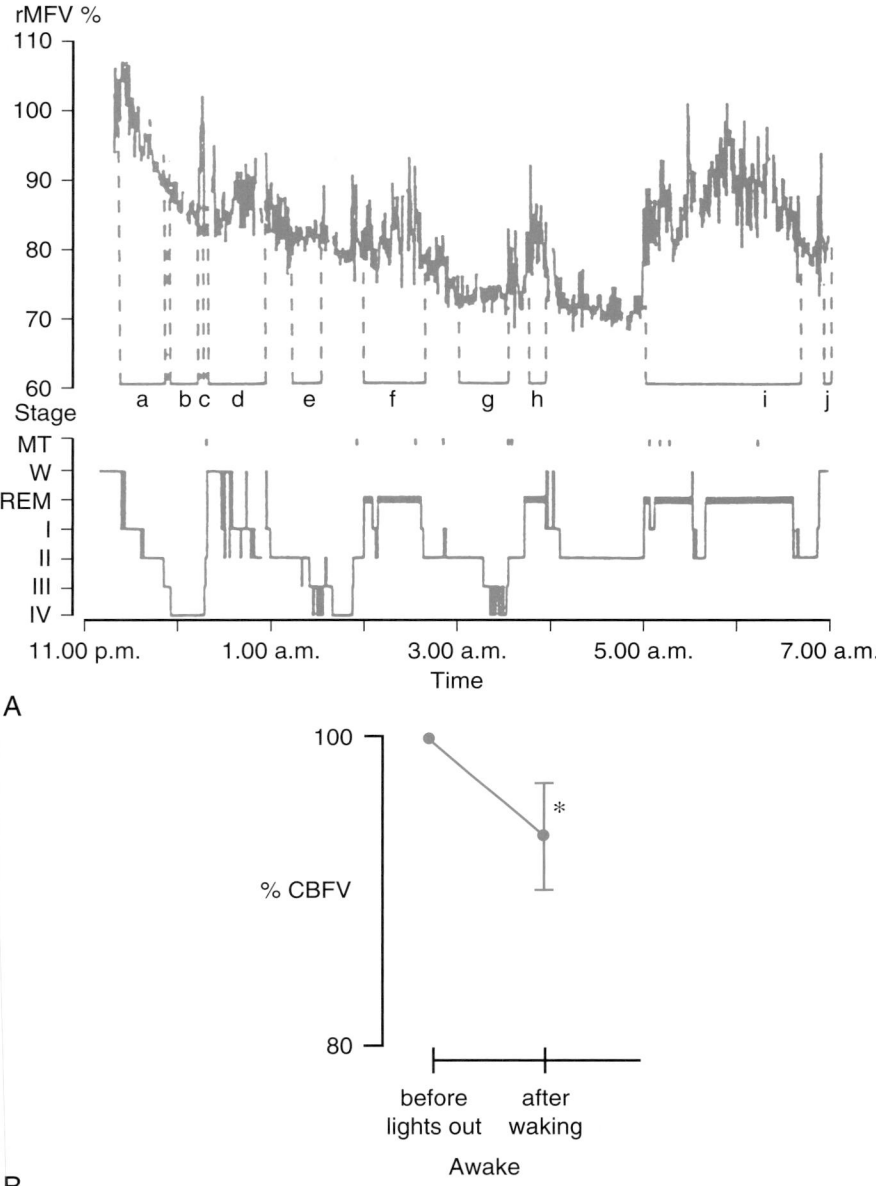

Figure 16–1. A, Relative mean flow velocity (rMFV) in the right middle cerebral artery and sleep profile of one healthy volunteer. (a) Progressive rMFV reduction during non–rapid eye movement (NREM) sleep; (b) continuous rMFV reduction during slow wave sleep (SWS); (c, j) movement artifact; (d) reduced rMFV during nighttime awakening; (e, g) constant mean level of rMFV during changes from sleep stage 2 to SWS; (f, h, i) rapid increase in rMFV during rapid eye movement (REM) sleep. MT, movement; W, wakefulness. (From Hajak G, Klingelhofer J, Schulz-Varszegi M, et al: Relationship between blood flow velocities and cerebral electrical activity in sleep. Sleep 1994;17:11-19.) rMFV can be considered a qualitative index of cerebral perfusion on the basis of the assumption of minimal caliber changes in large cerebral arteries in physiologic conditions in humans. A steady overall decrease in cerebral perfusion occurs during sleep, interrupted by pulsatile increments corresponding to each REM sleep episode. **B,** Percent cerebral blood flow velocity (CBFV) changes (mean ± SEM) for six subjects in the awake period before and after sleep. After-sleep CBFV was 6.6% lower than before sleep. *P < .05. (Modified from Kubayama T, Hori A, Sato T, et al: Changes in cerebral blood flow velocity in healthy young men during overnight sleep and while awake. Electroencephalogr Clin Neurophysiol 1997; 102:125-131, with permission.)

during REM sleep therefore remains to be proven. Comparison of presleep and postsleep brain glucose and O_2 metabolism[39] showed a greater decrease in glucose than in O_2 utilization. Reduced metabolism, reduced flow,[19,32,33] and reduced anaerobic glycolysis all agree with the concept of a restorative function of sleep. Wu et al.,[40] however, found no differences in mean cerebral glucose utilization during wakefulness before and after sleep deprivation. This discrepancy should be resolved, because it is central to the concept of a recovery function of sleep.

Finally, near infrared spectroscopy has been used to assess O_2 saturation and CBF changes during sleep. In the transition from wakefulness to NREM sleep, oxygenated hemoglobin is unchanged; in the transition from NREM to REM sleep, oxygenated hemoglobin is increased in accordance with a CBF increase.[41]

In conclusion, the cerebral metabolic rates for both glucose and O_2 increase during REM sleep; therefore, both glucose

and O_2 might act as mediators between metabolic and circulatory changes. However, the low extraction coefficient of glucose is inconsistent with the idea that it might couple flow and metabolism. On the other hand, the decreased arteriovenous O_2 difference in REM sleep indicated that the longitudinal O_2 gradient in the capillaries is reduced, so that a steeper transcapillary gradient is available to overcome the high resistance to O_2 diffusion from plasma to interstitium. This favors O_2 delivery. In addition, studies on brain microcirculation during sleep indicate that no capillary recruitment accompanies the sleep–wake cycle.[42] In the absence of capillary recruitment (relative to the endothelial surface area), the CBF increase during REM sleep is essential to maintaining the driving force for outward O_2 diffusion. Taken together, these data suggest that O_2 could be the coupling factor between cerebral activity and perfusion during REM sleep.[35]

Finally, the first study to probe the role of nitric oxide (NO) in CBF regulation during sleep by inhibiting NO synthase concluded that NO is the major determinant of CBF differences occurring across the sleep–wake states.[43]

Chemical Regulation

In NREM sleep, a slight hypercapnia develops (2 to 3 mm Hg). This counteracts the circulatory effects of the decreased cerebral metabolic rate and accounts for the small increase in CBF in some species (e.g., goat).[44] The response in any case is blunted by the decreased cerebral vascular reactivity to hypercapnia during NREM sleep.[45] $PaCO_2$ becomes an important determinant of CBF changes during sleep in pathologic conditions (e.g., sleep apnea).[46]

Autoregulation

Autoregulation has been shown to operate during sleep. In lambs, cerebral vasodilation in response to acute hypotension occurs in all behavioral states (wakefulness, NREM, and REM sleep, albeit with reduced efficacy in REM sleep).[28] The independence of CBF from systemic hemodynamics is further supported by the lack of correlation between BF increments in the brain and BF changes in the external carotid bed[47] or in other peripheral circulations (kidney, muscle, skin, splanchnic)[48]: CBF is not affected by the redistribution of regional flows occurring in REM sleep.

Conclusions and Implications for Future Research

The main conclusions from the reviewed data can be summarized as follows:

1. A stereotypic pattern of CBF and metabolic changes has been demonstrated during sleep in the central core of brainstem–thalamic structures with decrements in NREM and increments in REM sleep.[8,10,19] In contrast, greater fluctuations characterize the cortical circulatory and metabolic pattern; this may result from interindividual variability in small sample populations. Alternatively, it might be a true feature of cortical activation, especially during REM sleep, and even intraindividual activation variability might become apparent when longitudinal studies in the same subject become methodologically feasible. In general terms, associative cortices seem to be more affected by sleep than primary sensory areas (see Maquet et al.,[10] Andersson et al.,[13] and Braun et al.[19]).
2. The low metabolic cost of the synchronizing mode of operation in the thalamocortical circuits is now well established.[8,10,12,13,19]
3. An overall reduction of CBF (and presumably metabolism) occurs during the night, with postsleep values significantly lower than presleep values.[19,32-34] Points 2 and 3 favor the long-held view of a restorative function of sleep.
4. The study of brain microcirculation during sleep has just started.[42] It should shed light on the molecular traffic across the blood–brain barrier during sleep.[49]
5. Flow–metabolism coupling currently appears to be the principal mechanism controlling CBF changes during sleep. The other two regulatory mechanisms (chemical regulation and autoregulation) may be involved in adjusting CBF during sleep in pathophysiologic conditions (e.g., hypercapnia, hypotension).

SLEEP-DEPENDENT CHANGES IN EXTRACEREBRAL CIRCULATION

The evidence reviewed in the following paragraphs results from experiments on different animal species (rat, rabbit, cat, dog, sheep, humans) in which BF was measured with flowmeters or with radioactive microspheres.

Cutaneous Circulation

In the transition from wakefulness to NREM sleep, a decrease in set point temperature is responsible for thermolytic cutaneous vasodilation, which has been demonstrated across species (rat,[50] rabbit,[51,52] cat,[53] humans[54]). In REM sleep, on the other hand, skin BF changes result from the loss of appropriate thermoregulatory vasomotor responses.[21] Thus, in a cold environment, a BF increment results from the drop in neurogenic vasoconstriction[2]; in a warm environment, a BF reduction may result from a decrease in BP[53] or from a drop in neurogenic vasodilation.[50,52]

Renal Circulation

The few existing studies on renal circulation during sleep indicate that kidney BF is not state dependent.[55-57] When, however, renal vasoconstriction is an integrated part of the overall thermoregulatory vasomotor response to a thermal load, it wanes in REM sleep as does any other thermoregulatory effector response[2]; BF increases accordingly.[51]

Splanchnic Circulation

No significant BF changes occur in the splanchnic territory during sleep.[58,59] In liver, the constancy of total BF depends on a precise mixing of its arterial and portal components: an increase in hepatic arterial flow is compensated for by a decrease in portal flow, and vice versa. This entails a significant negative correlation between arterial and portal flow during wakefulness and NREM sleep; in REM sleep, the disappearance of this correlation[58] is an example of random *perturbations* (breathing irregularities, changes in abdominal pressure, cardiovascular variability) that interfere with a finely tuned regulatory mechanism.

Muscle Circulation

Muscle BF does not change significantly in the transition from wakefulness to NREM sleep. In REM sleep, it decreases in red fibers, whereas it increases, decreases, or remains unchanged in white fibers according to the species (rabbit,[60] cat,[61] rat,[62] respectively).

REM sleep entails both an increase in sympathetic tone in muscle blood vessels[63-65] and specific changes in muscle activity (atonia and twitches). The cumulative effect of the following factors determines BF changes in the two muscle fiber populations: (1) differences in basal BF in NREM sleep, which is high in red and low in white fibers; (2) vasodilator influences (local metabolic factors secondary to twitching activity); and (3) vasoconstrictor influences (both neural and local metabolic factors, secondary to atonia). Slight quantitative differences in the same vasodilator and vasoconstrictor mechanisms, acting on different levels of basal BF, may underlie the reported differences according to species and fiber type. Thus, muscle circulation exemplifies the complex way sleep affects vascular conductances both directly (via neural vasomotion changes) and indirectly (via activity changes).

Coronary Circulation

In the dog, left coronary BF decreases significantly from wakefulness to NREM sleep, and it increases in REM sleep.[66] During phasic REM sleep, BF surges are coupled with episodes of sinus tachycardia, suggesting that local metabolic control is responsible for reduced coronary vascular resistance.[67] However, in the transition from NREM to REM sleep, an increase in coronary BF follows a pause in heart rhythm. This increase in flow without a corresponding increase in cardiac metabolic activity has been attributed to neurogenic cholinergic vasodilation.[68] The sympathetic nervous system triggers the sequence of increased heart rate (HR) causing increased metabolism, which in turn leads to an increased blood flow. Both tachycardia and BF surges are eliminated by bilateral stellectomy.[66] In contrast, when a marked stenosis is induced by cuff inflation in the left circumflex coronary artery, HR increases in REM sleep are accompanied by a decrease in coronary BF. A reduced diastolic perfusion time may account for the flow decrement.[69]

These data emphasize the complex role of sympathovagal interactions in determining cardiac activity and coronary circulation changes during REM sleep.

Integrated Vasomotor Patterns

The circulatory system has control mechanisms hierarchically organized in levels of increasing complexity. At the hypothalamic level, the higher integrative control of autonomic functions can interfere with the physiologic control of the sleep cycle.[4] According to this model, the need to maintain an integrated autonomic pattern can hinder the natural progression from NREM to REM sleep, and, conversely, the entrance into REM sleep can disrupt the operating autonomic pattern. The model can be tested by applying a stimulus, for example, a thermal load or hemorrhage, that requires a complex cardiovascular response (compensatory distribution of regional flows).

The conflict arising between the maintenance of an adequate vasomotor pattern and the occurrence of REM sleep has been shown in experiments in which the intensity of vasoconstrictor sympathetic outflow was manipulated by abdominal cooling or by ligature of the common carotid arteries. The higher vasomotor tone caused by these manipulations hinders the transition from NREM to REM sleep, and it therefore positively correlates with the length of the NREM sleep episode.[70] Moreover, it has been shown that BP variability during REM sleep decreases at low ambient temperature (Fig. 16–2).[71] The wide range of fluctuations of physiologic variables is a distinguishing feature of REM sleep. The homeostatic control mechanism entrained by the thermal load may prevent attainment of the full-blown REM sleep episode at low ambient temperature, thus reducing spontaneous variability. On the other hand, integrated control mechanisms are altered during REM sleep in the following ways:

1. After hemorrhage,[72] the adaptive increase in peripheral vascular resistance is absent during REM sleep.
2. Exposure to a cold environment entails an adaptive increase in cardiac output during wakefulness and NREM sleep but not during REM sleep.[73] As far as the peripheral

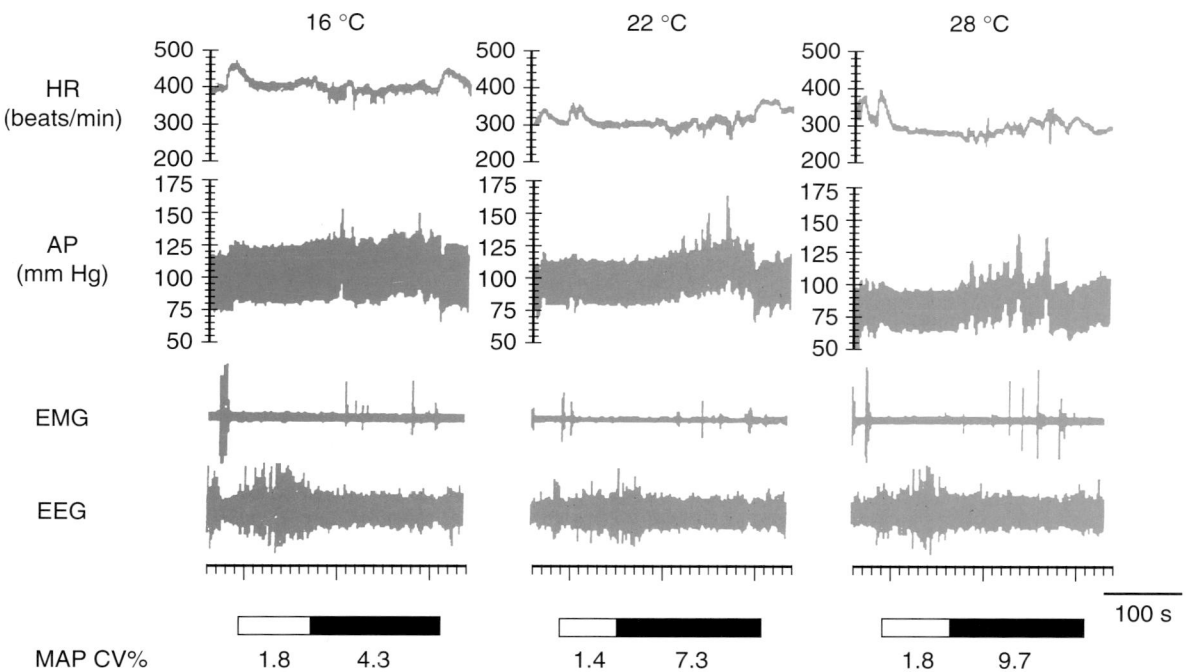

Figure 16–2. Representative computer-assisted digital recordings showing changes in heart rate (HR), arterial pressure (AP), electromyogram (EMG), and electroencephalogram (EEG) during successive non–rapid eye movement (NREM) sleep (indicated by horizontal *open columns* at bottom) and rapid eye movement (REM) sleep (indicated by horizontal *closed columns* at bottom) at three ambient temperatures. The coefficient of variation of mean arterial pressure (MAP CV%) decreased in REM sleep as the ambient temperature was lowered. (From Sei H, Morita Y: Effect of ambient temperature on arterial pressure variability during sleep in the rat. J Sleep Res 1996;5:37-41.)

circulation is concerned, the same thermoregulatory vasomotor adjustments occur in wakefulness and in NREM sleep. This BF redistribution abates in REM sleep: the compensatory modulation of peripheral resistances in response to a thermal load is lost.[51]

3. An acoustic impulsive stimulus differentially affects the integrated vasomotor response in NREM sleep, where homeostatic closed-loop mechanisms prevail, and in REM sleep, where nonhomeostatic, open-loop mechanisms prevail.[74]

Another vasomotor pattern—namely, the gradient of muscle vasoconstriction, increasing from superficial to deeper layers and corresponding to the reduction of the inner thermoregulated core in a cold environment—is similarly lost during REM sleep.[75]

This experimental evidence can be referred to the following scheme. REM sleep occurs when the responsible brainstem structures are freed from hypothalamic homeostatic control. This release is hindered by homeostatic challenges.[76] The release in turn results from an impairment of hypothalamic integrative activity during REM sleep. The hypothalamus is unresponsive to both thermal[77] and electrical[78] stimulation, and recordings of hypothalamic neurons show that cellular thermosensitivity is attenuated or abolished[79,80]; the modification at a central level entails the disorganization of complex adaptive vasomotor patterns at the periphery.

Control Mechanisms of the Extracerebral Circulation during the Wake–Sleep Cycle

Autonomic nervous system activity is a central issue in sleep physiology (see Parmeggiani and Morrison[81]). In recent years, two techniques—namely, spectral analysis of HR and BP variability in humans and other species, and sympathetic

nerve activity recordings in humans—have prompted a series of new studies. The results of these investigations and their congruence with previous reports are considered next.

Spectral Analysis of Heart Rate and Blood Pressure Variability

Oscillations in HR and BP result both from central commands and from the feedback operation of the regulatory loops. The frequency content of these fluctuations can be assessed by spectral analysis and can reflect changes in autonomic control of cardiac and vascular muscle cells (see Parati et al.[82] for a critical review).

In HR power spectra, the low-frequency (LF) band (less than 0.15 Hz in humans) has been associated with the modulation of sympathetic outflow, whereas the high-frequency (HF) band (greater than 0.15 Hz in humans) has been associated with the modulation of parasympathetic outflow.[83] The vast majority of spectral analysis studies during sleep have focused on HR spectra. Extrapolation of these results to the autonomic nervous system in general requires the assumption of a uniform "sympathetic tone." However, the concept of a uniform sympathetic tone has been challenged,[84] and regional differences have been demonstrated during sleep (Fig. 16–3).[64] On the other hand, BP power spectra, like BP itself, are affected by changes in both cardiac output and peripheral resistance. For these reasons, inferences about the nervous control of peripheral circulation drawn from spectral analysis data can overlook differences in autonomic output to the heart and to discrete peripheral beds. An exception occurs in specific pathophysiologic conditions in which a global increase in sympathetic tone may arise (e.g., sleep apnea,[85] fatal familial insomnia[86]; see also later).

Studies of HR power spectra during sleep (see Lenzi et al.[87] for a review) report reasonably concordant results: during NREM sleep, the LF (sympathetic) component decreases, and

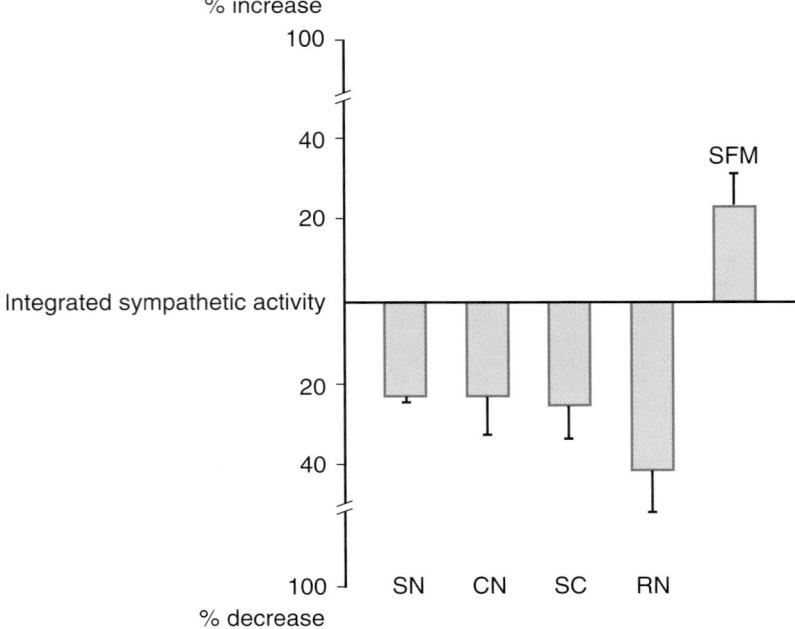

Figure 16–3. Regional differences in sympathetic tone in REM sleep. Histogram shows changes in integrated sympathetic nerve activity, expressed as a percentage of control values, during desynchronized sleeplike periods induced by physostigmine in 11 cats. CN, inferior cardiac nerve; RN, renal nerve; SC, lumbar sympathetic chain; SFM, sympathetic vasoconstrictor fibers to muscle; SN, greater splanchnic nerve. Standard error bars are shown. (Reprinted from Futuro-Neto HA, Coote JH: Changes in sympathetic activity to heart and blood vessels during desynchronized sleep. Brain Res 1982;252:259-268, with permission.)

the HF (parasympathetic) component increases, compared to wakefulness levels. During REM sleep, both the LF and the HF components return toward the wakefulness levels; overshoots and undershoots have been described, to maximal values of the LF components and to zero value of the HF components, respectively. The shift in HR precedes electroencephalographic (EEG) changes by several minutes except for sleep onset when the increase in parasympathetic activity does not anticipate sleep. The contribution of sympathetic and parasympathetic efferent activity to LF and HF power spectra, respectively, has been confirmed during sleep by experiments using selective pharmacologic blockade (propranolol, atropine).

Few studies have measured BP power spectra during sleep. In humans, the LF component decreases and the HF component increases during NREM sleep compared to wakefulness. In REM sleep, only the HF component returns toward the waking levels, whereas the LF component remains low. This contrasts with the increment of the LF components of HR variability and indicates that cardiac activity differs from vasomotor sympathetic activity during REM sleep. In the cat, the LF component was found to prevail during REM sleep. Further confirmation of the complexity of autonomic regulation during sleep comes from the work of Yang et al.[88,89]: both in rats and in humans, during NREM sleep, cardiac sympathetic regulation is negatively related to the depth of sleep, whereas vagal regulation is uncorrelated. In partial agreement, Furlan et al.[90] and Parati et al.,[91] with continuous 24-hour recordings of HR and BP in humans outside the laboratory setting, showed that by and large, power spectra related to sympathetic control decrease during the night, whereas power spectra related to parasympathetic activity increase. However, more complex circadian patterns have been described, casting doubt on reductive interpretations of power spectra changes as solely depending on autonomic control changes.[91] Moreover, ultradian changes in autonomic activity might mask the autonomic pattern related to the wake–sleep cycle.[92]

Sympathetic Nerve Activity Recordings

Multiunit recordings of sympathetic nerve vasomotor activity during sleep have been obtained in cats, rats, and humans. In renal nerves of the normal[93] and decerebrate[64] cat and of the normal rat,[94] sympathetic vasomotor activity decreases during REM sleep. In rats, this decrement parallels the decrease in HR, whereas BP increases, indicating regional differences in sympathetic outflow in REM sleep. During REM sleep in the decerebrate cat,[64] sympathetic vasomotor activity of splanchnic nerves decreases, whereas muscle nerve sympathetic vasomotor activity (MNSA) increases. In humans, MNSA decreases during NREM sleep and increases during REM sleep.[65] Cutaneous vasodilator activity is unchanged from wakefulness to NREM sleep, but it increases in REM sleep.[54]

In conclusion, these data favor differential sympathetic efferent control and do not support the idea of a global sympathetic tone during REM sleep (see Wallin and Elam[84] and Mancia[95]). Moreover, given the multiple hierarchic controls on the autonomic effector, a strict correspondence in efferent–effector activity is often lacking.[84] This is well exemplified in the control of muscle circulation during REM sleep: BF may increase, decrease, or remain unchanged in white fibers[60-62] in the face of a stereotypic increase in MNSA.

Patients with sleep apnea show a high level of MNSA during wakefulness and further increases during sleep. Therefore, in this disorder there is disruption of the sleep state–related profile of MNSA. It remains to be ascertained whether the increase in MNSA in sleep in these patients reflects an increase in overall sympathetic vasomotor tone or whether regional differences do remain.[96,97]

Finally, Tank et al.[98] attempted to relate K-complexes to MNSA and cardiovascular variables. They concluded that the increase in MNSA after the K-complex may depend on direct activation of sympathetic centers, reflecting the effect of arousal on MNSA.

CONCLUSIONS AND PATHOPHYSIOLOGIC IMPLICATIONS

An apparent contradiction emerges from the reviewed data. During REM sleep, major modifications in autonomic control entail relatively modest changes at the effector level of vascular smooth muscle. This reflects the redundancy of local and neural reflex control of peripheral circulation. However, studies investigating integrated vasomotor patterns show that when a complex adaptive adjustment is required in response to a perturbation (thermal,[51] volemic,[72] or acoustic[74]), a regulatory change is evident in REM sleep. Thus, in a pathophysiologic condition such as chronic heart failure, where the overall redistribution of peripheral BF is an indispensable adaptive mechanism, patients may face two equally risky alternatives:

1. Progression into REM sleep is hindered by the increased compensatory vasoconstriction resulting from hypoxia (see Yamashiro and Kryger[99]), thus contributing to selective sleep deprivation and the disruption of sleep architecture.[100,101]
2. Progression into REM sleep may result in pathologic cardiovascular events resulting from the loss of the adaptive pattern of peripheral vasoconstriction.[102,103]

> *Clinical Pearl*
>
> *Integrated control of peripheral vascular beds is impaired in REM sleep. Therefore, the clinician should regard REM sleep as a state of higher risk in pathophysiologic conditions when the control of peripheral resistances is an indispensable adaptive mechanism (e.g., in chronic heart failure).*

Acknowledgments

This work was supported by MIUR grants (Ministry of Education, Rome). The author thanks Professors P. Lenzi, P. L. Parmeggiani, and G. Zoccoli for their discussion of the manuscript. The graduate students V. Asti, T. Bojic, V. Ferrari, and A. Silvani helped generously with comments and references.

References

1. Parmeggiani PL: Behavioral phenomenology of sleep (somatic and vegetative). Experientia 1980;36:6-11.
2. Parmeggiani PL: Temperature regulation during sleep: A study in homeostasis. In Orem J, Barnes CD (eds): Physiology in Sleep. New York, Academic Press, 1980, pp 97-143.

3. Phillipson EA, Bowes G: Control of breathing during sleep. In Cherniack NS, Widdicombe JG (eds): The Respiratory System: Control of Breathing. Bethesda, Md, American Physiological Society, 1986, pp 649-689.

4. Franzini C, Zoccoli G, Cianci T, et al: Sleep-dependent changes in regional circulations. News Physiol Sci 1996;11:274-280.

5. Franzini C: Brain metabolism and blood flow during sleep. J Sleep Res 1992;1:3-16.

6. Maquet P: Functional neuroimaging of normal human sleep by positron emission tomography. J Sleep Res 2000;9:207-231.

7. Zoccoli G, Walker AM, Lenzi P, et al: The cerebral circulation during sleep: Regulation mechanisms and functional implications. Sleep Med Rev 2002;6:443-455.

8. Maquet P, Péters J-M, Aerts J, et al: Functional neuroanatomy of human rapid-eye-movement sleep and dreaming. Nature 1996;383:163-166.

9. Critchley HD, Corfield DR, Chandler MP, et al: Cerebral correlates of autonomic cardiovascular arousal: A functional neuroimaging investigation in humans. J Physiol 2000;523:259-270.

10. Maquet P, Degueldre C, Delfiore G, et al: Functional neuroanatomy of human slow wave sleep. J Neurosci 1997;17:2807-2812.

11. Kajimura N, Uchiyama M, Takayama Y, et al: Activity of midbrain reticular formation and neocortex during the progression of human non-rapid eye movement sleep. J Neurosci 1999;19:1065-1073.

12. Hofle N, Paus T, Reutens D, et al: Regional cerebral blood flow changes as a function of delta and spindle activity during slow wave sleep in humans. J Neurosci 1997;17:4800-4808.

13. Andersson JLR, Onoe H, Hetta J, et al: Brain networks affected by synchronized sleep visualized by Positron Emission Tomography. J Cereb Blood Flow Metab 1998;18:701-715.

14. Steriade M, Contreras D, Amzica F: Synchronized sleep oscillations and their paroxysmal developments. Trends Neurosci 1994;17:199-208.

15. Lugaresi E, Medori R, Montagna M, et al: Fatal familial insomnia and dysautonomia with selective degeneration of thalamic nuclei. N Engl J Med 1986;315:997-1003.

16. Alkire MT, Haier RJ, Fallon JH: Toward a unified theory of narcosis: Brain imaging evidence for a thalamocortical switch as the neurophysiologic basis of anesthetic-induced unconsciousness. Conscious Cogn 2000;9:370-386.

17. Fiset P, Paus T, Daloze T, et al: Brain mechanisms of propofol-induced loss of consciousness in humans: A positron emission tomographic study. J Neurosci 1999;19:5506-5513.

18. Balkin TJ, Braun AR, Wesensten NJ, et al: The process of awakening: A PET study of regional brain activity patterns mediating the re-establishment of alertness and consciousness. Brain 2002;125:2308-2319.

19. Braun AR, Balkin TJ, Wesensten NJ, et al: Regional cerebral blood flow throughout the sleep-wake cycle: An $H_2(^{15})O$ PET study. Brain 1997;120:1173-1197.

20. Bosinelli M: Mind and consciousness during sleep. Behav Brain Res 1995;69:195-201.

21. Czisch M, Wetter TC, Kaufmann C, et al: Altered processing of acoustic stimuli during sleep: reduced auditory activation and visual deactivation detected by a combined fMRI/EEG study. Neuroimage 2002;16:251-258.

22. Azzaroni A, Parmeggiani PL: Mechanisms underlying hypothalamic temperature changes during sleep in mammals. Brain Res 1993;632:136-142.

23. Parmeggiani PL, Azzaroni A, Calasso M: Systemic hemodynamic changes raising brain temperature in REM sleep. Brain Res 2002;940:55-60.

24. Lenzi P, Cianci T, Guidalotti PL, et al: Regional spinal cord blood flow during sleep-waking cycle in rabbit. Am J Physiol 1986;251:H957-H960.

25. Zoccoli G, Bach V, Nardo B, et al: Spinal cord blood flow changes during the sleep-wake cycle in rat. Neurosci Lett 1993;163:173-176.

26. Maquet P, Laureys S, Peigneux P, et al: Experience-dependent changes in cerebral activation during human REM sleep. Nat Neurosci 2000;3:831-836.

27. Grant DA, Franzini C, Wild J, et al: Continuous measurement of blood flow in the superior sagittal sinus of the lamb. Am J Physiol 1995;269:R274-R279.

28. Grant DA, Franzini C, Wild J, et al: Cerebral circulation in sleep: Vasodilatory response to cerebral hypotension. J Cereb Blood Flow Metab 1998;18:639-645.

29. Osborne PG: Hippocampal and striatal blood flow during behavior in rats: Chronic laser Doppler flowmetry study. Physiol Behav 1997;61:485-492.

30. Seno H, Sano A, Maita Y: Cerebral local blood flow with a laser-Doppler flowmetry in rat sleep. Tokushima J Exp Med 1995;42:1-4.

31. Gerashenko D, Matsumura H: Continuous recording of brain regional circulation during sleep/wake state transitions in rats. Am J Physiol 1996;270:R855-R863.

32. Droste DW, Berger W, Schler E, et al: Middle cerebral artery blood flow velocity in healthy persons during wakefulness and sleep: A transcranial Doppler study. Sleep 1993;16:603-609.

33. Hajak G, Klingelhofer J, Schulz-Varszegi M, et al: Relationship between blood flow velocities and cerebral electrical activity in sleep. Sleep 1994;17:11-19.

34. Kuboyama T, Hori A, Sato T, et al: Changes in cerebral blood flow velocity in healthy young men during overnight sleep and while awake. Electroencephalogr Clin Neurophysiol 1997;102:125-131.

35. Lenzi P, Zoccoli G, Walker AM, et al: Cerebral blood flow regulation in REM sleep: A model for flow-metabolism coupling. Arch Ital Biol 1999;137:165-179.

36. Chao CR, Hohimer AR, Bissonnette JM: The effect of electrocortical state on cerebral carbohydrate metabolism in fetal sheep. Dev Brain Res 1989;49:1-5.

37. Clapp JF, Szeto HH, Abrams R, et al: Physiological variability and fetal electrocortical activity. Am J Obstet Gynecol 1980;136:1045-1050.

38. Madsen PL: Blood flow and oxygen uptake in the human brain during various states of sleep and wakefulness. Acta Neurol Scand 1993;88(Suppl 148):1-27.

39. Boyle PJ, Scott JC, Krentz AJ, et al: Diminished brain glucose metabolism is a significant determinant for failing rates of systemic glucose utilization during sleep in normal humans. J Clin Invest 1994;93:529-535.

40. Wu JC, Gillin JC, Buchsbaum MS, et al: The effect of sleep deprivation on cerebral glucose metabolic rate in normal humans assessed with positron emission tomography. Sleep 1991;14:155-162.

41. Onoe H, Watanabe V, Tamura M, et al: REM-sleep associated hemoglobin oxygenation in the monkey forebrain studied using near-infrared spectrophotometry. Neurosci Lett 1991;129:209-213.

42. Zoccoli G, Lucchi ML, Andreoli E, et al: Brain capillary perfusion during sleep. J Cereb Blood Flow Metab 1996;16:1312-1318.

43. Zoccoli G, Grant DA, Wild J, et al: Nitric oxide inhibition abolishes sleep-wake differences in cerebral circulation. Am J Physiol 2001;280:H2598-H2606.

44. Santiago TV, Guerra E, Neubauer JA, et al: Correlation between ventilation and brain blood flow during sleep. J Clin Invest 1984;73:497-506.

45. Meadows GE, Dunroy HM, Morrell MJ, et al: Hypercapnic cerebral vascular reactivity is decreased, in humans, during sleep compared with wakefulness. J Appl Physiol 2003;94:2197-2202.

46. Hajak G, Klingelhofer J, Schulz-Varszegi M, et al: Sleep apnea syndrome and cerebral hemodynamics. Chest 1996;110:670-679.

47. Zoccoli G, Bach V, Cianci T, et al: Brain blood flow and extra-cerebral carotid circulation during sleep in rat. Brain Res 1994; 641:46-50.

48. Lenzi P, Cianci T, Guidalotti PL, et al: Brain circulation during sleep and its relation to extracerebral hemodynamics. Brain Res 1987;415:14-20.

49. Zoccoli G, Bojic T, Cianci T, et al: Blood-brain barrier permeability to glucose does not change with cerebral blood flow from wakefulness to REM sleep in unrestrained rats. J Cereb Blood Flow Metab 2003;23(Suppl 1):171.

50. Alfoldi P, Rubicsek G, Cserni G, et al: Brain and core temperatures and peripheral vasomotion during sleep and wakefulness at various ambient temperatures in the rat. Pflugers Arch 1990;417:336-341.

51. Cianci T, Zoccoli G, Lenzi P, et al: Loss of integrative control of peripheral circulation during desynchronized sleep. Am J Physiol 1991;261:R373-R377.

52. Franzini C, Lenzi P, Cianci T, et al: Neural control of vasomotion in rabbit ear is impaired during desynchronized sleep. Am J Physiol 1982;243:R142-R146.

53. Parmeggiani PL, Zamboni G, Cianci T, et al: Absence of thermoregulatory vasomotor responses during fast wave sleep in cats. Electroencephalogr Clin Neurophysiol 1977;42:372-380.

54. Noll G, Elam M, Kunimoto M, et al: Skin sympathetic nerve activity and effector function during sleep in humans. Acta Physiol Scand 1994;151:319-329.

55. Braaksma MA, Vos J, Dassel ACM, et al: Urine production rate and renal blood flow in near-term ovine fetus are not related to high and low voltage electrocortical activity. Pediatr Res 1998;43:121-125.

56. Mancia G, Baccelli G, Zanchetti A: Regulation of renal circulation during behavioral changes in the cat. Am J Physiol 1974; 227:536-542.

57. Oosterhof H, Lander M, Aanoudse JG: Behavioral states and Doppler velocimetry of the renal artery in the near term human fetus. Early Hum Dev 1993;33:183-189.

58. Cianci T, Zoccoli G, Lenzi P, et al: Regional splanchnic blood flow during sleep in the rabbit. Pflugers Arch 1990;415:594-597.

59. Mancia G, Adams DB, Baccelli G, et al: Regional blood flows during desynchronized sleep in the cat. Experientia 1969;25: 48-49.

60. Lenzi P, Cianci T, Leonardi GS, et al: Muscle blood flow changes during sleep as a function of fibre type composition. Exp Brain Res 1989;74:549-554.

61. Reis DJ, Moorhead D, Wooten GF: Differential regulation of blood flow to red and white muscle in sleep and defense behavior. Am J Physiol 1969;217:541-546.

62. Zoccoli G, Lalatta Costerbosa G, Bach V, et al: Muscle blood flow during the sleep-wake cycle in the rat. J Sleep Res 1994; 3(Suppl 1):283.

63. Baccelli G, Albertini R, Mancia G, et al: Central and reflex regulation of sympathetic vasoconstrictor activity to limb muscles during desynchronized sleep in the cat. Circ Res 1974;35: 625-635.

64. Futuro-Neto HA, Coote JH: Changes in sympathetic activity to heart and blood vessels during desynchronized sleep. Brain Res 1982;252:259-268.

65. Hornyak M, Cejnar M, Elam M, et al: Sympathetic muscle nerve activity during sleep in man. Brain 1991;114:1281-1295.

66. Kirby DA, Verrier RL: Differential effects of sleep stage on coronary hemodynamic function. Am J Physiol 1989;256: H1378-H1383.

67. Dickerson LW, Huang HA, Thurnher MM, et al: Relationship between coronary hemodynamic changes and the phasic events of REM sleep. Sleep 1993;16:550-557.

68. Dickerson LW, Huang AH, Nearing BD, et al: Primary coronary vasodilation associated with pauses in heart rhythm during sleep. Am J Physiol 1993;264:R186-R196.

69. Kirby DA, Verrier RL: Differential effects of sleep stage on coronary hemodynamic function during stenosis. Physiol Behav 1989;45:1017-1020.

70. Azzaroni A, Parmeggiani PL: Synchronized sleep duration is related to tonic vasoconstriction of thermoregulatory heat exchanges. J Sleep Res 1995;4:41-47.

71. Sei H, Morita Y: Effect of ambient temperature on arterial pressure variability during sleep in the rat. J Sleep Res 1996;5:37-41.

72. Fewell JE, Williams BJ, Hill DE: Behavioral state influences the cardiovascular response to hemorrhage in lambs. J Dev Physiol 1984;6:339-348.

73. Berger PJ, Horner RSC, Walker AM: Cardio-respiratory response to cool ambient temperature differs with sleep state in neonatal lambs. J Physiol 1989;412:351-363.

74. Silvani A, Bojic T, Cianci T, et al: Effects of acoustic stimulation on cardiovascular regulation during sleep. Sleep 2003;26:201-205.

75. Zoccoli G, Cianci T, Lenzi P, et al: Shivering during sleep: Relationship between muscle blood flow and fiber type composition. Experientia 1992;48:228-230.

76. Parmeggiani PL: Telencephalo-diencephalic aspects of sleep mechanisms. Brain Res 1968;7:350-359.

77. Parmeggiani PL, Franzini C, Lenzi P, et al: Threshold of respiratory responses to preoptic heating during sleep in free moving cats. Brain Res 1973;52:189-201.

78. Parmeggiani PL, Calasso M, Cianci T: Respiratory effects of preoptic-anterior hypothalamic electrical stimulation during sleep in cats. Sleep 1980;4:71-82.

79. Parmeggiani PL, Azzaroni A, Cevolani D, et al: Responses of anterior hypothalamic-preoptic neurons to direct thermal stimulation during wakefulness and sleep. Brain Res 1983; 269:382-385.

80. Glotzbach SF, Heller HC: Changes in the thermal characteristics of hypothalamic neurons during sleep and wakefulness. Brain Res 1984;309:17-26.

81. Parmeggiani PL, Morrison AR: Alterations in autonomic functions during sleep. In Loewy AD, Spyer KM (eds): Central Regulation of Autonomic Functions. Oxford, Oxford University Press, 1990, pp 367-386.

82. Parati G, Saul JP, Di Rienzo M, et al: Spectral analysis of blood pressure and heart rate variability in evaluating cardiovascular regulation: A critical appraisal. Hypertension 1995;25: 1276-1286.

83. Malliani A, Pagani M, Lombardi F, et al: Cardiovascular neural regulation explored in the frequency domain. Circulation 1991;84:482-492.

84. Wallin GB, Elam M: Insights from intraneural recordings of sympathetic nerve traffic in humans. News Physiol Sci 1994;9: 203-207.

85. Fletcher EC: Sympathetic activity and blood pressure in the sleep apnea syndrome. Respiration 1997;64(Suppl 1):22-28.

86. Cortelli P, Pierangeli G, Parchi G, et al: Power spectral analysis reveals sympathetic hyperactivity as an early feature of fatal familial insomnia (FFI). Neurology 1994;44(Suppl. 2):A363.

87. Lenzi P, Zoccoli G, Franzini C: Regulation of the cerebral and extracerebral circulation during the wake-sleep cycle. In Lugaresi E, Parmeggiani PL (eds): Somatic and Autonomic Regulation in Sleep: Physiological and Clinical Aspects. Milan, Springer-Verlag, 1997, pp 25-41.

88. Yang CC, Lai CW, Lai HY, et al: Relationship between electroencephalogram slow-wave magnitude and heart rate variability during sleep in humans. Neurosci Lett 2002;329:213-216.

89. Yang CC, Shaw FZ, Lai CJ, et al: Relationship between electroencephalogram slow-wave magnitude and heart rate variability during sleep in rats. Neurosci Lett 2003;336:21-24.

90. Furlan R, Guzzetti S, Crivellaro W, et al: Continuous 24-hour assessment of the neural regulation of systemic arterial pressure and RR variabilities in ambulant subjects. Circulation 1990; 81:537-547.

91. Parati G, Castiglioni P, Di Rienzo M, et al: Sequential spectral analysis of 24-hour blood pressure and pulse interval in humans. Hypertension 1990;16:414-421.

92. Ako M, Kawara T, Uchida S, et al: Correlation between electro-encephalography and heart rate variability during sleep. Psychiatry Clin Neurosci 2003;57:59-65.

93. Baust W, Weidinger H, Kirchner F: Sympathetic activity during natural sleep and arousal. Arch Ital Biol 1968;106:379-390.

94. Miki K, Kato M, Kajii S: Relationship between renal sympathetic nerve activity and arterial pressure during REM sleep in rats. Am J Physiol Regul Integr Comp Physiol 2003;284:R467-473.

95. Mancia G: Autonomic modulation of the cardiovascular system during sleep. N Engl J Med 1993;328:347-349.

96. Shimizu T, Takahashi Y, Kogawa S, et al: Muscle sympathetic nerve activity during apneic episodes in patients with obstructive sleep apnea syndrome. Electroencephalogr Clin Neurophysiol 1994;93:345-352.

97. Somers VK, Dyken ME, Clary MP, et al: Sympathetic neural mechanisms in obstructive sleep apnea. J Clin Invest 1995;96:1897-1904.

98. Tank J, Diedrich A, Hale N, et al: Relationship between blood pressure, sleep K-complexes, and muscle sympathetic nerve activity in humans. Am J Physiol 2003;285:R208-214.

99. Yamashiro H, Kryger MH: Review: Sleep in heart failure. Sleep 1993;16:513-523.

100. Hanly PJ, Millar TW, Steljes DG, et al: Respiration and abnormal sleep in patients with congestive heart failure. Chest 1989;96:480-488.

101. Schafer H, Koehler U, Ploch T, et al: Sleep-related myocardial ischemia and sleep structure in patients with obstructive sleep apnea and coronary heart disease. Chest 1997;111:387-393.

102. Cassano GB, Maggini C, Guazzelli M: Nocturnal angina and sleep. Progr Neuropsychopharmacol 1981;5:99-104.

103. Nowlin JB, Troyer WG, Collins WS, et al: The association of nocturnal angina pectoris with dreaming. Ann Intern Med 1965;63:1040-1046.

Respiratory Physiology: Central Neural Control

John Orem

Leszek Kubin

ABSTRACT

State-dependent changes in breathing are caused by nonrespiratory (tonic) inputs to the brainstem systems that control ventilation. In wakefulness, tonic excitatory inputs include those from the reticular formation, brainstem aminergic systems, and hypothalamic orexin-containing neurons. In non–rapid eye movement (NREM) sleep, decrements in these excitatory inputs can explain the features of breathing characteristic of this state. In patients with obstructive sleep apneas, these decrements facilitate upper airway obstructions because upper airway muscles fail to properly compensate for airway collapsing effects of the negative pressure generated by respiratory pump muscles. In rapid eye movement (REM) sleep, there are tonic excitatory inputs to the respiratory system that cause the irregularities and rapidity of breathing, as well as tonic and phasic inhibitory inputs that may cause periods of ineffective ventilation. The loss of excitation mediated by serotonin and norepinephrine contributes to the REM sleep–related hypotonia of motor neurons that innervate the genioglossus and possibly also other upper airway muscles.

The respiratory muscles are controlled by central neural systems that are influenced by feedback from chemical and mechanical sensors and by the sleep–waking state of the nervous system. This chapter deals with the mechanisms by which state of consciousness affects the respiratory system. We begin with non–rapid eye movement (NREM) sleep, a state in which the respiratory system seems to be in its most elemental configuration, and we then consider rapid eye movement (REM) sleep, in which there are both excitatory and inhibitory effects on the respiratory system. We will show that state-dependent effects are the result of either the presence or the absence of tonic inputs to the central respiratory controller.

RESPIRATORY ACTIVITY IN NON–RAPID EYE MOVEMENT SLEEP

Characteristics of Breathing in NREM Sleep

The frequency of breathing is lower and more regular in NREM sleep than in wakefulness.[1,2] Peak instantaneous airflow rate and the peak negative pressure developed against a narrowed airway decrease, whereas upper airway resistance increases. Tidal volume increases as the result of an increased duration of inspiration, but minute ventilation decreases and end-tidal carbon dioxide concentrations increase. Responses to carbon dioxide and low oxygen are intact (see Chapter 18). In humans, there may be periodic breathing, particularly at high altitude (see Chapter 20).[2]

Medullary Respiratory Neuronal Activity in NREM Sleep

There is a decrease in medullary respiratory neuronal activity in NREM sleep[3-6] (Fig. 17–1). The neurons affected are those in the ventral and dorsal respiratory groups. Some cells are affected more than others. Quantitative analysis shows that the effect of sleep on a respiratory neuron is proportional to the amount of nonrespiratory (tonic) activity in the activity of that cell. That is, the drive to a cell may be rhythmic (i.e., respiratory related) or it may be nonrhythmic (i.e., tonic). Respiratory cells whose activity depends primarily on tonic inputs and only weakly on respiratory-modulated inputs are affected more by sleep than respiratory cells whose activity depends primarily on rhythmic, respiratory-related inputs. Some upper airway motor neurons are in the former category of cells, and their activity decreases accordingly. In contrast, neurons whose activity is primarily determined by rhythmic, respiratory inputs do not show dramatic changes in activity in NREM sleep compared to relaxed wakefulness (Fig. 17–2). This indicates that sleep affects primarily neurons that receive large amounts of nonrespiratory inputs. Consistent with this is the finding that iontophoresis of glutamate onto silent and sleep-sensitive respiratory neurons reveals their respiratory activity pattern during sleep.[6] This indicates that respiratory-modulated inputs to these cells are not lost in sleep but become subthreshold because of a loss of state-dependent tonic excitatory inputs.

Pontine, Mesencephalic, and Telencephalic Respiratory Neuronal Activities

There are changes in the activities of pontine parabrachial respiratory-modulated neurons in NREM sleep. Increases and decreases are observed, but on average, decreases are minimal.[7-10] One study has found that respiratory activity in the pons is weak even in wakefulness and that with sleep there are few consistent changes.[11] The functional significance of these and other results showing state-related changes in the activity of respiratory cells in the amygdala, anterior cingulate gyrus, orbital frontal cortex, and mesencephalic central gray[12-14] is not known.

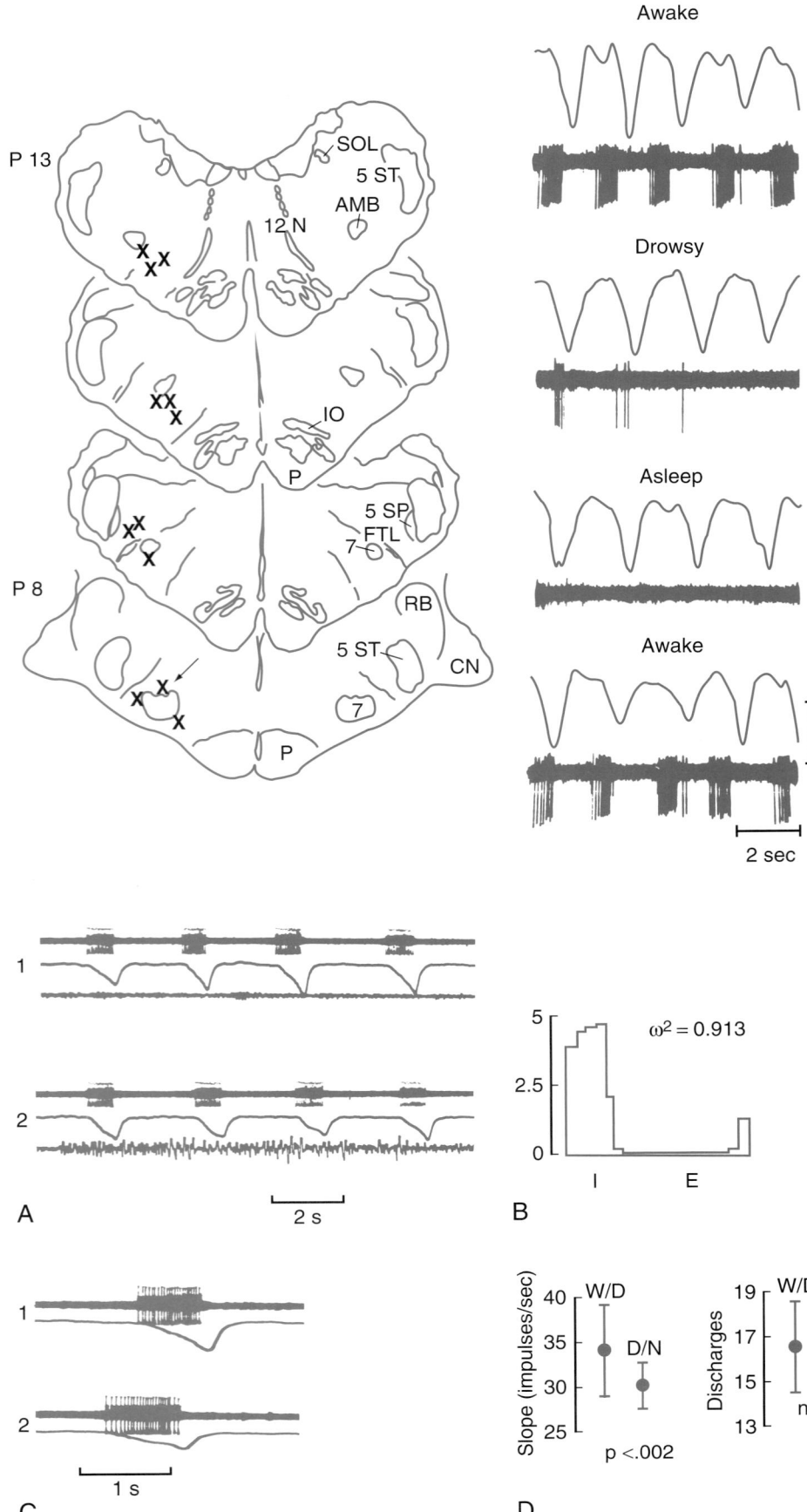

Figure 17–1. The activity of a sleep-sensitive respiratory neuron, and the locations of it and others like it. AMB, Nucleus ambiguus; CN, cochlear nucleus; FTL, lateral tegmental field; IO, inferior olive; P, pyramidal tract; RB, restiform body; SOL, solitary tract; 5 SP, nucleus of the spinal tract of V; 5 ST, spinal tract of V; 7, facial nucleus; 12 N, hypoglossal nerve. (From Orem J, Montplaisir J, Dement W: Changes in the activity of respiratory neurones during sleep. Brain Res 1974;82:309-315.)

Figure 17–2. The activity of an inspiratory cell during wakefulness and non–rapid eye movement (NREM) sleep. Action potentials and respiration (downward deflection signals inspiration) during wakefulness (**A**-1) and during NREM sleep (**A**-2). **B,** Cycle-triggered histogram of the activity. The omega-squared statistic (with a value of 0.913) expresses the high relationship of the activity to breathing. **C** and **D,** Although the numbers of discharges per breath were equivalent in wakefulness (C-1) and NREM sleep (C-2), the frequency of discharge (plotted as slope in **D**) was slightly, but significantly, lower in NREM sleep. This effect seemed related to the duration of inspiration and was observed for breaths of different durations within wakefulness, as well as between wakefulness and NREM sleep. D/N, Drowsiness/NREM sleep; E, expiration; I, inspiration; n.s., not significant; W/D, wakefulness/drowsiness. (Data from Orem J, Osorio I, Brooks E, et al: Activity of respiratory neurons during NREM sleep. J Neurophysiol 1985;54:1144-1156.)

State-Dependent Excitatory Inputs to Respiratory System That Decrease during NREM Sleep

Recordings from medullary respiratory neurons show that tonic inputs to them decrease in NREM sleep. Although all sources of these inputs are not known, the following have been implicated by various studies: (1) the brainstem reticular formation, (2) the collection of higher structures that exert behavioral control on the respiratory system, (3) the aminergic brainstem nuclei, and (4) the hypothalamic orexin-containing neurons. These systems all excite the respiratory system and may collectively constitute the wakefulness stimulus for breathing. Another major excitatory drive to breathe originates in central neurons sensitive to pH/CO_2. Although breathing remains under chemical control during NREM sleep, the contribution of some of these neurons may vary with the sleep–wake cycle.

Reticular Formation

Stimulation of the reticular formation excites the respiratory system.[15-24] Midbrain reticular stimulation causes a reduction in the duration of expiration and an increased rate of rise and amplitude of phrenic nerve activity. It also causes an increase in laryngeal abductor activity,[23] converting it from patterns characteristic of NREM sleep to those of wakefulness, and, like wakefulness, reticular stimulation preferentially facilitates the activity of the muscles of the upper airway rather than the muscles of the diaphragm.[23] Respiratory activation declines slowly after the cessation of reticular stimulation. These results imply that, during the transition from wakefulness to NREM sleep, the muscles of the upper airway may lose their tonic excitatory inputs to a greater extent than the diaphragm. This could lead to occlusive collapse of the airway during sleep. Other studies indicate that the neural systems driving upper airway motor neurons are more sensitive than those of phrenic motor neurons to the depressive effects of ethanol, diazepam, pentobarbital, halothane, hypocapnia, chemical stimuli, and thermal depression of neuronal activity near the ventral medullary surface.[25-30] Similarly, the systems controlling the upper airway muscles are more sensitive than those of the diaphragm to the excitatory effects of protriptyline, strychnine, cyanide, and doxapram.

There is a preferential activation of upper airway muscles on arousal to wakefulness in response to occlusion.[31] In cats, tracheal occlusions instituted during NREM sleep cause progressive augmentation of both laryngeal abductor and diaphragmatic activity, but increases in laryngeal activity exceed the increases in diaphragmatic activity. The greatest augmentations between one breath and the next were seen when the first occluded breath occurred in sleep and the next in wakefulness. This increase in activity at the transition from sleep to wakefulness was greater for the laryngeal abductors than for the diaphragm. Similarly, the progressive response of the genioglossus muscle to occlusion, as well as the response to hypoxia and hypercapnia, is quantitatively greater than the diaphragmatic response.[32,33] Other studies confirm the powerful effect of arousal on upper airway dilating activity and demonstrate that airway-dilating responses to occlusions and negative pressure during sleep are weak compared to those in wakefulness. It has been suggested that the weaker response in sleep may contribute to pharyngeal collapse in patients with obstructive sleep apnea.[34,35] According to this idea, occlusion is the result of failed compensation in sleep. The idea is supported by demonstrations of greater genioglossal muscle activity (compensatory activity) in wakefulness in patients with obstructive sleep apnea than in normal subjects.[35]

Behavioral Control

Behavioral control of breathing may be reflexive, as occurs in sneezing, coughing, vomiting, and eructation, or voluntary, as during speaking, breath holding, and playing a wind instrument. These behavioral acts require the integration of nonrespiratory inputs into circuits of the respiratory oscillator. Behavioral respiratory acts generally occur only in wakefulness. For example, mechanical and chemical stimulation of the larynx[36] and bronchopulmonary stimulation[37] cause coughing in wakefulness but not in sleep.[38] It is not known why these responses can occur in wakefulness but not sleep, but it may be that the readiness of behavioral control in wakefulness constitutes a stimulus for the respiratory system. The potential for behavioral controllers to affect breathing directly is clear in REM sleep, when they may act in association with dreams (see "Increased Respiratory Neuronal Activity in REM Sleep: Endogenous Excitatory Drives," later). In contrast, in NREM sleep, effects on breathing may be the result of the *absence* of behavioral control. This may be relevant to obstructive sleep apnea if what is lost in sleep is a wakefulness-dependent behavioral compensation for a high upper airway resistance.

The list of structures that can contribute to behavioral control of brainstem and spinal respiratory neurons includes structures from all levels of the neuraxis. The controls exerted by telencephalic structures, amygdala, and the central gray may occur in relation to emotional and volitional acts.[39-41] Many of these higher structures, such as the central nucleus of the amygdala, the anterior cingulate gyrus, the orbital frontal cortex, and the central gray, contain cells that have state-dependent respiratory activity.[12-14] Stimulation or inactivation of limbic,[13,14] subcortical,[42] and cerebellar[43] structures can influence the respiratory system. The site of behavioral control within the respiratory neuraxis varies depending on the behavioral act. It may be exerted directly on respiratory motor neurons, thus bypassing the central respiratory generator, or on medullary premotor and higher-order central respiratory neurons.

Aminergic Systems

Serotonin (5-hydroxytryptamine [5-HT])-containing and norepinephrine-containing neurons of the brainstem are an important source of sleep-related changes in breathing. Their activity decreases during sleep and they have extensive axonal projections to respiratory regions. Both central respiratory neurons and respiratory motor neurons have receptors for 5-HT and norepinephrine.

The activity of the neurons belonging to these two aminergic systems is highest during active wakefulness, declines during NREM sleep, and is minimal or absent during REM sleep.[44-46] Serotonin has excitatory effects on motor neurons, including those innervating the upper airway and respiratory pump muscles.[47-51] Antagonists of the excitatory effects of 5-HT reduce the spontaneous activity of XII motor neurons, thus showing the presence of an endogenous serotonergic excitatory drive.[52,53] Data from pharmacologic models of REM sleep (see "The Atonia of REM Sleep and the Carbachol Models," later) reveal that the suppression of XII motor neuron activity produced during the carbachol-induced REM sleep-like state is associated with silencing of medullary serotonergic cells and decrements in extracellular levels of 5-HT in the XII nucleus region[54,55] (Fig. 17–3). Likewise, norepinephrine levels are reduced in the XII motor nucleus region during the motor atonia elicited by electrical stimulation of the pontine REM sleep–triggering region.[56]

Like 5-HT, norepinephrine is predominantly excitatory to motor neurons, whereas its effect on medullary respiratory neurons is inhibitory.[51,57-60] The excitatory effects of 5-HT and norepinephrine on respiratory motor neurons may represent an important neurochemical substrate of the wakefulness stimulus. The magnitude of the excitatory effect of 5-HT on different groups of upper airway motor neurons varies,[61] and the same is likely to be the case for norepinephrine. These differences may contribute to major differences in the magnitude of the suppressant effect of sleep among different upper airway muscles.[62,63]

The activity of locus coeruleus neurons, which are often regarded as typical of norepinephrine-containing brainstem neurons, is more variable than that of the serotonergic neurons, with phasic bursts occurring in response to various peripheral stimuli, especially those perceived as novel or stressful.[64] Thus, in addition to its tonic effects related to the sleep-related decrements in noradrenergic cell activity, norepinephrine may have phasic effects on breathing during wakefulness, especially during states with emotional or sensory activation.

Hypothalamic Orexin-Containing Neurons

The hypothalamus exerts control over the respiratory system in relation to temperature regulation, metabolism, and motor activation. These original findings were recently refined by the discovery of a unique of group of hypothalamic neurons containing excitatory peptides, orexins (also known as hypocretins).[65] These cells, located exclusively in the perifornical region of the posterior hypothalamus, have widespread axonal projections that target all known wakefulness-related neuronal groups (serotonergic, noradrenergic, histaminergic, and cholinergic), as well as motor neurons and sympathetic preganglionic neurons.[66-71] The activity of orexin neurons and orexin release are maximal during wakefulness, especially in relation to motor activation.[72-75] Thus, orexins have the potential to enhance the respiratory output in a manner consistent with the concept of the wakefulness stimulus for breathing by their direct actions on motor neurons and indirectly by stimulation of the activity of brainstem aminergic neurons.

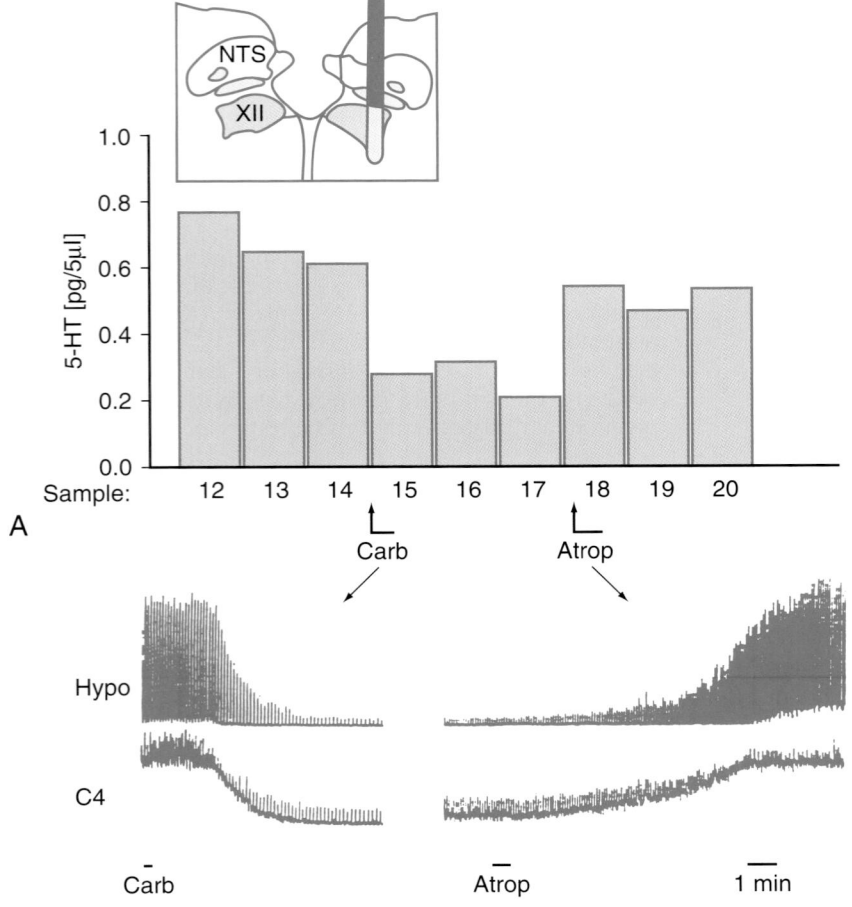

A

B

Figure 17–3. Extracellular level of 5-hydroxytryptamine (5-HT) is reduced in the region of the hypoglossal (XII) motor nucleus during the rapid eye movement (REM) sleep–like atonia produced by pontine injection of carbachol. **A,** 5-HT level in microdialysis samples collected in successive 20-minute intervals from the XII nucleus in a decerebrate, paralyzed, and artificially ventilated cat. At the end of collection of sample 14, carbachol was injected into the pons and produced a suppression of (fictive) postural and respiratory activity. One hour and three samples later, pontine microinjection of atropine was made to terminate the atonia. The level of 5-HT decreased in association with the onset of the atonia and then increased when the atonia was terminated. The *inset* shows the location of the dialysis probe in this experiment. NTS, Nucleus tractus solitarius; XII, hypoglossal motor nucleus. **B,** Moving averages of the activities recorded from the XII nerve (Hypo) and a cervical nerve branch innervating dorsal neck muscles (C4) at the times of transition into and out of the carbachol-induced atonia. The *bars* attached to the marker *arrows* in **A** indicate the position of the records in **B** relative to the changes in 5-HT level shown in **A**. (Modified from Kubin L, Reignier C, Tojima H, et al: Changes in serotonin level in the hypoglossal nucleus region during the carbachol-induced atonia. Brain Res 1994;645:291-302, with permission.)

Central pH/CO₂–Sensitive Sites

The level of O_2, CO_2, and acidity of the cerebrospinal fluid and blood are the major determinants of the drive to breathe. The chemical control of breathing is maintained during sleep.[76-78] However, end-tidal CO_2 increases in NREM sleep, and, in REM sleep, as in wakefulness, there are periods during which respiratory effort varies independently of the chemical drive.

The ventral medullary surface has three chemosensitive zones. The use of topical anesthetic agents or cold blockade of these zones eliminates respiratory responses to changes in the pH of the cerebrospinal fluid and reduces respiratory effort, but other regions of the medullary reticular formation also contain cells sensitive to extracellular pH and CO_2.[79,80] In vitro studies reveal that cells located near the ventral medullary surface, cells in the nucleus of the solitary tract, and serotonergic and noradrenergic brainstem neurons have pH/CO_2 sensitivity.[81-84] Also, ventral medullary cells, which may be involved in the generation of respiratory rhythm in the in vitro neonatal rat brainstem, are excited by a decrease in pH.[85] The connectivity with central respiratory neurons and excitability changes with the sleep–wake cycle, if any, remain to be determined for most known putative central chemosensors. Although the activity of aminergic cells is reduced during sleep, it is not known whether selective silencing of these neurons attenuates central respiratory chemosensitivity.

RESPIRATORY ACTIVITY IN RAPID EYE MOVEMENT SLEEP

Characteristics of Breathing in REM Sleep

In REM sleep, the frequency of breathing increases, tidal volumes decrease, and minute ventilation decreases.[1,2] In the cat, end-tidal CO_2 decreases, signifying hyperventilation, which is associated with a decrease in the rate of metabolism. In humans, however, metabolic rate increases in REM sleep, presumably because of a large increase in cerebral metabolism. The average peak inspiratory airflow rates are about 15% less than in NREM sleep or wakefulness. Ventilatory responses to chemical stimuli and other respiratory reflexes are impaired during phasic REM activity,[2] and laryngeal and diaphragmatic responses to occlusions are inconsistent and variable.[31] In cats[86] and adolescent humans,[87] but not in rats,[88] atonia of the intercostal muscles reduces or eliminates costal breathing in REM sleep. Many upper airway respiratory muscles are also atonic or hypotonic.[23,62] There is a decrease in postinspiratory diaphragmatic activity in REM sleep.[89] Both central apneas and hyperpneas occur as the extremes of very irregular breathing in REM sleep. The variable breathing pattern of REM sleep does not depend on variations in chemoreceptor,[90] vagal,[91-93] or thoracic[93,94] afferent activity.

Obstructive episodes are the longest, and blood oxygen desaturations most severe, during REM sleep in patients with obstructive sleep apnea. Similarly, oxygen desaturations are generally most severe during REM sleep in patients with lung disease.

Increased Respiratory Neuronal Activity in REM Sleep: Endogenous Excitatory Drives

Many results support the existence of excitatory drives to the respiratory system in REM sleep and indicate that these drives are of central origin. The first description of REM sleep noted the rapid breathing in that state, which has been confirmed many times since then.[1,2] In addition, with few exceptions, cells throughout the nervous system are more active in REM sleep than in NREM sleep. This generalized activation in REM sleep also includes parts of the respiratory system. Medullary respiratory neurons activated in REM sleep include augmenting and late inspiratory cells[95] (Fig. 17–4) and some

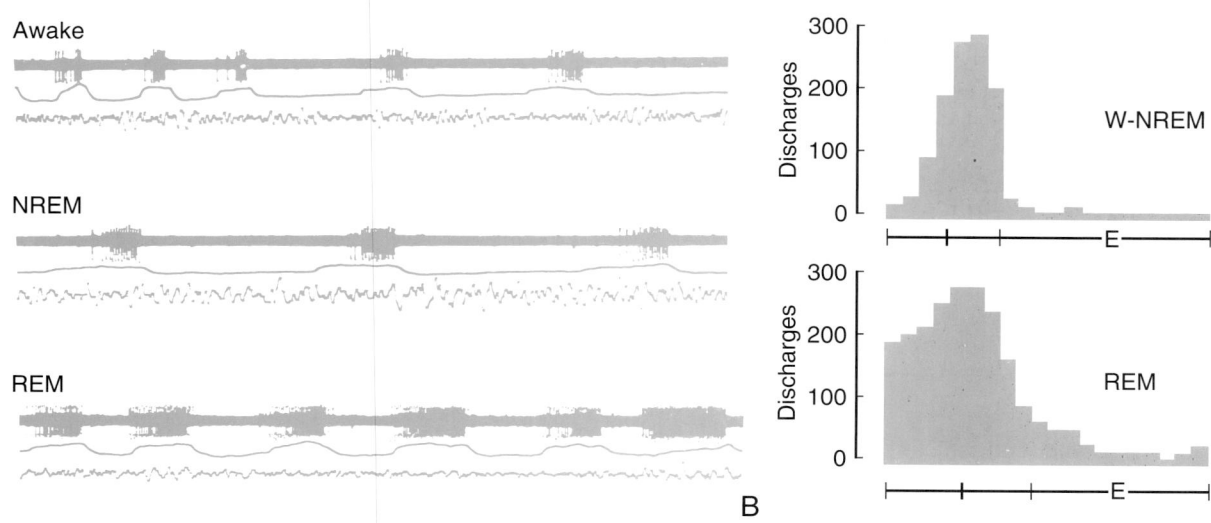

Figure 17–4. Increased and advanced activity of a late inspiratory neuron in rapid eye movement (REM) sleep. **A,** The cell discharges during the last part of inspiration in wakefulness and non–rapid eye movement (NREM) sleep but is active throughout inspiration during REM sleep. Traces from top to bottom for each section are the action potentials, intratracheal pressure (inspiration is signaled by an upward deflection), and the electroencephalogram. **B,** Cycle-triggered histograms constructed from 50 breaths in wakefulness/NREM sleep (W-NREM) and REM sleep. E, expiration. (Modified from Orem J: The activity of late respiratory cells during the behavioral inhibition of inspiration. Brain Res 1988;458:224-230.)

augmenting expiratory cells, which are active even during the very short expirations that occur during periods of irregular and rapid breathing.[96] Like medullary respiratory neurons, many, but not all, pontine parabrachial respiratory neurons show prominent increases in activity during REM sleep.[8] Similar changes occur in non–respiratory-modulated cells in this region.[8,10]

The excitation of respiratory neurons in REM sleep is apparently the result of endogenous processes. Excitation of respiratory neurons and respiratory pump muscles occurs during REM sleep even when mechanical variables (e.g., airway resistance, chest wall compliance) are removed or held constant by mechanical ventilation[97] (Fig. 17–5). This indicates that the excitatory drive has an internal source—an idea supported also by reported positive relationships between activity of some respiratory neurons and phasic REM sleep activity[98] and between the rate of breathing in REM sleep and the activity of REM sleep–specific neurons.[99] Little is known about the characteristics or sources of this endogenous excitatory drive. During apnea caused by mechanical hyperventilation, the drive is seen as the emergence of activity in respiratory muscles and neurons out of the background apnea (see Fig. 17–5). It has been suggested that the drive may account for the rapid and irregular breathing in this state.[97] The function of the drive is not known, but it may be that it produces the first respiratory movements in utero.

There has been the long-standing idea that the endogenous drive during REM sleep is related to behavioral mechanisms that are activated during the dream. Evidence of this comes from studies in which the dreamer is aroused and the pattern of breathing is related to the reported content of the dream. Just as eye movements have been related to a recalled dream involving visual scanning, the pattern of breathing might be appropriate to the content of the dream. One study found that the probability of a dream report and the vividness, emotional content, and amount of physical activity in the dream were higher when breathing rates were high and variable. They found also that specific respiratory content was twice as likely when the subject was awakened following apnea as compared to following other respiratory patterns.[100] Other authors found that highly variable rates of breathing were associated with reports of the sleeper having little active participation in the dream and of there being little physical aggression in it. However, large-amplitude breaths were associated with the sleeper having intense active participation in the dream, and variability in amplitude was associated with dreams containing a high degree of physical aggression.[101] These results support the idea that breathing patterns may parallel the content of the dream.

Other literature is less convincing. Hauri and Van de Castle[102] examined heart rate, the galvanic skin response, and breathing in relation to dream emotionality, physical activity in the dream, and dream intensity. Respiration rate was related to emotionality and to dream intensity, but these authors found that there was no significant relationship between physical activity in the dream and the rate of breathing.

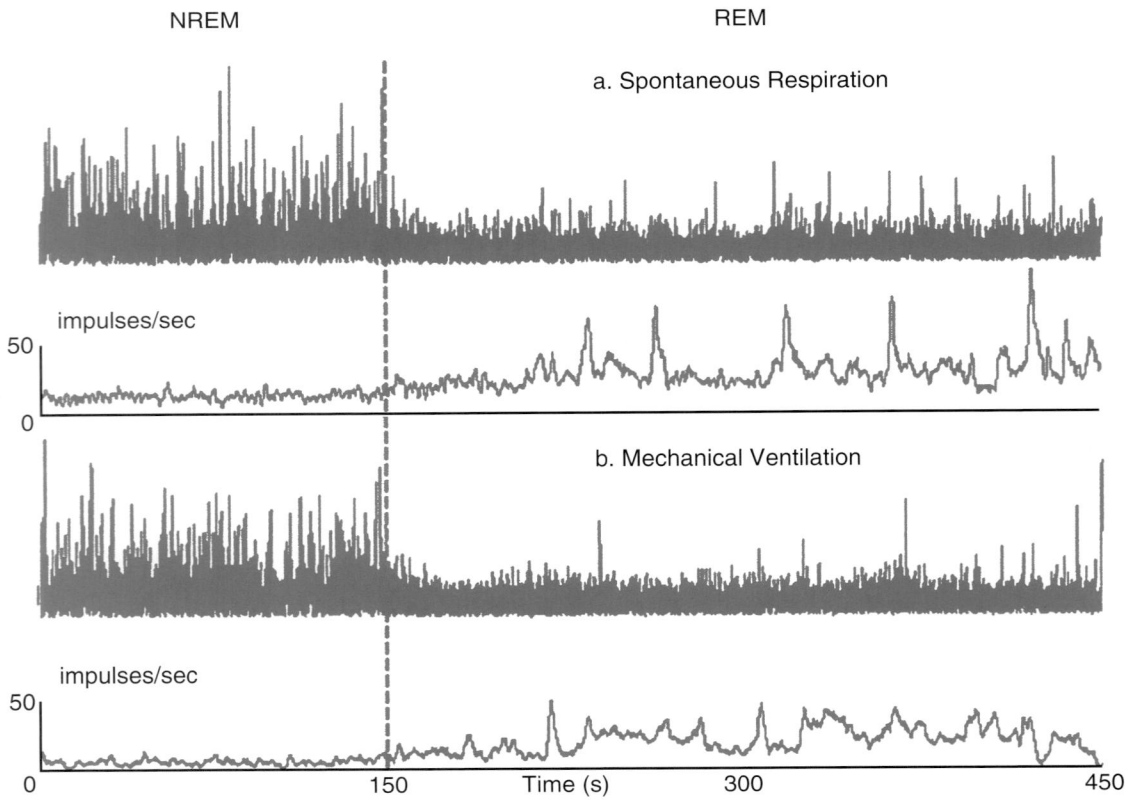

Figure 17–5. Half-wave rectified electroencephalograms and instantaneous discharge rate of an inspiratory neuron in non–rapid eye movement (NREM) and rapid eye movement (REM) sleep during spontaneous respiration (a) and during mechanical ventilation (b). The figure shows that in REM sleep, this neuron is driven by endogenous tonic inputs that account for much of the activity of the neuron during spontaneous breathing.

Others have argued that the irregular pattern of breathing in REM sleep is a byproduct of endogenous REM-sleep processes and does not have its origin in the content of the dream. According to this theory, there are REM-sleep processes that depend on the pons and that affect the entire nervous system. In support of this idea, discharge rates of medullary respiratory neurons in REM sleep are related positively to the frequency of ponto-geniculo-occipital (PGO) waves,[98] and the discharge rates of REM-specific cells are positively correlated with the rate of breathing.[99] Furthermore, brief inhibitions of diaphragmatic activity (lasting in the order of 80 msec) are associated with PGO waves.[103] These results support the idea that REM-specific processes affect central respiratory drive, but they do not refute the idea that they cause also the dream that then affects the respiratory system.

The endogenous drive may be clinically important. At times, it may be so intense that it causes a breathing pattern that can be characterized as respiratory fibrillation. Patients with lung disease desaturate in REM sleep and, in particular, during periods with intense rapid eye movements.

The Atonia of REM Sleep and the Carbachol Models

Intercostal and some accessory respiratory muscles innervated by spinal and cranial motor neurons are atonic or hypotonic in REM sleep. Patients with narrow and collapsible upper airways may experience upper airway obstructions, and those with lung disease may become hypoxemic because of the atonia. The loss of intercostal and accessory (scaleni and sternocleidomastoid) muscle activity may lead to severe oxygen desaturation in a patient whose diaphragm is compromised or ineffective. State-specific inhibitory actions and disfacilitation (i.e., withdrawal of excitatory inputs) contribute to the atonia. We review here the latter mechanism and the work in the carbachol models that led to its understanding.

Microinjections of agonists that stimulate muscarinic cholinergic receptors (e.g., carbachol, bethanechol) into the dorsal pontine reticular formation are used in experimental animals to induce a REM sleep–like state (see George et al.,[104] Baghdoyan et al.,[105] and Vanni-Mercier et al.[106]). Individual phenomena of REM sleep, such as postural atonia, hippocampal theta rhythm, and PGO waves, can be elicited this way from wide areas of the pons and midbrain,[106-110] but the site at which carbachol produces a state that best corresponds to natural REM sleep is discrete and localized in the dorsomedial pontine tegmentum.[106,110-113] Increases in acetylcholine release occur during natural REM sleep in this region.[114]

The ability to trigger a REM sleep–like state by pontine injections of muscarinic cholinergic receptor agonists has been used to study the mechanisms of respiratory changes characteristic of REM sleep in chronically instrumented cats,[9,10,115,116] decerebrate cats,[117-119] decerebrate rats,[109] and urethane-anesthetized rats.[110,113,120] Following pontine carbachol injections, medullary serotonergic cells are silenced[55] as they are in natural REM sleep, and so are noradrenergic neurons of the locus coeruleus and the A5 group,[113,121] the latter being particularly important for cardiorespiratory regulation (Fig. 17–6). Also as in REM sleep, pharyngeal motor neurons are profoundly suppressed, whereas phrenic and laryngeal motor neurons are relatively unaffected,[117-119] and the activity of medullary inspiratory neurons is minimally suppressed or even increased.[120,122] One notable difference is that the respiratory rate is reduced and regular in carbachol models, whereas it may be greatly accelerated during natural REM sleep.

To explain the absence of irregularities in the respiratory rate, Kimura et al.[117] proposed that they may be caused, at least in part, by rapidly changing levels of endogenous acetylcholine that are likely to occur during natural REM sleep but cannot be adequately mimicked by pontine carbachol microinjections. This, however, does not explain the large respiratory rate accelerations observed at times during natural REM sleep. Such respiratory rate increases must be mediated by pathways and mechanisms other than those activated by carbachol injections into the dorsal pontine tegmentum, whereas cholinergic stimulation within the dorsal pontine

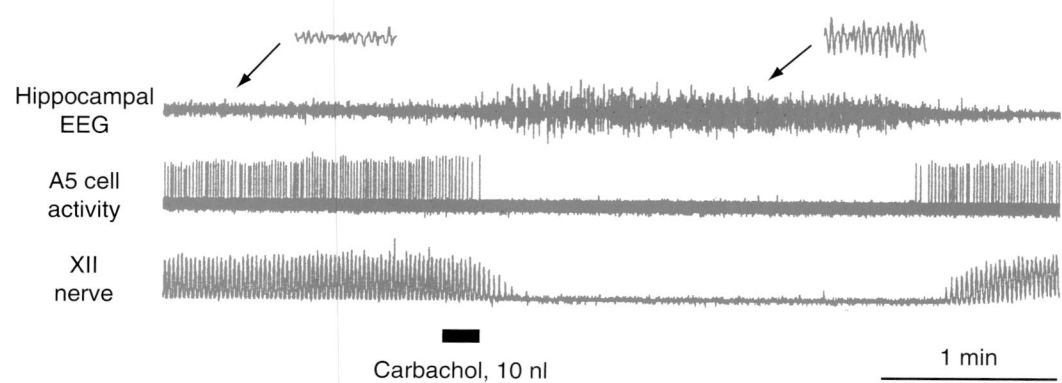

Figure 17–6. Noradrenergic cells of the pontine A5 group are silenced during the rapid eye movement (REM) sleep–like episodes elicited by pontine microinjections of carbachol in urethane-anesthetized, paralyzed and artificially ventilated rats. Silencing of these cells, which play an important role in cardiorespiratory regulation, shows that a withdrawal of noradrenergic influences may contribute to respiratory changes characteristic of REM sleep. The REM sleep–like episode is marked by a simultaneous appearance of the hippocampal theta rhythm (*top trace*, with 5-second *insets* showing portions of the trace at an expanded time scale) and a profound suppression of hypoglossal nerve activity (*bottom trace*, showing the moving average of the signal). The cell stops firing and then resumes activity just prior to the reappearance of hypoglossal nerve activity. (From Fenik V, Marchenko V, Janssen P, et al: A5 cells are silenced when REM sleep-like signs are elicited by pontine carbachol. J Appl Physiol 2002;93:1448-1456.)

reticular formation appears to activate those pathways that act to reduce the respiratory rate.

Carbachol models helped elucidate the mechanisms of REM sleep–related upper airway hypotonia. In the decerebrate cat model, the atonia of XII motor neurons is not caused by inhibitory amino acids such as glycine or gamma-aminobutyric acid (GABA).[123] Instead, a loss of serotonergic excitatory influences that impinge on motor neurons makes a major, albeit only partial, contribution to the observed decrements in their activity.[54,55,124] Thus, although inhibitory synaptic events occur in XII motor neurons in carbachol models of REM sleep,[125] their contribution to the suppression of motor activity appears to be small.

A major role of the withdrawal of aminergic excitation in the suppression of XII motoneuronal activity during REM sleep is further supported by studies in the urethane-anesthetized rat carbachol model. In this model, a combined antagonism of noradrenergic, serotonergic, GABAergic, and glycinergic receptors located in the XII nucleus region (by prazosin, methysergide, bicuculline, and strychnine, respectively) reversibly abolished the carbachol-induced, REM sleep–like decrements of XII motoneuronal activity.[126] It was then determined that neither the GABA$_A$ receptor antagonist, bicuculline, nor the glycinergic receptor antagonist, strychnine, was required to achieve this effect, whereas the combined antagonism of serotonergic and noradrenergic receptors was both necessary and sufficient to abolish the REM sleep–like depression of XII nerve activity.[127] These results suggest that the suppression of XII motoneuronal activity during REM sleep is primarily caused by a simultaneous withdrawal of serotonergic and noradrenergic excitation.

The results from the carbachol models are supported by recordings from upper airway muscles innervated by XII motor neurons in chronically instrumented, behaving animals. For example, antagonism of serotonergic excitatory effects during wakefulness reduced the activity of geniohyoid and sternohyoid muscles in the English bulldog, which is a natural model of obstructive sleep apnea,[53] and perfusion of the XII nucleus with 5-HT attenuated the suppression of genioglossal muscle activity during sleep in rats.[128] The applicability of these findings to the behavior of other upper airway motor neurons during natural REM sleep remains to be determined.

Animal studies have suggested that obstructive sleep apnea could be alleviated by increasing aminergic excitation of upper airway motor neurons during sleep. However, most clinical trials based on this hypothesis yielded weak results or proved ineffective. One reason for such an unsatisfactory outcome may be that most trials have not been designed to target appropriate combinations of aminergic receptors. The main receptors mediating the excitatory effects of 5-HT and norepinephrine in upper airway motor neurons have now been identified as type 5-HT$_{2A}$ and alpha$_{1B}$-adrenergic receptors, respectively.[129-132] Interestingly, in one study in the English bulldog, the results of a systemic treatment that had a partial preference towards 5-HT$_2$ receptors were more promising than in other trials.[133]

Nevertheless, the prospects for pharmacotherapy for obstructive sleep apnea are complicated by the fact that the same excitatory aminergic receptors that mediate wakefulness-related excitatory effects in upper airway motor neurons are also present in many other brain regions and subserve many other functions, including sleep. Thus, targeting selected combinations of receptors may be insufficient, and a successful therapeutic intervention may require new methods of selective drug delivery to the desired sites of their action.

Clinical Pearl

There is a wakefulness stimulus for breathing that, when lost in NREM sleep, allows occlusive collapse of the extrathoracic airway in patients with obstructive sleep apnea. This stimulus may involve multiple systems within the brain, including those that are serotonergic and noradrenergic. In REM sleep, there are both excitatory and suppressant influences on the respiratory system. Excitatory influences may cause rapid, irregular breathing and hypoventilation that, in patients with lung disease, leads to oxygen desaturation. Suppressant influences cause atonia of intercostal and accessory respiratory muscles, which in patients with lung disease or compromised upper airways can lead to hypoxemia and upper airway obstructions. In the carbachol model of REM sleep, suppression of the activity of hypoglossal motor neurons results primarily from the withdrawal of excitation mediated by serotonin and norepinephrine.

Acknowledgments

This work was made possible by grants HL21257, HL62589, and NS46062 (to J.O.) and grants HL47600, HL42236, and HL60287 (to L.K.) from the National Heart, Lung, and Blood Institute of the National Institutes of Health.

REFERENCES

1. Orem JA, Netick A, Dement WC: Breathing during sleep and wakefulness in the cat. Respir Physiol 1977;30:265-289.
2. Phillipson EA: Control of breathing during sleep. Am Rev Respir Dis 1978;118:909-939.
3. Orem J, Montplaisir J, Dement W: Changes in the activity of respiratory neurones during sleep. Brain Res 1974;82:309-315.
4. Orem J, Osorio I, Brooks E, et al: Activity of respiratory neurons during NREM sleep. J Neurophysiol 1985;54:1144-1156.
5. Puizillout JJ, Ternaux JP: Variations d'activités toniques, phasiques et respiratoires au niveau bulbaire pendant l'endormement de la préparation encéphale isolé. Brain Res 1974;66:67-83.
6. Foutz AS, Boudinot E, Morin-Surin M-P, et al: Excitability of "silent" respiratory neurons during sleep-waking states: An iontophoretic study in undrugged chronic cats. Brain Res 1987;171:135-141.
7. Lydic R, Orem J: Respiratory neurons of the pneumotaxic center during sleep and wakefulness. Neurosci Lett 1979;15:187-192.
8. Sieck GE, Harper RM: Pneumotaxic area neuronal discharge during sleep-waking states in the cat. Exp Neurol 1980;67:79-102.
9. Gilbert KA, Lydic R: Parabrachial neuron discharge in the cat is altered during the carbachol-induced REM sleep-like state (DCarb). Neurosci Lett 1990;120:241-244.
10. Gilbert KA, Lydic R: Pontine cholinergic reticular mechanisms cause state-dependent changes in the discharge of parabrachial neurons. Am J Physiol 1994;266:R136-R150.
11. Dick TE, Orem JM: Pontine respiratory neurons in unanesthetized cats. Soc Neurosci Abstr 1997;23:725.
12. Frysinger RC, Harper RM: Cardiac and respiratory relationships with neural discharge in the anterior cingulate cortex during sleep-waking states. Exp Neurol 1986;94:247-263.

13. Frysinger RC, Zhang J, Harper RM: Cardiovascular and respiratory relationships with neuronal discharge in the central nucleus of the amygdala during sleep-waking states. Sleep 1988;11:317-322.

14. Zhang J, Harper RM, Frysinger RC: Respiratory modulation of neuronal discharge in the central nucleus of the amygdala during sleep and waking states. Exp Neurol 1986;91:193-207.

15. Martin HN: The normal respiratory movements of the frog, and the influence upon its respiratory centre of stimulation of the optic lobes. J Physiol 1878;1:131-170.

16. Martin HN, Booker WD: The influence of stimulation of the midbrain upon the respiratory rhythm of the mammal. J Physiol 1878;1:370-376.

17. Ranson SW, Kabat H, Magoun HW: Autonomic responses to electrical stimulation of hypothalamus, preoptic region and septum. Arch Neurol Psych 1935;33:467-477.

18. Kabat H: Electrical stimulation of points in the forebrain and midbrain: The resultant alterations in respiration. J Comp Neurol 1936;64:187-208.

19. Baxter DW, Olszewski J: Respiratory responses evoked by electrical stimulation of pons and mesencephalon. J Neurophysiol 1955;18:276-287.

20. Hugelin A, Cohen MI; The reticular activating system and respiratory regulation in the cat. Ann N Y Acad Sci 1963;109:586-603.

21. Cohen MI, Hugelin A: Suprapontine reticular control of intrinsic respiratory mechanisms. Arch Ital Biol 1965;103:317-334.

22. Trouth CO, Loeschke HH, Berndt J: Topography of the respiratory responses to electrical stimulation of the medulla oblongata. Pflügers Arch 1973;339:153-170.

23. Orem J, Lydic R: Upper airway function during sleep and wakefulness: Experimental studies on normal and anesthetized cats. Sleep 1978;1:49-68.

24. Orem J, Lydic R, Norris P: Experimental control of the diaphragm and laryngeal abductor muscles by brain stem arousal systems. Respir Physiol 1979;38:203-221.

25. Bonora M, Shields GI, Knuth SL, et al: Selective depression by ethanol of upper airway respiratory motor activity in cats. Am Rev Respir Dis 1984;130:156-161.

26. Bonora M, St John WM, Bledsoe TA: Differential elevation by protriptyline and depression by diazepam of upper airway respiratory motor activity. Am Rev Respir Dis 1985;131:41-45.

27. Haxhiu MA, Mitra J, van Lunteren E, et al. Responses of hypoglossal and phrenic nerves to decreased respiratory drive in cats. Respiration 1986;50:130-138.

28. St John WM, Bledsoe TA: Comparison of respiratory-related trigeminal, hypoglossal and phrenic activities. Respir Physiol 1985;62:61-78.

29. St John WM: Influence of reticular mechanisms upon hypoglossal, trigeminal and phrenic activities. Respir Physiol 1986;66:27-40.

30. St John WM, Bartlett DJ, Knuth KV, et al: Differential depression of hypoglossal nerve activity by alcohol: Protection by pretreatment with medroxyprogesterone acetate. Am Rev Respir Dis 1986;133:46-48.

31. Orem J, Dick T, Norris P: Laryngeal and diaphragmatic responses to airway occlusion in sleep and wakefulness. Electroencephalogr Clin Neurophysiol 1980;50:151-164.

32. Brouillette RT, Thach BT: A neuromuscular mechanism maintaining extrathoracic airway patency. J Appl Physiol 1979;46:772-79.

33. Brouillette RT, Thach BT: Effects of chemoreceptors and pulmonary mechanoreceptors on the respiratory activity of the genioglossus muscle. Fed Proc 1979;38:1142.

34. Wheatley JR, Mezzanotte WS, Tangel DJ, White DP: Influence of sleep on genioglossus muscle activation by negative pressure in normal men. Am Rev Respir Dis 1993;148:597-605.

35. Mezzanotte WS, Tangel DJ, White DP: Waking genioglossal electromyogram in sleep apnea patients versus normal controls (a neuromuscular compensatory mechanism). J Clin Invest 1992;89:1571-1579.

36. Sullivan CE, Kozar LE, Murphy E, et al: Arousal, ventilatory, and airway responses to bronchopulmonary stimulation in sleeping dogs. J Appl Physiol 1978;45:681-689.

37. Sullivan CE, Zamel N, Kozar LE, et al: Regulation of airway smooth muscle tone in sleeping dogs. Am Rev Respir Dis 1979; 119:87-99.

38. Anderson CA, Dick TE, Orem J: Respiratory responses to tracheobronchial stimulation during sleep and wakefulness in the adult cat. Sleep 1996;19:472-478.

39. Plum F, Leigh RJ: Abnormalities of central mechanisms. In Hornbein TF (ed): Regulation of Breathing: Part 2. New York, Marcel Dekker, 1981, pp 989-1067.

40. Eldridge FL, Millhorn DE, Waldrop TG: Exercise hyperpnea and locomotion: Parallel activation from the hypothalamus. Science 1981;211:844-846.

41. Reis DJ, McHugh PR: Hypoxia as a cause of bradycardia during amygdala stimulation in monkey. J Appl Physiol 1968;214:601-610.

42. Bassal M, Bianchi AL: Effets de la stimulation des structures nerveuses centrales sur les activites respiratoires efferentes chez le chat: II. Responses a la stimulation sous corticale. J Physiol (Paris) 1981;77:754-777.

43. Lutherer LO, Williams JL: Stimulating fastigial nucleus pressor region elicits patterned respiratory responses. Am J Physiol 1986;250:R418-R426.

44. Trulson ME, Trulson VM: Activity of nucleus raphe pallidus neurons across the sleep-waking cycle in freely moving cats. Brain Res 1982;237:232-237.

45. Heym J, Steinfels GF, Jacobs BL: Activity of serotonin-containing neurons in the nucleus raphe pallidus of freely moving cats. Brain Res 1982;251:259-276.

46. Aston-Jones G, Bloom FE. Activity of norepinephrine-containing locus coeruleus neurons in behaving rats anticipates fluctuations in the sleep-waking cycle. J Neurosci 1981;1:876-886.

47. Schmid K, Böhmer G, Merkelbach S: Serotonergic control of phrenic motoneuronal activity at the level of the spinal cord of the rabbit. Neurosci Lett 1990;116:204-209.

48. Arita H, Ochiishi M: Opposing effects of 5-hydroxytryptamine on two types of medullary inspiratory neurons with distinct firing patterns. J Neurophysiol 1991;66:285-292.

49. Rasmussen K, Aghajanian GK: Serotonin excitation of facial motoneurons: receptor subtype characterization. Synapse 1990;5324-5332.

50. Ribeiro-do-Valle LE, Metzler CW, Jacobs BL: Facilitation of masseter EMG and masseteric (jaw-closure) reflex by serotonin in behaving cats. Brain Res 1991;550:197-204.

51. Al-Zubaidy ZA, Erickson RL, Greer JJ: Serotonergic and noradrenergic effects on respiratory neural discharge in the medullary slice preparation of neonatal rats. Pflugers Arch 1996;431:942-949.

52. Kubin L, Tojima H, Davies RO, et al: Serotonergic excitatory drive to hypoglossal motoneurons in the decerebrate cat. Neurosci Lett 1992;139:243-248.

53. Veasey SC, Panckeri KA, Hoffman EA, et al: The effect of serotonin antagonists in an animal model of sleep-disordered breathing. Am J Respir Crit Care Med 1996;153:776-786.

54. Kubin L, Reignier C, Tojima H, et al: Changes in serotonin level in the hypoglossal nucleus region during the carbachol-induced atonia. Brain Res 1994;645:291-302.

55. Woch G, Davies RO, Pack AI, et al: Behavior of raphe cells projecting to the dorsomedial medulla during carbachol-induced atonia in the cat. J Physiol 1996;490:745-758.

56. Lai YY, Kodama T, Siegel J: Changes in monoamine release in the ventral horn and hypoglossal nucleus linked to pontine inhibition of muscle tone: An in vivo microdialysis study. J Neurosci 2001;21:7384-7391.

57. Nishimura Y, Muramatsu M, Asahara T, et al: Electrophysiological properties and their modulation by norepinephrine in

the ambiguus neurons of the guinea pig. Brain Res 1995; 702: 213-222.

58. Funk GD, Smith JC, Feldman JL: Development of thyrotropin-releasing hormone and norepinephrine potentiation of inspiratory-related hypoglossal motoneuron discharge in neonatal and juvenile mice in vitro. J Neurophysiol 1994;72:2538-2541.

59. Larkman PM, Kelly JS: Ionic mechanisms mediating 5-hydroxy-tryptamine- and noradrenaline-evoked depolarization of adult rat facial motoneurones. J Physiol 1992;456:473-490.

60. Champagnat J, Denavit-Saubié M, Henry JL, et al: Catecholaminergic depressant effects on bulbar respiratory mechanisms. Brain Res 1979;160:57-68.

61. Fenik V, Kubin L, Okabe S, et al: Differential sensitivity of laryngeal and pharyngeal motoneurons to iontophoretic application of serotonin. Neuroscience 1997;81:873-885.

62. Kubin L, Davies RO: Mechanisms of airway hypotonia. In Pack AI (ed): Sleep Apnea: Pathogenesis, Diagnosis, and Treatment. New York, Dekker, 2002, pp 99-154.

63. Fenik V, Davies RO, Pack AI, et al: Differential suppression of upper airway motor activity during carbachol-induced, REM sleep-like atonia. Am J Physiol 1998;275:R1013-R1024.

64. Aston-Jones G, Rajkowski J, Kubiak P, et al: Role of the locus coeruleus in emotional activation. Progr Brain Res 1996;107: 379-402.

65. de Lecea L, Kilduff TS, Peyron C, et al: The hypocretins: Hypothalamus-specific peptides with neuroexcitatory activity. Proc Natl Acad Sci USA 1998;95:322-327.

66. Peyron C, Tighe DK, van den Pol AN, et al: Neurons containing hypocretin (orexin) project to multiple neuronal systems. J Neurosci 1998;18:9996-10015.

67. Trivedi P, Yu H, MacNeil DJ, et al: Distribution of orexin receptor mRNA in the rat brain. FEBS Lett 1998;438:71-75.

68. Marcus JN, Aschkenasi CJ, Lee CE, et al: Differential expression of orexin receptors 1 and 2 in the rat brain. J Comp Neurol 2001;435:6-25.

69. Hervieu GJ, Cluderay JE, Harrison DC, et al: Gene expression and protein distribution of the orexin-1 receptor in the rat brain and spinal cord. Neuroscience 2001;103:777-797.

70. Antunes VR, Brailoiu GC, Kwok EH, et al: Orexins/hypocretins excite rat sympathetic preganglionic neurons in vivo and in vitro. Am J Physiol 2001;281:R1801-R1807.

71. Volgin DV, Saghir M, Kubin L: Developmental changes in the orexin 2 receptor mRNA in hypoglossal motoneurons. Neuroreport 2002;13:433-436.

72. Estabrooke IV, McCarthy MT, Ko E, et al: Fos expression in orexin neurons varies with behavioral state. J Neurosci 2001;21:1656-1662.

73. Yoshida Y, Fujiki N, Nakajima T, et al: Fluctuation of extracellular hypocretin-1 (orexin A) levels in the rat in relation to the light-dark cycle and sleep-wake activities. Eur J Neurosci 2001;14:1075-1081.

74. Kiyashchenko LI, Mileykovskiy BY, Maidment N, et al: Release of hypocretin (orexin) during waking and sleep states. J Neurosci 2002;22:5282-5286.

75. Torterolo P, Yamuy J, Sampogna S, et al: Hypocretinergic neurons are primarily involved in activation of the somatomotor system. Sleep 2003;26:25-28.

76. Parisi RA, Edelman NH, Santiago TV: Central respiratory carbon dioxide chemosensitivity does not decrease during sleep. Am Rev Respir Dis 1992;145:832-836.

77. Issa FG, Bitner S: Effect of route of breathing on the ventilatory and arousal responses to hypercapnia in awake and sleeping dogs. J Physiol 1993;465:615-628.

78. Horner RL, Kozar LF, Kimoff RJ, et al: Effects of sleep on the tonic drive to respiratory muscle and the threshold for rhythm generation in the dog. J Physiol 1994;474:525-537.

79. Nattie E: CO_2, brainstem chemoreceptors and breathing. Progr Neurobiol 1999;59:299-331.

80. Ballantyne D, Scheid P: Central chemosensitivity of respiration: A brief overview. Respir Physiol 2001;129:5-12.

81. Dean JB, Lawing WL, Millhorn DE. CO_2 decreases membrane conductance and depolarizes neurons in the nucleus tractus solitarii. Exp Brain Res 1989;76:656-661.

82. Bradley SR, Pieribone VA, Wang W, et al: Chemosensitive serotonergic neurons are closely associated with large medullary arteries. Nat Neurosci 2002;5:401-402.

83. Oyamada Y, Ballantyne D, Muckenhoff K, et al: Respiration-modulated membrane potential and chemosensitivity of locus coeruleus neurones in the in vitro brainstem-spinal cord of the neonatal rat. J Physiol 1998;513:381-398.

84. Kita I, Sakamoto M, Arita H: Adrenergic cell group in rostral ventrolateral medulla of cat: Its correlation with central chemoreceptors. Neurosci Res 1994;20:265-274.

85. Onimaru H, Arata A, Homma I: Intrinsic burst generation of preinspiratory neurons in the medulla of brainstem-spinal cord preparations isolated from newborn rats. Exp Brain Res 1995;106:57-68.

86. Parmeggiani PL, Sabattini L: Electromyographic aspects of postural, respiratory and thermoregulatory mechanisms in sleeping cats. Electroencephalogr Clin Neurophysiol 1972;33:1-13.

87. Tabachnik E, Muller NS, Bryan AC, et al: Changes in ventilation and chest wall mechanics during sleep in normal adolescents. J Appl Physiol 1981;51:557-564.

88. Megirian D, Pollard MJ, Sherrey JH: The labile respiratory activity of ribcage muscles of the rat during sleep. J Physiol 1987;389:99-110.

89. Lovering AT, Dunin-Barkowski WL, Vidruk EH, Orem JM: Ventilatory response of the cat to hypoxia in sleep and wakefulness. J Appl Physiol 2003;95:545-554.

90. Gauzzi M, Freis ED: Sino-aortic reflexes pH, po_2, and pco_2 in wakefulness and sleep. Am J Physiol 1969;217:1623-1627.

91. Dawes GS, Fox HE, Leduc BM, et al: Respiratory movements and rapid eye movement sleep in the foetal lamb. J Physiol 1972;220:119-143.

92. Remmers JE, Bartlett D Jr, Putnam MD: Changes in the respiratory cycle associated with sleep. Respir Physiol 1976;28: 227-238.

93. Foutz AS, Netick A, Dement WC: Sleep state effects on breathing after spinal cord section and vagotomy in the cat. Respir Physiol 1979;37:89-100.

94. Netick A, Foutz AS: Respiratory activity and sleep-wakefulness in the deafferented paralyzed cat. Sleep 1980;3:1-12.

95. Orem J: Central respiratory activity in rapid eye movement sleep: Augmenting and late inspiratory cells. Sleep 1994; 17:665-673.

96. Orem J: Augmenting expiratory neuronal activity in sleep and wakefulness and in relation to duration of expiration. J Appl Physiol 1998;85:1260-1266.

97. Orem J, Lovering AT, Dunin-Barkowski W, Vidruk EH: Endogenous excitatory drive to the respiratory system in rapid eye movement sleep in cats. J Physiol 2000;527:365-376.

98. Orem J: Medullary respiratory neuron activity: Relationship to tonic and phasic REM sleep. J Appl Physiol 1980;48:54-65.

99. Netick A, Orem J, Dement W: Neuronal activity specific to REM sleep and its relationship to breathing. Brain Res 1977;120:197-207.

100. Hobson JA, Goldfrank F, Snyder F: Respiration and mental activity in sleep. J Psychiatr Res 1965;3:79-90.

101. Baust W, Engel R: The correlation of heart and respiratory frequency in natural sleep of man and their relation to dream content. Electroencephalogr Clin Neurophysiol 1971;30: 262-263.

102. Hauri P, Van de Castle RL: Psychophysiological parallels in dreams. Psychosom Med 1973;35:297-308.

103. Dunin-Barkowski WL, Orem JM: Suppression of diaphragmatic activity during spontaneous ponto-genicular-occipital waves in cat. Sleep 1998;21:671-675.

104. George R, Haslett WL, Jenden DJ: A cholinergic mechanism in the brainstem reticular formation: Induction of paradoxical sleep. Int J Neuropharmacol 1964;3:541-552.

105. Baghdoyan HA, Rodrigo-Angulo ML, McCarley RW, et al: Site-specific enhancement and suppression of desynchronized sleep signs following cholinergic stimulation of three brainstem regions. Brain Res 1984;306:39-52.

106. Vanni-Mercier G, Sakai K, Lin JS, et al: Mapping of cholinoceptive brainstem structures responsible for the generation of paradoxical sleep in the cat. Arch Ital Biol 1989;127:133-164.

107. Datta S, Calvo JM, Quattrochi J, et al: Cholinergic microstimulation of the peribrachial nucleus in the cat: I. Immediate and prolonged increases in ponto-geniculo-occipital waves. Arch Ital Biol 1992;130:263-284.

108. Vertes RP, Colm LV, Fortin WJ, et al: Brainstem sites for the carbachol elicitation of the hippocampal theta rhythm in the rat. Exp Brain Res 1993;96:419-429.

109. Taguchi O, Kubin L, Pack AI: Evocation of postural atonia and respiratory depression by pontine carbachol in the decerebrate rat. Brain Res 1992;595:107-115.

110. Kubin L: Carbachol models of REM sleep: Recent developments and new directions. Arch Ital Biol 2001;139:147-168.

111. Yamamoto K, Mamelak AN, Quattrochi JJ, et al: A cholinoceptive desynchronized sleep induction zone in the anterodorsal pontine tegmentum: Locus of the sensitive region. Neuroscience 1990;39:279-293.

112. Bourgin P, Escourrou P, Gaultier C, et al: Induction of rapid eye movement sleep by carbachol infusion into the pontine reticular formation in the rat. Neuroreport 1995;6:532-536.

113. Fenik V, Marchenko V, Janssen P, et al: A5 cells are silenced when REM sleep-like signs are elicited by pontine carbachol. J Appl Physiol 2002;93:1448-1456.

114. Kodama T, Takahashi Y, Honda Y: Enhancement of acetylcholine release during paradoxical sleep in the dorsal tegmental field of the cat brainstem. Neurosci Lett 1990;114:277-282.

115. Lydic R, Baghdoyan HA, Zwillich CW: State-dependent hypotonia in posterior cricoarytenoid muscles of the larynx caused by cholinoceptive reticular mechanisms. FASEB J 1989;3:1625-1631.

116. Lydic R, Baghdoyan HA: Cholinoceptive pontine reticular mechanisms cause state-dependent respiratory changes in the cat. Neurosci Lett 1989;102:211-216.

117. Kimura H, Kubin L, Davies RO, et al: Cholinergic stimulation of the pons depresses respiration in decerebrate cats. J Appl Physiol 1990;69:2280-2289.

118. Tojima H, Kubin L, Kimura H, et al: Spontaneous ventilation and respiratory motor output during carbachol-induced atonia of REM sleep in the decerebrate cat. Sleep 1992;15:404-414.

119. Fenik V, Davies RO, Pack AI, et al: Differential suppression of upper airway motor activity during carbachol-induced, REM sleep-like atonia. Am J Physiol 1998;275:R1013-R1024.

120. Woch G, Ogawa H, Davies RO, Kubin L: Behavior of hypoglossal inspiratory premotor neurons during the carbachol-induced, REM sleep-like suppression of upper airway motoneurons. Exp Brain Res 2000;130:508-520.

121. Fenik V, Ogawa H, Davies RO, et al: The activity of locus coeruleus neurons is reduced in urethane-anesthetized rats during carbachol-induced episodes of REM sleep-like suppression of upper airway motor tone. Soc Neurosci Abstr 1999;25:2144.

122. Kubin L, Kimura H, Tojima H, et al: Behavior of VRG neurons during the atonia of REM sleep induced by pontine carbachol in decerebrate cats. Brain Res 1992;592:91-100.

123. Kubin L, Kimura H, Tojima H, et al: Suppression of hypoglossal motoneurons during the carbachol-induced atonia of REM sleep is not caused by fast synaptic inhibition. Brain Res 1993;611:300-312.

124. Kubin L, Tojima H, Reignier C, et al: Interaction of serotonergic excitatory drive to hypoglossal motoneurons with carbachol-induced, REM sleep-like atonia. Sleep 1996;19:187-195.

125. Fung SJ, Yamuy J, Xi MC, et al: Changes in electrophysiological properties of cat hypoglossal motoneurons during carbachol-induced motor inhibition. Brain Res 2000;885:262-272.

126. Fenik V, Davies RO, Kubin L: Combined antagonism of aminergic excitatory and amino acid inhibitory receptors in the XII nucleus abolishes REM sleep-like depression of hypoglossal motoneuronal activity. Arch Ital Biol 2004;142:237-249.

127. Fenik VB, Davies RO, Kubin L: REM sleep-like atonia of XII motoneurons is caused by loss of noradrenergic and serotonergic inputs. Am J Resp Crit Care Med 2005; in press.

128. Jelev A, Sood S, Liu H, et al: Microdialysis perfusion of 5-HT into hypoglossal motor nucleus differentially modulates genioglossus activity across natural sleep-wake states in rats. J Physiol 2001;532:467-481.

129. Okabe S, Mackiewicz M, Kubin L: Serotonin receptor mRNA expression in the hypoglossal motor nucleus. Respir Physiol 1997;110:151-160.

130. Volgin DV, Mackiewicz M, Kubin L: Alpha$_{1B}$ receptors are the main postsynaptic mediators of adrenergic excitation in brainstem motoneurons, a single-cell RT-PCR study. J Chem Neuroanat 2001;22:157-166.

131. Volgin DV, Fay R, Kubin L: Postnatal development of serotonin 1B, 2A and 2C receptors in brainstem motoneurons. Eur J Neurosci 2003;17:1179-1188.

132. Fenik P, Veasey SC: Pharmacological characterization of serotonergic receptor activity in the hypoglossal nucleus. Am J Respir Crit Care Med 2003;167:563-569.

133. Veasey SC, Fenik P, Panckeri K, et al: The effects of trazodone with L-tryptophan on sleep-disordered breathing in the English bulldog. Am J Respir Crit Care Med 1999;160:1659-1667.

Respiratory Physiology: Control of Ventilation

Neil J. Douglas

ABSTRACT

Sleep is a time when the respiratory tranquility of resting wakefulness is replaced by marked respiratory variability due to changes in both the drive to the ventilatory pump muscles and the upper airway opening muscles. Breathing during wakefulness is controlled by several factors, including voluntary and behavioral elements, chemical factors (e.g., low oxygen levels, high carbon dioxide levels, and acidosis), and mechanical signals from the lung and chest wall. During sleep, there is loss of voluntary control and a decrease in the usual ventilatory response to both low oxygen and high carbon dioxide levels. Both hypoxemic and hypercapnic responses are most depressed in rapid eye movement (REM) sleep.

These blunted ventilatory responses during sleep are clinically important. They permit the marked hypoxemia that occurs during REM sleep in patients with lung or chest wall disease, and they may also be important in the pathogenesis of upper airway obstruction during sleep and particularly in the failure to arouse rapidly during apneas.

Sleep alters both breathing pattern and respiratory responses to many external stimuli. These changes permit the development of sleep-related hypoxemia in patients with respiratory disease and may contribute to the pathogenesis of apneas in patients with sleep apnea syndrome.

Many respiratory problems during sleep are related to an abnormal control of ventilation. Much is known about the control of breathing during wakefulness, but less is known about how breathing is controlled in the sleeping healthy person or in a patient with a sleep disorder. The major goal of the respiratory control system is homeostatis—that is, keeping blood gases in a tight range so that the metabolic functions of the body remain normal. This chapter reviews the control of ventilation in adults during sleep and its relevance to clinical problems.

Unlike the heart, the respiratory muscles do not have a built-in pacemaker. These muscles receive impulses from the medulla from a region that has been called the respiratory center, respiratory oscillator, respiratory signal generator, and respiratory pacemaker. For breathing to change as physiologic conditions change, the respiratory center receives and responds to three general types of information: chemical information (from chemoreceptors responding to pH and to the partial pressures of oxygen [PaO_2] and carbon dioxide [$PaCO_2$]), mechanical information (from receptors in the lung and chest wall), and behavioral information (from higher cortical centers). These aspects of awake control also have an impact on the control of breathing during sleep.

Chemical Information

The carotid body senses PaO_2, which sends impulses to the medulla via the ninth cranial nerve. Ventilation usually increases only when PaO_2 is less than 60 mm Hg. When PaO_2 drops acutely to less than 30 to 40 mm Hg, the medulla may be depressed by the hypoxemia and thus ventilation may decrease. CO_2 is sensed in both the carotid body and a region of the medulla called the central chemoreceptor. As $PaCO_2$ increases, there is a brisk linear increase in ventilation. Drugs that depress central nervous system (CNS) function may profoundly depress chemical drives to breathe.

Mechanical Information

In the presence of lung diseases or changes in the load of the respiratory system, receptors in the lung and chest wall send impulses to the medulla. Receptors in the lung are the best understood: they respond to irritation, inflation (stretch), deflation, and congestion of blood vessels. The information from these sensors travels centrally via the vagus nerve. The major result of stimulating these sensors is shortened inspiration and reduced tidal volume, causing a rapid, shallow breathing pattern.

Information from Higher Central Nervous System Centers

The respiratory system is used for many nonbreathing functions (e.g., singing, laughing, crying, speaking) that are directed by higher brain centers. The efferent pathways involved in these activities can bypass the respiratory center in the medulla and override the metabolic homeostatic function of the respiratory control system. Just as abnormal chemistry may increase the drive to breathe, there is a respiratory drive linked to wakefulness. As one sleeps, arouses, and dreams, there may be dramatic changes in the information from higher CNS centers.

PHYSIOLOGY OF VENTILATORY CONTROL DURING SLEEP

This chapter focuses on the effects of sleep on the mechanisms that control breathing.

Hypoxic Ventilatory Response during Sleep

In *adult humans*, the ventilatory response to hypoxia falls during sleep[1-4] (Fig. 18–1). The hypoxic ventilatory response was lower during non–rapid eye movement (NREM) sleep

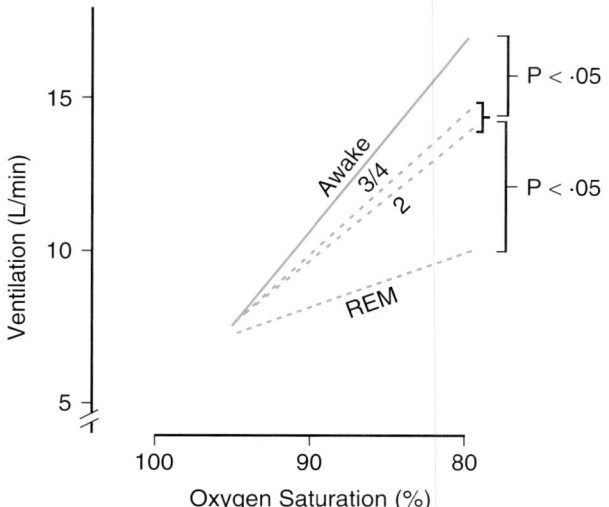

Figure 18–1. Mean relationship between expired ventilation and decreasing O_2 saturation in rapid eye movement (REM) sleep, in sleep stages 2 and 3/4, and awake, in 12 subjects, six men[1] and six women.[4] (From Douglas NJ: Control of ventilation during sleep. Clin Chest Med 1985;6:563.)

than during wakefulness when the study subjects were exclusively or mostly men,[1,2] but the responses were similar in wakefulness and in NREM sleep in the studies in which women predominated.[3-5] It is not clear why there is such a difference between the sexes in the effect of sleep on the hypoxic ventilatory response. Comparison of the results in men and women (Fig. 18–2) shows that the major sex difference is in the levels of ventilatory drives during wakefulness, which are much higher in men than in women.[4]

The hypoxic ventilatory response during rapid eye movement (REM) sleep is lower than in NREM sleep in both men and women.[1-4] The hypoxic ventilatory response during REM sleep was remarkably similar in all three directly comparable studies[1,2,4]: about 0.4 L/min per oxygen saturation (SaO_2) percentage (see Fig. 18–2).

In studies on *adult animals*, the isocapnic hypoxic ventilatory response has been found to be unchanged[6] or decreased[7]

during sleep in tracheostomized dogs and decreased[8] during sleep in goats.

Hypercapnic Ventilatory Response during Sleep

In *adult humans*, the hypercapnic ventilatory response is depressed during sleep (Fig. 18–3). Studies performed in either electroencephalogram-documented[9-12] or presumed[13-15] NREM sleep showed that the slope of the ventilation–CO_2 response line falls during NREM sleep compared with wakefulness. Two large studies[10,11] suggested that the decrease in response from wakefulness to NREM sleep is approximately 50%. Although Bülow[10] reported lower responses in stages 3 and 4 sleep than in stage 2 sleep, later researchers[11,16] found no such difference. In fact, Bülow did not apply statistics, and his data indicate considerable overlap (see Figs. 21, 26, and 27 in Bülow[10]). Indeed, no separation is evident until high CO_2 levels are reached, when the number of data points is small.

NREM sleep does not significantly change the position of the ventilation–CO_2 response line, as assessed by the rebreathing technique with extrapolation of the CO_2 response line to the intercept at zero ventilation.[11,16] However, as the slope of the response line decreases during NREM sleep, the CO_2 increment between the awake resting ventilatory set point and the ventilatory response line is increased significantly[10,11] (see Fig. 18–3).

Berthon-Jones and Sullivan[16] found that women did not change the hypercapnic ventilatory response from wakefulness to NREM sleep, a result consistent with the finding by Davis et al.[17] of higher ventilatory responses during sleep in women than in men. In contrast, neither Douglas et al.[11] nor Gothe et al.[18] identified any difference between the sexes in any stage.

Three groups measured the hypercapnic ventilatory response during REM sleep in adults. Douglas et al.[11] found that in 10 of 12 subjects, the hypercapnic response was lower in REM sleep than in either wakefulness or NREM sleep. The mean hypercapnic ventilatory response during REM sleep was 28% of the level during wakefulness (see Fig. 18–3). These authors were unable to accurately define the position of the hypercapnic ventilatory response line because some

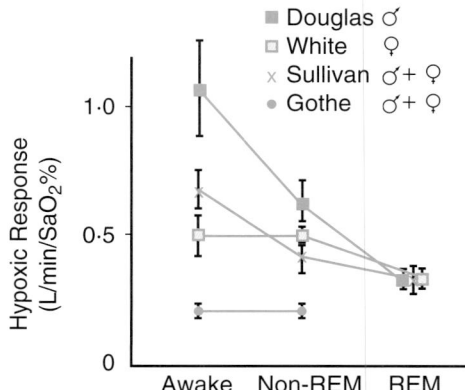

Figure 18–2. Comparison of hypoxic ventilatory responses in different sleep stages and awake in four studies,[1,3,5] indicating the unchanged responses in non–rapid eye movement (non-REM) sleep in women, and the similarity of responses in rapid eye movement (REM) sleep in all studies.

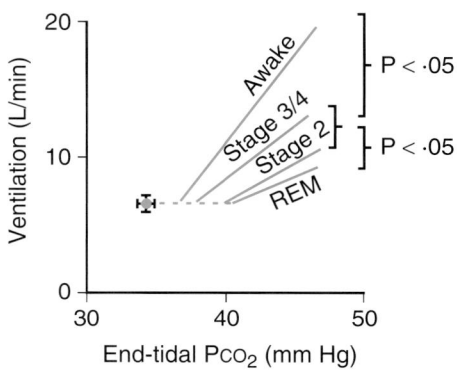

Figure 18–3. Mean relationship between expired ventilation and increasing end-tidal PCO_2 ($PETCO_2$) during wakefulness and sleep in 12 subjects, six men and six women, indicating the mean ± SE resting ventilation–CO_2 set point during wakefulness. REM, rapid eye movement. (From Douglas NJ: Control of ventilation during sleep. Clin Chest Med 1985;6:563.

responses during REM sleep had negative slopes. Berthon-Jones and Sullivan[16] and White[19] found a tendency for the lowest responses to occur during REM sleep.

Studies in *adult animals* showed that, as in adult humans, the hypercapnic ventilatory response is lower in NREM sleep than in wakefulness in dogs[20,21] and cats,[22] with a further drop in response from NREM to REM sleep.[20-23] Sullivan and colleagues[21] found that the hypercapnic ventilatory response was lower in phasic than in tonic REM sleep in dogs.

Ventilatory Response to Chemical Stimuli: Conclusions

There appear to be genuine sex and species differences in the effect of sleep on the hypoxic ventilatory response. Although there are no major species differences in the effect of sleep on the hypercapnic ventilatory response, there may be sex differences. In human adults, both responses are reduced during sleep and are at their lowest during REM sleep.

ADDED RESISTANCE AND AIRWAY OCCLUSION DURING SLEEP

In *adult humans,* sleep modifies the ventilatory response to added inspiratory resistance.[24-27] All agree that NREM sleep blunts the respiratory timing response to added resistance,[24-28] and some studies report a net effect on ventilation as well.[25,27,28] In adults with asthma, the ventilatory response to induced bronchoconstriction is not modified by sleep.[29] Issa and Sullivan[30] reported that, in response to airway occlusion, there was a progressive increase in respiratory effort during NREM sleep and rapid, shallow breathing during REM sleep.

Studies with *animals* have shown that, in both dogs[31,32] and cats,[22] ventilatory compensation for added loads is maintained during NREM sleep at the level found in wakefulness. However, when the respiratory system is further stressed by combining resistive loading with hypercapnia, the ventilatory and airway occlusion responses to loading are found to be impaired during both NREM and REM sleep.[22]

It is not yet clear precisely what effect increased airflow resistance has on ventilation during sleep, particularly during REM sleep, in adults.

AROUSAL RESPONSES

Isocapnic Hypoxia

In healthy subjects, isocapnic hypoxia is a poor stimulus to arousal (Fig. 18–4). Many subjects remain asleep with an SaO_2 as low as 70%[1,2,5] and no difference in arousal threshold between NREM and REM sleep. On the other hand, the arousal sensitivity to hypoxia is decreased in REM sleep in patients with obstructive sleep apnea and asphyxial hypoxia,[33] in dogs with isocapnic hypoxia,[6,7] and in cats with hypocapnic hypoxia.[34] Carotid body denervation reduces arousal sensitivity in dogs[7] but does not alter the arousal threshold in cats.[34]

Hypercapnia

Hypercapnia also produces arousal at variable levels,[3,9,11] but it awakens most subjects before the end-tidal CO_2 has risen to 15 mm Hg above the level in wakefulness.[3,9-11] Berthon-Jones and Sullivan[16] reported arousal thresholds up to 6 mm Hg higher in slow wave sleep than in either stage 2 or REM sleep in male but not in female subjects, whereas Douglas and associates[11] found no sex- or sleep stage–related differences. Hypoxia increases the sensitivity to CO_2 arousal.[35]

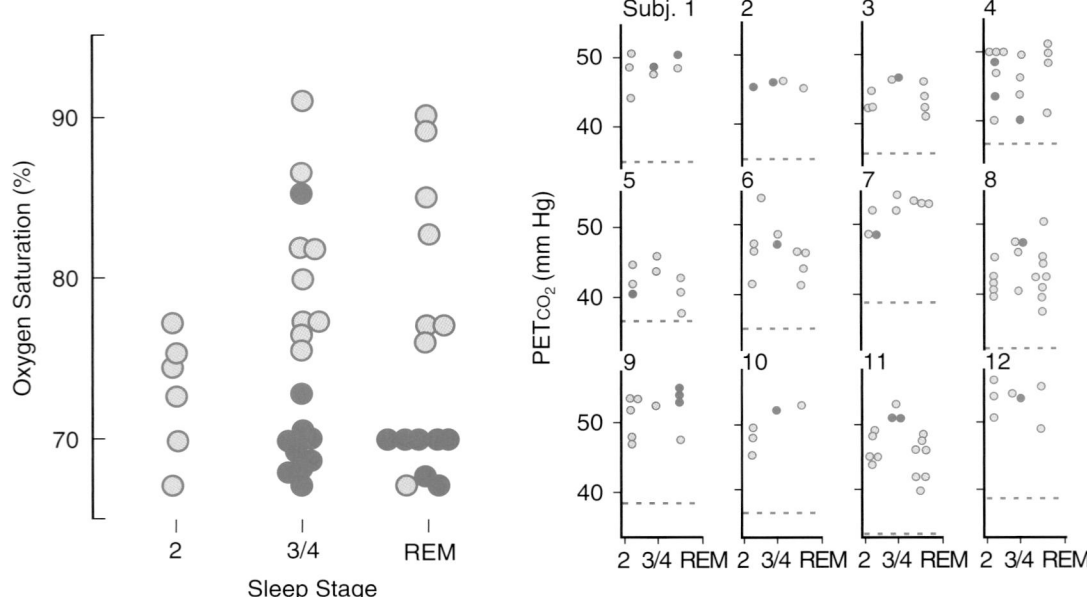

Figure 18–4. Arousal responses to hypoxia and hypercapnia[11] in different sleep stages, indicating whether the subjects remained asleep *(dark circles)* or aroused *(light circles)*. The hypoxic responses *(left)* are total data for nine subjects; the hypercapnic plots *(right)* are for each of 12 individuals, six women (1 through 6) and six men (7 through 12), and the *dotted line* indicates the mean $PETCO_2$ in wakefulness for each subject. (From Douglas NJ: Control of ventilation during sleep. Clin Chest Med 1985;6:563.)

Added Resistance

Humans tend to arouse from sleep after either the addition of an inspiratory resistance[26] or the occlusion of inspiration.[30] Added inspiratory resistance was found to produce similar percentages of increase in arousal frequency in stages 2 and 3/4 and in REM sleep.[24] However, the arousal frequency during control sleep periods was lowest in stage 3/4 sleep and remained significantly lower during slow wave sleep than in REM sleep after the addition of inspiratory resistance[22,23] (Fig. 18–5).

Arousal from REM sleep after airway occlusion[30,36] is far more rapid than arousal from NREM sleep (Fig. 18–6), whereas patients with obstructive apneas have longer apneas during REM sleep. Upper airway receptors would be exposed to respiratory pressure changes in healthy people with airway occlusion but not in patients with sleep apnea, but why these upper airway receptors should be more effective in REM sleep than in NREM sleep is unclear.

Arousal response to chemostimulation was found to occur at similar levels of ventilation regardless of stimulus.[16] The final common pathway for arousal from sleep after hypoxia, hypercapnia, or increased resistance may actually be the level of ventilatory effort.[37] This is compatible with the observation that patients with upper airway resistance syndrome tend to awaken at relatively reproducible levels of pleural pressure, and that this arousal occurs without the development of either significant hypoxemia or significant hypercapnia.

Bronchial Irritation

Sleep suppresses the cough response to inhaled irritants in humans,[38] dogs,[39] and cats,[40] with cough occurring only after arousal. Similarly, in patients with chronic bronchitis and emphysema, cough is suppressed during sleep.[41] There is no difference between NREM and REM sleep in the arousal response to inhaled citric acid in humans,[38] but in dogs, the arousal responses both to instilled water and to inhaled citric acid are markedly depressed during REM sleep.[42]

Ventilatory Response to Arousal

The reverse of considering which elements of respiration cause arousal is examining the effect of arousal on ventilation. Awakening from sleep, whatever the arousing response, leads to an increase in ventilation,[43,44] just as sleep onset is associated with a decrease in ventilation.

CONTROL OF BREATHING RHYTHM DURING SLEEP

Spontaneously occurring breathing irregularities during sleep are reviewed in Chapter 19, but a few points are relevant to this chapter.

In studies with *humans*, Bülow[10] found that the subjects who had the most irregular breathing during NREM sleep had the greatest CO_2 tolerance between the awake ventilation–CO_2 set point and the CO_2 response line. This CO_2 control laxity at sleep onset may be important in the pathogenesis of breathing irregularities, which are common at this time.[10,45] The induction of hypocapnia either alone or in conjunction with hypoxia can induce irregular breathing in healthy subjects during NREM sleep[46] and may lead to occlusive apneas, especially when an inspiratory resistance is added.[47] After airway occlusion in NREM sleep, ventilatory overshoot may occur, especially in those with high hypercapnic ventilatory responses,[12] and this could contribute to respiratory instability during sleep. More recently, it has been found that subjects with high hypoxic ventilatory responses have greater variability in ventilation during sleep.[48] During REM sleep, irregular breathing is the norm in adults, and neither isocapnic hypoxia nor hypercapnia regularizes this pattern.[1,11]

In mature *animals*, spontaneous irregular breathing is uncommon in NREM sleep. In REM sleep, irregular breathing is universal and is not regularized by hypoxia,[6] hyperoxia,[39] hypercapnia,[21] metabolic alkalosis,[39] carotid body resection,[49] or vagotomy,[50,51] and indeed respiratory irregularity may increase after vagotomy.[51]

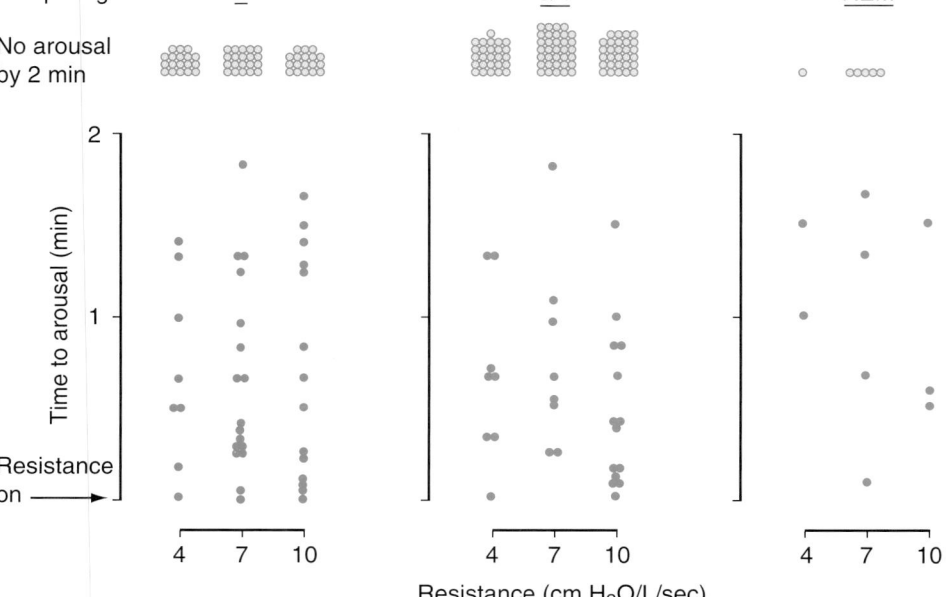

Figure 18–5. Timing of arousal after application of inspiratory resistance of 4, 7, or 10 cm H_2O/L/sec in stages 2 and 3/4 and in rapid eye movement (REM) sleep. *Dark circles* indicate occasions when arousal occurred within 2 minutes of addition of resistance. *Light circles* indicate occasions when arousal did not occur within 2 minutes. (From Gugger M, Molloy J, Gould GA, et al: Ventilatory and arousal responses to added inspiratory resistance during sleep. Am Rev Respir Dis 1989;140: 1301-1307.)

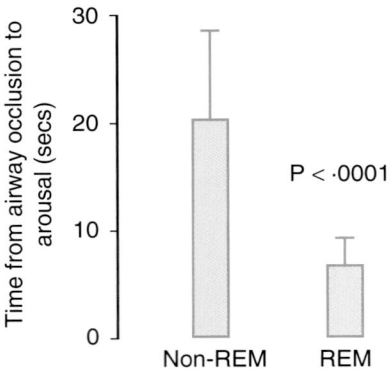

Figure 18–6. Time from airway occlusion to arousal (mean + SD) in 12 subjects, showing that arousal from rapid eye movement (REM) sleep is faster than that from non–rapid eye movement (non-REM) sleep.[30] (From Douglas NJ: Control of ventilation during sleep. Clin Chest Med 1985;6:563.)

UPPER AIRWAY–OPENING MUSCLES DURING SLEEP

In cats, the activity of upper airway opening muscles decreases during NREM sleep, with a further marked reduction during REM sleep.[52] During wakefulness, the activity of these muscles parallels that of the diaphragm during respiratory stimulation with either hypoxia or hypercapnia.[52,53] Both genioglossal tone[54] and palatal muscle tone[54,55] decrease during sleep in healthy humans. Decreases in genioglossal and palatal muscle activity occur immediately at alpha-to-theta transition in parallel with changes in diaphragm muscle tone.[56] These decreases are greater in older subjects.[57] Genioglossal activity is relatively insensitive to hypoxia, hypercapnia, or applied resistance during NREM sleep in adults.[58] Neither genioglossus nor tensor palatini activity increases in response to applied resistance during NREM sleep in men or women.[59]

FACTORS INFLUENCING RESPIRATORY CONTROL DURING SLEEP

The following mechanisms are likely to contribute to decreased ventilatory responses during sleep.

Decreased Basal Metabolic Rate

Basal metabolic rate falls during sleep, with no major differences between the levels in the different sleep stages.[60,61] Both ventilation and ventilatory responses are reduced when metabolic rate falls,[62] although the sensor for this is unclear. The decreased basal metabolic rate during sleep is probably a factor in the decreased chemosensitivity during sleep, but it cannot explain the further reduction in ventilatory response from NREM to REM sleep.

Relationship between Cerebral Blood Flow and Metabolism

Cerebral blood flow increases during sleep.[63-66] The 4% to 25% increase in brain blood flow in slow wave sleep over that in wakefulness is explicable on the basis of the mild

hypercapnia that results from hypoventilation.[65] Brain blood flow increases markedly during REM sleep; this increase was as large as 80% in one study.[64] In goats, Santiago et al.[65] found a 26% increase in brain blood flow during REM sleep, and an increase that was greater than could be explained by the increase in CO_2. They also found that brain metabolism in REM sleep was similar to that in wakefulness. This increase in the ratio of brain blood flow to brain metabolism would depress central chemoreceptor activity during REM sleep and might be a factor in reducing ventilatory responses during REM sleep. However, in humans, Madsen and colleagues[67] reported that changes in cerebral blood flow paralleled changes in cerebral oxygen metabolism during both slow wave and REM sleep.

Neurologic Changes during Sleep

Cortical activity can influence breathing, with mental concentration increasing both ventilation[68] and ventilatory responses.[10] It seems probable that the hypoventilation and decreased responses to chemical and mechanical stimuli in NREM sleep partially reflect the loss of the wakefulness drive to ventilation.[69]

During REM sleep, sensory and motor functions are impaired. There is both presynaptic and postsynaptic inhibition of afferent neurons,[70] which results in raised arousal thresholds to external stimuli[71] and in postsynaptic inhibition of motoneurons,[72] which produces the postural hypotonia typical of REM sleep.[73] This combination of decreased sensory and motor function probably contributes to the marked impairment of ventilatory responses during REM sleep.

It has been suggested that irregular breathing and impaired ventilatory responses during REM sleep result from alteration of the control of ventilation by behavioral factors.[69] However, evidence suggests that chemical stimuli are the most important factor during REM sleep in people.[74] Furthermore, at least in cats,[52] there seems to be a positive correlation between the activity of some medullary respiratory neurons during REM sleep and pontine-generated discharges termed ponto-geniculo-occipital waves. Ponto-geniculo-occipital waves are one of the basic electrophysiologic phenomena of REM sleep, and thus the dysrhythmic nature of breathing in REM sleep may relate directly to the dysrhythmic nature of REM sleep itself. This is supported by the observation that tidal volume is closely related to the density of eye movements during REM sleep in humans.[75]

Neuromechanical Factors

It has been suggested that a decreased ventilatory response in REM sleep results from hypotonia of the intercostal muscles. Although chest movement and levels seen on the intercostal electromyogram are decreased during REM sleep, as compared with NREM sleep, studies that included measurements during wakefulness show that chest movement contributes similar proportions to tidal volume in wakefulness and in REM sleep.[76-78] Further electromyogram studies are required, as are studies on the contribution of the chest to ventilation during the different components of REM sleep.[79]

Functional residual capacity is decreased during REM sleep.[80] Although this might contribute to the hypoxia in REM sleep, it is unlikely to contribute to the decreased ventilatory responses, because volume reduction usually increases these responses.[81]

Airflow resistance increases during sleep. The increase is maximal in NREM sleep in humans.[82,83] However, in cats, resistance seems to be highest during REM sleep.[53] This increased resistance results from hypotonia of the muscles that open the upper airway during sleep. Some of the diminution in ventilatory responses between wakefulness and NREM sleep may be caused by changes in upper airway resistance, because the occlusion pressure response to hypercapnia is well maintained during NREM sleep.[19] One study[84] looked at the threshold CO_2 level for respiratory muscle activation in intubated subjects, in whom upper airway resistance was thus kept constant. The authors suggested that there are sleep stage–related differences in the neuromuscular response to CO_2. The CO_2 level at which respiratory muscle augmentation occurred rose significantly from wakefulness to NREM sleep. The occlusion pressure response to hypercapnia is markedly reduced during REM sleep,[19] which indicates diminution of neuromuscular function.

Mechanism of Reduction in Ventilatory Responses: Conclusions

It is not possible with our current knowledge to apportion causes for the decrease in ventilatory responses during sleep. It seems likely that the major cause of the decrease in ventilatory responses during NREM sleep is the loss of the wakefulness drive to breathe coupled with the decrease in metabolic rate and increase in airflow resistance. The further reduction during REM sleep is likely to result from altered CNS function during REM sleep.

CLINICAL SEQUELAE OF ABNORMAL VENTILATORY RESPONSES

The impaired ventilatory responses permit the development of hypoventilation during sleep and of sleep-related hypoxemia in patients with hypoxic chronic bronchitis and emphysema[85-87] and other respiratory diseases that cause hypoxia.[88,89] In all of these conditions, the hypoxia is most marked in REM sleep, when the ventilatory responses are at their lowest. The remarkable insensitivity to external stimuli during sleep allows patients with all of these conditions to develop clinically significant hypoxia and hypercapnia before arousal occurs.

Instability of the control of breathing during sleep may contribute to the development of the obstructive sleep apnea/hypopnea syndrome in some patients.[90] Paradoxically, enhanced ventilatory responses may be present in some patients, which may destabilize ventilation and lead to periodic breathing.[91] This may be an important factor in the development of Cheyne-Stokes respiration in left ventricular heart failure.[92] In heart failure, central apnea during sleep may be initiated by an acute increase in ventilation and reduction in $PaCO_2$ following a spontaneous arousal.[93] When $PaCO_2$ falls below the threshold level required to stimulate breathing, the drive to respiratory muscles and airflow cease, and central apnea results. Apnea persists until $PaCO_2$ rises above the threshold required to stimulate ventilation. Prolonged circulation time appears not to play a key role in initiating central apneas, and indeed cardiac transplantation with normalization of cardiac function does not always prevent Cheyne-Stokes respiration.[94] The major influence of circulation time appears to be on the lengths of the hyperpneic phase and of the total periodic breathing cycle. Once triggered, the pattern of alternating hyperventilation and apnea is sustained by the combination of increased respiratory chemoreceptor drive, pulmonary congestion, arousals, and apnea-induced hypoxia, which cause oscillations in $PaCO_2$ above and below the apneic threshold. Inhalation of a CO_2-enriched gas to raise $PaCO_2$ abolishes Cheyne-Stokes respiration in heart failure.[95]

> *Clinical Pearl*
>
> *Decreased ventilatory responses to hypoxia, hypercapnia, and inspiratory resistance during sleep, particularly in REM sleep, permit REM hypoxemia in patients with chronic obstructive pulmonary disease, chest wall disease, and neuromuscular abnormalities affecting the respiratory muscles. They may also contribute to the development of the sleep apnea/hypopnea syndrome.*

REFERENCES

1. Douglas NJ, White DP, Weil JV, et al: Hypoxic ventilatory response decreases during sleep in normal men. Am Rev Respir Dis 1982;125:286-289.
2. Berthon-Jones M, Sullivan CE: Ventilatory and arousal responses to hypoxia in sleeping humans. Am Rev Respir Dis 1982;125:632-639.
3. Hedemark LL, Kronenberg RS: Ventilatory and heart rate responses to hypoxia and hypercapnia during sleep in adults. J Appl Physiol 1982;53:307-312.
4. White DP, Douglas NJ, Pickett CK, et al: Hypoxic ventilatory response during sleep in normal women. Am Rev Respir Dis 1982;126:530-533.
5. Gothe B, Goldman MD, Cherniack NS, et al: Effect of progressive hypoxia on breathing during sleep. Am Rev Respir Dis 1982;126:97-102.
6. Phillipson EA, Sullivan CE, Read DJC, et al: Ventilatory and waking responses to hypoxia in sleeping dogs. J Appl Physiol 1978;44:512-520.
7. Bowes G, Townsend ER, Kozar LF, et al: Effect of carotid body denervation on arousal response to hypoxia in sleeping dogs. J Appl Physiol 1981;51:40-45.
8. Santiago TV, Scardella AT, Edelman NH: Determinants of the ventilatory response to hypoxia during sleep. Am Rev Respir Dis 1984;130:179-182.
9. Birchfield RI, Sieker HO, Heyman A: Alterations in respiratory function during natural sleep. J Lab Clin Med 1959;54:216-222.
10. Bülow K: Respiration and wakefulness in man. Acta Physiol Scand 1963;59(Suppl 209):1-110.
11. Douglas NJ, White DP, Weil JV, et al: Hypercapnic ventilatory response in sleeping adults. Am Rev Respir Dis 1982;126:758-762.
12. Gleeson K, Zwillich CW, White DP: Chemosensitivity and the ventilatory response to airflow obstruction during sleep. J Appl Physiol 1989;67:1630-1637.
13. Magnussen G: Studies on the Respiration During Sleep: A Contribution to the Physiology of the Sleep Function. London, England, HK Lewis, 1944.
14. Ostergaard T: The excitability of the respiratory centre during sleep and during Evipan anaesthesia. Acta Physiol Scand 1944;8:1-15.
15. Robin ED, Whaley RD, Crump CH, et al: Alveolar gas tensions, pulmonary ventilation and blood pH during physiological sleep in normal subjects. J Clin Invest 1958;37:981-989.
16. Berthon-Jones M, Sullivan CE: Ventilation and arousal responses to hypercapnia in normal sleeping adults. J Appl Physiol 1984;57:59-67.

17. Davis JN, Loh L, Nodal J, et al: Effects of sleep on the pattern of CO_2 stimulated breathing in males and females. Adv Exp Med Biol 1978;99:79-83.

18. Gothe B, Altose MD, Goldman MD, et al: Effect of quiet sleep on resting and CO_2-stimulated breathing in humans. J Appl Physiol 1981;50:724-730.

19. White DP: Occlusion pressure and ventilation during sleep in normal humans. J Appl Physiol 1986;61:1279-1287.

20. Phillipson EA, Kozar LF, Rebuck AS, et al: Ventilatory and waking responses to CO_2 in sleeping dogs. Am Rev Respir Dis 1977;115:251-259.

21. Sullivan CE, Murphy E, Kozar LF, et al: Ventilatory responses to CO_2 and lung inflation in tonic versus phasic REM sleep. J Appl Physiol 1979;47:1304-1310.

22. Santiago TV, Sinha AK, Edelman NH: Respiratory flow-resistive load compensation during sleep. Am Rev Respir Dis 1981; 123:382-387.

23. Netick A, Dugger WJ, Symmons RA: Ventilatory response to hypercapnia during sleep and wakefulness in cats. J Appl Physiol 1984;56:1347-1354.

24. Gugger M, Molloy J, Gould GA, et al: Ventilatory and arousal responses to added inspiratory resistance during sleep. Am Rev Respir Dis 1989;140:1301-1307.

25. Hudgel DW, Mulholland M, Hendricks C: Neuromuscular and mechanical responses to inspiratory resistive loading during sleep. J Appl Physiol 1987;63:603-608.

26. Iber C, Berssenbrugge A, Skatrud JB, et al: Ventilatory adaptations to resistive loading during wakefulness and non-REM sleep. J Appl Physiol 1982;52:607-614.

27. Wiegand L, Zwillich CW, White DP: Sleep and the ventilatory response to resistive loading in normal men. J Appl Physiol 1988;64:1186-1195.

28. Gora J, Kay A, Colrain IM, et al: Load compensation as a function of state during sleep onset. J Appl Physiol 1998;84: 2123-2131.

29. Ballard RD, Tan WC, Kelly PL, et al: Effect of sleep and sleep deprivation on ventilatory response to broncho-constriction. J Appl Physiol 1990;69:490-497.

30. Issa FG, Sullivan CE: Arousal and breathing responses to airway occlusion in healthy sleeping adults. J Appl Physiol 1983;55: 1113-1119.

31. Bowes G, Kozar LF, Andrey SM, et al: Ventilatory responses to inspiratory flow-resistive loads in awake and sleeping dogs. J Appl Physiol 1983;54:1550-1557.

32. Phillipson EA, Kozar LF, Murphy E: Respiratory load compensation in awake and sleeping dogs. J Appl Physiol 1976;40: 895-902.

33. Sullivan CE, Issa FG: Pathophysiological mechanisms in obstructive sleep apnea. Sleep 1980;3:235-246.

34. Neubauer J, Santiago TV, Edelman NH: Hypoxic arousal in intact and carotid chemodenervated sleeping cats. J Appl Physiol 1981;51:1294-1299.

35. Gothe B, Cherniack NS, Williams L: Effect of hypoxia on ventilatory and arousal responses to CO_2 during non-REM sleep with and without flurazepam in young adults. Sleep 1986; 9:24-37.

36. Gugger M, Bogershausen S, Schaffler L: Arousal response to added inspiratory resistance during REM and non-REM sleep in normal subjects. Thorax 1993;48:125-129.

37. Gleeson K, Zwillich CW, White DP: The influence of increasing ventilatory effort on arousal from sleep. Am Rev Respir Dis 1990;142:295-300.

38. Jamal K, McMahon G, Edgell G, et al: Cough and arousal responses to inhaled citric acid in sleeping humans (Abstract). Am Rev Respir Dis 1983;127(Suppl):237.

39. Sullivan CE, Kozar LF, Murphy E, et al: Primary role of respiratory afferents in sustaining breathing rhythms. J Appl Physiol 1978;45:11-17.

40. Anderson CA, Dicke TE, Orem J: Respiratory responses to tracheobronchial stimulation during sleep and wakefulness in the adult cat. Sleep 1996;19:472-478.

41. Power JT, Stewart IC, Connaughton JJ, et al: Nocturnal cough in patients with chronic bronchitis and emphysema. Am Rev Respir Dis 1984;130:999-1001.

42. Sullivan CE, Kozar LF, Murphy E, et al: Arousal, ventilatory and airway responses to bronchopulmonary stimulation in sleeping dogs. J Appl Physiol 1979;47:17-25.

43. Badr MS, Morgan BJ, Finn L, et al: Ventilatory response to induced auditory arousal during non REM sleep. Sleep 1997;20: 707-714.

44. Carley DW, Applebaum R, Basner RC, et al: Respiratory and arousal responses to acoustic stimulation. Chest 1997;112: 1567-1571.

45. Douglas NJ, White DP, Pickett CK, et al: Respiration during sleep in normal man. Thorax 1982;37:840-844.

46. Skatrud JB, Dempsey JA: Interaction of sleep state and chemical stimuli in sustaining rhythmic ventilation. J Appl Physiol 1983; 55:813-822.

47. Onal E, Burrows DL, Hart RH, et al: Induction of periodic breathing during sleep causes upper airway obstruction in humans. J Appl Physiol 1986;61:1438-1443.

48. Dunai J, Kleiman J, Trinder J: Ventilatory instability during sleep onset in individuals with high peripheral chemo-sensitivity. J Appl Physiol 1999;87:661-672.

49. Guazzi M, Freis ED: Sinoaortic reflexes and arterial pH, PO_2 and PCO_2 in wakefulness and sleep. Am J Physiol 1969; 217:1623-1627.

50. Phillipson EA, Murphy E, Kozar LF: Regulation of respiration in sleeping dogs. J Appl Physiol 1976;40:688-693.

51. Remmers JE, Bartlett D, Putnam MD: Changes in the respiratory cycle associated with sleep. Respir Physiol 1976;28:227-238.

52. Orem J: Medullary respiratory neuron activity: Relationship to tonic and phasic REM sleep. J Appl Physiol 1980;48: 54-65.

53. Orem J, Netick A, Dement WC: Increased upper airway resistance to breathing during sleep in the cat. Electroencephalogr Clin Neurophysiol 1977;43:14-22.

54. Mezzanote WS, Tangel DJ, White DP: Influence of sleep onset on upper airway muscle activity in apnea patients versus normal controls. Am J Respir Crit Care Med 1996;153:1880-1887.

55. Tangel DJ, Mezzanote WS, White DP: Influence of sleep on tensor palatini EMG and upper airways resistance in normal man. J Appl Physiol 1991;70:2574-2581.

56. Worsnop C, Kay A, Pierce R, et al: Activity of respiratory pump and upper airway muscles during sleep onset. J Appl Physiol 1998;85:908-920.

57. Worsnop C, Kay A, Kim Y, et al: Effect of age on sleep onset-related changes in respiratory pump and upper airway muscle function. J Appl Physiol 2000;88:1831-1839.

58. Stanchina ML, Malhotra A, Fogel RB, et al: Genioglossus muscle responsiveness to chemical and mechanical stimuli during non-rapid eye movement sleep. Am J Respir Crit Care Med 2002; 165:945-949.

59. Pillar G, Malhotra A, Fogel R, et al: Airway mechanics and ventilation in response to resistive loading during sleep: Influence of gender. Am J Respir Crit Care Med 2000;162:1627-1632.

60. Brebbia DR, Altshuler KZ: Oxygen consumption rate and electroencephalographic stage of sleep. Science 1965;150: 1621-1623.

61. White DP, Weil JV, Zwillich CK: Metabolic rate and breathing during sleep. J Appl Physiol 1985;59:384-391.

62. Zwillich C, Sahn S, Weil J: Effects of hyper-metabolism on ventilation and chemosensitivity. J Clin Invest 1977;60:900-906.

63. Mangold R, Sokoloff K, Conner E, et al: The effects of sleep and lack of sleep on the cerebral circulation and metabolism of normal young men. J Clin Invest 1955;34:1092-1100.

64. Reivich M, Isaacs G, Evarts E, et al: The effect of slow wave sleep and REM sleep on regional cerebral blood flow in cats. J Neurochem 1968;15:301-306.

65. Santiago TV, Guerra E, Neubauer JA, et al: Correlation between ventilation and brain blood flow during sleep. J Clin Invest 1984;73:497-506.

66. Townsend RE, Prinz PN, Obrist WD: Human cerebral blood flow during sleep and waking. J Appl Physiol 1973;35:620-625.

67. Madsen PL, Schmidt JF, Wildschiodtz G, et al: Cerebral O_2 metabolism and cerebral blood flow in humans during deep and rapid-eye movement sleep. J Appl Physiol 1991;70:2597-2601.

68. Asmussen E: Regulation of respiration: "The black box." Acta Physiol Scand 1977;99:85-90.

69. Phillipson EA: Control of breathing during sleep. Am Rev Respir Dis 1978;118:909-939.

70. Pompeiano O: Mechanisms of sensorimotor integration during sleep. Prog Physiol Psychol 1973;3:1-179.

71. Steriade M, Hobson JA: Neuronal activity during the sleep-waking cycle. Prog Neurobiol 1976;6:155-376.

72. Nakamura Y, Goldberg LJ, Chandler SH, et al: Intra-cellular analysis of trigeminal motor neuron activity during sleep in the cat. Science 1978;199:204-207.

73. Pompeiano O: The control of posture and movements during REM sleep: Neurophysiological and neurochemical mechanisms. Acta Astronautica 1975;2:225-239.

74. Meza S, Giannouli E, Younes M: Control of breathing during sleep assessed by proportional assist ventilation. J Appl Physiol 1998;84:3-12.

75. Gould GA, Gugger M, Molloy J, et al: Breathing pattern and eye movement density during REM sleep in man. Am Rev Respir Dis 1988;138:874-877.

76. Mortola JP, Anch AM: Chest configuration in supine man: Wakefulness and sleep. Respir Physiol 1978;35:201-213.

77. Stradling JR, Chadwick GA, Frew AJ: Changes in ventilation and its components in normal subjects during sleep. Thorax 1985;40:364-370.

78. Tabachnik E, Muller NL, Bryan AC, et al: Changes in ventilation and chest wall mechanics during sleep in normal adults. J Appl Physiol 1981;51:557-564.

79. Millman RP, Knight H, Chung DC, et al: Changes in compartmental ventilation in association with eye movements during REM sleep. J Appl Physiol 1988;65:1196-1202.

80. Hudgel DW, Devadatta P: Decrease in functional residual capacity during sleep in normal humans. J Appl Physiol 1984;57:1319-1322.

81. Cherniack NS, Stanley NN, Tuteur PG, et al: Effect of lung volume changes on respiratory drive during hypoxia and hypercapnia. J Appl Physiol 1973;35:635-641.

82. Hudgel DW, Martin RJ, Johnson B, et al: Mechanics of the respiratory system and breathing pattern during sleep in normal humans. J Appl Physiol 1984;56:133-137.

83. Lopes JM, Tabachnik E, Muller NL, et al: Total airway resistance and respiratory muscle activity during sleep. J Appl Physiol 1983;54:773-777.

84. Ingrassia TS III, Nelson SB, Harris CD, et al: Influence of sleep state on carbon dioxide responsiveness: A study of the unloaded respiratory pump in man. Am Rev Respir Dis 1991;144: 1125-1129.

85. Douglas NJ, Calverley PMA, Leggett RJE, et al: Transient hypoxaemia during sleep in chronic bronchitis and emphysema. Lancet 1979;1:1-4.

86. Fleetham JA, Mezon B, West P, et al: Chemical control of ventilation and sleep arterial oxygen desaturation in patients with COPD. Am Rev Respir Dis 1980;122:583-589.

87. Koo KW, Sax DS, Snider GL: Arterial blood gases and pH during sleep in chronic obstructive pulmonary disease. Am J Med 1975;58:663-670.

88. Mezon BL, West P, Israels J, et al: Sleep breathing abnormalities in kyphoscoliosis. Am Rev Respir Dis 1980;122:617-621.

89. Muller NL, Francis PW, Gurwitz D, et al: Mechanism of hemoglobin desaturation during rapid-eye-movement sleep in normal subjects and in patients with cystic fibrosis. Am Rev Respir Dis 1980;121:463-469.

90. Younes M, Ostrowski M, Thompson W, et al: Chemical control stability in patients with obstructive sleep apnea. Am J Respir Crit Care Med 2001;163:1181-1190.

91. Cherniack NS: Apnea and periodic breathing during sleep. N Engl J Med 1999;341:985-987.

92. Javaheri S: A mechanism of central sleep apnea in patients with heart failure. N Engl J Med 1999;341:949-954.

93. Bradley TD, Floras JS: Sleep apnea and heart failure: Part II: central sleep apnea. Circulation 2003;107:1822-1826.

94. Mansfield DR, Solin P, Roebuck T, et al: The effect of successful heart transplant treatment of heart failure on central sleep apnea. Chest 2003;124:1675-1681.

95. Lorenzi-Filho G, Rankin F, Bies I, Douglas BT: Effects of inhaled carbon dioxide and oxygen on Cheyne-Stokes respiration in patients with heart failure. Am J Respir Crit Care Med 1999; 159:1490-1498.

Respiratory Physiology: Breathing in Normal Subjects

Jean Krieger

ABSTRACT

Sleep is associated with definite changes in respiratory function in normal humans. Whether these changes serve a specific function remains unclear and will probably not be clarified before the functions of sleep itself are better understood.

Drowsiness, or unsteady non–rapid eye movement (NREM), sleep is characterized in many subjects by a regularly oscillating, periodic breathing resulting in swings in the partial pressures of oxygen (PO_2) and carbon dioxide (PCO_2), with an overall moderate decrease in ventilation. These oscillations seem to result mainly from sleep instability during this stage, and the natural tendency of breathing regulation to be unstable probably aggravates this situation.

In steady NREM sleep, there occurs a regular pattern of breathing with more pronounced hypoventilation than during drowsiness. This hypoventilation seems to result from a combination of decreased ventilatory drive and a sleep-related defective compensation for an increased upper airway resistance. Ventilatory mechanics do not seem to be impaired during NREM sleep.

Rapid eye movement (REM) sleep is characterized by erratic, shallow breathing with irregularities both in amplitude and in frequency synchronous to REM bursts that are most probably of central origin and related to REM sleep processes. Hypoxemia equal to or greater than that during NREM sleep seems mainly to result from hypoventilation.

This chapter describes changes in spontaneous breathing during sleep in normal subjects and discusses possible mechanisms for these changes. This topic has become important because of the recognition of sleep breathing disorders.[1,2]

In sleep physiology as a whole, and the physiology of respiration during sleep in particular, a general, clearly established finding is that most major functions in non–rapid eye movement (NREM) sleep differ from those in rapid eye movement (REM) sleep (see Duron et al.[3] for a review). Therefore, respiration during sleep in normal humans is reviewed separately for these two sleep states.

Ventilation performs various secondary functions, such as speech and laughter in humans and thermoregulation in animals. For this reason, control systems and especially central nervous control systems are likely to be different in humans and in animals. In animal studies, the upper airways are usually bypassed in experiments; ventilation may then be altered during sleep because changes in upper airway resistance have a crucial role in breathing during sleep. Thus, in this chapter, reference to animal data is seldom made, although they may be used to replace missing human data or as sources for interpreting observations made in humans.

THE DEFINITION OF NORMALITY

The criteria of normality, whatever the field considered, depend on the methods used to assess the absence of abnormality. Thus, the composition of groups selected as "normal" will reflect these criteria, and their variability may result in variability in the observations made. The difficulty in establishing criteria for reference groups is of particular importance in the area of breathing during sleep, because breathing abnormalities during sleep have been related to such common conditions as male sex, increased age, excess weight, and snoring.

It must be kept in mind that respiratory measurement devices may alter breathing during sleep in at least two ways: (1) by direct effects on respiration and (2) by effects on sleep, and especially on sleep stability, which may in turn affect breathing stability.

NREM SLEEP

The four stages of NREM sleep are characterized by progressively slower electroencephalographic (EEG) activity associated with transients (spindles and K-complexes) in stages 2 and 3. Usually, NREM sleep is divided into light sleep (stages 1 and 2) and slow wave sleep (stages 3 and 4). When breathing during sleep is considered, it is more convenient to separate unsteady and steady sleep. At sleep onset, deep slow wave sleep is not attained immediately, but rather the level of vigilance oscillates from arousal to stages 1 and 2 for several minutes or tens of minutes before steady sleep in stage 2 and then stage 3 to 4 is reached. Thus, unsteady NREM sleep includes stage 1 and short periods of stage 2 interrupted by arousals, and steady NREM sleep includes stable stage 2 and stages 3 and 4.

Unsteady NREM Sleep

The irregularity of breathing at sleep onset struck early authors who studied breathing during sleep.[4] The irregularity was not random, however, but consisted of a regular waxing and waning of breathing amplitude. Thus, it was called periodic breathing (*periodische Athmung*).[4]

Periodic breathing at sleep onset and during drowsiness was later observed by many authors, but the most comprehensive study was that of Bülow.[5] *Periodic breathing* is defined as oscillations in breathing amplitude, which regularly decreases and increases. However, this definition is rather elastic, for the oscillations may be of low amplitude, resulting in alternating hyperventilation and hypoventilation, or of large amplitude, including apneas at the nadir of the oscillations. During the oscillations in amplitude, there are few if any changes in respiratory rate.[6] In different studies, the incidence of periodic breathing at sleep onset ranges from 40% to 80% of normal subjects. This variability may be related to the elastic definition of periodic breathing. Another possible explanation is the age of the subjects studied, because it has been suggested that the frequency of periodic breathing increases with age,[7,8] although this age relationship is not universally observed.[5] The pattern of periodic breathing (Fig. 19–1) resembles either Cheyne-Stokes respiration, with a progressive decrease and progressive increase in breathing amplitude before the apnea or hypopnea,[5,8] or Biot's breathing, with a progressive decrease in amplitude and then a brisk increase after the apnea, the first or second breath on breathing resumption being of maximal amplitude.[5]

The wavelength of periodic breathing is usually between 60 and 90 seconds[5] but has been found to range from 30 seconds[9] to 120 seconds.[8] The duration of the apnea itself ranges from 10 seconds[3,10] to 40 seconds[5,8] or more.[7] The apneas observed during drowsiness in normal subjects are generally of the central type,[6] meaning that the interruption (or decrease) of airflow is concomitant with an interruption (or decrease) of respiratory effort. However, obstructive apneas, during which

respiratory effort persists during the respiratory arrest, may occasionally be seen.[7]

Simultaneous EEG recordings have shown that the variations in breathing amplitude parallel variations in the level of vigilance.[5,11] The highest ventilatory levels are recorded during wakefulness or arousal; the progressive decrease in breathing amplitude is synchronous to falling asleep. Resumption of breathing, if it is sudden, usually corresponds to an arousal with reappearance of EEG alpha activity.

The duration of periodic breathing at sleep onset varies in length; it lasts from 10 to 20 minutes[5] up to 60 minutes.[8] Periodic breathing persists as long as sleep oscillates between arousal and stage 1 or 2; it disappears when stable stage 2 or deeper sleep is reached.[5] Because the respiratory system is controlled by negative feedback, it is prone to instability, the more so when the feedback loop gain (including the controller gain and the controlled system gain) or the delay between a change and its detection is high. An artificially increased, controlled system gain induces periodic breathing in normal subjects; periodic breathing was more likely to occur in men who had higher ventilatory responses to hypercapnia, an index of controller gain.[12] Because hypoxia induces an increase in the controller gain, this may be the mechanism of hypoxia-induced periodic breathing during sleep. Other theories have been proposed to explain the periodic breathing observed at

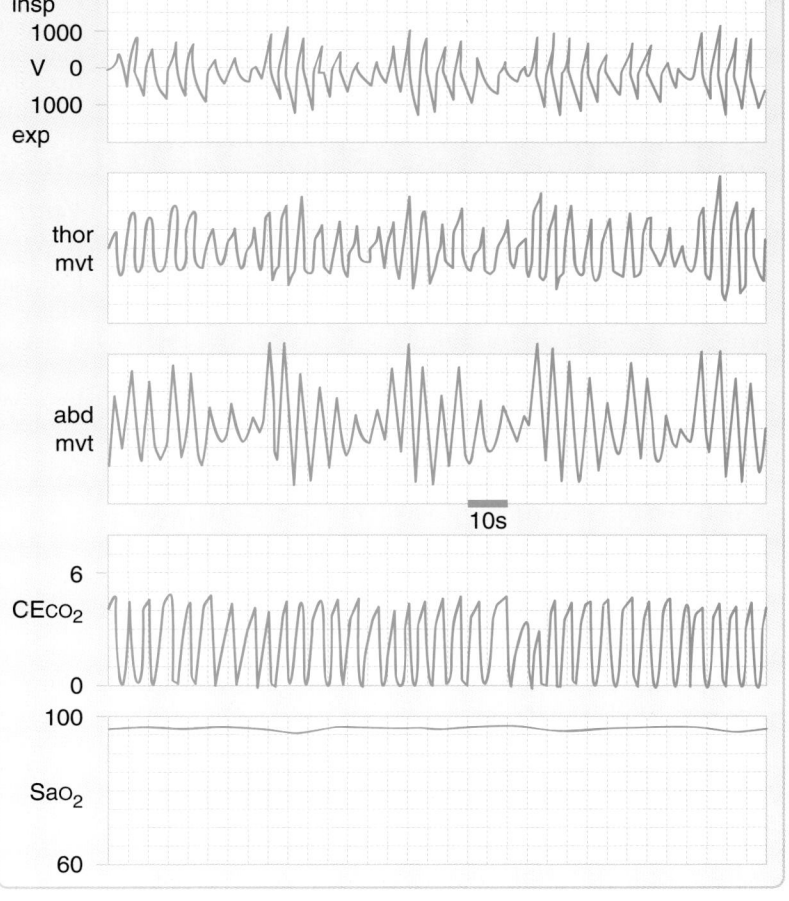

Figure 19–1. Typical breathing pattern during unsteady non–rapid eye movement sleep. CEco_2, CO_2 concentration (%) in the face mask; exp, expiration; insp, inspiration; Sao_2, oxygen saturation (%); thor mvt, abd mvt, thoracic and abdominal movements; V, ventilatory volumes (mL) obtained from a pneumotachograph attached to a face mask. (From Krieger J: Breathing during sleep in normal subjects. Clin Chest Med 1985;6:577-594.)

sleep onset.[13,14] Breathing instability at sleep onset would result from the combination of two factors:

1. The set point of regulation of ventilation is different in wakefulness and sleep, with a higher level of carbon dioxide partial pressure (PCO_2) and a lower ventilation during sleep.
2. Sleep onset is not immediate but rather oscillates between arousal, stage 1 sleep, and stage 2 sleep before stable stage 2 and then stages 3 and 4 sleep are reached.

Thus, falling asleep results in decreased ventilation and a higher PCO_2 adjusted to the sleep set point; on subsequent arousal, the increased PCO_2, above the wakefulness set point, constitutes an error signal that provokes hyperventilation until the wakefulness set point is reached. When the subject subsequently falls asleep, the level of PCO_2 will in turn be below the sleep set point, with resultant hypoventilation and so forth until stable sleep is reached.

According to this theory, breathing at sleep onset should be more unstable when (1) sleep is more unstable and the changes from arousal to sleep are sudden, (2) the difference between the wakefulness and sleep set points is greater, and (3) the ventilatory response to chemical stimuli is greater. These implications are in agreement with Bülow's observations.[5]

In other cases, especially in younger, healthy subjects, respiratory instability at sleep onset is aperiodic.[5,15] In those cases, the dependence of ventilatory instability on sleep–wake state has also been demonstrated;[15] the magnitude of sleep state–related fluctuations in ventilation increases over the sleep-onset period because of chemical amplification of sleep-state effects, and because of nonchemical factors.[16]

The waking state per se appears to stimulate breathing by a poorly understood mechanism. That this respiratory *wakefulness stimulus* is of crucial importance in sustaining breathing rhythmicity when chemical stimuli are reduced is suggested by posthyperventilation apnea, the occurrence of which is facilitated by falling asleep.[17,18] A threshold level of PCO_2 below which sleep apnea appears has been demonstrated.[14] Because of a delay between blood gas changes and the chemoreceptor response, hypercapnia and hypoxia can occur during periodic breathing. Models have shown that once hypoxia occurs during sleep, the intrinsic respiratory control mechanisms lead to breathing instability.[19,20] These models, although they fail to account for the initial disturbance resulting in the hypoxia that initiates periodic breathing, show that periodic breathing, once established, tends to be self-maintained. However, hypoxia does not have a key role in periodic breathing at sea level because periodic breathing is not suppressed by hyperoxic conditions.[5] Because hypoxia and hypercapnia are arousal stimuli,[21] sleep instability is further aggravated. Thus, sleep instability and intrinsic respiratory control mechanisms together create a vicious circle of breathing instability at sleep onset (for a review of the mechanisms of breathing instability at sleep onset, see Stradling et al.[22]). The increase in upper airway resistance related to sleep (see later) and the associated increase in respiratory effort probably contribute to this instability, because partial occlusion of the upper airways in normal subjects has been shown to produce central and obstructive apneas during sleep.[23] The information from the lungs to the centers does not seem to have a major role, because there is no difference in the occurrence of hypopneas and apneas or periodic

breathing between patients with heart–lung transplants and age-matched controls.[24] Stable sleep can be reached only if this vicious circle is somehow broken. It is likely that dampening systems, more probably neurogenic than chemical in nature, have a major role in allowing ventilation and sleep to reach a steady state.

Once instability is established, obstructive apneas may occur as a consequence of the different response of diaphragm and upper airway muscles to chemical stimuli.[24] A similar mechanism has been proposed to explain obstructive sleep apneas in sleep apnea syndromes, which suggests that these syndromes could result from an exaggeration of normal periodic breathing at sleep onset.[25,26] However, in normal subjects, auditory-induced arousals, although followed by transient hyperpnea, do not induce secondary hypopnea or apnea.[27]

Thus, breathing at sleep onset is physiologically unstable, but the magnitude of the instability is variable, ranging from small fluctuations in breathing amplitude, which result in increased indices of variability during light NREM sleep stages,[28] to severe periodic breathing with repeated apneas. The extremes of this range overlap with what may be called sleep apnea syndromes in regard to both duration and frequency of apneas.

Because of the instability of ventilation during light NREM sleep, these periods have often been disregarded in studies of ventilatory parameters during sleep, so little is known about them. On average, ventilation decreases and PCO_2 increases during periodic breathing.[5] In addition, there is oscillation in oxygen saturation (SaO_2) (see Fig. 19–1); however, the extent of these SaO_2 oscillations is not clear.

During periods of stage 1 sleep devoid of periodic breathing, minute ventilation decreases to a level intermediate between that of wakefulness and that of stage 2 sleep[14]; alveolar PCO_2 then increases by a mean of about 1 mm Hg.[14]

Steady NREM Sleep

Ventilation

During steady NREM sleep, breathing is remarkably regular in both amplitude and frequency,[5,10,29,30] resulting in the lowest indices of variability of all sleep stages[5] (Fig. 19–2). There is a decrease in minute ventilation during steady slow wave sleep, compared with wakefulness, although in some reports the changes are not statistically significant. The decrease in minute ventilation ranges from 0.4 to 1.5 L/min.

When all available data are averaged, the decrease in minute ventilation is about 13% of the wakefulness value in sleep stage 2 and about 15% in stage 3 to 4[31] (Fig. 19–3). Thus, ventilation appears to decrease progressively from stage 1 to stage 4,[32] which suggests that the decrease is not merely the consequence of the suppression of a wakefulness stimulus for breathing. It could be related to a progressive decrease in metabolic rate[33] with deepening of sleep, a possibility that is, however, contradicted by the progressive increase in PCO_2 with deepening of NREM sleep.[5] Thus, it is more likely that the decrease in minute ventilation during NREM sleep is linked to active sleep mechanisms.

It is unclear whether the decrease in minute ventilation is caused by a decrease in tidal volume or a decrease in respiratory frequency, or both. Most studies report a decrease in tidal volume that averages 16% in stage 2 and 18.5% in

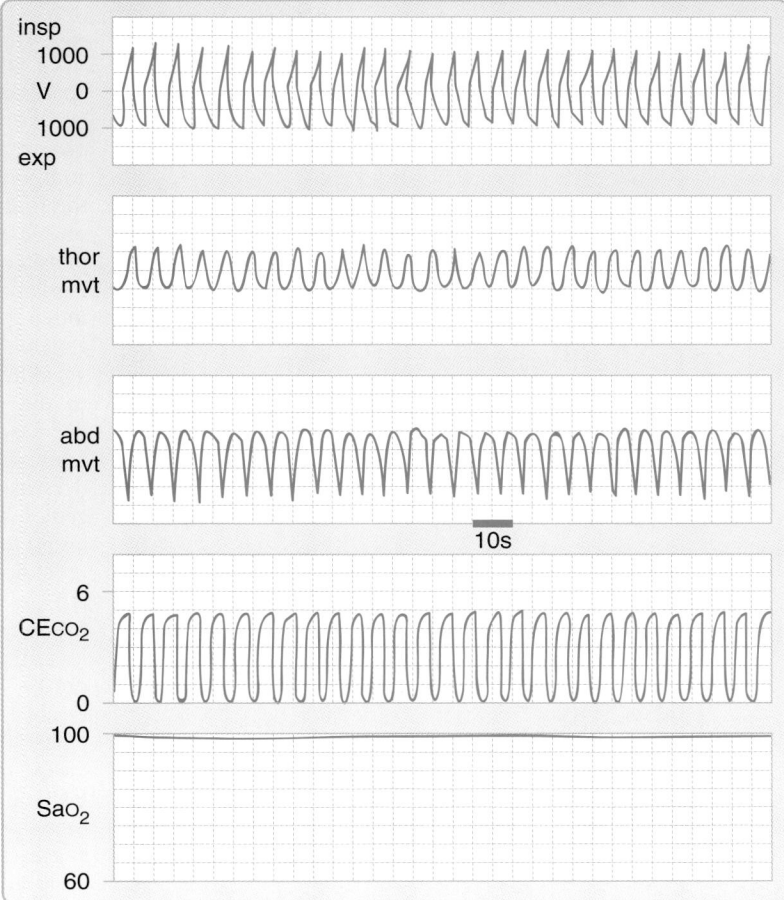

Figure 19–2. Typical breathing pattern during steady non–rapid eye movement sleep. CEco$_2$, CO$_2$ concentration (%) in the face mask; exp, expiration; insp, inspiration; Sao$_2$, oxygen saturation (%); thor mvt, abd mvt, thoracic and abdominal movements; V, ventilatory volumes (mL) obtained from a pneumotachograph attached to a face mask. (From Krieger J: Breathing during sleep in normal subjects. Clin Chest Med 1985;6:577-594.)

stage 3 to 4 (see Fig. 19–3). Generally, the greater the wakefulness tidal volume and the more invasive the respiratory device, the greater is the decrease in sleep tidal volume, which suggests that nonadaptation to the experimental conditions may have a role. In terms of minute ventilation, the decrease in tidal volume is aggravated or partially compensated for by a decrease or an increase in respiratory rate, depending on the study considered, but on average, changes in respiratory rate are minimal (see Fig. 19–3).

The changes in ventilation observed during NREM sleep in humans are different from those observed in animals,[2] in which the decrease in minute ventilation is the result of a decrease in respiratory rate incompletely compensated for by an increase in tidal volume. This fact emphasizes why the greatest care must be used in extrapolating results from animals to humans.

Respiratory timing has been less often analyzed during NREM sleep than have minute ventilation and tidal volume. Inspiratory and expiratory durations have been found to change diversely during sleep, compared with wakefulness.[22,28,34,35] As a result, the duty cycle of breathing (T_I/T_{TOT}) has been seen to increase,[6,36] to not change,[22] or to decrease.[34] None of these changes were statistically significant, which suggests that the fluctuations occur at random. In all of these studies, the mean inspiratory flow (V_I/T_I) decreased; the reduction ranged from 0.02 to 0.50 L/sec.

In conclusion, quantitative studies show that ventilation during steady NREM sleep is lower than during wakefulness, and the deeper the NREM sleep stages, the lower is the ventilation. Mean inspiratory flow is decreased, whereas there are no consistent changes in inspiratory duration and cycle duration; the result is a decreased tidal volume.

Rib Cage and Abdominal Contributions

Most studies of the thoracic and abdominal contributions to breathing during sleep report an increased rib cage contribution.[4,22,30,35,37,38] This increase involves mainly lateral expansion of the rib cage.

The increase in rib cage contribution to tidal volume is accompanied by an increase in the respiratory electromyographic (EMG) activity of the intercostal muscles,[3,35,39] diaphragmatic respiratory activity being a little increased[35] or unchanged[39] (but decreased when alveolar Pco$_2$ is maintained at a constant level).[40] The increased thoracoabdominal muscle activity results in increased esophageal pressure swings.[39] The contradiction between increased EMG activity and decreased flow rate suggests either impaired muscular efficiency or increased airway resistance.[3,39] Impaired muscular efficiency is unlikely because of the observation that transdiaphragmatic pressure is increased with no change in diaphragmatic activity.[39]

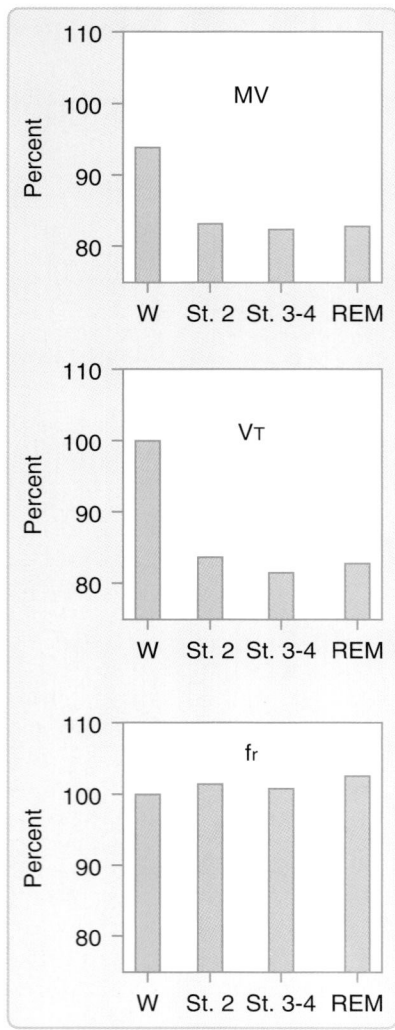

Figure 19–3. Changes in respiratory parameters during non–rapid eye movement sleep (stages 2 [St. 2] and 3/4 [St. 3-4]) and during rapid eye movement (REM) sleep. The data are computed (from references 5, 22, 28, 31, 34, 35, 37, 39, 55, 66, and 100) as the average percentage of the wakefulness (W) value of minute ventilation (MV) = 7.17 L·min^{-1}, tidal volume (VT) = 471 mL, and respiratory frequency (fr) = 15.4 cycles·min^{-1}.

Upper Airway Resistance

Contrary to early studies, a large increase (230%) has been shown to occur in total airway resistance during NREM sleep.[39] The resistance of the upper airway (above the retroepiglottic space) increases more than twofold,[41] whereas the elastic or flow-resistive properties of the lung are not altered. The sleep-related increase in upper airway resistance is much more important during mouth breathing than during nose breathing.[42] The site of the increased resistance is palatal or hypopharyngeal.[43]

The finding of an increased upper airway resistance during sleep is in keeping with changes in the EMG activity of upper airway muscles during sleep. Using transcutaneous recordings of suprahyoid and infrahyoid muscles, Berger[44] observed a continual discrete decrease in the EMG activity of "laryngeal" muscles from wakefulness to stage 2 sleep. Because of the

possible implications of the changes in upper airway muscle activity for the mechanism of upper airway obstruction during sleep apnea, many muscles have been investigated more specifically during sleep by use of wire electrodes.

Two aspects of muscle activity must be considered: the phasic activity, which occurs periodically, in phase with a component of the respiratory cycle, generally inspiration; and the tonic activity, which is the background activity on which phasic activity is superimposed.[45] Whereas the regulation of phasic activity is clearly related to respiratory regulation, the regulation of the tonic background is probably more or less independent of respiratory regulation and more related to the general muscle tone. Sleep-related changes in phasic activity are different in the various muscles investigated: unchanged in the geniohyoid,[46] increased in the genioglossus,[47] and decreased in the posterior cricoarytenoid.[48] The changes in tonic activity are more consistent, because it was found to decrease in the tensor veli palatini,[49] the genioglossus,[50] the geniohyoid,[46] and the posterior cricoarytenoid,[48] but it was found to be unchanged in the genioglossus in other studies.[49,51] It is noteworthy that the decrease in tonic activity of the tensor veli palatini was correlated with the increase in nasopharyngeal resistance.[49] Furthermore, the genioglossus is less responsive to chemical stimuli or resistive loading than during wakefulness,[52] and the negative pressure reflex, which is able to maintain genioglossus muscle activation during negative pressure ventilation during wakefulness, is unable to do so during sleep.[53] The contrast between the decreased EMG activity of upper airway muscles and the increased or maintained activity of intercostal and diaphragmatic muscles suggests different neural control of these muscle groups.

In addition to decreased EMG activity of dilating muscles, the decrease in lung volume that occurs during NREM sleep[54,55] probably concurs to increase upper airway resistance during sleep, because it has been shown that lung inflation decreases upper airway resistance.[56] The thoracic volume dependence of upper airway resistance does not seem to be mediated by a decrease in upper airway muscle activity.[57]

The resulting increase in upper airway resistance has a role in the decrease in ventilation during sleep. During wakefulness, an added external inspiratory resistance, similar in magnitude to the increase in upper airway resistance observed during NREM sleep, results in decreased mean inspiratory flow compensated for by changes in respiratory timing (increased inspiratory time and decreased expiratory time), which results in an increased tidal volume. Despite a decreased respiratory rate, minute ventilation is maintained, but at the expense of increased respiratory work.[58] The ability to maintain minute ventilation is reduced during NREM sleep, because the mouth occlusion pressure, a measure of the respiratory drive, which is markedly increased during wakefulness, is unchanged during NREM sleep under these loading conditions.[37] An acute resistive load of about 20 cm H_2O/L/sec (i.e., in the order of magnitude of the change in upper airway resistance during NREM sleep) has more effects on ventilation than during wakefulness[37,59]; after sustained loading of 12 cm H_2O/L/sec, tidal volume and minute ventilation returned to baseline values. However, a lower load of 4, 7, or 10 cm H_2O/L/sec decreased tidal volume and minute ventilation similarly during wakefulness and NREM sleep.[60]

The effect of increased upper airway resistance on ventilation during sleep is further demonstrated by the effects of preventing the physiologic increase in upper airway resistance with nasal continuous positive airway pressure (CPAP), which is followed by an increase in ventilation, even when end-tidal $PaCO_2$ is held constant,[61] a finding that was not confirmed in another similar work,[62] in which CPAP did not correct the sleep-related decrease in ventilation and increase in end-tidal PCO_2, although total pulmonary resistance returned to wake values. However, in this latter study, the subjects were selected for the absence of obesity and of snoring, and the sleep-related increase in pulmonary resistance was much less. Thus, it can be concluded that increased upper airway resistance is one factor contributing to decreased ventilation during sleep, especially when the increase in upper airway resistance is large. Recent data show that changes in upper airway resistance contribute to the decrease in ventilation early at sleep onset, whereas during stable NREM sleep, larger increases in upper airway resistance are compensated for, so that ventilation decreases less than upper airway resistance increases.[63] Data from otherwise normal, laryngectomized subjects show that increased upper airway resistance during sleep is not the only factor of decreased ventilation and CO_2 retention.[64]

In addition, a decreased respiratory drive has also been demonstrated: mouth occlusion pressure decreases during NREM sleep; furthermore, when compared at equal alveolar CO_2 levels, the EMG activities of intercostal and diaphragmatic muscles are lower during NREM sleep than during wakefulness.[65] Thus, the mechanisms of decreased ventilation during sleep involve both a decrease in ventilatory drive and an impaired efficacy of the respiratory pump due to increased upper airway resistance.

Arterial Blood Gases

Alveolar ventilation also decreases during NREM sleep, as reflected by higher alveolar and arterial PCO_2. Alveolar and arterial PCO_2 values increase by 3 to 7 mm Hg during NREM sleep.[5,10,17,29,34] A few studies found increases of 2 mm Hg or less, or no change.[6,14,66,67]

The reduction in alveolar ventilation decreases alveolar and arterial PO_2 (ranging from 3.5 to 9.4 mm Hg)[66] and SaO_2 (2% or less).[68] These changes occur despite a reduced metabolic rate, reflected by 10% to 20% decreases of O_2 consumption and CO_2 production.[5,33,69-71]

Pulmonary Arterial Pressure

Pulmonary arterial pressures have rarely been investigated during sleep in normal subjects. During light NREM sleep, periodic oscillations of pulmonary arterial pressure with a period of 20 to 30 seconds occurred in one of three subjects[9]; they occurred even during regular, steady breathing. On average, both diastolic and systolic pulmonary arterial pressures increased by 4 to 5 mm Hg during NREM sleep.[10]

Effects of Arousal

Induced transient arousal from NREM sleep (a brief change in EEG without awakening) results in an increase in EMG activity of the diaphragm (150% of wake level) and of upper airway dilating muscles (levator veli palatini, 250%; genioglossus, 150%),[72] together with an increase in maximum inspiratory flow and tidal volume (160%) and a decrease in upper airway

resistance,[27] but auditory stimuli without EEG arousal cause no change in ventilation.

REM SLEEP

Ventilation

When Aserinsky and Kleitman[73] first described a hitherto unidentified sleep stage characterized by low-voltage EEG activity and regularly occurring periods of ocular motility, they mentioned, among other associated periodic phenomena, an increased respiratory frequency. This sleep stage was called REM sleep and was identified as the stage during which dreams occur. Later, breathing during REM sleep was described as irregular (Fig. 19–4). The irregularity consists of sudden changes in both respiratory amplitude and frequency,[3,5,35,74-76] at times interrupted by central apneas lasting 10 to 30 seconds,[3,32] and is different from the regular periodic breathing at sleep onset. The breathing irregularities do not occur at random but are linked to bursts of rapid eye movements.[5,77,78] The first eye movement of a REM burst is associated with a sudden decrease in breathing amplitude, followed by a progressive increase even when the REM burst is prolonged.[77] Although it was first considered to be part of the emotional reaction to the dream content,[75] Aserinsky[77] later ascribed this breathing pattern to REM sleep processes per se. In animals, this irregular pattern persists during hypoxia, hypercapnia, and metabolic alkalosis, as well as after vagotomy and chemodenervation.[2] For these reasons, it has been suggested that the breathing pattern is not dependent on chemical regulation processes but is produced by activation of the behavioral respiratory control system by REM sleep processes.[13] Nevertheless, ventilation over prolonged periods (i.e., 3 to 25 minutes) was found to be highly correlated with O_2 consumption and CO_2 production in REM sleep, as well as in NREM sleep,[33] which indicates that the chemical regulation of ventilation is not abolished in REM sleep.

Quantitative measurements of ventilation in REM sleep in normal subjects show a variable decrease in minute ventilation, compared with that in wakefulness. However, the comparison with NREM ventilation reveals discrepancies: minute ventilation in REM sleep has been found to be increased,[5,33,35] slightly decreased,[22,28,32] markedly decreased,[66] or unchanged; in addition to reflecting the same methodologic problems as in NREM sleep, these discrepancies may be due to differences in the choice of the REM sleep period selected for analysis, because minute ventilation is lower during phasic REM sleep, when REM bursts are abundant, than during tonic REM sleep, when REM bursts are absent.[36] In addition, body movements, which frequently occur during REM sleep, may alter both the level of ventilation and the calibration of indirect measurement of ventilatory flow.[79] Parallel to reported discrepancies in minute ventilation changes, tidal volume changes also vary. Tidal volume has been found to be decreased, unchanged,[32,35,66] or increased[39] in REM sleep, compared with NREM sleep, and the respiratory frequency was either slightly increased[35,66] or slightly decreased.[32,39] V_I/T_I has been described as unchanged or increased.[6] All these studies, however, report an unchanged T_I/T_{TOT}. Thus, the available data on breathing during REM sleep in normal humans are somewhat discordant. Nevertheless, when all available data are averaged, minute ventilation, tidal volume, and respiratory rate during REM sleep differ little from those observed in NREM sleep (see Fig. 19–3).

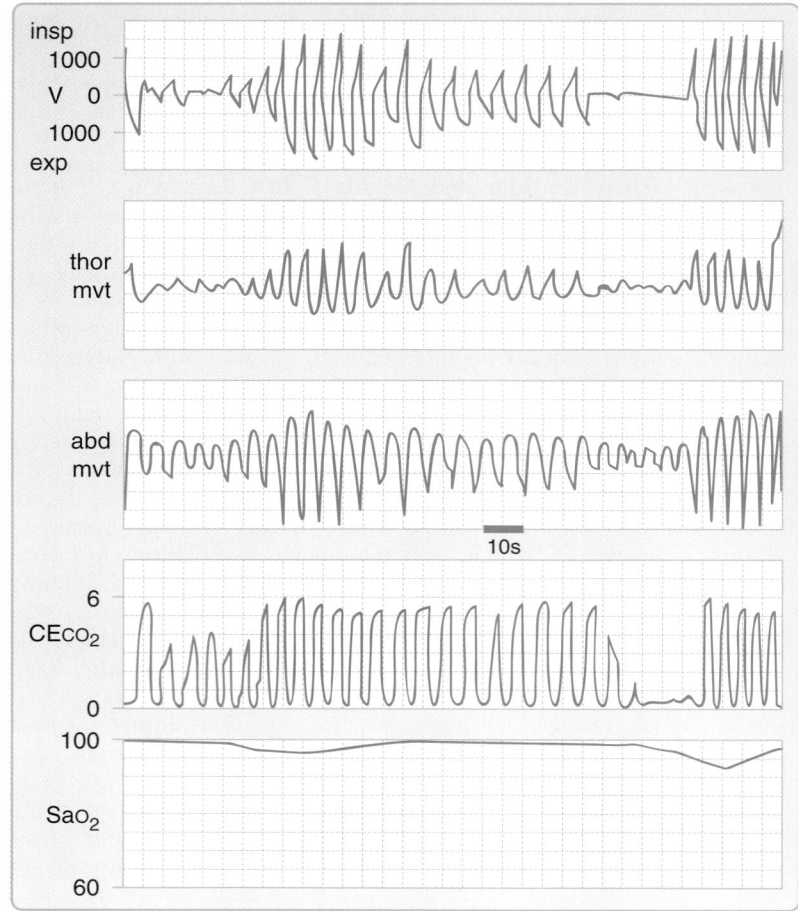

Figure 19–4. Typical breathing pattern during rapid eye movement sleep. $CEco_2$, CO_2 concentration (%) in the face mask; exp, expiration; insp, inspiration; Sao_2, oxygen saturation (%); thor mvt, abd mvt, thoracic and abdominal movements; V, ventilatory volumes (mL) obtained from a pneumotachograph attached to a face mask.

Rib Cage and Abdominal Contributions

In contrast to the increased rib cage contribution to breathing during NREM sleep, the rib cage contribution during REM sleep is found to be decreased,[3,6] owing to a marked reduction in intercostal muscle activity,[6,23] or to be unchanged.[22] Diaphragmatic activity, both tonic and phasic inspiratory[35,39] or only phasic,[68] is increased. In addition, even though paradoxical thoracoabdominal movements are not observed, thoracic and abdominal displacements are not exactly in phase.[3] Despite the increase in diaphragmatic activity, transdiaphragmatic pressure is decreased, which implies impaired muscle efficiency.[39] The decreased intercostal EMG activity is attributed to the REM-related supraspinal inhibition of the alpha motoneuron drive and the specific depression of fusimotor function.[73] Because the diaphragm's fusorial innervation is quite low, this muscle is relatively spared from the depressive effects described.[80]

Upper Airway Resistance

Airway resistance measurements during REM sleep are also contradictory. Total airway resistance was said to be lower during REM sleep than during NREM sleep, with large individual variations; but on average, airway resistance in REM sleep is similar to that of awake humans.[81] In contrast, other studies show an increase in upper airway resistance during REM sleep that is approximately the same as in NREM sleep, or intermediate between wakefulness and NREM sleep,[41]

whereas the lower airway resistance is unchanged. The upper airway resistance would be expected to be highest during REM sleep, because the muscular atonia of the upper airway is maximal during this sleep stage,[44,50] but this has been much less investigated than during NREM sleep.

Arterial Blood Gases

In contrast to the abundant literature concerning changes in oxygenation during REM sleep in patients with chronic obstructive pulmonary disease, data on oxygenation during REM sleep in normal subjects are surprisingly few. Some studies on blood oxygenation during sleep report an unchanged O_2 level during REM sleep compared with NREM sleep,[35] whereas others give lower values in REM than in NREM sleep.[36,68] REM values are always reported as lower than wakefulness values, including both a sustained[68] drop and further transient drops in Sao_2 in conjunction with REM-related hypoventilation.[68,77] Pco_2 is even more difficult to evaluate during REM sleep. End-tidal Pco_2 does not yield an approximation of alveolar Pco_2 because end-expiratory plateaus are seldom reached during the rapid, shallow breathing pattern characteristic of REM sleep. Because arterial values have been only occasionally measured during sleep in normal subjects, the lack of reliable information on Pco_2 is probably a cause of the controversy with respect to the mechanisms of hypoxemia during REM sleep. Some authors argue that no sustained hypoventilation can be demonstrated and instead incriminate impaired lung mechanics.[68] According to these hypotheses, loss of intercostal and, to a lesser extent, diaphragmatic tonic activity results in a decreased baseline position of rib cage and abdomen and thus in a decreased functional residual capacity, which leads to airway closure in the dependent lung regions and a consequent ventilation–perfusion mismatch. However, the measured decrease in functional residual capacity is too low, both in REM and in NREM sleep, to be likely to produce a significant ventilation–perfusion mismatch, at least in normal subjects.[55] Thus, it seems probable that the hypoxemia observed during REM sleep is the result of hypoventilation.

Conclusions

Drowsiness or unsteady NREM sleep is characterized in many subjects by a regularly oscillating periodic breathing that results in swings in partial pressure of oxygen (PO_2) and PCO_2, with an overall moderate decrease in ventilation (Table 19–1). These oscillations seem to be mainly due to sleep instability during this stage, and the natural tendency of breathing regulation to be unstable probably aggravates this situation.

In steady NREM sleep, there occurs a regular pattern of breathing with more pronounced hypoventilation than during drowsiness. This hypoventilation seems to result from a combination of decreased ventilatory drive and a sleep-related defective compensation of an increased upper airway resistance. Ventilatory mechanics do not seem to be impaired during NREM sleep.

REM sleep is characterized by erratic, shallow breathing with irregularities both in amplitude and in frequency synchronous to REM bursts that are most probably of central origin and related to REM sleep processes. Hypoxemia equal to or greater than that during NREM sleep seems mainly to result from hypoventilation.

RESPIRATION-RELATED EVENTS DURING SLEEP

Snoring

Snoring is reviewed in greater detail in Chapter 83. In a survey of 4713 people, it was found that 41% of men and 28% of women were occasional or habitual snorers.[82] After the age of 60 years, the figure rises to 60% of men and 40% of women. This high frequency, confirmed by other studies, may explain why snoring is considered to be normal, annoying only to the snorer's bedroom partner, who usually calls for treatment for the snorer.

Table 19–1. Summary of Breathing Patterns during Sleep in Normal Subjects

Breathing Pattern	Type of Sleep
Periodic	Unsteady NREM sleep
Regular	Steady NREM sleep
Mostly regular	"Tonic" REM sleep
Irregular; central apneas common	"Phasic" REM sleep

NREM, Non–rapid eye movement; REM, rapid eye movement.

Snoring may be more than an acoustic nuisance, however. Systemic hypertension, cardiac dysfunction, angina pectoris, and cerebral infarction are more frequent among habitual snorers,[82,83] even when the data are corrected for the effects of increased age, male sex, and obesity, which are more frequent among snorers[82] and are factors contributing to these diseases. The link between blood pressure and snoring seems to be close; Robin[84] had a patient who knew his blood pressure had increased when he was told he snored more heavily. The immediate rise in systemic blood pressure during snoring has been confirmed by polygraphic recordings.[85]

However, because sleep apnea syndromes are frequent in otherwise asymptomatic snorers (30% to 50%), it is not clear whether these diseases (hypertension, angina pectoris, and cerebral infarction) are a consequence of snoring by itself or of the associated obstructive sleep apnea syndrome. Nevertheless, even in nonapneic snorers, the resistance of the upper airways during sleep increases more than in nonsnorers, with resultant distortion of the rib cage, which might cause an increase in respiratory work or hypoventilation during sleep.[86] That snoring is by itself a factor contributing to hypoxemia is further demonstrated by the effects of nasal CPAP on patients with sleep apnea: the elimination of snoring by an increase in the applied pressure is regularly accompanied by an increase in oxyhemoglobin saturation. Snoring may be considered to be part of a continuum including normal, silent, unobstructed breathing; occasional snoring; habitual snoring with occasional obstructive sleep apneas; and, finally, an overt[81,87] obstructive sleep apnea syndrome. However, the male-to-female ratio of snoring, which is roughly 2:1, is fairly different from the male-to-female ratio of the obstructive sleep apnea syndrome, which is 9:1; this suggests that the link between obstructive sleep apnea and snoring is not as close as postulated.

Sighs

Sighs are deep breaths with higher-than-average tidal volumes. The function of the sigh during wakefulness is to open collapsed alveoli and hence to increase the pulmonary compliance and functional residual capacity,[88] thus preventing atelectasis. Sighing during sleep may thus be of crucial importance. Among normal sleeping subjects, wide intersubject variability was reported, ranging from 1 to 25 sighs per night.[89] Sighs occur in all sleep stages, including REM sleep, but with a higher frequency in light NREM sleep. Sighs are also often associated with arousals. Finally, sighs are often followed by apneas, hypoventilation, or a decreased respiratory frequency.[6,65]

FACTORS INFLUENCING BREATHING IN SLEEPING NORMAL SUBJECTS

Sex

None of the sleep studies, including quantitative measurement of breathing parameters, demonstrates a significant difference between sexes with respect to changes in minute ventilation, tidal volume, or respiratory rate. However, the increase in upper airway resistance is much more important in men than in women.[90] It has been suggested that female hormones have a significant effect on the upper dilator muscles, peaking during the luteal phase, lower during the follicular phase, and lowest after menopause.[91] A sex-related difference is also suggested by a greater frequency of episodes of O_2 desaturation during both NREM and REM sleep in normal men compared with normal women.[7] Yet, a greater frequency of disordered breathing has not been confirmed by other studies.[32,92] Because increased frequencies of desaturation episodes are also associated with excess weight, it was suggested that the male predominance of desaturation episodes during sleep could be an artifact resulting from poor body weight matching between sex groups.[92]

Age

Because of maturational differences in the central nervous system and muscle and osteochondral structures, the problems of respiration during sleep in newborns, infants, and children are different from those in adults (see Ferber and Kryger[93]). Adolescents' breathing patterns during sleep closely resemble those of young adults.[6] Tabachnik et al.,[35] however, noticed less marked O_2 desaturation during REM sleep in the adolescents they studied; they attributed this to the lower closing capacity in adolescents, which results in less ventilation–perfusion mismatching because of the decrease in the functional–residual capacity during REM sleep. In young adults of both sexes, no nocturnal desaturation was observed either.[94]

Studies of breathing during sleep in normal adults have demonstrated more periodic breathing[8] and episodes of O_2 desaturation among older subjects. Several investigations have focused specifically on ventilation during sleep in subjects older than 55 years who were in good health and had no sleep or respiratory complaints[86,92,95,96] or in randomly selected older subjects. Despite a variability among studies concerning the definition of sleep-related breathing disorders, there was striking agreement that among these normal subjects, 30% to 60% fulfilled the generally accepted criterion of sleep apnea syndrome—more than five apneas or episodes of sleep-disordered breathing per hour of sleep. Only one study found fewer than 2% of older subjects fulfilling this criterion.[97] However, in this study, snorers had been excluded, even when they were otherwise healthy. Given the high frequency of snorers, especially among older subjects, the sample studied was not representative of the general population of normal older subjects. This bias might explain the difference with respect to other studies.

Apneas in older sleeping subjects are of both the central and the obstructive type.[32,96] The mean number and duration of apneas do not differ between older subjects having more than five apneas per hour of sleep and subjects diagnosed as having obstructive sleep apnea syndrome.[95] In addition, they closely resemble typical patients with sleep apnea with respect to the number and depth of desaturation episodes.[96] This close similarity raises the important question of why sleep apneas in older subjects may have little effect on health. Not only did most of these subjects exhibit none of the symptoms associated with sleep apnea syndrome but also their future does not seem to be jeopardized by sleep apneas.[39,92]

The underlying mechanisms of sleep apneas in normal older subjects remain uncertain. No clear relationship to body weight, increased awake airway resistance, or chemoreceptor responses has been demonstrated.[96] Speculations include altered endocrine function, use of alcohol and hypnotic drugs,[96] and an aggravation of normal periodic breathing.[28,32] Physiologic periodic breathing at sleep onset may be aggravated by larger differences between the wakefulness and sleep ventilation set points, higher controller gain, increased circulatory delay from the lung to the chemoreceptors, or increased sleep instability.

The decrease in minute ventilation from wakefulness to sleep does not differ between older subjects with and those without high sleep apnea indices, or between older and younger subjects,[32] which suggests that the difference in the ventilation set points between wakefulness and sleep is not increased in older subjects with sleep apneas. The ventilatory response to chemical stimuli is not greater in these subjects.[96] A delayed circulatory time is not likely to occur in healthy older subjects, in whom blood velocity should be slightly increased because of stiffening of the arterial walls. Decrease in deep slow wave sleep stages and more awakening with increasing age have been demonstrated.[65,98] It has been suggested that a primary increase in sleep instability in older subjects could be a factor leading to increased breathing instability, which results in apneas of both the central and obstructive type.[28,32] This hypothesis is in keeping with the predominance of sleep-disordered breathing in older subjects during light slow wave sleep, and it is in keeping with the fact that the frequency of periodic breathing in younger subjects is similar to the frequency of high rates of apneas in older subjects. Furthermore, an increased rate of apneas could be merely a consequence of increased sleep instability resulting from the invasiveness of sleep recording techniques and the spontaneous fragility of sleep in older subjects. This hypothesis would explain the absence of repercussions of sleep-disordered breathing on the health of these subjects.

Aside from sleep-disordered breathing episodes, the ventilatory parameters in sleeping older subjects have been little investigated. Only Krieger et al.[95] and Shore et al.[28] have analyzed minute ventilation, tidal volume, and respiratory frequency quantitatively. They found a decrease in minute ventilation during steady NREM sleep that was similar in magnitude to that found in younger subjects.[32] It resulted from a smaller tidal volume despite a slightly higher ventilatory frequency.[95] In addition, in older subjects, the sleep-related decrease in the hypercapnic ventilatory response is not different from that seen in younger subjects.[99]

In middle-aged normal subjects, the occurrence of sleep-disordered breathing was intermediate between younger and older subjects, but the change in minute ventilation, tidal volume, and respiratory rate was of the same order of magnitude.[100]

Pregnancy

Because of a reduced functional residual capacity and residual volume, as well as a reduced cardiac output in the supine position, pregnant women could be exposed to more severe hypoxemia during sleep. A study of breathing during sleep in women at 36 weeks of gestation and postpartum did not show more severe hypoxemia during pregnancy. Indeed, hypopneas and apneas were less frequent during pregnancy, probably because of the respiratory stimulatory effects of progesterone.[101,102] However, these results, involving only normal women, may perhaps not be extended to pathologic conditions of pregnancy (see Chapter 109).

On the other hand, snoring is common in pregnancy,[103] and snoring women have an increased risk for growth retardation of the fetus.[103] They also have an increased rate of preeclampsia,[104,105] with its associated greater inspiratory flow limitation[105] and upper airway narrowing.[104]

Drugs

Many drugs probably interfere with breathing during sleep.[106] The effects of alcohol on ventilation in awake subjects are either depressive or stimulatory[107,108]; the effects on basic ventilatory parameters during sleep have not been studied. In a group of 20 asymptomatic men aged 20 to 65 years, alcohol significantly increased the number of apneas and the number of episodes of desaturation occurring in conjunction with, as well as independently of, episodes of hypoventilation; the mean duration of hypopneas and apneas was increased.[109] These effects of alcohol are observed in men but not in women (even postmenopausal women).[110] Similar effects of alcohol on obstructive sleep apneas have been shown in the sleep apnea syndrome.[111,112] Even though the type of apnea—central or obstructive—was not specified,[109] it can be speculated that alcohol exerts its deleterious effect on breathing during sleep through its depressive effects on upper airway muscle activity,[113] with resultant increased pharyngeal resistance. This opinion is reinforced by the observation that alcohol induces or aggravates snoring,[111] which results from an imbalance between an increased airflow and decreased upper airway tone. The alcohol-induced lengthening of apneas may be due to its depressive effects on arousal systems,[109,114] given that arousal probably has a key role in protective respiratory mechanisms during sleep.[21] These mechanisms, however, do not explain the aggravating effects of alcohol on desaturation episodes unrelated to obvious hypoventilation.

Benzodiazepines have effects on sleep apneas[86] and on snoring[115] similar to those of alcohol in normal subjects. These effects may be due to the depressive respiratory effects of benzodiazepines[86]; however, the same mechanisms as those suggested for alcohol—namely, upper airway muscle hypotonia and arousal depressant effects—may be involved in the effects of benzodiazepines on breathing during sleep.

Deleterious effects of alcohol and benzodiazepines are not observed in all subjects studied, which raises the question of whether the subjects sensitive to these drugs, even though asymptomatic, are normal, or whether they should be considered as having latent sleep apnea syndromes revealed by these drugs. The effects of alcohol and benzodiazepines, both of which are widely used, and their possible combination or potentiation may be hazardous. Sleep-disordered breathing may be one of the mechanisms of the reduced longevity associated with the use of these drugs.[116]

CONCLUSIONS

Sleep is associated with definite changes in respiratory function in normal humans. Whether these changes serve a specific function remains unclear and will probably not be clarified before the functions of sleep itself are better understood.

Ventilation during sleep appears to be fragile, being prone to instability, upper airway obstruction, hypoventilation, and ventilation–perfusion mismatch, thus jeopardizing the homeostatic function of CO_2 output and O_2 uptake that it is supposed to serve.

Although the other automatic homeostatic functions are executed by the autonomic nervous system (an important exception being the thermoregulatory function), ventilation, in addition to its homeostatic function, is also under voluntary control by the conscious nervous system. Voluntarily controlled ventilation gives rise to a conflict when consciousness is periodically abolished and motor control is subjected to central nervous system influences specific to sleep. This conflict is incompletely solved in humans. A possible solution would be to sleep like dolphins: alternately and independently with either cerebral hemisphere.[117]

Clinical Pearl

The clinician should keep in mind that there are normal changes in respiration associated with sleep, including an increase in upper airway resistance, and breathing instability in the form of periodic breathing at sleep onset and erratic breathing during REM sleep, which do not imply a breathing abnormality and do not require specific treatment. However, the frontier between normal sleep-associated changes and pathology requires further clarification.

Acknowledgments

I wish to thank Emmanuel Weitzenblum for his helpful advice and Marie-Rose Boh and Véronique Fehr for secretarial assistance.

References

1. Saunders NA, Sullivan CE (eds): Sleep and Breathing. New York, Marcel Dekker, 1984.
2. Sullivan CE: Breathing in sleep. In Orem J, Barnes CD (eds): Physiology in Sleep. New York, Academic Press, 1980, pp 214-272.
3. Duron B, Tassinari CA, Gastaut H: Analyse spirographique et électromyographique de la respiration au cours du sommeil contrôlé par l'EEG chez l'homme normal. Rev Neurol (Paris) 1966; 115:562-574.
4. Mosso A: Periodische Athmung and Luxusathmung. Arch Physiol 1886;(Suppl):37-116.
5. Bülow K: Respiration and wakefulness in man. Acta Physiol Scand Suppl 1963;209:1-110.
6. Duron B, Andrag C, Laval P: Ventilation pulmonaire globale, CO_2 alvéolaire et consommation d'oxygène au cours du sommeil normal. C R Seances Soc Biol Fil 1968;162:139-145.
7. Block AJ, Boysen PG, Wynne JW, et al: Sleep apnea, hypopnea and oxygen desaturation in normal subjects: A strong male predominance. N Engl J Med 1979;300:513-517.
8. Webb P: Periodic breathing during sleep. J Appl Physiol 1974; 37:899-903.
9. Lugaresi E, Coccagna G, Mantovani M, et al: Some periodic phenomena arising during drowsiness and sleep in man. Electroencephalogr Clin Neurophysiol 1972;32:701-705.
10. Lugaresi E, Coccagna G, Farnetti P, et al: Snoring. Electroencephalogr Clin Neurophysiol 1975;39:59-64.
11. de Groen JHM: Influence of diffuse brain stimulation (DBS) on human sleep: II. Sleep-induced periodic breathing with apnea. Electroencephalogr Clin Neurophysiol 1979;46:696-701.
12. Chapman KR, Bruce EN, Gothe B, Cherniack NS: Possible mechanisms of periodic breathing during sleep. J Appl Physiol 1988;64:1000-1008.

13. Phillipson EA: Control of breathing during sleep. Am Rev Respir Dis 1978;118:909-939.

14. Bülow K, Ingvar D: Respiration and state of wakefulness in normals, studied by spirography, capnography and EEG. Acta Physiol Scand 1961;51:230-238.

15. Trinder J, VanBeveren JA, Smith P, et al: Correlation between ventilation and EEG-defined arousal during sleep onset in young subjects. J Appl Physiol 1997;83:2005-2011.

16. Dunai J, Wilkinson M, Trinder J: Interaction of chemical and state effects on ventilation during sleep onset. J Appl Physiol 1996;81:2235-2243.

17. Mangin P, Krieger J, Kurtz D: Apnea following hyperventilation in man. J Neurol Sci 1982;57:67-82.

18. Plum F, Brown HW, Snoep E: Neurologic significance of post-hyperventilation apnea. JAMA 1962;181:1050-1055.

19. Khoo MC, Kronauer RE, Strohl KP, et al: Factors inducing periodic breathing in humans: A general model. J Appl Physiol 1982;53:644-659.

20. Longobardo GS, Gothe B, Goldman MD, et al: Sleep apnea considered as a control system instability. Respir Physiol 1982; 50:311-333.

21. Phillipson EA, Sullivan CE: Arousal: The forgotten response to ventilatory stimuli (Editorial). Am Rev Respir Dis 1978;118: 807-809.

22. Stradling JR, Chadwick GT, Frew AJ: Changes in ventilation and its components in normal subjects during sleep. Thorax 1985;40:364-370.

23. Lavie P, Fischer N, Zomer J, et al: The effects of partial and complete mechanical occlusion of the nasal passages on sleep structure and breathing in sleep. Acta Otolaryngol 1983;95: 161-166.

24. Sanders MH, Costantino JP, Owens GR, et al: Breathing during wakefulness and sleep after human heart-lung transplantation. Am Rev Respir Dis 1989;140:45-51.

25. Cherniack NS, Longobardo GS, Gothe B, et al: Interactive effects of central and obstructive apnea. Adv Physiol Sci 1981;10: 553-560.

26. Önal E, Lopata M: Periodic breathing and the pathogenesis of occlusive sleep apneas. Am Rev Respir Dis 1982;126:676-680.

27. Badr MS, Morgan BJ, Finn L, et al: Ventilatory response to induced auditory arousals during NREM sleep. Sleep 1997;20: 707-714.

28. Shore ET, Millman RP, Silage DA, et al: Ventilatory and arousal patterns during sleep in normal young and elderly subjects. J Appl Physiol 1985;59:1607-1615.

29. Magnussen G: Studies on the Respiration During Sleep: A Contribution to the Physiology of the Sleep Function. London, England, HK Lewis, 1944.

30. Reed CI, Kleitman N: Studies of the physiology of sleep: The effect of sleep on respiration. Am J Physiol 1926;75:600-608.

31. Skatrud JB, Dempsey JA: Airway resistance and respiratory muscle function in snorers during NREM sleep. J Appl Physiol 1985;59:328-335.

32. Krieger J, Mangin P, Kurtz D: Incidence of sleep disordered breathing in normal younger and older subjects: Correspondence analysis of related factors. In Sleep, 1982: Sixth European Congress on Sleep Research. Basel, Switzerland, Karger, 1983, pp 308-311.

33. White DP, Weil JV, Zwillich CW: Metabolic rate and breathing during sleep. J Appl Physiol 1985;59:384-391.

34. Gothe B, Altose MD, Goldman MD, et al: Effect of quiet sleep on resting and CO_2 stimulated breathing in humans. J Appl Physiol 1981;50:724-730.

35. Tabachnik E, Muller NL, Bryan AC, et al: Changes in ventilation and chest wall mechanics during sleep in normal adolescents. J Appl Physiol 1981;51:557-564.

36. Douglas NJ: Control of breathing during sleep. Clin Sci 1984; 67:465-472.

37. Iber C, Berssenbrugge A, Skatrud JB, et al: Ventilatory adaptations to resistive loading during wakefulness and non-REM sleep. J Appl Physiol 1982;52:607-614.

38. Naifeh KH, Kamiya J: The nature of respiratory changes associated with sleep onset. Sleep 1981;4:49-59.

39. Lopes JM, Tabachnik E, Muller NL, et al: Total airway resistance and respiratory muscle activity during sleep. J Appl Physiol 1983;54:773-777.

40. Robin ED, Whaley RD, Crump CC, et al: Alveolar gas tensions, pulmonary ventilation and blood pH during physiological sleep in normal subjects. J Clin Invest 1958;37:981-989.

41. Wiegand DA, Latz B, Zwillich CW, et al: Geniohyoid muscle activity in normal men during wakefulness and sleep. J Appl Physiol 1990;69:1262-1269.

42. Fitzpatrick MF, McLean H, Urton AM, et al: Effect of nasal or oral breathing route on upper airway resistance during sleep. Eur Respir J 2003;22:827-832.

43. Hudgel DW, Hendricks C: Palate and hypopharynx sites of inspiratory narrowing of the upper airway during sleep. Am Rev Respir Dis 1988;138:1542-1547.

44. Berger RJ: Tonus of extrinsic laryngeal muscles during sleep and dreaming. Science 1961;134:840.

45. Tangel DJ, Mezzanotte WS, Sandberg EJ, et al: Influences of NREM sleep on the activity of tonic vs inspiratory phasic muscles in normal men. J Appl Physiol 1992;73:1058-1066.

46. Wiegand DA, Latz B, Zwillich CW, et al: Upper airway resistance and geniohyoid muscle activity in normal men during wakefulness and sleep. J Appl Physiol 1990;69:1252-1261.

47. Basner RC, Ringler J, Schwartzstein RM, et al: Phasic electromyographic activity of the genioglossus increases in normals during slow-wave sleep. Respir Physiol 1991;83:189-200.

48. Kuna ST, Smickley JS, Insalaco G: Posterior cricoarytenoid muscle activity during wakefulness and sleep in normal adults. J Appl Physiol 1990;68:1746-1754.

49. Tangel DJ, Mezzanotte WS, White DP: Influence of sleep on tensor palatini EMG and upper airway resistance in normal men. J Appl Physiol 1991;70:2574-2581.

50. Harper RM, Sauerland EK: The role of the tongue in sleep apnea. In Guilleminault C, Dement WC (eds): Sleep Apnea Syndromes. New York, Alan R Liss, 1978, pp 219-234.

51. Sauerland EK, Harper RM: The human tongue during sleep: Electromyographic activity of the genioglossus muscle. Exp Neurol 1976;51:160-170.

52. Stanchina ML, Malhotra A, Fogel RB, et al: Genioglossus muscle responsiveness to chemical and mechanical stimuli during non-rapid eye movement sleep. Am J Respir Crit Care Med 2002; 165:945-949.

53. Fogel RB, Trinder J, Malhotra A, et al: Within-breath control of genioglossal muscle activation in humans: Effect of sleep-wake state. J Physiol (London) 2003;550:899-910.

54. Ballard RD, Irvin CG, Martin RJ, et al: Influence of sleep on lung volume in asthmatic patients and normal subjects. J Appl Physiol 1990;68:2034-2041.

55. Hudgel DW, Devadatta P: Decrease in functional residual capacity during sleep in normal humans. J Appl Physiol 1984;57: 1319-1322.

56. Begle RL, Badr S, Skatrud JB, et al: Effect of lung inflation on pulmonary resistance during NREM sleep. Am Rev Respir Dis 1990;141:854-860.

57. Aronson RM, Carley DW, Önal E, et al: Upper airway muscle activity and the thoracic volume dependence of upper airway resistance. J Appl Physiol 1991;70:430-438.

58. Daubenspeck JA: Influence of small mechanical loads on variability of breathing pattern. J Appl Physiol 1981;50: 299-306.

59. Hudgel DW, Mulholland M, Hendricks C: Neuromuscular and mechanical responses to inspiratory resistive loading during sleep. J Appl Physiol 1987;63:603-608.

60. Gugger M, Molloy J, Gould GA, et al: Ventilatory and arousal responses to added inspiratory resistance during sleep. Am Rev Respir Dis 1989;140:1301-1307.

61. Henke KG, Dempsey JA, Kowitz JM, et al: Effects of sleep-induced increases in upper airway resistance on ventilation. J Appl Physiol 1990;69:617-624.

62. Morrell MJ, Harty HR, Adams L, et al: Changes in total pulmonary resistance and P_{CO_2} between wakefulness and sleep in normal human subjects. J Appl Physiol 1995;78:1339-1349.

63. Kay A, Trinder J, Kim Y: Progressive changes in airway resistance during sleep. J Appl Physiol 1996;81:282-292.

64. Morrell MJ, Harty HR, Adams L, et al: Breathing during wakefulness and NREM sleep in humans without an upper airway. J Appl Physiol 1996;81:274-281.

65. Agnew HW, Webb WB, Williams RL: Sleep patterns in late middle age males: An EEG study. Electroencephalogr Clin Neurophysiol 1967;23:168-171.

66. Douglas NJ, White DP, Pickett CK, et al: Respiration during sleep in normal man. Thorax 1982;37:840-844.

67. Duron B: La fonction respiratoire pendant le sommeil physiologique. Bull Eur Physiopathol Respir 1972;8:1031-1057.

68. Muller NL, Francis PW, Gurwitz D, et al: Mechanism of hemoglobin desaturation during REM sleep in normal subjects and in patients with cystic fibrosis. Am Rev Respir Dis 1980; 121:463-469.

69. Ryan T, Mlynczak S, Erickson T, et al: Oxygen consumption during sleep: Influence of sleep stage and time of night. Sleep 1989;12:201-210.

70. Shapiro CM, Goll CC, Cohen GR, et al: Heat production during sleep. J Appl Physiol 1984;56:671-677.

71. Webb P, Hiestand M: Sleep metabolism and age. J Appl Physiol 1974;38:257-267.

72. Carlson DM, Carley DW, Onal E, et al: Acoustically induced cortical arousal increases phasic pharyngeal muscle and diaphragmatic EMG in NREM sleep. J Appl Physiol 1994;76:1553-1559.

73. Aserinsky E, Kleitman N: Regularly occurring periods of eye motility and concurrent phenomena during sleep. Science 1953;118:273-274.

74. Rohmer F, Schaff G, Collard M, et al: La motilité spontanée, la fréquence cardiaque et la fréquence respiratoire au cours du sommeil chez l'homme normal. In Fischgold M (ed): Le Sommeil de Nuit Normal et Pathologique. Paris, France, Masson & Cie, 1965, pp 192-205.

75. Snyder F, Hobson JA, Morrison DF, et al: Changes in respiration, heart rate and systolic blood pressure in human sleep. J Appl Physiol 1964;19:417-422.

76. Spreng LF, Johnson CL, Lubin A: Autonomic correlates of eye movement bursts during stage REM sleep. Psychophysiology 1968;4:311-323.

77. Aserinsky E: Periodic respiratory pattern occurring in conjunction with eye movements during sleep. Science 1965;150:763-766.

78. Gould GA, Gugger M, Molloy J, et al: Breathing pattern and eye movement density during REM sleep in humans. Am Rev Respir Dis 1988;138:874-877.

79. Zimmermann PV, Connellan SJ, Middleton MC, et al: Postural changes in rib cage and abdominal volume-motion coefficients and their effect on the calibration of a respiratory inductance plethysmograph. Am Rev Respir Dis 1983;127:209-214.

80. Parmeggiani PL, Sabattini L: Electromyographic aspect of postural respiratory and thermoregulatory mechanisms in sleeping cats. Clin Neurophysiol 1972;33:1-13.

81. Lugaresi E, Cirignotta F, Coccagna G, et al: Some epidemiological data on snoring and cardiocirculatory disturbances. Sleep 1980;3:221-224.

82. Lugaresi E, Coccagna G, Cirignotta F, et al: Breathing during sleep in man in normal and pathological conditions. In Fitzgerald R, Gautier H, Lahiri S (eds): The Regulation of Respiration During Sleep and Anesthesia. New York, Plenum, 1978, pp 35-45.

83. Koskenvuo M, Kapro J, Partinen M, et al: Snoring as a risk factor for hypertension and angina pectoris. Lancet 1985; 1:893-896.

84. Robin IG: Snoring. Proc R Soc Lond B Biol Sci 1968;61:575-582.

85. Lugaresi E, Coccagna G, Cirignotta F: Snoring and its clinical implications. In Guilleminault C, Dement WC (eds): Sleep Apnea Syndromes. New York, Alan R Liss, 1978, pp 13-21.

86. Carskadon MA, Dement WC: Respiration during sleep in the aged human. J Gerontol 1981;36:420-423.

87. Lugaresi E, Mondini S, Zucconi M, et al: Staging of heavy snorer's disease: A proposal. Bull Eur Physiopathol Respir 1983; 19:590-594.

88. Feris BG, Pollard DS: Effect of deep and quiet breathing on pulmonary compliance in man. J Clin Invest 1960;39:143.

89. Perez-Padilla R, West P, Kryger MH: Sighs during sleep in adult humans. Sleep 1983;6:234-243.

90. Trinder J, Kay A, Kleiman J, et al: Gender differences in airway resistance during sleep. J Appl Physiol 1997;83:1986-1997.

91. Manber R, Armitage R: Sex, steroids, and sleep: A review. Sleep 1999;22:540-555.

92. Catterall JR, Calverley PMA, Shapiro CM, et al: Breathing and oxygenation during sleep are similar in normal men and normal women. Am Rev Respir Dis 1985;132:86-88.

93. Ferber R, Kryger M (eds): Principles and Practice of Sleep Medicine in the Child. Philadelphia, Saunders, 1995.

94. Gimeno F, Peset R: Changes in oxygen saturation and heart frequency during sleep in young normal subjects. Thorax 1984;39:673-675.

95. Krieger J, Mangin P, Kurtz D: Les modifications respiratoires au cours du sommeil du sujet âgé normal. Rev Electroencephalogr Neurophysiol Clin 1980;10:177-185.

96. McGinty D, Littner M, Beahm E, et al: Sleep related breathing disorders in older men: A search for underlying mechanisms. Neurobiol Aging 1982;3:337-350.

97. Bixler EO, Kales A, Cadieux R, et al: Sleep apneic activity in older healthy subjects. J Appl Physiol 1985;58:1597-1601.

98. Feinberg I, Carlson VR: Sleep variables as a function of age in man. Arch Gen Psychiatry 1968;18:239-250.

99. Browne HAK, Adams L, Simonds AK, Morrell MJ: Ageing does not influence the sleep-related decrease in the hypercapnic ventilatory response. Eur Respir J 2003;21:523-529.

100. Krieger J, Maglasiu N, Sforza E, et al: Breathing during sleep in normal middle-aged subjects. Sleep 1990;13:143-154.

101. Brownell LG, West P, Kryger MH: Breathing during sleep in normal pregnant women. Annu Rev Respir Dis 1986;133:38-41.

102. Trakada G, Tsapanos V, Spiropoulos K: Normal pregnancy and oxygenation during sleep. Eur J Obstetr Gynecol Reprod Biol 2003;109:128-132.

103. Franklin KA, Holmgren PA, Jonsson F, et al: Snoring, pregnancy-induced hypertension, and growth retardation of the fetus. Chest 2000;117:137-141.

104. Izci B, Riha RL, Martin SE, et al: The upper airway in pregnancy and pre-eclampsia. Am J Respir Crit Care Med 2003;167:137-140.

105. Connolly G, Razak AR, Hayanga A, et al: Inspiratory flow limitation during sleep in pre-eclampsia: Comparison with normal pregnant and nonpregnant women. Eur Respir J 2001; 18:672-676.

106. Read DJ, Jeffery HE: Some neurochemical influences on breathing. In Saunders NA, Sullivan CE (eds): Sleep and Breathing. New York, Marcel Dekker, 1984, pp 201-220.

107. Johnstone RE, Reier CE: Acute respiratory effects of ethanol in man. Clin Pharmacol Ther 1973;14:501-508.

108. Zilm DH: Ethanol-induced spontaneous and evoked EEG, heart rate and respiration rate changes in man. Clin Toxicol 1981;18:549-563.

109. Taasan V, Block AJ, Boysen P, et al: Alcohol increases sleep apnea and oxygen desaturation in asymptomatic men. Am J Med 1981;71:240-245.

110. Block AJ, Hellard DW, Slayton PC: Minimal effect of alcohol ingestion on breathing during the sleep of postmenopausal women. Chest 1985;88:181-184.

111. Issa FG, Sullivan CE: Alcohol, snoring and sleep apnea. J Neurol Neurosurg Psychiatry 1982;45:353-359.

112. Scrima L, Broudy M, Nay KN, et al: Increased severity of obstructive sleep apnea after bedtime alcohol ingestion: Diagnostic potential and proposed mechanism of action. Sleep 1982;5:318-328.

113. Krol RC, Knuth SL, Bartlett D: Selective reduction of genioglossal muscle activity by alcohol in normal human subjects. Am Rev Respir Dis 1984;129:247-250.

114. Berry RB, Bonnet MH, Light RW: Effect of ethanol on the arousal response to airway occlusion during sleep in normal subjects. Am Rev Respir Dis 1992;145:445-452.

115. Cirignotta F, Mondini S, Zucconi M, et al: Snoring and sleep apnea: Effects of lorazepam and mazindol evaluated by means of snoring and sleep apnea monitoring. Bull Eur Physiopathol Respir 1982;18:113P-134P.

116. Kripke DF, Simons NR, Garfinkel L, et al: Short and long sleep and sleeping pills: Is increased mortality associated? Arch Gen Psychiatry 1979;36:103-116.

117. Mukhametov LM: Sleep in marine mammals. Exp Brain Res 1984;8(Suppl):227-238.

20

Respiratory Physiology: Sleep at High Altitudes

John V. Weil

ABSTRACT

Sleep disturbance is a frequent feature of an acute ascent to high altitude. The symptom is frequent awakening with a sense of suffocation. Objective observations indicate that sleep at altitude is associated with periodic breathing and frequent awakenings but relatively little change in total sleep time. Sleep stages are generally shifted from deeper toward lighter sleep stages.

Periodic breathing at altitude seems to reflect the respiratory dilemma of acute altitude ascent in which the stimulatory effects of hypoxia are opposed by the inhibitory action of hypocapnic alkalosis. The outcome is respiratory oscillation. Hypocapnic alkalosis induces apnea, which in turn lessens alkalotic inhibition and augments hypoxic stimulation. This triggers hyperpnea, which lessens respiratory stimulation by decreasing hypoxia and increasing alkalosis, leading to recurrent apnea. The occurrence of apnea with lessening of ventilatory stimuli is enhanced during sleep.

On balance, the poor subjective quality of sleep seems to reflect the fragmentation of sleep by frequent arousals linked to the marked changes in respiratory pattern of periodic breathing. Arousals commonly occur at the transition from the end of apnea to the onset of hyperpnea. Subsequent acclimatization to altitude is associated with lessening of periodic breathing and better-quality sleep.

The most common treatment is prophylactic administration of acetazolamide, an inhibitor of carbonic anhydrase, which likely works by reducing alkalotic ventilatory inhibition. The results of recent studies suggest that benzodiazepines may improve sleep quality without apparent adverse effects.

Sleep disturbance is a common cause of discomfort among the constellation of symptoms after ascent to high altitude. Subjectively, the sensation is that of a restless or sleepless night. Individuals commonly experience awakening from sleep with a feeling of suffocation, taking a deep breath, feeling much improved, and falling back to sleep. In this chapter, a few general, relevant aspects of acute physiologic adjustment to high altitude are briefly summarized; the characteristics of the sleep disturbance of altitude, its pathogenesis, and therapeutic interventions are then reviewed. Although much of the focus is on sleep after acute ascent to high altitude, alterations in sleep during long-term altitude exposure are also briefly mentioned.

PHYSIOLOGIC ADJUSTMENT TO HIGH ALTITUDE

Primary among the changes in physical environment that attend the ascent to altitude is a decrease in barometric pressure

such that although the fractional concentration of O_2 is similar to that at sea level, O_2 tension—the product of fractional concentration and barometric pressure—is reduced (Fig. 20–1). This decreased O_2 tension of ambient air presents a threat to arterial and tissue oxygenation and elicits a series of responses that may act to minimize tissue hypoxia. These consist of early increases in ventilation and cardiac output and, during more prolonged exposure, rises in circulating red cell concentration and changes in peripheral tissue, including increased spatial density of capillaries and mitochondria.

Increased Ventilation

Probably the earliest and best studied and one of the most important of these responses is increased ventilation, which acts to minimize the extent of alveolar hypoxia and arterial hypoxemia in the face of a decrease in ambient O_2 tension. The magnitude of the ventilatory response increases with increasing altitude, but it also varies considerably between individuals at a fixed altitude. This variability in part reflects intrinsic, interindividual differences in the strength of the basal (preascent) ventilatory response to hypoxia.[1] In addition, ventilation progressively increases over several days *after* ascent to high altitude. This gradual increase occurs despite the fact that the increasing ventilation is lessening hypoxia— the presumed stimulus to breathing—and increasing hypocapnic alkalosis—a ventilatory inhibitor. This is the phenomenon of ventilatory acclimatization to high altitude, which is manifested as a progressive decrease in arterial P_{CO_2} (Pa_{CO_2}) with increasing ventilation over several days. Although the mechanism of acclimatization is debated, studies in humans and animals suggest that increased hypoxic sensitivity of the carotid body may be a major contributor.[2] In any case, it is during the early phase of altitude adjustment, shortly after ascent, that sleep disturbances appear to be most marked; they tend to improve during the period of acclimatization.

Sleep Disturbances

The earliest systematic study of sleep at altitude was a report in 1970 of studies of subjects working in Antarctica, where a combination of geographic elevation and terrestrial spin produces decreased barometric pressure ranging from 485 to 525 mm Hg, equivalent to moderately high altitude. The men stationed there experienced a sleep disturbance termed *polar red-eye,* and electroencephalographic studies showed major disruption of sleep with a marked decrease in slow wave sleep (stages 3 and 4).[3] Although these changes were ascribed to hypobaric hypoxia, the effects of isolation and disturbances of light–dark cycle that are typical in persons living at the South Pole clouded their interpretation.

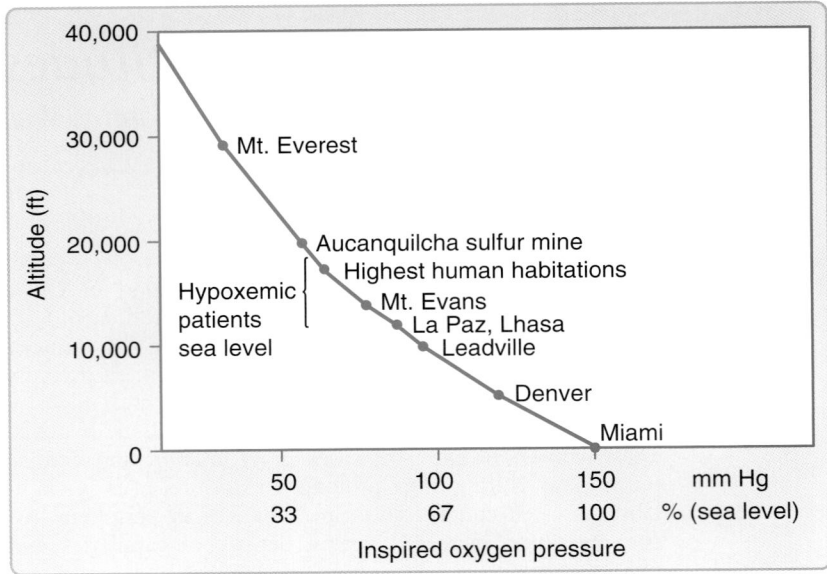

Figure 20–1. Relationship between altitude and inspired O$_2$ pressure. (From Kryger MH: Pathophysiology of Respiration. New York, John Wiley & Sons, 1981, with permission.)

As research at low altitude began to elucidate the close links between breathing and sleep and to show that sleep disruption was often closely linked to changes in respiratory rhythm, such as occurs in sleep apnea, studies were performed at high altitude with simultaneous monitoring of sleep state and respiratory pattern. Reite et al.[4] studied normal subjects at sea level and during a stay of several days on the summit of Pike's Peak (4300 m). On the initial night after ascent, most subjects exhibited periodic breathing that was present during roughly half the time asleep but varied among subjects from 0% to 93%. Sleep was characterized by significant decreases in stages 3 and 4, with an increased number of arousals (Fig. 20–2). In most but not all subjects who initially showed periodic breathing, this tended to decrease over subsequent nights, with a decreased number of arousals. Although there

was a trend toward more wakefulness, the duration of sleep (total sleep time) was not significantly reduced compared with that at sea level.

Although most of these subjects complained of difficulty in sleeping, this could not be related to abbreviated sleep, which, as mentioned, was of normal duration. Rather, it seemed associated with an increased number of awakenings. Many of these were synchronous to the transition from termination of apnea to onset of hyperpnea and thus were similar in some respects to the arousal seen in sleep apnea syndromes at low altitude. Although this suggests that periodic breathing, frequent awakenings, and poor-quality sleep are mechanistically interrelated, there must be some reservation about this because increased awakenings in one subject occurred in the absence of periodic breathing[4] and because oxygen administration abolishes

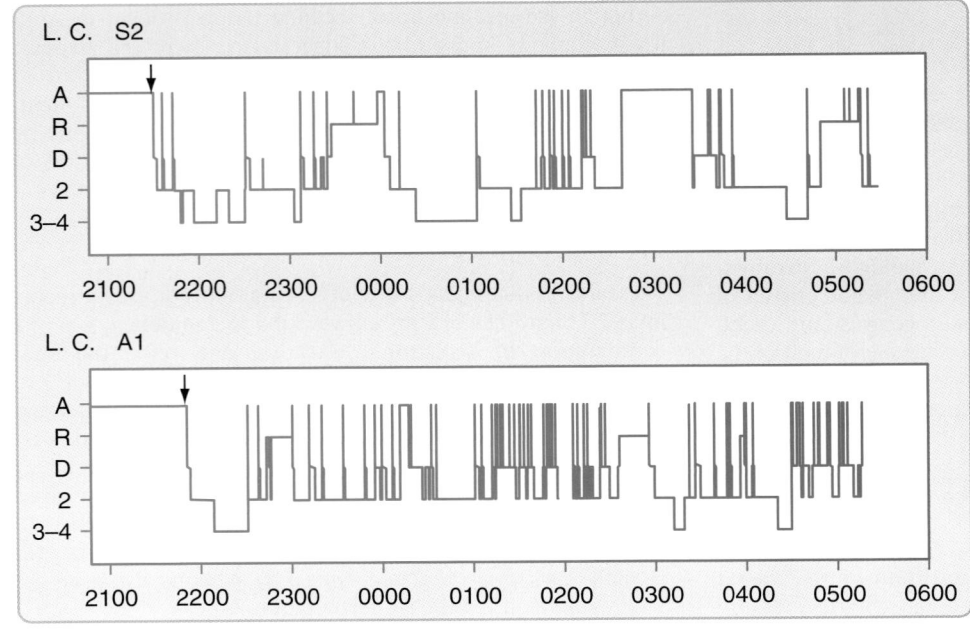

Figure 20–2. All-night sleep plots for a single subject during a night at sea level *(upper plot)* and the first night at altitude *(lower plot)*. Time in hours is plotted on the horizontal axis. Lights out occurred at the small vertical *arrow* in each plot. Sleep stage is shown on the vertical axis: A, awake; R, REM sleep; D, stage 1 sleep; 2, stage 2 sleep; 3-4, stages 3 and 4 sleep combined. Sleep at high altitude was associated with increased fragmentation by frequent awakenings and a reduction in stage 3/4 sleep. (Reprinted from Reite M, Jackson D, Cahoon RL, et al: Sleep physiology at high altitude. Electroencephalogr Clin Neurophysiol 1975;38:463-471, with permission.)

periodic breathing but not the increased frequency of awakenings.[4-7] It has been suggested that increased sleep fragmentation at altitude may be specifically related to the increased frequency of arousals that are temporally linked to apneas (as reviewed by Wickramasinghe and Anholm[8]).

Poor subjective quality of sleep might also reflect altitude-associated changes in sleep stage distribution. Most studies find that sleep at altitude is characterized by an increase in light sleep (stage 1) with a decrease in stage 2 sleep, and a relative paucity of deeper stages (3 and 4) of non–rapid eye movement (NREM) sleep. Total sleep time is usually unchanged, but there is a significant increase in time spent awake, and there is shortening of sleep epochs, which are fragmented by frequent arousals.[4-6,9] There seems to be no consistent change in the amount of rapid eye movement (REM) sleep, which is variably found to be either unchanged,[4,6] increased, or decreased[7,10] at altitude. The disparity between subjective evaluation of sleep quality and objective findings of normal sleep duration most likely reflects the importance of sleep continuity in the apparent subjective quality of sleep and suggests that sleep fragmentation despite normal cumulative duration might produce the impression of sleeplessness.[4,8,11,12]

As mentioned earlier, total sleep time is remarkably preserved or may even increase[13] in the face of the disruptive effect of periodic breathing. Perhaps this paradox is explained by the frequent but largely unstudied observation that ascent to altitude induces sleepiness, which is consistent, prompt, and often profound. Although this may be due to hypoxia, a study in normal subjects at low altitude showed marked sleepiness induced by brief voluntary hyperventilation, pointing to a potential role of hypocapnia.[14] Regardless of its cause, the hypnotic effect of altitude could contribute to the maintenance of total sleep duration. Hypocapnia may also suppress REM sleep—a study in sleeping cats at simulated altitude and during mechanical hyperventilation showed decreases in REM sleep that were reversed by CO_2 administration.[15]

Periodic Breathing

Occurrence

In the mid-19th century, Cheyne and Stokes described the crescendo–decrescendo breathing pattern in cardiac patients that now bears their names.[16] That periodic breathing is frequent during sleep in normal individuals at high altitude was observed shortly thereafter by Tyndall in 1857, by Egli-Sinclair and Mosso in 1893 and 1894, and by Douglas et al.[17] in 1913, and it continues to be a consistent finding in current studies of sleep after ascent to high altitude.[4,9,18-21] The respiratory dysrhythmia of sleep at altitude is one of machinery-like periodicity (Fig. 20–3) similar to that seen at low altitude in patients with heart failure (see Chapter 102) or with central nervous system disorders.

The temporal pattern of periodic breathing and its linkage to sleep stages show some night-to-night variation and considerable intersubject differences,[4,7,10,20,22-26] yet on balance, periodicity is usually evident early in sleep and during light stages. Periodic breathing at altitude may also occur in wakefulness, especially during periods of drowsiness.[27-29] The pattern, as mentioned, is similar to that of patients with central apnea at low altitude, but there is a relatively short cycle length ranging from 12 to 34 seconds, which progressively shortens with

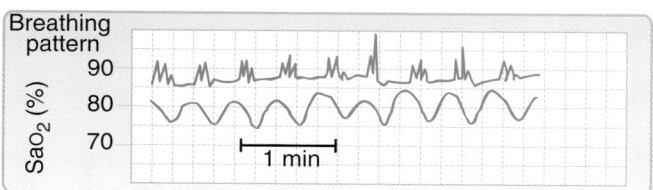

Figure 20–3. Breathing pattern and arterial oxygen saturation in a normal subject during sleep at high altitude (4300 m). Such a pattern is seen throughout much of sleep in most individuals after ascent. There is characteristic, monotonously repetitive, machinery-like periodic alternation of apnea and repetitive clusters of hyperpneic breaths. (From Weil JV, Kryger MH, Scoggin CH: Sleep and breathing at high altitude. In Guilleminault C, Dement WC [eds]: Sleep Apnea Syndromes. New York, Alan R Liss, 1978, pp 119-136.)

increasing altitude[30-32] and differs from the longer cycles of 40 to 90 seconds in patients with heart failure.[33] The most obvious aspect of this periodicity is the oscillation of tidal volume, and there is less obvious change in breathing frequency. However, there are subtle, but parallel, variations in frequency that produce a reinforcing effect on ventilatory oscillation.[30] Like periodic breathing at sea level, periodicity at altitude is often initiated by movement or a deeper breath with a transient increase in hypocapnia. Periodicity at altitude is also most prevalent in light, stage 1 or 2 sleep. Although deeper stages of NREM sleep are relatively rare after acute ascent, the propensity to periodic breathing seems much reduced at these times.

The most striking influence of sleep stage on periodic breathing is the observation in most,[4,6,23] but not all,[5,7] studies that REM sleep promptly and consistently terminates periodicity and restores regular breathing. However, periodicity seems to persist in REM sleep at altitudes greater than 4300 meters.[8]

During sleep, ventilation and oxygenation fall below waking values, and the relative decreases are similar at altitude and at sea level.[34] However, the important difference is that at altitude, basal (awake) oxygenation and P_{CO_2} are lower and thus closer to critical thresholds (Fig. 20–4). Oxygen tensions fall closer to the descending limb of the dissociation curve, where values are associated with desaturation and are nearer the threshold for stimulation of ventilation. Similarly, CO_2 tensions fall to values nearer the dog-leg below which CO_2 may lose its ventilatory stimulus potential, and they closely approach the P_{CO_2} apneic threshold below which breathing ceases during sleep.[35] As a result, small variations in gas tensions have much greater effects on ventilation at altitude.

It seems likely that the respiratory pauses in sleep at altitude are of central origin. They are usually unassociated with snoring or other noises suggestive of obstruction and are accompanied by an absence of rib cage and abdominal activity,[5,6,18,20,36] which suggests a nonobstructive cause, and there is no evident association with the usual risk factors for obstruction, such as obesity. However, at low altitude, many apneas are "mixed"—they have both central and obstructive features.[37,38] This is most likely a reflection of the phasic "respiratory" nature of many upper airway muscles such that loss of drive reduces activation of both classic inspiratory muscles and those responsible for maintenance of upper airway patency. Thus, increased upper airway resistance may contribute to periodic breathing at altitude but probably plays only a minor role.

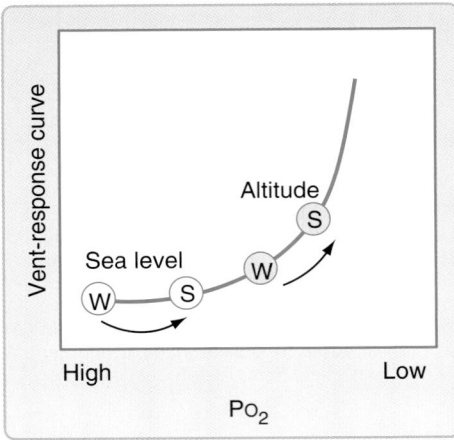 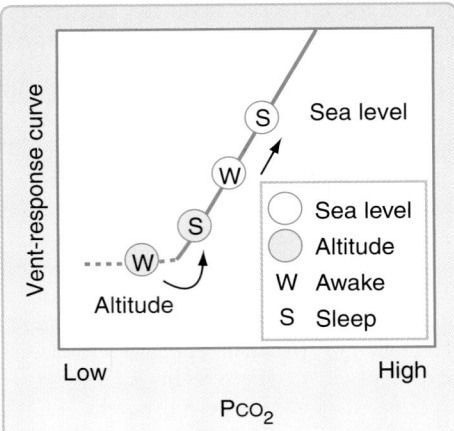

Figure 20-4. A schematic illustration of the relationship of blood gases to ventilatory responses during wakefulness and sleep at low and high altitude. At altitude, during wakefulness (W), arterial oxygen tensions move lower toward the steeper portion of the hypoxic ventilatory response curve—an effect that is augmented during sleep (S). Hyperventilation causes arterial CO_2 tensions during wakefulness and sleep to decrease and move closer to the dogleg of the CO_2 response curve, where the ventilatory response to P_{CO_2} is greatly reduced. The result is that during sleep at high altitude, small changes in the partial pressure of either oxygen (P_{O_2}) or carbon dioxide (P_{CO_2}) produce much greater changes in ventilation than at low altitude. This sets the stage for respiratory instability.

As mentioned, sleep disturbance and periodic breathing seem to be most pronounced during the first few nights after ascent to moderate altitude, with a tendency toward more regular breathing on subsequent nights. However, several studies describe the persistence of periodic breathing throughout sleep after 10 days to 5 weeks at altitudes greater than 4500 meters.[20,36,39,40]

Mechanisms

In the early 1900s, ingenious, deceptively simple experiments by Douglas and Haldane[41] at low altitude explored the physiologic mechanisms of periodic breathing and highlighted the importance of both hypoxia and hypocapnia. They were aware that during wakefulness, breathing was characterized by intrinsic momentum, a "flywheel" effect that caused breathing to continue despite brief hypocapnia. They also showed that respiratory periodicity could be readily induced in normal subjects by intense, sustained voluntary hyperventilation with room air, which produced apnea followed by Cheyne-Stokes respiration. When they produced hyperventilation with an O_2-enriched gas, they found that this induced only apnea, without periodic breathing, indicating the importance of hypoxia in the induction of periodicity. They also demonstrated the specific role of phasic hypoxia through the application of dead space containing the CO_2 absorber soda lime, which produced rebreathing-induced hypoxia without the usual attendant hypercapnia. When the resulting progressive hyperpnea produced an increase in tidal volume sufficient to bring in "fresh air" replete with O_2, the resolution of hypoxia produced apnea followed by recurrent rebreathing-induced hypoxia and perpetuation of the cycle. Their findings pointed to the combined roles of hypocapnia, which initiates apnea, and hypoxia, which stimulates hyperpnea, in the genesis of periodic breathing.

Similar principles apply at high altitude, as suggested by findings that the administration of O_2 or CO_2 abolishes periodic breathing.[4,18,24,36] Interpretation of the specific roles of

O_2 and CO_2 is complicated, first because O_2 administration improves oxygenation but also reduces ventilation and increases $PaCO_2$ with lessening of alkalosis. Second, the administration of CO_2 corrects respiratory alkalosis but also increases ventilation and improves oxygenation.

Despite this difficulty, considerable evidence suggests that although hypoxia may be contributory, hypocapnic alkalosis may have a particularly important role. Respiratory alkalosis is typical in patients with classic Cheyne-Stokes respiration at low altitude[42] and occurs in normal subjects in whom apneas during sleep have been noted to occur after transient episodes of decreased end-tidal P_{CO_2} and presumed increase in blood pH.[27] Important studies by Sullivan et al.[43] demonstrated that the withdrawal of classic stimuli to breathing by the administration of O_2, induction of metabolic alkalosis, or blockade of vagal afferents led to little change in respiratory rhythm during wakefulness but to profound pauses and slowing of breathing in sleep. This echoes the suggestion of Douglas and Haldane[29,41] that wakefulness acts in some fashion to sustain respiratory rhythm even in the absence of ventilatory stimuli, but that during sleep the maintenance of respiratory rhythm becomes critically dependent on such stimulation. Hyperventilation thus seems to be an excellent way to induce a respiratory pause in sleep because it simultaneously induces hyperoxia and withdrawal of hydrogen ion–CO_2 stimulation. Indeed, posthyperventilation apnea, which is variable in occurrence in wakefulness[44] but consistently found in sleep, is likely an example of such a relationship.[45] Indeed, Bulow[27] suggested that a stable and slightly elevated P_{CO_2} is necessary for stable rhythmic breathing during low-altitude sleep.

The critical role of hypocapnic alkalosis in periodic breathing in sleep at altitude is clearly evident in the study of Berssenbrugge et al.,[18] who showed that periodic breathing in NREM sleep at simulated altitude (barometric pressure of 455 mm Hg) was abolished by a selective increase in $PaCO_2$. This was achieved through the administration of low levels of CO_2 with added nitrogen to prevent the increase in oxygen saturation (SaO_2) that would be anticipated as a result of the stimulation of ventilation by a rising PaCO$_2$. They noted in one subject that in NREM sleep, the appearance of periodic breathing during the induction of hypoxia was temporally related more closely to the fall in end-tidal CO$_2$ than to the decrease in PO$_2$. Similarly, they showed that breathing was regular in NREM sleep in hypoxia when CO$_2$ was added to maintain isocapnia. However, when CO$_2$ administration was terminated, periodic breathing occurred when end-tidal CO$_2$ fell, although the extent of hypoxia remained constant. Furthermore, Skatrud and Dempsey[45] showed that apneas could be consistently produced at low altitude in NREM sleep through the induction of hypocapnia by passive positive-pressure hyperventilation against a background of either hypoxia or hyperoxia. Apnea tended to occur when the end-tidal CO$_2$ was lowered 1 to 3 mm Hg below levels observed during wakefulness (the apneic threshold). Thus, hypoxia alone seems insufficient to produce periodic breathing, for which a fall in PCO$_2$, below an apneic threshold, seems important (Fig. 20–5). Just as apneas at low altitude frequently follow sighs or breaths of increased tidal volume with a drop in PCO$_2$,[27] breaths of increased tidal volume with decreased end-tidal PCO$_2$ often trigger periodic breathing at altitude.[18,36] It thus appears that the events leading to periodic breathing at altitude begin with hypoxia, which stimulates hyperventilation, and the resulting hypocapnic alkalosis induces apnea, as illustrated in Figure 20–6. Apnea in turn leads to enhanced ventilatory stimulation by increasing hypoxemia and lessening hypocapnic alkalosis, which promotes subsequent hyperpnea and arousal. The ensuing increase in ventilation lessens hypoxia and restores hypocapnic alkalosis, promoting the recurrence of apnea.

Ventilatory oscillation in response to the rapidly changing arterial blood gases in periodic breathing points to an important

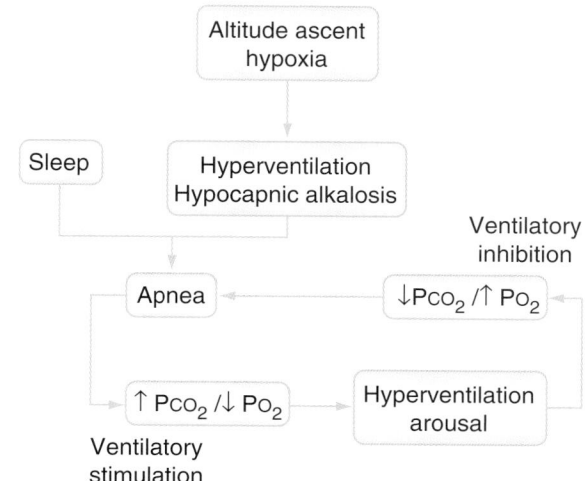

Figure 20–6. Schematic summary of mechanisms responsible for periodic breathing during sleep at altitude. Altitude-induced hypoxia stimulates increased ventilation. The resulting hypocapnic alkalosis together with the effects of sleep promotes apnea. During apnea, increasing hypoxemia and lessening hypocapnic alkalosis stimulate resumption of ventilation and arousal. This augments oxygenation and lessens hypocapnic alkalosis, permitting recurrence of apnea.

role for the fast-responding carotid body in the genesis of this respiratory periodicity. Recent studies in sleeping dogs with denervation or isolated perfusion of the carotid body show that carotid body chemoreception is necessary for induction of periodic breathing after a ventilatory overshoot induced by mechanical ventilation. The findings showed a surprising degree of carotid body sensitivity to changes in PCO$_2$ in the hypocapnic range, which may contribute to acute posthyperventilation apnea (see review by Smith et al.[35]).

This raises the question of the relative importance of decreased PCO$_2$ versus increased pH in the generation of apnea. It is clear that apneas at altitude are reversed by the administration of CO$_2$, but this also reverses alkalosis. Observations described later show the resolution of periodic breathing during acclimatization and its prevention by the use of inhibitors of carbonic anhydrase. In both instances, hypocapnia is accentuated whereas alkalosis is reduced.

The importance of hypocapnia and alkalosis in the genesis of periodic breathing suggests, in turn, a role for the strength of the ventilatory response to the hypoxia of high altitude, which is the primary cause of hyperventilation and hypocapnia after ascent. Theoretical considerations suggest that increased controller gain contributes to respiratory instability and periodicity.[46-48] These models emphasize the role of the curvilinear peripheral chemoreceptor response to hypoxia (for which the slope [gain] increases in hypoxia) and the steepening of the ventilatory response to hypercapnia by hypoxia. In a study of healthy subjects after acute ascent to high altitude, it was found that the extent of periodic breathing was greatest in subjects with the highest ventilatory responses to both hypoxia and hypercapnia measured before and after ascent.[34] Several subsequent studies have reaffirmed the association of high hypoxic ventilatory responses and periodic breathing in sleep at a high altitude[18,20,24,26,36,39] (Fig. 20–7), although some have found no relationship.[32,49] A steeper slope of ventilatory response to hypercapnia might imply a greater inhibitory action of

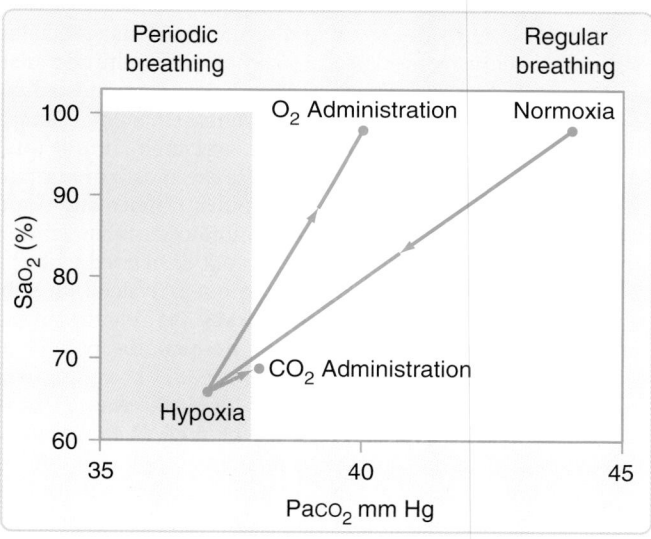

Figure 20–5. Relationship of respiratory pattern to arterial partial pressure of CO$_2$ (PaCO$_2$) and oxygen saturation (SaO$_2$). This figure is a schematic representation of data of Berssenbrugge et al.[18] and demonstrates that reduction in PCO$_2$ is a critical determinant of periodic breathing in normal human subjects during hypoxia. Even a small increase in PCO$_2$ after administration of either O$_2$ or CO$_2$ restores normal breathing. This effect seems largely independent of changes in SaO$_2$. (From Weil JV: Sleep at high altitude. Clin Chest Med 1985;6:615-621.)

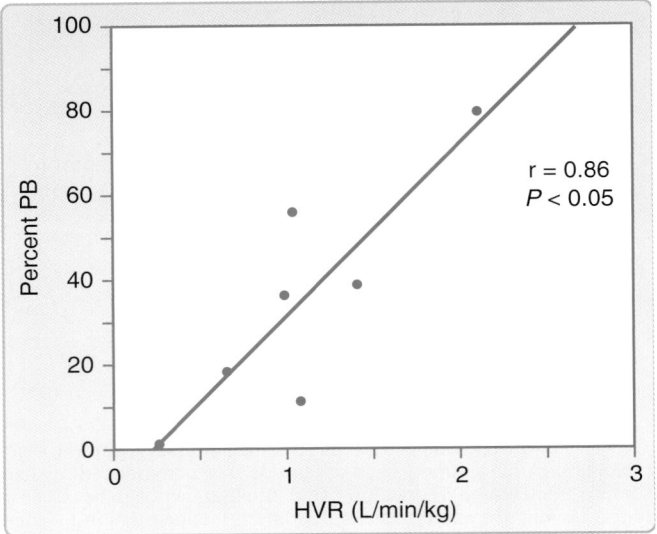

RELATION BETWEEN PERIODIC BREATHING
AND HYPOXIC VENTILATORY RESPONSE

$r = 0.86$
$P < 0.05$

Figure 20–7. Positive correlation of prevalence of periodic breathing (PB) in sleep at 6542 m and hypoxic ventilatory response (HVR). (From Goldenberg F, Richalet JP, Onnen I, et al: Sleep apneas and high altitude newcomers. Int J Sports Med 1992;13:S34-S36.)

hypocapnia. Two studies suggest an association of periodicity with increased hypercapnic ventilatory response,[20,34] but this is less consistent than the correlation with hypoxic response.

It is also apparent that the extent of periodic breathing shows a progressive decline over successive nights at moderate altitude, less than 4500 meters,[34] which suggests that the process of ventilatory acclimatization to altitude may act in some fashion to decrease the tendency toward periodic breathing. This is in some respects paradoxical, because the increased hypoxic ventilatory response and decreased P_{CO_2} and persistent alkalosis with acclimatization would be expected to increase periodic breathing. It may be that acclimatization acts to lessen the inhibitory effects of respiratory alkalosis on ventilation or produces local correction of alkalosis at some chemosensitive site and thus reduces the absolute value of Pa_{CO_2} required to produce an apnea (apneic threshold). At very high altitudes, severe hypoxia may override these effects of acclimatization. In studies of subjects over 4 weeks at a simulated altitude of 5050 meters, parallel increases were observed in hypoxic ventilatory response and periodic breathing during sleep.[40,50]

Consequences of Periodic Breathing

Fragmentation of sleep by frequent awakenings is an important probable byproduct of periodic breathing, which is, in turn, a contributor to the subjective sense of poor-quality sleep. As mentioned, arousals often occur in close synchrony to apnea termination—so close that it is unclear whether arousal stimulates resumption of breathing or the reverse occurs (resumption of breathing causes arousal). It also is unclear whether these arousals are triggered by chemosensory responses to apnea-induced asphyxia, by mechanical stimuli, or by central command signals associated with the abrupt resumption of breathing. Observations at low altitude suggest

that apnea-associated arousals correlate poorly with chemical variables but have a consistent relationship to mechanical stimuli, suggesting linkage to the resumption of ventilatory effort rather than to blood chemistry.[51] Regardless of the precise cause of arousal, it seems likely that the awakening or lightening of sleep stage contributes to periodicity by reversing the respiratory depressant influence of sleep and enhancing the postapneic hyperpnea. Although periodic breathing may contribute to the generation of arousals, as mentioned, a clear dissociation is seen with O_2 administration, which abolishes periodic breathing but fails to prevent arousals.[4] Factors responsible for this residual excess remain unknown.

The net influence of periodic breathing on average ventilation in sleep at altitude is incompletely understood. Although it has been suggested that the respiratory pauses may exaggerate nocturnal hypoxemia,[52] most studies show little effect on average ventilation. Indeed, when a difference is found, there appears to be better ventilation and oxygenation during periodic than during regular breathing, with a lesser incidence of symptoms of altitude adaptation that are linked to relative hypoventilation.[6,8,20,26] The association of periodic breathing with better ventilation may reflect the association of periodicity with increased chemosensitivity, which raises the level of overall ventilation. It may also be that periodic breathing is mechanically and energetically efficient. The high tidal volumes of the hyperpneic phase enhance relative alveolar versus dead space ventilation, and apneas conserve respiratory muscle work. Modeling suggests that optimal oxygenation, at least "pressure cost," is produced by clusters of two to four large breaths separated by apneas.[30,53] Such a pattern might be especially efficient at altitude, where decreased air density reduces the respiratory pressure cost.

Relationship of Sleep Disturbance and Periodic Breathing to Altitude Syndromes

In susceptible individuals, rapid altitude ascent is associated with two well-recognized syndromes of acute altitude maladaptation: acute mountain sickness (AMS; manifested by loss of appetite, nausea, vomiting, decreased mental acuity, insomnia, and, in rare cases, coma) and high-altitude pulmonary edema (HAPE). Although these are most common in the early postascent period when sleep disturbance and respiratory periodicity are also most pronounced, most studies find that periodic breathing in sleep is not correlated with the development or severity of these syndromes. Indeed, in subjects with pronounced symptoms of AMS, periodic breathing tends to be replaced by an irregular, nonperiodic pattern[5,26] (Fig. 20–8). However, in one study, periodic breathing was found to be more frequent in those with HAPE than in those with AMS or in control subjects.[54] This might be a result of stimulation of intrapulmonary afferents and ventilation–perfusion imbalance related to pulmonary edema with consequent exaggerated hypoxemia and hypocapnia. As mentioned, periodic breathing is linked to increased hypoxic ventilatory response, which may improve oxygenation and reduce the likelihood or severity of these maladaptive syndromes. In a study of high altitude expedition members, headache (a common feature of AMS) was largely unassociated with sleep, with only 26% occurring during sleep or on awakening, which suggested an absence of clear relationship to sleep-associated periodic breathing.[55] The well-known decline in daytime

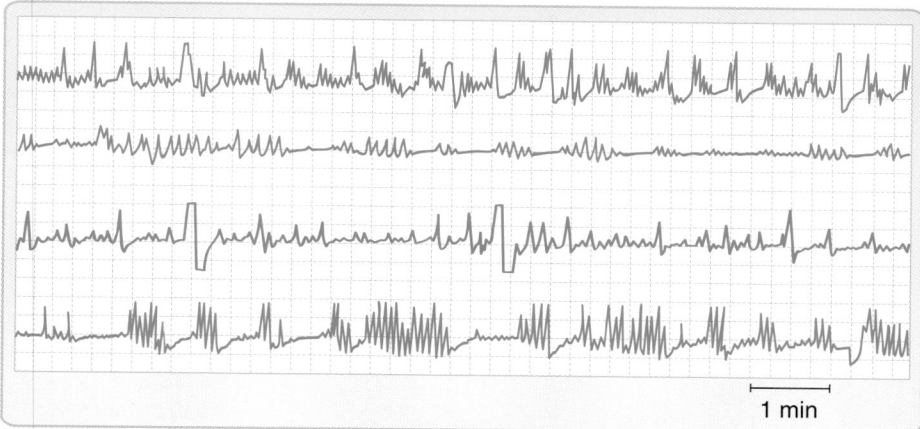

Figure 20–8. Impedance plethysmograms show irregular, nonperiodic, breathing during sleep at 2850 m in four subjects susceptible to high-altitude pulmonary edema. (From Fujimoto K, Matsuzawa Y, Hirai K, et al: Irregular nocturnal breathing patterns at high altitude in subjects susceptible to high-altitude pulmonary edema [HAPE]: A preliminary study. Aviat Space Environ Med 1989; 60:786-791.)

1 min

intellectual function at altitude most likely reflects in part the central nervous system effects of hypoxemia compounded by the cerebral vasoconstrictor effects of hypocapnia. However, sleep fragmentation of the sort encountered at altitude probably also contributes to this decline.[56]

TREATMENT

The treatment of, or prophylaxis for, periodic breathing and related sleep disturbance at high altitude is similar to that commonly used for control of the daytime syndrome of AMS. Staged, gradual ascent to altitude is an effective way to prevent or blunt sleep-related symptoms, but this may be inconvenient. Pharmacologic approaches are also useful and include inhibitors of carbonic anhydrase, benzodiazepines, stimulators of peripheral chemosensitivity, and progestational agents.

Carbonic Anhydrase Inhibitors

Acetazolamide is the most common and best studied agent used for amelioration of sleep disturbance at altitude; it has the advantage of also reducing symptoms of AMS.[57-60] This class of agents produces marked reductions in periodic breathing in sleep with higher and less oscillatory SaO_2[24,61] (Fig. 20–9). In two studies of sleep at altitude, acetazolamide markedly improved both the mean level and the stability of arterial oxygenation during sleep and reduced the proportion of sleep time during which periodic breathing occurred by roughly 50%[21,23] (Fig. 20–10). Awakenings that occur more frequently in sleep at high altitude are reduced and subjective and objective sleep quality is improved with augmentation of stage 2 sleep and decreased wakefulness.[62]

The primary action of these agents is the blockade of enzymatic hydration of CO_2 to carbonic acid with consequent induction of a bicarbonate diuresis and metabolic acidosis (Fig. 20–11). Blockade of carbonic anhydrase could also promote the accumulation of CO_2 in tissue, which might be responsible for the increase in cerebral blood flow induced by the intravenous administration of acetazolamide[63] and could stimulate central chemoreceptors. However, these central effects are minimal or absent with the relatively low doses used for symptom reduction at altitude,[64] and selective agents with action limited to the kidney seem as effective as acetazolamide in reducing periodic breathing.[57] Thus, the main mechanism of action is most likely the renal tubular effect

with induction of systemic metabolic acidosis. Reduction in respiratory periodicity with these agents may be in part the result of lessening of hypoxemia secondary to stimulation of ventilation by acidosis, but carbonic anhydrase inhibitors have a similar utility in eliminating central apneas at low altitude,[65,66] where hypoxemia is not a likely factor. This suggests that reduction of alkalosis, with possible lowering of the apneic threshold, is the major contribution. In sleeping dogs with mechanically induced ventilatory overshoot, acidosis lowers the apneic PCO_2 threshold relative to basal levels and thus increases the drop in PCO_2 required to induce apnea (the CO_2 reserve), an action that may contribute to the reduction of periodic breathing with acetazolamide.[35,67]

These agents raise ventilation with improved oxygenation and greater hypocapnia during wakefulness and sleep at altitude,[58,59] suggesting an effect on ventilatory control. Although hypoxic ventilatory responses are shifted upward (higher ventilation at all points), the steepness of the relationship is unchanged, indicating no potentiation of hypoxic sensitivity.[23,61,68,69] Effects on the hypercapnic response are variable, and, for uncertain reasons, findings differ for progressive

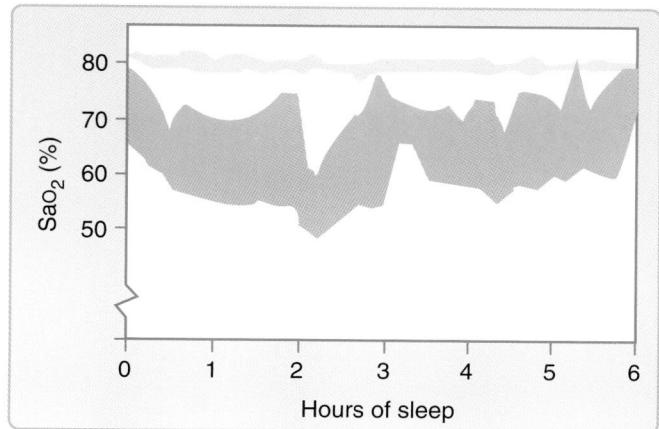

Figure 20–9. Average arterial oxygen saturation (SaO_2) in a sleeping subject at altitude (5360 m) without (*dark shaded area*) and with (*light shaded area*) acetazolamide. Treatment raised and stabilized arterial oxygen saturation. (From Sutton JR, Houston CS, Mansell AL, et al: Effect of acetazolamide on hypoxemia during sleep at high altitude. N Engl J Med 1979;301:1329-1331.)

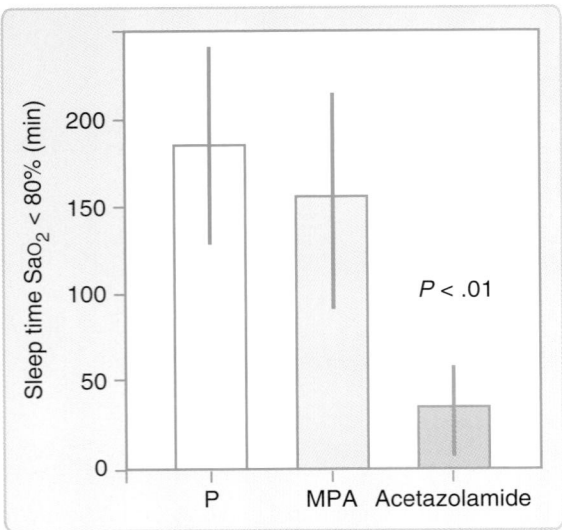

Figure 20–10. Length of time during which arterial oxygen saturation (SaO_2) is below 80% is used as an arbitrary index of the duration of severe hypoxemia. This was slightly and nonsignificantly reduced by medroxyprogesterone acetate (MPA), whereas acetazolamide led to marked improvement. (From Weil JV, Kryger MH, Scoggin CH: Sleep and breathing at high altitude. In Guilleminault C, Dement WC [eds]: Sleep Apnea Syndromes. New York, Alan R Liss; 1978, pp 119-136.)

versus steady-state measurements.[68] Overall, the findings suggest that these agents act primarily on the kidney to produce a metabolic acidosis, which drives ventilation without any clear effect on peripheral or central chemoreceptor sensitivity.

Benzodiazepines

These agents can substantially reduce hypoxic ventilatory responses[70] and were once thought to be hazardous respiratory

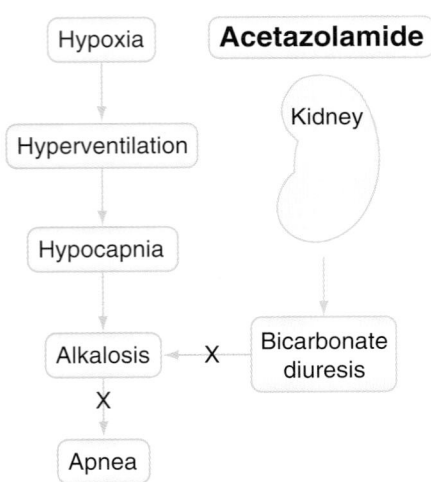

Figure 20–11. Schematic representation of potential mechanisms by which carbonic anhydrase inhibitors (e.g., acetazolamide) decrease periodic breathing during sleep at high altitude. These agents promote a bicarbonate diuresis, which lessens alkalosis and reduces apnea but augments hyperventilation and hypocapnia. This suggests that alkalosis may be more important than hypocapnia in the genesis of periodic breathing.

disorders of sleep. However, recent evidence suggests that in low doses they are relatively safe in such situations and seem to produce no increase in sleep-disordered breathing in older[71] or in nonselected patients with apnea.[72] In sleeping patients with chronic obstructive pulmonary disease, there is no clear increase in apnea or hypopnea or worsening of hypoxemia,[73,74] and little or no adverse effect is seen in patients with obstructive apnea.[75] In patients with heart failure, temazepam decreased microarousals and improved daytime alertness with no change in the extent of periodic breathing or oxygenation in sleep.[76]

Three studies suggest the safety and potential utility of these agents in the sleep disturbance of high altitude.[5,77,78] Shortened latency, decreased arousals, increased sleep efficiency, increased REM, and subjectively better sleep were evident with low-dose temazepam.[77] Benzodiazepines may also slightly reduce periodicity, augment slow wave sleep, and reduce wakefulness during acclimatization but not in early nights after ascent.[5] In a single-blinded, randomized protocol in subjects at 5300 meters, temazepam (10 mg) consistently improved subjective sleep quality, with quicker onset, fewer awakenings, and less awareness of periodic breathing than placebo. Subjects felt more rested the following day. Compared to placebo, mean SaO_2 in sleep was unchanged and oscillations in SaO_2 were reduced.[78]

Other Agents

Almitrine, which stimulates the carotid body and augments hypoxic ventilatory responses, augments arterial oxygenation during sleep but increases respiratory periodicity.[39] These effects would be expected to decrease the continuity and subjective quality of sleep, but this has not been directly studied.

Progestational agents such as medroxyprogesterone acetate substantially reduce periodic breathing with little change in oxygenation in sojourners,[23] but they have greater effects on oxygenation in long-term residents with chronic mountain sickness.[19]

Whether other agents that are used to treat HAPE (such as calcium channel blockers and glucocorticoids) affect breathing, oxygenation, and symptoms related to sleep remains unknown.

SLEEP AT HIGH ALTITUDE AFTER LONG-TERM ADAPTATION

Little is known about sleep and breathing in normal long-term residents of high altitude, although Kryger et al.[79] reported some data. In Leadville, Colorado, with an altitude of 3100 meters, normal subjects have sleep duration and distribution of stages comparable to those in subjects at lower altitude, but no direct comparisons were made. Although little or no prolonged sleep apnea was noted in such subjects, the majority did have various kinds of respiratory dysrhythmia, typically an undulant oscillation in depth of breathing without true apnea and associated with swings in SaO_2 (Fig. 20–12). Because these subjects were middle-aged men, in whom respiratory dysrhythmias are known to be common during sleep at low altitude, it is unclear to what extent the breathing in sleep at chronic high altitude truly differs from that at sea level. It is possible that arterial desaturation induced by high altitude shifts SaO_2 during sleep to the steeper portion of the dissociation curve and

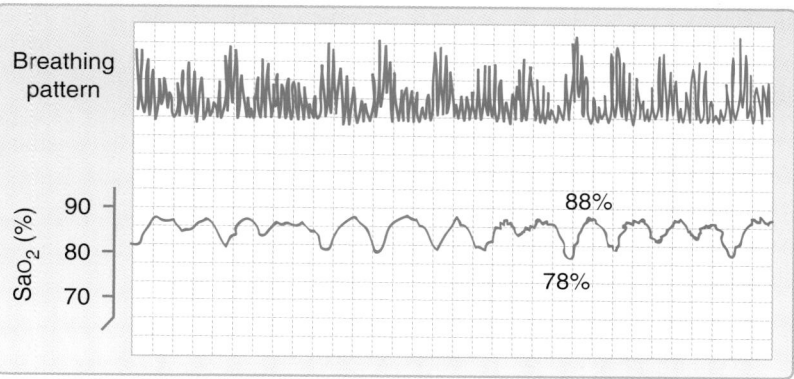

Figure 20–12. Breathing pattern and arterial oxygenation in a subject with chronic mountain polycythemia during sleep at his native altitude of 3100 m. The breathing pattern consists of an undulating depth of breathing with oscillation of arterial oxygen saturation (SaO$_2$). (From Kryger M, Glas R, Jackson D, et al: Impaired oxygenation during sleep in excessive polycythemia of high altitude: Improvement with respiratory stimulation. Sleep 1978;1:3-17, with permission.)

thereby amplifies the influence of ventilatory dysrhythmia on SaO$_2$.

Ventilatory and SaO$_2$ oscillations similar to those observed by Kryger et al.[79] have also been described at high altitude by Lahiri et al.[36] in Sherpas native to high altitude but not in Sherpas native to low altitude. The potential contribution of ethnic or genetic differences is suggested by a study comparing Tibetan and Chinese Han residents of 4000 meters. Sleep was studied in a hypobaric chamber at simulated altitudes of 2261 and 5000 meters. At the higher altitude, Tibetans had more periodic breathing, higher SaO$_2$, and better sleep structure than the Han subjects.[80]

Although decreased hypoxic ventilatory response during wakefulness has been observed in natives of Leadville[81] and in Sherpas native to high altitude,[82] it is unclear whether this contributes to respiratory dysrhythmia and hypoxemia in highlanders during sleep at altitude. However, improvement in hypoxemia during wakefulness and sleep in long-term residents at high altitude with use of the ventilatory stimulant medroxyprogesterone acetate suggests that decreased ventilatory drive may have a permissive role.[79,83]

CONCLUSIONS

The sensation of disrupted sleep after ascent to high altitude is associated with frequent awakenings, which in part probably reflect sleep fragmentation by respiratory dysrhythmia typically consisting of monotonously repetitive periodic breathing. This periodicity is produced by ventilatory inhibition by hypocapnic alkalosis alternating with stimulation by hypoxia, which terminates apnea and initiates hyperpnea with consequent hypocapnia, leading to perpetuation of periodicity. Sleep disruption and periodic breathing decrease with time at moderate altitude and are also considerably reduced by pretreatment with acetazolamide, which reduces alkalosis. In long-term residents of high altitude, less-distinctive, undulating respiratory dysrhythmias are described, with unstable and decreased arterial oxygenation.

The most common treatment is prophylactic administration of acetazolamide, an inhibitor of carbonic anhydrase, which likely works by reducing alkalotic ventilatory inhibition. Recent studies suggest that benzodiazepines may improve sleep quality without apparent adverse effects.

Clinical Pearl

Sleep at altitude is disturbed by the opposing influences of hypoxic stimulation and alkalotic inhibition which lead to periodic breathing and frequent associated arousals. Effective treatments include correction of alkalosis with acetazolamide or blunting of hypoxic stimulation with benzodiazepines.

REFERENCES

1. Moore LG, Harrison GL, McCullough RE, et al: Low acute hypoxic ventilatory response and hypoxic depression in acute altitude sickness. J Appl Physiol 1986;60:1407-1412.
2. Bisgard GE: Carotid body mechanisms in acclimatization to hypoxia. Respir Physiol 2000;121:237-246.
3. Joern AT, Shurley JT, Brooks RE, et al: Short-term changes in sleep patterns on arrival at the South Polar Plateau. Arch Int Med 1970;125:649-654.
4. Reite M, Jackson D, Cahoon RL, et al: Sleep physiology at high altitude. Electroencephalogr Clin Neurophysiol 1975;38:463-471.
5. Goldenberg F, Richalet JP, Onnen I, et al: Sleep apneas and high altitude newcomers. Int J Sports Med 1992;13:S34-36.
6. Normand H, Barragan M, Benoit O, et al: Periodic breathing and O$_2$ saturation in relation to sleep stages at high altitude. Aviat Space Environ Med 1990;61:229-235.
7. Mizuno K, Asano K, Okudaira N: Sleep and respiration under acute hypobaric hypoxia. Jap J Physiol 1993;43:161-175.
8. Wickramasinghe H, Anholm JD: Sleep and breathing at high altitude. Sleep Breath 1999;3:89-102.
9. Miller JC, Horvath SM: Sleep at altitude. Aviat Space Environ Med 1977;48:615-620.
10. Anholm JD, Powles AC, Downey RD, et al: Operation Everest: II. Arterial oxygen saturation and sleep at extreme simulated altitude. Am Rev Resp Dis 1992;145(Pt 1):817-826.
11. Bonnet MH: Performance and sleepiness as a function of frequency and placement of sleep disruption. Psychophysiol 1986;23:263-271.
12. Zielinski J, Koziej M, Mankowski M, et al: The quality of sleep and periodic breathing in healthy subjects at an altitude of 3,200 m. High Alt Med Biol 2000;1:331-336.
13. Netzer NC, Strohl KP: Sleep and breathing in recreational climbers at an altitude of 4200 and 6400 meters: Observational study of sleep and patterning of respiration during sleep in a group of recreational climbers. Sleep Breath 1999;3:75-82.

14. Ohi M, Chin K, Hirai M, et al: Oxygen desaturation following voluntary hyperventilation in normal subjects. Am J Resp Crit Care Med 1994;149(Pt 1):731-738.

15. Lovering AT, Fraigne JJ, Dunin-Barkowski WL, et al: Hypocapnia decreases the amount of rapid eye movement sleep in cats. Sleep 2003;26:961-967.

16. Ward M: Periodic respiration: A short historical note. Ann R Coll Surg Engl 1973;52:330-334.

17. Douglas C, Haldane J, Henderson Y, et al: Physiological observations made of Pikes Peak, Colorado, with special reference to adaptation to low barometric pressures. Phil Trans R Soc Lond 1913;203:185-381.

18. Berssenbrugge A, Dempsey J, Iber C, et al: Mechanisms of hypoxia-induced periodic breathing during sleep in humans. J Physiol 1983;343:507-526.

19. Kryger M, McCullough RE, Collins D, et al: Treatment of excessive polycythemia of high altitude with respiratory stimulant drugs. Am Rev Respir Dis 1978;117:455-464.

20. Masuyama S, Kohchiyama S, Shinozaki T, et al: Periodic breathing at high altitude and ventilatory responses to O_2 and CO_2. Jap J Physiol 1989;39:523-535.

21. Sutton JR, Houston CS, Mansell AL, et al: Effect of acetazolamide on hypoxemia during sleep at high altitude. N Engl J Med 1979;301:1329-1331.

22. Normand H, Vargas E, Bordachar J, et al: Sleep apneas in high altitude residents (3,800 m). Int J Sports Med 1992;13:S40-42.

23. Weil JV, Kryger MH, Scoggin CH: Sleep and breathing at high altitude. In Guilleminault C, Dement WC (eds): Sleep Apnea Syndromes. New York, Liss, 1978, pp 119-136.

24. Lahiri S, Barnard P: Role of arterial chemoreflex in breathing during sleep at high altitude. Prog Clin Biol Res 1983;136:75-85.

25. Lahiri S, Data PG: Chemosensitivity and regulation of ventilation during sleep at high altitudes. Int J Sports Med 1992;13:S31-33.

26. Fujimoto K, Matsuzawa Y, Hirai K, et al: Irregular nocturnal breathing patterns at high altitude in subjects susceptible to high-altitude pulmonary edema (HAPE): A preliminary study. Aviat Space Environ Med 1989;60:786-791.

27. Bulow K: Respiration and wakefulness in man. Acta Physiol Scand 1963;59:1-110.

28. Douglas C, Haldane J: Causes of periodic or Cheyne-Stokes breathing. J Physiol 1909;38:401-419.

29. Douglas CG, Haldane JS: Regulation of normal breathing. J Physiol 1909;38:420-440.

30. Brusil PJ, Waggener TB, Kronauer RE, et al: Methods for identifying respiratory oscillations disclose altitude effects. J Appl Physiol 1980;48:545-556.

31. Waggener TB, Brusil PJ, Kronauer RE, et al: Strength and cycle time of high-altitude ventilatory patterns in unacclimatized humans. J Appl Physiol 1984;56:576-581.

32. West JB, Peters R Jr, Aksnes G, et al: Nocturnal periodic breathing at altitudes of 6,300 and 8,050 m. J Appl Physiol 1986;61:280-287.

33. Naughton M, Benard D, Tam A, et al: Role of hyperventilation in the pathogenesis of central sleep apneas in patients with congestive heart failure [see comments]. Am Rev Resp Dis 1993;148:330-338.

34. White DP, Gleeson K, Pickett CK, et al: Altitude acclimatization: Influence on periodic breathing and chemoresponsiveness during sleep. J Appl Physiol 1987;63:401-412.

35. Smith CA, Nakayama H, Dempsey JA: The essential role of carotid body chemoreceptors in sleep apnea. Can J Physiol Pharmacol 2003;81:774-779.

36. Lahiri S, Maret K, Sherpa MG: Dependence of high altitude sleep apnea on ventilatory sensitivity to hypoxia. Resp Physiol 1983;52:281-301.

37. Fletcher EC: Recurrence of sleep apnea syndrome following tracheostomy: A shift from obstructive to central apnea. Chest 1989;95:205-209.

38. Badr MS, Toiber F, Skatrud JB, et al: Pharyngeal narrowing/occlusion during central sleep apnea. J Appl Physiol 1995;78:1806-1815.

39. Hackett PH, Roach RC, Harrison GL, et al: Respiratory stimulants and sleep periodic breathing at high altitude: Almitrine versus acetazolamide. Am Rev Resp Dis 1987;135:896-898.

40. Salvaggio A, Insalaco G, Marrone O, et al: Effects of high-altitude periodic breathing on sleep and arterial oxyhaemoglobin saturation. Eur Respir J 1998;12:408-413.

41. Douglas CG, Haldane JS, Henderson Y, et al: The physiological effects of low atmospheric pressures as observed on Pike's Peak, Colorado. J Physiol 1912;85:65-67.

42. Gotoh F, Meyer JS, Takagi Y: Cerebral venous and arterial blood gases during Cheyne-Stokes respiration. Am J Med 1969;47:534-545.

43. Sullivan C, Kosar L, Murphy E, et al: Primary role of respiratory afferents in sustaining breathing rhythm. J Appl Physiol 1978;45:11-17.

44. Tawadrous FD, Eldridge FL: Posthyperventilation breathing patterns after active hyperventilation in man. J Appl Physiol 1974;37:353-356.

45. Skatrud JB, Dempsey JA: Interaction of sleep state and chemical stimuli in sustaining rhythmic ventilation. J Appl Physiol 1983;55:813-822.

46. Cherniack N, Gothe B, Strohl K: Mechanisms for recurrent apneas at altitude. High Alt Man 1984:129-140.

47. Khoo MC, Kronauer RE, Strohl KP, et al: Factors inducing periodic breathing in humans: A general model. J Appl Physiol 1982;53:644-659.

48. Khoo MC, Anholm JD, Ko SW, et al: Dynamics of periodic breathing and arousal during sleep at extreme altitude. Respir Physiol 1996;103:33-43.

49. Powles AC, Sutton JR, Gray GW, et al: Sleep hypoxemia at altitude: Its relationship to acute mountain sickness and ventilatory responsiveness to hypoxia and hypercapnia. In: Folinsbee LJ, Wagner JA, Borgia JF (eds): Environmental Stress. New York, Academic Press, 1978, pp 373-381.

50. Insalaco G, Romano S, Salvaggio A, et al: Cardiovascular and ventilatory response to isocapnic hypoxia at sea level and at 5,050 m. J Appl Physiol 1996;80:1724-1730.

51. Berry RB, Gleeson K: Respiratory arousal from sleep: Mechanisms and significance. Sleep 1997;20:654-675.

52. Milledge JS: The ventilatory response to hypoxia: How much is good for a mountaineer? Postgrad Med J 1987;63:169-172.

53. Ghazanshahi SD, Khoo MC: Optimal ventilatory patterns in periodic breathing. Ann Biomed Eng 1993;21:517-530.

54. Eichenberger U, Weiss E, Riemann D, et al: Nocturnal periodic breathing and the development of acute high altitude illness. Am J Respir Crit Care Med 1996;154(Pt 1):1748-1754.

55. Silber E, Sonnenberg P, Collier DJ, et al: Clinical features of headache at altitude: A prospective study. Neurol 2003;60:1167-1171.

56. Bonnet MH: [Sleep fragmentation as the cause of daytime sleepiness and reduced performance]. Wien Med Wochenschr 1996;146:332-334.

57. Swenson ER: Carbonic anhydrase inhibitors and ventilation: A complex interplay of stimulation and suppression. Eur Respir J 1998;12:1242-1247.

58. Cain SM, Dunn JE 2d: Low doses of acetazolamide to aid accommodation of men to altitude. J Appl Physiol 1966;21:1195-1200.

59. Forwand SA, Landowne M, Follansbee JN, et al: Effect of acetazolamide on acute mountain sickness. N Engl J Med 1968;279:839-845.

60. Hackett PH, Rennie D: The incidence, importance, and prophylaxis of acute mountain sickness. Lancet 1976;2:1149-1155.

61. Sutton JR, Gray GW, Houston CS, et al: Effects of duration at altitude and acetazolamide on ventilation and oxygenation during sleep. Sleep 1980;3:455-464.

62. Nicholson AN, Stone BM: Hypnotics and transient insomnia. Acta Psychiatr Scand Suppl 1986;332:55-59.

63. Hauge A, Nicolaysen G, Thoresen M: Acute effects of acetazolamide on cerebral blood flow in man. Acta Physiol Scand 1983;117:233-239.

64. Huang SY, McCullough RE, McCullough RG. et al: Usual clinical dose of acetazolamide does not alter cerebral blood. Respir Physiol 1988;72:315-326.

65. White DP, Zwillich CW, Pickett CK, et al: Central sleep apnea: Improvement with acetazolamide therapy. Arch Intern Med 1982;142:1816-1819.

66. DeBacker WA, Verbraecken J, Willemen M, et al: Central apnea index decreases after prolonged treatment with acetazolamide. Am J Resp Crit Care Med 1995;151:87-91.

67. Nakayama H, Smith CA, Rodman JR, et al: Effect of ventilatory drive on carbon dioxide sensitivity below eupnea during sleep. Am J Respir Crit Care Med 2002;165:1251-1260.

68. Swenson ER, Leatham KL, Roach RC, et al: Renal carbonic anhydrase inhibition reduces high altitude sleep periodic breathing. Resp Physiol 1991;86:333-343.

69. Bashir Y, Kann M, Stradling JR: The effect of acetazolamide on hypercapnic and eucapnic/poikilocapnic hypoxic ventilatory responses in normal subjects. Pulm Pharm 1990;3:151-154.

70. Lakshminarayan S, Sahn SA, Hudson LD, et al: Effect of diazepam on ventilatory responses. Clin Pharmacol Ther 1976; 20:178-183.

71. Camacho ME, Morin CM: The effect of temazepam on respiration in elderly insomniacs with mild sleep apnea. Sleep 1995; 18:644-645.

72. Hoijer U, Hedner J, Ejnell H, et al: Nitrazepam in patients with sleep apnoea: A double-blind placebo-controlled study. Eur Resp J 1994;7:2011-2015.

73. Gentil B, Tehindrazanarivelo A, Lienhart A, et al: [Respiratory effects of midazolam in patients with obstructive sleep apnea syndromes.] Ann Fr Anesth Reanim 1994;13:275-279.

74. Steens RD, Pouliot Z, Millar TW, et al: Effects of zolpidem and triazolam on sleep and respiration in mild to moderate chronic obstructive pulmonary disease. Sleep 1993;16:318-326.

75. Berry RB, Kouchi K, Bower J, et al: Triazolam in patients with obstructive apnea. Am J Resp Crit Care Med 1995;151:450-454.

76. Biberdorf DJ, Steens R, Miller TW, et al: Benzodiazepines in congestive heart failure: Effects of temazepam on arousability and Cheyne-Stokes respiration. Sleep 1993;16:529-538.

77. Nicholson AN, Smith PA, Stone BM, et al: Altitude insomnia: Studies during an expedition to the Himalayas. Sleep 1988; 11:354-361.

78. Dubowitz G: Effect of temazepam on oxygen saturation and sleep quality at high altitude: Randomised placebo controlled crossover trial. BMJ 1998;316:587-589.

79. Kryger M, Glas R, Jackson D, et al: Impaired oxygenation during sleep in excessive polycythemia of high altitude: Improvement with respiratory stimulation. Sleep 1978;1:3-17.

80. Plywaczewski R, Wu TY, Wang XQ, et al: Sleep structure and periodic breathing in Tibetans and Han at simulated altitude of 5000 m. Respir Physiol Neurobiol 2003;136:187-197.

81. Weil JV, Byrne-Quinn E, Sodal IE, et al: Acquired attenuation of chemoreceptor function in chronically hypoxic man at high altitude. J Clin Invest 1971;50:186-195.

82. Hackett PH, Reeves JT, Reeves CD, et al: Control of breathing in Sherpas at low and high altitude. J Appl Physiol 1980;49:374-379.

83. Kryger M, Weil J, Grover R: Chronic mountain polycythemia: A disorder of the regulation of breathing during sleep? Chest 1978;73(Suppl):303-304.

21

Host Defense

James M. Krueger

Jeannine A. Majde

ABSTRACT

During the onset of infection, excess sleepiness is often experienced. This phenomenon was noted by Hippocrates, although it was not until the 1980s that sleep over the course of an infection was measured. Changes in sleep induced by microbes appear to be one facet of the acute phase response. Typically, soon after infectious challenge, animals exhibit excess non–rapid eye movement (NREM) sleep and decreased rapid eye movement (REM) sleep. The exact time course of sleep responses depends on the infectious agent, the route of administration, and the time of day the infectious challenge is given.

There is a common perception that sleep loss can render one vulnerable to infection. Many studies have combined sleep deprivation with measurement of one or more parameters of the immune response. Very few studies have combined sleep deprivation with infectious challenge. After sleep deprivation, several immune system parameters—for example, natural killer cell activity—change. Furthermore, after prolonged (2 to 3 weeks) sleep deprivation, rats become septicemic. Small amounts of sleep loss may help host defenses, whereas prolonged sleep loss is devastating.

The molecular mechanisms responsible for the changes in sleep associated with infection appear to be an amplification of a physiologic sleep regulatory biochemical cascade. This chain of events includes well-known immune response modifiers, such as interleukin-1, tumor necrosis factor, prostaglandins, nitric oxide, and adenosine. All these substances are normal constituents of brain and are involved in physiologic sleep regulation.

There is little direct evidence showing that sleep per se aids in recuperative processes. It most likely does, but it is difficult to directly test this notion.

Most individuals have experienced the intense desire to sleep that occurs at the onset of certain infections, and they have heard the advice to get plenty of rest to prevent or help recover from infectious diseases. These experiences suggest a connection between sleep and host defense systems. Indeed, Hippocrates and Aristotle acknowledged such a relationship. It is thus somewhat surprising that it is only within the past 15 years that modern science and medicine have systematically investigated whether sleep has anything to do with host defense systems. In this chapter, four questions related to this issue will be addressed:

1. Does sleep change after infectious challenge?
2. Does sleep loss affect immune function?
3. Do the sleep and immune systems share regulatory molecules?
4. Does sleep per se aid in recuperative processes?

Clear affirmative answers are at hand for the first three questions, and the evidence thus far is consistent with a role for sleep in recuperation.

SLEEP IS GREATLY ALTERED AFTER INFECTIOUS CHALLENGE

Viral Challenge

Viral diseases that cause central nervous system lesions or inflammation can affect sleep.[1,2] In his seminal paper, von Economo[3] related the location of virus-induced brain lesions to changes in sleep patterns. This work led to the concept that sleep was an active process, not simply the withdrawal of sensory stimuli, and to the idea that there was some degree of localization of neural networks regulating sleep. Despite the importance of this work, many years passed before the direct effects of viral infections on sleep were experimentally determined. During the early stages of human immunodeficiency virus infections, before the onset of acquired immunodeficiency disease syndrome (AIDS), patients have excess stage 4 non–rapid eye movement (NREM) sleep during the latter half of the night.[4-7] Another central nervous system viral disease, rabies, is also associated with disrupted sleep.[8,9] In these diseases, as was the case with von Economo's virus, it is difficult to distinguish whether the effects of the viral infection on sleep are direct or whether they result from virus-induced lesions.[2] Viral pathogenic mechanisms have also been implicated in several conditions that involve sleep disorders; the list includes infectious mononucleosis,[10] sudden infant death syndrome,[11] and chronic fatigue syndrome[12] (see review by Krueger and Majde[13]). However, the direct involvement of the viruses themselves in the sleep disorders associated with these syndromes has not been investigated.

The influenza virus, which localizes to the lungs during the early stage of disease, has been used in several sleep investigations. Smith[14] at the British Common Cold Unit reported that low doses of influenza in humans induce excess behavioral sleep and cognitive dysfunction; these symptoms appear after low viral doses that fail to induce the better-known characteristics of the acute phase response such as a fever. However, polysomnography was not used in Smith's study. More recently, animal studies of influenza viral infections have clearly shown that sleep is profoundly affected by infectious challenge. In a rabbit model, intravenous injections of influenza virus are associated with large increases in NREM sleep lasting 6 to 10 hours.[15] In rabbits, however, influenza virus can undergo only partial replication and the disease is thus limited in course because new virions cannot be formed. (The partial replication of the virus allows double-stranded viral RNA to be formed: the importance of double-stranded RNA in viral pathogenic mechanisms is explained later.)

Another animal model, the influenza-infected mouse, is more applicable to humans because in mice this virus can fully replicate. Mice challenged intranasally with influenza virus display profound increases in NREM sleep lasting 3 or more days, whereas rapid-eye movement (REM) sleep is inhibited[16-18] (Fig. 21–1). These sleep responses are much attenuated if the viral infection is confined to the upper airway.[18] When the initial viral challenge is limited to the upper airway, it takes about a week for the virus to move down the respiratory track; by then, the animals are able to mount an effective immune response. Different strains of mice respond differentially to viral challenge. Very large changes in sleep are observed in Swiss-Webster[16] and C57BL/6[17] strains, whereas influenza-induced sleep responses in BALB/c mice are much attenuated. This difference may result from the reduced ability of BALB/c mice[17] to produce and respond to[19] cytokines; later, we provide evidence that cytokines are involved in physiologic sleep regulation and in the sleep responses induced by infectious challenge.

The mechanism by which viruses induce sleep responses seems to involve viral double-stranded (ds) RNA induction of cytokines such as interferons and interleukin (IL)-1. Influenza virus is a negative-sense, single-stranded RNA virus. When influenza virus infects a cell, it forms the positive-sense RNA strand that can anneal to the negative-sense strand to form dsRNA. Viral dsRNA can be extracted from lungs of infected mice[20] and from supernates of cells infected in culture.[21] If rabbits are given the viral dsRNA extracted from mouse lungs, they exhibit sleep responses similar to those observed after injection of viable virus. RNA from healthy mouse lungs has no effect on sleep.[20] Similar responses are observed if rabbits are given a synthetic dsRNA, polyriboinosinic:polyribocytidylic (poly I:C), but not if given the corresponding single strands of poly I and poly C.[22]

Similarly, rabbits given short double-stranded oligomers corresponding to a portion of influenza gene segment 3 also exhibit large increases in NREM sleep.[23] Rabbits do not respond if given the single-stranded oligomers. Rabbits that are challenged on sequential days with influenza virus fail to express a fever or excess NREM sleep on day 2.[24] This same state of physiologic hyporesponsiveness to the virus on day 2 can be induced by injecting poly I:C, rather than virus, on day 1, suggesting that poly I:C can totally replace the viral stimulus in this system.[24] Rabbits challenged with viable virus or poly I:C have increased plasma antiviral activity that occurs concomitantly with the changes in sleep.[15] The antiviral activity is attributed to interferon-α and other cytokines. Injection of interferon-α into rabbits also induces sleep responses similar to those induced by virus, poly I:C, or the double-stranded oligomers.[25,26] High doses of interferon-α also stimulate NREM sleep in other species,[27,28] but lower doses inhibit both NREM and REM sleep in humans.[29] Mice genetically deficient for the receptor that binds both interferon-α and interferon-β still respond to poly I:C challenge with excess sleep and a hypothermic response similar to that induced by influenza virus (J. Krueger and J. Majde, unpublished results), suggesting that interferon-α does not mediate the viral acute phase response. Our current hypothesis is that other cytokines known to be somnogenic are likely to mediate the excess sleep response to influenza virus. The role of such cytokines in sleep regulation is discussed later.

Bacterial Challenge

Sleep responses are also observed after bacterial challenge. Indeed, results obtained after challenging rabbits with the gram-positive bacterium *Staphylococcus aureus* were the first to suggest that NREM sleep responses formed part of the acute phase response.[30] In those experiments, rabbits were given *S. aureus* intravenously to induce septicemia; within a few hours of the inoculation, large excesses in NREM sleep were observed. Associated with the increase in NREM sleep were increases in amplitude of slow waves on the electroencephalogram (EEG). EEG slow wave (0.5 to 4 Hz) amplitudes are thought to be indicative of the intensity of NREM sleep. This initial phase of increased duration and intensity of NREM sleep lasted about 20 hours; it was followed by a more prolonged phase of decreased duration of NREM sleep and decreased EEG slow wave amplitudes.[30] During both phases of the NREM sleep changes, REM sleep was inhibited and animals were febrile. Other changes characteristic of the acute

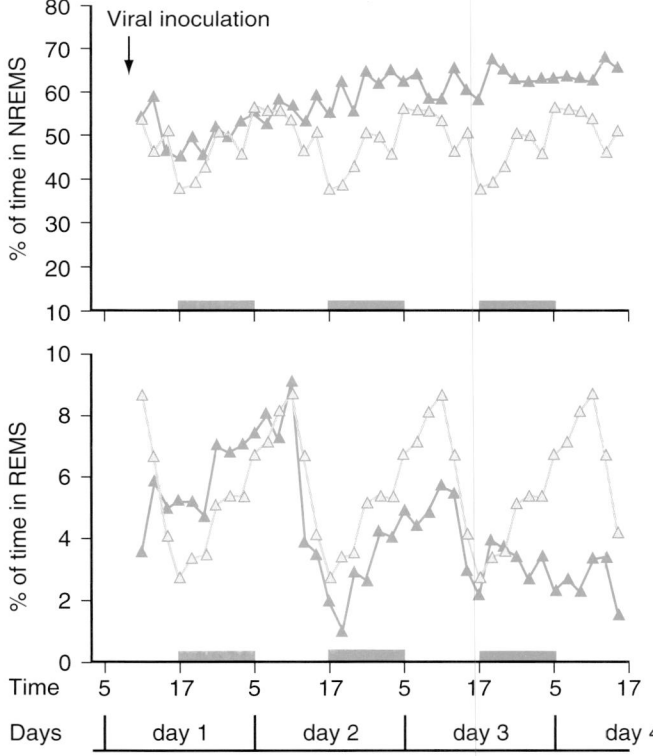

Figure 21–1. Influenza virus challenge induces prolonged increases in non–rapid eye movement (NREM) sleep *(top)* and decreases in rapid eye movement (REM) sleep *(bottom)* in mice. *Dark blue triangles* represent data collected after viral inoculation. *Light blue triangles* represent the averaged baseline data collected over a 3-day period just prior to viral inoculation. Horizontal *dark bars* show lights-off periods for each experimental day. (Data from Fang J, Sanborn CK, Renegar KB, et al: Influenza viral infections enhance sleep in mice. Proc Soc Exp Med Biol 1995;210:242-252.)

phase response (e.g., fibrinogenemia and neutrophilia) occurred concurrently with the changes in sleep.

In subsequent studies, gram-negative bacteria and other routes of administration were used, and a similar general pattern of biphasic NREM sleep responses and REM sleep inhibition was observed (see review by Krueger and Majde[13]). However, the timing of sleep responses depends on both bacterial species and the route of administration. For example, after intravenous administration of *Escherichia coli*, NREM sleep responses are rapid in onset, but the excess NREM sleep phase lasts only 4 to 6 hours.[31] The subsequent phase of reduced NREM sleep and reduced amplitude of EEG slow waves is sustained for relatively long periods. In contrast, if the gram-negative bacterium *Pasteurella multocida* (a natural pathogen in rabbits) is given intranasally, a different time course of sleep responses is observed.[32] In this case, the increased NREM sleep responses occur after a longer latency, and the magnitude of the increases in NREM sleep is less than the effects of this pathogen given by other routes of administration.[32]

Much is known about how bacteria induce sleep responses. Unlike for viruses, bacterial replication is not necessary. Injection of killed bacteria or purified bacterial cell walls induces excess NREM sleep, enhances EEG slow waves, and inhibits REM sleep (see review by Krueger and Majde[13]). Bacteria and bacterial cell walls are phagocytized by macrophages, which kill the bacteria, digest their cell walls, and secrete low-molecular-weight soluble components derived from these cell walls into the surrounding medium.[33-35] Some of these cell-wall–derived substances are effective stimulants of host defense systems and somnogenic (see review by Krueger and Majde[13]). This process is thought to provide a mechanism whereby the host can amplify its defenses. For example, muramyl peptides are the monomeric building blocks of bacterial peptidoglycan. Macrophages release muramyl peptides when they phagocytize bacterial cell walls, and the released substances are somnogenic.[33]

The sleep-promoting activity of muramyl peptides depends on their chemical structure. For example, the muramyl dipeptide N-actyl-muramyl-L-alanyl-D-isoglutamine (MDP-LD) is somnogenic (see, e.g., Krueger et al.[36]), whereas the stereoisomers MDP-LL and MDP-DD are not. Many muramyl peptides are also immunoadjuvants and pyrogenic, although the structural requirements for these biologic activities are distinct from those required for sleep-promoting activity (see review by Krueger and Majde[13]).

Muramyl peptides were first implicated in sleep regulation after a disaccharide-tetrapeptide, N-acetylglucosaminyl-1,6-anhydro-N-acetylmuramyl-alanyl-glutamyl-diaminopime-lyl-alanine, isolated from brain and urine, was shown to be somnogenic.[37] Muramyl peptides are probably not synthesized by mammals, because there are no known synthetic pathways in mammals for muramic acid or diaminopimelic acid. Nonetheless, muramyl peptides are readily available to mammals via the intestinal lumen, which contains large amounts of bacteria. We are constantly challenged by bacteria and their breakdown products through lymphatic drainage of the intestine. As mentioned, on entering the body, bacteria are phagocytized and digested, and somnogenic muramyl peptides are released in the process. This mechanism is viewed as operating at a low basal rate under normal conditions and amplified greatly during infection. It is also probably involved in sleep responses induced by sleep deprivation and excess food intake (see later). Furthermore, reduction of bacterial populations in the intestine is associated with a reduction of sleep.[38,39]

Another bacterial cell wall product that could be involved in sleep responses induced by gram-negative bacteria is endotoxin or lipopolysaccharide. Endotoxin and its biologically active moiety lipid A are somnogenic in animals and man (see review by Krueger and Majde[13]). Sleep responses induced by endotoxin are distinct from those induced by muramyl peptides. Muramyl peptides are somnogenic over a wide dose range and are relatively nontoxic in the sense that very large doses (e.g., for MDP, 10,000 times the minimal somnogenic dose) are not lethal. In contrast, the somnogenic dose range of endotoxin is more restricted, and small increases above the threshold somnogenic dose (about 10-fold) can induce shock. Modification of the lipid A structure alters somnogenic activity (e.g., conversion of diphosphoryl lipid A to monophosphoryl lipid A reduces its somnogenicity). Like dsRNA, endotoxin and muramyl peptides induce production of a wide variety of cytokines and hormones. Some of these substances are involved in physiologic sleep regulation, and the enhanced sleep responses observed during infection are believed to be manifestations of the amplification of the production of these substances (see later).

Humans inoculated with lipopolysaccharide and followed for 12 hours manifest sleep changes, fever, cytokine expression, and hormonal changes[40] somewhat similar to those seen in animals, although EEG changes are distinct from those seen in rabbits or rats, and NREM sleep increases require a higher dose of lipopolysaccharide than does REM sleep reduction.

Other microbes (e.g., fungal organisms such as *Candida albicans* or protozoans such as *Trypanosoma brucei brucei*) also have the capacity to induce sleep responses. Some of these microbe-induced sleep responses are quite interesting. Trypanosomiasis in rabbits is associated with recurrent bouts of enhanced NREM sleep occurring about every 7 days. Trypanosomes undergo antigenic variations in the host; the proliferating new antigenic variants stimulate the host immune response, and such periods are accompanied by excess NREM sleep.[41] Like bacteria and viruses, fungi and protozoans have the capacity to enhance cytokine production by the host.

Recently, an overarching theory has been articulated that explains why diverse microbial factors activate stereotypic host defense responses. This theory involves Toll-like receptors (TLRs), which are expressed primarily on macrophages and dendritic cells. TLRs were originally defined in fruit flies and were demonstrated to be essential for surviving certain infections.[42] Ten TLRs have been identified to date in mammals. For example, TLR2 recognizes peptidoglycans, fungal polysaccharides, and trypanosome components; TLR3 recognizes dsRNA; and TLR4 recognizes lipopolysaccharide.[42] Once a TLR binds its ligand, a series of complex signaling mechanisms activates induction of cytokines, which in turn induce host defenses such as fever and excess sleep.[42]

In summary, infectious challenge is associated with profound changes in sleep. The immune system has evolved receptors that recognize stable microbial components and initiate these sleep changes. These microbe-induced sleep responses are now considered part of the acute phase response and, like the other components of this response, sleep may be adaptive.

SLEEP LOSS AFFECTS IMMUNE FUNCTION

Answering the question of whether sleep loss affects immune function is difficult. For example, what measurement should one use to assess immune function? The important question is whether sleep loss renders the animal more vulnerable to infectious challenge, tumor formation, and systemic inflammation. (That sleep loss increases vulnerability to accidental injury is clear.) Unfortunately, only a very few studies have directly measured host outcomes. Instead, the approach most often used is to choose a parameter associated with the immune system (e.g., natural killer cell activity or a plasma cytokine level) and determine whether it changes after sleep deprivation. Often, such results leave the reader uninformed as to whether the outcome is adverse or beneficial for the host. In addition, it is very difficult in sleep deprivation studies to isolate sleep loss per se as the independent variable. Sleep deprivation is usually associated with stress, increased locomotor activity, changes in feeding patterns, hormonal changes, and changes in body temperature. Each of these variables is known to affect immune function. Despite these limitations, a picture is emerging that suggests that sleep loss does indeed influence the immune system. Paradoxically, it may be that short-term sleep deprivation can enhance host defenses, whereas long-term sleep loss is devastating.

Most people are under the impression that sleep loss renders one more vulnerable to infection. Yet in human experimental studies of sleep deprivation, there has been a failure to demonstrate an increased incidence of infection. Most of these studies are limited in that healthy young volunteers are used, environmental conditions are unchallenging, and the deprivation periods short. Some animal studies, using short-term sleep deprivation, are consistent with the human studies. Toth and colleagues[43] challenged rabbits with *E. coli* before or after 4 hours of sleep deprivation. They concluded that sleep deprivation failed to exacerbate the *E. coli*–induced clinical illness. Using rats partially deprived of sleep for several days and challenged with a subdermal allogeneic carcinoma, Bergmann and colleagues[44] concluded that host defenses were improved by sleep deprivation because the rats deprived of sleep had smaller tumors than those in control animals. In contrast, Brown and colleagues[45] deprived mice of sleep for 7 hours that were immunized against influenza virus and then rechallenged with influenza virus just prior to sleep deprivation. The sleep-deprived immunized mice, but not immunized control mice, failed to clear the virus from their lungs. These results strongly suggest that sleep loss is detrimental to host defenses. However, in a similar study by Renegar and colleagues,[46] sleep loss failed to alter preexisting mucosal and humoral immunity in either young or senescent mice.

The effects of long-term sleep deprivation on host defenses are more striking. If rats obtain only about 20% of their normal sleep, they die after a period of 2 to 3 weeks. Yoked control rats, which manage to achieve about 80% of their normal sleep during the deprivation period, survive. Everson[47] showed that the experimental rats, but not the yoked controls, develop septicemia. Bacteria cultured from the blood were primarily facultative anaerobes indigenous to the host and environment. Similar opportunistic infections plague patients with suppressed immune systems. Everson's results clearly suggest that host defenses are compromised by long-term sleep loss.

One source of possible invading microbes is bacterial translocation across the gut wall. In another study, after only a few days of partial sleep deprivation, viable bacteria could be cultured from mesenteric lymph nodes, although the blood of these animals remained sterile.[48] In another model of sleep deprivation in which rats were placed on a small pedestal in a pool of water, Landis and colleagues[49] obtained similar results. After 72 hours of REM sleep loss, they could culture bacteria from mesenteric lymph nodes. These results suggest that sleep loss very likely amplifies the normally occurring process of gut permeability to bacteria and bacterial products. As discussed later, food intake also affects gut permeability to bacteria and bacterial products[50] and also affects sleep. Small amounts of bacterial cell wall products, such as endotoxin and peptidoglycan, "prime" immunocytes and could thereby render them more effective for nonspecific host defenses (see review by Pabst et al.[51]). Thus, perhaps under appropriate experimental conditions, a small amount of sleep loss is associated with more effective priming, whereas after more prolonged sleep loss, the host is overwhelmed by microbial challenge.

Regardless of such speculation, an independent body of literature clearly indicates that sleep loss is associated with changes in parameters normally associated with the immune response. Cytokines, such as interferon, IL-1, and tumor necrosis factor (TNF), are well known for their roles as immune response modifiers. These substances are affected by sleep deprivation (see review by Obal and Krueger[52]). More than 25 years ago, Palmblad and colleagues[53] showed that after sleep deprivation, the ability of human lymphocytes to produce interferon is enhanced. More recently, many laboratories have obtained similar results. For example, sleep deprivation enhances TNF production in streptococcus-stimulated white blood cells. Other stressors, unlike sleep deprivation, fail to prime for systemic production of TNF,[54] whereas sleep loss increases the ability of endotoxin-stimulated monocytes to produce TNF.[55] The ability of cultures of whole blood to produce IL-1β and interferon-γ in response to endotoxin is maximal at the time of sleep onset.[56] In humans, sleep deprivation leads to enhanced nocturnal plasma levels of IL-1–like activity. Using rabbits, Opp and Krueger[57] reached a similar conclusion.

There are several reports that in normal people, plasma levels of cytokines are related to the sleep–wake cycle. Moldofsky et al.[58] first described such relationships in humans, showing that IL-1 activity was related to the onset of slow wave sleep. Darko and colleagues[59] showed that plasma levels of TNF vary in phase with EEG slow wave amplitudes. Gudewill et al.[60] and Covelli et al.[61] also described a temporal relationship between sleep and IL-1β activity. Several clinical conditions associated with sleepiness, such as sleep apnea, chronic fatigue syndrome, chronic insomnia, preeclampsia, postdialysis fatigue, psychoses, rheumatoid arthritis, and AIDS are associated with enhanced plasma levels of TNF and other cytokines (see review by Obal and Krueger[52]). In fact, when patients who have rheumatoid arthritis are treated with a TNF soluble receptor, their fatigue is reduced.[62]

Other facets of the immune response are also linked to sleep. Over 25 years ago, Casey et al.[63] demonstrated altered antigen uptake after sleep deprivation. Palmblad et al.[64] showed a decrease in lymphocyte DNA synthesis after 48 hours of sleep deprivation and, in an earlier study,[53] a decrease in phagocytosis after 72 hours of sleep deprivation. Moldofsky[58] described sleep deprivation–induced changes in mitogen responses (see review by Krueger and Majde[13]). In humans, circulating immune complexes fall during sleep and rise again just before getting out of bed, and in mice, sleep deprivation reduces IgG catabolism, resulting in elevated IgG levels (see review by Krueger and Majde[13]). In contrast, Benca et al.[65] failed to show an effect of sleep deprivation on spleen cell counts, lymphocyte proliferation, or plaque-forming cell responses to antigens in rats. In an extensive elegant study of humans deprived of sleep for 64 hours, Dinges and colleagues[66] also failed to show an effect of sleep deprivation on proliferative responses to mitogens. However, they did show a depression of CD4, CD16, CD56 and CD57 lymphocytes after 1 night of sleep loss, although CD56 and CD57 lymphocytes increased after 2 nights of sleep loss. Born et al.[67] also showed that a night of sustained wakefulness reduced counts of all lymphocyte subsets measured. Finally, Brown et al.[68] showed that 8 hours of sleep deprivation suppressed the secondary antibody response to sheep red blood cells in rats.

Two clinical studies have examined the effects of sleep deprivation on functional immunity by following antibody responses in human subjects to viral vaccines. Acute sleep deprivation for 1 whole night after immunization with hepatitis A vaccine at 0900 results in an antibody response at 4 weeks that is about half that seen in subjects that slept regularly from 2300 to 0700 on the night following the vaccination.[69] Sleeping subjects show increases in growth hormone, prolactin, and dopamine, but decreases in thyrotropin, norepinephrine, and epinephrine, compared to sleep-deprived subjects.[69] Another vaccination study was conducted in subjects restricted to 4 hours of sleep for 4 nights and then immunized with influenza vaccine.[70] Sleep deprivation continued for 2 more nights after the vaccination. Then subjects were allowed to sleep for 12 hours over 7 days to recover. Antibody determinations at 10 days after vaccination revealed that sleep-deprived subjects expressed influenza antibodies at less than half the level seen in controls. However, by 3 weeks after immunization, antibody titers were similar in both groups.[70] No analyses of cellular immunity, cytokine expression, or other immune parameters were conducted in these studies.

Changes in natural killer cell activity in conjunction with sleep and sleep loss have been measured by several laboratories. In several studies, natural killer cell activity decreased after sleep deprivation.[71,72] In contrast, Born et al.[67] and Dinges et al.[66] reported increased natural killer cell activity after sleep deprivation. In normal men and women, natural killer cell activity may decrease with sleep.[73] However, insomnia is associated with a reduction of natural killer cell activity.[74] It is likely that circulating natural killer cell activity as well as natural killer cell activity in a variety of tissue compartments are sensitive to sleep, although the exact tissue distribution of natural killer cell activity is likely to be dependent on the specific experimental conditions.

SLEEP REGULATORY MECHANISM AND THE IMMUNE SYSTEM SHARE REGULATORY MOLECULES

Associations between the nervous and immune systems are numerous. For example, there is neuronal innervation of lymphoid organs, and endocrines, such as growth hormone,

prolactin, and glucocorticoids, have the capacity to affect both sleep and immunocytes. Another class of substances, the cytokines, act as autocrines, juxtacrines, and paracrines and are well characterized as immune response modifiers (see reviews by Krueger and Majde[13] and Plata-Salaman[75]). Two of these cytokines, IL-1β and TNF-α, are especially well characterized as being involved in physiologic NREM sleep regulation (see review by Obal and Krueger[52]). The evidence for the involvement of IL-1β and TNF-α in NREM sleep regulation and in the sleep responses to infectious challenge is briefly reviewed here.

In addition to being immunocyte products whose production is amplified by viral and bacterial products, both IL-1β and TNF-α are also found in normal brain.[52,76] Both IL-1β mRNA and TNF-α mRNA have diurnal rhythms in the brain, and the highest values are associated with periods of maximal sleep (Fig. 21–2). TNF protein levels also have a sleep-associated diurnal rhythm in several brain areas, and IL-1 cerebrospinal fluid levels vary with the sleep–wake cycle.[77]

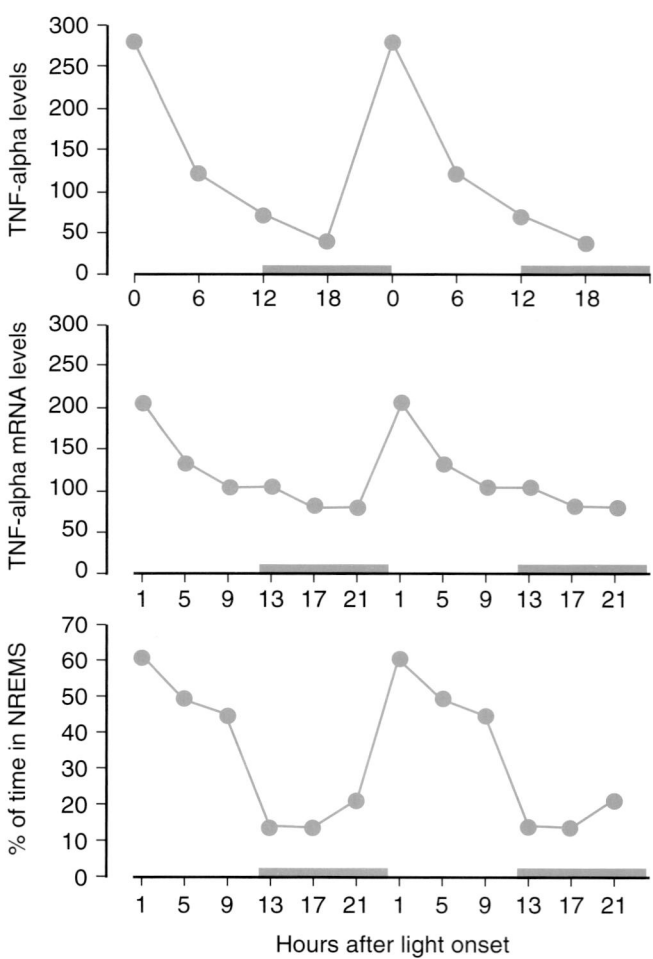

Figure 21–2. In rats, TNF bioactivity *(top)* and tumor necrosis factor (TNF)-α mRNA *(middle)* have diurnal rhythms. Peak levels of these substances occur at the beginning of daylight hours; during that period, duration of non–rapid eye movement (NREM) sleep is maximal in rats *(lower)*. Horizontal *dark bars* indicate the lights-off period; rats are nocturnal animals, thus sleep less during the night. *Top:* Values are picograms of TNF per gram of tissue. *Middle:* Values are relative densities of stained bands imaged from electrophoresis gels. *Bottom:* Values are percent of time spent in NREM sleep in 3-hour time blocks.

Both IL-1β and TNF-α belong to larger functional families of molecules (see review by Obal and Krueger[52]). All of the IL-1–associated and TNF-associated molecules are constitutively expressed in normal brain.

Administration of either IL-1β or TNF-α (or IL-1α or TNF-β, as well) promotes NREM sleep[78,79] (see review by Obal and Krueger[52]). The excessive NREM sleep occurring after either IL-1β or TNF-α injection appears to be physiologic in the sense that sleep remains episodic, sleep cycle length remains normal, and sleep is readily reversible if animals are disturbed. Furthermore, if IL-1β or TNF-α is given either intracerebroventricularly or intravenously, sleep intensity, as measured by the amplitude of EEG delta waves, is greater. The effects of IL-1 on sleep depend on dose and the time of day it is given. Low doses of IL-1β promote NREM sleep, whereas high doses inhibit NREM sleep.

The inhibition of either IL-1β or TNF-α inhibits spontaneous NREM sleep (see review by Obal and Krueger[52]). Thus, spontaneous NREM sleep is reduced after the administration of anti–IL-1 antibodies, anti-TNF antibodies, the soluble IL-1 receptor, the soluble TNF receptor, peptide fragments of the IL-1 or TNF soluble receptor, or the IL-1 receptor antagonist (see review by Obal and Krueger[52]). Furthermore, sleep is inhibited when animals are given substances that inhibit either the production or actions of IL-1 or TNF. Alpha melanocyte–stimulating hormone, corticotropin-releasing hormone, prostaglandin E$_2$, IL-4, IL-10, and glucocorticoids, all of which inhibit IL-1 or TNF, all inhibit spontaneous NREM sleep (see reviews by Krueger and Majde[13] and Obal and Krueger[52]). Finally, knockout strains of mice that lack either the type I IL-1 receptor or the 55-kd TNF receptor, sleep less than strain controls (see review by Obal and Krueger[52]).

Sleep deprivation, excessive food intake, and acute mild increases in ambient temperature are effective somnogens. The somnogenic actions of each of these manipulations are associated with enhanced production of either IL-1 or TNF. After sleep deprivation, brain levels of IL-1β mRNA increase (see review by Obal and Krueger[52]). The NREM sleep rebound that would normally occur after sleep deprivation is greatly attenuated if either IL-1 or TNF is blocked using antibodies or soluble receptors. In humans and rabbits, IL-1 plasma levels increase during sleep deprivation. Although the somnogenic effects of sleep deprivation seem to involve both IL-1 and TNF, the enhanced NREM sleep associated with mild increases in ambient temperature involves TNF but not IL-1.

Excessive food intake induces enhanced liver and brain production of IL-1β mRNA. The increased brain IL-1β mRNA is dependent on vagal afferent activity induced by liver IL-1β. Thus, rats presented with palatable food (cafeteria diet) display excess NREM sleep[80] and increased IL-1β mRNA levels in liver and brain.[81] The cafeteria diet–induced NREM sleep responses are blocked by vagotomy.[80] Similarly, intraperitoneal IL-1β induces excess NREM sleep and increased IL-1β mRNA in liver and brain; both effects are also lost if animals are vagotomized.[82] Vagal-associated paraganglia in the liver have IL-1 receptors,[83] and hepatoportal injection of IL-1β induces vagal afferent activity.[84]

The actions of cafeteria diet feeding on NREM sleep and liver and brain production of IL-1 represent physiologic change, yet they most likely involve the actions of bacterial cell wall products. Gut permeability to bacteria and bacterial products is influenced by dietary factors,[50] and endotoxin,

a gram-negative bacteria cell wall product, is a normal constituent of portal blood.[85] Endotoxin stimulates IL-1 production in liver and elsewhere. Other bacterial cell wall products (e.g., muramyl peptides) also have the capacity to stimulate IL-1 and TNF production (see review by Krueger and Majde[13]). Muramyl peptides also cross the intestinal wall into blood. NREM sleep responses induced by muramyl dipeptide are attenuated if animals are pretreated with either blockers of IL-1 or TNF (see reviews by Krueger and Majde,[13] Pabst et al.,[51] and Obal and Krueger[52]). As mentioned, prolonged sleep deprivation results in bacteremia. It thus seems likely that the interaction of those bacteria with liver macrophages results in the amplification of the physiologic processes that are also associated with excessive food intake. Other forms of infection are also likely to interact with these processes, resulting in the excess sleep associated with infection (see earlier).

The molecular steps by which IL-1 and TNF induce sleep are beginning to be understood, but there is yet much to learn. IL-1 and TNF act within a cascade of events that include parallel interacting pathways (Fig. 21–3). For example, both IL-1 and TNF stimulate nuclear factor kappa B (NFκB) production. NFκB is a DNA-binding protein involved in transcription. Other somnogenic cytokines, such as acidic fibroblast growth factor, epidermal growth factor, and nerve growth factor, also stimulate NFκB production. In contrast, several substances that inhibit NFκB activation (e.g., IL-4, IL-10 and glucocorticoids) all inhibit spontaneous sleep. NFκB promotes IL-1 and TNF production and thus forms a positive feedback loop; such a mechanism could be involved in the amplification of signals promoting sleep. Sleep deprivation is associated with the activation of NFκB in the cerebral cortex,[86] basal forebrain cholinergic neurons,[87] and the lateral hypothalamus.

Several NFκB downstream events also play a role in sleep regulation. Thus, inducible nitric oxide synthase DNA has several NFκB enhancer elements. Inhibition of nitric oxide synthase inhibits sleep, whereas nitric oxide donors promote sleep (see review by Obal and Krueger[52]). Adenosine, another substance implicated in sleep regulation,[88] augments IL-1β–induced nitric oxide synthase production.[89] Adenosine also induces astrocytes to produce nitric oxide.[90] Activation of NFκB also promotes IL-2, IL-6, IL-8, IL-15, and IL-18 production; all of these cytokines promote sleep in rats (see review by Obal and Krueger[52]).

Growth hormone–releasing hormone (GHRH) is probably involved in IL-1 promotion of NREM sleep. There is an independent literature implicating GHRH in sleep regulation (see review by Obal and Krueger[52]). Administration of GHRH promotes NREM sleep, and inhibition of GHRH inhibits spontaneous NREM sleep. Hypothalamic GHRH mRNA varies with the sleep–wake cycle, and sleep deprivation enhances GHRH mRNA in the hypothalamus. Microinjection of GHRH into the basal forebrain enhances NREM sleep. In contrast, microinjection of a GHRH antagonist inhibits NREM sleep. IL-1 induces growth hormone release; this action is mediated via hypothalamic GHRH.[52] If animals are pretreated with anti-GHRH antibodies and then given IL-1β, IL-1β–induced growth hormone release and increased NREM sleep are blocked,[91] suggesting that GHRH forms part of the IL-1 somnogenic pathway. Furthermore, there exists a population of hypothalamic gamma-aminobutyric acid–ergic (GABAergic) GHRH- and IL-1β–receptive neurons[92]; it seems likely these are involved

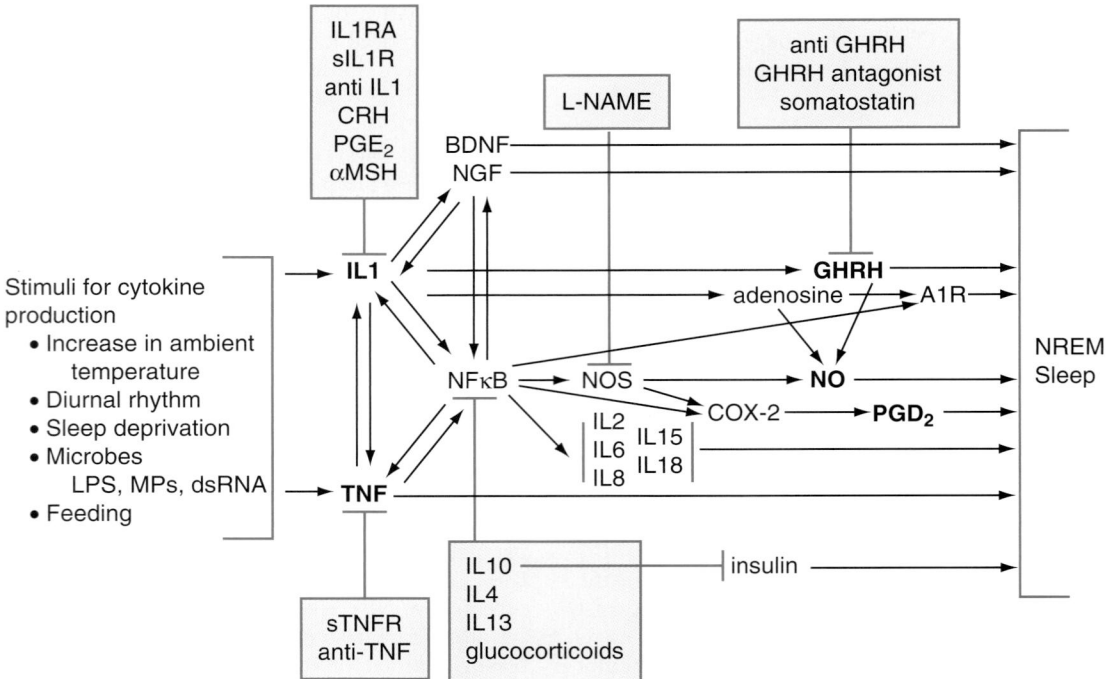

Figure 21–3. Interleukin (IL)-1β and tumor necrosis factor (TNF)-α are part of the brain cytokine network that includes several other endoge-nous somnogenic substances and sleep inhibitory substances. Substances in *boxes* inhibit non–rapid eye movement (NREM) sleep and inhibit either the production of, or the action of, substances in the somnogenic pathways. Inhibition of any one step does not result in complete sleep loss; animals probably compensate for the loss of any one step by relying on parallel somnogenic pathways. Such redundant pathways provide stability to the sleep regulatory system as well as alternative mechanisms by which a variety of sleep-promoting, or sleep inhibitory, stimuli may affect sleep. Our current knowledge of the biochemical events involved in sleep regulation is much more complicated than that shown here. For example, several laboratories have shown that acidic fibroblast growth factor enhances sleep. The receptor and intracellular signaling systems for all these substances are in neurons, and in some cases, these mechanisms are very complex. A1R, adenosine A1 receptor; anti IL1, anti-IL-1 anti-body; anti-TNF, anti-TNF antibody; BDNF, brain-derived neurotrophic factor; COX-2, cyclooxygenase-2; CRH, corticotropin-releasing hormone; dsRNA, double-stranded RNA; GHRH, growth hormone releasing hormone; IL1RA, IL-1 receptor antagonist; L-NAME, an arginine analogue; LPS, lipopolysaccharide; MPs, muramyl peptides; αMSH, alpha melanocyte–stimulating hormone; NFκB, nuclear factor κB; NGF, nerve growth factor; NOS, nitric oxide synthase; PGD$_2$, prostaglandin D$_2$; PGE$_2$, prostaglandin E$_2$; sIL1R, soluble IL-1 receptor; sTNFR, soluble TNF receptor; → indicates stimulation; ⊣ indicates inhibition.

in the somnogenic actions of these substances. The somno-genic actions of GHRH may also involve nitric oxide. GHRH-induced growth hormone release involves nitric oxide.[93]

There is a growing body of literature linking the somno-genic cytokines to more classical sleep mechanisms. IL-1β and TNF-α interact with a variety of neurotransmitter systems. The list includes glutamate, serotonin, acetylcholine, GABA, histamine, and dopamine (see reviews by Krueger and Majde,[13] Obal and Krueger,[52] and Plata-Salaman[75]). Little is known about the specificity of these interactions for sleep, although there are some promising investigations. For example, Imeri and colleagues[94] showed that depletion of brain serotonin blocks MDP-induced NREM sleep responses and attenuates IL-1–induced sleep responses. In another report, the same group directly measured medial preoptic serotonin metabolism after IL-1 treatment and concluded that serotonergic activation could play a role in mediating the effects of IL-1 on sleep.[95] Furthermore, injection of IL-1β into the dorsal raphe nucleus inhibits serotonergic neurons and enhances sleep.[96] These data are consistent with prior studies that showed that IL-1 can promote sleep if injected into the locus coeruleus.[97] Within the hypothalamus, IL-1β activates sleep-active neurons and inhibits wake-active neurons.[98] TNF-α promotes sleep if microinjected into the anterior hypothalamus, whereas

injection of a soluble TNF receptor into this area reduces sleep.[99] TNF-α is also somnogenic if injected into the locus coeruleus.[97] This latter observation likely relates to TNF-α interactions with α-2 adrenergic receptive mechanisms and norepinephrine release.[100] TNF-α also promotes glutamate receptor expression and activity, and these receptors have a role in EEG synchronization.[101-103] In neuroprotective doses, TNF also alters outward potassium currents.[104,105] Interestingly, TNF-α, if applied locally onto the surface of the cerebral cortex unilaterally, enhances EEG delta activity on the side to which it is applied but not the contralateral side.[106] On the other hand, application of the TNF soluble receptor uni-laterally onto the cortex of sleep-deprived rats attenuates sleep loss–induced EEG delta activity on the side injected but not on the opposite side. These latter data suggest that TNF-α acts locally within the cortex (in addition to its somnogenic actions in the hypothalamus) to enhance EEG synchroniza-tion and possibly sleep intensity.

In summary, sleep regulatory mechanisms and the immune system share regulatory molecules. The best characterized are IL-1 and TNF. These substances are involved in physiologic NREM sleep regulation and are key factors in the development of the acute phase response induced by infectious agents. During the initial response to infectious challenge, these proinflammatory cytokines are upregulated and thereby amplify physiologic sleep mechanisms leading to the acute phase sleep response.

> ### Clinical Pearl
>
> *Although physicians have always prescribed bed rest to aid in recuperation from bouts of infectious diseases and other maladies, there is, as yet, no direct evidence that sleep per se aids in recuperation. Nevertheless, physicians continue to prescribe bed rest, and often this is just what the patient wishes to do. It seems likely that such advice is beneficial. The only evidence relevant to this issue, of which we are aware, is consistent with the notion that sleep aids in recuperation. After infectious challenge, animals that have robust NREM sleep responses have a higher probability of survival than animals that fail to exhibit NREM sleep responses.[107] Although this evidence is strictly correlative in nature, it behooves those of us interested in sleep and sleep disorders to investigate this further. Perhaps our grandmothers' folk wisdom of the preventative and curative attributes of sleep is correct.*

Acknowledgments

This work was suggested in part by grants from the National Institutes of Health, NS-25378, NS-27250, NS-31453, and HD 36520.

References

1. Fu ZF, Weihe E, Zheng YM, et al: Differential effects of rabies and Borna disease viruses on immediate-early- and late-response gene expression in brain tissues. J Virol 1993;67:6674-6681.
2. Toth LA: Microbial modulation of sleep. In Lydic R, Baghdoyan H (eds): Handbook of Behavioral State Control: Cellular and Molecular Mechanisms. Boca Raton, CRC Press, 1999, pp 641-657.
3. Von Economo C: Sleep as a problem of localization. J Nerv Ment Dis 1930;71:249-259.
4. Norman SE, Chediak AD, Kiel M, et al: Sleep disturbances in HIV-infected homosexual men. AIDS 1990;4:775-781.
5. Norman SE, Chediak AD, Freeman C, et al: Sleep disturbances in men with asymptomatic human immunodeficiency (HIV) infection. Sleep 1992;15:150-155.
6. White JL, Darko DF, Brown SJ, et al: Early central nervous system response to HIV infection: Sleep distortion and cognitive-motor decrements. AIDS 1995;9:1043-1050.
7. Kubicki S, Henkes H, Terstegge K, et al: AIDS related sleep disturbances: A preliminary report. In Kubicki ST, Henkes H, Bienzle U, et al. (eds): HIV and the Nervous System. New York, Fischer, 1988, pp 97-105.
8. Gourmelon P, Biet D, Clarencon D, et al: Sleep alterations in experimental street rabies virus infection occur in the absence of major EEG abnormalities. Brain Res 1991;554:159-165.
9. Gourmelon P, Biet D, Court L, et al: Electrophysiological and sleep alterations in experimental mouse rabies. Brain Res 1986; 398:128-140.
10. Guilleminault C, Mondini S: Mononucleosis and chronic daytime sleepiness: A long-term follow-up study. Arch Intern Med 1986;146:1333-1335.
11. Hoffman HJ, Damus K, Hillman L, et al: Risk factors for SIDS: Results of the National Institute of Child Health and Human Development SIDS cooperative epidemiological study. Ann NY Acad Sci 1988;533:13-30.
12. Komaroff AL: Chronic fatigue syndromes: Relationships to chronic viral infections. J Virol Methods 1988;21:3-10.
13. Krueger JM, Majde JA: Microbial products and cytokines in sleep and fever regulation. Crit Rev Immunol 1994;14:355-379.
14. Smith A: Sleep, colds, and performance. In Broughton RJ, Ogilvie RD (eds): Sleep, Arousal and Performance. Boston, Birkhauser, 1992, pp 233-242.
15. Kimura-Takeuchi M, Majde JA, Toth LA, et al: Influenza virus-induced changes in rabbit sleep and acute phase responses. Am J Physiol 1992;263:R1115-R1121.
16. Fang J, Sanborn CK, Renegar KB, et al: Influenza viral infections enhance sleep in mice. Proc Soc Exp Med Biol 1995;210: 242-252.
17. Toth LA, Rehg JE, Webster RG: Strain differences in sleep and other pathophysiological sequelae of influenza virus infection in naive and immunized mice. J Neuroimmunol 1995;58:89-99.
18. Fang J, Tooley D, Gatewood C, et al: Differential effects of total and upper airway influenza viral infection on sleep in mice. Sleep 1996;19:337-342.
19. Pope M, Marsden PA, Cole E, et al: Resistance to murine hepatitis virus strain 3 is dependent on production of nitric oxide. J Virol 1998;72:7084-7090.
20. Majde JA, Brown RK, Jones MW, et al: Detection of toxic viral-associated double-stranded RNA (dsRNA) in influenza-infected lung. Microb Pathol 1991;10:105-115.
21. Majde JA, Guha-Thakurta N, Chen Z, et al: Spontaneous release of stable viral double-stranded RNA into the extracellular medium by influenza virus-infected MDCK epithelial cells: Implications for the viral acute phase response. Arch Virol 1998; 143:2371-2380.
22. Krueger JM, Majde JA, Blatteis CM, et al: Polyriboinosinic:polyribocytidylic acid (poly I:C) enhances rabbit slow-wave sleep. Am J Physiol 1988;255:R748-R755.
23. Bredow S, Fang J, Guha-Thakurta N, et al: Synthesis of an influenza double-stranded RNA-oligomer that induces fever and sleep in rabbits. Sleep Res 1995; 24A:101.
24. Kimura-Takeuchi M, Majde JA, Toth LA, et al: The role of double-stranded RNA in the induction of the acute phase response in an abortive influenza viral infection. J Infect Dis 1992;166: 1266-1275.
25. Krueger JM, Dinarello CA, Shoham S, et al: Interferon alpha-2 enhances slow-wave sleep in rabbits. Int J Immunopharmacol 1987;9:23-30.
26. Kimura M, Majde JA, Toth LA, et al: Somnogenic effects of rabbit and human recombinant interferons in rabbits. Am J Physiol 1994;267:R53-R61.
27. DeSarro GB, Masuda Y, Ascioti C, et al: Behavioral and ECoG spectrum changes induced by intracerebral infusion of interferons and interleukin-2 in rats are antagonized by naloxone. Neuropharmacology 1990;29:167-179.
28. Reite M, Landenslager M, Jones J, et al: Interferon decreases REMS latency. Biol Psychiatry 1987;22:104-107.
29. Späth-Schwalbe E, Lange T, Perras P, et al: Interferon-α acutely impairs sleep in healthy humans. Cytokine 2000;12:518-521.
30. Toth LA, Krueger JM: Alterations in sleep during *Staphylococcus aureus* infection in rabbits. Infect Immun 1988;56:1785-1791.
31. Toth LA, Krueger JM: Effects of microbial challenge on sleep in rabbits. FASEB J 1989;3:2062-2066.
32. Toth LA, Krueger JM: Somnogenic, pyrogenic and hematologic effects of experimental pasteurellosis in rabbits. Am J Physiol 1990;258:R536-R542.
33. Johannsen L, Wecke J, Obál F Jr, et al: Macrophages produce somnogenic and pyrogenic muramyl peptides during digestion of staphylococci. Am J Physiol 1991;260:R126-R133.
34. Vermeulen MW, Grey GR: Processing of *Bacillus subtilis* peptidoglycan by a mouse macrophage cell line. Infect Immun 1984; 46:476-483.
35. Smialowicz RJ, Schwab JH: Processing of streptococcal cell walls by rat macrophages and human monocytes in vitro. Infect Immun 1977;17:591-598.

36. Krueger JM, Walter J, Karnovsky ML, et al: Muramyl peptides: Variation of somnogenic activity with structure. J Exp Med 1984; 159:68-76.

37. Krueger JM, Karnovsky ML, Martin SA, et al: Peptidoglycans as promoters of slow-wave sleep: II. Somnogenic and pyrogenic activities of some naturally occurring muramyl peptides— Correlations with mass spectrometric structure determination. J Biol Chem 1984;259:12659-12662.

38. Brown R, Price RJ, King MG, et al: Are antibiotic effects on sleep behavior in the rat due to modulation of gut bacteria? Physiol Behav 1990;48:561-565.

39. Rhee YH, Kim HI: The correlation between sleeping-time and numerical range in intestinal normal flora in psychiatric insomnia patients. Bull Natl Sci Chungbuk Natl Univ 1987; 1:159-172.

40. Pollmacher T, Mullington J, Korth C, et al: Influence of host defense activation on sleep in humans. Adv Neuroimmunol 1995;5:155-169.

41. Toth LA, Tolley EA, Broady R, et al: Sleep during experimental trypanosomiasis in rabbits. Proc Soc Exp Biol Med 1994; 205:174-181.

42. Akira S, Hemmi H: Recognition of pathogen-associated molecular patterns by TLR family. Immunol Lett 2003; 85:85-95.

43. Toth LA, Opp MR, Mao L: Somnogenic effects of sleep deprivation and *Escherichia coli* inoculation in rabbits. J Sleep Res 1995; 4:30-40.

44. Bergmann BM, Rechtschaffen A, Gilliland MA, et al: Effect of extended sleep deprivation on tumor growth in rats. Am J Physiol 1996;271:R1460-R1464.

45. Brown R, Pang G, Husband AJ, et al: Suppression of immunity to influenza virus infection in the respiratory tract following sleep disturbance. Reg Immunol 1989;2:321-325.

46. Renegar KB, Floyd RA, Krueger JM: Effects of short-term sleep deprivation on murine immunity to influenza virus in young adult and senescent mice. Sleep 1998;21:241-248.

47. Everson CA: Sustained sleep deprivation impairs host defense. Am J Physiol 1993;265:R1148-R1154.

48. Everson CA, Toth LA: Systemic bacterial invasion induced by sleep deprivation. Am J Physiol 2000;278:R905-R916.

49. Landis C, Pollack S, Helton WS: Microbial translocation and NK cell cytotoxicity in female rats sleep deprived on small platforms. Sleep Res 1997;26:619.

50. Deitch EA: Bacterial translocation: The influence of dietary variables. Gut 1994;35:S23-S27.

51. Pabst MJ, Beranova-Giorgianni S, Krueger JM: A review of the effects of muramyl peptides on macrophages, monokines and sleep. Neuroimmunomodulation 1999;6:261-283.

52. Obal F Jr, Krueger JM: Biochemical regulation of sleep. Front Biosci 2003;8:520-550.

53. Palmblad J, Cantell K, Strander H, et al: Stressor exposure and immunological response in man: Interferon producing capacity and phagocytosis. Psychosom Res 1976;20:193-199.

54. Yamasu K, Shimada Y, Sakaizumi M, et al: Activation of the systemic production of tumor necrosis factor after exposure to acute stress. Eur Cytokine Netw 1992;3:391-398.

55. Uthgenannt D, Schoolmann D, Pietrowsky R, et al: Effects of sleep on the production of cytokines in humans. Psychosom Med 1995;57:97-104.

56. Hohagen F, Timmer J, Weyerbrock A, et al: Cytokine production during sleep and wakefulness and its relationship to cortisol in healthy humans. Neuropsychobiology 1993;28:9-16.

57. Opp MR, Krueger JM: Anti-interleukin-1β reduces sleep and sleep rebound after sleep deprivation in rats. Am J Physiol 1994;266:R688-R695.

58. Moldofsky H, Lue FA, Eisen J, et al: The relationship of interleukin-1 and immune functions to sleep in humans. Psychosom Med 1986;48:309-318.

59. Darko DF, Miller JC, Gallen C, et al: Sleep electroencephalogram delta frequency amplitude, night plasma levels of tumor necrosis factor α and human immunodeficiency virus infection. Proc Natl Acad Sci U S A 1995;92:12080-12086.

60. Gudewill S, Pollmacher T, Vedder H, et al: Nocturnal plasma levels of cytokines in healthy men. Eur Arch Psychiatry Clin Neurosci 1992;242:53-56.

61. Covelli V, D'Andrea L, Savastano S, et al: Interleukin-1 beta plasma secretion during diurnal spontaneous and induced sleeping in healthy volunteers. Acta Neurol (Napoli) 1994;16:79-86.

62. Franklin CM: Clinical experience with soluble TNF p75 receptor in rheumatoid arthritis. Semin Arthrit Rheum 1999;29:171-181.

63. Casey FB, Eisenberg J, Peterson D, et al: Altered antigen uptake and distribution due to exposure to extreme environmental temperatures or sleep deprivation. Reticuloendothel Soc J 1974; 15:87-90.

64. Palmblad J, Petrini B, Wasserman J, et al: Lymphocyte and granulocyte reactions during sleep deprivation. Psychosom Med 1979;41:273-278.

65. Benca RM, Kushida CA, Everson CA, et al: Sleep deprivation in the rat: VII. Immune function. Sleep 1989;12:47-52.

66. Dinges DF, Douglas SD, Zaugg L, et al: Leukocytosis and natural killer cell function parallel neurobehavioral fatigue induced by 64 hours of sleep deprivation. J Clin Invest 1994;93:1930-1939.

67. Born J, Lange T, Hansen K, et al: Effects of sleep and circadian rhythm on human circulating immune cells. J Immunol 1997; 158:4454-4464.

68. Brown R, Price RJ, King MG, et al: Interleukin-1β and muramyl dipeptide can prevent decreased antibody response associated with sleep deprivation. Brain Behav Immun 1989;3:320-330.

69. Lange T, Perras B, Fehm HL, et al: Sleep enhances the human antibody response to hepatitis A vaccination. Psychosom Med 2003;65:831-835.

70. Spiegel K, Sheridan JF, Van Cauter E: Effect of sleep deprivation on responses to immunization. JAMA 2002;288:1471-1472.

71. Irwin M, McClintick J, Costlow C, et al: Partial night sleep deprivation reduces natural killer and cellular immune responses in humans. FASEB J 1996;10:643-653.

72. Irwin M, Mascovich A, Gillin JC, et al: Partial sleep deprivation reduces natural killer cell activity in humans. Psychosom Med 1994;56:493-498.

73. Moldofsky H, Lue FA, Davidson J, et al: Comparison of sleep-wake circadian immune functions in women vs men. Sleep Res 1989;18:431.

74. Irwin M, Smith TL, Gillin JC: Electroencephalographic sleep and natural killer activity in depressed patients and control subject. Psychosom Med 1992;54:10-21.

75. Plata-Salaman CR: Immunoregulators in the nervous system. Neurosci Biobehav Rev 1991;15:185-215.

76. Vitkovic L, Bockaert J, Jacque C: "Inflammatory" cytokines: Neuromodulators in normal brain? J Neurochem 2000;74: 457-471.

77. Lue FA, Bail M, Jephthah-Ochola J, et al: Sleep and cerebrospinal fluid interleukin-1-like activity in the cat. Int J Neurosci 1988; 42:179-183.

78. Krueger JM, Walter J, Dinarello CA, et al: Sleep-promoting effects of endogenous pyrogen (interleukin 1). Am J Physiol 1984; 246:R994-R999.

79. Shoham S, Davenne D, Cady AB, et al: Recombinant tumor necrosis factor and interleukin-1 enhance slow-wave sleep. Am J Physiol 1987;253:R142-R149.

80. Hansen M, Kapás L, Fang J, et al: Cafeteria diet-induced sleep is blocked by subdiaphragmatic vagotomy in rats. Am J Physiol 1998;274:R168-R174.

81. Hansen MK, Taishi P, Chen Z, et al: Cafeteria-feeding induces interleukin-1β mRNA expression in rat liver and brain. Am J Physiol 1998;274:R1734-R1739.

82. Hansen MK, Taishi P, Chen Z, et al: Vagotomy blocks the induction of interleukin-1β mRNA in the brain of rats in response to systemic interleukin-1β. J Neurosci 1998;18:2247-2253.

83. Goehler LE, Relton JK, Dripps D, et al: Vagal paraganglia bind biotinylated interleukin-1 receptor antagonist: A possible mechanism for immune-to-brain communication. Brain Res Bull 1997;43:357-364.

84. Niijima A: The afferent discharges from sensors for interleukin-1β in the hepatoportal system in the anesthetized rat. J Auton Nerv Syst 1996;61:287-291.

85. Jacob AI, Goldberg PK, Bloom N, et al: Endotoxin and bacteria in portal blood. Gastroenterology 1977;72:1268-1270.

86. Chen Z, Fang J, Gardi J, et al: Sleep-deprivation induces activation of nuclear factor-κB. Soc Neurosci Abst 1997;23:792.

87. Basheer R, Rainnie DG, Porkka-Heiskanen T, et al: Adenosine, prolonged wakefulness, and A1-activated NF-kappaB DNA binding in the basal forebrain of the rat. Neuroscience 2001; 104:731-739.

88. Houston JP, Haas HL, Boix F, et al: Extracellular adenosine levels in neostriatum and hippocampus during rest and activity periods of rats. Neuroscience 1996;73:99-107.

89. Seo HG, Fujii J, Asahi M, et al: Roles of purine nucleotides and adenosine in enhancing NOS II gene expression in interleukin-1 beta-stimulated rat vascular smooth muscle cells. Free Rad Res 1997;26:409-413.

90. Janigro D, Wender R. Ransom G, et al: Adenosine-induced release of nitric oxide from cortical astrocytes. Neuroreport 1996; 7:1640-1643.

91. Obál F Jr, Fang J, Payne LC, et al: Growth hormone releasing hormone (GHRH) mediates the sleep promoting activity of interleukin-1 (IL1) in rats. Neuroendocrinology 1995;61:559-565.

92. De A, Churchill L, Obál F Jr, Simasko SM, et al: GHRH and IL1β increase cytoplasmic Ca^{2+} levels in cultured hypothalamic GABAergic neurons. Brain Res 2002;949:209-212.

93. Tena-Sempere M, Pinilla L, Gonzalez D, Aguilar E: Involvement of endogenous nitric oxide in the control of pituitary responsiveness to different elicitors of growth hormone release in prepubertal rats. Neuroendocrinology 1996;64:146-152.

94. Imeri L, Bianchi S, Mancia M: Muramyl dipeptide and IL1 effects on sleep and brain temperature following inhibition of serotonin synthesis. Am J Physiol 1997;273:R1663-R1668.

95. Gemma C, Imeri L, Grazia De Simoni M, et al: Interleukin-1 induces changes in sleep, brain temperature, and serotonergic metabolism. Am J Physiol 1997;272:R601-R606.

96. Manfredi A, Brambilla D, Bianchi S, et al: Interleukin-1β enhances non-rapid eye movement sleep when microinjected into the dorsal raphe nucleus and inhibits serotonergic neurons in vitro. Eur J Neurosci 2003;18:1-10.

97. De Sarro G, Gareri P, Sinopoli VA, et al: Comparative, behavioural and electrocortical effects of tumor necrosis factor-alpha and interleukin-1 microinjected into the locus ceruleus of rat. Life Sci 1997;60:555-564.

98. Alam N, McGinty D, Imeri L, et al: Effects of interleukin-1 beta on sleep- and wake-related preoptic anterior hypothalamic neurons in unrestrained rats. Sleep 2001;24:A59.

99. Kubota T, Li N, Guan Z, et al: Intrapreoptic microinjection of TNF α enhances non-REM sleep in rats. Brain Res 2002; 932:37-44.

100. Elenkov IJ, Kovacs K, Duda E, et al: Presynaptic inhibitory effect of TNF-alpha on the release of noradrenaline in isolated median eminence. J Neuroimmunol 1992;41:117-120.

101. De A, Krueger JM, Simasko S: TNFα increases cytosolic Ca^{++} responses to AMPA and KCl in primary cultures of fetal hippocampal neurons. Brain Res 2003;981:133-142.

102. Bazhenov M, Timofeev I, Steriade M, et al: Model of thalamo-cortical slow-wave sleep oscillations and transitions to activated states. J Neurosci 2002;22:8691-8704.

103. Beattie EC, Stellwagen D, Morishita W, et al: Control of synaptic strength by glial TNF alpha. Science 2002;295: 2282-2285.

104. Diem R, Meyer R, Weishaupt JH, et al: Reduction of potassium currents and phosphatidylinositol 3-kinase-dependent Akt phosphorylation by tumor necrosis factor-α rescues axotomized retinal ganglion cells from retrograde cell death in vivo. J Neurosci 2001;21:2058-2066.

105. Houzen S, Kikuchi S, Kanno M, et al: Tumor necrosis factor enhancement of transient outward potassium currents in cultured rat cortical neurons. J Neurosci Res 1997;50: 990-999.

106. Yoshida H, Peterfi Z, Garcia-Garcia F, et al: State-specific asymmetries in EEG slow wave activity induced by local application of TNFα. Brain Res 2004;1009:129-136.

107. Toth LA, Tolley EA, Krueger JM: Sleep as a prognostic indicator during infectious disease in rabbits. Proc Soc Exp Biol Med 1993;203:179-192.

22

Endocrine Physiology

Eve Van Cauter

ABSTRACT

Sleep exerts important modulatory effects on most components of the endocrine system. The secretion of growth hormone (GH) and prolactin (PRL) is markedly increased during sleep, whereas the release of cortisol and thyrotropin (TSH) is inhibited. Conversely, awakenings interrupting sleep inhibit nocturnal GH and PRL secretions and are associated with increased cortisol and TSH concentrations. The gonadotropic axis is also influenced by sleep, and, reciprocally, gonadal steroids affect sleep quality. Modulatory effects of sleep on endocrine release are not limited to the hormones of the hypothalamic-pituitary axes; these effects are also observed for the hormones controlling carbohydrate metabolism, appetite, and water and electrolyte balance. Sleep loss is associated with disturbances of hormone secretion and metabolism, which may have clinical relevance, particularly as voluntary partial sleep curtailment has become a highly prevalent behavior in modern society. Findings suggest that part of the constellation of hormonal and metabolic alterations that characterize normal aging may reflect the deterioration of sleep quality. Strategies to reverse decrements in sleep quality may have beneficial effects on endocrine and metabolic function.

MODULATION OF ENDOCRINE FUNCTION BY SLEEP-WAKE HOMEOSTASIS AND CIRCADIAN RHYTHMICITY

In healthy adults, reproducible changes of essentially all hormonal and metabolic variables occur during sleep and around wake-sleep and sleep-wake transitions. These daily events reflect the interaction of circadian rhythmicity and sleep-wake homeostasis (see Chapters 31 and 33). Thus, the dual control of sleep timing and quality by circadian processes (i.e., process C) and sleep-wake homeostasis (i.e., process S) is readily reflected in the modulatory effects exerted by sleep on endocrine and metabolic function. The relative contributions of circadian timing compared with homeostatic control in the regulation of the temporal organization of hormone release vary from one endocrine axis to another. Similarly, modulatory effects of the transitions between wake and sleep (and vice versa) and between non–rapid eye movement (NREM) and rapid eye movement (REM) stages also vary from one hormone to the other.

The impact of sleep on endocrine function and metabolism has been studied extensively in the human being, probably because methods of measurement, including repeated blood sampling at frequent intervals, sensitive assays of blood constituents, and polysomnographic (PSG) sleep recordings, are more readily available for people than for laboratory animals. Human sleep is normally consolidated in a single 6- to 9-hour period, whereas other mammals generally sleep in several fragmented periods. The detection of hormonal changes during sleep is thus hindered by the short duration of the sleep cycle in laboratory species. Possibly because of the consolidation of the sleep period, the wake-sleep and sleep-wake transitions in the human being are associated with hormonal and metabolic changes that are more marked than those in other mammals.

To differentiate between effects of circadian rhythmicity and those subserving sleep-wake homeostasis, researchers have used experimental strategies that take advantage of the fact that the circadian pacemaker takes several days to adjust to a large sudden shift of sleep-wake and light-dark cycles (such as occur in jet lag and shift work). Such strategies allow for the effects of circadian modulation to be observed in the absence of sleep and for the effects of sleep to be observed at an abnormal circadian time. Figure 22–1 illustrates mean profiles of plasma growth hormone (GH), plasma cortisol, plasma prolactin (PRL), plasma thyrotropin (TSH), plasma glucose, and insulin-secretion rates (ISR) observed in healthy subjects who were studied before and during an abrupt 12-hour delay of the sleep-wake and dark-light cycles. To eliminate the effects of feeding, fasting, and postural changes, the subjects remained recumbent throughout the study, and the normal meal schedule was replaced by intravenous glucose infusion at a constant rate.[1]

As shown in Figure 22–1, this drastic manipulation of sleep had only modest effects on the wave shape of the cortisol profile, in sharp contrast with the immediate shift of the GH and PRL rhythms that followed the shift of the sleep-wake cycle. The temporal organization of TSH secretion appears to be influenced equally by circadian and sleep-dependent processes. Indeed, the evening elevation of TSH levels occurs well before sleep onset and has been shown to reflect circadian phase. During sleep, an inhibitory process prevents TSH concentrations from rising further. Consequently, in the absence of sleep, the nocturnal TSH elevation is markedly amplified.[2] Both sleep and time of day clearly modulated glucose levels and insulin-secretion rates: Nocturnal elevations of glucose and ISR occurred even when the subjects were sleep-deprived, and recovery sleep at an abnormal circadian time was also associated with elevated glucose and ISR. This pattern of changes in glucose levels and ISR reflected changes in glucose use because, when glucose is infused exogenously, endogenous glucose production is largely inhibited.

In the first part of this chapter, the interactions between sleep and endocrine release in the hypothalamo-pituitary axes are reviewed. The roles of sleep in carbohydrate metabolism, appetite regulation, and hormone control of body-fluid

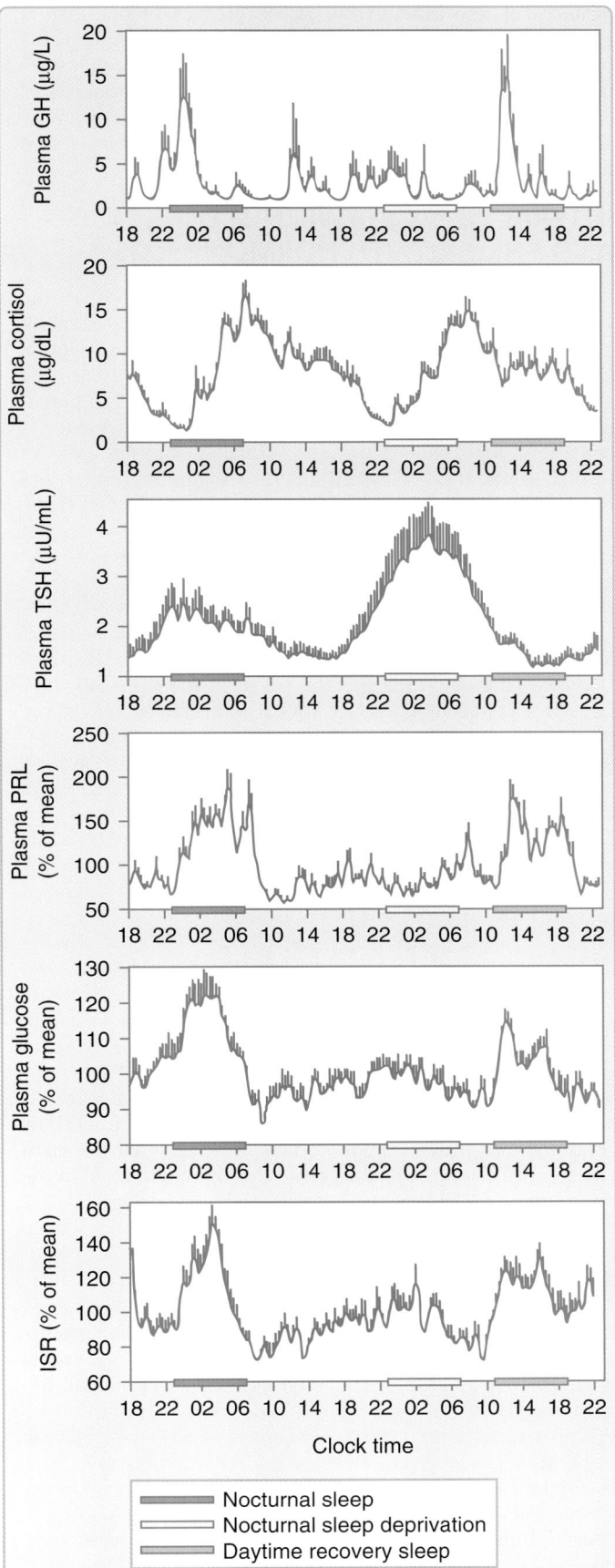

Figure 22–1. From *top* to *bottom*: Mean 24-hour profiles of plasma growth hormone (GH), cortisol, thyrotropin (TSH), prolactin (PRL), glucose, and insulin secretion rates (ISR) in a group of eight healthy young men (20 to 27 years old) studied during a 53-hour period including 8 hours of nocturnal sleep, 28 hours of sleep deprivation, and 8 hours of daytime sleep. The *vertical bars* on the tracings represent the standard error of the mean (SEM) at each time point. The *dark blue bars* represent the sleep periods. The *light blue bars* represent the period of nocturnal sleep deprivation. The *medium blue bars* represent the period of daytime sleep. Caloric intake was exclusively under the form of a constant glucose infusion. Shifted sleep was associated with an immediate shift of GH and PRL release. In contrast, the secretory profiles of cortisol and TSH remained synchronized to circadian time. Both sleep-dependent and circadian inputs can be recognized in the profiles of glucose and ISR. (Adapted from Van Cauter E, Spiegel K: Circadian and sleep control of endocrine secretions. In Turek FW, Zee PC [eds]: Neurobiology of Sleep and Circadian Rhythms. New York, Marcel Dekker, 1999; and Van Cauter E, Blackman JD, Roland D, et al: Modulation of glucose regulation and insulin secretion by sleep and circadian rhythmicity. J Clin Invest 1991;88:934-942.)

balance are also examined. The second part of the chapter summarizes the growing body of evidence linking decrements of sleep duration or quality, such as occur during sleep restriction or as a result of normal aging, and disturbances of endocrine and metabolic function. For a detailed review of sleep abnormalities in endocrine disease, the reader is referred to Chapter 105.

INTERACTIONS BETWEEN SLEEP AND THE GROWTH HORMONE AXIS

Pituitary release of GH is stimulated by hypothalamic GH-releasing hormone (GHRH) and inhibited by somatostatin. In addition, the acylated form of ghrelin, a peptide produced predominantly by the stomach, binds to the growth-hormone-secretagogue (GHS) receptor and is a potent endogenous stimulus of GH secretion.[3] Current evidence is consistent for a combined and probably synergic role of GHRH stimulation, elevated nocturnal ghrelin levels, and decreased somatostatinergic tone in the control of GH secretion during sleep. Although sleep clearly involves major stimulatory effects on GH secretion, the hormones of the somatotropic axis, including GHRH, ghrelin, and GH itself, in turn appear to be involved in sleep regulation. Indeed, studies in both humans and laboratory rodents have indicated that injections of GHRH and ghrelin stimulate slow wave sleep and slow wave activity (EEG spectral power in the delta range).[4-7] In contrast, injections of GH appear to enhance REM sleep, particularly in rodents,[5] and somatostatin injections impair sleep quality in older, but not in young, adults, presumably because endogenous GHRH activity is already decreased in old age.[6]

In healthy adult subjects, the 24-hour profile of plasma GH levels consists of stable low levels abruptly interrupted by bursts of secretion. Already in the late 1960s it was recognized that the most reproducible GH pulse occurs shortly after sleep onset.[8-14] In men, the sleep-onset GH pulse is generally the largest, and often the only, secretory pulse observed over the 24-hour span. In women, daytime GH pulses are more frequent, and the sleep-associated pulse, although still present in the vast majority of individual profiles, does not account for the majority of the 24-hour secretory output.

Sleep onset elicits a pulse in GH secretion whether sleep is advanced, delayed, or interrupted and reinitiated. In real-life conditions, a study of night workers indicated that the main GH secretory episode still occurred during the first half of the sleep period.[15] The mean GH profile shown in Figure 22–1 illustrates the maintenance of the relationship between sleep onset and GH release in subjects who underwent a 12-hour delay shift of the sleep-wake cycle.

Although the observation that GH is preferentially secreted during early sleep is now more than 30 years old, the mechanisms that underlie this robust relationship remain unclear. As noted by Obal and Krueger[5] the significance of this relationship is that anabolic processes in the body are synchronized to a state when behavioral rest occurs and when cerebral glucose use is at its lowest point. Sleep-onset GH secretion appears to be primarily regulated by GHRH stimulation occurring during a period of decreased somatostatin inhibition of somatotropic activity. Indeed, in humans, GH secretion during early sleep may be nearly totally suppressed by administration of a GHRH antagonist.[16] The late evening and nocturnal hours coincide with the trough of a diurnal variation in hypothalamic somatostatin tone[17] that is likely to facilitate nocturnal GH release. It is also possible that ghrelin plays a role in causing increased GH secretion during sleep since the normal 24-hour ghrelin profile shows a marked nocturnal increase peaking in the early part of the night.[18,19]

Well-documented studies published in the late 1960s concurred in indicating that there is a consistent relationship between the appearance of delta waves in the EEG and elevated GH concentrations.[10-12,20] These findings were confirmed and extended in later reports that examined GH secretory rates, rather than plasma GH levels.[21,22] Using this approach, a study with 30-second sampling of plasma GH during sleep indicated that maximal GH release occurs within minutes of the onset of slow wave sleep (SWS).[22] Furthermore, studies examining GH secretion in healthy young men of similar height and weight found that approximately 70% of GH pulses during sleep occurred during SWS and that there was a quantitative correlation between the amount of GH secreted during these pulses and the duration of the slow wave episode.[21]

Additional evidence for the existence of a robust relationship between slow wave activity and increased GH release has been obtained in studies using pharmacologic stimulation of SWS.[23,24] Reliable stimulation of SWS in normal subjects has been obtained with oral administration of low doses of gamma hydroxybutyrate (GHB), a drug used for the treatment of narcolepsy, as well as with ritanserin, a selective 5-hydroxytryptamine (5-HT$_2$) receptor antagonist. Both studies found an excellent correlation between increases in GH secretion and increases in slow wave sleep or slow wave activity, or both, following drug administration.[23,24] There is good evidence to indicate that stimulation of nocturnal GH release and stimulation of SWS reflect, to a large extent, synchronous activity of at least two populations of hypothalamic GHRH neurons.[5]

The upper panel of Figure 22–1 shows that the secretion of GH is increased during sleep independent of the circadian time when sleep occurs and that sleep deprivation results in greatly diminished release of this hormone. However, a slight increase may be observed during nocturnal sleep deprivation, indicating the existence of a weak circadian component that could reflect, as discussed above, lower somatostatin inhibition. However, since ghrelin levels increase during the nocturnal period, even when the subjects remain awake,[18] persistent low levels of GH release during nocturnal sleep deprivation could be driven by this gastric hormone. Following a night of total sleep deprivation, GH release is increased during the daytime such that the total 24-hour secretion is not significantly affected.[25] Again, the mechanisms underlying this compensatory daytime secretion are unknown, but they could involve decreased somatostatinergic tone or elevated ghrelin levels.

Marked rises in GH secretion before the onset of sleep have been reported by several investigators.[26-28] Such presleep GH pulses are likely to reflect a circadian rhythm in propensity to secrete GH, independent of the occurrence of sleep.[17] The short-term negative feedback inhibition exerted by GH on its own secretion may also explain observations of an absent GH pulse during the first slow wave period, when a secretory pulse occurred before sleep onset.

Although robust stimulatory mechanisms clearly activate GH secretion during NREM sleep, awakenings interrupting sleep have an inhibitory effect. In a study in which GH secretion was stimulated by the injection of GHRH at the beginning of the sleep period, it was found that whenever sleep was interrupted by a spontaneous awakening, the ongoing GH secretion was abruptly suppressed.[29] This inhibitory effect of awakenings on the GH response to GHRH was further demonstrated in a study in which sleeping subjects who had received a GHRH injection were awakened 30 minutes after the injection and then allowed to reinitiate sleep 30 minutes later.[30] A marked inhibition of the GH response was observed shortly after the awakening. These findings indicate that sleep fragmentation generally decreases nocturnal GH secretion.

INTERACTIONS BETWEEN SLEEP AND THE CORTICOTROPIC AXIS

Activity of the corticotropic axis—a neuroendocrine system associated with the stress response and behavioral activation—may be measured peripherally via plasma levels of the pituitary adrenocorticotropic hormone (ACTH) and of the adrenal hormone directly controlled by ACTH stimulation, cortisol. The plasma levels of these hormones decline from an early morning maximum throughout the daytime and are near the lower limit of most assays in the late evening and early part of the sleep period. Thus, sleep is normally initiated when corticotropic activity is quiescent. Reactivation of ACTH and cortisol secretion occurs abruptly a few hours before the usual waking time.

The mean cortisol profile shown in Figure 22–1 illustrates the remarkable persistence of this diurnal variation when sleep is manipulated. Indeed, the overall waveshape of the profile is not markedly affected by the absence of sleep or by sleep at an unusual time of day. Studies using similar experimental designs have therefore indicated that the 24-hour periodicity of corticotropic activity is primarily controlled by circadian rhythmicity.

Nevertheless, modulatory effects of the sleep or wake condition have been clearly demonstrated. Indeed, a number of studies have indicated that sleep onset is reliably associated with a short-term inhibition of cortisol secretion,[1,31-33] although this effect may not be detectable when sleep is initiated at the time of the daily maximum of corticotropic activity, that is, in the morning.[34] Under normal conditions, because cortisol secretion is already quiescent in the late evening, this inhibitory effect of sleep, which appears to be related to slow wave stages,[35-37] results in a prolongation of the quiescent period. Therefore, under conditions of sleep deprivation, the nadir of cortisol secretion is less pronounced and occurs earlier than under normal conditions of nocturnal sleep. Conversely, awakening at the end of the sleep period is consistently followed by a pulse of cortisol secretion.[1,30,38]

During sleep deprivation, these rapid effects of sleep onset and sleep offset on corticotropic activity are obviously absent, and, as may be seen in the profiles shown in Figure 22–1, the nadir of cortisol levels is higher than during nocturnal sleep (because of the absence of the inhibitory effects of the first hours of sleep), and the morning acrophase is lower (because of the absence of the stimulating effects of morning awakening). Overall, the amplitude of the rhythm is reduced by approximately 15% during sleep deprivation as compared to normal conditions.

Several studies have shown that awakenings interrupting the sleep period consistently trigger pulses of cortisol secretion.[30,39,40] In an analysis of cortisol profiles during daytime sleep, it was observed that 92% of awakenings interrupting sleep coincided with or were followed within 20 minutes by a significant cortisol pulse.[40] A study involving continuous experimentally induced arousals during sleep suggested that feedback inhibition of corticotropic activity is less effective during sleep than during wake.[30] Sleep fragmentation, as occurs in aging,[41] is thus associated with alterations of nocturnal corticotropic activity. A recent study[42] in patients with insomnia revealed that those with decreased total sleep time have higher cortisol levels across the night (Fig. 22–2). It is unclear whether this relative hypercortisolism is the result of sleep fragmentation and the associated sleep loss, or, alternatively, whether hyperactivity of the corticotropic axis is causing hyperarousal and insomnia.

In addition to the immediate modulatory effects of sleep-wake transitions on cortisol levels, even partial nocturnal sleep deprivation appears to affect corticotropic activity on the following evening.[43] Figure 22–3 summarizes the results from a study involving two groups of healthy young men studied before, during, and after a night of normal sleep or of total sleep deprivation. In the sleep-deprived group, in contrast to the group with a normal sleep period, evening cortisol levels were significantly higher on the day following sleep deprivation than on the previous day at the same time. Sleep loss thus appears to delay the normal return to evening quiescence of the corticotropic axis. This endocrine alteration is remarkably similar to that occurring in normal aging, where increases in evening cortisol levels of similar magnitude are consistently observed. It is possible that the elevated evening and nocturnal cortisol levels occurring in insomniacs with reduced total sleep time[42] reflect the impact of chronic partial sleep loss. This interpretation is consistent with findings in normal subjects submitted to recurrent partial sleep restriction, as discussed later.

THE THYROID AXIS DURING SLEEP AND SLEEP DEPRIVATION

Daytime levels of plasma TSH are low and relatively stable and are followed by a rapid elevation starting in the early evening and culminating in a nocturnal maximum occurring around the beginning of the sleep period.[37,44] The later part of sleep is associated with a progressive decline in TSH levels, and daytime values resume shortly after morning awakening. The first 24 hours of the study illustrated in Figure 22–1 are typical of the diurnal TSH rhythm. Because the nocturnal rise of TSH occurs well before the time of sleep onset, it probably reflects a circadian effect. However, a marked effect of sleep on TSH secretion may be seen during sleep deprivation (clearly seen in Fig. 22–1), when nocturnal TSH secretion is increased by as much as 200% over the levels observed during nocturnal sleep. Thus, sleep exerts an inhibitory influence on TSH secretions, and sleep deprivation relieves this inhibition.[37,45]

Interestingly, when sleep occurs during daytime hours, TSH secretion is not suppressed significantly below normal daytime levels. Thus, the inhibitory effect of sleep on TSH secretion appears to be operative when the nighttime elevation has taken place, indicating once again the interaction of the effects of circadian time and the effects of sleep. When the depth of sleep at the habitual time is increased by prior sleep deprivation, the nocturnal TSH rise is more markedly inhibited, suggesting that SWS is probably the primary determinant

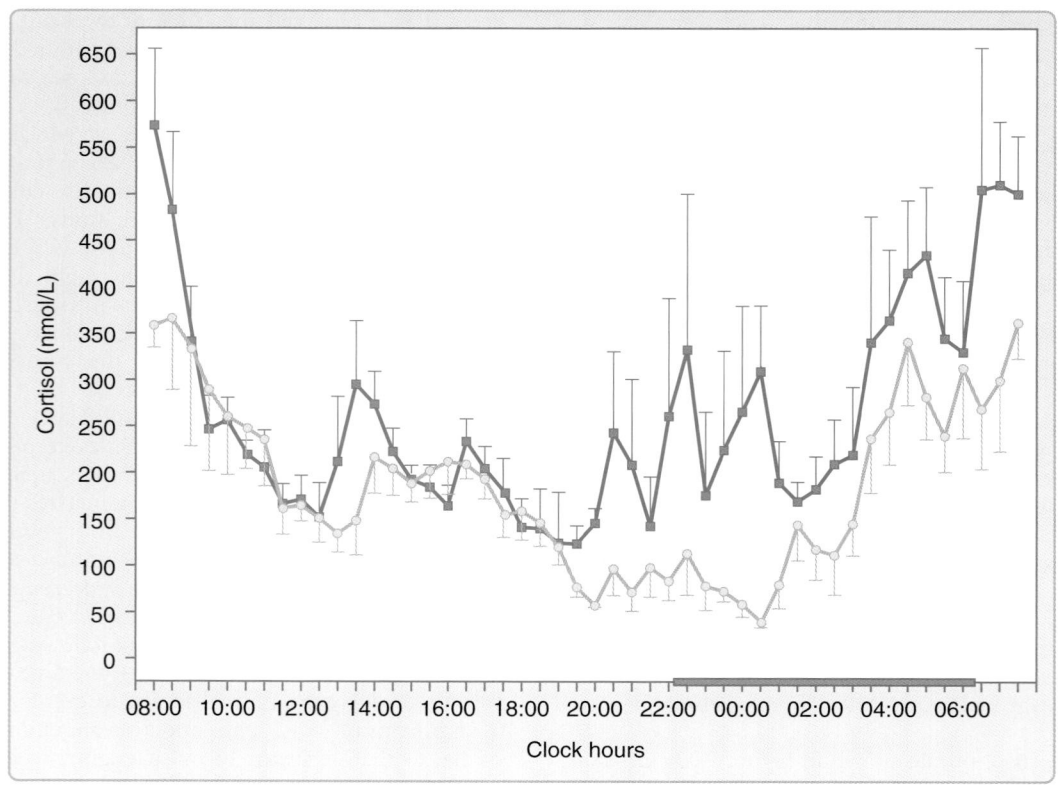

Figure 22–2. Mean 24-hour profiles of plasma cortisol in young insomniacs with low total sleep time *(dark blue squares)* as compared to young insomniacs with high total sleep time *(light blue circles)*. The *dark blue bar* indicates the sleep-recording period. The *error bars* indicate standard error of the mean (SEM). (From Vgontzas A, Bixler EO, Lin HM, et al: Chronic insomnia is associated with neurohumoral activation of the hypothalamo-pituitary-adrenal axis: Clinical implications. J Clin Endocrinol Metab 2001;86:3787-3794).

NORMAL SLEEP

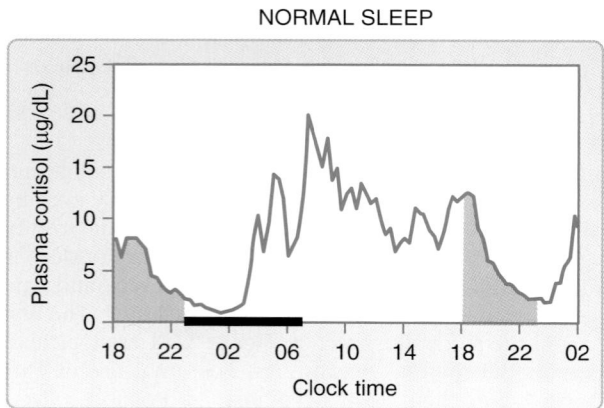

MEAN EVENING
CORTISOL LEVEL (µg/dL)

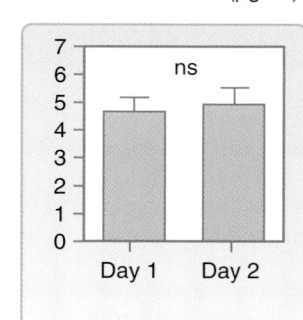

TOTAL SLEEP DEPRIVATION

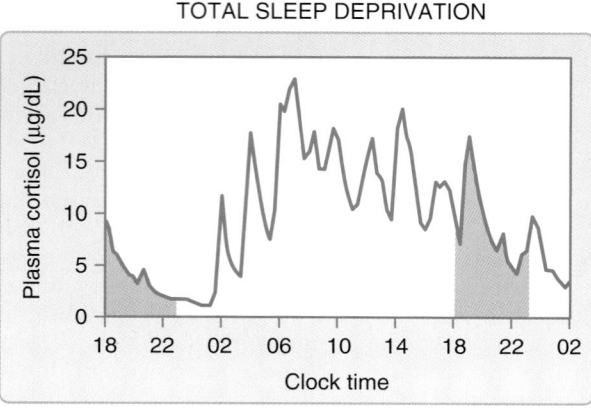

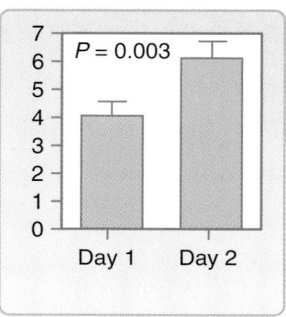

Figure 22–3. Mean profiles of plasma cortisol from two groups of healthy young subjects studied during a 32-hour period with normal sleep (bedtimes: 23:00 to 07:00, *top*) or total sleep deprivation *(bottom)*. The *black bar* represents the sleep period. The *blue shaded areas* highlight cortisol levels during the time interval 18:00 to 23:00 on day 1 and on day 2. Mean cortisol levels for the same time period before and after normal sleep *(top)* and before and after total sleep deprivation *(bottom)* are shown for the two groups on the right panels. One night of sleep loss thus results in increased cortisol levels on the following evening. (Data from Leproult R, Copinschi G, Buxton O, et al: Sleep loss results in an elevation of cortisol levels the next evening. Sleep 1997;20:865-870.)

of the sleep-associated fall.[37] Indeed, analyses of concomitant TSH profiles and sleep parameters has revealed a consistent association between descending slopes of TSH concentrations and slow wave stages and the existence of a negative cross-correlation between TSH fluctuations and relative spectral power in the delta range.[46,47] Awakenings interrupting nocturnal sleep appear to relieve the inhibition of TSH and are consistently associated with a short-term TSH elevation.

Circadian and sleep-related variations in thyroid hormones have been difficult to demonstrate, probably because these hormones are bound to serum proteins and thus their peripheral concentrations are affected by diurnal variations in hemodilution caused by postural changes. However, under conditions of sleep deprivation, the increased amplitude of the TSH rhythm may result in a detectable increase in plasma triiodothyronine (T_3) levels, paralleling the nocturnal TSH rise.[48] If sleep deprivation is continued for a second night, the nocturnal rise of TSH is markedly diminished as compared with that occurring during the first night.[48,49] It is likely that following the first night of sleep deprivation, the elevated thyroid hormone levels, which persist during the daytime period because of the prolonged half-life of these hormones, limit the subsequent TSH rise at the beginning of the next nighttime period. A well-documented study involving 64 hours of sleep deprivation demonstrated a more than 50% increase in the T_3 level measured at 11:00 PM across the study period without significant change in the concomitant thyroxin (T_4) concentration.[50] During the second night of sleep deprivation, a nocturnal increase in both T_3 and T_4 levels was observed, contrasting with the decreases seen during normal sleep.[50] These data suggest that prolonged sleep loss may be associated with an upregulation of the thyroid axis.

The inhibitory effects of sleep on TSH secretion are time dependent, and that may cause, under specific circumstances, elevations of plasma TSH levels that reflect the misalignment of sleep and circadian timing. For example, Figure 22–4 shows the mean profiles of plasma TSH and T_3 levels observed in a group of healthy young men in the course of adaptation to simulated jet lag, achieved by an abrupt 8-hour advance of the sleep-dark period.[51] In the course of adaptation to this 8-hour advance shift, TSH levels increased progressively because daytime sleep failed to inhibit TSH and nighttime wakefulness was associated with large circadian-dependent TSH elevations. As a result, mean TSH levels following awakening from the second shifted sleep period were more than twofold higher than during the same time interval following normal nocturnal sleep. This overall elevation of TSH levels was paralleled by a small increase in T_3 concentrations.[51] This study demonstrated that the subjective discomfort and fatigue often referred to as "jet-lag syndrome" are associated not only with a desynchronization of bodily rhythms but also with a prolonged elevation of a hormone concentration in the peripheral circulation.

INTERACTIONS BETWEEN SLEEP AND PROLACTIN SECRETION

The major role of sleep in stimulating PRL secretion has been recognized for more than three decades. Under normal conditions, PRL levels are minimal around noon, increase modestly during the afternoon, and then undergo a major nocturnal elevation starting shortly after sleep onset and culminating around midsleep. Decreased dopaminergic inhibition of PRL

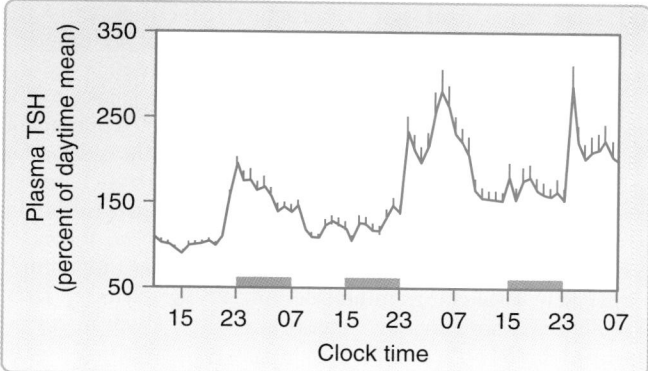

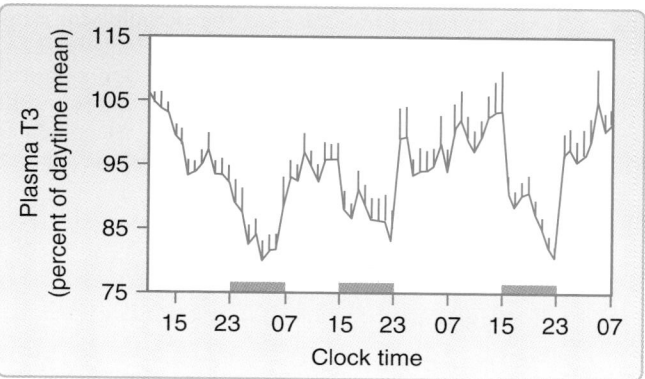

Figure 22–4. Mean (and standard error of the mean) profiles of plasma thyrotropin (TSH) and plasma T_3 from eight healthy young men who were submitted to an 8-hour advance of the sleep-wake and dark-light cycles (from 23:00 to 07:00 to 15:00 to 23:00). *Blue bars* indicate bedtime periods. Under these simulated advanced jet lag conditions, both TSH and T_3 increased during the course of adaptation. (Data from Hirschfeld U, Moreno-Reyes R, Akseki E, et al: Progressive elevation of plasma thyrotropin during adaptation to simulated jet lag: Effects of treatment with bright lights or zolpidem. J Clin Endocrinol Metab 1996;81:3270-3277.)

during sleep is likely to be the primary mechanism underlying this nocturnal PRL elevation. In adults of both sexes, the nocturnal maximum corresponds to an average increase of more than 200% above the minimum level.[52-54] Morning awakenings and awakenings interrupting sleep are consistently associated with a rapid inhibition of PRL secretion.[53,54]

Studies of the PRL profile during daytime naps or after shifts of the sleep period have consistently demonstrated that sleep onset, irrespective of the time of day, has a stimulatory effect on PRL release. This is well illustrated by the profiles shown in Figure 22–1, in which elevated PRL levels occur both during nocturnal sleep and during daytime recovery sleep, whereas the nocturnal period of sleep deprivation was not associated with an increase in PRL concentrations. However, sleep is not the sole factor responsible for the nocturnal elevation of PRL concentrations. Indeed, a number of experiments involving abrupt advances or delays of sleep times have shown that the sleep-related rise of PRL may still be present, although with a reduced amplitude, when sleep does not occur at the normal nocturnal time and that maximal stimulation is observed only when sleep and circadian effects are superimposed.[53-55] The sleep-independent circadian component of

PRL secretion is expressed as a progressive increase across the late afternoon and the hours preceding the usual bedtime and is much more pronounced in women than in men.[54]

Because of the marked effect that sleep onset has on PRL release, several studies have examined the possible relationship between pulsatile PRL release during sleep and the alternation of REM and NREM stages. When sleep structure is characterized using power spectral analysis of the electroencephalogram (EEG), a close temporal association between increased prolactin secretion and delta-wave activity is apparent.[56] Conversely, awakenings inhibit nocturnal PRL release.[56] Thus, fragmented sleep generally is associated with lower nocturnal prolactin levels.

Benzodiazepine (as well as nonbenzodiazepine) hypnotics taken at bedtime may cause an increase in the nocturnal PRL rise, resulting in concentrations near the pathological range for part of the night.[57,58] The upper panels of Figure 22–5 illustrate the effects of bedtime oral administration of triazolam (0.5 mg) compared with placebo on the 24-hour PRL profiles obtained in a group of six healthy men. Sleep-related PRL release was enhanced by triazolam, and in some subjects the PRL concentrations during the early part of the night were nearly threefold higher (although still in the physiological range) than with placebo.[57] The lower panels of Figure 22–5 show the similar effects of zolpidem (10 mg) in eight healthy women.[58] Neither triazolam nor zolpidem had any effect on the 24-hour profiles of cortisol, melatonin, or GH.

There is rapidly accumulating evidence from studies in rats and rabbits that PRL is involved in the humoral regulation of sleep.[59] The primary effect is a stimulation of REM sleep, which may be observed 1 to 2 h posttreatment. This stimulatory effect of PRL on REM sleep depends on time of day because it is only observed during the light (i.e., inactive) period, and this effect may be exerted by centrally released PRL rather than by pituitary PRL. There are no direct studies of the effects of PRL on sleep in the human being, although one study has used injections of vasoactive intestinal polypeptide to stimulate endogenous PRL secretion and has reported an enhancement of REM sleep. A role for PRL in the circadian regulation of REM sleep propensity has been hypothesized.[59] However, there is also evidence for an involvement of PRL in SWS regulation. In particular, SWS is enhanced in patients

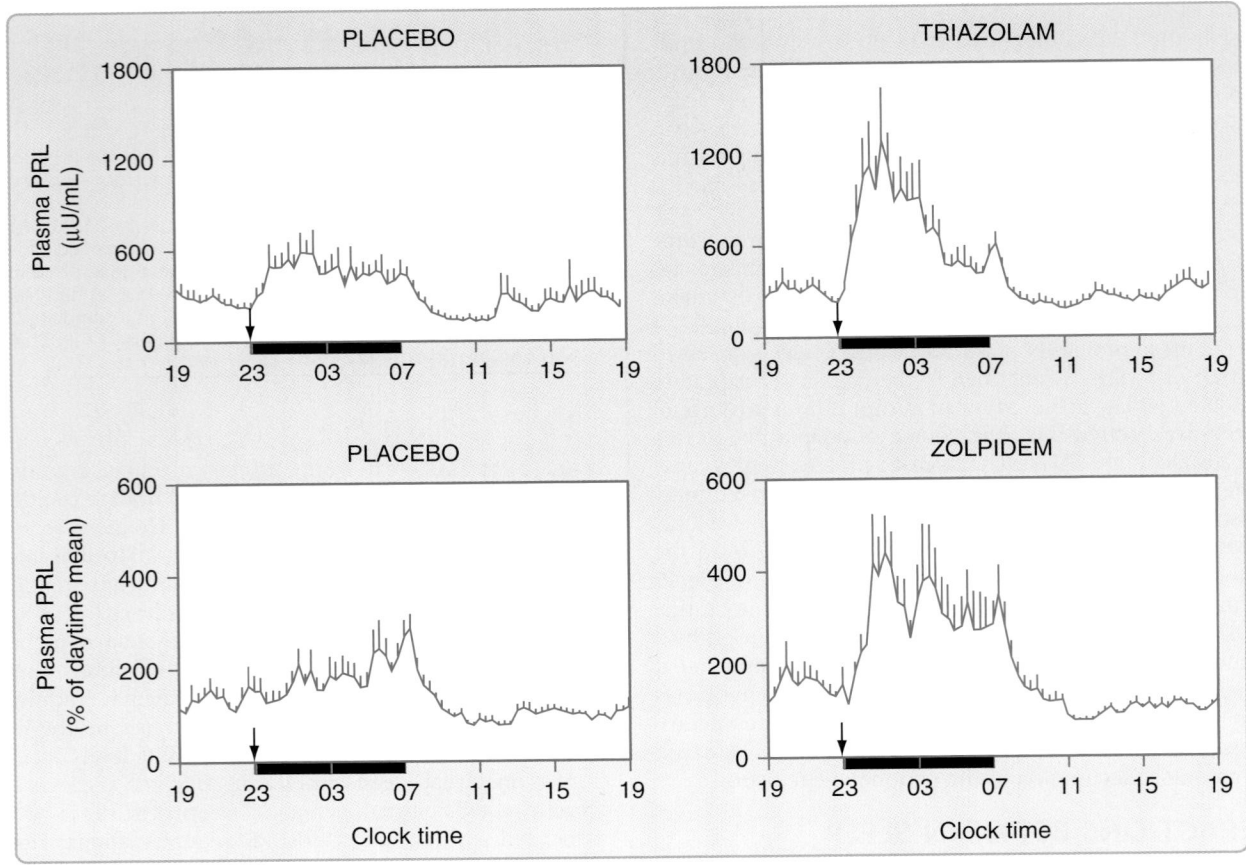

Figure 22–5. Effects of commonly used hypnotics on the 24-hour profile of plasma prolactin (PRL) in healthy young subjects. Data are mean plus standard error of the mean. Samples were collected at 15- to 20-minute intervals. Sleep was polygraphically recorded. *Top,* effects of bedtime administration of triazolam (0.5 mg). *Bottom,* effects of bedtime administration of zolpidem (10 mg). Both benzodiazepine and nonbenzodiazepine hypnotics cause transient hyperprolactinemia during the early part of sleep. Time in bed is denoted by the *black bars. Arrows* denote time of drug administration. (Data from Copinschi G, Van Onderbergen A, L'Hermite-Balériaux M, et al: Effects of the short-acting benzodiazepine triazolam taken at bedtime on circadian and sleep-related hormonal profiles in normal men. Sleep 1990;13:232-244; Copinschi G, Akseki E, Moreno-Reyes R, et al: Effects of bedtime administration of zolpidem on circadian and sleep-related hormonal profiles in normal women. Sleep 1995;18:417-424; and Van Cauter E, Spiegel K: Circadian and sleep control of endocrine secretions. In Turek FW, Zee PC [eds]: Neurobiology of Sleep and Circadian Rhythms. New York, Marcel Dekker, 1999.)

with hyperprolactinemia[60] and in women who breast-feed and have high prolactin levels as compared with women who bottle-feed their infants.[61]

INTERACTIONS BETWEEN SLEEP AND THE GONADAL AXIS

The relationship between the 24-hour patterns of gonadotropin release and gonadal steroid levels varies according to the stage of maturation, and it is gender dependent in young adulthood (for review see Van Cauter et al.[62]).

Prior to puberty, LH and FSH are secreted in a pulsatile pattern, and an augmentation of pulsatile activity is associated with sleep onset in a majority of both girls and boys. The increased amplitude of gonadotropin release during sleep is one of the hallmarks of puberty. Both sleep and circadian rhythmicity contribute to the nocturnal elevation of gonadotropin pulses in pubertal children. As the pubescent child enters adulthood, the daytime pulse amplitude increases as well, eliminating or diminishing the diurnal rhythm. In pubertal girls, a diurnal variation of circulating estradiol levels, with higher concentrations during the daytime instead of the nighttime, becomes apparent. It has been suggested that the lack of parallelism between gonadotropin and estradiol levels reflects an approximate 10-hour delay between gonadotropin stimulation and the subsequent ovarian response. In pubertal boys, a nocturnal rise of testosterone coincides with the elevation of gonadotropins.

In men, the day-night variation of plasma LH levels is dampened or even undetectable. During the sleep period, LH pulses appear to be temporally related to the REM-NREM cycle.[63] Despite the low amplitude of the nocturnal increase in gonadotropin release, a marked diurnal rhythm in circulating testosterone levels is present in young healthy men, with minimal levels in the late evening and maximal levels in the early morning.[64,65] Thus, the robust circadian rhythm of plasma testosterone may be partially controlled by factors other than LH. The nocturnal rise of testosterone appears temporally linked to the latency of the first REM episode,[66] as plasma levels continue to rise until the first REM episode occurs. A study involving experimental sleep fragmentation in young men by allowing only 7 minutes of sleep every 20 minutes showed that the nocturnal rise of testosterone was attenuated, particularly in subjects who did not achieve REM sleep during the experimental night.[67]

In women, the 24-hour variation in plasma LH is markedly modulated by the menstrual cycle.[68,69] In the early follicular phase, LH pulses are large and infrequent, and a marked slowing of the frequency of secretory pulses occurs during sleep. In the midfollicular phase, pulse amplitude is decreased, pulse frequency is increased, and the frequency modulation of LH pulsatility by sleep is less apparent. Pulse amplitude increases again by the late follicular phase. In the early luteal phase, the pulse amplitude is markedly increased, the pulse frequency is decreased, and nocturnal slowing of pulsatility is again evident. In the mid and late luteal phase, pulse amplitude and frequency are decreased and there is no modulation by sleep.

In older men, the amplitude of LH pulses is decreased[70,71] but the frequency is increased[72] and no significant diurnal pattern can be detected.[73] The circadian variation of testosterone is still present, although markedly dampened.[64,73] The sleep-related rise is still apparent in older men, but its amplitude

is lower and the relationship to REM latency is no longer apparent.[74] In post-menopausal women, gonadotropin levels are elevated, but they show no consistent circadian pattern.[75] A number of studies[76-78] have indicated that estrogen replacement therapy has modest beneficial effects on subjective and objective sleep quality, particularly in the presence of environmental disturbance[79] or sleep-disordered breathing.[76,77,80]

SLEEP AND GLUCOSE REGULATION

The consolidation of human sleep in a single 7- to 9-hour period implies that an extended period of fast must be maintained overnight. A large number of studies have sampled levels of glucose and insulin in subjects sleeping in the laboratory and have observed that despite the prolonged fasting condition, glucose levels remain stable or fall only minimally across the night.[81-87] In contrast, if subjects are awake and fasting in a recumbent position, in the absence of any physical activity, glucose levels fall by an average of 0.5 to 1.0 mmol/L (± 10 to 20 mg/dL) over a 12-hour period.[88] Thus, a number of mechanisms that operate during nocturnal sleep (reviewed later) must intervene to maintain stable glucose levels during the overnight fast.

Experimental protocols allowing for the study of nighttime glucose tolerance during sleep without awakening the subjects include constant intravenous glucose infusion and continuous enteral nutrition. Confounding effects of food ingestion and prolonged fasting are avoided by replacing the normal caloric intake with a constant input, thereby creating a steady-state condition with levels of glucose and insulin secretion within the physiologic range. Sleep has been polysomnographically recorded under both conditions, and normal sleep parameters have been observed following a period of habituation to the laboratory procedures. Thus, both constant glucose infusion and continuous enteral nutrition offer the possibility of examining glucose tolerance during the sleep state, although under conditions that are clearly artificial. In particular, prolonged glucose infusion results in a marked inhibition of endogenous glucose production.

Both experimental conditions have been used in extended studies in healthy subjects.[89-91] The lower panels of Figure 22–1 show profiles of blood glucose and insulin secretion rates (ISR) obtained in normal subjects who were studied under conditions of constant glucose infusion. A marked decrease in glucose tolerance (reflected in higher plasma glucose levels despite the constant rate of exogenous infusion) is apparent during nighttime and well as daytime sleep. A smaller elevation of glucose and insulin also occurs during nocturnal sleep deprivation, indicating an effect of circadian-dependent mechanisms.

During nocturnal sleep, the overall increase in plasma glucose ranged from 20% to 30%, despite the maintenance of rigorously constant rates of caloric intake. Maximal levels occur around the middle of the sleep period. During the later part of the night (i.e., at the time of the so-called dawn phenomenon), glucose tolerance begins to improve, and glucose levels progressively decrease toward morning values. The mechanisms underlying these robust variations in set-point of glucose regulation across nocturnal sleep are different in early sleep and late sleep.

Under conditions of constant glucose infusion, the decrease in glucose tolerance during the first half of the sleep period is reflected in a robust increase in plasma glucose, which is followed by a more than 50% increase in insulin secretion. Under these conditions, the major underlying cause of the glucose increase is decreased glucose use. It is estimated that about two thirds of the fall in glucose use during sleep is due to a decrease in brain glucose metabolism[92] related to the predominance of slow wave stages, which are associated with a 30% to 40% reduction in cerebral glucose metabolism as compared to the waking state. The last third of the fall would then reflect decreased peripheral use. Diminished muscle tone during sleep and rapid antiinsulin-like effects of the sleep-onset GH pulse[93] are both likely to contribute to decreased peripheral glucose uptake.

Under conditions of constant glucose infusion, during the later part of the sleep period, glucose levels and insulin secretion decrease to return to presleep values, and this decrease appears to be partially due to the increase in wake and REM stages.[94] Indeed, glucose use during the REM and wake stages is higher than during NREM stages.[92,95-98] In addition, several other factors may also contribute to the decline of glucose levels during late sleep. These include the hypoglycemic activity of previously secreted insulin during early sleep, the increased insulin-independent glucose disposal due to transient mild hyperglycemia, and the quiescence of GH secretion and thus the rapid attenuation of the short-term inhibitory effects of this hormone on tissue glucose uptake. Finally, the later part of the night appears to be associated with increased insulin sensitivity, reflecting a delayed effect of low cortisol levels during the evening and early part of the night.[99]

SLEEP AND APPETITE REGULATION

Sleep plays an important role in energy balance. In rodents, food shortage or starvation results in decreased sleep[100] and, conversely, total sleep deprivation leads to marked hyperphagia.[101] The identification of hypothalamic excitatory neuropeptides, referred to as hypocretins or orexins, that have potent wake-promoting effects and stimulate food intake, has provided a molecular basis for the interactions between the regulation of feeding and sleeping.[102] Hypocretin-containing neurons in the lateral hypothalamus project directly to the locus coeruleus and other brainstem and hypothalamic arousal areas, where they interact with the leptin-responsive neuronal network involved in balancing food intake and energy expenditure.

Leptin, a hormone released by the adipocytes, provides information about energy status to regulatory centers in the hypothalamus.[103] Circulating leptin concentrations in humans show a rapid decline or increase in response to acute caloric shortage or surplus, respectively.[104,105] These changes in leptin levels have been associated with reciprocal changes in hunger.[104] The 24-hour leptin profile shows a marked nocturnal rise, which is partly dependent on meal intake.[106] Nevertheless, a study using continuous enteral nutrition to eliminate the impact of meal intake showed the persistence of a sleep-related leptin elevation, although the amplitude was lower than during normal feeding conditions.[107] Prolonged total sleep deprivation results in a decrease in the amplitude of the leptin diurnal variation.[108] Systemic administration of leptin to normally fed rats results in an increase of SWS and a decrease in REM sleep. Prior food deprivation negated these effects of leptin on sleep regulation. In humans with narcolepsy, leptin levels are markedly decreased and the nocturnal rise is absent.[109]

Ghrelin, a peptide produced predominantly by the stomach, is also involved in regulating energy balance. However, in contrast to the anorexigenic effects of leptin, ghrelin stimulates appetite.[110] The 24-hour profile of ghrelin levels shows a marked nocturnal rise, which is only modestly dampened when subjects are sleep deprived.[18] Studies in both humans and laboratory rodents have indicated that ghrelin injections stimulate slow wave sleep and slow wave activity.[4]

It has been proposed that leptin and ghrelin "represent the 'yin-yang' of one regulatory system that has developed to inform the brain about the current energy balance state."[3] However, during the normal rest period, peripheral levels of both peptides are elevated, whereas their responses to feeding and fasting are in the opposite directions.

HORMONES CONTROLLING HYDROMINERAL BALANCE DURING SLEEP

Water and salt homeostasis is under the combined control of the posterior pituitary, the renin-angiotensin-aldosterone system, and the atrial natriuretic peptide. Urine flow and electrolyte excretion are higher during the day than during the night, and this variation partly reflects circadian modulation. In addition to this 24-hour rhythm, urine flow and osmolarity oscillate with the REM-NREM cycle. REM sleep is associated with decreasing urine flow and increasing osmolarity. During the 1990s, a series of elegant studies began to elucidate the endocrine control of the ultradian oscillations in hydromineral balance.[111]

Vasopressin release is pulsatile but without apparent relationship to sleep stages.[111] Levels of atrial natriuretic peptide are relatively stable and do not show fluctuations related to the sleep-wake or REM-NREM cycles.[112] Whether the levels of plasma atrial natriuretic peptide exhibit a circadian variation is still a matter of controversy.[112] A close relationship between the beginning of REM episodes and decreased activity has been consistently observed for plasma renin activity.[111,113-115] Figure 22–6 illustrates the 24-hour rhythm of plasma renin activity in a subject studied during a normal sleep-wake cycle and in a subject studied following a shift of the sleep period. A remarkable synchronization between decreased plasma renin activity and REM stages is apparent during both sleep periods.[116] This relationship was confirmed in studies with selective REM-sleep deprivation in healthy subjects.[117]

Increases in plasma renin activity parallel increases in slow wave EEG activity.[118] In conditions of abnormal sleep architecture (e.g., narcolepsy, sleeping sickness), the temporal pattern of plasma renin activity faithfully reflects the disturbances of the REM-NREM cycle.[111] A well-documented study[119] has delineated the mechanisms responsible for oscillations of plasma renin activity during sleep. The initial event is a reduction in sympathetic tone, followed by a decrease in mean arterial blood pressure and an increase in slow wave activity. The rise in plasma renin activity becomes evident a few minutes after the increase in slow wave activity. During REM sleep, sympathetic activity increases, whereas renin and slow wave activity decrease and blood pressure is highly variable.

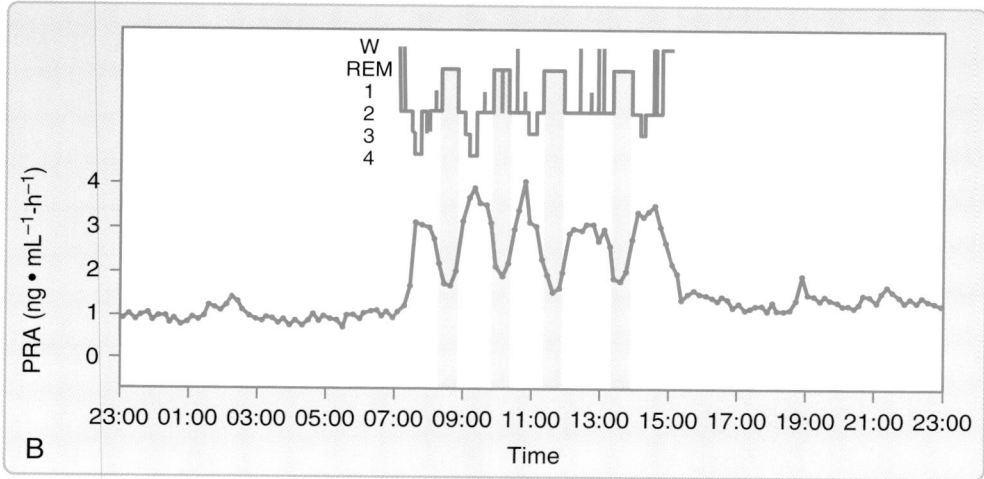

Figure 22–6. The 24-hour profiles of plasma renin activity sampled at 10-minute intervals in a healthy subject. **A,** Nocturnal sleep from 23:00 to 07:00. **B,** Daytime sleep from 07:00 to 15:00 after a night of total sleep deprivation. The temporal distribution of stages wake (W); REM; 1, 2, 3, and 4 are shown above the hormonal values. The oscillations of plasma renin activity are synchronized to the REM-NREM cycle during sleep. (From Brandenberger G, Follenius M, Goichot B, et al. Twenty-four hour profiles of plasma renin activity in relation to the sleep-wake cycle. J Hypertens 1994;12:277-283.)

The increased release of renin during sleep is associated with elevated levels of plasma aldosterone.[120] Acute total sleep deprivation dampens the nighttime elevation of plasma aldosterone and increases natriuresis.[121]

CHRONIC SLEEP RESTRICTION: IMPACT ON ENDOCRINE AND METABOLIC FUNCTION

During the last century, the availability of electricity has allowed an artificial extension of the light phase and the curtailment of bedtimes, which in turn allows people to extend the duration of activity. Additionally, the advent of the 24-hour society implies that millions of people work during the night and sleep during the day, and such schedules almost invariably result in substantial sleep loss.[122] Sleep loss due to voluntary bedtime curtailment has thus become a hallmark of modern society.[123] Today, many people are in bed 5 to 6 hours per night on a chronic basis,[124] particularly in the United States. Several laboratory studies involving extension of the bedtime period for prolonged periods of time have, however, provided evidence that an 8-hour night does not meet the sleep needs of healthy young adults, who may carry a substantial sleep debt even in the absence of obvious efforts at sleep curtailment.[125-127]

While the impact of various durations of acute total sleep deprivation on endocrine function has been extensively studied, the much more common condition of partial chronic sleep restriction has not received nearly as much attention. We review next the hormonal and metabolic patterns (illustrated in Fig. 22–7) observed after 6 days of partial sleep restriction to 4 hours per night as compared to 6 days of sleep extension to 12 hours per night in a group of healthy young men.[128-130]

The top panels in Figure 22–7 show the 24-hour plasma GH profiles after sleep curtailment as compared to the fully rested condition. The well-known GH pulse associated with sleep onset was observed in all individual profiles for both conditions. However, after chronic partial sleep restriction, all subjects exhibited a GH pulse prior to sleep onset. There was a negative correlation between presleep onset GH secretion and postsleep onset GH release. This profile of GH release is quite different from that observed during acute total sleep deprivation (top panels of Fig. 22–1), where minimal GH secretion occurred during prolonged wakefulness and a large secretory pulse followed the initiation of daytime recovery sleep.

The 24-hour cortisol profiles obtained in the same study are shown in the second panel from the top. The overall wave-shape of the 24-hour cortisol profile was similar under both bedtime conditions. However, when compared to the fully

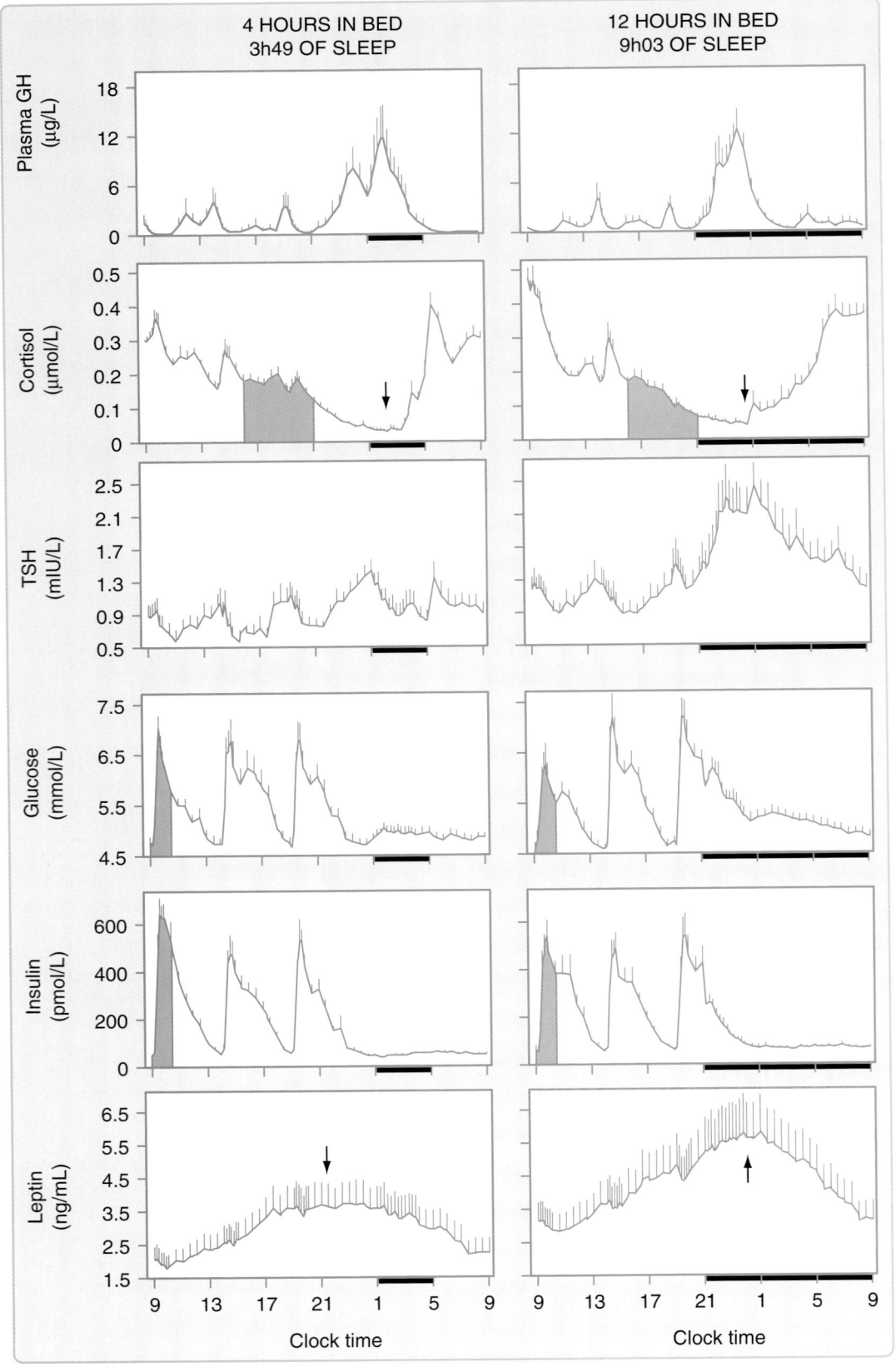

Figure 22–7. For legend see opposite page.

rested condition, the state of sleep debt was associated with alterations of the 24-hour profile of plasma cortisol, including a shorter quiescent period and elevated levels in the afternoon and early evening (shaded areas). This alteration was similar to that observed after acute total or partial sleep deprivation (see Fig. 22–3) and may reflect decreased efficacy of the negative feedback regulation of the HPA axis. Based on the analysis of the levels of free cortisol in saliva, the rate of decrease of free cortisol concentrations between 16:00 and 21:00 was indeed approximately six-fold slower during the sleep-debt condition than after full sleep recovery.[130]

Restriction and extension of sleep duration were also associated with clear changes in thyrotropic function. The nocturnal elevation of plasma TSH was markedly dampened in the sleep debt state as compared to the fully rested state, and the overall 24-hour mean TSH level was significantly reduced by 30%. Differences in TSH profiles between the two bedtime conditions are likely to be related to changes in thyroid hormone levels since the free thyroxin index (FT$_4$I) was significantly higher under sleep restriction than under sleep recovery.[130] Previous studies have demonstrated that total sleep deprivation is associated during the first night with a marked increase in TSH secretion (as illustrated in Fig. 22–1), which becomes smaller during the next two or three nights, presumably because of negative feedback effects from slowly rising levels of thyroid hormones.[49,131] Similar mechanisms are likely to underlie the elevated FT$_4$I values and depressed TSH concentrations observed after 6 nights of partial sleep restriction.

When bedtimes are curtailed to 6 hours per night for 6 days, the glucose response to ingestion of a carbohydrate-rich breakfast is higher than after 6 days of sleep extended to 12 hours per night, despite similar insulin secretory responses (lower panels of Fig. 22–7). The difference in peak glucose levels in response to breakfast between the sleep debt and fully rested conditions (i.e., ±15 mg/dL) translates into an approximate 20 mg/dL difference in glucose levels 120 minutes after the beginning of a standard glucose tolerance test, consistent with current diagnostic criteria for impaired glucose tolerance. The response to intravenous glucose tolerance testing (IVGTT) confirmed the clinically significant deterioration in glucose tolerance observed after ingestion of a high-carbohydrate breakfast following recurrent sleep restriction.[130] The rate of disappearance of glucose after injection (K$_G$) was indeed 40% slower in the sleep debt condition than after recovery sleep.

The lower panels of Figure 22–7 show the 24-hour leptin profiles under both bedtime conditions.[128] Despite identical caloric intake, similar levels of physical activity, and stable weight, mean leptin levels, acrophase, and amplitude of the diurnal variation were markedly reduced by 20% to 30% under sleep restriction as compared to sleep extension. The magnitude of this impact of sleep restriction on leptin levels is comparable to that occurring after three days of dietary restriction by approximately 900 kcal per day in young adults with normal sleep conditions.[104] Research in humans suggests that reduced sleep duration reduces leptin and raises ghrelin, resulting in increased hunger and thus is a risk factor for weight gain.[131a,131b] Decreased leptin levels have also been observed in rats submitted to sleep deprivation by the disk-over-water method.[132]

AGE-RELATED SLEEP ALTERATIONS: IMPLICATIONS FOR ENDOCRINE FUNCTION

Normal aging is associated with pronounced age-related alterations in sleep quality, which consist primarily of a marked reduction of SWS (stages 3 and 4), a reduction in REM stages, and an increase in the number and duration of awakenings interrupting sleep (see Chapter 3). There is increasing evidence that these alterations in sleep quality result in disturbances of endocrine function, suggesting the hypothesis that some of the hormonal and metabolic hallmarks of aging partly reflect the deterioration of sleep quality.

Several studies have shown that decreases in amount of SWS occur rapidly in adulthood (30 to 40 years of age) and precede the appearance of significant sleep fragmentation or declines in REM sleep. A retrospective analysis of sleep and concomitant profiles of plasma GH from 149 healthy men, ages 16 to 83 years, showed that the impact of aging on GH release occurred with a similar chronology characterized by major decrements from early adulthood to midlife (Fig. 22–8).[133] The statistical analysis further indicated that reduced amounts of SWS, and not age per se, is associated with reduced GH secretion in middle life and late life. The observation that in older adults, levels of insulin-like growth factor (IGF-1), the hormone secreted by the liver in response to stimulation by GH, are correlated with the amounts of SWS,[134] is consistent with this finding. Although the clinical implications of decreased SWS are still unclear, the relative GH deficiency of the elderly is associated with increased fat tissue and abdominal obesity, reduced muscle mass and strength, and reduced exercise capacity.[135-137] The persistence of a consistent relationship between SWS and GH secretion in older men suggests that drugs that reliably stimulate SWS in older adults may represent a novel strategy for GH replacement therapy.

In contrast to the rapid decline of SWS and GH secretion from young adulthood to midlife, the impact of age on REM sleep and sleep fragmentation does not become apparent until later in life. Aging is associated with an elevation of evening

Figure 22–7. The 24-hour profiles of plasma GH, plasma cortisol, plasma TSH, plasma glucose, serum insulin and plasma leptin levels in 11 healthy young men who were studied after 1 week of bedtime restriction to 4 hours per night (*left panels*) and 1 week of bedtime extension to 12 hours per night (*right panels*). The *black bars* represent the bedtime period. On the cortisol profiles, the *blue areas* show the increase in evening cortisol levels and the *arrows* indicate the timing of the nadir. On the glucose and insulin profiles, the *blue area* shows the response to the morning meal. On the leptin profiles, the *arrows* indicate the timing of the nocturnal acrophase. (From Spiegel K, Leproult R, Van Cauter E: Impact of a sleep debt on metabolic and endocrine function. Lancet 1999;354:1435-1439; Spiegel K, Leproult R, Colecchia E, et al: Adaptation of the 24-hour growth hormone profile to a state of sleep debt. Am J Physiol 2000;279:R874-R883; and Spiegel K, Leproult R, L'Hermite-Balériaux M, et al: Leptin levels are dependent on sleep duration: Relationships with sympathovagal balance, carbohydrate regulation, cortisol, and thyrotropin. J Clin Endocrinol Metab 2004;89:5762-5771.)

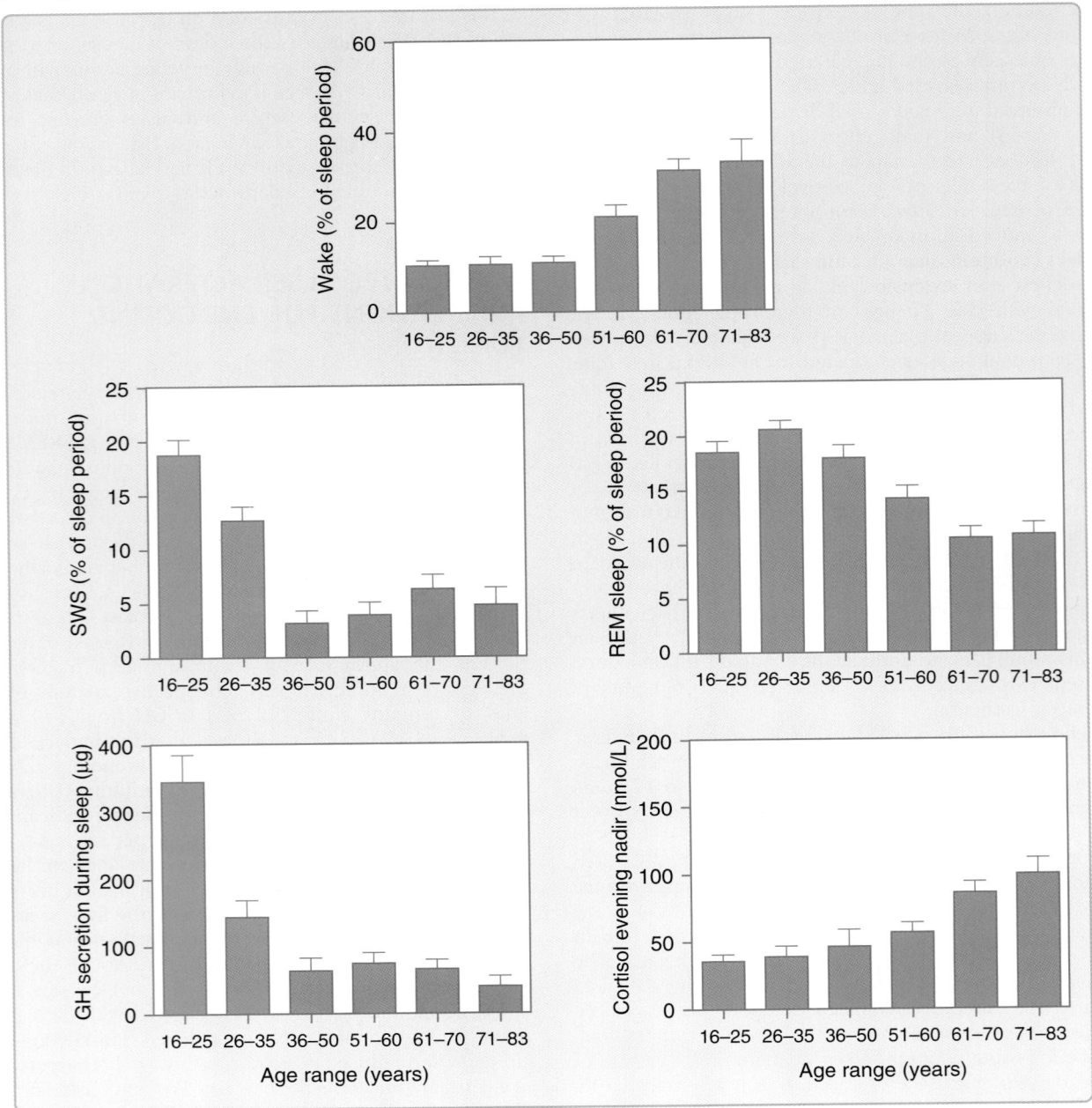

Figure 22–8. Mean (SEM) amounts of wake after sleep onset *(top panel)*, slow wave sleep (stages III + IV, *middle left panel)*, REM sleep *(middle right panel)*, GH secretion during sleep *(lower left panel)* and nadir of plasma cortisol concentrations *(lower right panel)* by age group in 149 healthy nonobese men. Sleep stages are expressed as a percentage of the sleep period, defined as the time interval between sleep onset and final morning awakening. (From Van Cauter E, Leproult R, Plat L: Age-related changes in slow wave sleep and REM sleep and relationship with growth hormone and cortisol levels in healthy men. JAMA 2000;284:861-868.)

cortisol levels, which follows the same chronology (i.e., no alteration until midlife, and then a steady rise from midlife to old age).[133] Analysis of variance indicates that this inability to achieve or maintain the quiescence of the corticotropic axis in aging partly reflects the loss of REM sleep in old age. Both animal and human studies have indicated that deleterious effects of HPA hyperactivity are more pronounced at the time of the trough of the rhythm than at the time of the peak.[138,139] Therefore, modest elevations in evening cortisol levels could

facilitate the development of central and peripheral disturbances associated with glucocorticoid excess, such as memory deficits and insulin resistance,[138,140] and further promote sleep fragmentation. Indeed, several studies have demonstrated that elevated corticosteroid levels result in increased propensity for awakenings.[141,142]

A nearly 50% dampening of the nocturnal PRL elevation is evident in healthy elderly subjects.[143] This diminished nocturnal rise in aging is associated with a decrease in the amplitude of the nocturnal secretory pulses.[144] Whether this age-related endocrine alteration partly reflects the increased number of awakenings (which inhibit PRL release) and decreased amounts of deep NREM stages (which stimulate PRL release) remains to be determined.

Clinical Pearl

Sleep exerts important modulatory effects on most components of the endocrine system. Sleep loss and alterations of sleep quality are associated with disturbances of hormone secretion and metabolism, which may be of clinical relevance. Findings suggest that part of the constellation of hormonal and metabolic alterations that characterize normal aging may reflect the deterioration of sleep quality. Strategies to reverse decrements in sleep quality may have beneficial effects on endocrine and metabolic function.

REFERENCES

1. Van Cauter E, Blackman JD, Roland D, et al: Modulation of glucose regulation and insulin secretion by circadian rhythmicity and sleep. J Clin Invest 1991;88:934-942.
2. Van Cauter E: Hormones and sleep. In Kales A (ed): The Pharmacology of Sleep. Berlin, Springer-Verlag, 1995, pp 279-306.
3. Muccioli G, Tschop M, Papotti M, et al: Neuroendocrine and peripheral activities of ghrelin: Implications in metabolism and obesity. Eur J Pharmacol 2002;440:235-254.
4. Weikel JC, Wichniak A, Ising M, et al: Ghrelin promotes slow-wave sleep in humans. Am J Physiol Endocrinol Metab 2003;284:E407-415.
5. Obal F Jr, Krueger JM: Biochemical regulation of non-rapid-eye-movement sleep. Front Biosci 2003;8:d520-d550.
6. Steiger A: Sleep and endocrinology. J Intern Med 2003;254:13-22.
7. Van Cauter E, Plat L, Copinschi G: Interrelations between sleep and the somatotropic axis. Sleep 1998;21:553-566.
8. Quabbe H, Schilling E, Helge H: Pattern of growth hormone secretion during a 24-hour fast in normal adults. J Clin Endocr Metab 1966;26:1173-1177.
9. Hunter WM, Rigal WM: The diurnal pattern of plasma growth hormone concentration in children and adolescents J Endocr 1966;34:147-153.
10. Takahashi Y, Kipnis DM, Daughaday WH: Growth hormone secretion during sleep. J Clin Invest 1968;47:2079-2090.
11. Sassin JF, Parker, DC, Mace JW, et al: Human growth hormone release: relation to slow-wave sleep and sleep-waking cycles. Science 1969;165:513-515.
12. Honda Y, Takahashi K, Takahashi S, et al: Growth hormone secretion during nocturnal sleep in normal subjects. J Clin Endocrinol Metab 1969;29:20-29.
13. Sassin JF, Frantz AG, Weitzman ED, et al: Human prolactin: 24-hour pattern with increased release during sleep. Science 1972;177:1205-1207.
14. Sassin J, Frantz A, Kapen S, et al: The nocturnal rise of human prolactin is dependent on sleep. J Clin Endocrinol Metab 1973;37:436-440.
15. Weibel L, Spiegel K, Gronfier C, et al: Twenty-four-hour melatonin and core body temperature rhythms: Their adaptation in night workers. Am J Physiol 1997;272:R948-R954.
16. Ocampo-Lim B, Guo W, DeMott Friberg R, et al: Nocturnal growth hormone (GH) secretion is eliminated by infusion of GH-releasing hormone antagonist. J Clin Endocrinol Metab 1996;81:4396-4399.
17. Jaffe C, Turgeon D, DeMott Friberg R, et al: Nocturnal augmentation of growth hormone (GH) secretion is preserved during repetitive bolus administration of GH-releasing hormone: Potential involvement of endogenous somatostatin—a clinical research center study. J Clin Endocrinol Metab 1995;80:3321-3326.
18. Dzaja A, Dalal M, Himmerich H, et al: Sleep enhances nocturnal plasma ghrelin levels in healthy subjects. Am J Physiol Endocrinol Metab 2004;286:963-967.
19. Cummings DE, Weigle DS, Frayo RS, et al: Plasma ghrelin levels after diet-induced weight loss or gastric bypass surgery. N Engl J Med 2002;346:1623-1630.
20. Parker DC, Sassin JF, Mace JW, et al: Human growth hormone release during sleep: electroencephalographic correlations. J Clin Endocrinol Metab 1969;29:871-874.
21. Van Cauter E, Kerkhofs M, Caufriez A, et al: A quantitative estimation of GH secretion in normal man: reproducibility and relation to sleep and time of day. J Clin Endocrinol Metab 1992;74:1441-1450.
22. Holl RW, Hartmann ML, Veldhuis JD, et al: Thirty-second sampling of plasma growth hormone in man: Correlation with sleep stages. J Clin Endocrinol Metab 1991;72:854-861.
23. Gronfier C, Luthringer R, Follenius M, et al: A quantitative evaluation of the relationships between growth hormone secretion and delta wave electroencephalographic activity during normal sleep and after enrichment in delta waves. Sleep 1996;19:817-824.
24. Van Cauter E, Plat L, Scharf M, et al: Simultaneous stimulation of slow-wave sleep and growth hormone secretion by gamma-hydroxybutyrate in normal young men. J Clin Invest 1997;100:745-753.
25. Brandenberger G, Gronfier C, Chapotot F, et al: Effect of sleep deprivation on overall 24 h growth-hormone secretion, Lancet 2000;356:1408.
26. Jarrett DB, Greenhouse JB, Miewald JM, et al: A reexamination of the relationship between growth hormone secretion and slow wave sleep using delta wave analysis. Biol Psychiatry 1990;27:497-509.
27. Mendlewicz J, Linkowski P, Kerkhofs M, et al: Diurnal hypersecretion of growth hormone in depression. J Clin Endocrinol Metab 1985;60:505-512.
28. Steiger A, Herth T, Holsboer F: Sleep-electroencephalography and the secretion of cortisol and growth hormone in normal controls. Acta Endocrinol 1987;116:36-42.
29. Van Cauter E, Caufriez A, Kerkhofs M, et al: Sleep, awakenings and insulin-like growth factor I modulate the growth hormone secretory response to growth hormone-releasing hormone. J Clin Endocrinol Metab 1992;74:1451-1459.
30. Spath-Schwalbe E, Gofferje M, Kern W, et al: Sleep disruption alters nocturnal ACTH and cortisol secretory patterns. Biol Psychiatry 1991;29:575-584.
31. Born J, Muth S, Fehm HL: The significance of sleep onset and slow wave sleep for nocturnal release of growth hormone (GH) and cortisol. Psychoneuroendocrinology 1988;13:233-243.
32. Weitzman ED, Zimmerman JC, Czeisler CA, et al: Cortisol secretion is inhibited during sleep in normal man. J Clin Endocrinol Metab 1983;56:352-358.
33. Spath-Schwalbe E, Uthgenannt D, Voget G, et al: Corticotropin-releasing hormone-induced adrenocorticotropin and cortisol secretion depends on sleep and wakefulness. J Clin Endocrinol Metab 1993;77:1170-1173.
34. Weibel L, Follenius M, Spiegel K, et al: Comparative effect of night and daytime sleep on the 24-hour cortisol secretory profile. Sleep 1995;18:549-556.
35. Gronfier C, Luthringer R, Follenius M, et al: Temporal relationships between pulsatile cortisol secretion and electroencephalographic activity during sleep in man. Electroencephalogr Clin Neurophysiol 1997;103:405-408.
36. Bierwolf C, Struve K, Marshall L, et al: Slow wave sleep drives inhibition of pituitary-adrenal secretion in humans. J Neuroendocrinol 1997;9:479-484.

37. Brabant G, Prank K, Ranft U, et al: Physiological regulation of circadian and pulsatile thyrotropin secretion in normal man and woman. J Clin Endocrinol Metab 1990;70:403-409.

38. Pruessner JC, Wolf OT, Hellhammer DH, et al: Free cortisol levels after awakening: a reliable biological marker for the assessment of adrenocortical activity. Life Sci 1997;61:2539-2549.

39. Follenius M, Brandenberger G, Bardasept J, et al: Nocturnal cortisol release in relation to sleep structure. Sleep 1992;15:21-27.

40. Van Cauter E, van Coevorden A, Blackman JD: Modulation of neuroendocrine release by sleep and circadian rhythmicity. In Yen S, Vale W (eds): Advances in Neuroendocrine Regulation of Reproduction. New York, Serono Symposia USA, Springer-Verlag, 1990, pp 113-122.

41. Bliwise DL: Normal Aging. In Kryger MH, Roth T, Dement WC (eds): Principles and Practice of Sleep Medicine. Philadelphia, WB Saunders, 1989.

42. Vgontzas AN, Bixler EO, Lin HM, et al: Chronic insomnia is associated with nyctohemeral activation of the hypothalamic-pituitary-adrenal axis: Clinical implications. J Clin Endocrinol Metab 2001;86:3787-3794.

43. Leproult R, Copinschi G, Buxton O, et al: Sleep loss results in an elevation of cortisol levels the next evening. Sleep 1997;20:865-870.

44. Veldhuis JD, Iranmanesh A, Johnson ML, et al: Twenty-four-hour rhythms in plasma concentrations of adenohypophyseal hormones are generated by distinct amplitude and/or frequency modulation of underlying pituitary secretory bursts. J Clin Endocrinol Metab 1990;71:1616-1623.

45. Parker DC, Rossman LG, Pekary AE, et al: Effect of 64-hour sleep deprivation on the circadian waveform of thyrotropin (TSH): further evidence of sleep-related inhibition of TSH release. J Clin Endocrinol Metab 1987;64:157-161.

46. Goichot B, Brandenberger G, Saini J, et al: Nocturnal plasma thyrotropin variations are related to slow-wave sleep. J Sleep Res 1992;1:186-190.

47. Gronfier C, Luthringer R, Follenius M, et al: Temporal link between plasma thyrotropin levels and electroencephalographic activity in man. Neurosci Lett 1995;200:97-100.

48. Van Cauter E, Aschoff J: Endocrine and other biological rhythms. In DeGroot LJ (ed): Endocrinology. Philadelphia, WB Saunders, 1989, pp 2658-2705.

49. Allan JS, Czeisler CA: Persistence of the circadian thyrotropin rhythm under constant conditions and after light-induced shifts of circadian phase. J Clin Endocrinol Metab 1994;79:508-512.

50. Gary KA, Winokur A, Douglas SD, et al: Total sleep deprivation and the thyroid axis: Efects of sleep and waking activity. Aviat Space Environ Med 1996;67:513-519.

51. Hirschfeld U, Moreno-Reyes R, Akseki E, et al: Progressive elevation of plasma thyrotropin during adaptation to simulated jet lag: effects of treatment with bright light or zolpidem. J Clin Endocrinol Metab 1996;81:3270-3277.

52. Van Cauter E, L'Hermite M, Copinschi G, et al: Quantitative analysis of spontaneous variations of plasma prolactin in normal man. Am J Physiol 1981; 241:E355–E363.

53. Spiegel K, Follenius M, Simon C, et al: Prolactin secretion and sleep. Sleep 1994;17:20-27.

54. Waldstreicher J, Duffy JF, Brown EN, et al: Gender differences in the temporal organization of prolactin (PRL) secretion: Evidence for a sleep-independent circadian rhythm of circulating PRL levels. A Clinical Research Center study. J Clin Endocrinol Metab 1996;81:1483-1487.

55. Desir D, Van Cauter E, L'Hermite M, et al: Effects of "jet lag" on hormonal patterns. III. Demonstration of an intrinsic circadian rhythmicity in plasma prolactin. J Clin Endocrinol Metab 1982;55:849-857.

56. Spiegel K, Luthringer R, Follenius M, et al: Temporal relationship between prolactin secretion and slow-wave electroencephalographic activity during sleep. Sleep 1995;18:543-548.

57. Copinschi G, Van Onderbergen A, L'Hermite-Balériaux M, et al: Effects of the short-acting benzodiazepine triazolam, taken at bedtime, on circadian and sleep-related hormonal profiles in normal men. Sleep 1990;13:232-244.

58. Copinschi G, Akseki E, Moreno-Reyes R, et al: Effects of bedtime administration of zolpidem on circadian and sleep-related hormonal profiles in normal women. Sleep 1995;18:417-424.

59. Roky R, Obal F, Valatx JL, et al: Prolactin and rapid eye movement sleep regulation. Sleep 1995;18:536-542.

60. Frieboes RM, Murck H, Stalla GK, et al: Enhanced slow-wave sleep in patients with hyperprolactinemia. J Clin Endocrinol Metab 1998;83:2706-2710.

61. Blyton DM, Sullivan CE, Edwards N: Lactation is associated with an increase in slow-wave sleep in women. J Sleep Res 2002;11:297-303.

62. Van Cauter E, Copinschi G, Turek F: Endocrine and other biological rhythms. In DeGroot L, Jameson J (eds): Endocrinology, 4th ed. Philadelphia, WB Saunders, 2001, pp 235-256.

63. Fehm HL, Clausing J, Kern W, et al: Sleep-associated augmentation and synchronization of luteinizing hormone pulses in adult men. Neuroendocrinology 1991;54:192-195.

64. Bremner WJ, Vitiello MV, Prinz PN: Loss of circadian rhythmicity in blood testosterone levels with aging in normal men. J Clin Endocrinol Metab 1983;56:1278-1280.

65. Lejeune-Lenain C, Van Cauter E, Desir D, et al: Control of circadian and episodic variations of adrenal androgens secretion in man. J Endocrinol Invest 1987;10:267-276.

66. Luboshitzky R, Herer P, Levi M, et al: Relationship between rapid eye movement sleep and testosterone secretion in normal men. J Androl 1999;20:731-737.

67. Luboshitzky R, Zabari Z, Shen-Orr Z, et al: Disruption of the nocturnal testosterone rhythm by sleep fragmentation in normal men. J Clin Endocrinol Metab 2001;86:1134-1139.

68. Reame N, Sauder SE, Kelch RP, et al: Pulsatile gonadotropin secretion during the human menstrual cycle: evidence for altered frequency of gonadotropin-releasing hormone secretion. J Clin Endocrinol Metab 1984;59:328-337.

69. Filicori M, Santoro N, Merriam GR, et al: Characterization of the physiological pattern of episodic gonadotropin secretion throughout the menstrual cycle. J Clin Endocrinol Metab 1986;62:1136-1144.

70. Vermeulen A, Deslypere JP, Kaukman JM: Influence of antiopioids on luteinizing hormone pulsatility in aging men. J Clin Endocrinol Metab 1989;68:68-72.

71. Veldhuis JD, Urban RJ, Lizarralde G, et al: Attenuation of luteinizing hormone secretory burst amplitude as a proximate basis for the hypoandrogenism of healthy aging in men. J Clin Endocrinol Metab 1992;75:52-58.

72. Mulligan T, Iranmanesh A, Gheorghiu S, et al: Amplified nocturnal luteinizing hormone (LH) secretory burst frequency with selective attenuation of pulsatile (but not basal) testosterone secretion in healthy aged men: Possible Leydig cell desensitization to endogenous LH signaling. A clinical research center study. J Clin Endocrinol Metab 1995;80:3025-3031.

73. Tenover JS, Matsumoto AM, Clifton DK, et al: Age-related alterations in the circadian rhythms of pulsatile luteinizing hormone and testosterone secretion in healthy men. J Gerontol 1988;43:M163-M169.

74. Luboshitzky R, Shen-Orr Z, Herer P: Middle-aged men secrete less testosterone at night than young healthy men. J Clin Endocrinol Metab 2003;88:3160-3166.

75. Turek FW, Van Cauter E: Rhythms in reproduction. In Knobil E, Neill JD (eds): The Physiology of Reproduction. New York, Raven Press, 1993, pp 1789-1830.

76. Saletu-Zyhlarz G, Anderer P, Gruber G, et al: Insomnia related to postmenopausal syndrome and hormone replacement therapy: sleep laboratory studies on baseline differences between patients and controls and double-blind, placebo-controlled investigations on the effects of a novel estrogen-progestogen combination (Climodien, Lafamme) versus estrogen alone. J Sleep Res 2003; 12:239-254.

77. Hays J, Ockene JK, Brunner RL, et al: Effects of estrogen plus progestin on health-related quality of life. N Engl J Med 2003;348:1839-1854.

78. Antonijevic IA, Stalla GK, Steiger A: Modulation of the sleep electroencephalogram by estrogen replacement in postmenopausal women. Am J Obstet Gynecol 2000;182:277-282.

79. Moe KE, Larsen LH, Vitiello MV, et al: Estrogen replacement therapy moderates the sleep disruption associated with nocturnal blood sampling. Sleep 2001;24:886-894.

80. Shahar E, Redline S, Young T, et al: Hormone replacement therapy and sleep-disordered breathing. Am J Respir Crit Care Med 2003;167:1186-1192.

81. Mauras N, Blizzard RM, Link K, et al: Augmentation of growth hormone secretion during puberty: Evidence for a pulse amplitude-modulated phenomenon. J Clin Endocrinol Metab 1987;64:596-601.

82. Polonsky KS, Given BD, Van Cauter E: Twenty-four-hour profiles and pulsatile patterns of insulin secretion in normal and obese subjects. J Clin Invest 1988;81:442-448.

83. Levy I, Recasens A, Casamitjana R, et al: Nocturnal insulin and C-peptide rhythms in normal subjects. Diabetes Care 1987; 10:148-151.

84. Clore JN, Nestler JE, Blackard WG: Sleep-associated fall in glucose disposal and hepatic glucose output in normal humans. Diabetes 1989;38:285-290.

85. Simon C, Brandenberger G, Follenius M: Absence of the dawn phenomenon in normal subjects. J Clin Endocrinol Metab 1988;67:203-205.

86. Garvey WT, Olefsky JM, Rubenstein AH, et al: Day-long integrated serum insulin and C-peptide profiles in patients with NIDDM. Diabetes 1988;37:590-599.

87. Kern W, Offenheuser S, Fehm HL: Entrainment of ultradian oscillations in the secretion of insulin and glucagon to the nonREM/REM sleep rhythm in humans. J Clin Endocrinol Metab 1996;81:1541-1547.

88. Van Cauter E, Polonsky KS, Scheen AJ: Roles of circadian rhythmicity and sleep in human glucose regulation. Endocr Rev 1997;18:716-738.

89. Simon C, Brandenberger G, Follenius M: Ultradian oscillations of plasma glucose, insulin, and C-peptide in man during continuous enteral nutrition. J Clin Endocrinol Metab 1987;64:669-674.

90. Van Cauter E, Desir D, Decoster C, et al: Nocturnal decrease in glucose tolerance during constant glucose infusion. J Clin Endocrinol Metab 1989;69:604-611.

91. Simon C, Brandenberger G, Saini J, et al: Slow oscillations of plasma glucose and insulin secretion rate are amplified during sleep in humans under continuous enteral nutrition. Sleep 1994;17:333-338.

92. Boyle PJ, Scott JC, Krentz AJ, et al: Diminished brain glucose metabolism is a significant determinant for falling rates of systemic glucose utilization during sleep in normal humans. J Clin Invest 1994;93:529-535.

93. Møller N, Jorgensen JOL, Schmitz O, et al: Effects of a growth hormone pulse on total and forearm substrate fluxes in humans. Am J Physiol 1990;258:E86-E91.

94. Scheen AJ, Byrne MM, Plat L, et al: Relationships between sleep quality and glucose regulation in normal humans. Am J Physiol 1996;271:E261-E270.

95. Buchsbaum MS, Gillin JC, Wu J, et al: Regional cerebral glucose metabolic rate in human sleep assessed by positron emission tomography. Life Sci 1989;45:1349-1356.

96. Maquet P, Dive D, Salmon E, et al: Cerebral glucose utilization during sleep-wake cycle in man determined by positron emission tomography and [18F]2-fluoro-2-deoxy-D-glucose method. Brain Res 1990;513:136-143.

97. Maquet P, Dive D, Salmon E, et al: Cerebral glucose utilization during stage 2 sleep in man. Brain Res 1992;571:149-153.

98. Maquet P: Positron emission tomography studies of sleep and sleep disorders. J Neurol 1997;244 (4 Suppl1):S23-S28.

99. Plat L, Byrne MM, Sturis J, et al: Effects of morning cortisol elevation on insulin secretion and glucose regulation in humans. Am J Physiol 1996;270:E36-E42.

100. Danguir J, Nicolaidis S: Dependence of sleep on nutrients' availability. Physiol Behav 1979;22:735-740.

101. Rechtschaffen A, Bergmann BM: Sleep deprivation in the rat by the disk-over-water method. Behav Brain Res 1995;69:55-63.

102. Taheri S, Zeitzer JM, Mignot E: The role of hypocretins (orexins) in sleep regulation and narcolepsy. Ann Rev Neurosci 2002;25:283-313.

103. Ahima RS, Saper CB, Flier JS, et al: Leptin regulation of neuroendocrine systems. Front Neuroendocrinol 2000;21:263-307.

104. Chin-Chance C, Polonsky KS, Schoeller D: Twenty-four hour leptin levels respond to cumulative short-term energy imbalance and predict subsequent intake. J Clin Endocrinol Metab 2000;85:2685-2691.

105. Kolaczynski JW, Considine RV, Ohannesian J, et al: Responses of leptin to short-term fasting and refeeding in humans: A link with ketogenesis but not ketones themselves. Diabetes 1996; 45:1511-1515.

106. Schoeller DA, Cella LK, Sinha MK, et al: Entrainment of the diurnal rhythm of plasma leptin to meal timing. J Clin Invest 1997;100:1882-1887.

107. Simon C, Gronfier C, Schlienger JL, et al: Circadian and ultradian variations of leptin in normal man under continuous enteral nutrition: Relationship to sleep and body temperature. J Clin Endocrinol Metab 1998;83:1893-1899.

108. Mullington JM, Chan JL, Van Dongen HP, et al: Sleep loss reduces diurnal rhythm amplitude of leptin in healthy men. J Neuroendocrinol 2003;15:851-854.

109. Kok SW, Meinders AE, Overeem S, et al: Reduction of plasma leptin levels and loss of its circadian rhythmicity in hypocretin (orexin)-deficient narcoleptic humans. J Clin Endocrinol Metab 2002;87:805-809.

110. Havel PJ: Peripheral signals conveying metabolic information to the brain: short-term and long-term regulation of food intake and energy homeostasis. Exp Biol Med 2001;226:963-977.

111. Brandenberger G, Charloux A, Grongier C, et al: Ultradian rhythms in hydromineral hormones. Horm Res 1998;49:131-135.

112. Follenius M, Brandenberger G, Saini J: Lack of diurnal rhythm in plasma atrial natriuretic peptide. Life Sci 1992;51:143-149.

113. Brandenberger G, Krauth MO, Ehrhart J, et al: Modulation of episodic renin release during sleep in humans. Hypertension 1990;15:370-375.

114. Brandenberger G, Follenius M, Muzet A, et al: Ultradian oscillations in plasma renin activity: their relationship to meals and sleep stages. J Clin Endocrinol Metab 1985;61:280-284.

115. Portaluppi F, Bagni B, Degli UB, et al: Circadian rhythms of atrial natriuretic peptide, renin, aldosterone, cortisol, blood pressure, and heart rate in normal and hypertensive subjects. J Hypertens 1990;8:85-95.

116. Brandenberger G, Follenius M, Goichot B, et al: Twenty-four hour profiles of plasma renin activity in relation to the sleep-wake cycle. J Hypertens 1994;12:277-283.

117. Brandenberger G, Follenius M, Simon C, et al: Nocturnal oscillations in plasma renin activity and REM-NREM sleep cycles in man: A common regulatory mechanism? Sleep 1988; 11:242-250.

118. Luthringer R, Brandenberger G, Schaltenbrand N, et al: Slow wave electroencephalographic activity parallels renin oscillations during sleep in humans. Electroencephalogr Clin Neurophysiol 1995;95:318-322.

119. Charloux A, Piquard F, Ehrhart J, et al: Time-courses in renin and blood pressure during sleep in humans. J Sleep Res 2002;11:73-79.

120. Charloux A, Gronfier C, Lonsdorfer-Wolf E, et al: Aldosterone release during the sleep-wake cycle in humans. Am J Physiol 1998;276:E43-E49.

121. Charloux A, Gronfier C, Chapotot F, et al: Sleep deprivation blunts the night time increase in aldosterone release in humans. J Sleep Res 2001;10:27-33.

122. Bliwise DL: Historical change in the report of daytime fatigue. Sleep 1996;19:462-464.

123. Johnson EO: Sleep in America: 2000. Washington, DC, National Sleep Foundation, 2000.

124. Jean-Louis G, Kripke D, Ancoli-Israel S: Sleep and quality of well-being. Sleep 2000;23:1115-1121.

125. Wehr T, Moul D, Barbato G, et al: Conservation of photoperiod-responsive mechanisms in humans. Am J Physiol 1993;265: R846-R857.

126. Roehrs T, Shore E, Papineau K, et al: A two-week sleep extension in sleepy normals. Sleep 1996:576-582.

127. Harrison Y, Horme JA: Long-term extension to sleep. Are we really chronically sleep deprived? Psychophysiology 1996; 33:22–30.

128. Spiegel K, Leproult R, L'Hermite-Balériaux M, et al: Leptin levels are dependent on sleep duration: Relationships with sympathovagal balance, carbohydrate regulation, cortisol, and thyrotropin. J Clin Endocrinol Metab 2004;89: 5762-5771.

129. Spiegel K, Leproult R, Colecchia EF, et al: Adaptation of the 24-h growth hormone profile to a state of sleep debt. Am J Physiol Regul Integr Comp Physiol 2000;279: R874-883.

130. Spiegel K, Leproult R, Van Cauter E: Impact of sleep debt on metabolic and endocrine function. Lancet 1999;354: 1435-1439.

131. Van Cauter E, Sturis J, Byrne MM, et al: Demonstration of rapid light-induced advances and delays of the human circadian clock using hormonal phase markers. Am J Physiol 1994;266: E953-E963.

131a. Spiegel K, Tasali E, Penev P, Van Cauter E: Sleep curtailment in healthy young men is associated with decreased leptin levels, elevated ghrelin levels, and increased hunger and appetite. Ann Intern Med 2004;141:846-850.

131b. Taheri S, Lin L, Austin D, Young T, Mignot E: Short sleep duration is associated with reduced leptin, elevated ghrelin, and increased body mass index. PLoS Med 2004;1(3):e62.

132. Everson CA, Crowley W: Reductions in circulating anabolic hormones induced by sustained sleep deprivation in rats. Am J Physiol Endocrinol Metab 2004;286:1060-1070.

133. Van Cauter E, Leproult R, Plat L: Age-related changes in slow-wave sleep and REM sleep and relationship with growth hormone and cortisol levels in healthy men. JAMA 2000; 284:861-868.

134. Prinz P, Moe K, Dulberg E, et al: Higher plasma IGF-1 levels are associated with increased delta sleep in healthy older men. J Gerontol 1995;50A:M222–M226.

135. Corpas E, Harman SM, Blackman MR: Human growth hormone and human aging. Endocrinol Rev 1993;14:20-39.

136. Cuneo RC, Salomon F, McGauley GA, et al: The growth hormone deficiency syndrome in adults. Clin Endocrinol 1992;37:387-397.

137. Rosen T, Hansson T, Granhed H, et al: Reduced bone mineral content in adult patients with growth hormone deficiency. Acta Endocrinol 1993;129:201-206.

138. Dallman MF, Strack AL, Akana SF, et al: Feast and famine: Critical role of glucocorticoids with insulin in daily energy flow. Front Neuroendocrinol 1993;14:303-347.

139. Plat L, Féry F, L'Hermite-Balériaux M, et al: Metabolic effects of short-term physiological elevations of plasma cortisol are more pronounced in the evening than in the morning. J Clin Endocrinol Metab 1999;84:3082-3092.

140. McEwen BS, Sapolsky RM: Stress and cognitive function. Curr Opin Neurobiol 1995;5:205-216.

141. Holsboer F, von Bardelein U, Steiger A: Effects of intravenous corticotropin-releasing hormone upon sleep-related growth hormone surge and sleep EEG in man. Neuroendocrinol 1988;48:32-38.

142. Born J, Späth-Schwalbe E, Schwakenhofer H, et al: Influences of corticotropin-releasing hormone, adrenocorticotropin, and cortisol on sleep in normal man. J Clin Endocrinol Metab 1989;68:904-911.

143. van Coevorden A, Mockel J, Laurent E, et al: Neuroendocrine rhythms and sleep in aging men. Am J Physiol 1991;260: E651-E661.

144. Greenspan SL, Klibanski A, Rowe JW, et al: Age alters pulsatile prolactin release: influence of dopaminergic inhibition. Am J Physiol 1990;258:E799-E804.

23

Gastrointestinal Physiology

William C. Orr

ABSTRACT

Gastrointestinal functioning shows significant changes associated with sleep. There is a diminution in esophageal peristaltic amplitude and a substantial decrease in the swallowing rate during sleep. Transient relaxations of the lower esophageal sphincter to the intragastric baseline have been shown to be decreased during sleep. The normal gastric electrical cycle at three cycles per minute has been shown to be markedly altered during NREM sleep. Basal gastric acid secretion is minimal between meals but appears to reach a peak between midnight and 2:00 AM. Intestinal motility is largely regulated via a sequence of contractions that occur periodically throughout the night in the form of a 90-minute cycle, albeit unrelated to the cycle of rapid eye movement (REM) sleep. This cycle does appear to be somewhat shorter during the sleeping interval. In general, there does appear to be diminished contractile activity and electrical activity in the colon during sleep. High peristaltic contractions of the colon, which are associated with defecation, are also markedly diminished during sleep but facilitated with arousals from sleep and on awakening in the morning. Resting anal canal pressure is substantially diminished during sleep, but spontaneous cyclic motor activity, including retrograde propagation, appears to be present to prevent the involuntary loss of rectal contents during sleep. Sleep does alter sensory motor functioning in the anal canal, resulting in an increase in the threshold of sensation for rectal distention, with the preservation of normal internal anal sphincter relaxation responses. The voluntary contractions of the external anal sphincter to rectal distention are markedly diminished during sleep.

Descriptions of the normal physiology of many organ systems rarely include the normal alterations of the systems during sleep. The impact of sleep-related or *circadian-related* changes on gastrointestinal (GI) physiology and pathophysiology are not widely known. This can be largely attributed to the inaccessibility of the luminal GI tract to measurement of its many functions. Monitoring any of the basic functions of the GI system requires invading an orifice, which is an unpleasant experience and one that would generally be assumed to be disruptive of normal sleep.

The functioning of the luminal GI tract (to which this review is confined) reflects the final common pathway of a complex interaction of the central nervous system (CNS) with both the autonomic nervous system (ANS) and the enteric nervous system (ENS). The latter is a complex neuronal network that is woven throughout the subserosal layers of the luminal GI tract. The ENS provides an autonomous source of GI motor activity. The movement through the GI tract is controlled and regulated by the ENS and the ANS, and the interaction of these two influences ultimately determines that appropriate movement, at an appropriate rate, occurs throughout the passage from mouth to anus.[1]

Alterations in GI functioning during sleep appear to be quite different depending on the particular organ studied and its function within the GI system. For example, spontaneous esophageal function is markedly reduced during sleep because there is no need for this organ to function except in the event of food being transmitted from the upper esophageal area. This rarely occurs without volitional swallowing, which is diminished significantly during sleep.[2] On the other hand, rectal motor activity persists during sleep, which appears to be a mechanism necessary to preserve continence during sleep.[3]

The ultimate description of GI functioning and its complex physiology requires that autonomic and central control be separated from the intrinsic control generated by the ENS. Because sleep essentially represents a state of reversible decortication, the study of GI motor functioning during sleep allows an assessment of autonomous activity without higher cortical influence. Thus, the study of GI motility during sleep allows the separation of CNS and ENS processes and a more clear understanding of what has been referred to as the *brain–gut axis*.

HISTORICAL ASPECTS

Interest in GI physiology during sleep preceded the development of sophisticated techniques for monitoring GI function by well over 50 years. For example, Friedenwald,[4] in 1906, described the secretory function of the stomach during sleep and reported that it was not appreciably altered. In 1924, Johnson and Washeim[5] reported a decrease in the volume of gastric juice secreted during sleep, and, in addition, they reported an increase in the acidity of the gastric juice. Henning and Norpoth[6] measured acidity hourly during sleep, and they reported that sleep was associated with a cessation of acid secretion and that only in patients with gastric ulcers did there appear to be continuous acid secretion. These results were confirmed nearly 20 years later.[7]

In 1915, Luckhardt[8] described the inhibition of gastric motility during periods of sleep, which, from his description, sounded remarkably like rapid eye movement (REM) sleep. His observations were made in dogs and were described in association with sonorous respiration (snoring?), irregular breathing, movements of the forelimbs and hindlimbs, and occasional "abortive yelps." Luckhardt stated, "I assumed that the dog was experiencing during sleep a form of cerebral excitation akin to or identical with the dreaming state in man."[8]

A few years later, in 1922, Wada[9] reported an extensive study of hunger and its relationship to gastric and somatic activity by use of simultaneous records of gastric contractions and body movements during sleep. Gastric contractions were reported that were often associated with body movements and reports of dreaming. The techniques used in these studies were clearly somewhat crude, but it is clear that interest in GI function during sleep was not a development of the more modern era of sleep investigation.

GASTRIC FUNCTION

Acid Secretion

Gastric acid secretion has been shown to exhibit a clear circadian rhythm in healthy subjects.[10,11] There is a peak in acid secretion occurring generally between 10 PM and 2 AM, whereas basal acid secretion in the waking state is minimal in the absence of meal stimulation.[11] Similar results have been described in patients who have duodenal ulcer (DU) disease with levels of acid secretion markedly enhanced throughout the circadian cycle.[12,13] Thus, there is an endogenous circadian rhythm of unstimulated basal acid secretion, but it is not clear that this is specifically altered in any way by sleep.

An interest in the pathogenesis of DU disease and the possible role of nocturnal gastric acid secretion in this process was further stimulated by research that analyzed hourly samples of acid secretion in both healthy subjects and patients with DU disease and that identified nearly continuous acid secretion throughout the night in healthy volunteers.[12,14] There was a considerable degree of night-to-night and subject-to-subject variation. In contrast, in patients with DU disease, there were increases in both volume and acid concentration during sleep. Patients with DU disease who tended to be high acid secretors were consistently high, and those who were low secretors were consistently low. These studies paved the way for more extensive investigations into the role of nocturnal acid secretion in the pathogenesis of DU disease. This research is at variance with other studies,[10] which did not find a substantial difference in nocturnal acid secretion between healthy subjects and patients with DU. These discrepant results may result from varying degrees of ulcer activity in the patients studied. Studies that used hourly collections of overnight acid secretion in healthy subjects and in patients with DU disease reported that the nocturnal acid secretion in patients with DU disease is 3 to 20 times greater than that in healthy subjects.[15] This greater secretion was abolished by vagotomy, which invariably produced prompt ulcer healing. These data were interpreted to be strong evidence in favor of a "nervous" origin for DU disease.

The first study to describe gastric acid secretion during polysomnographic (PSG) monitoring was reported in 1960.[16] Using relatively crude determinations of stages of sleep, no correlation between gastric acid secretion and sleep stages in healthy subjects was found. Subsequent research[17] reported the rather startling finding of a hypersecretion of acid during REM sleep in patients with DU disease. Both of these studies suffered from major methodologic flaws: the number of patients studied and the number of nights per patient were small, and drugs were used to induce sleep. As earlier studies had documented the considerable night-to-night variability in acid secretion, studying a patient or a healthy volunteer with a nasogastric tube for a single night would undoubtedly result in numerous awakenings and generally poor sleep, with correspondingly more variable acid secretion.

Another study[18] reported no significant differences in acid secretion during non–rapid eye movement (NREM) sleep and found that REM sleep was associated with an inhibition of acid secretion. This study, although avoiding the use of drugs to induce sleep, used a rather cumbersome technique for determining acid output that caused numerous disruptions in the patients' sleep.

To avoid these methodologic problems, acid production was measured in five healthy volunteers and five patients with DU disease, and each subject was studied for 5 consecutive nights in the sleep laboratory.[19] The study involved continuous aspiration of gastric contents, assessment of serum gastrin levels, and PSG monitoring. The results did not reveal any significant correlation between the sleep stage (REM or NREM) and acid concentration or total acid secretion. Furthermore, there was no relationship between any of these variables and serum gastrin levels. These data did show, however, that the patients with DU failed to inhibit acid secretion during the first 2 hours of sleep. This was consistent with previously reported studies[12] that suggested that acid secretion is poorly inhibited during sleep in patients with DU disease.

In conclusion, there is a clear-cut circadian rhythm in basal acid secretion, with a peak occurring in the early part of the normal sleep interval. However, there are no definitive data suggesting a major effect of sleep stage on this process. Acid secretion is extremely variable from night to night and from person to person, and for this reason definitive conclusions require numerous replications across and within a large number of subjects and patients. The extremely demanding logistics of sleep studies and the clearly aversive aspects of numerous nasal intubations to study participants make the acquisition of such data exceedingly difficult.

Motor Function

The motor function of the stomach serves to empty solids and liquids into the duodenum at an appropriate rate and pH. The stomach is functionally divided into two sections: the fundus of the stomach functions primarily to control liquid emptying into the duodenum, whereas the antrum controls emptying of solids.[20] Because liquids and solids are handled differently by the stomach, the regulation of gastric emptying is correspondingly complicated, involving intrinsic regulation of motor activity as well as specific alterations associated with the ingestion of liquids and solids. Thus, although gastric emptying itself can be regarded as the final common pathway reflecting the motor activity of the stomach, it should be kept in mind that the processes of liquid and solid emptying are regulated by quite different mechanisms.

There have been many reports of gastric motility during sleep, with contradictory results. Inhibition of gastric motility during sleep has been reported, and it was suggested that the "dream mechanism" was part of this inhibitory process.[21] A cortical inhibitory mechanism acting through the splanchnic nerve is the postulated mechanism. Other research done nearly 30 years later found that gastric motility was enhanced during sleep, as compared with waking.[22] Some research has described a marked enhancement in gastric motility during REM sleep,[23] but in other studies, a decrease in gastric motility during REM sleep was noted.[24] No consistent findings concerning alterations by sleep stage were noted in a study in unanesthetized and unrestrained cats.[25]

Gastric emptying during sleep has been reported in studies that required the patient to sleep with a nasogastric tube through which 750 mL of 10% glucose was administered.[26] After 30 minutes, the gastric contents were aspirated, and the residual volume was determined. Aspiration was followed by a washout meal of 150 mL of saline. This process was done during the presleep waking interval, during NREM and REM sleep, and during postsleep waking. These data suggested a more rapid gastric emptying during REM sleep and a slower emptying during the postsleep waking state. The emptying of a hypertonic solution is controlled by vagally mediated osmoreceptors in the duodenum. These data, therefore, suggest a possible anticholinergic action during REM and a cholinergic process during the postsleep waking state. These data represent only an approximation of the alterations in gastric emptying during sleep because these measurement techniques are relatively crude, and gastric emptying is a complex process.

In another study, a technique that permits the simultaneous assessment of acid secretion, water secretion, and the fractional rate of emptying was employed during sleep.[27] The results indicate that in healthy subjects, acid secretion, water secretion, and the fractional rate of emptying, all showed significant decrements during sleep.[28] There did not appear to be any differences between REM and NREM sleep, but all of these measures demonstrated a significant difference between presleep waking and REM sleep. Data obtained by use of radionuclide emptying assessments suggest that this difference may be a circadian, rather than a sleep-dependent, effect. Another study shows a marked delay in gastric emptying of solids in the evening compared with the morning.[29]

Gastric motor functioning is characterized by an endogenous electrical cycle generated by the gastric smooth muscle. The electrical rhythm is generated by a pacemaker located in the proximal portion of the greater curvature of the stomach.[30] The electrical cycle occurs at a frequency of approximately three per minute and represents the precursor to contractile activity of the stomach, which allows movement of gastric contents to the antrum and subsequent emptying into the duodenum.

The gastric electrical rhythm can be measured by surface electrodes placed in the periumbilical area. The identification of this basic motor function of the stomach requires highly sophisticated measurement, digital filtering, and spectral analysis to describe the parameters of this oscillation.[31] The noninvasive measurement of the gastric electrical rhythm is called electrogastrography. The progressive sophistication of the measurement and analytic techniques has allowed a reliable noninvasive technique to measure an important function of the GI system.

Analysis of gastric electrical activity has documented three fundamental characteristics of this electrical rhythm that determine its normal activity. First, the power in the frequency band is approximately three per minute. This is essentially a method of quantifying the extent to which the wave approximates a sinusoidal rhythm, and the power reflects the peak-to-peak amplitude of the cycle. Second, more sophisticated techniques have allowed a minute-by-minute characterization of the cycle.[32] This has permitted other parameters to describe the normal function of the gastric electrical rhythm. For example, 1-minute segments can be analyzed for 15 to 20 minutes and the percentage of 1-minute segments in which the peak amplitude is located at the dominant frequency can be calculated. "Normal" is approximately 70% or greater. Third, this technique of 1-minute segmental analysis, termed the *running spectrum,* also allows determination of the instability coefficient, which describes the variability of the center frequency of the cycle. A larger coefficient means greater instability of the endogenous oscillation.

It has been generally thought that the gastric electrical rhythm is a product of the endogenous functioning of the gastric electrical pacemaker and that it is generally without influence from the CNS. However, sleep studies from our laboratory have challenged this traditional belief. Initially, our studies showed a significant decline in the power in the three-per-minute cycle during NREM sleep.[33] There is a significant recovery of this toward the waking state during REM sleep. Further preliminary data from our laboratory have used running spectral analysis to describe a profound instability in the functioning of the basic electrical cycle during NREM sleep.[34] These two studies clearly suggest that NREM sleep is associated with a marked alteration or destabilization of the basic gastric electrical rhythm. It might be concluded from these results that higher cortical input or a degree of CNS arousal must be present to stabilize and promote normal gastric functioning and consequently normal gastric emptying.

It seems clear from these results that definitive statements concerning the alteration of gastric motor function and gastric emptying during sleep or specific sleep stages cannot be made. It would have to be concluded that gastric motor function appears to be retarded during sleep, but it is not clear whether this is specifically the result of altered gastric emptying attributable to sleep per se or whether this is simply a natural circadian rhythm independent of sleep.

SWALLOWING AND ESOPHAGEAL FUNCTION

Interest in esophageal function during sleep was stimulated by 24-hour esophageal pH studies, which documented the important role of nocturnal gastroesophageal reflux (GER) in the pathogenesis of reflux esophagitis.[35] GER may occur in healthy people even while upright and awake. This occurrence was identified primarily postprandially in healthy subjects and was associated with multiple episodes of reflux that were relatively rapidly (in less than 5 minutes) neutralized. Studies by these investigators and others have documented that in healthy individuals, sleep is relatively free of episodes of GER.[2,36] However, when reflux does occur during sleep, it is associated with a marked prolongation in the acid clearance time. Data from these studies suggest that the prolongation of acid clearance during sleep is caused by several factors. First, and perhaps most important, there is a delay in the conscious response to acid in the esophagus during sleep, and studies from our laboratory have documented that an arousal response almost invariably precedes the initiation of swallowing.[2,37]

In fact, a relatively predictable and inverse relationship has been described between the acid clearance time and the amount of time the individual spends awake during the acid clearance interval. That is, if an individual responds with an awakening and subsequent swallowing when acid is infused into the distal esophagus during sleep, clearance is substantially faster than if an individual has a prolonged latency to the initial arousal response.[2,37]

Another important aspect of complete neutralization of the acidic distal esophagus is salivary flow. The importance of saliva in the final neutralization of the acidic esophagus has been documented.[38] This finding is important because salivary flow stops completely with the onset of sleep, substantially retarding the acid neutralization.[39]

Swallowing initiates the acid clearance process and, in general, is considered a volitional act. Thus, one would expect that it would be substantially depressed during altered states of consciousness such as sleep. Studies have confirmed this supposition by showing a significant diminution in swallowing frequency during sleep.[40,41] Although the state of sleep certainly depresses the frequency of swallows, it appears that swallowing is usually associated with a brief arousal response.[2,42] Studies with healthy volunteers suggest that even though the swallowing frequency is substantially diminished during sleep, peristalsis appears to be completely normal.[2] This includes primary peristalsis, which is initiated by a swallow, and secondary peristalsis, which is not preceded by a swallow. However, in a study of cats, it has been shown that, although swallowing frequencies diminished during sleep as noted in humans, peristaltic amplitudes are hypotonic during REM sleep.[43] Thus, alterations in esophageal acid clearance during sleep are primarily the result of two factors: decreased swallowing frequency and absence of salivary flow.

A study has addressed the issue of esophageal function during sleep and has clearly shown that esophageal motor activity is sleep stage dependent.[44] This study showed that the frequency of primary contractions in the esophagus (peristaltic contractions preceded by a swallow) diminishes progressively from stage 1 to stage 4 sleep. Of interest is the fact that secondary peristaltic contractions (spontaneous contractions) showed a similar decline from waking to stage 4 sleep but showed a significant recovery during REM sleep. This suggests that spontaneous, or secondary, esophageal peristaltic contractions are perhaps more influenced by the endogenous level of CNS arousal. In agreement with previous studies, this study identified long periods of nocturnal esophageal motor quiescence with apparently random bursts of contractions.[45,46] In contrast to a previous study, secondary peristaltic contractions during sleep were noted to be of diminished amplitude and shorter duration when compared with primary contractions.[2,44] In addition, primary peristaltic contractions appeared to be of higher amplitude during sleep than during waking. This supports the notion that primary and secondary contractions may be controlled by different mechanisms and that awake CNS influences may inhibit primary peristaltic contractions.

The actual mechanism of GER during sleep has been addressed.[42] Via a specially designed monitoring device, the lower esophageal sphincter pressure was continuously monitored during sleep. In addition, a pH probe was placed in the distal esophagus to identify episodes of GER. This study determined that the majority of episodes of reflux occurred in association with a spontaneous decline in the lower esophageal sphincter pressure to close to the intragastric pressure. This pressure decline creates a common cavity between the stomach and the esophagus, and because there is a 5-mm Hg pressure gradient between the stomach and the midesophagus, a situation is created that is particularly conducive to the reflux of gastric contents into the esophagus. The majority of these episodes were associated with a brief arousal response, although they were identified in some cases without movement. Other reflux events were noted to occur when the lower esophageal sphincter pressure was clearly above the intragastric baseline, thereby creating a pressure barrier to reflux. Under these circumstances, reflux occurs mechanically by the creation of intraabdominal pressure that is sufficient to overcome the pressure barrier in the lower esophageal sphincter. Thus, reflux could occur under these circumstances during transient arousals from sleep associated with positional change, coughing, or swallowing.

The upper esophageal sphincter, created primarily by the cricopharyngeal muscle, serves as an additional protective barrier to prevent the aspiration of noxious material into the lungs. The upper esophageal sphincter is tonically contracted, and a pressure of between 40 and 80 mm Hg usually exists within this sphincter. Swallowing induces a reflex relaxation to allow the positioning of food and liquids in the upper esophagus, where the normal peristaltic mechanism transports these materials into the stomach. The tonic contraction of the upper esophageal sphincter therefore prevents the ingestion of material into the esophagus with a previous volitional swallow. A study[47] has documented relatively little change in the functioning of the upper esophageal sphincter during sleep, including REM sleep. Only a modest decline in the resting pressure was noted. This observation is somewhat surprising, because the cricopharyngeal muscle is a skeletal muscle, and if this finding can be verified, it would be one of the few skeletal muscles in the body that does not show a substantial inhibition during REM sleep. Clearly, persisting tone in the upper esophageal sphincter during REM sleep is advantageous because it protects the lungs from the aspiration of gastric contents. It should be pointed out that the subjects slept relatively poorly during this study, and, before any particular importance is ascribed to these findings, they should be replicated.

INTESTINAL MOTILITY

The primary functions of the small and large intestine are transport and absorption. These functions are intimately related, in that, for example, rapid transit through the colon results in poor absorption and loose, watery stools, whereas slow transit results in increased water absorption, slow transit of fecal material to the rectum, and the clinical consequence of infrequent defecation and complaints of constipation. Alterations in the motor function of the lower bowel are evident from clinical phenomena, such as the occurrence of nocturnal diarrhea in diabetics and nocturnal fecal incontinence, which is commonly noted in patients with ileoanal anastomosis.[48]

The accessibility of GI tract motility to monitoring decreases with distance from the oral cavity. The earliest attempts at measurement were purely observational via fluoroscopic surveillance of the progress of food through the intestines of the cat.[49] Similar observational techniques were employed by subsequent investigators to describe the differences in intestinal motility during waking and sleep.[50,51] These individuals exteriorized a small section of dog intestine and determined via visual observation that motility was relatively unaffected by sleep. In 1926, a similar fluoroscopic observation of exteriorized human intestine was made.[52] In agreement with the animal studies, these observations reported no change in intestinal motility during sleep.

Prolonged monitoring of the large and small bowel by a variety of sophisticated techniques, including telemetry, implanted microelectrodes, and suction electrodes, has allowed a more comprehensive description of intestinal motor activity. On the basis of these studies, tonic activity in the stomach and small bowel has been described as a basic electrical rhythm and as a more phasic phenomenon, such as the *migrating motor complex* (MMC), which is a wave of intestinal contraction beginning in the stomach and proceeding through the colon. The MMC consists of a dependent pattern of interdigestive motor phenomena. Subsequent to food ingestion, there is an interval of motor quiescence termed phase I. This is followed by a period of somewhat random contractions throughout the small bowel, called phase II. Phase III describes a coordinated peristaltic burst of contractile activity that proceeds distally throughout the small bowel. Food ingestion establishes a pattern of vigorous contraction throughout the distal stomach and small bowel. If no food enters the stomach, the MMC cycle has a period of about 90 minutes.[53]

In a more recent study, the activity of the MMC after a meal was assessed during waking and during subsequent sleep.[53] In addition, these authors assessed the behavior of a variety of regulatory peptides. They concluded that postprandial intestinal motor activity was substantially altered by sleep, primarily a reduction in the "fed" pattern of intestinal motility. Because there was little appreciable alteration in peptide levels, the authors concluded that the alteration in small bowel motility was most likely neurally mediated. They noted that responses were similar to those described after vagotomy in the waking state. This suggests that reduced levels of arousal result in diminished vagal modulation of the ENS.

In a study describing jejunal motor activity in 20 healthy subjects during sleeping and waking, no differences were found in the incidence of motor complexes.[54] In another study, it was found that sleep prolonged the interval between motor complexes in the small intestine.[55] A subsequent study revealed a sleep-related diminution in the number of contractions of a specific type in the jejunum.[56] These changes were seen in vagotomized patients with DU as well as in healthy subjects, which suggests that this phenomenon is independent of vagal control and unaffected by duodenal disease. The alteration of the MMC during sleep has been investigated.[57] Results showed a statistically significant relationship between REM sleep and the onset of MMCs originating in the duodenum.[57] A circadian rhythm in the propagation of the MMC, with the slowest velocities occurring during sleep, has been reported.[58] This finding appears to be the effect of a circadian rhythm rather than a true modulation by sleep. These results have been confirmed in a study that also noted that the esophageal involvement in the MMC was decreased during sleep, with a corresponding tendency for MMCs to originate in the jejunum at night.[59] In a study that examined the relationship between the MMC cycle and REM sleep, it was found that during sleep, there was a significant reduction in the MMC cycle length and in the duration of phase II of the MMC.[60] The MMCs were distributed equally between REM and NREM sleep, with no obvious alteration in the parameters of the MMC by sleep stage. These data give evidence of alteration in periodic activity in the gut during sleep, but they are also consistent with the notion that the two cycles (i.e., MMCs and REM sleep) are independent. The same group of investigators examined how the presence or absence of food in the GI tract alters small bowel motility during sleep.[61] A late evening meal restored phase II activity of the MMC, which is normally absent during sleep. These MMC changes during the sleeping interval have been substantially confirmed by subsequent ambulatory studies but without the benefit of PSG.[62,63]

Sleep, intestinal motility, and symptoms of abdominal pain have been studied in patients with irritable bowel syndrome. Striking differences between sleeping and waking small bowel motor activity have been described.[64] The marked increase in contractility seen in the daytime is notably absent during sleep. In a related study, it has also been noted that propulsive clusters of small bowel motility were somewhat enhanced in the daytime in patients with irritable bowel syndrome, and this distinguished them from controls.[65] Patients often had pain associated with these propulsive contractions, but there was no difference in small bowel activity during sleep between patients with irritable bowel syndrome and controls. Interestingly, an increase in REM sleep in patients with irritable bowel syndrome has been documented.[66] These authors proposed that this is evidence of a CNS abnormality in patients with this complex, enigmatic disorder.

With the development of more sophisticated electronic measuring and recording techniques, more accurate measures of intestinal motility have been possible in both animals and humans. Unfortunately, these studies have produced results that conflict with those noted earlier from direct observation. Decreases in small intestinal motility during sleep were reported in two separate studies conducted 20 years apart.[67,68] Specific duodenal recordings in humans have been conflicting, showing no change in one instance and an increase in duodenal motility during sleep in another.[22,69]

A different approach to duodenal recording recorded duodenal electromyographic (EMG) activity during various stages of sleep.[70] This study describes an inhibition of duodenal EMG activity during REM sleep and an increase in activity with changes from one sleep phase to another. In a subsequent study, a decrease in duodenal EMG activity during sleep was described by the same group.[71] An activity rhythm of 80 to 120 minutes per cycle that was impervious to the changes associated with the sleep–waking cycle was also noted.

EFFECT OF INTESTINAL MOTILITY ON SLEEP

Although this chapter has concentrated on the effects of sleep on GI motility, some fascinating studies have addressed the issue of how intestinal motility may affect sleep (see Chapter 107). A practical and provocative thought concerning this issue relates to the familiar experience of postprandial somnolence. There is some question about whether it actually exists. Could changes in the GI system with food ingestion produce a hypnotic effect? An intriguing observation was made in 1920 by Alverez,[72] who noted that distention of a jejunal balloon caused his human subject to drop off to sleep. The hypnotic effects of afferent intestinal stimulation have also been documented in animal studies. As an example, cortical synchronization has been observed in cats induced by both mechanical and electrical stimulation of the small bowel.[73] These results were interpreted to be the effect of rapidly adapting phasic afferent fibers from the small intestine carried to the CNS via the splanchnic nerve. These data strongly suggest the existence of a hypnogenic effect of luminal distention.

In a subsequent study, these same investigators reported an increase in the duration of slow wave sleep and an increase in the number of episodes of paradoxical sleep in cats subjected to low-level intestinal stimulation.[74] The possible hypnogenic role of intestinal hormones such as cholecystokinin was discussed. A study in which administration of intestinal hormones produced a pronounced increase in paradoxical sleep episodes provides support for this hypothesis.[75] The final common pathway of the afferent stimulation from the intestinal tract would presumably result in an increase in sleepiness subsequent to either luminal distention or hormonal secretion postprandially. In a fascinating study concerning neuronal processing during sleep, it was shown that neurons in the visual cortex, which usually respond to visual stimulation in the waking state, are activated during sleep by electrical stimulation of the stomach and small bowel.[76]

In an attempt to document the presence of postprandial sleepiness objectively, a study was undertaken to measure sleep onset latency both with and without a prior meal.[77] Statistically, the results of this test did not support the presence of postprandial sleepiness in 16 healthy volunteers. However, it was clear from these results that there was a small group of individuals in whom there was a substantial decrease in the sleep onset latency after ingestion of a meal. This phenomenon seems to be affected by many variables: the volume of the meal, the meal constituents, and the circadian cycle of the individual. A follow-up study tested the hypothesis that afferent stimulation from the gastric antrum would enhance postprandial sleepiness.[78] This was tested by comparing three conditions: a solid meal and a liquid meal of equal calories, and an equal distention of the stomach accomplished with water. Sleep onset latency was determined subsequent to each of these conditions. Because antral stimulation results from the digestion of a solid meal, sleep onset latency should be shorter after consumption of the solid meal, and this was confirmed: the sleep onset latency after the solid meal was significantly shorter than the equal-volume water condition. These results are compatible with the animal studies cited earlier and lend further support to the notion that contraction of the lumen of the GI tract produces afferent stimulation, which induces drowsiness.

COLONIC AND ANORECTAL FUNCTION

As noted, the colon has two main functions: transport and absorption. It is the motor activity of the colon that determines the rate of transport and, therefore, indirectly, the rate of absorption from the colonic lumen. Thus, alterations in colonic motility have significant consequences in terms of transit through the colon and water absorption, and ultimately clinical consequences such as constipation and diarrhea.

A decrease in colonic function during sleep has been reported.[79] These results have been confirmed by two other studies that included measurements of the transverse, descending, and sigmoid colon.[80,81] In one of these studies, a clear inhibition of colonic motility index is evident during sleep in the transverse, descending, and sigmoid colon segments, with a marked increase in activity on awakening.[81] Certainly, this explains the common urge to defecate on awakening in the morning. Neither of these studies attempted to document sleep with standard PSG. However, in a study that measured colonic activity from cecum to rectum continuously for 32 hours, a rather marked decrease in colonic motor activity during sleep was reported.[82] This study also described an interesting abolition in propagating waves during slow wave sleep. During REM sleep, the frequency of propagating events rose substantially. Other studies do not provide evidence for any significant change in colonic motility or variability in the rectosigmoid colon during sleep.[83,84] However, a study of colonic myoelectrical activity in humans suggested a decrease in spike activity during sleep.[85] Again, this study does not determine whether the results are accounted for on the basis of true physiologic sleep or simply reflect a circadian variation in colonic activity independent of sleep.

Collectively, these studies suggest an inhibition of colonic contractile and myoelectric activity during sleep, and other studies have documented the fact that there is diminished colonic tone during sleep.[86] Resumption of the waking state, and consequently increased CNS arousal, suggest two different effects on colonic motility. First, it appears that spontaneous awakening does induce high-amplitude peristaltic contractions, and this appears to be somewhat different than colonic motor activity induced by a sudden awakening from sleep. In another investigation, sudden awakening from sleep induced a pattern of segmental colonic contractions, rather than the propagating high-amplitude peristaltic contractions noted in previous studies.[87] These data are of considerable interest in that they demonstrate not only the influence of higher cortical functions on colonic motility but also the fact that these functions can affect the colon in rather subtle ways in terms of the induction of different patterns of colonic motility.

The striated muscle of the anal canal was evaluated during sleep in a 1953 study that included EEG documentation of sleep.[88] These investigators described a marked reduction in EMG activity during sleep. They concluded that this muscle is under voluntary control. In another study, anal canal pressure was measured continuously during sleep (but without PSG monitoring).[89] The results indicated a decrease in the minute-to-minute variation and the amplitude of spontaneous decreases in anal canal pressure during sleep. These results have been largely confirmed in a study involving the ambulatory monitoring of anorectal activity.[90] A decrease in anal canal resting pressure during sleep and alterations in rectal motor complexes were described and noted to be similar in waking and sleep in the mid-rectum. However, in the distal rectum, this motor pattern was found to be more prevalent during sleep. They also noted that during sleep, the anal canal resting pressure exceeded that of the rectal pressure, which would seem to be important in maintaining rectal continence during sleep. The structures of the rectum and anal canal are vital in maintaining normal bowel continence and ensuring normal defecation. In general, normal defecation is associated with sensory responses to rectal distention and appropriate motor responses of the muscles of the anal canal. These responses include a contraction of the external anal sphincter and a transient decrease in the internal anal sphincter pressure associated with rectal distention. It is thought that the high resting basal pressure in the internal anal sphincter of the anal canal and the response of the external anal sphincter to rectal distention are critical in maintaining continence.

To assess the effect of sleep on these anorectal sensorimotor responses, 10 healthy volunteers were studied during sleep with an anorectal probe in place.[91] This probe permits the transient distention of the rectum via a rectal balloon while the responses of the internal and external anal sphincters can be simultaneously monitored. This study documented a marked decrease—and, in most subjects, an abolition—of the external anal sphincter response to rectal distention. The internal anal sphincter response remained unaltered. In addition, there was no evidence of an arousal response with up to 50 mL of rectal distention during sleep. The normal threshold of response in the waking state is approximately 10 mL. These results confirm that the external anal sphincter response to rectal distention is most likely a learned response, whereas the internal anal sphincter response is clearly a reflex response to rectal distention because it persists during sleep.

The results also raise certain clinical questions with regard to the phenomenon of nocturnal diarrhea and the maintenance of fecal continence during sleep. In an ambulatory study of anorectal functioning, it was demonstrated that external anal sphincter contractions occurred periodically during sleep, and these periodic bursts of activity were followed by motor quiescence.[92] These spontaneous contractions were associated with a rise in the anal canal pressure, but internal anal sphincter contractions were shown to occur independently of external anal sphincter activity.[92] The *sampling reflex*, which is a spontaneous relaxation of the internal anal sphincter, occurred frequently in the waking state but was markedly reduced during sleep.

A more recent study has shed light on intrinsic anal–rectal functioning, which is altered during sleep.[3] The authors confirmed the presence of an endogenous oscillation in rectal motor activity, and they specifically noted that these bursts of cyclic rectal motor activity occupied approximately 44% of the overall recording time at night. They described the incidence of this motor activity to be nearly twofold greater at night than during the daytime. Of particular importance is the finding that the majority of contractions were propagated in a retrograde direction. Other studies have shown that rectal motor activity is not altered by REM sleep,[89] and still others that anal canal pressure is decreased during sleep.[93,94] Of particular interest is the fact that even though there was a diminution in anal canal pressure during sleep, anal canal pressure was always greater than rectal pressure, even in the presence of cyclic rectal motor activity.[92]

These studies collectively shed important light on the mechanisms of rectal continence during sleep. There appear to be at least two mechanisms that prevent the passive escape of rectal contents during sleep. First, rectal motor activity increases substantially during sleep, but the propagation is retrograde rather than anterograde. Furthermore, these physiologic studies have shown that, even under the circumstances of periodic rectal contractions, the anal canal pressure is consistently above that of the rectum. Both of these mechanisms would tend to protect against rectal leakage during sleep, and alterations in these mechanisms would explain loss of rectal continence during sleep in individuals with diabetes or who have undergone ileal–anal anastomosis.

CONCLUSIONS

This chapter has described a variety of basic findings concerning the GI system and sleep. It is evident that there are marked alterations in the GI system during sleep, and these have numerous consequences in normal digestive processes as well as in digestive disease (reviewed in Chapter 107). Our understanding of the modulation of GI function by sleep has

increased, and this has occurred in concert with substantially more sophisticated techniques for the measurement of smooth muscle functioning. Clearly, the past 50 years have shown a marked increase in interest in sleep and GI physiology, and this will undoubtedly continue as the importance of sleep physiology and pathophysiology is further revealed.

Clinical Pearl

Understanding gastrointestinal physiology during sleep allows a more complete description of basic intestinal functioning, and it provides a more thorough understanding of the pathogenesis of gastrointestinal disease. Alterations in the secretion of saliva in response to acid mucosal contact during sleep and the marked suppression in swallowing during sleep both lead to a prolongation in the neutralization of refluxed gastric contents that may occur during sleep. This results in an increase in hydrogen ion–backed diffusion and ultimate tissue damage. The state of sleep also facilitates the proximal migration of refluxed gastric contents, which increases the risk of pulmonary aspiration. Delayed gastric emptying during sleep may also facilitate the occurrence of acid reflux and delay intestinal transit and absorption. The alteration in intestinal motility during sleep may also contribute to delayed intestinal transit and absorption during sleep. The decrease in resting anal canal pressure during sleep creates a high risk of incontinence during sleep, but this appears to be prevented by retrograde rectal propulsions, which have been noted exclusively during sleep. Awareness of these alterations in basic physiologic functioning during sleep should enhance the clinician's ability to diagnose and treat gastrointestinal disease.

REFERENCES

1. Champion MC, Orr WC (eds): Evolving Concepts in Gastrointestinal Motility. Oxford, England, Blackwell Science, 1996.
2. Orr WC, Johnson LF, Robinson MG: The effect of sleep on swallowing, esophageal peristalsis, and acid clearance. Gastroenterology 1984;86:814-819.
3. Rao SS, Welcher K: Periodic rectal motor activity: The intrinsic colonic gatekeeper? Am J Gastroenterol 1996;91:890-897.
4. Friedenwald J: On the influence of rest, exercise and sleep on gastric digestion. Am J Med 1906;1:249-255.
5. Johnson RL, Washeim H: Studies in gastric secretion. Am J Physiol 1924;70:247-253.
6. Henning N, Norpoth L: Die Magensekretion waehrend des Schlafes. Dtsch Arch Klin Med 1932;172:558-562.
7. Banche M: La secrezione gastric notturna durante il sonno. Minerva Med 1950;1:428-434.
8. Luckhardt AB: Contributions to the physiology of the empty stomach. Am J Physiol 1915;39:330-333.
9. Wada T: Experimental study of hunger in its relation to activity. Arch Psychol 1922;8:1-65.
10. Sandweiss DJ, Friedman HF, Sugarman MH, et al: Nocturnal gastric secretion. Gastroenterology 1946;1:38-54.
11. Moore JG, Englert E: Circadian rhythm of gastric acid secretion in man. Nature 1970;226:1261-1262.
12. Levin E, Kirsner JB, Palmer WL, et al: A comparison of the nocturnal gastric secretion in patients with duodenal ulcer and in normal individuals. Gastroenterology 1948;10:952-964.
13. Feldman M, Richardson CT: Total 24-hour gastric acid secretion in patients with duodenal ulcer: Comparison with normal

subjects and effects of cimetidine and parietal cell vagotomy. Gastroenterology 1986;90:540-544.

14. Levin E, Kirsner JB, Palmer WL, et al: The variability and periodicity of the nocturnal gastric secretion in normal individuals. Gastroenterology 1948;10:939-951.

15. Dragstedt LR: A concept of the etiology of gastric and duodenal ulcers. Gastroenterology 1956;30:208-220.

16. Reichsman F, Cohen J, Colwill J, et al: Natural and histamine-induced gastric secretion during waking and sleeping states. Psychosom Med 1960;1:14-24.

17. Armstrong RH, Burnap D, Jacobson A, et al: Dreams and acid secretions in duodenal ulcer patients. N Physician 1965;33:241-243.

18. Stacher G, Presslich B, Starker H: Gastric acid secretion and sleep stages during natural night sleep. Gastroenterology 1975;68:1449-1455.

19. Orr WC, Hall WH, Stahl ML, et al: Sleep patterns and gastric acid secretion in duodenal ulcer disease. Arch Intern Med 1976;136:655-660.

20. Dubois A, Castell DO: Abnormal gastric emptying response to pentagastrin in duodenal ulcer disease. Dig Dis Sci 1981;26:292.

21. Scantlebury RE, Frick HL, Patterson TL: The effect of normal and hypnotically induced dreams on the gastric hunger movements of man. J Appl Physiol 1942;26:682-691.

22. Bloom PB, Ross DL, Stunkard AJ, et al: Gastric and duodenal motility, food intake and hunger measured in man during a 24-hour period. Dig Dis Sci 1970;15:719-725.

23. Baust W, Rohrwasser W: Das Verhalten von pH und Motilitat des Megens in naturlichen Schlaf des Menschen. Pflugers Arch 1969;305:229-240.

24. Yaryura-Tobias HA, Hutcheson JS, White L: Relationship between stages of sleep and gastric motility. Behav Neuropsychiatry 1970;2:22-24.

25. Fujitani Y, Hosogai M: Circadian rhythm of electrical activity and motility of the stomach in cats and their relation to sleep-wakefulness states. Tohoku J Exp Med 1983;141:275-285.

26. Hall WH, Orr WC, Stahl ML: Gastric function during sleep. In Brooks FP, Evers PW (eds): Nerves and the Gut. Thorofare, NJ, Slack, 1977, pp 495-502.

27. Dubois A, Van Eerdewegh P, Gardner JD: Gastric emptying and secretion in Zollinger-Ellison syndrome. J Clin Invest 1977;59:255.

28. Orr WC, Dubois A, Stahl ML: Gastric function during sleep. Sleep Res 1978;7:72.

29. Goo RH, Moore JG, Greenburg E, et al: Circadian variation in gastric emptying of meals in humans. Gastroenterology 1987;93:515-518.

30. Chen JZ, McCallum RW, Familoni BO: Validity of the cutaneous electrogastrogram. In Chen JZ, McCallum RW (eds): Electrogastrography: Principles and Applications. New York, Raven Press, 1994, pp 103-125.

31. Chen JZ, McCallum RW, Smout AJPM, et al: Acquisition and analysis of electrogastrographic data. In Chen JZ, McCallum RW (eds): Electrogastrography: Principles and Applications. New York, Raven Press, 1994, pp 3-30.

32. Chen JZ, McCallum RW, Lin Z: Comparison of three running spectral analysis methods. In Chen JZ, McCallum RW (eds): Electrogastrography: Principles and Applications. New York, Raven Press, 1994, pp 75-99.

33. Orr WC, Crowell MD, Lin B, et al: Sleep and gastric function in irritable bowel syndrome: Derailing the brain-gut axis. Gut 1997;41:20.

34. Elsenbruch S, Harnish MJ, Orr WC, et al: Disruption of normal gastric myoelectric functioning by sleep. Sleep 1999;22:453-458.

35. Johnson LF, DeMeester TR: Twenty-four-hour pH monitoring of the distal esophagus: A quantitative measure of gastroesophageal reflux. Am J Gastroenterol 1974;62:325-332.

36. DeMeester TR, Johnson LF, Joseph CJ, et al: Patterns of gastroesophageal reflux in health and disease. Ann Surg 1976;184:459-470.

37. Orr WC, Robinson MG, Johnson LF: Acid clearing during sleep in patients with esophagitis and controls. Dig Dis Sci 1981;26:423.

38. Helm JF, Dodds WJ, Hogan WJ, et al: Acid neutralizing capacity of human saliva. Gastroenterology 1982;83:69-74.

39. Schneyer LH, Pigman W, Hanahan L, et al: Rate of flow of human parotid, sublingual, and submaxillary secretions during sleep. J Dent Res 1956;35:109-114.

40. Lear CSC, Flanagan JB Jr, Moorees CFA: The frequency of deglutition in man. Arch Oral Biol 1965;10:83-96.

41. Lichter J, Muir RC: The pattern of swallowing during sleep. Electroencephalogr Clin Neurophysiol 1975;38:427-432.

42. Dent J, Dodds WJ, Friedman RH, et al: Mechanism of gastroesophageal reflux in recumbent asymptomatic human subjects. J Clin Invest 1980;65:256-257.

43. Anderson CA, Dick TE, Orem J: Swallowing in sleep and wakefulness in adult cats. Sleep 1995;18:325-329.

44. Castiglione F, Emde C, Armstrong D, et al: Nocturnal oesophageal motor activity is dependent on sleep stage. Gut 1993;34:1653-1659.

45. Armstrong D, Emde C, Bumm R, et al: Twenty-four-hour pattern of esophageal motility in asymptomatic volunteers. Dig Dis Sci 1990;35:1659.

46. Smout AJPM, Breedijk M, van der Zouw C, et al: Physiological gastroesophageal reflux and esophageal motor activity studied with a new system for 24-hour recording and automated analysis. Dig Dis Sci 1989;34:1659.

47. Kahrilas PJ, Dodds WJ, Dent J, et al: Effect of sleep, spontaneous gastroesophageal reflux, and a meal on upper esophageal sphincter pressure in normal human volunteers. Gastroenterology 1987;92:466-467.

48. Metcalf AM, Dozois RR, Kelly KA, et al: Ileal J pouch-anal anastomosis: Clinical outcome. Ann Surg 1985;202:735-739.

49. Cannon WB: The movements of the intestine studied by means of the roentgen rays. Am J Physiol 1902;6:275-276.

50. Barcroft J, Robinson CS: A study of some factors influencing intestinal movements. Am J Physiol 1929;67:211-220.

51. Douglas DM, Mann FG: An experimental study of the rhythmic contractions in the small intestine of the dog. Am J Dig Dis 1977;6:318-322.

52. Hines LE, Mead HCA: Peristalsis in a loop of small intestine. Arch Intern Med 1926;38:539.

53. Soffer EE, Adrian TE, Launspach J, et al: Meal-induced secretion of gastrointestinal regulatory peptides is not affected by sleep. Neurogastroenterol Motil 1997;9:7-12.

54. Archer L, Benson MJ, Green WJ, et al: Radiotelemetric measurement of normal human small bowel motor activity during prolonged fasting. J Physiol 1979;296:53.

55. Thompson DG, Wingate DL: Characterisation of interdigestive and digestive motor activity in the normal human jejunum. Gut 1979;20:A943.

56. Ritchie HD, Thompson DG, Wingate DL: Diurnal variation in human jejunal fasting motor activity. In Proceedings of the American Physiological Society, March 1980, pp 54-55.

57. Finch P, Ingram D, Henstridge J, et al: The relationship of sleep stage to the migrating gastrointestinal complex of man. In Christensen J (ed): Gastrointestinal Motility. New York, Raven Press, 1980, pp 261-265.

58. Kumar D, Wingate D, Ruckebusch Y: Circadian variation in the propagation velocity of the migrating motor complex. Gastroenterology 1986;91:926-930.

59. Kellow JE, Borody TJ, Phillips SF, et al: Human interdigestive motility: Variations in patterns from esophagus to colon. Gastroenterology 1986;91:386-395.

60. Kumar D, Idzikowski C, Wingate DL, et al: Relationship between enteric migrating motor complex and the sleep cycle. Am J Physiol 1990;259(Pt 1):G983-G940.

61. Kumar D, Soffer EE, Wingate DL, et al: Modulation of the duration of human postprandial motor activity by sleep. Am J Physiol 1989;256(Pt 1):G851-G855.

62. Wilson P, Perdikis G, Hinder RA, et al: Prolonged ambulatory antroduodenal manometry in humans. Am J Gastroenterol 1994;89:1489-1495.

63. Wilmer A, Andrioli A, Coremans G, et al: Ambulatory small intestinal manometry: Detailed comparison of duodenal and jejunal motor activity in healthy man. Dig Dis Sci 1997;42:1618-1627.

64. Kellow JE, Gill RC, Wingate DL: Prolonged ambulant recordings of small bowel motility demonstrate abnormalities in the irritable bowel syndrome. Gastroenterology 1990;98:1208-1218.

65. Kellow JE, Phillips SF: Altered small bowel motility in irritable bowel syndrome is correlated with symptoms. Gastroenterology 1987;92:1885-1893.

66. Kumar D, Thompson PD, Wingate DL, et al: Abnormal REM sleep in the irritable bowel syndrome. Gastroenterology 1992;103:12-17.

67. Helm JD, Kramer P, MacDonald RM, et al: Changes in motility of the human small intestine during sleep. Gastroenterology 1948;10:135-137.

68. Sadler HH, Orten AU: The complementary relationship between the emotional state and the function of the ileum in a human subject. Am J Psychiatry 1968;124:1377-1381.

69. Bloom PB, Ross DL, Stunkard AJ. et al: Gastric and duodenal motility, food intake and hunger measured in man during a 24-hour period. Dig Dis Sci 1970;15:719-725.

70. Spire JP, Tassinari CA: Duodenal EMG activity during sleep. Electroencephalogr Clin Neurophysiol 1971;31:179-183.

71. Tassinari CA, Coccagna G, Mantovani M, et al: Duodenal EMG activity during sleep in man. In Jovanovic UJ (ed): The Nature of Sleep. Stuttgart, Germany, Gustav Fischer Verlag, 1973.

72. Alverez WC: Physiologic studies on the motor activities of the stomach and bowel in man. Am J Physiol 1920;88:658-660.

73. Kukorelli T, Juhasz G: Sleep induced by intestinal stimulation in cats. Physiol Behav 1976;19:355-358.

74. Juhasz G, Kukorelli T: Modifications of visceral evoked potentials during sleep in cats. Act Nerv Super (Praha) 1977;19:212-214.

75. Rubenstein EH, Sonnenschein RR: Sleep cycles and feeding behavior in the cat: Role of gastrointestinal hormones. Acta Cient Venez 1971;22:125-128.

76. Pigarev IN: Neurons of visual cortex respond to visceral stimulation during slow wave sleep. Neuroscience 1994;62:1237-1243.

77. Stahl ML, Orr WC, Bollinger C: Postprandial sleepiness: Objective documentation via polysomnography. Sleep 1983;6:29-35.

78. Orr WC, Shadid G, Harnish MJ, et al: Meal composition and its effect on postprandial sleepiness. Physiol Behav 1997;62:709-712.

79. Adler HF, Atkinson AJ, Ivy AC: A study of the motility of the human colon: An explanation of dyssynergia of the colon, or of the unstable colon. Am J Dig Dis 1941;8:197-202.

80. Rosenblum MJ, Cummins AJ: The effect of sleep and of Amytal on the motor activity of the human sigmoid colon. Gastroenterology 1954;27:445-450.

81. Narducci F, Bassotti G, Gaburri M, et al: Twenty four hour manometric recording of colonic motor activity in healthy man. Gut 1987;28:17-25.

82. Furukawa Y, Cook IJ, Panagopoulos V, et al: Relationship between sleep patterns and human colonic motor patterns. Gastroenterology 1994;107:1372-1381.

83. Kerlin P, Zinsmeister A, Phillips S: Motor responses to food of the ileum, proximal colon, and distal colon of healthy humans. Gastroenterology 1983;84:762-770.

84. Posey EL, Bargen JA: Observations of normal and abnormal human intestinal motor function. Am J Med Sci 1951;221:10-20.

85. Frexinos J, Bueno L, Fioramonti J: Diurnal changes in myoelectric spiking activity of the human colon. Gastroenterology 1985;88:1104-1110.

86. Steadman CJ, Phillips SF, Camilleri M, et al: Variations of muscle tone in the human colon. Gastroenterology 1991;101:24.

87. Bassotti G, Bucaneve G, Betti C, et al: Sudden awakening from sleep: Effects on proximal and distal colonic contractile activity in humans. Eur J Gastroenterol Hepatol 1990;2:6.

88. Floyd WF, Walls EW: Electromyography of the sphincter and externus in man. J Physiol 1953;122:599-609.

89. Orkin BA, Hanson RB, Kelly KA, et al: Human anal motility while fasting, after feeding, and during sleep. Gastroenterology 1991;100:1016-1023.

90. Ronholt C, Rasmussen O, Christiansen J: Ambulatory manometric recording of anorectal activity. Dis Colon Rectum 1999;12:1551-1559.

91. Whitehead WE, Orr WC, Engel BT, et al: External anal sphincter response to rectal distention: Learned response or reflex. Psychophysiology 1981;19:57-62.

92. Kumar D, Waldron D, Williams NS, et al: Prolonged anorectal manometry and external anal sphincter electromyography in ambulant human subjects. Dig Dis Sci 1990;35:641-648.

93. Ferrara A, Pemberton JH, Levin KE, et al: Relationship between anal canal tone and rectal motor activity. Dis Colon Rectum 1993;36:337-342.

94. Enck P, Eggers E, Koletzko S, et al: Spontaneous variation of anal "resting" pressure in healthy humans. Am J Physiol 1991;261:G823-G826.

24

Temperature, Thermoregulation, and Sleep

H. Craig Heller

ABSTRACT

The properties of the autonomic thermoregulatory system vary with vigilance states and with time of day. Both human and animal studies have shown sleep-related and circadian changes in body temperatures and thermoregulatory responses. In addition, animal studies have revealed the underlying changes in feedback sensitivity of the central nervous thermoregulatory system that accompany changes in vigilance states and circadian phase.

Body temperature is regulated at a lower level during NREM sleep than during waking, and thermoregulation is inhibited during REM sleep. The circadian system influences thermoregulation independent of sleep and waking as well as through the timing of sleep. Thus, the regulation of body temperature is modulated by the circadian system and by sleep-control mechanisms. Conversely, body temperature and ambient temperature have strong influences on sleep expression and sleep architecture. Nonthermoneutral ambient temperatures disrupt sleep expression and especially REM sleep. Even within thermoneutrality, REM sleep is maximal at the upper end of the thermoneutral range. Core body temperatures above and below normal also disrupt sleep. If core and peripheral temperatures are manipulated in opposite directions, NREM sleep is seen to be a function of autonomic thermoregulatory drive, and REM sleep is a function of peripheral temperature regardless of thermoregulatory status of the animal, which probably reflects conscious sensation.

Although several hypotheses about sleep function involving thermoregulation have been advanced, none are supported by convincing evidence. Mammalian hibernation, however, is probably a clear example of natural selection favoring the downregulation of body temperature during NREM sleep as an adaptation for energy conservation. The relationships between sleep and thermoregulatory homeostasis have important implications for a variety of clinical problems ranging from sudden infant death syndrome to sleep disorders associated with the uncoupling of normally phase-linked circadian rhythms of sleep and body temperature.

This chapter is a review of the evidence of several features of temperature regulation in sleep. First, the decline in metabolic rate (MR) and body temperature (T_b) at the onset of sleep are not simply due to decreased motor and digestive activity but also are due to regulated lowering of metabolism or T_b, or both. Second, daily cycles of MR and T_b are caused by the separate but additive influences of circadian and sleep control systems on thermoregulation. Third, the effects of rapid eye movement (REM) and non-REM (NREM) sleep on thermoregulation are qualitatively different: NREM sleep is associated with a changed level of regulation and REM sleep is associated with an inhibition of regulation. Fourth, body temperature and ambient temperature have profound effects on arousal-state expression.

I shall focus on human studies wherever possible to address these issues; to review what is known about the relationship among temperature, temperature regulation, and arousal state control; and to discuss directions for further research and clinical applications in these areas. However, most of our insights into physiological mechanisms underlying the relationships between temperature and sleep come from animal studies, which therefore constitute an important body of information in this field. These topics have been covered in previous, extensive reviews.[1-5]

METABOLISM DECREASES DURING SLEEP RELATIVE TO WAKEFULNESS

The decline in MR during sleep cannot be simply a consequence of decreased motor and digestive activity because it occurs in fasted subjects, in patients on total bedrest, and even in paralyzed humans.[2] Also, the daily decline in MR cannot be due entirely to sleep because it occurs in subjects deprived of sleep.[6-8] Clearly, both sleep and circadian factors influence MR.

In humans, the mean drop in metabolism reported in different studies between wakefulness and the sleep minima is on the order of 5% to 17%[9-11]; however, there is considerable intersubject variability in these studies. Moreover, metabolic differences between waking and sleep increase at ambient temperatures (T_a) below thermoneutrality.[3] For example, Palca and coworkers reported a 40% drop in oxygen consumption during sleep in a naked subject at an ambient temperature of 21° C.[10] The reduction in regulated T_b is less likely to be reflected in a decrease in MR when the animal or human is under thermoneutral conditions.

Data on MR in sleeping humans as a function of arousal state are distinctly different from those of animal studies. The pioneering study of Brebbia and Altshuler[12] showed higher metabolism in REM sleep than in NREM sleep stages 3 and 4. This result has been confirmed,[10,13] but other studies have revealed no difference in MR when comparing REM-sleep and NREM-sleep episodes.[9,11,14] Studies that address this question must take into account circadian effects on MR when comparing MR in different sleep states. For example, in one study[10] MR in REM sleep was significantly higher than in NREM sleep when contiguous episodes were analyzed, but there was no significant difference between REM sleep and NREM sleep when data across the entire night were pooled. Another critical variable is T_a; there is a tendency for the difference between MRs measured in REM sleep and NREM sleep to be greater at lower T_a.[13]

Therefore, in adult humans, MR either shows no change or is elevated in REM sleep compared with NREM sleep.

In contrast, results from animal studies show a clear *decrease* in metabolic rate in REM sleep compared with NREM sleep. A possible explanation for the human-nonhuman difference in direction of MR change is the large contribution of brain metabolism to total MR in humans and the increase in cerebral blood flow and brain metabolism in humans during REM sleep.[15,16]

This explanation is supported in part by imaging techniques that have been used to measure brain metabolism and cerebral blood flow in animals and humans. Ramm and Frost[17] showed in cats significantly lowered levels of mean cerebral metabolism during NREM sleep, but they found no clear link between mean cerebral metabolism and REM sleep. In humans, both cerebral metabolic studies and cerebral blood flow studies[18] show a decided decrease in cerebral blood flow and metabolism during NREM sleep. The transition from NREM to REM sleep was marked by a global increase in cerebral blood flow[18] and areas of marked increase in metabolism.[19,20] Given these results and the significantly longer REM and NREM episodes in humans as compared to animals, it is possible that increases in brain metabolism during REM sleep contribute significantly to the increases in whole-body metabolism seen in humans when comparing REM sleep to NREM sleep.

THERMOREGULATORY RESPONSES DEPEND ON SLEEP STATE

Even before the use of electroencephalography, changes in T_b and thermoregulatory responses at sleep onset in humans suggested that T_b is actively regulated at a lower level in sleep than during wakefulness. Day's observation[21] that declines in rectal temperatures of napping children coincided with increased evaporative water loss and elevated skin temperatures at sleep onset provided strong evidence of a readjustment of the thermoregulatory system coincident with sleep. Decreases in rectal temperature or increases in skin temperature have been reported routinely at the onset of sleep in adult humans sleeping in neutral or cool environments.[22,23] In neutral or warm environments, an increase in sweat rate has been observed at sleep onset.[24,25] Studies on humans and animals in which sleep and wakefulness were measured with standard electrophysiological montages have extended earlier observations on the changes in thermoregulatory control during NREM sleep, compared to wakefulness, and have produced evidence that thermoregulation is disturbed during REM sleep.

It is commonly observed in animal studies that brain temperature (T_{br}) falls during NREM sleep compared to wakefulness, but it increases in REM sleep relative to NREM sleep (see Heller and Glotzbach[2] and Parmeggiani[26] for extensive reviews). Changes in T_{br} can be influenced by changes in the temperature of the blood perfusing the brain, changes in cerebral blood flow, and changes in cerebral metabolism. The temperature of the perfusing blood is affected by systemic changes in thermoregulatory responses, and the cerebral blood flow is affected by systemic changes in blood pressure, which in turn reflect thermoregulatory changes in peripheral vasomotor activity.

An extensive series of studies of these relationships by Parmeggiani and colleagues has produced general conclusions[5] that explain the diverse observations on sleep-related changes in brain temperature of mammals sleeping under different conditions. The T_{br} changes associated with the transition from waking to NREM sleep are always compatible with a downregulation of body temperature; however, the T_{br} changes that occur during the transitions from NREM to REM sleep reflect a relaxation or inhibition of whatever thermoregulatory responses had been active during the preceding NREM sleep episode. Thus, the direction of change in blood flow depends solely on the prevailing vasomotor state in NREM sleep prior to the transition.[27] Vasodilated vascular beds show decreased blood flow and constricted beds show increased flow in REM sleep compared to NREM sleep. In further support of the concept that vasomotor state reflects thermoregulatory status in NREM sleep but not in REM sleep, the intensity of the tonic vasoconstrictor sympathetic outflow to heat exchange vascular beds in cats was shown to be proportional to duration of NREM sleep episodes but showed no correlation to duration of REM sleep episodes.[28]

The contribution of neural activity to changes in cerebral metabolism is hard to assess. Increases in MR due to neuronal activity during REM sleep, for example, might be counteracted by the cooling effect of increased blood flow because carotid artery blood temperature is usually lower than brain temperature during REM sleep. Therefore, T_{br} rises during REM sleep despite an overall increase in cerebral blood flow; this has been interpreted as indirect evidence that cerebral heat production must be increasing in REM sleep.[29] There is another possibility, however. In both rabbits and cats, the transition from NREM to REM sleep has been shown to be accompanied by a decrease in carotid blood flow that is compensated for by an increase in blood flow through the vertebral artery.[27,30] The blood in the vertebral artery tends to be warmer than the blood in the carotid artery and might account for the rise in T_{br}.

Animal studies have demonstrated that thermoregulatory responses to changes in peripheral or core body temperatures are qualitatively different in NREM sleep compared to REM sleep. At high T_a, panting increases in cats and pigeons in NREM sleep compared with wakefulness, which suggests that the increase in heat loss in NREM sleep results from a decrease in the set point for heat loss responses at sleep onset.[31,32] In contrast, transitions from NREM sleep to REM sleep are characterized by a disruption of ongoing thermoregulation. Panting is inhibited in REM sleep,[26,33] although panting mechanisms continue to operate during REM sleep in cats at high T_a and the degree of panting is proportional to the heat load.[34] Shivering is present during NREM sleep at low T_a, but in REM sleep, ongoing shivering ceases.[7,33,35] In addition, the temperature of rat interscapular brown adipose tissue increases during cold exposure in NREM sleep, but it decreases in REM sleep.[36]

Thermoregulatory responses in humans are markedly inhibited during REM sleep. Shivering during sleep in cool environments is confined to NREM sleep stages 1 and 2 and is not seen in NREM sleep stages 3 or 4 or during REM sleep.[13,37] It is not known whether the thresholds for shivering are lowered during these latter stages or whether the stimulus to shiver is arousing, thus blocking those states. Evidence from skin and body temperature measurements in subjects selected for their ability to sleep in the cold has been interpreted as suggesting that some aspects of thermoregulatory control may remain intact during REM sleep.[10]

Disruption of thermal effector mechanisms in REM sleep is not limited to heat production; reduction of sweating during

REM sleep in subjects in neutral or warm ambient temperature indicates impairment of heat loss effector mechanisms as well.[38,39] The sharp declines in sweat rate associated with REM sleep often precede the onset of REM sleep by 2 to 3 minutes, which is consistent with the finding that some REM-sleep processes precede electrophysiologically defined REM sleep. Measurements of sweating from subjects at a warm T_a show that evaporative water loss declines sharply at the onset of REM sleep, reaches minimal levels in REM sleep, and rises sharply at the termination of REM sleep.[38,39] Cessation of sweating and increases in skin temperature were accompanied by elevations in rectal temperature of 0.2° C.[38] Evaporative water loss measured from sweat capsules placed on the chests of subjects sleeping in warm environments demonstrated a sleep-dependent change in evaporative water loss: Sweat rate was higher in NREM sleep stages 3 and 4 than in NREM sleep stages 1 and 2, and it was lowest in REM sleep.[40,41]

Buguet et al.[42] measured thermoregulatory adjustments during sleep in a patient with anhidrotic dysplasia, a congenital syndrome in which sweat glands are absent. Compared to a control subject, in whom sweating in a warm environment (32.2° C) decreased during REM sleep and T_b decreased during the night, the patient showed no sleep state–dependent change in evaporative water loss and had minimal changes in T_b. Although increased convective and radiative heat loss avenues were potentially available by virtue of a higher mean skin temperature, the patient exhibited disturbed sleep as indicated by increased wakefulness and stage 1 sleep, less REM sleep, and more state transitions compared to the control subject.

Although evaporative water loss reaches basal levels in REM sleep in subjects sleeping in a warm environment, increases in sweat rate occur during the phasic events of REM sleep, such as during bursts of rapid eye movements.[43] This finding raises the possibility that increases in evaporative water loss during REM sleep may be psychogenic (related to dream content) and not thermoregulatory. Alternatively, inhibition impinging on the thermoregulatory system may be released briefly during the phasic events of REM sleep. In addition, continuous measurements of chest sweat rates during sleep indicated that the inhibition of sweating gradually relaxed as the REM episode progressed.[39] Mean T_b was positively correlated with T_a in REM sleep (but not during stage 4 NREM sleep) during heat exposure, which indicates that changes in T_b occur passively in REM sleep in relation to the heat load.[44]

The studies cited in this discussion support the concept that thermoregulatory mechanisms are intact in NREM sleep and inhibited in REM sleep. However, results from numerous studies of changes in skin and body temperatures during REM sleep are extremely variable and do not always support this general conclusion. In evaluating these studies, it is necessary to remember that changes in blood pressure, blood flow, and peripheral vasomotor tone are under the influence of several systems interacting independently of or in concert with thermoregulation.[45] For example, skin temperature changes are influenced by heat transfer from the skin surface as well as convective and conductive transfer of heat to the surface from deeper tissues. The methods and sites of attaching thermistors and thermocouples to the skin and the amount of insulating covers are important variables that may affect experimental results.

AMBIENT AND BODY TEMPERATURES PROFOUNDLY INFLUENCE SLEEP STRUCTURE

Because thermoregulatory abilities differ with arousal state, one might expect thermal stress to elicit arousal or a shift in the distribution of sleep states. Indeed, environmental temperature has a prominent influence on both the amount and distribution of arousal states. Therefore, accurate comparisons of both interspecies and intraspecies sleep state distributions require information on the thermal environment *and* the thermal neutral zones of the subjects. Parmeggiani and colleagues[33,46] first showed in cats that total sleep time (TST) is maximum within the thermoneutral zone and decreases above and below the thermoneutral zone. Moreover, the NREM-sleep–to–REM-sleep ratio increases as T_a deviates from thermoneutrality, which is due primarily to a reduction in the number of epochs of REM sleep. These results have been subsequently confirmed and extended in several animal models.[47-49] Alfoldi et al.[49] found that the temperature effects on sleep were more prominent during the light phase compared with the dark phase of the diurnal cycle. These results underscore the importance of considering time-of-day effects on the relationship between temperature and sleep, which can be ascertained only by recordings that are substantially longer than a few hours.

REM sleep is influenced by peripheral temperature even within thermoneutrality. When both oxygen consumption and sleep distribution were measured in rats at T_a between 23° C and 33° C, NREM sleep did not vary in T_a between 23° C and 31° C, and MR was constant in T_a between 25° C and 31° C. However, the amount of REM sleep varied significantly in this range, peaking at a T_a of 29° C.[49a] A marked depression of REM sleep occurred at a T_a of 33° C. Previous work on rats showed a maximum REM-sleep propensity at a T_a closer to 33° C than to 29° C.[50,51] The reasons for these discrepancies are not clear, but they could be due to differences in heat tolerance, weight, or acclimation of the animals. Another important finding is that slow wave delta activity increases after relatively small elevations in ambient[52] and hypothalamic temperatures,[53] even when there is no significant change in the overall percentage of NREM sleep.

The studies just described were all conducted at a constant T_a, but acute changes in the thermal environment *during* NREM sleep can also influence the subsequent distribution of wakefulness and sleep. Rats sleeping at ambient temperatures above 34° C or below 23° C showed increased transitions into REM sleep if T_a was changed *toward* thermoneutrality during sleep; in contrast, if T_a was changed *away* from thermoneutrality, transitions into REM sleep were fewer and transitions to wakefulness increased, compared with control rats sleeping at a T_a of 29° C.[54]

The influence of T_a on sleep-state distribution has been studied in humans.[10,37,55,56] In a cold environment, there was an increase in wakefulness, sleep latency, and movement time, and the decrease in sleep time was due mostly to decreased REM sleep and stage 2 NREM sleep.[37,57] However, subjects selected for their claimed ability to sleep in the cold showed an increase in wakefulness and a decrease in NREM-sleep stage 2 but no decrease in REM sleep when tested at a cold (21° C) versus a neutral (29° C) ambient temperature.[10]

Increased wakefulness and reductions in both REM sleep and NREM sleep are seen during nocturnal sleep in warm environments.[44,58] When subjects were exposed to a range of ambient temperatures, TST, NREM-sleep stages 3 and 4, and REM sleep were maximal at thermoneutrality (T_a = 29° C), and progressively decreased as T_a deviated from thermoneutrality. REM-sleep duration also peaked in the thermoneutral zone, significantly decreasing outside of thermoneutrality.[55]

Fragmentation of sleep seen during the night at high temperatures can cause changes in sleep measures during recovery sleep. Libert and coworkers recorded changes in sleep before, during, and after continuous (24-hour), multi-day exposure of subjects to a warm (35° C) environment.[59] Although sleep was more fragmented at the warm T_a, as manifested by decreased total sleep time and increased wakefulness, there were no differences in the amount of delta sleep or REM sleep between the baseline (20° C) and experimental conditions. TST and stage 3 NREM sleep increased, and the number of epochs of wakefulness and the number of transient arousals in REM sleep decreased in recovery sleep only. In a follow-up study,[60] the combined influences of heat and noise on sleep organization confirmed that heat exposure significantly increased the number of transient arousals without clear changes in the overall amounts of SWS and REM sleep. Heat was more potent as a disrupter of sleep than was noise, and the disturbing effects of heat and noise were more prominent during the last third of the night. Finally, thermal stimulation *during* REM sleep was more likely to lead to a state change, especially in response to cooling, compared to NREM sleep.[61]

In summary, results from animal and human studies have shown that ambient temperature is an important determinant of both the quantity and quality of sleep. TST is greatest in thermoneutrality and decreases above and below the thermoneutral zone. REM sleep appears to be more sensitive than NREM sleep to deviations of air temperature outside of thermoneutrality. Because of the decrease in sleep efficiency in the elderly, more work needs to be done investigating how the relationship between T_a and sleep organization changes with age. For example, in both young and aged cats, sleep was disrupted as T_a decreased (range 35° C to 5° C), although transient arousals in NREM sleep were significantly higher in the aged group at temperature extremes.[62]

Exercise and passive heating of subjects have been used to examine the influence of elevated T_b on sleep. In one study,[63] trained subjects ran on a treadmill or were passively heated in a warm water tank during the afternoon such that core temperature rose 2° C above resting levels. Both passive heating and high-intensity exercise increased NREM sleep stages 3 and 4 and had no effect on REM sleep. These effects appeared to be due primarily to the influence of core temperature on sleep. This conclusion was further substantiated by recordings of sleep parameters after exercise with and without body cooling.[64] When the normal rise in core temperature of about 2° C during exercise was limited to 1° C by facilitating heat loss during running, nocturnal sleep parameters did not differ from baseline recordings. Horne and Reid[65] later measured the effects of passive heating (to increase core temperature 1.8° C) versus immersion in cooler water (which caused no change in T_b) on sleep in both fit and unfit subjects. Whereas the neutral condition caused no change in sleep parameters, passive heating in both groups of subjects resulted in an increase both in sleepiness at bedtime and in

stage 4 sleep. REM sleep decreased slightly, especially in the first REM sleep period.

Further studies have investigated the temporal relationship of imposed core temperature changes on sleep parameters in adult humans. Horne and Shackell[66] speculated that larger "doses" of heating are needed to increase slow wave sleep as the time between heating and bedtime increases. Circadian influences may play a role, however, because heatings given at 7.5 hours versus 2.5 hours before bedtime are at different phases in the circadian temperature rhythm. Pretreatment of the subjects with aspirin (600 mg) at the time of a "late" heating (2.5 hours before bedtime) neutralized the increase in slow wave sleep, even though the T_b rise *during the heating* was the same in aspirin-treated and experimental groups. Unfortunately, T_b measurements were not available during the sleep period. These authors speculate that aspirin blocks the heating-induced rise in brain prostaglandin levels, which have been shown to increase NREM sleep in rodents. In fact, prostaglandin synthesis inhibitors damp the core temperature rhythm in rats by reducing the nocturnal rise in T_b,[67] leading Horne and Shackell to speculate that the circadian rise in the threshold hypothalamic temperature (T_{set}) may be mediated by prostaglandins.

Bunnell and coworkers[68] also measured the relationship between passive body heating in the morning, afternoon, early evening, and late evening (immersion in water at 41° C for 1 hour) and subsequent sleep changes. Increases in slow wave sleep delta activity were seen only following the evening heating periods. Passive heating by a hot bath prior to bedtime may be useful in ameliorating insomnia in the elderly.[69]

Shapiro and colleagues[70] also noted changes in sleep following 4 hours' exposure to ambient temperatures of 15° C, 25° C, 35° C, or 45° C ending 90 minutes before bedtime. The young male subjects, who slept at T_as of 19° C to 26° C, had significantly reduced wakefulness and increased slow wave sleep after exposure to environments of 35° C and 45°C; REM sleep was highest after exposure to the thermoneutral (25° C) T_a.

There is some question about whether slow wave sleep parameters are related more to the body temperature at sleep onset[71] or to the rate of fall in T_b following sleep onset.[72] To address the question, Jordan and colleagues[73] repeated earlier passive heating protocols with the important addition of measuring rectal temperature *during the sleep period*. These investigators found that passive heating resulted in a sustained elevation of rectal temperature of about 0.2° C, compared with controls, throughout the night. In addition, both REM sleep and NREM sleep were significantly increased during the first part of the night in the experimental subjects in this study, and thus increases in NREM sleep were not due to a suppression of REM sleep. Finally, the increase in NREM sleep during the first 150 minutes of the sleep period could not be accounted for by the rate of change of T_b, which did not differ significantly from that of control subjects. These authors concluded that the amount of delta sleep is a function of the level of T_b at sleep onset, in agreement with previous studies by Berger's group.[71] Some recent studies have implicated the dynamics of T_b decline with the timing of sleep onset.[74,75]

It seems clear that body heating before bedtime increases NREM sleep, but how does body heating *during* the sleep period influence sleep? To investigate this question, the core temperatures of subjects were elevated during the late part of the night, when REM sleep propensity is high, stage 4 propensity is low, and T_b is normally at its circadian nadir.[76] Contrary to the expectation that body heating would suppress REM sleep when heating took place at the normal temperature nadir, REM sleep parameters following the 2.5° C elevation in core temperature did not change, but NREM sleep stages 2 through 4 increased significantly in the fourth NREM sleep cycle. Despite the differences in the timing and the duration of heating in this study and those that manipulated T_b before sleep onset, similar effects on sleep were obtained. Another observation that suggests a causative association between body warming and delta sleep is that the occurrence of hot flashes in menopausal women during sleep is correlated with increased stage 4 sleep.[77]

A more specific, albeit complicated, example of the effects of body temperature on sleep comes from studies of fever. In 1968, Karacan and colleagues[78] reported that fever had specific effects on nocturnal sleep, including an increase in wakefulness and NREM sleep stage 1 as well as dramatic decreases in both REM sleep and NREM sleep stage 4. Because administration of a pyrogen in some individuals did not alter body temperature or sleep, it was concluded that the effects of the pyrogens on sleep were not due to the pyrogens per se but rather to the ensuing rise in T_b. In apparent support of this view, daytime administration of aspirin (600 mg) to healthy subjects resulted in a 12% reduction in stage 4 NREM sleep,[79] and this reduction in slow wave sleep seemed linked to a small (0.1° C to 0.2° C) decrease in oral temperature seen three hours before sleep onset.[80]

The relationship between sleep and fever has been examined in more detail in the rat.[81] In this multiday study, the effects of a fungal infection on T_b and diurnal variations in sleep distribution were studied at two T_as. Fevers resulted in a short-term attenuation of the diurnal NREM sleep rhythm and an elimination of the REM sleep and T_b rhythms. At ambient temperatures of 20° C and 30° C, NREM sleep increased more during lights-off periods, owing primarily to an increase in the number of NREM-sleep bouts. Changes in REM sleep were more complex. Although REM sleep decreased during lights-on and increased during lights-off periods, the total amount of REM sleep increased at a T_a of 20° C and decreased at a T_a of 30° C, contrary to the usual relationship between T_a and REM sleep seen in previous studies. An important conclusion from these studies is that fever may cause changes in the diurnal organization of sleep.

Studies[82-84] have further characterized changes in sleep in rabbits in response to the administration of cytokines, as well as the associated effects on immune system function (see Clark and Lipton[96] for a review). Human endogenous pyrogen (interleukin-1 [IL-1]) leads to a dose-dependent increase in NREM sleep concomitant with a rise in T_{br}, but IL-1 still increases sleep after administration of the antipyretic anisomycin, which prevents IL-1 from elevating T_{br}. Therefore, the somnogenic effect of IL-1 is not secondary to its pyrogenic activity. In addition, IL-1 infusion is accompanied by an increase in the amplitude of delta electroencephalographic (EEG) activity and a decrease in the amount of REM sleep, although the T_{br} changes that normally occur at sleep-state transitions were not modified by the IL-1 in these febrile rabbits. Similar results have been obtained with muramyl peptides.[83]

Despite the close links between sleep and thermoregulatory processes, a variety of studies suggest that the response of these two control systems to various biochemical agents can be uncoupled. For example, studies of the effects of putative somnogens and pyrogens on sleep and temperature have revealed that administration of many of these agents results in an increase in NREM sleep, a decrease in REM sleep, and an increase in core temperature.[85,86] However, in most cases the sleep and temperature effects are temporally displaced and dose-dependent, and they depend upon the site and mode of injection and time of day.[85,87-89] In addition, some cytokines are pyrogenic without increasing sleep.[90]

Future studies that attempt to determine the efficacy of putative somnogenic agents or that involve any pharmacologic manipulations of sleep must continue to evaluate changes in sleep parameters resulting from temperature variations secondary to the drug treatment. An example that clearly illustrates this principle is shown in a study of the effects of phentolamine on sleep in rats.[91] Administration of this adrenergic receptor antagonist caused decreases in REM sleep and T_b. When changes in body temperature were minimized by testing rats in a warm (32° C) rather than a cool (20° C) T_a, "drug" effects disappeared. A comprehensive inventory of the effects of drugs and a wide variety of biochemical agents on T_b is available[92-97] and will be of general interest to all sleep researchers.

In conclusion, both ambient and core temperatures have prominent influences on sleep parameters. As discussed in the next section, sleep is influenced both by thermal sensation and by indirect effects operating through the thermoregulatory system (thermoregulatory drive). Moreover, thermal sensation and thermoregulatory drive are interactive. The intensity of a thermal sensation is a function of whether actual body temperature is above or below the "set points" of the thermoregulatory system. For proper evaluation of the diverse body of data on effects of temperature on sleep, it is essential to understand the properties of the thermoregulatory system.

INTERACTIONS BETWEEN SLEEP STATES AND CNS REGULATION OF BODY TEMPERATURE

The properties of the mammalian thermoregulatory system have been investigated extensively. In general, a dominant source of feedback information in this system is the temperature of the preoptic and anterior hypothalamic nuclei (POAH). A common technique for studying the thermoregulatory system in animals is to use chronically implanted, water perfused, stainless steel thermodes placed around the POAH to manipulate hypothalamic temperature (T_{hy}) while simultaneously measuring effector responses such as metabolic heat production or evaporative water loss. In this way, hypothalamic thermosensitivity can be quantitatively described in terms of thermoregulatory responses that alter thermal balance. For example, by heating and cooling the POAH of a resting mammal, a T_{hy} can be identified above which metabolic rate remains at basal levels and below which metabolic heat production increases with further cooling. This T_{hy} can then be defined as the threshold T_{hy} or T_{set} for the metabolic heat production response, and the slope of the response curve below T_{set} represents the gain for this response. Threshold T_{hy}s for thermoregulatory responses are sensitive to changes in skin and other body temperatures. It is not clear, however, whether thermoafferent information is integrated in the POAH as has been generally assumed[98] or lower in the neural axis as more recent research suggests.[99]

Direct thermal stimulation of the POAH, which evokes strong thermoregulatory responses in unanesthetized animals, provides quantitative evidence for changes in thermoregulation during sleep. In a series of experiments in which T_{hy} was manipulated by chronically implanted water-perfused thermodes during sleep and wakefulness,[100] both the gain and threshold of the metabolic heat production response decreased in NREM sleep compared to waking, suggesting a central nervous system mechanism to account for the changes in body temperatures and thermoregulatory responses associated with the transition from wakefulness to NREM sleep. Moreover, metabolic responses to thermal manipulation of the POAH were absent during REM sleep, which explains the inhibition of thermoregulatory responses during this state.

The lack of POAH thermosensitivity during REM sleep could be due to descending inhibition of effector systems, inhibition of afferent thermal information, or inhibition of POAH integrative circuits. Hendricks[101] showed that the inhibition of thermogenesis during REM sleep could not be simply attributed to the descending motor inhibition characteristic of REM sleep. Lesions of the pontine tegmentum result in REM sleep without atonia. In cats with such lesions, however, shivering is absent in the cold during REM sleep even though the motor neurons that would mediate shivering were permanently disinhibited. Further work demonstrated that such pontine lesions render cats more sensitive to thermal loads in wakefulness and that the absence of shivering in animals during REM sleep without atonia cannot be ascribed to an overall decrease in the threshold for heat gain responses due to the lesions.[102] Therefore the inhibition of thermoregulatory control during REM sleep must involve an inhibition of thermal afferent or central thermoregulatory mechanisms, or both. However, in contrast to the results on control of shivering, studies of panting in response to high (35° C) ambient temperatures showed panting during 90% of REM-sleep episodes in animals with pontine tegmental lesions, compared to 52% of REM-sleep episodes in control animals.[34] The mechanisms by which pontine tegmental lesions decrease thresholds for panting in REM sleep and, more generally, the differential manifestation of different effectors (shivering, panting, sweating) in REM sleep remain unexplained.

Clearly, the control-systems properties of the thermoregulatory system change with sleep states, and these changes can be summarized as a downward regulation of body temperature during NREM sleep and an inhibition or relaxation of thermoregulatory responses during REM sleep. Given these powerful influences of sleep on thermoregulation, the reciprocal question can be asked: Are the effects of ambient and body temperature on sleep, which were described above, mediated through the thermoregulatory system? To answer this question, we studied the separate and combined effects of hypothalamic and peripheral temperature manipulations on arousal-state distributions.[52] Water-perfused thermodes around the POAH were used to disassociate thermoregulatory drive from peripheral thermal stimulation. By first knowing the threshold hypothalamic temperature (T_{set}) for the metabolic heat production response at each T_a used in the study, we were then able to manipulate T_{hy} to maintain the same difference between T_{hy} and T_{set} (thermoregulatory drive) regardless of T_a.

The question was whether distributions of arousal states would follow peripheral temperature or thermoregulatory drive. The results were that total sleep time was a function of thermoregulatory drive. In other words, the animal in a cold environment had a TST equal to that seen in a warm environment if T_{hy} was warmed to reduce thermoregulatory drive, and hence the cold stimulus to the skin had no effect on TST other than its effect through the thermoregulatory system. Reciprocally, the TST of animals in warm environments was reduced by mild cooling of the POAH. The distribution of NREM sleep and REM sleep, however, was not a simple function of thermoregulatory drive. Either central or peripheral thermal stimulation characteristic of nonneutral conditions caused a reduction of the REM-sleep–to–NREM-sleep ratio regardless of thermoregulatory drive, a result that has been confirmed in the pigeon,[103] where spine temperature provides primary feedback, modulating thermoregulatory and arousal state control. These results argue for a direct effect of thermal afferents on mechanisms regulating transitions between NREM sleep and REM sleep in addition to the indirect influence of those afferents on transitions between wakefulness and NREM sleep via the thermoregulatory system.

The neural mechanisms underlying the interaction of sleep and thermoregulation may involve many areas of the CNS.[104-108] Much recent attention, however, has been given to the POAH, which contains populations of neurons that are involved in thermoregulation as well as populations of neurons that are involved in the regulation of sleep. The question is whether or not these two populations are totally separate and interact, or whether there are preoptic hypothalamic cells that serve both thermoregulation and sleep regulation. For example, POAH cholinergic mechanisms are important in the regulation of sleep and body temperature. Injection of the cholinergic agonist carbachol into the POAH results in increased arousal and decreased brain temperature,[109,110] but are these actions due to carbachol's effects on the same or on separate populations of POAH cells?

Single-unit studies clearly show that POAH neurons that are likely to be responsible for thermoregulation are influenced by arousal state.[111-113] First, neuronal thermosensitivity is generally suppressed in REM sleep,[104,105,108] which fits with the observations of inhibited thermoregulatory responses during REM sleep. However, one study shows that warm-sensitive neurons, in comparison to cold-sensitive neurons, may be less prone to loss of sensitivity during REM sleep.[112] Second, a wealth of single-unit data supports the concept of a downward resetting of hypothalamic thermoregulatory mechanisms during NREM sleep. The majority of warm-sensitive neurons in the hypothalamus increase spontaneous discharge during the transition from waking to NREM sleep, whereas cold-sensitive neurons decrease firing rate. In addition, changes in thermosensitivity paralleled changes in spontaneous firing rates, such that cells that showed an increased firing rate in NREM sleep relative to waking displayed an increase in thermosensitivity as well.[114]

Because we assume that POAH cells responsible for thermoregulation should be temperature sensitive, it is easy to interpret these single-unit studies as showing arousal-state influences on thermoregulatory networks. However, we could view the data in reverse as supporting the concept that POAH cells that cause arousal state are temperature sensitive.[4] This would explain the effects of changes in ambient and body temperature on sleep. In support of this view, a number of studies have shown that manipulations of POAH temperature can influence the activity of cells in non-POAH areas that are known to be involved in sleep-state control. As early as 1971, DeArmond and Fusco showed that warming the POAH of dogs suppressed sensory-evoked responses in the ascending reticular activating system.[116] In recent studies, warming of the POAH has been shown to suppress waking-related cell activity in the magnocellular basal forebrain and in the posterior lateral hypothalamus of cats[113,117] and in the dorsal raphe[118] and lateral hypothalamus[119] of rats. These results suggested that warm-sensitive POAH neurons may play a key role in the regulation of NREM sleep.[4,111,114,115]

The assignment of sleep-control function to POAH temperature-sensitive cells must be viewed as tentative because it is based on indirect evidence. First, it is difficult to assign a role for a neuron in thermoregulatory control on the basis of its thermosensitivity. For example, highly warm sensitive neurons have been found in the hypothalamus of the unanesthetized duck, even though thermal stimulation of this area fails to evoke the same types of responses seen in mammals.[120] Additionally, it can be argued that warm sensitivity, or, more specifically, a positive thermal coefficient, should be expected for neurons in general based on simple biophysical considerations. Moreover, firing rates and thermosensitivities of hypothalamic neurons recorded in anesthetized preparations or in in vitro preparations have been, as a whole, much higher than those in studies using unanesthetized preparations. Thus, despite the compelling evidence about the role of the POAH as a key site for both the regulation of body temperature and control of arousal state, the specific neuronal basis for the integration and interaction of sleep and thermoregulation remains elusive. We need to consider the possible roles of temperature-insensitive neurons (which typically compose about 70% to 80% of all POAH cells studied) and neurons that respond to changes in the rate or magnitude of variations in temperature with changes in discharge pattern.

In conclusion, sleep has a strong influence on homeostatic regulation of body temperature, and conversely, temperature influences sleep through both direct effects of thermal stimuli on centers controlling sleep and wakefulness and indirect effects through the thermoregulatory system. A challenging area for future investigations will be to characterize the neuronal networks at the POAH and at extrahypothalamic levels that mediate the interaction between sleep and thermoregulatory control. In this regard, it is important to examine the functional roles of the brainstem in thermoregulation and arousal-state control and the connections of these nuclei with the POAH.[121-123]

CIRCADIAN MODULATION OF SLEEP AND THERMOREGULATION

In addition to the variations in body temperatures and thermoregulatory responses associated with stages of sleep and wakefulness, there are daily cycles in the properties of the thermoregulatory system that are independent of arousal states. These daily changes in the thermoregulatory system and consequent changes in body temperature are under control of the circadian system, which also influences the organization of vigilance states (see Chapter 31). The daily core temperature rhythm is not a simple consequence of the daily activity cycle; paralyzed, bed-ridden subjects, as well as normal subjects kept inactive in bed, show continuing cycles of body temperature independent of levels of muscle activity.[124] Moreover, daily fluctuations in body temperature are primarily due to changes in thermal conductance rather than in changes in heat production.[125,126] The magnitude of the sleep-related declines in body temperature, which are considered "masking" components of the circadian T_b rhythm, depend on the phase of the T_b rhythm and are maximal (~0.5° C) on the descending phase.[127,128] Daily fluctuations in temperature continue during sleep deprivation,[6,115,124] and specific thermoregulatory responses in awake subjects vary with a daily rhythm.[129,130]

One study partitioning circadian versus sleep influences on central thermoregulatory feedback sensitivity showed that the spinal temperature thresholds for both shivering and thermal polypnea in pigeons were lower during the subjective night than during the subjective day in awake birds, and sleep caused an additional and equal decline in these thresholds.[32] In studies on rats, multiple regression analysis was used to determine the relative influence of sleep occurrence and the circadian system on the daily changes in T_b. The conclusion was that 84% of the daily change in T_b is due to a circadian influence and 16% is due to the occurrence of sleep-wake transitions.[131] This dominance of vigilance state over circadian modulation on T_b changes as seen in the rat does not apply to other species. In fact, in the euthermic ground squirrel, the circadian modulation of T_b appears far greater than the sleep-related changes.[132] Even though the strength of the circadian rhythm of T_b may differ between species, it is common in mammals and may result in direct thermal influences on sleep.

The daily rhythm of temperature in humans has strong influences on both the timing and duration of sleep. In environments devoid of time cues, the sleep-wake and body temperature cycles can uncouple and free-run with different circadian periodicities.[129,133-135] Under such conditions, the voluntary bedtime and sleep onset is most likely to occur near the T_b nadir.[134] When one uncoupled subject went to bed near his T_b minimum, waking usually occurred on the rising phase of his T_b rhythm, 7.8 hours later. If, on the other hand, he went to bed at his T_b maximum, he still woke up on the rising phase and his sleep time averaged 14.4 hours. This relationship between duration of sleep and the phase of the T_b rhythm when sleep onset occurs was confirmed on ten desynchronized subjects.[133]

The influence of the phase of the T_b cycle on sleep propensity was also determined in an experiment in which subjects were placed on a cycle of 2 hours of activity and 1 hour of imposed bed rest.[135] If bed rest coincided with the decline of or near the nadir of T_b, sleep propensity and especially REM sleep propensity were maximal. However, when bed rest occurred near the rising phase of the T_b rhythm, sleep was disturbed and REM sleep was absent. The timing and duration of minor sleep periods, or naps, also depends on the phase of the T_b cycle in free-running subjects. Naps occurring at temperature minima were shorter than major sleep periods but were longer than naps occurring halfway between minima.[136]

In free-running subjects with desynchronized cycles of T_b and bed rest activity, sleep parameters correlated with the

T_b cycle and not with length of prior wakefulness. A very strong influence of T_b on REM sleep is especially evident. REM-sleep latency was shortest, REM-sleep episode duration was longest, and the amount of REM sleep was greatest at the T_b minimum.[135] Results obtained from subjects entrained to a normal 24-hour day but sleep deprived for varying lengths of time before being permitted to sleep ad libitum, beginning at different points in the T_b cycle, have also shown that sleep parameters were more influenced by phase of the T_b cycle at bedtime than by length of prior wakefulness.[137] Several human studies suggest that sleep propensity[138] and REM-sleep propensity may have a bimodal distribution in relation to the T_b cycle.[134,135,139] A plot of REM-sleep propensity as a function of phase of the T_b cycle in subjects under a normal sleep schedule showed two distinct peaks in the occurrence of REM sleep across nights: One occurred at about 20 minutes and another at about 100 minutes after the temperature minimum.[139]

In summary, the daily T_b rhythm and the characteristics of thermoregulatory responses depend on both circadian and sleep-related influences. But in turn, circadian changes in body temperature influence the expression of vigilance states. Although body temperature has a strong influence on sleep architecture, it should be emphasized that the timing, duration, and quality of sleep result from the interaction of many factors.

The interaction of sleep and T_b rhythms has important implications for several clinical and applied problems. As discussed previously, when the synchrony between the daily rhythm of body temperature and the daily sleep-wake cycle is disrupted, there are prominent effects on sleep propensity and sleep architecture. Such uncoupling between T_b and sleep may contribute to disorders of initiating and maintaining sleep (DIMS). DIMS resulting from jet lag and shift work are related to changes in the phase angle between scheduled sleep and the circadian rhythm, as reflected in T_b changes. As a result of shift work or jet lag, scheduled bedtime can occur in the evening "wake maintenance" zone, about 8 hours before the T_b minimum, where it is extremely difficult to initiate sleep.[138]

Sleep-onset insomniacs were found to have a core temperature rhythm that was phase delayed several hours compared to normal subjects, placing their bedtimes within what the T_b rhythm would indicate to be the wake-maintenance zone.[140] Sleep *length* is also reduced in the day sleep of night-shift workers, the premature awakenings being correlated with the high or rising phase of the T_b cycle.[141] Treatment for these DIMS and for sleep disturbances resulting from primary affective disorders has included manipulation of sleep-wake scheduling[142] and photic stimulation to entrain the circadian rhythm,[143-146] and it involves a phase shift of the temperature rhythm relative to sleep. Photic stimulation has a direct and immediate effect on temperature, and this effect appears to be mediated by the retinohypothalamic tract.[147,148]

The T_b rhythms of the elderly[149,150] have been characterized by increased nocturnal T_b minima or a decrease in rhythm amplitude, or both. These changes in T_b rhythms may be related to the alterations of sleep timing and quality that occur in the elderly (such as increases in wakefulness and decreases in stages 3 and 4 and in REM sleep) and in females, as well as an association of shorter TST, poorer sleep quality, and earlier rising times with the phase-advance of the acrophase.[151]

Studies examining gender differences in sleep and T_b rhythms suggest that the acrophase in elderly women is phase-advanced about an hour, and the amplitude is higher relative to age-matched men.[151,152]

The T_b rhythms of depressed patients[153,154] are often characterized by increased nocturnal T_b minima. In a recent study that measured both temperature and sleep parameters in depressed patients,[155] the reduced REM-sleep latency typically reported in many depressed patients was correlated with a higher nocturnal mean temperature and a higher T_b at sleep onset. However, this reduced REM-sleep latency was not a simple consequence of a phase-advance of the core temperature rhythm. As pointed out by Avery and colleagues,[153] adequate consideration of age and gender effects in studies of sleep and depression is essential when comparing different studies. Further work is necessary to determine whether sleep disturbances in depression (decreased slow wave sleep and short REM-sleep latency) are secondary to alterations in thermoregulatory control or if the reduced amplitude of the T_b rhythm reflects increased nocturnal wakefulness, sleep fragmentation, or other modifications in sleep patterns.

In evaluating the causes and possible treatments for sleep disturbances associated with changes in the phase relationship or amplitude of the core body temperature rhythm relative to sleep, it will be important to understand if T_b modulates sleep independently of circadian control mechanisms. Conversely, it is possible that disrupted sleep alters the core T_b rhythm. It must be remembered that while both the circadian rhythms and temperature per se are important determinants of sleep propensity, these parameters act in concert with other physiologic factors, especially sleep homeostasis, to influence sleep timing and architecture.[156]

DOES SLEEP HAVE THERMOREGULATORY FUNCTIONS?

This chapter has presented studies that lead to the following conclusions:

- Body temperature is regulated at a lower level during NREM sleep than during waking, and this regulatory shift is in addition to circadian changes in body temperature.
- Thermoregulation is severely inhibited during REM sleep.
- Nonneutral thermal environments favor wakefulness and NREM sleep, due both to thermal sensation and to thermoregulatory error signals.
- Even within thermoneutrality, temperature influences sleep structure, with REM sleep being maximal at the upper end of the thermoneutral zone.

Given these strong interactions among temperature, thermoregulation, and sleep, hypotheses have been advanced about possible thermoregulatory functions of sleep.

One of the first hypotheses was that NREM sleep has the primary function of energy conservation.[3,157] This view was supported by the downregulation of body temperature during NREM sleep, by the coincidence of sleep and hypometabolism,[158] and by the fact that shallow torpor and deep hibernation—clear adaptations for energy conservation—are evolutionary extensions of NREM sleep.[159] Some birds and mammals that occupy certain ecological niches where energy conservation is highly adaptive may show more sleep than do other species. Many species, however, do not seem to be under heavy selection to conserve energy, yet sleep is also an essential aspect of their lives. Thus, whereas the energy-conservation hypothesis fits well into an evolutionary scenario for NREM sleep and for explaining some specialized adaptive extensions of NREM sleep, it seems unreasonable to expect that whole-body energy conservation is the major and obligatory general function of mammalian sleep.

Another hypothesis proposed that NREM sleep is a thermoregulatory adaptation to counter heat loads built up during waking.[160] Support for this hypothesis, as for the energy-conservation hypothesis, is circumstantial. There is an anatomic coincidence between thermoregulatory controls and hypnogenic functions in the basal forebrain, and as described earlier, gentle warming of the POAH and basal forebrain induces sleep. Furthermore, raising body temperature during the active period either passively or through exercise increases NREM sleep during the subsequent inactive period.[65,66] The "heat loss function of sleep" hypothesis is interesting, but it ignores the time constant for changes in body heat content. Small- to medium-sized animals, such as those used in sleep research, can dissipate enormous heat loads in minutes unless they are held at high ambient temperatures. If sleep were primarily a heat-loss adaptation, large animals should sleep more than small animals, and whereas the time course for changes in body heat content and sleep might be organized on a daily basis for an animal the size of an elephant, it would not be in a mouse that can alter its body heat content in only a few minutes. The hypothesis would also predict that animals in cold climates would sleep less than animals in warm climates and that whole-body cooling or hypothalamic cooling would reduce sleep need or would substitute for sleep. There is no evidence to support these predictions.

The extensive experiments of Rechtschaffen and colleagues on the effects of long-term sleep deprivation suggest that sleep may be essential for heat production rather than heat loss. Prior to death, chronically sleep-deprived rats become extremely hypothermic and behaviorally select very high ambient temperatures, although the cause of this thermoregulatory pathology is not known.[161] It is unlikely, however, that these thermoregulatory pathologies that appear only after at least a week of sleep deprivation are reflections of a sleep-specific thermoregulatory function that occurs in the time frame of the daily cycle of sleep and activity.

Thomas Wehr has proposed in a lengthy, scholarly review paper that a function of REM sleep is to warm the central nervous system.[162] He states that his argument is largely circumstantial, being based on such observations as the fact that in most studies brain metabolism and brain temperature have been seen to rise at the transition from NREM to REM sleep and REM sleep is accompanied by a variety of heat-producing events such as rapid eye movements and muscle twitches. He also notes that in humans, at least, more REM sleep occurs later in the rest period when the body temperature is at its lowest levels. The adaptive rationale that Wehr puts forward is that brain warming during REM sleep enables animals to sleep at low ambient temperatures without brain temperature falling to levels that would compromise ability to arouse periodically or in response to external stimuli. Several facts run counter to this brain-warming hypothesis: The thermoregulatory system is relatively unresponsive during REM sleep; there is not more REM sleep in smaller animals or in animals that live in cold climates; REM sleep is inhibited by

low ambient and low body temperatures; and in small animals sleeping in the cold, brain temperature falls during REM sleep.

Although there is no convincing evidence supporting a thermoregulatory function for sleep, two related areas of sleep research may be leading toward deeper understanding of sleep function. The first of these areas is the study of sleep homeostasis and the underlying neurochemical mechanisms, which indicates that a function of NREM sleep is the restoration of cerebral energy reserves.[163] The other area is the study of hibernation.

The rationale for the first hypothesis is that the most reliable quantitative relationship between prior wake duration and a sleep parameter is the amount of activity in the NREM-sleep EEG in the 0.5 to 4.5 Hz range—delta activity or delta power.[164] Adenosine agonists selective for the adenosine A1 receptor produce increases in delta power that resemble the increases seen after sleep deprivation; these findings suggest that adenosine is the feedback molecule that controls the relationship between delta power and prior wake duration. Since adenosine release by neurons and other cells is tightly coupled to the energy charge (ATP/ADP ratio) of the cells, it seems that compromise of cerebral energy during wakefulness could influence the intensity of subsequent NREM sleep. The adenosine hypothesis of sleep homeostasis suggests that regional depletion of cerebral glycogen reserves during wakefulness leads to transient declines in cell energy charge, and these declines produce increases in extracellular adenosine.

It is possible to see in this hypothesis a mechanism whereby higher body and hence brain temperatures could promote sleep. The metabolism of most cells increases with temperature, and therefore higher brain temperatures could contribute to reductions in brain energy charge with concomitant increases in extracellular adenosine. In fact, gentle warming of the POAH increases the EEG delta power during NREM sleep more than it does the duration of NREM sleep.[165] Thus, the restoration of brain energy reserves may be a function of sleep that could also offer some explanation for thermal effects on NREM sleep.

Mammalian hibernation is another area of sleep research that may hold clues for sleep function. It is a reasonable hypothesis that hibernation evolved in species exposed to

---

Clinical Pearls

Increases in slow wave sleep delta activity have been documented following evening heating periods. Passive heating by a hot bath prior to bedtime may be useful in ameliorating insomnia in the elderly. At the other end of the age spectrum, apneic events during sleep are common in infants during the first year of life, and they normally trigger arousal responses. However, interactions among the circadian, thermoregulatory, and sleep-control systems that are developing in parallel, but not necessarily in synchrony, could produce episodes of deep sleep with high arousal thresholds or prolonged REM bouts with low respiratory chemosensitivity. Coincidence of such an episode with an apneic event could result in SIDS. Attention to the thermal state of infants deemed at risk for SIDS is warranted.

seasonal food scarcity. In such species, natural selection would have favored the decreased body temperature and therefore decreased metabolism that is associated with sleep. Animals in deep hibernation are observed to be in almost continuous NREM sleep that lasts many days.

REFERENCES

1. Heller HC, Glotzbach SF: Thermoregulation during sleep and hibernation. Int Rev Physiol 1977;15:147-188.
2. Heller HC, Glotzbach SF: Thermoregulation and sleep. In Shitzer A, Eberhart RC (eds): Heat Transfer in Medicine and Biology—Analysis and Applications. New York, Plenum Press, 1985, pp 107-134.
3. Berger RJ, Phillips NH: Comparative physiology of sleep, thermoregulation and metabolism from the perspective of energy conservation. In (eds): Issa FG, Suratt PM, Remmers JE (eds): Sleep and Respiration: Progress in Clinical and Biological Research, Vol V. New York, Wiley-Liss, 1990, pp 41-52.
4. McGinty D, Szymusiak R: Hypothalamic regulation of sleep and arousal. Front Biosci 2003;8:1074-1083.
5. Parmeggiani PL: Thermoregulation and sleep. Front Biosci 2003;8:557-567.
6. Timbal J, Colin J, Boutelier C, Guieu JD: Bilan thermique en ambience controlée pendent 24 heures. Pfluegers Arch 1972; 335:97-108.
7. Kreider MB: Effects of sleep deprivation on body temperature. Fed Proc 1961;20:214.
8. Kleitman N: Studies of the physiology of sleep. I: The effects of prolonged sleeplessness on man. Am J Physiol 1923;66:67-72.
9. White DP, Weil JV, Zwillich CW: Metabolic rate and breathing during sleep. J Appl Physiol 1985;59:384-391.
10. Palca JW, Walker JM, Berger RJ: Thermoregulation, metabolism, and stages of sleep in cold-exposed men. J Appl Physiol 1986; 61:940-947.
11. Ryan T, Mlynczak S, Erickson T, et al: Oxygen consumption during sleep: Influence of sleep stage and time of night. Sleep 1989;12:201-210.
12. Brebbia DR, Altshuler KZ: Oxygen consumption rate and electroencephalographic stage of sleep. Science 1965;150:1621-1623.
13. Haskell EH, Palca JW, Walker JM, et al: Metabolism and thermoregulation during stages of sleep in humans exposed to heat and cold. J Appl Physiol 1981;51:948-954.
14. Webb P, Hiestand M. Sleep metabolism and age. J Appl Physiol 1975;38:257-262.
15. Ingvar DH, Rosen I, Johannesson G: EEG related to cerebral metabolism and blood flow. Pharmakopsychiat 1979;12: 200-209.
16. Townsend RE, Prinz PN, Obrist WD: Human cerebral blood flow during sleep and waking. J Appl Physiol 1973;35:620-625.
17. Ramm P, Frost BJ: Cerebral and local cerebral metabolism in the cat during slow wave and REM sleep. Brain Res 1986;365:112-124.
18. Braun AR, Balkin TJ, Wesensten NJ: Regional cerebral blood flow throughout the sleep-wake cycle. Brain 1997;120:1173-1197.
19. Nofzinger EA, Buysse DJ, Miewald JM, et al: Human regional cerebral glucose metabolism during non–rapid eye movement sleep in relation to waking. Brain 2002;125:1105-1115.
20. Maquet P, Dive D, Salmon E, et al: Cerebral glucose utilization during sleep-wake cycle in man determined by positron emission tomography and [^{18}F]2-fluoro-2-deoxy-D-glucose method. Brain Res 1990;513:136-143.
21. Day R: Regulation of body temperature during sleep. Am J Dis Child 1941;61:734-746.
22. Scholander PF, Hammel HT, Hart JS, et al: Cold adaptation in Australian Aborigines. J Appl Physiol 1958;13:211-218.
23. Kreider MB, Iampietro PF: Oxygen consumption and body temperature during sleep in cold environments. J Appl Physiol 1958;14:765-767.
24. Geschickter EH, Andrews PA, Bullard RW: Nocturnal body temperature regulation in man: A rationale for sweating in sleep. J Appl Physiol 1966;21:623-630.
25. Satoh T, Ogawa T, Takagi K: Sweating during daytime sleep. Jpn J Physiol 1965;15:523-531.
26. Parmeggiani PL: Temperature regulation during sleep: A study in homeostasis. In Orem J, Barnes CD (eds): Physiology in Sleep. New York, Academic Press, 1980:97-143.
27. Azzaroni A, Parmeggiani PL: Mechanisms underlying hypothalamic temperature changes during sleep in mammals. Brain Res 1993;632:136-142.
28. Azzaroni A, Parmeggiani PL: Changes in selective brain cooling across the behavioral states of the ultradian wake-sleep. Brain Res 1999;844:206-209.
29. Tachibana S: Relation between hypothalamic heat production and intra- and extracranial circulatory factors. Brain Res 1969;16:405-416.
30. Parmeggiani PL, Azzaroni A, Calasso M: Systemic hemodynamic changes raising brain temperature in REM sleep. Brain Res 2002;940:55-60.
31. Parmeggiani PL, Sabattini L: Electromyographic aspects of postural, respiratory and thermoregulatory mechanisms in sleeping cats. Electroencephalogr Clin Neurophysiol 1972;33: 1-13.
32. Heller HC, Graf R, Rautenberg W: Circadian and arousal state influences on thermoregulation in the pigeon. Am J Physiol 1983;245:R321-R328.
33. Parmeggiani PL, Rabini C: Sleep and environmental temperature. Arch Ital Biol 1970;108:369-387.
34. Amini-Sereshki L, Morrison AR: Release of heat-loss responses in paradoxical sleep by thermal loads and by pontine tegmental lesions in cats. Brain Res 1988;450:9-17.
35. Parmeggiani PL, Rabini C: Shivering and panting during sleep. Brain Res 1967;6:789-791.
36. Calasso M, Zantedeschi E, Parmeggiani PL: Cold-defense function of brown adipose tissue during sleep. Am J Physiol 1993;265: R1060-R1064.
37. Buguet AG, Livingstone SD, Reed LD: Skin temperature changes in paradoxical sleep in man in the cold. Aviat Space Environ Med 1979;50:567-570.
38. Henane R, Buguet A, Roussel B, Bittel J: Variations in evaporation and body temperatures during sleep in man. J Appl Physiol 1977;42:50-55.
39. Dewasmes G, Bothorel B, Candas V, Libert JP: A short-term poikilothermic period occurs just after paradoxical sleep onset in humans: Characterization changes in sweating effector activity. J Sleep Res 1997;6:252-258.
40. Libert JP, Candas V, Muzet A, Ehrhart J: Thermoregulatory adjustments to thermal transients during slow wave sleep and REM sleep in man. J Physiol (Paris) 1982;78:251-257.
41. Sagot JC, Amoros C, Candas V, Libert JP: Sweating responses and body temperatures during nocturnal sleep in humans. Am J Physiol 1987;252:R462-R470.
42. Buguet A, Bittel J, Gati R, et al: Thermal exchanges during sleep in anhidrotic ectodermal dysplasia. Eur J Appl Physiol 1990; 59:454-459.
43. Takagi K: Sweating during sleep. In Hardy JD, Gagge AP, Stolwijk JAJ (eds): Physiological and Behavioral Temperature Regulation. Springfield, Ill: Charles C Thomas, 1970, pp 669-675.
44. Lenzi P, Libert JP, Cianci T, Franzini C: Comparative aspects of the interaction between sleep and thermoregulation. In Horne J (ed): Sleep'90. Bochum, Germany: Pontenagel Press, 1990, pp 388-390.
45. Johnson JM: Non-thermoregulatory control of human skin blood flow. J Appl Physiol 1986;61:1613-1622.
46. Parmeggiani PL, Rabini C, Cattalani M: Sleep phases at low environmental temperature. Arch Sci Biol (Bologna) 1969;53: 277-290.

47. Sichieri R, Schmidek WR: Influence of ambient temperature on the sleep-wakefulness cycle in the golden hamster. Physiol Behav 1984;33:871-877.

48. Rosenthal MS, Vogel G: Prolonged temperature increase produces prolonged REM sleep increase in the rat. Sleep Res 1991;20A:513.

49. Alfoldi P, Rubicsek G, Cserni G, Obal F: Brain and core temperatures and peripheral vasomotion during sleep and wakefulness at various temperatures in the rat. Pflugers Arch 1990;417:336-341.

49a. Szymusiak R, Satinoff E: Maximal REM sleep time defines a narrower thermoneutral zone than does minimal metabolic rate. Physiol Behav 1981;26:687-690.

50. Schmidek WR, Hoshino K, Schmidek M, Timo IC: Influence of environmental temperature on the sleep-wakefulness cycle in the rat. Physiol Behav 1972;8:363-371.

51. Valatx JL, Roussel B, Cure M: Sleep and cerebral temperature in rat during chronic heat exposure. Brain Res 1973;55:107-122.

52. Sakaguchi S, Glotzbach SF, Heller HC: Influence of hypothalamic and ambient temperatures on sleep in kangaroo rats. Am J Physiol 1979;237:R80-R88.

53. Roussel B, Turrillot P, Kitahama K: Effect of ambient temperature on the sleep-waking cycle in two strains of mice. Brain Res 1984;294:67-73.

54. Szymusiak R, Satinoff E, Schallert T, Whishaw IQ: Brief skin temperature changes towards thermoneutrality trigger REM sleep in rats. Physiol Behav 1980;25:305-311.

55. Haskell EH, Palca JW, Walker JM, et al: The effects of high and low ambient temperatures on human sleep stages. Electroencephalogr Clin Neurophysiol 1981;51:494-501.

56. Sewitch DE, Kittrell EM, Kupfer DJ, Reynolds CF: Body temperature and sleep architecture in response to a mild cold stress in women. Physiol Behav 1986;36:951-957.

57. Buguet AC, Livingstone SD, Reed LD, Limmer RE: EEG patterns and body temperatures in man during sleep in arctic winter nights. Int J Biometeorol 1976;20:61-69.

58. Karacan I, Thornby JI, Anch AM, Williams RL, Perkins HM: Effects of high ambient temperature on sleep in young men. Aviat Space Environ Med 1978;49:855-860.

59. Libert JP, Di NJ, Fukuda H, et al: Effect of continuous heat exposure on sleep stages in humans. Sleep 1988;11:195-209.

60. Libert JP, Bach V, Johnson LC, et al: Relative and combined effects of heat and noise exposure on sleep in humans. Sleep 1991;14:24-31.

61. Candas V, Libert JP, Muzet A: Heating and cooling stimulations during SWS and REM sleep in man. J Therm Biol 1982;7:155-158.

62. Bowersox SS, Dement WC, Glotzbach SF: The influence of ambient temperature on sleep characteristics in the aged cat. Brain Res 1988;457:200-203.

63. Horne JA, Staff LH: Exercise and sleep: Body-heating effects. Sleep 1983;6:36-46.

64. Horne JA, Moore VJ: Sleep EEG effects of exercise with and without additional body cooling. Electroencephalogr Clin Neurophysiol 1985;60:33-38.

65. Horne JA, Reid AJ: Night-time sleep EEG changes following body heating in a warm bath. Electroencephalogr Clin Neurophysiol 1985;60:154-157.

66. Horne JA, Shackell BS: Slow wave sleep elevations after body heating: proximity to sleep and effects of aspirin. Sleep 1987;10:383-392.

67. Scales WE, Kluger MJ: Effect of antipyretic drugs on circadian rhythm of body temperature of rats. Am J Physiol 1987;253:R306-R313.

68. Bunnell DE, Agnew JA, Horvath SM, et al: Passive body heating and sleep: Influence of proximity to sleep. Sleep 1988;11:210-219.

69. Dorsey CM, Lukas SE, Teicher MH, et al: Effects of passive body heating on the sleep of older female insomniacs. J Geriatr Psychiatry Neurol 1996;9:83-90.

70. Shapiro CM, Allan M, Driver H, Mitchell D: Thermal load alters sleep. Biol Psychiatry 1989;26:736-740.

71. Berger RJ, Palca JW, Walker JM, Phillips NH: Correlations between body temperatures, metabolic rate and slow wave sleep in humans. Neurosci Lett 1988;86:230-234.

72. Sewitch DE: Slow wave sleep deficiency insomnia: a problem in thermo-downregulation at sleep onset. Psychophysiology 1987;24:200-215.

73. Jordan J, Montgomery I, Trinder J: The effect of afternoon body heating on body temperature and slow wave sleep. Psychophysiol 1990;27:560-566.

74. Murphy JP; Campbell SS: Nighttime drop in body temperature: A physiological trigger for sleep onset? Sleep 1997;20:505-511.

75. Campbell SS, Broughton RJ: Rapid decline in body temperature before sleep: Fluffing the physiological pillow? Chronobiology International 1994;11:126-131.

76. Bunnell DE, Horvath SM: Effects of body heating during sleep interruption. Sleep 1985;8:274-282.

77. Woodward S, Freedman RR: The thermoregulatory effects of menopausal hot flashes on sleep. Sleep 1994;17:497-501.

78. Karacan I, Wolff SM, Williams RL, et al: The effects of fever on sleep and dream patterns. Psychosomatics 1968;9:331-339.

79. Horne JA, Percival JE, Traynor JR: Aspirin and human sleep. Electroenceph Clin Neurophysiol 1980;49:409-413.

80. Horne JA: Aspirin and nonfebrile waking oral temperature in healthy men and women: Links with SWS changes? Sleep 1989;12:516-521.

81. Kent S, Price M, Satinoff E: Fever alters characteristics of sleep in rats. Physiol Behav 1988;44:709-715.

82. Krueger JM, Walter J, Dinarello CA, et al: Sleep-promoting effects of endogenous pyrogen (interleukin-1). Am J Physiol 1984;246:R994-R999.

83. Krueger JM, Kubillus S, Shoham S, Davenne D: Enhancement of slow-wave sleep by endotoxin and lipid A. Am J Physiol 1986;R251:R591-R597.

84. Walter J, Davenne D, Shoham S, et al: Brain temperature changes coupled to sleep states persist during interleukin 1-enhanced sleep. Am J Physiol 1986;250:R96-R103.

85. Krueger JM, Karnovsky ML: Sleep and the immune response. Ann N Y Acad Sci 1987;496:510-516.

86. Krueger JM, Majde JA: Sleep as a host defense: Its regulation by microbial products and cytokines. Clin Immun Immunopathol 1990;57:188-199.

87. Walter JS, Meyers P, Krueger JM: Microinjection of interleukin-1 into brain: Separation of sleep and fever responses. Physiol Behav 1989;45:169-176.

88. Opp MR, Obal FJ, Krueger JM: Interleukin 1 alters rat sleep: temporal and dose-related effects. Am J Physiol 1991;260:R52-R58.

89. Onoe H, Ueno R, Fujita I, et al: Prostaglandin D2, a cerebral sleep-inducing substance in monkeys. Proc Nat Acad Sci U S A 1988;85:4082-4086.

90. Opp M, Obal FJ, Cady AB, et al: Interleukin-6 is pyrogenic but not somnogenic. Physiol Behav 1989;45:1069-1072.

91. Kent S, Satinoff E: Influence of ambient temperature on sleep and body temperature after phentolamine in rats. Brain Res 1990;511:227-233.

92. Clark WG, Clark YL: Changes in body temperature after administration of adrenergic and serotonergic agents and related drugs including antidepressants. Neurosci Biobehav Rev 1980;4:281-375.

93. Clark WG, Clark YL: Changes in body temperature after administration of acetylcholine, histamine, morphine, prostaglandins and related agents. Neurosci Biobehav Rev 1980;4:175-240.

94. Clark WG, Clark YL: Changes in body temperature after administration of antipyretics, LSD, delta 9-THC, CNS depressants and stimulants, hormones, inorganic ions, gases, 2,4-DNP and miscellaneous agents. Neurosci Biobehav Rev 1981; 5:1-136.

95. Clark WG, Lipton JM: Changes in body temperature after administration of amino acids, peptides, dopamine, neuroleptics and related agents: II. Neurosci Biobehav Rev 1985;9: 299-371.

96. Clark WG, Lipton JM: Changes in body temperature after administration of acetylcholine, histamine, morphine, prostaglandins and related agents: II. Neurosci Biobehav Rev 1985;9:479-552.

97. Clark WG, Lipton JM: Changes in body temperature after administration of adrenergic and serotonergic agents and related drugs including antidepressants: II. Neurosci Biobehav Rev 1986;10:153-220.

98. Hammel HT, Heller HC, Sharp FR: Probing the rostral brainstem of anesthetized, unanesthetized, and exercising dogs and of hibernating and euthermic ground squirrels. Fed Proc 1973;32:1588-1597.

99. Berner NJ, Heller HC: Does the preoptic anterior hypothalamus receive thermoafferent information? Am J Physiol 1998;274: R9-R18.

100. Glotzbach SF, Heller HC: Central nervous regulation of body temperature during sleep. Science 1976;194:537-539.

101. Hendricks JC: Absence of shivering in the cat during paradoxical sleep without atonia. Exp Neurol 1982;75:700-710.

102. Amini-Sereshki L, Morrison AR: Effects of pontine tegmental lesions that induce paradoxical sleep without atonia on thermoregulation in cats during wakefulness. Brain Res 1986;384:23-28.

103. Graf R, Heller HC, Sakaguchi S, Krishna S: Influence of spinal and hypothalamic warming on metabolism and sleep in pigeons. Am J Physiol 1987;252:R661-R667.

104. Glotzbach SF, Heller HC: Changes in the thermal characteristics of hypothalamic neurons during sleep and wakefulness. Brain Res 1984;309:17-26.

105. Parmeggiani PL, Cevolani D, Azzaroni A, Ferrari G: Thermosensitivity of anterior hypothalamic-preoptic neurons during the waking-sleeping cycle: A study in brain functional states. Brain Res 1987;415:79-89.

106. Grahn DA, Radeke CM, Heller HC: Arousal state vs. temperature effects on neuronal activity in subcoeruleus area. Am J Physiol 1989;256:R840-R849.

107. Alam MN, McGinty D, Szymusiak R: Thermosensitive neurons of the diagonal band in rats: Relation to wakefulness and non–rapid eye movement sleep. Brain Res 1997;752:81-89.

108. Cevolani D, Parmeggiani PL: Responses of extrahypothalamic neurons to short temperature transients during the ultradian wake-sleep cycle. Brain Res Bull 1995;37:227-232.

109. Mallick BN, Joseph MM: Role of cholinergic inputs to the medial preoptic area in regulation of sleep-wakefulness and body temperature in freely moving rats. Brain Res 1997; 750:311-317.

110. Imeri L, Bianchi S, Angeli P, Mancia M: Stimulation of cholinergic receptors in the medial preoptic area affects sleep and cortical temperature. Am J Physiol 1995;269:R294-R299.

111. Alam MN, McGinty D, Szymusiak R: Neuronal discharge of preoptic/anterior hypothalamic thermosensitive neurons: relation to NREM sleep. Am J Physiol 1995;269:R1240-R1249.

112. Alam MN, McGinty D, Szymusiak R: Preoptic/anterior hypothalamic neurons: Thermosensitivity in rapid eye movement sleep. Am J Physiol 1995;269:R1250-R1257.

113. Alam N, Szymusiak R, McGinty D: Local preoptic/anterior hypothalamic warming alters spontaneous and evoked neuronal activity in the magno-cellular basal forebrain. Brain Res 1995; 696:221-230.

114. Alam MN, McGinty D, Szymusiak R: Preoptic/anterior hypothalamic neurons: Thermosensitivity in wakefulness and non rapid eye movement sleep. Brain Res 1996;718:76-82.

115. Kreider MB: Effects of sleep deprivation on body temperature. Fed Proc 1961;20:214.

116. DeArmond SJ, Fusco MM: The effect of preoptic warming on the arousal system in the mesencephalic reticular formation. Exp Neurol 1971;33:653-670.

117. Krilowicz BL, Szymusiak R, McGinty D: Regulation of posterior lateral hypothalamic arousal related neuronal discharge by preoptic anterior hypothalamic warming. Brain Res 1994; 668:30-38.

118. Guzman-Marin R, Alam MN, Drucker-Colin R, McGinty D: Discharge modulation of rat dorsal raphe neurons during sleep and waking: Effects of preoptic/basal forebrain warming. Brain Res 2000;875:23-34.

119. Methippara MA, Alam MN, Szymusiak R, McGinty D: Preoptic area warming inhibits wake-active neurons in the perifornical lateral hypothalamus. Brain Res 2003;960:165-173.

120. Simon E, Hammel HT, Oksche A: Thermosensitivity of single units in the hypothalamus of the conscious Pekin duck. J Neurobiology 1977;8:523-535.

121. Denoyer M, Sallanon M, Buda C, et al: The posterior hypothalamus is responsible for the increase of brain temperature during paradoxical sleep. Exp Brain Res 1991;84:326-334.

122. Denoyer M, Sallanon M, Buda C, et al: Neurotoxic lesion of the mesencephalic reticular formation and/or the posterior hypothalamus does not alter waking in the cat. Brain Res 1991;539:287-303.

123. Sallanon M, Denoyer M, Kitahama K, et al: Long-lasting insomnia induced by preoptic neuron lesions and its transient reversal by muscimol injection into the posterior hypothalamus in the cat. Neuroscience 1989;32:669-683.

124. Kleitman N: Sleep and Wakefulness. 2nd ed. Chicago, University of Chicago Press, 1963.

125. Aschoff J, Heise A: Thermal conductance in man: Its dependence on time of day and ambient temperature. Adv Clin Physiol 1972;20:334-348.

126. Smith RE: Circadian variations in human thermoregulatory responses. J Appl Physiol 1969;26:554-560.

127. Gillberg M, Akerstedt T: Body temperature and sleep at different times of day. Sleep 1982;5:378-388.

128. Mills JN, Minors DS, Waterhouse JM: The effect of sleep upon human circadian rhythms. Chronobiologia 1978;5:14-27.

129. Wever R: The circadian multi-oscillator system of man. Int J Chronobiol 1975;3:19-55.

130. Wenger CB, Roberts MF, Stolwijk JAJ, Nadel ER: Nocturnal lowering of thresholds for sweating and vasodilation. J Appl Physiol 1976;41:15-19.

131. Franken P, Tobler I, Borbely AA: Sleep and waking have a major effect on the 24 hr rhythm of cortical temperature in the rat. J Biol Rhythms 1992;7:341-352.

132. Larkin JE, Franken P, Heller HC: Loss of circadian organization of sleep and wakefulness during hibernation. Am J Physiol Regul Integr Comp Physiol 2002;282:R1086-R1095.

133. Zulley J, Wever R, Aschoff J: The dependence of onset and duration of sleep on the circadian rhythm of rectal temperature. Pflugers Arch 1981;391:314-318.

134. Czeisler CA, Weitzman ED, Moore EM, et al: Human sleep: its duration and organization depend on its circadian phase. Science 1980;210:1264-1267.

135. Czeisler CA, Zimmerman JC, Ronda JM, et al: Timing of REM sleep is coupled to the circadian rhythm of body temperature in man. Sleep 1980;2:329-346.

136. Campbell SS, Zulley J: Circasemidian distribution of human sleep/wake patterns during disentrainment. Sleep Res 1985;14:291.

137. Akerstedt T, Gillberg M: The circadian variation of experimentally displaced sleep. Sleep 1981;4:159-169.

138. Strogatz SH, Kronauer RE, Czeisler CA: Circadian pacemaker interferes with sleep onset at specific times each day: Role in insomnia. Am J Physiol 1987;253:R172-R178.

139. Carman GJ, Mealey L, Thompson ST, Thompson MA: Patterns in the distribution of REM sleep in normal human sleep. Sleep 1984;7:347-355.

140. Morris M, Lack L, Dawson D: Sleep-onset insomniacs have delayed temperature rhythms. Sleep 1990;13:1-14.

141. Akerstedt T, Gillberg M: Displacement of the sleep period and sleep deprivation. Implications for shift work. Hum Neurobiol 1982;1:163-171.

142. Czeisler CA, Richardson GS, Coleman RM, et al: Chronotherapy: Resetting the circadian clocks of patients with delayed sleep phase insomnia. Sleep 1981;4:1-21.

143. Czeisler CA, Allan JS, Strogatz SH, et al: Bright light resets the human circadian pacemaker independent of the timing of the sleep-wake cycle. Science 1986;233:667-671.

144. Lewy AJ, Sack RL, Miller LS, Hoban TM: Antidepressant and circadian phase-shifting effects of light. Science 1987;235:352-354.

145. Sack RL, Lewy AJ, Miller LS, Singer CM: Effects of morning versus evening bright light exposure on REM latency. Biol Psychiatry 1986;21:402-405.

146. Czeisler CA, Kronauer RE, Allan JS: Bright light induction of strong (Type 0) resetting of the human circadian pacemaker. Science 1989;244:1328-1333.

147. Dijk DJ, Cajochen C, Borbely AA: Effect of a single 3-hour exposure to bright light on core body temperature and sleep in humans. Neurosci Lett 1991;121:59-62.

148. Drennan M, Kripke DF, Gillin JC: Bright light can delay human temperature rhythm independent of sleep. Am J Physiol 1989;257:R136-R141.

149. Vitiello MV, Smallwood RG, Avery DH, et al: Circadian temperature rhythms in young adult and aged men. Neurobiol Aging 1986;7:97-100.

150. Weitzman ED, Moline ML, Czeisler CA, Zimmerman JC: Chronobiology of aging: Temperature, sleep-wake rhythms and entrainment. Neurobiol Aging 1982;3:299-309.

151. Campbell SS, Gillin JC, Kripke DF, et al: Gender differences in the circadian temperature rhythms of healthy elderly subjects: relationships to sleep quality. Sleep 1989;12:529-536.

152. Moe KE, Prinz PN, Vitiello MV, et al: Healthy elderly women and men have different entrained circadian temperature rhythms. J Am Geriatr Soc 1991;39:383-387.

153. Avery DH, Wildschiodtz G, Rafaelsen OJ: Nocturnal temperature in affective disorder. J Affective Disord 1982;4:61-71.

154. Souetre E, Salvati E, Wehr TA, et al: Twenty-four-hour profiles of body temperature and plasma TSH in bipolar patients during depression and during remission and in normal control subjects. Am J Psychiatry 1988;145:1133-1137.

155. Avery DH, Wildschiodtz G, Smallwood RG, et al: REM latency and core temperature relationships in primary depression. Acta Psychiatr Scand 1986;74:269-280.

156. Borbely AA: A two process model of sleep regulation. Hum Neurobiol 1982;1:195-204.

157. Berger RJ: Bioenergetic functions of sleep and activity rhythms and their possible relevance to aging. Fed Proc 1975;34:97-102.

158. Heller HC: Sleep and hypometabolism. Can J Zool 1988;66:61-69.

159. Berger RJ: Slow wave sleep, shallow torpor and hibernation: Homologous states of diminished metabolism and body temperature. Biol Psychol 1984;19:305-326.

160. Szymusiak RS, Satinoff E: Thermal influences on basal forebrain hypnogenic mechanisms. In McGinty DJ, Drucker-Colin R, Morrison A, Parmeggiani PL (eds): Brain Mechanisms of Sleep. New York, Raven Press, 1985, pp 301-319.

161. Prete FR, Bergmann BM, Holtzman P, et al: Sleep deprivation in the rat: XII. Effect on ambient temperature choice. Sleep 1991;14:109-115.

162. Wehr TA: A brain-warming function for REM sleep. Neurosci Biobehav Rev 1992;16:379-397.

163. Benington JH, Heller HC: Restoration of brain energy metabolism as the function of sleep. Prog Neurobiol 1995;45:347-360.

164. Endo T, Roth C, Landolt HP: Selective REM sleep deprivation in humans: Effects on sleep and sleep EEG. Am J Physiol 1998:274:R1186-R1194.

165. McGinty D, Szymusiak R, Thomson D: Preoptic/anterior hypothalamic warming increases EEG delta frequency activity within non-rapid eye movement sleep. Brain Res 1994;667:273-277.

Neural Mechanisms of Sleep-Related Penile Erections

Markus H. Schmidt

ABSTRACT

Penile erections are a characteristic phenomenon of paradoxical sleep (PS) or rapid eye movement sleep. Although the neural mechanisms of other classic PS-related events, such as muscle atonia, rapid eye movements, and cortical activation, are well studied, the neural control of penile erections during PS has been explored only recently. A new animal model for sleep-related erection research in freely behaving rats has provided many new insights.

The spinal control of penile erections is characterized by a complex interplay among parasympathetic, somatic motor, and sympathetic components. Although the supraspinal control is less well understood, numerous structures from the medulla to the telencephalon have been implicated in erectile mechanisms, including the medial preoptic area, which plays an essential role in copulatory behavior. Advances in erectile neurophysiology suggest that penile erections involve a descending oxytocinergic excitation of the spinal erection generator from the hypothalamic paraventricular nucleus (PVN) and the removal of a descending serotonergic inhibition from the medullary nucleus paragigantocellularis (nPGi).

The executive mechanisms of PS, as well as the subsystems that generate its tonic and phasic phenomena, are located in the pedunculopontine tegmentum and rostral medulla. Although these brainstem structures are sufficient for the generation of PS and its classic phenomena, the brainstem is not sufficient for the generation of PS-related erections, as demonstrated by brainstem transection experiments. An essential role of the forebrain in PS-related erectile control is confirmed by lesion experiments of the preoptic area. Neurotoxic lesions of the lateral preoptic area (LPOA) severely disrupt PS-related erections while leaving at least some types of waking-state erections intact, suggesting that the higher central mechanisms of erections are context specific. Similar lesions of the medial preoptic area have only minimal effects on sleep-related or waking-state erectile activity. Although it does not project to the spinal cord, the LPOA may modulate the spinal erection generator during PS through its relay connections with the PVN and nPGi. Although the source of brainstem control of forebrain erectile mechanisms in sleep was previously unknown, more recent work demonstrates the presence of putative cholinergic neurons in the lateral dorsal tegmental nucleus (LDT) that increase their firing rate directly in association with PS-related erectile activity. The LDT may modulate or trigger forebrain erectile mechanisms through their ascending projections, potentially by releasing acetylcholine into the LPOA during PS. Finally, sleep-related erections appear to be androgen sensitive because such erections are diminished in pathologically or experimentally induced

hypogonadal states. Since its discovery more than 3 decades ago, numerous hypotheses and assumptions regarding PS-related erectile mechanisms have been postulated and are reviewed in this chapter. Clinical implications and directions for future research also are discussed.

Penile erection cycles during sleep were first described in the early 1940s,[1] more than a decade before the discovery of paradoxical sleep (PS) or rapid eye movement (REM) sleep. These sleep-related erections (SREs) in human beings were found to occur at 85-minute intervals and to last approximately 25 minutes each.[1] After the discovery of PS, several authors hypothesized that erections in sleep may coincide with PS because the cyclicity and duration of these two phenomena are virtually identical. Fisher et al.[2] and Karacan et al.[3] later demonstrated a strong temporal association between the occurrence of penile erections and PS.

Penile tumescence cycles in sleep occur in all normal healthy males from early infancy, through adulthood, and into old age.[4] Similar clitoral erection cycles and increases in vaginal blood flow during PS have been described in females.[5] Although these erection cycles occur during dream sleep, PS erectile activity is not related to dream content.[6] Because of the consistent, involuntary, and autonomic nature of penile tumescence in sleep, SRE testing has been used as a clinical tool to differentiate "psychogenic" from "organic" impotence.

In addition to penile erections, PS is characterized by other classic tonic and phasic phenomena, including cortical desynchronization, rapid eye movements, ponto-geniculo-occipital (PGO) spikes, and a general muscle atonia. The executive mechanisms of PS and the neural subsystems generating its classic tonic and phasic events have been relatively well elucidated. In contrast, the neural mechanisms of PS-related erections, until recently, were not investigated, primarily because an animal model was not available for recording penile erections across behavioral states.

NEUROPHYSIOLOGY OF "WAKING-STATE" PENILE ERECTIONS

Anatomy and Hemodynamics

The penis is composed of two separate erectile tissue systems, the paired corpora cavernosa of the penis (CCP) and the single corpus spongiosum of the penis (CSP), which envelops the urethra. At the proximal portions, or base, of these erectile tissues, the paired CCP separate to form the crura of the CCP, which lie along the lateral border of the ischiopubic rami. In contrast, the most proximal portion of the CSP, known as the bulb of the CSP, lies between the two crura. The ischiocavernosus (IC) and bulbospongiosus (BS) muscles are located at the base of the penis and are closely associated with these two separate erectile tissue systems.

The erectile tissues are composed of a framework of smooth muscle bundles that, in the flaccid state, form collapsed vascular spaces known as cavernous sinuses. Blood is restricted from entering these vascular spaces when the penis is flaccid. With appropriate autonomic and local control during tumescence (see later), blood enters the cavernous sinuses after a relaxation of the smooth muscle cells in the arteries and trabecular framework. The penis becomes engorged and erect as blood expands the spongy erectile tissue. Reflex IC and BS muscle contractions subsequently compress the crura and bulb, respectively. Repetitive and phasic contractions of these perineal muscles appear to augment rigidity by producing intracavernous and intraspongious pressure peaks in excess of the systolic arterial blood pressure.[7]

Spinal Control

The neural control of penile erections involves the complex interplay of parasympathetic, sympathetic, and somatic components. These neural elements comprise what has been referred to as the *spinal generator* or *spinal pacemaker* controlling penile erections, in that erections may still occur after the removal of all descending input from higher brain structures. Indeed, because reflex-induced erections are facilitated by spinal transection,[8] it has long been assumed that the brain exhibits a tonic descending inhibition on this spinal generator.

Penile tumescence traditionally is viewed as a parasympathetic phenomenon causing vasodilation of the supplying arteries and relaxation of smooth muscle cells in the erectile tissues.[9] Release of acetylcholine and nitric oxide appears to play a major role in this local, vasodilatory process,[9,10] in part by stimulating the formation of cyclic guanosine monophosphate (GMP).[11] The first oral medication for the treatment of erectile dysfunction, sildenafil (Viagra), acts at the end-organ level by preventing the inactivation of cyclic GMP through an inhibition of its deactivating enzyme phosphodiesterase.[11]

Rigidity is augmented by an additional somatic motor component involving reflex skeletal muscle contractions of the IC and BS muscles.[7] In contrast, detumescence and the maintenance of the flaccid state is under primarily sympathetic control involving the release of norepinephrine, causing vasoconstriction of the supplying arteries and contraction of smooth muscles in the erectile tissues through alpha receptors.[9] Finally, although proerectile mechanisms primarily involve parasympathetic control, the temporal balance between parasympathetic and sympathetic output from the spinal cord to the penis may be of primary importance.[9] For example, the generation of an erection may be triggered if the summation of parasympathetic and sympathetic output from the spinal generator to the end organ tips the balance in favor of parasympathetic tone, potentially even if this balance to parasympathetic predominance results from a selective decrease in sympathetic activity.

Parasympathetic supply to the penis originates in the pelvic nerve,[9] whose preganglionic neurons are located in the sacral parasympathetic nucleus within L5 to S1 spinal cord segments in the rat[9,12] (Fig. 25–1). The pudendal nerve carries the

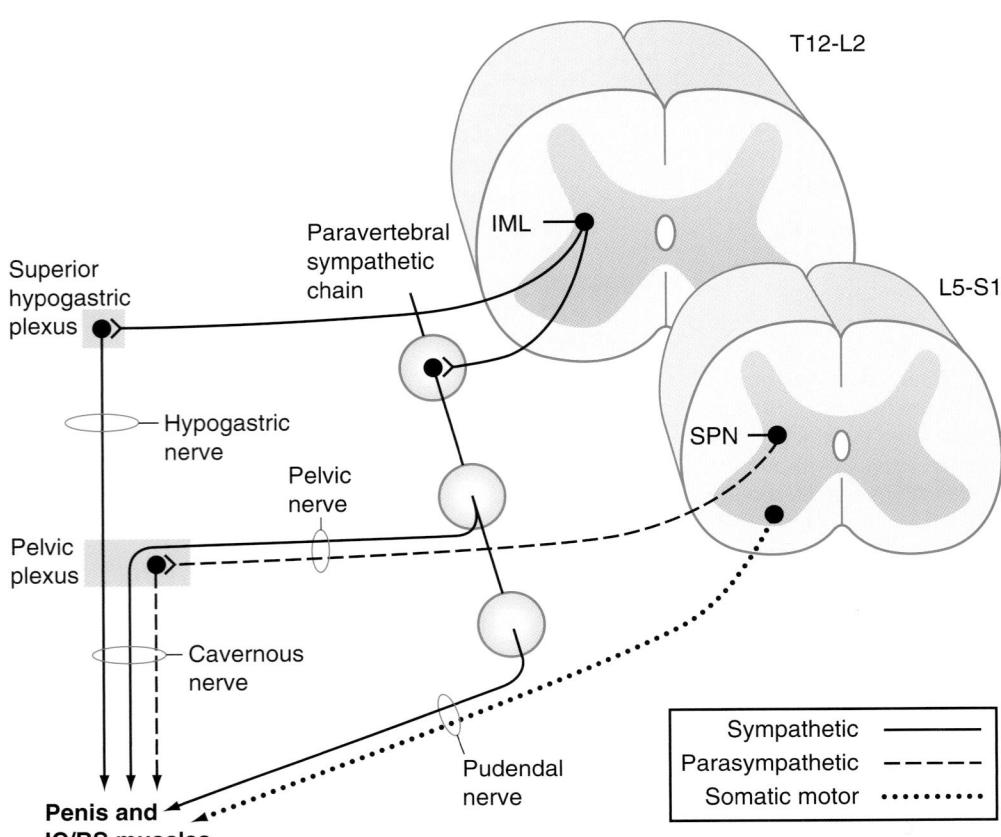

Figure 25–1. A schematic diagram demonstrating spinal erectile mechanisms, including parasympathetic, sympathetic, and somatic motor components. The somatic sensory afferents from the penis and surrounding skin are not depicted in this figure. See text for a detailed explanation. BS, bulbospongiosus; IC, ischiocavernosus; IML, intermediolateral cell column; SPN, sacral parasympathetic nucleus.

somatic motor supply to the IC and BS muscles, whose motoneurons are located in the dorsolateral and dorsomedial nucleus, respectively, in the ventral horn at levels L5 to L6 of the spinal cord in the rat[13] (see Fig. 25–1). These motoneurons are notable for their extensive, androgen-dependent dendritic arborizations,[14] which may play a role in the bilateral synchronization of IC and BS muscle bursts during penile erections.[15]

Much of the sympathetic innervation to the penis originates in the hypogastric nerve (see Fig. 25–1). Preganglionic sympathetic neurons are located primarily in the dorsal commissural nucleus and the intermediolateral columns of T12 to L2 spinal cord segments in the rat.[9,16] Although the hypogastric nerve carries much of the sympathetic innervation, sympathetic fibers are also found in the pelvic and pudendal nerves.[9,13]

The pelvic and hypogastric nerves join at the pelvic plexus on the lateral aspect of the rectum to form the cavernous nerve, which innervates the penis (see Fig. 25–1). Preganglionic parasympathetic fibers from the pelvic nerve synapse onto their postganglionic counterparts at this level. The cavernous nerve, therefore, carries postganglionic sympathetic and parasympathetic innervation to the penis.[9]

Afferent sensory fibers from the glans penis and surrounding skin travel through the dorsal nerve of the penis to join the pudendal nerve trunk. These sensory fibers innervate the spinal cord through the dorsal root ganglia of L6 to S1 spinal cord segments in the rat.[13]

Supraspinal Control

Although the spinal control of penile erections has been relatively well described, supraspinal mechanisms have only recently been elucidated. Many structures in the brain have been implicated in the control of either copulatory behavior or penile erections. Some of these structures, including the nucleus accumbens,[17] hippocampus,[18] and septum,[19] are considered to be potential candidates in reproductive mechanisms but are not examined in this review because their roles in erection neurophysiology remain unclear.

The Medial Preoptic Area and Dopaminergic Mechanisms

The medial preoptic area (MPOA) has long been implicated in the neural control of reproductive physiology. Bilateral electrolytic[20] or neurotoxic[21] lesions of the MPOA eliminate copulatory behavior in every species examined to date.[9] In contrast, electrical or chemical stimulation of the MPOA has been shown to augment copulatory behavior,[22] to increase intracavernous pressure in anesthetized rats,[23] and to remove a descending inhibition of penile reflexes.[24] Unit recordings of this structure demonstrate increases in unit activity associated with specific copulatory events.[25] Moreover, c-Fos expression in the MPOA has been found to increase after copulation in both male[26] and female[27] rats.

Dopaminergic mechanisms appear to play an important role in the afferent modulation of the MPOA. Indeed, dopamine has long been known to play an important role in erectile mechanisms because the systemic administration of dopaminergic agonists, such as apomorphine, induces penile erections.[9] Sexual activity in the male rat is associated with increased concentrations of dopamine in the MPOA.[28] Microinjections of dopaminergic agonists into the MPOA have

been shown to facilitate penile reflexes[29] and copulation[30] in this species. In contrast, the administration of dopaminergic antagonists into the MPOA impairs copulatory behavior, penile reflexes, and sexual motivation.[31] Although the source of dopaminergic modulation of the MPOA remains unknown, the incertohypothalamic dopaminergic system has been postulated to play such a role.[31] Finally, the efferent projections of the MPOA related to copulatory mechanisms remain poorly understood because the MPOA does not project to the spinal cord.

The MPOA has been hypothesized to play a role in the integration of information from other forebrain structures related to reproductive physiology. For example, the olfactory bulb,[32] amygdala[33] and bed nucleus of the stria terminalis (BNST)[34] are all implicated in copulatory mechanisms because lesioning of these structures disrupts aspects of sexual behavior. A general working hypothesis traditionally has been that the amygdala transmits olfactory and other limbic, copulatory-related input to the BNST through strial and nonstrial pathways.[35] The MPOA is thought to receive, integrate, and transmit information arising from the BNST and amygdala.[35] More recent data suggest that the MPOA is critical for copulatory behavior but is not essential for noncopulatory or noncontact erections because such erections are maintained after MPOA lesions.[34] Noncontact erections occur in male rats when in proximity to a receptive female, but the male rat is prevented from making contact with the female because of a physical barrier that is permeable to olfactory, visual, and auditory cues.

The Nucleus Paragigantocellularis and a Descending Serotonergic Inhibition

Serotonin (5-hydroxytryptamine [5-HT]) plays an inhibitory role in the production of penile erections, and data suggest that this inhibition occurs at the spinal level. Reflexive erections in awake rats are facilitated by the selective depletion of 5-HT in the lower lumbar spinal cord after local intrathecal application of the 5-HT neurotoxin 5,7-dihydroxytryptamine.[36] In contrast, intrathecal application of 5-HT at the lumbar level inhibits reflex-induced erections in rats during general anesthesia after upper spinal cord transection.[37] Reflexive erections can be induced under general anesthesia by urethral stimulation. This reflex, termed the urethrogenital reflex, is seen only after complete spinal transection above the lower thoracic level,[38] indicating the presence of a tonic descending inhibition in the intact animal. The intrathecal 5-HT–induced inhibition of this urethrogenital reflex in spinally transected rats is prevented by the systemic administration of methysergide, a general 5-HT receptor antagonist, given 5 to 20 minutes before the intrathecal 5-HT.[37]

The nucleus paragigantocellularis (nPGi) has been postulated to be a major supraspinal source of descending 5-HT erectile inhibition. Electrolytic or neurotoxic lesions with kainic acid of the rostral juxtafacial nPGi remove a tonic descending inhibition of penile erections during general anesthesia comparable with the effect of spinal transection.[39] Subsequent studies have found that lesions of the nPGi facilitate both mating behavior[40] and reflex-induced erections in the intact unanesthetized rat.[41] Finally, neuronal tracing studies indicate that the nPGi projects to spinal autonomic structures innervating the penis[12,37] and that a majority of these neurons in the nPGi contain 5-HT as their neurotransmitter.[37]

The involvement of medullary 5-HT structures in the excitation of the sympathetic nervous system[42] suggests that the descending 5-HT inhibition of penile erections may be mediated, in part, through its sympathoexcitatory function. Although the mechanism of this sympathoexcitation remains to be fully clarified, microiontophoretic application of 5-HT[43-45] or substance P,[46] which is colocalized in many serotonergic projections from the ventromedial medulla, may cause a concentration-dependent membrane depolarization of many sympathetic preganglionic neurons in the thoracolumbar spinal cord. Initial investigations showing an inhibitory role of raphe stimulation on sympathetic activity[47] may be due to the heterogeneity of this and other serotonergic brainstem structures. For example, sympathetic-related neurons in medullary raphe nuclei include nonserotonergic sympathoexcitatory and nonserotonergic sympathoinhibitory neurons that are influenced by baroreceptor reflexes.[42] Other raphe serotonergic neurons appear to exhibit a tonic discharge activity not related to baroreceptor input, which may influence the excitability of sympathetic preganglionic neurons.[48]

The Paraventricular Nucleus and a Descending Oxytocinergic Excitation

Is the simple removal of descending inhibition sufficient for the production of penile erections? This remains unclear because spinal transection, spinal block, and nPGi lesioning do not, in isolation, produce penile erections.[8,38] Excitatory input from peripheral sensory reflex activation or from higher brain structures may be necessary.

A candidate for such an excitatory role is a descending oxytocinergic excitation from the hypothalamic paraventricular nucleus (PVN). Intracerebroventricular (ICV) injection of oxytocin induces penile erections and yawning in rats.[49] In contrast, ICV injection of [Arg^8] vasopressin, which differs from oxytocin by only two amino acids, is unable to induce such an effect.[49] Oxytocin-induced penile erections are prevented by ICV injections of d(CH$_2$)$_5$Tyr(Me)-[Orn^8]vasotocin, an oxytocin antagonist.[50] Penile sexual responses are impaired after PVN lesioning[51] or after administration of muscimol, a gamma-aminobutyric acid–ergic agonist, into the PVN.[52] Finally, stimulation of the PVN with excitatory amino acids induces penile erection and yawning, and this effect is inhibited by systemic administration of an oxytocin antagonist.[53]

Neuroanatomic evidence is consistent with the hypothesis that oxytocinergic neurons in the PVN may play a proerectile role through its descending connections with the spinal erection generator. Immunohistochemical data demonstrate the presence of oxytocin-stained fibers making direct synaptic contacts, as demonstrated at both the microscopic and the ultrastructural levels, with retrogradely labeled preganglionic autonomic neurons in the spinal cord identified after pseudorabies virus injections into the penis.[54] Neuronal tracing studies indicate a strong projection from the parvocellular PVN to spinal autonomic structures innervating the penis[12,55] and to ventral horn motoneurons in the lumbar spinal cord that innervate the BS muscles of the penis.[54,56] The mechanism by which oxytocin may modulate spinal autonomic structures innervating the penis remains unclear. Although the effects of oxytocin agonists on parasympathetic preganglionic neurons in the sacral spinal cord remain to be explored, the PVN may theoretically play a proerectile role at

the spinal level by simultaneously inhibiting sympathetic output from the spinal cord while stimulating or augmenting parasympathetic tone destined to the penis. The PVN may also potentially modulate descending 5-HT inhibition of penile reflexes through its direct projection to the medullary nPGi.[57]

An Integrated Model of the Neural Control of Penile Erections

Penile erections are generated in different contexts and perhaps, as hypothesized, by different neural mechanisms.[58] For example, reflexive erections may be induced by tactile stimulation of the penis involving a direct reflex activation of the spinal generator without input from supraspinal structures. Moreover, psychogenic erections induced by memory or fantasy may involve higher central mechanisms that are different from penile erections induced by auditory, visual, or chemosensory input.[58] The MPOA appears to play a critical role in copulatory-related erectile mechanisms, whereas the olfactory bulbs and amygdala may be more involved in erectile mechanisms induced by olfactory cues.

The MPOA, as well as its functional association with the medial amygdala and BNST, has been one of the most investigated forebrain regions in reproductive physiology. Because few of these structures project to the spinal cord, the mechanisms by which the MPOA and related structures are able to influence the spinal generator controlling erections are unclear.

The missing link between these forebrain structures and descending erectile control may involve relay structures projecting to the spinal cord, a potential "final common path" from brain to spinal cord in erectile control, characterized by a descending oxytocinergic excitation from the PVN and a descending 5-HT inhibition from the nPGi (Fig. 25–2). It still remains to be determined how the various forebrain structures involved in context-specific erectile mechanisms may modulate this descending control. Indeed, the concept of a final common path from brain to spinal cord in erectile neurophysiology is likely an oversimplification in that it does not include a potential role of other ascending and descending systems between spinal and supraspinal structures in erectile mechanisms. However, this model provides a conceptual framework when designing experimental protocols regarding context-specific erectile mechanisms. A neural model of PS erectile control involving relay structures that project to the spinal cord is shown in Figure 25–2 and is discussed next.

ANIMAL MODEL FOR SLEEP-RELATED ERECTION RESEARCH

To elucidate SRE mechanisms, an animal model is essential. Although several early abstracts or anecdotal accounts reported erections visually observed during sleep in several nonhuman mammals,[59,60] these reports did not clarify whether such erections in nonhumans are simply occasional random events during sleep or if they are consistently associated with a specific sleep state. Indeed, a method of chronic penile erection recording in common laboratory animals such as the rat was not available. Previous animal erection data relied on visual observation or acute recording conditions under general anesthesia.

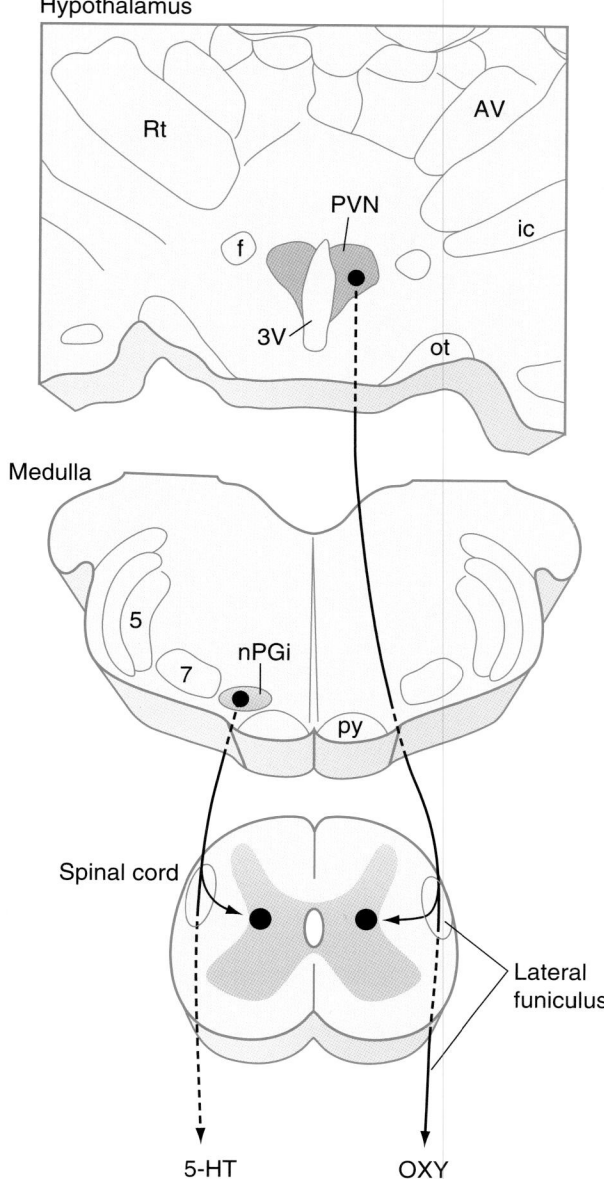

Figure 25–2. A potential final common path from brain to spinal cord in the descending control of the spinal erection generator. Serotonergic (5-HT) neurons in the medullary nucleus paragigantocellularis (nPGi) may exert an inhibitory effect on penile erection generation by increasing sympathetic tone, potentially through stimulation of sympathetic preganglionic neurons in the thoracolumbar spinal cord (*arrow* in spinal cord). Oxytocinergic (OXY) neurons in the hypothalamic paraventricular nucleus (PVN), on the other hand, may play a proerectile role in erectile mechanisms through a descending inhibition of sympathetic preganglionic outflow (*arrow* in spinal cord), as well as a simultaneous augmentation of parasympathetic tone by increasing parasympathetic preganglionic outflow from the sacral spinal cord to the penis. Although not shown in the figure, the parvocellular division of the PVN also projects to the nPGi and likely modulates this medullary inhibitory source of erectile activity. See text for a detailed explanation. AV, anteroventral thalamic nucleus; f, fornix; ic, internal capsule; ot, optic tract; py, pyramid; Rt, reticular thalamic nucleus; 3V, third ventricle; 5, spinal trigeminal nucleus; 7, facial nucleus.

A method of chronic penile erection monitoring in freely behaving rats has now been developed, involving pressure monitoring in the erectile tissues, as shown in Figure 25–3, and electromyography (EMG) of the IC and BS muscles.[61,62] Pressure monitoring in the erectile tissues without perineal muscle activity in freely moving rats has been reported by others.[63,64] Validation of this technique, which can be used for animal SRE research, demonstrates that erectile tissue pressure monitoring with perineal muscle activity both quantitatively and qualitatively records erectile events across behavioral states.[61,62]

This new technique definitively revealed for the first time that PS-related erections occur in nonhuman mammals.[61] PS erectile events in the rat are associated with an increase in baseline erectile tissue pressure and, concurrent with BS muscle bursts, suprasystolic CSP pressure peaks similar to visually confirmed erections during wakefulness and reflex induction[61,62] (Fig. 25–4). PS-related erections are found in approximately 30% of all PS phases in the rat, compared with 80% to 95% of PS phases in the human being.[2] Moreover, longer PS episodes are more likely to exhibit an erectile event.[61] Erectile activity in the rat is characterized by approximately 11 erections per hour of PS, 4 erections per hour of wakefulness, and a virtual absence of erections during slow wave sleep (SWS). Although the average PS erectile duration (mean 11 ± 7 seconds) usually is much shorter than the associated PS episode, this erectile event duration during PS is similar, if not longer in duration, to that typically observed during either coital or noncoital erections for this species.[62,63] Finally, no obvious relationships between erectile events and phasic PS phenomena

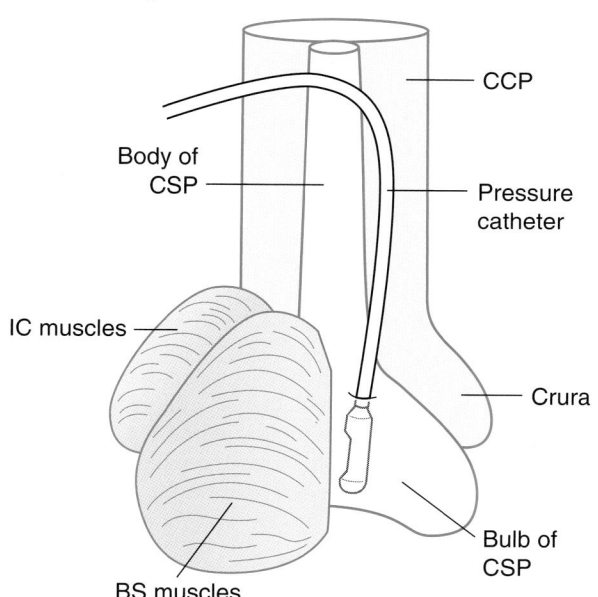

Figure 25–3. A schematic diagram of the proximal half of the rat penis demonstrating a method of chronic erectile tissue pressure monitoring. The ischiocavernosus (IC) and bulbospongiosus (BS) muscles have been removed on one side to expose the underlying erectile tissues. A microtip pressure transducer (outside diameter 1.2 mm) or an open-tip pressure catheter connected to a telemetric pressure transducer is implanted into the bulb of the corpus spongiosum of the penis (CSP) according to a method previously described.[62] Although not shown, the IC and BS muscles are implanted for perineal muscle recordings with bipolar Teflon-coated hook electrodes (0.002-inch uncoated diameter, multistranded stainless steel wire [AM-Systems]). CCP, corpora cavernosa of the penis.

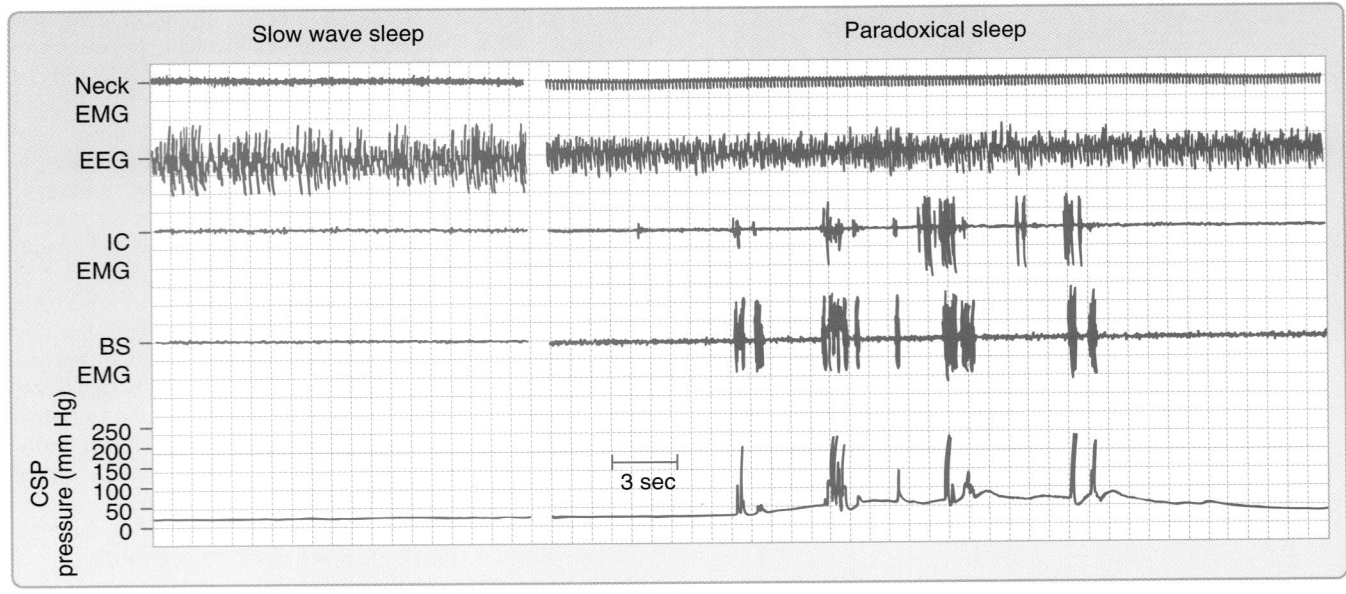

Figure 25–4. Slow wave sleep is characterized by an absence of erectile events. Specifically, corpus spongiosum of the penis (CSP) pressures remain stable, generally below 25 mm Hg, and there is an absence of ischiocavernosus (IC) and bulbospongiosus (BS) muscle bursts during high-amplitude slow waves. Paradoxical sleep, on the other hand, is associated with significant erectile activity, characterized by increases in baseline CSP pressure to 50 to 70 mm Hg and, concurrent with BS muscle bursts, large CSP pressure peaks that saturate the polygraph pens at 220 mm Hg. EEG, electroencephalogram; EMG, electromyogram. (From Schmidt MH, Valatx JL, Schmidt HS, et al: Experimental evidence of penile erections during paradoxical sleep in the rat. Neuroreport 1994;5:561-564.)

such as rapid eye movements were observed in the rat. These findings in the rat establish a new animal model for SRE research.

NEUROPHYSIOLOGY OF PARADOXICAL SLEEP-RELATED ERECTIONS

The neural mechanisms of penile tumescence in sleep have been investigated only recently. Our previous understanding of SRE neurophysiology was largely speculative and came entirely from human data. Moreover, the etiologies of organic impotence, as defined by clinical SRE criteria, have focused on the end-organ level. Although it is well documented that SREs may be adversely affected by diabetes,[65] depression,[66] cardiovascular disease,[67] and hypogonadal states,[68] potential neurogenic contributions to erectile dysfunction in these disease states are poorly understood. For example, diabetic impotence, generally presumed to be secondary to peripheral vascular or autonomic abnormalities, has been suggested to include a central dysregulation even before peripheral abnormalities are apparent.[65] Elucidation of both sleep-related and waking-state erectile mechanisms is essential for the eventual diagnosis and treatment of potential supraspinal neurogenic etiologies of impotence.

Numerous assumptions and speculations concerning PS erectile control have been postulated since its discovery in the mid-1960s. An early publication suggested that the neural mechanisms of both PS generation and PS-related erections are not completely interdependent, given the variable onset of tumescence relative to PS and the occasional occurrence of erections during slow wave sleep (SWS).[69] Schmidt et al.[61]

also speculated that PS mechanisms are not always linked functionally to the neural systems controlling tumescence because erections are observed in only 30% of PS episodes in the rat[61] and 80% to 95% of PS episodes in the human being,[2,3] unlike other tonic and phasic events such as muscle atonia and rapid eye movements, which occur during every PS episode.

Many authors have speculated about the role of the autonomic nervous system in the control of SREs because the pattern of autonomic nervous system activity during PS changes with respect to SWS and wakefulness. It has long been assumed that tumescence during PS is the result of a general increase in parasympathetic activity and a decrease in sympathetic tone.[70] The role of the autonomic nervous system in PS erectile control, however, is unknown and is complicated by the great variability in activity of the two autonomic divisions both within and among species, as well as by phasic alterations in autonomic activity during PS, which may have variable effects (parasympathetic versus sympathetic), depending on the effector organ involved.

It is commonly assumed that PS-related erections result from a decrease in descending erectile inhibition.[61,71] Reflex activation of local spinal erectile mechanisms has been suggested to coincide with this disinhibition. The source of this assumption may reside historically in the clinical appeal of SRE testing in that "psychogenic" impotence is characterized by normally occurring erections during sleep when psychological inhibitory influences are minimized. Although it is well established that the spinal generator controlling erections is under a tonic descending inhibition during wakefulness,[8] the level of inhibitory control during sleep remains to be explored. Finally, it is unknown if the simple removal of a descending inhibition is sufficient for the production of penile erection. Given the many structures from the brainstem reticular core to cortex that become active during PS, several authors have suggested that SRE control also may involve a descending activation or excitation.[70]

Androgens and Sleep-Related Erections

Androgens have long been thought to play a role in SRE neurophysiology. Testosterone administration can augment SREs in hypogonadal men,[72] whereas terminating testosterone replacement in such patients decreases the number of tumescence episodes, maximum penile circumference, and total tumescence time during sleep.[73] Administration of testosterone in normal healthy men augments penile rigidity during PS but has no effect on the frequency of erections or circumference changes.[74] Antiandrogens such as medroxyprogesterone acetate given to patients for deviant sexual behavior adversely affected SREs in several case studies.[75,76] Finally, the luteinizing hormone–releasing hormone agonist, leuprolide acetate, causes a severe reduction in serum testosterone levels, and, when administered to normal eugonadal men, it is associated with a significant decrease in total tumescence time during sleep.[68]

Although the aforementioned data appear compelling and the role of androgens in sexual desire, interest, and motivation is well documented,[77,78] the role of androgens in SRE physiology is unclear for several reasons. First, hypogonadal men show a reduction in SREs as described, yet exhibit normal erections in terms of latency and intensity (rigidity) compared with eugonadal men when watching erotic films.[79] This finding has led to speculation that PS-related erections are "androgen dependent," whereas visually induced erections are "androgen-independent" and that these context-specific erections may be mediated by different neurophysiologic mechanisms.[79] Second, although erections during sleep have been called androgen dependent, they may more appropriately be termed *androgen sensitive*.[80] Androgen deficiency may adversely affect erections during sleep as described, but such erections usually persist and, even in hypogonadal men, often remain within the normal range.[73] Third, the role of androgens in SREs is complicated further by the existence of such erections in infants[4] in the face of undetectable testosterone levels. Indeed, young children exhibit more total SRE activity than adults simply because children have more total REM sleep time.[4] Finally, the mechanism by which androgens may affect SREs currently is unknown. Because the frequency, duration, and magnitude of penile tumescence in sleep do not change when varying serum testosterone levels within the normal range,[81] it has been hypothesized that the integrity of such erections depends on a low threshold of serum testosterone level.[68]

Spinal Cord Transections

SREs are commonly thought to be disrupted by spinal cord injury, as described in two early abstract publications.[82,83] Although human data are limited, experiments in rats confirmed that mid-thoracic spinal transections virtually eliminate PS-related erections.[84] Moreover, any residual erectile activity observed during sleep after spinal cord transection occurs at random during SWS and PS, suggesting intermittent reflex activation below the transection. Sleep–wake parameters, in contrast, remain unchanged postlesion. The data clearly demonstrate that an intact spinal cord above the mid-thoracic level is critical for the integrity of PS erectile activity. It remains to be determined what PS erectile activity would remain after transections below the thoracolumbar level, leaving sympathetic innervation from the brain to the penis intact.

Brainstem Transections

The pons and rostral medulla contain the neural elements responsible for the various tonic and phasic phenomena characteristic of PS, including cortical desynchronization, rapid eye movements, PGO spikes, and muscle atonia.[85] Schmidt et al.[84] transected the rostral mesencephalon in the rat (Fig. 25–5) to determine if the brainstem is sufficient to generate PS-related erections, as it is sufficient to generate these other tonic and phasic events. Although PS persists posttransection in all rats, as seen by the rhythmic appearance of rapid eye movements and muscle atonia, penile erections during PS are severely disrupted in a *cerveau isolé* preparation (Fig. 25–6). These data suggest that although brainstem PS mechanisms persist in a *cerveau isolé* rat, neural structures rostral to the transection, as in the forebrain, are necessary for the production of PS-related erections.

A tonic descending erectile inhibition appears to be enhanced after mesencephalic transection.[84] Although spinal transection facilitates reflexive erections as seen by the significantly shorter latency to reflex induction relative to pretransection control animals,[8,84] mesencephalic transection, on the other hand, significantly increases the latency to reflex induction.[84] These data demonstrate that the descending inhibition after mesencephalic transection not only remains intact but may be enhanced posttransection, suggesting that the forebrain may play a role in erectile mechanisms at least in part through an inhibition of tonic brainstem inhibitory mechanisms. Such a disinhibitory role of the forebrain has been postulated by others.[24]

Forebrain Lesions

How does the forebrain control penile tumescence in sleep? As discussed earlier, numerous structures such as the MPOA, amygdala, BNST, and PVN have been implicated in reproductive physiology and, therefore, are potential forebrain candidates in PS erectile mechanisms.

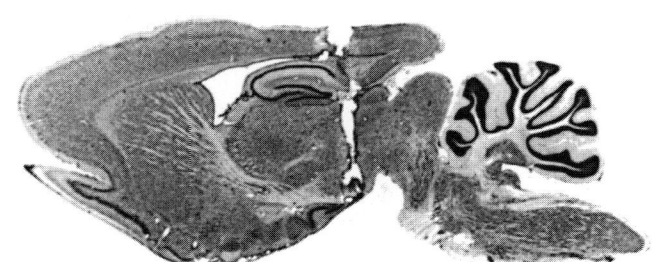

Figure 25–5. A photomicrograph of a sagittal section of the brain stained with cresyl violet demonstrating a typical mesencephalic transection at the level of the rostral superior colliculus. (From Schmidt MH, Sakai K, Valatx JL, et al: The effects of spinal or mesencephalic transections on sleep-related erections and ex-copula penile reflexes in the rat. Sleep 1999;22:409-418.)

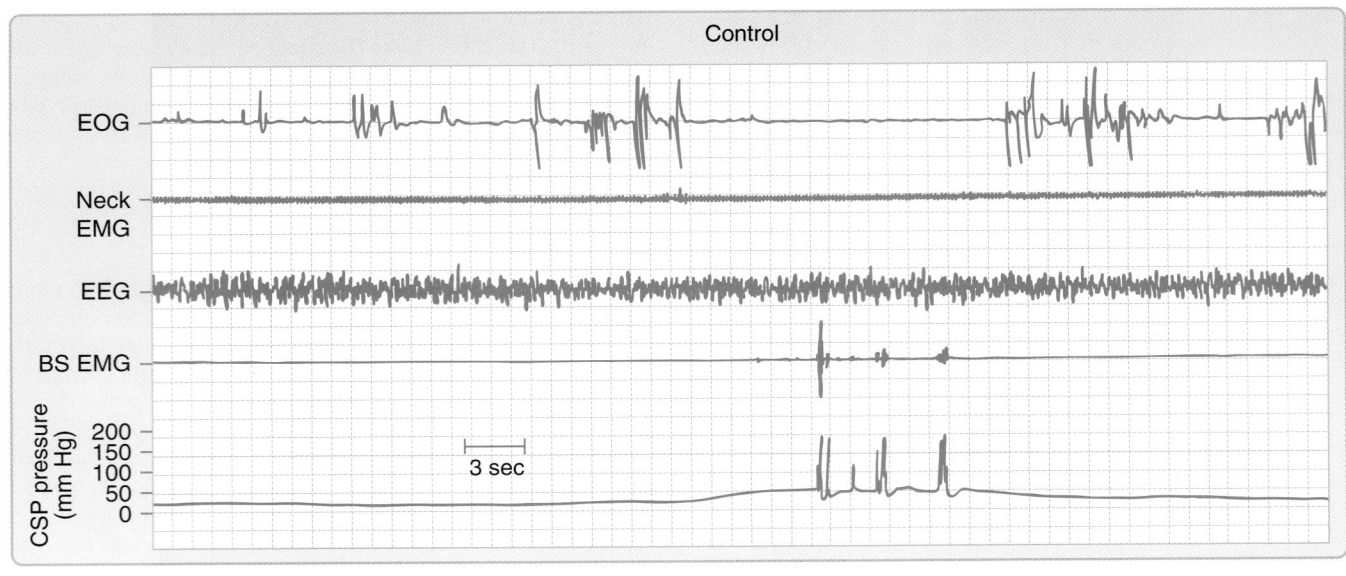

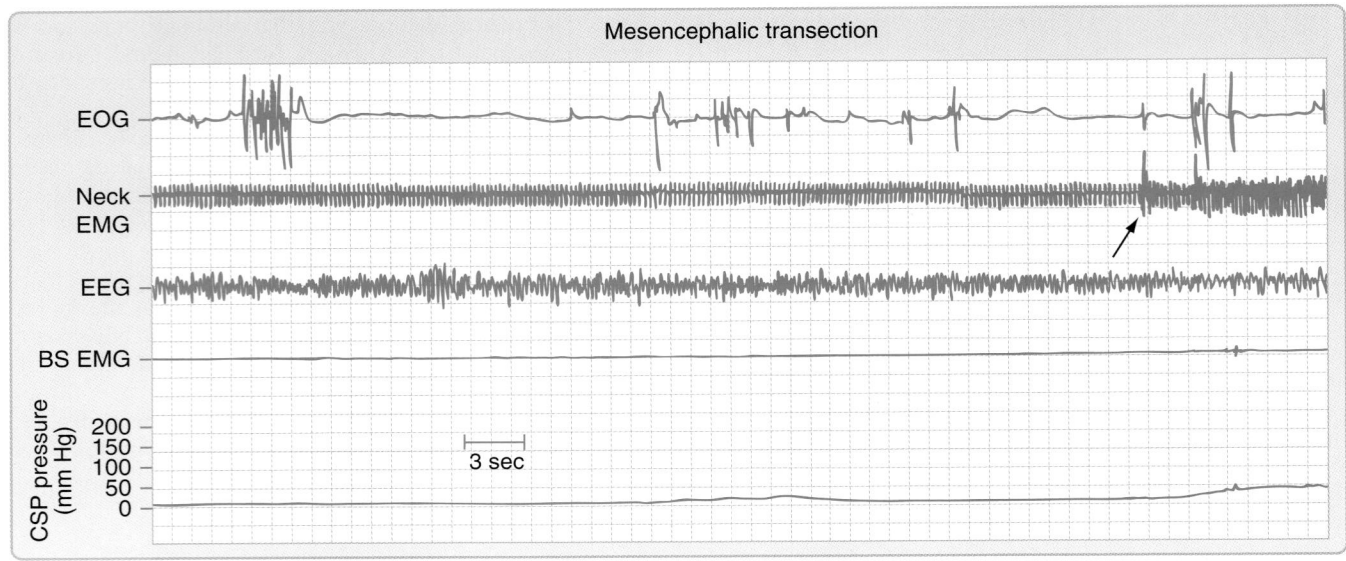

Figure 25–6. A polygraphic recording of paradoxical sleep (PS) before (*control*) and after mesencephalic transection. *Control*, A PS-related erectile event in the intact rat characterized by an increase in baseline corpus spongiosum of the penis (CSP) pressure and, with bulbospongiosus (BS) muscle bursts, and large pressure peaks. *Mesencephalic transection*, A PS episode after mesencephalic transection in the same rat. Note the simultaneous appearance of rapid eye movements in the electrooculogram (EOG) and muscle atonia in the neck electromyogram (EMG), which defines PS in the *cerveau isolé* rat. The *arrow* marks the end of the PS episode with a return of neck EMG activity. Activity seen in the neck EMG during the PS episode is electrocardiographic artifact on an otherwise atonic baseline. Although PS was found to persist after mesencephalic transection, PS erectile activity was severely disrupted, as seen by the absence of CSP pressure changes or BS muscle bursts. EEG, electroencephalogram. (From Schmidt MH, Sakai K, Valatx JL, et al: The effects of spinal or mesencephalic transections on sleep-related erections and ex-copula penile reflexes in the rat. Sleep 1999;22:409-418.)

The preoptic area may be a primary candidate in this regard given its dual role in both reproductive physiology and sleep generation. The role of the preoptic area as a "sleep center" is supported by numerous stimulation, lesion, and unit recording studies. Moreover, a set of neurons in this region has been demonstrated to exhibit a specific unitary activity during PS.[86] Finally, the MPOA has been identified to contain androgen-sensitive neurons important for reproductive physiology,[87,88] and, as noted earlier, SREs are thought to be androgen sensitive.

A series of cytotoxic lesions with ibotenic acid of the preoptic area suggest that this region plays an important role in PS

erectile control.[89] Lesions of the lateral preoptic area (LPOA), as in the lateral preoptic and medial preoptic–lateral preoptic groups in Figure 25–7, cause a severe and significant reduction in PS-related erections. In contrast, lesions of the entire rostrocaudal extent of the MPOA, as in the medial preoptic group in Figure 25–7, have no significant effects on SRE or waking-state erectile activity. Because the total PS duration, average PS episode duration, and number of PS phases did not significantly change postlesion in all groups, the decrease in PS erectile activity cannot be attributed to a disruption in PS architecture. Interestingly, the total number of erections during wakefulness, as well as the number of erections per

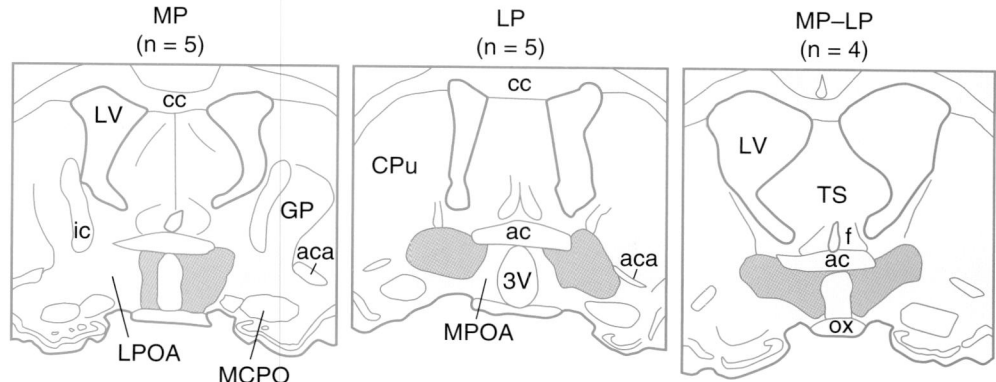

Figure 25-7. Three groups of rats with bilateral neurotoxic lesions of the preoptic area were identified. *MP*, Cytotoxic lesions were generally restricted to the medial preoptic area (MPOA) (*dark blue area*). *LP*, Bilateral lesions involved the lateral preoptic area (LPOA) (*dark blue area*) while leaving the MPOA intact. *MP-LP*, Neurotoxic lesions were more extensive in this group, involving both the MPOA and LPOA (*dark blue area*). ac, anterior commissure; aca, anterior commissure, anterior part; cc, corpus callosum; CPu, caudate putamen; f, fornix; GP, globus pallidus; ic, internal capsule; LP, lateral preoptic; LV, lateral ventricle; MCPO, magnocellular preoptic nucleus; MP, medial preoptic; MP-LP, medial preoptic–lateral preoptic; ox, optic chiasm; TS, triangular septal nucleus. (From Schmidt MH, Valatx JL, Sakai K, et al: Role of the lateral preoptic area in sleep-related erectile mechanisms and sleep generation in the rat. J Neurosci 2000;20:6640-6647.)

hour of wakefulness, were only minimally affected in all groups. These data confirm an essential role of the forebrain in PS erectile control, as was originally suggested from the brainstem transection experiments, and they identify a new region in erection neurophysiology.

DIRECTIONS FOR FUTURE RESEARCH

The executive structures of PS are located in the brainstem, as well as the subsystems that generate the classic tonic and phasic events of this sleep state. Although PS persists after mesencephalic transections or even after the complete removal of all neural elements rostral to the pons, an intact LPOA appears critical for the production of PS-related erections. Waking-state erections, however, appear minimally affected by LPOA lesioning. These findings raise several salient questions regarding SRE neurophysiology.

First, given the role of the brainstem in the generation of PS, how does the brainstem control forebrain erectile mechanisms during this sleep state? A potential source of ascending modulation of the LPOA from brainstem PS executive structures has recently been explored. Koyama et al.[90] performed single-unit recordings within the lateral dorsal tegmental nucleus (LDT) in unanesthetized head-restrained rats while simultaneously recording sleep–wake states and penile erections. These authors identified a group of putative cholinergic neurons in the LDT that significantly increase their firing rate in direct association with penile erections during PS, yet are not active during erections in wakefulness.[90] The presence of PS-erection-on neurons in the LDT would be consistent with the role of the LDT in the generation of both REM sleep and other tonic and phasic phenomena characteristic of this sleep state, including cortical activation and PGO spike wave generation. Given the major ascending projections from the LDT to the forebrain, Schmidt et al.[91] hypothesize that ascending cholinergic mechanisms may be involved in PS-related erectile control. These authors performed a series of iontophoretic injections involving carbachol, a potent cholinergic agonist, into the LPOA with a multibarrel micropipette assembly using the head-restrained rat model.

Carbachol administration into the LPOA was found significantly and consistently to trigger penile erections, whereas similar injections into neighboring forebrain regions were not effective.[91] The retrograde tracer cholera toxin B subunit was injected from an adjacent barrel of the micropipette assembly in sites where carbachol triggered penile erections. Double staining for choline acetyltransferase revealed that the LDT was the only source of cholinergic input to the LPOA. Although much research is needed to elucidate the role of the brainstem in modulating the LPOA and forebrain erectile mechanisms, these data would suggest that putative cholinergic PS-erection-on neurons in the LDT may generate erections during PS, at least in part, by releasing acetylcholine into the LPOA, as shown in Figure 25–8.

What is the role of the brainstem, if any, in the direct descending control of PS-related erections? Although results from mesencephalic transections suggest that the brainstem is not sufficient for PS erectile generation, the data do not exclude a potential role of the brainstem in the direct descending control of the spinal cord in PS-related erectile control. As described earlier, a major source of tonic descending inhibition of the spinal erection generator is located in the brainstem nPGi and involves 5-HT as a neurotransmitter. It is well established that brainstem serotonergic neurons generally cease firing during PS (PS-off neurons).[92] One may speculate, therefore, that a decrease in serotonergic inhibition from the brainstem could play an important role in the production of PS erectile activity.

How does the LPOA modulate the spinal erection generator during PS given that it does not project to the spinal cord? As shown in Figure 25–2, relay structures projecting to the spinal cord have been elucidated in erectile mechanisms, characterized by a descending oxytocinergic excitation from the PVN and the removal of a descending serotonergic inhibition from the nPGi. Microinjections of the anterograde tracer *Phaseolus vulgaris* leukoagglutinin into the LPOA demonstrate a strong projection from the LPOA to both the PVN and nPGi (Schmidt et al., unpublished data). As shown in Figure 25–8, the LPOA may play a role in sleep-related erectile control through its relay connections with the PVN and nPGi.

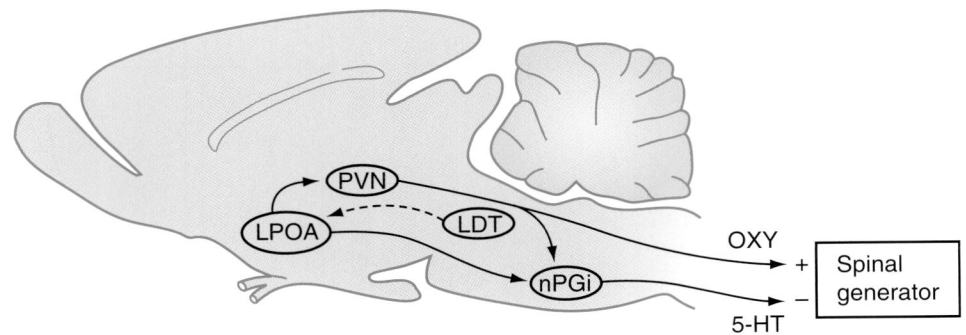

Figure 25–8. A working model of the neural control of sleep-related penile erections. The lateral preoptic area (LPOA) may play a role in paradoxical sleep (PS) erectile mechanisms by modulating a final common path from brain to spinal cord. The LPOA sends a strong projection to the paraventricular nucleus (PVN) and nucleus paragigantocellularis (nPGi; see text). The PVN and nPGi play an important role in descending excitation (+) and inhibition (−), respectively, of the spinal erection generator and may comprise a final common path in descending erectile control (see Fig. 25–2). The PVN also projects to the nPGi and may modulate this medullary source of descending erectile inhibition. Recent data demonstrate the presence of putative cholinergic neurons in the lateral dorsal tegmental nucleus (LDT) that increase their firing rate specifically in association with PS erectile events. The LDT may modulate LPOA PS erectile mechanisms through their ascending projections to the forebrain. See text for details. OXY, oxytocin; 5-HT, serotonin.

The neurotransmitter in the LPOA involved in efferent PS erectile control remains to be determined and would be purely a matter of speculation given the marked heterogeneity of this forebrain region.

Are sleep-related and waking-state erections generated by different neural mechanisms? LPOA lesioning, for example, selectively disrupts tumescence in sleep with only minimal effects on erectile activity during wakefulness.[89] In addition, hypogonadal states adversely affect SREs yet have little effect on erections induced by visual erotic stimulation during wakefulness.[79] The answer to this question is further complicated by data suggesting that neural mechanisms of waking-state erections may be context specific.[58] That is, waking-state erections may be generated by different higher central mechanisms depending on the context in which the erection occurs. For example, lesions of the BNST severely disrupt noncontact erections in male rats when in the vicinity of receptive females but cause only moderate deficits in copulation.[34] Similar lesions of the MPOA, in contrast, disrupt copulation yet leave noncontact erections intact.[34] Moreover, erections may be induced reflexively by stimulating the external genitalia without descending input from supraspinal structures. As noted earlier, stimulation of the hippocampus produces an erection,[18] and one may speculate that the hippocampus and cortex may be involved in psychogenic erections generated from memory or fantasy. The amygdala and olfactory bulbs, on the other hand, may be more involved in erections induced by olfactory stimuli.[35] The various forebrain structures involved in context-specific erectile control may possibly exert their influence on spinal mechanisms by modulating a final common pathway, or relay structures, from brain to spinal cord. Our data give further support to the hypothesis that context-specific erections, such as those generated during sleep, may involve specialized higher central mechanisms.

Finally, the function of penile tumescence in sleep remains an enigma. One may speculate that repetitive nocturnal erections from infancy to old age potentially play a role in both the development and maintenance of erectile neural circuitry from the end-organ to supraspinal levels, as well as perhaps in the daily "exercise" of skeletal perineal muscles essential for penile rigidity. Given the unpredictable nature of mating opportunities for many species, it is tempting to hypothesize that daily SRE activity since birth would confer a reproductive advantage in generating an erection relative to a competing male who may have never produced a penile erection before his first sexual encounter.

Although more than half a century has passed since the discovery of erection cycles during sleep, the neural mechanisms of such erections have only begun to be explored. Advances in our understanding of peripheral mechanisms have led to the development of the first oral medication for erectile dysfunction (i.e., sildenafil), which is hypothesized to exert its effect at the end-organ level.[11] Continued research is required to elucidate potential central mechanisms of human erectile dysfunction. For example, supraspinal etiologies of psychogenic impotence remain to be investigated. The hypothesis that context-specific erections may involve specialized higher central mechanisms would suggest that impotent men with normal SREs, commonly defined as psychogenic impotence, may suffer from context-specific "organic impotence." Central contributions to erectile dysfunction in common disease entities, such as diabetes, which has numerous peripheral consequences, are also poorly understood. These examples underscore the need to explore

---

Clinical Pearl

Penile erections are a robust physiologic phenomenon during paradoxical sleep (PS), also known as rapid eye movement sleep, from infancy to the elderly in all normal healthy males. Sleep-related erections are well documented to be adversely affected after androgen deficiency; however, such erections usually persist and often remain within the normal range in the face of low androgen levels. Although the brainstem is sufficient for the generation and maintenance of PS, the brainstem is not sufficient for the generation of penile erections during this sleep state. The lateral preoptic area in the forebrain plays an essential role in sleep-related erectile neurophysiology.

both central and peripheral etiologies of erectile failure. The development of an animal model for SRE research may stimulate much-needed basic and applied SRE research and help develop new directions for alternative treatments of erectile dysfunction.

Acknowledgments

Research was supported in part by the Ohio Sleep Medicine and Neuroscience Institute, the Sleep Medicine Research Foundation, INSERM U52, CNRS URA 1195, Claude Bernard University, and the Medical College of Ohio. Special thanks are given to Helmut S. Schmidt for introducing me to the field of sleep and for his ongoing input and critical review of this manuscript, to the laboratory of Professor Michel Jouvet for providing invaluable support for much of the research presented in this chapter, to Kevin McKenna for his review of portions of the chapter, and to Jason Davis and Esther Culp for their help in preparation of the manuscript.

References

1. Ohlmeyer P, Brilmayer H, Hüllstrung H: Periodische Vorgänge im Schlaf. Pflugers Arch 1944;248:559-560.
2. Fisher C, Gorss J, Zuch J: Cycle of penile erection synchronous with dreaming (REM) sleep: Preliminary report. Arch Gen Psychiatry 1965;12:29-45.
3. Karacan I, Goodenough DR, Shapiro A, et al: Erection cycle during sleep in relation to dream anxiety. Arch Gen Psychiatry 1966;15:183-189.
4. Karacan I, Salis PJ, Thornby JI, et al: The ontogeny of nocturnal penile tumescence. Waking Sleep 1976;1:27-44.
5. Fisher C, Cohen HD, Schiavi RC, et al: Patterns of female sexual arousal during sleep and waking: Vaginal thermo-conductance studies. Arch Sex Behav 1983;12:97-122.
6. Karacan I: The Effect of Exciting Presleep Events on Dream Reporting and Penile Erections During Sleep [dissertation]. Brooklyn, NY, Downstate Medical Center, State University of New York, 1965.
7. Schmidt MH, Schmidt HS: The ischiocavernosus and bulbospongiosus muscles in mammalian penile rigidity. Sleep 1993;16:171-183.
8. Sachs BD, Garinello LD: Spinal pacemaker controlling sexual reflexes in male rats. Brain Res 1979;171:152-156.
9. Giuliano F, Rampin O: Central neural regulation of penile erection. Neurosci Biobehav Rev 2000;24:517-533.
10. Wang R, Domer FR, Sikka SC, et al: Nitric oxide mediates penile erection in cats. J Urol 1994;151:234-237.
11. Goldstein I, Lue TF, Padma-Nathan H, et al: Oral sildenafil in the treatment of erectile dysfunction: Sildenafil Study Group. N Engl J Med 1998;338:1397-1404.
12. Marson L, Platt KB, McKenna KE: Central nervous system innervation of the penis as revealed by the transneuronal transport of pseudorabies virus. Neuroscience 1993;55:263-280.
13. McKenna KE, Nadelhaft I: The organization of the pudendal nerve in the male and female rat. J Comp Neurol 1986;248:532-549.
14. Sasaki M, Arnold AP: Androgenic regulation of dendritic trees of motoneurons in the spinal nucleus of the bulbocavernosus: Reconstruction after intracellular iontophoresis of horseradish peroxidase. J Comp Neurol 1991;308:11-27.
15. Rose RD, Collins WF III: Crossing dendrites may be a substrate for synchronized activation of penile motoneurons. Brain Res 1985;337:373-377.
16. Nadelhaft I, McKenna KE: Sexual dimorphism in sympathetic preganglionic neurons of the rat hypogastric nerve. J Comp Neurol 1987;256:308-315.
17. Louilot A, Gonzalez-Mora JL, Guadalupe T, et al: Sex-related olfactory stimuli induce a selective increase in dopamine release in the nucleus accumbens of male rats: A voltametric study. Brain Res 1991;553:313-317.
18. Chen KK, Chan JY, Chang LS, et al: Elicitation of penile erection following activation of the hippocampal formation in the rat. Neurosci Lett 1992;141:218-222.
19. Maeda N, Matsuoka N, Yamaguchi I: Possible involvement of the septo-hippocampal cholinergic and raphe-hippocampal serotonergic activations in the penile erection induced by fenfluramine in rats. Brain Res 1994;652:181-189.
20. Ginton A, Merari A: Long range effects of MPOA lesion on mating behavior in the male rat. Brain Res 1977;120:158-163.
21. Hansen S, Kohler C, Goldstein M, et al: Effects of ibotenic acid-induced neuronal degeneration in the medial preoptic area and the lateral hypothalamic area on sexual behavior in the male rat. Brain Res 1982;239:213-232.
22. Merari A, Ginton A: Characteristics of exaggerated sexual behavior induced by electrical stimulation of the medial preoptic area in male rats. Brain Res 1975;86:97-108.
23. Giuliano F, Rampin O, Brown K, et al: Stimulation of the medial preoptic area of the hypothalamus in the rat elicits increases in intracavernous pressure. Neurosci Lett 1996;209:1-4.
24. Marson L, McKenna KE: Stimulation of the hypothalamus initiates the urethrogenital reflex in male rats. Brain Res 1994;638:103-108.
25. Shimura T, Yamamoto T, Shimokochi M: The medial preoptic area is involved in both sexual arousal and performance in male rats: Re-evaluation of neuron activity in freely moving animals. Brain Res 1994;640:215-222.
26. Baum MJ, Everitt BJ: Increased expression of c-fos in the medial preoptic area after mating in male rats: Role of afferent inputs from the medial amygdala and midbrain central tegmental field. Neuroscience 1992;50:627-646.
27. Erskine MS: Mating-induced increases in FOS protein in preoptic area and medial amygdala of cycling female rats. Brain Res Bull 1993;32:447-451.
28. Mas M, Rodriguez DC, Guerra M, et al: Neurochemical correlates of male sexual behavior. Physiol Behav 1987;41:341-345.
29. Hull EM, Eaton RC, Markowski VP, et al: Opposite influence of medial preoptic D1 and D2 receptors on genital reflexes: Implications for copulation. Life Sci 1992;51:1705-1713.
30. Markowski VP, Eaton RC, Lumley LA, et al: A D1 agonist in the MPOA facilitates copulation in male rats. Pharmacol Biochem Behav 1994;47:483-486.
31. Warner RK, Thompson JT, Markowski VP, et al: Microinjection of the dopamine antagonist cis-flupentixol into the MPOA impairs copulation, penile reflexes and sexual motivation in male rats. Brain Res 1991;540:177-182.
32. Meisel RL, Lumia AR, Sachs BD: Effects of olfactory bulb removal and flank shock on copulation in male rats. Physiol Behav 1980;25:383-387.
33. Wood RI, Coolen LM: Integration of chemosensory and hormonal cues is essential for sexual behaviour in the male Syrian hamster: Role of the medial amygdaloid nucleus. Neuroscience 1997;78:1027-1035.
34. Liu YC, Salamone JD, Sachs BD: Lesions in medial preoptic area and bed nucleus of stria terminalis: Differential effects on copulatory behavior and noncontact erection in male rats. J Neurosci 1997;17:5245-5253.
35. Sachs BD, Meisel RL: The physiology of male sexual behavior. In Knobil E, Neill J (eds): The Physiology of Reproduction. New York, Raven Press, 1988, pp 1393-1485.
36. Marson L, McKenna KE: Serotonergic neurotoxic lesions facilitate male sexual reflexes. Pharmacol Biochem Behav 1994;47:883-888.
37. Marson L, McKenna KE: A role for 5-hydroxytryptamine in descending inhibition of spinal sexual reflexes. Exp Brain Res 1992;88:313-320.

38. McKenna KE, Chung SK, McVary KT: A model for the study of sexual function in anesthetized male and female rats. Am J Physiol 1991;261:R1276-R1285.

39. Marson L, McKenna KE: The identification of a brainstem site controlling spinal sexual reflexes in male rats. Brain Res 1990;515:303-308.

40. Yells DP, Hendricks SE, Prendergast MA: Lesions of the nucleus paragigantocellularis: Effects on mating behavior in male rats. Brain Res 1992;596:73-79.

41. Marson L, List MS, McKenna KE: Lesions of the nucleus paragigantocellularis alter ex copula penile reflexes. Brain Res 1992;592:187-192.

42. Morrison SF, Gebber GL: Raphe neurons with sympathetic-related activity: Baroreceptor responses and spinal connections. Am J Physiol 1984;246:R338-R348.

43. Ma RC, Dun NJ: Excitation of lateral horn neurons of the neonatal rat spinal cord by 5-hydroxytryptamine. Brain Res 1986;389:89-98.

44. Coote JH, Macleod VH, Fleetwood-Walker S, et al: The response of individual sympathetic preganglionic neurones to microelectrophoretically applied endogenous monoamines. Brain Res 1981;215:135-145.

45. McCall RB: Serotonergic excitation of sympathetic preganglionic neurons: A microiontophoretic study. Brain Res 1983;289:121-127.

46. Gilbey MP, McKenna KE, Schramm LP: Effects of substance P on sympathetic preganglionic neurones. Neurosci Lett 1983;41:157-159.

47. Gilbey MP, Coote JH, Macleod VH, et al: Inhibition of sympathetic activity by stimulating in the raphe nuclei and the role of 5-hydroxytryptamine in this effect. Brain Res 1981;226:131-142.

48. McCall RB, Clement ME: Identification of serotonergic and sympathetic neurons in medullary raphe nuclei. Brain Res 1989;477:172-182.

49. Argiolas A, Melis MR, Gessa GL: Oxytocin: An extremely potent inducer of penile erection and yawning in male rats. Eur J Pharmacol 1986;130:265-272.

50. Argiolas A, Melis MR, Vargiu L, et al: d(CH2)5Tyr(Me)-[Orn8]vasotocin, a potent oxytocin antagonist, antagonizes penile erection and yawning induced by oxytocin and apomorphine, but not by ACTH-(1-24). Eur J Pharmacol 1987;134:221-224.

51. Liu YC, Salamone JD, Sachs BD: Impaired sexual response after lesions of the paraventricular nucleus of the hypothalamus in male rats. Behav Neurosci 1997;111:1361-1367.

52. Melis MR, Succu S, Mascia MS, et al: The activation of gamma aminobutyric acid(A) receptors in the paraventricular nucleus of the hypothalamus reduces non-contact penile erections in male rats. Neurosci Lett 2001;314:123-126.

53. Melis MR, Stancampiano R, Argiolas A: Penile erection and yawning induced by paraventricular NMDA injection in male rats are mediated by oxytocin. Pharmacol Biochem Behav 1994;48:203-207.

54. Veronneau-Longueville F, Rampin O, Freund-Mercier MJ, et al: Oxytocinergic innervation of autonomic nuclei controlling penile erection in the rat. Neuroscience 1999;93:1437-1447.

55. Luiten PG, ter Horst GJ, Karst H, et al: The course of paraventricular hypothalamic efferents to autonomic structures in medulla and spinal cord. Brain Res 1985;329:374-378.

56. Wagner CK, Clemens LG: Projections of the paraventricular nucleus of the hypothalamus to the sexually dimorphic lumbosacral region of the spinal cord. Brain Res 1991;539:254-262.

57. Bancila M, Giuliano F, Rampin O, et al: Evidence for a direct projection from the paraventricular nucleus of the hypothalamus to putative serotoninergic neurons of the nucleus paragigantocellularis involved in the control of erection in rats. Eur J Neurosci 2002;16:1240-1248.

58. Sachs BD: Contextual approaches to the physiology and classification of erectile function, erectile dysfunction, and sexual arousal. Neurosci Biobehav Rev 2000;24:541-560.

59. Pearson OP: Reproduction in the shrew (*Blarina brevicaudasay*). Am J Anat 1944;75:39-93.

60. Snyder F: The REM State in a Living Fossil. Palo Alto, Calif, Association for the Psychophysiological Study of Sleep, 1964.

61. Schmidt MH, Valatx JL, Schmidt HS, et al: Experimental evidence of penile erections during paradoxical sleep in the rat. Neuroreport 1994;5:561-564.

62. Schmidt MH, Valatx JL, Sakai K, et al: Corpus spongiosum penis pressure and perineal muscle activity during reflexive erections in the rat. Am J Physiol 1995;269:R904-R913.

63. Giuliano F, Bernabe J, Rampin O, et al: Telemetric monitoring of intracavernous pressure in freely moving rats during copulation. J Urol 1994;152:1271-1274.

64. Bernabe J, Rampin O, Giuliano F, et al: Intracavernous pressure changes during reflexive penile erections in the rat. Physiol Behav 1995;57:837-841.

65. Nofzinger EA, Schmidt HS: An exploration of central dysregulation of erectile function as a contributing cause of diabetic impotence. J Nerv Ment Dis 1990;178:90-95.

66. Thase ME, Reynolds CF III, Glanz LM, et al: Nocturnal penile tumescence in depressed men. Am J Psychiatry 1987;144:89-92.

67. Rosen RC, Weiner DN: Cardiovascular disease and sleep-related erections. J Psychosom Res 1997;42:517-530.

68. Hirshkowitz M, Moore CA, O'Connor S, et al: Androgen and sleep-related erections. J Psychosom Res 1997;42:541-546.

69. Karacan I, Hursch CJ, Williams RL, et al: Some characteristics of nocturnal penile tumescence in young adults. Arch Gen Psychiatry 1972;26:351-356.

70. Hirshkowitz M, Moore CA: Sleep-related erectile activity. Neurol Clin 1996;14:721-737.

71. Fisher C, Schiavi P, Lear H, et al: The assessment of nocturnal REM erection in the differential diagnosis of sexual impotence. J Sex Marital Ther 1975;1:277-289.

72. O'Carroll R, Shapiro C, Bancroft J: Androgens, behaviour and nocturnal erection in hypogonadal men: The effects of varying the replacement dose. Clin Endocrinol (Oxf) 1985;23:527-538.

73. Cunningham GR, Hirshkowitz M, Korenman SG, et al: Testosterone replacement therapy and sleep-related erections in hypogonadal men. J Clin Endocrinol Metab 1990;70:792-797.

74. Carani C, Scuteri A, Marrama P, et al: The effects of testosterone administration and visual erotic stimuli on nocturnal penile tumescence in normal men. Horm Behav 1990;24:435-441.

75. Cooper AJ, Cernovovsky Z: The effects of cyproterone acetate on sleeping and waking penile erections in pedophiles: Possible implications for treatment. Can J Psychiatry 1992;37:33-39.

76. Cooper AJ, Losztyn S, Russell NC, et al: Medroxyprogesterone acetate, nocturnal penile tumescence, laboratory arousal, and sexual acting out in a male with schizophrenia. Arch Sex Behav 1990;19:361-372.

77. Schiavi RC, White D, Mandeli J, et al: Effect of testosterone administration on sexual behavior and mood in men with erectile dysfunction. Arch Sex Behav 1997;26:231-241.

78. Skakkebaek NE, Bancroft J, Davidson DW, et al: Androgen replacement with oral testosterone undecenoate in hypogonadal men: A double blind controlled study. Clin Endocrinol (Oxf) 1981;14:49-61.

79. Carani C, Bancroft J, Granata A, et al: Testosterone and erectile function, nocturnal penile tumescence and rigidity, and erectile response to visual erotic stimuli in hypogonadal and eugonadal men. Psychoneuroendocrinology 1992;17:647-654.

80. Sachs BD: Placing erection in context: the reflexogenic-psychogenic dichotomy reconsidered. Neurosci Biobehav Rev 1995;19:211-224.

81. Buena F, Swerdloff RS, Steiner BS, et al: Sexual function does not change when serum testosterone levels are pharmacologically varied within the normal male range. Fertil Steril 1993;59:1118-1123.

82. Karacan I, Dervent A, Salis PJ, et al: Spinal cord injuries and NPT. Sleep Res 1978;7:261.

83. Karacan I, Dimitrijevic M, Lauber A, et al: Nocturnal penile tumescence (NPT) and sleep stages in patients with spinal cord injuries. Sleep Res 1977;6:52.

84. Schmidt MH, Sakai K, Valatx JL, et al: The effects of spinal or mesencephalic transections on sleep-related erections and ex-copula penile reflexes in the rat. Sleep 1999;22:409-418.

85. Jones BE: Paradoxical sleep and its chemical/structural substrates in the brain. Neuroscience 1991;40:637-656.

86. Koyama Y, Hayaishi O: Firing of neurons in the preoptic/anterior hypothalamic areas in rat: Its possible involvement in slow wave sleep and paradoxical sleep. Neurosci Res 1994;19:31-38.

87. Anderson RH, Fleming DE, Rhees RW, et al: Relationships between sexual activity, plasma testosterone, and the volume of the sexually dimorphic nucleus of the preoptic area in prenatally stressed and non-stressed rats. Brain Res 1986;370:1-10.

88. Cherry JA, Tobet SA, DeVoogd TJ, et al: Effects of sex and androgen treatment on dendritic dimensions of neurons in the sexually dimorphic preoptic/anterior hypothalamic area of male and female ferrets. J Comp Neurol 1992;323:577-585.

89. Schmidt MH, Valatx JL, Sakai K, et al: Role of the lateral preoptic area in sleep-related erectile mechanisms and sleep generation in the rat. J Neurosci 2000;20:6640-6647.

90. Koyama Y, Schmidt MH, Takahashi K, et al: Cholinergic neurons in the laterodorsal tegmental nucleus regulate penile erections during paradoxical sleep. In Abstract Viewer/Itinerary Planner. San Diego, CA: Society for Neuroscience; 2001: Progr No 522.20.

91. Schmidt MH, Gervasoni D, Luppi PH, et al: Carbachol administration into the lateral preoptic area induces penile erections and wakefulness. In Abstract Viewer/Itinerary Planner. San Diego, CA: Society for Neuroscience; 2001: Progr No 522.19.

92. Sakai K: Neurons responsible for paradoxical sleep. In Wauquier A, Gaillard JM, Monti JM, Radulovacki M (eds): Sleep: Neurotransmitters and Neuromodulators. New York, Raven Press, 1985, pp 29-42.

Master Circadian Clock, Master Circadian Rhythm

Fred W. Turek
Christine Dugovic
Aaron D. Laposky

ABSTRACT

Studies over the past 3 decades have established that a master circadian clock resides in the bilaterally paired suprachiasmatic nucleus (SCN) in the anterior hypothalamus; the SCN clock controls the timing of most, if not all, circadian rhythms in mammals. The expression of many behavior and physiologic rhythms depends on the control of the diurnal rhythm of the sleep–wake cycle by the SCN, which in turn regulates the timing of rhythms that depend on the presence or absence of sleep and wake behaviors. Thus, the sleep–wake cycle can be considered to be the master circadian rhythm, regulating the expression of many diurnal rhythms. The circadian and sleep control centers have evolved together to ensure that the timing of internal events relative to one another, as well as to the external environment, are synchronized to maximize the survival of the organism.

One of the distinguishing characteristics of sleep in animals as diverse as insects, fish, and mammals is that the timing of sleep and wake for the vast majority of species is rigidly confined to certain times of the day or night. As detailed in a number of chapters in this section, the master biological clock regulating the timing of sleep and wake in mammals also regulates most, if not all, 24-hour (i.e., circadian) behavioral, physiologic, and biochemical rhythms. This master circadian clock is located in the bilaterally paired suprachiasmatic nucleus (SCN) in the anterior hypothalamus (see Chapter 28). Although it has recently been discovered that many tissues and organs can generate circadian rhythms independent of the SCN in vitro (Chapter 29), the SCN remains at the top of the hierarchy of the mammalian circadian clock system.

Similarly, one could argue that the sleep–wake cycle represents the "master circadian rhythm"; the SCN control of this rhythm in turn controls the timing and expression of a multitude of downstream rhythms. Although the expression of many 24-hour rhythms may be primarily under the control of the circadian clock in the SCN, many rhythms are largely dependent on whether the organism is asleep or awake, regardless of the circadian clock time.[1] Undoubtedly, the expression of most rhythms at the behavioral, physiologic, and biochemical levels are regulated by the integration of inputs from the circadian clock and the sleep–wake state of the animal. Indeed, it can be argued that the entire temporal organization of an organism represents some combined effect of circadian clock inputs and the sleep–wake state of the organism. Thus, the circadian and sleep control centers have evolved together to ensure that the timing of internal events relative to one another and to the external environment are coordinated in such a fashion as to maximize the survival of the species.

Indeed, the need to "rest" and the need to adjust to the daily changes in the physical environment that result from celestial mechanics certainly represented two darwinian pressures that have guided the evolution of living organisms since the beginning of time (it is thought that, at an earlier time in the history of the earth, the solar day was 18 hours; the change to the current 24-hour day occurred over millions of years, allowing plenty of time for clock genes to be altered, so the molecular circadian cycle stayed in synchrony with the solar day). As detailed in the rest of this chapter, the early linkage for the need to rest, and to rest at a specific phase (or at specific phases) of the daily external environment, may have resulted in the coevolution of the circadian clock and the sleep–wake cycle and their being integrated with one another at many different levels of organization.

THE INTEGRATION OF THE CIRCADIAN CLOCK AND SLEEP–WAKE SYSTEMS

The next four chapters in this section ("Chronobiology") of this book deal primarily with the circadian clock system, with a focus on the following:

1. The formal properties and "rules" that govern the generation of circadian rhythms (Chapter 27).

2. The anatomy of the neural clock system in mammals (Chapter 28).
3. The physiology of the mammalian circadian clock system (Chapter 29).
4. The molecular genetic bases for the actual circadian core machinery, which has been highly conserved at least from insects to mammals (Chapter 30).

The remaining five chapters then discuss from different vantage points how the circadian clock system is highly integrated with the sleep–wake regulatory system. Chapter 32 focuses on the still mysterious pineal gland hormone, melatonin. Although the synthesis and release of melatonin is under tight regulatory control via circadian neural signals from the SCN, melatonin itself can act as a "chronobiotic" and influence the timing of SCN-controlled rhythms, and it also appears to be a "hypnotic" that can directly influence the drive to sleep. Chapters 31, 33, and 34 focus specifically on how the circadian process and the homeostatic process work together and independently to regulate sleep. The complex nature of this interaction requires more of an introduction, and this will be provided here. Finally, the last chapter in this section (Chapter 35) focuses on how the circadian clock and sleep loss together, and independently, regulate neurobehavioral performances.

In the now classic two-process model of Borbely and colleagues, the timing of sleep and wake is a function of a homeostatic process that defines sleep need as being dependent on the previous amount of sleep and wake (process S), and on the circadian clock (process C) that modulates the timing and propensity of sleep (Chapter 33). However, as noted by Czeisler and coworkers (Chapter 31) the interactions between the circadian pacemaker and sleep homeostat should not be underestimated, and there is great difficulty in separating these two processes functionally. In addition, recent genetic and anatomic findings (Chapters 30 and 34) also tend to blur the distinction between the homeostatic and circadian inputs in the regulation of the sleep–wake cycle.

In the two-process model, the electroencephalographic slow wave activity in non–rapid eye movement (NREM) sleep serves as an indicator of sleep homeostasis either under baseline or after sleep deprivation conditions. Although substantial evidence indicates that sleep homeostasis, as defined by the slow wave activity during NREM sleep, is independent mechanistically from the circadian clock, it is not known how the two processes actually contribute to the overall sleep need of the organism, or what role the circadian clock may play in other homeostatically regulated sleep–wake events, such as total sleep time, NREM sleep time, or rapid eye movement (REM) sleep time under baseline or sleep deprivation conditions.

Evidence has accumulated for a critical role for mammalian circadian clock genes in sleep–wake regulation that goes beyond just the circadian timing of sleep. For example, in *Clock* mutant mice, NREM sleep is reduced by 1 to 2 hours per day under both light–dark and dark–dark conditions, and the rebound of REM sleep after sleep deprivation is attenuated.[2] Sleep time in mice with deletion of the Clock heterodimer partner, BMAL1, is increased (Chapter 30). Interestingly, Cry1,2 double-knockout mice have a severely attenuated sleep–wake rhythm and increased NREM baseline sleep time and NREM delta power, similar to BMAL1/KO mice, as well as decreased compensatory responses after sleep deprivation.[3] The variety of sleep phenotypes among these genetic models suggests unique roles for individual genes in the sleep regulatory system. Determining whether the mechanisms linking the circadian and sleep systems are specific to the circadian clock feedback-loop, or whether they extend to posttranslational and noncircadian pathways, remains to be determined. The finding of circadian clock gene expression in a variety of brain regions, including some that are involved in sleep regulation,[4] raises the possibility that changes in circadian clock gene expression (independent of SCN timing mechanisms) may underlie the wide-ranging effects of circadian clock genes on sleep architecture.

The fruit fly, *Drosophila*, has emerged as an important model for studying the molecular and genetic regulation of sleep. The identification of rest–activity patterns in flies that parallel properties of sleep–wake states in mice, including compensatory responses to rest deprivation, has led to evidence for the role of circadian clock genes in the homeostatic regulation of rest–activity in flies.[5] Thus, a body of literature is now accumulating from studies with flies and mice, suggesting the hypothesis that homologous genes identified as core elements of the circadian clock in these diverse species also influence sleep regulatory processes that are involved in the amount and consolidation of sleep and wake bouts, amount of sleep, sleep architecture, and the rebound response to sleep deprivation. The use of genetically altered flies and mice is expected to lead to new insights into the mechanisms governing circadian and sleep regulatory processes and how these processes have remained integrated with one another to regulate the overall temporal organization of diverse animals over millions of years of evolutionary time.

REGULATING SLEEP AMOUNT: A HOMEOSTATIC AND A CIRCADIAN INPUT

All phases of normal sleep and wake are under homeostatic control. That is, the longer one is awake or deprived of specific sleep stages (e.g., REM sleep deprivation), the greater will be the drive to recover the lost sleep or sleep stage. In addition, all phases of normal sleep and wake are under circadian control; the clock is doing more than saying wake up and go to sleep at specific times of day. An unanswered question is, what actually regulates the amount of sleep? Or, put another way, what are the relative contributions of the homeostatic control and of the circadian control to the actual amounts of time a given animal is awake and interacting with the external world or asleep and avoiding the external world? Studies in laboratory, zoo, and wild animals reveal that sleep times are unrelated to taxonomic classification, and, as noted by Siegel,[6] "The range of sleep times of different primates extensively overlaps that of rodents which overlaps that of carnivores, and so on across many orders of mammals." The total sleep time is correlated in a global sense to body size with, for example, the opossum sleeping 18 hours, the ferret 14.4 hours, the cat 12.5 hours, the dog 10.1 hours, humans 8 hours, and the elephant 3 hours.[6] Although on a global level, body size (and associated metabolic rate) is inversely related to total sleep time, there appear to be other factors regulating sleep time, as indicated by the fact that the smaller mouse sleeps about the same amount as the larger rat.[7-10] Indeed, there is considerable variability in sleep time among strains of mice: strains of mice that are of similar size and of the same species can show total sleep time differences of up to 2.5 hours.[9]

In the evolution of life on earth, there has been great pressure for organisms to (1) adapt their lifestyle to the external world, and (2) coordinate the internal temporal environment, so as to maximize the chances of survival and pass their genetic material on to the next generation. Total sleep time could be expected to be part of the survival strategy to ensure that animals were engaged as well as disengaged with the external environment at the appropriate times of day and night. Similarly, as noted at the beginning of this chapter, the sleep–wake cycle can be considered to be the master circadian rhythm, as the expression of so many behavioral and physiologic rhythms are tied to the sleep–wake/activity–rest cycle. Thus, the total amount of sleep and wake may have evolved in individual species, in part, to create an internal temporal framework, in conjunction with the circadian clock, to maximize survival and reproduction fitness.

Thinking about the circadian clock as a major determinant of the pressure to sleep and the ability to stay awake has

mechanistic indications on various neural, genetic, and molecular levels, as well as potentially important therapeutic implications for treating sleep–wake disorders. If the circadian clock is regulating not only the timing of sleep and wake, but also the propensity to sleep and to wake, then it becomes a target for interventions that could promote sleep and wakefulness that go beyond any interventions presently in use.

Clinical Pearl

The circadian clock may be sending an "alerting signal" at some times of the day, as well as a "sleep signal" at other times of the day. Thus, a disruption of these signals could lead to daytime sleepiness and/or nighttime insomnia. Alteration of the circadian clock at the molecular or systems level could lead to sleep disorders that go beyond just the abnormal timing of sleep relative to our social and work environment.

REFERENCES

1. Van Cauter E, Copinschi G, Turek FW: Endocrine and other biologic rhythms. In DeGroot LJ, Jameson JL (eds): Endocrinology, 4th ed. New York, WB Saunders, 2001, pp 235-256.
2. Naylor E, Bergmann BM, Krauski K, et al: The circadian Clock mutation alters sleep homeostasis in the mouse. J Neurosci 2000;20:8138-8143.
3. Wisor JP, O'Hara BF, Terao A, et al: A role for cryptochromes in sleep regulation. BMC Neurosci 2002;3:20.
4. Abe M, Herzog ED, Yamazaki S, et al: Circadian rhythms in isolated brain regions. J Neurosci 2002;22:350-356.
5. Hendricks JC: Sleeping flies don't lie: The use of *Drosophila melanogaster* to study sleep and circadian rhythms (Invited review). J Appl Physiol 2003;94:1660-1672; discussion, p 1673.
6. Siegel JM: Why we sleep. Sci Am 2003;289:92-97.
7. Dugovic C, Solberg LC, Redei E, et al: Sleep in the Wistar-Kyoto rat, a putative genetic animal model for depression. Neuroreport 2000;11:627-631.
8. Everson CA, Bergmann BM, Rechtschaffen A: Sleep deprivation in the rat: III. Total sleep deprivation. Sleep 1989;12:13-21.
9. Franken P, Malafosse A, Tafti M: Genetic determinants of sleep regulation in inbred mice. Sleep 1999;22:155-169.
10. Koehl M, Battle SE, Turek FW: Sleep in female mice: A strain comparison across the estrous cycle. Sleep 2003;26:267-272.

27

Circadian Rhythms in Mammals: Formal Properties and Environmental Influences

Ralph E. Mistlberger

Benjamin Rusak

ABSTRACT

Circadian rhythms are approximately 24-hour cycles of behavior and physiology that are generated by endogenous biological clocks (pacemakers or oscillators). Circadian rhythms persist ("free-run") with near 24-hour periods (cycle lengths) in time-free environments but normally are synchronized to the 24-hour day by environmental stimuli (zeitgebers or "time cues"). Synchrony is achieved by a process of entrainment, involving daily, stimulus-induced phase shifts that correct for the difference between the intrinsic period of the pacemaker and the period of the environmental cycle. Light is the dominant zeitgeber for most species and can induce phase shifts that vary in magnitude and direction depending on the circadian phase of exposure.

Circadian rhythms in some species can also be shifted and entrained by stimuli other than light, such as scheduled feeding, exercise, social interactions, and temperature variations. Entrainment to feeding schedules is mediated by a circadian pacemaker that is separate from the pacemaker mediating synchrony to light–dark cycles. Interactions between photic and nonphotic zeitgebers are complex; for example, light and exercise, depending on their relative timing and magnitude, may be synergistic or mutually inhibitory in producing phase shifts. Stable entrainment in natural environments therefore likely reflects integration of multiple zeitgebers by multiple, formally distinct pacemakers and oscillators.

Overt rhythms in behavior and physiology may emerge only weeks or months postnatally, but the circadian pacemaker responsible for entrainment to lighting cycles in adulthood is also entrained prenatally by maternal cues. Over the life span, circadian rhythms exhibit changes in period, amplitude, and responsiveness to zeitgebers. Some of these changes may lead to altered circadian organization in older people, which may contribute to disruptions in physiologic mechanisms, including those regulating sleep.

THE NATURE OF CIRCADIAN RHYTHMS

A salient characteristic of sleep in humans is its daily rhythmicity. A similar 24-hour rhythmicity characterizes the behavior, physiology, and biochemistry of most living organisms. Historically, daily rhythms were interpreted as innate or acquired responses to environmental stimuli, such as light, temperature, and humidity, that vary markedly with time of day. However, as early as 1729, it was reported that the daily rhythm of leaf movements of the heliotrope *Mimosa* does not depend on exposure to the day–night cycle, that is, the rhythm persists ("free-runs") in constant dark (DD). Many studies have since confirmed that daily rhythms in a great variety of species, including humans, free-run, often indefinitely and with impressive precision, despite housing in controlled environments that lack variations in lighting, temperature, food access, or other stimuli[1] (Figs. 27–1, 27–2, and 27–3).

Persistence of daily rhythms for many cycles in the apparent absence of environmental time cues suggests that organisms possess one or more endogenous clocklike timekeeping mechanisms. If these mechanisms were biochemical processes within organisms, they might reasonably be expected to show dependence of rate (= frequency, the reciprocal of which is cycle duration or period, represented by the Greek letter τ) on tissue temperature because chemical processes are almost universally temperature dependent. Yet, for these mechanisms to time behavior and physiology accurately, they must be capable of cycling at a constant rate, despite variations in tissue temperature caused by changes in metabolism (for homeothermic species) or environmental conditions (for heterothermic species). The evidence accumulated in the 1950s that daily rhythms in most organisms show an impressive stability of period across a range of temperatures fueled a debate over whether daily rhythms were truly endogenously generated, or whether they reflected a response of the organism to some unknown, periodic environmental "Factor X" associated with the earth's rotation on its axis (e.g., electromagnetic fields[2]).

Although the mechanism by which daily rhythms maintain a stable period at different temperatures remains to be fully elucidated, the evidence is now overwhelming that daily clocks are endogenously generated. The most compelling behavioral evidence in support of the endogenous clock concept is the observation that daily rhythms in constant conditions typically express stable τ's that deviate from the 24-hour periodicity of the solar day, and thus would rapidly slide out of phase with any geophysical correlate of planetary rotation. This "circadian" (Latin for "approximately a day") periodicity exhibits individual differences around a species-typical mean, usually within the range of 23 to 25 hours. Consequently, individual animals housed separately but under identical environmental conditions gradually drift out of synchrony with local time and with each other. Moreover, a short (less than 24 hours) or long (greater than 24 hours) circadian τ (reflecting a fast- or slow-running circadian clock, respectively) can be selected by breeding, induced by gene mutations (see Chapter 30), drugs, hormones, or certain environmental manipulations, and may accompany aging (discussed further later).

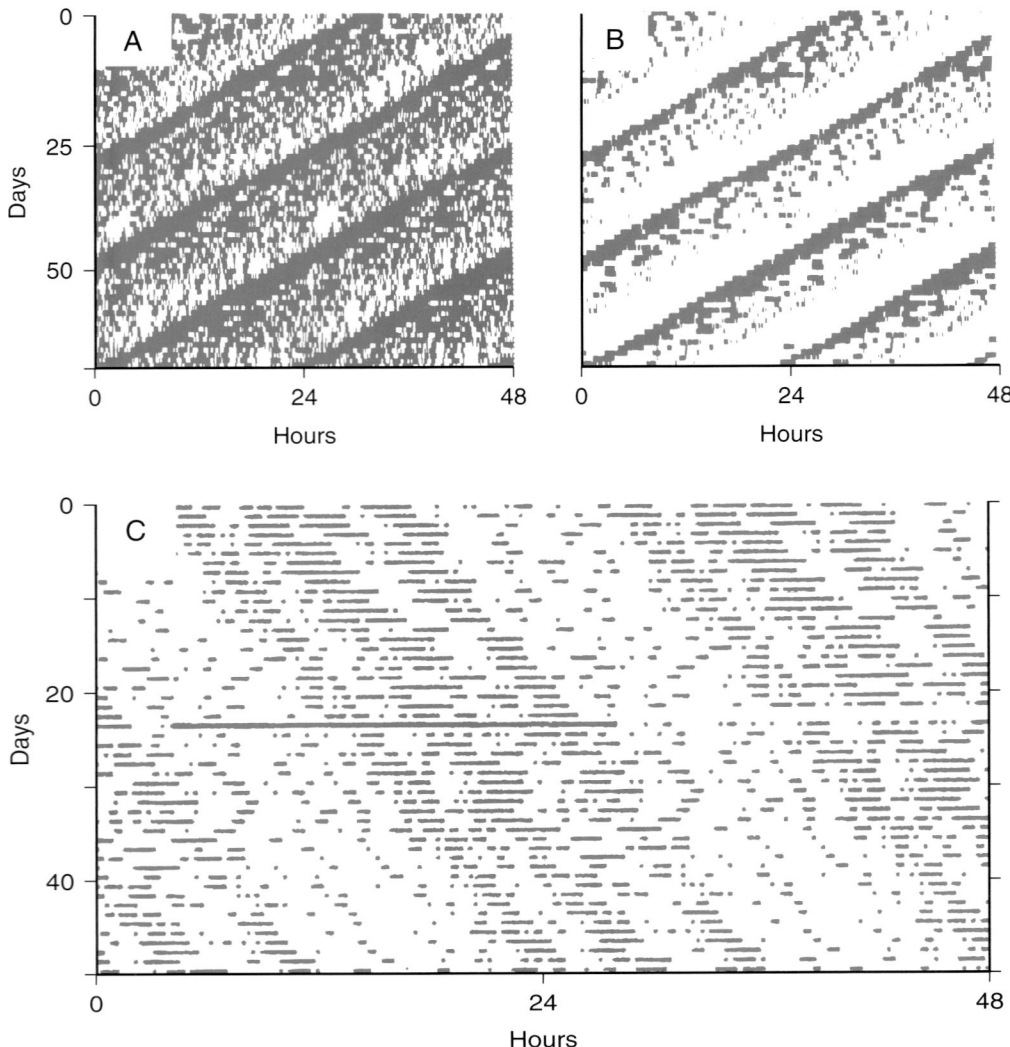

Figure 27–1. Circadian rhythms free-running in constant dark, plotted in conventional "actogram" format. **A,** The circadian rhythm of poly-graphically recorded wake time in a C57 mouse. Each line represents 48 consecutive hours, and consecutive days are aligned vertically (thus, the data are double-plotted, i.e., the right half of the chart is a duplicate of the left half, but is moved up one line). Data were collected in 6-min time bins, and a *blue bar* was assigned to those bins during which wake time accounted for more than 50% of the 6 min. This plotting format reveals at a glance that there is a bout of continuous waking lasting 2 to 3 hr each circadian cycle, and that this bout occurs slightly earlier each 24-hr day (i.e., the circadian cycle is <24 hr). **B,** The circadian rhythm of wheel-running activity from the same mouse. Note the precise onsets of the daily active period. In rodents, all circadian rhythms free-run in phase. **C,** The circadian rhythm of nonspecific locomotor activity in a rat, measured by photobeams. Note that activity onsets occur a little later each day (i.e., the circadian cycle is >24 hr). The *long blue line* on day 23 denotes a 24-hr period of forced activity in a rotating drum; this procedure did not perturb the free-running rhythm. (**A** and **B** modified from Welsh DK, Engel EM, Richardson GS, et al: Precision of circadian wake and activity onset timing in the mouse. J Comp Physiol [A] 1986;158: 827-834; **C** modified from Borbely AA: Sleep regulation: Circadian rhythm and homeostasis. Curr Top Neuroendocrinol 1982;1:83-103, with permission.)

All of these observations are consistent with the hypothesis that there is a genetically specified internal circadian clock that drives daily rhythms in behavior and physiology. Indeed, circadian rhythms are known to persist in constant conditions on space shuttles in orbit, completely removed from any hypothetical terrestrial Factor X.[3]

Over the past few decades, circadian clocks have been localized in the brains and other tissues of several species, and genes and proteins that comprise the "gears" of these clocks have now been identified in cyanobacteria, a fungus, insects, and mammals (for references, see Chapter 30). Thus, the focus of research in this area is no longer on whether circadian rhythms are generated by internal clocks but, rather, what the components and processes of these clocks are, how they control behavior and physiology, how are they synchronized to the environment, and what impact they have on a variety of medical conditions. In addition, a major current focus is on understanding how our internal clocks might be manipulated to treat problems related to circadian timing, such as the disturbances of sleep, arousal, and other physiologic processes associated with shift work, rapid transmeridian jet travel, blindness, and other conditions. An understanding of the functional properties of circadian clocks is essential to set the framework for the cellular and molecular analyses that

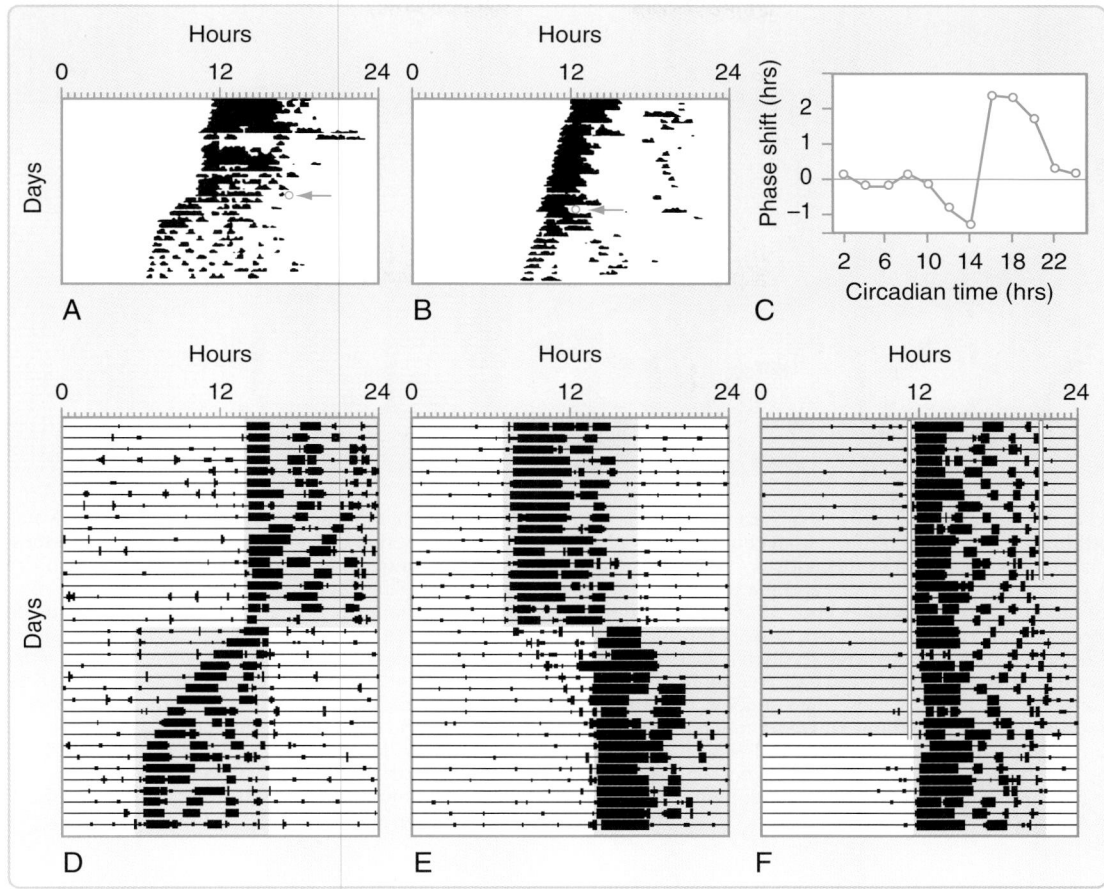

Figure 27–2. Phase shifting and entrainment by light. **A,** Circadian rhythm of wheel running recorded from a hamster in constant dark. On the day indicated by the *arrow*, the hamster was exposed to light for 30 min (*open circle*). The pulse was timed to occur at circadian time 20, which is 8 circadian hours (where 1 circadian hour = τ/24) after the daily onset of wheel running (denoted circadian time 12, by convention, and estimated by fitting a regression line to the activity onsets for 7 to 10 days before the day of light exposure). On the day after the light pulse, activity occurs earlier than predicted by extrapolation from the preceding free run. After several days of "transient" advancing cycles, a stable phase advance shift of several hours is revealed. Transients are by definition those cycles before completion of the full shift. **B,** In this experiment, the light pulse was presented at circadian time 14. This induced a small phase delay shift of approximately 1 hour, which was complete within one circadian cycle. Phase resetting without transients is typical of light-induced delay shifts. **C,** A full phase–response curve (PRC) depicting the relation between the circadian time (CT) of light exposure, and the magnitude and direction of the resulting phase shift. Delay shifts occur to light early in the subjective night (~CT10-15) and advance shifts to light late in the subjective night (CT15-24). **D,** An 8-hr phase advance of the light–dark (LD) cycle (dark period indicated by shading), illustrating gradual reentrainment by a series of approximately 1-hr phase advances each day (due to differential exposure of the delay and advance portions of the circadian pacemaker's PRC to light). Note inhibition of activity by light during the later portion of the hamster's active period, during the first few days after the LD shift. **E,** A 6-hr phase delay of the LD cycle, illustrating gradual reentrainment by delay shifts. Note inhibition of running early in the hamster's active period. **F,** Stable entrainment to a skeleton photoperiod in a hamster exposed to two daily 30-min pulses of light (denoted by the *vertical bars*), simulating dawn and dusk and defining a 14-hr "day" (diurnal rest period) and 10-hr "night" (nocturnal active period). The hamster's activity rhythm began to phase delay when the "morning" light pulse was omitted, and a stable phase was restored when a full 14:10 photoperiod was implemented. (**C** modified from Takahashi JS, DeCoursey PJ, Bauman L, et al: Spectral sensitivity of a novel photoreceptive system mediating entrainment of mammalian circadian rhythms. Nature 1984;308:186-188; **D** modified from Mistlberger RE, Nadeau J: Ethanol and circadian rhythms in the Syrian hamster: Effects on entrained phase, reentrainment rate and period. Pharmacol Biochem Behav 1992;43:159-165, with permission; **E** and **F,** R. E. Mistlberger, unpublished data.)

address these important questions. This chapter reviews the basic functional properties of circadian clocks, whereas subsequent chapters review the neurobiologic and molecular genetic analyses of these clocks.

PARAMETERS AND MEASUREMENT OF CIRCADIAN RHYTHMS

Overt circadian rhythms have phase and amplitude dimensions (Fig. 27–4). Phase (conventionally represented by the Greek letter φ) refers to any point in a cycle. An observable

phase (e.g., daily wake-up time) can be used as the hand of a clock to track its motion. The elapsed time between successive occurrences of a particular phase represents τ. The φ and τ of an observed circadian rhythm reflect parameters of the underlying circadian clock—namely, its current position and its rate of cycling, respectively. Amplitude refers to the range of values that an overt circadian rhythm can assume through the course of its cycle. One measure of amplitude is the difference between the peak value and the mean value of a purely sinusoidal circadian rhythm (the acrophase of a fitted cosine wave; e.g., Fig. 27–4). However, the amplitude of overt

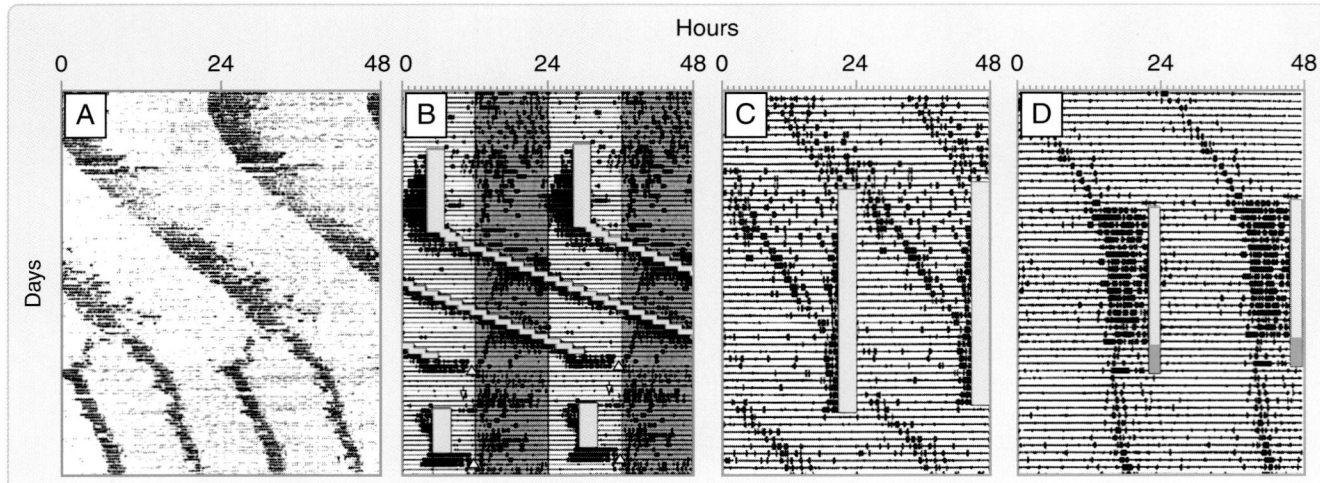

Figure 27–3. A, Wheel-running activity of a Syrian hamster in constant light. The rhythm "splits" into two components that free-run with different periods for approximately 10 days, then couple in "antiphase." Note that the period of the free-running rhythm shortens after the split, suggesting that τ in the coupled state depends on the phase relation between two underlying oscillators. **B,** Wheel-running rhythm of a rat entrained to a 12:12 light–dark cycle (light and shaded areas, respectively) during *ad libitum* feeding, restricted feeding (*open blue vertical bars*), and food deprivation. Food deprivation ends at *triangles*, begins at *arrowheads*. Running is primarily nocturnal during *ad libitum* feeding. A prominent bout of running anticipates a 3-hr daily mealtime, and remains coupled to mealtime when feeding intervals are extended from 24 to 26 hr. Activity persists at the predicted mealtime when food is withheld for 3 days (note heavy bouts of daytime running, and rapid reversion to nocturnal activity when food is restored). **C,** Free-running rhythm of a rat in constant light does not entrain to a restricted 3-hr daily mealtime, despite anticipatory activity. These data suggest that there are separate pacemakers driving free-running (light-entrainable) circadian rhythms and food-anticipatory rhythms. **D,** Free-running activity rhythm of a hamster in constant light entrains to a restricted daily feeding and drinking opportunity. (**A** from Pickard GE, Turek FW: The suprachiasmatic nuclei: two circadian clocks? Brain Res 1983;268:201-210; **B** from Mistlberger RE, Marchant EG: Computational and entrainment models of circadian food-anticipatory activity: Evidence from non-24 h feeding schedules. Behav Neurosci 1995;109:790-798, with permission; **C,** R. E. Mistlberger, unpublished data; **D** from Mistlberger RE: Effects of scheduled food and water access on circadian rhythms of hamsters in constant light, dark, and light:dark. Physiol Behav 1993;53:509-516, with permission.)

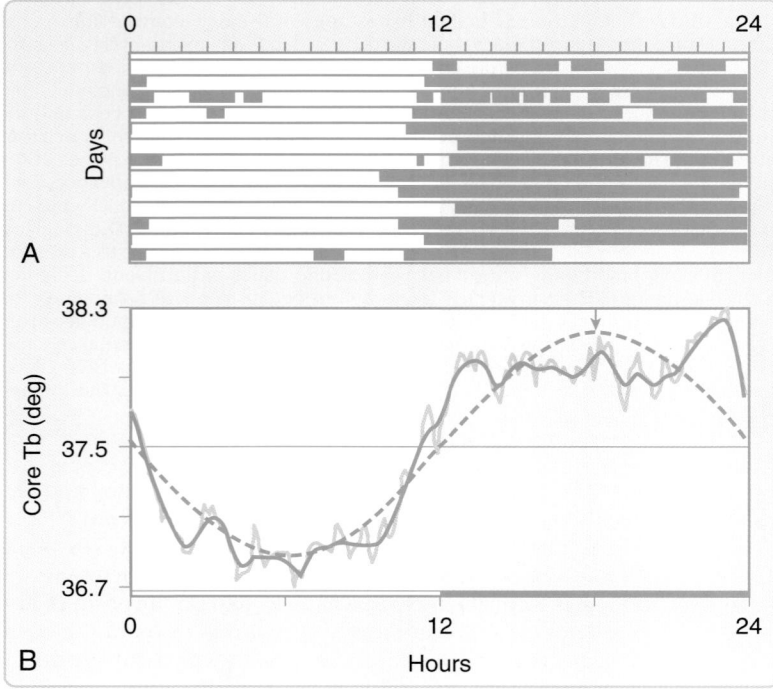

Figure 27–4. A, Circadian rhythm of core body temperature recorded from a rat by telemetry. The data are single-plotted (each line is 24 hr, with 5-min bins plotted left to right, and consecutive days aligned vertically). The interval with lights-off (12 hr) is denoted by the *shading*. **B,** Average waveform constructed from the data in **A**. The *light blue line* represents the raw data and the *dark blue line* a running average. A cosine function (*broken line*) was fit to the smoothed data, and the *arrow* denotes the peak (acrophase) of the function. Note that the waveform of the temperature rhythm in light–dark has a prominent square-wave component, evident particularly during the nocturnal segment; thus, a cosine function is not an optimal fit because the acrophase occurs approximately 6 hr before the true peak in the raw data. (R. E. Mistlberger, unpublished data.)

rhythms cannot be taken to represent a parameter of the underlying clock because many factors downstream from the clock can affect the level and range of particular observable behavioral or physiologic variables.

The experimental analysis of circadian rhythms has relied heavily on a few organisms that exhibit precise and easily measured circadian rhythms. The most popular model systems, and the favored rhythm for measurement, have included the bread mold *Neurospora* (daily rhythm of spore production), the fruit fly *Drosophila* (daily rhythm of activity or, for population studies, eclosion), the marine mollusc *Bulla* (compound action potentials recorded from the optic nerve), and several nocturnal rodents, particularly the Syrian hamster (daily rhythm of wheel running), the house mouse (wheel running), and the Norway rat (wheel running, body temperature, and sleep). Behavioral and physiologic data are typically acquired by sensors whose outputs are monitored continuously by computers. Data stored in digital format are amenable to time-series analyses (e.g., linear regression, spectral analysis) using a variety of established techniques to measure ϕ and τ, and curve-fitting procedures (e.g., cosinor analysis) to measure ϕ and amplitude.[4-6] Despite the broad range of species studied and variables monitored, the formal properties of circadian rhythms are remarkably general, a feature consistent with an ancient origin for circadian clocks. In this chapter, we refer primarily to the literature from studies of mammalian circadian rhythms.

ENVIRONMENTAL INFLUENCES

Photic Entrainment

Circadian clocks are thought to have several important functions that enhance reproductive fitness in natural environments. A primary function is to promote consolidated periods of sleep (or rest) and wakefulness (and activity), and to restrict these to appropriate phases of the solar day, resulting in relatively stable "nocturnal" (night-active), "diurnal" (day-active), or "crepuscular" (dawn- and dusk-active) chronotypes that are consistent with the sensory and other adaptations of a given species. A fundamental advantage of using an internal clock to regulate rest–activity cycles is that physiologic changes can be mobilized in anticipation of the transitions between day to night that herald the dramatic ecologic differences between these daily phases. This adaptation allows for the expression of an anticipatory, rather than reactive, regulation of physiology, thus ensuring that the organism is fully prepared for activity or rest at the correct time. Humans and other diurnal species thus exhibit a gradual increase in body temperature, plasma cortisol, and sympathetic autonomic tone beginning several hours before habitual wake onset, thereby facilitating a rapid switch from sleep to alert waking.[7] Similar preparatory processes occur in reverse to facilitate sleep onset (e.g., body temperature declines, melatonin secretion begins).

In at least some species, the circadian clock has been exploited not only as a device for driving daily rhythms (i.e., a pacemaker function), but as a true clock that can be continuously consulted to provide a sense of time. Evidence for this function is available from studies showing that some animals can discriminate time of day without external cueing, and thereby learn to associate the time and place of food availability.[8,9] Some species use this time sense to navigate using celestial

cues as a compass, which requires continuous adjustment of the angle of movement relative to the sun's apparent position in the sky.[10] The circadian clock is also used by many species to measure day length for the purposes of regulating reproduction, hibernation, and other seasonally varying functions.[11]

To achieve these adaptive functions, it is imperative that the circadian clock maintain an appropriate phase relation to local environmental time. This challenge is complicated by seasonal variations in day length; outside the equatorial zones, the hours of dawn and dusk shift systematically each day as the earth moves in its orbit around the sun. The circadian clock therefore has two tasks: It must generate a cycle to match approximately the period of the day–night cycle, and it must track a particular phase of the day–night cycle, so that diurnal animals become active near dawn, and nocturnal animals near dusk. The process by which this optimal synchronization occurs is called *entrainment*, defined as phase and period control of one oscillating process by another. In the case of the daily sleep–wake cycle and other circadian rhythms, entrainment to local environmental time is mediated by the actions of periodic environmental stimuli (so-called zeitgebers, German for "time-givers") on the circadian clock.

As might be expected, light is a virtually universal zeitgeber for the circadian rhythms displayed by most organisms, from cyanobacteria to mammals. The mechanism by which light entrains circadian rhythms has been investigated by assessing the effects of discrete applications of light on circadian rhythms free-running in DD.[12] Brief light pulses cause phase shifts of free-running rhythms, the magnitude and direction of which depend on when within the circadian cycle the light pulse is presented (see Fig. 27–2A and B). This phase dependence of light effects is illustrated graphically by plotting the size and direction of the phase shift against the circadian phase of light presentation, producing a phase–response curve (PRC) for light (see Fig. 27–2C).

The PRC for light pulses is universal in its general shape. Light exposure at the beginning of the "subjective night" (when nocturnal species are normally active and diurnal species are asleep), induces a "phase delay" shift, whereby the onset of the next "subjective day" (rest phase in nocturnal species, active phase in diurnal species) is reset to a later time, and the circadian cycle resumes its free-run from this new phase. Light exposure toward the end of the subjective night induces a shift in the opposite direction, a "phase advance," whereby the next subjective day begins earlier than usual. During most of the subjective day, light pulses have relatively little effect, defining a so-called dead zone on the PRC.

The shape of the PRC for light pulses suggests that entrainment can be accomplished by a phase-delaying action of light at dusk and a phase-advancing action at dawn, producing a net daily shift equal to the difference between τ of the circadian pacemaker and the period (T) of the light–dark (LD) cycle (24 hours in natural environments). Consistent with this hypothesis, known as the "discrete" (or nonparametric) model of entrainment,[13] organisms can be entrained to photoperiods consisting of only two brief light pulses in each 24-hour cycle, simulating dawn and dusk (e.g., Fig. 27–2F). Stable entrainment under such "skeleton" photoperiods has been documented in several species and appears to be similar in most respects to entrainment under a full photoperiod. In fact, studies of semifossorial nocturnal rodents in seminatural environments indicate that self-selected brief exposures to light at dawn or dusk may account fully for entrainment in these species.[14]

The τ of a circadian pacemaker and its circadian rhythm of sensitivity to light (summarized quantitatively in the PRC) determine several important properties of entrainment. One property is the limited range of entrainment. The circadian clock can entrain to LD cycles only if there is a relatively close match between τ and T of the LD cycle. For stable entrainment to occur, the difference between τ and T generally cannot exceed the maximum daily phase shift that can be induced by exposure to available light. Thus, entrainment of humans to the solar day on Mars (24.6 hours) is feasible (assuming a τ of 24.2 hours, this requires a 24-minute delay each day), whereas stable entrainment to the 18-hour duty cycle on an American submarine crew should be virtually impossible (a 6-hour advance being required each circadian cycle[15]).

In practice, the circadian range of entrainment can be extended if T of the LD cycle is changed gradually. This observation appears to be related to a partial modification of the intrinsic circadian τ toward the value of T. Thus, τ in DD tends to be longer after entrainment to T greater than 24 hours, and shorter after entrainment to T less than 24 hours.[16] These so-called after-effects on τ can persist for many weeks and suggest that entrainment limits are somewhat flexible because the intrinsic τ of the circadian clock can be modified by experience. Thus, for a given species there is a range of endogenous circadian periodicities that can be expressed, and observed τ depends on both the current and recent environmental conditions.

A second property of entrainment predictable from τ, T, and PRC shape is the phase relation between rhythm and zeitgeber during stable entrainment. The phase relation, or phase difference (abbreviated Ψ), is the difference in minutes or hours (or radial degrees, if expressed as a phase angle) between a definable circadian rhythm phase (e.g., wake onset) and a definable zeitgeber phase (e.g., sunrise, in which case the phase relation can be abbreviated Ψ_{LD}). The case can be made that Ψ_{LD} is the ultimate target of natural selection for the value of τ and the shape of the PRC, a premise summarized indirectly in the aphorism that it is the early bird that gets the worm.

How might a bird enhance its chances of getting the pick of the breakfast buffet? One strategy is to have a short τ. Recall that stable entrainment occurs at whatever Ψ_{LD} results in the photic stimulation that generates a net phase shift that precisely compensates for the difference between τ and T. If τ is less than 24 hours, then a net phase delay is required each circadian cycle. A larger net delay occurs when evening light stimulates more of the phase-delay portion of the PRC, and when morning light stimulates less of the phase-advance portion. This occurs if the PRC is shifted slightly to the left (i.e., advanced) relative to environmental time. Thus, a bird with a short circadian τ assumes a more advanced (positive) Ψ_{LD}, resulting in an earlier onset of activity at dawn. By contrast, if τ is greater than 24 hours, a net daily advance is required, stable entrainment occurs at a more negative Ψ_{LD}, and wake-up time occurs later relative to dawn. Within limits set by other factors (e.g., availability of light and prey for feeding), a short τ could confer an "early-bird" feeding advantage.

Individual differences in τ may also account for the "early-bird" and "night-owl" phenotypes that we recognize among humans. In fact, an extreme form of the early-bird phenotype (advanced sleep-phase syndrome) has been traced to a molecular change that affects the periodicity of the human circadian clock.[17] Note that differences in Ψ_{LD} can also occur as a result of small differences in PRC shape or in the strength of the zeitgeber (e.g., the duration, intensity, or wavelength of light exposure each day).

A third important property of entrainment predictable from τ and the PRC is the response of circadian rhythms to acute displacements of the LD cycle. If the LD cycle is advanced by 6 hours, simulating a rapid trip from North America to Europe, the circadian clock reentrains gradually, by small phase shifts (so-called transient cycles) over several days. The size and direction of these shifts is determined by τ, the intensity, wavelength, and precise timing of light, and the shape of the PRC (specifically, the area under the delay and advance portions and the phase at which resetting crosses over from delays to advances). Syrian hamsters, a favorite model species in chronobiology, have a species-typical τ very close to 24 hours and a relatively large advance-to-delay ratio of their PRC (Fig. 27–2C). Not surprisingly, they reentrain to an advance of the LD cycle by daily phase advances of approximately 1-hour magnitude (Fig. 27–2D), and to a delay of LD cycle by a series of approximately 1-hour daily delays. By contrast, Norway rats typically express a τ greater than 24 hours, and reentrain to an 8-hour LD advance by phase delaying 16 hours (R. E. Mistlberger, unpublished data). Endogenous τ in humans is slightly longer than 24 hours, which likely contributes to more rapid reentrainment after flying west (requiring a delay) than east (requiring an advance), and explains why humans may phase delay for many cycles to achieve a large phase advance.[18]

The experimental analysis of entrainment mechanisms in mammals has been based primarily on a few nocturnal rodent species that express very precise circadian rest–activity rhythms, enabling accurate measurement of even small phase shifts. Relatively little work has been done on diurnal mammals. Unlike their nocturnal cousins, diurnal animals are typically exposed to light for long durations each day. However, light pulse PRCs in the few diurnal mammals studied so far appear to be qualitatively similar to those for nocturnal rodents (see, e.g., Kas and Edgar[19]). Thus the mechanism of "discrete" entrainment by daily phase adjustments induced by light exposure at dawn and dusk appears to be available to diurnal as well as nocturnal species.

Evidence from studies of the European ground squirrel, however, suggest that in the natural environment this "discrete" entrainment may be only part of the entrainment mechanism in diurnal animals.[20] In its natural environment, this semifossorial diurnal rodent completely avoids dawn and dusk; it spends the night in a dark, enclosed burrow, emerges to forage approximately 4 hours after sunrise, returns to its burrow approximately 3 hours before sunset, and blocks the burrow entrance with soil before retiring to sleep. Light exposure is therefore self-selected and falls during the predicted dead zone of the photic PRC. Under these circumstances, the circadian clock should free-run, yet these animals exhibit a stable diurnal phase of entrainment without systematic drifts toward dawn or dusk. It is not yet clear how this is accomplished, but it suggests that light exposure during the day is modulating τ.

Recent studies of the human circadian pacemaker also indicate that it is sensitive to light throughout the subjective day,[21] with light apparently exerting a continuous action on the pacemaker. Entrainment might be accomplished without discrete phase shifts during lighting transitions by accelerating or slowing the angular motion of the pacemaker throughout the day, with the net result of a 24-hour τ and stable Ψ_{LD}. This model of a continuous action of light on pacemaker τ forms the basis of a "continuous" or "parametric" model of entrainment.

Support for this model derives from the observation that τ varies with the intensity of constant light (LL) exposure in most species.[22] In nocturnal rodents, LL slows the circadian clock (i.e., τ is lengthened), shortens the daily active phase, and reduces total daily activity (e.g., Fig. 27–5D). In diurnal animals, LL usually has the opposite set of effects, although there are more exceptions across species (and diurnal primates, in particular, tend not to conform). These empirical generalizations are collectively known as the "Circadian Rule"[22] and suggest that light could facilitate entrainment by continuous modulation of τ. Although this mechanism is not applicable to semifossorial nocturnal species that see little daylight, it may contribute to entrainment of diurnal species. It may also account for entrainment in animals at high latitudes that are exposed during mid-summer to continuous illumination with a sinusoidal variation in intensity. Modulation of τ in diurnal animals by total daily light may also have consequences for Ψ_{LD}, which would be particularly apparent at the extremes of winter and summer photoperiods.

It is also possible that extended daily light exposure in diurnal animals affects the amplitude of the circadian clock. A widely used model of the circadian clock treats it as a limit-cycle oscillator that has both phase and amplitude dimensions, and a preferred trajectory of oscillation between two or more state variables. When the phase of the oscillation is acutely shifted, the amplitude of oscillation may also transiently change before the preferred trajectory (the limit cycle) is reestablished. A continuous or very strong zeitgeber (e.g., critically timed bright light) may drive the state parameters to a low-amplitude trajectory, or even a point of singularity characterized by zero amplitude. When the amplitude of oscillation is small, a resetting stimulus of given intensity elicits larger phase shifts.[23,24] Such effects may underlie potentiated responses to phase shifting stimuli in Syrian hamsters after exposure to 2 days of LL (e.g., Fig. 27–5A,B).[25,26] If the long photoperiod of summer at high latitudes does affect the amplitude of the circadian clock, then this may also affect the Ψ_{LD} at which entrainment stabilizes. Such effects remain to be substantiated empirically.

Another influential heuristic model of the circadian clock postulates that the master, light-entrainable circadian pacemaker consists of two coupled oscillators, each with a full or partial PRC to light[13] (in mammals, this clock is located in the hypothalamic suprachiasmatic nucleus; SCN; see Chapters 28 and 29). When entrained to a natural photoperiod, the two oscillators are assumed to be coupled with a phase relation such that one is affected primarily by morning light, and the other primarily by evening light. This dual-oscillator model accounts successfully for many features of circadian rhythms observed under skeleton and non–24-hour LD cycles, and in response to LD shifts and light pulses.

Although the model was developed to explain photic entrainment and photoperiodic timing of annual rhythms, it was inspired by the observation that animals exposed to LL conditions for several weeks often exhibit splitting of their circadian rhythms (including those of activity, temperature, and hormones) into two components. In nocturnal hamsters, these features emerge after exposure to bright LL for many days. The two split components often free-run with different τ's for at least a few cycles before coupling stably in an antiphase relation (e.g., Fig. 27–3A). The components rapidly revert to normal coupling under standard photoperiods, but can be maintained in the split state by certain exotic photoperiods.[27] A two-oscillator organization appears to generalize to at least some diurnal organisms because perhaps the best examples of prolonged splitting are seen in diurnal tree shrews maintained in DD.[28] The two-oscillator formalism continues to stimulate debate and experiment in search of its cellular and molecular basis[29,30] (see also Chapter 29).

Although early evidence suggested that the circadian clock in humans was especially sensitive to social cues and less so to photic cues, it is now clear that humans can be entrained by LD cycles and exhibit phase shifts to light pulses with a PRC qualitatively similar to that for other organisms.[31,78] These and other properties of circadian regulation in humans are described in greater detail in Chapters 31 and 34).

Nonphotic Entrainment

Masking and Entrainment

An important distinction in chronobiology is that between "masking" and "entraining" effects of environmental stimuli. Light can entrain circadian rhythms in virtually every species that has been studied carefully. In many species, light also has direct effects on the expression of behavior and physiology. In nocturnal rodents, light at night inhibits locomotor activity and promotes sleep. Light in this case constitutes a "negative masking" stimulus because it suppresses a behavior at a circadian phase when that behavior is usually present, thereby "masking" the true phase of the circadian clock. An example of partial negative masking is illustrated in Figure 27–2D and E; activity early or late in the hamster's subjective night is strongly suppressed by light exposure after a delay or advance, respectively, of the LD cycle. In diurnal animals, light usually stimulates activity; at night this would constitute a "positive" masking effect. Another well-known masking effect of light is acute suppression of nocturnal pineal melatonin secretion,[32] a rapid response that is evident in nocturnal and diurnal animals.

These direct effects of environmental stimuli on physiology and behavior contribute to the waveform of daily rhythms in natural environments. They can also present interpretive difficulties in evaluating whether a periodic environmental stimulus functions as a true zeitgeber (i.e., affects the pacemaker rather than only overt behavior). A periodic signal may entrain a behavioral or physiologic rhythm, in which case it is functioning as a zeitgeber, or it may directly impose a rhythm without affecting an underlying oscillator, in which case it is functioning as a masking stimulus. The criteria for distinguishing

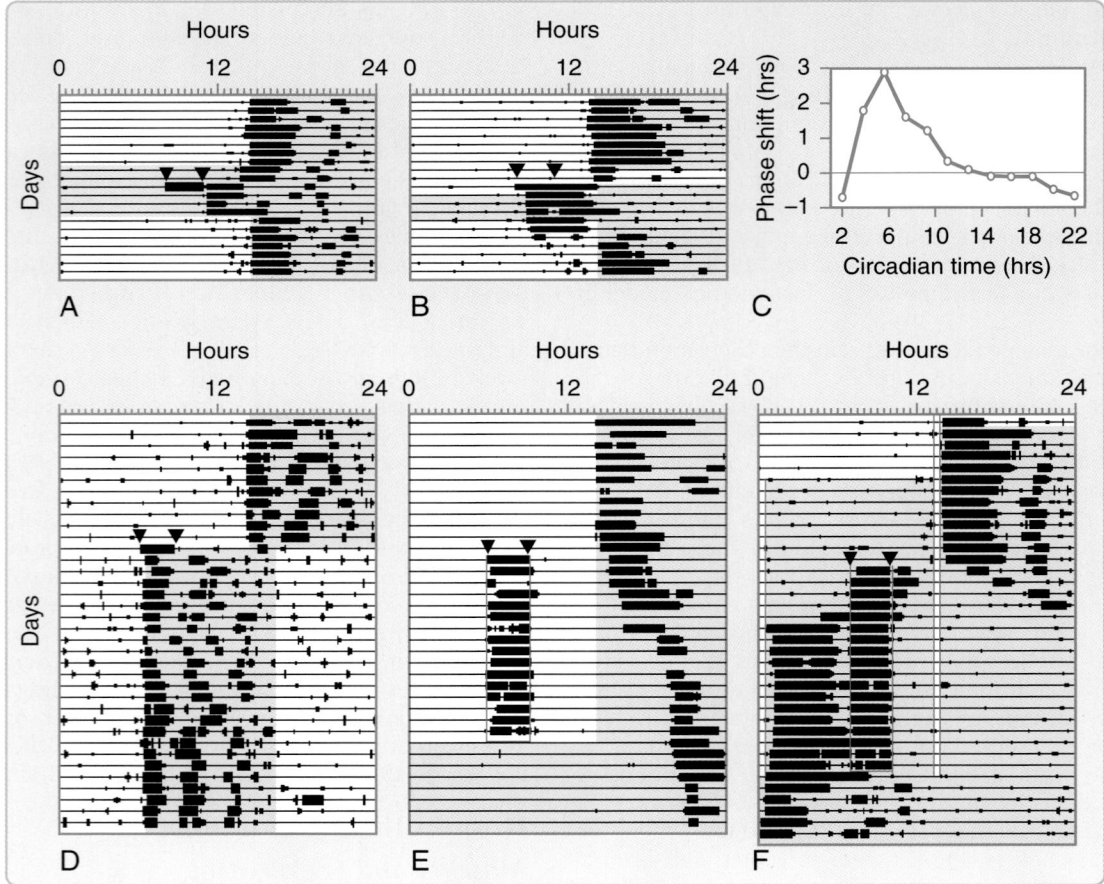

Figure 27–5. Phase shifting effects of 3-hr bouts of arousal (indicated by *arrowheads*) stimulated by confinement to a novel running wheel during the middle of the subjective day (rest period) in Syrian hamsters. Lights-off is indicated by *shading*. **A,** A 150-min phase advance was induced by running on the third day of constant dark. **B,** A 350-min phase advance was induced by running on the third day of constant light. Lights were turned off during running and left off for the next 3 days. **C,** Phase–response curve to 3-hr bouts of wheel running. **D,** An 8-hr phase shift of light–dark (LD), combined with 3 hr of stimulated running at the onset of darkness on the first night of the advanced LD cycle. The hamster reentrains to LD within one cycle (compare this with Fig. 27–2D, same hamster without stimulated running). **E,** Phase delay of nocturnal activity in a hamster entrained to LD and subjected to novelty-induced running each day. **F,** Inversion of the circadian activity rhythm in a hamster entrained to a skeleton photoperiod (two 30-min light pulses) and subjected to novelty-induced running. Such inversions are prevented by full photoperiods. (**A** and **B** from Mistlberger RE, Antle MC, Webb IC, et al: Circadian clock resetting by arousal: The role of stress and activity. Am J Physiol 2003;285:R917-R925; **C** modified from Mrosovsky N, Salmon PA, Menaker M, et al: Nonphotic phase-shifting in hamster clock mutants. J Biol Rhythms 1992;7:41-49; **D** modified from Mistlberger RE, Nadeau J: Ethanol and circadian rhythms in the Syrian hamster: Effects on entrained phase, reentrainment rate and period. Pharmacol Biochem Behav 1992;43:159-165; **E** from Sinclair SV, Mistlberger RE: Activity reorganizes circadian phase of Syrian hamsters under full and skeleton photoperiods. Behav Brain Res 1997;87:127-137, with permission.)

masking from entrainment are based on the properties of oscillator entrainment discussed in relation to photic cycles.

- An entrained rhythm should persist (free-run) in the absence of the periodic stimulus, just as photically entrained rhythms persist in constant lighting conditions, and the initial phase of the free-run should reflect the apparent phase of the rhythm during entrainment.
- An entrained rhythm should follow an environmental cycle over only a limited range of environmental periods.
- The phase relation between an entrained rhythm and an environmental cycle should vary depending on the values of τ and T.
- This phase relation should be reestablished if the environmental cycle is abruptly shifted. If the rhythm is a direct response to the environmental cycle, shifting is immediate. If, instead, it reflects entrainment of an underlying oscillator,

several transient cycles may be evident before the prior phase relation is reestablished.

As reviewed in the following sections, several nonphotic stimuli have been identified that meet these criteria and can therefore be said to entrain circadian rhythms.

Scheduled Feeding

Rats provided with food for only a few hours each day at a fixed time show changes in locomotor activity, body temperature, and other physiologic variables that anticipate the daily mealtime.[33] These anticipatory responses begin to emerge within several days of scheduled feeding, and appear to be generated independently of photically entrained rhythms. If the meal is provided in the middle of the light period, rats exhibit two main bouts of activity each day, an intense bout before mealtime, and at least some activity persisting during the usual nocturnal active period (Fig. 27–3B). If the photic cycle is replaced by LL or DD, photically entrained rest–activity rhythms free-run while premeal activity remains coupled to mealtime (Fig. 27–3C). It is common, then, to observe two circadian activity components in food-restricted rats in LL, one free-running with a period slightly different from 24 hours, and a second, food-anticipatory component with a period of exactly 24 hours.

Several models have been proposed to account for the emergence of food-anticipatory activity rhythms.[33] Most findings, however, are explained parsimoniously by the hypothesis that anticipatory activity is generated by circadian oscillators entrained by food availability:

- Anticipatory responses do not emerge when the period of the food cycle is outside a broad circadian range of approximately 22 to 33 hours.[34]
- The phase relation between anticipatory activity onset and mealtime becomes increasingly positive as the period of the feeding cycle is lengthened and less positive as it is shortened.[35]
- Phase shifting the feeding time is usually followed by gradual rather than immediate shifts of the activity peak to resynchronize to the mealtime.[36]
- When the period of the food availability cycle is abruptly shortened or lengthened from 24 hours to 22 or 30 hours, the meal-synchronized rhythm may dissociate from feeding time and free-run for many cycles.[34]
- When food is made freely available, the control exerted by these oscillators over behavior diminishes, resulting in a loss of overt activity related to the former mealtime. However, when the rat is subsequently food deprived for several days, activity reappears at the circadian phase previously associated with feeding time.[37]

Taken together, these observations provide strong evidence that a self-sustained oscillator is involved in generating meal-anticipatory activity, and indicate that its influence on behavior is gated by the animal's motivational state. Other studies show that rats can use food-entrainable oscillators to discriminate time of day, which may enable them to anticipate multiple feeding times and link these with multiple feeding places.[9] Dissociation of food-anticipatory rhythms from LD-entrained rhythms suggests separate food- and light-entrainable circadian clocks, and lesion studies have confirmed that the master light-entrainable circadian pacemaker (the SCN) is not necessary for food-entrained rhythms. Although food-anticipatory behavioral rhythms have been described in numerous species (reviewed in Mistlberger[33]), only in rats, hamsters, and mice have the appropriate studies been done to confirm mediation by a separate food-entrained clock.[38-40] The broad physiologic significance of such food-entrained rhythms may be related to the discovery that some peripheral organs and tissues express genes with a circadian rhythm that is entrained preferentially by feeding cycles rather than LD cycles[41,42] (see Chapter 29). However, the site of the circadian mechanisms that drive food-anticipatory behavioral rhythms has not yet been identified.

The stimuli associated with food acquisition and ingestion that provide the timing signals necessary to entrain circadian oscillators also are not well characterized. Rats can anticipate meals of any nutrient composition, provided that these meals represent a significant contribution to daily caloric intake.[43,44]

Similar results have been obtained in studies examining the ability of specific nutrients to shift food-anticipatory rhythms.[45,46] Observations of anticipatory behaviors to restricted schedules of water[47] or salt[48] access suggest that the range of effective stimuli may extend to any motivationally significant resource for which a rat must forage.

The use of separate pacemakers to mediate food and light entrainment in rats confers flexibility on the circadian organization of their behavior, and permits anticipation of a stable window of food availability at any time of day, without necessarily altering the phase of photically entrained activity rhythms. However, occasionally feeding schedules do entrain or markedly shift the entire circadian system in rats,[49] and in some species this may be the rule rather than the exception[40,50-52] (e.g., Fig. 27–3D). In these cases, it is not clear which stimuli associated with scheduled feeding serve as the zeitgeber for the light-entrainable circadian clock in the SCN. The SCN clock may, for example, be entrained indirectly as a result of its coupling relations with food-entrained oscillators located elsewhere. Alternatively, the SCN may be entrained by stimuli from specific ingested nutrients, metabolic hormones associated with their ingestion, or nonspecific stimuli, such as the arousal associated with anticipatory activity or the thermogenic consequences of digestion. The following sections consider the evidence that nonspecific, nonphotic stimuli can entrain circadian rhythms in mammals.

Temperature

Free-running rhythms in a variety of heterothermic species can be entrained by 24-hour cycles of ambient temperature.[53] However, responses of homeothermic animals to temperature cycles are more variable. In some species, temperature cycles failed to entrain various circadian rhythms,[54,55] whereas in other species, including squirrel monkeys,[56] pig-tailed macaques,[57] rats, and a marsupial mouse,[58] temperature cycles have clear entrainment effects in at least some individuals.

The mechanism by which temperature entrains circadian rhythms in mammals is unclear. The SCN circadian pacemaker, studied in vitro, can be phase shifted by temperature pulses (step changes from 34° C to 37° C), possibly by a direct effect on clock gene transcription or translation.[59] In homeothermic species in vivo, however, entrainment to temperature pulses would seem unlikely to involve a direct effect on circadian oscillators in the brain, assuming that brain temperature is defended homeostatically. However, some mammals can regularly sustain very low body temperatures, and in these cases significant changes in pacemaker temperature may have τ-modulating and phase-resetting effects.[60] It is also possible that temperature cycles affect the circadian clock indirectly, by inhibiting or facilitating sleep and wake. The neural and endocrine correlates of changes in sleep–wake states, and the obvious changes in food and water intake, activity, and light exposure they entail, may in turn have phase-modulating feedback effects on circadian oscillators. Conceivably, any stimulus that has potent effects on behavioral state may have significance as a circadian zeitgeber.

Activity and Arousal States

In an early description of the Circadian Rule, Aschoff noted that the relation between light intensity and τ might be mediated by changes in arousal states because bright LL both lengthens τ and suppresses activity in nocturnal rodents.[22] A later study provided some support for the idea that metabolism, arousal, or some correlate affected the circadian pacemaker, in that the free-running τ of activity rhythms (measured as general locomotor activity using photobeam interruptions) was longer in hamsters with access to running wheels.[61] More recent studies indicate that this effect is weak in hamsters,[62] but is robust in rats[63] and mice[64]: τ shortens when wheels are available, and lengthens when wheels are locked. Evidently, some correlate of spontaneous, clock-regulated wheel-running activity provides a feedback signal that alters the rate at which the circadian pacemaker cycles.

The effects of behavior on functional properties of the circadian pacemaker were not widely recognized until the late 1980s, when a series of studies demonstrated unequivocally that acutely stimulated locomotor activity and arousal can reliably induce large phase shifts in hamsters (Fig. 27–5A and B), and, if repeated on a daily basis, can entrain free-running rhythms in hamsters, rats, and mice.[65-69] The earliest of these studies showed that hamsters could be phase shifted or entrained simply by changing their litter or cages[65] or by the opportunity for a 30-minute daily bout of foraging activity in an open field, despite little or no eating at that time.[66] More robust phase shifts were reliably obtained by confining hamsters in DD to novel running wheels for 2 to 3 hours. Hamsters that ran continuously while in the wheel exhibited phase shifts of 2 to 3 hours or more.[67]

As with phase-shifting light stimuli, the magnitude and direction of the phase shifts evoked by activity depend on when the stimulus is scheduled. The shape of the associated PRC, however, is markedly different; running stimulated during the mid-subjective day (the dead zone for photic stimuli) induces large phase advance shifts, whereas running during the mid- to late subjective night (the advance zone for photic stimuli) induces small phase delays (Fig. 27–5C). These findings indicate that the circadian clock in mammals has distinct circadian rhythms of sensitivity to photic and nonphotic stimuli.

A variety of stimuli have been shown to induce phase shifts by stimulating activity; these include 3- to 6-hour "pulses" of darkness interrupting LL, injections of triazolam or morphine, cold exposure, and activity stimulated by an acute bout of food deprivation.[68-71] All of these stimuli also necessarily arouse animals, raising the possibility that phase shifts are due to being awake, rather than to intense or continuous running. Indeed, in Syrian hamsters, the phase-shifting effects of stimulated running can be fully mimicked by the sleep deprivation procedure of gentle handling, which is associated with only low levels of occasional activity in the home cage.[72] However, if locomotor activity is entirely prevented, by confining hamsters to a restraint tube or to a small platform over water, no phase shifts occur, even if arousal is confirmed by concurrent electroencephalographic or plasma cortisol measures.[71,73] Thus, locomotion does appear to be necessary for the induction of phase shifts in response to arousal procedures. It has not yet been definitively ruled out that neuroendocrine correlates of the stress of these procedures actually inhibit the phase-shifting effect of being awake in the usual rest period.

The conclusion that "nonphotic" stimuli cause phase shifts because they induce activity is clearly not universally applicable to all stimuli, nor to all species. Dark pulses, for example, phase shift sparrows even though darkness inhibits their activity,[74]

and shift rhythms of pineal cells cultured in vitro,[75] where the issue of mediation by activity is not relevant. Dark pulses in the "subjective night" in hamsters can also induce shifts by an apparent "antiphotic" mechanism independent of locomotor activity.[76] A variety of drugs have also been shown to induce phase advances during the subjective day that are either not associated with increased activity or are not blocked by procedures for preventing activity These pharmacologic manipulations may directly activate pathways (e.g., serotonin, neuropeptide Y) that mediate the effects of activity and arousal on the circadian clock.[76,77]

The adaptive significance of the phase-shifting effects of activity in hamsters is unclear, but it may represent a mechanism for modulating circadian activity patterns in response to biologically important events related, for example, to social or sexual interactions (for review, see Mistlberger and Skene[78]). The potential practical applications of this phenomenon are, however, notable. For example, a single 3-hour bout of appropriately scheduled wheel activity in hamsters can greatly accelerate reentrainment to a shifted LD cycle[79] (compare Fig. 27–2D with Fig. 27–5D), and repeated daily bouts can alter the phase of entrainment to an LD cycle.[80,81] Scheduled activity can shift circadian rhythms in humans, and may thus represent a useful tool for manipulating the circadian system to remedy acute disorders associated with travel across time zones, shift work,[82] or disorders of entrainment, such as are commonly experienced by the blind.[83]

Social Cues

Interactions between members of the same species are known to phase shift, entrain, or modify the period of free-running rhythms in several species.[78] However, interpreting these effects can be problematic because social interactions can have strong masking effects and may also determine the pattern of light exposure, thereby complicating attributions of causality. In most cases, social effects on circadian timing appear to be weak, and in many experiments, no effects were observed. For example, under standard laboratory housing, the circadian rhythms of rats, mice, and hamsters housed individually in adjacent cages typically do not become mutually synchronized despite auditory, olfactory, and visual contact. Hamsters housed in the same cage may fail to become mutually entrained,[84] although cohousing a resident dominant hamster with a subordinate for 3 hours in the middle of the usual rest period can result in very large phase advance shifts in one or both of the pair.[73] Blind humans may also display free-running sleep–wake and other rhythms despite exposure to the social cues of a 24-hour society.[83] The mechanisms by which social cues influence circadian timing are not known, but effects on arousal states are probably a necessary, if not sufficient, component of this mechanism.[78]

Interactions between Photic and Nonphotic Zeitgebers

The striking effects of spontaneous activity on free-running τ in rats and mice, and of stimulated activity on phase in free-running hamsters, suggest that the steady-state, entrained phase of circadian rhythms may reflect integration of photic and nonphotic stimuli. A number of studies, most using hamsters as subjects, have examined whether activity stimulated each day at a particular phase of the LD cycle can alter entrainment to LD cycles. The results of some of these studies suggest that photic and nonphotic inputs combine linearly, in accordance with their respective PRCs. For example, activity or arousal induced in the middle of the light period by triazolam injections, wheel confinement, social/sexual stimuli, or restricted feeding can advance the phase of nocturnal activity onset,[50,77] whereas activity induced late in the subjective night can delay the phase of activity onset.[73,80]

Other results indicate that under some circumstances photic and nonphotic stimuli may combine nonlinearly and produce phase changes that are not predictable from separate analyses of the photic and nonphotic PRCs. Two studies have shown that activity induced in the middle of the light period can in some cases significantly delay, rather than advance, nocturnal activity onset.[81,83] This apparent delay may reflect splitting of the activity rhythm into two components, one that delays with respect to dark onset, and another that advances and aligns with the midday wheel-running session.[27,81,85]

Other studies have examined the interactive effects of single pulses of photic and nonphotic stimuli in combination (for detailed review and references, see Challet and Pevet[77]). The results again suggest complex, nonlinear interactions. Phase advances induced by an activity bout in the mid–subjective day can be blocked by a subsequent light pulse, although the light pulse alone at that time produces no phase shift. Conversely, phase advances induced by a light pulse in the late subjective night can be significantly attenuated by a 45-minute bout of stimulated running, which alone does not induce phase shifts at this phase. Phase delay shifts to light early in the subjective night were not inhibited by concurrent running, but were attenuated by a 6-hour sleep deprivation procedure, in both hamsters and mice. Thus, all portions of the photic PRC are amenable to inhibition by manipulations of behavior, although the delay and advance zones may be differentially sensitive.

In other combinations, photic and nonphotic stimuli can show nonlinear synergy rather than mutual inhibition. Hamsters subjected to a 7-hour advance of the LD cycle reentrained within one or two cycles if they were induced to run for 3 hours at the beginning of the new dark period, compared with 6 to 10 days if they were left undisturbed[79] (Fig. 27–5D). The rapidity of phase shifting in this paradigm is clearly greater than that predicted by simple addition of the photic and nonphotic PRCs. The analysis of the rules of interaction between photic and nonphotic zeitgebers is still at an early stage but should benefit from progress made on the molecular basis of circadian clock resetting.

The study of nonphotic effects on circadian rhythms in the past decade has produced a number of surprising discoveries, one of which is the report that a neutral, nonphotic stimulus can acquire the phase-shifting properties of light by repeated pairing with light pulses. An air disturbance created by a fan that reliably preceded a daily, phase-shifting light pulse was reported to acquire the capacity to induce a phase shift similar to that induced by light in rats.[86] Although attempts to replicate this finding using modified conditions have not yet been successful,[87] it remains possible that both current and previous exposure to nonphotic stimuli can modify photic entrainment processes. Other studies have, for example, demonstrated that photic phase shifts can be inhibited in an environment previously conditioned to evoke fear.[88]

The neurochemical interactions that underlie such effects may be related to the mechanisms by which nonphotic and photic stimuli interact in the absence of conditioning.

CIRCADIAN RHYTHMS ACROSS THE LIFE SPAN

Assessment of biologic rhythmicity across the mammalian life span presents many methodologic and interpretive challenges. Nevertheless, a valid cross-species generalization is that circadian rhythms in behavioral, physiologic, or neural functions are first evident prenatally, stabilize and entrain to LD cycles within the first few weeks (e.g., in rodents) or months (e.g., in humans) postnatally, and may exhibit changes in phase, period, amplitude, and response to zeitgebers in old age, with considerable variability within and among species.

In rodents, behavioral rhythmicity is not apparent before the second week postnatally.[89,90] Extrapolation of the phase at which behavioral and physiologic rhythms emerge back to prenatal life indicates, however, that the circadian pacemaker is functioning at or before birth in rats, hamsters, and mice. 2-Deoxyglucose autoradiography has been used to confirm that the circadian pacemaker located in the SCN expresses a daily rhythm of glucose metabolism as early as day 19 of gestation, which is 2 to 3 days before birth and before significant synaptogenesis in the SCN.[91] Although the fetal pacemaker lacks most input and output pathways, its metabolic rhythm is synchronized to the dam by a mechanism that involves pacemaker sensitivity to endogenous dopamine and maternal melatonin. Postnatally, the pacemaker becomes sensitive to photic stimuli during days 2 to 6, at which time it loses sensitivity to dopamine.[92] Maternal coordination of the fetus in utero ensures that when the pacemaker becomes coupled to effector systems for behavior and physiology postnatally, the emerging rhythms in these functions are appropriately phased with respect to the day–night cycle, and to rhythms of the dam.

Studies of the human fetus in utero have revealed daily variations in fetal motility, heart rate, and other variables by 20 to 22 weeks' gestation.[93] Although these rhythms may be driven directly by maternal factors, evidence for circadian periodicities of various functions in premature infants suggests that humans can generate rhythms endogenously as early as 30 weeks of gestation.[94] Neonates tracked over the first year of life exhibit a gradual emergence of circadian rhythmicity that initially may appear to free-run, but which usually becomes synchronized to the day–night cycle within 2 to 3 months. The conditions under which infants are maintained (e.g., on-demand versus scheduled feeding) can greatly influence the temporal organization of sleep–wake states (reviewed in Reppert and Rivkees[93]). The extent to which maturation of masking and entrainment processes contributes to the appearance of synchronized rhythms early in life is unknown.

Poor sleep is a primary concern of the aged, and deterioration of circadian organization may be a significant contributing factor. The most widely observed change in circadian rhythmicity with age is a decrease in the amplitude of a variety of rhythms, including activity, temperature, and sleep–wake, under entrained and free-running conditions.[95] However, a reduced rhythm amplitude is difficult to interpret, and could reflect changes in intrinsic properties of the pacemaker (e.g., coupling among a population of cellular oscillators), or changes upstream or downstream from the molecular machinery of the circadian clock. Changes upstream from the pacemaker may include reductions in sensitivity to photic or nonphotic stimuli. There is evidence that phase shifts to light at low intensities are reduced in aged rodents, but that responses to saturating intensities are greatly enhanced, at least at the transition point between delays and advances on the photic PRC.[96] These effects are consistent with a reduced sensitivity to light at the receptor level, and reduced amplitude of oscillation at the pacemaker level. Phase-shift responses to nonphotic stimuli (e.g., triazolam injections, dark pulses) have also been reported to be reduced in aged rodents in some studies,[96] but not others,[97] and may to some extent be secondary to a reduced running response to the stimulus in old animals.

Daily rhythms of sleep in aged humans are commonly viewed as "fragmented," with less sleep at night and more napping during the day.[98] A reduced amplitude of circadian rhythms has been reported in entrained and free-running humans in many but not all studies.[95] Failure to observe differences between young and old subjects in some samples may reflect individual differences and illustrate limitations of cross-sectional studies because these of necessity include only survivors in the advanced age groups, whose circadian mechanisms may differ from those of others in the cohort. In addition, the unknown histories of light exposure and entrainment of subjects in these studies may contribute significantly to observed differences.

Another commonly observed effect of aging in rodents and humans is an advanced Ψ_{LD}.[95] This is consistent with reports that free-running τ shortens with age. This effect is consistently evident in studies using extended longitudinal, rather than cross-sectional, designs (e.g., Pittendrigh and Daan[99]). In other species τ may lengthen with age (e.g., Valentinuzzi et al.[100]). Detection of τ changes may depend on the use of sufficiently aged subjects (many studies have used middle-aged subjects), on the duration of recording (after-effects of previous photoperiods may obscure age-related changes), and on the recording method. In rats and mice, for example, wheel-running activity shortens τ, and its intensity is significantly attenuated with age. Any possible changes in τ intrinsic to an aging pacemaker might thus be obscured by changes secondary to a reduction of feedback signals from behavior, arousal, hormones, or other factors.

It has been suggested that loss of temporal order may be a contributing cause, rather than merely a consequence, of aging.[101] In aged rodents, loss of circadian rhythmicity is predictive of impending death,[102] and extended exposure to lighting schedules at the limits to entrainment can reduce life span in some invertebrate species.[103] Although loss of rhythmicity due to experimental ablation of the SCN circadian pacemaker is clearly not fatal to laboratory rodents, effects on mean and maximal life span have not been studied carefully. The empirical data base remains insufficient to draw strong conclusions about causal relations between altered circadian organization and the normal aging process.

CONCLUSION

This overview of the properties of circadian regulation of behavior and physiology highlights the complexity of the underlying circadian system. The circadian system in mammals is sensitive to light and nonphotic cues, and manipulations of these have revealed a multiplicity of circadian clocks and complex interactions among inputs to these clocks. Black-box models of the circadian system based on a vast descriptive literature have provided a framework for analyses at the neurobiologic and molecular level, and progress at these levels has been remarkable over the past decade. This work is reviewed in detail in Chapters 29 and 30.

Clinical Pearl

Circadian biology has provided insights that are fundamental to understanding normal and abnormal sleep. If rhythm generation or entrainment is disrupted, by aging, blindness, or other conditions, this can be expected directly to affect the consolidation or timing of sleep, producing such symptoms as sleep fragmentation, sleep-onset insomnia, early morning arousals, and daytime sleepiness. Lifestyles associated with abnormal exposure to zeitgebers, such as with shift work and transmeridian jet travel, are also associated with disrupted sleep because of the natural delays and impediments in resynchronizing circadian clocks to shifted behavioral and environmental cycles.

REFERENCES

1. Aschoff J (ed): Handbook of Behavioral Neurobiology, vol 4: Biological Rhythms. New York, Plenum Press, 1980.
2. Brown FA: Response to pervasive geophysical factors and the biological clock problem. Cold Spring Harb Symp Quant Biol 1960;25:57-72.
3. Sulzman FM, Ellman D, Fuller CA, et al: *Neurospora* circadian rhythms in space: A reexamination of the endogenous-exogenous question. Science 1984;225:232-234.
4. Enright JT: Data analysis. In Aschoff J (ed): Handbook of Behavioral Neurobiology, vol 4: Biological Rhythms. New York, Plenum Press, 1981, pp 21-40.
5. Van Cauter E, Huyberechts S: Problems in the statistical analysis of biological time series: The cosinor test and the periodogram. J Interdisc Cycle Res 1973;4:41-57.
6. Refinetti R: Laboratory instrumentation and computing: Comparison of six methods for the determination of the period of circadian rhythms Physiol Behav 1993;54:869-875.
7. Moore-Ede MC, Sulzman F: Internal temporal order. In Aschoff J (ed): Handbook of Behavioral Neurobiology, vol 4: Biological Rhythms. New York, Plenum Press, 1980, pp 215-241.
8. Biebach H, Falk H, Krebs JR: The effect of constant light and phase shifts on a learned time-place association in garden warblers (*Sylvia borin*): Hourglass or circadian clock? J Biol Rhythms 1991;6:353-365.
9. Mistlberger RE, de Groot MH, Bossert J, et al: Discrimination of circadian phase in intact and SCN ablated rats. Brain Res 1996;739:12-18.
10. Schmidt-Koenig K, Ganzhorn JU, Ranvaud R: Orientation in birds: The sun compass. EXS 1991;60:1-15.
11. Goldman BD: Mammalian photoperiodic system: Formal properties and neuroendocrine mechanisms of photoperiodic time measurement. J Biol Rhythms 2001;16:283-301.
12. DeCoursey PJ: Daily light sensitivity rhythm in a rodent. Science 1960;131:33-35.
13. Pittendrigh CS, Daan S: A functional analysis of circadian pacemakers in nocturnal rodents: IV. Entrainment: Pacemaker as clock. J Comp Physiol [A] 1976;106:291-331.
14. DeCoursey PJ: Circadian photoentrainment: Parameters of phase delaying. J Biol Rhythms 1986;1:171-186.

15. Kelly TL, Neri DF, Grill JT, et al: Nonentrained circadian rhythms of melatonin in submariners scheduled to an 18-hour day. J Biol Rhythms 1999;14:190-196.

16. Pittendrigh CS, Daan S: A functional analysis of circadian pacemakers in nocturnal rodents: I. The stability and lability of spontaneous frequency. J Comp Physiol [A] 1976;106:223-252.

17. Toh KL, Jones CR, He Y, et al: An hPer2 phosphorylation site mutation in familial advanced sleep phase syndrome. Science 2001;291:1040-1043.

18. Aschoff J, Wever R: The circadian system of man. In Aschoff J (ed): Handbook of Behavioral Neurobiology, vol 4: Biological Rhythms. New York, Plenum Press, 1980, pp 311-331.

19. Kas MJH, Edgar DM: Photic phase response curve in *Octodon degus*: Assessment as a function of activity phase preference. Am J Physiol 2000;278:R1385-R1389.

20. Hut RA, van Oort BE, Daan S: Natural entrainment without dawn and dusk: The case of the European ground squirrel (*Spermophilus citellus*). J Biol Rhythms 1999;14:290-299.

21. Jewett ME, Rimmer DW, Duffy JF et al: Human circadian pacemaker is sensitive to light throughout subjective day without evidence of transients. Am J Physiol 1997;273: R1800-R1809.

22. Aschoff J: Exogenous and endogenous components in circadian rhythms. Cold Spring Harb Symp Quant Biol 1960;25:11-26.

23. Lakin-Thomas PL: A beginner's guide to limit cycles, their uses and abuses. Biol Rhythm Res 1995;26:216-232.

24. Johnson CH, Elliott J, Foster R: Fundamental properties of circadian rhythms. In Dunlap JC, Loros J, DeCoursey PJ (eds): Chronobiology: Biological Timekeeping. Sunderland, Mass, Sinauer, 2004, pp 67-106.

25. Mistlberger RE, Belcourt J, Antle MC: Circadian clock resetting by sleep deprivation without exercise: Dark pulses revisited. J Biol Rhythms 2002;17:227-237.

26. Knoch M, Gobes S, Pavlovska I, et al: Brief exposure to constant light promotes strong (type 0) circadian phase resetting responses to nonphotic stimuli in Syrian hamsters. Eur J Neurosci 2004; 19:2779-90.

27. Gorman MR, Elliott JA: Entrainment of 2 subjective nights by daily light:dark:light:dark cycles in 3 rodent species. J Biol Rhythms 2003;18:502-512.

28. Meijer JH, Daan S, Overkamp GJ, et al: The two-oscillator circadian system of tree shrews (*Tupaia belangeri*) and its response to light and dark pulses. J Biol Rhythms 1990;5:1-16.

29. de la Iglesia HO, Meyer J, Carpino A Jr, et al: Antiphase oscillation of the left and right suprachiasmatic nuclei. Science 2000; 290:799-801.

30. Daan S, Albrecht U, van der Horst GT, et al: Assembling a clock for all seasons: Are there M and E oscillators in the genes? J Biol Rhythms 2001;16:105-116.

31. Czeisler CA: The effect of light on the human circadian pacemaker. Ciba Found Symp 1995;183:254-290.

32. Klein D, Weller J: Rapid light-induced decrease in pineal serotonin N-acetyltransferase activity. Science 1972;177:532-533.

33. Mistlberger R: Circadian food anticipatory activity: formal models and physiological mechanisms. Neurosci Biobehav Rev 1994;18:1-25.

34. Stephan F: Limits of entrainment to periodic feeding in rats with suprachiasmatic lesions. J Comp Physiol [A] 1981;143:401-410.

35. Aschoff J, von Goetz C, Honma K: Restricted feeding in rats: Effects of varying feeding cycles. Z Tierpsychol 1983;63:91-111.

36. Stephan F: Phase shifts of circadian rhythms in activity entrained to food access. Physiol Behav 1984;32:663-671.

37. Coleman GJ, Harper S, Clarke JD, et al: Evidence for a separate meal-associated oscillator in the rat. Physiol Behav 1982;29: 107-115.

38. Stephan FK, Swann JM, Sisk CL: Entrainment of circadian rhythms by feeding schedules in rats with suprachiasmatic lesions. Behav Neural Biol 1979;25:545-554.

39. Abe H, Rusak B: Anticipatory activity and entrainment of circadian rhythms in Syrian hamsters exposed to restricted palatable diets. Am J Physiol 1992;263:R116-R124.

40. Marchant EG, Mistlberger RE: Anticipation and entrainment to feeding time in intact and SCN-ablated C57Bl/6j mice. Brain Res 1997;765:273-282.

41. Balsalobre A: Clock genes in mammalian peripheral tissues. Cell Tissue Res 2002;309:193-199.

42. Damiola F, Le Minh N, Preitner N, et al: Restricted feeding uncouples circadian oscillators in peripheral tissues from the central pacemaker in the suprachiasmatic nucleus. Genes Dev 2000;14:2950-2961.

43. Stokkan KA, Yamazaki S, Tei H, et al: Entrainment of the circadian clock in the liver by feeding. Science 2001;291:490-493.

44. Mistlberger R, Houpt T, Moore-Ede M: Food-anticipatory rhythms under 24h schedules of limited access to single macronutrients. J Biol Rhythms 1990;5:35-46.

45. Mistlberger R, Rusak B: Palatable daily meals entrain anticipatory activity rhythms in free-feeding rats: Dependence on meal size and nutrient content. Physiol Behav 1987;41:219-226.

46. Stephan FK: Calories affect zeitgeber properties of the feeding entrained circadian oscillator. Physiol Behav 1997;62:995-1002.

47. Mistlberger RE: Anticipatory activity rhythms under daily schedules of water access in the rat. J Biol Rhythms 1992;7:149-160.

48. Rosenwasser AM, Schulkin J, Adler NT: Anticipatory appetitive behavior of adrenalectomized rats under circadian salt-access schedules. Anim Learn Behav 1988;16:324-329.

49. Stephan FK: The role of period and phase in interactions between feeding- and light-entrainable circadian rhythms. Physiol Behav 1986;36:151-158.

50. Mistlberger RE: Effects of scheduled food and water access on circadian rhythms of hamsters in constant light, dark, and light:dark. Physiol Behav 1993;53:509-516.

51. Kennedy GA, Coleman GJ, Armstrong SM: Restricted feeding entrains circadian wheel-running activity rhythms of the kowari. Am J Physiol 1991;261:R819-R827.

52. Abe H, Kida M, Tsuji K, et al: Feeding cycles entrain circadian rhythms of locomotor activity in CS mice but not in C57BL/6J mice. Physiol Behav 1989;45:397-401.

53. Sweeney B, Hastings J: Effects of temperature upon diurnal rhythms. Cold Spring Harb Symp Quant Biol 1960;25:87-104.

54. Hoffman K: Die relative Wirksamkeit von Zeitgebern. Oecologia 1969;3:184-206.

55. Stewart MC, Reeder WG: Temperature and light synchronization experiments with circadian activity in two color forms of the rock pocket mouse. Physiol Zool 1968;41:149-156.

56. Aschoff J, Tokura H: Circadian activity rhythms in squirrel monkeys: Entrainment by temperature cycles. J Biol Rhythms 1986;1:91-100.

57. Tokura H, Aschoff J: Effects of temperature on the circadian rhythm of pig-tailed macaques, *Macaca nemestrina*. Am J Physiol 1983;245:R800-R804.

58. Francis A, Coleman G: Ambient temperature cycles entrain the free-running circadian rhythms of the stripe-faced dunnart. J Comp Physiol [A] 1990;167:357-362.

59. Ruby NF, Burns DE, Heller HC: Circadian rhythms in the suprachiasmatic nucleus are temperature-compensated and phase-shifted by heat pulses in vitro. J Neurosci 1999;19: 8630-8636.

60. Lee TM, Holmes WG, Zucker I: Temperature dependence of circadian rhythms in golden-mantled ground squirrels. J Biol Rhythms 1990;5:25-34.

61. Aschoff J, Figala J, Poppel E: Circadian rhythms of locomotor activity in the golden hamster measured with two different techniques. J Comp Physiol Psychol 1973;85:20-28.

62. Mrosovsky N: Further experiments on the relationship between the period of circadian rhythms and locomotor activity levels in hamsters. Physiol Behav 1999;66:797-801.

63. Yamada N, Shimoda K, Ohi K, et al: Free-access to a running wheel shortens the period of free-running rhythm in blinded rats. Physiol Behav 1988;42:87-91.

64. Edgar DK, Martin CE, Dement WC: Activity feedback to the mammalian circadian pacemaker: Influence on observed measures of rhythm period length. J Biol Rhythms 1991;6:185-199.

65. Mrosovsky N: Phase-response curves for social entrainment. J Comp Physiol [A] 1988;162:35-46.

66. Rusak B, Mistlberger RE, Losier B, et al: Daily hoarding opportunity entrains the pacemaker for hamster activity rhythms. J Comp Physiol [A] 1988;64:165-171.

67. Reebs SG, Mrosovsky N: Effects of induced wheel running on the circadian activity rhythms of Syrian hamsters: Entrainment and phase-response curve. J Biol Rhythms 1989;4:39-48.

68. Marchant E, Mistlberger R: Morphine phase shifts circadian rhythms in mice: Role of behavioral activation. Neuroreport 1996;7:209-212.

69. Mistlberger RE, Marchant EG, Sinclair SV: Nonphotic phase shifting and the motivation to run: Cold exposure re-examined. J Biol Rhythms 1996;11:208-215.

70. Mistlberger RE, Sinclair SV, Marchant EG, et al: Circadian phase shifts to food deprivation and refeeding in the Syrian hamster are mediated by running activity. Physiol Behav 1997;61:273-278.

71. Van Reeth O, Turek F: Stimulated activity mediates phase shifts in the hamster circadian clock induced by dark pulses or benzodiazepines. Nature 1989;339:49-51.

72. Antle MC, Mistlberger RE: Circadian clock resetting by sleep deprivation without exercise in the Syrian hamster. J Neurosci 2000;20:9326-9332.

73. Mistlberger RE, Antle MC, Webb IC, et al: Circadian clock resetting by arousal: The role of stress and activity. Am J Physiol 2003;285:R917-R925.

74. Binkley S, Mosher K: Direct and circadian control of sparrow behaviour by light and dark. Physiol Behav 1985;35:785-798.

75. Zatz M, Mullen D, Moskal JR: Photoendocrine transduction in cultured chick pineal cells: Effects of light, dark, and potassium on the melatonin rhythm. Brain Res 1988;438:199-215.

76. Rosenwasser AM: Neurobiology of the mammalian circadian system: Oscillators, pacemakers and pathways. Prog Psychobiol Physiol Psychol 2003;18:1-38.

77. Challet E, Pevet P: Interactions between photic and nonphotic stimuli to synchronize the master circadian clock in mammals. Front Biosci 2003;8:s246-s257.

78. Mistlberger RE, Skene DJ: Social influences on circadian rhythms in man and animal. Biol Rev 2004;79:533-556.

79. Mrosovsky N, Salmon P: A behavioural method for accelerating re-entrainment of rhythms to new light-dark cycles. Nature 1987;330:372-373.

80. Mistlberger RE: Scheduled daily exercise or feeding alters the phase of photic entrainment in Syrian hamsters. Physiol Behav 1991;50:1257-1260.

81. Sinclair S, Mistlberger R: Activity reorganizes circadian phase of Syrian hamsters under full and skeleton photoperiods. Behav Brain Res 1997;87:127-137.

82. Buxton OM, Lee CW, L'Hermite-Baleriaux M, et al: Exercise elicits phase shifts and acute alterations of melatonin that vary with circadian phase. Am J Physiol 2003;284:R714-R724.

83. Klerman EB, Rimmer DW, Dijk DJ, et al: Nonphotic entrainment of the human circadian pacemaker. Am J Physiol 1998;274:R991-R996.

84. Refinetti R, Nelson DE, Menaker M: Social stimuli fail to act as entraining agents of circadian rhythms in the golden hamster. J Comp Physiol [A] 1992;170:181-187.

85. Mrosovsky N, Janik D: Behavioral decoupling of circadian rhythms. J Biol Rhythms 1993;8:57-65.

86. Amir S, Stewart J: Resetting of the circadian clock by a conditioned stimulus. Nature 1996;379:542-545.

87. de Groot MH, Rusak B: Responses of the circadian system of rats to conditioned and unconditioned stimuli. J Biol Rhythms 2000;157:277-291.

88. Amir S, Stewart J: The effectiveness of light on the circadian clock is linked to its emotional value. Neuroscience 1999;88:339-345.

89. Reppert SM: Circadian rhythms: Basic aspects and pediatric implications. In Styne DM, Brook CGD (eds): Current Concepts in Pediatric Endocrinology. New York, Elsevier, 1987, pp 91-125.

90. Reppert SM: Interaction between the circadian clocks of mother and fetus. Ciba Found Symp 1995;183;198-211.

91. Moore RY, Shibata S, Bernstein ME: Developmental anatomy of the circadian system. In Reppert SM (ed): Development of Circadian Rhythmicity and Photoperiodism in Mammals. Ithaca, NY, Perinatology Press, 1989, pp 1-23.

92. Weaver DR, Reppert SM: Definition of the developmental transition from dopaminergic to photic regulation of c-fos gene expression in the rat suprachiasmatic nucleus. Mol Brain Res 1995;33:136-148.

93. Reppert SM, Rivkees SA: Development of human circadian rhythms: Implications for health and disease. In Reppert SM (ed): Development of Circadian Rhythmicity and Photoperiodism in Mammals. Ithaca, NY, Perinatology Press, 1989, pp 245-259.

94. Mirmiran M, Lunshof S: Perinatal development of human circadian rhythms. Prog Brain Res 1996;111:217-225.

95. Myers BL, Badia P: Changes in circadian rhythms and sleep quality with aging: Mechanisms and interventions. Neurosci Biobehav Rev 1995;19:553-571.

96. Turek FW, Penev P, Zhang Y, et al: Alterations in the circadian system in advanced age. Ciba Found Symp 1995;183:212-234.

97. Duncan MJ, Deveraux AW: Age-related changes in circadian responses to dark pulses. Am J Physiol 2000;279:R586-R590.

98. Miles LE, Dement WC: Sleep and aging. Sleep 1980;3:119-220.

99. Pittendrigh C, Daan S: Circadian oscillations in rodents: A systematic increase in their frequency with age. Science 1974;186:548-550.

100. Valentinuzzi VS, Scarbrough K, Takahashi JS, et al: Effects of aging on the circadian rhythm of wheel-running activity in C57BL/6 mice. Am J Physiol 1997;273:R1957-R1964.

101. Samis HV: Aging: The loss of temporal organization. Perspect Biol Med 1968;12:95-102.

102. Pittendrigh C, Minis D: Circadian systems: Longevity as a function of circadian resonance in Drosophila melanogaster. Proc Natl Acad Sci U S A 1972;69:1537-1539.

103. Wax TM, Goodrick CL: Nearness to death and wheel running behavior in mice. Exp Gerontol 1978;13:233-236.

28

Anatomy of the Mammalian Circadian System

Joshua J. Gooley

Clifford B. Saper

ABSTRACT

Circadian rhythms in mammals, including sleep-wake cycles, are endogenously driven by the suprachiasmatic nucleus (SCN) in the anterior hypothalamus. The SCN consists of ventrolateral (SCNvl) and dorsomedial (SCNdm) components based on differences in chemoarchitecture, peptide phenotype, and afferent-efferent projection pattern, and this organizational scheme is conserved across mammalian species. The SCN is functionally subdivided to generate a coordinated circadian rhythm of neuronal activity in the SCN, to integrate photic and nonphotic time cues to reset the circadian phase of SCN neurons, and to transmit circadian output signals to effector systems to temporally coordinate genetic, physiologic, and behavioral rhythms with daily changes in the environment.

The near-24-hour rhythm of neuronal activity in the SCN is normally entrained to the 24-hour light-dark cycle prescribed by Earth's rotation. Photic information reaches the SCN directly via the retinohypothalamic tract (RHT) and indirectly through other retinorecipient structures including the intergeniculate leaflet (IGL) in the thalamic lateral geniculate nucleus (LGN). Visual photoreceptors (rods and cones) and intrinsically photosensitive melanopsin-containing retinal ganglion cells contribute to photic circadian entrainment, and RHT axons likely signal light information to the SCN by releasing glutamate and pituitary adenylate cyclase–activating polypeptide (PACAP).

The SCN also receives dense input from neuropeptide Y (NPY)- and gamma-aminobutyric acid (GABA)-containing neurons in the IGL and serotoninergic input from the median raphe nucleus (MRN). However, light versus NPY or 5-HT (serotonin) appear to have mutually antagonistic effects on SCN electrical activity and circadian phase shifting. The IGL and MRN are not essential for circadian entrainment or rhythmicity, but they appear to play a modulatory role in regulating light-induced circadian phase shifts and transmitting nonphotic information to the circadian clock.

Despite the widespread role of the SCN in regulating behavioral, physiologic, and genetic rhythms, SCN output is largely confined to the hypothalamus. The primary neuronal pathway underlying the circadian regulation of sleep-wake cycles involves a dense SCN efferent projection to the adjacent subparaventricular zone (SPZ), followed by a secondary projection to the dorsomedial hypothalamic nucleus (DMH), which projects to other brain regions critical for regulating sleep and wakefulness. The SCN also projects directly and indirectly to the paraventricular hypothalamic nucleus (PVH) to regulate corticosteroid secretion and synthesis of the hormone melatonin. Although SCN neuronal connectivity is required for maintenance of endocrine rhythms, diffusible SCN signals are sufficient to generate weak rhythms of rest-activity cycles and, likely, sleep-wake cycles.

Circadian rhythms are widely conserved and remarkably pervasive in determining daily patterns of behavior, physiology, and gene expression in animals, plants, fungi, and unicellular organisms. In mammals, the master circadian pacemaker in the SCN determines the period and phase of behavioral rhythms including sleep-wake cycles, and disruption of the circadian system is associated with deficits in sleep-wake behavior and cognitive performance. Identifying the neuronal pathways and neurotransmitters important for entrainment and maintenance of circadian rhythms is important for the development of pharmacologic and strategic approaches to improving the quality of sleep-wake cycles and performance, especially in persons afflicted with chronobiologic disorders.

In this chapter, we will describe the intrinsic organization, inputs, and outputs of the circadian clock in the SCN and provide in vitro and in vivo functional evidence for the role of specific pathways and neurotransmitters in the regulation of circadian rhythms. We will primarily discuss functional anatomy of the circadian system in rodents, which has been studied most extensively, but we will compare these findings to the organization of the primate circadian system. The discussion will emphasize the neuronal circuitry underlying the circadian control of sleep-wake and rest-activity cycles and how SCN afferent-efferent projections and neurotransmitters regulate behavioral output.

INTRINSIC ORGANIZATION OF THE SUPRACHIASMATIC NUCLEUS

The intrinsic organization of the SCN must allow it to generate a coordinated circadian rhythm of neuronal activity in the SCN and to integrate photic and nonphotic time cues to reset the circadian phase of SCN neurons. The SCN must also be organized to transmit circadian output signals to effector systems, to temporally coordinate genetic, physiologic, and behavioral rhythms with daily changes in the environment (i.e., the light-dark cycle and food availability), thus maximizing survival. In the following section we examine the intrinsic organization of the SCN and how this organizational scheme fulfills the aforementioned roles of the SCN. We begin with a basic histologic description of the SCN, including the neurotransmitter content and distribution, followed by an analysis of the functional role of these neurotransmitters in coordinating the circadian rhythm of neuronal activity within the SCN. In addition to classical neurotransmitter-mediated communication, we also explore alternative means by which SCN neurons reset or synchronize the circadian phase of neighboring SCN neurons. Potential mechanisms for light-dependent and circadian phase–dependent changes in SCN plasticity will also be discussed.

Cytoarchitecture

In Nissl-stained sections, the SCN is a conspicuous structure easily identified by its tightly compacted small-diameter neurons; it is located immediately dorsal to the optic chiasm and lateral to the third ventricle (Fig. 28–1A). In rats, the SCN measures less than 1 mm in the rostrocaudal axis and approximately 350 μm in diameter at the midlevel. Medially, the SCN is separated from the ependymal cells of the third ventricle by the periventricular nucleus, and ventrally the SCN indents the dorsal border of the optic chiasm. SCN neurons are among the smallest of the brain, and in rats each of the bilaterally paired SCN contains approximately 8000 to 10,000 neurons.[1] Based on neuronal morphology, ultrastructure, neurotransmitter phenotype, and afferent-efferent projections, the SCN can be divided into dorsomedial (SCNdm) and ventrolateral (SCNvl) components, commonly referred to as the shell and core, respectively.

The neurons in the SCNdm are smaller and more tightly compacted than those located in the SCNvl, and Golgi stains of SCN neurons show that the dendritic arbors of SCNvl neurons are more extensive than those of SCNdm neurons. Ultrastructural analysis of the SCN has revealed that SCNvl neurons have more organelles, rough endoplasmic reticulum, and nuclear invaginations, whereas soma-soma appositions are most frequently observed between neurons within the SCNdm.[1]

Neurotransmitters Synthesized in the Suprachiasmatic Nucleus

The SCNdm and SCNvl subdivisions can be easily distinguished by their neurotransmitter content. In the rat, SCNvl neurons contain vasoactive intestinal polypeptide (VIP; see Fig. 28–1B), peptide histidine isoleucine (PHI), gastrin-releasing peptide (GRP), and neurotensin (NT). VIP and PHI arise from the same precursor polypeptide and are therefore coexpressed in SCNvl neurons. The distribution of GRP-containing neurons largely overlaps that of VIP and PHI, but GRP-immunoreactive (ir) neurons are also located more laterally. The SCNdm is best defined by a population of arginine vasopressin (AVP)–containing neurons (see Fig. 28–1C). Angiotensin II–containing cells are also found throughout the SCNdm subdivision, and enkephalin (ENK)-ir neurons are located in more lateral regions of the SCNdm. Relatively few somatostatin (SOM)- and substance P (SP)-ir neurons are found in the SCNdm of rats, and they are typically found at the border of the SCNdm and SCNvl. The inhibitory neurotransmitter gamma-aminobutyric acid (GABA) is heavily expressed throughout both SCN subdivisions, and it is contained in most, if not all, SCN neurons.[2]

As in rodents, the monkey SCN region that receives the heaviest retinohypothalamic input is characterized by VIP immunoreactivity.[3] These VIP neurons are surrounded by an area of AVP-ir cells, suggesting that the SCNvl and SCNdm subdivisions are conserved in primates. Monkey SCN neurons in both subdivisions also express the synthetic enzyme glutamic acid decarboxylase (GAD), indicating that these neurons are GABAergic. In addition, NT-ir neurons are scattered throughout the monkey SCN, with a distribution much broader than that observed in rodents.

Consistent with other species, Nissl stains of the human hypothalamus reveal the SCN as a compact group of small-diameter cells dorsal to the optic chiasm and lateral to the third ventricle. Although the boundaries of the human SCN are sometimes difficult to discern in Nissl-stained material,[4] the human SCN can be readily identified and subdivided based on VIP and AVP immunoreactivity.[3] Similar to rodents, VIP-ir cells compose most of the ventral and central part of the SCN, whereas AVP-ir neurons surround the VIP cells in the caudal SCN. Preproenkephalin messenger RNA (mRNA) is expressed in the dorsal SCN,[5] partially overlapping the distribution of AVP-ir neurons, and scattered SOM-containing neurons are found in the medial SCN.[6] Postmortem tracing techniques suggest that human retinohypothalamic tract (RHT) fibers primarily contact NT-ir and VIP-ir neurons in the ventral SCN.[7]

However, there are notable differences in the human SCN compared to other species. An extensive population of NT-ir cells is found throughout the SCN, representing the largest known population of SCN neurons.[8] Also, neuropeptide Y

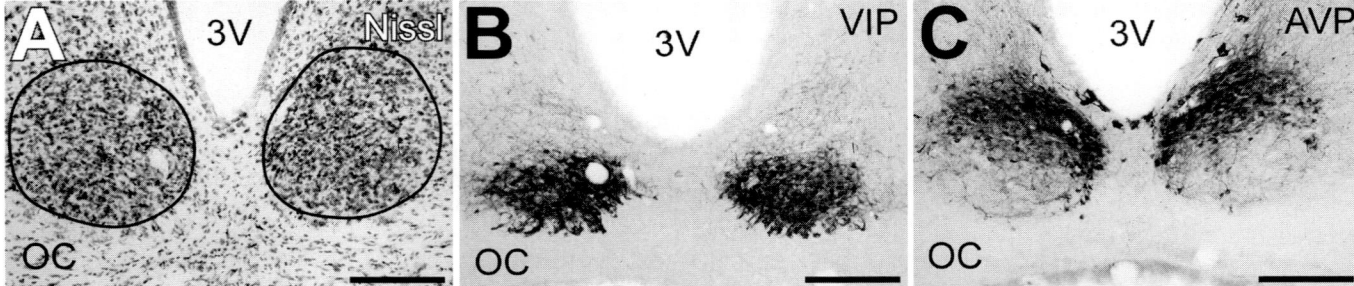

Figure 28–1. The suprachiasmatic nucleus (SCN) is composed of ventrolateral (SCNvl) and dorsomedial (SCNdm) subdivisions. In Nissl-stained coronal sections in rats **(A)**, the SCN can be identified by its tightly compacted small-diameter neurons located immediately dorsal to the optic chiasm and lateral to the third ventricle. VIP-immunoreactive (ir) perikarya are found in the SCNvl **(B)**, whereas AVP-ir cell bodies are found in the SCNdm **(C)**. 3V, third ventricle; AVP, arginine vasopressin; OC, optic chiasm; VIP, vasoactive intestinal polypeptide. Scale bars equal 200 μm.

(NPY)-ir neurons are found throughout the SCN, with the greatest density found in the central part of the nucleus, where they overlap with the distribution of VIP-ir cells. Because NPY-containing cells are absent in the rodent SCN, but a heavy afferent projection arises from NPY-ir neurons in the intergeniculate leaflet (IGL) of the lateral geniculate nucleus (LGN), it has been proposed that the NPY-ir cells in human SCN function similarly to the geniculohypothalamic tract (GHT) neurons in rodents.

It is currently unclear whether there is an IGL homologue in the human brain, but a population of NPY-ir neurons has been identified in the pregeniculate nucleus bordering the LGN.[9] It has yet to be determined whether the dense NPY-ir terminal plexus in the human SCN originates solely from NPY-ir perikarya within the boundaries of the nucleus or if there is an additional source of input from NPY-containing neurons in the pregeniculate nucleus.

In summary, the SCN can be subdivided into ventrolateral (core) and dorsomedial (shell) components based on neurotransmitter phenotype, and this organizational scheme is conserved across mammalian species. The relative distribution and projections (discussed later) of SCN neurons expressing VIP, AVP, and GABA are conserved in rodents and primates, and the bulk of retinal input is to the SCNvl. However, there are notable species-specific differences in the abundance and distribution of some SCN neurotransmitters. For example, the relative number of neurons in the human SCN that express NT or NPY far exceeds the number observed in other species. Therefore, the human SCN is likely functionally homologous to the SCN of other mammals, but the relative contributions and combinations of SCN neurotransmitters that regulate circadian rhythms may vary across species.

Inter– and Intra–Suprachiasmatic Nucleus Connectivity

Early anatomical studies of the SCN using the Golgi method suggested that SCN neurons are highly interconnected.[1] Subsequent studies using immunohistochemistry for SCN neurotransmitters, electron microscopy, and neuronal tracing confirm these results. Axonal terminals immunoreactive for AVP, angiotensin II, and ENK are primarily found in the SCNdm; SOM- and SP-containing fibers are predominantly found in the SCNvl; and VIP- and GRP-ir terminal boutons extend throughout both SCN subdivisions. Electron microscope studies of the SCN have shown that VIP-ir perikarya receive synaptic input from AVP- and SOM-ir axon terminals, AVP-ir cell bodies make synaptic contact with VIP- and SOM-ir axons, and VIP-, GRP-, SOM-, and AVP-ir neurons form synapses with cells containing the same peptide.[10,11] A caveat of these studies, however, is that the source of the terminals could not be determined.

Consistent with Golgi-stained material, some peptide-ir fibers from the SCN also cross the midline, and injection of retrograde tracer into one SCN results in retrogradely labeled neurons in the contralateral SCN, showing that the bilaterally paired SCN are interconnected. Tracing studies in rats using the transneuronal retrograde tracer pseudorabies virus (PRV; Bartha strain) showed that commissural connections primarily exist from SCNdm to SCNdm and SCNvl to SCNvl, and the flow of information in each SCN is predominantly unidirectional from the SCNvl to the SCNdm.[12] Likewise, unilateral intra-SCN injection of anterograde tracer into the dorsomedial or ventrolateral SCN of hamsters reveals a prominent projection from the SCNvl to the SCNdm and not vice versa.[13]

FUNCTIONAL ROLE OF SUPRACHIASMATIC NUCLEUS NEUROTRANSMITTERS IN REGULATING CIRCADIAN RHYTHMS

To coordinate the ensemble of circadian gene expression and electrical activity in the SCN, neurons of the circadian clock must communicate extensively with each other. The dense network of SCN neuron interconnectivity likely plays an important role in establishing stable phase relationships between SCN neurons. Upon exposure to light during the subjective night, retinorecipient neurons in the SCNvl appear to be chiefly responsible for resetting the circadian phase of neurons in the SCNdm. However, the mechanism by which SCN neurons phase shift or synchronize the circadian rhythm of other SCN neurons is poorly understood. In the following section, we will discuss the role of intra-SCN neurotransmission in the regulation of circadian rhythms and how the SCN is functionally divided to promote and maintain circadian rhythmicity within the SCN itself.

Vasoactive Intestinal Polypeptide

VIP-ir perikarya are found extensively throughout the SCNvl, overlapping with the heaviest region of RHT terminals. Retinal axons form synapses with VIP-ir neurons in the SCNvl, and light induces c-Fos (a transcription factor commonly used as a marker for cellular activity) in VIP-containing neurons during the subjective night. VIP-ir neurons project heavily to both subdivisions within the SCN, consistent with the distribution of VPAC$_2$ receptor (which binds both VIP and pituitary adenylate cyclase–activating polypeptide [PACAP] with equal affinity).[14] VIP-containing SCN neurons also send efferent projections beyond the borders of the SCN, and these projections are discussed later in this chapter.

VIP peptide and VIP mRNA content do not exhibit a circadian rhythm in constant darkness, but they do show a diurnal rhythm in a light-dark cycle, suggesting that VIP levels are predominantly regulated by light. Similar to the effects of VIP on SCN electrical activity in vitro, microinjection of VIP into the SCN region in vivo shifts the circadian rhythm of wheel-running activity similar to the way light does.[15] VIP knockout mice exhibit normal diurnal locomotor rhythms in a light-dark cycle, but they show a reduction in the circadian amplitude of wheel-running activity in constant darkness.[16] As in VIP–deficient mice, VPAC$_2$-receptor knockout mice can synchronize their behavior to the light-dark cycle (probably due to the masking effects of light on behavior) but have profoundly weakened locomotor activity rhythms in constant darkness.[17] Because clock gene expression and SCN electrical activity were not monitored across the circadian cycle in individual SCN neurons, it has yet to be established whether the loss of behavioral rhythmicity in VPAC$_2$-receptor–deficient mice is due to dampened circadian rhythms of clock gene expression in individual SCN neurons, or if the reduction in rhythmicity results from a loss of synchrony between SCN neurons in which the cellular rhythms of clock gene expression remain intact.

The aforementioned data are consistent with a model in which light regulates VIP expression in SCNvl neurons, and these neurons reset or synchronize the phase of other SCNvl and SCNdm neurons by VIP signaling through the VPAC$_2$ receptor. However, redundant or compensatory pathways appear to contribute to the maintenance of SCN rhythms, because a low-amplitude rest-activity rhythm is still evident in many VIP-receptor and VPAC$_2$-receptor–deficient mice.

Gastrin-Releasing Peptide

The distribution of GRP-expressing neurons largely overlaps the region of VIP immunoreactivity in the SCNvl, and many neurons contain both neurotransmitters. As expected, RHT terminals form synapses with GRP-ir neurons in the SCNvl, and light induces c-Fos in GRP-containing cells during the subjective night. Similar to VIP, GRP content exhibits a diurnal rhythm in a light-dark cycle, but not in constant darkness, suggesting that GRP levels are regulated by light. GRP receptor is predominantly found in the SCNdm, but low levels of GRP receptor expression are also found in the SCNvl. Consistent with the effects of GRP on SCN neuronal activity in vitro, microinjection of GRP into the SCN induces small phase shifts of locomotor activity, with phase-response properties similar to light-induced shifts of the rest-activity rhythm.[15]

GRP-induced phase shifts are also associated with induction of the clock genes mPer1 and mPer2 mRNA and c-Fos protein in the dorsal SCN, and these responses are absent in GRP-receptor–deficient mice.[18] Light-induced phase shifts of behavior and induction of mPer1, mPer2, and c-Fos are attenuated, but not absent, in GRP-receptor knockout mice. However, GRP-deficient mice show normal rest-activity rhythms in constant darkness, indicating that GRP signaling is not required for the expression of behavioral circadian rhythms. Therefore, light regulates GRP expression in the SCNvl, and GRP signaling plays a limited or redundant role in shifting the circadian phase of SCNdm neurons.

Neurotensin

Compared to the human SCN, there are relatively few NT-ir neurons in the SCN of rodents. In rats, the distribution of NT-ir neurons overlaps with the region of VIP immunoreactivity in the SCNvl, and neurotensin 1 receptor (NTS1) is specifically expressed in the SCNvl.[19] Although the limited in vitro data suggest that NT induces circadian phase shifts similar to dark pulses or NPY,[20] the physiologic relevance of NT in the regulation of circadian rhythms has not been tested in vivo. The distribution of NT and NTS1 receptor and the phase-shifting effects of NT in vitro suggest that NT signaling may play a role in resetting the circadian phase of neurons within the ventral SCN. However, it is unclear whether NT receptors in the SCNvl are activated by NT-containing neurons within the SCN, or if SCN afferent projections also contain NT. Based on the marked difference in the relative number of NT-ir neurons in rodents and humans, it is possible that NT plays a more prominent role in the expression of circadian rhythms in humans.

Somatostatin

SOM-containing neurons are primarily found along the boundary of the SCNvl and SCNdm, and the SOM receptors

SSTR1 and SSTR2 are predominantly expressed in the SCNvl.[21,22] In contrast to VIP and GRP, SOM content and SOM mRNA in the SCN show an endogenous circadian rhythm in constant darkness. In hypothalamic slices, application of SOM induces phase shifts in neuronal activity consistent with light-induced shifts of locomotor activity in vivo.[23] However, the role of SOM signaling in the SCN has not been tested in vivo. The SOM-containing neurons, which receive synaptic input from AVP-ir terminals that likely arise from SCNdm neurons, primarily send axons into the SCNvl, where SOM-ir terminals make synaptic contact with VIP-containing neurons.[24] Researchers have not tested, though, whether VIP and SOM receptors are coexpressed in SCNvl neurons. Nevertheless, SOM-containing neurons are positioned to receive indirect input from SCNvl neurons via SCNdm neurons and to provide rhythmic feedback to SCNvl neurons via SOM signaling.

Vasopressin

AVP and AVP V1a receptor mRNA are primarily found in the SCNdm, suggesting that AVP signaling within the SCN is largely restricted to the dorsomedial subdivision.[25] In addition to intra-SCN local projections, AVP-ir fibers from the SCN project to other hypothalamic areas including the medial preoptic area (MPOA), SPZ, DMH, and PVH, and to the paraventricular thalamic nucleus. Despite the abundance of AVP and AVP V1a receptor mRNAs in the SCNdm, AVP signaling appears to play a limited or redundant role in the regulation of circadian rhythms. AVP shows a circadian rhythm of gene expression in constant darkness,[26] but AVP-deficient Brattleboro rats show normal behavioral circadian rhythms,[27,28] indicating that AVP is not required for SCN rhythm generation or the output of rest-activity cycles. Furthermore, injection of AVP or V1 receptor antagonists into the SCN region does not alter the phase or period of locomotor activity,[29] and AVP does not shift SCN electrical activity in SCN slices.[23]

Gamma-Aminobutyric Acid

Most, if not all, neurons in both SCN subdivisions contain GABA, suggesting that the output of SCN neurons is principally inhibitory. GABA is found in approximately half of all presynaptic axons in the SCN,[30] and GABA- or GAD-ir axons form synapses with all types of neurons studied in the SCN.[11] GABAergic terminals in the SCN derive from SCN afferent projections and from GABA-containing neurons intrinsic to the circadian clock.

Histologic and functional studies indicate that GABA acts on both inotropic GABA$_A$ receptors and metabotropic GABA$_B$ receptors in the SCN. In situ hybridization and immunocytochemical studies have shown that several GABA$_A$ receptor subunits and the GABA$_{B1}$ receptor subunit are found in the SCN. Because the functional properties of GABA receptors are dependent on the subunit composition, and GABA$_A$ receptor subunits in the SCN are differentially distributed,[31] the effects of GABA on SCN neuronal activity may also be region specific. In cell cultures, GABA$_A$ or GABA$_B$ receptor agonists inhibit the firing rate of individual SCN neurons, but only GABA$_A$ receptor agonists induce circadian phase-dependent shifts of neuronal activity.[32] Thus, GABA induces phase shifts of neuronal firing in vitro by activating the GABA$_A$ receptor subtype. In dissociated cell culture, SCN neurons normally display independent and asynchronous circadian rhythms of neuronal firing, but daily administration of GABA synchronizes SCN neuronal electrical rhythms.[32] Thus, GABAergic signaling may play a role in coordinating the circadian phase of individual SCN cellular oscillators, but this has not been tested in vivo.

Similar to results in cell culture, GABA$_A$ receptor agonists inhibit neuronal and metabolic activity of SCN neurons in hypothalamic brain slices,[33,34] and the GABA$_B$ receptor agonist baclofen inhibits optic nerve–stimulated field potentials.[35] Consistent with in vitro data, light-induced phase shifts of locomotor activity are blocked by both GABA$_A$ and GABA$_B$ receptor agonists.[36,37] Collectively, these results suggest that GABAergic signaling within the SCN plays a pleiotropic role in the regulation of circadian rhythms.

Based on in vitro data, GABA may reset and coordinate the circadian rhythm of SCN electrical activity via GABA$_A$ receptor, while GABA$_A$ and GABA$_B$ receptors may be important for modulating RHT input to the SCN. As will be discussed later, GABAergic SCN afferent projections, especially from the IGL, may also be important in nonphotic resetting of circadian phase. In addition, SCN efferent projection neurons are GABAergic, suggesting that GABA may be the principle neurotransmitter of the circadian timing system.

ROLE OF CALCIUM-BINDING PROTEINS IN THE SUPRACHIASMATIC NUCLEUS

The circadian pacemaker exhibits a circadian rhythm in spontaneous firing in which SCN neurons are predominantly active during the subjective day and silent during the subjective night. SCN neurons exhibit spontaneous oscillations in membrane potential that are generated during the daytime by the diurnal regulation of L-type voltage-sensitive calcium channels.[38] The amplitude of the oscillation is sufficient to activate voltage-gated sodium channels, resulting in spontaneous firing during the subjective day. The amplitude of L-type Ca^{2+} currents in SCN neurons is highest during the daytime, corresponding to an increase in intracellular Ca^{2+} concentration.

In vivo, the diurnal entry of Ca^{2+} likely regulates light-induced and circadian phase–dependent changes in gene expression, including phosphorylation-dependent induction of the transcription factor cAMP (cyclic adenosine monophosphate) response element–binding protein (CREB), and the subsequent induction of the immediate-early gene *c-fos* in the SCN. Intracellular Ca^{2+} homeostasis is likely regulated by the Ca^{2+} binding proteins calbindin-D28K (CB) and calretinin (CAL), which are found in the SCN. In hamsters, RHT axons form synapses on CB-ir neurons, and light induces c-Fos in these cells.[39] CB-ir neurons define a distinct subregion in the caudal SCN, and many CB-containing neurons coexpress GRP or VIP.[40]

SCN lesion and transplantation studies suggest that the CB-ir subregion in hamsters may be important for the expression of locomotor activity rhythms.[41] Similar to other Ca^{2+} binding proteins, CB and CAL may function as cytosolic Ca^{2+} buffers to limit the availability of intracellular Ca^{2+}, thereby regulating Ca^{2+}-mediated signaling across the circadian cycle. In addition to hamsters and mice, CB-ir neurons have been described in the SCN of monkeys and humans,[6,42] but CB

immunoreactivity is conspicuously absent in the SCN of rats. CAL-ir neurons are also abundantly found in the SCN of rodents and monkeys,[42] but a functional role for CAL in the regulation of circadian rhythms has not been tested.

ROLES OF GLIA, GAP JUNCTIONS, NEUROTROPHINS, AND CELL ADHESION MOLECULES IN THE SUPRACHIASMATIC NUCLEUS

In addition to classical neuronal synaptic transmission, other modes of intercellular communication participate in synchronizing individual cellular oscillators and modulating the effects of light on SCN neuronal activity. Light-induced and circadian-modulated changes in synaptic plasticity appear to contribute to the circadian phase–dependent rhythm of sensitivity of the circadian clock to light and nonphotic zeitgebers. In the following sections, we will discuss the roles of glia, gap junctions, nerve growth factor signaling, and neural cell adhesion molecules in maintaining circadian rhythmicity and regulating the response of SCN neurons to light.

Glia and Gap Junctions

Cells immunoreactive for glial fibrillary acidic protein (GFAP), an astrocyte structural protein, are abundantly found in the SCN, and the distribution of GFAP immunoreactivity in hamster SCN fluctuates throughout the day in a light-dark cycle or in constant darkness.[43] In addition to functioning as insulators between SCN neurons, astrocytes may play a role in regulating the extracellular concentration of neurotransmitters such as glutamate released by RHT terminals. Transforming growth factor-alpha (TGF-α), a putative output molecule of the circadian clock (discussed later), has been identified primarily in GFAP-ir cells,[44] suggesting that SCN astrocytes may signal circadian phase to peri-SCN cells containing epidermal growth factor receptor (the receptor for TGF-α).

At the ultrastructural level, gap junctions are found between SCN astrocytes, which may serve to couple glia electrically or metabolically.[1] In vitro, glutamate or serotonin induces an increase in intracellular Ca^{2+} in SCN astrocytes, and Ca^{2+} oscillations are rapidly propagated to other glia, presumably via gap junctions.[45] The connexin subunits Cx32 and Cx43, which primarily constitute gap junctions in the plasma membranes of oligodendrocytes and astrocytes, respectively, have also been immunohistochemically identified throughout both SCN subdivisions, but the cellular phenotype of these cells has not been tested.

Some researchers have proposed that gap junctions act to synchronize electrical activity of SCN neurons, but there is only limited evidence suggesting that gap junctions exist between SCN neurons. This is primarily based on the observation that tracer from intracellularly injected SCN neurons spreads to other neurons, a process termed *dye-coupling*, which is thought to occur via gap junctions. However, electron microscope studies have failed to demonstrate the presence of gap junctions between SCN neurons, and connexin subunits have yet to be identified in SCN neurons. Furthermore, growing evidence suggests SCN neurons exhibit independently phased rhythms of neuronal firing and clock gene expression geographically across the SCN,[46] suggesting that electrical rhythms are not as tightly coupled as would be expected by gap junction communication. Nevertheless, it remains possible that SCN neurons contain low numbers of gap junctions that have eluded detection by electron microscopy, and gap junctions may serve to synchronize the neuronal firing rhythms of subsets of SCN neurons.

Neurotrophin Signaling

In addition to regulating neuronal survival, neurite outgrowth, and axonal pathfinding during embryonic and early postnatal development, neurotrophin signaling regulates neurotransmission, cytoskeletal changes, and synaptic plasticity in adulthood. Neurotrophins bind neurotrophin-specific tropomyosin-related kinase (trk) receptors and the common nerve growth factor receptor p75, or both. Conventionally, neurotrophins are thought to signal retrogradely by binding to nerve growth factor receptors on presynaptic terminals, but anterograde signaling also occurs in some contexts via neurotrophin receptors on postsynaptic dendrites.

Immunohistochemical studies indicate the p75 neurotrophin receptor (p75NTR) is the most abundant nerve growth factor in the adult SCN, and p75NTR-ir axonal fibers are primarily found in the SCNvl. Because in situ hybridization studies have failed to detect p75NTR mRNA in the SCN, it is likely that neurotrophin-containing SCN neurons signal retrogradely to afferent neurons containing p75NTR. Indeed, optic nerve transection results in a reduction of p75NTR immunoreactivity in the SCNvl and IGL, and some retrogradely labeled retinal ganglion cells from the SCN are p75NTR-ir, indicating that a subset of p75NTR-containing fibers in the SCN is of retinal origin.[47]

Thus far, the strongest candidate neurotrophin for nerve growth factor signaling in the mature SCN is brain-derived neurotrophic factor (BDNF). A circadian rhythm of BDNF has been reported in the SCN in vivo and in cell lines derived from the rat SCN.[48,49] Small numbers of fibers immunoreactive for tyrosine kinase receptor trkB, the receptor that preferentially binds BDNF, are found along the ventral border of the SCN above the optic chiasm, but it has not been tested whether these fibers are of retinal origin. Infusion of BDNF into the SCN region in vivo augments light-induced phase shifts of locomotor activity during the subjective day (when BDNF levels are normally low), but it does not affect phase shifts during the subjective night (when BDNF content is normally high).[50] Also, heterozygous BDNF mutant mice, which show reduced levels of BDNF and a dampened rhythm of SCN BDNF, show blunted light-induced phase shifts during the subjective night. Collectively, these data suggest that SCN neurons promote or enhance retinal neurotransmission during the subjective night by retrogradely activating p75 or trkB receptors, or both, on RHT terminals through BDNF signaling. BDNF has been reported to enhance glutamatergic neurotransmission in other brain regions, but the mechanisms by which BDNF regulates light-induced phase shifts in the SCN have not been examined.

VGF (not an acronym), which is regulated by nerve growth factor in vitro, is heavily expressed in both SCN subdivisions and also in the IGL.[51] In hamsters, VGF mRNA exhibits a circadian rhythm in constant darkness, and light induces expression of VGF during the subjective night in the caudal region of the SCN that receives the densest RHT input.[52] However, the role of VGF in the SCN and IGL is completely unknown, and VGF-deficient mice do not show overt deficits in circadian behavior.

Cell Adhesion Molecules

The polysialylated form of neural cell adhesion molecule (PSA-NCAM) has been implicated in activity-dependent remodeling of neuronal circuits and is thought to modulate cell-cell interactions by attenuating NCAM-mediated cell adhesion. As shown in hippocampal pyramidal neurons, PSA-NCAM can also promote activity-dependent plasticity by sensitizing neurons to BDNF. Polysialic acid (PSA) immunoreactivity is most intense in the SCNvl and exhibits a circadian rhythm in vivo and in in vitro hypothalamic slices.[53,54] In vivo, light increases PSA levels and induces c-Fos in PSA-ir neurons in the calbindin-containing subregion of the SCN in hamsters.[53]

Consistent with these results, in vitro application of glutamate increases PSA levels during the subjective night, and removal of PSA from NCAM by treatment with endoneuraminidase blocks glutamate- and optic nerve stimulation–induced phase delays in SCN neuronal activity.[54] Mice deficient in the NCAM-180 isoform that carries PSA show a reduction in circadian amplitude and eventual loss of the locomotor activity rhythm in constant darkness.[55]

These data suggest that PSA-NCAM plays an important role in mediating light-induced phase shifts and maintaining rhythmicity, perhaps via the reorganization of cell-cell interactions and synapses on SCN neurons. Consistent with this hypothesis, ultrastructural studies have shown that prolonged exposure to light reduces postsynaptic density and changes the relative number of asymmetrical and symmetrical synaptic appositions in the SCN.[56]

In summary, glia, neurotrophin signaling or PSA-NCAM–mediated cellular interactions, or both, may contribute to activity-dependent remodeling of SCN circuitry in response to light or nonphotic zeitgebers. SCN neuronal plasticity may also vary across the circadian cycle in accordance with the endogenous rhythm of SCN electrical activity, thereby influencing the circadian phase–dependent sensitivity of the circadian clock to zeitgebers and the coupling of SCN cellular oscillators.

SUPRACHIASMATIC NUCLEUS INPUTS

The endogenous circadian rhythm of neuronal activity in the circadian pacemaker is close to, but not exactly, 24 hours. Therefore, the circadian clock must be reset daily by extrinsic time cues to entrain the circadian rhythm of electrical activity in the SCN to the imposed solar day length. To coordinate behavioral, physiologic, and genetic circadian rhythms appropriately with diurnal changes in the environment, such as changes in the light-dark cycle or food availability, the circadian timing system processes both photic and nonphotic input.

The SCN is functionally divided such that the SCNvl receives dense input from the retina, IGL, and the midbrain raphe nuclei, whereas the SCNdm primarily receives projections from other hypothalamic areas, basal forebrain, limbic cortex, septal area, and brainstem (Fig. 28–2A).[57] Both SCN subdivisions, though, receive a dense afferent projection from the paraventricular thalamic nucleus (PVT). The SCN also receives small cholinergic projections from the basal forebrain and brainstem and histaminergic afferents from the tuberomammillary nucleus, but the role of these projections in the

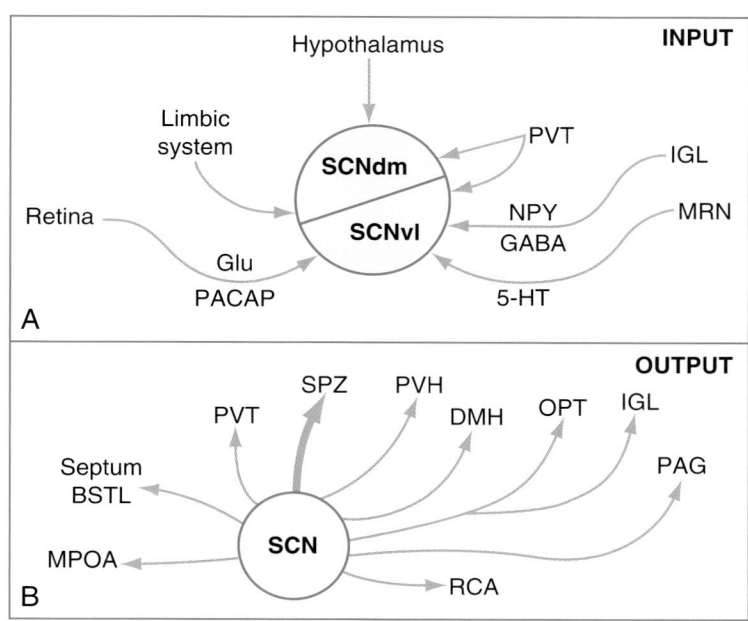

Figure 28–2. Afferent and efferent projections of the suprachiasmatic nucleus (SCN). SCN afferent projections terminate differentially in the SCNvl and SCNdm **(A)**. Neurotransmitters contained in these projections are shown next to the arrows. SCN efferent projections are primarily confined to the hypothalamus **(B)**. 5-HT, 5-hydroxytryptamine (serotonin); BSTL, bed nucleus of the stria terminalis; DMH, dorsomedial hypothalamic nucleus; GABA, gamma-aminobutyric acid; Glu, glutamate; IGL, intergeniculate leaflet; MPOA, medial preoptic area; MRN, median raphe nucleus; NPY, neuropeptide Y; OPT, olivary pretectal nucleus; PACAP, pituitary adenylate cyclase–activating polypeptide; PAG, periaqueductal gray matter; PVH, paraventricular hypothalamic nucleus; PVT, paraventricular thalamic nucleus; RCA, retrochiasmatic area; SCNdm, dorsomedial suprachiasmatic nucleus (shell); SCNvl, ventrolateral suprachiasmatic nucleus (core); SPZ, subparaventricular zone.

regulation of circadian rhythms remains controversial and requires further investigation. In the following sections we will examine the functional role of projections to the SCNvl in resetting and regulating the circadian clock, with particular emphasis on projections arising from the retina, IGL, and midbrain raphe nuclei.

Retina

The retinohypothalamic tract (RHT) is the densest input to the SCN and was first identified nearly 30 years ago by autoradiographic tracing methods.[58,59] In contrast to most other retinofugal projections, retinal efferents to the SCN are bilateral, with a slight to moderate contralateral predominance in most species (Fig. 28–3A). When retrograde tracers are injected into the SCN, a homogeneous population of small-diameter retinal ganglion cells (RGCs; ~13 µm diameter in the rat) that morphologically resemble type III (rat) or gamma (cat) RGCs is labeled in each retina, representing approximately 0.1% to 3% of all RGCs.[60,61] Although the RHT sends its densest projection to the SCNvl, the RHT sends smaller projections to the SCNdm, SPZ, anterior hypothalamic area (AHA), retrochiasmatic area (RCA), MPOA, ventrolateral preoptic nucleus (VLPO), and lateral hypothalamic area (LHA), especially in the region bordering the supraoptic nucleus.[62]

In contrast to most species, the retinohypothalamic projection in monkeys has been described as predominantly ipsilateral.[63] Similar to the rodent retina, the monkey retina projects most strongly to the ventral SCN, and scattered terminals are found throughout the dorsal SCN and extend into other hypothalamic areas including the AHA, especially dorsal to the SCN (equivalent to the SPZ defined in rodents), and the RCA.[3]

An intact RHT is required for photic circadian entrainment in mammals, but the classical photopigments (rhodopsin and cone opsins) are not required for entrainment to a light-dark cycle.[64] Recently, a novel invertebrate-like opsin termed melanopsin (Opn4) has been localized to the inner retina of mammals, including primates.[65] In rodents, melanopsin-expressing neurons are predominantly found in the RGC layer, and both anterograde and retrograde tracing strategies have been used to demonstrate that melanopsin-containing RGCs project heavily to the SCN.[66,67] Remarkably, melanopsin-containing RGCs that project to the SCN are intrinsically photosensitive and depolarize in response to light.[68,69] Consistent with the response properties of light-responsive SCN neurons, melanopsin-containing RGCs respond slowly to light, show sustained responses, and monotonically encode irradiance.[68]

A definitive role for melanopsin in circadian photoreception was shown in *Opn4* null mice, which show attenuated phase shifts of the rest-activity rhythm in response to bright light.[70,71] However, because these animals can still synchronize to a light-dark cycle, clearly there are redundant phototransduction pathways that mediate photic circadian entrainment. Bipolar cells in the eye form synapses with the dendrites and soma of melanopsin-containing neurons,[72] indicating that melanopsin-containing RGCs may receive indirect photic input from rods and cones. Recently, it was shown that photic circadian entrainment is abolished in mice lacking both the classical visual photopigments and melanopsin.[73,74] Thus, the presence of either melanopsin in RGCs or classical photoreceptors is sufficient for synchronizing daily rhythms to the solar cycle.

In addition to the SCN, melanopsin-expressing RGCs project to other brain areas that are involved in nonvisual photoreception including the VLPO, SPZ, olivary pretectal nucleus (OPT), and IGL[69,75] (see Fig. 28–3B). Some melanopsin-expressing RGCs send bifurcating axons to both the SCN and OPT,[75] and a subset of RGCs projects to both the SCN and IGL.[76] Each of these retinorecipient brain areas is interconnected with the SCN, suggesting that photic input from melanopsin-containing RGCs can modulate circadian rhythms via multiple routes. The projection to the sleep-promoting

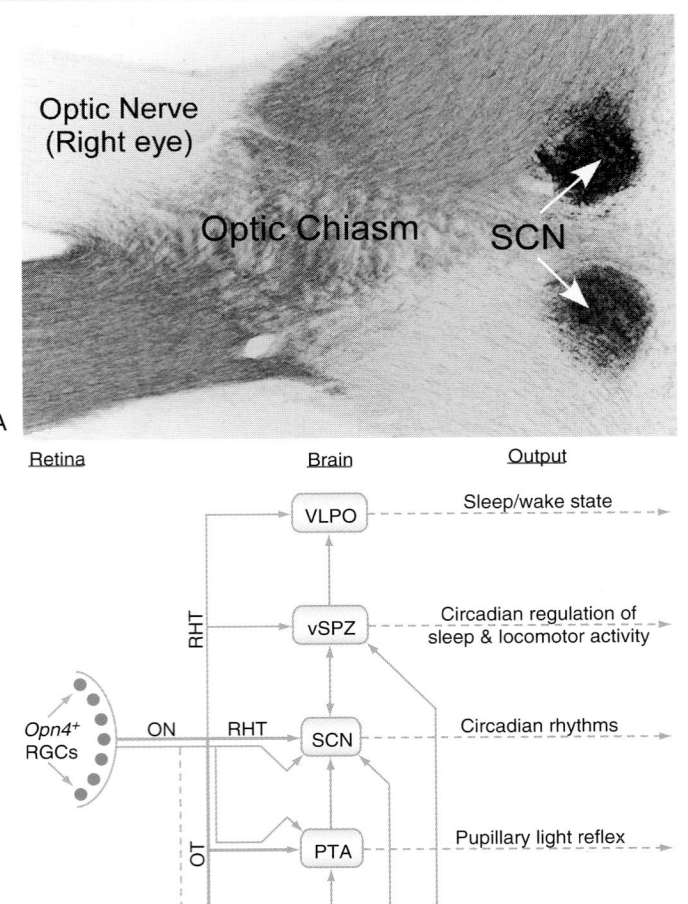

Figure 28–3. Retinal input to the circadian timing system from melanopsin-containing retinal ganglion cells. Following intraocular injection of cholera toxin B subunit into the left eye, anterogradely labeled axons project bilaterally to the SCN of rats, as shown in a horizontal section through the optic chiasm **(A)**. Melanopsin-containing retinal ganglion cells project to brain areas involved in processing nonvisual information, including the SCN and IGL **(B)**. The *branched solid arrow* to the SCN and PTA indicates collateralized projections, and the *branched dashed arrow* to the SCN and IGL indicates proposed axon collaterals. *Long dashed arrows* indicate physiologic and behavioral outputs of the targeted retinorecipient brain areas. Direct projections between brain areas are shown, but indirect projections are not shown for reasons of clarity. IGL, intergeniculate leaflet; *Opn4+* RGCs, melanopsin-positive retinal ganglion cells; ON, optic nerve; OT, optic tract; PTA, pretectal area; RHT, retinohypothalamic tract; SCN, suprachiasmatic nucleus; VLPO, ventrolateral preoptic nucleus; vSPZ, ventral subparaventricular zone. (**B**, Copyright 2003 by the Society for Neuroscience. From Gooley JJ, Lu J, Fischer D, et al: A broad role for melanopsin in nonvisual photoreception. J Neurosci 2003;23:7093-7106.)

VLPO could provide a direct substrate for the regulation of sleep-wake state, and the projection to the SPZ could modify circadian output from the SCN that determines the phase of the sleep-wake cycle (discussed later).

Several lines of evidence suggest that photic information is conveyed to the SCN via the release of excitatory amino acids such as glutamate from RHT terminals. Most light-responsive SCN neurons exhibit excitatory responses, and at the electron microscope level, RHT terminals predominantly form asymmetrical Gray's type-1 synapses on SCN neurons, presumed to be excitatory.[77] Glutamate and N-acetylaspartylglutamate (NAAG), which is metabolized to its constituent amino acids glutamate and aspartate, have been localized to RHT terminals in the SCN.[78,79] In a brain slice preparation, optic nerve stimulation induces the release of glutamate and aspartate in the SCN, but not GABA.[80] Glutamate mimics the effects of optic nerve stimulation on the circadian rhythm of SCN neuronal activity in vitro,[81] and microinjection of NMDA into the SCN region in vivo mimics the phase-shifting effects of light on rest-activity rhythms.[82] Similar to the effects of light, N-methyl-D-aspartate (NMDA) injected into the SCN region during the subjective night induces expression of *c-fos* in the SCN and acutely suppresses the synthesis of melatonin in the pineal gland.[83,84]

Consistent with pharmacologic studies implicating various glutamate receptor subtypes on SCN neuronal activity, receptor subunits from the NMDA-, AMPA-, and kainate-preferring classes of ionotropic glutamate receptors are found in the SCN, in addition to subunits from metabotropic glutamate receptors.[85] Most glutamate receptor subunits appear to be concentrated in the SCNvl, but the abundance and regional distribution of each glutamate receptor subunit varies. Because the physiologic properties of glutamate receptors depend on the subunit composition, the effects of glutamate on SCN neurons may differ with respect to the region-specific expression of glutamate receptor subunits.

RGCs that give rise to the RHT also express PACAP, and these PACAP-containing RGCs coexpress melanopsin.[67] At the electron microscope level, PACAP colocalizes with glutamate at RHT terminals, suggesting that both glutamate and PACAP transmit photic information to the circadian clock.[86] Both in vitro and in vivo studies indicate that the phase-shifting effects of PACAP are concentration dependent: High concentrations of PACAP induce phase advances during the subjective day similar to the effects of dark pulses or NPY, and low concentrations of PACAP yield phase shifts similar to those induced by light.[87] Also, PACAP binds the PAC1 receptor and VPAC2 receptor with equal affinity, both of which are expressed in the SCN.

Thus, determining the endogenous role of PACAP signaling in the SCNvl has presented a significant challenge. Mice deficient in the PAC1 receptor appear to entrain normally to a light-dark cycle, indicating that PAC1 signaling is not required for photic circadian entrainment.[88] However, PAC1−/− mice exhibit circadian phase-dependent deficits in light-induced phase shifts of behavior and light-induced gene expression in the SCN. Therefore, PACAP plays a role in resetting and regulating the circadian clock, but it appears to play a partially redundant role in transmitting photic information to the SCN.

Intergeniculate Leaflet

The IGL is a thin cellular layer sandwiched between the dorsal and ventral subdivisions of the LGN of the thalamus. Caudally, the IGL sweeps ventromedially at the lateral border of the medial geniculate nucleus, where it becomes contiguous with the zona incerta. In contrast to the dorsal and ventral LGN, which receive a predominantly contralateral projection from the eye, the IGL receives a dense bilateral projection,[89] with a slight to moderate contralateral predominance in most species. IGL neurons also receive dense afferents from the ipsilateral and contralateral IGL and RCA and smaller projections from the SCN, locus coeruleus, midbrain raphe, and brainstem cholinergic nuclei.[90] The IGL projects heavily to the SCNvl via the GHT and also sends efferents to hypothalamic areas adjacent to the SCN, including the SPZ and RCA. In addition, the IGL sends axons to the DMH, midline thalamus, pretectum, periaqueductal gray (PAG), superior colliculus, and the lateral and dorsal terminal nuclei of the accessory optic system.[91]

Most, if not all IGL neurons (~2000 on each side of the brain in rats) contain the inhibitory neurotransmitter GABA,[2] and the IGL is characterized by large populations of NPY- and ENK-containing neurons.[90,92] NPY-containing neurons in the IGL project heavily to the SCNvl subdivision, and GABA has been shown to colocalize with NPY in GHT terminals in the SCN,[2] indicating that these transmitters may be coreleased. NPY-ir terminals form synapses on VIP-containing neurons in the SCNvl, which also receive afferents from the retina. In rats, ENK-containing IGL neurons project to the contralateral IGL and not the SCN, but in hamsters enkephalinergic IGL neurons project to both the contralateral IGL and the SCN.[92]

As in the SCN, light-responsive neurons in the IGL are thought to encode changes in irradiance and show sustained responses to light, and some RGCs that project to the SCN send bifurcating axons to the IGL.[76] Unlike the dorsal LGN, which functions as a thalamic relay in image-formation processes, the IGL has a well-defined role in the regulation of circadian rhythms. Lesions of the IGL have been reported to result in a broad array of circadian phenotypes, including a slower rate of reentrainment following a shift in the photoperiod, a block in the lengthening of circadian period by constant light, elimination of NPY-type phase responses induced by novel wheel-induced locomotion, and a block in the ability of wheel running access to synchronize circadian rhythms.[93] Thus, the IGL transmits both photic and nonphotic information to the circadian clock. However, IGL-lesioned animals are clearly able to entrain to light-dark cycles, indicating that the IGL plays a modulatory, rather than principal, role in the regulation of photic circadian entrainment and rhythm generation.

The effects of NPY and photic stimuli on the circadian pacemaker appear to be mutually inhibitory. Consistent with the effects of NPY on SCN electrical activity in hypothalamic slices, microinjection of NPY into the SCN region induces phase advances in locomotor activity during the subjective day,[94] and NPY-induced phase shifts are attenuated by glutamate or light.[95,96] Conversely, glutamate-induced phase shifts in SCN electrical activity or light-induced phase advances in locomotor activity can be inhibited by NPY.[97] In vitro pharmacologic studies indicate that NPY inhibits neuronal discharge and NMDA-induced phase shifts via the Y5 receptor,[98] whereas NPY-induced phase shifts are mediated by the Y2 receptor.[99] Consistent with in vitro data, NPY attenuates light-induced phase shifts of rest-activity via Y1 or Y5 receptors, or both,[100] and NPY-induced phase shifts of locomotor activity appear to be mediated by the Y2 receptor.[101] Y1- and Y5-receptor mRNAs are highly expressed in the rat SCN, but surprisingly the Y2 receptor has yet to be detected.

Midbrain Raphe Nuclei

The SCN receives a dense serotoninergic input from neurons in the median raphe nucleus (MRN) and relatively sparse input from neurons in the dorsal raphe nucleus (DRN).[102] In contrast to the MRN, the DRN projects to the IGL and to the SPZ immediately dorsal to the SCN, with few fibers to the SCN itself. DRN projections to the forebrain are generally more widespread than projections from the MRN. Serotonin (5-HT)-ir axonal terminals in the SCNvl overlap extensively with the terminal fields of the RHT and GHT and form synapses with VIP-ir neurons.

Similar to NPY, the effects of 5-HT and photic stimuli on the circadian pacemaker appear to be mutually inhibitory. Light-induced, optic nerve-stimulated-induced, or glutamate-induced phase shifts are attenuated by administration of 5-HT during the subjective night, and 5-HT–induced phase advances during the subjective day are inhibited by glutamate agonists or optic chiasm stimulation.[103] The midbrain raphe nuclei are not required for photic circadian entrainment or the maintenance of circadian rhythmicity, but 5-HT clearly modulates photic and nonphotic input to the circadian clock. Lesions of the midbrain raphe nuclei have been reported to phase advance the locomotor activity onset, lengthen the activity phase, induce deficits in rhythmicity in constant light, and reduce the amplitude or clarity of circadian rhythms.[104]

Several 5-HT receptor subtypes have been described in the SCN of hamsters, mice, or rats,[104,105] but current functional evidence is strongest for 5-HT1B and 5-HT7 receptors in the regulation of circadian rhythms. In vitro and in vivo evidence suggest the 5-HT1B receptor mediates inhibitory effects of 5-HT on light-induced phase shifts and melatonin suppression.[106-108] In addition, electron microscopic studies have shown that 5-HT1B receptor immunoreactivity is predominantly found in presynaptic terminals of RHT and nonoptic axons, whereas the dendrites and cell bodies of SCN neurons contained relatively little 5-HT1B immunoreaction product.[109]

In vitro pharmacologic studies indicate the 5-HT7 receptor mediates 5-HT–induced phase advances in SCN neuronal firing during the subjective day and the inhibitory effects of 5-HT on SCN spontaneous discharge.[110,111] Consistent with in vitro data, 5-HT7 agonists induce phase advances in hamster behavioral circadian rhythms during the subjective day[112,113] and inhibit light-induced phase shifts and c-Fos in the SCN.[104,114] The 5-HT7 receptor has been localized to GABA-, VIP-, and AVP-ir dendrites in the SCN as postsynaptic receptors and also to presynaptic axonal terminals.[109]

In summary, the retinal projection to the SCNvl mediates photic circadian entrainment in mammals, and RHT axons are thought to transmit light information to the SCN via the release of glutamate and PACAP. Classical photoreceptors (rods and cones) or melanopsin-containing RGCs at the origin of the RHT are sufficient for photic circadian entrainment, but the absence of both types of photoreceptors abolishes entrainment to light-dark cycles. The SCNvl also receives dense input from NPY- and GABA-containing neurons in the IGL and serotoninergic input from the MRN. Light appears to have mutually antagonistic effects to NPY or 5-HT on SCN electrical activity and circadian phase shifting, but the IGL and MRN are not essential for circadian entrainment or rhythmicity. Thus, the IGL and MRN are thought to play a modulatory, rather than principal, role in regulating light-induced circadian phase shifts and transmitting nonphotic information to the SCN.

SUPRACHIASMATIC NUCLEUS OUTPUTS

The SCN plays a principal role in the circadian regulation of sleep-wake cycles and the diurnal release of endocrine factors, such as melatonin and corticosteroids, that influence behavioral state. In the following sections we discuss SCN efferent pathways, with particular emphasis on neuronal circuits regulating the circadian control of sleep. We will begin with a basic description of SCN efferent projections, including those critical for the circadian control of sleep and endocrine rhythms, followed by a discussion of the potential role for SCN diffusible factors in the regulation of circadian behavioral rhythms. Finally, we will address the hierarchical role of the SCN in determining circadian rhythms in peripheral tissues.

Considering the important role that the SCN plays in the regulation of circadian physiology and behavior, hormone regulation, and reproduction status, the number and density of SCN efferent pathways are surprisingly limited[115,116] (see Fig. 28–2B). The SCN projects rostrally to limbic structures, including the lateral septum and bed nucleus of the stria terminalis (BSTL), and to the MPOA and VLPO. The SCN sends dorsal projections to the midline thalamus, including the PVT and paratenial thalamic nuclei, and dorsocaudally to the SPZ, PVH, and DMH. A caudal projection from the SCN terminates in the RCA, and some fibers branch toward the supraoptic nucleus and the LHA. The SCN also sends a minor projection laterally to the IGL and small posterior projections to the OPT and central gray matter. Based on retrograde tracing studies in rats, the SCNdm projects more strongly to the MPOA, DMH, and BSTL, whereas the SCNvl projects more strongly to the lateral septum and tuberal hypothalamus.[115,117] However, the projections of the SCNdm and SCNvl partially overlap, and both SCN subdivisions project strongly to the SPZ and midline thalamus.

Local SCN projections have been mapped in primates by performing immunohistochemisty for VIP.[3,8] In monkeys, as in rats, VIP-ir axons project rostrally into the MPOA and dorsally into the SPZ and AHA ventral to the PVH. Some VIP-ir terminals

from the SCN are also observed in the PVH, LHA, and PVT. A dense VIP-containing projection extends caudally into the RCA, with some fibers continuing into the capsule of the VMH, DMH, and dorsal hypothalamic area. In humans, VIP-containing SCN neurons project most heavily into the region just dorsal to the SCN and extending to the area just ventral to the PVH, corresponding to the SPZ in rodents. Similar to monkeys, the SCN also sends a dense VIP-ir projection caudally into the RCA.

Sleep-Wake Rhythm

The densest output from the SCN is to the SPZ, which is located immediately dorsal to the SCN and extends dorsocaudally ventral to the PVH.[116] The projection to the SPZ has been demonstrated by conventional neuronal tracing techniques and by immunohistochemistry for SCN peptides such as AVP and VIP, which send axons dorsocaudally into the SPZ. Tracing studies have shown that the SCNvl projects more strongly to the lateral SPZ, whereas the SCNdm projects more densely to the medial SPZ.[117] Consistent with these results, AVP-ir axonal terminals are found medially in the SPZ, whereas VIP-ir terminals are found more laterally.

The SPZ innervates similar targets as the SCN but in much greater density, leading some to postulate that the SPZ functions as an amplifier of circadian output from the SCN. Cell-specific lesions of the SPZ eliminate circadian rhythms of sleep, locomotor activity, and core body temperature, suggesting that the SPZ is part of the primary neuronal pathway mediating the output of SCN-generated circadian rhythms.[118] Lesions in the ventral part of the SPZ abolish the circadian rhythms of sleep and locomotor activity, whereas lesions in the dorsal SPZ reduce the body temperature rhythm. The ventral SPZ, in turn, sends a strong caudal projection to the DMH. Cell-specific lesions of the DMH eliminate the circadian rhythms of sleep-wake, locomotor activity, feeding, and plasma corticosteroids, but not body temperature or plasma melatonin.[119] Hence, the major neuronal pathway mediating the SCN-generated circadian rhythm of sleep is through a first-order projection to the SPZ, followed by a second-order projection to the DMH.

As would be expected, the DMH projects to brain areas involved in the regulation of sleep-wakefulness including a primarily GABAergic projection to the VLPO, a sleep-active area in the anterior hypothalamus. The SCN and SPZ also send minor projections directly to the VLPO, but the projection originating from the DMH is much larger.[120] The VLPO, which contains the inhibitory neurotransmitters GABA and galanin, is thought to promote sleep via its projections to the ascending monoaminergic arousal system[121,122] (see Chapter 13). The DMH also sends a primarily glutamatergic projection to the lateral hypothalamus, which contains the wake-promoting population of orexin-expressing neurons.[119] Thus, the DMH receives circadian input directly from the SCN and indirectly via the SPZ and projects to the VLPO and LHA, which are critical in the regulation of sleep-wakefulness, defining a putative pathway for the circadian regulation of sleep and wakefulness (Fig. 28–4). The relay of SCN circadian signals in the SPZ and then the DMH may allow for modification of circadian rhythms by other inputs such as food availability, external temperature, or social cues.

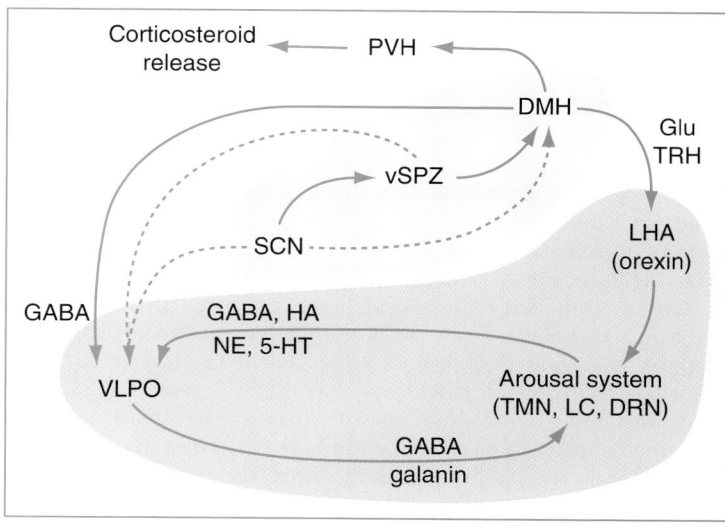

Figure 28–4. Circadian regulation of sleep-wakefulness. The neuronal pathway that regulates circadian sleep-wake cycles (SCN→vSPZ→DMH, indicated in *light blue*) directly interacts with arousal- and sleep-promoting brain regions (indicated in *darker blue*), providing a putative pathway for the circadian regulation of sleep-wakefulness. *Solid arrows* indicate prominent neuronal projections, and *dashed arrows* indicate relatively small projections. Neurotransmitters contained in these projections are shown next to the arrows. 5-HT, 5-hydroxytryptamine (serotonin); DMH, dorsomedial hypothalamic nucleus; DRN, dorsal raphe nucleus; GABA, gamma-aminobutyric acid; Glu, glutamate; HA, histamine; LC, locus coeruleus; LHA, lateral hypothalamic area; NE, norepinephrine; PVH, paraventricular hypothalamic nucleus; SCN, suprachiasmatic nucleus; TMN, tuberomammillary nucleus; TRH, thyrotropin-releasing hormone; VLPO, ventrolateral preoptic nucleus; vSPZ, ventral subparaventricular zone.

Circadian Regulation of Endocrine Rhythms

Melatonin Rhythm

Melatonin is a light- and circadian rhythm–regulated hormone that is thought to promote sleep in humans and regulates photoperiod-dependent effects on reproduction status in some rodents. The SCN is required for the circadian synthesis and release of melatonin in the pineal gland, which is regulated via a circuitous pathway.[123] A subset of SCN neurons projects directly to dorsal parvocellular neurons in the autonomic subdivision of the PVH. These PVH neurons send a glutamatergic projection to the sympathetic preganglionic neurons in the intermediolateral cell column (IML) in the upper thoracic spinal cord. The IML sends a cholinergic projection to the superior cervical ganglion (SCG), and the SCG postganglionic sympathetic neurons send a noradrenergic projection to the pineal gland. The release of noradrenalin activates alpha- and beta-adrenergic receptors in the pineal that stimulate the production of melatonin by control of the enzyme serotonin N-acetyltransferase.

The SCN is most active during the subjective day and inhibits tonic activity of PVH neurons, likely via GABAergic signaling, thereby resulting in a lower firing rate in the remainder of the pathway and promoting inhibition of melatonin synthesis. Thus, melatonin is produced during the subjective night, when SCN activity is low, and this is a common feature of both diurnal and nocturnal animals. Exposure to light during the subjective night activates SCN neurons via the retinohypothalamic tract, resulting in the inhibition of melatonin synthesis through the aforementioned pathway.

Melatonin can also provide direct feedback to the circadian system via melatonin receptors (MT1 and MT2) located in the SCN. Melatonin acutely inhibits SCN electrical activity, and this response is mediated by the MT1 receptor.[124] In vivo, the locomotor activity rhythm of rats can be entrained by periodic administration of melatonin as long as the SCN remains intact,[125] suggesting that melatonin receptor–signaling in the SCN is required for melatonin-induced entrainment. However, melatonin-induced phase shifts persist in MT1- or MT2-receptor

knockout mice, suggesting that melatonin receptor subtypes may play a redundant role in this response.[124,126] Melatonin has also been reported to phase shift circadian sleep-wake rhythms in humans, and daily administration of melatonin can entrain the circadian system of blind persons who show deficits in circadian photoreception.[127,128]

Corticosteroid Rhythm

Early lesion studies of the SCN showed loss of the circadian rhythm of adrenal corticosterone, the major glucocorticoid in rodents.[129] The circadian rhythm of corticosteroids rises sharply before the waking period presumably to promote a general state of readiness in anticipation of the myriad stressors associated with the active phase. SCN neurons project directly and indirectly to the DMH, which is critical for expression of the corticosteroid rhythm, and the DMH sends efferents to the PVH. By comparison with the circadian timing system controlling the sleep rhythm, it is likely that the ventral SPZ is also an obligate relay for corticosteroid rhythms, but this hypothesis remains to be tested. The SCN also sends a direct projection to the PVH, and some anterogradely labeled fibers from the SCN closely appose corticotropin-releasing hormone (CRH)-containing neurons in the parvocellular division of the PVH. However, this is a relatively weak projection, and in animals with DMH lesions it is not capable of maintaining corticosteroid rhythms.[119] The CRH-containing neurons in the PVH project to the median eminence, where CRH is released into the portal circulation and activates the release of adrenocorticotrophic hormone (ACTH) from the anterior pituitary gland. The SCN-driven release of ACTH into the blood results in the rhythmic induction of corticosteroid secretion from the adrenal gland.

Diffusible Suprachiasmatic Nucleus Output Signals

In SCN-lesioned hosts, transplantation of fetal SCN grafts in the third ventricle restores a low-amplitude circadian rest-activity rhythm with the period of the donor animal. However, photic entrainment, reproductive responses to photoperiod, estrous cycles, and corticosteroid and melatonin rhythms are not restored by SCN transplants. Polymer-encapsulated SCN transplants that prevent neuronal communication between host and donor tissue reinstate low levels of locomotor activity rhythms in SCN-lesioned hosts, suggesting that a diffusible factor can partially reconstitute the rest-activity cycle.[130] The distance of SCN transplants from the normal site of the SCN is an important factor for the recovery of the locomotor rhythm, indicating that a diffusible factor acts locally in a paracrine fashion.

Recently, candidate diffusible mediators have been identified in the SCN that may regulate the output of circadian behavioral rhythms including sleep-wake cycles. TGF-α is a secreted factor that is expressed rhythmically in the SCN with higher expression levels corresponding with the inactive phase in nocturnal animals (subjective day). Infusion of TGF-α into the third ventricle reversibly inhibits the circadian expression of wheel-running, sleep-wake, and body temperature rhythms, but it does not affect the underlying phase of the circadian clock.[131] However, recent data indicate that TGF-α is expressed mainly by astrocytes in the SCN, suggesting that a novel neural-glial interaction in the SCN may be involved in secreting TGF-α.[44] TGF-α functions through the epidermal growth factor (EGF) receptor, which has been described in the peri-SCN region and medial hypothalamus in rodents and monkeys. Mice with a hypomorphic EGF receptor mutation also show excessive activity during the daytime and fail to suppress locomotor behavior in response to light during the night, further implicating EGF receptor signaling in the control of rest-activity cycles.

Prokineticin 2 (PK2) is another secreted protein that functions as a putative output molecule of the circadian pacemaker.[132] PK2 is a clock-controlled gene that is rhythmically expressed in the SCN, with higher expression levels observed during the subjective day. Intracerebroventricular (ICV) injection of PK2 inhibits locomotor activity during the subjective night in rats (the active phase), suggesting that PK2 may regulate the circadian output of locomotor activity. PK2 receptor has also been described in many SCN output regions including the PVH, DMH, PVT, paratenial nucleus, lateral septum, and the SCN itself.

SYNCHRONIZATION OF PERIPHERAL OSCILLATORS

Recently, our view of the organization of the circadian timing system was changed considerably by the demonstration that peripheral circadian oscillators are present in nearly all tissues studied.[133] Apparently the SCN normally entrains these subordinate oscillators to ensure coordinated changes in physiology that are appropriately timed to the rest-activity cycle. As with the SCN, extra-SCN clocks show rhythmic clock gene expression and widespread rhythmic transcription of clock-controlled genes.[134-136] Circadian rhythms of gene expression in extra-SCN tissues can persist in vitro for several days, indicating that the SCN is not required for short-term maintenance of rhythmicity.[134] However, under normal conditions in vivo, the SCN determines the phase of clock gene expression in peripheral clocks, and SCN-lesioned animals show a loss of circadian gene expression in peripheral tissues.[137,138] Thus, the SCN is normally hierarchically dominant in determining circadian phase and maintaining long-term rhythmicity in peripheral clocks.

However, the phase of peripheral oscillators can become uncoupled from the SCN pacemaker. In animals that are exposed to circadian cycles of restricted food availability, circadian gene expression in tissues such as the liver, kidney, and heart entrain to the feeding cycle rather than to the phase of SCN activity or the light-dark cycle.[139,140] The mechanism(s) by which rhythmic SCN output or nonphotic zeitgebers synchronize peripheral oscillators is currently an area of intense interest.

In conclusion, the SCN regulates the circadian sleep-wake rhythm via a primary projection to the SPZ, followed by a secondary projection to the DMH. The DMH, in turn, projects to brain areas critical for promoting sleep or wakefulness, defining a putative pathway for the circadian regulation of sleep wake cycles. A direct projection from the SCN to the PVH mediates rhythmic control of melatonin secretion from the pineal gland, and an indirect projection from the SCN to the PVH via the DMH is critical for the circadian release of corticosteroids. Although SCN neuronal projections are required for photic entrainment and circadian control of endocrine rhythms, SCN-diffusible factors are sufficient to support a weak circadian rest-activity rhythm and, likely, sleep-wake cycles. Although candidate diffusible mediators of circadian phase have been recently identified, the pathways underlying nonneuronal SCN regulation of behavioral rhythms have yet to be determined, as are the SCN efferent pathways regulating the phase of circadian rhythms in peripheral tissues.

Clinical Pearl

The suprachiasmatic nucleus provides a 24-hour genetic clock, which allows daily scheduling of wake-sleep, feeding, corticosteroid secretion, and other bodily functions during a normal light-dark cycle. This cycle can be modified by light exposure or melatonin administration (which resets the suprachismatic clock), but new evidence suggests that feeding schedules and social interactions may reset the daily activity cycle by acting on circuits that are downstream of the clock. Thus, in patients with difficulty adjusting to shift work, jet lag, or other disruptions of their schedules, in addition to adjusting light exposure and taking melatonin, it is possible to adjust to a new schedule more quickly if the meal times, social interactions, and sleep-activity schedule of the new environment are adopted as soon as possible.

References

1. Van den Pol AN: The hypothalamic suprachiasmatic nucleus of rat: Intrinsic anatomy. J Comp Neurol 1980;191:661-702.
2. Moore RY, Speh JC: GABA is the principal neurotransmitter of the circadian system. Neurosci Lett 1993;150:112-116.
3. Moore RY: Organization of the primate circadian system. J Biol Rhythms 1993;8 Suppl:S3-S9.
4. Saper, CB: Hypothalamus. In Paxinos G, Mai JK (eds): The Human Nervous System, 2nd ed. New York, Academic Press, 2004, pp 513-549.
5. Sukhov RR, Walker LC, Rance NE, et al: Opioid precursor gene expression in the human hypothalamus. J Comp Neurol 1995; 353:604-622.
6. Mai JK, Kedziora O, Teckhaus L, et al: Evidence for subdivisions in the human suprachiasmatic nucleus. J Comp Neurol 1991;305:508-525.

7. Dai J, Van D, V, Swaab DF, et al: Human retinohypothalamic tract as revealed by in vitro postmortem tracing. J Comp Neurol 1998;397:357-370.

8. Moore RY: The fourth C.U. Ariens Kappers lecture. The organization of the human circadian timing system. Prog Brain Res 1992;93:99-115.

9. Moore RY: The geniculohypothalamic tract in monkey and man. Brain Res 1989;486:190-194.

10. Daikoku S, Hisano S, Kagotani Y: Neuronal associations in the rat suprachiasmatic nucleus demonstrated by immunoelectron microscopy. J Comp Neurol 1992;325:559-571.

11. Van den Pol AN, Gorcs T: Synaptic relationships between neurons containing vasopressin, gastrin-releasing peptide, vasoactive intestinal polypeptide, and glutamate decarboxylase immunoreactivity in the suprachiasmatic nucleus: Dual ultrastructural immunocytochemistry with gold-substituted silver peroxidase. J Comp Neurol 1986;252:507-521.

12. Leak RK, Card JP, Moore RY: Suprachiasmatic pacemaker organization analyzed by viral transsynaptic transport. Brain Res 1999;819:23-32.

13. Kriegsfeld LJ, Leak RK, Yackulic CB, et al: Organization of suprachiasmatic nucleus projections in Syrian hamsters (Mesocricetus auratus): An anterograde and retrograde analysis. J Comp Neurol 2004;468:361-379.

14. Sheward WJ, Lutz EM, Harmar AJ: The distribution of vasoactive intestinal peptide 2 receptor messenger RNA in the rat brain and pituitary gland as assessed by in situ hybridization. Neuroscience 1995;67:409-418.

15. Piggins HD, Antle MC, Rusak B: Neuropeptides phase shift the mammalian circadian pacemaker. J Neurosci 1995;15:5612-5622.

16. Colwell CS, Michel S, Itri J, et al: Disrupted circadian rhythms in VIP- and PHI-deficient mice. Am J Physiol Regul Integr Comp Physiol 2003;285:R939-R949.

17. Harmar AJ, Marston HM, Shen S, et al: The VPAC(2) receptor is essential for circadian function in the mouse suprachiasmatic nuclei. Cell 2002;109:497-508.

18. Aida R, Moriya T, Araki M, et al: Gastrin-releasing peptide mediates photic entrainable signals to dorsal subsets of suprachiasmatic nucleus via induction of Period gene in mice. Mol Pharmacol 2002;61:26-34.

19. Nicot A, Rostene W, Berod A: Neurotensin receptor expression in the rat forebrain and midbrain: A combined analysis by in situ hybridization and receptor autoradiography. J Comp Neurol 1994;341:407-419.

20. Meyer-Spasche A, Reed HE, Piggins HD: Neurotensin phase-shifts the firing rate rhythm of neurons in the rat suprachiasmatic nuclei in vitro. Eur J Neurosci 2002;16:339-344.

21. Beaudet A, Greenspun D, Raelson J, et al: Patterns of expression of SSTR1 and SSTR2 somatostatin receptor subtypes in the hypothalamus of the adult rat: Relationship to neuroendocrine function. Neuroscience 1995;65:551-561.

22. Breder CD, Yamada Y, Yasuda K, et al: Differential expression of somatostatin receptor subtypes in brain. J Neurosci 1992;12:3920-3934.

23. Hamada T, Shibata S, Tsuneyoshi A, et al: Effect of somatostatin on circadian rhythms of firing and 2-deoxyglucose uptake in rat suprachiasmatic slices. Am J Physiol 1993;265:R1199-R1204.

24. Maegawa M, Hisano S, Tsuruo Y, et al: Differential immunolabeling for electron microscopy of diverse peptidergic neurons. J Histochem Cytochem 1987;35:251-255.

25. Young WS, III, Kovacs K, Lolait SJ: The diurnal rhythm in vasopressin V1a receptor expression in the suprachiasmatic nucleus is not dependent on vasopressin. Endocrinology 1993;133:585-590.

26. Uhl GR, Reppert SM: Suprachiasmatic nucleus vasopressin messenger RNA: Circadian variation in normal and Brattleboro rats, Science 1986;232:390-393.

27. Groblewski TA, Nunez AA, Gold RM: Circadian rhythms in vasopressin deficient rats. Brain Res Bull 1981;6:125-130.

28. Peterson GM, Watkins WB, Moore RY: The suprachiasmatic hypothalamic nuclei of the rat. VI. Vasopressin neurons and circadian rhythmicity. Behav Neural Biol 1980;29:236-245.

29. Albers HE, Ferris CF, Leeman SE, et al: Avian pancreatic polypeptide phase shifts hamster circadian rhythms when microinjected into the suprachiasmatic region. Science 1984;223:833-835.

30. Decavel C, Van den Pol AN: GABA: A dominant neurotransmitter in the hypothalamus. J Comp Neurol 1990;302:1019-1037.

31. Gao B, Fritschy JM, Moore RY: GABAA-receptor subunit composition in the circadian timing system. Brain Res 1995;700:142-156.

32. Liu C, Reppert SM: GABA synchronizes clock cells within the suprachiasmatic circadian clock. Neuron 2000;25:123-128.

33. Liou SY, Shibata S, Albers HE, et al: Effects of GABA and anxiolytics on the single unit discharge of suprachiasmatic neurons in rat hypothalamic slices. Brain Res Bull 1990;25:103-107.

34. Mason R, Biello SM, Harrington ME: The effects of GABA and benzodiazepines on neurones in the suprachiasmatic nucleus (SCN) of Syrian hamsters. Brain Res 1991;552:53-57.

35. Jiang ZG, Allen CN, North RA: Presynaptic inhibition by baclofen of retinohypothalamic excitatory synaptic transmission in rat suprachiasmatic nucleus. Neuroscience 1995;64:813-819.

36. Gillespie CF, Mintz EM, Marvel CL, et al: GABA(A) and GABA(B) agonists and antagonists alter the phase-shifting effects of light when microinjected into the suprachiasmatic region. Brain Res 1997;759:181-189.

37. Tominaga K, Shibata S, Hamada T, et al: GABAA receptor agonist muscimol can reset the phase of neural activity rhythm in the rat suprachiasmatic nucleus in vitro. Neurosci Lett 1994;166:81-84.

38. Pennartz CM, de Jeu MT, Bos NP, et al: Diurnal modulation of pacemaker potentials and calcium current in the mammalian circadian clock. Nature 2002;416:286-290.

39. Bryant DN, LeSauter J, Silver R, et al: Retinal innervation of calbindin-D28K cells in the hamster suprachiasmatic nucleus: ultrastructural characterization. J Biol Rhythms. 2000;15:103-111.

40. LeSauter J, Kriegsfeld LJ, Hon J, et al: Calbindin-D(28K) cells selectively contact intra-SCN neurons. Neuroscience 2002;111:575-585.

41. LeSauter J, Silver R: Localization of a suprachiasmatic nucleus subregion regulating locomotor rhythmicity. J Neurosci 1999;19:5574-5585.

42. Fortin M, Parent A: Distribution of calretinin, calbindin-D28k and parvalbumin in the hypothalamus of the squirrel monkey. J Chem Neuroanat 1997;14:51-61.

43. Lavialle M, Serviere J: Circadian fluctuations in GFAP distribution in the Syrian hamster suprachiasmatic nucleus. Neuroreport 1993;4:1243-1246.

44. Li X, Sankrithi N, Davis FC: Transforming growth factor-alpha is expressed in astrocytes of the suprachiasmatic nucleus in hamster: Role of glial cells in circadian clocks. Neuroreport 2002;13:2143-2147.

45. Van den Pol AN, Finkbeiner SM, Cornell-Bell AH: Calcium excitability and oscillations in suprachiasmatic nucleus neurons and glia in vitro. J Neurosci 1992;12:2648-2664.

46. Yamaguchi S, Isejima H, Matsuo T, et al: Synchronization of cellular clocks in the suprachiasmatic nucleus. Science 2003;302:1408-1412.

47. Bina KG, Rusak B, Semba K: Sources of p75-nerve growth factor receptor-like immunoreactivity in the rat suprachiasmatic nucleus. Neuroscience 1997;77:461-472.

48. Liang FQ, Walline R, Earnest DJ: Circadian rhythm of brain-derived neurotrophic factor in the rat suprachiasmatic nucleus. Neurosci Lett 1998;242:89-92.

49. Earnest DJ, Liang FQ, Ratcliff M, et al: Immortal time: Circadian clock properties of rat suprachiasmatic cell lines. Science 1999;283:693-695.

50. Liang FQ, Allen G, Earnest D: Role of brain-derived neurotrophic factor in the circadian regulation of the suprachiasmatic pacemaker by light. J Neurosci 2000;20:2978-2987.

51. Van den Pol AN, Decavel C, Levi A, et al: Hypothalamic expression of a novel gene product. VGF: Immunocytochemical analysis. J Neurosci 1989;9:4122-4137.

52. Wisor JP, Takahashi JS: Regulation of the vgf gene in the golden hamster suprachiasmatic nucleus by light and by the circadian clock. J Comp Neurol 1997;378:229-238.

53. Glass JD, Watanabe M, Fedorkova L, et al: Dynamic regulation of polysialylated neural cell adhesion molecule in the suprachiasmatic nucleus. Neuroscience 2003;117:203-211.

54. Prosser RA, Rutishauser U, Ungers G, et al: Intrinsic role of polysialylated neural cell adhesion molecule in photic phase resetting of the Mammalian circadian clock. J Neurosci 2003;23:652-658.

55. Shen H, Watanabe M, Tomasiewicz H, et al: Role of neural cell adhesion molecule and polysialic acid in mouse circadian clock function. J Neurosci 1997;17:5221-5229.

56. Guldner FH, Bahar E, Young CA, et al: Structural plasticity of optic synapses in the rat suprachiasmatic nucleus: Adaptation to long-term influence of light and darkness. Cell Tissue Res 1997; 287:43-60.

57. Krout KE, Kawano J, Mettenleiter TC, et al: CNS inputs to the suprachiasmatic nucleus of the rat. Neuroscience 2002; 110:73-92.

58. Moore RY, Lenn NJ: A retinohypothalamic projection in the rat. J Comp Neurol 1972;146:1-14.

59. Hendrickson AE, Wagoner N, Cowan WM: An autoradiographic and electron microscopic study of retino-hypothalamic connections. Z Zellforsch Mikrosk Anat 1972;135:1-26.

60. Moore RY, Speh JC, Card JP: The retinohypothalamic tract originates from a distinct subset of retinal ganglion cells. J Comp Neurol 1995;352:351-366.

61. Murakami DM, Miller JD, Fuller CA: The retinohypothalamic tract in the cat: retinal ganglion cell morphology and pattern of projection. Brain Res 1989;482:283-296.

62. Levine JD, Weiss ML, Rosenwasser AM, et al: Retinohypothalamic tract in the female albino rat: A study using horseradish peroxidase conjugated to cholera toxin. J Comp Neurol 1991;306:344-360.

63. Tigges J, Bos J, Tigges M: An autoradiographic investigation of the subcortical visual system in chimpanzee. J Comp Neurol 1977;172:367-380.

64. Freedman MS, Lucas RJ, Soni B, et al: Regulation of mammalian circadian behavior by non-rod, non-cone, ocular photoreceptors. Science 1999;284:502-504.

65. Provencio I, Rodriguez IR, Jiang G, et al: A novel human opsin in the inner retina. J Neurosci 2000;20:600-605.

66. Gooley JJ, Lu J, Chou TC, et al: Melanopsin in cells of origin of the retinohypothalamic tract. Nat Neurosci 2001;4:1165.

67. Hannibal J, Hindersson P, Knudsen SM, et al: The photopigment melanopsin is exclusively present in pituitary adenylate cyclase-activating polypeptide-containing retinal ganglion cells of the retinohypothalamic tract. J Neurosci 2002;22:RC191.

68. Berson DM, Dunn FA, Takao M: Phototransduction by retinal ganglion cells that set the circadian clock. Science 2002; 295:1070-1073.

69. Hattar S, Liao HW, Takao M, et al: Melanopsin-containing retinal ganglion cells: Architecture, projections, and intrinsic photosensitivity. Science 2002;295:1065-1070.

70. Panda S, Sato TK, Castrucci AM, et al: Melanopsin (Opn4) requirement for normal light-induced circadian phase shifting. Science 2002;298:2213-2216.

71. Ruby NF, Brennan TJ, Xie X, et al: Role of melanopsin in circadian responses to light. Science 2002;298:2211-2213.

72. Belenky MA, Smeraski CA, Provencio I, et al: Melanopsin retinal ganglion cells receive bipolar and amacrine cell synapses. J Comp Neurol 2003;460:380-393.

73. Hattar S, Lucas RJ, Mrosovsky N, et al: Melanopsin and rod-cone photoreceptive systems account for all major accessory visual functions in mice. Nature 2003;424:76-81.

74. Panda S, Provencio I, Tu DC, et al: Melanopsin is required for non-image-forming photic responses in blind mice. Science 2003;301:525-527.

75. Gooley JJ, Lu J, Fischer D, et al: A broad role for melanopsin in nonvisual photoreception. J Neurosci 2003;23:7093-7106.

76. Pickard GE: Bifurcating axons of retinal ganglion cells terminate in the hypothalamic suprachiasmatic nucleus and the intergeniculate leaflet of the thalamus. Neurosci Lett 1985;55: 211-217.

77. Guldner FH, Wolff JR: Retinal afferents form Gray-type-I and type-II synapses in the suprachiasmatic nucleus (rat). Exp Brain Res 1978;32:83-89.

78. Castel M, Belenky M, Cohen S, et al: Glutamate-like immunoreactivity in retinal terminals of the mouse suprachiasmatic nucleus. Eur J Neurosci 1993;5:368-381.

79. de Vries MJ, Nunes Cardozo B, van der Want J, et al: Glutamate immunoreactivity in terminals of the retinohypothalamic tract of the brown Norwegian rat. Brain Res 1993;612:231-237.

80. Liou SY, Shibata S, Iwasaki K, et al: Optic nerve stimulation-induced increase of release of 3H-glutamate and 3H-aspartate but not 3H-GABA from the suprachiasmatic nucleus in slices of rat hypothalamus. Brain Res Bull 1986;16:527-531.

81. Shirakawa T, Moore RY: Glutamate shifts the phase of the circadian neuronal firing rhythm in the rat suprachiasmatic nucleus in vitro. Neurosci Lett 1994;178:47-50.

82. Mintz EM, Marvel CL, Gillespie CF, et al: Activation of NMDA receptors in the suprachiasmatic nucleus produces light-like phase shifts of the circadian clock in vivo. J Neurosci 1999; 19:5124-5130.

83. Ohi K, Takashima M, Nishikawa T, et al: N-methyl-D-aspartate receptor participates in neuronal transmission of photic information through the retinohypothalamic tract. Neuroendocrinology 1991;53:344-348.

84. Abe H, Rusak B, Robertson HA: Photic induction of Fos protein in the suprachiasmatic nucleus is inhibited by the NMDA receptor antagonist MK-801. Neurosci Lett 1991;127:9-12.

85. Ebling FJ: The role of glutamate in the photic regulation of the suprachiasmatic nucleus. Prog Neurobiol 1996;50:109-132.

86. Hannibal J, Moller M, Ottersen OP, et al: PACAP and glutamate are co-stored in the retinohypothalamic tract. J Comp Neurol 2000;418:147-155.

87. Harmar AJ: An essential role for peptidergic signalling in the control of circadian rhythms in the suprachiasmatic nuclei. J Neuroendocrinol 2003;15:335-338.

88. Hannibal J, Jamen F, Nielsen HS, et al: Dissociation between light-induced phase shift of the circadian rhythm and clock gene expression in mice lacking the pituitary adenylate cyclase activating polypeptide type 1 receptor. J Neurosci 2001;21: 4883-4890.

89. Hickey TL, Spear PD: Retinogeniculate projections in hooded and albino rats: an autoradiographic study. Exp Brain Res 1976;24:523-529.

90. Moore RY, Card JP: Intergeniculate leaflet: An anatomically and functionally distinct subdivision of the lateral geniculate complex. J Comp Neurol 1994;344:403-430.

91. Moore RY, Weis R, Moga MM: Efferent projections of the intergeniculate leaflet and the ventral lateral geniculate nucleus in the rat. J Comp Neurol 2000;420:398-418.

92. Morin LP, Blanchard J: Organization of the hamster intergeniculate leaflet: NPY and ENK projections to the suprachiasmatic nucleus. intergeniculate leaflet and posterior limitans nucleus. Vis Neurosci 1995;12:57-67.

93. Harrington ME: The ventral lateral geniculate nucleus and the intergeniculate leaflet: Interrelated structures in the visual and circadian systems. Neurosci Biobehav Rev 1997;21:705-727.

94. Albers HE, Ferris CF: Neuropeptide Y: Role in light-dark cycle entrainment of hamster circadian rhythms. Neurosci Lett 1984;50:163-168.

95. Biello SM, Golombek DA, Harrington ME: Neuropeptide Y and glutamate block each other's phase shifts in the suprachiasmatic nucleus in vitro. Neuroscience 1997;77:1049-1057.

96. Biello SM, Mrosovsky N: Blocking the phase-shifting effect of neuropeptide Y with light. Proc R Soc Lond B Biol Sci 1995; 259:179-187.

97. Weber ET, Rea MA: Neuropeptide Y blocks light-induced phase advances but not delays of the circadian activity rhythm in hamsters. Neurosci Lett 1997;231:159-162.

98. Gribkoff VK, Pieschl RL, Wisialowski TA, et al: Phase shifting of circadian rhythms and depression of neuronal activity in the rat suprachiasmatic nucleus by neuropeptide Y: Mediation by different receptor subtypes. J Neurosci 1998;18: 3014-3022.

99. Golombek DA, Biello SM, Rendon RA, et al: Neuropeptide Y phase shifts the circadian clock in vitro via a Y2 receptor. Neuroreport 1996;7:1315-1319.

100. Lall GS, Biello SM: Attenuation of circadian light induced phase advances and delays by neuropeptide Y and a neuropeptide Y Y1/Y5 receptor agonist. Neuroscience 2003;119: 611-618.

101. Huhman KL, Gillespie CF, Marvel CL, et al: Neuropeptide Y phase shifts circadian rhythms in vivo via a Y2 receptor. Neuroreport 1996;7:1249-1252.

102. Moga MM, Moore RY: Organization of neural inputs to the suprachiasmatic nucleus in the rat. J Comp Neurol 1997;389: 508-534.

103. Prosser RA: Glutamate blocks serotonergic phase advances of the mammalian circadian pacemaker through AMPA and NMDA receptors. J Neurosci 2001;21:7815-7822.

104. Morin LP: Serotonin and the regulation of mammalian circadian rhythmicity. Ann Med 1999;31:12-33.

105. Roca AL, Weaver DR, Reppert SM: Serotonin receptor gene expression in the rat suprachiasmatic nuclei. Brain Res 1993; 608:159-165.

106. Pickard GE, Weber ET, Scott PA, et al: 5HT1B receptor agonists inhibit light-induced phase shifts of behavioral circadian rhythms and expression of the immediate-early gene c-fos in the suprachiasmatic nucleus. J Neurosci 1996;16:8208-8220.

107. Rea MA, Pickard GE: A 5-HT(1B) receptor agonist inhibits light-induced suppression of pineal melatonin production. Brain Res 2000;858:424-428.

108. Pickard GE, Smith BN, Belenky M, et al: 5-HT1B receptor-mediated presynaptic inhibition of retinal input to the suprachiasmatic nucleus. J Neurosci 1999;19:4034-4045.

109. Belenky MA, Pickard GE: Subcellular distribution of 5-HT(1B) and 5-HT(7) receptors in the mouse suprachiasmatic nucleus. J Comp Neurol 2001;432:371-388.

110. Prosser RA: Serotonin phase-shifts the mouse suprachiasmatic circadian clock in vitro. Brain Res 2003;966:110-115.

111. Shibata S, Tsuneyoshi A, Hamada T, et al: Phase-resetting effect of 8-OH-DPAT, a serotonin 1A receptor agonist, on the circadian rhythm of firing rate in the rat suprachiasmatic nuclei in vitro. Brain Res 1992;582:353-356.

112. Mintz EM, Gillespie CF, Marvel CL, et al: Serotonergic regulation of circadian rhythms in Syrian hamsters. Neuroscience 1997;79:563-569.

113. Bobrzynska KJ, Godfrey MH, Mrosovsky N: Serotonergic stimulation and nonphotic phase-shifting in hamsters. Physiol Behav 1996;59:221-230.

114. Glass JD, Selim M, Rea MA: Modulation of light-induced C-Fos expression in the suprachiasmatic nuclei by 5-HT1A receptor agonists. Brain Res 1994;638:235-242.

115. Watts AG, Swanson LW: Efferent projections of the suprachiasmatic nucleus: II. Studies using retrograde transport of fluorescent dyes and simultaneous peptide immunohistochemistry in the rat. J Comp Neurol 1987;258:230-252.

116. Watts AG, Swanson LW, Sanchez-Watts G: Efferent projections of the suprachiasmatic nucleus: I. Studies using anterograde transport of Phaseolus vulgaris leucoagglutinin in the rat. J Comp Neurol 1987;258:204-229.

117. Leak RK, Moore RY: Topographic organization of suprachiasmatic nucleus projection neurons. J Comp Neurol 2001;433: 312-334.

118. Lu J, Zhang YH, Chou TC, et al: Contrasting effects of ibotenate lesions of the paraventricular nucleus and subparaventricular zone on sleep-wake cycle and temperature regulation. J Neurosci 2001;21:4864-4874.

119. Chou TC, Scammell TE, Gooley JJ, et al: Critical role of dorsomedial hypothalamic nucleus in a wide range of behavioral circadian rhythms. J Neurosci 2003;23:10691-10702.

120. Chou TC, Bjorkum AA, Gaus SE, et al: Afferents to the ventrolateral preoptic nucleus. J Neurosci 2002;22:977-990.

121. Sherin JE, Shiromani PJ, McCarley RW, et al: Activation of ventrolateral preoptic neurons during sleep. Science 1996; 271:216-219.

122. Sherin JE, Elmquist JK, Torrealba F, et al: Innervation of histaminergic tuberomammillary neurons by GABAergic and galaninergic neurons in the ventrolateral preoptic nucleus of the rat. J Neurosci 1998;18:4705-4721.

123. Teclemariam-Mesbah R, Ter Horst GJ, Postema F, et al: Anatomical demonstration of the suprachiasmatic nucleus-pineal pathway. J Comp Neurol 1999;406:171-182.

124. Liu C, Weaver DR, Jin X, et al: Molecular dissection of two distinct actions of melatonin on the suprachiasmatic circadian clock. Neuron 1997;19:91-102.

125. Cassone VM, Chesworth MJ, Armstrong SM: Entrainment of rat circadian rhythms by daily injection of melatonin depends upon the hypothalamic suprachiasmatic nuclei. Physiol Behav 1986;36:1111-1121.

126. Jin X, von Gall C, Pieschl RL, et al: Targeted disruption of the mouse Mel(1b) melatonin receptor. Mol Cell Biol 2003;23: 1054-1060.

127. Lockley SW, Skene DJ, James K, et al: Melatonin administration can entrain the free-running circadian system of blind subjects. J Endocrinol 2000;164:R1-R6.

128. Sack RL, Brandes RW, Kendall AR, et al: Entrainment of free-running circadian rhythms by melatonin in blind people. N Engl J Med 2000;343:1070-1077.

129. Moore RY, Eichler VB: Loss of a circadian adrenal corticosterone rhythm following suprachiasmatic lesions in the rat. Brain Res 1972;42:201-206.

130. Silver R, LeSauter J, Tresco PA, et al: A diffusible coupling signal from the transplanted suprachiasmatic nucleus controlling circadian locomotor rhythms. Nature 1996;382: 810-813.

131. Kramer A, Yang FC, Snodgrass P, et al: Regulation of daily locomotor activity and sleep by hypothalamic EGF receptor signaling. Science 2001;294:2511-2515.

132. Cheng MY, Bullock CM, Li C, et al: Prokineticin 2 transmits the behavioural circadian rhythm of the suprachiasmatic nucleus. Nature 2002;417:405-410.

133. Schibler U, Sassone-Corsi P: A web of circadian pacemakers. Cell 2002;111:919-922.

134. Yamazaki S, Numano R, Abe M, et al: Resetting central and peripheral circadian oscillators in transgenic rats. Science 2000;288:682-685.

135. Panda S, Antoch MP, Miller BH, et al: Coordinated transcription of key pathways in the mouse by the circadian clock. Cell 2002;109:307-320.

136. Storch KF, Lipan O, Leykin I, et al: Extensive and divergent circadian gene expression in liver and heart. Nature 2002; 417:78-83.

137. Akhtar RA, Reddy AB, Maywood ES, et al: Circadian cycling of the mouse liver transcriptome, as revealed by cDNA microarray, is driven by the suprachiasmatic nucleus. Curr Biol 2002;12:540-550.

138. Hara R, Wan K, Wakamatsu H, et al: Restricted feeding entrains liver clock without participation of the suprachiasmatic nucleus. Genes Cells 2001;6:269-278.

139. Stokkan KA, Yamazaki S, Tei H, et al: Entrainment of the circadian clock in the liver by feeding. Science 2001;291: 490-493.

140. Damiola F, Le Minh N, Preitner N, et al: Restricted feeding uncouples circadian oscillators in peripheral tissues from the central pacemaker in the suprachiasmatic nucleus. Genes Dev 2000;14:2950-2961.

29

Physiology of the Mammalian Circadian System

Alan M. Rosenwasser

Fred W. Turek

ABSTRACT

Our understanding of the physiology of the mammalian circadian system has increased enormously in just the past few years. Although it has been known for many years that the circadian clock has a period of approximately 24 hours (hence the name *circadian*, "about a day"), and that the light–dark cycle synchronizes ("entrains") the clock to the solar day through a special tract of nerves to the anterior hypothalamus, called the *retinohypothalamic tract*, only in the past few years have the functional retinal photoreceptors been identified as a unique subset of melanopsin-containing ganglion cells. Embedded in the hypothalamus are the bilaterally paired suprachiasmatic nuclei (SCN), first identified in the early 1970s as critical for the normal expression of circadian rhythms, and long considered to be the master circadian pacemaker in mammals. Only in the past few years, however, has the SCN given up the secret of how it generates circadian rhythmicity, a process that is now known to be intrinsic to individual SCN neurons and to involve a transcriptional–translational feedback loops (s) comprising a number of "clock genes" and their protein products. In addition to photic signals from the retina, the SCN also receives inputs from a number of other sources conveying functional information about various aspects of the internal and external environments that are integrated to regulate the overall temporal organization of the animal. Just as the mystery of the molecular timing mechanism is being unraveled, new findings have revealed that the circadian timing system at the organismal level is much more complex and interesting than previously thought. The circadian system is now seen as hierarchically organized, such that the master clock in the SCN synchronizes multiple circadian oscillators distributed throughout the brain and body. Indeed, most, if not all, tissues and organs of the body appear to contain the core molecular circadian clock machinery, such that the molecular clock in the SCN entrains similar molecular clocks throughout the body to ensure overall internal temporal organization. Thus, two revolutionary developments in the circadian clock field—(1) the elucidation of the core molecular clock machinery, and (2) the demonstration that most, if not all, tissues can themselves express the 24-hour molecular clock—have opened up an entirely new area of biomedical research on the importance of internal timing for health and disease. With hundreds and even thousands of genes oscillating in any given organ system, under the control of both central (i.e., SCN) and local (i.e., within the tissues) self-sustained circadian oscillations, the circadian clock system clearly plays a central role in regulating cellular function in many ways. Indeed, the balance between health and disease may be highly dependent on the proper synchrony within and between oscillating systems.

A great deal of new information has been obtained in just the past few years about the mammalian circadian timing system at the molecular, cellular, neural systems, and behavioral levels. These advances have led to improved understanding of the neuroanatomy, neurochemistry, and molecular neurobiology of the circadian pacemaker, how this pacemaker is synchronized (entrained) to the external environment, and how it regulates a variety of peripheral oscillating systems. This chapter reviews recent findings on the structure and function of the mammalian circadian timing system, with an emphasis on the newly emerging multioscillatory nature of this system, how the master circadian clock in the hypothalamus receives inputs from the internal and external environment, and how the clock regulates the wide diversity of biochemical, molecular, cellular, physiologic, and behavioral rhythms.

THE SUPRACHIASMATIC NUCLEUS, "STILL" THE MASTER CIRCADIAN PACEMAKER IN MAMMALS

As described later in this chapter, exciting new results demonstrating that the molecular circadian clock exists in many tissues and organs are revolutionizing our understanding of how the circadian clock system is organized in mammals. Nevertheless, there is still substantial evidence from a variety of different experiments that the hypothalamic suprachiasmatic nucleus (SCN) is the site of a "master" circadian clock in mammals that is responsible for regulating, directly or indirectly, most, if not all, circadian rhythms in mammals.[1,2] Over the years, a variety of studies involving SCN lesions, recordings of SCN neural activity in vivo and in vitro, functional metabolic mapping, fetal tissue transplantation, and molecular rhythm analysis, have revealed that the SCN not only is capable of sustained rhythmic activity, but is responsible for maintaining circadian rhythmicity in central and peripheral tissues.[3-5]

Although early mathematical models raised the possibility that the circadian pacemaker could be constructed from an ensemble of coupled, high-frequency (i.e., noncircadian) oscillatory units, it is now clear that the generation of circadian signals by the SCN is fundamentally a cellular process.

Studies using a variety of in vitro models, including long-term SCN cell culture,[6] simultaneous recording of multiple single units using multielectrode plates,[7-10] and optical monitoring of calcium flux[11] or gene expression[12] in individual SCN neurons, have now provided compelling evidence that circadian oscillation is indeed a cell-autonomous process, expressed in many, and possibly all, individual SCN neurons. Nevertheless, this multitude of cellular circadian oscillators normally interacts to produce coherent circadian patterns of behavior.[13] Although the mechanisms underlying intra-SCN oscillator coupling have not been identified completely, early studies using tetrodotoxin revealed that individual neuronal oscillators in the SCN apparently remain synchronized even in the absence of sodium-dependent action potentials, both in vivo and in vitro.[14,15] Thus, it has been suggested that gap junctions, glial coupling, calcium-dependent action potentials, or local diffusible signals may be responsible for maintaining interoscillator synchrony (for reviews, see Shirakawa et al.[16] and Miche and Colwell[17]).

Although early studies demonstrated that protein synthesis was involved in the generation of circadian signals,[18,19] analysis of the fundamental circadian oscillatory mechanism has more recently been extended to the molecular genetic level (see Chapter 30). The discovery of the first mammalian circadian clock gene, *Clock*,[20,21] was followed quickly by the identification of a number of other "core" clock genes, many of which showed clear homology to previously or later discovered circadian clock genes in the fruit fly.[22] At present, putative mammalian clock genes include three *Per* genes (*Per1*, *Per2*, *Per3*), *Tim*, *Clock*, *Bmal*, *CK1e*, and two plant cryptochrome gene homologs (*Cry1* and *Cry2*), all of which are expressed in SCN neurons.[23-25] These genes and their protein products interact to form interlocking autoregulatory transcription–translation feedback loops that define the molecular core of the circadian oscillator[26-28] (Fig. 29–1). These basic molecular feedback loops are modulated by posttranslational biochemical processes, leading eventually to the display of remarkably precise 24-hour rhythms in metabolic, physiologic, and behavioral processes.[24,25]

CLOCK and BMAL form protein heterodimers that exert positive drive on transcription of the *Per* and *Cry* genes, whereas the PER and CRY proteins form both homodimers and heterodimers that negatively regulate *Clock* and *Bmal* activity. This feedback loop results in rhythmic transcription of specific clock genes in the in vivo[29-31] and in vitro SCN.[32,33] In addition, molecular outputs from the core oscillator result in rhythmic expression of various clock-controlled genes (i.e., genes that are controlled by, but not part of, the core circadian oscillator loop), which in turn serve as the basis for rhythmic outputs to myriad other cellular processes.[28] Ultimately, these molecular processes are reflected in circadian behavioral rhythmicity, as amply documented by analysis of altered circadian pacemaker function in mice carrying a mutation of the *Clock* gene[20,34] or null or loss-of-function mutations of *Per* and *Cry* genes,[35-37] as well as in *tau*-mutant hamsters carrying a mutation of the *CK1e* gene.[38,39] Interestingly, mutation or deletion of circadian clock genes has also been shown recently to affect sleep–wake homeostasis, suggesting a possible molecular link between the circadian and sleep-regulatory systems.[40,41]

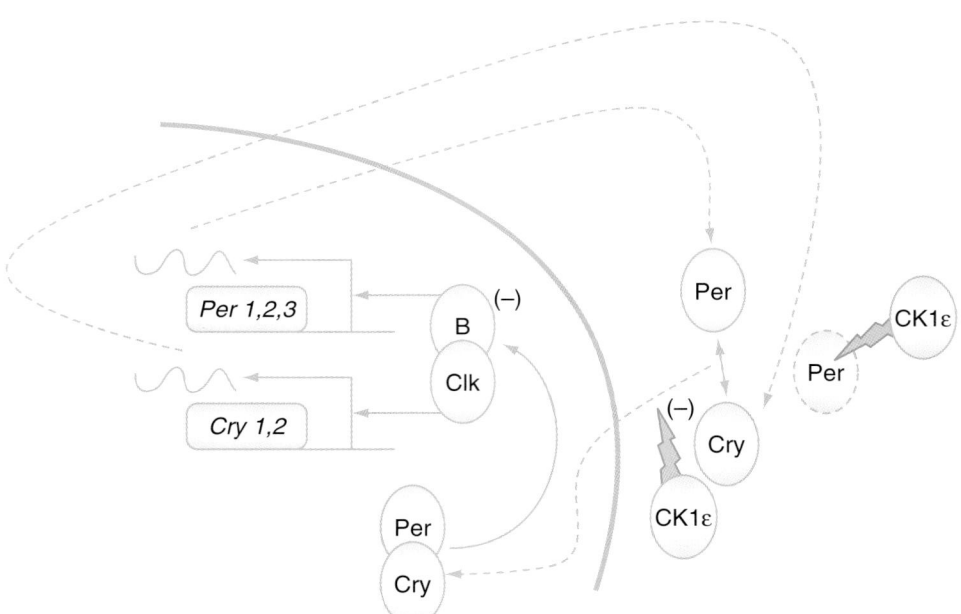

Figure 29–1. Essential elements of the core molecular loop underlying circadian timing at the cellular level in mammals. The transcription factors CLOCK (Clk) and BMAL1 (B) form protein heterodimers exerting positive drive on the transcription of several clock genes, including the *Per* ("period") genes *Per1*, *Per2*, and *Per3*, and the *Cry* (cryptochrome) genes *Cry1* and *Cry2*. The protein products of these genes dimerize in several different combinations, including PER-CRY (as shown here) and PER-PER pairings. After nuclear translocation, PER and CRY inhibit the transcriptional effects of CLOCK-BMAL1 through direct protein–protein interaction, and thus exert negative autoregulation of their own transcription. This negative feedback results in circadian expression of *Per* and *Cry* transcripts. CK1ε acts posttranslationally to degrade PER and inhibit its nuclear translocation, thus regulating the period of the rhythm. At the behavioral level, this model predicts (1) the shortening of free-running period seen in *tau*-mutant hamsters carrying a mutation of the *CK1ε* gene, (2) the lengthening of free-running period seen in *Clock*-mutant mice, and (3) the loss of coherent free-running rhythms seen in *Clock* mice and in *Per*- and *Cry*-knockout mice.

FUNCTIONAL NEUROANATOMY AND NEUROCHEMISTRY OF THE SUPRACHIASMATIC NUCLEUS

Traditionally, the SCN has been characterized as comprising distinct ventrolateral and dorsomedial subdivisions. Recently, however, this scheme has been reconceptualized to include SCN "core" and "shell" subnuclei, a concept that may better accommodate species differences in the anatomic distribution of neuropeptides and afferent terminal fields in the SCN[42,43] (Fig. 29–2). Although SCN neurons express a large number of neuropeptides, core and shell subnuclei have been most commonly identified by the concentration of arginine vasopressin–positive neurons in the SCN shell, and by vasoactive intestinal peptide– and gastrin-releasing peptide–positive neurons in the SCN core.[42,44] Beyond this basic organization, however, clear species differences have been noted, even among nocturnal rodents. For example, the hamster SCN core contains a very distinct and compact cluster of photoresponsive calbindin-positive cells, which is absent in the rat.[43]

Although the specific functions of these chemically defined SCN cell populations are not fully known, a reasonable heuristic is that the SCN core serves to collect and collate pacemaker inputs, whereas the shell is primarily responsible for generation of the circadian timing signal. These suggestions are consistent with findings that (1) major SCN efferent systems converge in the core subnucleus[42,44]; (2) spontaneous circadian rhythmicity in neuronal activity, neuropeptide release, and *cFos* and *Per* gene expression is seen more reliably in the SCN shell than in the core[45-49]; and (3) administration of SCN core peptides such as vasoactive intestinal peptide and gastrin-releasing peptide can mimic both light-induced phase shifting and *Per* gene expression in the SCN, in vivo and in vitro.[50-53] On the other hand, the view that SCN core and shell functions reflect circadian entrainment and circadian pacemaking functions, respectively, is probably too simplistic because (1) light-evoked responses are seen in SCN shell as well as in core neurons; (2) certain nonretinal SCN afferent systems converge within the SCN shell; and (3) in vitro studies have revealed independent circadian rhythmicity in secretion of both SCN core and SCN shell peptides, which may free-run with different periods in the same tissue, implicating separate core and shell oscillators.[49,54]

LIGHT INPUT TO THE PACEMAKER: THE RETINOHYPOTHALAMIC TRACT

Numerous studies have established that a specialized retinal projection system, referred to as the *retinohypothalamic tract*

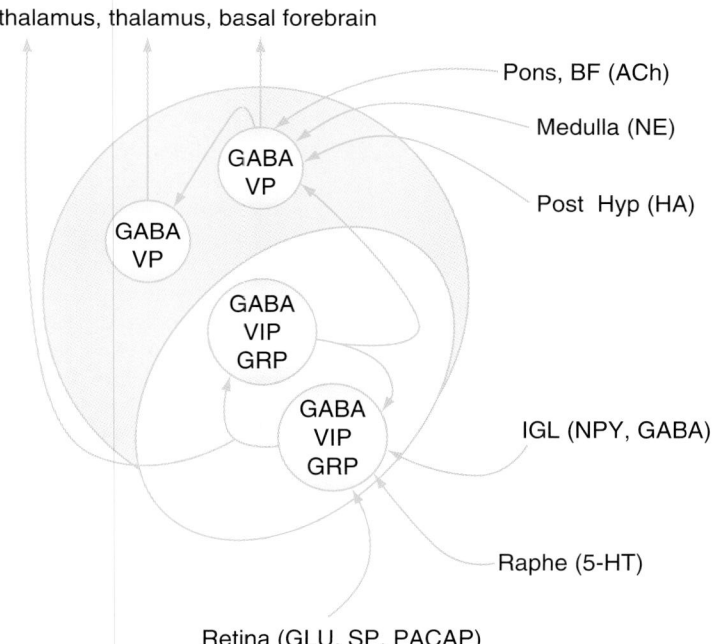

Figure 29–2. Core and shell organization of the suprachiasmatic nucleus (SCN). The vast majority of SCN neurons release the inhibitory amino acid transmitter gamma-aminobutyric acid (GABA). In the SCN core (*light blue*), GABA is commonly colocalized with one or more neuropeptides, including vasoactive intestinal polypeptide (VIP) and gastrin-releasing peptide (GRP), whereas neurons of the SCN shell (*darker blue*) frequently contain GABA colocalized with arginine vasopressin (VP). SCN core neurons project to other core neurons, to SCN shell neurons, and to extra-SCN targets, most prominently in the diencephalon and basal forebrain; SCN shell neurons project to other shell neurons, and to extra-SCN targets, but not to SCN core neurons. This anatomic organization implies that the flow of information within the SCN is generally from core to shell. Consistent with this suggestion, the three best-characterized SCN afferent systems, originating in the retina, the intergeniculate leaflet of the thalamus (IGL), and the mesencephalic raphe nuclei, converge in the SCN core. Retinal afferents contain the excitatory amino acid transmitter glutamate (GLU) as well as the neuropeptides substance P (SP) and pituitary adenyl cyclase–activating peptide (PACAP); raphe afferents contain 5-hydroxytryptamine (5-HT; serotonin); and IGL afferents contain neuropeptide Y (NPY) and GABA. Beyond these core afferents, several less well-characterized afferent systems converge in the SCN shell, including acetylcholine (ACh)-containing projections from the basal forebrain (BF) and pons, medullary norepinephrine (NE)-containing projections, and histamine (HA)-containing projections from the posterior hypothalamus (Post Hyp). A number of other anatomically identified but functionally uncharacterized SCN afferent systems have been omitted from this figure, and are not discussed in the chapter.

(RHT), is both necessary and sufficient for photic entrainment of the circadian pacemaker.[55] The RHT originates from a distinct subset of retinal ganglion cells separate from those giving rise to the primary visual pathways,[56] and terminates mainly in the SCN, as well as more sparsely in the antero-lateral hypothalamus, subparaventricular zone, and supra-optic region.[57,58] In addition, RHT axon collaterals also project to the thalamic intergeniculate leaflet (IGL; Fig. 29–3), which, as discussed later, is itself an important component of the circadian system.

Remarkably, retinally degenerate strains of mice, in which nearly all classic photoreceptors (i.e., rods and cones) are lost by early adulthood, exhibit normal circadian responses to light.[59] More recently, similar findings have been reported in genetically engineered mice with a total developmental absence of both rods and cones, demonstrating conclusively that circadian light entrainment can be mediated by a novel, nonrod, noncone photoreceptor system.[60] Recent studies indicate that the protein melanopsin, found specifically within the small subset of retinal ganglion cells giving rise to the RHT, serves as a circadian photoreceptor molecule in a novel popu-lation of photosensitive RHT retinal ganglion cells.[61-63] Thus, light entrainment of the circadian pacemaker is mediated by a dedicated system of photoreceptors, retinal neurons, and central pathways, entirely distinct from those mediating visual perception: a startling finding still not appreciated by most of the biomedical community outside of the fields of sleep and circadian rhythmicity.

Although these surprising findings represent the first evidence for non–rod/cone-mediated photic input to the mammalian nervous system, it has been known for many years that the circadian clock of *non*-mammalian vertebrates could be entrained even in the absence of the eyes, and that such extraretinal entrainment is mediated by both pineal and "deep-brain" (encephalic) photoreceptors.[64] Even though non–rod/cone-mediated entrainment in the mammalian system is nevertheless based on a retinal photoreceptor, the recent findings on the nature of these photoreceptors do high-light the evolutionary continuity between nonmammalian and mammalian vertebrates, and reveal that circadian entrainment depends on "nonvisual" photoreceptive mechanisms in all vertebrates.

RHT terminals release the excitatory amino acid neuro-transmitter, glutamate, in response to photic stimulation. Extensive evidence from in vivo and in vitro studies indicates that glutamate acts through both N-methyl-D-aspartate (NMDA) and non-NMDA receptors and a variety of intra-cellular signaling molecules (e.g., Ca^{2+}, nitric oxide, calmodulin/calmodulin kinase, protein kinase C, protein kinase G, cyclic adenosine monophosphate–responsive element-binding protein [CREB], and others)[65] and immediate early-response genes including *c-fos*,[66] leading to increased expression of *Per1* and *Per2*, and possibly other core clock genes.[67,68] The protein products of these genes represent state variables of the molec-ular oscillator, such that alterations in their transcription levels, when superimposed on the ongoing circadian tran-scription cycle, correspond functionally to phase shifts of the oscillator[69] (Fig. 29–4).

In addition to glutamate, RHT terminals also release two identified peptide cotransmitters, substance P (SP) and pitu-itary adenyl cyclase–activating peptide (PACAP). SP appears to play an important role in RHT transmission because selective SP antagonists block light-induced phase shifting and early-response gene expression in vivo,[70-72] as well as glutamate receptor–mediated phase shifting in vitro.[73] By itself, SP can mimic at least one component of the photic phase–response curve (phase delays during early subjective night) both in vivo and in vitro.[74,75] At least in vitro, the phase-shifting effects of SP appear to depend on SP-evoked glutamate release, and can be blocked by the NMDA antagonist, MK-801.[74] In contrast, PACAP administration has been reported either to antagonize or mimic the effects of glutamate on circadian phase shifting and *Per* gene expression in vitro, depending on dose and on circadian phase.[76-80] Specifically, when administered at relatively high doses, PACAP blocks the effects of glutamate during subjective night and evokes phase advances during subjective day, but when administered at much lower doses, PACAP actually mimics or potentiates the effects of glutamate on the SCN pacemaker.

OTHER FUNCTIONAL INPUTS TO THE CIRCADIAN CLOCK

An additional major SCN afferent system arises from the IGL, a distinct retinorecipient region of the lateral geniculate complex, intercalated between the dorsal and ventral lateral geniculate nucleus.[81-83] The projection from the IGL to the SCN is referred to as the *geniculohypothalamic tract* (GHT),

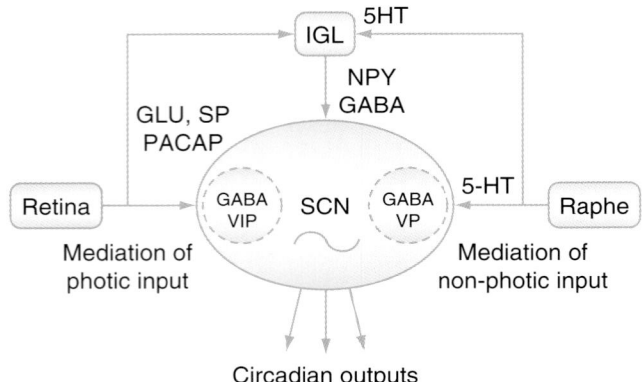

Figure 29–3. Overview of functional neuroanatomic pathways in the mammalian circadian system. Major suprachiasmatic nucleus (SCN) afferent systems originating in the retina and raphe nuclei also target the intergeniculate leaflet of the thalamus (IGL), which in turn projects to the SCN. Retinal projections to the SCN and IGL mediate photic input to the circadian system, raphe projections to the SCN and IGL mediate the effects of certain nonphotic, behavioral state–related signals, and IGL-SCN projections are involved in mediation of both photic and nonphotic signaling to the SCN pacemaker. As described in the text, photic and nonphotic pathways generally interact to produce mutually antagonistic effects on the circadian pacemaker. Thus, photic signals evoke circadian phase shifting during subjective night and antagonize nonphotic phase shifting during sub-jective day, whereas signals related to arousal and wakefulness evoke phase shifting during subjective day and antagonize photic phase shifting during subjective night. These antagonistic interactions are mediated in part at the level of the SCN, but the scheme presented here suggests that the IGL is also a probable locus for interaction between photic and nonphotic signals—a hypothesis that is largely unexplored. GABA, gamma-aminobutyric acid; GLU, glutamate; 5-HT, 5-hydroxytryptamine (serotonin); NPY, neuropeptide Y; PACAP, pituitary adenyl cyclase–activating peptide; SP, substance P; VIP, vasoactive intestinal polypeptide.

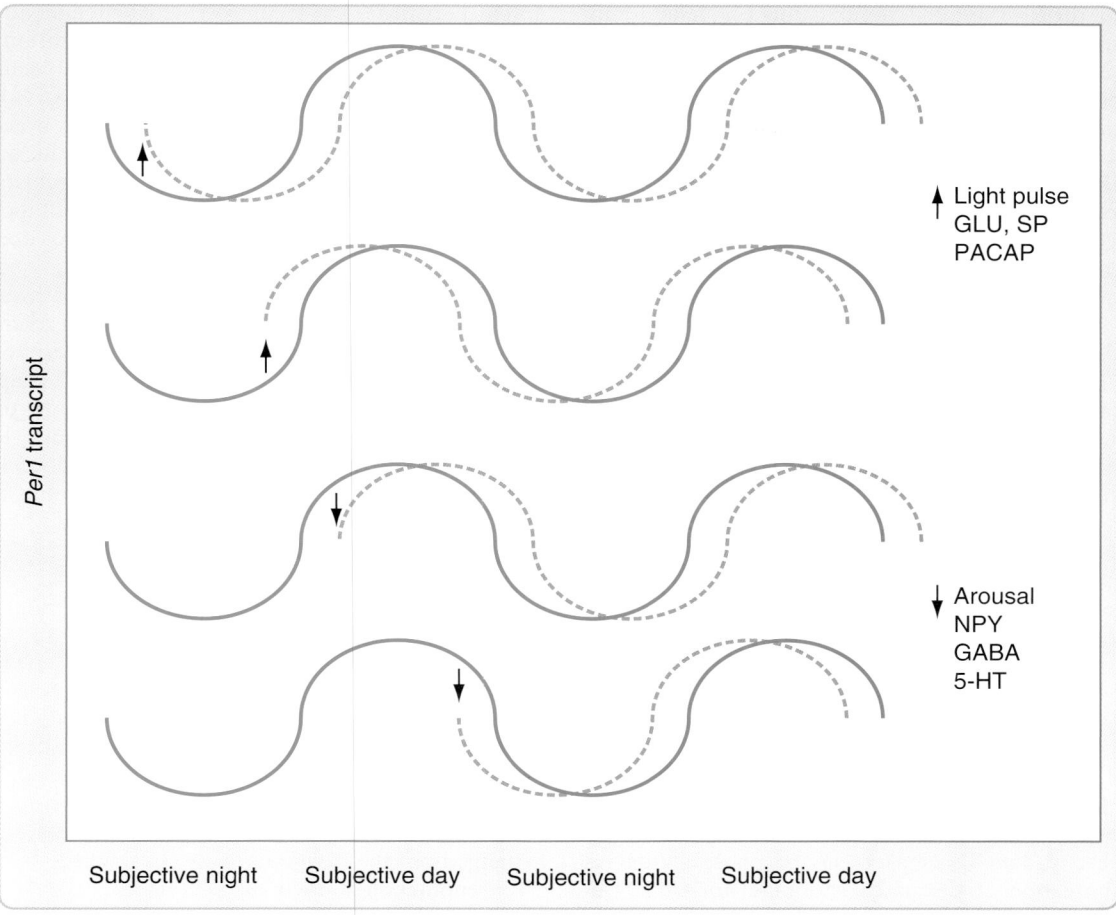

Light pulse
GLU, SP
PACAP

Arousal
NPY
GABA
5-HT

Subjective night   Subjective day   Subjective night   Subjective day

Figure 29–4. A simple qualitative-molecular model for circadian phase shifting by photic and nonphotic signals, and for their mutually antagonistic interaction. In this "phase-only" model, amplitude is fixed and the underlying state variable (here, *Per1* transcript level) can oscillate only within predetermined upper and lower bounds, such that the *Per1* level represents the phase of the molecular oscillator. During the subjective night, *Per1* levels are relatively low (*solid line*), and light pulses (or corresponding neurotransmitters or intracellular messengers) induce an abrupt increase in transcript level (*arrow*). Early in the night, when *Per1* levels are normally decreasing, this increase in transcription essentially forces the oscillator to repeat part of its normal trajectory, and is thus equivalent to resetting the oscillator to an earlier phase, resulting in a permanent phase delay (*dashed line*). In contrast, late in the night, *Per1* levels are normally increasing, such that a light-induced increase in transcription forces the oscillator to omit part of its normal trajectory, equivalent to resetting the oscillator to a later phase, and resulting in a permanent phase advance. Opposite to light pulses, arousal-related signals (or corresponding neurotransmitters or intracellular messengers) induce abrupt *decreases* in *Per1* transcription, resulting in phase delays during early subjective day and phase advances during late subjective day. Thus, the model predicts that photic and nonphotic phase–response curves (PRCs) should have essentially identical shapes, but should be phase-displaced by 180 degrees (12 circadian hours) along the horizontal axis; these predictions are at least roughly consistent with experimental observations.[69] Further, this model accounts for the general insensitivity of the circadian pacemaker to photic phase shifting during mid-subjective day and to nonphotic phase shifting during mid-subjective night: Because the underlying state variable can vary only within a predetermined range, stimuli that increase *Per1* transcription are ineffective when transcript levels are already maximal, and stimuli that decrease *Per1* transcription are ineffective when transcript levels are already minimal. Nevertheless, despite these periods of insensitivity, nonphotic signals would remain capable of counteracting light-evoked increases in transcription, and photic signals would remain capable of counteracting arousal-evoked decreases in transcription. Finally, the exact waveform and phasing of the photic and nonphotic PRCs would obviously depend on the exact waveform and phasing of the underlying spontaneous transcription cycle, here presented arbitrarily as two interlocking circular arcs centered over mid-subjective day and mid-subjective night. GABA, gamma-aminobutyric acid; GLU, glutamate; 5-HT, 5-hydroxytryptamine (serotonin); NPY, neuropeptide Y; PACAP, pituitary adenyl cyclase–activating peptide; SP, substance P.

and GHT neurons release both neuropeptide Y and gamma-aminobutyric acid (see Fig. 29–3). Retinal signals are conveyed to the IGL in part by axon collaterals of RHT neurons,[84] and GHT and RHT terminal fields are largely coextensive within the SCN core.[42,44] It is thus not surprising that early functional studies emphasized the possible role of the IGL/GHT system in providing a secondary, indirect pathway for photic entrainment of the circadian pacemaker.[81] Although the IGL is clearly not necessary for photic entrainment, lesions of the IGL/GHT do produce subtle modifications in

the ability of light signals to effect phase and period control of the circadian clock.[81]

In addition to its role as a secondary source of photic signaling to the circadian clock, the IGL also plays a preeminent role in the nonphotic regulation of the circadian system. Thus, IGL lesions abolish the phase-shifting effects of novelty-induced wheel running[85,86] and benzodiazepine administration in hamsters,[87-91] as well as the period-shortening effect of running-wheel access in rats[92] and the entrainment effect of scheduled daily treadmill activity in mice.[93] Further studies on the role of the RHT and IGL in mediating photic and non-photic inputs to the SCN are reviewed in Rosenwasser.[5]

Another major SCN afferent system converging on the SCN core originates from the serotonergic midbrain raphe, especially the median raphe nucleus.[94,95] In addition, ascending serotonergic projections originating in the dorsal raphe nucleus innervate the IGL, providing a second potential route for serotonergic regulation of the SCN circadian pacemaker (see Fig. 29–3). Extensive evidence has implicated serotonergic projections to the SCN (and IGL) in two distinct functions: (1) modulation of photic effects on the circadian pacemaker during the subjective night,[94-96] and (2) mediation of nonphotic, behavioral state–related effects on the pacemaker during subjective day.[97-100] In addition, whereas light during the middle of the subjective day is normally thought to have no effects on the circadian clock, light at this time can block the phase-shifting effects of a 5-hydroxytryptamine (5-HT; serotonin) agonist.[101] These latter results indicate that in addition to 5-HT inputs having a modulatory effect on light input to the SCN, the reverse is also true.

During the subjective night, photic effects on the circadian pacemaker are attenuated by electrical stimulation of the raphe nuclei or by systemic or intra-SCN administration of serotonergic agonists active at the $5-HT_{1A}$, $5-HT_7$, or $5-HT_{1B}$ receptors, whereas conversely, photic signaling in the SCN is potentiated by neurotoxic lesions of serotonin projections or by targeted serotonin antagonists.[94,95] In addition, photic entrainment is inhibited in the presence of high levels of arousal or locomotor activity, apparently through arousal-related release of endogenous serotonin.[97] During the subjective day, the circadian pacemaker can be phase shifted by electrical stimulation of the midbrain raphe nuclei[102,103] as well as by in vivo[104,105] or in vitro[106] administration of $5-HT_{1A}/5-HT_7$ receptor agonists. The ability of direct 5-HT application to the in vitro SCN to evoke circadian phase shifts indicates that stimulation of intra-SCN 5-HT receptors is sufficient to phase shift the pacemaker. Nevertheless, in vivo experiments using direct intracerebral 8-OH-DPAT [8-hydroxy-2-(di-N-propylamino)tetralin] administration have identified several potential loci in the circadian system for serotonergic phase shifting, including the SCN, the IGL, and the median and dorsal raphe nuclei.[71,104,107]

The phase-shifting effects evoked by serotonergic stimulation closely resemble those seen with other nonphotic phase-shifting stimuli, including novelty-induced activity, sleep deprivation, and benzodiazepine and neuropeptide Y administration.[5,108] Thus, several studies have directly examined the potential role of serotonergic afferents to the SCN and IGL in mediating the effects of behavioral state on the circadian pacemaker. Arousal, wakefulness, and motor activity are all associated with increased forebrain serotonin release,[109-111] and serotonin content in the rat SCN is correlated positively with spontaneous activity level and negatively with free-running period.[112] Indeed, state-dependent variations in serotonin release appear to mediate (1) the effects of activity level on free-running period,[111] (2) phase-shifting by activity or sleep deprivation,[110] (3) entrainment by restricted daily running wheel access[113] or scheduled daily treadmill activity,[93] and (4) activity-dependent inhibition of photic phase shifting in hamsters.[114]

Several other chemically identified pathways provide afferent input to the circadian system, including noradrenergic projections from the locus coeruleus, cholinergic projections from the basal forebrain and pontine tegmentum, and histaminergic projections from the posterior hypothalamus.[95,115,116] The cholinergic inputs, and their unknown function, are particularly intriguing because it was studies with the cholinergic agonist, carbachol, that were among the first to use a pharmacologic approach to study the neurochemistry of the circadian clock.[117] However, the significance of the cholinergic system in the circadian organization is still not understood. In addition, noradrenergic and cholinergic projections both innervate the IGL, providing an alternate pathway by which these transmitter systems could alter SCN circadian pacemaker function. Unlike the retinal, geniculate, and raphe projections described previously, which form generally overlapping terminal fields in the SCN core, these afferents target preferentially the SCN shell[42,44] (see Fig. 29–2). Although less studied than the SCN core afferents, sufficient data exist to suggest that these SCN shell afferents also contribute to circadian pacemaker regulation.

MULTIPLE OSCILLATOR NATURE OF CIRCADIAN SYSTEM

To this point, the review of current circadian neurobiology presented in this chapter has treated the SCN as the locus of *the* circadian pacemaker, but in fact, the circadian system comprises a multiplicity of circadian oscillators and pacemakers. As reviewed earlier,[118,119] circadian systems may exhibit complex dissociations among multiple rhythmic subcomponents. For example, two or more discrete daily activity epochs may emerge from the single normally consolidated activity period, a phenomenon known as *splitting*.[120,121] Such phenomena at the behavioral and endocrine level strongly imply the existence of an underlying multioscillatory neurobiologic circadian system. Interest in these complex phenomena appears to have been deprioritized for several years, coincident with the ongoing maturation of molecular approaches to the core pacemaker mechanism. However, in the last few years, these same molecular approaches, and especially the finding that mammalian clock genes are expressed not only in the SCN but in other brain regions[122] and in many peripheral tissues as well,[123,124] have spurred renewed interest in the identification and functions of multiple circadian oscillators in the circadian timing system.

At the level of the SCN itself, the observation that individual SCN neurons express the molecular mechanisms responsible for generating a circadian time signal demonstrates that the SCN pacemaker is *itself* composed of numerous, potentially autonomous but normally coupled, cellular circadian oscillators. Further, the clock genes *Per1*, *Per2*, and *Per3* exhibit a significant degree of functional specialization in the SCN,[37,125-127] and according to one hypothesis, *Per1* and *Per2* may represent state variables of Pittendigh's "morning" and "evening" oscillators, respectively.[128,129] Ultimately, it may be possible to integrate this molecular model with other recent findings suggesting that morning and evening oscillators may be represented by different subpopulations of SCN neurons.[49,130] In addition, it is not known if hypothesized intra-SCN morning and evening oscillators are related to the separate intra-SCN oscillators capable of driving independent secretion of core and shell peptide rhythms.[54] An important challenge for circadian biologists over the next few years will be to integrate modern insights into the molecular nature of the circadian clock with the earlier and equally important era of the field when many of the formal properties and basic principles underlying circadian organization were initially defined.[131,132]

Outside the SCN, recent evidence suggests that several non-SCN neural and neuroendocrine tissues are capable of expressing autonomous (although generally damped) circadian oscillations. Thus, cultured mammalian retinae display persisting circadian rhythmicity in melatonin secretion,[133] whereas more recent studies have demonstrated self-sustaining oscillations of *Per* gene expression in cultured endocrine tissues (pineal, pituitary), diencephalic nuclei (e.g., hypothalamic arcuate and paraventricular nuclei, thalamic paraventricular nucleus), and the olfactory bulbs[122] as well. Although the relationships between these extra-SCN neural oscillators and the SCN pacemaker have not been fully elucidated, it appears that at least certain types of behavioral rhythm splitting may involve dissociations between intra-SCN and extra-SCN central clocks.[134,135]

Similar techniques have also been used to reveal rhythmic *Per* expression in liver, lung, kidney, and other peripheral tissues.[136-138] Initial studies found these peripheral rhythms to be highly damped, and dependent on periodic input from the SCN for their continuous expression.[136,139] However, a more recent and highly elegant series of studies using mice with a reporter gene that could measure real-time circadian dynamics[124] revealed that circadian oscillations could persist for many days in peripheral tissues in vivo (Fig. 29–5). In addition, tissues from different SCN-lesioned animals were found to be rhythmic in vitro, although no longer in phase with one another as they are when taken from SCN-intact animals entrained to a light–dark cycle, indicating that the SCN synchronizes rather than drives these peripheral rhythms (see Fig. 29–5). Peripheral oscillators may also dissociate from the SCN pacemaker under certain conditions, such as after light–dark cycle phase shifts (i.e., simulated jet lag)[123] or during restricted feeding schedules, which entrain peripheral but not SCN *Per* gene oscillations.[4] These observations indicate that the SCN pacemaker normally serves to entrain both central and peripheral secondary oscillations generated by a broadly distributed population of autonomous cellular oscillators, but that under certain conditions, these downstream

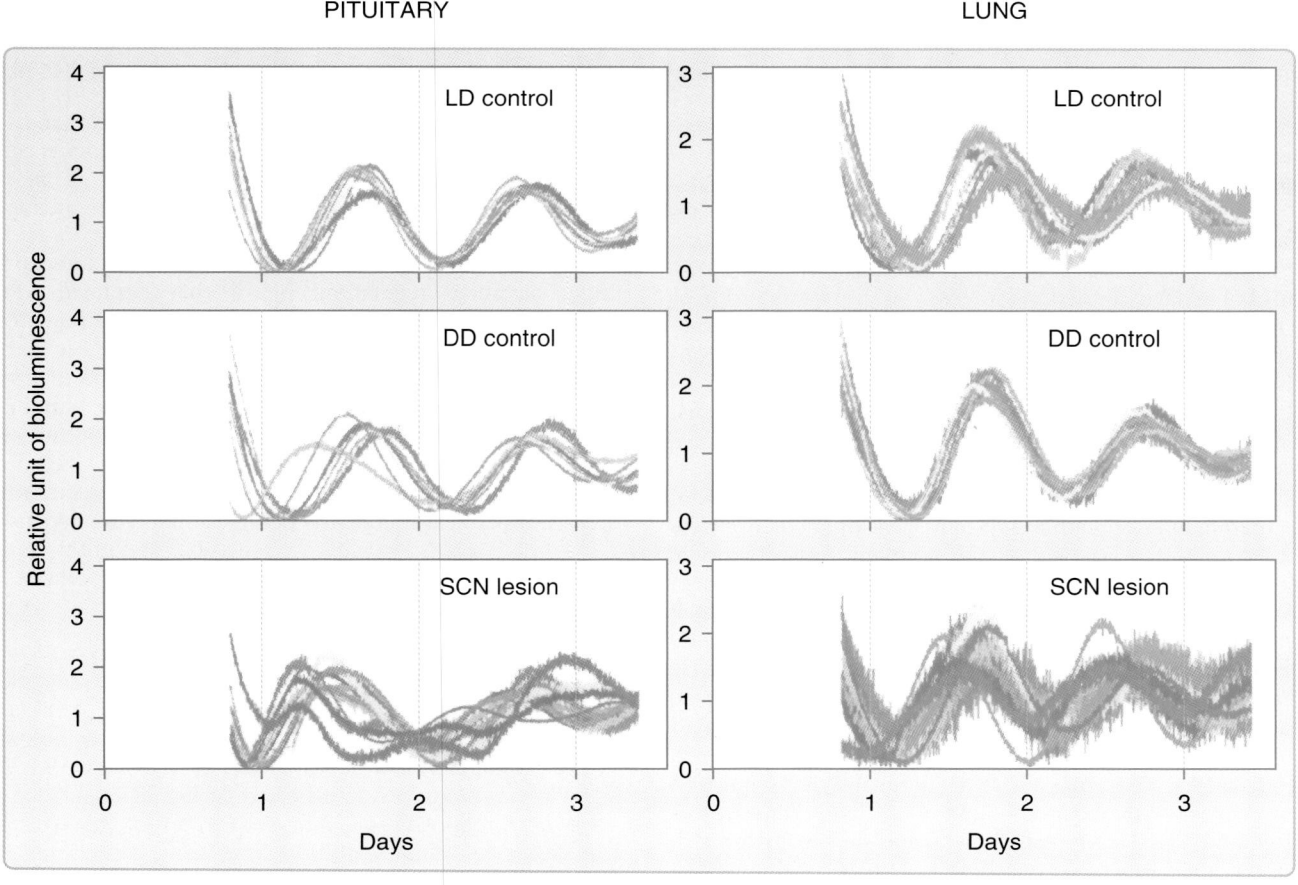

Figure 29–5. Superimposed plots of bioluminescent data from pituitary and lung tissues from individual animals that were intact and maintained on a light–dark cycle (LD controls) or in constant darkness (DD controls), as well as from suprachiasmatic nucleus (SCN)-lesioned animals. The tissue was maintained in vitro and made use of a Period2:Luciferase fusion protein as a real-time reporter of circadian dynamics. The first three cycles in culture are represented; each animal's record is a different shade. Although tissues collected from individual animals on an LD cycle, and relative to activity onset in DD control animals, were in phase with one another, phase desynchronization is evident in individual records of the SCN-lesioned animals for both tissues. (From Yoo SH, Yamazaki S, Lowrey PL, et al: PERIOD2:LUCIFERASE real-time reporting of circadian dynamics reveals persistent circadian oscillations in mouse peripheral tissues. Proc Natl Acad Sci U S A 2004;101:5339-5346.)

oscillators are capable of adaptive (as well as maladaptive?) disengagement from SCN control.

With the thought-provoking title "Circadian lessons from peripheral clocks: Is the time of the mammalian pacemaker up?," Brandstaetter suggested that perhaps "...the hypothalamic SCN of a rodent has to resign from its major function."[140] To paraphrase from a "live speech" of the American humorist, Mark Twain, "The recent announcement of my death is premature." We maintain that the death of the SCN is premature. For years the clock community has referred to the SCN as a "master pacemaker," and many speculated that such a pacemaker may drive circadian rhythms or regulate "slave oscillators."[131,141] Although it is now clear that many (most, all?) tissues and organs can produce circadian rhythms (using the same or similar molecular clock machinery as the SCN cells) in the absence of the SCN (e.g., in vitro), that does not mean these slave oscillators are independent of the SCN. Indeed, what is emerging in the field is the hypothesis that the SCN is still (in 2004) the "master oscillator" regulating all circadian rhythms either directly or indirectly. Rhythms are regulated directly when circadian information from the SCN directly controls a particular rhythm (presumably, by imposing circadian timing on the neural and physiologic systems regulating that function). However, "indirect" control is also important, as, for example, when the SCN's direct control of behavioral rhythms (e.g., feeding, sleep–wake cycle) sets in motion various metabolic, endocrine, and physiologic processes, which in turn control (entrain?) downstream rhythms. Indeed, many circadian rhythms are controlled by the behavioral states of sleep and wake in that the circadian expression of many rhythms depends on whether the animal is awake or asleep.[141] In animals, direct and indirect control of circadian rhythms by the SCN are normally in synchrony with each other. After all, it is only humans (and perhaps their live-in domestic pets) that routinely override their biologic clock with respect to the control of behavioral rhythms such as the sleep–wake cycle or the feeding cycle. Only humans sleep (or eat) at inappropriate times with respect to the adaptively appropriate environmental time. Whether direct or indirect, the SCN in mammals still appears to control the expression of all circadian rhythms, and in 2004 it is not time (yet) for the SCN pacemaker to give up its preeminent role in the circadian timing system.

This enriched appreciation of the multioscillatory nature of the mammalian circadian system has opened up new approaches for understanding the temporal organization of mammalian physiology and behavior, and raises a number of questions about the adverse effects associated with lack of normal synchronization between central and peripheral oscillations. Although such circadian dysregulation rarely occurs in nature, it certainly occurs quite often in humans, who can override their circadian clock and exert substantial volitional control over their sleep–wake cycles. Under such circumstances, abnormal phase relationships are expressed between sleep–wake behaviors (and other rhythmic processes tightly linked to sleep or wake states) and the circadian clock (and rhythmic processes tightly linked to it). Although the internal desynchronies that occur with jet lag and shift work may be the most dramatic, they are not the only examples of such dyschrony. Regardless of work or travel schedules, humans in our modern, around-the-clock society are becoming increasingly nocturnal despite millions of years of evolutionary pressure to be diurnal.

SUMMARY AND CONCLUSIONS

The primary pacemaker for the mammalian circadian system is contained in the SCN, and the mechanisms underlying the pacemaker function of this structure are rapidly being elucidated at the molecular, cellular, and neuroanatomic levels. The SCN contains a large number of normally coupled but potentially autonomous cellular oscillators that generate a circadian time base through the expression of a complex molecular feedback loop. The activity of the core molecular loop results in the circadian expression of a large number of clock-controlled genes, which in turn regulate coordinated circadian rhythms in the metabolism, electrical activity, and neurotransmitter and neuropeptide release of SCN neurons. These processes result in the transmission of circadian timing signals to both passive targets and inherently rhythmic secondary oscillators throughout the brain and periphery.

The core molecular loop is entrained by a number of convergent SCN afferent pathways. Photic signals are transmitted from a specialized set of photoreceptive retinal ganglion cells by a dedicated neural pathway (the RHT) to the SCN, and activity in this pathway results in the release of glutamate as well as multiple peptidergic cotransmitters. Other major SCN afferents arise from the IGL and raphe nuclei, which form terminal fields that largely overlap the RHT terminal field in the SCN core. These afferents serve to regulate photic signaling in the SCN during subjective night and to mediate the phase-shifting effects of nonphotic stimuli, including behavioral activity and arousal, during subjective day.

Two revolutionary developments in the circadian clock field—(1) the elucidation of the core molecular clock machinery, and (2) the demonstration that most, if not all, tissues/organs can themselves generate the 24-hour molecular clock—when coupled with recent studies indicating that 5% to 10% of all genes being expressed in any particular tissue/organ are under circadian regulation,[123,142,143] have opened up an entirely new area of biomedical research on the importance of internal timing for health and disease. Indeed, it can be argued that we are at the beginning of a new era in understanding human health and disease. With hundreds and even thousands of genes oscillating in most, if not all, tissues and organs that are under the control of central (i.e., SCN) and local (i.e., within the tissues) self-sustained circadian oscillations, normal health and well-being undoubtedly depend on

---

Clinical Pearl

Most, if not all, organs/tissues contain the core molecular circadian clock machinery, and can produce circadian rhythms in vitro. This greatly heightens the theoretical importance of internal synchronization for normal physiologic function. Abnormal circadian timing between and within tissue/organ systems could be just as important as the overproduction or underproduction of key cellular processes to overall health. Internal temporal dysfunction may thus be at the root of many physical and mental diseases. Although jet lag and shift work have been the primary ways in which circadian dyschrony were thought to occur (see Section 8, this volume), it is probable that dyschrony may turn out to play an important role in many human pathologic processes as well.

internal synchronization. Further, this internal synchronization can occur on two levels, between separate oscillating systems and within each self-sustained system, and the balance between health and disease is likely to be highly dependent on proper synchrony at both levels.

Recent findings that there are different alleles of circadian clock genes that can influence the timing of human sleep and wake[144,145] surely represent the early understanding of human variability in the molecular clock machinery. The importance of this variability at the level of the organism, as well as at the tissue/organ level, and the implications of this variability for different human populations and for understanding disease states are not known, but surely will be the subject of extensive future research.

Acknowledgments

Preparation of this manuscript was in part supported by National Institutes of Health grants R01 AG 18200, R-01 HL-59598, and P01-AG11412. The National Aeronautics and Space Administration also supported this work through a NASA Cooperative Agreement NCC 9-58 with the National Space Biomedical Research Institute. Portions of this review have appeared in Rosenwasser,[5] with permission.

REFERENCES

1. Hofman MA: The brain's calendar: Neural mechanisms of seasonal timing. Biol Rev Camb Philos Soc 2004;79:61-77.
2. Takahashi JS, Turek FW, Moore RY (eds): Handbook of Behavioral Neurobiology, vol 12: Circadian Clocks. New York, Kluwer Academic/Plenum, 2001, p 770.
3. Klein DC, Moore RY, Reppert SM: Suprachiasmatic Nucleus: The Mind's Clock. New York, Oxford University Press, 1991.
4. Stokkan KA, Yamazaki S, Tei H, et al: Entrainment of the circadian clock in the liver by feeding. Science 2001;291:490-493.
5. Rosenwasser AM: Neurobiology of the mammalian circadian system: Oscillators, pacemakers, and pathways. Prog Psychobiol Physiol Psychol 2003;18:1-38.
6. Mirmiran M, Koster-Van Hoffen GC, Bos NP: Circadian rhythm generation in the cultured suprachiasmatic nucleus. Brain Res Bull 1995;38:275-283.
7. Welsh DK, Logothetis DE, Meister M, Reppert SM: Individual neurons dissociated from rat suprachiasmatic nucleus express independently phased circadian firing rhythms. Neuron 1995;14:697-706.
8. Herzog ED, Geusz ME, Khalsa SB, et al: Circadian rhythms in mouse suprachiasmatic nucleus explants on multimicroelectrode plates. Brain Res 1997;757:285-290.
9. Shirakawa T, Honma S, Katsuno Y, et al: Synchronization of circadian firing rhythms in cultured rat suprachiasmatic neurons. Eur J Neurosci 2000;12:2833-2838.
10. Nakamura W, Honma S, Shirakawa T, Honma K: Clock mutation lengthens the circadian period without damping rhythms in individual SCN neurons. Nat Neurosci 2002;5:399-400.
11. Colwell CS: Circadian modulation of calcium levels in cells in the suprachiasmatic nucleus. Eur J Neurosci 2000;12:571-576.
12. Kuhlman SJ, Quintero JE, McMahon DG: GFP fluorescence reports Period 1 gene regulation in the mammalian biological clock. Neuroreport 2000;11:1479-1482.
13. Low-Zeddies SS, Takahashi JS: Chimera analysis of the Clock mutation in mice shows that complex cellular integration determines circadian behavior. Cell 2001;105:25-42.
14. Schwartz W, Gross RA, Morton MT: The suprachiasmatic nuclei contain a tetrodotoxin-resistant circadian pacemaker. Proc Natl Acad Sci U S A 1987;84:1694-1698.
15. Shibata S, Moore RY: Tetrodotoxin does not affect circadian rhythms in neuronal activity and metabolism in rodent suprachiasmatic nucleus in vitro. Brain Res 1993;606:259-266.
16. Shirakawa T, Honma S, Honma K: Multiple oscillators in the suprachiasmatic nucleus. Chronobiol Int 2001;18:371-387.
17. Miche S, Colwell CS: Cellular communication and coupling within the suprachiasmatic nucleus. Chronobiol Int 2001;18:579-600.
18. Takahashi JS, Turek FW: Anisomycin, an inhibitor of protein synthesis, perturbs the phase of a mammalian circadian pacemaker. Brain Res 1987;405:199-203.
19. Inouye ST, Takahashi JS, Wollnik F, Turek FW: Inhibitor of protein synthesis phase shifts a circadian pacemaker in the mammalian SCN. Am J Physiol 1988;255:R1055-R1058.
20. King DP, Zhao Y, Sangoram AM, et al: Positional cloning of the mouse circadian Clock gene. Cell 1997;89:641-653.
21. Antoch MP, Song E, Chang A, et al: Functional identification of the mouse circadian Clock gene by transgenic BAC rescue. Cell 1997;89:655-667.
22. Hendricks JC, Seghgal A: Why a fly? Using *Drosophila* to understand the genetics of circadian rhythms and sleep. Sleep 2004;27:334-342.
23. Barnes JW, Tischkau SA, Barnes JA, et al: Requirement of mammalian Timeless for circadian rhythmicity. Science 2003;302:439-442.
24. Lowrey PL, Takahashi JS: Genetics of the mammalian circadian system: Photic entrainment, circadian pacemaker mechanisms and posttranslational regulation. Annu Rev Genet 2000;34:533-562.
25. Van Gelder RN: Recent insights into mammalian circadian rhythms. Sleep 2004;27:166-171.
26. Dunlap JC: Molecular bases for circadian clocks. Cell 1999;96:271-290.
27. Young MW: Life's 24-hour clock: molecular control of circadian rhythms in animal cells. Trends Biochem Sci 2000;25:601-606.
28. Shearman LP, Sriram S, Weaver DR, et al: Interacting molecular loops in the mammalian circadian clock. Science 2000;288:1013-1019.
29. Shearman LP, Zylka MJ, Weaver DR, et al: Two period homologs: Circadian expression and photic regulation in the suprachiasmatic nuclei. Neuron 1997;19:1261-1269.
30. Miyamoto Y, Sancar A: Circadian regulation of cryptochrome genes in the mouse. Brain Res Mol Brain Res 1999;71:238-243.
31. Okano T, Sasaki M, Fukada Y: Cloning of mouse BMAL2 and its daily expression profile in the suprachiasmatic nucleus: A remarkable acceleration of Bmal2 sequence divergence after Bmal gene duplication. Neurosci Lett 2001;300:111-114.
32. Wilsbacher LD, Yamazaki S, Herzog ED, et al: Photic and circadian expression of luciferase in mPeriod1-luc transgenic mice in vivo. Proc Natl Acad Sci U S A 2002;99:489-494.
33. Asai M, Yamaguchi S, Isejima H, et al: Visualization of mPer1 transcription in vitro: NMDA induces a rapid phase shift of mPer1 gene in cultured SCN. Curr Biol 2001;11:1524-1527.
34. Vitaterna MH, King DP, Chang A-M, et al: Mutagenesis and mapping of a mouse gene, Clock, essential for circadian behavior. Science 1994;264:719-725.
35. Thresher RJ, Vitaterna MH, Miyamoto Y, et al: Role of mouse cryptochrome blue-light photoreceptor in circadian photoresponses. Science 1998;282:1490-1494.
36. Van der Horst GT, Muijtjens M, Kobayashi K, et al: Mammalian Cry1 and Cry2 are essential for maintenance of circadian rhythms. Nature 1999;398:627-630.
37. Albrecht U, Zheng B, Larkin D, et al: MPer1 and mper2 are essential for normal resetting of the circadian clock. J Biol Rhythms 2001;16:100-104.
38. Ralph MR, Menaker M: A mutation of the circadian system in golden hamsters. Science 1988;241:1225-1227.

39. Lowrey PL, Shimomura K, Antoch MP, et al: Positional syntenic cloning and functional characterization of the mammalian circadian mutation tau. Science 2000;288:483-492.

40. Naylor E, Bergmann BM, Krauski K, et al: The circadian Clock mutation alters sleep homeostasis in the mouse. J Neurosci 2000;20:8138-8143.

41. Tafti M, Franken P: Functional genomics of sleep and circadian rhythm. Invited review: Genetic dissection of sleep. J Appl Physiol 2002;92:1339-1347.

42. Moore RY: Entrainment pathways and the functional organization of the circadian system. Prog Brain Res 1996;111:103-119.

43. Moore RY, Silver R: Suprachiasmatic nucleus organization. Chronobiol Int 1998;15:475-487.

44. Moore RY: Chemical neuroanatomy of the mammalian circadian system. In Redfern P, Lemmer B (eds): Physiology and Pharmacology of Biological Rhythms. New York, Springer, 1997, pp 79-93.

45. Inouye ST: Circadian rhythms of neuropeptides in the suprachiasmatic nucleus. Prog Brain Res 1996;111:75-90.

46. Sumova A, Travnickova Z, Mikkelsen JD, Illnerova H: Spontaneous rhythm in c-Fos immunoreactivity in the dorsomedial part of the rat suprachiasmatic nucleus. Brain Res 1998;801:254-258.

47. Yan L, Takekida S, Shigeyoshi Y, Okamura H: Per1 and Per2 gene expression in the rat suprachiasmatic nucleus: Circadian profile and the compartment-specific response to light. Neuroscience 1999;94:141-150.

48. Hamada T, LeSauter J, Venuti JM, Silver R: Expression of Period genes: Rhythmic and nonrhythmic compartments of the suprachiasmatic nucleus pacemaker. J Neurosci 2001;21:7742-7750.

49. Nakamura W, Honma S, Shirakawa T, Honma K: Regional pacemakers composed of multiple oscillator neurons in the rat suprachiasmatic nucleus. Eur J Neurosci 2001;14:666-674.

50. Albers HE, Liou SY, Stopa EG, Zoeller RT: Interaction of colocalized neuropeptides: Functional significance in the circadian timing system. J Neurosci 1991;11:846-851.

51. Piggins HD, Antle MC, Rusak B: Neuropeptides phase shift the mammalian circadian pacemaker. J Neurosci 1995;15:5612-5622.

52. McArthur AJ, Coogan AN, Ajpru S, et al: Gastrin-releasing peptide phase-shifts suprachiasmatic nuclei neuronal rhythms in vitro. J Neurosci 2000;20:5496-5502.

53. Nielsen HS, Hannibal J, Fahrenkrug J: Vasoactive intestinal polypeptide induces per1 and per2 gene expression in the rat suprachiasmatic nucleus late at night. Eur J Neurosci 2002;15:570-574.

54. Shinohara K, Honma S, Katsuno Y, et al: Two distinct oscillators in the rat suprachiasmatic nucleus in vitro. Proc Natl Acad Sci U S A 1995;92:7396-7400.

55. Johnson RF, Moore RY, Morin LP: Loss of entrainment and anatomical plasticity after lesions of the hamster retinohypothalamic tract. Brain Res 1988;460:297-313.

56. Moore RY, Speh JC, Card JP: The retinohypothalamic tract originates from a distinct subset of retinal ganglion cells. J Comp Neurol 1995;352:351-366.

57. Johnson RF, Morin LP, Moore RY: Retinohypothalamic projects in the hamster and rat demonstrated using cholera toxin. Brain Res 1988;462:301-312.

58. Levine JD, Weiss ML, Rosenwasser AM, Miselis RR: Retinohypothalamic tract in the female albino rat: A study using horseradish peroxidase conjugated to cholera toxin. J Comp Neurol 1991;306:344-360.

59. Foster RG, Argamaso S, Coleman S, et al: Photoreceptors regulating circadian behavior: A mouse model. J Biol Rhythms 1993;8(Suppl):S17-S23.

60. Freedman MS, Lucas RJ, Soni B, et al: Regulation of mammalian circadian behavior by non-rod, non-cone, ocular photoreceptors. Science 1999;284:502-504.

61. Hannibal J, Hindersson P, Knudsen SM, et al: The photopigment melanopsin is exclusively present in pituitary adenylate cyclase-activating polypeptide-containing retinal ganglion cells of the retinohypothalamic tract. J Neurosci 2002;22:RC191.

62. Hattar S, Liao HW, Takao M, et al: Melanopsin-containing retinal ganglion cells: Architecture, projections, and intrinsic photosensitivity. Science 2002;295:1065-1070.

63. Berson DM, Dunn FA, Takao M: Phototransduction by retinal ganglion cells that set the circadian clock. Science 2002;295:1070-1073.

64. Underwood H: Circadian organization in nonmammalian vertebrates. In Takahashi JS, Turek FW, Moore RY (eds): Handbook of Behavioral Neurobiology, Vol 12. New York, Kluwer Academic/Plenum, 2001, pp 111-135.

65. Gillette MU: Regulation of entrainment pathways by the suprachiasmatic circadian clock: Sensitivities to second messengers. Prog Brain Res 1996;111:121-132.

66. Kornhauser JM, Ginty DD, Greenberg ME, et al: Light entrainment and activation of signal transduction pathways in the SCN. Prog Brain Res 1996;111:133-146.

67. Shigeyoshi Y, Taguchi K, Yamamoto S, et al: Light-induced resetting of a mammalian circadian clock is associated with rapid induction of the mPer1 transcript. Cell 1997;91:1043-1053.

68. Moriya T, Horikawa K, Akiyama M, Shibata S: Correlative association between N-methyl-D-aspartate receptor-mediated expression of period genes in the suprachiasmatic nucleus and phase shifts in behavior with photic entrainment of clock in hamsters. Mol Pharmacol 2000;58:1554-1562.

69. Rosenwasser AM, Dwyer SM: Circadian phase shifting: Relationships between photic and nonphotic phase-response curves. Physiol Behav 2001;73:175-183.

70. Abe H, Honma S, Shinohara K, Honma K: Substance P receptor regulates the photic induction of Fos-like protein in the suprachiasmatic nucleus of Syrian hamsters. Brain Res 1996;708:135-142.

71. Challet E, Naylor E, Metzger JM, et al: An NK1 receptor antagonist affects the circadian regulation of locomotor activity in golden hamsters. Brain Res 1998;800:32-39.

72. Challet E, Dugovic C, Turek FW, Van Reeth O: The selective neurokinin 1 receptor antagonist R116301 modulates photic responses of the hamster circadian system. Neuropharmacology 2001;40:408-415.

73. Kim DY, Kang HC, Shin HC, et al: Substance P plays a critical role in photic resetting of the circadian pacemaker in the rat hypothalamus. J Neurosci 2001;21:4026-4031.

74. Hamada T, Yamanouchi S, Watanabe A, et al: Involvement of glutamate release in substance P-induced phase delays of suprachiasmatic neuron activity rhythm in vitro. Brain Res 1999;836:190-193.

75. Piggins HD, Rusak B: Effects of microinjections of substance P into the suprachiasmatic nucleus region on hamster wheel-running rhythms. Brain Res Bull 1997;42:451-455.

76. Hannibal J, Ding JM, Chen D, et al: Pituitary adenylate cyclase-activating peptide (PACAP) in the retinohypothalamic tract: A potential daytime regulator of the biological clock. J Neurosci 1997;17:2637-2644.

77. Chen D, Buchanan GF, Ding JM, et al: Pituitary adenylate cyclase-activating peptide: A pivotal modulator of glutamatergic regulation of the suprachiasmatic circadian clock. Proc Natl Acad Sci U S A 1999;96:13468-13473.

78. Harrington ME, Hoque S, Hall A, et al: Pituitary adenylate cyclase activating peptide phase shifts circadian rhythms in a manner similar to light. J Neurosci 1999;19:6637-6642.

79. Nielsen HS, Hannibal J, Knudsen SM, Fahrenkrug J: Pituitary adenylate cyclase-activating polypeptide induces period1 and period2 gene expression in the rat suprachiasmatic nucleus during late night. Neuroscience 2001;103:433-441.

80. Hannibal J, Jamen F, Nielsen HS, et al: Dissociation between light-induced phase shift of the circadian rhythm and clock gene expression in mice lacking the pituitary adenylate cyclase activating polypeptide type 1 receptor. J Neurosci 2001;21: 4883-4890.

81. Moore RY, Card JP: Intergeniculate leaflet: An anatomically and functionally distinct subdivision of the lateral geniculate complex. J Comp Neurol 1994;344:403-430.

82. Morin LP: The circadian visual system. Brain Res Rev 1994;67: 102-127.

83. Harrington ME: The ventral lateral geniculate nucleus and the intergeniculate leaflet: Interrelated structures in the visual and circadian systems. Neurosci Biobehav Rev 1997;21:705-727.

84. Pickard GE: Bifurcating axons of retinal ganglion cells terminate in the hypothalamic suprachiasmatic nucleus and in the intergeniculate leaflet of the thalamus. Neurosci Lett 1982; 55:211-217.

85. Wickland CR, Turek FW: Lesions of the thalamic intergeniculate leaflet block activity-induced phase shifts in the circadian activity rhythm of the golden hamster. Brain Res 1994;660: 293-300.

86. Janik D, Mrosovsky N: Intergeniculate leaflet lesions and behaviorally-induced shifts of circadian rhythms. Brain Res 1994;651:174-182.

87. Johnson R, Smale L, Moore RY, Morin LP: Lateral geniculate lesions block circadian phase-shift responses to a benzodiazepine. Proc Natl Acad Sci U S A 1988;85:5301-5304.

88. Meyer EL, Harrington ME, Rahmani T: A phase-response curve to the benzodiazepine chlordiazepoxide and the effect of geniculo-hypothalamic tract ablation. Physiol Behav 1993;53: 237-243.

89. Maywood ES, Smith E, Hall SJ, Hastings MH: A thalamic contribution to arousal-induced, non-photic entrainment of the circadian clock of the Syrian hamster. Eur J Neurosci 1997;9: 1739-1747.

90. Biello SM, Harrington ME, Mason R: Geniculo-hypothalamic tract lesions block chlordiazepoxide-induced phase advances in Syrian hamsters. Brain Res 1991;552:47-52.

91. Schuhler S, Pitrosky B, Saboureau M, et al: Role of the thalamic intergeniculate leaflet and its 5-HT afferences in the chronobiological properties of 8-OH-DPAT and triazolam in Syrian hamster. Brain Res 1999;849:16-24.

92. Kuroda H, Fukushima M, Nakai M, et al: Daily wheel running activity modifies the period of free-running rhythm in rats via intergeniculate leaflet. Physiol Behav 1997;61:633-637.

93. Marchant EG, Watson NV, Mistlberger RE: Both neuropeptide Y and serotonin are necessary for entrainment of circadian rhythms in mice by daily treadmill running schedules. J Neurosci 1997;17:7974-7987.

94. Meyer-Bernstein EL, Morin LP: Differential serotonergic innervation of the suprachiasmatic nucleus and the intergeniculate leaflet and its role in circadian rhythm modulation. J Neurosci 1996;16:2097-2111.

95. Moga MM, Moore RY: Organization of neural inputs to the suprachiasmatic nucleus in the rat. J Comp Neurol 1997;389: 508-534.

96. Penev PD, Turek FW, Zee PC: Monoamine depletion alters the entrainment and the response to light of the circadian activity rhythm in hamsters. Brain Res 1993;612:156-164.

97. Morin LP: Serotonin and the regulation of mammalian circadian rhythmicity. Ann Med 1999;31:12-33.

98. Rea MA, Pickard GE: Serotonergic modulation of photic entrainment in the Syrian hamster. Biol Rhythm Res 2000; 31:284-314.

99. Mistlberger RE, Antle MC, Glass JD, Miller JD: Behavioral and serotonergic regulation of circadian rhythms. Biol Rhythm Res 2000;31:240-283.

100. Penev P, Zee PC, Turek FW: Monoamine depletion blocks triazolam-induced phase advances of the circadian clock in hamsters. Brain Res 1994;637:255-261.

101. Penev PD, Zee PC, Turek FW: Serotonin in the spotlight. Nature 1997;385:123.

102. Meyer-Bernstein EL, Morin LP: Electrical stimulation of the median or dorsal raphe nuclei reduces light-induced FOS protein in the suprachiasmatic nucleus and causes circadian activity rhythm phase shifts. Neuroscience 1999;92: 267-279.

103. Glass JD, DiNardo LA, Ehlen JC: Dorsal raphe nuclear stimulation of SCN serotonin release and circadian phase-resetting. Brain Res 2000;859:224-232.

104. Ehlen JC, Grossman GH, Glass JD: In vivo resetting of the hamster circadian clock by 5-HT7 receptors in the suprachiasmatic nucleus. J Neurosci 2001;21:5351-5357.

105. Penev PD, Turek FW, Wallen EP, Zee PC: Aging alters the serotonergic modulation of light-induced phase advances in golden hamsters. Am J Physiol 1997;272:R509-R513.

106. Prosser RA: Serotonergic actions and interactions on the SCN circadian pacemaker: In vitro investigations. Biol Rhythm Res 2000;31:315-339.

107. Mintz EM, Gillespie CF, Marvel CL, et al: Serotonergic regulation of circadian rhythms in Syrian hamsters. Neuroscience 1997; 79:563-569.

108. Turek FW, Scarbrough K, Penev P, et al: Aging of the mammalian circadian system. In Takahashi JS, Turek FW, Moore RY (eds): Circadian Clocks. New York, Kluwer Academic/Plenum, 2001, pp 292-317.

109. Jacobs BL, Fornal CA: Activity of serotonergic neurons in behaving animals. Neuropsychopharmacology 1999; 21(2 Suppl):9S-15S.

110. Grossman GH, Mistlberger RE, Antle MC, et al: Sleep deprivation stimulates serotonin release in the suprachiasmatic nucleus. Neuroreport 2000;11:1929-1932.

111. Mistlberger RE, Bossert JM, Holmes MM, Marchant EG: Serotonin and feedback effects of behavioral activity on circadian rhythms in mice. Behav Brain Res 1998;96:93-99.

112. Shioiri T, Takahashi K, Yamada N, Takahashi S: Motor activity correlates negatively with free-running period, while positively with serotonin content in SCN of free-running rats. Physiol Behav 1991;49:779-786.

113. Edgar DM, Reid MS, Dement WC: Serotonergic afferents mediate activity-dependent entrainment of the mouse circadian clock. Am J Physiol 1997;273:R265-R269.

114. Mistlberger RE, Antle MC: Behavioral inhibition of light-induced circadian phase resetting is phase and serotonin dependent. Brain Res 1998;786:31-38.

115. Panula P, Pirvola U, Auvinen S, Airaksinen MS: Histamine-immunoreactive nerve fibers in the rat brain. Neuroscience 1989;28:585-610.

116. Bina KG, Rusak B, Semba K: Localization of cholinergic neurons in the forebrain and brainstem that project to the suprachiasmatic nucleus of the hypothalamus in rat. J Comp Neurol 1993;335:295-307.

117. Earnest DJ, Turek FW: Role of acetylcholine in mediating effects of light on reproduction. Science 1983;219:77-79.

118. Rosenwasser AM, Adler NT: Structure and function in circadian timing systems: Evidence for multiple coupled circadian oscillators. Neurosci Behav Rev 1986;10:431-448.

119. Turek FW: Circadian neural rhythms in mammals. Annu Rev Physiol 1985;47:49-64.

120. Pickard GE, Turek FW, Sollars PJ: Light intensity and splitting in the golden hamster. Physiol Behav 1993;54:1-5.

121. Swann JM, Turek FW: Multiple circadian oscillators regulate the timing of behavioral and endocrine rhythms in female golden hamsters. Science 1985;228:898-900.

122. Abe M, Herzog ED, Yamazaki S, et al: Circadian rhythms in isolated brain regions. J Neurosci 2002;22:350-356.

123. Storch KF, Lipan O, Leykin I, et al: Extensive and divergent circadian gene expression in liver and heart. Nature 2002; 417:78-83.

124. Yoo SH, Yamazaki S, Lowrey PL, et al: PERIOD2:LUCIFERASE real-time reporting of circadian dynamics reveals persistent circadian oscillations in mouse peripheral tissues. Proc Natl Acad Sci U S A 2004;101:5339-5346.

125. Albrecht U, Sun ZS, Eichele G, Lee CC: A differential response of two putative mammalian circadian regulators, mper1 and mper2, to light. Cell 1997;91:1055-1064.

126. Bae K, Jin X, Maywood ES, et al: Differential functions of mPer1, mPer2, and mPer3 in the SCN circadian clock. Neuron 2001;30:525-536.

127. Zheng B, Albrecht U, Kaasik K, et al: Nonredundant roles of the mPer1 and mPer2 genes in the mammalian circadian clock. Cell 2001;105:683-694.

128. Daan S, Albrecht U, van der Horst GT, et al: Assembling a clock for all seasons: Are there M and E oscillators in the genes? J Biol Rhythms 2001;16:105-116.

129. Steinlechner S, Jacobmeier B, Scherbarth F, et al: Robust circadian rhythmicity of Per1 and Per2 mutant mice in constant light, and dynamics of Per1 and Per2 gene expression under long and short photoperiods. J Biol Rhythms 2002;17: 202-209.

130. Jagota A, de la Iglesia HO, Schwartz WJ: Morning and evening circadian oscillations in the suprachiasmatic nucleus in vitro. Nat Neurosci 2000;3:372-376.

131. Pittendrigh CS: Circadian rhythms and the circadian organization of living organisms. Cold Spring Harb Symp Quant Biol 1960;25:159-184.

132. Aschoff J: Exogenous and endogenous components in circadian rhythms. Cold Spring Harb Symp Quant Biol 1960;25:11-18.

133. Tosini G, Menaker M: Circadian rhythms in cultured mammalian retina. Science 1996;272:419-421.

134. Abe H, Honma S, Namihira M, et al: Clock gene expressions in the suprachiasmatic nucleus and other areas of the brain during rhythm splitting in CS mice. Brain Res Mol Brain Res 2001;87:92-99.

135. Abe H, Honma S, Namihira M, et al: Behavioural rhythm splitting in the CS mouse is related to clock gene expression outside the suprachiasmatic nucleus. Eur J Neurosci 2001;14:1121-1128.

136. Zylka MJ, Shearman LP, Weaver DR, Reppert SM: Three period homologs in mammals: Differential light responses in the suprachiasmatic circadian clock and oscillating transcripts outside of brain. Neuron 1998;20:1103-1110.

137. Sakamoto K, Nagase T, Fukui H, et al: Multitissue circadian expression of the rat period homolog (rPer2) mRNA is governed by the mammalian circadian clock, the suprachiasmatic nucleus in the brain. J Biol Chem 1998;273: 27039-27042.

138. Yamazaki S, Numano R, Abe M, et al: Resetting central and peripheral circadian oscillators in transgenic rats. Science 2000;288:682-685.

139. Fukuhara C, Tosini G: Role of peripheral oscillators in mammals. Front Biosci 2003;8:642-651.

140. Brandstaetter R: Circadian lessons from peripheral clocks: is the time of the mammalian pacemaker up? Proc Natl Acad Sci U S A 2004;101:5699-5700.

141. Van Cauter E, Copinschi G, Turek FW: Endocrine and other biologic rhythms. In DeGroot LJ, Jameson JL (eds): Endocrinology, 4th ed. Philadelphia, WB Saunders, 2001, pp 235-256.

142. Akhtar RA, Reddy AB, Maywood ES, et al: Circadian cycling of the mouse liver transcriptome, as revealed by cDNA microarray, is driven by the suprachiasmatic nucleus. Curr Biol 2002;12:540-550.

143. Panda S, Antoch MP, Miller BH, et al: Coordinated transcription of key pathways in the mouse by the circadian clock. Cell 2002;109:307-320.

144. Reid KJ, Chang AM, Dubocovich ML, et al: Familial advanced sleep phase syndrome. Arch Neurol 2001;7:1089-1094.

145. Toh KL, Jones CR, He Y, et al: An hPer2 phosphorylation site mutation in familial advanced sleep phase syndrome. Science 2001;291:1040-1043.

Molecular Genetic Basis for Mammalian Circadian Rhythms

Martha Hotz Vitaterna

Lawrence H. Pinto

Fred W. Turek

ABSTRACT

Circadian (near-24-hour) rhythms can be produced by individual cells in a self-sustaining manner. These rhythms result from coordinated daily oscillations in the levels of several clock component proteins. In mammals, central to the generation of these cycles are the levels of the proteins PER and CRY, which feed back to inhibit transcription of their own genes. This inhibition is exerted on the enhancement of transcription that results from binding of the CLOCK and BMAL1 proteins to E-box elements of the promoter regions of the *Per* and *Cry* genes. Additional interactions between circadian clock proteins may slow the time course of this feedback, achieving the near-24-hour interval: the phosphorylation of PER by CKIε may lead to its degradation, and the association with BMAL1 appears needed for CLOCK to be present in the nucleus. Rhythmic transcription of *Bmal1* appears to result from regulation via the protein REV-ERBα, its transcription regulated by CLOCK-BMAL1 binding to E-box elements. Finally, it appears that rhythms in histone acetylation contribute to the circadian expression pattern of some core circadian genes. Additional genes have been identified on the basis of altered circadian rhythms in mutants, although the roles of these genes in the circadian system remain to be determined. The importance of these central circadian clock genes in regulation of sleep and metabolism, as well as in human health, is beginning to be defined.

Over the past three decades, remarkable progress has been made in elucidating the physiologic substrates that underlie the generation of 24-hour rhythms in mammals. Such rhythms are now known to be produced by a circadian system with a "master" biologic clock located in the bilaterally paired suprachiasmatic nuclei (SCN) of the hypothalamus that acts to coordinate oscillators in tissues throughout the organism. Although normally coordinated, individual tissues and cells are capable of producing sustained rhythms in isolation. These rhythms are the result of oscillations of expression of a core set of interrelated circadian genes. This chapter describes the genes expressed in the SCN and other oscillators and the proteins they encode that are responsible for this daily rhythmicity. Readers not familiar with some of the terms used in genetics research should refer to the websites http://www.biologytext.com/ and http://www.biochem.northwestern.edu/holmgren/Glossary/Definitions/Def-A/Index-A.html, which contain glossaries of terms used in genetics.

ORGANIZATION OF THE MAMMALIAN CIRCADIAN SYSTEM

Beginning in the 1970s, several lines of evidence pointed to the suprachiasmatic nucleus (SCN) as the site of the master circadian pacemaker. Destruction of the SCN abolishes circadian oscillations in the plasma concentration of cortisol[1] and in locomotion and drinking.[2] These oscillations are independent of inputs from the eye,[1] although an autonomous circadian clock has been demonstrated to exist within the eye that controls, among other functions, the shedding of rod outer segment discs.[3] Normal circadian rhythms can be restored to an SCN-lesioned animal by transplantation of fetal SCN tissue, but not by transplantation of fetal tissue from other regions of the brain.[4] Transplantation into an SCN-lesioned animal of fetal tissue from the SCN of a circadian mutant animal confers the short period of the donor,[5] indicating that the properties of the rhythm are determined by the SCN rather than other tissues or brain regions. Thus, several lines of evidence point to the SCN as the site driving or controlling circadian behavior for mammals (see Chapter 29 for review).

Recent studies of rhythms in gene expression have indicated that persistent rhythms can be observed in tissues throughout the organism, even in tissue explants kept in culture for extended periods of time.[6,7] The phase of these peripheral tissue rhythms differs from that of the SCN but nonetheless appears to be coordinated by the SCN. In SCN-lesioned animals, these peripheral rhythms persist but no longer exhibit the consistent phase seen in un-lesioned animals.[7] Some environmental manipulations, such as temperature cycles or restricted feeding, can alter the phase of peripheral rhythms.[8,9] In addition, studies confirm the presence of oscillations in gene expression throughout the body, with different phases in different tissues.[10-13] Loss of many of these rhythms is reported with SCN lesions. However, it is important to note that these studies cannot discriminate between a loss of rhythmicity by individual animals and a loss of synchronicity among the individuals. Thus, the roles of the SCN and of the peripheral oscillators in the mammalian circadian system continue to be defined.

How does the SCN communicate and coordinate oscillations throughout the body? This is another question that is only beginning to be addressed. It appears that information from the SCN may take the form of a diffusible signal.[14] The transforming growth factor alpha (TGFα) peptide was identified in a screen for SCN factors that might inhibit locomotor activity; when infused into the third ventricle, this peptide inhibits locomotor activity. Mice with targeted mutations of the epidermal growth factor receptor (the receptor likely to bind TGFα) also display disruption of activity rhythms.[15]

There are several ways in which the neurons of the SCN might produce oscillatory activity. One way would be for the individual neurons to have intrinsic oscillatory behavior. Alternatively, no one neuron may possess oscillatory behavior, but rather the ensemble of neurons oscillates because of the intrinsic properties and connections of the ensemble. Several lines of evidence point to the oscillations being intrinsic to individual SCN neurons. Blockade of action potentials by injection of the sodium channel blocker TTX into the SCN does not stop the circadian oscillator, although blockade does prevent inputs and outputs from being transmitted to and from the SCN.[16] In addition, synaptogenesis in the SCN occurs after the development of circadian rhythms.[17] These two findings demonstrate that the oscillations do not depend on communication between SCN neurons. Indeed, the periods of individual SCN cells studied in slices vary widely, and the circadian period of an animal appears to reflect the mean of the periods of many SCN neurons.[18] Finally, individual, dissociated SCN neurons in culture demonstrate oscillations with periods that differ from cell to cell, indicating that these neurons possess an intrinsic oscillatory mechanism.[19] The remainder of this chapter will focus on the mechanism by which individual cells generate oscillations with a period of about 1 day.

GENE EXPRESSION DRIVES THE CIRCADIAN OSCILLATOR

How do individual cells generate rhythmic activity with a period of about 1 day? Many pacemaker neurons generate oscillatory activity, such as rhythmic patterns of action potentials, and these relatively rapid oscillations can be explained by the concerted action of a small number of ion channels. However, the much slower oscillations of the individual SCN neurons are not likely to involve the same mechanisms. In fact, the finding that nonneuronal tissues can produce sustained circadian rhythms, as well as the prevalence of circadian rhythms in plants and unicellular organisms would argue against a neural process underlying circadian rhythm generation. Indeed, it appears that the synthesis of proteins by each SCN neuron is central to the mechanism for the generation of 24-hour rhythms. The initial evidence for this is that application of protein synthesis inhibitors in the region of the SCN shifts the circadian phase of activity of animals by an amount and in a direction that depends on the time at which the inhibition is imposed.[20,21] A similar shift in the phase of vasopressin release from explanted SCN also results from inhibition of protein synthesis.[22] Thus, gene expression is central to the generation of circadian oscillations.

THE *period* GENE OF THE CIRCADIAN CLOCK

The first identified gene that encodes a clock component, *period*, denoted with the symbol *per*, was discovered in 1971 in *Drosophila* using a forward genetic approach consisting of chemically inducing random mutations in the genome, and detecting those mutations that affect circadian rhythms by screening the progeny of the mutagenized individuals for altered rhythmicity.[23] This approach has the advantage that no assumptions are made about the nature of the genes or gene products involved, but it is based on the presumption that there exist genes that, when mutated, will alter rhythms in a detectable manner. At the time, this presumption of the existence of genes that regulate a complex behavior was considered radical, but it has proven to have been a field-defining moment.

Initially, three alleles of the *per* gene were identified by the process of mutagenesis and screening. Either these alleles had no apparent rhythm in eclosion (emergence from the pupal case) or locomotion, or they had long (e.g., 29 hours) or short periods (e.g., 19 hours) for the rhythms of eclosion and locomotor activity.[23] It is important to note that the finding of three alleles with three different phenotypes made it possible to have confidence in the conclusion that the *per* gene encodes a protein that is a clock component. Had only an arrhythmic mutant been found, then the alternative explanation could be proposed that the lack of circadian behavior was secondary to another primary defect that did not lie in a clock component. It should also be noted that the approach of mutagenesis and screening has also been successful in identifying circadian clock genes in other organisms such as *Neurospora crassa*,[24] plants,[25] and cyanobacteria.[26] However, a discussion of these important findings is outside the scope of this chapter.

Confirmation of the importance of the *per* gene as a central circadian clock component was provided by the rescue of the mutant phenotype after introduction of the wild-type allele of the *per* gene into mutant flies.[27,28] The level of the mRNA transcript encoded by the *per* gene was shown to oscillate in a circadian fashion[29] as a result of transcriptional regulation,[30] and the levels of the PER protein were shown to lag the *per* mRNA levels.[31] In fact, shifts in the circadian phase can be evoked by the induction of PER protein under the control of a noncircadian promoter.[32] Thus, many lines of evidence indicate that the *per* gene encodes a protein that is a clock component. Three orthologs of the *per* gene, *mPer1*, *mPer2*, and *mPer3*, have now been identified in the mouse and the levels of their mRNA have also been shown to oscillate with a circadian period.[33-37]

THE MAMMALIAN *Clock* GENE

Because no mammalian orthologs (genes with both functional and sequence homology) to *Drosophila* circadian clock genes had been identified by the early 1990s, and no other genes in mammals had been identified as even possible candidate circadian clock genes in genetically accessible organisms, we undertook mutagenesis and screening in mice in an effort to identify mammalian circadian clock genes. For this, we used the C57BL/6J mouse strain, in which wild-type mice show robust entrainment to a light–dark cycle and have a circadian period between 23.6 and 23.8 hours under free-running conditions in constant darkness (DD) (Fig. 30–1). In a screen for dominant or semidominant mutations of over 300 progeny of mutagen-treated mice, we found one animal that had a free-running period of about 24.8 hours, more than six standard deviations longer than the mean.[38] In the homozygous condition, this mutation results in a dramatic lengthening of the period to about 28 hours, which is usually followed by the eventual loss of circadian rhythmicity (i.e., arrhythmicity)

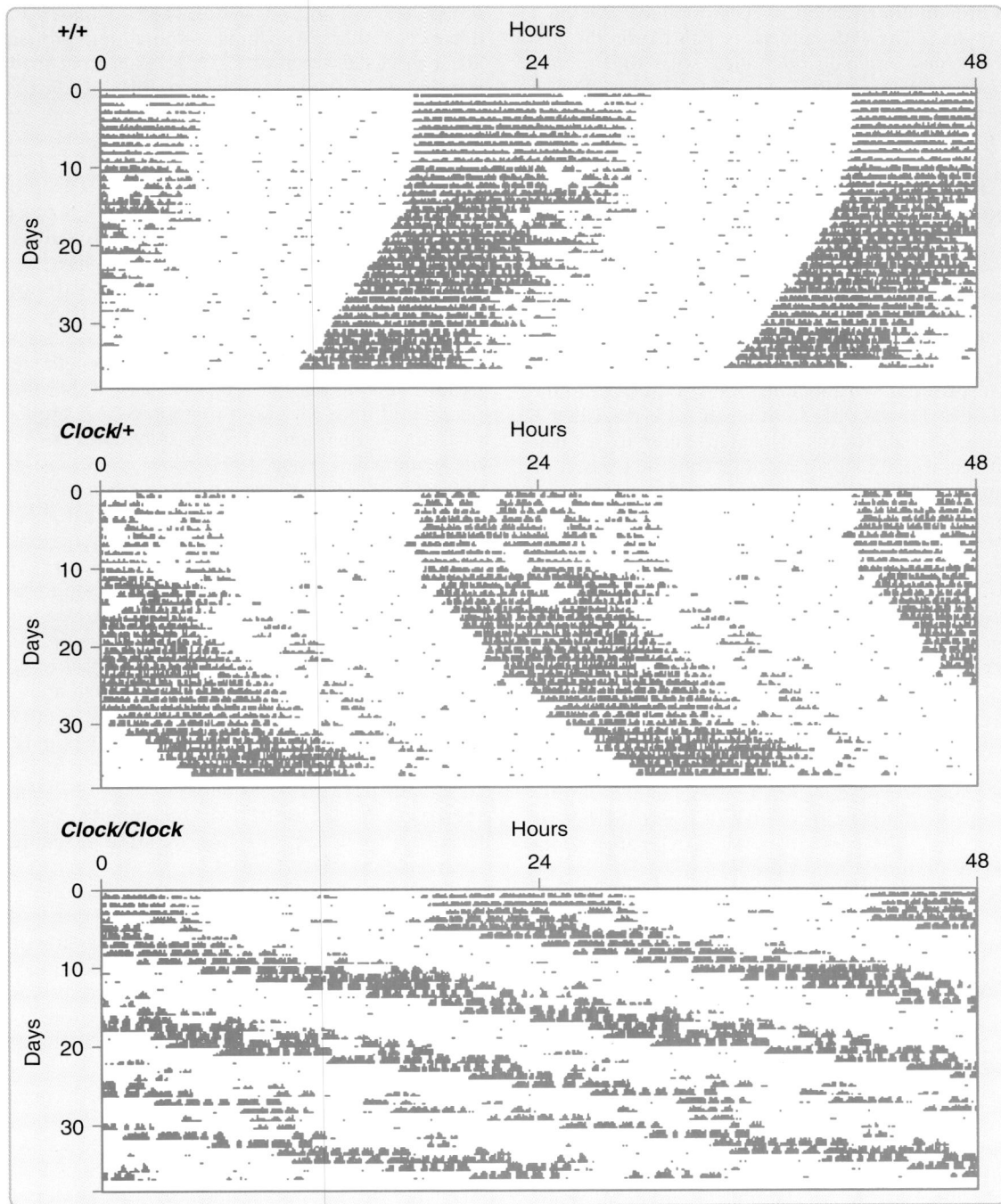

Figure 30–1. Activity records of mice. Each record is double-plotted according to convention, so that each day's data are presented both to the right of and beneath the day preceding. Times of wheel-running activity are indicated by *dark blue*. On days 1 to 6, mice were maintained under a 12-hours-light, 12-hours-dark light cycle. Mice were then transferred to continuous darkness by allowing lights to go out at the usual time and then to remain off through the remaining days of data collection. **Top:** Activity record of a wild-type C57BL/6J mouse, with a free-running period of approximately 23.7 hours. **Middle:** Activity record of a *Clock*/+ heterozygote C57BL/6J mouse, with a free-running period that lengthened over time to approximately 24.8 hours. **Bottom:** Activity record of a homozygous *Clock/Clock* mutant C57BL/6J mouse, with a free-running period of approximately 28 hours.

after about 1 to 3 weeks in DD. The affected gene was mapped to mouse chromosome 5 and named *Clock*.[38,39] We cloned the *Clock* gene by a combination of genetic rescue and positional cloning techniques. *Clock/Clock* mutant mice were phenotypically rescued by a bacterial artificial chromosome (BAC) transgene that contained the *Clock* gene, allowing for

functional identification of the gene.[40] The *Clock* gene encodes a transcriptional regulatory protein having a basic helix-loop-helix DNA-binding domain, a PAS dimerization domain, and a Q-rich transactivation domain. The mutant form of the CLOCK protein (CLOCK Δ19) lacks a portion of the activation domain found in wild-type protein, and thus, although it is capable of protein dimerization, transcriptional activation is diminished or lost. The PAS domain is named for the first letters of the genes originally identified with this protein dimerization domain, *per*, *ARNT*, and *sim*. *Clock* mRNA is expressed in the SCN as well as other tissues, but it has not been found to oscillate in a circadian fashion.[41]

INTERACTIONS OF *Clock* WITH *period* AND *Bmal1* GENES

The presence of the PAS dimerization domain in CLOCK protein suggested that it may form a heterodimer similar to that of PER and the protein product of another *Drosophila* clock gene, TIM.[42] A screen for potential partners for the CLOCK protein using the yeast two-hybrid system revealed that a protein of unknown function, BMAL1 (for brain and muscle ARNT-like 1), was able to dimerize with the CLOCK protein.[43] Next, the ability of this heterodimer to regulate transcription was tested using a reporter construct based on the upstream regulatory elements of the *per* gene. The *per* gene of *Drosophila* contains an upstream regulatory element, the "clock control region," within which is contained a sequence needed for positive regulation of transcription, the E-box element (CACGTG).[44] CLOCK-BMAL1 heterodimers were found to activate transcription of the *mPer* gene in a process that requires binding to the E-box element.[43] However, CLOCK Δ19 mutant protein was not able to activate transcription, consistent with the finding that exon 19, which is skipped in *Clock* mutant animals,[41] is necessary for transactivation. Thus, CLOCK protein interacts with the regulatory regions of the *per* gene to allow transcription of the *per* mRNA and eventual translation of PER protein. A similar activation of transcription of the *tim* gene by the CLOCK:BMAL1 heterodimer also occurs.[45] However, this positive regulation alone will not produce an oscillation in *per* mRNA levels, which is known to be responsible for the oscillation in PER protein levels.[30] The finding that the *Clock* mutation dramatically decreases *per* genes' expression also confirms the positive regulation of CLOCK:BMAL1 on *per* transcription in situ.[46]

Creation of mice harboring a null allele of *Bmal1* (also referred to as *MOP3*) demonstrated the critical role of this gene in circadian rhythm generation. These mutant mice, while displaying light–dark responsive differences in activity level, become arrhythmic immediately upon release in constant darkness.[47] Mice with null mutations of *mPer1*, *mPer2*, or *mPer3* display altered circadian periods,[48,49] whereas mice with both *mPer1* and *mPer2* null mutations also lose rhythmicity. *mPer3* null mutant mice exhibit only a subtle alteration in rhythmicity, and *mPer1/mPer3* or *mPer2/mPer3* double mutants are not substantially distinct from the *mPer1* or *mPer3* single mutants. These findings suggest there may be some compensation of function among the different mammalian *per* genes, and they raise the question of how significant the role played by *mPer3* may be.

Recently, additional actions of the CLOCK:BMAL1 heterodimer have become clear. Although *Clock* mRNA does not oscillate, its protein's nuclear (as opposed to cytoplasmic) localization does.[50] By studying the intracellular localization of CLOCK and BMAL1 in fibroblasts of mouse embryos with mutations in different clock genes, and ectopically expressing the proteins, it was found that nuclear accumulation of CLOCK was dependent on formation of the CLOCK:BMAL1 dimer, as was phosphorylation of the complex and its degradation.[50] Other PAS domain–containing proteins failed to affect the localization of CLOCK, indicating that these posttranslational events are specific to the CLOCK:BMAL dimer.

THE *Cryptochromes*

Cryptochromes are blue light–responsive flavoprotein photopigments related to photolyases, so named because their function was cryptic when they were first identified. In mammals, two cryptochrome genes, *Cry1* and *Cry2*, have been identified and were found to be highly expressed in the ganglion cells and inner nuclear layer of the retina and the SCN,[51] and their mRNA expression levels oscillate in these tissues. Targeted mutant mice lacking *Cry2* exhibit a lengthened circadian period, whereas mice lacking *Cry1* have a shortened circadian period and mice with both mutations have immediate loss of rhythmicity upon transfer to constant darkness.[52-54] Thus, like the mammalian *period* genes, the *cryptochrome* genes appear to have both distinct (given their opposite effects on circadian period) and compensatory (given that either gene can sustain rhythmicity in the absence of the other) functions.

Because of their expression pattern, the *cryptochromes* were thought to be the long-unidentified mammalian circadian photoreceptors (see later), and thus light responses were examined in characterizing the null mutants. *Cry2* mutant mice exhibit altered phase-shifting responses to light pulses.[52] *Cry1/Cry2* double mutants exhibit impaired light induction of *mPer1* in the SCN, whereas light induction of *mPer2* in double mutants remains.[53,55] Neither *mPer1* nor *mPer2* exhibits persistent oscillations in expression in the SCN in constant conditions in *Cry1/Cry2* double mutants.[53,55] Thus, although the *cryptochromes* are not the mammalian circadian photoreceptor, they do appear to play a central role in the generation of circadian signals.

Further evidence for a central clock function is the finding that the *cryptochromes* appear to share a number of regulatory features with the *period* genes. In *Clock* mutant mice, the mRNA levels of *Cry1* and *Cry2* are reduced in the SCN and in skeletal muscle,[56] suggesting that the *cryptochromes* also are induced by CLOCK:BMAL1 transactivation. Using mammalian (NIH 3T3 or COS7) cell lines, CRY1 and CRY2 were found by coimmunoprecipitation to interact with mPER1, mPER2, and mPER3, leading to nuclear localization of the CRY:PER dimer as indicated by cotransfection assays with epitope-tagged proteins.[56] Luciferase assays indicate that CRY:CRY or CRY:PER complexes were capable of inhibiting CLOCK:BMAL1 transactivation of *mPer1* or vasopressin transcription.[56] Thus, the CRYs as well as the PERs are capable of a negative feedback function, inhibiting CLOCK:BMAL1-induced transcription.

MELANOPSIN—THE MAMMALIAN CIRCADIAN PHOTOPIGMENT

The circadian rhythms of many humans who are blind, with no conscious perception of light, are nevertheless able to be entrained by light.[57] This and other findings early on raised the question, What are the photoreceptors and the neural pathways for entraining the circadian clock? A great deal of progress has been made toward an answer to this question in the past few years.

Classical rod and cone photoreceptor cells with their opsin-based pigments cannot be solely responsible for light entrainment. In experiments employing mouse mutations that result in degeneration of rods[58] or both rods and cones,[59] light entrainment of the circadian rhythm was preserved.[60] However, the eye must be the site of the light-entraining pathways in mammals because enucleated mammals are not capable of light entrainment.[58] Indeed, a morphologically distinct set of retinal ganglion cells projects to the SCN via the retinohypothalamic tract.[61] Ablation of the SCN abolishes circadian rhythmicity, and ablation of the retinohypothalamic tract abolishes light entrainment.[62] Thus, the light signal responsible for light entrainment enters the SCN via a unique axonal pathway from the eye.

Two recently discovered photopigments found in the eye, the cryptochromes have been suggested to serve light entrainment[51]: and melanopsin.[63-66] Whereas the cryptochromes, CRY1 and CRY2, are expressed in both inner retinal neurons and the SCN,[51] as noted earlier, studies in double *Cry1/Cry2* mutants demonstrated the cryptochromes were not necessary for photoentrainment.[53,54]

Ocular melanopsin, a member of the opsin family of photopigments was first found in the inner retina[63] and later found to be expressed in the somata and dendrites of retinal ganglion cells of the retinohypothalamic tract.[65] Neurons that contribute axons to the retinohypothalamic tract were found to express the marker pituitary adenylate cyclase-activating polypeptide (PACAP)[65]; when PACAP was used as a marker for rat retinohypothalamic tract neurons, every PACAP-positive neuron was found to express melanopsin and every melanopsin-positive neuron was PACAP positive.[65] Most of the double-labeled cells were found in the retinal ganglion cell layer, but some were also found in the inner layers of the inner nuclear layer, where both displaced ganglion cells and amacrine cells are found. The SCN-projecting neurons of the retinohypothalamic tract can also be retrogradely labeled by injection of microspheres into the SCN; these retrogradely labeled ganglion cells were found to be responsive to light under conditions in which synaptic transmission was inhibited by incubation in solutions containing Co(II),[64] a treatment that eliminated synaptic inputs originating with rods and cones. The action spectrum of these ganglion cells was determined, and a Dartnall nomogram with lambda max of 484 nm best fitted the spectral data; this value is consistent with the wavelength for maximal sensitivity for phase shifting of the behavioral response.[67] These recordings were consistent with behavioral observations of the phase shift in another way: the threshold irradiance for the response to light was within the range of irradiance required for phase shifting the activity rhythm.

Further evidence confirming the role of melanopsin as the phase-shifting pigment has come from genetically engineered mice in which the gene encoding melanopsin was disrupted.[68,69] Two behavioral measures of circadian rhythm responses to light were altered in these mice: the phase-shifting response to a discrete light pulse was of lesser amplitude in the knockout mice than in wild-type mice, and the free-running periods of the knockout mice were lengthened less by exposure to constant light than the periods of wild-type mice. However, the phase of onset of activity when the mice were placed in constant darkness did not differ between the melanopsin knockout and the wild-type mice. A much stronger case for the involvement of melanopsin in entraining the circadian clock was obtained from experiments using double-mutant mice in which the rods were eliminated with the *pde4rd* mutation and melanopsin expression was eliminated by disrupting the *Opn4* gene.[70] The activity rhythm of these double-mutant mice was unable to be entrained to a light–dark cycle, and their activity was not able to be suppressed by treatment with a 2-hour-long pulse of white light, a treatment that suppresses the activity of wild-type mice and mice with a single mutation in either the *Opn4* or *pde4* genes. Taken together, these results indicate that melanopsin-expressing cells of the retinohypothalamic tract are capable of mediating a change in phase of the circadian rhythm when they are stimulated by light, and that these signals can replace the signals that are generated by the rod and cone photoreceptors that are needed for visual perception. Two important questions about circadian phase shifting still need to be addressed more completely: the interaction between phase-shifting signals that originate from rods, cones, and melanopsin-containing ganglion cells, and the mechanism by which phase-shifting signals impinge on the molecular oscillator that is present in neurons of the SCN.

Timeless

How is the level of the PER protein regulated by the circadian clock? The first hint came from the identification of the *timeless* gene *tim*, which when mutated produces abnormal circadian rhythms in *Drosophila*.[71] The levels of the mRNA encoded by the *tim* gene oscillate with a time course that is indistinguishable from those of *per* mRNA.[72] The levels of the TIM protein lag behind those of *tim* mRNA by several hours,[73] something also found with *per* mRNA and PER protein. The PER and TIM proteins form heterodimers[74] that are transported to the nucleus.[75] The finding that the heterodimer is transported to the nucleus suggested that it might be involved in the regulation of transcription of the *per* or *tim* genes. Indeed, recent experiments have shown that the transcription of the *per* and *tim* genes is repressed by the PER:TIM protein heterodimer.[45] This finding is very important because it demonstrates that the production of mRNA encoded by a clock component gene, the delayed accumulation of the encoded protein, and the later feedback to the clock gene's promoter in the nucleus are able to explain the basic features of the circadian clock in *Drosophila*.

However, PER–TIM interactions are not sufficient, and the basic mechanism does not become clear until one adds interactions with other clock genes. In experiments using a luciferase reporter assay, the luminescent luciferase protein was expressed under the control of the promoter regions of the *Drosophila per* and *tim* genes. It was found that the fly homolog of *Clock*, *dClock*,[76] was capable of driving expression of luciferase[45] in cells that have high endogenous levels of the *Drosophila* homolog of BMAL1, CYC (for *cycle*). The effect of the PER:TIM heterodimer on the ability of the dCLOCK:CYC heterodimer to drive the transcription of the *per* and *tim* genes was tested by cotransfecting the encoding genes into the cells that expressed the luciferase reporter gene. Indeed, it was found that the expressions of both the *per* and *tim* genes were reduced by their own protein products. This negative feedback has recently been found for a mammalian heterodimer consisting of homolog of the TIMELESS and mPER1 proteins.[77]

Whether the mammalian *tim* homologue identified[77,78] actually represents an orthologous gene has been called into question.[79] This issue has been difficult to resolve, as gene targeting to create a null mutant resulted in early embryonic lethality. Differences in results obtained by different groups examining the oscillation of *mTim* expression could result from both a full-length and a truncated protein being expressed, with only the full-length form oscillating.[80] Using antisense oligodeoxynucleotides directed against *Timeless* in rat SCN slice preparations disrupts neuronal oscillations in vitro, suggesting that a role in rhythmicity may exist.[80] However, true functional homology of *Timeless* in mammals remains to be demonstrated.

THE *tau* MUTATION

The *tau* mutation of the hamster arose spontaneously in a laboratory stock.[81] The mutation is semidominant and shortens the period from 24 to 22 hours in heterozygotes and to 20 hours in homozygotes. This mutation has been of great importance for several reasons:

1. The mutation predated the *Clock* mutation and demonstrated that single gene mutations could profoundly alter the circadian clock in mammals, just as in flies and *Neurospora*.
2. *Tau* mutants display several other physiologic phenotypes, such as alteration of the responses of males to photoperiod length[82] and effects of the estrous cycles in females,[83] which gave further insights into the importance of the circadian clock for other biologic cycles.
3. The evidence that the SCN is indeed the site of the master circadian oscillator (see earlier) was demonstrated unequivocally using transplantation of the SCN that employed the *tau* mutation.

These manipulations also gave rise to the evidence necessary to conclude that the *tau* mutation encodes a protein that is a clock component. Unfortunately, the genetic tools needed for cloning this important and interesting gene were not available for the hamster, and thus its molecular identity could not be determined by conventional genetic mapping/positional cloning.

Lowrey and colleagues were able to identify a genomic region of conserved synteny (a grouping of genes together on a chromosome) in hamsters, mice, and humans, that encompassed the *tau* mutation.[84] *Tau* was thus identified as being a mutation in the *casein kinase I epsilon* (CKIε) gene, the mammalian ortholog of the *Drosophila doubletime* gene. Sequencing of the gene identified a point mutation that leads to altered enzyme dynamics and an autophosphorylation state. In vitro assays demonstrated that *CKIε* can phosphorylate PER proteins, and that the *tau* mutant enzyme is deficient in this ability. Thus, CKIε may lead to degradation of PERs, slowing the accumulation of PER in the nucleus and thus repression of CLOCK:BMAL1.

ADDING MORE LOOPS TO THE CYCLE

Although the negative feedback of PER and CRY proteins on their own CLOCK:BMAL1-induced transcription constitutes a form of negative feedback and may be sufficient to explain the

oscillations in expression of *mPer* and *Cry* genes, the rhythmic expression of *Bmal1* with an opposite phase is not explained by this feedback. What regulatory elements produced the rhythmic transcription of *Bmal1*, with an anti-phase relationship to the *Pers*? *Rev-erb alpha*, an orphan nuclear receptor, may act as the missing link. Its promoter region contains three E-boxes, and transcription is thus positively regulated by CLOCK and BMAL1.[85] Its transcription is negatively regulated by PER and CRYs and is at a minimum when mPER2 is at a maximum, and it is constitutively expressed at intermediate levels in *Cry1/Cry2* or *Per1/Per2* double knockouts. REV-ERBα protein appears to drive the circadian oscillation in *Bmal1* transcription: the *Bmal1* promoter includes two RORE sequences (enhancer sequences that recognize members of the REV-ERB and ROR orphan nuclear receptor families), and *Bmal1* expression is drastically reduced in *Rev-erbα* null mutants.[85] Thus *Rev-erb alpha* may act to link the positive and negative regulatory signals of other clock genes to the transcription of *Bmal1*.

The differences between the phase of *Cry1* mRNA rhythms relative to other clock genes whose transcription is enhanced by CLOCK:BMAL binding to E-boxes may also be attributable to *Rev-erbα*. The *Cry1* gene has three candidate REV-ERB/ROR binding sites[86]; in vitro assays indicate that REV-ERBα binds to two of these sites. Luciferase reporter assays indicate that REV-ERBα protein can inhibit transcription of *Cry1* through binding at these two sites.

There is also evidence of regulation of clock gene transcription via rhythms in acetylation of H3 histone: CRY proteins may inhibit H3 acetylation.[86] The *Per1*, *Per2*, and *Cry1* promoters have rhythms in H3 acetylation. The *Per1*, *Per2*, and *Cry1* promoters have rhythms in RNA polymerase II binding. These promoter rhythms are in phase with mRNA levels. P300, a histone acetyltransferase, immunoprecipitates together with CLOCK in liver nuclear preparations, with a peak at CT 6 and minimum at CT 18.[86] P300 may be part of the CLOCK:BMAL1 coactivator complex; a *Per1* promoter-driven luciferase reporter assay indicates that CRY proteins can disrupt this. Hence, inhibition of histone acetylation by P300 provides a potential separate mechanism by which CRY proteins can preclude CLOCK:BMAL1 transactivation of *Per* and *Cry* genes.

A MOLECULAR MODEL FOR THE CIRCADIAN CLOCK

Our current knowledge of the molecular genetic interactions of circadian clock genes provides for a basic mechanism involving multiple feedback loops of clock proteins on transcription of clock genes. These core interactions are summarized in Figure 30–2. These and other suspected circadian clock gene interactions are listed in Table 30–1.

Undoubtedly, additional clock genes will be part of the mechanism, and additional transcriptional, translational, and posttranslational interactions among these genes and their proteins will be identified.

OTHER GENES AND MUTATIONS

Four additional mammalian genes have been proposed to play roles in the circadian system, because mutations in these genes result in alterations in circadian rhythms. The *Rab3α*

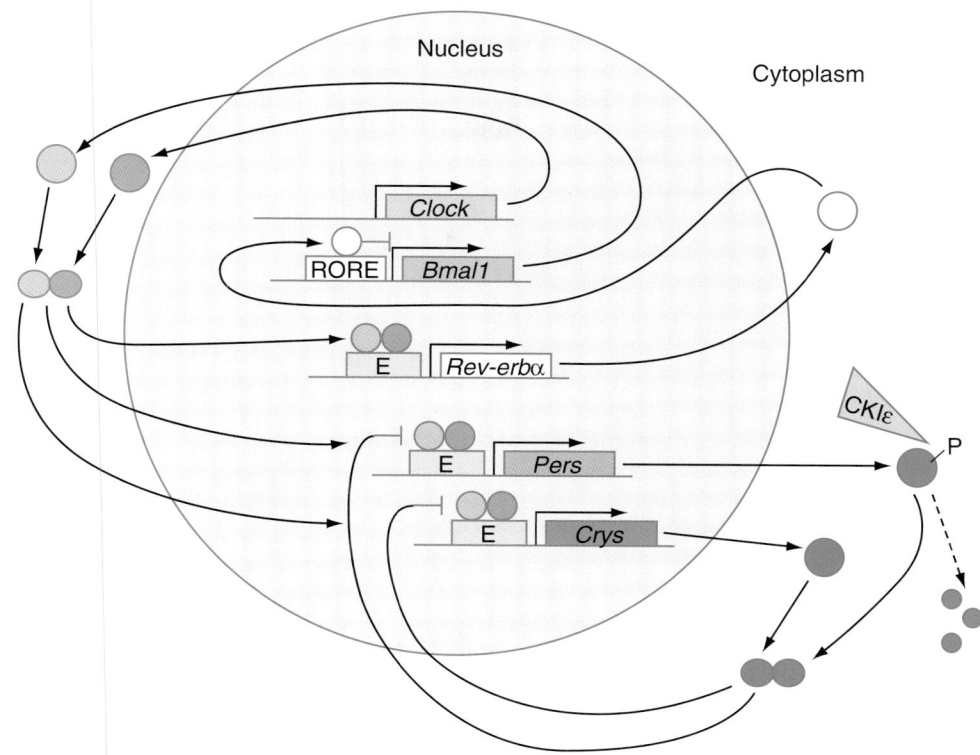

Figure 30–2. Molecular model of the core circadian oscillator. CLOCK and BMAL1 proteins *(light gray)* form heterodimers in the cytoplasm and, on nuclear entry, bind to E-box promoter elements in the *Rev-erbα, Per,* and *Cry* genes to drive transcription of these genes. REV-ERBα *(white)* binds to a retinoic acid–related orphan receptor response element (RORE) to inhibit transcription of *Bmal1*. PER proteins are phosphorylated by CKIε (casein kinase I ε *[triangle]*), possibly leading to its degradation. PER and CRY proteins form heterodimers *(dark blue)* and enter the nucleus to repress CLOCK:BMAL1-driven transcription of *Rev-erbα, Per,* and *Cry* genes.

Table 30–1.   Ten Steps to Build a Circadian Pacemaker

Step	Action	Effect
1	CLOCK and BMAL1 form protein heterodimers.	CLOCK is phosphorylated and CLOCK:BMAL1 dimers enter the nucleus.
2	CLOCK:BMAL1 binds to E-box enhancer elements of *Pers, Crys,* and *Rev-Erbα.*	Positive and rhythmic drive of expression of these circadian genes.
3	PER and CRY proteins form homodimers and heterodimers in the cytoplasm.	CRY:CRY and CRY:PER dimers enter the nucleus.
4	PER is phosphorylated by CKIε.	PER protein is degraded, nuclear accumulation is slowed.
5	PER:CRY and CRY:CRY represses CLOCK:BMAL1-driven transcription of *Pers* and *Crys.*	Negative feedback of PER and CRY proteins on their own transcription.
6	PER:TIM can repress *Per* transcription.	Mammalian *timeless* may have function orthologous to *Drosophila tim,* acting in a negative feedback.
7	PER:CRY represses *Rev-Erbα* transcription.	*Rev-Erbα* is regulated by negative feedback of PER:CRY, resulting in a similar oscillation in expression.
8	REV-ERBα enhances *Bmal1* and represses *Cry1* transcription.	REV-ERBα modulation of transcription produces different phases in expression of *Bmal1* and *Cry1.*
9	CRY proteins inhibit H3 histone acetylation by P300.	CRY proteins can modulate transcription via modulations in histone acetylation.
10	The histone acetyl transferase P300 works together with CLOCK:BMAL in promoting *mPer1, mPer2,* and *Cry1* transcription.	H3 histone acetylation rhythms in the promoter regions of *mPer1, mPer2,* and *Cry1* may regulate timing of the transcription of these genes.

gene was identified in a mutagenesis screen (*earlybird*) on the basis of an advanced phase angle of entrainment and shortened circadian period. Null mutant mice display a similar phenotype.[87] The *DBP* gene has E-box elements in its promoter, and it exhibits robust oscillations in expression in the SCN and the liver. *DBP* null mutant mice display alterations in circadian period as well.[88] *NPAS2* is another bHLH PAS family member that forms heterodimers with BMAL1. Null mutant mice for this gene display alterations in the pattern of their activity rhythms.[89] Mice that lack the peptide receptor VPAC2 show abnormal entrainment and disrupted rhythms, indicating that VIP signaling in the SCN may be necessary for normal expression and coordination of rhythms.[90] Although these genes should be considered as possible mammalian clock genes because their mutations affect expression of circadian rhythms, their roles in the circadian timekeeping mechanism remain equivocal. Further studies are needed to define their roles, if any, in the core molecular circadian clock. Thus, although the story of clock genes is certainly not complete, it now appears that the core of the mammalian molecular clock has been identified.

SLEEP IN CIRCADIAN CLOCK MUTANT ANIMALS

The discovery of circadian genes and the use of animal genetic models have been instrumental in understanding how molecular components of the circadian clock influence the multiple output rhythmic systems under their control. In particular, recent studies in both mice and flies have found that deletion or mutation in core clock genes induces unexpected alterations in sleep amount, sleep architecture, and compensatory responses to sleep deprivation.[91-94] These results have led to the hypothesis that circadian clock genes may also be central to sleep regulatory processes beyond just the circadian timing of sleep. For example, mutation in the mammalian circadian gene, *Clock,* induces a decrease in non–rapid eye movement (NREM) sleep time and an attenuated rapid eye movement sleep recovery after sleep deprivation.[91] A mutation in the fly homologue of this gene, *dClock,* reduces consolidated rest time and leads to alterations in response to rest deprivation.[92,94] Cryptochrome (*Cry1/Cry2*) double-knockout mice have increases in baseline amounts of NREM sleep, consolidation of NREM episodes, and NREM delta power over wild-type control levels, and they lack the normal compensatory response in sleep amount and NREM delta power after sleep deprivation.[93] Interestingly, a mutation in the *Drosophila* gene *timeless* leads to an impaired recovery response to short-term rest deprivation in flies.[92,94] In addition, deletion of *Bmal1* in mice and the fly homologue *cycle* also leads to altered sleep–wake/rest activity amounts under baseline conditions, as well as after sleep deprivation.[92,94,95]

The finding that mutation or deletion of canonical circadian clock genes can induce major effects on the sleep–wake cycle that go beyond just the timing of this rhythm, may be just the beginning of a new way of thinking about how the circadian clock regulates a multitude of physiologic and behavioral rhythms. It may well be that once the central circadian input to a particular output rhythmic system has been disrupted, that downstream rhythm may now be disrupted or altered in many different ways as a result of the loss of normal temporal organization. Indeed, the recent discovery that *Clock* mutant animals show a wide range of metabolic abnormalities lends support to the hypothesis that a disrupted molecular circadian clock can have far-reaching implications for physiology and pathophysiology.[96] Whether such disruptions in physiology and behavior are the result of altered circadian information from the SCN or of local tissue-specific changes in the molecular circadian clock is not known. Regardless of the mechanisms, such results point to a very central role of circadian clock genes in regulating biochemical, metabolic, and physiologic processes at many different levels of organization.

CIRCADIAN CLOCK GENES IN HUMANS

The discovery of circadian clock genes in mice led almost immediately to the search for homologous genes in humans. In addition to searching for human orthologues of the murine clock genes based on sequence similarities, a number of laboratories are attempting to link specific clock gene alleles with two of the major recognized altered circadian phenotypes in humans, delayed sleep phase syndrome (DSPS) and advanced sleep phase syndrome (ASPS), either in large populations or in small families demonstrating genetic linkage with these syndromes (see Chapter 58). DSPS has been associated with a dominant mode of inheritance[97,98] and has been linked to polymorphisms in circadian clock and related genes including *hPER3, arylalkylamine N-acetyltransferase,* and *hCLOCK.*[99-102] Similarly, several families have also been identified in which ASPS shows a clear autosomal dominant mode of inheritance,[103-105] with a genetic polymorphism in *hPER2* being identified in one ASPS family.[106] Although Katzenberg and coworkers[107] found that subjects with a preference for "eveningness" based on the Horne-Ostberg test carried a specific allele of *hCLOCK,* subsequent studies did not find such linkage.[101,108]

The finding that different circadian phenotypes may be linked to different circadian clock genes, or may result from different allelic forms of any given clock gene, may be the rule and not the exception. Indeed, pre-"molecular era" findings that DSPS may increase at northern latitudes[109] and that a human psychiatric disorder linked to human rhythms (seasonal affective disorder) is also associated with latitude, raise the intriguing possibility that throughout human evolution, there may have been subtle changes in human clock genes that enabled humans to fine-tune their temporal relationship to the environment as they migrated into every possible environmental habitat on earth. Indeed, the circadian clock genome may gave greatly diversified as humans successfully invaded and adapted to such extreme environments as polar regions, deserts, and high mountains that required changes in the phase relationship of daily life to the harsh but often predictable changes in the daily environment. With so many clock genes (at least 10 and counting) and their possible allelic variations, it will be perhaps not surprising to find that there are many, many circadian genotypes in the human population.

Linking circadian genotype with human circadian phenotypes in the modern world may provide a much deeper understanding of health and disease. Disorders of circadian temporal organization come in two general varieties: those imposed by the lifestyle of the individual (e.g., jet lag and shift work) and those that arise from endogenous alterations in normal rhythmicity.[110,111] Elucidating the genetic basis of human circadian rhythmicity holds promise for new therapeutic approaches for both the "voluntary" and the "involuntary" disruption of normal circadian function. It will also be of great interest, from both a scientific and a medical perspective, to determine if the expression of human clock genes is altered under various pathophysiologic conditions or in advanced age. The effects of aging are of particular interest because it has been associated with abnormal circadian timekeeping.[112]

The potential richness of the circadian genotype for human health and disease takes on possible special significance in view of two "relatively recent" developments. First, humans in modern society rarely live in the temporal lifestyle in which their circadian clock genes/alleles evolved. Although there is for good reason a great interest in how human metabolic genes, which evolved over millions of years to survive a feast-and-famine way of life, are now influencing feeding behavior and metabolism in a modern society of plenty, it may well be of similar importance to understand how humans are attempting to navigate our round-the-clock modern society with circadian genes adapted for another time. The second "relatively recent" development is the surprising finding that although the SCN circadian clock may be the master pacemaker, most, if not all, tissues/organs of the body may contain the molecular circadian clock machinery, and, furthermore, hundreds if not thousands of genes may be under circadian control (see Chapter 29). This multi-oscillatory nature of the circadian timing system may require very fine timing for normal physiologic function, and it is likely that different allelic forms of the circadian clock genes may have evolved for tissue- or organ-specific, as well as whole-organism, phase preference for internal as well as external synchronization.

CONCLUSIONS

The core circadian oscillator is autonomous to individual neurons of the SCN and is the result of the daily oscillation in the levels of several clock component proteins. The basis for this oscillation in mammals, as in other organisms, lies in rhythmic feedback regulation of transcription of the genes encoding these proteins. The levels of the PER and CRY proteins alter the rate of transcription of their own genes. This alteration is achieved by inhibition of the enhancement of transcription that results from binding of the CLOCK:BMAL1 heterodimer to the E-box element of the promoter region of the *per* and *Cry* genes. Additional interactions between circadian clock proteins may slow the time course of this feedback, achieving the near-24-hour interval; the phosphorylation of PER by CKIε may lead to its degradation, and the association with BMAL1 appears needed for CLOCK to be present in the nucleus. Rhythmic transcription of *Bmal1* appears to result from regulation via REV-ERBα, itself regulated by E-box elements. Finally, it appears that rhythms in histone acetylation contribute to the circadian expression pattern of some core circadian genes. Additional genes have been identified on the basis of altered circadian rhythms in mutants, although the roles of these genes in the circadian system remain to be determined.

It is of interest that the majority of the core genes have been identified in mice or in flies by forward genetics, in which mutations were induced in the genome randomly, and those mutations that specifically affect the circadian oscillator

were identified with carefully crafted circadian phenotypic screens. Now that these clock component proteins have been identified, it will be easier to find the proteins that serve the input and output pathways of the circadian oscillator, and to identify the components that are out of order in disease states that affect circadian rhythms. It is fortuitous that the unraveling of the molecular basis for circadian rhythmicity is occurring at a time when the general public is becoming aware of the importance of normal circadian timekeeping for human health, safety, performance, and productivity, as detailed in Section 8 of this volume.

> ### Clinical Pearl
>
> *In recent years, findings from a number of different laboratories have added considerably to our understanding of the molecular components of the mammalian circadian clock. It has become clear that a number of genes are involved and multiple complex interactions among the genes and their products have been identified. Even though the mammalian circadian clock genes have only recently been discovered, they are already being implicated in circadian sleep phase disorders such as advanced and delayed sleep phase syndromes (see Chapter 58). In addition, recent studies in mice indicate that alterations of clock genes can lead to altered amounts of sleep, metabolic abnormalities, and reproductive dysfunction. The door is now open to examine the role of alterations in circadian clock genes in human pathophysiology.*

Acknowledgments

Preparation of this manuscript was in part supported by National Institutes of Health cooperative agreement U01 MH 61915, and grant numbers R01 AG 18200, P01 AG11412, and R01 HL 59598.

References

1. Moore RY, Eichler VB: Loss of a circadian adrenal corticosterone rhythm following suprachiasmatic lesions in the rat. Brain Res 1972;42:201-206.
2. Stephan FK, Zucker I: Circadian rhythms in drinking behavior and locomotor activity of rats are eliminated by hypothalamic lesions. Proc Natl Acad Sci U S A 1972;69:1583-1586.
3. Tosini G, Menaker M: Circadian rhythms in cultured mammalian retina. Science 1996;272:419-421.
4. Lehman MN, Silver R, Gladstone WR, et al: Circadian rhythmicity restored by neural transplant: Immunocytochemical characterization of the graft and its integration with the host brain. J Neurosci 1987;7:1626-1638.
5. Ralph MR, Foster RG, Davis FC, Menaker M: Transplanted suprachiasmatic nucleus determines circadian period. Science 1990;247:975-978.
6. Yamazaki S, Numano R, Abe M, et al: Resetting central and peripheral circadian oscillators in transgenic rats. Science 2000;288:682-685.
7. Yoo SH, Yamazaki S, Lowrey PL, et al: PERIOD2::LUCIFERASE real-time reporting of circadian dynamics reveals persistent circadian oscillations in mouse peripheral tissues. Proc Natl Acad Sci U S A 2004;101:5339-5346.
8. Brown SA, Zumbrunn G, Fleury-Olela F, et al: Rhythms of mammalian body temperature can sustain peripheral circadian clocks. Curr Biol 2002;12:1574-1583.

9. Stokkan KA, Yamazaki S, Tei H, et al: Entrainment of the circadian clock in the liver by feeding. Science 2001;291:490-493.

10. Panda S, Antoch MP, Miller BH, et al: Coordinated transcription of key pathways in the mouse by the circadian clock. Cell 2002;109:307-320.

11. Akhtar RA, Reddy AB, Maywood ES, et al: Circadian cycling of the mouse liver transcriptome, as revealed by cDNA microarray, is driven by the suprachiasmatic nucleus. Curr Biol 2002;12:540-550.

12. Storch KF, Lipan O, Leykin I, et al: Extensive and divergent circadian gene expression in liver and heart. Nature 2002;417:78-83.

13. Duffield GE, Best JD, Meurers BH, et al: Circadian programs of transcriptional activation, signaling, and protein turnover revealed by microarray analysis of mammalian cells. Curr Biol 2002;12:551-557.

14. Silver R, LeSauter J, Tresco PA, Lehman MN: A diffusible coupling signal from the transplanted suprachiasmatic nucleus controlling circadian locomotor rhythms. Nature 1996;382:810-813.

15. Kramer A, Yang FC, Snodgrass P, et al: Regulation of daily locomotor activity and sleep by hypothalamic EGF receptor signaling. Science 2001;294:2511-2515.

16. Schwartz WJ, Gross RA, Morton MT: The suprachiasmatic nuclei contain a tetrodotoxin-resistant circadian pacemaker. Proc Natl Acad Sci U S A 1987;84:1694-1698.

17. Moore RY, Bernstein ME: Synaptogenesis in the rat suprachiasmatic nucleus demonstrated by electron microscopy and synapsin I immunoreactivity. J Neurosci 1989;9:2151-2162.

18. Liu C, Weaver DR, Strogatz SH, Reppert SM: Cellular construction of a circadian clock: Period determination in the suprachiasmatic nuclei. Cell 1997;91:855-860.

19. Welsh DK, Logothetis DE, Meister M, Reppert SM: Individual neurons dissociated from rat suprachiasmatic nucleus express independently phased circadian firing rhythms. Neuron 1995;14:697-706.

20. Takahashi JS: Molecular neurobiology and genetics of circadian rhythms in mammals. Annu Rev Neurosci 1995;18:531-553.

21. Inouye SIT, Takahashi JS, Wollnik F, Turek FW: Inhibitor of protein synthesis phase shifts a circadian pacemaker in the mammalian SCN. Am J Physiol 1988;255:R1055-R1058.

22. Watanabe K, Katagai T, Ishida N, Yamaoka S: Anisomycin induces phase shifts of circadian pacemaker in primary cultures of rat suprachiasmatic nucleus. Brain Res 1995;684:179-184.

23. Konopka RJ, Benzer S: Clock mutants of Drosophila melanogaster. Proc Natl Acad Sci U S A 1971;68:2112-2116.

24. Dunlap JC: Genetics and molecular analysis of circadian rhythms. Annu Rev Genet 1996;30:579-601.

25. Millar AJ, Carre IA, Strayer CA, et al: Circadian clock mutants in Arabidopsis identified by luciferase imaging. Science 1995;267:1161-1163.

26. Kondo T, Tsinoremas NF, Golden SS, et al: Circadian clock mutants of cyanobacteria. Science 1994;266:1233-1236.

27. Bargiello TA, Jackson FR, Young MW: Restoration of circadian behavioural rhythms by gene transfer in Drosophila. Nature 1984;312:752-754.

28. Zehring WA, Wheeler DA, Reddy P, et al: P-element transformation with period locus DNA restores rhythmicity to mutant, arrhythmic Drosophila melanogaster. Cell 1984;39:369-376.

29. Hardin PE, Hall JC, Rosbash M: Feedback of the Drosophila period gene product on circadian cycling of its messenger RNA levels. Nature 1990;343:536-540.

30. Hardin PE, Hall JC, Rosbash M: Circadian oscillations in period gene mRNA levels are transcriptionally regulated. Proc Natl Acad Sci U S A 1992;89:11711-11715.

31. Edery I, Zwiebel LJ, Dembinska ME, Rosbash M: Temporal phosphorylation of the Drosophila period protein. Proc Natl Acad Sci U S A 1994;91:2260-2264.

32. Edery I, Rutila JE, Rosbash M: Phase shifting of the circadian clock by induction of the Drosophila period protein. Science 1994;263:237-240.

33. Albrecht U, Sun ZS, Eichele G, Lee CC: A differential response of two putative mammalian circadian regulators, mper1 and mper2, to light. Cell 1997;91:1055-1064.

34. Shearman LP, Zylka MJ, Weaver DR, et al: Two period homologs: Circadian expression and photic regulation in the suprachiasmatic nuclei. Neuron 1997;19:1261-1269.

35. Sun ZS, Albrecht U, Zhuchenko O, et al: RIGUI, a putative mammalian ortholog of the Drosophila period gene. Cell 1997;90:1003-1011.

36. Tei H, Okamura H, Shigeyoshi Y, et al: Circadian oscillation of a mammalian homologue of the Drosophila period gene. Nature 1997;389:512-516.

37. Zylka MJ, Shearman LP, Weaver DR, Reppert SM: Three period homologs in mammals: Differential light responses in the suprachiasmatic circadian clock and oscillating transcripts outside of brain. Neuron 1998;20:1103-1110.

38. Vitaterna MH, King DP, Chang AM, et al: Mutagenesis and mapping of a mouse gene, Clock, essential for circadian behavior. Science 1994;264:719-725.

39. King DP, Vitaterna MH, Chang AM, et al: The mouse Clock mutation behaves as an antimorph and maps within the W19H deletion, distal of Kit. Genetics 1997;146:1049-1060.

40. Antoch MP, Song EJ, Chang AM, et al: Functional identification of the mouse circadian Clock gene by transgenic BAC rescue. Cell 1997;89:655-667.

41. King DP, Zhao Y, Sangoram AM, et al: Positional cloning of the mouse circadian clock gene. Cell 1997;89:641-653.

42. Huang ZJ, Edery I, Rosbash M: PAS is a dimerization domain common to Drosophila period and several transcription factors. Nature 1993;364:259-262.

43. Gekakis N, Staknis D, Nguyen HB, et al: Role of the CLOCK protein in the mammalian circadian mechanism. Science 1998;280:1564-1569.

44. Hao H, Allen DL, Hardin PE: A circadian enhancer mediates PER-dependent mRNA cycling in Drosophila melanogaster. Molec Cell Biol 1997;17:3687-3693.

45. Darlington TK, Wager-Smith K, Ceriani MF, et al: Closing the circadian loop: CLOCK-induced transcription of its own inhibitors per and tim. Science 1998;280:1599-1603.

46. Shearman LP, Weaver DR: Photic induction of Period gene expression is reduced in Clock mutant mice. Neuroreport 1999;10:613-618.

47. Bunger MK, Wilsbacher LD, Moran SM, et al: Mop3 is an essential component of the master circadian pacemaker in mammals. Cell 2000;103:1009-1017.

48. Bae K, Jin X, Maywood ES, et al: Differential functions of mPer1, mPer2, and mPer3 in the SCN circadian clock. Neuron 2001;30:525-536.

49. Zheng B, Albrecht U, Kaasik K, et al: Nonredundant roles of the mPer1 and mPer2 genes in the mammalian circadian clock. Cell 2001;105:683-694.

50. Kondratov RV, Chernov MV, Kondratova AA, et al: BMAL1-dependent circadian oscillation of nuclear CLOCK: Posttranslational events induced by dimerization of transcriptional activators of the mammalian clock system. Genes Dev 2003;17:1921-1932.

51. Miyamoto Y, Sancar A: Vitamin B_2-based blue-light photoreceptors in the retinohypothalamic tract as the photoactive pigments for setting the circadian clock in mammals. Proc Natl Acad Sci U S A 1998;95:6097-6102.

52. Thresher RJ, Vitaterna MH, Miyamoto Y, et al: Role of mouse cryptochrome blue-light photoreceptor in circadian photoresponses. Science 1998;282:1490-1494.

53. Vitaterna MH, Selby CP, Todo T, et al: Differential regulation of mammalian period genes and circadian rhythmicity by

cryptochromes 1 and 2. Proc Natl Acad Sci U S A 1999;96: 12114-12119.

54. van der Horst GT, Muijtjens M, Kobayashi K, et al: Mammalian Cry1 and Cry2 are essential for maintenance of circadian rhythms. Nature 1999;398:627-630.

55. Okamura H, Miyake S, Sumi Y, et al: Photic induction of mPer1 and mPer2 in cry-deficient mice lacking a biological clock. Science 1999;286:2531-2534.

56. Kume K, Zylka MJ, Sriram S, et al: mCRY1 and mCRY2 are essential components of the negative limb of the circadian clock feedback loop. Cell 1999;98:193-205.

57. Czeisler CA, Shanahan TL, Klerman EB, et al: Suppression of melatonin secretion in some blind patients by exposure to bright light. N Engl J Med 1995;332:6-11.

58. Foster RG, Provencio I, Hudson D, et al: Circadian photoreception in the retinally degenerate mouse (rd/rd). J Comp Physiol (A) 1991;169:39-50.

59. Freedman MS, Lucas RJ, Soni B, et al: Regulation of mammalian circadian behavior by non-rod, non-cone, ocular photoreceptors. Science 1999;284:502-504.

60. von Schantz M, Provencio I, Foster RG: Recent developments in circadian photoreception: More than meets the eye. Invest Ophthalmol Vis Sci 2000;41:1605-1607.

61. Moore RY, Lenn NJ: A retinohypothalamic projection in the rat. J Comp Neurol 1972;146:1-14.

62. Johnson RF, Moore RY, Morin LP: Loss of entrainment and anatomical plasticity after lesions of the hamster retinohypothalamic tract. Brain Res 1988;460:297-313.

63. Provencio I, Jiang G, De Grip WJ, et al: Melanopsin: An opsin in melanophores, brain, and eye. Proc Natl Acad Sci U S A 1998; 95:340-345.

64. Berson DM, Dunn FA, Takao M: Phototransduction by retinal ganglion cells that set the circadian clock. Science 2002;295: 1070-1073.

65. Hannibal J, Hindersson P, Knudsen SM, et al: The photopigment melanopsin is exclusively present in pituitary adenylate cyclase-activating polypeptide-containing retinal ganglion cells of the retinohypothalamic tract. J Neurosci 2002;22:RC191.

66. Hattar S, Liao HW, Takao M, et al: Melanopsin-containing retinal ganglion cells: Architecture, projections, and intrinsic photosensitivity. Science 2002;295:1065-1070.

67. Nelson DE, Takahashi JS: Sensitivity and integration in a visual pathway for circadian entrainment in the hamster (*Mesocricetus auratus*). J Physiol 1991;439:115-145.

68. Panda S, Sato TK, Castrucci AM, et al: Melanopsin (Opn4) requirement for normal light-induced circadian phase shifting. Science 2002;298:2213-2216.

69. Ruby NF, Brennan TJ, Xie X, et al: Role of melanopsin in circadian responses to light. Science 2002;298:2211-2213.

70. Panda S, Provencio I, Tu DC, et al: Melanopsin is required for non-image-forming photic responses in blind mice. Science 2003;301:525-527.

71. Sehgal A, Price JL, Man B, Young MW: Loss of circadian behavioral rhythms and per RNA oscillations in the *Drosophila* mutant timeless. Science 1994;263:1603-1606.

72. Sehgal A, Rothenfluh-Hilfiker A, Hunter-Ensor M, et al: Rhythmic expression of timeless: A basis for promoting circadian cycles in period gene autoregulation. Science 1995;270: 808-810.

73. Hunter-Ensor M, Ousley A, Sehgal A: Regulation of the *Drosophila* protein timeless suggests a mechanism for resetting the circadian clock by light. Cell 1996;84:677-685.

74. Gekakis N, Saez L, Delahaye-Brown AM, et al: Isolation of timeless by PER protein interaction: Defective interaction between timeless protein and long-period mutant PERL. Science 1995;270:811-815.

75. Saez L, Young MW: Regulation of nuclear entry of the *Drosophila* clock proteins period and timeless. Neuron 1996;17:911-920.

76. Allada R, White NE, So WV, et al: A mutant *Drosophila* homolog of mammalian Clock disrupts circadian rhythms and transcription of period and timeless. Cell 1998;93:791-804.

77. Sangoram AM, Saez L, Antoch MP, et al: Mammalian circadian autoregulatory loop: A Timeless ortholog and mPer1 interact and negatively regulate CLOCK-BMAL1-induced transcription. Neuron 1998;21:1101-1113.

78. Tischkau SA, Barnes JA, Lin FJ, et al: Oscillation and light induction of timeless mRNA in the mammalian circadian clock. J Neurosci 1999;19:RC15.

79. Gotter AL, Manganaro T, Weaver DR, Kolakowski LF Jr, et al: A time-less function for mouse timeless. Nat Neurosci 2000; 3:755-756.

80. Barnes JW, Tischkau SA, Barnes JA, et al: Requirement of mammalian Timeless for circadian rhythmicity. Science 2003;302: 439-442.

81. Ralph MR, Menaker M: A mutation of the circadian system in golden hamsters. Science 1988;241:1225-1227.

82. Shimomura K, Menaker M: Light-induced phase shifts in tau mutant hamsters. J Biol Rhythms 1994;9:97-110.

83. Refinetti R, Menaker M: Evidence for separate control of estrous and circadian periodicity in the golden hamster. Behav Neural Biol 1992;58:27-36.

84. Lowrey PL, Shimomura K, Antoch MP, et al: Positional syntenic cloning and functional characterization of the mammalian circadian mutation tau. Science 2000;288:483-492.

85. Preitner N, Damiola F, Lopez-Molina L, et al: The orphan nuclear receptor REV-ERBalpha controls circadian transcription within the positive limb of the mammalian circadian oscillator. Cell 2002;110:251-260.

86. Etchegaray JP, Lee C, Wade PA, Reppert SM: Rhythmic histone acetylation underlies transcription in the mammalian circadian clock. Nature 2003;421:177-182.

87. Kapfhamer D, Valladares O, Sun Y, et al: Mutations in Rab3a alter circadian period and homeostatic response to sleep loss in the mouse. Nat Genet 2002;32:290-295.

88. Lopez-Molina L, Conquet F, Dubois-Dauphin M, Schibler U: The DBP gene is expressed according to a circadian rhythm in the suprachiasmatic nucleus and influences circadian behavior. EMBO J 1997;16:6762-6771.

89. Dudley CA, Erbel-Sieler C, Estill SJ, et al: Altered patterns of sleep and behavioral adaptability in NPAS2-deficient mice. Science 2003;301:379-383.

90. Harmar AJ: An essential role for peptidergic signalling in the control of circadian rhythms in the suprachiasmatic nuclei. J Neuroendocrinol 2003;15:335-338.

91. Naylor E, Bergmann BM, Krauski K, et al: The circadian clock mutation alters sleep homeostasis in the mouse. J Neurosci 2000;20:8138-8143.

92. Shaw PJ, Tononi G, Greenspan RJ, Robinson DF: Stress response genes protect against lethal effects of sleep deprivation in *Drosophila*. Nature 2002;417:287-291.

93. Wisor JP, O'Hara BF, Terao A, et al: A role for cryptochromes in sleep regulation. BMC Neurosci 2002;3:20.

94. Hendricks JC, Lu S, Kume K, et al: Gender dimorphism in the role of cycle (BMAL1) in rest, rest regulation, and longevity in *Drosophila melanogaster*. J Biol Rhythms 2003;18:12-25.

95. Laposky AD, Easton AE, Bradfield CA, et al: Null allele mice for the MOP-3 gene have increased sleep time and altered sleep consolidation. Sleep 2003;26:A110.

96. Kohsaka A, Joshu C, McDearmon D, et al: Role of the transcription factor, CLOCK, in feeding and energy balance. 9th Meeting of the Society for Research on Biological Rhythms, 2004.

97. Alvarez B, Dahlitz MJ, Vignau J, Parkes JD: The delayed sleep phase syndrome: Clinical and investigative findings in 14 subjects. J Neurol Neurosurg Psychiatry 1992;55: 665-670.

98. Ancoli-Israel S, Schnierow B, Kelsoe J, Fink R: A pedigree of one family with delayed sleep phase syndrome. Chronobiol Int 2001;18:831-840.

99. Archer SN, Robilliard DL, Skene DJ, et al: A length polymorphism in the circadian clock gene Per3 is linked to delayed sleep phase syndrome and extreme diurnal preference. Sleep 2003;26:413-415.

100. Hohjoh H, Takasu M, Shishikura K, et al: Significant association of the arylalkylamine N-acetyltransferase (AA-NAT) gene with delayed sleep phase syndrome. Neurogenetics 2003;4:151-153.

101. Iwase T, Kajimura N, Uchiyama M, et al: Mutation screening of the human Clock gene in circadian rhythm sleep disorders. Psychiatry Res 2002;109:121-128.

102. Takahashi Y, Hohjoh H, Matsuura K: Predisposing factors in delayed sleep phase syndrome. Psychiatry Clin Neurosci 2000;54:356-358.

103. Jones CR, Campbell SS, Zone SE, et al: Familial advanced sleep-phase syndrome: A short-period circadian rhythm variant in humans. Nat Med 1999;5:1062-1065.

104. Reid KJ, Chang AM, Dubocovich ML, et al: Familial advanced sleep phase syndrome. Arch Neurol 2001;58:1089-1094.

105. Satoh K, Mishima K, Inoue Y, et al: Two pedigrees of familial advanced sleep phase syndrome in Japan. Sleep 2003;26:416-417.

106. Toh KL, Jones CR, He Y, et al: An hPer2 phosphorylation site mutation in familial advanced sleep phase syndrome. Science 2001;291:1040-1043.

107. Katzenberg D, Young T, Finn L, et al: A CLOCK polymorphism associated with human diurnal preference. Sleep 1998;21:568-575.

108. Robilliard DL, Archer SN, Arendt J, et al: The 3111 Clock gene polymorphism is not associated with sleep and circadian rhythmicity in phenotypically characterized human subjects. J Sleep Res 2002;11:305-312.

109. Lingjaerde O, Bratlid T, Hansen T: Insomnia during the "dark period" in northern Norway: An explorative, controlled trial with light treatment. Acta Psychiatr Scand 1985;71:506-512.

110. Turek FW, Pénev P, Zhang Y, et al: Alterations in circadian system in advanced age. In Circadian Clocks and their Adjustment. London, Pitman Press, 1994.

111. Czeisler C, Cajochen C, Turek FW, eds: Melatonin in the regulation of sleep and circadian rhythms. In Kryger MH, Roth T, Dement WC (eds): Principles and Practice of Sleep Medicine, 3rd ed., Philadelphia, Saunders, 2000, pp 400-406.

112. Turek FW, Scarborough K, Penev P, et al: Aging of the mammalian circadian system. In Takahashi JS, Turek FW, Moore RY (eds): Handbook of Behavioral Neurobiology, vol. 12: Circadian Clocks. New York, Kluwer Academic/Plenum, 2001, pp 292-317.

The Human Circadian Timing System and Sleep-Wake Regulation

Charles Andrew Czeisler

Orfeu M. Buxton

Sat Bir Singh Khalsa

ABSTRACT

The circadian pacemaker (or biological clock) confers endogenous rhythmicity with a period just slightly greater than 24 hours, persists independent of periodic changes in the external environment, and has timing or phase relative to the time of day that is genetically conferred and can be modified or reset by environmental inputs. Melatonin, body temperature, and many other physiologic processes can be used to assess circadian phase or biological clock time. Although environmental light-dark schedules are the primary synchronizer, other nonphotic stimuli such as exercise can shift circadian phase. The circadian pacemaker interacts with sleep-wake regulatory processes to influence many physiologic variables including hormone levels, autonomic nervous system activity, neurobehavioral performance, and the propensity, timing, and internal structure of sleep. Environmental, social, behavioral, genetic, pharmacologic, and age factors influence all elements of this system.

The circadian pacemaker (or biological clock) is phylogenetically ubiquitous, having been found in nearly all species from prokaryotes to humans. Circadian pacemakers have several defining characteristics including endogenous rhythmicity that persists independent of periodic changes in the external environment, a period that is very close to 24 hours (hence the term *circadian* from "circa" meaning "about" and "dies" referring to a "day"), and the ability to have the timing or phase of the rhythm modified or reset by environmental inputs.[1-3]

The purpose of this chapter is to provide an overview of the human circadian timing system, including the pacemaker and its inputs and outputs, and to describe how this pacemaker interacts with sleep-wake regulatory processes to influence many physiologic variables including hormone levels, autonomic nervous system activity, neurobehavioral performance, and the propensity, timing, and internal structure of sleep. From this perspective, it is important to consider the relative influence of episodic and daily recurring behavior, including the occurrence of sleep itself, on these physiologic variables relative to that of the endogenous circadian pacemaker.

IDENTIFICATION OF THE MAMMALIAN CIRCADIAN PACEMAKER

Localization

In mammals, the suprachiasmatic nucleus (SCN) in the hypothalamus serves as the central neural pacemaker of the circadian timing system. Based upon an assembly of carefully taken patient histories that were characterized by disruptions of the timing of the sleep-wake cycle (e.g., insomnia, reversal of the sleep-wake schedule), Fulton and Bailey[4] postulated in 1929 that there was a region in the anterior hypothalamus that regulated not the occurrence of sleep itself but the timing of sleep within the 24-hour day.

However, it was not until 1972 that the SCN of the anterior hypothalamus was identified as the site of the mammalian circadian pacemaker,[5,6] and further research has conclusively established that the SCN is a principal source of endogenous rhythmicity in mammals.[7] Physiologic studies have revealed that multiple distributed circadian oscillators must drive daily rhythms in peripheral systems.[8] Molecular research has confirmed the presence of peripheral clocks that use the same molecular machinery as the central circadian pacemaker located in the SCN. Pacemakers like the SCN serve to convey internal synchrony to these distributed oscillators.

INFLUENCE OF SLEEP AND CIRCADIAN RHYTHMS ON HUMAN PHYSIOLOGY

The discovery of the functional role of the SCN as a central circadian pacemaker set the stage for understanding how it drives the prominent daily fluctuations in a wide array of physiologic functions in human subjects who are synchronized to the 24-hour day and on a normal sleep-wake schedule[9-17] (Figure 31–1, left panels). Core body temperature is lowest and melatonin levels (not shown) are highest[11,17,18] during night sleep. Cortisol is low at the time of habitual sleep onset but then is high at the habitual morning wake time. The temporal profile of each of these different parameters during entrainment to the 24-hour day exhibits a characteristic fingerprint that is the result of a combination of drives from the timing of the sleep-wake state, the endogenous circadian pacemaker, and responses evoked by other factors such as posture, mood, exercise, and environmental lighting.[16,19,20]

In an effort to isolate the circadian pacemaker–driven component of a diurnal temporal profile from the effects of sleep-wake state, behavior, posture, periodic environmental stimuli, and so on, the constant-routine protocol originally proposed by Mills's group[21] has been refined and extended.[22] In the constant routine, subjects typically undergo continuous enforced wakefulness throughout day and night in a constant posture at a constant level of inactivity and in a constant, relatively dim level of ambient illumination.[23] Under such

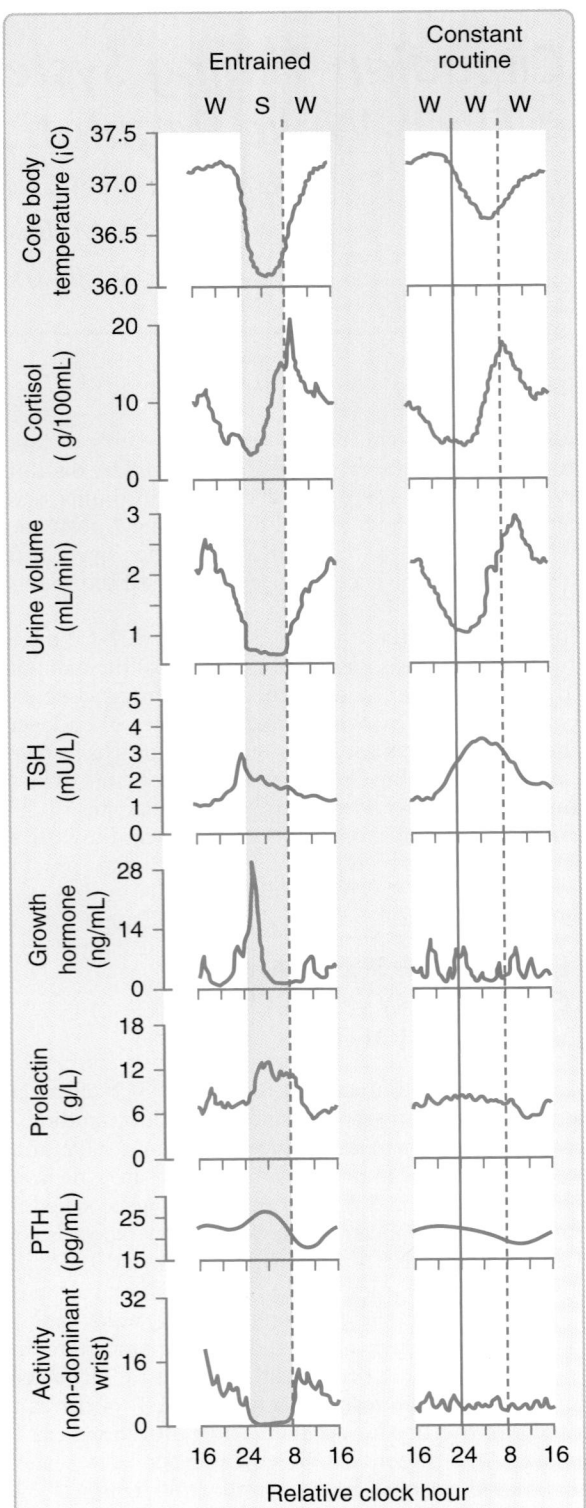

Figure 31–1. Comparison of temporal profiles of an array of physiologic and behavioral variables from subjects studied under baseline conditions while maintaining a regular schedule of nocturnal sleep *(shaded area)* and daytime wakefulness at their habitual times *(left panels)* as compared with profiles from those subjects under constant routine conditions while maintaining a schedule of continuous wakefulness in a constant semirecumbent posture *(right panels)*. Vertical dashed line indicates habitual wake time during the week prior to study, when subjects were required to maintain a regular sleep-wake schedule. All data are from healthy young men, 18 to 30 years old,

conditions, the temporal profiles of many physiologic variables are significantly altered, and it becomes possible to isolate the component that is driven by the endogenous circadian pacemaker from the components that reflect changes in the sleep-wake state, posture, or the periodic external environment.[22]

Circadian Variation of Temperature and Hormones

It has long been recognized that there is a drop in body temperature during sleep.[24-26] In comparing the profile of core body temperature recorded from individuals on a normal sleep-wake schedule with that in constant-routine conditions (see Fig. 31–1, right panels), it is apparent that the sleep episode itself (including the associated change in posture, light intensity, and activity level) generates a drop in body temperature relative to wakefulness.[8,26-30] Therefore, on a normal sleep-wake schedule, the sleep episode–induced temperature drop combines with the circadian-driven temperature drop (which exhibits a nadir during the latter half of the habitual nocturnal sleep episode) to yield a larger apparent amplitude than that of the endogenous circadian component alone (as measured on the constant routine) (see Fig. 31–1, first row). Urine volume is an example of another variable that exhibits a robust oscillation under constant-routine conditions but is also influenced by sleep-wake state (see Fig. 31–1, third row).[11,31]

Rhythmicity in some variables appears to be nearly independent of the sleep-wake state. The temporal profile of melatonin is relatively unchanged whether a person is asleep or awake all night on a constant routine,[32] although posture has been reported to influence circulating melatonin concentrations to a small degree.[33] The temporal profile of cortisol is also relatively unchanged whether people sleep on their habitual schedule or remain awake all night, although cortisol levels are elevated upon awakening/lights on and during the following afternoon and evening (see Fig. 31–1, second row).[34] Plasma cortisol concentrations can be suppressed if sleep onset occurs at the crest of the cortisol rhythm rather than at the nadir.[35]

A number of other hormones are very sensitive to the sleep-wake state. Sleep opposes the circadian rhythm regulating thyroid stimulating hormone (TSH), inhibiting the endogenous circadian rhythm of TSH release, which would otherwise peak in the middle of the night.[12,15,36-38] Under entrained conditions, that nocturnal peak is blunted by the timing of sleep so that TSH levels are highest just before sleep onset and continue to be suppressed during the remainder of

studied under similar conditions. For a given variable, data in the *left panel* are from the same subjects as data in the *right panel*; however, all variables were not monitored in the same subjects. Activity data were measured using a wrist actigraph (Vitalog Monitoring Inc., Redwood City, Calif) worn on the nondominant wrist. TSH, thyroid stimulating hormone; PTH, parathyroid hormone. (TSH data reproduced from Allan JS, Czeisler CA, Persistence of the circadian thyrotropin rhythm under constant conditions and after light-induced shifts of circadian phase. J Clin Endocrinol Metab 1994;79:508-512, copyright 1994 The Endocrine Society; prolactin data reproduced from Waldstreicher J, Duffy JF, Brown EN, et al: Gender differences in the temporal organization of prolactin (PRL) secretion: Evidence for a sleep-independent circadian rhythm of circulating PRL levels—A clinical research center study. J Clin Endocrinol Metab 1996;81:1483-1487, copyright 1996 The Endocrine Society; PTH data reproduced from El Hajj Fuleihan G, Klerman EB, Brown EN, et al: Parathyroid hormone circadian rhythm is truly endogenous. J Clin Endocrinol Metab 1997;82:281-286, copyright 1997 The Endocrine Society.)

the sleep episode (see Fig. 31–1, fourth row).[12] This inhibitory effect of sleep on TSH secretion has been closely associated with both slow wave sleep[39] and, more recently, with relative delta power in the sleep EEG.[40] Growth hormone, prolactin, and parathyroid hormone all show a prominent sleep-dependent increase in their levels (see Fig. 31–1, rows 5-7).[14,20,37,41] In the case of growth hormone, this sleep-related increase has been associated with both slow wave sleep[42] and relative delta power of the sleep EEG,[43] whereas in the case of prolactin, such associations have been controversial.[44-46]

Ultradian variations in the release of renin from the kidney—a key factor in blood pressure control—are closely linked to the timing of the REM-NREM sleep cycle.[47,48] This association remains evident even among patients with disturbed sleep, whose plasma renin profiles reflect pathologic changes in sleep structure. Increased relative delta power in the sleep EEG is associated with increased levels of plasma renin activity, whereas decreased slow wave activity was associated with a decrease in plasma renin activity.[49]

In 1979, Aschoff pointed out that there is some evidence for an endogenously rhythmic component even among so-called sleep-dependent hormones, particularly with respect to the magnitude of the response evoked by sleep.[50] In fact, using the constant-routine protocol, it has been shown that in the absence of sleep, prolactin and parathyroid hormone also have an endogenous circadian component that exhibits a low point a few hours after habitual wake time (see Fig. 31–1, sixth row).[13,14] A study involving repeated injections of growth hormone releasing hormone (GHRH) across the day demonstrated elevated peak growth hormone responses in the evening, suggesting that the diurnal variation in growth hormone secretion reflects in part circadian rhythmicity.[51]

The effects of the interaction between sleep-dependent and circadian factors on these hormones may have significant importance when the sleep-wake schedule is not synchronized with the circadian pacemaker. In the case of shift workers who must acutely remain awake on the first night shift, for example, one would expect a substantial increase in TSH release relative to that secreted under normal sleep-wake conditions during entrainment (see Fig. 31–1, fourth row). On the other hand, these shift workers would be deprived of their normally higher levels of growth hormone, prolactin, and parathyroid hormone during the waking night. Such alterations of the profiles of a variety of hormones have been documented in laboratory studies of night-shift workers.[52]

Circadian Variation of Alertness and Neurobehavioral Performance

The circadian pacemaker has a significant influence on a variety of neurobehavioral and cognitive functions.[53-58] Under constant routine conditions, subjects display a circadian variation in short-term memory, cognitive performance, and alertness that is tightly coupled to the timing of the body temperature rhythm (Fig. 31–2).[59] During the constant routine, these cognitive functions tend to be at their nadir at a clock time that is 1 to 3 hours after habitual wake time. However, because subjects are undergoing prolonged wakefulness during the constant routine, the profiles of these variables are determined not only by the drive from the circadian pacemaker but also by a contribution from the consequences of sleep deprivation. This point will be discussed more extensively later.

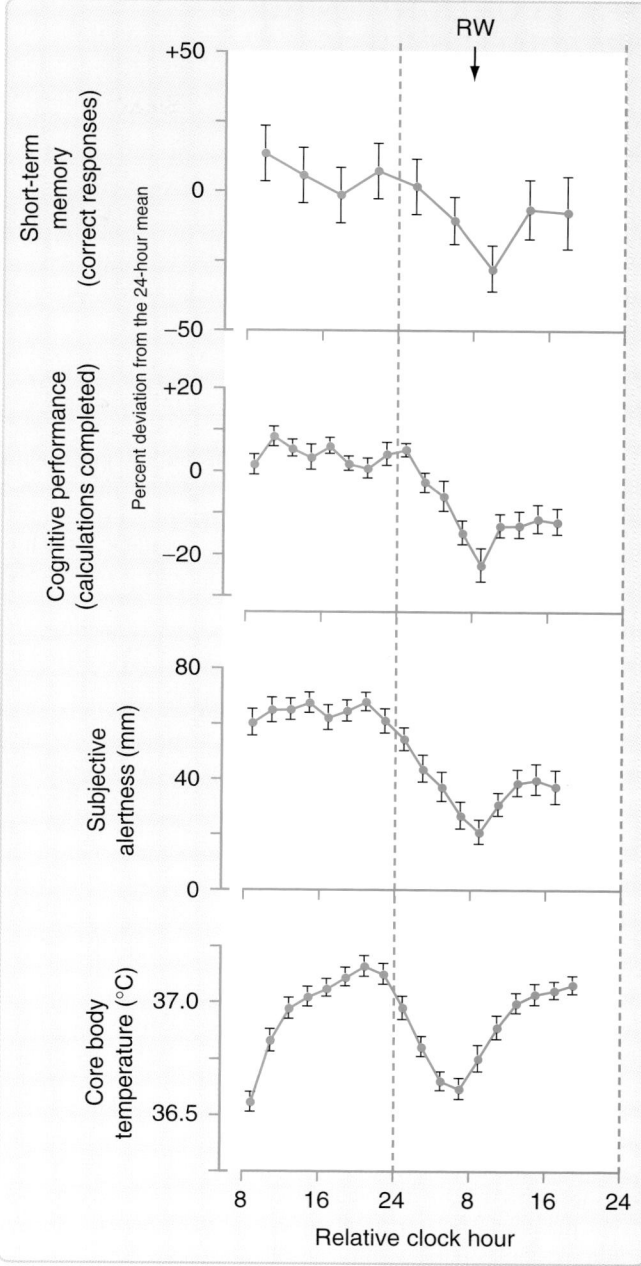

Figure 31–2. Daily patterns of short-term memory, cognitive performance, subjective alertness (mm), and core body temperature (°C) averaged across 18 subjects during a 36-hour constant routine. Data collection times are normalized with respect to each subject's regular wake time (assigned a reference value of 08:00 hours and indicated by the *downward arrow*). The extent to which memory and performance scores deviated from the subject's 24-hour mean is averaged across subjects. These data are expressed as the percentage by which these absolute deviations differed from the subjects' overall 24-hour mean score (assigned a reference value of zero). Each point is the centered mean (SEM) of all determinations made across a 2-hour interval for performance, alertness, and temperature and across a 4-hour interval for short-term memory. (Reproduced from Johnson MP, Duffy JF, Dijk D-J, et al: Short-term memory, alertness and performance: A reappraisal of their relationship to body temperature. J Sleep Res 1992;1:24-29.)

EFFECTS OF LIGHT ON HUMAN CIRCADIAN RHYTHMS

A biological clock is only useful if it can be set appropriately to local time. The primary synchronizing agent for circadian systems in a wide array of species, including humans, is the environmental light-dark cycle.[1,11,60,61]

There are two modes of photoreception. First, there is visual photoreception, which provides us with a spatiotemporal image of the environment. Second, there is nonvisual, or nonimage-forming, photoreception, which affects—among other things—the circadian system.

Retinal Input to the Suprachiasmatic Nucleus

The SCN receives direct retinal input via the retinohypothalamic tract (RHT), a monosynaptic pathway by which information about the environmental light-dark cycle reaches the SCN.[62-65] Although the experimental techniques used to establish the link between circadian rhythmicity and the SCN in other species cannot be used in humans, postmortem studies reveal that the human brain contains the same key structural elements—the SCN and RHT—as that of other mammals.[65-67] Furthermore, neuropathologic studies indicate that damage to these structures is associated with marked abnormalities in the timing of the sleep-wake cycle and other circadian rhythms.[68,69]

In the past decade, rapid progress has been made in this quest. Recently it was demonstrated in rodents and humans that the three-cone system and rods, the visual photoreceptors, are not required for transmitting the light signal to the circadian system.[70-75] Furthermore, a distinct set of ganglion cells in the inner retinal layer were demonstrated to project to the SCN.[64] Retinal ganglion cells were thought only to pass on information from the rods and cones.

However, researchers have demonstrated that the subset of these retinal ganglion cells that project to the SCN are intrinsically photosensitive. Only those ganglion cells that project from retina to SCN selectively contain the newly discovered vitamin A–based photoreceptor molecule melanopsin.[76,77] Furthermore, animal studies determining the action spectrum show that blue light (450-480 nm) is the most potent in shifting the phase of the circadian rhythm.[74,78] This action spectrum matches the sensitivity peak of melanopsin. Recent studies have revealed a similar peak sensitivity for melatonin suppression by light in humans,[70,71,75] consistent with recent data on phase shifting responses in humans.[75,79]

Together, these discoveries indicate that within the specific set of retinal ganglion cells, melanopsin may be one of the crucial circadian photoreceptor molecules, although additional photoreceptor molecules may also participate in circadian photoreception, resulting in more redundancy of circadian photoreception.[80,81] A neural output pathway of the SCN passes through the intermediate-lateral cell column of the upper thoracic spinal cord, to the superior cervical ganglion, and then provides sympathetic input into the pineal gland.[82,83]

Photic Suppression of Melatonin Secretion

The neural pathway from the SCN to the pineal provides for the regulation of the pineal output of melatonin by the suprachiasmatic nucleus.[84] The release of this hormone is inhibited by retinal exposure to light by the circuitous pathway from the eye to the pineal.[64,82,83,85] This inhibition of melatonin by light in humans[86] can therefore be used as an assay for the functional input of light into the circadian system.[87]

The nocturnal increase in melatonin is illustrated in the upper panel of Figure 31–3 for a normally sighted subject on a constant routine.[87] During a second peak of melatonin on the next night, a bright light stimulus yielded an acute suppression of melatonin levels, which returned to elevated nighttime levels after the light exposure was terminated. In the lower panel of Figure 31–3, the bright light–induced suppression of melatonin still occurs even in a person who is totally blind and who has no conscious light perception, no pupillary light reflexes, and a negative electroretinogram. This is not the case in all such blind persons. The loss of conscious light

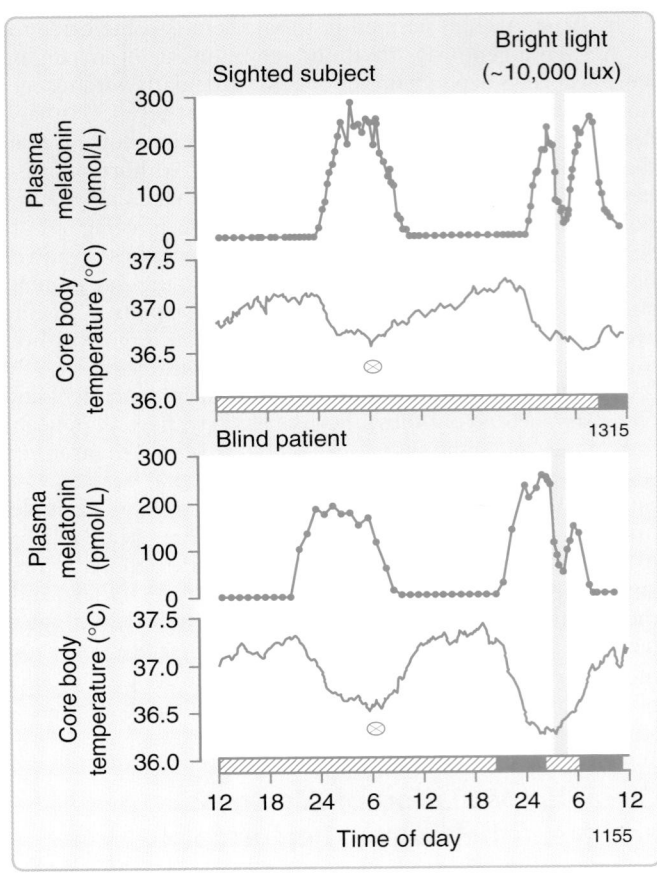

Figure 31–3. Melatonin-suppression test in a healthy sighted subject *(upper panel)* and a blind patient *(lower panel)*. In each, plasma melatonin *(upper traces)* and temperature *(lower traces)* were measured repeatedly during a constant routine *(hatched bar)* and subsequent episode(s) of sleep *(solid bars)*. The light intensity was ~10 to ~15 lux during the constant routines, less than ~0.02 lux during the sleep episodes, and ~10,000 lux during 90 to 100 minutes of exposure to bright light *(shaded columns)* 22 to 23 hours after the initial fitted temperature minimum (encircled × 's). In both subjects, plasma melatonin concentrations decreased markedly in response to bright light and then increased after the return to dim light. (Reproduced from Czeisler CA, Shanahan TL, Klerman EB, et al: Suppression of melatonin secretion in some blind patients by exposure to bright light. N Engl J Med 1995;332:6-11 Copyright © 1995 Massachusetts Medical Society. All rights reserved.)

perception does not necessarily indicate the loss of photic input to the circadian timing system.[87] In fact, there are two distinct visual systems, one for image-forming perception and a separate circadian visual system for the purpose of detecting environmental illuminance levels and synchronizing the circadian pacemaker in the suprachiasmatic nucleus.[64,70-79,88,89]

Human Phase Response Curves to Light

In circadian biology, the phase response curve is used to characterize the synchronizing effects of light on a circadian pacemaker.[1,3,23,60,90] To construct a phase response curve,[16] discrete light stimuli are applied systematically over the entire circadian cycle; the magnitudes of the light-induced phase shifts are then plotted as a function of circadian phase at which the organism is exposed to the stimuli. In human experiments, the constant routine has been used to estimate both the initial circadian phase of the pacemaker prior to a stimulus and then the final poststimulus circadian phase. The difference between the initial and final circadian phases therefore represents the light-induced phase shift.

All circadian systems exhibit a characteristic photic phase response curve in which the largest light-induced phase shifts are generated in the subjective night of the circadian cycle. Phase delays are generated to light stimuli in the late subjective day or early subjective night, and phase advances are generated in the late subjective night or early subjective day.[1,3,23,60,90] Figure 31–4 illustrates the phase response curve to a single pulse of light. The human phase response curve to a single light pulse[92] exhibits the classic pattern of light phase response curves observed in many organisms,[1] including both phase advances and phase delays. In humans, phase delays were observed in response to bright light pulses applied prior to the time of the minimum of the core body temperature cycle, which occurred on average about 2.3 hours before the habitual wake time. Phase advances were observed when light was applied after the time of the core body temperature minimum.

The response to light during the subjective day of both the one-pulse PRC illustrated in Figure 31–4 and the three-pulse phase response curve illustrated in Figure 31–5 reveals that the human circadian pacemaker is responsive to light throughout the subjective day.[93] This characteristic of the human phase response curve has also been reported for other species, especially diurnal ones,[1] and suggests that it is possible to shift the phase of the human circadian pacemaker not just during the night but also in the morning and late afternoon or evening with appropriate light intensities. This possibility has important clinical implications for the use of phototherapy to reset circadian phase in delayed or advanced sleep phase syndrome, for example.

Photic Resetting of the Pineal Melatonin Rhythm

Because circadian rhythms are expressed in many physiologic and neurobehavioral variables, the phase of the pacemaker can be ascertained by using any of these variables as a marker. In humans, the core body temperature rhythm has often been a preferred marker of circadian phase because it can provide an accurate representation of the underlying pacemaker's characteristics under certain conditions.

Melatonin is also an accurate circadian marker.[11,32,87,91,92,94,95] Melatonin is less heavily influenced by sleep or posture than is the core body temperature rhythm.[33,94] Furthermore, it has been shown in humans to reflect the phase of the underlying pacemaker following light-induced phase shifts even better than the endogenous component of the core body temperature rhythm measured during a constant routine.[11] Both of these rhythms shift by an equivalent amount regardless of whether the rhythm is shifted to an earlier or a later hour.[11,95]

Studies have demonstrated that the endogenous circadian melatonin rhythm can be reset to any desired phase within 2 or 3 days by properly timed light exposure.[95] Furthermore, photic stimuli designed to suppress the amplitude of the

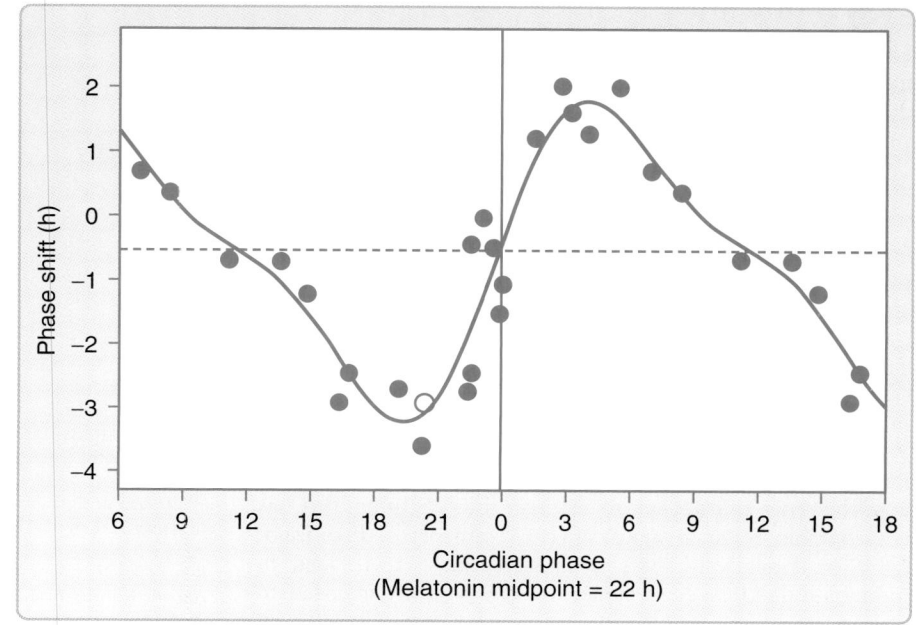

Figure 31–4. Phase response curve to 1-hour light pulses in human subjects. Phase shift in hours is plotted for a light pulse centered at different times relative to the initial endogenous circadian phase of the timing of melatonin secretion. By convention, phase advances to an earlier time are depicted as positive numbers, phase delays as negative. *Filled circles:* determinations of circadian phase from plasma melatonin profiles. *Open circle:* determination of circadian phase from salivary melatonin profiles. (Reproduced from Khalsa SB, Jewett ME, Cajochen C, Czeisler CA. A phase response curve to single bright light pulses in human subjects. J Physiol 2003;549:945-952.)

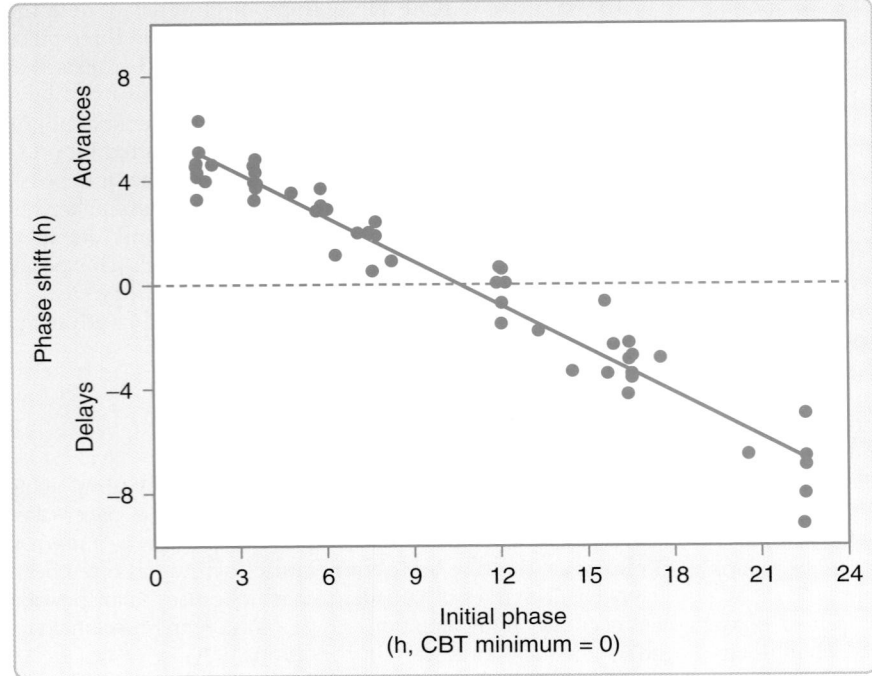

Figure 31–5. The phase response curve to a stimulus of three consecutive daily 5-hour pulses of bright light, centered on the subjective day. Initial phase is the number of hours after the fitted minimum of the endogenous core body temperature rhythm at which the center of the light stimulus occurred. Phase shift is the difference between the time of the pre- and post-stimulus temperature minima. A regression line has been fitted to the data points. (Adapted from Jewett ME, Rimmer DW, Duffy JF, et al: The human circadian pacemaker is sensitive to light throughout subjective day without evidence of transients. Used with permission, Am J Physiol 1997;273:R1800-R1809.)

endogenous circadian temperature cycle also lead to suppression of the amplitude of the endogenous circadian melatonin rhythm.[95]

The use of the rhythm in melatonin levels as a circadian marker has additional practical advantages. The demonstrated melatonin rhythm in human saliva, which correlates well with the rhythm in plasma,[96] together with recent advances in melatonin assay techniques, are making it possible to evaluate circadian phase in patients or research subjects in a relatively noninvasive manner.[96,97]

Human Dose Response Curve to Circadian Phase Resetting Effects of Light

The degree of light-induced phase shift also depends upon the intensity of the light stimulus and the number of consecutive days of exposure. Three consecutive daily pulses of light can generate a larger phase shift than does a single light pulse. This intensity relationship also applies to the brightness or illuminance level of the light to which the retina is exposed. Following 5-hour, 3-cycle, bright light stimuli of different light intensities applied at a circadian phase known to generate a phase advance, an increase in the resetting response is seen at an intensity of 50 lux, with a maximum slope at 100 lux and maximum shifts at approximately 500 lux. The light intensity versus resetting response relationship is clearly nonlinear (Fig. 31–6)[98] and can be predicted using a mathematical model.[99,100]

These data also show that even lower levels of light (~180 lux) have a very substantial phase-shifting effect. Since ~180 lux is in the range of intensity of ordinary room lighting, this has considerable practical significance. We are exposed to bright light for a relatively short time each day.[101-103] In fact, in modern industrialized societies we are typically exposed to ordinary indoor room light for a greater number of hours each

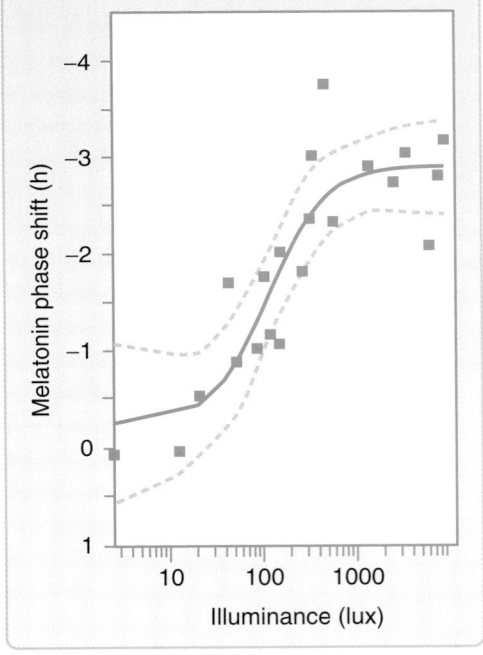

Figure 31–6. Illuminance-response curve of the phase-shifting effect of light on the human circadian pacemaker administered outside the critical region. The shift in the phase of the melatonin rhythm following a 6.5 hour pulse of light as assessed on the day following the photic stimulus has been fitted with a four-parameter logistic model using a nonlinear least squares analysis. The logistic models predict an inflection point of the curve (i.e., the sensitivity of the system) at ~120 lux, and phase shifts saturate at ~550 lux. Individual subjects are represented by the *closed boxes*, the model by the *solid line*, and the 95% confidence intervals by the *dashed lines*. (Adapted from Zeitzer JM, Dijk DJ, Kronauer RE, et al: Sensitivity of the human circadian pacemaker to nocturnal light: Melatonin phase resetting and suppression. J Physiol [Lond] 2000; 526:695-702.).

day than we are exposed to bright light. This predominance of exposure to ordinary room light probably has a greater impact on our circadian system than the few minutes to which we are typically exposed to bright light each day.

The simple schema in Figure 31–7 illustrates the influence of the circadian pacemaker and the sleep-wake state on the various physiologic variables and the influence of light input via the eye to the circadian pacemaker. The feedback loop from the sleep-wake state back to the eye in this schema represents the effects of exposure to the environmental light cycle. The sleeping state in humans is usually associated with eyelid closure and self-selected exposure to darkness, which is achieved by drawing window shades and switching off artificial light sources. The waking state in humans is usually associated with opening of the eyelids and retinal light exposure via self-selected use of artificial light or self-selected exposure to outdoor light during waking hours. Under conditions of a strict sleep-wake and light-exposure schedule, the timing of the pacemaker will be consistent from day to day. However, if sleep were to be initiated late or terminated early, or a waking episode were to occur within a sleep episode, the associated light exposure may reset the pacemaker. This association between waking and light exposure, together with the fact that low levels of light intensity can exert a significant resetting effect on the pacemaker, is relevant on a practical level for routine sleep-wake scheduling.

NONPHOTIC CIRCADIAN PHASE RESETTING AND REENTRAINMENT

The nonphotic input to the human circadian system is less well characterized than the photic input. Early studies focused on social cues such as gong sounds or regularly scheduled performance tests, meals, and bedtimes.[104,133] The results of these early studies were confounded by the limitations of the phase measures used and self-selected lighting conditions.

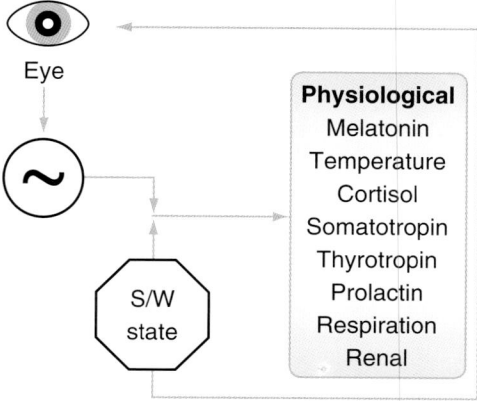

Figure 31–7. Schema illustrating the influence of both the circadian pacemaker *(circle with oscillator symbol)* and sleep-wake (S/W) state *(octagon)* on a number of physiologic variables. Under normal conditions, the circadian pacemaker and sleep-wake state each influence these variables; the relative contribution and nature of the interaction (i.e., synergistic or oppositional) of each depends upon the variable observed. Also illustrated is the influence of the environmental illumination on the human circadian clock via the eye, as well as the influence of the sleep-wake state, in determining the timing of this illumination via both behavioral action (i.e., switching off artificial indoor room lights and drawing bedroom window shades at bedtime) and eyelid closure during sleep and eyelid opening during waking.

Several studies have demonstrated that exposure of healthy young men to nocturnal exercise of 1 to 3 hours in duration results in a phase delay of the onset of nocturnal melatonin secretion on the following day.[105,106] These phase delays appeared to be more consistent when the subjects were submitted to a 3-hour session of moderate-intensity exercise than when they performed a 1-hour session of high-intensity exercise.[107] Early evening 1-hour high-intensity exercise sessions (at approximately 18:30) resulted on the following day in relative *phase advances* significantly different from the phase delays observed in response to morning, afternoon, and nocturnal exercise and in no-exercise subjects who did not exercise. Figure 31–8 depicts results from a series of these studies.

In a study of the facilitation of reentrainment to a delay-shifted sleep-wake episode in extremely dim light (to control for ambient light during exercise), exercise during the biological night resulted in phase delays compared to no exercise.[106] Taken together, these findings support the hypothesis that appropriately timed nonphotic stimuli such as exercise or other forms of arousal could facilitate adaptation to acute changes in the light-dark cycle.

Evidence supporting the hypothesis that appropriately timed exposure to exercise could also result in phase advances has been obtained in a study that demonstrated partial entrainment to a 23.5-hour light-dark and sleep-wake schedule in healthy volunteers exercising at a moderate intensity twice daily (at midday and late afternoon) over 2 weeks.[108] Subjects exercising daily in the late afternoon exhibited partial entrainment, advancing on average 10 minutes per day more than control subjects who did not exercise, consistent with phase-advancing effects of late afternoon or early evening exercise on the human circadian clock. Given the slightly greater than 24-hour endogenous period of humans and the net daily phase advance required for stable entrainment, evening exercise, particularly repeated daily exposure, could result in daily phase advances leading to nonphotic entrainment of the human circadian system if the timing and intensity of the exercise stimulus were optimized.

Exercise per se may not be the relevant stimulus. An interaction of exercise with the homeostatic regulation of sleep has been suggested by a study in hamsters that indicated that the phase-shifting effects of nonphotic stimuli may be due solely to the maintenance of wake during the normal sleep episode.[2,109] Maintenance of wakefulness by gentle handling in the absence of substantial activity elicited phase shifts comparable to sustained wheel-running. Because a smaller number of required rousing interventions predicted greater phase shifting, the authors speculated that the arousing nature of the stimulus may be the most salient component of phase-shifts elicited by increased physical activity during the sleep episode.[109] Further studies are needed to determine the relevance of these sleep deprivation findings for human circadian regulation.

INVESTIGATING CIRCADIAN AND SLEEP-WAKE DEPENDENT MODULATION

Separation from 24-hour Environmental and Behavioral Cues

Nathaniel Kleitman was the first investigator to conduct an experiment in which humans were studied in the absence of

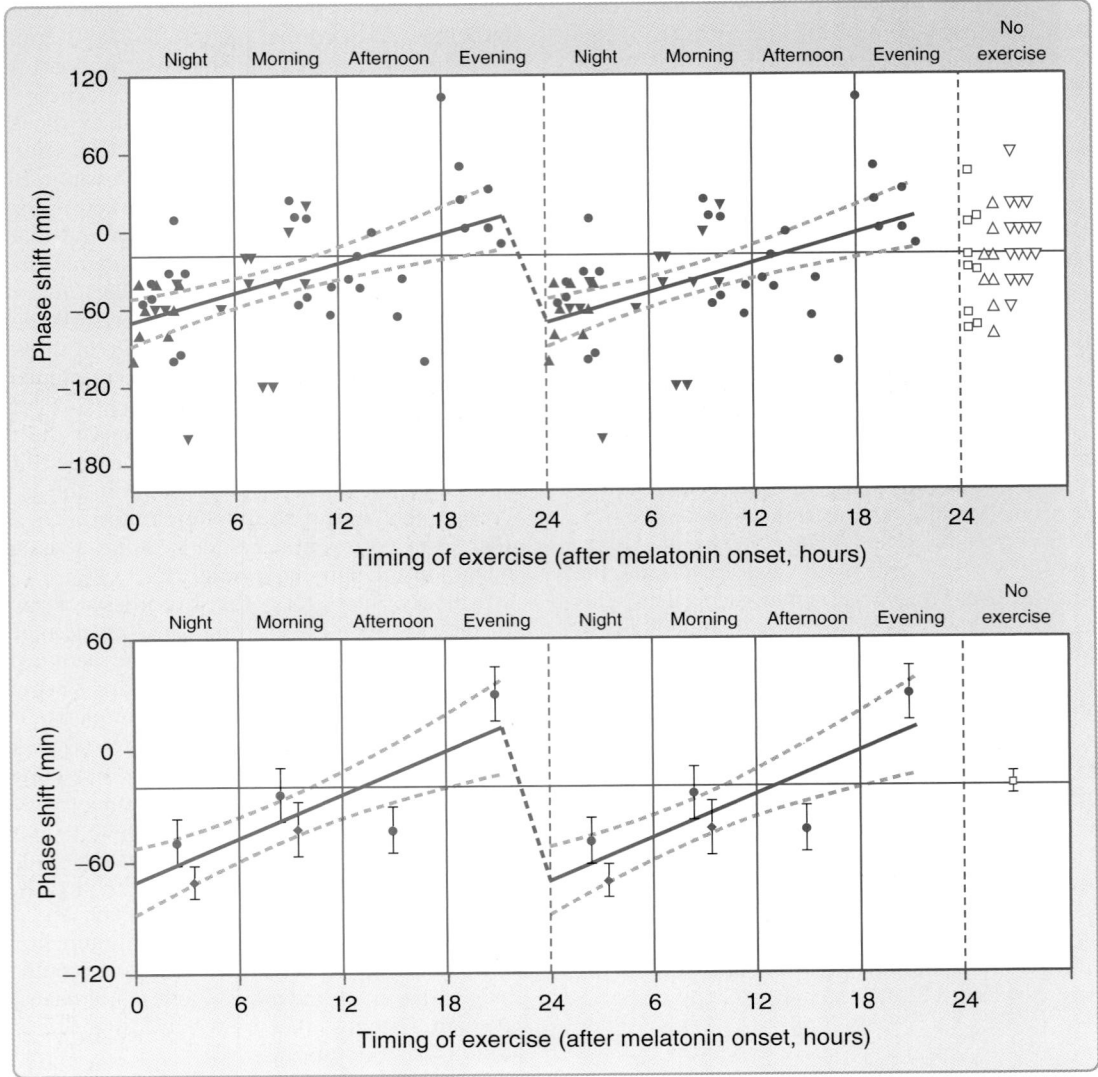

Figure 31–8. Phase response curves observed in response to exercise at different circadian times of day. Phase *delays* are observed in responses to nocturnal exercise, phase *advances* are observed in response to exercise performed during the late afternoon or early evening. Phase shifts in response to high-intensity, 1-hour nocturnal exercise and daytime exercise are shown by *closed circles*. Phase shifts in response to low-intensity, 3-hour exercise sessions are depicted by *upward triangles* and *downward triangles* in the top panel and by *diamonds* in the bottom panel. *Solid line* depicts significant relationship between phase shifts and circadian time of exercise ($R^2 = 0.28$, $P = 0.0003$; slope significantly different from zero). *Dashed curves* depict 95% confidence intervals of the slope of the line.[105] (Reproduced from Buxton OM, Lee CW, L'Hermite-Balériaux M, et al: Exercise elicits phase shifts and acute alterations of melatonin levels that vary with circadian phase. Am J Physiol 2003;284:R714-R724. © 2003 American Physiological Society, used with permission.)

periodic 24-hour cues in the external environment (Fig. 31–9).[56] Figure 31–10 shows core body temperature records from one of the two human subjects he studied in Mammoth Cave, Kentucky, in 1938 while undergoing a 28-hour imposed sleep-wake schedule, compared with laboratory data collected at the University of Chicago from the same subject living on a 24-hour routine.[56] On the 24-hour schedule, there were 7 cycles of the body temperature rhythm, as one would expect over the course of a one-week recording (Fig. 31–10, lower panel). On the imposed 28-hour schedule, there were also 7 cycles of the body temperature rhythm, although there were only 6 sleep-wake cycles over the course of the week (Fig. 31–10, upper panel). Despite the confounding effect of

sleep itself on the core body temperature (as noted above, see Fig. 31–1), this experimental protocol could still separate the influence of the timing of the sleep-wake schedule from that of the circadian pacemaker—at least in this subject.

This imposed desynchrony between the sleep-wake schedule and the output of the circadian pacemaker driving the temperature rhythm occurs under conditions in which the non–24-hour sleep-wake schedule is outside the range of entrainment or range of capture of the circadian system. This protocol has been termed the *forced desynchrony protocol* and is an extremely useful tool in evaluating the influence of the circadian pacemaker on many physiologic variables, because it allows separation of the confounding effect of the sleep-wake schedule from the output of the endogenous circadian pacemaker.[56]

Figure 31–11 illustrates a raster plot of a forced desynchrony experiment incorporating core body temperature and wakefulness data for a subject living on a 28-hour day in a laboratory shielded from external time cues.[30,110] The waking episodes in this protocol were 18 hours and 40 minutes long followed by sleep episodes of 9 hours and 20 minutes. Core body temperature exhibited a period of 24.3 hours in this subject and was therefore desynchronized from both the 24-hour day and the timing of the imposed 28-hour sleep-wake schedule.

Separating Circadian and Sleep-Wake–Dependent Modulation

The constant routine protocol does not allow for a complete and unconfounded separation of the circadian and homeostatic influences on neurobehavioral and physiologic variables. However, in the Kleitman forced desynchrony protocol, sleep and wakefulness are distributed much more evenly over the entire circadian cycle during the course of the experiment. It is thus possible to average data either over successive circadian cycles or over successive sleep-wake episodes and to thereby separate these two components. This averaging serves to isolate the circadian profile of the variable of interest by removing the contribution of the confounding sleep-wake–dependent contribution in the averaging process. Conversely, the temporal portion of the sleep-wake–dependent profile can be isolated from the confounding circadian influence. This averaging process is similar to that of cortical evoked potential

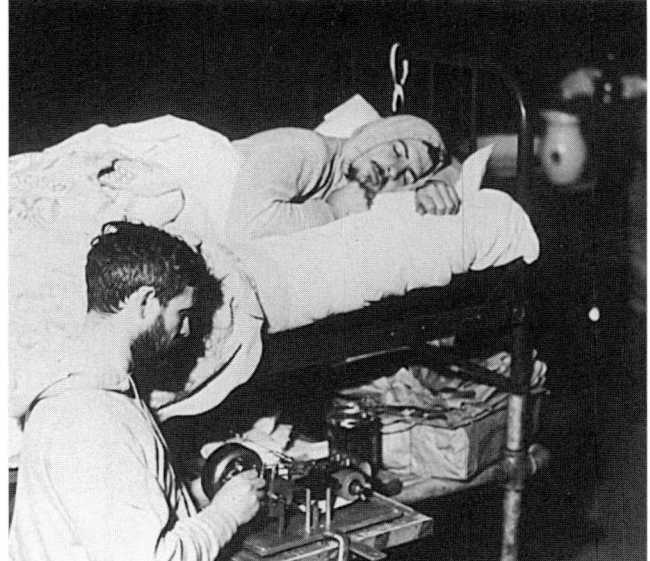

Figure 31–9. Professor Nathaniel Kleitman *(left)* attends to experimental equipment while fellow research subject Bruce Richardson lies in bed deep within Mammoth Cave in Kentucky where, for the first time, human subjects were studied while shielded from periodic environmental changes on Earth's surface. The two pioneers lived on an imposed 28-hour sleep-wake schedule in these quarters from June 4 to July 6, 1938, in an effort to approximate uniform environmental and behavioral conditions, free from the influence of Earth's 24-hour day. In a 60-foot wide chamber free from any external environmental sounds, the temperature remained at 54° F (±1°), humidity approached complete vapor saturation, and darkness was absolute when the artificial light used during waking hours was shut off. The Mammoth Cave Hotel provided daily meals, which were consumed upon awakening and after the 7th and 13th hour of each 19-hour waking day. (Photo courtesy of National Park Service, Mammoth Cave National Park, Mammoth, Kentucky; description adapted from Kleitman N: Sleep and Wakefulness. Chicago, University of Chicago Press, 1963, pp 178-179).

Figure 31–10. Weekly body temperature rhythms of a subject under two different routines of sleep and wakefulness. *Upper panel:* data from subject K on a 28-hour daily routine consisting of 19 hours of wakefulness and 9 hours of sleep during Professor Nathaniel Kleitman's historic forced desynchrony protocol carried out in Mammoth Cave, Kentucky. *Lower panel:* laboratory data recorded at the University of Chicago from subject K on a customary daily 24-hour routine consisting of 17 hours of wakefulness and 7 hours of sleep. *Shaded areas* represent time spent in bed, attempting to sleep. Data in the *upper panel* are based on the last three weeks of data collected in Mammoth Cave. Data in the *lower panel* iare based on five weeks of following the 24-hour routine of living. Each weekly record shows seven body-temperature waves, within the minima in the *shaded areas* on the customary 24-hour routine, but not on the artificial 28-hour sleep-wakefulness schedule. In the subject shown, the endogenous circadian temperature cycle maintained a near-24-hour oscillation, despite the 28-hour day length to which the subject's sleep-wake cycle was scheduled. However, it was reported that temperature data from subject R (not shown) showed adaptation to this non-24-hour routine.

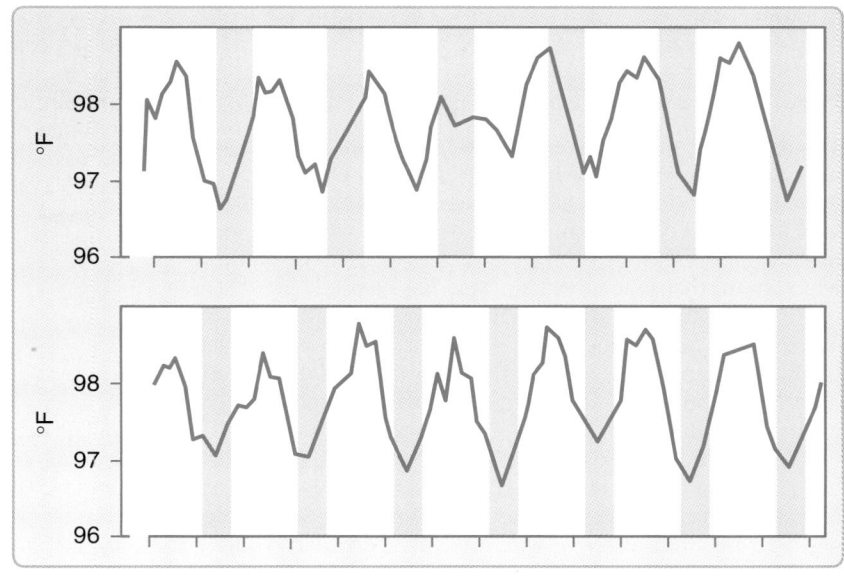

Such adaptation has not been observed in more recent forced desynchrony studies. Interindividual differences in the strength of the endogenous versus the evoked component of the body temperature rhythm may account for what appeared to be circadian adaptation observed during the forced desynchrony conducted in subject R of Kleitman's experiment. (Figure and parts of legend adapted from Kleitman N, Sleep and Wakefulness. Chicago, University of Chicago Press, 1963; © 1963 by the University of Chicago.)

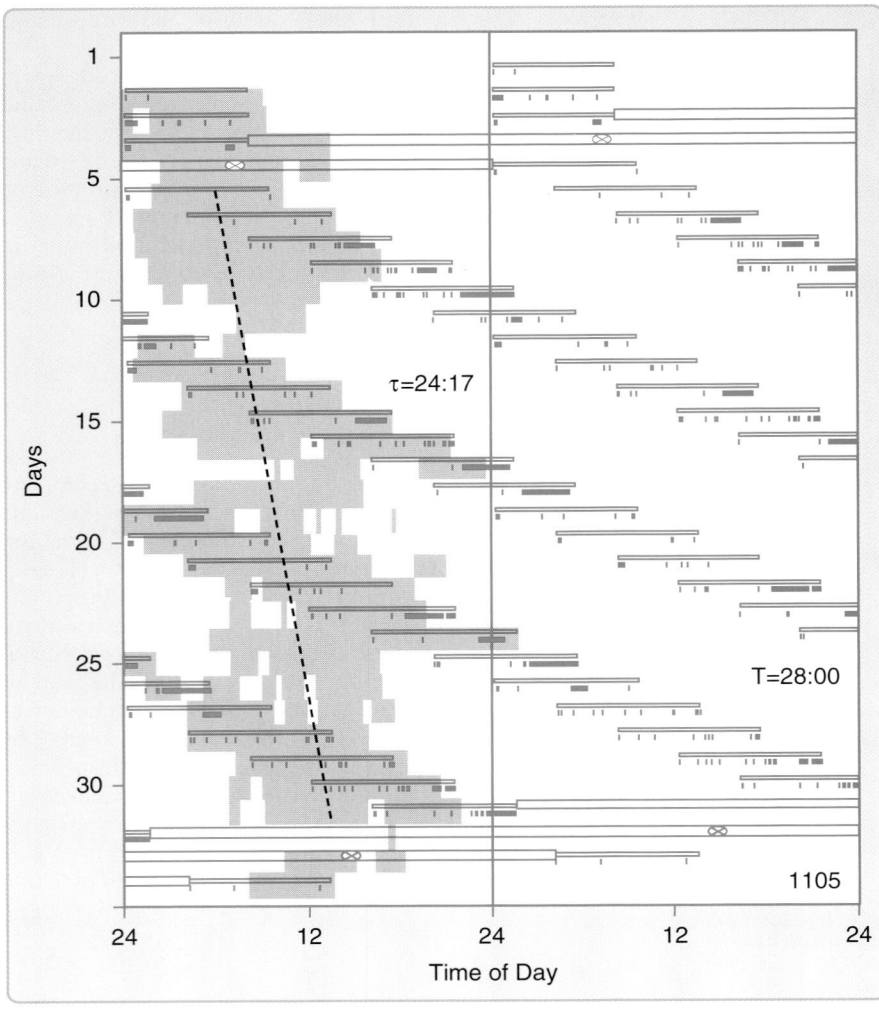

Figure 31–11. Double plot of the 28-hour forced desynchrony protocol. Successive days are plotted both next to and beneath each other. Scheduled sleep episodes *(open narrow bars)*, polysomnographically determined wakefulness within each sleep episode *(black tick marks* below the narrow open bars), and intervals during which core body temperature was below the mean *(stippled area)* are indicated. An intrinsic temperature cycle period of 24.3 hours from the data of this subject was estimated by a nonparametric spectral analysis of the core body temperature data during the forced desynchrony part of the protocol. The phase of the minimum of the circadian temperature rhythm, as estimated by this nonparametric spectral analysis, is indicated by the *broken line.* The minimum of the endogenous circadian rhythm of core body temperature as unmasked by a 40-hour constant routine protocol is indicated by an *encircled* ×. (Reproduced from Dijk D-J, Czeisler CA: Paradoxical timing of the circadian rhythm of sleep propensity serves to consolidate sleep and wakefulness in humans. Neurosci Lett 1994;166:63-68. Copyright 1994, with permission from Elsevier.)

recordings that effectively subtract background noise that is not temporally related to the evoked response.[111]

Neurobehavioral Functions

To predict the time course of neurobehavioral function, it is necessary to recognize the influence of the sleep-wake state on what has been termed a *sleep homeostat* driving neurobehavioral functions. This becomes apparent when one examines these variables during a longer course of sleep deprivation in which more than one circadian cycle has elapsed.[31,59,112] The cyclic contribution of the circadian pacemaker in influencing alertness and performance is superimposed on an overall decline in function during the course of the experiment, as described in models that incorporate both the homeostatic and circadian influences in the regulation of sleep and wakefulness.[113,114]

Using a 20-hour forced desynchrony protocol, researchers have determined the temporal profiles of cognitive performance and subjective sleepiness as a function of circadian phase and as a function of elapsed time in the scheduled day (Fig. 31–12).[115] These data suggest that the overall magnitudes of the circadian and wake-dependent drives are similar during the course of a typical waking day.

From the timing of the circadian and sleep-dependent profiles, it is possible to reconstruct qualitatively the separate contributions of each toward the maintenance of alertness and performance over the course of the normal waking day (see Fig. 31–12). The first half of the day following wake time shows little homeostatic sleep drive because it has just been discharged by the prior sleep episode, and so both alertness and cognitive performance are high. In the latter half of the waking episode, when the homeostatic sleep drive would otherwise cause alertness and cognitive performance to decline, the circadian drive becomes elevated and opposes that decline in alertness and performance and thereby sustains a high, stable level of alertness throughout the normal waking day.

Sleep and Wakefulness

Similar dynamics apply for reconstructing the respective circadian and homeostatic contributions to sleep and wakefulness.[30,110,116] From the raster plot of the forced desynchrony experiment in Figure 31–11, it is apparent that almost all wakefulness within a scheduled sleep episode occurs when the subject's sleep episode is not in phase with the body temperature nadir. This observation was first quantified by Kleitman, based on his data recorded in Mammoth Cave.[56] Averaging polysomnographically recorded sleep data from free-running subjects on a self-selected cycle and in an environment

Figure 31–12. Double plots of the main effects of circadian phase relative to the minimum of core body temperature *(left panels)* and duration of prior scheduled wakefulness *(right panels)* on neurobehavioral measures. Plotted points show deviation from mean values during the forced desynchrony section of the protocol and their respective standard errors of the mean. For all panels, values plotted lower in the panel represent impairment on that neurobehavioral measure. Addition Task ADD **(A)**, Digit Symbol Substitution Task DSST **(B)**, and Probe Recall Memory (PRM) **(C)** scores are derived from the total number of correct responses. Psychomotor Vigilance Task (PVT) results represent the median reaction time **(D)** and the total number of lapses (**E**, reaction times >500 msec). Karolinska Sleepiness Scale (KSS) scores **(F)** represent responses on this 1 through 9 Likert-type scale. (Reproduced from Wyatt JK, Ritz-De Cecco A, Czeisler CA, Dijk DJ. Circadian temperature and melatonin rhythms, sleep, and neurobehavioral function in humans living on a 20-h day. Am J Physiol 1999;277:R1152-R1163, used with permission.)

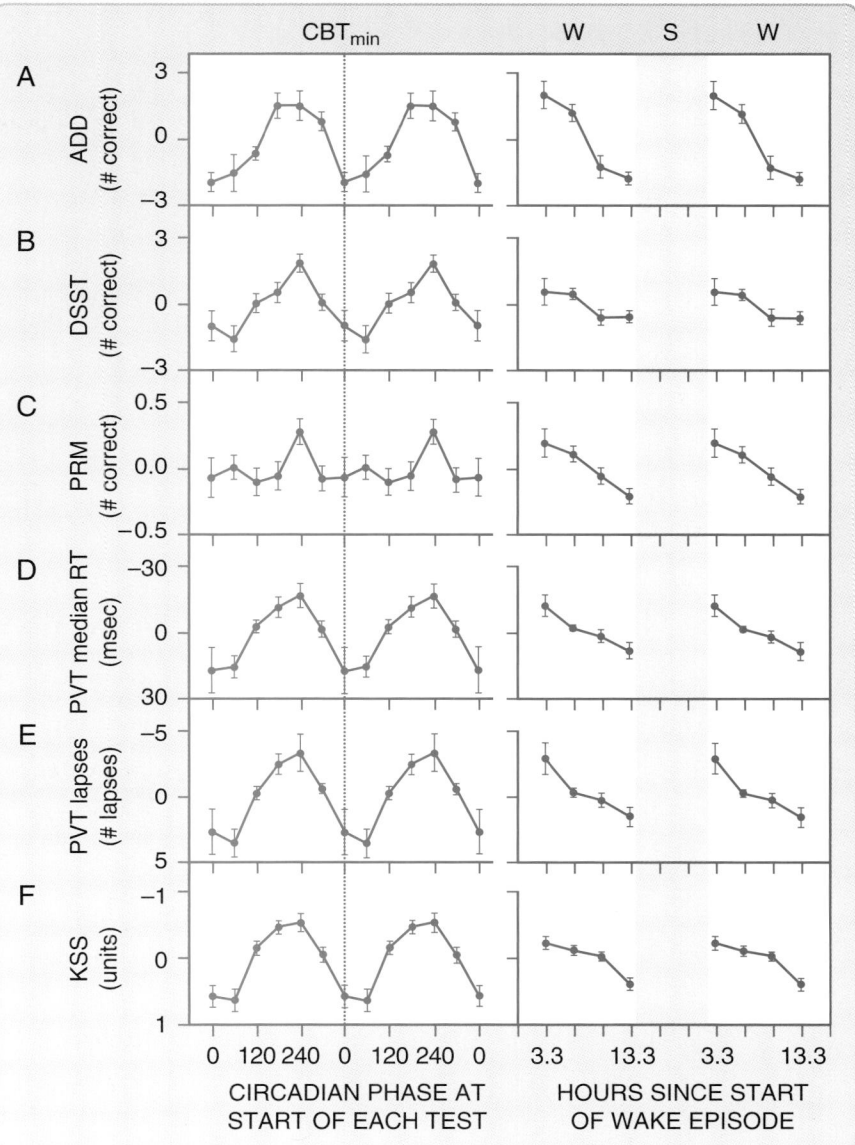

free of time cues yields the data in Figure 31–13. These data show the temporal profiles of sleep parameters as a function of circadian phase.[117] The circadian contribution to REM sleep timing is robust, and it exhibits a maximum that is centered just after the core body temperature nadir.

Figure 31–14 depicts sleep-dependent changes in the propensity for wakefulness as a function of the circadian phase at which a sleep episode is initiated. Under entrained conditions, a consolidated bout of sleep is maintained with minimal wakefulness during the scheduled sleep episode by initiating the sleep episode at the end of the wake maintenance zone. However, when sleep is initiated in the early morning hours (as is the case for a shift worker after the first night shift), a high percentage of time would be spent in wakefulness during the latter half of this intended sleep episode. During entrained conditions, homeostatic drive for sleep is greatest after an extended bout of wakefulness at sleep onset and facilitates sleep in the first half of the night. In the latter half of the sleep episode, as the homeostatic drive declines,

the circadian drive for sleep becomes greatest, thus maintaining elevated sleep drive through the end of the sleep episode. Together these two components act to generate consolidated sleep throughout the night.

The three-dimensional representation in Figure 31–15 combines the temporal profiles of circadian and sleep-dependent drives to illustrate their respective contributions in maintaining wakefulness.[160] A maximum in sleepiness quantified by slow rolling eye movements occurs at 0 degrees. The sleep-dependent contribution exhibits an increasing profile over the course of the wake episode, with the greatest propensity for slow eye movements near the end of the wake episode. When this combines with an adverse circadian phase, the drive for sleep is so great that slow eye movements and lapses of attention intrude involuntarily during wakefulness.

The circadian and sleep-wake modulation of sleep-wake propensity and neurobehavioral function are shown simply in the schema in Figure 31–16. Experimental evidence indicates that a simple additive model is not adequate to account for

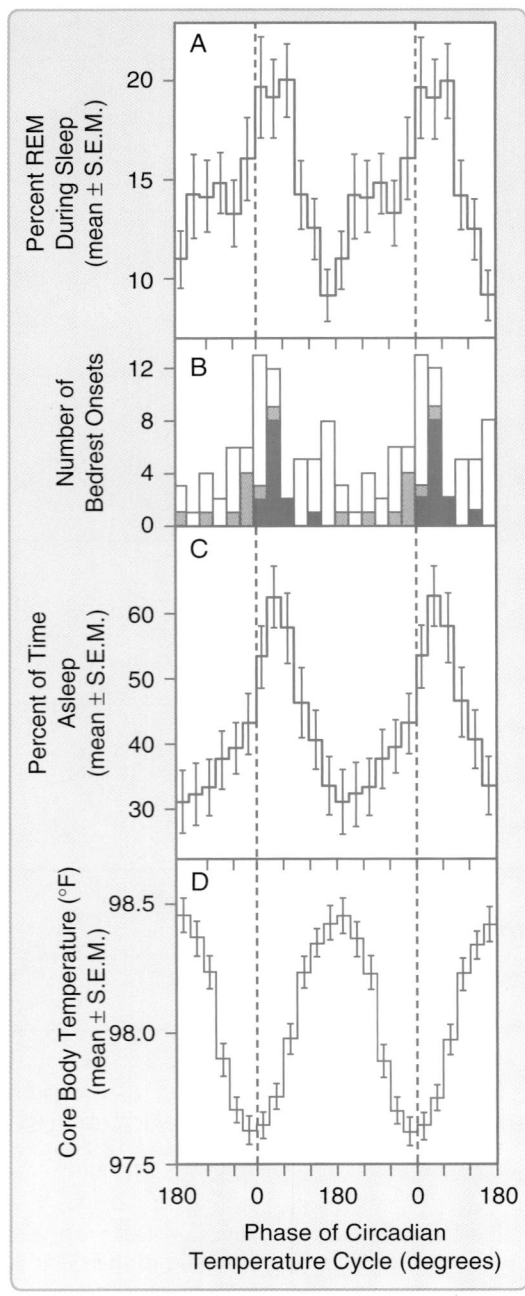

Figure 31–13. Variations in the occurrence and internal organization of sleep with the circadian temperature cycle phase. Data are shown for 94 days from 4 subjects. In *panel B,* bed rests in which REM-sleep episodes occurred within 10 minutes after bed-rest onset are *shaded dark blue;* those in which REM-sleep episodes occurred within 30 minutes after bed-rest onset are *light blue.* (Republished with permission of American Academy of Sleep Medicine. Czeisler CA, Zimmerman JC, Ronda JM, et al: Timing of REM sleep is coupled to the circadian rhythm of body temperature in man. Sleep 1980;2:329-346.)

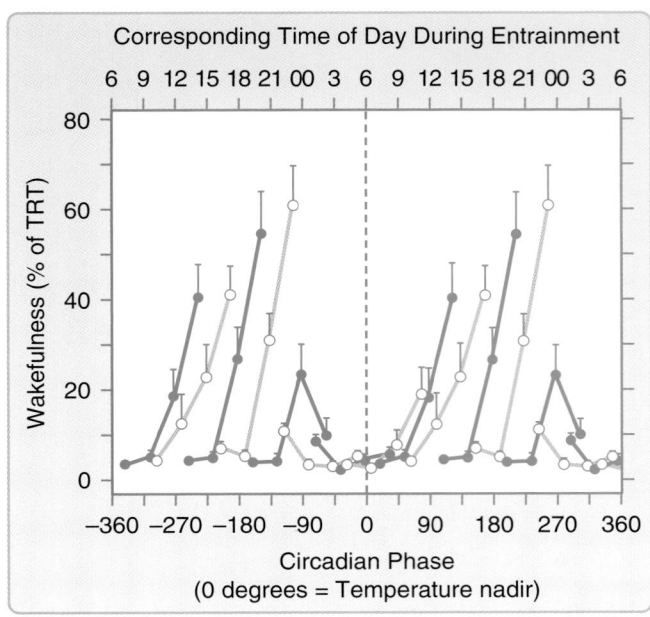

Figure 31–14. Wakefulness during scheduled sleep episodes (expressed as a percentage of recording time) as a function of circadian temperature phase. Sleep episodes were assigned to 12 30-degree bins based on the circadian phase at lights out with 0 degrees on the abscissa scale corresponding to the endogenous circadian temperature rhythm nadir. (Adapted from Dijk DJ, Czeisler CA: Contribution of the circadian pacemaker and the sleep homeostat to sleep propensity, sleep structure, electroencephalographic slow waves, and sleep spindle activity in humans. J Neurosci 1995;15:3526-3538. Copyright 1995 by the Society for Neuroscience.)

variations observed in alertness and cognitive performance data.[53,58,59,118] In fact, there is relatively little circadian variation in various waking neurobehavioral measures in the first few hours of wakefulness when averaged across all circadian phases, and the circadian contribution increases as a function of the number of hours awake, suggesting that the homeostatic and circadian drives are not independent. These data suggest that there is a nonadditive interaction between the homeostatic and circadian systems that drive alertness and cognitive performance.[119]

Internal Sleep Structure

It has long been recognized that REM sleep propensity varies with circadian phase.[120] Studies in which nap opportunities were evenly distributed throughout day and night every 1½ to 3 hours were the first to establish the REM sleep propensity rhythm in a protocol that did not involve concomitant variations in prior wake length.[117,121,122] It was then shown that REM-sleep latency, the rate of REM-sleep accumulation, REM episode duration, and REM-sleep propensity all varied with the phase of the endogenous circadian temperature cycle in free-running subjects whose self-selected rest-activity cycle spontaneously desynchronized from the timing of the endogenous circadian temperature cycle (see Fig. 31–13).[117,123]

The peak of the endogenous circadian rhythm in REM-sleep propensity found in these free-running desynchronized subjects was just after the nadir of the endogenous component of the circadian temperature cycle, coincident with the circadian peak of sleepiness and sleep propensity.[117] Furthermore, during such spontaneous desynchrony, when free-running subjects elected to go to bed near the peak of the REM-sleep propensity rhythm, they usually exhibited sleep-onset REM episodes,[117,123] (see Fig. 31–13) an otherwise rare phenomenon normally diagnostic of narcolepsy. Interestingly, under these conditions the density of rapid eye movements per minute of REM sleep exhibits a sleep-dependent variation

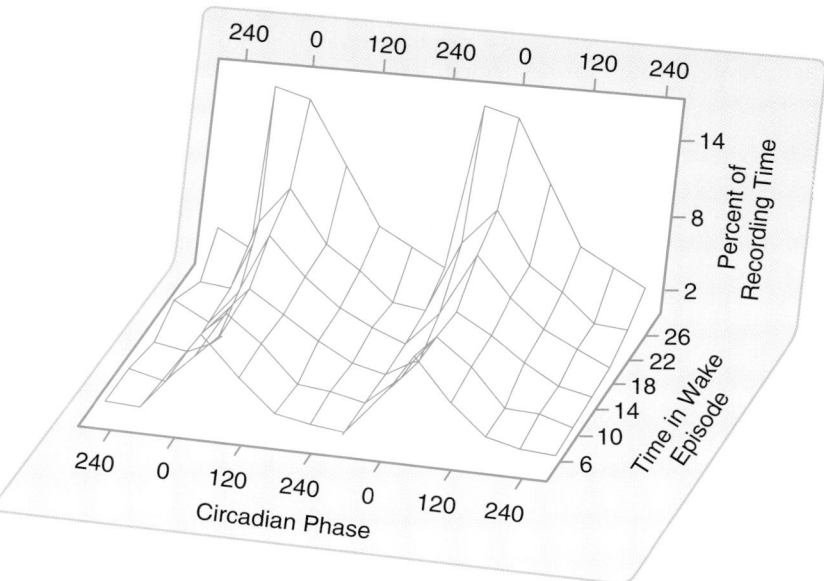

Figure 31–15. Quasi three-dimensional plot of slow rolling eye movements (SREMs) within scheduled wake episodes relative to circadian temperature phase and time elapsed since start of wake episode. 0 degrees on the abscissa scale corresponds to the endogenous circadian temperature rhythm nadir. Data were assigned to 12 circadian-phase bins (30 degrees each) and 6 bins of time since start of the wake episode (112 min each). Each point represents SREMs expressed as percentage of recording time in a bin. (Adapted from Cajochen C, Wyatt JK, Bonikowska M, et al: Non-linear interaction between circadian and homeostatic modulation of slow eye movements during wakefulness in humans. J Sleep Res 2000;9:58. Reprinted with permission.)

that appears to be dissociated from the REM-sleep propensity rhythm itself.[124]

These findings on the timing of the circadian REM-sleep propensity rhythm have since been confirmed and extended using polysomnography data from subjects studied in the forced desynchrony protocol.[30,110] Because sleep episodes in the forced desynchrony protocol always begin after a fixed duration of enforced wakefulness, the results were less confounded by the effects of systematic variations in prior wake durations characteristic of spontaneous desynchrony. Furthermore, since subjects were scheduled to remain in bed for a fixed interval on the forced desynchrony protocol, the results were not confounded by self-selected termination of the sleep episode, although the circadian variations in sleep efficiency prevent complete elimination of this confounding factor.

Nonetheless, under such conditions, the twofold circadian variation in REM sleep propensity was again found to peak just after the nadir in the endogenous circadian component of the body temperature rhythm. Moreover, on average this was found to be the case within each fifth of the scheduled sleep episode, notwithstanding the average sleep-dependent

increase in REM-sleep propensity. A sleep-dependent increase in REM sleep propensity that was not dependent on circadian phase was also quantified. A significant nonadditive interaction between circadian phase and time since the start of the sleep episode was found from the REM sleep data collected during forced desynchrony.[30]

Using the forced desynchrony protocol, significant and substantial circadian and sleep-dependent variations in NREM-sleep propensity were also observed, whereas the robust sleep-dependent decline in slow wave activity was associated with only a small but statistically significant variation of slow wave activity as a function of circadian phase.[30] Similar circadian variations in internal sleep structure have been documented in a blind patient whose circadian pacemaker was not synchronized to the 24-hour day, even though he had maintained a very regular sleep-wake schedule for decades.[125] Such blind patients are, in essence, living in society on the biological equivalent of a forced desynchrony protocol, since the 24-hour day is outside the range of entrainment of their circadian pacemaker.

More recently, quantitative analysis of the sleep EEG has revealed circadian variations in the electroencephalographic activity during both NREM sleep and REM sleep,[126] with low-frequency sleep spindle activity in NREM sleep paralleling the endogenous circadian melatonin rhythm. Overall, these data indicate that the timing and internal structure of sleep are profoundly dependent on an interaction between robust circadian and homeostatic regulatory factors, with circadian factors predominant in the regulation of REM sleep and with sleep-dependent factors predominant in the regulation of slow wave sleep.

Potential Feedback Pathways

As is typical of physiologic regulatory systems, feedback pathways play a significant role in this system. The neurobehavioral variables influenced by the circadian pacemaker and the sleep homeostat can affect the sleep-wake state because wakefulness and sleep propensity influence determination

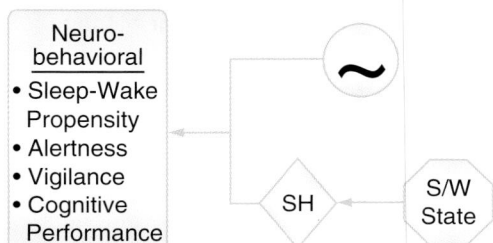

Figure 31–16. A schema illustrating the combined influence of the circadian clock (oscillator symbol in the circle) and sleep-wake (S/W) state on neurobehavioral variables (sleep-wake propensity, alertness, vigilance, and cognitive performance). The sleep-wake state influence is illustrated by the intermediary of the sleep homeostat (SH in the diamond).

of sleep and wake times. For example, a sleep episode is more likely to be initiated following a rise in sleep propensity to a high level during an extended waking episode, and a sleep episode is more likely to be terminated following a decline in sleep propensity to a low level over the course of a sleep episode. This influence on behavior in turn influences the level of the sleep homeostat and, due to associated changes in light exposure and activity, may affect the phase or amplitude, or both, of the circadian pacemaker.

There may be another important feedback pathway in this system. Studies demonstrating that melatonin receptors can be found on cells within the human suprachiasmatic nucleus have drawn attention to a potential feedback pathway from the pineal gland to the SCN via circulating melatonin. Several physiologic studies have suggested that exogenous melatonin may exert a phase-resetting effect on the human circadian pacemaker, and both a phase-response curve and dose-dependent phase shifting have been reported. However, none of these studies has thoroughly controlled for retinal light exposure, confounding interpretation of the results. There has also been a great interest in the potential efficacy of melatonin as a hypnotic; however, the reliability and degree of both of these effects remain to be fully established (see Chapter 32 for a review of this literature).

Examination of the temporal profile of endogenous melatonin secretion during the forced desynchrony protocol reveals that the daily circadian increase in melatonin levels coincides with a decrease in wakefulness (Fig. 31–17).[126] This melatonin rise may open a gate that allows sleep to occur.[127,128] Taken as a whole, these data provide suggestive evidence that there may be feedback from the pineal gland both to the circadian pacemaker and to neurobehavioral variables involved in regulating the sleep-wake state.[129] It is likely that other physiologic systems also affect sleep-regulating mechanisms; for example, some evidence suggests an effect of growth hormone[130,131] on sleep.

Intrinsic Period of the Human Circadian Pacemaker

Numerous studies have been performed in the absence of environmental synchronizers in human subjects, and based on these studies, it was initially concluded that the average period of the human circadian pacemaker averaged about 25 hours. However, many of the early experiments designed to evaluate the characteristics of the human circadian system incorporated self-selected exposure to ordinary room light. In these experiments, which had been done deep within caves and in laboratories shielded from periodic cues from the external environment, the subjects were permitted to illuminate their living quarters when they were awake and to switch off the lighting when they were asleep, because these experiments were predicated on the strongly entrenched belief that ordinary room light had no effect on the human circadian system.[132,133] The results of these studies were therefore systematically compromised by the profound effects of this light exposure.[60,61,95,134]

Recognition of this confounding effect of room light on prior attempts to estimate circadian period using a protocol involving self-selected timing of sleep in darkness and wakefulness in artificial room light led to the suggested use of Kleitman's forced desynchrony protocol to assess the intrinsic

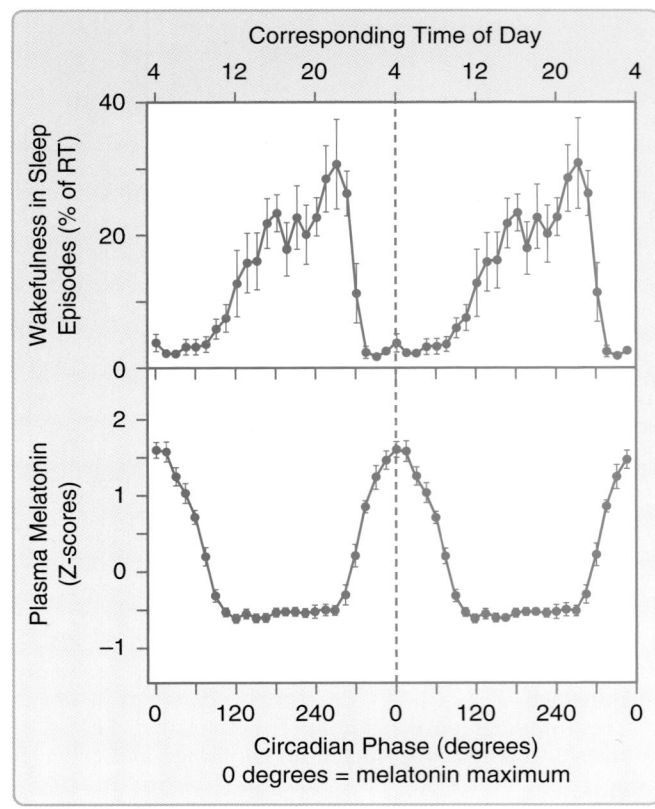

Figure 31–17. Phase relationships between the endogenous circadian rhythms of wakefulness and plasma melatonin as assessed during a forced desynchrony protocol. Data are plotted against circadian phase of the plasma melatonin rhythm (0 degrees on the *lower abscissa scale* corresponds to the fitted melatonin maximum). To facilitate comparison with the entrained conditions, the *upper abscissa scale* indicates the approximate clock time corresponding to the circadian melatonin rhythm during the first day of the forced desynchrony protocol (i.e., immediately on release from entrainment). Plasma melatonin data are expressed as Z-scores to correct for interindividual differences in mean values. Wakefulness is expressed as a percentage of recording time (RT). Data are double plotted (i.e., all data plotted left from the dashed vertical line are repeated to the right of this vertical line). (Adapted from Dijk D-J, Shanahan TL, Duffy JF, et al: Variation of electroencephalographic activity during non–rapid eye movement and rapid eye movement sleep with phase of circadian melatonin rhythm in humans. J Physiol [Lond]. 1997;505:851-858.)

period of the human circadian pacemaker.[135] In fact, using simulations based on Kronauer's mathematical model of the effect of light on the circadian system, it was found that under conditions in which room lighting was self-selected, the observed period of the circadian temperature rhythm would be 25 hours even when an actual circadian input period of 24.1 to 24.2 hours was employed in the simulations.[134]

Subsequent studies using the forced desynchrony protocol have been done controlling the intensity of background illumination and the timing of the exposure to the light-dark cycle. Using this forced desynchrony protocol with subjects living in dim light (~10-15 lux) on either a 28-hour or a 20-hour schedule, the average intrinsic period of the circadian pacemaker has been estimated to be much closer to 24 hours, with an average period of about 24.2 hours[136] rather than 25 hours (Fig. 31–18). This circadian period was consistent

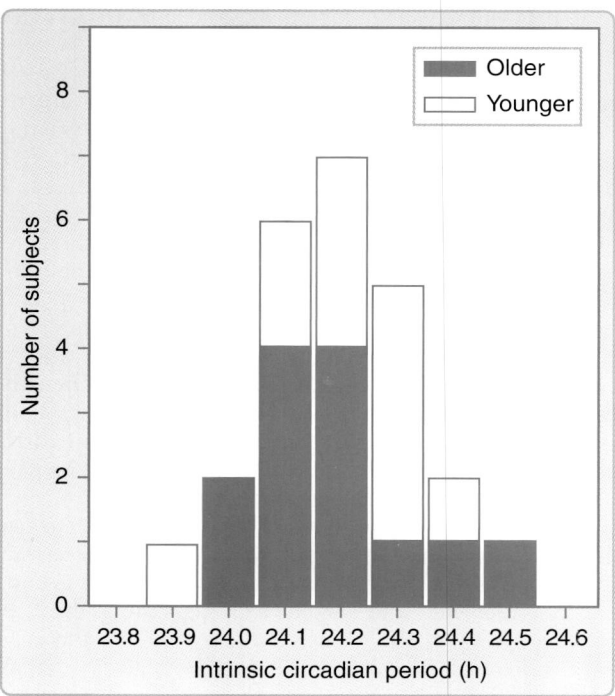

Figure 31–18. Histogram of intrinsic circadian period estimates derived from young and older subjects. Intrinsic circadian period estimates of older subjects are indicated by *solid bars;* those of young adults are indicated by *open bars.* Each subject's estimated intrinsic circadian period is reported as the average of the estimated periods from his or her core body temperature, melatonin, and cortisol rhythms. (Reproduced from Czeisler CA, Duffy JF, Shanahan TL, et al: Stability, precision, and near-24-hour period of the human circadian pacemaker. Science 1999;284:2177-2181.)

for all of the circadian markers tested: core body temperature, melatonin, and cortisol.

This value for the period of the human circadian pacemaker is also consistent with the results of other recent studies performed under a variety of differing protocols.[137-140] Moreover, entrainment studies have functionally confirmed the intrinsic circadian period in humans to be near 24 hours, because a weak synchronizing stimulus (candlelight during the scheduled day and darkness or sleep during the scheduled night) can entrain most people to a light-dark cycle with an imposed period of 24.0 hours, but not an imposed period of 23.5 hours or 24.6 hours.[141]

AGING AND CIRCADIAN SLEEP-WAKE REGULATION

The process of aging is another factor that has a pervasive influence on many aspects of the circadian and sleep-wake regulating system.[142-150] The prevalence of disrupted sleep complaints is much greater in older people than it is in young people. In fact, 57% of people in the United States who are older than 65 years complain of at least one chronic sleep problem, 43% complain of difficulty initiating or maintaining sleep, and 19% complain of awakening too early in the morning.[151] A key question in examining the basis for these complaints is the extent to which the circadian pacemaker or the sleep homeostat, or both, may play a role in these age-related changes.

In experiments using a constant routine protocol, the minima of the core body temperature rhythm in young subjects tended to fall later than in healthy older subjects, and it exhibited a higher amplitude of their core body temperature rhythm (Fig. 31–19).[144,152] However, in forced desynchrony experiments with healthy young and older subjects, the circadian period was not observed to be different between these two groups.[136,153] Although this does not rule out the possibility that circadian period may differ in older people who have sleep disorders or compromised health, it does suggest that a change in period is not a necessary consequence of aging.

The results from the forced desynchrony study confirmed those of the earlier constant routine study, which showed that circadian phase of older subjects is set to an earlier hour and older subjects exhibit a lower amplitude of the body temperature and melatonin rhythms. More importantly, other results from this study suggest that young subjects are able to sleep over a much wider range of circadian phases than are older subjects, and older subjects also wake up at an earlier internal circadian phase.[152,154] This waking at an earlier phase may also explain why their circadian system is shifted to an earlier hour, because if they wake up spontaneously at an earlier circadian phase, they are going to be exposed to light at an earlier hour, which will, in turn, reset their pacemaker to an earlier hour and essentially exacerbate this problem.

INFLUENCE OF SOCIETAL FACTORS

The independent self-selection of sleep and wake times in humans is another important factor in the sleep-regulatory system. Although the circadian and homeostatic drives for

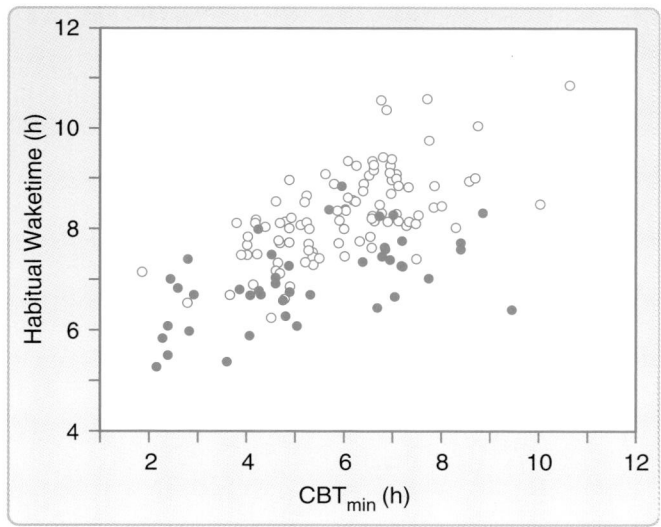

Figure 31–19. Habitual wake time versus endogenous circadian phase of young and older individuals. Symbols represent average self-reported wake time from the week before the study versus the phase of the endogenous fitted core body temperature minimum (CBT_{min}) for each individual subject. *Filled circles* indicate older subjects (N = 44); *open circles* indicate young subjects (N = 101). The relationship between the groups was significant (slope of older subjects, 0.266 ± 0.06; slope of young subjects, 0.471 ± 0.05). (Reproduced from Duffy JF, Dijk DJ, Klerman EB, Czeisler CA. Later endogenous circadian temperature nadir relative to an earlier wake time in older people. Am J Physiol 1998;275:R1478-R1487, used with permission.)

sleep exert an influence on the choice of sleep and wake times via a feedback pathway, societal factors are often an overriding influence. This is in stark contrast to laboratory animal behavior, in which independent self-selection does not appear to contribute significantly, and the observed times of activity and sleep are predictable enough to be used as a marker of the time of day.

Humans, especially since the advent of alarm clocks and artificial lighting, can and do override the signals from the circadian and sleep-wake regulating system and freely decide to stay awake because of job or school requirements or for recreational and social events. One of the consequences is that humans in modern times may be more sleep deprived than their ancestors and exhibit self-determined sleep and wake schedules.[155] The long-term consequences of this recent trend in industrialized society are unknown. However, recent studies have indicated that the modern consolidated sleep episode shows significant differences from that observed under more naturalistic conditions in which the sleep episode was determined by the longer length of darkness in the natural environment during winter.[155,156]

The most conspicuous example of this self-selection is the phenomenon of rotating shift work, when the choice is made to work in direct opposition to the modulation of the circadian and homeostatic regulatory systems at the cost of internal temporal dissociation, fragmented sleep, and impaired wakefulness. Therefore, any realistic model of the human circadian and sleep-wake regulating system must take into account this environmental and societal factor.

CONCLUSION

An overall schema of the entire system can now be assembled from those presented above and further updated to incorporate the feedback pathway of neurobehavioral variables on the sleep-wake state and the putative feedback pathways from melatonin and other physiologic variables onto the circadian pacemaker and neurobehavioral function (Fig. 31–20). This schema also incorporates the global influence of environmental, social, behavioral, genetic, pharmacologic, and age factors on all elements of this system.

Another addition to this final schema relates to the clear decrements in neurobehavioral performance and alertness that immediately follow the transition from sleep to waking, a phenomenon called sleep inertia. The time course of this underappreciated phenomenon has been characterized and it has been demonstrated that sleep inertia persists for as long as several hours after a long sleep episode.[157-159] This schema incorporates much of what is known concerning the role of the circadian pacemaker in the regulation of sleep. It is not intended to be a complete representation of the factors involved in the system regulating sleep, because that would be beyond the scope of this chapter. Nevertheless, the strength of this schema is that it serves as a useful tool in understanding the interplay between the circadian and homeostatic drives, and it perhaps also serves as a useful framework from which future scientific inquiry can be initiated.

The complexity of the interactions of the circadian pacemaker and the sleep homeostat to regulate the sleep-wake cycle should not be underestimated. Furthermore, it is important to understand the difficulty in separating these two processes functionally. Under ordinary circumstances, in which individuals are sleeping during the night in darkness and awake during the day in daylight, it is not possible to distinguish the relative contributions of the sleep homeostat from that of the circadian pacemaker to a given recurrent daily characteristic, symptom or disorder of sleep or wakefulness (e.g., narcolepsy, delayed sleep phase syndrome). The occurrence of a pathologic event, such as a nocturnal seizure, at the same time each night may be driven by the circadian pacemaker, the sleep homeostat, a specific sleep stage, or some combination of these processes.

It is currently possible, though difficult, to experimentally dissociate these factors for research purposes (e.g., using either the forced desynchrony protocol in human subjects or suprachiasmatic lesions in animal studies). Although clinically feasible techniques, such as the use of dim-light salivary melatonin onset, may provide limited information about

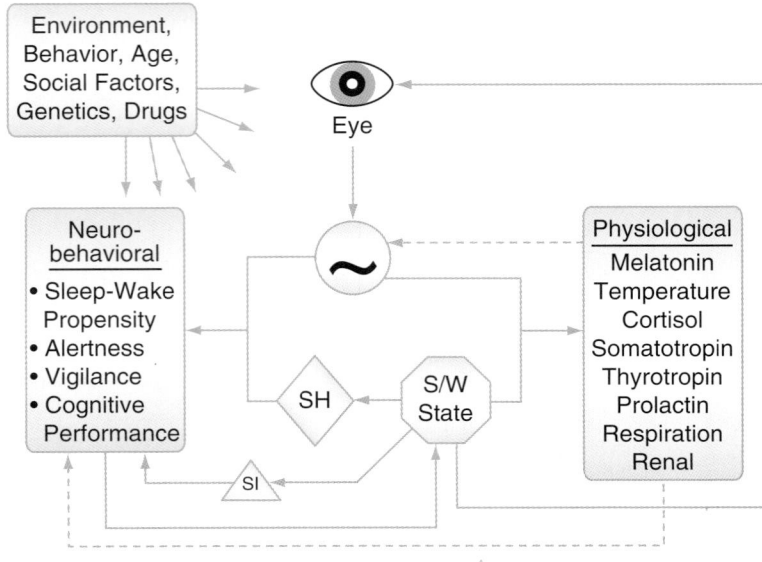

Figure 31–20. An overall schema coalescing the potential influence of physiologic variables (e.g., melatonin, body temperature) on neurobehavioral variables or the circadian clock (oscillator symbol) is indicated by the *dashed arrows,* the feedback influence of neurobehavioral variables on sleep-wake (S/W) state is indicated by a *solid arrow,* and the influence of sleep-wake state on neurobehavioral variables through sleep inertia (SI) is indicated by *solid arrows.* The global influence of environment, behavior, age, social factors, genetics, and drugs on virtually all elements contributing to sleep-wake regulation is also represented.

circadian phase, a routine complete clinical assessment of whether a disorder is circadian or homeostat-dependent awaits the results of continued basic and clinical research.

> ### Clinical Pearl
>
> *The circadian timing system is disrupted by shift work, travel across time zones, and the activities of the round-the-clock society. This disruption has an adverse effect on many physiologic variables, including hormone levels, autonomic nervous system activity, neurobehavioral performance, and the propensity, timing, and internal structure of sleep. Such disruption could result in patient complaints of insomnia or excessive daytime sleepiness and may impair overall health.*

Acknowledgments

The research conducted by the Division of Sleep Medicine has been supported by grants NIA-1-RO1-AG06072, NIA-PO1-AG09975 and NIA-1-U01-12642 from the National Institute on Aging; grant NIMH-1-RO1-MH45130 from the National Institute of Mental Health; grant RO1-HL52992 from the National Heart, Lung, and Blood Institute; grants NAG9-524 and NAG5-3952 from the National Aeronautics and Space Administration; the National Aeronautics and Space Administration through the NASA Cooperative Agreement NCC 9-58 with the National Space Biomedical Research Institute; and General Clinical Research Center Grant NCRR-GCRC-MO1-RR02635 from the National Center for Research Resources; and by the Brigham and Women's Hospital.

REFERENCES

1. Johnson CH: An atlas of phase response curves for circadian and circatidal rhythms. Nashville, Tenn, Department of Biology, Vanderbilt University, 1990.
2. Edmunds LN Jr: Cellular and Molecular Bases of Biological Clocks: Models and Mechanisms for Circadian Timekeeping. New York, Springer-Verlag, 1988.
3. Pittendrigh CS: Circadian systems: Entrainment. In Aschoff J (ed): Handbook of Behavioral Neurobiology: Biological Rhythms. New York, Plenum Press, 1981, pp 95-124.
4. Fulton JF, Bailey P: Tumors in the region of the third ventricle: Their diagnosis and relation to pathological sleep. J Nerv Ment Dis 1929;69:1-25, 145-164.
5. Moore RY, Eichler VB: Loss of a circadian adrenal corticosterone rhythm following suprachiasmatic lesions in the rat. Brain Res 1972;42:201-206.
6. Stephan FK, Zucker I: Circadian rhythms in drinking behavior and locomotor activity of rats are eliminated by hypothalamic lesions. Proc Natl Acad Sci U S A 1972;69:1583-1586.
7. Ralph MR, Foster RG, Davis FC, Menaker M: Transplanted suprachiasmatic nucleus determines circadian period. Science 1990;247:975-978.
8. Aschoff J, Wever R: Human circadian rhythms: A multioscillatory system. Fed Proc 1976;35:2326-2332.
9. Weitzman ED, Boyar RM, Kapen S, Hellman L: The relationship of sleep and sleep stages to neuroendocrine secretion and biological rhythms in man. Recent Prog Horm Res 1975;31:399-441.
10. Aschoff J, Wever R: The circadian system of man. In Aschoff J (ed): Biological Rhythms: Handbook of Behavioral Neurobiology. New York, Plenum Press, 1981, pp 311-331.
11. Shanahan TL, Czeisler CA: Light exposure induces equivalent phase shifts of the endogenous circadian rhythms of circulating plasma melatonin and core body temperature in men. J Clin Endocrinol Metab 1991;73:227-235.
12. Allan JS, Czeisler CA: Persistence of the circadian thyrotropin rhythm under constant conditions and after light-induced shifts of circadian phase. J Clin Endocrinol Metab 1994;79:508-512.
13. Waldstreicher J, Duffy JF, Brown EN, et al: Gender differences in the temporal organization of prolactin (PRL) secretion: Evidence for a sleep-independent circadian rhythm of circulating PRL levels—a clinical research center study. J Clin Endocrinol Metab 1996;81:1483-1487.
14. El Hajj Fuleihan G, Klerman EB, Brown EN, et al: Parathyroid hormone circadian rhythm is truly endogenous. J Clin Endocrinol Metab 1997;82:281-286.
15. Brandenberger G, Gronfier C, Weibel L, Spiegel K: Modulatory role of sleep on hormonal pulsatility. In Hayaishi O, Inoue S (eds): Sleep and Sleep Disorders: From Molecule to Behavior. Tokyo, Academic Press, 1997, pp 195-208.
16. Van Cauter E, Copinschi G, Turek FW: Endocrine and other biologic rhythms. In DeGroot LJ, Jameson JL (eds): Endocrinology, 4th ed. Philadelphia, WB Saunders, 2001, pp 235-256.
17. Van Cauter E, Turek FW: Endocrine and other biological rhythms. In DeGroot LJ (ed): Endocrinology, 3rd ed. Philadelphia, WB Saunders, 1995, pp 2487-2548.
18. Leproult R, Van Reeth O, Byrne MM, et al: Sleepiness, performance, and neuroendocrine function during sleep deprivation: Effects of exposure to bright light or exercise. J Biol Rhythms 1997;12:245-258.
19. Czeisler CA: Human Circadian Physiology: Internal Organization of Temperature, Sleep-Wake, and Neuroendocrine Rhythms Monitored in an Environment Free of Time Cues [thesis]. Palo Alto, Stanford University, 1978.
20. Buxton OM, Spiegel K, Van Cauter E: Modulation of endocrine function and metabolism by sleep and sleep loss. In Lee-Chiong M, Carskadon M, Sateia M (eds): Sleep Medicine. Philadelphia, Hanley and Belfus, 2002, pp 59-69.
21. Mills JN, Minors DS, Waterhouse JM: Adaptation to abrupt time shifts of the oscillator(s) controlling human circadian rhythms. J Physiol (Lond) 1978;285:455-470.
22. Duffy JF, Dijk DJ: Getting through to circadian oscillators: Why use constant routines? J Biol Rhythms 2002;17:4-13.
23. Czeisler CA, Kronauer RE, Allan JS, et al: Bright light induction of strong (type 0) resetting of the human circadian pacemaker. Science 1989;244:1328-1333.
24. Hunter J: Of the heat of animals and vegetables. Philos Trans R Soc Lond 1778;68:7-49.
25. Benedict FG: Studies in body-temperature I. Influence of the inversion of the daily routine: The temperature of night-workers. Am J Physiol 1904;11:145-169.
26. Kleitman N, Doktorsky A: Studies on the physiology of sleep. VII. The effect of the position of the body and of sleep on rectal temperature in man. Am J Physiol 1933;104:340-343.
27. Mills JN, Minors DS, Waterhouse JM: The effect of sleep upon human circadian rhythms. Chronobiologia 1978;5:14-27.
28. Wever RA: The circadian system of man: Results of experiments under temporal isolation. New York, Springer-Verlag, 1979.
29. Zulley J, Wever RA: Interaction between the sleep-wake cycle and the rhythm of rectal temperature. In Aschoff J, Daan S, Groos G (eds): Vertebrate Circadian Systems. Berlin, Springer-Verlag, 1982, pp 253-261.
30. Dijk DJ, Czeisler CA: Contribution of the circadian pacemaker and the sleep homeostat to sleep propensity, sleep structure, electroencephalographic slow waves, and sleep spindle activity in humans. J Neurosci 1995;15:3526-3538.
31. Czeisler CA, Johnson MP, Duffy JF, et al: Exposure to bright light and darkness to treat physiologic maladaptation to night work. N Engl J Med 1990;322:1253-1259.

32. Shanahan TL, Kronauer RE, Duffy JF, et al: Melatonin rhythm observed throughout a three-cycle bright-light stimulus designed to reset the human circadian pacemaker. J Biol Rhythms 1999; 14:237-253.

33. Deacon S, Arendt J: Posture influences melatonin concentrations in plasma and saliva in humans. Neurosci Lett 1994;167: 191-194.

34. Leproult R, Copinschi G, Buxton OF, Van Cauter E: Sleep loss results in an evaluation of cortisol levels the next evening. Sleep 1997;20:865-870.

35. Weitzman ED, Zimmerman JC, Czeisler CA, Ronda J: Cortisol secretion is inhibited during sleep in normal man. J Clin Endocrinol Metab 1983;56:352-358.

36. Brabant G, Prank K, Ranft U, et al: Physiological regulation of circadian and pulsatile thyrotropin secretion in normal man and woman. J Clin Endocrinol Metab 1990;70:403-409.

37. Czeisler CA, Klerman EB: Circadian and sleep-dependent regulation of hormone release in humans. Recent Prog Horm Res 1999;54:97-132.

38. Baumgartner A, Dietzel M, Saletu B, et al: Influence of partial sleep deprivation on the secretion of thyrotropin, thyroid hormones, growth hormone, prolactin, luteinizing hormone, follicle stimulating hormone, and estradiol in healthy young women. Psychiatry Res 1993;48:153-178.

39. Goichot B, Brandenberger G, Saini J, et al: Nocturnal plasma thyrotropin variations are related to slow-wave sleep. J Sleep Res 1992;1:186-190.

40. Gronfier C, Luthringer R, Follenius M, et al: Temporal link between plasma thyrotropin levels and electroencephalographic activity in man. Neurosci Lett 1995;200:97-100.

41. Chapotot F, Gronfier C, Spiegel K, et al: Relationships between intact parathyroid hormone 24-hour profiles, sleep-wake cycle, and sleep electroencephalographic activity in man. J Clin Endocrinol Metab 1996;81:3759-3765.

42. Holl RW, Hartman ML, Veldhuis JD, et al: Thirty-second sampling of plasma growth hormone in man: Correlation with sleep stages. J Clin Endocrinol Metab 1991;72:854-861.

43. Gronfier C, Luthringer R, Follenius M, et al: A quantitative evaluation of the relationships between growth hormone secretion and delta wave electroencephalographic activity during normal sleep and after enrichment in delta waves. Sleep 1996;19:817-824.

44. Parker DC, Rossman LG, Vanderlaan EF: Relation of sleep-entrained human prolactin release to REM–non-REM cycles. J Clin Endocrinol Metab 1974;38:646-651.

45. Van Cauter E, Desir D, Refetoff S, et al: The relationship between episodic variations of plasma prolactin and REM–non-REM cyclicity is an artifact. J Clin Endocrinol Metab 1982;54:70-75.

46. Spiegel K, Luthringer R, Follenius M, et al: Temporal relationship between prolactin secretion and slow-wave electroencephalic activity during sleep. Sleep 1995;18:543-548.

47. Brandenberger G, Follenius M, Muzet A, et al: Ultradian oscillations in plasma renin activity: Their relationships to meals and sleep stages. J Clin Endocrinol Metab 1985;61:280-284.

48. Brandenberger G, Follenius M, Simon C, et al: Nocturnal oscillations in plasma renin activity and REM-NREM sleep cycles in humans: A common regulatory mechanism? Sleep 1988; 11:242-250.

49. Luthringer R, Brandenberger G, Schaltenbrand N, et al: Slow wave electroencephalic activity parallels renin oscillations during sleep in humans. Electroenceph Clin Neurophysiol 1995;95:318-322.

50. Aschoff J: Circadian rhythms: General features and endocrinological aspects. In Krieger DT (ed): Endocrine Rhythms. New York, Raven Press, 1979, pp 1-62.

51. Jaffe CA, Turgeon DK, DeMott-Friberg R, et al: Nocturnal augmentation of growth hormone (GH) secretion is preserved during repetitive bolus administration of GH-releasing hormone: Potential involvement of endogenous somatostatin—a clinical research center study. J Clin Endocrinol Metab 1995;80:3321-3326.

52. Weibel L, Brandenberger G: Disturbances in hormonal profiles of night workers during their usual sleep and work times. J Biol Rhythms 1998;13:202-208.

53. Babkoff H, Mikulincer M, Caspy T, Kempinski D: The topology of performance curves during 72 hours of sleep loss: A memory and search task. Q J Exp Psychol 1988;40A:737-756.

54. Folkard S, Hume KI, Minors DS, et al: Independence of the circadian rhythm in alertness from the sleep/wake cycle. Nature 1985;313:678-679.

55. Folkard S, Wever RA, Wildgruber CM: Multi-oscillatory control of circadian rhythms in human performance. Nature 1983;305: 223-226.

56. Kleitman N: Sleep and Wakefulness. Chicago, University of Chicago Press, 1963.

57. Monk TH, Buysse DJ, Reynolds III CF, et al: Circadian rhythms in human performance and mood under constant conditions. J Sleep Res 1997;6:9-18.

58. Boivin DB, Czeisler CA, Dijk DJ, et al: Complex interaction of the sleep-wake cycle and circadian phase modulates mood in healthy subjects. Arch Gen Psychiatry 1997;54:145-152.

59. Johnson MP, Duffy JF, Dijk DJ, et al: Short-term memory, alertness and performance: A reappraisal of their relationship to body temperature. J Sleep Res 1992;1:24-29.

60. Czeisler CA: The effect of light on the human circadian pacemaker. In Waterhouse JM, (ed): Circadian Clocks and Their Adjustment. Chichester, UK (Ciba Foundation Symposium 183), John Wiley and Sons, 1995, pp 254-302.

61. Czeisler CA, Wright Jr. KP: Influence of light on circadian rhythmicity in humans. In Turek FW, Zee PC (eds): New York, Marcel Dekker, 1999, pp 149-180.

62. Moore RY: Retinohypothalamic projection in mammals: A comparative study. Brain Res 1973;49:403-409.

63. Moore RY, Lenn NJ: A retinohypothalamic projection in the rat. J Comp Neurol 1972;146:1-14.

64. Moore RY, Speh JC, Card JP: The retinohypothalamic tract originates from a distinct subset of retinal ganglion cells. J Comp Neurol 1995;352:351-366.

65. Sadun AA, Schaechter JD, Smith LE: A retinohypothalamic pathway in man: Light mediation of circadian rhythms. Brain Res 1984;302:371-377.

66. Dai J, van der Vliet J, Swaab DF, Buijs RM: Human retinohypothalamic tract as revealed by in vitro postmortem tracing. J Comp Neurol 1998;397:357-370.

67. Friedman DI, Johnson JK, Chorsky RL, Stopa EG: Labeling of human retinohypothalamic tract with the carbocyanine dye, DiI. Brain Res 1991;560:297-302.

68. Schwartz WJ, Busis NA, Hedley-Whyte ET: A discrete lesion of ventral hypothalamus and optic chiasm that disturbed the daily temperature rhythm. J Neurol 1986;233:1-4.

69. Cohen RA, Albers HE: Disruption of human circadian and cognitive regulation following a discrete hypothalamic lesion: A case study. Neurology 1991;41:726-729.

70. Brainard GC, Hanifin JP, Rollag MD, et al: Human melatonin regulation is not mediated by the three cone photopic visual system. J Clin Endocrinol Metab 2001;86:433-436.

71. Brainard GC, Hanifin JP, Greeson JM, et al: Action spectrum for melatonin regulation in humans: Evidence for a novel circadian photoreceptor. J Neurosci 2001;21:6405-6412.

72. Lucas RJ, Freedman MS, Muñoz M, et al: Regulation of the mammalian pineal by non-rod, non-cone, ocular photoreceptors. Science 1999;284:505-507.

73. Lucas RJ, Foster RG: Neither functional rod photoreceptors nor rod or cone outer segments are required for the photic inhibition of pineal melatonin. Endocrinology 1999;140: 1520-1524.

74. Thapan K, Arendt J, Skene DJ: An action spectrum for melatonin suppression: Evidence for a novel non-rod, non-cone photoreceptor system in humans. J Physiol 2001;535:261-267.

75. Lockley SW, Brainard GC, Czeisler CA: High sensitivity of the human circadian melatonin rhythm to resetting by short wavelength light. J Clin Endocrinol Metab 2003;88:4502-4505.

76. Gooley JJ, Lu J, Chou TC, et al: Melanopsin in cells of origin of the retinohypothalamic tract. Nature Neurosci 2001;4:1165.

77. Berson DM, Dunn FA, Takao M: Phototransduction by retinal ganglion cells that set the circadian clock. Science 2002;295:1070-1073.

78. Takahashi JS, DeCoursey PJ, Bauman L, Menaker M: Spectral sensitivity of a novel photoreceptive system mediating entrainment of mammalian circadian rhythms. Nature 1984;308:186-188.

79. Warman VL, Dijk DJ, Warman GR, et al: Phase advancing human circadian rhythms with short wavelength light. Neurosci Lett 2003;342:37-40.

80. Selby CP, Thompson C, Schmitz TM, et al: Functional redundancy of cryptochromes and classical photoreceptors for nonvisual ocular photoreception in mice. Proc Natl Acad Sci U S A 2000;97:14697-14702.

81. Hattar S, Lucas RJ, Mrosovsky N, et al: Melanopsin and rod-cone photoreceptive systems account for all major accessory visual functions in mice. Nature 2003;424:75-81.

82. Watts AG: The efferent projections of the suprachiasmatic nucleus: Anatomical insights into the control of circadian rhythms. In Klein DC, Moore RY, Reppert SM (eds): Suprachiasmatic Nucleus: The Mind's Clock, 1st ed. New York, Oxford University Press, 1991, pp 77-106.

83. Klein DC, Moore RY, Reppert SM (eds): Suprachiasmatic Nucleus: The Mind's Clock. New York, Oxford University Press, 1991.

84. Illnerová H: The suprachiasmatic nucleus and rhythmic pineal melatonin production. In Klein DC, Moore RY, Reppert SM (eds): Suprachiasmatic Nucleus: The Mind's Clock. New York, Oxford University Press, 1991, pp 197-216.

85. McIntyre IM, Norman TR, Burrows GD, Armstrong SM: Human melatonin suppression by light is intensity dependent. J Pineal Res 1989;6:149-156.

86. Wetterberg L: Melatonin in humans—physiological and clinical studies. J Neural Transm 1978;13:289-310.

87. Czeisler CA, Shanahan TL, Klerman EB, et al: Suppression of melatonin secretion in some blind patients by exposure to bright light. N Engl J Med 1995;332:6-11.

88. Provencio I, Cooper HM, Foster RG: Retinal projections in mice with inherited retinal degeneration: Implications for circadian photoentrainment. J Comp Neurol 1998;395:417-439.

89. Moore RY: Vision without sight. N Engl J Med 1995;332:54-55.

90. Hastings JW, Sweeney BM: A persistent diurnal rhythm of luminescence in Gonyaulax polyedra. Biol Bull 1958;115:440-458.

91. Van Cauter E, Buxton M: Circadian modulation of endocrine secretion. In Takahashi J, Turek FW, Moore RY (eds): Handbook of Behavioral Neurobiology. New York, Plenum, 2001, pp 685-714.

92. Khalsa SB, Jewett ME, Cajochen C, Czeisler CA: A phase response curve to single bright light pulses in human subjects. J Physiol (Lond) 2003;549(Pt 3):945-952.

93. Jewett ME, Rimmer DW, Duffy JF, et al: Human circadian pacemaker is sensitive to light throughout subjective day without evidence of transients. Am J Physiol 1997;273:R1800-R1809.

94. Lewy AJ, Cutler NL, Sack RL: The endogenous melatonin profile as a marker for circadian phase position. J Biol Rhythms 1999;14:227-236.

95. Shanahan TL, Zeitzer JM, Czeisler CA: Resetting the melatonin rhythm with light in humans. J Biol Rhythms 1997;12:556-567.

96. Voultsios A, Kennaway DJ, Dawson D: Salivary melatonin as a circadian phase marker: Validation and comparison to plasma melatonin. J Biol Rhythms 1997;12:457-466.

97. Wirz-Justice A, Graw P, Krauchi K, et al: "Natural" light treatment of seasonal affective disorder. J Affect Disord 1996;37:109-120.

98. Zeitzer JM, Dijk DJ, Kronauer RE, et al: Sensitivity of the human circadian pacemaker to nocturnal light: Melatonin phase resetting and suppression. J Physiol (Lond) 2000;526:695-702.

99. Kronauer RE: A quantitative model for the effects of light on the amplitude and phase of the deep circadian pacemaker, based on human data. In Horne J (ed): Sleep '90, Proceedings of the Tenth European Congress on Sleep Research. Dusseldorf, Pontenagel Press, 1990, pp 306-309.

100. Jewett ME, Kronauer RE: Interactive mathematical models of subjective alertness and cognitive throughput in humans. J Biol Rhythms 1999 Dec;14:588-597.

101. Cole RJ, Kripke DF, Wisbey J, et al: Seasonal variation in human illumination exposure at two different latitudes. J Biol Rhythms 1995;10:324-334.

102. Okudaira N, Kripke DF, Webster JB: Naturalistic studies of human light exposure. Am J Physiol 1983;245:R613-R615.

103. Hébert M, Dumont M, Paquet J: Seasonal and diurnal patterns of human illumination under natural conditions. Chronobiol Int 1998;15:59-70.

104. Aschoff J: Circadian rhythms within and outside their ranges of entrainment. In Assenmacher I, Farner DS (eds): Environmental Endocrinology. Berlin, Springer-Verlag, 1978, pp 172-181.

105. Buxton OM, Lee CW, L'Hermite-Balériaux M, et al: Exercise elicits phase shifts and acute alterations of melatonin that vary with circadian phase. Am J Physiol Regul Integr Comp Physiol 2003;284:R714-R724.

106. Barger LK, Wright KP Jr, Hughes RJ, Czeisler CA: Daily exercise facilitates phase delays of circadian melatonin rhythm in very dim light. Am J Physiol Regul Integr Comp Physiol 2004;286(6):R1077-1084.

107. Buxton OM, L'Hermite-Balériaux M, Hirschfeld U, Van Cauter E: Acute and delayed effects of exercise on human melatonin secretion. J Biol Rhythms 1997;12:568-574.

108. Miyazaki T, Hashimoto S, Masubuchi S, et al: Phase-advance shifts of human circadian pacemaker are accelerated by daytime physical exercise. Am J Physiol Regul Integr Comp Physiol 2001;281:R197-R205.

109. Antle MC, Mistlberger RE: Circadian clock resetting by sleep deprivation without exercise in the Syrian hamster. J Neurosci 2000;20:9326-9332.

110. Dijk DJ, Czeisler CA: Paradoxical timing of the circadian rhythm of sleep propensity serves to consolidate sleep and wakefulness in humans. Neurosci Lett 1994;166:63-68.

111. Chiappa KH: Evoked Potentials in Clinical Medicine, 3rd ed. Philadelphia, Lippincott-Raven, 1997.

112. Åkerstedt T: Sleepiness as a consequence of shift work. Sleep 1988;11:17-34.

113. Borbély AA: A two process model of sleep regulation. Hum Neurobiol 1982;1:195-204.

114. Åkerstedt T, Folkard S, Portin C: Predictions from the three-process model of alertness. Aviat Space Environ Med 2004;75(3 Suppl):A75-83.

115. Wyatt JK, Ritz–De Cecco A, Czeisler CA, Dijk DJ: Circadian temperature and melatonin rhythms, sleep, and neurobehavioral function in humans living on a 20-h day. Am J Physiol 1999;277:R1152-R1163.

116. Czeisler CA, Dijk DJ: Human circadian physiology and sleep-wake regulation. In Takahashi JS, Turek FW, Moore RY (eds): Handbook of Behavioral Neurobiology: Circadian Clocks. New York, Plenum Publishing, 2001, 531-569.

117. Czeisler CA, Zimmerman JC, Ronda JM, et al: Timing of REM sleep is coupled to the circadian rhythm of body temperature in man. Sleep 1980;2:329-346.

118. Dijk DJ, Duffy JF, Czeisler CA: Circadian and sleep/wake dependent aspects of subjective alertness and cognitive performance. J Sleep Res 1992;1:112-117.

119. Dijk DJ, Edgar DM: Circadian and homeostatic control of wakefulness and sleep. In Turek FW, Zee PC, eds. Regulation of Sleep and Wakefulness. New York, Marcel Dekker, 1999, pp 111-147.

120. Czeisler CA, Guilleminault C: REM Sleep: Its Temporal Distribution. New York, Raven Press, 1980.

121. Carskadon MA, Dement WC: Sleep studies on a 90-minute day. Electroenceph Clin Neurophysiol 1975;39:145-155.

122. Weitzman ED, Nogeire C, Perlow M, et al: Effects of a prolonged 3-hour sleep-wake cycle on sleep stages, plasma cortisol, growth hormone, and body temperature in man. J Clin Endocrinol Metab 1974;38:1018-1030.

123. Czeisler CA, Weitzman ED, Moore-Ede MC, et al: Human sleep: Its duration and organization depend on its circadian phase. Science 1980;210:1264-1267.

124. Zimmerman JC, Czeisler CA, Laxminarayan S, et al: REM density is dissociated from REM sleep timing during free-running sleep episodes. Sleep 1980;2:409-415.

125. Klein T, Martens H, Dijk DJ, et al: Chronic non-24-hour circadian rhythm sleep disorder in a blind man with a regular 24-hour sleep-wake schedule. Sleep 1993;16:333-443.

126. Dijk DJ, Shanahan TL, Duffy JF, et al: Variation of electro-encephalographic activity during non-rapid eye movement and rapid eye movement sleep with phase of circadian melatonin rhythm in humans. J Physiol (Lond) 1997;505.3:851-858.

127. Lavie P: MelatonIn Role in gating nocturnal rise in sleep propensity. J Biol Rhythms 1997;12:657-665.

128. Shochat T, Luboshitzky R, Lavie P: Nocturnal melatonin onset is phase locked to the primary sleep gate. Am J Physiol 1997;273:R364-R370.

129. Dawson D, van den Heuvel CJ: Integrating the actions of melatonin on human physiology. Ann Med 1998;30:95-102.

130. Wu RH, Thorpy MJ: Effect of growth hormone treatment on sleep EEGs in growth hormone-deficient children. Sleep 1988;11:425-429.

131. Mendelson WB, Slater S, Gold P, Gillin JC: The effect of growth hormone administration on human sleep: A dose-response study. Biol Psychiatry 1980;15:613-618.

132. Aschoff J, Fatranská M, Giedke H, et al: Human circadian rhythms in continuous darkness: entrainment by social cues. Science 1971;171:213-215.

133. Wever R: Zur Zeitgeber-Stärke eines Licht-Dunkel-Wechsels für die circadiane Periodik des Menschen. Eur J Physiol 1970;321:133-142.

134. Klerman EB, Dijk DJ, Kronauer RE, Czeisler CA: Simulations of light effects on the human circadian pacemaker: implications for assessment of intrinsic period. Am J Physiol 1996;270:R271-R282.

135. Czeisler CA, Allan JS, Kronauer RE: A method for assaying the effects of therapeutic agents on the period of the endogenous circadian pacemaker in man. In Montplaisir J, Godbout R (eds): Sleep and Biological Rhythms: Basic Mechanisms and Applications to Psychiatry. New York, Oxford University Press, 1990, pp 87-98.

136. Czeisler CA, Duffy JF, Shanahan TL, et al: Stability, precision, and near-24-hour period of the human circadian pacemaker. Science 1999;284:2177-2181.

137. Campbell SS, Dawson D, Zulley J: When the human circadian system is caught napping: Evidence for endogenous rhythms close to 24 hours. Sleep 1993;16:638-640.

138. Middleton B, Arendt J, Stone BM: Complex effects of melatonin on human circadian rhythms in constant dim light. J Biol Rhythms 1997;12:467-477.

139. Middleton B, Arendt J, Stone BM: Human circadian rhythms in constant dim light (8 lux) with knowledge of clock time. J Sleep Res 1996;5:69-76.

140. Hiddinga AE, Beersma DG, van den Hoofdakker RH: Endogenous and exogenous components in the circadian variation of core body temperature in humans. J Sleep Res 1997;6:156-163.

141. Wright KP Jr, Hughes RJ, Kronauer RE, et al: Intrinsic near-24-hour pacemaker period determines limits of circadian entrainment to a weak synchronizer in humans. Proc Natl Acad Sci U S A 2001;98:14027-14032.

142. Campbell SS, Murphy PJ: Relationships between sleep and body temperature in middle-aged and older subjects. J Am Geriatr Soc 1998;46:458-462.

143. Copinschi G, Van Cauter E: Effects of ageing on modulation of hormonal secretions by sleep and circadian rhythmicity. Horm Res 1995;43:20-24.

144. Czeisler CA, Dumont M, Duffy JF, et al: Association of sleep-wake habits in older people with changes in output of circadian pacemaker. Lancet 1992;340:933-936.

145. Touitou Y, Bogdan A, Haus E, Touitou C: Modifications of circadian and circannual rhythms with aging. Exp Gerontol 1997;32:603-614.

146. Myers BL, Badia P: Changes in circadian rhythms and sleep quality with aging: Mechanisms and interventions. Neurosci Biobehav Rev 1995;19:553-571.

147. Bliwise DL: Sleep in normal aging and dementia. Sleep 1993;16:40-81.

148. Haimov I, Lavie P: Circadian characteristics of sleep propensity function in healthy elderly: A comparison with young adults. J Sleep Res 1996;5:82.

149. Monk TH, Buysse DJ, Reynolds III CF, et al: Subjective alertness rhythms in elderly people. J Biol Rhythms 1996;11:268-276.

150. Monk TH, Buysse DJ, Reynolds III CF, et al: Circadian temperature rhythms of older people. Exp Gerontol 1995;30:455-474.

151. Foley DJ, Monjan AA, Brown SL, et al: Sleep complaints among elderly persons: An epidemiologic study of three communities. Sleep 1995;18:425-432.

152. Duffy JF, Dijk DJ, Klerman EB, Czeisler CA: Later endogenous circadian temperature nadir relative to an earlier wake time in older people. Am J Physiol 1998;275:R1478-R1487.

153. Czeisler CA, Duffy JF, Shanahan TL, et al: Reassessment of the intrinsic period (τ) of the human circadian pacemaker in young and older subjects [abstract]. Sleep Res 1995;24A:505.

154. Dijk DJ, Duffy JF, Riel E, et al: Ageing and the circadian and homeostatic regulation of human sleep during forced desynchrony of rest, melatonin and temperature rhythms. J Physiol (Lond) 1999;516.2:611-627.

155. Wehr TA, Moul DE, Barbato G, et al: Conservation of photoperiod-responsive mechanisms in humans. Am J Physiol 1993;265:R846-R857.

156. Wehr TA, Giesen HA, Moul DE, et al: Suppression of men's responses to seasonal changes in day length by modern artificial lighting. Am J Physiol 1995;269:R173-R178.

157. Folkard S, Åkerstedt T: A three-process model of the regulation of alertness-sleepiness. In Broughton RJ, Ogilvie RD (eds): Sleep, Arousal, and Performance. Boston, Birkhäuser, 1992, pp 11-26.

158. Achermann P, Werth E, Dijk DJ, Borbély AA: Time course of sleep inertia after nighttime and daytime sleep episodes. Arch Ital Biol 1995;134:109-119.

159. Jewett ME, Wyatt JK, Ritz–De Cecco A, et al: Time course of sleep inertia dissipation in human performance and alertness. J Sleep Res 1999;8:1-8.

160. Cajochen C, Wyatt JK, Czeisler CA, et al: Non-linear interaction between the circadian and homeostatic modulation of slow eye movements during wakefulness in humans. J Sleep Res 2000;9(Suppl 1):29.

Melatonin in the Regulation of Sleep and Circadian Rhythms

Frank A. Scheer

Christian Cajochen

Fred W. Turek

Charles A. Czeisler

ABSTRACT

The pineal hormone melatonin is secreted primarily during the hours of darkness in all mammalian species. Melatonin secretion, which is driven by the suprachiasmatic nucleus, can be thought of as a neuroendocrine transducer of the light–dark cycle. In human beings, high levels of melatonin are present in the bloodstream during the normal time of sleep at night and low levels are present during the waking day. The endogenous circadian rhythm of melatonin secretion is closely associated with the endogenous rhythm of sleep propensity. Coupled with reports that exogenous melatonin administration can have sleep-promoting and phase-shifting effects, this has led to the hypothesis that melatonin might be useful in the treatment of insomnia and in the readjustment of daily rhythms. The purpose of this chapter is to summarize the current state of the scientific literature with respect to the use of melatonin for these purposes.

Insomnia—difficulty falling asleep or difficulty staying asleep—is likely to occur when individuals voluntarily choose to alter the timing of their sleep–wake schedule; in such cases, this can be due to rapid travel across time zones, inducing what is known as the *jet lag syndrome* (see Chapters 31 and 55), or to shift work schedules that require work at their usual sleep time, leaving only their usual wake time for sleep (see Chapters 31, 56, and 57).

The sleep–wake cycle is regulated primarily by two processes (see Chapters 31 and 33). The *circadian process* involves an internal near–24-hour clock (i.e., the circadian clock) that regulates the timing of sleep. The *homeostatic process* depends on the duration of prior wakefulness and the quality and duration of sleep episodes. Thus, an effective agent for the treatment of insomnia due to misalignment of circadian phase would be one that could (1) induce sleep when the homeostatic drive to sleep is insufficient to induce or maintain normal sleep (i.e., a *hypnotic* agent); (2) inhibit the drive for wakefulness emanating from the circadian pacemaker during the wake-propensity phase of the cycle (i.e., a *chronohypnotic* agent); or (3) induce phase shifts in the circadian clock regulating the sleep–wake cycle such that the circadian phase of increased sleep propensity occurs at a new, desired time (i.e., a *chronobiotic* agent). The evidence that melatonin can act as a hypnotic, a chronohypnotic, or a chronobiotic and the significance of this evidence for the use of melatonin to treat insomnia, shift work–related sleep difficulties, or jet lag are described in this chapter. The clinical pharmacology of melatonin and melatonin analogues is reviewed in Chapter 37.

CLINICAL IMPLICATIONS OF MELATONIN REGULATION

Nocturnal melatonin secretion from the pineal gland is under control of the suprachiasmatic nucleus (SCN), the circadian pacemaker, through a multisynaptic projection that includes the sympathetic nervous system.[1] Light at night causes a rapid suppression of melatonin concentrations.[2,3] It has recently been demonstrated that even ordinary room light (approximately 100 lux) can have a robust suppressive effect on plasma melatonin concentrations[4] (Fig. 32–1). These effects of light can be of direct clinical relevance; for example, even the seemingly innocuous behavior of reading in bed when unable to sleep may suppress endogenous melatonin[4] and may even lead to further disruption of sleep.[5] In addition to light, various drugs can influence the levels of melatonin at night. Beta-blockers, commonly used in the treatment of hypertension and cardiac arrhythmias, block sympathetic signaling not only to the heart but to the pineal gland. Beta-blockers can thus suppress nighttime melatonin levels, which might be involved in some of their side effects.[6,7] Drugs interacting with the metabolism of melatonin, such as fluvoxamine, can affect plasma melatonin levels.[8,9]

USE OF MELATONIN AS A SLEEP-PROMOTING AGENT

Evidence that treatment with melatonin can have sleep-promoting properties has come from studies on healthy volunteers to whom melatonin was administered (1) just before scheduled naps during the normal wake time (when endogenous melatonin levels are very low), or (2) several hours before the subjects' habitual bedtimes, during the circadian wake-maintenance zone[10,11] that occurs just before the nocturnal rise in endogenous melatonin levels (see Fig. 31–17 in Chapter 31; for reviews, see references 12 through 18).

Melatonin Effects on Sleep during the Biologic Day

There is a general consensus that melatonin in doses ranging from 0.3 to 80 mg has *somnogenic* properties when ingested

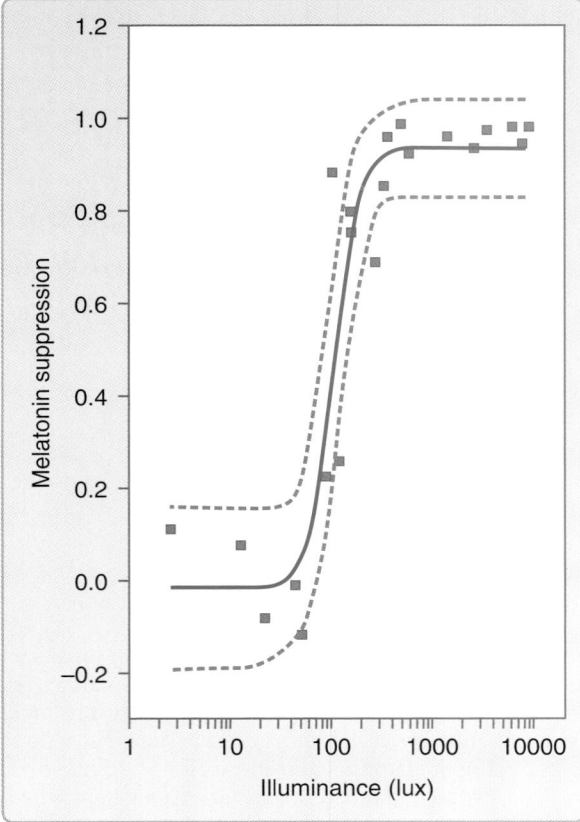

Figure 32–1. Illuminance–response curve for the acute suppression of plasma melatonin is demonstrated during a 6.5-hour pulse of light. Data have been fit with a four-parameter logistic model using a non-linear least-square analysis. The logistic models predict an inflection point of the curve (i.e., the sensitivity of the system) at ~200 lux. Individual subjects are represented by the *boxes*, the model by the *solid line*, and the 95% confidence intervals by the *dotted lines*. (Reproduced with permission from Zeitzer JM, Dijk DJ, Kronauer R, et al: Sensitivity of the human circadian pacemaker to nocturnal light: Melatonin phase resetting and suppression. J Physiol [Lond] 2000;526:695-702.)

throughout the biologic day, that is, during the entire phase in which endogenous melatonin levels are low.[15,17,19-22] Even when a low (0.3 mg) dose of melatonin was administered 1 hour before sleep episodes scheduled to begin at the peak of the circadian wake propensity rhythm, just several hours before habitual bedtime, sleep latency was significantly shortened.[23] Because of the high individual variability in the pharmacokinetics of melatonin, it is difficult to determine which of the aforementioned doses induces physiologic or supraphysiologic levels in a particular individual. In young subjects without sleep complaints, daytime melatonin administration increased self-rated sleepiness and improved sleep initiation as indexed by a reduction in polysomnographically measured sleep latency. This effect was dose dependent and paralleled by hypothermia.[21,24-26] Therefore, some investigators have suggested that melatonin-induced hypothermia may underlie a sleep-promoting action.[20,21,26-28] However, others have reported that the sleep-promoting influence of melatonin

is not just a secondary result of the suppression of core temperature.[29]

Most studies on the sleep-promoting effects of melatonin have been performed while subjects were lying down. However, body posture affects the somnogenic impact of melatonin. The effects of melatonin on both subjective and objective sleepiness are decreased when standing compared with lying down.[19]

In studies investigating the effects of daytime melatonin administration, the scheduled sleep durations have usually been short naps. For example, when subjects were not sleep deprived before a 2-hour nap, melatonin (3 and 6 mg) increased the amount of total sleep time in polygraphically recorded sleep episodes.[22,30] However, this effect appears to have resulted primarily from a decrease in sleep latency during this short nap. To assess the effects of exogenous melatonin on *sleep consolidation*, longer sleep opportunities (4 to 9 hours) are required. Improved sleep efficiency was observed during the last hour of a 4-hour daytime nap after 10 and 40 mg of melatonin.[21]

Some studies have investigated the effects of melatonin on *sleep architecture* during daytime sleep (i.e., the contribution of rapid eye movement [REM] sleep and non-REM [NREM] sleep to total sleep time). A number of studies have reported the suppression of daytime slow wave sleep (SWS, stages 3 and 4 of NREM sleep) after melatonin ingestion in doses of 1 to 250 mg.[21,31] This effect has been observed primarily in daytime sleep when melatonin was administered near the beginning of the scheduled sleep episode.

Quantitative analysis of the sleep electroencephalogram (EEG) has revealed that 5 mg of melatonin given shortly before a daytime sleep episode suppresses low-frequency EEG components and increases EEG activity in the sleep-spindle frequency range.[30,32] The effects of melatonin are, to some extent, similar to the changes induced by benzodiazepine hypnotics.[30,32] However, the effects of melatonin on sleep EEG spectra could not be blocked by flumazenil, which may indicate that the effects are not mediated by the gamma-aminobutyric acid type A receptor complex.

Melatonin Effects on Sleep during the Biologic Night

Inconsistent results have been obtained from studies on the effects of melatonin administered before sleep onset during the biologic night, when endogenous melatonin levels are normally elevated. A single dose of melatonin (5 mg) administered to healthy volunteers at 8:40 PM significantly enhanced not only *subjective sleepiness* during the wake-maintenance zone, but reduced *sleep latency* in the subsequent sleep episode at midnight. In contrast, when melatonin (1 and 5 mg) was administered later in the evening at 10:45 PM, 15 minutes before the lights were turned off, no reduction in sleep latency was observed.[33]

Several recent studies have investigated the effect of melatonin administration on nighttime *sleep consolidation*, with conflicting results. In subjects with primary insomnia, and older subjects with sleep-maintenance insomnia but without melatonin deficiency, 1 to 4 weeks of 0.3 to 5 mg near bedtime had no influence on actigraphic or polygraphic measures of sleep.[34,35] Also in a recent multicenter trial in 157 patients with Alzheimer's disease, no significant effect of 8 weeks of melatonin (1 hour before bedtime, 10 mg or 2.5 mg slow release) was found on actigraphic sleep measures, although trends were found for increased nocturnal total sleep time and reduced wake after sleep onset.[36] However, in studies in older subjects with insomnia and low endogenous melatonin concentrations, 1 to 3 weeks of supplementation 2 hours before bedtime with 2 mg immediate-release melatonin caused a shortening of sleep onset, whereas 2 mg of slow-release melatonin caused a reduction in wake after sleep onset[37] or an improvement of sleep maintenance.[38] The recent discovery of neurotransmitter disturbances of the SCN in patients with essential hypertension,[39] together with the earlier finding of a blunted melatonin rhythm in patients with coronary artery disease,[40] later replicated under more controlled light conditions,[41] led to the investigation of the potential beneficial effect of nighttime melatonin administration in patients with hypertension. A randomized, double-blinded, placebo-controlled, crossover study demonstrated that 3 weeks of nighttime melatonin (1 hour before bedtime, 2.5 mg) increased total sleep time and sleep efficiency as assessed by actigraphy in subjects with untreated essential hypertension.[42] Interestingly, a single melatonin administration was unable to influence sleep. Similarly, in an earlier study, a longer duration of melatonin treatment (2 months) resulted in a significant additional improvement in sleep quality and sleep onset latency compared with a shorter duration (1 week) of treatment in older patients with insomnia and low endogenous melatonin levels.[38] Furthermore, it has been shown that melatonin can have a carryover effect, in that sleep quality is improved several days to weeks after discontinuation of melatonin treatment.[43] Together, these data indicate that nighttime melatonin administration does not lose its efficacy after repeated use from the development of tolerance, as happens with some conventional hypnotics (e.g., benzodiazepine),[44] and that *nighttime* melatonin administration may rather gain in efficacy after repeated use.

A number of studies have investigated the effects of melatonin on *sleep architecture* during the biologic night. In general, during nocturnal sleep, melatonin administration resulted in an increase in REM sleep duration. After melatonin (5 mg) administration either 5 or 3 hours before nocturnal sleep, the first REM sleep episode was markedly lengthened.[5,45] These effects are consistent with earlier experiments in which higher doses of melatonin were administered (for a review, see Zhdanova and Wurtman[18]). A potential clinical value of this effect was recently indicated in a study in which 3 mg melatonin between 22:00 and 23:00 for 4 weeks significantly increased the REM sleep percentage in patients with reduced REM sleep duration.[43] For SWS at the biologic nighttime, 5 mg melatonin administered 3:20 hours before scheduled bedtime in healthy subjects caused an initial suppression during the first NREM sleep episode, followed by a rebound increase in SWS during the second NREM sleep episode.[5]

REM sleep propensity, but not SWS propensity, is mainly under circadian control, peaking around the time of the core body temperature minimum.[46] Whether the specific REM sleep–stimulating effect of melatonin might be related to effects of melatonin directly on the circadian pacemaker is not known.

The effects of melatonin on quantitative sleep EEG, as seen during the biologic day, were not observed when melatonin (5 mg) was administered 5 hours before the nighttime sleep episode in healthy subjects,[19] even though melatonin levels were pharmacologically high at the time of sleep onset.

Implications

Melatonin is a natural hormone that partially fits the definition of a hypnotic because it induces sleepiness and facilitates sleep. Unlike the benzodiazepine hypnotics, melatonin is not a tranquilizer in the classic sense of a sedative drug, and there is little evidence for any anxiolytic characteristics. Some have even considered melatonin to be a *soporific* (to make drowsy, sleepy, preparing for sleep) rather than a hypnotic per se.[47] This may be because the hypnotic effects of melatonin are time dependent, showing stronger efficacy during the daytime. Furthermore, as discussed, *nighttime* melatonin administration may gain in efficacy after repeated daily use, in contrast to benzodiazepine hypnotics. Evidence from studies in both day-active animals[48] and humans[46,49] that the circadian pacemaker promotes wakefulness at certain times of day, together with evidence that mammalian SCN neuronal firing is inhibited by SCN mel1a receptor–specific melatonin binding,[50] have led to the hypothesis that melatonin may act to facilitate sleep by inhibiting the circadian drive for waking that emanates from the SCN.[15,17,51] If this hypothesis were proven to be correct, we propose that it would be more appropriate to classify the action of melatonin as a chronohypnotic, rather than as simply a hypnotic.

Of course, if the sleep-promoting action of melatonin were indeed stronger during sleep episodes in the biologic daytime, when endogenous melatonin levels are low, than during sleep episodes in the biologic nighttime, when endogenous melatonin levels are normally higher, this would call for a tailored approach when applying melatonin administration as a treatment of insomnia.

Older subjects complaining of insomnia have reduced motor activity at night after daily treatment with both high and low doses of melatonin just before bedtime.[37,52,53] The potential use of melatonin for treating sleep–wake disorders in older people is a particularly attractive hypothesis because disturbed sleep becomes more prevalent with age,[54-56] and melatonin levels may be significantly lower in older insomniac patients than in age-matched control subjects.[52] These findings call for further polysomnographic studies to investigate the potential beneficial effects of nighttime melatonin administration on the quality and quantity of sleep in older subjects with insomnia.

Recently, a number of polysomnographic sleep studies have been performed to investigate the effects of melatonin as a hypnotic or chronohypnotic in people with insomnia. In older subjects with sleep-maintenance insomnia, 0.5 mg melatonin taken either 30 minutes before bedtime (as an immediate-release or controlled-release formula) or 4 hours after bedtime for 2 weeks, all reduced sleep onset latency, without effect on other sleep parameters.[57] In addition, in subjects older than 50 years of age with insomnia and low endogenous melatonin levels, 0.1, 0.3, and 3 mg melatonin 30 minutes before bedtime for a week significantly increased sleep efficiency but had no effects on sleep onset latency or total sleep time.[29]

If insomniac patients or even a subset of them prove to be melatonin deficient, as has been reported,[29,58,59] then there would at least be a rationale for nocturnal melatonin administration. Although there is no clear link between low endogenous melatonin levels and insomnia per se,[29,57] melatonin may be most promising in treating insomnia associated with reduced nocturnal melatonin secretion due to age, disease, or medication,[29,37,59a] and may even be able to facilitate discontinuation of chronic benzodiazepine use.[60]

In children with various developmental disorders, melatonin (0.3 to 5.0 mg) has also been reported to promote sleep.[61-63] Sleep onset especially was found to be improved, which may be due to the chronohypnotic effect of melatonin. However, the phase advance of the endogenous melatonin rhythm[63] and the continuation of improved sleep after discontinuation of melatonin in some children[62] provide support for the involvement of a chronobiotic effect of melatonin, resetting the circadian pacemaker.

Overall, melatonin may be most effective in inducing sleep during the biologic day. Acutely (after single administration), the *chronohypnotic* effect of melatonin administration may facilitate sleep during the biologic day, whereas repeated administration near the desired bedtime may facilitate entrainment to the light–dark cycle because of its *chronobiotic* effect (see next section). This may be desirable for people experiencing jet lag, during shift work, for individuals with delayed sleep phase syndrome, and blind people who are not entrained to the light–dark cycle. In all of these conditions, the biologic night does not coincide with the desired sleep episode. Melatonin may facilitate daytime sleep for night shift workers, as indicated by a simulated night shift study in which 1.8 mg slow-release melatonin facilitated polysomnographic sleep during the first daytime sleep opportunity after an 8-hour night shift, although it was ineffective during the second daytime sleep opportunity.[64] Also in misaligned blind subjects, it has recently been shown that a single administration of 5 mg melatonin 1 hour before schedule bedtime could increase total sleep time, sleep efficiency, and REM sleep, together with a normalization of the adrenocorticotropic hormone and cortisol rhythm.[65] The combination of both sleep-promoting and phase-shifting effects (discussed later) may make melatonin especially promising in the treatment of sleep disorders due to circadian misalignment.

As noted previously, although a number of studies have examined the effects of melatonin as a hypnotic under a variety of different conditions and dosing regimes, large-scale, carefully controlled studies have not been performed. The lack of such studies is due in part to the fact that melatonin cannot be patented. As a result, a few promising melatonin agonists have been developed and are in various stages of clinical testing for their hypnotic and chronobiotic properties.

USE OF MELATONIN AS A CHRONOBIOTIC

A *chronobiotic* is defined as a chemical substance capable of therapeutically reentraining short-term dissociated or long-term desynchronized circadian rhythms or prophylactically preventing their disruption after an environmental insult.[66] It has been known for a number of years that treatment with melatonin in a variety of animal species can induce phase shifts and entrain the circadian clock underlying the expression of multiple 24-h rhythms (for reviews, see Czeisler et al.[12] and Redman[67]). In addition, melatonin is a major entraining signal for the circadian systems of fetal and neonatal mammals (for a review, see Davis[68]). Daily exposure to circulating

melatonin allows fetuses to be synchronized with each other and with their mother long before they are able directly to perceive the environmental light–dark cycle. Overall, the animal literature does support a role of melatonin as a chronobiotic. The next concern is whether melatonin administration can shift circadian phase or entrain circadian rhythms in human beings.

Phase Shifting

The findings that the human SCN contains a high concentration of melatonin receptors[69] and that melatonin exerts circadian actions at the SCN in vitro[70] support the possibility that melatonin may have direct phase-shifting effects on the human circadian clock. There are intriguing studies showing that a single or repeated daily treatment with a near-physiologic dose of melatonin can induce phase delays or phase advances in human circadian rhythms, with the direction for the phase shift dependent on the time of administration.[71-73] This has led to a number of hypotheses regarding the possible use of melatonin for treating disorders of circadian timekeeping, including those related to insomnia and jet lag. Unfortunately, light exposure, known to exert a phase-shifting effect on the circadian pacemaker, which is an order of magnitude more powerful than that reported for melatonin, was not controlled or too high (greater than 50 lux) during (part of) the wake periods in those resetting trials. However, in a double-blinded, placebo-controlled, crossover study in which subjects were studied under dim light (less than 10 lux) and constant posture conditions, a single melatonin dose (5 mg) administered at 6:00 PM induced an advance of the circadian nocturnal decline in core body temperature, heart rate, and the dim light melatonin onset as assessed on the second day (more than 24 hours) after melatonin administration.[74] Furthermore, a double-blinded, crossover study in dim light in which daytime administration of 1.5 mg melatonin at the start of scheduled 16-hour sleep opportunities (4 PM until 8 AM) for 8 days resulted in a phase advance of both melatonin and cortisol (by approximately 5 and 4 hours, respectively).[75] The simultaneous phase shifting of various different circadian-regulated variables lends strong support to the notion that melatonin actually shifts the phase of the circadian pacemaker itself.

Conflicting results on melatonin's capacity to induce phase *delays* have been found between two randomized, double-blinded, placebo-controlled trials under controlled light conditions. At 7:00 AM, melatonin in doses between 0.05 and 5 mg caused a dose-dependent phase delay of the onset of melatonin secretion in one study,[76] whereas no effect was found in a study with a 5-mg melatonin administration at 7:00 AM.[77] The authors of the latter study also suggest that the use of 5 mg of melatonin may have resulted in plasma melatonin remaining high for many hours, leading to "spillover" into the phase advance portion for melatonin, which could counteract any phase delay. This may explain why a clear phase delay was found with a 0.5-mg melatonin dose.[73] On the other hand, uncontrolled light conditions in most studies complicate interpretation. Well-controlled studies under dim light conditions are needed to establish the effects of melatonin at different circadian phases, thus creating a phase–response curve, and to establish conclusively the ability of melatonin to phase delay the circadian pacemaker.

Overall, melatonin seems more reliably to elicit phase advances than phase delays.

Entrainment

From algae to humans, periodic environmental stimuli normally synchronize (or entrain) the non–24-hour intrinsic period of endogenous circadian rhythms to a period of exactly 24 hours. In contrast to the periodic light–dark cycle—which is the primary signal by which the human circadian pacemaker is synchronized—melatonin obviously does not represent a periodic external environmental stimulus. However, melatonin feeds back onto melatonin receptors in the SCN,[69] the brain site of the circadian clock, and therefore may play an important role as a synchronizer of the internal environment and in modulating the synchronizing effects of the light–dark cycle.

It has been demonstrated that daily melatonin treatment can entrain totally blind people who are not entrained to the 24-hour-day while living in society. The first convincing demonstration of entrainment by melatonin was by a placebo-controlled, single-blinded study in which three of seven subjects entrained to a 5-mg fast-release dose administered at 21:00 hours[78] (Fig. 32–2). This finding was later confirmed in a placebo-controlled, single-blinded study using a 10-mg dose administered approximately 1 hour before bedtime.[79] In the latter study, it was furthermore demonstrated that once the subject was entrained, the melatonin dose could be gradually reduced to 0.5 mg without disrupting entrainment. More recent studies have shown that de novo 0.5-mg doses of melatonin in the late evening are as effective as 5- or 10-mg doses in entraining free-running circadian rhythms.[80-82]

Because most totally blind people free-run with a period longer than 24 hours,[83] melatonin should be timed to induce a phase advance in order to entrain (i.e., between approximately 8 hours before to 4 hours after the plasma melatonin onset). This critical time window may explain the earlier

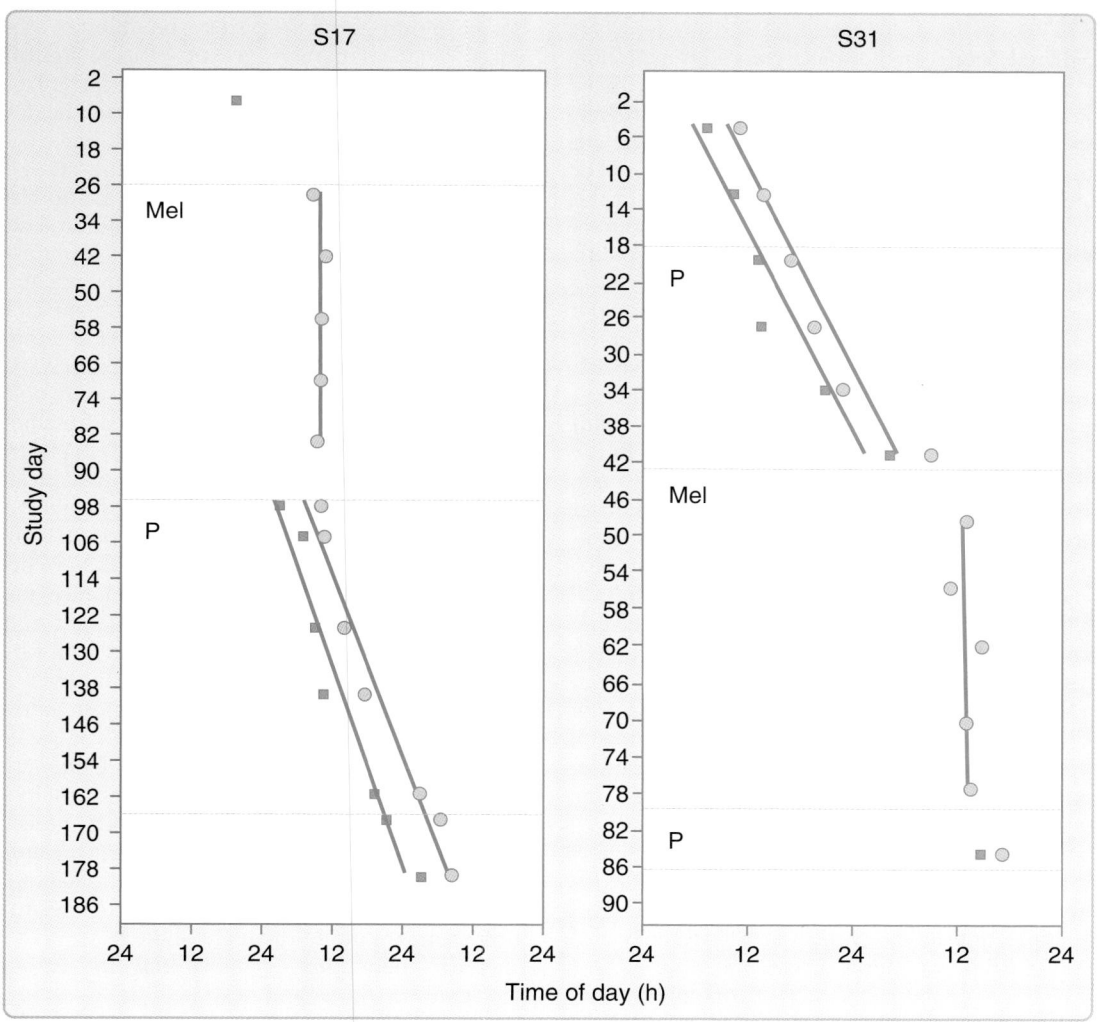

Figure 32–2. Melatonin can entrain the circadian rhythm in blind people. Peak times of the circadian phase markers are shown for two subjects who entrained during melatonin treatment (S17, S31). Melatonin was administered at 21:00. Study days are shown on the vertical axis and the time of day is shown as a continuous sequence along the horizontal axis. Best-fit regression lines during each treatment are plotted for the 6-sulfatoxy melatonin (*filled squares*) and cortisol (*circles*) data. Duration of the placebo (P) and melatonin (Mel) treatment is shown by the *horizontal lines*. (Reproduced with permission from Lockley SW, Skene DJ, James K, et al: Melatonin administration can entrain the free-running circadian system of blind subjects. J Endocrinol 2000;164:R1-R6.)

variability of success in entraining free-running individuals with melatonin application.[12,84] Whether the timing of the *initial* dose of melatonin affects subsequent entrainment has been the matter of some debate,[78,81,85] and may be related to dose. Previous failures to entrain with higher doses (5 to 20 mg) have been ascribed to a spillover effect of higher doses remaining in circulation during both the advance and delay zones of the melatonin phase–response curve, thereby reducing the net phase shift and compromising entrainment.[85,86]

Whereas light can be used in most circadian rhythm disorders to realign circadian rhythms to the desired sleep–wake schedule (such as in jet lag, delayed sleep phase syndrome, and shift work), it cannot be used as such in those blind people who lack photic input to the SCN. Therefore, melatonin may be of special value for the treatment of circadian misalignment in the blind. Indeed, the ability of melatonin to entrain the circadian rhythms of some blind people has convincingly been demonstrated.[78,79] The implications for other circadian sleep disorders are discussed in the next section.

Implications

As discussed, there is evidence that melatonin administration alone is able to elicit phase advances in various circadian rhythm markers, including its own endogenous rhythm, although the phase-resetting effects of the light–dark cycle are more powerful than those observed thus far for melatonin. For the chronobiotic properties of melatonin to be useful in the treatment of insomnia, the underlying cause of the insomnia would need to be due to an abnormal timing of sleep with respect to circadian phase.

Such abnormal timing occurs in what is known as the *delayed sleep phase syndrome* (DSPS), in which sleep occurs at a delayed clock time relative to the light–dark cycle and social, economic, and family demands[87] (see Chapter 58). Although originally described in adults,[88] DSPS often begins in childhood and is relatively common among adolescents.[89,90] In the first use of melatonin in patients with DSPS, melatonin (5 mg, 5 hours before sleep onset for 4 weeks) advanced sleep onset and wake times compared with placebo.[91] Although the sample size in this study was small ($N = 8$), a similar study, also with a small sample size ($N = 7$), produced similar results.[92] A study with a larger sample size confirmed the result of the first placebo-controlled study[91] in showing that melatonin induces an advance in sleep onset in patients with DSPS.[93] In a recent placebo-controlled polysomnographic study in patients with DSPS, it was further shown that 4 weeks administration of 5 mg melatonin in the evening not only shortened sleep onset latency and increased total sleep time, but suppressed the feeling of fatigue and sleepiness during the wake episode.[94] These initial studies indicate that melatonin may be an effective treatment for this specific sleep disorder. Furthermore, as reported for blind people, the therapeutic effectiveness of melatonin administration in the patient with DSPS may also be due to its acute sleep-promoting effects.

In contrast to the timing of sleep in DSPS, one of the most common sleep complaints in older people is that the timing of sleep onset or offset is advanced.[95] In principle, if melatonin were effective in delaying the circadian clock that times the sleep–wake cycle, it could perhaps normalize the timing of sleep in older insomniac patients who have an advanced circadian cycle; however, to date, no such studies have been reported.

However, as discussed, the evidence for the phase-delaying capacity of melatonin is inconclusive. More important, the predicted phase delays would require melatonin administration in the morning. Thus, treatment of older subjects who have a phase-advanced sleep–wake cycle with melatonin in the morning hours might be counterproductive if it were to act also as a chronohypnotic or as a soporific at wake time. There clearly are many issues that relate to the appropriate timing of melatonin treatment for its use in insomnia associated with alterations in the timing of the sleep–wake cycle in older people that need to be addressed in large clinical trials before any recommendations can be made for its use in such patients.

A number of studies have attempted to use melatonin to alleviate the perceived effects of jet lag (primarily sleep disturbances; see also Chapter 55). Indeed, one laboratory has reported that in a population of 474 subjects taking melatonin versus 112 subjects taking placebo (both placebo-controlled and uncontrolled with no statistical difference between these), there is an overall 50% reduction in self-rated jet lag, and it was hypothesized that at least part of the beneficial effects of melatonin for jet lag may be due to a phase-shifting effect.[71,96,97] In a more recent placebo-controlled, double-blinded trial on the effect of melatonin on jet lag symptoms in 257 physicians, no beneficial effects could be demonstrated.[98] The absence of a significant effect might have been due to the absence of full entrainment before the start of this study. Indeed, in a recent review of 10 randomized, placebo-controlled trials on the efficacy of melatonin to alleviate jet lag symptoms, a clear beneficial effect was demonstrated in 8 of the 10 trials.[99] The authors conclude that melatonin was most effective when taken after an eastward flight and at the target bedtime of the destination. Furthermore, a 5-mg dose seemed to be more effective than a 0.5-mg dose, without further improvement at higher dosages. However, objective assessment of circadian phase markers or of sleep efficiency was not conducted in most jet lag studies, and it is not clear whether the beneficial effect evident from the subjective data was due to a hypnotic, chronohypnotic, or chronobiotic effect of melatonin. Nevertheless, based on the reported phase–response curve to melatonin, elaborate timetables have been developed to advise travelers when they should take melatonin after eastward and westward travel over different numbers of time zones.[96,97] One difficulty in using melatonin for jet lag is that its use as a chronobiotic may require administration at times when it will have undesired (chrono)hypnotic properties (i.e., after a westward flight).[96,97,100]

Similar to reentrainment to the light–dark cycle of a different time zone, melatonin may also help in facilitating reentrainment to a different work shift. Indeed, in a night work–simulating study, 0.5 mg and 3 mg melatonin for 4 days taken at a 7-hour–advanced bedtime facilitated the phase adjustment of the circadian rhythm of melatonin and core body temperature to the night shift.[101]

With the ability of melatonin to entrain misaligned circadian rhythms and also to amplify blunted circadian rhythms,[72,102,103] melatonin may be applicable for diseases with an underlying circadian disturbance. Recently, it has been shown that levels of three important SCN neurotransmitters, including vasopressin, are suppressed by 50% in patients with hypertension compared with normotensive subjects, suggesting functional impairment of the SCN in people with hypertension.[39] Together with the recent demonstration that the SCN is involved in the regulation of the cardiovascular system through the autonomic nervous system[104-107] (for a review, see Scheer et al.[108]), this led to the investigation of whether repeated bedtime melatonin administration might lower blood pressure in patients with essential hypertension. In a randomized, double-blinded, placebo-controlled, crossover study it was demonstrated that 3-week administration of 2.5 mg 1 hour before schedule bedtime caused a significant reduction in nighttime blood pressure of 6 mm Hg systolic and 4 mm Hg diastolic in 16 patients with untreated essential hypertension[42] (Fig. 32–3). Interestingly, a single melatonin capsule 1 hour before bedtime had no effect on blood pressure during the following 24 hours. This indicates that melatonin has a different mode of action than directly acting vasodilator drugs (e.g., alpha-adrenergic receptor antagonists) that cause an acute drop in blood pressure. As discussed earlier, 3-week melatonin administration also caused a significant increase in total sleep time and sleep efficiency as assessed by actigraphy in these patients.[42] No correlation was found between the change in sleep parameters and the change in nocturnal blood pressure assessed during the same nights of recording. Still, long-term changes in sleep quality may have participated in a reduction in blood pressure. Before its clinical use can be justified, larger studies will

be required to define the characteristics of the patients who would benefit most from nighttime melatonin application. Studies applying circadian protocols could also reveal whether a change in the autonomic or neuroendocrine circadian rhythm output of the SCN underlies the observed changes in sleep and blood pressure.

CONCLUSIONS

Data from studies in human beings indicate that melatonin has sleep-inducing properties that are less consistent when administration follows the evening endogenous melatonin rise. There also is evidence that melatonin may induce phase shifts in human circadian rhythms. If this were the case, melatonin could be useful for the treatment of insomnia and jet lag. In addition, it has recently been suggested that melatonin might also be used to amplify circadian rhythms. Indeed, the combined circadian and chronohypnotic effects of melatonin could make it an attractive candidate for the treatment of sleep disorders related to inappropriate circadian timing. Carefully controlled clinical trials that focus on the possible beneficial effects of melatonin on specific sleep and circadian rhythm disorders are urgently needed. Furthermore, issues that relate to dose of melatonin, method of delivery, time of delivery, number of deliveries, pharmacologic profile, and the

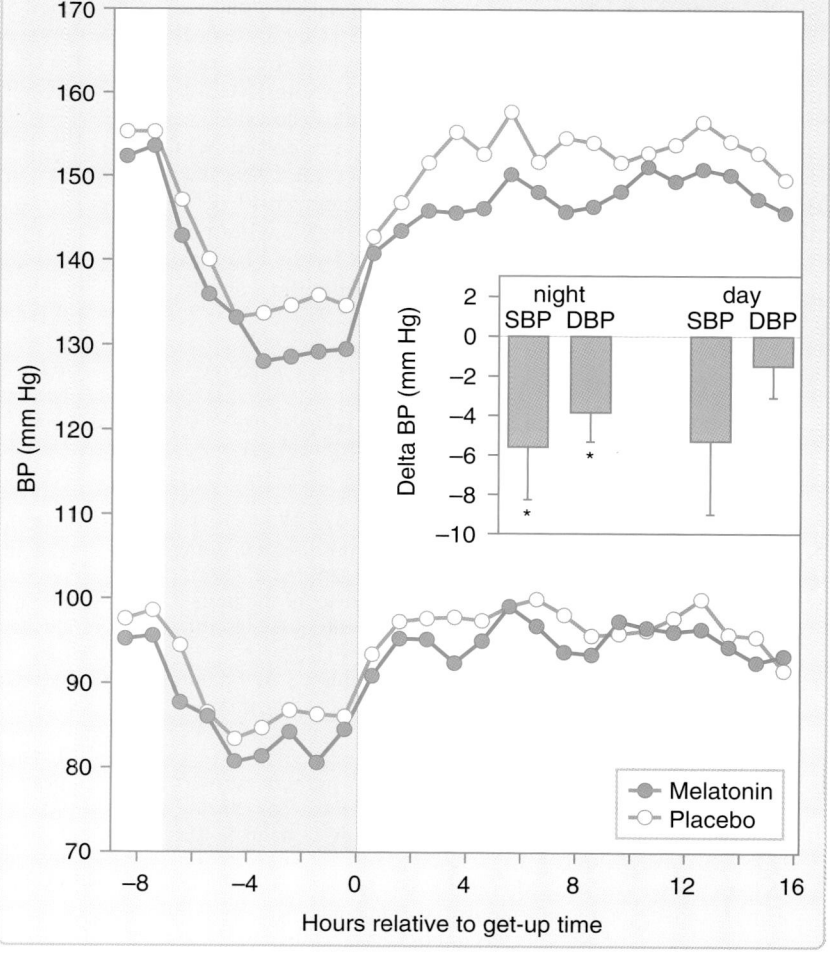

Figure 32–3. Daily nighttime melatonin reduces blood pressure (BP) in hypertensive subjects. Hourly means of systolic (SBP) and diastolic (DBP) ambulatory blood pressure are plotted relative to get-up time (vertical line) after 3-week melatonin and 3-week placebo administration in 16 patients with essential hypertension. Melatonin/placebo was administered 1 hour before schedule bedtime in a double-blinded, crossover design. The light blue background indicates the average period in bed (7.1 hours ± 44 minutes). Inset: Effect of repeated melatonin administration on SBP and DBP at night and during the day. Zero values indicate the levels assessed after placebo. *Significant difference compared with placebo treatment. (Modified from Scheer FAJL, Van Montfrans GA, van Someren EJW, et al: Daily nighttime melatonin reduces nighttime blood pressure in male patients with essential hypertension. Hypertension 2004;43:192-197.)

like should be examined because they are relevant to specific sleep and circadian rhythm disorders. The availability of newly developed melatonin agonists that are being tested in large-scale clinical trials may lead to improved understanding of how effective and safe melatonin-related agonists are for the treatment of sleep or circadian disorders.

> ### Clinical Pearls
>
> *During the daytime, physiologic and pharmacologic doses of melatonin have somnogenic properties, whereas during the nighttime, the effects of melatonin are inconsistent, and may depend on dose, time, and number of deliveries, type of insomnia, and endogenous melatonin production.*
>
> *Melatonin can phase advance the circadian pacemaker when administered during the evening, whereas the phase-delaying properties of melatonin when administered in the morning are disputed.*
>
> *Melatonin can serve as a primary entrainment factor in blind people who cannot be entrained by light. Melatonin can also facilitate reentrainment to a new sleep–wake schedule (i.e., shift work and jet lag after eastward flight).*

Acknowledgments

The authors thank Dr. Rod J. Hughes for his helpful comments on this manuscript. This work was supported in part by grants from the National Institute on Aging (NIA-P01-AG09975 and NIA-1-U01-12642), the National Aeronautics and Space Administration, and the National Space Biomedical Research Institute. Frank A. Scheer was supported by a grant from the National Heart, Lung, and Blood Institute (NHLBI-R01-HL64815) and by a Cephalon Clinical Fellowship in Circadian Medicine. Christian Cajochen was supported by a Swiss National Science Foundation postdoctoral fellowship (823A-046640). Some portions of a White Paper entitled "Is Melatonin a Treatment for Insomnia and Jet Lag?," written by C. A. Czeisler and F. W. Turek and published by the National Sleep Foundation, are included here with permission from the publisher.

References

1. Teclemariam-Mesbah R, Ter Horst GJ, Postema F, et al: Anatomical demonstration of the suprachiasmatic nucleus-pineal pathway. J Comp Neurol 1999;406:171-182.
2. Klein DC, Weller JL: Rapid light-induced decrease in pineal serotonin N-acetyltransferase activity. Science 1972;177:532-533.
3. Lewy AJ, Wehr TA, Goodwin FK, et al: Light suppresses melatonin secretion in humans. Science 1980;210:1267-1269.
4. Zeitzer JM, Dijk DJ, Kronauer RE, et al: Sensitivity of the human circadian pacemaker to nocturnal light: Melatonin phase resetting and suppression. J Physiol (Lond) 2000;526:695-702.
5. Cajochen C, Kräuchi K, Danilenko KV, Wirz-Justice A: Evening administration of melatonin and bright light: Interactions on the EEG during sleep and wakefulness. J Sleep Res 1998;7:145-157.
6. Arendt J, Bojkowski C, Franey C, et al: Immunoassay of 6-hydroxymelatonin sulfate in human plasma and urine: Abolition of the urinary 24-hour rhythm with atenolol. J Clin Endocrinol Metab 1985;60:1166-1172.
7. VanDen Heuvel CJ, Reid KJ, Dawson D: Effect of atenolol on nocturnal sleep and temperature in young men: Reversal by pharmacological doses of melatonin. Physiol Behav 1997;61:795-802.
8. Facciolá G, Hidestrand M, von Bahr C, Tybring G: Cytochrome P450 isoforms involved in melatonin metabolism in human liver microsomes. Eur J Pharmacol 2001;56:881-888.
9. Härtter S, Grözinger M, Weigmann H, et al: Increased bioavailability of oral melatonin after fluvoxamine coadministration. Clin Pharmacol Ther 2000;67:1-6.
10. Lavie P: Ultrashort sleep-waking schedule: III. "Gates" and "forbidden zones" for sleep. Electroencephalogr Clin Neurophysiol 1986;63:414-425.
11. Strogatz SH, Kronauer RE, Czeisler CA: Circadian pacemaker interferes with sleep onset at specific times each day: Role in insomnia. Am J Physiol 1987;253:R172-R178.
12. Czeisler CA, Turek FW: Melatonin, sleep, and circadian rhythms: Current progress and controversies. J Biol Rhythms 1997;12:485-708.
13. Cajochen C, Kräuchi K, Wirz-Justice A: Role of melatonin in the regulation of human circadian rhythms and sleep. J Neuroendocrinol 2003;15:432-437.
14. Dijk DJ, Cajochen C: Melatonin and the circadian regulation of sleep initiation, consolidation, structure, and the sleep EEG. J Biol Rhythms 1997;12:627-635.
15. Lavie P: Melatonin: Role in gating nocturnal rise in sleep propensity. J Biol Rhythms 1997;12:657-665.
16. Mendelson WB: Efficacy of melatonin as a hypnotic agent. J Biol Rhythms 1997;12:651-656.
17. Sack RL, Hughes RJ, Edgar DM, Lewy AJ: Sleep-promoting effects of melatonin: At what dose, in whom, under what conditions, and by what mechanisms? Sleep 1997;20:908-915.
18. Zhdanova IV, Wurtman RJ: Efficacy of melatonin as a sleep-promoting agent. J Biol Rhythms 1997;12:644-650.
19. Cajochen C, Kräuchi K, Wirz-Justice A: The acute soporific action of daytime melatonin administration: Effects on the EEG during wakefulness and subjective alertness. J Biol Rhythms 1997;12:636-643.
20. Dawson D, Encel N: Melatonin and sleep in humans. J Pineal Res 1993;15:1-12.
21. Hughes RJ, Badia P: Sleep-promoting and hypothermic effects of daytime melatonin administration in humans. Sleep 1997;20:124-131.
22. Nave R, Peled R, Lavie P: Melatonin improves evening napping. Eur J Pharmacol 1995;275:213-216.
23. Zhdanova IV, Wurtman RJ, Morabito C, et al: Effects of low oral doses of melatonin, given 2-4 hours before habitual bedtime, on sleep in normal young humans. Sleep 1996;19:423-431.
24. Dollins AB, Zhdanova IV, Wurtman RJ, et al: Effect of inducing nocturnal serum melatonin concentrations in daytime on sleep, mood, body temperature, and performance. Proc Natl Acad Sci U S A 1994;91:1824-1828.
25. Deacon S, Arendt J: Melatonin-induced temperature suppression and its acute phase-shifting effects correlate in a dose-dependent manner in humans. Brain Res 1995;688:77-85.
26. Kräuchi K, Cajochen C, Wirz-Justice A: A relationship between heat loss and sleepiness: Effects of postural change and melatonin administration. J Appl Physiol 1997;83:134-139.
27. Holmes AL, Gilbert SS, Dawson D: Melatonin and zopiclone: The relationship between sleep propensity and body temperature. Sleep 2002;25:301-306.
28. Badia P, Myers BL, Murphy PJ: Melatonin and thermoregulation. In Reiter RJ, Yu HS (eds): Melatonin: Biosynthesis, Physiological Effects, and Clinical Applications. Boca Raton, Fla, CRC Press, 1992, pp 349-364.
29. Zhdanova IV, Wurtman RJ, Regan MM, et al: Melatonin treatment for age-related insomnia. J Clin Endocrinol Metab 2001;86:4727-4730.
30. Nave R, Herer P, Haimov I, et al: Hypnotic and hypothermic effects of melatonin on daytime sleep in humans: Lack of antagonism by flumazenil. Neurosci Lett 1996;23:123-126.

31. Anton-Tay F, Diaz J, Fernandez-Guardiola A: On the effect of melatonin upon human brains possible therapeutic implications. Life Sci 1971;10:841-850.

32. Dijk DJ, Roth C, Landolt HP, et al: Melatonin effect on daytime sleep in men: Suppression of EEG low frequency activity and enhancement of spindle frequency activity. Neurosci Lett 1995;201:13-16.

33. James SP, Mendelson WB, Sack DA, et al: The effect of melatonin on normal sleep. Neuropsychopharmacology 1987;1:41-44.

34. Baskett JJ, Broad JB, Wood PC, et al: Does melatonin improve sleep in older people? A randomised crossover trial. Age Ageing 2003;32:164-170.

35. Almeda Montes LG, Ontiveros Uribe MP, CortésSotres J, Heinze Martin G: Treatment of primary insomnia with melatonin: A double-blind, placebo-controlled, crossover study. J Psychiatry Neurosci 2003;28:191-196.

36. Singer C, Tractenberg RE, Kaye J, et al: A multicenter, placebo-controlled trial of melatonin for sleep disturbance in Alzheimer's disease. Sleep 2003;26:893-901.

37. Garfinkel D, Laudon M, Nof D, Zisapel N: Improvement of sleep quality in elderly people by controlled-release melatonin. Lancet 1995;346:541-544.

38. Haimov I, Lavie P, Laudon M, et al: Melatonin replacement therapy of elderly insomniacs. Sleep 1995;18:598-603.

39. Goncharuk VD, van Heerikhuize J, Dai JP, et al: Neuropeptide changes in the suprachiasmatic nucleus in primary hypertension indicate functional impairment of the biological clock. J Comp Neurol 2001;431:320-330.

40. Brugger P, Marktl W, Herold M: Impaired nocturnal secretion of melatonin in coronary heart disease. Lancet 1995;345:1408.

41. Sakotnik A, Liebmann PM, Stoschitzky K, et al: Decreased melatonin synthesis in patients with coronary artery disease. Eur Heart J 1999;20:1314-1317.

42. Scheer FA, Van Montfrans GA, Van Someren EJ, et al: Daily nighttime melatonin reduces blood pressure in male patients with essential hypertension. Hypertension 2004;43:192-197.

43. Kunz D, Mahlberg R, Müller C, et al: Melatonin in patients with reduced REM sleep duration: Two randomized controlled trials. J Clin Endocrinol Metab 2004;89:128-134.

44. Gilbert SS, Burgess HJ, Kennaway DJ, Dawson D: Attenuation of sleep propensity, core hypothermia, and peripheral heat loss after temazepam tolerance. Am J Physiol 2000;279:R1980-R1987.

45. Cajochen C, Kräuchi K, Möri D, et al: Melatonin and S-20098 increase REM sleep and wake-up propensity without modifying NREM sleep homeostasis. Am J Physiol 1997;272:R1189-R1196.

46. Dijk DJ, Czeisler CA: Contribution of the circadian pacemaker and the sleep homeostat to sleep propensity, sleep structure, electroencephalographic slow waves, and sleep spindle activity in humans. J Neurosci 1995;15:3526-3538.

47. Wirz-Justice A, Armstrong SM: Melatonin: Nature's soporific? Sleep Res 1996;5:137-141.

48. Edgar DM, Dement WC, Fuller CA: Effect of SCN lesions on sleep in squirrel monkeys: Evidence for opponent processes in sleep-wake regulation. J Neurosci 1993;13:1065-1079.

49. Dijk DJ, Czeisler CA: Paradoxical timing of the circadian rhythm of sleep propensity serves to consolidate sleep and wakefulness in humans. Neurosci Lett 1994;166:63-68.

50. Liu C, Weaver DR, Jin X, et al: Molecular dissection of two distinct actions of melatonin on the suprachiasmatic circadian clock. Neuron 1997;19:91-102.

51. Barinaga M: How jet-lag hormone does double duty in the brain. Science 1998;277:480.

52. Haimov I, Lavie P: Potential of melatonin replacement therapy in older patients with sleep disorders. Drugs Aging 1995;7:75-78.

53. Wurtman RJ, Zhdanova I: Improvement of sleep quality by melatonin. Lancet 1995;346:1491.

54. Bliwise DL: Normal aging. In Kryger MH, Roth T, Dement WC (eds): Principles and Practice of Sleep Medicine, 2nd ed. Philadelphia, WB Saunders, 1994, pp 26-39.

55. Dement WC, Miles LE, Carskadon MA: "White paper" on sleep and aging. J Am Geriatr Soc 1982;30:25-50.

56. Prinz PN: Sleep and sleep disorders in older adults. J Clin Neurophysiol 1995;12:139-146.

57. Hughes RJ, Sack RL, Lewy AJ: The role of melatonin and circadian phase in age-related sleep-maintenance insomnia: Assessment in a clinical trial of melatonin replacement. Sleep 1998;21:52-68.

58. Haimov I, Laudon M, Zisapel N, et al: Sleep disorders and melatonin rhythms in elderly people. BMJ 1994;309:167.

59. Hajak G, Rodenbeck A, Staedt J, et al: Nocturnal plasma melatonin levels in patients suffering from chronic primary insomnia. J Pineal Res 1995;19:116-122.

59a. Eitzer JM, Daniels JE, Duffy JF, et al: Do plasma melatonin concentrations decline with age? Am J Med 1999;107:432-436.

60. Garfinkel D, Zisapel N, Wainstein J, Laudon M: Facilitation of benzodiazepine discontinuation by melatonin: A new clinical approach. Arch Intern Med 1999;159:2456-2460.

61. Zhdanova IV, Wurtman RJ, Wagstaff J: Effects of a low dose of melatonin on sleep in children with Angelman syndrome. J Pediatr Endocrinol Metab 1999;12:57-67.

62. Pillar G, Shahar E, Peled N, et al: Melatonin improves sleep-wake patterns in psychomotor retarded children. Pediatr Neurol 2000;23:225-228.

63. Smits MG, van Stel HF, van der Heijden K, et al: Melatonin improves health status and sleep in children with idiopathic chronic sleep-onset insomnia: A randomized placebo-controlled trial. J Am Acad Child Adolesc Psychiatry 2003;42:1286-1293.

64. Sharkey KM, Fogg LF, Eastman CI: Effects of melatonin administration on daytime sleep after simulated night shift work. J Sleep Res 2001;10:181-192.

65. Fischer S, Smolnik R, Herms M, et al: Melatonin acutely improves the neuroendocrine architecture of sleep in blind individuals. J Clin Endocrinol Metab 2003;88:5315-5320.

66. Short RV, Armstrong SM: Method for minimizing disturbances in circadian rhythms and bodily performance and function. Australia Patent Application PG 1984;4737.

67. Redman JR: Circadian entrainment and phase shifting in mammals with melatonin. J Biol Rhythms 1997;12:581-587.

68. Davis FC: Melatonin: Role in development. J Biol Rhythms 1997;12:498-508.

69. Reppert SM, Weaver DR, Rivkees SA, Stopa EG: Putative melatonin receptors in a human biological clock. Science 1988;242:78-81.

70. Gillette MU, McArthur AJ: Circadian actions of melatonin at the suprachiasmatic nucleus. Behav Brain Res 1996;73:135-139.

71. Lewy AJ, Sack RL, Blood ML, et al: Melatonin marks circadian phase positions and resets the endogenous circadian pacemaker in humans. Ciba Found Symp 1995;183:303-321.

72. Zaidan R, Geoffriau M, Brun J, et al: Melatonin is able to influence its secretion in humans: Description of a phase-response curve. Neuroendocrinology 1994;60:105-112.

73. Lewy AJ, Bauer VK, Ahmed S, et al: The human phase response curve (PRC) to melatonin is about 12 hours out of phase with the PRC to light. Chronobiol Int 1998;15:71-83.

74. Kräuchi K, Cajochen C, Möri D, et al: Early evening melatonin and S-20098 advanced circadian phase and nocturnal regulation of core body temperature. Am J Physiol 1997;272:R1178-R1188.

75. Rajaratnam SM, Dijk DJ, Middleton B, et al: Melatonin phase-shifts human circadian rhythms with no evidence of changes in the duration of endogenous melatonin secretion or the 24-hour production of reproductive hormones. J Clin Endocrinol Metab 2003;88:4303-4309.

76. Deacon S, English J, Arendt J: Sensitivity of the human circadian pacemaker to melatonin timed phase delay: A dose response study [abstract]. Chronobiol Int 1997;14(Suppl 1):41.

77. Wirz-Justice A, Werth E, Renz C, et al: No evidence for a phase delay in human circadian rhythms after a single morning melatonin administration. J Pineal Res 2002;32:1-5.

78. Lockley SW, Skene DJ, James K, et al: Melatonin administration can entrain the free-running circadian system of blind subjects. J Endocrinol 2000;164:R1-R6.

79. Sack RL, Brandes RW, Kendall AR, Lewy AJ: Entrainment of free-running circadian rhythms by melatonin in blind people. N Engl J Med 2000;343:1070-1077.

80. Lewy AJ, Bauer VK, Hasler BP, et al: Capturing the circadian rhythms of free-running blind people with 0.5 mg melatonin. Brain Res 2001;918:96-100.

81. Hack LM, Lockley SW, Arendt J, Skene DJ: The effects of low-dose 0.5-mg melatonin on the free-running circadian rhythms of blind subjects. J Biol Rhythms 2003;18:420-429.

82. Lewy AJ, Emens JS, Bernert RA, Lefler BJ: Eventual entrainment of the human circadian pacemaker by melatonin is independent of the circadian phase of treatment initiation: Clinical implications. J Biol Rhythms 2004;19:68-75.

83. Lockley SW, Skene DJ, Arendt J, et al: Relationship between melatonin rhythms and visual loss in the blind. J Clin Endocrinol Metab 1997;82:3763-3770.

84. Arendt J, Skene DJ, Middleton B, et al: Efficacy of melatonin treatment in jet lag, shift work, and blindness. J Biol Rhythms 1997;12:604-617.

85. Lewy AJ, Emens JS, Bernert RA, Lefler BJ: Eventual entrainment of the human circadian pacemaker by melatonin is independant of the circadian phase of treatment initiation: Clinical implications. J Biol Rhythms 2004;19:68-75.

86. Lewy AJ, Emens JS, Sack RL, et al: Low, but not high, doses of melatonin entrained a free-running blind person with a long circadian period. Chronobiol Int 2002;19:649-658.

87. Parkes JD: Melatonin and sleep. In Fraschini F, Reiter RJ, Stankov B (eds): The Pineal Gland and Its Hormones: Fundamentals and Clinical Perspectives. New York, Plenum Press, 1995, pp 183-197.

88. Weitzman ED, Czeisler CA, Coleman RM, et al: Delayed sleep phase syndrome: A chronobiological disorder associated with sleep onset insomnia. Arch Gen Psychiatry 1981;38:737-746.

89. Thorpy MJ, Korman E, Spielman AJ: Delayed sleep phase syndrome in adolescents. Adolesc Health Care 1988;9:22-27.

90. Pelayo RP, Thorpy MJ, Glovinsky P: Prevalence of delayed sleep phase syndrome among adolescents. Sleep Res 1988;17:391.

91. Dahlitz M, Alvarez B, Vignau J, et al: Delayed sleep phase syndrome response to melatonin. Lancet 1991;337:1121-1124.

92. Oldani A, Ferini-Strambi I, Zucconi M, et al: Melatonin and delayed sleep phase syndrome: Ambulatory polygraphic evaluation. Neuroreport 1994;6:132-134.

93. Nagtegaal JE, Kerkhof GA, Smits MG, Swart ACW: Delayed sleep phase syndrome: A placebo-controlled cross-over study on the effects of melatonin administered five hours before the individual dim light melatonin onset. J Sleep Res 1998;7:135-143.

94. Kayumov L, Brown G, Jindal R, et al: A randomized, double-blind, placebo-controlled crossover study of the effects of exogenous melatonin on delayed sleep phase syndrome. Psychosom Med 2001;63:40-48.

95. Van Coevorden A, Mockel J, Laurent E, et al: Neuroendocrine rhythms and sleep in aging men. Am J Physiol 1991;260: E651-E661.

96. Arendt J, Deacon S, English J, et al: Melatonin and adjustment to phase shift. J Sleep Res 1995;4(Suppl 2):74-79.

97. Arendt J, Aldhous M, Marks V: Alleviation of jet lag by melatonin: Preliminary results of controlled double blind trial. BMJ 1986;292:1170.

98. Spitzer RL, Terman M, Williams JBW, et al: Jet lag: Clinical features, validation of a new syndrome-specific scale, and lack of response to melatonin in a randomized, double-blind trial. Am J Psychiatry 1999;156:1392-1396.

99. Herxheimer A, Petrie KJ: Melatonin for the prevention and treatment of jet lag. Cochrane Database Syst 2002; CD001520:1.

100. Lino A, Silvy S, Condorelli L, Rusconi AC: Melatonin and jet lag: Treatment schedule. Biol Psychiatry 1993;34:587-588.

101. Sharkey KM, Eastman CI: Melatonin phase shifts human circadian rhythms in a placebo-controlled simulated night-work study. Am J Physiol 2002;282:R454-R463.

102. Depres-Brummer P, Metzger G, Levi F: Pharmacologic restoration of suppressed temperature rhythms in rats by melatonin, melatonin receptor agonist, S20242, or 8-OH-DPAT. Eur J Pharmacol 1998;347:57-66.

103. Bothorel B, Barassin S, Saboureau M, et al: In the rat, exogenous melatonin increases the amplitude of pineal melatonin secretion by a direct action on the circadian clock. Eur J Neurosci 2002;16:1090-1098.

104. Scheer FA, Van Doornen LJ, Buijs RM: Light and diurnal cycle affect autonomic cardiac balance in human: Possible role for the biological clock. Auton Neurosci 2004;110:44-48.

105. Scheer FAJL, van Doornen LJP, Buijs RM: Light and diurnal cycle affect human heart rate: Possible role for the circadian pacemaker. J Biol Rhythms 1999;14:202-212.

106. Scheer FAJL, Ter Horst GJ, van der Vliet J, Buijs RM: Physiological and anatomic evidence for regulation of the heart by suprachiasmatic nucleus in rats. Am J Physiol 2001;280: H1391-H1399.

107. Sly DJ, Colvill L, McKinley MJ, Oldfield BJ: Identification of neural projections from the forebrain to the kidney, using the virus pseudorabies. J Auton Nerv Syst 1999;77:73-82.

108. Scheer FAJL, Kalsbeek A, Buijs RM: Cardiovascular control by the suprachiasmatic nucleus: Neural and neuroendocrine mechanisms in human and rat. Biol Chem 2003;384: 697-709.

Sleep Homeostasis and Models of Sleep Regulation

Alexander A. Borbély

Peter Achermann

ABSTRACT

Sleep homeostasis denotes a basic principle of sleep regulation. A sleep deficit elicits a compensatory increase in the intensity and duration of sleep, and excessive sleep reduces sleep propensity. It is as though "sleep pressure" is maintained within a range delimited by an upper and a lower threshold. Sleep homeostasis is represented in the two-process model of sleep regulation by process S, which increases during waking and declines during sleep. The timing and propensity of sleep are also modulated by a circadian process. Electroencephalographic (EEG) slow wave activity (SWA) serves as an indicator of sleep homeostasis in non–rapid eye movement (NREM) sleep. The level of SWA, a correlate of sleep intensity, is determined by the duration of prior sleep and waking. Power in the range of sleep spindles (spindle frequency activity, SFA) shows in part an inverse relationship to SWA.

This observation can be accounted for by neurophysiologic mechanisms. Thalamocortical neurons exhibit oscillations in the range of sleep spindles at an intermediate level of hyperpolarization (corresponding to superficial NREM sleep), and they exhibit slow oscillations at a high level of hyperpolarization (corresponding to deep NREM sleep). In the waking EEG, theta activity may serve as a marker of process S. In contrast to SWA, it exhibits a marked circadian modulation. The rise rate of theta activity during prolonged waking is correlated with the increase of SWA during recovery sleep. Therefore, a common homeostatic process may be evident in the EEG in both waking and sleep.

Advanced versions of the two-process model were applied to simulate the SWA pattern in a variety of experimental schedules. Rapid eye movement (REM) sleep was incorporated as a separate process that periodically interrupts the occurrence of SWA.

There is recent evidence for a local, use-dependent facet of sleep regulation. In humans and animals, the selective unihemispheric regional cerebral activation during waking gives rise to a predominant increase in sleep intensity in the previously activated hemisphere as reflected by SWA.

Three distinct processes underlie sleep regulation. A homeostatic process, whose level is a function of prior sleep and waking, plays a major role in sleep regulation. Sleep is also modulated by a circadian process, a clocklike mechanism that is independent of prior sleep and waking (see Chapters 31 and 34). An ultradian process occurs within sleep and is represented by the alternation of the two basic sleep states: non–rapid eye movement (NREM) sleep and rapid eye movement (REM) sleep.

This chapter focuses on "sleep homeostasis." *Homeostasis* has been defined as "the coordinated physiological processes, which maintain most of the steady states in the organism."[1] The term *sleep homeostasis*[2] refers to the sleep-wake balance of sleep regulation, as homeostatic mechanisms counteract deviations from an average "reference level" of sleep. These mechanisms augment sleep propensity when sleep is curtailed or absent, and they reduce sleep propensity in response to excess sleep.

The interest in the modeling approach to sleep regulation has increased over the past decade. Models help delineate the processes involved in regulating sleep and thereby offer a conceptual framework for analyzing existing and new data.[3] An international symposium was devoted to the analysis of various mathematical models of sleep regulation and related topics[4] and in another recent workshop, the state of the art of biomathematical modeling of fatigue and performance was discussed.[5]

HOMEOSTATIC REGULATION OF SLEEP

Electroencephalographic Slow Wave Activity: A Physiologic Indicator of NREM Sleep Homeostasis

Slow Wave Sleep and Slow Wave Activity

NREM sleep is not a homogeneous substate of sleep, but it can be subdivided according to the predominance of electroencephalographic (EEG) slow waves. The percentage of slow waves (frequency, 0 Hz to 2 Hz; minimum peak-to-peak value, 75 µV) is the major criterion for categorizing (or scoring) human NREM sleep into stages 2, 3, or 4.[6] Stages 3 and 4 are commonly referred to as slow wave sleep (SWS). However, the conventional sleep-scoring method is inadequate for a quantitative analysis, because the sleep stages are based on general and arbitrary criteria. Currently, EEG parameters are increasingly assessed by computer-aided methods of signal analysis. One of the most important functional EEG parameters is referred to as "slow wave activity" (SWA). It is equivalent to "delta activity" and encompasses components of the EEG signal in the frequency range of approximately 0.5 Hz to 4.5 Hz as obtained by spectral analysis.[7]

In addition to delta waves, a low-frequency component with a mean peak value of 0.7 Hz to 0.8 Hz is present in the EEG power spectrum of NREM sleep.[8,9] The typical decline in delta activity from the first to the second NREM-sleep episode was not present at frequencies below 2 Hz.[8] Periodicities at even lower frequencies include the recurrence of sleep spindles at 4-second intervals[8,10] and the tendency of slow waves to recur at 20- to 30-second intervals.[8]

Slow Waves and Sleep Intensity

It was recognized as early as 1937 that sleep intensity is reflected by the predominance of slow waves in the sleep EEG.[11] Subsequent studies confirmed that the responsiveness to stimuli decreases as EEG slow waves become more predominant.[12] Under physiologic conditions, this EEG parameter can be regarded therefore as an indicator of "sleep depth" or "sleep intensity" (for sleep intensity in animals see Chapter 7).

Global Time Course of Slow Wave Activity During Sleep

Figure 33–1 illustrates the conventionally scored sleep stages and SWA of a young subject. Note that SWS provides a rough indication of the prevalence of SWA. However, this EEG parameter shows a continuous rise from sleep onset to stage 4, a change that is only grossly reflected by the stepwise transitions of the sleep stages. In general, the measure derived directly from the EEG signal shows the variations of the NREM-REM sleep cycle and the fluctuations within NREM-sleep episodes in much greater detail than the sleep profile. Moreover, the EEG parameter lends itself to a quantitative analysis from which inferences can be made regarding the underlying processes.

It is a plausible assumption that "sleep need" is high during the initial part of the sleep episode and gradually declines with the progression of sleep. In accordance with this notion, early studies reported that both the arousal threshold and the

predominance of slow waves in the EEG were high in the initial part of sleep and then progressively decreased.[11] Thus SWS, the high-intensity part of NREM sleep, appeared to be a good candidate for a physiologic indicator of sleep homeostasis. The predominance of SWS in the early part of the sleep episode was confirmed in subsequent studies.[12-14]

All-night spectral analysis of the sleep EEG made it possible to quantify SWA and to delineate its time course during sleep.[7] Its mean value per cycle plotted for consecutive NREM-REM sleep cycles showed a monotonic decline over the first three cycles.

Figure 33–2 (left panel) shows the changes of mean EEG power density over four cycles for the frequency range between 0.25 Hz and 20 Hz. The values of each frequency bin are expressed relative to the reference level of cycle 4 (100%). Note that although the largest changes occur in the low-delta range, they encompass frequencies up to the theta band.

Nap Studies

The analysis of daytime naps is useful for assessing the level of SWA after various durations of waking. Naps taken later in the day contained more SWS than naps taken early in the day. In a detailed study of daytime naps scheduled at 2-hour intervals throughout the day, direct evidence for a monotonic rise of SWA was obtained.[15-17]

If naps reverse the rising trend of slow wave propensity, a reduction of SWA in the subsequent nighttime sleep can be expected. This prediction was borne out by the results of several experiments (see Werth et al.[18] for literature references). When the duration of nighttime sleep was shortened, SWA in a subsequent morning nap was enhanced.[19,20]

Effect of Sleep Deprivation

It has been repeatedly shown that partial or total sleep deprivation gives rise to increased SWS in the recovery night

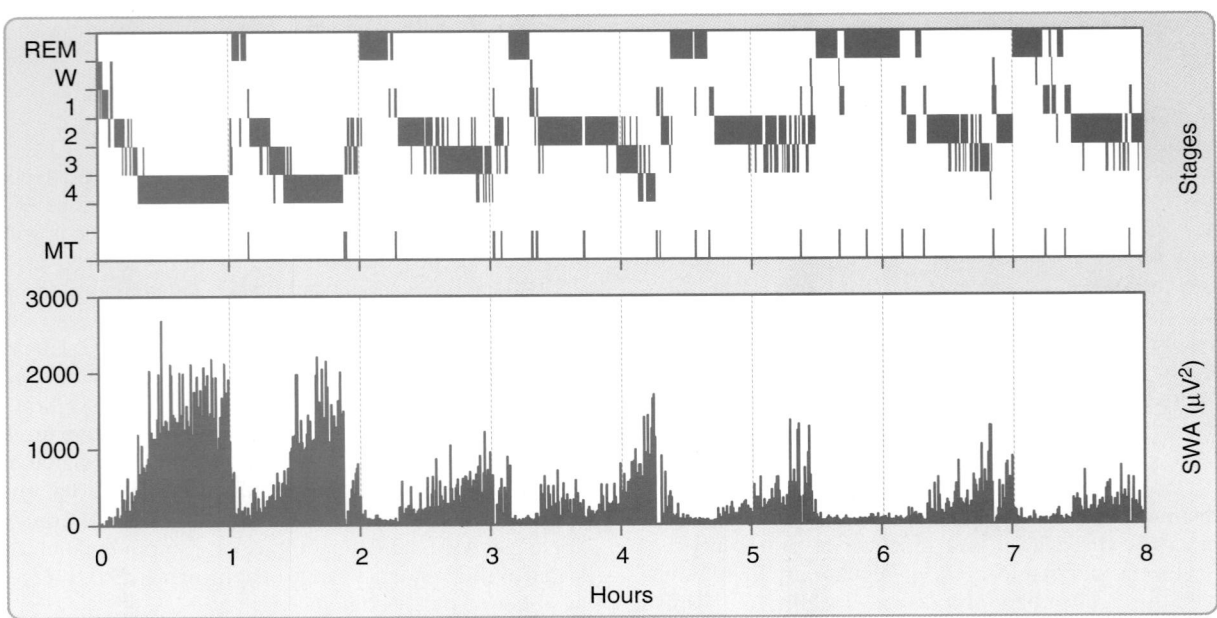

Figure 33–1. Sleep stages and slow wave activity. Sleep stages were scored for 20-second epochs. Slow wave activity (electroencephalographic [EEG] power in the 0.75- to 4.5-Hz band) was calculated for 20-second epochs. MT, movement time; REM, rapid eye movement sleep; SWA, slow wave activity; W, waking; 1-4, NREM sleep stages 1 to 4.

Figure 33–2. *Left,* Changes of relative spectral power density over the first four NREM-REM sleep cycles of a baseline night (N = 8; curves for consecutive cycles are indicated by corresponding numbers). In each frequency bin, the data are expressed relative to the value in the fourth cycle (100%; horizontal line). *Right,* Effect of sleep deprivation (40.5-hour waking) on spectra of the sleep electroencephalogram (EEG). In each frequency bin, the values of the first two recovery nights are plotted relative to the baseline night (100%). The upper and lower horizontal bars below the abscissa indicate *(left)* significant differences between cycles 1 and 2 and between cycles 2 and 3, respectively, and *(right)* between recovery 1 and baseline and between recovery 2 and baseline, respectively. (Modified from Borbély AA, Baumann F, Brandeis D, et al: Sleep deprivation: Effect on sleep stages and EEG power density in man. Electroencephalogr Clin Neurophysiol 1981;51:483-493.)

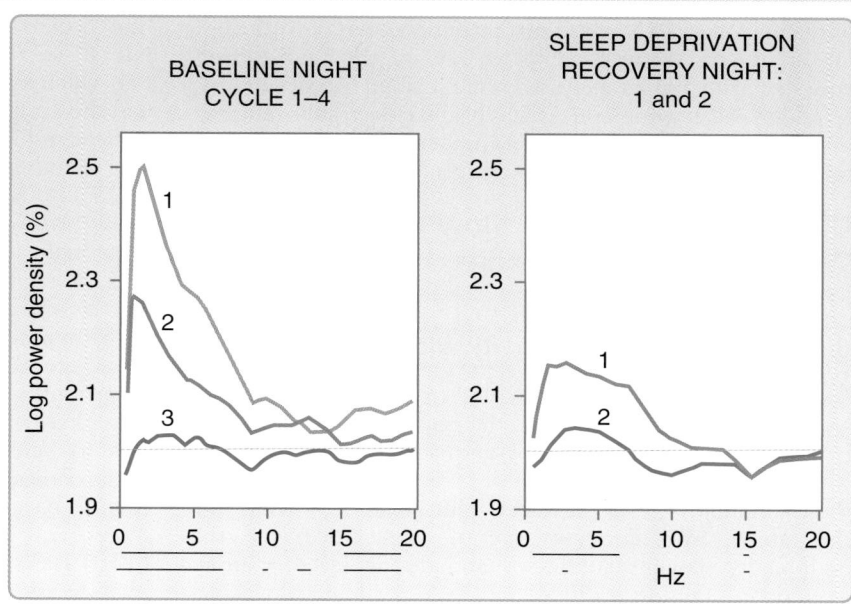

(see Borbély[21] for a review of the older literature). Webb and Agnew[14] presented compelling evidence that SWS increases as a function of prior waking. The quantitative assessment of SWA by all-night spectral analysis revealed that a night without sleep (i.e., 40.5 hours of wakefulness) resulted in an enhancement of this EEG parameter during recovery sleep.[7] Figure 33–2 (right panel) illustrates the changes of power density in the two recovery nights relative to the baseline level (100%). In the first recovery night, the largest increase was present in the low-delta range, the part of the spectrum undergoing the largest changes in the course of baseline sleep (see Fig. 33–2, left panel).

Figure 33–3 depicts the global trend as well as the ultradian dynamics of SWA over successive NREM-REM sleep cycles. The prolongation of the waking period causes a prominent rise of SWA during recovery sleep. A declining trend over three to four cycles is evident in both records. Note that the peaks are at a steady low level during the last four cycles of recovery sleep.

The enhancement of SWA by sleep deprivation was confirmed in several studies[22,23] (for studies before 1992, see Borbély and Achermann[24]; for animal studies, see Chapter 7). The extent of the increase was shown to be a function of the duration of prior waking.[17,25]

Intranight Rebound after Selective Slow Wave Deprivation

The propensity of SWA does not necessarily dissipate rapidly during sleep but may persist at an elevated level if SWS is prevented. Thus suppression of slow waves by acoustic stimuli during the first 3 hours of sleep resulted in a prominent rise of SWA after discontinuation of the stimuli.[26] In another study, daytime sleep episodes with and without SWS deprivation

Figure 33–3. Time course of slow wave activity (power in the 0.75- to 4.5-Hz band, *lower curves*) and activity in the spindle frequency range (13.25- to 15.0-Hz band, *upper curves*) recorded under baseline conditions and after sleep deprivation (36 hours of wakefulness). NREM sleep episodes were subdivided into 20 equal intervals and REM sleep episodes into 5 intervals. Mean values per interval were calculated prior to averaging across subjects (N = 8, except for cycle 8 of recovery sleep, where N = 6) and were expressed relative to the mean level in baseline NREM sleep (100%). The mean timing of REM sleep episodes is delimited by vertical lines and horizontal bars above the abscissa. (Reanalysis of the data from Dijk DJ, Brunner DP, Borbély AA: Time course of EEG power density during long sleep in humans. Am J Physiol 1990;258:R650-R651, by D. Aeschbach.)

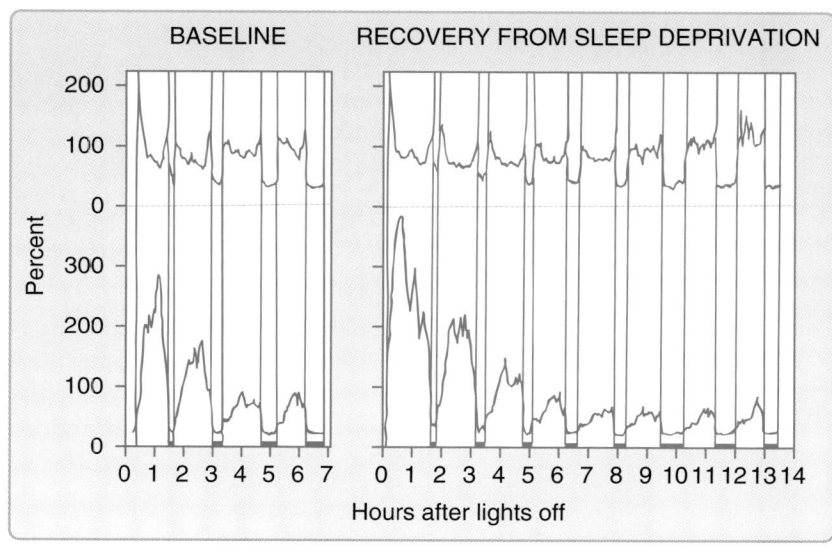

were compared.[27] The experimental suppression of SWS during an interval corresponding to 90% of the undisturbed episode resulted in an increased accumulation of SWS and an extension of sleep duration. Taken together, the results indicate that slow waves are not merely an epiphenomenon of sleep but reflect major sleep-regulating mechanisms.

Ultradian Dynamics of Slow Wave Activity and Spindle Frequency Activity

Buildup of Slow Wave Activity within NREM Sleep Episodes

Not only are the mean level and the peak of SWA determined by the duration of prior waking and sleep, but the rise rate within single NREM sleep episodes is also determined by these durations.[28-30] It is evident from Figure 33–3 that the rise rate of SWA decreases over the first three episodes both under baseline conditions and during recovery from sleep deprivation. In addition, the effect of prolonged waking manifests itself in a steeper buildup (of SWA) within NREM sleep episodes.[22,23,30]

Slow-Wave Activity and Spindle Frequency Activity

The term *spindle frequency activity* (SFA) is used to denote the power in the frequency range of sleep spindles (12 to 15 Hz). There is a close correspondence between this measure and measures based on the occurrence of sleep spindles.[22]

The time courses of SWA and SFA differ in several respects. The global decline of SWA does not occur in the spindle frequency range. Within NREM sleep episodes, SFA shows a bimodal pattern with an initial and a terminal peak. This gives rise to a U-shaped curve within the episode and a partly inverse relationship to SWA[22,31-36] (see Fig. 33–3). This inverse relationship becomes less prominent with age.[37] The age-related decline of SWA and SFA were similar.[38]

Within the 12- to 15-Hz range, low-frequency (12 Hz to 13 Hz) and high-frequency (14 Hz to 15 Hz) activity exhibited opposite circadian variations.[33,39,40] An analysis of sleep-dependent and circadian components of sleep spindles and their regional distribution was recently published.[41,42] Sleep spindles in the 13- to 14-Hz band are remarkable because of their high intrahemispheric and interhemispheric coherence.[43,44] This raises the question whether this episodic, high-coherence activity is of functional significance for sleep and whether sleep spindles may represent carrier frequencies upon which some relevant information is modulated (see Achermann and Borbély[43] for a further discussion). Sejnowski and Destexhe[45] hypothesized that molecular events that occur in conjunction with sleep spindles may serve to promote neural plasticity and memory consolidation. Recently, it was reported that the density of sleep spindles was significantly higher after a learning task than after a nonlearning control task.[46]

Relationship to Neurophysiology

In recent years it has become increasingly evident that the typical oscillations in the sleep EEG are closely associated with cellular changes at the level of thalamic and cortical neurons.[47-50] The progressive hyperpolarization of thalamocortical neurons

that occurs during the progression from waking to deep NREM sleep[51] results in fluctuations in the membrane potential, which are initially in the frequency range of sleep spindles and then in the range of delta waves.[47]

Synchronized oscillations appear to arise from the progressive recruitment of neurons, and their spontaneous cessation results from a hyperpolarization-activated cation conductance.[52] In 1993 a new type of slow oscillation was reported to occur in the thalamocortical system.[47,48] Its frequency (less than 1 Hz) was lower than that of the delta rhythm (1 Hz to 4 Hz). This slow oscillation originating in cortical networks consisted of rhythmical depolarizing components separated by prolonged (0.2 seconds to 0.8 seconds) hyperpolarizations, which grouped the thalamically generated spindles and the delta waves in slowly recurring sequences.[50] Long-lasting hyperpolarizations were associated with prolonged-depth positive waves in the cortical EEG. The cortical generating mechanisms derive from a balance of excitatory and inhibitory influences.[53,54] A low-frequency component with a mean peak value of 0.7 Hz to 0.8 Hz is also present in the power spectrum of NREM sleep.[8,9] Its frequency corresponded to the 0.7- to 0.9-Hz oscillation that has been reported in the sleeping cat.

Sleep oscillations and their possible functional significance have been recently reviewed.[55] Taken together, these advances in electrophysiology indicate that not only sleep mechanisms per se but also the regulatory processes will be open for investigation at the cellular level.

NREM-Sleep versus REM-Sleep Homeostasis

Effect of NREM-Sleep Pressure on REM-Sleep Homeostasis

During recovery from total sleep deprivation, SWS and EEG SWA exhibit an immediate rebound, whereas the increase in REM sleep is delayed to subsequent nights or does not occur at all. Selective REM-sleep deprivation augments "REM-sleep pressure," which is manifested by the increasing number of interventions required to prevent REM-sleep episodes (for the older literature, see references in Borbély[21]). However, a REM-sleep rebound during recovery sleep is smaller than expected on the basis of the deficit.[56] This suggests that REM sleep is not as finely regulated as SWA.

However, this notion is contradicted by partial sleep-deprivation studies. A REM-sleep deprivation in the first 5 hours of sleep induced a REM-sleep rebound in the subsequent 2.25 hours.[57] A curtailment of sleep duration during 2 or 4 nights, which induced a substantial REM-sleep deficit, was followed by a REM-sleep rebound in the 2 recovery nights.[58,59] In these experiments, the REM-sleep rebound occurred at a time when slow wave pressure either was low at the end of sleep[57] or was much less increased than "REM-sleep pressure."[58,59] These results also suggest that REM sleep is regulated but that the manifestation of REM-sleep homeostasis is hampered by an elevated slow wave pressure.

Effect of REM-Sleep Pressure on the REM-Sleep EEG

An electrophysiologic indicator of an intensity dimension of human REM sleep, comparable to SWA in NREM sleep, has not been identified. The density of rapid eye movements (REM density) is not associated with REM-sleep pressure[60] but is inversely related to slow wave propensity.[18,23,61-63] This relation is further supported by a study conducted with the forced desynchrony protocol in which REM density showed an inverse relationship to sleep pressure.[64] Selective REM-sleep deprivation gave rise to a reduction of power in the alpha band in the REM-sleep EEG during recovery sleep.[56,65] This effect was most pronounced in the first recovery night and then gradually subsided.

A progressive and persistent attenuation of alpha activity in REM sleep has been observed previously during recovery from total sleep deprivation[7] as well as in a 4-day partial sleep deprivation protocol that induced a preferential deficit in REM sleep.[59] Such a relationship, however, is not invariably observed. Nevertheless, alpha activity in REM sleep seems to be inversely related to REM sleep pressure. This conclusion is supported by a forced desynchrony study in which the circadian rhythm of alpha activity in REM sleep and the REM-sleep fraction of total sleep showed an inverse relationship.[40]

Effect of REM-Sleep Pressure on the NREM-Sleep EEG

In accordance with the notion of a mutual inhibitory interaction of the factors controlling SWA and REM sleep,[21] REM sleep is inhibited by "slow wave pressure," and slow wave activity is inhibited by REM-sleep pressure. Thus, selective REM-sleep deprivation led to a significant reduction in the low-frequency activity of the NREM-sleep EEG,[57] an observation that was also made in an animal experiment.[66] The rise in REM-sleep pressure induced by repeated partial sleep deprivation suppressed the typical low-delta peak in the NREM-sleep spectrum.[58,59] However, this effect was not seen after selective REM-sleep deprivation.[56]

Homeostatic Marker in the Waking EEG

Early studies had shown that power in the theta band (theta activity) and alpha activity of the waking EEG is associated with sleepiness[67,68] and that total[68] or partial[59] sleep deprivation enhanced the power in these frequency bands. A saturating exponential function with a time constant of 18.18 hours was reported to fit the rise of theta activity in the waking EEG.[69] Spectral analysis showed that the largest changes occurred in the theta band.[70,71] These undergo a circadian modulation in addition to the waking time–related changes.[71-75] During prolonged wakefulness, subjective sleepiness correlated positively with theta activity with a focus in frontal derivations and negatively with alpha activity at all derivations.[76] A forced desynchrony study with a scheduled waking episode of 28 hours showed a monotonic rise of delta and beta activity in the fronto-central derivation.[75] An analysis of persons subjected to sleep deprivation revealed that the rise rate of theta activity in the waking EEG is correlated with the increase of SWA in the first NREM-sleep episode of recovery sleep (Fig. 33–4A and B).[71] Moreover, both effects were largest in frontal areas (Fig. 33–4C). In summary, theta activity in waking and SWA in sleep may be markers of a common homeostatic sleep process.

Independence and Interactions of Homeostatic and Circadian Processes

There is evidence that homeostatic and circadian facets of sleep regulation can be independently manipulated and therefore may be controlled by separate mechanisms. Thus, throughout a 72-hour sleep-deprivation period, the subjective alertness ratings continued to show a prominent circadian rhythm.[77] Conversely, in a study in which the phase of the circadian process (as indexed by body temperature and plasma melatonin) was shifted by bright light in the morning, the time course of SWA remained unaffected.[78]

A powerful experimental paradigm is the forced desynchrony schedule, in which the homeostatic and circadian facets of sleep can be separately analyzed (see Chapters 31 and 34). In this long-term protocol, the scheduled sleep episodes occur at different circadian phases. Various claims of the two-process model were supported by the results obtained in a forced desynchrony paradigm.[39] Thus, SWA proved to be determined mainly by homeostatic (i.e., sleep-wake–dependent) factors, whereas the REM/NREM sleep ratio is controlled by both homeostatic and circadian factors. Furthermore, a previously postulated sleep-related disinhibition of REM sleep[21] was confirmed.

MODELS OF SLEEP REGULATION

Models help delineate the processes involved in the regulation of sleep and thereby offer a conceptual framework for analyzing existing and new data. In addition, they inspire new experiments to test the predictions of the model. A synopsis of the major models discussed in this chapter is provided in Table 33–1.[3,24,70,79,80]

Two-Process Model and Related Models

The relationship between SWS and the duration of prior waking has been documented by Webb and Agnew[14] and placed into a theoretical framework by Feinberg.[81] The two-process model, originally proposed to account for sleep regulation in the rat,[2,82] postulates that a homeostatic process (process S) rises during waking and declines during sleep, and it interacts with a circadian process (process C) that is independent of sleep and waking. The time course of the homeostatic variable S was derived from EEG SWA (Fig. 33–5A). Various aspects of human sleep regulation were addressed in a qualitative version of the two-process model.[21] An elaborated, quantitative version of the model was established in which process S varied between an upper and a lower threshold that are both modulated by a single circadian process.[83,84] This model was able to account for such diverse phenomena as recovery from sleep deprivation, circadian phase dependence of sleep duration, sleep during shift work, sleep fragmentation during continuous bed rest, and internal desynchronization in the absence of time cues.[84]

The two-process model triggered numerous experimental studies to test its predictions and was used to predict the response of habitual short and long sleepers to sleep deprivation.[23,73] The researchers concluded that short sleepers live under a higher NREM-sleep pressure than long sleepers and

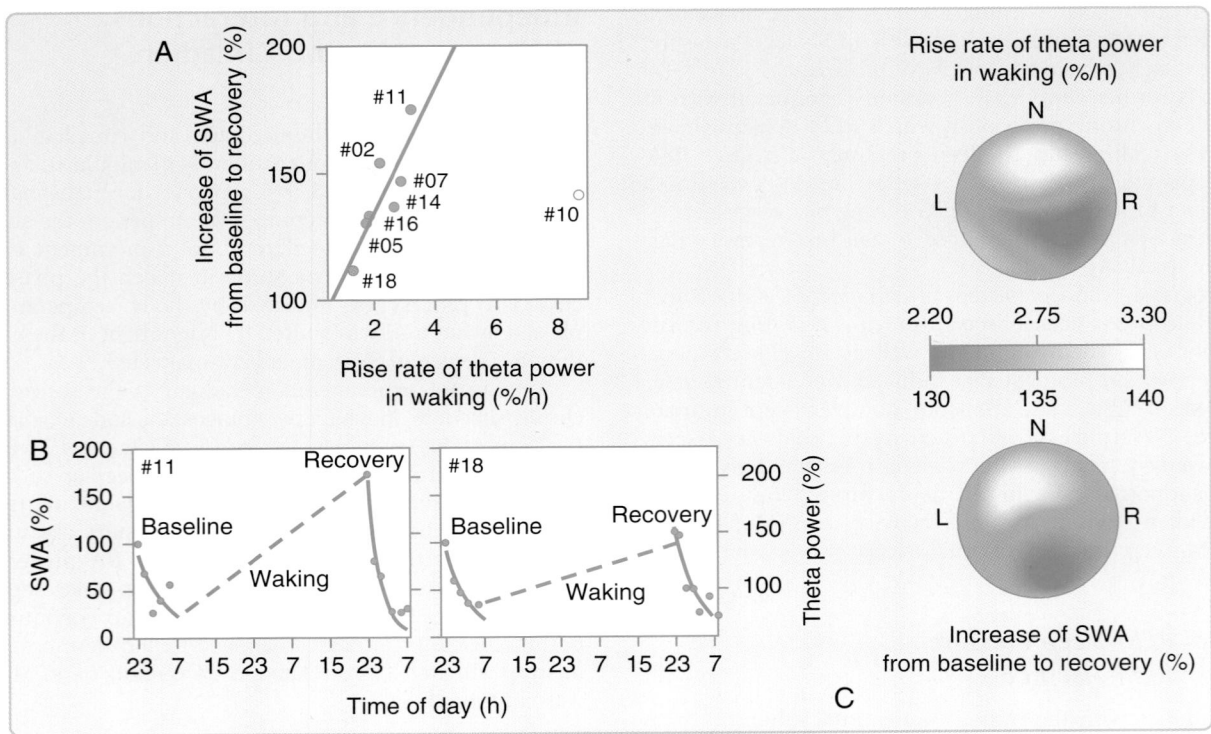

Figure 33–4. **A**, Relationship between homeostatic markers of the sleep electroencephalogram (EEG) and waking EEG. Increase (%) of slow wave activity (SWA; power in the 0.75- to 4.5-Hz range) in the first NREM sleep episode from baseline to recovery sleep is plotted as a function of the rise rate (%/h) of theta power (5.0 to 8.0 Hz) in waking. The linear regression line fitted through 7 data points is indicated (r = .851, r^2 = .724, P = .015). Subject #10 was excluded from the regression. **B**, Association between rise of SWA in sleep and theta activity in waking illustrated for two subjects. Mean SWA per NREM sleep episode is plotted at the beginning of each episode and expressed relative to the baseline value of the first NREM sleep episode (100%). Exponential functions were fitted through the data points (*solid curves*). The regression line represents theta power in waking (*interrupted line*). **C**, Topographic distribution of the rise rate of theta power (*top panel*) during waking and of the increase of SWA (*bottom panel*) in the first NREM-sleep episode from baseline to recovery sleep. Maps are based on 27 EEG derivations (average reference, extended 10-20 systems). Values are plotted on a blue scale at the corresponding position on the planar projection of the hemispheric scalp model. Values between electrodes were linearly interpolated. NREM, non–rapid eye movement; REM, rapid eye movement. (Adapted from Finelli LA, Baumann H, Borbély AA, Achermann P: Dual electroencephalogram markers of human sleep homeostasis: Correlation between theta activity in waking and slow wave activity in sleep. Neuroscience 2000;101:523-529.)

that the two groups do not differ with respect to the homeostatic regulatory mechanisms. However, the circadian pacemaker differed between the two groups in that long sleepers exhibited a longer "biological night" and were more sensitive to the circadian drive for sleep.[85]

In a later version of the model (proposed by Beersma et al.[15] and Dijk et al.[26] and formalized by Achermann and Borbély[86]), it is the change of S, and not its level, that is proportional to the momentary amount of SWA. The elaborated model addressed not only the global changes of SWA as represented by process S but also the changes within NREM-sleep episodes. The magnitude of the intranight rebound after selective SWS deprivation in the first 3 hours of sleep was in accordance with the prediction.[86]

A further elaborated version of the model was subjected to an optimization procedure.[87] In general, a close fit was obtained between the simulated and empirical SWA data and their time course (Fig. 33–5D). In particular, the occurrence of late SWA peaks during extended sleep could be simulated (Fig. 33–5C). The simulations demonstrated that the model accounts in quantitative terms for empirical data and predicts the changes induced by the prolongation of waking or sleep. This version of the model was used to simulate the dynamics

of SWA in an experimental protocol with an early evening nap[18] and the effect of changes in REM sleep latency on the time course of SWA.[88]

Finally, the data analysis showed that not only the timing of sleep but also the changes in daytime vigilance are governed by the interaction of processes S and C, as simulated by Daan and coworkers.[84] The rising homeostatic sleep pressure during waking seems to be compensated for by the declining circadian sleep propensity.[84,89-91] Conversely, during sleep the rising circadian sleep propensity may serve to counteract the declining homeostatic sleep pressure, thereby ensuring the maintenance of sleep.[92]

Based on a similar concept, the changes of subjective sleepiness/alertness ratings were simulated by a combined action of a homeostatic process (S), a circadian process (C), and a process representing sleep inertia (W) ("three-process model"; see Table 33–1).[93,94]

Jewett and Kronauer[95] (see Table 33–1) proposed interactive mathematical models of subjective alertness and cognitive throughput in humans. A homeostatic component (H) falls in a sigmoidal manner during waking and rises in a saturating exponential manner during sleep. The rise of H during sleep is determined by the circadian phase. H interacts with a

Table 33–1. Models of Sleep Regulation

Designation	Assumption	Description/Comment
	Two-Process Model and Related Models	
Two-process model[21,83,84]	Sleep propensity is determined by a homeostatic process (S) and circadian process (C). The interaction of S and C determines the timing of sleep and waking.	Time course of S derived from EEG slow-wave activity; phase position and shape (skewed sine wave) of C derived from sleep duration data obtained at various times of the 24-hour cycle.
Model of ultradian variation of slow-wave activity[86-88]	Derived from the two-process model. The level of S determines the buildup rate and the saturation level of slow-wave activity within NREM sleep episodes.	In contrast to the original two-process model, the change of S, not the level of S, corresponds to slow-wave activity; i.e., the decline of S is proportional to the amount of slow-wave activity. A REM-sleep oscillator triggers the decline of slow-wave activity prior to REM sleep.
Three-process model of the regulation of sleepiness and alertness[93,94]	Sleepiness and alertness are simulated by the combined action of a homeostatic process, a circadian process, and a sleep inertia process (W). Extension to include performance, sleep latency, and sleep length.	Parameters derived from rated sleepiness during sleep-wake manipulations. Alertness nomogram for sleep-related safety risks.
Interactive mathematical models of alertness and cognitive throughput[95]	Alertness and cognitive throughput are determined by a nonlinear interaction of a homeostatic (H) and C. In addition, sleep inertia is included. H shows a sigmoidal decline during waking and a saturating exponential increase during sleep at a rate determined by the circadian phase.	Parameters derived from sleep inertia studies, sleep deprivation studies initiated across all circadian phases, and 28-hour forced desynchrony studies.
	Models of the NREM-REM Sleep Cycle	
Reciprocal interaction model[143]	NREM-REM sleep cycle generated by two coupled cell populations in the brainstem with self-excitatory and self-inhibitory connections according to the Lotka-Volterra model.	Simulation of data: Discharge rate of cholinergic FTG (or LDT/PPT) cells in the cat. The role of postulated cell populations in the control of REM sleep and their interactions have undergone revisions.
Limit cycle reciprocal interaction model: Original version[144]	NREM-REM sleep cycle generated by the reciprocal interaction of two coupled cell populations (REM-on and REM-off).	Main features of reciprocal interaction model maintained; assumption of a stable limit cycle oscillation that is independent of initial conditions. Introduction of a circadian term that determines mode of approach to limit cycle.
	Combined Models	
Composite model of sleep regulation[111]	Combination of model of ultradian variation of slow-wave activity,[87] limit cycle reciprocal interaction model,[144] model of the circadian pace maker,[114] and sleep inertia.	Different models proposed to account for processes underlying the regulation of sleep and alertness are considered "modules" and have been integrated into a combined model.
Limit cycle reciprocal interaction model: Extended version[112]	As above; incorporation of sleep homeostasis and arousal events.	Assumption of first-order decay dynamics for the arousal system. Arousal as a stochastic process.

EEG, electroencephalographic; FTG, gigantocellular tegmental field; LDT, laterodorsal tegmental nucleus; NREM, non–rapid eye movement; PPT, pedunculopontine tegmental nucleus; REM, rapid eye movement.

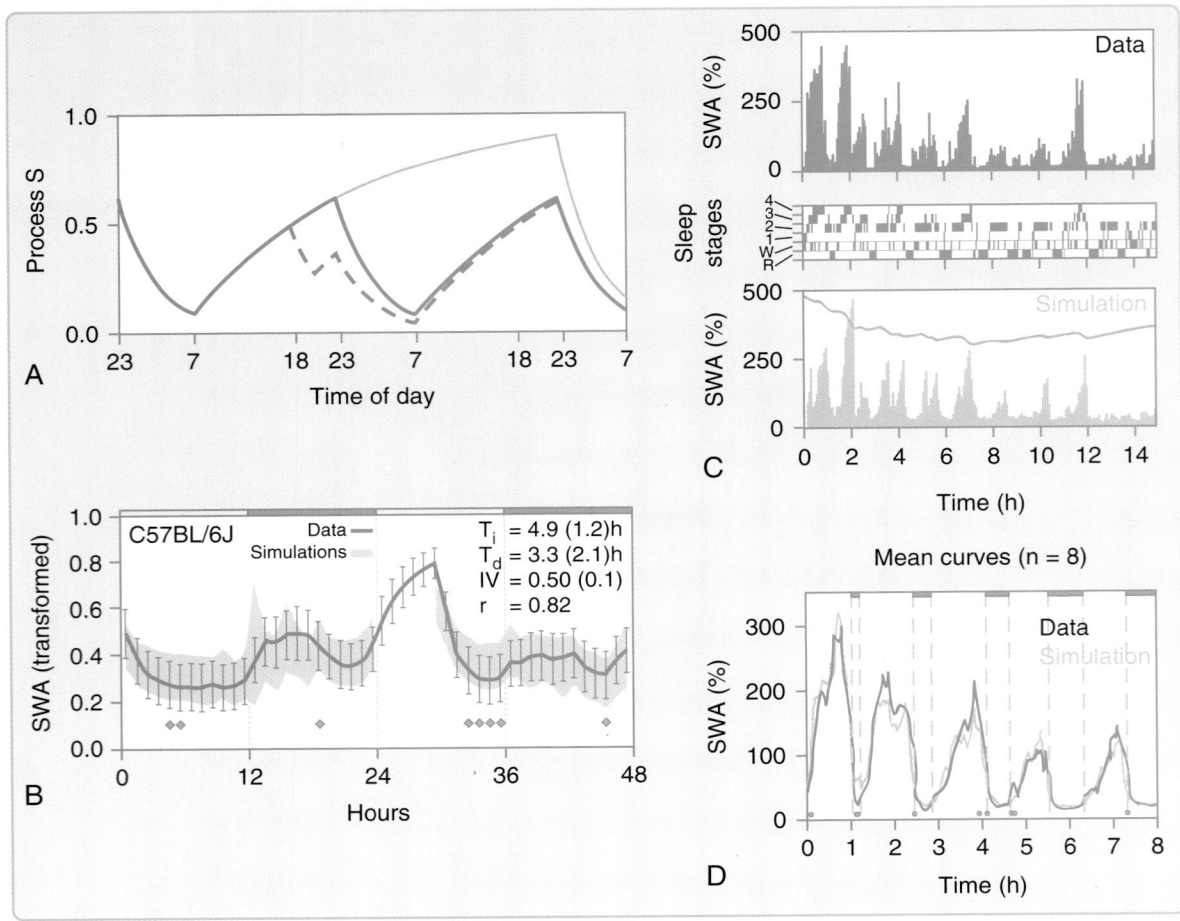

Figure 33–5. Two-process model of sleep regulation. **A,** Simulations of the homeostatic process S according to different experimental conditions. *Heavy line* indicates the baseline condition with an 8-hour sleep episode; *thin line* indicates sleep deprivation (40 hours wakefulness) and recovery sleep; *dashed line* indicates the effect of a 2-hour daytime nap at 6:00 PM. **B,** Sleep regulation in the mouse. Time course of slow wave activity (SWA) and simulation with the optimized time constants for the increase (T_i), decrease (T_d), and initial value (IV) of process S for C57BL/6J mice ($N = 8$). *Curves* and *shaded* areas connect 1-hour mean values (±SEM) for 24-hour baseline, 6-hour sleep deprivation, and 18-hour recovery. The close fit between the simulation of process S (*blue areas*) and time course of empirical SWA (*solid line*) indicates that the model can predict SWA from the temporal organization of sleep. *Diamonds* indicate differences between simulation and data ($P < .05$, two-tailed paired t-test). For the comparison between SWA and S, SWA was transformed according to a linear regression. Inset legend shows mean values of T_i, T_d and IV (SEM) and the mean r-value of the fit between SWA and S. **C,** Empirical SWA *(top)*, sleep stages *(middle)* and simulation of SWA and process S *(bottom)* of an individual extended baseline sleep episode starting at 0 hours (prior waking: 17 hours). Empirical and simulated SWAs were standardized with respect to the mean value of the first 7 hours of sleep. Values are plotted for 1-minute intervals. **D,** Mean empirical *(dark blue line)* and simulated SWA *(light blue line)* ($N = 8$) of an extended baseline experiment (analysis of first 8 hours). Significant differences are indicated by *black dots* (paired t test; $P < .05$). *Bars* on top and the *interrupted vertical lines* indicate REM-sleep episodes (mean values). (**B** modified from Huber R, Deboer T, Tobler I: Effects of sleep deprivation on sleep and sleep EEG in three mouse strains: Empirical data and simulations. Brain Res 2000;857:8-19. **C** and **D** modified from Achermann P, Dijk DJ, Brunner DP, Borbély AA: A model of human sleep homeostasis based on EEG slow-wave activity: Quantitative comparison of data and simulations. Brain Res Bull 1993;31:97-113.)

circadian component[96] (C), accounting for the effect of light on the circadian pacemaker. The amplitude of C depends on the level of H. In addition, a sleep inertia component (W) is included. In contrast to the two- and three-process models, a nonlinear interaction is assumed. Whether the interaction is linear or nonlinear is still unresolved.[97,98] A statistical approach to test for nonlinear interactions was recently proposed[99] and is based on a comparison of model predictions and empirical data. Chronic sleep restriction experiments demonstrated that the homeostatic sleep drive is not associated with neurobehavioral performance.[100] Neurobehavioral performance showed a cumulative impairment with a considerable degree of individual variability.

Although the qualitative version of the two-process model originated from animal data,[2,82] the quantitative version of the model was elaborated on the basis of findings from human studies. In the meantime, quantitative simulations of NREM-sleep homeostasis were also performed in rats[101-103] and mice[104,105] (see Fig. 33–5B). SWA of consecutive 4-second epochs in a 24-hour baseline, a 6-hour sleep deprivation, and 18-hour recovery period[104] served as the database for the simulation in mice. As in the original human version of the model, process S was assumed to decrease exponentially in NREM sleep and to increase according to a saturating exponential function in waking. Unlike in the human model, an increase of S was assumed to occur also in REM sleep.

After optimizing the initial value (IV) of S as well as its time constants (time increase, T_i; time decrease, T_d), a close fit was obtained between the hourly mean values of SWA in NREM sleep and the prediction of process S (see Fig. 33–5B and Chapter 7).

Modeling REM Sleep

Whereas models have focused on NREM-sleep homeostasis, on the interaction of NREM and REM sleep, and on the circadian oscillator, REM-sleep homeostasis has been largely ignored. In the context of a selective REM-sleep deprivation experiment,[56] two salient observations were made that were difficult to reconcile. On the one hand, REM-sleep deprivation necessitated a dramatic increase in the frequency of interventions during the night to prevent this sleep state. On the other hand, there was a modest rise in the number of interventions across the three consecutive deprivation nights, and the 40% REM-sleep rebound in the first recovery night by no means compensated for the amount of REM sleep lost.

Two hypotheses were advanced. In the first, it is assumed that the homeostatic drive is strong, which is reflected by the dramatic increase in interventions during the deprivation nights. Waking may in part substitute for REM sleep, thereby accounting for the moderate night-to-night increase in interventions and the small REM-sleep rebound. According to the second hypothesis, the homeostatic drive for REM sleep is weak and the rising trend in the number of interventions is attributed to circadian factors as well as to a sleep-dependent disinhibition of REM-sleep propensity. The second hypothesis could explain the limited savings from one night to the other as well as the modest rebound.

In a selective REM-sleep deprivation study starting in the morning, the limited increase in interventions was attributed to declining circadian REM-sleep propensity, which was partly offset by the homeostatic drive and the sleep-dependent disinhibition of REM sleep.[106] Franken[107] proposed, on the basis of animal studies, that the initiation and maintenance of REM sleep could be controlled by separate processes and that the former may be accounted for by a rise in REM-sleep propensity during NREM sleep, as postulated by Benington and Heller.[108] Further experiments are required to resolve this issue.

A novel facet of REM-sleep regulation was revealed in a recent selective REM-sleep deprivation study.[109] Muscle atonia, the hallmark of REM sleep, was shown to occur also in NREM sleep. Its distribution exhibited features suggesting an association with REM-sleep regulation. Thus atonia in NREM sleep showed a bimodal pattern after sleep onset: a declining trend when sleep began in the morning and an initial enhancement after selective REM-sleep deprivation. The results suggested the possibility that the NREM-sleep state characterized by atonia may contribute to the compensation of a REM-sleep deficit.

Further Models

The limit cycle reciprocal interaction model accounts for the NREM-REM sleep cycle on the basis of interacting neuronal systems (see Table 33–1; for its most recent version and for the activation-synthesis model see Pace-Schott and Hobson[110]). Attempts were made to integrate various concepts into a combined model[111,112] (see Table 33–1).

Kronauer's two-oscillator model had been originally applied to sleep[113] but was then used mainly to simulate effects of light on the circadian system.[114] Various experimental protocols were simulated[115] and the model has been refined.[96,116] The generation of circadian rhythms was also modeled at the genetic level[117] as well as on the basis of coupled oscillators.[118,119]

Various mathematical models have been proposed to account for aspects of sleep regulation and circadian rhythms, both at the macroscopic (systemic) and microscopic (cellular) level. To investigate the possible role of different oscillations such as sleep spindles, computational models of neuronal networks were developed to simulate cellular activity in different sleep states.[53,120-122] One of the attractive features of the modeling approach is that it can be applied at different levels of analysis.

In conclusion, models help delineate the regulating processes underlying such a complex and little-understood phenomenon as sleep, and they thereby offer a conceptual framework for the analysis of existing and new data. The major models have already inspired a considerable number of experiments. The modeling approach has become particularly attractive because it is possible to use quantitative physiologic measures in human beings for testing the predictions of a model. Thus EEG SWA represents the key parameter in the investigation of NREM-sleep homeostasis, and the "unmasked" core body temperature and plasma melatonin are valuable indicators of the circadian process. Another positive feature of the modeling approach is its universality: The regulatory processes postulated are not restricted to a single species but probably represent basic mechanisms that are common to vertebrates and invertebrates (see Chapter 7).

SLEEP: A LOCAL, USE-DEPENDENT BRAIN PHENOMENON?

Recently the question arose whether sleep represents a global or a local brain process. The dolphin does not exhibit deep SWS in both hemispheres simultaneously, and the selective deprivation of unihemispheric sleep gives rise to a unihemispheric SWS rebound[123]; these observations show that the sleep process is not necessarily present in the entire brain. There is evidence from studies in monkeys that the process of falling asleep may not occur synchronously in the entire brain.[124]

Two hypotheses have been advanced that imply that regional increases in neuronal activity and metabolic demand during wakefulness may result in selective changes in EEG synchronization of these neuronal populations during NREM sleep.[125,126] Benington and Heller[126] proposed that adenosine, which is released upon increased metabolic demand via facilitated transport by neurons and glia cells throughout the central nervous system (CNS), promotes slow EEG potentials. Thus a use-dependent, local mechanism would underlie the sleep deprivation–induced changes in the sleep EEG. There is evidence from microdialysis studies that the adenosine level in the brain rises during waking and declines during sleep.[127,128]

The theory of a local, use-dependent increase of sleep intensity was tested by investigating whether a local activation of a particular brain region during wakefulness affects the EEG recorded from the same site during sleep.[129] An intermittent vibratory stimulus was applied to the left or right hand during the 6-hour period prior to sleep to activate the contralateral somatosensory cortex. Stimulation of the right (dominant) hand resulted in a shift of power in the NREM-sleep EEG toward the left hemisphere. This effect was most prominent in the delta range, was limited to the first hour of sleep, and was restricted to the central derivation situated over the somatosensory cortex.[129]

An interhemispheric asymmetry of the NREM-sleep EEG in the delta band was induced by sleep deprivation.[130] This may reflect a functional asymmetry between the dominant and nondominant hemisphere. A similar finding was obtained in the rat: The interhemispheric asymmetry of the NREM-sleep EEG in the low-frequency range varies as a function of sleep pressure[131] (see Chapter 7).

Topographical analyses of the sleep EEG revealed regional differences also along the anteroposterior axis. In particular, a sleep-dependent hyperfrontality of SWA was demonstrated.[132,133] Thus in the initial two NREM-sleep episodes, the power in the 2-Hz band was dominant at the frontal derivation, whereas in the second part of sleep the anteroposterior gradient vanished. An increase of frontal predominance of the low-frequency EEG was shown to occur after partial[134] and total sleep deprivation.[135]

These initial findings were confirmed and extended in subsequent studies.[42,71,136] A detailed topographic analysis was performed on the basis of power maps.[137] Hallmarks were the frontal predominance in the delta and alpha bands, the occipital predominance in the theta band, and the sharply delineated vertex maximum in the sigma band. Prolonged waking induced an increase in power in the low-frequency range, which was largest over the frontal region (see Fig. 33–4C), and a decrease in power in the sigma band, which was most pronounced over the vertex. The regional specificity of the homeostatic sleep drive was evident from the similarity of the topographic pattern of the recovery-to-baseline power ratio and the power ratio between the first and second halves of the baseline night. It was proposed that the predominant increase of low-frequency power in frontal areas may be due to a high "recovery need" of the frontal heteromodal association areas of the cortex. This proposition is supported by positron emission tomography (PET) studies showing a selective deactivation of frontal areas in NREM sleep[138,139] and prolonged waking.[140]

Experiments reported in 2000 have shown that a sleep deficit impairs primarily high-level cognitive skills, which depend on frontal lobe function.[141] Patients with lesions of the prefrontal cortex suffer from deficits that include distraction by irrelevant stimuli, diminished word fluency, flat intonation of speech, impaired divergent thinking, apathy, and childish humor.[142] Subjects forgoing sleep exhibit similar symptoms. Therefore, it may be more than a coincidence that the prevalence of slow waves is maximal at frontal EEG derivations in the initial part of sleep. This finding is consistent with the notion that the sleep process may occur in a topographically graded manner by preferentially involving those neuronal populations that have been most activated during waking.

One could speculate that the progressive anteroposterior shift in power in the low-frequency range reflects a high "need for recovery" in frontal parts of the cortex, which seem to exhibit the largest activity during wakefulness. In the framework of the two-process model, the results indicate that process S may decline in the anterior region of the brain at a steeper rate than in posterior regions and that therefore the homeostatic NREM sleep regulating process may exhibit regional differences. Experiments involving a specific manipulation of daytime activity are required to test this possibility.[142a]

> *Clinical Pearl*
>
> *The common experience that a good night's sleep dissipates fatigue and tiredness and regenerates energy points to a specific restorative function of sleep that cannot be achieved by merely resting. Sleep homeostasis denotes a basic principle of sleep regulation that can lead to a better understanding of sleep pathologies. Deficient sleep homeostasis may account for the altered sleep architecture in depression, and the transient normalization of sleep propensity can explain the antidepressant effect of sleep deprivation.*[61] *The elucidation of sleep homeostasis at the cellular and molecular levels is likely to open new avenues for the pharmacologic therapy of sleep disorders.*

Acknowledgments

This work was supported by the Swiss National Science Foundation and the Human Science Frontier Program. The comments of Drs. Irene Tobler and Hanspeter Landolt are gratefully acknowledged.

REFERENCES

1. Cannon WB: The Wisdom of the Body. New York, WW Norton, 1939.
2. Borbély AA: Sleep: circadian rhythm versus recovery process. In Koukkou M, Lehmann D, Angst J (eds): Functional states of the brain: Their determinants. Amsterdam, Elsevier, 1980, pp 151-161.
3. Achermann P, Borbély AA: Mathematical models of sleep regulation. Front Biosci 2003;8:683-693.
4. Jewett ME, Borbély AA, Czeisler CA: Proceedings of the workshop on biomathematical models of circadian rhythmicity, sleep regulation, and neurobehavioural function in humans. J Biol Rhythms 1999;14:429-630.
5. Neri D: Proceedings of the fatigue and performance modeling workshop. Aviat Space Environ Med 2004;75:A1-A200.
6. Rechtschaffen A, Kales A: A manual of standardized terminology, techniques and scoring system for sleep stages of human subjects. Bethesda, Md, National Institutes of Health, 1968.
7. Borbély AA, Baumann F, Brandeis D, et al: Sleep deprivation: Effect on sleep stages and EEG power density in man. Electroencephalogr Clin Neurophysiol 1981;51:483-493.
8. Achermann P, Borbély AA: Low-frequency (<1 Hz) oscillations in the human sleep EEG. Neuroscience 1997;81:213-222.
9. Amzica F, Steriade M: The K-complex—its slow (<1-Hz) rhythmicity and relation to delta waves. Neurology 1997;49:952-959.
10. Evans BM, Richardson NE: Demonstration of a 3-5 s periodicity between the spindle bursts in NREM sleep in man. J Sleep Res 1995;4:196-197.
11. Blake H, Gerard RW: Brain potentials during sleep. Am J Physiol 1937;119:692-703.
12. Williams HL, Hammack JT, Daly RL, et al: Responses to auditory stimulation, sleep loss and the EEG stages of sleep. Electroencephalogr Clin Neurophysiol 1964;16:269-279.
13. Dement W, Kleitman N: Cyclic variations in EEG during sleep and their relation to eye movements, body motility, and dreaming. Electroencephalogr Clin Neurophysiol 1957;9:673-690.

14. Webb WB, Agnew Jr. HW: Stage 4 sleep: Influence of time course variables. Science 1971;174:1354-1356.

15. Beersma DGM, Daan S, Dijk DJ: Sleep intensity and timing: A model for their circadian control. In Carpenter GA (ed): Some Mathematical Questions in Biology: Circadian Rhythms. Lectures on Mathematics in the Life Sciences. Providence, RI: American Mathematical Society, 1987, pp 39-62.

16. Dijk DJ, Beersma DGM, Daan S: EEG power density during nap sleep: Reflection of an hourglass measuring the duration of prior wakefulness. J Biol Rhythms 1987;2:207-219.

17. Dijk DJ: EEG slow waves and sleep spindles: Windows on the sleeping brain. Behav Brain Res 1995;69:109-116.

18. Werth E, Dijk DJ, Achermann P, et al: Dynamics of the sleep EEG after an early evening nap: Experimental data and simulations. Am J Physiol 1996;271:R501-R510.

19. Åkerstedt T, Gillberg M: Sleep duration and the power spectral density of the EEG. Electroencephalogr Clin Neurophysiol 1986;64:119-122.

20. Gillberg M, Åkerstedt T: The dynamics of the first sleep cycle. Sleep 1991;14:147-154.

21. Borbély AA: A two process model of sleep regulation. Hum Neurobiol 1982;1:195-204.

22. Dijk DJ, Hayes B, Czeisler CA: Dynamics of electroencephalographic sleep spindles and slow wave activity in men: Effect of sleep deprivation. Brain Res 1993;626:190-199.

23. Aeschbach D, Cajochen C, Landolt HP, et al: Homeostatic sleep regulation in habitual short sleepers and long sleepers. Am J Physiol 1996;270:R41-R53.

24. Borbély AA, Achermann P: Concepts and models of sleep regulation: An overview. J Sleep Res 1992;1:63-79.

25. Dijk DJ, Brunner DP, Beersma DGM, et al: Electroencephalogram power density and slow wave sleep as a function of prior waking and circadian phase. Sleep 1990;13:430-440.

26. Dijk DJ, Beersma DGM, Daan S, et al: Quantitative analysis of the effects of slow wave sleep deprivation during the first 3 h of sleep on subsequent EEG power density. Eur Arch Psychiatry Neurol Sci 1987;236:323-328.

27. Gillberg M, Anderzén I, Åkerstedt T: Recovery within day-time sleep after slow wave sleep suppression. Electroencephalogr Clin Neurophysiol 1991;78:267-273.

28. Sinha AK, Smythe H, Zarcone VP, et al: Human sleep-electroencephalogram: A damped oscillatory phenomenon. J Theor Biol 1972;35:387-393.

29. Achermann P, Borbély AA: Dynamics of EEG slow wave activity during physiological sleep and after administration of benzodiazepine hypnotics. Hum Neurobiol 1987;6:203-210.

30. Dijk DJ, Brunner DP, Borbély AA: Time course of EEG power density during long sleep in humans. Am J Physiol 1990;258:R650-R661.

31. Aeschbach D, Borbély AA: All-night dynamics of the human sleep EEG. J Sleep Res 1993;2:70-81.

32. Aeschbach D, Dijk DJ, Trachsel L, et al: Dynamics of slow-wave activity and spindle frequency activity in the human sleep EEG: effect of midazolam and zopiclone. Neuropsychopharmacology 1994;11:237-244.

33. Aeschbach D, Dijk DJ, Borbély AA: Dynamics of EEG spindle frequency activity during extended sleep in humans: Relationship to slow-wave activity and time of day. Brain Res 1997;748:131-136.

34. Uchida S, Maloney T, March JD, et al: Sigma 12-15 Hz and delta 0.3-3 Hz EEG oscillate reciprocally within NREM sleep. Brain Res Bull 1991;27:93-96.

35. Uchida S, Atsumi Y, Kojima T: Dynamic relationships between sleep spindles and delta waves during a NREM period. Brain Res Bull 1994;33:351-355.

36. Merica H, Blois R: Relationship between the time courses of power in the frequency bands of human sleep EEG. Neurophysiol Clin 1997;27:116-128.

37. Landolt HP, Dijk DJ, Achermann P, et al: Effect of age on the sleep EEG: Slow-wave activity and spindle frequency activity in young and middle-aged men. Brain Res 1996;738:205-212.

38. Landolt HP, Borbély AA: Age-dependent changes in sleep EEG topography. Clin Neurophysiol 2001;112:369-377.

39. Dijk DJ, Czeisler CA: Contribution of the circadian pacemaker and the sleep homeostat to sleep propensity, sleep structure, electroencephalographic slow waves, and sleep spindle activity in humans. J Neurosci 1995;15:3526-3538.

40. Dijk DJ, Shanahan TL, Duffy JF, et al: Variation of electroencephalographic activity during non–rapid eye movement and rapid eye movement sleep with phase of circadian melatonin rhythm in humans. J Physiol (Lond) 1997;505:851-858.

41. Knoblauch V, Martens W, Wirz-Justice A, et al: Regional differences in the circadian modulation of human sleep spindle characteristics. Eur J Neurosci 2003;18:155-163.

42. Knoblauch V, Kräuchi K, Renz C, et al: Homeostatic control of slow-wave and spindle frequency activity during human sleep: Effect of differential sleep pressure and brain topography. Cereb Cortex 2002;12:1092-1100.

43. Achermann P, Borbély AA: Coherence analysis of the human sleep electroencephalogram. Neuroscience 1998;85:1195-1208.

44. Achermann P, Borbély AA: Temporal evolution of coherence and power in the human sleep electroencephalogram. J Sleep Res 1998;7:36-41.

45. Sejnowski TJ, Destexhe A: Why do we sleep? Brain Res 2000; 886:208-223.

46. Gais S, Molle M, Helms K, et al: Learning-dependent increases in sleep spindle density. J Neurosci 2002;22:6830-6834.

47. Steriade M, Contreras D, Amzica F: Synchronized sleep oscillations and their paroxysmal developments. Trends Neurosci 1994;17:199-208.

48. Steriade M, McCormick DA, Sejnowski TJ: Thalamocortical oscillations in the sleeping and aroused brain. Science 1993;262:679-685.

49. McCormick DA, Bal T: Sleep and arousal: Thalamocortical mechanisms. Ann Rev Neurosci 1997;20:185-215.

50. Steriade M: The corticothalamic system in sleep. Front Biosci 2003;8:D878-D899.

51. Hirsch JC, Fourment A, Marc ME: Sleep-related variations of membrane potential in the lateral geniculate body relay neurons of the cat. Brain Res 1983;259:308-312.

52. Bal T, McCormick DA: What stops synchronized thalamocortical oscillations. Neuron 1996;17:297-308.

53. Sanchez-Vives MV, McCormick DA: Cellular and network mechanisms of rhythmic recurrent activity in neocortex. Nat Neurosci 2000;3:1027-1034.

54. Shu Y, Hasenstaub A, McCormick DA: Turning on and off recurrent balanced cortical activity. Nature 2003;423:288-293.

55. Steriade M, Timofeev I: Neuronal plasticity in thalamocortical networks during sleep and waking oscillations. Neuron 2003; 37:563-576.

56. Endo T, Roth C, Landolt HP, et al: Selective REM sleep deprivation in humans: Effects on sleep and sleep EEG. Am J Physiol 1998;274:R1186-R1194.

57. Beersma DGM, Dijk DJ, Blok CGH, et al: REM sleep deprivation during 5 hours leads to an immediate REM sleep rebound and to suppression of non-REM sleep intensity. Electroencephalogr Clin Neurophysiol 1990;76:114-122.

58. Brunner DP, Dijk DJ, Tobler I, et al: Effect of partial sleep deprivation on sleep stages and EEG power spectra: Evidence for non-REM and REM sleep homeostasis. Electroencephalogr Clin Neurophysiol 1990;75:492-499.

59. Brunner DP, Dijk DJ, Borbély AA: Repeated partial sleep deprivation progressively changes the EEG during sleep and wakefulness. Sleep 1993;16:100-113.

60. Antonioli M, Solano L, Torre A, et al: Independence of REM density from other REM sleep parameters before and after REM deprivation. Sleep 1981;4:221-225.

61. Borbély AA, Wirz-Justice A: Sleep, sleep deprivation and depression. A hypothesis derived from a model of sleep regulation. Hum Neurobiol 1982;1:205-210.

62. Feinberg I, Floyd TC, March JD: Effects of sleep loss on delta (0.3-3 Hz) EEG and eye movement density: New observations and hypotheses. Electroencephalogr Clin Neurophysiol 1987;67:217-221.

63. Barbato G, Barker C, Bender C, et al: Extended sleep in humans in 14 hour nights (LD 10:14): Relationship between REM density and spontaneous awakening. Electroencephalogr Clin Neurophysiol 1994;90:291-297.

64. Khalsa SB, Conroy DA, Duffy JF, et al: Sleep- and circadian-dependent modulation of REM density. J Sleep Res 2002;11:53-59.

65. Roth C, Achermann P, Borbély AA: Alpha activity in the human REM sleep EEG: Topography and effect of REM sleep deprivation. Clin Neurophysiol 1999;110:632-635.

66. Endo T, Schwierin B, Borbély AA, et al: Selective and total sleep deprivation: Effect on the sleep EEG in the rat. Psychiatry Res 1997;66:97-110.

67. Åkerstedt T, Torsvall L, Gillberg M: Sleepiness in laboratory and field experiments. In Koella WP, Rüther E, Schulz H (eds): Sleep '84. Stuttgart: Gustav Fischer Verlag, 1985, pp 125-126.

68. Torsvall L, Åkerstedt T: Sleepiness on the job: Continuously measured EEG changes in train drivers. Electroencephalogr Clin Neurophysiol 1987;66:502-511.

69. Cajochen C, Brunner DP, Kräuchi K, et al: Power density in theta/alpha frequencies of the waking EEG progressively increases during sustained wakefulness. Sleep 1995;18:890-894.

70. Borbély AA, Achermann P: Sleep homeostasis and models of sleep regulation. J Biol Rhythms 1999;14:557-568.

71. Finelli LA, Baumann H, Borbély AA, et al: Dual electroencephalogram markers of human sleep homeostasis: Correlation between theta in waking and slow-wave activity in sleep. Neuroscience 2000;101:523-529.

72. Aeschbach D, Matthews JR, Postolache TT, et al: Dynamics of the human EEG during prolonged wakefulness: Evidence for frequency-specific circadian and homeostatic influences. Neurosci Lett 1997;239:121-124.

73. Aeschbach D, Postolache TT, Sher L, et al: Evidence from the waking electroencephalogram that short sleepers live under higher homeostatic sleep pressure than long sleepers. Neuroscience 2001;102:493-502.

74. Cajochen C, Knoblauch V, Kräuchi K, et al: Dynamics of frontal EEG activity, sleepiness and body temperature under high and low sleep pressure. Neuroreport 2001;12:2277-2281.

75. Cajochen C, Wyatt JK, Czeisler CA, et al: Separation of circadian and wake duration-dependent modulation of EEG activation during wakefulness. Neuroscience 2002;114:1047-1060.

76. Strijkstra AM, Beersma DG, Drayer B, et al: Subjective sleepiness correlates negatively with global alpha (8-12 Hz) and positively with central frontal theta (4-8 Hz) frequencies in the human resting awake electroencephalogram. Neurosci Lett 2003;340:17-20.

77. Åkerstedt T, Fröberg JE: Psychophysiological circadian rhythms in women during 72 h of sleep deprivation. Waking Sleeping 1977;1:387-394.

78. Dijk DJ, Beersma DGM, Daan S, et al: Bright morning light advances the human circadian system without affecting NREM sleep homeostasis. Am J Physiol 1989;256:R106-R111.

79. Beersma DGM: Models of human sleep regulation. Sleep Med Rev 1998;2:31-43.

80. Achermann P: The two-process model of sleep regulation revisited. Aviat Space Environ Med 2004;75:A37-A43.

81. Feinberg I: Changes in sleep cycle patterns with age. J Psychiatr Res 1974;10:283-306.

82. Borbély AA: Sleep regulation: Circadian rhythm and homeostasis. In Ganten D, Pfaff D (eds): Current Topics in Neuroendocrinology, vol 1. Sleep: Clinical and Experimental Aspects. Berlin, Springer-Verlag, 1982, pp 83-103.

83. Daan S, Beersma D: Circadian gating of human sleep-wake cycles. In Moore-Ede MC, Czeisler CA (eds): Mathematical Models of the Circadian Sleep-Wake Cycle. New York, Raven Press, 1984, pp 129-155.

84. Daan S, Beersma DGM, Borbély AA: Timing of human sleep: Recovery process gated by a circadian pacemaker. Am J Physiol 1984;246:R161-R178.

85. Aeschbach D, Sher L, Postolache TT, et al: A longer biological night in long sleepers than in short sleepers. J Clin Endocrinol Metab 2003;88:26-30.

86. Achermann P, Borbély AA: Simulation of human sleep: Ultradian dynamics of electroencephalographic slow-wave activity. J Biol Rhythms 1990;5:141-157.

87. Achermann P, Dijk DJ, Brunner DP, et al: A model of human sleep homeostasis based on EEG slow-wave activity: Quantitative comparison of data and simulations. Brain Res Bull 1993;31:97-113.

88. Beersma DGM, Achermann P: Changes of sleep EEG slow-wave activity in response to sleep manipulations: To what extent are they related to changes in REM sleep latency? J Sleep Res 1995;4:23-29.

89. Borbély AA, Achermann P, Trachsel L, et al: Sleep initiation and initial sleep intensity: Interactions of homeostatic and circadian mechanisms. J Biol Rhythms 1989;4:149-160.

90. Edgar DM, Dement WC, Fuller CA: Effect of SCN lesions on sleep in squirrel monkeys: Evidence for opponent processes in sleep-wake regulation. J Neurosci 1993;13:1065-1079.

91. Achermann P, Borbély AA: Simulation of daytime vigilance by the additive interaction of a homeostatic and a circadian process. Biol Cybern 1994;71:115-121.

92. Dijk DJ, Czeisler CA: Paradoxical timing of the circadian rhythm of sleep propensity serves to consolidate sleep and wakefulness in humans. Neurosci Lett 1994;166:63-68.

93. Folkard S, Åkerstedt T, Macdonald I, et al: Beyond the three-process model of alertness: Estimating phase, time on shift, and successive night effects. J Biol Rhythms 1999;14:577-587.

94. Folkard S, Åkerstedt T: A three-process model of the regulation of alertness-sleepiness. In Broughton RJ, Ogilvie RD (eds): Sleep, arousal, and performance. Boston: Basel, Birkhäuser Verlag, 1992, pp 11-26.

95. Jewett ME, Kronauer RE: Interactive mathematical models of subjective alertness and cognitive throughput in humans. J Biol Rhythms 1999;14:588-597.

96. Jewett ME, Forger DB, Kronauer RE: Revised limit cycle oscillator model of human circadian pacemaker. J Biol Rhythms 1999;14:493-499.

97. Achermann P: Technical note: A problem with identifying nonlinear interactions of circadian and homeostatic processes. J Biol Rhythms 1999;14:602-603.

98. Dijk DJ, Jewett ME, Czeisler CA, et al: Reply to technical note: Nonlinear interactions between circadian and homeostatic processes: Models or metrics? J Biol Rhythms 1999;14:604-605.

99. Van Dongen HP, Dinges DF: Investigating the interaction between the homeostatic and circadian processes of sleep-wake regulation for the prediction of waking neurobehavioural performance. J Sleep Res 2003;12:181-187.

100. Van Dongen HPA, Maislin G, Mullington JM, et al: The cumulative cost of additional wakefulness: Dose-response effects on neurobehavioral functions and sleep physiology from chronic sleep restriction and total sleep deprivation. Sleep 2003;26:117-126.

101. Franken P, Tobler I, Borbély AA: Sleep homeostasis in the rat: Simulation of the time course of EEG slow-wave activity [erratum in Neurosci Lett 1991;132:279]. Neurosci Lett 1991;130:141-144.

102. Franken P, Tobler I, Borbély AA: Sleep and waking have a major effect on the 24-hr rhythm of cortical temperature in the rat. J Biol Rhythms 1992;7:341-352.

103. Tobler I, Franken P, Trachsel L, et al: Models of sleep regulation in mammals. J Sleep Res 1992;1:125-127.

104. Huber R, Deboer T, Tobler I: Effects of sleep deprivation on sleep and sleep EEG in three mouse strains: Empirical data and simulations. Brain Res 2000;857:8-19.

105. Franken P, Chollet D, Tafti M: The homeostatic regulation of sleep need is under genetic control. J Neurosci 2001;21:2610-2621.

106. Werth E, Cote KA, Gallmann E, et al: Selective REM sleep deprivation during daytime: I. Time course of interventions and recovery sleep. Am J Physiol 2002;283:521-526.

107. Franken P: Long-term vs. short-term processes regulating REM sleep. J Sleep Res 2002;11:17-28.

108. Benington JH, Heller HC: Does the function of REM sleep concern non-REM sleep or waking? Prog Neurobiol 1994;44:433-449.

109. Werth E, Achermann P, Borbély AA: Selective REM sleep deprivation during daytime: II. Muscle atonia in non-REM sleep. Am J Physiol 2002;283:527-532.

110. Pace-Schott EF, Hobson JA: The neurobiology of sleep: Genetics, cellular physiology and subcortical networks. Nat Rev Neurosci 2002;3:591-605.

111. Achermann P, Borbély AA: Combining different models of sleep regulation. J Sleep Res 1992;1:144-147.

112. Massaquoi SG, McCarley RW: Extension of the limit cycle reciprocal interaction model of REM cycle control. An integrated sleep control model. J Sleep Res 1992;1:138-143.

113. Kronauer RE, Czeisler CA, Pilato SF, et al: Mathematical model of the human circadian system with two interacting oscillators. Am J Physiol 1982;242:R3-R17.

114. Kronauer RE: A quantitative model for the effects of light on the amplitude and phase of the deep circadian pacemaker, based on human data. In Horne J (ed): Sleep '90. Bochum, Pontenagel Press, 1990, pp 306-309.

115. Klerman EB, Dijk DJ, Kronauer RE, et al: Simulations of light effects on the human circadian pacemaker: Implications for assessment of intrinsic period. Am J Physiol 1996;270:R271-R282.

116. Jewett ME, Kronauer RE: Refinement of a limit cycle oscillator model of the effects of light on the human circadian pacemaker. J Theor Biol 1998;192:455-465.

117. Goldbeter A: Computational approaches to cellular rhythms. Nature 2002;420:238-245.

118. Achermann P, Kunz HP: Modeling circadian rhythm generation in the suprachiasmatic nucleus with locally coupled self-sustained oscillators: Phase shifts and phase response curves. J Biol Rhythms 1999;14:460-468.

119. Kunz HP, Achermann P: Simulation of circadian rhythm generation in the suprachiasmatic nucleus with locally coupled self-sustained oscillators. J Theor Biol 2003;224:63-78.

120. Destexhe A, Sejnowski TJ: Thalamocortical Assemblies. How Ion Channels, Single Neurons and Large-Scale Networks Organize Sleep Oscillations. Oxford, Oxford University Press, 2001.

121. Compte A, Sanchez-Vives MV, McCormick DA, et al: Cellular and network mechanisms of slow oscillatory activity (<1 Hz) and wave propagations in a cortical network model. J Neurophysiol 2003;89:2707-2725.

122. Hill SL, Habeck CG, Edelman GM, et al: The dynamics of sleep and waking in a large-scale computer model of the thalamocortical system. Sleep 2001;24:A156-A157.

123. Oleksenko AI, Mukhametov LM, Polyakova IG, et al: Unihemispheric sleep deprivation in bottlenose dolphins. J Sleep Res 1992;1:40-44.

124. Pigarev IN, Nothdurft HC, Kastner S: Evidence for asynchronous development of sleep in cortical areas. Neuroreport 1997;8:2557-2560.

125. Krueger JM, Obál F Jr: A neuronal group theory of sleep function. J Sleep Res 1993;2:63-69.

126. Benington JH, Heller HC: Restoration of brain energy metabolism as the function of sleep. Prog Neurobiol 1995;45:347-360.

127. Porkka-Heiskanen T, Strecker RE, Thakkar M, et al: Adenosine: A mediator of the sleep-inducing effects of prolonged wakefulness. Science 1997;276:1265-1268.

128. Porkka-Heiskanen T, Alanko L, Kalinchuk A, et al: Adenosine and sleep. Sleep Med Rev 2002;6:321-332.

129. Kattler H, Dijk DJ, Borbély AA: Effect of unilateral somatosensory stimulation prior to sleep on the sleep EEG in humans. J Sleep Res 1994;3:159-164.

130. Achermann P, Finelli LA, Borbély AA: Unihemispheric enhancement of delta power in human frontal sleep EEG by prolonged wakefulness. Brain Res 2001;913:220-223.

131. Vyazovskiy VV, Borbély AA, Tobler I: Interhemispheric sleep EEG asymmetry in the rat is enhanced by sleep deprivation. J Neurophysiol 2002;88:2280-2286.

132. Werth E, Achermann P, Borbély AA: Brain topography of the human sleep EEG: Antero-posterior shifts of spectral power. Neuroreport 1996;8:123-127.

133. Werth E, Achermann P, Borbély AA: Fronto-occipital EEG power gradients in human sleep. J Sleep Res 1997;6:102-112.

134. Werth E, Achermann P, Borbély AA: Regional differences in the sleep EEG: Functional implications. Sleep 1998;21:207.

135. Cajochen C, Foy R, Dijk DJ: Frontal predominance of a relative increase in sleep delta and theta EEG activity after sleep loss in humans. Sleep Res Online 1999;2:65-69.

136. Ferrara M, De Gennaro L, Curcio G, et al: Regional differences of the human sleep electroencephalogram in response to selective slow-wave sleep deprivation. Cereb Cortex 2002;12:737-748.

137. Finelli LA, Borbély AA, Achermann P: Functional topography of the human nonREM sleep electroencephalogram. Eur J Neurosci 2001;13:2282-2290.

138. Maquet P: Functional neuroimaging of normal human sleep by positron emission tomography. J Sleep Res 2000;9:207-231.

139. Finelli LA, Landolt HP, Buck A, et al: Functional neuroanatomy of human sleep states after zolpidem and placebo: A $H_2^{15}O$-PET study. J Sleep Res 2000;9:161-173.

140. Thomas M, Sing H, Belenky G, et al: Neural basis of alertness and cognitive performance impairments during sleepiness. I. Effects of 24 h of sleep deprivation on waking human regional brain activity. J Sleep Res 2000;9:335-352.

141. Harrison Y, Horne JA: The impact of sleep deprivation on decision making: A review. J Exp Psychol Appl 2000;6:236-249.

142. Horne JA: Human sleep, sleep loss and behaviour. Implications for the prefrontal cortex and psychiatric disorder. Br J Psychiatry 1993;162:413-419.

142a. Huber R, Ghilardi MF, Massimini M, Tononi G: Local sleep and learning. Nature 2004;430:78-81.

143. McCarley RW, Hobson JA: Neuronal excitability modulation over the sleep cycle: A structural and mathematical model. Science 1975;189:58-60.

144. McCarley RW, Massaquoi SG: A limit cycle mathematical model of the REM sleep oscillator system. Am J Physiol 1986;251:R1011-R1029.

34

Interaction of Sleep Homeostasis and Circadian Rhythmicity: Dependent or Independent Systems?

Derk-Jan Dijk

Paul Franken

ABSTRACT

Circadian rhythmicity and sleep homeostasis both contribute to sleep timing and sleep structure in animals and humans. The circadian process and the sleep homeostat interact to consolidate the sleep-wake cycle. The circadian process generates a sleep-wake propensity rhythm that is timed to oppose homeostatic changes in sleep drive. In humans, circadian sleep propensity reaches its nadir just prior to bedtime and its crest just prior to wake time, in opposition to the wake-dependent increase and sleep-dependent dissipation of sleep drive. Elimination of the circadian sleep-wake propensity rhythm through lesions of the neuroanatomic locus of the circadian pacemaker, the suprachiasmatic nuclei (SCN), leads to fragmentation of wakefulness and sleep and may lead to an increase in sleep time in some species but does not eliminate the homeostatic response to sleep loss as indexed by the increase in slow wave activity (SWA). In humans, SWA declines during sleep episodes nearly, but not completely, independent of circadian phase. Elimination of the circadian sleep-wake propensity by ablation of some of the canonical clock genes alters the homeostatic regulation of SWA, suggesting that the independence of circadian rhythmicity and sleep homeostasis does not extend to all molecular components of circadian rhythm generation.

The impact of circadian rhythmicity on sleep propensity depends on homeostatic sleep pressure; when homeostatic sleep pressure is low, the influence of the circadian pacemaker on sleep initiation and consolidation is much stronger than when homeostatic sleep pressure is high. This may explain why aging, which is associated with a reduction in SWA and misalignment between the circadian pacemaker and the sleep-wake cycle, leads to a greater disruption of sleep consolidation than in younger people. The nonadditive and fine-tuned interaction between circadian rhythmicity and sleep homeostasis implies that minor changes in either of these processes can contribute significantly to normal and pathological variation in sleep timing and duration.

Circadian rhythmicity and sleep homeostasis are two major physiologic principles contributing to sleep-wake phenomenology. Endogenous circadian rhythmicity—rhythmicity driven by innate biological clocks with a period of approximately 1 day—is observed in many organisms and at many different levels of organization. Sleep-wake cycles are considered closely related to circadian cycles, and human sleep-wake rhythms are among the most frequently mentioned examples of circadian rhythmicity. Rest-activity cycles are commonly used as markers of circadian rhythmicity and of sleep-wake cycles, and in the popular science literature, the terms sleep-wake cycles, rest-activity cycles, and circadian rhythmicity are habitually used interchangeably.

From a phylogenetic perspective, circadian rhythmicity is, however, much more ubiquitous than sleep (see Chapters 7 and 27) and from a physiologic and neuroanatomic perspective, regulation of circadian rhythmicity and sleep are to a large extent separate (see Chapters 11 and 28). Sleep-wake cycles and rest-activity cycles can exhibit variable phase relationships to other circadian rhythms and can even desynchronize from these rhythms as first described by Aschoff et al.[1]

Homeostasis refers to regulatory mechanisms that maintain the constancy of the internal milieu. This concept is applicable to sleep regulation because sleep loss leads to compensatory sleep responses, indicating that constancy of internal parameters are defended. The neuroanatomic basis and functional domains of circadian rhythmicity and sleep homeostasis are thought to be very different and indeed separate. However, homeostasis and circadian rhythmicity both contribute to the regulation of sleep-wake behavior, and therefore these two systems must interact somewhere in the central nervous system (CNS).

How can the relative contribution of these two processes be separated, and how do these two main organizational principles interact? Is the separation of these two processes applicable to different levels of description—that is, at the level of sleep function, sleep neuroanatomy, and sleep and circadian genetics? Approaches to disentangle and quantify this interaction contribute to the understanding of normal and pathologic variation in sleep timing and duration, age-related changes in sleep, the effects of sleep displacement on sleep and waking performance, and the interpretation of the effects of "clock" and "sleep" genes on sleep patterns.

HOMEOSTASIS, HOURGLASSES, AND CLOCKS: DEFINITIONS

The discussion about the contribution of sleep homeostasis and circadian rhythmicity, as well as their interaction with sleep regulation, requires generally accepted definitions of these terms.[2]

From a functional perspective, circadian rhythmicity serves the appropriate timing of sleep and wakefulness relative to external (light-dark) cycles, and sleep homeostasis serves the appropriate duration and structure relative to the history of sleep and wakefulness. From a systems approach, a circadian clock may be defined as a system generating near 24-hour rhythms independent of the processes and behavior it drives; for example, the circadian clock will continue to oscillate even in the absence of sleep-wake rhythms, such as during sleep deprivation.

Sleep homeostatic systems are defined as those systems that respond to changes in the timing or history of sleep. Sleep-wake behavior itself is therefore the main determinant of the sleep homeostat, which keeps track of sleep debt; in other words, sleep-wake behavior generates rhythmicity in sleep drive and sleep structure.

The sleep-homeostat is an oscillator, although the extent to which it is self-sustaining remains unclear; it is also referred to as an hourglass oscillator or homeostat (see Chapter 33).[3,4] These latter terms are preferred over the term *homeostasis* because it can be argued that homeostasis, at least in the long run, is also served by circadian processes. The term *sleep homeostasis* is sometimes used to refer to direct effects of the presence or absence of sleep on physiologic and endocrine variables, but *evoked effects* may be the more appropriate term in that context.

THE BASIC PROBLEM: SLEEP HOMEOSTAT AND CIRCADIAN CLOCK OSCILLATE SIMULTANEOUSLY AND IN SYNCHRONY

An assessment of the contribution of circadian rhythmicity and the sleep homeostat is not easily obtained on the basis of sleep data collected under baseline conditions. Under these conditions, sleep onset occurs at a specific phase of the circadian cycle (Fig. 34–1).[5] In humans, sleep onset occurs approximately 1 to 2 hours after the onset of nocturnal melatonin secretion from the pineal, 6 hours before the nadir of the core body temperature rhythm, and 8 hours before the crest of the cortisol rhythm, which are all driven by the suprachiasmatic nuclei (SCN).[6-8] Sleep onset also occurs after 16 hours of wakefulness. Thus, sleep may be initiated because we are at the circadian phase of sleep initiation, because we have been awake for 16 hours, or because of an interaction between a circadian process and a process linked to the duration of wakefulness.

Slow wave sleep (SWS) and slow wave activity (SWA) decline in the course of a nocturnal sleep episode (see Fig. 34–1 and Chapter 33). This decline could be driven by the time spent asleep or alternatively by the change in circadian phase that occurs in the course of a sleep episode. We go through one third of a complete circadian cycle in the course of one nocturnal sleep episode. The increase in the duration of the REM episodes in the course of a nocturnal sleep episode could be related to the progression of the sleep process or the progression of circadian phase. Similar arguments apply to other aspects of human sleep, such as the increase in the density of rapid eye movements (REMs) in REM sleep and the increase in sleep spindle activity in the course of a nocturnal sleep episode.

Assessment of daytime sleep propensity by the multiple sleep latency test (MSLT) also necessarily confounds the contribution of time awake (the sleep homeostat) and circadian phase. We go through two thirds of a circadian cycle every 16-hour waking episode and simultaneously accumulate a sleep debt associated with 16 hours of wakefulness. An MSLT profile reflects the interaction of circadian phase and time awake on the ability to initiate sleep. A short sleep-latency may be caused either by a very high homeostatic sleep pressure or by a very weak wake-promoting signal generated by the circadian pacemaker.

The changes in sleep across the 24-hour cycle observed in animals are also the result of the combined influence of sleep-wake history and circadian phase. In many animals, and small rodents in particular, the sleep-wake cycle is polyphasic (see Chapters 7 and 8). This short-term alternation between sleep and wakefulness is superimposed on a night-day difference in sleep propensity.

The assessment of the relative contribution of sleep homeostasis and circadian rhythmicity is therefore not straightforward. The interpretation of sleep-wake characteristics in animals, and under some circumstances in humans, is further complicated by the presence of a light-dark cycle. Variation in sleep parameters across the 24-hour day may be caused by nonuniform distribution of sleep and wakefulness (i.e., the sleep homeostat), a circadian effect, or the direct effects of light. These interactions are illustrated schematically in Figure 34–2.[11]

The circadian clock and the sleep homeostat are the major determinants of the sleep-wake cycle. The sleep homeostat is driven entirely by the sleep-wake behavior. The clock is affected by light and may be affected by feedback of the sleep-wake cycle. One pathway by which the sleep-wake cycle affects the clock is through its effect on light input to the clock: We close our eyes when we go to sleep.

Only the sleep-wake cycle can be observed directly; the challenge has been to estimate the separate contribution of the homeostat, circadian clock, and light input to sleep-wake characteristics. Such an assessment nearly always requires laboratory experiments, because in the real world the timing of the sleep-wake cycle is to a large extent driven by social demands such as work hours, family, and social activities.

QUANTIFYING THE INTERACTION OF SLEEP HOMEOSTASIS AND CIRCADIAN RHYTHMICITY

Studies in which the spontaneous timing of sleep was studied in volunteers living without knowledge of clock time in environments shielded from external light-dark cycles provided insights into the interaction of circadian rhythmicity and the sleep-wake cycle. Under these conditions, the sleep-wake cycle continues to oscillate in synchrony with, or desynchronizes from, other rhythms, such as the body temperature rhythm. Such studies of synchronized and desynchronized free-running subjects demonstrated that the phase relationship between the sleep-wake cycle and other circadian rhythms may change and that the duration and structure of sleep depend on the circadian phase at which sleep occurs.[9,10]

The contribution of sleep homeostasis and circadian rhythmicity to sleep phenomenology has been quantified in ultrashort sleep-wake cycle protocols and forced desynchrony protocols.

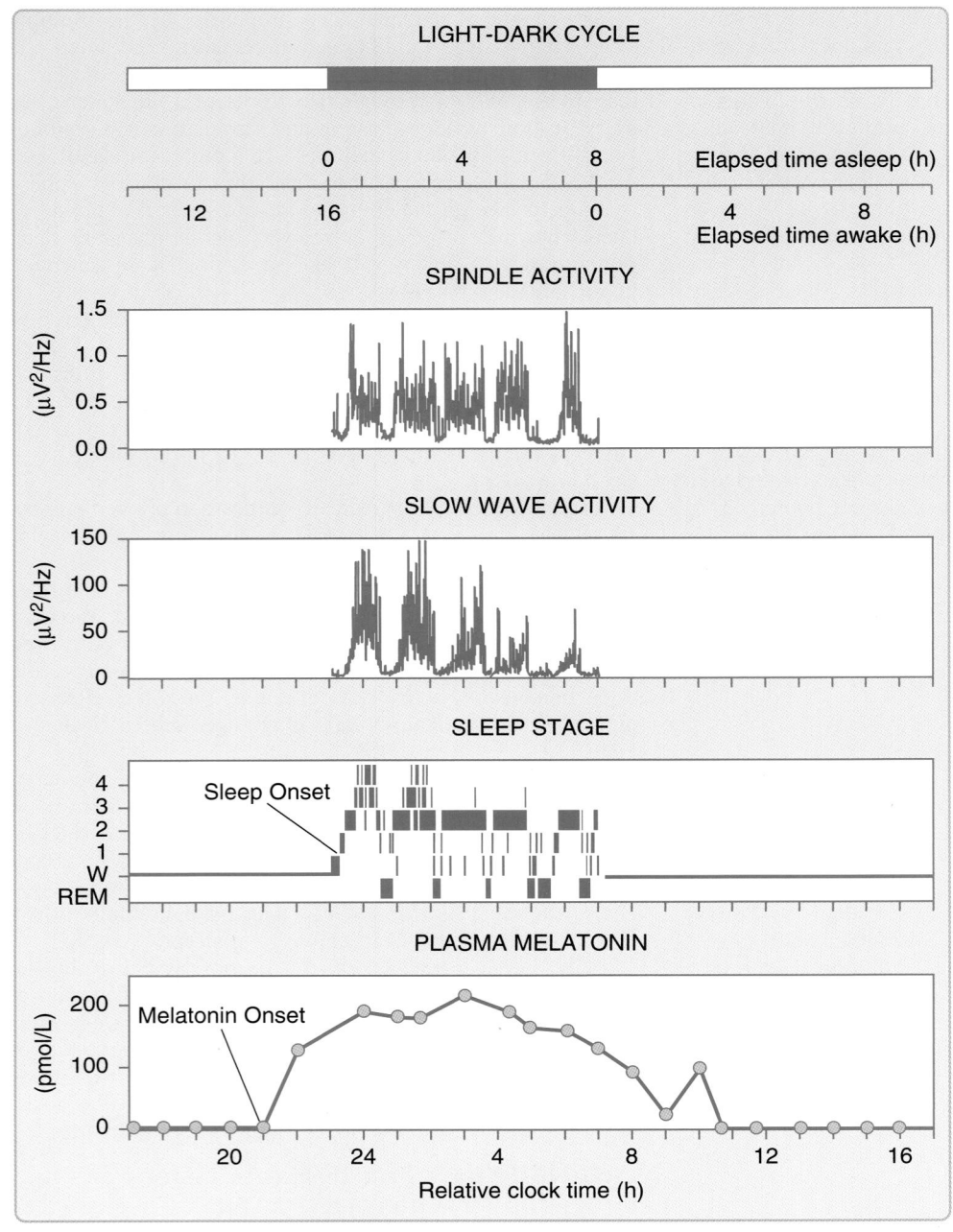

Figure 34–1. Time course of sleep stages, slow wave activity, and sleep spindle activity during a nocturnal sleep episode, relative to the plasma melatonin rhythm. The *top panel* indicates the artificial light-dark cycle and the elapsed time awake and asleep. Data are plotted against relative clock time, such that 23:00 corresponds to habitual bedtime. (Modified from Waterhouse JM, Decoursey PJ: Human circadian organization. In Dunlap JC, Loros JJ, DeCoursey PJ [eds]: Chronobiology: Biological Timekeeping. Sunderland, Mass, Sinauer Associates, 2004, pp 291-323.)

In these protocols, sleep is scheduled to occur at many circadian phases, while the scheduled wake to sleep ratio is held constant at 2:1. Some of the sleep-wake cycles that have been imposed were 20 minutes,[12] 90 minutes,[13] 180 minutes,[14] 225 minutes,[15] 20 hours,[16,17] 28 hours,[4] and even 42.85 hours.[18] In these experiments, when the light levels during scheduled wake episodes are low, markers of the circadian pacemaker such as core body temperature, plasma melatonin, and cortisol all oscillate with a near 24-hour periodicity,[19] and they appear only slightly modulated by the imposed sleep-wake cycle.[20]

These protocols generate many combinations of circadian phase and sleep homeostasis coordinates (Fig. 34–3).[4,21] When sufficient data have been collected, simple data analysis techniques can extract the main effects of circadian rhythmicity

and sleep homeostasis in a way that is somewhat similar to the estimation of main effects in an analysis of variance. The contribution of circadian rhythmicity is estimated by folding the data of the variable under study at the period of the circadian rhythm. The contribution of the sleep homeostat is estimated by folding the data at the period of the sleep-wake cycle.

Results from such protocols, conducted over a time span of approximately three decades in many different laboratories and inspired by many different theoretical models, are both remarkably consistent and informative about the contribution of the circadian pacemaker and sleep homeostat to sleep phenomenology. These experiments also provided insights into the functional significance of the normal phase relationship between the sleep-wake oscillator and the circadian process.

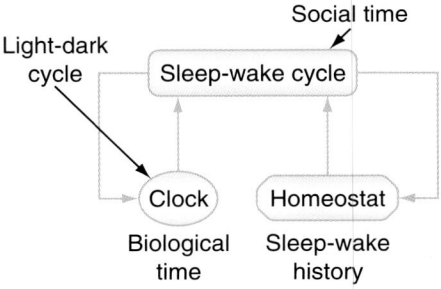

Figure 34–2. Interactions among major determinants of the sleep-wake cycle. The circadian clock and the sleep homeostat both contribute to sleep-wake propensity, but social factors are another major determinant of the timing of sleep. The sleep homeostat is driven by the sleep-wake cycle. The circadian clock is self-sustained and synchronized to the external world by the light-dark cycle. The sleep-wake cycle modulates this light input and might provide additional feedback to the clock. (Modified from Dijk DJ, Lockley SW: Integration of human sleep-wake regulation and circadian rhythmicity. J Appl Physiol 2002;92:852-862.)

Circadian Variation in the Ability to Initiate Sleep in the Absence of the Homeostatic Confound

Sleep can be initiated at all circadian phases, provided that the homeostatic pressure for sleep is sufficient. The latency to sleep onset varies significantly even in the absence of variation in prior wakefulness. Shortest sleep latencies are invariably observed at or shortly after the nadir of the body temperature rhythm (Fig. 34–4). Thereafter they increase gradually, with a plateau phase at approximately 12 hours after the temperature nadir, followed by a steep increase and longest sleep latencies during the wake maintenance zone,[22] which is close to habitual bedtime. This zone, also called the "forbidden zone for sleep,"[12] is followed by a rapid dissipation of the drive for wakefulness just after the nocturnal rise in plasma melatonin.[23,24] This time course of the circadian variation in sleep propensity is observed in all protocols in which the confounding effects of prior wakefulness are controlled for.

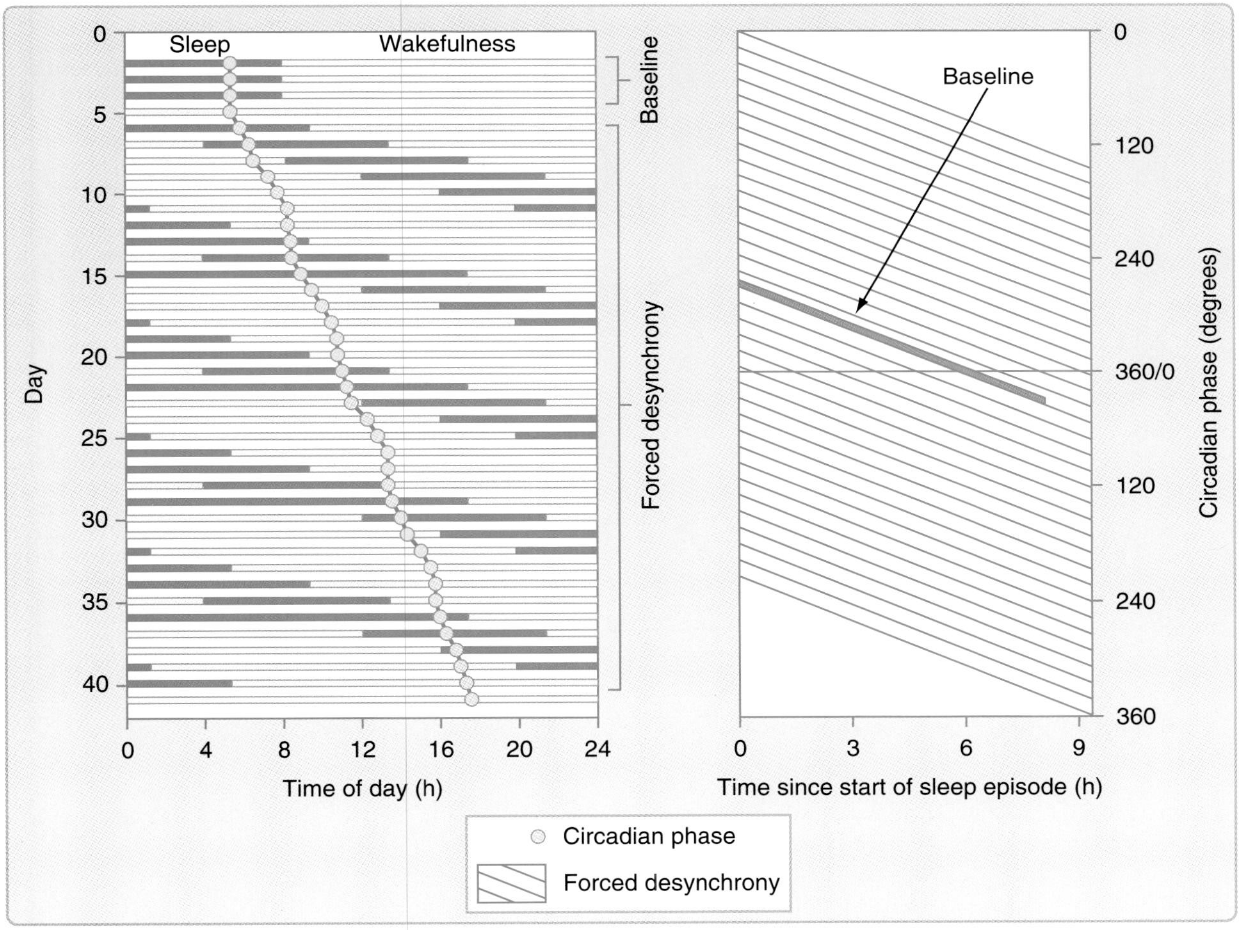

Figure 34–3. Timing of sleep (*dark blue bars*) and wake episodes (*open bars*) during baseline conditions and a 28-hour forced desynchrony protocol. *Left panel,* After 3 baseline days and a constant routine, the volunteer is scheduled to a 28-hour sleep-wake cycle. The timing of a circadian phase marker (nadir of core body temperature) is indicated by the *open circles. Right panel,* Under baseline conditions (*solid blue line*) sleep is initiated at approximately 6 hours before the body temperature nadir. This corresponds to 270 degrees in a circadian cycle, for which 360/0 degrees is defined to coincide with the core body temperature nadir. Sleep ends 2 hours after the body temperature nadir (30 degrees). During baseline conditions, only a very limited number of combinations of circadian phase and the sleep homeostat (time since start of sleep episode) occur. During forced desynchrony, many combinations occur, and this makes it possible to separate the contribution of the clock and the homeostat. (*Left panel,* Modified from Klerman EB, Dijk DJ, Kronauer RE, Czeisler CA: Simulations of effects of light on the human circadian pacemaker: Implications for assessment of intrinsic period. Am J Physiol 1996; 270:R271-R282.)

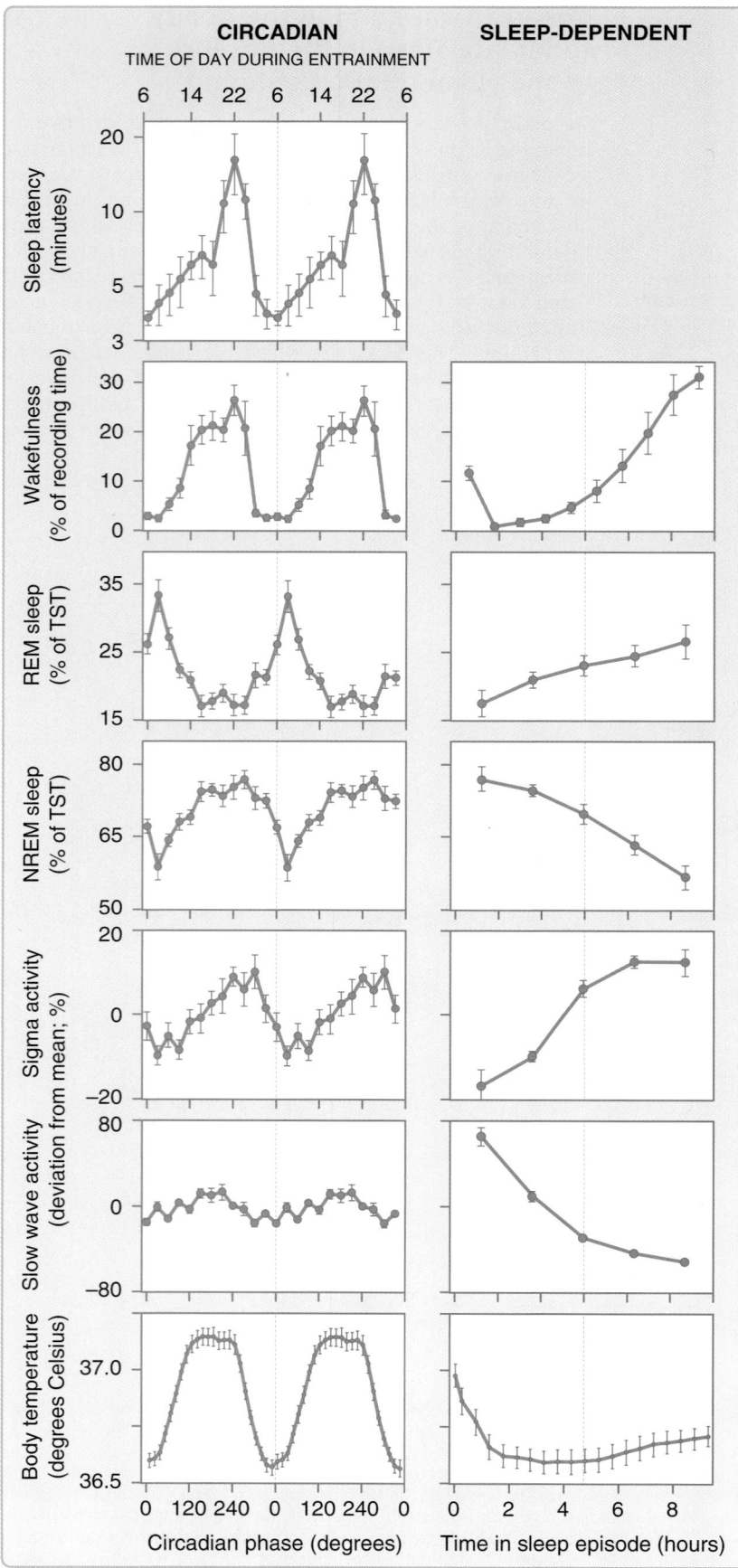

Figure 34–4. Circadian and sleep-dependent or homeostatic contributions to sleep propensity and structure. The main effects of circadian phase and sleep homeostasis on sleep structure were analyzed by aligning the data relative to the circadian component of the body temperature cycle *(left panels)* or the beginning of the sleep opportunity *(right panels)*. Slow wave activity shows weak circadian and strong sleep-dependent modulation; sigma (sleep spindle) activity shows strong circadian and sleep-dependent modulation. Non–rapid eye movement (NREM) sleep % shows equal circadian and sleep-dependent component. Rapid eye movement (REM) sleep % shows marked circadian maximum just after the temperature nadir and sleep-dependent increase (disinhibition). Wakefulness in scheduled sleep episodes shows the circadian drive for wakefulness is maximal 7 to 9 hours before temperature nadir, which is 1 to 3 hours before habitual bedtime; there is a strong wake-dependent increase. Sleep latency shows strong circadian modulation; the longest sleep latencies occur 7 to 9 hours before the body temperature nadir, and the shortest sleep latencies occur at the body temperature nadir. TST, total sleep time. (Modified from Dijk DJ, Czeisler CA: Contribution of the circadian pacemaker and the sleep homeostat to sleep propensity, sleep structure, electroencephalographic slow waves and sleep spindle activity in humans. J Neurosci 1995;15:3526-3538; and Dijk DJ, Czeisler CA: Paradoxical timing of the circadian rhythm of sleep propensity serves to consolidate sleep and wakefulness in humans. Neurosci Lett 1994;166:63-68.)

The midafternoon increase in sleep propensity often observed under normal entrained conditions,[25] when time awake and circadian phase are confounded, is not observed in the circadian sleep propensity rhythm derived from forced desynchrony protocols.

Sleep Duration and Sleep Consolidation

Total sleep time within scheduled sleep episodes varies across the circadian cycle in all protocols in which the circadian variation has been assessed. A specific problem related to the analysis of sleep time concerns the choice of the circadian reference marker. When the beginning of the sleep episode is selected as the phase reference point, sleep duration will be longest when sleep is initiated near the maximum of the body temperature rhythm. This analysis has, however, led to the suggestion that sleep propensity is highest when body temperature is high, in contrast to the conclusion from sleep latency data, which suggest that sleep propensity is highest when body temperature is at its nadir. The apparent paradox disappears when the midpoint of the sleep episode is taken as the phase reference point.

When sleep consolidation is considered, and the probability to be awake within a scheduled sleep opportunity is plotted as a function of circadian phase, a waveform similar to that for sleep latency emerges. Sleep consolidation is highest when close to the body temperature nadir, declines in the course of the biologic day to reach a crest in the late evening hours, then subsides rapidly, shortly after the nocturnal increase in plasma melatonin (see Fig. 34–4). Thus sleep propensity is highest when body temperature is low and wake propensity is highest close to the crest of the temperature rhythm.

Analyses of the duration and frequency of awakening within these scheduled sleep episodes demonstrated that the circadian variation in sleep consolidation is primarily mediated by a circadian variation in the duration, rather than frequency, of awakenings.[26] The circadian waveforms of the duration of awakenings in humans and squirrel monkeys are remarkably consistent, suggesting that indeed the duration of awakenings is driven by a circadian signal that increases in strength in the course of the biologic day and then suddenly dissipates, nearly coinciding with the increase in plasma melatonin.[24,27,28]

REM Sleep, REM Latency, and the Density of Rapid Eye Movements

The crest of the circadian REM sleep propensity rhythm is located at or shortly after the temperature nadir and is particularly pronounced when SWS pressure is low (see Fig. 34–4).[4,21] During normal entrained conditions, the circadian promotion of REM sleep in combination with sleep-dependent disinhibition leads to a very high REM propensity close to habitual wake time. From a functional perspective, this is consistent with REM sleep's role as a gate to wakefulness. Analyses of spontaneous awakenings during entrainment, synchronized free-running, desynchronized free-running, and forced desynchrony have all shown that most awakenings occur from REM sleep (reviewed by Barbato et al.[29]).

The circadian variation of the rapid eye movements during REM sleep is less robust and was thought to be virtually nonexistent,[30] which implies that the nocturnal increase in the density of rapid eye movements during REM sleep is more related to the progression of sleep than to circadian phase. Separation of the sleep-dependent and circadian component of REM density has revealed a circadian modulation when sleep pressure is low. Surprisingly, the crest of the circadian rhythm in REM density dissociates from the crest for REM-sleep duration and REM latency and is located near the wake-maintenance zone, which is 6 to 8 hours before the temperature nadir rather than at or shortly after the temperature nadir.[31]

Slow Wave Sleep, Slow Wave Activity, Sleep Spindle Activity, and Other EEG Frequencies

Analyses of the time course of SWS during spontaneous desynchrony established that the circadian variation of SWS is minor; that is, SWS declined in all sleep episodes.[32] This observation is consistent with results obtained in early sleep displacement studies during entrainment in humans,[33-35] squirrel monkeys,[36] and rats.[37] During forced desynchrony, SWA declines in the course of sleep at all circadian phases, suggesting independence of this homeostatic marker from circadian rhythmicity (see Fig. 34–4). A weak but significant circadian variation is, however, observed such that the nadirs of both SWS and SWA are located close to the crest of the sleep-propensity rhythm.[4] A similar weak circadian modulation is observed for all electroencephalogram (EEG) frequencies in the 0.75-Hz to 8.0-Hz range.

A strong circadian modulation of the EEG in non-REM (NREM) sleep is observed in the frequency range of sleep spindles (12 to 15 Hz; see Fig. 34–4). This circadian modulation entails an increase in high-frequency spindle activity during the biologic day and an increase in low-frequency spindle activity during the biologic night. This variation is associated with the plasma melatonin rhythm,[24] dissociates from the rhythm of core body temperature,[38] and includes circadian variation in the frequency, amplitude, and incidence of sleep spindles.[39] Whether this variation, in part, reflects differential circadian modulation of two types of sleep spindles (i.e., the fast and slow sleep spindles, which are dominant in more caudal and frontal regions, respectively[40]) remains to be firmly established, although it appears that parietal spindles are strongly modulated by the circadian pacemaker.[41] In REM sleep, circadian modulation of the EEG is most prominent in the alpha range (8 to 12 Hz), with a circadian nadir coinciding with the circadian crest of the REM-sleep propensity rhythm.[24] Circadian modulation of high-frequency EEG activity during sleep has also been observed in rodents.[42]

CONTRIBUTION OF THE INTERACTION OF CIRCADIAN RHYTHMICITY AND SLEEP HOMEOSTASIS TO PERFORMANCE AND THE EEG DURING WAKEFULNESS

Researchers have separated the contribution of the circadian process and the sleep homeostat for waking performance on 20 hours and 42.85 hours of forced-desynchrony protocols.[16,18] Forced desynchrony of the wake-sleep episode of the circadian rhythms uncovered a remarkable sensitivity of performance to elapsed time awake (Fig. 34–5). When the circadian contribution to alertness and performance is controlled for, wake episodes with durations as short as 13 hours lead to a significant deterioration of alertness and performance. This deterioration is monotonic for wake duration up to 28.6 hours. Performance measures that were analyzed include cognitive throughput, psychomotor vigilance, and probed recall memory. The progression of time awake is associated with a progressive increase in low-frequency components in the wake EEG (1 to 4.5 Hz),[43] as well as a progressive increase in slow eye movements during wakefulness.[18]

For all variables mentioned, as well as for mood,[44,45] circadian phase exerts a significant influence. Invariably, the nadir of performance is located during the biologic night, often close to the temperature nadir (see Fig. 34–5). The crest of performance and alertness is located during the biologic day, with minor differences in the precise location of the crest (see Fig. 34–5). For probed recall memory, the circadian peak performance is located close to the wake maintenance zone, whereas for cognitive throughput measures this crest may occur somewhat earlier. Slow eye movements and the EEG during wakefulness are all modulated by circadian phase.

The homeostatic and circadian modulation of the EEG during wakefulness is dependent on the location of EEG electrodes and EEG frequency; low-frequency activity in frontal areas is most sensitive to changes in the sleep homeostat.[43] Alpha activity exhibits a prominent circadian rhythm, with a nadir close to the melatonin maximum and temperature nadir and a crest 12 to 15 hours earlier, in both frontal and

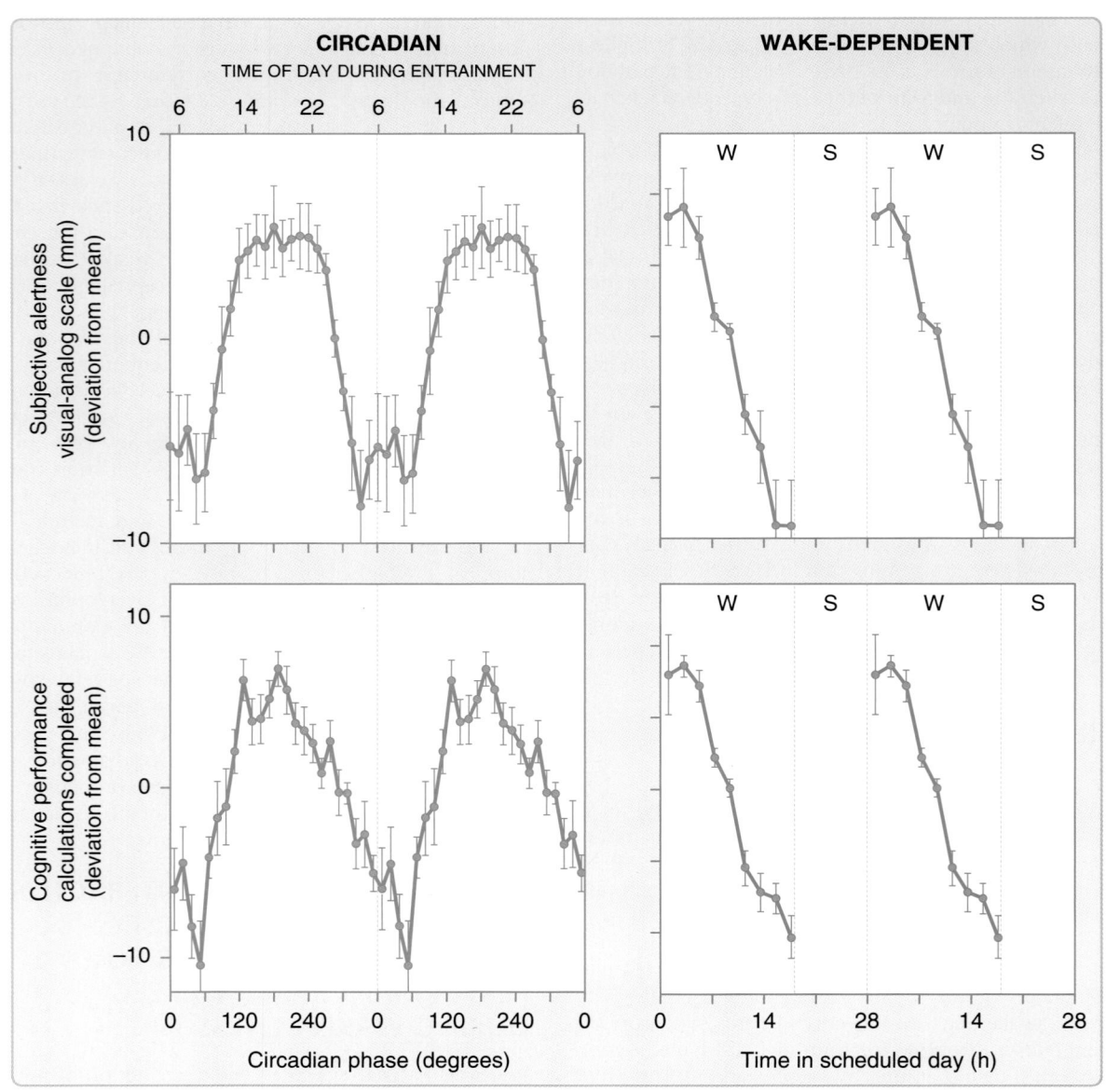

Figure 34–5. Circadian and wake-dependent (homeostatic) modulation of alertness and cognitive throughput. (Modified from Dijk DJ, Duffy JF, Czeisler CA: Circadian and sleep/wake dependent aspects of subjective alertness and cognitive performance. J Sleep Res 1992;1:112-117, with permission.)

occipital derivations. In the frequencies below and above the alpha range, similar yet smaller-amplitude circadian modulations are present. Thus, while both circadian and homeostatic factors influence EEG activity during wakefulness, a functional interpretation of the topographical differences remains elusive.

CIRCADIAN AND HOMEOSTATIC PROCESSES: THEY DON'T ADD UP!

The separation of circadian and homeostatic influences is in essence a description of the main effects of these two factors. The interaction of these two factors is, however, more relevant to everyday life because the circadian clock and the sleep homeostat change in synchrony. In most current models for the circadian and homeostatic regulation of waking performance, the effects of the two factors are additive (see Chapter 33). Quantitative analyses of these interactions have, however, shown that for many performance measures the two factors interact, they do not simply add up.[16,18,46] This implies that the amplitude of the observed circadian modulation depends on homeostatic sleep pressure. For example, when sleep pressure is relatively low, the circadian variation in performance is relatively small. Even at the circadian performance nadir, performance levels are not markedly impaired. However, when sleep pressure increases, the amplitude of the circadian modulation grows, and performance is now markedly impaired at the circadian performance nadir (Fig. 34–6).

Similar changes in circadian amplitude in association with variation in sleep pressure have been observed for sleep spindle activity, sleep consolidation, REM density in REM sleep, slow eye movements during wakefulness, the EEG during wakefulness, subjective sleepiness, and mood (see Fig. 34–6). This nonadditive nature of the interaction is unlikely to be an artifact of the characteristics of the scales on which these variables are measured.[47]

The main implication of this nonadditive interaction is that relatively minor changes in circadian phase can have a major

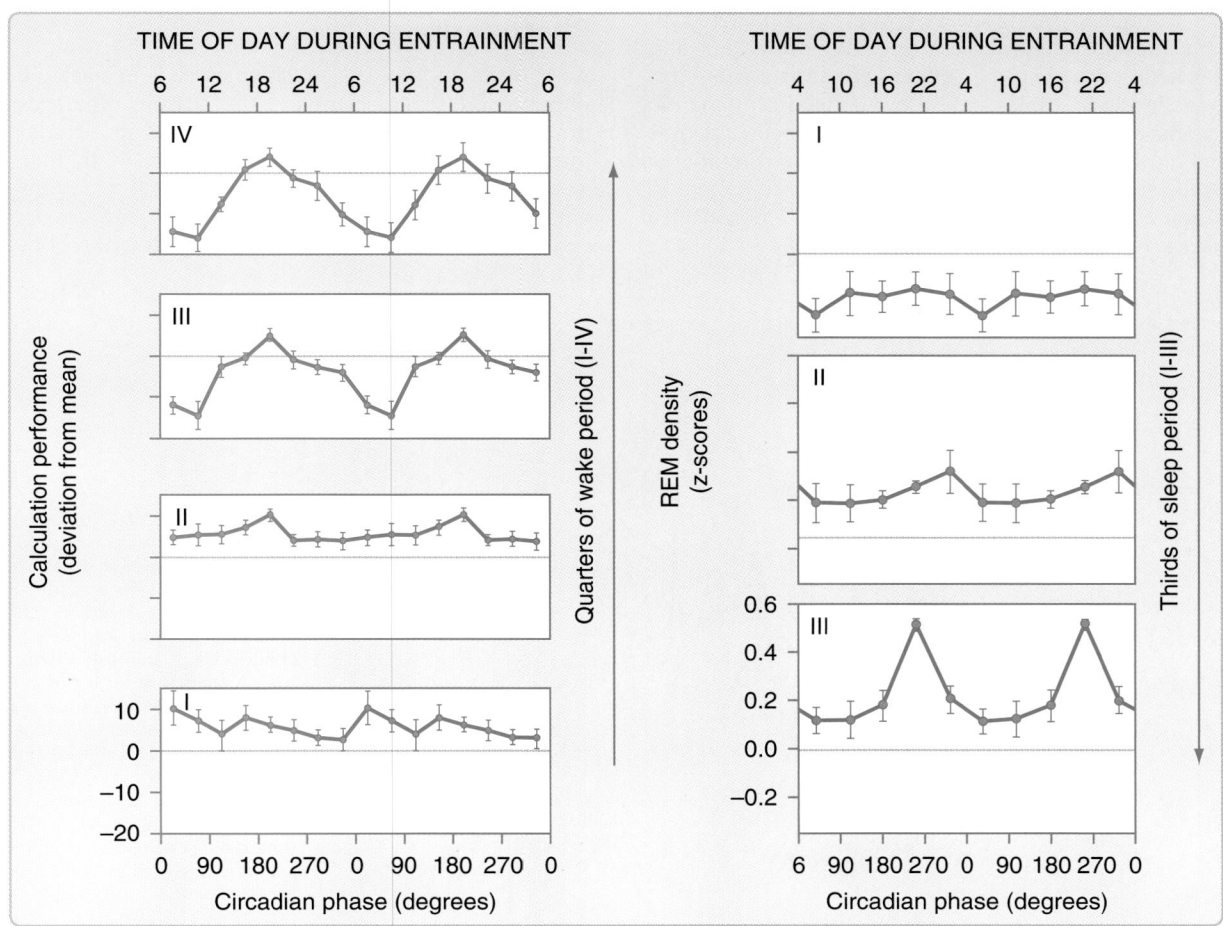

Figure 34–6. Interaction of homeostatic sleep pressure and circadian rhythmicity during wakefulness and sleep. *Left panel,* Circadian modulation of calculation performance during the first (low homeostatic sleep pressure) to final quarter (high homeostatic sleep pressure) of wake episodes lasting 18 hours 40 minutes during forced desynchrony. Note the increase in circadian amplitude and decline in average performance with increasing sleep pressure. *Horizontal dotted line* indicates average performance under baseline conditions. *Right panel,* Circadian modulation of the density of rapid eye movements (REMs) during REM sleep during the first (high homeostatic sleep pressure) through final third (low homeostatic sleep pressure) of sleep episodes lasting 9 hours 20 minutes during forced desynchrony. (*Left panel,* Modified from Dijk DJ, Duffy JF, Czeisler CA: Circadian and sleep/wake dependent aspects of subjective alertness and cognitive performance. J Sleep Res 1992;1:112-117. *Right panel,* Modified from Khalsa SBS, Conroy DA, Duffy JF, et al: Sleep- and circadian-dependent modulation of REM density. J Sleep Res 2002;11:53-59.)

impact on a given variable provided that sleep pressure is high. It also implies that the impact of changes in circadian phase is relatively minor provided that sleep pressure is low. The nonadditive nature of the interaction between circadian rhythmicity and sleep homeostasis has considerable implications for everyday life. For example, recommendation on maximum duty hours should take into consideration the circadian phase during which the duties are carried out.

FUNCTIONAL SIGNIFICANCE OF THE PHASE RELATIONSHIP BETWEEN THE HOMEOSTATIC AND CIRCADIAN SLEEP PROPENSITY RHYTHM

Figure 34–7 illustrates sleep consolidation as a function of both circadian phase and time since start of sleep episode. Trajectories that are traversed during a normal nocturnal sleep episode and during a sleep episode initiated a few hours after the temperature nadir, which is a typical scenario in night shift work, are indicated. Obviously, only when sleep is initiated close to the wake maintenance zone can sleep consolidation be maintained for 8 hours or more. Likewise, maintenance of optimal performance during a wake episode is critical depending on the trajectory followed. During the normal day shift, work is scheduled during the optimal combination of circadian phase and time awake—in other words, during the biologic day and with the duration of wakefulness being relatively short. In contrast, for the night-shift worker, the combination of the two factors is worst: Performance is jeopardized because the duration of wakefulness is relatively long and the circadian pacemaker promotes sleep rather than wakefulness.

The functional significance of the fine-tuned paradoxical phase relationship between the circadian pacemaker and the sleep homeostat (in which sleep is initiated shortly after the crest of the circadian drive for wakefulness, and wakefulness is initiated shortly after the crest of the circadian drive for sleep) is to maintain consolidated wakefulness and sleep. This is consistent with a model for the control of sleep and performance by the SCN, in which a signal from the SCN opposes homeostatic drive for sleep during the biologic day. In the absence of this signal, sleep-wake behavior is no longer consolidated and becomes fragmented, and adequate performance can no longer be maintained beyond a few hours of wakefulness (Fig. 34–8).

CIRCADIAN RHYTHMICITY AND SLEEP HOMEOSTASIS

The interaction between the sleep homeostat and circadian rhythmicity can be studied in natural models such as the changes associated with variation in day length, long and short sleepers, and aging.

Interaction during Long and Short Photoperiods

A major function of the circadian clock is to track changes in photoperiod that accompany the seasons. Changes in the duration of photoperiod lead to changes in circadian waveforms, such as the waveform of melatonin. Many humans live in temperate areas where marked annual variations in day length occur. Most humans living in industrialized societies can, however, maintain a near-constant duration of daily light

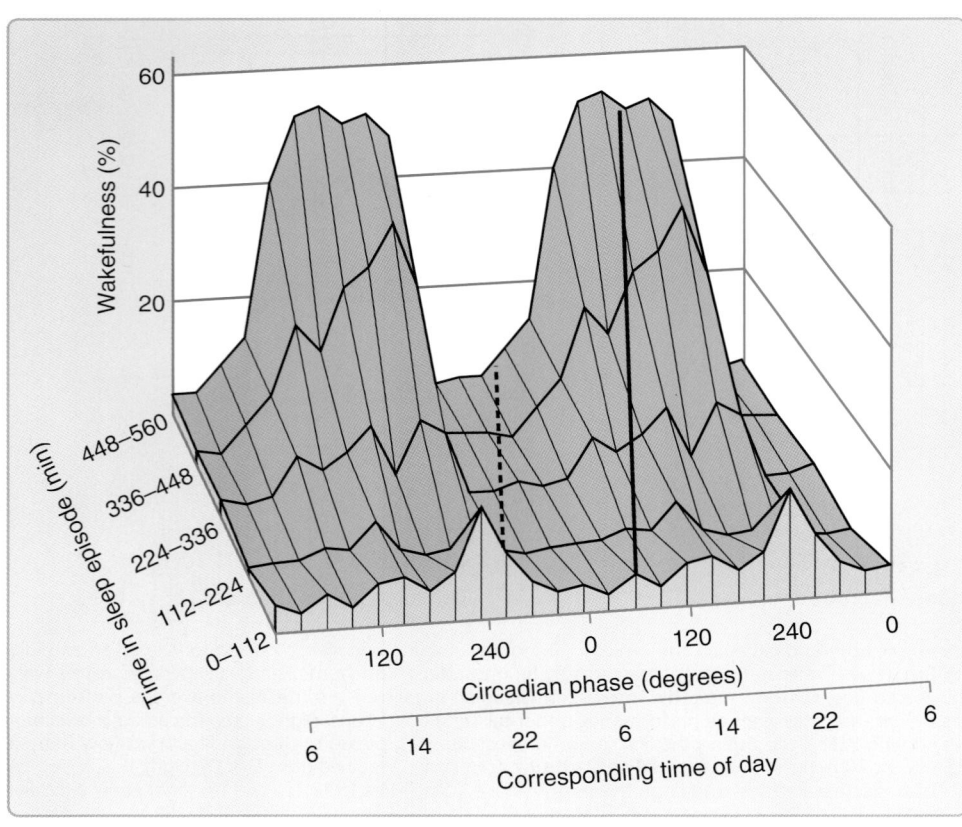

Figure 34–7. Wakefulness in scheduled sleep episodes as a simultaneous function of circadian phase and time since start of sleep episode. During a sleep episode, circadian phase and time since start of sleep episode change simultaneously along a trajectory. A trajectory for a nocturnal sleep episode *(dashed line)* initiated at 270 degrees *(approximately midnight)* and a diurnal sleep episode *(solid line)* initiated at 60 degrees *(approximately 10:00 AM)* are indicated. (Modified from Dijk DJ, Czeisler CA: Paradoxical timing of the circadian rhythm of sleep propensity serves to consolidate sleep and wakefulness in humans. Neurosci Lett 1994;166:63-68.)

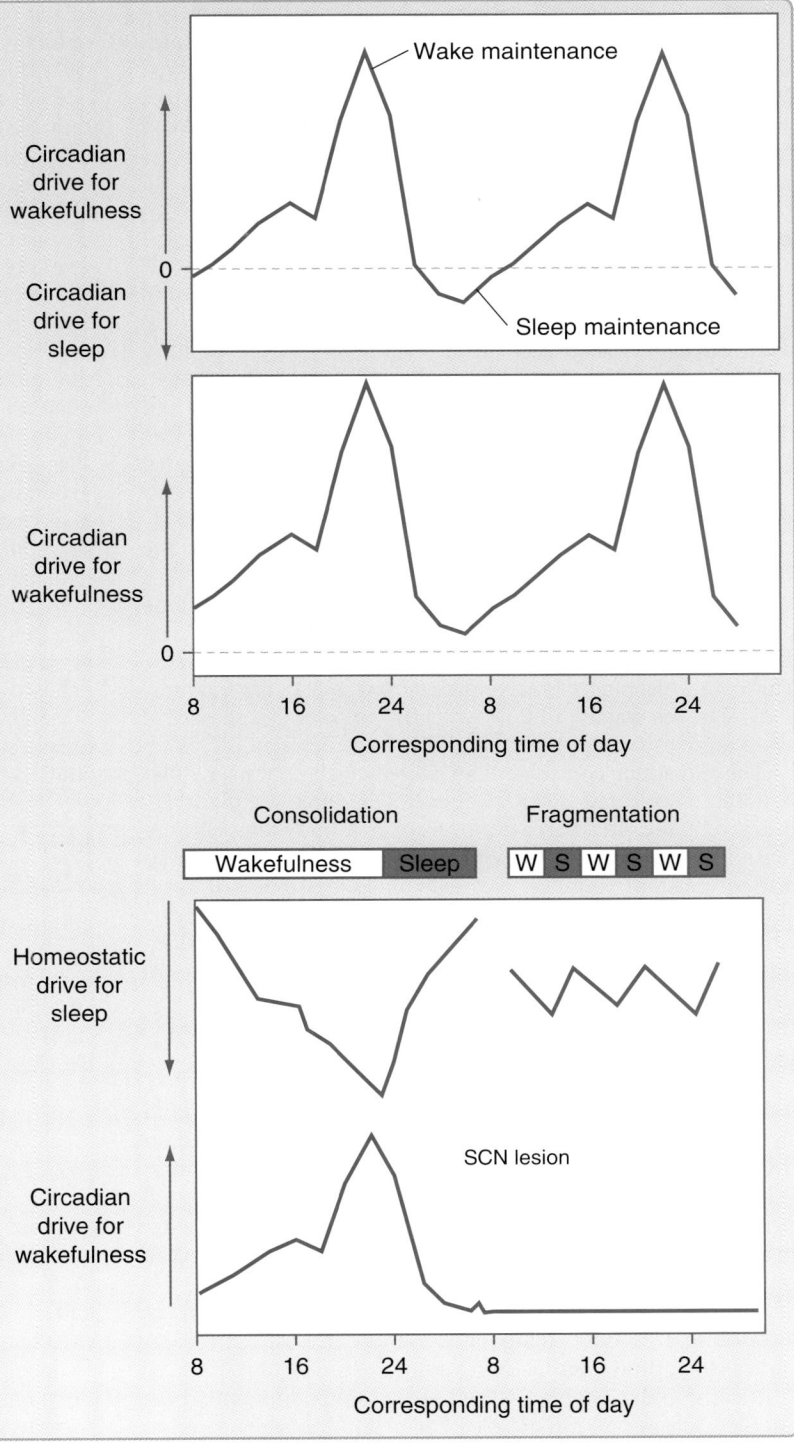

Figure 34–8. Circadian modulation of total sleep time in young and older people. Total sleep time *(top panel)* in a 9-hour, 20-minute sleep episode, and wakefulness in the last quarter of the sleep episode *(middle panel),* plotted relative to the circadian melatonin rhythm *(bottom panel).* Note that total sleep time is shorter in older people than in young people at all circadian phases. The onset of melatonin secretion is associated with a rapid increase in sleep propensity in both young and older people. In the last quarter of the sleep episode, young people can maintain high sleep efficiency (little wakefulness) for several hours after the crest of the melatonin rhythm, whereas in older people there is much wakefulness when the last quarter of the sleep episode occurs after the crest of the melatonin rhythm. TRT, total recording time. (Modified from Dijk DJ, Duffy JF, Riel E, et al: Ageing and the circadian and homeostatic regulation of human sleep during forced desynchrony of rest, melatonin and temperature rhythms. J Physiol [Lond] 1999; 516.2:611-627.)

exposure by the use of artificial light, which we now know to be of sufficient intensity to affect the human circadian pacemaker.[48,49]

The impact of photoperiod on circadian organization and sleep-wake timing has been investigated in experimental studies in which healthy subjects were scheduled to remain in darkness and in bed for 14 hours per day for several weeks. The duration of nocturnal melatonin secretion lengthens under such a short-day photoperiod.[50] Sleep onset and sleep

termination remain closely associated with the melatonin rhythm and sleep period time; that is, the period between sleep onset and the final awakening increases.

When subjects were scheduled to bed rest in darkness for 14 hours, the duration of the endogenous biologic night increased; however, total sleep time stabilized to 8.25 hours after approximately 4 weeks of exposure to these long dark periods.[51] This remarkably small change in total sleep time is consistent with previous polysomnographic recordings of diurnal[52] and nocturnal rodents[53,54] under different photoperiods. Despite marked changes in multiple circadian waveforms, only minor changes in total sleep time are observed and the homeostatic regulation of SWA is not affected, providing further evidence for the independence of the circadian rhythm and the sleep homeostat.

INTERACTION IN SHORT AND LONG SLEEPERS

Habitual short and long sleepers provide another natural model for studying the interaction of homeostatic and circadian aspects of sleep regulation. Parameters of the buildup and dissipation of sleep need as indexed by the time course of theta activity in the waking EEG during sleep deprivation and the time course of SWA in the sleep EEG during baseline and recovery sleep were quantified. Quantification revealed no differences between the short and long sleepers.[55,56] Thus the differences in sleep-wake timing are not easily explained by differences in the parameters describing the kinetics of the homeostatic aspect of sleep.

Because short sleepers sleep less than long sleepers and the parameters for the buildup and dissipation of SWA are similar, short sleepers carry a higher sleep debt than long sleepers. This higher sleep debt is accompanied by a higher level of theta activity in the waking EEG,[56] which is considered a marker of sleep homeostasis in the waking EEG (see Chapter 33).[57]

The circadian component of sleep regulation may differ between short and long sleepers. The biologic night, as indexed by the circadian waveforms of core body temperature, plasma melatonin, cortisol, and subjective sleepiness assessed during constant routines, is longer in long sleepers than in short sleepers.[58] This change in circadian organization may be either the cause or the consequence of the differences in sleep duration, because sleep is associated with a near cessation of light input to the circadian pacemaker.

INTERACTION IN AGING

Aging is associated with major changes in sleep timing and sleep quality, and the separate contributions of circadian rhythmicity and sleep homeostasis have been considered. When older subjects, who have been living with a habitual sleep-wake schedule, are studied under constant conditions, the onset of melatonin secretion and the nadir of the core body temperature rhythm are advanced by 1 hour or less.[59,60] Several other studies have reported that circadian rhythms of melatonin, core body temperature, and cortisol occur at an earlier clock time than in young adults.[61]

Healthy older people without sleep complaints and without sleep disorders initiate sleep at nearly the same internal phase of melatonin rhythm and body temperature rhythm as young subjects (Fig. 34-9). However, habitual wake time has been shown to occur earlier relative to the core body temperature and melatonin rhythm in the older subjects.[60,61] This internal circadian phase advance persists for both subjective[59] and polysomnographically defined awakening during forced desynchrony protocols (see Fig. 34-9).[62]

When studied during forced desynchrony or ultrashort sleep-wake cycles, the circadian regulation of sleep appears robust in healthy older people.[62,63] Some age-related changes in the circadian aspect of sleep regulation include a reduction in the circadian modulation of sleep spindle activity[39] and a reduced sleep propensity as indexed by sleep latency in the early morning.[62] The homeostatic aspect of sleep is markedly altered. SWS is reduced at all circadian phases, and total sleep time obtained in sleep opportunities that are of equal duration in young and older people is reduced at all circadian phases (see Fig. 34-9). These data, as well as the observed attenuation of inhibition of REM sleep in the initial part of sleep episodes, are consistent with the hypothesis that homeostatic sleep pressure is lower in older people than in young adults. Whether this reflects a reduced need for sleep or a reduced ability to sleep is currently debated.[64]

One consequence of reduced homeostatic sleep pressure is that older people become very susceptible to sleep disruption related to misalignment of the sleep-wake cycle and circadian rhythmicity. Whereas young adults can maintain consolidated sleep even when sleeping several hours after the melatonin maximum, older people cannot maintain sleep at this circadian phase (see Fig. 34-9). These age-related changes in the susceptibility to circadian phase misalignment, as well as the reduction in SWS, are already present in middle-aged people.[65-67]

Further evidence for the hypothesis that age-related changes are primarily related to a noncircadian process was reported in animals. In the rat, age-related changes in sleep persist when the SCN are ablated.[68]

Separation of circadian and homeostatic aspects and quantification of their interaction is a powerful approach in the study of age-related changes in sleep.

EFFECTS OF ELIMINATING CIRCADIAN RHYTHMICITY ON SLEEP

Elimination and disruption of circadian rhythmicity are alternative approaches to investigating the interdependency of circadian rhythmicity and sleep homeostasis. Surgical ablation of the SCN (SCNx) can be applied to investigate whether sleep homeostasis and circadian rhythmicity are neuroanatomically separable. Targeted gene mutations aimed at the canonical circadian clock genes *clock*, *bmal1*, *period*, and the *cryptochromes* allow the study of the impact of clock genes on the sleep homeostat.

Effects of SCN Ablation

In intact mice,[69] rats,[70] and squirrel monkeys,[71] sleep need that accumulates during the active period is manifested early in the subsequent rest period by high levels of SWA and sleep and by increased sleep consolidation. SCNx animals lack circadian organization of sleep and wakefulness and thus lack a consolidated active period. As a consequence, high levels of sleep need are never reached under baseline conditions. This is evident by the higher prevalence of lighter stages of NREM sleep, increased sleep fragmentation, and lower average levels of SWA observed in SCNx rats,[72-74] mice,[75] and squirrel monkeys.[28] In rats and mice, SCNx leaves the daily sleep time largely unchanged, although small increases in NREM sleep time have been reported.[68] In contrast, ablation of the SCN in the squirrel monkey leads to a marked increase in NREM sleep time.[28] The latter results gave rise to the view that an SCN-dependent process actively promotes wakefulness, thereby suppressing sleep at specific times of day (see Fig. 34-9). If the SCN promotes not only wakefulness but also sleep, then the effects of lesioning the SCN may reflect variation in

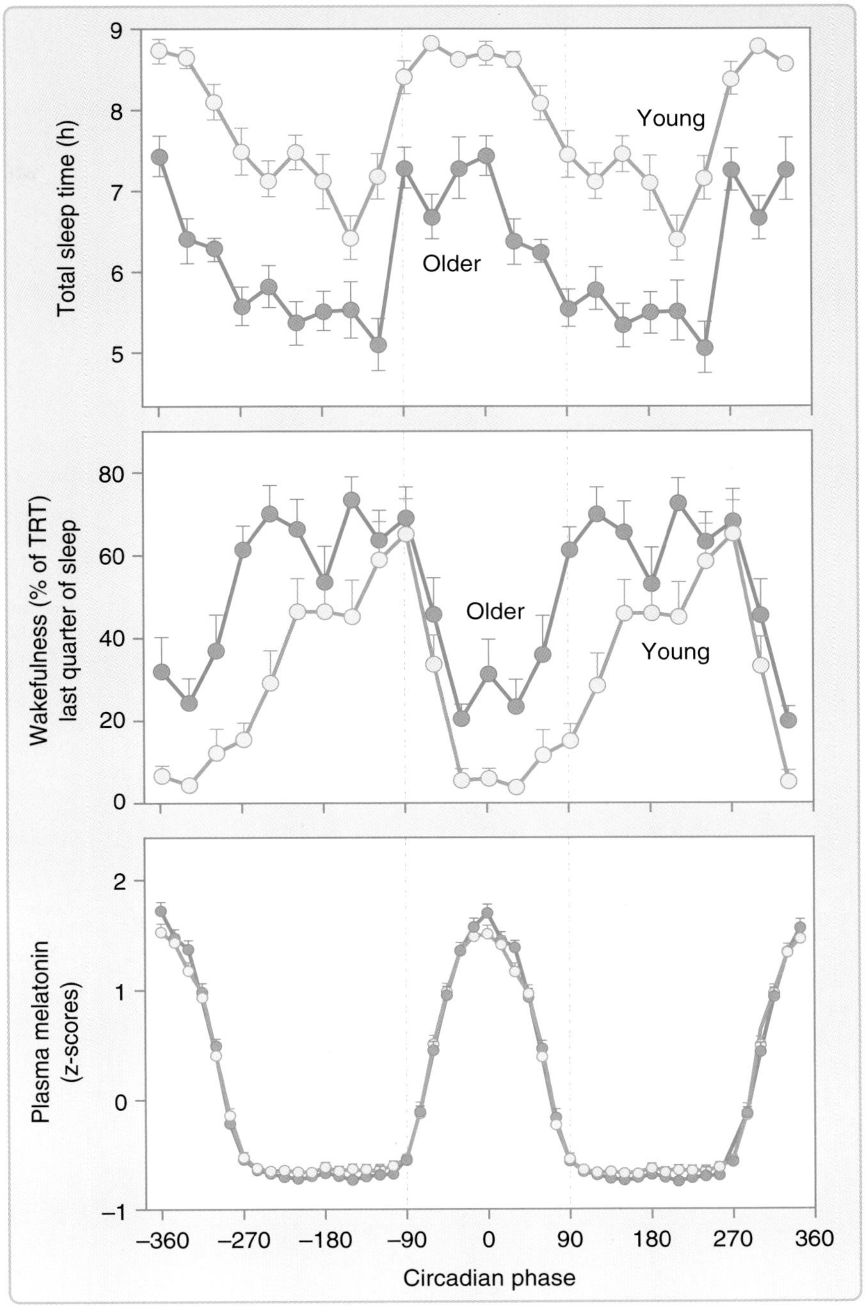

Figure 34–9. Circadian regulation of sleep through opposing processes. **A,** Two views of the way the suprachiasmatic nucleus (SCN) regulates sleep: The SCN promotes wakefulness,[28] and the SCN promotes both wakefulness and sleep. These two views yield slightly different predictions of the effects of SCN lesion on sleep. In both views, SCN lesions lead to fragmentation of the sleep-wake cycle because there is no longer a signal to oppose changes in homeostatic sleep drive **(B)**. If the SCN only promotes wakefulness, SCN lesions lead to an increase in total sleep time and a reduction in wakefulness, whereas in the case of SCN-dependent promotion of sleep and wakefulness, total sleep time might not change.

relative magnitude of wake- and sleep-promoting influences. Evidence for an active promotion of sleep by the circadian pacemaker has been demonstrated for REM sleep in the rat.[76]

Changes in sleep duration after SCNx do not constitute evidence that homeostatic sleep regulation is altered. Indeed, in all species investigated, sleep deprivation leads to an increase in SWA and sleep duration even in the absence of the SCN. These data suggest a neuroanatomical separation of the circadian and homeostatic regulation of sleep.

Ablation of "Clock" Genes

At the cellular-molecular level, circadian rhythms are generated by a network of transcriptional regulators (see Chapter 30).

In humans, some cases of delayed and advanced sleep-wake syndrome, as well as the normal variation in sleep timing,[77-79] have been associated with alterations in clock genes, but sleep homeostasis has not been studied extensively in these populations. In animal models, circadian rhythms can be disrupted with targeted gene mutations aimed at clock genes. Such disruptions offer an alternative to surgical destruction of the SCN, which often damages adjacent tissue and thereby may not exclusively affect the circadian pacemaker. The use of transgenic model organisms is, however, also not without limitations. Loss of gene function is not restricted to the adult SCN but is present throughout development and throughout the body. This widespread expression suggests that clock genes are pleiotropic and thus could affect other than circadian regulatory pathways.

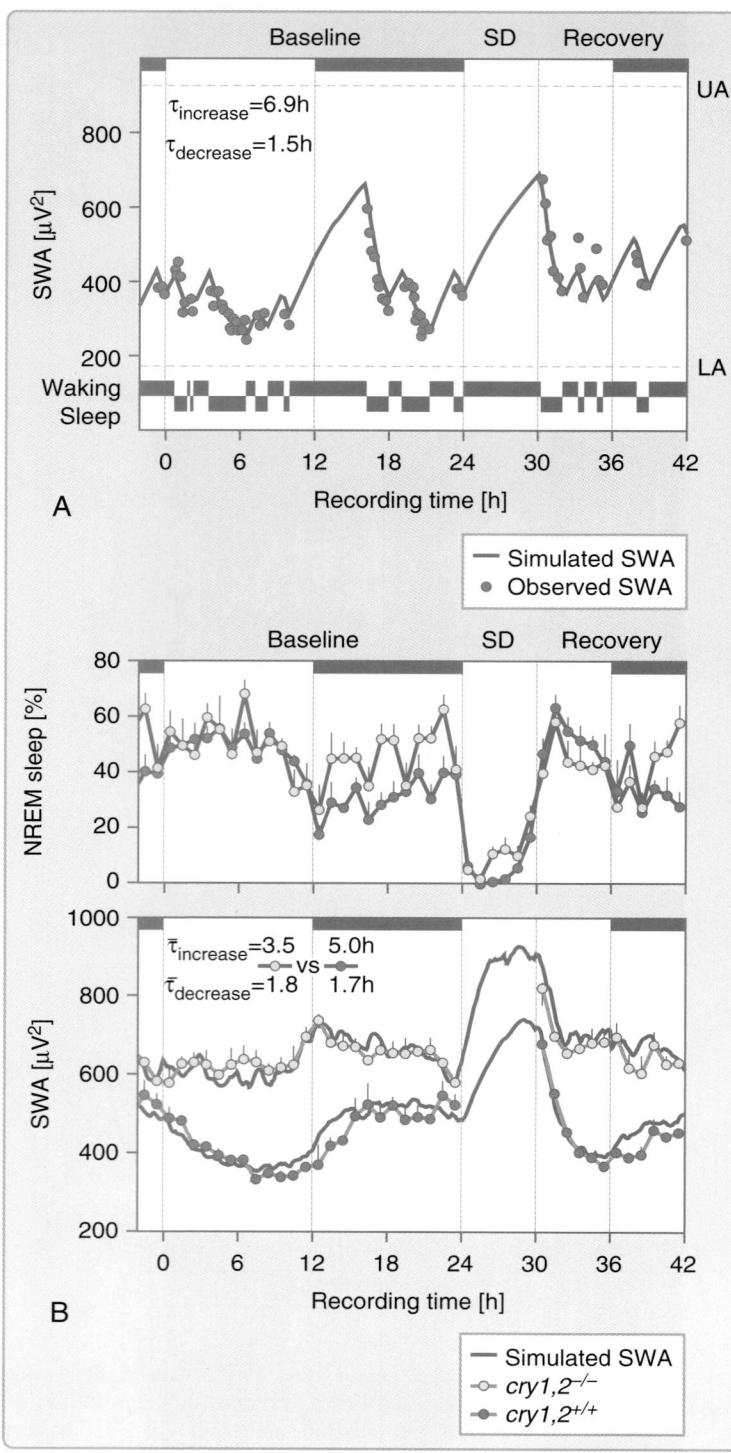

Figure 34–10. Sleep homeostasis is altered in mice lacking the clock genes *cryptochrome 1* and *2* (*cry1,2*⁻/⁻). **A,** Quantification of the relationship between the sleep-wake distribution (simplified hypnogram) and homeostatic sleep pressure indexed by the level of slow wave activity (SWA) in discrete non–rapid eye movement (NREM) sleep episodes in an individual mouse. A simulated time course of sleep pressure was derived from the hypnogram by assuming that sleep pressure increases during wakefulness and dissipates during sleep according to exponential functions with upper (UA) and lower (LA) asymptotes, respectively. The combination of time constants (τ) that describe the increase and decrease, respectively, that yielded the best fit between simulated and observed SWA levels for this mouse is indicated in the figure (see Franken et al.[69] for details). **B,** In baseline, NREM sleep time was increased, especially in the dark or active period, and SWA was maintained at higher levels in *cry1,2*⁻/⁻ mice. Simulation analysis demonstrated that although SWA still varied according to the sleep-wake distribution, the buildup of homeostatic sleep pressure was significantly faster (i.e., shorter τ) in *cry1,2*⁻/⁻ mice, which might have contributed to their higher overall level of sleep pressure in baseline and the reduced compensatory rebound after sleep deprivation (SD). (Modified from Wisor JP, O'Hara BF, Terao A, et al: A role for cryptochromes in sleep regulation. BMC Neurosci 2002;3:20.)

Circadian rest-activity rhythms are severely disrupted in *clock* mutant mice[80] and are altogether absent in mice lacking both *per1* and *per2* or both *cry1* and *cry2*.[81,82] This lack of circadian rhythmicity is not associated with a major change in sleep time during baseline conditions in *per1* and *per2* single- and double-mutant mice, and it is not associated with a major change in the sleep deprivation–induced increase in SWA.[83,84] These authors therefore concluded that the clock genes *per1* and *per 2* are not part of the sleep homeostat.

In *clock* mutant mice, NREM sleep time and consolidation of NREM sleep are reduced compared to those in wild-type mice. Sleep deprivation elicited a similar increase in NREM sleep time but an attenuated REM sleep response in mutant compared with control mice.[85] The reduction in baseline sleep time and the differential effect of sleep deprivation on REM sleep may suggest that sleep homeostasis is affected when circadian organization is altered by the *clock* mutation. Quantification of sleep homeostasis through dose-response experiments can strengthen this interpretation because a differential response to a single sleep deprivation in the presence of baseline differences in sleep time can only be taken as evidence for an effect on sleep homeostasis if the dose-response relation is strictly linear.

In mice lacking both *cry1* and *cry2*, circadian rhythmicity is absent. In these mice, NREM sleep time is increased and SWA is higher than in wild-type mice (Fig. 34–10).[86] These sleep characteristics are opposite to those observed in SCN-lesioned mice and rats, in which sleep duration does not noticeably change, sleep is more fragmented, and SWA is maintained at lower levels. In addition, the response to sleep deprivation is altered in mice lacking both *cryptochrome* genes; NREM sleep time and consolidation do not increase and the increase in SWA is attenuated compared to wild-type controls. Estimation of the parameters of the homeostatic regulation of SWA through computer modeling revealed that per unit of time spent awake, sleep need increased at a faster rate in mice lacking *cryptochromes* (see Fig. 34–10). Together, these observations provide evidence that the *cryptochromes* affect sleep homeostasis and that the separation of circadian rhythmicity and sleep homeostasis does not extend all molecular components of circadian rhythm generation.

Analyses of the time course of clock gene expression in the brain, notably in areas outside the SCN, in relation to rest-activity and sleep-wake cycles have provided some further insights into the association between clock gene expression and sleep homeostasis. In intact wild-type animals, *per1* and *per2* expression in the cerebral cortex is high at times when NREM sleep propensity is high, independent of the circadian oscillation of *per* expression in the SCN. Thus in both nocturnal and diurnal species, *per* expression in the cerebral cortex is maximal in conjunction with the major waking episode whereas in the SCN *per* levels are high in the (subjective) light phase.[87,88] This phase difference is reminiscent of the phase difference in multiple-unit activity (MUA) recorded from inside the SCN and extra-SCN areas.[89]

Under conditions where the phase or distribution of locomotor activity is altered through methamphetamine administration[90] or restricted feeding,[91,92] *per* expression in the cortex parallels the overt rhythm of wakefulness, leaving the circadian *per* expression in the SCN unaffected. Manipulation of the sleep homeostat through sleep deprivation leads to a selective increase of *per1* and *per2* expression in the cortex of rats and mice.[86,93] Thus, in contrast to their expression in the SCN, expression of clock genes in the cortex appear to follow the sleep-wake history[94] according to an "hourglass" oscillation, which is consistent with their suggested role in sleep homeostasis.[86,95] This leads to the suggestion that both the circadian rhythm and the sleep homeostat might be emergent properties of oscillations set up by the same transcriptional regulators that are nevertheless neuroanatomically distinct.

DOES SLEEP TALK BACK TO THE CLOCK?

Sleep regulation is often viewed as emanating from an interaction of sleep regulatory centers and the circadian clock, whereby the clock is self-sustained, synchronized by the external light-dark cycle, and imposing its output signals onto the rest of the CNS. Does sleep influence the clock? Sleep displacement or nap studies are the obvious approach to answer this question. Changes in light exposure associated with sleep are, however, a potential confound in such studies. In addition, changes in posture and the associated physiologic and autonomic nervous system changes are other possible mediators of effects on the clock.

In recent years a number of studies, in which these potential confounds were controlled for, have provided some evidence that sleep talks back to the clock. Scheduling of sleep can synchronize the circadian rhythms of some blind persons.[96] Sleep deprivation in dim light modulates the phase of the melatonin rhythm, and this modulation is significantly larger than predicted from models for the effect of light on the human circadian pacemaker.[97] Gradual shifts of the timing of sleep within an episode of near darkness leads to small changes in the phase of circadian markers such as body temperature and melatonin.[98]

Animal experiments have also provided evidence for effects of sleep on the clock. For example, in the Syrian hamster, sleep deprivation without exercise causes the circadian rhythms to phase shift and suppresses expression of the immediate early gene *c-fos*.[99] The most compelling evidence that the behavioral state itself feeds back onto the clock has been derived from simultaneous recordings of EEG activity from the cortex and MUA from the SCN in the rat.[100] During NREM sleep with high values of SWA, MUA was low; during REM sleep and wakefulness, MUA was high. These associations persisted during selected SWS deprivation, indicating that the EEG correlates of NREM sleep, REM sleep, and wakefulness are influencing MUA in the clock. Whether these effects on the electrical activity of the clock also affect the molecular machinery of the clock remain to be established. Nevertheless, these data indicate that the sleep and circadian systems are interrelated even more closely than was previously recognized and that the interactions between these systems are bidirectional.

> ### Clinical Pearl
>
> Circadian rhythmicity and sleep homeostasis contribute to many aspects of sleep-wake phenomenology. The fine-tuned interaction between these two oscillatory processes enables prolonged optimal waking performance and sleep consolidation. Relatively minor changes in either of these processes may lead to performance decrements and clinically significant sleep disruption as observed in shift work, jet lag, aging, narcolepsy, the blind, and delayed and advanced sleep-wake syndrome. Disentanglement of the contributions of these two processes to sleep disruption is not accomplished easily, but procedures to characterize the interaction between circadian rhythmicity and sleep-wake cycles in the field have been developed. Assessment of the timing of the onset of nocturnal melatonin secretion through the dim light melatonin onset procedure[101] can detect abnormalities in the timing of the circadian component of sleep regulation such as may occur in advanced and delayed sleep phase syndrome, non–24-hour sleep-wake syndrome, the blind, and shift work. Abnormalities in the timing of the sleep-wake cycle relative to the circadian component of sleep regulation can be detected through long-term actigraphic recordings and sleep diaries in combination with assessment of the plasma melatonin rhythm[102] or the rhythm of melatonin's major metabolite in urine, 6-sulfatoxy melatonin.[103]

REFERENCES

1. Aschoff J, Gerecke U, Wever R: Desynchronization of human circadian rhythms. Jpn J Physiol 1967;17:450-457.

2. Daan S: Clocks and hourglass timers in behavioural cycles. In Hiroshige T, Honma K-I (eds): Comparative aspects of circadian clocks. Sapporo, Hokkaido University Press, 1987, pp 42-54.

3. Daan S, Beersma DGM, Borbély AA: Timing of human sleep: Recovery process gated by a circadian pacemaker. Am J Physiol 1984;246:R161-R178.

4. Dijk DJ, Czeisler CA: Contribution of the circadian pacemaker and the sleep homeostat to sleep propensity, sleep structure, electroencephalographic slow waves and sleep spindle activity in humans. J Neurosci 1995;15:3526-3538.

5. Waterhouse JM, Decoursey PJ: Human circadian organization. In Dunlap JC, Loros JJ, DeCoursey PJ (eds): Chronobiology: Biological Timekeeping. Sunderland, Mass, Sinauer Associates, 2004, pp 291-323.

6. Tzischinsky O, Shlitner A, Lavie P: The association between the nocturnal sleep gate and nocturnal onset of urinary 6-sulfatoxymelatonin. J Biol Rhythms 1993;8:199-209.

7. Czeisler CA, Dumont M, Duffy JF, et al: Association of sleep-wake habits in older people with changes in output of circadian pacemaker. Lancet 1992;340:933-936.

8. Duffy JF, Dijk DJ, Hall EF, Czeisler CA: Relationship of endogenous circadian melatonin and temperature rhythms to self-reported preference for morning or evening activity in young and older people. J Investig Med 1999;47:141-150.

9. Czeisler CA, Weitzman ED, Moore-Ede MC, et al: Human sleep: Its duration and organization depend on its circadian phase. Science 1980;210:1264-1267.

10. Zulley J, Wever R, Aschoff J: The dependence of onset and duration of sleep on the circadian rhythm of rectal temperature. Pflugers Arch 1981;391:314-318.

11. Dijk DJ, Lockley SW: Integration of human sleep-wake regulation and circadian rhythmicity. J Appl Physiol 2002;92:852-862.

12. Lavie P: Ultrashort sleep-waking schedule III. "Gates" and "forbidden zones" for sleep. Electroenceph Clin Neurophysiol 1986;63:414-425.

13. Carskadon MA, Dement WC: Sleep studies on a 90-minute day. Electroenceph Clin Neurophysiol 1975;39:145-155.

14. Weitzman ED, Nogeire C, Perlow M, et al: Effects of a prolonged 3-hour sleep-wake cycle on sleep stages, plasma cortisol, growth hormone, and body temperature in man. J Clin Endocrinol Metab 1974;38:1018-1030.

15. Cajochen C, Knoblauch V, Krauchi K, et al: Dynamics of frontal EEG activity, sleepiness and body temperature under high and low sleep pressure. Neuroreport 2001;12:2277-2281.

16. Wyatt JK, Ritz-De Cecco A, Czeisler CA, Dijk DJ: Circadian temperature and melatonin rhythms, sleep, and neurobehavioral function in humans living on a 20-h day. Am J Physiol 1999; 277:R1152-R1163.

17. Koorengevel KM, Beersma DG, Den Boer JA, van den Hoofdakker RH: Sleep in seasonal affective disorder patients in forced desynchrony: An explorative study. J Sleep Res 2002; 11:347-356.

18. Wyatt JK, Cajochen C, Ritz-De Cecco A, et al: Low dose, repeated caffeine administration for circadian-phase dependent performance degradation during extended wakefulness. Sleep 2004;27:374-381.

19. Czeisler CA, Duffy JF, Shanahan TL, et al: Stability, precision, and near-24-hour period of the human circadian pacemaker. Science 1999;284:2177-2181.

20. Klerman EB, Dijk DJ, Kronauer RE, Czeisler CA: Simulations of effects of light on the human circadian pacemaker: Implications for assessment of intrinsic period. Am J Physiol 1996;270:R271-R282.

21. Akerstedt T, Hume K, Minors D, Waterhouse J: Experimental separation of time of day and homeostatic influences on sleep. Am J Physiol 1998;274:R1162-R1168.

22. Strogatz SH, Kronauer RE, Czeisler CA: Circadian pacemaker interferes with sleep onset at specific times each day: Role in insomnia. Am J Physiol 1987;253:R172-R178.

23. Lavie P: Melatonin: Role in gating nocturnal rise in sleep propensity. J Biol Rhythms 1997;12:657-665.

24. Dijk DJ, Shanahan TL, Duffy JF, et al: Variation of electroencephalographic activity during non–rapid eye movement and rapid eye movement sleep with phase of circadian melatonin rhythm in humans. J Physiol (Lond) 1997;505:851-858.

25. Richardson GS, Carskadon MA, Orav EJ, Dement WC: Circadian variation of sleep tendency in elderly and young adult subjects. Sleep 1982;5:S82-S94.

26. Dijk DJ, Duffy JF, Czeisler CA: Age-related increase in awakenings: Impaired consolidation of NREM sleep at all circadian phases. Sleep 2001;24:565-577.

27. Dijk DJ, Czeisler CA: Paradoxical timing of the circadian rhythm of sleep propensity serves to consolidate sleep and wakefulness in humans. Neurosci Lett 1994;166:63-68.

28. Edgar DM, Dement WC, Fuller CA: Effect of SCN lesions on sleep in squirrel monkeys: Evidence for opponent processes in sleep-wake regulation. J Neurosci 1993;13:1065-1079.

29. Barbato G, Barker C, Bender C, et al: Extended sleep in humans in 14 hour nights (LD 10:14): Relationship between REM density and spontaneous awakening. Electroenceph Clin Neurophysiol 1994;90:291-297.

30. Zimmerman JC, Czeisler CA, Laxminarayan S, et al: REM density is disassociated from REM sleep timing during free-running sleep episodes. Sleep 1980;2:409-415.

31. Khalsa SBS, Conroy DA, Duffy JF, et al: Sleep- and circadian-dependent modulation of REM density. J Sleep Res 2002;11:53-59.

32. Weitzman ED, Czeisler CA, Zimmerman JC, Ronda JM: Timing of REM and stages 3 and 4 sleep during temporal isolation in man. Sleep 1980;2:391-407.

33. Webb WB, Agnew HW Jr, Williams RL: Effect on sleep of a sleep period time displacement. Aerospace· Med 1971;42:152-155.

34. Åkerstedt T, Gillberg M: The circadian variation of experimentally displaced sleep. Sleep 1981;4:159-169.

35. Dijk DJ, Brunner DP, Borbély AA: EEG power density during recovery sleep in the morning. Electroenceph Clin Neurophysiol 1991;78:203-214.

36. Klerman EB, Boulos Z, Edgar DM, et al: Circadian and homeostatic influences on sleep in the squirrel monkey: Sleep after sleep deprivation. Sleep 1999;22:45-59.

37. Trachsel L, Tobler I, Borbely AA: Sleep regulation in rats: Effects of sleep deprivation, light, and circadian phase. Am J Physiol 1986;251:R1037-R1044.

38. Dijk DJ: Circadian variation of EEG power spectra in NREM and REM sleep in humans: Dissociation from body temperature. J Sleep Res 1999;8:189-195.

39. Wei HG, Riel E, Czeisler CA, Dijk DJ: Attenuated amplitude of circadian and sleep-dependent modulation of electroencephalographic sleep spindle characteristics in elderly human subjects. Neurosci Lett 1999;260:29-32.

40. Anderer P, Klosch G, Gruber G, et al: Low-resolution brain electromagnetic tomography revealed simultaneously active frontal and parietal sleep spindle sources in the human cortex. Neuroscience 2001;103:581-592.

41. Knoblauch V, Martens WLJ, Wirz-Justice A, et al: Regional differences in the circadian modulation of human sleep spindle characteristics. Eur J Neurosci 2003;18:155-163.

42. Trachsel L, Tobler I, Borbely AA: Electroencephalogram analysis of non–rapid eye movement sleep in rats. Am J Physiol 1988;255:R27-R37.

43. Cajochen C, Wyatt JK, Czeisler CA, Dijk DJ: Separation of circadian and wake duration–dependent modulation of EEG activation during wakefulness. Neuroscience 2002;114:1047-1060.

44. Boivin DB, Czeisler CA, Dijk DJ, et al. Complex interaction of the sleep-wake cycle and circadian phase modulates mood in healthy subjects. Arch Gen Psychiatry 1997;54:145-152.

45. Koorengevel KM, Beersma DG, Den Boer JA, van den Hoofdakker RH: Mood regulation in seasonal affective disorder patients and healthy controls studied in forced desynchrony. Psychiatry Res 2003;117:57-74.

46. Dijk DJ, Duffy JF, Czeisler CA: Circadian and sleep/wake dependent aspects of subjective alertness and cognitive performance. J Sleep Res 1992;1:112-117.

47. van Dongen HPA, Dinges DF: Investigating the interaction between the homeostatic and circadian processes of sleep-wake regulation for the prediction of waking neurobehavioural performance. J Sleep Res 2003;12:181-187.

48. Wehr TA, Giesen HA, Moul DE, et al: Suppression of men's responses to seasonal changes in day length by modern artificial lighting. Am J Physiol 1995;269:R173-R178.

49. Zeitzer JM, Dijk DJ, Kronauer RE, et al: Sensitivity of the human circadian pacemaker to nocturnal light: Melatonin phase resetting and suppression. J Physiol (Lond) 2000;526:695-702.

50. Wehr TA, Aeschbach D, Duncan WC: Evidence for a biological dawn and dusk in the human circadian timing system. J Physiol (Lond) 2001;535:937-951.

51. Wehr TA: The impact of changes in night length (scotoperiod) on human sleep. In Turek FW, Zee PC (eds): Regulation of Sleep and Circadian Rhythms. New York, Marcel Dekker, 1999, pp 263-285.

52. Dijk DJ, Daan S: Sleep EEG spectral analysis in a diurnal rodent: *Eutamias sibiricus.* J Comp Physiol A 1989;165:205-215.

53. Franken P, Tobler I, Borbely AA: Varying photoperiod in the laboratory rat: Profound effect on 24-h sleep pattern but no effect on sleep homeostasis. Am J Physiol 1995;268:R1365-R1373.

54. Deboer T, Tobler I: Shortening of the photoperiod affects sleep distribution, EEG and cortical temperature in the Djungarian hamster. J Comp Physiol A 1996;179:483-492.

55. Aeschbach D, Cajochen C, Landolt H-P, Borbély AA: Homeostatic sleep regulation in habitual short sleepers and long sleepers. Am J Physiol 1996;270:R41-R53.

56. Aeschbach D, Postolache TT, Sher L, et al: Evidence from the waking electroencephalogram that short sleepers live under higher homeostatic sleep pressure than long sleepers. Neuroscience 2001;102:493-502.

57. Finelli LA, Baumann H, Borbely AA, Achermann P: Dual electroencephalogram markers of human sleep homeostasis: Correlation between theta activity in waking and slow-wave activity in sleep. Neuroscience 2000;101:523-529.

58. Aeschbach D, Sher L, Postolache TT, et al: A longer biological night in long sleepers than in short sleepers. J Clin Endocrinol Metab 2003;88:26-30.

59. Duffy JF, Dijk DJ, Klerman EB, Czeisler CA: Later endogenous circadian temperature nadir relative to an earlier wake time in older people. Am J Physiol 1998;275:R1478-R1487.

60. Duffy JF, Zeitzer JM, Rimmer DW, et al: Peak of circadian melatonin rhythm occurs later within the sleep of older subjects. Am J Physiol Endocrinol Metab 2002;282:E297-E303.

61. Yoon IY, Kripke DF, Elliott JA, et al: Age-related changes of circadian rhythms and sleep-wake cycles. J Am Geriatr Soc 2003;51:1085-1091.

62. Dijk DJ, Duffy JF, Riel E, et al: Ageing and the circadian and homeostatic regulation of human sleep during forced desynchrony of rest, melatonin and temperature rhythms. J Physiol (Lond) 1999;516.2:611-627.

63. Haimov I, Lavie P: Circadian characteristics of sleep propensity function in healthy elderly: A comparison with young adults. Sleep 1997;20:294-300.

64. Drapeau C, Carrier J: Fluctuation of waking electroencephalogram and subjective alertness during a 25-hour sleep-deprivation episode in young and middle-aged subjects. Sleep 2004;27:55-60.

65. Gaudreau H, Morettini J, Lavoi HB, Carrier J: Effects of a 25-h sleep deprivation on daytime sleep in the middle-aged. Neurobiol Aging 2001;22:461-468.

66. Carrier J, Land S, Buysse DJ, et al: The effects of age and gender on sleep EEG power spectral density in the middle years of life (ages 20-60 years old). Psychophysiology 2001;38:232-242.

67. Campbell SS, Murphy PJ: Relationships between sleep and body temperature in middle-aged and older subjects. J Am Geriatr Soc 1998;46:458-462.

68. Mendelson WB, Bergmann BM, Tung A: Baseline and post-deprivation recovery sleep in SCN-lesioned rats. Brain Res 2003;980:185-190.

69. Franken P, Chollet D, Tafti M: The homeostatic regulation of sleep need is under genetic control. J Neurosci 2001;21:2610-2621.

70. Borbély AA, Neuhaus HU: Sleep-deprivation: Effects on sleep and EEG in the rat. J Comp Physiol 1979;133:71-87.

71. Klerman EB, Boulos Z, Edgar DM, et al: EEG delta activity during undisturbed sleep in the squirrel monkey. Sleep Research Online 2000;3:113-119.

72. Eastman CI, Mistlberger RE, Rechtschaffen A: Suprachiasmatic nuclei lesions eliminate circadian temperature and sleep rhythms in the rat. Physiol Behav 1984;32:357-368.

73. Trachsel L, Edgar DM, Seidel WF, et al: Sleep homeostasis in suprachiasmatic nuclei-lesioned rats: Effects of sleep deprivation and triazolam administration. Brain Res 1992;589:253-261.

74. Tobler I, Borbely AA, Groos G: The effect of sleep deprivation on sleep in rats with suprachiasmatic lesions. Neurosci Lett 1983;42:49-54.

75. Ibuka N, Nihonmatsu I, Sekiguchi C: Sleep-wakefulness rhythms in mice after suprachiasmatic nucleus lesions. Waking Sleeping 1980;4:167-173.

76. Wurts SW, Edgar DM: Circadian and homeostatic control of rapid eye movement (REM) sleep: Promotion of REM tendency by the suprachiasmatic nucleus. J Neurosci 2000;20:4300-4310.

77. Toh KL, Jones CR, He Y, et al: An hPer2 phosphorylation site mutation in familial advanced sleep phase syndrome. Science 2001;291:1040-1043.

78. Ebisawa T, Uchiyama M, Kajimura N, et al: Association of structural polymorphisms in the human period3 gene with delayed sleep phase syndrome. EMBO Rep 2001;2:342-346.

79. Archer SN, Robilliard DL, Skene DJ, et al: A length polymorphism in the circadian clock gene *Per3* is linked to delayed sleep phase syndrome and extreme diurnal preference. Sleep 2003;26:413-415.

80. Vitaterna MH, King DP, Chang AM, et al: Mutagenesis and mapping of a mouse gene, *Clock*, essential for circadian behavior. Science 1994;264:719-725.

81. Vitaterna MH, Selby CP, Todo T, et al: Differential regulation of mammalian period genes and circadian rhythmicity by cryptochromes 1 and 2. Proc Natl Acad Sci U S A 1999;96:12114-12119.

82. Van Der Horst GTJ, Muijtjens M, Kobayashi K, et al: Mammalian cry1 and cry2 are essential for maintenance of circadian rhythms. Nature 1999;398:627-630.

83. Kopp C, Albrecht U, Zheng B, Tobler I: Homeostatic sleep regulation is preserved in mPer1 and mPer2 mutant mice. Eur J Neurosci 2002;16:1099-1106.

84. Shiromani PJ, Xu M, Winston EM, et al: Sleep rhythmicity and homeostasis in mice with targeted disruption of mPeriod genes. Am J Physiol Regul Integr Comp Physiol 2004;287:R47-57.

85. Naylor E, Bergmann BM, Krauski K, et al: The circadian clock mutation alters sleep homeostasis in the mouse. J Neurosci 2000;20:8138-8143.

86. Wisor JP, O'Hara BF, Terao A, et al: A role for *cryptochromes* in sleep regulation. BMC Neuroscience 2002;3:20.

87. Abe H, Honma S, Namihira M, et al: Behavioural rhythm splitting in the CS mouse is related to clock gene expression outside the suprachiasmatic nucleus. Eur J Neurosci 2001;14:1121-1128.

88. Mrosovsky N, Edelstein K, Hastings MH, Maywood ES: Cycle of period gene expression in a diurnal mammal (*Spermophilus tridecemlineatus*): Implications for nonphotic phase shifting. J Biol Rhythms 2001;16:471-478.

89. Inouye ST, Kawamura H: Persistence of circadian rhythmicity in a mammalian hypothalamic "island" containing the suprachiasmatic nucleus. Proc Natl Acad Sci U S A 1979;76: 5962-5966.

90. Masubuchi S, Honma S, Abe H, et al: Clock genes outside the suprachiasmatic nucleus involved in manifestation of locomotor activity rhythm in rats. Eur J Neurosci 2000;12:4206-4214.

91. Dudley CA, Erber-Sieler C, Estill SJ, et al: Altered patterns of sleep and behavioral adaptability in *NPAS2*-deficient mice. Science 2003;301:379-383.

92. Wakamatsu H, Yoshinobu Y, Aida R, et al: Restricted-feeding–induced anticipatory activity rhythm is associated with a phase-shift of the expression of *mPer1* and *mPer2* mRNA in the cerebral cortex and hippocampus but not in the suprachiasmatic nucleus of mice. Eur J Neurosci 2001;13:1190-1196.

93. Cirelli C, Gutierrez CM, Tononi G: Extensive and divergent effects of sleep and wakefulness on brain gene expression. Neuron 2004;41:35-43.

94. Abe H, Herzog ED, Yamazaki S, et al: Circadian rhythms in isolated brain regions. J Neurosci 2002;22:350-356.

95. Shaw PJ, Franken P: Perchance to dream: Solving the mystery of sleep through genetic analysis. J Neurobiol 2003;54:179-202.

96. Klerman EB, Rimmer DW, Dijk DJ, et al: Nonphotic entrainment of the human circadian pacemaker. Am J Physiol 1998;43: R991-R996.

97. Cajochen C, Jewett ME, Dijk DJ: Human circadian melatonin rhythm phase delay during a fixed sleep-wake schedule interspersed with nights of sleep deprivation. J Pineal Res 2003;35: 149-157.

98. Danilenko KV, Cajochen C, Wirz-Justice A: Is sleep per se a zeitgeber in humans? J Biol Rhythms 2003;18:170-178.

99. Antle MC, Mistlberger RE: Circadian clock resetting by sleep deprivation without exercise in the Syrian hamster. J Neurosci 2000;20:9326-9332.

100. Deboer T, VanSteensel MJ, Detari L, Meijer JH: Sleep states alter activity of suprachiasmatic nucleus neurons. Nat Neurosci 2003;6:1086-1090.

101. Lewy AJ: Melatonin as a marker and phase-resetter of circadian rhythms in humans. Adv Exp Med Biol 1999;460: 425-434.

102. Uchiyama M, Shibui K, Hayakawa T, et al: Larger phase angle between sleep propensity and melatonin rhythms in sighted humans with non–24-hour sleep-wake syndrome. Sleep 2002; 25:83-88.

103. Lockley SW, Skene DJ, Tabandeh H, et al: Relationship between napping and melatonin in the blind. J Biol Rhythms 1997;12:16-25.

35

Circadian Rhythms in Sleepiness, Alertness, and Performance

Hans P. A. Van Dongen

David F. Dinges

ABSTRACT

The biological clock in the suprachiasmatic nuclei regulates our behavior as it changes over the day. Consequently, a circadian rhythm can be detected in almost all variables describing sleepiness and neurobehavioral performance. This explains why people are less alert in the early morning or late at night, even when they had sleep beforehand. A variety of factors (e.g., posture, background noise) can mask the circadian profile of neurobehavioral functioning, making it important to study the circadian rhythmicity of neurobehavioral functions under strictly controlled laboratory conditions. Even if all masking influences are controlled, however, measurements of the endogenous circadian rhythmicity in sleepiness and cognitive performance still reflect the interaction of the biological clock with the homeostatic regulation of sleep. It can also be argued that certain masking influences (e.g., sensory stimulation, body movement) are an integral part of the system regulating waking neurobehavioral functions. A better understanding of their interactions with the biological clock will help to predict accurately the occurrence of cognitive performance deficits across the circadian cycle.

Both wakefulness and sleep are modulated by an endogenous regulating system, the biological clock, located in the suprachiasmatic nuclei of the hypothalamus. The impact of the biological clock goes beyond compelling the body to fall asleep and to wake up again. The biological clock also modulates hour-to-hour waking behavior, as reflected in sleepiness and cognitive performance, generating circadian rhythmicity in almost all neurobehavioral variables investigated.

Before focusing on circadian rhythmicity in waking functions, it is appropriate to give a brief description of some variables capturing aspects thereof, because differences of opinion exist about their meaning. We use *sleepiness* here for subjective reports of sleepiness or the desire to sleep. By *alertness* we mean selective and sustained attention. *Performance* refers to cognitive functions ranging in complexity from psychomotor vigilance and working memory to logical reasoning and complex thought.

The term *sleepiness* expresses the relationship between behavioral alertness and cognitive performance during wakefulness on the one hand and sleep on the other hand. The interaction of the circadian and sleep–wake systems in regulating sleepiness and performance is described in the second part of this chapter. Sleep propensity[1,2] is not covered in this chapter, however; the focus is rather on effortful cognitive performance and its corresponding subjective states.

CIRCADIAN RHYTHMS

Self-Report Measures of Sleepiness and Alertness

Many different techniques are available for the detection of circadian rhythmicity in neurobehavioral variables. Successful results have been reported in studies with a wide variety of subjective measures of sleepiness and alertness. These include an array of visual analogue scales (VAS)[3]; Likert-type rating scales such as the Stanford Sleepiness Scale (SSS)[4] and the Karolinska Sleepiness Scale (KSS)[5]; the Activation-Deactivation Adjective Check List (AD-ACL)[6]; and the Profile of Mood States (POMS).[7] Subjective measures of sleepiness and alertness are vulnerable to numerous confounding influences, however, that can "mask" their circadian rhythmicity.

Masking is a critical concept with regard to the assessment of circadian rhythms in neurobehavioral variables. Masking refers to the evoked effects of noncircadian factors on the measurements of circadian rhythmicity. The *context* in which such measurements are taken (i.e., the environmental and experimental conditions) is a major source of masking effects. Masking can alter or obscure a circadian rhythm, or create the appearance of a circadian rhythm. Masking factors may include the following: demand characteristics of the experiment,[8] distractions by environmental stimuli and noise,[9] boredom and motivational factors,[10-12] stress,[13] food intake,[14,15] posture and activity,[16,17] ambient temperature,[11] lighting conditions,[18,19] and drug intake (e.g., caffeine).[20]

Physical, mental, and social activities can be masking factors as well. This is illustrated in Figure 35–1, where the effects of performing cognitive tests on subjective estimates of alertness are apparent at certain circadian phases during sleep deprivation. Subjects report feeling less alert after being challenged to perform. This indicates that prior activity can influence subjective estimates, and that it can interact with circadian effects if not properly controlled when measuring the rhythmicity in subjective states.

Sleep and wakefulness can also be considered masking factors when it comes to observing circadian rhythmicity in neurobehavioral variables. Sleep and sleep loss have significant effects on alertness and performance. These issues are illustrated in the second half of the chapter. Despite potential masking effects and their interactions, subjective scales have been used to index circadian rhythmicity, by applying them repeatedly across the day under carefully controlled conditions.[21,22]

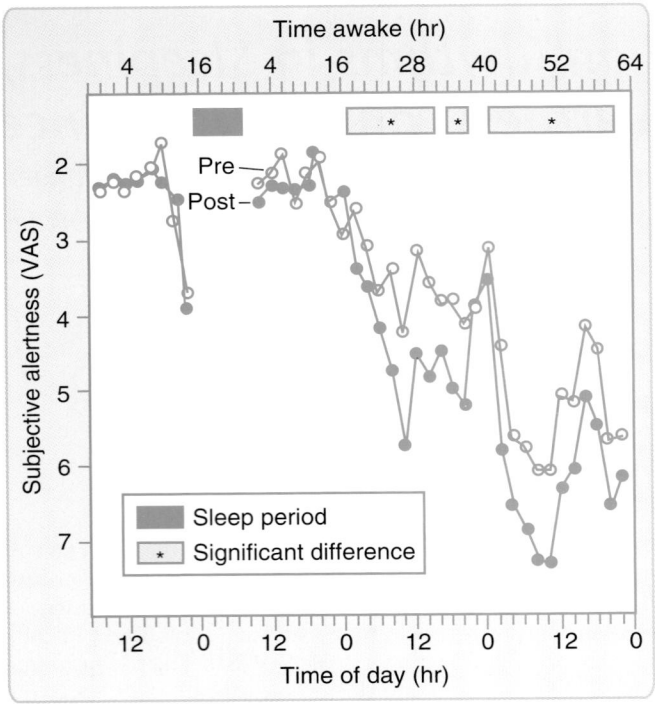

Figure 35–1. Average (with standard error of the mean) subjective alertness ratings (visual analogue scale [VAS]) in 24 healthy adults during 64 hr of wakefulness, after 8 hr of sleep (*dark blue bar*) from 11:30 PM until 7:30 AM. In this experiment, subjects were tested on a 35-min performance and mood neurobehavioral battery every 2 hr when awake. Alertness ratings are shown for two conditions: (1) ratings made just before each 35-min performance test bout (*open circles*); and (2) ratings made directly after each 35-min performance test bout (*closed circles*). No graphic or statistical differences between prebout and postbout alertness ratings were evident during the 16-hr baseline day, or during the first 16 hr of wakefulness in the sleep deprivation period. However, for most of the time from 2 AM on the first night awake until 10 PM after 62 hr awake, postbout alertness ratings were statistically significantly lower (*P* ≤ .05) than prebout ratings (times involving statistically significant differences are shown with boxes containing asterisks at the top of the graph). Only near the circadian peak in body temperature (i.e., from 8 PM until 10 PM) did these prebout versus postbout differences disappear during sleep deprivation. Such data highlight the masking effect of activity-based factors on subjective ratings of alertness, and the circadian rhythm therein, when there is a heightened pressure for sleep.

Cognitive Performance Measures

Rather than relying on subjective measures, many studies of circadian rhythms have relied on objective performance measures. For example, studies have used search-and-detection tasks[23] and simple and choice reaction time tasks[24] to obtain objective measures of circadian variation in performance. Typically, the speed and the accuracy of responses to a series of repetitive stimuli are analyzed.

There are many performance outputs that have been conceptually distinguished, including simple sorting,[25] logical reasoning,[26] memory access,[27] and more complex activities such as meter reading accuracy[28] and school performance.[29] Various tasks have been used to study circadian variation in these different aspects of performance. A number of studies concluded that different tasks[30,31] and different task outcomes[32,33] may yield

different peak phases of circadian rhythmicity. This has led to the speculation that there are many different circadian rhythms and many different clock mechanisms controlling them.[34,35]

Under strictly controlled laboratory conditions, most of the intertask differences disappear.[36,37] As illustrated in Figure 35–2, it can generally be stated that under such conditions, the circadian rhythms of neurobehavioral performance variables covary with subjective sleepiness. Furthermore, these rhythms mimic the circadian rhythm of core body temperature, a conventional marker of the biological clock. Roughly, high and low body temperature values correspond to good and poor performance, respectively.[37-39] In addition, for tasks with multiple outcome measures (e.g., response speed and response accuracy), performance outcomes may be subject to task-specific relationships (e.g., speed/accuracy tradeoff; see Osman et al.[40]).

The Mid-Afternoon Dip

In some individuals, there appears to be a short-term afternoon dip in the circadian profiles of neurobehavioral variables and core body temperature, which is called the mid-afternoon, siesta, postlunch, or postprandial dip. This dip has been observed in field studies (e.g., see Bjerner et al.[28]) and in controlled laboratory experiments (e.g., see Monk et al.[41]) independently of food intake. However, the mid-afternoon dip is not consistently found.[42,43]

Field studies of human performance have been used as evidence supporting the existence of a mid-afternoon dip,[44] but such data cannot be considered definitive evidence because of the uncontrolled influence of differential amounts of activity by varying numbers of people over time (i.e., exposure). The most compelling evidence for the existence of a mid-afternoon dip comes from studies on sleep propensity[45,46] and on the natural timing of daytime naps.[47] Nevertheless, because of the inconsistent appearance of the mid-afternoon dip, the phenomenon is poorly understood and its relationship with the biological clock remains unknown.

The Practice Effect and Other Artifacts

A problem that limits the reliability of performance on many cognitive tasks for the assessment of circadian rhythmicity in alertness is the well-known practice effect. This is illustrated in Figure 35–3, which shows cognitive performance improving across three consecutive days. The practice effect is difficult to distinguish from the circadian rhythm. This dilemma might be circumvented by testing subjects in different orders across times of day—the practice effect is then balanced out by averaging over subjects. This assumes that the practice effect and the circadian rhythm are additive and have the same relationship in every subject. Because this assumption has remained untested, it is unclear whether practice effects on cognitive tests can be averaged out reliably. A better way to deal with this problem is by training subjects to asymptotic performance levels before attempting to assess circadian rhythmicity in cognitive performance.

Practice effects are not the only masking factors that may hide, accentuate, or otherwise distort circadian rhythmicity in task results. Many of the same variables that serve to mask circadian rhythmicity in subjective estimates of sleepiness and alertness can also mask circadian variation in performance. The effects of masking vary from distortions of the range of circadian variation to changes in the shape of the circadian

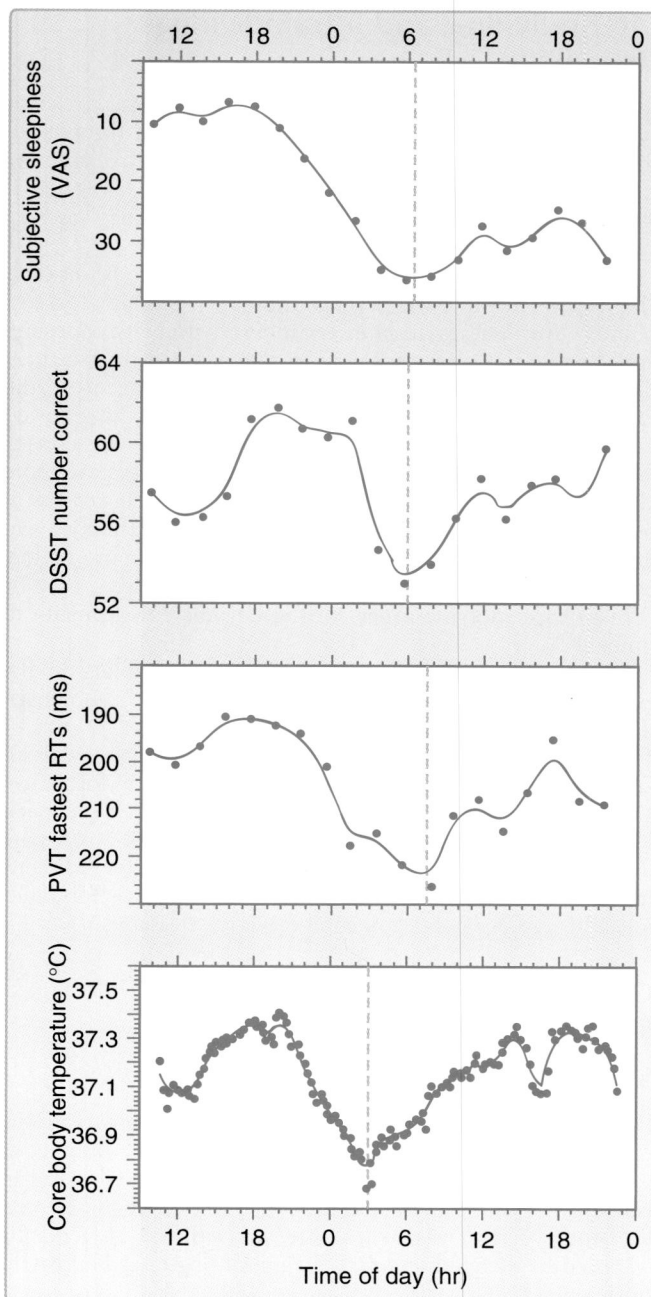

Figure 35–2. Circadian covariation of changes in subjective sleepiness as assessed by (reversed) visual analogue scale (VAS); in cognitive performance as assessed by the digit symbol substitution task (DSST); in 10% fastest reaction times (RT) as assessed by the psychomotor vigilance task (PVT); and in core body temperature (CBT) as assessed by means of a rectal probe. Data shown are the mean values from five subjects who remained awake in dim light, in bed, in a constant routine protocol, for 36 hr consecutively (a distance-weighted least-squares function was fitted to each variable). The circadian trough is evident in each variable (marked by *vertical broken lines*). A phase difference is also apparent, such that all three neurobehavioral variables had their average minimum between 3.0 hr and 4.5 hr after the time of the body temperature minimum. This phase delay in neurobehavioral functions relative to CBT has been observed in many protocols, but remains unexplained. Although body temperature reflects predominantly the endogenous circadian clock, neurobehavioral functions are also affected by the homeostatic pressure for sleep, which escalates with time awake and which may contribute to the phase delay through interaction with the circadian clock. This explanation is

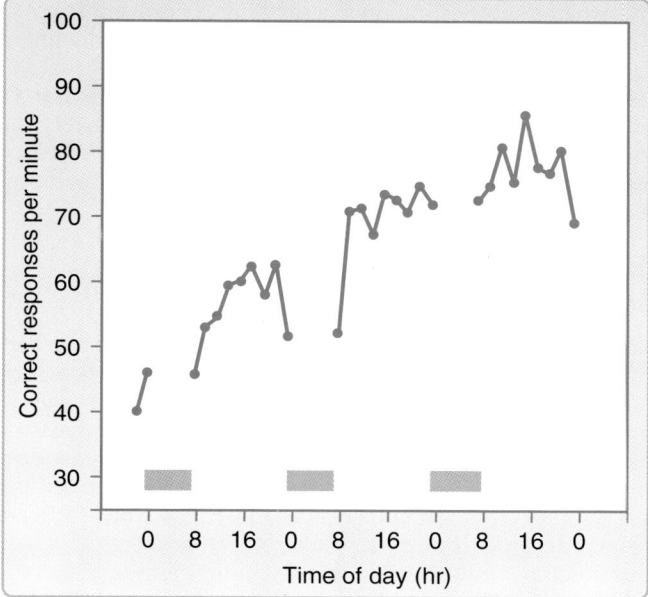

Figure 35–3. Practice effect in average cognitive throughput performance for 29 healthy adult subjects tested every 2 hr from 7:30 AM until 11:30 PM each day, during a 3-day period in which they were allowed up to 8 hr of sleep per night (*blue bars*). The performance task was the serial addition/subtraction test, which is part of the Walter Reed performance assessment battery.[100] In this task, subjects were presented with a rapid sequence of two single digits (0 to 9) followed by an operator (plus or minus), and they were to enter only the least-significant single digit of the algebraic sum, unless the result was negative, in which case 10 was to be added to the answer first. Note the substantial learning curve (i.e., practice effect) across days, resulting in a doubling of the mean correct responses within 25 trials. This effect dominates the performance profile, obscuring circadian changes within the days. Practice effects "contaminate" nearly all tasks that involve mental operations.

curve; even total concealment of the circadian rhythm is possible (as shown in Fig. 35–3, where sleep prevents measurement of nocturnal performance and the practice effect obscures circadian variation in diurnal performance). Thus, it is not easy to extract meaningful information about the amplitude (i.e., magnitude) and the phase (i.e., timing) of the circadian rhythm in performance measures without understanding the masking effects that influence these variables.

Compared with subjective sleepiness and alertness, circadian rhythmicity in cognitive performance is more complicated to assess. Not only is performance often affected by learning, aptitude, and other masking factors (e.g., lighting, background noise, demand characteristics, as listed above), but it is affected by the multiplicity of the brain processes that regulate performance. As an example, it has been reported that subjects may change their performance strategy on a task

not universally supported by the available data, but at the very least it is necessary to correct the common misconception that alertness and performance are worst at the body temperature minimum. Neurobehavioral functions usually do show the circadian decline at night as observed in CBT, but they appear to continue their decline after CBT has begun to rise, making the subsequent 2- to 6-hr period (i.e., clock time approximately 6 AM to 10 AM) a zone of maximum vulnerability to loss of alertness and performance failure.

by invoking subvocalization in a rhythmic, circadian pattern.[48] Thus, it can be difficult to distinguish the circadian rhythm in task performance per se from that of simultaneous changes in performance strategy. The same applies to compensatory effort (that is, increased effort to keep up performance). The effect of compensatory effort may be especially notable if subjects are informed about their results during a performance task (i.e., performance feedback).

Electroencephalographic and Ocular Measures

The circadian rhythm in task performance is believed to reflect functional changes in the brain. The brain potentials associated with the reaction to a stimulus—evoked potentials or event-related potentials (ERPs)—have been used to measure alertness. Many ERP measurements must be taken consecutively (i.e., many stimuli must be offered) to average out the background electroencephalogram (EEG). Therefore, ERPs are usually recorded during repetitive search-and-detection and reaction time tasks. Diurnal changes in the amplitude and the location of ERP waves have been interpreted as reflecting circadian variations in alertness.[49,50] Hemispheric differences have been detected,[51] suggesting separate circadian rhythms for the left and right hemispheres. However, masking from a variety of sources presents a problem in the interpretation of ERP data (e.g., see Geisler and Polich[52]).

Circadian variations in alertness have also been associated with changes in the background EEG during wakefulness. The amounts of theta and alpha activity (i.e., EEG activity in the frequency bands from 4 to 8 Hz and from 8 to 12 Hz, respectively) in the resting EEG with eyes held either open or closed (to avoid artifacts from blinking) have been observed to be related to the level of alertness.[53-55] However, difficulties in the recording and analysis of the waking EEG[56,57] have limited its interpretability. Furthermore, significant effects in the EEG occur primarily when alertness is much lower than what is normally encountered at the trough of circadian variation—such as when subjects are sleep deprived.[58]

Another way in which the EEG has been used is to measure the latency with which subjects fall asleep (as a measure of sleep propensity) at various times of day. These sleep latency tests include the Multiple Sleep Latency Test (MSLT) and the Maintenance of Wakefulness Test (MWT) as well as variations on these paradigms. Sleep latency tests are covered in other chapters in this volume.

Slow eyelid closures have been found to be related to sleepiness.[59] Similar findings have been reported for slow-rolling eye movements (SEMs) and other ocular variables.[5,60-62] Pupil diameter is related to autonomic tone (i.e., pupils dilate with greater sympathetic dominance), and autonomic tone has been shown to covary with sleep pressure.[63] Pupillometry may therefore also yield estimates of sleepiness, but only if environmental light and other confounding influences on pupil diameter are strictly controlled. The various ocular measures of sleepiness have been investigated primarily under conditions of considerable sleep loss, when the observed effects are more substantial than across the circadian cycle. Whether ocular measures can be used reliably for detecting circadian fluctuations in sleepiness thus remains to be determined.

Interindividual and Intraindividual Variability

Interindividual differences in circadian amplitude, circadian phase, and mean performance level are reported throughout the literature. Interindividual differences in the free-running circadian period have been reported as well,[64] although it should be emphasized that under normal, entrained circumstances the circadian period equals 24 hours.

Morningness/eveningness (i.e., the tendency to be an early "lark" or a late "owl") is perhaps the most substantial source of interindividual variation in circadian rhythmicity. Morning- and evening-type individuals differ endogenously in the circadian phase of their biological clock.[65] This is echoed in the diurnal course of their neurobehavioral variables (as reviewed in Kerkhof[66] and Van Dongen[67])—some people are consistently at their best in the morning, whereas others are more alert and perform better in the evening. There is reason to believe that this difference in circadian phase preference and its reflection in neurobehavioral functions is a more or less enduring trait. To the extent that this is the case, it may be seen as a phenotypic aspect of the circadian rhythmicity in humans.[68]

Age is also a source of interindividual variability in the circadian rhythm of alertness and performance.[69] No consistent relevance of sex has been found.

Decreased alertness during the circadian trough is associated with increased intraindividual variability in performance. This is evidenced by intermittent lapsing,[70] which has been hypothesized to reflect *wake state instability*.[71] The wake state instability hypothesis posits that sleep-initiating mechanisms may interfere with wakefulness, making sustained performance unstable and dependent on compensatory mechanisms.[71]

CIRCADIAN RHYTHMICITY VERSUS SLEEP AND WAKE

Sleep Deprivation

Considerable research effort has been put into *unmasking* the circadian rhythm, that is, eliminating sources of extraneous variance to expose the endogenous circadian rhythm in variables of interest, including alertness and cognitive performance. The constant routine procedure[72] is generally regarded as the gold standard for measuring circadian rhythmicity. By keeping subjects awake with a fixed posture in a constant laboratory environment for at least 24 hours, circadian rhythms in a variety of physiologic and neurobehavioral variables can be recorded (Fig. 35–2). Indeed, for body temperature, the circadian rhythm is believed to be free of masking effects under constant routine.

When neurobehavioral variables are considered, the elimination of sleep (i.e., sleep deprivation) and the stimuli delivered to sustain wakefulness can constitute masking factors. In constant routine experiments, these untoward masking effects have become evident in subjective measures of sleepiness and alertness.[65,73] Figure 35–2 shows the somewhat reduced values for subjective alertness as well as cognitive and psychomotor performance after 30 hours awake under constant routine, compared with the values of these variables 24 hours earlier (i.e., at the same circadian phase but without sleep deprivation).

Typically, superimposed on the circadian rhythm in a neurobehavioral variable there is also a progressive change that is associated with the time spent awake (e.g., see Åkerstedt et al.[74]). When total sleep deprivation is continued for several days (whether in a constant routine procedure or an experimental design involving ambulation), the detrimental effects on alertness and performance grow, and although the circadian process can thus be exposed,[75] it is overlaid on a continuing (nearly linear) change reflecting increasing homeostatic pressure for sleep (e.g., see Bohlin and Kjellberg[76]). This is illustrated in Figure 35–4 for performance lapses on a psychomotor vigilance task.

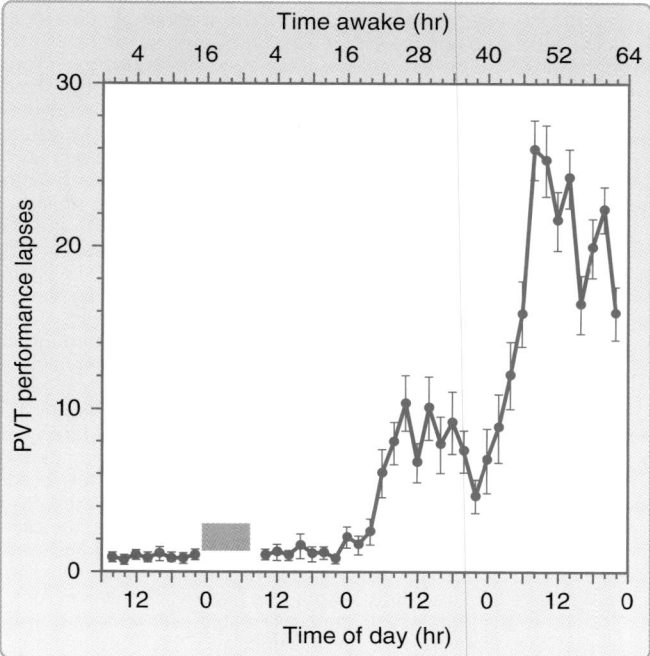

Figure 35–4. Average (with standard error of the mean) frequency of performance lapses (reaction times longer than 500 msec) on a 10-min psychomotor vigilance task (PVT) in 24 healthy adults during 64 hr of wakefulness, after 8 hr of sleep (*blue bar*) from 11:30 PM until 7:30 AM. In this experiment, subjects were tested on a 35-min neurobehavioral assessment battery that included the PVT, every 2 hr when awake. As is evident in the figure, there is little variation in PVT lapses during the 16-hr baseline day, or during the first 16 hr of wakefulness in the sleep deprivation period. Lapses are relatively rare events within this range of wakefulness duration and during this largely diurnal portion of the circadian cycle (i.e., from 7:30 AM until 11:30 PM). However, from 18 hr awake (at 2 AM on the first sleepless night) to 62 hr awake (at 10 PM before the third sleepless night), PVT lapses are clearly evident, indicating a substantial increase in neurobehavioral dysfunction. There appears to be circadian modulation of lapsing within days, superimposed on a steady increase in lapses across days. The interaction makes it difficult to estimate the relative contributions of the circadian versus homeostatic influences on performance over time. Mathematical deconvolution of the two influences, even if statistically sound, does not resolve this problem owing to nonlinearity of the interaction.[85] Nevertheless, all neurobehavioral performance and subjective alertness variables that show circadian variation also respond to sleep loss, and vice versa. The combined effect of the two processes typically takes the form of a rough staircase function, as seen in this figure (compare with Fig. 35–1).

Sleep–Wake Regulation

The apparent superposition of circadian modulation of alertness and performance on monotonic change during sleep deprivation has prompted efforts to model mathematically the regulatory processes involved. The two-process model of sleep regulation has been applied to describe the temporal profiles of sleep[77,78] and wakefulness.[79] The model consists of a *homeostatic* process (process S) and a *circadian* process (process C), which combine to determine the timing of the onset and offset of sleep. The homeostatic process represents the drive for sleep that increases during wakefulness (as can be felt when wakefulness is maintained beyond the habitual bedtime into the night and subsequent day) and decreases during sleep (symbolizing recuperation obtained from sleep). When the "homeostat" increases above a certain threshold, sleep is triggered; when it decreases below another threshold, wakefulness is invoked. The circadian process represents daily oscillatory modulation of these threshold levels. It has been suggested that the circadian system actively promotes wakefulness more than sleep,[80] although this hypothesis is not universally accepted. The circadian drive for wakefulness may be experienced as the spontaneously enhanced alertness in the early evening even after a sleepless night (Fig. 35–2).

The homeostatic and circadian processes are thought to interact to determine waking neurobehavioral functions as expressed in alertness and performance.[81] This is clearly seen in sustained sleep deprivation experiments (Figs. 35–1 and 35–4). For alertness and performance, sleep and sleeplessness are not only masking factors, but dynamic biologic forces that interact with the circadian system.

Forced Desynchrony

The forced desynchrony protocol[82,83] is an experimental procedure especially suitable for studying the interaction of the circadian and homeostatic processes.[36,43,84] In this protocol, a subject stays in an isolated laboratory in which the times for sleep and waking are scheduled to deviate from the normal 24-hour day (for instance, 20- or 28-hour days have been used), to such an extent that the subject's biological clock is unable to synchronize to this schedule. The subject experiences two distinct influences simultaneously: the schedule of predetermined sleep and waking times (i.e., time awake) representing the homeostatic system, and the rhythm of the subject's unsynchronized (i.e., free-running) circadian system. Neurobehavioral variables can be recorded when the subject is in the waking periods of the schedule. By folding the data over either the free-running circadian rhythm or the imposed sleep–wake cycle, the other component can be balanced out. Thus, insight is gained into the separate effects of the circadian rhythm and the wake duration (i.e., homeostatic drive for sleep) on recorded variables.

Not surprisingly, it has been observed in forced desynchrony studies that both the circadian and homeostatic processes influence sleepiness and performance. The interaction of the two seems to be oppositional during natural diurnal wake periods (from approximately 7 AM until 11 PM), such that a relatively stable level of alertness and performance can be maintained throughout the day.[43,83] This may explain why often in studies of alertness and performance, very little temporal variation is seen during the waking portion of a normal day.

The interaction of the homeostatic and circadian processes has been found to be nonlinear (i.e., nonadditive).[85] Therefore, the separation of circadian and homeostatic influences on neurobehavioral variables presents a conceptual and mathematical problem, and it is difficult, if not impossible, to quantify the relative importance of the two influences on neurobehavioral functions. Moreover, their relative contributions may vary across different experimental conditions[36,43] and among subjects (e.g., see Lenné et al.[86]).

Ultradian Days

The importance of taking into account sleep when studying alertness and performance has led to the design of paradigms with very short (i.e., ultradian) artificial days. Such paradigms seek to redistribute the opportunities for sleep and wakefulness across the natural 24-hour day, to sample waking behavior across the circadian cycle without significantly curtailing the total amount of sleep allowed. Studies have been performed with the "90-minute day" schedule,[87] which alternately allows subjects to sleep for 30 minutes and forces them to stay awake for 60 minutes, and with the "7/13-minute sleep–waking" schedule,[2] which alternately allows subjects to sleep for 7 minutes and forces them to stay awake for 13 minutes. With respect to objective measures, studies with very short days have primarily focused on sleep propensity rather than alertness and performance. However, subjective sleepiness scores have been recorded in both the 90-minute day schedule[87] and the 7/13-minute sleep–waking schedule.[88] After 24 hours of 7/13-minute sleep–waking cycles, the level of subjective sleepiness is elevated with respect to the initial level 24 hours earlier (which does not seem to be the case in the 90-minute day schedule). Thus, at least with respect to subjective sleepiness, the sleep obtained across 24 hours of the 7/13-minute sleep–waking schedule may not have the same recovery potential as natural nighttime sleep.

Cognitive performance was assessed in one experiment using the 7/13-minute sleep–waking schedule.[89] A clear circadian rhythm emerged for the response time on a choice reaction time task. Furthermore, a movement time component was recorded, which showed a circadian rhythm as well, but also an overall gradual increase over time. This may reflect a growing homeostatic pressure for sleep across the ultradian days. This study shows that even in paradigms with very short artificial days it is difficult to separate the circadian and homeostatic influences on neurobehavioral functions.

Sleep inertia is another problem that may be expected to interfere with the assessment of alertness and performance in these studies. Sleep inertia is the cognitive performance impairment, feeling of disorientation, grogginess, and tendency to return to sleep experienced immediately after awakening.[90,91] Sleep inertia may affect alertness and performance on every artificial day of a study with ultradian days. There are some indications that the circadian and homeostatic influences interact with sleep inertia, varying its impact across artificial days[92] and complicating estimation of its effect.

CONCLUSION

Figure 35–5 schematically shows how the circadian drive for wakefulness, the homeostatic drive for sleep, the sleep inertia effect, and various endogenous and exogenous "masking" factors

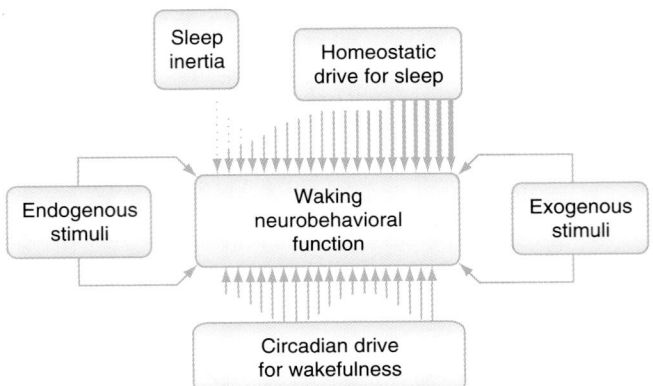

Figure 35–5. Schematic representation of the (speculative) oppositional interplay of circadian and homeostatic drives in the regulation of alertness, performance, and related neurobehavioral functions. This representation was inspired by a number of theoretical conceptualizations, but it does not necessarily reflect their authors' original intentions. Included are the two-process model of sleep regulation[77,78] and the opponent-process model of sleep–wake regulation[80]; the three-process model of the endogenous neurobiological regulation of subjective sleepiness[81,101]; and results of a study on the effects of postural, environmental, cognitive, and social stimulation (masking) on neurobehavioral functions at different circadian phases during sleep deprivation.[102] The schematic is necessarily simplified (e.g., the nonlinear interaction between the circadian and homeostatic drives[85] and the systematic interindividual differences in these two processes[65,103,104] are not represented here). As illustrated in the upper part of the figure, wakefulness typically begins with rapidly dissipating sleep inertia, which suppresses neurobehavioral functioning for a brief period after awakening. The homeostatic drive for sleep accumulates throughout wakefulness, and progressively downregulates neurobehavioral performance and alertness (while increasing subjective sleepiness). Unlike the circadian system, which is limited by its amplitude, the homeostatic drive for sleep can accumulate far beyond the levels typically encountered in a 24-hr day (illustrated by the increasing density of *downward arrows*). In opposition to these downward influences on performance and alertness is the endogenous circadian rhythmicity of the biological clock. Through its promotion of wakefulness, the circadian system modulates the enhancement of performance and alertness. The improvement in waking neurobehavioral functions by the circadian drive is an oscillatory output that periodically involves robust opposition to the homeostatic drive, alternated with periods of withdrawal of the circadian drive for wakefulness. Critical modulators of neurobehavioral functions other than the sleep and circadian drives are subsumed in the schematic under the broad categories of *endogenous* and *exogenous* stimulation. Although common in the real world, these factors are considered masking factors in most laboratory experiments. They can include endogenous (e.g., anxiety) or exogenous (e.g., environmental light) wake-promoting processes that oppose the homeostatic drive for sleep. Alternatively, they can include endogenous (e.g., narcolepsy) or exogenous (e.g., rhythmic motion) sleep-promoting processes that oppose the circadian drive for wakefulness either directly, or indirectly by exposing the previously countered sleep drive.[1,105] The neurobiologic underpinnings of these exogenous and endogenous processes are undoubtedly diverse, and few of their interactions with the circadian and homeostatic systems have been studied systematically (e.g., see Sharafkhaneh and Hirshkowitz[106]).

simultaneously affect neurobehavioral functioning. When alertness and performance are considered, masking factors cannot be regarded as mere undesirable influences that should be ignored or controlled (compare Cluydts et al.[93]). Rather, they are an integral part of the regulation of neurobehavioral functions and the interaction of the human being with his or her environment. Manipulation of endogenous and exogenous stimuli may affect the circadian and homeostatic systems through mechanisms that cannot yet be accurately quantified.

Understanding of circadian rhythmicity in neurobehavioral functions is important when either the sleep–wake rhythm is displaced, as is the case during night-shift work,[94] or when the circadian rhythm is displaced, as is the case after transmeridian flights.[95] In such situations, the interaction of the circadian and homeostatic influences decreases alertness and performance. This problem is compounded when sleep is lost on a chronic basis. Eventually, performance deficits and sleepiness reach considerable levels,[96,97] inducing opportunities for accidents.[98,99]

Clinical Pearl

Clinicians should realize that 24-hour profiles of sleepiness and performance combine the effects of the endogenous circadian rhythmicity, the homeostatic regulation of sleep, sleep inertia, and a variety of endogenous and exogenous stimuli or "masking" influences. Distinguishing these factors is important for proper diagnosis and treatment of sleep disorders involving excessive daytime sleepiness and/or circadian irregularities.

REFERENCES

1. Carskadon MA, Dement WC: The multiple sleep latency test: What does it measure? Sleep 1982;5:S67-S72.
2. Lavie P: The 24-hour sleep propensity function (SPF): Practical and theoretical implications. In Monk TH (ed): Sleep, Sleepiness and Performance. Chichester, United Kingdom, John Wiley & Sons, 1991, pp 65-93.
3. Monk TH, Embrey DE. A visual analogue scale technique to measure global vigor and affect. Psychiatry Res 1989;27:89-99.
4. Hoddes E, Zarcone V, Smythe H, et al: Quantification of sleepiness: A new approach. Psychophysiology 1973;10: 431-436.
5. Åkerstedt T, Gillberg M: Subjective and objective sleepiness in the active individual. Int J Neurosci 1990;52:29-37.
6. Thayer RE: Factor analytic and reliability studies on the Activation-Deactivation Adjective Check List. Psychol Rep 1978;42:747-756.
7. McNair DM, Lorr M, Druppleman LF: EITS Manual for the Profile of Mood States. San Diego, Calif, Educational and Industrial Test Services, 1971.
8. Orne MT: On the social psychology of the psychological experiment: With particular reference to demand characteristics and their implications. Am Psychol 1962;17:776-783.
9. Landström U, Englund K, Nordström B, Åström A: Laboratory studies of a sound system that maintains wakefulness. Percept Mot Skills 1998;86:147-161.
10. Minors DS, Waterhouse JM: Circadian rhythm amplitude: Is it related to rhythm adjustment and/or worker motivation? Ergonomics 1983;26:229-241.
11. Mavjee V, Horne JA: Boredom effects on sleepiness/alertness in the early afternoon vs. early evening and interactions with warm ambient temperature. Br J Psychol 1994;85:317-333.
12. Hull JT, Wright KP Jr, Czeisler CA: The influence of subjective alertness and motivation on human performance independent of circadian and homeostatic regulation. J Biol Rhythms 2003;18: 329-338.
13. Orr WC, Hoffman HJ, Hegge FW: The assessment of time-dependent changes in human performance. Chronobiologia 1976;3:293-305.
14. Paz A, Berry EM: Effect of meal composition on alertness and performance of hospital night-shift workers. Ann Nutr Metab 1997;41:291-298.
15. Wells AS, Read NW, Idzikowski C, Jones J: Effects of meals on objective and subjective measures of daytime sleepiness. J Appl Physiol 1998;84:507-515.
16. Kräuchi K, Cajochen C, Wirz-Justice A: A relationship between heat loss and sleepiness: Effects of postural change and melatonin administration. J Appl Physiol 1997;83:134-139.
17. Johns MW: Sleep propensity varies with behaviour and the situation in which it is measured: The concept of somnificity. J Sleep Res 2002;11:61-67.
18. Cajochen C, Zeitzer JM, Czeisler CA, Dijk D-J: Dose-response relationship for light intensity and ocular and electroencephalographic correlates of human alertness. Behav Brain Res 2000;115:75-83.
19. Phipps-Nelson J, Redman JR, Dijk D-J, Rajaratnam SMW: Daytime exposure to bright light, as compared to dim light, decreases sleepiness and improves psychomotor vigilance performance. Sleep 2003;26:695-700.
20. Åkerstedt T, Ficca G: Alertness-enhancing drugs as a countermeasure to fatigue in irregular work hours. Chronobiol Int 1997;14:145-158.
21. Monk TH, Leng VC, Folkard S, Weitzman ED: Circadian rhythms in subjective alertness and core body temperature. Chronobiologia 1983;10:49-55.
22. Babkoff H, Caspy T, Mikulincer M: Subjective sleepiness ratings: The effects of sleep deprivation, circadian rhythmicity and cognitive performance. Sleep 1991;14:534-539.
23. Colquhoun WP: Circadian variations in mental efficiency. In Colquhoun WP (ed): Biological Rhythms in Human Performance. London, Academic Press, 1971, pp 39-107.
24. Kleitman N: Sleep and Wakefulness. Chicago, University of Chicago Press, 1963.
25. Kleitman N: Diurnal variation in performance. Am J Physiol 1933;104:449-456.
26. Folkard S: Diurnal variation in logical reasoning. Br J Psychol 1975;66:1-8.
27. Folkard S, Monk TH: Circadian rhythms in human memory. Br J Psychol 1980;71:295-307.
28. Bjerner B, Holm A, Swensson A: Diurnal variation in mental performance: A study of three-shift workers. Br J Ind Med 1955;12:103-110.
29. Laird DA: Relative performance of college students as conditioned by time of day and day of week. J Exp Psychol 1925;8: 50-63.
30. Hockey GRJ, Colquhoun WP: Diurnal variation in human performance: A review. In Colquhoun WP (ed): Aspects of Human Efficiency: Diurnal Rhythm and Loss of Sleep. London, English Universities Press, 1972, pp 1-23.
31. Gillooly PB, Smolensky MH, Albright DL, et al: Circadian variation in human performance evaluated by the Walter Reed performance assessment battery. Chronobiol Int 1990;7: 143-153.
32. Monk TH, Leng VC: Time of day effects in simple repetitive tasks: Some possible mechanisms. Acta Psychol 1982;51: 207-221.
33. Kirkcaldy BD: Performance and circadian rhythms. Eur J Appl Physiol Occup Physiol 1984;52:375-379.
34. Folkard S, Wever RA, Wildgruber CM: Multi-oscillatory control of circadian rhythms in human performance. Nature 1983;305:223-226.
35. Monk TH, Weitzman ED, Fookson JE, et al: Task variables determine which biological clock controls circadian rhythms in human performance. Nature 1983;304:543-545.
36. Johnson MP, Duffy JF, Dijk D-J, et al: Short-term memory, alertness and performance: A reappraisal of their relationship to body temperature. J Sleep Res 1992;1:24-29.
37. Monk TH, Buysse DJ, Reynolds CF III, et al: Circadian rhythms in human performance and mood under constant conditions. J Sleep Res 1997;6:9-18.

38. Kleitman N, Jackson DP: Body temperature and performance under different routines. J Appl Physiol 1950;51:309-328.

39. Blake MJF: Time of day effects on performance in a range of tasks. Psychon Sci 1967;9:349-350.

40. Osman A, Lou L, Muller-Gethmann H, et al: Mechanisms of speed-accuracy tradeoff: Evidence from covert motor processes. Biol Psychol 2000;51:173-199.

41. Monk TH, Buysse DJ, Reynolds CF III, Kupfer DJ: Circadian determinants of the postlunch dip in performance. Chronobiol Int 1996;13:123-133.

42. Folkard S: Diurnal variation. In Hockey GRJ (ed): Stress and Fatigue in Human Performance. New York, John Wiley & Sons, 1983, pp 245-272.

43. Dijk D-J, Duffy JF, Czeisler CA: Circadian and sleep/wake dependent aspects of subjective alertness and cognitive performance. J Sleep Res 1992;1:112-117.

44. Mitler MM, Miller JC: Methods of testing for sleeplessness. Behav Med 1996;21:171-183.

45. Richardson GS, Carskadon MA, Flagg W, et al: Excessive daytime sleepiness in man: Multiple sleep latency measurement in narcoleptic and control subjects. Electroencephalogr Clin Neurophysiol 1978;45:621-627.

46. Lavie P: To nap, perchance to sleep: Ultradian aspects of napping. In Dinges DF, Broughton RJ (eds): Sleep and Alertness: Chronobiological, Behavioral, and Medical Aspects of Napping. New York, Raven Press, 1989, pp 99-120.

47. Dinges DF: Nap patterns and effects in human adults. In Dinges DF, Broughton RJ (eds): Sleep and Alertness: Chronobiological, Behavioral, and Medical Aspects of Napping. New York, Raven Press, 1989, pp 171-204.

48. Folkard S, Monk TH: Time of day and processing strategy in free recall. Q J Exp Psychol 1979;31:461-475.

49. Münte T-F, Heinze H-J, Kunkel H, Scholz M: Human event-related potentials and circadian variations in arousal level. Prog Clin Biol Res 1987;227B:429-437.

50. Stolz G, Aschoff JC, Born J, Aschoff J: VEP, physiological and psychological circadian variations in humans. J Neurol 1988;235:308-313.

51. Corbera X, Grau C, Vendrell P: Diurnal oscillations in hemispheric performance. J Clin Exp Neuropsychol 1993;15:300-310.

52. Geisler MW, Polich P: P300 and time of day: Circadian rhythms, food intake, and body temperature. Biol Psychol 1990;31:117-136.

53. Bjerner B: Alpha depression and lowered pulse rate during delayed actions in a serial reaction test. Acta Physiol Scand 1949;19(Suppl 65).

54. Cajochen C, Knoblauch V, Kräuchi K, et al: Dynamics of frontal EEG activity, sleepiness and body temperature under high and low sleep pressure. Neuroreport 2001;12:2277-2281.

55. Strijkstra AM, Beersma DGM, Drayer B, et al: Subjective sleepiness correlates negatively with global alpha (8-12 Hz) and positively with central frontal theta (4-8 Hz) frequencies in the human resting awake electroencephalogram. Neurosci Lett 2001;340:17-20.

56. Gale A, Harpham B, Lucas B: Time of day and the EEG: Some negative results. Psychon Sci 1972;28:269-271.

57. Jones D, Gale A, Smallbone A: Short-term recall of nine-digit strings and the EEG. Br J Psychol 1979;70:97-119.

58. Cajochen C, Brunner D, Kräuchi K, et al: Power density in theta/alpha frequencies of the waking EEG progressively increases during sustained wakefulness. Sleep 1995;18:890-894.

59. Wierwille WW, Ellsworth LA: Evaluation of driver drowsiness by trained raters. Accid Anal Prev 1994;26:571-581.

60. Torsvall L, Åkerstedt T: Extreme sleepiness: quantification of EOG and spectral EEG parameters. Int J Neurosci 1988;38:435-441.

61. Cajochen C, Khalsa SBS, Wyatt JK, et al: EEG and ocular correlates of circadian melatonin phase and human performance decrements during sleep loss. Am J Physiol 1999;277:R640-R649.

62. Caffier PP, Erdmann U, Ullsperger P: Experimental evaluation of eye-blink parameters as a drowsiness measure. Eur J Appl Physiol 2002;89:319-325.

63. Holmes AL, Burgess HJ, Dawson D: Effects of sleep pressure on endogenous cardiac autonomic activity and body temperature. J Appl Physiol 2002;92:2578-2584.

64. Czeisler CA, Duffy JF, Shanahan TL, et al: Stability, precision, and near-24-hour period of the human circadian pacemaker. Science 1999;284:2177-2181.

65. Kerkhof GA, Van Dongen HPA: Morning-type and evening-type individuals differ in the phase position of their endogenous circadian oscillator. Neurosci Lett 1996;218:153-156.

66. Kerkhof GA: Inter-individual differences in the human circadian system: A review. Biol Psychol 1985;20:83-112.

67. Van Dongen HPA: Inter- and Intra-individual Differences in Circadian Phase. PhD thesis, Leiden University. Leiden, the Netherlands, 1998.

68. Van Dongen HPA, Kerkhof GA, Dinges DF: Human circadian rhythms. In Sehgal A (ed): Molecular Biology of Circadian Rhythms. New York, John Wiley & Sons, 2004, pp 255-269.

69. Duffy JF, Dijk D-J, Klerman EB, Czeisler CA: Later endogenous circadian temperature nadir relative to an earlier wake time in older people. Am J Physiol 1998;275:R1478-R1487.

70. Williams HL, Lubin A, Goodnow JJ: Impaired performance with acute sleep loss. Psychol Monogr Gen Appl 1959;73:1-26.

71. Doran SM, Van Dongen HPA, Dinges DF: Sustained attention performance during sleep deprivation: Evidence of state instability. Arch Ital Biol 2001;139:253-267.

72. Mills JN, Minors DS, Waterhouse JM: Adaptation to abrupt time shifts of the oscillator(s) controlling human circadian rhythms. J Physiol (Lond) 1978;285:455-470.

73. Monk TH, Carrier J: Speed of mental processing in the middle of the night. Sleep 1997;20:399-401.

74. Åkerstedt T, Gillberg M, Wetterberg L: The circadian covariation of fatigue and urinary melatonin. Biol Psychiatry 1982;17:547-554.

75. Babkoff H, Mikulincer M, Caspy T, et al: The implications of sleep loss for circadian performance accuracy. Work Stress 1989;3:3-14.

76. Bohlin G, Kjellberg A: Self-reported arousal during sleep deprivation and its relation to performance and physiological variables. Scand J Psychol 1973;14:78-86.

77. Borbély AA: A two-process model of sleep regulation. Hum Neurobiol 1982;1:195-204.

78. Daan S, Beersma DGM, Borbély AA: Timing of human sleep: Recovery process gated by a circadian pacemaker. Am J Physiol 1984;246:R161-R178.

79. Achermann P, Borbély AA: Simulation of daytime vigilance by the additive interaction of a homeostatic and a circadian process. Biol Cybern 1994;71:115-121.

80. Edgar DM, Dement WC, Fuller CA: Effect of SCN lesions on sleep in squirrel monkeys: Evidence for opponent processes in sleep-wake regulation. J Neurosci 1993;13:1065-1079.

81. Folkard S, Åkerstedt T: Towards the prediction of alertness on abnormal sleep/wake schedules. In Coblentz A (ed): Vigilance and Performance in Automated Systems. Dordrecht, the Netherlands, Kluwer Academic, 1989, pp 287-296.

82. Kleitman N, Kleitman E: Effect of non-twenty-four-hour routines of living on oral temperature and heart rate. J Appl Physiol 1953;6:283-291.

83. Dijk D-J, Czeisler CA: Paradoxical timing of the circadian rhythm of sleep propensity serves to consolidate sleep and wakefulness in humans. Neurosci Lett 1994;166:63-68.

84. Monk TH, Moline ML, Fookson JE, Peetz SM: Circadian determinants of subjective alertness. J Biol Rhythms 1989;4:393-404.

85. Van Dongen HPA, Dinges DF: Investigating the interaction between the homeostatic and circadian processes of sleep-wake

regulation for the prediction of waking neurobehavioural performance. J Sleep Res 2003;12:181-187.

86. Lenné MG, Triggs TJ, Redman JR: Interactive effects of sleep deprivation, time of day, and driving experience on a driving task. Sleep 1998;21:38-44.

87. Carskadon MA, Dement WC: Sleepiness and sleep state on a 90-min schedule. Psychophysiology 1977;14:127-133.

88. Lavie P: Modelling sleep propensity: A need for rethinking. J Sleep Res 1992;1:99-102.

89. Lavie P, Gopher D, Wollman M: Thirty-six hour correspondence between performance and sleepiness cycles. Psychophysiology 1987;24:430-438.

90. Dinges DF: Are you awake? Cognitive performance and reverie during the hypnopompic state. In Bootzin RR, Kihlstrom JF, Schacter DL (eds): Sleep and Cognition. Washington, DC, American Psychological Association, 1990, pp 159-175.

91. Van Dongen HPA, Price NJ, Mullington JM, et al: Caffeine eliminates psychomotor vigilance deficits from sleep inertia. Sleep 2001;24:813-819.

92. Wilkinson RT, Stretton M: Performance after awakening at different times of night. Psychon Sci 1971;23:283-285.

93. Cluydts R, De Valck E, Verstraeten E, Theys P: Daytime sleepiness and its evaluation. Sleep Med Rev 2002;6:83-96.

94. Folkard S, Totterdell P, Minors D, Waterhouse J: Dissecting circadian performance rhythms: Implications for shiftwork. Ergonomics 1993;36:283-288.

95. Wegmann HM, Klein KE: Jet-lag and aircrew scheduling. In Folkard S, Monk TH (eds): Hours of Work: Temporal Factors in Work-Scheduling. Chichester, United Kingdom, John Wiley & Sons, 1985, pp 263-276.

96. Belenky G, Wesensten NJ, Thorne DR, et al: Patterns of performance degradation and restoration during sleep restriction and subsequent recovery: A sleep dose-response study. J Sleep Res 2003;12:1-12.

97. Van Dongen HPA, Maislin G, Mullington JM, Dinges DF: The cumulative cost of additional wakefulness: Dose-response effects on neurobehavioral functions and sleep physiology from chronic sleep restriction and total sleep deprivation. Sleep 2003;26:117-126.

98. Mitler MM, Carskadon MA, Czeisler CA, et al: Catastrophes, sleep, and public policy: Consensus report. Sleep 1988;11:100-109.

99. Dinges DF: An overview of sleepiness and accidents. J Sleep Res 1995;4:4-14.

100. Thorne DR, Genser SG, Sing GC, Hegge FW: The Walter Reed performance assessment battery. Neurobehav Toxicol Teratol 1985;7:415-418.

101. Åkerstedt T, Folkard S: The three-process model of alertness and its extension to performance, sleep latency, and sleep length. Chronobiol Int 1997;14:115-123.

102. Dijkman M, Sachs N, Levine E, et al: Effects of reduced stimulation on neurobehavioral alertness depend on circadian phase during human sleep deprivation. Sleep Res 1997;26:265.

103. Aeschbach D, Postolache TT, Sher L, et al: Evidence from the waking electroencephalogram that short sleepers live under higher homeostatic sleep pressure than long sleepers. Neuroscience 2001;102:493-502.

104. Van Dongen HPA, Rogers NL, Dinges DF: Sleep debt: Theoretical and empirical issues. Sleep Biol Rhythms 2003;1:5-13.

105. Dinges DF: The nature of sleepiness: Causes, contexts, and consequences. In Stunkard AJ, Baum A (eds): Eating, Sleeping, and Sex. Hillsdale, NJ, Lawrence Erlbaum, 1989, pp 147-179.

106. Sharafkhaneh A, Hirshkowitz M: Contextual factors and perceived self-reported sleepiness: A preliminary report. Sleep Med 2003;4:327-331.

5 Pharmacology
Wallace B. Mendelson

36

Hypnotic Medications: Mechanisms of Action and Pharmacologic Effects

Wallace B. Mendelson

ABSTRACT

All currently available hypnotics induce sleep by acting at various moieties of the gamma-aminobutyric acid$_A$–benzodiazepine receptor complex. It is one of the family of ligand-gated receptors, comprised of several glycoprotein subunits, each of which appears in multiple isoforms. Microinjection studies indicate that a common neuroanatomic site of action of hypnotics from a variety of pharmacologic classes is the preoptic area of the anterior hypothalamus. The inputs to the preoptic area from the forebrain and brainstem, and the integrative nature of the anterior hypothalamus, help explain the mechanism by which sleep—and drugs that affect sleep—interact with a variety of physiologic systems. Several hypnotic agents with novel mechanisms of action are under development and likely to be available clinically in the next few years.

At the time of this writing, the clinically used sedative/hypnotics in the United States include five benzodiazepines ("Valium-like" compounds) available in both proprietary and generic forms, and three nonbenzodiazepines (zolpidem zaleplon, and eszopiclone) available as prescription agents (Table 36–1). (See Chapter 63 for a description of the clinical use of these agents.) This represents a large market, involving approximately 27 million prescriptions, the value of which in 2002 was approximately $1.2 billion. During the same year, approximately the same number of prescriptions were written for nonhypnotics prescribed for purposes of aiding sleep; the largest among these was the antidepressant trazodone, which alone accounted for roughly 10 million prescriptions.*

Although in one sense this amount of prescription hypnotics sounds quite large, to put it in perspective, in 2002 there were approximately 118 million prescriptions for statin drugs for lowering cholesterol, costing approximately $12 billion. The two leading antipsychotic drugs, Zyprexa and Risperdal, cost consumers $2.29 billion and $1.38 billion, respectively.[1]

Indeed, one could make a case that in the population at large, prescription hypnotics are taken relatively infrequently by people with insomnia. In a survey of over 7000 enrollees in

five large health maintenance organizations (HMOs),[2] patients with insomnia were divided into those with only sleep complaints (Level 1) and those who believed that their sleep difficulties had an adverse effect on their daytime functioning (Level 2). The percentages of patients with Level 1 insomnia taking prescription and nonprescription hypnotics were 5.5% and 11.2%, respectively; comparable values for patients with Level 2 insomnia were 11.6% and 21.4%, respectively. Many patients, of course, receive other classes of prescription drugs given for purposes of helping sleep. One study of primary care patients in an HMO indicated that 13% of patients with insomnia who were not considered to have affective disorder were receiving antidepressant medications.[3] Many people also self-medicate with alcohol; a recent telephone survey of approximately 1000 representative adults in the general population found that 10% had done so in the past year.[4] A survey in the Detroit area reported that during the past year, 13% had used alcohol to aid sleep, whereas 18% used medication (either prescription or over the counter), and 5% had taken both.[5] Alcohol use to help sleep is thus common even though it exposes the patient to the risk of ethanol dependence, and it is also relatively ineffective. Although orally administered ethanol has some sleep-inducing properties, it often promotes sleep disturbance as the night progresses.[6]

MECHANISM OF ACTION

GABA$_A$ Agonists: Benzodiazepines and the Newer Nonbenzodiazepines

When the benzodiazepines first gained prominence in the 1960s, most theories of how they might act were inherited from previous studies of ethanol and barbiturates, and involved possible alterations in membrane phospholipid integrity and energy metabolism. With the discovery of the "benzodiazepine receptor" (now generally referred to as the gamma-aminobutyric acid$_A$ [GABA$_A$]–benzodiazepine receptor complex) in the late 1970s, attention was focused on the possibility that the pharmacologic effects of these compounds result from their saturable, stereospecific binding to a specific recognition site.[7,8] The receptor complex is part of a group of ligand-gated ion channel complexes that also includes

---

*Data on file, Elan Biopharmeuticals, courtesy of Dr. S. P. James.

Table 36–1.   Pharmacokinetic Properties and Dosages of Some Hypnotic Drugs Used in the Treatment of Insomnia

Hypnotic Drugs*	Half-life (hr)	Onset of Action (min)†	Pharmacologically Active Metabolites	Dose (mg)
Benzodiazepine hypnotics				
Quazepam (Doral)	48-120	30	N-desalkyl (flurazepam)	7.5-15
Flurazepam (Dalmane)	48-120	15-45	N-desalkyl (flurazepam)	15-30
Triazolam (Halcion)	2-6	2-30	None	0.125-0.25
Estazolam (ProSom)	8-24	Intermediate	None	1-2
Temazepam‡ (Restoril)	8-20	45-50	None	15-30
Loprazolam§ (Dormonoct)	4.6-11.4	—	None	1-2
Flunitrazepam§ (Rohypnol)	10.7-20.3	Short	N-desmethyl (flunitrazepam)	0.5-1
Lormetazepam§ (Loramet)	7.9-11.4	—	None	1-2
Nitrazepam§ (Alodorm)	25-35	Intermediate	None	5-10
Nonbenzodiazepine hypnotics				
Eszopiclone (Lunesta)	5-7	Intermediate	None	2-3 adult, 1 elderly
Zolpidem (Ambien)	1.5-2.4	Rapid	None	5-10 (age >65 yr) 10-20 (age <65 yr)
Zopiclone§ (Imovane)	5-6	Intermediate	None	3.75 (age >65 yr) 7.5 (age <65 yr)
Zaleplon (Sonata)	1	Rapid	None	5-10
Nonhypnotics sometimes used to aid sleep‖				
Clonazepam (Klonopin)	30-40	—	4-Amino derivative	0.5-3¶
Diazepam (Valium)	30-100	Rapid	N-desmethyl	2-10¶
Chlordiazepoxide (Librium)	24-28	Intermediate	N-desmethyl (chlordiazepoxide, demoxepam, oxazepam)	10-25¶

*Citations for kinetic information are found in Maczaj.[63]

†Derived from Smith CM, Reynard AM: Essentials of Pharmacology. Philadelphia, WB Saunders, 1995, p 228, and other sources.

‡Originally formulated as a hard capsule in the United States, concerns with kinetics and efficacy led to reformulation of the preparation to a soft gelatin capsule with characteristics comparable with those of other marketed benzodiazepines of its class.[64,65]

§Not available in the United States.

‖Drugs that do not have U.S. Food and Drug Administration (FDA) indications for aiding sleep.

¶Because there is not an FDA indication for sleep, there is no FDA-recommended dose for this purpose. Doses stated here are approximations of those often used in clinical practice.

the glycine, serotonin-3, neuronal nicotinic acetylcholine, and other receptors.[9] It functionally comprises three moieties, a benzodiazepine recognition site, a GABA$_A$ recognition site, and a chloride ionophore. Molecular cloning studies indicate that structurally it consists of at least five different glycoprotein subunits (Fig. 36–1). The actual binding site for benzodiazepines appears to be located at the junction of the α and γ subunits. Each of the subunits may have multiple isoforms.[10] There appear to be as many as six α, three β, and three γ isoforms. Studies using "knock-in" technology in mice suggest that the α$_1$ subunit may mediate both sedation and memory effects of benzodiazepines.[11] This suggests that we will be unlikely to develop a hypnotic that acts at this site and that will have sleep-promoting, but not amnesic, properties.

Two particular combinations of isoforms that are often noted are the type I configuration (α$_1$, β$_2$, γ$_2$) and type II (α$_3$, β$_2$, γ$_2$). The former, the most common type and representing roughly 40% of GABA$_A$ receptors, are found in most areas of the brain, and localized in interneurons of the hippocampus and cortex. The latter, perhaps half as common, are found dominantly in spinal cord motoneurons and hippocampal

pyramidal neurons. Most traditional benzodiazepine hypnotics bind to both types. Some of the newer nonbenzodiazepine agents, including zolpidem and zaleplon, bind with relatively greater specificity to the type I receptor. Whether this selective binding translates into more specific pharmacologic properties continues to be studied.

The end result of a benzodiazepine agonist binding to its specific site is that, as an outcome of a complex interaction with the GABA recognition site, the flow of negatively charged chloride ions into the neuron is enhanced, changing the postsynaptic membrane potential and altering input resistance such that the postsynaptic neuron is less likely to achieve an action potential. This inhibitory mechanism is a very potent one in the central nervous system (CNS) because the GABA$_A$ receptor is the most widespread receptor mechanism in inhibitory synapses, comprising up to 30% of all synapses in the CNS. One of the intriguing features of this view is that it provides a beginning for understanding a long-standing puzzle: how hypnotic medications of many different pharmacologic classes may have relatively similar effects on the process of inducing sleep. As mentioned previously, the newer

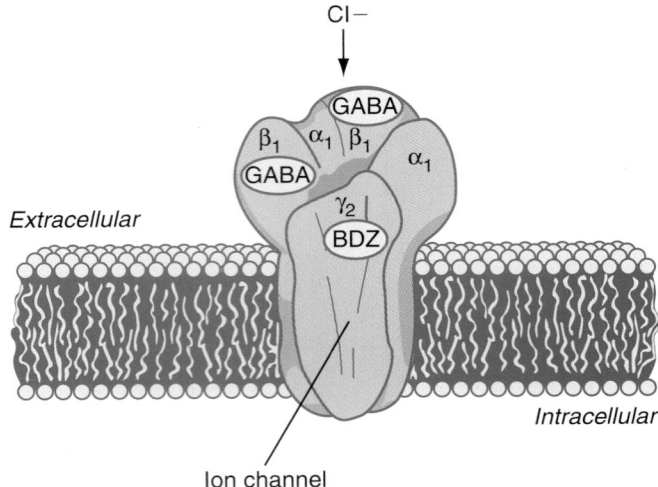

Figure 36–1. Schematic representation of the gamma-aminobutyric acid (GABA$_A$)–benzodiazepine (BDZ) receptor complex. (From Zorumski CF, Isenberg KE: Insights into the structure and function of GABA-benzodiazepine receptors: ion channels and psychiatry. Am J Psychiatr 1991;48:162-173. Copyright 1991, the American Psychiatric Association. Reprinted by permission.)

nonbenzodiazepine agents such as zolpidem and zaleplon bind to a subclass of benzodiazepine recognition sites, ethanol has profound effects on chloride channel function,[6] and barbiturates bind to a distinct site.[12] Barbiturates, for instance, may cause chloride channels to open for prolonged periods,[13] whereas benzodiazepines may increase the frequency of opening.[14] Similarly, the active metabolite of chloral hydrate[9] and the anesthetic propofol[15] modulate GABA$_A$ receptor function. Several lines of evidence have also suggested that the hypnotic effects of benzodiazepines may also involve presynaptic effects mediated by alterations in potential-dependent calcium channel activity.[16]

The original characterization of the receptor complex indicated that it mediates the anxiolytic, muscle relaxant, and anticonvulsant effects of benzodiazepines.[7,8] That it also mediates the sleep-inducing effects was demonstrated in a series of studies showing, for instance, that some β-carboline compounds that act as receptor inverse agonists induce increased wakefulness, and at low doses block sleep induction by benzodiazepines,[16] and that the binding of benzodiazepines is stereospecific, such that an enantiomeric form (the "B$_{10}$" compounds) has opposite effects, one inducing sleep whereas the other promotes wakefulness.[6,16]

Neuroanatomic Considerations

In contrast to the growing understanding of the interaction of benzodiazepine agonists at a molecular level, the anatomic sites at which they act to induce sleep are less well understood. The most parsimonious view would be that hypnotics act at loci thought to be important in sleep regulation on the basis of lesion or stimulation studies (a general review of the neuroanatomy of sleep is found in Chapter 11). Using that approach, Mendelson and Martin[17] microinjected triazolam into a number of such sites. One of the most striking findings was how in many areas injections produced no effect on sleep (e.g., the locus coeruleus, the gigantocellular tegmental fields,

the basomedial nucleus of the amygdala) or actually enhanced wakefulness (the dorsal raphe nuclei). In contrast, injections into the medial preoptic area (MPA) of the anterior hypothalamus consistently enhanced sleep, an anatomically very specific effect insofar as injections into nearby structures (the lateral preoptic area, the horizontal limb of the diagonal band of Broca) had no effect. The basal forebrain and anterior hypothalamus have long been thought to have an important role in sleep regulation. The MPA is a complex structure that receives afferents from many areas in the forebrain and brainstem. Among these are projections from various areas of the hypothalamus, as well as serotonergic fibers from the dorsal raphe nuclei and noradrenergic projections.[18] Cell bodies and fibers of different parts cross-react in immunohistochemical studies with a number of neurotransmitters, such as substance P and neuropeptide Y.[19] Push-pull cannula studies have reported release of catecholamines, GABA, and glutamate.[20] GABA is uniformly distributed throughout the hypothalamus, and its synthetic enzyme is found in high concentrations in the preoptic area.[21] GABA–benzodiazepine receptors appear in significant concentrations here,[22] suggesting that benzodiazepines might inhibit neuronal activity. The preoptic area also contains cells that are responsive to temperature, osmolarity, glucose, and steroids,[23] and receives afferents from various sensory systems.[18] The basal forebrain contains neurons that increase firing during non–rapid eye movement (NREM) sleep compared with waking ("sleep-active neurons"), although higher concentrations are found in the lateral preoptic area and diagonal band of Broca.[24] There are also neurons that selectively increase or decrease firing rates during REM sleep and NREM sleep.[25] Thus, the preoptic area in general, and the MPA in particular, appears to have a role in coordinating various systems involved in reproductive and homeostatic functions.[18] Given the bidirectional interactions of sleep with cardiovascular, thermoregulatory, endocrine, and sensory systems,[26] it seems likely that the preoptic area might be involved in coordinating sleep with other systems. It may be, then, that the preoptic area is among the loci at which benzodiazepine agonists act to induce sleep.

Other Neurotransmitters

Subsequent studies have also indicated that microinjections of pentobarbital,[27] ethanol,[28] adenosine,[29] and propofol[30] into the MPA enhance sleep. Indeed, looking at a somewhat broader area, adenosine has been shown to accumulate extracellularly in the basal forebrain cholinergic region,[31] which in turn has efferents to cortical and thalamic systems involved in arousal; it has been suggested that alteration in functioning of this cholinergic area may be the mechanism by which the propensity to sleep is enhanced by prolonged wakefulness. Similarly, it may be that possible sleep-promoting effects of antihistamines and some antidepressants (many of which have significant anticholinergic properties) might be mediated by alterations of cholinergic neurons in the basal forebrain. The histaminergic system, centered in the tuberomammillary nucleus of the posterior hypothalamus, sends efferents to the preoptic area,[32] as well as the perifornicular area[33,34] and the cortex, so it also seems possible that sedative effects of antihistamines might be mediated by altering the influence of the tuberomammillary nuclei on these centers. There has been increasing interest in the hypocretin/orexin system, centered in the perifornicular region of the posterior and lateral hypothalamus as a mechanism of arousal, as well as evidence that various defects in this system are associated with the genesis of narcolepsy (see Chapter 65). Microinjection of triazolam into this area shortens sleep latency and increases total sleep time in rats, raising the possibility that such hypnotics reduce wakefulness, either by direct action at the perifornicular area or indirectly through GABAergic outputs from the preoptic area.[35] In summary, the manner in which hypnotics may function to induce sleep is not fully elucidated, but a number of findings suggest that the basal forebrain/anterior hypothalamus will be among the crucial areas to consider.

CLINICAL EFFECTS

Moving from the neuroanatomic to the clinical level, less is understood about the mechanism by which hypnotics act. One approach raises the possibility that, among their actions, hypnotics alter the *perception* of sleep and wakefulness.[36] This notion grew out of the classic observation by Rechtschaffen[37] that poor sleepers, when experimentally awakened early in stage 2 sleep, tend to report that they had been awake, whereas good sleepers tend to report that they had been asleep. Later studies by Mendelson[38,39] replicated this observation and demonstrated that after administration of triazolam or zolpidem, patients with insomnia were more likely to report that they believed they had been asleep compared with when they were given placebo. In contrast, when zolpidem was given to normal subjects, this effect was not evident.[40] One interpretation of these data is that hypnotics such as triazolam and zolpidem may correct a misperception of sleep in some insomniac individuals, such that their experience of whether they are awake or asleep becomes more like that of good sleepers.

Other Sleep-Inducing Agents

Most over-the-counter hypnotics are first-generation *antihistamines*, including diphenhydramine and doxylamine. Although they possess to varying degrees other properties, including anticholinergic effects, their common quality is inhibition of the histamine-1 receptor. (Later generations of antihistamines are more hydrophilic, and in principle enter the CNS less readily, thus producing less sedation.) Tolerance to daytime sleepiness appears to develop rapidly, in approximately 4 days.[41] As discussed earlier, antihistamines produce drowsiness by inhibiting the histaminergic pathways centered in the tuberomammillary nucleus of the posterior hypothalamus, which enhance wakefulness. A study from the author's laboratory indicates that microinjections of histamine into the perifornicular region of the posterior hypothalamus increases wakefulness in rats, suggesting that one aspect of the mechanism by which histamine enhances wakefulness (and antihistamines promote drowsiness) may be by altering function of the orexin/hypocretin system centered in the perifornicular region (A. D. Laposky and W. B. Mendelson, unpublished data).

Although there is debate about the effectiveness and range of side effects of melatonin as a hypnotic,[42] newer agents that act as selective agonists for the melatonin-1 receptor are being examined as possible hypnotics. It has been hypothesized that melatonin and its agonists might act to affect circadian systems through effects on melatonin receptors in the suprachiasmatic nucleus, but the ways in which it might alter sleep have not been well understood. One possibility is that these effects are GABAergic. Melatonin administration is known to raise GABA concentrations in the rat hypothalamus, as well as ^{3}H-diazepam binding in the forebrain.[43] Similarly, decreases in motor activity produced by melatonin in the hamster are prevented by the benzodiazepine receptor blocker flumazenil.[44] The author's laboratory has reported that microinjections of melatonin into the MPA of the rat hypothalamus enhance sleep, suggesting that its site of action may be similar to that of benzodiazepines, barbiturates, adenosine, and ethanol, as described earlier.[45]

Although the topic of anesthetics is beyond the scope of this chapter, we briefly mention the intravenous agent propofol, which has made it much more practicable to induce anesthesia for prolonged periods in, for instance, intensive care unit settings. Neurochemically, its mechanism of action has not been fully elucidated, although it is known to interact with the GABA$_A$–benzodiazepine receptor complex, with resultant decreases in acetylcholine release from the frontal cortex and hippocampus, and also to increase functional activity of dopamine and serotonin in the cortex. Interestingly, microinjection of propofol into the MPA of rats induces sleep, and this effect is blocked by the benzodiazepine receptor blocker flumazenil.[46]

PHARMACOKINETICS

Benzodiazepines

With the possible exception of temazepam, the benzodiazepines used as hypnotics are rapidly and completely absorbed, with most achieving peak plasma levels in 1 to 1.5 hours. Some, notably flurazepam, are detectable primarily only in the form of their active metabolites, and many display kinetics that reflect enterohepatic circulation.[47] In general, oral administration is more reliable and complete than intramuscular injection. Although there is significant protein binding, there are few or no cases in which displacement of other protein-bound drugs is clinically relevant. Most are very lipophilic, and rapidly enter the CNS, where concentrations reflect unbound drug in plasma. Whereas the older, longer-acting agents are metabolized to active compounds, the shorter-acting agents such as triazolam are broken down into inactive substances (see Table 36–1). The elimination half-lives vary widely, from the relatively short-acting triazolam to intermediate agents such as temazepam to long-acting substances such as flurazepam (see Table 36–1). Accumulation of the agents with longer elimination half-lives taken nightly has significant bearing on one major clinical issue—the appearance of daytime residual sedation (Fig. 36–2). Because of their lipophilicity, many are rapidly redistributed, which may play as important a role in the decline in CNS effects as does their metabolism. Another implication of the high lipophilicity is that the volume of distribution is often increased in the elderly (who tend to have a higher ratio of lipid to muscle), resulting in an increased half-life. Most are broken down by hepatic microsomal systems and excreted as conjugated glucuronides. There is no stimulation of the hepatic microsomal systems, and hence no enhancement of the rate of breakdown of other drugs that undergo the same metabolic processes. Their own metabolism may be inhibited by some compounds such as cimetidine and some steroids, and may be accelerated in smokers.

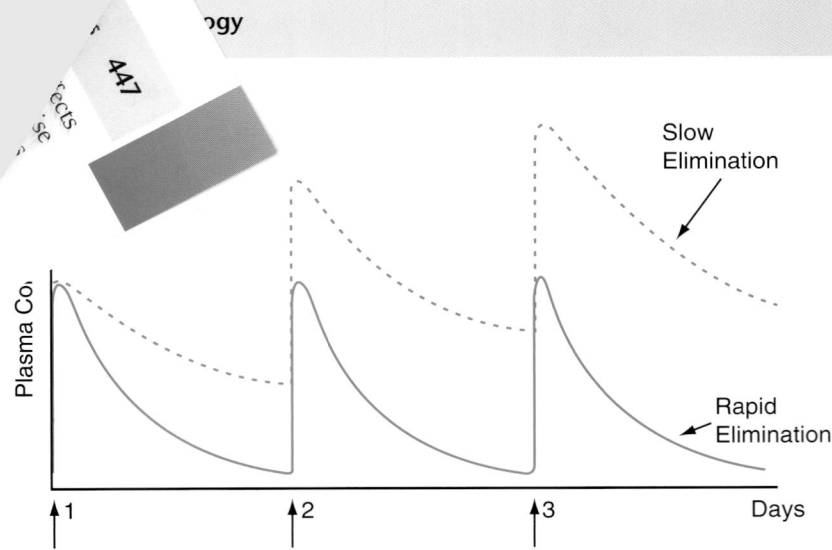

Figure 36–2. A hypnotic with a relatively long elimination half-life (e.g., >24 hr; *broken blue line*) will accumulate during nightly use, in contrast to an agent with relatively short elimination half-life (e.g., 6 hr; *solid blue line*). (From Nicholson AN: Hypnotics: Clinical pharmacology and therapeutics. In Kryger MH, Roth T, Dement WC [eds]: Principles and Practice of Sleep Medicine, 2nd ed. Philadelphia, WB Saunders, 1989, pp 355-363.)

Zolpidem

Zolpidem, an imidazopyridine compound with relative selectivity for the type I $GABA_A$–benzodiazepine receptor, is rapidly absorbed; because of first-pass metabolism, it has a bioavailability of 67% after oral administration of doses up to 20 mg.[48] Peak concentrations are reached after 1.6 hours. Total protein binding is approximately 92%. Absorption is slightly decreased when taken on a full stomach. It has no pharmacologically active metabolites, and is eliminated primarily by renal excretion.

Zopiclone

Zopiclone, which is not on the market in the United States, is a cyclopyrrolone that acts at the $GABA_A$–benzodiazepine receptor complex, but possibly at a binding domain or producing different conformational changes from the benzodiazepines.[49] It is rapidly absorbed, with peak plasma concentrations occurring in 0.5 to 2 hours.[49] Bioavailability is approximately 80%, implying that the first-pass effect is relatively small.[50] It is very lipophilic and enters rapidly into the CNS. Protein binding is approximately 45%. It has two major metabolites, the *N*-oxide, which has lower pharmacologic activity, and the inactive *N*-desmethyl derivative, which along with various minor metabolites are excreted primarily by the kidneys and lungs.[49] At the time of this writing, an isomerically pure derivative, eszopiclone, is under development, and has been reported to sustain efficacy over 6 months of nightly use.[51]

Zaleplon

A pyrazolopyrimidine that binds selectively to the benzodiazepine-1 receptor, zaleplon is rapidly absorbed after oral administration, with peak concentrations being reached in 1 hour, and has an elimination half-life of approximately 1 hour. Protein binding is approximately 60%. It is rapidly metabolized to inactive forms, with approximately 71% of labeled compound recovered in the urine and 17% in feces. Recommendations for administration in the United States include taking it immediately before bedtime, or after the patient has gone to bed and has experienced difficulty falling asleep. In the latter case, it should be taken at least 4 hours before time of arising to avoid any possible memory difficulties.

PHARMACOLOGIC PROPERTIES

Although the hypnotic benzodiazepines are given for purposes of aiding sleep, they share a spectrum of pharmacologic properties with agents given as daytime sedatives or anxiolytics; indeed, some authors have suggested that the designation of some benzodiazepines as hypnotics is as much a marketing plan as it has been a pharmacologic decision. Among their effects are anxiolytic, myorelaxant, and anticonvulsant properties. Many, particularly the longer-acting agents, have mild respiratory depressant properties,[52,53] which are much less evident in shorter-acting agents.[54] There is even some limited evidence that triazolam may improve sleep-disturbed respiration in central sleep apnea,[55] although whether this is related to direct respiratory effects or secondary to decreasing the number of arousals during sleep is not clear. Even for the longer-acting agents, however, respiratory depression is much milder than for the older nonbenzodiazepine hypnotics, such as the barbiturates. In practical terms, there is no significant effect in patients with normal ventilation, although it may become evident when there is preexisting compromised respiration, such as in patients with chronic obstructive pulmonary disease or persons with unrecognized sleep-disordered breathing. The newer nonbenzodiazepines appear to have very few respiratory effects. One recent study of clinically used doses of zaleplon, for instance, found minimal effects on measures of sleep-disturbed respiration in patients with mild to moderate obstructive sleep apnea.* In most cases, the preceding generalizations in this section apply as well to zolpidem. There is some evidence from animal studies that it possesses a greater separation of hypnotic and sedative doses. It has been reported to have no respiratory depressant properties up to doses of 10 mg, and to exhibit very mild inhibition of mean inspiratory drive at 20 mg.[56] Zopiclone in therapeutic doses appears to have no significant effect on

---

*Data on file, Elan Biopharmaceuticals, courtesy of Dr. S. P. James.

sleep-disordered breathing in patients with chronic obstructive pulmonary disease.[57]

In general, adverse reactions to hypnotics are relatively rare and mild; one review of 3 years' experience in a 1000-bed teaching hospital found the median rate of reported adverse events to be 0.01% (1 in 10,000 doses administered), and ran as high as 0.05%.[27] The rate for triazolam was 0.02%.

Unlike older hypnotics such as the barbiturates, the hypnotic benzodiazepines are relatively benign in overdose when taken alone by a medically healthy individual. They may be very toxic, however, when taken in combination with other CNS depressants such as alcohol, and because a significant portion of overdoses involve a combination of drugs,[58] it is wise to treat them as potentially toxic or even lethal agents. In practice, this translates into being very conscious of the possibility that a patient seeking help for sleep disturbance may be suffering from unrecognized depressive illness, and if it is present, initiating appropriate antidepressant therapy.

EFFECTS ON SLEEP

Polygraphic studies of benzodiazepines indicate that, consistent with their clinical effects, sleep latency and wake time after sleep onset are usually reduced, and total sleep time increased.[6] As with barbiturates and ethanol, spindle activity may be increased. REM sleep time may be reduced mildly, in contrast to the very potent REM suppression induced by barbiturates. In the early years after the introduction of benzodiazepines into the U.S. market, much was made of this observation, which was interpreted to mean that they somehow produced a more "natural" sleep. With hindsight, many investigators recognize that the psychological effects of REM deprivation are much less clear than originally thought, and that indeed in the case of depressed patients, REM deprivation may even be therapeutic (see Chapter 112), so whether having only mild REM-suppressant properties translates into some clinical advantage seems uncertain. The benzodiazepines are, however, in contrast to the barbiturates, potent suppressors of slow wave sleep. The same dilemma that arises with regard to REM sleep appears once again: Because the function of slow wave sleep has not been determined, the clinical significance of pharmacologically suppressing this stage remains uncertain. The nonbenzodiazepine zolpidem shares with the benzodiazepines the very mild effects on REM sleep, but in contrast does not alter slow wave sleep, which may even increase toward more expected values in some insomniac individuals with low baseline levels.

Clinical efficacy studies indicate that virtually all these agents potently improve polygraphic measures of sleep and result in better subjective ratings of sleep quality during short-term use. One of the few distinctions among the benzodiazepines is that the longer-acting agents such as flurazepam may not have as much effectiveness on sleep latency until the second night of administration.[59] One concern that was initially raised about the short-acting agents such as triazolam was the possibility that their relatively rapid metabolism might lead to sleep disturbance after several hours; later studies analyzing awakening in the latter part of the night have in general found no evidence that this is the case.[60,61]

Another pharmacologic property to consider is the potential for dependence. A recent review of this topic by a panel from academia, industry, and government concluded that the dependence potential of currently available hypnotics in patients without a history of substance abuse is minimal.[62] A variety of other issues at a clinical level include determination of whether tolerance develops during long-term nightly administration, and the effectiveness of nonnightly use, which are considered in Chapter 63.

FUTURE HYPNOTICS

This is a very fruitful time in the development of hypnotics because several new agents are under development. Among compounds that act at the GABA$_A$ receptor are a new non-benzodiazepine selective GABA$_A$ agonist and an isomer of a currently available nonbenzodiazepine hypnotic. Agents with novel mechanisms of action are also being developed. These include compounds that act as antagonists to specific serotonin receptor subtypes, and agonists for the melatonin-1 receptor, as mentioned earlier. Advances in medicinal chemistry are enabling the development of hypnotics that may come in multiple preparations that vary in duration of action. There has been interest in other mechanisms, including alterations in substance P function, and novel modes of administration, including an intranasal technique. All in all, it will be exciting to see what will happen by the next edition of this book!

> ### Clinical Pearl
>
> Virtually all currently available hypnotics induce sleep by acting on various moieties of the GABA$_A$–benzodiazepine receptor complex; knock-in studies of the α_1 subunit suggest that it is unlikely that hypnotics that act by this mechanism can be developed that will have sleep-inducing, but not amnesic, properties. Hypnotics with novel mechanisms of action are likely to be available for clinical use within a few years.

REFERENCES

1. Editors: Antipsychotics worth billions in sales. Psychiatr Times July 4, 2003.
2. Hatoum HT, Kania CM, Kong SX, et al: Prevalence of insomnia: A survey of the enrollees at five managed care organizations. Am J Managed Care 1998;4:79-86.
3. Simon GE, VonKorff M: Prevalence, burden, and treatment of insomnia in primary care. Am J Psychiatry 1997;154:1417-1423.
4. National Sleep Foundation: 1998 Omnibus Sleep in America Poll. Washington, DC, National Sleep Foundation, 1998.
5. Johnson EO, Roehrs T, Roth T, Breslau N: Epidemiology of alcohol and medication as aids to sleep in early adulthood. Sleep 1998;21:178-186.
6. Mendelson WB: Human Sleep: Research and Clinical Care. New York, Plenum Press, 1987.
7. Mohler H, Okada T: Benzodiazepine receptor: Demonstration in the central nervous system. Science 1977;198:849-851.
8. Squires RF, Braestrup C: Benzodiazepine receptors in rat brain. Nature 1977;266:732-734.
9. Krasowski MD, Finn SE, Ye Q, Harrison NL: Trichloroethanol modulation of recombinant GABA-A, glycine, and GABA p1 receptors. J Pharmacol Exp Ther 1998;284:934-942.
10. Whiting PJ, McKernan RM, Wager-Srdar SA: Structure and pharmacology of vertebrate GABA-A receptor subtypes. Int Rev Neurobiol 1995;38:95-138.

11. Rudolph U, Crestani F, Benke D, et al: Benzodiazepine actions mediated by specific GABA-A receptor subtypes. Nature 1999; 401:796-800.

12. Harrison N, Mendelson W, de Wit H: Barbiturates. In Watson SJ (ed): Psychopharmacology: Fourth Generation of Progress, 1998 edition CD/ROM, p 113. Philadelphia, ACNP/Lippincott-Raven, 1998. Also available at http://www.acnp.org/citations/GN401000173.

13. MacDonald RL, Rogers CJ, Twyman RE: Barbiturate regulation of kinetic properties of the GABA-A receptor channel of mouse spinal neurones in culture. J Physiol (Lond) 1989;417:483-500.

14. Study RE, Barker JL: Diazepam and (-)pentobarbital: Fluctuation analysis reveals different mechanisms for potentiation of gamma-aminobutyric acid responses in cultured neurons. Proc Natl Acad Sci U S A 1981;78:7180-7184.

15. Krasowski MD, O'Shea SM, Rick CEM, et al: Alpha subunit isoform influences GABA-A receptor modulation by propofol. Neuropharmacology 1997;36:941-949.

16. Mendelson WB: Neuropharmacology of sleep induction by benzodiazepines. Crit Rev Neurobiol 1992;6:221-232.

17. Mendelson WB, Martin JV: Characterization of the hypnotic effects of triazolam microinjections into the medial preoptic area. Life Sci 1992;50:1117-1128.

18. Simerly RB, Swanson LW: The organization of neural inputs to the medial preoptic nucleus of the rat. J Comp Neurol 1985; 246:312-342.

19. Simerly RB, Gorski RA, Swanson LW: Neurotransmitter specificity of cell and fibers in the medial preoptic nucleus: An immunohistochemical study in the rat. J Comp Neurol 1986;246: 343-363.

20. Demling J, Fuchs E, Baumert M, Wuttke W: Preoptic catecholamine, GABA, and glutamate release in ovariectomized estrogen-primed rats utilizing a push-pull cannula technique. Neuroendocrinology 1985;41:212-218.

21. Tappaz ML, Brownstein MJ, Kopin IJ: Glutamate decarboxylase (GAD) and gamma-aminobutyric acid (GABA) in discrete nuclei of hypothalamus and substantia nigra. Brain Res 1977;125: 109-121.

22. Unnerstall JR, Niehoff DL, Kuhar MJ, Palacios JM: Quantitative receptor autoradiography using 3H-ultrofilm: Application to multiple benzodiazepine receptors. J Neurosci 1982;6:59-73.

23. Boulant JA, Silva NL: Neuronal sensitivities in preoptic tissue slices: Interactions among homeostatic systems. Brain Res Bull 1988;20:871-878.

24. Szymusiak R, McGinty DJ: Sleep-related neuronal discharge in the basal forebrain of cats. Brain Res Bull 1986;17:82-92.

25. Koyama Y, Hayaishi O: Firing of neurons in the preoptic/anterior hypothalamic areas in rat: Its possible involvement in slow wave sleep and paradoxical sleep. Neurosci Res 1994;19:31-38.

26. McGinty D: Brain mechanisms of sleep. In McGinty D, Morrison A, Drucker-Colin R, Parmeggiani PL (eds): Brain Mechanisms of Sleep. New York, Raven Press, 1985:361-384.

27. Mendelson WB, Thompson C, Franko T: Adverse reactions to sedative/hypnotics: Three years' experience. Sleep 1996;19: 702-706.

28. Ticho SR, Stojanovic M, Lekovic G, Radulovacki M: Effects of ethanol injection to the preoptic area on sleep and temperature in rats. Alcohol 1992;9:275-278.

29. Ticho SR, Radulovacki M: Role of adenosine in sleep and temperature regulation in the preoptic area of rats. Pharmacol Biochem Behav 1991;40:33-40.

30. Tung A, Bluhm B, Mendelson WB: Sleep inducing effects of propofol microinjection into the medial preoptic area are blocked by flumazenil. Brain Res 2001;908:155-160.

31. Porkka-Heiskanen T, Strecker RE, Thakkar M, et al: Adenosine: A mediator of the sleep-inducing effects of prolonged wakefulness. Science 1997;276:1265-1268.

32. Lin JS, Sakai K, Vanni-Mercier G, Jouvet M: Hypothalamo-preoptic histaminergic projections in sleep-wake control in the cat. Eur J Neurosci 1994;66:618-625.

33. Inagaki N, Toda K, Taniuchi I, et al: An analysis of histaminergic efferents of the tuberomammillary nucleus to the medial preoptic area and inferior colliculus of the rat. Exp Brain Res 1990;80: 374-380.

34. Panula P, Pirvola U, Auvinen S, Airaksinen MS: Histamine-immunoreactive nerve fibers in the rat brain. Neuroscience 1989;28:585-610.

35. Mendelson WB, Laposky AD: Effects of triazolam microinjections into the peri-fornicular region on sleep in rats. Sleep Hypnosis 2003;5:154-162.

36. Mendelson WB: Clinical neuropharmacology of sleep. Neurol Clin 1990;8:153-160.

37. Rechtschaffen A: Polygraphic aspects of insomnia. In Gastaut H, Lugaresi L, Berti G, Coccagano C, eds. The Abnormalities of Sleep in Man. Bologna, Italy, Gaggi, 1968, pp 109-125.

38. Mendelson WB: Pharmacologic alteration of the perception of being awake or asleep. Sleep 1993;16:641-646.

39. Mendelson WB: Effects of flurazepam and zolpidem on the perception of sleep in insomniacs. Sleep 1995;18:92-96.

40. Mendelson WB: Effects of flurazepam and zolpidem in the perception of sleep in normal volunteers. Sleep 1995; 18:88-91.

41. Richardson GS, Roehrs TA, Rosenthal L, et al: Tolerance to daytime effects of sedative H1 antihistamines. J Clin Psychopharmacol 2002;22:511-515.

42. Mendelson WB: A critical evaluation of the hypnotic efficacy of melatonin. Sleep 1997;20:916-919.

43. Rosenstein RE, Cardinali DP: Melatonin increases in vivo GABA accumulation in rat hypothalamus, cerebellum, cerebral cortex and pineal gland. Brain Res 1986;398:403-406.

44. Golombek DA, Escolar E, Cardinali DP: Melatonin-induced depression of locomotor activity in hamsters: Time-dependency and inhibition by the central-type benzodiazepine antagonist Ro 15-1788. Physiol Behav 1991;49:1091-1097.

45. Mendelson WB: Melatonin microinjection into the preoptic area increases sleep in the rat. Life Sci 2002;71:2067-2070.

46. Tung A, Bluhm B, Mendelson WB: Flumazenil blocks the increase in sleep after propofol microinjection into the medial preoptic area of the rat. Anesthesiology 2000;93:A803-A803.

47. Hobbs WR, Rall TW, Verdoorn TA: Hypnotics and sedatives; ethanol. In Hardman JG, Limbird LE, Molinoff PB, et al (eds): The Pharmacological Basis of Therapeutics, 7th ed. New York, McGraw-Hill, 1996, pp 361-396.

48. Langtry HD, Benfield P: Zolpidem: A review of its pharmacodynamic and pharmacokinetic properties and therapeutic potential. Drugs 1990;40:291-313.

49. Noble S, Langtry HD, Lamb HM: Zopiclone: An update of its pharmacology, clinical efficacy and tolerability in the treatment of insomnia. Drugs 1998;55:277-302.

50. Hindmarch IE: Zopiclone monograph. Manchester, United Kingdom, Adis Press International, 1990.

51. Krystal A, Walsh J, Roth T, et al: The sustained efficacy and safety of eszopiclone over six months of nightly treatment: A placebo-controlled study in patients with chronic insomnia. Sleep 2003;26(Suppl):A310.

52. Rudolf M, Geddes DM, Turner JA, Saunders KB: Depression of central respiratory drive by nitrazepam. Thorax 1978;33: 97-100.

53. Dolly FR, Block AJ: Effect of flurazepam on sleep-disordered breathing and nocturnal oxygen desaturation in asymptomatic patients. Am J Med 1982;73:239-243.

54. Mendelson WB: Drugs which alter sleep and sleep-related respiration. In Kuna ST (ed): Sleep and Respiration in Aging Adults. New York, Elsevier, 1991, pp 49-54.

55. Bonnet MH, Dexter JR, Arand DL: The effect of triazolam on arousal and respiration in central sleep apnea patients. Sleep 1990;13:31-41.

56. Cohn MA: Effects of zolpidem, codeine phosphate and placebo on respiration: A double-blind, crossover study in volunteers. Drug Safe 1993;9:312-319.

57. Muir JF, Defouilloy C, Broussier PM, et al: Incidence of zopiclone vs placebo on sleep-disordered breathing in COPD patients. Rev Respir Dis 1988;13:12-14.

58. Mendelson WB, Rich CL: The use of sedative/hypnotics in completed suicides: The San Diego study [abstract]. Sleep Res 1992;21:62.

59. Kripke DF, Hauri P, Ancoli-Israel S, et al. Sleep evaluation in chronic insomniacs during 14-day use of flurazepam and midazolam. J Clin Psychopharmacol 1990;10:32S-43S.

60. Roehrs T, Zorick F, Wittig R, Roth T: Efficacy of a reduced triazolam dose in elderly insomniacs. Neurobiol Aging 1985;6:293-296.

61. Kales A, Bixler EO, Vela-Bueno A, et al: Comparison of short and long half-life benzodiazepine hypnotics: Triazolam and quazepam. Clin Pharmacol Ther 1986;49:378-386.

62. Mendelson WB, Roth T, Cassella J, et al: The treatment of chronic insomnia: Drug indications, chronic use and abuse liability: Summary of a 2001 New Clinical Drug Evaluation Unit (NCDEU) meeting symposium. Sleep Med Rev 2003;8:7-17.

63. Maczaj M: Pharmacological treatment of Insomnia. Drugs 1993;45:44-45.

64. Roehrs T, Vogel G, Vogel F, et al: Dose effects of temazepam tablets on sleep. Drugs Exp Clin Res 1986;12:693-699.

65. Physicians' Desk Reference. Montvale, NJ, Medical Economics, 1998.

37

Clinical Pharmacology of Other Drugs Used as Hypnotics

Daniel J. Buysse

Paula K. Schweitzer

Douglas E. Moul

ABSTRACT

A variety of drugs other than benzodiazepine receptor agonists are used as hypnotics. These include drugs originally developed as antidepressants, anticonvulsants, and antipsychotics, as well as hormones and other "natural" substances. Understanding the pharmacokinetics, pharmacodynamics, sleep effects, and side effects of these drugs is essential for clinical practice. Sedating tricyclic and other antidepressant drugs show considerable heterogeneity in terms of half-lives (ranging from 2 to 30 hours), receptor pharmacology, and sleep effects. They act primarily through serotonin, norepinephrine, and histamine receptor effects. Evidence for their positive effects on sleep continuity comes mainly from studies of depressed patients. Some of these drugs also increase slow wave sleep and reduce rapid eye movement sleep. Melatonin has a very short duration of action. Its sleep effects are probably mediated by effects on melatonin receptors in the suprachiasmatic nucleus. Its most consistent sleep effect is reducing sleep latency. Antihistamines antagonize central histamine receptors in the posterior hypothalamus. They are widely used because of their clear effects on subjective sedation. A limited amount of evidence exists regarding their effects on nocturnal sleep, and, like antidepressants, they can have potentially serious side effects. Valerian extracts have uncertain pharmacokinetics and mechanisms of action. They appear to affect primarily sleep latency, although some studies also show increased slow wave sleep. Small numbers of studies suggest that the sedating antipsychotic drugs, tiagabine, gabapentin, and γ-hydroxybutyrate may all increase slow wave sleep and improve sleep continuity. These drugs have a wide variety of receptor effects, and the mechanisms of their effects on human sleep are poorly understood. Few human sleep studies have been conducted with any of these agents, particularly with regard to their use as hypnotic agents. Further study is needed to understand the appropriate role of these drugs in the treatment of sleep disorders.

Benzodiazepine receptor agonists (BzRAs) are the only drugs currently approved by the U.S. Food and Drug Administration (FDA) for treatment of insomnia. However, no class of drugs is universally efficacious for any condition, and other classes of drugs have been used for the treatment of insomnia. Persistent concerns regarding potential side effects of BzRAs such as tolerance, dependence, and abuse have also led clinicians to investigate other classes of drugs for insomnia treatment.

Finally, the search for other drugs to treat insomnia is warranted by the complexity of neurochemical regulation of sleep–wake states and the complexity of insomnia itself, which presents with different symptoms and likely has multiple causes.

Pharmacoepidemiology data indicate that prescribers often use non-BzRA drugs to treat insomnia. Data from the National Disease and Therapeutic Index between 1986 and 1996 show that benzodiazepine hypnotic prescriptions fell by almost 50%, whereas the use of antidepressant drugs to treat insomnia increased by 146%.[1] Most of this increase was accounted for by prescription of trazodone. In fact, trazodone was the most commonly prescribed drug to treat insomnia in 1996.

Unlike BzRAs, other drugs used to treat insomnia do not share consistent chemical structures, receptor activities, or other pharmacologic properties. Some argue that use of non-BzRA drugs to treat insomnia is inappropriate because their hypnotic activity is a "side effect" rather than a "therapeutic" effect. However, many drug effects can be considered therapeutic or adverse, depending on the intended action. For instance, the first antidepressants, monoamine oxidase inhibitors, were originally developed for the treatment of tuberculosis, and the prototype tricyclic antidepressant (TCA), imipramine, was actually discovered during a search for sedatives and antipsychotic agents.[2] Benzodiazepines were themselves developed as anxiolytics rather than hypnotics. Thus, the use of drugs that are not approved by the FDA as hypnotic medications is not necessarily inappropriate. A more realistic limitation is that most nonapproved hypnotic drugs have not been rigorously evaluated with regard to their sleep effects, leaving uncertainties regarding appropriate dose, demonstrated efficacy, and side effects.

This chapter addresses the clinical pharmacology of prescription and over-the-counter drugs used as hypnotics that do not have pharmacologic activity at the benzodiazepine receptor. For each drug or drug class, we review pharmacokinetics (how the body acts on drugs, with particular reference to absorption, distribution, metabolism, and elimination); pharmacodynamics (how the drug acts on the body, particularly the brain); effects on human sleep (both subjective and polysomnographic [PSG] measures); and side effects.

SEDATING ANTIDEPRESSANTS

Overview

In 2003, over 20 drugs were marketed as antidepressants in the United States, but only a few of these have been used

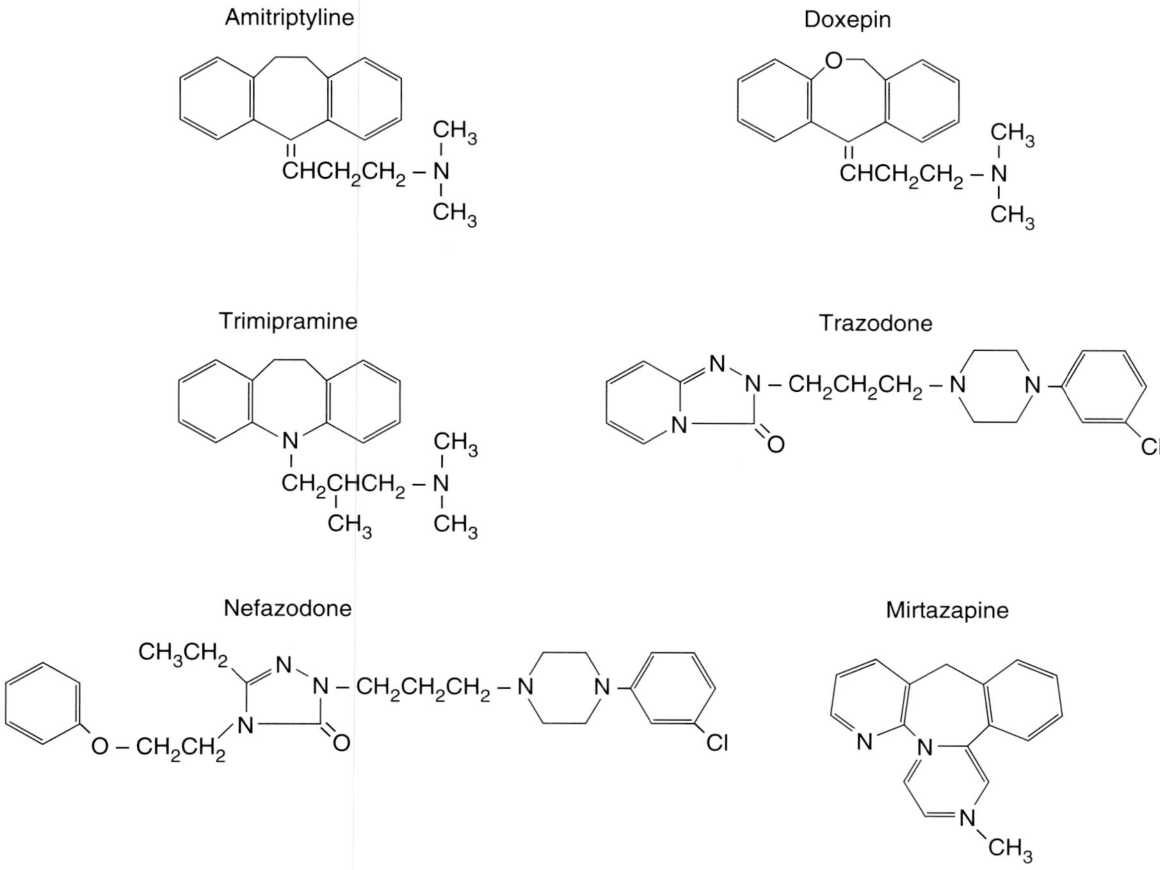

Amitriptyline

Doxepin

Trimipramine

Trazodone

Nefazodone

Mirtazapine

Figure 37–1. Chemical structures of sedating antidepressant drugs.

specifically for the treatment of insomnia. These include the TCAs doxepin, trimipramine, and amitriptyline, as well as trazodone, nefazodone, and mirtazapine. Their chemical structures are shown in Figure 37–1, and pharmacokinetic properties are summarized in Table 37–1.

Antidepressant drugs are thought to exert their beneficial effects on mood primarily through effects at serotonin (5-hydroxytryptamine [5-HT]) and norepinephrine (NE) receptors. Many antidepressants inhibit 5-HT and NE reuptake, and have a variety of agonist and antagonist effects at presynaptic and postsynaptic 5-HT and NE receptors. Serotonin neuropharmacology is quite complex; at least seven subtypes of 5-HT receptors have been identified. Furthermore, antidepressants have effects at multiple receptors other than 5-HT and NE. Consequently, it is not possible to specify their exact mechanism of action with regard to sleep effects. However, the most likely mechanisms of action for sedating antidepressant drugs include a combination of histamine type 1 (H_1) and serotonin type 2 (5-HT_2) receptor antagonism, possibly in combination with alpha-adrenergic type 1 (alpha$_1$) receptor antagonism. Receptor effects of sedative antidepressants are summarized in Table 37–2.

The majority of data regarding the effects of antidepressant drugs on human sleep come from studies in patients with depression. In many of these studies, the doses of drugs used were higher than those typically used for treatment of insomnia. Formal dose-ranging studies have not been conducted to determine optimal hypnotic doses. Sleep effects of

sedating antidepressant drugs have been discussed elsewhere,[3] and are summarized in Table 37–3.

Sedative antidepressants can have a variety of systemic and central nervous system (CNS) side effects, summarized in Table 37–4. Like their sleep effects, many of the side effects of antidepressants are derived from clinical trials investigating relatively high doses of these drugs used as antidepressants. Some of the side effects of antidepressants are dose related, but others are not.

Tricyclic Antidepressant Drugs

TCAs share a core cyclic structure, and differ from one another in their specific side chains (Fig. 37–1). TCAs are often subgrouped according to side chain structures as tertiary or secondary amines. Tertiary amine TCAs are metabolized to secondary amine TCAs. Both the parent drugs and their metabolites have measurable blood levels and pharmacologic activity. For example, amitriptyline is metabolized to nortriptyline. Tertiary TCAs are more sedating than secondary TCAs.

Pharmacokinetics

TCAs are rapidly absorbed from the gastrointestinal (GI) tract, with maximum concentrations occurring at 2 to 6 hours postdose. They undergo extensive (30% to 90%) first-pass metabolism and are extensively protein bound (up to 95%). Consequently, bioavailability is low after oral administration.[2,4,5] TCAs are very lipophilic, ensuring large volumes of

Table 37–1.   Pharmacokinetic Properties of Sedating Antidepressant Drugs

Drug	Drug Class	t_{max} (hr)	Metabolism (CYP Enzymes)	$t_{1/2}$ in Hours (Range)	Usual Dose (mg) Antidepressant	Hypnotic*
Doxepin	Tricyclic	2-8	Major: 2D6, 2C19; Minor: 1A2, 3A4	20 (10-30)	100-300	25-150
Amitriptyline	Tricyclic	2-8	Major: 2D6, 2C19; Minor: 1A2, 3A4	30 (5-45)	100-300	25-150
Trimipramine	Tricyclic	2-8	Major: 2D6, 2C19; Minor: 1A2, 3A4	25 (15-40)	100-300	25-150
Trazodone	Phenylpiperazine	1-2	3A4, 2D6	9 (3-14)	200-600	25-150
Nefazodone	Phenylpiperazine	1	3A4, 2D6, 2C19	2-4 (6-18 for active metabolites)	150-450	50-150
Mirtazapine	Noradrenergic and specific serotonergic antidepressant	1-3	3A4, 2D6, 1A2	25 (13-40)	15-45	15-30

*Hypnotic doses are based on published studies and common clinical practice. No formal dose-ranging studies for this indication have been published.

t_{max}, Time to maximal concentration; $t_{1/2}$, elimination half-life; CYP, cytochrome P-450 (individual letters and numbers in table represent specific CYP enzymes).

Data from references 2, 4, 5, 24, 25, and 100.

distribution and high concentrations in the brain. TCAs have half-lives of approximately 15 to 30 hours, leading to high concentrations during sleep after nighttime administration, but also posing risks for residual daytime sedation. Active metabolites of TCAs have slightly longer half-lives than the parent compounds.[6]

TCAs undergo extensive hepatic metabolism, the most important pathways being oxidative demethylation of the side chains and hydroxylation of the ring structure.[4-6] After oxidation, TCAs are conjugated with glucuronic acid to form inactive hydrophilic metabolites that are renally excreted. Hepatic oxidative metabolism is accomplished by enzymes of

Table 37–2.   Receptor Pharmacology of Sedating Antidepressant Drugs

Drug	NE Reuptake	5-HT Reuptake	5-HT$_2$ Receptor Antagonism	Receptor Effects* Alpha$_1$ Antagonism	M$_1$ Antagonism (Anticholinergic)	H$_1$ Antagonism (Antihistaminic)	Other Effects
Doxepin	+	0/+	+	+++	++	+++	
Amitriptyline	+	++	+	+++	+++	++	
Trimipramine	0	0	+	+++	++	+++	
Trazodone	0	+	++	++	0	0/+	5-HT$_{1A}$, 5-HT$_{1C}$, and alpha$_2$ antagonism
Nefazodone	0	++	++	++	0	+	
Mirtazapine	0/+	0	++	+	+	+++	Alpha$_2$ and 5-HT$_1$ antagonism

*"+" Indicates strength of effect relative to other antidepressant drugs; "0" indicates no significant effect.

NE, norepinephrine; 5-HT, serotonin; M, muscarinic cholinergic receptor; H, histamine receptor. Numbers after receptor abbreviations indicate specific receptor subtype.

Data from Richelson E: Synaptic effects of antidepressants. J Clin Psychopharmacol 1996;16(3, Suppl 2):1S-9S, and references 2, 5, 24, and 100.

Table 37–3.   Polysomnographic Effects of Sedating Antidepressant Drugs on Sleep*

Drug	Sleep Latency	Sleep Continuity[†]	Stage 3/4 NREM Sleep Amount (Percentage)	REM Sleep	Other
Doxepin	↓	↑	↔	↓ Amount (percentage) of REM ↑ Phasic eye movements (REM density)	↓ Sleep apnea (minor effect); ↔ or ↑ periodic limb movements; ↑ restless legs symptoms; may induce eye movements during NREM sleep
Amitriptyline	↓	↑	↔	↓ Amount (percentage) of REM ↑ Phasic eye movements (REM density)	
Trimipramine	↓	↑	↔	↔ Amount (percentage) of REM	
Trazodone	↓	↔ to ↑	↑	↔ Amount (percentage) of REM (↓ to ↑ in individual studies)	
Nefazodone	↔	↑	↔	↔	
Mirtazapine	↓	↑	↔	↔	

*Reported effects are based on preponderance of evidence from published studies (see text for details). Many effects are inconsistent between individual studies. "↑" Indicates increase from pretreatment baseline; "↓" indicates decrease from pretreatment baseline; "↔" indicates no change from pretreatment baseline.

[†]Sleep continuity refers to the proportion of sleep relative to wakefulness after sleep onset, as reflected by measures such as sleep efficiency. Other indicators of sleep continuity, such as wakefulness after sleep onset or number of awakenings, would have opposite signs. Thus, "↑" indicates improvement in overall sleep continuity.

REM, rapid eye movement; NREM, non-REM.

the cytochrome P-450 (CYP) system. CYP enzymes metabolize a large number of lipophilic endogenous and exogenous substances, including 40% to 50% of all medications, into more hydrophilic substances.[7] Demethylation of TCAs is accomplished primarily by CYP2C19, and hydroxylation by CYP2D6; CYP1A2 and CYP3A4 are also involved.[2,4,6] At usual doses, metabolism of TCAs follows linear kinetics, meaning that drug blood levels (and metabolism) are proportional to dose. At higher doses, however, metabolic enzymes can become saturated, leading to nonlinear pharmacokinetics (i.e., higher blood levels than predicted by dose alone).[6] Furthermore, there is wide interindividual variability in metabolism and steady-state levels of TCAs, largely because of population variability in intrinsic CYP2D6 activity.[7] Polymorphisms in CYP2D6 are well recognized, and are responsible for differences between "poor metabolizers," who are at risk for increased toxicity, and "extensive metabolizers," who may require larger doses to achieve a therapeutic effect. Age is associated with decreased metabolic clearance by CYP3A4, but not CYP2D6, and with decreased renal clearance.[4,5]

Other medications can have important interactions with TCAs. For instance, cimetidine and diltiazem can decrease hepatic blood flow and first-pass metabolism, leading to increased TCA levels. CYP3A4 can be induced by drugs such as barbiturates and tamoxifen, leading to reduced TCA levels, whereas CYP2D6 can be inhibited by drugs such as antipsychotic drugs, methylphenidate, fluoxetine, and paroxetine,

leading to increased TCA levels.[6] Grapefruit juice is another common, if unsuspected, inhibitor of CYP3A4.

Pharmacodynamics and Receptor Pharmacology

Doxepin and amitriptyline inhibit both serotonin and NE reuptake transporters, whereas trimipramine has minimal reuptake effects. Tertiary TCAs, including amitriptyline and doxepin, have relatively more pronounced effects on serotonin than NE reuptake, whereas their secondary amine metabolites have more pronounced effects on NE reuptake.[6,8] After chronic dosing, additional effects on serotonergic and noradrenergic neurotransmission are also observed: desensitization of presynaptic 5-HT$_{1A}$ autoreceptors; upregulation (sensitization) of postsynaptic 5-HT$_{1A}$ receptors; and both downregulation and antagonism of postsynaptic 5-HT$_2$ receptors.[9] At 5-HT$_2$ receptors, antagonism of the 5-HT$_{2C}$ subtype is more strongly associated with increasing slow wave sleep than antagonism of 5-HT$_{2A}$ receptors.[3] The net effect of the TCAs' receptor effects is an enhancement of serotonin effects in the CNS. Noradrenergic effects of TCAs include desensitization of presynaptic alpha$_2$ autoreceptors and a compensatory downregulation of postsynaptic beta receptors,[5] with a net effect of increasing noradrenergic neurotransmission. Sedating TCAs also antagonize peripheral alpha$_1$- and alpha$_2$-adrenergic receptors, which accounts for their cardiovascular effects.

Table 37–4. Sedating Antidepressant Drug Side Effects

Drug	Side Effects
Doxepin, amitriptyline, trimipramine	Sedation Anticholinergic: dry mouth, constipation, urinary retention, increased perspiration, exacerbation of narrow angle glaucoma Antihistamine: dry mouth, increased appetite, weight gain Alpha$_1$ antagonism: orthostatic hypotension, falls Other: cardiac conduction delay (quinidine-like effect), prolonged QRS complex and corrected QT interval duration
Trazodone	Sedation Orthostatic hypotension, lightheadedness, weakness Premature ventricular contractions Weight gain Priapism
Nefazodone	Sedation Dry mouth Orthostatic hypotension, lightheadedness, weakness Hepatotoxicity
Mirtazapine	Sedation Dry mouth Increased appetite, weight gain

Sedating TCAs also antagonize M$_1$ muscarinic cholinergic and H$_1$ histamine receptors. Amitriptyline is the most anticholinergic of all antidepressants, and doxepin is a more potent antihistamine than many drugs marketed as antihistamines, including diphenhydramine.

The effects of TCAs on serotonin and NE transporters, and on cholinergic, histaminergic, and peripheral adrenergic receptors, occur immediately. The other effects on serotonin and NE receptors described previously occur over a period of days or weeks. The sedative effects of TCAs are seen immediately, whereas antidepressant effects are typically delayed, and more closely follow the time course of the secondary receptor effects. Therefore, the mechanisms of the hypnotic and antidepressant effects of TCAs are likely to be different.

Effects on Human Sleep

Subjectively, tertiary TCAs are perceived as sedating, associated with reports of decreased sleep latency and wakefulness during the sleep period, and improved sleep quality. Secondary TCAs such as desipramine are less sedating, and may even be subjectively alerting. In studies of patients with insomnia, low doses of doxepin and trimipramine have been associated with improved overall subjective sleep quality and daytime well-being compared with placebo.[10-12]

The PSG effects of sedating TCAs in depression have been studied extensively. Reduced sleep latency, reduced wakefulness during sleep, and increased sleep efficiency have been reported in depressed patients treated with amitriptyline,[13-15] doxepin,[16] and trimipramine,[17,18] and patients with primary insomnia treated with doxepin[10,11] and trimipramine.[12] By contrast, secondary TCAs such as desipramine and nortriptyline have little or no effect on sleep onset and continuity measures in depressed patients.[14,19]

Doxepin and amitriptyline have consistent effects on sleep stage architecture, including reductions in rapid eye movement (REM) sleep percentage, and increases in phasic REM activity and REM sleep latency.[13,15,16,20,21] Trimipramine differs from most TCAs in its effects on REM sleep, which has been reported to increase, decrease, or remain unchanged during treatment.[12,15,17,18] Doxepin, amitriptyline, and trimipramine have inconsistent effects on stage 3/4 non-REM (NREM) sleep, which has been reported to increase in some studies,[21] but not in most others.[11,15,17,18] TCAs more consistently increase the amount of electroencephalographic (EEG) delta wave activity, especially during the first NREM period relative to subsequent NREM periods, which has been termed the *delta ratio*.[20] The effects of a TCA on PSG sleep are illustrated in Figure 37–2.

Other effects of TCAs on PSG sleep can include increases in periodic limb movements during sleep, and the appearance of eye movements during NREM sleep; such effects are particularly noted with strongly serotonergic TCAs such as clomipramine. TCAs do not worsen sleep apnea, and may have a small beneficial effect.[20] Finally, the acute effects of TCAs on sleep in depression appear to be maintained over 1 to 3 years of maintenance treatment.[20,22] Rebound insomnia, indicated by decreased sleep time and sleep efficiency, has been noted on discontinuation of sedating TCAs.[23]

Side Effects

Anticholinergic side effects of doxepin and amitriptyline include dry mouth, increased perspiration, constipation, and urinary retention. More serious effects include precipitation of ocular crises in patients with narrow-angle glaucoma, seizures, and anticholinergic delirium. These last two side effects are dose related and typically occur at blood levels greater than 300 ng/mL.[5] Side effects related to antihistaminic properties include sedation and weight gain.

Side effects related to alpha$_1$ antagonism include orthostatic hypotension with attendant risks of lightheadedness, syncope, and falls. TCAs have potentially serious cardiac effects. In particular, TCAs typically increase heart rate and slow cardiac electrical conduction, the latter because of their type I antiarrhythmic (quinidine-like) activity. Thus, TCAs can produce conduction delays and heart block, a particular concern among patients with bundle branch conduction defects. TCA effects on cardiac conduction include prolongation of the QRS duration and PR and QT intervals. Their lethality in overdose is largely due to their cardiovascular toxicity, which can occur at doses as low as 10 times the therapeutic antidepressant daily dose. On the other hand, TCAs have no effect on cardiac contractility, and they can suppress atrial and ventricular ectopy.[5]

Trazodone and Nefazodone

Pharmacokinetics

Trazodone is rapidly absorbed, with peak plasma concentrations occurring 1 to 2 hours after oral doses. Like TCAs, it is

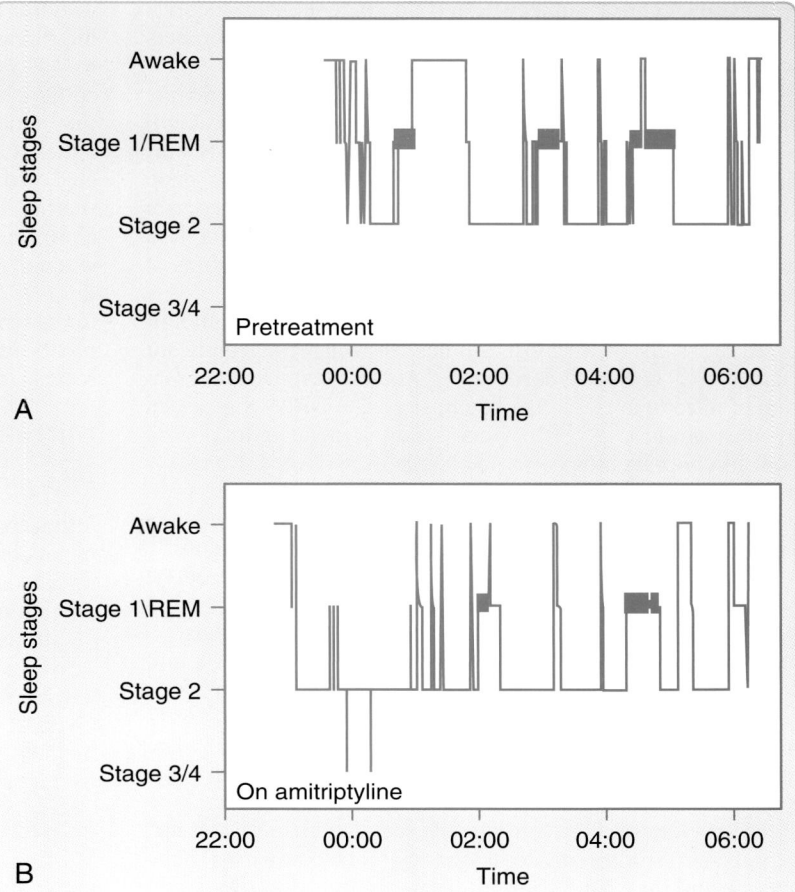

Figure 37–2. Effects of amitriptyline on electroencephalographic sleep in a 54-year-old depressed woman. **A,** Baseline sleep histogram during acute depressive episode showing prolonged sleep latency, reduced sleep efficiency, and reduced stage 3/4 sleep. **B,** Sleep histogram after treatment with amitriptyline for 24 days (final dose, 200 mg) and remission of symptoms. Compared with baseline, the histogram during treatment shows reduced sleep latency, improved sleep efficiency, reduced rapid eye movement (REM) sleep, and prolonged REM sleep latency.

highly (85% to 95%) protein bound. Nefazodone is rapidly and completely absorbed but rapidly metabolized, resulting in low bioavailability (approximately 20%). Trazodone and nefazodone have short half-lives of approximately 5 to 9 hours and 2 to 4 hours, respectively. However, active metabolites of nefazodone have slightly longer half-lives.[24,25]

The major metabolic pathway for trazodone and nefazodone is N-dealkylation to produce meta-chlorophenylpiperazine (mCPP), an active metabolite that possesses serotonergic activity.[2,24] Both drugs also undergo oxidation. Trazodone and mCPP are substrates for CYP2D6, and trazodone is also metabolized to a lesser extent by CYP3A4. Nefazodone is oxidized by CYP3A4 and CYP2C19. Drugs that inhibit CYP3A4, such as ketoconazole, inhibit trazodone and nefazodone metabolism and decrease mCPP formation.[24] Nefazodone and hydroxynefazodone themselves can also inhibit the activity of CYP3A4, thereby impairing the clearance of other drugs metabolized by the same route, including alprazolam, diazepam, and triazolam. In practice, this can lead to large increases in plasma levels of these benzodiazepines.[26] Nefazodone metabolism and hepatic clearance are also reduced by age and liver impairment.

Pharmacodynamics and Receptor Pharmacology

Trazodone is a relatively weak but specific inhibitor of the serotonin reuptake transporter with minimal affinity for NE or dopamine reuptake. Trazodone also inhibits 5-HT$_{1A}$, 5-HT$_{1C}$, and 5-HT$_2$ receptors. It has essentially no affinity for M$_1$ receptors, but it does have moderate H$_1$ receptor antagonism. Finally, trazodone is a relatively weak antagonist of alpha$_2$-adrenergic receptors, and a somewhat more potent antagonist of alpha$_1$ receptors.[2,24]

Like trazodone, nefazodone is a 5-HT$_2$ receptor antagonist and a weak inhibitor of both serotonin and NE reuptake. Unlike trazodone, nefazodone shows little affinity for 5-HT$_{1A}$ receptors, adrenergic alpha$_1$, alpha$_2$, or beta receptors, H$_1$ receptors, or M$_1$ receptors.[24]

The active metabolite mCPP inhibits serotonin reuptake and is a partial agonist at postsynaptic 5-HT$_{2C}$ receptors. These actions can lead to increased side effects from trazodone and nefazodone among individuals who are "poor metabolizers" with CYP2D6, or who are taking inhibitors of CYP2D6, such as fluoxetine.[25] Nefazodone shows nonlinear pharmacokinetics, resulting in greater-than-proportional plasma levels after higher doses.[24]

Effects on Human Sleep

Studies of trazodone effects on human sleep have been limited by small sample sizes; only three published studies have included sample sizes greater than 12 subjects. In addition, most studies have not included double-blinded, placebo-controlled, randomized study designs. Sedation is a commonly reported effect from trazodone in the treatment of depression, reported by over 40% of patients. When specifically assessed, subjective sleep quality is improved by trazodone in healthy control subjects[27] and in patients with depression.[28-30] However, some negative studies with small numbers of depressed subjects have also been reported.[31]

Trazodone has relatively consistent effects of improving sleep latency, sleep efficiency, total sleep time, and wakefulness during sleep in older control subjects[27] and patients with depression.[29,32,33] Some negative studies with regard to sleep continuity have also been reported in younger healthy control subjects,[34] where ceiling effects may have been an issue, and in some studies of depressed patients with small numbers of subjects.[28,31]

Unlike most TCAs, trazodone has little effect on the amount of REM sleep, with most studies showing no significant change[29,32-34] or a small decrease.[27,31] Another distinguishing feature of trazodone is the increase in stage 3/4 NREM sleep seen in most studies.[27-29,33,34] In one study, a small reduction in apnea-hypopnea index and no change in periodic limb movements were noted.[29] Although no information has been published regarding its long-term effects on sleep, rebound insomnia has been noted on discontinuation after several weeks of use.[27]

Only one study has been published on the effects of trazodone in primary insomnia, compared with both placebo and zolpidem.[35] Compared with placebo, trazodone 50 mg was associated with reduced subjective sleep latency, awakenings, and wake time during sleep, and increased subjective sleep time, ease of falling asleep, and sleep quality. These findings were noted only during the first of 2 study weeks owing to late improvements in the placebo condition, and were comparable in magnitude with those seen with zolpidem 10 mg.

Nefazodone is less consistently sedating than trazodone. A series of studies in depressed patients comparing nefazodone and fluoxetine showed that both drugs improved subjective sleep disturbance, but nefazodone had a significantly greater effect.[36-38] Nefazodone was associated with increased PSG sleep efficiency, decreased wakefulness during sleep, and no change in sleep latency. REM sleep was increased in two of the studies and unchanged in one, and stage 3/4 NREM sleep was decreased in two studies and increased in one. Thus, nefazodone appears to have somewhat less potent effects on either sleep continuity or slow wave sleep than trazodone. No published studies have specifically examined nefazodone in patients with primary insomnia.

Side Effects

Trazodone can produce side effects such as orthostatic hypotension, lightheadedness, and weakness.[24] Unlike TCAs, trazodone does not have anticholinergic side effects, but it can have antihistaminic effects such as weight gain. Case reports suggest a potential for ventricular tachyarrhythmias.[39] A potentially serious effect of trazodone is priapism, sustained, painful erections in men.[40] Although uncommon, priapism can be serious, requiring prompt surgical treatment. The risk appears to be greatest early in the course of treatment, and can occur even at low doses. The incidence of abnormal erections during trazodone treatment is approximately 1 per 6000 male patients treated. Fatalities have been reported with overdoses of trazodone, although most of these occurred in conjunction with other drug ingestion.

Common side effects associated with nefazodone include dry mouth, somnolence, dizziness, nausea, blurred vision, and postural hypotension.[24] Nefazodone has recently been associated with serious hepatic toxicity, in some cases leading to fulminant hepatic failure and death.[41] The reported rate of life-threatening liver failure is estimated at 1 case per 250,000 to 300,000 patient-years of exposure. This risk led to nefazodone being withdrawn from the market in some countries; the brand name Serzone has been discontinued in the United States. On the other hand, nefazodone has not been associated with fatal toxicity in overdose. There has been concern that mCPP, the metabolite of trazodone and nefazodone, can contribute to the development of the "serotonin syndrome" when this drug is used in combination with other serotonergic drugs such as selective serotonin reuptake inhibitors. The serotonin syndrome includes symptoms of confusion or delirium, restlessness similar to akathisia, muscular irritability, hyperreflexia, and autonomic instability, including hypotension.

Mirtazapine

Pharmacokinetics

Mirtazapine is rapidly absorbed, undergoes extensive first-pass metabolism, and is approximately 85% protein bound, yielding a bioavailability of approximately 50%.[42,43] Mirtazapine has an elimination half-life of approximately 20 to 40 hours.

Mirtazapine undergoes N-demethylation (producing an active metabolite) and N-oxidation, followed by conjugation and excretion. CYP2D6 and, to a lesser extent, CYP3A4 and CYP1A2 are the major enzymes involved in mirtazapine metabolism. Mirtazapine follows linear pharmacokinetics, but its metabolism is affected by both age and sex; metabolic clearance is reduced in women and in older adults, as well as those with liver disease.[42] Although mirtazapine itself does not strongly inhibit or induce hepatic enzymes, mirtazapine blood levels are decreased by medications such as carbamazepine that induce CYP enzymes, and increased by medications such as fluoxetine that inhibit CYP enzymes.

Pharmacodynamics and Receptor Pharmacology

Mirtazapine is a very weak inhibitor of noradrenergic reuptake, and has no effect on serotonin reuptake.[44] However, similar to TCAs, it increases serotonergic and noradrenergic neurotransmission through blockade of alpha$_2$ autoreceptors and heteroreceptors.[25] It also has prominent antagonist activity at 5HT$_1$, 5HT$_2$, H$_1$, and alpha$_1$-adrenergic receptors.[44] Each of these may contribute to its hypnotic effects.

Effects on Human Sleep

Mirtazapine is reported to be subjectively sedating in clinical studies of depression. In a PSG study in healthy adults, mirtazapine decreased sleep latency, awakenings, and stage 1 NREM sleep and increased stage 3/4 sleep.[45] In a study of six depressed patients, mirtazapine had similar effects, decreasing sleep latency, increasing sleep efficiency and sleep time, and having no significant effect on REM or stage 3/4 sleep.[46] Thus, although potentially promising, mirtazapine has not yet been adequately evaluated as a hypnotic.

Side Effects

In addition to causing sedation, mirtazapine is associated with increased appetite, weight gain, and dry mouth, probably related to its antihistaminic properties. Clinical observations suggest that mirtazapine may be less sedating at doses greater

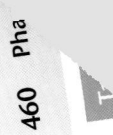
than 30 mg/day than at lower doses. This is hypothesized to be related to greater noradrenergic effects relative to antihistaminic and serotonergic effects at lower doses.[43] Mirtazapine has not been associated with serious toxicity or death in overdose.

OTHER DRUGS USED TO TREAT INSOMNIA

A summary of the pharmacologic characteristics of the other non-BzRA drugs used to treat insomnia is provided in Table 37–5, and their PSG effects are outlined in Table 37–6.

Melatonin and Melatonin Analogues

Biosynthesis, Physiologic Regulation, and Specific Compounds

Unlike most hypnotic agents, melatonin is a hormone endogenously produced in the pineal gland, retina, and intestinal tract. Melatonin is synthesized from serotonin (Fig. 37–3) and is very lipid soluble. Melatonin is normally secreted at night, with blood levels rising at dusk, reaching peak levels of 0.04

to 0.48 pmol/L in the middle of the dark̶ ping at dawn. The nocturnal secretion p̶ raises the possibility that melatonin may̶ humans. However, the same nocturnal se̶ occurs in night-active species, and is obs̶ of sleep and wakefulness. Melatonin se̶ suppressed by light stimulation of the retina. ̶̶noradrenergic sympathetic nervous system, acting through the superior sympathetic ganglion, stimulates pineal melatonin production at night. Specifically, beta$_1$ stimulation with alpha$_1$ amplification leads to increased availability of N-acetyltransferase, the rate-limiting enzyme in melatonin biosynthesis.[47] Hence, beta- and alpha-adrenergic antagonists may affect melatonin synthesis.

A synthetic melatonin receptor agonist, ramelteon, has been approved by the FDA for the treatment of insomnia.[48] Ramelteon decreased PSG sleep latency and increased total sleep time in a study of healthy adults during an adaptation model of transient insomnia. No adverse effects were noted on psychomotor performance. Other compounds being tested include agomelatine (S-20098), a serotonergic/melatonergic antidepressant.[49,50]

Table 37–5. Summary of Other Drugs Used to Treat Insomnia

Drug	Drug Type	t_{max} (hr)	Metabolism	$t_{1/2}$ (hr)	Mechanism of Action
Melatonin	Hormone	20-60 min	Conjugation; oxidation by CYP enzymes	40-60 min	Agonist at melatonin type 1 and type 2 receptors
Ramelteon	Melatonin Receptor agonist	0.3 hrs	Extensive first-pass metabolism; hepatic oxidation primarily via CYP1A2; active metabolite M-II	1.2 (2-5 hours for M-II)	Agonist at melatonin MT$_1$ and MT$_2$ receptors
Diphenhydramine	Ethanolamine antihistamine	2-2.5	Hepatic demethylation, oxidation	4-8	Antagonizes H$_1$ receptors
Doxylamine	Ethanolamine antihistamine	2-3	Majority excreted unchanged in urine; some hepatic metabolism	10	Antagonizes H$_1$ receptors
Valerian	Plant extract	Uncertain owing to multiple constituents	Uncertain owing to multiple constituents	Uncertain owing to multiple constituents	Uncertain; may increase GABA formation, interact with L-amino acid transporter receptor, or act as adenosine receptor agonist
Gabapentin	Anticonvulsant (structural analogue of GABA)	3-3.5	Renal excretion (unchanged)	5-9	Uncertain; may affect GABA release or interact with L-amino acid transporter protein
Tiagabine	Anticonvulsant	1-1.5	CYP3A4	8	Inhibits GABA transporter GAT-1
Choral hydrate	Two-carbon molecule	Short	Converted to trichloroethanol, which undergoes conjugation	5-10 (for trichloroethanol)	Barbiturate-like effect at GABA$_A$ receptors
Olanzapine	Thienobenzodiazepine antipsychotic	4-6	CYP1A2, CYP2D6	20-54	Antagonizes H$_1$, alpha$_1$, alpha$_2$, M$_1$, 5-HT$_2$, D$_2$ receptors
Quetiapine	Dibenzothiazepine antipsychotic	1-2	CYP 3A4	6	Antagonizes H$_1$, alpha$_1$, M$_1$, 5-HT$_2$, D$_2$ receptors
Gamma-hydroxybutyrate	Endogenous four-carbon molecule	30-45 min	Metabolized to GABA, succinic semialdehyde, H$_2$O and CO$_2$	20-70 min	May act directly as neurotransmitter, increases brain dopamine levels

Data compiled from sources indicated in text.

t_{max}, Time to maximal concentration; $t_{1/2}$, elimination half-life; CYP, cytochrome P-450 system (individual letters and numbers represent CYP families); H$_1$, histamine type 1 receptor; GABA, gamma-aminobutyric acid; 5-HT, 5-hydroxytryptamine (serotonin); M$_1$, muscarinic cholinergic type 1 receptor; D$_2$, dopamine type 2 receptor.

Table 37–6. Polysomnographic Effects of Other Drugs Used to Treat Insomnia*

Drug	Sleep Latency	Sleep Continuity†	Stage 3/4 NREM Sleep Amount (Percentage)	REM Sleep	Other
Melatonin	↓	↔ to ↑	↔	↔	
Ramelteon	↓	↔ to ↑	↔	↔	
Diphenhydramine	↓	↔ to ↑	↔ to ↑	↓	
Valerian	↓	↔ to ↑	↔ to ↑	↔ to ↑	Inconsistent effects on sleep continuity, stage 3/4 across studies
Gabapentin	↔	↔ to ↑	↑	↔	Reduced periodic limb movements
Tiagabine	↔	↑	↑	↔	Results based on single study
Chloral hydrate	↓	↑	↔	↔ to ↓	Rapid tolerance may develop
Olanzapine	↔ to ↓	↑	↑	↔ to ↓	Reports of increased periodic limb movements, sleep-eating
Gamma-hydroxybutyrate	↔ to ↓	↑	↑	↔ to ↓	↓ Alpha NREM intrusions in patients with fibromyalgia

*Reported effects are based on preponderance of evidence from published studies [see Buysse[81] and text for details]. Many effects are inconsistent between individual studies. "↑" Indicates increase from pretreatment baseline; "↓" indicates decrease from pretreatment baseline; "↔" indicates no change from pretreatment baseline.

†Sleep continuity refers to the proportion of sleep relative to wakefulness after sleep onset, as reflected by measures such as sleep efficiency. Other indicators of sleep continuity, such as wakefulness after sleep onset or number of awakenings, would have opposite signs. Thus, "↑" indicates improvement in overall sleep continuity.

REM, rapid eye movement; NREM, non-REM.

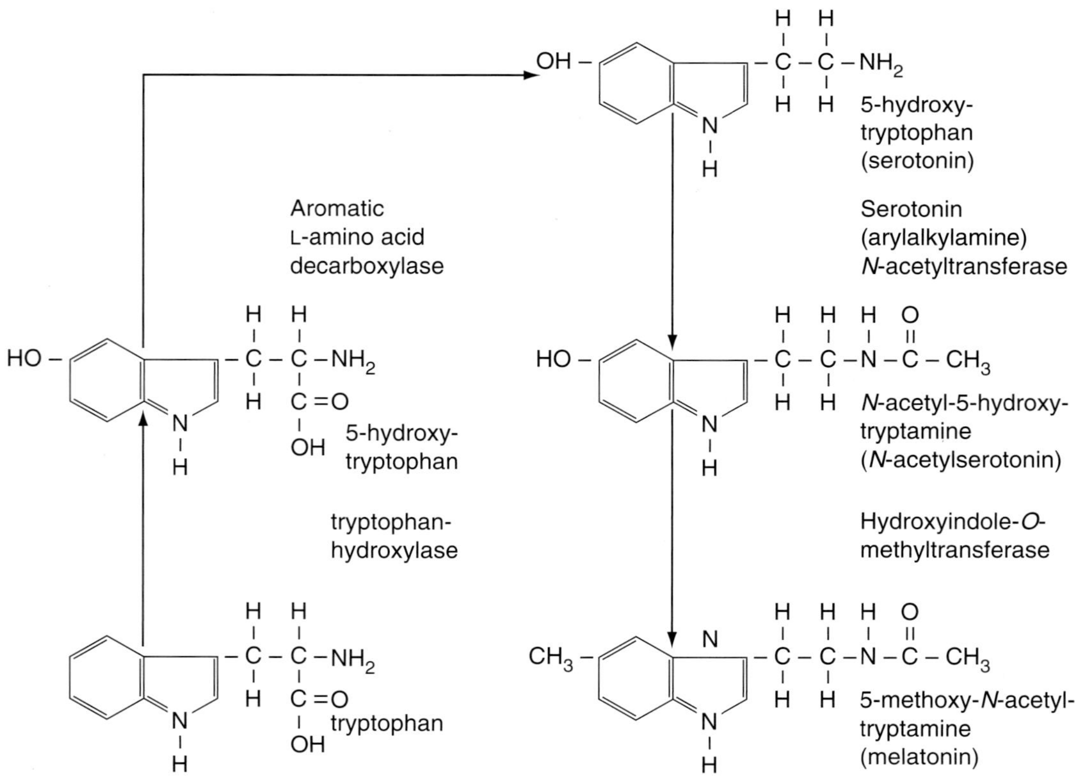

Figure 37–3. Biosynthetic pathway for melatonin. Activity of *N*-acetyltransferase is the rate-limiting step governing melatonin production in the pineal gland.

than 30 mg/day than at lower doses. This is hypothesized to be related to greater noradrenergic effects relative to antihistaminic and serotonergic effects at lower doses.[43] Mirtazapine has not been associated with serious toxicity or death in overdose.

OTHER DRUGS USED TO TREAT INSOMNIA

A summary of the pharmacologic characteristics of the other non-BzRA drugs used to treat insomnia is provided in Table 37–5, and their PSG effects are outlined in Table 37–6.

Melatonin and Melatonin Analogues

Biosynthesis, Physiologic Regulation, and Specific Compounds

Unlike most hypnotic agents, melatonin is a hormone endogenously produced in the pineal gland, retina, and intestinal tract. Melatonin is synthesized from serotonin (Fig. 37–3) and is very lipid soluble. Melatonin is normally secreted at night, with blood levels rising at dusk, reaching peak levels of 0.04

to 0.48 pmol/L in the middle of the dark period, then dropping at dawn. The nocturnal secretion pattern of melatonin raises the possibility that melatonin may promote sleep in humans. However, the same nocturnal secretion pattern also occurs in night-active species, and is observed independent of sleep and wakefulness. Melatonin secretion is acutely suppressed by light stimulation of the retina. The noradrenergic sympathetic nervous system, acting through the superior sympathetic ganglion, stimulates pineal melatonin production at night. Specifically, beta$_1$ stimulation with alpha$_1$ amplification leads to increased availability of N-acetyltransferase, the rate-limiting enzyme in melatonin biosynthesis.[47] Hence, beta- and alpha-adrenergic antagonists may affect melatonin synthesis.

A synthetic melatonin receptor agonist, ramelteon, has been approved by the FDA for the treatment of insomnia.[48] Ramelteon decreased PSG sleep latency and increased total sleep time in a study of healthy adults during an adaptation model of transient insomnia. No adverse effects were noted on psychomotor performance. Other compounds being tested include agomelatine (S-20098), a serotonergic/melatonergic antidepressant.[49,50]

Table 37–5. Summary of Other Drugs Used to Treat Insomnia

Drug	Drug Type	t_{max} (hr)	Metabolism	$t_{1/2}$ (hr)	Mechanism of Action
Melatonin	Hormone	20-60 min	Conjugation; oxidation by CYP enzymes	40-60 min	Agonist at melatonin type 1 and type 2 receptors
Ramelteon	Melatonin Receptor agonist	0.3 hrs	Extensive first-pass metabolism; hepatic oxidation primarily via CYP1A2; active metabolite M-II	1.2 (2-5 hours for M-II)	Agonist at melatonin MT$_1$ and MT$_2$ receptors
Diphenhy-dramine	Ethanolamine antihistamine	2-2.5	Hepatic demethylation, oxidation	4-8	Antagonizes H$_1$ receptors
Doxylamine	Ethanolamine antihistamine	2-3	Majority excreted unchanged in urine; some hepatic metabolism	10	Antagonizes H$_1$ receptors
Valerian	Plant extract	Uncertain owing to multiple constituents	Uncertain owing to multiple constituents	Uncertain owing to multiple constituents	Uncertain; may increase GABA formation, interact with L-amino acid transporter receptor, or act as adenosine receptor agonist
Gabapentin	Anticonvulsant (structural analogue of GABA)	3-3.5	Renal excretion (unchanged)	5-9	Uncertain; may affect GABA release or interact with L-amino acid transporter protein
Tiagabine	Anticonvulsant	1-1.5	CYP3A4	8	Inhibits GABA transporter GAT-1
Choral hydrate	Two-carbon molecule	Short	Converted to trichloroethanol, which undergoes conjugation	5-10 (for trichloro-ethanol)	Barbiturate-like effect at GABA$_A$ receptors
Olanzapine	Thienobenzo-diazepine antipsychotic	4-6	CYP1A2, CYP2D6	20-54	Antagonizes H$_1$, alpha$_1$, alpha$_2$, M$_1$, 5-HT$_2$, D$_2$ receptors
Quetiapine	Dibenzothiazepine antipsychotic	1-2	CYP 3A4	6	Antagonizes H$_1$, alpha$_1$, M$_1$, 5-HT$_2$, D$_2$ receptors
Gamma-hydroxy-butyrate	Endogenous four-carbon molecule	30-45 min	Metabolized to GABA, succinic semialdehyde, H$_2$O and CO$_2$	20-70 min	May act directly as neurotransmitter, increases brain dopamine levels

Data compiled from sources indicated in text.

t_{max}, Time to maximal concentration; $t_{1/2}$, elimination half-life; CYP, cytochrome P-450 system (individual letters and numbers represent CYP families); H$_1$, histamine type 1 receptor; GABA, gamma-aminobutyric acid; 5-HT, 5-hydroxytryptamine (serotonin); M$_1$, muscarinic cholinergic type 1 receptor; D$_2$, dopamine type 2 receptor.

Table 37–6.   Polysomnographic Effects of Other Drugs Used to Treat Insomnia*

Drug	Sleep Latency	Sleep Continuity†	Stage 3/4 NREM Sleep Amount (Percentage)	REM Sleep	Other
Melatonin	↓	↔ to ↑	↔	↔	
Ramelteon	↓	↔ to ↑	↔	↔	
Diphenhydramine	↓	↔ to ↑	↔ to ↑	↓	
Valerian	↓	↔ to ↑	↔ to ↑	↔ to ↑	Inconsistent effects on sleep continuity, stage 3/4 across studies
Gabapentin	↔	↔ to ↑	↑	↔	Reduced periodic limb movements
Tiagabine	↔	↑	↑	↔	Results based on single study
Chloral hydrate	↓	↑	↔	↔ to ↓	Rapid tolerance may develop
Olanzapine	↔ to ↓	↑	↑	↔ to ↓	Reports of increased periodic limb movements, sleep-eating
Gamma-hydroxybutyrate	↔ to ↓	↑	↑	↔ to ↓	↓ Alpha NREM intrusions in patients with fibromyalgia

*Reported effects are based on preponderance of evidence from published studies [see Buysse[81] and text for details]. Many effects are inconsistent between individual studies. "↑" Indicates increase from pretreatment baseline; "↓" indicates decrease from pretreatment baseline; "↔" indicates no change from pretreatment baseline.

†Sleep continuity refers to the proportion of sleep relative to wakefulness after sleep onset, as reflected by measures such as sleep efficiency. Other indicators of sleep continuity, such as wakefulness after sleep onset or number of awakenings, would have opposite signs. Thus, "↑" indicates improvement in overall sleep continuity.

REM, rapid eye movement; NREM, non-REM.

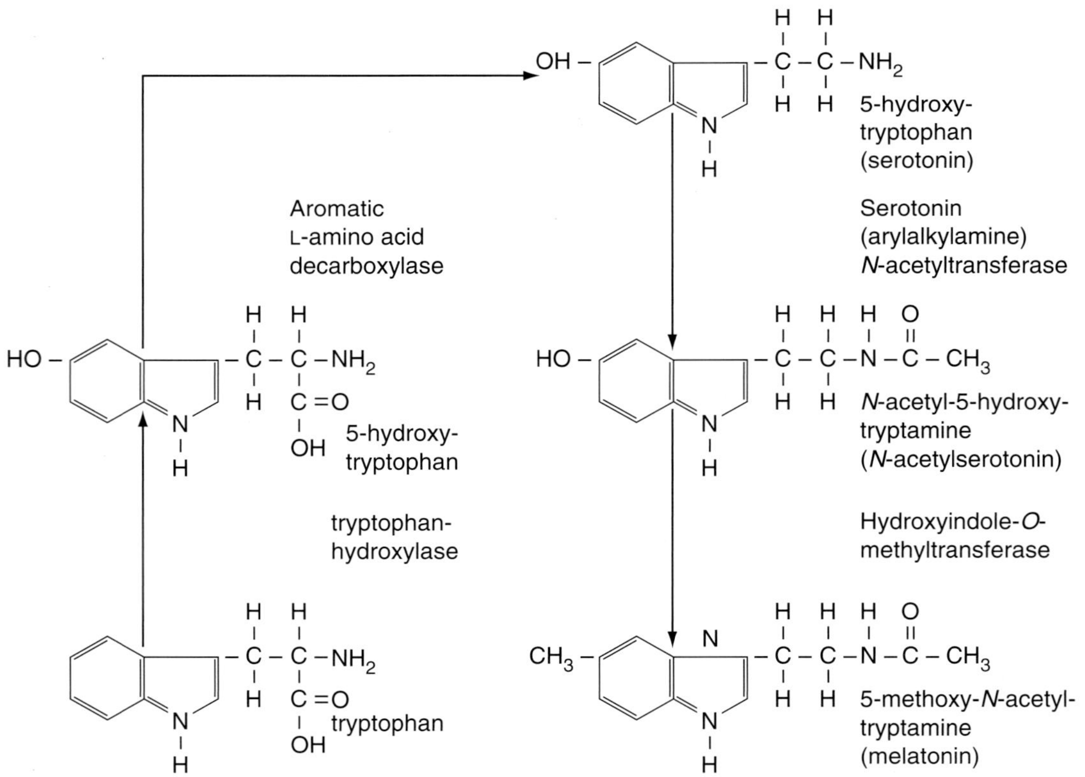

Figure 37–3. Biosynthetic pathway for melatonin. Activity of *N*-acetyltransferase is the rate-limiting step governing melatonin production in the pineal gland.

Pharmacokinetics

Exogenous melatonin is rapidly absorbed, with peak levels occurring in approximately 20 to 30 minutes. It has a 40- to 60-minute elimination half-life.[51] When complexed with an absorption-retarding binder, systemic availability can be prolonged to mimic the normal period of nocturnal secretion.[52,53] Approximately 85% of an oral dose is removed by hepatic first-pass metabolism, the predominant product being 6-sulfatoxymelatonin. Metabolism includes oxidation by CYP1A2 and CYP2C19 isotypes, followed by glucuronate and sulfate conjugation and renal excretion.[54] Melatonin is secreted in breast milk. The melatonin receptor agonist ramelteon has a half-life of 1.5 to 2.5 hours.

Pharmacodynamics and Receptor Effects

Three melatonin membrane receptor subtypes have been described[55]: mt1, MT2, and MT3. Both mt1 and MT2 receptors act through inhibitory G-protein pathways to lower cyclic adenosine monophosphate levels. Melatonin receptors have been identified in the suprachiasmatic nucleus (mt1 and MT2 subtypes), the retina (mt1 and MT2 subtypes), reproductive organs, immune cells, vasculature, and a variety of other organs. In the suprachiasmatic nucleus, MT2 receptors appear to mediate phase-shift responses. Melatonin receptor function in the pituitary plays a role in the reproductive cycles of seasonal breeding animals, but may also help regulate the timing of sexual maturity. In the vasculature, mt1 receptors apparently mediate vasoconstriction, whereas MT2 receptors mediate vasodilation. In lymphocytes, melatonin counteracts the inhibitory effect of prostaglandin E_2 on interleukin-2 production.[56] Similar effects of melatonin may be present in the hypothalamus to lower body temperature. Melatonin has been proposed to have roles in regulating retinal light sensitivity, systemic immunity, and cancer cell growth.

Ramelteon is a selective melatonin agonist with an estimated 15-fold greater affinity for mt1 receptors than melatonin itself. The receptor affinities of the melatonin agonists agomelatine and BMS-214778 have not been described.

Effects on Human Sleep

In humans, melatonin has been studied both as a chronobiotic (where the indication is to phase shift circadian rhythms) and as a hypnotic (where the indication is to induce or maintain sleep). Its use as a chronobiotic is discussed elsewhere in this volume. Part of the appeal of melatonin may be its availability as a "dietary supplement." Subjects in studies of its potential hypnotic actions have included healthy adults,[57,58] adults and children with insomnia,[59,60] older adults with insomnia,[52] patients with dementia,[53,61] medically ill adults,[62] and patients with affective disorders.[63] Drawing conclusions about melatonin's hypnotic effects is further complicated by the heterogeneity of the doses and schedules used.[64-65a] Doses exceeding 0.5 mg at bedtime are supraphysiologic, and have been used in a number of studies. However, across studies involving patients with an insomnia complaint, a dose–response effect has not been obvious above physiologic dosing.

A number of studies have shown that melatonin results in self-reports of improved sleep latency and greater quality of sleep. Effects on sleep maintenance and duration are less consistent. In middle-aged patients with insomnia, one study supported increased total sleep time using 75 mg,[66] whereas two other studies[67,68] using other doses found no major effect. In a study of older adults with sleep problems, 5 mg of melatonin did not alter self-reported sleep parameters.[69] In a mixed sample of medically ill patients, a modal dose of 6 mg decreased sleep latency and increased total sleep time.[62]

A variety of studies have used actigraphy and PSG outcomes. In two pediatric studies, melatonin increased total sleep time.[59,60] A few studies suggest a small improvement in sleep latency. In studies of older adults, melatonin therapy is often conceptualized as a hormone replacement where the hypnotic and chronobiotic actions synergize to reduce sleep latency and overall lower the activity rate of adults with dementia. However, sleep effects do not appear to be robust using 2.5- to 10-mg doses of melatonin in the elderly.[53,61]

A variety of studies also indicate that exogenous melatonin is associated with reductions in sleep latency by PSG measures.[52,70] Among patients with insomnia, consistent effects in other sleep parameters have not been observed, yet studies in normal volunteers suggest that sleep can be more broadly affected by melatonin. Effects on REM sleep have been inconsistent, although anecdotally some patients complain of nightmares when placed on melatonin. When taken during the daytime, melatonin increases theta/alpha activity and sleepiness,[71] and decreases neurobehavioral performance.[72] Paradoxically, melatonin may act preferentially as a hypnotic in situations of low homeostatic drive for sleep, such as during the daytime period of low endogenous secretion.[73]

Side Effects

Exogenous melatonin causes dramatic physiologic effects in species with seasonally regulated physiologies, leading to some concern that melatonin consumption might pose serious consequences in humans. However, individuals have taken gram quantities without immediately obvious problems, and despite widespread use of melatonin at low doses, no obvious public health risk has yet emerged. Nonetheless, the actual risks of protracted melatonin consumption remain unknown. The most common side effect reported from taking melatonin is headache. Acutely, increased sleepiness and fatigue might contribute to the loss of vigilance in critical work situations. Melatonin is nonaddicting. Because exogenous melatonin has been shown to affect blood pressure in humans[74] and to affect blood pressure responses of hypertensive patients on a calcium channel blocker,[75] it is possible that melatonin affects blood pressure in specific patient populations. Isolated case reports have described side effects including disorientation, seizures, nausea, and dyspnea, but the frequency of such effects appears to be quite low. An additional concern is that commercial sources of melatonin sometimes contain indoline contaminants[76] that were associated with the development of eosinophilia-myalgia syndrome in tryptophan consumers. However, exposure to this contaminant at the usual doses of melatonin is 1000-fold less than occurred with tryptophan use. Side effects associated with melatonin receptor agonists have not yet been described in large clinical trials.

Antihistamines

Specific Agents

Antihistamine drugs used in the treatment of insomnia are reversible antagonists of histamine H_1 receptors. Antihistamines are a diverse group of drugs broadly divided clinically into two groups based on their sedative potential.[77] First-generation agents include doxepin (discussed earlier in the section on antidepressants), diphenhydramine, doxylamine, chlorpheniramine, hydroxyzine, meclizine, promethazine, and cyproheptadine. Essentially all of the over-the-counter antihistamine drugs marketed for insomnia treatment include diphenhydramine, the prototype of this class, or doxylamine. Second-generation, nonsedating antihistamine drugs are used primarily for treatment of seasonal, environmental, and other allergic reactions, and are not used for the treatment of insomnia.

Pharmacokinetics

Antihistamines are well absorbed from the GI tract and widely distributed throughout the body, including the CNS. Most first-generation antihistamines, including diphenhydramine, have 4- to 6-hour durations of action, although specific agents such as hydroxyzine and meclizine may last for up to 24 hours. The plasma elimination half-life of diphenhydramine is 4 to 8 hours. Diphenhydramine is extensively metabolized by CYP enzymes.[78]

Pharmacodynamics and Receptor Pharmacology

Histamine is widely present throughout the CNS and the body. Three types of histamine receptors have been described, labeled H_1, H_2, and H_3. Histamine is synthesized from histidine by the action of L-histidine decarboxylase, and is metabolized by methylation and oxidative deamination.[77] In most tissues, histamine is stored in mast cells, which mediate allergic responses. In the CNS, histamine serves as a neurotransmitter primarily localized to the tuberomammillary nucleus of the posterior hypothalamus. Histaminergic neurons project widely to the brainstem and cerebral cortex, and promote wakefulness.[79] Histaminergic neurons fire actively during wakefulness and are inhibited during sleep by the activity of gamma-aminobutyric acid (GABA)–ergic projections from the ventrolateral preoptic area.[80]

Histamine has a variety of effects in the periphery, including H_1 receptor–mediated vasodilation, increased capillary permeability, bronchoconstriction, and contraction of the gut. Histamine also promotes gastric acid secretion, an effect mediated by H_2 receptors and blocked by H_2 antihistamines such as cimetidine, ranitidine, famotidine. H_2 receptor antagonists have essentially no CNS activity, and are not used as hypnotics. H_3 receptors serve as presynaptic autoreceptors that mediate feedback inhibition of histamine synthesis and release.

H_1 receptor antagonists have a variety of CNS and systemic effects. Well-described CNS effects include sedation, decreased alertness, decreased reaction times, and sleepiness.[81] Paradoxically, a minority of patients respond with CNS activation, including restlessness, anxiety, and increased alertness. Such reactions may also be seen in overdoses. Systemic effects of antihistamines include inhibition of immediate hypersensitivity reactions mediated by mast cell release of histamine. In addition, H_1 antagonists decrease capillary permeability, thus inhibiting edema and wheal reactions as well as the flare and itch response. H_1 antihistamines also have minor effects on antagonizing respiratory smooth muscle, relaxing bronchospasm, and promoting vasodilation.[77]

Many of the early sedating antihistamines, including diphenhydramine, have muscarinic anticholinergic effects similar to atropine. In addition, diphenhydramine increases serotonergic neurotransmission and antagonizes alpha-adrenergic receptors. The "nonsedating" H_1 antagonists have very little CNS effect because of their inability to penetrate the blood–brain barrier. Thus, their actions are restricted to those peripheral actions described previously.

Effects on Human Sleep

Older antihistamines such as diphenhydramine and doxylamine are associated with subjective drowsiness and sleepiness, leading to their widespread use as over-the-counter hypnotic agents. However, their efficacy has not been well studied. Clinical trials using doses of 12.5 to 50 mg have shown subjective improvements in sleep latency, nocturnal awakenings, sleep duration, and sleep quality.[82-84] PSG studies have largely been confined to daytime studies comparing sedating and nonsedating antihistamines. These studies confirm the hypnotic effect of drugs such as diphenhydramine, while showing no significant sedation with nonsedating drugs such as astemizole, loratadine, or cetirizine.[85-87]

Side Effects

The CNS actions described previously constitute the usual intended therapeutic effect of H_1 antihistamines. However, sedation can often be experienced as a side effect. Impairment of psychomotor performance with diphenhydramine has been well documented.[81] Epidemiologic studies have also suggested cognitive impairment associated with diphenhydramine use in the elderly.[88] Other side effects related to CNS activity include dizziness, fatigue, and tinnitus. Peripheral side effects can include decreased appetite, nausea, vomiting, diarrhea, and constipation, as well as weight gain. A number of case reports have also documented potentially serious side effects of doxylamine, including coma, and rhabdomyolysis with resultant kidney failure.[89]

Valerian Preparations

Pharmacokinetics

Valerian preparations include extracts derived from the roots of the plants genus *Valeriana*. Most of the more than 400 extracts available in the United States and Europe are derived specifically from the species *Valeriana officinalis*. These extracts contain a number of chemicals with CNS activity, including sesquiterpenes, valepotriates, valerianic acid, and various other alkaloids. All commercial preparations include a combination of these chemicals in unknown proportions.[90]

The pharmacokinetics of valerian preparations have not been well described, which is not surprising given the multiple chemicals that constitute therapeutic extracts. Doses used in clinical studies have typically ranged from 400 to 900 mg/day.

Pharmacodynamics and Receptor Pharmacology

The exact mechanism of action of valerian preparations is also unknown. The GABA-like activity of valerian extracts is suggested by their sedative, anxiolytic, myorelaxant, and possible anticonvulsant effects.[91] Valerian extracts contain a small amount of GABA, but GABA is not transported across the blood–brain barrier. Valerianic acid may inhibit brain GABA metabolism. Valerian extracts do not act on benzodiazepine receptors.

Other potential mechanisms of action include serotonin receptor activity and adenosine receptor antagonism. Finally, some components of valerian, including valepotriates, may act as prodrugs transformed into homobaldrinal, a compound that inhibits motor activity in mice.[90]

Effects on Human Sleep

The effects of valerian extracts on sleep in humans have been investigated in healthy young adults, as well as middle-aged and older adults with insomnia. Duration of treatment has ranged from 1 to 14 days, and outcome measures have included self-reports, actigraphy, and PSG. Subjective effects of valerian preparations include decreased sleep latency, improved sleep quality, and decreased awakenings.[92,93] Effects on PSG sleep include increased stage 3/4 and reduced stage 1 NREM sleep.[94,95] Although improved sleep latency and sleep efficiency have been observed in some PSG studies, sleep continuity effects of valerian are inconsistent.[95-97]

Side Effects

Side effects associated with valerian have been reported to be few and mild, and include headache and weakness. Morning sleepiness is an infrequent side effect.[90]

Other Agents Used as Hypnotics

Gabapentin

Gabapentin was initially developed and marketed as an anti-convulsant drug, but it has subsequently found more widespread use in treating neuropathic pain, periodic limb movement disorder, bipolar mood disorder, and insomnia. Typical daily doses range from 300 to 2100 mg, taken in divided doses, with larger doses in the evening hours. Gabapentin has bioavailability of 35% to 60%, with lower availability at higher doses. It is distributed extensively, has an elimination half-life of 5 to 9 hours, and is excreted unchanged in urine. The mechanism of action of gabapentin is not well understood. Although it does not block GABA uptake, it may promote formation of GABA in the CNS.[98,99] Other potential mechanisms of action include antagonizing N-methyl-D-aspartate receptors, decreasing glutamate levels, and interacting with the L-amino acid transporter receptor.[100]

Gabapentin has been used clinically as a hypnotic because of its sedative effects in patients with various medical conditions. It has not been well investigated in the study of insomnia per se. In addition to subjective sensation, one study demonstrated decreased awakenings in stage 1 sleep, as well as increased REM sleep and slow wave sleep in patients with epilepsy.[101] In patients with restless legs syndrome, gabapentin has been associated with improved sleep continuity, increased stage 3/4 sleep, and reduced periodic limb movements.[102] No published studies have formally evaluated gabapentin in insomnia. Side effects associated with gabapentin include sedation and fatigue, as well as dizziness, ataxia, and a less common risk of leukopenia. However, in most clinical scenarios, gabapentin is well tolerated.

Tiagabine

Tiagabine was initially developed as an adjuvant anticonvulsant drug. It inhibits the GABA transporter GAT-1, thereby reducing GABA reuptake into presynaptic neurons and glia and increasing GABA's inhibitory actions in the CNS.[98] When used for insomnia, tiagabine is typically prescribed in doses of 4 to 16 mg, although dose-ranging studies have not been conducted. The doses typically used for sleep disorders are much lower than the dose of up to 56 mg used in epilepsy. Tiagabine is rapidly absorbed and extensively protein bound. It is metabolized by CYP3A4, and has a terminal elimination half-life of approximately 8 hours. Tiagabine is subjectively sedating, although individuals who have experienced benzodiazepines describe the effect as different from that of classic BzRA hypnotics. The effects of tiagabine in patients with insomnia have not been investigated in controlled, published studies. One study in healthy adults demonstrated increased slow wave sleep and delta EEG activity, as well as improved sleep efficiency,[103] leading to speculation that it may be efficacious for insomnia as well.

Chloral Hydrate

Chloral hydrate is an old compound that has been used primarily as a hypnotic and as a sedative in children undergoing clinical procedures. It is rapidly converted by alcohol dehydrogenase in the liver to the active compound trichloroethanol. Therefore, chloral hydrate technically acts as a prodrug. Trichloroethanol acts at the barbiturate site on $GABA_A$ receptors. Metabolism of trichloroethanol occurs through hepatic conjugation, with a half-life of approximately 5 to 10 hours. Sleep effects include subjective and objective reduction in sleep latency and improvement in sleep continuity, with little effect on stage 3/4 sleep or REM sleep.[81] Because chloral hydrate is a skin and mucous membrane irritant, it can have side effects of unpleasant taste, GI distress, nausea, and vomiting. Other potential side effects include light-headedness, nightmares, and ataxia. More serious potential side effects include hepatic injury. Fatal overdoses are possible and chronic use can result in severe withdrawal.

Chloral hydrate is only of historic interest as a hypnotic, although it continues to be used for sedation in children. It is not indicated for treatment of insomnia in adults or children, given its low therapeutic index and the availability of safer alternative drugs.

Sedative Antipsychotic Drugs

Several of the newer antipsychotic drugs have been used in the treatment of insomnia, particularly among patients with severe depression, bipolar disorder, and psychotic disorders, but occasionally among patients without serious psychiatric conditions as well. Although many different antipsychotic drugs have sedative effects, the most widely used drugs for this purpose are olanzapine and quetiapine. Typically, olanzapine is administered in doses of 2.5 to 20 mg and quetiapine in doses of 25 to 200 mg at bedtime.

Unlike older antipsychotic drugs, which antagonize primarily dopamine receptors, olanzapine and quetiapine have a variety of receptor effects.[100,104] Olanzapine's receptor effects include serotonin 5-HT$_{2A}$ antagonism, as well as activity at 5-HT$_{2C}$, 5-HT$_3$, and 5-HT$_6$ receptors. It also has antimuscarinic, antihistaminic, and alpha$_1$-adrenergic antagonist properties. Quetiapine, like olanzapine, is an antagonist of 5-HT$_{2A}$ receptors. It has somewhat more potent dopamine D$_2$ receptor antagonist, but its dopamine-binding is rapidly reversible.

It also acts as an H_1 and alpha$_1$ antagonist. Olanzapine is structurally similar to benzodiazepines.

Olanzapine is rapidly absorbed, but a significant portion of the drug is metabolized in first-pass circulation. Its peak concentration occurs at approximately 6 hours, and it has a terminal elimination half-life of 20 to 54 hours. It is metabolized through the activity of CYP1A2 and CYP2D6. Quetiapine is also rapidly absorbed, but reaches peak concentration in approximately 1.5 hours and has a terminal elimination half-life of approximately 6 hours. Quetiapine is also metabolized in the liver, primarily through CYP3A4.

Both of these antipsychotic drugs have a much lower incidence of extrapyramidal side effects compared with traditional antipsychotic drugs such as haloperidol. However, both can cause hypotension. In addition, olanzapine has been associated with weight gain and glucose intolerance, as well as neurocognitive impairment at higher doses. Quetiapine has been associated with prolongation of the corrected QT interval on electrocardiography.

Both olanzapine and quetiapine are subjectively sedating. PSG studies with limited numbers of subjects indicate that olanzapine is associated with decreased wakefulness, stage 1 sleep, and REM sleep, and increased stage 3/4 and stage 2 NREM sleep and subjective sleep quality.[105-107] No published studies have reported on the PSG effects of quetiapine, or on its efficacy specifically for insomnia. Given their potentially significant neurologic side effects, these drugs are best reserved for treatment of individuals with major psychiatric disorders and coexisting insomnia.

Gamma-Hydroxybutyrate

Gamma-hydroxybutyrate (GHB) is FDA approved for the treatment of cataplexy in patients with narcolepsy. GHB may act directly as a neurotransmitter, but is unusual because it crosses the blood–brain barrier after oral administration. It is administered as a liquid. The exact mechanism of action of GHB is unclear, but some evidence suggests that it may modulate dopamine activity, specifically by increasing the availability of cerebral dopamine. GHB's effects on the CNS include sedation and, in higher doses, coma. GHB has also been investigated as an anesthetic agent.[108] When used in this way, GHB has few effects on cardiovascular or respiratory systems.

GHB is absorbed rapidly after oral administration, particularly because it is administered as a liquid. Peak concentrations occur approximately 30 to 60 minutes after administration. GHB is not bound to plasma protein. It is metabolized to a limited extent to GABA. GHB is also decomposed to water and carbon dioxide and exhaled. The mean half-life is quite short, ranging from 20 to 70 minutes (mean, 53 minutes).[108]

GHB is subjectively sedating. When administered to patients with narcolepsy, its PSG effects include reduced REM sleep latency and increased stage 3/4 sleep and sleep efficiency.[109] In healthy subjects, GHB increases stage 3/4 sleep, decreases stage 1 sleep, and reduces REM sleep latency.[110,111] A study in patients with fibromyalgia showed similar results, with reduced sleep latency and REM sleep, increased stage 3/4 sleep, and a reduction in alpha EEG intrusion during NREM sleep.[112] GHB has not been formally assessed for its hypnotic properties in patients with other types of insomnia.

The rapid sedative effects of GHB have led to its abuse as a so-called "date rape" drug. Other side effects of GHB include excess salivation, increased dreaming, sleepwalking, and GI effects such as vomiting. It is also associated with amnesia, similar to other BzRA hypnotic agents. In overdoses, GHB can be associated with acute delirium.[108] High-dose recreational users of GHB have been described as having a withdrawal syndrome characterized by insomnia, tremor, and anxiety.

SUMMARY AND CONCLUSIONS

A variety of drugs that do not act at benzodiazepine receptors have been used as hypnotics. These drugs represent a wide variety of drug classes, and differ widely in terms of their pharmacokinetics, pharmacodynamics, specific sleep effects, and side effects. In almost all cases, very limited empirical evidence is available specifically to address their effects as hypnotic agents. The largest amount of data is available for sedating TCAs, melatonin, and valerian preparations. An appreciation of the clinical pharmacology of these drugs is important for designing research studies and clinical interventions.

> *Clinical Pearl*
>
> *Although antidepressants, antihistamines, and other drugs are often considered to be safer alternatives to BzRAs for treatment of insomnia, their efficacy has not been well demonstrated, and they can have clinically important side effects.*

Acknowledgments

Supported by National Institutes of Health grants MH24652, AG15138, and AG20677.

REFERENCES

1. Walsh JK, Schweitzer PK: Ten-year trends in the pharmacological treatment of insomnia. Sleep 1999;22:371-375.
2. Baldessarini RJ: Drugs and the treatment of anxiety disorders: Depression and anxiety disorders. In Hardman JG, Limbird LE (eds): Goodman and Gilman's the Pharmacologic Basis of Therapeutics, 10th ed. New York, McGraw-Hill, 2001, pp 447-483.
3. Sharpley AL, Cowen PJ: Effect of pharmacologic treatments on the sleep of depressed patients. Biol Psychiatry 1995;37:85-98.
4. Rudorfer MV, Potter WZ: Pharmacokinetics of antidepressants. In Meltzer HY (ed): Psychopharmacology: The Third Generation of Progress. New York, Raven Press, 1987, pp 1353-1363.
5. Nelson JC: Tricyclic and tetracyclic drugs. In Schatzberg A, Nemeroff C (eds): The American Psychiatric Publishing Textbook of Psychopharmacology, 3rd ed. Washington, DC, American Psychiatric Publishing, 2004, pp 207-230.
6. Rudorfer MV, Potter WZ: Metabolism of tricyclic antidepressants. Cell Mol Neurobiol 1999;19:373-409.
7. Rogers JF, Nafziger AN, Bertino JS: Pharmacogenetics affects dosing, efficacy, and toxicity of cytochrome P450-metabolized drugs. Am J Med 2002;113:746-750.
8. Richelson E, Nelson A: Antagonism by antidepressants of neurotransmitter receptors of normal human brain in vitro. J Pharmacol Exp Ther 1984;230:94-102.
9. Tatsumi M, Groshan K, Blakely RD, Richelson E: Pharmacological profile of antidepressants and related compounds at human monoamine transporters. Eur J Pharmacol 1997;340:249-258.
10. Hajak G, Rodenbeck A, Adler L, et al: Nocturnal melatonin secretion and sleep after doxepin administration in chronic primary insomnia. Pharmacopsychiatry 1996;29:187-192.

11. Hajak G, Rodenbeck A, Voderholzer U, et al: Doxepin in the treatment of primary insomnia: A placebo-controlled, double-blind, polysomnographic study. J Clin Psychiatry 2001;62:453-463.

12. Hohagen F, Montero RF, Weiss E, et al: Treatment of primary insomnia with trimipramine: An alternative to benzodiazepine hypnotics? Eur Arch Psychiatry Clin Neurosci 1994;244(2):65-72.

13. Kupfer DJ, Spiker DG, Coble P, McPartland RJ: Amitriptyline and EEG sleep in depressed patients: I. Drug effect. Sleep 1978; 1:149-159.

14. Shipley JE, Kupfer DJ, Griffin SJ, et al: Comparison of effects of desipramine and amitriptyline on EEG sleep of depressed patients. Psychopharmacology (Berl) 1985;85:14-22.

15. Dunleavy DLF, Brezinova V, Oswald I, et al: Changes during weeks in effects of tricyclic drugs on the human sleep brain. Br J Psychiatry 1972;120:663-672.

16. Roth T, Zorick F, Wittig R, et al: The effects of doxepin HCl on sleep and depression. J Clin Psychiatry 1982;43:366-368.

17. Feuillade P, Pringuey D, Belugou JL, et al: Trimipramine: acute and lasting effects on sleep in healthy and major depressive subjects. J Affect Disord 1992;24:135-145.

18. Ware JC, Brown FW, Moorad PJ, et al: Effects on sleep: A double-blind study comparing trimipramine to imipramine in depressed insomniac patients. Sleep 1989;12:537-549.

19. Kupfer DJ, Spiker DG, Rossi A, et al: Nortriptyline and EEG sleep in depressed patients. Biol Psychiatry 1982;17:535-546.

20. Buysse DJ, Reynolds CF, Hoch CC, et al: Longitudinal effects of nortriptyline on EEG sleep and the likelihood of recurrence in elderly depressed patients. Neuropsychopharmacology 1996; 14:243-252.

21. Hartmann E, Cravens J: The effects of long term administration of psychotropic drugs on human sleep: III. The effects of amitriptyline. Psychopharmacologia (Berl) 1973;33:185-202.

22. Kupfer DJ, Ehlers CL, Frank E, et al: Persistent effects of antidepressants: EEG sleep studies in depressed patients during maintenance treatment. Biol Psychiatry 1994;35:781-793.

23. Gillin JC, Wyatt RJ, Fram D: The relationship between changes in REM sleep and clinical improvement in depressed patients treated with amitriptyline. Psychopharmacology (Berl) 1978; 59:267-272.

24. Golden RN, Dawkins K, Nicholas L: Trazodone and nefazodone. In Schatzberg A, Nemeroff C (eds): The American Psychiatric Publishing Textbook of Psychopharmacology, 3rd ed. Washington, DC, American Psychiatric Publishing, 2004, pp 315-325.

25. Caccia S: Metabolism of newer antidepressants. Clin Pharmacokinet 1998;34:281-302.

26. Rickels K, Schweizer E, Case WG, et al: Nefazodone in major depression: Adjunctive benzodiazepine therapy and tolerability. J Clin Psychopharmacol 1998;18:145-153.

27. Montgomery I, Oswald I, Morgan K, Adam K: Trazodone enhances sleep in subjective quality but not in objective duration. Br J Clin Pharmacol 1983;16:139-144.

28. Parrino L, Spaggiari MC, Boselli M, et al: Clinical and polysomnographic effects of trazodone CR in chronic insomnia associated with dysthymia. Psychopharmacology (Berl) 1994;116:389-395.

29. Saletu-Zyhlarz G, Abu-Bakr M, Anderer P, et al: Insomnia in depression: Differences in objective and subjective sleep awakening quality to normal controls and acute effects of trazodone. Neuropsychopharmacol Biol Psychiatry 2002;26:249-260.

30. Davey A, Moon CA: The efficacy and residual effects of trazodone (150 mg nocte) and mianserin in the treatment of depressed general practice patients. Psychopharmacology (Berl) 1988;95: S7-S13.

31. van Bemmel AL, Havermans RG, van Diest R: Effects of trazodone on EEG sleep and clinical state in major depression. Psychopharmacology (Berl) 1992;107:569-574.

32. Scharf MB, Sachais BA: Sleep laboratory evaluation of the effects and efficacy of trazodone in depressed insomniac patients. J Clin Psychiatry 1990;51:13-17.

33. Mouret J, Lemoine P, Minuit MP, et al: Effects of trazodone on the sleep of depressed subjects: A polygraphic study. Psychopharmacology (Berl) 1988;95:37-43.

34. Ware JC, Pittard JT: Increased deep sleep after trazodone use: a double-blind placebo- controlled study in healthy young adults. J Clin Psychiatry 1990;51(Suppl):18-22.

35. Walsh JK, Erman M, Erwin CW, et al: Subjective hypnotic efficacy of trazodone and zolpidem in DSMIII-R primary insomnia. Hum Psychopharmacol 1998;13:191-198.

36. Gillin JC, Rapaport M, Erman MK, et al: A comparison of nefazodone and fluoxetine on mood and on objective, subjective, and clinician-rated measures of sleep in depressed patients: A double-blind, 8-week clinical trial. J Clin Psychiatry 1997;58: 185-192.

37. Armitage R, Yonkers K, Cole D, Rush AJ. A multi-center, double-blind comparison of the effects of nefazodone and fluoxetine on sleep architecture and quality of sleep in depressed outpatients. J Clin Psychopharmacol 1997;17:161-168.

38. Rush AJ, Armitage R, Gillin JC, et al: Comparative effects of nefazodone and fluoxetine on sleep in outpatients with major depressive disorder. Biol Psychiatry 1998;44:3-14.

39. Janowsky D, Curtis G, Zisook S, et al: Ventricular arrhythmias possibly aggravated by trazodone. Am J Psychiatry 1983;140: 796-797.

40. Thompson JWJ, Ware MR, Blashfield BK: Psychotropic medication and priapism: A comprehensive review. J Clin Psychiatry 1990;51:430-433.

41. Schirren CA, Baretton G: Nefazodone-induced acute liver failure. Am J Gastroenterol 2000;95:1596-1597.

42. Timmer CJ, Ad Sisten JM, Delbressine LP: Clinical pharmacokinetics of mirtazapine. Clin Pharmacokinet 2000;38:461-474.

43. Flores BH, Schatzberg AF: Mirtazapine. In Schatzberg A, Nemeroff C (eds): The American Psychiatric Publishing Textbook of Psychopharmacology, 3rd ed. Washington, DC, American Psychiatric Publishing, 2004, pp 341-347.

44. De Boer T: The pharmacologic profile of mirtazapine. J Clin Psychiatry 1996;57(Suppl 4):19-25.

45. Ruigt GS, Kemp B, Groenhout CM, Kamphuisen HA: Effect of the antidepressant Org 3770 on human sleep. Eur J Clin Pharmacol 1990;38:551-554.

46. Winokur A, Sateia MJ, Hayes JB, et al: Acute effects of mirtazapine on sleep continuity and sleep architecture in depressed patients: a pilot study. Biol Psychiatry 2000;48:75-78.

47. Korf HW, Schomerus C, Stehle JH: The Pineal Organ, Its Hormone Melatonin, and the Photoneuroendocrine System. New York, Springer, 1998.

48. Roth T, Stubbs C, Walsh JW. Ramelteon (TAK-375), A Selective Mt1/Mt2-Receptor Agonist, Reduces Latency to Persistent Sleep in a Model of Transient Insomnia Related to Novel Sleep Environment. Sleep, 28(3):303-307, 2005.

48a. Cajochen C. TAK-375 Takeda. Current Opinion in Investigational Drugs, 6(1):114-121, 2005.

49. Cajochen C, Kräuchi K, Mori D, et al: Melatonin and S-20098 increase REM sleep and wake-up propensity without modifying NREM sleep homeostasis. Am J Physiol 1997;272:1189-1196.

50. Lôo H, Hale A, D'haenen H: Determination of the dose of agomelatine, a melatoninergic agonist and selective 5-HT(2C) antagonist, in the treatment of major depressive disorder: A placebo-controlled dose range study. Int Clin Psychopharmacol 2002;17:239-247.

51. DeMuro RL, Nafziger AN, Blask DE, et al: The absolute bioavailability of oral melatonin. J Clin Pharmacol 2000;40:781-784.

52. Hughes RJ, Sack RL, Lewy AJ: The role of melatonin and circadian phase in age-related sleep-maintenance insomnia: Assessment in a clinical trial of melatonin replacement. Sleep 1998;21:52-68.

53. Singer C, Tractenberg RE, Kaye J, et al: A multicenter, placebo-controlled trial of melatonin for sleep disturbance in Alzheimer's disease. Sleep 2003;26:893-901.

54. von Bahr C, Ursing C, Yasui N, et al: Fluvoxamine but not citalopram increases serum melatonin in healthy subjects: An indication that cytochrome P450 CYP1A2 and CYP2C19 hydroxylate melatonin. Eur J Clin Pharmacol 2000;56:123-127.

55. Dubocovich ML, Masana MI, Benloucif S: Molecular pharmacology and function of melatonin receptor subtypes. In Olcese J (ed): Melatonin after Four Decades: An Assessment of its Potential. New York, Kluwer Academic/Plenum, 1999, pp 181-190.

56. Carrillo-Vico A, Garcia-Maurino S, Calvo JR, Guerrero JM: Melatonin counteracts the inhibitory effect of PGE2 on IL-2 production in human lymphocytes via its mt1 membrane receptor. FASEB J 2003;17:755-757.

57. Zhdanova IV, Wurtman RJ, Morabito C, et al: Effects of low oral doses of melatonin, given 2-4 hours before habitual bedtime, on sleep in normal young humans. Sleep 1996;19:423-431.

58. Waldhauser F, Saletu B, Trinchard-Lugan I: Sleep laboratory investigations on hypnotic properties of melatonin. Psychopharmacology (Berl) 1990;100:222-226.

59. Zhdanova IV, Wurtman RJ, Wagstaff J: Effects of a low dose of melatonin on sleep in children with Angelman syndrome. J Pediatr Endocrinol Metab 1999;12:57-67.

60. Smits MG, Nagtegaal EE, van der Heijden J, et al: Melatonin for chronic sleep onset insomnia in children: A randomized placebo-controlled trial. J Child Neurol 2001;16:86-92.

61. Serfaty M, Kennell-Webb S, Warner J, et al: Double blind randomised placebo controlled trial of low dose melatonin for sleep disorders in dementia. Int J Geriatr Psychiatry 2002;17:1120-1127.

62. Andrade C, Srihari BS, Reddy KP, Chandramma L: Melatonin in medically ill patients with insomnia: A double-blind, placebo-controlled study. J Clin Psychiatry 2001;62:41-45.

63. Dalton EJ, Rotondi D, Levitan RD, et al: Use of slow-release melatonin in treatment-resistant depression. J Psychiatry Neurosci 2000;25:48-52.

64. Sack RL, Hughes RJ, Edgar DM, Lewy AJ: Sleep-promoting effects of melatonin: At what dose, in whom, under what conditions, and by what mechanisms? Sleep 1997;20:908-915.

65. Mendelson WB: Efficacy of melatonin as a hypnotic agent. J Biol Rhythms 1997;12:651-656.

65a. Buscemi N, Vandermeer B, Pandya R, et al: Melatonin for Treatment of Sleep Disorders: Summary, Evidence Report/Technology Assessment No. 108. AHRQ Publication No. 05-E002-1. Rockville, MD, Agency for Healthcare Research and Quality, November 2004.

66. MacFarlane JG, Cleghorn JM, Brown GM, Streiner DL: The effects of exogenous melatonin on the total sleep time and daytime alertness of chronic insomniacs: A preliminary study. Biol Psychiatry 1991;30:371-376.

67. James SP, Sack DA, Rosenthal NE, Mendelson WB: Melatonin administration in insomnia. Neuropsychopharmacology 1990;3: 19-23.

68. Ellis CM, Lemmens G, Parkes JD: Melatonin and insomnia. J Sleep Res 1996;5:61-65.

69. Baskett JJ, Broad JB, Wood PC, et al: Does melatonin improve sleep in older people? A randomised crossover trial. Age Ageing 2003;32:164-170.

70. Zhdanova IV, Wurtman RJ: Efficacy of melatonin as a sleep-promoting agent. J Biol Rhythms 1997;12:644-650.

71. Cajochen C, Kräuchi K, von Arx MA, et al: Daytime melatonin administration enhances sleepiness and theta/alpha activity in the waking EEG. Neurosci Lett 1996;207:209-213.

72. Rogers NL, Kennaway DJ, Dawson D: Neurobehavioural performance effects of daytime melatonin and temazepam administration. J Sleep Res 2003;12:207-212.

73. Cajochen C, Kräuchi K, Wirz-Justice A: Role of melatonin in the regulation of human circadian rhythms and sleep. J Neuroendocrinol 2003;15:432-437.

74. Lusardi P, Preti P, Savino S, et al: Effect of bedtime melatonin ingestion on blood pressure of normotensive subjects. Blood Press Monit 1997;2:99-103.

75. Lusardi P, Piazza E, Fogari R: Cardiovascular effects of melatonin in hypertensive patients well controlled by nifedipine: A 24-hour study. Br J Clin Pharmacol 2000;49:423-427.

76. Naylor S, Johnson KL, Williamson BL, et al: Structural characterization of contaminants in commercial preparations of melatonin by on-line HPLC-electrospray ionization-tandem mass spectrometry. In Huether G, Kochen W, Simat TJ, Steinhart H (eds): Tryptophan, Serotonin, and Melatonin: Basic Aspects and Applications. New York, Kluwer Academic/Plenum, 1999, pp 769-777.

77. Brown NJ, Roberts LJ: Histamine, bradykinin, and their antagonists. In Hardman JG, Limbird LE (eds): Goodman and Gilman's the Pharmacological Basis of Therapeutics, 10th ed. New York, McGraw-Hill, 2001, pp 645-667.

78. Simons FE, Simons KJ: The pharmacology and use of H1-receptor-antagonists drugs. N Engl J Med 1994;330:1663-1670.

79. Schwartz JC, Arrang JM: Histamine. In Davis KL, Charney D, Coyle JT, Nemeroff C (eds): Neuropsychopharmacology: The Fifth Generation of Progress. Philadelphia, Lippincott Williams & Wilkins, 2002, pp 179-190.

80. Saper CB, Chou TC, Scammell TE: The sleep switch: Hypothalamic control of sleep and wakefulness. Trends Neurosci 2001;24:726-731.

81. Buysse DJ: Drugs affecting sleep, sleepiness and performance. In Monk TH (ed): Sleep, Sleepiness and Performance. Chichester, United Kingdom, John Wiley & Sons, 1991, pp 249-306.

82. Kudo Y, Kurihara M: Clinical evaluation of diphenhydramine hydrochloride for the treatment of insomnia in psychiatric patients: A double-blind study. J Clin Pharmacol 1990;30: 1041-1048.

83. Rickels K, Morris RJ, Newman H, et al: Diphenhydramine in insomniac family practice patients: A double-blind study. J Clin Pharmacol 1983;23:234-242.

84. Meuleman JR, Nelson RC, Clark RL: Evaluation of temazepam and diphenhydramine as hypnotics in a nursing-home population. Drug Intell Clin Pharm 1987;21:716-720.

85. Roth T, Roehrs T, Koshorek G, et al: Sedative effects of antihistamines. J Allergy Clin Immunol 1987;80:94-98.

86. Schweitzer PK, Muehlbach MJ, Walsh JK: Sleepiness and performance during three-day administration of cetirizine or diphenhydramine. J Allergy Clin Immunol 1994;94:716-724.

87. Gengo FM, Gabos C: Antihistamines, drowsiness, and psychomotor impairment: Central nervous system effect of cetirizine. Ann Allergy 1987;59:53-57.

88. Basu R, Dodge H, Stoehr GP, Ganguli M: Sedative-hypnotic use of diphenhydramine in a rural, older adult, community-based cohort: Effects on cognition. Am J Geriatr Psychiatry 2003; 11:205-213.

89. Koppel C, Tenczer J, Ibe K: Poisoning with over-the-counter doxylamine preparations: An evaluation of 109 cases. Hum Toxicol 1987;6:355-359.

90. Houghton PJ: The scientific basis for the reputed activity of valerian. J Pharm Pharmacol 1999;51:505-512.

91. Krystal AD, Ressler I: The use of valerian in neuropsychiatry. CNS Spectrums 2001;6:841-847.

92. Leathwood PD, Chauffard F, Heck E, Munoz-Box R: Aqueous extract of valerian root (Valeriana officinalis L.) improves sleep quality in man. Pharmacol Biochem Behav 1982; 17:65-71.

93. Lindahl O, Lindwall L: Double blind study of a valerian preparation. Pharmacol Biochem Behav 1989;32:1065-1066.

94. Schulz H, Stolz C, Muller J: The effect of valerian extract on sleep polygraphy in poor sleepers: A pilot study. Pharmacopsychiatry 1994;27:147-151.

95. Donath F, Quispe S, Diefenbach K, et al: Critical evaluation of the effect of valerian extract on sleep structure and sleep quality. Pharmacopsychiatry 2000;33(2):47-53.

96. Schulz H, Stolz C, Muller J: The effect of valerian extract on sleep polygraphy in poor sleepers: A pilot study. Pharmacopsychiatry 1994;27(4):147-151.

97. Balderer G, Borbély AA: Effect of valerian on human sleep. Psychopharmacology (Berl) 1985;87:406-409.

98. McNamara JO: Drugs effective in the therapy of epilepsies. In Hardman JG, Limbird LE (eds): Goodman and Gilman's the Pharmacological Basis of Therapeutics, 10th ed. New York, McGraw-Hill, 2001, pp 521-547.

99. Rose MA, Kam CA: Gabapentin: Pharmacology and its use in pain management. Anaesthesia 2002;57:451-462.

100. Stahl SM: Essential Pharmacology: Neuroscientific Basis and Practical Application, 2nd ed. New York, Cambridge University Press, 2000.

101. Foldvary-Schaefer N, De Leon Sanchez I, Karafa M, et al: Gabapentin increases slow-wave sleep in normal adults. Epilepsia 2002;43:1493-1497.

102. Garcia-Borreguero D, Larrosa O, de la Llave Y, et al: Treatment of restless legs syndrome with gabapentin: A double-blind, cross-over study. Neurology 2002;59:1573-1579.

103. Mathias S, Wetter TC, Steiger A, Lancel M: The GABA uptake inhibitor tiagabine promotes slow wave sleep in normal elderly subjects. Neurobiol Aging 2001;22:247-253.

104. Baldessarini RJ, Tarazi FI: Drugs and the treatment of anxiety disorders: Psychosis and Mania. In Hardman JG, Limbird LE (eds): Goodman and Gilman's the Pharmacological Basis of Therapeutics, 10th ed. New York, McGraw-Hill, 2001, pp 485-520.

105. Sharpley AL, Vassallo CM, Cowen PJ: Olanzapine increases slow-wave sleep: Evidence for blockade of central 5-HT$_{2C}$ receptors in vivo. Biol Psychiatry 2000;47:468-470.

106. Salin-Pascual RJ, Herrera-Estrella M, Galicia-Polo L, Laurrabaquio MR: Olanzapine acute administration in schizophrenic patients increases delta sleep and sleep efficiency. Biol Psychiatry 1999;46:141-143.

107. Lindberg N, Virkkunen M, Tani P, et al: Effect of a single-dose of olanzapine on sleep in healthy females and males. Int Clin Psychopharmacol 2002;17:177-184.

108. Meredith B, Cupp MJ, Tracy TS: γ-Hydroxybutyric acid (GHB), γ-butyrolctone (GBL), and 1,4-butanediol (BD). In Cupp MJ, Tracy TS (eds): Forensic Science: Dietary Supplements: Toxicology and Clinical Pharmacology. Totowa, NJ, Humana Press, 2003, pp 173-195.

109. Scrima L, Hartman PG, Johnson FH Jr, et al: The effects of gamma-hydroxybutyrate on the sleep of narcolepsy patients: A double-blind study. Sleep 1990;13:479-490.

110. Lapierre O, Montplaisir J, Lamarre M, Bedard MA: The effect of gamma-hydroxybutyrate on nocturnal and diurnal sleep of normal subjects: Further considerations on REM sleep-triggering mechanisms. Sleep 1990;13:24-30.

111. Van Cauter E, Plat L, Scharf MB, et al: Simultaneous stimulation of slow-wave sleep and growth hormone secretion by gamma-hydroxybutyrate in normal young men. J Clin Invest 1997;100:745-753.

112. Scharf MB, Baumann M, Berkowitz DV: The effects of sodium oxybate on clinical symptoms and sleep patterns in patients with fibromyalgia. J Rheumatol 2003;30: 1070-1074.

Wake-Promoting Medications: Basic Mechanisms and Pharmacology

Seiji Nishino

Emmanuel Mignot

ABSTRACT

Central nervous system stimulants used in sleep medicine include amphetamine-like compounds (L- and D-amphetamine and methamphetamine, methylphenidate, pemoline), mazindol, modafinil, some antidepressants with stimulant properties (e.g., bupropion), and caffeine. The effects of most of these drugs on wakefulness is primarily mediated through an inhibition of dopamine reuptake/transport and in some cases through increased dopamine release. An exception is caffeine, a compound with adenosine receptor antagonistic effects. Biogenic amine transporters (for dopamine [DA], norepinephrine [NE], and serotonin [5-hydroxytryptamine, 5-HT]) are located at nerve terminals, and are important in terminating transmitter action and maintaining transmitter homeostasis. In the past decade, monoamine transporters have been cloned and their molecular mechanisms have been elucidated. Genetically engineered mice lacking these molecules (knockout mice) have also become available. In parallel with these discoveries, potent and selective ligands for DA, NE, and 5-HT transporters have been developed. The results of pharmacologic studies using these new ligands in narcoleptic dogs and DA transporter knockout mice models suggest the importance of the DA transporter (as opposed to the adrenergic transporter) for the mode of action of amphetamines, amphetamine-like compounds, and bupropion on wakefulness. Importantly, however, the various stimulants also have differential effects on dopamine storage (through vascular monoamine transporter-2 inhibition) or release, and in most cases have effects on other monoaminergic systems. The mode of action of modafinil, a more recent compound used as a first-line treatment for excessive daytime sleepiness, is controversial. Dopamine reuptake inhibition may or may not be involved in modafinil's primary mechanism of action.

CENTRAL NERVOUS SYSTEM STIMULANTS: DEFINITION

Although widely used, *central nervous system (CNS) stimulant* is a loosely defined scientific term. In *Drugs and the Brain*,[1] stimulants are "drugs that have an alerting effect; they improve the mood and quicken the intellect." In *Handbook of Sleep Disorders*,[2] CNS stimulation implies "an increase in neuronal activity due to enhanced excitability, with a change in the normal balance between excitatory and inhibitory influences. This may result from blockage of inhibition, enhancement of excitation, or both." In *A Primer of Drug Action*,[3] the term "psychomotor stimulants (psychostimulants)" is used, and "psychostimulants" are said to induce excitement, alertness, euphoria, a reduced sense of fatigue, and increased motor activity. "Psychostimulants" include dopamine (DA) uptake blockers, DA-releasing agents, adenosine receptor blockers, and acetylcholine receptor stimulants. In *The Pharmacological Basis of Therapeutics*,[4] "indirect sympathomimetic amines" is used to refer to amphetamines, the "most potent compounds with respect to stimulation of the CNS."

In this chapter, the generic term *CNS stimulants* is used for wake-promoting compounds of potential use in the treatment of excessive daytime sleepiness (EDS; see Chapters 39 and 51 for the classification of EDS disorders and see Chapters 64-66 for the indications for CNS stimulants for patients with sleep disorders). EDS is a common symptom in patients with sleep disorders and in the general population at large. CNS stimulants are usually effective for this symptom regardless of its underlying cause. They should be used cautiously because of their potential for abuse and misuse. In this chapter, we review the neurochemical, neurophysiologic, and neuropharmacologic properties of the CNS stimulants most commonly used in sleep medicine.

AMPHETAMINES AND AMPHETAMINE-LIKE COMPOUNDS

Historical Perspective

Amphetamine was first synthesized in 1897, but its stimulant effects were not recognized until 1929 by Alles.[5] Alles wanted to find a synthetic substitute for the recently banned ephedrine, a compound isolated from the *Ephedra vulgaris* plant in 1925. Amphetamine increases energy, elevates mood, prevents fatigue, increases vigilance and prevents sleep, stimulates respiration, and causes electrical and behavioral arousal from natural- or drug-induced sleep. It was rapidly shown to be a safer and cheaper alternative to ephedrine as a stimulant. In World War II, amphetamine was supplied to paratroopers and commandos. British troops alone were issued 72 million tablets.[2] In Japan, methamphetamine, initially used for munition factory workers, flooded the civilian market at the end of the war; 5% of the Japanese population between the ages of 16 and 25 years became dependent on the drug (see Seijun[6]). More than 50 "amphetamine" preparations containing amphetamine or derivatives, alone or in combination with other drugs (most notably barbiturates), were on the market after the war.[7]

Narcolepsy was probably the first condition for which amphetamine was used clinically.[8] It revolutionized therapy for the condition, although it was not curative. The piperazine derivative of amphetamine, methylphenidate, was introduced in 1959 by Yoss and Daly.[9] The use of amphetamine in treating parkinsonism dates back to 1937, when it was first used to alleviate muscular rigidity and postencephalitis parkinsonism. By 1968, its use in the treatment of this condition was largely suspended owing to the use of more effective dopaminergic agents.[7] Until the dangers of amphetamine dependence and abuse became recognized, amphetamine was widely used in the treatment of obesity. It was also prescribed in the treatment of sedative abuse and alcoholism to offset sleepiness and lethargy.

Bradley and Bowen were the first to report on the use of amphetamine to modify antisocial behavior in children[10]: "when children are withdrawn or lethargic, the amphetamine tended to make them more alert, more accessible to persons and the environment." A paradoxical calming effect was noted in some children and aggressive adults. Most notably, some children who were "hyperactive" tended to move more quietly and to be calmer and less quarrelsome after being treated with amphetamine. In 1958, methylphenidate was introduced to treat hyperactivity in children (see Anders and Ciaranello[11]). These observations preceded reports on the effects of amphetamine and methylphenidate in the hyperkinetic child (children diagnosed with what is now called attention-deficit/hyperactivity disorder [ADHD]).[11]

Although no controlled trials have investigated the use of stimulants in depression, many case series suggest effectiveness in treatment-resistant cases.[12,13] The use of stimulants with monoamine oxidase inhibitors (MAOIs) is generally not advised but has not been reported to induce significant hypertension or hyperthermia. The combination of amphetamines with low doses of tricyclic antidepressants is often prescribed in narcolepsy-cataplexy without any significant adverse effects, and combining these substances in depression may be helpful. Part of the beneficial effects of amphetamine on depression may be due to a reduction of fatigue and apathy, rather than a genuine antidepressant effect.[14] In an open-label trial in depressive patients with cancer, both amphetamine and methylphenidate were reported to improve depression rapidly (within 2 days).[15]

From a historical perspective, the number of indications for amphetamine stimulants has narrowed considerably over the years to include primarily narcolepsy, ADHD, and treatment-resistant depression. The rationale for this change has been the realization of the risk of abuse and dependence with these compounds. The introduction of other effective therapies for these conditions (e.g., modafinil for narcolepsy, atomoxetine for ADHD) has also led to narrower indications, although many new formulations and isomer-specific preparations have been recently developed and are increasingly used, mostly for the treatment of ADHD.

Structure–Activity Relationships and Major Chemical Entities

Phenylisopropylamine (amphetamine) has a simple chemical structure that resembles endogenous catecholamines (Fig. 38–1). This scaffold forms the template for a wide variety of pharmacologically active substances. Although amphetamine possesses strong central stimulant effects, minor modifications can result in agents having a broad spectrum of effects, including nasal decongestion, anorexia, vasoconstriction, antidepressant effects (for the MAOI tranylcypromine), or hallucinogenic properties (MDMA [methylenedioxymethamphetamine] and MDA [methylenedioxyamphetamine]).[16]

The phenylisopropylamine molecule can be divided into three structural components: (1) the aromatic nucleus, (2) the terminal amine, and (3) the isopropyl side chain. Substitution on the aromatic nucleus usually produces less potent, if not inactive CNS stimulants.[16] The substitution of two or more methoxy groups plus addition of ethyl, methyl, or bromine groups on the aromatic nucleus creates hallucinogens of various potencies. "Ecstasy" (MDMA) is built on a methamphetamine backbone, with a dimethoxy ring extending from the aromatic group. If this hallucinogen is designed with a primary amine (without the methyl group), the result is "love" (MDA). Substitution at the amine group is the most common alteration. Methamphetamine, which is characterized by an additional methyl group attached to the amine, making secondary substituted amines, is more potent than amphetamine, probably because of increased CNS penetration.[17] An intact isopropyl side chain appeared to be necessary to maintain stimulant efficacy. Changing the propyl to an ethyl side chain, for example, creates phenylethylamine, an endogenous neuroamine, which has mood- and energy-enhancing properties but is less potent and has a much shorter half-life than amphetamine.[18]

The pharmacologic effects of most amphetamine derivatives are isomer-specific. D-Amphetamine, for example, is a far more potent stimulant than the L-derivative. In electroencephalographic (EEG) studies, D-amphetamine is four times more potent in inducing wakefulness than L-amphetamine.[19] Not all effects are stereospecific, however. For example, both enantiomers are equipotent at suppressing rapid eye movement (REM) sleep in humans and rats[19] and at producing amphetamine psychosis.[20] The relative effects of the D- and L-isomers of amphetamine on norepinephrine (NE) and DA transmission may explain some of these differences (for details, see the section on presynaptic modulation of the DA system).

Amphetamine-like compounds, such as methylphenidate, pemoline, and fencamfamin, are structurally similar to amphetamines; all compounds include a benzene core with an ethylamine group side chain (see Fig. 38–1). Both methylphenidate and pemoline were commonly used for the treatment of EDS in narcolepsy, but pemoline has been withdrawn from the market in several countries because of liver toxicity (Table 38–1). The most commonly used commercially available form of methylphenidate is a racemic mixture of both a D- and L-enantiomer, but D-methylphenidate mainly contributes the clinical effects, especially after oral administration. This is because L-methylphenidate, but not D-methylphenidate, undergoes a significant first-pass metabolism (by deesterification to L-ritalinic acid). A single-isomer form of D-methylphenidate is also marketed under the brand name of Focalin.

Cocaine also mediates its psychostimulant effects by blocking catecholamine reuptake (mainly DA), but its structure is different from amphetamine-like compounds (see Fig. 38–1).

Amphetamines are highly lipid-soluble molecules that are well absorbed by the gastrointestinal tract. Peak levels are achieved approximately 2 hours after oral administration, with rapid tissue distribution and brain penetration. Protein binding is highly variable, with an average volume of distribution (V_d) of 5 L/kg.

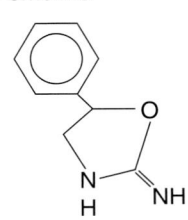

Figure 38–1. Chemical structures of amphetamine-like stimulants, modafinil, cocaine, and caffeine (a xanthine derivative), compared with dopamine and norepinephrine.

Both hepatic catabolism and renal excretion are involved in the inactivation of amphetamine. Amphetamine can be metabolized in the liver by either aromatic or aliphatic hydroxylation, yielding parahydroxyamphetamine or norephedrine, respectively, both of which are biologically active.[21] The metabolism of amphetamine and amphetamine-like compounds is pH dependent. Amphetamine is metabolized into benzoic acid (23%), which is subsequently converted to hippuric acid or to parahydroxyamphetamine (2%). This in turn is converted to parahydroxynorephedrine (0.4%). Thirty-three percent of the oral dose is excreted unchanged in the urine. Urinary excretion of amphetamine and many amphetamine-like stimulants is greatly influenced by urinary pH. At urinary pH 5.0, the elimination half-life of amphetamine is short, approximately 5 hours, but at pH 7.3 it increases to 21 hours.[22] Sodium bicarbonate delays excretion of amphetamine and prolongs its clinical effects, whereas ammonium chloride shortens amphetamine action (and can possibly induce toxicity).

Methylphenidate is almost totally absorbed after oral administration. Methylphenidate has low protein binding (15%) and is fairly short acting; the effects last approximately 4 hours, with a half-life of 3 hours. The primary means of clearance is through the urine, in which 90% is excreted.

Molecular Targets of Amphetamine Action

The molecular targets mediating amphetamine-like stimulant effects are complex and vary depending on the specific analogue/isomer and the dose administered. Amphetamine per se increases catecholamine (DA and NE) release and inhibits reuptake. These effects are mediated by specific catecholamine transporters[23,24] (Fig. 38–2). Axelrod and colleagues first demonstrated that epinephrine could be rapidly and selectively taken up by the heart, spleen, and glandular organs, each of which has significant sympathetic innervation.[25] It was subsequently discovered that NE-containing neurons bind and take up NE against a concentration gradient, suggesting the existence of selective transporters. Further experiments also found that these transporters not only can carry catecholamine back into nerve terminals but can release them.

The molecules responsible, the DA transporter (DAT) and the NE transporter (NET), have now been cloned and characterized.[26-28] The DAT and NET proteins are approximately 620–amino-acid proteins with 12 putative membrane-spanning regions. Amphetamine derivatives inhibit the uptake and enhance the release of DA, NE, or both by interacting with

Table 38–1.   Commonly Used Pharmacologic Compounds for Excessive Daytime Sleepiness

Stimulant Compound	Usual Daily Doses*	Side Effects and Notes
Amphetamine and Amphetamine-like CNS Stimulants		
D-Amphetamine sulfate	5–60 mg (15, 100 mg)	Irritability, mood changes, headaches, palpitations, tremors, excessive sweating, insomnia
Methamphetamine HCl	5–60 mg (15, 80 mg)	Same as D-amphetamine May have greater central over peripheral effects than D-amphetamine[†]
Methylphenidate HCl	10–60 mg (30, 100 mg)	Same as amphetamines, better therapeutic index than D-amphetamine, with less reduction of appetite or increase in blood pressure Short duration of action
Pemoline	20–115 mg (37.5, 150 mg)	Less sympathomimetic effect, milder stimulant Slower onset of action, a tendency for drug buildup Occasionally produces liver toxicity Pemoline is not a controlled substance
Dopamine/Norepinephrine Uptake Inhibitor		
Mazindol[‡]	2–6 mg (NA)	Weaker CNS stimulant effects, anorexia, dry mouth, irritability, headaches, gastrointestinal symptoms Mazindol is reported to have less potential for abuse
Other Agents for Treatment of Excessive Daytime Sleepiness		
Modafinil	100–400 mg (NA)	No peripheral sympathomimetic action, headaches, nausea Modafinil is reported to have less potential for abuse
Monoamine Oxidase Inhibitor with Alerting Effect		
Selegiline[‡]	5–40 mg (NA)	Low abuse potential Partial (10–40%) interconversion to amphetamine
Xanthine Derivative		
Caffeine[§]	100–200 mg (NA)	Weak stimulant effect, 100 mg of caffeine roughly equivalent to one cup of coffee Palpitations, hypertension

*Dosages recommended by the American Sleep Disorders Association are listed in parentheses (usual starting dose and maximal dose recommended).

[†]Methamphetamine is reported to have more central effects and may predispose more to amphetamine psychosis. The widespread misuse of methamphetamine has led to severe legal restriction on its manufacture, sale, and prescription in many countries. L-Amphetamine (dose range 20–60 mg) is not available in the United States, but probably has no advantage over D-amphetamine in the treatment of narcolepsy (slightly weaker stimulant).

[‡]Demonstrated anticataplectic effects in humans.

[§]Caffeine can be bought without prescription in the form of tablets (No Doz, 100 mg; Vivarin, 200 mg caffeine) and is used by many patients with narcolepsy before diagnosis.

CNS, central nervous system; NA, not applicable.

these molecules. The DAT and NET normally move DA and NE, respectively, from the outside to the inside of the cell. This process is sodium dependent; sodium and chloride bind to DAT and NET to immobilize them at the extracellular surface and to alter the conformation of the DA/NE binding site, thereby facilitating substrate binding. Substrate binding allows movement of the carrier to the intracellular surface of the neuronal membrane, driven by sodium concentration gradients. In the presence of some drugs such as amphetamine, the direction of transport appears to be reversed (see Fig. 38–2). DA and NE are moved from the inside of the cell to the outside through a mechanism called *exchange diffusion*, which occurs at low doses (1 to 5 mg/kg) of amphetamine.

At higher dose, other effects are involved. Increased serotonin (5-hydroxytryptamine [5-HT]) release is also observed. Moderate to high doses of amphetamine (more than 5 mg/kg) also interact with vascular monoamine transporter-2 (VMAT2;

see Seiden et al.[23] and Kuczenski and Segal[24]). The vesicularization of the monoamines (DA, NE serotonin, and histamine) in the CNS depends on VMAT2; VMAT2 regulates the size of the vesicular and cytosolic DA pools. Amphetamine is highly lipophilic and easily enters nerve terminals by diffusing across plasma membranes. Once inside, amphetamine depletes vesicular monoamine stores by several mechanisms. First, it binds directly, albeit with low affinity, to VMAT2, thereby inhibiting vesicular uptake.[29] Second, amphetamine, a weak base, diffuses across the vesicular membrane in its uncharged (lipophilic) form and accumulates in the granules in its charged form (because of the lower pH of the synaptic vesicle interior). As vesicular amphetamine concentration increases, the buffering capacity of the catecholamine-containing vesicle is lost. The vesicular pH gradient diminishes,[30,31] a loss of the free energy necessary for monoamine sequestration occurs, and vesicular monoamine uptake decreases. In addition, the

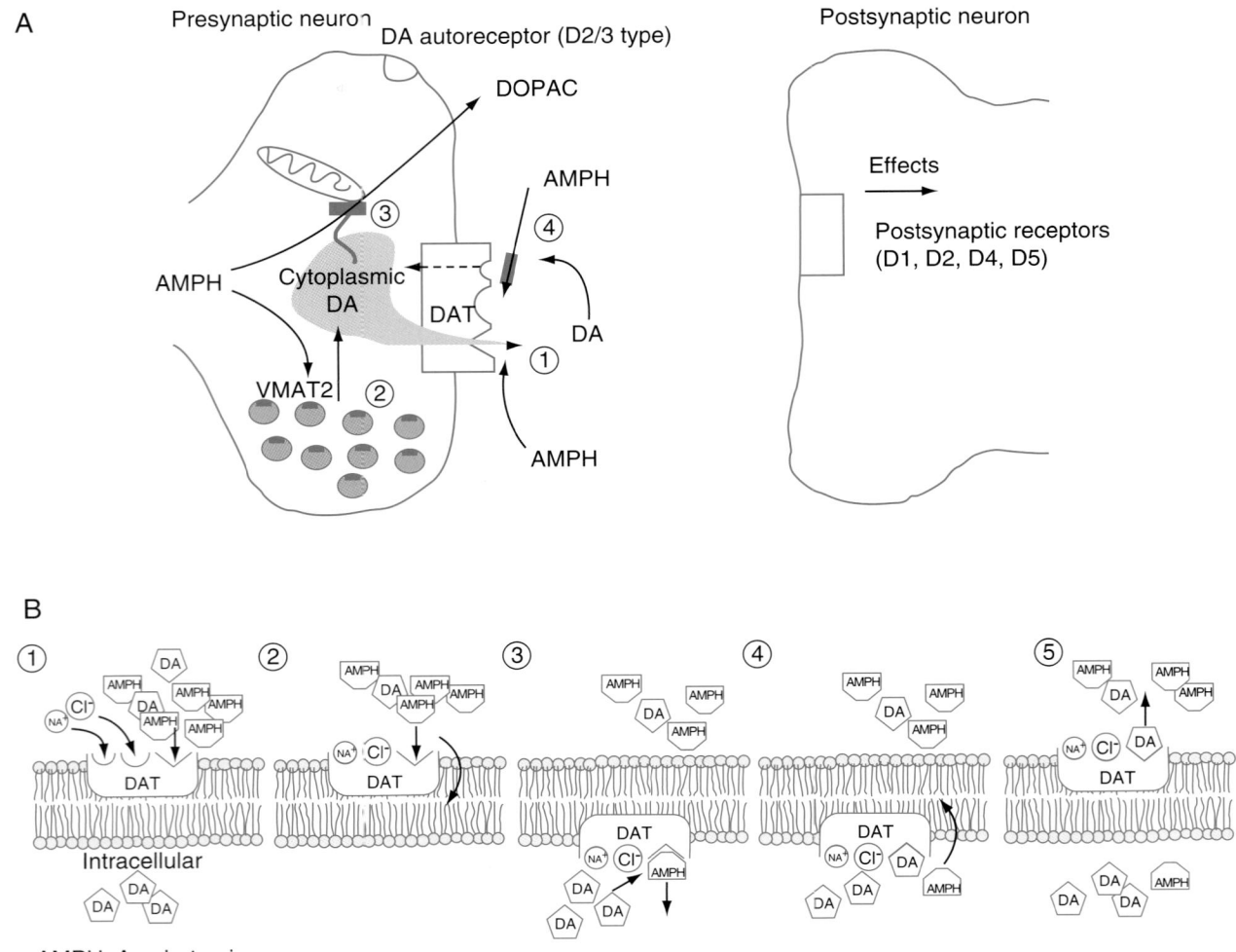

AMPH: Amphetamine

Figure 38–2. Effects of amphetamines at the dopaminergic nerve terminal **(A)** and a schematic model of the exchange diffusion process in relation to the mode of action of amphetamines **(B)**. **A,** (1) Amphetamine (AMPH) interacts with the dopamine (DA) transporter (DAT) to facilitate DA release from the cytoplasm through an exchange diffusion mechanism. At higher intracellular concentrations, amphetamine also (2) disrupts vesicular storage of DA, and (3) inhibits monoamine oxidase (MAO). Both these actions increase cytoplasmic DA concentrations. (4) Amphetamine also inhibits DA uptake by virtue of its binding to and transport by the DAT. DOPAC, dihydroxyphenylacetic acid. **B,** (1) Sodium and chloride bind to the DAT to immobilize it at the extracellular surface. This alters the conformation of the DA binding site on the DAT to facilitate substrate binding. (2) Amphetamine, in competition with extracellular DA, binds to the transporter. Substrate binding allows the movement of the carrier to the intracellular surface of the neuronal membrane, driven by the sodium and amphetamine concentration gradients, resulting in a reversal of the flow of DA uptake. (3) Amphetamine dissociates from the transporter, making the binding site available to cytoplasmic DA. (4) DA binding to the transporter enables the movement of the transporter to the extracellular surface of the neuronal membrane, as driven by the favorable DA concentration gradient. (5) DA dissociates from the transporter, making the transporter available for amphetamine, and thus another cycle. (Adapted from Kuczenski R, Segal DS: Neurochemistry of amphetamine. In Cho AK, Segel DS [eds]: Psychopharmacology, Toxicology and Abuse, pp 81-113. San Diego, Academic Press, 1994.)

collapse of the gradient purportedly results in a competition for protons between the native monoamines and amphetamine, thereby increasing uncharged vesicular neurotransmitter concentrations. All these mechanisms lead to a diffusion of the native monoamines out of the vesicles into the cytoplasm along a concentration gradient.[30] Amphetamine can therefore be viewed as a physiologic VMAT2 antagonist that releases the vascular DA/NE loaded by VMAT2 into the cytoplasm. These mechanisms, as well as the reverse transport and the blocking of DA/NE reuptake by amphetamine, all lead to an increase in NE and DA synaptic concentrations.[23,24]

Various amphetamine derivatives have slightly different effects on all these systems. For example, methylphenidate also binds to NET and DAT and enhances catecholamine release. However, it has less effect on the VMAT2 granular storage site than native amphetamine. Similarly, D-amphetamine has proportionally more releasing effect on the DA versus the NE system compared with L-amphetamine. MDMA has more effect on 5-HT release than on catecholamine release. Other antidepressant medications acting on monoaminergic systems, including DA, NE, and 5-HT (e.g., bupropion or mazindol; see later), tend to exert their actions by simply blocking the reuptake mechanism.

Some, but not all, amphetamines have neurotoxic effects on monoaminergic systems. This is well established for MDMA and serotoninergic systems in both humans and animals.

Similarly, amphetamine derivatives with strong effects on monoamine release (typically methamphetamine but not derivatives with simple monoamine reuptake inhibition effects) have neurotoxic effects on DA systems at high doses in animal studies, especially in the context of repeated administration that mimics binges of stimulant abuse.

Presynaptic Modulation of the Dopaminergic System Mediates Electroencephalographic Arousal Effects

How amphetamines and other stimulants increase EEG arousal has been explored using a canine model of narcolepsy and DAT knockout mouse models. Canine narcolepsy is a naturally occurring animal model of the human disorder.[32,33] Similar to human patients, narcoleptic dogs are excessively sleepy (i.e., shorter sleep latency), have fragmented sleep patterns, and display cataplexy.[34,35] Although amphetamine-like compounds are well known to stimulate catecholaminergic transmission, the exact mechanism by which they promote EEG arousal is still uncertain. Stimulation of either or both

adrenergic or dopaminergic transmission has been suggested to play a role.[2,36,37]

To address this question, the effects of ligands specific for DAT (GBR-12909, bupropion, and amineptine), NET (nisoxetine and desipramine) or both DAT and NET (mazindol and nomifensine), as well as amphetamine and a nonamphetamine stimulant, modafinil, were studied in narcoleptic and control Dobermans.[38] As shown in Figure 38–3, DA uptake inhibitors such as GBR-12909 and bupropion dose-dependently increased EEG arousal in narcoleptic dogs, whereas nisoxetine and desipramine, two potent NE uptake inhibitors, had no effect on EEG arousal at doses that almost completely suppressed REM sleep and cataplexy (see Nishino and Mignot[34] and Nishino et al.[38]). Most strikingly, the EEG arousal potency of various DA uptake inhibitors correlated tightly with in vitro DAT binding affinities (see Fig. 38–3), whereas a reduction in REM sleep correlated with in vitro NET binding affinities.[38] These results strongly suggest that DA uptake inhibition is critical for the EEG arousal effects of these compounds.

D-Amphetamine has a relatively low DAT binding affinity but potently (i.e., at a low dose) promotes alertness (see Fig. 38–3). It is also generally considered more efficacious (i.e., can produce more alertness at a high dose) than pure DA uptake inhibitors

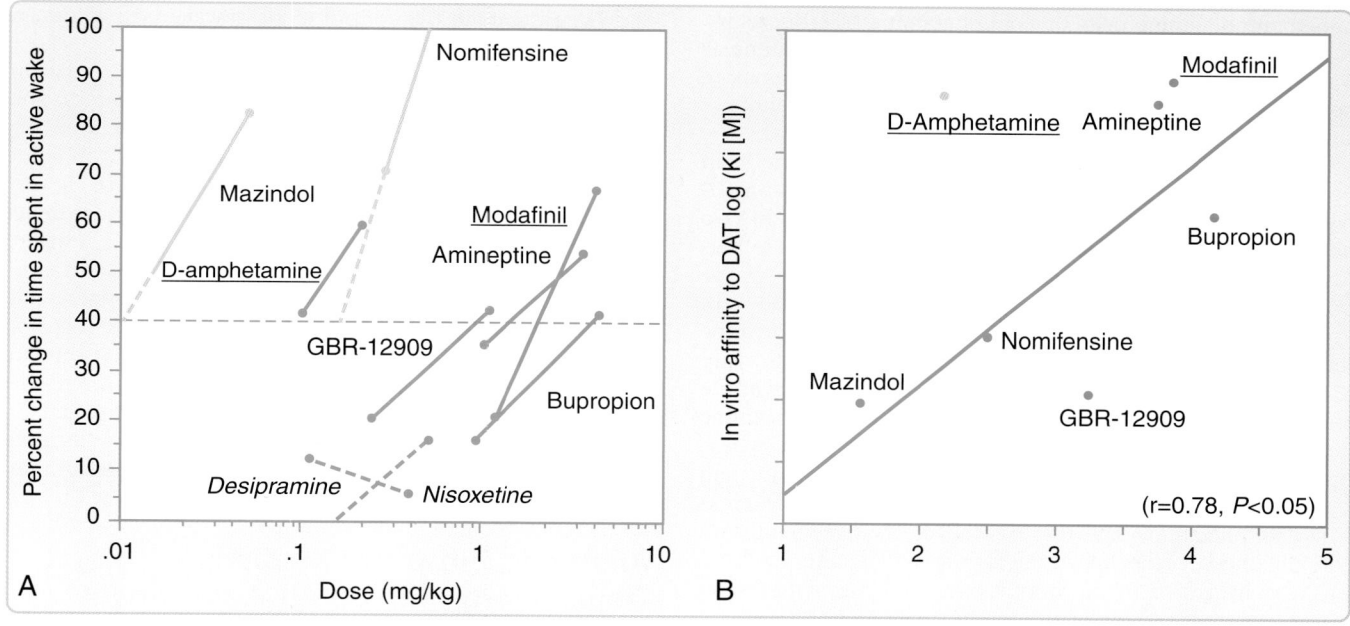

Figure 38–3. Effects of various dopamine (DA) and norepinephrine (NE) uptake inhibitors and amphetamine-like stimulants on the electroencephalographic (EEG) arousal of narcoleptic dogs **(A)** and correlation between in vivo EEG arousal effects and in vitro DA transporter binding affinities **(B)**. **A,** The effects of various compounds on daytime sleepiness were studied using 4-hr daytime polygraphic recordings (10:00–14:00) in four or five narcoleptic animals. Two doses were studied for each compound. All DA uptake inhibitors and central nervous system stimulants dose-dependently increased EEG arousal and reduced slow wave sleep compared with vehicle treatment. In contrast, nisoxetine and desipramine, two potent NE uptake inhibitors, had no significant effect on EEG arousal at doses that completely suppressed cataplexy (see Nishino and Mignot[34]). Compounds with both adrenergic and dopaminergic effects (nomifensine, mazindol, D-amphetamine) were active on both EEG arousal and cataplexy. The effects of the two doses studied for each stimulant were used to approximate a dose–response curve; the drug dose that increased the time spent in wakefulness by 40% above baseline (vehicle session) was estimated for each compound. The order of potency of the compounds obtained was, in decreasing order of potency, mazindol, amphetamine, nomifensine, GBR-12909, amineptine, modafinil, and bupropion. **B,** In vitro DA transporter (DAT) binding onto canine caudate membranes was performed using [³H]-WIN 35,428. Affinity for the various DA uptake inhibitors tested varied widely between 6.5 nM and 3.3 mM. In addition, it was also found that both amphetamine and modafinil have a low, but significant, affinity (same range as amineptine) for the DAT. A significant correlation between in vivo and in vitro effects was observed for all five DA uptake inhibitors and modafinil. Amphetamine, which had potent EEG arousal effects, has a relatively low DAT binding affinity, suggesting that other mechanisms, most probably monoamine releasing effects or monoamine oxidase inhibition, are involved. In contrast, there was no significant correlation between in vivo EEG arousal effects and in vitro NE transporter binding affinities for DA and NE uptake inhibitors.[38] These results suggest that presynaptic enhancement of DA transmission is the key pharmacologic property mediating the EEG arousal effects of most wake-promoting central nervous system stimulants.

in promoting wakefulness. As described in the section on the molecular targets of amphetamine action, however, D-amphetamine not only inhibits DA reuptake, it enhances DA release (at lower doses by exchange diffusion and at higher doses by antagonistic action against VMAT2) and inhibits monoamine oxidation to prevent DA metabolism. The DA-releasing effects of amphetamine likely explain the unusually high potency and efficacy of amphetamine in promoting EEG arousal.

To differentiate further between the involvement of the DA and NE systems in the mode of action of amphetamine derivatives, the effects of various amphetamine analogues (D-amphetamine, L-amphetamine, and L-methamphetamine) on EEG arousal and their in vivo effects on brain extracellular DA levels in narcoleptic dogs were compared.[39] In vitro studies have demonstrated that the potency and selectivity for enhancing release or inhibiting uptake of DA and NE vary between amphetamine analogues and isomers.[22,40-42] Amphetamine derivatives thus offer a unique opportunity to study the pharmacologic control of alertness in vivo. Hartmann and Cravens previously reported that D-amphetamine is four times more potent in inducing EEG arousal than is L-amphetamine, but that both enantiomers are equipotent at suppressing REM sleep in humans and rats.[19] Enantiomer-specific effects have also been reported with methamphetamine; L-methamphetamine is much less potent as a stimulant than either D-methamphetamine or L- or D-amphetamine (see Kuczenski et al.[40]). Similarly, in canine narcolepsy, D-amphetamine is 3 times more potent than L-amphetamine and 12 times more potent than L-methamphetamine in increasing wakefulness and reducing slow wave sleep[39] (Fig. 38–4A).

To study further what mediates these differences in potency, the effects of these amphetamine derivatives on DA release were examined in freely moving animals using in vivo microdialysis. Amphetamine derivatives (100 μM) were perfused locally for 60 minutes through a dialysis probe implanted in the caudate of narcoleptic dogs[39] (Fig. 38–4B). Local perfusion of D-amphetamine raised DA levels to nine times baseline. L-Amphetamine also increased DA levels by up to seven times, but peak DA release was obtained only at the end of the 60-minute perfusion period. L-Methamphetamine did not change DA levels under these conditions. These results suggest that D-amphetamine is more potent than L-amphetamine in increasing caudate DA levels, whereas L-methamphetamine had the least effect, in agreement with data obtained in other species using the same technique.[40] NE was also measured in the frontal cortex during perfusion of D-amphetamine, L-amphetamine and L-methamphetamine. Although all compounds increased NE efflux, no significant difference in potency was detected among the three analogues (Fig. 38–4C).

The fact that the potency of amphetamine derivatives on EEG arousal correlates with effects on DA efflux in the caudate of narcoleptic dogs further suggests that the enhancement of DA transmission by presynaptic modulation mediates the wake-promoting effects of amphetamine analogues. This result is also consistent with data obtained with DA transporter blockers (see Fig. 38–3). Given that other amphetamine-like stimulants, such as methylphenidate and pemoline, also inhibit DA uptake and enhance release of DA, presynaptic enhancement of DA transmission is likely to be the key pharmacologic property mediating wake promotion for all amphetamines and amphetamine-like stimulants.

The role of the DA system in sleep regulation was further assessed using mice lacking the DAT gene. Consistent with a role of DA in the regulation of wakefulness, these animals have reduced non-REM sleep time and increased wakefulness consolidation (independent from locomotor effects).[43] DAT knockout mice have also proven to be a powerful tool to help dissect the molecular mechanisms mediating the effects of nonselective monoaminergic compounds. Using these animals, DAT was shown to be involved in mediating locomotor activation after amphetamine and cocaine administration. Indeed, no locomotor stimulation is observed in these mice after cocaine or amphetamine,[44,45] although, interestingly, the deletion of DAT alone does not fully eliminate cocaine reward.[46] NET knockout mice are more sensitive to the locomotor stimulation of amphetamine, suggesting that NET may play a feedback control role in amphetamine-induced dopaminergic effects.[47] With regard to sleep, the most striking finding was that DAT knockout mice were completely unresponsive to the wake-promoting effects of methamphetamine, GBR-12909 (a selective DAT blocker), and modafinil. These results further confirm the critical role of DAT in mediating the wake-promoting effects of amphetamines and modafinil[43] (see Figs. 38–3 and 38–4; also see section on modafinil). DAT knockout animals were also found to be more sensitive to caffeine,[43] suggesting functional interactions between adenosine and DA systems in the control of sleep/wake (see section on caffeine).

The VMAT2 gene has been cloned and mice lacking VMAT2 have been produced.[48,49] Although homozygous VMAT2 knockout mice (VMAT2 –/–) are nonviable, heterozygous animals (VMAT2 +/–) survive and express a 50% reduction of VMAT2 concentration. VMAT2 +/– mice have a significant deficit of DA transmission but normal noradrenergic and serotonergic neurotransmission.[48,49] VMAT2 heterozygous knockout mice are supersensitive to amphetamine locomotor stimulation, but have an attenuated amphetamine-conditioned behavioral reward.[48,49] Recent results in our laboratory suggest that methamphetamine and modafinil similarly promote wakefulness in both VMAT2 +/– and VMAT2 +/+ animals. This suggests that VMAT blockade by amphetamine is not required for its wake-promoting effect. The results are in contrast to the absence of any wake-promoting effects of these drugs in DAT knockout mice.

Anatomic Substrates Mediating Dopaminergic Effects on Wakefulness

Anatomic studies have demonstrated two major subdivisions of the ascending DA projections from mesencephalic DA nuclei (ventral tegmental area [VTA], substantia nigra (SN), and retrorubral nucleus [A8]): (1) The mesostriatal system originates in the SN and retrorubral nucleus and terminates in the dorsal striatum (principally the caudate and putamen).[50] (2) The mesolimbocortical DA system consists of the mesocortical and mesolimbic DA systems. The mesocortical system originates in the VTA and the medial SN and terminates in the limbic cortex (medial prefrontal, anterior cingulated, and entorhinal cortices). DA reuptake is of physiologic importance for the elimination of DA in cortical hemispheres, limbic forebrain, and striatum, but not in midbrain DA neurons.[51] It is thus possible that DA uptake inhibitors (and amphetamine and modafinil) act mostly on DA terminals of the cortical

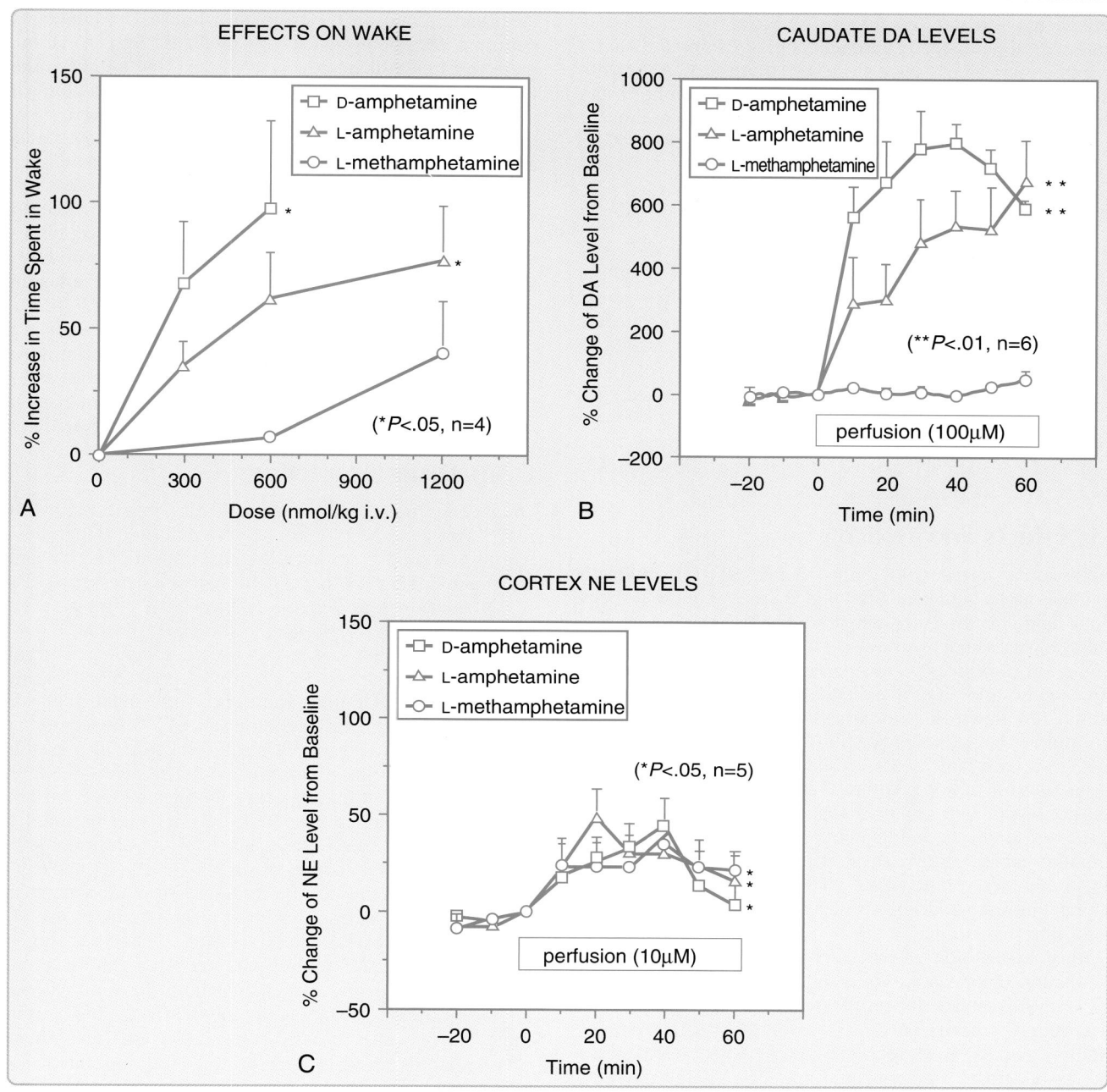

Figure 38–4. Effect of D-amphetamine, L-amphetamine, and L-methamphetamine on time spent in wake during 6-hr polygraphic recordings in narcoleptic Dobermans **(A)**; and effects of local perfusion of D-amphetamine, L-amphetamine, and L-methamphetamine on caudate dopamine (DA) **(B)** and cortex norepinephrine (NE) **(C)** release in narcoleptic Dobermans. **A,** Polygraphic recordings in canine narcolepsy demonstrated that D-amphetamine was approximately 3 times more potent than L-amphetamine, and 12 times more potent than L-methamphetamine in increasing wakefulness. **B,** Amphetamine derivatives (100 μM) were perfused locally for 60 min through a dialysis probe implanted in the caudate of narcoleptic dogs (n = 4). The local perfusion of D-amphetamine raised DA levels nine times above baseline. L-Amphetamine also increased DA levels by up to seven times, but peak DA release was obtained only at the end of the 60-min perfusion period. L-Methamphetamine did not change DA levels under these conditions. **C,** Amphetamine derivatives were perfused for 60 min (10 μM) through the dialysis probes in the frontal cortex. Amphetamine derivatives all significantly increased cortex NE levels above baseline, and there was no significant difference between the potencies of the three derivatives on NE efflux.

hemispheres, limbic forebrain, and striatum to induce wakefulness. Local perfusion experiments of DA compounds in rat and canine narcolepsy have suggested that the VTA, but not the SN, is critically involved in EEG arcusal regulation.[52,53] DA terminals of the mesolimbocortical DA system may thus be important in mediating wakefulness after DA-related CNS stimulant coadministration.

Indications

Amphetamine and methylphenidate are primarily indicated for narcolepsy, idiopathic hypersomnia, and ADHD. Other therapeutic uses are controversial because of their abuse potential. As a result, amphetamine is classified as a schedule II substance, and methylphenidate is classified as a schedule III substance under the Controlled Substances Act of 1970. Moreover, certain states (e.g., Wisconsin) have passed even more restrictive legislation limiting the use of these substances to specific indications (see also Piscopo[54]). The use of these compounds is highly regulated and, in the United States, requires triplicate prescription and monthly renewal.

Side Effects and Toxicology

Amphetamine releases not only DA but NE. NE indirectly stimulates alpha- and beta-adrenergic receptors, a profile common to all indirectly acting sympathomimetic compounds. This results in significant cardiovascular effects. Alpha-adrenergic stimulation produces vasoconstriction, thereby increasing both systolic and diastolic blood pressure. Heart rate may slightly slow down in reflex (this effect is more pronounced than indirect beta-adrenergic stimulation on heart rate at low doses) but, with large doses, cardiac dysrhythmia may occur. Cardiac output is not modulated by therapeutic doses, and cerebral blood flow is unchanged.[55] In general, smooth muscles respond to amphetamine as they do with other sympathomimetic drugs. There is a contractile effect on the urinary bladder sphincter, an effect that has been used in treating enuresis and incontinence. Pain and difficulty in micturition may occur.

Other acute side effects include mild gastrointestinal disturbance, anorexia, dryness of the mouth, tachycardia, cardiac dysrhythmias, insomnia and restlessness, headaches, palpitations, dizziness, and vasomotor disturbances. Agitation, confusion, dysphoria, apprehension, and delirium may also occur. Other documented side effects include flushing, pallor, excessive sweating, and muscular pains. Tiredness and sleepiness as well as lethargy and listlessness may occur when the effects wear off, together with a mild depression of mood. For common side effects of CNS stimulant drugs in narcoleptic patients, refer to Table 38–1.

Common side effects occurring during long-term treatment in narcolepsy include irritability, headache, bad temper, and profuse sweating (reported by over one third of subjects). Other, less common side effects include anorexia, gastric discomfort, nausea, talkativeness, insomnia, orofacial dyskinesia, nervousness, palpitations, muscle jerking, chorea, and tremor. Psychiatric symptoms such as delusions or hallucinations may also occur, but are rather rare in narcoleptic patients who receive amphetamine.

Methamphetamine (and to a lesser extent amphetamine) can be neurotoxic at high doses. This effect is mediated by a free radical increase, causing mitochondrial damage and decreasing adenosine triphosphate synthesis. In dopaminergic neurons, the neurotoxicity is mediated by formation of peroxynitrite, which can be reduced by antioxidants or L-carnitine.[56] L-Carnitine is needed to transport long-chain fatty acids into mitochondria for fatty acid oxidation, preventing the generation of free radicals and peroxynitrite. MDMA, another amphetamine derivative with a preferential effect (and toxicity) on serotoninergic neurons, appears also to decrease glutathione and vitamin E in the brain. Mice deficient in vitamin E were found to have greater susceptibility to both MDMA neurotoxicity and hepatic necrosis, a finding further supporting a free radical mechanism for amphetamine toxicity.[57]

The side effect profile of methylphenidate is similar to that of amphetamine and includes nervousness, insomnia, and anorexia, as well as dose-related systemic effects such as increased heart rate and blood pressure. Methylphenidate overdose may lead to seizures, dysrhythmias, or hyperthermia.

Drug–Drug Interactions

Drug–drug interactions with amphetamine and methylphenidate are generally pharmacodynamic/neurochemical in nature.[58] A small portion of the metabolism of amphetamine and methylphenidate occurs through the cytochrome P-450 (CYP) enzyme CYP2D6, and drugs that inhibit CYP2D6 metabolism can theoretically increase plasma levels of amphetamine. This is, however, rarely a significant problem with therapeutic doses. Tricyclic antidepressant drugs inhibit the metabolism of amphetamine and amphetamine-like stimulants and enhance their behavioral effects.[59-61] The combination of amphetamine with tricyclics could theoretically raise blood pressure further (because of the combined effects of NE reuptake and release), but in practice amphetamine 10 to 16 mg (and also methylphenidate 10 to 60 mg, and mazindol 2 to 12 mg), have been safely given with imipramine and clomipramine 10 to 100 mg to treat narcolepsy-cataplexy.[60,61] The dosage of amphetamine required to control narcolepsy may be reduced by one third by the simultaneous use of tricyclic drugs.[62] MAO-A inhibitors (e.g., nialamide, pargyline, and tranylcypromine) inhibit the removal of amphetamine by the liver and greatly potentiate the behavioral effects of amphetamine.[62] Coadministration of MAOIs and amphetamine derivatives is usually contraindicated. In contrast to tricyclic antidepressants and MAO-A inhibitors, haloperidol, reserpine, and atropine have no effect on amphetamine hydroxylation in the animal liver, although they may reduce the central effects of amphetamine.[2] Chlorpromazine, trifluoperazine, perphenazine, and thioproperazine increase the half-life of amphetamine in the brain but inhibit its central behavioral effects, such as stereotyped behavior in animals and euphoria in humans.[2]

Hypnotic drugs prevent many behavioral effects of amphetamines, although chlordiazepoxide and diazepam increase amphetamine tissue levels.[2]

NONAMPHETAMINE STIMULANTS

Modafinil

Modafinil (2-[(diphenylmethyl)sulfinyl]acetamide) is a chemically unique compound (see Fig. 38–1). It was developed in France and has been available in Europe since 1986.

Modafinil has recently been approved in the United States for the treatment of narcolepsy, essential hypersomnia, and shift work disorder, and for the treatment of residual sleepiness in treated patients with the sleep apnea syndrome. Modafinil is a primary metabolite of adrafinil, a vigilance-promoting compound developed in France in the 1970s. Modafinil lacks adrafinil's terminal amide hydroxy group (see Fig. 38–1) and is better tolerated.

Modafinil is rapidly absorbed but slowly cleared. It has fairly high protein binding and a V_d of 0.8 L/kg. Its half-life is 11 to 14 hours. Up to 60% of modafinil is converted into modafinil acid and modafinil sulfone, both of which are inactive metabolites. Metabolism primarily occurs through CYP3A4/5, but the compound has also been reported to induce CYP2C19 in vitro.[63] Modafinil is available as a racemic mixture of two active isomers. The elimination profile of the two isomers is reversed in rats versus humans. In humans, the D-isomer is cleared three times faster than L-isomer, and women clear modafinil faster than do men.[64] The two isomers may also have slightly different pharmacodynamic properties, and the longer-acting isomer is currently under development.

Modafinil is one of the few compounds that have been specifically developed for the treatment of narcolepsy. Early clinical trials in France and Canada have shown that 100 to 300 mg modafinil is effective in improving daytime sleepiness in narcolepsy and hypersomnia without interfering with nocturnal sleep, but has limited efficacy on cataplexy and other symptoms of abnormal REM sleep.[65-67] Pharmacologic experiments in canine narcolepsy also demonstrated that modafinil has no effects on cataplexy, although it significantly increases time spent in wakefulness.[68] A recent double-blinded trial in 18 centers in the United States on 283 narcoleptic subjects revealed that 200 mg and 400 mg of modafinil significantly reduced EDS and improved the patients' overall clinical condition. Modafinil is well tolerated. The most frequent reported side effects are headache and nausea.[69]

Several factors make modafinil an attractive alternative to amphetamine-like stimulants. First, animal studies suggest that the compound does not affect blood pressure as much as amphetamines do.[70] Modafinil administration is only rarely associated with high blood pressure and tachycardia, generally at high doses (>800 mg/day).[71] This suggests that modafinil might be useful for patients with a heart condition or high blood pressure. Second, data obtained to date suggest that tolerance and dependence are limited with this compound,[65,72] although a recent animal study suggested cocaine-like discriminative stimulus and reinforcing effects of modafinil in rats and monkeys, respectively.[73] Third, modafinil has few effects on the neuroendocrine system. A comparison of healthy volunteers who were sleep deprived for 36 hours with those who received modafinil during sleep deprivation found no difference in cortisol, melatonin, or growth hormone levels.[74] Fourth, clinical experience suggests that the alerting effects of modafinil might be qualitatively different from those observed with amphetamine.[65] In general, patients feel less irritable or agitated with modafinil than with amphetamines,[65] and do not experience severe rebound hypersomnolence once modafinil is eliminated. This differential profile is substantiated by animal experiments. In rats and dogs, modafinil does not increase locomotion beyond the effect expected in association with increased wakefulness.[68,75] Similarly, modafinil acutely decreases both REM and non-REM sleep in rats for up to 5 to 6 hours,

but the effect is not followed by a rebound hypersomnolence. This profile contrasts with the intense recovery sleep seen after amphetamine-induced wakefulness.[76] Considering the many advantages of modafinil over amphetamine treatment (fewer cardiovascular side effects, lower abuse potential and tolerance, and less rebound sleepiness when the drug effects are waning), modafinil has replaced amphetamine-like stimulants as a first-line treatment for EDS.

Current indications for modafinil include narcolepsy and hypersomnia. It has also been recently approved by the U.S. Food and Drug Administration for the treatment of shift work disorder and residual sleepiness in treated patients with sleep apnea (usually with continuous positive airway pressure). There are several reports suggesting that modafinil is also effective for treatment of ADHD,[77,78] fatigue in multiple sclerosis,[79] and EDS in myotonic dystrophy[80] or Prader-Willi syndrome. Modafinil is also being used in the treatment of periodic hypersomnia, where treatment immediately after initiation of the episode may be critical.

The mechanism of action of modafinil is highly debated. An interaction or involvement of alpha$_1$-adrenergic systems was initially suggested by the ability of the alpha$_1$ antagonist, prazosin, to antagonize modafinil-induced increases in motor activity in mice[81] and wakefulness in cats.[82] However, modafinil does not bind to alpha$_1$ receptors in vivo (Ki greater than 10^{-3} M, obtained from prazosin binding using canine cortex; see Shelton et al.[68]). Furthermore, previous studies in the canine model of narcolepsy have shown that alpha$_1$-adrenergic agonists are potent anticataplectic agents[83-85] and have a significant acute hypertensive effect.[85] The facts that modafinil has no anticataplectic activity and lacks hypertensive effects rather suggest that its alerting properties are not derived from alpha$_1$-adrenergic stimulation.

A serotoninergic 5-HT2 receptor–mediated change in gamma-aminobutyric acid (GABA)–ergic transmission was next suggested.[86] Modafinil increases 5-HT metabolism in the striatum and reduces GABA flow to the cortex.[86] The effect on GABA release is blocked by ketanserin (a 5-HT2 antagonist) but not by prazosin.[86] Furthermore, muscimol, a GABAergic agonist, blocks the effect of modafinil on wakefulness in cats.[82] Although serotonergic/GABAergic interaction may be involved in the mode of action of modafinil, the effects described may be indirect and additional work is needed to substantiate this hypothesis. As for the 5-HT2 receptor, modafinil does not bind serotoninergic receptors in vitro.

In 1993, it was observed that selective dopaminergic reuptake inhibitors have no effect on canine cataplexy, yet these compounds seem to increase alertness selectively.[87] Modafinil had a similar profile. It was subsequently found that modafinil has a low but selective affinity for the DAT.[38,88] The EEG-promoting effects of dopamine reuptake inhibitors were later found to correlate with in vitro affinity for DAT (see Fig. 38–3). As mentioned earlier, modafinil (as well as amphetamine) has no wake-promoting effects in DAT knockout mice, clearly demonstrating that an intact DAT molecule is required for mediating modafinil's arousal effect.[43]

Other investigators have shown, however, that modafinil can be distinguished pharmacologically from most other compounds with presynaptic dopaminergic activity. For example, modafinil does not produce stereotypic behavior at high doses.[81] In addition, agents that inhibit dopaminergic function, such as D$_1$ blockers, D$_2$ blockers, and tyrosine hydroxylase blockers, have no effects on modafinil's locomotor-enhancing effects in mice.[89] Finally, an in vitro voltametric study found that modafinil did not increase the catechol oxidation peak height (an indirect measure of dopaminergic activity), suggesting a lack of presynaptic dopaminergic involvement of modafinil activity.[90] Ferraro et al.,[91] however, reported that systemic administration of modafinil (30 to 300 mg/kg) dose-dependently increased DA release in the nucleus accumbens in rats, but these authors claimed that the DA-releasing action of modafinil was most likely secondary to its ability to reduce local GABAergic transmission.

Not only is the exact molecular target of modafinil action uncertain, but there is much debate regarding modafinil's neuroanatomic site of action. Anatomic studies coupled with functional markers of neuronal activity (i.e., the immediate early gene product, c-Fos) have been used to determine activation patterns induced by modafinil in comparison with other stimulants.[92] In cats, amphetamine and methylphenidate induce c-Fos throughout the cortex, striatum, and other brain regions. In contrast, modafinil induces a much more restricted pattern of neuronal activation, with marked expression of c-Fos in neurons of the anterior hypothalamus area and SCN, brain regions that have been implicated in sleep and circadian regulation.[92] Modafinil also increases c-Fos expression in hypocretin cells[93,94] and histaminergic cells of the tuberomammillary nucleus; these effects have been suggested to mediate the wake-promoting effects of modafinil. At higher doses, the striatum and cingulate cortex are also activated.[94] However, it is likely that the stimulation of hypocretin cells is not essential to induce wakefulness because both hypocretin receptor-2–mutated canine narcolepsy and hypocretin-ligand–deficient human narcolepsy (90% of patients with narcolepsy-cataplexy) respond well to modafinil treatment. More probably, activation of these cell groups is secondary to the expression of increased wakefulness because c-Fos expression in these cell groups increases in naturally occurring wakefulness.

Gallopin and colleagues recently reported that modafinil inhibits the sleep-active neurons of the ventrolateral preoptic area (VLPO), a sleep-promoting network of neurons, by facilitating adrenergic neurotransmission.[95] In this study, modafinil potentiated the inhibitory effects of NE on VLPO neurons in a slice preparation. Surprisingly, modafinil did not potentiate the inhibitory effects of dopamine or serotonin on VLPO neurons. Nisoxetine, a potent NET inhibitor with low affinity to DAT,[38] had a similar effect, and the response to the two drugs was not additive, suggesting they might work through the same biochemical pathways. Because modafinil does not bind to the NET[38] and NE uptake inhibitors do not possess strong wake-promoting effects, modafinil may modulate NE/DA uptake mechanisms through novel mechanisms. In this case, modafinil may work on both the DA and NE system to promote wakefulness,[96] and adrenergic/DAT interactions may be involved. However, very high modafinil concentrations (usually 200 μM, the maximum that can be dissolved) were used in this study in vitro. It may also be that at this very high dose, small effects on adrenergic uptake undetectable with usual radioligand receptor binding assays could occur.

Further studies of the action of modafinil are needed to clarify the aforementioned discrepancies regarding its modes of action and may lead to new and interesting insights regarding the mode of action of stimulant medications in general.

Mazindol

Mazindol (2 to 6 mg/day) is rarely used in the United States. At these dosages, mazindol produces central stimulation, a reduction in appetite, and an increase in alertness, but has little or no effect on mood or the cardiovascular system.[97-100] Mazindol is a weak releasing agent for DA that also blocks both DA and NE reuptake. Mazindol has a high affinity for DAT and NET (see Nishino et al.[38]) yet, interestingly, this compound has a low abuse potential. This compound is effective for the treatment of both EDS and cataplexy in humans[101] and for canine narcolepsy,[102] possibly because of its dual dopaminergic and noradrenergic effects.[38] Problematically, however, mazindol often causes significant side effects, including anorexia, gastrointestinal discomfort, insomnia, nervousness, dry mouth, nausea, constipation, urinary retention, and occasionally angioneurotic edema, vomiting, and tremor.[103] The relatively poor tolerance at higher dosages may explain its lack of popularity and lower abuse potential.

Bupropion

Bupropion is a DA reuptake inhibitor that may be useful for the treatment of EDS associated with narcolepsy.[38,104] It may be especially useful in cases associated with atypical depression.[104] Bupropion was synthesized in 1966 by a group seeking new antidepressants chemically related to tricyclic antidepressants but without any significant sympathomimetic, cholinolytic, and MAO inhibitory properties. Bupropion is classified as a monocyclic phenylbutylamine of the aminoketone group. It selectively blocks DA uptake, and is 6 times more potent than imipramine and 19 times more potent than amitriptyline in blocking DA reuptake. The selectivity of bupropion for DAT is not absolute. Bupropion is a weak competitive inhibitor of NE reuptake (65-fold less potent than imipramine). Very limited serotoninergic effects are also observed (200-fold less potent than imipramine).

Selegiline (L-Deprenyl)

Selegiline is a methamphetamine derivative and a potent, irreversible, MAO-B–selective inhibitor primarily used for the treatment of Parkinson's disease.[105,106] Low doses of selegiline do not necessitate dietary restriction, as is usually required with other irreversible MAOIs. Ten milligrams of selegiline daily has no effect on the symptoms of narcolepsy, but 20 to 30 mg improves alertness and mood and reduces cataplexy, an effect comparable to D-amphetamine at the same dose.[107-110] Selegiline may be an interesting alternative to the use of more classic stimulants because its potential for abuse has been reported to be very low.[109]

The fact that this compound is often considered as a simple MAO-B inhibitor rather than an amphetamine precursor deserves special mention. Selegiline not only inhibits MAO-B irreversibly, it also metabolizes into amphetamine (20% to 60% in urine) and methamphetamine (9% to 30% in urine).[106] In the canine model of narcolepsy, selegiline (2 mg/kg orally) was demonstrated to be an effective anticataplectic agent, but this effect was found to be mediated by its amphetamine metabolites rather than through MAO-B inhibition.[111] Several trials in human narcolepsy have demonstrated a good therapeutic efficacy of selegiline on both sleepiness and cataplexy with relatively few side effects.[107-110]

Caffeine

Caffeine may be the most popular and widely consumed CNS stimulant in the world. An average cup of coffee contains 50 to 150 mg of caffeine. Tea, cola drinks, chocolate, and cocoa all contain significant amounts of caffeine. Caffeine can also be bought over the counter (No Doz, 100 mg caffeine; Vivarin, 200 mg caffeine), and is commonly used by narcoleptic patients before diagnosis.

Taken orally, caffeine is rapidly absorbed. The half-life of caffeine is 3.5 to 5 hours. The behavioral effects of caffeine include increased mental alertness, a faster and clearer flow of thought, wakefulness, and restlessness.[112] Fatigue is reduced and sleep onset delayed.[112] The physical effects of caffeine include palpitations, hypertension, increased gastric acid secretion, and increased urine output.[112] Heavy consumption (12 or more cups per day, or 1.5 g of caffeine) causes agitation, anxiety, tremors, rapid breathing, and insomnia.[112]

Caffeine is a xanthine derivative. The mechanism of action of caffeine on wakefulness involves nonspecific adenosine receptor antagonism. Adenosine is an endogenous sleep-promoting substance with neuronal inhibitory effects. In animals, sleep can be induced after administration of metabolically stable adenosine analogues with adenosine A_1 receptor (A1R) or A_{2A} receptor (A2AR) agonistic properties, such as N-6-L-(phenylisopropyl)-adenosine, adenosine-5′-N-ethylcarboxamide, and cyclohexyladenosine.[113,114] Adenosine content is increased in the basal forebrain after sleep deprivation. Adenosine has thus been proposed to be a sleep-inducing substance accumulating in the brain during prolonged wakefulness.[115]

Most studies in the area of sleep and adenosinergic effects have focused on A1R-mediated effects.[116,117] The rationale for this focus is that A1Rs are widely distributed in the CNS, whereas A2ARs are discretely localized in the striatum, nucleus accumbens, and olfactory bulb. Sleep–wake patterns and response to sleep deprivation were recently examined in A1R knockout mice and found to be generally unaltered, suggesting that the constitutional lack of A1R does not prevent homeostatic regulation of sleep. In contrast, the sleep-inhibitory effect of 8-cyclopentyltheophylline (a selective A1R antagonist) was abolished in these animals, indicating A1R mediation of stimulant effects with this compound.

Recent experiments using several selective A1R and A2AR agonists, and A2AR knockout mice indicate that A2AR may play an important role in sleep regulation.[118] Prostaglandin D_2, a somnogenic prostanoid highly concentrated in the brain, mediates its sleep-enhancing effects indirectly through an A2AR-sensitive pathway.[119] A2AR also interacts strongly with dopaminergic transmission. A2AR forms a heterodimer with dopamine D_2 receptors, and A2AR knockout mice have been shown to have reduced amphetamine-induced locomotor simulation and reward.[120-122]

FUTURE STIMULANT TREATMENTS

As discussed in Chapters 64 through 66, the sleep disorder narcolepsy is caused by alterations of hypocretin (orexin) transmission in animal models and humans.[93,123] Most notably, human narcolepsy is caused by a dramatic decrease in hypocretin levels in the brain and the cerebrospinal fluid.[124-129] This raises the possibility that hypocretin-based stimulant therapies may be designed in the future. Hypocretin-1 and hypocretin-2 are produced by a small group of neurons localized in the lateral hypothalamus. The neurons project to the olfactory bulb, cerebral cortex, thalamus, hypothalamus, and brainstem, particularly the locus coeruleus, VTA, and raphe nucleus, and to cholinergic nuclei and cholinoceptive sites (such as the pontine reticular formation) thought to be important for sleep regulation.[130]

A series of studies have shown that the hypocretin system is a major excitatory system that controls the activity of monoaminergic and cholinergic systems with major effects on vigilance states.[131,132] Hypocretins potently excite most monoaminergic neurons, including the adrenergic locus coeruleus, dopaminergic VTA, serotonergic raphe, and histaminergic tuberomammillary neurons.[133-136] It is thus likely that a deficiency in hypocretin neurotransmission induces an imbalance between these classic neurotransmitter systems, with primary effects on sleep state organization and vigilance.

The potential effect of hypocretin injections on wakefulness has been explored by several groups. Whereas the effects of peripherally administered hypocretins is controversial,[137,138] central administration of hypocretin-1 (more stable than hypocretin-2) strongly promotes wakefulness in animals.[137,139,140] Recent experiments in canine narcolepsy (receptor-mutated and ligand-deficient) suggest that stable and centrally active hypocretin analogues (possibly nonpeptide synthetic hypocretin ligands) will need to be developed to be effective peripherally.[137] This is also substantiated by a recent study that found normalization of sleep–wake patterns and behavioral arrest episodes (equivalent to cataplexy and REM sleep onset) in orexin/hypocretin-deficient mice knockout models supplemented by central administration of hypocretin-1.[141]

Histaminergic compounds represent another potential for drug development in the area of wake promotion. Histamine has long been implicated in the control of vigilance, and H_1 receptor antagonists are strongly sedative. The downstream effects of hypocretins on the histaminergic system (excitatory effects through hypocretin receptor 2 stimulation) are likely to be important in mediating the wake-promoting properties of hypocretin.[133,142,143] In fact, brain histamine and cerebrospinal fluid histamine contents are reduced in narcoleptic subjects.[144,145] Although centrally injected histamine or histaminergic H_1 agonists promote wakefulness, systemic administration of these compounds induces various unacceptable side effects through peripheral H_1 receptor stimulation. In contrast, the histaminergic H_3 receptors are regarded as inhibitory autoreceptors, and are enriched in the CNS.[146] H_3 antagonists enhance wakefulness in normal rats and cats[147,148] and in narcoleptic mice models.[149] Histaminergic H_3 antagonists might be a useful as wake-promoting compounds for the treatment of EDS or as cognitive enhancers and are under study at several pharmaceutical companies.

Other pathways with possible applications in the development of novel stimulant medications include the adenosinergic system (see earlier), the adrenergic system (e.g., some NE reuptake inhibitors), the GABAergic system (e.g., inverse benzodiazepine agonists), the glutamatergic system (ampakines), thyrotropin-releasing hormone analogues,[150,151] and some other classes of compounds.[152]

CONCLUSION

Amphetamine-like stimulants have been used in the treatment of narcolepsy and various other conditions for decades, yet only recently has the mode of action of these drugs on vigilance been characterized. In almost all cases, the effects on vigilance were found to be mediated by effects on the DAT. This has led to the widely accepted hypothesis that wake-promoting effects will be impossible to differentiate from abuse potential effects for these compounds. However, the various mediations available have differential effects and potency on the DAT and on monoamine storage/release. The various available stimulants are more or less selective for DA versus other amines. Even if much work remains to be done in this area, it appears more and more likely that complex properties, such as the ability to release DA rather than simply block reuptake, plus the combined effects on other monoamines (such as serotonin), may be important to explain abuse potential. Differential binding properties on the DAT itself may also be involved, together with drug potency and compound solubility. The lack of solubility of some low-potency compounds may, for example, result in an inability to administer the drug by snorting or intravenous injection. Finally, lower abuse potential for these compounds has long been suspected in patients with narcolepsy-cataplexy, either because of the biochemical hypocretin abnormality or because of the social aspects of treating narcolepsy as a disease.

The mode of action of modafinil remains controversial and may involve dopaminergic or nondopaminergic effects, or both. Whatever its mode of action, the compound is in general found to be safer and to have a lower abuse potential than amphetamine stimulants. Its favorable side effect profile has led to its increasing use for indications other than narcolepsy, most recently in the context of shift work disorder and residual sleepiness in patients with treated sleep apnea. This recent success exemplifies the need for developing novel wake-promoting compounds with low abuse potential. A need for treating daytime sleepiness extends well beyond the relatively rare indication of narcolepsy-cataplexy.

> *Clinical Pearl*
>
> Almost all the currently available medications used to treat EDS (amphetamines, amphetamine-like stimulants, and modafinil) act presynaptically to increase dopaminergic transmission, either by stimulating dopamine release or by blocking dopamine reuptake. These effects are believed to be critically involved in the mediation of the wake-promoting effects of these compounds. Caffeine is a nonselective adenosine receptor blocker. The potency and efficacy of caffeine are too low to provide substantial relief in the treatment of narcolepsy. When using stimulants for the treatment of sleepiness, it is suggested that compounds with minimal effects on dopamine release (e.g. modafinil) be started first, followed by dopamine releasing agents without effects on dopamine storage (e.g. methylphenidate). Drugs with strong effects on dopamine storage and release (e.g. amphetamine and methamphetamine) should be used only when the other compounds are not effective. In contrast to methyphenidate and amphetamine, modafinil has been shown to have limited or no abuse potential.

Acknowledgment

This work is partially supported by National Institutes of Health grant NS-23724.

REFERENCES

1. Snyder SH: Drugs and the Brain. New York, Scientific American Library, 1986.
2. Parkes JD: Central nervous system stimulant drugs. In Thorpy M (ed): Handbook of Sleep Disorders. New York, Marcel Dekker, 1990, pp 755-778.
3. Julien RM: A Primer of Drug Action: A Concise, Nontechnical Guide to the Actions, Uses, and Side Effects of Psychoactive Drugs, 7th ed. New York, WH Freeman, 1995.
4. Weiner N: Norepinephrine, epinephrine, and the sympathomimetic amines. In Gilman AG, Goodman LS, Theodore WR, Murad F (eds): The Pharmacological Basis of Therapeutics, 7th ed. New York, Macmillan, 1985, pp 145-180.
5. Alles GA: The comparative physiological actions of d 1-beta-phenylisopropylamines: Pressor effects and toxicity. J Pharmacol Exp Ther 47:339-354, 1933.
6. Seijun T: Metamphetamine psychosis. In Ellinwood EH, Cohen S (eds): Current Concepts on Amphetamine Abuse. Rockville, Md, National Institute of Mental Health, 1970, pp 159-161.
7. Connell PH: Amphetamine Psychosis. London, Oxford University Press, 1958.
8. Prinzmetal M, Bloomberg W: The use of benzedrine for the treatment of narcolepsy. JAMA 1935;105:2051-2054.
9. Yoss RE, Daly DD: Treatment of narcolepsy with Ritalin. Neurology 1959;9:171-173.
10. Bradley C, Bowen M: Amphetamine (benzedrine) therapy of children's behavior disorders. Am J Orthopsychiatry 1941;11:92-103.
11. Anders TF, Ciaranello RD: Pharmacologic treatment of minimal brain dysfunction syndrome. In Barchas JD, Berger PA, Ciaranello RD (eds): Psychopharmacology: From Theory to Practice. New York, Oxford University Press, 1977, pp 425-435.
12. Fawcett J, Kravitz HM, Zajecka JM, Schaff MR: CNS stimulant potentiation of monoamine oxidase inhibitors in treatment-refractory depression. J Clin Psychopharmacol 1991;11:127-132.
13. Feighner JP, Herbstein J, Damlouji N: Combined MAOI, TCA, and direct stimulant therapy of treatment-resistant depression. J Clin Psychiatry 1985;46:206-209.
14. Masand PS, Anand VS, Tanquary JF: Psychostimulant augmentation of second generation antidepressants: a case series. Depress Anxiety 1998;7:89-91.
15. Olin J, Masand P: Psychostimulants for depression in hospitalized cancer patients. Psychosomatics 1996;37:57-62.
16. Glennon RA: Psychoactive phaenylisopropylamines. In Meltzer HY (ed): Psychopharmacology: The Third Generation of Progress. New York, Raven Press, 1987, p 1627.
17. Fujimori M. Himwich HE: Electroencephalographic analyses of amphetamine and its methoxy derivatives with reference to their sites of EEG alerting in the rabbit brain. Int J Neuropharmacol 1969;8:601-613.
18. Janssen PA, Leysen JE, Megens AA, Awouters FH: Does phenylethylamine act as an endogenous amphetamine in some patients? Int J Neuropsychopharmacol 1999;2:229-240.
19. Hartmann A, Cravens J: Sleep: Effect of D- and L-amphetamine in man and rat. Psychopharmacology 1976;50:171-175.
20. Angrist BM, Shopsin B, Gershon S: Comparative psychotomimetic effects of stereoisomers of amphetamine. Nature 1971;234:152-153.
21. Williams RT, Caldwell RJ, Dreng LG: Comparative metabolism of some amphetamines in various species. In Schneider SH, Esdin E (eds): Frontiers of Catecholamine Research. Oxford, Pergamon, 1973, 927-932.
22. Beckett AH, Rowland M, Turner P: Influence of urinary pH on excretion of amphetamine. Lancet 1965;1:303.

23. Seiden L, Sabol KE, Ricaurte GA: Amphetamine: Effects on catecholamine systems and behavior. Annu Rev Pharmacol Toxicol 1993;32:639-677.

24. Kuczenski R, Segal DS: Neurochemistry of amphetamine. In Cho AK, Segel DS (eds): Psychopharmacology, Toxicology and Abuse. San Diego, Academic Press, 1994, pp 81-113.

25. Axelrod J, Weil-Malherbe H, Tomchik R: The physiological disposition of 3H-epinephrine and its metabolite metanephrine. J Pharmacol Exp Ther 1959;127:251-256.

26. Shimada S, Kitayama S, Lin C-L: Cloning and expression of a cocaine-sensitive dopamine transporter complementary DNA. Science 1991;254:576-578.

27. Kilty JE, Lorang D, Amara SG: Cloning and expression of a cocaine-sensitive rat dopamine transporter. Science 1991;254:578-580.

28. Pacholczyk T, Blakely RD, Amara SG: Expression cloning of a cocaine- and antidepressant-sensitive human noradrenaline transporter. Nature 1991;350:350-354.

29. Gonzalez AM, Walther D, Pazos A, Uhl GR: Synaptic vesicular monoamine transporter expression: distribution and pharmacologic profile. Brain Res Mol Brain Res 1994;22:219-226.

30. Sulzer D, Rayport S: Amphetamine and other psychostimulants reduce pH gradients in midbrain dopaminergic neurons and chromaffin granules: A mechanism of action. Neuron 1990;5:797-808.

31. Sulzer D, Chen TK, Lau YY, et al: Amphetamine redistributes dopamine from synaptic vesicles to the cytosol and promotes reverse transport. J Neurosci 1995;15:4102-4108.

32. Baker TL, Dement WC: Canine narcolepsy-cataplexy syndrome: Evidence for an inherited monoaminergic-cholinergic imbalance. In McGinty DJ, Drucker-Colin R, Morrison A, Parmeggiani PL (eds): Brain Mechanisms of Sleep. New York, Raven Press, 1985, pp 199-233.

33. Baker TL, Foutz AS, McNerney V, et al: Canine model of narcolepsy: Genetic and developmental determinants. Exp Neurol 1982;75:729-742.

34. Nishino S, Mignot E: Pharmacological aspects of human and canine narcolepsy. Prog Neurobiol 1997;52:27-78.

35. Nishino S, Okura M, Mignot E: Narcolepsy: Genetic predisposition and neuropharmacological mechanisms. Sleep Med Rev 2000;4:57-99.

36. Nicholson AN, Pascoe PA: Dopaminergic transmission and the sleep-wakefulness continuum in man. Neuropharmacology 1990;29:411-417.

37. Monti JM: Catecholamines and the sleep-wake cycle: I. EEG and behavioral arousal. Life Sci 1982;30:1145-1157.

38. Nishino S, Mao J, Sampathkumaran R, et al: Increased dopaminergic transmission mediates the wake-promoting effects of CNS stimulants. Sleep Res Online 1998;1:49-61. Available at http://www.sro.org/1998/Nishino/1949.

39. Kanbayashi T, Nishino S, Honda K, et al: Differential effects of D- and L-amphetamine isomers on dopaminergic transmission: Implication for the control of alertness in canine narcolepsy. Sleep Res 1997;26:383.

40. Kuczenski R, Segal DS, Cho A, Melega W: Hippocampus norepinephrine, caudate dopamine and serotonin and behavioral responses to the stereoisomers of amphetamine and methamphetamine. J Neurosci 1995;15:1308-1317.

41. Chiueh CC, Moore KE: Relative potencies of D- and L-amphetamine on the release of dopamine from cat brain in vivo. Res Commun Chem Pathol Pharmacol 1974;7:189-199.

42. Ferris RM, Tang FLM, Maxwell RA: A comparison of the capacities of isomers of amphetamine, deoxypiperadrol and methylphenidate to inhibit the uptake of tritiated catecholamines into rat cerebral cortex slices, synaptosomal preparations of rat cerebral cortex, hypothalamus and striatum and into adrenergic nerves of rabbit aorta. J Pharmacol Exp Ther 1972;181:407-416.

43. Wisor JP, Nishino S, Sora I, et al: Dopaminergic role in stimulant-induced wakefulness. J Neurosci 2001;1:1787-1794.

44. Giros B, Jaber M, Jones SR, et al: Hyperlocomotion and indifference to cocaine and amphetamine in mice lacking the dopamine transporter. Nature 1996;379:606-612.

45. Gainetdinov RR, Jones SR, Caron MG: Functional hyperdopaminergia in dopamine transporter knock-out mice. Biol Psychiatry 1999;46:303-311.

46. Sora I, Wichems C, Takahashi N, et al: Cocaine reward models: Conditioned place preference can be established in dopamine- and in serotonin-transporter knockout mice. Proc Natl Acad Sci U S A 1998;95:7699-7704.

47. Xu F, Gainetdinov RR, Wetsel WC, et al: Mice lacking the norepinephrine transporter are supersensitive to psychostimulants. Nat Neurosci 2000;3:465-471.

48. Uhl GR, Li S, Takahashi N, et al: The VMAT2 gene in mice and humans: Amphetamine responses, locomotion, cardiac arrhythmias, aging, and vulnerability to dopaminergic toxins. FASEB J 2000;14:2459-2465.

49. Takahashi N, Miner LL, Sora I, et al: VMAT2 knockout mice: heterozygotes display reduced amphetamine-conditioned reward, enhanced amphetamine locomotion, and enhanced MPTP toxicity. Proc Natl Acad Sci U S A 1997;94:9938-9943.

50. Björklund A, Lindvall O: Dopamine-containing systems in the CNS. In Björklund A, Hökfelt T (eds): Handbook of Chemical Neuroanatomy, vol 2: Classical Transmitters in the CNS, Part I. Amsterdam, Elsevier, 1984, pp 55-121.

51. Nissbrandt N, Engberg G, Pileblad E: The effects of GBR 12909, a dopamine re-uptake inhibitor, on monoaminergic neurotransmission in rat striatum, limbic forebrain, cortical hemispheres and substantia nigra. Naunyn Schmiedebergs Arch Pharmacol 1991;344:16-28.

52. Honda K, Riehl J, Mignot E, Nishino S: Dopamine D3 agonists into the substantia nigra aggravate cataplexy but do not modify sleep. Neuroreport 1999;10:3717-3724.

53. Bagetta G, De Sarro G, Priolo E, Nistico G: Ventral tegmental area: site through which dopamine D2-receptor agonists evoke behavioural and electrocortical sleep in rats. Br J Pharmacol 1988;95:860-866.

54. Piscopo A: The impact of prescription drug diversion control systems on medical practice and patient care. In National Institute on Drug Abuse Technical Review Meeting, 1991. Bethesda, Md, 1991.

55. Hoffman BB, Lefkowitz RJ: Catecholamine and sympathomimetic drugs. In Gilman AG, Goodman LS, Rall TW, Murad F (eds): The Pharmacological Basis of Therapeutics, 8th ed. New York, Macmillan, 1993, pp 187-220.

56. Virmani A, Gaetani F, Imam S, et al: The protective role of L-carnitine against neurotoxicity evoked by drug of abuse, methamphetamine, could be related to mitochondrial dysfunction. Ann NY Acad Sci 2002;965:225-232.

57. Johnson EA, Shvedova AA, Kisin E, et al: d-MDMA during vitamin E deficiency: Effects on dopaminergic neurotoxicity and hepatotoxicity. Brain Res 2002;933:150-163.

58. Markowitz JS, Patrick KS: Pharmacokinetic and pharmacodynamic drug interactions in the treatment of attention-deficit hyperactivity disorder. Clin Pharmacokinet 2001;40:753-772.

59. Burrell JM, Black M, Wharton RN, et al: Inhibition of imipramine metabolism by methylphenidate. Fed Proc 1969;28:418.

60. Cooper TB, Simpson GM: Concomitant imipramine and methylphenidate administration: A case report. Am J Psychiatry 1973;130:6.

61. Wharton RN, Perel JM, Dayton PG, et al: A potential clinical use for methylphenidate with tricyclic antidepressants. Am J Psychiatry 1971;127:1619-1625.

62. Carlton PL: Potentiation of the behavioural effects of amphetamines by imipramine. Psychopharmacologia 1961;2:364-376.

63. Robertson P, DeCory HH, Madan A, Parkinson A: In vitro inhibition and induction of human hepatic cytochrome P450 enzymes by modafinil. Drug Metab Dispos 2000;28:664-671.

64. Wong YN, King SP, Simcoe D, et al: Open-label, single-dose pharmacokinetic study of modafinil tablets: Influence of age and gender in normal subjects. J Clin Pharmacol 1999;39:281-288.

65. Bastuji H, Jouvet M: Successful treatment of idiopathic hypersomnia and narcolepsy with modafinil. Prog Neuropsychopharmacol Biol Psychiatry 1988;12:695-700.

66. Besset A, Tafti M, Villemine E, Billiard M: Effect du modafinil (300mg) sur le sommeil, la somnolence et la vigilance du narcoleptique. Neurophysiol Clin 1993;23:47-60.

67. Boivin DB, Montplaisir J, Petit D, et al: Effect of modafinil on symptomatology of human narcolepsy. Clin Neuropharmacol 1993;16:46-53.

68. Shelton J, Nishino S, Vaught J, et al: Comparative effects of modafinil and amphetamine on daytime sleepiness and cataplexy of narcoleptic dogs. Sleep 1995;18:817-826.

69. U.S. Modafinil in Narcolepsy Multicenter Study Group: Randomized trial of modafinil for the treatment of pathological somnolence in narcolepsy. Ann Neurol 1998;43:88-97.

70. Hermant JF, Rambert FA, Deuteil J: Lack of cardiovascular effects after administration of modafinil in conscious monkeys. Fundam Clin Pharmacol 1991;5:825.

71. Wong YN, Simcoe D, Hartman LN, et al: A double-blind, placebo-controlled, ascending-dose evaluation of the pharmacokinetics and tolerability of modafinil tablets in healthy male - volunteers. J Clin Pharmacol 1999;39:30-40.

72. LaGarde D: Sustained/continuous operations subgroup of the department of defense human factors engineering technical group: Program Summary and Abstracts from the 9th Semiannual Meeting. In 1990 March: Pensacola, Fla, Naval Aerospace Medical Research Laboratory, 1990, pp 90-91.

73. Gold LH, Balster RH: Evaluation of the cocaine-like discriminative stimulus effects and reinforcing effects of modafinil. Psychopharmacology 1996;126:286-292.

74. Brun J, Chamba G, Khalfallah Y, et al: Effect of modafinil on plasma melatonin, cortisol and growth hormone rhythms, rectal temperature and performance in healthy subjects during a 36 h sleep deprivation. J Sleep Res 1998;7:105-114.

75. Edgar DM, Seidel WF, Contreras P, et al: Modafinil promotes EEG wake without intensifying motor activity in the rat. Can J Physiol Pharmacol 1994;72(Suppl 1):362.

76. Edgar DM, Seidel WF: Modafinil induces wakefulness without intensifying motor activity or subsequent rebound hypersomnolence in the rat. J Pharmacol Exp Ther 1997;283:757-769.

77. Rugino TA, Copley TC: Effects of modafinil in children with attention-deficit/hyperactivity disorder: An open-label study. J Am Acad Child Adolesc Psychiatry 2001;40:230-235.

78. Rugino TA, Samsock TC: Modafinil in children with attention-deficit hyperactivity disorder. Pediatr Neurol 2003;29:136-142.

79. Rammohan KW, Rosenberg JH, Lynn DJ, et al: Efficacy and safety of modafinil (Provigil) for the treatment of fatigue in multiple sclerosis: A two centre phase 2 study. J Neurol Neurosurg Psychiatry 2002;72:179-183.

80. Damian MS, Gerlach A, Schmidt F, et al: Modafinil for excessive daytime sleepiness in myotonic dystrophy. Neurology 2001; 56:794-796.

81. Duteil J, Rambert FA, Pessonnier J, et al: Central α1-adrenergic stimulation in relation to the behaviour stimulating effect of modafinil: Studies with experimental animals. Eur J Pharmacol 1990;180:49-58.

82. Lin JS, Roussel B, Akaoka H, et al: Role of catecholamines in modafinil and amphetamine induced wakefulness: A comparative pharmacological study. Brain Res 1992;591:319-326.

83. Nishino S, Fruhstorfer B, Arrigoni J, et al: Further characterization of the alpha-1 receptor subtype involved in the control of cataplexy in canine narcolepsy. J Pharmacol Exp Ther 1993;264: 1079-1084.

84. Mignot E, Guilleminault C, Bowersox S, et al: A role of central alpha-1 adrenoceptor in canine narcolepsy. J Clin Invest 1988; 82:885-894.

85. Renaud A, Nishino S, Dement WC, et al: Effect of SDZ NVI-085, a putative subtype selective alpha-1 agonist on canine cataplexy. Eur J Pharmacol 1991;205:11-16.

86. Tanganelli S, Fuxe K, Ferraro L, Jansen AM: Inhibitory effects of the psychoactive drug modafinil on gamma-aminobutyric acid outflow from the cerebral cortex of the awake freely moving guinea pig. Arch Pharmacol 1992;345:461-465.

87. Mignot E, Renaud A, Nishino S, et al: Canine cataplexy is preferentially controlled by adrenergic mechanisms: Evidence using monoamine selective uptake inhibitors and release enhancers. Psychopharmacology 1993;113:76-82.

88. Mignot E, Nishino S, Guilleminault C, Dement WC: Modafinil binds to the dopamine uptake carrier site with low affinity. Sleep 1994;17:436-437.

89. Simon P, Hemet C, Ramassamy C, Costentin J: Non-amphetaminic mechanism of stimulant locomotor effect of modafinil in mice. Eur Neuropsychopharmacol 1995;5:509-514.

90. De Séréville JE, Bore C, Rambert FA, Duteil J: Lack of presynaptic dopaminergic involvement in modafinil activity in anaesthetized mice: In vivo voltammetry studies. Neuropharmacology 1994;33:755-761.

91. Ferraro L, Tananelli S, O'Connor WT, et al: The vigilance promoting drug modafinil increases dopamine release in the rat nucleus accumbens via the involvement of a local GABAergic mechanism. Eur J Pharmacol 1996;306:33-39.

92. Lin JS, Hou Y, Jouvet M: Potential brain neuronal targets for amphetamine-, methylphenidate-, and modafinil-induced wakefulness, evidenced by c-fos immunocytochemistry in the cat. Proc Natl Acad Sci U S A 1996;93:14128-14133.

93. Chemelli RM, Willie JT, Sinton CM, et al: Narcolepsy in orexin knockout mice: Molecular genetics of sleep regulation. Cell 1999;98:437-451.

94. Scammell TE, Estabrooke IV, McCarthy MT, et al: Hypothalamic arousal regions are activated during modafinil-induced wakefulness. J Neurosci 2000;20:8620-8628.

95. Gallopin T, Luppi PH, Rambert FA, et al: Effect of the wake-promoting agent modafinil on sleep-promoting neurons from the ventrolateral preoptic nucleus: An in vitro pharmacologic study. Sleep 2004;27:19-25.

96. Saper CB, Scammell TE: Modafinil: A drug in search of a mechanism. Sleep 2004;27:11-12.

97. Gogerty JJ, Trapold JH: Chemistry and pharmacology of mazindol. Triangle 1976;15:25-36.

98. Parkes JD, Shachter M: Mazindol in the treatment of narcolepsy. Acta Neurol Scand 1979;60:250-254.

99. Vespignani H, Barroche G, Escaillas JP, Weber M: Importance of mazindol in the treatment of narcolepsy. Sleep 1984;7:274-275.

100. Maclay WP, Wallace MG: A multicentre general practice trial of mazindol in the treatment of obesity. Practitioner 1977;218: 431-440.

101. Iijima S, Sugita Y, Teshima Y, Hishikawa Y: Therapeutic effects of mazindol on narcolepsy. Sleep 1986;9:265-268.

102. Nishino S, Mao J, Sampathkumaran R, et al: Adrenergic, but not dopaminergic, uptake inhibition reduces REM sleep and cataplexy concomitantly. Sleep Res 1997;26:445.

103. Wallace AG: AN 448 Sandoz (mazindol) in the treatment of obesity. Med J Aust 1976;1:343.

104. Rye DB, Dihenia B, Bliwise DL: Reversal of atypical depression, sleepiness, and REM-sleep propensity in narcolepsy with bupropion. Depress Anxiety 1998;7:92-95.

105. Golbe LI: Deprenyl as symptomatic therapy in Parkinson's disease. Clin Neuropharmacol 1988;11:387-400.

106. Reynolds GP, Elsworth JD, Blau K, et al: Deprenyl is metabolized to methamphetamine and amphetamine in man. Br J Clin Pharmacol 1978;6:542-544.

107. Hublin C, Partinen M, Heinonen EH, et al: Selegiline in the treatment of narcolepsy. Neurology 1994;44:2095-2101.

108. Reinish LW, McFarlane JG, Sandor P, Shapiro CM: REM changes in narcolepsy with selegiline. Sleep 1995;18:362-367.

109. Roselaar SE, Langdon N, Lock CB, et al: Selegiline in narcolepsy. Sleep 1987;10:491-495.

110. Mayer G, Meier E, Hephata K: Selegiline hydrochloride in narcolepsy: A double-blind placebo-controlled study. Clin Neuropharmacol 1995;18:306-319.

111. Nishino S, Arrigoni J, Kanbayashi T, et al: Comparative effects of MAO-a and MAO-b selective inhibitors on canine cataplexy. Sleep Res 1996;25:315.

112. Rall TR: Central nervous system stimulants. In Gilman AG, Goodman LS, Rall TW, Murad F (eds): The Pharmacological Basis of Therapeutics, 7th ed. New York, Pergamon Press, 1985, pp 345-382.

113. Radulovacki M, Virus RM, Djuricic-Nedelson M, Green RD: Adenosine analogs and sleep in rats. J Pharmacol Exp Ther 1984;228:268-274.

114. Radulovacki M, Miletich RS, Green RD: N6 (L-phenylisopropyl) adenosine (L-PHA) increases slow-wave sleep (S2) and decreases wakefulness in rats. Brain Res 1982;246:178-180.

115. Porkka-Heiskanen T, Strecker RE, Thakkar M, et al: Adenosine: A mediator of the sleep-inducing effects of prolonged wakefulness. Science 1997;276:1265-1268.

116. Porkka-Heiskanen T, Kalinchuk A, Alanko L, et al: Adenosine, energy metabolism, and sleep. Sci World J 2003;3:790-798.

117. Strecker RE, Morairty S, Thakkar MM, et al: Adenosinergic modulation of basal forebrain and preoptic/anterior hypothalamic neuronal activity in the control of behavioral state. Behav Brain Res 2000;115:183-204.

118. Urade Y, Eguchi N, Qu WM, et al: Minireview: Sleep regulation in adenosine A(2A) receptor-deficient mice. Neurology 2003;61(11 Suppl 6):S94-S96.

119. Satoh S, Matsumura H, Suzuki F, Hayaishi O: Promotion of sleep mediated by the A2a-adenosine receptor and possible involvement of this receptor in the sleep induced by prostaglandin D2 in rats. Proc Natl Acad Sci U S A 1996;93:5980-5984.

120. Chen JF, Beilstein M, Xu YH, et al: Selective attenuation of psychostimulant-induced behavioral responses in mice lacking A(2A) adenosine receptors. Neuroscience 2000;97:195-204.

121. Chen JF, Moratalla R, Impagnatiello F, et al: The role of the D(2) dopamine receptor (D(2)R) in A(2A) adenosine receptor (A(2A)R)-mediated behavioral and cellular responses as revealed by A(2A) and D(2) receptor knockout mice. Proc Natl Acad Sci U S A 2001;98:1970-1975.

122. Chen JF, Moratalla R, Yu L, et al: Inactivation of adenosine A2A receptors selectively attenuates amphetamine-induced behavioral sensitization. Neuropsychopharmacology 2003;28:1086-1095.

123. Lin L, Faraco J, Li R, et al: The sleep disorder canine narcolepsy is caused by a mutation in the hypocretin (orexin) receptor 2 gene. Cell 1999;98:365-376.

124. Nishino S, Ripley B, Overeem S, et al: Hypocretin (orexin) deficiency in human narcolepsy. Lancet 2000;355:39-40.

125. Nishino S, Ripley B, Overeem S, et al: Low CSF hypocretin (orexin) and altered energy homeostasis in human narcolepsy. Ann Neurol 2001;50:381-388.

126. Mignot E, Lammers GJ, Ripley B, et al: The role of cerebrospinal fluid hypocretin measurement in the diagnosis of narcolepsy and other hypersomnias. Arch Neurol 2002;59: 1553-1562.

127. Nishino S: The hypocretin/orexin system in health and disease. Biol Psychiatry 2003;54:87-95.

128. Peyron C, Faraco J, Rogers W, et al: A mutation in a case of early onset narcolepsy and a generalized absence of hypocretin peptides in human narcoleptic brains. Nat Med 2000;6:991-997.

129. Thannickal TC, Moore RY, Nienhuis R, et al: Reduced number of hypocretin neurons in human narcolepsy. Neuron 2000;27: 469-474.

130. Peyron C, Tighe DK, van den Pol AN, et al: Neurons containing hypocretin (orexin) project to multiple neuronal systems. J Neurosci 1998;18:9996-10015.

131. Willie JT, Chemelli RM, Sinton CM, Yanagisawa M: To eat or to sleep? Orexin in the regulation of feeding and wakefulness. Annu Rev Neurosci 2001;24:429-458.

132. Taheri S, Zeitzer JM, Mignot E: The role of hypocretins (orexins) in sleep regulation and narcolepsy. Annu Rev Neurosci 2002; 25:283-313.

133. Eriksson KS, Sergeeva O, Brown RE, Haas HL: Orexin/hypocretin excites the histaminergic neurons of the tuberomammillary nucleus. J Neurosci 2001;21:9273-9279.

134. Korotkova TM, Sergeeva OA, Eriksson KS, et al: Excitation of ventral tegmental area dopaminergic and nondopaminergic neurons by orexins/hypocretins. J Neurosci 2003;23:7-11.

135. Brown RE, Sergeeva O, Eriksson KS, Haas HL: Orexin A excites serotonergic neurons in the dorsal raphe nucleus of the rat. Neuropharmacology 2001;40:457-459.

136. Nakamura T, Uramura K, Nambu T, et al: Orexin-induced hyperlocomotion and stereotypy are mediated by the dopaminergic system. Brain Res 2000;873:181-187.

137. Fujiki N, Ripley B, Yoshida Y, et al: Effects of IV and ICV hypocretin-1 (orexin A) in hypocretin receptor-2 gene mutated narcoleptic dogs and IV hypocretin-1 replacement therapy in a hypocretin ligand deficient narcoleptic dog. Sleep 2003; 6:953-959.

138. John J, Wu MF, Siegel JM: Systemic administration of hypocretin-1 reduces cataplexy and normalizes sleep and waking durations in narcoleptic dogs. Sleep Res Online 2000;3:23-28. http:www.sro.org/2000/John/23/

139. Piper DC, Upton N, Smith MI, Hunter AJ: The novel brain neuropeptide, orexin-A, modulates the sleep-wake cycle of rats. Eur J Neurosci 2000;12:726-730.

140. Hagan JJ, Leslie RA, Patel S, et al: Orexin A activates locus coeruleus cell firing and increases arousal in the rat. Proc Natl Acad Sci U S A 1999;96:10911-10916.

141. Mieda M, Willie JT, Hara J, et al: Orexin peptides prevent cataplexy and improve wakefulness in an orexin neuron-ablated model of narcolepsy in mice. Proc Natl Acad Sci U S A, 2004;101: 4649-4654.

142. Huang ZL, Qu WM, Li WD, et al: Arousal effect of orexin A depends on activation of the histaminergic system. Proc Natl Acad Sci U S A 2001;98:9965-9970.

143. Yamanaka A, Tsujino N, Funahashi H, et al: Orexins activate histaminergic neurons via the orexin 2 receptor. Biochem Biophys Res Commun 2002;290:1237-1245.

144. Nishino S, Fujiki N, Ripley B, et al: Decreased brain histamine contents in hypocretin/orexin receptor-2 mutated narcoleptic dogs. Neurosci Lett 2001;313:125-128.

145. Nishino S, Sakurai E, Nevisimalova S, et al: CSF histamine content is decreased in hypocretin-deficient human narcolepsy. Sleep 2002;25(Suppl):A476.

146. Leurs R, Blandina P, Tedford C, Timmerman H: Therapeutic potential of histamine H3 receptor agonists and antagonists. Trends Pharmacol Sci 1998;19:177-183.

147. Monti JM, Jantos H, Ponzoni A, Monti D: Sleep and waking during acute histamine H3 agonist BP 2.94 or H3 antagonist carboperamide (MR 16155) administration in rats. Neuropsychopharmacology 1996;15:31-35.

148. Lin JS, Sakai K, Vanni-Mercier G, et al: Involvement of histaminergic neurons in arousal mechanisms demonstrated with H3-receptor ligands in the cat. Brain Res 1990;523:325-330.

149. Shiba T, Fujiki N, Wisor J, et al: Wake promoting effects of thioperamide, a histamine h3 antagonist in orexin/ataxin-3 narcoleptic mice. Sleep 2004;(Suppl):A241-242.

150. Nishino S, Arrigoni J, Kanbayashi T, et al: TRH and its analogs significantly reduce canine cataplexy. Sleep Res 1995; 24A:352.

151. Riehl J, Honda K, Kwan M, et al: Chronic oral administration of CG-3703, a thyrotropin releasing hormone analog, increases wake and decreases cataplexy in canine narcolepsy. Neuropsychopharmacology 2000;23:34-45.

152. Mignot E, Taheri S, Nishino S: Sleeping with the hypothalamus: Emerging therapeutic targets for sleep disorders. Nat Neurosci 2002;5(Suppl):1071-1075.

39

Wake-Promoting Medications: Efficacy and Adverse Effects

Merrill M. Mitler

Mary B. O'Malley

ABSTRACT

There are a variety of wake-promoting medications used to treat excessive sleepiness, ranging from over-the-counter caffeine, to schedule II amphetamine-like compounds. Each has a potential role in the clinical treatment of excessive sleepiness due to sleep disorders. Because their pharmacologic profiles are diverse, the clinician may guide selection of the agent based on a variety of factors: time of onset, length of activity, degree of tolerance in chronic use, side effects expected, and abuse liability. Although the traditional stimulants have been prescribed most widely for disorders such as narcolepsy, modafinil, a nonsympathomimetic compound, is now considered a first-line wake-promoting agent for this disorder. Modafinil has also recently received U.S. Food and Drug Administration approval for treatment of excessive sleepiness due to shift work sleep disorder and in patients with obstructive sleep apnea whose sleepiness fails to remit despite optimal treatment with nasal continuous positive airway pressure. Understanding the underlying pharmacology of the range of alerting agents available may also clarify the qualitative aspects of wakefulness that they affect.

Wake-promoting medications fall into three chemical classes: (1) direct-acting sympathomimetics, such as the alpha$_1$-adrenergic agonist phenylephrine; (2) indirect-acting sympathomimetics, such as methylphenidate, amphetamine, mazindol, and pemoline; and (3) the "nonstimulants" that are not sympathomimetics, and have different mechanisms of action, such as modafinil and caffeine. The pharmacology of sympathomimetics is reviewed in Chapter 38. This chapter focuses on the clinical use of alerting medications.

THE HISTORY OF WAKE-PROMOTING MEDICATIONS

Psychostimulants have been used for centuries in tonics and other preparations to allay fatigue and treat a variety of ailments (for reviews, see Haddad[1] and Angrist and Sudilovsky[2]). One of the oldest and most ubiquitous psychostimulants is caffeine. As early as 1672, coffee, along with leaves of sage or rosemary, was prescribed for disorders associated with sleepiness. The effect of coffee on sleepiness stems from caffeine. It has been consumed in some form for much of human history, but was not officially discovered until 1819. The native peoples of Peru and Bolivia used cocaine, a crystalline alkaloid derived from the leaves of the coca plant, for pleasure and to increase stamina. From 1886 to 1905, cocaine was an ingredient in Coca-Cola. The medicinal use of cocaine was advocated by Freud.[3] However, cocaine's profound potential for abuse and addiction soon limited the role of this stimulant in modern medicine.

The treatment of narcolepsy underwent a dramatic change with the introduction of ephedrine. In 1931, Doyle and Daniels[4] and Janota[5] described the use of ephedrine to treat sleepiness. Despite its clinically noteworthy efficacy, it was soon apparent that side effects, incomplete patient acceptance, rapid development of tolerance, and cost limited its usefulness. In 1935, Prinzmetal and Bloomberg[6] suggested that amphetamine sulfate would be appropriate treatment for narcolepsy because of its close relationship to ephedrine and epinephrine, its low toxicity and low cost, its prolonged action, and its lack of pronounced sympathomimetic side effects. In their first report, nine patients noted complete relief from sleep attacks and practically complete relief from cataplexy. They noted that insomnia and restlessness were potential problems and that the medication should not be given late in the day. They recommended 10-mg doses initially with a gradual increase until an optimal effect was obtained.

By 1949, amphetamines, racemic B-phenylisopropylamine, in one or another of the several oral preparations as a phosphate or sulfate, had become the treatment of choice for excessive sleepiness due to narcolepsy, with a typical initial treatment of 10 mg three times daily, followed by gradual increases until sleepiness was controlled. Methylphenidate, a piperidine derivative, was introduced in the 1950s as a milder stimulant. After 1956, methylphenidate came into broad use, as suggested by Yoss and Daly.[7] Pemoline, an oxazolidine compound, was later introduced as a mild central nervous system (CNS) stimulant. Mazindol, an imidazoline derivative, is another mild stimulant marketed as an appetite suppressant. Since the 1970s, the treatment of narcolepsy has been modified by the introduction of rapid eye movement sleep–suppressing antidepressants to treat cataplexy and the reintroduction of psychological and sleep hygiene advice.

Modafinil (2-iphenylmethylsulfinyl acetamide) is a racemic compound unrelated to the amphetamines or other CNS stimulants. Of all the alerting agents, modafinil has the most specific and selective wake-promoting properties, and usually has minimal side effects. Modafinil began to appear on the world market for the indication of narcolepsy and CNS hypersomnia in the early 1990s, and is now considered a first-line agent for treatment of these conditions.[8] The recent additional U.S. Food and Drug Administration (FDA)–approved indications for modafinil—treatment of excessive sleepiness due to shift work sleep disorder (SWSD) and in patients with

Table 39–1.   Caffeine Content of Popular Ingestibles

Product	Serving Size	Caffeine Content (mg)	Product	Serving Size	Caffeine Content (mg)
*Coffees**			*Soft Drinks (cont'd)*		
Coffee	8 oz	110	Caffeine-free Pepsi or Diet Pepsi	12 oz	0
Coffee, decaf	8 oz	5	Minute Maid Orange Soda	12 oz	0
Starbucks Coffee, grande	16 oz	550	*Caffeinated Waters*		
Starbucks Coffee, short	8 oz	250	Java Water	500 mL	125
Starbucks Coffee, tall	12 oz	375	Krank 20	500 mL	100
Espresso	1 oz	90	Aqua Blast	500 mL	90
Espresso, decaf	1 oz	10	Water Joe	500 mL	60-70
Instant coffee	8 oz	75	Aqua Java	500 mL	50-60
Caffe Latte	6 oz	90	Red Bull	250 mL	80
Arizona Blue Luna Iced Coffees	8 oz	40-50	Red Eye Gold	250 mL	48
Arizona Iced Coffees	8 oz	40-50	*Chocolate*		
Coffee Ice Cream	8 oz	58	Baker's chocolate	1 oz	26
*Teas**			Chocolate milk beverage	8 oz	5
Arizona Iced Tea, Black Tea	8 oz	16	Chocolate-flavored syrup	1 oz	4
Arizona Iced Tea, Green Tea	8 oz	7.5	Cocoa beverage	8 oz	6
Arizona Iced Tea, Rx Power and Energy	8 oz	30	Dark chocolate, semisweet	1 oz	20
Brewed, Imported Brands	8 oz	60	Milk chocolate	1 oz	6
Brewed, Major U.S. Brands	8 oz	40	*Medications*		
Lipton Brisk Iced Tea	8 oz	6	Anacin	2 tablets	26
Mistic Teas	8 oz	17 (avg.)	Aqua Ban	1 tablet	100
Snapple Iced Tea, all kinds	8 oz	21	Cafergot	1 tablet	100
Soft Drinks			Caffedrine	2 capsules	200
Josta	12 oz	58	Coryban-D	1 tablet	30
Mountain Dew	12 oz	55.5	Darvon Compound	1 tablet	32
Surge	12 oz	52.5	Dexatrim	1 tablet	200
Diet Coke	12 oz	46.5	Dristan	1 tablet	30
Coca-Cola	12 oz	34.5	Excedrin, max. strength	2 tablets	130
Dr. Pepper, regular or diet	12 oz	42	Fiorinal	1 tablet	40
Sunkist Orange Soda	12 oz	42	Midol	1 tablet	32
Pepsi-Cola	12 oz	37.5	Migralam	1 tablet	100
Diet Pepsi	12 oz	36	Neo-Synephrine	1 tablet	15
Diet RC	12 oz	54	NoDoz, max. strength; Vivarin	1 tablet	200
Tab	12 oz	70	NoDoz, regular strength	1 tablet	100
Barqs Root Beer	12 oz	22.5	Percodan	1 tablet	32
Barqs Diet Root Beer	12 oz	0	Permathene Water Off	1 tablet	100
7-Up or Diet 7-Up	12 oz	0	Pre-Mens Forte	1 tablet	50
Sprite or Diet Sprite	12 oz	0	Prolamine	1 tablet	140
Mug Root Beer	12 oz	0	Triaminicin	1 tablet	30
Caffeine-free Coke or Diet Coke	12 oz	0	Vanquish	1 tablet	33

*Note: The listed caffeine content is average for a standard brewed cup of coffee or tea; certain brewing methods may increase or decrease the average caffeine content per cup.

From Etherton GM, Kochar MS: Coffee: Facts and controversies. Arch Fam Med 1993;2:317-322.

obstructive sleep apnea (OSA) to augment nasal continuous positive airway pressure (CPAP)—have helped fuel discussion of the more general need for assessment and treatment of pathologic sleepiness in clinical practice.

CAFFEINE

Mechanism of Action

Caffeine can be extracted from plants such as coffee and tea or synthetically produced. The most popular drinks in the world, coffee, tea, and cola, contain caffeine (Table 39–1). Caffeine is also an important CNS-active constituent of chocolate. Caffeine's main mechanism of action on the CNS is antagonism of adenosine receptors.

Adenosine-releasing neurons are found in the hypothalamus, and project to cells in the cortex, basal forebrain, and hypothalamus and to cells of the reticular activating system. It is known that endogenous adenosine levels rise with continued wakefulness and may be a fundamental part of the homeostatic sleep mechanism.[9] Exogenous adenosine promotes slow wave sleep, whereas xanthines, including caffeine, block the A_1 adenosine receptors, thereby inhibiting sleep onset and maintenance. Caffeine inhibits sleep in other mammals and insects through similar mechanisms.[10,11] At high doses, caffeine stimulates the medullary vagal, vasomotor, and respiratory centers, as well as skeletal muscles, giving rise to the common side effects: gastric stimulation, diarrhea, flushing, sweating, increased heart and respiratory rates, and muscle tension and tremor.

Alerting Effects

Caffeine has widely recognized and used effects on alertness, mood, and cognitive performance. The usual dose in tablet form is 50 to 200 mg, and beverages contain amounts within this range as well (see Table 39–1). Caffeine shows peak blood levels 30 minutes to 1 hour after ingestion, and has a half-life typically of 3 to 5 hours. If taken before sleep, caffeine clearly postpones sleep onset, and reduces the amount of stages 3 and 4 sleep.[12] Its disruptive effects on sleep are also well known: Typically, sleep efficiency declines with caffeine consumption taken within a few hours of bedtime. The sleepiness of sleep deprivation in young, healthy, non–caffeine-dependent volunteers can clearly be attenuated both subjectively and objectively using caffeine supplements. In doses of 600 mg of a sustained-release preparation, caffeine reduced slow wave activity on the electroencephalogram and improved psychomotor performance tasks after up to 36 hours of sleep deprivation.[13] Similarly, two 300-mg doses of sustained-release caffeine significantly improved both vigilance and performance during 64 hours of continued wakefulness.[14] In a study of U.S. Navy SEALs randomly assigned to receive 100, 200, or 300 mg caffeine or placebo after 72 hours of sleep deprivation and continuous exposure to other stressors, caffeine at 200 mg or above clearly improved tests of vigilance, alertness, and reaction time. However, it did not improve marksmanship, a task that requires fine motor control that tends to be worsened further by caffeine.[15]

Because it is such a widely available alerting agent, caffeine stands in a unique position to help improve the safety of drivers and shift workers, if used correctly. That is, if used in sufficient doses (usually at least 200 mg), ideally in individuals not already moderately caffeine dependent, it may significantly improve the alertness and cognitive skills that become impaired by sleepiness. The effectiveness is greater in the sustained-release form of 600-mg daily dose, which clearly extends the benefit of short naps for a partially sleep-deprived driver.[16] Caffeine has been shown to substantially improve alertness in a simulated night shift.[17] In regular practice, night shift workers do consume more caffeine than day workers, and yet continue to be at risk of accidents both on the road and at the work place.[18] Clearly, there are multiple factors, including the timing of driving home with the circadian nadir, that compromise the ability of any alerting agent to mitigate severe sleepiness. However, caffeine's potential benefits for alertness may be lost because (1) it may not be consumed in adequate doses; (2) acute benefits are relatively short-lived, and so it must be taken at the right time; and (3) a background of caffeine dependence may reduce its overall ability to be effective. No doubt an educational program to acquaint people with these facts would help center their efforts to become more alert.

In standard daily practice, 85% of Americans use caffeine, many to foster wakefulness on arising from sleep.[19] This culturally accepted truism has been examined, and it is clear that caffeine effectively eliminates the cognitive fog of sleep inertia on psychomotor tasks.[20] This suggests that sleep inertia may be an effect of sustained increased levels of adenosine in the brain, and these levels are successfully antagonized by caffeine's action on the adenosine receptors. It is also commonly assumed that someone intoxicated with alcohol will "sharpen up" by taking strong coffee. In a recent study, a 150-mg dose of caffeine was demonstrated to reverse the effects of modest ethanol consumption (blood alcohol content 0.04%) in normal volunteers on the multiple sleep latency test (MSLT), as well as tests of memory and psychomotor performance, although the dizziness and other somatic changes due to alcohol remained.[21] It is unclear how helpful caffeine would be in cases of greater intoxication.

Compared with the potency of other alerting medications, caffeine is judged to be a moderately effective alerting agent when taken on an intermittent basis. Parkes and Dahlitz estimated that a dose of six cups of strong coffee has about the same effect as 5 mg dextroamphetamine.[22] High doses of caffeine may approximate the efficacy of low doses of stimulants, or of standard doses of modafinil in maintaining alertness and performance during sleep deprivation.[23] In one study, young, healthy adults remained awake for 54.5 hours, and were given placebo, modafinil (100 mg, 200 mg, 400 mg), or caffeine (600 mg). There was similar performance improvement over placebo in subjects treated with caffeine or modafinil at the higher doses, with the best performance being demonstrated by the subjects on modafinil 400 mg. A low incidence of adverse side effects was seen in all conditions. These results suggest that for young, healthy people (such as enlisted recruits), caffeine can be an effective countermeasure to prolonged wakefulness. However, testing over repeated conditions would be necessary to assess the efficacy of caffeine after tolerance had time to develop because the benefits typically diminish quickly in dependent individuals. As such, caffeine is ineffective as a daily treatment for the severe sleepiness of sleep disorders such as narcolepsy and idiopathic CNS hypersomnia.

Side Effects, Dependence, and Withdrawal

The most common side effect of caffeine use is disrupted nighttime sleep. Caffeine reduces slow wave sleep and decreases total sleep time. Individual sensitivity to this varies, and usually those most sensitive to caffeine's effects are acutely aware of it. However, because its effects are often underestimated once tolerance begins to develop, moderate, regular caffeine use in the late afternoon or evening is a frequently overlooked cause of a patient's complaints of sleeplessness. The decline in metabolic rate with age makes caffeine an increasingly likely contributor to sleep fragmentation in the elderly.

Because regular caffeine use is so prevalent in our culture, many studies include it as a variable in looking at the health costs, if any, associated with other health outcomes. So far, moderate to heavy coffee use has been causally associated only with the development of bladder cancer and an increased risk of miscarriage during pregnancy.[24,25] Coffee may also exacerbate several disorders such as fibrocystic breast disease, irritable bowel syndrome, and peptic ulcer disease. Controversy continues concerning the risk of long-term adverse cardiovascular effects.[26] In general, it appears caffeine in moderation appears safe to use if side effects are not apparent.

Caffeine can produce strong CNS and somatic side effects at high doses (above 4 mg/kg body weight). Most common side effects are nervousness, nausea, diarrhea, muscle twitches and cramps, and sleeplessness. Although the lethal level of caffeine is quite high—more than 10 g for an adult, the equivalent of 100 cups of coffee—overdoses have occurred with fatal outcomes to those who submitted to the unorthodox practice of coffee enemas.

Caffeine in moderate daily doses has been shown to produce a withdrawal syndrome after abrupt cessation. In one double-blinded, placebo-controlled study, an average of 235 mg/day was consumed. On discontinuation, subjects reported headache, increased sleepiness, reduced vigor, and worsened mood. These symptoms were seen by the second day after caffeine cessation (20 hours post-caffeine use).[27] Although there are clearly both physical and mental changes associated with withdrawal, an expectation of symptoms may also increase the likelihood that they emerge.[28]

SYMPATHOMIMETIC ALERTING AGENTS

Mechanism of Action

As discussed in detail in Chapter 38, the amphetamines work by directly or indirectly increasing the activity in dopaminergic and noradrenergic CNS systems. The primary effect on alertness is mediated through increased efficacy of the dopaminergic ventral tegmental area and the noradrenergic locus coeruleus, which both project widely throughout the brain. The additional activation of other non–wake-promoting areas (e.g., striatum, nucleus accumbens) accounts for the side effects typical of the sympathomimetics, such as tics and abuse liability.

Alerting Effects

The clinical treatment of excessive sleepiness due to narcolepsy originated with the traditional stimulants, and the dosing guidelines have changed little since their development in the first part of the last century. Early reports described the benefits of dextroamphetamine,[29] methamphetamine,[30] and the use of up to 80 mg of amphetamine sulfate to achieve control of sleepiness.[31] Daly and Yoss, who introduced methylphenidate as a treatment for narcolepsy, reported their experience in using daily doses of methylphenidate ranging from 20 to 200 mg.[7,32] For patients who did not respond well to methylphenidate, Yoss subsequently recommended methamphetamine at a daily dose of up to 40 mg. In Daly and Yoss' 1974 summary[33] of their experience, they advocated that patients be given initial trials of low to moderate dosages of methamphetamine or methylphenidate, with gradual increases in doses to as much as 200 mg of either drug if needed to control sleep attacks. Several preparations of amphetamine have been subsequently developed as oral compounds that vary in terms of the concentration of the dextro-isomer and whether a phosphate or sulfate salt is used. The wide variety of available preparations offer a range of half-lives, and therefore dosing strategies to treat sleepiness.

Side Effects

When used in the treatment of narcolepsy or other conditions, stimulants commonly produce side effects, including irritability, talkativeness, and sympathomimetic side effects such as sweating, particularly at higher doses. The reported frequency of side effects of stimulants in clinical practice and in clinical trials varies from 0% to 73% (references from Table 39–2); the extreme variation reflects, at least in part, differences in methods of determining side effects and the definition of a side effect. Common side effects include headaches, irritability, nervousness or tremulousness, anorexia, insomnia, gastrointestinal complaints, dyskinesias, and palpitations.[7,34,47] Available studies show a wide range of reported side effects, although at high doses, side effects as well as disturbed nocturnal sleep are experienced by most patients.[34,36,48] Pemoline use has been associated with hepatocellular liver damage[49-52]; the mechanism appears to be idiosyncratic and metabolic rather than immunologic.[53] Given the potential for serious side effects, the role of pemoline in the treatment of sleepiness is thus problematic. Because of these concerns, pemoline has been withdrawn from the market in Canada. Side effects with selegiline 20 to 30 mg/day are comparable with those with dextroamphetamine at a similar dose.[45]

Psychiatric complications with the use of sympathomimetics are dose dependent, and more likely to occur in patients with coexisting or preexisting psychiatric conditions.[54-58] Psychosis and hallucinations are rare in narcoleptic patients treated with stimulants.[48,59] In four series totaling 243 patients, there were two cases of amphetamine psychosis, two of hallucinations, and three of addiction.[34,60-62] There is no evidence that different agents confer a greater or lesser risk for psychotic symptoms, although the use of short-acting forms lends itself to mood swings and irritability.

Cardiac and vascular complications due to prescribed sympathomimetics have been reported only rarely in people with narcolepsy. They do not appear to cause a clinically significant increase in blood pressure at commonly used doses in normotensive individuals.[7,34,63] Isolated cases of severe disease such as stroke, cardiomyopathy, and ischemic vascular complications have been reported in the context of chronic use of sympathomimetics, especially at high doses. These complications must be assessed in light of the many narcoleptic patients who have taken stimulants on a regular basis for decades, often into the seventh or eighth decade of life, without experiencing cardiovascular disturbances. Although advanced cardiovascular disease is a reasonable contraindication to sympathomimetic therapy, there are no systematic studies indicating that well-controlled hypertension is exacerbated by moderate doses of stimulants.

Dependence, Abuse, and Withdrawal

Amphetamines and related compounds have a high abuse potential and can produce dependence. Although most users (more than 90%) do not become addicted, controlled use may become compulsive use, especially when the drug is readily available or when a rapid route of administration is used. A sequence of euphoria, dysphoria, paranoia, and psychosis can occur after a single exposure to a high dose or with chronic exposure to low doses. During a binge, the user characteristically administers the drug repeatedly for up to several days, foregoing sleep. After a binge, there is the "crash": extreme exhaustion, often with depression, anxiety, and an intense desire to sleep. The subsequent withdrawal phase is characterized by apathy, anhedonia, and strong drug craving. Episodic craving gradually diminishes over weeks and months.

Sustained use of high doses of amphetamines and related compounds can lead to cognitive and behavioral pathology. In healthy volunteers, repetitive oral administration of 5 to 10 mg of dextroamphetamine produces paranoid delusions, often with blunted affect, after a cumulative dose of 55 to 75 mg.[64] Other symptoms of amphetamine abuse are motor tics, stereotypic movements, and perseveration: repetitive thoughts or organized, goal-directed, but meaningless activity[65] such as repetitive cleaning, elaborate sorting of small objects, or endless disassembly and reassembly of such items as clocks and radios. A variety of complications can occur with intravenous, intranasal, or oral amphetamine or methamphetamine abuse.[66-74] In young adults, the relative risk for stroke is estimated to be 6.5 times greater for drug abusers compared with nonabusers,[72] with amphetamines implicated in a substantial proportion of young drug abusers with stroke.[72,73]

Tolerance to the Alerting Effects of Sympathomimetics

In people with narcolepsy, tolerance to alerting effects appears to occur with variable frequency. In one review, 10 of 100 patients had discontinued stimulants owing to failure to respond, tolerance, or side effects, and 31 others had required doubling of dosage over a 1-year period for the same control of symptoms.[34] Other studies have found a similar or higher amount of tolerance evident clinically in patients using sympathomimetic agents.[59,62] On the other hand, Honda et al.[75] observed no tolerance in 106 narcoleptic patients treated with methylphenidate for up to several years. Tolerance to stimulants appears to be more likely, or at least more evident in patients taking high doses.[76-79] There is little evidence that the incidence of tolerance and side effects is less in people with narcolepsy than others taking sympathomimetics.[80] Further, it does not appear that tolerance reported by some patients is an effect of inadequate nocturnal sleep rather than true tolerance,[81] or that tolerance and other side effects are less likely to occur with methylphenidate than with dextroamphetamine.[33,77]

MODAFINIL

Mechanism of Action

Modafinil is a novel medication chemically unrelated to the amphetamines or other sympathomimetic agents, sometimes referred to as a somnolytic.[82-84] The precise mechanism through which modafinil enhances wakefulness remains unclear. However, progress has been made in the last several years in defining its pharmacologic effects. A carefully designed study in rats demonstrated that low to moderate doses of modafinil increase c-Fos activation in specific brain areas: (1) histaminergic cells in the tuberomammillary nucleus (TMN); (2) hypocretin (orexin)-containing cells in the perifornical area of the posterior lateral hypothalamus; and (3) a portion of the central nucleus of the amygdala.[85] The TMN and hypocretin cell groups are both thought to facilitate wakefulness by virtue of their widespread projections throughout the brain. In addition, modafinil treatment prompted decreased activity in the sleep-promoting ventrolateral preoptic area, most likely secondary to the increased inhibitory input from TMN cells. At higher doses of modafinil, some activation of the striatum and many cortical areas could also be detected. Modafinil did not activate many brain areas known to be activated by amphetamines, including the ventral tegmental area, autonomic control areas, and the nucleus accumbens. The authors comment that all of the modafinil-activated brain areas identified are known to receive both gamma-aminobutyric acid (GABA)–ergic as well as dopaminergic afferents, and so suggest that modafinil may somehow selectively increase dopaminergic or decrease GABAergic neurotransmission in areas known to regulate sleep and wakefulness. Although orexin cell activation may play an important role in wake state control, modafinil-induced wakefulness in narcoleptic humans and animals deficient in orexin suggests that their activation is not essential for the wake-promoting effects of modafinil.

Extensive studies to define further modafinil's mechanism of action have so far failed to identify the specific receptor or other ligand through which modafinil exerts its effects.[86] That is, modafinil does not bind to any known receptor or ligand except for very weak binding at the dopamine transporter.[87] There is conflicting evidence on the role, if any, of dopamine in the mechanism of modafinil's alerting effect. Modafinil does not activate dopaminergic neurons (e.g., the ventral tegmental area), and modafinil-induced wakefulness is not blocked by the catecholamine synthesis inhibitor α-methylparatyrosine or by dopamine receptor blockers; however, dopamine transporter knockout mice appear to be insensitive to modafinil.[84] Clearly, modafinil does not act like an amphetamine to evoke widespread catecholaminergic activity throughout the brain. Moreover, the subcortical effects typical of amphetamines (e.g., stimulation of motor and reward/abuse systems) are largely absent with modafinil treatment. On the other hand, weakly inhibiting the dopamine transporter may become physiologically relevant in certain brain areas like the prefrontal cortex, where there is a paucity of dopamine catabolic systems, and lead to focal enhancement of dopamine-mediated brain functions, especially at higher doses.

To complicate the picture further, a recent in vitro study in rodents has demonstrated that modafinil enhances the activity of norepinephrine on neurons of the ventrolateral preoptic area, causing inhibition of this sleep-promoting brain area.[88] This in vitro activity mimics that of another norepinephrine reuptake inhibitor, nisoxetine, suggesting that modafinil may somehow interact with the norepinephrine transporter to enhance norepinephrine activity. However, when given in vivo, nisoxetine and other norepinephrine transporter inhibitors (e.g., atomoxetine) show only modest enhancement of wakefulness, and demonstrate changes in sleep architecture not seen with modafinil.[89] It is certainly possible that, like other CNS medications that interact with multiple receptor systems (e.g., the atypical antipsychotics), modafinil may have a unique pharmacologic profile that adjusts neuronal activity through a number of biochemical mechanisms to exert its effects on hypothalamic sleep and wakefulness centers.

Alerting Effects

Although in some individuals, 100 mg of modafinil is sufficient to sustain alertness for several hours, most patients with excessive sleepiness require doses of 200 mg/day or higher. In two large populations of narcoleptic patients on 200 to 400 mg/day, alertness measures (Maintenance of Wakefulness Test [MWT], Epworth Sleepiness Scale [ESS], Clinical Global Impression of Change) gradually increased over 9 weeks of double-blinded treatment.[41,42] Clinical and subjective self-assessments of efficacy remained stable for most of those patients who enrolled in open-label studies taking the same dose of modafinil for 3 years.[39,42,90] Some individuals with severe sleepiness may require modafinil at 600 to 800 mg/day in divided doses (morning and noon) for effective control of their symptoms.[91,92] Although these doses are significantly above the FDA-indicated guidelines, if lower doses are well tolerated but ineffective it is reasonable carefully to titrate up to higher doses.

Recently, modafinil has been approved by the FDA for the treatment of excessive daytime sleepiness due to SWSD, and for patients with OSA who continue to have disabling sleepiness despite treatment of airway obstruction during sleep with mechanical treatments such as nasal CPAP. This expanded labeling for modafinil represents the first time that pathologic sleepiness has been more broadly defined as a symptom warranting treatment across a range of disorders.

Nasal CPAP treatment has been clearly demonstrated to improve alertness in patients with OSA,[93] and it may reverse the comorbid cardiovascular effects associated with OSA. However, a significant portion of patients with OSA continue to experience pathologic sleepiness while adhering to CPAP treatment. Some studies have estimated this population to comprise 35% of CPAP-treated patients with OSA.[94] In a large, double-blinded, placebo-controlled study of patients with OSA reporting residual excessive sleepiness while on CPAP, modafinil at doses of 400 mg improved alertness by 2.6 points on the ESS above placebo-treated patients, and more than half the modafinil-treated patients reported normal ESS values (score of less than 10) by the study end point. Further, adjunctive modafinil treatment improved objective measures of alertness on the MSLT (8.6 minutes compared with 7.4 minutes at baseline) without adversely affecting compliance with CPAP.[95] Subsequent studies have also demonstrated the efficacy of modafinil in daily doses of 200 to 400 mg for improving alertness in CPAP-treated patients with OSA with residual sleepiness, and confirmed a relative absence of adverse consequences in this patient population.[95-97] The use of modafinil as adjunctive therapy in the patient with OSA certainly requires adequate education of the patient and proper follow-up to ensure compliance with mechanical treatments that are essential to preventing the cardiovascular morbidity and mortality of OSA. In our experience, the most frequent cause of residual sleepiness in patients with OSA is their failure to sleep with CPAP on for a full 8 hours of sleep per day. However, even with optimal mechanical therapy, chronic sleepiness is clearly a problem for some patients with OSA, perhaps because of the effect of hypoxic episodes before therapy.[98] For appropriate patients, this strategy appears to be a reasonable and safe measure to improve their safety and quality of life.

Another large, ill-defined population of people with chronic, problematic sleepiness is the millions of adults who keep nonstandard work hours. Although many shift workers adapt adequately to the constraints of their schedule, there are many more who suffer at least transiently from the effects of both sleep deprivation and circadian misalignment. Further, it is estimated that approximately 25% of the adults working nonstandard hours have persistent complaints of excessive sleepiness or insomnia consistent with the diagnosis of SWSD (T. Roth, personal communication). A recent, double-blinded, placebo-controlled study of over 200 night-shift workers demonstrated this group to be pathologically sleepy at baseline (MSLT approximately 2 minutes), with significant cognitive impairment (as measured by psychomotor vigilance task), as well as numerous mistakes, near-misses, or accidents at work or while driving home after work. All these measures improved substantially after treatment with 200 mg modafinil taken at the beginning of their night shift. Further, this treatment did not interfere with their ability to sleep during time off duty.[99] On the basis of this and other evidence, the FDA approved modafinil for the treatment of excessive sleepiness due to SWSD in 2004. Together with a program of nonpharmacologic measures to protect sleep time and sleep ability in this patient population, this represents a potentially life-saving treatment for these adults.

Side Effects and Tolerance to Modafinil

Side effects are less frequent with modafinil than with sympathomimetics. The most common adverse event in the initial modafinil trials was a headache, which increased in frequency if the modafinil dose was high or increased too quickly.[41] There have been no significant cardiovascular adverse effects from modafinil treatment in the clinical trials to date, including among patients with OSA.[95] So far, it appears that only patients with a history of sensitivity to activating medications (e.g., those with mitral valve prolapse) experienced cardiovascular side effects from modafinil (e.g., palpitations, chest pain), and these symptoms reversed when the medication was discontinued. The use of modafinil has so far been reported to cause infrequent complaints of insomnia or nervousness, and these symptoms are usually transient and dose dependent. Psychotic symptoms have developed rarely, and only at high doses of modafinil.[100] Modafinil appears to have a very low, or idiosyncratic occurrence of tolerance.

COMPARATIVE CLINICAL EFFICACY OF PRESCRIPTION ALERTING AGENTS

The initial evaluations of the effectiveness of stimulants for the treatment of sleepiness and sleep attacks in narcolepsy were based on clinical assessment.[4-6,29] Yoss and colleagues, the first to apply pupillography[101] to the assessment of sleepiness, measured pupil diameter and stability of pupil diameter to evaluate the response of individual patients to alerting drugs.[81,102] More recently, the MSLT[103] and the MWT (see Chapter 120)[104] have been used to assess sleepiness in a variety of sleep disorders[105] and to evaluate pharmacotherapeutic efficacy.[36,37,106-110] Because the average MSLT or MWT sleep latency can be regarded as a single numeric measure of sleep tendency, some determinations of relative efficacy of pharmacotherapeutic agents have been calculated[111] (Table 39-2). On the whole, patients who are medicated for excessive sleepiness are still monitored primarily by clinical assessment of their ability to remain alert during sedentary activities, with medication selection and dosing decisions adjusted accordingly.

On the basis of available publications, it is impossible objectively to measure the relative efficacy of alerting agents.

Table 39–2.   Efficacy of Alerting Agents for Treatment of Sleepiness in Narcolepsy

Reference	Year of Report	Type of Study	No. of Subjects	Medications	Daily Dose	Efficacy	Side Effects
Daly and Yoss[32]	1956	Case series	25	Methylphenidate	40–240 mg	Good to excellent in 84%	Nervousness and tremulousness (35%), anorexia (22%), insomnia (17%), palpitations (3%)
Yoss and Daly[7]	1959	Case series	60	Methylphenidate	40–80 mg*	Good to excellent in 68%	
Parkes et al.[34]	1975	Case series	63	Dextroamphetamine	5–150 mg	Moderate to good in 73%	Side effects (73%) Irritability (49%) Headache (48%) Palpitations (24%) Jitteriness (24%) Muscle jerks (22%) Insomnia (11%) Dyskinesias (5%) Hallucinations (3%) Psychosis (1.6%)
Honda et al.[35]	1960	Case series	80	Methamphetamine Methylphenidate Dextroamphetamine	5–15 mg 20–80 mg ?? mg	Disappearance of sleep attacks	Disturbed nocturnal sleep
Mitler et al.[36]	1993	Sleep laboratory	8	Methamphetamine	20–60 mg	Improved by MSLT	
Mitler et al.[37]	1990	Sleep laboratory	13	Methylphenidate	10–60 mg	Improved by MWT	
Mitler et al.[37]	1990	Sleep laboratory	5	Dextroamphetamine	30–60 mg	Improved by MWT	
Mitler et al.[37]	1990	Sleep laboratory	14	Pemoline	19–113 mg	Improved by MWT at 113 mg	
Laffont et al.[38]	1987	Placebo controlled	19†	Modafinil	200 mg	Decreased sleep attacks	Side effects in less than 10%
Bastuji and Jouvet[39]	1988	Clinical trial	42‡	Modafinil	200–500 mg	Improvement in 71% with narcolepsy and 83% with idiopathic hypersomnia	Side effects in less than 10%
Broughton et al.[40]	1997	Placebo-controlled, crossover clinical trial	75	Modafinil	200–400 mg	Improved by MWT, clinical and self-report criteria	Side effects not significantly different from placebo
U.S. Modafinil Study Group[41]	1998	Placebo-controlled, parallel-groups clinical trial	283	Modafinil	200–400 mg	Improved by MSLT, MWT, clinical and self-report criteria	Side effects not significantly different from placebo
U.S. Modafinil Study Group[42]	2000	Placebo-controlled, parallel-groups clinical trial	271	Modafinil	200–400 mg	Improved by MSLT, MWT, clinical and self-report criteria	Side effects not significantly different from placebo
Alvarez et al.[43]	1991	Clinical retrospective review	41	Mazindol	1–16 mg	Moderate to good in 78%	39%—Mainly gastrointestinal
Shindler et al.[44]	1985	Placebo-controlled clinical trial	20	Dextroamphetamine Mazindol Fencamfamin	10–30 mg 4 mg 60 mg	Sleep attacks reduced by 36–52%	Side effects similar to placebo
Roselaar et al.[45]	1987	Clinical trial	7	Selegiline	20–30 mg	Sleep attacks reduced by 30%	Similar to dextroamphetamine
Saletu et al.[46]	1989	Placebo-controlled clinical trial	10§	Modafinil Dextroamphetamine	100–200 mg 10–20 mg		Disturbed nocturnal sleep with dextroamphetamine but not with modafinil

*One took 300 mg.

†Twelve with narcolepsy; seven with idiopathic hypersomnia.

‡Twenty-four with narcolepsy; 18 with idiopathic hypersomnia.

§Elderly nonnarcoleptic subjects.

MSLT, Multiple Sleep Latency Test; MWT, Maintenance of Wakefulness Test.

Among the most important problems hampering quantitative comparisons of stimulants are the following: (1) Investigators have used different outcome measures (e.g. clinical assessment, MSLT, MWT); (2) among published reports, subject samples varied widely in the baseline level of sleepiness; (3) some investigators have studied multiple doses, thereby providing a basis for estimating the dose–response curve, whereas others have not; and (4) there is little correlation between oral doses and blood levels of methylphenidate and probably of other traditional stimulants.[112] One approach to the relative efficacy problem applied a normalization technique to published data for a number of possible pharmacotherapies for narcolepsy.[111] Clinical trials for the following drugs were reviewed: codeine, gamma-hydroxybutyrate, ritanserin, viloxazine, pemoline, modafinil, protriptyline, dextroamphetamine, and methylphenidate. The greatest effect of each drug, as measured by mean MSLT or MWT sleep latency, was normalized in terms of the degree to which the sleep latencies of narcoleptic patients treated with the drug approached normal values. Later, using this same normalization technique, Mitler et al.[113] focused on the following treatment and testing conditions because the published articles reported both statistically significant efficacy and what was judged to be clinically meaningful therapeutic effects: pemoline, 112.5 mg using the MWT[37]; modafinil, 200 and 400 mg using the MWT[40,41]; dextroamphetamine, 60 mg using the MWT[37]; methylphenidate, 60 mg using the MWT[37]; and methamphetamine, 40 to 60 mg using the MSLT.[36] Sleep latencies measured during drug-free baseline and appropriate treatment phases of each study were then expressed as a percentage of published values for normal subjects[37] for either the MSLT (13.4 minutes) or the MWT (18.9 minutes). Results are summarized in Figure 39–1.

Quantitative comparisons among these treatments cannot be made with this normalization technique. There are other important limitations: First, only the single end point of percentage change in average sleep latency was considered. Other important end points not considered are the number of subjects who did respond versus the number who did not, subjective alertness, and psychomotor performance.

Second, because of the small number of subjects, no interdrug statistical tests were performed. For quantitative assessment of the relative efficacy of medications, parallel-group, placebo-controlled designs are necessary. For example, in one parallel-group study of modafinil versus dextroamphetamine, there was no statistically significant difference between the efficacy of the two active drugs.[114] More such studies are needed.

The data in Figure 39–1 are useful in establishing a framework with which a patient's treatment response can be viewed. Limitations notwithstanding, one can appreciate that each drug did produce a clinically significant change above baseline toward normal levels. The drugs studied in these trials did not, however, normalize sleepiness, and it is not possible to predict whether treatment with higher doses of these drugs would normalize sleepiness. Clinicians treat individual patients based on their particular therapeutic needs and abilities to tolerate side effects. Nevertheless, some narcoleptic patients report satisfactory control of sleepiness with doses of alerting agents higher than the usually recommended range.

Idiopathic hypersomnia has not been studied as extensively as narcolepsy and there are few controlled studies that objectively evaluate the efficacy of any pharmacologic or nonpharmacologic treatment for idiopathic hypersomnia. The sleepiness of idiopathic hypersomnia appears to respond to alerting agents in substantially the same manner as does the sleepiness of narcolepsy.[115] In one series, 15 of 21 patients (71%) with idiopathic hypersomnia had a good subjective response to sympathomimetic compounds.[116]

Is All Wakefulness the Same?

An additional aspect of efficacy is the subjective experience of wakefulness that each medication supports. That is, sympathomimetic-induced wakefulness may not feel the same, or in fact be the same, as the wakefulness produced by caffeine or modafinil. It has been suggested that although several neurotransmitter systems facilitate alertness through their extensive projections throughout the cortex, these systems may not be simply redundant, but rather support different aspects of wakefulness.[117] In particular, the monoaminergic projections

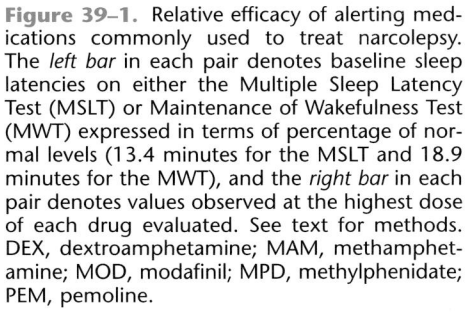

Figure 39–1. Relative efficacy of alerting medications commonly used to treat narcolepsy. The *left bar* in each pair denotes baseline sleep latencies on either the Multiple Sleep Latency Test (MSLT) or Maintenance of Wakefulness Test (MWT) expressed in terms of percentage of normal levels (13.4 minutes for the MSLT and 18.9 minutes for the MWT), and the *right bar* in each pair denotes values observed at the highest dose of each drug evaluated. See text for methods. DEX, dextroamphetamine; MAM, methamphetamine; MOD, modafinil; MPD, methylphenidate; PEM, pemoline.

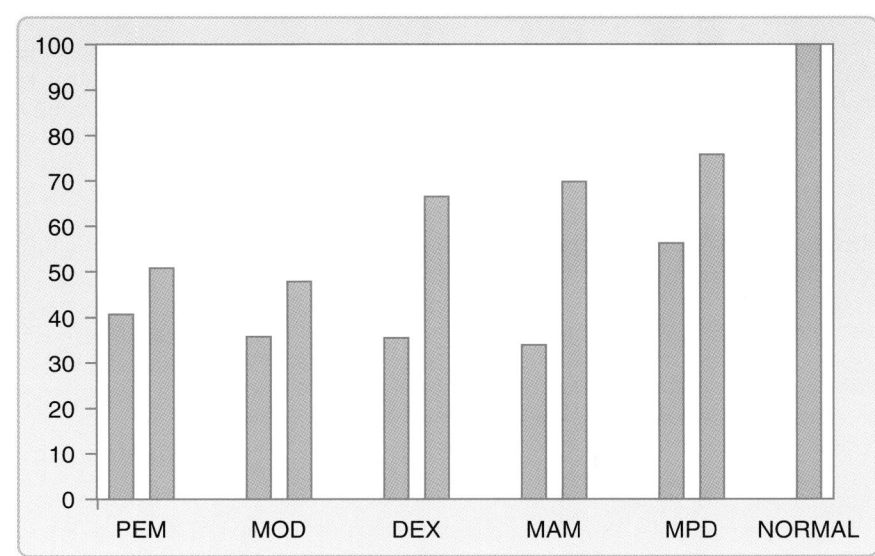

of the ascending reticular activating system may mediate a sort of "guard duty"—an externally directed vigilance or awareness of one's surroundings—whereas the hypothalamic arousal regions (TMN and orexin systems) may perhaps support a form of internally directed vigilance—attention, motivation, insight, and planning. Normally, a healthy balance of activity from these systems should allow a person to focus on a task, while being aware of the surrounding milieu. This hypothesis stems in part from the observation that the excess dopamine and norepinephrine release after administration of high-dose amphetamines provokes a state of exaggerated hypervigilance, or paranoia, and executive functions, including judgment and insight, are impaired.[64] In our experience, patients using modafinil often report a sense of being "simply awake," compared with the experience of being "stimulated" on sympathomimetics. The comparison of relative efficacy on cognitive benefits may be more difficult, however, because sleepy patients frequently judge their level of wakefulness not by the degree of mental alertness present, but rather by the autonomic arousal that sympathomimetics generate. Certainly, the cognitive roles of the neurotransmitters that enhance alertness and vigor are not all clearly understood, but consideration of the varied mechanisms of alerting medications may be useful in understanding clinical outcomes.

INDICATIONS FOR PRESCRIBING MEDICATIONS TO TREAT EXCESSIVE SLEEPINESS

Although numerous disorders and diseases lead to excessive somnolence,[118] multicenter surveys based on standardized diagnostic techniques and criteria[119,120] indicate that more than 80% of individuals who present with this symptom have sleep apnea, narcolepsy, idiopathic hypersomnia, or insufficient sleep.[121,122] Although the sleepiness associated with sleep apnea usually resolves or improves with effective treatment of the apnea, and that associated with insufficient sleep syndrome improves with increased amounts of sleep, narcolepsy and idiopathic hypersomnia are chronic CNS disorders, and the sleepiness caused by these two conditions usually requires pharmacologic interventions. Illnesses not typically viewed as sleep disorders, such as Parkinson's disease,[123] may also cause chronic pathologic sleepiness, and the primary care practitioner may require collaboration with a sleep clinician to provide adequate assessment and effective treatment strategies.

Few drugs have FDA approval for the indication of narcolepsy: methylphenidate, dextroamphetamine, and modafinil. The only alerting agent approved to treat sleepiness due to sleep disorders other than narcolepsy is modafinil. Most of the alerting medications now prescribed by sleep specialists for the control of sleepiness were introduced into the market for weight loss or the treatment of attention-deficit/hyperactivity disorder (ADHD). Amphetamine was first used in the 1930s as a bronchodilator, respiratory stimulant, and analeptic. Modafinil was developed to treat the sleepiness of narcolepsy, and this was its initial indication.[40,41] The use of alerting medications that do not have specific indications to treat sleepiness is considered "off-label," though may be standard clinical practice (e.g., pemoline).

For many patients, controlling excessive sleepiness is critically important to allow adequate functioning at home, while driving, or in the workplace. Furthermore, sleepiness and fatigue, stemming either from sleep disorders or from sleep deprivation, create major safety problems.[124] However, because the classic psychomotor stimulants have significant potential for abuse and side effects, clinicians have had to weigh the patient's need for adequate treatment, and the personal and social risks of inadequate treatment, against the potential for toxic side effects and abuse. In general, the vast majority of patients use their medications responsibly, but the potential for abuse makes clinicians and patients wary. On the other hand, modafinil carries little, if any, risk of abuse,[125,126] and so offers an important addition to the armamentarium of alerting medications that are available to treat excessive daytime sleepiness.

SPECIFIC USE OF WAKE-PROMOTING MEDICATIONS

In Children

Side effects of sympathomimetics in children with narcolepsy have not been studied in detail; much of the available data concern the use of these agents for children with ADHD. The potential side effect of greatest concern is growth retardation.[127] For example, deficits in weight gain and height increase may occur after treatment of ADHD with pemoline, dextroamphetamine, or methylphenidate.[128-131] The growth retardation effects of the sympathomimetic agents are due to drug-induced anorexia and the reduction of slow wave sleep and attendant suppression of growth hormone release. The growth deficits may be reversed during summers off medication,[132,133] and with these drug holidays, there is little or no evidence of long-term effects on growth. Obviously, the need for drug holidays to circumvent the effects on growth means that during treatment interruptions, the child may suffer disabling symptoms that hamper functioning socially and at home. Motor tics can also occur in children taking sympathomimetics,[134] and may limit dosing. Typical initial doses of these agents for treatment of ADHD in children are methylphenidate 0.3 mg/kg; dextroamphetamine 0.15 mg/kg; or pemoline 37.5 mg, followed by dose titration to achieve optimal effects.[134] The safety in narcoleptic children of higher doses than those currently recommended for ADHD (e.g. methylphenidate 60 mg/day) is unknown.

Modafinil appears to be safe to use in children.[135] The half-life of modafinil in children appears to be significantly shorter (6.6 hours) compared with that in adults (15 hours), so higher or more frequent doses may be required to maintain wakefulness across the day. The side effects of modafinil in children 6 to 18 years of age are minimal, the most common being headache. The incidence of effects on mood and behavior is similar to that with placebo. Because modafinil does not degrade nighttime sleep and does not affect appetite, growth retardation is not a hazard of treatment; therefore, in contrast to the sympathomimetic agents, drug holidays are not indicated for treatment regimens with modafinil. For this reason, modafinil should be considered a first-line agent for treatment of sleepiness due to narcolepsy in children.

In Pregnancy

The risk of teratogenicity with commonly used alerting medications is uncertain because well-controlled studies of their use by pregnant women are unavailable. Based on limited evidence, all alerting agents are listed as pregnancy category C, except pemoline, which is pregnancy category B. A threefold to sevenfold increase in amphetamine content in breast milk compared with plasma in a nursing mother with narcolepsy[136] suggests that amphetamines should be used cautiously or not at all in nursing mothers. Although pemoline is so far the only alerting medication listed as a pregnancy category B, it has also been associated with elevated liver enzymes and rarely with hepatic failure. Liver functions should therefore be monitored before and during therapy. Given the uncertainties, the benefits for any given patient must be weighed carefully against the potential risks. For many patients, it may be advisable to reduce or discontinue alerting agents during attempts at conception and for the duration of pregnancy. The efficacy of medications for treatment of narcolepsy during pregnancy is probably similar to efficacy at other times.

In Sustained Military Operations

In military operations during World War II, pilots and other members of the allied forces were issued dextroamphetamine to reduce the effects of fatigue during sustained operations. During the 1991 Persian Gulf War, and during the American-led occupation of Iraq, armed forces were issued modafinil for the same purpose (S. Lubin, personal communication). Although there are few controlled studies, in a study of U.S. Army helicopter pilots engaged in flight simulation after prolonged periods of wakefulness, dextroamphetamine 10 mg, compared with placebo, improved aviator simulator control on descents and turns. Performance was facilitated most noticeably after 22, 26, and 34 hours of continuous wakefulness. Alertness was sustained significantly by dextroamphetamine—there was reduced slow wave electroencephalographic activity and improved rating of vigor and fatigue. No adverse behavioral or physiologic effects were observed.[137,138] Comparable results on performance have also been demonstrated with modafinil during 64 hours of sustained mental work.[114] Interestingly, the recovery sleep after extended periods of modafinil treatment shows a lack of the rebound hypersomnolence characteristic of post–amphetamine treatment recovery sleep.[83,139] This difference suggests that modafinil exerts its alerting effects in a novel way, without invoking a rise in the homeostatic sleep drive.

The Use of Wake-Promoting Agents for Sleepiness Due to Insufficient Sleep: Is There a Role?

Insufficient sleep, beyond the military situation, arises in many circumstances. Common among these circumstances are jet lag and shift work. Modafinil has recently been approved for the treatment of sleepiness in SWSD. The prospective use of alerting agents to enhance the alertness and performance among resident physicians has become a focus of discussion.[140,141] Some argue that such use would foster improved safety as well as learning for physicians in training. This use of alerting medications is problematic for many physicians, and active debate continues. The key points of this debate center on the relative importance of the potential benefit for safety and performance, especially when a high degree of vigilance is required, and the potential for abuse and dependency associated with these agents. The demand for alerting medications in these circumstances is likely to increase

as our society continues to depend on 24-hour operations in the manufacturing, transportation, and service industries.

DISCONTINUATION

There are no systematic studies of the advantages and disadvantages of abrupt discontinuation versus gradual dose reduction before discontinuation of alerting medications. However, practitioners have found few problems with abrupt discontinuation for patients taking any of the alerting medications within the dose ranges discussed in this chapter. Some patients who can remember the severity of their symptoms before pharmacotherapy with the traditional stimulants may report that, for some days after discontinuation, sleepiness was more profound than before stimulant therapy began. This rebound hypersomnolence characterizes the withdrawal from all sympathomimetics, and may persist for several days. This, in addition to changes in sleep architecture effected by sympathomimetics, mandates that sleep testing not be performed unless adequate time off medication (usually 3 weeks) has passed. Marked cardiovascular sequelae such as hypotension have not been reported with abrupt discontinuation of sympathomimetic therapy. However, in patients taking higher doses (e.g., over 100 mg dextroamphetamine per day), it is wise, before abrupt discontinuation, to reduce successively the daily dose by half every 3 to 7 days until the highest dose range recommended by the manufacturer is reached.

There are no rebound phenomena associated with the abrupt discontinuation of modafinil.[42] Sleepiness returns to levels present before treatment. Because there are no effects of modafinil on sleep architecture during treatment or withdrawal, cessation of treatment before nocturnal polysomnographic or daytime sleep studies can be shortened to five half-lives (3 to 4 days), rather than the 3 weeks necessary after withdrawal of sympathomimetics. Appropriate arrangements to ensure the safety of the patient or people in their care (e.g., abstinence from driving) need to be addressed before the discontinuation of any alerting medication.

CHANGING OR COMBINING MEDICATIONS

For most patients, abrupt replacement of one alerting agent with another should present few problems. However, as discussed previously, for patients taking high doses of sympathomimetic medications, a gradual weaning period may be prudent. Further, if the patient is switching from a traditional stimulant to modafinil the qualitative difference in their alerting effects—and difference in peripheral side effects—usually necessitates a 3- to 4-week adjustment period during which the stimulant withdrawal effects dissipate, and the patient begins to experience what he or she feels like on modafinil alone. Titration toward optimum control of alertness can then be done more clearly.

There are no systematic studies of chronic treatment with more than one alerting agent at a time. Some patients report satisfactory management with combinations such as methylphenidate and pemoline or modafinil, using one agent for long-lasting effects and small doses of an agent like methylphenidate on an as-needed basis. There are no known drug–drug interactions that would preclude this practice; however, in some patients, hypertension may develop or be exacerbated by the coadministration of modafinil with a prescribed or over-the-counter sympathomimetic (M. O'Malley, personal communication), so appropriate blood pressure monitoring is indicated during treatment.

In patients who require treatment for cataplexy as well as treatment for excessive sleepiness, it is usually best to select a nonsedating antidepressant agent as an anticataplectic (e.g., protriptyline or fluoxetine). Both the alerting agent and the anticataplectic may be taken in the morning with possible additional dosing of an alerting agent throughout the day. It is rarely necessary to divide the dose of any antidepressant when it is used as an anticataplectic agent. If a sedating antidepressant is selected (e.g., imipramine), this drug should be taken at bedtime. Studies of the nighttime anticataplectic agent sodium oxybate were conducted in narcoleptic patients on concurrent alerting medications, and no clinical or laboratory adverse effects were seen; in some patients, higher doses of sodium oxybate may also reduce subjective levels of sleepiness.[142]

RECOMMENDATIONS

Current practices in the use of alerting medications vary considerably. Recommendations for medications are summarized in Table 39–3. Although many authorities recommend temporary withdrawal of sympathomimetic medications or reduction of dose for 1 to 28 days if tolerance occurs (i.e., drug holidays),[59,79,143,144] this recommendation appears to be based on clinical experience. There are no published studies demonstrating the efficacy of drug holidays. One should also consider the effect of drug holidays on patient safety and quality of life.

Another factor that probably influences clinical practice is whether an alerting medication has been placed on Schedule II by the U.S. Drug Enforcement Agency. Because of the extra paperwork required in some states to prescribe Schedule II agents, Schedule IV drugs such as pemoline and modafinil may be preferentially prescribed. Gamma-hydroxybutyrate has been listed as a Schedule III prescription agent, but if diverted from clinical use (i.e., the patient gives it to others for recreational use), it carries the federal penalties of a Schedule I agent (such as cocaine). This liability issue has mandated a centralized pharmacy and education system to ensure patient and prescriber access to the medication with less opportunity for abuse.

The criteria for determining drug dose vary. Many authorities recommend a goal of obtaining maximum alertness at selected times of the day, such as during work or school hours and while driving, and using scheduled naps to help maintain alertness. Others recommend a goal of maximal or "normal" alertness throughout conventional waking hours. Unfortunately, available data in patients with narcolepsy, for example, indicate that although daytime sleep episodes can be reduced in most, they cannot be completely abolished in all patients.

TREATMENT PLANNING

Alerting medications, however prescribed, represent only part of a comprehensive therapeutic approach to excessive somnolence. Sound sleep hygiene, attention to other substances and drugs that may disrupt the sleep–wake cycle, and periodic reassessment of symptom severity and of the need for and adequacy of treatment modalities are other important aspects of management. The physician should consider the following points in establishing the proper dose of an alerting drug and structuring a management plan.

1. *Diagnosis.* It is important to define as carefully as possible the factors that contribute to a patient's excessive sleepiness. Differentiating an insidious and lifelong condition such as narcolepsy from sleepiness due to shift work is essential for both the patient and the clinician. When possible, a work schedule change (such as a switch to daytime work hours) may be the best alternative to fully restore alertness. Unfortunately, many people do not have the ability to control their schedule directly, and must continue to cope with their current situation. In this case, the clinician must support the patient's need for alertness without imposing his or her judgment about the need for lifestyle changes.
2. *Education.* Clarify the goals of treatment, side effects, risks, and benefits. This process involves discussions with the patient and, perhaps, the patient's spouse or companions. Normal alertness throughout the day may not be attainable in many patients because of the disease process, drug side effects, work schedules, and other idiosyncratic circumstances.
3. *Dosing.* Begin with a low to moderate dose of a wake-promoting agent and match the drug and dosage to the patient. For most patients, aim for enough treatment to provide even alertness throughout the day. Modafinil, long-acting sympathomimetics, or pemoline provide advantages in this respect. Short-acting sympathomimetics may be useful especially for someone who needs rapid alertness on arising from sleep (e.g., in order to drive). Short-acting medications also provide opportunities for napping between

Table 39–3.	Published Recommendations of Alerting Medication Dosages for Treatment of Narcolepsy	
Medication	**Daily Dose Range**	**References**
Methylphenidate (Ritalin)	Up to 60 mg	47,48,59,76,78,79,143–150
	Up to 80 mg	7,35,80,81,148,150–152
	Occasional use of up to 100-300 mg	
	Up to 40-60 mg in children	
Dextroamphetamine (Obetrol, Biphetamine)	Up to 60 mg	35,37,81
Methamphetamine (Desoxyn)	5–100 mg	36
Pemoline (Cylert)	112.5 mg	37,47
Mazindol (Mazanor, Sanorex)	2–8 mg	59
Levoamphetamine (not available in United States)	20–60 mg	145
Fencamfamin (Reactivan; not available in United States)	20–30 mg	59
Modafinil (Provigil)	200–600 mg	40-42,91,92

doses, but also unprotected sleepiness. For patients starting on modafinil, it is best to start 100 mg for the first 4 days, and then 200 mg if sleepiness is still present. Doses may be increased by 100 mg every week as needed until optimal alertness is effected. This titration schedule helps minimize headache, and allows the patient adequate time to assess the impact of treatment on his or her functioning. To start sympathomimetics, it is often easiest to start low doses of long-acting preparations, but if side effects are limiting (e.g., anxiety, palpitations), short-acting forms can be used first to screen which formulation is preferred.

4. *Follow-up*. Initially, pharmacologic management should be guided by regular (e.g., weekly) contact with the patient. If prescribing sympathomimetics, it is wise to measure growth (height/weight) periodically in children, and pulse and blood pressure in adults. After a patient has begun to adjust to the medication, follow up every 3 to 4 weeks, then again in 2 to 3 months. Once the dose is stable, see the patient every 6 to 12 months. Under circumstances where the patient's safety or the safety of others depends on adequate control of excessive somnolence, laboratory confirmation of therapeutic efficacy with the MSLT or MWT is helpful. Such laboratory documentation may not be possible in certain health care settings.

5. Emphasize *sleep hygiene*; consider short (30-minute), prophylactic naps. The effect of sleep inertia must be factored in if naps are used in the work setting. The use of light therapy (or dark sunglasses on the morning ride home), melatonin, or other modalities should be considered as well if appropriate.

6. *Adjust dosages* based on clinical information. Narcolepsy and idiopathic hypersomnia are usually stable conditions that do not progressively worsen. For a patient who has been on a stable dose for some time (years) and now appears to require more, consider other possible causes of increased sleepiness, such as: (a) interval development of sleep apnea (a common scenario in our experience); (b) tolerance to medication; (c) change in schedule (such as a change in job shift, causing less sleep at night); (d) change in life situation (such as a new baby causing sleep disruption) or a new job that requires greater vigilance, hence the patient notes his or her sleepiness interferes more often; (e) stress, anxiety, or depression; and (f) unrealistic expectations. Thus, evaluation should include a detailed history covering the aforementioned possibilities as well as a review of the sleep schedule and napping.

7. Recommend *counseling* and *long-term support*. A suddenly awake person may evoke strong feelings from family members not used to their active participation. Or, patients may become depressed or grieve the time "lost to sleep" before treatment once the degree of their prior impairment becomes clear to them. Available evidence suggests that patients tend to take less, not more, of their prescribed stimulant.[145] Although the reasons for such noncompliance are undoubtedly complex and incompletely understood, it is important that the patient understand the long-term nature of his or her condition and the benefits that can be obtained with regular use of alerting medications.

CONCLUSIONS

The potentially disabling symptom of sleepiness occurs in many sleep disorders. When this sleepiness does not resolve with nonpharmacologic approaches, the use of alerting medications is appropriate. Caffeine is widely available and consumed by most adults in many countries. As an alerting agent, caffeine is most effective when used intermittently at doses of 200 mg or more. Severe or chronic sleepiness is best treated with one of the variety of prescription alerting medications. Such drugs produce behavioral activation and increased wakefulness, enhanced alertness, decreased sense of fatigue, and increased performance. Treatment of excessive sleepiness associated with narcolepsy or idiopathic hypersomnia with alerting medications is almost always indicated to allow wakefulness when sustained vigilance is necessary, especially for individual and public safety. Pharmacologic treatment with modafinil is now also indicated for severe sleepiness in patients with SWSD and in patients with OSA who remain sleepy despite compliance with nasal CPAP. All alerting medications improve daytime alertness in the majority of studied patients; these medications vary in the extent to which lack of efficacy, tolerance, and side effects are reported to occur. Side effects (headaches, nervousness, anxiety, palpitations, and insomnia) are most common with the sympathomimetic agents. These are dose related, and may require discontinuation of therapy. Headache is the most common side effect with modafinil treatment. Because the risk for teratogenicity associated with alerting agents' use is uncertain, these drugs in general should be avoided in pregnancy unless the benefits associated with their use are likely to outweigh the risks. Severe psychiatric complications are rare with use of alerting medications, but they are more likely to occur with high doses of sympathomimetic compounds and in patients with coexisting psychiatric illness. Although the safety and added efficacy of modafinil or traditional stimulants at doses higher than those recommended by the manufacturers are not well established with controlled clinical trials, some patients obtain added benefit with higher doses without ill effects.

> *Clinical Pearl*
>
> *The main goal of the treatment of pathologic sleepiness is to address and correct the underlying sleep disorder. When sleepiness remains an issue despite nonpharmacologic treatment (such as in narcolepsy, SWSD, and some patients with OSA using CPAP), prescription alerting medications should be considered for the patient's safety and quality of life. Modafinil is a first-line agent in patients with excessive sleepiness due to these disorders because it prompts wakefulness without many side effects or rebound hypersomnia. A broad array of sympathomimetic compounds are also available to treat sleepiness, but their risk of abuse, tolerance, and side effects makes them second-line agents in treating narcolepsy or for treatment of other sleep disorders "off-label." Caffeine is a useful alerting agent only when used on an as-needed basis, at doses of 200 mg or higher, because of the rapid development of tolerance when taken daily.*

Acknowledgments

This chapter is based in part on a review of the literature done by a taskforce (Mitler MM, Aldrich MS, Koob GF, et al. Narcolepsy and its treatment with stimulants: ASDA standards of practice. Sleep 1994;17:352-371).

REFERENCES

1. Haddad LM: 1978: Cocaine in perspective. J Am Coll Emerg Physicians 1979;8:374-376.
2. Angrist B, Sudilovsky A: Central nervous system stimulants: Historical aspects and clinical effects. In Iversen LL, Iversen SD, Snyder SH (eds): Handbook of Psychopharmacology, vol 11. New York, Plenum Press, 1976, pp 99-165.
3. Byck R: Cocaine papers by Sigmund Freud. New York, Stonehill, 1974.
4. Doyle JB, Daniels LE: Symptomatic treatment for narcolepsy. JAMA 1931;96:1370-1372.
5. Janota O: Symptomatische Behandlung der pathologischen Schlafsucht, besonders der Narkolepsie. Med Klin 1931;27:278-281.
6. Prinzmetal M, Bloomberg W: Use of benzedrine for the treatment of narcolepsy. JAMA 1935;105:2051-2054.
7. Yoss RE, Daly DD: Treatment of narcolepsy with Ritalin. Neurology 1959;9:171-173.
8. American Academy of Sleep Medicine Standards of Practice Committee: Practice parameters for the treatment of narcolepsy: An update for 2000. Sleep 2001;24:451-466.
9. Porkka-Heiskanen T, Strecker RE, Thakkar M, et al: Adenosine: A mediator of the sleep-inducing effects of prolonged wakefulness. Science 1997;276:1265-1268.
10. Hendricks JC, Finn SM, Panckeri KA, et al: Rest in *Drosophila* is a sleep-like state. Neuron 2000;25:129-138.
11. Shaw PJ, Cirelli C, Greenspan RJ, et al: Correlates of sleep and waking in *Drosophila melanogaster*. Science 2000;287:1834-1837.
12. Roehrs T, Merlotti L, Halpin D, et al: Effects of theophylline on nocturnal sleep and daytime sleepiness/alertness. Chest 1995;108:382-387.
13. Patat A, Rosenzweig P, Enslen M, et al: Effects of a new slow release formulation of caffeine on EEG, psychomotor and cognitive functions in sleep-deprived subjects. Hum Psychopharmacol 2000;15:153-170.
14. Beaumont M, Batejat D, Pierard C, et al: Slow release caffeine and prolonged (64-h) continuous wakefulness: Effects on vigilance and cognitive performance. J Sleep Res 2001;10:265-276.
15. Lieberman HR, Tharion WJ, Shukitt-Hale B, et al: Effects of caffeine, sleep loss, and stress on cognitive performance and mood during U.S. Navy SEAL training. Sea-Air-Land. Psychopharmacology (Berl) 2002;164:250-261.
16. De Valck E, De Groot E, Cluydts R: Effects of slow-release caffeine and a nap on driving simulator performance after partial sleep deprivation. Percept Mot Skills 2003;96:67-78.
17. Muehlbach MJ, Walsh JK: The effects of caffeine on simulated night-shift work and subsequent daytime sleep. Sleep 1995;18:22-29.
18. Richardson GS, Miner JD, Czeisler CA: Impaired driving performance in shiftworkers: The role of the circadian system in a multifactorial model. Alcohol Drugs Driving 1989;5-6:265-273.
19. National Sleep Foundation: 2001 "Sleep in America" Poll. Washington, DC, National Sleep Foundation, 2001.
20. Van Dongen HP, Price NJ, Mullington JM, et al: Caffeine eliminates psychomotor vigilance deficits from sleep inertia. Sleep 2001;24:813-819.
21. Drake CL, Roehrs T, Turner L, et al: Caffeine reversal of ethanol effects on the multiple sleep latency test, memory, and psychomotor performance. Neuropsychopharmacology 2003;28:371-378.
22. Parkes JD, Dahlitz M: Amphetamine prescription. Sleep 1993;16:201-203.
23. Wesensten NJ, Belenky G, Kautz MA, et al: Maintaining alertness and performance during sleep deprivation: modafinil versus caffeine. Psychopharmacology (Berl) 2002;159:238-247.
24. Etherton GM, Kochar MS: Coffee: Facts and controversies. Arch Fam Med 1993;2:317-322.
25. Nawrot P, Jordan S, Eastwood J, et al: Effects of caffeine on human health. Food Addit Contam 2003;20:1-30.
26. Frishman WH, Del Vecchio A, Sanal S, et al: Cardiovascular manifestations of substance abuse: Part 2. Alcohol, amphetamines, heroin, cannabis, and caffeine. Heart Dis 2003;5:253-271.
27. Silverman K, Evans SM, Strain EC, et al: Withdrawal syndrome after the double-blind cessation of caffeine consumption. N Engl J Med 1992;327:1109-1114.
28. Dews PB, O'Brien CP, Bergman J: Caffeine: Behavioral effects of withdrawal and related issues. Food Chem Toxicol 2002;40:1257-1261.
29. Prinzmetal M. Alles GA: The central nervous system stimulant effects of dextro-amphetamine sulphate. Am J Med Sci 1940;200:665-673.
30. Eaton LM: Treatment of narcolepsy with desoxyephedrine hydrochloride. Staff Meet Mayo Clin 1943;7:262-264.
31. Brock S, Wiesel B: The narcoleptic-cataplectic syndrome—and excessive and dissociated reaction of the sleep mechanism—accompanying mental states. J Nerv Ment Dis 1941;94:700-712.
32. Daly DD, Yoss RE: The treatment of narcolepsy with methyl phenylpiperidylacetate: A preliminary report. Proc Staff Meet Mayo Clin 1956;31:620-625.
33. Daly D, Yoss R: Narcolepsy. In Magnus O, Lorentz de Haas A (eds): The Epilepsies, vol 15, Handbook of Clinical Neurology. Amsterdam, North Holland Publishing, 1974, pp 836-852.
34. Parkes JD, Baraitser M, Marsden CD, et al: Natural history, symptoms and treatment of the narcoleptic syndrome. Acta Neurol Scand 1975;52:337-353.
35. Honda Y, Akimoto H, Takahashi Y: Pharmacotherapy in narcolepsy. Dis Nerv Syst 1960;21:1-3.
36. Mitler MM, Hajdukovic R, Erman MK: Treatment of narcolepsy with methamphetamine. Sleep 1993;16:306-317.
37. Mitler MM, Hajdukovic R, Erman M, et al: Narcolepsy. J Clin Neurophysiol 1990;7:93-118.
38. Laffont F, Cathala HP, Kohler F: Effect of modafinil on narcolepsy and idiopathic hypersomnia. Sleep Res 1987;16:377.
39. Bastuji H, Jouvet M: Successful treatment of idiopathic hypersomnia and narcolepsy with modafinil. Prog Neuropsychopharmacol Biol Psychiatry 1988;12:695-700.
40. Broughton RJ, Fleming JA, George CF, et al: Randomized, double-blind, placebo-controlled crossover trial of modafinil in the treatment of excessive daytime sleepiness in narcolepsy. Neurology 1997;49:444-451.
41. U.S. Modafinil in Narcolepsy Multicenter Study Group: Randomized trial of modafinil for the treatment of pathological somnolence in narcolepsy. Ann Neurol 1998;43:88-97.
42. U.S. Modafinil in Narcolepsy Multicenter Study Group: Randomized trial of modafinil as a treatment for the excessive daytime somnolence of narcolepsy. Neurology 2000;54:1166-1175.
43. Alvarez B, Dahlitz M, Grimshaw J, et al: Mazindol in long-term treatment of narcolepsy. Lancet 1991;337:1293-1294.
44. Shindler J, Schachter M, Brincat S, et al: Amphetamine, mazindol and fencamfamin in narcolepsy. BMJ 1985;290:1167-1170.
45. Roselaar SE, Langdon N, Lock CB, et al: Selegiline in narcolepsy. Sleep 1987;10:491-495.
46. Saletu B, Frey R, Krupka M, et al: Differential effects of a new central adrenergic agonist modafinil and d-amphetamine on sleep and early morning behavior in elderlies. Arzneimittelforschung 1989;39:1268-1273.
47. Honda Y: Clinical features of narcolepsy. In Honda T, Juji T (eds): HLA in Narcolepsy. Berlin, Springer-Verlag, 1988, pp 24-57.
48. Regestein QR, Reich P, Mufson MJ: Narcolepsy: An initial clinical approach. J Clin Psychiatry 1983;44:166-172.
49. Tolman KG, Freston JW, Berenson MM, et al: Hepatotoxicity due to pemoline: Report of two cases. Digestion 1973;9:532-539.
50. Elitsur Y: Pemoline (Cylert)-induced hepatotoxicity [letter]. J Pediatr Gastroenterol Nutr 1990;11:143.
51. Pratt DS, Dubois RS: Hepatotoxicity due to pemoline (Cylert): A report of two cases. J Pediatr Gastroenterol Nutr 1990;10:239-241.

52. Jaffe SL: Pemoline and liver function [letter]. J Am Acad Child Adolesc Psychiatry 1989;28:457-458.

53. Nehra A, Mullick F, Ishak KG, et al: Pemoline-associated hepatic injury. Gastroenterology 1990;99:1517-1519.

54. Young D, Scoville WB: Paranoid psychosis in narcolepsy and the possible danger of benzedrine treatment. Med Clin North Am 1938;22:637-646.

55. Cadieux RJ, Kales JD, Kales A, et al: Pharmacologic and psychotherapeutic issues in coexistent paranoid schizophrenia and narcolepsy: A case report. J Clin Psychiatry 1985;46:191-193.

56. Leong GB, Shaner AL, Silva JA: Narcolepsy, paranoid psychosis and analeptic abuse. Psychiatr J Univ Ottawa 1989;14:481-483.

57. Pfefferbaum A, Berger PA: Narcolepsy, paranoid psychosis, and tardive dyskinesia: A pharmacological dilemma. J Nerv Ment Dis 1977;164:293-297.

58. Schrader G, Hicks EP: Narcolepsy, paranoid psychosis, major depression and tardive dyskinesia. J Nerv Ment Dis 1984;172:439-441.

59. Parkes JD: Sleep and Its Disorders. London, WB Saunders, 1985.

60. Guilleminault C, Carskadon M, Dement WC: On the treatment of rapid eye movement narcolepsy. Arch Neurol 1974;30:90-93.

61. Akimoto H, Honda Y, Takahashi Y: Pharmacotherapy in narcolepsy. Dis Nerv Syst 1960;21:704-706.

62. Passouant P, Billiard M: Evolution of narcolepsy with age. In Guilleminault C, Dement WC, Passouant P (eds): Narcolepsy. New York, Spectrum, 1976, pp 179-196.

63. Simpson LL: The effects of behavioral stimulant doses of amphetamine on blood pressure. Arch Gen Psychiatry 1976;33:691-695.

64. Griffith J, Oates JA, Cavanaugh JH: Paranoid episodes induced by drug. JAMA 1968;205:39.

65. Rylander G: Stereotype behaviour in man following amphetamine abuse. In De SB, Baker C (eds): The Correlation of Adverse Effects in Man with Observations in Animals. Amsterdam, Excerpta Medica, 1971, pp 28-31.

66. Alldredge BK, Lowenstein DH, Simon RP: Seizures associated with recreational drug abuse. Neurology 1989;39:1037-1039.

67. Conci F, D'Angelo V, Tampieri D, et al: Intracerebral hemorrhage and angiographic beading following amphetamine abuse. Ital J Neurol Sci 1988;9:77-81.

68. Harrington H, Heller HA, Dawson D, et al: Intracerebral hemorrhage and oral amphetamine. Arch Neurol 1983;40:503-507.

69. Olsen ER: Intracranial hemorrhage and amphetamine usage: Review of the effects of amphetamines on the central nervous system. Angiology 1977;28:464-471.

70. Rothrock JF, Rubenstein R, Lyden PD: Ischemic stroke associated with methamphetamine inhalation. Neurology 1988;38:589-592.

71. Margolis MT, Newton TH: Methamphetamine ("speed") arteritis. Neuroradiology 1971;2:179-182.

72. Kaku DA, Lowenstein DH: Emergence of recreational drug abuse as a major risk factor for stroke in young adults. Ann Intern Med 1991;113:821-827.

73. Grant I, Mohns L: Chronic cerebral effects of alcohol and drug abuse. Int J Addict 1975;10:883-920.

74. Michel R, Adams AP: Acute amphetamine abuse: Problems during general anaesthesia for neurosurgery. Anaesthesia 1979;34:1016-1019.

75. Honda Y, Hishikawa Y, Takahashi Y: Long-term treatment of narcolepsy with Ritalin (methylphenidate). Curr Ther Res 1979;25:288-298.

76. Zarcone VP: Narcolepsy. N Engl J Med 1973;288:1156-1166.

77. Billiard M: Narcolepsy: Clinical features and aetiology. Ann Clin Res 1985;17:220-226.

78. Dement WC, Carskadon MA, Guilleminault C, et al: Narcolepsy: Diagnosis and treatment. Prim Care 1976;3:609-623.

79. Thorpy MJ, Goswami M: Treatment of narcolepsy. In Thorpy MJ (ed): Handbook of Sleep Disorders. New York, Marcel Dekker, 1990, pp 235-258.

80. Soldatos CR, Kales A, Cadieux RJ: Treatment of sleep disorders: II. Narcolepsy. Ration Drug Ther 1983;17(3):1-7.

81. Yoss RE: Treatment of narcolepsy. Mod Treat 1969;6:1263-1274.

82. Sawynok J: Pharmacological rationale for the clinical use of caffeine. Drugs 1995;49:37-50.

83. Edgar DM, Seidel WF: Modafinil induces wakefulness without intensifying motor activity or subsequent rebound hypersomnolence in the rat. J Pharmacol Exp Ther 1997;283:757-769.

84. Wisor JP, Nishino S, Sora I, et al: Dopaminergic role in stimulant-induced wakefulness. J Neurosci 2001;21:1787-1794.

85. Scammell TE, Estabrooke IV, McCarthy MT, et al: Hypothalamic arousal regions are activated during modafinil-induced wakefulness. J Neurosci 2000;20:8620-8628.

86. Ballas C, Kim D, Baldassano C, et al: Modafinil: Past, present and future. Neurotherapeutics 2002;2:449-457.

87. Mignot E, Nishino S, Guilleminault C, et al: Modafinil binds to the dopamine uptake carrier site with low affinity. Sleep 1994;17:436-437.

88. Gallopin T, Luppi PH, Rambert FA, et al: Effect of the wake-promoting agent modafinil on sleep-promoting neurons from the ventrolateral preoptic nucleus: An in vitro pharmacologic study. Sleep 2004;27:19-25.

89. Python A, Charnay Y, Mikolajewski R, et al: Effects of nisoxetine, a selective noradrenaline transporter blocker, on sleep in rats. Pharmacol Biochem Behav 1997;58:369-372.

90. Mitler MM, Harsh J, Hirshkowitz M, et al: Long-term efficacy and safety of modafinil (PROVIGIL) for the treatment of excessive daytime sleepiness associated with narcolepsy. Sleep Med 2000;1:231-243.

91. Schwartz FN Jr, Bogan RK, Nelson MT, Hughes RJ: Dosing regimen effects of modafinil for improving daytime wakefulness in patients with narcolepsy. Clin Neuropharmacol 2003;26:252-257.

92. Schwartz JR, Nelson MT, Schwartz ER, et al: Effects of modafinil on wakefulness and executive function in patients with narcolepsy experiencing late-day sleepiness. Clin Neuropharmacol 2004;27(2):74-79.

93. Patel SR, White DP, Malhotra A, et al: Continuous positive airway pressure therapy for treating sleepiness in a diverse population with obstructive sleep apnea: Results of a meta-analysis. Arch Intern Med 2003;163:565-571.

94. Gaddy JR, Dogharmji K: Daytime sleepiness after nCPAP treatment. Sleep Res 1991;20:245.

95. Kingshott RN, Vennelle M, Coleman EL, et al: Randomized, double-blind, placebo-controlled crossover trial of modafinil in the treatment of residual excessive daytime sleepiness in the sleep apnea/hypopnea syndrome. Am J Respir Crit Care Med 2001;163:918-923.

96. Black J, Hirshkowitz M, Earl CQ: Modafinil adjunctive therapy improves excessive sleepiness and quality of life in obstructive sleep apnea: A 12-month open-label extension study [abstract]. Sleep 2003;26:A270-A271.

97. Schwartz JR, Hirshkowitz M, Erman MK, et al: Modafinil as adjunct therapy for daytime sleepiness in obstructive sleep apnea: A 12-week, open-label study. Chest 2003;124:2192-2199.

98. Veasey SC, Davis CW, Fenik P, et al: Long-term intermittent hypoxia in mice: Protracted hypersomnolence with oxidative injury to sleep-wake brain regions. Sleep 2004;27:194-201.

99. Wright K: Modafinil as a treatment for shift work sleep disorder. Sleep 2005 (in press).

100. Bassetti C: Narcolepsy. Curr Treat Options Neurol 1999;1:291-298.

101. Lowenstein O, Loewenfeld I: Electronic pupillography: A new instrument and some clinical applications. Arch Ophthalmol 1958;59:352-363.

102. Yoss RE, Moyer NJ, Ogle KN: The pupillogram and narcolepsy: A method to measure decreased levels of wakefulness. Neurology 1969;19:921-928.

103. Richardson GS, Carskadon MA, Flagg W, et al: Excessive daytime sleepiness in man: Multiple sleep latency measurement in narcoleptic and control subjects. Electroencephalogr Clin Neurophysiol 1978;45:621-627.

104. Mitler MM, Gujavarty KS, Browman CP: Maintenance of wakefulness test: A polysomnographic technique for evaluation treatment efficacy in patients with excessive somnolence. Electroencephalogr Clin Neurophysiol 1982;53:658-661.

105. Thorpy MJ: Report from the Amzerican Sleep Disorders Association: The clinical use of the multiple sleep latency test. Sleep 1992;15:268-276.

106. Scrima L, Hartman PG, Johnson FH, et al: Effects of gamma-hydroxybutyrate (GHB) on sleep of narcolepsy patients: A double blind study. Sleep 1990;13:479-490.

107. Fry JM, Pressman MR, DiPhillipo MA, et al: Treatment of narcolepsy with codeine. Sleep 1986;9:269-274.

108. Scrima L, Hartman PG, Johnson FH, et al: Effects of gamma-hydroxybutyrate (GHB) on multiple sleep latency test (MSLT) in narcolepsy patients: A long term study. Sleep Res 1990;19:288.

109. Guilleminault C, Mancuso J, Salva MA, et al: Viloxazine hydrochloride in narcolepsy: A preliminary report. Sleep 1986;9:275-279.

110. Lammers GJ, Arends J, Declerk AC, et al: Ritanserin, a 5-HT2 receptor blocker, as add-on treatment in narcolepsy. Sleep 1991;14:130-132.

111. Mitler MM, Hajdukovic R: Relative efficacy of drugs for the treatment of sleepiness in narcolepsy. Sleep 1991;14:218-220.

112. Gualtieri CT, Wargin W, Kanoy R, et al: Clinical studies of methylphenidate serum levels in children and adults. J Am Acad Child Psychiatry 1982;21:19-26.

113. Mitler MM, Aldrich MS, Koob GF, et al: Narcolepsy and its treatment with stimulants: ASDA standards of practice. Sleep 1994;17:352-371.

114. Pigeau R, Naitoh P, Buguet A, et al: Modafinil, d-amphetamine and placebo during 64 hours of sustained mental work: I. Effects on mood, fatigue, cognitive performance and body temperature. J Sleep Res 1995;4:212-228.

115. Guilleminault C: Idiopathic central nervous system hypersomnia. In Kryger MH, Roth T, Dement WC (eds): Principles and Practice of Sleep Medicine. Philadelphia, WB Saunders, 1989, pp 347-350.

116. Bassetti C, Aldrich MS: Idiopathic hypersomnia: A series of 42 patients. Brain 1997;120:1423-1435.

117. Stahl SM: Awakening to the psychopharmacology of sleep and arousal: Novel neurotransmitters and wake-promoting drugs. J Clin Psychiatry 2002;63:467-468.

118. American Sleep Disorders Association: International Classification of Sleep Disorders, revised: Diagnostic and Coding Manual. Rochester, Minn, American Sleep Disorders Association, 1997.

119. Guilleminault C: Sleeping and Waking Disorders: Indications and Techniques. Menlo Park, Calif, Addison-Wesley, 1982.

120. Association of Sleep Disorders Centers: Diagnostic Classification of Sleep and Arousal Disorders, First Edition. Prepared by the Sleep Disorders Classification Committee, H.P. Roffwarg, chairman. Sleep 1979;2:1-137.

121. Coleman RM, Roffwarg HP, Kennedy SJ, et al: Sleep-wake disorders based on a polysomnographic diagnosis: A national cooperative study. JAMA 1982;247:997-1003.

122. Coleman RM: Diagnosis, treatment, and follow-up of about 8,000 sleep/wake disorder patients. In Guilleminault C, Lugaresi E (eds): Sleep/Wake Disorders: Natural History, Epidemiology, and Long-Term Evolution. New York, Raven Press, 1983, pp 87-98.

123. Rye DB: Sleepiness and unintended sleep in Parkinson's disease. Curr Treat Options Neurol 2003;5:231-239.

124. Mitler MM, Erman M, Hajdukovic R: The treatment of excessive somnolence with stimulant drugs. Sleep 1993;16:203-206.

125. Warot D, Corruble E, Payan C, et al: Subjective effects of modafinil, a new central adrenergic stimulant in healthy volunteers: A comparison with amphetamine, caffeine, and placebo. Eur Psychiatry 1993;8:201-208.

126. Rush CR, Kelly TH, Hays LR, et al: Acute behavioral and physiological effects of modafinil in drug abusers. Behav Pharmacol 2002;13:105-115.

127. Croche AF, Lipman RS, Overall JE, et al: The effects of stimulant medication on the growth of hyperkinetic children. Pediatrics 1979;63:847-850.

128. Friedmann N, Thomas J, Carr R, et al: Effect on growth in pemoline-treated children with attention deficit disorder. Am J Dis Child 1981;135:329-332.

129. Satterfield JH, Cantwell DP, Schell A, et al: Growth of hyperactive children treated with methylphenidate. Arch Gen Psychiatry 1979;36:212-217.

130. Mattes JA, Gittelman R: Growth of hyperactive children on maintenance regimen of methylphenidate. Arch Gen Psychiatry 1983;40:317-321.

131. Golinko BE: Side effects of dextroamphetamine and methylphenidate in hyperactive children: A brief review. Prog Neuropsychopharmacol Biol Psychiatry 1984;8:1-8.

132. Klein RG, Landa B, Mattes JA, et al: Methylphenidate and growth in hyperactive children: A controlled withdrawal study. Arch Gen Psychiatry 1988;45:1127-1130.

133. Safer DJ, Allen RP, Barr E: Growth rebound after termination of stimulant drugs. J Pediatr 1975;86:113-116.

134. Stevenson RD, Wolraich ML: Stimulant medication therapy in the treatment of children with attention deficit hyperactivity disorder. Pediatr Clin North Am 1989;36:1183-1197.

135. Guilleminault C, Pelayo R: Narcolepsy in children: a practical guide to its diagnosis, treatment and follow-up. Paediatr Drugs 2000;2:1-9.

136. Steiner E, Villen T, Halberg M, et al: Amphetamine secretion in breast milk. Eur J Clin Pharmacol 1984;27:123-124.

137. Caldwell JA, Caldwell JL, Crowley JS, et al: Sustaining helicopter pilot performance with Dexedrine during periods of sleep deprivation. Aviat Space Environ Med 1995;66:930-937.

138. Caldwell JA Jr: Effects of operationally effective doses of dextroamphetamine on heart rates and blood pressures of army aviators. Mil Med 1996;161:673-678.

139. Buguet A, Montmayeur A, Pigeau R, et al: Modafinil, d-amphetamine and placebo during 64 hours of sustained mental work: II. Effects on two nights of recovery sleep. J Sleep Res 1995;4:229-241.

140. Jockovich M, Cosentino D, Cosentino L, et al: Effect of exogenous melatonin on mood and sleep efficiency in emergency medicine residents working night shifts. Acad Emerg Med 2000;7:955-958.

141. Halbach MM, Spann CO, Egan G: Effect of sleep deprivation on medical resident and student cognitive function: A prospective study. Am J Obstet Gynecol 2003;188:1198-1201.

142. U.S. Xyrem Multicenter Study Group: A randomized, double blind, placebo-controlled multicenter trial comparing the effects of three doses of orally administered sodium oxybate with placebo for the treatment of narcolepsy. Sleep 2002;25:42-49.

143. Aldrich MS: Narcolepsy. N Engl J Med 1990;323:389-394.

144. Mitler MM, Nelson S, Hajdukovic R: Narcolepsy: Diagnosis, treatment, and management. Psychiatr Clin North Am 1987;10:593-606.

145. Rogers AE, Aldrich MS, Berrios AM, et al: Compliance with stimulant medications in patients with narcolepsy. Sleep 1997;20:28-33.

146. Parkes JD, Fenton GW: Levo(−)amphetamine and dextro(+) amphetamine in the treatment of narcolepsy. J Neurol Neurosurg Psychiatry 1973;36:1076-1081.

147. Kales A, Vela-Bueno A, Kales JD: Sleep disorders: Sleep apnea and narcolepsy. Ann Intern Med 1987;106:434-443.

148. Richardson JW, Fredrickson PA, Lin S-C: Narcolepsy update. Mayo Clin Proc 1990;65:991-998.

149. Dahl RE: The pharmacologic treatment of sleep disorders. Psychiatr Clin North Am 1992;15:161-178.

150. Yoss RE, Daly DD: On the treatment of narcolepsy. Med Clin North Am 1968;52:781-787.

151. Yoss RE, Daly DD: Narcolepsy. Med Clin North Am 1960;44:953-968.

152. Yoss RE, Daly DD: Narcolepsy in children. Pediatrics 1960;25:1025-1033.

40

Drugs That Disturb Sleep and Wakefulness

Paula K. Schweitzer

ABSTRACT

Insomnia and sedation are some of the unwanted effects of many medications. Disturbed sleep as well as daytime sleepiness or decreased cognitive functioning may also be features of the illness being treated with medications.

The first-generation antidepressants (tricyclics and monoamine oxidase inhibitors) tend to be sedating primarily because of histamine blockade. Newer antidepressants are more receptor specific and, depending on the receptor activity, less likely to be sedating. These drugs include the selective serotonin reuptake inhibitors as well as a number of other compounds that have differential effects on serotonin, norepinephrine, and dopamine. Except for trazodone and mirtazapine, which are sedating, these newer drugs are more likely to be associated with insomnia. An increase in periodic limb movements has been reported with the tricyclics as well as some of the newer compounds.

Among antihypertensive drugs, the beta-adrenergic antagonists, alpha$_2$ agonists, and catecholamine depleters have been associated with insomnia and nightmares. Several hypolipidemic compounds have been associated with insomnia and decreased cognitive or psychomotor performance. Antiarrhythmic drugs are frequently associated with fatigue.

Patients with Parkinson's disease have multiple complaints relating to sleep, including insomnia, fatigue, and nightmares; these complaints may be the result of the disease or of drug treatment. Low doses of levodopa and dopaminergic agonists tend to improve sleep, whereas higher doses are likely to disrupt sleep. Drug-related improvement in Parkinson's symptoms may outweigh the sleep-disrupting effects of the drug, resulting in an improvement in sleep overall. Dopaminergic agonists have been linked to daytime sleepiness and sudden "sleep attacks." Whether the sleepiness is related to the pathologic process of Parkinson's disease or the specific drugs is unclear.

Sedation is one of the most common adverse effects of the older antiepileptic drugs such as phenobarbital and carbamazepine. Newer drugs such as gabapentin and tiagabine appear to be much less sedating but may also improve sleep; they are being studied off-label for their use as hypnotics. Antipsychotics, histamine antagonists, corticosteroids, theophylline, and anorectic agents all have effects on the nervous system and might cause sleep complaints. Opioids are sedating but their most serious adverse effect is respiratory depression, which is of particular concern in patients with pulmonary disease or obstructive sleep apnea.

This chapter reviews drugs that are used for common medical and psychiatric conditions and that have unintended effects on sleep or wakefulness. Drugs not classified as hypnotics but sometimes used for their sedating effects to treat insomnia (e.g., trazodone, tricyclic antidepressants [TCAs], melatonin, first-generation antihistamines) are reviewed in Chapter 37. Benzodiazepines used as hypnotics are covered separately in Chapter 36, whereas benzodiazepines used as anxiolytics are covered briefly in this chapter. Stimulant medications (including caffeine), as well as drugs of abuse (including alcohol and nicotine), are discussed in Chapters 38, 39, and 115.

Numerous prescription drugs act in the central nervous system (CNS) and have the potential to affect sleep or daytime functioning. Insomnia, sleepiness, sedation, and fatigue are some of the listed side effects of many prescription and over-the-counter medications. Although such side effects can be problematic, they may not occur in all patients, their severity can vary considerably, and in some situations failure to provide treatment may be more disruptive of sleep or wakefulness than these side effects. In some instances, the desired action of a drug (e.g., sedation to treat insomnia or stimulation to treat sleepiness) becomes an undesirable action when the effect carries over into daytime or nighttime hours, respectively. In other cases, the desired action of a drug may be produced by effects at specific receptor sites and undesired actions occur because of concomitant effects at other receptor sites. In addition, undesired actions (e.g., unwanted sedation) may be the result of a discontinuation or withdrawal effect (i.e., a reflection of declining plasma levels after a period of stimulation such as might occur with the use of caffeine). Thus, understanding the mechanisms of action as well as the pharmacokinetics of a drug can help determine when a desired action might become an undesired action or when desired actions may be accompanied by undesirable actions.

In this chapter the effects of widely used drugs on sleep and wakefulness are presented, generally in the following order: (1) subjective data, including clinical trials; (2) polysomnographic (PSG) data; (3) objective data on sleepiness/alertness (primarily Multiple Sleep Latency Test [MSLT] data); and (4) objective performance data. In many cases, there are few PSG or MSLT data available. Drug withdrawal effects are not addressed.

ANTIDEPRESSANT AGENTS

Antidepressant drugs can improve or disturb sleep, as well as have effects on waking function. Evaluation of the effects of these drugs on sleep and wakefulness is complicated by the fact that many individuals with depression have disturbed sleep[1] as well as daytime complaints such as fatigue, sleepiness, somatic complaints, and decreased cognitive and psychomotor functioning.[2-4] In addition, PSG evidence of disturbed nocturnal sleep does not always correlate with the subjective reports of patients and is not related to the efficacy of these drugs in the treatment of depression.

The first-generation antidepressants (TCAs [see Chapter 37] and monoamine oxidase inhibitors [MAOIs]) have multiple mechanisms of action, some of which are believed to mediate the antidepressant response (e.g., through effects on serotonin, norepinephrine, or dopamine) and others that mediate side effects such as sedation (through histamine blockade), dry mouth (through cholinergic blockade), orthostatic hypotension (alpha-adrenergic receptors), and so on. Currently available antidepressants include a number of drugs that are more receptor specific. These compounds include the selective serotonin reuptake inhibitors (SSRIs; e.g., fluoxetine), the dual serotonin and norepinephrine reuptake inhibitor venlafaxine, the norepinephrine and dopamine reuptake inhibitor bupropion, the serotonin type 2 receptor antagonist and reuptake inhibitors (e.g., nefazodone, trazodone), and noradrenergic and specific serotonergic antidepressants such as mirtazapine (see Chapter 37). Table 40–1 summarizes the effects of these drugs on sleep and waking behavior. For a

Table 40–1. Antidepressants: Effects on Sleep and Waking Behavior

Class/Drug	Primary Neurotransmitter/ Receptor Activity	Subjective Data (Placebo-Corrected %)	PSG Data	Performance/ MSLT Data
TCAs				
(See Chapter 37) (amitriptyline, doxepin, imipramine, trimipramine, clomipramine, desipramine, nortriptyline, protriptyline)	NE, 5-HT uptake inhibition; acetylcholine, H₁, H₂ blockade; inhibition of fast sodium channels	Improves sleep; may be sedating during the daytime, but effects may lessen with time; doxepin, trimipramine, amitriptyline, imipramine more sedating than others	Generally ↑ TST, ↓ W, ↓↓ REM, ↑ PLMs	Most data on amitriptyline and imipramine: generally ↓↓ cognitive and psychomotor performance, at least with acute use in healthy subjects, but there is some evidence that effects lessen with time; decrements may be more likely in elderly; effects on depressed patients are variable; no MSLT data
MAOIs				
Classic: phenelzine tranylcypromine	Inhibit MAO enzymes that metabolize NE, 5-HT, DA Inhibit both MAO-A and MAO-B	Insomnia, daytime sedation	Generally ↑ W, ↓ TST, ↓↓↓ REM	Limited data; no MSLT data
Selective, reversible: moclobemide brofaromine	Inhibit only MAO-A	Insomnia ~2-4%	No clear effects on REM	Some evidence of improved performance; no MSLT data
SSRIs				
	5-HT uptake inhibition	Variable; may worsen sleep or cause sedation; questionable differential effects among drugs	Generally ↑ W, ↓ TST, ↓ REM, may ↑ PLMs	No effect or mild ↑ performance; no MSLT data
Fluoxetine		Insomnia: 5-22%; daytime sedation: 5-6%, up to 21%	↓ TST, ↑ W, ↑ S1, ↓ REM, ↓ SWS, ↑ SEMs, ↑ PLMs	Usually no change or mild ↑ in performance; ↑ SL on modified MSLT
Paroxetine		Subjective ratings show improved sleep but in clinical trials insomnia reported in 6-14% and daytime sedation in 2-21%	↑ W, ↓ TST, ↑ S1, ↑ SL, ↓ REM	Mixed results: mild ↑ performance, ↓ memory; ↓ in performance noted on abrupt discontinuation; no MSLT data

Continued

Table 40–1. Antidepressants: Effects on Sleep and Waking Behavior—cont'd

Class/Drug	Primary Neurotransmitter/Receptor Activity	Subjective Data (Placebo-Corrected %)	PSG Data	Performance/ MSLT Data
SSRIs—cont'd				
Sertraline		Insomnia ~7-16%; daytime sedation ~7-13%	↑ SL, ↓ TST, ↓ REM	No change or mild ↑ performance
Fluvoxamine		Ratings show no sedation; clinical trials show sedation ~6-40% & insomnia ~4-15%	↓ TST, ↑ W, ↑ S1, ↑ SL, ↓ REM	No impairment in performance; no change in MSLT
Citalopram		Daytime sedation 5-18%, dose-dependent insomnia 2-18%	No change in TST, W	No impairment in performance; no MSLT data
Escitalopram	(s-Enantiomer of citalopram)	Insomnia 0-5%; sedation 0-5%; dose-dependent	No data	No data
SNRIs	Dual 5-HT and NE uptake inhibition			
Venlafaxine	Predominantly 5-HT uptake inhibition at low doses, NE uptake inhibition at higher doses, also weakly inhibits DA uptake	Insomnia: 8-32%; sedation: ~13-31%	↓ TST, ↑ W, ↑ PLMs, ↓↓ REM	↑ Performance in healthy subjects; no MSLT data
Milnacipran (not marketed in United States)	Equipotent reuptake inhibition of both 5-HT and NE		No data	Limited data; no cognitive/performance impairment
SARIs				
(See Chapter 37)	5-HT$_{2A}$ antagonist/reuptake inhibition			
Trazodone	Primarily 5-HT$_{2A}$ antagonist but also alpha$_1$, H$_1$ blockade	Improves sleep; daytime sedation 15-49%	↑ TST, ↓ SL, ↓ W, ? ↑ SWS, minimal ↓ REM	Limited data; ↓ performance in one study on elderly; no MSLT data
Nefazodone	Much weaker alpha$_1$ blockade than trazodone; no H$_1$ affinity	Dose-dependent daytime sedation 6-24%	Variable, may ↑ TST, ↓ W, ↑ REM	↑ Performance in one study; no impairment of driving; some impairment of cognition and memory especially with ↑ dose or duration; may be "alerting" after single dose but not repeated dosing; two MSLT studies: ↑ SL
NDRI				
Bupropion	Dual NE and DA uptake inhibition	Insomnia: ~5-22%, vivid dreaming, nightmares	Minimal data: may ↑ REM, ↑ sleep efficiency, ↓ SWS, ↓ PLMs	Usually no performance impairment; no MSLT data

Continued

Table 40–1. **Antidepressants: Effects on Sleep and Waking Behavior—cont'd**

Class/Drug	Primary Neurotransmitter/Receptor Activity	Subjective Data (Placebo-Corrected %)	PSG Data	Performance/ MSLT Data
NaSSA				
Mirtazapine (see Chapter 37)	NE, 5-HT$_2$, 5-HT$_3$ blockade but also alpha$_2$, H$_1$ blockade	Improves sleep; daytime sedation 9-54%	↑ TST, ↓ SL, ↓ S1	Minimal data, may ↓ performance acutely; no MSLT data
NaRI				
Reboxetine (not available in United States)	Selective NE reuptake inhibition	Insomnia 11%	↓ REM, no change in TST	No impairment, possible improvement in psychomotor, cognitive function
Miscellaneous				
Maprotiline	NE uptake inhibition; H$_1$ blockade	Sedation	Minimal data	Minimal data, no impairment?
Amoxapine	5-HT$_2$ blockade; NE uptake inhibition; H$_1$, alpha$_1$ blockade	Sedation	Minimal data	Insufficient data
Mianserin (not available in United States)	5-HT$_2$, alpha$_1$, alpha$_2$, H$_1$ blockade	Sedation	↑ TST in depressed patients	Impairs performance
Lithium				
		Improves nocturnal sleep, increases daytime sleepiness		No MSLT studies, prolongs reaction times, decreases vigilance, other cognitive impairment

DA, dopamine; H, histamine; 5-HT, 5-hydroxytryptamine (serotonin); MAOI, monoamine oxidase inhibitor; MSLT, Multiple Sleep Latency Test; NaRI, selective norepinephrine reuptake inhibitor; NaSSA, noradrenergic and specific serotonergic blocker; NDRI, norepinephrine and dopamine reuptake inhibitor; NE, norepinephrine; PLM, periodic limb movement; PSG, polysomnographic; REM, rapid eye movement; S1, stage 1; SL, sleep latency; SARI, serotonin type 2 receptor antagonist/reuptake inhibitor; SEM, slow eye movement; SNRI, dual serotonin and norepinephrine reuptake inhibitor; SSRI, selective serotonin reuptake inhibitor; SWS, slow wave sleep; TCA, tricyclic antidepressant; TST, total sleep time; W, wake.

review of their pharmacology and a comparison of their side effects, see references 5 through 10. The PSG effects of many of these drugs are reviewed in Obermeyer and Benca,[11] Gursky and Krahn,[12] and Winokur et al.[13] Performance effects are also reviewed in a number of articles.[13-15]

Monoamine Oxidase Inhibitors

MAOIs inhibit the action of MAO enzymes, which metabolize serotonin, norepinephrine, and dopamine. The classic MAOIs (e.g., isocarboxazid, phenelzine, tranylcypromine) irreversibly inhibit both MAO-A and MAO-B enzymes. Insomnia and daytime sedation are commonly reported side effects (up to 62% and 42% of patients, respectively),[16] but there are no placebo-controlled studies. The most impressive PSG finding is a marked decrease in rapid eye movement (REM) sleep, including almost complete abolishment of REM.[17] Total sleep time (TST) is also decreased. Although MSLT studies are lacking, actigraphic monitoring in a small group of patients confirmed periods of decreased daytime activity coincident with reported episodes of napping, possibly associated with poor nighttime sleep. Cognitive and psychomotor performance do not appear to be influenced by the classic MAOIs, but data are limited.

Unlike the classic MAOIs, the newer MAOIs reversibly and selectively inhibit the MAO-A enzyme, resulting in fewer severe adverse effects. Drugs of this type include moclobemide, befloxatone, and brofaromine. Sleep disturbance is commonly reported in clinical trials of these drugs, with a reported incidence of up to 67%, but these studies lack a placebo control. PSG data suggest that the degree of sleep disturbance may depend on both duration of treatment and dosage.[18] A study on brofaromine demonstrated increased waking during sleep (compared with baseline) for up to 4 weeks of treatment. However, several studies of moclobemide showed no significant effect on sleep, including REM sleep.[19] Moclobemide may enhance cognitive function in depressed outpatients.[20] In psychomotor performance studies of healthy subjects, moclobemide, brofaromine, and befloxatone in general do not differ from placebo, whereas trazodone, mianserin, doxepin, and amitriptyline result in decreased performance.[21,22]

Selective Serotonin Reuptake Inhibitors

Clinical trials of SSRIs show placebo-adjusted rates of insomnia ranging from 5% to 35% in depressed patients.[6,23] Fluoxetine causes insomnia in a dose-dependent fashion; insomnia typically emerges within the first few weeks of treatment and is likely to persist. Trazodone is frequently added to manage

SSRI-induced insomnia.[24,25] Sedation has also been reported in a number of clinical trials of SSRIs, more commonly with fluvoxamine (up to 26% of patients) and paroxetine (up to 24%).[6,23] There are few data directly comparing SSRIs with one another; however paroxetine may be more sleep disturbing than fluvoxamine in healthy normal individuals.[26]

PSG studies show that fluoxetine decreases TST and increases wake time and stage 1 sleep in both normal subjects during single-night studies with doses of 20 to 60 mg[27] and in depressed patients with doses of 20 to 80 mg for up to 1 year.[28] Fluoxetine has been associated with the presence of prominent slow eye movements in non-REM (NREM) sleep,[29] the significance of which is unknown. SSRIs are also associated with increased frequency of periodic limb movements during sleep (PLMs) as well as REM sleep without atonia.[30] Paroxetine (15 to 30 mg) decreases TST and increases awakenings in normal subjects with 1- to 2-day dosing.[31] There also is evidence of increased awakenings and sleep fragmentation after 5 weeks of paroxetine treatment in depressed inpatients.[32] Fluvoxamine has had similar effects on the sleep architecture of depressed patients.[33] Citalopram produced the typical decrease in REM sleep but no changes in sleep latency (SL) or TST during 5 weeks of treatment in one study of depressed patients.[34]

SSRIs usually do not negatively affect daytime performance or cognitive functioning and may actually improve functioning in some patients. However, paroxetine has been associated with memory impairment,[33,35] whereas abrupt discontinuation of paroxetine has been associated with impairment in cognitive and psychomotor performance as well as worsened sleep.[36] A single nighttime dose of fluvoxamine in healthy subjects showed increased daytime sleep latencies compared with dothiepin, but no change compared with placebo in a modified MSLT study.[37] Low doses (50 to 100 mg) of sertraline have been reported to improve cognitive function,[38] whereas very high doses (200 to 400 mg) have shown detrimental effects.

Selective Serotonin and Norepinephrine Reuptake Inhibitors

Venlafaxine and milnacipran (not available in the United States) inhibit reuptake of both norepinephrine and serotonin. Insomnia has been reported by 4% to 18% of patients taking venlafaxine, whereas somnolence occurs in a dose-dependent manner in approximately 12% to 31% of patients.[39] In normal subjects, 75 to 150 mg of venlafaxine produced increased waking and stage 1 sleep; in addition, in six of the eight subjects, frequent PLMs (more than 25 per hour) were noted.[40] In depressed inpatients treated for 1 month, venlafaxine (maximum dose 225 mg/day) increased PSG-recorded waking after sleep onset by approximately 30 minutes compared with placebo.[41] There are no studies that objectively evaluate daytime sleepiness and alertness. Single doses of venlafaxine improved performance and cognitive function in healthy subjects, particularly 6 to 8 hours after dosing.[42]

Serotonin Antagonist and Reuptake Inhibitors

Trazodone and nefazodone are in this drug class (see Chapter 37 for additional information). Drowsiness is the most commonly reported side effect of trazodone.[39] Because of its sedation, trazodone is currently more likely to be used as a h... than as an antidepressant. Nefazodone is structurally r... to trazodone but is a much less potent alpha$_1$-blocker and... no affinity for histamine type 1 (H$_1$) receptors.[43] Neverthele... drowsiness is one of its major side effects, with placeb... adjusted incidence rates ranging from approximately 6% to 24% and dependent on dose.

One study in normal individuals demonstrated an increase in MSLT mean latency (i.e., decreased sleepiness) after 16 days of nefazodone treatment.[44] Trazodone impairs performance in healthy individuals,[21] but data on depressed individuals are inconclusive. Cognitive and performance studies of nefazodone in general show no impairment or even slight improvement in psychomotor performance and memory in middle-aged and elderly healthy subjects.[45,46]

Norepinephrine and Dopamine Reuptake Inhibitors

Bupropion, which inhibits the uptake of dopamine and norepinephrine, is associated with insomnia in 5% to 19% of patients in clinical trials.[6] In a PSG study of seven depressed patients, after 4 weeks of treatment bupropion did not affect SL or TST but did decrease REM latency and increase REM sleep percentage.[46] In a study of depressed patients with PLMs, bupropion SR decreased PLMs, possibly because of its effects on dopamine reuptake.[47] Bupropion is not usually associated with cognitive or psychomotor performance impairment.[21,48]

Norepinephrine and Specific Serotonin Antagonists

Mirtazapine is a noradrenergic and specific serotonin antagonist that also has affinity for the H$_1$ receptor, which likely accounts for its sedating effect. See Chapter 37 for more information.

Selective Norepinephrine Reuptake Inhibitors

Reboxetine, not currently available in the United States, is a selective norepinephrine reuptake inhibitor. Clinical trials indicate an incidence of insomnia of approximately 10%.[49] A single PSG study showed a decrease in REM sleep and increased REM latency but no change in TST.[50] Reboxetine resulted in improved cognitive function in one study of depressed patients.[51]

Miscellaneous Antidepressants

Amoxapine, a dibenzoxazepine tricyclic, and maprotiline and mianserin, both tetracyclic compounds (the latter is not available in the United States), have sedative profiles similar to that of the TCAs, likely because of their high affinity for H$_1$ receptors.[5] Amoxapine and maprotiline are not commonly used because of other serious side effects, namely seizures in the case of maprotiline and dopamine-blocking side effects with amoxapine. There are no studies objectively measuring sleepiness. There appears to be little cognitive impairment with maprotiline,[20] although minimal data are available. In healthy individuals, mianserin impaired driving and tracking performance, as well as reaction time and other psychomotor measures.[14,21]

...rily in the treatment of manic- ...ctively associated with improved ...ncreased daytime sleepiness, at least ...turbance is a prominent feature of mania ...ysomnographically to that observed in major ... There are no objective studies evaluating the ...n lithium on daytime sleepiness. In healthy volunteers, ...ium administered for 1 to 3 weeks produced cognitive and psychomotor deficits, including prolonged reaction times, decreased vigilance, and impairment of semantic reasoning.[52] Similar deficits have been shown in psychiatric patients taking lithium for periods of time ranging from 2 weeks to longer than 3 months,[53] although it is difficult to determine whether the deficits seen in the patient population are caused by the medication or their psychiatric illness. A comparison group of healthy subjects taking lithium for at least 3 months did not show the same psychomotor deficits as did the patient group. As age, severity of disease, or lithium concentration increases, so does the degree of cognitive deficit in patients on long-term lithium.

ANTIPSYCHOTIC AGENTS

Evaluation of the effects of antipsychotic medications is complicated by difficulty with sleep onset, sleep maintenance, and cognitive impairment in schizophrenia.[54] Reported findings such as decreased slow wave sleep (SWS), decreased REM sleep latency, and increased REM sleep density may reflect prior neuroleptic treatment rather than the pathophysiology of the disorder.

Sedation is a common side effect of the traditional antipsychotics, although extrapyramidal symptoms and tardive dyskinesia may be more troublesome.[55] However, the incidence of sedation varies considerably among drugs, probably as a function of variation in affinity for cholinergic and histaminic receptors as well as blockade of alpha$_1$ adrenoreceptors.[56] Among the older neuroleptics, chlorpromazine and thioridazine tend to be more sedating than haloperidol. The newer agents (clozapine, risperidone, olanzapine, sertindole, quetiapine, and ziprasidone) have unique pharmacologic profiles.[57,58] Risperidone, sertindole, and quetiapine are dopamine (D$_2$ receptor), serotonin, and norepinephrine (alpha$_1$ receptor) antagonists, whereas clozapine and olanzapine also bind to cholinergic, histaminergic, and D$_1$ receptors. Aripiprazole, a third-generation novel antipsychotic, is a dopamine D$_2$ receptor partial agonist with partial agonist activity at serotonin 5-hydroxytryptamine-1A (5-HT$_{1A}$) receptors and antagonist activity at 5-HT$_{2A}$ receptors,[59] while having very low affinity for alpha$_1$, histamine, and muscarinic receptors. These newer drugs appear to be less likely to produce extrapyramidal symptoms, although there is some controversy over this subject.[60] Clinical studies show a high incidence of sedation with clozapine (with transient sedation reported by 54% of patients, persistent sedation by 46%, and sedation requiring drug discontinuation by 24%).[61] Olanzapine and quetiapine appear to be more sedating than risperidone and sertindole but to a much lesser extent than clozapine. Both olanzapine and quetiapine have been investigated for their hypnotic use (see Chapter 37 for more information.) PSG studies show that clozapine increases TST,[62] and olanzapine increases both TST and SWS in schizophrenic patients[63] and healthy individuals.[64]

There are no MSLT or other studies that objectively evaluate daytime sleepiness.

Although neuroleptics cause cognitive impairment in healthy subjects,[65] these drugs in patient populations either have no demonstrable effect[66] or may actually improve cognitive function.[67] Clozapine, in particular, despite its significant sedation, has been associated with improvement in various aspects of cognitive function in schizophrenic patients.[68]

ANXIOLYTIC AGENTS

Benzodiazepines

Benzodiazepines, which are used to treat anxiety, are also sometimes used for their sleep-inducing effects. It is not surprising that the most common side effect of these drugs is sedation.[69] In a placebo-controlled study of healthy subjects, daytime administration of alprazolam and diazepam produced decreased SLs as measured by MSLT on both day 1 and day 7 of treatment, with alprazolam producing greater sleepiness than diazepam on the first day of treatment.[70] Performance impairment, including impairment of actual driving performance,[71] is common with benzodiazepines in studies of normal subjects and patient groups for treatment periods of up to 3 weeks, particularly at higher doses.[69] Well-controlled studies are needed to determine whether longer-term use of benzodiazepine anxiolytics results in tolerance to these performance-impairing effects and whether there are differential effects between younger and older individuals.

Nonbenzodiazepines

SSRIs as well as a number of the other second- and third-generation antidepressants have been shown to be efficacious in anxiety disorders. Their effects on sleep, sedation, and performance are described in the antidepressant section of this chapter.

Buspirone

Buspirone does not have the hypnotic, anticonvulsant, and muscle relaxant properties of the benzodiazepines. The anxiolytic efficacy of buspirone is similar to that of the benzodiazepines, but its onset of action is much slower, requiring up to 3 to 4 weeks.[72] This delay in onset of action as well as the possibility that patients may inappropriately equate subjective feelings of sedation with efficacy may partially account for decreased use of this drug compared with benzodiazepine use in the treatment of anxiety. Although its mechanism of action is unknown, buspirone appears to act primarily as a 5-HT$_{1A}$ partial agonist, but also has effects on D$_2$ receptors.[73] It has no affinity for the benzodiazepine receptors and does not affect gamma-aminobutyric acid binding. In clinical studies of anxious patients, buspirone was comparable with placebo in the frequency of subjective reports of sedation.[74] In non–placebo-controlled clinical trials, reports of sleepiness or drowsiness were much more frequent with diazepam (34% to 45%), chlorazepate (26% to 33%), alprazolam (43% to 45%), and lorazepam (58% to 65%) than with buspirone (8% to 16%), despite similar efficacy.

In a study of 12 patients with chronic insomnia, alertness as measured by MSLT was not impaired by 20 mg/day buspirone in divided doses over a 3-day period.[75] In addition, the effects of buspirone on quantitative electroencephalography

(EEG) were indistinguishable from placebo. Compared with benzodiazepine anxiolytics, buspirone appears to have few negative effects on psychomotor, cognitive, or driving performance in healthy volunteers receiving short-term treatment or patients treated for up to 4 weeks.[71,75]

CARDIOVASCULAR DRUGS

There are numerous reviews on the effects of cardiovascular drugs, particularly antihypertensive medications, on sleep and waking function.[69,76-78] This section focuses primarily on antihypertensive medications because of their widespread use (including use for heart failure or arrhythmias) and because many have CNS side effects associated with sleep–waking function. In addition, a number of different classes of antihypertensive agents are available; these data are summarized in Table 40–2.

Antihypertensive Agents

Beta Antagonists

Information on pharmacologic characteristics of beta antagonists relevant to CNS sleep–waking function is given in Table 40–3. CNS side effects that have been reported to occur with beta-blockers include tiredness, fatigue, insomnia, nightmares and vivid dreams, depression, mental confusion, and psychomotor impairment.[76] Both age of the patient and dose contribute to the frequency of side effects, which may diminish with time. The incidence of sleep disturbance has been reported to be 2% to 4.3%. In general, sleep disturbance appears to be more common with the lipophilic drugs (e.g., propranolol) than with the hydrophilic drugs (e.g., atenolol) in both subjective reports and PSG studies. The data are not straightforward, however. Pindolol, which is less lipophilic than propranolol, appears to be more disruptive of sleep.[79] Even atenolol, the most hydrophilic of the beta-blockers, has been shown to increase total wake time, at least acutely, in normal subjects.[80] Thus, although lipophilicity may be a primary determinant of the CNS effects of these drugs, other factors are also likely involved, such as the relative affinity for beta$_2$ or 5-HT receptors, plasma catecholamine levels, molecule-specific structural details, plasma concentration, or the degree of melatonin suppression. There are reports that pindolol may hasten the antidepressant response of SSRIs, probably because of selective blockade of 5-HT$_{1A}$ receptors. The combination of pindolol with paroxetine produced longer latency to REM sleep and less SWS than either placebo or paroxetine alone.[81]

Complaints of tiredness, fatigue, and daytime sleepiness may be the consequences of disturbed nocturnal sleep or a direct action of the drugs themselves. There are no studies that have differentially evaluated these hypotheses, nor are there published reports using the MSLT or other measures to evaluate objectively daytime sleepiness in either healthy subjects or hypertensive patients.

Reviews on the effects of beta-blockers on cognitive and psychomotor performance[74,75,78,79] indicate that these drugs produce few consistent neuropsychological deficits. Decrements in performance appear to be more likely to occur with more complex cognitive or psychomotor tasks and have been reported more often with lipophilic beta-blockers than with hydrophilic drugs, although results are not always consistent.

Deficits in cognitive function may be more likely with older than with younger patients. In a review of 55 studies, Dimsdale et al.[78] concluded that beta-blockers improved cognitive function in 16% of subjects, worsened it in 17%, and caused no change in 67%, with no significant difference between lipophilic and nonlipophilic drugs.

Beta Antagonists with Alpha$_1$-Blocking Activity

Beta-blocking drugs that also have vasodilating properties (e.g., carvedilol, labetalol) have been associated with fatigue and somnolence (3% to 11% of patients taking labetalol and 1% to 4% of patients taking carvedilol). Insomnia has occasionally been reported.[82] Objective studies of sleep, sleepiness and alertness, and performance are lacking.

Alpha$_2$ Agonists

Sedation is the most common side effect of both clonidine and methyldopa, occurring in 30% to 75% of patients, but the severity apparently diminishes with time.[83] There also are some reports of insomnia and nightmares. In a double-blinded, placebo-controlled crossover study, hypertensive men aged 31 to 59 years who were given 0.1 to 0.3 mg of clonidine twice daily showed significantly decreased TST compared with placebo after 3 months of use.[84] Healthy subjects, however, given clonidine acutely showed increases in TST.[85] No MSLT studies exist to quantify daytime sedation objectively. However, one study of a single morning dose of clonidine in young healthy subjects demonstrated microsleeps in six of eight subjects despite efforts of study personnel to keep them awake.[86] In that study, subjective ratings of sleepiness were also higher with clonidine compared with placebo. Few well-controlled studies exist that evaluate the effects of these drugs on performance. Verbal memory impairment and poorer workplace performance[87] have been reported in patients receiving methyldopa.

5-Hydroxytryptamine Type 2 Antagonists

Ketanserin, which is not available in the United States, is a selective 5-HT$_2$ antagonist that acts primarily at peripheral sites; it also has affinity for alpha$_1$ adrenoreceptors, H$_1$ receptors, and dopamine receptors. After 1 to 3 months of use, ketanserin was more frequently associated with fatigue (11%) than was propranolol (6%).[88] There are no published PSG, MSLT, or performance studies.

Ritanserin, which blocks central 5-HT$_2$ receptors, has not been associated with subjective reports of insomnia or fatigue. Ritanserin increases SWS in normal subjects,[89] poor sleepers,[90] dysthymic patients,[91] and narcoleptic patients[92] without affecting SL or TST. The addition of ritanserin to the usual medication in patients with narcolepsy did not affect MSLT latency. No performance studies exist.

Other Antihypertensives

Except for reserpine, which can cause fatigue, sedation, and nightmares, particularly at higher doses, the remaining drugs used for the control of hypertension in general have few negative effects on sleep or wakefulness, although there are limited objective data for some of these drugs. The angiotensin receptor antagonist losartan is rarely associated with insomnia.[93]

Table 40–2.   Antihypertensive Drugs: Effects on Sleep and Waking Behavior

Drug Class	Example	Subjective Data	Polysomnographic Data	Performance Data
Beta antagonists	Propranolol metoprolol atenolol (see Table 40–3)	Insomnia, nightmares possibly more common with lipophilic drugs	Lipophilic drugs more likely to ↑ W, TWT, and S1, ↓ REM, SWS, and TST, but plasma concentration, receptor selectivity, and other factors may also be important in determining the degree of sleep disruption	Few consistent effects, but many methodologic problems in these studies
Alpha₂ agonists	Clonidine	Sedation, insomnia, mental slowing, ↓ concentration; nightmares	↓ REM; ↑ TST acutely in healthy subjects; ↓ TST in hypertensive patients	No impairment (one study)
	Methyldopa	Sedation; insomnia, nightmares; reports of poor workplace performance and lower QOL	↑ REM; ↑ TST, ↓ SWS	Memory impairment
Catecholamine depleters	Reserpine	Sedation, insomnia, nightmares, depression, difficulty concentrating	↑ REM and ↓ SWS initially; ↑ stage shifts	No studies
Beta antagonists with alpha₁-blocking activity	Carvedilol, labetalol	Fatigue, somnolence, insomnia	No studies	No studies
Calcium antagonists	Verapamil, nifedipine, diltiazem, amlodipine	One report of increased agitation with nifedipine	No polysomnographic studies; one report of increased alpha activity in waking electroencephalogram with nifedipine	No studies
Angiotensin-converting enzyme inhibitors	Captopril, cilazapril	No negative effects on sleep; improvement in QOL	No disturbance	Improved psychomotor performance
Angiotensin II receptor antagonists	Irbesartan, losartan	Rare insomnia	No studies	No studies
Alpha₁ antagonists	Prazosin, terazosin, doxazosin	Transiently sedating?	No studies in humans	Prazosin: no change in performance (one study)
Vasodilators	Hydralazine	?Anxiety, depression, insomnia	No studies	Hydralazine: no change in performance (one study)
Diuretics	Hydrochloro-thiazide, chlorthalidone, indapamide	Central nervous system effects unlikely; one report of subjective-rated worsening of work performance; one report of improved sleep with indapamide	No studies	No evidence of impairment
5-Hydroxytryp-tamine₂ antagonists (not yet available in United States)	Ketanserin (acts peripherally)	Fatigue, insomnia	No studies ↑ SWS, ↓ REM, no effects on SL or TST	No studies
	Ritanserin (blocks central receptors)	No negative effects reported		
Imidazoline agonists (not available in United States)	Moxonidine, rilmenidine	Rare sedation with low doses; increased sedation with higher doses but less than with clonidine	No studies	Little effect on psychomotor performance; slight decrements in vigilance and memory

QOL, quality of life; REM, rapid eye movement; S1, stage 1; SWS, slow wave sleep; TST, total sleep time; TWT, total wake time; W, wake.

Table 40–3. **Beta Antagonists: Selected Pharmacologic Characteristics**

Drug	Lipid Solubility	Selectivity	Relative Affinity for 5-Hydroxytryptamine Receptors
Propranolol	High	None	High
Timolol	High	None	High
Pindolol	Moderate	None	High
Acebutolol	Moderate	Beta$_1$	Low
Metoprolol	Moderate	Beta$_1$	Low
Bisoprolol	Moderate	Beta$_1$	Low
Nadolol	Low	None	High
Carvedilol	Low	None	High
Atenolol	Low	Beta$_1$	Low
Sotalol	Low	Beta$_1$	Low

Beta$_1$ receptors are located primarily in cardiac muscle, whereas beta$_2$ receptors are primarily in bronchial and vascular musculature. The nonselective beta-blocking agents have higher affinity for 5-hydroxytryptamine (5-HT) receptors.

Lipophilic compounds appear to be more disruptive of sleep than hydrophilic compounds, but high affinity for 5-HT receptors may be equally important in determining the effect on sleep.

The imidazoline agonists moxonidine and rilmenidine, which are not yet available in the United States, belong to a class of centrally active antihypertensives with greater selectivity for the imidazoline receptor relative to the alpha$_2$ adrenoreceptor, which theoretically results in fewer central adverse effects while maintaining central antihypertensive properties.[94] Compared with clonidine in clinical studies, both rilmenidine and moxonidine have had a much lower incidence of sedation. There is some evidence of slightly increased incidence of sedation at higher doses.[89,90,93,94]

The alpha$_1$ antagonists (e.g., prazosin, terazosin) are sometimes associated with transient sedation. There are no reports of sleep disturbance or wake dysfunction with the calcium channel blockers (e.g., verapamil, nifedipine); however, these drugs decrease the effectiveness of hypnotics and potentiate the effects of stimulants, at least in studies in animals.[95] Angiotensin-converting enzyme inhibitors (e.g., captopril, cilazapril) reportedly have a low incidence of central side effects. Vasodilators (e.g., hydralazine) and diuretics do not appear to disrupt sleep,[83] although one might expect more frequent awakenings for micturition with diuretics.

Among the aforementioned drugs, PSG data exist only for the angiotensin-converting enzyme inhibitors. In healthy individuals, PSG-recorded sleep was not affected by 14-day administration of cilazapril compared with the positive control, metoprolol, which produced increased awakenings.[96]

There are no objective evaluations of daytime sleepiness for these drugs, but they do not appear to affect daytime function negatively. Patients treated with captopril for 24 weeks demonstrated improvement in quality of life and cognitive function compared with patients treated with methyldopa or propranolol.[87] Studies on prazosin and hydralazine show no change in performance. Although performance impairment appears unlikely with diuretics, there is one report showing worsened scores on indices of subject-rated work performance and general well-being.[97] The imidazoline agonists do not affect psychomotor performance, although there may be minor decrements in vigilance and memory.[98]

Hypolipidemic Drugs

Available data on the effects of hypolipidemic drugs on sleep and waking are summarized in Table 40–4. Atorvastatin and lovastatin have been associated with subjective reports of insomnia. However, placebo-controlled clinical trials of lovastatin, simvastatin, and pravastatin have in general failed to

Table 40–4. **Hypolipidemic Drugs: Effects on Sleep and Waking Behavior**

Drug	U.S. Trade Name	Subjective Data	Polysomnographic Data	Performance Data
Atorvastatin	Lipitor	Insomnia >2% in clinical trials	No data	No data
Lovastatin	Mevacor	Insomnia per case reports	Conflicting results; some evidence for increased waking and stage 1 sleep	Conflicting results
Fluvastatin	Lescol	No effects	No data	No data
Pravastatin	Pravachol	No effects	No changes	No negative effects
Rosuvastatin	Crestor	No data	No data	No data
Simvastatin	Zocor	Insomnia per case reports	No changes	No data
Cholestyramine	Questran	Insomnia 1.3% in clinical trials	No data	No data
Clofibrate	Atromid	Fatigue, drowsiness	No data	No data
Colestipol	Colestid	Infrequent insomnia	No data	No data
Gemfibrozil	Lopid	Reports of sleepiness	No data	No data

show increased sleep disturbance.[99,100] PSG evidence of sleep disruption is conflicting as well. Roth et al.[101] demonstrated performance decrements with lovastatin even though nocturnal sleep and daytime sleep tendency (measured by MSLT) were not affected. There have been case reports of short-term memory loss associated with statin use. However, randomized studies using neuropsychological testing and a meta-analysis of observational studies suggest that these drugs may actually lower the odds for development of cognitive impairment.[102,103]

Antiarrhythmic Drugs

Subjective data on antiarrhythmic drugs are summarized in Table 40–5. Fatigue is the most common CNS complaint of patients taking these drugs, with placebo-adjusted incidence from clinical trials of up to 10%,[104] except for the beta antagonists, for which rates may be higher (see separate section on these drugs). Digoxin has been associated with cognitive abnormalities as well as insomnia, lethargy and fatigue.[105] There are few objective data available.

HISTAMINE TYPE 1 RECEPTOR ANTAGONISTS

The effects of the first-generation H_1 antihistamines are covered in Chapter 37. These drugs are lipophilic and easily cross the blood–brain barrier. In addition, these drugs demonstrate poor receptor selectivity as characterized by antagonism of muscarinic cholinergic, alpha-adrenergic, and tryptaminergic receptors. The second-generation H_1 antihistamines are large, hydrophilic molecules and do not easily penetrate the CNS; they have high affinity for H_1 receptors and little affinity for other amine receptors. Unlike the first-generation agents, the second-generation H_1 antihistamines do not appear to be sedating and are much less likely to impair performance.

MSLT studies in normal subjects and atopic individuals generally confirm that cetirizine, loratadine, and terfenadine are not sedating. Cetirizine, however, has been classified as sedating by the U.S. Food and Drug Administration (FDA). Indeed, there are a number of studies (primarily studies using high doses of cetirizine or cetirizine in combination with alcohol)

that suggest cetirizine, which is a metabolite of hydroxyzine, is not completely without sedating effects.[106] However, a number of well-controlled studies with objective evaluations of sleepiness and performance indicate that cetirizine in recommended doses of 5 to 10 mg does not differ from placebo.[107,108]

Controlled studies that evaluate psychomotor skills, memory and cognition, attention, visual processing, and actual driving performance generally confirm that the newer compounds do not impair performance.[109] A review[110] of studies with both positive and placebo controls concluded that the risk of performance impairment was minimal and similar for astemizole, cetirizine, terfenadine, azatadine, and loratadine (all second-generation compounds).

HISTAMINE TYPE 2 RECEPTOR ANTAGONISTS

H_2 antagonists (e.g., cimetidine, ranitidine, famotidine, and nizatidine) are unlikely significantly to impair CNS function because these compounds do not easily cross the blood–brain barrier, although there is some evidence of CNS penetration. Insomnia and somnolence usually occur in less than 2% of individuals involved in clinical trials. Although such side effects may be infrequent, they are apparently reproducible in susceptible individuals.[111] Moreover, the nature of these side effects and the widespread use of H_2 antagonists suggest that physicians should be aware of their potential occurrence. Side effects have been most frequently reported with cimetidine, possibly because it has been on the market longer than any of the other compounds. In addition, cimetidine slows the clearance of some benzodiazepines, which may make carryover effects of hypnotics more of a problem. Similarly, cimetidine has been shown to increase levels of theophylline, carbamazepine, and beta-blockers with resultant increases in the CNS effects of these drugs. Ranitidine has produced some of the same effects, although not to the extent seen with cimetidine.[112]

One crossover study comparing 1-week administration of cimetidine, famotidine, ranitidine, and placebo in normal subjects reported no differences in nocturnal sleep or daytime MSLT latencies, although cimetidine produced a slight increase in subjective estimates of sleepiness.[113] This study is

Table 40–5.   Antiarrhythmic Drugs: Effects on Sleep and Waking Behavior

Class*	Drug	Common U.S. Trade Name	Subjective Data†
IA	Disopyramide	Norpace	Fatigue: 3-10%
	Procainamide	Procanbid	None reported
	Quinidine	Quinaglute	Fatigue: 2.9%
1B	Mexiletine	Mexitil	Drowsiness: 7%; insomnia, memory impairment
	Moricizine	Ethmozine	Fatigue: 0.5%
	Tocainide	Tonocard	Fatigue: 0.8-2%
1C	Flecainide	Tambocor	Fatigue: 5-10%; insomnia: 1-3%
	Propafenone	Rythmol	None reported
II	Beta antagonists	various	See Table 40–2 and section on beta-antagonists in text
III	Amiodarone	Cordarone	Fatigue: 5-10%; nightmares, insomnia: 1-3%
IV	Diltiazem	Cardizem	Fatigue: 10%; insomnia, abnormal dreams, sleepiness
	Verapamil	Calan	Fatigue: 2%

*Vaughan-Williams classification
†Percentages indicate placebo-adjusted rates from clinical trials.

weakened by the lack of a positive control but, more important, by the fact that on placebo, these subjects were quite sleepy (mean SL, 6.6 minutes). H_2 antagonists do not appear to affect psychomotor performance. However, because H_2 antagonists are widely used, often in combination with other drugs and frequently in older individuals, additional data are needed to determine the extent of their CNS effects in specific populations and situations. For example, both cimetidine[114] and ranitidine administered in conventional doses have been associated with an increased incidence of lethargy, somnolence, and confusion in patients with renal impairment. In addition, benzodiazepine-produced impairment of psychomotor and cognitive function was significantly prolonged with concomitant administration of cimetidine and was somewhat prolonged with concomitant administration of ranitidine in healthy volunteers.[115]

CORTICOSTEROIDS

Corticosteroids are widely believed to disrupt sleep, but the results of objective studies are inconsistent. Differences in receptor affinities between synthetic and endogenous corticosteroids, dosage, methodologic issues associated with the study of patient populations, and the variety of organ systems affected by corticosteroids, as well as the variety of side effects reported,[116] all contribute to this confusion.

In patient populations, corticosteroids have frequently been associated with sleep disturbance. Approximately 50% of patients treated with prednisone for optic neuritis reported sleep disturbance, compared with 20% on placebo,[117] whereas patients taking prednisone for oral inflammatory ulcerative disease reported a dose-related incidence of insomnia ranging from 12% to 71%.[118] Parent ratings of sleep disturbance increased when steroids were added to the chemotherapy regimen of children with leukemia or other types of cancer.[119] Insomnia has also been reported more frequently in patients with asthma receiving steroid medications.[120] In addition, numerous anecdotal and case reports exist implicating systemic corticosteroid use with insomnia. Behavioral observations of 12 healthy subjects given prednisone 80 mg/day for 5 days showed decreased sleep in 25% and mild hypomania in 67%.[121] Inhaled glucocorticoids do not appear to have the same negative effects, but there have been case reports of hyperactivity, insomnia, and psychosis with these drugs as well.

The most consistent effect of corticosteroids on PSG-recorded sleep in normal subjects is a marked decrease in REM sleep.[122] Although less consistent, there is good evidence for increased waking during the night with cortisol, dexamethasone, and prednisone. Dexamethasone, administered before bedtime, resulted in increased daytime alertness the next day as measured with MSLT.[123]

In a single study evaluating performance, prednisone 80 mg/day given to 11 healthy subjects for 5 days produced increased frequency of errors of commission on a verbal memory task.[124]

THEOPHYLLINE

Theophylline, a respiratory stimulant and bronchodilator, is chemically related to caffeine. Peak plasma concentration is usually reached within 2 hours, but the half-life varies by preparation and is typically shorter in children (3.5 hours) and longer in adults (8 to 9 hours). Absorption is lower at night than in the morning[125] and may be greatly affected by food.[126]

Disturbed sleep is a common complaint among patients taking theophylline. In a prospective study, patients with asthma treated with theophylline were more likely to complain of sleep maintenance difficulty (55%) than were patients treated with other asthma medications (31%),[127] and in a retrospective study of treated patients with asthma, 46% of whom complained of insomnia, only theophylline or corticosteroid therapy was associated with the complaint of insomnia.[120] Most of the studies purporting that theophylline does not adversely affect sleep are limited by the lack of a placebo group or condition or other methodologic difficulties. Because theophylline improves asthma-related symptoms, there have also been reports of improved sleep continuity and decreased nocturnal awakenings associated with its use.[128]

Theophylline, administered for up to 3 weeks, has been shown to disturb PSG-recorded sleep in healthy subjects,[129] patients with asthma,[130] children with cystic fibrosis,[131] and patients with sleep apnea[132] or chronic obstructive pulmonary disease.[133]

There are few well-controlled studies that evaluate the effect of theophylline on cognitive performance. In a double-blinded study, asthmatic children were more likely to exhibit behavioral or attentional problems when receiving sustained-release theophylline for 4 weeks than when on placebo.[134] However, a meta-analysis of 12 studies of theophylline did not indicate any impairment in cognition or behavior.[135] Furthermore, academic achievement did not differ between 72 asthmatic patients who were treated with theophylline and siblings without asthma.[136]

ANTIPARKINSONIAN DRUGS

Patients with Parkinson's disease have multiple complaints relating to sleep, including insomnia, hypersomnia, fatigue, and, in some cases, vivid dreaming or nightmares.[137] These complaints may be the result of the degenerative processes associated with the disease; accompanying symptoms such as nighttime stiffness, pain, difficulty in turning, and nocturia; or the medications used for treatment. PSG studies confirm prolonged SLs and increased awakenings in untreated patients. Dopamine replacement is the primary treatment for Parkinson's disease.

Types of drugs used to treat Parkinson's disease (Table 40–6) include (1) combinations of a synthetic dopamine precursor with a dopamine decarboxylase inhibitor (levodopa/carbidopa); (2) dopaminergic agonists, including the ergot agonists apomorphine, bromocriptine, cabergoline, lisuride, piribedil, and pergolide, and nonergot agonists pramipexole and ropinirole; (3) the MAO-B inhibitor selegiline; (4) the presynaptic releasing agent amantadine; catechol-O-methyltransferase (COMT) inhibitors (entacapone, tolcapone); and (5) anticholinergics (hyoscyamine, benztropine). COMT inhibitors prolong the duration of the effect of levodopa, which may cause an initial worsening of levodopa-induced side effects.[138]

Sleep-related complaints have been reported in up to 75% of patients receiving levodopa.[139] The effects of levodopa on sleep appear to be related to dose, timing, and duration of drug administration, as well as to disease severity. Actigraphic,[137] PSG,[140] and subjective[141] studies indicate that low doses tend to improve sleep, whereas higher doses are likely to disrupt sleep, particularly when administered in the evening. In more severely affected patients, drug-related improvement in

Table 40–6.　Antiparkinsonian Drugs: Effects on Sleep and Waking Behavior

Drug Class	Example	Subjective Data*	PSG Data	MSLT Data	Cognitive/ Performance Data
Synthetic dopamine precursor + dopamine decarboxylase inhibitor	Levodopa/carbidopa	Low doses may improve sleep; higher doses disrupt sleep; nightmares, hallucinations, vocalizations, daytime sleepiness	↑ REM, ↓ REM ↑ REM density ↓ SWS, mixed results	None	Impairment of cognitive function and memory
Dopaminergic agonists					
Ergot agonists	Apomorphine, bromocriptine, cabergoline, lisuride, piribedil, pergolide	Daytime sleepiness; may be dose related		↓ MSLT with higher doses	
Nonergot agonists	Pramipexole, ropinirole	Daytime sleepiness, questionable "sleep attacks"; however, overall dopaminergic dose likely accounts for ↑ sleepiness	↑ TST in patients with restless legs syndrome	↓ MSLT with higher doses	Improved reaction time in healthy subjects
Monoamine oxidase-B inhibitors	Selegiline	Insomnia	↑ W, ↓ REM in healthy subjects; ↓ SL in patients		? Improved vigilance
Presynaptic releasing agents	Amantadine	Insomnia, confusion, hallucinations			
Catechol-O-methyl-transferase inhibitors	Entacapone, tolcapone	Prolong duration of levodopa so may increase effects on sleep	No data	No data	No data
Anticholinergic drugs	Hyoscyamine, benztropine	Similar to other anticholinergic drugs	↓ REM	No data	No data

MSLT, Multiple Sleep Latency Test; PSG, polysomnography; REM, rapid eye movement; SL, sleep latency; SWS, slow wave sleep; TST, total sleep time; W, wake.

parkinsonian symptoms may outweigh the sleep-disrupting effects of the drug, resulting in an improvement in sleep overall.[137] PSG studies have shown mixed results, including both increased and decreased REM sleep and decreased SWS. Nightmares and visual hallucinations are not uncommon and may be associated with increased ocular activity in REM sleep. The effects on sleep of the remaining drugs used to treat Parkinson's disease are less well studied. Insomnia has been reported in 10% to 32% of patients taking selegiline,[142] which preferentially oxidizes dopamine and phenylethylamine and is metabolized to L-methamphetamine and L-amphetamine. As with levodopa, low doses of selegiline are less likely to worsen sleep than are higher doses. Forty-two percent of patients taking pergolide reported insomnia.[143] Fourteen percent of patients receiving amantadine, either alone or in combination with other medications, reported insomnia.[144]

Daytime sleepiness in Parkinson's disease is common. In one controlled study, excessive daytime sleepiness was reported in 76% of patients with Parkinson's disease compared with 47% of control subjects, and sleep episodes while driving were reported by 21% of patients compared with 6% of control subjects.[145] Although the nonergot dopaminergic agonists have been specifically associated with increases in daytime sleepiness, including sudden "sleep attacks,"[146-148] there is some controversy as to whether the sleepiness is related to the pathologic process of Parkinson's disease or the specific drugs.[149,150] Although ropinirole decreased mean MSLT latency in healthy subjects,[151] total dopaminergic dose was the best predictor of daytime sleepiness in patients with Parkinson's disease taking pramipexole, ropinirole, bromocriptine, or pergolide.[152] In that study, although almost 19% of patients showed pathologic sleep latencies on MSLT, overall MSLT and Maintenance of Wakefulness Test latencies were within normal limits and did not differ among drugs.

Cognitive and motor deficits are common in Parkinson's disease. Only the anticholinergic drugs have been demonstrated to produce worsening of cognitive function, primarily in the areas of memory function.[153] Such impairment is more common in older patients and is reversible with discontinuation of medication. Ropinirole in healthy subjects resulted in improved fine motor activity and reaction time.[154] Behavioral symptoms that may affect cognitive function, such as hallucinations, delusions, confusion, mania, and anxiety, have been reported in 15% to 30% of patients treated with dopaminergic agents.[155]

ANTIEPILEPTIC AGENTS

Patients with epilepsy frequently complain of daytime fatigue and sleepiness and occasionally complain of disturbed nocturnal sleep. In addition, cognitive deficits have been reported to be common in these patients. These problems may result from sleep disruption secondary to seizures or interictal EEG activity, as well as from effects of antiepileptic drugs.

There are many antiepileptic drugs available for use, including a number of medications recently approved, primarily for use as adjunctive therapy. Findings regarding the effects of these medications on sleep and waking are summarized in Table 40–7. The mechanisms of action and pharmacokinetics of antiepileptic drugs are reviewed in several publications.[156,157] Compared with the classic antiepileptic compounds, the newer drugs have a variety of mechanisms of action, specifically gamma-aminobutyric acid–related mechanisms. Gabapentin, topiramate, lamotrigine, and vigabatrin have the greatest variety of mechanisms, which has led to their evaluation and use in other neurologic and psychiatric conditions.

Subjectively, sedation is one of the most common adverse effects of the older antiepileptic drugs, particularly phenobarbital.[158] Sedation is typically dose dependent and more likely to be experienced acutely, with some tolerance possibly developing with chronic use. The incidence of sedation with the older antiepileptic drugs is unclear because there are few placebo-controlled studies. The frequency of sedation has been reported to be as high as 70% with acute use of phenobarbital, 42% with carbamazepine and valproate, and 33% with phenytoin and primidone. In a prospective study of 509 patients treated with a variety of older anticonvulsant medications for more than 3 months, somnolence was the most common complaint (10%) and was most frequently associated with the use of phenobarbital or primidone.[159] Among the newer antiepileptic drugs, the incidence of reported sedation in placebo-controlled clinical trials is 5% to 15% for gabapentin, lamotrigine, levetiracetam, vigabatrin, and zonisamide, 15% to 27% for topiramate, and is generally more prevalent during the initial treatment.[160,161] The incidence of sedation with tiagabine was no different from that for placebo in placebo-controlled studies, but it was 25% in open-label, long-term studies.[162] Both sedation and insomnia have been reported with felbamate.

PSG studies of established antiepileptic drugs in general show these drugs produce shorter SL and increase TST.[163] The newer drugs show variable effects on sleep architecture. However, both gabapentin and tiagabine show increased SWS, whereas lamotrigine shows decreased SWS.[164,165] See Chapter 37 for additional information on gabapentin and tiagabine, which are being evaluated for their use as hypnotics.

There are several objective studies of the effects of these drugs on daytime sleepiness, but none with a placebo control. Patients treated with phenobarbital[166] or carbamazepine[167]

had lower mean MSLT latencies than did healthy control subjects. In a 6-minute test of ability to maintain wakefulness, patients receiving chronic stable doses of carbamazepine, phenytoin, phenobarbital, or valproate demonstrated increased duration of drowsiness (100.7 seconds) compared with healthy control subjects (12.0 seconds) and untreated patients with epilepsy (0.8 second).[157] However, drug-naive patients with partial epilepsy on topiramate showed no change in MSLT latencies compared with healthy control subjects either at baseline or 2 months later.[168]

Cognitive impairment appears to be more common with phenobarbital than with other drugs, more common when multiple medications are used, and more common in children than in adults. Phenobarbital and phenytoin have most frequently been associated with impaired neuropsychological function, particularly in the areas of short-term memory, concentration, and attention.[166,169] Carbamazepine and valproate appear to be less impairing. Gabapentin, vigabatrin, and tiagabine used as "add-on" therapy were no different from placebo in tests of cognitive and psychomotor function, whereas topiramate as monotherapy in partial epilepsy showed no impairment in simple and choice reaction time.[168] Patients who were changed from other antiepileptic agents to tiagabine alone demonstrated improvements in mental ability.[170]

ANORECTIC AGENTS

Drugs used to treat obesity can be divided into three groups: drugs that reduce food intake, drugs that alter metabolism, and drugs that increase thermogenesis.[171] Drugs that reduce food intake include the norepinephrine releasers amphetamine, methamphetamine, benzphetamine, phendimetrazine, and diethylpropion; the norepinephrine reuptake inhibitor, phentermine; the serotonin and norepinephrine reuptake inhibitor sibutramine; and the noradrenergic agonist phenylpropanolamine. Amphetamine and methamphetamine are rarely used because of their drug abuse potential. Only sibutramine is approved for long-term use. Insomnia is a side effect of all of these drugs. Drugs that influence serotonin release (fenfluramine and dexfenfluramine) as well as SSRIs (e.g., fluoxetine) have been used in obese patients. Fenfluramine and dexfenfluramine, both removed from the market in 1997 after reports of valvular heart disease, have been associated with insomnia. Peptides that reduce food intake such as leptin, antagonists to neuropeptide Y, and cholecystokinin are currently under development. Their effects on sleep are yet to be determined. Orlistat is the only anorectic drug approved by the FDA that alters metabolism. It is not absorbed to any significant degree and therefore does not appear to have any CNS effects. The only widely tested drug combination that increases energy expenditure is ephedrine plus caffeine. Both compounds have been associated with insomnia. Recent reports of serious adverse events with ephedrine have prompted prohibition of its sale in dietary supplements by the FDA.

PSEUDOEPHEDRINE AND PHENYLPROPANOLAMINE

Pseudoephedrine and phenylpropanolamine share the pharmacologic properties of ephedrine but have less potent CNS-stimulating effects. These drugs are used extensively as

Table 40–7.   Antiepileptic Drugs: Effects on Sleep and Waking Behavior

Drug or Class	U.S. Trade Name	Subjective Data*	PSG Data	MSLT Data	Cognitive/Performance Data
Established Antiepileptic Drugs					
Benzodiazepines	e.g., Klonopin, Valium	Sedation	↓ SL, ↓ SWS, ↓ REM	↓ SL	Mild impairment
Carbamazepine	Tegretol	Sedation	?↓ SL, ?↑ TST, ↓ REM, ↑ SWS	↓ SL	Mild impairment
Ethosuximide	Zarontin	Sedation	↑ S1	No data	No data
Phenobarbital	Phenobarbital	Sedation	↓ SL, ↓ #W, ↑ TST, ↓ REM	↓ SL	Significant impairment
Phenytoin	Dilantin	Sedation	↓ SL, ↑ S1, ↑ SWS	No data	Moderate impairment
Primidone	Mysoline	Sedation	↓ SL	No data	No data
Valproic acid	Depakene	Sedation	↑ TST, ↓ #W, ↑ S1	No negative effect	Mild impairment
Newer Antiepileptic Drugs					
Felbamate	Felbatol	Insomnia 10%, sedation 12%	No data	No data	No data
Fosphenytoin	Cerebyx	Sedation	No data	No data	No data
Gabapentin	Neurontin	Sedation 5-15%	↑ SWS, ↑ REM, ↑ TST, ↓ S1, ↓ #W	No data	No impairment as add-on treatment
Lamotrigine	Lamictal	Sedation 4-13%; insomnia 4%	↓ SWS	No data	No data
Levetiracetam	Keppra	Sedation 7%	↑ REM?		
Tiagabine	Gabitril	Sedation 0-5%; up to 25% in open-label studies	↑ TST, ↑ SWS	No data	No impairment as add-on treatment; improved performance when patients switched from other drug to tiagabine alone
Topiramate	Topamax	Sedation 15-27%	No data	No data	No data
Vigabatrin	Sabril	Sedation 7-12%	No effects	No change as add-on to carbamazepine	No impairment as add-on treatment
Zonisamide	Zonegran	Sedation 9-13%	No data	No data	No data

*Placebo-adjusted incidence of sedation listed for the new antiepileptic drugs; placebo-adjusted rates are not available for the older drugs.

MSLT, Multiple Sleep Latency Test; PSG, polysomnography; REM, rapid eye movement; S1, stage 1; SL, sleep latency; SWS, slow wave sleep; TST, total sleep time; #W, number of awakenings.

nasal decongestants and are available in a wide variety of over-the-counter cold preparations; phenylpropanolamine is also available in over-the-counter diet aids. Although similar in chemical structure to amphetamine, phenylpropanolamine is much less lipophilic and thus has much less potent CNS effects. Phenylpropanolamine, however, has been reported to increase plasma caffeine levels,[172] possibly adding to the stimulant effect of caffeine. These drugs have been reported to cause insomnia. In one study, 27% of patients given 120 mg of extended-release pseudoephedrine for 2 weeks for the treatment of allergic or vasomotor rhinitis complained of insomnia. In a PSG study, the administration of pseudoephedrine in the evening (as part of either a 60-mg four-times-daily or sustained-release, 120-mg twice-daily dosing regimen) produced increased wake time during sleep compared with the morning administration of a once-daily controlled-release formulation (240 mg).[173] Further objective evaluation of dosage, timing, and duration of treatment of these drugs would be useful.

ANTINEOPLASTIC AGENTS

Patients with cancer frequently experience fatigue, restless legs, insomnia, and excessive sleepiness.[174] These complaints may be a function of disease, psychophysiological factors, treatment, or a combination of factors. Chemotherapeutic agents have been associated with chronic pain, abnormal EEGs, and cognitive deficits. Chronotherapy, or circadian cancer therapy, is a research area in which timing of chemotherapy is targeted to maximize antitumor activity and minimize drug toxicity and side effects, including sleep-disrupting effects.[175,176]

ANALGESICS

Nonsteroidal Antiinflammatory Drugs

Nonsteroidal antiinflammatory drugs (NSAIDs) may affect sleep because they decrease the synthesis of prostaglandin D_2, suppress the normal nocturnal surge in melatonin synthesis, and attenuate the normal nocturnal decrease in body temperature.[177] NSAIDs inhibit cyclooxygenase (COX), blocking the synthesis of inflammatory prostaglandins. The classic NSAIDs inhibit both COX-1 (thereby accounting for their gastrointestinal toxicity) and COX-2 isoenzymes, whereas the newer NSAIDs selectively inhibit COX-2 (found primarily in the CNS, renal cortex, and vas deferens).[178] Acutely administered aspirin and ibuprofen have been shown to decrease sleep efficiency and increase waking in healthy subjects.[177,179] However there are no well-controlled PSG studies with the numerous other NSAIDs or in individuals experiencing pain. Subjective reports suggest an improvement in sleep quality with use of NSAIDs, presumably because of a reduction in pain. Cognitive deficits are apparently rare with NSAIDs, but may be a problem in older adults.[180]

Opioids

Opioids act at a variety of receptors, the major ones being mu, kappa, and delta. All three of these receptor subtypes appear to be involved in the analgesic effect of opioids, whereas the mu subtype plays a larger role compared with the kappa subtype in respiratory depression. Sedation is mediated by both mu and kappa receptors.[180] Sedation is a common side effect of opioid medication.[181,182] Degree of sedation may depend on the specific drug, dosage, and duration of use, as well as severity of the underlying disease,[183] but there is evidence that sedation may be persistent.[184] In addition, older adults appear to have increased pharmacodynamic sensitivity to opioids.[178] Although there is widespread belief that tolerance to the sedating effects of opioids develops with chronic use, there are no objective data to support this claim. Cognitive and psychomotor function are impaired, at least initially, with opioids,[181,183,185] but there are no well-controlled studies to confirm whether these effects improve over time. The limited PSG data available indicate that opioids decrease REM sleep and SWS.[186,187] Subjective quality of sleep is improved, presumably because of improved pain control.[188]

The most serious adverse effect of opioids is respiratory depression, particularly during sleep or after surgery. Opioids act directly on the brainstem respiratory centers through mu and delta receptors and at chemoreceptors through mu receptors, resulting in a shift to the right and a change in slope of the carbon dioxide response curve.[180] Opioids depress the pontine and medullary centers involved in the regulation of respiratory rhythmicity. Respiratory depression increases with increase in opioid dose. Clinically significant respiratory depression rarely occurs with standard opioid doses in healthy individuals,[189] although sleep itself also produces a decrease in the sensitivity of the brainstem to carbon dioxide, and the effects of opioids and sleep are additive. Individuals with pulmonary disease or obstructive sleep apnea are at greater risk for sustained hypoxemia during sleep.[190] Concomitant use of other sedatives, in particular, sleep aids, increases the risk for potentially fatal respiratory depression. After surgery, individuals with obstructive sleep apnea receiving intravenous morphine have been shown to have pronounced oxygen desaturation, paradoxical breathing, and slow ventilation.[191]

Adjunctive Drugs

Antidepressants, antihistamines, antiepileptics, and benzodiazepines are used as adjunctive treatment for pain. Certain antiepileptic drugs, in particular, are useful in suppression of neuropathic pain. Sedation is a common side effect of drugs such as gabapentin, tiagabine, and lamotrigine, drugs which are also under study as sleep aids. See Chapter 37 for additional information.

Clinical Pearl

Numerous neurotransmitter systems are involved in sleep–wake regulation. Thus, drugs that act on the central nervous system have the potential to affect sleep or daytime functioning. Knowledge of the mechanisms of action and pharmacokinetics of a drug can help determine whether the drug may disturb sleep or result in daytime side effects.

REFERENCES

1. Benca RM, Obermeyer WH, Thisted RA, et al: Sleep and psychiatric disorders: A meta-analysis. Arch Gen Psychiatry 1992; 49:651-668.
2. Claghorn JL, Mathew RJ, Weinman ML, et al: Daytime sleepiness in depression. J Clin Psychiatry 1981;42:342-343.
3. Newman AB, Enright PL, Manolio TA, et al: Sleep disturbance, psychosocial correlates, and cardiovascular disease in 5201 older adults: The Cardiovascular Health Study. J Am Geriatr Soc 1997;45:1-7.
4. Nebes RD, Pollock BG, Houck PR, et al: Persistence of cognitive impairment in geriatric patients following antidepressant treatment: A randomized, double-blind clinical trial with nortriptyline and paroxetine. J Psychiatr Res 2003;37:99-108.
5. Frazer A: Pharmacology of antidepressants. J Clin Psychopharmacol 1997;17(Suppl 1):2S-18S.

6. Preskorn SH: Comparison of the tolerability of bupropion, fluoxetine, imipramine, nefazodone, paroxetine, sertraline, and venlafaxine. J Clin Psychiatry 1995;56(Suppl 6):12-21.

7. Pacher P, Kohegyi E, Kecskemeti V, et al: Current trends in the development of new antidepressants. Curr Med Chem 2001; 8:89-100.

8. Kent JM: SNaRIs, NaSSAs, and NaRIs: New agents for the treatment of depression. Lancet 2000;335:911-918.

9. Thase ME: Treatment issues related to sleep and depression. J Clin Psychiatry 2000;61(Suppl 11):46-50.

10. Vaswani M, Linda FK, Ramesh S: Role of selective serotonin reuptake inhibitors in psychiatric disorders: A comprehensive review. Prog Neuropsychopharmacol Biol Psychiatry 2003; 27:85-102.

11. Obermeyer WH, Benca RM: Effects of drugs on sleep. Neurol Clin 1996;14:827-840.

12. Gursky JT, Krahn LE: The effects of antidepressants on sleep: A review. Harv Rev Psychiatry 2000;8:298-306.

13. Winokur A, Gary KA, Rodner S, et al: Depression, sleep physiology, and antidepressant drugs. Depress Anxiety 2001;14:19-28.

14. Volz H-P, Sturm Y: Antidepressant drugs and psychomotor performance. Neuropsychobiology 1995;31:146-155.

15. van Laar MW, Volkerts ER, Vertaten MN, et al: Differential effects of amitriptyline, nefazodone and paroxetine on performance and brain indices of visual selective attention and working memory. Psychopharmacology 2000;162:351-363.

16. Remick RA, Froese C, Keller FD: Common side effects associated with monoamine oxidase inhibitors. Prog Neuropsychopharmacol Biol Psychiatry 1989;13:497-504.

17. Wyatt RJ, Fram DH, Kupfer DJ, et al: Total prolonged drug-induced REM sleep suppression in anxious-depressed patients. Arch Gen Psychiatry 1971;24:145-155.

18. Monti JM, Alterwain P, Monti D: The effects of moclobemide on nocturnal sleep of depressed patients. J Affect Disord 1990; 20:201-208.

19. Bonnet U. Moclobemide: Evolution, pharmacodynamic, and pharmacokinetic properties. CNS Drug Rev 2002;8:283-308.

20. Allain H, Lieury A, Brunet-Bourgin F, et al: Antidepressants and cognition: Comparative effects of moclobemide, viloxazine and maprotiline. Psychopharmacology 1992;106:S56-S61.

21. Hindmarch I, Kerr J: Behavioural toxicity of antidepressants with particular reference to moclobemide. Psychopharmacology 1992;106:S49-S55.

22. Tiller JWG: Antidepressants, alcohol and psychomotor performance. Acta Psychiatr Scand Suppl 1990;360:13-17.

23. Oberndorfer A, Saletu-Zyhlarz G, Saletu B: Effects of selective serotonin reuptake inhibitors on objective and subjective sleep quality. Pharmacopsychiatry 2000;42:59-81.

24. Dording CM, Mischoulon D, Peterson TJ, et al: The pharmacologic management of SSRI-induced side effects: A survey of psychiatrists. Ann Clin Pract 2002;14:143-147.

25. Clark NA, Alexander B: Increased rate of trazodone prescribing with bupropion and selective serotonin-reuptake inhibitors versus tricyclic antidepressants. Ann Pharmacother 2000;34:1007-1012.

26. Silvestri R, Pace-Schott EF, Gersh T, et al: Effects of fluvoxamine and paroxetine on sleep structure in normal subjects: A home-based Nightcap evaluation during drug administration and withdrawal. J Clin Psychiatry 2001;62:642-652.

27. Nicholson AN, Pascoe PA: Studies on the modulation of the sleep-wakefulness continuum in man by fluoxetine, a 5-HT uptake inhibitor. Neuropharmacology 1988;27:597-602.

28. Kerkhofs M, Rielaert C, de Maertelaer V, et al: Fluoxetine in major depression: Efficacy, safety and effects on sleep polygraphic variables. Int Clin Psychopharmacol 1990;5:253-260.

29. Schenck CH, Mahowald MW, Kim SW, et al: Prominent eye movements during NREM sleep and REM sleep behavior disorder associated with fluoxetine treatment of depression and obsessive-compulsive disorder. Sleep 1992;15:226-235.

30. Winkelman J, James L: Serotonergic antidepressants are associated with REM sleep without atonia. Sleep 2004;27:317-321.

31. Sharpley AL, Williamson DJ, Attenburrow MEJ, et al: The effects of paroxetine and nefazodone on sleep: A placebo controlled trial. Psychopharmacology 1996;126:50-54.

32. Staner L, Kerkhofs M, Detroux D, et al: Acute, subchronic and withdrawal sleep EEG changes during treatment with paroxetine and amitriptyline: A double-blind randomized trial in major depression. Sleep 1995;18:470-477.

33. Kupfer DJ, Perel JM, Pollock BG, et al: Fluvoxamine versus desipramine: Comparative polysomnographic effects. Biol Psychiatry 1991;29:23-40.

34. van Bemmel AL, van den Hoofdakker RH, Beersma DG, et al: Changes in sleep polygraphic variables and clinical state in depressed patients during treatment with citalopram. Psychopharmacology 1993;113:225-230.

35. Schmitt JAJ, Kruizinga MJ, Riedel WJ: Non-serotonergic pharmacological profiles and associated cognitive effects of serotonin reuptake inhibitors. J Psychopharmacol 2001;15:173-179.

36. Hindmarch I, Kimber S, Cockle SM: Abrupt and brief discontinuation of antidepressant treatment: effects on cognitive function and psychomotor performance. Int Clin Psychopharmacol 2000;15:305-318.

37. Wilson SJ, Bailey JE, Alford C, et al: Sleep and daytime sleepiness the next day following single night-time dose of fluvoxamine, dothiepin and placebo in normal volunteers. J Psychopharmacol 2000;14:378-386.

38. Schmitt JA, Kruizinga MJ, Riedel WJ: Non-serotonergic pharmacological profiles and associated cognitive effects of serotonin reuptake inhibitors. J Psychopharmacol 2001;15:173-179.

39. Cunningham LA, Borison RL, Carman JS, et al: A comparison of venlafaxine, trazodone, and placebo in major depression. J Clin Psychopharmacol 1994;14:99-106.

40. Salin-Pascual RJ, Galicia-Polo L, Drucker-Colin R: Sleep changes after 4 consecutive days of venlafaxine administration in normal volunteers. J Clin Psychiatry 1997;58:348-350.

41. Luthringer R, Toussaint M, Schaltenbrand N, et al: A double-blind, placebo-controlled evaluation of the effects of orally administered venlafaxine on sleep in inpatients with major depression. Psychopharmacol Bull 1996;32:637-646.

42. Saletu B, Grunberger J, Anderer P, et al: Pharmacodynamics of venlafaxine evaluated by EEG brain mapping, psychometry and psychophysiology. Br J Clin Pharmacol 1992;33:589-601.

43. Goldberg RJ: Antidepressant use in the elderly: Current status of nefazodone, venlafaxine and moclobemide. Drugs Aging 1997;11:119-131.

44. Vogel G, Cohen J, Mullis D, et al: Nefazodone and REM sleep: How do antidepressant drugs decrease REM sleep? Sleep 1998; 21:70-77.

45. Frewer LJ, Lader M: The effects of nefazodone, imipramine, and placebo, alone and combined with alcohol, in normal subjects. Int Clin Psychopharmacol 1993;8:13-20.

46. Nofzinger EA, Reynolds CF, Thase ME, et al: REM sleep enhancement by bupropion in depressed men. Am J Psychiatry 1995;152:274-276.

47. Nofzinger EA, Fasiczka A, Berman S, et al: Bupropion SR reduces periodic limb movements associated with arousals from sleep in depressed patients with periodic limb movement disorder. J Clin Psychiatry 2000;61:858-862.

48. Paul MA, Gray G, Kenny G, et al: The impact of bupropion on psychomotor performance. Aviat Space Environ Med 2002;73: 1094-1099.

49. Scates AC, Doraiswamy PM: Reboxetine: A selective norepinephrine reuptake inhibitor for the treatment of depression. Ann Pharmacother 2000;34:1302-1312.

50. Farina B, Della Marca G, Mennuni G, et al: The effects of reboxetine on human sleep architecture in depression: Preliminary results. J Affect Disord 2002;71:273-275.

51. Ferguson JM, Wesnes KA, Schwartz GE: Reboxetine versus paroxetine versus placebo: Effects on cognitive functioning in depressed patients. Int Clin Psychopharmacol 2003;18:9-14.

52. Linnoila M, Rudorfer MV, Dubryoski KV, et al: Effects of one-week lithium treatment on skilled performance, information processing, and mood in healthy volunteers. J Clin Psychopharmacol 1986;6:356-359.

53. Hatcher S, Sims R, Thompson D: The effects of chronic lithium treatment on psychomotor performance related to driving. Br J Psychiatry 1990;157:275-278.

54. Lauer CJ, Schreiber W, Pollmacher T, et al: Sleep in schizophrenia: A polysomnographic study on drug-naive patients. Neuropsychopharmacology 1997;16:51-60.

55. Casey DE: The relationship of pharmacology to side effects. J Clin Psychiatry 1997;58(Suppl 10):55-62.

56. Gerlach J, Peacock L: New antipsychotics: The present status. Int Clin Psychopharmacol 1995;10(Suppl 3):39-48.

57. Casey DE: Side effect profiles of new antipsychotic agents. J Clin Psychiatry 1996;57(Suppl 11):40-45.

58. Fernandez HH, Trieschmann ME, Friedman JH: Treatment of psychosis in Parkinson's disease: Safety considerations. Drug Saf 2003;26:643-659.

59. Tamminga CA, Carlsson A: Partial dopamine agonists and dopaminergic stabilizers, in the treatment of psychosis. Curr Drug Target CNS Neurol Disord 2002;1:141-147.

60. Leucht S, Wahlbeck K, Hamann J, et al: New generation antipsychotics versus low-potency conventional antipsychotics: A systematic review and meta-analysis. Lancet 2003;361:1581-1589.

61. Fitton A, Heel RC: Clozapine: A review of its pharmacological properties and therapeutic use in schizophrenia. Drugs 1990;40:722-747.

62. Wetter TC, Lauer CJ, Gillich G, Pollmacher T: The electroencephalographic sleep pattern in schizophrenic patients treated with clozapine or classical antipsychotic drugs. J Psychiatr Res 1996;30:411-419.

63. Salin-Pascual RJ, Herrera-Estrella M, Galicia-Polo L, Laurrabaquio MR: Olanzapine acute administration in schizophrenic patients increased delta sleep and sleep efficiency. Biol Psychiatry 1999;46:141-143.

64. Sharpley AL, Vassallo CM, Cowen PJ: Olanzapine increases slow-wave sleep: Evidence for blockade of central 5-HT(2C) receptors in vivo. Biol Psychiatry 2000;47:468-470.

65. Vitiello B, Martin A, Hill J, et al: Cognitive and behavioral effects of cholinergic, dopaminergic, and serotonergic blockade in humans. Neuropsychopharmacology 1997;16:15-24.

66. Cassens G, Inglis AK, Appelbaum PS, et al: Neuroleptics: Effects on neuropsychological function in chronic schizophrenic patients. Schizophr Bull 1990;16:477-499.

67. Goldberg TE, Weinberger DR: Effects of neuroleptic medications on the cognition of patients with schizophrenia: A review of recent studies. J Clin Psychiatry 1996;57(Suppl 9):62-65.

68. Buchanan RW, Holstein C, Breier A: The comparative efficacy and long-term effect of clozapine treatment on neuropsychological test performance. Biol Psychiatry 1994;36:717-725.

69. Buysse DJ: Drugs affecting sleep, sleepiness, and performance. In Monk TH (ed): Sleep, Sleepiness and Performance. New York, John Wiley & Sons, 1991, pp 249-306.

70. Seidel WF, Cohen SA, Wilson L, et al: Effects of alprazolam and diazepam on the daytime sleepiness of non-anxious subjects. Psychopharmacology 1985;87:194-197.

71. O'Hanlon JF, Vermeeren A, Uiterwijk MMC, et al: Anxiolytics' effects on the actual driving performance of patients and healthy volunteers in a standardized test. Neuropsychobiology 1995;31:81-88.

72. Goa KL, Ward A: Buspirone: A preliminary review of its pharmacological properties and therapeutic efficacy as an anxiolytic. Drugs 1986;32:114-129.

73. Eison AS, Temple DL: Buspirone: Review of its pharmacology and current perspectives on its mechanism of action. Am J Med 1986;80(Suppl 3):61-68.

74. Newton RE, Casten GP, Alms DR, et al: The side effect profile of buspirone in comparison to active controls and placebo. J Clin Psychiatry 1982;43:100-102.

75. Seidel WF, Cohen SA, Bliwise NG, et al: Buspirone: An anxiolytic without sedative effect. Psychopharmacology 1985;87:371-373.

76. McAinsh J, Cruickshank JM: Beta-blockers and central nervous system side effects. Pharmacol Ther 1990;46:163-197.

77. Yamada Y, Shibuya F, Hamada J, et al: Prediction of sleep disorders induced by β-adrenergic receptor blocking agents based on receptor occupancy. J Pharmacokinet Biopharm 1995;23:131-145.

78. Dimsdale J, Newton R, Joist T: Neuropsychologic side effects of beta blockers. Arch Intern Med 1989;149:514-525.

79. Rosen RC, Kostis JB: Biobehavioral sequelae associated with adrenergic-inhibiting antihypertensive agents: A critical review. Health Psychol 1985;4:579-604.

80. van den Heuvel C, Reid K, Dawson D: Effect of atenolol on nocturnal sleep and temperature in young men: Reversal by pharmacological doses of melatonin. Physiol Behav 1997;61:795-802.

81. Bell C, Wilson S, Rich A, et al: Effects on sleep architecture of pindolol, paroxetine and their combination in healthy volunteers. Psychopharmacology 2003;166:102-110.

82. Pearce CJ, Wallin JD: Labetalol and other agents that block both alpha- and beta-adrenergic receptors. Cleve Clin J Med 1994;61:59-69.

83. Paykel ES, Fleminger R, Watson JP: Psychiatric side effects of antihypertensive drugs other than reserpine. J Clin Psychopharmacol 1982;2:14-39.

84. Kostis JB, Rosen RC, Holzer BC, et al: CNS side effects of centrally-active antihypertensive agents: A prospective, placebo-controlled study of sleep, mood state, and cognitive and sexual function in hypertensive males. Psychopharmacology 1990;102:163-170.

85. Kanno O, Clarenbach P: Effects of clonidine and yohimbine on sleep in man: Polygraphic study and EEG analysis by normalized slope descriptors. Electroencephalogr Clin Neurophysiol 1985;60:478-484.

86. Carskadon MA, Cavallo A, Rosekind MR: Sleepiness and nap sleep following a morning dose of clonidine. Sleep 1989;12:338-344.

87. Croog SH, Levine S, Testa MA, et al: The effects of antihypertensive therapy on the quality of life. N Engl J Med 1986;314:1657-1664.

88. Staessen J, Fagard R, Lijnen P, et al: Double-blind comparison of ketanserin and propranolol in hypertensive patients. J Cardiovasc Pharmacol 1988;12:718-725.

89. Idzikowski C, Mills FJ, James RJ: A dose-response study examining the effects of ritanserin on human slow wave sleep. Br J Clin Pharmacol 1991;31:193-196.

90. Adam K, Oswald I: Effects of repeated ritanserin on middle-aged poor sleepers. Psychopharmacology 1989;99:219-221.

91. Paiva T, Arriaga F, Wauquier A, et al: Effects of ritanserin on sleep disturbances of dysthymic patients. Psychopharmacology 1988;96:395-399.

92. Lammers GJ, Arends J, Declerck AC, et al: Ritanserin, a 5-HT2 receptor blocker, as add-on treatment in narcolepsy. Sleep 1991;14:130-132.

93. Reid JL: New therapeutic agents for hypertension. Br J Clin Pharmacol 1996;42:37-41.

94. Yu A, Frishman WH: Imidazoline receptor agonist drugs: A new approach to the treatment of systemic hypertension. J Clin Pharmacol 1996;36:98-111.

95. Monti J: Minireview: Disturbances of sleep and wakefulness associated with the use of antihypertensive agents. Life Sci 1987;41:1979-1988.

96. Dietrich B, Herrmann WM: Influence of cilazapril on memory functions and sleep behaviour in comparison with metoprolol and placebo in healthy subjects. Br J Clin Pharmacol 1989;27(Suppl 2):249S-261S.

97. Williams GH, Croog SH, Levine S, et al: Impact of antihypertensive therapy on quality of life: effect of hydrochlorothiazide. J Hypertens 1987;5(Suppl 1):S29-S35.

98. Wesnes K, Simpson PM, Jansson B, et al: Moxonidine and cognitive function: Interactions with moclobemide and lorazepam. Eur J Clin Pharmacol 1997;52:351-358.

99. Bradford RH, Shear CL, Chremos AN, et al: Expanded Clinical Evaluation of Lovastatin (EXCEL) study results: I. Efficacy in modifying plasma lipoproteins and adverse event profile in 8245 patients with moderate hypercholesterolemia. Arch Intern Med 1991;151:43-49.

100. Keech AC, Armitage JM, Wallendszus, et al: Absence of effects of prolonged simvastatin therapy on nocturnal sleep in a large randomized placebo-controlled study. Br J Clin Pharmacol 1996;42:483-490.

101. Roth T, Richardson GR, Sullivan JP, et al: Comparative effects of pravastatin and lovastatin on nighttime sleep and daytime performance. Clin Cardiol 1992;15:426-432.

102. Wagstaff LR, Mitton MW, Arvik BM, et al: Statin-associated memory loss: Analysis of 60 case reports and review of the literature. Pharmacotherapy 2003;23:871-880.

103. Etminan M, Gill S, Samii A: The role of lipid-lowering drugs in cognitive function: A meta-analysis of observational studies. Pharmacotherapy 2003;23:726-730.

104. Kruyer WB, Hickman JR Jr: Medication-induced performance decrements: Cardiovascular medications. J Occup Med 1990;32:342-349.

105. Keller S, Frishman WH: Neuropsychiatric effects of cardiovascular drug therapy. Cardiol Rev 2003;11:73-93.

106. Ramaekers JG, Uiterwijk MM, O'Hanlon JF: Effects of loratadine and cetirizine on actual driving and psychometric test performance, and EEG during driving. Eur J Clin Pharmacol 1992;42:363-369.

107. Schweitzer PK, Muehlbach MJ, Walsh JK: Sleepiness and performance during three-day administration of cetirizine or diphenhydramine. J Allergy Clin Immunol 1994;94:716-724.

108. Seidel WF, Cohen S, Bliwise NG, et al: Cetirizine effects on objective measures of daytime sleepiness and performance. Ann Allergy 1987;59:58-62.

109. Betts T, Markham D, Debenham S, et al: Effects of two antihistamine drugs on actual driving performance. BMJ 1984;288:281-282.

110. Hindmarch I: Psychometric aspects of antihistamines. Allergy. 1990;50:48-54.

111. Berlin RG. Effects of H2-receptor antagonists on the central nervous system. Drug Dev Res 1989:17:97-108.

112. Lipsy RJ, Fennerty B, Fagan T: Clinical review of histamine2 receptor antagonists. Arch Intern Med 1990;150:745-751.

113. Orr WC, Duke, JC, Imes NK, et al: Comparative effects of H2-receptor antagonists on subjective and objective assessments of sleep. Aliment Pharmacol Ther 1994;8:203-207.

114. Schentag JJ: Cimetidine-associated mental confusion: further studies in 36 severely ill patients. Ther Drug Monit 1980;78:791-795.

115. Sanders LD, Whitehead C, Gildersleve CD, et al: Interaction of H2-receptor antagonists and benzodiazepine sedation. Anaesthesia 1993;48:286-292.

116. Searle JP, Compton MR: Side-effects of corticosteroid agents. Med J Aust 1986;144:139-142.

117. Chrousos GA, Kattah JC, Beck RW, et al: Side effects of glucocorticoid treatment: Experience of the optic neuritis treatment trial. JAMA 1993;269:2110-2112.

118. Lozada F, Silverman S, Migliorati C: Adverse side effects associated with prednisone in the treatment of patients with oral inflammatory ulcerative diseases. J Am Dent Assoc 1984;109:269-270.

119. Harris JC, Carel CA, Rosenberg LA, et al: Intermittent high dose corticosteroid treatment in childhood cancer: Behavioral and emotional consequences. J Am Acad Child Adolesc Psychiatry 1988;27:720-725.

120. Bailey WC, Richards JM, Manzella BA, et al: Characteristics and correlates of asthma in a university clinic population. Chest 1990;98:821-828.

121. Wolkowitz OM, Rubinow D, Doran AR, et al: Prednisone effects on neurochemistry and behavior: Preliminary findings. Arch Gen Psychiatry 1990;47:963-968.

122. Born J, Zwick A, Roth G, et al: Differential effects of hydrocortisone, fluocortolone, and aldosterone on nocturnal sleep in humans. Acta Endocrinol 1987;116:129-137.

123. Rosenthal L, Folkerts M, Helmus T, et al: Administration of dexamethasone and its effects on sleep and daytime alertness. Sleep Res 1995;24:58.

124. Wolkowitz OM, Reus VI, Weingartner H, et al: Cognitive effects of corticosteroids. Am J Psychiatry 1990;147:1297-1303.

125. Scott PH, Tabachnik E, MacLeod S, et al: Sustained release theophylline for childhood asthma: Evidence for circadian variation of theophylline pharmacokinetics. J Pediatr 1981;99:476-479.

126. Hendeles L, Massanari M, Weinberger M: Update on the pharmacodynamics and pharmacokinetics of theophylline. Chest 1985;88(Suppl):103S-111S.

127. Janson C, Gislason T, Boman G, et al: Sleep disturbances in patients with asthma. Respir Med 1990;84:37-42.

128. Kraft M, Wenzel SE, Bettinger CM, et al: The effect of salmeterol on nocturnal symptoms, airway function, and inflammation in asthma. Chest 1997;111:1249-1254.

129. Kaplan J, Fredrickson PA, Renaux SA, et al: Theophylline effect on sleep in normal subjects. Chest 1993;103:193-195.

130. Rhind GB, Connaughton JJ, McFie J, et al: Sustained release choline theophyllinate in nocturnal asthma. BMJ 1985;291:1605-1607.

131. Avital A, Sanchez I, Holbrow J, et al: Effect of theophylline on lung function tests, sleep quality, and nighttime SaO_2 in children with cystic fibrosis. Am Rev Respir Dis 1991;144:1245-1249.

132. Saletu B, Oberndorfer S, Anderer P, et al: Efficiency of continuous positive airway pressure versus theophylline therapy in sleep apnea: Comparative sleep laboratory studies on objective and subjective sleep and awakening quality. Neuropsychobiology 1999;39:151-159.

133. Mulloy E, McNicholas WT: Theophylline improves gas exchange during rest, exercise, and sleep in severe chronic obstructive pulmonary disease. Am Rev Respir Dis 1993;148:1030-1036.

134. Rachelefsky GS, Wo J, Adelson J, et al: Behavior abnormalities and poor school performance due to oral theophylline use. Pediatrics 1986;78:1133-1138.

135. Stein MA, Krasowski M, Leventhal BL, et al: Behavioral and cognitive effects of methylxanthines: A meta-analysis of theophylline and caffeine. Arch Pediatr Adolesc Med 1996;150:284-288.

136. Lindgren S, Lokshin B, Stronmquist A, et al: Does asthma or treatment with theophylline limit children's academic performance? N Engl J Med 1992;327:926-903.

137. van Hilten B, Hoff JI, Middelkoop MA, et al: Sleep disruption in Parkinson's disease. Arch Neurol 1994;51:922-928.

138. Kaakkola S: Clinical pharmacology, therapeutic use and potential of COMT inhibitors in Parkinson's disease. Drugs 2000;59:1233-1250.

139. Nausieda PA, Glantz R, Weber S, et al: Psychiatric complications of levodopa therapy of Parkinson's disease. Adv Neurol 1984;40:271-277.

140. Askenasy JJM, Yahr MD: Reversal of sleep disturbance in Parkinson's disease by antiparkinson therapy. Neurology 1985; 35:527-532.

141. Leeman AL, O'Neill CJA, Nicholson PW, et al: Parkinson's disease in the elderly: Response to and optimal spacing of night time dosing with levodopa. Br J Clin Pharmacol 1987;24:637-643.

142. Chrisp P, Mammen GJ, Sorkin EM: Selegiline: A review of its pharmacology, symptomatic benefits and protective potential in Parkinson's disease. Drugs Aging. 1991;1:228-248.

143. Lavie P, Wajsbort J, Youdim MBH: Deprenyl does not cause insomnia in parkinsonian patients. Commun Psychopharmacol 1980;4:303-307.

144. Vardi J, Glaubman H, Rabey J, et al: EEG sleep patterns in parkinsonian patients treated with bromocriptine and L-dopa: A comparative study. J Neural Transm 1979;45:307-316.

145. Brodsky MA, Godbold J, Roth T, et al: Sleepiness in Parkinson's disease: A controlled study. Move Disord 2003;18:668-672.

146. Ondo WG, Dat Vuong K, Khan H, et al: Daytime sleepiness and other sleep disorders in Parkinson's disease. Neurology 2001; 57:1392-1396.

147. Etminan M, Samii A, Takkouche B, et al: Increased risk of somnolence with the new dopamine agonists in patients with Parkinson's disease: A meta-analysis of randomised controlled trials. Drug Saf 2001;24:863-868.

148. Paus S, Brecht HM, Koster J, et al: Sleep attacks, daytime sleepiness, and dopamine agonists in Parkinson's disease. Move Disord 2003;6:659-667.

149. Chaudhuri KR, Pal S, Brefel-Courbon C: "Sleep attacks" or "unintended sleep episodes" occur with dopamine agonists: Is this a class effect? Drug Saf 2002;25:473-483.

150. Homann CN, Wenzel K, Suppan K, et al: Sleep attacks in patients taking dopamine agonists: review. BMJ 2002;324: 1483-1487.

151. Ferreira JJ, Galitzky M, Thalamas C, et al: Effect of ropinirole on sleep onset: A randomized, placebo-controlled study in healthy volunteers. Neurology 2002;58:460-462.

152. Razmy A, Lang AE, Chapiro CM: Predictors of impaired daytime sleep and wakefulness in patients with Parkinson disease treated with older (ergot) vs newer (nonergot) dopamine agonists. Arch Neurol 2004;61:97-102.

153. Cooper JA, Sagar HJ, Doherty SM, et al: Different effects of dopaminergic and anticholinergic therapies on cognitive and motor function in Parkinson's disease. Brain 1992;115: 1701-1725.

154. Saletu B, Gruber G, Saletu M, et al: Sleep laboratory studies in restless legs syndrome patients as compared with normals and acute effects of ropinirole: 1. Findings on objective and subjective sleep and awakening quality. Neuropsychobiology 2000; 41:181-189.

155. Kieburtz K, McDermott M, Como P, et al: The effect of deprenyl and tocopherol on cognitive performance in early untreated Parkinson's disease. Neurology 1994;44:1756-1759.

156. Blum DE: New drugs for persons with epilepsy. In French J, Leppik I, Dichter MA (eds): Antiepileptic Drug Development (Advances in Neurology vol 76). Philadelphia: Lippincott Williams & Wilkins, 1998, pp 57-87.

157. Sammaritano M, Sherwin A: Effect of anticonvulsants on sleep. Neurology 2000;54:S16-S24.

158. Brodie MJ, Dichter MA: Established antiepileptic drugs. Seizure 1997;6:159-174.

159. Malow BA, Bowes RJ, Lix X: Predictors of sleepiness in epilepsy patients. Sleep 1997;20:1105-1110.

160. Salinsky MC, Oken BS, Binder LM: Assessment of drowsiness in epilepsy patients receiving chronic antiepileptic drug therapy. Epilepsia 1996;37:181-187.

161. Leppik IE: Antiepileptic drugs in development: prospects for the near future. Epilepsia 1994;35(Suppl 4):S29-S40.

162. Chadwick D, Leiderman DB, Sauermann W, et al: Gabapentin in generalized seizures. Epilepsy Res 1996;25:191-197.

163. Marson AG, Kadir ZA, Hutton JL, et al: The new antiepileptic drugs: A systematic review of their efficacy and tolerability. Epilepsia 1997;38:859-880.

164. Bazil CW: Effects of antiepileptic drugs on sleep structure: Are all drugs equal? CNS Drugs 2003;17:719-728.

165. Sammaritano M, Sherwin A: Effect of anticonvulsants on sleep. Neurology 2000;54:S16-S24.

166. Roeder-Wanner UU, Noachter S, Wolf P: Response of polygraphic sleep to phenytoin treatment for epilepsy: A longitudinal study of immediate, short- and long-term effects. Acta Neurol Scand 1987;76:157-167.

167. Palm L, Anderson H, Elmqvist D, et al: Daytime sleep tendency before and after discontinuation of antiepileptic drugs in preadolescent children with epilepsy. Epilepsia 1992;33: 687-691.

168. Bonanni E, Galli R, Maestri M, et al: Daytime sleepiness in epilepsy patients receiving topiramate monotherapy. Epilepsia 2004;45:333-337.

169. Manni R, Ratti MT, Perucca E, et al: A multiparametric investigation of daytime sleepiness and psychomotor function in epileptic patients treated with phenobarbital and sodium valproate: A comparative controlled study. Electroencephalogr Clin Neurophysiol 1993;86:322-328.

170. Provinciali L, Bartolini M, Mari F, et al: Influence of vigabatrin on cognitive performances and behaviour in patients with drug-resistant epilepsy. Acta Neurol Scand 1996;94:12-18.

171. Bray GA: A concise review on the therapeutics of obesity. Nutrition 2000;16:953-960.

172. Lake CR, Rosenberg DB, Gallant S, et al: Phenylpropanolamine increases plasma caffeine levels. Clin Pharmacol Ther 1990; 47:675-685.

173. Bertrand B, Jamart J, Arendt C: Cetirizine and pseudoephedrine retard alone and in combination in the treatment of perennial allergic rhinitis: A double-blind multicentre study. Rhinology 1996:34:91-96.

174. Ancoli-Israel S, Moore PJ, Jones V: The relationship between fatigue and sleep in cancer patients: A review. Eur J Cancer Care 2001;10:245-255.

175. Novak M, Shapiro CM: Drug-induced sleep disturbances: Focus on nonpsychotropic medications. Drug Saf 1997;16: 133-149.

176. Levi F: From circadian rhythms to cancer chronotherapeutics. Chronobiol Int 2002;19:1-19.

177. Murphy P, Badia P, Myers B, et al: Nonsteroidal anti-inflammatory drugs affect normal sleep patterns in humans. Physiol Behav 1994;55:1063-1066.

178. Nikolaus T, Zeyfang A: Pharmacological treatments for persistent non-malignant pain in older persons. Drugs Aging 2004;21:19-41.

179. Horne J, Percival J, Traynor J: Aspirin and human sleep. Electroencephalogr Clin Neurophysiol 1980;49:409-413.

180. Schug S, Garrett W, Gillespie G: Opioid and non-opioid analgesics. Best Pract Res Clin Anaesthesiol 2003;17:91-110.

181. Nicholson B: Responsible prescribing of opioids for the management of chronic pain. Drugs 2003;63:17-32.

182. Inturrisi C: Clinical pharmacology of opioids for pain. Clin J Pain 2002;18:S3-S13.

183. Clemons M, Regnard C, Appleton T: Alertness, cognition and morphine in patients with advanced cancer. Cancer Treat Rev 1996;122:451-468.

184. Meuser T, Pietruck C, Radbruch L, et al: Symptoms during cancer pain treatment following WHO-guidelines: A longitudinal follow-up study of symptom prevalence, severity and etiology. Pain 2001;93:247-257.

185. Sjogran P: Psychomotor and cognitive functioning in cancer patients. Acta Anaesthesiol Scand 1997;41:159-161.

186. Cronin A, Keifer J, Davies M, et al: Postoperative sleep disturbance: Influences of opioids and pain in humans. Sleep 2001;24:39-44.

187. Walder B, Tramer M, Blois R: The effects of two single doses of tramadol on sleep: A randomized, cross-over trial in healthy volunteers. Eur J Anaesthesiol 2001;18:36-42.

188. Caldwell J, Rapoport R, Davis J, et al: Efficacy and safety of a once-daily morphine formulation in chronic, moderate-to-severe osteoarthritis pain: Results from a randomized placebo-controlled, double-blind trial and an open-label extension trial. J Pain Symptom Manage 2002;23:278-291.

189. Robinson R, Zwillich C, Bixler E, et al: Effects of oral narcotics on sleep-disordered breathing in healthy adults. Chest 1987;91:197-203.

190. Farney R, Walker J, Cloward T, Rhondeau S: Sleep-disordered breathing associated with long-term opioid therapy. Chest 2003;123:632-639.

191. Catley D, Thornton C, Jordan C, et al: Pronounced, episodic oxygen desaturation in the postoperative period: Its association with ventilatory pattern and analgesic regimen. Anesthesiology 1985;63:20-28.

Psychobiology and Dreaming

Robert Stickgold

Introduction to Dreams and Their Pathology

Robert Stickgold

Since the mid-1990s, the study of dreams and dreaming has made remarkable progress, but it is still a relatively immature area of science. In its defense, it is in the unenviable position of being a subfield of the study of consciousness and shares with the larger topic several problematic features: It is only poorly defined, and there is no consensus on a definition; it has no consistent physiologic correlates, and hence its biologic basis is largely unknown; it has no behavioral correlates and hence has no known function; and its existence in species other than humans is a matter of conjecture, making more invasive studies of its mechanism and function impossible. In short, we don't know the cause, nature, or consequence of dreaming, a remarkably sad state of affairs! It is, however, absolutely clear that dreaming is a highly robust human experience that is most likely experienced by the vast majority of humans every night and that our understanding of it is growing rapidly.

DEFINITION

Given our ignorance of underlying biologic mechanisms and functions, it is perhaps not surprising that a clear definition of dreaming has evaded us. Most definitions in science refer either to physical objects or to processes that are defined by their underlying mechanisms or by their measurable consequences. We have none of these references for dreaming. Indeed, a recent publication based on discussion groups of the Association of Professional Sleep Societies and the Association for the Study of Dreams concluded that a "single definition for dreaming is most likely impossible given ... the diversity in currently applied definitions."[1] Everyone does agree that dreaming is phenomenological, that is, the definition refers to a state of mind rather than to a physiologic state (although there may yet be an unidentified physiologic state that corresponds to this mental state). But individual researchers restrict what they count as dreaming, and hence which reports are counted and analyzed as dreams, based on when they occur or what they contain, or both. Table 41–1 lists some of the criteria that have been applied.

For these reasons, some authors have eschewed the use of the term altogether, referring instead to "sleep mentation." Unlike the term *dreaming,* this phrase can be simply defined. *Sleep mentation* is defined as all perceptions, thoughts, and emotions experienced during sleep, or the process of perceiving, thinking, and emoting during sleep. Thus, it combines the sense of the words *dream* and *dreaming.* It is this concept, sleep mentation, that is more properly the subject of this section on dreaming.

METHODOLOGY

It is important to understand that researchers do not study dreams directly. Rather, they study dream reports that have been written, dictated, or, on rare occasions, drawn or acted out after a subject has awakened from sleep. (For those who include waking daydreams and fantasies within their definition of dreaming, real time reporting is possible, at least in theory, although such states are outside the scope of this book.)

In one sense, studying the artifact rather than the dream itself is not as big a problem as it is often considered. All scientific measurements are derivative. Until recently, blood pressure could only be measured with a pressure cuff applied externally, and the clinician listened with a stethoscope for the sounds produced by the movement of blood through arteries in the arm. Determination of the actual value of the blood pressure then depended on the conscious perception of the moment at which the intensity of these sounds dropped below the clinician's threshold of auditory perception. Yet no one questions the legitimacy of the technique. It certainly is not accurate to more than two decimal places at best, and it is a far derivative of the pressure developed in the heart during contraction, but it's good enough. And there may be no one at all who can explain the complete set of transformations that lead from an increase in neuronal activity in a region of the brain to the appearance of a bright red spot in the equivalent location on a functional magnetic resonance imaging statistical parametric mapping analysis.

The difference between dream reports and blood pressure measurements is in the concept of "good enough." Researchers confirmed the validity of using pressure cuffs by monitoring blood pressure with indwelling catheters in parallel with pressure cuff measurements, thus confirming the reliability of the pressure cuff technique. There is no way to tell whether or not a given dream report, or dream reports in general, are good enough, and it is not clear that it will ever be possible to record dreams (or any other conscious experiences) with the same level of confidence, precision, and reliability that exists for most other measurements in the biologic sciences.

Table 41–1. Restrictions of Dream Definitions

Any mentation recalled from sleep
Any "dreamlike" mentation from waking or sleep
Any mentation from REM sleep
Any hallucinatory mentation from sleep
Any hallucinatory, narrative, emotional mentation
  from sleep

REM, rapid eye movement.

Given that we study dream reports, the bigger question is how our data collection procedures affect the data. Table 41–2 outlines some of the parameters of dream collection that vary from one laboratory to the next.

For each of these parameters, changes in the methodology are known to affect dream reporting, with differences in report frequency, length, bizarreness, and emotional content being notable. But arguments continue in most cases over whether the difference reflects a difference in dreaming or just in the reporting of dreaming. Even in the case of laboratory awakenings from rapid eye movement (REM) and non-REM (NREM) sleep, arguments continue over how much of the difference in reporting seen between the two sleep stages reflects diminished dreaming during NREM sleep as opposed to diminished recall on awakening from NREM sleep. Since a given pair of studies can conceivably differ on all nine of these parameters

Table 41–2. Parameters of Dream Collection

Parameter	Common Values
Location	Home (monitored or unmonitored)
	Laboratory (monitored)
Awakening	Spontaneous
	Evoked
Timing	Morning (end of night)
	Naps
	Nocturnal (middle of night)
Sleep stage	REM
	Stage 1
	Stage 2
	SWS
Time in stage	Constant
	Random
	Spontaneous
	Later in stage (especially REM) later in the night
Time of night	Constant
	Variable
Nights	One
	Consecutive
	Fixed schedule (e.g., weekly)
	Ad libitum
Report style	Written
	Audio recordings
Probes	None
	Fixed
	Semistructured

REM, rapid eye movement; SWS, slow wave sleep.

(allowing several thousand distinct protocols), it is not surprising that disagreements are found in the literature over report frequencies, lengths, and features. It thus behooves the reader, both in interpreting the literature and in considering the interpretations of others, to gain clarity on the values of these parameters for each study under consideration.

DESCRIPTION

A proper description of dreaming (defined now as sleep mentation) should describe the nature of the perceptions, thoughts, and emotions experienced by the dreamer, as well as how these change with condition. The first chapters in this section focus on this question. Unfortunately these chapters provide only a partial answer. The vast majority of studies of dreaming focus on dream perceptions—the highly visual, narratively complex, and delusional hallucinations that we all think of when we think of dreaming. A smaller body of research has looked at the emotions of dreams, and almost no studies have looked at the thoughts of dreams.

Even in the area of dream perception, what is studied varies dramatically from number of words to number of characters and objects, to classification of characters (family, friends, strangers), to identification of bizarreness (on any of a number of ad hoc scales), to measures of "latent content." Thus, it is not uncommon for two studies of "dream content" to lack a single common outcome measure. As a result, two studies may be looking at different aspects of a different subset of mentation reports (see Table 41–1) from different parts of the night (see Table 41–2).

Individual and group differences are also poorly understood. Aside from clinical populations and very limited case studies (often from a psychoanalytic perspective), the best data on subpopulations relate to dreaming in children and to the question of whether some individuals do not dream at all.

Probably the greatest amount of investigation of variability in dreaming relates to the question of REM versus NREM dreaming, and even here huge chasms of disagreement exist. At this time, all that can be safely stated is that the two extreme positions, namely that dreaming occurs only during REM or, conversely, that there is no difference between REM and NREM dreaming, no longer appear to have any champions. But between these two extremes, almost every imaginable niche is occupied.

MECHANISMS

Efforts to explain how we dream date back to antiquity, when gods and indigestion were major contenders for the origins of dreams. Over the last 150 years, efforts at finding a brain-mind basis for dreaming have progressed slowly. At the moment, one can discern several schools of thought, which generally fall into the fields of neurophysiology, psychology, psychoanalysis, and, more recently, cognitive neuroscience. At their best, each of these takes an inclusive view, acknowledging the contributions of the other fields but focusing on their own. At their worst, they reject the usefulness of other fields, with the usefulness of at least neurophysiology and psychoanalysis explicitly rejected by some groups. We have tried to represent most, if not all, of these approaches in the chapters that follow.

FUNCTIONS

Theories of the function of dreaming abound. But it is often unclear what is actually being explained, whether it is the phenomenological experience of dreaming or the biologic processes that underlie it. This distinction is only important because some researchers state their belief that dreaming per se has no function, whereas the biologic processes that underlie it have very important functions. For example, these researchers would argue, the activation of neural networks within association cortex during REM sleep might lead to important, long-term changes in network connectivity and could also fleetingly create a dream, but the dream and the process of dreaming itself would be unimportant to the production of these changes. Other researchers believe that the phenomenological dream experience (with or without subsequent waking recall) is the critical element in the functionality of the dream and that the underlying biology is important only insofar as it is necessary to create the dream experience. Still others find the distinction unimportant or meaningless.

This range of theories should not be surprising, since it exactly parallels discussions of the functionality of consciousness in general. Philosophers and neurobiologists alike struggle to understand how to even think and talk about such functionality. Some reject any such functionality; others take it as a given; still others believe the issue reflects a poorly formed question, that consciousness and its underlying brain basis are the same. For the purpose of this section, we will collapse the two questions, talking about the function of dreaming and its underlying brain mechanisms as if they were interchangeable. While we are not claiming that they are, it appears safe to say that we do not know how to measure their effects independently.

Theories of the function of dreaming (or lack thereof) go hand in hand with the approaches taken to studying the mechanisms underlying dreaming. Thus, physiologic models tend to see little function in dreaming, while psychoanalytic models ascribe highly complex functions to it. Psychological and cognitive neuroscience models tend to lie somewhere in between, ascribing various levels of complexity to dream function. In the chapters that follow, some authors propose specific functions for dreaming, others assume that it has no functions, and still others fail to even discuss it.

CONCLUSION

In the end, we are left with a field that is very much a work in progress. There is no more than a hint of a complete brain-based model for dream construction, and there is limited experimental evidence that dreaming plays any functional role. But that being said, the last ten years have shown a resurgence of interest in and research on dreaming, and brain imaging studies during sleep have fueled the development of new models of dream construction and function. It is hoped that this section will provide a snapshot of the state of the field at this time, a warning of the questions so far unanswered, and a guide to how dream research will progress over the next decade.

Reference

1. Pagel JF, Blagrove M, Levin R, et al: Definitions of dream: A paradigm for comparing field descriptive specific studies of dream. Dreaming 2001;11:195-202.

42

The Content of Dreams: Methodologic and Theoretical Implications

G. William Domhoff

ABSTRACT

Drawing on both laboratory and nonlaboratory studies, this chapter reports on what is known and generally agreed upon about the nature of dream content in the general adult population in industrialized democracies, suggesting that for the most part dreams are a reasonable simulation of waking life in terms of characters, social interactions, activities, and settings. However, there is no consensus on the degree to which dreams are characterized by emotionality or bizarreness, owing to methodologic problems in studying these issues. There are developmental changes in dream content until late adolescence, when dream content becomes surprisingly stable and consistent throughout adulthood and old age. There are relatively few differences between the dreams of mental patients and normal adults, except for the low levels of friends and friendly interactions in the dreams of some patient groups. Samples of dreams from societies all over the world, including many nonindustrial ones, find that there are more similarities than differences in dream content, but there are also large individual differences that have been linked to the dreamer's concerns and interests in waking life. The several methodologic pitfalls in doing replicable studies of dream content are discussed. The ways clinical research could contribute to a better theoretical understanding of dreams are mentioned.

This chapter reviews systematic findings on normative dream content to provide baselines and methodologic strategies for future research in clinical and nonclinical settings. It begins with what is known about dream content from quantitative studies of rapid eye movement (REM) reports collected after awakenings in the sleep laboratory, briefly mentions the similarities and differences between REM and non-REM (NREM) reports, and then considers results based on several different comparisons of laboratory and home dream reports. The lab-home comparisons set the stage for an examination of dream reports collected from large samples of young adults outside the laboratory setting, which in turn provides a basis for discovering any differences based on age, mental health status, and culture. It is then possible to analyze the wide range of individual variation in dream content that is revealed through quantitative studies of individual dream series and to relate these variations to waking thought and behavior. Highly atypical dreams, such as those that make a lasting impression on the dreamer, also can be best assessed within this normative context. The methodologic implications of these general findings for future studies are presented at relevant places throughout the chapter, and the implications for theories of dreaming are briefly considered in the final section.

Since the emphasis of this chapter is on replicated findings where there is widespread agreement, studies using small sample sizes, samples of uncertain quality, or rating scales of unknown reliability and validity are not considered. Critiques of these and other shortcomings in the literature on dream content can be found elsewhere.[1,2] However, despite the focus on generally accepted findings, disparate results due to unresolved methodologic problems are addressed for two content categories of importance to theories of dreaming—those for coding emotions and those for coding dream elements that are unusual or unrealistic by waking standards (often called "bizarre" elements in the dream literature).

There is no consensus on what distinguishes "dreaming" from other cognitive processes, such as thinking or daydreaming, nor on what constitutes "dream content."[3] For purposes of this chapter, dreaming is defined as a sequence of perceptions, thoughts, and emotions during sleep that is experienced as a series of actual events; the nature of these events, the dream content, can be known to investigators only in the form of a verbal or written report. The kind of empirical studies discussed in this chapter reveal that the events of a dream always include the dreamer as an observer or participant and that they almost always include at least one other character besides the dreamer (either a person or an animal). In addition, the dreamer or the other characters in the dreams are invariably engaged in one or another activity (e.g., looking, walking, running) or a social interaction. Thus, the sense of participation in an event, along with characters, activities, and social interactions, is what distinguishes dreams from the more fleeting, fragmented, and/or thoughtlike forms of sleep mentation.

DREAM REPORTS FROM LABORATORY AWAKENINGS

Perhaps the most comprehensive study of REM dream content in the sleep laboratory is based on 635 dream reports collected "for a variety of experimental purposes" in a series of investigations over a period of seven years between 1960 and 1967 (see Snyder,[4] p. 127).[5] The 58 young men and women who participated in these studies were awakened on 250 nights in two different laboratories, one at the National Institute of Mental Health in Bethesda, the other at the Downstate Medical Center in Brooklyn. Owing to the varying purposes of the original investigations, some participants were simply asked to report anything they remembered upon awakening. Others were questioned in detail about what they recalled, a procedure that tended to produce longer dream reports. Still others, 20 male students taking part in an investigation of the sequence of dream emotions, were questioned at each awakening for details about any emotional accompaniments of the dream.

The investigators defined a dream report by specifying that "the subject's words must clearly convey an experience of complex and organized perceptual imagery," which also must have "undergone some temporal process or change" (see Snyder,[4] p. 129). They thereby excluded the isolated visual images, fragmented auditory recall, and thoughts that are also part of the more general category of sleep mentation. This definition is very similar to the one adopted for the purposes of this chapter. Based on this definition, 75% of the awakenings led to dream recall. The reports were divided into short (less than 150 words), medium (150-300 words), and long (more than 300 words) sets as a control for length.

Although there were some small differences due to word length, the overall finding was that "dreaming consciousness" is "a remarkably faithful replica of waking life" (see Snyder,[4] p. 133). For example, 38% of the settings were familiar to the dreamers, and another 43% were similar to places they knew (the remaining 19% of reports, most of them short, did not mention a setting). Of the identified settings, only 5% were "exotic," in the sense of highly unusual or out of the ordinary, and less than 1% were "fantastic," in the sense of unrealistic (see Snyder,[4] p. 134). Ninety-five percent of the dreams contained at least one other character in addition to the dreamer. The most frequent activity was talking, which appeared in 86% of the medium-length reports and 100% of the long reports. By contrast, "active exertion" (e.g., running, playing a sport, fighting) occurred in only 15% to 20%. Using a conservative standard to guard against imputing any emotions to the dreamers, specific emotions were judged to be present in only 30% to 35% of the reports, with unpleasant emotions outnumbering pleasant ones by 2 to 1. Anxiety and anger were the most frequent types of emotions; erotic feelings occurred in only 8 of the 635 reports (1.3%) (see Snyder,[4] p. 141).

The investigators made a series of ratings for coherence (does the narrative hold together as a story), dramatic quality (are the events outside the ordinary gamut of waking life), credibility (are the events conceivable, even if unlikely), and bizarreness (are any events "outside the conceivable expectations of waking life"). They found that 60% to 80% were highly coherent on a three-point scale, as compared with less than 5% that were rated low on coherence. Three fourths had a "nil" or "low" degree of drama on a four-point scale, and less than 10% were high on drama. Fully 65% of the dream reports were rated highly credible, and another 25% were rated of medium credibility; about 8% were rated low on credibility and 2% as having no credibility. In keeping with the findings on credibility, the dreams were rated as having a low degree of bizarreness. Focusing here on the longest reports because they were more frequently rated bizarre, 50% were rated as having no bizarreness, 30% as having a low degree of bizarreness, 8% as having a medium degree, and 2% as having a high degree (see Snyder,[4] p. 133).

The researchers also made a search for "typical" dreams, which are defined by certain common themes that many people, in response to questionnaires, report they have experienced, such as failing an examination, appearing partially dressed in public (with feelings of great embarrassment), suddenly losing teeth, flying under one's own power, falling through space, and finding money.[6] They discovered that typical dreams were not very frequent in their sample: Only 11 dreams related to examinations, none of which involved failure, and only 10 mentioned any degree of nudity, none of which included any embarrassment. The loss of teeth occurred in three dreams, and flying, falling, and finding money made one appearance each (see Snyder,[4] p. 148).

Based on their wide range of findings, the authors conclude that dreams as they have defined them are very different from what is commonly believed in psychiatry and popular culture. They characterized a prototypical REM dream report as a "clear, coherent, and detailed account of a realistic situation involving the dreamer and other people caught up in very ordinary activities and preoccupations, and usually talking about them" (see Snyder,[4] p. 148). Overall, they believe that as many as "90% would have been considered credible descriptions of everyday experience" (see Snyder,[5] p. 375).

The apparent lack of highly unusual dream content in REM reports was investigated in more detail in a study of 16 young women who each spent two consecutive nights in the lab and answered questions about the familiarity and likelihood of specific dream elements after an average of four REM awakenings per night.[7] Based on the categories of the Hall–Van de Castle coding system, which was designed specifically for the study of dream content, the contents were categorized as physical surroundings (settings and objects), characters (humans, animals, and creatures), activities (physical, expressive, verbal, and cognitive), and social interactions (aggressive, friendly, and sexual).[8] Then each type of element was placed in one of six nominal categories for types of "novelty." Three of the categories ranged from the exact replication of the dreamers' reality to large but plausible differences from their waking experience; the other three categories ranged from previously unexperienced but realistic elements to elements that are fantastic or improbable. Using the percentage of perfect agreement between two coders as their measure of reliability for these difficult judgments, the reliability for their novelty scale was 94.6% for characters, 84.5% for physical surroundings, 64.3% for activities and social interactions, and 53.1% for ratings of the overall dream (see Dorus et al.,[7] p. 366).

The investigators concluded that their results "emphasize the rarity of the bizarre in dreams" because major distortions of actual waking experiences reach a high of only 16.7% of all the activities and social interactions and a high of 6.2% and 7.8% for all characters and physical surroundings (see Dorus et al.,[7] p. 367). The figures for the most improbable category of event never experienced by the dreamer in waking life were 4.9% of all physical surroundings, 1.3% of all characters, and 6.8% of all activities and social interactions. When they carried out global ratings of each dream for overall novelty, they found that 25.8% showed large but plausible differences from previous waking experiences and that 8.9% were highly improbable by waking standards.

The issue of emotions, initially addressed in the Bethesda-Brooklyn study, was first investigated in great depth in the sleep lab in a study of 17 young adults (9 women, 8 men) over two nonconsecutive nights, with a mean of 6 REM awakenings per participant. The participants were quizzed in detail after each awakening about the presence of emotions and the appropriateness of the emotion to the content. Drawing on ratings by both participants and naive judges, the investigators concluded that about 70% of the dream reports had at least some affect,[9] a much higher figure than in the

Bethesda-Brooklyn study, but one that is supported in later studies of REM reports.[10,11] The type of emotion, or lack thereof, was appropriate to the dream situation in 60% of the dreams. However, there was no emotion in 17% of the cases where there would have been some in a similar waking situation, and there was dream emotion in 3.2% where there would have been none in waking life. The investigators concluded that emotions are generally appropriate in dreams, with the major anomaly being the absence of emotion when it would have been present in waking life.

Another comprehensive laboratory investigation of emotions used 500 REM dream reports from 44 participants (26 women, 18 men), who spent a total of 161 nights in the laboratory. Participants were asked after each awakening about the presence of any specific emotions and the nature of the overall feeling or mood of the dream. Specific emotions were present in 50% of the reports, a general mood was present in 23%, and no emotion was present in 26%. In terms of the specific emotions, negative feelings appeared twice as often as positive ones, but a positive feeling tone was 2.5 times more frequent in those dreams with an overall mood (see Strauch and Meier,[11] p. 93). This disparity between the negativity of specific emotions, as judged by content analysts, and the positive (pleasant) nature of general feeling tone, as rated by the dreamers themselves, will be encountered again later in the chapter.

Taken together, these detailed descriptive studies provide a consistent picture of REM dream reports as portraying a reasonable simulation of the dreamer's waking world. The dream scenario is original, but not usually fantastic, and the emotions are generally appropriate to the situation when they are present. This picture is supported by other studies that will be discussed later in the chapter when the results of studies comparing laboratory and home dream reports are presented.

Several laboratory studies have probed for any changes that might occur in dream content from REM period to REM period, uncovering very few replicable differences. Ratings by the dreamers themselves in one study found there is some increase in clarity, intensity, and vividness from the brief first REM period to later REM periods (see Foulkes,[12] pp. 92-94). A study with five participants found one difference among many comparisons: more references to the past in late-night REM periods.[13] However, that result could not be replicated in a large-scale study based on 332 REM reports from 11 young men.[14] Another study reported there may be somewhat more bizarre elements in later REM periods,[7] but that result was not supported in a larger study of 342 REM reports that found no differences through the first four sleep cycles of the night.[15]

Employing categories for settings, characters, activities, social interactions, and emotions, both quantitative and qualitative analyses find few or no differences from REM period to REM period when corrections are made for the length of report.[10,16] In the most comprehensive study of this issue, there were two minor differences among 26 analyses employing Hall–Van de Castle categories for the first four REM periods, whether they were nights with single or multiple awakenings, and there were no differences with spontaneously recalled dreams that came from night or morning REM self-awakenings.[14] However, there may be some degree of thematic continuity from REM to REM on a few nights. In a study of 36 nights of REM reports from 24 participants, for example, six nights contained a repeated theme (see Strauch and Meier,[11] p. 206).

REM and NREM Dream Reports

As is well known, there were indications in early laboratory studies that dreaming occurs almost exclusively in REM, but since then there have been many comparisons of REM and NREM reports that seem to contradict that initial assumption.[17-22] Most of these studies have been summarized in several places, including Chapter 47 in this volume.[23,24] These comparisons agree that dreams, when defined in much the same way as they are for purposes of this chapter, are more frequent and longer during REM periods. Most studies conclude that many NREM reports seem to be "thoughts," not dreams. In fact, NREM reports are more often a continuation of waking thoughts and memories, whereas there are few episodic memories in REM or home dream reports.[25,26]

However, three caveats need to be added to this quick characterization. First, most—although probably not all—of these differences disappear when there is a control for length.[17,19,27] Second, the differences that remain relate to a greater character density in REM reports, which in turn leads to the possibility of social interactions.[19,28] Third, there is evidence that NREM reports late in the sleep period are more similar to REM reports than are NREM reports from the first few hours of sleep (see Domhoff and Schneider,[28] p. 149).[29,30] In the most recent study of this kind, the thoughtlike nature of NREM decreased by 56% and the hallucinatory nature increased by 62%, leading to the conclusion that "as the night progresses NREM approaches the neurocognitive characteristics of REM" (see Fosse et al.,[31] p. 302).

The similarities in dream content between REM and late-night NREM reports, when combined with the fact that there are similarities in dream content from REM period to REM period, suggest that a representative sample of people's dream life, as defined in this chapter, can be collected at any time beginning with the third REM period, when participants are more likely to be alert and cooperative upon awakening. This suggestion is also supported by a study showing a high degree of recall from NREM awakenings at the end of the sleep period.[30] This is a highly useful conclusion because it makes the collection of dream reports in the laboratory less stressful and also more efficient in terms of good recall.

LABORATORY AND HOME DREAM COMPARISONS

The credible nature of most laboratory dream reports raises the possibility that there might be substantial differences between them and more bizarre dreams remembered at home—perhaps owing to an inhibitory effect from the laboratory setting or to the differences in method of reporting in the two settings (spoken versus written), or selective recall at home (forgetting small details and highlighting emotionally salient or anomalous elements), or some combination of these factors. However, several careful investigations reveal that there are relatively few differences between home and laboratory dream reports even when these differences are not perfectly controlled.[11,28,32,33] Furthermore, most of these differences disappear when the proper controls are introduced.[34,35] The one exception to this generalization seems to be hostile and aggressive dream elements, which occur more frequently in the home dream reports of young adults in three different studies.[28,35,36]

The largest and most detailed comparison of lab and home reports used written reports from home, which are usually shorter than transcribed lab reports. However, with corrections for length using the Hall–Van de Castle indicators for 21 categories of dream content, there were only 4 statistically significant differences between 120 home dreams and 272 lab dreams from 8 young men who recalled at least 34 lab dreams and 15 home dreams. The percentage of characters that were animals was higher in the home dreams, as were three aggression indicators. More specifically in terms of aggression, there was a higher percentage of dream reports with at least one instance of aggression; a higher rate of aggressions per character; and a higher percentage of aggressions that were physical, as defined by destruction of personal property, chases, physical attacks, and murders. The effect sizes for these statistically significant differences were in the small or medium range, except in the case of the physical aggressions percentage, which showed a large difference.[28]

The higher frequency of aggression in home dream reports supports the concern that there is some selective recall in everyday dream reports. Even here, however, it is noteworthy that 44% of the dreams did not contain any form of aggression, whether physical or nonphysical, and 72% were without any physical aggression. These findings are fairly similar to those from a normative sample of home dreams from young men (discussed later), where 53% of the reports had no form of aggression and 74% had no physical aggression.[8] If home dream reports have a strong bias for atypical elements, then it might be predicted that there would be a much larger number of sexual dreams, but only 9% of the home reports in this study contained as much as a sensual hug or kiss, as compared with 5% of the laboratory reports.

These findings on the relatively small differences between home and laboratory dreams may be explainable in terms of the results from laboratory studies that compare what is reported from REM awakenings with what is still remembered in the morning.[37-39] Such studies reveal that recency and length of report are the primary factors in later recall, which at home would lead to a representative sample of nightly dream content given the lack of content differences from REM period to REM period and between early REM periods and late-night NREM periods. However, some of these studies also show that intensity can be a tertiary factor in morning recall, which suggests there is some selection bias toward the everyday recall of more emotionally salient content.

All in all, the findings presented in this section demonstrate that new ideas can be tested with representative samples of dream content collected outside the laboratory, but it also must be stressed that empirical studies show there are numerous obstacles to obtaining such reports. They have to be collected with a standardized reporting form, and participants must be given ample time to respond. Otherwise, participants often provide brief and hasty reports consisting of a phrase or a few sentences. Systematic comparisons with longer reports suggest that reports of less than 50 words, far below the average laboratory report length, are usually too brief to describe dream content adequately and are often discarded before any analysis is made (see Domhoff,[40] pp. 79-84). In addition, it takes at least 75 to 125 reports from a group or individual for good quantitative studies because some dream elements appear too infrequently for adequate statistical analysis with fewer reports.

For normative studies of groups, it is essential to ask for the "most recent dream" people can recall to keep samples comparable to laboratory dream reports. If recency is not emphasized, the sample is likely to include many recurrent or highly memorable dreams, some of which may stem from childhood (see Domhoff,[1] p. 67). Such dreams are interesting, but it is first necessary to have a solid picture of everyday dream life in order to understand them more fully.

The collection of dream reports outside the laboratory also can be facilitated by the use of the Nightcap,* a computer-based home awakening system that uses the presence of eye movements and absence of head movements to detect REM sleep and then sends an awakening auditory signal to the dreamer. It already has proved useful in a study of 16 participants over a period of 14 nights each.[10,31]

NORMATIVE DREAM CONTENT IN HOME DREAMS

As might be expected from the results of the laboratory-home comparisons, studies of large samples of dream content collected from young college-educated adults outside the laboratory show many similarities with the laboratory results when the same or comparable content categories are employed. This point was first demonstrated as early as the 1890s in careful investigations of their own dreams by academic psychologists of the introspectionist school.[41,42] As the lead investigator in the Bethesda-Brooklyn laboratory investigation of 635 REM dream reports concluded, their findings "only confirm the findings of Calkins in 1893" (see Snyder,[4] p. 150).

The most systematic research on large samples of this kind has been done using the same Hall–Van de Castle coding categories employed in several of the laboratory investigations described earlier. The system, which has 10 general categories that cover characters, types of activities, and such descriptive elements as intensity, size, and temperature, relies on the nominal level of measurement owing to problems of both reliability and psychological validity with rating scales. The raw frequencies are analyzed using percentages and ratios to correct for the varying length of dream reports from sample to sample. Normative findings with 500 dream reports from 100 men and another 500 from 100 women reveal a pattern of gender differences that need to be taken into account when doing studies of individuals.[8]

For instance, men and women differ in the percentage of gendered characters who are male or female, with men having a 67:33 male-to-female ratio and women 48:52. Aggression, defined as a desire, intention, or action to annoy or harm some other character, is the most frequent type of social interaction in dreams, occurring at least once in 47% of men's dreams and 44% of women's. Although men and women are about the same in terms of the percentage of dreams in which aggression occurs, men have a higher rate of aggressions per character, and a much higher percentage of their aggressions are physical. The magnitude of these and other differences is calculated with the h statistic, which corrects for the fact that

---

*The Nightcap was manufactured by Healthdyne Technologies of Marietta, GA. It has since been acquired by Respironics, Inc. of Murrysville, PA. Its name has been changed to REMView.

standard deviations cannot be determined with data expressed in percentages (see Domhoff,[1] Appendix D). The dream reports used in creating the normative sample, as well as the codings for them, are available to researchers through www.dreambank.net.[43]

Emotions, which are placed into five categories (apprehension, anger, sadness, confusion, and happiness), can be coded only if they are explicitly expressed. By this strict criterion, emotions are present in 41% of men's dreams and 57% of women's. This figure is somewhat larger than what was reported in the Bethesda-Brooklyn study,[4] but it is well below the figure of 70% to 75% for three REM-based studies mentioned earlier in the chapter.[9-11] The most frequent of these emotions for both men and women is apprehension, which accounts for just over a third of all dream emotions, followed by happiness and confusion, which each account for about a fifth of all emotions. Overall, a great majority of the specific emotions in dream reports are negative for both men and women, a conclusion that has been replicated in four studies.[11,44-46]

The general Hall–Van de Castle norms can be used with confidence for a variety of purposes because they have been replicated for men and women at the University of Richmond in 1981, for women at the University of California at Berkeley in 1985, for women at Salem College in the late 1980s, and for women at the University of California at Santa Cruz in the early 1990s.[1,46-48] The results with these predominantly Anglo students also seem to generalize to Mexican-American college students in the Southwest according to three studies in the 1970s and 1990s.[49-51] Although two of these three studies used their own rating systems, not the Hall–Van de Castle system, they found a similar pattern of gender similarities and differences on key elements. Generally speaking, then, there is reason to believe that there has been little or no change in the dream life of American college students over the past 50 years.

The findings also are broadly similar to what has been reported in investigations of Canadian, Dutch, Swiss, and German college-educated adults, although there are fewer physical aggressions in the dreams of the Dutch and Swiss samples.[11,52-55] Dream content is also more similar than different for college students in two large industrialized societies outside of Europe and North America: India and Japan.[56-58]

Typical dreams, those with themes common to many people, have been studied in large samples outside the laboratory, where they turn out to be as rare as they are in the laboratory. A canvas of 983 dream reports from two-week journals provided by 126 students at the University of California at Santa Cruz discovered that virtually none of 10 typical dreams occurred more than a few times. For example, there were only five flying dreams in the two-week sample, 0.5% of the total. The figures for several other typical dreams were even lower. Two people dreamed of finding money, two became lost, two were taking an examination, one lost his teeth, and one fell (see Domhoff,[1] p. 198). A study based on 1910 dream reports from students at the University of North Carolina at Chapel Hill reported a similar low figure for flying dreams: 17 participants reported 22 flying dreams, 1.2% of the total dream report sample.[59] The similarity of these findings to those reported in laboratory studies is further evidence that carefully collected home dream reports can provide samples reasonably similar to those obtained from awakenings in the sleep laboratory.

PROBLEMS IN STUDYING EMOTIONS IN DREAMS

Although there is widespread agreement with the Hall–Van de Castle findings on the extent to which various settings, characters, social interactions, activities, and objects appear in dreams, there are disagreements over both the pleasantness and frequency of emotions in dreams, owing to methodologic difficulties alluded to at the beginning of the chapter. As already noted, several different studies using blind coders find that negative emotions outnumber positive ones.[44-46,48] However, very different results emerge when the dreamers themselves make a global rating of each of their dream reports on a pleasant-unpleasant dimension. Such studies regularly find that the dreamers rate the emotions in their dreams at least equally pleasant and unpleasant, and sometimes more pleasant than unpleasant.

This contrast is demonstrated in one of the earliest studies using both approaches. The content analyst concluded that 64% of the explicitly expressed emotions in a sample of 1000 home dream reports were negative or unpleasant and that only 18% expressed happiness, but the dreamers rated their dreams more pleasant than unpleasant by a margin of 41% to 25%, with 11% judged to be mixed (see Hall,[60] p. 62). Significantly, the dreamers also said that 23% of the dreams were without feeling tone, which is not much lower than the finding of no affect in 30% and 26% of the dreams in three REM-based studies mentioned earlier.[9-11] The contrast between the two types of findings in this early home study is similar to the findings in a more recent laboratory study of 500 REM dreams cited earlier, which showed that the specific emotions were negative by 2:1 according to coders but were positive in general mood according to the dreamers themselves by 2.5:1.[11] Later studies report the same tendency for dreamers to rate their home dreams as more pleasant than unpleasant.[10,61-63] There is no ready explanation for these contrasting results with the two different methods, which has been a hindrance in drawing theoretical conclusions about emotions in dreams.

Dreamers also tend to attribute many more emotions to their home dreams than do blind judges when the dreamers are asked to recall the emotions that accompanied the report they have written down.[44,62,63] However, based on the REM-report finding that only about 70% to 75% of dream reports have any affect, we must study whether or not this greater amount of emotions in self-ratings of home dream reports is the result of two extrinsic factors: the demand characteristics of such a rating task and the waking-life assumption that certain emotions would logically be present in many of the situations experienced in the dream. This may be especially the case where the dreams and ratings were obtained as part of "a graded class exercise," even though students were told that they could obtain dreams from the instructor if they did not remember their dreams (see Kahn et al.,[62] p. 35).[63] Perhaps it will prove useful to do both blind analyses and dreamer self-ratings for emotions in future studies, but it needs to be clear that so far the two approaches yield different results.

PROBLEMS IN STUDYING BIZARRENESS IN DREAMS

Content analysts also disagree about an issue not addressed by the Hall–Van de Castle coding system: the extent to which bizarreness is a facet of dreaming. In studies that focus on clearly impossible events, the figure is 10% or less for large samples of both REM and home dreams.[4,7,28] When sudden scene changes, uncertainties, and small distortions are included, the figure rises to between 30% and 60%, which is somewhat comparable to the finding for overall ratings for the most unusual elements in the detailed laboratory study of bizarreness discussed earlier in the chapter.[7,64-66] With a six-point rating scale based on the degree to which any dimension of the dream differs from waking experience and behavior, including such deviations from social norms as murder and leaving the scene of an accident, 75% of 500 REM reports from young men and women had at least one bizarre aspect, as compared with 7% to 8% that were bizarre in three or more ways (see Strauch and Meier,[11] pp. 95-103). Given these widely disparate results, there is not much chance of resolving these differences until there is agreement on categories that can be used with higher reliability than has been achieved with most bizarreness scales.

GROUP DIFFERENCES: AGE, MENTAL PATIENTS, AND SMALL NONINDUSTRIAL SOCIETIES

The findings on the dream content of young college-educated adults in industrialized societies provide a normative basis for a variety of group comparisons concerning age, mental health, and membership in the small nonindustrial societies studied by anthropologists.

Age Differences

There appear to be major changes in dream content from the preschool to teen years but few changes from the late teens to old age. Dream content thus seems to parallel cognitive and emotional development during childhood, as well as the stability of adult personality.

Much of what is known in a systematic way about children's dreams comes from a classic longitudinal laboratory study of children between the ages of 3 and 15, supplemented by a cross-sectional laboratory replication a few years later with children ages 5 to 8.[67,68] More recently, a 5-year longitudinal laboratory study of Swiss children ages 9 to 15 has provided additional supporting information.[69] However, as shown shortly when the home-reported dreams of children are discussed, there are larger differences between the lab and home dreams of children than there are for adults.

The first longitudinal study involved two groups of children who slept in the laboratory every other year for nine nonconsecutive nights over a 5-year period. The first group was between 3 and 4 years of age when the study started. The second group was between 9 and 10. The study began with a total of 30 children in the two groups; six boys ages 11 to 12 were added at the start of the third year, and seven girls ages 7 to 8 were added at the start of the fifth year. In all, 46 children were studied—26 for all 5 years, 34 for at least 3 years, and 43 for at least 1 complete year. The investigator made 2711 awakenings over the 5-year period.

The most unexpected finding was the low amount of recall from REM periods in the 3 to 5 year olds (only 27% of the REM awakenings yielded any recall that could reasonably be called a dream), and the static, bland, and underdeveloped content of the few reports that were obtained. The reports became more "dreamlike" (in terms of characters, themes, and actions) in the 5 to 7 year olds, but it was not until the children were 11 to 13 years old that their dreams began to resemble those of adult laboratory participants in frequency, length, emotions, and overall structure or to show any relationship to personality (see Foulkes,[67] p. 217).

Animals were the primary characters in the dreams of the preschool children; they also appeared in 38% of the REM reports from 5 to 7 year olds, with a gradual decline to the low levels of adulthood beginning at ages 7 to 9 years. With the people who did appear, the same differences in male-to-female ratio found in young adults were present from the outset—70:30 for boys between 3 and 9 years old, 51:49 for girls in the same age range.[70] "Hostile attacks" were virtually absent from the dreams of the preschoolers and were present in only one of four dream reports for both boys and girls between ages 5 and 7. All but one of these attacks were initiated by some character other than the dreamer, and the dreamer was rarely the victim. The same low level of attacks was found at age 7 to 9 years, although some of the acts were now initiated by the dreamer in 9% of the girls' dreams and 4% of the boys'.[67]

During the preadolescent and adolescent years, there was a general decline in dreaming about family members for both genders, but the girls' dreams tended to have home or residential settings more often than the boys' did. Between ages 11 and 13 years, positive social interactions outweighed "antisocial" interactions by 2:1, with a slight increase in antisocial interactions between ages 13 and 15 and with girls showing a greater amount of victimization in such interactions.

The cross-sectional replication study focused on 10 boys and 10 girls within 1 month of their fifth, sixth, seventh, and eighth birthdays because the most dramatic changes in the longitudinal study seemed to occur during this age period. These 80 children were awakened 10 times each over a period of 3 nonconsecutive nights for a total of 800 awakenings. All of the main original findings were supported. The median rate of reporting was only 20% for all age groups. The imagery in the dreams was more static than dynamic until age 7, and the child's "self" character did not tend to take an active role in the dreams until age 8.[68] As with young adults' dreams, there were more characters in the girls' dreams, and there was the same gender difference in the ratio of male to female characters. There were no failures, few negative emotions, and very few misfortunes. There were few aggressive or friendly interactions, with more friendliness in the girls' reports (see Domhoff,[1] p. 94).

The recent longitudinal study of Swiss children ages 9 to 15 involved 12 boys and 12 girls who slept in the laboratory for three nonconsecutive nights every other year and provided a total of 551 REM reports. The results were generally similar to those for preadolescents and adolescents in the earlier longitudinal study, and there were only relatively small changes in most categories over the 6-year period. Except for a decline in the animal percentage, there was consistency over time in most character categories, such as the percentage of familiar characters, along with the usual gender differences in the male-to-female percentage ratio. The percentage of dreams with at least one instance of aggression fluctuated between 24 and 28 for the boys and increased from 18 to 31 for the girls. The percentage of dreams with at least one instance of friendliness increased from 16 to 18 to 24 for the boys and varied from 28 to 20 to 23 for the girls. The largest change was a decline in bizarreness for both boys and girls, as defined by degrees of deviation from waking experience and social norms; just over 60% of the dream reports had at least some degree of bizarreness at ages 9 to 11 and 11 to 13, but the figure fell to 41% at ages 13 to 15.[69]

When these laboratory findings for children and teenagers are compared with those from studies of home reports provided by children,[71-73] there are far greater differences in terms of unusual characters, aggression, and unlikely events than is the case in comparisons of laboratory and home dreams for adults. This generalization includes the home dream reports that were collected as part of the longitudinal study of 9- to 15-year-old children in Switzerland, which had significantly more instances of friendliness, aggression, and bizarreness than did the laboratory reports.[69] However, the original longitudinal study of young children did include a separate study where children slept in the laboratory but were not awakened, as well as a home versus laboratory dream comparison, which together led to the conclusion that any differences were due to selective recall of more salient dreams from spontaneous morning recall in the lab or at home.[34]

In contrast to the apparent changes in dream content from childhood to adolescence, dream content is extremely stable in terms of characters, social interactions, and most other dream elements after age 18 according to cross-sectional studies in the United States, Canada, and Switzerland.[74-79] The elderly recalled fewer dreams in one large longitudinal study,[80] but their dream content remained generally the same—except perhaps in terms of aggression, where three studies suggest a decline.[74,76,79] A comparison of the results from two studies of how college-age and elderly (59 to 87 years) women rated the emotionality of their dream reports supports the idea that there is a decline in aggressive or hostile dream content in older adults.[81,82] Both sets of women wrote down five dreams over a period of 6 weeks and rated each dream on a 10-item emotional checklist. Anger-rage and fear-terror were checked less often in relation to the dream reports of the elderly; enjoyment-joy accounted for a higher proportion of emotions related to the dream reports of the elderly.

The Dream Reports of Mental Patients

There have been many studies of dream content in various psychiatric populations since the early 20th century, but most of them are anecdotal, use untested coding systems, or include only small numbers of patients, so there are few consistent findings.[83] There are several likely reasons for why the findings on psychiatric patients have been so meager and inconsistent. There may be variation from hospital to hospital in how illnesses are diagnosed and patients are classified. Patients within the same diagnostic categories may have been in different phases of their illnesses. The possible effects of medication or hospitalization on dream content usually are not controlled. Most of all, patients may be too heavily medicated, withdrawn, or resistant to provide full and accurate accounts of their dreams.

Moreover, there may not be very many large differences between normal dream content and what mental patients dream about, as seen in a study of 211 dream reports collected from 50 male patients who were grouped into four diagnostic categories: 5 patients who were both schizophrenic and alcoholic, 20 patients who were schizophrenic, 15 patients who were alcoholic, and 10 patients with a variety of other diagnoses. The dream reports of the four groups were compared with each other and with the Hall–Van de Castle male norms for characters, social interactions, success and failure, misfortune and good fortune, and eating and drinking. The differences among the patient groups were few and unrevealing: Dream reports from schizophrenics were shorter, for example, and there were more instances of drinking alcohol and fewer sexual interactions in the alcoholics' dream narratives. Moreover, there were only two differences between the 50 patients as a whole and the Hall–Van de Castle norms: a lower male-to-female ratio and a very low rate of friendly interactions, especially with women.[84]

Low rate of friendliness also was a striking outcome in a study of 27 hospitalized female patients, 15 of whom suffered from schizophrenia and 12 from other types of psychoses.[85] A similar result is reported in a study of female outpatients who suffered from high anxiety states.[86] Findings in a comparison of dream reports from depressed and schizophrenic patients studied in the laboratory reveal a lack of friends in patient dreams as well as a low rate of friendly interactions.[87] There were more strangers in the schizophrenics' dream reports and more family members in the depressed patients' reports, but the striking commonality is that both groups had a low number of friends as a percentage of all the human characters in the dreams: 18% for schizophrenics and 22% for depressives, as compared with 31% for men and 37% for women in the Hall–Van de Castle norms.

Although the study of four groups of male patients did not reveal any differences in instances of aggression, three studies of female patients suggest they may more often be victims of aggression in their dreams than other women. The study of hospitalized psychotic women just mentioned in terms of low rates of friendliness found that they were more likely to be victims in aggressive interactions, as did the study of anxious women outpatients. In addition, a study of 30 hospitalized female schizophrenics presents evidence for a high degree of both aggression and victimization in a patient population. The patients were mostly new admissions in an acute phase of their illness. None had received electroshock within the previous 3 months. They ranged in age from 15 to 39, with a median age of 19. Compared with dream reports by a control group of college women in the same age range, the schizophrenics' reports contained more aggression, especially physical aggression against the dreamers.[88]

Dream Reports from Small Nonindustrial Societies

Good anthropologic evidence reveals that interest in dreams and the uses to which they are put in religious and medicinal ceremonies vary greatly from culture to culture, with hunting and gathering societies putting more emphasis on dreams than agricultural ones.[89] However, contrary to culturalist expectations, there may be as many similarities as differences in dream content, according to several solid studies based on a wide range of cultures.

A detailed ethnographic study of a Mehinaku Indian village of about 80 to 85 people in the Amazon rain forests of central Brazil provides the best in-depth look at the dream reports of nonindustrial men and women known personally to the content analyst. Moreover, the traditional Mehinaku way of life was essentially undisturbed when they were studied in the 1970s, and the people liked to remember their dreams and tell them to each other. It was therefore very easy to collect dream reports from them, and most of the adult population of the village participated. Men contributed 276 dreams, women 109. The dream reports were coded for physical aggressions and sexuality with categories fairly similar to those in the Hall–Van de Castle system. They were also coded for the degree of activity or passivity, as determined by whether the dreamer initiated actions (active) or only observed or reacted to the actions of other dream characters (passive).

There is more physical aggression in these dreams than in American dream reports, especially with animals, but the gender differences are the same in that men report more physical aggressions than women. Mehinaku are also more likely than Americans to be victims of aggression, but in keeping with the Hall–Van de Castle norms, women are more likely than men to be victims. Sexual thoughts or interactions were present in 13% of the men's reports, which is virtually identical with the Hall–Van de Castle norms, and in 12% of the women's, which is three times higher. In men's sexual dreams there is sometimes a fear of assault by jealous male rivals or angry female lovers. Women's dream reports often express a fear of rape and other violent encounters with sexually aggressive men. Sixty-one percent of the men's dream reports were judged active and 39% passive. By way of contrast, 42% of women's dream reports were judged active and 58% passive.

The ethnographer concluded that his findings correspond with the waking life of the Mehinaku. There is threat from a wide range of animals and insects, and there is conflict and competition among the men. Most men and women have several lovers as well as a spouse, and women do fear sexual pressures and attacks from men. Moreover, the higher passivity in women's dreams corresponds with their situation in a highly patriarchal social order, where men dominate in the home as well as in the public aspects of village life. At the same time, there are similarities with the Hall–Van de Castle norms, especially in terms of gender similarities and differences, that led to the hypothesis that "with additional cross-cultural data it may be possible to show that the dream experience is less variant than other aspects of culture" (see Gregor,[90] p. 389).

This hypothesis is supported in an analysis of all the dream reports collected through the first six decades of the 20th century by American and British anthropologists. In more than a dozen cultures that are famous in the anthropology literature, including Alor, Baiga, Hopi, Ifaluk, Kwakiutl, Navajo, Tinguians, Truk, and Yir Yoront, there are more similarities than differences. In the case of characters, men always dream more of males than females, and women tend to dream equally of both genders. There are always more single than plural characters, more humans than animals, and more familiar than unfamiliar characters. In the realm of social interactions, the rate of aggression per character is higher than the rate of friendliness per character, with one exception; dreamers everywhere are more often victims of aggression, with two exceptions; and there is usually more physical than nonphysical aggression. Misfortunes outnumber good fortunes, and there are more negative than positive emotions (see Domhoff,[1] p. 119).

However, there are a few large differences that make sense in terms of the variations from culture to culture. For example, the animal percentage ranged from a high of 34% and 31% for the men in two hunting and gathering groups, the Baiga and Yir Yoront, to a low of 6% for Hopi women, who are sedentary agriculturalists, but it was always higher for small nonindustrial societies than it is in any industrialized society. There were also significant variations in the percentage of all aggressions that were physical; for male dreamers, the figure ranged from 92% for the Yir Yoront to 86% for the Baiga, 77% for the Navajo, and 40% for the Hopi (the figure is 50% for American men and 29% for Swiss men).

INDIVIDUAL CASE STUDIES

Within the context of the many well-established group findings, individual case studies can be of great value for both research and possible clinical applications because detailed comparisons can be made between specific aspects of dream content and waking thought or behavior. The collection of many such series has been rendered more feasible by the availability of the Nightcap for home awakenings.[10,91] Case studies also can be based on blind analyses of extant dream journals kept by individuals for their own reasons—personal, intellectual, or artistic. Such dream journals are a form of personal document long recognized in psychology as having the potential for providing new insights concerning motivation and personality.[92,93] They have value as nonreactive measures that have not been influenced by the purposes of the investigators who later analyze them. The conclusions drawn from nonreactive archival data are considered most reliable and useful when they are based on a diversity of archives likely to have different sources of potential bias.[94]

Studies of several different dream journals first proved their usefulness for scientific purposes by revealing an unexpected consistency in dream content that stretches from the late teens to old age. People's dream lives vary from day to day and week to week, but consistency in both themes and Hall–Van de Castle coding categories manifests itself through comparisons of hundreds of dream reports and with time spans of months and years (see Domhoff,[1] Chapter 7). The short-term variation in dream content, when combined with the fact that most recalled dreams are soon forgotten, may contribute to the belief that dream contents are unsystematic or highly responsive to daily events.

Analyses of dream journals reveal three kinds of consistency: absolute (the frequency or percentage with which an element appears remains the same year after year), relative (the incidence of one element always exceeds the incidence of another element, even though they both may increase or decrease in frequency), and developmental (there is a consistent increase or decrease from one period of time to the next). Relative consistency is the most frequent kind of consistency in dream series. Absolute consistency occurs slightly less often. Developmental regularities are much less common than the first two.

Absolute constancy over decades is best demonstrated in a study of the male-to-female ratio in the early and late dream reports in 11 different dream journals (eight from men, three from women), where there was great consistency for periods ranging from a few months to 32 years. The only exception is a woman who wrote down many of her dreams out of personal interest for a period of 50 years; her male-to-female ratio instead showed a developmental regularity, changing from 53:47 in 1912-1933 to 39:61 in 1960-1962, when she was in her 70s, lived in a women's retirement home, and had fewer contacts with men (see Domhoff,[1] p. 150).

Although the male-to-female percentage ratio showed a gradual decline for the woman in the retirement home, the themes in the first 600 of her dream reports remained quite constant. She is eating, preparing to eat, preparing a meal, buying or seeing food, watching someone eat, or mentioning she is hungry in 21% of the dreams. The loss of an object, usually her purse, occurs in 17%. She is in a small or disorderly room or her room is being invaded by others in 10% of the dreams, and another 10% involve the dreamer and her mother. She is trying to go to the toilet in 8%, usually being interrupted in the process, and she is late, concerned about being late, or missing a bus or train in 6%. These six themes account for at least part of the content in almost 75% of her dreams (see Domhoff,[1] p. 206).

Three separate studies of discontinuous dream series show that the consistency revealed in continuous dream journals is not the result of practice effects. The largest and most ambitious of the three involved a comparison of 2 or 3 dreams from each of 21 women ages 30 to 55 with dreams they had written down for researchers 10, 15, or 17 years earlier. In all, each sample contained 50 dream reports. Using several different scales, including the major Hall–Van de Castle categories, there were no differences.[95] Similar results were obtained in a small-scale study of the dream reports of a young man who wrote down 40 dreams at age 17, 20 at age 21, and 50 at age 24. The three most unusual features of his dream content—a low male-to-female ratio, a low rate of aggressions per character, and a low physical aggressions percentage—were consistent over all three time periods.[96]

The third study compared dream reports written down 34 years apart by a woman who recorded nearly 100 of her dreams out of personal interest when she was young and single between 1923 and 1932 and then several hundred more beginning in 1966, when she was a widow living in a small town in the West, several thousand miles from where she was born and raised. In terms of Hall–Van de Castle categories, the frequencies for most categories were similar in both sets of dreams. However, despite the quantitative similarities in the major character categories, the actual cast of characters changed almost completely, except for members of her family of origin. As in other dream series that have been studied, she dreamed about people with whom she was in contact at the time, even if it was only by correspondence. For all the similarities in the two sets of reports, there were some changes as well. The percentage of unfamiliar characters was higher in the 1960s than the 1920s, for example. Although her rate of aggressive interactions was low in both sets, she dreamed more often of being a victim of aggression, especially at the hands of males, when she was in her 20s, whereas in her 60s she was more often the aggressor (see Domhoff,[1] p. 146).

Blind analyses of dream journals also have led, through the formulation of inferences that can be accepted or rejected by the dreamer and other respondents, to the conclusion that much dream content is continuous with the dreamers' waking conceptions, concerns, and interests. That is, as already seen in the cross-cultural studies discussed earlier in the chapter, what people dream about is also what they think about or do when they are awake. The most direct continuities involve the main people in a dreamer's life and the nature of the social interactions with them. There also is good continuity for many of the dreamer's main interests and activities. Still, this general finding has to be qualified in three ways.

First, the continuity is not with day-to-day events but with general concerns. Three studies that tried to match detailed waking reports of daily concerns with dream reports, two based on REM awakenings and one based on morning recall at home, found that blind judges could not reliably match records of daily concerns or events with dream content. The content of the dreams often revolved around daily life, such as family, friends, and school, but if the actual events of the day were incorporated in any specific way, it was not understandable to independent raters.[97-99] This finding is consistent with studies showing low levels of episodic memory in dreams.[25,26]

Second, the continuity usually is with both thought and behavior, but sometimes it is only with one or the other. For example, people who have highly aggressive dreams are not always aggressive people in waking life, but they usually admit to many aggressive thoughts and fantasies during the day. Similarly, people who have frequent sex dreams are not always sexually active in reality, but they tend to entertain the same thoughts in waking life and sometimes practice frequent masturbation to the accompaniment of their sexual fantasies.

Third, not all dream elements are continuous with waking conceptions and concerns. It is these anomalous aspects of dream content that may be the products of figurative thinking, as some theorists assert, or impaired cognitive functioning, as other theorists claim.

The most complete study of a lengthy dream journal is based on 3118 dream reports over a 22-year period from a woman who was later interviewed over a 2-day period, as were four of her friends, about those aspects of her life that appear in her dreams (see Domhoff,[40] pp. 111-133). A blind analysis of social interactions with family members and friends showed that the dream enactments were continuous with her waking thoughts and concerns in terms of the frequency of their appearance and the balance of aggressive and friendly interactions with them. For example, the continuing anger and turmoil the dreamer felt in relation to her ex-husband were expressed in the dreams through repeated negative interactions with him over the first 15 years of the series, many of which dramatized their past waking conflicts. However, there was a significant (but not complete) change in the balance of aggressive and friendly interactions in her dreams at about the time when, according to both the dreamer and her friends, she could think or talk about him in waking life without becoming upset.

To take an example at the other extreme, her dreams over a 2-year period involving a man for whom she developed a great infatuation contained at the outset numerous portrayals of sexual interactions. Later on they presented a picture of betrayal and rejection by him. In reality, she had never had anything but a friendly social relationship with this person, who was several years younger and, according to her friends, had no romantic interest in her. This example demonstrates very clearly that continuity is sometimes with waking thought, but not waking behavior. In dreaming life, she imagined a love affair and then she imagined that he had rejected her for another woman, but she knew better in waking life.

The dreamer's great involvement in the theater as a playwright, actor, and director is revealed by the frequency with which she dreams of these activities. Her theater-related dreams portray moments of great triumph—such as when she is acknowledged for her underappreciated talents—but they also include an equal number of misfortunes, failures, and rejections that are consistent with what she and her friends say are her fears and anxieties in regard to this area of interest.

However, there are also aspects of her dreams where inferences based on the assumption of continuity were disconfirmed, which opens up new avenues for adding depth and complexity to the understanding of dreams. For instance, the appearance of cats that are underfed, lost, or deformed does not reflect any waking concerns in regard to her great affection for cats. She rides horses fearlessly in her dreams, but was on a horse only a handful of times in waking life and fears them. Her dreams also give the impression that she probably learned to shoot when she was growing up and enjoys doing so, but neither inference proved to be accurate.

Similar results appeared in an exhaustive study of 1368 dream reports from a convicted child molester in his mid-30s (see Domhoff,[1] pp. 166-171). Many of them were written on paper bags and laundry lists for his own personal reasons over a period of a few years while he was in a mental institution. A complete Hall–Van de Castle coding of the dream reports revealed that he differed from the norms in only a few ways, but most of those differences turned out to be continuous with his waking thoughts or behavior. In particular, the character patterns in his dream reports have many unusual features, with his mother appearing four times more often than would be expected from the norms and his sister appearing ten times more often. On the other hand, there are no mentions of his father.

Beyond female family members, he dreams primarily of unknown males and unknown females. The percentage of characters who are friends of the dreamer is only 9%, far below the male normative figure of 31%, and there is an especially low incidence of female friends and acquaintances. As for the male characters who are known to him, they are usually his fellow inmates, not friends of long standing (see Domhoff,[1] p. 166). However, the patient's dreams did not have an unusually low percentage of friendly interactions, because in his dreams he had generally positive interactions with his mother and sister and also often befriended or helped children and teenagers.

The patient had a typical number of dreams with at least one sexual thought or interaction, but his sexual dreams differ from those of other men in terms of the variety of characters with whom he is erotically involved and the types of interactions that occur. Whereas heterosexual men have erotic encounters almost exclusively with peer female characters, he is involved in or witnesses sexuality in his dreams with men as well as women and with children as well as adults. He is also unusual in the range of sexual acts in which he engages. Most of all, his dream reports contain more sexual fantasies and less sexual intercourse than the male norms.

These dream findings fit with the reality of his waking life, where he was very dependent on his highly controlling mother and his supportive sister, whom he said were the two most positive influences in his life. His father, often absent in his early years, was pushed out of the house by the patient's mother when the patient was 12, and he died a few years later. The patient had no friends and preferred to be around children. As in his dreams, he had had sex with other males and at least once with an animal. His main sexual outlet, however, was the same compulsive voyeurism present in his dream reports. He wrote that he had always had "a morbid yet fascinating curiosity about the female genitals" (see Domhoff,[1] p. 170). In his teens and early adulthood, his child molesting did consist primarily of looking at children's genitals, but later it included fondling on several occasions and exposure of himself at least once.

There were also some informative differences between the dream content and his waking behavior. Although he masturbated frequently in his dreams, leading to the inference that he was a compulsive masturbator in waking life, he reported that he did not masturbate for weeks at a time because he thought masturbation was wrong and often felt depressed afterwards. He used meditation and an interest in spirituality to help him control this urge, suggesting that an analysis of dream content may not always reveal how people actually deal with their desires in waking life. On the other hand, he claimed that his masturbation fantasies were heterosexual, unlike many of the sexual activities in his dreams, and that he thought of himself as heterosexual. However, his adult behavior showed a pattern that corresponded to his dreams. As already noted, he had experienced sex with men, children, and animals. Here it is relevant to add that he had never engaged in "petting" or sexual intercourse with a woman, which makes the point that his dreams are continuous with his waking behavior but not with his waking self-conceptions on the issue of his sexual orientation.

The possibilities for using individual dream journals in controlled pre- and posttreatment studies in clinical settings are demonstrated in a pilot study with a young woman. She first recorded her dreams at age 18 when she went into psychotherapy, which she quit after a year because she did not think it was helping her. A year later she began taking 25 mg of sertraline (Zoloft) to deal with generalized anxiety disorder and panic attacks, working up to 100 mg before the panic attacks stopped. One year after that, 21 years old and still taking medication, she resumed her journal for purposes of this comparison, but without any knowledge of the Hall–Van de Castle coding system. Based on pre- and posttreatment samples of 33 and 40 dream reports, she moved closer to the female norms on several categories. She had large declines in her rate of aggressions per character, familiar settings percentage, and elements from the past, as well as large increases in her friends percentage and rate of friendliness per character.[100]

IMPLICATIONS FOR THEORIES OF DREAMING

The array of systematic results presented in this chapter suggests that a considerable amount of psychological information can be extracted from dream reports. This conclusion provides support for the core idea of all 20th-century dream theories. At the same time, it must be stressed that much dream content is not yet understood. There is no convincing evidence regarding whether such dream elements may be the meaningful metaphoric products of figurative thinking or relatively meaningless random filler or a mixture of both. Obviously, much research work remains to be done.

The findings also suggest that a significant percentage of dream content focuses on a handful of personal concerns revolving around social interactions with family, friends, and coworkers. There are few age differences once young adulthood is reached, and there are many cross-cultural similarities. The greatest variability in dream content seems to concern the appearance of aggression, especially physical aggression. Differences in aggression are the biggest difference between laboratory and home dream reports. Aggression also varies greatly owing to age, with relatively little aggression in the dreams of children and elderly adults compared with young and middle-aged adults. In addition, there are large individual, gender, and cultural differences. This variability suggests that aggression might be valuable in developing a better theory of dreams because it might be especially sensitive to drug effects, brain lesions, or life-changing events (see Domhoff,[40] Chapter 1).

Despite the originality and creativity that are displayed in the cognitive production of dreams, and even given the aspects of dream content that are not understood, most dreams are more realistic and based in everyday life than is suggested by any traditional dream theory. In addition, much dream content seems more transparent than might be expected by clinical theories that emphasize disguise and symbolism in understanding dreams. Finally, a significant minority of dreams may not be as emotionally based as all traditional theories imply, especially before the adolescent years.

These conclusions can be used to focus future research, but uncertainties about the extent of emotionality and bizarreness must be resolved before the findings on dream content can constrain theorizing about dreams even more fully than they should now. Still, the generally accepted results do set the stage for seeing how the effects of various medications and brain lesions on dream content might contribute to theory construction. For example, such studies might provide the basis for linking the psychological findings on dream content to the neurologic substrate that is active during dreaming.[40] It may even be possible that new theorizing can be based in part on detailed case studies of unique individual patients who are brought to a variety of clinical settings, including sleep disorder clinics. Clinical studies would be especially valuable if the patient had been keeping a dream journal that could serve as a baseline for comparison with postmedication or posttrauma dreams.

At the most general level, the findings based on systematic content research suggest that dreams are first and foremost the embodiment of thoughts through dramatizations of life concerns and interests. They almost always involve the dreamer and they are usually intensely interpersonal. Dreams as they have been defined for the purposes of this chapter seem to be more similar to plays than any other waking-life analogue. Perhaps dreams are therefore best understood as enactments of various "scripts" in both the cognitive and playwright senses of that term. Hypotheses such as these might be fruitfully explored in the future in both clinical and nonclinical settings using the combined tools of content analysis, neuropsychology, and brain imaging.

Clinical Pearl

It is unlikely on the basis of systematic content studies that any one dream from an individual or any few from a group can establish any form of psychopathology.

REFERENCES

1. Domhoff GW: Finding Meaning in Dreams: A Quantitative Approach. New York, Plenum Publishing, 1996.
2. Domhoff GW: New directions in the study of dream content using the Hall and Van de Castle coding system. Dreaming 1996;9:115-137.
3. Pagel JF, Blagrove M, Levin R: Definitions of dream: A paradigm for comparing field descriptive specific studies of dream. Dreaming 2001;11: 195-202.
4. Snyder F: The phenomenology of dreaming. In Madow L, Snow L (eds): The Psychodynamic Implications of the Physiological Studies on Dreams. Springfield, Ill, Charles C Thomas, 1970, pp 124-151.
5. Snyder F, Karacan I, Tharp V, Scott J: Phenomenology of REM dreaming. Psychophysiology 1968;4:375.
6. Nielsen T, Zadra A, Simard V, et al: The typical dreams of Canadian university students. Dreaming 2004;13:211-235.
7. Dorus E, Dorus W, Rechtschaffen A: The incidence of novelty in dreams. Arch Gen Psychiatry 1971;25:364-368.
8. Hall C, Van de Castle R: The Content Analysis of Dreams. New York, Appleton-Century-Crofts, 1966.
9. Foulkes D, Sullivan B, Kerr N, Brown L: Appropriateness of dream feelings to dreamed situations. Cogn Emotion 1988;2: 29-39.
10. Fosse R, Stickgold R, Hobson JA: The mind in REM sleep: Reports of emotional experience. Sleep 2001;24:947-955.
11. Strauch I, Meier B: In Search of Dreams: Results of Experimental Dream Research. Albany, NY, State University of New York Press, 1996.
12. Foulkes D: The Psychology of Sleep. New York, Charles Scribner's Sons, 1966.
13. Verdone P: Temporal reference of manifest dream content. Percept Mot Skills 1965;20:1253-1268.
14. Hall C: Studies of dreams collected in the laboratory and at home. In Institute of Dream Research Monograph Series. Santa Cruz, Calif, privately printed, 1966.
15. Natale V, Esposito M: Bizarreness across the first four cycles of sleep. Sleep Hypnosis 2001;3:18-21.
16. Domhoff GW, Kamiya J: Problems in dream content study with objective indicators: III. Changes in dream content throughout the night. Arch Gen Psychiatry 1964;11:529-532 .
17. Antrobus J: REM and NREM sleep reports: Comparisons of word frequencies by cognitive classes. Psychophysiology 1983;20:562-568.
18. Foulkes D: Dream reports from different states of sleep. J Abnorm Social Psychol 1962;65:14-25.
19. Foulkes D, Schmidt M: Temporal sequence and unit comparison composition in dream reports from different stages of sleep. Sleep 1983;6:265-280.
20. Herman J, Ellman S, Roffwarg H: The problem of NREM dream recall reexamined. In Arkin A, Antrobus J, Ellman S (eds): The Mind in Sleep: Psychology and Psychophysiology. Mahwah, NJ, Erlbaum, 1978, pp 59-62.
21. Kamiya J: Behavioral, subjective, and physiological aspects of drowsiness and sleep. In Fiske DW, Maddi SR (eds): Functions of Varied Experience. Homewood, Ill, Dorsey, 1961, pp 145-174.
22. Rechtschaffen A, Verdone P, Wheaton J: Reports of mental activity during sleep. Can Psychiatr Assoc J 1963;8:409-414.

23. Foulkes D: Dreaming: A Cognitive-Psychological Analysis. Mahwah, NJ, Erlbaum, 1985.
24. Nielsen T: A review of mentation in REM and NREM sleep: "Covert" REM sleep as a possible reconciliation of two opposing models. Behav Brain Sci 2000;23:851-866.
25. Baylor G, Cavallero C: Memory sources associated with REM and NREM dream reports throughout the night: A new look at the data. Sleep 2001;24:165-170.
26. Fosse M, Fosse R, Hobson JA, Stickgold R: Dreaming and episodic memory: A functional dissociation? J Cog Neurosci 2003;15:1-9.
27. Hobson JA, Pace-Schott EF, Stickgold R: Dreaming and the brain: Toward a cognitive neuroscience of conscious states. Behav Brain Sci 2000;3:793-842.
28. Domhoff GW, Schneider A: Much ado about very little: The small effect sizes when home and laboratory collected dreams are compared. Dreaming 1999;9:139-151.
29. Antrobus J, Kondo T, Reinsel R: Summation of REM and diurnal cortical activation. Conscious Cogn 1995;4:275-299.
30. Cicogna P, Natale V, Occhionero M, Bosinelli M: A comparison of mental activity during sleep onset and morning awakening. Sleep 1998;21:462-470.
31. Fosse R, Stickgold R, Hobson JA: Thinking and hallucinating: Reciprocal changes in sleep. Psychophysiology 2004;41:298-305.
32. Heynick F, deJong M: Dreams elicited by the telephone. In Koella W, Ruther E, Schulz H (eds): Sleep '84. New York, Gustav Fischer Verlag, 1985, pp 341-343.
33. Hunt H, Ogilvie R, Belicki K, et al: Forms of dreaming. Percept Mot Skills 1982;54:559-633.
34. Foulkes D: Home and laboratory dreams: Four empirical studies and a conceptual reevaluation. Sleep 1979;2:233-251.
35. Weisz R, Foulkes D: Home and laboratory dreams collected under uniform sampling conditions. Psychophysiology 1970;6:588-596.
36. Domhoff GW, Kamiya J: Problems in dream content study with objective indicators: I. A comparison of home and laboratory dream reports. Arch Gen Psychiatry 1964;11:519-524.
37. Baekland F, Lasky R: The morning recall of rapid eye movement period reports given earlier in the night. J Nerv Ment Dis 1968;147:570-579.
38. Meier C, Ruef H, Zeigler A, Hall C: Forgetting of dreams in the laboratory. Percept Mot Skills 1968;26:551-557.
39. Trinder J, Kramer M: Dream recall. Am J Psychiatry 1971;128:296-301.
40. Domhoff GW: The Scientific Study of Dreams: Neural Networks, Cognitive Development, and Content Analysis. Washington, DC, American Psychological Association Press, 2003.
41. Calkins M: Statistics of dreams. Am J Psychol 1893;5:311-343.
42. Weed S, Hallam F: A study of dream-consciousness. Am J Psychol 1896;7:405-411.
43. Schneider A, Domhoff GW: DreamBank. http://www.dreambank.net.
44. Merritt J, Stickgold R, Pace-Schott E, et al: Emotion profiles in the dreams of men and women. Conscious Cogn 1994;3:46-60.
45. Roussy F, Raymond I, De Koninck J: Affect in REM dreams: Exploration of a time-of-night effect. Sleep 2000;23:A174-A175.
46. Tonay V: California women and their dreams: A historical and sub-cultural comparison of dream content. Imagination Cognition Personality 1990/1991;10:83-97.
47. Dudley L, Swank M: A comparison of the dreams of college women in 1950 and 1990. ASD Newsl 1990;7:3.
48. Hall C, Domhoff GW, Blick K, Weesner K: The dreams of college men and women in 1950 and 1980: A comparison of dream contents and sex differences. Sleep 1982;5:188-194.
49. Brenneis C, Roll S: Dream patterns in Anglo and Chicano young adults. Psychiatry 1976;39:280-290.
50. Kane CM, Mellen RR, Patten P, Samano I: Differences in the manifest dream content of Mexican, Mexican American, and Anglo American college women: A research note. Hispanic J Behav Sci 1993;15:134-139.
51. Kern C, Roll S: Object representations in dreams of Chicanos and Anglos. Dreaming 2001;11:149-166.
52. Schredl M, Sahin V, Schaefer G: Gender differences in dreams: Do they reflect gender differences in waking life? Pers Individ Differences 1998;25:433-442.
53. Waterman D, Dejong M, Magdelijns R: Gender, sex role orientation and dream content. In Sleep '86, Koella W (ed). New York, Gustav Fischer Verlag, 1988, pp 385-387.
54. Lortie-Lussier M, Simond S, Rinfret N, De Koninck J: Beyond sex differences: Family and occupational roles' impact on women's and men's dreams. Sex Roles 1992;26:79-96.
55. Rinfret N, Lortie-Lussier M, De Koninck J: The dreams of professional mothers and female students: An exploration of social roles and age impact. Dreaming 1991;1:179-191.
56. Prasad B: Content analysis of dreams of Indian and American college students: A cultural comparison. J Indian Psychol 1982;4:54-64.
57. Bose VS: Unpublished manuscript, Department of Psychology (Andhra University, Andhra, India, 1983).
58. Yamanaka T, Morita Y, Matsumoto J: Analysis of the dream contents in college students by REM-awakening technique. Folia Psychiatr Neurol Jpn 1982;36:33-52.
59. Barrett D: Flying dreams and lucidity: An empirical test of their relationship. Dreaming 1991;1:129-134.
60. Hall C: What people dream about. Sci Am 1951;184:60-63.
61. Schredl M, Doll E: Emotions in diary dreams. Conscious Cogn 1998;7:634-646.
62. Kahn D, Pace-Schott E, Hobson JA: Emotion and cognition: Feeling and character identification in dreaming. Conscious Cogn 2002;11:34-50.
63. Kahn D, Hobson JA: Stereotypic gender-based emotions are not detectable in dream reports. Dreaming 2002;12:209-222.
64. Bonato RA, Moffitt AR, Hoffmann RF, Cuddy MA: Bizarreness in dreams and nightmares. Dreaming 1991;1:53-61.
65. Revonsuo A, Salmivalli C: A content analysis of bizarre elements in dreams. Dreaming 1995;5:169-187.
66. Rittenhouse C, Stickgold R, Hobson J: Constraint on the transformation of characters, objects, and settings in dream reports. Conscious Cogn 1994;3:100-113.
67. Foulkes D: Children's Dreams. New York, Wiley, 1982.
68. Foulkes D, Hollifield M, Sullivan B, et al: REM dreaming and cognitive skills at ages 5-8: A cross-sectional study. Int J Behav Devel 1990;13:447-465.
69. Strauch I: Träume im Übergang von der späten Kindheit ins Jugendalter. Ergebnisse einer Langzeitstudie. Bern, Huber, 2003.
70. Hall C: A ubiquitous sex difference in dreams, revisited. J Pers Soc Psychol 1984;46:1109-1117.
71. Avila-White D, Schneider A, Domhoff GW: The most recent dreams of 12-13 year-old boys and girls: A methodological contribution to the study of dream content in teenagers. Dreaming 1999;9:163-171.
72. Saline S: The most recent dreams of children ages 8-11. Dreaming 1999;9:173-181.
73. Resnick J, Stickgold R, Rittenhouse C, Hobson J: Self-representation and bizarreness in children's dream reports collected in the home setting. Conscious Cogn 1994;3:30-45.
74. Brenneis C: Developmental aspects of aging in women: A comparative study of dreams. Arch Gen Psychiatry 1975;32:429-434.
75. Cote L, Lortie-Lussier M, Roy M, DeKoninck J: The dreams of women throughout adulthood. Dreaming 1996;6:187-199.

76. Hall C, Domhoff GW: Aggression in dreams. Int J Soc Psychiatry 1963;9:259-267.

77. Hall C, Domhoff GW: Friendliness in dreams. J Soc Psychol 1964;62:309-314.

78. Strauch I: Traume im alter. In Boothe B, Ugolino B (eds): Lebenshorizont Alter. Zurich, Hochschulverlag AG an der ETH, 2003, pp 171-187.

79. Zepelin H: Age differences in dreams: I. Men's dreams and thematic apperceptive fantasy. Int J Aging Hum Dev 1980;12:171-186.

80. Giambra L, Jung R, Grodsky A: Age changes in dream recall in adulthood. Dreaming 1996;6:17-31.

81. Stairs P, Blick K: A survey of emotional content of dreams recalled by college students. Psychol Rep 1979;45:839-842.

82. Howe JB, Blick K: Emotional content of dreams recalled by elderly women. Percept Mot Skills 1983;56:31-34.

83. Kramer M, Roth T: Dreams in psychopathology. In Wolman B (ed): Handbook of Dreams. New York, Van Nostrand Reinhold, 1979, pp 361-367.

84. Hall C: A comparison of the dreams of four groups of hospitalized mental patients with each other and with a normal population. J Nerv Ment Dis 1966;143:135-139.

85. Schnetzler J, Carbonel B: Etude thématique des recits de rêves de sujets normaux, schizophrènes et autres psychotiques. Ann Med Psychol (Paris) 1976;3:367-380.

86. Gentil M, Lader M: Dream content and daytime attitudes in anxious and calm women. Psychol Med 1978;8:297-304.

87. Kramer M, Roth T: Comparison of dream content in laboratory dream reports of schizophrenic and depressive patient groups. Compr Psychiatry 1973;14:325-329.

88. Carrington P: Dreams and schizophrenia. Arch Gen Psychiatry 1972;26:343-350.

89. D'Andrade R: Anthropological studies in dreams. In Hsu F (ed): Psychological Anthropology. Homewood, Ill, Dorsey Press, 1961, pp 296-332.

90. Gregor T: A content analysis of Mehinaku dreams. Ethos 1981;9:353-390.

91. Fosse R, Stickgold R, Hobson JA: Brain-mind states: Reciprocal variation in thoughts and hallucinations. Psychol Sci 2001;12:30-36.

92. Allport G: The Use of Personal Documents in Psychological Science. New York, Social Science Research Council, 1942.

93. Baldwin A: Personal structure analysis: A statistical method for investigating the single personality. J Abnorm Soc Psychol 1942;37:163-183.

94. Webb E, Campbell D, Schwartz R, et al: Nonreactive Measures in the Social Sciences. Chicago, Rand McNally, 1981.

95. Lortie-Lussier M, Cote L, Vachon J: The consistency and continuity hypotheses revisited through the dreams of women at two periods of their lives. Dreaming 2000;10:67-76.

96. Schneider A, Domhoff GW: The quantitative study of dreams. www.dreamresearch.net, interesting findings section (1995).

97. Roussy F: Testing the notion of continuity between waking experience and REM dream content. Dissertation Abstracts Int (B) 2000;61:1106.

98. Roussy F, Brunette M, Mercier P, et al: Daily events and dream content: Unsuccessful matching attempts. Dreaming 2000; 10:77-83.

99. Roussy F, Camirand C, Foulkes D: Does early-night REM dream content reliably reflect presleep state of mind? Dreaming 1996; 6:121-130.

100. Kirschner N: Medication and dreams: Changes in dream content after drug treatment. Dreaming 1999;9:195-200.

43

Chronobiology of Dreaming

Tore A. Nielsen

ABSTRACT

A review of the scientific literature clarifies several chronobiologic features of dreaming. The literature supports the conclusions that dreaming intensity, and to a lesser extent dreamlike quality, is modulated by a sinusoidal, 90-minute ultradian oscillation, a "switchlike" circadian oscillation, a 12-hour circasemidian rhythm, and a 28-day circatrigintan rhythm (for women). Further, access to dream memory sources appears to be modulated by a 7-day circaseptan clock. Greater clarification of these rhythmic influences on dreaming may help to explain diverse and often contradictory findings in the dream research literature, to better relate dreaming to waking-state cognitive processes, to better explain relationships between disturbed phase relationships and dream disturbances, and to shed new light on the problems of dreaming's function and biologic markers.

In the 50 years since discovery of a link between dreaming and the endogenous biorhythmic events defining rapid eye movement (REM) sleep[1] there has occurred strikingly little convergence between chronobiology and the study of dreaming—despite a vast accumulation of research in both domains. While many of the findings in one of these domains have clear implications for understanding basic and applied questions in the other, there still is no comprehensive theory that links chronobiologic concepts and findings to the processes of dreaming. This chapter is intended to redress this situation by reviewing evidence that is pertinent to the chronobiologic nature of dreaming. Five sections review chronobiologic processes of different types: ultradian, circasemidian, circadian, circaseptan, and circatrigintan.

In this chapter, the term *dreaming* is used in an inclusive sense equivalent to that of *sleep mentation*, in other words, the occurrence of any subjectively experienced cognitive events during sleep.

ULTRADIAN RHYTHMS

Transitions between REM and non-REM (NREM) sleep are widely viewed as "switchlike," flipping abruptly from one type of sleep to the other. Some measures, such as delta electroencephalograph (EEG) power, do in fact display marked switchlike transitions at the onset and offset of REM sleep. However, studies of multiple physiologic systems indicate that REM-NREM transitions are much more sinusoidal than typically acknowledged.[2] For example, the polarity of neurons driving REM sleep onset demonstrates a more graduated, oscillatory fluctuation that begins well before EEG-defined REM sleep onset.[3,4] It could be argued that the switchlike versus oscillatory nature of REM and NREM dreaming has been under debate for several decades among authors who contend that REM and NREM dreaming differ qualitatively (i.e., the transition is switchlike) versus those who insist the difference is quantitative (i.e., the transition is oscillatory).

In fact, research that has sampled dreaming at multiple points within and between REM and NREM sleep suggests that dreaming more closely conforms to a sinusoidal, oscillatory phenomenon than a switchlike one. This is the case for dependent measures implicating the frequency and length of recalled dreams and the quality of dream reports. These measures are discussed in separate sections later.

Frequency and Length of Recalled Dreams

Within-Stage Changes

The length of a dream report is typically assessed either by its total recall count (TRC)[5] or by the number of temporal units (TUs) composing the report.[6,7] TRC is typically defined as the number of nonredundant, content-bearing words in a report, excluding hesitations, speech errors, repeated words, and commentary[5]; TRC is log-transformed to minimize the effect of extremely long reports $(\log[\text{TRC}] + 1)$. TUs are identified based upon reported activities; synchronously occurring activities define a single TU. Whenever a character performs a new activity, responds to another character, or changes topics in a conversation, a new TU is scored.[6,8] Report length is widely thought to measure cortical activation and, thus, the overall "quantity" of output of a dream mentation generator.

By either measure, REM sleep reports are consistently longer than NREM reports. These measures also suggest that dream output over consecutive REM and NREM episodes oscillates in an ultradian pattern. When relationships between report length and time elapsed in REM or NREM sleep are assessed, report length fluctuates sinusoidally over time (Fig. 43–1).[9] For dreams from REM sleep (dark blue bars), length estimates are lowest 0-15 and 45-60 minutes after REM onset and highest for times in between. For dreams from NREM sleep (light blue bars), an *opposite* pattern is observed. A similar sinusoidal pattern was found in a second study.[10] These results complement earlier work that sampled dreaming at either 5 or 15 minutes into the REM period and found longer reports in the latter condition.[11]

The results in Figure 43–1 are highly suggestive of a sinusoidal function and thus of an ultradian oscillation in report length that is active both within and between sleep stages. The findings are also consistent with several additional studies that assessed dream length as a function of increasing distance from prior REM sleep. In four studies,[12-15] NREM dream reports were either more probable or of longer length when sampled in close proximity to (all at 5 minutes) rather than more distally from (10 minutes, 30 minutes, 12 minutes, and 15 minutes, respectively) prior REM sleep. Also consistent

REPORT LENGTHS DURING NREM AND REM CYCLES

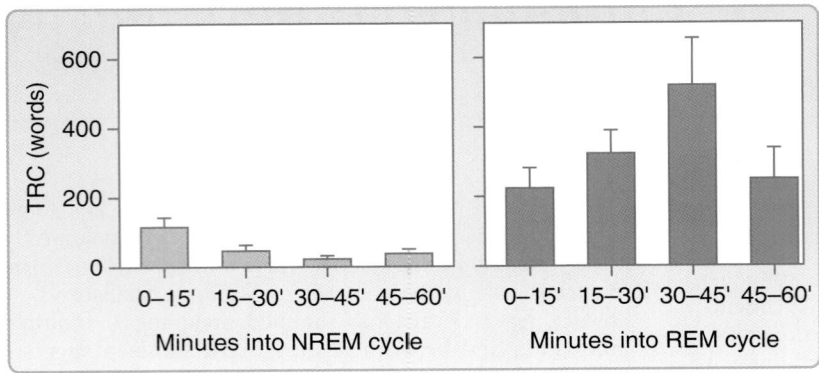

Figure 43–1. Report lengths for dream reports from rapid eye movement (REM) and non-REM (NREM) periods of different durations. Mean (SEM) report length as a function of elapsed time in stage for 88 REM and 61 NREM reports. TRC, total recall count. (From Hobson JA, Pace-Schott E, Stickgold R: Dreaming and the brain: Towards a cognitive neuroscience of conscious states. Behav Brain Sci 2000;23: 793-842.)

with the preceding, a fifth study[16] demonstrated that duration of NREM sleep preceding an awakening correlated negatively with report length.

The likelihood that report length reflects an ultradian oscillatory process may explain the seemingly nonconfirmatory finding[17] that report length differences for REM periods of 5 and 10 minutes' duration are small ($P = .114$). This result may reflect random variation in measurements that are sampled too close together on an ultradian curve, thus minimizing the chances of detecting a gradual change.

Between-Stage Changes

REM and NREM dream reports presumably reflect activity of an imagery generator functioning at the opposite extremes of its ultradian period. Large differences in dream recall frequency and length would thus be anticipated. In fact, increased probabilities and lengths of dream reports sampled after REM as compared with after NREM awakenings are among the most highly replicated findings in the dream research literature (see reviews in Nielsen[4] and Hobson et al.[2]). Figure 43–2 illustrates the marked differences in levels of dream recall from REM and NREM sleep in 39 studies conducted between 1953 and 2004. Two recent studies[18,19] are noteworthy because the very low probabilities of recall from NREM sleep are possibly

due to the use of procedures that minimize the influence of prior REM sleep on NREM dream recall.

Paralleling the differences in Figure 43–2 are similarly large REM-NREM differences in dream report length; REM-to-NREM ratios in TRC vary from 2:1 to as high as 5:1.[10] Much of the variability observed for both measures of recall and length may occur because experimental protocols have not consistently controlled for phase relationships between REM and NREM sampling points.

The use of a constant time-in-stage preawakening delay for both REM and NREM sleep (e.g., 10 minutes for each) guarantees neither similar phase relationships to the ultradian acrophase (for REM) and nadir (for NREM) nor constant phase relationships between the REM and NREM samples for several reasons. First, REM and NREM sleep occupy different proportions of the sleep cycle (e.g., 20% REM, 80% NREM); second, the proportions of REM and NREM sleep change across the night; and third, the periodicity of the 90-minute REM-NREM cycle is highly variable.[20] Further, the common procedure of sampling mentation with progressive temporal delay into stage (PTDIS) protocols—for example, 5 minutes into the first REM, 10 minutes into the second REM, 15 minutes into the third REM, and so on—further confounds ultradian phase with time-of-night (see also later).

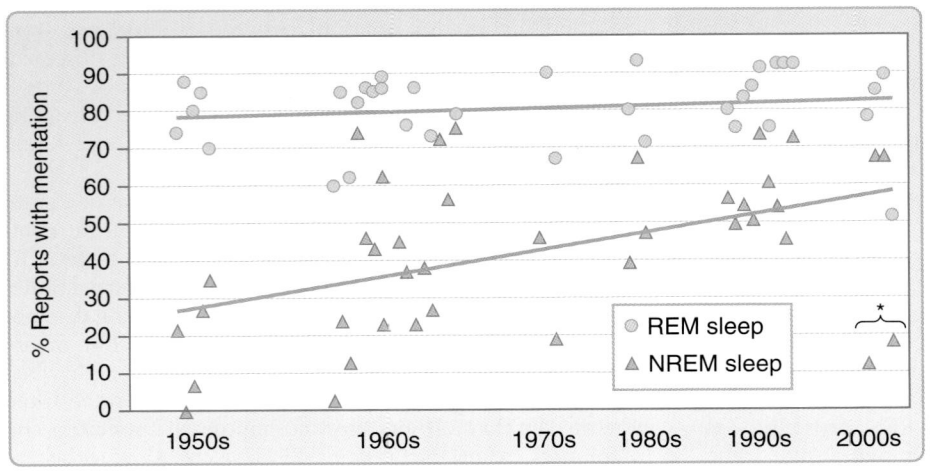

Figure 43–2. Percent recall of dreaming from rapid eye movement (REM) and non-REM (NREM) sleep awakenings in 39 studies from 1953 to 2004. Variation in recall from NREM sleep is attributable in part to changing definitions of dreaming, in part to nonstandardized choice of awakening times for dream sampling, and in part to uncontrolled sleep stage interactions. Flagged values (see *asterisk*) for very low NREM recall in 2001 and 2004 studies reflect use of the sleep interruption technique[19] and an ultrashort sleep–wake schedule,[18] both of which minimize possible influences on dreaming of prior sleep other than from the target stage.

Quality of Dream Reports

Within-Stage Qualitative Changes

As is the case for measures of dream recall frequency and length, much evidence indicates that the vividness, intensity, dreamlikeness, and other qualities of dream imagery increase progressively within REM sleep periods, whereas other evidence suggests that these qualities may decrease within NREM episodes. Unlike the findings for recall and length, however, clear sinusoidal variation of these measures has not yet been established.

For REM sleep, subject ratings indicate that dream reports from long REM sleep episodes (9 minutes or more) are more dreamlike in several respects than those from short episodes (1 minute or less).[21] Long REM sleep reports are more active, distorted, dramatic, emotional, anxious, unpleasant, and clear or vivid, and they contain more different scenes, more scenes with clear visualization, and more socially unacceptable content (violence or hostility) than short REM sleep reports. Consistent results were obtained when dreams were sampled from REM periods of several different lengths.[22-24] In the latter study, four male college students were each awakened twice from both REM 2 and REM 4 periods for each of six conditions—0.5, 2.5, 5, 10, 20, and 30 minutes after REM onset—and asked to rate 12 qualities of their dreams. *Recall, emotion, anxiety, pleasantness,* and *clarity* showed linear increases over time. Three of these measures (emotion, anxiety, pleasantness) had additional trend components, suggesting possible ultradian modulation, with two major peaks at 10 and 30 minutes.[23] Others[25,26] report that plausibility and sensibleness of dreams in relation to daily life do not change as a function of REM length. The possibility that some qualities of dreaming are subject to ultradian modulation while others are not is consistent with Kramer's[24] claim that an "affective surge" arises during REM sleep and is "contained" or processed by other dream content. The hypothesized surge function may be chronobiologically modulated, whereas the dream container may not.

For NREM sleep, evidence again points to relationships that are *opposite* in direction to those observed for REM sleep and thus suggests that measures reflect activity on the descending slope of an ultradian oscillation. In one study,[27] dreamlike fantasy (Df) scale* scores were lower (P <.10) for reports from 20-minute NREM (stage 4) episodes than for 5-minute NREM episodes, even though the reports were matched within subjects and for time of night. In a second study,[14] NREM (stage 2) reports obtained 12 minutes after the end of REM sleep episodes were rated less dreamlike (M rating = 4.17) than were NREM reports obtained 5 minutes after REM sleep episodes (M = 4.73, P < .001).

Between-Stage Qualitative Changes

A large body of research[2,4] demonstrates that REM sleep reports are consistently more perceptual, hallucinatory, emotional, dramatic, physically involving, and rich with characters and visual scenes than are NREM reports, whereas the latter are more conceptual, thoughtlike, and mundane.[21] However, these highly replicable findings are not easily interpreted as caused by ultradian processes because of their possible confounding by differences in report length described earlier. Because REM reports are consistently longer than NREM reports, it has been argued that the two may be compared only if this difference is removed or statistically controlled, for example, by comparing reports of equal length, by calculating proportions with a common metric (e.g., TU), or by removing report length as a covariate. The use of such procedures has caused significant qualitative differences between REM and NREM dream reports to disappear in some studies.

Most length control procedures have been criticized on methodologic grounds,[2,4,30] and there is evidence that the qualitative nature of sleep mentation changes as a function of the REM-NREM cycle, even with report length controlled.[4] In brief, even with length controls, REM dream reports surpass NREM dream reports on measures of self-reflectiveness,[31] bizarreness,[32,33] visual and verbal imagery,[5,32,34] movement imagery,[35] characters and self-involvement,[6,36] self-representation,[6] psycholinguistic structure,[37] and narrative linkage.[38]

MEMORY SOURCES OF DREAMING

Memory sources that subjects are requested to furnish in association to their dreams are another form of evidence that REM and NREM dream reports differ, although it remains unknown whether these differences are attributable to an ultradian oscillator. Results from several studies indicate that NREM dream sources are primarily biographic episodes (episodic memories), whereas REM sources are a mixture of episodic and semantic memories.[39-41] The predominance of episodic sources for NREM dreams is maintained regardless of time of night and independent of correction for report length.[8,39,41-43] It is thus possible that ultradian oscillations in memory access (e.g., episodic versus semantic) partially determine the content of REM and NREM dreams. Within-stage oscillations in memory sources have not yet been demonstrated, however.

In sum, most results from quantitative and qualitative assessments can be explained as due to oscillatory ultradian modulation of dreaming processes. REM and NREM dream reports reflect the output of a generator that is sampled at varying points along its rising and descending slopes. It remains unknown whether different components of dreaming, such as memory access, quality of content, or intensity of emotion, are modulated by the same or different ultradian processes. It is also not yet known what effects the desynchronization of such processes might have on the presence or form of dreaming. Further study that controls and avoids confounding time-in-stage and time-of-night sources of variation is clearly needed.

Basic Rest–Activity Cycle Hypothesis

Kleitman's ultradian basic rest–activity cycle (BRAC) hypothesis[44] has been a stimulating heuristic that conceptually links the 90-minute REM-NREM rhythm with circadian oscillations. One study of BRAC and dreaming suggested a continuation of the REM-NREM cycle and dreaming during the daytime in the form of fantasy fluctuations. Results for a series of individual

---

*The dreamlike fantasy scale is an eight-item scale: 0 = no recall (mind was blank); 1 = no recall (mind not blank, but forgets); 2 = content is conceptual (no sensory imagery), everydayish; 3 = content is conceptual, bizarre; 4 = content is perceptual (sensory imagery), nonhallucinatory (did not believe it was real), everydayish; 5 = content is perceptual, nonhallucinatory, bizarre; 6 = content is perceptual, hallucinatory (believed it was real), everydayish; 7 = content is perceptual, hallucinatory, bizarre.[28,29]

subjects and a separate group of normal subjects indicated that the intensity of daytime fantasy fluctuates with a 90-minute periodicity.[45] When these results were pooled with results from three additional experiments and assessed with superior statistical procedures, the effect was not clearly replicated; only a 200-minute ultradian rhythm was demonstrated.[46] On the other hand, there is ample support for the existence of daytime ultradian fluctuations in cognitive performance.[46-48] Correlations between daytime imagery abilities and dream recall frequency have also been reported.[49] Existing procedures could be adapted to assess whether rhythmicities in dreaming possess waking-state counterparts in a manner predicted by the BRAC hypothesis.

CIRCASEMIDIAN RHYTHMS

Broughton[20] has argued convincingly for the existence of 12-hour, or circasemidian, rhythms that are either distinct from 24-hour circadian rhythms or are subcomponents of their expression. Accumulating evidence supports the 12-hour rhythm in sleep propensity (postlunch sleepiness), slow wave sleep expression,[50] EEG power,[51] and other processes.[20] Although this rhythm explains the global human tendency to nap in the early afternoon, research examining circasemidian characteristics of dreaming are few. A single study[18] using an ultrashort (20 min/40 min) sleep–wake schedule with dream sampling at each awakening over three consecutive days provides some support for a circasemidian oscillation in dream intensity (see the discussion in "Experimental Desynchronization of Circadian Factors" later). While the scale employed (0 = none, 1 = a little, 2 = a moderate amount, 3 = a lot) to the question "how much did you dream?" might have produced a ceiling effect for REM sleep reports, for NREM reports both an acrophase at 8:00 AM and a secondary peak at 4:00 PM are visible in the time-plotted results.

Because of the problem of undersampling, many results described in the next section could be explained as due to the influence of circasemidian—rather than circadian—factors.

CIRCADIAN RHYTHMS

Circadian features of dreaming are difficult to validate because their measurement is typically limited to the nocturnal portion of the sleep–wake cycle. Either a waking counterpart of dreaming such as spontaneous fantasy or a 24-hour physiologic marker of dream propensity[18,52] is needed to convincingly demonstrate circadian oscillations in dreaming. Nonetheless, trends across the night can be assessed for whether they conform to known circadian influences. Such trends can be further evaluated for their temporal relationships to fluctuations in waking-state processes that may be dreaming counterparts, such as spontaneous fantasy or hemispherically lateralized processes.

The following sections summarize several converging lines of research that support a circadian mediation interpretation. First, research on across-the-night changes in dream length, content, organization, and memory sources demonstrates progressive increases or decreases consistent with a sinusoidal 24-hour rhythm in some cases, and exponential or switchlike changes[53] between reports from the first third of the night and all later sample points in others (Table 43–1). Second, these findings are complemented by evidence for increased dream vividness in conditions of circadian phase advance, e.g., forced desynchrony protocols, depression, and PTSD jet lag. Third, circadian mediation is suggested by evidence of continuity between sleep and wake states on measures of left hemisphere (LH) and right hemisphere (RH) processes.

Recall and Report Length Changes Across the Night

Measures of dream report length described earlier have also been applied to studies of dreaming across the night and provide information about potential circadian characteristics.

REM Sleep Effects

A study that experimentally varied both ultradian and circadian factors[17] found that dream reports from early REM periods (REM 2) were half the length (TRC) of those from later periods (REM 4), whether awakenings occurred 10 minutes into REM sleep ($P = .001$) or 5 minutes into REM sleep ($P = .07$). Similarly, a study of young adults' dream reports found an exponential lengthening in TRC from early (0.0 to 2.5 hours) to middle (2.5 to 5.0 hours) to late (5.0 to 7.5 hours) night awakenings—all conducted 4.8 to 5.0 minutes into REM sleep.[5,54] For older subjects, the increase in length occurred only in the middle-to-late comparison.

The previous effect was replicated[55] with mentation sampled from the first four REM periods in a study controlling for ultradian factors (awakenings all 9 minutes into each REM period). Time-of-night effects for several "story structure" measures included the number of statements in the event structure ($P < .001$) and the number of episodes per story ($P < .001$). For the former measure, REM 1 dreams possessed fewer statements than REM 2 to REM 4 dreams; for the latter measure, the order of means was REM 1 < REM 2 < REM 3, REM 4. No effect was obtained for the number of statements describing settings.

These findings are consistent with results from our study of 40 healthy subjects awakened from various REM sleep periods.[56] Measures of both probability of recall and mean TRC ($N = 135$ reports total) were lower for REM 1 than for REM 2 to REM 5 (Fig. 43–3A). Since REM awakenings were implemented with a PTDIS protocol (5 minutes into REM 1; 10 minutes into REM 2; 15 minutes into REM 3; 20 minutes into REM 4 and REM 5), findings may be confounded by ultradian factors.

NREM Sleep Effects

Findings for NREM sleep mentation parallel those for REM sleep. In a study[57] with four NREM awakenings per night, the percentage of awakenings bearing some mental content was low for NREM 1 (45%), rose dramatically for NREM 2 (70%), and remained relatively high for NREM 3 (70%) and NREM 4 (74%; see Fig. 43–3B). Similarly, in a study described earlier[5,54] in which dream reports were evaluated for early, middle, and late NREM (stage 2) awakenings, NREM report length increased linearly across the three sample times for young subjects. For older subjects, however, length was uniformly high for early and middle samples and then dropped sharply in the late sample.

Table 43–1. Studies Showing Quantitative and/or Qualitative Changes in Sleep Mentation across the Night

Study; Sleep Stage	No. of Subjects	Methods and Awakenings	Quantitative Findings	Qualitative Findings
Domhoff and Kamiya (1964)[58]; REM	22 college students (14 male, 8 female)	Total N = 219 reports (73/R)		R1 > R2, R3 (characters, aggression/misfortune, buildings as settings); R1 > R2, R3 (terrain/country as settings); R1, R2 > R3 (room settings); R1, R2 < R3 (sexual acts, food elements)
Foulkes (1966),[21] Foulkes and Rechtschaffen (1964)[59]; REM	22	PTDIS schedule (5R1, 10R2, 20R3)		R1 < R2, R3 (perceptual content)
Pivik and Foulkes (1968)[57]; NREM	20 male college students	2 consecutive nights 4 WU/night-SO30, 30NR1-30NR3	NR1 < NR2, NR3, NR4 (recall %)	NR1 < NR2, NR3, NR4 (Df score)
Van de Castle (1970)[64]; REM	15 male college students	Multiple series: 273 reports/R Single series: 196 reports for R1-R4		Multiple series: R1-R3 < R4-R8 (clarity, misfortunes, bizarreness, female characters, color elements) Single series: R1 = R2 = R3 = R4 (all measures) $NR_{EARLY} < NR_{LATE}$ (Df scale)
Tracy and Tracy (1974)[27]; NREM	11 male, 10 female young adults (mean age = 21 yr)	3 nonconsecutive nights 5-min samples each of descending stage 2 and stage 4 sleep; also 20 samples of stage 4		LH processes: dream recall quality, presence of verbal activity, high ego functioning, positive emotion, active participation RH processes: music, spatial salience, bizarre events, negative emotion
Cohen (1977)[63]; REM	10-23 male college students			5 replication studies LH: increase across night in all studies RH: few or inconsistent changes in all studies
Arkin et al. (1978)[14]; NREM	40 male college students (18-26 yr)	1 night each NR (S_2) reports during R deprivation and NR-control deprivation, first and second halves of night		$NR_{EARLY} < NR_{LATE}$ (DLQ)
Kramer et al. (1980)[60]; REM	25 (14 male, 11 female; 20-25 yr)	20 consecutive nights WU at "end" of R1-R4		Hall and Van de Castle (1966) frequency scales R1 to R2: Increase in 15/41 variables R2 to R3: Increase in 6/41 variables R3 to R4: Increase in 7/41 variables

Continued

Table 43–1. Studies Showing Quantitative and/or Qualitative Changes in Sleep Mentation across the Night—cont'd

Study; Sleep Stage	No. of Subjects	Methods and Awakenings	Quantitative Findings	Qualitative Findings
Waterman et al. (1992, 1993)[5,54]; REM	24 males: 12 elderly (mean age 65.1 yr), 12 young (mean age 22.9 yr)	4 consecutive nights 4.8–5.0 min into all R nights 3 and 4 = three WU/night: early (0.0–2.5 hr), middle (2.5–5.0 hr), late (5.0 hr)	Young subjects: $R_{EARLY} < R_{MIDDLE}, R_{LATE}$ (TRC) $NR_{EARLY} < NR_{MIDDLE} < NR_{LATE}$ (TRC) Elderly subjects: $R_{EARLY}, R_{MIDDLE} < R_{LATE}$ (TRC) $NR_{EARLY}, NR_{MIDDLE} > NR_{LATE}$ (TRC)	Young subjects: $R_{EARLY} < R_{MIDDLE}, R_{LATE}$ (visual imagery) $NR_{EARLY} < NR_{MIDDLE} < NR_{LATE}$ (visual imagery) Elderly subjects: $R_{EARLY}, R_{MIDDLE} < R_{LATE}$ (visual imagery) $NR_{EARLY}, NR_{MIDDLE} > NR_{LATE}$ (visual imagery)
Rosenlicht et al. (1994)[17]; REM	22 (12 male, 10 female, 19–27 yr)	2 consecutive nights 3 WU/night in SO, R2, R4 5 or 10 min into REM, counterbalanced across nights	R2 < R4 (TRC)	
Casagrande et al. (1996)[32]; REM, NREM	20 right-handed college students (4 female, 16 male, 20–27 yr)	5 consecutive nights; 4, 5 for dream recall: 5R2 (R_{EARLY}), 5R3 (R_{LATE}), 5S$_2$ (NR_{EARLY}), 5S$_4$ (NR_{LATE})	$R_{EARLY} < R_{LATE}$ (% recall) $NR_{EARLY} < NR_{LATE}$ (log TRC)	$R_{EARLY} = R_{LATE}$ (visual imagery) $NR_{EARLY} < NR_{LATE}$ (visual imagery)
Cipolli et al. (1998)[55]; REM	16 male college students (19–24 yr)	5 nights Nights 2, 3, 4 = 4 WU/night (9 min into R1–R4)	R1 < R2, R4 (no. statements in event structure) R1 < R2 < R3, R4 (no. episodes/story) R1 = R2 = R3 = R4 (no. setting statements)	
Agargun and Cartwright (2003)[62]; REM	26 (10 male, 16 female) with major depression (13 suicidal, 13 nonsuicidal)	3 consecutive nights night 2: baseline night 3: PTDIS schedule (5R1, 10R2, 15R3, 20R4)	Increase in DLQ from early to late half of the night	Suicidal: $R_{EARLY} < R_{LATE}$ (freq. negative affect) $R_{EARLY} > R_{LATE}$ (freq. positive affect); more DLQd, i.e., Df decrease R_{EARLY} to R_{LATE} Nonsuicidal: more DLQd+

Df, dreamlike fantasy; DLQ, dreamlike quality; DLQd, dreamlike quality difference; LH, left hemisphere; NR, NREM period; NREM, non-REM; PTDIS, progressive temporal delay into stage; R, REM period (5R1, 5 min into first REM period); REM, rapid eye movement; RH, right hemisphere; SO, sleep onset; S_2, stage 2; TRC, total recall count; WU, wake up.

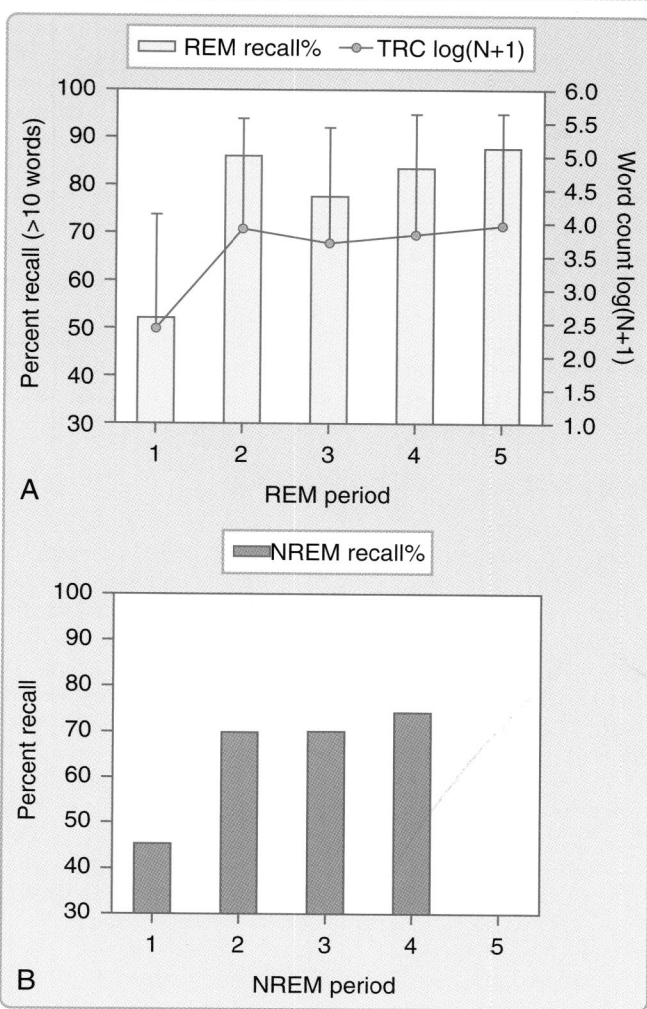

Figure 43–3. Percent recall and mean total recall count (TRC) for dream reports collected across the night from rapid eye movement (REM) sleep (**A**) and non-REM (NREM) sleep (**B**). Exponential ("switchlike") increases from first to second sleep cycles appear in both graphs. Values for NREM period 5 are not available. (**B**, Adapted from Pivik T, Foulkes D: NREM mentation: Relation to personality, orientation time, and time of night. J Consult Clin Psychol 1968; 32:144-151.)

Quality of Report Changes across the Night

Much research indicates that dreaming is more subjectively realistic and engaging in later sleep cycles and that dreams sampled in the first or second sleep cycles differ markedly from those in subsequent cycles. These qualitative changes are typically confounded by changes in report length, and the same caveats about length described earlier for ultradian rhythms also apply.

Qualitative REM Sleep Effects

An early study[58] of 73 dreams collected from each of the first three REM periods found REM 2 and REM 3 reports differed from REM 1 reports for several scales: Dream reports from later REM stages had more characters, more aggression and misfortune elements, more buildings, and fewer terrain settings. For some scales, a change occurred only from REM 2 to REM 3: REM 3 dreams had more sexual acts, more food elements, and fewer room settings.

Several groups have conceptually replicated these types of across-night changes. First, there are positive correlations between time of night of the REM period awakening and ratings of mentation vividness ($P = .01$) and emotionality ($P = .05$).[26] Second, subject ratings on several variables reveal that REM 1 dream reports differ more from REM 2 reports than the latter do from REM 3 reports.[21,59] Third, dream reports from young adults show marked changes from REM 1 to REM 2 (increases in 15 of 41 variables) and less-marked changes from REM 2 to REM 3 (6 of 41 variables) and REM 3 to REM 4 (7 of 41 variables).[60] Fourth, the dream reports of healthy volunteers increase in dreamlike quality (DLQ)* from early (REM 1 and REM 2) to late (REM 3 and later) sleep,[62] including an increase in *strongly emotional* content (from 16.7% to 23.1%) and *positive emotion* (from 15.4% to 38.5%) and a decrease in *neutral emotion* (69.2% to 46.1%).

Ultradian factors confound the preceding results, which unfortunately limits their generality. Two studies[21,62] confounded REM period order with prior stage duration due to a PTDIS protocol (waking 5 minutes into REM 1, 10 minutes into REM 2, and 20 minutes into REM 3 and later). Another study[60] likely confounded REM period order with length because all awakenings targeted the "end" of the REM episodes (early REM episodes are shorter than later ones). In another study,[26] a partial PTDIS protocol was used: REM 1 awakenings were always short (i.e., at 5 minutes), whereas all other REM awakenings were counterbalanced between short and long (i.e., 5 minutes versus 12 minutes).

Despite potential confounding factors in these studies, their results are consistent with findings from studies that have controlled for such factors. When the ultradian confounding factor was controlled by conducting awakenings 4.8 to 5.0 minutes into each REM period,[5] a visual imagery (VI) measurement—a count of visual nouns, action words, modifiers, and spatial relations—clearly increased across the night, with marked changes for the early- to middle-night comparison but not for the middle- to late-night comparison. Confounding effects are also mitigated by evidence[34] that circadian and ultradian factors do not interact statistically in subjective ratings of dream vividness and other features (see later).

Another early series of five replication studies[63] that minimized ultradian confounding factors (awakenings all 5 to 10 minutes into REM sleep) reported a within-night pattern of increases in LH, but not in RH, processes. In all studies of the series, a combined LH score increased significantly across the night. The pattern is consistent with the influence of a LH circadian process with an early morning acrophase, whereas the lack of variation in RH processes suggests either no circadian variation or a possible rise and acrophase later in the day. The latter case would imply that LH and RH influences on dreaming are modulated by separate circadian oscillators.

---

*Dreamlike quality is measured on a five-point scale: 1 = no recall; 2 = a nonperceptual report; 3 = a single visual image; 4 = two or more images with some story connecting them; and 5 = two or more images with an elaboration of detail and a well-developed narrative.61

Mixed support for circadian effects is found in a study[64] of male college students. A "multiple" series of dream reports (N = 273) collected after every REM period for several nights indicated change over REM periods using both objective and subjective measures: Later REM dreams had more lone female characters, had more misfortunes, had more clarity, were easier to recall, were more bizarre, and had more color elements. In contrast, a "single" series of reports collected from subjects (N = 196) awakened only once per night for the first four REM periods gave no comparable evidence of change. These findings might question whether the within-night changes seen in laboratory studies are artifacts induced by multiple awakening schedules; however, the methods of the study remain unpublished and cannot be evaluated for rigor and potential confounding variables.

Two studies[32,34] that showed no differences between "early" and "late" REM dreams on measures of visual and auditory imagery and bizarreness sampled "early" REM dreams only from REM 2 and "late" dreams only from REM 3. These studies therefore may have failed to detect the switch-like change found to occur prior to REM 2 in other studies. Another possible confounding variable in laboratory studies[34] (see also later) is that the vividness of some dreams is more pronounced when sleep onset is delayed by 3 hours—presumably because dreaming is forced farther along the rising edge of a circadian activation process. Thus, to the extent that a subject's normal bedtime is inadvertently delayed by electrode installation, equipment calibration, questionnaire administration, and other routine tasks, dream vividness may be affected proportionally.

Qualitative NREM Sleep Effects

Within-night patterns similar to those reported for REM sleep have been observed for NREM reports in several studies that control ultradian confounding factors. First,[57] Df ratings are low in NREM 1 compared with NREM 2 through NREM 4. Second, there is an increase in NREM (stage 2) DLQ from the first to the second half of the night in male college students' dreams.[14] Third, NREM (stage 2) visual imagery scores in healthy young adults increase linearly across early, middle, and late thirds of the night.[5] Fourth, visual imagery ratings of NREM (stage 2) reports are higher in NREM 4 than in NREM 2—even after covarying report length.[32]

Memory Sources

Memory source studies provide additional information about possible circadian influences on dream formation. Studies use either objective markers of memory sources, such as laboratory incorporations, or subjective markers, such as subject associations to recalled contents. The memory features most often evaluated are informational quality of the sources (semantic versus episodic) and temporal recency of the sources (recent versus remote events).

INFORMATION QUALITY OF MEMORY SOURCES

In one study[42] dreams were reported after 5 minutes into REM 1 and REM 3 and after an unspecified time into NREM 1 and NREM 3 while dream sources were elicited and rated by judges as being strict episodes, semantic knowledge, or abstract self-references.* For REM reports, only semantic sources were less frequent for early (16.4%) than for late (31.9%) awakenings (P = .027), even when report length was controlled. However, when the raw data from this study were combined with those from other studies, this effect disappeared,[41] whereas the absence of other effects (episodic, self-reference) was confirmed. Further, a significant within-night effect for NREM sleep reports was observed (P = .014), but its morphology was unfortunately not specified. Finally, a stage difference in episodic sources (NREM greater than REM) was found to be constant throughout the night.

These studies provide conflicting evidence for modulation of access to semantic memory sources across the night, but they concur in supporting an *absence* of such modulation for either episodic or self-reference source types.

TEMPORAL RECENCY OF MEMORY SOURCES

Studies evaluating the timing of memory sources provide findings discordant with those assessing their informational quality. Several early studies indicate that memory sources referring to temporally recent (presumably episodic) events are preferentially associated with early-night (versus late-night) dream reports. For example, a case study[65] reported that early-night dreams often refer to the laboratory experiment, whereas later dreams refer to early childhood or adolescent memories.

Two studies confirmed this finding. In one,[66] subjects associated recent memory elements to their early-night REM dreams and remote elements to their late-night REM dreams. In another,[26] recent elements were associated with dreams from the first 3.5 hours of sleep, remote elements to dreams from 3.5 to 7.5 hours, and moderately recent elements to dreams from later than 7.5 hours. Temporal remoteness of associations was also correlated with body temperature.

A subsequent study[67] (Table 43–2, second study) confirmed these findings among subjects who wore red-tinted goggles over 5 consecutive days and reported dreams after multiple REM period awakenings. On the first postexposure night, colors from the red end of the spectrum ("goggle" incorporations) occurred only in REM 1 dreams. On subsequent nights (nights 2 and 3), incorporations spread to REM 2 and REM 3 dreams, and on nights 4 and 5 they spread to REM 4 and REM 5 dreams. Thus, incorporations of new experiences were restricted to *early* REM periods; progressively older experiences were processed in *later* REM periods.

In contrast to the preceding, negative findings were reported[58] in an assessment of "elements from the past" among 219 dreams from 22 subjects. Although the proportion of elements increased in the expected direction from REM 1 to REM 3 (11%, 18%, 19%), the change was not statistically significant. However, later REM periods were not sampled and statistical tests were admittedly too conservative.

---

*The ratings are defined as: strict episode = discrete episode in the life of the dreamer, with precise spatial and/or temporal coordinates; abstract self-reference = memories not connected to any particular spatiotemporal context, referring to the dreamer's general knowledge of him- or herself and his or her own habits; semantic knowledge = elements of general knowledge of the world, including episodes from the biographies of others (adapted from Cavallero et al.[42]).

Table 43–2. Studies Showing Circaseptan Factor in Dream Memory Sources

Study	No. of Subjects	Mean Ages (SD)	Stimulus	No. of Dreams	Design	Peak Incorporations Identified
Jouvet (1979)[103]	1 researcher	Not specified	Retrospectively identified events (unspecified type) Change surroundings (Leave on trip or return from trip)	400 total	Within subject	On day 9 following event 7.8 days after leaving on trip 6.5 days after returning from trip
Roffwarg et al. (1978)[67]	9 (3 male, 6 female) 18-28 students	Not specified	Goggles with red filters for 5 consecutive days	Not specified (605 to 640-μm bandpass)	Within subject	On day 1 after first wearing goggles 5 days after first wearing goggles
Nielsen and Powell (1989 study 1)[98]	69 undergrads	Not specified	Retrospective self-selection of most significant events of prior week	55, 43, 41, 31, 14, 8 (days 1 to 7)	Within subjects	On days 1 and 6 after event
Nielsen and Powell (1989 study 2)[98]	34 undergrads	Not specified	Overnight stay in sleep laboratory	24, 20, 27, 22, 17, 21, 22 (days 1 to 7)	Within subjects	On days 1 and 6 after event
Nielsen and Powell (1992)[99]	84 undergrads	Not specified	Daily self-selection of emotionally meaningful events	Range: 59 (day 1) to 11 (day 14); mean: 34.9/day	Within subjects	On days 1, 6, and 12 after negative event
Powell et al. (1995)[102]	10 male, 9 female undergrads	Total: 24.9 (8.4)	30-min water buffalo sacrifice film with friends on 21-inch TV	Range: 17 (day 1) to 13 (day 7)	Within subjects	On days 1 and 7 after film for high incorporators
Nielsen and Powell (1995)[100]	9 male, 12 female undergrads	Female: 21.4 (2.4) Male: 22.8 (2.8)	30-min water buffalo sacrifice film alone in lab bedroom on 21-inch TV	Range: 10-16; mean: 12.2/day	Within subjects	On days 4 and 11 after film
Nielsen et al. (2004)[101]	212 undergrads	Male: 20.4 (7.4) Female: 20.1 (5.0)	Self-selection of events from one specific day	50, 38, 26, 25, 27, 26, 20	Between subjects	On days 1 and 7 after event for women; day 1 for men

Experimental and Pathologic Desynchronization of Circadian Factors

Some of the most compelling evidence for the existence of circadian influences on dreaming is found in studies in which relationships between circadian factors and dreaming are desynchronized by experimental design, by pathologic factors such as depression and posttraumatic stress disorder (PTSD), or by jet lag or aging. In all cases, dreaming becomes atypically intensified early in the sleep episode, and circadian rhythms appear to be phase-advanced relative to the habitual sleep period. These findings underline the potential value of forced desynchrony protocols for investigating circadian factors in dreaming.

Experimental Desynchronization of Circadian Factors

A study[34] using partial forced desynchrony created a phase delay of dreaming relative to a hypothesized circadian influence by delaying sleep onset and offset by 3 hours. REM and NREM dreaming both occurred 3 hours later than usual—coincident with the rising phase of the circadian influence (Fig. 43–4). Comparison of REM and NREM dream reports from the phase-delayed condition with control reports from nondelayed sleep revealed the relative contributions of an ultradian factor (early versus late awakenings) and a circadian factor (control versus delayed sleep). Sleep-delayed dream reports were longer and more visually intense, especially when collected later at night. Habitual REM greater than NREM differences were also shown, but REM and NREM reports were both affected by the circadian factor independent of this stage difference. For a visual imagery measure, the circadian effect size (.23, or small) was about 30% of the ultradian effect size (.70, or large). The results prompted the authors to claim that ultradian and circadian sources of cortical and subcortical activation are independent but combine to enhance dreaming, as in this study.

This finding was subsequently replicated by the same group[34a] using a more precise estimate of circadian phase. The effect size of the expected difference in this case was much larger (.51) than that for the sleep stage difference (.40).

One study[18] (described earlier) that employed 20-minute sleep/40-minute awake schedules to sample dream content from REM and NREM naps provides even more convincing evidence for circadian oscillation in dreaming propensity (Fig. 43–5). Subjective dreaming scores elicited for NREM reports were distributed sinusoidally across the 24-hour day, with an acrophase at 8:00 AM. REM report scores were elevated for the entire diurnal period of 6:00 AM to 4:00 PM, followed by a marked drop. Whereas REM dream scores likely reflect a ceiling effect on the four-point scale used, the fact that the curve for NREM dreaming parallels the curve for REM (but not NREM) sleep propensity and is robustly correlated with it (r = .87, P < 0.0001) suggests that dreaming propensity for REM and NREM sleep is influenced by the same underlying circadian oscillator.

Depression

In many depressed patients there may be a disruption of circadian factors affecting the REM-NREM sleep cycle[68,69] and

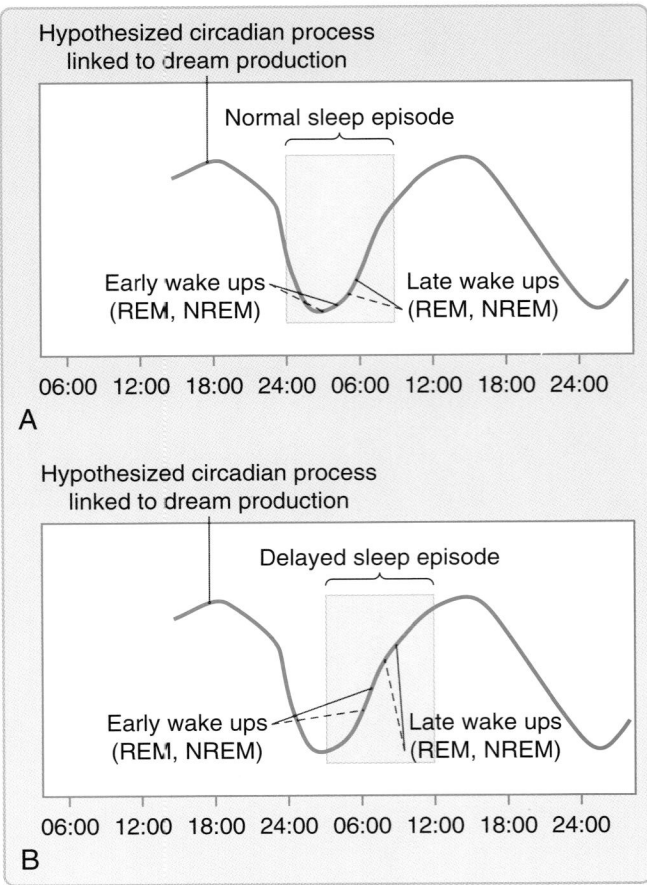

Figure 43–4. Theoretical model underlying partial forced asynchrony protocol used to manipulate hypothesized circadian influences on dream formation. Awakenings for report collection in the normal sleep, no delay condition (**A**) were made early and late in the sleep episode. Awakenings in the delayed sleep condition (**B**) were made at the same times relative to sleep onset and thus at different phase relationships to the hypothesized circadian process (i.e., on its rising phase). As predicted, dream vividness was increased for the late-night reports in the delayed condition. REM, rapid eye movement; NREM, non-REM. (Adapted from Antrobus J, Kondo T, Reinsel R, et al: Dreaming in the late morning: Summation of REM and diurnal cortical activation. Conscious Cogn 1995;4:275-299.)

accompanying dreaming.[62] For dream content, this disruption is a reversal of the normal increase in DLQ within a night. In one study,[62] all nondepressed subjects displayed the expected DLQ increase within the night for REM reports, but 46% of suicidal subjects displayed a DLQ decrease (P = .015). This "reversed DLQ" pattern may signal an abnormal phase advance of circadian processes. Similarly, Wehr's *internal coincidence* model of depression[70] stipulates that mood in depressed persons is affected by a phase-angle discrepancy between a phase-advanced circadian clock and the sleep–wake cycle. Manipulations of the sleep–wake cycle, such as sleep deprivation or phase advance of the sleep period, may alleviate depression symptoms.[71] A circadian-based explanation of depression is still contentious, and alternative models could account for the early-night changes in dreaming among the depressed. Some alternatives propose a deficiency in sleep need or "process S"[72] or, even more specifically, a diminution of the "delta sleep ratio."[73]

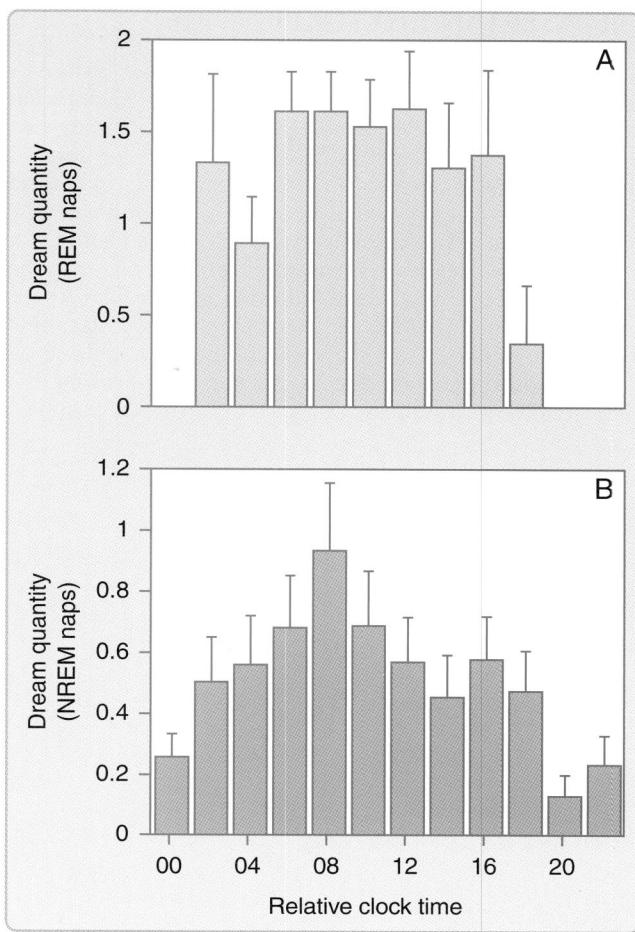

Figure 43–5. Dreaming scores for subjects on a 20-min sleep/40-min awake schedule for 3 consecutive days, with dream sampling at each awakening. Three-day means are displayed by 2-hour blocks time-locked to the onset of melatonin release (11:00 PM). Dream scores for non–rapid eye movement (NREM) sleep reports (*panel B*) clearly conform to a circadian oscillation with an acrophase at 8:00 AM, whereas scores for rapid eye movement (REM) sleep reports (*panel A*) remain elevated from 6:00 AM to 4:00 PM, possibly a ceiling effect for the rating scale used. Interestingly, the NREM dream score acrophase coincides with the acrophase of mean REM (but not NREM) stage duration. A further, circasemidian, component is suggested by the secondary NREM peak at 4:00 PM. (Adapted from Suzuki H, Uchiyama M, Tagaya H, et al: NREM dreaming in the absence of prior REM sleep. Sleep 2004;27:1486-1490.

Posttraumatic Stress Disorder

An imbalance of early versus late sleep like that observed in depression also appears to characterize PTSD; there is an apparent phase advance in dreaming such that vivid nightmares, which in nightmare disorder usually occur in late REM sleep, occur in PTSD patients also early in the sleep episode[74] and even during NREM sleep.[75-77] A circadian phase advance is also suggested by sleep anomalies such as reduced REM latency, increased REM density,[78] circadian phase–specific hypocortisolemia,[79] and increased autonomic responsivity during both REM and NREM in the first versus the second half of the night.[80] These changes all suggest that there has

occurred a shift in the circadian regulator of REM sleep and dreaming such that their intensification takes place much earlier in the night than is normally the case.

Jet Lag

In a similar manner, transmeridian travel may affect dreaming by desynchronizing dream-related circadian processes and sleep time. This possibility is consistent with the observation that jet lag produces more frequent sleep paralysis episodes,[81] which are usually accompanied by vivid, frightening dream images. Further, the physiologic prerequisite for sleep paralysis, sleep-onset REM (SOREM),[82] is more probable when REM sleep pressure is elevated, as it may be when the circadian propensity for REM sleep is phase advanced. Thus, the frequency of sleep-onset REM, sleep paralysis, and intensified frightful dreaming should all be increased immediately after east-to-west transmeridian travel that induces a temporary phase delay of the sleep episode and thus a relative phase advance of the circadian oscillator. Research is lacking on this question, but a report on two travelers who both underwent long transatlantic flights and both experienced anxious, isolated sleep paralysis events[81] is consistent with this suggestion.

Aging

Evidence that circadian rhythms are phase advanced in older subjects[83] may similarly explain a resurgence in sleep paralysis events among 40 to 80 year olds[84] as well as a decrease in retrospectively estimated dream recall with advanced age.[85] If dream intensification is phase advanced, then spontaneous morning recall of dreams (the presumed basis for retrospective recall) should be lower. Patterns of dream vividness within a night among older subjects[5,54] partially support this notion. The vividness of older subjects' NREM dreams peaks early then decreases—a pattern opposite to that of younger subjects and consistent with a phase advance. However, a similar vividness pattern for REM-sleep dreams is not observed, possibly because circadian variation of REM and NREM dreaming is more dissociable with age (see Yoon et al.[83] and Broughton[86] for reviews).

Continuity of Processes across Sleep–Wake States

Just as the propensity for REM sleep continues into wakefulness,[87] circadian factors affecting dreaming may also continue to influence waking-state processes that may be functionally related to dreaming. Studies[63] described earlier demonstrate within-night increases in LH content but no changes in RH content, a pattern that suggests LH processes may reach a peak in the morning, concomitant with REM sleep propensity, while RH processes reach a peak only later in the day. In fact, during wakefulness, LH processes such as spelling proficiency are more engaged in the early morning,[88] whereas RH processes such as consonant-vowel voicings and melodies are more engaged only later in the day.[89,90] Such LH-RH phase discrepancies are true of physiologic systems more generally.[91,92] Thus, although some aspects of dream production, such as total dream output, may have a single circadian oscillator, other more specific aspects may be modulated by separate circadian oscillators.

Alternative Explanations

Some of the evidence for circadian mediation of dreaming could be explained by alternative, nonoscillator models, such as the possibility that dream vividness is an inverse function of sleep propensity across the night. For example, delta EEG power, a common marker of sleep propensity, decreases clearly between the first and second NREM periods but much less so between the second and subsequent NREM periods. Dream vividness changes follow an inverse pattern. Nonetheless, an "inverse sleep propensity" explanation does not easily account for all the experimental and pathophysiologic findings reviewed earlier, nor does it easily explain why the changes in a process tied to NREM sleep should affect *both* NREM and REM dreaming.

CIRCASEPTAN RHYTHMS

Accumulating evidence implicates circaseptan factors in processes of dream formation. Circaseptan oscillators have been described for several biologic systems, including heart rate, blood pressure, and body weight,[93] and for cognitive phenomena such as reaction time.[94] Similarly, circaseptan interval timers (also known as hourglass clocks) that are reactive to endogenous or exogenous events have been identified for several adaptive and compensatory responses,[95] including changes in sleep architecture following learning.[96,97] At least seven studies indicate that the memory sources of sleep mentation are modulated by circaseptan factors (see Table 43–2).

Six studies were conducted by our group using both within- and between-subjects designs.[98-102] In the within-subjects

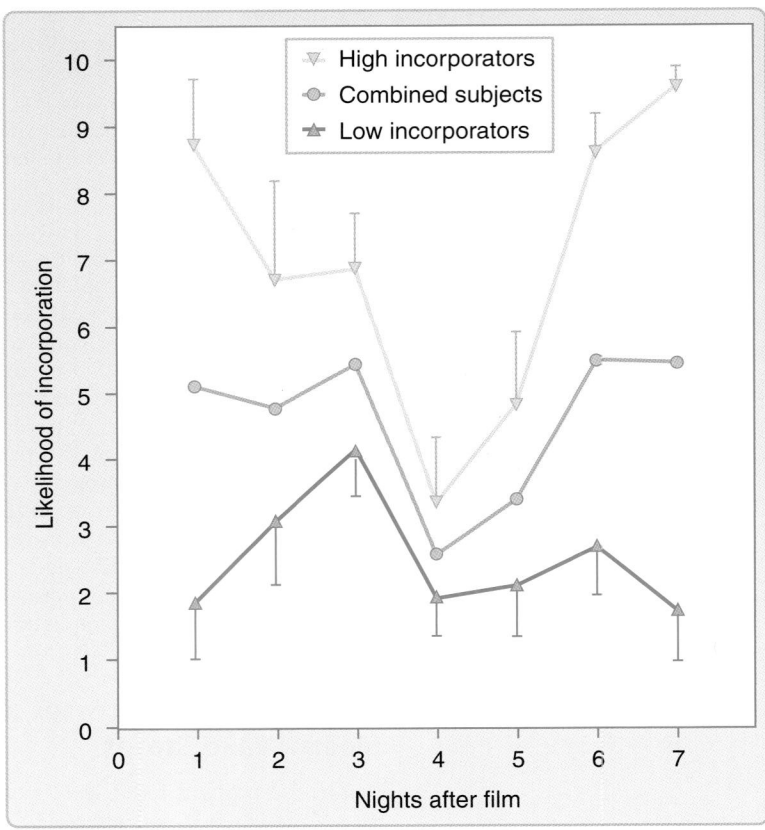

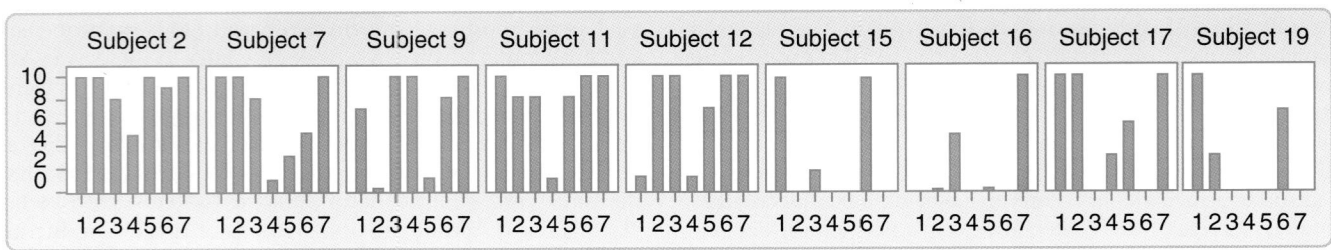

HIGH INCORPORATORS

Figure 43–6. Mean (SEM) judge ratings of likelihood that film elements were incorporated into dreams for high (*N* = 9) and low (*N* = 10) incorporating subjects. The U-shaped circaseptan effect is apparent only for high incorporating subjects. *Bottom panel* illustrates the U-shaped curve for ratings for these nine subjects. (From Powell RA, Nielsen TA, Cheung JS, et al: Temporal delays in incorporation of events into dreams. Percept Mot Skills 1995;81:95-104.)

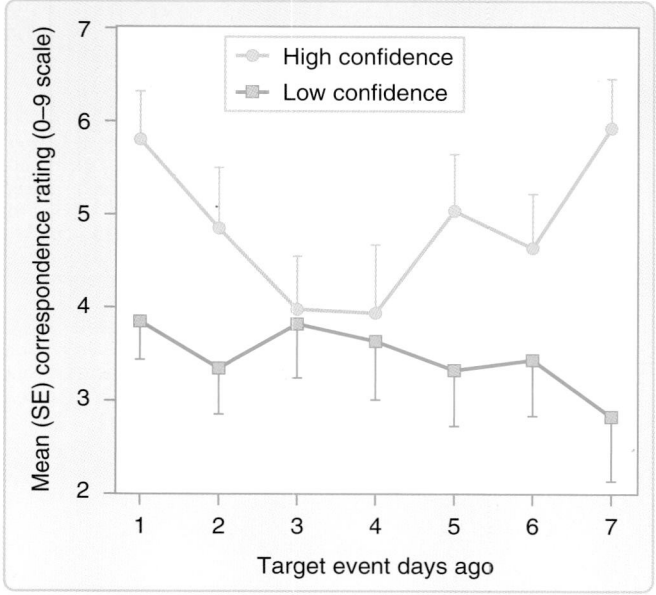

Figure 43–7. Mean (SEM) subject ratings of likelihood that prior events correspond to some element of the target dream for each target day for low (*squares*) and high (*circles*) confidence groups. The typical U-shaped curve is apparent only for the high confidence group. (From Nielsen TA, Kuiken D, Alain G, et al: Immediate and delayed incorporation of events into dreams: Further replication and implications for dream function. J Sleep Res [2004;13:327-336]).

design, dreams recorded for 7 to 12 days are rated by judges for their correspondence with a recent, traceable memory source, such as a current concern, a disturbing film, or a laboratory stayover. When correspondence ratings are plotted against days prior to the dream of the memory source, a sinusoidal U-shaped curve is observed. Peak scores occur for dreams following the source by 1 day (day-residue effect) and by 6 to 7 days ("dream-lag" effect; Fig. 43–6). The latter is consistent with a circaseptan hourglass clock.

In the between-subjects design,[101] subjects randomly distributed into groups are asked to find memory sources for a selected dream on a single specific day prior to the dream. They evaluate their certainty of recall and the correspondence between memory sources and the dream. This design again produces a clear U-shaped curve in dream-memory correspondence for subjects who are relatively certain of their recall (Fig. 43–7). Randomization and other controls minimize the possibility of confounding by the 7-day societal schedule and other factors.

Evidence consistent with the previous findings—and thus with a circaseptan influence on dream memory sources—was reported by Jouvet[103] in an analysis of 400 of his personal dreams. One analysis of 130 dreams and their memory sources revealed a sinusoidal U-shaped curve with peak correspondences occurring for memories 1 day (34.6%) and 9 days (10%) prior to the dream. A second analysis of 270 dreams recorded during and after travel abroad revealed that spatial elements of the new environments began to appear in recorded dreams on average 7.8 days after leaving on the trip and ceased occurring 6.5 days after returning home. Jouvet suggested that the delayed incorporations into dreams demonstrated a process responsible for spatial memory of environments, a suggestion that we subsequently confirmed.[101,104]

The "goggles" study[67] described earlier, in which subjects wore red-tinted goggles for a 5-day period, also supports a circaseptan process in dream memory access. The "goggle effect" (percentage of dream objects containing red, orange, or yellow) was most apparent for the first REM episode of each night and—for these episodes—was sinusoidally distributed over nights in a circaseptan fashion.

Our group also has evidence that the circaseptan pattern of memory access may be implicated in dream function.[101] On the one hand, delayed incorporations into dreams treat spatial location preferentially[103] relative to immediate incorporations. On the other hand, delayed incorporations are related to interpersonal problem solving—specifically, interpersonal relationships, positive emotions, and resolved problems.

CIRCATRIGINTAN RHYTHMS

Circatrigintan influences on dreaming are feasible in light of observed circatrigintan modulation of the menstrual cycle, including changes in sleep parameters (see reviews in Carrier[105] and in Driver and Baker[106]). The possibility is also consistent with the demonstration of monthly fluctuations in, for example, implicit memory,[107] person perception,[108] and spatial ability.[109] These changes are for the most part linked to circatrigintan oscillations in the hormones estrogen and progesterone.[107,110]

Although the research is not completely consistent, changes in dream recall and content have been reported for different temporal positions in the menstrual cycle. Several studies converge in suggesting that dream emotion is modulated on a monthly basis, with an intensification occurring during menses. One early study[111] revealed that dreams recalled during menses displayed more expressed emotional conflict than midcycle dreams. A second study[112] with 11 weekly polysomatographic (PSG) recordings replicated this finding: Specifically, manifest sexuality and overt hostility in dreams were both more frequent during menses; however, dream imaginativeness did not vary with menstrual cycle phase. The finding for sexual content, but not for hostility, was replicated in a case study.[113] Finally, a study of more than 450 dreams from 50 first-year nursing students[114] revealed changes during menses consistent with the prior studies: increased references to blood visible on females, increased aggressions toward males, and increased initiation of social interactions of all types.

Two other studies reported changes with menstrual phase that are not necessarily consistent with the previous findings.[115,116] Dreams with active sexual and libidinal impulses were correlated with preovulatory estrogen dominance, whereas dreams with passive receptivity and preoccupations with the self were correlated with postovulatory progesterone dominance. A reanalysis[117] revealed a further link between estrogen dominance and an enhanced capacity to retrieve and communicate concrete, specific, and clear dream images (Fig. 43–8).

Negative findings have also been reported[118] suggesting that conclusions about circatrigintan rhythms in dreaming should be drawn cautiously. Although relationships may exist between hormonal fluctuations and dreaming that parallel relationships for the waking state (see earlier), it remains unclear whether dream changes are due to the biologic fluctuations, to concomitant changes in self-perception, stress, and mood, or to both types of factors. Additionally, this type of research so far is limited to female subjects.

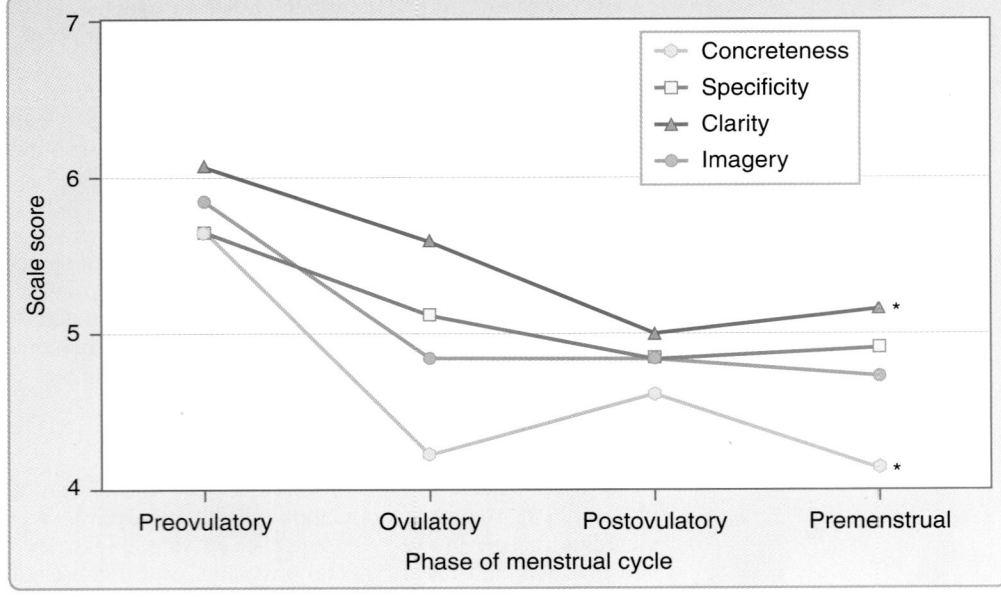

Figure 43–8. Mean scores for four psycholinguistically based dream content scales for dreams reported at four phases of the menstrual cycle; *asterisks* indicate significant effects for menstrual phase. (Adapted from Severino SK, Bucci W, Creelman ML: Cyclical changes in emotional information processing in sleep and dreams. J Am Acad Child Adolesc Psychiatry 1989;17:555-577.)

Clinical Pearl

Atypical recall of vivid dreams from early in the sleep period may be a marker of underlying phase advance of circadian processes implicated in dreaming.

REFERENCES

1. Aserinsky E, Kleitman N: Regularly occurring periods of eye motility, and concomitant phenomena during sleep. Science 1953;118:273-274.
2. Hobson JA, Pace-Schott E, Stickgold R: Dreaming and the brain: Towards a cognitive neuroscience of conscious states. Behav Brain Sci 2000;23:793-842.
3. McCarley RW: Dreams and the biology of sleep. In Kryger MH, Roth T, Dement WC (eds): Principles and Practice of Sleep Medicine, 2nd ed. Philadelphia, WB Saunders, 1994, pp 373-383.
4. Nielsen TA: A review of mentation in REM and NREM sleep: "Covert" REM sleep as a possible reconciliation of two opposing models. Behav Brain Sci 2000;23:851-866.
5. Waterman D, Elton M, Kenemans JL: Methodological issues affecting the collection of dreams. J Sleep Res 1993;2:8-12.
6. Foulkes D, Schmidt M: Temporal sequence and unit composition in dream reports from different stages of sleep. Sleep 1983;6:265-280.
7. Antrobus J: REM and NREM sleep reports: Comparison of word frequencies by cognitive classes. Psychophysiology 1983;20:562-568.
8. Cavallero C, Cicogna P, Natale V, et al: Slow wave sleep dreaming. Sleep 1992;15:562-566.
9. Stickgold R, Paceschott E, Hobson JA: A new paradigm for dream research—mentation reports following spontaneous arousal from REM and NREM sleep recorded in a home setting. Conscious Cogn 1994;3:16-29.
10. Stickgold R, Malia A, Fosse R, et al: Brain-mind states: I. Longitudinal field study of sleep/wake factors influencing mentation report length. Sleep 2001;24:171-179.
11. Dement W, Kleitman N: The relationship of eye movement during sleep to dream activity: An objective method for the study of dreaming. J Exp Psychol 1957;53:339-346.
12. Wolpert EA, Trosman H: Studies in psychophysiology of dreams. I. Experimental evocation of sequential dream episodes. Arch Neurol Psychiatr 1958;79:603-606.
13. Goodenough DR, Lewis HB, Shapiro A, et al: Dream reporting following abrupt and gradual awakenings from different types of sleep. J Pers Soc Psychol 1965;2:170-179.
14. Arkin AM, Antrobus JS, Ellman SJ, et al: Sleep mentation as affected by REM deprivation. In Arkin AM, Antrobus JS, Ellman SJ (eds): The Mind in Sleep: Psychology and Psychophysiology. Hillsdale, NJ, Erlbaum, 1978, pp 459-484.
15. Antrobus JS, Fein G, Jordan L, et al: Measurement and design in research on sleep reports. In Ellman SJ, Antrobus J (eds): The Mind in Sleep: Psychology and Psychophysiology. New York, Wiley, 1991, pp 83-122.
16. Nielsen TA: Covert REM sleep effects on NREM mentation: Further methodological considerations and supporting evidence. Behav Brain Sci 2000;23:1040-1057.
17. Rosenlicht N, Maloney T, Feinberg I: Dream report length is more dependent on arousal level than prior REM duration. Brain Res Bull 1994;34:99-101.
18. Suzuki H, Uchiyama M, Tagaya H, et al: NREM dreaming in the absence of prior REM sleep. Sleep 2004;27:1486-1490.
19. Takeuchi T, Miyasita A, Inugami M, et al: Intrinsic dreams are not produced without REM sleep mechanisms: Evidence through elicitation of sleep onset REM periods. J Sleep Res 2001;10:43-52.
20. Broughton RJ: SCN controlled circadian arousal and the afternoon "nap zone." Sleep Res Online 1998;1:166-178.
21. Foulkes D: The Psychology of Sleep. New York, Scribners, 1966.
22. Czaya J, Kramer M, Roth T: Changes in dream quality as a function of time into REM. Sleep Res 1973;2:122.
23. Kramer M, Roth T, Czaya J: Dream development within a REM period. In Levin P, Koella WP (eds): Sleep 1974, Second European Congress on Sleep Research, Rome, 1974. Basel, Karger, 1974, pp 406-408.
24. Kramer M: The selective mood regulatory function of dreaming: An update and revision. In Moffitt A, Kramer M, Hoffman R (eds): The functions of dreaming. Albany, State University of New York, 1993, pp 139-196.
25. Foulkes D: Dream reports from different stages of sleep. J Abnorm Soc Psychol 1962;65:14-25.
26. Verdone P: Temporal reference of manifest dream content. Percept Mot Skills 1965;20:1253-1268.
27. Tracy RL, Tracy LN: Reports of mental activity from sleep stages 2 and 4. Percept Mot Skills 1974;38:647-648.
28. Foulkes D: The dreamlike fantasy (Df) scale: A rating manual. Psychophysiology 1970;7:335-336.

29. Winget C, Kramer M: Dimensions of Dreams. Gainesville, University of Florida, 1979.

30. Hunt H, Ruzycki-Hunt K, Pariak D, et al: The relationship between dream bizarreness and imagination: Artifact or essence? Dreaming 1993;3:179-199.

31. Purcell S, Mullington J, Moffitt A, et al: Dream self-reflectiveness as a learned cognitive skill. Sleep 1986;9:423-437.

32. Casagrande M, Violani C, Lucidi F, et al: Variations in sleep mentation as a function of time of night. Int J Neurosci 1996; 85:19-30.

33. Porte H, Hobson JA: Bizarreness in REM and NREM reports. Sleep Res 1986;15:81.

34. Antrobus J, Kondo T, Reinsel R, et al: Dreaming in the late morning: Summation of REM and diurnal cortical activation. Conscious Cogn 1995;4:275-299.

34a. Wamsley EJ, Hirota Y, Tucker MA, et al: Circadian influences on sleep mentation. Sleep 2004;27(Suppl).

35. Porte HS, Hobson JA: Physical motion in dreams—one measure of three theories. J Abnorm Psychol 1996;105:329-335.

36. Strauch I, Meier B: In Search of Dreams. Results of Experimental Dream Research. Albany, State University of New York Press, 1996.

37. Casagrande M, Violani C, Bertini M: A psycholinguistic method for analyzing two modalities of thought in dream reports. Dreaming 1996;6:43-55.

38. Nielsen TA, Kuiken D, Hoffmann R, et al: REM and NREM sleep mentation differences: A question of story structure? Sleep Hypn 2001;3:9-17.

39. Cavallero C, Cicogna P: Memory and dreaming. In Cavallero C, Foulkes D (eds): Dreaming as Cognition. New York, Harvester Wheatsheaf, 1993, pp 38-57.

40. Cicogna P, Cavallero C, Bosinelli M: Differential access to memory traces in the production of mental experience. Int J Psychophysiol 1986;4:209-216.

41. Baylor GW, Cavallero C: Memory sources associated with REM and NREM dream reports throughout the night: A new look at the data. Sleep 2001;24:165-170.

42. Cavallero C, Foulkes D, Hollifield M, et al: Memory sources of REM and NREM dreams. Sleep 1990;13:449-455.

43. Cicogna P, Cavallero C, Bosinelli M: Cognitive aspects of mental activity during sleep. Am J Psychol 1991;104:413-425.

44. Kleitman N: The nature of dreaming. In Wostenholme GEW, O'Connor M (eds): The Nature of Sleep. London, J&A Churchill, 1961, pp 349-364.

45. Kripke DF, Sonnenschein D: A biological rhythm in waking fantasy. In Pope KS, Singer JL (eds): Scientific Investigations into the Flow of Human Experience. New York, Plenum, 1978, pp 321-332.

46. Kripke DF, Mullaney FPA: Ultradian rhythms during sustained performance. In Schulz H, Lavie P (eds): Ultradian Rhythms in Physiology and Behavior. Berlin, Springer-Verlag, 1985, pp 201-216.

47. Kleitman N: Basic rest-activity cycle—22 years later. Sleep 1982;5:311-317.

48. Shannahoff-Khalsa DS, Gillin JC, Yates FE, et al: Ultradian rhythms of alternating cerebral hemispheric EEG dominance are coupled to rapid eye movement and non–rapid eye movement stage 4 sleep in humans. Sleep Med 2001;2:333-346.

49. Okada H, Matsuoka K, Hatakeyama T: Dream-recall frequency and waking imagery. Percept Mot Skills 2000;91:759-766.

50. Hayashi M, Morikawa T, Hori T: Circasemidian 12 h cycle of slow wave sleep under constant darkness. Clin Neurophysiol 2002;113:1505-1516.

51. Miller JC: Quantitative analysis of truck driver EEG during highway operations. Biomed Sci Instrum 1997;34:93-98.

52. Esposito MJ, Nielsen TA, Paquette T: Reduced alpha power associated with the recall of mentation from stage 2 and stage REM sleep. Psychophysiology 2004;41:288-297.

53. Wehr TA, Aeschbach D, Duncan WC Jr: Evidence for a biological dawn and dusk in the human circadian timing system. J Physiol 2001;535:937-951.

54. Waterman D: Rapid Eye Movement Sleep and Dreaming. Studies of Age and Activation [dissertation]. Amsterdam, University of Amsterdam, 1992.

55. Cipolli C, Bolzani R, Tuozzi G: Story-like organization of dream experience in different periods of REM sleep. J Sleep Res 1998;7:13-19.

56. Nielsen TA, Germain A, Zadra AL, et al: Physiological correlates of dream recall vary across REM periods: Eye movement density vs heart rate. Sleep Res 1997;26:249.

57. Pivik T, Foulkes D: NREM mentation: Relation to personality, orientation time, and time of night. J Consult Clin Psychol 1968;32:144-151.

58. Domhoff B, Kamiya J: Problems in dream content study with objective indicators: III. Changes in dream content throughout the night. Arch Gen Psychiatry 1964;11:529-532.

59. Foulkes D, Rechtschaffen A: Presleep determinants of dream content: Effects of two films. Percept Mot Skills 1964;19: 983-1005.

60. Kramer M, McQuarrie E, Bonnet M: Dream differences as a function of REM period position. Sleep 1980;9:155.

61. Brown JN, Cartwright RD: Locating NREM dreaming through instrumental responses. Psychophysiology 1978;15:35-39.

62. Agargun MY, Cartwright R: REM sleep, dream variables and suicidality in depressed patients. Psychiatry Res 2003;119:33-39.

63. Cohen DB: Changes in REM dream content during the night: Implications for a hypothesis about changes in cerebral dominance across REM periods. Percept Mot Skills 1977;44: 1267-1277.

64. Van de Castle RL: Temporal patterns of dreams. Int Psychiatry Clin 1970;7:171-181.

65. Offenkrantz W, Rechtschaffen A: Clinical studies of sequential dreams I. A patient in psychotherapy. Arch Gen Psychiatry 1963;8:497-508.

66. Verdone P: Variables Related to the Temporal Reference of Manifest Dream Content [dissertation]. Chicago, University of Chicago,1963, pp 1253-1268.

67. Roffwarg HP, Herman JH, Bowe-Anders C, et al: The effects of sustained alterations of waking visual input on dream content. In Arkin AM, Antrobus JS, Ellman SJ (eds): The Mind in Sleep. Hillsdale, NJ, Erlbaum, 1978, pp 295-349.

68. Wirz-Justice A, Van den Hoofdakker RH: Sleep deprivation in depression: What do we know, where do we go? Biol Psychiatry 1999;46:445-453.

69. Riemann D, Berger M, Voderholzer U: Sleep and depression— results from psychobiological studies: An overview. Biol Psychol 2001;57:67-103.

70. Wehr TA, Wirz-Justice A: Internal coincidence model for sleep deprivation and depression. In Koella WP (ed): Sleep 1980. Fifth European Congress of Sleep Research, Amsterdam, 1980. Basel, Karger, 1981, pp 26-33.

71. Berger M, van Calker D, Riemann D: Sleep and manipulations of the sleep-wake rhythm in depression. Acta Psychiatr Scand (Suppl) 2003;108:S83-S91.

72. Borbély AA, Wirz-Justice A: Sleep, sleep deprivation and depression: A hypothesis derived from a model of sleep regulation. Hum Neurobiol 1982;1:205-210.

73. Kupfer DJ, Frank E, McEachran A, Grochosinski VJ: Delta sleep ratio: A biological correlate of early recurrence in unipolar affective disorder. Arch Gen Psychiatry 1990;47:1100-1105.

74. van der Kolk B, Blitz R, Burr W, et al: Nightmares and trauma: A comparison of nightmares after combat with lifelong nightmares in veterans. Am J Psychiatry 1984;141:187-190.

75. Hefez A, Metz L, Lavie P: Long-term effects of extreme situational stress on sleep and dreaming. Am J Psychiatry 1987; 144:344-347.

76. Kramer M, Kinney L: Sleep patterns in trauma victims with disturbed dreaming. Psychiatr J Univ Ott 1988;13:12-16.

77. Schlosberg A, Benjamin M: Sleep patterns in three acute combat fatigue cases. J Clin Psychiatry 1978;39:546-549.

78. Dow BM, Kelsoe JR Jr, Gillin JC: Sleep and dreams in Vietnam PTSD and depression. Biol Psychiatry 1996;39:42-50.

79. Bremner JD, Vythilingam M, Anderson G, et al: Assessment of the hypothalamic-pituitary-adrenal axis over a 24-hour diurnal period and in response to neuroendocrine challenges in women with and without childhood sexual abuse and posttraumatic stress disorder. Biol Psychiatry 2003;54:710-718.

80. Kramer M, Kinney L: Vigilance and avoidance during sleep in US Vietnam war veterans with posttraumatic stress disorder. J Nerv Ment Dis 2003;191:685-687.

81. Snyder S: Isolated sleep paralysis after rapid time zone change ("jet lag") syndrome. Chronobiology 1983;10:377-379.

82. Takeuchi T, Miyasita A, Sasaki Y, et al: Isolated sleep paralysis elicited by sleep interruption. Sleep 1992;15:217-225.

83. Yoon IY, Kripke DF, Elliott JA, et al: Age-related changes of circadian rhythms and sleep-wake cycles. J Am Geriatr Soc 2003;51:1085-1091.

84. Wing YK, Chiu H, Leung T, et al: Sleep paralysis in the elderly. J Sleep Res 1999;8:151-155.

85. Stenstrom PM, Nielsen TA, Zadra T, et al: Age and gender differences in dream recall estimated from a web-based questionnaire. Sleep 2003;26(Suppl):A94.

86. Broughton RJ: Three central issues concerning ultradian rhythms. In Schulz H, Lavie P (eds): Ultradian Rhythms in Physiology and Behavior. Berlin, Springer-Verlag, 1985, pp 217-233.

87. Czeisler C, Dijk DJ: Contribution of the circadian pacemaker and the sleep homeostat to sleep propensity, sleep structure, electroencephalographic slow waves, and sleep spindle activity in humans. J Neurosci 1995;15:3526-3538.

88. Morton LL, Diubaldo D: Circadian differences in hemisphere-linked spelling proficiencies. Int J Neurosci 1995;81:101-110.

89. Morton LL, Wojtowicz MJ, Williams NH, et al: Time-of-day-induced priming effects on verbal and nonverbal dichotic tasks in male and female adult subjects. Int J Neurosci 1992;64:83-96.

90. Morton LL, Diubaldo D: Circadian differences in the dichotic processing of voicing. Int J Neurosci 1993;68:43-52.

91. Corbera X, Grau C, Vendrell P: Diurnal oscillations in hemispheric performance. J Clin Exp Neuropsychol 1993;15:300-310.

92. Zimmermann P, Gortelmeyer R, Wiemann H: Diurnal periodicity of lateral asymmetries of the visual evoked potential in healthy volunteers. Neuropsychobiol 1983;9:178-181.

93. Cornelissen G, Engebretson M, Johnson D, et al: The week, inherited in neonatal human twins, found also in geomagnetic pulsations in isolated Antarctica. Biomed Pharmacotherapy 2001;55(Suppl 1):32s-50s.

94. Beau J, Carlier M, Duyme M, et al: Procedure to extract a weekly pattern of performance of human reaction time. Percept Mot Skills 1999;88:469-483.

95. Hildebrandt G: Reactive modifications of the autonomous time structure in the human organism. J Physiol Pharmacol 1991;42:5-27.

96. Leconte P: Sommeil et activité cognitive. In Pélicier Y (ed): La serrure et le songe. L'activité mentale du sommeil. Paris, Editions Economica, 1983, pp 41-60.

97. Smith C, Lapp L: Prolonged increases in both PS and number of REMS following a shuttle avoidance task. Physiol Behav 1986;36:1053-1057.

98. Nielsen TA, Powell RA: The "dream-lag" effect: A 6-day temporal delay in dream content incorporation. Psychiatr J Univ Ott 1989;14:561-565.

99. Nielsen TA, Powell RA: The day-residue and dream-lag effects: A literature review and limited replication of two temporal effects in dream formation. Dreaming 1992;2:67-77.

100. Nielsen TA, Powell RA: Temporal delays in dream content incorporation of a distressful film: A replication. Sleep Res 1995;24A:259.

101. Nielsen TA, Kuiken D, Alain G, et al: Immediate and delayed incorporation of events into dreams: Further replication and implications for dream function. J Sleep Res 2004;13:327-336.

102. Powell RA, Nielsen TA, Cheung JS, et al: Temporal delays in incorporation of events into dreams. Percept Mot Skills 1995;81:95-104.

103. Jouvet M: Memories and "split brain" during dream. 2525 memories of dream (in French). Rev Prat 1979;29:27-32.

104. Alain G, Nielsen TA, Stenstrom PM, et al: Qualitative differences in events incorporated into dreams either immediately or after a one-week delay. Sleep 2004; 27(Suppl 1):A65.

105. Carrier J: Sommeil et hormones sexuelles. Douleur et Analgésie 2003;2:99-104.

106. Driver HS, Baker FC: Menstrual factors and sleep. Sleep Med Rev 1998;2 213-229.

107. Maki PM, Rich JB, Rosenbaum RS: Implicit memory varies across the menstrual cycle: Estrogen effects in young women. Neuropsychology 2002;40:518-529.

108. Macrae CN, Alnwick KA, Milne AB, et al: Person perception across the menstrual cycle: Hormonal influences on social-cognitive functioning. Psychol Sci 2002;13:532-536.

109. Hampson E: Estrogen-related variations in human spatial and articulatory-motor skills. Psychoneuroendocrinology 1990;15:97-111.

110. Hausmann M, Becker C, Gather U, et al: Functional cerebral asymmetries during the menstrual cycle: A cross-sectional and longitudinal analysis. Neuropsychology 2002;40:808-816.

111. Hertz DG, Jensen MR: Menstrual dreams and psychodynamics: Emotional conflict and manifest dream content in menstruating women. Br J Med Psychol 1975;48:175-183.

112. Swanson EM, Foulkes D: Dream content and the menstrual cycle. J Nerv Ment Dis 1967;145:358-363.

113. Lewis SA, Burns M: Manifest dream content: Changes with the menstrual cycle. Br J Med Psychol 1975;48:375-377.

114. Van de Castle RL: Our Dreaming Mind: A Sweeping Exploration of the Role that Dreams Have Played in Politics, Art, Religion, and Psychology, from Ancient Civilizations to the Present Day. New York, Ballantine Books, 1994.

115. Benedek T, Rubenstein B: The correlations between ovarian activity and psychodynamic processes: I. The ovulation phase. Psychosom Med 1939;1:245-270.

116. Benedek T, Rubenstein B: The correlations between ovarian activity and psychosomatic processes: II. The menstrual phase. Psychosom Med 1939;1:461-485.

117. Severino SK, Bucci W, Creelman ML: Cyclical changes in emotional information processing in sleep and dreams. J Am Acad Child Adolesc Psychiatry 1989;17:555-577.

118. Schultz KJ, Koulack D: Dream affect and the menstrual cycle. J Nerv Ment Dis 1980;168:436-438.

44

The Neurobiology of Dreaming

Edward F. Pace-Schott

ABSTRACT

Dreaming, a universal human state of consciousness, is notable for its lack of insight and for its spontaneous generation of both familiar and wholly novel perceptual experiences and temporally ordered scenarios. As in waking consciousness, such experiences in both rapid eye movement (REM) and non-REM (NREM) sleep are believed to be associated with activation of forebrain structures by ascending arousal systems of the brainstem and diencephalon. Characteristic differences in forebrain activation patterns between waking and REM sleep, as revealed by positron emission tomography (PET) neuroimaging, suggest possible bases for phenomenological differences between these two states of consciousness. In REM sleep compared to waking, there is relatively more activation of limbic subcortex (e.g., amygdala, basal forebrain) and cortex (e.g., anterior cingulate) and relative deactivation of multimodal association cortices subserving executive functions (e.g., dorsolateral prefrontal cortex). Pharmacologic data indicate that a variety of neuromodulatory systems can influence dream quality and quantity or induce nightmares, or both. Such systems include the neuromodulators acetylcholine, dopamine, serotonin, and norepinephrine along with the ubiquitous amino acid neurotransmitters participating in their proximal effects on the forebrain.

Dream phenomenology bears a striking formal similarity to neuropsychiatric symptom complexes such as complex hallucinosis and spontaneous confabulation as well as to syndromes such as delirium and various misidentification syndromes. Lesion studies complement neuroimaging findings in suggesting key roles for limbic, prefrontal, visual association, and inferior parietal areas in dream construction. At present, descriptive models of dreaming link conscious awareness with ascending activation from the brainstem and diencephalon; pseudosensory experience with cortical activation of unimodal association cortices via thalamic intermediaries; affective salience with subcortical and cortical limbic activity; fictive movement with basal ganglia and cerebellar activity; experience of extrapersonal space with inferior parietal activity; executive deficits with lateral prefrontal deactivation; and mnemonic deficits with state-dependent alterations of interactions between hippocampal complex structures and cortical areas. Neurocognitive models of dreaming will evolve with emerging technologies in human experimental and clinical neuroscience.

COGNITIVE NEUROSCIENCE AND DREAMING

In this chapter, we will consider the relationship of dreaming with behavioral state, brain structures and networks, specific neuromodulatory systems, and neuropsychiatric models. The neuroscientific significance of the study of dreams becomes apparent by considering just two of the many remarkable aspects of this universally human mental state.

The first, dreaming's "singlemindedness and isolation," was eloquently described by Rechtschaffen[1] and refers to the dreamer's absorption in the dream world and plot without awareness of an alternate reality in waking—a condition that describes all but the most lucid of dreams. However, upon awakening from a dream one more or less abruptly switches from *sole* awareness of a dream reality to an awareness of external reality while, at the same time, retaining memory of the prior dream *as a dream*. This switch represents change from a condition of partial insight at best to one of full ability to conceptualize the possibility and nature of alternate states of mind and to decide which of these one is currently experiencing.

The second is the occurrence in dreams of entirely de novo imagery, plots, personages, and even motor skills (e.g., flying), emotion (e.g., numinosity), and memory (e.g., deja vu). In the case of visual images, perception by the waking brain is a neural transformation of extrinsically patterned templates of radiant energy. After its initial processing in the retina, thalamus, and primary sensory cortex, extracted information directs construction of endogenously organized representations in visual association cortices.[2] No such retinotopically organized information is available in dreaming, and yet we "see" endogenously patterned representations. Moreover, although transformations of our personal semantic and, to a lesser extent, our episodic memory[3] certainly compose *some* elements of our dreams, not *all* dream elements are memories, as exemplified by the novelty of dream plots.

Perhaps most remarkably, no extrinsically imposed chronology governs dreaming, yet dreams are organized into multidimensional virtual experience temporally sequenced into a coherent plot of causally linked events. Therefore, while dreaming may be phenomenologically more or less "like waking,"[4] it is *not* waking itself but a remarkable, imprecise experiential simulacrum of waking. And it results from neurobiologic processes that differ in many ways from those that generate waking consciousness.

THE ASSOCIATION OF DREAMING WITH BEHAVIORAL STATE

Early speculation that REM was the exclusive physiological substrate of dreaming,[5] which was followed by awakening studies showing substantial recall of mentation from NREM sleep,[6] has led to an ongoing controversy about whether REM and NREM dreams differ qualitatively or "only" quantitatively.[7] Nonetheless, REM reports are consistently found to be more frequent, longer, more bizarre, more visual, more motoric, and more emotional than NREM reports (see reviews in Hobson et al.[8]). For example, in a review of 29 studies, an estimated NREM recall rate of 42.5% has been contrasted with a REM recall rate of 81.8%.[9] Nielsen's theory that various NREM brain activation processes occur in the absence of polysomnographically scored REM ("covert REM") has been the most thorough and successful attempt to account for these discrepancies.[9] This review takes the position that dreaming is quantitatively and qualitatively associated with REM and that the study of REM physiology can powerfully inform the study of dream phenomenology, and it works from the hypothesis that what is unique physiologically in REM is likely related to what is enhanced during dreaming in REM.

Recent Electrophysiological Findings

Only a sample of five particularly intriguing new findings on the electrophysiology of sleep and dreaming are presented here, and undoubtedly there are many more. Hobson et al.[8] gives a comprehensive treatment of older reports.

Fast and Slow Oscillations and Dreaming

REM sleep shows much more gamma frequency (30 to 80 Hz) fast neuronal oscillations than does NREM sleep, as measured by electroencephalography (EEG)[10] and magnetoencephalography (MEG).[11] These fast oscillations are associated with attention to stimuli and other forms of active cognition in waking[12] and have been hypothesized to also be associated with the temporal binding of dream imagery.[13] An important related finding has been the desynchronization of gamma frequency oscillation between the frontal cortex and posterior perceptual areas during REM sleep.[14] This differs from the anteroposterior synchronization seen in waking. Perez-Garcia et al. have hypothesized that this REM-related desynchrony represents a disconnection of posterior cortical areas from frontal executive control and may contribute to the bizarreness of REM dreaming.

In contrast to REM, human slow wave sleep, which shows very little gamma activity, is associated with an abundance of slower rhythms (e.g., spindles and delta waves), including the cortical slow (<1 Hz) oscillation[15] originally described in the cat.[16] It has been suggested that these intrinsic thalamocortical rhythms may interfere with ongoing mental activity during NREM, leading to the lower frequency of dreaming seen in this state.[8]

Experimental Manipulation of Sleep Stage and Dreaming

Takeuchi and colleagues have used a sleep interruption technique to elevate the frequency of sleep onset REM periods (SOREMPs) in normal subjects.[17] Dreams elicited from SOREMPs were more bizarre and had different EEG correlates than NREM dreams occurring at similar circadian phases and preceded by similar sleep-wake durations.[17] For example, whereas SOREMP dreams were correlated with the amount of rapid eye movement in a sleep period and the absence of alpha frequency in the EEG spectrum, NREM dreams were correlated with the presence of arousals and the persistence of alpha rhythms.[17]

Dreaming and Phasic Activity in Sleep

The relationship between phasic components of sleep and dreaming continues to be studied.[18,19] Using induced eye movement as an awakening criterion, audiovisual stimuli applied below waking threshold during stage 2 NREM sleep were found to elevate the frequency of reports of visual imagery to a level comparable to those from REM awakenings,[18] although they did not elevate these rates in REM sleep. These authors initially hypothesized that stimulation was inducing a human NREM equivalent of the feline ponto-geniculo-occipital (PGO) wave, which, in turn, induced dream-like imagery. However, the increase in alpha activity following stimulation suggested, alternatively, that the increase in imagery may result from transient arousals.[18]

Since early EEG investigations of possible human equivalents of the feline PGO wave,[20] there have been numerous suggestive findings but none conclusive (see the review in Hobson et al.[8] and see Peigneux et al.[21]). Conduit and coworkers[19] sought such a human PGO sign in eyelid movements by correlating their occurrence with a suite of other phasic muscle movements that have been suggested to be PGO correlates (e.g., periorbital integrated potentials). Naturally occurring eyelid movements followed the pattern of PGOs predicted from animal studies, occurring maximally in REM sleep, least in NREM sleep, and at an intermediate rate just prior to REM sleep. In addition, they found well-above-chance correlations of eyelid movements with other phasic skeletal muscle movements. Based on these correlations, which are also present during arousals, these authors suggested an indirect link between eyelid movements and PGOs, reflecting a generalized central nervous system alerting or attentional mechanism similar to the startle response observed in waking.[19] Most recently, this group has shown that, in stage 2 NREM, awakenings following eyelid movements result in an enhanced frequency of visual imagery reports.[21a]

Experimental Evidence of State-Dependent Differences in Cognitive Processing

Evoked response potentials observed in waking (such as the P300 brainwave evoked in response to deviance in external stimuli) can also be elicited during REM sleep and light NREM sleep in response to changes in external auditory stimuli such as a deviant auditory tone or a highly salient stimulus occurring within a series of less salient stimuli (see review in Perrin et al.[22]). Exploiting this fact, Perrin et al.[22] studied the N400 brainwave in REM sleep. This evoked response potential can be elicited in waking by semantic incongruities such as pseudowords occurring among congruent words. They found that, unlike in waking and NREM sleep, the N400 elicited by pseudowords is attenuated in REM sleep and does not much differ from the evoked response potential elicited by congruent words. These authors conclude that the sleeper fails to detect the difference between real words and pseudowords in REM sleep, since other forms of stimulus enhancement (incongruous real words and primed words) continue to elicit the N400, albeit with a lesser amplitude than in waking. They relate this failure to detect nonwords in REM sleep to findings by Stickgold and colleagues[23] on the semantic priming effect following awakenings from REM sleep. In waking, the semantic priming effect is greater for strongly than for weakly associated words, whereas this priming effect is reversed (i.e., weakly associated greater than strongly associated) following awakenings from REM sleep. Both Stickgold and colleagues[23] and Perrin and colleagues[22] suggest that their respective findings may correspond to the loosening of associations and uncritical acceptance of bizzarreness in dreams.

A DISTINCTIVE PATTERN OF NEURAL ACTIVATION IN REM SLEEP

Alterations in regional glucose and oxygen use seen in positron emission tomography (PET) imaging studies are taken as indicators of changes in regional brain activation. During NREM sleep, PET studies have identified significant regional declines in activity (relative to waking) subcortically in the pons, thalamus, hypothalamus, and caudate as well as in certain lateral and medial prefrontal cortical regions.[24,25] This pattern of decreased brainstem, thalamic, and association cortex activity accompanying the onset and deepening of NREM sleep has now been widely replicated.[26,27,28]

During REM sleep, there is a prominent increase relative to NREM of neural activity in subcortical brain regions, including the pons, midbrain and thalamus,[25,29] amygdala,[29] hypothalamus, and basal ganglia.[25] The anterior cingulate as well as portions of the ventromedial, limbic-related prefrontal cortices have also been shown to reactivate in REM sleep following their deactivation in NREM sleep.[25,29,30,31,32] However, dorsolateral prefrontal areas do not participate in this reactivation, remaining, as in NREM sleep, less active than in waking.[25,29,33]

When REM sleep is compared to waking, there is relative deactivation of the dorsolateral prefrontal cortex[25,29] but greater activation of limbic and paralimbic regions.[25,29,30] Nofzinger and colleagues[30,31] have termed this area the "anterior paralimbic REM activation area" and describe it as a "bilateral confluent paramedian zone which extends from the septal area into ventral striatum, infralimbic, prelimbic, orbitofrontal and anterior cingulate cortex"[30] (p 192). PET researchers have interpreted these findings in terms of selective processing, during REM sleep, of emotionally influenced memories[29,34] or the integration during this sleep stage of neocortical functions with basal forebrain and hypothalamic motivational and reward mechanisms.[30] Figure 44–1 schematically illustrates

brain areas found in multiple studies that are activated or deactivated in REM sleep relative to waking.

Recent studies have also shed light on a possible human equivalent of phasic activation signals seen in feline REM sleep. Quantitative EEG techniques in humans have shown PGO wave–like activity involving the pons, midbrain, thalamus, hippocampus, and visual cortex.[35] Similarly, a recent $H_2^{15}O$ PET study in humans has shown REM-density correlations with activation of the lateral geniculate nucleus, thalamus and primary occipital cortex.[21] Lastly, MEG tomographic evidence of activity suggestive of PGO waves in the human brainstem has recently been reported.[35a] Thus, it appears likely that a human correlate of the feline PGO wave does exist.

DREAMING AND THE DEACTIVATION OF LATERAL PREFRONTAL CORTICES IN SLEEP

Deactivation of frontal cortices is one of the first physiologically measurable signs of human sleep, whether measured by quantitative EEG,[36,37] $H_2^{15}O$ PET,[24,25,27] or [18]FDG (2-deoxy-2[^{18}F] fluorodeoxyglucose) PET.[28] Global cerebral activity, and presumably also activity of frontal areas, further declines with deepening NREM sleep,[38] and a deactivated frontal cortex is maintained after the transition from NREM sleep to REM sleep as shown by $H_2^{15}O$ PET,[25,29,33] single photon emission computed tomography (SPECT),[39] and fMRI.[40] Further evidence that frontal deactivation is a general characteristic of sleep comes with the discovery that frontal reactivation lags behind that of the rest of the brain following awakening.[41] Notably, whether one views dreaming as a state of consciousness most fully and characteristically expressed during REM sleep[8,9,17] or as a state subserved more generally by sleep itself,[42,43,44,45] neuroimaging evidence now shows that lateral prefrontal deactivation remains a feature of any sleep state under consideration. This conclusion is reinforced by the fact that lesions of the lateral prefrontal cortices do not cause cessation or attenuation of dreaming.[45,46]

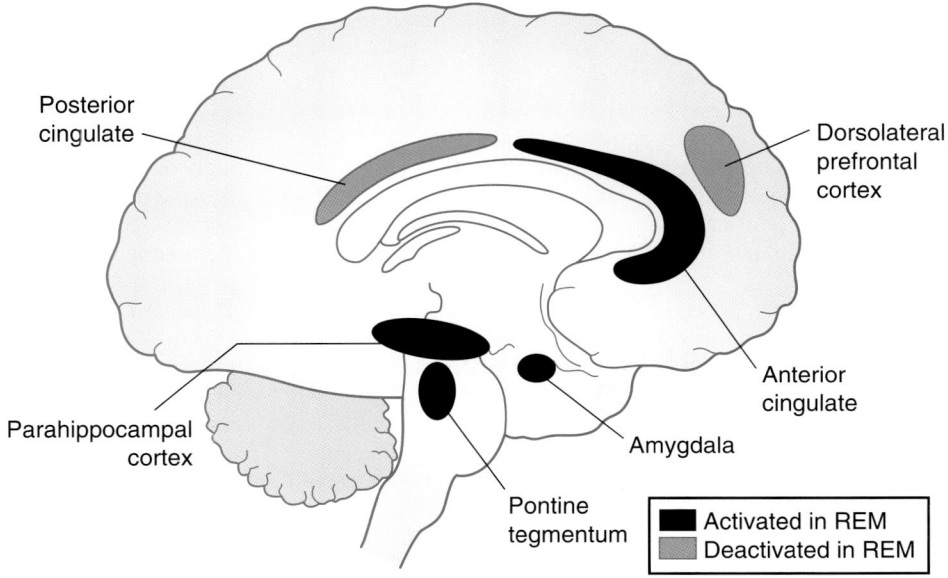

Figure 44–1. Schematic sagittal view of the human brain identifying areas that showed relative activation or deactivation in REM sleep compared to waking and/or NREM sleep in two or more of three PET studies.[25,29,30] A realistic morphology is not implied, only those areas that could be easily matched between two or more studies are depicted, and considerably more extensive areas of activation and deactivation are reported in individual studies. The depicted areas are, therefore, representative portions of larger areas subserving similar functions. (From Hobson JA, Stickgold R, Pace-Schott EF: The neuropsychology of REM sleep dreaming. Neuroreport 1998;9: R1-R14.)

Posterior cingulate

Dorsolateral prefrontal cortex

Anterior cingulate

Amygdala

Parahippocampal cortex

Pontine tegmentum

■ Activated in REM
▨ Deactivated in REM

During waking, the prefrontal cortex serves an executive role, regulating "the selection, timing, monitoring, and interpretation of behavior rather than the formation of the constituent percepts and movements"[47] (p 25), and it does so through the top-down modulation of other brain systems. For example, the frontal cortex regulates and recruits posterior sensory cortices for such specific purposes as novelty detection or sensory processing.[48] With the diminished frontal activation during sleep, frontal regulation of neural circuits subserving attention (fronto-parietal)[2] and memory encoding and retrieval (fronto-temporal)[49] is presumably weakened, and indeed, both attentional and memory processes appear impaired during dreaming.

THE NEUROCHEMISTRY OF DREAMING

Three major hypotheses have been put forward to explain differences between dreaming and waking consciousness in terms of their underlying neurochemistry. The activation-synthesis and AIM (activation-input-modulation) models, proposed by Hobson and colleagues, suggest that the massive increase in cholinergic (relative to noradrenergic and serotonergic) activation in the ascending reticular activating system (ARAS) during REM sleep contributes strongly to the unique nature of dream consciousness.[8,50] A second, neo-Freudian hypothesis, proposed by Solms, suggests that in all stages of sleep, ascending mesocortical and mesolimbic stimulation of limbic reward networks and prefrontal structures by dopaminergic projections from the midbrain ventral tegmental area (VTA) generates motivational impulses that initiate a dream consciousness based upon reward seeking.[45] A third hypothesis, proposed by Gottesmann, suggests that maintained dopaminergic stimulation of the cortex during REM, in the absence of the inhibitory serotonergic and noradrenergic modulation present in waking, allows emergence of the hallucinatory, delusional, and other psychotomimetic aspects of dream consciousness.[51] Pharmacologic influences on dreaming and related states (e.g., hallucinosis) suggest that neuromodulatory systems modulate dream consciousness. Not surprisingly, these systems are also those intimately involved in behavioral state control.

Acetylcholine

The activation-synthesis[50] and AIM[8] models of dreaming suggest that the forebrain activation underlying REM sleep dreaming originates in ascending activation of the thalamus by mesopontine cholinergic nuclei. Thalamic acetylcholine (ACh) of mesopontine origin is present in higher concentrations during waking and REM sleep than in NREM sleep,[52] and a REM-specific increase of ACh in the lateral geniculate body has also been observed.[53] Numerous studies have shown that cholinergic stimulation potentiates REM sleep when microinjected into animal ARAS brainstem nuclei or when systemically administered to humans (for a review, see Hobson et al.[8]). Moreover, cholinergic stimulation with the cholinesterase inhibitor physostigmine has been shown to induce REM sleep with dreaming,[54] and cholinesterase inhibitors such as donepezil have been associated with increased nightmares[55] and hypnogogic hallucinations.[56]

Similarly, nightmares accompany alcohol and benzodiazepine withdrawal,[57] which is associated with REM sleep rebound[8] in which, assuming similarity to normal REM, the major activating influences on the forebrain are cholinergic and dopaminergic.[51,58] Moreover, the most parsimonious explanation for nightmares induced by beta-blockers[59] is disinhibition of cholinergic brainstem REM-generating mechanisms.[57,60]

Nonetheless, the most common pharmacologic trigger for hallucinations is the *hypo*cholinergic state accompanying antimuscarinic delirium or intoxication.[57,61] Similarly, extensive cholinergic deficits may be the cause of visual hallucinations seen in Lewy body dementia.[61] The association of waking hallucinosis with anticholinergic agents and of REM dreaming with a higher ratio of cholinergic to aminergic ARAS activation[8] initially appears paradoxical. However, two lines of evidence suggest that dream and anticholinergic hallucinations may arise from different sources.

First, cholinergic effects, particularly at the cortical level, are complex, regionally specific, and interactive with other neuromodulatory systems. For example, it has long been known that ACh can have either excitatory or inhibitory effects on cortical pyramidal cells.[62] Cholinergic excitation of cortical pyramidal neurons occurs via M1 receptors located on the pyramidal cells, whereas these same neurons are inhibited by ACh via M2 receptors on inhibitory GABAergic (gamma aminobutyric acid–ergic) interneurons.[62]

In this context, Perry and Perry[61] suggest that cortical cholinergic neuromodulation from the basal forebrain (nucleus basalis) excites cortical GABAergic interneurons, increasing inhibition of pyramidal neurons. In contrast, the effects of mesopontine cholinergic modulation on thalamic GABAergic interneurons is inhibitory, resulting in the disinhibition of thalamocortical relay neurons.[61] Indeed, ascending mesopontine cholinergic modulation has been shown to both inhibit GABAergic thalamic reticular neurons and excite thalamocortical relay neurons.[63] Therefore, in waking, ACh increases inhibition of cortical neurons and improves the signal-to-noise ratio at their synapses. In contrast, a reduction in cortical ACh may lead to intrusion of weaker inputs, leading to hallucinosis. Cholinergic activation of the thalamus in REM increases activity in excitatory thalamocortical projections which, in the absence of perceptual input to the cortex, may also favor hallucinosis.[61] Direct cholinergic modulation of excitatory nicotinic receptors, which are more prevalent on thalamocortical than cortical projection neurons, may similarly increase corticopetal activation in REM sleep,[61] and excitation of these thalamic receptors may account for the intensification of dreaming seen in some individuals using nicotine patches for smoking cessation.[64]

In a second line of evidence, Furey et al.[65] found that cholinergic enhancement by physostigmine increased recruitment of posterior (extrastriate) working memory areas while, at the same time, decreasing recruitment of dorsal prefrontal "executive" working memory areas. They suggested that this is due to reduced demand, resulting from cholinergic enhancement of the efficiency of upstream posterior areas. Therefore, during dreaming, a cholinergic bias might enhance extrastriate activity while diminishing frontal activity, as has been noted in neuroimaging studies of REM.[25,29,33] Such conditions would thus contribute to both hallucinosis (extrastriate activation) and deficient insight (frontal deactivation) in REM.

Dopamine

Because dopamine (DA) release does not vary dramatically in phase with the REM-NREM cycle,[66] it has been studied less by sleep and dream researchers. However, given the key role assigned to DA in reward-based[45] and psychotomimetic[51] theories of dreaming, elucidation of this important CNS catecholamine's role in sleep might well have major implications for theories of dream biology. Only recently have behavioral state–related activities of dopamine neurons and their receptors begun to be reported.[67] DA-ACh interactions may also mediate DA's effects on sleep and dreaming. For example, mesopontine cholinergic neurons have been shown to enhance mesolimbic DA release.[68]

Although the dream effects of some dopaminergic drugs can be quite striking, this is by no means the case for all dopamine enhancers.[60] Parkinson's disease patients receiving chronic dopaminergic treatment show intensification of dreams and induction of nightmares, and L-dopa enhances dreaming in persons without Parkinson's, as do certain dopamine agonists and bupropion in clinical patients.[45,59,60] However, the powerful DA reuptake–inhibiting psychostimulants are not associated with dream enhancement; the D2 antagonist neuroleptics do not prevent dreaming; and there are dopamine agonists that reduce dreaming and antagonists that enhance it.[60] Thus it would appear that dopamine's effects on sleep and dreaming are complex, being at least dependent on receptor types and, most likely, on receptor location as well.

Serotonin

Possible effects of serotonin on dreaming are emerging from clinical and experimental reports of the dream intensity–enhancing effects of the selective serotonin reuptake inhibitors (SSRIs).[69] A variety of explanations can be made for this phenomenon, including within-night cholinergic REM rebound, generalized or regional brain activation, de-differentiation of REM-NREM sleep stages, and memory enhancement.[69]

Aghajanian and Marek[70] recently described a mechanism of action of serotonergic hallucinogens. Their work suggests that low or fluctuating cortical serotonin levels, or both, may induce cortical output activity conducive to hallucinosis,[70] and the same may be true of dreaming. The main site of action for indoleamine and phenethylamine hallucinogens is believed to be $5HT_{2A}$ (serotonin-2a) receptors in middle layers of cerebral cortex, where these drugs act as partial serotonin agonists.[70] These hallucinogens are believed to activate presynaptic $5HT_{2A}$ receptors located on excitatory glutamatergic inputs to apical dendrites of layer V neurons, promoting an "asynchronous" release of glutamate from presynaptic terminals.[70] The release develops slowly, after the larger action-potential mediated ("synchronous") release has occurred. This late slow release of glutamate induces prolonged excitatory postsynaptic potentials (EPSPs), which are hypothesized to underlie the cognitive-perceptual effects of the hallucinogens.[70]

While hallucinogens acting upon $5HT_{2A}$ receptors promote asynchronous neurotransmitter-release mediated EPSPs, 5-HT itself does not, presumably due to its actions at other inhibitory sites such as $5HT_1$ receptors.[70] However, under conditions of decreasing 5-HT concentration (as in Aghajanian and Marek's in vivo washout of iontophoretically applied 5-HT), such EPSPs do emerge. These authors speculate that conditions of low 5-HT may generally favor asynchronous transmitter release–evoked EPSPs.[70] The naturally occurring lowest levels of 5-HT occur during REM, whereas fluctuations of 5-HT release occur during sleep stage transitions.[8] Thus, these conditions may promote the natural occurrence of hallucinosis during dreaming.

Multiple Neuromodulatory Systems may Interact in Dreaming

Forebrain activation is maintained and modulated by multiple ascending systems[71,72] and it is most unlikely that global changes in levels of only one neuromodulator can account for any particular state of consciousness. For example, multifactorial etiologies at the neurochemical level are currently invoked for delirium,[57] hallucinosis,[73] and drug-induced nightmares.[59] All of the above modulators may participate in dream biology; given the multitude of pharmacologic agents with dream effects,[59] it is likely that multiple neurochemical systems are involved in the initiation, maintenance, and cessation of dreaming.

NEUROPSYCHIATRIC SYNDROMES THAT INFORM THE STUDY OF DREAMING

Despite striking differences between dreaming and waking experience, the same brain subserves both of these states.[8] It is therefore worthwhile to examine the brain bases of alterations of waking consciousness that shift particular dimensions of waking experiences in the direction of dream experience. This can be done by comparing the phenomenology of dreams with specific neuropsychiatric syndromes,[74] by comparing functional images of the sleeping brain with those of altered waking states,[75] or by comparing waking effects of anatomically localized brain lesions with their effects on dream phenomenology.[45] Table 44–1 illustrates alterations of waking cognition that may help explain certain formal characteristics of dreaming.[58] To exemplify this approach, I will focus upon analogies between dream plots and waking confabulation and between dream hallucinosis and complex visual hallucinations in waking.

Spontaneous Confabulation in Waking and Dreaming

Spontaneous confabulation is associated with lesions involving posterior medial orbitofrontal cortex and its direct and indirect connections with the basal forebrain, amygdala, mediodorsal thalamic nucleus, and hypothalamus.[76] Schneider's theory of the functional neuroanatomy and neuropsychology of such confabulation proposes a reality-monitoring function performed by the caudal medial orbitofrontal cortex and its subcortical limbic connections.[76] This region is hypothesized to preconsciously identify and suppress spontaneously activated memories that do not pertain to the "present" reality (i.e., temporally current facts, plans, and stimuli). Damage to this area would then result in a formal thought disorder in which evoked memories of past experiences are consciously perceived as related to the present and are spoken of (confabulation) and also acted upon as such.

Table 44-1. Neuropsychiatric Syndromes Which Inform the Study of Dreaming

Dream Phenomenon, Symptom, or Syndrome	Waking Symptomatology Resembling Dream Feature	Representative Syndromes Expressing Symptomatology	Brain Substrates of Symptomatology	W: Waking symptom described D: Dreaming phenomenon or symptom described (Reference no.)
Complex, realistic visual hallucinations	Complex visual hallucinosis	Peduncular hallucinosis Charles Bonnet syndrome Hallucinogen intoxication	ARAS/diencephalon Retino-geniculo-striate visual pathway Visual association cortex Serotonergic pathways Cholinergic pathways	W: Manford & Andermann 1998 (73) W: Agajanian & Marek 1999 (70) D: Hobson 2001 (58)
Narrative form with delusionality, disorientation, lost insight, & poor self monitoring	Spontaneous confabulation Disorientation to time	Amnesia with anterior limbic pathology Traumatic brain injury Delirium	Caudomedial OPFC Subcallosal cingulate Basal forebrain Chemical homeostasis	W: Schnider 2003 (76)
Recognition with episodic memory deficits	Relative preservation of recognition memory	Amnesias: Medial temporal Diencephalic	Hippocampal complex Parahippocampal cortices Diencephalic pathways	W: Brown & Aggleton 2001 (91) D: Fosse et al 2003 (3)
Emotional alterations Intensification Blunting	Lability/reactivity, apathy/hypoemotionality	Dorsolateral PFC or OPFC lesion Psychosis Mood disorders Anxiety disorders	Caudomedial OPFC Subcallosal cingulate Amygdala Dorsolateral PFC	W: Liotti et al 2000 (104) D: Hobson et al 2000 (8)
Visual distortions	Visual distortions: Micro/macropsia, polyopsia, achromatopsia	Visual cortex lesions	Visual association cortices Anterior occipital Inferior temporal Feature specific (V4, MT)	D, W: Schwartz & Maquet 2002 (74)
Nonvisual dreams	Visual irreminiscence	Temporo-occipital lesion	Visual association cortices	D, W: Solms 1997 (45)
Erroneous identification Visual hallucinosis Delusionality	Misidentification of person or place	Capgras delusion Fregoli syndrome, reduplicative paramnesia	Ventral temporal cortex Fusiform face area Prefrontal cortex Limbic system (e.g., amygdala)	D, W: Schwartz & Maquet 2002 (74)
Reciprocal frequency of thought and hallucination	Acute hallucinosis and disorientation	Delirium Acute psychosis Epileptic ictus	Chemical homeostasis Visual association cortices ARAS/diencephalon Limbic subcortex Prefrontal cortex	D: Fosse et al 2000 (105)
Bizarreness Incongruity Discontinuity Ad-hoc explanation	Impaired working memory and attention Delusion-based logic	Dorsolateral PFC lesion Psychosis	Dorsolateral PFC PGO system Mesocortical DA system	D: Hobson et al 2000 (8) Hobson 1988 (50)

ARAS, ascending reticular activating system; DA, dopamine system; MT, motion specific visual association area; PFC, prefrontal cortex; OPFC, orbital prefrontal cortex; PGO, ponto-geniculo-occipital wave; V4, color specific visual association area.

This failure to suppress elements of memory salient to past, rather than current, experiences has been demonstrated in spontaneous confabulators using continuous recognition tasks.[76] Experimental findings support clinical observation that errors made by spontaneous confabulators are almost always linked to past experiences admixing with current events and that their belief in the veracity of their errors is unshakable.[76] When lesions extend into ventromedial prefrontal cortex and adjacent subcortical structures, wake-dream confusional states can accompany the spontaneous confabulation.[45]

There are obvious formal similarities between the lack of insight in spontaneous confabulation and the observations, in dreaming, of single-mindedness and isolation,[1] disorientation to time, and delusional acceptance of the dream as reality.[8,50,58] However, there are additional "positive symptoms" in dreams. Unlike spontaneous confabulation, dreaming involves actual hallucinosis of its pseudosensory elements and wholly novel elements,[50] whereas spontaneous confabulation invariably relates to patients' past experience.[76]

Paradoxically, the brain areas whose damage leads to spontaneous confabulation broadly overlap with Nofzinger's anterior paralimbic REM activation area[30,31] and with limbic and paralimbic structures showing enhanced activity in REM.[25,29] Thus, *hyper*activation of these anterior limbic areas in REM may also alter their reality-monitoring functions in ways similar to those resulting from anterior limbic damage in confabulatory[76] and dream-wake confusional[45] syndromes. Indeed, abnormal activation of anterior limbic structures can profoundly alter consciousness.[77] One possible explanation of this apparent paradox is that the predominantly cholinergic nature of the ascending REM activation, together with the absence of the monoaminergic modulation normally present in waking, impairs the reality-testing capability of anterior limbic regions.

Visual Hallucinosis in Waking and Dreaming

There is a striking overlap between the anatomical regions implicated in dreaming and those associated with complex visual hallucinosis in waking. In a recent review, Manford and Andermann[73] note three conditions resulting in complex visual hallucinations: disruption of primary visual pathways (e.g., retina or V1), disruption of ascending upper brainstem reticular activation pathways, and irritative (e.g., epileptic) influences impinging on visual association areas. A common mechanism for the first two of these is the abnormal release of visual association cortices from restraints acting upon them, a release caused either by disruption of exogenous sensory inputs or by alteration of rostral brainstem serotonergic and cholinergic inputs to the thalamus and cortex.[73]

Manford and Andermann[73] suggest that a common target for all causes of complex visual hallucinosis is the ventral stream visual association cortices in the inferior occipital and temporal lobes. These regions have been shown to be more active in REM than in either NREM or postsleep waking,[25,33] and they are hypothesized to be a major source of dream imagery in two current neurobiologic models of dreaming.[8,45]

There is clear evidence for parallel mechanisms of hallucinosis during REM, corresponding to each of Manford and Andermann's mechanisms. In their first case, damage to the primary visual pathway can result in complex visual hallucinosis in waking, an outcome seen with Charles Bonnet syndrome, striate cortex lesions, and lesions of other portions of the retino-geniculo-striate pathway.[73] In dreaming, there is no retinal input to the geniculate, producing a condition similar to those described earlier, in which only pseudosensory visual inputs can reach visual cortices.[50] Furthermore, in REM sleep, primary visual cortices are deactivated relative to waking,[33] perhaps producing a condition akin to that seen in waking with striate cortex lesions.

Their second case is exemplified by peduncular hallucinosis, in which lesions of the rostral brainstem and diencephalon disrupt ascending reticular arousal systems, including the serotonergic and cholinergic projections from mesopontine nuclei.[73] The resulting pathological imbalances between these systems may predispose patients with rostral brainstem lesions to peduncular hallucinosis in waking.[73] The normal firing of serotonergic raphe neurons is at its naturally occurring minimum during REM sleep, when mesopontine cholinergic systems have reactivated to near waking levels.[8] This altered serotonergic-cholinergic balance during REM sleep relative to waking may therefore favor hallucinosis by mechanisms similar to those active during waking in peduncular hallucinosis.

Finally, irritative excitatory influences acting directly on the extrastriate cortex during waking produce complex hallucinosis in epilepsy,[73] and visual association areas are also active during waking hallucinations in Charles Bonnet syndrome.[78] During REM sleep, the visual cortex of the cat is indirectly activated by ponto-geniculo-occipital (PGO) waves originating in the mesopontine brainstem,[8] and similar waves probably occur during REM sleep in humans.[21,35,35a] These ascending PGO waves simultaneously activate many regions of the cerebral cortex,[79] most likely including visual association areas. Thus PGO waves could directly provoke complex hallucinosis,[73] especially in REM sleep, when there is both diminished striate input to extrastriate regions[33] and altered serotonergic-cholinergic balance,[8] two additional hallucinogenic conditions.[73]

DESCRIPTIVE MODEL OF NEURONAL NETWORKS GENERATING DREAM PHENOMENOLOGY

Behavioral states and cognitive capacities are physically instantiated in widely distributed networks with distinct epicenters of critical control in a pattern of "selectively distributed processing."[2] A working model of neurobiological structures and networks subserving REM-sleep dream phenomenology[8] is described here. These putative REM-active networks may also help explain NREM dreaming, and such elements relevant to NREM dreaming are emphasized in the first two sections. The following description refers to specific brain areas depicted in Figure 44–2.

Ascending Arousal Systems

Activation of the forebrain in REM sleep, as in waking, occurs through the ascending arousal systems of the brainstem ARAS,[63] basal forebrain,[80] and hypothalamus (areas 1 and 2 in Figure 44–2).[72] However, unlike in waking, ascending activation in REM sleep is primarily facilitated by cholinergic systems, whereas serotonergic, noradrenergic, and histaminergic neuromodulation are all drastically attenuated.[8,72]

FOREBRAIN PROCESSES IN NORMAL DREAMING-INTEGRATED MODEL

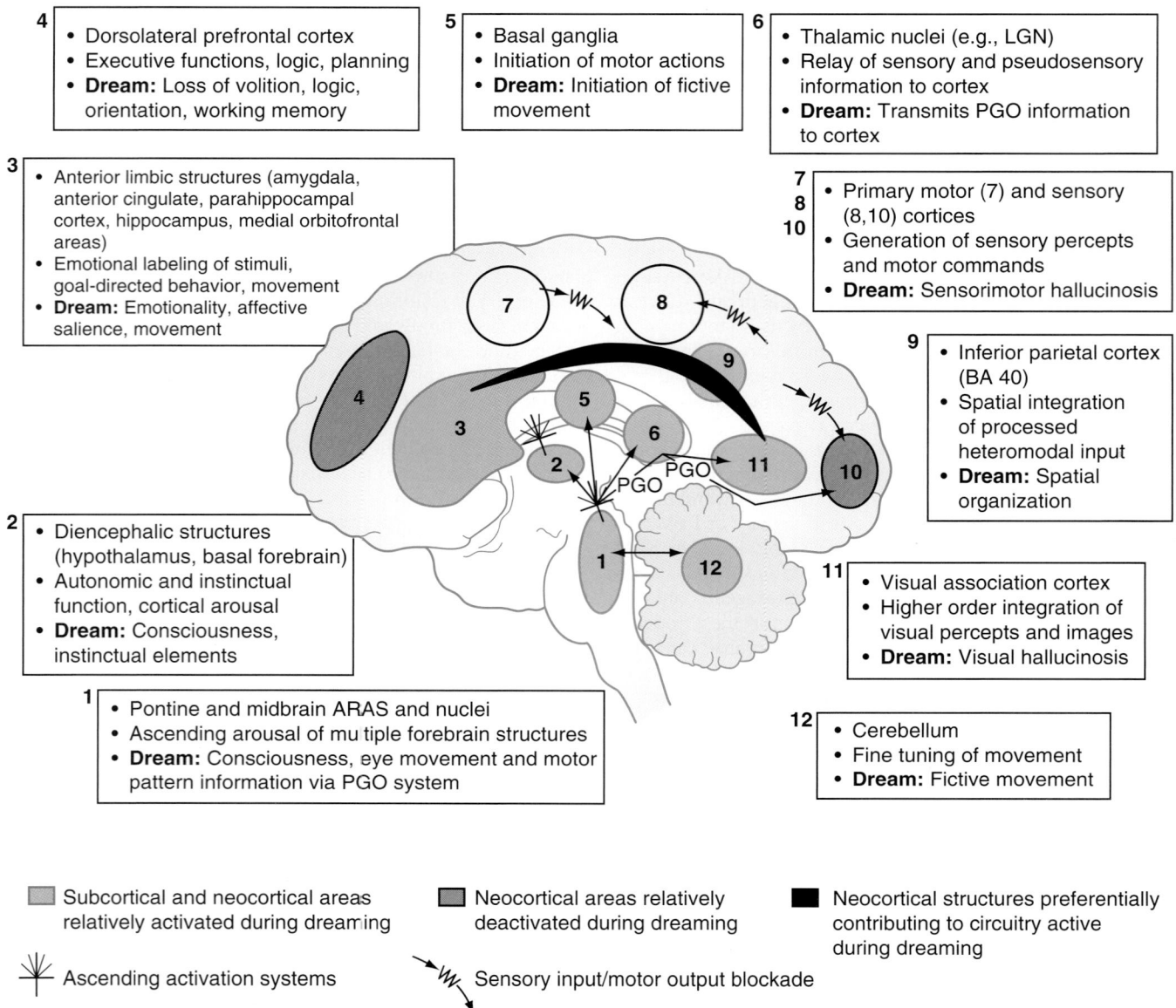

4
- Dorsolateral prefrontal cortex
- Executive functions, logic, planning
- **Dream:** Loss of volition, logic, orientation, working memory

5
- Basal ganglia
- Initiation of motor actions
- **Dream:** Initiation of fictive movement

6
- Thalamic nuclei (e.g., LGN)
- Relay of sensory and pseudosensory information to cortex
- **Dream:** Transmits PGO information to cortex

3
- Anterior limbic structures (amygdala, anterior cingulate, parahippocampal cortex, hippocampus, medial orbitofrontal areas)
- Emotional labeling of stimuli, goal-directed behavior, movement
- **Dream:** Emotionality, affective salience, movement

7 8 10
- Primary motor (7) and sensory (8,10) cortices
- Generation of sensory percepts and motor commands
- **Dream:** Sensorimotor hallucinosis

9
- Inferior parietal cortex (BA 40)
- Spatial integration of processed heteromodal input
- **Dream:** Spatial organization

2
- Diencephalic structures (hypothalamus, basal forebrain)
- Autonomic and instinctual function, cortical arousal
- **Dream:** Consciousness, instinctual elements

11
- Visual association cortex
- Higher order integration of visual percepts and images
- **Dream:** Visual hallucinosis

1
- Pontine and midbrain ARAS and nuclei
- Ascending arousal of multiple forebrain structures
- **Dream:** Consciousness, eye movement and motor pattern information via PGO system

12
- Cerebellum
- Fine tuning of movement
- **Dream:** Fictive movement

Subcortical and neocortical areas relatively activated during dreaming

Neocortical areas relatively deactivated during dreaming

Neocortical structures preferentially contributing to circuitry active during dreaming

Ascending activation systems

Sensory input/motor output blockade

Figure 44–2. Forebrain processes in normal dreaming, an integration of neurophysiologic, neuropsychological, and neuroimaging data. Regions 1 and 2, ascending arousal systems; region 3, subcortical and cortical limbic and paralimbic structures; region 4, dorsolateral prefrontal executive association cortex; region 5, motor initiation and control centers; region 6, thalamocortical relay centers and thalamic subcortical circuitry; region 7, primary motor cortex; region 8, primary sensory cortex; region 9, inferior parietal lobe; region 10, primary visual cortex; region 11, visual association cortex; region 12, cerebellum. (From Hobson JA, Pace-Schott EF, Stickgold R: Consciousness: Its vicissitudes in waking and sleep. In Gazzaniga M [ed]: The New Cognitive Neurosciences, 2nd ed. Cambridge, Mass, MIT Press, 2000, pp 1341-1354.)

The deepening of NREM sleep, characterized by the progressive slowing of EEG frequencies and decreases in global brain metabolism,[81] has been shown in animals to be accompanied by decreased firing rate of ARAS neurons in the locus coeruleus, raphe, pedunculopontine tegmental (PPT) nucleus, and laterodorsal tegmental (LDT) nucleus.[82] Hence, ARAS supports consciousness in both waking and REM sleep, and it may also transiently do so during NREM sleep. Phasic increases either in endogenous and exogenous stimuli or in autonomic activity might transiently enhance ARAS activity, stimulating the same rostral networks activated by ARAS activity in REM sleep and waking. Recent PET data have shown NREM-related metabolic increases in some of the same subcortical limbic areas that become highly active in REM sleep.[28] Hence, just as the ARAS supports consciousness in waking and REM sleep, it may also transiently do so in NREM sleep, the subjective manifestation of which may be NREM dreaming.

Thalamocortical Relay Centers and Thalamic Subcortical Circuitry

During REM sleep, activated thalamic nuclei (area 6 in Figure 44–2) transmit endogenous stimuli to the cortex, leading to the sensory phenomena of dreaming. In NREM sleep, intrinsic thalamocortical oscillations suppress but do not completely extinguish perception and mentation.[83]

During NREM sleep, both tonic (e.g., delta and slow rhythms) and phasic (e.g., spindles and K-complexes) oscillatory rhythms represent endogenous activity of corticocortical and thalamocortical circuits.[63] The slow cortical oscillations reflect the alternation of prolonged hyperpolarization and intense firing of spike trains among cortical neurons.[63] Steriade has suggested that when this oscillatory pattern is impinged upon by phasic thalamocortical bursts, such as the isolated PGO waves during the period leading up to REM sleep, transient elevations of regional activity may lead to vivid visual imagery outside REM sleep.[84] Activation in NREM sleep of striate[33,38] and extrastriate[28] areas may be manifestations of such a process.

Any phasic thalamocortical signal can, theoretically, produce a regional impact on the slowly oscillating burst-primed cortex, which may explain the experimental induction of NREM imagery by visual and auditory stimulation.[18] Such thalamocortical signaling may be interpreted as incoming sensory stimuli (as proposed in the original activation synthesis model), may evoke local activation of stored cognitive representations (hallucinosis of known entities), or may evoke generation of novel representations in association cortices (as in dream bizarreness). Such events may occur with greater relative frequency in REM sleep than in NREM sleep (as is known to be the case for PGO waves) and therefore evoke more frequent or sustained dreaming in REM sleep than in NREM sleep. Such phasic, transient elevations of reticulo-thalamo-cortical arousal may be prime examples of Nielsen's covert REM.[9]

Subcortical and Cortical Limbic and Paralimbic Structures

Medial forebrain structures, especially limbic and paralimbic areas of the cortex and subcortex (area 3 in Figure 44–2), are selectively activated during REM sleep.[25,29,30,33] This activation may underlie dream emotionality[8,25,34] and explain the highly social nature of dreaming.[75,85] Activated limbic structures include the amygdala, which affectively labels stimuli,[86] and the anterior cingulate cortices, which participate in emotional cognition, error detection, conflict monitoring, and affect-related premotor functions.[87] Portions of the medial orbitofrontal and insular cortices are also activated.[25,30]

The role of medial anterior limbic areas in confabulatory behavior was described in detail earlier. It is worth noting here that these ventromedial prefrontal areas are also recruited during emotional and social cognition.[88,89] Anecdotal reports suggest that "theory of mind," a complex aspect of social cognition,[89] is preserved in dreaming in the face of notable degradation of physicalistic reasoning.[75]

The hippocampal formation collaborates with the amygdala to mediate storage of emotional memories in waking,[90] and reactivation of these areas may allow readout of emotionally salient memory fragments in REM sleep. Specific veridical episodic memories have been shown to be remarkably rare in dreams and account for less than 2% of dream elements retrospectively ascribed to waking experience by the dreamer.[3] In REM, a cholinergically mediated informational barrier between cortex and hippocampus,[3] possibly combined with impaired episodic retrieval associated with prefrontal hypoactivity (see ref. 49), may underlie this phenomenon.

Despite this inaccessibility of episodic memory in dreams, another aspect of declarative memory, "familiarity" or "recognition,"[91] is ubiquitous in dreams. For example, up to 40% of dream characters are identified on the basis of "just knowing."[85] Schwartz and Maquet[74] liken this common dream phenomenon to a waking neurologic disorder, Fregoli's syndrome, and hypothesize that a sleep-related disconnection of temporal face recognition from prefrontal reality monitoring areas underlies this dream phenomenon.

Alternatively, frequent experiences of familiarity in the absence of veridical episodic memories in dreams may reflect activity of recognition memory mechanisms in anterior perirhinal cortices (Brodman area [BA] 35, 36), where recognition memory-related activation has been shown in human fMRI studies.[91] Since these perirhinal areas are proximal to the anterior paralimbic REM-activation area[30] and a delusional sense of familiarity occurs both in dreaming and in brain-damaged patients (reduplicative paramnesia),[74] altered activity in these systems during REM sleep may produce a dissociation between episodic recall (hippocampal) and recognition (perirhinal) components of declarative memory.

Motor Initiation and Control Centers

Strong activation of the basal ganglia[25] (area 5 in Figure 44–2) may mediate the ubiquitous fictive motion of dreams.[92] The basal ganglia are extensively connected with REM regulatory areas in the mesopontine tegmentum,[93] which contain gait circuitry and other motor-pattern generators.[8] Activation of brainstem vestibular nuclei and the associated cerebellar vermis[25] during REM fictive movement (double-head arrow between areas 1 and 12 in Fig. 44–2) may additionally contribute vestibular sensations interpreted as flying or falling as well as to a sense of motor control. In a similar manner, hypothalamic-brainstem circuits may initiate instinctively salient behavior in dreaming,[94] which may, in turn, recruit additional forebrain regions to enact appetitive[45] or other behaviors that have adaptive significance in waking.[94]

Visual Association Cortex

Occipito-temporal visual association cortices (area 11 in Figure 44–2) are activated in REM sleep,[25,33] and may generate the visual imagery of dreams.[8,45] As in waking, specific areas of the visual association cortex may process specific visual characteristics of dreaming. For example, the fusiform gyrus both mediates waking face recognition[95] and is selectively activated in REM sleep.[25,30,33] Braun and coworkers[33] suggest that REM constitutes a unique cortical condition of internal information processing (between extrastriate and limbic cortices) that is functionally isolated from input (via striate cortex) or output (via frontal cortex) to the external world. As noted earlier, reticular activation of thalamic and basal forebrain cholinergic nuclei may transmit ascending reticular activation to diverse targets in occipital, temporal, and inferior parietal visual and heteromodal association areas, contributing to formation of dream images.

Inferior Parietal Lobe

The supramarginal and angular gyri of the inferior parietal lobe (BA 40, 39; area 9 in Figure 44–2), especially in the right hemisphere, are essential for visuospatial awareness.[2]

These areas may, therefore, generate the fictive dream space necessary for the organized hallucinatory experience of dreaming.[45] Destruction of these areas alone is sufficient to produce global cessation of dreaming.[45,46] It is notable that the right inferior parietal cortex is relatively activated in REM sleep[29] and is also the area where the brain is most vulnerable to persistent dream cessation following damage.[45]

Posterior association cortices may, by themselves, be able to generate hallucinatory story-like material with organized plots integrated with visuospatial imagery. Posterior cortical activation may result, as in waking, from ascending ARAS and diencephalic arousal systems (pontine and midbrain ARAS, basal forebrain), which are known to increase their activity in REM sleep.[25,29] The subsequent integration of dream elements from activated unimodal sensory association cortices may take place, as in waking, in heteromodal association cortices of the inferior parietal cortex. Thus, there would appear to be no need for the back-projection of appetitive impulses hypothesized by Solms.[45]

Therefore, the widespread deactivation of prefrontal regions seen in REM sleep[25,29] may play a *permissive* role in the generation of dreams. Regulation of posterior sensory cortices is a widely accepted "executive" function of the prefrontal cortices,[47,48] which are reciprocally connected with all such posterior regions.[96] The sensory and narrative aspects of dreaming may thus, in part, result from the *disconnection, release,* or *disinhibition* of these posterior cortical regions.

Dorsolateral Prefrontal Executive Association Cortex

The dorsolateral prefrontal cortex (DLPFC; area 4 in Figure 44–2) and the more ventral portions of the frontal convexity are deactivated relative to waking at sleep onset and during NREM sleep.[24,25,27,33,38] Unlike the more medial proisocortical regions, which reactivate during REM sleep, these areas remain deactivated in REM sleep.[25,29,33] This maintained deactivation of isocortical areas of the frontal convexity could explain the prominent executive deficiencies of dream mentation, which include disorientation, illogic, impaired working memory, and amnesia for dreams.[8]

Hypothesized Dynamic Interactions of Brain Regions during REM Dreaming

In summary, ascending reticulo-thalamic, thalamocortical, and basal forebrain–cortical arousal systems activate the forebrain regions involved in dream construction in a manner that is chemically and anatomically different from waking. In REM sleep, such activation may be more frequent, be more sustained, and, perhaps, proceed via different or more diverse pathways than in NREM sleep. Cortical circuits activated in REM dreaming are medial circuits linking posterior association and paralimbic areas (central crescent in Figure 44–2) but not the primary sensory and lateral frontal executive cortical regions, which are active in waking.[33] Therefore, dreaming is emotionally salient (amygdala?), often conflictual (anterior cingulate?), and social (ventromedial prefrontal areas?) while also displaying profoundly deficient working memory, orientation, and logic (DLPFC deactivation?).

Subcortical circuits involving the limbic structures, basal ganglia, diencephalon, and brainstem regions are selectively activated in REM. These may contribute to dreaming's emotional (limbic subcortex), motoric (basal ganglia, brainstem, cerebellum), instinctual (hypothalamus), and motivational (midbrain-ventral striatum) properties, and probably to many other dream elements as well.

Activity patterns that differentiate REM sleep from waking, such as the anterior paralimbic REM activation area[30,31] and selective limbic and extrastriate activity,[33] reflect differential activity in REM sleep and waking of cortico-cortical and cortico-subcortical networks. These are networks that are intimately involved in the cognitive functions that show marked differences between waking and dreaming.

Based upon dream phenomenology, PET images of the human brain during REM sleep, and animal studies in sleep and waking, the following dream-wake differences in cortico-subcortical circuits might be hypothesized:

- DLPFC deactivation may reflect underactivity of the "cognitive" fronto-striatal-thalamo-cortical circuit (linking DLPFC with dorsal striatum) relative to "affective" (orbitofrontal–ventral caudate) and "motivational" (anterior cingulate–nucleus accumbens) circuits.[97]
- Interactions between the amygdala and orbitofrontal cortex, which serve as an integrated unit in the processing and regulation of affect in waking,[98] may be relatively disinhibited or facilitated during dreaming.
- The imbalance of recognition over recall memory in dreams suggests that perirhinal interactions with orbitofrontal areas may be more active than hippocampal interactions with these same areas during dreaming.[91]
- In dreaming, cortico-ponto-cerebello-thalamo-cortical loops[99] involving limbic cortices may be relatively more active than circuits involving other association cortices (e.g., DLPFC).

As one network example, Stickgold[100] suggests that the anterior cingulate, which elevates noradrenergic alerting of the DLPFC by the locus coeruleus in the face of conflict in waking, cannot similarly increase attentional effort during REM sleep, and therefore dream bizarreness is not detected but affective salience is maintained.

Prefrontal areas themselves are intimately interconnected,[96] as they are with diverse areas of the posterior sensory and limbic cortex.[96] This interconnectivity, combined with the known role of prefrontal cortices in regulating posterior regions,[47,48] suggests that the release of posterior cortices (e.g., visual association cortex) from frontal inhibition may be a prerequisite of dreaming.

REM PHYSIOLOGY AND MODELS OF DREAMING

In recent decades, a variety of cognitive and neurocognitive models of dreaming have been advanced that specifically question theories based upon observations of REM sleep physiology in animals and humans such as activation-synthesis and AIM.[42,43,44,45] Such critiques usually focus on the non-exclusive relationship between REM sleep and dreaming, and they propose instead more rostrally based dream initiation mechanisms varying from the midbrain[45] to the cerebral cortex itself.[42]

But one can embrace the activation-synthesis model's approach of studying REM sleep physiology to inform dream theory while simultaneously acknowledging that dreaming *can* occur in NREM sleep and that the forebrain *is* required for dreams to occur. One approach to such a reconciliation is the "covert REM" hypothesis of Nielsen,[9] which suggests that various elements of REM processing occur transiently in NREM sleep, supporting NREM dreaming.

A second approach emphasizes that brainstem circuits controlling the alternation of REM and NREM sleep are not proposed to be the sole *informational source* of dream mentation even in the original activation synthesis model of Hobson and McCarley.[101] Instead, activation-synthesis–based models, such as the one described above, propose that in dreaming, just as in waking, the brainstem ARAS and closely associated hypothalamic and basal forebrain nuclei activate the forebrain both generally and in region-specific and modality-specific patterns.

Given these caveats, the neural pathways of REM sleep that contribute to dreaming can be summarized as follows. Cortical activation in REM sleep is preceded by cholinergic activation of the diencephalon, since the Ch5 (pedunculo-pontine) and Ch6 (laterodorsal tegmental) mesopontine cholinergic neurons project to the thalamus but not to the cortex itself.[102] Activation of the thalamus in REM sleep also results from cholinergic inhibition of GABAergic reticular nucleus neurons, which inhibit other nonspecific and relay thalamic nuclei.[63] Therefore, much of thalamocortical activation in REM sleep (as in waking) is glutamatergic.

The lateral geniculate component of the PGO wave is only one modality-specific relay pathway by which the cholinergically excited thalamus might activate its cortical targets in REM sleep.[63,79] In addition to relay pathways of other sensory modalities, thalamocortical activation in REM sleep might involve nonrelay, modality-specific projections from the pulvinar to extrastriate cortex, limbic-related projections from mediodorsal nucleus to prefrontal targets, or widespread activating projections of intralaminar and midline nuclei.

Separate from these thalamic pathways, ascending reticular activation in REM sleep may proceed via a ventral cholinergic route leading from the brainstem to the basal forebrain as suggested by Braun et al.[25] Extensive bidirectional connectivity exists from the LDT and PPT to basal forebrain nuclei, such as the nucleus basalis[80] which, in turn, projects cholinergically to regionally specific areas of the cortex.[61,102]

Finally, midbrain VTA sources of mesolimbic and mesocortical dopamine are also recruited by ascending cholinergic activation (see earlier). This extensive mesopontine-diencephalic connectivity, along with the especially dense cholinergic innervation of limbic cortex and subcortex,[61] is anatomically consistent with the anterior paralimbic REM activation area.[30,31] Moreover, this REM activation area encompasses, but is by no means restricted to, the ventral striatal (e.g., nucleus accumbens) areas that Solms[45] suggests are involved in dream instigation.

CONCLUSION AND SYNTHESIS

From both a phenomenological and neurobiological perspective, dreaming is multidimensional and can be seen from many divergent theoretical viewpoints. Among cognitive theories, dreaming can simultaneously be seen as the complex cognitive process developing over the lifespan invoked by Foulkes,[44] the multilayered, nondegenerate consciousness argued by Kahan and LaBerge[103] *and* the profoundly altered, nonwake-like and psychotomimetic conscious state described by Hobson and colleagues.[8,50,58] Among neurocognitive theories, dreaming is *both* the product of ascending activation of the cortex by brainstem and diencephalic reticulo-thalamic and basal forebrain influences,[8] as well as the neocortical networks that elaborate its actual conscious experience.[42,45] With the explosive growth of neuroimaging technologies,[35a] the cognitive neurosciences, and behavioral neurology, any dream model must continually transform and evolve as new discoveries emerge.

> *Clinical Pearl*
>
> *The physician prescribing selective serotonin reuptake inhibitors, transdermal nicotine, beta-blockers, dopaminergic agents, or a variety of other medications*[59] *should be alert for possible dream intensification or nightmare induction. Although the percentage risks of such side effects for each particular medication are uncertain, patient reports are not uncommon. Other choices within the same class or a different class of medication may need to be considered if the patient finds such side effects intolerable.*

Acknowledgment

The author acknowledges support for this research from the National Institute on Drug Abuse DA11744.

References

1. Rechtschaffen A: The single-mindedness and isolation of dreams. Sleep 1978;1:97-109.
2. Mesulam M-M: From sensation to cognition. Brain 1998;121:1013-1052.
3. Fosse M, Fosse R, Hobson JA, et al: Dreaming and episodic memory: A functional dissociation? J Cog Neurosci 2003;15:1-9.
4. Dorus E, Dorus W, Rechtschaffen A: The incidence of novelty in dreams. Arch Gen Psychiatry 1971;25:364-368.
5. Dement W, Kleitman N: The relation of eye movements during sleep to dream activity: An objective method for the study of dreaming. J Exp Psychol 1957;53:339-346.
6. Foulkes D: Dream reports from different stages of sleep. J Abnorm Soc Psychol 1962;65:14-25.
7. Antrobus JS: REM and NREM sleep reports: Comparison of word frequencies by cognitive classes. Psychophysiol 1983;20:562-568.
8. Hobson JA, Pace-Schott EF, Stickgold R: Dreaming and the brain: Toward a cognitive neuroscience of conscious states. Behav Brain Sci 2000;23:793-842.
9. Nielsen TA: Mentation in REM and NREM sleep: A review and possible reconciliation of two models. Behav Brain Sci 2000;23:851-866.
10. Gross DW, Gotman J: Correlation of high-frequency oscillations with the sleep-wake cycle and cognitive activity in humans. Neuroscience 1999;94:1005-1018.
11. Llinas R, Ribary U: Coherent 40-Hz oscillation characterizes dream state in humans. Proc Nat Acad Sci U S A 1993;90:2078-2081.
12. Tallon-Baudry C, Bertrand O: Oscillatory gamma activity in humans and its role in object representation. Trend Cog Sci 1999;3:151-162.

13. Kahn D, Pace-Schott EF, Hobson JA: Consciousness in waking and dreaming: The roles of neuronal oscillation and neuromodulation in determining similarities and differences. Neuroscience 1997;78:13-38.

14. Perez-Garcia E, del Rio-Portilla Y, Guevara MA, et al: Paradoxical sleep is characterized by uncoupled gamma activity between frontal and perceptual cortical regions. Sleep 2001;24:118-126.

15. Achermann P, Borbely AA: Low frequency (<1 Hz) oscillations in the human sleep electroencephalogram. Neuroscience 1997;81:213-222.

16. Steriade M, Contreras D, Dossi C, et al: The slow (<1 Hz) oscillation in reticular thalamic and thalamocortical neurons: Scenario of sleep rhythm generation in interacting thalamic and neocortical networks. J Neurosci 1993;13:3284-3299.

17. Takeuchi T, Ogilvie RD, Murphy TI, et al: EEG activities during elicited sleep onset REM and NREM periods reflect diferent mechanisms of dream generation. Clin Neurophysiol 2003; 114:210-220.

18. Conduit R, Bruck D, Coleman G: Induction of visual imagery during NREM sleep. Sleep 1997;20:948-956.

19. Conduit R, Crewther SG, Bruck D, et al: Spontaneous eyelid movements during human sleep: A possible ponto-geniculo-occipital analogue? J Sleep Res 2002;11:95-104.

20. McCarley RW, Winkelman JW, Duffy H: Human cerebral potentials associated with REM sleep rapid eye movements: Links to PGO waves and waking potentials. Brain Res 1983;274:359-364.

21. Peigneux P, Laureys S, Fuchs S: Generation of rapid eye movements during paradoxical sleep in humans. Neuroimage 2001; 14:701-708.

21a. Conduit R, Crewther SG, Coleman G: Spontaneous eyelid movements (ELMS) during sleep are related to dream recall on awakening. J Sleep Res 2004;13:137-144.

22. Perrin F, Bastuji H, Garcia-Larrea L: Detection of verbal discordances during sleep. Neuroreport 2002;13:1345-1349.

23. Stickgold R, Scott L, Rittenhouse et al: Sleep induced changes in associative memory. J Cog Neurosci 1999;11:182-193.

24. Maquet P, Degueldre C, Delfiore G. et al: Functional neuroanatomy of human slow wave sleep. J Neurosci 1997;17:2807-2812.

25. Braun AR, Balkin TJ, Wesensten NJ, et al: Regional cerebral blood flow throughout the sleep-wake cycle. Brain 1997;120:1173-1197.

26. Kajimura N, Uchiyama M, Takayama Y, et al: Activity of midbrain reticular formation and neocortex during the progression of human non-rapid eye movement sleep. J Neurosci 1999;19: 10065-10073.

27. Kjaer TW, Law I, Wiltschiotz G, et al: Regional cerebral blood flow during light sleep—a $H_2^{15}O$-PET study. J Sleep Res 2002; 11:201-207.

28. Nofzinger EA, Buysse DJ, Miewald JM, et al: Human regional cerebral glucose metabolism during non-rapid eye movement sleep in relation to waking. Brain 2002;125:1105-1115.

29. Maquet P, Peters JM, Aerts J, et al: Functional neuroanatomy of human rapid-eye-movement sleep and dreaming. Nature 1996; 383:163-166.

30. Nofzinger EA, Mintun MA, Wiseman MB, et al: Forebrain activation in REM sleep: An FDG PET study. Brain Res 1997; 770:192-201.

31. Nofzinger EA, Nichols TE, Meltzer CC, et al: Changes in forebrain function from waking to REM sleep in depression: Preliminary analysis of [18F] FDG PET studies. Psychiat Res Neuroimag.1999;91:59-78.

32. Wu J, Buchsbaum MS, Gillin JC, et al: Prediction of antidepressant effects of sleep deprivation by metabolic rates in the ventral anterior cingulate and the medial prefrontal cortex. Am J Psychiat 1999;56:1149-1158.

33. Braun AR, Balkin TJ, Wesensten NJ, et al: Dissociated pattern of activity in visual cortices and their projections during human rapid eye-movement sleep. Science 1998;279:91-95.

34. Maquet P, Franck G: REM Sleep and the amygdala. Mol Psychiatry 1997;2:195-196.

35. Inoue S, Saha UK, Musha T: Spatio-temporal distribution of neuronal activities and REM sleep. In Mallick BN, Inoue S (eds): Rapid Eye Movement Sleep. New York, Marcel Dekker, 1999, pp 214-220.

35a. Ioannides AA, Corsi-Cabrera M, Fenwick PBC, et al: MEG tomography of human cortex and brainstem activity in waking and REM sleep saccades. Cereb Cortex 2004;14:56-72.

36. Finelli LA, Borbely AA, Achermann P: Functional topography of the human nonREM sleep electroencephalogram. Eur J Neurosci 2001;13:2282-2290.

37. Werth E, Achermann P, Borbely AA: Fronto-occipital EEG power gradients in human sleep. J Sleep Res 1997;6: 102-112.

38. Hofle N, Paus T, Reutens D, et al: Regional cerebral blood flow changes as a function of delta and spindle activity during slow wave sleep in humans. J Neurosci 1997;17: 4800-4808.

39. Madsen PC, Holm S, Vorstup S, et al: Human regional cerebral blood flow during rapid eye movement sleep. J Cereb Blood Flow Met 1991;11:502-507.

40. Lovblad KO, Thomas R, Jakob PM, et al: Silent functional magnetic resonance imaging demonstrates focal activation in rapid eye movement sleep. Neurology 1999;53:2193-2195.

41. Balkin TJ, Braun AR, Wesensten NJ, et al: The process of awakening: A PET study of regional brain activity patterns mediating the reestablishment of alertness and consciousness. Brain 2002;125:2308-2319.

42. Antrobus JS: The neurocognition of sleep mentation: Rapid eye movements, visual imagery, and dreaming. In Bootzin R, Kihlstrom J, Schacter D (eds): Sleep and Cognition. Washington, DC, American Psychological Association, 1990, pp 3-24.

43. Domhoff GW: A new neurocognitive theory of dreams. Dreaming 2001;11:13-33.

44. Foulkes D: Dream research 1953-1993. Sleep 1996;19: 609-624.

45. Solms M: The Neuropsychology of Dreams: A Clinico-Anatomical Study. Mahwah, NJ, Erlbaum, 1997.

46. Doricchi F, Violani C: Dream recall in brain-damaged patients: A contribution to the neuropsychology of dreaming through a review of the literature. In Antrobus JS, Bertini M (eds): The Neuropsychology of Sleep and Dreaming. Mahwah, NJ, Erlbaum, 1992, pp 99-143.

47. Mesulam M-M: The human frontal lobes: Transcending the default mode through contingent encoding. In Stuss DT, Knight RT (eds): Principles of Frontal Lobe Function. New York, Oxford, 2002, pp 8-30.

48. Stuss DT, Alexander MP, Floden D, et al: Fractionalization and localization of distinct frontal lobe processes: Evidence from focal lesions in humans. In Stuss DT, Knight RT (eds). Principles of Frontal Lobe Function. New York, Oxford, 2002, pp 392-407.

49. Fletcher PC, Henson RN: Frontal lobes and human memory: Insights from functional neuroimaging. Brain 2001; 124:849-881.

50. Hobson JA: The Dreaming Brain. New York, NY, Basic Books, 1988.

51. Gottesmann C: The neurochemistry of waking and sleeping mental activity: The disinhibition-dopamine hypothesis. Psychiat Clin Neurosci 2002;56:345-354.

52. Williams JA, Comisarow J, Day J, et al: State-dependent release of acetylcholine in rat thalamus measured by microdialysis. J Neurosci 1994;14:5236-5242.

53. Kodama T, Honda Y: Acetylcholine releases of mesopontine PGO-on cells in the lateral geniculate nucleus in sleep-waking cycle and serotonergic regulation. Prog Neuro-Psychopharm Biol Psychiat. 1996;20:1213-1227.

54. Sitaram N, Moore AM, Gillin JC: The effect of physostigmine on normal human sleep and dreaming. Arch Gen Psychiatry 1978; 35:1239-1243.

55. Ross JS, Shua-Haim JR: Aricept-induced nightmares in Alzheimer's disease: 2 case reports. J Am Geriatr Soc 1998;46: 119-120.

56. Yorston GA, Gray R: Hypnopompic hallucinations with donepezil. J Psychopharm 2000;14:303-304.

57. Ashton H: Delirium and hallucinations. In Perry E, Ashton H, Young Y (eds): Neurochemistry of Consciousness: Transmitters in Mind. Amsterdam, John Benjamins, 2002, pp 181-203.

58. Hobson JA: The Dream Drug Store. Cambridge, Mass, MIT Press, 2001.

59. Pagel JF, Helfter P: Drug induced nightmares—an etiology based review. Hum Psychopharm 2003;18:59-67.

60. Hobson JA, Pace-Schott EF: Reply to Solms, Braun and Reiser. Neuropsychoanalysis 1999;1:206-224.

61. Perry EK, Perry RH: Acetylcholine and hallucinations: Disease-related compared to drug-induced alterations in human consciousness. Brain Cogn 1995;28:240-258.

62. McCormick D, Prince A: Two types of muscarinic response to acetylcholine in mammalian cortical neurons. Proc Nat Acad Sci U S A 1985;82:6344-6348.

63. Steriade M: Corticothalamic resonance, states of vigilance and mentation. Neuroscience 2000;101:243-276.

64. Aubin HJ: Tolerability and safety of sustained release bupropion in the management of smoking cessation. Drugs 2002; 62(suppl):45-52.

65. Furey ML, Pietrini P, Haxby JV: Cholinergic enhancement and increased selectivity of perceptual processing during working memory. Science 2000;290:2315-2319.

66. Miller JD, Farber J, Gatz P, et al: Activity of mesencephalic dopamine and non-dopamine neurons across stages of sleep and waking in the rat. Brain Res 1983;273:133-141.

67. Keating GL, Rye DB: Where you least expect it: Dopamine in the pons and modulation of sleep and REM sleep. Sleep 2003; 26:788-789.

68. Oakman SA, Faris PL, Cozzari C, et al: Characterization of the extent of pontomesencephalic cholinergic neurons' projections to the thalamus: Comparison with projections to midbrain dopaminergic groups. Neuroscience 1999;94:529-547.

69. Pace-Schott EF, Gersh T, Silvestri-Hobson R. et al: SSRI treatment suppresses dream recall frequency but increases subjective dream intensity in normal subjects. J Sleep Res 2001;10:129-142.

70. Aghajanian GK, Marek GJ: Serotonin and hallucinations. Neuropsychopharmacol 1999;21:16S-23S.

71. Pace-Schott EF, Hobson JA: The neurobiology of sleep: genetic mechanisms, cellular neurophysiology and subcortical networks. Nat Rev Neurosci 2002;3:591-605.

72. Saper CB, Chou TC, Scammell TE: The sleep switch: Hypothalamic control of sleep and wakefulness. Trend Neurosci 2001;24:726-731.

73. Manford M, Andermann F: Complex visual hallucinations: Clinical and neurobiological insights. Brain 1998;121:1819-1840.

74. Schwartz S, Maquet P: Sleep imaging and the neuropsychological assessment of dreams. Trend Cog Sci 2002;6:23-30.

75. Pace-Schott EF: Recent findings on the neurobiology of sleep and dreaming. In Pace-Schott EF, Solms M, Blagrove M, Harnad S (eds): Sleep and Dreaming: Scientific Advances and Reconsiderations. Cambridge, UK, Cambridge University Press, 2003, 335-350.

76. Schneider A: Spontaneous confabulation and the adaptation of thought to ongoing reality. Nat Rev Neurosci 2003;4: 662-671.

77. Servan-Schreiber D, Perlstein WM: Pharmacologic activation of limbic structures and neuroimaging studies of emotions. J Clin Psychiat 1997;58(Suppl);16:13-15.

78. Ffytche DH, Howard RJ, Brammer MJ, et al: The anatomy of conscious vision: An fMRI study of visual hallucinations. Nat Neurosci 1998;1:738-742.

79. Amzica F, Steriade M: Progressive cortical synchronization of ponto-geniculo-occipital potentials during rapid eye movement in sleep. Neuroscience 1996;2:309-314.

80. Semba K: The mesopontine cholinergic system: A dual role in REM sleep and wakefulness. In Lydic R, Baghdoyan HA (eds): Handbook of Behavioral State Control: Molecular and Cellular Mechanisms. Boca Raton, Fla, CRC Press, 1999, pp 161-180.

81. Maquet P: Sleep function(s) and cerebral metabolism. Behav Brain Res 1995;69:75-83.

82. Hobson JA, McCarley RW, Wyzinki PW: Sleep cycle oscillation: Reciprocal discharge by two brainstem neuronal groups. Science 1975;189:55-58.

83. Hobson JA, Pace-Schott EF: The cognitive neuroscience of sleep: Neuronal systems, consciousness and learning. Nat Rev Neurosci 2002;3:679-693.

84. Steriade M: Neuronal basis of dreaming and mentation during slow wave (non-REM) sleep. Behav Brain Sci 2000;23: 1009-1011.

85. Kahn D, Stickgold R, Pace-Schott EF, Hobson JA: Dreaming and waking consciousness: A character recognition study. J Sleep Res 2000;9:317-325.

86. LeDoux JE: The Emotional Brain. New York, Simon and Schuster, 1996.

87. Paus T: Primate anterior cingulate cortex: Where motor control, drive and cognition interface. Nat Rev Neurosci 2001;2: 417-424.

88. Damasio AR, Grabowski TJ, Bechara A, et al: Subcortical and cortical brain activity during the feeling of self-generated emotions. Nat Neurosci 2000;3:1049-1056.

89. Siegal M, Varley R: Neural systems involved in "Theory of Mind." Nat Rev Neurosci 2002;3:463-471.

90. Cahill L, McGough JL: Mechanisms of emotional arousal and lasting declarative memory. Trend Neurosci 1998;21:294-299.

91. Brown MW, Aggleton JP: Recognition memory: What are the roles of the perirhinal cortex and hippocampus. Nat Rev Neurosci 2001;2:51-61.

92. Porte HS, Hobson JA: Physical motion in dreams: One measure of three theories. J Abnorm Psychol 1996;105:329-335.

93. Rye DB: Contributions of the peduculopontine region to normal and altered REM sleep. Sleep 1997;20:757-788.

94. Jouvet M: The Paradox of Sleep: The Story of Dreaming. Cambridge, Mass, MIT Press, 1999.

95. Haxby JV, Hoffman EA, Gobbini MI: The distributed human neural system for face perception. Trend Cog Sci 2000;4: 223-233.

96. Petrides M, Pandya DN: Association pathways of the prefrontal cortex and functional observations. In Stuss DT, Knight RT (eds): Principles of Frontal Lobe Function. New York, Oxford, 2002, pp 31-50.

97. Saint-Cyr JA, Bronstein YI, Cummings JL: Neurobehavioral consequences of neurosurgical treatments and focal lesions of frontal-subcortical circuits. In Stuss DT, Knight RT (eds): Principles of Frontal Lobe Function. New York, Oxford, 2002, pp 408-427.

98. Barbas H: Connections underlying the synthesis of cognition, memory and emotion in primate prefrontal cortices. Brain Res Bull 2000;52:319-330.

99. Middleton FA, Strick PL: Cerebellar projections to the prefrontal cortex of the primate. J. Neurosci 2001;21:700-712.

100. Stickgold R: Memory, cognition and dreaming. In Maquet P, Smith C, Stickgold R (eds): Sleep and Brain Plasticity. Cambridge, UK, Oxford University Press, 2003, pp 17-39.

101. Hobson JA, McCarley RW: The brain as a dream-state generator: An activation-synthesis hypothesis of the dream process. Am J Psychiatry 1977;134:1335-1348.

102. Mesulam M-M: Cholinergic pathways and the ascending reticular activating system of the human brain. Annals N Y Acad Sci 1995;757:169-179.

103. Kahan TL, LaBerge S: Lucid dreaming as metacognition: Implications for cognitive science. Conscious Cogn 1994; 3:246-264.

104. Liotti M, Mayberg HS, Brannan SK, et al: Differential limbic-cortical correlates of sadness and anxiety in healthy subjects: Implications for affective disorders. Biol Psychiatry 2000; 48:30-42.

105. Fosse R, Stickgold R, Hobson JA: Brain-mind states: Reciprocal variation in thoughts and hallucinations. Psychol Sci 2001; 12:30-36.

45

Dreaming as a Mood Regulation System

Rosalind Cartwright

ABSTRACT

This chapter reviews the recent literature in support of one of the many hypothesized functions of dreaming: It processes, off-line, the emotional component of recent waking experience and does so sequentially within sleep. Further, this regular downloading of affect into associated memory networks weakens the impact of disruptive emotion and prepares the sleeper for more adaptive waking behavior. This proposal suggests that under normal circumstances, there is some interaction among the various mind-brain states characteristic of the 24-hour circadian cycle: waking-sleeping-dreaming-waking. Further, there are not only "day residues," which can be traced from waking into non–rapid eye movement (NREM) sleep and then on into rapid eye movement (REM) sleep and dreaming, but also "dreaming residues" that have an effect on subsequent waking mood and thus on behavior.

This chapter reviews studies of healthy adults and of patients who experience abnormal levels of disturbed affect. These show that dreaming as a psychological process has a developmental course parallel to that of waking cognition and that there are specific dysfunctional changes associated with various clinical disorders. One such example is the reduced recall of dreams and absence of dream affect in many patients suffering from an episode of major depression. There are also other pathologies of dreaming: the aggressive dreams acted out in REM behavior disorder (RBD), the delayed dreaming secondary to an arousal from the first NREM in the parasomnias, and the repetitive dreams characteristic of posttraumatic stress disorder (PTSD).

All of these dysfunctions suggest that if dreaming has an active self-regulatory role in emotional modulation, that role can be disrupted due to various trait and state variables and their interactions. Illustrations of some of these are the association of RBD with degenerative neurologic disorders that release dreaming from the normally protective muscle atonia, the genetic bias to behavioral arousals from NREM sleep in the parasomnias, and the stress responsivity of those vulnerable to the nightmares of PTSD. Some personality traits, hormonal changes, circadian rhythm disturbances, and effects of various medications or other substances can disrupt a putative function of normal dreaming.

The major current psychological theories of dreaming of Antrobus,[1] Breger,[2] Foulkes,[3,4] Hartmann,[5] Kramer,[6] Palombo,[7] and Reiser[8] are considered in the light of evidence from recent research. Testing the various proposed functions of dreaming has been spurred by increasing methodologic and technologic sophistication.

CURRENT THEORIES OF DREAMING

In general, we feel better after a good night of sleep. A major focus of modern sleep research has been to investigate why this is so. What is it about sleep that restores us both physiologically and psychologically? This became an even more puzzling question as the paradoxes of the rapid eye movement (REM) sleep state were identified.[9] Dreaming largely occurs during this regularly appearing complex state of high brain activation, during which there are motor inhibition, a shut down of afferent input, and visual hallucinations.[1]

Many psychological functions of this state have been proposed. The classic theories were summarized in an early review by Dallett,[10] and the newer theoretical statements are well covered by Moffitt, Kramer, and Hoffman.[11] Too often these viewpoints are well argued but lack empirical support. However, many of these theories suggest that a key element in understanding dreaming as a psychological process is recognizing its connection with emotion. Foulkes[4] states, "In dreaming, feeling is a kind of knowing, a knowing of myself and knowing of my environment" (p. 18). Also, "it makes more sense to look for meanings over a series of dreams from the same dreamer. The recurrence of patterns suggests that more than random mnemonic activation is involved. They [the recurrent patterns] can index what the dreamer knows of her or his self and how she or he tends to conceptually organize life experiences" (p. 208).

Hartmann[12] suggests how the particular memory material comes to be selected for dreaming display. "The emotional concerns of the dreamer are what is most important in guiding or determining the images in the dreams" (p. 68). Later, he states, "dreams make connections more broadly than in waking and these connections produce a calming effect" (p. 119). Breger,[2] too, links dreaming not only to presleep affect but also to postsleep adaptation. Dreaming, "serves a unique function in the assimilation and mastery of aroused material into 'solutions' embodied in existing memory systems" (p. 1). New emotional experiences are mapped onto these previously stored "solutions" during sleep.

The brain activation of REM sleep may be random, but, as Foulkes[3] reminds us, "the system being activated is not. Activation spreads according to pre-existing patterns in symbolic memory" (p. 151). Reiser[8] supports this point of view and spells it out a little further: "Emotion plays a role in generating and shaping both the process and content of dreaming. Networks of memories encoded by images perceived during significant emotional life experiences may appear later in dreams when they serve as mnemonic references to those meaningful experiences organized by emotion" (p. 355).

DATA SOURCES FOR TESTING THE THEORY

There are several sources of information that can be searched for evidence in support of this proposed emotion-dream connection. These include the "home" dreams as they are recalled spontaneously by many people, the "office" dreams reported by patients during psychotherapy, the areas of the brain activated and deactivated during REM sleep as revealed by brain imaging studies and their correlation to known functions of these areas, and the "laboratory" dreams retrieved by sleep researchers and sleep disorder clinicians by awakening sleepers from each of the three to five REM periods of the night in turn.

FUNCTION OF DREAMING

People have always had considerable interest in understanding the experience of being in another mode of mental life while asleep, one that is beyond their own power to control or even to understand. This has led to a good deal of myth-making to fill in the knowledge gap. One prominent belief is that dreams contain important information about the future, particularly warnings of disease, deaths, droughts, and disasters. Such dreams that forecast negative events carry with them negative affect, primarily anxiety. Gluckman[13] asserts that this predictive power of dreams is of particular importance to the psychotherapist. "Dreams," he states, "may serve as an early warning" not of outside trouble but signs of internal turmoil and disintegration, "of suicidality, homocidality, ego disintegration, psychosis, and acting out behavior" (p. 222). To date, no special prescient ability of dreams has received any support from research. The posting of dreams on the Internet by laypersons, along with the date of the dream, may be of use in testing this belief.

Whether or not this idea turns out to have any validity, the fact that dreams that are spontaneously remembered are often accompanied by anxiety or other negative feelings has been substantiated in many studies. One is Snyder's[14] landmark report on the content analysis of the dreams of 250 healthy adults collected in the sleep laboratory. Of the emotions mentioned, his data show unpleasant affect predominating at a ratio of 2:1, with fear, anxiety, and anger the most commonly identified.

Some dreams are, in fact, sufficiently unpleasant to abort sleep and awaken the sleeper prematurely with vivid frightening dream recall. This is the usual definition of a nightmare. Nightmares have been studied for their frequency and their association with measures of mental health. Zarda and Donderi[15] tested a hypothetical dimension of negative affect in dreaming. In this model, nightmares are at one extreme, and bad dreams that do not wake the sleeper are at a midpoint. At the opposite end are presumably neutral or more pleasant dreams. The authors report that the frequency of the two types of unpleasant dreams correlate negatively with self-report measures of well-being.

A further understanding of the association of feeling and dreaming comes from the work of Ernest Hartmann.[16] He has linked frequent nightmare experience to a personality dimension he has called "boundaries of the mind." This concept refers to the ability to make clear distinctions between thoughts and feelings, reality and fantasy, and other such categories. Although persons with "thin" boundaries, as measured by the Boundaries Questionnaire (see Hartmann,[12] pp. 251-267), may benefit from this trait of fluidity of affective associations by being more artistically creative, they are also more likely to be subject to the invasion of troubling dreams that they vividly recall.

In sum, the dreams recalled spontaneously by many healthy people often have a negative affective tone. There are individual differences, with some people having a specific personality trait associated with more frequent recall of their dreams, and these dreams also have more intense negative affect. Their disturbing dreams will, on occasion, exceed the capacity of sleep to contain them.

The next step in assessing the putative mood-regulatory function is to examine the impression that dreams are most frequently negative to see if that impression is due to a sampling bias, because dreams we recall tend to be those that wake us. But most dreaming does *not* result in an awakening. Since we usually feel better in the morning, perhaps these unremembered dream sequences are normally successful in regulating the typical range of presleep affect, except when the waking degree of affect does not require any regulation. In either case, waking in a good mood would be expected. The possibility that dreaming is the mechanism responsible for this improved mood requires testing of three propositions basic to this mood regulatory theory:

1. Dreaming varies systematically with the degree and kind of presleep emotional state.
2. When the level of negative affect is elevated prior to sleep, the sequence of dreams within the night shows a progressive reduction of this affect.
3. The change in morning mood is related to both of the first two propositions, namely the degree of presleep negative emotion and the extent of its downregulation from REM to REM.

Dreaming Varies with Presleep Emotional State

Evidence related to the first proposition, the input part of this equation, comes from studies of dreams following natural disasters and personal traumas. These studies show that when presleep negative affect is unusually high, dream quality and content are responsive to emotion-evoking waking events. Following the 1989 earthquake in San Francisco, nightmares were reported at high levels in those sampled who were most exposed (37%) or living in the area (40%) but at low levels (5%) in a control group living at a physical distance.[17]

A traumatic event plus helplessness to cope with it were conditions implicated in the persistence of nightmares over four or more years in a group of children who had been kidnapped and buried in an abandoned quarry for two days.[18] On the basis of theories such as Breger's,[2] the long delay in dream adaptation might reflect the children's lack of experience with such an event. Their long-term emotional memory did not contain the stored solutions necessary to provide helpful dream images.

In a study by Berger et al.,[19] dreams of a small group of subjects were recorded in the sleep laboratory before and after elective surgery. The content of these dreams demonstrated the importance of knowing the personal meaning of a traumatic event. The positive or negative emotional impact of the surgery on the dreamer's sense of integrity could be predicted from the content of their dreams, but metaphorically rather than directly.

Marital separation and divorce is another disturbing life event that has been the subject of sleep laboratory investigation.[20] The 40 volunteers for this study were in a major depression episode secondary to the breakup of a marriage. None was being treated for depression. Those who were able to structure and report well-developed dreams when awakened from the first REM sleep period were more likely to be in remission when reevaluated one year later. In contrast, the depressed subjects who had little recall from the first REM period or who could report only short, static dreams were more likely to remain depressed at the follow-up point.

Data from these various life-event studies support the first proposition, that dreaming is generally responsive to new emotion-evoking situations requiring adaptation. These data also show, however, that there are individual differences in this response. Some persons who are less able to compartmentalize experience, such as those with thin boundaries, may increase dream intensity to levels that disrupt sleep, whereas others, such as the depressed, reduce dreaming amount and dampen dream affect. Both high- and low-affect responders display less mood regulation following sleep.

Normal Dreaming Reduces Aroused Negative Affect

Next we examine studies relevant to the second proposition: that aroused negative affect is progressively reduced when dreaming is functioning normally. A corollary to this proposition is that the sequence of dream affect within one night may not be progressive and that such inefficient mood regulation patterns may be corrected. To examine this proposition, we turn to studies of dreams in psychotherapy and to treatment programs undertaken to change dysfunctional emotional response patterns by the interpretation of the emotional meaning of patients' dreams.

Dreaming in Psychotherapy

Psychotherapists who encourage their patients to report their dreams do so to obtain information they believe will further their treatment goals. The assumption is that dreams give the therapist access to information about the emotional life that patients are unable or unwilling to verbalize directly, that dreams provide a shortcut to those affective-cognitive organizational patterns underlying the irrational anxieties and behavior choices that have brought patients to seek help. Here the emphasis is on how dreams reveal the way a patient's past affective learning history influences present behavior in a detrimental manner.

Schredle et al.[21] surveyed psychotherapists engaged in private practice about their use of dreams in treatment. They found that both psychoanalytic and humanistic therapists report they work on dreams in 28% of their sessions. Moreover, 70% of those therapists believed this work to be beneficial to their patients. With few exceptions,[22,23] there is no evidence from hypothesis-driven research that therapeutic work with dreams provides a direct benefit to the patient. Support of this practice rests on abundant case reports illustrating that dream interpretation furthers the insight of the therapist into the patient. Evidence that it promotes more or better use of the therapy hours by the patient, is instrumental in changing dysfunctional dreaming patterns, or is responsible for changes in waking emotional adaptation is, at best, correlational.

Palombo[7] proposes a mechanism to explain how dream interpretation "has a special efficacy in the building of those intrapsychic structures which restore and renew the incomplete self." Further, he views dream interpretation as a collaboration between the patient's inherent adaptive dream function and the analyst's work interpreting the patient's dreams.

The work during sessions on interpreting dreams leads the patient to have a "corrective" dream. A corrective dream theoretically melds the original dream and the therapist's interpretation of it into permanent memory at the same brain location as the original dream (paraphrased from Palombo,[7] p 14). The assumption is that the patient responds emotionally to the therapist's interpretation with the same affect that prompted the production of the original dream. This stimulates the same dream memory network, which incorporates the interpreted changes, producing a corrective dream now ready for response to a similar but new emotion-evoking experience.

Cartwright, Tipton, and Wicklund[22] tested the idea that becoming conscious of what one is dreaming is helpful to emotionally dysfunctional patients. In the study, subjects slept in the sleep laboratory over a two-week period. The subjects were waiting to begin psychotherapy and had been evaluated by the intake worker as being poor risks for successful treatment. They were judged to be uninsightful and to have poor skills for self-understanding and self-disclosure, and they were predicted to drop out of treatment before gaining any benefit.

There were one experimental group and two control groups. Researchers awakened the experimental subjects from each REM sleep period to collect their dreams and prompted their recall in the morning. Those in the first control group were awakened and asked for reports an equal number of times but only from episodes of NREM sleep, and the second control group went directly into therapy without preparation in therapy-appropriate behavior.

The criteria of benefit from this intervention of dream recall practice were remaining in treatment for at least ten sessions, engaging in therapy-appropriate behavior such as discussing their feelings, and showing improvement in self-understanding as judged by a review of the first and tenth tape-recorded treatment hours. The results were generally supportive of the hypotheses. Increasing the patients' access to their dreams, and practice in recalling and discussing them, helped the experimental patients stay in treatment and engage in productive psychotherapy.

There were two interesting sidelights of this study. One was the observation that some of these alexythymic patients, the emotionally dampened type, were unable to report well-constructed dreams even with the help of the experimental REM awakenings. The other was that a few of the control subjects who had only NREM awakenings produced reports that were judged to be dreams and derived the same benefits from treatment expected only for the REM-awakening experimental group. Although the therapists involved in this study had no training in working with dreams, those patients who were "clued in" to their emotional issues through dream retrieval, whether from REM or NREM sleep, progressed well in their treatment.

Hill and her colleagues carried the Cartwright et al.[22] study forward in a series of studies developing and testing a program for working with dreams, the Hill Cognitive-Experiential Dream Model.[24] This is a three-stage approach: exploration, insight, and action. The method is designed to elicit the feelings of the dreamer in relation to the dream images by having the dreamer retell a recalled dream using the present tense and to search with the therapist for links between the dream and the waking experience.

Several studies using this technique are summarized in a recent paper.[25] Although many of these studies involve large numbers of subjects, they also have several limitations. One is the level of experience of the therapists, who were often graduate students in training. The clients, too, are often student volunteers, and the experimental dream "therapy" is limited to one or only a few sessions of work on a single dream recalled from home sleep. Not having the opportunity to see the recalled dream in the context of a series of dreams occurring during the same night limits the applicability of this method to the question of within-sleep progressive mood regulation. Nevertheless, the model has potential for formalizing dream work and testing the effectiveness of practice in dream recall on improving waking mood regulation.

Evidence from Brain and Behavior Studies

The third data source for understanding the function of dreaming comes from the brain and behavior scientists who have investigated how and where in the brain dreams are formed and who only then began to speculate about their function. Winson,[26] Hobson,[27] Solms,[28] Braun,[29] Maquet,[30] and Nofzinger[31] have all have contributed to this work. Winson[26] set up a model from his animal studies that states, "dreams are a window on the neural processes whereby, from early childhood on, strategies of behavior are being set down, modified or consulted" (p. 209).

Recently, the application of brain-imaging technology has mapped the location of those areas in which there is increased brain activation and deactivation during REM sleep. The consensus of this work is that there is increased activation in the integrative visual cortex and the limbic and paralimbic systems and decrease in the dorso-lateral prefrontal and parietal cortices during REM sleep, in comparison to the patterns during waking and NREM sleep. This evidence supports the hypothesis that REM dreaming displays emotional concerns in visual terms in nonlogical structure.

Gottesman[32] summarized the neuroanatomic and neurochemical uniqueness of the REM state. He states that the noradrenergic and histaminergic neurons are turned off but the dopaminegeric neurons continue to fire, and this combination is what is responsible for the dream qualities of fantasy and irrationality. Solms[33] has tracked the correlation between the sites of brain damage and the characteristic changes in the dream experience reported by patients. He, too, suggests that an intact dopaminergic circuit of the ventromesial forebrain is basic to maintaining normal dreaming. This work has added to our knowledge base of how dreams are made but not why.

Evidence from Sleep Laboratory Studies of Dreaming

Sleep researchers and sleep disorder clinicians have used online sleep monitoring technology to study dreaming during REM and NREM sleep by healthy subjects and by patients presenting with various sleep complaints. The regular 90-minute cycling of REM sleep, originally established by Dement and Kleitman,[34] and its high correlation with the presence of visual narratives of dreaming has been confirmed in many studies throughout the world. Foulkes[35] extended this work to show that the development of dreaming in children is a cognitive skill that parallels waking cognitive development. His recording of the REM and NREM reports of children from preschool though early adolescence is a landmark in developmental psychology.

Another landmark is Snyder's study,[14] mentioned earlier, on the components of the laboratory-recorded dreams of 250 healthy adults. The conclusion—that ordinary people have ordinary dreams—was somewhat disappointing to those who expected dreams to show more bizarreness. With respect to emotion, Snyder found little direct mention of emotion in the REM reports of well-functioning adults. When a feeling was specified, the negatives outweighed the positives.

To date, the evidence suggests that under most circumstances, dreaming runs smoothly, but when presleep disturbing feelings are strong enough, they activate an emotional memory network selected to match the current concern, and further processing into a dream story takes place. This processing is constrained by the structure of that network, which continues to produce related images and associations from memory throughout the night. If only unsuccessful solutions are stored in long-term emotional memory, the dreams will have negative affect, and if no matching images and associations are available in the stimulated network, dreaming may not succeed in downregulating mood within the night. Not all dreaming is successful. Presumably additional more-positive waking experiences may be what is needed to restore well-functioning dreaming.

Dreaming in Depression

The finding that the classic timing of REM sleep is shifted to occur earlier in those who are suffering from a major mood disorder was pointed out by several early sleep investigators.[36,37] Wehr et al.[38] modeled this shift as a phase advance of REM sleep; others interpreted it as perhaps an attempt to respond to the prevailing dysphoric mood.[20] There are other abnormalities of sleep in the depressed, including an increased fragmentation of sleep, particularly of the REM periods. Hauri and Hawkins[37] pointed out that the percentage of rapid eye movements themselves is a good indicator of the general emotional or motivational turmoil in both schizophrenic and depressed patients. The density of the rapid eye movements during the REM episodes is more variable in depressed subjects than in controls. These patients show periods when the eye movements are very sparse and periods when there are eye movement storms.

These sleep abnormalities suggest an explanation for the difficulty experienced by the depressed in developing and reporting coherent dreams and consequently their failure to regulate mood. This explanation is based on a dream-construction hypothesis proposed by Molinari and Foulkes.[39] It suggests that dreams are formed by the interplay of two components of REM sleep, the tonic and the phasic events. The phasic rapid eye movements trigger visual images, and during the intervening tonic periods, associations to these images occur. This sequence of image-then-association allows the visual components to be woven into a dream story within a REM episode.

As we have noted, the dream recall in the depressed state is poor. Even when depressed subjects are awakened from REM sleep, their reports are typically short; usually only a few words are used to describe a single image with flat affect.[40,41,42] This poverty of dreaming may be due to the frequent interruptions of REM sleep or to the dysregulation of the release of rapid eye movements, allowing too few movements to supply the images or too many to allow time for the associations that are necessary to construct a dream scenario. Nofzinger et al.[43] reported that patients in remission from depression, following a cognitive behavior psychotherapy intervention, show a reduction in eye movement density.

Other aspects of sleep in depression prove to be more stable. Two of these—the poor quality of sleep and early onset of REM sleep—typically remain after remission.[37,42,44,45]

The most robust of these REM markers, the reduced latency to the first REM period, appears to represent a genetic vulnerability to depressive episodes in family members.[46] A PET imaging study of depressed and control subjects indicates that patients show altered patterns of activation in the limbic and paralimbic systems in waking relative to their first REM period.[47] The lack of an increase in activation of the anterior cingulate in the depressed patients was interpreted as perhaps related to the blunted responsiveness of these patients to emotionally salient information.

Effect on Morning Mood

The failure of many depressed patients to feel in a better mood following sleep and their well-documented REM sleep and dream abnormalities has prompted testing of the third proposition of the mood-regulatory function of dreaming: that dreaming has an effect on morning mood. Kramer[6] set the model for these studies by using a standardized mood scale, the Clyde Mood Scale,[48] before and after sleep in healthy subjects. These subjects show a significant overnight reduction in the "unhappy" mood scale scores. This improvement was not related to REM sleep time but to the dream content—specifically, the number of characters and their roles in the dreams.

Cartwright et al.[49] also tested the impact of dreaming on mood in a group of 60 high-functioning healthy subjects who were screened to eliminate those with psychopathology. This study supported Kramer's findings. Here the depression scale (D scale) of the Profile of Mood States (POMS)[50] was the measure used before and after sleep. The D-scale score was significantly reduced in the morning following both a night of uninterrupted sleep and a consecutive night in which REM periods were interrupted for dream collections. Again, there was no correlation between the amount of downregulation of negative mood and any REM sleep variable in this sample. Because the screening criteria resulted in truncating the range of D scores, few subjects had any elevation on this scale.

To examine whether morning mood change followed a within-sleep change in dream affect, the subjects were divided into two groups. Group 1 ($N = 50$) had zero or low D scores before sleep, and group 2 ($N = 10$) had some modest elevation in their depressed mood. The first group reported dreams with more positive than negative affect throughout the night. The second showed a different pattern: When asked about the feeling in each dream at the time of the REM awakenings, subjects

reported predominantly negative feelings for the first two REM periods, whereas feelings associated with the last two REM periods shifted to predominantly positive (Figure 45–1). In sum, healthy subjects who have some need to regulate even a modest degree of depressed mood did so within sleep, while those whose mood was not disturbed showed no within-sleep change in dream affect. This finding supports the second mood-regulation proposition: When presleep mood is dysphoric, dreaming shows a progressive reduction of negative content.

We turn now to studies applying this finer-grained analysis of sequential changes in REM sleep and dreaming in clinical samples. Studies have examined the within-the-night changes of the depression sleep "markers," the content and affect of the dreams, and the relation of these to the output, changes in waking mood. For two consecutive nights, Indrusky and Rotenberg[51] studied 23 patients meeting diagnostic criteria for major depression. Mood change was based on the patients' self-report of whether their morning mood was worse than, the same as, or better than it was before sleep. When morning mood was "better," the eye movement density was low in the first REM period and increased across the night to be highest in the last REM period. This is similar to the eye movement distribution pattern of healthy subjects. In contrast, those whose mood either did not change or worsened overnight had high eye movement density in the first REM period and a slow decrease from REM period to REM period. This is opposite to that of nondepressed sleepers. Thus depressed patients whose within-night sequence of rapid eye movement density resembles that of nondepressed subjects are more likely to feel an improvement of mood on awakening. This is consistent with the findings of mood improvement in healthy subjects reported by Kramer[6] and by Cartwright and colleagues[49] mentioned earlier and relates this to a specific REM sleep variable.

In another study[52] of the effects of divorce on sleep and dreaming, 70 volunteers, 30 of whom were not depressed and 40 of whom met clinical diagnostic criteria for major depression, were studied in the laboratory. At one-year follow-up, 61 of these subjects returned, 22 of those who were not depressed (group 1) and 39 who initially were clinically depressed. Twenty-two of the depressed were in remission, (group 2) and 17 remained unimproved (group 3) (Figure 45–2). Comparing the dream affect patterns observed in the two studies—those of the high-functioning nondepressed volunteers[49] and of the divorcing subjects—interesting similarities were noted. Group 1 subjects in both studies, the divorcing who were not

Figure 45–1. Percentage of positive and negative dream affect by half night in normal volunteers. Group 1 = depressed score not elevated; group 2 = depressed score elevated.

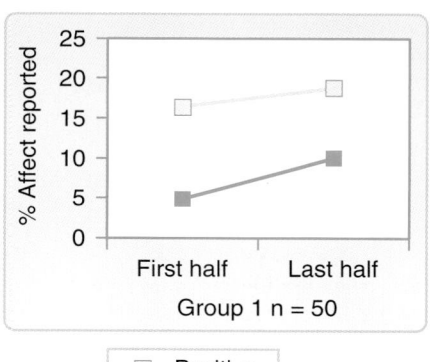

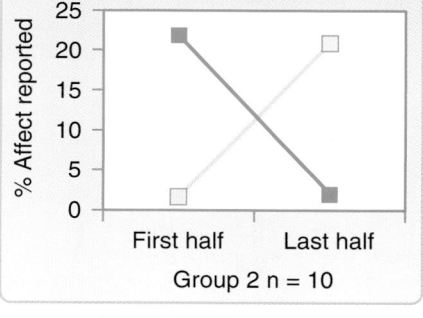

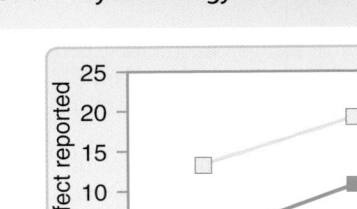
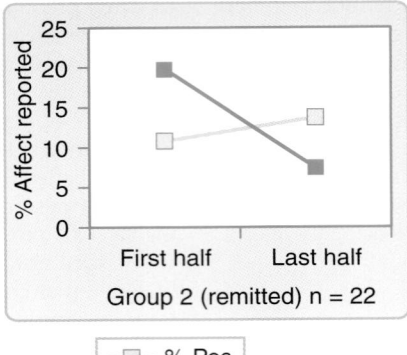
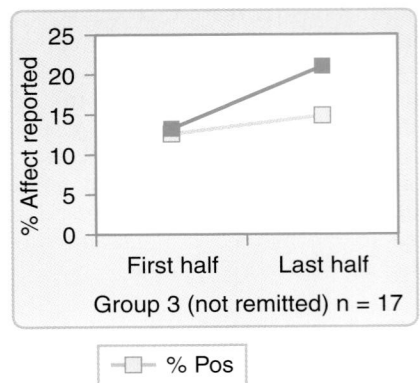

Figure 45–2. Percentage of positive and negative dream affect by half night in divorced volunteers.

depressed and the high-functioning healthy volunteers who had no elevation of depressed mood before sleep, show the predominance of positive affect in dreams throughout the night. Group 2 subjects in both studies, the depressed divorce subjects who later remitted and the healthy subjects who had some elevation on their presleep POMS depression scores, show the dominance of negative affect in dreams reported in the first half of the night and a marked decrease in the second half. It appears that presleep negative mood is being regulated from REM period to REM period in both groups of subjects. It is group 3, the depressed subjects who did not remit, and who also showed the high eye-movement density depression marker, who are of interest. Their REM reports of the initial night show a dominance of negative affect in the second half of the night, a failure of mood to be regulated within the night. It appears that some of those who are untreated while depressed can, and some cannot, "do it themselves." To get a better understanding of the role of REM sleep and dreaming on the output side of the mood regulation function hypothesis, the effect on the mood next day, required further study.

The next study in this series[53] again involved a sample of untreated depressed divorcing volunteers who were studied more frequently, for two nights at three time periods spread over five months. POMS D scores were again obtained before and after each night of laboratory sleep at months 1, 2, and 4 of the study. There were therefore four scores to plot at each of the three monthly sleep laboratory visits: before and after a sleep-through night and before and after the next night of REM-interruption sleep. At month 5 there was a repeat diagnostic evaluation that divided the group into those now in remission ($N = 12$) from those who failed to remit ($N = 8$) (Figure 45–3). Plotting the month-by-month before-and-after sleep POMS D scores, those in remission (R), show a reduction in depressed mood after sleep (morning 1), which is maintained during the day. The nonremitting group (NR) shows a consistent failure to maintain their sleep-related mood improvement, regressing during the day to their pre-sleep levels.

A regression analysis identified four variables associated with remission from untreated depression: (1) the initial severity of self-reported depression symptoms on the Beck Depression Inventory,[54] (2) the degree of downregulation of morning mood following REM-interruption nights, (3) the diurnal mood variability reported at screening (whether they felt better, worse, or the same following sleep), and (4) the ability to report well-constructed dreams on the first night of REM-interruption awakenings. These four variables accounted for 64% of the variance in remission. Those who were more depressed initially on a self-report measure, who could not report well-constructed dreams, who had less reduction of depressed mood following REM interruptions, and who identified themselves at intake as feeling at their worst on awakening were less likely to remit from depression without a treatment intervention. The modest degree of REM-sleep deprivation that resulted from the interruptions to collect dreams significantly increased the number of REM attempts on these nights. This intervention gave those able to construct REM dreams more opportunities to complete affect processing within the night. This study is additional support for the proposal that those more severely depressed have a poorer ability to produce well-organized dreaming and thus to regulate mood progressively during sleep. Waking up in a state of unregulated negative mood has an impact on the next day's waking experience.

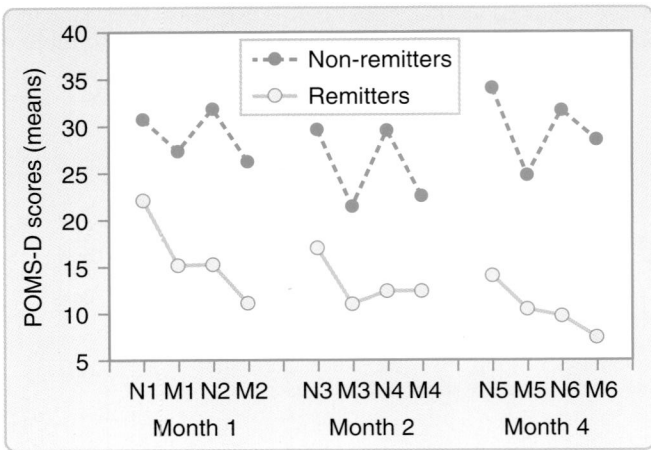

Figure 45–3. Overnight (night, morning) change in depressed mood in nonremitters and remitters, months 1, 2, and 4.

DREAMING IN OTHER CLINICAL DISORDERS

The research literature in support of a mood-regulatory function of dreaming is strongest from the studies comparing healthy sleepers to those with major depression. Although the dreaming patterns in other clinical disorders have not been studied in the same detail, there are indications of support also from the dreams acted out by the REM behavior disorder patients.[55] The patients explain their behavior, which is often aggressive, as responding to their perceived need to defend themselves or to attack others on the basis of a dream scenario. Similarly the NREM parasomnia patients may attack someone, even a loved one, in the behavioral arousal that occurs just prior to REM.[56] This suggests that an affective charge is being carried over into NREM sleep that normally would stimulate a relevant memory network and initiate a mood-regulatory process if REM were not aborted.

Although most NREM parasommia sleepwalking events are benign, these may become violent when interfered with, and sleep terrors are models of overwhelming fear. In neither of these cases is dreaming taking place to process affect and dampen the affect displayed in these events. It is reported that the higher the level of presleep stress, the more likely an NREM parasomnia event is to occur in one who is genetically prone to have difficulty in the transition from NREM sleep to REM sleep. The nightmares in PTSD are another example of nonprogressive affect reduction. These are often described as repetitive and as referring to some previous trauma that has left powerful images in long-term emotional memory, which then code a current problem as if it, too, were life threatening.[57]

CLINICAL APPLICATIONS

Dreaming has been an area neglected in recent years by sleep medicine clinicians. The legitimacy of this topic for patient care has been greatly enhanced by the recent neuropsychological and brain imaging studies. These have anchored dreaming in science by locating the REM activation areas and by relating the sites of brain damage to distortions of dream experience. Research designs have become more sophisticated as well. It is now clear that if the phenomenon of dreaming is to take its place in our understanding of ourselves and our patients, we must take into account that the mind works a 24-hour day. Therefore it is important to examine the normal functions and the dysfunctions of the sleeping mind and its interactions with waking feeling and behavior. To do this, there must be careful attention to the presleep variables that affect dreaming: the stable traits and the current state of the patient. Dreaming should be sampled in both REM and NREM sleep and examined in both its physiological characteristics (does REM come too early, are the eye movements too sparse) and psychological components (are the dreams well constructed, do they awaken the patient prematurely in an anxious state). Then the effect on the waking state that follows must be examined.

Patients suffering from PTSD nightmares, REM interruption insomnia, REM behavior disorder, the NREM parasomnias, brain injury, neurologic impairment, or depression all need the attention and understanding of sleep clinicians. Both we and they will profit from this. We will learn more about the mind, and they will be better cared for.

PITFALLS AND CONTROVERSIES

This review has not addressed some of the long-term debates in this field. One of these debates is whether dreaming is confined to REM sleep or occurs in NREM sleep as well. There is much evidence that the NREM reports of some individuals, perhaps those with thin boundaries, are indistinguishable from their REM reports. In others, NREM dreaming follows an increase in waking anxiety, which produces a higher level of cortical activation. It appears that dreaming, while not confined solely to REM sleep, is most consistently retrievable from this state. Solms[33] has pointed out that REM can occur without dreaming and dreaming can occur without REM. Other pitfalls stem from the noncomparability of data on dreaming from spontaneously recalled dreams and those derived from REM-sleep awakenings. The first are subject to unknown sampling bias and the second to experimenter effects.

> **Clinical Pearl**
>
> *Dreaming has a mood-regulatory effect except when presleep anxiety levels are high, resulting in frightening dreams that abort sleep, or when depression is severe, interfering with dream plot construction and the successful processing of dream affect.*

REFERENCES

1. Antrobus J: Dreaming: Cognitive processes during cortical activation and high afferent thresholds. Psychol Rev 1991;98:96-121.
2. Breger L: Function of dreams. J Abnorm Psychol (monograph) 1967;72:1-28.
3. Foulkes D: Dreaming: A cognitive-psychological analysis. Hillsdale, NJ, Erlbaum, 1985.
4. Foulkes D: Data constraints on theorizing about dream function. In Moffitt A, Kramer M, Hoffman R. (eds): The Functions of Dreaming. albany, State University of New York Press, 1993, pp 11-20.
5. Hartmann E: Dreaming. In Lee-Chiong T, Sateia M, Carskadon M, (eds): Sleep Medicine. Philadelphia, Hanley and Belfus, 2002, pp 93-98.
6. Kramer M: The selective mood regulatory function of dreaming: An update and revision. In Moffitt A, Kramer M, Hoffmann R (eds): The Functions of Dreaming. Albany, State University of New York Press, 1993, pp 139-195.
7. Palombo S: Dreaming and Memory: A New Information Processing Model. New York, Basic Books, 1978.
8. Reiser M: The dream in contemporary psychiatry. Am J Psychiatry 2001;158:351-359.
9. Jouvet M: Paradoxical sleep: A study of its nature and mechanisms. Prog Brain Res 1965;18:20-57.
10. Dallett J: Theories of dream function. Psychol Bull 1973;79:408-416.
11. Moffitt A, Kramer M, Hoffman R (eds): The Functions of Dreaming. Albany, State University of New York Press, 1993.
12. Hartmann E: Dreams and Nightmares: The New Theory on the Origin and Meaning of Dreams. New York, Plenum Press, 1998.
13. Glucksman M: The dream: A psychodynamically informative instrument. J Psychother Pract Res 2001;10:223-230.
14. Snyder F: The phenomenology of dreaming. In Madow L, Snow L: (eds): The Psychodynamic Implications of the Physiological Studies on Dreams. Springfield, Ill, Charles C Thomas, 1970, pp 124-151.
15. Zarda A, Donderi D: Nightmares and bad dreams: Their prevalence and relationship to well-being. J Abnorm Psychol 2000;109:273-281.

16. Hartmann E: Boundaries in the Mind: A New Psychology of Personality. New York, Basic Books, 1991.

17. Wood J, Bootzin R, Rosenhan D, et al: Effects of the 1989 San Francisco earthquake on frequency and content of nightmares. J Abnorm Psychol 1992;101:219-224.

18. Terr L: Chowchilla revisited: The effects of psychic trauma four years after a school-bus kidnapping. Am J Psychiatry 1983; 140:1543-1550.

19. Breger L, Hunter I, Lane R: The effect of stress on dreams. Psychological Issues, Monograph 27. Guilford, Conn, International Universities Press, 1971, pp 1-214.

20. Cartwright R, Lloyd S: Early REM sleep: A compensatory change in depression? Psychiatry Res 1994;51:245-252.

21. Schredl M, Bohusch C, Kahl J, et al: The use of dreams in psychotherapy: A survey of psychotherapists in private practice. J Psychother Pract Res 2000;9:81-87.

22. Cartwright R, Tipton L, Wicklund J: Focusing on dreams: A preparation program for psychotherapy. Arch Gen Psychiatry 1980;37:275-277.

23. Hill CE, Zack J, Wonnell T, et al: Structured brief therapy with a focus on dreams or loss for clients with troubling dreams and recent loss. J Counseling Psychol, 2000;47:90-101.

24. Hill C (ed): Dream Work in Therapy: Facilitating Exploration, Insight and Action. Washington, DC, American Psychological Assoc. 2004.

25. Hill C: Working with dreams: A road to self-discovering. Counseling Psychologist, 2003;31:362-372.

26. Winson J: Brain and Psyche. New York, Anchor Press, 1985, p 209.

27. Hobson A, Pace-Schott E, Stickgold R: Dreaming and the brain: Toward a cognitive neuroscience of conscious states. In Pace-Schott E, Solms M, Blagrove M, Hardad S (eds): Sleep and Dreaming: Scientific Advances and Reconsiderations. Cambridge, UK, Cambridge University Press, 2003, pp 1-50.

28. Solms M: Dreams and REM sleep are controlled by different brain mechanisms. In Pace-Schott E, Solms M, Blagrove M, Harnad S (eds): Sleep and Dreaming: Scientific Advances and Reconsiderations. Cambridge, UK, Cambridge University Press, 2003, pp 51-58.

29. Braun A, Blakin T, Wesenstein N, et al: Regional blood flow throughout the sleep-wake cycle. Brain 1997;120:1173-1197.

30. Maquet P, Peters JM, Aerts J, et al: Functional neuroanatomy of human rapid eye-movement sleep and dreaming. Nature 1996;383:163-166.

31. Nofzinger E, Mintun M, Wiseman M, et al: Forebrain activation in REM sleep: A FDG PET study. Brain Research 1997;770:192-201.

32. Gottesmann, C: Hypothesis for the neurophysiology of dreaming. Sleep Research Online, 2000;3:1-4.

33. Solms M: The Neuropsychology of Dreams: A Clinico-Anatomical Study. Mahwah, NJ, Erlbaum,1997.

34. Dement W, Kleitman N: Cyclic variations in EEG during sleep and their relation to eye movements, body motility, and dreaming. Electroencephalogr Clin Neurophysiol Suppl 1957;9:673-690.

35. Foulkes D: Children's Dreams: Longitudinal Studies. New York, Wiley, 1982.

36. Mendels J, Hawkins, D: Sleep and depression: A controlled EEG study. Arch Gen Psychiatry 1967;16:344-353.

37. Hauri P, Hawkins D: Phasic REM, depression, and the relationship between sleeping and waking. Arch Gen Psychiatry 1971;25:56-63.

38. Wehr T, Wirz-Justice A, Goodwin F, et al: Phase advance of the circadian sleep-wake cycle as an anti-depressant. Science 1979;206:710-713.

39. Molinari S, Foulkes D: Tonic and phasic events during sleep: Psychological correlates and implications. Percept Mot Skills 1969;29:343-368.

40. Armitage R, Rochlen A, Fitch T, et al: Dream recall and major depression: A preliminary report. Dreaming 1995;5: 189-198.

41. Reimann D, Weigand M, Majer-Trendel K, et al: Dream recall and dream content in depressive patients, patients with anorexia nervosa and normal controls. In Koella W, Obal F, Schulz H, et al (eds): Sleep '86. Stuttgart, Gustav Fischer Verlag, 1988, pp 373-375.

42. Beauchemin K, Hays D: Dreaming away depression: The role of REM sleep and dreaming in affective disorders. J Affec Disord 1996;41:125-1331.

43. Nofzinger E, Schwartz R, Reynolds C, et al: Affect intensity and phasic REM sleep in depressed men before and after treatment with cognitive-behavioral therapy. J Consulting Clin Psychol 1994;62:83-91.

44. Cartwright R: Rapid eye movement sleep characteristics during and after mood disturbing events. Arch Gen Psychiatry 1983;40:197-201.

45. Cartwright R, Kravitz H, Eastman C, et al: REM latency and the recovery from depression: Getting over divorce. Am J Psychiatry 1991;148:1530-1535.

46. Giles D, Roffwarg H, Rush AJ: REM latency concordance in depressed family members. Biol Psychiatry 1987;22:910-914.

47. Nofzinger E, Nichols T, Meltzer C, et al: Changes in forebrain function from waking to REM sleep in depression: Preliminary analyses of [18f] FDG PET studies. Psychiatry Res: Neuroimaging 1999;91:59-78.

48. Clyde D: Manual for the Clyde-Mood Scale. Coral Gables, Fla., Biometric Laboratory, University of Miami, 1963.

49. Cartwright R, Luten A, Young M, et al: Role of REM sleep and dream affect in overnight mood regulation: A study of normal volunteers. Psychiatry Res 1998; 81:1-8.

50. McNair D, Lorr M, Droppleman L: Profile of Mood States. San Diego, Education and Industrial Testing Service, 1981.

51. Indrusky P, Rotenberg V: Change of mood during sleep and REM sleep variables. Int J Psychiatry Clin Pract 1998;2: 47-51.

52. Cartwright R, Young M, Mercer P, et al: Role of REM sleep and dream variables in the prediction of remission from depression. Psychiatry Res 1998;80:249-255.

53. Cartwright R, Baehr E, Kirkby J, et al: REM sleep reduction, mood regulation and remission in untreated depression. Psychiatry Res 2003;121:159-167.

54. Beck A: Depression: Clinical, Experimental and Theoretical Aspects. New York, Harper & Row, 1967, pp 339-344.

55. Schneck C, Bundle S, Patterson A, et al: Rapid eye movement sleep behavior disorder: A treatable parasomnia affecting older adults. JAMA 1987;257:1786-1789.

56. Cartwright R: Sleep-related violence: Does the polysomnogram help establish the diagnosis? Sleep Med 2000;1:331-335.

57. Kramer M: Nightmares in Vietnam veterans. J Am Acad Psychoanal 1987;15:67-81.

46

Dreams and Nightmares in Posttraumatic Stress Disorder

Thomas A. Mellman

Wilfred R. Pigeon

ABSTRACT

Posttraumatic stress disorder develops in a significant minority of individuals who are exposed to severely threatening trauma. Trauma-related nightmares appear to be specific to PTSD and can be a persisting and distressing symptom. Not all dream content reported by individuals with PTSD is a direct representation of trauma memories, however. Stress and trauma appear to acutely affect the thematic content of dreams irrespective of whether the dreamer goes on to experience continuing emotional distress. Dreams that more specifically replicate the memory of the trauma during the early aftermath of exposure have been associated with the development of PTSD. In addition to indicating that stressful experiences are incorporated into dream content, findings from experimental and naturalistic studies further suggest that dreams can positively influence adaptation to stress and trauma. Persisting trauma-related nightmares may represent a failure of adaptive mechanisms.

Findings from polysomnographic studies of PTSD have not been entirely consistent. More recent studies suggest that the majority of nightmare episodes of study subjects with PTSD arise from REM sleep, although they can also be preceded by NREM sleep. A more fragmented pattern of REM sleep during the month following trauma was associated with the development of PTSD.

In contrast to normal dreams, dreams in persons with PTSD often incorporate actual memories of frightening experiences. These features have implications for understanding dreams' neurocognitive substrates. There is evidence that pharmacologic antagonism of noradrenergic receptors ameliorates nightmares in PTSD. A treatment approach that uses cognitive restructuring of nightmare content has yielded promising results.

REPLICATIVE-TRAUMA NIGHTMARES: HALLMARK OF A DISORDER?

PTSD is a psychiatric condition that develops in some but not all individuals who experience severely threatening traumatic experiences. (See also Chapters 78 and 111.) The diagnosis is based on persisting symptoms that include reexperiencing the trauma with intrusive images, flashbacks or nightmares, emotional numbing and avoidance behaviors, and heightened arousal. The course of PTSD can be self-limited, but in approximately a third of cases it persists for many years and it often manifests with comorbid psychiatric disorders.[1]

The fourth edition of the Diagnostic and Statistical Manual (DSM-IV) specifically delineates "recurrent distressing dreams of the event" among reexperiencing symptoms, describing them as dreams during which the traumatic event is "replayed."[2] In an influential review and theoretical paper, Ross and colleagues emphasized the occurrence of "repetitive replicas" of trauma scenes as a feature of dreams that is virtually specific to PTSD, further referring to trauma nightmares as a "hallmark of the disorder."[3]

Treating patients with PTSD often leaves the clinician impressed with the impact of distressing dreams featuring traumatic experiences. Several studies support the specificity of the relationship between trauma-related nightmares and PTSD proposed by Ross et al.[3] Van der Kolk and colleagues[4] reported that patients with combat-related PTSD were more likely to indicate that their nightmares exactly or almost exactly replicated an actual event as compared with nightmare sufferers who did not have PTSD. Mellman et al.[5] surveyed combat veterans from clinical and nonclinical settings and found that nightmares about combat experiences were more specifically associated with PTSD than were nightmares on other topics. In an analysis of a large epidemiologic database from Vietnam veterans, a measure that combined instances of nightmares related to military experiences and of distress from dreaming was strongly associated with PTSD.[6]

Thus there is consistent support for the theory that continuing representation of trauma memories in dreams is a feature of PTSD but not necessarily of trauma exposure absent the diagnosis. The aforementioned studies relied on retrospective and global, categorical assessments of dreams. Esposito and coworkers[7] performed content analysis of dreams elicited from morning diaries in a group of combat veterans receiving treatment for PTSD. About half of subjects' dreams contained direct references to combat experiences, and almost all of the dreams featured threat. The majority of dreams were also not unlike normal dream reports in terms of containing implausible elements that were not representations of actual memories. Elicitation of reports of mental activity upon awakening in a sleep laboratory is the most sensitive method for capturing dream content. Kramer et al.[8] also found in a symptomatic combat veteran group that about half of the dreams elicited after awakenings in the laboratory setting referred to military experiences. These studies all focused on combat veterans many years after their combat experiences.

Several studies have examined the influence of trauma on dream content during an acute phase following the traumatic event. In the two months following Hurricane Iniki, dream questionnaires from 22 primary care patients were compared to a larger sample surveyed prior to the hurricane ($N = 265$). A significantly higher percentage of the posthurricane subjects reported that their dreams were related to general stressors (74% versus 48%) and to "especially stressful life experiences" (67% versus 37%), although only 13% reported dreams specific to the hurricane.[9] Similarly, evacuees of the East Bay fire were more likely to have recorded dreams in their home diaries with content related to death, disasters, and fires than were controls.[10] Incorporation of trauma content in the dreams of recently traumatized children was reported by all 23 children kidnapped and buried underground in a trailer,[11] in 8 of 10 who witnessed rapes,[12] and in 63% of those on a playground during a sniper attack.[13] Unfortunately, these studies did not relate dream content to PTSD or acute stress disorder status, although the study of the sniper attack did document higher rates of trauma dreams as a function of proximity to the threat.

Mellman et al.[14] elicited dream content from study participants during the acute aftermath of traumatic injury. A subgroup of the sample described dreams that were distressing and "highly similar" to the traumatic experience (17% of the sample; 56% of those who reported dreams). This group had more severe concurrent PTSD symptom ratings than the groups with other categories of dreams, and they had higher subsequent PTSD severity than the group that did not recall dream content.[14]

Thus, exposed populations tend to report dreams with specific trauma-related or thematically related content during the acute aftermath of disasters and other traumas, and dreams that are similar to the memory of the actual traumatic event are associated with the development of PTSD. Chronic PTSD is associated with recurring dreams that represent specific memories of a traumatic experience. However, the more comprehensive evaluations of dreams during chronic phases of PTSD document that salient dream content is not limited to representations of traumatic memories.

DREAM CONTENT WITH STRESS AND TRAUMA: BEYOND REPLICATION

While the issue of trauma replication has received the most attention, there are descriptions of other aspects of content in the literature on dreaming, nightmares, and PTSD. The boundaries of traumatic stress are not always clear, and the topic seems embedded in broader questions of stress and dreaming, including observations of the impact of stressful experiences on dreams, the influence of dreams on adaptation to stressful experiences, and content themes related to trauma exposure and PTSD beyond trauma replication.

Stress and Dream Content

A number of studies of naturalistic stressors have suggested an impact of stressful waking experiences on dream content. For example, health-related stressors have been evidenced in the home dream content of patients awaiting surgery[15] and in hospitalized burn patients.[16] Dreams in pregnancy have been interpreted as reflecting concerns about the body and about the ability to mother and nurture.[17] In addition, the dreams of women with stressful menstruation are more likely to contain emotional content and relationship themes during the peak hormonal phase compared with other days in the menstrual cycle.[18]

Academic and occupational stress might also influence dream content. Duke and Davidson[19] found increased dream recall in a preexam week compared with a control week in college students. In contrast, Delorme, Lortie-Lussier, and De Koninck[20] found no difference in dream content involving exams or negative emotions 10 days before and after exam periods, although the authors failed to find a difference in the students' reported stress levels between the two periods. During one of the worst weekly performances of the Dow Jones Industrial Average, significant correlations were found between stockbrokers' stress levels and negative dream features, including recurrent nightmares, being chased, and falling.[21]

It has been noted that recurring dreams, which have more negative content than nonrecurring dreams,[22] tend to be activated by stressful life experiences.[23,24] In a community sample, subjects with active recurring dreams reported greater life stress in the prior six months and had more negative dream content than both former recurrent dreamers and dreamers who had never had recurrent dreams.[23] These findings were replicated in two college student samples.[25,19]

In addition to these naturalistic observations, studies have used experimental induction of stress and examined dream content. Disturbing movies,[26,27] sham intelligence exams,[28,29] deprivation of liquids,[30] and experimentally induced pain[31] have all been incorporated into dreams collected in the sleep laboratory. Overall, experimental stressors are associated with subsequent dreams that are characterized by a negative tone.

This almost uniform support for incorporation of stressful experiences into dream content contrasts somewhat with the debate and mixed findings around the broader question of whether dreams tend to incorporate recent experiences and waking concerns.[32-36] Although there is evidence that relatively innocuous daytime events and concerns can be incorporated into dreams, it seems reasonable to infer from the studies we have reviewed that stressful waking experiences are more likely to be incorporated into dreams and have an impact on dream emotional content. This relationship of dream incorporation to emotional saliency has led researchers to invoke an emotional information processing function for dreaming.[22,37-40] Although this contention is difficult to confirm, several lines of evidence support a relationship between dreams and adaptations to emotional stress.

Dreams and Adaptation to Stress

Two experimental studies suggest that dream content is related to adaptation to stress. In the study of liquid deprivation, subjects who had their thirst quenched in their dreams were less thirsty in the morning than those who had liquid in their dreams and remained unquenched or who had unrelated dreams.[30] In one of the experiments that used viewing a disturbing film as a probe, subjects experimentally deprived of REM sleep were subsequently more distressed by the film than either a NREM-sleep interruption group or an uninterrupted sleep group.[26] Naturalistic studies suggesting that dream incorporation can aid adaptive processing include several that found that references to drugs and alcohol in dreams are a positive predictor of abstinence,[41-44] including smoking cessation.[45] Cartwright and colleagues[38] elicited dream reports following laboratory awakenings from REM sleep in men and women going through divorce near the time of the initial breakup and one year later. Those who incorporated the ex-spouse into their dreams at the time of the breakup were less depressed and better adjusted at 12-month follow-up than those who did not. These two sets of observations might initially seem to contradict the observations reviewed earlier of an association between trauma-replicating dreams and the outcome of PTSD. The observations just reviewed, however, refer to incorporation of a reference or representation of a stressful situation and not necessarily the replication of events.

For dreaming to influence emotional adaptation to stress, the neurocognitive activity of sleep must have an enduring influence on memory representations. Although the theory remains controversial, there is increasing support for a role for sleep in the consolidation and reprocessing of memory (i.e., learning) that is reviewed in preceding chapters of this text.

Trauma, PTSD, and Content Themes

Dow et al.[46] studied depressed combat veterans with and without PTSD. They examined dreams collected from both groups in the sleep laboratory after awakenings from REM sleep. The PTSD group's dreams were rated higher for anxiety and were more likely to have been set in the past. Another laboratory study of veterans found more frequent aggression in the dreams of subjects with combat-related PTSD compared to the dreams of healthy controls.[47] Ratings for anxiety, aggression, and interpersonal conflicts were greater in the dreams of a symptomatic subgroup of Holocaust survivors.[48] In a study of combat-related PTSD using diary records of dreams that were spontaneously recalled, threatening content was observed in the majority of dreams (83%) with and without the presence of combat references.[7] In contrast, while the dreams from five female college students with PTSD were found to be more vivid and descriptive than dreams from five matched controls, they were not more negative, repetitive, or oriented to the past.[49]

Studies relating dreams to trauma exposure in children have also described content themes beyond representation of the trauma. The dreams of Palestinian children exposed to ongoing civil and military violence, elicited by home diaries, contained more themes of aggression, persecution, and negative emotions than dreams recorded by children living in a more peaceful region.[50] Kurdish children with trauma exposure evidenced more dreams with threat and aggression than either a nonexposed group or a control group from a peaceful country.[51] Unfortunately, neither of these studies determined the PTSD status of their subjects.

In our own study of patients with recent traumatic injuries, dreams contained less friendliness and sexuality compared with dreams from a normative sample of dreamers.[52] The dreams of those who developed PTSD had more content related to general and physical misfortune, as well as more negative emotions, than those who did not develop PTSD. Thus, compared to other dreams, dreams after trauma have more general negative emotions, anxiety, threat, and aggression, and these appear to be most pronounced with PTSD.

POLYSOMNOGRAPHIC CORRELATES OF NIGHTMARES IN PTSD

There is an association, albeit not an absolute one, between dreams—particularly those with content that is more elaborate, visual, emotional, and bizarre—and the REM-sleep stage.[53] Conversely, other sleep phenomena, such as night terrors and related parasomnias, arise from NREM-sleep stages, particularly slow wave sleep.[54] Due to the atypical aspects of dreams from patients with PTSD, there has been interest in determining their relationships to stages of sleep. It has been asserted that nightmares in PTSD are associated with NREM sleep. In one study, body movement occurred during stage 2 sleep when nightmares were reported in the morning.[4] In another study, Kramer and Kinney[55] studied a group of 24 subjects in the sleep laboratory and identified a subgroup of 8 combat veterans with nightmare symptoms who reported the majority of their nightmares after awakening from stage 2 sleep.

In contrast, the one spontaneous nightmare awakening that occurred during sleep recordings in a study by Ross et al.[3] and three of the three recorded by Mellman et al.[14] were preceded by REM sleep. Hefez et al.[56] described a pattern of "REM interruption insomnia" in a PTSD group with nightmares. The largest sample of polysomnographically recorded spontaneous nightmares (N=17) for PTSD patients was reported in an abstract by Woodward and colleagues.[57] They indicated that the probability of REM sleep occurring in the 10 minutes preceding spontaneous awakenings with nightmares was 57%, whereas only 17% of total sleep was REM. The probability of sleep preceding nightmares featuring stage 2 (27%) was less than its percentage of total sleep. None of the nightmares emerged from slow wave sleep. Thus on balance it seems that nightmares in PTSD tend to be preceded by the REM sleep stage but sometimes emerge from other sleep stages (1 and 2). This association (at least in part) with REM sleep underscores the characteristics of nightmares in PTSD that contrast with normative features of dreams associated with REM sleep, such as a lack of correspondence to actual events, bizarreness, and mixing of time frames and contexts.[53,58]

The observations reviewed in previous sections of this chapter suggest that associative memory functions linked to REM sleep may facilitate emotional adaptation. We have previously described a relationship between dreams that were rated as being very similar to the trauma memory and the development of PTSD. Another aim of our study of acute trauma was to evaluate characteristics of REM sleep and their relationship to outcome following trauma by obtaining polysomnographic recordings close to the time of medical and surgical stabilization in patients receiving treatment for traumatic injuries. The injured patients who developed PTSD did not differ from those who did not develop PTSD with respect to general measures of sleep maintenance, amount of REM sleep, and increased eye-movement density (compared with uninjured controls). The group developing PTSD, however, spent significantly less continuous time in REM sleep before shifting to waking or other EEG sleep stages. We hypothesized that this observed fragmentation of REM sleep may compromise REM sleep's potentially adaptive memory processing functions.[59]

SUMMARY AND IMPLICATIONS

The representation of the memory of a traumatic experience in dreams is a distinguishing feature of PTSD. While having characteristics different from those generally ascribed to dreams from the REM sleep stage, PTSD dreams appear most often to be preceded by REM sleep, although they do emerge from stage 1 and 2 as well. Traumatic and stressful experiences appear to influence dream content whether or not people are successfully adapting emotionally.

Recent data suggest that the more replicative-trauma nightmare is associated with the development of PTSD. When PTSD enters a chronic phase, trauma memories continue to be represented in recurring nightmares. Dream content of patients with established PTSD is not limited to trauma memories and may reflect the negative and restricted emotional state of the dreamer in other ways as well. The literature on stress and dreaming suggests that dream content reflects the emotional processing of the dreamer and that dreams potentially have a positive influence on emotional adaptation. In contrast, recurring nightmares in PTSD patients appear to reinforce the memory of the trauma and contribute to the individual's distress. The distinguishing feature of replicating or representing the memory of the trauma over time may provide important clues as to what is not working in the dream life and the more general emotional memory processing of people with PTSD.

Fosse et al.[60] have recently reported that dreams recalled by healthy college students frequently contained references to recent experiences, but the events' representation in the dreams rarely corresponded to the actual events. The researchers concluded that normal dreams are not episodic memories. Noncorrespondence to coherent whole memory representations and other characteristics of dream mentation are thought to be consequent to the selective activation of neural structures during REM sleep. In the generally accepted model of sleep state regulation, neural activation during REM sleep is mediated by firing of cholinergic brainstem nuclei and is further facilitated by inhibition of noradrenergic firing.[58]

As has been discussed, the dreams that characterize PTSD are not necessarily unaltered replays of the traumatic event. Yet there is a tendency for dreams occurring with PTSD to contain representations of events that include or are closer to unaltered memories (of traumatic events) than are normal dreams. Experimental evidence indicates that declarative memory for emotionally arousing stimuli is mediated by noradrenergic mechanisms.[61] Therefore, impaired inhibition of noradrenergic tone during sleep could be a mechanism underlying the presence of episodic-like, fear-enhanced memories in dreams. Direct support for this hypothesis comes from recent evidence that pharmacologic blockade of nor-adrenergic stimulation with prazosin, an alpha-1 noradrenergic antagonist, ameliorates nightmares in PTSD.[62]

There is a further consideration regarding an adaptive memory-processing function for REM sleep and REM dreaming that may be impaired with PTSD. Normal dream mentation has a "hyper-associative" quality: Characters, places, and sequences that are not typically linked in waking conscious thought tend to be juxtaposed in dreams.[58] Foa and colleagues[63] have suggested that one of the mechanisms of successful emotional processing during exposure therapy is the development of a new network of associations to the traumatic memories. Such a process may be facilitated by the normal neurocognitive characteristics of REM sleep and impaired by a more selective activation of trauma memories.

TREATMENT OF POSTTRAUMATIC NIGHTMARES AND RELATED SLEEP DISTURBANCES

A number of treatments, particularly selective serotonin reuptake inhibitor antidepressants and cognitive behavior psychotherapies, have recently been documented to be effective for treating PTSD.[64] Reports of the treatment studies typically indicate reduction of the severity of reexperiencing symptoms but do not specifically parcel out the treatment effects on nightmares. It is likely that nightmares tend to decrease in frequency and intensity as PTSD generally improves. Clinical experience and literature on the treatment of residual nightmare symptoms, however, suggest that nightmare symptoms can be inadequately responsive to first-line interventions for PTSD.

Formulations discussed in preceding sections suggest pharmacological and psychotherapeutic approaches for targeting PTSD nightmares. There is now clinical research evidence that supports efficacy of treatment strategies that are consistent with the previously stated theoretical formulations. Raskind et al.[62] followed up their initially more-anecdotal observations suggesting amelioration of nightmare symptoms with noradrenergic blockade. They evaluated prazosin treatment in 10 patients with combat-related PTSD using a randomized, double-blind, cross-over design. The medication was dosed aggressively (average dose of 10 mg), with initial daily titration, monitoring of orthostatic blood pressure, and use of late-afternoon dosing to supplement nighttime administration if doses exceeded 6 mg. The authors reported highly significant treatment effects on ratings of distressing dreams as well as benefits to insomnia and other PTSD symptoms.

A therapeutic effect of postsynaptic blockade of noradrenergic neurotransmission is consistent with the role for noradrenergic activity in mediating traumatic nightmares that was postulated in the previous section. Evaluations of other pharmacological approaches to target nightmare symptoms of PTSD have mostly not been controlled. Anecdotal descriptions of benefits to nightmares have been made for other nor-adrenergic suppressing agents (e.g. guanfacine),[65] novel antipsychotic medications,[66] antidepressants that feature postsynaptic serotonin antagonism (trazodone and nefazodone),[67,68] and the serotonin antagonist cyproheptadine,[69] although a subsequent double-blind evaluation of cyproheptadine failed to confirm a decrease in nightmares.[70]

The idea that dreams are related to both successful and impaired patterns of emotional processing suggests that recurrent nightmares related to trauma might respond to psychotherapeutic interventions. Krakow and colleagues[71] recently reported a trial of imagery-rehearsal therapy. In this technique, patients with recurring nightmares are instructed to write the content of their dream with an altered ending and to image the altered dream scenario before going to sleep. In their treatment study of women with PTSD related to sexual assault and recurring nightmares, 114 participants received followup assessment. There were highly significant reductions in nightmare severity and frequency in the treatment group compared to their baseline severity and compared to controls, as well as improvements in insomnia and other symptoms of PTSD. At present this approach cannot be recommended as a first-line comprehensive treatment for PTSD because the dropout rate was fairly high, end-of-study ratings for PTSD reflected significant severity of symptoms, and the results have not been replicated. However, imagery-rehearsal therapy is a practical brief treatment that appears particularly effective in targeting nightmare symptoms and can be applied as a stand-alone intervention or as an adjunct to other treatments.

The technique of imagery-rehearsal therapy appears consistent with principles from the established cognitive behavior treatments of PTSD that apply exposure or cognitive restructuring, or both, to trauma memories.[64] That such techniques can be effectively applied directly to nightmare content (which in PTSD often features trauma memories) has important implications. One is that clinicians can be realistically hopeful about the potential for alleviating distressing nightmare symptoms. We have previously referred to the apparent paradox that stress-related references in dreams are associated with positive outcome, whereas trauma-replicating nightmares are associated with PTSD. This paradox may be reconciled if the former dreams represent an adaptive emotional processing, possibly related to modification of associative networks, and the latter represent a failure of such a process. Studies of imagery rehearsal suggest that conscious exposure to the content of recurring distressing dreams, along with instruction to modify the dream scenario, facilitates movement toward the more adaptive response.

That benefits of nightmare-focused interventions generalize to other symptom domains lends support to the idea of continuity between waking emotional life and dreaming. Dreams may also offer clinicians a unique window into individuals' emotional adaptation to trauma and stress along with the status of their processing of traumatic memories. The apparently robust association between PTSD and replays or representations of trauma memories in dreams further provides an important clue to understanding abnormalities of emotional memory processing that differentiate those who suffer with PTSD and those who are more resilient to adverse psychobiological consequences of trauma.

Clinical Pearl

The phenomenon of trauma-replication in dreams is a distinguishing feature of posttraumatic stress disorder that has implications for understanding alterations of memory processing functions.

References

1. Kessler RC, Sonnega A, Bromet E, et al: Posttraumatic stress disorder in the National Comorbidity Survey. Arch Gen Psychiatry 1995;52:1048-1060.
2. Frances A, Pincus HA, First M, et al (eds): Diagnostic and Statistical Manual of Mental Disorders, 4th ed. Washington, DC, American Psychiatric Association, 1994.
3. Ross RJ, Ball WA, Sullivan KA, et al: Sleep disturbance as the hallmark of posttraumatic stress disorder. Am J Psychiatry 1989;146:697-707.
4. van der Kolk B, Blitz R, Burr W, et al: Nightmares and trauma: A comparison of nightmares after combat with lifelong nightmares in veterans. Am J Psychiatry 1984;141:187-190.
5. Mellman TA, Kulick-Bell R, Ashlock LE, et al: Sleep events in combat-related post-traumatic stress disorder. Am J Psychiatry 1995;152:110-115.
6. Neylan TC, Marmar CR, Metzler TJ, et al: Sleep disturbances in the Vietnam generation: Findings from a nationally representative sample of male Vietnam veterans. Am J Psychiatry 1998; 155:929-933.
7. Esposito K, Benitez A, Barza L, et al: Evaluation of dream content in combat-related PTSD. J Traumatic Stress 1999;12: 681-687.
8. Kramer M, Schoen LS, Kinney L: The dream experience in dream disturbed Vietnam veterans. In van der Kolk (ed): Posttraumatic Stress Disorders: Psychological and Biological Sequelae. Washington, DC, American Psychiaric Association, 1984, pp 82-95.
9. Pagel JF, Vann BH, Altomare CA: Reported association of stress and dreaming: Community background levels and changes with disaster (Hurricane Iniki). Dreaming 1995;5:43-50.
10. Siegel A: Dreams of firestorm survivors. In Barrett D (ed): Trauma and Dreams. Harvard University Press, 1996.
11. Terr LC: Children of Chowchilla: A study of psychic trauma. Psychoanalytic Study Child 1979;34:547-623.
12. Pynoos RS, Nader K: Children who witness the sexual assaults of their mothers. J Am Acad Child Adolesc Psychiatry 1988;27:567-572.
13. Nader K, Pynoos R, Fairbanks L, et al: Children's PTSD reactions one year after a sniper attack at their school. Am J Psychiatry 1990;147:1526-1530.
14. Mellman TA, David D, Bustamante V, et al: Dreams in the acute aftermath of trauma and their relationship to PTSD. J Traumatic Stress 2001;14:241-247.
15. Berger L, Hunter I, Lane RW: The Effect of Stress on Dreams. New York, International University Press, 1971.
16. Raymond I, Nielsen TA, Lavigne G, et al: Incorporation of pain in dreams of hospitalized burn victims. Sleep 2002; 25: 765-770.
17. Maybruck P: Pregnancy and Dreams. Los Angeles, Jeremy Tarcher, 1989.
18. Bucci W, Creelman ML, Severino SK: The effects of menstrual cycle hormones on dreams. Dreaming 1991;1:263-276.
19. Duke T, Davidson J: Ordinary and recurrent dream recall of active, past and non-recurrent dreamers during and after academic stress. Dreaming 2002;12:185-197.
20. Delorme M, Lortie-Lussier M, De Koninck J: Stress and coping in the waking and dreaming states during an examination period. Dreaming 2002;12:171-183.
21. Kroth J, Thompson L, Jackson J, et al: Dream characteristics of stock brokers after a major market downturn. Psychol Rep 2002;90:1097-1100.
22. Zadra AL: Recurrent dreams: their relation to life events. In Barrett D (ed): Trauma and Dreams. Cambridge, Mass, Harvard University Press, 1996, pp 231-267.
23. Brown RJ, Donderi DC: Dream content and self-reported well-being among recurrent dreamers, past recurrent dreamers, and nonrecurrent dreamers. J Pers Soc Psych 1986;50:612-623.
24. Cartwright RD: The nature and function of repetitive dreams: A survey and speculation. Psychiatry 1979;42:131-137.
25. Zadra AL, O'Brien S, Donderi DC: Dream content, dream recurrence, and well-being: A replication with a younger sample. Imagination Cog Pers 1998;17:293-311.
26. Greenberg R, Pillard R, Pearlman C: The effect of dream (stage REM) deprivation on adaptation to stress. Psychosom Med 1972; 34:257-262.
27. De Koninck JM, Koulac D: Dream content and adaptation to a stressful situation. J Abnorm Psych 1975;84:250-260.
28. Koulac D, Prevost F, De Koninck JM: Sleep, dreaming, and adaptation to a stressful intellectual activity. Sleep 1985;8: 244-253.

29. Stewart DW, Koulack D: The function of dreams in adaptation to stress over time. Dreaming 1993;3:259-268.

30. Bokert E: The effects of thirst and a related stimulus on dream reports. Dissertation Abstracts 1967;28:4753B.

31. Nielsen TA, McGregor DL, Zadra A, et al: Pain in dreams. Sleep 1993;16:490-498.

32. Roussy F, Camirand C, Foulkes D, et al: Does early-night REM dream content reliably reflect presleep state of mind? Dreaming 1996;6:121-130.

33. Roussy F, Brunette M, Mercier P, et al: Daily events and dream content: Unsuccessful matching attempts. Dreaming 2000; 10:77-83.

34. Rados R, Cartwright RD: Where do dreams come from? A comparison of presleep and REM sleep thematic content. J Abnorm Psych 1982;91:433-436.

35. Marquardt CJG, Bonato RA, Hoffmann RF: An empirical investigation into the day-residue and dream-lag effects. Dreaming 1996;6:57-65.

36. Saredi R, Baylor GW, Meier B, et al: Current concerns and REM-dreams: A laboratory Study of dream incubation. Dreaming 1997;7:195-208.

37. Breger L: Function of dreams. J Abnorm Psych Monograph 1969;72:1-28.

38. Cartwright RD: Dreams that work: The relation of dream incorporation to adaptation to stressful events. Dreaming 1991;1:3-9.

39. Hartmann E: Nightmares after trauma as paradigm for all dreams: A new approach to the nature and function of dreaming. Psychiatry 1998;61:223-238.

40. Van de Castle RL: Our Dreaming Mind. New York, Ballantine Books, 1993.

41. Choi SY: Dreams as a prognostic factor in alcoholism. Am J Psychiatry 1973;130:699-702.

42. Christo G, Franey C: Addicts' drug-related dreams: Their frequency and relationship to six-month outcomes. Subst Use Misuse 1996;31:1-15.

43. Reid SD, Simeon DT: Progression of dreams of crack cocaine abusers as a predictor of treatment outcome: A preliminary report. J Nerv Ment Dis 2001;189:854-857.

44. Hajek P, Belcher M: Dream of absent-minded transgression: An empirical study of a cognitive withdrawal symptom. J Abnorm Psychol 1991;100:487-491.

45. Persico AM: Predictors of smoking cessation in a sample of Italian smokers. Int J Addict 1992;27:683-695.

46. Dow BM, Kelsoe JR, Gillin JC: Sleep and dreams in Vietnam PTSD and depression. Biol Psychiatry 1996, 39:42-50.

47. Lavie P, Katz N, Pillar G, et al: Elevated awaking thresholds during sleep: Characteristics of chronic war-related posttraumatic stress disorder patients. Biol Psychiatry 1998;44:1060-1065.

48. Lavie P, Kaminer H: Dreams that poison sleep: Dreaming in Holocaust survivors. Dreaming 1991;1:11-21.

49. Vinent MH, Smith CT: REM sleep processes and dream content in posttraumatic stress disorder. Sleep 2000; 23(S2):A101.

50. Punamaeki R: The relationship of dream content and changes in daytime mood in traumatized vs. non-traumatized children. Dreaming 1999;9:213-233.

51. Valli K, Revonsuo A, Palkas, et al: The threat simulation theory of the evolutionary function of dreaming: Evidence from dreams of traumatized children. Conscious Cogn 2004; in press.

52. Pigeon WR, Mellman TA: Dream content in recently hospitalized trauma patients. Proceedings of the International Society of Trauma and Stress Studies, p 45, 2002. Available at: www.istss.org.

53. Foulkes WD: Dream reports from different stages of sleep. J Abnormal Social Psychology 1969;65:14-25.

54. Fisher C, Kahn E, Edwards A, et al: A psychophysiological study of nightmares and night terrors: The suppression of stage 4 night terrors with diazepam. Arch Gen Psychiatry 1973;28:253-259.

55. Kramer M, Kinney L: Sleep patterns in trauma victims with disturbed dreaming. Psychiatr J Univ Ott 1988;13:12-16.

56. Hefez A, Metz L, Lavie P: Long-term effects of extreme situational stress on sleep and dreaming: Am J Psychiatry 1987;144:344-347.

57. Woodward SH, Arsenault NJ, Michel GE, et al: Polysomnographic characteristics of trauma-related nightmares. Sleep 2000; 23(S2):A356.

58. Hobson JA, Stickgold R, Pace-Schott EF: The neuropsychology of REM sleep dreaming. Neuroreport 1998; 9:R1-R14.

59. Mellman TA, Bustamante V, Fins AI, et al: REM sleep and the early development of posttraumatic stress disorder. Am J Psychiatry 2002;159:1696-1701.

60. Fosse MJ, Fosse R, Hobson JA, et al: Dreaming and episodic memory: A functional dissociation? J Cog Neurosci 2003; 15:1-9.

61. Cahill L, Prins B, Weber M, et al: β-Adrenergic activation and memory for emotional events. Nature 1994; 371:702-704.

62. Raskind MA, Peskind ER, Kanter ED, et al: Reduction of nightmares and other PTSD symptoms in combat veterans by prazosin: A placebo-controlled study. Am J Psychiatry 2003; 160:371-373.

63. Foa EB, Kozak MJ: Emotional processing of fear: Exposure to corrective information. Psych Bull 1986; 99: 20-35.

64. Foa E, Keane TM, Friedman MJ (eds): Effective treatments for PTSD : Practice guidelines from the International Society for Traumatic Stress Studies. New York, NY, Guilford Press, 2000.

65. Horrigan JP: Guanfacine for PTSD nightmares. J Am Acad Child Adolesc Psychiatry 1996;35: 975-976.

66. Leyba CM, Wampler TP: Risperidone in PTSD. Psychiatr Serv 1998;49:245-246.

67. Ashford JW, Miller TW: Effects of Trazodone on sleep in patients diagnosed with post-traumatic stress disorder (PTSD). J Contemporary Psychotherapy 1996; 26(3):221-233.

68. Mellman TA, David D, Barza L: Nefazodone treatment and dream reports in chronic PTSD. Depress Anxiety 1999;9(3):146-148.

69. Brophy MH: Cyproheptadine for combat nightmares in posttraumatic stress disorder and dream anxiety disorder. Military Med 1991;156:100-101.

70. Jacobs-Rebhun S, Schnurr PP, Friedman MJ, et al: Posttraumatic stress disorder and sleep difficulty. Am J Psychiatry 2000;157:1525-1526.

71. Krakow B, Hollifield M, Johnston L, et al: Imagery rehearsal therapy for chronic nightmares in sexual assault survivors with posttraumatic stress disorder: A randomized controlled trial. JAMA 2001;286:537-545.

47

Why We Dream

Robert Stickgold

ABSTRACT

Historical models of dreaming have failed to achieve scientific validation. New models, built from studies in the cognitive neuroscience, are now being proposed. These are based on (1) patterns of reactivation of local brain circuits during sleep in humans and rats; (2) patterns of regional brain activation during wake, non–rapid eye movement (NREM), and REM sleep in humans; (3) sleep-dependent learning and memory consolidation; and (4) cognitive performance in humans immediately after awakenings from NREM and REM sleep. They suggest that dreaming represents the conscious experiencing of brain mechanisms that perform off-line memory reprocessing during sleep. At the same time, novel dream studies also suggest the nature of memory reprocessing occurring during sleep, and that a multiplicity of memory functions regulate the sleep state–dependent differences in the formal properties and content of dreams. Together, these findings suggest both a mechanism and function for dreaming.

The search for an understanding of dreaming is thousands of years old. Three publications over the last 100 years have formed the core of most of the scientific discussion of this question. These include Freud's *Interpretation of Dreams*, at the end of the 19th century,[1] the report of a correlation between dreaming and the newly discovered rapid eye movement (REM) sleep in the 1950s,[2] and the proposal of the activation-synthesis model of dreaming in the 1970s,[3] which argued that dreaming was initiated by random neural activity in the brainstem during REM sleep. But as we enter the 21st century, there is precious little on which dream researchers agree.

One relatively new approach has been to consider dreaming within a larger neurocognitive framework of offline memory processing during sleep. The rationale for this approach is that dreaming must reflect the activity of the brain, and specifically an activity that includes the reactivation of memories and emotions from earlier experiences. Because neural activity in the brain invariably leaves the activated networks altered, dreaming must modify the networks storing memories and emotions. Dreaming then becomes the conscious experiencing of these activated networks in the process of being modified.

BRAIN ACTIVITY DURING SLEEP

To understand how dreams might be produced, and the functions they may serve, it is important to understand how brain activity differs in wake and REM and non-REM (NREM) sleep. Over the last several years, a series of positron emission tomography studies have shown that patterns of human brain activation differ across the states of waking, REM sleep, and NREM sleep. Whereas most brain regions are relatively inactive during slow wave sleep (SWS), entry into REM sleep leads to reactivation of some regions, along with further deactivation of others. The pattern seen suggests a shift in global brain function in REM sleep away from conscious executive control (further decrease in dorsolateral prefrontal cortex activity) and toward hallucinatory (increased activity in sensory association cortices) and emotional (increased amygdala, anterior cingulate, and medial orbitofrontal cortex activity) processing.[4-6]

In addition to these changes in patterns of brain activity, cognitive testing performed immediately after awakenings from REM and NREM sleep suggest that the brain is biased toward less common associations and more flexible cognitive processing.[7-9]

In both humans and rats, patterns of brain activity observed during waking appear to be replayed during sleep. In rats, simultaneous recordings from large numbers of hippocampal neurons have shown that specific patterns and sequences of neuronal firings observed as the rats sought out food on a circular track were replayed during subsequent REM and NREM sleep, with rates and delays distinctly different between the two sleep states.[9,10] In humans, positron emission tomography studies have shown that brain regions activated during learning of a task were selectively reactivated during the next night's REM sleep.[11] These findings of reactivation of brain networks involved in prior waking experiences is paralleled by a growing body of evidence for sleep-dependent memory consolidation.

SLEEP-DEPENDENT MEMORY CONSOLIDATION

One interpretation of these changes during sleep is that they reflect a *homeostatic* process, working to restore the brain to the state it was in at the start of the previous day. This "rest" or "restorative" model of sleep argues that sleep serves to reverse deleterious changes that inevitably accrue across the day. But a more powerful, *progressive* model suggests that these changes reflect *off-line processing* of information obtained during the prior day, consolidating, integrating, and even, if appropriate, actively reversing changes that occurred during waking. Dreaming may serve similar processes. For example, Freud proposed a restorative model of dreaming, specifically considering, but then rejecting any progressive model.[1] In contrast, others have questioned[12] or rejected[13] any evolutionary purpose for dreaming.

Although the question of the function of dreaming remains unresolved, there is a growing consensus that sleep serves a function of offline memory processing (for reviews, see Maquet[4] and Walker and Stickgold[14]). Sleep has been shown to enhance prior learning of perceptual and motor skills,[15,16] paired word associates,[17,18] and emotionally charged episodic memories,[19] and even to enhance mathematical insight.[20]

But in relation to learning and memory consolidation, not all sleep is equal. For example, improvement on a motor skill task has been reported to correlate with amounts of late-night light (stage 2) NREM sleep,[16] but improvement on a visual perception task to correlate with both late-night REM sleep and early-night SWS[15,21,22]; others have found paired word associate learning to depend on early night sleep,[17,18] and emotional declarative memory on late sleep (for reviews, see Walker and Stickgold[14] and Wagner et al.[19]).

Thus, brain mechanisms are clearly in place that would permit dreaming to serve a similar function, namely, participating in the reprocessing of memories from daytime experiences. Such a claim is reminiscent of Freud's claim that "in every dream we may find some reference to the experiences of the *preceding day* (original emphasis),"[1] although in some cases this reprocessing, identified by sleep-dependent learning enhancements, has been shown to continue for several nights after an initial learning experience (see, e.g., Stickgold et al.[23]), and lesser, incremental enhancements might even continue for years.[24]

SLEEP STAGES AND DREAM CONTENT

If memory processes active during sleep are differentially activated across sleep stages, and dreaming at least parallels, and possibly contributes to, these memory processes, then one would expect to see changes in the content of dream reports collected from different sleep states. In its simplest form, this is exactly what is seen. Reports are more frequent after awakenings from REM sleep,[25-28] and both REM and NREM reports are more common when awakenings occur later in the night. Among those reports obtained, reports from REM are longer,[29-31] more vivid, more story-like, and more bizarre.[27,28,32,33] Although it has been suggested that some of these differences reflect poorer recall after NREM awakenings, little objective evidence supports such a claim, and other REM–NREM differences are not amenable to such an explanation. For example, hallucinations are more prevalent in reports from REM sleep, whereas directed thinking is more common in NREM sleep, a pattern that cannot be explained simply by poorer recall from one stage or another.[34]

Even at this level of analysis, there is a striking homology between dream content and memory function in sleep. In REM sleep, dreams are (1) hallucinatory, (2) emotional, and (3) narrative, with (4) frequent fictive movements (for review, see Hobson et al.[28]), and REM is thought to facilitate consolidation of visual perceptual and emotional memories.[14] In contrast, NREM sleep is more thoughtlike and less hallucinatory,[34,35] and is implicated in simple memorization of word pair lists.[17] Although there are notable exceptions (e.g., improvement on a motor task correlates with late-night NREM sleep, but REM dreams are decidedly more motoric), the argument can be made that differences in memory functions across sleep stages are reflected in differences in dream content.

DREAMS AND MEMORY SYSTEMS

All models of dreaming assume that dreams are constructed from our memories. But they also recognize that this construction need not involve the direct incorporation of memories into the dream scenario. Freud, for example, emphasized that actual memories, events, and their associated emotions underwent "condensation" and "displacement" before appearing in dreams. Although he elaborated a complex theory of "dream work" to explain the cause of these alterations, modern cognitive neuroscience provides a much simpler and more straightforward explanation, namely that dream construction does not include incorporation of hippocampally mediated episodic memories (memories of events), but rather of semantic (facts and general information) and representational memories (sensorimotor images) stored in and directly accessed in the neocortex.[36]

Memory sources appear to differ by sleep stage. Subjects ascribed episodic memory sources for dream elements more frequently after awakenings from sleep onset or NREM sleep than after REM awakenings.[38] This differential rate parallels the decline in directed thinking reported as subjects move from sleep onset to stage 2 NREM and then into REM sleep.[35,37] At the same time, the frequency of "generic semantic memory sources" was greater in dreams from REM than NREM sleep (Baylor and Cavallero,[38] p. 165).

But although episodic memory sources were identified in reports from both REM and NREM sleep, it appears that episodic memories themselves are not replayed during dreaming. In a subsequent study, subjects identified waking antecedents for 364 dream elements in 299 dream reports. When the extent of congruence between these dream element and their purported waking source was analyzed,[39] only 12 of the 364 dream elements identified had the same location, characters, and actions as the waking event, and only 5 to 8 of these appeared to judges as possible replays of the waking events, representing only 1% to 2% of the identified dream elements. Only this 1% to 2% arguably reflects the same presumably hippocampally mediated processes of episodic memory recall that occur in waking. The remaining 98% to 99% of dream elements related to waking thoughts and events appears to result from the priming of neocortical memory systems, in much the same way as implicit memory tasks provide access to often consciously inaccessible cortical memories,[36] and not from the activation of episodic memories. Thus, "we dream *about* what happened, but not what actually occurred" (Stickgold,[37] p. 24).

What is most striking in this study is that although specific episodic memories do not appear to be replayed, they are nonetheless confidently identified by the dreamer as the source of dream elements. What then, is the basis of this association? Unlike the characteristics of an episodic memory, the features that showed highest congruence between dream element and putative waking source were (1) theme, (2) emotion, and (3) characters.[39] Although the last of these is consistent with episodic memory replay, the first two decidedly are not. Thematic congruence reflects the activity of the nonhippocampally mediated, strongly associatively linked, semantic memory system. It is with this memory system, for example, that themes are identified and stored as associated memories sharing common features.

But the lack of episodic replay raises new questions. Although episodic memories are memories of events that unfold over time, semantic memories are not. Instead, semantic memories appear as isolated facts and images, usually without a temporal component. Although semantic memories of motor actions (how to swing a bat or tie a shoe) have such temporal aspects, it is unclear how the process of dream construction might go about putting elements of semantic memory together into an unfolding dream narrative occurring over time.

At an even more fundamental level, it becomes unclear how objects, characters, and actions would be brought together within such a scenario. If episodic memories are simply not accessible to the dreaming brain, perhaps because of an absence of outflow from the hippocampus to the neocortex during REM[40] or because of a generalized deactivation of dorsolateral prefrontal cortex across all sleep states,[6,41-43] it would suggest that insofar as Freud's "latent content" exists, it is absent from the dream not because of a censorship of intolerable desires, but because of an inaccessibility of all waking episodic memories. In the absence of such episodic memories, which normally bind together the individual features of an event—the persons, places, things, and actions that make up the event—the brain must look elsewhere for mechanisms of finding elements from which to construct a dream. "Condensation" and "displacement" would then be the natural consequence of these associative processes. It is to the nature of these associative processes that we now turn our attention.

ASSOCIATIVE PROCESSING DURING SLEEP

From a modern, cognitive neuroscience perspective, the questions of dream censorship, condensation, displacement, and latent and manifest content come together in a single question of how emotional and associative memory processes function during dream construction. Whether viewing dreams as arising from a hidden, perhaps forbidden, wish[1] or from the random firing of neurons in the pontine brainstem,[3] the subsequent development of the dream must occur through the activation of an admixture of random and associative memories, and insofar as dreams are at all coherent in space and time, associative memories must dominate in the construction process. What, then, of the nature of these associative processes?

One approach to this question is to perform standard cognitive tests of associative memory immediately after awakening from REM and NREM sleep in the middle of the night, during the period of "sleep inertia" that precedes the return to full wakefulness,[44] when the brain and mind still display properties of the previous sleep condition (see Dinges[45] for review), and regional brain activation has not yet returned to waking levels.[46,47]

Two such studies have found a bias toward the activation of less common associations after awakenings from REM sleep. In the first of these, subjects performed a semantic priming test within 2 to 3 minutes after being awakened from REM or stage 2 NREM sleep. In the task, subjects see a "priming" word for 200 msec, followed by a target letter string which may or may not be a word, and must press one of two keys indicating whether or not the target string is a word, responding as quickly and accurately as possible. When reaction times for words (as opposed to nonwords) are analyzed, the speed of response is found to be proportional to the degree of relationship between the prime and target words.[48-50] Thus, the response time to the target word "mouse" would be faster when preceded by a strongly related prime, such as "cat," than a weakly related prime, such as "fur," and faster yet than to an unrelated prime, such as "mop." This enhancement in response rate is thought to reflect the automatic spread of activation from neural ensembles representing the prime word to other ensembles representing the target word, a process that proceeds without intent or conscious awareness.[51-53] The lesser enhancement seen with "weak" primes presumably reflects the reduced spread of activation to these less strongly associated neural ensembles.

But when the efficacy of such weak and strong primes was measured after awakenings from REM sleep, weak priming increased reaction speed by 24 msec (compared with unrelated primes), whereas strong priming increased them only by a nonsignificant 3 msec, significantly less than the weak priming.[8] The implication of these findings is that the spread of activation among neural ensembles is altered during REM sleep, such that normally weak associations become more readily activated than normally strong associations. Such an inversion of the normal pattern might be expected to have two effects on cognitive processes during sleep. First, insofar as the associative networks control the development of dream scenarios, one would expect dreams to develop in bizarre and unpredictable ways, as is in fact the case. But such a shift in activation patterns would also foster creative processes, which act through the novel juxtaposition of known facts.

Just such an effect was found in the second study, where subjects awakened from REM or NREM sleep attempted to solve anagram puzzles, unscrambling such letter strings as "resmad" to discover a scrambled word, in this case the word "dreams." When awakened from REM sleep, subjects were able to solve 32% more anagrams in the allotted time than after awakening from stage 2 NREM sleep,[7] a finding consistent with the results of the semantic priming study.

In an even more dramatic example of sleep's ability to foster creative thinking, subjects taught a rote mathematical process were more than twice as likely to discover a shortcut that dramatically reduced the time required to complete the task if they were allowed a night of sleep between initial training and follow-up testing, than if they were given an equivalent amount of wake time either during the day or across a night.[20] Perhaps most important, this discovery was made in the absence of any suggestion that there was a shortcut to be found. Thus, the sleeping brain appears to be able to search out and find potentially valuable new associations without prior knowledge that such associations are to be found. Still, none of these studies actually studied dream content, to determine whether there was even a correlation between such changes in cognitive processing and dream content.

One source of information about how associative processes function in dreaming is to look at the actual associations found in dreams, and there may be no better place to look than in the bizarreness of dreams, one of the most broadly studied of all dream features.[1,33,54-56] In one description, bizarreness has been divided into three main categories: incongruities, discontinuities, and uncertainties.[57-59] Within this construct, discontinuities provide a useful insight into the nature of bizarre dream associations. In a study of bizarre discontinuities involving the sudden and unexpected transformation of one object into another, judges were asked to match the original dream objects with their transformation products.

When presented with the transformation pairs in scrambled lists (Table 47-1), judges could reliably identify the

Table 47–1. Scrambled Object Transformations

Object 1	Object 2
Bag	Georgia home
Bed	Burlap sack
Boston home	Bike
Building	Half-size bed
Car	School bus
Cash machine	Beach
Pool	Car wheels and frame
Car	Building
City bus	Lion (really a bed)
Flowers	Intense combat video game
Statue of a lamb	Figures

Transformations involved the sudden and discontinuous change of objects in column 1 into those in column 2. Judges were instructed to match each initial object with its transformed product.

From Rittenhouse CD, Stickgold R, Hobson JA: Constraint on the transformation of characters and objects in dream reports. Conscious Cogn 1994;3:100-113.

original transformations[60] (Table 47–2). Thus, although the transformations were sudden, unexpected, and bizarre, the related objects could be readily identified.

But perhaps of more interest is the nature of the relationships. Such transformations could be related by similarity of form or function, or by learned associations. For example, fire trucks and buses are related by similarity, whereas fire trucks and fire fighters are related by learned association. When the 11 transformations listed in Table 47–2 were analyzed, all

Table 47–2. Scores for Identification of Object Transformations by Judges

Object 1	Object 2	Correct Scores	Percentage Correct*
Bag	Burlap sack	6	100%
Bed	Half-size bed	6	100%
Boston home	Georgia home	6	100%
Building	Building	6	100%
Car	Bike	6	100%
Cash machine	Intense combat video game	6	100%
Pool	Beach	6	100%
Car	Car wheels and frame	5	83%
City bus	School bus	5	83%
Flowers	Figures	5	83%
Statue of a lamb	Lion (really a bed)	5	83%
Total		**62**	**94%**

*All P < .0001

"Correct scores" is the number of judges (of six) who correctly matched the initial and transformed objects.

From Rittenhouse CD, Stickgold R, Hobson JA: Constraint on the transformation of characters and objects in dream reports. Conscious Cogn 1994;3:100-113.

object pairs (with the possible exception of flowers–figures) were clearly related by similarity of form or function, and none by learned association. Thus, at least in the case of such transformations, the nature of the associative processes involved appear to be partially identified.

DECLARATIVE MEMORY PROCESSING DURING SLEEP

Sleep does not, in general, show robust enhancement of declarative, episodic memory, and early studies found relatively little evidence for sleep playing a role in declarative memory consolidation (for review, see Smith[61]). Simple recall of word lists or paired-associate lists showed no deterioration after total or REM sleep deprivation.[62-67] In addition, the Rey-Osterrieth task, a nonverbal declarative memory task, similarly showed no sleep dependence.[68] More recent reports,[18,69] however, using the same paired-associates task, have suggested that SWS may mediate declarative memory consolidation. Although at first glance these findings appear to contradict the earlier ones, these more recent studies have used a distinctly different flavor of paired-associates task.

In the paired-associates task, subjects are presented with perhaps 40 word pairs, one after another, for a fixed amount of time, such as 5 seconds, each. After the entire list has been presented, subjects are shown the first word of each pair, and asked to recall the second word. For example, for the word pair "book–car," subjects would be shown the word "book" and asked for its paired associate, "car." During this initial review, subjects are told after each trial whether their answer was correct, and, if not, are shown the correct word pair (book–car) again. This process of review is typically repeated until a target percentage correct, such as 60%, is achieved. This may take a single review of the list, or as many as 10. Once the target percentage is reached, training stops. Subjects are then retested at a later time, in these studies most commonly after a night with or without sleep.

What differed in these most recent studies, which showed sleep-dependent enhancement, is that rather than using unrelated word pairs (e.g., book–car), the researchers used "semantically related" (Gais and Born,[70] p. 2140) word pairs (e.g., mother–child; Table 47–3).

Although no studies have directly compared paired-associate lists with semantically related and unrelated word pairs, the various studies would be brought into agreement if memories for related, but not unrelated, word pairs were enhanced by sleep. Such a distinction would represent another example where memories that require hippocampal mediation (random word pairs lacking a previously learned associations) are unaffected by posttraining sleep, whereas memories that use hippocampally independent mechanisms of recall (semantically related word pairs) are enhanced.

By now, a pattern has begun to emerge. Forms of memory and memory processing that can be shown by cognitive testing to be facilitated by sleep, or even specific sleep stages, are also found to be used in the dream construction process, while forms of memory that do not appear to benefit from sleep fail to appear in the content of dreams. This is also seen in an exception to the rule that novel episodic declarative memories are not enhanced by sleep.

Table 47–3.	**Semantically Related Paired Associates Used by Gais and Born**		
school–board	tower–bell	sea–tide	family–marriage
newspaper–interview	sonata–joy	flag–camp	tendency–increase
mother–child	insect–caterpillar	river–ship	coast–beach
gun–bullet	blacksmith–metal	dwelling–room	building–hall
rain–flooding	avenue–thicket	decency–truth	regulation–answer
diamond–hardness	result–effect	occupation–butcher	book–story
attack–course of events	cat–soul	doll–cradle	episode–luck
railway–steam	kitchen–pot	landscape–moorland	musician–pianist
industry–factory	clothes–head cloth	car–headlight	prison–gangster
gale–breath of wind	bouquet–bloom	bottle–toast	group–person
crisis–emergency	girl–engagement	port–crane	garden–flower bed

Word pairs are English translations from the original German list.

From Gais S, Born J: Low acetylcholine during slow-wave sleep is critical for declarative memory consolidation. Proc Natl Acad Sci U S A 2004;101:2140-2144, Web supplement.

EMOTIONAL MEMORY PROCESSING DURING SLEEP

Wagner et al.[19] have reported that recall of emotionally charged story elements was selectively enhanced after periods of sleep rich in REM sleep. The story was told as a series of slides depicting the events of the story was shown, and subjects were later tested on their recall of details from the slides. Two different stories were told for the same set of slides. In the emotional version of the story, the middle third of the slides described a serious accident, whereas the neutral version of the story contained no emotional descriptions. At retest after sleep rich in REM sleep, the subjects who heard the emotional version of the story displayed enhanced recall, but only for the slides accompanied by the emotional description.

These findings are in agreement with numerous studies that have suggested that dreaming represents a highly complex analysis and recasting of both memories and emotions,[71-77] and suggest that dreaming acts to process the emotional content of events in an individual's life.[78]

The best-known example of emotional processing during sleep is perhaps also the least understood. This is the phenomenon of "sleeping on a problem," involving situations where a difficult decision must be made. Vast numbers of anecdotal cases indicate that people can go to bed at night with such a problem on their mind, and wake up the next morning with a clear choice in their mind. There are several features of this phenomenon that are worth noting. First, it is a remarkably robust effect, with most people casually surveyed believing that, as often as not, it successfully yields results overnight. Second, the decision normally becomes apparent without an explicit rationale. People report knowing at a "gut level" that they have come to the correct decisions, but without a clear and rational justification for it. Third, there is usually considerable confidence that the decision reached is the correct one, and little sense that further deliberation would be of any added benefit. At the same time, the process does not appear to be useful for the recall of forgotten information, such as a phone number or address. Rather, it serves to analyze available information and come to a decision based on some sort of weighing of the relevant information. Although these features of the process are clear from anecdotal observations, it must be made clear that, to our knowledge, no objective studies of the phenomenon have been made. Perhaps the closest we have at this time is the study of mathematical insight, described previously.[20]

INCORPORATION OF WAKING EVENTS INTO DREAMS

Although many the studies of dreaming described previously reflect the incorporation of waking events into dreams, few involved experimental manipulations of waking events with the goal of influencing subsequent dream content (for review, see Lauer et al.[77]). A new line of research investigating this process has focused on hypnagogic dreams, which occur at sleep onset. In the first of these studies,[79] subjects spent 2 to 3 hours per day playing the video game, Tetris, for 2 or 3 days. Three groups of subjects were studied—12 subjects with no prior Tetris experience ("novices"), 10 with extensive Tetris experience ("experts"), and 5 subjects with dense amnesia with extensive medial temporal lobe damage resulting from anoxia or encephalitis ("amnesiacs"). The game involves manipulating game pieces as they "fall" from the top of the computer screen to the bottom in a central "play window." Players can move pieces to the left or right and rotate them as they fall. Their goal is to rotate and position the pieces so that they fill the space at the bottom of the screen without leaving gaps between pieces. On the evening of each day of game play, subjects were awakened repeatedly during the first hour of the night, always within 3 minutes of sleep onset, and asked to report any thoughts, feelings, or images from the prior sleep period. Nine of the novices (75%) and five of the experts (50%) reported visual images of the game in 9.8% and 4.8% of their sleep onset reports, respectively. Taken together, 64% of the subjects reported instances of game imagery during the hypnagogic period, with images reported in 7.2% of all reports.

Subjects reported remarkably similar imagery, seeing Tetris pieces falling in front of their eyes, occasionally rotating and fitting them into empty spaces. Among the 27 reports of imagery, there were no reports of seeing the larger picture surrounding the play window, the scoreboard, or the keyboard, or of typing on the keyboard. There were only two reports of seeing a computer screen and none of seeing the desk or room. Thus the imagery was limited to those aspects of the experience that were most salient and to which subjects presumably paid the most attention, and none had the characteristics of episodic memories.

But more objective evidence of the lack of episodic memories participating in the construction of these dreams came from the five densely amnesic patients. Three of these reported hypnagogic Tetris images despite being unable to recall playing the game before or after the night's sleep. Not only did this represent the same frequency of subjects reporting (60% of amnesic versus 64% of normal subjects), but the same percentage of reports (7.4% for amnesic versus 7.2% for normal subjects). Even more striking was the similarity in actual report content. Although unable to recall having played the game (or even to recognize the experimenter from session to session), patients nonetheless reported, for example, "little squares coming down on a screen," and in one case, the subject explicitly stated that she had no knowledge of the source of the images. Thus she was able to produced dream images of events for which she had no declarative knowledge.

Also of note is that two of the five Tetris "experts" reporting Tetris images explicitly reported images from earlier versions of the game, which they had not played in the last year, with one of the subjects reporting that she had not played her older, Nintendo version of the game since she had been in high school, 5 years earlier. Thus, game imagery need not be a simple replay of recent sensory input, but instead can reflect older, strongly associated memories.

These last two findings, of Tetris images in the dreams of amnesic subjects and of images of previously played versions of the game, bear a striking resemblance to aspects of Freudian dream theory. Freud's belief that dream construction involved the reactivation, by events of the day, of memories from childhood finds support in the imagery of previously played versions of Tetris reported after a day with game play. But there is nothing of a negative, suppressed, forbidden, or sexual nature in the recalled and replayed memories seen in the dream. A more straightforward interpretation would be that associative processes, primed by the recently formed memories resulting from 2 to 3 hours of play earlier that day, reactivated strongly associated memories from childhood. This is what would be predicted based on a progressive, associative model of dream construction, which served to enhance the strength of such association, allowing more information from the earlier memories to be made available for use while performing the newer version of the game.

So also for the findings with amnesic subjects. Here, in perhaps the clearest form possible, dreams provide a royal path to the unconscious. With their inability to form new declarative memories, any incorporation of Tetris images into the dreams of these patients must reflect activation of memory systems that are not accessible through conscious search. Indeed, at least one patient explicitly reported a lack of knowledge of the waking source of the dream imagery. The fact that normal subjects produce similar images at similar rates, suggests that, even in normal subjects, these hypnagogic dream images are being recalled from memory systems unavailable to directed conscious recall. This is in keeping with our hypothesis that access to hippocampally mediated episodic memories is not available during sleep. But although this model implies dream access to "the unconscious," it is a very different unconscious from that proposed by Freud, one

not fraught with forbidden memories and desires, but rather one that evolved to provide us with general semantic knowledge of the world around us, rather than specific episodic memories from our past.

This fact is driven home even more forcefully by a study in which subjects were taught three nonsense sentences across a night, one immediately before going to sleep, and two more after awakening from REM sleep.[80] The nonsense sentences (translated from the original Italian) are (1) "In the bathroom the raven is painting a fish on a radio and spinning a bust on the custard"; (2) "In the embers a poster is fining a parcel along the bridge and betting a tooth in the game"; and (3) "In a liter a cock is tricking a ruble from a palm and nursing a ball in a tub." Subjects were instructed to memorize the sentences, and after hearing each one twice, repeated them back as accurately as possible. When dream reports were collected after awakening from the next REM period, dream content was frequently judged to be related to the previously memorized sentence. For example, after hearing the first sentence, with its reference to "painting a fish," one subject reported "walking with a friend on the seashore."

Of course, such apparent associations can be spurious. Indeed, when judges, blind to the source of reports, scored dream reports from a control night, before subjects had heard any of the sentences, apparent associations were again found. But the experimental design allowed for the use of these rates of "pseudoincorporation," obtained from the control night, to correct for such spurious associations, and when this was done, over a third of all REM reports collected on the experimental night contained actual incorporations of elements from the learned sentence (72% of reports on the experimental night versus 39% on the control night; $P < .01$).

Two features of these results are particularly striking. First, the simple act of intentional memorization seems to be sufficient to tag a memory for potential incorporation into subsequent dream content, even when the memory itself has no meaning. Second, as with the previously described study of the incorporation of waking memories into nocturnal dreams,[39] these incorporations are never in the form episodic memories, such as a report of memorizing a sentence. Instead, the brain seems simply to extract key elements of the memorized sentence (single words) and incorporate them is into an unrelated scenario. In fact, not only is the scenario changed, the object is as well, so that the actual word from the memorized sentence (e.g., the fish) is replaced by a semantically related word (e.g., the seashore). This is different from what was seen in the hypnagogic Tetris dreams,[79] but additional studies of sleep-onset imagery bridge this difference.

When subjects trained during the day on the arcade game Alpine Racer II, a downhill skiing simulation, 88% of subjects reported images from the game in their subsequent hypnagogic dreams, including places where they frequently crashed, or a particularly steep slope, but again without seeing the arcade game itself, or themselves playing it.[81,82] In agreement with the findings of the Tetris study, 5 of 10 subjects with prior downhill skiing experience also reported seeing images related not to the arcade game, but to actual skiing experiences from their past. This initial study thus extended the Tetris findings to a second game.

However, quite different results were obtained in a second study. In this case, subjects were allowed 2 hours of uninterrupted sleep at the start of each night, before being awakened and then, as they fell back asleep, awakened for hypnagogic dream reports. In this "delayed awakening" protocol, subjects no longer reported skiing images. Instead, they gave reports, for example, of "falling down a hill" or of "moving through some kind of forest" with their "entire upper body ... incredibly straight."[37] Thus, the more directly related images of skiing had been replaced with more weakly associated images, reminiscent of the apparent transformation of "fish" into "seashore" in the memory study described earlier,[80] and suggesting that the process of dream construction may be similar in REM sleep and at sleep onset.

A NEUROCOGNITIVE MODEL OF DREAM CONSTRUCTION AND FUNCTION

When memories are activated, they are inevitably altered. This is one of the most striking findings of cognitive neuroscience in the last decade. Indeed, it might be true that no neural circuits in the brain are ever activated without being at least subtly altered. This is true regardless of whether the activation of a particular circuit is perceived by the conscious mind. Thus, every time a child hears a sentence spoken, neural circuits are activated that, over time, will extract rules of grammar that will allow her to speak with near-perfect use of the grammar, even though she may never explicitly know those rules or even be consciously aware that they exist. This is a hallmark of the brain's construction—that it extracts similarities and rules without even knowing that they exist. And this is exactly what was seen in the study of mathematical insight,[20] in which sleep was shown to facilitate this process dramatically.

Of course, such activation can also occur in conscious experience, as is the case as you read and consider the arguments presented here. Just as there are distinct memory systems in the brain, some accessible to consciousness and some not,[36] so also are there distinct mechanisms for activating and manipulating these memories, some of which are amenable to conscious control and some of which are not. So it should come as no surprise when I suggest, first, that dreaming must inevitably alter the memories accessed in the process of dream construction, and, perhaps more important, that dreaming may simply be a byproduct of mechanisms that evolved to facilitate sleep-dependent memory consolidation and integration.

As in waking, these mechanisms would often activate systems that remain outside of our awareness. This presumably is the case when visual texture discrimination skills[15] or learning of a finger-tapping motor sequence[16] are consolidated during sleep. But at other times (or even at the same time, in parallel processes), these mechanisms would activate systems in ways that bring their contents into conscious awareness. When this happens we dream, observing the flow of images, thoughts, and feelings that occurs during this memory reactivation. But, critically, we do not see the changes in the memory systems that result from this reactivation, and thus we see the content of dreams, but neither their underlying purpose nor their ultimate effects. Thus, if one chose to, one could describe the dream content as "manifest content" and the underlying changes in memory systems as "latent consequences."

The question of the function of dreaming can now be reduced to a question of the function of that sleep-dependent memory processing that results in the conscious experience of dreaming, which is itself a subset of the more general question of the function of sleep-dependent memory processing. It is our belief that sleep has, as one of its most critical functions, the incremental improvement of cortical networks. Such a model has recently been put forward in some detail by others.[83] Because sleep has been shown to enhance (1) genetically preprogrammed but experientially controlled modification of visual circuitry during early development,[84] (2) visual and motor skill learning,[15,16] (3) emotional memories,[19] (4) some simple declarative memories,[17] and (5) mathematical insight,[20] it would appear that sleep's role in such processing spans an impressively wide range of brain circuits and functions. The question of dream function now becomes the question of which of these circuits and functions, when activated, enter our conscious awareness.

Which circuits might be critical? Based on studies of patients with neurologic disorders, several discrete regions have been proposed[85] as responsible for consciousness, including several brainstem nuclei (including monoaminergic and cholinergic nuclei involved in control of the REM cycle), the hypothalamus, superior colliculus, thalamus, somatosensory cortices (including the insula and medial parietal cortex), and the cingulate cortex. Brain imaging studies provide evidence that many, if not all, of these areas are specifically activated during REM sleep.[5] I propose that when these regions are sufficiently activated, consciousness arises in sleep as it does in waking, resulting in the phenomenon of dreaming. Thus, from one perspective, we dream because the necessary brain regions are appropriately activated, but from another perspective, dreaming *is* the appropriate activation of these regions. They become two levels of description of the same biologic event.

What function might be served by these circuits? We have proposed elsewhere[37] that dreaming occurs as the brain evaluates the potential value of novel forms of behavior, using, during REM sleep, the weak cortical associations preferentially activated in this state,[8] in the absence of dorsolateral prefrontal cortex (DLPFC)[6,41,43] or hippocampal[40,86] feedback, but in the presence of active error detection circuits in the anterior cingulate cortex (ACC),[87] and affective evaluation of such errors by the amygdala and medial orbitofrontal cortex (OFC). (Whether NREM dreaming involves separate circuitry carrying out separate functions remains unknown.)

How would such a circuitry function? The inability of the DLPFC to allocate attentional resources (and the dreaming brain classically pays little attention to bizarre incongruities in dreams) would be compounded by the inability of hippocampally mediated episodic memories to be reactivated in cortex.[40] As a result, dreamed responses would have to be constructed from those primarily weak neocortical associations available during REM sleep,[8] without the help of the directed (DLPFC) recall of episodic (hippocampal) memories. Although the process of incorporation of these weak associates into the dream narrative remains unknown, associated emotions, mediated by both the amygdala and the OFC, could play an important role. These responses would then, in turn, be reanalyzed by the ACC error detection circuitry. The consequences of this repeated modification and reanalysis of potential behaviors are twofold. First, at the brain level, we would see novel associations being activated within neocortical networks and being tested by an error detection system that could adjust the strengths of these associations based on the affective response to the imagined behavioral outcomes. At the conscious level, however, we would see classic REM dream construction. Situations would arise in the dream narrative without the dreamer appearing to participate in planning the course of events (DLPFC inactive), with the dreamer instead appearing simply to respond emotionally to each turn of events (ACC, OFC, amygdala), not paying attention (DLPFC) to incongruous or impossible twists in the plot (weak associations). The frequent perplexity that the dreamer experiences surrounding dream behavior suggests that, as in waking, "the ACC seems to come into play when rehearsed actions are not sufficient to guide behavior."[88]

In the end, then, we propose that dreaming is simply the conscious perception of the stream of images, thoughts, and feelings evoked in the brain by one of many forms of off-line learning and memory processing that occur during sleep. At the same time, however, it reflects one of the most sophisticated forms of processing that the brain performs, the analysis and interpretation of the events of our lives in a manner that provides meaning to these events and guides our future behavior. Whether assessing the chances in a sexual gambit or the choices in a complex moral dilemma, the mechanism is the same, and it is quintessentially human.

> **Clinical Pearl**
>
> *Dreaming may be the conscious awareness of underlying processes of off-line learning and memory consolidation and integration that occur during sleep, but without awareness of the underlying changes in memory systems that are the purpose of these brain processes.*

REFERENCES

1. Freud S: The Interpretation of Dreams. Strachey J (transl). New York, Basic Books, 1955.
2. Dement WC, Kleitman N: Cyclic variations in EEG during sleep and their relation to eye movements, body motility, and dreaming. Electroencephalogr Clin Neurophysiol 1957;9:673.
3. Hobson JA, McCarley RW: The brain as a dream-state generator: An activation-synthesis hypothesis of the dream process. Am J Psychiatry 1977;134:1335-1348.
4. Maquet P: The role of sleep in learning and memory. Science 2001;294:1048-1052.
5. Hobson JA, Stickgold R, Pace-Schott EF: The neuropsychology of REM sleep dreaming. Neuroreport 1998;9:R1-R14.
6. Nofzinger EA, et al: Forebrain activation in REM sleep: An FDG PET study. Brain Res 1997;770:192-201.
7. Walker MP, et al: Cognitive flexibility across the sleep-wake cycle: REM-sleep enhancement of anagram problem solving. Cogn Brain Res 2002;14:317-324.
8. Stickgold R, et al: Sleep induced changes in associative memory. J Cogn Neurosci 1999;11:182-193.
9. Wilson MA, McNaughton BL: Reactivation of hippocampal ensemble memories during sleep. Science 1994;265:676-679.
10. Louie K, Wilson MA: Temporally structured replay of awake hippocampal ensemble activity during rapid eye movement sleep. Neuron 2001;29:145-156.
11. Maquet P, et al: Experience-dependent changes in cerebral activation during human REM sleep. Nat Neurosci 2000;3:831-836.
12. Hobson JA: The Dreaming Brain. New York, Basic Books, 1988.
13. Flanagan O: The Dreaming Soul. New York, Oxford University Press, 2000.
14. Walker M, Stickgold R: Sleep-dependent learning and memory consolidation. Neuron 2004;44:121-133.
15. Stickgold R, et al: Visual discrimination task improvement: A multi-step process occurring during sleep. J Cogn Neurosci 2000;12:246-254.
16. Walker M, et al: Practice with sleep makes perfect: Sleep dependent motor skill learning. Neuron 2002;35:205-211.
17. Plihal W, Born J: Effects of early and late nocturnal sleep on declarative and procedural memory. J Cogn Neurosci 1997; 9:534-547.
18. Plihal W, Pietrowsky R, Born J: Dexamethasone blocks sleep induced improvement of declarative memory. Psychoneuroendocrinology 1999;24:313-331.
19. Wagner U, Gais S, Born J: Emotional memory formation is enhanced across sleep intervals with high amounts of rapid eye movement sleep. Learn Mem 2001;8:112-119.
20. Wagner U, et al: Sleep inspires insight. Nature 2004;427:352-355.
21. Karni A, et al: Dependence on REM Sleep of overnight improvement of a perceptual skill. Science 1994;265:679-682.
22. Gais S, et al: Early sleep triggers memory for early visual discrimination skills. Nat Neurosci 2000;3:1335-1339.
23. Stickgold R, James L, Hobson JA: Visual discrimination learning requires post-training sleep. Nat Neurosci 2000;2:1237-1238.
24. McClelland JL, McNaughton BL, O'Reilly RC: Why there are complementary learning systems in the hippocampus and neocortex: Insights from the successes and failures of connectionist models of learning and memory. Psychol Rev 1995; 102:419-457.
25. Aserinsky E, Kleitman N: Regularly occurring periods of ocular motility and concomitant phenomena during sleep. Science 1953;118:361-375.
26. Dement W, Kleitman N: Cyclic variations in EEG during sleep and their relation to eye movements, body mobility and dreaming. Electroencephalogr Clin Neurophysiol 1955;9: 673-690.
27. Nielsen TA: Mentation during sleep: The NREM/REM distinction. In Lydic R, Baghdoyan HA (eds): Handbook of Behavioral State Control: Cellular and Molecular Mechanisms. Boca Raton, Fla, CRC Press, 1999, pp 101-128.
28. Hobson JA, Pace-Schott EF, Stickgold R: Dreaming and the brain: Toward a cognitive neuroscience of conscious states. Behav Brain Sci 2000;23:793-842.
29. Antrobus JS: REM and NREM sleep reports: Comparison of word frequencies by cognitive classes. Psychophysiology 1983; 20:562-568.
30. Foulkes D, Schmidt M: Temporal sequence and unit composition in dream reports from different stages of sleep. Sleep 1983; 6:265-280.
31. Stickgold R, Pace-Schott E, Hobson JA: A new paradigm for dream research: Mentation reports following spontaneous arousal from REM and NREM sleep recorded in a home setting. Conscious Cogn 1994;3:16-29.
32. Antrobus JS, et al: Brightness and clarity of REM and NREM imagery: Photo response scale. Sleep Res 1987;16:240.
33. Cavallero C, et al: Slow wave sleep dreaming. Sleep 1992;15:562-566.
34. Fosse R, Stickgold R, Hobson JA: Thinking and hallucinating: Reciprocal changes in sleep. Psychophysiology 2004;41: 298-305.
35. Fosse R, Stickgold R, Hobson JA: Brain mind states: Reciprocal variation in thoughts and hallucinations. Psychol Sci 2001; 12:30-36.
36. Schacter DL, Tulving E: Memory Systems 1994. Cambridge, Mass, MIT Press, 1994.
37. Stickgold R: Memory, cognition, and dreams. In Maquet P, Smith C, Stickgold R (eds): Sleep and Plasticity. New York, Oxford University Press, 2003, pp 17-40.
38. Baylor GW, Cavallero C: Memory sources associated with REM and NREM dream reports throughout the night: A new look at the data. Sleep 2001;24:165-170.

39. Fosse MJ, et al: Dreaming and episodic memory: A functional dissociation? J Cogn Neurosci 2003;15:1-10.

40. Buzsáki G: The hippocampo-neocortical dialogue. Cereb Cortex 1996;6:81-92.

41. Braun AR, et al: Regional cerebral blood flow throughout the sleep-wake cycle. Brain 1997;120:1173-1197.

42. Maquet P, et al: Functional neuroanatomy of human slow wave sleep. J Neurosci 1997;17:2807-2812.

43. Maquet P, et al: Functional neuroanatomy of human rapid-eye-movement sleep and dreaming. Nature 1996;383:163.

44. Lubin A, et al: Effects of exercise, bedrest, and napping on performance decrement during 40 hours. Psychophysiology 1976;13:334-339.

45. Dinges DF: Are you awake? Cognitive performance and reverie during the hypnopompic state. In Bootzin R, Kihlstrom J, Schacter D (eds): Sleep and Cognition. Washington, DC, American Psychological Association, 1990, pp 159-178.

46. Balkin TJ, et al: The process of awakening: A PET study of regional brain activity patterns mediating the re-establishment of alertness and consciousness. Brain 2002;125:2308-2319.

47. Balkin TJ, et al: Bi-directional changes in regional cerebral blood flow across the first 20 minutes of wakefulness. Sleep Res Online 1999;2(Suppl 1):6.

48. Meyer DE, Schvaneveldt RW: Facilitation in recognizing pairs of words: Evidence of a dependence between retrieval operations. J Exp Psychol 1971;90:227-234.

49. Neely JH: Semantic priming and retrieval from lexical memory: Roles of inhibitionless spreading activation and limited-capacity attention. J Exp Psychol 1977;106:226-254.

50. Neely JH: Semantic priming effects in visual word recognition: A selective review of current findings and theories. In Besner D, Humphreys GW (eds): Basic Processes in Reading: Visual Word Recognition. Hillsdale, NJ, Erlbaum, 1991, pp 264-336.

51. Cañas JJ: Associative strength effects in the lexical decision task. Q J Exp Psychol 1990;42A:121-145.

52. Collins JJ, Chow CC, Imhoff TT: Stochastic resonance without tuning. Nature 1995;376:236-238.

53. Posner MI, Snyder RR: Attention and cognitive control: Information processing and cognition. In RL Solso (ed.): The Loyola Symposium. Hillsdale, NJ, Erlbaum, 1975, pp 55-85.

54. Casagrande M, et al: Variations in sleep mentation as a function of time of night. Int J Neurosci 1996;85:19-30.

55. Foulkes D: Dream reports from different stages of sleep. J Abnorm Soc Psychol 1962;65:14-25.

56. Molinari S, Foulkes D: Tonic and phasic events during sleep: Psychological correlates and implications. Percept Mot Skills 1969;29:343-368.

57. Hobson JA, et al: Dream bizarreness and the activation-synthesis hypothesis. Hum Neurobiol 1987;6:157-164.

58. Mamelak AN, Hobson JA: Dream bizarreness as the cognitive correlate of altered neuronal behavior in REM sleep. J Cogn Neurosci 1989;1:201-222.

59. Williams J, et al: Bizarreness in dreams and fantasies: Implications for the activation-synthesis hypothesis. Conscious Cogn 1992;1:172-185.

60. Rittenhouse CD, Stickgold R, Hobson JA: Constraint on the transformation of characters and objects in dream reports. Conscious Cogn 1994;3:100-113.

61. Smith C: Sleep states, memory processes and synaptic plasticity. Behav Brain Res 1996;78:49-56.

62. Ekstrand BR, et al: Spontaneous recovery and sleep. J Exp Psychol 1971;88:142-144.

63. Ekstrand BR: To sleep, perchance to dream (about why we forget). In Duncan CP, Sechrest L (eds): Human Memory: Festchrift in Honor of Benton J. Underwood. New York, Appleton-Century-Crofts, 1972, pp 59-82.

64. Empson JAC, Clarke PRF: Rapid eye movements and remembering. Nature 1970;227:287-288.

65. Lewin I, Glaubman H: The effect of REM deprivation: Is it detrimental, beneficial or neutral? Psychophysiology 1975;12:349-353.

66. McGrath MH, Cohen DB: REM sleep facilitation of adaptive waking behavior: A review of the literature. Psychiatr Bull 1978;85:24-57.

67. Smith C: REM sleep and learning: Some recent findings. In Moffitt A, Kramer M, Hoffman R (eds): The Functions of Dreaming. New York, SUNY Press, 1993, pp 341-361.

68. Conway J, Smith C: REM sleep and learning in humans: A sensitivity to specific types of learning tasks. J Sleep Res 1994;3:48.

69. Plihal W: Differential Effects of Early and Late Nocturnal Sleep on the Consolidation of Declarative and Nondeclarative Memory. Frankfurt, Germany, Peter Lang, 1996.

70. Gais S, Born J: Low acetylcholine during slow-wave sleep is critical for declarative memory consolidation. Proc Natl Acad Sci U S A 2004;101:2140-2144.

71. Berger M, Riemann D, Lauer C: The effect of presleep stress on subsequent sleep EEG and dreams in healthy subjects and the depressed. In Poella WP, et al (eds): Sleep '86. New York, Gustav Fischer Verlag, 1988, pp 84-86.

72. Cartwright R: Dreams that work: The relation of dream incorporation to adaptation to stressful events. Dreaming 1991;1:3-9.

73. Cartwright R, Newell P, Mercer P: Dream incorporation of a sentinel life event and its relation to waking adaptation. Sleep Hypnosis 2001;3:25-32.

74. Greenberg R, Pearlman CA: Cutting the REM nerve: An approach to the adaptive function of REM sleep. Perspect Biol Med 1974;17:513-521.

75. van der Kolk B, et al: Nightmares and trauma: A comparison of nightmares after combat with lifelong nightmares in veterans. Am J Psychiatry 1984;141:187-190.

76. Rothbaum BO, Mellman TA: Dreams and exposure therapy in PTSD. J Trauma Stress 2001;14:481-490.

77. Lauer C, et al: Shortened REM latency: A consequence of psychological strain. Psychophysiology 1987;24:263-271.

78. Stickgold R: EMDR: A putative neurobiological mechanism of action. J Clin Psychol 2002;58:61-75.

79. Stickgold R, et al: Replaying the game: Hypnagogic images in normals and amnesiacs. Science 2000;290:350-353.

80. Cipolli C, et al: Active processing of declarative knowledge during REM-sleep dreaming. J Sleep Res 2001;10:277-284.

81. Emberger KM: To sleep perchance to ski: The involuntary appearance of visual and kinesthetic imagery at sleep onset following play on the Alpine Racer II. In Psychology. Cambridge, Mass, Unpublished honors thesis, Harvard University, 2001.

82. Stickgold R, et al: Sleep learning and dreams: Off-line memory reprocessing. Science 2001;294:1052-1057.

83. Paller KA, Voss JL: Memory reactivation and consolidation during sleep. Learn Mem 2004;11:662-670.

84. Frank MG, Issa NP, Stryker MP: Sleep enhances plasticity in the developing visual cortex. Neuron 2001;30:275-287.

85. Damasio AR: The Feeling of What Happens. New York, Harcourt, Brace, 1999.

86. Chrobak JJ, Buzsáki G: Selective activation of deep layer (V-VI) retrohippocampal cortical neurons during hippocampal sharp waves in the behaving rat. J Neurosci 1994;14:1660-1670.

87. Carter CS, et al: Anterior cingulate cortex, error detection, and the online monitoring of performance. Science 1998;280:747-749.

88. Paus T: Primate anterior cingulate cortex: Where motor control, drive and cognition interface. Nat Rev Neurosci 2001;2:417-424.

Approach to the Patient with Disordered Sleep
Beth A. Malow

ABSTRACT

The evaluation of a patient with disordered sleep begins with the chief complaint, which can be classified into insomnia, daytime sleepiness, episodic nocturnal movements or behaviors, or a combination of these concerns. A thorough characterization of these concerns, coupled with a comprehensive sleep history that includes the daily schedule, the bedtime routine, and morning and daytime symptoms, forms the foundation for diagnosis. As in other fields of medicine, it is essential to consider other medical and psychiatric conditions, medication use, family history, social history including the psychosocial situation, review of systems, and the physical examination before formulating a differential diagnosis and performing diagnostic studies. This systematic approach allows for accurate diagnosis and specific interventions for many treatable sleep disorders.

Sleep disorders are common in the general population. They can contribute to impaired academic or occupational performance, accidents at work or while driving, and disturbances of mood and social adjustment. Marriages and relationships may be adversely affected by the disordered sleep of a spouse or bed partner. In addition, sleep disorders may lead to or exacerbate serious medical, neurologic, and psychiatric problems. The clinician should therefore take sleep complaints from a patient seriously and approach the evaluation of such problems in an orderly and systematic fashion.

Patients who complain of disturbed sleep usually describe one or more of three types of problems: insomnia; abnormal movements, behaviors, or sensations during sleep or during nocturnal awakenings; or excessive daytime sleepiness. These sleep complaints are not mutually exclusive, and a given sleep disorder may be associated with more than one type. For example, patients with sleep apnea may complain of insomnia, excessive daytime sleepiness, choking or gasping during the night, or all three. Those with narcolepsy may complain of

sleep paralysis and hallucinations at sleep onset or on awakening, disrupted sleep, and daytime sleepiness.

The foundation for the diagnosis of sleep disorders is the history of the sleep complaint. Ideally, the evaluation includes a history from the patient's bed partner. Many sleep problems are not evident to the patient, and it is often the bed partner who has persuaded the patient to seek evaluation. The bed partner can comment on the intensity of snoring and the presence of nocturnal behaviors or events. Rounding out the clinical evaluation are the past medical history, family history, social history, review of systems, and physical examination.

An assessment is then made on the basis of the clinical evaluation. In many cases, it is possible to make a definitive diagnosis and begin treatment, whereas in others, the diagnosis is presumptive and must be confirmed or excluded by diagnostic studies. If the diagnosis is uncertain, a differential diagnosis is formulated and a plan is developed to determine a definitive diagnosis, if possible. The elements of the evaluation of patients with disordered sleep are reviewed in this chapter, and signs and symptoms that may point to a particular diagnosis are emphasized.

CHIEF COMPLAINT AND HISTORY

Evaluation begins with the chief complaint, which provides a focus for delineating the patient's concerns and eliciting the history. It is often useful to ask why the patient is seeking help at the present time, particularly if the problem has been of long standing. If the chief complaint is from the spouse or bed partner, it is important to determine whether the patient recognizes the problem, is unaware of it, or denies its existence. Many clinicians also obtain a brief patient profile during the interview that includes the patient's age, sex, occupational or academic status, marital status, and living arrangements.

There are two kinds of nighttime symptoms: those that occur during sleep, and those that occur during nocturnal awakenings. Symptoms that occur during sleep concern movements or behaviors and often are reported by the spouse or bed partner because the patient may be unaware of the episodes.

Examples include snoring, cessation of breathing, twitching or kicking of the legs or arms, chewing movements, sleepwalking, sleeptalking, screams, and violent behavior. Complaints that occur during nocturnal awakenings concern sensations or events that are evident to the patient and include headaches, wheezing or shortness of breath, palpitations, heartburn, leg cramps, or feelings of paralysis, numbness, or tingling.

Once the chief complaint is delineated, details concerning the sleep problem are sought, including its duration, the circumstances at its onset, the factors that lead to exacerbation or improvement, and any associated symptoms.

The patient's daily schedule is reviewed, including the usual bedtime and estimated time to sleep onset, the number and timing of awakenings, and the time of final awakening. Particularly in children, the bedtime routine, or lack thereof, should be assessed; this information may suggest *limit-setting sleep disorder*. The method of awakening should be determined: spontaneous, with an alarm, or by a family member. The usual waking schedule should also be determined, including times of work, school, meals, and exercise. It is important to obtain detailed sleep–wake schedules in shift workers. A comparison of the patient's weekday and weekend schedules may reveal significant variations in sleep timing that suggest a *circadian rhythm sleep disorder* (see Chapter 58) or *insufficient sleep syndrome* (see Chapter 6).

Morning symptoms should be elicited, such as increased nasal congestion or dry mouth or morning headaches. These symptoms may support a diagnosis of obstructive sleep apnea. Daytime symptoms, including activities that tend to provoke sleepiness, should be investigated to characterize the severity of sleepiness. A comprehensive sleep history also includes questions about the frequency and duration of daytime naps and the presence or absence of cataplexy, hypnic hallucinations, sleep paralysis, and automatic behavior.

Questions assessing the sleep setting may elicit information about factors that cause or aggravate sleep problems. Noise, extreme temperature, uncomfortable sleep surfaces, and frequently changing sleep conditions may all adversely affect sleep continuity and suggest an *environmental sleep disorder*.

For patients with medical or psychiatric diseases, the degree of sleep disturbance usually varies with the severity of the underlying illness. For example, in patients with congestive heart failure, the degree of insomnia may correlate with the severity of orthopnea and paroxysmal nocturnal dyspnea. Similar relationships may occur in patients with sleep disturbance related to depression, asthma, gastroesophageal reflux, and arthritis. In patients with sleep apnea, daytime sleepiness may correlate with seasonal allergies, alcohol use, or other factors that worsen apnea.

Insomnia

Patients with insomnia usually complain that their nocturnal sleep is inadequate in some way. They may describe difficulty falling asleep, frequent awakening, or early morning awakening with inability to return to sleep. It is important to distinguish among these patterns of insomnia because they may have different causes. For example, awakenings from sleep due to obstructive sleep apnea may result in sleep maintenance insomnia but would not result in a patient complaining of

lying awake for hours not being able to fall asleep. The description of insomnia and its course may help determine cause. For example, insomnia that began in early childhood and continues with few remissions may suggest *idiopathic insomnia* (see Chapter 51). The relation of insomnia to stress is also important. If the cause of the stress is clear, such as the recent death of a family member, the diagnosis is likely to be *adjustment sleep disorder* (see Chapter 51). In other patients, however, the nature of the stress may not be immediately apparent. Positive life events, such as a promotion at work or recent marriage, may not be recognized by the patient as stressful. Medical conditions, such as cancer and its treatment (see Chapter 103), pain syndromes (see Chapter 106), or gastrointestinal disease (see Chapter 107), may also cause or contribute to insomnia.

Specific questions may reveal maladaptive behaviors and thought patterns that contribute to sleep difficulties. People with insomnia may become aroused and anxious when they are preparing for sleep and may worry about their insomnia and its effects on performance at work or at home the following day. Some may sleep better in an unfamiliar sleep setting, which suggests the presence of heightened arousal, frustration, or anxiety in attempting to sleep in the usual environment; these characteristics suggest *psychophysiological insomnia* (see Chapter 51). Irregular bedtimes, late night exercise, caffeine use in the afternoon or evening, watching television in bed, or going from work directly to bed may interfere with sleep and suggest *inadequate sleep hygiene* (see Chapter 61).

Systematic inquiry into the behaviors and thoughts that accompany nocturnal awakenings is useful and may reveal conscious or unconscious "rewards" for poor sleep. Awakenings followed by inability to return to sleep without eating or drinking alcohol suggest the *nocturnal eating syndrome* (see Chapter 114) or *alcohol-dependent sleep disorder* (see Chapter 115). Patients who report "resting" for up to 8 hours at night without sleeping or leaving the bed may have *sleep state misperception*.

Excessive Sleepiness

Patients with daytime sleepiness typically complain of drowsiness that interferes with daytime activities, unavoidable napping, or both. Falling asleep while driving or at other particularly inappropriate or dangerous times is often the impetus that brings the patient to the clinician. Some of these patients complain that they need more sleep at night or that daytime drowsiness occurs regardless of how much sleep is obtained at night. Patients may also complain of difficulty with concentration or memory, or increased irritability. Children may exhibit hyperactivity rather than sleepiness.

The situations associated with drowsiness and spontaneous sleep episodes help determine the severity of the problem. Drowsiness and naps either may be limited to sedentary situations in which falling asleep is socially acceptable, such as watching television or reading at home, or may occur at work, while driving, in conversation, sitting on the toilet, or even during sexual intercourse.

The differential diagnosis of excessive daytime sleepiness ranges from insufficient sleep to sufficient sleep that is disrupted by pathologic events such as apneas or neurologic disorders such as narcolepsy. Inquiring about sleep routines and bedtimes/wake times is essential in excluding insufficient sleep as a cause for sleepiness. Asking patients who complain of sleepiness about other associated symptoms provides essential information. Loud snoring, gasping, snorting, and episodes of apnea suggest the diagnosis of *obstructive sleep apnea syndrome* (see Chapter 87). The relationship of snoring to body position should be determined; snoring may occur in all positions or only in the supine position. A history of episodic muscle weakness with buckling of the knees, laxity of the neck or jaw muscles, or complete loss of muscle tone associated with laughter, anger, or hearing or telling a joke suggests cataplexy and a diagnosis of *narcolepsy*[1] (see Chapter 65). Episodes of partial or total paralysis at the onset or termination of sleep (sleep paralysis) and dreamlike auditory, visual, or tactile hallucinations occurring at sleep onset or on awakening (hypnagogic and hypnopompic hallucinations) also suggest narcolepsy. Questions assessing mood are needed to identify patients with *sleep disorder associated with mood disorders* (see Chapter 112).

The sleep–wake schedule may also provide clues to the diagnosis. Short nocturnal sleep time, longer sleep on weekends or days off, and fewer symptoms during vacations when the sleep period is longer suggest the *insufficient sleep syndrome*.

Circadian rhythm sleep disorders should be considered in patients with complaints of nocturnal insomnia and daytime sleepiness. Patients with *delayed sleep phase syndrome* (see Chapter 58) frequently complain of difficulty waking up, morning sleepiness and sluggishness, and difficulty falling asleep at night. Symptoms are worse on days when the patient must awaken by a set time to be at school or work. Patients with *advanced sleep phase syndrome* (see Chapter 58) may complain of evening sleepiness and early morning awakening. The patient's occupation and social schedule may suggest diagnoses of *shift work sleep disorder* (see Chapter 57) or *jet lag syndrome* (see Chapter 55).

Nocturnal Movements, Behaviors, and Sensations

Information from collateral sources is needed for evaluating episodic movements and behaviors during sleep. The bed partner should be asked to describe behaviors and vocalizations during the episodes, to relate episodes to sleep onset and time of night, and to note the degree of the patient's responsiveness during the episode. The patient's ability to recall the events is also significant. Episodes of inconsolable screaming and amnesia during the first third of the night suggest *sleep terrors* (see Chapter 74); episodes of dream-enacting behavior associated with dream recall that occur toward the end of the sleep cycle suggest the *rapid eye movement (REM) sleep behavior disorder* (see Chapter 75). Epileptic seizures may occur at any time of the night, and should be strongly considered if a history of stereotyped behavior or dystonic posturing is elicited (see Chapter 72).

In patients whose symptoms occur during nocturnal awakenings, the relations to evening activities and medical or psychiatric conditions are often illuminating. Repeated awakenings from sleep with chest discomfort may suggest *sleep-related gastroesophageal reflux*, *sleep disorder due to peptic ulcer disease* (see Chapter 107), or *nocturnal cardiac ischemia* (see Chapter 104), depending on associated symptoms and underlying diseases. Similarly, complaints of choking during sleep may

suggest *obstructive sleep apnea syndrome* when they are accompanied by snoring or *sleep-related gastroesophageal reflux* when they are accompanied by heartburn and a sour taste in the mouth.

MEDICATION USE AND PAST MEDICAL HISTORY

Assessment of medication use is critical because of the wide variety of medications that alter sleep and wakefulness (see Chapter 40). Some medications, such as theophylline and other bronchodilators, directly affect sleep; others, such as diuretics, have indirect effects. Chronic sedative or hypnotic use raises the possibility of *hypnotic-dependent sleep disorder* (Table 48–1). Because cold preparations, appetite suppressants, antihistamines, and nonprescription sedatives and stimulants affect sleep, it is important to ask specifically about nonprescription as well as prescription medications, as well as herbal supplements. Herbal supplements have a variety of sedating and stimulating effects on sleep, and patients often omit mention of them during a medical evaluation.[2] In addition, illicit drugs, such as ecstasy, can cause insomnia and altered mood in teenagers and young adults.[3] Many illicit drugs affect sleep by acting on adrenergic, gamma-aminobutyric acid–ergic, and other receptors.[4]

The history of current or past medical, surgical, and psychiatric illnesses is a source of important information. Seizure disorders, parkinsonism and dementia, arthritic conditions, asthma, ischemic heart disease, migraine or cluster headache, compressive neuropathies, obstructive uropathy, and almost any painful illness can cause significant sleep disturbance. A variety of medical conditions, including hypothyroidism, acromegaly, Cushing's syndrome, allergic rhinitis, and some of the mucopolysaccharidoses, may contribute to the development of *obstructive sleep apnea syndrome*. Anemia and renal disease may cause or exacerbate *restless legs syndrome* or *periodic limb movement disorder*. In infants and toddlers, milk and other food allergens may cause insomnia. Head trauma may lead to the postconcussion syndrome, often accompanied by disrupted sleep continuity. Information about tonsillectomy, cleft palate repair, nasal trauma or

Table 48–1.	Sleep Disorders/Concerns Associated with Medical Disorders Encountered in the Review of Systems
System (Symptom)	**Sleep Disorder or Concern**
Constitutional (weight gain)	Obstructive sleep apnea
Head, eyes, ears, nose, throat (hypothyroidism)	Obstructive sleep apnea
Lungs (nocturnal dyspnea)	Sleep disruption
Heart (nocturnal angina)	Sleep disruption
Gastrointestinal (reflux)	Nocturnal choking
Genitourinary (nocturia)	Sleep disruption
Musculoskeletal (joint pain)	Insomnia, sleep disruption
Neurologic (neuropathic pain)	Insomnia, sleep disruption, restless legs syndrome
Psychiatric (anxiety or depression)	Insomnia, sleep disruption

surgery, and other orofacial surgery is essential in patients with suspected obstructive sleep apnea syndrome.

Anxiety disorders, including panic disorder, and mood disorders are psychiatric disturbances that are often accompanied by insomnia, and some patients with depression complain of excessive daytime sleepiness. Exacerbation of schizophrenia and other psychotic disorders is frequently associated with severe sleep disruption.

FAMILY HISTORY

A history of disordered sleep in family members is important information. Specific inquiry should be made about the existence in family members of previously diagnosed sleep disorders or symptoms suggestive of narcolepsy, obstructive sleep apnea, periodic limb movements, enuresis, sleep terrors or sleepwalking, or insomnia. There is a strong genetic contribution to the development of narcolepsy (see Chapter 64), and genetic and familial influences sometimes have a role in the development and expression of obstructive sleep apnea (see Chapter 84) and some of the parasomnias.[5]

SOCIAL HISTORY

Assessment of psychosocial, occupational, and academic functioning as well as of satisfaction with personal relationships can yield valuable information about the impact of disordered sleep on the patient's life. When the chief complaint comes from the spouse or bed partner, the patient may have one of the many sleep disorders whose symptoms may not be noticed by the patient. However, the possibility of marital or relationship difficulties should also be considered and explored. In patients complaining of excessive sleepiness, potential occupational hazards should be assessed, and special attention should be paid to the assessment of social and occupational functioning of shift workers. The ability of the work environment to provide support for the patient should be evaluated. For children and adolescents, school performance should be determined.

Alcohol, caffeine, nicotine, and illicit drug use should be determined. Alcohol use or abuse may intensify snoring and obstructive sleep apnea, may be a contributor to insomnia, or may produce long-lasting changes in sleep patterns. Patients who drink heavily on the weekend may complain of sleepiness primarily during the early part of the week. Caffeine use produces significant sleep disturbance in susceptible persons, and nicotine dependency may lead to nocturnal awakenings. Cocaine, amphetamines, barbiturates, and opiates can be associated with major disruption of sleep architecture. Illicit drugs, such as ecstasy, may be the cause of an altered mood or sleep schedule in a teenager.

REVIEW OF SYSTEMS

The review of systems may uncover symptoms of medical illnesses that can cause or contribute to sleep disorders (Table 48–1). Recent weight gain or increase in collar size increases the likelihood of obstructive sleep apnea syndrome. Particular attention should be paid to the cardiovascular and pulmonary systems because of their relation to breathing and oxygenation during sleep. Angina, orthopnea, paroxysmal nocturnal dyspnea, and wheezing may indicate that sleep disturbance is due to cardiac or pulmonary disease. Heartburn and reflux of gastric contents into the throat when the patient is recumbent may cause nocturnal choking episodes. Leg cramps and neuropathic pain may be accompanied by sleep disruption. Nocturia is a common cause of disturbed sleep, particularly in older men. Depression or anxiety can contribute to insomnia.

PHYSICAL EXAMINATION

Physical examination of the patient with disordered sleep begins with observation. Body habitus often provides clues to potential etiologic factors of sleep complaints; thus, obesity with distribution of fat around the neck or midriff suggests the diagnosis of obstructive sleep apnea. Psychomotor slowing, poor hygiene, downcast eyes, blunted affect, or sad facies may suggest major depression and its associated sleep disturbance.

Examination of the head and neck is particularly important in patients with suspected obstructive sleep apnea. Mandibular hypoplasia, craniosynostosis, retrognathia, and other craniofacial abnormalities may indicate the presence of Pierre Robin syndrome, Treacher Collins syndrome, Crouzon's disease, achondroplasia, or other skeletal disorders that are associated with an increased incidence of sleep-related respiratory disturbances. Boggy, edematous nasal mucosa in patients with allergies or deviation of the nasal septum after trauma may compromise nasal patency and predispose the patient to obstructive sleep apnea syndrome. Oropharyngeal findings suggestive of obstructive sleep apnea include an elongated soft palate and uvula; edema and erythema of the peritonsillar pillars, uvula, soft palate, or posterior oropharynx; redundant pharyngeal mucosa; enlarged tongue; and enlarged tonsillar tissue. Examination of the neck may reveal an enlarged thyroid or prominent fatty infiltration suggesting the likelihood of excess retropharyngeal adipose tissue.

Auscultation of the chest may reveal expiratory wheezes in patients with nocturnal asthma attacks. Thoracic abnormalities such as kyphoscoliosis may compromise ventilatory capacity, leading to hypoventilation and nocturnal breathing difficulties. Patients with severe obstructive sleep apnea may have findings consistent with right-sided heart failure, including hepatomegaly, ascites, and ankle edema. Cardiac complications of disordered breathing during sleep may be indicated by a cardiac thrust at the left sternal border as a result of right ventricular enlargement or in the left second intercostal space adjacent to the sternum as a result of pulmonary hypertension. Auscultation may reveal a prominent fourth heart sound originating from the enlarged right ventricle and murmurs of pulmonary or tricuspid valve insufficiency.

On abdominal examination, hepatomegaly may suggest that alcohol abuse is contributing to sleep disturbance or, in conjunction with other findings, that congestive heart failure is a factor. Examination of the extremities may reveal joint swelling or deformity, decreased range of motion across affected joints, and thickening of synovial tissue in patients with disordered sleep due to arthritis.

Findings on mental status testing and neurologic examination may indicate the presence of a psychiatric or neurologic disease that causes or contributes to disturbed sleep. Impairment of short-term memory, judgment, language functions, and abstract reasoning suggests the presence of a dementing illness that may cause insomnia or nocturnal confusion. Assessment of mood may suggest the presence of mania or depression, either of which may be associated with insomnia. Delusional thoughts and agitation may indicate that acute psychosis is the cause of insomnia. Reduced alertness with slurred speech and nystagmus may be signs of hypnotic or sedative abuse. Impaired sensation and reduced or absent tendon reflexes may indicate peripheral neuropathy, sometimes accompanied by nocturnal paresthesias or burning pain.

FORMULATION AND DIAGNOSTIC STUDIES

Once the initial evaluation is complete, the clinician generates a differential diagnosis. The International Classification of Sleep Disorders-2 provides a comprehensive diagnostic approach and is discussed in detail in Chapter 51. On the basis of the relative likelihood of the diagnostic possibilities, appropriate diagnostic studies are ordered (see Chapter 50). Even when the diagnosis is clear, laboratory tests may be required to determine the severity of the condition before the clinician decides on the appropriate treatment.

Additional diagnostic information can be obtained through the use of laboratory or radiologic investigations, sleep logs, and sleep laboratory studies. Radiologic and laboratory tests may clarify or refine the diagnosis or may indicate its severity. Thyroid function tests or pulmonary function tests may be indicated in some patients with suspected obstructive sleep apnea. If the diagnosis of narcolepsy is under consideration, tissue typing for specific human leukocyte antigens implicated in the genetics of narcolepsy is sometimes helpful. Uremia, anemia, iron deficiency, or other metabolic abnormalities may be present in patients with suspected periodic limb movement disorder or restless legs syndrome. Iron-deficiency anemia contributing to restless legs syndrome may be due to low body stores of iron.[6] Repeat blood donation has been associated with restless legs syndrome and periodic limb movements of sleep,[7] perhaps because of reduced iron stores. A urine toxicology screen may be diagnostic in cases of insomnia or hypersomnia due to substance abuse.

The sleep log is particularly useful in patients with insomnia or suspected circadian rhythm disturbances. Although a variety of sleep logs exist, a 2-week log in which the patient records bedtime, approximate time of sleep onset, times and durations of awakenings during the sleep period, final awakening time, and nap times during the day is commonly used. The sleep log may provide a new perspective on the sleep problem for both the clinician and the patient; some patients are surprised and relieved to note that their sleep is better than they believed.

Polysomnography can provide confirmatory diagnostic evidence in cases of sleep apnea, narcolepsy, periodic limb movements, nocturnal seizures, and sleep terrors and helps determine the severity of these conditions. Its use in the evaluation of insomnia is somewhat controversial but may be beneficial, especially when sleep apnea, periodic limb movements, or sleep state misperception is suspected. The multiple sleep latency test, described in Chapters 50 and 120, can confirm the presence of excessive sleepiness, quantify its severity, and determine the presence of pathologically early onset of REM sleep. This test is used the day after polysomnography. Ambulatory sleep–wake recordings, wrist actigraphy, portable monitoring devices that record esophageal acidity, electrocardiography, and extended electroencephalography with video monitoring are useful in selected patients.

CONCLUSIONS

Sleep disorders are prevalent in the general population and are common in patients who consult with physicians and other health care providers. Patients with complaints of sleep disturbance often present a diagnostic challenge to the clinician because of the many possible causes for symptoms and the patients' inability to describe accurately events occurring during sleep. A systematic evaluation usually yields a provisional diagnosis or a set of diagnostic possibilities that can be confirmed or excluded with specific diagnostic tests. With accurate diagnosis and specific interventions, most sleep disorders are treatable.

Clinical Pearl

A complete sleep and medical history often yields a specific cause of the patient's sleep complaint. For example, in patients complaining of excessive daytime sleepiness, the etiology can often be pinpointed by close attention to the patient's (and bed partner's) account of nighttime symptoms, bedtime/wake time schedules, medications, and coexisting medical disorders.

REFERENCES

1. Anic-Labat S, Guilleminault C, Kraemer HC, et al: Validation of a cataplexy questionnaire in 983 sleep-disorders patients. Sleep 1999;22:77-87.
2. Gyllenhall C, Merritt SL, Peterson SD, et al: Efficacy and safety of herbal stimulants and sedatives in sleep disorders. Sleep Med Rev 2000;4:229-251.
3. Yates KM, O'Connor A, Horsley CA: "Herbal ecstasy": A case series of adverse reactions. N Z Med J 2000;113:315-317.
4. Giannini AJ: An approach to drug abuse, intoxication, and withdrawal. Am Fam Physician 2000;61:2763-2774.
5. Hublin C, Kaprio J: Genetic aspects and genetic epidemiology of parasomnias. Sleep Med Rev 2003;7:413-421.
6. Kryger MH, Otake K, Foerster J: Low body stores of iron and restless legs syndrome: A correctable cause of insomnia in adolescents and teenagers. Sleep Med 2002;2002:127-132.
7. Kryger MH, Shepertycky M, Foerseter J, Manfreda J: Sleep disorders in repeat blood donors. Sleep 2003;26:625-626.

49

Cardinal Manifestations of Sleep Disorders

Bradley V. Vaughn

O'Neill F. D'Cruz

ABSTRACT

Sleep disorders produce a wide range of manifestations that impair health and quality of life. The fundamental symptoms of sleep disorders include insomnia, hypersomnia, and unusual sleep-related behaviors, but more subtle signs and symptoms may also provide clues to the presence of an underlying sleep dysfunction. Insomnia, a symptom of difficulty initiating or maintaining sleep with daytime sequelae, can be related to many contributing factors. Features that predispose, precipitate, and perpetuate insomnia can be identified in individuals who have primary and secondary insomnias. Insomnia can have an intricate relationship to other medical and psychiatric disorders. Excessive daytime sleepiness is the propensity to enter sleep at inappropriate times. Other symptoms such as snoring and apnea may indicate sleep-related breathing disorders or other medical problems. Cataplexy, as a symptom of sudden loss of muscle tone in relation to an emotional trigger, in combination with excessive sleepiness, should prompt an evaluation for narcolepsy. Patients or bed partners may also complain of movements before or during sleep. Restless legs syndrome is a set of complex symptoms related to discomfort of the extremities during periods of inactivity that is relieved with movement. Periodic limb movements in sleep can occur in association with restless legs syndrome and may involve movements of the upper or lower extremities. This movement may not disrupt the sleep of the patient, but disturb the bed partner. Other parasomnias, such as sleepwalking, sleep terrors, and dream enactment, require detailed description of the sleep-related behaviors to help differentiate potential causes.

Sleep is essential to health. The restorative properties of sleep promote wakefulness and a sense of well-being. However, disturbance of sleep frequently disrupts this sense of well-being and can produce a wide range of systemic and psychological symptoms. As we realize the connection of sleep with good health, we also recognize that sleep disruption may exacerbate symptoms of other diseases. The challenge for physicians is to recognize these manifestations and appropriately delineate them as related to dysfunction of sleep. The vast majority of patients referred to sleep centers present with one or a combination of three classic complaints: excessive sleepiness, difficulty attaining or sustaining sleep, or unusual events associated with sleep. These symptoms can be easily recognized as related to sleep and are not mutually exclusive. Patients may note more than one problem, such as difficulty sleeping at night and excessive sleepiness during the day. Each of these symptoms conveys clues to the underlying pathologic process. In this chapter, we review the cardinal manifestations of sleep disorders and address some of the key features that guide the clinician in pursuing further diagnostic evaluations.

SLEEP DISORDERS AND SYMPTOMS

Insomnia

Many individuals complain of an occasional night fraught with difficulty falling asleep.[1] Insomnia, however, is the complaint of difficulty initiating or maintaining sleep combined with adverse daytime consequences. These daytime manifestations of insomnia may take the form of excessive fatigue, impairment of performance, or emotional change. Individual sleep needs can vary significantly. Some people may feel fine and note no impairment of performance with 5 hours of sleep per night, whereas others may need greater than 9 hours to preserve daytime functioning. Thus, the requirement of daytime sequelae differentiates individual sleep need from the complaint of insomnia.

These patients frequently give historical clues that explain the mechanisms causing their insomnia. Insomnia may be due to an underlying disorder related to primary failure of the sleep mechanism, or the sleep disruption may be the byproduct of another disorder. Patients rarely have just one factor responsible for their chronic insomnia. Most patients have several factors that create a foundation for insomnia, initiate the insomnia, and perpetuate the insomnia. The division of predisposing, precipitating, and perpetuating factors suggests that insomnia is an ongoing process, and clinicians need to search for these issues to provide effective therapeutic management.

Individual features that predispose patients to insomnia include sex, age, lower socioeconomic status, poor education, and psychiatric or chronic medical illness. Behavioral traits such as obsessive-compulsive nature, frequent rumination, poor coping strategies, and "hyperalertness" appear to have a correlation with greater risk for insomnia. Patients with insomnia frequently describe themselves as tense, anxious, nervous, tired, irritable, unable to relax, obsessively worried, and depressed. Many of these traits may predate the onset of the insomnia.

Insomnia may be initiated by sudden changes in environment or challenges to the body or mind. These challenges may come in the form of acute medical illness, psychological or psychiatric events, a shift in schedule, or changes in medications or supplements. Initiating events may play little role in the patient's current ongoing process, but give important clues to preventing further recurrence of the insomnia.

In an attempt to improve the poor sleep, many patients adopt behaviors that help perpetuate the insomnia. During this evolution, the patient may make changes in his or her sleep schedule, become dependent on certain somnogenic substances, or develop secondary medical or psychological issues. Many of these behaviors conflict with typical sleep hygiene practices. Such maladaptive practices may occur during the day or night and include heavy caffeine or alcohol use, watching television or playing video games while in bed, or even eating or exercising during the usual sleep period. Some patients actually fear going to bed or have performance anxiety over the oncoming sleep period. This expectation of poor sleep promotes the apprehension toward sleep and may perpetuate counter productive sleep rituals. These maladaptive behaviors become the predominant feature of psychophysiological insomnia.

Timing of the insomnia during the sleep period may also be helpful. Circadian rhythm disorders can masquerade as complaints of insomnia or excessive sleepiness, and circadian rhythm dysfunction may develop in patients with insomnia. Difficulty with the onset of sleep suggests an underlying delayed sleep phase or occasionally depression in younger adults. Insomnia with early morning arousal raises the possibility of underlying depression or advanced sleep phase. History of schedule changes such as from jet lag or shift work also provides important clues. Sleep diaries of bedtime and wake time can be useful in determining potential links to schedule or circadian rhythm issues.

As a symptom, insomnia is directly related to the patient's perception of poor sleep. Perception of sleep is an important factor in evaluating the complaint of insomnia. Some patients exaggerate their symptoms, whereas other patients may not perceive they are asleep. Although results of sleep studies may be entirely normal, the patients may not recognize that they have slept. Sleep misperception state is one of the primary insomnias. Patients may also have unrealistic expectations or goals. Patients may assume that sleep should not be interrupted by any arousals or that one must sleep a set number of hours. Thus, the clinician should ask the patient about personal beliefs regarding sleep. Another primary insomnia, idiopathic insomnia, is associated with no clear inciting factors. These individuals usually have lifelong difficulty with sleep and may have a significant family history. The primary insomnias are discussed further in Chapter 59.

Insomnia may also be a complaint produced by medical or neurologic disorders. Derangement of almost any system in the body can disrupt sleep. Patients with diseases affecting the nervous system, heart, liver, kidneys, gastrointestinal tract, lungs, and skin may complain of insomnia. These are discussed elsewhere in this volume.

Pain can disturb sleep and promote insomnia. Musculoskeletal discomfort may become worse with periods of rest. Pain from entrapment neuropathies such as carpal tunnel syndrome is typically worse at night, and headaches such as cluster headache and even pain related to increased intracranial pressure or brain mass lesions can become more intense during sleep. Restless legs produce significant discomfort, and are classically worse in the evening, before the onset of sleep. Arthritis and other rheumatologic disorders frequently can disrupt sleep through increased nighttime pain and stiffness.

Nearly all of the psychiatric illnesses have some link to poor sleep. Patients with depression or anxiety disorders may have insomnia years before the presentation of the affective component. Insomnia may also herald the onset of psychosis or mania. Although cause and effect are still debated, physicians should question their patients for symptoms of potential underlying psychiatric disorders.

Patients with other sleep disorders may complain of insomnia or disturbed sleep. Individuals with obstructive sleep apnea, restless legs syndrome, or even narcolepsy describe fragmentation or difficulty with maintenance of their sleep. Further questioning may identify individuals who potentially have another underlying sleep disorder.

The clinician may uncover few physical findings in patients with insomnia. Anxious or hyperalert individuals may demonstrate mild tachycardia, rapid respiratory rate, or cold hands. These individuals may startle easily or be easily distracted during the interview. The clinician should look carefully for signs of obstructive sleep apnea, narrow airway, or obesity because these too can present as insomnia. Signs of Cushing's syndrome (round face and buffalo hump) or hyperthyroidism (tachycardia and excessive sweating) are important clues to an endocrine contribution. Each patient with insomnia should have a complete neurologic examination to look for potential neurologic lesions impairing sleep. This examination should include an assessment of cognition, mood, and affect. The Mini-Mental Status Examination is one tool that helps assess cognitive abilities and can be followed over time.[2] Clinicians can also use the Minnesota Multiphasic Personality Inventory to identify personality and affect issues.

Excessive Daytime Sleepiness

Sleepiness is a common symptom noted by 5% to 15% of individuals.[3,4] Defined as the propensity to enter sleep, most people can relate some instances of falling asleep when they intended to be awake. Sleepiness is a normal feeling as one approaches a typical sleep period or after prolonged wakefulness. Excessive sleepiness, however, is defined as a condition in which one enters sleep at an inappropriate time or setting. Patients who complain of excessive sleepiness usually describe episodes of unintentional sleep. Excessive sleepiness can occur in degrees. In mild sleepiness, a person might fall asleep while reading a book or while sitting quietly. Greater degrees of sleepiness may be associated with bouts of irresistible sleep or sleep attacks that intrude on such activities as driving, having a conversation, or eating meals. This degree of sleepiness may place the patient at significant risk for accidents, and have a major impact on the person's health and sense of well-being.

As with other subjective symptoms, a person's perception of sleepiness influences the information being relayed. Some patients may overreport their degree of sleepiness and note sleepiness even during periods of normal wakefulness. Other individuals may underreport periods of sleepiness, but describe periods of lapse of attention or diminished cognitive abilities. Patients may note missing an exit on the highway or a brief delay in performing a task. Perception of sleepiness is also reduced with continued sleep deprivation. People who are chronically sleep deprived become accustomed to their impairment and are less likely to recognize their degree of sleepiness.

Clinicians should always question their hypersomniac patients for clues to potential sleep debt, dyssomnia, medication use, or medical or psychiatric causes. Sleep deprivation is common in our society, and patients should be asked about their schedule during the week and weekends. Information regarding sleep habits and environment may disclose other important contributing factors.

Excessive sleepiness may result from a wide range of medical disorders and medications. Patients with heart, kidney, or liver failure or rheumatologic, endocrinologic, or neurologic disorders may note sleepiness and fatigue as a result of the disease process or treatment. Sleepiness is frequently the cardinal symptom of many sleep disorders. Patients with sleep apnea, narcolepsy, restless legs syndrome–periodic limb movements, and even parasomnias may note excessive daytime sleepiness as their main complaint. Historical features of snoring, observed apneas, morning headaches, cataplexy, sleep paralysis, hypnagogic hallucinations, or confusion on arousal suggest contributions of specific sleep disorders. Individuals with idiopathic hypersomnolence have unrelenting daytime sleepiness despite prolonged periods of sleep, which differentiates it from sleep deprivation.

Physical findings are few in patients with sleepiness. Frequent pauses, slowed responses, drooping eyelids, and repetitive yawning support the complaint of sleepiness. Patients may be asleep when the clinician enters the examination room, and some patients may show signs of chronic sleepiness such as dark circles under the eyes. The patient's neurologic examination may show findings of inattentiveness or even brief "microsleeps."

Sleepiness can be quantified subjectively by questionnaires or by physiologic measures such as a multiple sleep latency test (MSLT). The Epworth Sleepiness Scale is one example of a quantifiable subjective measure of sleepiness[5] (Table 49–1). In this scale, the person is asked to rate on a scale of 0 to 3 (0 no chance, 3 high likelihood) the chance of dozing in a series of eight situations. This score has a modest correlation with physiologic measures of sleep, but has a better correlation with the respiratory disturbance index in patients with obstructive sleep apnea (Table 49–2). The MSLT quantifies objective sleepiness based on the time to onset of physiologic changes that mark sleep. The MSLT quantifies the propensity to enter sleep and thus is a reliable objective marker. This test is covered in more detail in Chapters 50 and 120.

Fatigue

Many patients with excessive daytime sleepiness note fatigue and decreased energy. The complaint of fatigue is a complex symptom related to the perception of lack of energy. Patients may confuse the lack of energy with excessive sleepiness, but do not have an increased ability to fall asleep. Frequently they believe that a good night's sleep would improve their fatigue. Distinguishing sleepiness from fatigue can be difficult even for the most careful clinicians, but the MSLT can be helpful. Fatigue is a common complaint in patients with insomnia and is also associated with a wide range of medical and psychiatric disorders. Endocrinologic and metabolic disorders such as diabetes mellitus and cardiac, renal, or liver failure; status post-organ transplantation; and psychiatric disease such as depression can be associated with fatigue without sleepiness.

Snoring

Snoring is the sound created by turbulent airflow vibrating upper airway soft tissue, and occurs in approximately 32% of adults and over 3% of children.[6,7] Many adults have little knowledge or recognition of their snoring habits, and accounts from bed partners may be more helpful to the clinician. Snoring is usually worse in the supine position, after sleep deprivation or alcohol ingestion. Loud snoring may not disturb sound

---

Table 49–1. **The Epworth Sleepiness Scale**

Name: _____

Today's date: _____ Your age (years): _____

Your sex (male = M; female = F): _____

How likely are you to doze off or fall asleep in the following situations, in contrast to feeling just tired? This refers to your usual way of life in recent times. Even if you have not done some of these things recently, try to work out how they would have affected you. Use the following scale to choose the *most appropriate number* for each situation:

0 = would *never* doze
1 = *slight* chance of dozing
2 = *moderate* chance of dozing
3 = *high* chance of dozing

Situation*	Chance of Dozing
Sitting and reading	_____
Watching TV	_____
Sitting, inactive in a public place (e.g., a theater or a meeting)	_____
As a passenger in a car for an hour without a break	_____
Lying down to rest in the afternoon when circumstances permit	_____
Sitting and talking to someone	_____
Sitting quietly after a lunch without alcohol	_____
In a car, while stopped for a few minutes in traffic	_____
Thank you for your cooperation	

*The numbers for the eight situations are added together to give a global score between 0 and 24.

Table 49–2 shows scores for various conditions.

From Johns MW: A new method for measuring daytime sleepiness: The Epworth Sleepiness Scale. Sleep 1991;14:540-545.

Table 49–2. Ages and Epworth Sleepiness Scale Scores of Experimental Subjects

Subjects/Diagnoses	Total Number of Subjects (M/F)	Age in Years (Mean ± SD)	Epworth Sleepiness Scale Scores (Mean ± SD)	Range
Healthy control subjects	30 (14/16)	36.4 ± 9.9	5.9 ± 2.2	2-10
Primary snoring	32 (29/3)	45.7 ± 10.7	6.5 ± 3.0	0-11
Obstructive sleep apnea syndrome	55 (53/2)	48.4 ± 10.7	11.7 ± 4.6	4-23
Narcolepsy	13 (8/5)	46.6 ± 12.0	17.5 ± 3.5	13-23
Idiopathic hypersomnia	14 (8/6)	41.4 ± 14.0	17.9 ± 3.1	12-24
Insomnia	16 (6/12)	40.3 ± 14.6	2.2 ± 2.0	0-6
Periodic limb movement disorder	18 (16/2)	52.5 ± 10.3	9.2 ± 4.0	2-16

SD, standard deviation.

From Johns MW: A new method for measuring daytime sleepiness: The Epworth Sleepiness Scale. Sleep 1991;14:540-545.

sleepers, but some patients may receive complaints from family members and even neighbors. Witnesses may be able to account for snore-associated gasps, choking, body jerks, and movements, and patients occasionally recall being awakened by their own gasps. These associated symptoms are classic features of obstructive sleep apnea syndrome, but the absence of snoring does not exclude the diagnosis of apnea. Some patients have airway dynamics that are not conducive to snoring. This is especially true in patients who have had upper airway surgical procedures that eliminated flaccid tissue that can vibrate. Other individuals, such as those with neuromuscular disorders, may not generate enough force to produce turbulent airflow.

Sleep Apnea

Apnea is the absence of ventilation. The patient's bed partner notes that breathing has stopped or that the individual "holds their breath." The events are aborted with a loud gasp, snort, or the resumption of breathing. Some patients may have hundreds of events in a single night and are unable to obtain good-quality sleep because of the frequent arousals. These individuals are typically unaware of the arousals, but some may report occasional awakening with a gasp, snorts, or symptoms of gastroesophageal reflux. Sleep apnea is classified into two major forms: obstructive and central.

Obstructive apnea is the most common form of sleep apnea. These apneas occur because of obstruction in the upper airway. *Obstructive sleep apnea syndrome* is the cluster of features caused by the repetitive apneas. Snoring is a frequently associated complaint, but a wide variety of symptoms may be present. Some questionnaires such as the Sleep Apnea portion of the Sleep Disorder Questionnaire (SA/SDQ) or the Berlin Questionnaire inventory a combination of items regarding snoring, witnessed apneas, body habitus, and associated disorders such as hypertension[8,9] (Table 49–3). These questionnaires provide a summary score that correlates with presence of obstructive sleep apnea, but the questionnaires have been tested only in selected populations. Thus, the questionnaires themselves require further study and may not be appropriate for broad clinical use. The topics inventoried, however, are important and provide basic information intrinsic to formulating the diagnosis. Astute clinicians should not exclude patients on the basis of a low score on a questionnaire. The physical examination may show structural evidence for airway obstruction. Many patients are obese and have a large neck or crowded upper airway, yet some have a normal body habitus. Common structural abnormalities such as narrow nasal passage, long soft palate, large tonsils, or retroflexed mandible leading to a small airway contribute to airway obstruction. These features are discussed in greater detail in Chapters 82 and 87.

Central apnea is the absence of ventilation due to an absence of effort. Central apneas can be caused by a neurologic abnormality in the brainstem or other areas involved in regulation of respiration. Cheyne-Stokes breathing can have features of both central and obstructive apnea. The classic pattern of crescendo-decrescendo breathing with central apnea can be seen in patients with heart failure, neurologic lesions, and metabolic or toxic encephalopathies. This pattern may be present only in sleep, but may be found during wakefulness as well. Apneas may follow other neurologic events such as nocturnal seizures and strokes. Central apnea is reviewed in Chapter 81.

Morning Headache

Morning headache is a common symptom. Over 70% of the population has occasional headache; this symptom is relatively nonspecific. Morning headache has been suggested to be linked to sleep dysfunction. Characteristics of the headache, such as location, quality and nature of pain, and potential associations, can aid in determining the etiology. Approximately half of patients with obstructive sleep apnea and hypoventilation note morning headache that is usually dull and generalized. Patients with chronic obstructive pulmonary disease and obstructive sleep apnea may experience morning headache from the increase in carbon dioxide, low oxygen saturation, or changes in the trigeminal vascular complex. Headache that awakens patients from sleep should always raise the possibility of further evaluation, potentially including head imaging. Patients with brain tumors frequently note worsening of headache at night. Patients with sinus disorders, muscle contraction headache, recent alcohol intake, and withdrawal from medication (rebound headache) may all have distinct headache patterns. Cluster headaches are noted to occur in rapid eye movement (REM) sleep. Hypnic headaches are brief, sharp pains that awaken the patient.[10] Headaches in sleep are discussed in greater detail in Chapter 73.

Cataplexy

Cataplexy is the abrupt loss of muscle tone triggered by strong emotional stimuli or physical exercise. Patients are aware of

Table 49–3.	Key Features of the Berlin Questionnaire
Height	Age
Weight	Gender
Has your weight changed in the last 5 years?	Increased Decreased No change
Do you snore?	Yes No Do not know
Your snoring is	Slightly louder than breathing As loud as talking Louder than talking Very loud
How often do you snore?	Nearly every day 3 to 4 times per week 1 to 2 times per week 1 to 2 times per month Never or almost never
Has your snoring bothered other people?	Yes No
Has anyone noticed that you quit breathing during your sleep?	Almost every day 3 to 4 times per week 1 to 2 times per week 1 to 2 times per month Never or almost never
Are you tired or fatigued after your sleep?	Nearly every day 3 to 4 times per week 1 to 2 times per week 1 to 2 times per month Never or almost never
During your wake time do you feel tired, fatigued, or not up to par?	Nearly every day 3 to 4 times per week 1 to 2 times per week 1 to 2 times per month Never or almost never
Have you ever fallen asleep while driving?	Yes No If so, how often does it occur? Nearly every day 3 to 4 times per week 1 to 2 times per week 1 to 2 times per month Never or almost never
Do you have high blood pressure?	Yes No Do not know

Adapted from: From the Editors: Reprinting of the Berlin Questionnaire. Sleep and Breathing 2000;4:187-192. Permission was granted from Kingman P. Strohl.

their surroundings and have clear memory of the events. Events can be triggered by a joke, surprise, anger, fear, or athletic endeavors. Individual experiences vary from a mild feeling of weakness to severe falls. The clinician should ask about episodes of feeling weak or heaviness that appear during laughter or surprise. Cataplectic attacks are usually brief, lasting less than 5 minutes. Patients then regain their muscle control and have no postictal confusion or deficits. Longer events may be ended with the patient entering sleep and then awakening. The combination of excessive daytime sleepiness and cataplexy is nearly always related to narcolepsy. Cataplexy can rarely be seen as an isolated symptom suggesting an underlying neurologic disorder. Examination of the patient during the cataplectic attack demonstrates paralysis with diffuse hypotonia, absence of deep tendon reflexes, diminished corneal reflexes, preserved pupillary responses, and phasic muscle twitching. Phasic muscle twitching can occur as single jerks or repetitive muscle twitching and is most frequently seen in the face. Maintenance of consciousness and memory help differentiate these events from most seizures and syncope.

Sleep Paralysis

Sleep paralysis is an inability to move during the transition into or out of sleep. The association with intentional sleep distinguishes these events from cataplexy. Patients may describe complete awareness of their surroundings or feeling half asleep with awareness but unable to move even their fingers or speak. Patients may try to scream but produce only a whisper. Some individuals describe a feeling of suffocation and being able to resume breathing only when the event has passed. Patients frequently describe a strong feeling of impending doom, having to escape imminent danger, or a feeling that someone else is in the room. Auditory and tactile hallucinations may accompany the events, and patients may recount dramatic stories. These events can be emotionally profound and leave a lasting memory that patients vividly recall years later. Clinicians may find that describing a sleep paralysis event may help the patient recall specific incidents. Most sleep paralysis episodes last a few minutes and usually end after the patient is touched or is alerted to a sound. If the event is allowed to persist, the patient usually reenters sleep and awakens later. These events are experienced by many people after severe sleep deprivation, schedule disruption, or ingestion of alcohol, and may be more frequently seen in patients with narcolepsy or depression.

Hypnagogic and Hypnopompic Hallucinations

Hallucinations can occur with sleep onset (hypnagogic) or at the end of sleep (hypnopompic). These relatively brief hallucinations occur at the transition between wake and sleep and may include visual, auditory, or tactile components. The events can be relatively pleasant or very terrifying and difficult to distinguish from reality. Patients may note a feeling of weightlessness, falling, flying, or out-of-body–like experiences, and the event may sometimes terminate with a sudden jerk (hypnic jerk). Visual hallucinations may be described as poorly formed colors or shapes to well-formed images of people or animals. The events are aborted once the patient awakens. These events may be repetitive but are not usually stereotypic. Many patients are unwilling to talk about the symptoms and clinicians should ask the patient, "when falling asleep, do you see or hear things that are not there?" Individuals may experience these events after sleep deprivation, a change in sleep schedule, or ingestion of alcohol.

Automatic Behavior

Automatic behavior is purposeful but inappropriate activity that occurs with the patient partially asleep. Patients relay stories of putting milk containers in the microwave oven, cereal bowls in the dryer, or even missing an exit on the highway.

Patients appear drowsy during the event and are usually partially or totally amnestic for the actual happenings. Events may last minutes to hours. They are more common in people with idiopathic hypersomnolence or narcolepsy but are also common in patients with delayed sleep phase. Most events are associated with non-REM (NREM) sleep, but REM activity is witnessed in patients with narcolepsy. Patients with sleep-related automatic behavior appear sleepy, but can be alerted and answer questions appropriately.

Excessive Movement in Sleep or Parasomnias

Parasomnias are undesirable physical or behavioral phenomena that occur predominantly during sleep. Bed partners may complain or note concern over frequent movement during the sleep period. This is a common complaint among patients with insomnia or sleep apnea. The category of parasomnias includes disorders of arousals, such as sleepwalking or night terrors; sleep–wake transition disorders, such as sleeptalking, rhythmic movement disorder (e.g., head banging); and REM parasomnias, such as REM sleep behavior disorder (RBD). These behavioral events may mimic epileptic seizures or other psychiatric events. Key historical features of age of onset, time of night of the events, characteristics of the behavior, memory for the events, and family history are important in distinguishing the etiology. The parasomnias are covered in greater detail in Chapters 74 to 80.

Sleeptalking

Sleeptalking is a relatively frequent event consisting of any vocalization ranging from isolated utterances to coherent conversation during sleep. This usually occurs in the lighter stages of NREM sleep, but can occur in REM sleep. The patients have no memory of the events and may convey information with little resemblance to the truth. Sleeptalking may occur more frequently during periods of stress, fever, or disturbed sleep, but in the absence of other sleep disturbances is of little medical concern.

Sleepwalking

Sleepwalking events are partial arousals, typically from slow wave sleep, occurring during the first half of the sleep period. The events can be minor behaviors or include very elaborate behaviors, including dressing, unlocking locks, and driving. Patients usually have no memory for the events or recall various impressions with rare imagery. Accounts from witnesses of the behavior are essential to the clinical evaluation. The patients do not exhibit significant tachycardia, sweating, or expression of fear. This lack of autonomic features differentiates sleepwalking from sleep terrors. Any disorder evoking arousals may increase the likelihood of these events, and thus both children and adults should be carefully questioned for signs of other sleep disorders. Patients typically have normal results on neurologic examinations during wakefulness.

Sleep Terrors

Sleep terrors are a form of disorder of arousal with a predominance of autonomic expression. Witnesses may describe a piercing scream or cry and the behavioral manifestations of intense fear.[11] The onset of the event is abrupt and patients have tachycardia, tachypnea, flushing, diaphoresis, and mydriasis. During events, patients appear confused and disoriented, and attempts to intercede may prolong the event. Patients can become violent, resulting in injury to the patient and bed partners. These events typically occur in the first third of the night and patients are amnestic for the events. Patients have normal results on diurnal neurologic examination, and should be questioned for the presence of other sleep disorders.

Confusional Arousals and Sleep Drunkenness

Confusional arousals can occur during any arousal from NREM sleep. These events are characterized by disorientation, slow speech and mentation, or inappropriate behavior. The patients have memory impairment for the event and the events can be induced with forced arousal. The course of these events usually becomes less frequent with age but may remain stable in adulthood.

Sleep drunkenness refers to inability to attain full alertness after an extended time of sleep. Patients are drowsy and disoriented, and show signs of poor coordination. Patients experiencing these events may note poor ability to concentrate and automatic behavior. This can be associated with dysfunction of the arousal system, such as is seen in idiopathic hypersomnolence.

Dream-Related Movement

REM sleep is characterized by diffuse muscle atonia, but some individuals enact dream-related behavior. These behaviors can include punching, kicking, leaping, running, talking, and yelling. Bed partners are frequently injured, and patients may go to great lengths to prevent injury to themselves or bed partners. In RBD, patients usually have vivid recall of the actual dreams that correlate to the witnessed behavior. These events occur more commonly in the latter half of the night, but can occur any time that the patient enters REM sleep. Most cases begin in late adulthood, but children with symptoms of RBD have been reported. RBD can be induced by medications such as tricyclic antidepressants, monoamine oxidase inhibitors, and serotonin reuptake inhibitors, and can also occur during alcohol withdrawal. As described in Chapter 75, the chronic form of RBD has been linked to several neurologic disorders, and patients should have a complete neurologic evaluation to look for the cardinal signs of these processes.[12]

Rhythmic Movement Disorder

Rhythmic movement disorder can present as a variety of behaviors occurring before sleep onset. The stereotyped movements usually involve large muscles, and may be sustained into light sleep. Movements may include head banging, body rocking, leg rolling, humming, and chanting. Family members may hear the rhythmic movements or chanting. Some patients are unaware of the movement, and others describe the movement as a calming compulsion before sleep. This behavior is frequently seen in infants and young children, and diminishes with age. Movements are more commonly seen in individuals with mental challenges or autism, and are more prevalent in boys. Emotional stress may provoke them. Patients can be easily alerted during the events.

Bruxism

Sleep-related bruxism can also occur as a rhythmic or repetitive movement during sleep.[13] Bed partners may complain of the loud clicking, grinding, bizarre sounds, and even rare vocalization. Patients may have abnormal wear of the teeth, jaw pain, headache, facial pain, or tooth pain. The events increase with emotional stress and may occur hundreds of times per night.

Restless Legs Syndrome and Periodic Movements of Sleep

Patients may complain of an unpleasant crawling, deep-aching sensation in the legs or arms that is improved by motion of the extremities. Others note that their legs move or dance on their own accord. These movements and uncomfortable sensations appear worse in the evening and characterize the *restless legs syndrome*. Diagnostic criteria focusing on the main symptoms have been established.[14] Patients with restless legs syndrome may relay that the discomfort can be debilitating at times and even drive some of them to pursue extreme measures to decrease the symptoms. Most patients experience the symptoms while sitting or lying down and may complain of the need to walk or have continuous movement of their legs.

Restless legs syndrome usually occurs with periodic movements of sleep. Patients or bed partners may complain of kicking or arm movements at night. These movements may occur as periodic events or appear random. *Periodic movements of sleep* are repetitive, stereotyped movements of the lower extremities that occur during sleep, consisting of extension of the great toe with dorsiflexion of the ankle and flexion of the knee and hip. Movements can also occur in the arms and axial muscles. Although most individuals with restless legs have periodic limb movements of sleep, only a minority of patients with periodic movements of sleep have excessive daytime sleepiness or insomnia. Factors that provoke periodic limb movements similarly increase the likelihood of restless legs syndrome. Periodic movements of sleep have been associated with uremia, peripheral vascular disease, anemia, arthritis, peripheral neuropathy, spinal cord lesions, antidepressants, and caffeine use.

SYSTEMIC FEATURES

The relationship of sleep disorders to systemic illness offers the clinician another opportunity to uncover underlying disordered sleep in patients. The systemic effects of sleep may be threefold: (1) sleep disorders may primarily cause physiologic changes that result in systemic disease, (2) sleep disorders may exacerbate a preexisting disorder, and (3) the systemic disease and sleep disorder may share a common pathophysiologic mechanism. Sleep disorders resulting in systemic manifestations are clearly seen with obstructive sleep apnea. Sleep apnea with oxygen desaturation decreases systemic vascular relaxation and promotes hypertension, and potentially other vascular disorders. Physicians must question patients with high-risk disorders, including hypertension, vascular disease, heart disease, neurologic disorders, diabetes mellitus, and obesity, for symptoms of sleep dysfunction that may indicate a sleep disorder acting as a cofactor. Sleep disorders may also exacerbate underlying conditions; for example, obstructive sleep apnea may worsen congestive heart failure, epilepsy, and depression. Therefore, the clinician must recognize the exacerbation of a medical, neurologic, or psychiatric disorder as a clue to disordered sleep. Patients may diminish the importance of their sleep symptoms, unaware of the connection between sleep and their other medical problems. Patients also may have a systemic illness that shares a common pathophysiologic mechanism with a sleep disorder. In patients with anemia and restless legs, iron deficiency may be the common link, and thus appropriate treatment of the underlying cause may improve both. Although these symptoms may not be considered the typical cardinal manifestations of sleep disorders, they do represent an important aspect of sleep and an entry point into the medical system for patients.

PEDIATRIC CARDINAL MANIFESTATIONS

Symptoms of sleep disorders in children can be strikingly different from those in adults and are likely to be overlooked or misinterpreted. Children can present with a range of physical and behavioral manifestations. In young children, sleep disturbances may present as poor growth, persistent fussiness, inconsolability, or increased oppositional behavior. School-aged children may exhibit suboptimal academic performance, and inattentive, hyperactive, or day-dreaming behavior in sedentary settings. Adolescents fall asleep in class and may present with affective symptoms that need to be differentiated from primary psychiatric disorders. In all ages, unrefreshing nocturnal sleep is often a clue to sleep disturbance. Although many of these symptoms are nonspecific, the clinician must discern the role of sleep dysfunction in the genesis of the symptoms.

SUMMARY

The restorative powers of sleep improve our wakefulness and ability to attain a higher level of functioning, whereas poor sleep has a negative impact on health, sense of well-being, and performance. Obvious manifestations of poor sleep such as daytime sleepiness, insomnia, and sleep-related events are the hallmark indications for further investigation. Clinicians must pay attention to the obvious and discrete signs that suggest that a sleep disorder is present. Through insight into the connection between sleep and the body, we will expand our recognition of the cardinal manifestations of sleep disorders. Identification of individuals who need further evaluation and application of appropriate therapies as described in the following chapters will aid not only these patients, but also society.

Clinical Pearl

The most common presenting symptoms of sleep disorders are insomnia and excessive daytime sleepiness. By determining the presence or absence of additional symptoms, such as snoring, observed apnea, hypnagogic hallucinations, sleep paralysis, cataplexy, or abnormal behaviors, and the presence of other medical or psychiatric conditions, the clinician usually is able to develop a comprehensive differential diagnosis, a critical step in managing the patient.

REFERENCES

1. Balter MB, Uhlenhuth EH: New epidemiologic findings about insomnia and its treatment. J Clin Psychiatry 1992;53(12 Suppl):34-39.
2. Bleecker ML, Bolla-Wilson K, Kawas C, Agnew J: Age-specific norms for the Mini-Mental State Exam. Neurology 1988;38:1565-1568.
3. Hublin C, Kaprio J, Partinen M, et al: Daytime sleepiness in an adult Finnish population. J Intern Med 1996;239:417-423.
4. Ohayon MM, Caulet M, Philip P, et al: How sleep and mental disorders are related to complaints of daytime sleepiness. Arch Intern Med 1997;157:2645-2652.
5. Johns MW: A new method for measuring daytime sleepiness: The Epworth Sleepiness Scale. Sleep 1991;14:540-545.
6. Young T, Palta M, Dempsey J, et al: The occurrence of sleep disordered breathing among middle aged adults. N Engl J Med 1993; 328:1230-1235.
7. Gislason T, Benediktsdottir B: Snoring, apneic episodes and nocturnal hypoxemia among children 6 months to 6 years old: An epidemiological study of the lower limit of prevalence. Chest 1995;107:963-966.
8. Douglass AB, Bornstein R, Nino-Murcia G, et al: The Sleep Disorders Questionnaire: I. Creation and multivariate structure of SDQ. Sleep 1994;17:160-167.
9. Netzer NC, Stoohs RA, Netzer CM, et al: Using the Berlin Questionnaire to identify patients at risk for the sleep apnea syndrome. Ann Intern Med 1999;131:485-491.
10. Dalessio DJ, Lipton RB, Silberstein SD (eds): Wolff's Headache and Other Pain, 7th ed. New York, Oxford University Press, 2001.
11. Hublin C, Kaprio J, Partinen M, Koskenvuo M: Limits of self-report in assessing sleep terrors in a population survey. Sleep 1999;22:89-93.
12. Schenck CH, Mahowald MW: Polysomnographic, neurologic, psychiatric, and clinical outcome report on 70 consecutive cases with the REM Sleep Behavior Disorder (RBD): Sustained clonazepam efficacy in 89.5% of 57 treated patients. Cleve Clin J Med 1990;57:S10-S24.
13. Ohayon MM, Li KK, Guilleminault C: Risk factors for sleep bruxism in the general population. Chest 2001;119:53-61.
14. Walters AS: Toward a better definition of the restless legs syndrome: The International Restless Legs Syndrome Study Group. Mov Disord 1995;10:634-642.

50

Use of Clinical Tools and Tests In Sleep Medicine

Ronald D. Chervin

ABSTRACT

A clinician confronted with a sleep-related complaint combines symptoms, signs, and test results to make a diagnostic assessment that will best serve the patient. When available, information about test performance characteristics, such as sensitivity, specificity, and predictive value, can be used more formally to decide on optimal approaches. Evaluations for obstructive sleep-disordered breathing start with a history and physical examination, which generate valuable information, although mathematical symptom-based models usually show inadequate specificity. Laboratory-based nocturnal polysomnography is the gold standard, but not infallible. Final diagnostic decisions should be based on integration of multiple clinical and objective data points, rather than any specific cutoff for one specific variable such as the apnea/hypopnea index. Evaluation for hypersomnolence also relies on historical symptoms, collected during an interview or using a questionnaire. Objective testing with a multiple sleep latency test or one of its variants is particularly useful when a short mean sleep latency confirms excessive daytime sleepiness. Results must be interpreted carefully, especially when negative, because of potential confounds. The multiple sleep latency test is also useful in an assessment for narcolepsy, particularly in the absence of cataplexy. Evaluation for insomnia usually relies solely on historical information. Sleep logs also can be helpful, and polysomnography is indicated when sleep-disordered breathing, periodic leg movements, or other occult sleep disorders may underlie the insomnia. Evaluation for parasomnia often starts with a thorough history, obtained whenever possible from a bed partner in addition to the patient. Polysomnography may confirm a diagnosis or distinguish between several possibilities, though few data on test performance in these settings are published.

This chapter focuses on the comparative value of different approaches to clinical assessment of sleep-related problems. The symptoms, signs, and test results relevant to particular sleep disorders are described in detail in other parts of this volume. This chapter, instead, highlights the clinical reasoning process by which a clinician challenged with a sleep complaint can combine information from different sources, appropriately weigh available evidence, and arrive at sound diagnoses and treatment plans. The first section reviews methods used to judge the value of diagnostic information. Subsequent sections review data on the value of test results in evaluations of four common clinical problems: suspected obstructive sleep-disordered breathing, hypersomnolence, insomnia, and parasomnias. Then, formal clinical decision-making techniques and cost-effectiveness analyses are introduced. The chapter concludes with a discussion of remaining challenges in the development of diagnostic methods in sleep medicine.

The Standards of Practice Committee of the American Academy of Sleep Medicine periodically reviews data on the value of clinical tests. Published evidence-based practice parameters and reviews can be accessed at http://www.aasmnet.org/practiceparameters.htm (Box 50–1). These documents are strongly recommended to supplement overviews presented in this chapter.

DIAGNOSTIC VALUE

The value of a diagnostic tool depends on both test-specific characteristics and the patient sample to be assessed. Sensitivity and specificity, however, are test specific. The sensitivity of a test represents the probability that the test will be positive given that the disorder is present. The specificity represents the probability that the test will be negative given that the disorder is absent. Sensitivity and specificity can be determined when another test is considered a gold standard. A test with both high sensitivity and specificity is optimal, but sometimes tests with imbalanced performance may still be useful. For example, to screen for a rare but serious disorder, a quick, inexpensive test with high sensitivity but low specificity might be useful to identify patients who require more extensive testing.

The prevalence of a disorder in a tested population also affects the value of a test, as reflected by the positive predictive value (PPV) and negative predictive value (NPV). Information on prevalence, sensitivity, and specificity can be used with Bayes' Theorem to calculate the PPV, which is the probability that a patient with a positive test actually has the disorder, and the NPV, which is the probability that a patient with a negative test is truly free of the disorder.[1] The equations can be expressed as:

$$PPV = prev \times sens/[prev \times sens + (1 - prev) \times (1 - spec)]$$

$$NPV = (1 - prev) \times spec/[(1 - prev) \times spec + prev \times (1 - sens)]$$

where prev = prevalence, sens = sensitivity, and spec = specificity. Although prevalence has a strong effect on predictive values, a test with a high sensitivity tends to have a high NPV and a test with a high specificity tends to have a high PPV.

After a clinician's interview, examination, and initial diagnostic formulation, the usefulness of a test depends on the pretest probability of disease, rather than the prevalence, and on the posttest or posterior probability should the test prove positive or negative.[2] Tests are valuable to the extent that the

---

Box 50–1.   Practice Parameters and Reviews

Practice parameters and reviews, published in *Sleep* by the Standards of Practice Committee of the American Academy of Sleep Medicine, are available at http://www.aasmnet.org/PracticeParam.aspx.* Examples include:

- *Clinical Use of the Multiple Sleep Latency Test and the Maintenance of Wakefulness Test*
  Published January 2005
- *Dopaminergic Treatment of Restless Legs Syndrome and Periodic Limb Movement Disorder*
  Published May 2004
- *Use of Portable Monitoring Devices in the Investigation of Suspected Obstructive Sleep Apnea in Adults*
  Published November 2003
- *Using Polysomnography to Evaluate Insomnia: An Update*
  Published September 2003
- *The Role of Actigraphy in the Study of Sleep and Circadian Rhythms*
  Published May 2003
- *Use of Auto-Titrating Continuous Positive Airway Pressure Devices for Titrating Pressures and Treating Adult Patients with Obstructive Sleep Apnea Syndrome*
  Published March 2002
- *Use of Laser-Assisted Uvulopalatoplasty (Update—2000)*
  Published August 2001
- *Treatment of Narcolepsy: An Update for 2000*
  Published June 2001
- *Evaluation of Chronic Insomnia*
  Published March 2000
- *Nonpharmacologic Treatment of Chronic Insomnia*
  Published December 1999
- *Use of Light Therapy in the Treatment of Sleep Disorders*
  Published August 1999
- *Indications for Polysomnography and Related Procedures*
  Published September 1997
- *Treatment of Obstructive Sleep Apnea in Adults: The Efficacy of Surgical Modifications of the Upper Airway*
  Published March 1996
- *Treatment of Snoring and Obstructive Sleep Apnea with Oral Appliances*
  Published September 1995
- *Use of Laser-Assisted Uvulopalatoplasty*
  Published December 1994
- *Use of Stimulants in the Treatment of Narcolepsy*
  Published June 1994

*Practice parameters from other organizations can be found at: http//www.guideline.gov/

---

posterior probability of disease is significantly lower or higher than the pretest probability.

Other concepts important in evaluation of diagnostic tools include validity and reliability. Valid tests measure the construct they are intended to measure; reliable tests yield results that are repeatable. The validity of a test can be supported in many different ways: by theory; intuition; agreement of experts; comparison with a gold standard, outcome, or other sign; convergence with expectations based on related findings; or ability to distinguish differences between conditions. The overall reliability of a test is supported by test–retest reliability, interrater reliability, and internal consistency.[3]

EVALUATION FOR OBSTRUCTIVE SLEEP-DISORDERED BREATHING

History and Questionnaires

The value of interview and questionnaire information has been studied with respect to polysomnographically confirmed diagnoses of obstructive sleep apnea syndrome (OSAS) and, to a much lesser extent, upper airway resistance syndrome (UARS). For primary snoring, no objective measure has been shown to be better than subjective reports.[4]

Subjective clinical impressions of OSAS tend to have inadequate sensitivity and specificity.[5,6] Combinations of some symptoms can have sensitivity above 0.90, but specificity is usually poor (Table 50–1). Performance of these models in clinical practice can be worse than originally reported.[7] Most studies do not report the PPV and NPV, but sensitivity and specificity data suggest that the NPV of some symptom combinations may be good, whereas the PPV is probably poor, especially when the prevalence of OSAS in the tested population is not high.[8] Accordingly, patients without a history suggestive of OSAS usually do not receive further testing for it. Among patients referred for suspected OSAS, models based on historical information may accurately classify a minority as apnea-free without further tests.[9,10] However, patients who do have symptoms of OSAS usually are tested.

Although in general the PPV of symptoms alone is not high, a minority of patients have a clinical presentation that is essentially diagnostic. The International Classification of Sleep Disorders lists a strongly positive history as adequate to fulfill minimal criteria for a diagnosis of OSAS.[11] In these cases, tests may be more useful to define the severity of OSAS than to confirm the diagnosis. In such patients, the diagnosis should still be suspected when it is not initially confirmed by oximetry, ambulatory cardiorespiratory sleep studies, or even

Table 50–1. Value of Historical or Questionnaire-Derived Diagnostic Information in the Diagnosis of Obstructive Sleep Apnea at Sleep Centers: Representative Studies

Reference	Subjects	Gold-Standard	Model	Sensitivity	Specificity	Other Results Provided
Kapuniai et al., 1988[143]	53 Sleep center patients	AHI > 10 on PSG	Observed apneas, loud snoring	0.78	0.67	
Crocker et al., 1990[144]	105 Sleep center patients	AHI > 15 on PSG	Observed apneas, hypertension, BMI, age	0.92	0.51	
Viner et al., 1991[145]	410 Patients referred for suspected sleep apnea	AHI > 10 on PSG	Age, BMI, male sex, snoring.	0.94*	0.28*	PPV* = 0.75 with pre-test probability of OSA = 0.46
			Subjective impression Usually has…	0.52	0.70	
Bliwise et al., 1991[146]	1409 Patients referred for sleep-related problems	AHI ≥ 10	Any snoring	Men, 0.97; women, 0.82	Men, 0.47; women, 0.79	
			Disruptive snoring	Men, 0.89; women, 0.71	Men, 0.71; women, 0.89	
			Nocturnal breathholding	Men, 0.70; women, 0.47	Men, 0.88; women, 0.96	
Haraldsson et al., 1992[147]	42 Patients referred for snoring	AI > 10	Habitual snoring, sleep disturbances, sleepiness	0.91	0.74	PPV = 0.56 with pretest probability of OSA = .26 NPV = 0.96 with pretest probability of no OSA = .74
Hoffstein and Szalai 1993[6]	594 Patients referred for suspected sleep apnea	AHI > 10 on PSG	Age, sex, BMI, observed apneas, pharyngeal examination.			Regression model explained 36% of variability in square root-transform of AHI
Rauscher et al., 1993[148]	116 Patients referred for heavy snoring	AHI > 10	Subjective impression	0.60	0.63	
			Weight, height, sex, observed apneas, falling asleep while reading	0.94	0.45	
Flemons et al., 1994[149]	180 Patients suspected of having sleep apnea	AHI > 10	Habitual snoring, observed gasping/ choking, neck circumference, hypertension			PPV* = 0.81 with pretest pretest probability of OSA = .45 Model explained 34% of the variation in AHI
Dealberto et al., 1994[150]	129 Adults referred for nocturnal PSG	AHI ≥ 10	Loud habitual snoring, observed apneas, sex, age, BMI	0.82	0.68	

Study	Sample	Criteria	Variables			PPV/NPV
Douglass et al., 1994[151]	435 Patients with specified sleep disorders and 84 normal control subjects	Followed International Classification of Sleep Disorders[11] criteria and had PSG, but PSG criteria not otherwise specified	Several snoring questions, observed apneas, sweat at night, history of hypertension, nasal obstruction, weight, years of smoking, age, BMI	Men, 0.85; women, 0.88	Men, 0.76; women, 0.81	Men: PPV = 0.72, NPV = 0.87 with pretest probability of OSAS = .42 Women: PPV = 0.31, NPV = 0.99 with pretest probability of OSAS = .09
Deegan and McNicholas, 1996[10]	250 Patients referred for suspected SDB	AHI ≥ 15	Observed apneas Snoring Falls asleep driving Predominant sleep position is supine			PPV = 0.64, NPV = 0.53 PPV = 0.63, NPV = 0.56 PPV = 0.70, NPV = 0.51 PPV = 0.77, NPV = 0.47 with pretest probability of OSA = .54 and pretest probability of no OSA = .46
Netzer et al., 1999[152]	744 Primary care patients	AHI > 5 on cardiorespiratory portable monitor	Weight change, snoring, snoring loudness, snoring frequency, bothersome snoring, observed apneas, tiredness, tired after sleeping, falling asleep while driving, high blood pressure	0.86	0.77	PPV = 0.89 with pretest probability of OSA = .69
Kirby et al., 1999[153]	255 Patients referred for suspected SDB (training set); 150 similar patients (model testing)	AHI > 10 on PSG	23 Variables, including age, sex, frequent awakening, witnessed apneas, reported sleepiness, hypertension, alcohol use, smoking, BMI, blood pressure, pharynx crowding	0.99	0.80	PPV = 0.88, NPV = 0.98 with pretest probability of OSA = .65 Area under receiver operating curve = 0.94 This study trained a neural network to predict OSA based on 23 clinical variables
Martinez Garcia et al., 2003[154]	207 Patients referred for suspected SDB (model development); 102 similar patients (model testing)	AHI > 30 on automatically-titrating continuous positive airway pressure unit	Hypertension, observed apneas, Epworth Sleepiness Scale score, BMI	0.83	0.91	PPV = 0.87, NPV = 0.85 with 87% of patients correctly classified, pretest probability of OSA = .38, and pretest probability of no OSA = .62

*Depended on cutoff chosen for model results.

AHI, apnea-hypopnea index (number of apneas or hypopneas per hour of sleep); AI, apnea index; BMI, body mass index; OSA, obstructive sleep apnea; PSG, polysomnography; PPV, positive predictive value; NPV, negative predictive value; SDB, sleep-disordered breathing.

single-night polysomnograms (PSGs), which are not infallible (see later).

The diagnostic values of specific symptoms are difficult to judge based on studies with significant methodologic differences. The author's clinical impressions are listed in Table 50–2, with reference to adults referred for sleep evaluations. These data are not quantitative, but they illustrate how PPV and NPV for the same symptom may differ substantially. Clinical value may be quite different in other populations. For example, among patients referred specifically for possible OSAS, the symptom of excessive daytime sleepiness (EDS) may[12] or may not[13] be useful in making the diagnosis, and a history of hypertension may be better than a report of snoring as an indication that OSAS is present.[14] In the community, the symptom with the highest predictive value for OSAS is habitual snoring, although EDS and observed apneas are also useful.[15]

Little is known about the ability of historical symptoms to identify UARS and distinguish it from OSAS or primary snoring. The probability of UARS rather than OSAS may be increased by youth, female sex, sleep-onset insomnia, functional somatic complaints, resting hypotension, and normal neck circumference.[16-20] The probability of UARS rather than primary snoring is increased by the presence of EDS or insomnia and may be increased by a history of insomnia, hypertension, hypotension, dysmenorrhea, chronic fatigue syndrome, or bruxism.[17,21,22] The likelihood of UARS rather than no sleep-disordered breathing is increased by a history of snoring, but the absence of snoring may not diminish the probability of UARS as much as it does the probability of OSAS.[21]

Table 50–2.	Estimated Clinical Values of Specific Symptoms in the Diagnosis of Obstructive Sleep Apnea Syndrome, with Reference to Patients Referred to a Sleep Clinic

	Effect on Probability of Obstructive Sleep Apnea Syndrome	
Symptom	Symptom Present	Symptom Absent
Habitual snoring	↑↑	↓↓↓
Loud snoring	↑↑↑	↓↓
Observed apneas	↑↑↑	↓
Sleepy while driving	↑↑	↓
Sleepy while reading	↑	↓↓
Morning headaches	↑	↓
Dry mouth on awakening	↑↑	↓
Nocturia (>1 episode/night)	↑↑	↓
Excessive sweating at night	↑	↓
Nocturnal reflux	↑↑	↓
Sleep maintenance insomnia	↑↑	↓↓
Nocturnal restlessness	↑	↓↓
History of hypertension	↑↑	↓
History of stroke	↑↑	↓

↑↑↑, Large increase; ↑↑, moderate increase; ↑, little or no increase; ↓↓↓, large decrease; ↓↓, moderate decrease; ↓, little or no decrease.

Physical Examination

Among variables related to body weight, neck circumference and body mass index (BMI, equal to weight in kilograms divided by height in meters squared) correlate well with the presence and severity of OSAS in the community.[23] Among patients referred for possible OSAS, these variables still may be useful, but their predictive value is not large except in extreme ranges.[6,10,24-30] Patients with OSAS who are not obese often have pharyngeal crowding, obstructed nasal passages, or other craniofacial abnormalities associated with narrowing of the upper airway.[31,32] However, reports of oropharyngeal examination findings are often subjective and seldom cite predictive values.

One quantitative model to aid in the diagnosis of OSAS is based on BMI, neck circumference, and bedside craniofacial measurements that include palatal height, maxillary intermolar distance, mandibular intermolar distance, and overjet.[33] Among 300 sleep center patients, the model showed a sensitivity of 98% and a specificity of 100% for obstructive sleep apnea. The PPV was 100% and the NPV was 89%. A second model is based on a modified Mallampati grade (for pharyngeal size), tonsil size, and BMI.[34] This model showed a PPV of 90% and an NPV of 67%. A third model is based on simple neck profile, pharyngeal, and overbite scores: obstructive sleep apnea was identified with 40% sensitivity and 96% specificity, which produced a PPV of 95% and an NPV of 49%.[35] The neck profile measurement alone accurately excluded OSAS in approximately one fourth of referred patients. Direct comparison of these three models is difficult because the studies used different recording techniques and criteria for OSAS. None of the studies addressed UARS.

Some physical findings other than craniofacial features and obesity also have value in the diagnosis of OSAS. High blood pressure increases the chance that OSAS will be present, especially among those persons who are less obese.[36] Signs of neuropathy or neuromuscular disease also may increase the likelihood of OSAS.

Nocturnal Polysomnography

A nocturnal, laboratory-based PSG is the most commonly used test in the diagnosis of OSAS. The PSG often is considered the gold standard for OSAS diagnosis, assessment of severity, and identification of some other sleep disorders that can accompany OSAS. The PSG allows direct monitoring and quantification of respiratory events and physiologic consequences—such as hypoxemia, arousals, and awakenings—that are believed to cause daytime symptoms. A single-night PSG is usually sufficient to diagnose or exclude OSAS.[37] However, the test is not infallible. Accuracy may be reduced by variability in biologic severity, laboratory equipment, human scoring, or scoring protocols. Night-to-night variability may be particularly high in subjects with low but clinically significant rates of apneas and hypopneas during sleep.[38,39] In one study, when 11 patients thought likely to have OSAS on clinical grounds were restudied after initial negative PSGs, 6 had OSAS.[40]

In contrast to widely accepted standards for scoring normal sleep,[41] standards for scoring sleep-related breathing abnormalities are not uniform between laboratories. When research shows what types and severities of sleep-related breathing disorders cause symptoms and morbidity, clearer standards may emerge. Until that time, however, the clinician must be aware of variations in practice that make interpretation of unfamiliar reports more difficult. Most important, the definition of an hypopnea varies considerably between laboratories.[42] Recommendations for scoring hypopneas have been published,[43] but whether they have led to more uniformity among sleep laboratories is not known.

The definition of an apnea also varies; some laboratories require complete cessation of airflow, whereas others allow for a small percentage (e.g., 20%) of the original airflow signal. Some laboratories score respiratory effort–related arousals, defined by nasal or esophageal pressure monitoring, in the absence of apneas or hypopneas.[44] Most laboratories report a summary measure, called the apnea-hypopnea index (AHI) or the respiratory disturbance index, which represents the sum total of apneas, hypopneas, and—sometimes in the second case— respiratory effort–related arousals per hour of sleep. An index of this type is often given the most weight in interpretation of whether the study shows significant sleep-disordered breathing. Other commonly used results, the extent and frequency of oxygen desaturations, are also tallied and reported in differing formats. The result is that interpretation of PSG reports is complicated, requiring both training and experience. The PSG may not be definitive, especially in borderline cases, without clinical information about the patient.

Despite researchers' tendency to use a specified AHI threshold to define OSAS, the clinician cannot succumb to the same temptation. An individual patient with an AHI of 40 is at risk for EDS and cardiovascular morbidity, but may not have either. Conversely, a patient with an AHI of 2 may still have OSAS (e.g., because of night-to-night variability in test results) or may have UARS with associated sleepiness and morbidity.[21,22] Interpretation of a PSG without knowledge of the patient's clinical presentation can lead to serious underdiagnosis and overdiagnosis. Many clinicians believe that an AHI above 5 suggests OSAS, but a large, population-based epidemiologic study found that only 22.6% of women and 15.5% of men who met this criterion clearly complained of daytime hypersomnolence.[23] Some patients who meet polysomnographic criteria for OSAS but do not complain of hypersomnolence have little to gain from treatment.[45]

Further research is needed to define and improve the ability of PSGs to measure those aspects of sleep-disordered breathing that most affect health and daytime sleepiness. The AHI and minimum oxygen saturation do not correlate strongly with daytime sleepiness,[46,47] although AHI may correlate better with cardiovascular morbidity.[43,48] Many patients with UARS have, by definition, EDS in the absence of a significant AHI. Esophageal pressure monitoring, the gold standard in assessment of respiratory effort,[44] facilitates the diagnosis of UARS and is particularly helpful when sleep-disordered breathing is evaluated in patients who lack obvious symptoms and signs.[17,49] However, criteria for abnormal esophageal pressure recordings, as defined by association with poor outcomes, are not yet well known. Nasal pressure monitoring may provide a well-tolerated alternative,[50] but identification of more apneic events by this sensitive measure of airflow is not necessarily a diagnostic advantage: Studies have yet to demonstrate improved prediction of outcomes, and initial comparisons with thermistor results show correlations high enough (e.g., 0.90 or higher[51]) to suggest redundancy of information.

Other polysomnographic measures that may (or may not) prove to enhance the ability of PSGs to predict outcomes of sleep-disordered breathing include end-tidal or transcutaneous carbon dioxide monitoring,[52,53] pulse transit time,[54] peripheral arterial tonometry,[55] scoring of arousals,[56] and analysis of respiratory cycle–related electroencephalographic changes.[57,58]

In short, the PSG is the single most useful and definitive test in the diagnosis of sleep-related breathing disorders, but the information it provides cannot be reliably interpreted by persons without experience in sleep medicine, summarized by any single number, or applied to patient care without careful use of additional clinical data. Failure to recognize these limitations, by health care policy makers or clinicians, could trigger unnecessary intervention or deprive a patient of effective treatment.

Modified Forms of the Polysomnogram

Compared with the standard PSG, daytime nap studies and split-night studies may reduce costs and expedite evaluation. Studies of daytime PSGs have sometimes found a high NPV, with lower PPV, but inconsistent results and the lack of sufficient data explain why daytime PSGs are not generally recommended.[8,59] A successful split-night study may save a patient from a second night in the sleep laboratory. Initial studies of diagnostic accuracy and treatment outcomes appear promising.[60] However, no prospective, double-blinded trials have compared split-night and traditional two-night protocols, and split-night studies are considered acceptable alternatives only in specific circumstances.[61]

Portable Recording

The wide range of recordings that can be performed during sleep in a patient's home are designed primarily to test for OSAS, although a portable esophageal catheter has been developed that may offer the potential to diagnose UARS.[62] Portable recordings are less costly than laboratory-based PSGs and patients usually prefer home studies over laboratory studies. However, the diagnostic value of unattended portable monitoring is reduced by the inability to make behavioral observations, standardize recording conditions, address technical problems, or make interventions during the night. Portable studies that do not monitor sleep stages or leg movements may show respiratory events that cannot be assumed to have occurred during sleep and may fail to demonstrate disorders other than OSAS.

Consensus committee reviews of portable monitoring systems have noted that relevant research has focused on many different recording systems, reducing the adequacy of data for any one system.[62] Few studies have compared portable monitors used at home, rather than the laboratory, with laboratory-based PSGs. Several cardiorespiratory recording devices have sensitivities of 95% or more but have lower specificities. Predictive values have rarely been reported. Portable monitoring therefore is not recommended, except under some specific circumstances[63]: (1) urgent evaluation of patients with severe symptoms when laboratory polysomnography is not readily available, (2) evaluation of patients unable to be studied in a sleep laboratory, and (3) evaluation of response to therapy once the diagnosis has been established and especially if multiple subsequent evaluations will be necessary. Recent re-review of available evidence did not change the recommendation that unattended monitoring be avoided, although attended portable cardiorespiratory monitoring may assist, in limited circumstances, in confirmation that OSAS is present or absent.[64]

Despite limited validation data for many portable recording devices, those that have low costs, high sensitivities, and high specificities have convinced some clinicians that portable studies are cost-effective compared with PSGs. However, cost-effectiveness analyses have been scarce (see later). The need for full laboratory-based studies may be less convincing when pretest probability is particularly high, or perhaps when pretest probability is low.[64,65] In other situations, portable monitoring could increase costs if it delays confirmatory laboratory testing, leads to treatment of patients who do not truly have OSAS, or allows development of medical morbidity from undiagnosed and therefore untreated OSAS.

Studies of Airway Morphology

Although imaging of the upper airway for research purposes has led to a better understanding of the pathophysiologic process of OSAS, such studies are not routinely performed in diagnostic evaluations of patients, in part because findings that predict OSAS or its severity with sufficient accuracy have not been identified. However, cephalometric radiography and pharyngoscopy may be useful in preoperative identification of sites of obstruction and in selection of appropriate surgical procedures.[66-70] The diagnostic value of cephalometrics may be limited in part because only sagittal plane dimensions are provided, and coronal plane dimensions or volume may by more pertinent to OSAS.[71,72] Pharyngoscopy allows three-dimensional anatomic characterization, but whether airway collapse with Mueller's maneuver predicts response to uvulopalatopharyngoplasty is debated.[73-75] Pharyngoscopy may be particularly valuable if performed during supine sleep.[76]

Computed tomography and magnetic resonance imaging studies can show upper airway morphology[71,72,77,78] and some authors suggest the potential for clinical usefulness,[79] but the value of these techniques in the clinical setting is not well defined. In particular, it is uncertain that imaging techniques more sophisticated and expensive than cephalometric radiographs and pharyngoscopy provide additional, valuable clinical information.

EVALUATION OF HYPERSOMNOLENCE

History and Questionnaires

The history provides important clues to the severity of hypersomnolence. Direct inquiry about sleepiness can be supplemented by questions about sleepiness in sedentary situations, such as driving, desk work, reading, or watching television. However, patients may report little of the EDS suggested by family members, clinical signs, or objective tests.[80] Words other than "sleepiness" are often used by patients with sleep disorders to describe the chief complaint. Among 190 apneic patients in one study, preferred terms included "lack of energy" (40%), "tiredness" (20%), "fatigue" (18%), and "sleepiness" (22%).[81] Patients' opinions about their own sleepiness sometimes show no significant association with results of the multiple sleep latency test (MSLT).[82]

Questionnaires such as the Epworth Sleepiness Scale and the Stanford Sleepiness Scale provide a more formal and perhaps reliable measure of EDS.[83-85] The impact of sleepiness on activities of daily living can be assessed with the Functional Outcomes of Sleep Questionnaire.[86] Epworth Sleepiness Scale results correlate reasonably well with patients' self-ratings for overall sleepiness, but not well with MSLT results.[82,85,87,88] Although the Epworth and Stanford Sleepiness Scales can have clinical utility, for example when monitoring response to treatment over time, they do not substitute for well-validated objective measures of sleepiness. Unfortunately, the ability of subjective or objective tests of sleepiness to predict future health outcomes is essentially unknown.

Physical Examination

Although the alerting effect of an examination obscures physical signs of sleepiness in most patients, overt signs of sleepiness—such as the inability to stay awake or keep eyes open in the examination room—have high PPV and may obviate the need for additional tests. The examination may also help to distinguish severe sleepiness from stupor due to neurologic impairment or drugs.

Nocturnal Polysomnography

Many patients referred to sleep centers for EDS have nocturnal sleep disorders, and polysomnography is often more notable for the manifestations of such disorders than for signs of EDS. Patients whose EDS is due to insufficient sleep can show shorter sleep latencies, increased sleep efficiency, decreased stage 1 sleep, and increased amounts of deep non–rapid eye movement (NREM) sleep and REM sleep. The single polysomnographic variable that best reflects sleepiness, as measured by the mean sleep latency on an MSLT, is nocturnal sleep latency.[46] Polysomnographic measures of sleep disorder, such as the AHI and minimum oxygen saturation, show only low magnitudes of correlation with MSLT results.[46,89]

Multiple Sleep Latency Test

The mean sleep latency on the MSLT (see Chapter 120) is the most commonly used objective measure in assessment of daytime sleepiness. The MSLT often contributes to diagnosis but is usually not sufficient, alone, to establish a diagnosis. The mean sleep latency is most useful when it is clearly abnormally low. A patient with a mean sleep latency of 2 minutes on a properly performed MSLT[90] is unlikely to be exaggerating a complaint of EDS, to suffer from fatigue rather than sleepiness, or to be free of any sleep disorder. The MSLT can help to determine the clinical significance of a sleep disorder or to assess response to treatment.

As a general guideline, many clinicians consider mean sleep latencies of 5 to 8 minutes or shorter to be consistent with EDS; 10 to 12 minutes or more to be normal; and middle values to represent a "gray zone." However, proper interpretation of MSLT results requires integration of other factors, and especially knowledge of the limitations of this test.

Results may be misleading if they are affected by youth (different criteria apply for children), noise, anxiety, or atypical sleep on the previous night.[90-93] Use of medications such as stimulants or antidepressants, their recent discontinuance, or inability to wean off them well before testing can prevent administration of an MSLT or complicate interpretation of results. Sleep apnea and other sleep disorders may make sleep onset more difficult and thereby interfere with the test. In general, the NPV of a long mean sleep latency is less than the PPV of a particularly short mean sleep latency. When MSLT results are normal, clinicians must carefully consider other possible explanations before telling subjectively sleepy patients that they do not have objective evidence of EDS. When MSLT results fall between extremes, the data tend to be less useful because their interpretation varies among both researchers and clinicians. Formal studies of outcomes associated with different mean sleep latencies are still needed, but until such data are available, clinicians should realize that MSLT results form a continuum without strictly interpretable cutoffs. Like most other physiologic tests, the MSLT is subject to test–retest biologic variation: A patient's mean sleep latency may be 4 minutes on one day and 7 minutes on another without any intervening therapy. High test–retest reliability among normal subjects[94] does not necessarily generalize to patients.[95] Interrater reliability can be excellent[96] but adds another source of potential variation in test results.

Finally, interpretation of the mean sleep latency on the MSLT must take into account available data on validity of the test. The most consistent data in support of the validity of the MSLT were generated in experiments with sleep deprivation, restriction, or fragmentation.[97-100] However, in clinical practice, polysomnographic measures of the severity of sleep disorders may show small[89,101-103] or insignificant[46,104,105] correlation with MSLT results. A clinician should not be surprised when a patient with 8 apneic events per hour of sleep has a lower mean sleep latency than a patient who has 50 such events per hour of sleep. Furthermore, despite clear clinical improvement demonstrated by patients with sleep apnea and other patients treated for their sleep disorders, the MSLT does not always reflect the improvement.[21,104,106-110]

Evidence that mean sleep latency on the MSLT does not necessarily parallel other measures of sleepiness or reflect patient symptoms may mean that the MSLT does not measure sleepiness precisely. However, the same evidence can also be used to support the importance of the MSLT, which provides unique data not generated by other methods. Sleepiness may have several aspects, some of which are measured better by the MSLT and some by other means.[111] The investigators who developed the MSLT originally described it as a measure of physiologic sleep tendency rather than a direct measure of sleepiness.[112] The narrower concept may define an important part of the neurophysiologic state of sleepiness without capturing the entire concept.

Use of the Multiple Sleep Latency Test in the Diagnosis of Narcolepsy

The MSLT criteria for narcolepsy—two or more sleep-onset REM periods (SOREMPs) and a short mean sleep latency—were once thought to have high sensitivity and specificity, in part because original series suggested all narcoleptic patients

and no normal control subjects had two or more SOREMPs.[113,114] Subsequent analyses of two larger groups of patients showed that none of the 63 sleepy, nonnarcoleptic patients met this criterion[115] or that only 1 of 83 nonnarcoleptic patients did so.[116] In the latter study, the PPV of two or more SOREMPs for the diagnosis of narcolepsy was 98% and the NPV was 89%.

More recent studies did not find the SOREMP criteria to provide such diagnostic accuracy, partly because the most common reasons for sleep laboratory referral evolved. Two or more SOREMPs were found in 25% of 187 patients with sleep apnea,[117] 17% of 139 normal subjects,[118] and only 83% of 200 narcoleptic patients who had cataplexy.[119] Among 2083 patients evaluated with MSLTs at one sleep center, the PPV of two or more SOREMPs was 57% and the NPV was 98%.[120] Other combinations of MSLT and polysomnographic criteria may have additional utility,[120] but MSLT results cannot be used alone to diagnose narcolepsy: The presence of SOREMPs must be interpreted in conjunction with other clinical and polysomnographic findings. In particular, the criterion of two or more SOREMPs cannot be used to diagnose narcolepsy when the patient has untreated OSAS, UARS, or other sleep disorders associated with SOREMPs.

The International Classification of Sleep Disorders has been newly revised (see Chapter 51). The new edition classifies narcolepsy with cataplexy separately from narcolepsy without cataplexy, in part because hypocretin deficiencies in the former, but not most of the latter patients, suggest a different pathogenesis for the two conditions. With adoption of the new criteria, MSLT SOREMPs have become irrelevant to a diagnosis of narcolepsy with cataplexy, but they are required for a diagnosis of narcolepsy without cataplexy.

Variations of the Multiple Sleep Latency Test and Other Physiologic Tests

Results on the Maintenance of Wakefulness Test (MWT) can differ markedly from those of the MSLT,[121] but whether the MWT results are more predictive of adverse effects of sleepiness in daily life remains unknown. The MWT results correlate with measures of sleep apnea severity to approximately the same extent as MSLT results,[122] but may better reflect improvement with treatment.[121] However, until more evidence accrues that information from the MWT differs in a clinically meaningful way from that generated with the MSLT, the MSLT will continue to offer the advantages of more published experience, familiarity among clinicians, and relevance to the diagnosis of narcolepsy.

Other MSLT modifications, for which limited validity data exist, include the assignment of a simple performance task during the nap attempts[91]; a formula to combine quantities of sleep stages attained on naps into an overall polygraphic score of sleepiness[123]; calculation of mean wake efficiencies (100% time asleep during nap attempt) as an alternative to mean sleep latencies[124]; definition of sleep onset by a subject's failure to respond to an intermittent light signal[125]; and use of survival analysis methods that incorporate information from nap attempts on which no sleep was obtained.[126] In the clinical setting, none of these modifications has a well-established role in the evaluation of hypersomnolence, and neither do a range of other physiologic tests, including pupillometry[127,128] and brainstem auditory evoked potentials.[129] A variety of performance-based tests are used, usually in research settings, to assess variables related to sleepiness. Examples are the Psychomotor Vigilance Task[130] and the Steer Clear driving simulation test.[131]

EVALUATION OF INSOMNIA

Like EDS, the complaint of inadequate, insufficient, or non-restorative sleep can have many different causes. Unlike causes of hypersomnia, however, sleep disorders that cause insomnia are most often diagnosed by history alone.[132-134] In part because the gold standard is not a physiologic test, few data are available with which to assess the relative value of individual symptoms. Predictive values for some symptoms are likely to be high because symptoms define the disorders. When a history does not reveal a cause for the insomnia, polysomnography may be useful (see later), but referral to an appropriate specialist for further history taking and evaluation is sometimes necessary. For example, if the sleep clinician cannot thoroughly evaluate a patient for depression, a psychiatrist or psychologist may be better able to establish a diagnosis and treatment regimen that will lead to resolution of the patient's insomnia. Psychometric tests can reveal cognitive differences between insomniac patients and normal control subjects,[135] but these tests are not commonly used for diagnostic purposes in the clinical sleep medicine setting.

Sleep logs are an important tool in the evaluation of insomnia,[136] but data on their predictive value have not been published. Logs are not necessary to establish the presence of insomnia, but can help define severity and facilitate identification of causes such as inadequate sleep hygiene, delayed sleep phase syndrome, or psychophysiologic insomnia.

The physical and mental status examinations may provide clues that the cause of a patient's insomnia is an underlying medical or psychiatric illness such as hyperthyroidism, asthma, benign prostatic hypertrophy, painful lumbar radiculopathy, arthritis, depression, or anxiety. The importance and focus of an examination vary depending on what is learned from the history. In patients with psychiatric causes of insomnia, the mental status examination may reveal valuable diagnostic clues such as pressured speech, thought disorders, depressed affect, or nervousness.

A patient's history and physical examination sometimes suggest that insomnia may be due to sleep-disordered breathing, periodic limb movement disorder, or uncertain causes. In such cases, polysomnography can be an important aid to diagnosis.[133,134] If insomnia fails to respond to treatment for initial diagnoses, polysomnography also may be useful. Polysomnography may be indicated for patients who have precipitous arousals with violent or injurious behavior.[134] Polysomnography may also be useful in some cases when sleep state misperception is suspected. However, injudicious use of polysomnography can sometimes enhance an insomniac patient's conviction that symptoms are due to physical rather than behavioral causes or lead to diagnoses that eventually prove irrelevant to the main complaint. Polysomnography is not indicated for routine evaluation of insomnia that is transient or chronic, due to psychiatric disorders, associated with dementia, or found in the many conditions such as fibromyalgia that are associated with the alpha-delta sleep pattern.[134]

EVALUATION FOR SUSPECTED PARASOMNIAS

Parasomnias often are diagnosed by history alone,[11] but information obtained from a bed partner may contribute more than that obtained from the patient. Classic descriptions can be diagnostic for disorders such as sleep terrors, rhythmic movement disorder, sleep paralysis, sleep bruxism, and sleep enuresis. However, the history in such cases occasionally can be misleading, as when one patient's nocturnal behaviors and bed-wetting episodes were shown by polysomnography to occur only during wakefulness.[137] Furthermore, some parasomnia presentations commonly lead to a differential diagnosis that frequently requires clarification by polysomnography. For example, the differential diagnosis for a middle-aged adult who presents with behavioral episodes at night may include REM sleep behavior disorder, sleepwalking, and complex partial seizures.

The physical examination of patients evaluated for parasomnias can be useful but its value is not well quantified. Some signs may suggest sleep apnea as an underlying trigger for confusional arousals, sleepwalking, sleep terrors, REM sleep behavior disorder, or nocturnal enuresis. Worn occlusive surfaces of molars can provide key evidence of sleep bruxism. The urogenital examination is important in patients suspected to have impaired sleep-related penile erections, sleep-related painful erections, or sleep enuresis. Endocrine, cardiac, vascular, and neurologic examination findings can also show a cause for erectile dysfunction. A neurologic examination may suggest a primary cause of sleep enuresis or REM sleep behavior disorder. Similarly, appropriate laboratory findings may be helpful in some cases; for example, a urinalysis may reveal the cause of sleep enuresis.

Few studies have examined the predictive value of polysomnography for parasomnia diagnoses. When the behavior in question occurs during polysomnography, the diagnostic value of the test is likely to be high, especially if appropriate additional recording devices, such as extra electroencephalography leads, extra surface electromyography leads, or video monitoring are used.[138] Unfortunately, polysomnography often fails to document the behavior—especially in cases of suspected REM sleep behavior disorder, sleepwalking, night terrors, and epilepsy—either because the behavior does not occur on most nights or perhaps because the sleep laboratory is not an environment familiar to the patient. However, other findings during polysomnography can have good PPV. Examples would include excessive limb twitching during REM sleep in a patient tested for REM sleep behavior disorder, or spike-and-wave complexes in the electroencephalogram of a patient suspected to have epilepsy. The NPV of a completely normal study result is less clear. In one series of 122 patients with suspected parasomnias, 1 to 2 nights of polysomnography with video monitoring contributed useful diagnostic information in more than 50% of the cases.[138]

BEYOND SENSITIVITY, SPECIFICITY, AND PREDICTIVE VALUE: DECISION AND COST-EFFECTIVENESS ANALYSES

Data on sensitivity, specificity, pretest probability, and utility of outcomes can be used to construct a decision analysis. A clinical decision analysis typically models a choice between diagnostic or therapeutic alternatives. Logical rules are used to weigh information and make the best decision for an individual patient.[2] Decision analysis may be useful, for example, when one procedure has a high probability of a small benefit while an alternative has a low probability of a large benefit. Physicians often attempt a similar mental process, but do not usually make optimal use of their own beliefs about probabilities and values of outcomes. Although decision analyses are becoming more common, they have rarely been used in sleep medicine.

Economic pressures have expanded evaluations of diagnostic procedures beyond utility to include cost and cost-effectiveness. Economic analyses can include cost studies, cost-effectiveness analyses that compare different methods to achieve the same end, cost-utility analyses that compare costs per common unit of utility (often quality-adjusted life years), and cost-benefit analyses that compare monetary costs with monetary gains.[139] Such studies require quantitative information on costs and outcomes, data that are not abundant for sleep disorders.[140,141]

In one relevant cost-utility analysis, investigators modeled the decision of whether to diagnose OSAS with the aid of a PSG, portable cardiorespiratory monitor, or no ancillary test.[142] The model used published figures for the utility of OSAS treatment, mortality rates without treatment, and performance of one of the more effective home study devices. Polysomnography generated higher utility than the other diagnostic options, even when the pretest probability of OSAS was varied between .35 and .95. Moreover, the magnitude of the advantage of polysomnography easily justified the added initial expense. This result appeared to reflect the high utility of an OSAS diagnosis, and the high costs of treatment for OSAS relative to the costs of an accurate diagnosis. Diagnostic mistakes are expensive. These findings highlight the importance of performing decision and cost-utility analyses before conclusions are made about relative values of diagnostic tests. Health care managers and policy makers increasingly rely on such data to make decisions about allocation of scarce resources.

Clinical Pearl

Evaluation of common sleep complaints is based on symptoms, signs, and test results, combined with an understanding of the diagnostic value that each type of data contributes.

REFERENCES

1. Woolson RF: Statistical Methods for the Analysis of Biomedical Data. New York, John Wiley & Sons, 1987.
2. Weinstein MC, Fineberg HV, Elstein AS, et al: Clinical Decision Analysis. Philadelphia, WB Saunders, 1980.
3. DeVellis RF: Scale Development: Theory and Applications. Newbury Park, Calif, Sage, 1991.
4. Hoffstein V: Snoring. Chest 1996;109:201-222.
5. Viner S, Szalai JP, Hoffstein V: Are history and physical examination a good screening test for sleep apnea? Ann Intern Med 1991;115:356-359.
6. Hoffstein V, Szalai JP: Predictive value of clinical features in diagnosing obstructive sleep apnea. Sleep 1993;16:118-122.
7. Rowley JA, Aboussouan LS, Badr MS: The use of clinical prediction formulas in the evaluation of obstructive sleep apnea. Sleep 2000;23:929-938.
8. Chesson AL, Ferber RA, Fry JM, et al: The indications for polysomnography and related procedures. Sleep 1997;20:423-487.
9. Viner S, Szalai JP, Hoffstein V: Are history and physical examination a good screening test for sleep apnea? Ann Intern Med 1991;115:356-359.
10. Deegan PC, McNicholas WT: Predictive value of clinical features for the obstructive sleep apnoea syndrome. Eur Respir J 1996;9:117-124.
11. American Sleep Disorders Association: International Classification of Sleep Disorders, Revised: Diagnostic and Coding Manual. Rochester, Minn, American Sleep Disorders Association, 1997.
12. Dealberto MJ, Ferber C, Garma L, et al: Factors related to sleep apnea syndrome in sleep clinic patients. Chest 1994;105:1753-1758.
13. Flemons WW, Whitelaw WA, Brant R, Remmers JE: Likelihood ratios for a sleep apnea clinical prediction rule. Am J Respir Crit Care Med 1994;150:1279-1285.
14. Crocker BD, Olson LG, Saunders NA, et al: Estimation of the probability of disturbed breathing during sleep before a sleep study. Am Rev Respir Dis 1990;142:14-18.
15. Young T, Hutton R, Finn L, et al: The gender bias in sleep apnea diagnosis: Are women missed because they have different symptoms? Arch Intern Med 1996;156:2445-2451.
16. Guilleminault C, Kim Y, Stoohs R: Upper airway resistance syndrome. Oral Maxillofac Surg Clin North Am 1995;7:243-256.
17. Guilleminault C, Stoohs R, Kim Y, et al: Upper airway sleep-disordered breathing in women. Ann Intern Med 1995;122:493-501.
18. Guilleminault C, Black JE, Palombini L, Ohayon M: A clinical investigation of obstructive sleep apnea syndrome (OSAS) and upper airway resistance syndrome (UARS) patients. Sleep Med 2003;1:51-56.
19. Guilleminault C, Faul JL, Stoohs R: Sleep-disordered breathing and hypotension. Am J Respir Crit Care Med 2001;164:1242-1247.
20. Gold AR, Dipalo F, Gold MS, O'Hearn D: The symptoms and signs of upper airway resistance syndrome. Chest 2003;123:87-95.
21. Guilleminault C, Stoohs R, Clerk A, et al: A cause of excessive daytime sleepiness: the upper airway resistance syndrome. Chest 1993;104:781-787.
22. Guilleminault C, Stoohs R, Shiomi T, et al: Upper airway resistance syndrome, nocturnal blood pressure monitoring, and borderline hypertension. Chest 1996;109:901-908.
23. Young T, Palta M, Dempsey J, et al: The occurrence of sleep-disordered breathing among middle-aged adults. N Engl J Med 1993;328:1230-1235.
24. Flemons WW, Whitelaw WA, Brant R, Remmers JE: Likelihood ratios for a sleep apnea clinical prediction rule. Am J Respir Crit Care Med 1994;150:1279-1285.
25. Viner S, Szalai JP, Hoffstein V: Are history and physical examination a good screening test for sleep apnea? Ann Intern Med 1991;115:356-359.
26. Kump K, Whalen C, Tishler PV, et al: Assessment of the validity and utility of a sleep-symptom questionnaire. Am J Respir Crit Care Med 1994;150:735-741.
27. Dealberto MJ, Ferber C, Garma L, et al: Factors related to sleep apnea syndrome in sleep clinic patients. Chest 1994;105:1753-1758.
28. Stradling JR, Crosby JH: Predictors and prevalence of obstructive sleep apnoea and snoring in 1001 middle aged men. Thorax 1991;46:85-90.
29. Crocker BD, Olson LG, Saunders NA, et al: Estimation of the probability of disturbed breathing during sleep before a sleep study. Am Rev Respir Dis 1990;142:14-18.
30. Davies RJ, Ali NJ, Stradling JR: Neck circumference and other clinical features in the diagnosis of the obstructive sleep apnoea syndrome. Thorax 1992;47:101-105.

31. Liistro G, Rombaux P, Belge C, et al: High Mallampati score and nasal obstruction are associated risk factors for obstructive sleep apnea. Eur Respir J 2003;21:248-252.

32. Ferguson KA, Ono T, Lowe AA, et al: The relationship between obesity and craniofacial structure in obstructive sleep apnea. Chest 1995;108:375-381.

33. Kushida CA, Efron B, Guilleminault C: A predictive morphometric model for the obstructive sleep apnea syndrome. Ann Intern Med 1997;127:581-587.

34. Friedman M, Tanyeri H, La Rosa M, et al: Clinical predictors of obstructive sleep apnea. Laryngoscope 1999;109:1901-1907.

35. Tsai WH, Remmers JE, Brant R, et al: A decision rule for diagnostic testing in obstructive sleep apnea. Am J Respir Crit Care Med 2003;167:1427-1432.

36. Young T, Peppard P, Palta M, et al: Population-based study of sleep-disordered breathing as a risk factor for hypertension. Arch Intern Med 1997;157:1746-1752.

37. American Thoracic Society, Medical Section of the American Lung Association: Indications and standards for cardiopulmonary sleep studies. Am Rev Respir Dis 1989;139:559-568.

38. Wittig RM, Romaker A, Zorick FJ, et al: Night-to-night consistency of apneas during sleep. Am Rev Respir Dis 1984;129:244-248.

39. Chediak AD, Acevedo-Crespo JC, Seiden DJ, et al: Nightly variability in the indices of sleep-disordered breathing in men being evaluated for impotence with consecutive night polysomnograms. Sleep 1996;19:589-592.

40. Meyer TJ, Eveloff SE, Kline LR, Millman RP: One negative polysomnogram does not exclude obstructive sleep apnea. Chest 1993;103:756-760.

41. Rechtschaffen A, Kales A: A Manual of Standardized Terminology, Techniques and Scoring System for Sleep Stages of Human Subjects. Los Angeles, Brain Information Service/Brain Research Institute, UCLA, 1968.

42. Moser NJ, Phillips BA, Berry DTR, Harbison L: What is hypopnea, anyway? Chest 1994;105:426-428.

43. Meoli AL, Casey KR, Clark RW, et al: Clinical Practice Review Committee: Hypopnea in sleep-disordered breathing in adults. Sleep 2001;24:469-470.

44. American Academy of Sleep Medicine Task Force: Sleep-related breathing disorders in adults: Recommendations for syndrome definition and measurement techniques in clinical research. Sleep 1999;22:667-689.

45. Barbe F, Mayoralas LR, Duran J, et al: Treatment with continuous positive airway pressure is not effective in patients with sleep apnea but no daytime sleepiness: A randomized, controlled trial. Ann Intern Med 2001;134:1015-1023.

46. Chervin RD, Kraemer HC, Guilleminault C: Correlates of sleep latency on the multiple sleep latency test in a clinical population. Electroencephalogr Clin Neurophysiol 1995;95:147-153.

47. Gottlieb DJ, Whitney CW, Bonekat WH, et al: Relation of sleepiness to respiratory disturbance index: The Sleep Heart Health Study. Am J Respir Crit Care Med 1999;159:502-507.

48. Young T, Peppard P, Palta M, et al: Population-based study of sleep-disordered breathing as a risk factor for hypertension. Arch Intern Med 1997;157:1746-1752.

49. Guilleminault C, Pelayo R, Leger D, et al: Recognition of sleep-disordered breathing in children. Pediatrics 1996;98:871-882.

50. Ayappa I, Norman RG, Krieger AC, et al: Non-Invasive detection of respiratory effort-related arousals (RERAs) by a nasal cannula/pressure transducer system. Sleep 2000;23:763-771.

51. Serebrisky D, Cordero R, Mandeli J, et al: Assessment of inspiratory flow limitation in children with sleep-disordered breathing by a nasal cannula pressure transducer system. Pediatr Pulmonol 2002;33:380-387.

52. American Thoracic Society, Medical Section of the American Lung Association: Standards and indications for cardiopulmonary sleep studies in children. Am J Respir Crit Care Med 1996;153:866-878.

53. Morielli A, Desjardins D, Brouillette RT: Transcutaneous and end-tidal carbon dioxide pressures should be measured during pediatric polysomnography. Am Rev Respir Dis 1993;148:1599-1604.

54. Bennett LS, Barbour C, Langford B, et al: Health status in obstructive sleep apnea: Relationship with sleep fragmentation and daytine sleepiness, and effects of continuous positive airway pressure treatment. Am J Respir Crit Care Med 1999;159:1884-1890.

55. O'Donnell CP, Allan L, Atkinson P, Schwartz AR: The effect of upper airway obstruction and arousal on peripheral arterial tonometry in obstructive sleep apnea. Am J Respir Crit Care Med 2002;166:965-971.

56. Bennett LS, Langford BA, Stradling JR, Davies RJO: Sleep fragmentation indices as predictors of daytime sleepiness and nCPAP response in obstructive sleep apnea. Am J Respir Crit Care Med 1998;158:778-786.

57. Chervin RD, Burns JW, Subotic NS, et al: Method for detection of respiratory cycle-related EEG changes in sleep-disordered breathing. Sleep 2004;27:110-115.

58. Chervin RD, Burns JW, Subotic NS, et al: Correlates of respiratory cycle-related EEG changes in children with sleep-disordered breathing. Sleep 2004;27:116-120.

59. Redline S, Tishler PV, Hans MG, et al: Racial differences in sleep-disordered breathing in African-Americans and Caucasians. Am J Respir Crit Care Med 1997;155:186-192.

60. Rodway GW, Sanders MH: The efficacy of split-night sleep studies. Sleep Med Rev 2003;7:391-401.

61. American Sleep Disorders Association Standards of Practice Committee: Practice parameters for the indications for polysomnography and related procedures. Sleep 1997;20:406-422.

62. Tvinnereim M, Mateika S, Cole P, et al: Diagnosis of obstructive sleep apnea using a portable transducer catheter. Am J Respir Crit Care Med 1995;152:775-779.

63. American Sleep Disorders Association: Practice parameters for the use of portable recording in the assessment of obstructive sleep apnea. Sleep 1994;17:372-377.

64. Chesson AL, Berry RB, Pack AI: Practice parameters for the use of portable monitoring devices in the investigation of suspected obstructive sleep apnea in adults. Sleep 2003;26:907-913.

65. Strohl KP: Timing, number and complexities of sleep studies. Sleep Breathing 1997;2:45-49.

66. Riley RW, Powell NB, Guilleminault C: Obstructive sleep apnea syndrome: A review of 306 consecutively treated surgical patients. Otolaryngol Head Neck Surg 1993;108:117-125.

67. Guilleminault C, Riley R, Powell N: Obstructive sleep apnea and abnormal cephalometric measurements. Implications for treatment. Chest 1984;86:793-794.

68. Sher AE, Schechtman KB, Piccirillo JF: The efficacy of surgical modifications of the upper airway in adults with obstructive sleep apnea syndrome. Sleep 1996;19:156-177.

69. Woodson BT, Conley SF: Prediction of uvulopalatopharyngoplasty response using cephalometric radiographs. Am J Otolaryngol 1997;18:179-184.

70. Hans MG, Goldberg J: Cephalometric examination in obstructive sleep apnea. Oral Maxillofac Surg Clin North Am 1995;7:269-281.

71. Schwab RJ, Gefter WB, Hoffman EA, et al: Dynamic upper airway imaging during awake respiration in normal subjects and patients with sleep disordered breathing. Am Rev Respir Dis 1993;148:1385-1400.

72. Schwab RJ, Pasirstein M, Pierson R, et al: Identification of upper airway anatomic risk factors for obstructive sleep apnea with volumetric magnetic resonance imaging. Am J Respir Crit Care Med 2003;168:522-530.

73. Woodson BT: Examination of the upper airway. Oral Maxillofac Surg Clin North Am 1995;7:257-267.

74. Sher AE, Thorpy MJ, Shprintzen RJ, et al: Predictive value of Muller maneuver in selection of patients for uvulopalatopharyngoplasty. Laryngoscope 1985;95:1483-1487.

75. Skatvedt O: Localization of site of obstruction in snorers and patients with obstructive sleep apnea syndrome: A comparison of fiberoptic nasopharyngoscopy and pressure measurements. Acta Otolaryngol 1993;113:206-209.

76. Pringle MB, Croft CB: A grading system for patients with obstructive sleep apnoea—based on sleep nasendoscopy. Clin Otolaryngol 1993;18:480-484.

77. Schwab RJ, Gupta KB, Gefter WB, et al: Upper airway and soft tissue anatomy in normal subjects and patients with sleep-disordered breathing: Significance of the lateral pharyngeal walls. Am J Respir Crit Care Med 1995;152:1673-1689.

78. Pevernagie DA, Stanson AW, Sheedy PF, et al: Effects of body position on the upper airway of patients with obstructive sleep apnea. Am J Respir Crit Care Med 1995;152:179-185.

79. Suto Y, Matsuda E, Inoue Y, et al: Sleep apnea syndrome: comparison of MR imaging of the oropharynx with physiologic indexes. Radiology 1997;201:393-398.

80. Dement WC, Carskadon MA, Richardson G: Excessive daytime sleepiness in the sleep apnea syndrome. In Guilleminault C, Dement WC (eds): Sleep Apnea Syndromes. New York, Alan R. Liss, 1978, pp 23-46.

81. Chervin RD: Sleepiness, fatigue, tiredness, and lack of energy in obstructive sleep apnea. Chest 2000;118:372-379.

82. Chervin RD, Aldrich MS, Pickett R, Guilleminault C: Comparison of the results of the Epworth Sleepiness Scale and the multiple sleep latency test. J Psychosom Res 1997;42:145-155.

83. Hoddes E, Dement W, Zarcone V: The development and use of the Stanford Sleepiness Scale (SSS). Psychophysiology 1972;9:150.

84. Herscovitch J, Broughton R: Sensitivity of the Stanford Sleepiness Scale to the effects of cumulative partial sleep deprivation and recovery oversleeping. Sleep 1981;4:83-92.

85. Johns MW: A new method for measuring daytime sleepiness: The Epworth Sleepiness Scale. Sleep 1991;14:540-545.

86. Weaver TE, Laizner AM, Evans LK, et al: An instrument to measure functional status outcomes for disorders of excessive sleepiness. Sleep 1997;20:835-843.

87. Johns MW: Sleepiness in different situations measured by the Epworth Sleepiness Scale. Sleep 1994;17:703-710.

88. Chervin RD, Aldrich MS: The Epworth Sleepiness Scale may not reflect objective measures of sleepiness or sleep apnea. Neurology 1999;52:125-131.

89. Chervin RD, Aldrich MS: The relation between MSLT findings and the frequency of apneic events in REM and NREM sleep. Chest 1998;113:980-984.

90. Carskadon MA, Dement WC, Mitler MM, et al: Guidelines for the multiple sleep latency test (MSLT): A standard measure of sleepiness. Sleep 1986;9:519-524.

91. Naitoh P, Kelly TL: Modification of the multiple sleep latency test. In Ogilvie RD, Harsh JR (eds): Sleep Onset: Normal and Abnormal Processes. New York, John Wiley & Sons, 1995, pp 327-338.

92. American Sleep Disorders Association: The clinical use of the multiple sleep latency test. Sleep 1992;15:268-276.

93. Hoban TF, Chervin RD: Assessment of sleepiness in children. Semin Pediatr Neurol 2001;8:216-228.

94. Zwyghuizen-Doorenbos A, Roehrs T, Schaefer M, Roth T: Test-retest reliability of the MSLT. Sleep 1988;11:562-565.

95. Roehrs T, Roth T: Multiple sleep latency test: Technical aspects and normal values. J Clin Neurophysiol 1992;9:63-67.

96. Benbadis SR, Qu Y, Perry MC, et al: Interrater reliability of the multiple sleep latency test. Electroencephalogr Clin Neurophysiol 1995;95:302-304.

97. Carskadon MA, Dement WC: Sleep tendency: an objective measure of sleep loss. Sleep Res 1977;6:200.

98. Carskadon MA, Dement WC: Effects of total sleep loss on sleep tendency. Percept Mot Skills 1979;48:495-506.

99. Carskadon MA, Dement WC: Nocturnal determinants of daytime sleepiness. Sleep 1982;5:S73-S81.

100. Roehrs T, Merlotti L, Petrucelli N, et al: Experimental sleep fragmentation. Sleep 1994;17:438-443.

101. Guilleminault C, Partinen M, Quera-Salva MA, et al: Determinants of daytime sleepiness in obstructive sleep apnea. Chest 1988;94:32-37.

102. Roehrs T, Zorick F, Wittig R, et al: Predictors of objective level of daytime sleepiness in patients with sleep-related breathing disorders. Chest 1989;95:1202-1206.

103. Aldrich MS: Sleep continuity and excessive daytime sleepiness in sleep apnea. Sleep Res 1990;19:178.

104. Roth T, Hartse M, Zorick F, Conway W: Multiple naps and the evaluation of daytime sleepiness in patients with upper airway sleep apnea. Sleep 1980;3:425-439.

105. Cheshire K, Engleman H, Deary I, et al: Factors impairing daytime performance in patients with sleep apnea/hypopnea syndrome. Arch Intern Med 1992;152:538-541.

106. Lamphere J, Roehrs T, Wittig R, et al: Recovery of alertness after CPAP in apnea. Chest 1989;96:1364-1367.

107. Engleman HM, Martin SE, Deary IJ, Douglas NJ: Effect of continuous positive airway pressure treatment on daytime function in sleep apnoea/hypopnoea syndrome. Lancet 1994;343:572-575.

108. Engleman HM, Cheshire KE, Deary IJ, Douglas NJ: Daytime sleepiness, cognitive performance and mood after continuous positive airway pressure for the sleep apnoea/hypopnoea syndrome. Thorax 1993;48:911-914.

109. Sangal RB, Thomas L, Mitler MM: Disorders of excessive sleepiness: Treatment improves ability to stay awake but does not reduce sleepiness. Chest 1992;102:699-703.

110. Phillips BA, Schmitt FA, Berry DT, et al: Treatment of obstructive sleep apnea: A preliminary report comparing nasal CPAP to nasal oxygen in patients with mild OSA. Chest 1990;98:325-330.

111. Chervin RD, Guilleminault C: Assessment of sleepiness in clinical practice. Nat Med 1995;1:1252-1253.

112. Carskadon MA, Dement WC: The multiple sleep latency test: what does it measure? Sleep 1982;5:S67-S72.

113. Mitler MM, Van den Hoed J, Carskadon MA, et al: REM sleep episodes during the multiple sleep latency test in narcoleptic patients. Electroencephalogr Clin Neurophysiol 1979;46:479-481.

114. Richardson GS, Carskadon MA, Flagg W, et al: Excessive daytime sleepiness in man: Multiple sleep latency measurement in narcoleptic and control subjects. Electroencephalogr Clin Neurophysiol 1978;45:621-627.

115. Mitler MM: The multiple sleep latency test as an evaluation for excessive daytime sleepiness. In Guilleminault C (ed): Sleeping and Waking Disorders: Indications and Techniques. Menlo Park, Calif, Addison-Wesley, 1982, pp 145-153.

116. Amira SA, Johnson TS, Logowitz NB: Diagnosis of narcolepsy using the multiple sleep latency test: analysis of current laboratory criteria. Sleep 1985;8:325-331.

117. Biniaurishvili RG, Fry JM, DiPhillipo MA, Goldberg R: MSLT REM sleep episodes, excessive daytime sleepiness and sleep structure in obstructive sleep apnea patients [abstract]. Sleep Res 1994;23:231.

118. Bishop C, Rosenthal L, Helmus T, et al: The frequency of multiple sleep onset REM periods among subjects with no excessive daytime sleepiness. Sleep 1996;19:727-730.

119. Moscovitch A, Partinen M, Guilleminault C: The positive diagnosis of narcolepsy and narcolepsy's borderland. Neurology 1993;43:55-60.

120. Aldrich MS, Chervin RD, Malow BA: Value of the multiple sleep latency test (MSLT) for the diagnosis of narcolepsy. Sleep 1997;20:620-629.

121. Sangal RB, Thomas L, Mitler MM: Maintenance of Wakefulness Test and multiple sleep latency test: Measurement of different abilities in patients with sleep disorders. Chest 1992;101: 898-902.

122. Poceta JS, Timms RM, Jeong DU, et al: Maintenance of Wakefulness Test in obstructive sleep apnea syndrome. Chest 1992;101:893-897.

123. Roth B, Nevsimalova S, Sonka K, Docekal P: An alternative to the multiple sleep latency test for determining sleepiness in narcolepsy and hypersomnia: Polygraphic score of sleepiness. Sleep 1986;9:243-245.

124. Pollak CP: How should the multiple sleep latency test be analyzed? Sleep 1997;20:34-39.

125. Bennett LS, Stradling JR, Davies RJ: A behavioural test to assess daytime sleepiness in obstructive sleep apnoea. J Sleep Res 1997;6:142-145.

126. Punjabi NM, O'Hearn DJ, Neubauer DN, et al: Modeling hypersomnolence in sleep-disordered breathing. Am J Respir Crit Care Med 1999;159:1703-1709.

127. Yoss RE, Moyer NJ, Hollenhorst RW: Pupil size and spontaneous pupillary waves associated with alertness, drowsiness, and sleep. Neurology 1970;20:545-554.

128. O'Neill WD, Oroujeh AM, Keegan AP, Merritt SL: Neurological pupillary noise in narcolepsy. J Sleep Res 1996;5: 265-271.

129. Sangal RB, Sangal JM: Measurement of P300 and sleep characteristics in patients with hypersomnia: Do P300 latencies, P300 amplitudes, and multiple sleep latency and maintenance of wakefulness tests measure different factors? Clin Electroencephalogr 1997;28:179-184.

130. Kribbs NB, Pack AI, Kline LR, et al: Effects of one night without nasal CPAP treatment on sleep and sleepiness in patients with obstructive sleep apnea. Am Rev Respir Dis 1993;147: 1162-1168.

131. Findley L, Unverzagt M, Guchu R, et al: Vigilance and automobile accidents in patients with sleep apnea or narcolepsy. Chest 1995;108:619-624.

132. American Sleep Disorders Association: Practice parameters for the use of polysomnography in the evaluation of insomnia. Sleep 1995;18:55-57.

133. Reite M, Buysse D, Reynolds C, Mendelson W: The use of polysomnography in the evaluation of insomnia. Sleep 1996;18:58-70.

134. Littner M, Hirshkowitz M, Kramer M, et al: Practice parameters for using polysomnography to evaluate insomnia: An update. Sleep 2003;26:754-760.

135. Hauri PJ: Cognitive deficits in insomnia patients. Acta Neurol Belg 1997;97:113-117.

136. Spielman AJ, Nunes J, Glovinsky PB: Insomnia. Neurol Clin 1996;14:513-543.

137. Molaie M, Deutsch GK: Psychogenic events presenting as parasomnias. Sleep 1997;20:402-405.

138. Aldrich MS, Jahnke B: Diagnostic value of video-EEG polysomnography. Neurology 1991;41:1060-1066.

139. Crawford B: Clinical economics and sleep disorders. Sleep 1997;20:829-834.

140. Rodenstein DO: Sleep apnoea syndrome: The health economics point of view. Monaldi Arch Chest Dis 2003;55:404-410.

141. Martin SA, Aikens JE, Chervin RD: Toward cost-effectiveness analysis in the diagnosis and treatment of insomnia. Sleep Med Rev 2004;8:63-72.

142. Chervin RD, Murman DL, Malow BA, Totten V: Cost-utility of three approaches to the diagnosis of sleep apnea: Polysomnography, home testing, and empirical therapy. Ann Intern Med 1999;130:496-505.

143. Kapuniai LE, Andrew DJ, Crowell DH, Pearce JW: Identifying sleep apnea from self-reports. Sleep 1988;11:430-436.

144. Crocker BD, Olson LG, Saunders NA, et al: Estimation of the probability of disturbed breathing during sleep before a sleep study. Am Rev Respir Dis 1990;142:14-18.

145. Viner S, Szalai JP, Hoffstein V: Are history and physical examination a good screening test for sleep apnea? Ann Intern Med 1991;115:356-359.

146. Bliwise DL, Nekich JC, Dement WC: Relative validity of self-reported snoring as a symptom of sleep apnea in a sleep clinic population. Chest 1991;99:600-608.

147. Haraldsson PO, Carenfelt C, Knutsson E, et al: Preliminary report: Validity of symptom analysis and daytime polysomnography in diagnosis of sleep apnea. Sleep 1992;15:261-263.

148. Rauscher H, Popp W, Zwick H: Model for investigating snorers with suspected sleep apnoea. Thorax 1993;48:275-279.

149. Flemons WW, Whitelaw WA, Brant R, Remmers JE: Likelihood ratios for a sleep apnea clinical prediction rule. Am J Respir Crit Care Med 1994;150:1279-1285.

150. Dealberto MJ, Ferber C, Garma L, et al: Factors related to sleep apnea syndrome in sleep clinic patients. Chest 1994;105: 1753-1758.

151. Douglass AB, Bornstein R, Nino-Murcia G, et al: The sleep disorders questionnaire I: Creation and multivariate structure of SDQ. Sleep 1994;17:160-167.

152. Netzer NC, Stoohs RA, Netzer CM, et al: Using the Berlin Questionnaire to identify patients at risk for the sleep apnea syndrome. Ann Intern Med 1999;131:485-491.

153. Kirby SD, Danter W, George CFP, et al: Neural network prediction of obstructive sleep apnea from clinical criteria. Chest 1999;116:409-415.

154. Martinez Garcia MA, Soler Cataluna JJ, Roman Sanchez P, et al: Clinical predictors of sleep apnea-hypopnea syndrome susceptible to treatment with continuous positive airway pressure. Arch Bronconeumol 2003;39:449-454.

51

Classification of Sleep Disorders

Michael J. Thorpy

ABSTRACT

The classification of sleep disorders is necessary to discriminate between disorders and to facilitate an understanding of symptoms, etiology, pathophysiology, and treatment. The earliest classification systems were largely organized according to the major symptoms (insomnia, excessive sleepiness, and abnormal events that occur during sleep), as the pathophysiologic basis for many of the sleep disorders was unknown. These three categories provide a classification system that is easily understood by physicians and that is useful for developing a differential diagnosis. With the development of modern sleep research, some categories can now be based on pathophysiology. The *International Classification of Sleep Disorders,* version 2 (ICSD-2), published in 2004, combines a symptomatic presentation (e.g., insomnia) with one organized in part on pathophysiology (e.g., circadian rhythms) and in part on body systems (e.g., breathing disorders). This organization is necessary because of the varied nature of the sleep disorders and because the pathophysiology for many of the disorders is unknown. The ICSD-2 is not just a listing of the sleep disorders but is a manual that lists relevant information on the diagnostic features and epidemiology to help the reader more easily differentiate between the disorders.

The classification of sleep disorders has been of particular interest to clinicians ever since sleep disorders were first recognized. The first major classification, the Diagnostic Classification of Sleep and Arousal Disorders, published in 1979,[1] organized the sleep disorders into categories that formed the basis of the current classification systems. In 1990, the International Classification of Sleep Disorders (ICSD) was produced after a 5-year process, initiated by the American Sleep Disorders Association (ASDA), that involved the three major international sleep societies at that time—the European Sleep Research Society, the Japanese Society of Sleep Research, and the Latin American Sleep Society. It resulted in the production of a diagnostic and coding manual, the *International Classification of Sleep Disorders: Diagnostic and Coding Manual.*[2] The ICSD classification, developed primarily for diagnostic, epidemiologic, and research purposes, has been widely used by clinicians and has allowed better international communication in sleep disorder research. In 2003, the American Academy of Sleep Medicine, formerly the ASDA, initiated the process of a complete revision and update of the ICSD. The resulting text, the *International Classification of Sleep Disorders,* version 2 (ICSD-2), to be published in 2005 (Table 51–1).[3] This review discusses the ICSD-2 as of May 2004, before publication, and may contain content that is changed in the final version. The reader is referred to the published manual for the final version of the classification.

The ICSD-2 classification lists 85 sleep disorders, each presented in detail and with a descriptive diagnostic text that includes specific diagnostic criteria. The ICSD-2 has eight major categories:

1. The insomnias.
2. The sleep-related breathing disorders.
3. The hypersomnias not due to a breathing disorder.
4. The circadian rhythm sleep disorders.
5. The parasomnias.
6. The sleep-related movement disorders.
7. Isolated symptoms, apparently normal variants and unresolved issues.
8. Other sleep disorders.

INSOMNIAS

The insomnias are defined by a repeated difficulty with sleep initiation, duration, consolidation, or quality that occurs despite adequate time and opportunity for sleep, and they result in some form of daytime impairment (see Chapters 59 to 63). Insomnia complaints typically include difficulty initiating and/or maintaining sleep, and they usually include extended periods of nocturnal wakefulness and/or insufficient amounts of nocturnal sleep. Occasionally, insomnia complaints are characterized by the perception of poor quality, or nonrestorative, sleep, even when the amount and quality of the usual sleep episode is perceived to be "normal" or adequate.

The insomnias can be either primary or secondary. Secondary forms can occur when the insomnia is a symptom of a medical or psychiatric illness, another sleep disorder, or substance abuse. Primary insomnias may have both intrinsic and extrinsic factors involved in their etiology, but they are not regarded as being secondary to another disorder.

There are six types of primary insomnia. *Psychophysiological insomnia*[4,5] is a common form of insomnia that is present for at least 1 month and is characterized by a heightened level of arousal with learned sleep-preventing associations. There is an overconcern with the inability to sleep. *Paradoxical insomnia* (formerly known as *sleep state misperception*),[6,7] is a complaint of severe insomnia that occurs without evidence of objective sleep disturbance and without daytime impairment to the extent that would be suggested by the amount of sleep disturbance reported. The patient often reports little or no sleep on most nights. It is thought to occur in up to 5% of insomniac patients. *Adjustment sleep disorder*[8,9] is insomnia that is associated with a specific stressor. The stressor can be psychological, physiologic, environmental, or physical. This disorder exists for a short period of time, usually days to weeks, and usually resolves when the stressor is no longer present. *Inadequate sleep hygiene*[10,11] is a disorder associated with common daily activities that are inconsistent with good-quality

Table 51-1. ICSD-2 Sleep Disorder Categories and Individual Sleep Disorders

Insomnias	ICD-9	ICD-10
Adjustment Sleep Disorder (Acute Insomnia)	307.41	F 51.01
Psychophysiological Insomnia	307.42	F 51.03
Paradoxical Insomnia (formerly Sleep State Misperception)	307.42	F 51.02
Idiopathic Insomnia	780.52	F 51.04
Insomnia due to mental disorder (Code also the associated mental disorder)	307.42	F 51.05
Inadequate Sleep Hygiene (Code also any associated insomnia [F51.0-, G47.0-])	307.41	Z72.821
Behavioral Insomnia of Childhood	307.42	Z73.81
Sleep-onset Association Type	—	Z73.810
Limit-setting Sleep Type	—	Z73.811
Combined Type	—	Z73.812
Unspecified Type	—	Z73.819
Insomnia due to a medical condition (Code also the associated medical condition)	780.52	G 47.03
Insomnia due to a drug or substance (Code first [T36-T65 with 6th character 1-4] to identify drug or substance, and use additional code [T36-T50 with 6th character 5] to identify adverse effect of drug). Use F10-F19 codes when there is associated drug abuse or dependence.	291.89	G 47.02
Insomnia not due to a substance or known physiological condition, unspecified (Nonorganic Insomnia, NOS)	307.42	F 51.00
Physiological (organic) insomnia, unspecified; (Organic Insomnia, NOS)	780.52	G 47.00
Sleep-Related Breathing Disorders		
Central Sleep Apnea Syndromes		
Primary Central Sleep Apnea	780.51	G 47.31
Other Central Sleep Apnea due to a medical condition	780.57	G 47.39
Cheyne Stokes Breathing Pattern	—	—
High Altitude Periodic Breathing	—	—
Central Sleep Apnea due to a medical condition, not Cheyne Stokes or High Altitude	—	—
Central Sleep Apnea due to a drug or substance	995.2	G 47.36
Other Sleep-Related Breathing Disorder due to a drug or substance	—	—
Primary Sleep Apnea of Infancy (formerly Primary Sleep Apnea of Newborn)	770.81	P 28.3
Obstructive Sleep Apnea Syndromes		
Obstructive Sleep Apnea, Adult	780.53	G 47.32
Obstructive Sleep Apnea, Pediatric	780.53	G 47.32
Sleep-Related Hypoventilation/Hypoxemic Syndromes		
Sleep-Related Non-obstructive Alveolar Hypoventilation, Idiopathic	780.57	G 47.34
Congenital Central Alveolar Hypoventilation Syndrome	780.57	G 47.35
Sleep-Related Hypoventilation/Hypoxemia due to a medical condition	780.57	G 47.37
Sleep-Related Hypoventilation/Hypoxemia due to pulmonary parenchymal or vascular pathology	—	—
Sleep-Related Hypoventilation/Hypoxemia due to lower airways obstruction	—	—
Sleep-Related Hypoventilation/Hypoxemia due to neuromuscular or chest wall disorders	—	—
Other Sleep-Related Breathing Disorder		
Sleep Apnea/Sleep-Related Breathing Disorder, unspecified (Sleep-Related Breathing Disorder, NOS)	780.57	G 47.30
Hypersomnias Not Due to a Sleep-Related Breathing Disorder		
Narcolepsy		
Narcolepsy with Cataplexy	347.01	G 47.41
Narcolepsy without Cataplexy	347.00	G 47.42
Narcolepsy due to a medical condition	347.1	G 47.43
Narcolepsy, unspecified	347	G 47.0
Other Hypersomnias		
Recurrent Hypersomnia	780.54	G 47.11
Kleine-Levin Syndrome	—	—
Menstrual-Related Hypersomnia	—	—
Idiopathic Hypersomnia with long sleep time	780.54	G 47.12
Idiopathic Hypersomnia without long sleep time	780.54	G 47.13
Behaviorally Induced Insufficient Sleep Syndrome	307.44	F 51.11
Hypersomnia due to a medical condition	780.54	G 47.15
Hypersomnia due to a drug or substance	995.2	G 47.14

Table 51–1.   ICSD-2 Sleep Disorder Categories and Individual Sleep Disorders—cont'd

	ICD-9	ICD-10
Other Hypersomnias—cont'd		
Hypersomnia not due to a substance or known physiological condition (Nonorganic Hypersomnia, NOS)	307.44	F 51.10
Physiological (Organic) Hypersomnia, unspecified (Organic Hypersomnia, NOS)	780.54	G 47.10
Circadian Rhythm Sleep Disorders		
Primary Circadian Rhythm Sleep Disorders		
Circadian Rhythm Sleep Disorder, Delayed sleep phase type	780.55	G 47.21
Circadian Rhythm Sleep Disorder, Advanced sleep phase type	780.55	G 47.22
Circadian Rhythm Sleep Disorder, Irregular sleep-wake type	780.55	G 47.23
Circadian Rhythm Sleep Disorder, Free running (non-entrained) type	780.55	G 47.24
Circadian Rhythm Sleep Disorders due to a medical condition	780.55	G 47.26
Primary (Organic) Circadian Rhythm Sleep Disorders, unspecified other physiological (organic) circadian rhythm, unspecified (organic circadian rhythm disorder, NOS)	780.55	G 47.20
Behaviorally Induced Circadian Rhythm Sleep Disorders		
Circadian Rhythm Sleep Disorder not due to a substance or known physiological condition, jet lag type	307.45	F 51.21
Circadian Rhythm Sleep Disorder not due to a substance or known physiological condition, shift work type	307.45	F 51.22
Circadian Rhythm Sleep Disorder not due to a substance or known physiological condition, delayed sleep phase type	307.45	F 51.23
Circadian Rhythm Sleep Disorder not due to a substance or known physiological condition, unspecified (Nonorganic circadian rhythm sleep disorder, NOS)	307.45	F 51.20
Other Circadian Rhythm Sleep Disorder not due to a substance or known physiological condition	307.45	F 51.29
Other Circadian Rhythm Sleep Disorder due to a drug or substance	291.89	G 47.25
Parasomnias		
Disorders of Arousal (From Non-REM Sleep)		
Confusional Arousals	780.56	G 47.51
Sleepwalking	307.46	F 51.3
Sleep Terrors	307.46	F 51.4
Parasomnias Usually Associated with REM Sleep		
REM Sleep Behavior Disorder	780.56	G 47.52
Parasomnia Overlap Disorder	—	—
Status Dissociatus	—	—
Recurrent Isolated Sleep Paralysis	780.56	G 47.53
Nightmare Disorder	307.47	F 51.5
Other Parasomnias		
Sleep-Related Dissociative Disorder	300.15	F 44.9
Sleep-Related Enuresis	788.36	N 39.44
Sleep-Related Groaning (Catathrenia)	780.56	G 47.50
Exploding Head Syndrome	780.56	G 47.50
Sleep-Related Hallucinations	307.49	R 29.81
Sleep-Related Eating Disorder	780.56	G 47.59
Parasomnia, unspecified	780.56	G 47.50
Parasomnia due to a drug or substance	780.56	G 47.54
Parasomnia due to a medical condition	780.56	G 47.55
Sleep-Related Movement Disorders		
Restless Legs Syndrome (including Sleep-Related Growing Pains)	333.99	G 47.61
Periodic Limb Movement Sleep Disorder	780.58	G 47.62
Sleep-Related Leg Cramps	780.58	G 47.63
Sleep-Related Bruxism	780.58	G 47.64
Sleep-Related Rhythmic Movement Disorder	780.58	G 47.65
Sleep-Related Movement Disorder, unspecified (no text)	780.58	G 47.60
Sleep-Related Movement Disorder due to a drug or substance (no text)	291.89	G 47.66
Sleep-Related Movement disorder due to a medical condition	780.58	G 47.67

Continued

Table 51–1. ICSD-2 Sleep Disorder Categories and Individual Sleep Disorders—cont'd

Isolated Symptoms, Apparently Normal Variants, and Unresolved Issues

Long Sleeper	307.49	R 29.81
Short Sleeper	307.49	R 29.81
Snoring	786.09	R 06.5
Sleeptalking	307.49	R 29.81
Sleep Starts, Hypnic Jerks	781.01	R 25.8
Benign Sleep Myoclonus of Infancy	781.01	R 25.8
Hypnagogic Foot Tremor and Alternating Leg Muscle Activation during Sleep	781.01	R 25.8
Propriospinal Myoclonus at Sleep Onset	781.01	R 25.8
Excessive Fragmentary Myoclonus	781.01	R 25.8

Other Sleep Disorders

Other Physiological (Organic) Sleep Disorder	780.50	G 47.8
Physiological (Organic) Sleep Disorder, unspecified	780.50	G 47.8
Other Sleep Disorder not due to a substance or physiological condition	307.40	F 51.8
Environmental Sleep Disorder	—	—
Sleep Disorder not due to a substance or physiological condition, unspecified	307.40	F 51.9

APPENDIX A: Sleep Disorders Associated with Conditions Classifiable Elsewhere

Fatal Familial Insomnia	046.8	A 81.8
Fibromyalgia	729.1	M 79.0
Sleep-Related Epilepsy	345	G 40.5
Sleep-Related Headaches	784.0	R 51
Sleep-Related Gastroesophageal Reflux Disease	530.1	K 21.9
Sleep-Related Coronary Artery Ischemia	411.8	I 25.6
Sleep-Related Cardiac Arrhythmias	427	I 49.9
Sleep-Related Abnormal Swallowing, Choking, and Laryngospasm	787.2	R 13.1

APPENDIX B: Other Psychiatric/Behavioral Disorders Frequently Encountered in the Differential Diagnosis of Sleep Disorders

Mood Disorders	—	—
Anxiety Disorders	—	—
Selected Somatoform Disorders (Somatization Disorder, Hypochondriasis)	—	—
Schizophrenia and other Psychotic Disorders	—	—
Selected Disorders Usually First Diagnosed in Infancy, Childhood, or Adolescence (Mental Retardation, Pervasive Developmental Disorders, Attention Deficit/Hyperactivity Disorder)	—	—
Personality Disorder	—	—

ICD-9, International Classification of Diseases, Ninth Revision; ICD-10, International Classification of Diseases, Tenth Revision; ICSD-2, International Classification of Sleep Disorders, Revised.

Courtesy of the American Academy of Sleep Medicine, Chicago, Ill.

sleep and full daytime alertness. Such activities include irregular sleep onset and wake times, stimulating and alerting activities before bedtime, and substances (e.g., alcohol, caffeine, cigarette smoke) ingested around sleep time. These practices do not necessarily cause sleep disturbance in other people. For example, an irregular bedtime or wake time that produces insomnia in one person may not be important in another. *Idiopathic insomnia*[12,13] is a long-standing form of insomnia that appears to date from childhood and has an insidious onset. Typically, there are no factors associated with the onset of the insomnia, which is persistent and without periods of remission. *Behavioral insomnia of childhood*[14,15] includes *limit-setting sleep disorder* and *sleep-onset association disorder*. Limit-setting sleep disorder is a stalling or a refusing to go to sleep that is eliminated once a caretaker enforces limits on sleep times and other sleep-related behaviors. Sleep-onset association disorder occurs when there is reliance on inappropriate sleep associations, such as rocking, watching television, holding a bottle or other object, or requiring environmental conditions such as a lighted room or an alternative place to sleep.

The ICSD-2 classification lists several secondary insomnias. *Insomnia due to a medical condition*[16,17] is applied when a medical or neurologic disorder gives rise to the insomnia. The medical disorder and the insomnia type are given when a patient is diagnosed. *Insomnia due to a drug or substance*[18,19] is applied when there is dependence on or excessive use of a substance such as alcohol, a recreational drug, or caffeine that is associated with the occurrence of the insomnia. The insomnia may be associated with the ingestion or discontinuation of the substance. Excessive use or dependency is not a feature of this diagnosis. *Other insomnia not due to a substance or known physiological condition*[22,23] (formerly "associated with other mental/behavioral factors") is the diagnosis applied when an underlying mental disorder is associated with the occurrence of the insomnia, and when the insomnia constitutes a distinct complaint or focus of treatment.

Differentiation between two diagnoses (*inadequate sleep hygiene* and *other insomnia due to a substance*) requires some elaboration. Caffeine ingestion in the form of coffee or soda can produce a disorder of *inadequate sleep hygiene* if the intake amount is normal and within the limits of common use but the timing of ingestion is inappropriate. On the other hand, ingestion of caffeine in an amount that is considered excessive by normal standards can lead to a diagnosis of *other insomnia due to a substance*.

SLEEP-RELATED BREATHING DISORDERS

The disorders in this group are characterized by disordered respiration during sleep (see Chapters 81 to 95). *Central apnea disorders*[24,25] include those in which respiratory effort is diminished or absent in an intermittent or cyclical fashion as a result of central nervous system dysfunction. *Other central sleep apnea* forms are associated with underlying pathologic or environmental causes, such as *Cheyne-Stokes breathing*[26,27] or *high-altitude periodic breathing.*[28,29]

Primary central sleep apnea is a disorder of unknown cause characterized by recurrent episodes of cessation of breathing during sleep without associated ventilatory effort. A complaint of excessive daytime sleepiness, insomnia, or difficulty breathing during sleep is reported. The patient must not be hypercapnic (PCO_2 greater than 45 mm Hg). This diagnosis requires that five or more apneic episodes per hour of sleep be seen by polysomnography. *Other central sleep apnea including Cheyne-Stokes breathing pattern* is characterized by recurrent apneas and/or hypopneas alternating with prolonged hyperpnea in which tidal volume waxes and wanes in a crescendo–decrescendo pattern. This pattern is characteristically seen in non–rapid eye movement (NREM) sleep and does not occur in rapid eye movement (REM) sleep. The pattern is typically seen in medical disorders such as heart failure, cerebrovascular disorders, and renal failure. *Other central sleep apnea, including high-altitude periodic breathing,*[30,31] is characterized by sleep disturbance that is caused by acute mountain sickness. Apnea and hyperpnea cycle without ventilatory effort during the apnea. The cycle length is typically between 12 and 34 seconds. Five or more central apneas per hour of sleep are required to make the diagnosis. Most people will have this ventilatory pattern at elevations greater than 7600 meters, and some at lower altitudes.

A secondary form of *central sleep apnea due to a substance (substance abuse)*[30,32] is most commonly associated with users of long-term opioid use. The substance causes a respiratory depression by acting on the mu-receptors of the ventral medulla. A central apnea index of greater than 5 is required for the diagnosis. *Primary sleep apnea of infancy*[31,33] is a disorder of respiratory control most often seen in preterm infants (apnea of prematurity), but it can occur in predisposed infants (apnea of infancy). This may be a developmental pattern, or it may be secondary to other medical disorders. Respiratory pauses of 20 seconds or longer are required for the diagnosis.

The *obstructive sleep apnea disorders* include those in which there is an obstruction in the airway resulting in increased breathing effort and inadequate ventilation. Upper airway resistance syndrome has been recognized as a manifestation of obstructive sleep apnea syndrome and therefore is not included as a separate diagnosis. Adult and pediatric forms of obstructive sleep apnea syndrome are discussed separately because the disorders have different methods of diagnosis and treatment. *Obstructive sleep apnea, adult*[34,35] is characterized by repetitive episodes of cessation of breathing (apneas) or partial upper airway obstruction (hypopneas). These events are often associated with reduced blood oxygen saturation. Snoring and sleep disruption are typical and common. Excessive daytime sleepiness or insomnia can result. Five or more respiratory events (apneas, hypopneas, or respiratory effort–related arousals) per hour of sleep are required for diagnosis. Increased respiratory effort occurs during the respiratory event. *Obstructive sleep apnea, pediatric*[36,37] is characterized by features similar to those seen in the adult, but cortical arousals may not occur, possibly because of a higher arousal threshold. At least one obstructive event, of at least two respiratory cycles duration, per hour of sleep is required for diagnosis.

Other sleep-related breathing disorder due to a known physiologic condition and *sleep-related hypoxemia related to pulmonary parenchymal or vascular pathology*[38,39] are disorders with significant oxygen desaturation and lung parenchymal disease such as that seen in chronic obstructive pulmonary disease, cystic fibrosis, and interstitial lung disease.

Hypoventilation/hypoxemic disorders are related to elevated arterial carbon dioxide tension ($PaCO_2$). *Sleep-related hypoventilation/hypoxemic syndrome, unspecified*[40-45] is seen in patients with lower airway disease such as emphysema, bronchiectasis, or cystic fibrosis, neuromuscular disease or kyphoscoliosis, and *congenital central alveolar hypoventilation syndrome*[46,47] is a failure of automatic central control of breathing in infants who do not breathe spontaneously or who breathe shallowly and erratically.

HYPERSOMNIA NOT DUE TO A SLEEP-RELATED BREATHING DISORDER

The hypersomnia disorders are those in which the primary complaint is daytime sleepiness and the cause of the primary symptom is not disturbed nocturnal sleep or misaligned circadian rhythms. Daytime sleepiness is defined as the inability to stay alert and awake during the major waking episodes of the day, resulting in unintended lapses into sleep. Other sleep disorders may be present, and they must first be effectively treated.

Narcolepsy with cataplexy[48,49] requires the documentation of a definite history of cataplexy (see Chapters 64 and 65). *Narcolepsy without cataplexy*[50,51] is the diagnosis when cataplexy is not present but when there are sleep paralysis, hypnagogic hallucinations, and supportive evidence in the form of a positive multiple sleep latency test with a mean sleep latency of less than 8 minutes and two or more sleep-onset REM periods. *Narcolepsy, unspecified*[52,53] is the diagnosis applied to a patient with sleepiness who has a significant neurologic or medical disorder that accounts for the daytime sleepiness. *Recurrent hypersomnia,*[54,55] also known as periodic hypersomnia or Kleine-Levin syndrome, is associated with episodes of sleepiness together with binge eating, hypersexuality, or mood changes. *Idiopathic hypersomnia with long sleep time*[56,57] is the classic form of idiopathic hypersomnia, characterized by a major sleep episode that is at least 10 hours in duration, whereas *idiopathic hypersomnia without long sleep time*[58,59] is the commonly seen disorder of excessive sleepiness with unintended naps that are typically unrefreshing (see Chapter 66). *Behaviorally induced insufficient sleep syndrome*[60,61] occurs in patients who have a habitual short sleep episode and who sleep considerably longer when the habitual sleep episode is not maintained.

Other organic hypersomnia[62,63] is hypersomnia that is caused by a medical or neurologic disorder. Cataplexy or other diagnostic features of narcolepsy are not present. *Other hypersomnia due to a substance (substance abuse)*[64-67] is diagnosed when the complaint is believed to be secondary to current or past use of drugs. *Other hypersomnia not due to a substance or physiological condition*[68,69] is excessive sleepiness that is temporally associated with a psychiatric diagnosis.

CIRCADIAN RHYTHM SLEEP DISORDERS

The circadian rhythm sleep disorders share a common underlying chronophysiologic basis. The major feature of these disorders is a persistent or recurrent misalignment between the patient's sleep pattern and the pattern that is desired or regarded as the societal norm (see Chapters 54 to 58). Maladaptive behaviors influence the presentation and severity of the circadian rhythm sleep disorders. The underlying problem in the majority of the circadian rhythm sleep disorders is that the patient cannot sleep when sleep is desired, needed, or expected. The wake episodes can occur at undesired times as a result of sleep episodes that occur at inappropriate times; therefore, the patient may complain of insomnia or excessive sleepiness. For several of the circadian rhythm sleep disorders, once sleep is initiated, the major sleep episode is of normal duration with normal REM-NREM cycling.

Delayed sleep phase type,[70,71] which is more commonly seen in adolescents, is characterized by a delay in the phase of the major sleep period in relation to the desired sleep time and wake time, whereas *advanced sleep phase type,*[72,73] which is more commonly seen in older adults, is characterized by an advance in the phase of the major sleep period in relation to the desired sleep time and wake-up time. The *irregular sleep-wake type,*[74,75] a disorder that involves a lack of a clearly defined circadian rhythm of sleep and wakefulness, is most often seen in institutionalized older adults and is associated with a lack of synchronizing agents such as light, activity, and social activities. The *free running type*[75,77] (formerly known as the *non-24-hour sleep-wake syndrome*) occurs because there is a lack of entrainment to the 24-hour period, and the sleep pattern often follows that of the underlying free-running pacemaker with a sequential shift in the daily sleep pattern.

Organic circadian rhythm sleep disorders, unspecified[78,79] is related to an underlying primary medical or neurologic disorder. A disrupted sleep–wake pattern leads to complaints of insomnia or excessive daytime sleepiness. *Circadian rhythm sleep disorder not due to a substance or known physiological condition, jet lag type*[80,81] is related to a temporal mismatch between the timing of the sleep–wake cycle generated by the endogenous circadian clock produced by a rapid change in time zones. The severity of the disorder is influenced by the number of time zones crossed and the direction of travel, with eastward travel usually being more disruptive. *Circadian rhythm sleep disorder not due to a substance or known physiological condition*[82,83] is characterized by complaints of insomnia or excessive sleepiness that occur in relation to work hours that are scheduled during the usual sleep period.

Circadian rhythm sleep disorder not due to a substance or known physiological condition[84,85] is a form of delayed sleep phase type that is predominantly either caused by the individual's choice to remain awake late into the night or associated with social or professional demands. *Other circadian rhythm sleep disorder not due to a known physiological condition* is an irregular or unconventional sleep–wake pattern that can be the result of social, behavioral, or environmental factors. Noise, lighting, or other factors can predispose an individual to developing this disorder.

The appropriate timing of sleep within the 24-hour day can be disturbed in many other sleep disorders, particularly those associated with the complaint of insomnia. Patients with narcolepsy may have a pattern of sleepiness that is identical to that described as being caused by an irregular sleep–wake type. However, because the primary sleep diagnosis is narcolepsy, the patient should not receive a second diagnosis of a circadian rhythm sleep disorder unless the disorder is unrelated to the narcolepsy. For example, a diagnosis of jet lag type could be stated along with a diagnosis of narcolepsy, if appropriate. Similarly, patients with mood disorders or psychoses can, at times, have a sleep pattern similar to that of delayed sleep phase type. A diagnosis of delayed sleep phase type would be coded only if the disorder is not directly associated with the psychiatric disorder.

Some disturbance of sleep timing is a common feature in patients who have a diagnosis of inadequate sleep hygiene. Only if the timing of sleep is the predominant cause of the sleep disturbance and is outside the societal norm would the patient be given a diagnosis of a circadian rhythm sleep disorder. Limit-setting sleep disorder is also associated with an altered time of sleep within the 24-hour day. If the setting of limits is a function of the caretaker, then the sleep disorder is more appropriately diagnosed as a limit-setting sleep disorder.

PARASOMNIAS

The parasomnias are undesirable physical or experiential events that accompany sleep (see Chapters 74 to 80). These sleep disorders are not abnormalities of the processes responsible for sleep and awake states per se but are undesirable phenomena that occur predominantly during sleep. The parasomnias consist of abnormal sleep-related movements, behaviors, emotions, perceptions, dreaming, and autonomic nervous system functioning. They are disorders of arousal, partial arousal, and sleep-stage transition. Many of the parasomnias are manifestations of central nervous system activation. Autonomic nervous system changes and skeletal muscle activity are the predominant features. The parasomnias often occur in conjunction with other sleep disorders such as obstructive sleep apnea syndrome. It is not uncommon for several parasomnias to occur in one patient.

Three parasomnias have typically been associated with arousal from non-REM sleep. *Confusional arousals*[86,87] are characterized by mental confusion or confusional behavior that occurs during or after arousal from sleep. These arousals are common in children and can occur not only from nocturnal sleep but also from daytime naps. They sometimes occur in association with obstructive sleep apnea syndrome. *Sleepwalking*[88,89] is a series of complex behaviors that occur from sudden arousals from slow wave sleep and result in walking behavior during a state of altered consciousness. *Sleep terrors*[90,91] also occur from slow wave sleep and are associated with a cry or piercing scream accompanied by autonomic system activation and behavioral manifestation of intense fear. Individuals may be difficult to arouse from the episode and when aroused can be confused and subsequently amnestic for the episode. These two disorders, sleep walking and sleep terrors, often coexist together, and sometimes one form blends into the other or is difficult to distinguish from the other.

Several parasomnias are typically associated with the REM sleep stage. Some common underlying pathophysiologic mechanism related to REM sleep may underlie these disorders. *REM sleep behavior disorder*[92,93] involves abnormal behaviors that occur in REM sleep and result in injury or sleep disruption. The behaviors are often violent with dream enactment that is action filled. The disorder can occur in narcolepsy, and many patients with Parkinson's disease have REM sleep behavior disorder. The delayed emergence of a neurodegenerative disorder can occur, especially in men older than 50 years. *Recurrent isolated sleep paralysis*[94,95] can occur at sleep onset or on awakening and is characterized by an inability to perform voluntary movements. Ventilation is usually unaffected. Hallucinatory experiences often accompany the paralysis. *Nightmare disorder*[96,97] is characterized by recurrent nightmares that occur in REM sleep and result in an awakening with intense anxiety, fear, or other negative feelings.

Sleep-related dissociative disorders[98,99] involve a disruption of the integrative features of consciousness, memory, identity, or perception of the environment. This disorder can occur in the transition from wakefulness to sleep or after an awakening from stage 1 or 2 sleep. A history of physical or sexual abuse is common in such patients. These patients fulfill the Diagnostic and Statistical Manual of Mental Disorders, Fourth Edition (DSM-IV) criteria for dissociative disorder. *Sleep-related enuresis*[100,101] is recurrent involuntary voiding that occurs during sleep. Enuresis is considered primary in a child who has never been dry for 6 months or longer; otherwise, it is called secondary. *Sleep-related groaning (catathrenia)*[102,103] is an unusual disorder in which there is a chronic, often nightly, expiratory groaning that occurs during sleep. The affected person is often unaware of the groaning. The disorder is rare and the pathophysiology, unknown. *Exploding head syndrome*[104,105] is characterized by a loud imagined noise or sense of a violent explosion that occurs in the head as the patient is falling asleep or during waking in the night. *Sleep-related eating disorder*[106,107] involves recurrent eating and drinking episodes during arousals from nocturnal sleep. The eating behavior is uncontrollable and often the patient is unaware of the behavior until the next morning. It can be associated with sleepwalking and can be medication induced.

Organic parasomnia, unspecified[108,109] is the manifestation of a parasomnia associated with an underlying medical or neurologic disorder. *Other parasomnia due to a substance*[110] is a parasomnia that has a close temporal relationship between exposure to a drug, medication, or biologic substance. *Other parasomnia not due to a substance or known physiological condition (psychiatric disorders)*[111,112] is a parasomnia that occurs as a manifestation of an underlying psychiatric disorder.

SLEEP-RELATED MOVEMENT DISORDERS

The sleep-related movement disorders are characterized by relatively simple, usually stereotyped movements that disturb sleep (see Chapter 70). Disorders such as periodic limb movement disorder and restless legs syndrome are classified in this section.

Restless legs syndrome[113,114] is characterized by a complaint of a strong, nearly irresistible urge to move the legs. The sensations are worse at rest and occur more frequently in the evening or during the night. Walking or moving the legs relieves the sensation. *Periodic limb movement sleep disorder*[115,116] is often associated with restless legs syndrome but can occur as an independent disorder. In this condition, repetitive, highly stereotyped limb movements occur during sleep. *Sleep-related leg cramps*[117,118] are painful sensations that cause sudden intense muscle contractions, usually of the calves or small muscles of the feet. Episodes commonly occur during the sleep period and can lead to disrupted sleep. Relief is usually obtained by stretching the affected muscle. *Sleep related bruxism*[119,120] is characterized by clenching of the teeth during sleep and can result in arousals. Often the activity is severe or frequent enough to result in symptoms of temporomandibular joint pain or wearing down of the teeth. *Sleep-related rhythmic movement disorder*[121,122] is a stereotyped, repetitive rhythmic motor behavior that occurs during drowsiness or light sleep and results in large movements of the head, body, or limbs. Typically seen in children, the disorder can also be seen in adults. Head and limb injuries can result from violent movements. Rhythmic movement disorder can also occur during full wakefulness and alertness, particularly in individuals who are mentally retarded.

Other sleep-related movement disorders not due to a substance or known physiological disorder are movement disorders that occur during sleep that are diagnosed before a psychiatric disorder can be ascertained. *Organic sleep-related movement disorder* is a sleep disorder not specified elsewhere that appears to have a physiologic or medical basis. *Sleep-related movement disorder due to a substance* is a sleep disorder not specified elsewhere that appears to have a substance as its basis.

OTHER SLEEP DISORDERS

These disorders are difficult to fit into any other classification section. *Environmental sleep disorder*[123,124] is a sleep disturbance that is caused by a disturbing environmental factor that disrupts sleep and leads to a complaint of either insomnia or excessive sleepiness.

ISOLATED SYMPTOMS, APPARENTLY NORMAL VARIANTS, AND UNRESOLVED ISSUES

This section lists sleep-related symptoms that are in the borderline between normal and abnormal sleep. Sleep length and snoring are two examples.

Long sleeper[125,126] is a person who sleeps more in the 24-hour day than the typical person. Sleep is normal in architecture and quality. Usually, sleep lengths of 10 hours or greater qualify for this diagnosis. Symptoms of excessive sleepiness occur if the person does not get that amount of sleep. A *short sleeper*[125,126] is a person with a routine pattern of obtaining 5 hours or less of sleep in a 24-hour day. In children, this sleep length can be 3 hours or less than the norm for the age group. *Snoring*[127,128] is diagnosed when a respiratory sound is disturbing to the patient, a bed partner, or others. This diagnosis is made when the snoring is not associated with either insomnia or excessive sleepiness. Not only can snoring lead to impaired health but also it may be a cause of social embarrassment and can disturb the sleep of a bed partner. Snoring associated with obstructive sleep apnea syndrome is not diagnosed as snoring.

Sleeptalking[129,130] can be either idiopathic or associated with other disorders such as REM sleep behavior disorder, or sleep-related eating disorder. *Sleep starts (hypnic jerks)*[131,132] are sudden brief contractions of the body that occur at sleep onset. These movements are associated with a sensation of falling, a sensory flash, or a sleep-onset dream. *Benign sleep myoclonus of infancy*[133,134] is a disorder of myoclonic jerks that occur during sleep in infants. It typically occurs from birth to age 6 months and is benign and resolves spontaneously. *Hypnagogic foot tremor and alternating leg muscle activation*[135,136] occurs at the transition between wake and sleep or during light NREM sleep. It is demonstrated by recurrent EMG potentials in one or both feet that are in the myoclonic range of greater than 250 msec. *Propriospinal myoclonus at sleep onset*[137,138] is a disorder of recurrent sudden muscular jerks in the transition from wakefulness to sleep. The disorder may be associated with severe sleep-onset insomnia. *Excessive fragmentary myoclonus*[139,140] is small muscle twitches in the fingers, toes, or the corner of the mouth that do not cause actual movements across a joint. The myoclonus is often a finding during polysomnography that is often asymptomatic or can be associated with daytime sleepiness or fatigue.

APPENDIX A: OTHER ORGANIC DISORDERS FREQUENTLY ENCOUNTERED IN THE DIFFERENTIAL DIAGNOSIS OF SLEEP DISORDERS

Fatal familial insomnia[141,142] is a progressive disorder characterized by difficulty in falling asleep and maintaining sleep that develops into enacted dreams or stupor. Autonomic hyperactivity with pyrexia, excessive salivation, and hyperhidrosis leads to cardiac and respiratory failure. The disease is caused by a prion and it leads eventually to death. *Sleep-related epilepsy*[143,144] is the diagnosis when epilepsy occurs during sleep. Several epilepsy types are associated with sleep, including nocturnal frontal lobe epilepsy, benign epilepsy of childhood with centrotemporal spikes, and juvenile myoclonic epilepsy. *Sleep-related headaches*[145,146] are headaches that occur during sleep or on awakening from sleep. Chronic paroxysmal hemicrania, hypnic headache, or cluster headaches can all occur during sleep. *Sleep-related gastroesophageal reflux*[147,148] is characterized by regurgitation of stomach contents into the esophagus during sleep. Shortness of breath or heartburn can result, but occasionally the disorder is asymptomatic. *Sleep-related coronary artery ischemia*[149,150] is ischemia of the myocardium that occurs at night.

APPENDIX B: OTHER PSYCHIATRIC/BEHAVIORAL DISORDERS FREQUENTLY ENCOUNTERED IN THE DIFFERENTIAL DIAGNOSIS OF SLEEP DISORDERS

This final section of the ICSD-2 lists the psychiatric diagnoses that are often encountered during an evaluation of sleep complaints. Many psychiatric disorders are associated with disturbances of sleep and wakefulness. The main sleep-related features are presented. Psychiatric diagnoses that are discussed include mood disorders, anxiety disorders, somatoform disorders, schizophrenia and other psychotic disorders, disorders first diagnosed in childhood or adolescence, and personality disorders.[151]

> ### *Clinical Pearls*
>
> *The classification of sleep disorders allows accurate diagnosis, improved communication between physicians, and the standardization of data for research purposes. New sleep disorders have been recognized and previous sleep disorders have been clarified with a better understanding of their diagnostic and epidemiologic features. The International Classification of Sleep Disorder version 2 increases the refinement of sleep disorder diagnoses because of recent advances in sleep research. Referral to the ICSD-2 will help clinicians establish a rational differential diagnosis when evaluating patients.*

REFERENCES

1. Association of Sleep Disorders Centers: Diagnostic Classification of Sleep and Arousal Disorders, prepared by the Sleep Disorders Classification Committee, Roffwarg HP, Chairman. Sleep 1979; 2:1-137.
2. Diagnostic Classification Steering Committee, Thorpy MJ, Chairman: International Classification of Sleep Disorders: Diagnostic and Coding Manual. Rochester, Minn, American Sleep Disorders Association, 1990.
3. American Academy of Sleep Medicine: International Classification of Sleep Disorders: Diagnostic and Coding Manual, 2nd ed. Westchester, Ill, American Academy of Sleep Medicine, 2005.
4. Hauri PJ, Fischer J: Persistent psychophysiological (learned) insomnia. Sleep 1986;9:38-53.
5. Reynolds CF, Taska LS, Sewitch DE, et al: Persistent psychophysiologic insomnia: Preliminary research diagnostic criteria and EEG sleep data. Am J Psychiatry 1984;141:804-805.
6. Edinger JD, Fins A: The distribution and clinical significance of sleep time misperceptions. Sleep 1995;18:232-239.
7. Salin-Pascual RJ, Roehrs TA, Merlotti LA, et al: Long-term study of the sleep of insomnia patients with sleep state misperception and other insomnia patients. Am J Psychiatry 1992;149:904-908.
8. Haynes SN, Adams A, Franzen M: The effects of pre-sleep stress on sleep-onset insomnia. J Abnorm Psychol 1981;90:601-606.
9. Morin CM, Rodriquez S, Ivers H: Role of stress, arousal and coping skills in primary insomnia. Psychosom Med 2003;65: 259-267.
10. Spielman AJ: Assessment of insomnia. Clin Psychol Rev 1986;6: 11-25.
11. Morin CM, Hauri PJ, Espie CA, et al: Nonpharmacologic treatment of chronic insomnia. An American Academy of Sleep Medicine Review. Sleep 1986;22:1134-1156.
12. Hauri PJ, Olmsted E: Childhood onset insomnia. Sleep 1980;3: 59-65.
13. Bastien CB, Morin CM: Familial incidence of insomnia. J Sleep Res 2000;9:49-54.
14. Ferber R: Clinical assessment of child and adolescent sleep disorders. Child Adolesc Psychiatr Clin North Am 1996;5:569-579.
15. Gaylor EE, Goodlin-Jones BL, Anders TF: Classification of young children's sleep problems. J Am Acad Child Adolesc Psychiatry 2001;40:60-67.

16. Buysse DJ, Reynolds CF 3rd, Kupfer DJ, et al: Clinical diagnoses in 216 insomnia patients using the International Classification of Sleep Disorders (ICSD), DSM-IV and ICD-10 categories: A report from the APA/NIMH DSM-IV field trial. Sleep 1994;17: 630-637.

17. Gislason T, Almqvist M: Somatic disease and sleep complaints: An epidemiological study of 3201 Swedish men. Acta Med Scand 1987;221:475-581.

18. Shirlow MJ, Mathers CD: A study of caffeine consumption and symptoms: Indigestion, palpitations, tremor, headache and Insomnia. Int J Epidemiol 1985;14:239-248.

19. Gillin JC, Drummond SPA: Medication and substance abuse. In Kryger MH, Roth T, Dement WC (eds): Principles and Practice of Sleep Medicine, 3rd ed. Philadelphia, WB Saunders, 2000, pp 1176-1196.

20. Schweitzer PK: Drugs that disturb sleep and wakefulness. In Kryger MH, Roth T, Dement WC (eds): Principles and Practice of Sleep Medicine, 3rd ed. Philadelphia, WB Saunders, 2000, pp 441-462.

21. Kahn A, Mozin MJ, Casimir G, et al: Insomnia and cow's milk allergy in infants. Pediatrics 1985;76:880-884.

22. Nofzinger EA, Buysse DJ, Reynolds CF, Kupfer DJ: Sleep disorders related to another mental disorder (nonsubstance/primary): A DSM-IV literature review. J Clin Psychiatry 1993;54:244-255.

23. Ohayon MM: Prevalence of DSM-IV diagnostic criteria of insomnia: Distinguishing insomnia related to mental disorders from sleep disorders. J Psychiatr Res 1997;31:333-346.

24. Bradley TD, McNicholas WT, Rutherford R, et al: Clinical and physiological heterogeneity of the central sleep apnea syndrome. Am Rev Respir Dis 1986;134:217-221.

25. Guilleminault C, Robinson A: Central sleep apnea. Neurol Clin 1996;14:611-628.

26. Hall MJ, Xie A, Rutherford R, et al: Cycle length of periodic breathing in patients with and without heart failure. Am J Respir Crit Care Med 1996;154:376-381.

27. Naughton MT, Benard D, Tam A, et al: The role of hyperventilation in the pathogenesis of central sleep apnea in patients with congestive heart failure. Am Rev Respir Dis 1993;148: 330-338.

28. Nicholson AN, Smith PA, Stone BM, et al: Altitude insomnia: Studies during an expedition to the Himalayas. Sleep 1988;11: 354-361.

29. Weil JV: Sleep at high altitude. In Kryger M, Roth T, Dement WC (eds): Principles and Practice of Sleep Medicine. Philadelphia, WB Saunders, 1989, pp 269-275.

30. Teichtahl H, Prodromidis A, Miller B, et al: Sleep-disordered breathing in stable methadone programme patients: A pilot study. Addiction 2001;96:395-403.

31. Durand M, Cabal L, Gonzalez F, et al: Ventilatory control and carbon dioxide response in preterm infants with idiopathic apnea. Am J Dis Child 1985;139:717-720.

32. Farnery R, Walker J, Cloward T, Rhondeau S: Sleep-disordered breathing associated with long-term opioid therapy. Chest 2003; 123:632-639.

33. National Institutes of Health: Consensus Development Conference on Infantile Apnea and Home Monitoring, Sept 29 to Oct 1, 1986. Pediatrics 1987;79:292-299.

34. The Report of an American Academy of Sleep Medicine Task Force: Sleep-related breathing disorders in adults: Recommendations for syndrome definition and measurement techniques in clinical research. Sleep 1999;22:667-689.

35. Strohl KP, Redline S: Recognition of obstructive sleep apnea. Am J Respir Crit Care Med 1996;154:279-289.

36. American Thoracic Society: Standards and indications for cardiopulmonary sleep studies in children. Am J Respir Crit Care Med 1996;153:866-878.

37. Brouillette RT, Fernbach SK, Hunt CE: Obstructive sleep apnea in infants and children. J Pediatr 1982;100:31-40.

38. Bradley S, Solin P, Wilson J, et al: Hypoxemia and hypercapnia during exercise and sleep in patients with cystic fibrosis. Chest 1999;116:647-654.

39. Douglas N, Flenley D: Breathing during sleep in patients with obstructive lung disease. Am Rev Respir Dis 1990;141:1055-1070.

40. Plum F, Leigh RJ: Abnormalities of central mechanisms. In Hornbein TF (ed): Regulation of Breathing: II, vol 17. Lung Biology in Health and Disease. New York, Marcel Dekker, 1981, pp 989-1067.

41. Sullivan CE, Issa FG, Berthon-Jones M, et al: Pathophysiology of sleep apnea. In Saunders NA, Sullivan CE (eds): Sleep and Breathing, vol 21: Lung Biology in Health and Disease. New York, Marcel Dekker, 1984, pp 299-364.

42. Sanders MH, Newman AB, Haggerty CL, et al: Sleep and sleep-disordered breathing in adults with chronic obstructive pulmonary disease. Am J Respir Crit Care Med 2003;167:7-14.

43. Fletcher EC, Levin DC: Cardiopulmonary hemodynamics during sleep in subjects with chronic obstructive pulmonary disease: The effect of short- and long-term oxygen. Chest 1984;85:6-14.

44. Martin TJ, Sanders MH: Chronic alveolar hypoventilation: A review for clinicians. Sleep 1995;18:617-634.

45. Labanowski M, Schmidt-Nowara W, Guilleminault C: Sleep and neuromuscular disease: Frequency of sleep-disordered breathing in a neuromuscular disease clinic population. Neurology 1996; 47:1173-1180.

46. Gozal D, Marcus CL, Shoseyov D, Keens TG: Peripheral chemoreceptor function in children with the congenital central hypoventilation syndrome. J Appl Physiol 1993;74:379-387.

47. Paton JY, Swaminathan S, Sargent CW, et al: Hypoxic and hypercapneic ventilatory responses in awake children with congenital central hypoventilation syndrome. Am Rev Respir Dis 1989;140: 368-372.

48. Overeem S, Mignot E, van Dijk JG, Lammers GJ: Narcolepsy: Clinical features, new pathophysiologic insights, and future perspectives. J Clin Neurophysiol 2001;18:78-105.

49. Anic-Labat S, Guilleminault C, Kraemer HC, et al: Validation of a cataplexy questionnaire in 983 sleep-disorders patients. Sleep 1999;22:77-87.

50. Mignot E, Lammers GJ, Ripley B, et al: The role of cerebrospinal fluid hypocretin measurement in the diagnosis of narcolepsy and other hypersomnias. Arch Neurol 2002;59:1553-1562.

51. Silber MH, Krahn LE, Olson EJ, Pankratz VS: The epidemiology of narcolepsy in Olmsted County, Minnesota: A population-based study. Sleep 2002;15;25:197-202.

52. Guilleminault C, Yuen KM, Gulevich MG, et al: Hypersomnia after head-neck trauma: A medico-legal dilemma. Neurology 2000;54:653-659.

53. Kanbayashi T, Abe M, Fujimoto S, et al: Hypocretin deficiency in Niemann-Pick type C with cataplexy. Neuropediatrics 2003;34: 52-53.

54. Billiard M, Guilleminault C, Dement WC: A menstruation-linked periodic hypersomnia: Kleine-Levin syndrome or new clinical entity? Neurology 1975;25:436-443.

55. Takahashi Y: Clinical studies of periodic somnolence: Analysis of 28 personal cases. Psychiatr Neurol (Jpn) 1965;67:853-889.

56. Bassetti C, Aldrich MS: Idiopathic hypersomnia: A series of 42 patients. Brain 1997;120:1423-1435.

57. Billiard M, Dauvillier Y: Idiopathic hypersomnia. Sleep Med Rev 2001;5:351-360.

58. Aldrich MS: The clinical spectrum of narcolepsy and idiopathic hypersomnia. Neurology 1996;46:393-401.

59. Roth B: Narcolepsy and hypersomnia: Review and classification of 642 personally observed cases. Schweiz Arch Neurol Neurochir Psychiat 1976;119:31-41.

60. Carskadon MA, Dement WC: Effects of total sleep loss on sleep tendency. Percept Mot Skills 1979;48:495-506.

61. Roehrs T, Zorick F, Sicklesteel J, et al: Excessive daytime sleepiness associated with insufficient sleep. Sleep 1983;6:319-325.

62. Martinez-Rodriguez JE, Lin L, Iranzo A, et al: Decreased hypocretin-1 (Orexin-A) levels in the cerebrospinal fluid of patients with myotonic dystrophy and excessive daytime sleepiness. Sleep 2003;26:287-290.

63. Overeem S, van Hilten JJ, Ripley B, et al: Normal hypocretin-1 levels in Parkinson's disease patients with excessive daytime sleepiness. Neurology 2002;58:498-499.

64. Guilleminault C, Brooks SN. Excessive daytime sleepiness: A challenge for the practicing neurologist. Brain 2001;124:1282-1291.

65. Gault FP: A review of recent literature on barbiturate addiction and withdrawal. Bol Estud Med Biol 1976;29:75-83.

66. Blum DE: New drugs for persons with epilepsy. Adv Neurol 1998;76:57-87.

67. Buffett-Jerrott SE, Stewart SH: Cognitive and sedative effects of benzodiazepine use. Curr Pharm Des 2002;8:45-58.

68. Billiard M, Dolenc L, Aldaz C, et al: Hypersomnia associated with mood disorders: A new perspective. J Psychosom Res 1994;38:41-47.

69. Vgontzas AN, Bixler EO, Kales A, et al: Differences in nocturnal and daytime sleep between primary and psychiatric hypersomnia: Diagnosis and treatment implications. Psychosom Med 2000;62:220-226.

70. Thorpy MJ, Korman E, Spielman AJ, et al: Delayed sleep phase syndrome in adolescents. J Adolesc Health Care 1988;9:22-27.

71. Weitzman ED, Czeisler CA, Coleman RM, et al: Delayed sleep phase syndrome: A chronobiological disorder with sleep-onset insomnia. Arch Gen Psychiatry 1981;38:737-746.

72. Kamei R, Hughes L, Miles L, et al: Advanced-sleep phase syndrome studied in a time isolation facility. Chronobiologia 1979;6:115.

73. Moldofsky H, Musisi S, Phillipson EA: Treatment of advanced sleep phase syndrome by phase advance chronotherapy. Sleep 1986;9:61-65.

74. Pollak CP, Stokes PE: Circadian rest-activity rhythms in demented and non-demented older community residents and their caregivers. J Am Geriatr Soc 1997;45:446-452.

75. Witting W, Kwa IH, Eikelenboom P, et al: Alterations in the circadian rest-activity rhythm in aging and Alzheimer's disease. Biol Psychiatry 1990;27:563-572.

76. Kokkoris CP, Weitzman ED, Pollak CP, et al: Longterm ambulatory monitoring in a subject with a hypernychthemeral sleep–wake cycle disturbance. Sleep 1980;2:347-354.

77. Weber AL, Cary MS, Conner N, et al: Human non-24-hour sleep-wake cycles in an everyday environment. Sleep 1980;2:347-354.

78. Ancoli-Israel S, Parker L, Sinaee R, et al: Sleep fragmentation in patients from a nursing home. J Gerontol 1989;44:M18-21.

79. Bliwise DL, Watts RL, Rye DB, et al: Disruptive nocturnal behavior in Parkinson's disease and Alzheimer's disease. J Geriatr Psychiatry Neurol 1995;8:107-110.

80. Arendt J, Marks V: Physiological changes underlying jet lag. BMJ 1982;284:144-146.

81. Spitzer RL, Terman M, Williams JB, et al: Jet lag: Clinical features, validation of a new syndrome specific scale, and lack of response to melatonin in a randomized, double blind trial. Am J Psychiatry 1999;156:1392-1396.

82. Akerstedt T: Shift work and disturbed sleep/wakefulness. Occup Med (Lond) 2003;53:89-94.

83. Torsvall L, Akerstedt T: Sleepiness on the job: Continuously measured EEG changes in train drivers. Electroencephalogr Clin Neurophysiol 1987;66:502-511.

84. Regestein QR, Monk TH: Delayed sleep phase syndrome: A review of its clinical aspects. Am J Psychiatry 1995;152:602-608.

85. Yamadera H, Takahashi K, Okawa M: A multicenter study of sleep wake rhythm disorders: Clinical features of sleep-wake cycle rhythm disorders. Psychiatry Clin Neurosci 1996;50:195-201.

86. Ferber R: Sleep disorders in infants and children. In Riley TL (ed): Clinical Aspects of Sleep and Sleep Disturbance. Boston, Butterworths, 1985, pp 113-158.

87. Broughton RJ: Sleep disorders: Disorders of arousal? Science 1968;159:1070-1078.

88. Crisp AH: The sleepwalking/night terrors syndrome in adults. Postgrad Med J 1996;72:599-604.

89. Kales A, Soldatos CR, Bixler EO, et al: Hereditary factors in sleep walking and night terrors. Br J Psychiatry 1980;137:111-118.

90. Fisher C, Kahn E, Edwards A, et al: A psychophysiological study of nightmares and night terrors: Physiological aspects of the stage 4 night terror. J Nerv Ment Dis 1973;157:75-98.

91. Crisp AH, Matthews BM, Oakey M, Crutchfield M: Sleepwalking, night terrors, and consciousness. BMJ 1990;300:360-362.

92. Schenck CH, Bundlie SR, Ettinger MG, et al: Chronic behavioral disorders of human REM sleep: A new category of parasomnia. Sleep 1986;9:293-306.

93. Olson E, Boeve B, Silber M: Rapid eye movement sleep behavior disorder: Demographic, clinical, and laboratory findings in 93 cases. Brain 2000;123:331-339.

94. Goode GB: Sleep paralysis. Arch Neurol 1962;6:228-234.

95. Ohayon MM, Zulley J, Guilleminault C, Smirne S: Prevalence and pathologic associations of sleep paralysis in the general population. Neurology 1999;52;1194-1200.

96. Fisher CJ, Byrne J, Edwards T, et al: A psychophysiological study of nightmares. J Am Psychoanal Assoc 1970;18:747-782.

97. Levin R, Fireman G: Nightmare prevalence, nightmare distress, and self-reported psychological disturbance. Sleep 2002;25:205-212.

98. Agargun MY, Kara H, Ozer OA, et al: Characteristics of patients with nocturnal dissociative disorders. Sleep Hypnosis 2001;3:131-134.

99. Rice E, Fisher C: Fugue states in sleep and wakefulness: A psychophysiological study. J Nerv Ment Dis 1976;163:79-87.

100. Mikkelsen EJ, Rapoport JL: Enuresis: Psychopathology, sleep stage, and drug response. Urol Clin North Am 1980;7:361-377.

101. Yeung CK: Nocturnal enuresis (bedwetting). Curr Opin Urol 2003;13:337-343.

102. De Roeck J, Van Hoof E, Cluydts R: Sleep-related expiratory groaning: A case report. Sleep Res 1983;12:237.

103. Vetrugno R, Provini F, Plazzi G, et al: Catathrenia (nocturnal groaning): A new type of parasomnia. Neurology 2001;56:681-683.

104. Pearce JMS: Clinical features of the exploding head syndrome. J Neurol Neurosurg Psychiatry 1989;52:907-910.

105. Sachs C, Svanborg E: The exploding head syndrome: Polysomnographic recordings and therapeutic suggestions. Sleep 1991;14:263-266.

106. Birketvedt GS, Florholmen J, Sundsfjord J, et al: Behavioral and neuroendocrine characteristics of the night-eating syndrome. JAMA 1999;282:657-663.

107. Schenck CH, Mahowald MW: Review of nocturnal sleep-related eating disorders 1994;15:343-356.

108. Lugaresi E, Provini F: Agrypnia excitata: Clinical features and pathophysiological implications. Sleep Med Rev 2001;5:313-322.

109. Silber MH, Hansen MR, Girish M: Complex nocturnal visual hallucinations. Sleep 2002;25:484.

110. Plazzi G, Montagna P, Meletti S, Lugaresi E: Polysomnographic study of sleeplessness and oneiricisms in the alcohol withdrawal syndrome. Sleep Med 2002;3:279-282.

111. Ohayon MM, Priest RG, Caulet M, Guilleminault C: Hypnagogic and hypnopompic hallucinations: Pathological phenomena? Br J Psychiatry 1996;169:459-467.

112. Schenck CH, Mahowald MW: On the reported association of psychopathology with sleep terrors in adults. Sleep 2000;23:448-449.

113. Ekbom KA: Restless legs syndrome. Neurology 1960;10:868-873.

114. Earley CJ: Restless legs syndrome. N Engl J Med 2003;348: 2103-2109.

115. Symonds CP: Nocturnal myoclonus. J Neurol Neurosurg Psychiatry 1953;16:166-171.

116. Picchietti DL, Walters AS: Moderate to severe periodic limb movement disorder in childhood and adolescence. Sleep 1999;22:297-300.

117. Layzer RB, Rowland LP: Cramps. N Engl J Med 1971;285:31-40.

118. Saskin P, Whelton C, Moldofsky H, Akin F: Sleep and nocturnal leg cramps. Sleep 1988;11:307-308.

119. Lavigne GJ, Kato T, Kolta A, Sessle BJ: Neurobiological mechanisms involved in sleep bruxism. Crit Rev Oral Biol Med 2003; 14:30-46.

120. Ware JC, Rugh J: Destructive bruxism: Sleep stage relationship. Sleep 1988;11:172-181.

121. Dyken ME, Lin-Dyken DC, Yamada T: Diagnosing rhythmic movement disorder with video-polysomnography. Pediatr Neurol 1997;16:37-41.

122. Sallustro F, Atwell CW: Body rocking, head banging and head rolling in normal children. J Pediatr 1978;93:704-708.

123. Roth T, Kramer M, Trinder J: The effect of noise during sleep on the sleep patterns of different age groups. Can Psychiatr Assoc J 1972;17:SS197-SS201.

124. Thiessen GJ, Lapointe AC: Effect of continuous traffic noise on percentage of deep sleep, waking, and sleep latency. J Acoust Soc Am 1983;73:225-229.

125. Hartmann E, Baekeland F, Zwilling GR: Psychological differences between short and long sleepers. Arch Gen Psychiatry 1972;26:463-468.

126. Webb WB: Are short and long sleepers different? Psychol Rep 1979;44:259-264.

127. Dalmasso F, Prota R: Snoring: Analysis, measurements, clinical implications and applications. Eur Respir J 1996;9:146-159.

128. Jennum P, Hein HO, Suadicani P, et al: Snoring, family history, and genetic markers in men. The Copenhagen Male Study. Chest 1995;107:1289-1293.

129. Arkin AM: Sleep talking: A review. J Nerv Ment Dis 1966;143: 101-122.

130. Hublin C, Kaprio J, Partinen M, Koskenvuo M: Sleeptalking in twins: Epidemiology and psychiatric comorbidity. Behav Genet 1998;28:289-298.

131. Broughton R: Pathological fragmentary myoclonus, intensified sleep starts and hypnagogic foot tremor: Three unusual sleep-related disorders. In Koella WP (ed): Sleep 1986. New York, Fischer-Verlag, 1988, pp 240-243.

132. Oswald I: Sudden bodily jerks on falling asleep. Brain 1959; 82:92-93.

133. Coulter DL, Allen RJ: Benign neonatal sleep myoclonus. Arch Neurol 1982;39:191-192.

134. Resnick TJ, Moshe SL, Perotta L, et al: Benign neonatal sleep myoclonus: Relationship to sleep states. Arch Neurol 1986;43: 266-268.

135. Chervin RD, Consens FB, Kutluay E: Alternating leg muscle activation during sleep and arousals: A new sleep-related motor phenomenon? Mov Disord 2003;18:551-559.

136. Wichniak A, Tracik F, Geisler P, et al: Rhythmic feet movements while falling asleep. Mov Disord 2001;16:1164-1170.

137. Montagna P, Provini F, Plazzi G, et al: Propriospinal myoclonus upon relaxation and drowsiness: A cause of severe insomnia. Mov Disord 1997;12:66-72.

138. Tison F, Arne P, Dousset V, et al: Propriospinal myoclonus induced by relaxation and drowsiness. Rev Neurol (Paris) 1998;154:423-425.

139. Broughton R, Tolentino MA, Krelina M: Excessive fragmentary myoclonus in NREM sleep: A report of 38 cases. Electroencephalogr Clin Neurophysiol 1985;61:123-309.

140. Vetrugno R, Plazzi G, Provini F, et al: Excessive fragmentary hypnic myoclonus: Clinical and neurophysiological findings. Sleep Med 2002;3:73-76.

141. Lugaresi E, Medori R, Montagna P, et al: Fatal familial insomnia and dysautonomia with selective degeneration of thalamic nuclei. N Engl J Med 1986;315:997-1003.

142. Montagna P, Gambetti P, Cortelli P, Lugaresi E: Familial and sporadic fatal Insomnia. Lancet Neurol 2003;2:167-176.

143. Provini F, Plazzi G, Tinuper P, et al: Nocturnal frontal lobe epilepsy: A clinical and polygraphic overview of 100 consecutive cases. Brain 1999;122:1017-1031.

144. Scheffer IE, Bhatia KP, Lopes-Cendes I, et al: Autosomal dominant nocturnal frontal lobe epilepsy: A distinctive clinical disorder. Brain 1995;118:61-73.

145. Dexter JD: Relationship between sleep and headaches. In Thorpy MJ (ed): Handbook of Sleep Disorders. New York, Marcel Dekker, 1990, pp 663-671.

146. Evers S, Goadsby PJ: Hypnic headache-clinical features, pathophysiology, and treatment. Neurology 2003;60:905-909.

147. Nebel OT, Fornes MF, Castell DO: Symptomatic gastroesophageal reflux: Incidence and precipitating factors. Am J Dig Dis 1976;21:953-956.

148. Orr WC: Gastrointestinal functioning during sleep. In Lee-Chiong TL, Sateia MJ, Carskadon MA (eds): Sleep Medicine. Philadelphia, Hanley & Belfus, 2002, pp 463-470.

149. Nowlin JB, Troyer WG Jr, Collins WS, et al: The association of nocturnal angina pectoris with dreaming. Ann Intern Med 1965;63:1040-1046.

150. Verrier RL, Muller JE, Hobson JA: Sleep, dreams, and sudden death: The case for sleep as an autonomic stress test for the heart. Cardiovasc Res 1996;31:181-211.

151. Benca RM: Sleep in psychiatric disorders. Neurol Clin 1996;14:739-764.

52

Epidemiology of Sleep Disorders

Markku Partinen

Christer Hublin

ABSTRACT

Sleep disorders are common. At least 10% of the population suffers from a sleep disorder that is clinically significant and of public health importance. Insomnia is the most common sleep disorder, followed by sleep-disordered breathing and restless legs syndrome. Sleep disorders are interrelated with medical and psychiatric disorders such as arterial hypertension, cardiovascular and cerebrovascular diseases, diabetes, and depression. More epidemiologic studies are needed to understand the ethnic differences that exist in the prevalence sleep disorders.

Sleep disorders such as sleep apnea, insomnia, and restless legs syndrome (RLS) fulfill the criteria of a public health disease. In the 1980s, the large epidemiologic studies on sleep disorders were based on the 1979 sleep disorders classification.[1] In 1990, a new *International Classification of Sleep Disorders* (ICSD) was published and it was recently revised. It is currently the most widely used classification system on sleep disorders.[2] Other international classifications include the *International Classification of Diseases, 10th Revision* (ICD-10) published by the World Health Organization, and the *Diagnostic and Statistical Manual of Mental Disorders, Fourth Edition* (DSM-IV), published by the American Psychiatric Association.

From the public health viewpoint, the most important sleep problems are insomnia, sleep-related breathing disorders, RLS, and excessive daytime sleepiness (EDS); these are discussed in this chapter. Discussions of the prevalence of specific sleep disorders may be found in the corresponding chapters of this textbook.

For a general review of epidemiology, the reader is referred to some excellent sources.[3] Many clinical epidemiologists, as well as economists, believe in the importance of *evidence-based medicine*. In a critical article, Wright et al.[4] claimed that very little is known about the health effects of sleep apnea, implying that much of the research in this field does not meet the standards of evidence-based medicine. New data have been published since 1997, but additional studies are needed, especially from randomized clinical trials. In large-scale surveys, the data must often be collected by postal questionnaires, structured personal interviews, or telephone. Many different questionnaires and methods have been used to obtain data regarding sleep disorders.[5-12]

EARLY STUDIES

The oldest epidemiologic studies of sleep length date from the end of the 18th century. Classic studies include those by Clement Dukes from England about the need for sleep in young children. Other well-known early studies are by Hertel from Denmark, Bernhard from Germany, and Claparéde from France. According to the reports of that time, 6-year-old children should sleep 10.5 to 13.5 hours per night, 15-year-olds should sleep 9 to 10 hours per night, and adults should sleep 8 to 8.5 hours per night.

Sleep disturbances increase with age. Already in 1931, Laird reported that slightly more than 90% of subjects 25 years of age have uninterrupted sleep at night, but at the age of 95 years, 100% have some wakefulness each night.[12a] More than 70% of 509 elderly men reported some difficulty in going to sleep, and more than 40% reported wakefulness during the night. Difficulty going to sleep increased with age. Most men used special techniques to aid them in falling asleep; reading was used by 25%, and relaxation techniques with or without the aid of warm drinks were used by 18%. The author was surprised that 3% used drugs other than alcohol to help them sleep, and 2% used alcohol. This figure should be compared with modern times, when hypnotics are sometimes prescribed too easily.

Many epidemiologic studies of sleeping habits have been performed since 1960. In these studies, the average length of sleep varied between 7 and 8 hours. In a questionnaire survey by Bixler et al., 7.4% of 1278 University of Florida students reported less than 6.5 hours of sleep at night, and 13.4% reported more than 8.5 hours. Recent studies have confirmed many of the earlier findings.[13]

INSOMNIA AND USE OF HYPNOTIC AGENTS

Insomnia is the most common sleep–wake-related complaint, and sleeping pills are among the most commonly prescribed drugs in clinical practice at the primary health care level. Insomnia can be a symptom of an underlying condition, for which there are dozens of candidates, or it can be a primary disease. Many of the insomnia diagnoses are relatively new diagnostic entities, and there are few or no studies of their prevalence. We concentrate here on studies dealing with insomnia in general, its three main manifestations (i.e., trouble falling asleep, trouble staying asleep, and early morning awakening), and the use of hypnotic agents.

Table 52–1 presents studies on insomnia in general. The heterogeneity of the definitions and methods used is striking, but some clear trends can be seen.

First, insomnia increases with age. Approximately one third of subjects older than 65 years of age have more or less continuous insomnia, although at very old age, the levels may be lower. In Australia, insomnia was persistent in 16.2% of the

Table 52–1. Occurrence of Insomnia in General

Reference	N	Study Population (Age Range, Yr)	Definition	Methods	Occurrence, %
Saarenpää-Heikkilä et al. (1995)[101]	574	School-age children (7–17)	Sleeplessness	Questionnaire	Often or always: 4 (m), 5 (f) Sometimes: 61 (m), 57 (f)
Tynjälä et al. (1993)[102]	40,202	School-age children (11–16)	Inability to fall asleep twice a week	Questionnaire (in nine countries)	11–12 yr: 16.4–33.2 13–14 yr: 11.5–25.3 15–16 yr: 10.8–26.6
Lugaresi et al. (1983)[103]	5713	Population sample (3–94)	Sleeping badly always or almost always	Questionnaire	9.9 (m), 16.8 (f)
Cirignotta et al. (1985)[104]					<20 yr: 1.6 20–44 yr: 11.9 45–54 yr: 20 (m), increase from 20 to 40 (f) >60 yr: increase from 20 to 30 (m)
Smirne et al. (1983)[105]	2518	Inpatients (6–92; >90% adults)	Current complaint of insomnia	Questionnaire	12.8
Partinen and Rimpelä (1982)[106]	2016	Population sample (15–64)	Insomnia daily or several times weekly	Telephone interview	7 (m), 9 (f) 15–24 yr: 5 25–44 yr: 6 45–64 yr: 14
Yeo et al. (1996)[107]	2418	Chinese and Malays in Singapore (15–55)	Having insomnia for the past year	Interview at home	12.9 (m) 17.5 (f) Chinese 14.2 Malay 18.6
Hohagen et al. (1991)[108]	1500	Outpatients (18–65)	Severe insomnia including daytime impairment (DSM-III-R)	Questionnaire	19 18–35 yr: 11 35–50 yr: 21 51–65 yr: 27
Ford and Kamerow (1989)[109]	7954	Population sample (18–65+)	Ever a period of 2 weeks or longer with trouble falling asleep, staying asleep, or waking up too early	Direct structured interview using Diagnostic Interview Schedule[109]	7.9 (m), 12.1 (f)
Weissman et al. (1997)[110]	10,533	Population sample (18+)	During the past year, ever having a period of 2 weeks or more with trouble falling asleep, staying asleep, or waking	Direct structured interview using Diagnostic Interview Schedule[109]	All types: 11.9 Uncomplicated: 4.9 Complicated: 3.6
Dodge et al. (1995)[111]	1667	Population sample (18–64+)	Current trouble falling asleep, trouble staying asleep, or waking up too early	Questionnaire and interview	18–44 yr: 22.8 (m), 30.0 (f) 45–64 yr: 31.5 (m), 43.8 (f) >64 yr: 36.4 (m), 47.6 (f)
Husby and Lingjaerde[15]	14,667	Population sample (20–54)	Sleeplessness (yes/no)	Questionnaire	Men: 29.9 Women: 41.0
Morgan and Clarke (1997)[112]	1042	Primary care patients (65–80+)	Sleeping problems often or all the time	Questionnaire	65–69 yr: 33.2 (m), 44.1 (f) 70–74 yr: 39.4 (m), 44.4 (f) 75–79 yr: 11.2 (m), 30.8 (f)
Ohayon and Partinen (2002)[16]	982	Population sample (18+)	Insomnia (DSM-IV)	Telephone survey using Sleep-EVAL	DSM-IV: 11.7 Any type: 37.6
Kim et al. (2000)[113]	3030	Population sample (20+)	Insomnia of any type	Interview at home	22.3 (m), 20.5 (f) 20–39 yr: 18.1 40–59 yr: 18.9 60+ yr: 29.5 No stress: 15.9 Stress: 25.8

DSM, Diagnostic and Statistical Manual of Mental Disorders; f, female; m, male.

community-dwelling population and 12.2% of institutional residents. Altogether, 14.5% of elderly subjects living in the community were using hypnotics regularly, whereas the corresponding figure was 39.7% among institutional residents.[14] In a large U.S. population-based study,[13] the prevalence of insomnia was 7.5%, and that of difficulty sleeping an additional 22.4%. In children and adolescents, the prevalence of frequent insomnia is quite variable; in several studies, it is higher than 10%. In middle-aged populations, the frequency of long-standing insomnia seems to be approximately 10%. Table 52–2 shows that trouble falling asleep seems to be the most common manifestation in younger age groups, whereas trouble staying asleep is the most frequent form of insomnia in middle-aged and elderly people.

Second, there is a clear sex difference, with insomnia occurring approximately 1.5 times more often in women than in men; this is especially true in menopausal and postmenopausal women compared with middle-aged men.

Third, seasonal differences, probably due to light exposure, can be seen, and the results are consistent in Nordic countries.[15,16] In northern Norway, 41.7% of women and 29.9% of men had occasional insomnia.[15] As a whole, complaints of insomnia were more common during the dark period of year than during other times of the year. In the Tromsø study, occurrence of insomnia during the midnight sun period (summer insomnia) decreased with age, whereas the other seasonal types of insomnia increased with age.[15]

Fourth, the association of psychiatric disorders, especially depression, with insomnia is well known. Primary insomnia and insomnia related to mental disorders are the two most common DSM-IV insomnia diagnoses.[17] The differential diagnosis may be difficult. In a large U.S. community survey by Weissman et al.,[110] the prevalence of insomnia uncomplicated by psychiatric disorders was 4.9%. Among those with complicated insomnia in the past year, 25% had major depression, 19% abused alcohol, 12% had dysthymia, 9% had panic disorder, 8% abused drugs, 8% had schizophrenia, and 2% had somatization disorder. In a World Health Organization collaborative study, 25,916 primary health care attendees were evaluated.[17a] Sleep problems were present in 27% of the patients. Of the patients with insomnia, 51% had a well-defined ICD-10 mental disorder, mainly depression or anxiety, or abused alcohol, or a combination. Use of alcohol and over-the-counter medications to control insomnia is common. Also, somatic and psychological complaints as well as psychological stress are associated with a higher prevalence of insomnia.

Fifth, social and occupational factors are important contributors to insomnia, as are medical illnesses. Being unemployed or unmarried is associated with a higher prevalence of insomnia complaints in Japan and other countries. Insomnia is a frequent complaint among patients with various respiratory symptoms. In a study by Dodge et al.,[111] the prevalence of insomnia was 31.8% to 52.4% among adults with cough, dyspnea, or wheezing; among adults without respiratory symptoms, the prevalence was 25.3% to 26.2%. In a questionnaire survey of 6268 adults in 40 different occupations, 18.9% of bus drivers complained of having some or very much difficulty falling asleep. Among male managers and male physicians, the respective percentages were 3.7% and 4.9%. Disturbed nocturnal sleep was complained of the most often by male laborers (28.1% waking up at least three times

a night) and female cleaners (26.6%). Disturbed nocturnal sleep was rare among male physicians (1.6%), male managers (7.4%), female head nurses (8.9%), and female social workers (9.4%).[18] Symptoms of work-related stress and mental exhaustion are associated with insomnia. Simple methods, such as the five-item version of the Mental Health Index and some other questions, may be used effectively to screen workers with mental health and sleep problems.[19]

Table 52–3 lists some studies on the use of hypnotic agents. In a nationally representative probability sample survey of non-institutionalized adults, 3161 people 18 to 79 years of age were surveyed.[20] Insomnia affected 35% of all adults during the course of 1 year. During the year before the survey, 2.6% of adults had used a medically prescribed hypnotic agent; 0.3% of all adults and 11% of all users of hypnotic agents reported using the medication regularly for 1 year or longer. When anxiolytic and antidepressant agents were excluded, 4.3% of adults had used a medically prescribed hypnotic for sleep and 3.1% had used an over-the-counter sleeping pill. Since that time, the use of hypnotic agents has continued to increase.[21]

In Sweden, 10,216 members of the Swedish Pensioners' Association were surveyed.[22] Hypnotic agents were used by 13.5% of the men and 22.3% of the women. Of the men younger than 70 years of age, 7.9% were receiving such treatment; of those 70 to 80 years of age, 14.4% were using hypnotic agents; and of those 80 years of age or older, 21.8% were taking hypnotic agents ($P < .0001$). The corresponding frequencies among women were 15.0%, 23.0%, and 34.9%, respectively ($P < .0001$). Hypnotic agents are used by many institutionalized elderly subjects even without insomnia. This is problematic, and it raises an ethical question because the chronic use of hypnotic agents is associated with excessive mortality rates.[23]

An excellent way of tracking the use of hypnotic medication of a population is to count unit defined daily doses (DDD) from the sales statistics of pharmacies and hospitals. When one knows the assumed average dose per day for each drug, sales per year, and population of the country, one can calculate DDDs per 1000 inhabitants per day. In Finland, for all hypnotic agents, the rate in 1994 was 38 DDD/1000 inhabitants/day. In 2002 the rate had increased to 53.4 DDD/1000 inhabitants/day. Benzodiazepines are available in all Scandinavian countries, and in 2001, the consumption of benzodiazepines (in DDD/1000 inhabitants/day) was 14.9 in Denmark, 21.5 in Finland, 20.8 in Iceland, 13.1 in Norway, and 11.7 in Sweden.[21] Respectively, the consumption of cyclopyrrolones was 17.7 in Denmark, 29.5 in Finland, 34.5 in Iceland, 20.9 in Norway, and 24.3 in Sweden.[21]

SHORT AND LONG SLEEPERS

Healthy people sleeping less than 6 or 6.5 hours per night are called "natural short sleepers" and those sleeping more than 9.5 hours of sleep "natural long sleepers." In a cross-sectional study of 5419 adult men in Finland, a higher prevalence of diagnosed myocardial infarction was found among those who slept more than 9 hours, whereas those sleeping less than 6 hours per night had more symptomatic coronary heart disease. This relationship held after controlling for age, sleep quality, use of sleeping pills and tranquilizers, smoking, alcohol use, type A score, neuroticism, use of cardiovascular drugs,

Table 52–2. Main Manifestations of Insomnia

Reference	N	Study Population (Age Range, yr)	Methods	Trouble Falling Asleep, %	Trouble Staying Asleep, %	Early Morning Awakening, %
Blader et al. (1997)[114]	987	School-age children (5–12)	Questionnaire	1–2 nights/week: 12.9; ≥3 nights/week: 11.3	1–2 nights/weeks: 6.0; ≥3 nights/week: 6.5	
Morrison et al. (1992)[115]	943	Cohort (15)	Interview	≥4 nights/week: 9.1 (m), 10.0 (f)	≥4 nights/week: 1.5 (m), 3.0 (f)	>4 nights/week: 2.5 (m), 4.4 (f)
Ohayon (1996)[16]	5622	Population sample (>15)	Telephone interview using the Sleep-EVAL expert system		Regularly 32.8 (m), 45.0 (f)	
Ohayon et al. (1997)[17]	4972	Population sample (>15)	Telephone interview using the Sleep-EVAL expert system	Currently: 10.5 (m), 15.3 (f)	Currently: 16.4 (m), 24.8 (f)	Currently: 13.7(m), 17.8 (f)
Bixler et al. (1979)[117]	1006	Population sample (>18)	Questionnaire	Currently: 14.4 (about two thirds women)	Currently: 22.9 (about two thirds women)	Currently: 13.8 (about two thirds women)
Karacan et al. (1983)[118]	2347	Population sample (18–65+)	Interview	Often or always (no age effect): 6.0 (m), 11.2 (f)	Often or always (significant increase with age): 12.9 (m), 17.4 (f)	Often or always (significant increase with age): 6.2 (m), 8.0 (f)
Ganguli et al. (1996)[119]	1050	Population sample (66–97)	Questionnaire	Sometimes or usually: 26.7 (m), 44.1 (f)	Sometimes or usually: 19.2 (m), 35.8 (f)	Sometimes or usually: 13.6 (m), 23.3 (f)
Blazer et al. (1995)[20]	3976	Population sample (≥65; EPESE)	Interview using a questionnaire	Blacks: 14.8; Whites: 16.3	Blacks: 19.9; Whites: 33.8	Blacks: 12.9; Whites: 16.0
Foley et al. (1995)[121]	9282	Population sample (≥65; EPESE)	Interview using a questionnaire	Most of the time: 19.2	Most of the time: 29.7	Most of the time: 18.8
Henderson et al. (1995)[14]	869	Population sample (≥70)	Home interview, use of a computer algorithm	Nearly every night over the previous 2 weeks: 5.1	NA	Nearly every night over the previous 2 weeks: 2.6
Liljenberg et al. (1988)[122]	1763 m 1794 f	Population sample	Questionnaire	5.1(m) 7.1 (f)	7.7 (m) 8.9 (f)	NA NA
Kim et al. (2000)[113]	3030	Population sample (20+)	Home interviews	7.0 (m) 9.4 (f) No stress: 4.1 Stress; 11.6	20–39 yr: 11.1 40–59 yr: 13.6 60+ yr: 22.6 No stress: 11.2 Stress: 18.3	20–39 yr: 5.1 40–59 yr: 6.7 60+ yr: 13.3 No stress: 6.0 Stress: 9.4
Ohayon and Partinen[16] (2002)	982	Population sample (18+)	Telephone survey using Sleep-EVAL	(≥3 nights/week) 10.4 (m) 13.2 (f)	(≥3 nights/week) 30.2 (m) 33.0 (f)	(≥3 nights/week) 9.7 (m) 12.2 (f)

EPESE, Established Populations for Epidemiologic Studies in the Elderly; f, female; m, male; NA, not applicable.

Table 52–3.   Use of Hypnotics

Reference, Country	N (Age Ranges, yr)	Definition of Use	Users, %
Kirmil-Gray et al. (1984),[123] United States	277 (13–17)	Used medication at least once for disturbed sleep	14.9
Lack (1986),[124] Australia	211 (16–50; median, 19)	At least occasionally	4.7
Janson et al. (1996),[125] Iceland, Sweden, Belgium	2394 (20–45)	At least once weekly	1.3
Ohayon (1996),[116] France	5622 (>15)	Current use	6.8 (m), 12.7 (f)
Simen et al. (1996),[126] Germany	1653 (14–65)	At least once weekly	1
	344 (>65)	At least once weekly	10
Johnson et al. (1998),[127] United States	2181 (18–45)	Use of sleep aids at least some time during the past year	Sleep medication: 18 (36% using for >1 mo) Alcohol: 13 (15% for >1 mo) Any substance: 26
Karacan et al. (1983),[118] United States	2347 (18–65+)	Sometimes Often or always	3.8 (m), 6.8 (f) 3.3 (m), 4.0 (f)
Partinen et al. (1983),[128] Finland	30,142 (18–69)	For more than 2 mo the preceding year	18–29 yr: 0.4 (m), 0.3 (f) 30–39 yr: 1.1 (m), 1.0 (f) 40–49 yr: 2.3 (m), 2.3 (f) 50–59 yr: 3.3 (m), 3.9 (f) 60–69 yr: 3.8 (m), 7.5 (f)
Mellinger et al. (1985),[20] United States	3161 (18–79)	Hypnotic use in the past year Hypnotic use regularly for longer than 1 yr	2.6 0.3 of all adults, 11 of all users of hypnotics (35% of all adults complained of insomnia)
Lopez et al. (1955),[129] Mexico	1000 (18–84)	Use to sleep	5 (50% of men and 14% of women did not report insomnia)
Hyyppä and Kronholm (1987),[130] Finland	1099 (29–79)	Frequently Sometimes Often Almost every evening	1.4 10.7 (m), 15.4 (f) 1.9 (m), 3.3 (f) 1.7 (m), 3.5 (f)
Morgan et al. (1988),[131] Great Britain	1020 (>65)	Sometimes Often All the time	3 1 12
Asplund (1955),[22] Sweden	10,216 (pensioners; >65)	Taking hypnotics	<70 yr: 7.9 (m), 15.0 (f) 70–80 yr: 14.4 (m), 23.0 (f) 80+ yr: 21.8 (m), 34.9 (f)
Henderson et al. (1995),[14] Australia	Community: 874 Institutions: 59 (≥70)	Taking hypnotics nearly every night over the previous 2 wk	Community: 14.5 (10.3% among those with no insomnia) Institutions: 39.7 (36.5% among those with no insomnia)

f, female; m, male.

and history of hypertension. Kripke et al. have published several studies showing a relationship between short sleep and mortality.[23] A population-based Japanese cohort of 5322 inhabitants from Gifu has been followed for more than 11 years.[24] Both longer and shorter sleep, compared with 7- to 8-hour sleep, were related to a significantly increased risk of total mortality in men but not in women. The relationship between longer sleep and mortality may arise because people may sleep longer if they feel fatigued owing to some underlying disease. However, it may also be that for most adults there is no need to sleep more than 8 hours per night.

INSUFFICIENT SLEEP

Insufficient sleep is the most common cause of daytime fatigue and sleepiness. In a population-based study in Japan[25] among 3030 subjects aged 20 years and older, 29% slept less than 6 hours per night, and 23% reported having insufficient sleep. Short sleep duration was the strongest predictor of EDS.[25] The findings are comparable with those reported in Western countries.[26] In Sweden, 12% of adults had persistent and considerable chronic sleep loss. One half of these also reported concomitant sleeping difficulties. In subjects without sleeping difficulties, the most common cause of insufficient sleep was too little time for sleep.[27] In Finland, the prevalence of insufficient sleep, defined as a difference of at least 1 hour between reported need of sleep and obtained sleep length, was 20.4% (16.2% in men and 23.9% in women). Almost half of those with insufficient sleep continued to have it 9 years later. One third of the liability to chronic insufficient sleep was attributed to genetic influences.[26]

DAYTIME SLEEPINESS

Daytime sleepiness is a common complaint (Table 52–4). The most common causes of daytime sleepiness are insufficient sleep (poor quality of sleep or sleep loss) and sleep-related breathing disorders. The use of hypnotic agents, other sleeping difficulties, and irregular sleep–wake schedule are also related to daytime sleepiness. Obstructive sleep apnea syndrome (OSAS) is the most common cause of sleepiness diagnosed in U.S. and European sleep laboratories. In sleep laboratory populations, approximately 75% of patients with daytime sleepiness have sleep-related breathing disorders (most commonly OSAS), 20% have narcolepsy, and 5% have restless legs, periodic movements in sleep, or other sleep disorders causing daytime sleepiness.

Definition of Daytime Sleepiness

The feeling of not being alert is common, occurring both as a physiologic everyday phenomenon and as a symptom of sleep disorders.[1,2] In spoken language, this feeling is probably most often called "sleepiness," but the actual meaning varies. By definition, "sleepiness" implies an increased risk of falling asleep,[2] but the complaint of sleepiness is sometimes used to describe physical tiredness, fatigue, and loss of mental alertness without an increase in sleep behavior—conditions often associated with a decreased ability to fall asleep, contrary to true sleepiness.

Our own studies exemplify these problems. Among those reporting daytime sleepiness every or almost every day, approximately 20% of women and 40% of men were habitual

snorers, 25% had scores suggesting moderate to severe depression, 25% had insomnia at least every other day, 10% were regular hypnotic or tranquilizer users, and 10% reported insufficient sleep. Thus, a "tired" or "sleepy" (in the patient's words) person may have insomnia and not EDS or hypersomnia. In a multiple sleep latency test study, the patients may have great difficulty falling asleep, contrary to the experience of hypersomniac and narcoleptic patients. A proper term for such an insomniac person is "fatigued." In practice, it must be remembered that descriptions of the symptoms are related to the person's feelings, emotions, level of education, and cultural background. These facts must also be taken into consideration when using just one or two items about sleepiness in a questionnaire. However, the issue is even more complex because other studies that use more extensive screening instruments provide similar results.[9,28] Sleep researchers usually talk about "sleepiness" when referring to poor vigilance, lack of alertness, and tendency to fall asleep, but traffic researchers often talk about "fatigue" or "drowsiness."

Occurrence of Daytime Sleepiness

Table 52–4 provides a summary of studies on daytime sleepiness. Depending on the wording, there is approximately a 100-fold difference in occurrence, ranging from 0.3% to more than 30% (see Table 52–4), and in most of the studies the range is from 5% to 15%. The prevalence is lowest for hypersomnialike states (more sleep per 24 hours than normal). Sleep attacks (involuntary sleep episodes during wake) are reported on average in 5% to 10% of subjects up to middle age, and in older persons, the frequency seems to increase to 20% to 30%, without a clear sex difference. Frequent or excessive (subjective) daytime sleepiness occurs in approximately 10% to 15%, and occurs more often in school-aged children or young adults than in middle-aged adults and more often in female than in male subjects. Results are contradictory regarding occurrences in middle-aged and older adults.

The variability of the results in different studies can be explained by differences in the definition of sleepiness and by other methodologic aspects, but there probably also are real differences in different populations. The differences in definitions of EDS lead to low comparability of the results. One problem is how "excessive" is characterized in different studies. In questionnaires, the word "excessive" is subjective, and it should be compared with something that the responder considers normal for her or him.

NARCOLEPSY AND NARCOLEPSY-LIKE SYMPTOMS

The most commonly stated prevalence of narcolepsy (see Chapter 65) is approximately 0.05%, or 50 per 100,000 population. However, large differences exist in its reported occurrence. The highest figures are from Japan (Table 52–5). Honda et al.[146,147] interviewed symptomatic Japanese school-aged children selected by questionnaire and found "a suspect of narcolepsy" in 160 per 100,000. The lowest frequency, 0.23 per 100,000 population, is found among Israeli Jews.

Studies using polygraphic confirmation of narcolepsy or including only cataplectic patients have provided lower frequency rates. However, the 95% confidence intervals (CIs) for the frequencies overlap in most studies. Thus, given the

Table 52–4.   Occurrence of Daytime Sleepiness

Reference	N (Sex)	Study Population (Age Range, yr)	Definition of Sleepiness (Wording of Questions)	Methods	Occurrence, %
Hypersomnia-Like States					
Karacan et al. (1976)[132]	1645 (?)	Population sample (18–70)	Too much sleep	Questionnaire	0.3
Bixler et al. (1979)[117]	1006 (m, f)	Population sample (18–80)	Sleeping too much	Questionnaire	7.1 (current, 4.2)
Ford and Kamerow (1989)[109]	7954 (m, f)	Population sample (18–65+)	Ever a period of 2 wk or longer sleeping too much	Direct structured interview using Diagnostic Interview Schedule	2.8 (m), 3.5 (f)
Sleep Attacks					
Saarenpää-Heikkilä et al. (1995)[101]	574 (m, f)	School-age children (7–17)	Sleeping in lessons often or always	Questionnaire (both subject and parents)	3 (m), 0 (f)
Partinen (1982)[133]	2537 (m)	Army draftees (17–29)	Falling asleep at work	Questionnaire	6.4
Partinen and Rimpelä (1982)[106]	2016 (m, f)	Population sample (15–64)	Involuntary sleep attacks daily or almost daily	Telephone interview	3.4 (m), 2.5 (f)
Billiard et al. (1987)[134]	58,162 (m)	Army draftees (17–22)	Daily sleep episodes	Questionnaire	4.9
Schmidt-Nowara et al. (1991)[135]	1278 (?)	Population sample (?)	Falling asleep often or always	Direct interview using a validated questionnaire	5.7 (inactive in a public place) 13.3 (as passenger in a vehicle) 2.4 (at work)
Klink and Quan (1987)[136]	2187 (?)	Population sample (18–64)	Falling asleep during the day	Questionnaire	12
Johns and Hocking (1997)[28]	331 (m, f)	Australian workers (22–59)	Chance of dozing (ESS > 10)	Questionnaire including ESS	10.9 (no gender difference) 29.1 (in 71-year-olds)
Hyyppä and Kronholm (1987)[130]	1099 (m, f)	Population sample (29–79)	Falling asleep	Questionnaire	7.9 (m), 4.9 (f) (as a passenger often or almost always) 10.9 (m), 7.5 (f) (often or daily in tasks requiring accuracy)
Hays et al. (1996)[137]	3962 (m, f)	Population sample (65–85+)	Most of the time sleepiness, forcing to take a nap	Interview	25.2
Ganguli et al. (1996)[19]	1050 (m, f)	Population sample (66–97)	Ever becoming uncontrollably sleepy so cannot help falling asleep	Interview	18.9 (no gender difference)

Daytime Sleepiness

Study	Sample	N	Definition	Method	Prevalence (%)
Saarenpää-Heikkilä et al. (1995)[101]	School-age children (7–17)	574 (m, f)	Daytime sleepiness always or often	Questionnaire (both subject and parents)	20 (m), 22 (f)
Berg Kelly et al. (1991)[138]	Students (13–18)	3543 (m, f)	Tiredness	Questionnaire	29.3
Partinen (1982)[133]	Army draftees (17–29)	2537 (m)	Excessive daytime sleepiness often or always	Questionnaire	35.8
Partinen and Rimpelä (1982)[106]	Population sample (15–64)	2016 (m, f)	Sleepier than fellow persons	Telephone interview	10 (m), 14 (f)
Lugaresi et al. (1983)[103]	Population sample (3–94)	5713 (m, f)	Sleepiness independent of meal times	Direct interview	8.7
Hyyppä and Kronholm (1987)[130]	Population sample (29–79)	1099 (m, f)	Daytime sleepiness often or always	Questionnaire	17.0 (m), 17.3 (f)
Janson et al. (1996)[125]	Population sample (20–44)	2394 (m, f)	Feeling drowsy in the daytime three times per week	Questionnaire	16.0
Martikainen et al. (1992)[139]	Population sample (36, 41, 46, 50)	1190 (m, f)	Tiredness/sleepiness indicated by (1) more tired than fellow persons, (2) daily compulsory desire to sleep, or (3) feeling tired every day	Questionnaire	6.9 (m), 12.0 (f)
Hublin et al. (1996)[140]	Population sample (33–60)	11,354 (m, f)	Daytime sleepiness daily or almost daily	Questionnaire	6.7 (m), 11.0 (f)
Ohayon et al. (1997)[141]	Population sample (15–100)	4952 (m, f)	Feeling sleepy during the day on a daily basis at least 1 mo greatly (severe sleepiness) or moderately (moderate sleepiness)	Telephone interview using the Sleep-EVAL expert system	Severe: 4.4 (m), 6.6 (f) Moderate: 15.2

?, not known, not exactly stated; ESS, Epworth Sleepiness Scale; f, female; m, male.

Table 52–5. Prevalence Studies on Narcolepsy

Reference	Frequency (per 100,000)	95% Confidence Interval*	Base Population (Age Range, yr)[†] Country	Methods
Solomon (1945)[142]	20 (190)[‡]	0–48	10,000 (16–34)[§] United States (blacks)	Male population sample
Solomon (1945)[142]	3[‖]	0.6–5.7	189, 196 (?)[§] United States (whites)	Male population sample
Roth (1962), (1980)[143]	13–20[¶**] 20–30[‡¶]	NC	? (?) Czechoslovakia	Patient material Electroencephalography/polygraphy
Dement et al. (1972)[144]	50[††]	NC	169 (?)[‡‡] United States	Population sample Newspaper ad[§§] Telephone interview
Dement et al. (1973)[145]	67[‖‖]	NC	113 (?)[‡‡] United States	Population sample TV ad[§§] Telephone interview
Honda (1979),[146] Honda et al. (1983)[147]	160	9–230	12,469 (12–16) Japan	Population sample Questionnaire[§§] Personal interview
Partinen (1982)[133]	79	6–287	2537 (?)[§] Finland	Male population sample Questionnaire Polygraphy
Franceschi et al. (1982)[148]	40[¶]	0–118	2518 (6–92) Italy	Unselected inpatients Questionnaire[§§] Polygraphy
Wilner et al. (1988)[149]	0.23[¶]	NC	1800 (30–57) Israel (Jews)	Patient material Polygraphy HLA typing
Martikainen et al. (1992)[139]	168[‖]	18–604	1190 (36, 41, 46, 50) Finland	Population sample Questionnaire
Tashiro et al. (1992)[150]	590	369–816	4559 (17–59) Japan	Population sample Questionnaire
al Rajeh et al. (1993)[151]	4[‡]	0–13	23,227 (all ages) Saudi Arabia	Population sample Personal interview Neurologic examination HLA typing
Hublin et al. (1994)[29]	26	0–56	11,354 (33–60) Finland	Population sample Questionnaire[§§] Telephone interview Polygraphy HLA typing
Ohayon et al. (1996)[152]	40	0–96	4972 (15–100) United Kingdom	Population sample, Telephone interview (using the Sleep-EVAL expert system)
Silber et al. (2002)[153]	56.3	NC	97,667 Minnesota, Olmstead County	Census data, record linkage covering 1960–1989
Wing et al. (2002)[30]	34	10–117	9851 (Chinese) Hong Kong	Population sample, telephone interview, Ullanlinna Narcolepsy Scale, clinical examination, polygraphy, HLA typing
Ohayon et al. (2002)[154]	47	NC	18,980 Five European countries	Telephone survey using the Sleep-EVAL system and International Classification of Sleep Disorders criteria

*95% confidence interval for the frequency of narcolepsy per 100,000 (NC, cannot be computed).
[†]Number of subjects studied.
[‡]Reported total narcolepsy frequency (including also noncataplectic cases) or no information on the cataplexy status given.
[§]Army recruits.
[‖]Not reported whether with or without cataplexy.
[¶]Estimated population prevalence based on patient material.
[**]Approximately 35% of the patients had only one symptom (sleep attacks, cataplexy, or sleep paralysis).
[††]Estimated from the following data: San Francisco Bay area population (4 million), the newspaper circulation (1.2 million), the number of respondents (196) and interview-confirmed narcolepsy cases (114), and the number of persons seeing/not seeing and responding/not responding to a control advertisement.
[‡‡]Number of subjects interviewed.
[§§]Used as a screening method.
[‖‖]Estimated from the following data: number of television homes in Los Angeles area (2,290,200), rating of the number of viewers of the advertisement (56,576), number of respondents (165), and interview-confirmed narcolepsy cases (35); 30% sampling error and errors in making the diagnosis.
HLA, human leukocyte antigen.

low prevalence rate of the disorder and the relatively small numbers of cases in each study, most of the wide variation in the reported frequencies can be attributed to sample variation.

A simple screening method called the Ullanlinna Narcolepsy Scale (UNS) for population studies has been developed and validated.[8] The UNS consists of 11 items assessing cataplexy-like symptoms and the tendency to fall asleep. Using the UNS (excluding more than 99% of the study population), telephone interviews, and polygraphic confirmation of the diagnosis, the prevalence of narcolepsy with clinically significant cataplexy was found to be 26 per 100,000 population in adult Finns.[29] Using the validated Chinese version of UNS, the prevalence rate of narcolepsy in southern (Hong Kong) Chinese was found to be 34 per 100,000, or 0.034% (95% CI, 0.010% to 0.117%). All narcoleptic subjects were human leukocyte antigen DRB1-1501 positive and 50% were DQB1-0602 positive.[30]

Although typical cataplexy is pathognomonic of narcolepsy, mild forms are difficult to separate from similar physiologic phenomena. As mentioned, reports of EDS in the population are common. In Finland, 29.3% of the people reported (at least once during his or her lifetime) feelings of limb weakness associated with emotions.[29] If this is considered as evidence of cataplexy and combined with the occurrence of daytime sleep episodes at least 3 days per week, 6.5% of the population would have "fulfilled" the minimal diagnostic criteria for narcolepsy of the ICSD.[2,29] Therefore, using only questionnaires in population studies risks results in which narcolepsy prevalence rates are too high.

SNORING

Snoring is an inspiratory noise caused by vibration of the soft palate and posterior faucial pillars (see Chapter 83). Snoring corresponds to partial obstruction of the upper airways, and complete obstruction is followed by apnea. Habitual (almost every night or every night) snoring is practically always present in patients with OSAS. Some of the prevalence rates of snoring are shown in Table 52–6. In the first large-scale epidemiologic study on snoring, approximately 24% of San Marino men and 14% of San Marino women were reported to snore habitually (see Table 52–6). In Finland, 9% of adult men and 3.6% of adult women reported snoring always or almost always when asleep.[31]

SLEEP-DISORDERED BREATHING–SLEEP APNEA SYNDROME

A Syndrome or a Disease?

OSAS is a public health problem. It is the most common organic sleep disorder causing EDS. Sleep-related breathing disorders and sleep-disordered breathing usually refer to the same clinical disorder (see Chapter 51). In this chapter, we use the term OSAS, although hypopneas are now included in the syndrome.

According to various cross-sectional studies, the lowest rates for the prevalence of OSAS among adult men are 1% to 4%. There is an age relationship, so the prevalence of OSAS among men 40 to 59 years of age may be greater than 4% to 8%.[32] OSAS is less common in younger and older age groups. After menopause, up to the age of 65 years, OSAS is almost as common among women as among men.

Obstructive sleep apneas are part of the complex of "heavy snorer's disease" as defined by Lugaresi et al.[33] Heavy snoring (i.e., partial upper airway obstruction) even without apneas may influence pulmonary arterial pressure, and it may cause daytime sleepiness, arterial hypertension, insulin resistance, or other health consequences.[34-37] On the other hand, we know that some heavy snorers have been snoring from childhood until the age of 60 years or older, and they are healthy. Nonetheless, habitual heavy snoring and sleep apnea, independent of obesity, can now be considered as potential determinants of risk at least for cardiovascular disease and insulin resistance. In all epidemiologic studies on these diseases, habitual snoring and sleep apnea also should be included among the potential risk factors.

The etiologic problem arises in many situations. Is a morbidly obese patient with a body mass index (BMI) of 44 kg/m² called a patient with OSAS? The proper diagnosis may be morbid obesity with obstructive sleep apnea. Morbid obesity is a disease, and it is a risk factor for cardiovascular disease even without sleep apneas. Another example is acromegaly with sleep apnea. Such patients do not have essential OSAS but rather symptomatic sleep apnea. The disease (acromegaly) may be treated with pituitary adenomectomy, but the consequence (sleep apnea) often necessitates nasal continuous positive airway pressure (CPAP) or upper airway surgery. This is analogous to a patient with a brain tumor who has symptomatic epilepsy. The primary diagnosis is brain tumor (e.g., glioma), and epilepsy is a secondary symptom caused by the brain tumor.

Sleep apnea should be properly quantified, not only by an apnea index (AI; or apnea-hypopnea index [AHI]) but by the number of oxygen desaturations, limitation of air flow, and cardiac manifestations associated with the breathing events. It is also necessary to quantify impact of sleep apnea on daytime alertness, and some notion about this should be recorded (e.g., the Epworth Sleepiness Scale score).[7] An AI of 5 events per hour of sleep or an AHI of 10 is commonly used as a criterion of OSAS. The diagnostic criteria should be adjusted for age. Bixler et al.[38] studied 20- to 100-year-old men. The criteria for OSAS were an AHI of at least 10 in the sleep laboratory and clinical criteria fulfilled with the presence of daytime symptoms. OSAS was found in 3.3% of the sample, with its maximum prevalence among 45- to 64-year-old men. It may also be that although the prevalence of sleep apnea increases with age, its clinical meaningfulness decreases.

Prevalence

In Israel, Lavie estimated in a cross-sectional study that the prevalence of the syndrome among male industrial workers is at least 1% (Table 52–7). In Bologna, Italy, 2.5% of 30- to 69-year-old men had heavy snorer's disease of stage 1 or higher. The minimal prevalence of sleep apnea in that population was 2.7%, considering an AHI of 10 or more to be pathologic. In the United States, the first large epidemiologic polysomnographic study was conducted in Madison, Wisconsin.[32] The authors estimated that 2% of women and 4% of men in the middle-aged workforce met the minimal diagnostic criteria for the sleep apnea syndrome, defined as an AHI of 5 and daytime hypersomnolence.[32] Up to 9% of women and 24% of men had an AHI of 5 without daytime somnolence. On examination of the subgroup of patients between the ages of 50 and 60 years, 4% of women and 9.1%

Table 52-6. Occurrence of Habitual Snoring

Reference, Population	Methods	Definition/Wording of Habitual Snoring	Sex	N	Age (yr)	Prevalence, %
Lugaresi et al. (1980)[55] San Marino general population	Interview	"Every night" (alternatives: no, sometimes, every night)*	m f	2858 2855	3–94 3–94	24.1 13.8
Partinen (1982)[133] Army recruits	Questionnaire, clinical studies	Snoring always or almost always Snoring often or always	m	2537	18–29	2.9 9.5
Koskenvuo et al. (1985)[31] Finnish population sample	Postal questionnaire	"Snoring always or almost always"†	m f	3847 3864	40–69 40–69	9 3.6
Norton and Dunn (1985)[155] Canadian population sample	Questionnaire filled during a medical visit	Snoring every night (reported by spouses)	m f	1411 1211	3rd to 8th decade	13.2 5.6
Billiard et al. (1987)[134] French army draftees	Questionnaire completed under supervision	Snoring habitually	m	58,162	17–22	13.6
Gislason et al. (1987)[57] Swedish men	Postal questionnaire	"Loud and disturbing snoring" very often	m	4064	30–69	15.5
Cirignotta et al. (1989)[156] Italian adults	Postal questionnaire	Snoring always (alternatives: never, rarely, sometimes, often, always)	m	1170 890 304	30–69 40–69 50–59	10.1 all 11.5 15.5
Corbo et al. (1989)[157] Italian primary school-age children	Questionnaire filled by parents	Snoring often	Total m f	1615 810 815	6–13 6–13 6–13	7.3 7.3 7.3
Schmidt-Nowara et al. (1990)[158] Hispanic-American adults	Interview using a questionnaire	"Regular and loud snoring" always (every night)	m f	482 724	18 or older	10.2 5.4
Young et al. (1993)[32] State employees in Wisconsin	Postal questionnaire (first stage of the Sleep Cohort study)	Almost every night or every night snoring	m f	1670 1843	30–60 30–60	35 28
Ohta et al. (1993)[159] Subjects from four Japanese cities	Questionnaire given during a regular medical checkup	"Habitual snoring"	m, f	3243	Mean, 50	12.8–16
Jennum and Sjol (1994)[160] Danish population sample, part of Dan-MONICA II project	Interview and clinical examinations	Snoring nightly (every night)	m f	Total 1504	30–60 30–60	19.1 7.9
Teculescu et al. (1992)[161] France, children in nine kindergartens	Questionnaire, interview, and clinical examination	Habitual snoring	m, f	190	5–6	10; 95% CI: 5.7–14.3
Kayukawa et al. (2000)[162] Japan, new outpatients from 11 centers	Questionnaire, outpatient clinic visit	Habitual snoring	m, f	6445	Adults	m: 16.0 f: 6.5

*In the San Marino study, there were four alternatives: "no," "I don't know," "yes, sometimes," and "yes, every night."
†In the Finnish studies, five alternatives were used: "I don't know," "never," "sometimes," "often," and "almost always or always."

CI, confidence interval; f, female; m, male.

Table 52–7.   Occurrence of Obstructive Sleep Apnea and Obstructive Sleep Apnea Syndrome

Reference, Country	Methods	Subjects, N	Age (yr)	Criteria	Prevalence, %
Lavie (1983),[163] Israel	Questionnaire. PSG recordings and clinical examination for potential patients	1262 (m)	18–67	AI > 10, symptomatic	1.0–5.9
Peter et al. (1985),[164] Germany	Questionnaire. PSG recordings and clinical examination for potential patients	354 (m)	25–55	AI > 10, symptomatic	2.3
Telakivi et al. (1987),[42] Finland	Questionnaire. PSG recordings and clinical examination for potential patients	1939 (m)	30–69	Snoring, EDS, and RDI > 10	0.4–1.4
Gislason et al. (1988),[41] Sweden	Questionnaire. PSG recordings and clinical examination for potential patients	3201 (m)	30–69	Snoring, EDS, and AHI > 10	0.7–1.9
Cirignotta et al. (1989),[156] Italy	Questionnaire, telephone survey. PSG recordings and clinical examination for potential patients	1170 (m)	30–39 40–59 60–69	AI > 10, symptomatic AI > 10, symptomatic AI > 10, symptomatic	0.2–1.0 3.4–5.0 0.5–1.1
Stradling and Crosby (1991),[165] Great Britain	Ambulatory oximetry recordings at home	893 (m)	35–65	$ODI_4 > 20$, symptomatic $ODI_4 > 10$ $ODI_4 > 5$	0.3 1.0 4.6
Haraldsson et al. (1992),[166] Sweden	Questionnaire. PSG recordings and clinical examination for potential patients	846 (m)	30–69	Positive history and verification of OSAS in PSG	2.8–5.5
Young et al. (1993),[32] Wisconsin, United States	A sample of state employees. PSG recordings and clinical examination for potential patients	352 (m) 250 (f)	30–60 30–60	Hypersomnia and RDI ≥ 5	4.0 (m) 2.0 (f)
Gislason et al.(1993),[167] Iceland	Questionnaire. PSG recordings and clinical examination for potential patients	2016 (f)	40–59	Habitual snoring, EDS, and verification of OSAS in PSG	>2.5
Olson et al. (1995),[168] Australia	Questionnaire and home sleep recordings	1233 (m) 969 (f)	35–69	AHI ≥ 15 AHI ≥ 10 AHI ≥ 5	4–18 7–35 14–69
Bearpark et al. (1995),[169] Australia	Ambulatory home sleep recordings (MESAM IV). Estimation of sleep-disordered breathing. Collection of medical history	294 (m)	40–65	RD ≥ 10 Subjective EDS and RDI ≥ 5	10.0 ≥3.0
Gislason and Benediktsdottir (1995),[49] Iceland	Questionnaire. PSG and examination for suspected patients with habitual snoring or reported apneic episodes	555 children	6 mo to 6 yr	Habitual snoring or apneic episodes, and $ODI_4 > 3$	>2.9
Esnaola et al. (1995),[170] Spain	Questionnaire. PSG recordings and clinical examination for potential patients	1077 (m)	30–70	AHI ≥ 5 AHI ≥ 10 AHI ≥ 5 and EDS	15.3 13.4 6.5–9.1

Continued

Table 52-7. Occurrence of Obstructive Sleep Sleep Apnea and Obstructive Sleep Apnea Syndrome—cont'd

Reference, Country	Methods	Subjects, N	Age (yr)	Criteria	Prevalence, %
Ohayon et al. (1997),[171] Great Britain	Telephone interview (Sleep-EVAL). A sample of the general population. No examinations. No sleep recordings	2078 (m) 2894 (f)	35–64 35–64	NA NA	2.4–4.6 (m) 0.8–2.2 (f)
Kripke et al. (1997),[172] San Diego, United States	Telephone interview. A random sample of 40–64-year-olds living in San Diego. Home interview, home plus oximeter, and snoring recording	165 (m) 190 (f)	40–64 40–64	$ODI_4 > 20$ $ODI_4 > 20$	5.4–13.2 (m) 2.1–8.3 (f)
Bixler et al. (1998),[38] United States	Telephone survey. Random sample of men aged 20–100 yr. A sleep laboratory evaluation of a survey subsample	4364 (m) Subsample: 741	20–100	AHI > 10 and clinical criteria fulfilled with daytime symptoms	All: 3.3 45–64 yr: 47
Marin et al. (1997),[43] Spain	Personal interview, clinical examination, home oximetry. A representative population sample	597 (m) 625 (f)	>18	Loud snoring + excessive daytime sleepiness + abnormal home oximeter recording	2.2 (m) 0.8 (f)
Hui et al. (1999),[173] Hong Kong, China	Questionnaire and MESAM IV ambulatory sleep recordings	Students, 1306 male and 1757 female	Students, mean age 19.4	RDI >5 and daytime sleepiness	0.1% of all (2 students)
Bixler et al. (2001),[39] United States	Telephone survey. Random sample of men and women. A sleep laboratory study (PSG) for a subsample	12,219 women of whom 1000 had PSG; and 4346 men, 741 with PSG	20–100	AHI > 10 and clinical criteria fulfilled with presence of daytime symptoms	Women overall: 1.2 Premenopausal women: 0.6 Premenopausal women without HRT: 2.7 Postmenopausal women with HRT: 0.5 Men overall: 3.9

AHI, apnea-hypopnea index; AI, apnea index; EDS, excessive daytime sleepiness; f, female; HRT, hormone replacement therapy; m, male; NA, not applicable; ODI₄, oxygen desaturation index (≥4% desaturation); OSAS, obstructive sleep apnea syndrome; PSG, polysomnography; RDI, respiratory disturbance index.

of men were found to have an AHI exceeding 15.[32] The results from a larger U.S. population-based study[38,39] are close to these figures. For clinically defined sleep apnea (AHI of 10 or more and daytime symptoms), men had a prevalence of 3.9% and women, 1.2%. The peak prevalence, 4.7% (95% CI, 3.1% to 7.1%), was found, supporting other studies, among men 45 to 64 years of age. Among the 20- to 44-year-olds and those older than 65 years, the prevalence was 1.7%.[38] Among women, the average prevalence was 1.2.[39]

In women, the prevalence of sleep-disordered breathing increases after menopause, and hormone replacement therapy is associated with a lower incidence of sleep-disordered breathing.[39,40] In the study by Bixler et al.,[39] the prevalence of clinically defined sleep apnea among premenopausal women was 0.6%. Among postmenopausal women with hormone replacement therapy, the prevalence was also quite low (0.5%).[39]

In the Scandinavian countries, the prevalence figures have been lower. Gislason et al.[41] reported a prevalence of 1.3% in a Swedish 30- to 69-year-old male population. The prevalence of OSAS among 40- to 50-year-old Finnish men is between 0.4% and 1.4%[42] (see Table 52–5). The criteria have been rather strict in the Scandinavian studies. Presence of clinical symptoms was used to select subjects for sleep recordings. Hence, some people with sleep apnea may have been excluded from the study, giving lower figures of occurrence than in the U.S. studies, where objective sleep recordings were done independently of the clinical symptoms.

In the Zaragoza, Spain, metropolitan area, 0.8% of women and 2.2% of men met the minimal criteria of sleep apnea syndrome.[43] In an Italian study, 13.7% of the 349 monitored subjects had more than 10 desaturations of at least 4% per hour.[44]

The prevalence depends on the base populations. OSAS is most common in people 40 to 65 years of age. One can safely estimate that the prevalence of OSAS in that age group is approximately 4% (3% to 8%) in men and 2% in women, and that the absolute minimum prevalence of clinically significant OSAS is 1%. Among obese subjects, hypertensive patients, patients with adult-onset diabetes, and many patient groups with abnormal facial anatomy, the prevalences are significantly higher.

Role of Obesity as a Risk Factor for Snoring and Sleep Apnea

Obesity is an important risk factor for snoring and sleep apnea. Obesity may be measured by the BMI, which is calculated as weight in kilograms divided by the square of height in meters. Adults with a BMI of more than 27 kg/m^2 are considered obese. Several lines of evidence show that central and upper body obesity in particular is related to increased risk of cardiovascular disease. The same may be true for heavy snoring and sleep apnea. Using multivariate analysis, Katz et al.[45] reported that neck size is more closely related to severity of sleep apnea than is BMI. Neck size may be easily measured, and it is a useful indicator of upper body obesity. The frequency of snoring increases with obesity in all published epidemiologic reports on snoring and sleep-disordered breathing. Habitual snoring was found to occur in 7% of men and 2.8% of women with a BMI of less than 27 kg/m^2 and in 13.9% and 6.1%, respectively, of those with a BMI above this level.[45]

Alcohol increases upper airway resistance and tends to induce obstructive sleep apnea in healthy people and especially among chronic snorers, and it increases the duration and frequency of occlusive episodes in patients with obstructive sleep apnea. This is probably due to the acute centrally depressing effects of alcohol. However, OSAS seems not to be significantly more common among past alcoholic patients than among nonalcoholic subjects.

Practically any cause that can obstruct the upper airways poses a risk factor for heavy snoring and sleep apnea. These risk factors include large adenoids or tonsils, rhinitis, and other abnormalities in upper airways, such as those found in different syndromes of dysmorphia and in the mentally disabled. Acromegaly[46,47] and amyloidosis[48] are among reported risk factors.

Snoring and Sleep Apnea in Children

Upper airway obstruction with snoring or obstructive sleep apnea is commonly seen in children of all ages. In Italy, 1615 children 6 to 13 years of age were categorized according to whether they snored often, occasionally apart from with colds, only with colds, or never. One hundred eighteen children (7.3%) were habitual snorers. Rhinitic children were more than twice as likely to be habitual snorers than were others. There is also a positive correlation between parental smoking and the presence of snoring in children. In Iceland,[49] 3.2% of 555 children 6 months to 6 years of age snored often or always at sleep. The estimated minimal prevalence of obstructive sleep apnea in that age group was 3.2%. In another study, significant sleep and breathing disorders occurred in approximately 0.7% of 4- to 5-year-olds.[50] The prevalence of sleep-disordered breathing among adolescents aged 12 to 16 years is similar to that reported for younger children. Adenotonsillar hypertrophy is the most common cause of upper airway obstruction in infants and children.

Sleep Apnea among Older People

The prevalence of habitual snoring seems to decrease after the age of 65 or 70 years. According to Ancoli-Israel et al.,[51] 62% of older people have a respiratory disturbance index (RDI) of 10 or more. Because of its high prevalence in older people, sleep apnea has been suggested as one mechanism contributing to sleep-related death. This does not mean that older persons with an RDI of 10 or more have sleep apnea syndrome. The clinical significance of the high frequency of sleep apnea among older people remains to be seen. Bixler has emphasized the need to adjust the criteria for OSAS in older persons.[39]

A cohort of 198 noninstitutionalized older individuals (mean age at entry, 66 years) was followed for periods up to 12 years after initial polysomnography.[52] The mortality ratio for sleep apnea, defined as an RDI of more than 10 events per sleep hour, was 2.7 (95% CI, 0.95 to 7.47). These results raise the possibility that "natural" death during sleep in older people may be associated with disordered breathing during sleep or with other pathologic events during sleep. However, in a cohort of 426 older people, those with an RDI of 30 had significantly shorter survivals, but the RDI was not an independent predictor of death among the elderly subjects during 5 years of follow-up when age, cardiovascular disease, and pulmonary disease were included in the model.[53]

Other Patient Groups

Snoring is common among infants and children with Pierre Robin syndrome and among infants with nasal obstruction. Snoring and obstructive sleep apnea are also common in men with acromegaly. Many other syndromes or diseases exist in which upper airways are narrowed; the prevalence of snoring and sleep apnea is increased in all such situations.[54]

Arterial Hypertension

An association between always or almost-always snoring and arterial hypertension has been found in several cross-sectional studies.[55-57] In the San Marino study,[55] the relation was particularly significant in the age group of 41 to 60 years; hypertension was present in 15.2% of habitual snorers and in 7.5% of nonsnorers. In the Finnish study, the odds ratio for hypertension between habitual snorers and nonsnorers was 1.94 for men ($P < .0001$).[56] The association remained significant when BMI and age were adjusted. These results have been confirmed in a large U.S. cross-sectional study belonging to the Sleep Heart Health Study[58] and in prospective follow-up studies. Sleep-disordered breathing in the form of habitual snoring or sleep apnea is a determinant of risk of arterial hypertension, but occasional snoring is not associated with an increased risk.[37,59]

Sleep apnea is a risk factor for arterial hypertension. Case–control studies have shown that the prevalence of sleep apnea among patients with essential hypertension is approximately 30%. In a case–control study by Worsnop et al.,[60] 38% of the hypertensive subjects and 4% of the normotensive subjects had an AHI higher than 5. In middle-aged adults with drug-resistant hypertension, the prevalence of OSAS may be over 80%.[61] Prospective cohort studies have confirmed these results, indicating that habitual snoring and sleep apnea are risk factors for development of arterial hypertension.[37,59]

The relationship among arterial hypertension, cardiovascular disease, and OSAS is strongest among middle-aged adults. In elderly persons, the clinical significance of OSAS becomes weaker. Obstructive sleep apnea is a common finding among patients with arterial hypertension. According to all of these studies, the prevalence of sleep apnea among patients with essential hypertension is so high (25% or higher) that patients with arterial hypertension should always be queried about their snoring history and possible sleep apnea. The cost of monitoring and treatment of sleep apnea should be weighed against beneficial health effects.

Snoring, Sleep Apnea, and Heart Disease

An association of habitual snoring with electrocardiographic changes and arrhythmias has been reported.[62] In one of our early case–control studies, the odds ratio for myocardial infarction of "often" or "always" snorers compared with "never" or "sometimes" snorers was 5.5 (Yates' corrected $\chi^2 = 7.93$; 95% CI for odds ratio, 1.7 to 18). The association of snoring and ischemic heart disease was tested in a population consisting of 3847 men and 3664 women 40 to 69 years of age. Reported angina pectoris was associated with habitual snoring among men (risk ratio, 1.9) but not among women (risk ratio, 1.2). Reported myocardial infarction and ischemic heart disease were also associated with habitual snoring. The association

was also found after adjustment for arterial hypertension and BMI.[56] These results were confirmed in a prospective follow-up study of 4388 men 40 to 69 years of age. The age-adjusted risk ratio of ischemic heart disease between "often" or "always" snorers and nonsnorers was 1.91. The 95% CI was 1.18 to 3.09. An additional adjustment for BMI, history of arterial hypertension, smoking, and alcohol use decreased the risk ratio slightly to 1.71 (95% CI, 0.96 to 3.05).[63] Other studies also have confirmed that there is an association between habitual snoring, sleep apnea, and ischemic heart disease[64,65] or congestive heart failure.[66]

In a case–control study with 50 patients with myocardial infarction and 100 control subjects, snoring every night was associated with myocardial infarction. The odds ratio was 2.35 (95% CI, 1.18 to 4.67) when patients were compared with both hospital control and population control subjects. The effect of snoring every night was independent of smoking, arterial hypertension, diabetes mellitus, and alcohol consumption.[67] In Australia, 101 male patients with myocardial infarction and 53 male control subjects were investigated.[68] A significant association of sleep apnea with myocardial infarction was found. The association was independent of age, BMI, arterial hypertension, smoking, and cholesterol level. There was an increase in adjusted risk of myocardial infarction with increasing levels of sleep apnea. Men with an AI of more than 5.3 had 23.3-fold (95% CI, 3.9 to 139.9) the risk of myocardial infarction than did men with an AI of less than 0.4. The mean AI was 6.9 in patients with myocardial infarction versus 1.4 in the control subjects.[68]

Fifty patients 61 ± 6 years of age who were diagnosed as having coronary artery disease by coronary angiography were investigated prospectively. In 25 patients (50%), the AI was more than 10 per hour of sleep. EDS was exhibited by 8 of the 25 patients.[69] The minimum prevalence of OSAS among patients with coronary disease can be estimated as approximately 16%.

Excessive use of alcohol is associated with increased coronary death. Snoring could be a cofactor because alcohol tends to induce snoring and obstructive sleep apnea and to increase the duration and frequency of occlusive episodes in patients with obstructive sleep apnea.

Smoking is also associated with coronary disease. Habitual snorers smoke more than do occasional or never snorers. These two factors may be additive, so a habitually snoring smoker is at greater risk for coronary disease than is a habitual snorer who does not smoke.

Snoring, Sleep Apnea, and Brain Infarction

The most important factors associated with brain infarction are age, male sex, arterial hypertension, various abnormal cardiac conditions, diabetes mellitus, and cigarette smoking. In addition to these established risk factors, however, there is increasing evidence that suggests a link also between habitual, every-night snoring, OSAS, and stroke.

An association between cerebral infarction and habitual snoring has been found in many studies. In a case–control study of 50 male patients with brain infarction and 100 male control subjects,[70] the risk ratio for brain infarction between habitual or frequent snorers and occasional or never snorers was 2.8. Between habitual snorers and occasional or never snorers, the risk ratio for stroke was 10.3. The independent contribution of snoring as a risk factor for brain infarction was confirmed in another case–control study[71] of 177 male patients and control subjects matched for age and sex. After adjustment for several confounding variables, the independent odds ratio relating to snoring and stroke remained at 2.13.[71] Other studies have provided supporting results. In a study by Smirne et al.,[72] the adjusted (age, sex, obesity, diabetes, dyslipidemia, smoking, use of alcohol, hypertension) odds ratio for "often or always snoring" in relation to ischemic brain infarction was 1.9 (95% CI, 1.2 to 2.9). Neau et al.[73] studied 133 patients 45 to 75 years of age and 133 control subjects matched for age and sex. The prevalence of habitual snoring was 23.3% among patients with stroke and 8.3% among the control subjects. The odds ratio for habitual snoring was 3.4 (95% CI, 1.5 to 7.6). The odds ratio for "often or always snoring" was 1.7 (95% CI, 1.03 to 2.93). Even after adjustment for age, sex, arterial hypertension, cardiac arrhythmia, and obesity, the odds ratio of habitual snoring for stroke remained statistically significant (2.9; 95% CI, 1.3 to 6.8). The risk for ischemic stroke seems to be especially high among habitually snoring men with arterial hypertension.[73]

The physiologic rise in blood pressure after awakening in the morning may temporarily disturb the autoregulation of cerebral blood flow. In normal conditions, nothing happens, but under unfavorable conditions, an infarction may follow. Arterial hypertension is common among patients with sleep apnea. The association of snoring and brain infarction could in part be explained by the high prevalence of habitual snoring and obstructive sleep apnea in patients with arterial hypertension, which is a known risk factor for stroke. However, there is an increasing amount of evidence that the effects of habitual snoring and sleep apnea remain as risk factors for stroke even after adjustment for arterial hypertension. The exact reasons for the relationship are not well understood.[74]

Snoring and Sudden Death

An autopsy was performed in 460 consecutive cases of sudden death among 35- to 76-year-old men. The closest cohabiting person to each deceased was interviewed. The mean age was 55.4 years, and the mean BMI was 26.3 kg/m². Among the obese snorers ($N = 82$), apneas had been observed "occasionally," "often," or "habitually" in 49 cases. Death was classified as cardiovascular in 186 cases (40.4%). Cardiovascular cause of death was more common among the habitual and frequent snorers than among occasional or never snorers. Habitual snorers died more often while sleeping. Habitual snoring was found to be a risk (odds ratio, 4.07; 95% CI, 1.45 to 11.45) for cardiovascular early morning death between 4 and 8 AM.[75]

In a follow-up study of 34 obese men, history of obstructive sleep apnea was a strong risk factor for sudden cardiovascular death. On autopsy, the degree of atherosclerosis was found to be moderate in all cases.[76] Thus, factors other than atherosclerotic coronary heart disease seem to be important as a cause of premature death in obese subjects. Habitual snoring with partial upper airway obstruction and OSAS are among these factors.

Snoring and Dementia

The occurrence of snoring was studied in 46 patients with Alzheimer's disease, in 37 patients with multiinfarct dementia, and in a random sample of 124 elderly community residents.[77]

The demented patients snored twice as frequently as did the control subjects. No difference in the occurrence of snoring was found between the two types of dementia. Vitiello and Prinz[78] studied 24 female patients with Alzheimer's disease and 26 control subjects. The mean AHIs among the female control subjects and the patients with Alzheimer's disease were 2 ± 0.4 and 9 ± 3, respectively. An association between the apolipoprotein E epsilon-4 allele and sleep apnea[79] may have some importance in the association of dementia and sleep-disordered breathing.

Evolution of Obstructive Sleep Apnea Syndrome

Evolution of OSAS and the effects of treatment are discussed in greater detail elsewhere in this book. OSAS may be a lethal disease if not treated. There are several studies showing an increased risk of cardiovascular complications and death in patients with at least moderate (AI > 20) or severe (AI > 40) OSAS.[80-82] The increased risk is found especially among middle-aged people with sleep-disordered breathing, but not in the elderly,[83,84] where several other risk factors for cardiovascular disease and death coexist with OSAS. In a Swedish study of 3100 men aged 30 to 69 years followed for 10 years, 213 men died, 88 of cardiovascular diseases. In that study isolated snoring or EDS displayed no significantly increased mortality, but the combination of snoring and EDS was associated with a significant increase in mortality. The relative rates decreased with increasing age, as in other studies.[85] Men younger than the age of 60 years with both snoring and EDS had an age-adjusted total death rate that was 2.7 times higher than men with no snoring or EDS (95% CI, 1.6 to 4.5). The corresponding age-adjusted hazard ratio for cardiovascular mortality was 2.9 (95% CI, 1.3 to 6.7) for subjects with both snoring and EDS. Further adjustment for BMI and reported hypertension, cardiac disease, and diabetes reduced the relative mortality risk associated with the combination of snoring and EDS to 2.2 (95% CI, 1.3 to 3.8) and the relative risk of cardiovascular mortality to 2.0 (95% CI, 0.8 to 4.7).[85] CPAP (see Chapter 89) is an effective treatment of OSAS and can reduce mortality rates. Weight loss may also be effective.[86] Although CPAP is highly regarded as an effective and even life-saving treatment for severe sleep-disordered breathing, well-done prospective epidemiologic studies are lacking regarding the long-term effect of CPAP in mild OSAS. There are no studies showing benefit of CPAP in simple snoring. Different surgical methods are used to treat snoring and sleep apnea, but there are only a few studies with acceptable epidemiologic methodology. Janson et al.[87] studied the long-term effects of uvulopalatopharyngoplasty in 34 patients with OSAS. Response to treatment was defined as a 50% or greater reduction in AHI and a postoperative AHI of 10 or less. Sixty-four percent were responders at 6 months and 48% were responders at 4 to 8 years after surgery. None of the seven patients with an initial AHI of more than 40 were responders.[87] More randomized, controlled trials are needed, as advocated by Wright et al.[4] Their systemic review of the CPAP literature demonstrated the lack of many good studies showing that sleep-disordered breathing is associated with cardiovascular disease among middle-aged subjects and that at least severe OSAS must be treated efficiently. Recent randomized trials show a modest CPAP effect on moderate and severe sleep apnea, especially if there are no symptoms of daytime sleepiness.[88-92]

OSAS is an important disease. It has also many economic consequences.[93,94] Much research, however, is needed before sleep researchers can convince others that OSAS and other sleep-related breathing disorders are important medical problems.

PARASOMNIAS

The parasomnias have been identified as a major category of sleep disorders (see Chapters 74-80). They represent a group of physiologic and behavioral phenomena that occur

Table 52–8.   Prevalence of Restless Legs Syndrome

Reference, Country	Population (N)	Methods, Criteria	Prevalence, %
Ekbom (1945),[174] Sweden	Patients in a physician's practice (500)	Presence of restless legs (original description)	5
Oboler et al. (1991),[175] Germany	Elderly veteran outpatients (515)	Reported restless legs	29
O'Keefe et al. (1993),[176] Ireland	Acute-care geriatric service patients (317)	Presence of restless legs	5 31% of the patients with RLS had S-ferritin level <18 ng/mL vs. 6% in subjects without RLS
Lavigne et al. (1994),[177] Canada	Population sample, age 18 yr+ (2019)	Leg restlessness at bedtime, face-to-face interviews	10–15
Phillips et al. (2000),[178] United States	Kentucky random population sample, men and women, aged ≥18 yr (1803)	Telephone interview, presence of restless legs five or more times/month At least once per month	18–29 yr: 3 30–79 yr: 10 80+ yr: 19 All ages: 19.4
Rothdach et al. (2000),[179] Berger et al. (2002),[180] Germany	German elderly population sample, age 65–83 yr (369)	RLS criteria and neurologic examination; IRLSSG criteria	Overall: 9.8 Men: 6.1 Women: 13.9 65–69 yr: 9.8 70–74 yr: 12.75 75+ yr: 7.4
Tan et al. (2001),[181] Singapore	General population sample subjects aged ≥55 yr (157), and 1000 consecutive patients aged ≥21 yr in a health center	IRLSSG criteria	0.6 in the population 0.1 among the patients
Ulfberg et al. (2001),[182] Sweden	A random male population sample in central Sweden (4000)	IRLSSG criteria	5.8
Ulfberg et al. (2001),[183] Sweden	Random sample of women in central Sweden, aged 18–64 yr (200)	IRLSSG criteria	11.4
Ohayon and Roth (2002),[184] Five European countries	United Kingdom, Germany, Italy, Portugal, and Spain; 18,980 subjects, aged 15–100 yr	Telephone survey, Sleep-EVAL with International Classification of Sleep Disorders criteria	RLS: 5.5 Periodic leg movements during the day: 3.9
Sevim et al. (2003),[185] Turkey	Turkish population, adults (3234)	IRLSSG criteria, face-to-face personal interviews	3.19
Bhowmik et al. (2003),[186] India	Case–control study, 121 hemodialysis patients and 99 control patients	Questionnaire with RLS criteria; electroneuromyography	Patients on hemodialysis: 6.6 Control patients: 0.0
Nichols et al. (2003),[187] United States	A primary care patient population seen by family physicians (2099)	IRLSSG criteria, examined by family physicians	All four symptoms present: 24.0 Symptoms present at least weekly: 15.3
Suzuki et al. (2003),[188] Japan	Japanese pregnant women (16,528)	Questionnaire survey in 500 maternity services	19.9

IRLSSG, International Restless Legs Syndrome Study Group; RLS, restless legs syndrome.

predominantly during sleep. The parasomnias are disorders of arousal, partial arousal, and sleep stage transition.[2]

The reader is asked to refer to the previous edition of this book for a table on parasomnia and further references on the epidemiology of parasomnias. See also Chapters 74-80 in this edition.

It is not easy to obtain reliable prevalences for parasomnias. One major problem is the definition of different parasomnias and the wording in questionnaires. It seems probable that sleep terror as a medical entity is largely unknown to people, and different types of nocturnal attacks of unpleasant nature (nightmares, panic attacks, and so on) may be reported as "sleep terrors." One additional problem is the obvious risk that the parasomnias occur without being noticed. Unless a cohabiting person reports, the subject may be unaware of the symptoms of sleeptalking or bruxism or of sleepwalking or sleep terror. Recall bias in retrospective questionnaire studies may also be a major factor that affects the results. Genetic factors also play an important role in different parasomnias.[95]

RESTLESS LEGS SYNDROME

RLS or Ekbom's syndrome is a neurologic disorder characterized by paresthesias in the limbs associated with an irresistible urge to move. The symptoms are provoked by rest and interfere with the ability to fall asleep or stay asleep, leading to chronic sleep deprivation. The pathophysiologic process of RLS is unknown, but it is hypothesized that the condition results from a deficiency in or dysfunction of dopaminergic transmission related to abnormalities of iron transport and storage.[96] Recent epidemiologic studies have verified that the condition is common in populations derived from the north and west of Europe,[97] and have begun to uncover some of the genetic substrate of the disorder. New instruments have been developed to facilitate diagnosis and assessment of severity.[98,99] Those are described elsewhere in this book (see Chapter 70).

RLS is common (Table 52–8). In general, the prevalence varies between 5% and 15%. The prevalence is higher among elderly people. In some patients groups, such as patients with end-stage renal disease, the prevalence may be higher than 20%. Also, more than 20% of pregnant women suffer from restless legs,[100] with different degrees of severity. RLS during pregnancy is related to low ferritin and folate levels.[100]

Clinical Pearl

Sleep disorders are among the most common complaints by patients seen by general practitioners. Insomnia, sleep apnea, and restless legs syndrome are of major public health importance. It is probable that nobody becomes totally exhausted or "burned out" as long as he or she sleeps well. Physicians should always ask questions at least about the quality and amount of sleep, daytime sleepiness, snoring history, and possible breathing pauses, and about feelings of restless legs.

REFERENCES

1. American Sleep Disorders Association: Diagnostic classification of sleep and arousal disorders. Sleep 1979;2:1-137.

2. American Academy of Sleep Medicine. International Classification of Sleep Disorders: Diagnostic and Coding Manual, 2nd ed. Westchester, Ill, American Academy of Sleep Medicine, 2005.

3. Feinstein A: Clinical Epidemiology: The Architecture of Clinical Research. Philadelphia, WB Saunders, 1985.

4. Wright J, Johns R, Watt I, et al: Health effects of obstructive sleep apnoea and the effectiveness of continuous positive airways pressure: A systematic review of the research evidence. BMJ 1997;314:851-860.

5. Torsvall L, Akerstedt T: A diurnal type scale: Construction, consistency and validation in shift work. Scand J Work Environ Health 1980;6:283-290.

6. Buysse D, Reynolds C III, Monk T, et al: The Pittsburgh Sleep Quality Index: A new instrument for psychiatric practice and research. Psychiatr Res 1989;28:193-213.

7. Johns MW: A new method for measuring daytime sleepiness: The Epworth Sleepiness Scale. Sleep 1991;14:540-545.

8. Hublin C, Kaprio J, Partinen M, et al: The Ullanlinna Narcolepsy Scale: Validation of a measure of symptoms in the narcoleptic syndrome. J Sleep Res 1994;3:52-59.

9. Partinen M, Gislason T: Basic Nordic Sleep Questionnaire (BNSQ): A quantitated measure of subjective sleep complaints. J Sleep Res 1995;4(Suppl 1):150-155.

10. Jenkinson C, Stradling J, Petersen S, et al: Comparison of three measures of quality of life outcome in the evaluation of continuous positive airways pressure therapy for sleep apnoea. J Sleep Res 1997;6:199-204.

11. Flemons WW, Reimer MA: Development of a disease-specific health-related quality of life questionnaire for sleep apnea. Am J Respir Crit Care Med 1998;158:494-503.

12. Chesson A, Hartse K, Anderson WM, et al: Practice parameters for the evaluation of chronic insomnia. An American Academy of Sleep Medicine report. Standards of Practice Committee of the American Academy of Sleep Medicine. Sleep 2000;23: 237-241.

12a. Laird D: The sleep habits of 509 men of distinction. Am Med 1931;37:271-275.

13. Bixler EO, Vgontzas AN, Lin HM, et al: Insomnia in central Pennsylvania. J Psychosom Res 2002;53:589-592.

14. Henderson S, Jorm AF, Scott LR, et al: Insomnia in the elderly: Its prevalence and correlates in the general population. Med J Aust 1995;162:22-24.

15. Husby R, Lingjaerde O: Prevalence of reported sleeplessness in northern Norway in relation to sex, age and season. Acta Psychiatr Scand 1990;81:542-547.

16. Ohayon M, Partinen M: Insomnia and global sleep dissatisfaction in Finland. J Sleep Res 2002;11:339-346.

17. Ohayon MM, Caulet M, Priest RG, Guilleminault C: DSM-IV and ICSD-90 insomnia symptoms and sleep dissatisfaction. Br J Psychiatry 1997;171:382-388.

17a. Costa e Silva JA, Chase M, Sartorius N, et al: Special report from a symposium held by the World Health Organization and the World Federation of Sleep Research Societies: An overview of insomnias and related disorders—recognition, epidemiology, and rational management. Sleep 1996;19:412-416.

18. Partinen M, Eskelinen L, Tuomi K: Complaints of insomnia in different occupations. Scand J Work Environ Health 1984; 10(6 Spec No):467-469.

19. Berwick D, Murphy J, Goldman P, et al: Performance of a five-item mental health screening test. Med Care 1991;29:169-176.

20. Mellinger GD, Balter MB, Uhlenhuth EH: Insomnia and its treatment: Prevalence and correlates. Arch Gen Psychiatry 1985; 42:225-232.

21. NOMESCO: Health Statistics in the Nordic Countries 2001. Copenhagen, NOMESCO, 2001.

22. Asplund R: Sleep and hypnotics among the elderly in relation to body weight and somatic disease. J Intern Med 1995;238:65-70.

23. Kripke DF, Klauber MR, Wingard DL, et al: Mortality hazard associated with prescription hypnotics. Biol Psychiatry 1998; 43:687-693.

24. Kojima M, Wakai K, Kawamura T, et al: Sleep patterns and total mortality: A 12-year follow-up study in Japan. J Epidemiol 2000;10:87-93.

25. Liu X, Uchiyama M, Kim K, et al: Sleep loss and daytime sleepiness in the general adult population of Japan. Psychiatry Res 2000;93:1-11.

26. Hublin C, Kaprio J, Partinen M, Koskenvuo M: Insufficient sleep: A population-based study in adults. Sleep 2001;24: 392-400.

27. Broman JE, Lundh LG, Hetta J: Insufficient sleep in the general population. Neurophysiol Clin 1996;26:30-39.

28. Johns M, Hocking B: Daytime sleepiness and sleep habits of Australian workers. Sleep 1997;20:844-849.

29. Hublin C, Kaprio J, Partinen M, et al: The prevalence of narcolepsy: An epidemiological study of the Finnish Twin Cohort. Ann Neurol 1994;35:709-716.

30. Wing YK, Li RH, Lam CW, et al: The prevalence of narcolepsy among Chinese in Hong Kong. Ann Neurol 2002;51:578-584.

31. Koskenvuo M, Partinen M, Kaprio J: Snoring and disease. Ann Clin Res 1985;17:247-251.

32. Young T, Palta M, Dempsey J, et al: The occurrence of sleep-disordered breathing among middle-aged adults. N Engl J Med 1993;328:1230-1235.

33. Lugaresi E, Mondini S, Zucconi M, et al: Staging of heavy snorers' disease: A proposal. Bull Eur Physiopathol Respir 1983;19:590-594.

34. Tiihonen M, Partinen M, Närvänen S: The severity of obstructive sleep apnoea is associated with insulin resistance. J Sleep Res 1993;2:56-61.

35. Grunstein RR: Metabolic aspects of sleep apnea. Sleep 1996; 19(10 Suppl):S218-S220.

36. Lavie P, Herer P, Hoffstein V: Obstructive sleep apnoea syndrome as a risk factor for hypertension: Population study. BMJ 2000; 320:479-482.

37. Peppard PE, Young T, Palta M, Skatrud J: Prospective study of the association between sleep-disordered breathing and hypertension. N Engl J Med 2000;342:1378-1384.

38. Bixler EO, Vgontzas AN, Ten Have T, et al: Effects of age on sleep apnea in men: I. Prevalence and severity. Am J Respir Crit Care Med 1998;157:144-148.

39. Bixler EO, Vgontzas AN, Lin HM, et al: Prevalence of sleep-disordered breathing in women: Effects of gender. Am J Respir Crit Care Med 2001;163:608-613.

40. Dancey DR, Hanly PJ, Soong C, et al: Impact of menopause on the prevalence and severity of sleep apnea. Chest 2001;120:151-155.

41. Gislason T, Almqvist M, Eriksson G, et al: Prevalence of sleep apnea syndrome among Swedish men: An epidemiological study. J Clin Epidemiol 1988;41:571-576.

42. Telakivi T, Partinen M, Koskenvuo M, et al: Periodic breathing and hypoxia in snorers and controls: Validation of snoring history and association with blood pressure and obesity. Acta Neurol Scand 1987;76:69-75.

43. Marin JM, Gascon JM, Carrizo S, Gispert J: Prevalence of sleep apnoea syndrome in the Spanish adult population. Int J Epidemiol 1997;26:381-386.

44. Ferini-Strambi L, Zucconi M, Palazzi S, et al: Snoring and nocturnal oxygen desaturations in an Italian middle-aged male population: Epidemiologic study with an ambulatory device. Chest 1994;105:1759-1764.

45. Katz I, Stradling J, Slutsky S, et al: Do patients with obstructive sleep apnea have thick necks? Am Rev Respir Dis 1990; 141:1228-1231.

46. Pekkarinen T, Partinen M, Pelkonen R, Iivanainen M: Sleep apnoea and daytime sleepiness in acromegaly: Relationship to endocrinological factors. Clin Endocrinol 1987;27:649-654.

47. Rosenow F, Reuter S, Deuss U, et al: Sleep apnoea in treated acromegaly: Relative frequency and predisposing factors. Clin Endocrinol 1996;45:563-569.

48. Kiuru S, Nieminen T, Partinen M: Obstructive sleep apnoea syndrome in hereditary gelsolin-related amyloidosis. J Sleep Res 1999;8:143-149.

49. Gislason T, Benediktsdottir B: Snoring, apneic episodes, and nocturnal hypoxemia among children 6 months to 6 years old: An epidemiologic study of lower limit of prevalence. Chest 1995;107:963-966.

50. Ali N, Pitson D, Stradling J: Snoring, sleep disturbance, and behaviour in 4-5 year olds. Arch Dis Child 1993;68:360-366.

51. Ancoli-Israel S, Kripke DF, Klauber MR, et al: Sleep-disordered breathing in community-dwelling elderly. Sleep 1991;14:486-495.

52. Bliwise D, Bliwise N, Partinen M, et al: Sleep apnea and mortality in an aged cohort. Am J Public Health 1988;78:544-547.

53. Ancoli-Israel S, Kripke DF, Klauber MR, et al: Morbidity, mortality and sleep-disordered breathing in community dwelling elderly. Sleep 1996;19:277-282.

54. Kryger MH, Roth T, Dement WC (eds): Principles and Practice of Sleep Medicine, 3rd ed. Philadelphia, WB Saunders, 2000.

55. Lugaresi E, Cirignotta F, Coggagna G, Piana C: Some epidemiological data on snoring and cardiocirculatory disturbances. Sleep 1980;3:221-224.

56. Koskenvuo M, Kaprio J, Partinen M, et al: Snoring as a risk factor for hypertension and angina pectoris. Lancet 1985;1: 893-896.

57. Gislason T, Aberg H, Taube A: Snoring and systemic hypertension: An epidemiological study. Acta Med Scand 1987;222:415-421.

58. Nieto FJ, Young TB, Lind BK, et al: Association of sleep-disordered breathing, sleep apnea, and hypertension in a large community-based study: Sleep Heart Health Study. JAMA 2000;283:1829-1836.

59. Hu FB, Willett WC, Colditz GA, et al: Prospective study of snoring and risk of hypertension in women. Am J Epidemiol 1999;150:806-816.

60. Worsnop CJ, Naughton MT, Barter CE, et al: The prevalence of obstructive sleep apnea in hypertensives. Am J Respir Crit Care Med 1998;157:111-115.

61. Logan AG, Perlikowski SM, Mente A, et al: High prevalence of unrecognized sleep apnoea in drug-resistant hypertension. J Hypertens 2001;19:2271-2277.

62. Shepard JJ: Hypertension, cardiac arrhythmias, myocardial infarction, and stroke in relation to obstructive sleep apnea. Clin Chest Med 1992;13:437-458.

63. Koskenvuo M, Kaprio J, Telakivi T, et al: Snoring as a risk factor for ischaemic heart disease and stroke in men. BMJ 1987; 294:16-19.

64. Olson L, King M, Hensley M, Saunders N: A community study of snoring and sleep-disordered breathing. Health outcomes. Am J Respir Crit Care Med 1995;152:717-720.

65. Franklin K, Nilsson J, Sahlin K, et al: Sleep apnea and nocturnal angina. Lancet 1995;345:1085-1087.

66. Javaheri S, Parker TJ, Liming JD, et al: Sleep apnea in 81 ambulatory male patients with stable heart failure: Types and their prevalences, consequences, and presentations. Circulation 1998;97:2154-2159.

67. D'Alessandro R, Magelli C, Gamberini G, et al: Snoring every night as a risk factor for myocardial infarction: A case-control study. BMJ 1990;300:1557-1558.

68. Hung J, Whitford E, Parsons R, Hillman D: Association of sleep apnoea with myocardial infarction in men. Lancet 1990;336: 261-264.

69. Andreas S, Schulz R, Werner GS, Kreuzer H: Prevalence of obstructive sleep apnoea in patients with coronary artery disease. Coron Artery Dis 1996;7:541-545.

70. Partinen M, Palomäki H: Snoring and cerebral infarction. Lancet 1985;2:1325-1326.

71. Palomäki H: Snoring and the risk of ischemic brain infarction. Stroke 1991;22:1021-1025.

72. Smirne S, Palazzi S, Zucconi M, et al: Habitual snoring as a risk - factor for acute vascular disease. Eur Respir J 1993;6:1357-1361.

73. Neau J, Meurice J, Paquereau J, et al: Habitual snoring as a risk factor for brain infarction. Acta Neurol Scand 1995;92:63-68.

74. Neau JP, Paquereau J, Meurice JC, et al: Stroke and sleep apnoea: Cause or consequence? Sleep Med Rev 2002;6:457-469.

75. Seppälä T, Partinen M, Penttilä A, et al: Sudden death and sleeping history among Finnish men. J Intern Med 1991; 229:23-28.

76. Rossner S, Lagerstrand L, Persson H, Sachs C: The sleep apnoea syndrome in obesity: Risk of sudden death. J Intern Med 1991;230:135-141.

77. Erkinjuntti T, Partinen M, Sulkava R, et al: Snoring and dementia. Age Ageing 1987;16:305-310.

78. Vitiello M, Prinz P: Sleep/wake patterns and sleep disorders in Alzheimer's disease. In Thorpy MJ (ed): Handbook of Sleep Disorders. New York, Marcel Dekker, 1990, pp 703-718.

79. Foley DJ, Masaki K, White L, Redline S: Relationship between apolipoprotein E epsilon4 and sleep-disordered breathing at different ages. JAMA 2001;286:1447-1448.

80. He J, Kryger M, Zorick F, et al: Mortality and apnea index in obstructive sleep apnea. Chest 1988;94:9-14.

81. Partinen M, Jamieson A, Guilleminault C: Long-term outcome for obstructive sleep apnea syndrome patients: Mortality. Chest 1988;94:1200-1204.

82. Partinen M, Guilleminault C: Daytime sleepiness and vascular morbidity at seven-year follow-up in obstructive sleep apnea patients. Chest 1990;97:27-32.

83. Lavie P, Herer P, Peled R, et al: Mortality in sleep apnea patients: A multivariate analysis of risk factors. Sleep 1995;18:149-157.

84. Noda A, Okada T, Yasuma F, et al: Prognosis of the middle-aged and aged patients with obstructive sleep apnea syndrome. Psychiatry Clin Neurosci 1998;52:79-85.

85. Lindberg E, Janson C, Svardsudd K, et al: Increased mortality among sleepy snorers: A prospective population based study [see comments]. Thorax 1998;53:631-637.

86. Kajaste S, Brander P, Telakivi T, et al: A cognitive-behavioral weight reduction program in the treatment of obstructive sleep apnea syndrome with or without initial nasal CPAP: A randomized study. Sleep Med 2004;5:125-131.

87. Janson C, Gislason T, Bengtsson H, et al: Long-term follow-up of patients with obstructive sleep apnea treated with uvulopalatopharyngoplasty. Arch Otolaryngol Head Neck Surg 1997;123:257-262.

88. Lojander J, Maasilta P, Partinen M, et al: Nasal-CPAP, surgery, and conservative management for treatment of obstructive sleep apnea syndrome: A randomized study. Chest 1996; 110:114-119.

89. Engleman HM, Kingshott RN, Wraith PK, et al: Randomized placebo-controlled crossover trial of continuous positive airway pressure for mild sleep apnea/hypopnea syndrome. Am J Respir Crit Care Med 1999;159:461-467.

90. Dimsdale JE, Loredo JS, Profant J: Effect of continuous positive airway pressure on blood pressure: A placebo trial. Hypertension 2000;35:144-147.

91. Barbe F, Mayoralas LR, Duran J, et al: Treatment with continuous positive airway pressure is not effective in patients with sleep apnea but no daytime sleepiness: A randomized, controlled trial. Ann Intern Med 2001;134:1015-1023.

92. Montserrat JM, Ferrer M, Hernandez L, et al: Effectiveness of CPAP treatment in daytime function in sleep apnea syndrome: A randomized controlled study with an optimized placebo. Am J Respir Crit Care Med 2001;164:608-613.

93. Kryger MH, Roos L, Delaive K, et al: Utilization of health care services in patients with severe obstructive sleep apnea. Sleep 1996;19(9 Suppl):S111-S116.

94. Ronald J, Delaive K, Roos L, et al: Health care utilization in the 10 years prior to diagnosis in obstructive sleep apnea syndrome patients. Sleep 1999;22:225-229.

95. Hublin C, Kaprio J: Genetic aspects and genetic epidemiology of parasomnias. Sleep Med Rev 2003;7:413-421.

96. Allen RP: Race, iron status and restless legs syndrome. Sleep Med 2002;3:467-468.

97. Desautels A, Turecki G, Montplaisir J, et al: Identification of a major susceptibility locus for restless legs syndrome on chromosome 12q. Am J Hum Genet 2001;69:1266-1270.

98. Allen RP, Picchietti D, Hening WA, et al: Restless legs syndrome: Diagnostic criteria, special considerations, and epidemiology: A report from the restless legs syndrome diagnosis and epidemiology workshop at the National Institutes of Health. Sleep Med 2003;4:101-119.

99. Hening WA, Allen RP: Restless legs syndrome (RLS): The continuing development of diagnostic standards and severity measures. Sleep Med 2003;4:95-97.

100. Lee KA, Zaffke ME, Baratte-Beebe K: Restless legs syndrome and sleep disturbance during pregnancy: The role of folate and iron. J Womens Health Gend Based Med 2001;10:335-341.

101. Saarenpää-Heikkilä O, Rintahaka P, Laippala P, Koivikko M: Sleep habits and disorders in Finnish schoolchildren. J Sleep Res 1995;4:173-182.

102. Tynjälä J, Kannas L, Välimaa R: How young Europeans sleep. Health Educ Res 1993;8:69-80.

103. Lugaresi E, Cirignotta F, Zucconi M, et al: Good and poor sleepers: An epidemiological survey of the San Marino population. In Guilleminault C, Lugaresi E (eds): Sleep/Wake Disorders: Natural History, Epidemiology, and Long-Term Evolution. New York, Raven Press, 1983, pp 1-12.

104. Cirignotta F, Mondini S, Zucconi M, et al: Insomnia: An epidemiological survey. Clin Neuropharmacol 1985;8(Suppl 1): S49-S54.

105. Smirne S, Franceschi M, Zamproni P, et al: Prevalence of sleep disorders in an unselected inpatient population. In Guilleminault C, Lugaresi E (eds): Sleep/Wake Disorders: Natural History, Epidemiology, and Long-Term Evolution. New York, Raven Press, 1983, pp 61-71.

106. Partinen M, Rimpelä M: Sleeping habits and sleep disorders in a population of 2,016 Finnish adults. In The Yearbook of Health Education Research 1982. Helsinki, Finland, The National Board of Health, 1982, pp 253-260.

107. Yeo BK, Perera IS, Kok LP, Tsoi WF: Insomnia in the community. Singapore Med J 1996;37:282-284.

108. Hohagen F, Grabhoff U, Ellringmann D, et al: The prevalence of insomnia in different age groups and its treatment modalities in general practice. In Smirne S, Franceschi M, Ferini-Strambi L (eds): Sleep and Ageing. Milan, Masson, 1991, pp 205-215.

109. Ford D, Kamerow D: Epidemiologic study of sleep disturbances and psychiatric disorders: An opportunity for prevention? JAMA 1989;262:1479-1484.

110. Weissman MM, Greenwald S, Nino-Murcia G, Dement WC: The morbidity of insomnia uncomplicated by psychiatric disorders. Gen Hosp Psychiatry 1997;19:245-250.

111. Dodge R, Cline MG, Quan SF: The natural history of insomnia and its relationship to respiratory symptoms. Arch Intern Med 1995;155:1797-1800.

112. Morgan K, Clarke D: Risk factors for late-life insomnia in a representative general practice sample. Br J Gen Pract 1997; 47:166-169.

113. Kim K, Uchiyama M, Okawa M, et al: An epidemiological study of insomnia among the Japanese general population. Sleep 2000;23:41-47.

114. Blader JC, Koplewicz HS, Abikoff H, Foley C: Sleep problems of elementary school children: A community survey. Arch Pediatr Adolesc Med 1997;151:473-480.

115. Morrison DN, McGee R, Stanton WR: Sleep problems in adolescence. J Am Acad Child Adolesc Psychiatry 1992;31:94-99.

116. Ohayon M: Epidemiological study on insomnia in the general population. Sleep 1996;19(3 Suppl):S7-S15.

117. Bixler EO, Kales A, Soldatos CR, et al: Prevalence of sleep disorders in the Los Angeles metropolitan area. Am J Psychiatry 1979;136:1257-1262.

118. Karacan I, Thornby J, Williams R: Sleep disturbance: A community survey. In Guilleminault C, Lugaresi E (eds): Sleep/Wake Disorders: Natural History, Epidemiology, and Long-Term Evolution. New York, Raven Press, 1983, pp 37-60.

119. Ganguli M, Reynolds CF, Gilby JE: Prevalence and persistence of sleep complaints in a rural older community sample: The MoVIES project. J Am Geriatr Soc 1996;44:778-784.

120. Blazer DG, Hays JC, Foley DJ: Sleep complaints in older adults: A racial comparison. J Gerontol A Biol Sci Med Sci 1995; 50:M280-M284.

121. Foley DJ, Monjan AA, Brown SL, et al: Sleep complaints among elderly persons: An epidemiologic study of three communities. Sleep 1995;18:425-432.

122. Liljenberg B, Almqvist M, Hetta J, et al: The prevalence of insomnia: The importance of operationally defined criteria. Ann Clin Res 1988;20:393-398.

123. Kirmil-Gray K, Eagleston J, Gibson E, Thoresen CE: Sleep disturbance in adolescents: Sleep quality, sleep habits, beliefs about sleep, and daytime functioning. J Youth Adolesc 1984;13:375-384.

124. Lack L: Delayed sleep and sleep loss in university students. J Am Coll Health 1986;35:105-110.

125. Janson C, De Backer W, Gislason T, et al: Increased prevalence of sleep disturbances and daytime sleepiness in subjects with bronchial asthma: A population study of young adults in three European countries. Eur Respir J 1996;9:2132-2138.

126. Simen S, Rodenbeck A, Schlaf G, et al: Sleep complaints and hypnotic use by the elderly: Results of a representative survey in West Germany. Wien Med Wochenschr 1996; 146:306-309.

127. Johnson EO, Roehrs T, Roth T, Breslau N: Epidemiology of alcohol and medication as aids to sleep in early adulthood. Sleep 1998;21:178-186.

128. Partinen M, Kaprio J, Koskenvuo M, Langinvainio H: Sleeping habits, sleep quality and use of sleeping pills: A population study of 31,140 adults in Finland. In Guilleminault C, Lugaresi E (eds): Sleep/Wake Disorders: Natural History, Epidemiology, and Long-Term Evolution. New York, Raven Press, 1983, pp 29-35.

129. Lopez AT, Sanchez EG, Torres FG, et al: Hábitos y trastornos del dormir en residentes del área metropolitana de Monterrey. Salud Mental 1995;18:14-22.

130. Hyyppä M, Kronholm E: How does Finland sleep? Sleeping habits of the Finnish adult population and the rehabilitation of sleep disturbances [in Finnish]. Publ Soc Insurance Inst Finland 1987;ML:68:110.

131. Morgan K, Dalloso H, Ebrahim S, et al: Prevalence, frequency, and duration of hypnotic drug use among the elderly living at home. BMJ 1988;296:601-602.

132. Karacan I, Thornby JI, Anch M, et al: Prevalence of sleep disturbance in a primary urban Florida county. Soc Sci Med 1976;10:239-244.

133. Partinen M: Sleeping habits and sleep disorders on Finnish men before, during and after military service. Ann Med Milit Fenn 1982;57(Suppl 1):1-96.

134. Billiard M, Alperovitch A, Perot C, Jammes A: Excessive daytime somnolence in young men: Prevalence and contributing factors. Sleep 1987;10:297-305.

135. Schmidt-Nowara WW, Wiggins CL, Walch JK: Sleepiness in an adult population: Prevalence, validity and correlates. In Peter JH, Podszus T, von Wichert P (eds): Sleep and Health Risk. Berlin, Springer-Verlag, 1991, pp 78-83.

136. Klink M, Quan SF: Prevalence of reported sleep disturbances in a general adult population and their relationship to obstructive airway diseases. Chest 1987;91:540-546.

137. Hays JC, Blazer DG, Foley DJ: Risk of napping: excessive daytime sleepiness and mortality in an older community population. J Am Geriatr Soc 1996;44:693-698.

138. Berg Kelly K, Ehrver M, Erneholm T, et al: Self-reported health status and use of medical care by 3500 adolescents in Western Sweden. Acta Pediatr Scand 1991;80:837-843.

139. Martikainen K, Hasan J, Urponen H, et al: Daytime sleepiness: A risk factor in community life. Acta Neurol Scand 1992;86: 337-341.

140. Hublin C, Kaprio J, Partinen M, et al: Daytime sleepiness in an adult, Finnish population. J Intern Med 1996;239:417-423.

141. Ohayon MM, Caulet M, Philip P, et al: How sleep and mental disorders are related to complaints of daytime sleepiness. Arch Intern Med 1997;157:2645-2652.

142. Solomon P: Narcolepsy in Negroes. Dis Nerv Syst 1945; 6:179-183.

143. Roth B: Narcolepsy and Hypersomnia. Basel, Karger, 1980.

144. Dement W, Zarcone V, Varner V, et al: The prevalence of narcolepsy. Sleep Res 1972;1:148.

145. Dement W, Carskadon M, Ley R: The prevalence of narcolepsy: II. Sleep Res 1973;2:147.

146. Honda Y: Census of narcolepsy, cataplexy and sleep life among teen-agers in Fujisawa City. Sleep Res 1979;8:191.

147. Honda Y, Asaka A, Tanimura M, Furusho T: A genetic study of narcolepsy and excessive daytime sleepiness in 308 families with a narcolepsy or hypersomnia proband. In Guilleminault C, Lugaresi E (eds): Sleep/Wake Disorders: Natural History, Epidemiology, and Long-Term Evolution. New York, Raven Press, 1983, pp 187-199.

148. Franceschi M, Zamproni P, Crippa D, Smirne S: Excessive daytime sleepiness: A 1-year study in an unselected inpatient population. Sleep 1982;5:239-247.

149. Wilner AS, Lavie L, Peled P, et al: Narcolepsy-cataplexy in Israeli Jews is associated exclusively with the HLA DR2 haplotype. Hum Immunol 1988;21:15-22.

150. Tashiro T, Kanbayashi T, Iijima S, Hishikawa Y: An epidemiological study on prevalence of narcolepsy in Japanese. J Sleep Res 1992;1(Suppl 1):228.

151. al Rajeh S, Bademosi O, Ismail H, et al: A community survey of neurological disorders in Saudi Arabia: The Thugbah Study. Neuroepidemiology 1993;12:164-178.

152. Ohayon MM, Priest RG, Caulet M, Guilleminault C: Hypnagogic and hypnopompic hallucinations: Pathological phenomena? Br J Psychiatry 1996;169:459-467.

153. Silber MH, Krahn LE, Olson EJ, Pankratz VS: The epidemiology of narcolepsy in Olmsted County, Minnesota: A population-based study. Sleep 2002;25:197-202.

154. Ohayon MM, Priest JH, Zulley J, et al: Prevalence of narcolepsy, symptomatology and diagnosis in the European general population. Neurology 2002;58:1826-1833.

155. Norton PG, Dunn EV: Snoring as a risk factor for disease: An epidemiological survey. BMJ 1985;291:630-632.

156. Cirignotta F, D'Alessandro R, Partinen M, et al: Prevalence of every night snoring and obstructive sleep apnoeas among 30–69-year-old men in Bologna, Italy. Acta Neurol Scand 1989; 79:366-372.

157. Corbo G, Fuciarelli F, Foresi A, De Benedetto F: Snoring in children: Association with respiratory symptoms and passive smoking. BMJ 1989;299:1491-1494.

158. Schmidt-Nowara WW, Coultas DB, Wiggins C, et al: Snoring in a Hispanic-American population: Risk factors and association with hypertension and other morbidity. Arch Intern Med 1990; 150:597-601.

159. Ohta Y, Okada T, Kawakami Y, et al: Prevalence of risk factors for sleep apnea in Japan: A preliminary report. Sleep 1993; 16(8 Suppl):S6-S7.

160. Jennum P, Sjol A: Self-assessed cognitive function in snorers and sleep apneics: An epidemiological study of 1,504 females and males aged 30-60 years: The Dan-MONICA II Study. Eur Neurol 1994;34:204-208.

161. Teculescu DB, Caillier I, Perrin P, et al: Snoring in French preschool children. Pediatr Pulmonol 1992;13:239-244.

162. Kayukawa Y, Shirakawa S, Hayakawa T, et al: Habitual snoring in an outpatient population in Japan. Psychiatry Clin Neurosci 2000;54:385-391.

163. Lavie P: Sleep apnea in industrial workers. In Guilleminault C, Lugaresi E (eds): Sleep/Wake Disorders: Natural History, Epidemiology, and Long-Term Evolution. New York, Raven Press, 1983, pp 127-135.

164. Peter J, Siegrist J, Podszus T, et al: Prevalence of sleep apnea in healthy industrial workers. Klin Wochenschr 1985;63: 807-811.

165. Stradling J, Crosby J: Predictors and prevalence of obstructive sleep apnoea and snoring in 1001 middle age men. Thorax 1991;46:85-90.

166. Haraldsson PO, Carenfelt C, Tingvall C: Sleep apnea syndrome symptoms and automobile driving in a general population. J Clin Epidemiol 1992;45:821-825.

167. Gislason T, Benediktsdottir B, Bjornsson J, et al: Snoring, hypertension, and the sleep apnea syndrome: An epidemiologic survey of middle-aged women. Chest 1993;103: 1147-1151.

168. Olson L, King M, Hensley MJ, Saunders NA: A community study of snoring and sleep-disordered breathing: Prevalence. Am J Respir Crit Care Med 1995;152:711-716.

169. Bearpark H, Elliott L, Grunstein R, et al: Snoring and sleep apnea: A population study in Australian men. Am J Respir Crit Care Med 1995;151:1459-1465.

170. Esnaola S, Duran J, Rubio R, Iztueta A: Prevalence of obstructive sleep apnea in the male population of Vittoria-Gasteiz, Spain. In European Seminar on Sleep Disordered Breathing, February 1995 (abstract).

171. Ohayon MM, Guilleminault C, Priest RG, Caulet M: Snoring and breathing pauses during sleep: Telephone interview survey of a United Kingdom population sample. BMJ 1997;314: 860-863.

172. Kripke DF, Ancoli-Israel S, Klauber MR, et al: Prevalence of sleep-disordered breathing in ages 40-64 years: A population-based survey. Sleep 1997;20:65-76.

173. Hui DS, Chan JK, Ho AS, et al: Prevalence of snoring and sleep-disordered breathing in a student population. Chest 1999; 116:1530-1536.

174. Ekbom K: Restless legs. Acta Med Scand Suppl 1945; 158:1-123.

175. Oboler SK, Prochazka AV, Meyer TJ: Leg symptoms in outpatient veterans [see comments]. West J Med 1991;155: 256-259.

176. O'Keeffe S, Noel J, Lavan JN: Restless legs syndrome in the elderly. Postgrad Med J 1993;69:701-703.

177. Lavigne GJ, Montplaisir JY: Restless legs syndrome and sleep bruxism: Prevalence and association among Canadians. Sleep 1994;17:739-743.

178. Phillips B, Young T, Finn L, et al: Epidemiology of restless legs symptoms in adults. Arch Intern Med 2000;160: 2137-2141.

179. Rothdach AJ, Trenkwalder C, Haberstock J, et al: Prevalence and risk factors of RLS in an elderly population: The MEMO Study. Memory and Morbidity in Augsburg Elderly. Neurology 2000;54:1064-1068.

180. Berger K, von Eckardstein A, Trenkwalder C, et al: Iron metabolism and the risk of restless legs syndrome in an elderly general population: The MEMO Study. J Neurol 2002;249: 1195-1199.

181. Tan EK, Seah A, See SJ, et al: Restless legs syndrome in an Asian population: A study in Singapore. Mov Disord 2001; 16:577-579.

182. Ulfberg J, Nystrom B, Carter N, Edling C: Prevalence of restless legs syndrome among men aged 18 to 64 years: An association with somatic disease and neuropsychiatric symptoms. Mov Disord 2001;16:1159-1163.

183. Ulfberg J, Nystrom B, Carter N, Edling C: Restless legs syndrome among working-aged women. Eur Neurol 2001; 46:17-19.

184. Ohayon MM, Roth T: Prevalence of restless legs syndrome and periodic limb movement disorder in the general population. J Psychosom Res 2002;53:547-554.

185. Sevim S, Dogu O, Camdeviren H, et al: Unexpectedly low prevalence and unusual characteristics of RLS in Mersin, Turkey. Neurology 2003;61:1562-1569.

186. Bhowmik D, Bhatia M, Gupta S, et al: Restless legs syndrome in hemodialysis patients in India: A case controlled study. Sleep Med 2003;4:143-146.

187. Nichols DA, Allen RP, Grauke JH, et al: Restless legs syndrome symptoms in primary care: A prevalence study. Arch Intern Med 2003;163:2323-2329.

188. Suzuki K, Ohida T, Sone T, et al: The prevalence of restless legs syndrome among pregnant women in Japan and the relationship between restless legs syndrome and sleep problems. Sleep 2003;26:673-677.

53

Sleep Medicine, Public Policy, and Public Health

James K. Walsh

William C. Dement

David F. Dinges

ABSTRACT

A sizable body of knowledge comprises the sleep medicine field and a significant proportion relates to public health in a number of ways. The prevalence of sleep disorders and the widespread occurrence of sleep deprivation in modern society affect the public through industrial and transportation accidents, and in reduced performance in the workplace and in educational settings. Sleep disturbances also may contribute to epidemic societal levels of hypertension and cardiovascular disease, obesity, and diabetes. In part, the failure of the biomedical community to translate research advances into educational messages, interventional research, individual lifestyle changes, and institutional and public policies underlies the heavy public health burden. The minimal responsiveness of policy makers in many industries and the government also contributes to the impact on public health. Health professionals in general, and sleep specialists specifically, are encouraged to participate in the translation of sleep medicine advances for the betterment of society.

Sleep is among the most basic of human needs. Waking brain function and behavioral capability depend on obtaining adequate sleep quality and quantity each day. As amply illustrated throughout this book, a person's sleep can be disrupted not only by pathologic processes but also by a person's lifestyle and by societal demands on the sleep–wake schedule.[1] When sleep disruption occurs, regardless of the reason, the consequences for the individual and in some circumstances for society can be serious. At present there is only limited recognition of this fundamental fact because of failure to translate advances in sleep science and medicine into educational programs and institutional action directed toward improved public health and safety.

Sleep medicine constitutes an important public health resource because of the widespread and diverse ways in which sleep and sleepiness are related to public health and safety. Health professionals have always had a major role in decisions regarding public health issues. One does not have to look far to find cogent examples of behavioral and societal changes that were initiated by and through the health care system that reduced the prevalence of catastrophic outcomes. Physicians advanced the knowledge of linkages between "unseen" microbes and disease, which led to improvements in food preparation and waste disposal. Pulmonologists led the way in reducing cigarette smoking. Emergency department physicians helped

implement mandatory seatbelt laws. These and many other public health initiatives have saved millions of lives, and improved the quality of life for many more. It can be argued that sleep loss and sleepiness are other "unseen" threats to public health. It is now appropriate and necessary to develop similar educational and regulatory approaches to improve society's understanding of sleep and sleep disorders, and to modernize public policies that affect the quantity and quality of sleep. By communicating what has been learned about the effects of sleep disturbances, sleep loss, and sleepiness on public health and safety, health care professionals can contribute to the formulation of behaviors and public policies that promote healthy sleep and prevent sleepiness on the job and during other safety-sensitive activities such as driving.[2-4]

The purpose of this chapter is to review aspects of sleep science and sleep medicine from a societal perspective and to facilitate translation of that knowledge into behaviors and practices that will have a positive impact on public health. The public health benefits of enhanced application of research findings in various biomedical fields have recently received increased attention.[5]

SLEEP IN MODERN SOCIETY

Sleep, like many other aspects of human activity, has been irrevocably altered by the industrial revolution and its attendant artificial light and affordable energy. Around-the-clock operations are now commonplace and the time traditionally allocated to sleep has given way to expanded hours for business, long commutes, recreation, and so on. As societies make the transition from agrarian economies to industrial economies, some of the more dramatic changes that occur involve sleep. For example, the transition to industrialization typically involves elimination of daytime siesta and implementation of shift work.[6-8] The advent of highly technological societies has made inadequate daily sleep and substandard levels of waking alertness commonplace for many people. As a result, there is a risk of sleepiness-related human errors in many segments of society, such as public transportation, energy plants, security and public safety, and military operations. Errors in situations such as these can have catastrophic consequences. When such catastrophes have occurred on the night shift, such as the event at Three Mile Island nuclear power plant and the grounding of the *Exxon Valdez* oil tanker, public trust in these industries has been undermined.[2]

Technological advances have markedly reduced or eliminated many sources of accidents, but sleep deprivation and its consequent fatigue and human error continue to contribute to performance failures and accidents throughout society.[8] Automation has potentiated the negative effects of reduced alertness by increasing the monotony involved in many jobs, leaving people to stand vigil—an activity that is especially susceptible to elevated sleep pressure and sleepiness.[9,10] At present, human error causes the majority (60% to 90%) of all industrial and transportation accidents.[2,9] Although the proportion that is directly related to sleep loss, fatigue, and sleepiness is unknown, the economic and human impact is undoubtedly substantial.

Unfortunately and ironically nearly 100 years of technological advances aimed at improving life has been accompanied by a parallel reduction in societal priority for adequate sleep. For example, in 1913, 8- to 12-year-old schoolchildren slept an average of 10.5 hours per night[11]; by 1964, the average had dropped to 9.2 hours per night.[12] In 1994, 13- to 14-year-olds averaged 7.7 hours on school nights and 9.5 hours on weekends.[13] Failure to understand the effect of inadequate sleep on the entire 24-hour cycle has created a public health problem. Even modest amounts of daily sleep loss accumulate as a *sleep debt* that is manifest as an increasing tendency to fall asleep[14,15] and a reduced level of neurobehavioral function.[15,16] Although most people can resist this tendency under normal circumstances, when physical activity is low and circadian alerting effects are minimal, the likelihood of a lapse in vigilance, a "microsleep," or a longer sleep episode can become high. People who are directly responsible for public health and safety, including but not limited to doctors and nurses, often work night shifts and long hours that make them prone to sleepiness-related errors.[17] In work environments where sustained attention is necessary for safety, the probability of an accident rises and falls along with the biologic tendency to fall asleep.[18] Thus, catastrophic accidents related to sleepiness and fatigue do not occur at random throughout the day. Rather, they are more likely at times when human beings are most prone to sleep, between midnight and 8 AM and between 1 and 3 PM.[19-21]

THE CHALLENGE

Most people, including many involved in public health and public policy, do not know the fundamentals of homeostatic sleep need and circadian physiology; and most remain unaware of, or choose to ignore, important relationships between sleepiness and human waking performance capacity. Societal ignorance about the importance of sleep stems in part from the relative recency of scientific and medical advances in this area. In addition, our educational systems have been slow to integrate into course work even the most fundamental principles of the field, such as that the effects of chronic sleep restriction on the ability to perform are cumulative (see Chapter 6), or that adolescents require much more sleep than they routinely obtain,[22] or that driving while sleepy is as risky as driving while impaired by alcohol.[23] Rather, if any sleep material is presented it tends to focus on descriptive information that is largely irrelevant to public health, such as sleep stages or dreaming.

The challenge sleep specialists face is to develop methods to translate the body of sleep medicine knowledge into messages and strategies directed toward reducing or resolving the economic, social, health, and safety issues associated with insufficient or disrupted sleep. Such translation is essential if the knowledge of sleep science is positively to influence public health. Lessons from other areas of medicine that led to major societal policy and behavior changes, and subsequently to improved public health, are instructive. For example, changes in societal behavior and institutional policies have now made it possible to limit the public health impact of communicable diseases. Similarly, changes in public policy have reduced motor vehicle crash fatalities and injuries due to alcohol. Fighting the most common cause of lung cancer required public health programs to warn consumers about the dangers of smoking and policies to create smoke-free environments. Considering the various areas of life in the 21st century that are especially vulnerable to sleepiness, it is apparent that untoward outcomes caused by sleepiness will persist until key scientific principles are translated into action for the betterment of public health.

Sleep researchers and clinicians must encourage many components of society to promote individual and institutional behavior change (e.g., increasing habitual sleep duration, planning work schedules with consideration of human biology). Also, research efforts must be hastened to provide detailed information on the prevalence of sleep-related mishaps and on the economic and personal consequences of inadequate sleep. This information is vital for designing approaches and targeting resources where they will be most likely to advance public health and safety. Much of what we know or suspect about the role of sleep and sleepiness in public and private catastrophes is gleaned inferentially from retrospective studies and time-of-day data. Some prospective efforts to obtain data on sleepiness-related catastrophes are underway, in parallel with attempts to define the biologic limits sleep places on the alertness and safety of operators in certain occupations.[4,24,25]

KEY AREAS FOR TRANSLATION

A number of sleep research areas have progressed to the degree that research findings can lead to improved public health if adequately translated to various segments of society, and, if necessary, into improved public policy.

Cardiovascular Disease

Two lines of investigation implicate an association of cardiovascular disease and habitual sleep duration. First, acute periods of experimental sleep restriction produce increased blood pressure and heightened sympathetic nervous system activity,[26,27] as well as elevated levels of inflammatory markers associated with cardiovascular risk.[28] After recovery sleep, these physiologic measures return to baseline levels, suggesting a role for sleep in maintaining physiologic homeostasis. Second, an epidemiologic study of over 71,000 female nurses found that both short and long self-reported sleep durations are associated with the risk of coronary heart disease during a 10-year follow-up period.[29] Consistent with the latter finding are studies demonstrating that either short or long habitual self-reported sleep lengths are associated with an increase in all-cause mortality rates.[29-35]

Distinct from sleep duration per se, there is also convincing evidence that sleep-disordered breathing is a contributing factor to hypertension.[36,37] Less well established are apparent associations between sleep-disordered breathing and coronary artery disease and heart failure.[38,39]

The likelihood of suffering a myocardial infarction varies significantly across time of day, with a peak between 8 and 10 AM, which is 2 hours later than the morning peak for disease-related mortality.[40,41] Circadian regulation may underlie the shape of the 24-hour pattern in disease-related mortality. Direct observations of platelet aggregability show diurnal variation with a prominent morning peak.[42,43] Moreover, disease-related mortality closely approximates the two-peak pattern throughout the 24-hour day that has been described for sleep tendency.[40,44] Circadian and sleep-related increases in plasma concentrations of molecules that potentiate blood clotting or vasospasm may play a role in these temporal relationships, since aspirin reduces mortality due to myocardial infarct primarily during the morning peak, which suggests that the morning peak may be related to heightened platelet aggregability.[42,43]

Sleep-disordered breathing may also play a role in the early morning mortality peak of cardiovascular morbidity.[45] Jennum et al.[46] found that morning awake arterial blood pressure and nocturnal arterial blood pressure decreased with nasal continuous positive airway pressure treatment and concluded that these hemodynamic changes were associated with a treatment-related decrease in the number of sleep apnea events, a decrease in sympathetic activity, and an increase in parasympathetic activity. More evidence for the putative role of sleep apnea in the timing of deaths comes from work by Ancoli-Israel and colleagues, who reported that 24% of people over age 65 years had more than 5 apneic events per hour of sleep, and 62% had more than 10 respiratory disturbances per hour of sleep.[47] The high prevalence of sleep apnea in older people may contribute to the shape of the 24-hour pattern in disease-related mortality.

Metabolism, Obesity, and Diabetes

Impaired glucose tolerance has been described in healthy subjects after 6 nights of restriction of sleep to approximately 4 hours per night.[26] Combined with higher evening cortisol levels, and reduced leptin secretion, the results suggest endocrine changes with acute sleep loss that are consistent with the development of diabetes. A growing body of evidence also supports a link between sleep-disordered breathing and insulin resistance, independent of degree of obesity.[48-50] Thus, both short sleep and disrupted sleep associated with sleep-disordered breathing appear to be associated with endocrine and metabolic changes that may promote obesity and diabetes. Consistent with that interpretation is the observation of decreased nocturnal leptin levels during 3 consecutive nights of total sleep deprivation.[51]

An epidemiologic study found a relationship of shorter reported sleep durations and a diagnosis of diabetes, although when controlling for body mass index, the association was no longer significant.[52] The authors speculated that because sleep deprivation reduced leptin levels, sleep loss may affect diabetes risk through weight gain. Further, sleep restriction predicted symptomatic diabetes, even after controlling for body weight, suggesting that sleep loss may be more closely associated with more severe forms of diabetes.

Transportation Safety

It is known that sleepiness represents a significant risk to driving safety and may pose as great a risk to driving safety as does alcohol.[23,53] That sleep loss increases vehicular crash risk is evident in studies showing that crashes were more likely in sleepy patients with untreated obstructive sleep apnea,[54,55] and in people sleeping less than 6 hours per night.[56] Moreover, motor vehicle accidents do not occur randomly throughout the 24-hour day but tend to peak during early morning and mid-afternoon, in accordance with times of increased sleep propensity.[19,21,57-59] One study in Great Britain estimated that 27% of drivers who lost consciousness behind the wheel fell asleep, as opposed to fainting, having a seizure, or having a heart attack.[60] Moreover, this 27% of motor vehicle accidents accounted for 83% of the fatalities. Other investigators have also observed a high rate of fatality in sleep-related accidents.[21,61] The increased fatality rate is likely due to a combination of reduced vigilance, slowed reaction times, and loss of steering control (i.e., drift out of lane). Once a driver is sufficiently inattentive due to sleepiness, or has transitioned to sleep, there is little or no attempt to brake or otherwise avoid collision.[21]

Comparisons have been made between the behavioral impairment similarities of driving while excessively sleepy and driving under the influence of alcohol. In fact, if authorities determine that impairment from sleep deprivation has caused an accident, the driver can be considered negligent and held liable for civil and criminal penalties. However, the parallel with alcohol ends there. In contrast to measurement of breath or blood alcohol levels, accident investigators have no reliable objective measurement of the degree of sleepiness. Thus, errors due to falling asleep or impaired performance due to sleep deprivation must be inferred from the nature of the accident and the operator's prior sleep–wake schedule.

Impairment due to alcohol is heightened by sleep deprivation.[22] It is not yet fully appreciated how great a contributory role sleepiness may have in the overall number of transportation accidents involving drug and alcohol use. In a study of fatal-to-the-driver truck accidents, the National Transportation Safety Board (NTSB) found that fatigue plus alcohol or drugs accounted for a large proportion of lethal accidents.[57,58] We may speculate that sleepy individuals operating a vehicle may be very susceptible to further impairment from consumption of even modest quantities of alcohol (or other depressant drugs).

The first law to specifically criminalize drowsy driving was enacted by the state of New Jersey in 2003. Specifically, this legislation allows law enforcement officials to charge individuals with vehicular homicide if, after not sleeping for 24 hours or more, they cause a fatal accident. The legislation was termed "Maggie's Law" after Maggie McDonnell, who was killed in a head-on collision in 1997 by a driver who had gone without sleep for 30 hours.

Historically, the trucking industry has been a focus of regulation to prevent driving while fatigued. Each year in the United States there are approximately 4800 fatal crashes involving trucks, and many more nonfatal crashes. The NTSB reported a probable cause of fatigue in 57% of accidents that led to a truck driver's death,[57,58] although this percentage is not universally accepted by all public and private entities concerned with trucking safety. The term *fatigue* has been used throughout federal agencies to describe human performance failure attributable to a variety of factors. It is clear from the NTSB's texts that their intended meaning of the term *fatigue* is most congruent with what sleep specialists mean by the term *sleepiness*.[2]

When a truck driver dies in a crash, three to four other people are usually also killed.[59] Depending on the involvement of other vehicles and the nature of the cargo, associated damages may be substantial. The mean cost of a crash involving a single large vehicle has been calculated to be $51,000, but when fatalities result, the cost per crash is estimated at $2.7 million.[62] The trucking industry employs approximately 2.5 million drivers, operates 1 million motor carriers, and accounts for 10 billion miles per year of travel on U.S. highways. Trucks deliver products and materials to every segment of society, from local deliveries through transcontinental long hauls. There are economic incentives for driving long hours in some segments of the trucking industry. Several major studies on the quality and quantity of sleep in commercial truck drivers were completed in recent years.[63-65] These studies show that sleep of truck drivers is often inadequate to ensure stable alertness and performance. In one study of 80 long-haul truck drivers operating on North American routes with four demanding driving schedules, drivers slept an average of only 4.8 hours per day.[63]

Despite general recognition of the effects of chronically inadequate sleep on performance and safety, federal regulations promulgated in 1939 remained unaltered for years. Perhaps the complexity of the problem and the understandable fear of harming such a vital industry delayed initiation of research and the revision of hours of service regulations directed toward the reduction of accidents due to sleepiness in truck drivers.[64]

In April, 2003, a revised Hours-of-Service Rule was announced by the Department of Transportation's Federal Motor Carrier Safety Administration[66] in response to a Congressional mandate in 1995. This new legislation allows long-haul drivers (i.e., those who do not routinely return to their home base after each driving shift) to drive a maximum of 11 hours per day after 10 consecutive off-duty hours—the old rule required only 8 hours off-duty for sleep and recovery. In addition, in the new rule drivers are prohibited from driving after 14 hours on duty during a single shift, whereas the old rule allowed 15 hours on duty. Thus, the new rule allows more off-duty time for sleep and personal time (i.e., 14 hours on duty and 10 hours off duty), in contrast to the 23-hour pattern of the old rule (i.e., 15 hours on duty and 8 hours off duty). Finally, as in the earlier regulation, drivers may not drive after being on-duty for 60 hours in a 7-consecutive-day period, or after 70 hours in an 8-day period. Enforcement of the new rule begins January 4, 2004, and undoubtedly the impact on trucking safety will be closely monitored. Many in the sleep field contributed to the formulation of these new regulations—tangible evidence that we can and do have a public policy impact, which it is hoped will benefit public health.

In addition to regulatory approaches, prevention of the dangers of driving while impaired by sleepiness will require research on countermeasures such as drowsy-driving detection technologies,[67-70] roadside signs, safe sleeping areas, and tests to assess sleepiness. Advances in these areas may then require public policy changes and education. In addition, recognition and treatment of sleep apnea and other sleep disorders is crucial if the total health and economic impact is to be reduced. Recent projections suggest that more than 800,000 drivers were involved in sleep apnea–related vehicle crashes in the year 2000, and that those events cost $15.8 billion and 1400 lives that year.[71] Further, treating all drivers having sleep apnea with continuous positive airway pressure would produce a net savings of approximately $11 million and save 960 lives each year.

Many of the same issues pertaining to the role of work schedules and sleep in trucking safety are common to other commercial transportation modes. Sleep-related catastrophic accidents on the railroad have been identified, for example. The NTSB concluded that sleep deprivation with its related impairment was a primary cause in at least four catastrophic railroad accidents between 1987 and 1992.[72]

Maritime transportation typically involves 24-hour operations, and sleep deprivation has been the cause of several catastrophes. One of the most dramatic involved the grounding of the supertanker *Exxon Valdez* on Bligh Reef in Prince William Sound, Alaska, in March 1989. The NTSB determined that a "probable cause of the grounding of the Exxon Valdez was the failure of the third mate to properly maneuver the vessel because of fatigue and excessive work load... (p v)."[73] The grounding of the oil tanker *World Prodigy* off the coast of Rhode Island is another example of a major maritime accident involving fatigue due to sleep deprivation.[74] The NTSB determined that the probable cause was the master's impaired judgment from acute fatigue. The master had been awake for 36 hours at the time of the accident. There have been other summaries of fatigue-related performance failures in transportation modes that resulted in catastrophic outcomes.[75]

In each of these transportation areas, little research has been conducted to identify effective measures to counter sleep-based fatigue. Impetus to begin such countermeasure research will be enhanced as more public attention focuses on human error accidents and as top management integrates the real costs of accidents due to sleepiness-based error into their overall plans for risk management. This has begun in many of these industries, under the aegis of "fatigue management."[76,77] As the essential principles and practices of fatigue management develop, it will be important for sleep scientists to translate research findings into policies and practices that limit sleep debt, and provide maximal opportunity for recovery sleep. Moreover, sleepiness countermeasures should be data based, as well as reasonably feasible for the industry/occupation of concern.

An area of fatigue management that has received growing federal attention in recent years concerns the development of technologies that detect or prevent sleepiness on the job. Fatigue management technologies fall into four broad categories: (1) biomathematical models of human performance,[78] (2) readiness-to-perform and fitness-for-duty, (3) work-based performance technologies, and (4) on-line operator status monitoring technologies. Although such efforts have a long history, they have increased markedly recently owing to the prevalence and seriousness of fatigue-related crashes, the unreliability of subjective estimates of sleepiness or impairment, the potential of drowsiness detection technologies as alternatives (in part or in whole) to proscriptive hours of service, and the fact that technological advances have made the goal of on-line drowsiness detection feasible.[79] As these technologies continue to develop, the sleep field should take an active role to ensure they meet stringent criteria for scientific validity, reliability, sensitivity, and specificity. In addition, there are substantive public policy questions that will have to be addressed concerning privacy, liability, and related legal issues in the use of sleepiness prevention and drowsiness detection technologies.

Relieving Sleepiness with Naps: Aviation as a Case Study

Although accidents caused by sleep-based fatigue imperil all modes of transportation, aviation is one mode that has a history of research on the nature of fatigue and on developing countermeasures, primarily through research initiatives at the National Aeronautics and Space Administration (NASA) Ames Research Center. One example of this work serves to illustrate how sleep science can be used to address policy (i.e., research undertaken to investigate job-specific strategies to reduce sleepiness in the work place). However, this example also serves to highlight the significant challenges involved in gaining acceptance of viable sleepiness countermeasures by government, industry, labor, and the public.

For transmeridian flight crews, inadequate sleep has been a major source of fatigue.[80,81] A multidisciplinary research effort was undertaken to evaluate the benefits to long-haul flight crews of preplanned naps while in the air.[82] The results indicated not only that crew members could safely rotate, taking a brief (40-minute) nap period in flight, but also that the naps enhanced alertness of crews during transmeridian flights. Interestingly, the brief naps did not totally eliminate the cumulative sleep debt of crews, but they did provide transient relief from in-flight fatigue, especially on night flights. Such a clear example of an evidenced-based approach to mitigating sleepiness on the job also exposes a problem in translating science into public policy. Although many European and Asian transcontinental air carriers have adopted planned cockpit napping, the Federal Aviation Administration, because of political concerns, has not yet approved it for U.S. carriers. Public policy change requires both evidence of the need and benefits of the proposed change, as well as the acceptance of evidenced-based research as the standard for implementing organizational change. Absence of the latter prevented U.S. policy makers from incorporating a viable fatigue countermeasure in long-haul flight operations.

Health Care Workers

Health care workers can be on duty for extended shifts ranging in duration from 12 to 24 hours, with day and night shifts alternating as frequently as every few days. In any work situation, a tired and sleepy worker is less effective and at some point at higher risk for an error or accident. The nature of the risk depends on the nature of the work. When 24-hour operations are involved, the likelihood of cumulative sleep deprivation and working at an adverse circadian phase are considerable. The associated risks for diminished productivity, errors, and accidents are also higher.

In 1984, Libby Zion, an 18-year-old college freshman, died in a hospital in New York City. A grand jury found that her death was due to an undiagnosed infection and blamed inadequate supervision of residents and resident fatigue for the failure to institute proper treatment.[83] As a result, New York enacted laws to reduce the total number of hours that residents are permitted to work. The state of New Jersey followed in 2002 with a bill limiting residents' work hours. More recently, the Accreditation Council for Graduate Medical Education (ACGME) implemented in July, 2003, standard requirements for work hours for all resident physicians.[84] In brief, the ACGME regulations prescribe no more than an 80-hour work week, a maximum shift duration of 24 hours, at least 10 hours off between shifts, 1 day off per week, and overnight on-call assignment no more than every third night. Compared with traditional schedules, shorter shifts by interns in intensive care units result in more sleep, substantially fewer serious medical errors, and fewer attentional failures.[84a,84b]

Although regulation is one possible approach to manage resident sleepiness, it is likely that multiple interventions will be needed significantly to reduce sleep-related risk. Approaches such as providing brief sleep opportunities during prolonged work periods are also likely to be necessary to limit the effects of fatigue even within the ACGME duty limits. While the costs and benefits of restricting work hours for physicians are being evaluated, we should note that the medical community has often used scientific knowledge as the basis for new policies and guidelines for physician behavior relative to improved public health. The widespread use of sterile technique in surgery and the modern emphasis on preventive medicine through smoking cessation are two of many examples of evidenced-based behavior changes.

Hazardous Workplaces

Sleep is inexorably intertwined with a large number of occupations that have a potential impact on public safety and health. It is not possible here to provide an exhaustive discussion, but some obvious examples other than those already mentioned include emergency operations and military conflict. Although the need to sustain wakefulness for prolonged periods of time may be obvious in a national disaster, the consequences of human error due to sleepiness and fatigue can be particularly serious in essential but nonemergency hazardous work environments that operate around the clock (e.g., nuclear power plants and plants producing hazardous or toxic chemicals). The early morning human errors that led to the on-site disaster at Three Mile Island[85] and the environmental disaster at Chernobyl[86,87] bear all the earmarks of sleepiness-related accidents. The sequence of decisions leading up to the space shuttle *Challenger* accident in 1986 is an example of sleep deprivation being contributory, if not causal, according to a supplemental report to the investigation.[88] The senior manager's decision to launch was based not on engineering or safety judgments but rather on other factors, including public image and preset schedules—the latter also was found to be contributory in the official investigation of the space shuttle *Columbia* investigation. In the case of the loss of *Challenger*, a Presidential Commission concluded that specific key managers had slept less than 2 hours the night before and had been on duty since 1 AM on the day of the launch. The report stated that "time pressure, particularly that caused by launch scrubs and turnarounds, increased the potential for sleep loss and judgment errors" and that working "excessive hours, while admirable, raises serious questions when it jeopardizes job performance, particularly when critical management decisions are at stake" (p G5).[88] Such a cogent example serves to illustrate that any workplace in which the consequences of a human error can be catastrophic economically, environmentally, or physically must consider the role of sleep need in maintaining safe and effective functioning.

Adolescents and Young Adults

The prevalence of significant sleepiness associated with insufficient sleep is particularly high among adolescents and young adults. The adolescent years are accompanied by decreasing parental control, growing academic challenges, increasing social activities, and more employment opportunities. All of these forces tend to push sleep to a lower priority in time management. The net result is that few adolescents obtain adequate sleep, especially during the school week. The resultant sleepiness increases the risk for fatigue-related motor vehicle accidents, contributes to negative mood, impairs memory and other measures of cognition, and increases use of stimulants and alcohol.[89,90] Up to 40% of high school and college students are sleep deprived, and laboratory studies have documented performance impairments in them due to sleep loss.[13,90] This age group is also heavily represented among those who have drowsy driving crashes.[21] In addition, tired students are likely to have impaired motivation and unintended sleep episodes.[91,92] Students earning Cs or below report obtaining less sleep and having more irregular sleep schedules than do students with higher grades, although a causal relationship has not been established.[13,93] In an effort to address the problem of sleep-deprived adolescents, a recent study[94] reported that delaying high school start times from 7:15 AM to 8:40 AM, for a Minneapolis School District, resulted in students obtaining an hour more sleep per night, and improved attendance rates. In response to growing concerns, Congresswoman Zoe Lofgren introduced to the U. S. House of Representatives the "Z's to A's Bill" (H.R. 1313) to draw the attention of policy makers to this important issue.

MAKING SLEEP A MATTER OF PUBLIC HEALTH AND PUBLIC POLICY

As discussed earlier, scientific advances in understanding sleep, sleepiness, and the impact of sleepiness on behavior and health need to be interpreted and communicated in ways that are useful to society. Without dissemination of the necessary knowledge and concepts, it is difficult to influence public consciousness and behavior. In some instances, our society faces problems related to sleep loss and sleepiness without the knowledge to formulate solutions.

There have been some important milestones in the history of federal policy regarding sleep medicine and research. Many came about through effective communication of scientific knowledge by individuals or appointed representatives of the sleep research community to federal authorities, who then acted in the interests of the public.

From the early 1970s, when the U.S. Food and Drug Administration developed guidelines for the evaluation of hypnotic medications, and moving to the present activities of the National Center for Sleep Disorders Research (NCSDR), our history has been one of activism and progress. Here we mention only a few of the important milestones.

In 1979, the Surgeon General's office created Project Sleep to focus further governmental attention on sleep research and sleep disorders.

In 1984, the American Sleep Disorders Association created an active government affairs committee. The committee's mandate was to provide all three branches of the government with up-to-date information on sleep physiology and current sleep research. Committee members gave congressional testimony and worked with regulatory and investigative agencies.

In 1990, the Institute of Medicine prepared a research briefing entitled "Basic Sleep Research." The briefing was prompted, in part, by the Institute of Medicine's recognition that the continuation of basic sleep research in the United States was being threatened by limited training of young researchers, limited research funding, and attacks by animal rights groups on several basic sleep research programs.

In an independent but complementary effort stimulated by the heightened federal interest in the impact of the sleep–wake cycle on society, the Office of Technology Assessment of the U.S. Congress conducted a major review of biologic rhythms and their impact in the workplace.[95]

The National Sleep Foundation (NSF; www.sleepfoundation. org), an independent nonprofit organization whose mission includes improving public health and safety by achieving understanding of sleep and sleep disorders, was established by the American Academy of Sleep Medicine (AASM) in 1990. The NSF's programs have contributed to a heightened public awareness of the importance of sleep for public health.

The National Commission for Sleep Disorders Research, established by Congress, completed its comprehensive report of its findings in 1993.[72] In the Executive Summary, the Commission called for permanent and concerted government efforts in expanding basic and clinical research on sleep disorders as well as in improving public awareness of the dangers of inappropriate sleepiness. The NCSDR was subsequently created within the National Heart, Lung, and Blood Institute at the National Institutes of Health. The NCSDR's mandate has been to conduct and support research, training, health information dissemination, and other activities with respect to sleep disorders, including biologic and circadian rhythm research, basic understanding of sleep, and chronobiology, and to coordinate the sleep activities of other federal agencies. The legislation also mandated development of a National Sleep Disorders Research Plan. This plan was recently updated, and provides an excellent presentation of the progress in sleep research over the last several years, as well as detailing the key research and training recommendations for the future. The plan is available from www.nhlbisupport.com/sleep/research/research-a.htm, and a summary was recently published.[96] Since the establishment of the NCSDR, total National Institutes of Health funding for sleep research has grown steadily; with the latest estimates showing an increase from $75 million to more than $175 million during the period 1996 to 2002.

Recognition of sleep medicine as a medical subspecialty has been significantly advanced through the efforts of the AASM. For example, in recent years the AASM has gained official recognition in the American Medical Association House of Delegates (1996); received approval of the ACGME for accreditation of sleep fellowship training programs (2003); and entered discussions with the American Board of Medical Specialties regarding the acceptance of a sleep medicine board examination.

CONCLUSION

Sleepiness and inattention related to sleep loss and circadian rhythms adversely affect workers in many industries, as well as the general public, and lead to public health and safety problems.

Evidence is accumulating that sleep disorders and restriction may be contributing factors not only to many errors and accidents, but also to certain highly prevalent disease states that are major public health concerns, such as diabetes, obesity, and hypertension. For each of these societal concerns, sleep science must be translated to the general public, biomedical researchers, and to those in policy positions for wiser public policy and the betterment of public health. Just as massive epidemics in crowded cities of 19th century thrust the notion of disease-carrying microbes into public consciousness, industrial and transportation catastrophes of the 20th and 21st centuries should be forcing the morbidity of sleepiness and sleep loss into the public consciousness.

Education and recognition of true risk are necessary first steps toward improved public health and formulation of wise public policy. Elementary and secondary level health and science classes clearly should include the critical messages of our field. The health impact of inadequate or disrupted sleep should be known as well as the negative effects of poor nutrition or smoking. All opportunities for translation of sleep science to engender behavior change of the general public should be taken. Communication of sleep science to researchers in other biomedical areas is also necessary to encourage the interdisciplinary approaches most likely to produce rapid advances in understanding sleep-related morbidity and its prevention.

There is also ample precedent for health professionals to assume responsibility, both individually and collectively through their professional organizations, to take action to improve the health and safety of the public. This includes societal health in its broadest sense: the reduction of risk and the enhancement of quality of life. Indeed, the special expertise of sleep medicine professionals confers a unique and heightened set of obligations to address and to shape rational public policy. It is axiomatic that public policy does not change by itself. It is also axiomatic that public policy can change in a manner that is counterproductive or that poses a threat to the health of the public. There may be economic incentives involved in maintaining or increasing the risks associated with sleep deprivation. It is the responsibility of health professionals and biomedical organizations to foster knowledge transfer to the public, to industry, to policy makers, and to others in a position to influence public health and safety. By translating the scientific body of knowledge about sleep and its disorders, we may promote behavior change and the formulation of good public policy, and as a result improve public health.

Acknowledgments

Merrill M. Mitler, PhD, contributed substantially to prior versions of this chapter. Dr. Mitler chose not to continue authorship of this chapter in his current position at the National Institute of Neurological Disease and Stroke, National Institutes of Health.

REFERENCES

1. American Sleep Disorders Association: International Classification of Sleep Disorders, Revised: Diagnostic and Coding Manual. Rochester, Minn, American Sleep Disorders Association, 1997.
2. Dinges DF, Graeber RC, Carskadon MA, et al: Attending to inattention. Science 1989;245:342.
3. Kribbs NB, Getsy J, Dinges DF: Investigation and management of daytime sleepiness in sleep apnea. In Saunders NA, Sullivan CE (eds): Sleep and Breathing, vol 2. New York, Marcel Dekker, 1992, pp 575-604.
4. Buysse DJ, Barzansky B, Dinges DF, et al: Sleep, fatigue, and medical training: Setting an agenda for optimal learning and patient care. A report from the conference "Sleep, Fatigue and Medical Training: Optimizing Learning and the Patient Care Environment." Sleep 2003;3:218-225.
5. Lenfant C: Clinical research to clinical practice—lost in translation? N Engl J Med 2003;349:868-874.
6. Berwick DM: Disseminating innovations in health care. JAMA 2003;289:1969-1975.
7. Webb WB, Dinges DF: Cultural perspectives on napping and the siesta. In Dinges DF, Broughton RJ (eds): Sleep and Alertness: Chronobiological, Behavioral and Medical Aspects of Napping. New York, Raven Press, 1989, pp 247-266.
8. Dinges DF, Broughton RJ (eds): Sleep and Alertness: Chronobiological, Behavioral and Medical Aspects of Napping. New York, Raven Press, 1989.
9. Dinges DF: An overview of sleepiness and accidents. J Sleep Res 1995;4:4-11.
10. Kribbs NB, Dinges DF: Vigilance decrement and sleepiness. In Harsh JR, Ogilvie RD (eds): Sleep Onset Mechanisms. Washington, DC, American Psychological Association, 1994, pp 113-125.
11. Terman LM, Hocking A: The sleep of school children: Its distribution according to age and its relation to physical and mental efficiency. J Educ Psychol 1913;4:138-147.
12. O'Connor AL: Questionnaire Responses about Sleep. Master's thesis, University of Florida. Gainesville, Fla, University of Florida, 1964.
13. Wolfson AR, Carskadon MA: Sleep schedules and daytime functioning in adolescents. Child Dev 1998;69:875-887.
14. Rosenthal L, Roehrs TA, Rosen A, et al: Level of sleepiness and total sleep time following various time in bed conditions. Sleep 1993;16:226-232.
15. Belenky G, Wesensten N, Thorne D, et al: Patterns of performance degradation and restriction during sleep restriction and subsequent recovery: A sleep dose-response study. J Sleep Res 2003;12:1-12.
16. Van Dongen H, Maislin G, Mullington J, et al: The cumulative cost of additional wakefulness: Dose-response effects on neurobehavioral functions and sleep physiology from chronic sleep restriction and total sleep deprivation. Sleep 2003;26:117-126.
17. Howard S, Caba D, Smith B, et al: Simulation study of rested versus sleep-deprived anesthesiologists. Anesthesiology 2003;98:1345-1355.
18. Van Dongen, HPA, Dinges, DF: Circadian rhythms in fatigue, alertness and performance. In Kryger MH, Roth T, Dement WC (eds): Principles and Practice of Sleep Medicine, 4th ed. Philadelphia, Elsevier, 2004.
19. Mitler MM, Carskadon MA, Czeisler CA, et al: Catastrophes, sleep, and public policy: Consensus report. Sleep 1988;11:100-109.
20. Mitler MM, Miller JC: Methods of testing for sleepiness. Behav Med 1996;21:171-183.

Clinical Pearl

Clinicians and researchers should contribute their knowledge and expertise to the development of public and institutional policies that will serve to improve public health and safety in areas such as educational systems, public utilities, transportation, and workplace safety. In the near future there may be an increasing role for sleep specialists in dealing with major public health issues such as obesity, hypertension, and diabetes.

21. Pack AI, Pack AM, Rodgman E, et al: Characteristics of crashes attributed to the driver having fallen asleep. Accid Anal Prev 1995;27:769-775.

22. Carskadon MA, Acebo C: Regulation of sleepiness in adolescents: Update, insights, and speculation. Sleep 2002;25:453-460.

23. Roehrs T, Beare D, Zorick F, et al: Sleepiness and ethanol effects on simulated driving. Alcohol Clin Exp Res 1994;18:154-158.

24. Dinges DF, Graeber RC, Rosekind MR, et al: Principles and Guidelines for Duty and Rest Scheduling in Commercial Aviation. NASA Technical Memorandum Report no. 110404. Washington, DC, NASA, 1996, pp 1-10.

25. Rosekind MR, Neri DF, Dinges DF: From laboratory to flight-deck: Promoting operational alertness. Presented at the Royal Aeronautical Society's Symposium on Fatigue and Duty Time Limitations: An International Review, London, September 16, 1997.

26. Spiegel K, Leproult R, Van Cauter E: Impact of sleep debt on metabolic and endocrine function. Lancet 1999;23:1435-1439.

27. Tochibuko O, Ikeda A, Miyajima E, et al: Effects of insufficient sleep on blood pressure monitored by a new multibiomedical recorder. Hypertension 1996;27:1318-1324.

28. Meier Ewert HK, Ridker PM, Rifai N, et al: Effect of sleep loss on C-reactive protein, an inflammatory marker of cardiovascular risk. J Am Coll Cardiol 2004;43:678-683.

29. Ayas NT, White DP, Manson JE, et al: A prospective study of sleep duration and coronary heart disease in women. Arch Intern Med 2003;163:205-209.

30. Appels A, de Yos Y, van Diest R, et al: Are sleep complaints predictive of future myocardial infarction? Activ Nerv Super 1987;29:147-151.

31. Eaker ED, Pinsky J, Castelli WP: Myocardial infarction and coronary death among women: Psychosocial predictors from a 20-year follow-up of women in the Framingham Study. Am J Epidemiol 1992;135:854-864.

32. Schwartz SW, Cornoni-Huntley J, Cole SR, et al: Are sleep complaints an independent risk factor for myocardial infarction? Ann Epidemiol 1998;8:384-392.

33. Newman AB, Spiekerman CF, Enright P, et al: Daytime sleepiness predicts mortality and cardiovascular disease in older adults. J Am Geriatr Soc 2000;48:115-123.

34. Kripke DF, Garfinkel L, Wingard DL, et al: Mortality associated with sleep duration and insomnia. Arch Gen Psychiatry 2002;59:131-136.

35. Liu Y, Tanaka H: The Fukuoka Heart Study Group: Overtime work, insufficient sleep, and risk of non-fatal acute myocardial infarction in Japanese men. Occup Environ Med 2002;59:447-451.

36. Nieto FJ, Young TB, Lind BK, et al: Association of sleep-disordered breathing, sleep apnea, and hypertension in a large community-based study. Sleep Heart Health Study. JAMA 2000; 283:1829-1836.

37. Peppard PE, Young T, Palta M, et al: Prospective study of the association between sleep-disordered breathing and hypertension. N Engl J Med 2000;342:1378-1384.

38. Shahar E, Whitney CW, Redline S, et al: Sleep-disordered breathing and cardiovascular disease: Cross-sectional results of the Sleep Heart Health Study. Am J Respir Crit Care Med 2001; 163:19-25.

39. Javaheri S, Parker T, Liming J, et al: Sleep apnea in 81 ambulatory male patients with stable heart failure. Circulation 1996;97: 2154-2159.

40. Mitler MM, Hajdukovic RM, Shafor R, et al: When people die: Cause of death versus time of death. Am J Med 1987;82:266-274.

41. Müller JE, Stone PH, Turi ZG, et al: Circadian variation in the onset of acute myocardial infarction. N Engl J Med 1985;313: 1315-1322.

42. Smolensky M, Halberg F, Sargent F: Chronobiology of the life sequence. In Ito S, Ogata K, Yoshimura H (eds): Advances in Climatic Physiology. Tokyo, Igaku Shoin, 1972, pp 281-318.

43. Ridker PM, Manson JE, Buring JE, et al: Circadian variation of acute myocardial infarction and the effect of low-dose aspirin in a randomized trial of physicians. Circulation 1990;82:897-902.

44. Tofler GH, Brezinski D, Schafer Al, et al: Concurrent morning increase in platelet aggregability and the risk of myocardial infarction and sudden cardiac death. N Engl J Med 1987;316: 1514-1518.

45. Mitler MM, Dawson A, McNally E: Sleep disorders and coronary disease. In Zipes DP, Rowlands DJ (eds): Progress in Cardiology, vol 4/2. Philadelphia, Lea & Febiger, 1991, pp 99-113.

46. Jennum P, Wildschidtz G, Christensen NJ, et al: Blood pressure, catecholamines and pancreatic polypeptide in obstructive sleep apnea with and without nasal continuous positive airway pressure (nCPAP). Am J Hypertens 1989;2:847-852.

47. Ancoli-Israel S, Kripke DF, Klauber MR, et al: Sleep-disordered breathing in community-dwelling elderly. Sleep 1991;14:486-495.

48. Punjabi NM, Sorkin JD, Katzel L, et al: Sleep-disordered breathing and insulin resistance in middle aged and overweight men. Am J Respir Crit Care Med 2002;165:677-682.

49. Ip SM, Lam B, Ng M, et al: Obstructive sleep apnea is independently associated with insulin resistance. Am J Respir Crit Care Med 2002;165:670-676.

50. Vgontzas AN, Papanicolaou DA, Bixler EO, et al: Sleep apnea and daytime sleepiness and fatigue: Related to visceral obesity, insulin resistance, and hypocytokinemia. J Clin Endocrinol Metab 2000;85:1151-1158.

51. Mullington JM, Chan JL, Van Dongen HPA, et al: Sleep loss reduces diurnal rhythm amplitude of leptin in healthy men. J Neuroendocrinol 2003;15:851-854.

52. Ayas NT, White DP, Al-Delaimy WK, et al: A prospective study of self-reported sleep duration and incident diabetes in women. Diabetes Care 2003;26:380-384.

53. Dawson D, Reid K: Fatigue, alcohol and performance impairment. Nature 1997;388:235.

54. Findley L, Suratt P: Serious motor vehicle crashes: The cost of untreated apnoea. Thorax 2001;56:505.

55. George C, Smiley A: Sleep apnea and automobile crashes. Sleep 1999;22:790-795.

56. Stutts J, Wilkins J, Osberg J, et al: Driver risk factors for sleep-related crashes. Accid Anal Prev 2003;35:321-331.

57. National Transportation Safety Board: Safety Study: Fatigue, Alcohol, Other Drugs, and Medical Factors in Fatal-to-the-Driver Heavy Truck Crashes, vol 1. Washington, DC, National Transportation Safety Board, 1990.

58. National Transportation Safety Board: Safety Study: Fatigue, Alcohol, Other Drugs, and Medical Factors in Fatal-to-the-Driver Heavy Truck Crashes, vol 2. Washington, DC, National Transportation Safety Board, 1990.

59. U.S. Congress Office of Technology Assessment: Gearing up for Safety: Motor Carrier Safety in a Competitive Environment. Publication OTA-SET-382. Washington, DC, U.S. Government Printing Office, 1988.

60. Parsons M: Fits and other causes of loss of consciousness while driving. QJM 1986;58:295-303.

61. Maycock G: Sleepiness and driving: the experience of U.K. drivers. Accid Anal Prev 1997;29:453-462.

62. U.S. Department of Transportation: The Costs of Highway Crashes. Washington, DC, Federal Highway Administration, 1991.

63. Mitler MM, Miller JC, Lipsitz JJ, et al: The sleep of long-haul truck drivers. N Engl J Med 1997;337:755-761.

64. Wylie D, Miller JC, Shultz T, et al: Commercial Driver Fatigue, Loss of Alertness, and Countermeasures. Washington, DC, U.S. Department of Transportation, 1996.

65. Dingus T, Neale V, Wierwille W, et al: Impact of Sleeper Berth Usage on Driver Fatigue. Federal Motor Carrier Safety Administration Report no. DOT-RT-02-050. Washington DC, Federal Motor Carrier Safety Administration, 2001.

66. Department of Transportation's Federal Motor Carrier Safety Administration: Docket number FMCSA-97-2350. Federal Register 2003;68(81). Available at http://dms.dot.gov.

67. Dinges DF: Technology/scheduling approaches. In Proceedings: Managing Fatigue in Transportation: Promoting Safety and Productivity. Washington, DC, National Transportation Safety Board and NASA-Ames Research Center, 1995, pp 53-58.

68. Dinges DF: Validation of psychophysiological monitors. In Proceedings: Technical Conference on Enhancing Commercial Motor Vehicle Driver Vigilance. Washington, DC, American Trucking Associations, Federal Highway Administration, National Highway Traffic Administration, 1996, pp 35-41.

69. Dinges DF: The promise and challenges of technologies for monitoring operator vigilance. In Proceedings: An International Perspective on Managing Fatigue in Transportation: What We Know and Promising New Directions for Reducing the Risks. Washington, DC, American Trucking Associations, 1997, pp 77-86.

70. Dinges DF, Mallis MM: Managing fatigue by drowsiness detection: Can technological promises be realized? In Hartley L (ed): Managing Fatigue in Transportation: Proceedings of the 3rd Fatigue in Transportation Conference, Fremantle, Western Australia, February 1998. Oxford, Pergamon, 1998, pp 209-229.

71. Sassani A, Findley LJ, Kryger M, et al: Reducing motor vehicle collisions, costs, and fatalities by treating obstructive sleep apnea. Sleep 2004;27:453-458.

72. National Commission on Sleep Disorders Research: Report of the National Commission on Sleep Disorders Research: Wake Up America: A National Sleep Alert. Washington, DC, U.S. Department of Health and Human Services, 1993.

73. National Transportation Safety Board: Marine Accident Report: Grounding of the U.S. Tankship EXXON VALDEZ on Bligh Reef, Prince William Sound, Near Valdez, Alaska, March 24, 1989. NTSB/MAR-90/04. Washington, DC, National Transportation Safety Board, 1990.

74. National Transportation Safety Board: Marine Accident Report: Grounding of the Greek Tankship, World Prodigy off the Coast of Rhode Island, June 23, 1989. Washington, DC, National Transportation Safety Board, 1991.

75. Lauber JK, Kayten PJ: Sleepiness, circadian dysrhythmia, and fatigue in transportation system accidents. Sleep 1988;11:503-512.

76. Hartley L (ed): Managing Fatigue in Transportation: Proceedings of the 3rd Fatigue in Transportation Conference, Fremantle, Western Australia, February 1998. Oxford, Pergamon, 1998.

77. National Transportation Safety Board, NASA Ames Research Center. 1996 Fatigue Symposium Proceedings, November 1-2, 1995. Washington, DC, National Transportation Safety Board.

78. Mallis MM, Mejdal MS, Nguyen TT, et al: Summary of the key features of seven biomathematical models of human fatigue and performance. Aviat Space Environ Med 2004;75(3 Suppl):A4-A14.

79. Dinges DF, Mallis MM: Managing fatigue by drowsiness detection: Can technological promises be realized? In Hartley L (ed): Managing Fatigue in Transportation: Proceedings of the 3rd

80. Graeber RC, Dement WC, Nicholson AN, et al: International cooperative study of aircrew layover sleep: Operational summary. Aviat Space Environ Med 1986;57:B10-B13.

81. Graeber PC, Lauber JK, Connell LJ, et al: International aircrew sleep and wakefulness after multiple time zone flights: A cooperative study. Aviat Space Environ Med 1986;57:B3-B9.

82. Rosekind MR, Graeber PC, Dinges DF, et al: Crew Factors in Flight Operations: IX. Effects of Planned Cockpit Rest on Crew Performance and Alertness in Long-Haul Operations. Moffett Field, Calif, NASA Ames Research Center, 1994.

83. Asch DA, Parker RM: Sounding board: The Libby Zion case. N Engl J Med 1988;318:771-775.

84. Accreditation Council for Graduate Medical Education: Common Duty Hour Standards for Programs. Chicago, Accreditation Council for Graduate Medical Education, 2002. Available at http://www.acgme.org/.

84a. Landrigan CP, Rothschild JM, Cronin JW, et al: Effect of reducing interns' work hours on serious medical errors in intensive care units. N Engl J Med 2004;351:1838-1848.

84b. Lockley SW, Cronin JW, Evans EE, et al: Effect of reducing interns' weekly work hours on sleep and attentional failures. N Engl J Med 2004;351:1829-1837.

85. Moss TH, Sills DL: The Three Mile Island nuclear accident: Lessons and implications. Ann N Y Acad Sci 1981;365:1-341.

86. U.S. Nuclear Regulatory Commission: Report on the Accident at the Chernobyl Nuclear Power Station. Washington, DC, U.S. Government Printing Office, 1987.

87. United States Senate Committee on Energy and Natural Resources: The Chernobyl Accident. Washington, DC, U.S. Government Printing Office, 1986.

88. Presidential Commission: Report of the Presidential Commission on the Space Shuttle Challenger Accident, vol 2, appendix G. Washington, DC, U.S. Government Printing Office, 1986.

89. Carskadon MA: Patterns of sleep and sleepiness in adolescents. Pediatrician 1990;17:5-12.

90. Carskadon MA, Dement WC: Cumulative effects of sleep restriction on daytime sleepiness. Psychophysiology 1981;18:107-113.

91. Strauch I, Meier B: Sleep need in adolescence: A longitudinal approach. Sleep 1988;11:378-386.

92. Morrison DN, McGee R, Stranton WW: Sleep problems in adolescence. J Am Acad Child Adolesc Psychiatry 1992;31:94-99.

93. Drake C, Nickel C, Burduvali E, et al: The Pediatric Daytime Sleepiness Scale (PDSS): Sleep habits and school outcomes in middle-school children. Sleep 2003;26:455-458.

94. Wahlstrom K, Davidson ML, Choi J, et al: School Start Time Study—Executive Summary, August, 2001. Available at http://education.umn.edu/CAREI/Programs/start-time.

95. U.S. Congress Office of Technology Assessment: Biological Rhythms: Implications for the Worker. Washington, DC, U.S. Government Printing Office, 1991.

96. 2003 National Sleep Disorders Research Plan. Sleep 2003;26:253-257.

Introduction: Disorders of Chronobiology

Fred W. Turek

The four other chapters in this section focus on sleep disorders in which the timing of sleep and wake is abnormal relative to either the internal 24-hour circadian clock or the normal time for sleep and wake relative to the time when most of the rest of society is asleep and awake. That is, sleep and wake are out of phase with the internal or external environment. It is perhaps worth noting that from an evolutionary perspective, the circadian clock has one major role to play in ensuring the survival of the individual and the species: to regulate the phase of a multitude of circadian rhythms such that specific phase points of these rhythms occur at optimal times relative to each other (*internal synchronization*) or relative to the external environment (*external synchronization*), in order to optimize the chances that the organism will survive and contribute to the gene pool of future generations. Internal circadian clocks are found in all eukaryotic and at least some prokaryotic organisms,[1] indicating that natural selection has placed a high premium from the beginning of life on earth on maintaining proper phase relationships within the internal and between the internal and external environments.

As noted by Monk in Chapter 56, "Working at night must therefore be regarded as an inherently unnatural act." How very true. Indeed, human beings, unlike all other species, are routinely awake when their internal biological clocks are telling them it is time to sleep, and human beings are often trying to sleep when the circadian clock is sending signals throughout the brain and body that it is time to be awake. Human beings are clearly not slaves to their biological clocks and have the ability cognitively to override the temporal signals. Of course, fooling Mother Nature is not easily accomplished, and has its price. It can be difficult to perform, either physically or mentally, anywhere near one's capacity at times when the circadian clock is signaling the brain and body it is time to sleep, and trying to sleep at abnormal biological clock times often leads to poor and shortened sleep. This decrease in the quality and quantity of sleep itself leads to more deficits in alertness and performance during wake times. The combination of sleep loss, being awake at times of diminished capabilities, and the possible abnormal phasing of internal rhythms relative to one another, either on an acute or chronic basis, can have serious adverse effects on human health, safety, performance, and productivity.[2]

Whereas Chapter 56 discusses the basic principles underlying the causes and consequences of shift work–related problems, Chapter 57 by Rosekind offers a number of practical interventions that can be used to mitigate the adverse effects on health, safety, and performance that are associated with shift work. Although the adverse effects of shift work have been recognized for many years,[2] only recently has a more aggressive approach been taken not only to recognize the serious consequences of shift work on human health and safety, but to try to alleviate the consequences. A recent National Sleep Foundation Workshop, Shift-Work Sleep Disorders,[3] stressed the importance of new drugs coming on the market that will be indicated to alleviate the two fundamental physiologic problems associated with shift work: (1) trying to sleep when our circadian clock is telling the body it is time to be awake, and (2) trying to be awake when the biological clock is telling the body it is time to sleep. New hypnotics that can be taken for long periods (e.g., months) will allow workers to obtain more sleep even when sleep is occurring at an abnormal circadian time. In addition, the recent approval of an "alerting drug" for the treatment of shift work sleep disorder is undoubtedly just the beginning of a new era in which a number of drugs will be developed to help maintain alertness when there is a need to stay awake even though one is fatigued. Shift work sleep disorder is essentially a disorder of "circadian timing" that results in circadian dysregulation in conjunction with inadequate sleep owing to attempts to sleep at an abnormal circadian time. As we continue to develop into an around-the-clock global society, this "circadian disorder" will become more prevalent.

As reviewed by Arendt and colleagues in Chapter 55, a second "voluntary" circadian sleep–wake disorder occurs when humans move rapidly across time zones, an extremely unnatural act that humans have never experienced throughout their history until very recently. Although perhaps only a minor nuisance for the occasional long-distance tourist, "jet lag" can be very disruptive to the frequent business traveler, and even dangerous for the individuals who are responsible for moving the planes and people rapidly across time zones. As more and more drugs are developed as "lifestyle"-enhancing drugs, one may expect to see "chronohypnotic" lifestyle drugs being used for the treatment of jet lag, as well as shift work sleep disorder.

In contrast to the situations of jet lag and shift work, in which human beings choose to create temporal disorganization for themselves, there are situations in which such temporal disorganization, with respect either to internal or external time, occurs on an involuntary basis. Some of these phase "disorders" are reviewed by Reid and Zee in Chapter 58 in this section. I put the word *disorders* in quotation marks because these phase disorders are a problem only if the external environment cannot be phase controlled or phase ignored. For example, an individual with delayed sleep phase syndrome may have a major problem if he needs to start work early and thus does not obtain sufficient sleep, whereas the same individual may have no problem if his job requires him to be awake late at night and there are no constraints on when he needs to be awake in the morning. Indeed, although an individual may have problems in one society that places a premium on early morning awakening, she may have little, or no problem at all, if she is living in a society where the "phase of living" is different.

One final comment is in order. It can be argued that we have only just begun to understand how disorders of chronobiology, or disorders of the circadian clock system, affect sleep. Although most of the discussion about chronobiology disorders has focused on the abnormal timing of sleep and wake, the circadian input into sleep–wake regulatory mechanisms may include inputs that do much more than control the phase of sleep and wake. There is now considerable evidence to indicate that disrupting the normal sleep–wake cycle has feedback effects on the phase of the circadian clock,[4] and data in mice indicate that a mutation in a key genetic component of the circadian clock can influence the duration of sleep.[5] The hypothesis of Edgar et al.[6] that the master circadian clock located in the hypothalamic suprachiasmatic nucleus (SCN) may produce an "alerting" factor is consistent with the idea that the circadian clock may provide more than just phase information to the sleep–wake system. Indeed, new data cited elsewhere in this book from different genetic models indicate that the SCN may produce "sleep-inducing" as well as "wake-promoting" signals (see Chapter 26). Thus, many sleep disorders (e.g., insomnia) that normally are not considered as "circadian" disorders may in fact be due to abnormal sleep–wake signals from the circadian clock that affect the amount of sleep and not just the timing of sleep. Looking at the circadian clock in the SCN not only as a "timer" of the sleep–wake cycle, but a promoter or inhibitor of sleep or wake, opens up a new era for the development of drugs that would target possible circadian clock sleep- and wake-promoting output signals.

Finally, in many chapters of this book, numerous examples are provided in which chronobiologic disorders may have indirect adverse effects on sleep. For example, circadian abnormalities in metabolic, respiratory, endocrine, or behavioral rhythms can have severe negative consequences for normal sleep and wake. Thus, at many different levels, improving overall temporal organization may have beneficial effects in improving sleep and wake functions as well as overall health and well-being.

REFERENCES

1. Takahashi JS, Turek FW, Moore RY (eds): Handbook of Behavioral Neurobiology, vol 12: Circadian Clocks. New York, Kluwer Academic/Plenum, 2001.
2. Office of Technology Assessment: Biological Rhythms: Implications for the Worker. Publication OTA-BA-463. Washington, DC, Office of Technology Assessment, U.S. Congress, 1991.
3. National Sleep Foundation Workshop: Shift-Work Sleep Disorders. Washington, DC, March 4-5, 2004.
4. Turek FW, Scarbrough K, Penev P, et al: Aging of the mammalian circadian system. In Takahashi JS, Turek FW, Moore RY (eds): Handbook of Behavioral Neurobiology, vol 12: Circadian Clocks. New York, Kluwer Academic/Plenum, 2001, pp 292-317.
5. Naylor E, Bergmann BM, Krauski K, et al: The circadian *Clock* mutation alters sleep homeostasis in the mouse. J Neurosci 2000;20:8138-8143.
6. Edgar DM, Dement WC, Fuller CA: Effect of SCN lesions on sleep in squirrel monkeys: Evidence for opponent processes in sleep-wake regulation. J Neurosci 1993;13:1065-1079.

Sleep Disruption in Jet Lag and Other Circadian Rhythm–Related Disorders

Josephine Arendt

Barbara Stone

Debra J. Skene

ABSTRACT

Situations leading to sleep disorder, including jet lag and shift work, are common and likely to become more so. The temporary mismatch of internal clock timing with external time cues and behavioral requirements is primarily responsible for acute problems and, in shift workers, possible long-term health consequences. Non–24-hour sleep-wake disorder, frequently seen in blind people with no conscious or unconscious light perception, is a life-long problem: The circadian clock "free runs" in and out of phase with the 24-hour day without the strong time cues of visual and nonvisual light perception, leading to a state that is essentially intermittent jet lag.

Strategies to address the acute sleep problems of jet lag and shift work include attention to sleep hygiene; quiet, dark sleeping quarters; suitably timed naps; possible use of hypnotics with a short half-life; exposure to light of suitable intensity; and spectral composition during "biological night" to increase alertness and performance. Alertness drugs such as modafinil may also have a role. Where circadian adaptation is desirable (not for brief sojourns in a new time zone or for fast rotating shift schedules), patients may find it helpful to avoid light-countering adaptation of the circadian clock and to expose themselves to light timed to favor adaptation.

The hormone melatonin, administered at the correct circadian time, can shift circadian rhythms in the desired direction, particularly when followed by recumbency and very dim light or darkness. It has proved beneficial in most studies of jet lag. With increased attention to timing the dose, recent controlled studies have confirmed early observations that melatonin is useful for facilitating daytime sleep in shift work, and it can speed adaptation when this is desirable. Melatonin can synchronize and entrain free-running rhythms in most blind subjects and consistently improves sleep in non–24-hour sleep-wake disorder of blindness. In the latter case it is probably the treatment of choice.

Circadian rhythm abnormality as an underlying cause of sleep disorder has achieved greater recognition in recent years. A major influence is undoubtedly the so-called 24-hour society consequent upon mass air travel, 24-hour services, and globalization. Worldwide, approximately 500,000 people are reported to be airborne at any given time, and many of them will be crossing large numbers of time zones. A substantial fraction (probably 20% to 25%) of the working population of any industrialized country works during the biological night without fully (or often even partially) adapting their internal physiology to these shift-work conditions. Recent advances in dissecting the molecular machinery of circadian rhythm generation may well lead to a greater understanding of individual differences in adaptability to, and tolerance of, night-shift work and time-zone transition.

In general, the chaotic time cues of present-day society, in which exposure to natural bright light is probably insufficient, may well be an unidentified source of sleep problems. The extreme case is that of blind subjects with no conscious light perception, who frequently manifest non–24-hour sleep-wake disorder—effectively, intermittent jet lag. This chapter will consider these three conditions of circadian-rhythm disorder and discuss the possible therapeutic interventions.

WHAT IS JET LAG?

The preceding sections of this book have laid the foundations for understanding the phenomenon of jet lag and for appreciating the various countermeasures that can be taken to minimize this problem. Rapid travel across time zones leads to a mismatch or lack of synchrony between the activity of internal rhythm-generating systems and the local time cues, whether social or environmental.[1,2]

The internal circadian clock adapts slowly to abrupt changes of time cues. It has often been reported that on average, the clock shifts approximately 1 hour per day without countermeasures and that it will take 1 day for each hour of time zone change for adaptation to be complete. This is an oversimplification because the rate of adaptation varies with the individual, with the direction of time zone change , and with the course of adaptation. In general, adaptation is slower toward the east, and the rate of shift is usually faster in the initial than in the final stages.

In addition, it is relatively common for travelers to adapt in the "wrong" direction, such as by delaying 16 hours instead of advancing 8 hours. Figure 55–1 illustrates the highly individual nature of circadian adaptation after abrupt shifts of time cues. Reentrainment by "partition," in which some rhythms advance and some delay, has also been reported. In this case, the data may need reevaluation because immediate effects of the environment (masking) may have strongly influenced the parameters measured in early studies.

Possibly one third of all travelers do not experience jet lag. Those who do may experience symptoms such as daytime tiredness, inability to get to sleep at night (after an eastward flight) or early awakening (after a westward flight), disturbed

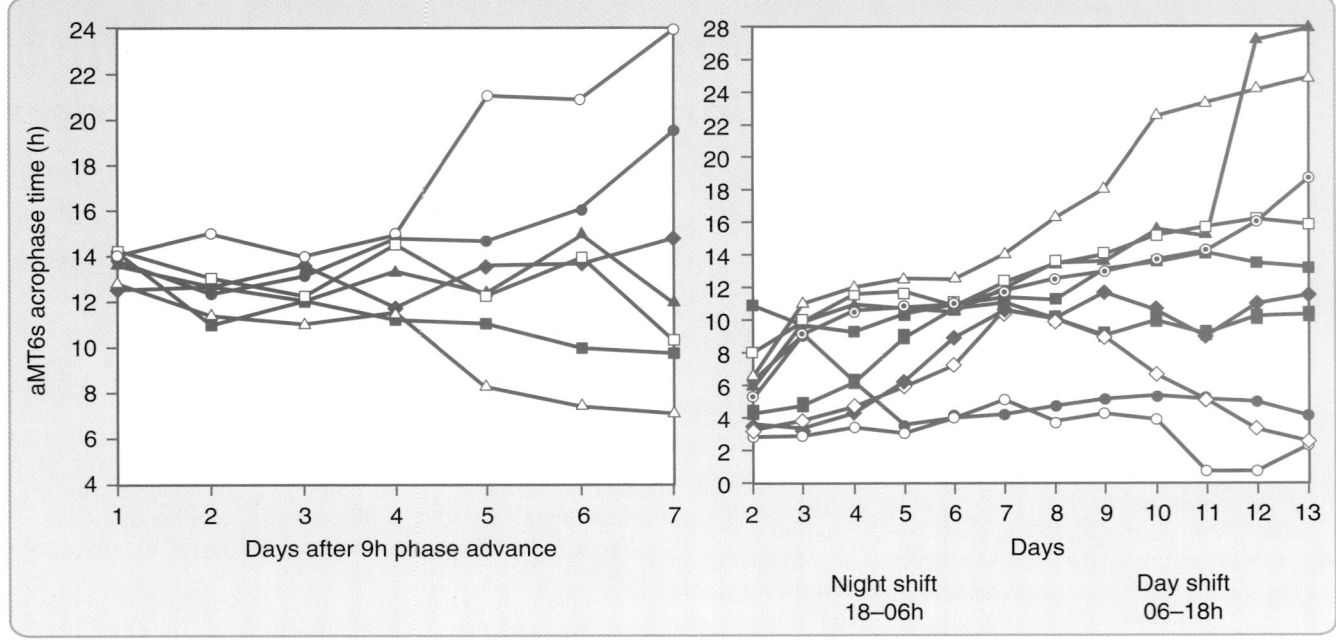

A

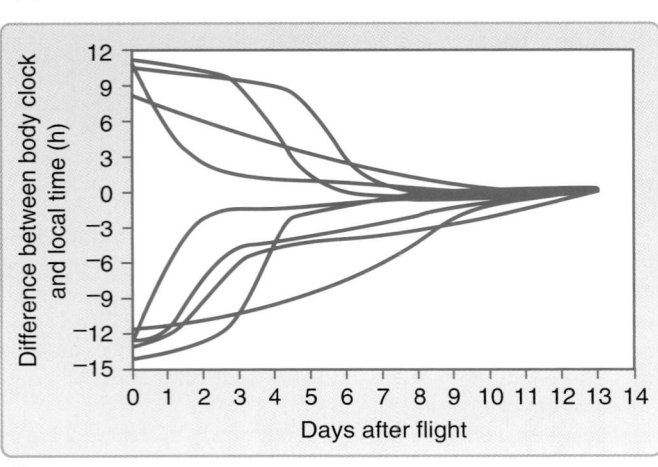

B

Figure 55–1. Individual differences in circadian adaptation to abrupt change of time cues. **A** *(left panel),* simulated jet lag with a forced 9-hour phase advance. Timing of the 6-sulfatoxymelatonin (aMT6s) rhythm in seven subjects in the days following phase shift. *Right panel,* real shift work on an offshore oil rig. Timing of the aMT6s rhythm in 11 subjects working 7 nights followed by 7 days. **B,** Real jet lag. Adaptation of the core body temperature rhythm in nine subjects following a 10-hour eastward transition. (A [*left panel*] redrawn from Deacon S, Arendt J: Adapting to phase shifts, II: Effects of melatonin and conflicting light treatment. Physiol Behav 1995;39:675-682, by permission. **B** from Spencer MB, Rogers AS, Pascoe PA: The effect of a large eastward time zone change on sleep, performance and circadian rhythms. DRA Report/CHS/A&N/CR/95/011, 1995.)

nighttime sleep, impaired daytime alertness and performance, disorientation, gastrointestinal problems, loss of appetite, inappropriate timing of defecation, and excessive need to urinate during the night. These symptoms may be just a nuisance for the first few days for a vacationer but may seriously impair the business traveler's ability to function. Aircrew, both civil and military, are of course more exposed than the general population to time zone change; their ability to perform is crucial, and much time has been devoted to developing strategies to combat jet lag in this population.[3,4] Models that assess the alertness associated with particular flight schedules take into account the impaired alertness and disturbed sleep associated with time zone change.[5]

All of the above symptoms may be ascribed in large part to temporary desynchronization of circadian rhythms. However, the circadian system may also be responsible for the organization of the menstrual cycle: female flight attendants may have more menstrual problems than women in the general population.[6] Meals eaten out of phase with the internal clock may give

rise to inappropriate pancreatic and metabolic responses, some of which may be long-term risk factors for heart disease.[7] Although to our knowledge there is little evidence that frequent time zone travel affects human life expectancy, there certainly is evidence from other forms of life (e.g., fruit flies, hamsters) that life span can be shortened with frequent phase shifting.[8,9]

Several attempts have been made to describe what exactly is meant by jet lag and how it may be measured. Simple subjective visual analogue scales have been used based on the assumption that subjects perceive as "jet lag" this complex of interrelated symptoms. The Surrey jet-lag scale correlates significantly with subjective sleep quality and latency[10,11] and the very similar Liverpool jet-lag scale[12] correlates closely with self-rated fatigue. More complex evaluations[13] add extra dimensions, which are of interest for in-depth studies. Performance measurements are of particular importance if optimal function is required immediately after flight, for example in some military operations and for business travelers. Abnormal timing of sleep and bowel functions ("gut lag") is more obvious than decrements in performance and abnormally timed hormone rhythms (for example). This is no doubt why they are the most frequently reported problems and should be targeted for therapeutic intervention.

CONDITIONS RELATED TO JET LAG

Shift Work

Health problems associated with night shift work are similar to those of jet lag, although travelers adapt with the help of local time cues, whereas shift workers are constantly living at odds with local time cues. Just as with jet lag, the cluster of problems associated with shift work has not been properly defined, although a new term, *shift-work sleep disorder* (SWSD), has now come into being. Perhaps the mere fact of attributing a simple name to a complex condition will help public understanding (as well as that of employers and funding agencies).

Most night-shift workers never fully adapt their internal clocks to the imposed sleep and work schedule.[14,15] This is especially true of workers in "fast rotation" schedules, such as 1 to 5 days of night shift interspersed with periods of day shift and rest days. Even permanent night-shift workers may not be fully adapted to their schedule, as it is common practice on rest days to revert to daytime living. Many of the night-shift workers in isolated situations, such as on oil rigs and in the Antarctic, do adapt, however.[16-18] Depending on the schedule, these subjects can fully adapt to a 12-hour shift within 4 to 7 days. Such situations are free of the social demands of, for example, family life and entertainment; sleeping quarters are usually quiet and dark; and exposure to natural light is minimized. However, if the work schedule leads to light exposure countering adaptation,[19] full adaptation does not occur, suggesting that factors other than light are less important.

Similarly, there is good evidence that exposure to morning light during the return home after a period of night shift counters the adaptive delay of circadian rhythms that might otherwise occur[20] and that avoidance of this light by wearing sunglasses or goggles can significantly help adaptation when it is desirable.[21] In a recent report,[22] subjects who had an identified evening preference ("owls" on the Horne-Ostberg scale) and who avoided morning light adapted by delay to a simulated night work schedule as fast as those who underwent other interventions. These observations emphasize the importance of exposure to time cues that may or may not aid adaptation depending on the timing of exposure.

For the majority, shift work is a lifetime experience of living out of phase at regular intervals. Many major accidents have been attributed to poor performance during an unadapted night shift. Night-shift workers may be more susceptible to accidents on the way home. This safety factor, coupled with the increased incidence of sleep problems, gastrointestinal disorders, metabolic syndrome, heart disease, and cancer,[23,24] indicates that for economic and health reasons, countermeasures should be developed. Considerable publicity has attended the reported increase in cancer in night-shift workers,[24] one hypothesis being that exposure to light at night is detrimental. It is worth noting that increased light during the night shift increases alertness, performance, and rate of adaptation.[25] Increasing nighttime light is already promoted to employers, but clearly it requires reevaluation if it is a possible factor in the development of major disease. Shift work is treated in detail in Chapters 56 and 57.

Circadian Sleep-Wake Disorders of Blindness

The light-dark cycle is the major synchronizer of human circadian rhythms. Without this time cue, many blind persons, especially those with no light perception at all, cannot remain on a 24-hour circadian clock. Some cannot remain synchronized to the 24-hour day-night cycle and "free run" with their own endogenous periodicity (τ); others take up an abnormal phase position of the internal clock so that, for example, they consistently have a peak of melatonin production and a trough in core body temperature during the daytime instead of at night.[26-28] The overt consequence often is a strong propensity to nap during the day and sleep poorly at night when the clock is out of phase.

The tendency to experience these circadian sleep disorders is strongly related to the degree of light perception and to whether a subject with no conscious light perception has no eyes or one or two remaining eyes. However, not all subjects with no conscious or unconscious[29] light perception show circadian desynchrony with or without a sleep disorder. In these cases, time cues other than light must be responsible for synchronization, or the endogenous periodicity must be very close to 24 hours. Very little is known of other possible circadian-related disorders, such as gastrointestinal disturbance and metabolic abnormalities, in the blind.

MECHANISMS UNDERLYING STRATEGIC COUNTERMEASURES

General

Circadian rhythms are probably internally generated from the central pacemaker, which is located in the suprachiasmatic nuclei (SCN) in the hypothalamus. Most circadian rhythms also have an exogenous component due to direct interaction with the environment (e.g., suppression of melatonin secretion by light) or with sleep times (sleep acutely lowers core body temperature) or exercise (which raises core body temperature). Thus, the overt manifestation of a rhythm is the sum of both exogenous and endogenous influences. The exogenous influence is usually known as masking.[30] The problems of jet lag, shift work, and blindness are probably caused by the endogenous component of the rhythm. The direct effects of the environment and of behavior can in principle (but often not in practice) be controlled. To hasten adaptation when it is desirable, it is sensible to exploit the acute effects of the environment, of behavior, and of drugs along with the strategies designed to hasten adaptation of the internal clock.

Sleep, Alertness, and Performance

Sleep is normally initiated on the rising phase of the melatonin rhythm and on the falling phase of the core body temperature rhythm in the evening (see Chapters 31 and 32). Sleep attempted on the rising phase of temperature and falling or baseline melatonin is shorter and associated with more awakenings.[14] This situation can occur with transitions over more than three or four time zones and is inevitable over a large number of time zones.

There have been many studies of sleep after transmeridian flights.[3,4,31,32] In general, the severity of sleep disturbance after a time zone change depends on the direction of travel and the number of time zones crossed and is influenced by the timing of the flight itself. After an eastward journey, when sleep is scheduled in advance of the "home" bedtime, there may be difficulty in falling asleep accompanied by increased wakefulness during the early part of the night, although these changes may not be apparent on the first night in the new time zone if the flight involves overnight travel without sleep. Sleep problems may continue for several days after the flight, with reductions in rapid eye movement (REM) sleep and possibly slow-wave sleep, and there may be a compensatory increase in REM sleep several nights later. Sleep disturbance after a westward flight is usually less persistent, lasting perhaps 2 or 3 days. Sleep is likely to be of good quality in the early part of the night, with increased slow-wave activity on the first night due to the long period without sleep. On subsequent nights, when the pressure for slow-wave sleep is less, there may be an increase in REM sleep as bedtime corresponds with early morning in the home time zone, when REM sleep predominates and body temperature begins to rise. Awakenings may be evident toward the end of the night at the time corresponding to daytime in the home time zone.

The decrements in performance and alertness that arise after a transmeridian flight can be attributed at least in part to the reduction in both the quality and quantity of sleep that occurs as a result of the requirement to sleep at an inappropriate circadian phase. One approach to optimizing performance and alertness is to preserve sleep as much as possible. There are several approaches, such as through the application of sleep-promoting techniques, attention to the circumstances surrounding sleep, the use of hypnotic agents, and the use of chronobiotics, which are drugs that shift the internal clock.[33,34] Other methods of treatment that may result in improved sleep for aircrew include, for example, changing duty schedules.

Other Physiologic Functions

Compared with sleep, alertness, and performance, far less is known of the precise manifestations of circadian desynchrony with respect to other physiologic systems. Any system under control of the circadian pacemaker will be affected by abrupt changes in time cues. Among the functions that merit much closer attention are the cardiovascular, immune, and reproductive systems, all of which are strongly rhythmic.[35] A start has been made in characterizing pancreatic and metabolic responses with respect to the influence of the endogenous clock and exogenous factors such as diet and sleep. Available information suggests that all three factors influence the enteroinsular axis.[7,36-38]

Recent reports concerning the adaptation of gene expression determining circadian phase (in rats) indicate that peripheral rhythm-generating genes (e.g., in the liver) can adapt very rapidly to a new light-dark and feeding schedule, whereas the central machinery (in the SCN) lags behind.[39] Thus by a rather large speculative jump it appears that much previous advice to travelers to behave according to their new time zone in terms of meal times (as well as attempted sleep times) may well be correct and may have a molecular explanation for its efficacy.

In principle, however, if it were possible to instantly and reliably shift the circadian clock(s) by any means, all problems due to the endogenous clock(s) would be countered. There is no one solution, although several approaches have met with some success. Two of the major problems in this area are the uncontrollable nature of field studies on jet lag and the fact that so far it has not been possible to simulate time zone change in the laboratory taking into account all the factors that may arise in the field.

COUNTERMEASURES

Sleep Hygiene

It is evident from studies in blind subjects and tolerant shift workers that, at least for some people, it is quite possible to sleep out of phase without perceived problems. Thus, the initial strategy to alleviate jet lag must be to ensure adequate sleep. Among the techniques or strategies that may be applied to promote sleep are those that aim to ensure that the sleeping environment is optimal: Whatever the circadian phase, sleep will be more disturbed if the bedroom environment is noisy and light. If the sleeping environment is not ideal, earplugs and eyeshades can be used to screen unwanted external stimuli. These strategies are frequently used by airline pilots when sleeping in hotels or when they have to obtain rest in the bunk facilities on board the aircraft on long-range flights.[32]

Caffeine and alcohol are known to have detrimental effects on sleep,[32,40,41] although alcohol may initially promote sleep onset. It has been suggested that a "jet-lag diet" will speed the adaptation of sleep and other rhythms. With this diet, an evening meal rich in carbohydrates provides a source of tryptophan for serotonin synthesis to assist sleep, and protein-rich meals in the morning provide tyrosine to enhance catecholamine levels and increase alertness during the day.[42] One review of this field of research concludes that there is no evidence to support this idea.[43] However, in view of the observations concerning peripheral clock genes, perhaps some reconsideration is required. Minor changes in phase after an evening carbohydrate meal have been recently reported; the mechanism of action is probably an effect on a peripheral oscillator.[44] The administration of tryptophan has been reported to increase total sleep time on the first night after transmeridian travel westward, although its effects on sleep are considered to be limited.

Specifically timed naps before, during, or after a flight can in theory and in practice markedly increase alertness.[45] Computer programs are available that enable a prediction of alertness as a function of nap timing.[45] However, napping is frequently not possible either before or during a flight. It is often recommended that the traveler not nap in the destination time zone but instead schedule sleep to be in synchrony with the new environment. This advice may be hard to follow after a long, sleepless flight. Passengers in first, club, and business class have more opportunity to sleep during the flight because the size and angle of the seats, as well as the footrests, are more conductive to sleep.[32] Sleep during flight should be taken as far as possible during the future night time in the destination time zone. The effect of napping is confounded by reduction of photic input when a person shuts the eyes. Naps timed to avoid light exposure and hasten adaptation could thus have a dual "therapeutic" effect.

Hypnotic Agents

Another approach to the preservation of sleep involves the use of drugs, and there have been numerous studies on the effects of hypnotic agents.[32-34] The largest class of hypnotic agents—the benzodiazepines—is known to speed sleep onset, reduce awakenings, and increase total sleep time in normal sleepers and in those with transient or chronic insomnia. In addition, these medications may modify sleep architecture by delaying the appearance of REM sleep, reducing slow-wave sleep, and enhancing sleep spindles. The imidazopyridine zolpidem and the cyclopyrrolone zopiclone have effects on the electroencephalogram similar to those of the benzodiazepines except that they may increase slow-wave sleep. The overriding factor when considering the potential use of a hypnotic agent is the drug's duration of action.[32]

Clearly, the benefits associated with improved sleep may be masked if use of the hypnotic agent leads to unwanted side effects that diminish alertness after the sleep period. After a transmeridian flight, hypnotic agents with a duration of action of around 3 to 5 hours may be useful to sustain sleep during the adaptation phase without producing adverse effects on performance. In such situations, the agents are likely to be effective due to their sleep-promoting properties rather than via an effect on shifting circadian rhythms.[46] However, because light is avoided during sleep, the lack of light may hasten or delay readaptation depending on when sleep is taken.

In addition to the use of hypnotic agents on arrival in a new time zone, passengers may consider the use of medication on the flight to assist in taking sleep timed to coincide with the nocturnal rest period at the destination. However, any increase in immobility may have implications for deep vein thromboses, and the ability to respond to an emergency situation is also likely to be impaired. One strategy for business travelers that (anecdotally) appears to be quite successful when traveling from the United Kingdom to the West Coast of the United States is to sleep early on arrival (with the use of a hypnotic agent), conduct meetings on the next morning, and return on the next evening.

Light

Laboratory Studies

The light-dark cycle is the principal time cue for resetting human circadian rhythms.[47] The most effective intensity, duration, and spectral composition in a given situation cannot yet be defined completely. The mechanisms underlying circadian photoreception are currently being dissected[48] and involve a novel "circadian" photoreceptor system. Following two demonstrations that the most effective wavelength for suppression of melatonin lies in the short wavelength 460- to 465-nm (blue) range,[49,50] it has become clear that the phase shifting potency of blue light is also very much greater than that of white[51] or 555-nm light.[52] The present discussion may well have to be updated when the widespread applications of these important observations have been evaluated.

Correctly timed white light of suitable intensity and duration will both phase advance and phase delay circadian rhythms according to a phase-response curve.[47,53,54] Broadspectrum white light of 3000 to 10,000 lux applied soon after the minimum of core body temperature (or the maximum of plasma melatonin) is attained will advance the internal clock; light scheduled soon before the core temperature minimum will delay it. Phase-response curves describing these interactions enable theoretical predictions to be made concerning the timing of light treatment to adapt to phase shift. It is also possible to induce large phase changes of the circadian system with light centered on the core temperature minimum, but this procedure appears to be somewhat unpredictable. It is clearly impractical to expose subjects to light in the middle of the night before departure, although in principle this would be possible during flight through the use of either carefully chosen window seats or artificial means. In addition to its phase-shifting ability, bright light also has immediate alertness-increasing and temperature-raising properties[25] that may, in part, be related to melatonin suppression.[55,56]

Bright light and avoidance of bright light[20,21,57] appear to be useful in helping to facilitate phase shifts of circadian rhythms, although very little research has been conducted in real-life settings. Phase shifts have been produced, however, in laboratory studies that simulate jet-lag and shift-work situations.[21,22,57-61] A few laboratory studies have measured circadian phase after exposure to bright light (more than 2000 lux) or dim light during the imposed wake time. The general finding has been that circadian rhythms shifted about 1 hour per day in the dim-light conditions and as much as 2 to 3 hours per day in the bright-light conditions.[57,58] Sleep problems abated as body temperature shifted to align with sleep time. With strict scheduling of sleep and darkness, even domestic-intensity light appears to be an effective phase-shifting agent.[61]

The importance of scheduled sleep and darkness cannot be overestimated. One study suggested that both 3- and 6-hour exposures to bright light are equally effective in shifting the temperature rhythm. Others suggest that only the initial part of the light treatment is necessary for effective shifting and also that intermittent exposure to light can be almost as effective as continuous exposure.[62] Thus, extremely long bright-light durations throughout the wake period may not be necessary, making the procedure more convenient and feasible. Some laboratory studies have compared different timings of bright light after large, abrupt phase advances of the sleep-wake schedule, but there is little consistency in the results. In some cases, there was little difference between the conditions predicted to enhance phase shifting and the conditions predicted to inhibit the phase shift.[58]

The use of a "nudging" technique, whereby periods of bright-light treatment are shifted on a daily basis to later or earlier times, has been very successful in adjusting circadian timing in the laboratory.[21,60] For example, 9 hours of moderately bright white light (1200 lux) followed by imposed darkness and sleep applied on a shifting schedule (3 hours per day, delay or advance) will reliably advance or delay all circadian rhythms, with no detrimental effects on sleep, mood, or performance. Unfortunately this nudging technique is impractical in many respects but has been used in some specific situations.[21]

Field Studies

The number of field studies of the use of light for jet lag and shift work is small. However, the results are increasingly consistent. In general, with the appropriate timing of light exposure, a modest acceleration in the rate of adaptation of circadian rhythms to the new sleep-wake schedule is observed.

It is worth noting that except during scheduled light treatments, the subjects in the early field studies were free to engage in activities of their choice, and no attempt was made to limit their exposure to bright light at times when such exposure might hinder reentrainment. Bright light administered under more controlled laboratory conditions after transmeridian flights appeared to speed up reentrainment.[58]

Additional field studies have examined the effects of morning bright-light treatment on postflight sleep patterns. For example, exposure to bright white or dim red light for 2 to 3 hours on awakening in the morning (centered around 9:30 AM local time) for 3 days after a 6.5- to 10-hour advance flight yielded no differences between the groups in any subjective sleep measure. In a second study with objective sleep electroencephalographic recordings after an 8-hour advance flight, subjects exposed for 3 days to bright light (3:00 to 6:00 AM local time) showed higher sleep efficiency than those exposed to dim light, with the latter exhibiting prolonged wakefulness during the first half of the night. A review by Samel and Wegmann in 1997[58] summarized available data. Their conclusion was that there is some evidence that correctly timed bright light may have been effective in accelerating reentrainment. More recently the use of timed light treatment to adapt to work schedules on offshore oil rigs has shown beneficial effects. In fact the greatest benefit was shown using light to adapt back to home time after adapting to offshore night shift.[63] With careful evaluation of phase in a laboratory setting, further evidence of the usefulness of timed light treatment has been presented.[59]

Many questions remain, particularly with regard to jet lag, including determination of optimal times for light exposure and avoidance on the first and subsequent treatment days and whether a given fixed light exposure time is likely to benefit a majority of travelers, or whether light treatment should instead be scheduled according to an individual circadian phase marker. A number of computer programs or calculators provide the times of exposure and avoidance of bright light for travelers based on the phase-response curve for light as a function of direction of flight, number of time zones crossed, and arrival time (for example MidnightSun[120] and New Light on Jet Lag, www.lightboxco.com).

Avoiding natural bright light may be the most important consideration. As previously mentioned, shift workers adapt to night shift when shielded from natural light and social time cues. There is good evidence that exposure to natural light when returning home in the early morning after a night shift opposes the delay required to sleep well during the day.[20] When traveling east over more than four or five time zones and arriving in the early morning, subjects experience light opposed to their adaptation, particularly if seated in sunlight by a window in the plane before and during the descent. (Other situations and predicted light avoidance and treatment times can be found in publicly available instructions as above.)

For aircrew scheduled to return to home base after a brief layover, remaining on home time may be preferable to trying to adjust to local time, eliminating the need for readjustment after the return flight. Indeed, a large proportion of flight personnel report going to bed early after a westward transatlantic flight. In such cases, bright light treatment may be used to maintain entrainment to home time rather than to accelerate reentrainment to new local times.

In addition to effects on alertness, temperature, heart rate, melatonin levels, and circadian phase shifting, there is a small amount of evidence that bright light can acutely modify some hormonal and metabolic responses, for example, elevation of luteinizing hormone and cortisol levels as a function of timing of exposure.[64,65]

Melatonin

In most respects, melatonin can be considered a "darkness hormone." It is normally produced at night, and the duration of secretion reflects the length of the night. It appears to serve similar functions in all life forms so far studied, acting as a time signal for the organization of daily and annual rhythms.[66] In animals that use day-length changes to time their seasonal cycles, melatonin indicates the length of the night. For example, a long night of melatonin induces sheep to start breeding in autumn and hamsters (who breed in the summer) to stop breeding. Other seasonal variations, such as coat growth, are also timed by melatonin.

There is some published information concerning the possible inhibitory effects of melatonin on human reproduction. However, one early and two recent studies have shown no effect of medium- to long-term melatonin use on the secretion of reproductive hormones in normal men.[67-69]

In some species, especially some lower vertebrates and birds, melatonin is essential for the organization of daily (circadian) rhythms. In mammals, it is not essential for circadian organization but appears to reinforce behavior associated with darkness, such as sleep in human beings. Taken during the "biological day" (when endogenous melatonin is low), it has rapid, transient, mild sleep-inducing effects and lowers alertness and body temperature during the 3 to 4 hours after low doses (0.05 to 5 mg). These effects are opposite to the acute effects of bright light. In the same dose range, it can shift the timing of the internal clock (including the sleep-wake cycle) to both later and earlier times when the administration is appropriately timed[67,70,71] and is particularly effective if treatment is associated with recumbency and darkness.[68]

For light treatment, the appropriate timing can be predicted from a phase-response curve in subjects whose body clock phase is known. The phase-response curve for melatonin is reported to be the reverse of that for light.[71,72] Studies show that melatonin administered from about 5 to 13 hours before core temperature minimum will phase advance, and melatonin administered during a 3- to 6-hour window beginning about 1 to 2 hours after core temperature minimum will phase delay the circadian system, although there are some discrepancies between authors and substantial scatter in the data (Figure 55-2). There remains some controversy concerning phase delays.[73] Taken to phase advance on a daily basis, melatonin can maintain entrainment to 24 hours in sighted subjects.[72] Importantly, it is able to resynchronize most free-running blind subjects,[74,75] and in this case it is possible that low doses (0.5 mg or less) are more effective than higher doses (5 to 10 mg).[76,77] In subjects synchronized to a normal 24-hour environment, the timing of desired phase shifts is relatively simple and can to some extent be judged by habitual sleep times. Optimal timing is not so simple after time zone travel, in shift workers, and in blind subjects unless circadian phase is determined prior to treatment. This is an

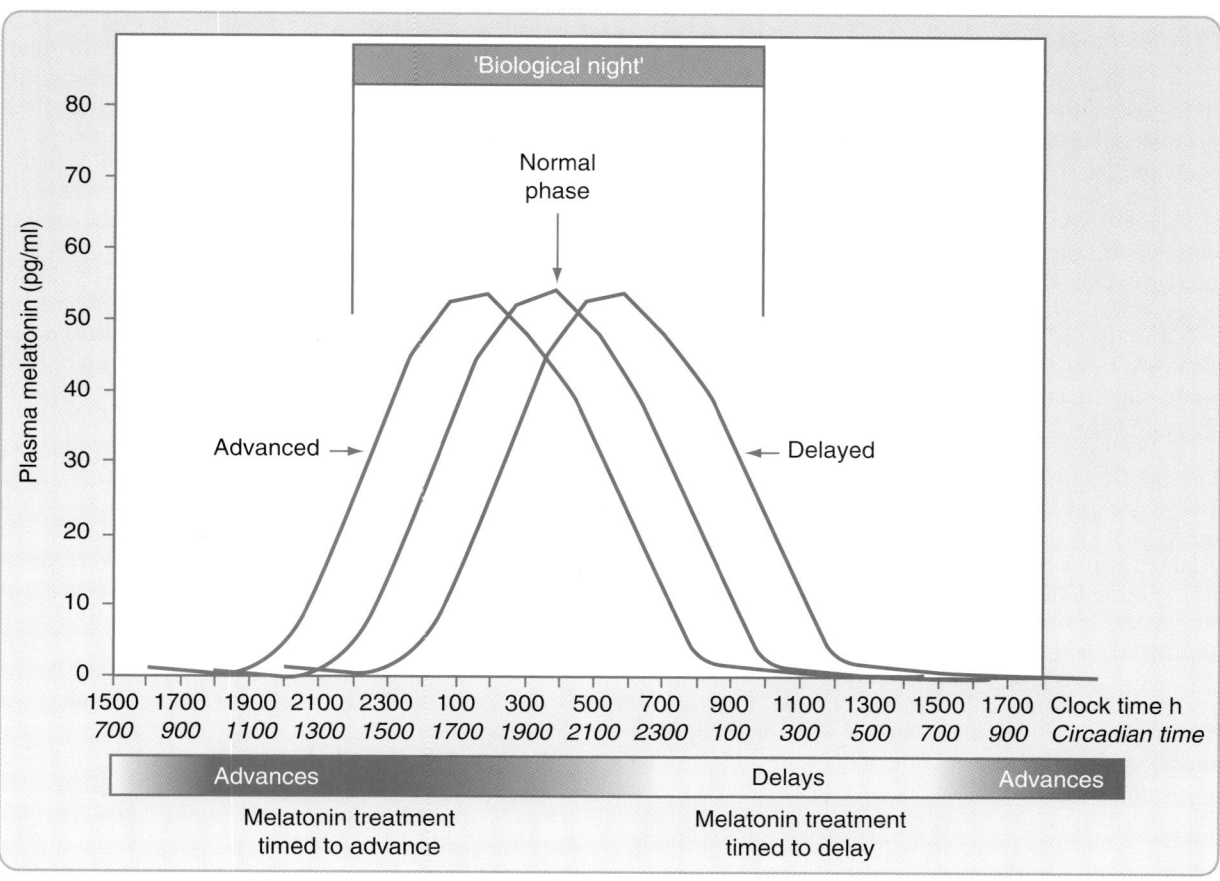

Figure 55–2. Diagram of the direction of phase shifts induced by melatonin treatment at different times in relation to "biological night" (the period of endogenous melatonin secretion). (From Arendt J, Skene DJ: Melatonin as a chronobiotic. Sleep Med Rev 2004;9:25-39.

onerous undertaking and impractical (at present) in clinical use. Melatonin is available in the United Kingdom from a licensed manufacturer on prescription; availability varies in other countries. Only licensed preparations have guaranteed content and purity.

Simulated Phase Shifts

At least four studies of melatonin have addressed its possible ability to hasten adaptation to simulated phase shift.[22,78-80] In environmental isolation, a simulated advanced phase shift and suitably timed treatment (5 mg) showed an increase in the rate of reentrainment of endogenous rhythms[78] but with inconsistent effects on sleep. Melatonin appeared to be able to specify the direction of reentrainment to advance rather than delay. During a simulated acute 9-hour delay of sleep time, the effectiveness of bright light (4 hours, 4000 to 7000 lux) for 3 days during the first half of the night-shift period, dim red light (50 lux) for the same period, and melatonin or placebo just before and during desired sleep time has been compared. Essentially, only the group receiving bright light showed significant circadian adaptation and improvements in performance, whereas both melatonin and bright light improved sleep.[79]

After a simulated rapid 9-hour phase advance, we investigated the ability of melatonin with or without conflicting bright light treatment to hasten adaptation. Melatonin (5 mg

fast release) or placebo was taken at 11:00 PM on the first night after the shift and for two additional nights at the same time. Conflicting light (white, 1200 lux) exposure occurred from 8:00 AM through noon during the first 3 days after the shift. Melatonin treatment was timed to be just within a phase-advance window, and light treatment was timed to phase delay. Melatonin rapidly and consistently improved sleep (quality, duration, and night awakenings) compared with placebo even in the presence of inappropriate light, and this was independent of the direction of phase shift.[80] Daily mean alertness and performance efficiency were higher for all treatments compared with placebo.

The effects of melatonin were apparent before phase adaptation occurred. They are likely to result from the combination of acute effects on behavior and temperature reinforced by a hastening of phase adaptation. The latter, however, did not appear to play a major role, at least during the first post phase shift days. However, it must be emphasized that simulations of this sort do not fully mimic field conditions. For example, sleep problems last longer in comparable field studies. In a recent crossover study of simulated phase shift, carefully timed melatonin was very effective in hastening adaptation to the new schedule.[22] In comparisons with hypnotics as an aid to sleep in short-term sleep displacement, melatonin had no impact on performance and was an effective sleep aid.[81,82]

Field Studies on Jet Lag

At least 13 placebo-controlled field studies[13,83-96] have reported the use of melatonin to alleviate perceived jet lag. Of these, 10 were successful in the sense that subjective (and, in one case, objective) measures of sleep and alertness improved compared with placebo. The first study,[83,84] over eight time zones eastward, used a time sequence of administration (5 mg melatonin daily) designed to initiate an eastward phase shift before departure by early evening administration (6:00 PM) for 3 days before flight and to reinforce the advance by bedtime (11:00 PM) administration in the new local time zone for 4 days. The results indicated that both subjective jet lag ratings and objective parameters (actigraphic sleep parameters, subjective sleep, alertness, endogenous melatonin, and cortisol) showed more rapid adaptation in the melatonin-treated group (N = 8) than in the placebo group (N = 9). Subjective jet lag was significantly correlated with sleep quality and latency.

In a larger population (N = 52) of subjects traveling to Australia from the United Kingdom and back, melatonin was timed to phase advance (early evening) for 2 days before departure and 4 days after arrival (at bedtime) eastward and westward for 4 days at local bedtime. The design was crossover, with melatonin outward and placebo on return or vice versa in subjects remaining in Australia for longer than 14 days. Again, a highly significant improvement in subjective jet lag with melatonin was seen,[85] with the caveat, however, that four subjects felt worse on melatonin. With the use of a very similar protocol and dose, subjective measures were improved in 20 subjects flying from New Zealand to the United Kingdom and back.[86]

With no preflight treatment, in a placebo-controlled crossover design after flight over 6, 9, and 11 time zone changes, 5 mg melatonin at bedtime accelerated adaptation of the cortisol rhythm with a consistent, but not significant, improvement of subjective jet lag both eastward and westward in 36 subjects.[87] The effect on cortisol was more significant with a greater number of time zones. Preflight treatment at 10:00 PM and then daily for 3 days after the flight at bedtime (8 mg) led to improved sleep and subjective jet lag in 37 subjects traveling eastward from the United States and Canada to France.[88]

Comperatore et al.[89] used melatonin treatment (10 mg daily) timed just within a theoretical phase-advance window and combined with other countermeasures (timed avoidance and exposure to bright light, preflight shift of bedtimes) to adapt to an 8-hour advance but with unusual bedtimes (4:00 AM local time) at the destination. The melatonin treatment led to improved sleep duration and cognitive performance compared with the placebo group. Interestingly, given the large dose of 10 mg, mild sleepiness and fatigue were reported only occasionally after ingestion and never after awakening. This dose of melatonin will not be fully cleared from the circulation after an 8-hour sleep, and thus such "high" doses, consistent with our experience with 5 mg and that of Waldhauser and colleagues[90] with 80 mg, do not appear to lead to hangover effects.

The largest controlled study reported to date involved a total of 320 subjects treated after their flight at bedtime for 4 days after an eastward flight (six to eight time zones). Melatonin (5 mg fast release) was strikingly efficient in improving sleep latency, sleep quality, daytime sleepiness, and fatigue compared with placebo. A lower dose (0.5 mg) of fast-release preparation was less effective, as was a slow-release preparation.[91] These same authors assessed the effectiveness of melatonin compared to zolpidem.[92] Although zolpidem appeared to be more effective than melatonin, it had undesirable side effects. Very few such comparative studies exist—one evaluated the use of caffeine compared to melatonin, concluding that they were equally effective.[93] However, these conclusions were based on single time-point saliva samples for phase assessment. A very small study (six subjects), distinguished by the use of full plasma melatonin profiles to determine phase, reported faster resynchronization with melatonin at 11:00 PM after travel from Tokyo to Los Angeles, in spite of uncontrolled exposure to natural light.[94]

These positive reports are in contrast to the results of three other studies. Petrie et al.[95] used aircrew (N = 52) traveling from Auckland to Los Angeles and returning to Auckland via London. The last leg of the journey was used for the trial. They reported problems with preflight (3 days) melatonin administration but improvement in subjective measures with only postflight treatment. In another large controlled study (249 subjects in four groups) in which 5 or 0.5 mg melatonin was taken at bedtime and 0.5 mg was taken on a shifting schedule to phase advance (New York to Oslo), melatonin was completely ineffective at alleviating subjective symptoms of jet lag.[13]

It should be noted that the successful studies involved subjects demonstrably or probably synchronized to the local environment before treatment. In the latter study, as with long-haul aircrew, the circadian state of the subjects was unknown before departure, and it is unlikely that 4 days was sufficient for full synchronization to New York time. Because the timing of melatonin is fairly critical, it is possible that the subjects received the treatment at an inappropriate circadian phase before the flight. A further study with athletes traveling to Australia from the United Kingdom used apparently inappropriate treatment times (phase delay timing when a phase advance was required.)[96] No beneficial effects were reported. A method for rapid assessment of circadian phase, suitable for use with minimum analytical training, would be highly desirable.

In both controlled and uncontrolled field studies on the traveling public since 1986,[97,98] we have observed an overall 50% reduction in subjective assessment of jet lag symptoms (N = 474) using 5 mg fast-release melatonin. For eastward travel, we suggest a single phase-advancing preflight early evening treatment, followed by treatment at bedtime for 4 days after arrival (Box 55–1). For westward travel, we advise subjects to take melatonin for 4 days at bedtime (11:00 PM or later for a phase delay time over more than six time zones) in the new time zone. This timing enables the exploitation of both sleep-inducing and phase-shifting effects (see Figures 55–2 and 55–3). The subjective improvement increases with the number of time zones crossed. Short layovers require specific instructions, and little evidence exists for efficacy in these circumstances.

A Cochrane review has been published[99] with a meta-analysis of those published studies considered suitable for analysis. The authors concluded that melatonin was indeed effective at alleviating jet lag if properly timed. There is a need to explore the limitations of the treatment and to make further comparisons with, for example, benzodiazepine hypnotics. There is little information on optimal dose or formulation.

Box 55–1.	**Experimental Use of Melatonin to Alleviate Jet Lag**

East

When going east, take one capsule of melatonin (lowest effective dose, licensed for human experimental use) on departure day, if necessary on the flight, between 6 and 7 PM local time. On arrival take a capsule at local bedtime, 10 to 11 PM, for 4 days. If your stopovers are fewer than 4 days, on the evening preceding your next departure, do not take a capsule at bedtime but instead at 6 to 7 PM local time. On arrival, take a capsule daily at the local bedtime 10 to 11 PM for 4 days.

West

When going west, take 1 capsule daily at the local bedtime (11 PM) or later for 4 days after arrival at each stopover and at the destination. If you are awake in the very early morning (before 4 AM), you may take another capsule. Be aware that taken as late as this, melatonin may make you sleepy in the morning. Do not take capsules before the flight if going west, except, of course, if your stopover is less than 4 days, when you will be taking them at bedtime on the night before departure.

Please Note

Melatonin can induce sleepiness and lowered alertness. You are advised not to drive or operate heavy or dangerous machinery, or perform equivalent tasks requiring alertness for 4 to 5 hours after taking the medication. Melatonin is most effective at shifting sleep timing and circadian rhythms if taken just prior to a period of recumbency and dim light. Thus, where possible, lie down in dim light for at least 5 hours after the dose.

Exclusion Criteria for Participation in the Jet Lag Studies of Arendt et al.:

You must have permission from your physician to take part. You may not participate in the study if you are a long-haul pilot or aircrew or shift worker (this is due to potential difficulties with timing the dose); you or a close blood relative have a psychiatric condition or migraine headaches; you are younger than 18 years old; you know (or suspect) that you are pregnant or intend to become pregnant; you are lactating; you are taking any medication other than minor analgesics or oral contraceptives; and/or you have any diseases.

Possible side effects of melatonin treatment are sleepiness (desirable), headache (infrequent), and nausea (very infrequent).

Modified from Arendt J, Deacon S: Treatment of circadian rhythm disorders-melatonin. Chronobiol Int 1997;14:185-204, courtesy of Marcel Dekker, Inc. Instructions used in field experiments by the authors. Preflight treatment eastward may not be important, but no comparative data are available.

The pharmacokinetics of fast-release melatonin is extremely variable among individuals, and the question of individual sensitivity has not been addressed. There is no information on long-term safety, although no significant problems have been reported in healthy adults.[100] Successful treatment appears to be associated with the use of subjects synchronized to the local environment before departure. It is a matter for discussion and further experiment whether preflight administration confers any advantages. In the authors' opinion, preflight treatment if traveling eastwards (as in the first study) is likely to be important, particularly as melatonin can specify the direction of reentrainment,[78] and this must be done before possible exposure to natural bright light or other time cues acting counter to the most rapid direction of reentrainment (Figure 55–3).

The "avoidance" of endogenous melatonin through the suppression of production by bright light or drugs or, in the future, the use of melatonin receptor antagonists is another important consideration. One report suggests that the suppression of melatonin with a beta-adrenergic antagonist (atenolol) facilitated phase shifts to bright light.[101]

Field Studies on Shift Work

The use of melatonin in adapting to night shift has been reported in several field studies.[102-104] Two initial studies used 7-day rotating shift workers, and both involved administering melatonin at the desired bedtime after the night shift. Early-morning melatonin administration, designed to phase delay, significantly improved daytime sleep duration and quality and night-shift alertness. Its effects on various performance tasks were variable. In the other study, melatonin improved the synchrony between endogenous circadian rhythms and daytime sleep. Some subsequent studies have shown no significant effects.[104] However, a simulated and carefully controlled shift-work study (referred to earlier) showed very clear benefits of melatonin treatment.[22]

In situations (fast rotation) where adaptation is undesirable, melatonin may be used in other ways to facilitate out-of-phase sleep. Taken in the late afternoon just before a period of recumbency and very dim light, it is clearly very effective at facilitating sleep[68,105-107] and has been considered a hypnotic in these circumstances.[106] However, with an extended sleep opportunity (16 hours following the dose) it is evident that melatonin does not increase total sleep time but, as observed many years ago, changes the timing of sleep.[67,68,107] Shift workers complain that it is difficult to sleep in the early evening, prior to night work, and thereby reduce sleep deprivation. Use of melatonin in this context might well be helpful. Melatonin can also facilitate daytime sleep in the short term without necessarily shifting circadian phase.

It will be important to ascertain whether or not the use of melatonin is accompanied by consistent changes in work-related performance. However, melatonin clearly shows promise in the context of shift work.

Sleep Disorder of Blindness

In an epidemiologic study in the United Kingdom, 60% of the registered blind subjects who were studied appeared to have a sleep disorder as assessed by use of the Pittsburgh Sleep Quality Index, with greater prevalence in individuals with no conscious light perception.[27,28,108] Similar statistics have been reported in other studies in the United States, Switzerland, and France. These sleep disturbances vary from delayed-sleep-phase syndrome to irregular phase position to free-running circadian rhythms in a normal environment (non–24-hour sleep-wake disorder). In most blind subjects, poor sleep corresponds to the antiphase of the endogenous melatonin rhythm.[27,109] Daytime napping is associated with the peak of melatonin production occurring during the day (this constitutes

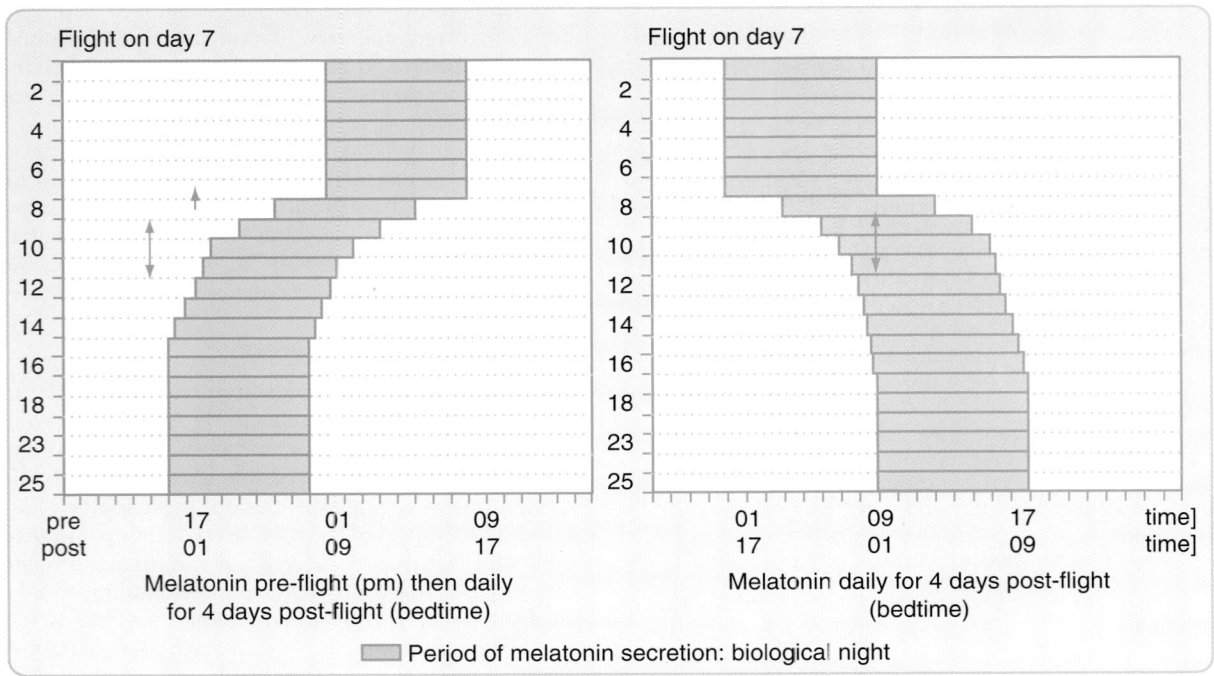

PRESUMED PHASE SHIFTS

Figure 55–3. Diagram of presumed phase shifts with melatonin treatment (timing shown by the *arrows*) to aid adaptation to an 8-hour eastward or westward time zone transition. Note that acute sleepiness or sleep is induced by melatonin during "biological day" as well as phase shifts. Note also that this is a highly simplified conception and that large individual differences (see Fig. 53–1) are evident. (From Arendt J, Skene DJ: Melatonin as a chronobiotic. Sleep Med Rev 2004;9:25-39.

some of the best evidence for a physiologic role for endogenous melatonin in human sleep). The situation thus is analogous to jet lag and shift work, in which subjects intermittently must sleep at an inappropriate circadian phase. In blind persons, this is a life-long problem, and there is an urgent need for further investigation of treatment strategies.

For subjects who retain a circadian response to light, appropriately timed bright light is the treatment of choice. When there is no response to light, techniques using nonphotic time cues (e.g., timed melatonin, exercise, caffeine) must be exploited. Timed melatonin is the treatment of choice at present. It is likely that combinations of scheduled sleep time, exercise, caffeine, and meal times with melatonin treatment will be even more effective.

Suitably timed administration of melatonin has provided positive results in stabilizing and consolidating sleep, greatly reducing daytime naps, and improving mood parameters in the vast majority of blind patients.[75-77,109-112] Recent important data from two independent laboratories indicate that in addition, melatonin can fully entrain the circadian system to the solar day in most blind persons.[74-77] In the past, entrainment of free-running circadian rhythms by melatonin has been the subject of intense debate. The early reports of melatonin treatment in the blind, using 5- to 10-mg fast-release preparations, were unable to show synchronization or entrainment despite treatment timing designed to exploit the phase-advancing properties of melatonin.[109-112]

At present the debate[113,114] over the most efficient approach to treatment centers on both the dose and the timing of administration (according to circadian phase). It is possible that lower doses (0.5 mg or less) are more effective for long-term entrainment[76,77] as opposed to acute phase shifts. It is also possible that a very long free-running circadian period cannot be entrained, melatonin instead producing a shortening of period (τ). In this situation, combinations of nonphotic time cues are well worth exploring. Even if their circadian periods cannot be entrained, however, nearly all blind patients derive some benefit from the treatment. One subject, studied by our group on numerous occasions, has slept well (in his estimation and when objectively assessed) without circadian entrainment for 15 years by taking 5 mg melatonin at bedtime nightly. He showed no evidence of addiction, tolerance, or toxicity when assessed after 10 years of treatment.[100]

In the clinical situation, the most common approach is probably to instruct subjects to take the melatonin dose approximately 1 hour before desired bedtime (Prof. A. Bird, personal communication). With large differences in individual pharmacokinetics and, probably, sensitivity, dose adjustment to increase effectiveness and avoid any possible "hangover" effects may well be required. In general, as for all other situations, the lowest effective dose is to be recommended.

Melatonin has also been effective when taken at bedtime to treat sleep-wake disorders in multiply disabled children with or without visual loss.[115] These patients have major behavioral problems during the day as well as during the night. Melatonin was found to consolidate sleep to the nighttime and to alleviate daytime problems. Better mood, alertness, and, in some cases, fewer seizures were reported. Many of the patients had tried a number of sedatives without success before becoming stabilized on melatonin. However, there are no data on the circadian status of these subjects, and the mechanism of action has yet to be elucidated.

OTHER STRATEGIES

There is some evidence that timed exercise can shift the human circadian system.[116,117] The use of vitamin B_{12} may sensitize the circadian system to light-induced phase shifts.[118] No controlled field studies have yet shown the effectiveness of these approaches in alleviating jet lag; however, it makes sense to combine behavioral strategies with any light or pharmacologic measures. Preadaptation to night shift or time zone change by shifting sleep timing, light exposure, and so on in the desired direction is, of course, a useful, if inconvenient, strategy.

SUMMARY AND FUTURE

Much research now demonstrates unequivocally that timed exposure to light and to melatonin is an effective means of manipulating the circadian timing system. Many questions remain, notably the numerous issues necessary to develop safe, effective, reliable, and practical treatment strategies. Concerns such as optimal light intensity, light-spectrum composition, duration and timing of light exposure, individual differences in response to light, and age effects must be addressed. Similarly, timed melatonin enhances adaptation to simulated and real night shifts; improves sleep, circadian adaptation, and subjectively perceived jet lag in most field studies; and greatly improves sleep in blind subjects without necessarily entraining all circadian rhythms. Melatonin and light may act in concert to maintain endogenous circadian synchronization in sighted individuals. Their combined use should provide optimal phase-shifting strategies, although a great deal of further research is needed.

Several major advances in our knowledge of the circadian system regarding rhythm generation and control have taken place in the last 5 years. Blue light for optimal phase shifting,[49-52] melatonin entrainment of the human circadian system,[72,74,75] and the genetics of the circadian clock are of primary importance. Dissection of the molecular machinery of rhythm generation has led to identification of a human polymorphism in the coding region of the clock gene *hPer3* associated with diurnal preference and delayed-sleep-phase syndrome.[119] As knowledge of human clock genes progresses, we shall be better equipped to identify the reasons for large individual differences in adapting to time zone transition and shift work. It is likely that advice can be given in the future, based on genotype, regarding how we should choose our work schedules and travel possibilities. New pharmacologic treatments to shift the circadian clock will be developed and may well make light and melatonin redundant.

RECOMMENDATIONS FOR TRAVELERS

- Where possible, choose daytime flights to minimize the loss of sleep and fatigue.
- Travel business or first class, if possible.
- Avoid large high-fat meals out of phase and caffeine and alcohol during the night.

- Drink a lot of water.
- Avoid making critical decisions or attending important meetings on the first day after arrival.
- Avoid driving long distances on the first day after arrival.
- Avoid or seek bright light according to the recommendations of, for example, Houpt et al.[120]
- Consider the use of short-acting hypnotic agents during the flight (to sleep during the destination nighttime) and for the first few days after arrival.
- Consider, with the advice of your physician, the use of correctly timed melatonin if a licensed, quality-controlled preparation and use instructions (see Box 55–1) are available. Use the lowest effective dose. Be aware that there are very few short-term and no long-term safety data available.

Clinical Pearls

To hasten adaptation when this is desirable, it is sensible to exploit the acute effects of the environment, of behavior, and (if necessary) of medication, together with the strategies designed to hasten adaptation of the internal clock.

The importance of scheduled sleep and darkness cannot be overestimated.

Avoiding natural bright light at the wrong time may be the most important consideration.

Correctly timed melatonin should be considered if a licensed, quality-controlled preparation and use instructions are available. Use the lowest effective dose. Be aware that there are very few short-term and no long-term safety data available.

Acknowledgments

This review was written during the tenure of grants from the Health and Safety Executive (UK), the Institute of Petroleum (UK), the Antarctic Funding Initiative, the Biotechnology and Biological Sciences Research Council, the European Union, Framework 5 (QLK6-CT-2000-00499), and the National Grid plc (UK).

REFERENCES

1. Klein KE, Wegmann HM: Significance of circadian rhythms in aerospace operations. Neuilly sur Seine, France, AGARD, 1980; No. 247.
2. Arendt J, Marks V: Physiological changes underlying jet-lag. BMJ 1982;284:144-146.
3. Samel A, Wegmenn HM, Vejvoda M: Jet lag and sleepiness in aircrew. J Sleep Res 1995;4:30-36.
4. Nicholson AN, Pascoe PA, Spencer MB, et al: Nocturnal sleep and daytime alertness of aircrew after transmeridian flights. Aviat Space Environ Med 1986;57(suppl 12):B43-B52.
5. Belyavin AJ, Spencer MB: Modelling performance and alertness: the QinetiQ approach. Aviat Space Environ Med 2004; 75(Suppl):A93-A103.
6. Vogel M: Self-reported menstrual concerns of U.S. Air Force and U.S. Army rated women aircrew. Milit Med 1996;161: 10614-10615.
7. Hampton SM, Morgan LM, Lawrence N, et al: Postprandial hormone and metabolic responses in simulated shift work. J Endocrinol 1996;151:259-267.
8. Aschoff I, von Saint Paul U, Wever R: Lifetime of flies under influence of time displacement. Naturwissenschaften 1971; 58:574.
9. Penev PD, Kolker DE, Zee PC, et al: Chronic circadian desynchronization decreases the survival of animals with cardiomyopathic heart disease. Am J Physiol 1998;275:H2334-H2337.

10. Arendt J, Aldhous, M, Marks V: Alleviation of jet-lag by melatonin: Preliminary results of controlled double-blind trial. BMJ 1986;292:1170.

11. Arendt J, Aldhous M, Marks M, et al: Some effects of jet-lag and their treatment by melatonin. Ergonomics 1987;30; 1379-1393.

12. Waterhouse J, Nevill A, Edwards B. et al: The relationship between assessments of jet lag and some of its symptoms. Chronobiol Int 2003;20:1061-1074.

13. Spitzer RL, Terman M, Williams IBW, et al: Jet lag: Clinical features, validation of a new syndrome-specific scale, and lack of response to melatonin in a randomized double-blind trial. Am J Psychiatry 1999;156:1392-1396.

14. Akerstedt T: Adjustment of physiological circadian rhythms and the sleep wake cycle to shift work. In Folkard S, Monk TH (eds): Hours of Work: Temporal Factors in Work Scheduling. New York, John Wiley & Sons, 1985, pp 185-198.

15. Rosa RR, Bonnet MH, Bootzin RR, et al: Intervention factors for promoting adjustment to nightwork and shiftwork. Occup Med 1990;5:391-415.

16. Barnes R, Arendt I, Forbes M: 6-Sulphatoxymelatonin rhythm in shiftworkers on offshore oil installations during a 2-week 12-h night shift. Neurosci Lett 1998;241:9-12.

17. Midwinter M and Arendt J: Adaptation of the melatonin rhythm in human subjects following night-shift work in Antarctica. Neurosci Lett 1991;122:195-198.

18. Ross IK, Arendt J, Horne J, et al: Night-shift work during Antarctic winter: Sleep characteristics and adaptation with bright light treatment. Physiol Behav 1995;57:1169-1174.

19. Barnes RG, Forbes MJ, Arendt J: Shift type and season affect adaptation of the 6-sulphatoxymelatonin rhythm in offshore oil rig workers. Neurosci Lett 1998;252:179-182.

20. Koller M, Harma M, Laitinen JT, et al: Different patterns of light exposure in relation to melatonin and cortisol rhythms and sleep of night workers. J Pineal Res 1994;16:127-135.

21. Burgess HJ, Sharkey KM, Eastman CI: Bright light, dark and melatonin can promote circadian adaptation in night shift workers. Sleep Med Rev 2002;6:407-420.

22. Crowley SJ, Lee C, Tseng CY, et al: Combinations of bright light, scheduled dark, sunglasses, and melatonin to facilitate circadian entrainment to night shift work. J Biol Rhythms 2003;18: 513-523.

23. Boggild H, Knutsson A: Shift work, risk factors and cardiovascular disease. Scand J Work Environ Health 1999;25:85-99.

24. Schernhammer ES, Laden F, Speizer FE, et al: Rotating night shifts and risk of breast cancer in women participating in the nurses health study. J Nat Cancer Inst 2001;93:1563-1568.

25. Badia P, Myers B, Boecker M, et al: Bright light effects on body temperature, alertness, EEG, and behaviour. Physiol Behav 1991;50:583.

26. Sack R, Lewy A, Blood M, et al: Circadian rhythm abnormalities in totally blind people: Incidence and clinical significance. J Clin Endocrinol Metab 1992;75:127-134.

27. Lockley SW, Skene DJ, Tabandeh H, et al: Relationship between napping and melatonin in the blind. J Biol Rhythms 1997; 12:16-25.

28. Lockley SW, Skene DJ, Arendt J, et al: Relationship between melatonin rhythms and visual loss in the blind. J Clin Endocrinol Metab 1997;82:3763-3770.

29. Czeisler CA, Shanahan TL, Klerman EB, et al: Suppression of melatonin secretion in some blind patients by exposure to bright light. N Engl J Med 1995;332:6-11.

30. Minors DS, Waterhouse JM: Masking in humans: The problem and some attempts to solve it. Chronobiol Int 1989;6:29-53.

31. Graeber RC, Sing HC, Cuthbert BN: The impact of transmeridian flight on deploying soldiers. In Johnson LC, Tepas DI, Colquhoun WP, et al (eds): Biological Rhythms, Sleep and Shiftwork. Lancaster, England, MTP Press, 1981, pp 513-537.

32. Stone BM, Turner C: Promoting sleep in shiftworkers and international travelers. Chronobiol Int 1997;14:133-144.

33. Redfern PH: Can pharmacological agents be used effectively in the alleviation of jet-lag? Drugs 1992;43:146-153.

34. Redfern PH, Minors D, Waterhouse J: Circadian rhythms, jet lag, and chronobiotics: An overview. Chronobiol Int 1994;11: 253-265.

35. Touitou Y, Haus E (eds): Biologic Rhythms in Clinical and Laboratory Medicine. Berlin, Springer-Verlag, 1992.

36. Morgan L, Arendt J, Owens D, et al: Effects of the endogenous clock and sleep time on melatonin, insulin, glucose and lipid metabolism. J Endocrinol 1998;157:443-451.

37. Van Cauter E, Blackman D, Roland D, et al: Modulation of glucose regulation and insulin secretion by circadian rhythmicity and sleep. J Clin Invest 1991;88:934-942.

38. Morgan L, Hampton S, Gibbs M, et al: Circadian aspects of postprandial metabolism. Chronobiol Int 2003;20:795-808.

39. Stokkan KA. Yamazaki S, Tei H, et al: Entrainment of the circadian clock in the liver by feeding. Science 2001;291: 490-493.

40. Stone BM: Sleep and low doses of alcohol. Electroencephalogr Clin Neurophysiol 1980;48:706-709.

41. Walsh IK, Muehlbach MJ, Schweitzer PK: Hypnotics and caffeine as countermeasures for shiftwork-related sleepiness and sleep disturbance. J Sleep Res 1995;4(suppl 2):80-83.

42. Ehret CF, Scanlon LW: Overcoming Jet Lag. New York, Berkley, 1983.

43. Leathwood P: Circadian rhythms of plasma amino acids, brain neurotransmitters and behaviour. In Arendt J, Minors DS, Waterhouse JM (eds): Biological Rhythms in Clinical Practice. London, Butterworth, 1989, pp 136-159.

44. Krauchi K, Cajochen C, Werth E, et al: Alteration of internal circadian phase relationships after morning versus evening carbohydrate-rich meals in humans. J Biol Rhythms 2002;17: 364-376.

45. Akerstedt T, Folkard S: The three process model of alertness and its extension to performance, sleep latency, and sleep length. Chronobiol Int 1997;14:115-123.

46. Buxton OM, Copinschi G, Van Onderbergen A, et al: A benzodiazepine hypnotic facilitates adaptation of circadian rhythms and sleep-wake homeostasis to an eight hour delay shift simulating westward jet lag. Sleep 2000;23:915-927.

47. Czeisler CA: The effect of light on the human circadian pacemaker. In Ciba Foundation Symposium No. 183. Circadian Clocks and their Adjustment. Chichester, England: John Wiley & Sons, 1995, pp 254-302.

48. Foster RG, Hankins MW: Non-rod, non-cone photoreception in the vertebrates. Prog Retin Eye Res 2002;21:507-27.

49. Brainard GC, Hanifin JP, Greeson JM, et al: Action spectrum for melatonin regulation in humans: Evidence for a novel circadian photoreceptor. J Neurosci 2001;21:6405-6412.

50. Thapan K, Arendt J, Skene DJ: An action spectrum for melatonin suppression: Evidence for a novel non-rod, non-cone photoreceptor system in humans. J Physiol 2001;535:261-7.

51. Warman VL, Dijk D-J, Warman GR, et al: Phase advancing human circadian rhythms with short wavelength light. Neurosci Lett 2003;342:37-40.

52. Lockley SW, Brainard GC, Czeisler CA: High sensitivity of the human circadian melatonin rhythm to resetting by short wavelength light. J Clin Endocrinol Metab 2003;88: 4502-4505.

53. Minors DS. Waterhouse JM, Wirz-Justice A: A human phase response curve to light. Neurosci Lett 1991;133:36-40.

54. Boivin DB, Czeisler CA: Resetting of circadian melatonin and cortisol rhythms in humans by ordinary room light. Neuroreport 1998;9:779-782.

55. Lewy AJ, Wehr TA, Goodwin FK, et al: Light suppresses melatonin secretion in humans. Science 1980;210:1267.

56. Strassman RJ, Qualls CR, Lisansky EJ, et al: Elevated rectal temperature produced by all-night bright light is reversed by melatonin infusion in men. J Appl Physiol 1991;71:2178-2182.

57. Czeisler CA, Johnson PI, Duffy JF, et al: Exposure to bright light and darkness to treat physiologic maladaptation to nightwork. N Engl J Med 1990;322:1253-1259.

58. Samel A, Wegmann HM: Bright light: A countermeasure for jet lag? Chronobiol Int 1997;14:173-184.

59. Boivin DB, James FO: Circadian adaptation to night-shift work by judicious light and darkness exposure. J Biol Rhythms 2002; 17:556-567.

60. Deacon S, Arendt J: Adapting to phase-shifts, I: An experimental model for jet lag and shift work. Physiol Behav 1996;59: 665-673.

61. Zeitzer JM, Dijk DJ, Kronauer R, et al: Sensitivity of the human circadian pacemaker to nocturnal light: Melatonin phase resetting and suppression. J Physiol 2000;526:695-702.

62. Rimmer DW, Boivin DB, Shanahan TL, et al: Dynamic resetting of the human circadian pacemaker by intermittent bright light. Am J Physiol Regul Integr Comp Physiol 2000;279: R1574-R1579.

63. Bjorvatn B, Kecklund G, Akerstedt T: Bright light treatment used for adaptation to night work and re-adaptation back to day life. A field study at an oil platform in the North Sea. J Sleep Res 1999;8:105-112.

64. Leproult R, Colecchia EF, L'Hermite-Baleriaux M, et al: Transition from dim to bright light in the morning induces an immediate elevation of cortisol levels. J Clin Endocrinol Metab 2001;86:151-157.

65. Yoon I-Y, Kripke DF, Elliot JA, et al: Luteinising hormone following light exposure in healthy young men. Neurosci Lett 2003;341:25-28.

66. Arendt J: Melatonin and the Mammalian Pineal Gland. London, Chapman Hall, 1995.

67. Arendt J, Bojkowski C, Folkard S, et al: Some effects of melatonin and the control of its secretion in humans. Ciba Found Symp 1985;117:266-283.

68. Rajaratnam SM, Dijk DJ, Middleton B, et al: Melatonin phase-shifts human circadian rhythms with no evidence of changes in the duration of endogenous melatonin secretion or the 24-hour production of reproductive hormones. J Clin Endocrinol Metab 2003;88:4303-4309.

69. Luboshitzky R, Levi M, S.hen Orr Z, et al: Long-term melatonin administration does not alter pituitary-gonadal hormone secretion in normal men. Hum Reprod 2000;15:60-65.

70. Arendt J, Deacon S: Treatment of circadian rhythm disorders—melatonin. Chronoduidol Int 1997;14:185-204.

71. Lewy AJ, Saeeduddin A, Latham-Jackson JM, et al: Melatonin shifts human circadian rhythms according to a phase response curve. Chronobiol Int 1992;9:380-392.

72. Middleton B, Arendt I, Stone B: Complex effects of melatonin on human circadian rhythms in constant dim light. J Biol Rhythms 1997;12:467-475.

73. Wirz-Justice A, Werth E, Renz C, et al: No evidence for a phase delay in human circadian rhythms after a single morning melatonin administration. J Pineal Res 2002;32:1-5.

74. Lockley SW, Skene DJ, James K, et al: Melatonin administration can entrain the free-running circadian system of blind subjects. J Endocrinol 2000;164:R1-R6.

75. Sack RL, Brandes RW, Kendall AR, et al: Entrainment of free-running circadian rhythms by melatonin in blind people. N Engl J Med 2000;343:1070-1077.

76. Lewy AJ, Bauer VK, Hasler BP, et al: Capturing the circadian rhythms of free-running blind people with 0.5 mg melatonin. Brain Res 2001;918:96-100.

77. Hack LM, Lockley SW, Arendt J, et al: The effects of low-dose 0.5-mg melatonin on the free-running circadian rhythms of blind subjects. J Biol Rhythms 2003;18:420-429.

78. Samel A, Wegman HM, Vejvoda M, et al: Influence of melatonin treatment on human circadian rhythmicity before and after a simulated 9 hour time shift. JBiol Rhythms 1991;6;235-248.

79. Dawson D, Encel N, Lushington K: Improving adaptation to simulated night-shift: Timed exposure to bright light versus day-time melatonin administration. Sleep 1995;18:11-21.

80. Deacon S, Arendt J: Adapting to phase shifts, II: Effects of melatonin and conflicting light treatment. Physiol Behav 1995; 39:675-682.

81. Paul MA, Brown G, Buguet A, et al: Melatonin and zopiclone as pharmacologic aids to facilitate crew rest. Aviation, Space and Environmental Medicine 2001;72:974-984.

82. Paul MA, Gray G, Kenny G, et al: Impact of melatonin, zaleplon, zopiclone and temazepam on psychomotor performance. Aviat Space Environ Med 2003;74:1263-1269.

83. Arendt J, Aldhous M, Marks V: Alleviation of jet-lag by melatonin: Preliminary results of controlled double-blind trial. BMJ 1986;292:1170.

84. Arendt I, Aldhous M, Marks M, et al: Some effects of jet-lag and their treatment by melatonin. Ergonomics 1987;30:1379-1393.

85. Skene DJ, Aldhous M, Arendt J: Melatonin, jet-lag and the sleep-wake cycle. In Horne J (ed): Sleep '88. Basel, Karger, 1989, pp 39-41.

86. Petrie K, Conaglen JV, Thompson L, et al: Effect of melatonin on jet-lag after long haul flights. BMJ 1989;298:705-707.

87. Nickelsen T, Lang A, Bergau L: The effect of 6-, 9- and 11-hour time shifts on circadian rhythms: Adaptation of sleep parameters and hormonal patterns following the intake of melatonin or placebo. Adv Pineal Res 1991;5:301-306.

88. Claustrat B, Brun I, David M, et al: Melatonin and jet-lag: Confirmatory result using a simplified protocol. Biol Psychiatry 1992;32:703-711.

89. Comperatore CA, Lieberman HR, Kirby AW, et al: Melatonin efficiency in aviation missions requiring rapid deployment and night operations. Aviat Space Environ Med 1996;67:520-524.

90. Waldhauser F, Saletu B, Trinchard-Lugan I: Sleep laboratory investigations on hypnotic properties of melatonin. Psycho-pharmacol 1990;100:222-226.

91. Suhner A, Schlagenhauf P, Johnson R, et al: Comparative study to determine the optimal melatonin dosage form for the alleviation of jet lag. Chronobiol Int 1998;15:655-666.

92. Suhner A, Schlagenhauf P, Hofer I, et al: Effectiveness and tolerability of melatonin and zolpidem for the alleviation of jet lag. Aviat Space Environ Med 2001;72: 638-646.

93. Pierard C, Beaumont M, Enslen M, et al: Resynchronisation of hormonal rhythms after an eastbound flight in humans: Effects of slow release caffeine and melatonin. Eur J Appl Physiol 2001;85:144-150.

94. Takahashi T, Sasaki M, Itoh H, et al: Melatonin alleviates jet lag symptoms caused by an 11-hour eastward flight. Psychiatry Clin Neurosci 2002;56:301-302.

95. Petrie K, Dawson, AG, Thompson L, et al: A double blind trial of melatonin as a treatment for jet lag in international cabin crew. Biol Psychiatry 1993;33:526-530.

96. Edwards B J, Atkinson G, Waterhouse J, et al: Use of melatonin in recovery from jet-lag following an eastward flight across 10 time-zones. Ergonomics 2000;43:1501-1513.

97. Arendt I, Skene DJ, Middleton B, et al: Efficacy of melatonin treatment in jet lag, shift work and blindness. J Biol Rhythms 1997;12:604-618.

98. Arendt J, Deacon S: Treatment of circadian rhythm disorders: Melatonin. Chronobiol Int 1997;14:185-204.

99. Herxheimer A, Petrie KJ: Melatonin for the prevention and treatment of jet lag [review]. London, The Cochrane Database of Systematic Reviews, The Cochrane Library, 2002. Available at http://www.mediscope.ch/cochrane-abstracts/ab001520.htm.

100. Arendt J: Safety of melatonin in long term use. J Biol Rhythms 1997;12:673-682.

101. Deacon S, English J, Tate J, et al: Atenolol facilitates light-induced phase shifts in humans. Neurosci Lett 1998;242:53-56.

102. Folkard S, Arendt J, Clark M: Can melatonin improve shift workers' tolerance of the night shift? Some preliminary findings. Chronobiol Int 1993;10:315-320.

103. Sack RL, Blood ML, Lewy AJ: Melatonin administration promotes circadian adaptation to shift work. Sleep Res 1994;23:509.

104. Jockovich M, Cosentino D, Cosentino L, et al: Effect of exogenous melatonin on mood and sleep efficiency in emergency medicine residents working night shifts. Acad Emerg Med 2000;7:955-958.

105. Deacon S, Arendt J: Melatonin-induced temperature suppression and its acute phase-shifting effects correlate in a dose-dependent manner in humans. Brain Res 1995;688:77-85.

106. Stone BM, Turner C, Mills SL, et al: Hypnotic activity of melatonin. Sleep 2000;23:663-669.

107. Rajaratnam SMW, Dijk D-J, Middleton B, et al: Rapid and persistent phase advance of human sleep and biological rhythms by melatonin in a 16-h night/8-h day protocol [abstract]. Sleep 2002;(suppl 25):A188-A189.

108. Tabandeh H, Lockley SW, Buttery R, et al: Disturbances of sleep in blindness. Am J Ophthalmol 1998;126:707-712.

109. Arendt J, Aldhous M, Wright J: Synchronisation of a disturbed sleep-wake cycle in a blind man by melatonin treatment. Lancet 1988;1:772-773.

110. Aldhous ME, Arendt J: Melatonin rhythms and the sleep wake cycle in blind subjects. J Interdisciplin Cycle Res 1991;22:84-85.

111. Sack RL, Lewy AJ, Blood ML, et al: Melatonin administration to blind people: Phase advances and entrainment. J Biol Rhythms 1991;6:249-261.

112. Folkard S, Arendt I, Aldhous M, et al: Melatonin stabilises sleep onset time in a blind man without entrainment of cortisol or temperature rhythms. Neurosci Lett 1990;113:193-198.

113. Arendt J: Melatonin, sleep and circadian rhythms. Editorial. N Engl J Med 2000;343:1114-1116.

114. Arendt J, Skene DJ: Melatonin as a chronobiotic. Sleep Med Rev 2004;9:25-39.

115. Jan IE, Espezel H, Appleton RE: The treatment of sleep disorders with melatonin. Dev Med Child Neurol 1994;36:97-107.

116. Buxton OM, L'Hermite-Baleriaux M, Hirschfeld U, et al: Acute and delayed effects of exercise on human melatonin secretion. J Biol Rhythms 1997;12:568-574.

117. Mistleberger R, Skene DJ: Social influences on mammalian circadian rhythms: Animal and human studies. Biol Rev 2004;79:533-556.

118. Honma K, Kohsaka M, Fukuda N, et al: Effects of vitamin B12 on plasma melatonin rhythm in humans: Increased light sensitivity phase advances the circadian dock? Experientia 1992;48:716-720.

119. Archer SN, Robilliard DL, Skene DJ, et al: A length polymorphism in the circadian clock gene Per3 is linked to delayed sleep phase syndrome and extreme diurnal preference. Sleep 2003;26:413-215.

120. Houpt TA, Boulos Z, Moore-Ede MC: MidnightSun: Software for determining light exposure phase-shifting schedules during global travel. Physiol Behav 1996;39:561-568.

56

Shift Work: Basic Principles

Timothy H. Monk

ABSTRACT

The term shift work is used to describe regular employment outside of the normal "day work" hours. Human beings are diurnal creatures for whom it is biologically unnatural to work at night, thus leading to the potential for impairments in work alertness and interference with daytime sleep. Society expects evenings and weekends to be free for social, religious, and recreational activities, thus placing shift workers at a disadvantage when they are required to be at work during evenings, overnight, or on weekends. This chapter discusses shift work coping ability in terms of an interactive three-factor model: circadian rhythms, sleep, and social/domestic factors. It is argued that patients who are shift workers need to be treated with a broad range of behavioral, educational, and perhaps pharmacological approaches addressing the three factors of the model.

Approximately one fifth of all employees are engaged in some form of work that requires their presence outside of the "standard" 7 AM to 6 PM working day on a regular basis, and can thus be regarded as "shift workers." This figure is expected to rise as second jobbing and mandatory overtime increase.[1] The fastest-growing sector of most Western economies is the service sector, and people are increasingly demanding and receiving around the clock availability of such services. Even in the production sector, plant machinery has become so expensive and so quickly obsolete that it has to be run 24 hours a day, 7 days a week, to be profitable. Also, many nations have adopted taxation and business evaluation strategies (e.g., in assessing profitability) that encourage employers to squeeze as many work hours per year as possible from their existing employees, rather than hiring new ones, as the volume of business increases. This leads to extended work weeks and fewer different work teams covering each 24-hour day. Physicians are thus increasingly confronted with patients whose conditions may be exacerbated by a failure to cope with the repeated changes in schedule that shift work requires.

Several social and demographic trends in Europe and North America make it increasingly likely for a shift worker to appear as a patient in the physician's office.[2] First, there is the social trend away from the "standard family" of one breadwinner and one homemaker. In most households there is now no longer a full-time homemaker to run the household and raise children. This inevitably places extra stresses on working parents, particularly mothers, who often bear a disproportionate share of childrearing and housekeeping responsibilities in addition to their career commitments.[3] Second, with regard to demographics, the post-war baby boom generation is reaching their fifties—precisely the age at which significant shift work coping problems start to develop, even in those who had hitherto coped comparatively well.[4]

Some people cope well with shift work, others poorly. At the extreme, Moore-Ede[5] and others have referred to a shift work maladaptation syndrome in those failing to cope. Several international classifications also refer to a sleep disorder associated with abnormal work hours. The International Classification of Sleep Disorders[6] formally lists shift work sleep disorder as one of the circadian rhythm sleep disorders. The *Diagnostic and Statistical Manual of Mental Disorders*[7] lists shift work type as a subtype of circadian rhythm sleep disorder (307.45). Thus, there is increasing acceptance that the difficulties some people experience with shift work should properly be regarded as a disorder worthy of medical diagnosis and treatment.

Although listed within circadian rhythm–related sleep disorders, shift work intolerance is a problem that should not be regarded as *solely* a circadian rhythm ("biological clock") issue, or a sleep-disorder issue, or a social and domestic issue.[8] Rather, it is a complex interaction of these three factors, with each factor influencing both of the other factors and the final outcome of shift work tolerance.[9] Shift work coping problems stem from factors within the individual (Box 56–1) and from factors relating to work systems (Box 56–2). The long-term health consequences of shift work have been reviewed extensively elsewhere.[10-13] Results have sometimes been contradictory, but in addition to sleep disorders, the major complaints implicated have been gastrointestinal dysfunction, depression, cancer, and cardiovascular disease, and patients should be encouraged to abstain from behavior (such as unwise dietary choices) that might further exacerbate such risks. The aim of this chapter is not to duplicate such reviews but rather to introduce a general conceptual framework within which shift work coping ability may be considered so that the physician can better understand the various factors that are involved.

Box 56–1. Factors within an Individual That Are Likely to Cause Problems Coping with Shift Work

History of gastrointestinal complaints
Age older than 50 years
Working second job for pay ("moonlighting")
Heavy domestic workload
"Morning-type" orientation ("lark")
History of sleep disorders
Psychiatric illness
History of alcohol or drug abuse
Epilepsy
Diabetes
Heart disease

From Tepas DI, Monk TH: Work schedules. In: Salvendy G (ed): Handbook of Human Factors. New York, John Wiley & Sons, 1987, pp 819-843. Reprinted by permission of John Wiley & Sons, Ltd.

Practical issues regarding the management of work schedules and sleep are covered in Chapter 57.

Shift work coping ability can be considered the product of a mutually interactive triad of factors (Figure 56–1). Circadian factors stem from the individual's biological clock, which has been shown to be endogenous and self-sustaining under conditions of temporal isolation.[14] Sleep factors are, of course, intimately bound up with the circadian ones, but they have a greater significance for shift workers themselves and are thus more likely to appear in presenting symptoms.[15] Domestic factors (including social and community aspects) are often neglected in terms of clinical research,[16] but they can be equally important as determinants of ability to cope with shift work, and they certainly influence the behavior of the shift worker in relation to the other two factors.[17] The three factors

are discussed in the following sections, and emphasis is placed on interactions and interrelationships.

CIRCADIAN FACTORS

One could argue that circadian factors constitute the essential determinant of ability to cope with shift work. Without an endogenous circadian system, sleep could simply be taken "at will," and society would probably be structured in a much less day-oriented fashion. Unfortunately, it is quite clear that, like it or not, *Homo sapiens* is a diurnal species, biologically hard-wired to be active during the day and sleepy at night. Working at night must therefore be regarded as an inherently unnatural act. Thus, much as the deep-sea diver is working in an unnatural *physical* environment, the shift worker is working in an unnatural *temporal* environment. In both cases, both employer and employee must understand the basic physiologic principles involved so that adverse health and safety consequences can be avoided.

Thus, one might argue that educational initiatives and regulatory protections available to deep sea divers in their domain should also be available to shift workers in their domain.[18] However, one must avoid the temptation of regarding the shift worker's problems as being *exclusively* physiologic in origin and blindly applying "chronohygiene" principles (perhaps derived from laboratory animal models) without recognizing all the social and behavioral complexities that are peculiar to the human being. Circadian factors are an important determinant of shift work coping ability, but they are not the only determinant.

The prime negative influence of the circadian system stems from its inability to adjust instantaneously to the changes in routine that shift work schedules require.[19,20] Figure 56–2 illustrates the process of circadian system realignment (as measured by the phase of the circadian temperature rhythm) in two young volunteers who worked 21 consecutive night shifts.[21] As in the jet-lag situation (see Chapter 55), the process is a slow one, with about a week elapsing before complete

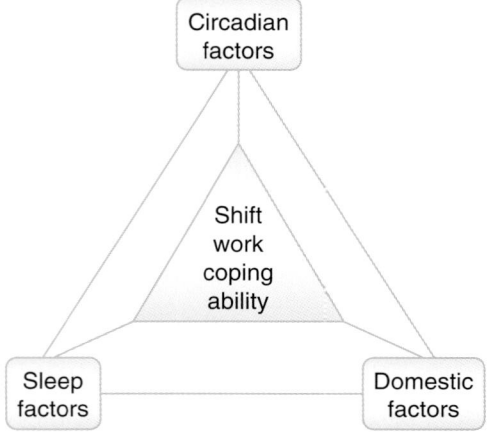

Figure 56–1. Schematic model of the interactive triad of factors influencing shift work coping ability.

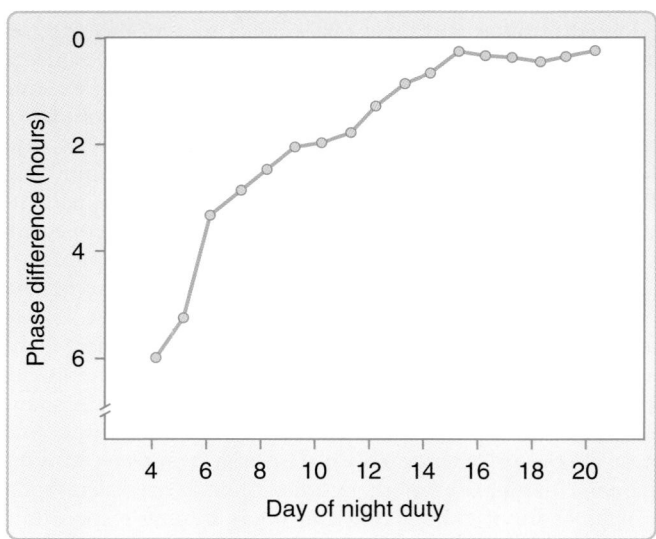

Figure 56–2. Pattern of phase adjustment of the circadian temperature rhythm in two young volunteers working 21 consecutive night shifts. (Data from Monk TH, Knauth P, Folkard S, et al.: Memory based performance measures in studies of shift work. Ergonomics 1978;21:819-826.)

circadian realignment occurs. Using subjects working on a socially isolated oil rig, Barnes and colleagues[22] have shown that the rate of phase adjustment of the circadian system to night work (as measured by the urinary melatonin sulfate rhythm) was about 90 minutes of phase delay per day. Thus, 5 or 6 days were needed before the melatonin onset achieved its desired timing, just prior to the (day) sleep episode. In most work situations, however, this would bring the individual to an off-duty break when a reversion to a diurnal pattern would likely ensue—see later.

One reason that the circadian realignment of shift workers can take longer than that associated with jet lag is the difference between the two situations in zeitgeber (time cue giver) influence. For the transmeridian traveler, both physical (daylight-darkness) and social (e.g., mealtimes and traffic noise) zeitgebers are *encouraging* the realignment of the circadian system. For the shift worker, however, the physical zeitgebers are resolutely *opposed* to a nocturnal alignment, as are most of the social zeitgebers stemming from a day-oriented society. Much research has thus focused on enhancing the zeitgebers that are encouraging a nocturnal circadian orientation.

The discovery of the strong zeitgeber effects of bright lights led to a series of studies using very bright artificial light to assist in changing the phase of the circadian system. Typically, the bright-light exposure regimens (e.g., of Czeisler[24] or of Campbell[37]) required at least three hours of >3000 lux exposure from a bank of fluorescent tubes in a light box. Eastman[23] conducted a careful series of experiments using both student volunteers and real shift workers to assess the utility of bright artificial light in helping shift workers to cope. As with other investigations, however,[24] these studies indicated that darkness during the sleep period was as important as the light during the awake period. Thus, complete bedroom lightproofing was required, and (more problematically), Eastman and colleagues[25] showed convincingly that dark sunglasses or welder's goggles usually needed to be worn during the morning commute home from night work for the required circadian system phase delay to be accomplished, a procedure that might sometimes compromise traffic safety.

The case can still be made quite strongly, however, for workplace lighting to be increased in brightness. Several studies have shown that bright light on the night shift definitely increases alertness *even when the light is of insufficient intensity to induce a strong resetting of the circadian system*. It appears plausible that this increase in alertness is, at least partially, associated with suppression of melatonin. Also, several authors (e.g. Boivin and colleagues,[26] Martin and Eastman[27]) have shown that even moderate levels of night-shift illumination can phase shift the circadian system, albeit less strongly than the phase shift achieved by very bright light.

Another way of enhancing circadian adjustment is by taking melatonin pills—a strategy used by many night workers following the attention given to that hormone in the popular press. Whereas there is some laboratory evidence for the effectiveness of melatonin as a chronobiotic,[28] its effects are comparatively weak compared to those of daylight and are likely to be washed out for many shift workers. Slightly different is the concept of using melatonin pills to facilitate daytime sleep (without necessarily changing the timing of the circadian pacemaker). However, although there is good laboratory evidence for such facilitation, double-blind studies of melatonin's effects in actual shift workers have resulted in few definitive improvements in the quality or duration of daytime sleep.[29,30] Concerns also remain regarding chronic use of melatonin pills whose safety and purity cannot always be guaranteed.

In all but the most socially isolated shift workers, attention must be paid to behavior during off-duty ("weekend-type") breaks. The process of circadian realignment for the night worker can be likened to a salmon leaping up a waterfall; it is difficult to achieve a nocturnal orientation (i.e., reach the top of the waterfall), but easy indeed to fall back down to a diurnal orientation, because that is the natural state for the human organism. That asymmetry becomes vitally important when social and domestic influences during days off lead to daytime activity, particularly when it is outdoors, resulting in daylight exposure. Few parents would forgo attending their child's Saturday morning sports game simply to preserve their nocturnal orientation. Thus, although a worker may be a permanent night worker as far as the company is concerned, in reality the individual may be alternating between nocturnal and diurnal orientations simply because of social and domestic requirements. In a reanalysis of field data, I have shown that on the first night after a weekend break, even permanent night workers may have a totally diurnal circadian orientation in their temperature and subjective alertness rhythms.[31]

During the process of circadian realignment, three mechanisms can adversely affect mood, well-being, and performance efficiency. First, sleep will be disrupted, and the individual will be in a state of partial sleep deprivation.[32] Second, the new time of wakefulness is likely to tap into the "down phases" of various psychological functions that are normally coincident with sleep in the day-oriented individual.[12,33] Third, the various individual components of the circadian system will be in a state of disarray, with the normal harmony of appropriate phase relationships destroyed.[34] A good analogy with the biological clock is a symphony orchestra, with a conductor on the rostrum making sure that the various instruments are brought in at the right time. For the night worker, it is as if a second conductor appears on the rostrum, beating at a different time. The rate at which the different instruments switch to the new conductor varies, and until they all do, there is a cacophony, with all harmony lost. In circadian terms, we speak of this cacophony as "desynchronosis" or "internal dissociation" because the component circadian rhythms no longer have appropriate phase relationships to each other. In addition to poor sleep, the symptoms of desynchronosis include malaise, gastrointestinal dysfunction, and performance decrements.

Individual differences in circadian system characteristics may also have a role in determining shift work coping ability. Individuals who are "night owls," or "late phasers," in their circadian system often find shift work considerably easier to cope with than do "morning larks," or "early phasers."[35] This may be because zeitgeber influences are less potent for late phasers (an advantage for shift workers), or it may be because late phasers have a longer natural free-running period (coping more easily with forward shift rotations), or for the prosaic reason that they can sleep well during the morning (something that night workers often do, because they usually take their recreation after sleep, rather than before it).

Phase differences may also explain why late-middle-aged people often find shift work difficult. A typical case is that of a 50-year-old patient who has hitherto been fairly happy with shift work but now finds it increasingly difficult to cope with.

In some ways, this is paradoxical, given that he has had many decades of learning shift work coping strategies and that he probably has a quieter house now that his children have grown up and he can afford better housing. The reason for the problem may be that he has become more of a "morning lark" in circadian phase orientation. Carrier and colleagues[36] have shown that many of the sleep decrements seen in the progression through the middle years of life (even in day workers) can be attributed to the age-related changes in morningness versus eveningness that can occur through a person's forties and fifties. Also, Campbell[37] has shown that circadian manipulations designed to improve night work tolerance may work much better for young adults than for those in middle age.

Before the discussion of circadian factors is concluded, the question must be addressed whether circadian realignment is actually desirable, given all the caveats regarding the weekend regression to a diurnal orientation mentioned before.[18] In Europe, many companies are switching to "rapidly rotating" systems in which only one or two shifts are worked at a time, before a different one is worked.[38] Thus, for example, on the "continental" rotation, employees work two morning shifts, two evening shifts, and two night shifts, followed by two days off. Most European experts favor such systems because they allow the circadian system to retain its diurnal orientation, thus eliminating problems of desynchronosis. Because only one or two night shifts are worked before time off is given, sleep loss and fatigue are minimized. The drawbacks of rapid rotation are the circadian-related fatigue experienced during the night shifts, which, for some tasks, may render the approach undesirable, and the workers' difficulties in predicting when they will be at work. However, there are undoubtedly many situations in which rapid rotation is worthy of consideration.

SLEEP FACTORS

Sleep is the major preoccupation of most shift workers. In both Europe[39] and the United States,[40] surveys have indicated that night workers get about 10 hours less sleep per week than their day-working counterparts. Thus, people who happen to need 9 hours of sleep per 24 hours in order to feel well rested very often find shift work extremely difficult to cope with. In his survey of field and laboratory shift work sleep studies, Akerstedt[41,42] concluded that the shortening in a night worker's day sleep comes primarily from a reduction in stage 2 and rapid eye movement (REM) sleep, with slow wave sleep relatively unaffected. Not surprisingly, given the prolonged levels of partial sleep deprivation involved, sleep latency can be somewhat reduced in night workers, and some studies have found shorter REM latencies to occur. Essentially, the problem is usually one of sleep-maintenance insomnia rather than sleep-onset insomnia. Although there are many social and domestic negatives to *evening* shift work, from a sleep point of view such shifts are much preferable to night shifts, and even preferable to daylight shifts, particularly when the latter have early start times.

A shift worker's sleep loss is sometimes partially recouped on days off and by taking naps, but it does represent a chronic state of partial sleep deprivation that undoubtedly affects the mood and performance abilities of the patient. Several well-controlled studies document the pathologic sleepiness levels exhibited by many shift workers, both at work[43] and on the drive home after work.[44] Indeed, one could argue that the latter represents the most dangerous activity that most shift workers ever engage in and one that, in the aggregate, represents a major public safety concern involving significant loss of life.[45]

Many shift workers assert that if only they could solve their sleep problem, then everything else would be quite tolerable. However, because of the impact of the circadian system on sleep, disrupted sleep may be as much a *symptom* of shift work maladjustment as a *cause* of it. This idea is demonstrated clearly in a study by Walsh and colleagues,[46] who brought actual shift workers into a sound-attenuated, electrically shielded bedroom for their sleep periods, with the subjects commuting to their work from the laboratory rather than from home. Even in this closely protected environment, there was a highly significant difference in duration between the day sleep of night workers and the night sleep of day workers (306 minutes versus 401 minutes, respectively). In addition, there were reliable differences between the polysomnographic characteristics of the sleep, with a smaller amount of REM sleep and a greater proportion of slow wave sleep for the night workers. Thus, even if it were economically feasible, the complete soundproofing and lightproofing of all shift workers' bedrooms would not eradicate the problem of sleep for shift workers.

Circadian factors are not the only ones having an impact on a shift worker's sleep, however. Domestic and social factors (see the next section) are also crucial in determining the patient's sleep quality and duration. First, the sleep of the shift worker is not as protected by society's taboos as that of a day worker; for example, no one would think of phoning a day worker at 2:00 AM, but few would have qualms about phoning a night worker at 2:00 PM. Similarly, unless the shift worker is in a well-adjusted household, his or (more especially) her sleep is liable to be truncated by the demands of childcare, shopping, and household management. In viewing the sleep of shift workers, one must therefore consider both endogenous and exogenous factors that are going to limit sleep time.

Sleep demands may also be as much of an *influence* on the other two factors in the triad as a *product* of their influence. Much domestic disharmony can be attributed to the shift worker's need for sleep at a time when households are usually rather noisy, and impaired mood is a classic symptom of partial sleep loss.[47] Prescribed circadian-rhythm coping strategies may not work because the weary shift worker may be asleep when he or she would ideally be experiencing bright light and activity.

Finally, in discussing the sleep of shift workers, one must address the issue of hypnotics. In a study of rotating shift workers, Walsh and colleagues[48] found that 0.5 mg triazolam could improve the quality and duration of day sleep. However, the study was also important in demonstrating that the drug had no significant "phase-resetting" effects. Thus, on the third- and fourth-day sleeps in a run of night duty, for which no medication was given, there were no significant differences between those who had been given triazolam on day sleeps 1 and 2 and those who had been given placebo. Moreover when drug and placebo groups were compared in terms of nighttime alertness and performance, no reliable differences emerged, even on the days in which medication was given.[49] One must therefore recognize that hypnotics will probably ameliorate only the *sleep* factor of the triad.

As a general rule, the use of hypnotics is thus inadvisable for shift workers because problems of tolerance and dependence are likely to occur. Moreover, the recently available short-acting hypnotics such a zaleplon are unlikely to be helpful to the shift worker who is usually suffering from a sleep-maintenance rather than a sleep-onset insomnia. One situation in which hypnotics might be more appropriate is in rapidly rotating shift systems, in which the occasional day sleep may be improved by hypnotics and no phase resetting is required.

DOMESTIC FACTORS

Human beings are essentially social creatures, and one could argue, as Walker[50] and others[51] have done, that the social and domestic factors are at least as important in shift work as the biological ones. Certainly, if a shift worker's domestic and social life is unsatisfactory, then the individual will not be coping satisfactorily, however well adjusted the sleep and circadian rhythm factors may be. More usually, however, poor domestic adjustment adversely affects the other two factors of the triad. A common example concerns the childcare and household management tasks that can be expected of a female shift worker. Unlike her male colleagues, she is often expected by her spouse to continue to run the household and can thus find herself completely unable to comply with the routine that good sleep hygiene and circadian adjustment might require.

This situation is illustrated by a comparison study[52] between full-time (four nights per week) and part-time (two nights per week) female night nurses. Few (36%) of the full-timers had children living with them at home, compared with the part-timers (96%). The study took place over the first two nights of a run of duty after some time off. From the sleep records of the two groups shown in Figure 56–3, it is clear that the full-timers were able to make more of a commitment to night work than were the part-timers in their ability to "sleep in" later in the morning, to take afternoon naps before coming on shift, and to sleep between the two shifts. Indeed, some of the part-timers remained so diurnal in their circadian orientation that they even took brief naps during their "lunch" hour, in the middle of the night shift.

Another aspect of domestic disruption concerns the role of the male shift worker as husband and parent. With regard to the former, three major spouse roles are affected: sexual partner, social companion, and protector-caregiver. All three roles are compromised. Perhaps as a consequence, shift work has been shown in a longitudinal follow-up study to increase the risk of divorce by 57%.[53] Although some of the problems are sexual in origin, many spring from the spouse's inability to be there when needed. Feelings of loneliness and insecurity in a wife left alone at home every night, for example, can represent a much more chronic and insoluble problem than that connected with the timing of lovemaking. Similarly, the evening shift, which has minimal impact on the sleep and circadian factors, can have a crushing impact on the role of the shift worker as social companion. With regard to the family role of parent, the evening shift is again the most disruptive. Often during the school week the shift worker may only get to see his or her children when they are asleep in bed. In addition, both spouse and parent roles are heavily disrupted when the shift worker is required to work on weekends.

In addition to disrupted family roles, the shift worker often suffers from social isolation from day-working friends and from religious and community organizations that work under the expectation that evenings or weekends will be free for meetings and activities. One might advance the view that perhaps a shift worker who is denied access to community meetings and social and political associations is as much disadvantaged as a handicapped person who is denied wheelchair access to a museum.

COPING STRATEGIES

As in many fields of endeavor, the task of enumerating all the *problems* connected with shift work is considerably less difficult than that of suggesting the *solutions*, which, in turn, is less difficult than the task of actual *implementation*. The solvency of companies and the livelihood of individuals are at stake, and one must be careful to avoid being too dogmatic or too theoretical in one's suggestions for improvement. As this chapter has sought to demonstrate, the area is a complicated

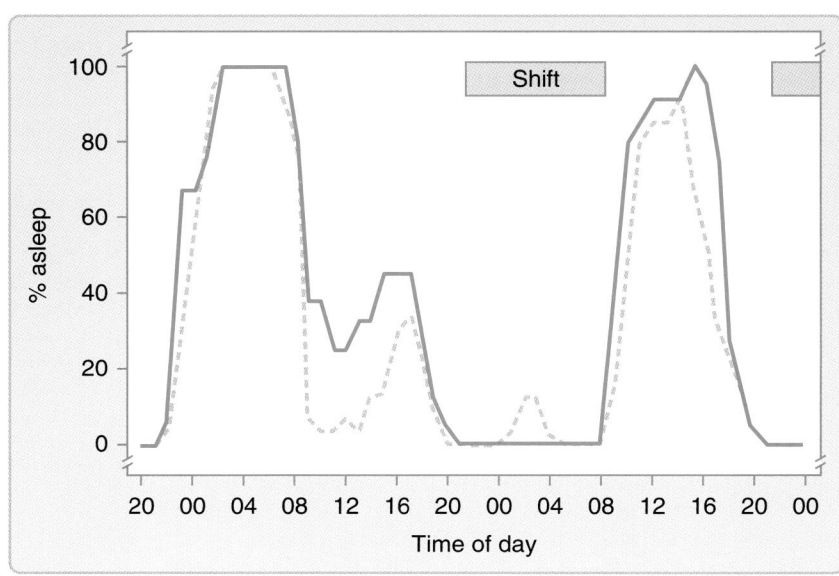

Figure 56–3. Percentage of full-time *(solid line)* and part-time *(dotted line)* night nurses asleep before, during, and after the first of a period of successive night shifts. (Data from Monk TH, Folkard S: Individual differences in shift work adjustment. In: Folkard S, Monk TH [eds]: Hours of Work—Temporal Factors in Work Scheduling. New York, John Wiley, 1985, pp 227-237. Reprinted by permission of John Wiley & Sons, Ltd.)

one, with a host of interrelated forces and pressures, many of them impossible to simulate in the laboratory.

Detailed practical suggestions regarding the management of work and rest are given in Chapter 57. In general terms, the approach required is one that involves both management and the work force.[8] Corporate safety officers and medical officers can be extremely helpful in this regard because they are skilled at bridging the gap between workers and managers and at developing long-running education and awareness programs. Management should realize that it has not only a *moral* but also a *financial* obligation to be sensitive to issues of shift work tolerance in the training of its employees and in the selection of shift schedules. Increasing medical, recruiting, and retraining costs dictate that poor employee morale, higher job turnover, and increased accident, ill-health, and absenteeism rates resulting from shift work intolerance can become a financial burden to the company or organization.

Employee education programs should emphasize the way circadian, sleep, and domestic factors can influence shift work coping ability. Workers should be taught good sleep hygiene practice and advised how they can manipulate zeitgebers to their advantage, enhancing those that are acting in their favor and attenuating those acting against them. They should also be taught the benefit of prophylactic naps. In some cases, family counseling may be indicated to discuss solutions to some of the social and domestic problems. The creation of self-help networks can often be of benefit, lessening some of the social and community isolation that many shift workers feel. When educational strategies fail and the shift schedule cannot be changed, the patient may require a change to a day-working job.

The main task with regard to management education is that of first convincing managers that there *is* a problem and that shift work concerns cannot simply be swept under the carpet or dismissed as a problem confined to sick or disgruntled employees who are simply not trying hard enough. Second, management must be informed of the wide range of different shift systems that are available, including the rapidly rotating systems so popular in Europe. Third, managers must be taught to recognize the factors (e.g., type of job, nature of work force, average commuting time, male-to-female ratio, and preponderance of moonlighting) that should influence the selection of the optimal schedule for that work group in that situation. For management, the "carrot" is a happy, healthy, and productive work force; the "stick" is the specter of human error failures, such as that at the Three Mile Island nuclear power plant, and of litigation from a work force that might consider inappropriately selected work schedules to have adversely affected their health or their safety. Such litigation may grow as the applicability of the Americans With Disabilities Act to shift workers is tested in the courts and as the United States grows increasingly out of step with the fairly restrictive legislation in place elsewhere in the world (e.g., Europe) for the protection of shift workers.[1]

A recent tool that might help management create a more "shift worker–tolerant" environment is the mathematical model. Several authors (e.g., Folkard and Akerstedt[54]) have developed models incorporating both circadian and sleep loss effects as determinants of on-shift alertness and performance. Such models are currently in the early stages of development and need considerable refinement. Eventually, though, they might allow for the effects of different shift schedule choices to be evaluated in computer simulations before they are actually imposed on the hapless shift worker.

CONCLUSIONS

Although some people cope well with shift work, many others have significant problems that can adversely affect their health and well-being. These problems can become a shift work sleep disorder, which can be quite debilitating to the patient. Shift work problems can be usefully understood with a multifaceted approach that recognizes the interaction of circadian rhythms, sleep, and social and domestic factors in determining shift work coping ability.

Clinical Pearl

Working at night is unnatural to human beings from a biologic point of view. Working evenings and weekends is unnatural from a social point of view. Shift worker patients need to be treated with a broad range of behavioral, educational, and perhaps pharmacologic approaches. Physicians should recognize that shift work tolerance is the result of a mutually interactive triad of factors (sleep, circadian, social/domestic). Besides sleep disorders, health consequences of shift work can include gastrointestinal and cardiovascular complaints, cancer, depression, and substance abuse.

REFERENCES

1. U.S. Congress, Office of Technology Assessment: Biological Rhythms: Implications for the Worker (OTA-BA-463). Washington, DC, U.S. Government Printing Office, 1991.
2. Presser HB: Work shifts of full-time dual earner couples: Patterns and contrasts by sex of spouse. Demography 1987;24:99-112.
3. Gadbois C: Women on night shift: Interdependence of sleep and off-the-job activities. In Reinberg A, Vieux N, Andlauer P (eds): Night and Shift Work: Biological and Social Aspects. Oxford, Pergamon Press, 1981.
4. Foret J, Bensimon G, Benoit O, et al: Quality of sleep as a function of age and shift work. In Reinberg A, Vieux N, Andlauer P (eds): Night and Shift Work: Biological and Social Aspects. Oxford, Pergamon Press, 1981.
5. Moore-Ede MC: Jet lag, shift work, and maladaption. NIPS 1986;1:156-160.
6. ICSD: International Classification of Sleep Disorders: Diagnostic and Coding Manual. Rochester, Minn, American Sleep Disorders Association, 1990.
7. American Psychiatric Association: Diagnostic and Statistical Manual of Mental Disorders. Washington, DC, American Psychiatric Association, 1994.
8. Knauth P, Hornberger S: Preventive and compensatory measures for shift workers. Occup Med (Lond) 2003;53:109-116.
9. Monk TH: Coping with the stress of shift work. Work Stress 1988;2:169-172.
10. Rutenfranz J, Colquhoun WP, Knauth P, et al: Biomedical and psychosocial aspects of shift work: A review. Scand J Work Environ Health 1977;3:165-182.
11. Scott AJ, LaDou J: Shiftwork: Effects on sleep and health with recommendations for medical surveillance and screening. Occup Med 1990;5:273-299.
12. Monk TH, Carrier J: Shift worker performance. Occup Env Med 2003;3:209-229.
13. Costa G: Shift work and occupational medicine: An overview. Occup Med (Lond) 2003;53:83-88.

14. Moore RY: The suprachiasmatic nucleus and the organization of a circadian system. Trends Neurosci 1982;5:404-407.

15. Tepas DI, Carvalhais AB: Sleep patterns of shiftworkers. Occup Med 1990;5:199-208.

16. Akerstedt T, Gillberg M: Night and Shift Work: Biological and Social Aspects. Oxford, Pergamon Press, 1990.

17. Tepas DI: Shift worker sleep strategies. J Hum Ergol 1982; 11(Suppl):325-326.

18. Monk TH: What can the chronobiologist do to help the shift worker? J Biol Rhythms 2000;15:86-94.

19. Aschoff J, Hoffman K, Pohl H, et al: Re-entrainment of circadian rhythms after phase-shifts of the zeitgeber. Chronobiologia 1975;2:23-78.

20. Roach GD, Burgess H, Lamond N, et al: A week of simulated night work delays salivary melatonin onset. J Hum Ergol (Tokyo) 2001;30:255-260.

21. Monk TH, Knauth P, Folkard S, et al: Memory based performance measures in studies of shiftwork. Ergonomics 1978; 21:819-826.

22. Barnes RG, Deacon SJ, Forbes MJ, et al: Adaptation of the 6-sulphatoxymelatonin rhythm in shiftworkers on offshore oil installations during a 2-week 12-h night shift. Neurosci Lett 1998;241:9-12.

23. Eastman CI: Squashing versus nudging circadian rhythms with artificial bright light: Solutions for shift work? Perspect Biol Med 1991;34,2:181-195.

24. Czeisler CA, Johnson MP, Duffy JF, et al: Exposure to bright light and darkness to treat physiologic maladaptation to night work. N Engl J Med 1990;322:1253-1259.

25. Eastman CI, Stewart KT, Mahoney MP, et al: Dark goggles and bright light improve circadian rhythm adaptation to night-shift work. Sleep 1994;17:535-543.

26. Boivin DB, Duffy JF, Kronauer RE, et al: Dose-response relationships for resetting of human circadian clock by light. Nature 1996;379:540-542.

27. Martin SK, Eastman CI: Medium-intensity light produces circadian rhythm adaptation to simulated night-shift work. Sleep 1998;21:154-165.

28. Sack RL, Lewy AJ: Melatonin as a chronobiotic: Treatment of circadian desynchrony in night workers and the blind. J Biol Rhythms 1997;12:595-603.

29. Jorgensen KM, Witting MD: Does exogenous melatonin improve day sleep or night alertness in emergency physicians working night shifts? Ann Emergency Med 1998;31:699-704.

30. James M, Tremea MO, Jones JS, et al: Can melatonin improve adaptation to night shift? Am J Emergency Med 1998;16:367-370.

31. Monk TH: Advantages and disadvantages of rapidly rotating shift schedules—a circadian viewpoint. Hum Factors 1986; 28:553-557.

32. Weitzman ED, Kripke DF, Goldmacher D, et al: Acute reversal of the sleep-waking cycle in man. Arch Neurol 1970;22:483-489.

33. Folkard S, Monk TH: Shiftwork and performance. Hum Factors 1979;21:483-492.

34. Wever RA: The Circadian System of Man: Results of Experiments under Temporal Isolation. New York, Springer-Verlag, 1979.

35. Monk TH, Folkard S: Individual differences in shiftwork adjustment. In Folkard S, Monk TH (eds): Hours of Work—Temporal Factors in Work Scheduling. New York, John Wiley, 1985.

36. Carrier J, Monk TH, Buysse DJ et al: Sleep and morningness-eveningness in the "middle" years of life (20y-59y). J Sleep Res 1997;6:230-237.

37. Campbell SS: Effects of timed bright-light exposure on shift-work adaptation in middle-aged subjects. Sleep 1995;18:408-416.

38. Knauth P, Rutenfranz J, Schulz H, et al: Experimental shift work studies of permanent night, and rapidly rotating, shift systems. II. Behaviour of various characteristics of sleep. Int J Occup Environ Health 1980;46:111-125.

39. Knauth P, Landau K, Droge C, et al: Duration of sleep depending on the type of shift work. Int J Occup Environ Health 1980; 46:167-177.

40. Tasto DL, Colligan MJ: Health consequences of shift work (Project UR11-4426). Menlo Park, Calif: Stanford Research Institute, 1978.

41. Akerstedt T: Adjustment of physiological circadian rhythms and the sleep-wake cycle to shiftwork. In Folkard S, Monk TH (eds): Hours of Work: Temporal Factors in Work scheduling. New York, Wiley, 1985.

42. Akerstedt T: Shift work and disturbed sleep/wakefulness. Occup Med (Lond) 2003;53:89-94.

43. Akerstedt T, Torsvall L, Gillberg M: Sleepiness and shift work: Field studies. Sleep 1982;5(Suppl 2):S95-S106.

44. Richardson GS, Miner JD, Czeisler CA: Impaired driving performance in shiftworkers: The role of the circadian system in a multifactorial model. Alcohol Drugs Driving 1989-1990; 5-6:265-273.

45. Pack AI, Pack AM, Rodgman E, et al: Characteristics of crashes attributed to the driver having fallen asleep. Accid Anal Prev 1995;27:769-775.

46. Walsh JK, Tepas DI, Moss PD: The EEG sleep of night and rotating shift workers. In: Johnson LC, Tepas DI, Colquhoun WP, et al (eds): The Twenty-four Hour Workday: Proceedings of a Symposium on Variations in Work-Sleep Schedules.Cincinnati, Ohio, Department of Health and Human Services (NIOSH), 1981.

47. Horne J: Why We Sleep: The Functions of Sleep in Humans and other Mammals. Oxford, Oxford University Press, 1988.

48. Walsh JK, Muehlbach MJ, Schweitzer PK: Acute administration of triazolam for the daytime sleep of rotating shift workers. Sleep 1984;7:223-229.

49. Walsh JK, Schweitzer PK, Anch AM, et al: Sleepiness/alertness on a simulated night shift following sleep at home with triazolam. Sleep 1991;14:140-146.

50. Walker JM: Social problems of shift work. In Folkard S, Monk TH (eds): Hours of Work—Temporal Factors in Work Scheduling. New York, Wiley, 1985.

51. Colligan MJ, Rosa RR: Shiftwork effects on social and family life. Occup Med 1990;5:315-322.

52. Folkard S, Monk TH, Lobban MC: Short and long-term adjustment of circadian rhythms in "permanent" night nurses. Ergonomics 1978;21:785-799.

53. White L, Keith B: The effect of shift work on the quality and stability of marital relations. J Marriage Fam 1990;52(May): 453-462.

54. Folkard S, Akerstedt T: Trends in the risk of accidents and injuries and their implications for models of fatigue and performance. Aviat Space Environ Med 2004;75:A161-A167.

57

Managing Work Schedules: An Alertness and Safety Perspective

Mark R. Rosekind

ABSTRACT

Around-the-clock activities ranging from essentials such as health care and public safety to conveniences like shopping are pervasive in modern society. These activities create significant physiologic challenges for workers in providing safe and productive operations. Humans are biologically designed to be awake during the day and to sleep at night. Work schedules that oppose this natural biologic rhythm generate physiologic disruptions that lead to significantly degraded performance and increased risks to health and safety. Such effects of continuous work schedules on individuals, organizations, and the public are frequently underestimated, contributing to incidents, accidents, and societal disasters. Still, some scientific and real-world considerations illustrate the intricacies of managing work schedules, including individual differences, organizational culture, and economic factors. Effectively addressing these risks is a complex and often contentious issue that requires a comprehensive and programmatic approach.

In many studies, workers in around-the-clock occupations report obtaining less than adequate amounts of sleep and experiencing sleepiness on the job. Approaches to address this issue must occur at all levels, from individuals to corporations to society. Individuals can obtain information on the topics of sleep, circadian rhythms, and alertness strategies, and organizations and society can facilitate such education. Organizations can also encourage the use of certain alertness strategies (such as naps) with support facilities and by institution of policy, and they can use scientifically based scheduling practices to minimize risks related to work schedules.

Individuals, organizations, and society all have important roles to play in the diagnosis and treatment of sleep disorders, many of which go unidentified. Effectively managing modern work schedules, and their associated sleep and circadian factors, offers an opportunity for sleep medicine to improve the health and safety of millions of individuals, corporations, and society.

Modern society has evolved into a world filled with around-the-clock activities that range from essentials such as health care, public safety, and power to conveniences such as shopping. These activities create significant physiologic challenges for the humans who must provide safe and productive operations. Human beings have evolved to be active during the day and to sleep at night. Therefore, any work schedule that opposes this natural biological programming will create physiologic disruptions that can lead to significantly degraded alertness, performance, and safety. These risks affect individuals, organizations, and the public and are frequently underestimated, leading to the potential for incidents, accidents, and societal disasters. Effectively addressing these risks is a complex and often contentious task that requires a comprehensive and programmatic approach.

First, a context will be provided to demonstrate why managing work schedules is both a health and safety issue and to show the extremely large number of people affected by these concerns. Next, effective approaches to address this issue will be outlined from both individual and organizational perspectives. Finally, the complexity of managing work schedules will be illustrated by identifying some scientific and real-world considerations that remain challenges to improving health and safety in around-the-clock settings.

WORK SCHEDULES AFFECT SLEEP, ALERTNESS, AND SAFETY

In work settings, it's all about safety. Obviously, the focus of a text on sleep medicine is health as it relates to the prevalence, risks, diagnosis, treatment, and other aspects of sleep disorders. Even "basic" research is presented in the context of clinical sleep medicine and its relevance to sleep disorders. However, although health and its promotion have become broadly acknowledged and integrated into work settings, the primary reason that occupational environments focus on work schedules is related to safety. This is the paramount concern in any work environment, and especially in safety-sensitive settings such as transportation, health care, and public safety. Even in life-threatening situations, where "getting the job done" is critical, the safety of everyone, especially the individual operator or provider, is a primary concern.[1] This book superbly addresses the health consequences of sleep loss, sleep disorders, and shift work. Therefore, the emphasis here will be on how work schedules affect sleep, alertness, and ultimately safety.

Any work not done in daytime, in standard working hours, or on a regular schedule has the potential to significantly affect both sleep and circadian rhythms. The operational issues are complex and are related to a variety of factors, such as the creation of acute sleep loss prior to a work period, the accumulation of a sleep debt across consecutive days, extended work periods or on-call schedules, and other issues to be outlined later. Some examples from transportation, health care, and public safety demonstrate how work schedules can create acute and cumulative sleep loss.

A variety of National Aeronautics and Space Administration (NASA) studies have examined the sleep and circadian disruption of commercial airline pilots.[2] For example, in one study, long-haul international pilots averaged 7.3 hours of sleep during a home baseline period prior to a trip. However, while on their trip, these pilots averaged 5.3 hours of sleep during a primary sleep period that was supplemented by naps for a total of 6.5 hours of sleep per 24 hours.[3] Short-haul domestic pilots who had a 12.5 hour layover or off-duty period averaged 6.7 hours of sleep.[4] Overnight cargo pilots averaged 4.6 hours of sleep in their primary sleep period, which was supplemented to a total of 6.3 hours of total sleep per 24 hours. This was in comparison to the 7.5 hours of home baseline sleep that they obtained.[5] Overall, 85% of the pilots studied in different flight environments accumulated a sleep debt across their trip schedules. Their sleep debt ranged from 8 hours on short-haul schedules to 16 hours on long-haul flight schedules.[6]

The sleep-wake schedules of truck drivers in different operations also have been studied.[7] In one large study of commercial drivers operating on different schedules, the drivers averaged 3.8 to 5.4 hours of total sleep. For example, after 10 hours of day driving, the drivers averaged 5.4 hours of sleep during their 10.7 hours off-duty. After a 13-hour night drive, the drivers averaged 3.8 hours of sleep during the 8.6 hour off-duty period; after a 13-hour day drive, the drivers averaged 5.1 hours of sleep during their 8.9 hour off-duty period.

In a study of train engineers conducted by the Federal Railroad Administration, the crews averaged 6.1 hours of sleep with an off-duty period of 12 hours and only 4.6 hours of sleep with a 9.3-hour off-duty period.[8]

The sleep-wake schedules of health care providers have been studied with an increased interest in how this affects patient safety.[1,9,10] For example, emergency department attending physicians averaged 5.5 hours of sleep after a night shift compared to 8.3 hours of sleep after a day shift.[11] A study of surgical residents found that they averaged 5 to 6 hours of sleep while they were on call, whether the schedule was every other night, every third night, or every fourth night.[12] Eighty-nine percent of OB/GYN residents reported less than 4 hours of sleep while on call, and a group of anesthesiologists reported an average of 4.8 hours of sleep while on call.[13,14] In a recent study, hospital staff nurses reported getting 6.5 hours of sleep on workdays compared to 7.8 hours on days off.[15]

Police officers have been found to average 6.2 hours of sleep while working an 8-hour shift and 6.5 hours when on a 12-hour shift. In one survey, 53% of officers reported an average of 6.5 hours of sleep or less.[16,17] Firefighters averaged 5.1 hours of sleep when working on a night shift schedule compared to 7.1 hours when working on a day shift schedule.[18]

These examples from transportation, health care, and public safety demonstrate the acute sleep loss and cumulative sleep debt experienced in these work settings. In fact, the amount of sleep typically averaged on work days is significantly less than the adult average requirement of about 8 hours. This becomes a relevant safety issue because acute and cumulative sleep loss lead to decreased alertness and performance.[19-21] Laboratory research has clearly established this relationship. One integrated demonstration of these findings showed that 5 hours of sleep across 7 consecutive nights created significantly increased physiologic sleepiness, and these decrements were highly correlated with decreased psychomotor performance.[22] Recently, varying amounts of acute sleep loss (2, 4, 6, and 8 hours) were found to increase sleepiness more than ethanol and had effects comparable to those of ethanol on degrading psychomotor performance.[23] In this study, 2 hours of sleep

loss equated to a breath ethanol concentration (BrEC) of .045%, which is the equivalent of ingesting 2 or 3 12-ounce beers. Four hours of sleep loss equated to a .095% BrEC, the equivalent of ingesting 5 or 6 12-ounce beers.

The acute and cumulative sleep loss found in various work settings has been associated with sleepiness on the job. In NASA studies, 80% of regional pilots and 71% of corporate and business aviation pilots reported "nodding off" in the cockpit during a flight.[24,25] In another NASA study of long-haul pilots, 154 occurrences of physiologic microevents (i.e., alpha or theta electroencephalogram [EEG] or slow eye movements) were recorded during the last 90 minutes of a 9-hour flight.[26] A study of air traffic controllers conducted by the Federal Aviation Administration (FAA) found that 48% report "they often fell asleep unintentionally."[27]

Police officers also report falling asleep on duty. For example, 80% report dozing off at a stop light once a week,[28] 26% nod off during daytime activities, and 41% fall asleep during a night shift.[29] An Alertness Solutions survey found that 85% of officers reported "unintentionally" nodding off while on duty (unpublished findings).

In a multiple sleep latency test (MSLT) study of anesthesia residents, the residents were found to have an average postcall sleep latency of 5.5 minutes.[30] However, their average baseline (no-call condition) sleep latency was 6.5 minutes, and difference between postcall and no-call MSLT, was not statistically significant. This demonstrated that both the acute (post-call) and cumulative (chronic) effects of sleep loss (baseline, no-call condition) created significant physiologic sleepiness in these residents. With increased total sleep, the residents' average sleep latency increased to a normal range (12.8 minutes).

Overall, 60% to 70% of shift workers report difficulty with sleep, sleepiness on the job, or actually falling asleep unintentionally while at work.[31]

This sleep loss and decreased alertness degrades safety, the real-world outcome of most significance. Incidents and accidents due to sleep loss, fatigue, and circadian disruption have been identified in every mode of transportation and most around-the-clock operational environments. An extensive literature describing these fatigue-related, sleep-loss, and circadian-based incidents and accidents is available, including in this text.[9,32-38] These include major societal disasters such as the grounding of the *Exxon Valdez,* the Three Mile Island nuclear accident, the space shuttle *Challenger* accident, and more.[36,39-41] Other data also demonstrate the associated safety risks. For example, in one study 41% of medical trainees reported having made a fatigue-related error.[14] In Alertness Solutions surveys of health care providers, 19% reported worsening a patient's condition and 30% reported injuring themselves because of fatigue. In a survey of police officers, Alertness Solutions found that 44% reported acting in an unsafe manner or taking unnecessary risks because of fatigue (unpublished findings). Extended work hours have been associated with a threefold increase in on-the-job accident and injury rates, and workers with sleepiness complaints had a more than twofold increased risk for an occupational injury.[42,43]

WHO IS AFFECTED?

Data regarding the number of people who are affected by these issues typically are discussed in the context of "shift work."

Traditionally, this has focused on the number of individuals working variable hours, nonfixed day shift, or alternate shifts. For example, one study of 1997 data published in 2000 indicated that 28% of the U.S. workforce, about 25 million people, worked variable hours.[44] In a September 2002 study, 22.2% of men and 21.4% of women worked schedules other than fixed day shifts.[45] In this analysis, to count as occurring in one of the four shift categories, at least half the hours worked had to fall into the criteria times for the reference week. Therefore, it is possible that 49% of the hours could have occurred outside the specific "shift" category. In another report, 14.5%, or 14.5 million full-time wage and salary workers, were categorized as working an "alternate" shift.[46] This percentage was reduced from a report 10 years earlier that found 18% working an alternate shift.[46]

Shift work has evolved from longstanding views related to swing- and night-shift work that occurred primarily as a result of the Industrial Revolution. Historically, electric lighting and machines made it possible for manufacturing and assembly line operations to expand into around-the-clock activities. However, the modern workforce has evolved far beyond these traditional views of shift work. Box 57–1 identifies some of the common schedule factors that affect the modern workforce and that can create sleep and circadian disruption, with subsequent effects on alertness and safety.

Even a cursory consideration of the factors identified in Box 57–1 clearly shows that the issues associated with modern work schedules extend far beyond traditional perspectives. In fact, many occupational settings that would have never been previously identified as "shift-work" environments do have to confront the physiologic challenges posed by the issues in Box 57–1. For this reason, it is unlikely that we have any accurate or relevant data to determine how many workers in the United States must confront the known sleep and circadian disruptions that can be associated with managing modern work schedules. One poignant example of this workforce evolution is the extensive amount of air travel that is now commonplace in many occupational settings. Whereas traditional "shift work" activities were generally ground based, the sleep and circadian disruptions associated with domestic and international travel can have similar physiologic outcomes. People in the United States take more than 161 million domestic trips on airplanes every year, and 47% of these trips are likely to be business or work related.[47,48]

No data are available on how many people have work schedules affected by the factors identified in Box 57–1. Therefore, there are no reliable estimates of the number of Americans who experience sleep and circadian disruptions related to their work schedules. However, some extrapolation from existing data sources suggests that significantly more people are affected than generally considered. A 2001 American Work Force report identified approximately 135 million workers in the United States in 2000.[49] If roughly 78% are on a fixed day schedule, then 30 million workers would be working outside this 9-to-5 day.[45] Since only 50% of the work hours had to fit this category, then the other 50% could have been outside this fixed day schedule. This could represent another 53 million workers for a total of 83 million people who are working outside a standard, fixed day schedule. Of course, data on who works these schedules regularly, occasionally, or on demand is also unknown.

Any discussion of who is affected by work schedules must also include the diverse entities that assume the cost of outcomes. Traditionally, discussions regarding shift work focused on the issues related to the individual worker. However, it is clear that work schedules affect individuals, employers, and the public. The primary focus on individuals has typically been related to health issues, such as increased risk for gastrointestinal and cardiovascular diseases, reproductive health problems, and cancer.[50-53] The organizational focus is usually on safety and work hours, and the public interest is safety for individuals and for society more generally. This is an expanded and critical perspective because it emphasizes that the organizational and societal roles in effectively managing work schedules equal that of the individual. It is this "shared responsibility" approach that offers an opportunity to bring disparate entities together for constructive change regarding these issues rather than deteriorate into finger pointing and blame. No one entity alone—individual, organization, or society—can fully or effectively manage the challenges posed by modern work schedules. The need for a comprehensive approach that involves shared responsibility is further highlighted by the complexity of real-world operational environments.

THERE IS NO MAGIC BULLET

Effectively managing the sleep and circadian disruption associated with work schedules is a complex, and often contentious, endeavor. Five factors illustrate the complexity of addressing this issue. First, there are diverse operational requirements both across work settings and within specific environments. For example, aviation environments include domestic and short-haul, international, air cargo, corporate, and on-demand flying; fixed-wing craft and helicopters; and other flight activities. Second, there are individual differences among the operators, such as age, experience, and sleep need. Third, sleep and circadian physiology is complex, as clearly illustrated by the content of this book. Fourth, historical and cultural factors affect work schedules; one such factor is the classic attitude, "that is how I learned it" or "it has always been done that way."

Box 57–1.   Work-Schedule Factors That Affect Sleep, Circadian Rhythms, and Alertness

Early start times
Extended work periods
Amount of work time within a shift or duty period
Less than 8 hours off between work periods
Number of consecutive work periods
Insufficient recovery time off between consecutive work periods
Night work through window of circadian low
Daytime sleep periods
Day-to-night or night-to-day transitions (schedule stability)
Changing work periods (e.g., starting and ending times, cycles)
On-call or reserve status
Schedule predictability (i.e., available in advance)
Time zone changes
Unplanned work extensions

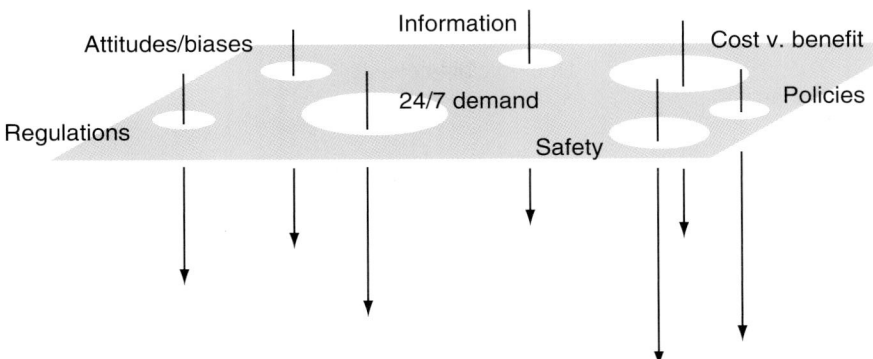

Figure 57–1. Alertness Risk Management (ARM) Model: Risk factors associated with society. Copyright Alertness Solutions 2004.

Fifth, economics can be a powerful consideration for all parties involved in defining work schedules. For individuals, the work schedule will affect income level, quality of life, and family relations. For the organization, work schedules can define workforce size and requirements (i.e., fixed personnel costs), productivity and output, and operational flexibility to meet changing corporate needs.

Together these five factors demonstrate the complexity of effectively managing the sleep and circadian disruption associated with work schedules. This complexity precludes a simple or single solution or a one-size-fits-all approach to managing fatigue in operational settings.

To expand further on this real-world complexity, an Alertness Risk Management (ARM) model based on Reason[54] is portrayed in Figures 57–1 to 57–5. It illustrates some examples of the risks associated with different levels of alertness, the complexity of their interaction, and how, when the factors coincide, an alertness-related incident or accident can occur.

The initial five factors identified and the expanded risk examples portrayed in the ARM clearly demonstrate the need for a comprehensive approach to effectively managing the sleep and circadian disruptions associated with modern work schedules. A comprehensive alertness management program (AMP) to address these issues would include education, alertness strategies, scheduling, healthy sleep, and policies and scientific foundation.[9,55-57] An overview of how to apply this comprehensive approach to individual, organizational, and societal issues related to managing work schedules is outlined next.

ALERTNESS MANAGEMENT

An Individual Perspective

Education

Perhaps the most crucial starting point for individuals is to become educated about the personal health and safety risks associated with sleep and circadian disruption. Previous National Sleep Foundation data have shown that generally people are uninformed and hold misconceptions about even the most basic sleep knowledge.[58] It is important for individuals to know the basics of sleep need, cumulative sleep debt, circadian windows of alertness and performance vulnerability, effects of sleep loss, and more. This knowledge-based education

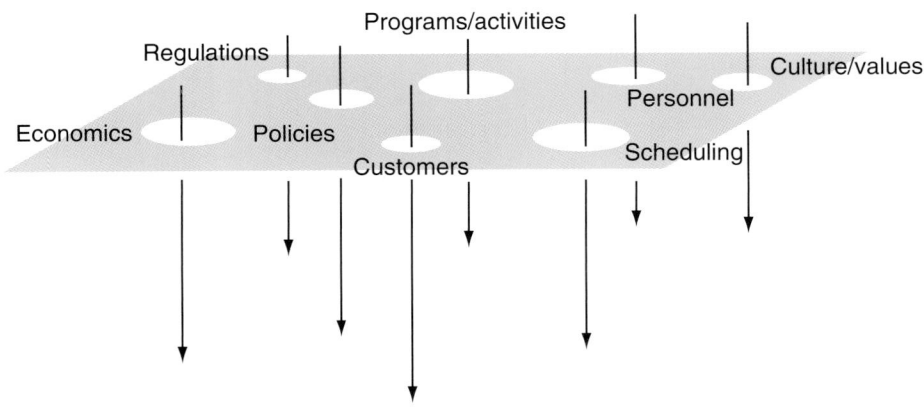

Figure 57–2. Alertness Risk Management (ARM) Model: Risk factors associated with organizations or corporations. Copyright Alertness Solutions 2004.

Operations

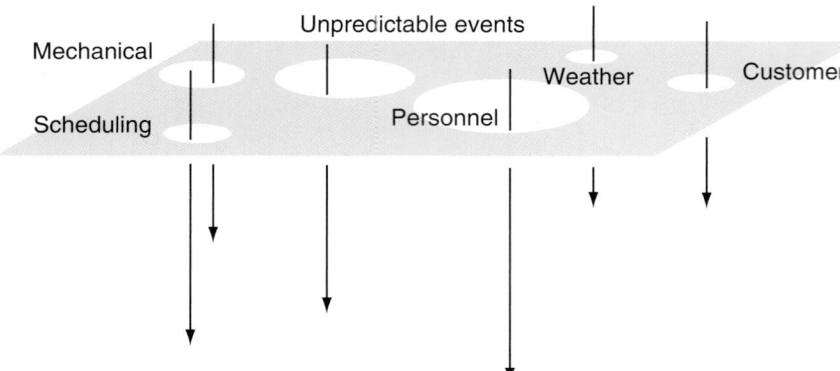

Figure 57–3. Alertness Risk Management (ARM) Model: Risk factors associated with operational demands. Copyright Alertness Solutions 2004.

should be complemented by a tailored personal identification of the signs and symptoms experienced as a result of sleep and circadian disruptions. There is a critical transition from identifying a sign and symptom to taking action.

Alertness Strategies

A variety of strategies have been empirically studied and shown to increase alertness and performance. These strategies include planned naps, caffeine, good sleep habits, managing the sleep environment, exercise, light and dark exposure, activity breaks, diet, sedative-hypnotic and stimulant medications, and sleep scheduling.[9,57,59] The effective use of these strategies requires that individuals understand the specifics of each one—for example, the length of naps, the doses of caffeine that boost alertness and the amounts in different drinks and food, what constitutes good sleep habits versus those that will disrupt sleep, potential benefits and adverse effects of prescription medications, and the timing of exposure to light and dark. Once people are knowledgeable about the effective use of these alertness strategies, they must take two important implementation steps. First, individuals should test the strategy at home, outside the work settings, to find out what works best for them.

Second, an "alertness strategies plan" can be developed that involves proactively determining when and how to use strategies to manage the challenges of a specific work schedule.

Scheduling

Scheduling can be the greatest challenge from an individual perspective, depending on the amount of control that the worker has in determining his or her own specific schedule. The tremendous number of external factors that determine work needs can leave little individual flexibility in choices. However, one basic choice available to someone is whether to work in a particular setting that has schedules that create significant individual disruption. In some cases, especially due to economic needs, individuals have minimal choices. In some circumstances, seniority, specific job skills, rotating positions, and changing corporate requirements do provide choice and even input to schedule design.

Any work environment has workers with average hours and those who work less or more. Sleep and circadian rhythm can be disrupted by considerable overtime, extended hours, minimal vacation, and other work "opportunities" that can represent increased income for an individual as well as increased risks

Individual

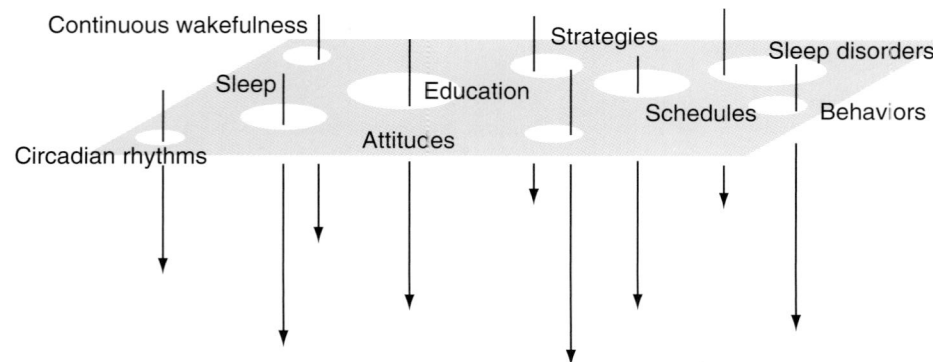

Figure 57–4. Alertness Risk Management (ARM) Model: Risk factors associated with the individual operator. Copyright Alertness Solutions 2004.

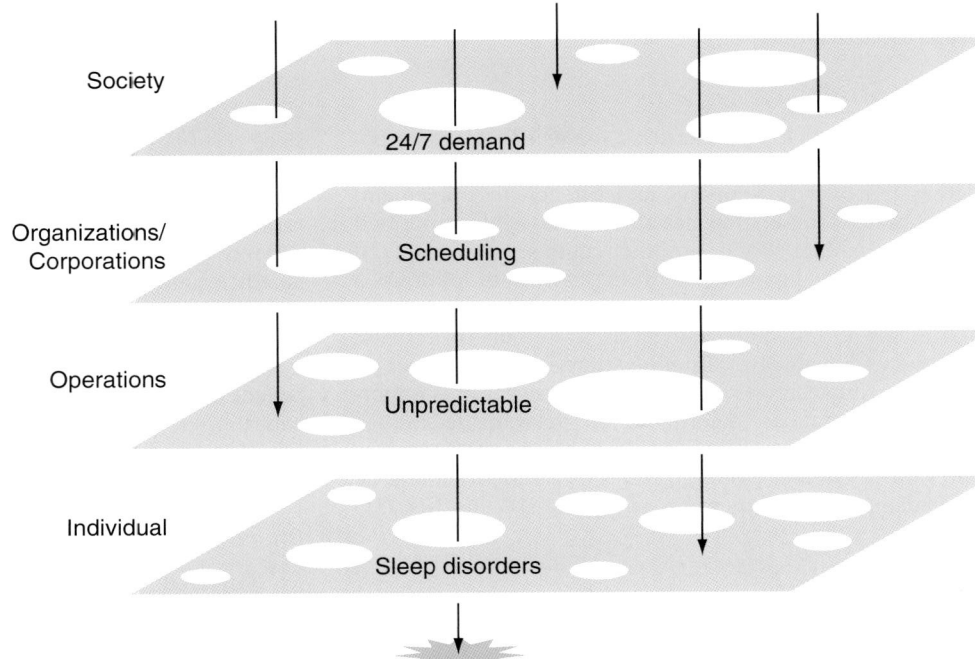

Figure 57–5. Alertness Risk Management (ARM) Model: An accident or incident can occur when the risk factors "line up." Copyright Alertness Solutions 2004.

to alertness, health, and safety. Shared responsibility is critical: An individual worker can seek every opportunity to increase work hours and income, and an organization or corporation can limit these opportunities in order to reduce potential health and safety risks. Conversely, in busy or emergency situations, individuals who are willing to work beyond schedule requirements can represent a significant resource for a corporation.

Healthy Sleep

This text outlines the prevalence, signs and symptoms, diagnosis, and treatment of known sleep disorders. Primary symptoms of these disorders include disturbed sleep and increased waking sleepiness, with subsequent effects on performance, health, and safety. In spite of their prevalence, many of these sleep disorders are undiagnosed or misdiagnosed. Therefore, many individuals have existing, undiagnosed sleep disorders known to affect waking alertness and performance. The associated signs and symptoms of these disorders are exacerbated when these individuals work schedules that further disrupt their sleep and circadian rhythms. It is critical that individuals learn about potential sleep disorders that may affect them and seek help from accredited sleep medicine professionals to identify and treat underlying causes of sleepiness.

Policies and Scientific Foundation

Individuals should seek information on appropriate policies that affect these alertness-management issues. For example, are there corporate policies on the use of planned naps or how work status is affected for employees with sleep apnea? Without explicit policies in these alertness-management areas, employees may hesitate to use strategies or seek diagnosis and treatment. It also is important that individuals use information and strategies that have a known scientific foundation. When exploring sleep, sleep disorders, alertness, and work schedules,

people can be overwhelmed by the claims for an "easy fix" or the latest "cure." Each claim should be examined or researched for appropriate scientific data that substantiate its safety and effectiveness.

Family and Support Network

Persons managing the challenges of work schedules should incorporate family and friends into a support network that provides another asset for their efforts. This could take the form of family education about sleep and circadian rhythms, participation in planning alertness strategies, or support in protecting an identified sleep opportunity. Rather than only viewed as another "stress" associated with challenging work schedules, family and friends can be another asset for effectively managing schedules.

An Organizational Perspective
Education

The most important foundation for any alertness management program is education. This education should be provided to everyone in the organization. Although there is a natural tendency to focus on the operational personnel (e.g., drivers, pilots, officers, nurses), it is critical that all members of the organization share a common knowledge and appreciation for the health and safety issues associated with work schedules. This provides a shared information base among operational personnel, managers, schedulers, and other employees who are either affected by or have an effect on work schedules. The alertness management education activities should be implemented through different corporate forums and in varied formats. Programs viewed as just another "safety issue of the month" will have little substantial effect on individual behavior or corporate activities. The organization must determine whether this education is voluntary or required and what evaluation mechanisms might be used to assess the effectiveness of the educational activities.

Alertness Strategies

Several activities related to alertness strategies require corporate attention. The organization must identify alertness strategies that it explicitly supports and intends to implement. Once identified, these strategies should be visibly supported through appropriate policies or other actions. For example, if planned naps are encouraged during breaks or prior to a commute home, are there appropriate facilities to support this strategy? If adjusting light levels in certain operational environments is part of a corporate strategy, defining responsibility for facility changes and oversight is critical. It is important that corporations determine any relevant federal or industry policies that affect organizational efforts. Any disconnection or conflict among policies can undermine efforts to implement corporate alertness strategies.

Scheduling

Organizations can assess their output or operational needs as a determining factor for designing work schedules. This can lead to identifying personnel requirements, coverage needs, productivity objectives, and so on.

An organization has a range of work schedule options available to consider for meeting its identified needs. These options include fixed schedules and rotation shifts. Fixed schedules include permanent day, evening, and night shifts. Rotating shifts can rotate fast or slow and forward or backward (day, swing/evening, night or night, swing/evening, day). It is critical that an organization examines the full range of scheduling factors that can affect sleep and circadian physiology. Often the emphasis is on the duty or shift length (8 or 10 or 12 hours). Although shift length is one important factor that can affect fatigue and safety, many more factors also should be considered in designing the schedule. A list of some core work-schedule factors are presented in Box 57–2.

These schedule-design factors, while not all-inclusive, do demonstrate that sleep and circadian physiology are affected by much more than just how long an employee is on duty. The complexity and challenges of designing a schedule is fully illustrated when considering how to merge organizational requirements with these core schedule factors that can affect sleep and circadian rhythms.

Box 57–2. Factors in Work Schedule Design

Minimum opportunity for rest or off-duty sleep
Shift length
Work time within duty period
Consecutive work days
Recovery opportunities
Work cycles of days on and days off
Duty time of day versus night
Start and end times of duty periods
Day-to-night duty transitions
Overtime or extended-duty periods
On-call or reserve status and procedures
Duty and recovery opportunities over extended periods

Healthy Sleep

Undiagnosed sleep disorders represent significant health and safety risks for corporations. At a minimum, corporations should provide information about the signs and symptoms of sleep disorders, assistance in locating accredited sleep medicine professionals, and help in determining health insurance coverage for evaluation and treatment. More direct and significant benefits can be obtained by having the corporation support healthy sleep activities. For example, a corporate health promotion program that focuses on sleep apnea can provide individual as well as organizational health and safety benefits. A corporation should determine what activities might be voluntary and which operational personnel would benefit from focused efforts. For these activities to succeed, it is critical that explicit corporate policies be determined and communicated. These organizational policies should be consistent with federal regulations and industry standards.

Policies and Scientific Foundation

As described in the sections on alertness strategies and healthy sleep, any aspect of a corporation's AMP that can be supported with explicit policies should be. If alertness management activities are unclear, unsupported, or interpreted as potentially negatively affecting personnel, there will be little progress toward change. However, clear policies that are communicated broadly and visibly supported will provide tremendous support for a corporation's AMP. It may be that areas of a corporation's AMP will require the corporation to develop a policy because none currently exists. This represents an opportunity to be proactive and potentially create best practices that could lead to industry standards.

It is also critical that a corporation's AMP be based on appropriate scientific data where appropriate. To determine what program elements to implement, management can refer to neutral and objective scientific data. However, it is also crucial to acknowledge that data do not exist to address every operational environment or contingency. Therefore, scientific knowledge can be used to guide operational decisions and actions but may not always address the specific issue in question.

Family and Support Network

Corporations should consider mechanisms that extend the organizational activities into the home. Providing AMP activities that involve family and friends will support individual efforts to engage these networks as an asset in managing work schedules. These activities can include education events, outreach efforts, and corporate communications. Some of the benefits of these activities are clear: Consider the opportunity to have family informed of the signs and symptoms of sleep disorders (e.g., snoring) and their role in encouraging diagnosis and treatment.

A Societal Perspective

Education

Significant progress has been made in providing health information on the importance of diet, exercise, smoking, and other issues, but education on sleep, circadian rhythms, and sleep disorders severely lags behind. For society to benefit from the already extensive knowledge available in these areas, an explicit effort must be made to integrate activities into all levels of the education system. These efforts should support alertness-education efforts in all aspects of society, beyond formal educational institutions to work settings and all relevant settings confronted by these issues.

Alertness Strategies

Strategies known to effectively promote alertness and performance should be supported and explicitly encouraged. Societal acknowledgment and clear encouragement for addressing work-schedule issues will provide sanctions and permission to overtly engage alertness strategies.

Scheduling

A challenging problem confronts modern society: Around-the-clock activities must be conducted in a safe and productive manner. It would be heresy to consider ceasing night or around-the-clock operations given modern society's reliance on these activities for the most basic of requirements. Yet the health and safety risks posed by these work schedules are not fully appreciated and certainly not widely addressed in occupational settings. However, this disconnection between need, acknowledgement, and action results in significant societal costs to health and safety for individuals, organizations, and society. Future efforts can focus on aligning societal needs with managing work schedules that will promote alertness, health, and safety in the context of around-the-clock operational requirements.

Healthy Sleep

Like education and alertness strategies, healthy sleep is another area where a societal priority needs to be established that will promote the diagnosis and treatment of sleep disorders. All aspects of this issue should be addressed, for example, educating health care providers, providing insurance coverage for diagnostic procedures and treatment, developing new treatment approaches, conducting research to determine the most effective treatments, and pursuing innovative activities that will identify and treat the significant numbers of undiagnosed individuals.

Policies and Scientific Foundation

Extensive scientific knowledge currently exists regarding the health and safety issues related to managing work schedules. This scientific knowledge can lead societal change, as it has in many other health-related areas, and should be a guide for the specific actions undertaken. Knowledge gaps should be addressed by appropriate research, although application of the formidable existing scientific literature should be a priority. Wherever possible, explicit policies that support alertness management activities and cultural change should be established, visibly enacted, and integrated into ongoing around-the-clock operations. At some point, society will have to confront the liability issues (broadly defined) associated with the work schedules currently required by around-the-clock demands.

ONGOING SCIENTIFIC AND OPERATIONAL CONSIDERATIONS

There is extensive scientific information available to guide effective management of work schedules, but many remaining relevant issues have received minimal attention. The following examples of these ongoing considerations demonstrate the need for further research and operational evaluation of these diverse issues.

Compressed Schedules

The general societal tendency is to compress work schedules for more time off. Although compressed schedules are attractive to workers as a means for having more "home time," the effects on sleep and circadian factors have not been examined. One example is the "quick change over" used typically at the end of a work cycle. In a backwards shift rotation there is a minimum rest period followed by the final duty period of the cycle. Although this can provide more time off, one study found an average of 5.1 hours of sleep obtained during the 8 hours off between the quick change.[60]

Long-Term Effects of Chronic Sleep Loss and Circadian Disruption

Most studies of work schedules involve either short periods of study or laboratory simulations. Of course, individuals work these schedules for months and years over the course of their lives. Although there are some data on long-term health effects of shift work, the potential outcomes from chronic sleep loss and circadian disruption associated with modern work schedules remain generally unknown.

Prescription Medications

There are two obvious applications for the use of prescription medications in addressing work schedule issues: promoting sleep and promoting wakefulness. There are safe, effective short-acting sedative/hypnotic medications (see Chapter 37) that can provide improved sleep in challenging circumstances. For example, workers with day sleep periods or during off-duty transitions between schedules could benefit from increased quantity and quality of sleep by using a prescription sleep medication. The use of a sleep medication could reduce the amount of acute sleep loss experienced prior to a work period. Currently, none of the prescription sleep medications has an indication for use in managing work schedules or specifically to treat shift work sleep disorder.

The first U.S. Food and Drug Administration (FDA)-approved medication for treating shift work sleep disorder is modafinil, which promotes wakefulness. The product insert suggests a dose of 200 mg to be taken 1 hour before the start of the shift. Given the extensive number of work schedule factors that can affect sleep, circadian rhythms, alertness, and performance (see Box 57–1 and Box 57–2), a safe, effective prescription medication that promotes wakefulness could have beneficial applications in many settings and circumstances. For example, unforeseen circumstances that extend work periods, on-call situations, or significant circadian disruption represent opportunities for a wakefulness-promoting medication to improve alertness and performance.

The issue of using prescription medications to address sleep and alertness issues related to work schedules is a prime example of the ongoing scientific and operational considerations that need attention. With the available scientific literature as a foundation, more clinical research is required to establish the safety and effectiveness of prescription medications in operational use. Future research efforts in this area should reflect actual work scenarios and operational complexity, so that findings can guide safe, effective, and responsible use of prescription medications. Appropriate cautions should be fully acknowledged, and every possible strategy that can promote alertness, performance, and safety should be given consideration and, where suitable, used to its full benefit.

Subjective Disconnection

The current scientific literature clearly demonstrates that there is usually a discrepancy between subjective reports of sleep, alertness, and performance compared to objective measures.[61-63] Generally, people are by objective measures less alert and have more reduced performance compared to their subjective report. This is important because people report that their performance and alertness are better than their actual levels. This disconnection can inhibit a decision to engage an alertness strategy: "don't need it, doing fine." Therefore, the role of sleep loss and circadian disruption and the effects of fatigue will be underestimated and workers will be at risk.

Worker as Patient

Most individuals do not perceive their work experience as making them a patient. There are, of course, many occupational health issues that are known and addressed. However, although many people are significantly affected by sleep loss and circadian disruption from the work-schedule factors in Box 57-1 on a daily basis, few seek intervention for these issues in the health care system. Of course, many of these work-related scheduling issues would not be amenable to a health care intervention. The combination of not perceiving these factors as health and safety risks and the subjective disconnection previously described is the primary reason that workers, organizations, and society continue to be at risk for incidents, accidents, and illnesses.

Sleep Apnea

Sleep apnea is one example of a well-established health and safety risk that is generally ignored in occupational settings. Estimates indicate that of the possible 18 million people with sleep apnea in the United States, less than 10% to 20% are identified and treated.[32,64] Every day, these individuals suffer the personal health consequences of not having their sleep apnea diagnosed, and thus they extend the safety risks to themselves, their coworkers, and the general public.

Drowsy Driving

The data are overwhelmingly clear that drowsy driving poses a significant safety risk for society. In particular, drowsy driving related to work schedules—whether going to work, on the job, or driving home—deserves to be examined more closely and addressed. Alertness Solutions surveys have found alarming levels of drowsy driving on the job: 41% of health care workers reported nodding off while driving and 39% reported a near-miss or accident due to being tired; 20% of a corporate fleet reported nodding off and 14% reported a near-miss or accident; and 45% of police officers reported nodding off and 30% reported a near-miss or accident. These reports were in relation to driving to and from work and specifically involved fatigue or being tired. Occupational settings should consider how work schedules contribute to this significant safety risk and actions that can lead to improving the safety of its workforce.

CONCLUSION

Modern work schedules have evolved dramatically from their roots as traditional shift work to meet historical manufacturing and line operations. There are few data to estimate the actual number of workers challenged by the sleep and circadian disruption engendered by the many modern work-schedule factors that affect these physiologic systems. Current data likely underestimate an issue that could affect 30 to 80 million people in the United States. The sleep loss and circadian disruption associated with today's work schedules create significant health and safety risks for individuals, organizations, and society. The complexity of these issues is best addressed through a comprehensive alertness management approach that involves a shared responsibility among all stakeholders. This approach can be applied to individuals, corporations, and society and provide an opportunity to effectively manage the health and safety risks associated with around-the-clock operations. There remain many challenges as further data are needed to address known work-schedule issues and as current scientific knowledge is more extensively applied to existing risks. Effectively managing modern work schedules and their associated sleep and circadian factors offers an opportunity for sleep medicine to improve the health and safety of millions of workers, corporations, and society.

Clinical Pearl

At least one quarter of American workers have schedules that disrupt sleep and circadian rhythms and lead to reduced alertness, performance, safety, and health. Evaluating individuals with sleep and alertness complaints related to their work schedules should include assessment of at least the following: their knowledge about sleep, circadian rhythms, and fatigue-related safety risks; their use and the effectiveness of alertness strategies (e.g., caffeine, naps); specifics of their schedule and work-rest pattern; and the potential of undiagnosed sleep disorders (e.g., sleep apnea). An effective clinical intervention may involve actions focused on each of these areas for optimal outcomes.

REFERENCES

1. Institute of Medicine, Committee on Quality of Health Care in America: To Err is Human: Building a Safer Health System. Washington, DC, National Academy Press, 1999.
2. Crew factors in flight operations: The initial NASA-Ames field studies on fatigue. Aviat Space Environ Med 1998;69(9 Suppl): B1-B60.

3. Gander PH, Gregory KB, Miller DL, et al: Flight crew fatigue V: Long-haul air transport operations. Aviat Space Environ Med 1998; 69:B37-B48.

4. Gander PH, Gregory KB, Graeber RC, et al: Flight crew fatigue II: Short-haul fixed-wing air transport operations. Aviat Space Environ Med 1998;69:B8-B15.

5. Gander PH, Gregory KB, Connell LJ, et al: Flight crew fatigue IV: Overnight cargo operations. Aviat Space Environ Med, 1998; 69:B26-36.

6. Gander PH, Rosekind MR, Gregory KB: Flight crew fatigue VI: A synthesis. Aviat Space Environ Med 1998;69:B49-B60.

7. Mitler MM, Miller JC, Lipsitz JJ, et al: The sleep of long-haul truck drivers. N Engl J Med 1997;337:755-761.

8. Thomas G, Raslear T, Kuehn G: The effects of work schedule on train handling performance and sleep of locomotive engineers: A simulator study. (No. DOT/FRA/ORD-97-09). Washington, DC, U.S. Department of Transportation, Federal Railroad Administration, 1997.

9. Howard SK, Rosekind MR, Katz JD, et al: Fatigue in anesthesia: Implications and strategies for patient and provider safety. Anesthesiology 2002;97:1281-1294.

10. Gaba DM, Howard SK: Patient safety: Fatigue among clinicians and the safety of patients. N Engl J Med 2002;347:1249-1255.

11. Smith-Coggins R, Rosekind MR, Hurd S, et al: Relationship of day versus night sleep to physician performance and mood. Ann Emerg Med 1994;24:928-934.

12. Sawyer RG, Tribble CG, Newberg DS, et al: Intern call schedules and their relationship to sleep, operating room participation, stress, and satisfaction. Surgery 1999;126:337-342.

13. Defoe DM, Power ML, Holzman GB, et al: Long hours and little sleep: Work schedules of residents in obstetrics and gynecology. Obstet Gynecol 2001;97:1015-1018.

14. Gaba DM, Howard SK, Jump B: Production pressure in the work environment. California anesthesiologists' attitudes and experiences. Anesthesiology 1994;81:488-500.

15. Rogers AE, Scott LD, Hwang WT, et al: Sleep durations reported by 392 hospital staff nurses. In The Paradox of Sleep: An Unfinished Story. An International Meeting in Honor of Michel Jouvet. Abstracts for Symposia, Round Tables and Posters. September 3-4, 2003, Lyon, France. 2003.

16. Peacock B, Glube R, Miller M, et al: Police officers' responses to 8 and 12 hour shift schedules. Ergonomics 1983;26:479-493.

17. Vila B: Tired cops: The importance of managing police fatigue. Washington, DC, Police Executive Research Forum, 2000.

18. Paley MJ, Tepas DI: Fatigue and the shiftworker: Firefighters working on a rotating shift schedule. Hum Factors 1994;36: 269-284.

19. Bonnet MH: Sleep deprivation. In Kryger MH, Roth T, Dement WC (eds): Principles and Practice of Sleep Medicine. Philadelphia, WB Saunders, 2000, pp 53-71.

20. Roehrs T, Carskadon MA, Dement WC, et al: Daytime sleepiness and alertness. In Kryger MH, Roth T, Dement WC (eds): Principles and Practice of Sleep Medicine. Philadelphia, WB Saunders, 2000, pp 43-52.

21. Van Dongen HPA, Dinges DF: Circadian rhythms in fatigue, alertness, and performance. In Kryger MH, Roth T, Dement WC (eds): Principles and Practice of Sleep Medicine. Philadelphia, WB Saunders, 2000, pp 391-399.

22. Dinges DF, Pack F, Williams K, et al: Cumulative sleepiness, mood disturbance, and psychomotor vigilance performance decrements during a week of sleep restricted to 4-5 hours per night. Sleep 1997;20:267-277.

23. Roehrs T, Burduvali E, Bonahoom A, et al: Ethanol and sleep loss: A "dose" comparison of impairing effects. Sleep 2003; 26:981-985.

24. Rosekind MR, Co EL, Gregory KB, et al: Crew Factors in Flight Operations XIII: A Survey of Fatigue Factors in Corporate/ Executive Aviation Operations. NASA Technical Memorandum #2000-209610. Moffett Field, Calif, NASA Ames Research Center, 2000.

25. Co EL, Gregory KB, Johnson MJ, et al: Crew Factors in Flight Operations XI: A Survey of Fatigue Factors in Regional Airline Operations. NASA Technical Memorandum #208799. Moffett Field, Calif, NASA Ames Research Center, 1999.

26. Rosekind MR, Graeber RC, Dinges DF, et al: Crew Factors in Flight Operations IX: Effects of Planned Cockpit Rest on Crew Performance and Alertness in Long-Haul Operations. NASA Technical Memorandum #108839. Moffett Field, Calif, NASA, 1994.

27. FAA Air Traffic Control Shiftwork Survey Results. Alexandria, Va: Human Resources Research Organization, 2001.

28. Maas JB, Wherry ML, Axelrod DJ, et al: Power Sleep. New York, Random House, 1998, p 110.

29. Cochrane G: The effects of sleep deprivation. FBI Law Enforcement Bulletin 2001;70:22-25.

30. Howard SK, Gaba DM, Rosekind MR, et al: The risks and implications of excessive daytime sleepiness in resident physicians. Acad Med 2002;77:1019-1025.

31. Akerstedt T, Torsvall L: Shift work. Shift-dependent well-being and individual differences. Ergonomics 1981;24:265-273.

32. Wake Up America: A National Sleep Alert. Executive Summary and Executive Report. Washington, DC, National Commission on Sleep Disorders Research, 1993.

33. National Transportation Safety Board. Evaluation of U.S. Department of Transportation. Efforts in the 1990s to Address Operator Fatigue (No. SR-99/01). Washington, DC, National Transportation Safety Board, 1999.

34. Dinges DF: An overview of sleepiness and accidents. J Sleep Res 1995;4:4-14.

35. Mitler MM, Carskadon MA, Czeisler CA, et al: Catastrophes, sleep, and public policy: Consensus report. Sleep 1988;11:100-109.

36. Mitler MM, Dement WC, Dinges DF: Sleep medicine, public policy, and public health. In Kryger MH, Roth T, Dement WC (eds): Principles and Practice of Sleep Medicine. Philadelphia, WB Saunders, 2000, pp 580-588.

37. Lauber JK, Kayten PJ: Sleepiness, circadian dysrhythmia, and fatigue in transportation system accidents. Sleep 1988;11:503-512.

38. Rosekind MR, Neri DF, Dinges DF: From laboratory to flight-deck: Promoting operational alertness. In Fatigue and Duty Time Limitations—An International Review. London, Royal Aeronautical Society, 1997, pp 7.1-7.14.

39. National Transportation Safety Board. Marine Accident Report—Grounding of the U.S. Tankship EXXON VALDEZ on Bligh Reef, Prince William Sound, Near Valdez, Alaska, March 24, 1989 (No. NTSB/MAR-90/04). Washington, DC, National Transportation Safety Board, 1990.

40. Presidential Commission. Report of the Presidential Commission on the Space Shuttle Challenger Accident, vol. 2, Appendix G. Washington, DC, U.S. Government Printing Office, 1986.

41. Moss TH, Sills DL: The Three Mile Island nuclear accident: Lessons and implications. Ann N Y Acad Sci 1981;365:1-341.

42. Akerstedt T: Work injuries and time of day—National data. Proceedings of a Consensus Development Symposium entitled "Work Hours, Sleepiness and Accidents." Stockholm, Sweden, 8-10 Sept. 1994, p 106.

43. Melamed S, Oksenberg A: Excessive daytime sleepiness and risk of occupational injuries in non-shift daytime workers. Sleep 2002;25:315-322.

44. Beers TM: Flexible schedules and shift work: Replacing the "9-to-5" workday? Monthly Labor Review 2000;123:33-40.

45. Presser HB, Altmanhe B: Work shifts and disability: A national view. Monthly Labor Review, 2002;125:11-24.

46. Bureau of Labor Statistics: U.S. Department of Labor. Workers on Flexible and Shift Schedules in 2001 Summary. Available at: http://www.bls.gov/news.release/flex.nr0.htm. Accessed February 5, 2004.

47. Bureau of Transportation Statistics: 1995 American Travel Survey. Washington, DC, U.S. Department of Transportation, 1997.

48. Air Transport Association: Air Travel Survey. Washington, DC, Air Transport Association, 1998.

49. U.S. Department of Labor: Report on the American Work Force. Washington, DC, U.S. Department of Labor, 2001.

50. Davis S, Mirick DK, Stevens RG: Night shift work, light at night, and risk of breast cancer. J Natl Cancer Inst 2001;93:1557-1562.

51. Nurminen T: Shift work and reproductive health. Scand J Work Environ Health 1998;24(Suppl 3):28-34.

52. Knutsson A: Health disorders of shift workers. Occup Med (Lond) 2003;53:103-108.

53. Scott AJ, LaDou J: Shiftwork: Effects on sleep and health with recommendations for medical surveillance and screening. Occup Med 1990;5:273-299.

54. Reason J: Human Error. New York, Cambridge University Press, 1990.

55. Rosekind MR, Flower DJC, Gregory KB, et al: General occupational implications of round-the-clock operations. In Kushida CA (ed): Sleep Deprivation. New York, Marcel Dekker, in press.

56. Rosekind MR, Gander PH, Gregory KB, et al: Managing fatigue in operational settings. 2: An integrated approach. Behav Med 1996;21:166-170.

57. Rosekind MR, Boyd JN, Gregory KB, et al: Alertness management in 24/7 settings: Lessons from aviation. Occup Med 2002;17:247-259.

58. National Sleep Foundation: 1998 Omnibus Sleep in America Poll. Washington, DC, National Sleep Foundation, 1998.

59. Rosekind MR, Gander PH, Connell LJ, et al: Crew Factors in Flight Operations X: Alertness Management in Flight Operations (No. NASA/TM-1999-208780). Moffett Field, Calif, National Aeronautics and Space Administration, 1999.

60. Totterdell P, Folkard S: The effects of changing from a weekly rotation to a rapidly rotating shift schedule. In Costa G, Cesana GC, Wedderburn A, Kogi K (eds): Shiftwork: Health, Sleep, and Performance. Frankfurt am Main, Peter Lang Verlag, 1990.

61. Carskadon MA, Dement WC: Effects of total sleep loss on sleep tendency. Percept Mot Skills 1979;48:495-506.

62. Howard SK, Gaba DM, Smith BE, et al: Simulation study of rested versus sleep-deprived anesthesiologists. Anesthesiology 2003;98:1345-1355.

63. Sasaki M, Kurosaki Y, Mori A, et al: Patterns of sleep-wakefulness before and after transmeridian flight in commercial airline pilots. Aviat Space Environ Med 1986;57:B29-B42.

64. Young T, Evans L, Finn L, et al: Estimation of the clinically diagnosed proportion of sleep apnea syndrome in middle-aged men and women. Sleep 1997;20:705-706.

58

Circadian Disorders of the Sleep–Wake Cycle

Kathryn J. Reid

Phyllis C. Zee

ABSTRACT

Circadian rhythm sleep disorders are primarily caused by alterations of the circadian time-keeping system or a misalignment between the endogenous circadian rhythm and external factors that affect the timing or duration of sleep. In this chapter, the diagnostic criteria for circadian rhythm sleep disorders and their subtypes are similar to the criteria published in the International Classification of Sleep Disorders, Revised (ICSD-2). In clinical practice, the most commonly encountered primary circadian rhythm sleep disorders are delayed sleep phase type (DSPT) and advanced sleep phase type (ASPT). DSPT is characterized by bedtimes and wake times that are usually delayed (DSPT) or advanced (ASPT) 3 or more hours relative to desired or socially acceptable sleep and wake times. Nonentrained sleep–wake type occurs predominantly in blind individuals and is characterized by a steady daily drift of the major sleep period with a period that is usually longer than 24 hours. When the nonentrained circadian clock is out of phase with the timing of conventional sleep and wake times, individuals complain of insomnia and excessive daytime sleepiness. Irregular sleep–wake type is characterized by a lack of well-defined circadian rhythms of sleep and waking and is seen in association with neurodegenerative disorders.

Although the basic pathophysiology of these disorders is an alteration in the endogenous circadian timing system, the clinical picture is often complicated by behavioral and environmental factors. Therefore, a comprehensive treatment approach for these disorders needs to address both the circadian misalignment and behavioral or environmental factors that affect the timing of sleep. Timed exposure to circadian synchronizing agents, such as bright light and melatonin, together with adequate attention to sleep hygiene have been shown to be effective treatment for circadian rhythm sleep disorders. Further advances in our understanding of the pathophysiology of the various types of circadian rhythm sleep disorders will lead to improvements in both diagnostic and therapeutic approaches for their clinical management.

The timing and duration of the sleep–wake cycle depends on the synchronization of the endogenous circadian clock with external environmental cues. The sleep–wake cycle becomes perturbed when these two rhythms become desynchronized (change their phase in relation to each other). These dyssynchronous states fall into two categories: (1) the terrestrial light–dark (LD) cycle may change relative to circadian timekeeping (shift work type and jet lag), or (2) circadian timekeeping may change relative to the terrestrial LD cycle (delayed sleep phase type, advanced sleep phase type, nonentrained sleep–wake type, and irregular sleep–wake type). The first circumstance occurs in the presence of a normal circadian timekeeping system and is generally self-limited or resolves with environmental change. The latter circumstance is believed to occur because of chronic alteration(s) in the circadian system which results in the inability of the circadian pacemaker to achieve a conventional phase relationship with the external world. This chapter will focus on the second group of disorders. Because circadian variation in wakefulness and sleep propensity is the most apparent of the many behavioral and physiologic outputs of the circadian pacemaker, it is not surprising that the first circadian rhythm disorders to be recognized involved the sleep–wake cycle.[1] Disruptions in the timing of sleep and wakefulness are often associated with symptoms of insomnia and/or excessive sleepiness that cause patients to seek medical attention.

Advances in the understanding of basic human circadian biology have created new clinical tools for the diagnosis and treatment of several circadian sleep disorders. Increasingly detailed knowledge about how the circadian system responds to photic as well as to nonphotic entraining agents is increasing the number of practical therapies that can be used in "real life" clinical settings.

ENTRAINMENT OF CIRCADIAN RHYTHMS

The suprachiasmatic nucleus (SCN), in the anterior hypothalamus, is responsible for the generation of circadian rhythmicity in animals.[2] Animals and humans removed from the external LD cycle and other time cues (zeitgebers) exhibit a continuing endogenous cycle of sleep and wakefulness as well as many other physiologic and hormonal parameters. The length of this cycle of oscillation or free-running period is largely genetically determined, with species and slight individual variation. In the mouse[3] and the hamster,[4] genes have been identified that lengthen[3] and shorten[4,5] the free-running period. The mammalian circadian period is generally slightly longer than 24 hours in diurnal animals, and slightly shorter than 24 hours in nocturnal animals. In humans, the average circadian period has been estimated to be approximately 24.18 hours[6] and must therefore be synchronized or entrained on a regular basis to the 24-hour terrestrial day by external influences.

Entrainment by Light

Light is the major external time cue in mammals. Light reaches the SCN by afferent projections from the retina via the retinohypothalamic tract.[2] Recent evidence indicates that the primary circadian photoreceptors are the melanopsin-containing retinal ganglion cells rather than the rods and cones.[7,8]

Although circadian rhythms can be entrained to LD cycles that are not exactly 24 hours in duration, entrainment is restricted to cycles with periods that are close to 24 hours in duration.[9] The range of entrainment can vary from species to species, and it is dependent on the experimental conditions (e.g., intensity of the LD cycle, whether period of the LD cycle is changed gradually or rapidly), but in general, animals do not entrain readily to LD cycles that are more than a few hours shorter or longer than the period of the endogenous circadian rhythm. If the period of the LD cycle is too short or too long for entrainment to occur, the circadian rhythm will free-run with a period of the endogenous pacemaker.

One of the most widely used methods to examine how the LD cycle influences the circadian system has been to expose animals and humans maintained in constant conditions to pulses of light. The effects of the light pulse on a phase reference point of a circadian rhythm (e.g., onset of melatonin, minimum of body temperature) in subsequent cycles is then determined. The direction and magnitude of the phase shifts are strongly dependent on the circadian time at which the light pulse occurs. A phase–response curve (PRC) is a plot of the magnitude and direction of the time shift induced by an environmental perturbation as a function of the circadian time at which the perturbation is given. Light pulses presented near the onset of the subjective night (the part of the circadian cycle that occurs during the dark or nighttime) delay circadian rhythms, whereas light pulses presented in the late subjective night or early subjective day (the part of the circadian cycle that occurs during the light or daytime) phase advance circadian rhythms. Czeisler and his colleagues[10,11] have carried out extensive studies in humans demonstrating that the LD cycle can entrain human rhythms, and that bright light can be used to manipulate human rhythms under a variety of experimental conditions. Although bright light (with intensities approximating that of sunlight) is a very strong and reliable entraining agent of the circadian system,[11,12] there is evidence that lower intensities, such as those encountered in ordinary room lighting, can also affect the timing of human circadian rhythms.[13] The recent discovery, that in humans, both light-induced phase shifts and melatonin suppression are most sensitive to short-wavelength light of approximately 460 nm,[14,15] provides an exciting new avenue for the development of light therapies to treat circadian rhythm sleep disorders.

Entrainment by Nonphotic Signals

The role of activity and social cues as synchronizing agents for the human circadian system has been recognized since the early 1970s. Studies by Aschoff and coworkers[16] showed that scheduled bedtimes, mealtimes, and various timed social cues could entrain circadian rhythms. More recent studies indicate that sleep and social schedules may also phase shift the circadian clock.[17] In addition, physical exercise during the night can produce a phase delay in human circadian rhythms.[18,19] These findings raise the possibility that social and physical activity may be useful tools to manipulate circadian rhythms in humans.

Melatonin

Melatonin is an important modulator of circadian rhythms,[20] and it can induce phase shifts of these rhythms in animals[21] and humans.[22] The circadian rhythm of melatonin release is controlled by the SCN via an indirect pathway, a noradrenergic synapse from the superior cervical ganglion to the pineal gland.[23] The PRC for melatonin in humans indicates that administration of exogenous melatonin to humans in the early evening advances the phase of the circadian rhythms, whereas administration in the early morning delays the phase, with the strongest phase-shifting effects of exogenous melatonin occurring during the evening, just preceding the increase in endogenous melatonin levels.[24,25] In addition to its phase-resetting properties, evidence supports a role for melatonin in sleep modulation by increasing evening sleep propensity and reduction in core body temperature.[20]

The potential importance of melatonin for regulating the sleep–wake cycle has led to interest in its use for treatment of insomnia and circadian rhythm sleep disorders. Indeed, there is good evidence that melatonin may be effective for entraining circadian rhythms in blind people with non–24-hour sleep–wake cycles.[26] Another potential use for melatonin has been suggested from the role of the circadian system in maintaining consolidation of sleep during the early morning hours in older adults.[27]

CIRCADIAN RHYTHM SLEEP DISORDER, DELAYED SLEEP PHASE TYPE

Clinical Features

Circadian rhythm sleep disorder, delayed sleep phase type (DSPT) (or delayed sleep phase syndrome), is characterized by sleep onset and wake times that are usually delayed 3 to 6 hours relative to conventional sleep–wake times (Fig. 58–1). The patient typically finds it difficult to initiate sleep before sometime between 2 and 6 AM and, when free of societal constraints, prefers a wake time that is between 10 AM and 1 PM. Sleep itself is reported to be normal for the person's age.[28,29] These symptoms are chronic, usually of at least 3 months'—and quite often of many years'—duration. The clinical picture may be similar to sleep-onset insomnia. Patients are unable to advance their sleep times despite repeated attempts, and they may report a history of prolonged sedative or hypnotic drug use, bedtime use of alcohol, behavioral interventions, or psychotherapy.[30] Patients often report feeling most alert in the late evening, and they score highly as night people on a morningness-eveningness scale.[31,32] Enforced "conventional" wake times may result in chronically insufficient sleep and excessive daytime sleepiness. Sleepiness is greatest in the morning and lessens as the circadian drive for wakefulness peaks in the late afternoon. In adolescents, the syndrome may be associated with daytime irritability and poor school performance,[33] whereas in adulthood, the syndrome may be associated with impaired job performance and associated financial difficulty, as well as with marital problems.[34] DSPT may be mistaken for depression, in which the sleep–wake cycle may also be delayed (or advanced). Several studies, generally from psychiatric clinics, have emphasized an association between DSPT and mood and personality disorders.[34,35]

Epidemiology

DSPT has been reported in preadolescents and in patients older than 60 years.[34] Although the actual prevalence in the general population is unknown, it is more common in adolescents and

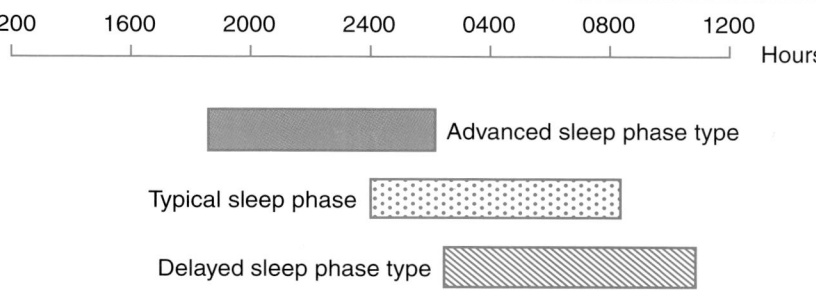

Figure 58–1. Schematic representation of the temporal distribution of sleep and wake in patients with circadian rhythm sleep disorders. Patients with advanced sleep phase type typically complain of evening sleepiness and either early-morning awakening or sleep disruption. Patients with delayed sleep phase type complain of difficulty initiating sleep, usually before 2 AM, and have difficulty awakening in the morning.

young adults, with a reported prevalence of 7%.[36] In middle-aged adults, the prevalence may be one tenth of that, or 0.7%.[37] In a sleep disorders clinic, 6.7%[29] to 16%[35] of patients seen for a primary complaint of insomnia were determined to have DSPT. There are no known sex differences in prevalence.

Pathogenesis

The tendency for late sleeping is not simply a function of the interaction between the circadian drive for wakefulness and the sleep homeostat but is analogous to eating and other behaviors that are mandated by physiology but overlaid by varying individual emotional, social, and medical states.[35] Although the exact cause of DSPT is not known, several mechanisms, involving both behavioral and physiologic factors, have been proposed. Behavioral preference may play a major role in some cases of DSPT, particularly when bedtimes and rise times are not enforced. Late wake times will delay exposure to light in the morning and may prevent active advancement of the circadian clock, allowing it to drift to a new phase relation with external clock time. In addition, recent evidence shows that under certain conditions (a background of dim light), ambient artificial light (as low as 100 lux) at night may be of sufficient intensity to affect circadian phase.[13] Therefore, light exposure later in the evening may also perpetuate and exacerbate the phase delay.

However, symptoms often persist despite severe social or professional consequences,[38] and DSPT has a high rate of relapse despite initially successful therapy,[30,39] suggesting that behavioral factors alone do not explain this disorder. There is considerable evidence that DSPT is the result of alterations in the endogenous circadian system. For example, many physiologic markers of circadian phase persist in a delayed pattern despite enforced sleep–wake times,[40] and there is also evidence that some individuals with DSPT have a hypersensitivity to nighttime suppression of melatonin by bright light.[41] Reduced sensitivity of the oscillator to photic entrainment (i.e., a reduction in the amplitude of the advance portion of the PRC to light) has also been hypothesized, as has a prolonged free-running period length of the circadian cycle.[30] Furthermore, the duration and timing of environmental light and dark exposure may play a role in the expression of the DSPT phenotype. For example, the prevalence of DSPT may be increased at extreme latitudes.[42] There is also evidence for a genetic basis to DSPT. In some cases, the syndrome may be familial, presenting with an autosomal dominant mode of inheritance.[34,43] Further support for a genetic basis for DSPT derives from reports of polymorphisms in circadian genes such as *hPer3*, arylalkylamine *N*-acetyltransferase gene, HLA genes, and *Clock*.[44-47]

Although it is commonly accepted that DSPT is predominantly a result of alterations in circadian timing, there is recent evidence that alterations in the homeostatic regulation of sleep may also play an important role.[48,49] Polysomnographic recordings of sleep in individuals with DSPT have shown that sleep architecture is not disrupted after the initiation of sleep when subjects are allowed to sleep until their desired wake times.[33,34,50] However, after 24 hours of sleep deprivation, subjects with DSPT, when compared to controls, show a decreased ability to compensate for sleep loss during the subjective day and the first hours of subjective night.[48,51] Therefore, it is likely that both alterations in circadian timing and impaired sleep recovery contribute to symptoms of insomnia and excessive sleepiness in DSPT.

Diagnosis

The diagnosis of DSPT is usually made on the basis of the patient's history of chronic or recurrent complaints of symptoms of insomnia resulting from a stable delay in the timing of the major sleep and wake periods.[52,53] The sleep disturbance is associated with impairment of social, occupational, or other areas of functioning. Sleep log or actigraphy monitoring should be performed for at least 7 days to demonstrate a stable delay in the timing of the habitual sleep period. Actigraphy is a practical tool for assessing sleep–wake cycles relative to clock time, and it has become more widely available clinically (Fig. 58–2A). A morningness-eveningness scale, such as provided by the Horne-Ostberg questionnaire, is also useful to gauge the patient's best time of performance.[31]

To make the diagnosis, medical, mental, or sleep disorders that may cause alterations in the sleep–wake cycle, insomnia, or excessive sleepiness should be excluded or adequately treated. Nocturnal polysomnography (PSG) is sometimes necessary to exclude other sleep-disrupting pathology. When performed during conventional sleep laboratory hours, PSG often shows a prolonged sleep-onset latency as well as a prolonged rapid eye movement sleep latency, and this may sometimes, in conjunction with an antecedent sleep log, be a clue to the diagnosis.

The use of other physiologic markers of circadian timing, such as a continuous recording of body temperature[54] or dim-light (plasma) melatonin onset (DLMO),[55] may also aid in determining the phase relationship between circadian and terrestrial time, although routine clinical availability remains limited. DLMO is probably the most useful marker for circadian pacemaker output.[56,57] In individuals with DSPT, the DLMO times usually occur after 10 PM[55] (Fig. 58–3A). Determination of DLMO can be made by measurements of melatonin from plasma or saliva. Commercially available

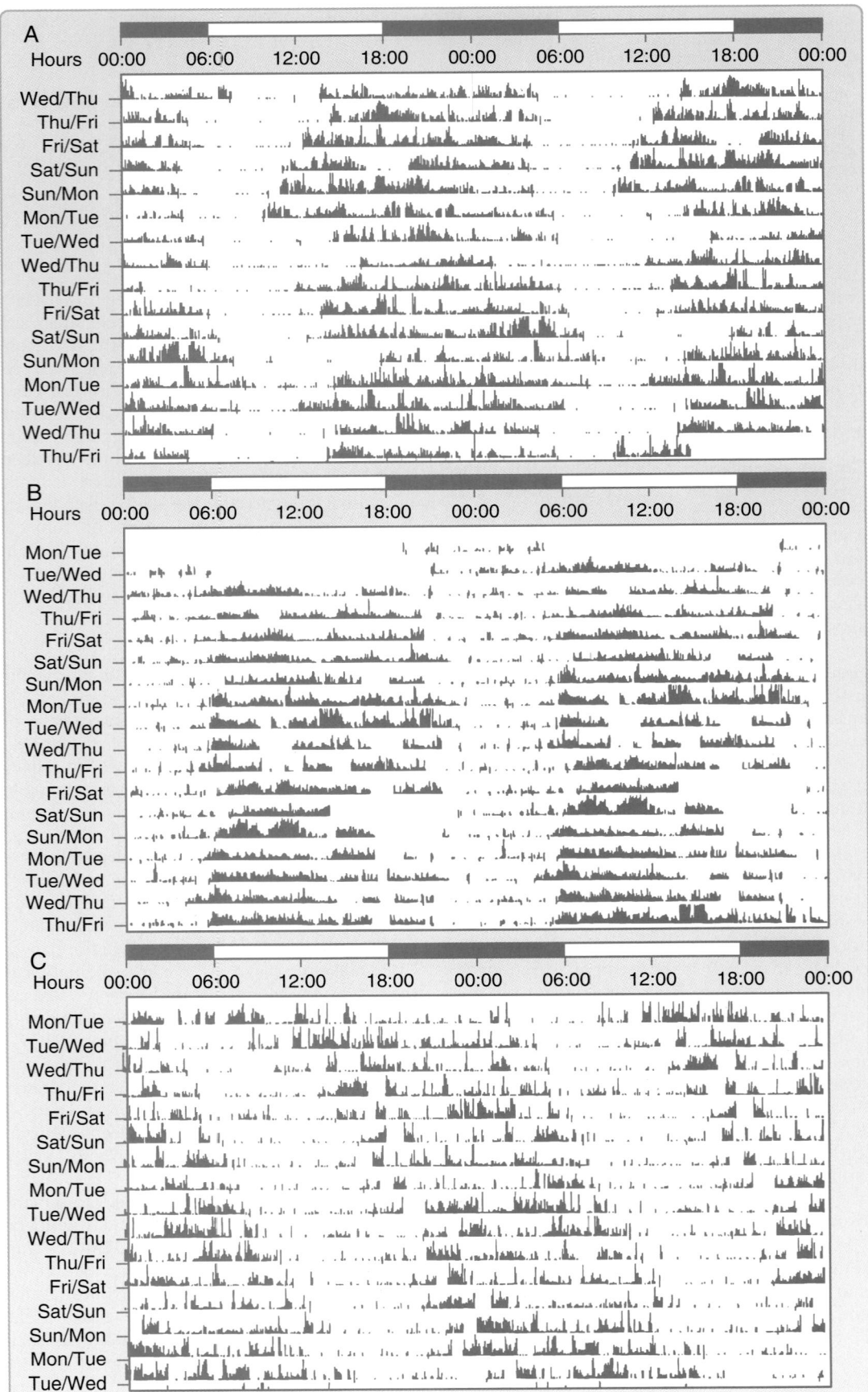

Figure 58–2. For legend see opposite page.

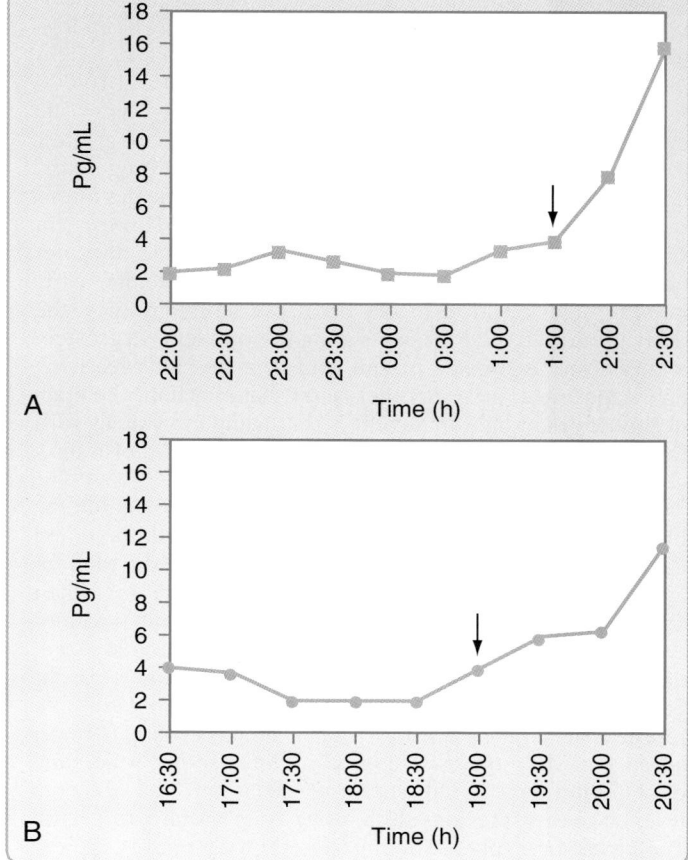

Figure 58–3. Dim-light melatonin profiles of an individual with advanced sleep phase type and a dim-light melatonin onset (DLMO) at 7 PM (**A**) and an individual with delayed sleep phase type with a DLMO at 1:30 PM (**B**). The *arrows* indicate the DLMO calculated as two standard deviations above the mean of baseline.

salivary determination of DLMO for clinical use may be feasible in the near future.

Treatment

The goal of therapy is to resynchronize the circadian clock with the desired 24-hour LD cycle. Richardson and Malin[1] noted that treatment of DSPT is the same whether it is the result of a primary behavioral or a primary physiologic process. The use of chronotherapy has been successful in a small group of patients in a laboratory setting.[30] Chronotherapy requires a successive delay of sleep times by 3 hours daily over a 5- to 6-day period until the desired sleep time is achieved. This shift is followed by rigid adherence to a set sleep–wake schedule and good sleep hygiene practices. However, outside the laboratory setting, the potential confounding effects of light exposure at the wrong circadian time may limit the effectiveness and practicality of this approach.[1]

As described earlier, light plays a major role in resetting the human circadian pacemaker.[10,11,58] Therapy with bright light in the morning (the advance portion of the human PRC) should advance the phase of circadian rhythms in DSPT and may be more practical than chronotherapy.[59,60] Although a

number of reports of successful application of bright light therapy in DSPT exist,[61,62] large, randomized, placebo-controlled studies to determine the intensity, duration, and overall effectiveness are still needed. Rosenthal and colleagues[63] found that 2 hours of bright light exposure (2500 lux) in the morning (7 to 9 AM), together with light restriction in the evening, successfully phase advanced (by 1.4 hours) circadian rhythms of core body temperature and multiple sleep latencies in 20 patients chosen prospectively after meeting clinical criteria for DSPT. In contrast, a retrospective report from a referral sleep clinic found that only 7 of 20 patients with DSPT treated with bright light alone were able to entrain reliably to a desired sleep schedule.[35]

Clinical application of bright light therapy remains empiric and there are no standard criteria for its use in DSPT. However, practice parameters have been suggested by the American Academy of Sleep Medicine.[64] The human PRC to a single 3-hour bright light pulse suggests that a light pulse given slightly before the time of body temperature minimum will result in a maximal phase delay, whereas a pulse given slightly after the minimum will cause a maximal phase advance (each about 2 hours).[58] When light pulses over three successive cycles were used, larger shifts (of 4 to 7 hours) can be produced.

Figure 58–2. Representative rest–activity cycles recorded with wrist actigraphy monitoring of patients with circadian rhythm sleep disorders. **A,** Delayed sleep phase type with sleep-onset time of approximately 4 to 6 AM and wake time of 10 AM to 2 PM. **B,** Advanced sleep phase type with sleep onset between 8 and 10 PM and wake time of 5 to 6 AM. **C,** Nonentrained type in a sighted individual. Sleep onset is later on each consecutive day, and sleep is initiated sometime between midnight and 1 AM for the 16 days represented in this actogram.

Because body temperature minimum is not routinely measured clinically, light therapy is usually timed using sleep logs to estimate the patient's endogenous circadian phase. A light pulse of 1 to 2 hours' duration and between 2500 and 10,000 lux is usually administered toward the end of the sleep–wake cycle. Because the portion of the PRC at which the greatest phase advance can be achieved occurs during sleeping hours, light is usually given immediately on awakening in the morning, which results in a smaller phase advance. However, in severely delayed individuals, the sleep–wake cycle does not necessarily correlate with circadian phase; therefore, early morning light could in theory be inadvertently given on the delay portion of the PRC, worsening the problem. Regenstein and Pavlova[65] reported a patient who slept later after receiving light exposure at 6 AM. Another factor that may limit the practicality of bright light treatment is that many individuals with DSPT may find it difficult to wake in time for administration of bright light therapy.

Administration of exogenous melatonin also shifts the phase of the endogenous circadian clock. It should be noted that the PRC for melatonin is nearly opposite to the PRC for light exposure: melatonin delays circadian rhythms when administered in the morning and advances them when administered in the afternoon or early evening.[24] In a randomized, double-blind, placebo-controlled crossover study of eight patients with DSPT, 5 mg of melatonin administered at 10 PM resulted in a phase advance in all subjects, with a mean advance of sleep onset time of 82 minutes and of wake time of 117 minutes.[66] On stopping melatonin, all patients reverted to their previous sleep–wake cycle within 2 to 3 days. The physiologic (phase shifting) dose of melatonin is approximately 0.1 to 0.5 mg or one tenth to one fiftieth of commercially available preparations.[67] Side effects of melatonin at these dose ranges are minimal, although sedative effects occur at higher (80-mg) doses. Although several studies have demonstrated the potential effectiveness of melatonin administered in the evening,[66,68-70] the relatively small number of clinical studies and the variability in dose and time of administration have been limiting factors in the development of a standardized approach for treatment with melatonin. The combination of morning bright light and early evening melatonin may be even more efficacious in creating a phase advance, although clinical data are lacking.

In summary, the clinical approach to a patient with DSPT should initially include assessment of circadian sleep phase by sleep diary or actigraphy measures for a period of at least 7 days. Behavioral interventions such as a structured sleep–wake schedule, good sleep hygiene practices and avoidance of exposure to bright light in the evening should be prescribed for all patients. In addition, exposure to bright light in the morning (1 to 2 hours shortly after awakening) or administration of melatonin in the evening (5 to 6 hours before habitual sleep time) can advance the timing of the sleep–wake cycle. Note that melatonin has not been approved for this indication.

Behaviorally Induced Delayed Sleep Phase Type

Individuals (usually adolescents and young adults) with behaviorally induced delayed sleep phase share many of the characteristics of individuals with primary DSPT, but they differ in that the delayed sleep phase pattern is predominantly the result either of an individual's choice to remain awake late into the night or of social, school, or professional demands. Individuals usually complain not of insomnia but of excessive daytime sleepiness and functional impairment associated with sleep curtailment. Voluntary behaviors such as staying awake late at night and waking up late in the morning or afternoon may result in an abnormal relationship between the two factors that regulate sleep and wakefulness: endogenous circadian rhythm and the sleep homeostatic process. A clear distinction between primary DSPT and behaviorally induced DSPT is often difficult in clinical practice, as both physiologic and behavioral factors are present in both types.

Structuring the sleep–wake schedule and using behavioral approaches can advance the timing of sleep hours and improve daytime behaviors. Behaviorally induced sleep curtailment together with the increased need for sleep in adolescence result in marked excessive daytime sleepiness and behavioral problems at school or work. The common use of stimulants to treat symptoms of sleepiness during normal waking hours may lead to further delay in sleep time and substance use. In adolescents, social maladjustment, family dysfunction, school avoidance, and affective disorders should be considered in the differential diagnosis.

CIRCADIAN RHYTHM SLEEP DISORDER, ADVANCED SLEEP PHASE TYPE

Clinical Features

Circadian rhythm sleep disorder, advanced sleep phase type (ASPT) (or advanced sleep phase syndrome) is characterized by habitual and involuntary sleep and wake times that are usually more than 3 hours earlier than societal means (see Fig. 58–1). Sleep itself is normal for the person's age. Individuals often complain of persistent and even irresistible sleepiness in the late afternoon or early evening, which may prevent their participation in desired evening activities. Because their circadian drive for wakefulness begins to rise prematurely, they may complain of involuntary early morning awakening (2 to 5 AM), which occurs even if sleep onset is voluntarily delayed. Because of professional or social obligations, later bedtimes can lead to chronically insufficient sleep and excessive daytime sleepiness. In general, individuals with ASPT have less difficulty adjusting to the earlier schedule than those with DSPT, because societal constraints on sleep time are less rigid than on wake time. Individuals with ASPT may gravitate to professions that are in phase with their endogenous circadian clock. Because of the early morning awakening, a diagnosis of depression may be erroneously made.

Epidemiology

ASPT is less frequently reported[71,72] than DSPT, possibly because affected individuals may not perceive it to be pathologic. The prevalence of ASPT in the general population is unknown. It has been estimated to be about 1% in middle-aged adults,[37] and it increases with age. Both sexes appear to be equally affected.

Pathogenesis

As with DSPT, the etiology of ASPT is unknown, although several hypotheses have been proposed. An abnormal PRC to light exhibiting an increased area under the advance portion of the curve could in theory result in a persistent phase advance. ASPT may also be the result of a shortened endogenous period. Evidence of a shortened free-running period of less than 24 hours has been demonstrated in a 66-year-old woman who had advanced sleep and wake times and intact or even enhanced responsiveness to photic entrainment,[10] and in a single member of a familial case of ASPT.[73]

Several familial cases of ASPT have been reported in the literature.[73-76] These families show a clear autosomal dominant mode of inheritance of ASPT. Genetic analysis of these familial cases indicates that there is heterogeneity of this disorder between and even within large families. Gene polymorphisms have been identified in the circadian clock gene *hPer2* in a large family with ASPT.[77]

Diagnosis

A diagnosis of ASPT is made primarily on the basis of the clinical history. Individuals have a chronic or recurrent complaint of difficulty staying awake until the desired time in the evening and inability to remain asleep until the desired and socially acceptable time for awakening. The sleep disturbance is associated with impairment of social, occupational, or other areas of functioning. When allowed to choose their preferred schedule, patients exhibit normal sleep quality and duration for their age and maintain an advanced but stable phase of entrainment to the 24-hour day. A sleep log should be kept or actigraphy monitoring (this is frequently helpful; see Fig. 58–2B) should be performed for at least 7 days to confirm a stable advance in the timing of the habitual sleep period.

Other medical, mental, or sleep disorders that may cause alterations in the sleep–wake cycle, insomnia, or excessive sleepiness should be excluded or adequately treated. Major affective disorders should be carefully excluded. PSG is sometimes necessary to confirm that sleep is normal, and that sleep-disordered breathing, periodic limb movements, or other causes of sleep disruption are not present. PSG should ideally be performed during the patient's normal sleep period. If it is carried out at conventional laboratory hours, a shortened or normal sleep onset latency and an early wake time may be seen. Early rapid eye movement sleep latency is not typically seen. If present, it may suggest depression, or other sleep disorders such as narcolepsy.[72,78]

When the diagnosis is in question, additional physiologic measures of circadian timing, such as continuous ambulatory monitoring of body temperature or collection of salivary melatonin samples to determine DLMO (see Fig. 58–3A) may be clinically useful to confirm the advance in circadian phase. Patients with ASPT have been reported to have a DLMO that is advanced several hours compared to controls.[74,75]

Treatment

Several therapeutic approaches are used to treat ASPT, each with practical limitations. A chronotherapeutic approach—advancing bedtime by 3 hours every 2 days until the desired bedtime was reached—has been reported,[72] although relapse occurred quickly.[78] Bright light therapy during the delay portion of the PRC (early evening) is usually tried, although the data on its use in ASPT are limited. Bright light from 7 to 9 PM in older adults with sleep maintenance complaints resulted in a phase advance and reduced awakenings.[79]

Melatonin given in the early morning, usually on awakening, could in theory result in a phase delay, although no data exist on its use in this situation.[67] The sedating effects of melatonin, which can be variable in patients, may limit its usefulness in this regard.

CIRCADIAN RHYTHM SLEEP DISORDER, NONENTRAINED TYPE

Clinical Features

Circadian rhythm sleep disorder, nonentrained type (or non–24-hour sleep–wake syndrome, free-running circadian sleep disorder, hypernychthemeral syndrome) is thought to be the result of a circadian pacemaker that has no stable phase relationship to the 24-hour LD cycle. Because most individuals must maintain a regular sleep–wake schedule, the clinical picture is of periodically recurring problems with sleep initiation, sleep maintenance, and rising, as the circadian cycle of wakefulness and sleep propensity moves in and out of synchrony with a fixed sleep period time.[80] Without social constraints, sleep onset and wake times are often successively delayed each day (see Fig. 58–2C). This is analogous to the free-running state created when all zeitgebers are removed.[81,82] Because the duration and quality of sleep depends on when it occurs in relation to the circadian cycle,[54] phase jumps between two physiologically permissive periods for sustained sleep can be observed.[83-85]

Epidemiology

Nonentrained sleep–wake pattern is rare in sighted people, occurring most often in totally blind individuals.[80,82,86-89] In one series, 50% of totally blind persons had free-running plasma melatonin rhythms[90]; in another, 73% were not entrained to a 24-hour sleep–wake rhythm.[91] A few cases of nonentrained type have also been reported in sighted individuals.[81,92]

Pathogenesis

The etiology in blind people is most likely either a reduction in or an absence of the entraining effects of light, although nonphotic time cues, such as an externally imposed 24-hour sleep–wake cycle and social activity, appear insufficient to entrain some individuals.[80] The melatonin rhythm may be damped[93] or nonexistent,[94] or it may be normal but delayed.[81,89] Coexistent mental retardation, which could make it difficult to process social time cues, may contribute to the symptoms in some individuals.[87] In some cases, totally blind persons without conscious perception of light nevertheless exhibit normal suppression of melatonin when exposed to very bright light and do not appear to have sleep difficulties.[91]

The etiology in sighted individuals is unknown. It has been postulated that sighted individuals may have a reduced sensitivity to the phase-resetting effects of light,[81] or that they may have an increased incidence of psychiatric conditions such as depression or certain personality disorders, which could precipitate the development of the syndrome by changing or removing social time cues.[81]

Nonentrained sleep–wake cycles have developed after chronotherapy for apparent delayed sleep phase type,[81,95] prompting the proposal that such therapy could prolong the free-running period to the point where it becomes non-entrainable to a 24-hour LD cycle.[95] However, free-running periods that are too short (less than 23 hours) or too long (greater than 27 hours)[11] for stable entrainment to a 24-hour cycle have never been demonstrated in humans. Because persons with DSPT tend to receive more light exposure in the delay (evening) portion of their PRCs than during the advance portion (early morning), progressive phase delays may sometimes be observed and mistaken for a nonentrained pattern.[1,81]

Diagnosis

The diagnosis is made primarily by a clinical history of insomnia or excessive sleepiness related to abnormal synchronization between the 24-hour LD cycle and the endogenous circadian rhythm of sleep and wake propensity. The pattern of sleep and wake times typically delays each day with a period longer than 24 hours. The pattern is present for at least 1 month and can be confirmed by sleep diary or actigraphy for at least 7 days (but preferably longer) to establish the progressive daily drift in the timing of sleep and wake times (see Fig. 58–2C). Close analysis of the sleep–wake cycle may reveal two distinct sleep–wake cycle periods, and alternation between them can be shown by phase jumps.[84,85] The sleep disturbance should be accompanied by impairment of social, occupational, or other areas of functioning.

It is important to exclude or adequately treat any other medical, mental, or sleep disorder that may cause alterations in the sleep–wake cycle, insomnia, or excessive sleepiness. If the diagnosis is in question, PSG may be useful to evaluate for other types of sleep disorders. PSG, when performed at the appropriate circadian time, is usually normal.[81] Overriding behavioral factors predisposing to irregular sleep–wake cycles (substance abuse, dementia, personality or affective disorders) should also be considered in the evaluation.

Treatment

Melatonin appears to be emerging as the initial treatment of choice in blind and sighted individuals with a nonentrained type.[22,81,82,87-89] Administration is started when the patient's free-running period approaches the normal or desired phase (i.e., sleep onset times of 10 to 11 PM). Doses sufficient for phase shifting (0.1 to 0.5 mg) are then given at 8 to 9 PM, or near the expected time of DLMO.[81,88] Initiating evening dosing when the free-running period is not in the "normal" phase could result in an inappropriate delay or advance of circadian phase and prolong the time to entrainment. Bright light entrainment is an option in sighted individuals and in blind individuals who exhibit intact photic suppression of melatonin.[96] Vitamin B_{12} has been anecdotally reported to be effective in treating nonentrained type,[97,98] although the mechanism is unknown. Benzodiazepines have not been systematically studied, although several anecdotal reports of their possible effectiveness exist.[97,98] Entrainment by non-photic stimuli (e.g., structured social cues) alone have not been successful.

IRREGULAR SLEEP–WAKE TYPE

Irregular sleep–wake type (or irregular sleep–wake disorder) is characterized by the absence of a well-defined circadian sleep–wake cycle. There is typically no major sleep period. Rather, patients present with three or more sleep episodes of varying length during a 24-hour period. Diagnosis of this disorder requires a complaint of insomnia and/or excessive sleepiness associated with multiple irregular sleep bouts or naps during a 24-hour period.[52,53] Despite irregular and fragmented sleep periods, the total sleep time per 24-hour period is usually normal for the person's age.

The prevalence of the irregular sleep–wake type in the general population is unknown but estimated to be rare.[99] This disorder is most often seen in association with neurologic dysfunction, such as brain injury, dementia, and in children with psychomotor retardation. In these individuals, the alterations in sleep–wake patterns may result from dysfunction of the central processes responsible for the generation of circadian rhythms.[100,101] In institutionalized older adults and those with dementia, reduced exposure to bright light and irregular social schedules have been suggested as contributing factors to the development and maintenance of irregular sleep–wake patterns.[102,103] Therefore, both dysfunction of circadian regulation and reduced exposure to environmental signals are probably involved in the etiology of irregular or arrhythmic sleep and wake patterns.

In addition to a clinical history, useful diagnostic tools include actigraphy and a sleep log, with continuous monitoring of sleep and wake activity for a minimum of 2 weeks. Actigraphic recordings show disturbed or low-amplitude circadian rhythm with loss of the normal diurnal sleep–wake pattern. Irregular sleep–wake type should be distinguished from poor sleep hygiene and voluntary maintenance of irregular sleep schedules, as seen with shift work.

The aim of clinical management is to improve the amplitude of circadian rhythms and their alignment with the external environment. Increasing exposure to synchronizing agents, such as bright light and structured social and physical activities, has been used to consolidate sleep–wake cycles.[43,104-106] A study using a combination of bright light, chronotherapy, vitamin B_{12}, and hypnotics was successful in 45% of patients with irregular sleep cycles.[99] In children with psychomotor retardation, evening administration of melatonin has been used to improve sleep–wake patterns.[107] Despite the potential utility of both behavioral and pharmacologic interventions, treatment may be difficult and outcomes variable.

CONCLUSION

Disorders of the sleep–wake cycle attributed to the disruption of the circadian timing system are characterized by an abnormal temporal distribution of the major sleep period within the 24-hour day. Although there is evidence that many of these disorders are the result of alterations in the circadian clock, more studies are needed to confirm this theory. The impact of these disorders is probably larger than estimated in terms of numbers, misdiagnoses, and health consequences. Most sleep clinics do not yet provide specific diagnostic tools to assess circadian rhythm profiles. Furthermore, many of the proposed therapies, including light, are often considered experimental by the health insurance industry. Application of our expanding knowledge of basic human circadian and sleep physiology to clinical practice remains an important challenge. There is a need for clinical practice parameters for circadian rhythm sleep disorders.

Clinical Pearls

Circadian rhythm sleep disorders should be considered in the differential diagnosis of patients presenting with symptoms of insomnia or excessive sleepiness. Furthermore, circadian rhythm sleep disorders, such as delayed sleep phase type and advanced sleep phase type, may be comorbid with other types of sleep disorders, making the diagnosis and treatment even more challenging. For effective management of circadian rhythm sleep disorders, one must obtain as accurate a measure of circadian timing as possible. Sleep onset time (determined by sleep diary or actigraphy) can be useful to determine circadian phase (dim-light melatonin onset occurs approximately 2 hours after sleep onset) in the clinical setting.

Behavioral interventions such as sleep hygiene, particularly enforcement of stable sleep and wake times, exposure to light at the correct time of day, and avoidance of exposure at the wrong time of day, are the basic approach for all patients. For the treatment of DSPT and nonentrained type, administration of melatonin may be useful. However, the use of melatonin for the treatment of circadian rhythm sleep disorders has not been approved by the U.S. Food and Drug Administration, and vascular and endocrine adverse effects need to be taken into account, particularly in patients who are at increased risk.

Acknowledgments

We acknowledge the contribution of the late Steven K. Baker to the original version of this chapter. We also thank Dr. Erik Naylor for his comments on the current version of this chapter. Support for this manuscript was provided by the National Aeronautics and Space Administration through NASA Cooperative Agreement NCC 9-58 with the National Space Biomedical Research Institute, NHBLI K07HL03891 and RO1HL69988.

References

1. Richardson G, Malin HV: Circadian rhythm sleep disorders: Pathophysiology and treatment. J Clin Neurophysiol 1996;13:17-31.
2. Klein D, Moore R, Reppert S: Suprachiasmatic Nucleus: The Mind's Clock. New York, Oxford University Press, 1991.
3. Vitaterna MH, King DP, Chang AM, et al: Mutagenesis and mapping of a mouse gene, Clock, essential for circadian behavior. Science 1994;264:719-725.
4. Ralph MR, Menaker M: A mutation of the circadian system in golden hamsters. Science 1988;241:1225-1227.
5. Zheng B, Larkin DW, Albrecht U, et al: The mPer2 gene encodes a functional component of the mammalian circadian clock. Nature 1999;400:169-173.
6. Czeisler CA, Duffy JF, Shanahan TL, et al: Stability, precision, and near-24-hour period of the human circadian pacemaker. Science 1999;284:2177-2181.
7. Ruby NF, Brennan TJ, Xie X, et al: Role of melanopsin in circadian responses to light. Science 2002;298:2211-2213.
8. Freedman MS, Lucas RJ, Soni B, et al: Regulation of mammalian circadian behavior by non-rod, non-cone, ocular photoreceptors. Science 1999;284:502-504.
9. Pittendrigh CS: Circadian organization and the photoperiodic phenomena. In Follett BK, Follett DE (eds): Biological Clocks in Seasonal Reproductive Cycles. Bristol, John Wright and Sons, 1981.
10. Czeisler CA, Allan JS, Strogatz SH, et al: Bright light resets the human circadian pacemaker independent of the timing of the sleep-wake cycle. Science 1986;233:667-671.
11. Czeisler CA, Kronauer RE, Allan JS, et al: Bright light induction of strong (type 0) resetting of the human circadian pacemaker. Science 1989;244:1328-1333.
12. Lewy AJ, Wehr TA, Goodwin FK, et al: Light suppresses melatonin secretion in humans. Science 1980;210:1267-1269.
13. Zeitzer JM, Dijk DJ, Kronauer R, et al: Sensitivity of the human circadian pacemaker to nocturnal light: Melatonin phase resetting and suppression. J Physiol 2000;526(pt 3):695-702.
14. Warman VL, Dijk DJ, Warman GR, et al: Phase advancing human circadian rhythms with short wavelength light. Neurosci Lett 2003;342:37-40.
15. Lockley SW, Brainard GC, Czeisler CA: High sensitivity of the human circadian melatonin rhythm to resetting by short wavelength light. J Clin Endocrinol Metab 2003;88:4502-4505.
16. Aschoff J, Fatranska M, Giedke H, et al: Human circadian rhythms in continuous darkness: Entrainment by social cues. Science 1971;171:213-215.
17. Honma K, Honma S, Nakamura K, et al: Differential effects of bright light and social cues on reentrainment of human circadian rhythms. Am J Physiol 1995;268:R528-R535.
18. Buxton OM, Frank SA, L'Hermite-Balériaux M, et al: Roles of intensity and duration of nocturnal exercise in causing phase-shifts of human circadian rhythms. Am J Physiol (Endocrinol Metab) 1997;273:E536-542.
19. Baehr EK, Eastman CI, Revelle W, et al: Circadian phase-shifting effects of nocturnal exercise in older compared with young adults. Am J Physiol Regul Integr Comp Physiol 2003;284:R1542-1550.
20. Cajochen C, Krauchi K, Wirz-Justice A: Role of melatonin in the regulation of human circadian rhythms and sleep. J Neuroendocrinol 2003;15:432-437.
21. Redman J, Armstrong S, Ng KT: Free-running activity rhythms in the rat: Entrainment by melatonin. Science 1983;219:1089-1091.
22. Sack RL, Lewy AJ, Blood ML, et al: Melatonin administration to blind people: Phase advances and entrainment. J Biol Rhythms 1991;6:249-261.
23. Moore RY: Neural control of the pineal gland. Behav Brain Res 1996;73:125-130.
24. Lewy AJ, Ahmed S, Jackson JML, et al: Melatonin shifts human circadian rhythms according to a phase-response curve. Chronobiol Int 1992;9:380-392.
25. Lewy AJ, Bauer VK, Ahmed S, et al: The human phase response curve (PRC) to melatonin is about 12 hours out of phase with the PRC to light. Chronobiol Int 1998;15:71-83.
26. Sack RL, Brandes RW, Kendall AR, et al: Entrainment of free-running circadian rhythms by melatonin in blind people. N Engl J Med 2000;343:1070-1077.
27. Dijk D-J, Cajochen C: Melatonin and the circadian regulation of sleep initiation, consolidation, structure and the sleep EEG. J Biol Rhythms 1997;12:627-635.
28. Weitzman E, Czeisler CA, Coleman RM: Delayed sleep phase syndrome: A biological rhythm sleep disorder. Sleep Res 1979;8:221.
29. Weitzman ED, Czeisler CA, Coleman RM, et al: Delayed sleep phase syndrome: A chronobiological disorder with sleep-onset insomnia Arch Gen Psychiatry 1981;38:737-746.
30. Czeisler CA, Richardson GS, Coleman RM, et al: Chronotherapy: Resetting the circadian clock of patients with delayed sleep phase insomnia. Sleep 1981;4:1-21.
31. Horne JA, Ostberg O: A self-assessment questionnaire to determine morningness-eveningness in human circadian rhythms. Int J Chronobiol 1976;4:97-110.
32. Chang A, Orbeta L, Gourineni R, et al: Relationship between circadian phase, sleep, and diurnal preference in patients with ASPS and DSPS. Sleep 2003;26(Suppl):A108.

33. Thorpy MJ, Korman E, Spielman AJ, et al: Delayed sleep phase syndrome in adolescents. J Adolesc Health Care 1988;9:22-27.

34. Alvarez B, Dahlitz M, Vignau J: The delayed sleep phase syndrome: Clinical and investigative findings in 14 subjects. J Neurol Neurosurg Psychiatry 1992;55:665-670.

35. Regestein QR, Monk TH: Delayed sleep phase syndrome: A review of its clinical aspects. Am J Psychiatry 1995;152:602-608.

36. Pelayo R, Thorpy MJ, Govinski P: Prevalence of delayed sleep phase syndrome among adolescents. Sleep Res 1988;17:392.

37. Ando K, Kripke DF, Ancoli-Israel S: Estimated prevalence of delayed and advanced sleep phase syndromes. Sleep Res 1995;24:509.

38. deBeck TW: Delayed sleep phase syndrome: Criminal offense in the military? Mil Med 1990;155:14-15.

39. Ito A, Ando K, Hayakawa T, et al: Long-term course of adult patients with delayed sleep phase syndrome. Jpn J Psychiatry Neurol 1993;47:563-567.

40. Czeisler CA, Richardson GS, Zimmerman JC, et al: Entrainment of human circadian rhythms by light-dark cycles: A reassessment. Photochem Photobiol 1981;34:239-247.

41. Aoki H, Ozeki Y, Yamada N: Hypersensitivity of melatonin suppression in response to light in patients with delayed sleep phase syndrome. Chronobiol Int 2001;18:263-271.

42. Lingjaerde O, Bratlid T, Hansen T: Insomnia during the "dark period" in northern Norway: An explorative, controlled trial with light treatment. Acta Psychiatr Scand 1985;71:506-512.

43. Ancoli-Israel S, Schnierow B, Kelsoe J, et al: A pedigree of one family with delayed sleep phase syndrome. Chronobiol Int 2001;18:831-840.

44. Archer SN, Robilliard DL, Skene DJ, et al: A length polymorphism in the circadian clock gene Per3 is linked to delayed sleep phase syndrome and extreme diurnal preference. Sleep 2003;26:413-415.

45. Hohjoh H, Takasu M, Shishikura K, et al: Significant association of the arylalkylamine N-acetyltransferase (AA-NAT) gene with delayed sleep phase syndrome. Neurogenetics 2003;4:151-153.

46. Iwase T, Kajimura N, Uchiyama M, et al: Mutation screening of the human Clock gene in circadian rhythm sleep disorders. Psychiatry Res 2002;109:121-128.

47. Takahashi Y, Hohjoh H, Matsuura K: Predisposing factors in delayed sleep phase syndrome. Psychiatry Clin Neurosci 2000;54:356-358.

48. Uchiyama M, Okawa M, Shibui K, et al: Poor recovery sleep after sleep deprivation in delayed sleep phase syndrome. Psychiatry Clin Neurosci 1999;53:195-197.

49. Watanabe T, Kajimura N, Kato M, et al: Sleep and circadian rhythm disturbances in patients with delayed sleep phase syndrome. Sleep 2003;26:657-661.

50. Uchiyama M, Okawa M, Shirakawa S, et al: A polysomnographic study on patients with delayed sleep phase syndrome (DSPS). Jpn J Psychiatry Neurol 1992;46:219-221.

51. Uchiyama M, Okawa M, Shibui K, et al: Poor compensatory function for sleep loss as a pathogenic factor in patients with delayed sleep phase syndrome. Sleep 2000;23:553-558.

52. American Academy of Sleep Medicine. International Classification of Sleep Disorders: Diagnostic and Coding Manual, 2nd ed. Westchester, Ill, American Academy of Sleep Medicine, 2005.

53. American Psychiatric Association: Diagnostic and Statistical Manual of Mental Disorders, 4th Edition, Text Revision. Washington, DC, 2000.

54. Czeisler CA, Weitzman E, Moore-Ede MC, et al: Human sleep: Its duration and organization depend on its circadian phase. Science 1980;210:1264-1267.

55. Shibui K, Uchiyama M, Okawa M: Melatonin rhythms in delayed sleep phase syndrome. J Biol Rhythms 1999;14:72-76.

56. Lewy AJ, Sack RL: The dim light melatonin onset as a marker for circadian phase position. Chronobiol Int 1989;6:93-102.

57. Lewy AJ: The dim light melatonin onset, melatonin assays and biological rhythm research in humans. Biol Signals Recept 1999;8:79-83.

58. Minors DS, Waterhouse JM, Wirz-Justice A: A human phase-response curve to light. Neurosci Lett 1991;13:36-40.

59. Lewy AJ, Sack RL, Singer CM: Treating phase typed chronobiologic sleep and mood disorders using appropriately timed bright artificial light. Psychopharmacol Bull 1985;21:368-372.

60. Lewy AJ, Sack RL, Singer CM: Melatonin, light and chronobiological disorders. Ciba Found Symp 1985;117:231-252.

61. Weyerbrock A, Timmer J, Hohagen F, et al: Effects of light and chronotherapy on human circadian rhythms in delayed sleep phase syndrome: Cytokines, cortisol, growth hormone, and the sleep-wake cycle. Biol Psychiatry 1996;40:794-797.

62. Akata T, Sekiguchi S, Takahashi M, et al: Successful combined treatment with vitamin B_{12} and bright artificial light of one case with delayed sleep phase syndrome. Jpn J Psychiatry Neurol 1993;47:439-440.

63. Rosenthal NE, Joseph-Vanderpool JR, Levendosky AA, et al: Phase-shifting effects of bright morning light as treatment for delayed sleep phase syndrome. Sleep 1990;13:354-361.

64. Chesson AL Jr, Littner M, Davila D, et al: Practice parameters for the use of light therapy in the treatment of sleep disorders. Standards of Practice Committee, American Academy of Sleep Medicine. Sleep 1999;22:641-660.

65. Regestein QR, Pavlova M: Treatment of delayed sleep phase syndrome. Gen Hosp Psychiatry 1995;17:335-345.

66. Dahlitz M, Alvarez B, Vignau J, et al: Delayed sleep phase syndrome response to melatonin. Lancet 1991;337:1121-1124.

67. Lewy AJ, Ahmed S, Sack RL: Phase shifting the human circadian clock using melatonin. Behav Brain Res 1996;73:131-134.

68. James SP, Sack DA, Rosenthal NE, et al: Melatonin administration in insomnia. Neuropsychopharmacology 1990;3:19-23.

69. Oldani A, Ferini-Strambi L, Zucconi M, et al: Melatonin and delayed sleep phase syndrome: Ambulatory polygraphic evaluation. Neuroreport 1994;6:132-134.

70. Nagtegaal JE, Kerkhof GA, Smits MG, et al: Delayed sleep phase syndrome: A placebo-controlled cross-over study on the effects of melatonin administered five hours before the individual dim light melatonin onset. J Sleep Res 1998;7:135-143.

71. Kamei R, Hughes L, Miles L, et al: Advanced sleep phase syndrome studied in a time isolation facility. Chronobiologia 1979;6:115.

72. Moldofsky H, Musisi S, Phillipson EA: Treatment of a case of advanced sleep phase syndrome by phase advance chronotherapy. Sleep 1986;9:61-65.

73. Jones CR, Campbell SS, Zone SE, et al: Familial advanced sleep-phase syndrome: A short-period circadian rhythm variant in humans. Nat Med 1999;5:1062-1065.

74. Reid KJ, Chang AM, Dubocovich ML, et al: Familial advanced sleep phase syndrome. Arch Neurol 2001;58:1089-1094.

75. Ondze B, Espa F, Ming LC, et al: [Advanced sleep phase syndrome.] Rev Neurol (Paris) 2001;157(pt 2):S130-134.

76. Satoh K, Mishima K, Inoue Y, et al: Two pedigrees of familial advanced sleep phase syndrome in Japan. Sleep 2003;26:416-417.

77. Toh KL, Jones CR, He Y, et al: An hPer2 phosphorylation site mutation in familial advanced sleep phase syndrome. Science 2001;291:1040-1043.

78. Wagner DR: Disorders of the circadian sleep-wake cycle. Neurol Clin 1996;14:651-670.

79. Campbell SS, Dawson D, Anderson MW: Alleviation of sleep maintenance insomnia with timed exposure to bright light. J Am Geriatr Soc 1993;41:829-836.

80. Klein T, Martens H, Dijk DJ, et al: Circadian sleep regulation in the absence of light perception: Chronic non-24-hour circadian

rhythm sleep disorder in a blind man with a regular 24-hour sleep-wake schedule. Sleep 1993;16:333-343.

81. McArthur AJ, Lewy AJ, Sack RL: Non-24-hour sleep-wake syndrome in a sighted man: Circadian rhythm studies and efficacy of melatonin treatment. Sleep 1996;19:544-553.

82. Lapierre O, Dumont M: Melatonin treatment of a non-24-hour sleep-wake cycle in a blind retarded child. Biol Psychiatry 1995;38:119-122.

83. Kokkoris CP, Weitzman ED, Pollak CP, et al: Long-term ambulatory temperature monitoring in a subject with a hypernychthemeral sleep–wake cycle disturbance. Sleep 1978;1:177-190.

84. Wollman M, Lavie P: Hypernychthemeral sleep-wake cycle: Some hidden regularities. Sleep 1986;9:324-334.

85. Uchiyama M, Okawa M, Ozaki S: Delayed phase jumps of sleep onset in a patient with non-24-hour sleep-wake syndrome. Sleep 1996;19:637-640.

86. Sack RL, Lewy AJ, Blood ML, et al: Circadian rhythm abnormalities in totally blind people: Incidence and clinical significance. J Clin Endocrinol Metab 1992;75:127-134.

87. Palm L, Blennow G, Wetterberg L: Correction of non-24-hour sleep/wake cycle by melatonin in a blind retarded boy. Ann Neurol 1991;29:336-339.

88. Tzischinsky O, Pal I, Epstein R, et al: The importance of timing in melatonin administration in a blind man. J Pineal Res 1992;12:105-108.

89. Palm L, Blennow G, Wetterberg L: Long-term melatonin treatment in blind children and young adults with circadian sleep-wake disturbances. Dev Med Child Neurol 1997;39:319-325.

90. Sack RL, Lewy AJ, Blood ML, et al: Circadian rhythm abnormalities in totally blind people: Incidence and clinical significance. J Clin Endocrinol Metab 1992;75:127-134.

91. Czeisler CA, Shanahan TL, Klerman EB, et al: Suppression of melatonin secretion in some blind patients by exposure to bright light. N Engl J Med 1995;332:6-11.

92. Boivin DB, James FO, Santo JB, et al: Non-24-hour sleep-wake syndrome following a car accident. Neurology 2003;60:1841-1843.

93. Nakamura K, Hashimoto S, Honma S, et al: A sighted man with non-24-hour sleep-wake syndrome shows damped plasma melatonin rhythm. Psychiatry Clin Neurosci 1997;51:115-119.

94. Tomoda A, Miike T, Uezono K, et al: A school refusal case with biological rhythm disturbance and melatonin therapy. D Dev 1994;16:71-76.

95. Oren DA, Wehr TA: Hypernychthemeral syndrome after chronotherapy for delayed sleep phase syndrome. N Engl J Med 1992;327:1762.

96. Hoban TM, Sack RL, Lewy AJ, et al: Entrainment of a free-running human with bright light? Chronobiol Int 1989;6:347-353.

97. Okawa M, Mishima K, Nanami T, et al: Vitamin B_{12} treatment for sleep-wake rhythm disorders. Sleep 1990;13:15-23.

98. Kamgar-Parsi B, Wehr TA, Gillin JC: Successful treatment of human non-24-hour sleep-wake syndrome. Sleep 1983;6:257-264.

99. Yamadera H, Takahashi K, Okawa M: A multicenter study of sleep-wake rhythm disorders: Clinical features of sleep-wake rhythm disorders. Psychiatry Clin Neurosci 1996;50:195-201.

100. Witting W, Kwa IH, Eikelenboom P, et al: Alterations in the circadian rest-activity rhythm in aging and Alzheimer's disease. Biol Psychiatry 1990;27:563-572.

101. Hoogendijk WJ, van Someren EJ, Mirmiran M, et al: Circadian rhythm-related behavioral disturbances and structural hypothalamic changes in Alzheimer's disease. Int Psychogeriatr 1996;8(Suppl 3):245-252; discussion, 269-272.

102. Pollak CP, Stokes PE: Circadian rest-activity rhythms in demented and nondemented older community residents and their caregivers. J Am Geriatr Soc 1997;45:446-452.

103. van Someren EJ, Hagebeuk EE, Lijzenga C, et al: Circadian rest-activity rhythm disturbances in Alzheimer's disease. Biol Psychiatry 1996;40:259-270.

104. Van Someren EJ, Swaab DF, Colenda CC, et al: Bright light therapy: Improved sensitivity to its effects on rest-activity rhythms in Alzheimer patients by application of nonparametric methods. Chronobiol Int 1999;16:505-518.

105. Naylor E, Penev PD, Orbeta L, et al: Daily social and physical activity increases slow-wave sleep and daytime neuropsychological performance in the elderly. Sleep 2000;23:87-95.

106. Ancoli-Israel S, Martin JL, Kripke DF, et al: Effect of light treatment on sleep and circadian rhythms in demented nursing home patients. J Am Geriatr Soc 2002;50:282-289.

107. Pillar G, Shahar E, Peled N, et al: Melatonin improves sleep-wake patterns in psychomotor retarded children. Pediatr Neurol 2000;23:225-228.

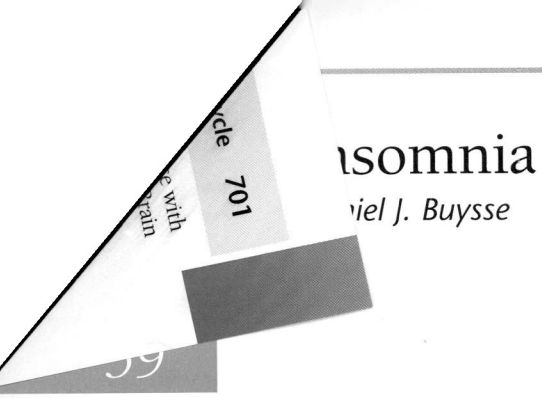

Overview of Insomnia: Definitions, Epidemiology, Differential Diagnosis, and Assessment

Jack D. Edinger

Melanie K. Means

ABSTRACT

Insomnia is by far the most common form of sleep disturbance, yet health care providers and the general public remain naïve about the nature, prevalence, and consequences of this condition. Most typically, insomnia has been defined as the symptom of difficulty initiating or maintaining sleep and more rarely as an inability to obtain restorative sleep. However, a set of more specific insomnia disorders has been defined according to the International Classification of Sleep Disorders and other classification systems. Insomnia disorders are most often classified as either primary or secondary to other sleep, psychiatric, or medical conditions, although it is often difficult in practice to determine true causality. The prevalence of isolated insomnia symptoms in the general population is approximately 30% to 50%, and approximately 9% to 15% report significant daytime impairments as a result of chronic insomnia problems. Increasing age, female sex, and psychiatric and medical disorders are consistent risk factors for insomnia. Insomnia is associated with significant consequences including impaired function and quality of life, increased risk for psychiatric disorders, and increased health care costs. The clinical assessment of insomnia is based on a careful clinical interview, often supplemented by questionnaires, psychological testing, and sleep logs. Polysomnography is indicated only when specific sleep pathologies are suspected.

Weary with toil I haste me to my bed,
The dear repose for limbs with travel tired,
But then begins a journey in my head
To work my mind when body's work's expired;
For then my thoughts, from far where I abide,
intend a zealous pilgrimage to thee,
And keep my drooping eyelids open wide, …
Lo, thus, by day my limbs, by night my mind,
For thee and for myself no quiet find.

William Shakespeare
Sonnet XXVII

As suggested by this Shakespearean passage, insomnia has long been recognized as a common, annoying, and potentially debilitating human malady. Over the past 50 years, sleep research and sleep medicine practice have served only to confirm that insomnia complaints are highly prevalent and too often associated with considerable morbidity. Moreover, insomnia places a considerable economic burden on its sufferers, their employers, the health care system, and society. Nonetheless, the nature, ubiquity, significance, and myriad causes of this sleep difficulty remain poorly understood by health care providers and the general public. Accordingly, a large proportion of insomnia sufferers go undiagnosed by their health care providers, and many of these incur considerable personal, vocational, and health-related consequences as a result.

This chapter highlights the nature and significance of insomnia, as well as the range of considerations facing clinicians who evaluate patients with insomnia. In the initial sections we consider the variety of definitions and classification approaches used to characterize this sleep difficulty. Subsequently, we review epidemiologic findings concerning insomnia's prevalence, factors that enhance its risk of occurrence, and its long-term consequences. Finally, we provide guidelines for a differential diagnosis of patients who present insomnia complaints and discuss common methods used in their assessment.

INSOMNIA DEFINITIONS

Symptom-Focused Definitions

The extensive clinical and research literature devoted to insomnia provides numerous definitions for this phenomenon. Most include descriptions of sleep-specific symptoms alone or sleep symptoms with associated daytime complaints.[1-5] Definitions focused on sleep symptoms typically describe insomnia as a difficulty initiating sleep, a difficulty maintaining sleep, a final awakening that occurs much earlier than desired, or sleep that is nonrestorative or of generally poor quality. When symptoms such as difficulty initiating or maintaining sleep or waking too early are described, it is implied, although often not stated, that such difficulties occur in the context of an adequate opportunity or sufficient time period allotted for sleep.[2] In contrast, terms such as non-restorative or poor quality are used when sleep is subjectively "shallow" and unrefreshing despite being apparently normal in length and continuity.

Whereas sleep-specific symptoms are generally considered essential to definitions of insomnia, such symptoms considered in isolation may have limited clinical significance. Ohayon et al.,[7] for example, found that over 10% of a large representative community sample reported satisfaction with their sleep despite reporting one or more of the symptoms of insomnia just described. In contrast, 6% of this sample had no insomnia symptoms yet reported sleep dissatisfaction. Furthermore, the complaint of "nonrestorative sleep" was not significantly more prevalent among those who reported sleep dissatisfaction than among those who were satisfied with their sleep. Hence, insomnia definitions that focus exclusively on sleep-specific symptoms may be inadequate to identify a clinically important syndrome.

As a consequence of these shortcomings, insomnia definitions in the clinical and research literature have increasingly highlighted both the sleep and waking symptoms of this condition. Typically, such definitions include reports of one or more of the previously mentioned sleep-related symptoms, along with such associated daytime complaints as fatigue, sleepiness, mood disturbance, cognitive difficulties, and social or occupational impairment.[1-4] An insomnia definition that includes consideration of the consequences of observed or reported sleep-related symptoms is more clinically useful because it connotes more global sleep/wake dysfunction. Moreover, well-designed epidemiologic studies have shown that persons with sleep disturbance and associated daytime consequences are more prone to report general sleep dissatisfaction and seek treatment for their sleep/wake complaints than are those with solely sleep-specific symptoms.[8,9]

Despite its appeal, the qualitative nature of this definition is problematic. It allows considerable variability in case identification, which leads to substantial inconsistency in clinical practice and research findings. To remedy this situation, Lichstein et al.[10] derived a quantitative definition based on the modal practice they observed in behavioral/psychological insomnia treatment studies and by testing several versions of severity criteria in prospective sensitivity–specificity analyses. On the basis of their findings, these authors suggest that a reported sleep onset latency (i.e., the time it takes to initially fall asleep) or wake time after sleep onset (i.e., the amount of time awake in the middle of the night) of greater than 31 minutes occurring at least three times per week for at least 6 months is the most defensible quantitative definition for insomnia.

This definition improves on exclusively qualitative definitions by providing precise severity, frequency, and duration criteria for defining the sleep-specific symptoms of persistent insomnia. However, it provides no quantitative guidelines for those patients who complain mainly of waking too early or getting poor-quality sleep, nor does it include quantitative guidelines for ascertaining the presence or absence of insomnia-related daytime complaints. This definition also excludes persons who have less frequent, intermittent, or shorter-term sleep onset or maintenance difficulties that confound daytime functioning. Hence, additional efforts to develop comprehensive operational insomnia definitions currently appear warranted.

Insomnia Classification

Over the past 30 years, considerable clinical and research experience has shown that insomnia complaints arise from varied causes including primary sleep disorders, medical diseases, psychiatric illnesses, medication/substance abuse, and a host of behavioral and environmental factors.[1-5,11,12] This experience has also shown that the sleep/wake symptom-based insomnia definitions we have discussed communicate little about causative factors. This realization, in turn, has spawned several diagnostic classification systems that provide more precise definition and differentiation of insomnia subtypes by means of detailed, subtype-specific diagnostic criteria.[1-3,13-15] In practice, the increased descriptive specificity of these nosologies facilitates communication among practitioners, aids decision making in treatment, and helps standardize subject selection for insomnia research.[16]

Currently, the three most widely used insomnia classification schemes are those included in the International Classification of Sleep Disorders (ICSD and ICSD-2),[1,2] the fourth edition of the American Psychiatric Association's Diagnostic and Statistical Manual (DSM-IV),[3] and the World Health Organization's International Classification of Diseases (ICD-9CM and ICD-10).[14,15] The original ICSD included over 40 diagnostic categories that could be applied to insomnia sufferers. This number has been reduced slightly in the ICSD-2 system, but this nosology continues to provide a high degree of specificity in the subtyping of insomnia disorders. In contrast, the DSM-IV[3] and ICD[14,15] nosologies include substantially fewer and more global diagnostic categories for insomnia. The first versions of the ICSD and the DSM-IV systems list insomnias that are primary sleep/wake disturbances or *dyssomnias* along with those so-called *secondary* insomnias that arise as a function of psychiatric conditions, medical diseases, or substance abuse. In contrast, the ICD system lists a limited number of *disorders of sleep of nonorganic origin* and *sleep disturbances* with a presumed organic basis. ICSD-2 includes insomnia disorders as one of six major categories of sleep disorders. Both the "primary" and "secondary" forms of insomnia are listed in this section. Table 59-1 provides a comparison of the ICSD-2, DSM-IV, and current ICD systems for classifying insomnia subtypes. Due to recent collaborative efforts between the American Academy of Sleep Medicine and the World Health Organization, forthcoming versions of the ICD are likely to include the majority of the ICSD-2 insomnia categories.

These insomnia classification schemes have their merits, but each has its limitations. The ICSD has been criticized for being too specific,[17,18] whereas the DSM-IV and ICD fail to provide diagnostic categories for certain insomnia subtypes (e.g., restless legs syndrome) that are widely recognized.[19] Additionally, the ICD's distinction between organic and nonorganic insomnia subtypes appears overly simplistic and inconsistent with current conceptualizations of many recognized insomnia phenotypes. In practice, clinicians within a setting show only modest agreement in their assignment of

Table 59–1. **Comparison of Insomnia Diagnoses of the DSM-IV, ICSD-2, and ICD-9-CM Nosologies**

ICSD-2 Insomnia Categories	
I. Insomnias	
F51.01	Adjustment Sleep Disorder
F51.03	Psychophysiologic Insomnia
F51.02	Paradoxical Insomnia
F51.04	Insomnia due to a mental disorder
G47.01	Idiopathic Insomnia
Z72.821	Inadequate Sleep Hygiene
Z3.81	Behavioral Insomnia of Childhood
G47.02	Insomnia due to a drug or substance
G47.03	Insomnia due to a medical condition
F51.00	Other insomnia not due to a substance or physiological condition, unspecified
G47.00	Organic insomnia, unspecified
II. Sleep-Related Breathing Disorders	
G47.31	Primary Central Sleep Apnea
G47.39	Other Central Sleep Apnea due to a medical condition
G47.32	Obstructive Sleep Apnea, Adult
G47.34	Sleep-Related Non-obstructive Alveolar Hypoventilation, Idiopathic
G47.37	Other Sleep-Related Hypoventilation/ Hypoxemia due to a medical condition
III. Circadian Rhythm Sleep Disorders	
G47.21	Delayed sleep phase type
G47.22	Advanced sleep phase type
G47.23	Irregular sleep–wake type
G47.24	Free-running type
G47.26	Due to a medical condition
F51.21	Jet lag type
F51.22	Shift work type
F51.23	Behaviorally-induced delayed sleep phase type
F51.29	Other not due to a substance or known physiological condition
G47.25	Other due to a drug or substance
IV. Sleep-Related Movement Disorders	
G47.61	Restless Legs Syndrome
G47.62	Periodic Limb Movement Sleep Disorder

G47.63	Sleep-Related Leg Cramps
G47.65	Sleep-Related Rhythmic Movement Disorder
G47.66	Sleep-Related Movement Disorder due to a drug or substance
G47.67	Sleep-Related Movement Disorder due to a medical condition
V. Parasomnias	
F51.50	Nightmare Disorder
G47.59	Sleep-Related Eating Disorder
G47.50, G47.54, G47.55	Other Parasomnias (n = 3)

DSM-IV Insomnia Categories	
I. Dyssomnias	
307.42	Primary Insomnia
780.59	Breathing-Related Sleep Disorder
307.45	Circadian Rhythm Sleep Disorder
307.47	Dyssomnia Not Otherwise Specified
II. 307.42	**Insomnia Related to Another Mental Disorder**
III. 780.52	**Sleep Disorder Due to a General Medical Condition, Insomnia Type**
IV. 291.89/292.89	**Substance-Induced Sleep Disorder, Insomnia Type**

ICD-9-CM Insomnia Diagnoses	
I. 307.4	**Specific Disorders of Sleep of Nonorganic Origin**
307.40	Nonorganic Sleep Disorder, Unspecified
307.41	Transient Disorder of Initiating or Maintaining Sleep
307.42	Persistent Disorder of Initiating or Maintaining Sleep
307.45	Phase-Shift Disruption of 24-Hour Sleep–Wake Cycle
307.49	Other
II. 780.5	**Sleep Disturbances**
780.51	Insomnia with Sleep Apnea
780.52	Other Insomnia
780.55	Phase-Shift Disruption of 24-Hour Sleep–Wake Cycle

Included are diagnoses that most likely would apply to insomnia patients in each of these three classification systems. Not shown are the diagnoses in these classification schemes that are for other types of sleep disorders (e.g., narcolepsy, selected parasomnias).

DSM-IV, Diagnostic and Statistical Manual of Mental Disorders, 4th Edition; ICD-9-CM, International Classification of Diseases, 9th Revision; ICSD-2, International Classification of Sleep Disorders, 2nd edition.

DSM-IV and ICSD insomnia diagnoses, and notable site biases are obvious when comparing diagnostic assignment patterns across settings.[20] Field applications[21,22] also highlight the markedly discordant results occurring when separate insomnia nosologies are applied to the same group of patients. The findings[21] reproduced in Figure 59–1, for example, show that many patients assigned an insomnia diagnosis derived from the initial ICSD[1] would not be assigned any corresponding insomnia diagnosis in the DSM-IV. Finally, when purely empirical techniques such as cluster analyses have been used to cross-validate insomnia nosologies, results provided only partial support for systems such as the DSM and original ICSD.[23] Notwithstanding the conceptual and empirical concerns raised herein, each of these nosologies provides a definitional specificity that improves on the purely symptom-focused insomnia definitions discussed here. As a result, each of these systems has proved of value in clinical and research venues.

EPIDEMIOLOGY

Prevalence

Like headaches, nausea, and the common cold, insomnia is a malady that falls within the experience of most individuals.

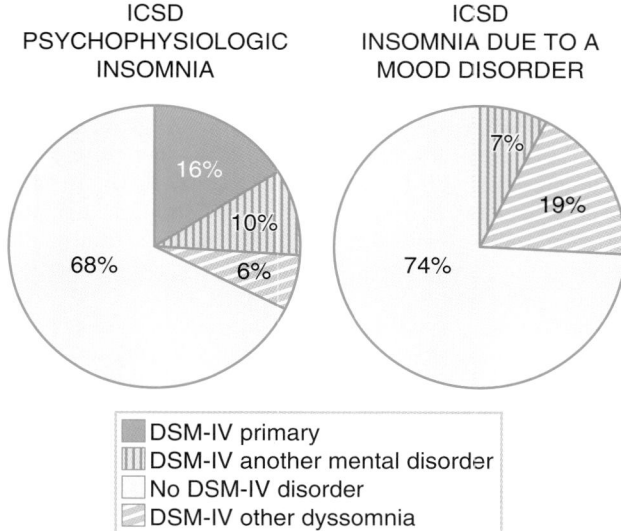

Figure 59–1. Concordance of DSM-IV insomnia diagnoses with the two ICSD diagnoses of Psychophysiologic Insomnia and Insomnia Due to a Mood Disorder. As the figure illustrates, a sizable proportion of individuals assigned an ICSD diagnosis of Psychophysiologic Insomnia or Insomnia Due to a Mood Disorder would not meet DSM-IV criteria for any insomnia diagnosis. Findings shown are from Ohayon MM, Roberts RE: Comparability of sleep disorders diagnoses using DSM-IV and ICSD classifications with adolescents. Sleep 2001;24:920-925.

Table 59–2.	Effect of Insomnia Definitions on Estimates of the Prevalence of Insomnia in the General Population

Insomnia Definition	Prevalence Estimate Range (%)
Sleep-Related Insomnia Symptoms only	30-48
Sleep-Related Insomnia Symptoms occurring ≥3 times/week or "often" or "always"	16-21
"Moderate" or "Severe" Sleep-Related Insomnia Symptoms	10-28
Insomnia Symptoms + Daytime Consequences	9-15
Dissatisfaction with Sleep Quantity or Quality	8-18
Insomnia Diagnosis (DSM-IV)	4.4-11.7

DSM-IV, Fourth Edition of the Diagnostic and Statistical Manual of the American Psychiatric Association. Prevalence estimates from summary findings reported in Ohayon MM: Epidemiology of insomnia: What we know and what we still need to learn. Sleep Med Rev 2002;6:97-111; and data reported by Ohayon MM, Partinen M: Insomnia and sleep dissatisfaction in Finland. J Sleep Res 2002;11:339-346.

A 1979 Gallup poll[24] showed that 95% of a randomly selected adult sample reported having experienced insomnia at some time during their lives. For most, however, insomnia represents a transient problem that resolves quickly when precipitating circumstances (stress, sudden schedule changes, transient illnesses) abate. Of more consequence are chronic forms of insomnia that persist over time and contribute to various types of dysfunction. Results of epidemiologic studies generally suggest that chronic or persistent forms of insomnia are relatively common in most western societies, but the prevalence estimates obtained in these studies have varied widely.

In a recent review of these studies, Ohayon[5] observed that prevalence estimates for chronic insomnia ranged from a low of 4.4%[7] to a high of 48%[25] across the numerous studies he reviewed. Various factors including geographic and sociocultural characteristics of study samples most likely account for some of this variability. Yet Ohayon's[5] findings, summarized by Table 59–2, suggest that much of this variability is attributable to the insomnia definitions used in case ascertainment. The largest prevalence estimates come from studies[25,26] that employed liberal symptom-based insomnia definitions without criteria to delineate the frequency or severity of such symptoms. When indices of sleep dissatisfaction (e.g., reported dissatisfaction with quality/quantity of sleep; self-labeling as an insomnia sufferer or poor sleeper) or insomnia symptoms are combined with daytime complaints, prevalence estimates appear more modest, ranging from 8% to 18%.[5] Finally, when strict DSM-IV diagnostic criteria for insomnia have been applied, prevalence estimates have been even lower, ranging from a low of 4.4%[7] to a high of 11.7%.[27] Nonetheless, a sizable proportion of individuals who either report insomnia symptoms and sleep dissatisfaction or use medications to improve their sleep do not meet DSM-IV criteria for an insomnia diagnosis. Consequently, use of strict DSM-IV diagnostic criteria

in prevalence surveys may lead to underestimates of those with clinically important sleep difficulties.

Risk Factors

Ideally, assessment of risk for a particular disease comes from longitudinal studies in which the emergence of that disease over time is statistically related to individuals' premorbid characteristics. Unfortunately, in the case of insomnia, much of what is known about risk factors comes from cross-sectional studies in which the presence or absence of insomnia has been related to coincident demographic traits, health status, occupation, or social functioning. This sort of research approach provides no information about the timing of insomnia onset vis-à-vis those characteristics found to predict the presence of insomnia. For a limited set of characteristics (e.g., sex), it is possible to assume risk when such characteristics predict insomnia. However, in the case of most acquired characteristics found to predict insomnia, such studies imply possible risk but do not confirm it. Nonetheless, there is enough consistency across much of this research that presumptions about many of the risk factors that will be discussed later seem reasonable.

Among the demographic characteristics studied, sex and age have received greatest scrutiny. No matter how insomnia is defined, the pertinent research has clearly demonstrated that women are more prone to present with insomnia complaints than are men.[9,26,28-32] Reasons for this difference are not entirely clear, although such findings may be the result of sex differences in proneness to report health complaints or a greater tendency for women to develop other important risk factors for insomnia. It is clear that insomnia symptoms are related to aging. Older adults are more prone to report these symptoms than are younger adults.[7,8,25,26] However, when more stringent insomnia definitions are used and/or other important comorbidities are statistically controlled, age does not correlate with the presence or absence of insomnia.[7-9,30,33,34] Thus, aging, per se, does not appear to increase the risk for clinically significant insomnia.

In addition to sex and age, several other demographic characteristics have been studied, including marital status, income, education, work status, and specific work-related stressors, as risk factors for insomnia. Most studies suggest that divorced/separated or widowed individuals are at increased risk for insomnia compared with married individuals, although this trend is more pronounced for women than for men.[7-9,30,35] Various studies[29,30,36] suggest limited education and low income may enhance insomnia risk, but these findings may be spurious, because studies that statistically controlled other important predictors failed to support this conclusion.[7,8] Several studies have suggested that those who are unemployed are significantly more likely to report insomnia than are those who are employed.[9,28,30,37] Yet, this sort of finding cannot be overgeneralized, because the unemployed groups most prone to insomnia are retirees and homemakers, whereas electively unemployed groups such as students do not appear at increased risk for insomnia.[5,8] Among employed groups, those subjected to rotating or variable work shifts and those who report overinvolvement in their jobs appear more prone to report insomnia symptoms.[38-40]

Research concerning the effect of race or ethnicity on insomnia risk has provided mixed results. Studies[41-43] of older-aged cohorts have shown that insomnia symptoms or complaints are less prevalent among African Americans than among age-matched European Americans. Among young college student samples, the reverse of this trend appears to be the case.[44,45] The apparent interaction between age and race implied by these studies, however, is complicated by additional findings showing (1) a higher prevalence of insomnia symptoms among U.S.-born African Americans than among Caribbean-born persons of the same race,[41] and (2) a higher incidence of insomnia among older African American women (19%) than among both African American men (12%) and European Americans (14%).[43] These mixed results imply that the influence of race or ethnicity on insomnia risk is complex and probably moderated by age, comorbidities, sex, and several sociocultural factors.

In contrast, studies concerning the effects of health status provide a fairly consistent view of the influence of poor health on insomnia risk. Several studies[30,37] have shown that the perception of poor health is associated with increased risk for insomnia. Moreover, individuals with documented digestive, respiratory, arthritic, vascular/circulatory, or cardiac disorders, or, among men, prostate disorders, are at greater risk for sleep-specific insomnia symptoms than are those without such conditions.[30,37,46-48] Mental or emotional disorders also appear to enhance insomnia risk. In particular, the presence of depression or anxiety disorders increases the likelihood that insomnia symptoms will be present as well.[28-30,46-49] Of course, insomnia may not represent a separate disorder in the context of the medical and mental conditions mentioned. These conditions may all adversely affect sleep and produce insomnia as one of their many symptoms. However, as discussed later, such secondary insomnias may warrant separate treatment attention, so it is prudent to recognize the medical and psychiatric conditions most commonly associated with this sleep disturbance.

Various behavioral and environmental factors may also enhance risk for insomnia. A stressful lifestyle,[30,37] physical inactivity,[30,34,37] irregular bedtimes,[50] alcohol dependence,[28,33] and heavy caffeine use[51] all predict insomnia symptoms. Cigarette smoking also appears to be a risk factor for insomnia symptoms,[52] and smoking cessation has been shown to predict insomnia remission.[33] Social relationships may also be an important consideration inasmuch as one study[34] showed older adults who were satisfied with their social lives were at relatively low risk for insomnia symptoms. Exposure to traffic noise during the sleeping period also enhances insomnia risk, as one recent study[50] showed insomnia complaints were highest among respondents living closest to busy highways. Finally, one study[53] showed sleep onset problems and associated daytime impairment increased in southern Norway from summer to winter whereas, the opposite seasonal pattern was observed in this country's northern-most regions. Thus, seasonal changes may interact with latitudinal variations to influence insomnia risk.

Little is known about genetic factors involved in insomnia. With the exception of fatal familial insomnia, research exploring the genetic basis of insomnia has been extremely limited. Nonetheless, some studies imply a genetic basis for insomnia. McCarren et al.,[54] for example, found that heritability of insomnia was higher in monozygotic than in dizygotic twins drawn from a Vietnam era military veteran population. More recently, Yves et al.[55] found that 48.8% of 256 insomnia sufferers reported that one or more first-degree relatives had insomnia, whereas only 23.5% of 90 individuals without insomnia reported insomnia in a first-degree relative. Family aggregation appeared highest among primary insomnia sufferers, in that 72.7% of such individuals reported familial insomnia, with 32% of relatives affected. In contrast, family aggregation was lowest among those with sleep apnea syndrome, in that only 26.9% of those with this diagnosis reported a family history of insomnia. Considered collectively, these findings suggest there may be a genetic vulnerability for insomnia. However, more research is needed, both to confirm this assumption and to identify specific genes that may be involved.

Morbidity

There is little doubt that persistent insomnia has a pronounced negative effect on perceptions of daytime functioning and general well-being. Compared to those without sleep/wake complaints, those with persistent insomnia report a greater sense of daytime fatigue, poorer mood, more anxiety or stress, less vigor, greater coping difficulties, less ability to complete tasks, and greater impairment of family or social functioning.[56-59] Those with persistent insomnia also report significantly poorer quality of life than do those free of insomnia.[8,60] Furthermore, persistent and severe insomnia may significantly influence perceptions of general health status. In fact, recent findings,[61] summarized in Figure 59-2, show that severe insomnia has as pronounced adverse effects on health-related quality-of-life perceptions as do such conditions as congestive heart failure and clinical depression.

Additionally, insomnia may significantly enhance risks for daytime hazards and mental or psychiatric disorders. Compared to those without sleep/wake complaints, insomnia sufferers report a greater tendency to suffer work-related or traffic accidents.[62,63] Furthermore, several studies have shown that the presence of insomnia at the time of an initial interview

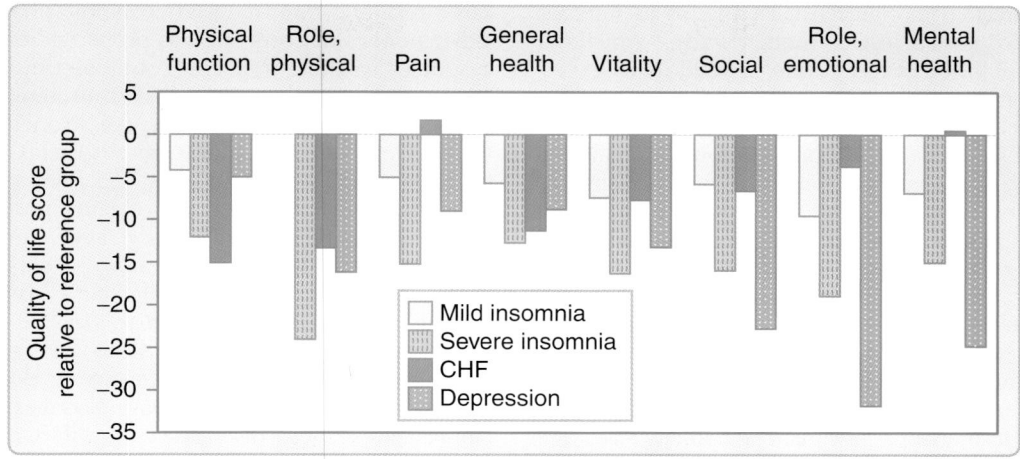

Figure 59–2. Mean deviations in Health-Related Quality of Life (HRQOL) Scale scores for individuals with mild insomnia, severe insomnia, congestive heart failure (CHF), and clinical depression (*N* = 3445). Average deviations in HRQOL scores are statistically controlled for demographic factors, health habits, obesity, other chronic conditions, severity of disease, and study location. All HRQOL raw scores are on a scale from 0 to 100. The reference group consisted of 1073 patients with mild hypertension and no other significant medical conditions or insomnia. The deviation scores shown are relative to the reference group. For example, a deviation score of –12 reflects a score that is 12 points lower than the score obtained by the reference group. Data derived from Katz DA, McHorney CA: The relationship between insomnia and health-related quality of life in patients with chronic illness. J Fam Pract 2002;51:229-235.

enhances risk for a major depressive disorder occurring between 1 and 3.5 years after that interview.[64-66] Perhaps most impressive are the longitudinal data of Chang et al.,[67] summarized in Figure 59–3. In this study of over 1000 male medical students, those who reported insomnia while in medical school showed an increased risk for a major depressive episode up to 30 years after their graduation. Additionally, longitudinal data have shown that insomnia sufferers are at risk for anxiety/panic disorders and substance abuse problems as well.[65] Finally, laboratory research[68] has shown that insomnia sufferers manifest more impairment of semantic memory than do controls, whereas a recent longitudinal study showed older men with insomnia were at increased risk for cognitive decline over a 3-year time span than were age-matched men without insomnia.[69]

Mortality

A very limited number of studies have examined the effects of insomnia and its treatment on risk for mortality. One recent study[33] showed that the presence of severe insomnia reported during an initial contact increased risk of mortality over a 10-year follow-up period. However, this study failed to control

Figure 59–3. Cumulative incidence of clinical depression over 40 years of follow-up in male medical students with and without insomnia during medical school. Reproduced from Chang PP, Ford DE, Mead LA, et al.: Insomnia in young men and subsequent depression. The Johns Hopkins Precursors Study. Am J Epidemiol 1997;146: 105-114.

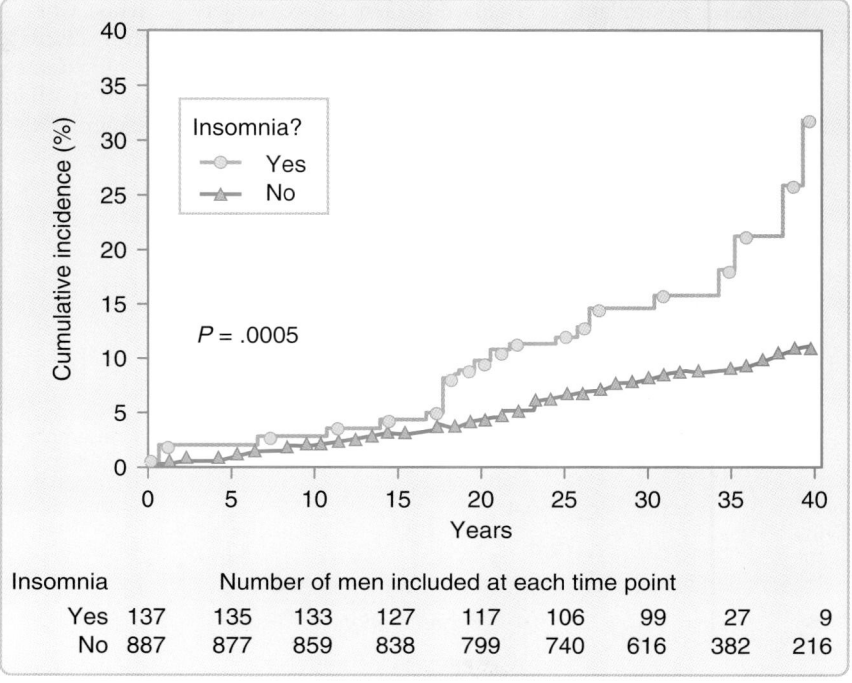

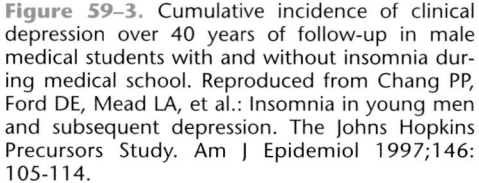

Insomnia	Number of men included at each time point								
Yes	137	135	133	127	117	106	99	27	9
No	887	877	859	838	799	740	616	382	216

for other health-related mortality risk factors, so its findings cannot be regarded as conclusive. Another study,[70] which did statistically control for other risk factors, showed that "severe" insomnia among men was related to increased risk for mortality during a 3-year follow-up period. In contrast, three other studies[71-73] that used similar statistical prediction models failed to find a significant relationship between the presence/absence or frequency of insomnia and subsequent mortality over 4- to 6-year follow-up periods. However, one[72] of these studies did find that mortality risk was significantly related to incident insomnia during the follow-up period. Another longitudinal study[74] showed that mortality risk over a 6-year follow-up period was significantly elevated in older adults who used medications other than traditional hypnotics to aid their sleep. Yet, given the inconsistent findings of these various studies, it remains questionable whether insomnia per se enhances mortality risk.

Health Care Utilization and Costs

Given the prevalence and potential seriousness of insomnia, it is not surprising that insomnia sufferers place a significant burden on both the health care system and their employers. Several studies[9,62,65] have shown that insomnia sufferers make significantly more visits to practitioners in both the medical and psychiatric sectors than do those without any sleep complaints. Furthermore, this increased health care utilization is shown not only by those presenting with insomnia complicated by comorbid conditions, but also by those with uncomplicated, primary forms of insomnia. Weissman et al.,[65] for example, found that insomnia sufferers with or without recent histories of psychiatric disorders were significantly more prone to access medical and psychiatric care providers during a 1-year observation period than were individuals with neither sleep nor psychiatric disorders. Insomnia sufferers who enter the workforce may represent a significant fiscal burden because of not only the health costs they confer to employers but also their high rate of absenteeism.[62,75] In fact, insomnia alone may account for as many as 3.5 disability days per month, a level of work impairment similar to that caused by Generalized Anxiety Disorder and Somatoform Disorder.[75]

Determining the total economic burden placed on society by insomnia is a complex task. Such efforts require consideration of insomnia's direct, treatment-related costs, its indirect costs resulting from reduced economic productivity, and its other nonhealth costs such as property damage and wasted resources resulting from this condition. Admittedly, accurate estimates, particularly of the cost of insomnia unrelated to its treatment, are difficult to ascertain. Nonetheless, in 1994, Stoller[76] estimated the annual total societal cost of insomnia to be between $92.45 and $107.53 billion. However, these estimates were based on a relatively high projected prevalence rate (33%) and included costs related more specifically to daytime sleepiness than to insomnia per se.

More recently, Walsh and Engelhardt[77] provided estimates for the direct costs of insomnia by considering costs of prescription and nonprescription sleep aids, outpatient health provider services, insomnia treatment during periods of hospitalization, and nursing home placements resulting from unmanageable sleep disturbances in the home setting. Using cost information drawn from a number of sources, these authors estimated the total direct costs for insomnia treatment in the United States during 1995 alone was $13,926,110,000. Figure 59–4 provides an itemized accounting of the costs contributing to this estimate. Perhaps the most controversial aspect to this projection is its inclusion of nursing home costs, because sleep disturbance is often only a symptom of the actual disorder (e.g., dementia) leading to nursing home placement. However, even if nursing home costs are excluded from this projection, the residual direct, treatment-related 1995 costs for insomnia still exceed $3 billion. This latter figure matches well with 1995 cost estimates of over $2 billion provided by Leger et al.[78] for treatment of insomnia in France. Thus, even after excluding nursing home costs, this form of sleep difficulty represents a significant financial burden to society.

Despite the sizable health care costs related to insomnia, a substantial proportion of insomnia sufferers remain untreated. This observation, in part, seems to be because a large percentage of insomnia sufferers do not actively seek treatment for their sleep problems. A 1991 Gallup poll, for example, showed that only 5% of all insomnia sufferers surveyed saw their physicians specifically for their sleep problems, whereas only 30% of all insomnia sufferers surveyed ever discussed their sleep problems with their doctors.[36] Unfortunately, health care providers confound this problem, as they often fail to detect insomnia symptoms among their patients.[9,79] Too often, health care providers either do not

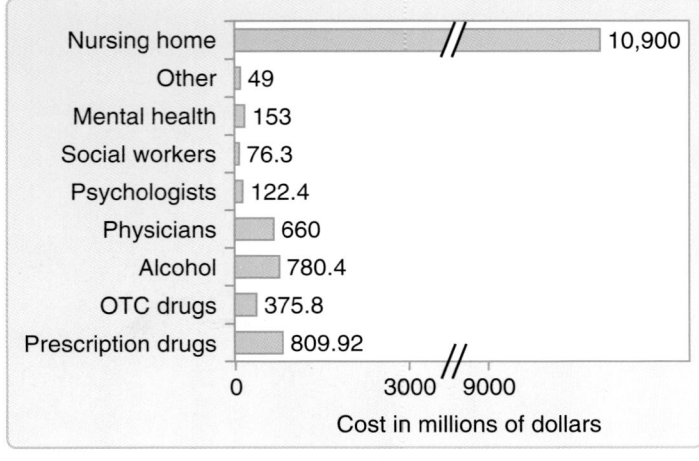

Figure 59–4. Direct treatment-related costs (in millions) for insomnia in the United States in 1995. OTC, over-the-counter. Estimates shown were obtained from estimates cited in Walsh JK, Engelhardt CL: The direct economic costs of insomnia in the United States for 1995. Sleep 1999;22:S386-S393.

question their patients sufficiently about their sleep or fail to recognize symptoms suggestive of an insomnia problem.[79] Given such observations, the remainder of the chapter will consider important diagnostic issues to consider in evaluating patients with insomnia and will review the range of methods that might be used in assessing their complaints.

DIFFERENTIAL DIAGNOSIS

Because insomnia can arise from varied causes (e.g., psychiatric, medical, substance use, cognitive, behavioral) and is often secondary to some other disease process,[22,80] consideration of differential diagnoses is a critical element in successful treatment planning. This section briefly reviews the range of insomnia diagnoses commonly encountered in clinical practice. An extensive list of diagnoses associated with a complaint of insomnia is provided by Sateia et al.[81]

Given the high comorbidity between insomnia and psychiatric disorders, it is essential to differentiate insomnia from these disorders. Approximately half of individuals with chronic insomnia have a current psychiatric diagnosis or past psychiatric history,[82] and "insomnia related to a mental disorder" is the most prevalent insomnia diagnosis assigned by sleep clinicians.[22] In addition, insomnia is part of the symptom profile of many psychiatric disorders, such as mood disorders, posttraumatic stress disorder, generalized anxiety disorder, and substance use disorders.[3] Often, insomnia appears as a prodromal symptom heralding the onset of a psychiatric disorder.[83] For example, one recent population-based study[82] found that the symptom of insomnia appeared before the onset of a first episode of mood disorder in 41% of cases and before the onset of an anxiety disorder in 18% of cases. These findings underscore the importance of conducting a thorough psychiatric history as part of an insomnia evaluation.

Various sleep pathologies also can present clinically as an insomnia complaint. Primary sleep disorders[1,2] such as periodic limb movement disorder, restless legs syndrome, and sleep-related breathing disorders can cause sleep onset difficulties, sleep fragmentation, and nocturnal awakenings that lead to insomnia complaints. Insomnia is also a prominent symptom of most circadian rhythm disorders.[1-3] Parasomnias less commonly present as a complaint of insomnia, but they should be routinely considered in the evaluation.

In many patients, insomnia problems are complex and multifactorial. For example, a patient whose insomnia initially arose during a mood episode may continue to experience sleep problems caused by poor sleep habits even once the depression is successfully treated. Similarly, a patient with another sleep disorder (e.g., sleep apnea) is not immune from developing insomnia independent of the initial sleep disorder. Alternatively, a patient may have chronic pain that delays sleep onset and occult sleep-disordered breathing that contributes to sleep maintenance difficulties. These more complicated cases illustrate the importance of a sophisticated and thorough assessment.

ASSESSMENT

Insomnia is a clinically challenging disorder that requires a comprehensive assessment to determine the appropriate diagnosis and formulate a treatment plan. Evaluation of an insomnia complaint centers on the clinical interview but can be enhanced by a number of complementary methodologies.

Because insomnia is a subjective complaint, the use of subjective assessment methods such as self-report questionnaires and sleep logs is warranted. However, objective methodologies such as actigraphy and polysomnography (PSG) also play an important role in diagnostic decisions. A typical strategy for the clinician is to combine the clinical interview and sleep logs with additional assessment approaches as indicated. This section briefly reviews various assessment techniques for evaluating insomnia.

Clinical Interview

The clinical interview is the most important component of an insomnia assessment because it is the springboard from which the clinician formulates hypotheses regarding etiologic factors and bases treatment decisions. In addition to a comprehensive assessment of the insomnia complaint and sleep history, the clinical interview should include evaluation of medication and substance use and medical and psychiatric issues.

Essential elements of a sleep assessment are outlined in Box 59–1 and reviewed in greater detail elsewhere.[81,84-86] A sleep history questionnaire,[87] completed by the patient prior to the interview, gathers pertinent information in a standardized manner. Semistructured interviews designed specifically for insomnia[85,88] focus on relevant issues and help guide the clinician's inquiries. The Structured Interview for Sleep Disorders[89] assists the clinician in determining a specific sleep disorder diagnosis. In addition, interviewing the patient's bed partner about the patient's sleep pattern and habits can reveal important diagnostic information such as symptoms of other sleep disorders.

Medical history should include a review of systems most commonly associated with sleep difficulties, such as rheumatologic (e.g., arthritis, fibromyalgia) pulmonary (e.g., asthma, chronic obstructive pulmonary disease), cardiac (e.g., heart disease), gastrointestinal (e.g., reflux, peptic ulcer disease), neurologic (e.g., seizure disorder), and endocrine (e.g., hyperthyroidism) disorders. The presence of chronic pain and its influence on sleep should also be assessed. In middle-aged women, menopausal status should be considered as a potential contributor to sleep difficulties, whereas in middle-aged and older men, prostate disease should be considered as a possible cause of sleep disruption. Results of a medical history and examination may uncover the need for laboratory testing (e.g., thyroid function, prostate-specific antigen, ferritin levels in suspected sleep movement disorders).

A psychiatric history is necessary to determine the influence of psychological factors on the insomnia complaint. Symptoms of depression and anxiety are most commonly encountered, and the clinician should query patients about their perceived level of stress. Although brief psychological screening is usually sufficient, in some cases the clinician may consider further interviewing or psychometric testing to identify and evaluate psychiatric issues.

Because insomnia is a side effect of many medications (e.g., stimulants, steroids, antihypertensives, antidepressants), current medication usage should be evaluated. Some antidepressants can exacerbate periodic limb movements and associated insomnia.[1,2] Patients' attempts to discontinue sedative or hypnotic medications can create a rebound insomnia.[1,2] Many patients resort to self-help remedies (e.g., melatonin, alcohol, antihistamines) to promote sleep. Finally, patients should be questioned about use of illicit substances.

Box 59–1   Components of a Clinical Interview for Insomnia

Sleep History and Assessment
- Nature of complaint (pattern, onset, history, course, duration, severity)
- Predisposing and precipitating factors
- Factors that exacerbate insomnia or improve sleep pattern
- Etiologic factors
- Sleep–wake pattern
- Daytime symptoms (sleepiness, hyperarousal)
- Perceived impact (consequences, impairment)
- Maladaptive conditioning to bedroom environment
- Physiologic or cognitive arousal at bedtime
- Beliefs about sleep and cause of insomnia
- Symptoms of other sleep disorders
- Sleep environment (bedtime routines, sleep-incompatible behaviors)
- Sleep hygiene practices
- Lifestyle (daily activity, exercise pattern)
- Treatment history (self-help attempts, coping strategies, response to previous treatments)
- Treatment expectations

Medication and Substance Use
- Sleep medication, home or herbal remedies
- Prescription medications
- Over-the-counter medications (diet pills, antihistamines)
- Alcohol, tobacco, caffeine
- Illicit substances

Medical History and Examination
- Medical disorders associated with sleep disruption
- Chronic pain
- Menopausal status (women)
- Prostate disease (men)
- Laboratory testing if indicated

Psychiatric History
- Depression
- Anxiety
- Other mental health disorders
- Stress level

Self-Report Questionnaires

A variety of self-report sleep questionnaires have been developed to measure the following insomnia-related factors: hyperarousal, daytime sleepiness, sleep hygiene behaviors, sleep quality, satisfaction with sleep, functional impairment, sleep-related beliefs and attitudes, and insomnia severity.[81,88] Comprehensive reviews of these questionnaires are provided by Sateia et al.[81] and Savard and Morin.[88] Although many of these questionnaires enjoy widespread research use, their contribution in the clinical setting is less clear. As Sateia[84] notes, the value of such questionnaires in diagnosing insomnia or measuring treatment outcome for patients with clinical insomnia remains to be determined. These questionnaires are not immune to subjective biases inherent in self-report methodology, and their utility is maximized when combined with other methods such as sleep logs or actigraphy.

Psychological Testing

Because of the prevalence of mood and anxiety symptoms among patients with insomnia, routine psychological screening is recommended. Brief psychological questionnaires such as the Beck Depression Inventory,[90] the Spielberger State-Trait Anxiety Inventories,[91] the Profile of Mood States,[92] and the Brief Symptom Inventory[93] are easily administered. Although they have limited value when used in isolation, these questionnaires may provide important supplemental information not apparent from the clinical interview.

In some cases, it may be necessary to conduct a more thorough psychological assessment. The Minnesota Multiphasic Personality Inventory-2 (MMPI-2)[94] is an extensive psychological questionnaire that produces personality profiles for a wide range of psychopathology. Validity scales provide information on response biases such as patients' attempts to either deny or exaggerate psychopathologic symptoms. Individuals with insomnia produce specific MMPI-2 profiles characterized by depression, anxiety, and somatization of emotional conflict.[81] Although some sleep disorders centers routinely administer the MMPI-2 to all patients as part of the intake evaluation, it is a lengthy questionnaire that requires interpretation by a trained psychologist.

Sleep Log

The sleep log or diary provides a subjective record of an individual's perceived sleep pattern and has become an indispensable tool in the assessment of insomnia. It contains questions that allow easy calculation of sleep onset latency, total wake and sleep time, number of awakenings, sleep efficiency, time in bed, and sleep quality. Additional information such as napping behavior, sleep medication use, and alcohol consumption can be easily obtained. Although no standardized format exists, numerous examples are readily available.[84,86,88,95] In addition to being simple and inexpensive, sleep logs provide more accurate information about insomnia severity and variability, sleep scheduling, and sleep–wake patterns than a patient's retrospective report.[84] This information may reveal important diagnostic issues such as circadian changes, insufficient sleep, or perpetuating factors.[88] Furthermore, sleep logs provide a reliable measurement of sleep changes and can be used over long time periods to assess treatment effects.[95] To reduce measurement variability, sleep logs should be completed for a minimum of 1 to 2 weeks.[81,84,96] New electronic versions on computerized hand-held devices (e.g., personal data assistants) promote accuracy and can be used to monitor compliance.[97]

Polysomnography

Although PSG is the only method that provides a comprehensive measurement of sleep and is essential in diagnosing many sleep disorders, it is not usually necessary in the assessment of an insomnia complaint. By definition, insomnia entails a subjective component relating to the perception of poor sleep, which may or may not be supported by the objective evaluation of sleep via PSG. Recent practice parameters for the evaluation of insomnia published by the American Academy of Sleep Medicine (see p. 239 of Chesson et al.[98]) state that PSG "is not indicated for the routine evaluation of chronic insomnia," unless there exists "valid indication and clear rationale."

PSG should be considered in situations where the patient presents with pathologic levels of sleepiness, reports symptoms of other sleep pathologies (e.g., sleep-disordered breathing, periodic limb movements, parasomnias. narcolepsy), or does not respond to insomnia treatment.[84]

Actigraphy

Actigraphy produces sleep estimates based on measurements of body movement from a wristwatch-sized recording device and is described in detail in Chapter 124. Its main advantage is the ability to inexpensively and unobtrusively collect sleep–wake data in the home environment over extended periods. Like PSG, actigraphy is not recommended for the routine diagnostic evaluation of insomnia.[99] However, when combined with information from a clinical interview and sleep log, actigraphy contributes additional objective data regarding sleep phase changes and variability of sleep patterns over time. This information can be used to assist in diagnosis, to document severity of an insomnia problem, to measure treatment outcome, and to monitor patient compliance to treatment recommendations.[99,100] Studies using actigraphy with insomnia samples have found the most benefit for assessing relative changes in night-to-night sleep variability.[100] Multiple nights of actigraphic monitoring may also provide information about patients' average nocturnal sleep and wake time, but such measures may vary somewhat from similar measures derived from PSG.[97,100] Current standards of practice recommend a minimum recording period of 3 days with concurrent use of a sleep log to assist in determining sleep periods.[99]

Summary

In summary, the evaluation of insomnia is a complex process that relies on multiple assessment procedures. To guide the clinician in this process, we offer the following practice guidelines:

- The *clinical interview,* the central component of an insomnia evaluation, is used to determine etiologic factors and to formulate diagnostic impressions. It should cover a history and assessment of the sleep complaint as well as medical, psychiatric, and substance use issues.
- Insomnia assessment should routinely include a *sleep log* completed for 1 to 2 weeks.
- *Psychological screening tests* are often useful to rule out depression and anxiety as causes of insomnia.
- *Self-report sleep questionnaires* are of questionable clinical utility but may be helpful, particularly when combined with other assessment methods.
- *Polysomnography* should be considered only in cases with symptoms of other sleep pathologies, pathologic levels of daytime sleepiness, or failure to respond to insomnia treatment.
- Although not a mandatory component of an insomnia assessment, *actigraphy* contributes information about sleep phase and variability of sleep patterns.

CONCLUSIONS

Insomnia is the most common sleep problem. Its heterogeneity is characterized by a variety of causes, definitions, classificatory schemes, and assessment methods. Insomnia impacts functioning in many areas of an individual's daily life and confers a significant economic burden on society. Chapters 60 to 63 present current knowledge regarding the management and treatment of this disorder.

Clinical Pearl

Insomnia is a prevalent and debilitating form of sleep disturbance that results in considerable morbidity and financial burden to both its sufferers and society. Because insomnia may arise from myriad causes, patients who present with insomnia complaints require a comprehensive assessment to determine appropriate diagnoses and treatment needs.

REFERENCES

1. American Sleep Disorders Association: International Classification of Sleep Disorders—Revised. Rochester, Minn, American Sleep Disorders Association, 1997.
2. American Academy of Sleep Medicine: International Classification of Sleep Disorders: Diagnostic and Coding Manual, 2nd ed. Westchester, Ill, American Academy of Sleep Medicine, 2005.
3. American Psychiatric Association: Diagnostic and statistical manual of mental disorders, 4th ed. Washington DC, American Psychiatric Association, 1994.
4. Ohayon MM, Roth T: What are the contributing factors for insomnia in the general population? J Psychosom Res 2001;51:745-755.
5. Ohayon MM: Epidemiology of insomnia: What we know and what we still need to learn. Sleep Med Rev 2002;6:97-111.
6. Leger D, Guilleminault C, Dreyfus JP, et al: Prevalence of insomnia in a survey of 12,778 adults in France. J Sleep Res 2000;9:35-42.
7. Ohayon MM, Caulet M, Guilleminault C: How a general population perceives its sleep and how this relates to the complaint of insomnia. Sleep 1997;20:715-723.
8. Ohayon MM, Caulet M, Priest RG, et al: DSM-IV and ICSD-90 insomnia symptoms and sleep dissatisfaction. Br J Psychiatry 1997;171:382-388.
9. Hajak G, SINE Study Group, Study of Insomnia in Europe: Epidemiology of severe insomnia and its consequences in Germany. Eur Arch Psychiatry Clin Neurosci 2001;251:49-56.
10. Lichstein KL, Durrence HH, Taylor DJ, et al: Quantitative criteria for insomnia. Behav Res Ther 2003;41:427-445.
11. Mellinger GD, Balter MB, Uhlenhuth EH: Insomnia and its treatment: Prevalence and correlates. Arch Gen Psychiatry 1985;42:225-232.
12. Vollrath M, Wicki W, Angst J: The Zurich study: VIII. Insomnia: Association with depression, anxiety, somatic syndromes, and course of insomnia. Eur Arch Psychiatry Neurol Sci 1989;239:113-124.
13. Association of Sleep Disorders Centers and the Association for the Psychophysiological Study of Sleep: Diagnostic classification of sleep and arousal disorders, 1st edition. Sleep 1979;2:1-154.
14. World Health Organization: ICD-9-CM: International classification of diseases, clinical modification, 4th ed, 9th rev. Salt Lake City, Utah, Medicode, 1994.
15. World Health Organization: The ICD-10 classification of mental and behavioural disorders. Geneva, World Health Organization, 1993.
16. Buysse DJ, Young T, Edinger JD, et al: Clinicians' use of the International Classification of Sleep Disorders: Results of a national survey. Sleep 2003;26:48-51.
17. Reynolds CF 3rd, Kupfer DJ, Buysse DJ, et al: Subtyping DSM-III-R primary insomnia: A literature review by the DSM-IV Work Group on Sleep Disorders. Am J Psychiatry 1991;148:432-438.
18. Vgontzas AN, Kales A, Bixler EO, et al: Sleep disorders related to another mental disorder (nonsubstance/primary): A DSM-IV literature review: Commentary. J Clin Psychiatry 1993;54:256-259.

19. Walters AS: Toward a better definition of the restless legs syndrome. The International Restless Legs Syndrome Study Group. Mov Disord 1995;10:634-642.

20. Buysse DJ, Reynolds CF 3rd, Hauri PJ, et al: Diagnostic concordance for DSM-IV sleep disorders: A report from the APA/NIMH DSM-IV field trial. Am J Psychiatry 1994;151:1351-1360.

21. Ohayon MM, Roberts RE: Comparability of sleep disorders diagnoses using DSM-IV and ICSD classifications with adolescents. Sleep 2001;24:920-925.

22. Buysse DJ, Reynolds CF 3rd, Kupfer DJ, et al: Clinical diagnoses in 216 insomnia patients using the International Classification of Sleep Disorders (ICSD), DSM-IV and ICD-10 categories: A report from the APA/NIMH DSM-IV field trial. Sleep 1994;17:630-637.

23. Edinger JD, Fins AI, Goeke JM, et al: The empirical identification of insomnia subtypes: A cluster analytic approach. Sleep 1996;19:398-411.

24. The Gallup Organization: The Gallup study of sleeping habits. Princeton, NJ, Gallup Organization, 1979.

25. Quera-Salva MA, Orluc A, Goldenberg F, et al: Insomnia and use of hypnotics: Study of a French population. Sleep 1991;14:386-391.

26. Klink ME, Quan SF, Kaltenborn WT, et al: Risk factors associated with complaints of insomnia in a general adult population: Influence of previous complaints of insomnia. Arch Intern Med 1992;152:1634-1637.

27. Ohayon M, Partinen M: Insomnia and global sleep dissatisfaction in Finland. J Sleep Res 2002;11:339-346.

28. Li RH, Wing YK, Ho SC, et al: Gender differences in insomnia: A study in the Hong Kong Chinese population. J Psychosom Res 2002;53:601-609.

29. Bixler EO, Vgontzas AN, Lin HM, et al: Insomnia in central Pennsylvania. J Psychosom Res 2002;53:589-592.

30. Sutton DA, Moldofsky H, Badley EM: Insomnia and health problems in Canadians. Sleep 2001;24:665-670.

31. Bazargan M: Self-reported sleep disturbance among African-American elderly: The effects of depression, health status, exercise, and social support. Int J Aging Hum Dev 1996;42:143-160.

32. Dodge R, Cline MG, Quan SF: The natural history of insomnia and its relationship to respiratory symptoms. Arch Intern Med 1995;155:1797-1800.

33. Janson C, Lindberg E, Gislason T, et al: Insomnia in men: A 10-year prospective population based study. Sleep 2001;24:425-430.

34. Ohayon MM, Zulley J, Guilleminault C, et al: How age and daytime activities are related to insomnia in the general population: Consequences for older people. J Am Geriatr Soc 2001;49:360-366.

35. Ohayon M: Epidemiological study on insomnia in the general population. Sleep 1996;19:S7-S15.

36. Ancoli-Israel S, Roth T: Characteristics of insomnia in the United States: Results of the 1991 National Sleep Foundation Survey: I. Sleep 1999;22:S347-S353.

37. Kim K, Uchiyama M, Okawa M, et al: An epidemiological study of insomnia among the Japanese general population. Sleep 2000;23:41-47.

38. Ohayon MM, Lemoine P, Arnaud-Briant V, et al: Prevalence and consequences of sleep disorders in a shift worker population. J Psychosom Res 2002;53:577-583.

39. Harma M, Tenkanen L, Sjoblom T, et al: Combined effects of shift work and life-style on the prevalence of insomnia, sleep deprivation and daytime sleepiness. Scand J Work Environ Health 1998;24:300-307.

40. Tachibana H, Izumi T, Honda S, et al: A study of the impact of occupational and domestic factors on insomnia among industrial workers of a manufacturing company in Japan. Occup Med 1996;46:221-227.

41. Jean-Louis G, Magai CM, Cohen CI, et al: Ethnic differences in self-reported sleep problems in older adults. Sleep 2001;24:926-933.

42. Whitney CW, Enright PL, Newman AB, et al: Correlates of daytime sleepiness in 4578 elderly persons: The Cardiovascular Health Study. Sleep 1998;21:27-36.

43. Blazer DG, Hays JC, Foley DJ: Sleep complaints in older adults: A racial comparison. J Gerontol A Biol Sci Med Sci 1995;50:M280-M284.

44. DiPalma J, Jean-Louis G, Zizi F, et al: Self-reported sleep duration among college students: Consideration of ethnic differences. Sleep 2001;24:A430.

45. Hicks RA, Lucero-Gorman K, Bautista J, et al: Ethnicity, sleep duration, and sleep satisfaction. Percept Mot Skills 1999;88:234-235.

46. Katz DA, McHorney CA: Clinical correlates of insomnia in patients with chronic illness. Arch Intern Med 1998;158:1099-1107.

47. Foley DJ, Monjan A, Simonsick EM, et al: Incidence and remission of insomnia among elderly adults: An epidemiologic study of 6,800 persons over three years. Sleep 1999;22:S366-S372.

48. Foley DJ, Monjan AA, Brown SL, et al: Sleep complaints among elderly persons: An epidemiologic study of three communities. Sleep 1995;18:425-432.

49. Hohagen F, Rink K, Kappler C, et al: Prevalence and treatment of insomnia in general practice: A longitudinal study. Eur Arch Psychiatry Clin Neurosci 1993;242:329-336.

50. Kageyama T, Kabuto M, Nitta H, et al: A population study on risk factors for insomnia among adult Japanese women: A possible effect of road traffic volume. Sleep 1997;20:963-971.

51. Shirlow MJ, Mathers CD: A study of caffeine consumption and symptoms: Indigestion, palpitations, tremor, headache and insomnia. Int J Epidemiol 1985;14:239-248.

52. Wetter DW, Young TB: The relation between cigarette smoking and sleep disturbance. Prev Med 1994;23:328-334.

53. Pallesen S, Nordhus IH, Nielsen GH, et al: Prevalence of insomnia in the adult Norwegian population. Sleep 2001;24:771-779.

54. McCarren M, Goldberg J, Ramakrishnan V, et al: Vietnam era veteran twins: Influence of genes and combat experience. Sleep 1994;17:456-461.

55. Yves E, Morin C, Cervena K, et al: Family studies in insomnia. Sleep 2003;26:A304.

56. The Gallup Organization: Sleep in America. Princeton, NJ, Gallup Organization, 1995.

57. Bonnet MH, Arand DL: 24-Hour metabolic rate in insomniacs and matched normal sleepers. Sleep 1995;18:581-588.

58. Morin CM, Gramling SE: Sleep patterns and aging: Comparison of older adults with and without insomnia complaints. Psychol Aging 1989;4:290-294.

59. Edinger JD, Fins AI, Glenn DM, et al: Insomnia and the eye of the beholder: Are there clinical markers of objective sleep disturbances among adults with and without insomnia complaints? J Consult Clin Psychol 2000;68:586-593.

60. Zammit GK, Weiner J, Damato N, et al: Quality of life in people with insomnia. Sleep 1999;22:S379-385.

61. Katz DA, McHorney CA: The relationship between insomnia and health-related quality of life in patients with chronic illness. J Fam Pract 2002;51:229-235.

62. Leger D, Guilleminault C, Bader G, et al: Medical and socio-professional impact of insomnia. Sleep 2002;25:625-629.

63. Ohayon MM, Zulley J: Correlates of global sleep dissatisfaction in the German population. Sleep 2001;24:780-787.

64. Ford DE, Kamerow DB: Epidemiologic study of sleep disturbances and psychiatric disorders: An opportunity for prevention? JAMA 1989;262:1479-1484.

65. Weissman MM, Greenwald S, Nino-Murcia G, et al: The morbidity of insomnia uncomplicated by psychiatric disorders. Gen Hosp Psychiatry 1997;19:245-250.

66. Breslau N, Roth T, Rosenthal L, et al: Sleep disturbance and psychiatric disorders: A longitudinal epidemiological study of young adults. Biol Psychiatry 1996;39:411-418.

67. Chang PP, Ford DE, Mead LA, et al: Insomnia in young men and subsequent depression. The Johns Hopkins Precursors Study. Am J Epidemiol 1997;146:105-114.

68. Mendelson WB, Garnett D, Gillin JC, et al: The experience of insomnia and daytime and nighttime functioning. Psychiatry Res 1984;12:235-250.

69. Cricco M, Simonsick EM, Foley DJ: The impact of insomnia on cognitive functioning in older adults. J Am Geriatr Soc 2001; 49:1185-1189.

70. Pollak CP, Perlick D, Linsner JP, et al: Sleep problems in the community elderly as predictors of death and nursing home placement. J Community Health 1990;15:123-135.

71. Kripke DF, Garfinkel L, Wingard DL, et al: Mortality associated with sleep duration and insomnia. Arch Gen Psychiatry 2002;59:131-136.

72. Morgan K, Clarke D: Longitudinal trends in late-life insomnia: Implications for prescribing. Age Ageing 1997;26:179-184.

73. Althuis MD, Fredman L, Langenberg PW, et al: The relationship between insomnia and mortality among community-dwelling older women. J Am Geriatr Soc 1998;46:1270-1273.

74. Rumble R, Morgan K: Hypnotics, sleep, and mortality in elderly people. J Am Geriatr Soc 1992;40:787-791.

75. Simon GE, VonKorff M: Prevalence, burden, and treatment of insomnia in primary care. Am J Psychiatry 1997;154:1417-1423.

76. Stoller MK: Economic effects of insomnia. Clin Ther 1994;16: 873-897.

77. Walsh JK, Engelhardt CL: The direct economic costs of insomnia in the United States for 1995. Sleep 1999;22:S386-S393.

78. Leger D, Levy E, Paillard M: The direct costs of insomnia in France. Sleep 1999;22:S394-S401.

79. Chevalier H, Los F, Boichut D, et al: Evaluation of severe insomnia in the general population: Results of a European multinational survey. J Psychopharmacol 1999;13:S21-S24.

80. McCrae CS, Lichstein KL: Secondary insomnia: A heuristic model and behavioral approaches to assessment, treatment, and prevention. Appl Prev Psychol 2001;10:107-123.

81. Sateia MJ, Doghramji K, Hauri PJ, et al: Evaluation of chronic insomnia. Sleep 2000;23:243-308.

82. Ohayon MM, Roth T: Place of chronic insomnia in the course of depressive and anxiety disorders. J Psychiatr Res 2003;37:9-15.

83. Harvey AG: Insomnia: Symptom or diagnosis? Clin Psychol Rev 2001;21:1037-1059.

84. Sateia MJ: Epidemiology, consequences, and evaluation of insomnia. In Lee-Chiong TL, Sateia MJ, Carskadon MA (eds): Sleep Medicine. Philadelphia, Hanley and Belfus, 2002, pp 151-160.

85. Spielman AJ, Anderson MW: The clinical interview and treatment planning as a guide to understanding the nature of insomnia. The CCNY Insomnia Interview. In Chokroverty S (ed): Sleep

86. Disorders Medicine: Basic Science, Technical Con and Clinical Aspects, 2nd ed. Boston, Butterworth-He 1999, pp 385-426.

86. Spielman AJ, Glovinsky PB: The diagnostic interview and ferential diagnosis for complaints of insomnia. In Pressman M Orr WC (eds): Understanding Sleep: The Evaluation and Treatment of Sleep Disorders. Washington, DC, American Psychological Association Press, 1997, pp 125-160.

87. Spielman AJ, Yang C, Glovinsky PB: Assessment techniques for insomnia. In Kryger MH, Roth T, Dement WC (eds): Principles and Practice of Sleep Medicine, 3rd ed. Philadelphia, WB Saunders, 2000, pp 1239-1250.

88. Savard J, Morin C: Insomnia. In Antony MM, Barlow DH (eds): Handbook of Assessment and Treatment Planning for Psychological Disorders. New York, Guilford, 2002, pp 523-555.

89. Schramm E, Hohagen F, Grasshoff U, et al: Test-retest reliability and validity of the Structured Interview for Sleep Disorders according to the DSM-III-R. Am J Psychiatry 1993;150: 867-872.

90. Beck AT, Rush AJ, Shaw BF, et al: Cognitive therapy of depression. New York, Guilford, 1979.

91. Spielberger CD: Manual for the state-trait anxiety inventory. Palo Alto, Calif, Consulting Psychologists Press, 1983.

92. McNair DM, Lorr M, Droppleman LF: EDITS manual for the Profile of Mood States. San Diego, Calif, EDITS, 1971.

93. Derogatis LR, Melisatoros N: The Brief Symptom Inventory: An introductory report. Psychol Med 1983;13:595-605.

94. Butcher JN, Dahlstrom WG, Graham JR, et al: Minnesota Multiphasic Personality Inventory-2 (MMPI-2): Manual for administration and scoring. Minneapolis, Minn, University of Minnesota Press, 1989.

95. Espie CA: Assessment and differential diagnosis. In Lichstein KL, Morin CM (eds): Treatment of Late-Life Insomnia. Thousand Oaks, Calif, Sage, 2000.

96. Lacks P, Morin CM: Recent advances in the assessment and treatment of insomnia. J Consult Clin Psychol 1992;60: 586-594.

97. Edinger JD, Means MK, Stechuchak KM, Olsen MK: A pilot study of inexpensive sleep assessment devices. Behav Sleep Med 2004;2:41-49.

98. Chesson A Jr, Hartse K, Anderson WM, et al: Practice parameters for the evaluation of chronic insomnia: An American Academy of Sleep Medicine report. Standards of Practice Committee of the American Academy of Sleep Medicine. Sleep 2000;23:237-241.

99. Standards of Practice Committee of the American Academy of Sleep Medicine: Practice parameters for the role of actigraphy in the study of sleep and circadian rhythms: An update for 2002. Sleep 2003;26:337-341.

100. Ancoli-Israel S, Cole R, Alessi C, et al: The role of actigraphy in the study of sleep and circadian rhythms. Sleep 2003;26: 342-392.

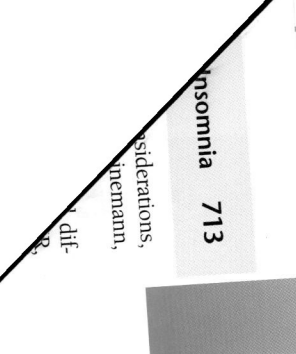

d Pathophysiology of Insomnia

ABSTRACT

Insomnia is perhaps the only sleep disorder where there has been a substantial amount of top-down theorization. This may be the case because a framework is required to comprehend a disorder that has multiple causes and an insidious and progressive course. In this chapter, four general models of the etiology and pathophysiology of insomnia are summarized and critically evaluated. In particular, we review how each model characterizes the hyperarousal that is thought to be responsible for disturbing sleep continuity. Additional information is provided on how sleep homeostasis and circadian considerations may mediate, moderate, or interact with the hyperarousal.

Insomnia is often considered a disorder of hyperarousal; that is, the patient has a level of arousal that is incompatible with the initiation or maintenance of sleep. The concept of hyperarousal is, however, likely to be quite complex. What is meant by arousal? How does it become elevated? Is hyperarousal a tonic phenomenon, and if not, what factors mediate or moderate its occurrence or intensity? Is arousal a singular construct, and are hyperarousal and sleep necessarily mutually exclusive?

In this chapter, we review physiologic, cognitive, behavioral, and neurocognitive models of insomnia. Each of these will be summarized as it pertains to primary insomnia and sleep state misperception insomnia (paradoxical insomnia). These models may also be relevant to the extrinsic or secondary insomnias, which, when chronic, have a great deal in common with primary insomnia.[1,2] In addition to reviewing the four models, we also summarize how sleep homeostasis and circadian considerations mediate, moderate, or interact with hyperarousal. Finally, we review a recent hypothesis that suggests that hyperarousal may be better conceptualized as a failure of wakefulness inhibition.

PHYSIOLOGIC MODEL OF INSOMNIA

The physiologic model suggests that chronic insomnia may be understood as a condition in which the patient has a trait level of arousal, or a level of arousal prior to or during the preferred sleep period, that is incompatible with good sleep continuity. This model assumes that physiologic arousal and sleep are mutually exclusive. Studies evaluating physiologic arousal in insomnia have used a variety of techniques, including basic psychophysiologic measures, whole-body metabolic rate, heart rate variability, caffeine-induced insomnia, neuroendocrine measures, and functional neuroimaging. The studies in the next section support the general concept of physiologic

hyperarousal but have yet to be integrated into a formal model that explains how insomnia develops and how arousal effects promote sleeplessness (Fig. 60–1).

Psychophysiolgic Measures of Arousal

Early studies comparing elevated physiologic arousal between poor sleepers and good sleepers were based on electrophysiologic measures of heart rate, respiration rate, skin and core body temperature, muscle tone, skin conductance and resistance, and peripheral blood flow or vasoconstriction.[3-8] Overall, these studies showed that poor sleepers exhibit increased physiologic arousal, and in the case of ECG measures of heart rate, this arousal was particularly evident at sleep onset.

Several methodologic difficulties limit the interpretation of these studies. First, subjects in these investigations would not necessarily meet current definitions for primary insomnia, and the inclusion of subjects with other types of insomnia (e.g., sleep phase delay disorder or insomnia secondary to major depression) could have influenced the findings. Second, it is not clear whether these studies carefully excluded short episodes of sleep prior to consolidated sleep onset or short awakenings after sleep onset. The failure to do so could account for some of the sleep onset and nocturnal findings regarding hyperarousal.

Third, most of the early studies did not distinguish between state and trait hyperarousal. This distinction is important in order to determine whether physiologic hyperarousal is a 24-hour phenomenon or whether it occurs only at night, only during the sleep period, or only in association with sleep-related stimuli. Of the early studies that provided data regarding this last issue, the results varied based on the measures and protocols adopted.[6,7] When examining body temperature, Adam and colleagues found persistent effects across the day.

PHYSIOLOGIC MODEL

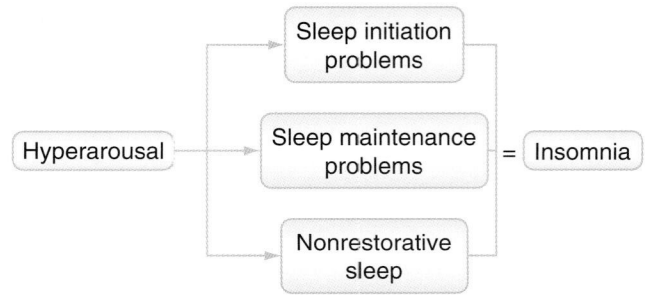

Figure 60–1. The physiologic model.

When examining heart-rate data, neither Stepanski nor Adam found evidence of hyperarousal outside the sleep period.

In addition to time-of-day effects, it is also possible that hyperarousal may vary in response to situational factors such as stress. Challenge paradigms have also provided mixed results. In one study, there was no evidence that acute stress prior to sleep onset increased physiologic arousal or sleep latency in insomnia subjects.[8] In a second study, patients with insomnia did not exhibit hyperarousal in the morning hours, but they were found to be more physiologically reactive than good sleepers.[7]

Whole Body Metabolic Rate

More recently, Bonnet and Arand undertook two studies to assess arousal using a measure of oxygen consumption ($\dot{V}O_2$), an index of whole-body metabolic rate, in patients with insomnia. In both studies, data were collected during the day and during sleep. In the first study, patients with primary insomnia exhibited significantly higher metabolic rate than good-sleeper controls across the 24-hour day and during the sleep interval.[9] In the second study, patients with sleep state misperception insomnia (paradoxical insomnia) also had higher $\dot{V}O_2$ compared to good-sleeper controls across the 24-hour day.[10] The increased metabolic activity during the night was not significantly correlated with the degree of sleep state misperception.

A major strength of these studies, in addition to sampling across 24-hour periods, is that the data were not confounded by state interactions (i.e., data from wake intervals included only wakefulness and data from sleep included only sleep). A limitation of these studies is that the $\dot{V}O_2$ measure is strongly influenced by the physical fitness of the individual and by caloric intake, so it is possible that the observed 24-hour effects could have been related to reduced physical fitness of patients with primary insomnia. The negative results of the correlational analyses in the patients with sleep state misperception insomnia are somewhat puzzling and suggest that the subjective-objective discrepancies in these patients are not simply related to physiologic hyperarousal.

Heart Rate Variability

Heart-rate variability is regulated by sympathetic and parasympathetic nervous system activity and therefore provides another measure of arousal in insomnia. In particular, sympathetic activity is reflected in low-frequency heart-rate variability. To date, this measure has been applied in only one published investigation of primary insomnia. In a 36-hour study, heart period was decreased (i.e., heart rate was increased) and heart-rate variability was decreased in all stages of sleep in patients with insomnia compared with good sleepers.[11] Specifically, spectral analysis of the R-R interval revealed significantly increased low-frequency power (reflecting sympathetic activity) and decreased high-frequency power (reflecting parasympathetic activity) in the insomnia patients across all stages of sleep.

Caffeine-Induced Hyperarousal and Insomnia

Increased endogenous sympathetic nervous system activity may be mimicked by the effects of caffeine, making caffeine administration a potentially useful model for hyperarousal in insomnia. In one study,[12] 400 mg caffeine was provided to good-sleeper subjects three times daily for 7 days. Caffeine administration increased whole body metabolic rate, reduced total sleep time and sleep efficiency, and increased sleep latency, wake after sleep onset, and multiple sleep latency test (MSLT) values. Subjects did not complain of daytime fatigue. By the end of the experimental week the metabolic and sleep continuity effects were reduced. Thus, caffeine-induced hyperarousal appears to be an adequate model of acute insomnia but not necessarily of chronic insomnia. In addition, it is not clear whether the magnitude and specific characteristics of caffeine-induced arousal or the behavioral, mood, and neuropsychological consequences are similar to those seen in primary insomnia.

Neuroendocrine Measures of Physiologic Arousal

Activation of the hypothalamic-pituitary-adrenal (HPA) axis may provide further evidence that insomnia involves, or results from, chronic activation of the stress response system. Other neuroendocrine measures, including norepinephrine and melatonin, have also been examined as potential correlates of insomnia.

Urinary Measures

An early study of urinary free 11-hydroxycorticosteriods in young adult good and poor sleepers found that the mean 24-hour rate of 11-hydroxycorticosteroid excretion over three days was significantly higher in the poor sleepers.[13] A subsequent study of urinary cortisol and epinephrine in middle-aged good and poor sleepers found no significant differences, although poor sleepers showed a trend toward higher urinary cortisol and epinephrine.[6] More recently, Vgontzas et al.[14,15] collected 24-hour urine specimens for urinary free cortisol, catecholamines (DHPG [dihydroxyphenylglycol] and DOPAC [3,4-dihydroxyphenylacetic acid]), and growth hormone and correlated these measures with polysomnographic (PSG) measures of sleep continuity and sleep architecture in subjects with primary insomnia. Urinary free cortisol levels were positively correlated with total wake time, and DHPG and DOPAC measures were positively correlated with stage 1 sleep percentage and wake after sleep-onset time. Although not statistically significant, norepinephrine levels tended to correlate positively with stage 1 percentage and wake after sleep onset, and they tended to correlate negatively with slow wave sleep percentage. These data suggest that HPA axis and sympathetic nervous system activity is associated with objective sleep disturbance.

Plasma Measures

Plasma measures of adrenocorticotropic hormone (ACTH) and cortisol have also been compared among patients with primary insomnia and matched good sleepers. In one study, patients with insomnia had significantly higher mean levels of ACTH and cortisol over the course of the 24-hour day, with the largest group differences observed in the evening and first half of the night.[14,15] Patients with a high degree of sleep disturbance (sleep efficiency <70%) secreted higher amounts of cortisol than patients with less sleep disturbance. In contrast to these findings, a recent study of patients with primary insomnia and age- and gender-matched good sleepers found no differences in the mean amplitude or area under the curve for cortisol secretion over a 16-hour period (7 PM to 9 AM).[16]

Like the psychophysiologic studies reviewed earlier, some of the neuroendocrine findings in insomnia could be explained by intrusion of wakefulness into the measured sleep period. This is a particular concern for studies using urinary measures, which integrate biologic activity over long periods of time. This possibility is important when considering causes of insomnia: whether increased HPA activity leads to insomnia, or whether insomnia leads to increased HPA activity.

Although findings from various studies are not entirely consistent, the elevations in ACTH and cortisol prior to and during sleep in insomnia patients may help to shed light on the intimate association between insomnia and major depression, which is also associated with activation of the HPA axis. Specifically, insomnia is a risk factor for,[17-25] a prodromal symptom of,[26] and a ubiquitous[27,28] and persistent symptom of major depression.[28] The common link may be that acute stress leads to both an activation of the HPA axis and insomnia, and that chronic insomnia in turn leads to a persistent activation of the HPA axis.

Functional Imaging and CNS Arousal

Functional neuroimaging methods such as single photon emission computed tomography (SPECT) and positron emission tomography (PET) may be used to identify regional brain blood flow or metabolic activity associated with particular tasks or states. Functional imaging techniques have been used to identify regional brain metabolic changes associated with sleep and sleep stages, and these techniques have recently been applied to the study of insomnia. To date, two studies have been undertaken, one using ^{99m}Tc-HMPAO SPECT and one using fluoro-deoxyglucose PET.

In the SPECT study, imaging was conducted around the sleep-onset interval of patients with primary insomnia and of good-sleeper controls. Contrary to expectation, patients with insomnia exhibited a consistent pattern of hypoperfusion across eight preselected regions of interest, with the most prominent effect observed in the basal ganglia.[29] The medial frontal, occipital, and parietal cortices also showed significant decreases in blood flow compared to those of good sleepers.

In the PET study, imaging data were acquired from patients with chronic insomnia and from control subjects for an interval during wakefulness and during consolidated non–rapid eye movement (NREM) sleep. Patients with insomnia exhibited increased global cerebral glucose metabolism during wakefulness and NREM sleep.[30] In addition, patients with insomnia exhibited smaller declines in relative glucose metabolism from wakefulness to sleep in wake-promoting regions including ascending reticular activating system, hypothalamus, and thalamus. A smaller decrease was also observed in areas associated with cognition and emotion, including the amygdala, hippocampus, and insular cortex as well as in the anterior cingulate and medial prefrontal cortices.

Although results from these studies appear to be inconsistent, numerous methodologic differences may help to explain differences in the findings. For instance, the SPECT study, with its short time resolution, may have captured a more transient phenomenon that occurs when subjects with chronic and severe insomnia first achieve persistent sleep. The PET study, with its longer time resolution, may have captured a more stable phenomenon that occurs throughout NREM sleep in subjects with moderate insomnia. In addition to the temporal resolution issues, the PET study used a sample of insomnia patients who did not show objective sleep-continuity disturbances in the laboratory, whereas the SPECT study included patients with objective sleep continuity disturbances. Thus, the samples may have differed with respect to the type of insomnia, the degree of partial sleep deprivation, and the degree of sleep-state misperception. Although further studies are needed, these preliminary investigations clearly demonstrate the feasibility of using functional neuroimaging methods in the study of insomnia, and they suggest that insomnia complaints may indeed have a basis in altered brain activity.

COGNITIVE MODELS OF INSOMNIA

Like the physiologic model of insomnia, the cognitive model suggests that insomnia occurs in association with arousal and that arousal and sleep are mutually exclusive. Unlike the physiologic perspective, the central tenet of these models is that cognitive arousal in the form of rumination and worry predisposes the individual to insomnia, precipitates acute episodes, and perpetuates the chronic form of the disorder. The "three-factor" framework (predisposing, precipitating, and perpetuating factors), although not an explicit part of any of the cognitive models, is applied here for its heuristic value (Fig. 60–2).

Worry and Rumination

Predisposing Factor

The tendency to ruminate and worry serves as a predisposing factor for insomnia in at least one of two ways. First, individuals given to rumination or worry are more likely to be reactive to life stressors. Second, individuals with high trait levels of cognitive arousal may require less activation to reach the level of arousal that is incompatible with sleep. Put differently, individuals prone to worry and rumination are more likely to react to life events, and less of a reaction is required to trigger a level of arousal that is incompatible with sleep.

Support for this position is found in patients with chronic insomnia who exhibit higher scores on instruments measuring personality factors related to trait worry.[31-33] These data are consistent with the possibility that worry and rumination are predisposing factors for insomnia. Only longitudinal studies, however, will be able to determine whether stable premorbid traits for worry and rumination actually predispose the individual to insomnia, or whether these features appear as a state-related characteristic during bouts of insomnia.

Precipitating Factor

Worry and rumination may also act as precipitating factors for insomnia. In this instance, life stress (acting alone or in combination with premorbid personality factors) triggers both physiologic and cognitive activation. The former presumably serves as the biologic basis for the "fight or flight" response that inhibits sleep. The latter is also thought to result in sleep-continuity disturbance but via a more subtle process.

COGNITIVE MODEL (GENERAL)

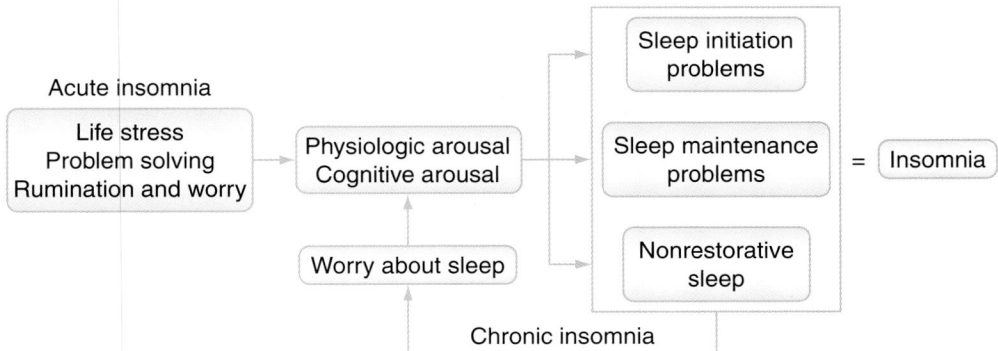

Figure 60–2. The cognitive model (general). Whether physiologic arousal and cognitive arousal independently contribute, or interact, to produce sleep continuity disturbance is often not well delineated within the cognitive perspective. This schematic allows for both types of arousal but does not distinguish between the two constructs.

Life stress presumably initiates an increase in problem solving. During the day, such a response is adaptive. During the night, such a response may be adaptive but has the consequence of sleeplessness. The effects of sleepiness, sleep loss, and sleep inertia on cognitive function may in turn increase the probability that effective problem solving will give way at night to rumination and worry, setting the stage for persistent cognitive activation and chronic insomnia.[1]

Empirical data support the role of life stress as a precipitating factor for insomnia. Patients with chronic insomnia report that life stress events often precede and precipitate their insomnia,[34,35] and epidemiologic studies show that job stress is related to sleep disturbance.[36] Insomnia patients also attribute their insomnia to cognitive activation more often than somatic arousal.[37-39] Finally, good sleepers in experimental stress paradigms show increased worry and sleep disruption.[7,40,41] Such data prospectively support the links among stress, cognitive activation, and sleep disturbance.

Perpetuating Factors

Worry and rumination may serve as perpetuating factors for insomnia. When insomnia becomes chronic, worry and rumination may acquire a different focus; that is, a person worries about the inability to sleep and the consequences of sleep loss. This shift in content may be one of the most important etiologic factors for chronic insomnia, setting up a self-perpetuating cycle wherein insomnia fuels worry and worry fuels the insomnia.[42] Although there are no longitudinal studies to demonstrate that patients actually shift the content of their worry in the transition from acute to chronic insomnia, empirical data do support the hypothesis that worry in chronic insomnia is often "worry about sleep." For instance, studies that sample thought content around sleep onset in chronic insomnia patients[38,43] and studies that differentiate between good and poor sleepers' presleep cognitions[44] show that the worry content of insomnia patients is indeed focused on sleep-related issues including worry about not falling or staying asleep and concerns about the next day's performance or the catastrophic consequences of extended sleep loss.

Individual attitudes and beliefs about sleep may also moderate the propensity for worry.[45,46] For example, if the individual believes that 8 hours of sleep are necessary for optimal daytime function, then when faced with the prospect of getting less than 8 hours of sleep, the individual is more prone to worry. In fact, patients with insomnia endorse more dysfunctional attitudes about sleep, and they believe them more strongly than subjects without insomnia.[46] Treatment outcomes for these patients are related to reductions in negative attitudes and beliefs about sleep.[45,47]

Reconceptualization of the Cognitive Model

Harvey has proposed that the self-perpetuating nature of insomnia may not be related solely to the persistent occurrence, and the shift in the content focus, of rumination and worry. Instead, she has hypothesized that worry about sleep may engage cognitive processes and behavior that mediate the occurrence and severity of chronic insomnia.[48] According to this model, acute insomnia occurs in association with life stress, subchronic insomnia occurs with worry about sleep, and chronic insomnia is maintained by selective attention and monitoring, distorted perceptions of daytime deficits, and counterproductive safety behaviors (Fig. 60–3).

Selective Attention

Some patients selectively monitor the environment for sleep-related threats, including both the internal environment (e.g., monitoring mental alertness or body sensations) and the external environment (e.g., monitoring the bedroom clock or the environment for noise). This selective attention is not conscious but automatic, and it increases the chance of perceiving random environmental events as sleep threats. Increased detection of relevant and random cues, in turn, increases both cognitive and physiologic arousal and reinforces monitoring behavior. Thus, a self-perpetuating cycle is established.

Distorted Perception of Daytime Deficits

Some people with insomnia exhibit increased attention or sensitivity to the consequences of poor sleep. They may worry that they have not obtained sufficient sleep, which causes them to selectively attend to daytime problems such as fatigue, sleepiness, and performance deficits. As with monitoring for sleep-related threats, monitoring for daytime deficits also increases the chance of detecting both occasional relevant cues and random cues. Unlike the monitoring that occurs at night, the detection of fatigue, sleepiness, and performance deficits prompts the patient to engage in safety behaviors. Examples of safety behavior include avoiding work and social

COGNITIVE MODEL (HARVEY MODEL)

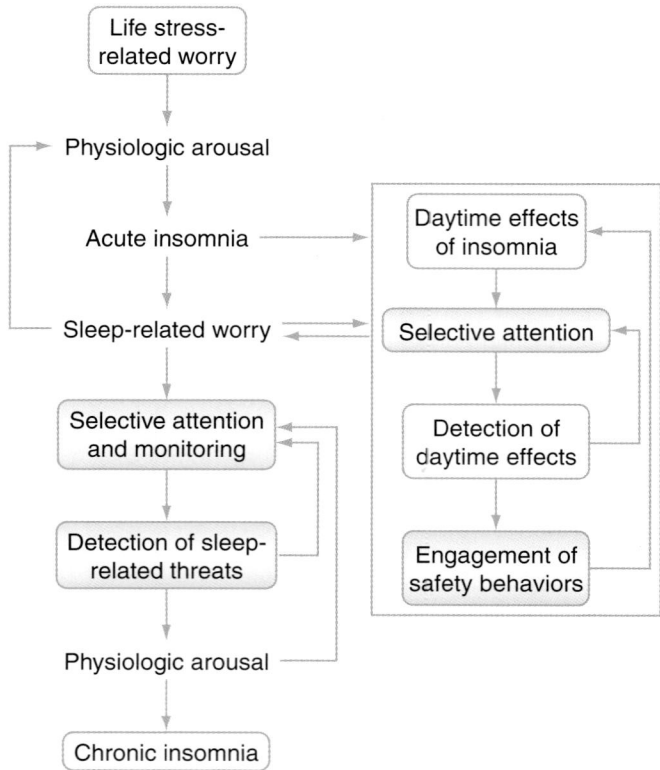

Figure 60–3. The cognitive model (Harvey model). The regions shaded in *light blue* represent the unique contribution of the Harvey model to the cognitive perspective.

tasks perceived to be too physically or mentally taxing. Such avoidance is thought to reinforce worry and cognitive arousal.

Consistent with this reconceptualization of the cognitive model of insomnia, patients with insomnia do indeed appear to excessively monitor their sleep environment, selectively attend to sleep-related stimuli,[49,50] and engage in daytime safety behaviors.[51] Whether the cognitive and behavioral factors delineated by this perspective represent the primary perpetuating factors for insomnia remains to be demonstrated.

BEHAVIORAL MODELS OF INSOMNIA

In general, the behavioral perspective suggests that although a variety of biopsychosocial factors may precipitate acute insomnia, chronic insomnia results from behaviors that disrupt sleep. A number of specific behavioral models have been proposed, most of which are closely tied to specific treatment techniques.

Sleep Hygiene Model

Sleep hygiene refers to the notion that specific kinds of behavior are conducive to or incompatible with sleep and that modifying behavior may alleviate insomnia. The earliest systematic reference to sleep hygiene can be found in Kleitman's *Sleep and Wakefulness*,[52] which includes a chapter entitled, "The Hygiene of Sleep and Wakefulness." Kleitman reviews evidence

regarding factors such as sleep duration, bedtime rituals, sleep surface, ambient temperature, sleep satiety, and body position. The chapter is discursive and in no way resembles the list of do's and don'ts of good sleep that exist today as sleep hygiene instructions. As for the validity of this perspective, poor sleep hygiene apparently is neither necessary nor sufficient for the occurrence of insomnia. Patients with primary insomnia do not necessarily engage in more poor sleep hygiene practices than good sleepers,[53] and monotherapy with sleep hygiene instructions does not reliably produce significant benefit.[54,55]

Stimulus Control Model

Stimulus control, as originally described by Bootzin and colleagues,[56] is based on the behavioral principle that one stimulus may elicit a variety of responses, depending on the conditioning history. A simple conditioning history, wherein a stimulus is always paired with a single kind of behavior, yields a high probability that the stimulus will yield only one response. A complex conditioning history, wherein a stimulus is paired with a variety of reactions, yields a low probability that the stimulus will yield only one response.

In persons with insomnia, the normal cues associated with sleep (e.g., bed, bedroom, bedtime) are often paired with activities other than sleep. For instance, in an effort to cope with insomnia, the patient may spend a large amount of time in the bed and bedroom doing something other than sleeping. Insomnia-related coping strategies appear to the patient to be both reasonable (staying in bed at least permits the patients to get "rest") and reasonably successful (engaging in alternative activities in the bedroom sometimes appears to end the insomnia). These practices, however, set the stage for stimulus dyscontrol, the lowered probability that sleep-related stimuli will elicit the desired response of sleepiness and sleep.

Stimulus control therapy for insomnia is one of the most widely used behavioral treatments, and its efficacy has been demonstrated consistently.[57-59] The therapy, however, includes active components that are not based solely on learning or behavioral theory. For instance, the treatment specifies that the patient should spend awake time somewhere other than the bed, and that the sleep schedule should be fixed. These two interventions also influence the homeostatic and circadian regulation of sleep. Thus, the efficacy of stimulus control therapy does not necessarily provide strong evidence for the stimulus control model. In fact, one investigation found that the reverse of stimulus control instructions also improved sleep continuity.[60]

The Spielman Model

Spielman's model,[61] alternatively referred to as the three-factor model or the three-P model, is a stress-diathesis model that has an additional behavioral component to account for how acute insomnia becomes chronic. A schematic representation of this model is presented in Figure 60–4.

In brief, this model posits that insomnia occurs acutely in relation to both traits (predisposing factors) and life stresses (precipitating factors) and that the chronic form of the disorder is maintained by maladaptive coping strategies (perpetuating factors). Thus, a person may be prone to insomnia due to trait characteristics, may experience acute episodes because

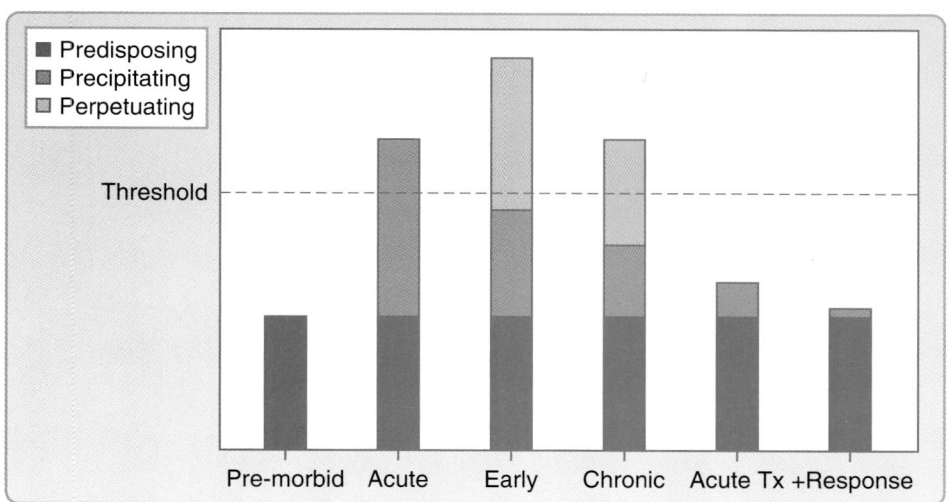

Figure 60–4. The traditional Spielman model does not extend to what occurs with treatment. The model is usually represented as ending with the chronic phase. The "Acute Tx" and "+ Response" intervals are included here so that the reader may appreciate the differences between the three-factor and four-factor models. +, positive; Tx, theories.

of precipitating factors, and may suffer from a chronic form of the disorder because of behavioral factors.

Predisposing factors extend across the entire biopsychosocial spectrum. Biologic factors include trait hyperarousal (e.g., elevated metabolic rate, stably elevated levels of cortisol) and hyperreactivity (elevated startle response or diminished capacity to recover following startle, or both). Psychological factors include worry or the tendency to ruminate excessively. Social factors, although rarely a focus at the theoretical level, include a sleep schedule incompatible with the bed partner's or social pressures to sleep according to a nonpreferred sleep schedule (e.g., child rearing).

Precipitating factors, as the name implies, are acute occurrences that interrupt sleep. The primary "triggers" are thought to be related to medical and psychiatric illness and stressful life events.

Perpetuating factors refer to the strategies that the patient adopts to compensate for sleep loss. Research and treatment have focused on two kinds of perpetuating factors: the practice of staying in bed while awake and the tendency to extend sleep opportunity. The stimulus control perspective speaks mainly to the former. The Spielman model focuses primarily on the latter. Extending sleep opportunity refers to the tendency of patients to compensate for sleep loss by going to bed earlier or by getting up later, or both. Such strategies are intended to "recover what has been lost." These strategies, however, lead to mismatch between *sleep opportunity* and *sleep ability*. The greater the mismatch, the greater the chance the person will spend more time awake during the given sleep period.

Perhaps the most compelling evidence for the validity of behavioral models is the success of treatments based on its principles. Multicomponent therapies composed of sleep restriction and stimulus control reliably produce significant pre-post change[57-59] and effects that are comparable to[62] and may be more durable than pharmacotherapy.[63] The central tenets of the stimulus control model and the Spielman model, however, have never been evaluated empirically. Such an evaluation would require an experimental or a prospective study. Obviously, a human experimental model to produce chronic insomnia is

not viable. A prospective study, while possible, has yet to be undertaken. Such a study would require that subjects at risk for acute insomnia be identified and then studied longitudinally in a way that allows for an assessment of which, if any, of the behavioral factors predict the occurrence of chronic insomnia.

Finally, neither the stimulus control model nor the Spielman model addresses the concept of conditioned arousal. Both models focus on the instrumental side of the behavioral equation—in other words, how behavior fuels insomnia. Neither model addresses the possibility that being awake in bed (for long periods of time and on frequent occasions) may directly elicit arousal responses via classical conditioning. Such conditioned arousal may contribute independently to the self-perpetuating nature of insomnia, even when the original maladaptive strategies are no longer operational.

Taking into account conditioned arousal as a possible perpetuating factor can help to explain two reliable findings from the treatment outcome literature. First, cognitive behavior therapy (CBT) for insomnia produces about a 50% reduction in symptoms during the acute treatment phase.[57-59] If only the traditional behavioral factors are responsible for chronic insomnia, a more complete response to treatment might be expected. Second, patients treated with CBT continue to improve over follow-up periods as long as 24 months.[63,64] If only behavioral factors are responsible for chronic insomnia, no additional improvements would be expected beyond the acute treatment phase.

While any number of unaccounted-for factors may be responsible for these clinical phenomena, allowing for the additional behavioral factor of conditioned arousal may help explain why treatment response during therapy is incomplete and why treatment gains appear to occur with time. In the case of the former, acute treatment with CBT may only reduce insomnia severity to the extent that it eliminates the behavioral tendency to extend sleep opportunity, leaving the part of the insomnia ascribable to conditioned arousal in play. In the case of the latter, successful treatment with CBT in the short term may result in counterconditioning in the long term because repeated pairing of sleep-related cues with sleep over

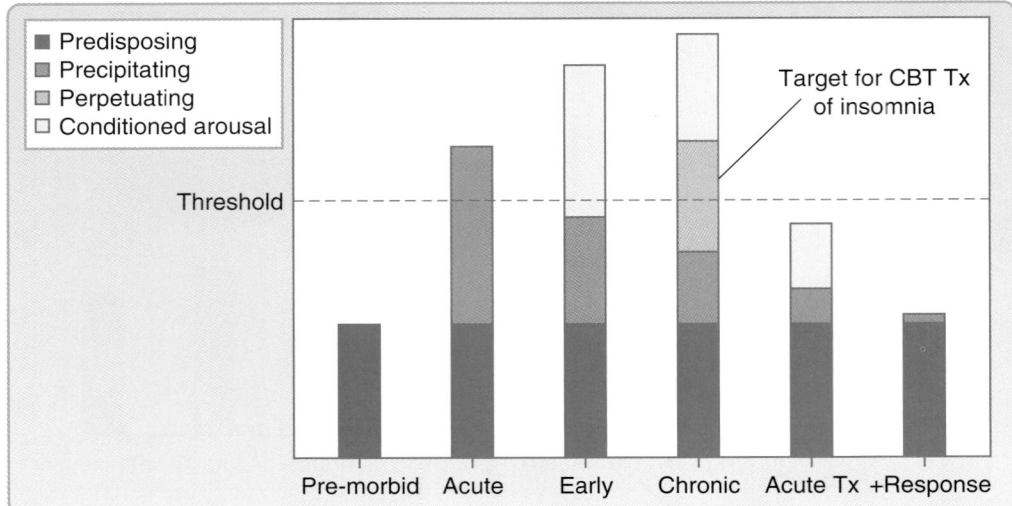

4 FACTOR MODEL

Legend:
- ■ Predisposing
- ■ Precipitating
- ▫ Perpetuating
- ☐ Conditioned arousal

Target for CBT Tx of insomnia

Threshold

Pre-morbid   Acute   Early   Chronic   Acute Tx   +Response

Figure 60–5. The four-factor model. CBT, cognitive behavior therapy; +, positive; Tx, theories.

time extinguishes the conditioned arousal. A version of the Spielman model that includes a conditioned arousal component is shown in Figure 60–5.

NEUROCOGNITIVE MODEL OF INSOMNIA

Central to the neurocognitive model is the view that *acute insomnia* occurs in association with cognitive and behavioral factors and *chronic insomnia* is a reversible central nervous system disorder that occurs in part in relation to behavioral factors and in part as a result of classical conditioning. Accordingly, the neurocognitive perspective[65,66] represents a position counter to the pure cognitive perspective and is an extension of the behavioral model (Fig. 60–6).

As a position contrary to the pure cognitive perspective, the neurocognitive model suggests that rumination and worry may extend wakefulness, but they are not responsible for the inability to initiate or maintain sleep. That is, individuals with chronic insomnia are not awake because they are worrying, but rather they are worrying because they are awake. As an extension of the behavioral model, the neurocognitive perspective acknowledges the role of behavioral factors and attempts both to define arousal and to specify precisely how arousal may interfere with sleep initiation, sleep maintenance, or the perception of sleep.

The neurocognitive model considers arousal along three intersecting dimensions (somatic, cognitive, and cortical) and focuses on the measurement and the consequences of conditioned cortical arousal. Cortical arousal, it is argued, occurs as a result of classical conditioning and may be observed in patients with primary insomnia as high-frequency EEG activity (14 Hz to 45 Hz) at or around sleep onset and during NREM sleep.[65,66] Cortical arousal, it is hypothesized, allows for abnormal levels of sensory and information processing and for the increased formation of long-term memory. These phenomena, in turn, are directly linked to sleep continuity disturbance and sleep state misperception.

Specifically, enhanced sensory processing around sleep onset and during NREM sleep is thought to make the patient particularly vulnerable to perturbation by environmental stimuli, which interferes with sleep. *Enhanced information processing during NREM sleep* may blur the phenomenological distinction between sleep and wakefulness. That is, one cue for "knowing" that one is asleep is the lack of awareness of events occurring during sleep. Enhanced information processing may therefore account for the tendency in insomnia to judge polysomnographically defined sleep as wakefulness.[67-73] Finally, *enhanced long-term memory* around sleep onset and during NREM sleep may interfere with the subjective experience of sleep initiation and duration. Normally, subjects cannot recall information from periods immediately prior to sleep,[74-77] during sleep,[78-80] or during brief arousals from sleep.[81,82] An enhanced ability to encode and retrieve information in insomnia would be expected to influence judgments about sleep latency, wakefulness after sleep onset, and sleep duration.

Several components of the neurocognitive model have been empirically evaluated. First, patients with primary insomnia exhibit more NREM high-frequency EEG activity than either good sleepers[83-89] or patients with insomnia secondary to major depression.[88] Second, patients with sleep state misperception disorder exhibit more beta EEG activity than good sleepers or patients with primary insomnia.[89] Third, correlational analyses provide evidence that beta activity is negatively associated with the perception of sleep quality[90,91] and is positively associated with the degree of subjective-objective discrepancy.[88] Taken together, these three lines of evidence suggest that CNS arousal may occur uniquely in association with primary insomnia (versus secondary insomnia) and suggests that this form of arousal is associated with the tendency toward misperception of sleep state.

In addition to these findings, there is also evidence that increased high-frequency activity appears to be limited to the beta and gamma portions of the EEG spectrum and that patients with chronic insomnia, as compared with good sleepers, have heightened recognition recall in the morning for words presented at sleep onset and from awakenings during the night.[92] The former suggests that the primary source potential for the signal is electroencephalographic, not

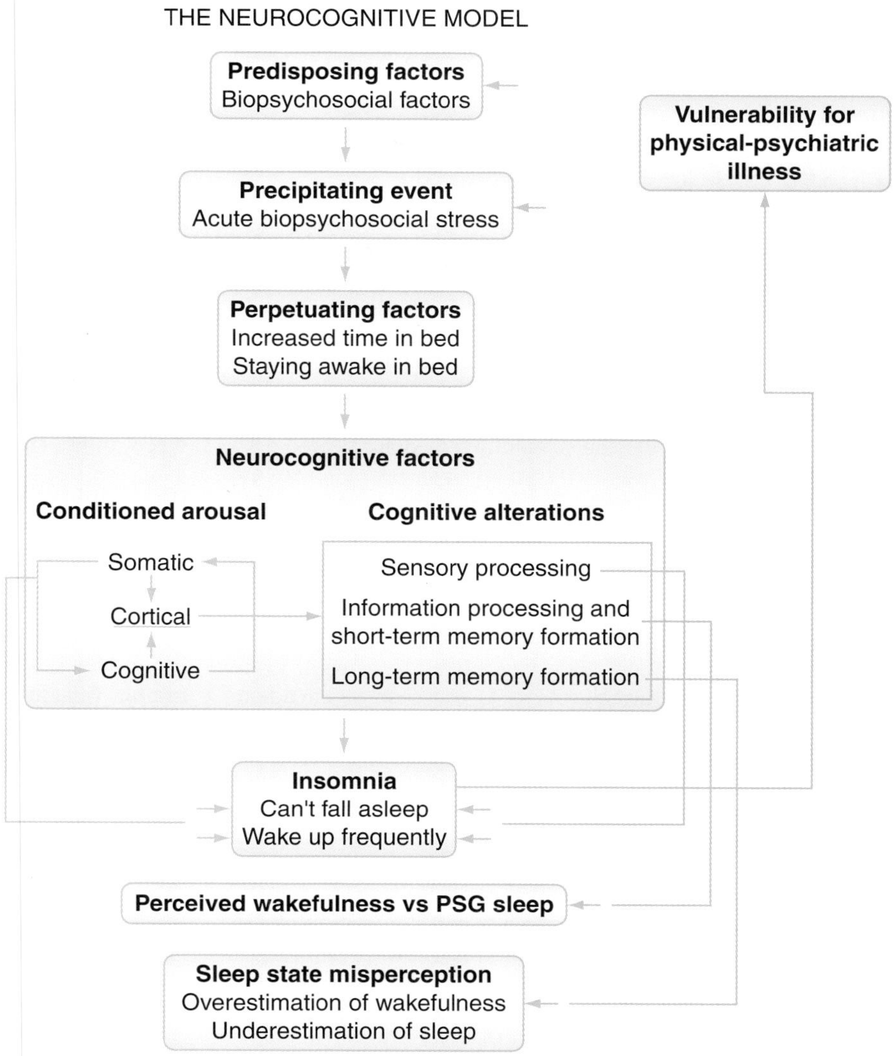

THE NEUROCOGNITIVE MODEL

Figure 60–6. This version of the neurocognitive model is slightly different from the schematic representations previously published. The primary differences are that this model explicitly incorporates the three-factor model; long-term memory formation is explicitly linked to the phenomenon of sleep-state misperception; and sleep-state misperception itself is allowed to be related to either the overestimation of wakefulness or the underestimation of sleep, or both.

electromyographic, and that therefore cortical and somatic arousal may be distinct phenomena. The latter provides support for the hypothesis that there is an attenuation in the normal mesograde amnesia that accompanies sleep in patients with primary insomnia.

The major strength of the neurocognitive model is that it provides for an integrated perspective on primary insomnia, allowing for behavior, neuropsychological function, and neurobiologic considerations to be taken into account as contributing to the etiology and pathogenesis of insomnia. The primary limitations of the model are that it does not account for the importance of homeostatic and circadian influences on sleep or for the likely possibility that cortical arousal may constitute a permissive factor for worry, rumination, and monitoring behavior.

FACTORS THAT MAY MEDIATE, MODERATE, OR INTERACT WITH HYPERAROUSAL

All of the models so far discussed provide good frameworks for understanding the nature of the hyperarousal that produces poor sleep continuity. None of the models, however, address factors that may mediate, moderate, or interact with hyperarousal. Such factors may explain heterogeneity among insomnia patients. For instance, some factors must account for how hyperarousal results in initial insomnia in some individuals, middle insomnia in others, and late insomnia in still others. Moreover, some factors must account for how these forms of insomnia occur variably within the individual. The two most likely factors are related to sleep homeostasis and the circadian control of sleep and wakefulness.

Sleep Homeostasis and Physiologic Arousal

Although a number of investigators have suggested that impaired sleep homeostasis may be an important etiologic factor in insomnia,[29,93-95] few empirical studies have addressed this factor. Only one investigation supports the possibility that patients with primary insomnia exhibit reduced slow wave sleep,[96] although decreased delta activity has been observed in insomnia secondary to major depression[27,97-99] and chronic pain.[100]

Impaired sleep homeostasis in patients with insomnia would also be supported by evidence of reduced levels of sleepiness following sleep deprivation in comparison with healthy subjects. Stepanski and colleagues[101] demonstrated that patients with primary insomnia and good sleepers had similar responses to sleep deprivation on the MSLT, suggesting that the sleep homeostat may be functioning normally, at least with respect to generating daytime sleepiness.

Finally, impaired sleep homeostasis in insomnia would be supported by smaller increases in total sleep time or in amount of slow wave sleep following sleep deprivation in comparison with healthy subjects. Two experimental studies have shown that compared to healthy control subjects, insomnia patients had similar increases in total sleep time during recovery from sleep deprivation, but they had smaller increases in slow wave sleep percentage or delta power.[95,101] These results, as well as the efficacy of sleep restriction treatments for insomnia, suggest that homeostatic dysregulation may be an important feature of primary insomnia.

Circadian Dysrhythmia and Physiologic Arousal

Sleep initiation and maintenance problems may result from circadian rhythm abnormalities, as is the case in circadian rhythm sleep disorders. It is less clear whether circadian rhythm factors may also contribute to the occurrence or severity of primary insomnia. Normal developmental phase shifts and acute phase shifts occurring as a part of jet lag or shift work may act as precipitating factors for acute episodes of insomnia and set the stage for the development of a chronic form of the disorder, as suggested in the Spielman model.

The more substantive question is whether chronobiologic factors contribute to chronic insomnia. Lack and colleagues[102,103] found that primary insomnia patients exhibit phase shifts that are consistent with their presenting complaint: Patients with sleep-onset insomnia exhibit a phase delay of the core body temperature rhythm,[102] and patients with early-morning awakening exhibit a phase advance of the core body temperature rhythm.[104,105] In addition to, and consistent with, these data are the studies that suggest that elderly patients with insomnia exhibit attenuated melatonin levels.[106] Taken together, these observations suggest that, at least for some patients with chronic insomnia, hyperarousal may not be a constant phenomenon but may have a specific temporal patterning that reflects the influence of circadian factors.

While it seems likely that circadian factors play a role in the etiology and pathogenesis of primary insomnia, it is perplexing that phase shifts have not been observed in the numerous studies of physiologic arousal using such measures as core body temperature and cortisol. One possible explanation is that most studies include samples of patients with either sleep-onset insomnia, sleep-maintenance insomnia, or mixed symptoms, rather than with one symptom profile alone. Combining subjects with different insomnia phases would obscure circadian phase shifts among individuals. That is, if patients with initial insomnia are phase delayed and patients with late insomnia are phase advanced, averaging across the two samples could yield a 24-hour oscillation that appears relatively normal. Failure to control for the masking influences of posture, activity, and light could also obscure circadian abnormalities in studies of insomnia. Protocols such as the 90-minute-day and constant routine could help to address potential circadian abnormalities in primary insomnia.

Finally, behavioral factors are likely to interact with normal circadian functioning to produce circadian abnormalities that in turn perpetuate and exacerbate primary insomnia. Individuals with acute insomnia caused by factors other than circadian ones may alter the way they are exposed to light, and this may have phase-shifting effects. For example, when people compensate for sleep loss by "sleeping in" or napping, they reduce their exposure to light during the diurnal phase. One or both of these compensatory strategies may cause a phase delay that reinforces the initial and middle insomnia problems. In this way, individuals with chronic insomnia could have observable circadian dysfunction without an inherent defect in the circadian system.

INHIBITION OF WAKEFULNESS VERSUS HYPERAROUSAL

The majority of insomnia models conceptualize insomnia as a disorder of hyperarousal. Espie,[107,108] however, has proposed an important alternative point of view, suggesting that insomnia occurs, at least initially, in association with the failure to inhibit wakefulness. This psychobiologic inhibition model suggests that in the early stages of chronic insomnia, problems with sleep initiation or sleep maintenance may occur because of dysfunction in the neurobiologic mechanisms that normally inhibit wakefulness and permit sleep to occur.

The failure to inhibit wakefulness is thought to result from two cognitive phenomena. First, when people are unable to sleep, their attention is drawn to an otherwise automatic process. The very process of attending, in turn, prevents perceptual and behavioral disengagement and sleep initiation. Second, when people are unable to sleep, effort is expended "trying" to fall asleep, and this effort, like enhanced attention, serves only to extend wakefulness. This increased attention and intention result in sustained wakefulness, which undermines what is normally an automatic process and sets the stage for additional cognitive and behavioral changes as discussed earlier.

Additional findings from other areas of research suggest the utility of the psychobiologic inhibition model. Merica and colleagues propose that cortical arousal may occur in insomnia patients as a failure to downregulate normal levels of cerebral activity before and during NREM sleep. Cortical arousal may indicate that the "wake off" system is not functioning properly,[66,109] the result being an intermediate state in which the dominant mode is consistent with sleep, but with neuronal groups related to the wake state still active.

Saper and colleagues[110] have proposed a similar idea that may be more closely related to the occurrence of PSG wakefulness. These investigators propose that homeostatic and circadian regulatory systems are regulated by a "flip flop circuit" in the ventrolateral preoptic area of the hypothalamus. The wake-promoting and sleep-promoting halves of the circuit each strongly inhibit the other, creating a bi-stable feedback loop that reinforces wakefulness and sleep and prevents intermediate states. The failure to inhibit wakefulness in insomnia could be related to a defect in the "sleep switch," favoring the occurrence of wakefulness relative to sleep both at the beginning and during the middle of the sleep period.

Distinguishing between hyperarousal and the failure to inhibit wakefulness may allow for better definitions of insomnia, greater precision in the search for the neurobiologic basis of insomnia, and better understanding of treatment mechanisms. The distinction between these two constructs, however, requires further clarification.

CONCLUSION

While each model of insomnia provides us with a deeper appreciation for the fact that insomnia is a complex and multiply determined disorder, it is unlikely that any one of these models is entirely correct or that all are equally correct. In the final analysis, if there ever is a unified theory of insomnia, it will likely be the case that physiologic, cognitive, and cortical arousal each play a role in the etiology of insomnia and that these factors are mediated or moderated by homeostatic and circadian considerations.

Clinical Pearls

The factors responsible for acute and chronic insomnia are different, and acute insomnia does not necessarily result in the chronic form of the disorder. This suggests that early detection and treatment may have substantial prophylactic value.

Hyperarousal is not likely to be a single factor, but rather a construct comprised of several factors including the somatic, cognitive, and cortical domains. In addition, homeostatic and circadian influences probably moderate and/or mediate the extent to which somatic, cognitive, and cortical arousal produce insomnia symptoms. Taking into account these concepts may help the clinician tailor treatment to the individual.

REFERENCES

1. Perlis M, Jungquist C, Smith MT, Posner D: The Cognitive Behavioral Treatment of Insomnia: A Treatment Manual. Contract pending 2003.
2. McCrae CS, Lichstein KL: Secondary insomnia: Diagnostic challenges and intervention opportunities. Sleep Med Rev 2001; 5:47-61.
3. Monroe LJ: Psychological and physiological differences between good and poor sleepers. J Abnorm Psychol 1967;72:255-264.
4. Haynes SN, Follingstad DR, McGowan WT: Insomnia: Sleep patterns and anxiety level. J Psychosom Res 1974;18:69-74.
5. Freedman RR, Sattler HL: Physiological and psychological factors in sleep-onset insomnia. J Abnorm Psychol 1982;91: 380-389.
6. Adam K, Tomeny M, Oswald I: Physiological and psychological differences between good and poor sleepers. J Psychiatr Res 1986; 20:301-316.
7. Stepanski E, Glinn M, Zorick F, et al: Heart rate changes in chronic insomnia. Stress Med 1994;10:261-266.
8. Haynes SN, Adams A, Franzen M: The effects of pre-sleep stress on sleep-onset insomnia. J Abnorm Psychol 1981;90:601-606.
9. Bonnet MH, Arand DL: 24-Hour metabolic rate in insomniacs and matched normal sleepers. Sleep 1995;18:531-588.
10. Bonnet MH, Arand DL: Physiological activation in patients with sleep state misperception. Psychosom Med 1997;59:533-540.
11. Bonnet MH, Arand DL: Heart rate variability in insomniacs and matched normal sleepers. Psychosom Med 1998;60:610-615.
12. Bonnet MH, Arand DL: Caffeine use as a model of acute and chronic insomnia. Sleep 1992;15:526-536.
13. Johns MW: Relationship between sleep habits, adrenocortical activity and personality. Psychosom Med 1971;33:499-508.
14. Vgontzas AN, Tsigos C, Bixler EO, et al: Chronic insomnia and activity of the stress system: A preliminary study. J Psychosom Res 1998;45:21-31.
15. Vgontzas AN, Bixler EO, Lin HM, et al: Chronic insomnia is associated with nyctohemeral activation of the hypothalamic-pituitary-adrenal axis: Clinical implications. J Clin Endocrinol Metab 2001;86:3787-3794.
16. Riemann D, Klein T, Rodenbeck A, et al: Nocturnal cortisol and melatonin secretion in primary insomnia. Psychiatry Res 2002; 113:17-27.
17. Ford DE, Kamerow DB: Epidemiologic study of sleep disturbances and psychiatric disorders. An opportunity for prevention? [see comments]. JAMA 1989;262:1479-1484.
18. Dryman A, Eaton WW: Affective symptoms associated with the onset of major depression in the community: Findings from the US National Institute of Mental Health Epidemiologic Catchment Area Program. Acta Psychiatr Scand 1991;84:1-5.
19. Breslau N, Roth T, Rosenthal L, Andreski P: Sleep disturbance and psychiatric disorders: A longitudinal epidemiological study of young adults. Biol Psychiatry 1996;39:411-418.
20. Chang PP, Ford DE, Mead LA, et al: Insomnia in young men and subsequent depression. The Johns Hopkins Precursors Study. Am J Epidemiol 1997;146:105-114.
21. Livingston G, Blizard B, Mann A: Does sleep disturbance predict depression in elderly people? A study in inner London [see comments]. Br J Gen Pract 1993;43:445-448.
22. Mallon L, Broman JE, Hetta J: Relationship between insomnia, depression, and mortality: A 12-year follow-up of older adults in the community. Int Psychogeriatr 2000;12:295-306.
23. Roberts RE, Shema SJ, Kaplan GA, Strawbridge WJ: Sleep complaints and depression in an aging cohort: A prospective perspective. Am J Psychiatry 2000;157:81-88.
24. Vollrath M, Wicki W, Angst J: The Zurich study. VIII. Insomnia: Association with depression, anxiety, somatic syndromes, and course of insomnia. Eur Arch Psychiatry Neurol Sci 1989;239: 113-124.
25. Weissman MM, Greenwald S, Nino-Murcia G, Dement WC: The morbidity of insomnia uncomplicated by psychiatric disorders. Gen Hosp Psychiatry 1997;19:245-250.
26. Perlis ML, Giles DE, Buysse DJ, et al: Self-reported sleep disturbance as a prodromal symptom in recurrent depression. J Affect Disord 1997;42:209-212.
27. Perlis ML, Giles DE, Buysse DJ, et al: Which depressive symptoms are related to which sleep electroencephalographic variables? Biol Psychiatry 1997;42:904-913.
28. Thase ME: Antidepressant treatment of the depressed patient with insomnia. J Clin Psychiatry 1999;60(Suppl):28-31.
29. Smith MT, Perlis ML, Chengazi VU, et al: Neuroimaging of NREM sleep in primary insomnia: A Tc-99-HMPAO single photon emission computed tomography study. Sleep 2002;25:325-335.
30. Nofzinger EA, Buysse DJ, et al: Functional imaging evidence for hyperarousal in insomnia. Am J Psychiatry 2004;161:2126-2131.
31. Dorsey CM, Bootzin RR: Subjective and psychophysiologic insomnia: An examination of sleep tendency and personality. Biol Psychiatry 1997;41:209-216.
32. Kales A, Caldwell A, Preston T: Personality patterns in insomnia. Arch Gen Psychiatry 1976;33:1128-1134.
33. Kales A, Caldwell AB, Soldatos CR, et al: Biopsychobehavioral correlates of insomnia. II. Pattern specificity and consistency with the Minnesota Multiphasic Personality Inventory. Psychosom Med 1983;45:341-356.
34. Morgan K, Healey DW, Healey PJ: Factors influencing persistent subjective insomnia in old age: A follow-up study of good and poor sleepers aged 65 to 74. Age Ageing 1989;18:117-122.

35. Bastien C, Vallieres A, Morin C: Precipitating factor of insomnia. Behav Sleep Med 2004;2:50-62.

36. Nakata A, Haratani T, Takahashi M, et al: Job stress, social support at work, and insomnia in Japanese shift workers. J Hum Ergol (Tokyo) 2001;30:203-209.

37. Lichstein K, Rosenthal T: Insomniacs' perceptions of cognitive versus somatic determinants of sleep disturbance. J Abnorm Psychol 1980;89:105-107.

38. Harvey AG: Pre-sleep cognitive activity: A comparison of sleep-onset insomniacs and good sleepers. Brit J Clin Psychol 2000;39:275-286.

39. Nicassio P, Mendlowicz M, Fussell J, Petras L: The phenomenology of the pre-sleep state: the development of the pre-sleep arousal scale. Behav Res Ther 1985;23:263-271.

40. Gross R, Borkovec T: Effects of cognitive intrusion manipulation on the sleep-onset latency of good sleepers. Behav Ther 1982; 13:112-116.

41. Hall M, Buysse DJ, Reynolds CF, et al: Stress-related intrusive thoughts disrupt sleep onset and continuity. Sleep Res 1996; 25:163.

42. Morin CM. Insomnia: Psychological Assessment and Management. New York, Guilford Press, 1993.

43. Kuisk LA, Bertelson AD, Walsh JK: Presleep cognitive hyper-arousal and affect as factors in objective and subjective insomnia. Percept Mot Skills 1989;69:1219-1225.

44. Smith MT, Perlis ML, Smith MS, Giles DE: Pre-sleep cognitions in patients with insomnia secondary to chronic pain. J Behav Med 2001;24:93-114.

45. Morin CM, Blais F, Savard J: Are changes in beliefs and attitudes about sleep related to sleep improvements in the treatment of insomnia? Behav Res Ther 2002;40:741-752.

46. Morin CM, Stone J, Trinkle D, et al: Dysfunctional beliefs and attitudes about sleep among older adults with and without insomnia complaints. Psychol Aging 1993;8:463-467.

47. Edinger JD: Does cognitive-behavioral insomnia therapy alter dysfunctional beliefs about sleep? Sleep 2001;24:599.

48. Harvey AG: A cognitive model of insomnia. Behav Res Ther 2002;40:869-893.

49. Semler CN, Harvey AG: Monitoring of sleep-related threat: A pilot study of the sleep associated monitoring index (SAMI). Psychosom Med 2004;66:242-250.

50. Neitzert-Semler C, Harvey AG: Monitoring of sleep-related threat in primary insomnia: Development and validation of the sleep associated monitoring inventory (SAMI). Psychosom Med 2004;66:242-250.

51. Harvey AG: Identifying safety behaviors in insomnia. J Nerv Ment Dis 2002;190:16-21.

52. Kleitman N: Sleep and Wakefulness. Chicago, University of Chicago Press, 1987.

53. Harvey AG: Sleep hygiene and sleep-onset insomnia. J Nerv Ment Dis 2000;188:53-55.

54. Chesson AL Jr, Anderson WM, Littner M, et al: Practice parameters for the nonpharmacologic treatment of chronic insomnia. An American Academy of Sleep Medicine report. Standards of Practice Committee of the American Academy of Sleep Medicine. Sleep 1999;22:1128-1133.

55. Stepanski EJ, Wyatt JK: Use of sleep hygiene in the treatment of insomnia. Sleep Med Rev 2003;7:215-225.

56. Bootzin RR: Stimulus control treatment for insomnia. Programs and abstracts of the 80th Annual Convention of the American Psychological Association; September 2, 1972; Honolulu, Hawaii.

57. Morin CM, Culbert JP, Schwartz SM: Nonpharmacological interventions for insomnia: A meta-analysis of treatment efficacy. Am J Psychiatry 1994;151:1172-1180.

58. Murtagh DR, Greenwood KM: Identifying effective psychological treatments for insomnia: A meta-analysis. J Consult Clin Psychol 1995;63:79-89.

59. Smith MT, Perlis ML, Park A, et al: Comparative meta-analysis of pharmacotherapy and behavior therapy for persistent insomnia. Am J Psychiatry 2002;159:5-11.

60. Davies R, Lacks P, Storandt M, Bertelson AD: Countercontrol treatment of sleep-maintenance insomnia in relation to age. Psychol Aging 1986;1:233-238.

61. Spielman A, Caruso L, Glovinsky P: A behavioral perspective on insomnia treatment. Psychiatr Clin North Am 1987;10:541-553.

62. Smith MT, Perlis ML, Park A, et al: Comparative meta-analysis of pharmacotherapy and behavior therapy for persistent insomnia. Am J Psychiatry 2002;159:5-11.

63. Morin CM, Colecchi C, Stone J, et al: Behavioral and pharmacological therapies for late-life insomnia: A randomized controlled trial [see comments]. JAMA 1999;281:991-999.

64. Edinger JD, Wohlgemuth WK, Radtke RA, et al: Cognitive behavioral therapy for treatment of chronic primary insomnia: A randomized controlled trial. JAMA 2001;285:1856-1864.

65. Perlis ML, Giles DE, Mendelson WB, et al: Psychophysiological insomnia: The behavioural model and a neurocognitive perspective. J Sleep Res 1997;6:179-188.

66. Perlis ML, Merica H, Smith MT, Giles DE: Beta EEG in insomnia. Sleep Med Rev 2001;5:365-376.

67. Borkovec T, Lane T, van Oot P: Phenomenology of sleep among insomniacs and good sleepers: Wakefulness experience when cortically asleep. J Abnorm Psychol 1981;90:607-609.

68. Coates T, Killen J, Silberman S, et al: Cognitive activity, sleep disturbance, and stage specific differences between recorded and reported sleep. Psychophysiology 1983;20:243.

69. Coates TJ, Killen J, George J, et al: Estimating sleep parameters: A multitrait-multimethod analysis. J Consult Clin Psychol 1982;50:345-352.

70. Mendelson W, James S, Garnett D, et al: A psychophysiological study of insomnia. Psychiatry Res 1986;19:267-284.

71. Mendelson W, Martin J, Stephens H, et al: Effects of flurazapam on sleep, arousal threshold, and perception of being asleep. Psychopharmacology (Berlin) 1988;95:258-262.

72. Engle-Friedman M, Baker E, Bootzin R: Reports of wakefulness during EEG identified stages of sleep. Sleep Res 1985;14:152.

73. Mercer JD, Bootzin RR, Lack LC: Insomniacs' perception of wake instead of sleep. Sleep 2002;25:564-571.

74. Wyatt JK, Allen JJBA, Bootzin RR, Anthony JL: Mesograde amnesia during the sleep onset transition: Replication and electrophysiological correlates. Sleep 1997;20:512-522.

75. Wyatt J, Bootzin R, Anthony J, Bazant S: Sleep onset is associated with retrograde and anterograde amnesia. Sleep 1994;17:502-511.

76. Guilleminault C, Dement W: Amnesia and disorders of excessive daytime sleepiness. In Drucker-Colin R, McGaugh J (eds): Neurobiology of Sleep and Memory. New York, Academic Press, 1977, pp 439-456.

77. Portnoff G, Baekeland F, Goodenough DR, et al: Retention of verbal materials perceived immediately prior to onset of non-REM sleep. Percept Mot Skills 1966;22:751-758.

78. Wood J, Bootzin R, Kihlstrom J, Schachter D: Implicit and explicit memory for verbal information presented during sleep. Psychol Sci 1992;3:236-239.

79. Bootzin R, Fleming G, Perlis M, et al: Short and long term memory for stimuli presented during sleep. Sleep Res 1991;20:258.

80. Koukkou M. Lehmann D: EEG and memory storage experiments with humans. Electroencephalogr Clin Neurophysiol 1968;25:455-462.

81. Goodenough D, Sapan J, Cohen H: Some experiments concerning the effects of sleep on memory. Psychophysiology 1971;8:749-762.

82. Bonnet M: Memory for events occurring during arousal from sleep. Psychophysiology 1983;20:81-87.

83. Freedman R: EEG power in sleep onset insomnia. Electroencephalogr Clin Neurophysiol 1986;63:408-413.

84. Merica H, Gaillard JM: The EEG of the sleep onset period in insomnia: A discriminant analysis. Physiol Behav 1992;52:199-204.

85. Merica H, Blois R, Gaillard JM: Spectral characteristics of sleep EEG in chronic insomnia. Eur J Neurosci 1998;10:1826-1834.

86. Lamarche CH, Ogilvie RD: Electrophysiological changes during the sleep onset period of psychophysiological insomniacs, psychiatric insomniacs, and normal sleepers. Sleep 1997;20:724-733.

87. Jacobs GD, Benson H, Friedman R: Home-based central nervous system assessment of a multifactor behavioral intervention for chronic sleep-onset insomnia. Behav Ther 1993;24:159-174.

88. Perlis ML, Smith MT, Orff HJ, et al: Beta/gamma EEG activity in patients with primary and secondary insomnia and good sleeper controls. Sleep 2001;24:110-117.

89. Krystal AD, Edinger JD, Wohlgemuth WK, Marsh GR: NREM sleep EEG frequency spectral correlates of sleep complaints in primary insomnia subtypes. Sleep 2002;25:630-640.

90. Hall M, Buysse DJ, Nowell PD, et al: Symptoms of stress and depression as correlates of sleep in primary insomnia. Psychosom Med 2000;62:227-230.

91. Nofzinger EA, Price JC, Meltzer CC, et al: Towards a neurobiology of dysfunctional arousal in depression: The relationship between beta EEG power and regional cerebral glucose metabolism during NREM sleep. Psychiatry Res 2000;98:71-91.

92. Perlis ML, Smith MT, Orff HJ, et al: The mesograde amnesia of sleep may be attenuated in subjects with primary insomnia. Physiol Behav 2001;74:71-76.

93. Stepanski EJ: Behavioral therapy for insomnia. In Kryger MH, Roth TG, Dement WC (eds): Principles and Practice of Sleep Medicine. Philadelphia, WB Saunders, 2000, pp 647-656.

94. Bonnet MH, Arand DL: Hyperarousal and insomnia. Sleep Med Rev 1997;1:97-108.

95. Besset A, Villemin E, Tafti M, Billiard M: Homeostatic process and sleep spindles in patients with sleep-maintenance insomnia: Effect of partial sleep deprivation. Electroencephalogr Clin Neurophysiol 1998;107:122-132.

96. Schneider-Helmert D: Insomnia and alpha sleep in chronic non-organic pain as compared to primary insomnia. Neuropsychobiology 2001;43:54-58.

97. Benca R: Mood disorders. In Kryger M, Roth T, Dement W (eds): Principles and Practice of Sleep Medicine. Philadelphia, WB Saunders, 1994, pp 899-913.

98. Benca RM, Obermeyer WH, Thisted RA, Gillin JC: Sleep and psychiatric disorders: A meta-analysis. Arch Gen Psychiatry 1992;49:651-668.

99. Kupfer DJ, Frank E, McEachran A, Grochocinski V: Delta sleep ratio: A biological correlate of early recurrence in unipolar affective disorder. Arch Gen Psychiatry 1989;47:1100-1105.

100. Harding SM: Sleep in fibromyalgia patients: Subjective and objective findings. Am J Med Sci 1998;315:367-376.

101. Stepanski E, Zorick F, Roehrs T, Roth T: Effects of sleep deprivation on daytime sleepiness in primary insomnia. Sleep 2000;23:215-219.

102. Morris M, Lack L, Dawson D: Sleep-onset insomniacs have delayed temperature rhythms. Sleep 1990;13:1-14.

103. Lack LC, Bootzin RR: Circadian rhythm factors in insomnia and their treatment. In Perlis ML, Lichstein KL (eds): Treating Sleep Disorders: Principles and Practice of Behavioral Sleep Medicine. Hoboken, NJ: John Wiley and Sons, 2003, pp 305-343.

104. Lack L, Wright H: The effect of evening bright light in delaying the circadian rhythms and lengthening the sleep of early morning awakening insomniacs. Sleep 1993;16:436-443.

105. Lack LC, Mercer JD, Wright H: Circadian rhythms of early morning awakening insomniacs. J Sleep Res 1996;5:211-219.

106. Riemann D, Klein T, Rodenbeck A, et al: Nocturnal cortisol and melatonin secretion in primary insomnia. Psychiatry Res 2002;113:17-27.

107. Leger D, Laudon M, Zisapel N: Nocturnal 6-sulfatoxymelatonin excretion in insomnia and its relation to the response to melatonin replacement therapy. Am J Med 2004;116:91-95.

108. Espie CA: Insomnia: Conceptual issues in the development, persistence, and treatment of sleep disorder in adults. Annu Rev Psychol 2002;53:215-243.

109. Merica H, Fortune RD: A neuronal transition probability model for the evolution of power in the sigma and delta frequency bands of sleep EEG. Physiol Behav 1997;62:585-589.

110. Saper CB, Chou TC, Scammell TE: The sleep switch: Hypothalamic control of sleep and wakefulness. Trends in Neurosciences 2001;24:726-731.

Psychological and Behavioral Treatments for Primary Insomnia

Charles M. Morin

ABSTRACT

Insomnia is a prevalent and costly health problem associated with a significant burden for the individual and society. Insomnia can be triggered by a variety of precipitating events, but when it becomes a persistent problem, psychological and behavioral factors are almost always involved in perpetuating or exacerbating sleep disturbances over time. Effective management of persistent insomnia must address these factors, which may involve poor sleep habits, irregular sleep–wake schedules, hyperarousal, and faulty beliefs and attitudes about sleep. Psychological and behavioral therapies for primary insomnia include sleep restriction, stimulus control therapy, relaxation training, cognitive strategies, and a combination of those methods, referred to as cognitive behavior therapy. Evidence from controlled clinical trials indicates that 70% to 80% of patients with primary insomnia benefit from treatment. Although only 20% to 30% of patients become "good sleepers" (i.e., symptom free), the majority of them achieve significant symptom reductions on sleep onset latency and on wake after sleep onset, with the absolute values of those parameters returning to below or near the 30-minute cutoff criterion typically used to define insomnia. Total sleep time is increased by a modest 30 to 45 minutes, but treatment increases sleep satisfaction and reduces psychological symptoms and hypnotic usage. Sleep improvements are well maintained up to 2 years after treatment completion. Treatment outcomes have been documented primarily with prospective sleep diaries, and some recent studies have also validated those outcomes with polysomnography and actigraphy. Despite evidence showing psychological and behavioral approaches to be efficacious and acceptable, such therapies are not readily available and are infrequently used by health care practitioners. An important challenge that remains is to disseminate more effectively those evidence-based therapies and increase their availability to patients and clinicians. Preliminary evidence suggests that the use of trained nurse clinicians, self-help materials, brief consultation models, and the Internet are cost-effective ways to enhance treatment access and facilitate its implementation in clinical practice.

SIGNIFICANCE OF INSOMNIA

Insomnia is among the most common health complaints in medical practice and the most prevalent of all sleep disorders in the general population. Epidemiologic estimates indicate that 6% of the adult population presents with an insomnia disorder, 12% report insomnia symptoms with daytime consequences, and an additional 15% are dissatisfied with their sleep.[1] In primary care medicine, about 20% of patients report significant sleep disturbances.[2,3] Persistent insomnia can be an important burden for the individual and for society, as evidenced by reduced quality of life, increased absenteeism and reduced productivity at work, and higher health care costs.[3,4] Persistent insomnia is also associated with increased risks of depression and chronic use of hypnotics and, among older adults with cognitive impairments, it may hasten placement in a nursing home facility.[3,5,6]

Despite its high prevalence and negative impact, insomnia often goes unrecognized and remains untreated, with less than 15% of those with severe insomnia receiving any treatment.[4] Most patients who initiate treatment do so without professional consultation and often resort to a host of alternative remedies (herbal or dietary supplements) of unknown risks and benefits. When insomnia is brought to professional attention, typically to a primary care physician, treatment is often limited to medication. Although hypnotic medications are clinically indicated and useful in selected situations, psychological and behavioral factors are almost always involved in perpetuating sleep disturbances, and these factors should be addressed in the clinical management of insomnia.[7-9] Significant advances have been made in the psychological and behavioral management of insomnia in the past decade, and although these approaches are well accepted by patients, they are not widely available and remain underutilized by health care practitioners.

This chapter addresses the treatment of primary insomnia with psychological and behavioral interventions. The first section describes validated interventions and their rationale, the second summarizes evidence regarding their efficacy and generalizability, and the last section discusses clinical and practical issues related to treatment implementation and feasibility.

PSYCHOLOGICAL AND BEHAVIORAL TREATMENTS

Treatment options for insomnia include basic sleep hygiene education, psychological and behavioral interventions, pharmacotherapy, and a variety of complementary and alternative therapies. The focus of this chapter is on the nonpharmacologic therapies and, more specifically, on psychological and behavioral interventions that have been validated in controlled clinical trials for primary insomnia. These methods include sleep restriction, stimulus control therapy, relaxation-based interventions, cognitive strategies, and combined cognitive and behavioral therapy. A summary of those interventions is provided below and in Table 61–1; more extensive descriptions are available in other sources.[8]

The main objectives of psychological and behavioral approaches are to target those factors (psychological, behavioral,

Table 61–1.   Psychological and Behavioral Treatments for Primary Insomnias

Therapy	Description
Stimulus control therapy	A set of instructions designed to reassociate the bed/bedroom with sleep, and to reestablish a consistent sleep–wake schedule: Go to bed only when sleepy; get out of bed when unable to sleep; use the bed/bedroom for sleep only (e.g., no reading, watching TV); arise at the same time every morning; no napping.
Sleep restriction therapy	A method to curtail time in bed to the actual sleep time, thereby creating mild sleep deprivation, which results in more consolidated and more efficient sleep.
Relaxation training	Clinical procedures aimed at reducing somatic tension (e.g., progressive muscle relaxation, autogenic training) or intrusive thoughts (e.g., imagery training, meditation) interfering with sleep.
Cognitive therapy	Psychotherapeutic method aimed at changing faulty beliefs and attitudes about sleep, insomnia, and the next-day consequences. Other cognitive strategies are used to control intrusive thoughts at bedtime and prevent excessive monitoring of the daytime consequences of insomnia.
Sleep hygiene education	General guidelines about health practices (e.g., diet, exercise, substance use) and environmental factors (e.g., light, noise, temperature) that may promote or interfere with sleep.

cognitive) that perpetuate or exacerbate sleep disturbances. Such features may include poor sleep habits, irregular sleep–wake schedules, misconceptions and excessive worrying about sleep, and hyperarousal. Although numerous factors can precipitate insomnia, when it becomes a persistent problem, psychological and behavioral factors are almost always involved in perpetuating it over time—hence the need to target those factors directly in treatment.[9] Another goal of treatment is to teach patients self-management skills to cope more adaptively with residual sleep disturbances that may persist even after therapy. Treatment does not, however, seek to alter the underlying personality structure of the patient with insomnia. Insight-oriented psychotherapy focusing on such predisposing variables of insomnia may be useful in some patients, but there has been no controlled evaluation of its efficacy specifically for insomnia.

Sleep Restriction

There is a natural tendency among poor sleepers to increase the amount of time spent in bed in an effort to provide more opportunity for sleep, a strategy that is more likely to result in fragmented and poor-quality sleep. Sleep restriction therapy consists of curtailing the amount of time spent in bed to the actual amount of time asleep.[10] Time in bed is subsequently adjusted on the basis of sleep efficiency (SE; ratio of total sleep time per time in bed × 100%) for a given period of time (usually the preceding week). For example, if a person reports sleeping an average of 6 hours per night out of 8 hours spent in bed, the initial prescribed sleep window (i.e., from initial bedtime to final arising time) would be 6 hours. The subsequent allowable time in bed is increased by about 15 to 20 minutes for a given week when SE exceeds 85%, decreased by the same amount of time when SE is lower than 80%, and kept stable when SE falls between 80% and 85%. Adjustments are made periodically (weekly) until optimal sleep duration is achieved. Changes to the prescribed sleep window can be made at the beginning of the night (i.e., postponing bedtime), at the end of the sleep period (i.e., advancing arising time), or at both ends. Variations in implementing this procedure may involve changing the time in bed on the basis of a moving average of the SE (e.g., the past 3 to 5 days), or changing it on a weekly basis regardless of changes in SE.[11] This procedure, or some variation of it, improves sleep continuity through a mild sleep deprivation and a reduction of sleep anticipatory anxiety. To prevent excessive daytime sleepiness, time in bed should not be reduced to less than 5 hours per night. Such precautions are particularly indicated for those whose jobs require operation of motor vehicles or heavy machinery or who have duties in which drowsiness may be a danger to the patient or others.

Stimulus Control Therapy

Stimulus control therapy[12] consists of a set of five instructions designed to reassociate temporal (bedtime) and environmental (bed and bedroom) stimuli with rapid sleep onset and to establish a regular circadian sleep–wake rhythm. The following instructions are given:

- Go to bed only when sleepy—not just fatigued, but sleepy.
- Get out of bed when unable to sleep (e.g., after 20 min), go to another room, and return to bed only when sleep is imminent.
- Curtailing all sleep-incompatible activities (overt and covert); no eating, TV watching, radio listening, planning or problem solving in bed.
- Arise at a regular time every morning regardless of the amount of sleep the night before.
- Avoid daytime napping.

The rationale of stimulus control therapy is that repeated and unsuccessful sleep attempts eventually lead to a negative association between the presleep rituals and the bedroom environment. This conditioning process may take place over several weeks or months, unrecognized by the patient. Over time, the presleep rituals become cues or stimuli for apprehension and arousal rather than for relaxation and sleep. In some cases, formerly benign habits such as watching television or reading in bed may also reduce the stimulus value of the bed and bedroom for sleep and may further exacerbate the sleep problem. This may explain why some individuals with insomnia report improved sleep in novel settings where conditioned environmental cues are absent. In addition, many insomniacs display poor sleep habits that initially emerge as a means of coping with sleep disturbances. For example, poor sleep at night may lead to daytime napping or sleeping late on weekends in an effort to catch up on lost sleep. Such individuals may lie in bed for prolonged periods trying to force sleep, only to find themselves becoming more awake.

Stimulus control is one of the most widely used interventions for insomnia (Table 61–2). It may appear quite simple, but the challenge is to foster strict compliance with all of the instructions for a few weeks. Also, there may be no need to follow some of those instructions (e.g., getting out of bed when unable to sleep) when time in bed is substantially reduced during the initial compression of time spent in bed; however, as time in bed is gradually increased, these procedures become more relevant and must be implemented systematically.

Relaxation-Based Interventions

As stress, tension, and anxiety are frequent contributing factors to sleep disturbances, relaxation is the most commonly used nondrug therapy for insomnia. The goal of this treatment is to reduce arousal at bedtime or on nighttime awakening. Among the different relaxation interventions, some methods (e.g., progressive muscle relaxation, autogenic training) focus primarily on reducing somatic arousal, whereas attention-focusing procedures (e.g., imagery training, meditation, thought stopping) target mental arousal in the form of worries, intrusive thoughts, or a racing mind.[13-16] Biofeedback is designed to train patients to control some physiologic parameters (e.g., frontalis tension, using electromyography) through visual or auditory feedback; despite its popularity in the 1980s, this method is not often used today (see Table 61–2), perhaps because of the equipment necessary to provide feedback to patients.

Although most relaxation procedures are equally effective for treating insomnia, they are not necessarily indicated for all individuals with insomnia. Some people, perhaps the more perfectionist ones, may have a paradoxical response and actually become more anxious when trying to relax. The most critical issue is to ensure diligent and daily practice of the selected method for at least 2 to 4 weeks, and to keep the focus on reducing arousal rather than on inducing sleep. Professional guidance is often necessary in the initial phase of training. Sometimes, it may be necessary to implement a more comprehensive stress management program involving relaxation and other therapeutic components such as time management and problem-solving training.

Cognitive Therapy

Insomnia is often exacerbated by excessive preoccupation with sleep and by apprehensions and monitoring of the next-day consequences, all of which can heighten arousal and interfere with sleep.[17] Cognitive restructuring therapy seeks to alter dysfunctional sleep cognitions (e.g., beliefs, attitudes, expectations, attributions). The basic premise of this approach is that appraisal of a given situation (sleeplessness) can trigger negative emotions (fear, anxiety) that are incompatible with sleep. For example, when a person is unable to sleep at night and begins thinking about the possible consequences of sleep loss on the next day's performance, a spiral reaction is set off that feeds into a vicious cycle of insomnia, emotional distress, and more sleep disturbance. Cognitive therapy is designed to short-circuit the self-fulfilling nature of this vicious cycle. Treatment targets include unrealistic expectations ("I must get

my 8 hours of sleep every night"), faulty causal attributions ("My insomnia is entirely caused by a biochemical imbalance"), and amplification of the consequences of insomnia ("Insomnia may have serious consequences on my health").[17] In addition, patients often perceive themselves as victims of insomnia and as having few resources to cope with sleep difficulties and their daytime consequences. Cognitive therapy is useful to teach patients coping skills to prevent or minimize recurrence of sleep disturbances after treatment.[18,19] The main therapeutic message to communicate to patients is as follows:

- Keep realistic expectations.
- Do not blame insomnia for all daytime impairments.
- Never try to sleep.
- Do not give too much importance to sleep.
- Do not catastrophize after a poor night's sleep.
- Develop some tolerance to the effects of insomnia.

A more didactic cognitive approach can be used to provide basic information about normal sleep, individual differences in sleep needs, and changes in sleep physiology over the course of the life span. This information is useful to help some patients distinguish clinical insomnia from short-sleep or from normal (age-related) sleep disturbances. Such knowledge can prevent excessive worry and concern, which can themselves lead to clinical insomnia. Cognitive therapy has become a fairly standard therapeutic component to most insomnia treatment programs, although its specific contribution to overall outcomes has not yet been evaluated.

In addition to cognitive restructuring therapy, several other cognitive strategies may be useful in treating insomnia.[8] For instance, paradoxical intention is a clinical procedure designed to eliminate performance anxiety. In the context of insomnia, any attempt to control or induce sleep voluntarily is likely to generate performance anxiety and to delay sleep onset. With paradoxical intention, the patient is instructed to remain passively awake and to give up any effort (intention) to fall asleep, the rationale being that good sleepers do not make any effort to fall asleep. Other cognitive control techniques can be helpful to minimize mental activity at bedtime and in the bedroom surroundings. This can be facilitated by simply asking the patients to set aside a time and a place (other than bedtime and the bedroom) to write down thoughts or worries of the day and plans for the next day. Imagery techniques can also be a useful complement to block out such unwanted presleep thoughts.[20]

Sleep Hygiene Education

Sleep hygiene education is intended to provide information about lifestyle (diet, exercise, substance use) and environmental factors (light, noise, temperature) that may either interfere with or promote better sleep.[15,21] It may also include general sleep-facilitating recommendations, such as allowing enough time to relax before bedtime, and information about the benefits of maintaining a regular sleep schedule. The following instructions are guidelines:

- Avoid stimulants (e.g., caffeine, nicotine) for several hours before bedtime.
- Avoid alcohol around bedtime, as it fragments sleep.
- Exercise regularly (especially in late afternoon or early evening).
- Allow at least a 1-hour period to unwind before bedtime.
- Keep the bedroom environment quiet, dark, and comfortable.
- Maintain a regular sleep schedule.

Table 61-2.   Studies of Psychological and Behavioral Treatments for Primary Insomnia

Authors, Reference (Date)	Patients: N % Female Mean Age	Treatment Methods	Treatment: Weeks/Hours; Follow-Up (mo)	Outcomes
Backhaus et al.[13] (2001)*	20 65.0 43.0	CBT and a self-help manual (stimulus control, relaxation, cognitive restructuring)	6/9; 24	Treatment increased TST and SE, and it reduced SOL, negative sleep-related cognitions, and depressive and anxiety symptoms. Treatment effects persisted up to 36-month FU.
Edinger et al.[14] (2001)	75 46.7 55.8	CBT (sleep restriction, stimulus control, cognitive therapy/education) Progressive muscle relaxation Placebo therapy	6/6; 6	CBT produced larger subjective reductions of WASO (54%) than relaxation training (16%) or placebo (12%). PSG changes were smaller but CBT was also more effective. Sleep changes maintained at 6-month FU.
Edinger and Sampson[35] (2003)	20 10 51.0	CBT (abbreviated version) Sleep hygiene information	2/1; 3	Six of 10 patients treated with CBT obtained at least a 50% reduction in WASO, compared with none among the 10 patients in the minimal sleep hygiene group.
Espie et al.[28] (2001)	139 68.3 51.4	CBT (stimulus control, sleep restriction, relaxation, cognitive therapy) Wait-list control	6/5	Significant reductions of SOL (61 to 28 min) and WASO in CBT but not in control group. Significant increase of TST at FU; 84% of patients initially using hypnotics remained drug free.
Guilleminault et al.[32] (1995)	30 56.3 44.0	Stimulus control/sleep hygiene Stimulus control/sleep hygiene/exercise Stimulus control/sleep hygiene/bright light	4/NA; 9-12	All three conditions improved on measures of SOL and TST, but only the bright light condition showed statistically significant changes over time. Outcome corroborated with actigraphy.
Hryshko-Mullen et al.[62] (2000)	42 53.6 52	CBT (sleep hygiene education, stimulus control, stress management, relaxation)	6/NA	Treatment reduced SOL by 52% and WASO by 40% from baseline values, with an increase of 30 min in TST.
Hauri[15] (1997)	26 73.1 47.7	Sleep hygiene/relaxation Sleep hygiene/relaxation/medication Waiting list	6/6; 10	The two treatments were more effective than control after treatment. At FU, subjects treated with the behavioral approach alone had a higher SE (83%) than the combined intervention (79%). Actigraphy used to document outcome.
Jacobs et al.[16] (1996)*	102 61.0 39.3	CBT (sleep restriction, modified stimulus control, relaxation, education, cognitive restructuring, medication withdrawal)	10/14; 6	58% of patients reported significant sleep improvement, 33% moderate, and 9% slight improvement. 91% of hypnotic users eliminated or reduced medication. 90% of patients maintained or enhanced their sleep at FU.
Lichstein et al.[41] (1999)*	40 57.5 52	Medication withdrawal plus relaxation Medication withdrawal alone Wait-list control	2/2; 2	Sleep medication reduced by nearly 80%. Participants who received relaxation therapy obtained additional benefits in sleep efficiency, sleep quality, and reduced withdrawal symptoms.

Continued

Table 61-2. Studies of Psychological and Behavioral Treatments for Primary Insomnia—cont'd

Authors, Reference (Date)	Patients: N, % Female, Mean Age	Treatment Methods	Treatment: Weeks/Hours; Follow-Up (mo)	Outcomes
Lichstein et al.[11] (2001)	74 72.6 68.03	Relaxation Sleep restriction Placebo desensitization	6/5; 12	All three conditions improved subjective but not PSG-defined sleep parameters. Sleep restriction was the most effective treatment.
Mimeault and Morin[42] (1999)	54 59.2 50.8	Self-help CBT manual Self-help CBT manual plus weekly phone consultation Wait-list control	NA/6; 3	The two treatments showed significant changes on SE and TWT, whereas the control did not. The addition of a phone consultation provided a slight advantage during treatment but not at follow-up.
Morin et al.[29] (1994)*	100 64.0 45.1	CBT (stimulus control, sleep restriction, cognitive therapy, education, medication withdrawal)	14/NA; 24	Reported SE improved from 68% to 80% for the total sample. Significant reductions in usage of sleep aids (46% to 28% medicated nights).
Morin et al.[30] (1999)	78 64.0 65.0	CBT (stimulus control, sleep restriction, sleep hygiene, cognitive therapy) Pharmacotherapy Combined CBT plus pharmacotherapy Placebo	8/12; 24	The three active treatments were more effective than placebo after treatment. The combined approach improved sleep more than either of its two single components. CBT participants sustained their clinical gains at FU, whereas those treated with medication alone did not.
Perlis et al.[49] (2000)*	116 57 39.2	CBT (sleep restriction, stimulus control, sleep hygiene, cognitive therapy, relaxation)	4-9/NA	61% of patients completed therapy and reported significant global improvements. Subjects who completed minimal treatment reduced their SOL (65%) and WASO (47%) and increased their TST (13%).
Riedel et al.[60] (1995)	75 65.6 67.4	Education/sleep restriction (video) Education/sleep restriction (video/therapist guidance) Waiting list	Video: 2/30 min Therapist: 2/4; 2	Treatment administered via videotape only yielded reductions in WASO (92 to 63 min), but the addition of therapist guidance enhanced outcome on SOL and WASO (68 to 37 min).
Riedel et al.[55] (1998)*	41 54 56.6	Stimulus control Stimulus control plus medication withdrawal Medication withdrawal Wait-list control	2/2; 2	Stimulus control participants, unlike controls, showed improvements at FU for TST, SE, and sleep quality. Nonmedicated patients showed a more positive response to stimulus control therapy than medicated participants.
Verbeek et al.[37] (1999)*	86 65.1 49.6	CBT (sleep hygiene, relaxation, cognitive therapy, behavioral techniques)	6/5-6; 1	Reductions of subjective SOL and WASO and increase in SE; 19% of patients became good sleepers.

*Use of sleep medication upon entering treatment was permissible.

CBT, cognitive behavior therapy; FU, longest available follow-up; NA, information not available; PSG, polysomnography; SE, sleep efficiency; SOL, sleep onset latency; TST, total sleep time; TWT, total wake time; WASO, wake after sleep onset.

Although inadequate sleep hygiene is rarely the primary cause of insomnia, it may potentiate sleep difficulties caused by other factors, or interfere with treatment progress. Even when patients with insomnia are well informed about the detrimental impact of poor sleep hygiene, they may not maintain good sleep hygiene practices. Thus, it is important to directly address these factors in therapy. On the other hand, although sleep hygiene education may be helpful for mild insomnia, it is rarely sufficient for more severe and chronic forms, which often require more directive and potent behavioral interventions.[22]

Multifaceted Cognitive Behavior Therapy

The different interventions described to this point are not incompatible with each other and can easily be combined. As can be seen from Table 61–2, multicomponent therapy is becoming the standard approach to treating insomnia. This approach typically includes a behavioral (stimulus control, sleep restriction, and, sometimes, relaxation), a cognitive (cognitive restructuring therapy), and an educational component (sleep hygiene), hence the term cognitive behavior therapy (CBT). This multimodal approach is appealing because it addresses different facets of insomnia and is consistent with a multidimensional etiologic model of primary insomnia.[7-9]

Complementary and Alternative Therapies

Several additional alternative and nonpharmacologic therapies have been used in the treatment of primary insomnia. These include acupuncture, hypnosis, and electrosleep therapy. Although potentially useful in practice, those methods have not been evaluated as extensively in controlled studies as the other interventions described.

TREATMENT OUTCOME EVIDENCE

Table 61–2 provides a list of some of the most recent treatment studies evaluating the efficacy of psychological and behavioral treatments for primary insomnia. Only studies published in the last decade (1994-2003) are listed (although the remainder of this text refers to earlier studies as well). For each study in the table, patients' demographics, types of treatment, and outcomes are summarized.

Evidence for Efficacy

Findings from more than 50 clinical trials (more than 2000 patients) conducted in the 1980s and early 1990s and evaluating nonpharmacologic interventions for insomnia have been summarized in at least three meta-analyses[22-24] and in a review/practice parameters paper commissioned by the American Academy of Sleep Medicine.[25] Evidence from these different sources shows that psychological and behavioral treatments produce reliable changes in several sleep parameters (Fig. 61–1), including sleep onset latency (average effect size, 0.88), number of awakenings (0.53 to 0.63), duration of awakenings (0.65), total sleep time (0.42 to 0.49), and sleep quality ratings (0.94). Based on Cohen's criteria, the magnitude of those therapeutic effects is large (i.e., Cohen's effect size $d > 0.8$) for sleep latency and sleep quality, and moderate (i.e., $d > 0.5$) for other sleep parameters. These effect sizes are similar to those obtained for benzodiazepine-receptor agonists,[24,26] with a slight advantage for psychological treatment on measures of sleep onset latency and sleep quality, and for pharmacotherapy on total sleep time. When transformed into a percentile rank, these data indicate that approximately 70% to 80% of patients with insomnia benefit from psychological and behavioral treatments.

In terms of absolute changes, treatment reduces subjective sleep-onset latency from an average of 60 to 65 minutes at baseline to about 35 minutes after treatment. The duration of awakenings is decreased from an average of 70 minutes at baseline to about 38 minutes after treatment. Total sleep time is increased by 30 minutes, from 6 hours to 6.5 hours after treatment, and ratings of sleep quality are enhanced with treatment. Thus, for the average patient with insomnia, treatment effects may be expected to reduce sleep onset latency and wake after sleep onset by an average of about 50% and to bring the absolute values of those sleep parameters below or near the 30-minute cutoff criterion initially used to define sleep-onset or sleep-maintenance insomnia. Treatment effects are similar for sleep-onset and sleep-maintenance problems, although fewer studies have targeted the latter type and

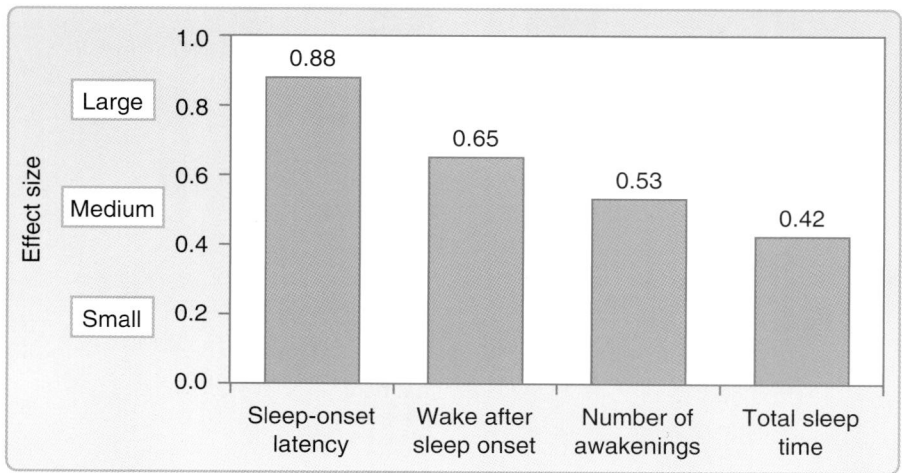

Figure 61–1. Efficacy of psychological and behavioral therapies for insomnia. Mean effect size (reported as a standardized z score) across sleep parameters. These effect sizes are averaged across all nonpharmacologic interventions evaluated in 59 treatment studies (N = 2102). (From Morin CM, Culbert JP, Schwartz SM: Nonpharmacological interventions for insomnia: A meta-analysis of treatment efficacy. Am J Psychiatry 1994;151:1172-1180.)

particularly early morning awakening problems. Overall, findings from meta-analyses represent fairly conservative estimates of treatment effects, as they are based on averages computed across all psychological and behavioral interventions and insomnia diagnoses (i.e., primary and secondary). On the other hand, although the majority of patients benefit from treatment, it appears that only a small proportion (20% to 30%) of them achieve full remission and that the majority continue to experience residual sleep disturbances.[27-29]

Treatment outcome has been documented primarily with prospective daily sleep diaries. Several studies have complemented those findings with data from polysomnography (PSG)[14,30,31] and from actigraphy.[15,28,32] Although the magnitude of improvements is usually smaller on those objective measures, they parallel clinical changes reported in daily sleep diaries. For example, in a study of older adults with sleep maintenance insomnia[30] (Fig. 61–2), average baseline values for wake after sleep onset were 62 minutes for diaries and 73 minutes for PSG measures. Posttreatment values were 29 minutes for the diary and 35 minutes for PSG, yielding improvement rates of 54% and 51%, respectively, for the two assessment methods. In a study of sleep onset insomnia,[31] baseline sleep latencies were 77 minutes (diary) and 84 minutes (PSG); after treatment, these values had decreased to 19 minutes and 21 minutes, respectively, by both measurement methods. In another study,[14] sleep efficiency increases of 8% and 12% were obtained for PSG and diary measures, respectively, after CBT. Collectively, these findings indicate that treatment not only alters sleep perception on daily diaries but also produces objective changes on PSG sleep continuity measures. Except for a modest increase in stages 3 and 4 after sleep restriction, there is little evidence of changes in sleep stages with psychological and behavioral treatment.

Comparative Efficacy of Therapies

Comparative studies of monotherapies have shown that stimulus control and sleep restriction therapies are slightly more effective than relaxation or paradoxical intention.[11,22,23,25,33,34] Sleep restriction tends to produce better outcomes than stimulus control in terms of sleep efficiency and continuity, but it also decreases total sleep time during the initial treatment period. Relaxation methods focusing on cognitive arousal (e.g., reducing intrusive thoughts at bedtime) yield slightly greater improvements than those targeting somatic arousal. Sleep hygiene education produces little impact on sleep when used as the only intervention.[35] Formal cognitive therapy has not been evaluated yet as a single treatment modality, although it is increasingly incorporated as a key component in multifaceted interventions.[13,14,28-30] Also, there is no evidence of differential treatment efficacy as a function of insomnia subtypes (e.g., sleep onset versus sleep maintenance).

Treatment Specificity and Mechanisms of Changes

Although there is evidence supporting the *efficacy* of psychological and behavioral treatment for insomnia, there is still little information about the *specificity* of this treatment modality and the active therapeutic mechanisms responsible for sleep improvements. With a few notable exceptions, which have used attention–placebo conditions,[11,14] most clinical trials of behavioral approaches have used wait-list control groups, precluding the unequivocal attribution of treatment effects to any specific ingredient of psychological and behavioral treatment. The lack of a pill-placebo control equivalent in psychological outcome research makes it difficult to determine what percentage of the variance in outcomes is the result of specific therapeutic ingredients (e.g., restriction of time in bed, cognitive restructuring), the measurement process (e.g., self-monitoring), or to nonspecific factors (e.g., therapist attention, patients' expectations).

A few studies have addressed this issue of treatment specificity by examining the mechanisms of changes. In a follow-up study of patients who had completed CBT for insomnia, Harvey and colleagues[36] found that the most critical ingredients associated with long-term sleep improvements were stimulus control and sleep restriction, followed by cognitive restructuring. Relaxation was the most frequently endorsed component (79% of respondents), but it did not predict improvement in any of the sleep outcome variables. Other studies have examined the association between changes in sleep beliefs and attitudes and sleep improvements. Reductions of dysfunctional sleep cognitions during treatment were correlated with sleep improvements after treatment, and fewer dysfunctional cognitions after treatment were associated with better maintenance of sleep changes over time.[18,19]

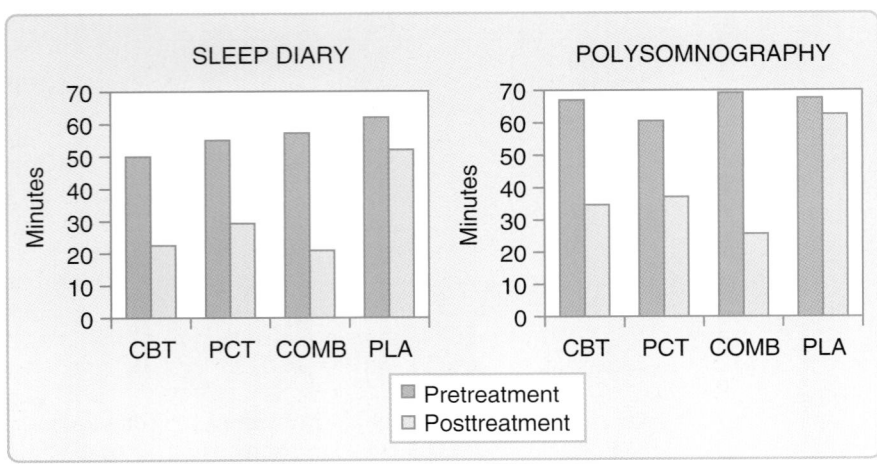

Figure 61–2. Changes in wake after sleep onset from pretreatment to posttreatment as measured by sleep diaries (subjective) and nocturnal polysomnography (objective). Sleep diary data are based on 2 weeks of self-monitoring at baseline (Pretreatment) and the last 2 weeks of treatment (Posttreatment). Polysomnographic data are based on nights 2 and 3 before (Pretreatment) and nights 5 and 6 after (Posttreatment) treatment. CBT, cognitive behavior therapy; PCT, pharmacotherapy; COMB, combined CBT and PCT; PLA, placebo. (From Morin CM, Colecchi C, Stone J, et al: Behavioral and pharmacological therapies for late-life insomnia: A randomized clinical trial. JAMA 1999;281:991-999.)

In their clinical series of 89 patients with mixed primary and secondary insomnias, Verbeek and colleagues[37] found that there were more treatment responders among those who received the cognitive therapy component (83%) than among those who did not receive it (56%). With increasing evidence that central nervous system hyperarousal is implicated in primary insomnia, there is a need for greater attention to identify the biologic, as well as the psychological, mechanisms responsible for sleep changes.

Initial Treatment Response versus Long-Term Outcome

A fairly robust finding across studies is that psychological and behavioral treatment produce stable changes in sleep patterns over time.[22,23] Most studies with follow-up data indicate that changes in sleep latency and wake after sleep onset observed after treatment are well maintained up to 12, 24, and even 36 months later.[13,28,30] Although interventions that restrict the amount of time spent in bed may yield only modest increases (and even a reduction) of sleep time during the initial treatment period, this parameter is usually improved at follow-up, with total sleep time often exceeding 6.5 hours. Long-term outcome must be interpreted cautiously, however, as few studies report long-term follow-up and, among those that do, attrition rates increase substantially over time. In addition, it is important to keep in mind that a substantial proportion of those patients with chronic insomnia who benefit from short-term therapy may remain vulnerable to recurrent episodes of insomnia in the long term.[38,39] There is a need to develop and evaluate the effects of long-term maintenance therapies to prevent or minimize the frequency and severity of those episodes.[40]

Clinical Significance of Treatment Outcome

Despite reliable changes noted on several sleep parameters, few studies have been able to document the extent to which treatment improves other important domains such as daytime functioning, alertness, mood, psychological well-being, and quality of life. Several recent studies have incorporated a variety of self-report measures to assess changes on those collateral variables, but only a few have actually shown reductions of some of those symptoms (e.g., anxiety, depression) with insomnia treatment.[13,28,41,42] Because studies of primary insomnia typically exclude patients with clinically significant depressive or anxious symptoms, there may be little room to show improvement among patients enrolled in those studies. Likewise, performance-based measures currently used to document cognitive functions such as attention, concentration, and memory are not sensitive enough to show deficits at baseline, and hence to detect changes with treatment. Despite these limitations, it is imperative to document outcome beyond symptom reductions. Insomnia is more than a sleep problem, and patients often seek treatment because of the perceived consequences of insomnia rather than because of the sleep problem per se. In the future, a core assessment battery should be developed that would incorporate multiple outcomes including sleep, functional impairments, psychological symptoms, and quality of life.[43]

Combined Behavioral and Pharmacologic Approaches

Combined behavioral and drug interventions should theoretically optimize treatment outcome by capitalizing on the more immediate and potent effects of medication and the more sustained effects of behavioral therapy. Only a few studies have directly evaluated the combined or differential effects of behavioral and pharmacologic therapies for insomnia.[15,30,44-46] Collectively, the evidence from those studies and from a meta-analysis[24] indicates that both treatment modalities are effective in the short term, with drug therapy producing quicker and slightly better results in the acute phase (the first week) of treatment, whereas behavioral and drug therapies are equally effective in the short-term interval (within 4 to 8 weeks). Combined interventions appear to have a slight advantage over single treatment modality during the initial course of treatment, but it is unclear whether a combined approach produces a better long-term outcome than behavioral therapy alone. For instance, sleep improvements are well sustained after behavioral treatment, and those obtained with hypnotic drugs are quickly lost after discontinuation of the medication (Fig. 61–3).

The long-term effects of combined behavioral and pharmacologic approaches are more equivocal. Some patients treated with a combined approach retain their initial sleep improvements over time, whereas others return to their baseline values. Thus, despite the intuitive appeal of combining drug and nondrug interventions, it is not entirely clear when, how, and for whom the combination of behavioral and drug treatments is indicated for insomnia. In light of the mediating role of psychological factors in chronic insomnia, behavioral and attitudinal changes appear essential to sustain improvements in sleep patterns. When behavioral and drug therapies are combined, patients' attributions of the initial benefits may be critical in determining long-term outcomes. Attribution of therapeutic benefits to the drug alone, without integration of self-management skills, may place a patient at greater risk for insomnia recurrence after the drug is discontinued. Additional research is needed to evaluate the effects of combined treatments for insomnia and to examine the mechanisms that mediate short- and long-term outcomes.[47]

Generalizability of Treatment Outcomes

Most treatment studies have focused on primary insomnia in otherwise healthy and medication-free patients. An important question that often arises is whether the findings obtained in those studies generalize to patients with comorbid medical or psychiatric disorders. Findings from clinical case series[16,29,48,49] suggest that patients with medical and psychiatric conditions can also benefit from insomnia-specific treatment, even though the outcome with those patients is more modest than with those who suffer from primary insomnia. Recent controlled studies have also shown that cognitive behavior therapy is effective for treating insomnia associated with chronic pain,[50] with cancer,[51] and with various medical conditions in older adults.[52-54] In general, the findings from secondary insomnia studies indicate that baseline and posttreatment scores on insomnia symptom measures are usually more severe among

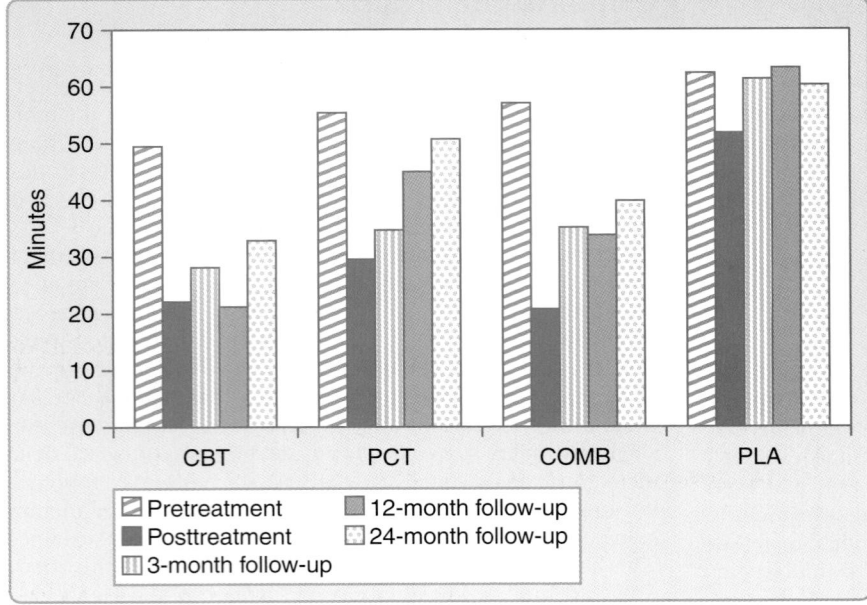

Figure 61–3. Changes in wake after sleep onset, as measured by sleep diaries, over long-term assessment periods. CBT, cognitive behavior therapy; PCT, pharmacotherapy; COMB, combined CBT and PCT; PLA, placebo. (From Morin CM, Colecchi C, Stone J, et al: Behavioral and pharmacological therapies for late-life insomnia: A randomized clinical trial. JAMA 1999;281: 991-999.)

patients with comorbid psychiatric and medical disorders, but the absolute changes on those outcomes during treatment are comparable to those among patients with primary insomnia (reviewed in Chapter 62). Behavioral treatment is also beneficial for medicated as well as for unmedicated patients with insomnia.[29,55] Two clinical trials have also shown that a supervised, structured, and time-limited withdrawal program, with or without cognitive behavior therapy, can facilitate discontinuation of hypnotic medications among older adults with insomnia who are prolonged users.[56,57]

TREATMENT FEASIBILITY AND IMPLEMENTATION

Applicability in Clinical Practice

Because the main entry point for professional insomnia treatment is typically in primary care medicine, an important question is the extent to which treatment validated in academic research centers is also effective in purely clinical settings. This issue was tackled in an innovative clinical effectiveness trial[28,58] in which nurse practitioners were trained to provide group CBT to patients with insomnia seen in primary care practices. The results showed an average reduction of sleep onset latency from 61 minutes to 28 minutes after treatment, with similar improvements on time awake after sleep onset. In addition, 84% of patients initially using hypnotics remained drug free at a 1-year follow-up.[58] Another study conducted in Germany[13] showed that group CBT was also effective in treating patients referred by their primary care physicians to a sleep clinic. The benefits of brief consultation models involving one or two consultations have been documented in both primary care[35] and specialty sleep clinics.[59]

Self-help approaches using printed materials or videotapes have also been shown to be useful in the treatment of insomnia.[42,60] For example, Mimeault and Morin[42] reported that a self-help treatment program, consisting of six printed booklets mailed weekly to participants was effective to reduce total wake time and to improve sleep efficiency; the addition of

professional guidance in the form of brief (15-minute) telephone consultation added to the initial outcomes. One recent study from Sweden also demonstrated the benefits of an Internet-based intervention.[61] Finally, the benefits and feasibility of insomnia treatment provided in behavioral sleep medicine clinics have been shown in several clinical replication series.[13,16,29,49,62] Collectively, the evidence indicates that psychological and behavioral treatments for insomnia are effective not only in the context of controlled research studies but also in various clinical settings such as in primary care clinics and in behavioral sleep medicine clinics. The use of nurse clinicians, self-help materials, brief consultations, and even the Internet, can enhance treatment access and facilitate its implementation in clinical practice.

Clinical and Practical Issues

Psychological and behavioral approaches to treating primary insomnia are time limited, structured, and sleep focused.[8] General clinical guidelines are outlined in Box 61–1. For typical patients with primary insomnia, direct consultation time varies between 4 and 6 hours per patient, which is usually spread over a treatment period of 6 to 8 weeks.[63] The amount of direct clinical contact and the number of follow-up visits is likely to vary as a function of several factors (insomnia severity, comorbidity, use of hypnotic medications, and patient's motivation and education). This treatment period is considerably shorter than for other forms of psychotherapy, and shorter than behavioral approaches applied to other health and psychological problems (e.g., chronic pain, anxiety, depression), yet it may still not be feasible for some practitioners to spend that much time with a single patient. Although milder forms of insomnia may require less time, it would be unrealistic to expect to treat every patient with insomnia in a single session. Even for highly motivated patients, adequate time is necessary to conduct a detailed clinical evaluation, and to explain the nature of the intervention, its rationale, and the essential role played by the patients.

Box 61–1 Clinical Guidelines for the Management of Primary Insomnia

Evaluation

- Complete a detailed sleep history, addressing the nature of the insomnia (initial, middle, late); typical sleep schedule (bedtime, arising time); onset, duration, and course of the insomnia; exacerbating/facilitating factors; medical, psychiatric, and substance use factors; use of sleep medication; prior therapies; and outcomes.
- Obtain baseline sleep diary monitoring and psychological screening assessment for anxiety and depressive symptoms.

Treatment

- Explain the nature of behavioral treatment, its rationale, and the importance of the patient's involvement in and compliance with the treatment. Discuss the patient's expectations and provide realistic outcome expectations.
- Provide a conceptual framework (predisposing, precipitating, and perpetuating factors) to explain how insomnia may have evolved into a persistent problem over time (Spielman's model).[9]
- Introduce sleep restriction; prescribe initial "sleep window" based on baseline diary data; revise this sleep window periodically as a function of sleep efficiency and total sleep time.
- Introduce stimulus control procedures and emphasize the need to implement all instructions in a systematic fashion.
- Examine and assist patients in revising common misconceptions about sleep expectations and attributions of insomnia as the only cause of daytime impairments.
- Consider relaxation training and use of commercially available audiotapes.
- Review basic sleep hygiene principles.
- Discontinue hypnotic medications among chronic users; consider adding medication if patient is nonresponsive to behavioral treatment.
- Urge the patient to continue daily sleep diary monitoring throughout treatment; review these data to evaluate insomnia severity, to monitor treatment compliance and progress, and to involve patient in the treatment.
- Schedule periodic follow-up visits to address compliance issues and to monitor treatment progress.

The success of psychological and behavioral approaches depends largely on the patients' willingness to comply with the recommended self-management procedures. For this reason, it is particularly important to schedule follow-up visits after the initial evaluation to address compliance issues. Although treatment is generally well accepted by patients, it is more time consuming and requires more efforts than drug therapy, both for clinicians and patients. Thus, compliance may not always be optimal. For example, a recent study[64] found a difference of 28 minutes between recommended time in bed and actual time spent in bed after treatment. Greater consistency in bedtime and arising time predicted a better outcome.

Given the multifactorial nature of primary insomnia, it is often necessary and useful to combine several psychological and behavioral procedures. Sleep restriction is almost always relevant for any patient with insomnia, and the use of this procedure early in therapy is likely to produce rapid therapeutic benefits, which may serve as an incentive for the patient to remain in treatment. Some stimulus control procedures (e.g., getting out of bed when unable to sleep) may not be necessary early on when the initial sleep window is restricted to 5 to 6 hours per night, but those procedures become particularly relevant as the sleep window is increased. Relaxation is helpful for those individuals with elevated tension or anxiety; however, caution is needed as some individuals may have a paradoxical response and become more anxious. Cognitive therapy is particularly helpful to challenge some misconceptions about sleep, to alleviate emotional distress, and to minimize recurrence of sleep disturbances over time. For mild forms of insomnia, basic sleep hygiene education may be sufficient, whereas more severe and persistent forms of insomnia often require multimodal interventions and more frequent follow-up visits.

Who should treat insomnia? Although psychological and behavioral treatments have traditionally been implemented by clinical psychologists, some of those procedures (e.g., sleep restriction, stimulus control instructions) can also be implemented successfully by trained nurse practitioners[28] or through self-help manuals with some therapist guidance.[42,60] Other procedures (e.g., relaxation, cognitive therapy) may require more time in treatment or therapists with specialized training. Group therapy is a very cost-effective treatment for the management of insomnia,[13,37,65] as is self-help treatment,[42] although this latter approach is appropriate only for highly motivated individuals. Therapist guidance is almost always necessary for more complicated cases and, in the presence of significant comorbidity, it is preferable to refer to a behavioral sleep medicine specialist.

CONCLUSION

Significant advances have been made over the last decade in the conceptualization, diagnosis, and treatment of insomnia. Despite this progress and increasing recognition that insomnia is a prevalent and costly health problem, there is still a significant gap between research-based evidence and clinical practices.[66] Important challenges for investigators will be to validate insomnia therapies with patients actually seen in clinical practice and for the professional sleep community and health-decision makers to promote wider dissemination and utilization of such evidenced-based therapies for primary insomnia.

Clinical Pearl

Poor sleep habits, irregular sleep schedules, hyperarousal, and misconceptions about sleep are important contributing factors to primary insomnia. Effective clinical management of insomnia must consider those perpetuating factors and incorporate psychological and behavioral therapies such as sleep restriction, stimulus control, relaxation, and cognitive therapy.

Acknowledgment

Preparation of this chapter was supported in part by grants from the National Institute of Mental Health (MH-60413) and from the Canadian Institutes of Health Research (MT-42504).

REFERENCES

1. Ohayon M: Epidemiology of insomnia: What we know and what we still need to learn. Sleep Med Rev 2002;6:97-111.
2. Hohagen F, Rink K, Kappler C, et al: Prevalence and treatment of insomnia in general practice: A longitudinal study. Eur Arch Psychiatry Clin Neurosci 1993;242:329-336.
3. Simon G, VonKorff M: Prevalence, burden, and treatment of insomnia in primary care. Am J Psychiatry 1997;154:1417-1423.
4. Mellinger GD, Balter MB, Uhlenhuth EH: Insomnia and its treatment: Prevalence and correlates. Arch Gen Psychiatry 1985;42:225-232.
5. Breslau N, Roth T, Rosenthal L, Andreski P: Sleep disturbance and psychiatric disorders: A longitudinal epidemiological study of young adults. Biol Psychiatry 1996;39:411-418.
6. Ford DE, Kamerow DB: Epidemiologic study of sleep disturbances and psychiatric disorders: An opportunity for prevention? JAMA 1989;262:1479-1484.
7. Espie CA: Insomnia: Conceptual issues in the development, persistence, and treatment of sleep disorders in adults. Annu Rev Psychol 2002;53:215-243.
8. Morin CM, Espie CA: Insomnia: A Clinical Guide to Assessment and Treatment. New York, Kluwer Academic/Plenum, 2003.
9. Spielman AJ, Glovinsky PB: The varied nature of insomnia. In Hauri P (ed): Case Studies in Insomnia. New York, Plenum Press, 1991, pp 1-15.
10. Spielman AJ, Saskin P, Thorpy MJ: Treatment of chronic insomnia by restriction of time in bed. Sleep 1987;10:45-56.
11. Lichstein KL, Riedel BW, Wilson NM, et al: Relaxation and sleep compression for late-life insomnia: A placebo-controlled trial. J Consult Clin Psychol 2001;69:227-239.
12. Bootzin RR, Epstein D, Wood JM: Stimulus control instructions. In Hauri P (ed): Case Studies in Insomnia. New York, Plenum Press, 1991, pp 19-28.
13. Backhaus J, Hohagen F, Voderholzer U, Riemann D: Long-term effectiveness of a short-term cognitive-behavioral group treatment for primary insomnia. Eur Arch Psychiatry Clin Neurosci 2001;251:35-41.
14. Edinger JD, Wohlgemuth WK, Radtke RA, et al: Cognitive behavioral therapy for treatment of chronic primary insomnia: A randomized controlled trial. JAMA 2001;285:1856-1864.
15. Hauri PJ: Insomnia: Can we mix behavioral therapy with hypnotics when treating insomniacs? Sleep 1997;20:111-118.
16. Jacobs GD, Benson H, Friedman R: Perceived benefits in behavioral-medicine insomnia program: A clinical report. Am J Med 1996;100:212-216.
17. Morin CM, Insomnia: Psychological Assessment and Management. New York, Guilford Press, 1993.
18. Edinger JD, Wohlgemuth WK, Radtke RA, et al: Does cognitive-behavioral insomnia therapy alter dysfunctional beliefs about sleep? Sleep 2001;24:591-599.
19. Morin CM, Blais FC, Savard J: Are changes in beliefs and attitudes about sleep related to sleep improvements in the treatment of insomnia? Behav Res Ther 2002;40:741-752.
20. Harvey AG, Payne S: The management of unwanted pre-sleep thoughts in insomnia: Distraction with imagery versus general distraction. Behav Res Ther 2002;40:267-277.
21. Riedel BW: Sleep hygiene. In Lichstein KL, Morin CM (eds): Treatment of Late-Life Insomnia. Thousand Oaks, Calif, Sage, 2000, pp 125-146.
22. Morin CM, Culbert JP, Schwartz SM: Nonpharmacological interventions for insomnia: A meta-analysis of treatment efficacy. Am J Psychiatry 1994;151:1172-1180.
23. Murtagh DRR, Greenwood KM: Identifying effective psychological treatments for insomnia: A meta-analysis. J Consult Clin Psychol 1995;60:79-89.
24. Smith MT, Perlis ML, Park A, et al: Comparative meta-analysis of pharmacotherapy and behavior therapy for persistent insomnia. Am J Psychiatry 2002;159:5-11.
25. Morin CM, Hauri PJ, Espie CA, et al: Nonpharmacologic treatment of chronic insomnia. Sleep 1999;22:1134-1156.
26. Nowell PD, Mazumdar S, Buysse DJ, et al: Benzodiazepines and zolpidem for chronic insomnia: A meta-analysis of treatment efficacy. JAMA 1997;278:2170-2177.
27. Lacks P, Powlishta K: Improvement following behavioral treatment for insomnia: Clinical significance, long-term maintenance, and predictors of outcome. Behav Ther 1989;20:117-134.
28. Espie CA, Inglis SJ, Tessier S, Harvey L: The clinical effectiveness of cognitive behaviour therapy for chronic insomnia: Implementation and evaluation of a sleep clinic in general medical practice. Behav Res Ther 2001;39:45-60.
29. Morin CM, Stone J, McDonald K, Jones S: Psychological management of insomnia: A clinical replication series with 100 patients. Behav Ther 1994;25:291-309.
30. Morin CM, Colecchi C, Stone J, et al: Behavioral and pharmacological therapies for late-life insomnia: A randomized clinical trial. JAMA 1999;281:991-999.
31. Jacobs GD, Benson H, Friedman R: Home-based central nervous system assessment of a multifactorial behavioral treatment of chronic sleep-onset insomnia. Behav Ther 1993;24:159-174.
32. Guilleminault C, Clerk A, Black J, et al: Nondrug treatment trials in psychophysiological insomnia. Arch Intern Med 1995;155:838-844.
33. Friedman L, Bliwise D, Yesavage JA, Salom SR: A preliminary study comparing sleep restriction and relaxation treatments for insomnia in older adults. J Gerontol 1991;46:1-8.
34. Jacobs GD, Rosenberg PA, Friedman R, et al: Multifactorial behavioral treatment of chronic sleep-onset insomnia using stimulus control and the relaxation response: A preliminary study. Behav Modif 1993;17:498-509.
35. Edinger JD, Sampson WS: A primary care "friendly" cognitive behavioral insomnia therapy. Sleep 2003;26:177-182.
36. Harvey L, Inglis SJ, Espie CA: Insomniacs' reported use of CBT components and relationship to long-term clinical outcome. Behav Res Ther 2002;40:75-83.
37. Verbeek I, Schreuder K, Declerck G: Evaluation of short-term nonpharmacological treatment of insomnia in a clinical setting. J Psychosom Res 1999;47:369-383.
38. Mendelson WB: Long-term follow-up of chronic insomnia. Sleep 1995,18:698-701.
39. Vollrath M, Wicki W, Angst J: The Zurich study: VII. Insomnia: Association with depression, anxiety, somatic syndromes, and course of insomnia. Eur Arch Psychiatry Neurol Sci 1989;239:113-124.
40. Jindal RD, Buysse DJ, Thase ME: Maintenance treatment of insomnia: What can we learn from the depression literature? Am J Psychiatry 2004;161:19-24.
41. Lichstein KL, Peterson BA, Riedel BW, et al: Relaxation to assist sleep medication withdrawal. Behav Modif 1999;23:379-402.
42. Mimeault V, Morin CM: Self-help treatment for insomnia: Bibliotherapy with and without professional guidance. J Consult Clin Psychol 1999;67:511-519.
43. Morin CM: Measuring outcome in randomized clinical trials of insomnia therapies. Sleep Med Rev 2003;7:263-279.
44. McClusky HY, Milby JB, Switzer PK, et al: Efficacy of behavioral versus triazolam treatment in persistent sleep-onset insomnia. Am J Psychiatry 1991;148:121-126.
45. Milby JB, Williams V, Hall JN, et al: Effectiveness of combined triazolam-behavioral therapy for primary insomnia. Am J Psychiatry 1993;150:1259-1260.
46. Rosen RC, Lewin DS, Goldberg RL, Woolfolk RL: Psychophysiological insomnia: Combined effects of pharmacotherapy and relaxation-based treatments. Sleep Med 2000;1:279-288.
47. Stepanski E, Wyatt JK: Controversies in the treatment of primary insomnia. Sleep Med 2000;1:259-261.

48. Dashevsky B, Kramer M: Behavioral treatment of chronic insomnia in psychiatrically ill patients. J Clin Psychiatry 1998; 59:693-399.

49. Perlis M, Aloia M, Millikan A, et al: Behavioral treatment of insomnia: A clinical case series study. J Behav Med 2000;23: 149-161.

50. Currie SR, Wilson KG, Pontefract AJ, deLaplante L: Cognitive-behavioral treatment of insomnia secondary to chronic pain. J Consul Clin Psychol 2000;68:407-416.

51. Quesnel C, Savard J, Simard S, et al: Efficacy of cognitive-behavioral therapy for insomnia in women treated for non-metastatic breast cancer. J Consul Clin Psychol 2003;71: 189-200.

52. Rybarczyk B, Lopez M, Benson R, et al: Efficacy of two behavioral treatment programs for comorbid geriatric insomnia. Psychol Aging 2002;17:288-298.

53. Lichstein KL, Morin CM (eds): Treatment of Late-Life Insomnia. Newberry Park, Calif, Sage, 2000.

54. Lichstein KL, Wilson NM, Johnson CT: Psychological treatment of secondary insomnia. Psychol Aging. 2000;15:232-240.

55. Riedel B, Lichstein KL, Peterson BA, et al: A comparison of the efficacy of stimulus control for medicated and nonmedicated insomniacs. Behav Modif 1998;22:3-28.

56. Baillargeon L, Landreville P, Verreault R, et al: Discontinuation of benzodiazepines among older insomniac adults treated through cognitive-behavioral therapy combined with gradual tapering: A randomized trial. CMAJ 2003;169:1015-1020.

57. Morin CM, Bastien C, Guay B, et al: Insomnia and chronic use of benzodiazepines: A randomized clinical trial of supervised tapering, cognitive-behavioral therapy, and a combined approach to facilitate benzodiazepine discontinuation. Am J Psychiatry 2004;161:332-342.

58. Espie CA, Inglis SJ, Harvey L: Predicting clinically significant response to cognitive behavior therapy for chronic insomnia in general medical practice: Analyses of outcome data at 12 months posttreatment. J Consul Clin Psychol 2001;69:58-66.

59. Hauri PJ: Consulting about insomnia: A method and some preliminary data. Sleep 1993;16:344-350.

60. Riedel BW, Lichstein KL, Dwyer WO: Sleep compression and sleep education for older insomniacs: Self-help versus therapist guidance. Psychol Aging 1995;10:54-63.

61. Ström S, Pettersson R, Andersson G: Internet-based treatment for insomnia: A controlled evaluation. J Consult Clin Psychol 2004;72:113-120.

62. Hryshko-Mullen AS, Broeckl LS, Haddock K, Peterson AL: Behavioral treatment of insomnia: The Wilford Hall Insomnia Program. Mil Med 2000;165:200-207.

63. Edinger JD, Wohlgemuth WK, Radtke RA, Marsh GR: Dose response effects of behavioral insomnia therapy. Sleep 2000; 23:310.

64. Riedel BW, Lichstein KL: Strategies for evaluating adherence to sleep restriction treatment for insomnia. Behav Res Ther 2001; 39:201-12.

65. Bastien C, Morin, CM, Ouellet MC, et al: Cognitive-behavior therapy for insomnia: Comparison of individual therapy, group therapy, and telephone consultations. J Consult Clin Psychol 2004 (in press).

66. National Institutes of Health: NIH releases statement on behavioral and relaxation approaches for chronic pain and insomnia. Am Fam Physician 1996;53:1877-1880.

Psychological and Behavioral Treatments for Secondary Insomnias

Kenneth L. Lichstein

Sidney D. Nau

Christina S. McCrae

Kristen C. Stone

ABSTRACT

Secondary insomnia, late-life insomnia, and hypnotic-dependent insomnia may be collectively referred to as secondary insomnias because external agents or disease processes are commonly implicated in the sleep disturbance. Relying mainly on a behavioral/psychological perspective (also known as behavioral sleep medicine), this chapter reviews treatment procedures, assessment and diagnostic strategies, clinical outcomes, and mechanisms of action associated with these forms of insomnia.

With all three types of insomnia, the bulk of the literature related to clinical outcome strongly suggests that some variety of cognitive behavior therapy is effective, and this optimistic literature has emerged mostly in the past 10 to 15 years. With secondary insomnia, research shows that regardless of its origin, the insomnia becomes functionally independent and is self-sustaining, so that supposed secondary insomnia can be expected to respond as well as primary insomnia to cognitive behavior therapy. Indeed, evidence is emerging that successful treatment of secondary insomnia may bring therapeutic relief to the primary condition, arguing for a reciprocal rather than a unidirectional causal model of secondary insomnia. With late-life insomnia, prevalence and comorbidity sharply increase compared with insomnia in younger age groups, but here too, cognitive behavior therapies (in particular, stimulus control, sleep restriction/sleep compression, and cognitive therapy) have demonstrated clinical efficacy. With hypnotic-dependent insomnia, sleep medication consumption increases substantially among older adults, the group most vulnerable to drug side effects. In regard to prescription hypnotics that have lost therapeutic potency but still control patients by dependency, several studies have shown that slow, scheduled drug weaning combined with cognitive behavior therapies achieves sleep improvement and substantial reduction in medication use while avoiding potent insomnia and anxiety rebound.

Thus, these forms of secondary insomnia are amenable to cognitive behavior therapy, and health providers should not hesitate to treat these forms of sleep disturbance. Robust cognitive behavior therapy treatment exposure usually does not exceed 10 sessions, unless drug weaning is also required, and multicomponent treatments are often preferred to unitary interventions.

This chapter will address three insomnia variants: secondary insomnia (SI), late-life insomnia, and hypnotic-dependent insomnia (HDI). Collectively, these account for the majority of the population of people with insomnia. Although seemingly disparate, a moderate stretch of reasoning supports the argument that HDI and late-life insomnia are special cases of SI. Substance-induced insomnia is a common variety of SI. In the case of HDI, the substance is a hypnotic and the insomnia is sustained by its continued use. The precipitous rise in insomnia prevalence in older adults supports the conclusion that insomnia is secondary to aging, regardless of whether the mechanism is biologic or behavioral/emotional.

SECONDARY INSOMNIA

When poor sleep is thought to arise from conditioned aversion to the bedroom or from subclinical emotional/cognitive/physiologic turmoil, the disturbance may be termed primary insomnia. However, when poor sleep is associated with a psychiatric disorder, medical condition, or medication/substance, the term SI or comorbidity applies.

The diagnosis of SI is conferred if the offending agent, termed the primary condition, is believed to have a causal relationship with the insomnia, such that the primary condition instigated and sustains poor sleep. A corollary of this definition presumes the insomnia will resolve when the primary condition is successfully treated. However, if the suspect agent shares a reciprocal or parallel relationship with the insomnia, the term comorbid insomnia is more appropriate than SI. We will review SI with an emphasis on a deeper understanding of its diagnosis and implications for treatment.

Epidemiology

Sleep is reactive to a broad range of psychiatric disorders, medical conditions, and substances.[1] Estimating the prevalence of SI is difficult because epidemiologic studies rarely collect sufficient information to distinguish SI from comorbidity. This important constraint notwithstanding, rough estimates of SI prevalence can be achieved. Epidemiologic research typically finds comorbidity rates around 50% between insomnia and serious psychiatric disorders.[2] Ohayon[3] found a 65% rate of SI using the most extensive interviews to date to establish this diagnosis. A review[4] of diagnostic data from six sleep disorders centers found that nearly 75% of their patients presenting with insomnia were diagnosed as having SI.

Pathogenesis

There are four paths by which the primary condition can alter sleep. Insomnia can be induced by *direct effects* (e.g., neurologic diseases that produce muscle tremors and stiffness that disrupt sleep[5]), *physical side effects* (e.g., pain associated with a wide range of disorders[6]), *psychological side effects* (e.g., stress associated with cancer[7]), and *medications/substances* (including a broad range of nonprescription [e.g., caffeine and alcohol[8]] and prescription [e.g., energizing antidepressants, antihypertensives, bronchodilators, diuretics, and corticosteroids[1]] drugs).

Clinical Features

SI may present with the same constellation of symptoms as primary insomnia. Evidence is emerging from basic research that shows that the polysomnography profile,[9] subjective sleep disturbance,[10] and presleep cognitive arousal[11] associated with SI do not significantly differ from those associated with primary insomnia. Therefore, the nature of the sleep disturbance in SI appears similar to that in primary insomnia, and these findings are consistent with the idea that SI would be responsive to the same interventions used for primary insomnia.

Diagnosis

Discriminating SI and comorbid insomnia is difficult. The critical issue distills down to the philosophy of science question of causal inference. To assert that A (the primary condition) causes B (insomnia), one must at least show that A precedes B, and that variations in A and B covary. These conditions can be established by interview, although the longer the presumed SI endures, the more difficult it is to obtain reliable historical information. Establishing the presence of a causal relationship between the primary condition and the insomnia is the weak link in SI theory and diagnosis.

A recently introduced heuristic diagnostic model of SI[4] specified three SI states: *absolute, partial,* and *specious.* Absolute SI reflects the common use of the term SI. That is, a primary condition instigated and now sustains the poor sleep.

Two varieties of partial SI can be discerned. First, partial SI can occur when poor sleep followed the onset of the primary condition, but the insomnia subsequently acquired part or full functional independence. Regardless of the source, sustained insomnia is an engine producing sleep-incompatible cognitions and arousing conditioning experiences that promote insomnia autonomy. Second, the insomnia could have existed before the onset of the primary condition, but subsequently the course of the insomnia partially or fully responded to variations in the severity of the primary condition.

Specious SI refers to cases of apparent absolute or partial SI, but nevertheless there is no SI, only comorbidity. This occurs when the patient's historical account, the main source of diagnostic information, is unreliable. Health care professionals commonly encounter this problem, although it is not always obvious that the patient is providing an inaccurate report.

It is important to appreciate the complexity of the diagnosis of SI, because it directly invites behavioral intervention.

The premise that absolute, partial, and specious SI usually cannot be distinguished illuminates the reality that clinicians never really know what they are treating. Absolute SI would be a poor candidate for direct behavioral intervention, because, indeed, the primary condition would replenish the treated insomnia. However, partial SI would be expected to show at least a moderate treatment response, and specious SI should respond as well as primary insomnia.

Treatment

Several reviews have provided an adequate summary of behavioral treatment for SI.[1,4,12] In the following abbreviated review, three randomized studies with strong methodologies are presented.

A mixed-age sample of 30 cancer patients with insomnia were randomly assigned to usual medical care or usual care plus three sessions of progressive relaxation.[13] Latency to sleep was dramatically improved in the progressive relaxation group only, going from 124 minutes at pretreatment to 29 minutes after treatment. Sleep improvement was maintained at the 3-month follow-up.

Two decades later, Currie and colleagues[14] evaluated cognitive behavior therapy (CBT) for SI in 60 patients having chronic pain from a variety of sources. Participants were randomized to CBT (sleep restriction, stimulus control, cognitive restructuring, and relaxation) or to a wait list control. Compared with the wait list control, CBT participants demonstrated significant improvement from baseline to 3-month follow-up on self-reported sleep onset latency (54.7 to 27.8 minutes), wake time after sleep onset (88.9 to 51.6 minutes), sleep efficiency (72% to 84%), and sleep quality (Pittsburgh Sleep Quality Index score of 13.6 to 7.9).

Last, our group[15] reported a randomized study of SI in older adults. Forty-four volunteers were randomized to four sessions of combined hybrid passive relaxation, stimulus control, and sleep hygiene instructions or to a wait list control. Our sample was evenly divided between insomnia secondary to psychiatric disorders and insomnia secondary to medical disorders. There was significantly greater improvement at posttreatment and 3-month follow-up for the treated group on three self-report sleep measures: wake time after sleep onset, sleep efficiency percent, and rated quality of sleep (from 1 [very poor] to 5 [excellent]). From baseline to follow-up for the treated group, wake time went from 87.3 minutes to 56.4 minutes, sleep efficiency went from 66.7% to 77.7%, and rated quality of sleep went from 2.7 to 3.2. Participants with medical and psychiatric SI did not differentially respond.

Combining data from Currie et al.[14] and Lichstein et al.[15] in Figure 62–1 dramatically reveals the consistency of treatment effects in the management of SI. In the figure, the sleep efficiency for both studies was flat across treatment phases in the control groups, and it improved in unison in the treatment groups. (Data from Cannici et al.[13] were not included because this early study reported minimal sleep data.)

Clinical Course and Prevention

SI tends to be a persistent rather than a short-lived disorder,[16] but the role of the primary condition and the insomnia may transform over time. For delimited periods, it may be clear that the primary condition is affecting the insomnia, the insomnia is affecting the primary condition, or neither is affecting the other.

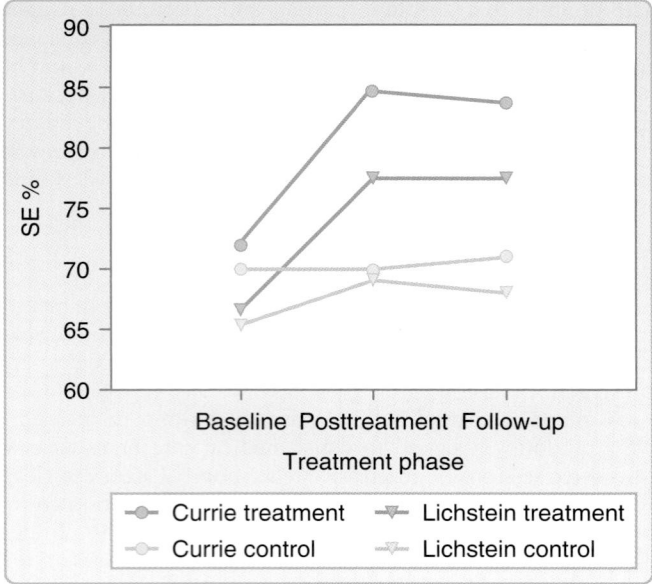

Figure 62–1. Sleep efficiency (SE) compared in two clinical trials of treatment for secondary insomnia. *Medium blue circles* represent the group treated with sleep restriction, stimulus control, cognitive restructuring, and relaxation (Currie et al.). *Medium blue triangles* represent the group treated with passive relaxation, stimulus control, and sleep hygiene instructions (Lichstein et al.). *Light blue circles and triangles* represent the corresponding controls. (Data from Currie SR, Wilson KG, Pontefract AJ, et al.: Cognitive-behavioral treatment of insomnia secondary to chronic pain. J Consult Clin Psychol 2000;68:407-416; and Lichstein KL, Wilson NM, Johnson CT: Psychological treatment of secondary insomnia. Psychol Aging 2000;15:232-240.)

Numerous clinical reports show SI influencing the primary condition.[15,17-19] Similarly, insomnia is a health risk factor for drug abuse, depression, and anxiety.[20]

There is no intervention literature on prevention of SI, but we have suggested adaptations[12,21] of relapse prevention methods[22] and stress inoculation[23] that appear well suited for insomnia prevention. Insomnia is predictable in chronic pain (50% to 70% prevalence[24,25]), depression (40% to 90% prevalence[26]), and cancer (20% to 50% prevalence[27]). Primary prevention and early intervention are advisable for these and other disorders, but the efficacy of this recommendation awaits testing.

Pitfalls and Controversies

Once diagnosed, SI may cause the clinician to pause before treating the insomnia. Such hesitancy never intrudes in the management of the identified primary disorder, which always commands robust treatment. It is only when the primary condition becomes chronic that SI emerges as a therapeutic issue. Such reasoning rests on the faulty assumptions that the relationship between illness and sleep is static over time and that it is unidirectional.

Unidimensional conceptions of SI fail to appreciate the role of comorbidity, lead to overdiagnosis of SI, and result in lost opportunities for effective insomnia intervention. When considering the SI diagnosis, the health provider is obliged to scrutinize the relationship between the primary condition and the sleep disturbance. There may evolve an upward-spiraling,

reciprocal relationship between insomnia and the primary disorder, whereby each aggravates the other, and each subsequently suffers as the other worsens.[19,25] A downward-spiraling, beneficial version of this reciprocity has also been reported.[15,18] At other times, the insomnia may precede and instigate the "primary" disorder.[2,19]

LATE-LIFE INSOMNIA

Safe and effective psychological treatments are available for late-life insomnia. Early studies suggested that treatment gains were not as great for older adults as they were for younger adults (reviewed in Lichstein et al.[28]). However, research has since demonstrated not only that psychological therapies for insomnia are clinically effective in older adults but indeed that the treatment gains are similar to those in younger adults.[28]

Sedative medications are the most common treatments for insomnia,[29] but they carry tolerance and dependency risks. Psychological treatments for insomnia provide an opportunity to resolve the problem without the drawbacks of side effects and dependency.

Epidemiology and Risk Factors

The high prevalence of insomnia is well documented; population surveys estimate that one third of all adults have one or more episodes each year.[30] As people age, insomnia complaints increase—a trend that accelerates after age 40.[30] Insomnia is common enough in late life to be one of the negative changes that characterize the experience of aging. In a recent U.S. poll, 67% of adults older than 55 years reported having symptoms of sleep disorders at least a few nights a week, but only 8% had been diagnosed with a sleep disorder, and fewer received treatment.[31]

Insomnia in older adults is more common and more likely to be treated with medication than insomnia in younger people. Clinically significant insomnia prevalence in older people is estimated at 25% and higher,[32] and this is 30% to 50% higher than the rate for younger adults in life-span survey samples. Older adults with insomnia are more likely to have medical illness, physical disability, and elevated anxiety or symptoms of depression than older adults without an insomnia complaint.[32]

Older adults are at an increased risk for hypnotic-dependent insomnia. Older adults with insomnia receive treatment with sedative/hypnotic medication at a disproportionately high rate (as high as 20% for those age 75 and older, and 17% for those age 65 to 74, compared with 5% among younger adults[29]), risking drug interactions, daytime sedation, and worsening of sleep apnea. Metabolic changes of aging slow down elimination of hypnotic compounds, potentiating and exacerbating side effects. Ray et al.[33] found that older adults using long half-life benzodiazepines have a significantly higher rate of hip fractures than nonusers. Among nonbenzodiazepine alternatives, zolpidem may produce psychomotor and memory deficits comparable to deficits produced by benzodiazepines.[34]

Clinical Features

Primary insomnia and insomnia associated with psychiatric disorders are common during late life.[35] In addition, late-life insomnia includes sleep-related physiologic disorders (such as sleep apnea), insomnia associated with medical and neurologic disorders, substance use disorders, and circadian rhythm disorders. There are over 30 adult sleep disorders that often present with an insomnia complaint, and most are more common in older adults.[36] Many of these disorders increase sharply after age 40; some appear first in late life (e.g., insomnia associated with parkinsonism typically starts around age 50 to 60).

Assessment Methods and Diagnosis

The assessment approach for older adults with insomnia is similar to that used with other patients. It begins with a clinical interview. Then a daily sleep diary is often used to collect a pattern sample that supplements global sleep pattern estimates obtained in the interview. Psychiatric interview is a standard element of insomnia screening. There are screening assessments to check for physical disorders that could be contributing to the insomnia complaint. Finally, the treatment plan is prepared.

Differential diagnosis is especially important in older adults because the prevalence of sleep disorders other than primary insomnia is higher in this age group. Sleep apnea and periodic limb movement disorder are two sleep disorders that may mimic primary insomnia. Polysomnography is not routinely indicated for evaluation of late-life insomnia, except when sleep disturbance by a physiologic factor, such as apnea or periodic limb movement disorder, is strongly suspected.[37]

Treatment

Psychological treatments are often applied to late-life insomnia. The individual treatment methods are often combined into a package of behavioral techniques, termed cognitive behavior therapy.

Relaxation

Progressive relaxation (PR) is the most widely researched treatment for insomnia. Passive relaxation is an alternative to PR. Its procedures omit the sequential muscle tensing of PR and employ passive body focusing. The literature suggests that passive relaxation techniques are more consistently effective for older adults with insomnia than PR, possibly because they are less physically demanding and procedurally simpler. For a description of relaxation procedures, see Lichstein.[38]

Stimulus Control

Stimulus control emerged from the hypothesis that insomnia may be the result of bedtime and the bedroom becoming poor discriminative stimuli for sleep. The goals of stimulus control are to help the person with insomnia learn to fall asleep quickly at bedtime and learn to maintain sleep. This is accomplished by strengthening the bed and bedroom as cues for sleep, weakening them as cues for activities that might interfere with sleep, and helping the person to acquire a consistent sleep rhythm. Description of the procedures for stimulus control is available in Bootzin and Epstein.[39]

Sleep Restriction Therapy and Sleep Compression Therapy

The goals of sleep restriction therapy (SRT)[40] and sleep compression therapy (SCT)[41] are a decrease in awake time during the night and an increase in the restorative benefits of sleep. The treatments aim to consolidate sleep by restricting the amount of time the patient is allowed to be in bed. SCT gradually reduces the time allowed in bed, and SRT abruptly reduces the time.

Cognitive Therapy

In its application to insomnia treatment, cognitive therapy is used to alleviate insomnia-causing anxiety that arises from undue worrying and exaggerated fears related to sleep. Its therapeutic goal is to interrupt the vicious cycle of distress over poor sleep–provoking dysfunctional cognitions, leading to more sleep disturbance. Cognitive therapy seeks to replace faulty beliefs and attitudes about sleep.[42] The treatment begins with learning the patient's dysfunctional sleep cognitions, then challenging their validity, and then achieving resolution by replacing them with more adaptive alternatives.

Treatment Outcome

Table 62–1 presents a large sample of treatment trials[43-57] for chronic primary insomnia in older adults. Its objective is to briefly summarize all published studies (with a minimum of seven patients) that have tested behavioral treatment for older adults with insomnia. Clinical trials and case series are included. For each study, the methodology and a summary of outcomes are reported. The outcome measures include one or more of the following: sleep onset latency, number of awakenings or combined duration of awakenings, sleep efficiency, total sleep time, and ratings of sleep quality.

The 16 studies are sorted into five treatment categories (CBT, stimulus control, relaxation therapy, SRT/SCT, and sleep hygiene instruction). Half of the 16 studies tested more than one treatment; when this occurred, the summary information for that study appears in more than one category, up to a maximum of three categories. For example, Engle-Friedman et al.[48] appears in three categories: stimulus control treatment, relaxation treatment, and sleep hygiene.

The "Outcomes" column of Table 62–1 is the most important column; it presents global treatment efficacy conclusions, reached by abstracting and boiling down the significant and the nonsignificant quantitative outcomes for each study. The conclusions are stated in a condensed form that depends heavily on abbreviations. The reader should begin by reading the first footnote in the table legend, which includes a teaching example that explains the highly condensed way of summarizing the outcomes for each study.

Overall, Table 62–1 shows strong improvement and consistent results for most of the commonly tested behavioral treatments for older adults with insomnia (stimulus control, SRT, SCT, and multicomponent treatments). The exceptions, relaxation therapies and sleep hygiene education, exhibit less-consistent outcomes but do nevertheless produce favorable results.

A 1994 quantitative review of psychological treatments for insomnia found stimulus control and SRT to be the most effective treatments for improving sleep, with age unrelated to outcome.[58] Stimulus control is effective for onset insomnia[51] and maintenance insomnia,[47] and it may be particularly well suited for older adults with insomnia, as it has been consistently effective for maintenance insomnia. SRT[59] and SCT[57] are also effective for both types of late-life insomnia. Maintenance insomnia is more common than onset insomnia among older adults. In recent clinical trials, CBT has shown the largest

Table 62–1.   Treatment Outcomes for Primary Insomnia in Older Adults

Study, Reference (Date)	Design	Treatment Groups	FU	Bias	Outcomes*
Cognitive Behavior Therapy Treatment Package Studies					
Alperson & Biglan[43] (1979)†	RCT	REL + SC; back exercises + in-bed activities (young); WL	2 mo	Small sample, short FU	At FU, older adults did not significantly improve with REL + SC.
Edinger et al.[44] (1992)	CRS	Two-step package: (1) REL with posttest, then (2) CBT (SC, SRT, sleep education), then CBT posttest	3 mo	No control group, small sample	CBT > REL.
Morin et al.[45] (1993)	RCT	CBT (SC, SRT, CT, sleep education); WL	1 yr	—	CBT > WL. This conclusion supported by PSG data.
Morin et al.[46] (1999)†	RCT	CBT (SC, SRT, CT, HYG, sleep education); MED; CBT + MED; PL	2 yr	—	At POST, CBT = MED = CBT + MED. At FU, CBT > MED and CBT > CBT + MED. PSG improvement at POST.
Stimulus Control Studies					
Davies et al.[47] (1986)	RCT	Countercontrol (similar to SC); WL	1 yr	Most FU was short term	Countercontrol > WL. Improvement uncorrelated with age.
Engle-Friedman et al.[48] (1992)	RCT	HYG; REL + HYG; SC + HYG; WL	2 yr	—	At FU, SC + HYG > REL + HYG and SC + HYG > HYG. At POST, all 3 treatment groups > WL. No significant PSG changes.
Morin & Azrin[49] (1988)†	RCT	SC; IT; WL	1 yr	Small sample	SC > IT; SC and IT > WL
Pallesen et al.[50] (2003)†	RCT	SC + HYG; REL + HYG; WL	6 mo	—	Improvement at POST and FU. No between-group differences for SC + HYG vs. REL + HYG.
Puder et al.[51] (1983)	RCT	SC; WL	1.5 mo	Small sample, short FU	SC > WL.
Relaxation Studies					
Edinger et al.[44] (1992)	CRS	Two-step package: (1) REL with posttest, then (2) CBT (SC, SRT, sleep education), then CBT posttest	3 mo	No control group, small sample	CBT > REL.
Engle-Friedman et al.[48] (1992)	RCT	HYG; REL + HYG; SC + HYG; WL	2 yr	—	At FU, SC + HYG > REL + HYG and SC + HYG > HYG. At POST, all 3 treatment groups > WL. No significant PSG changes.
Friedman et al.[52] (1991)†	RCT	SRT; REL	3 mo	No control group	SRT and REL improved. SRT > REL.
Lichstein et al.[41] (2001)	RCT	REL + HYG; SCT + HYG; PL + HYG	1 yr	—	SCT + HYG > REL + HYG > PL. No significant PSG changes.

Study	Study design	Treatment groups			Outcomes
Lichtstein & Johnson[53] (1993)[†]	NRCT	REL for three different subject groups	1.5 mo	Short FU	REL most effective for unmedicated group.
Lick & Heffler[54] (1977)[†]	RCT	REL; REL + tape for practice; PL; WL	1 mo	Short FU, small sample	REL > WL. Improvement negatively correlated with age.
Morin & Azrin[49] (1988)[†]	RCT	SC; IT; WL	1 yr	Small sample	SC > IT. SC and IT > WL.
Nicassio & Bootzin[55] (1974)	RCT	REL; self-REL; WL	6 mo	Mixed-age sample	REL > WL. Improvement negatively correlated with age.
Pallesen et al.[50] (2003)[†]	RCT	SC + HYG; REL + HYG; WL	6 mo	—	Improvement at POST and FU. No between-group differences for SC + HYG vs. REL + HYG.
Sleep Restriction and Sleep Compression Studies					
Friedman et al.[52] (1991)[†]	RCT	SRT; REL	3 mo	No control group	SRT and REL improved. SRT > REL.
Friedman et al.[56] (2000)	RCT	SRT + HYG; nap modification of SRT + HYG; HYG	3 mo	—	At FU, all treatments improved. No between-group effects at POST or FU.
Lichtstein et al.[41] (2001)	RCT	REL + HYG; SCT + HYG; PL + HYG	1 yr	—	SCT + HYG > REL + HYG > PL. No significant PSG changes.
Riedel et al.[57] (1995)	RCT	HYG video; SCT + HYG video; WL	2 mo	Short FU	HYG video = SCT + HYG video, and SCT + HYG video > HYG video for different measures.
Sleep Hygiene Studies					
Engle-Friedman et al.[48] (1992)	RCT	HYG; REL + HYG; SC + HYG; WL	2 yr	—	At FU, SC + HYG > REL + HYG and SC + HYG > HYG. At POST, all 3 treatment groups > WL. No significant PSG changes.
Friedman et al.[56] (2000)	RCT	SRT + HYG; nap modification of SRT + HYG; HYG	3 mo	—	At FU, all treatments improved. No between-group effects at POST or FU.
Riedel et al.[57] (1995)	RCT	HYG video; SCT + HYG video; WL	2 mo	Short FU	HYG video = SCT + HYG video, and SCT + HYG video > HYG video for different measures.

*The comparison statements under "Outcomes" present treatment efficacy conclusions based on a distillation of the study's statistical results. Conclusions represent effects with most or main sleep measures. The efficacy conclusions are in a highly abbreviated format. For example, Morin and Azrin (1988) results showed "SC > IT. SC and IT > WL." These abbreviated statements mean first, that the overall improvement was greater after stimulus control therapy than it was after imagery training therapy, and second, that both treatments showed results superior to the waiting list condition.

[†]Use of sleep medication upon entering treatment was permissible.

Study designs: CRS, clinical replication series; NRCT, nonrandomized clinical trial; RCT, randomized clinical trial.

Treatment groups: CBT, cognitive behavior therapy; CT, cognitive therapy; HYG, sleep hygiene; IT, imagery training; MED, pharmacologic therapy; PL, placebo (either pill or behavioral); REL, various methods of relaxation; SC, stimulus control; SCT, sleep compression therapy; SRT, sleep restriction therapy; WL, waiting list.

Treatment phases: FU, follow-up evaluation; POST, posttreatment outcome evaluation.

Sleep measures: PSG, polysomnography. If not otherwise indicated, the sleep measure was self-reported.

improvement for late-life maintenance insomnia.[45,46] CBT packages, however, have not always generated larger treatment effects than stimulus control or SRT used as single treatments.[58]

Studies with older adults show that PR has been at times moderately effective in reducing sleep onset latency (e.g., see Engle-Friedman et al.[48] and Friedman et al.[52]) and at times mildly to moderately effective in reducing wake time after sleep onset (e.g., see Friedman et al.[52]). Overall, however, the effects of PR have been inconsistent, with some studies failing to show significant improvement among older adults. Passive relaxation techniques for geriatric insomnia have been investigated in three published studies[41,49,53] and have shown consistent, mild to moderate improvement in sleep onset latency, wake time after sleep onset, and total sleep time. Passive forms of relaxation have been more consistently effective than PR for older adults with insomnia.

CBT treatment packages typically include cognitive therapy among the treatments. Multicomponent CBT was judged to be effective and it was recommended as a treatment option in the 1999 American Academy of Sleep Medicine practice parameters on insomnia treatment.[60] Two large trials of CBT with late-life insomnia (using a package of stimulus control, SRT, cognitive therapy, and sleep hygiene) demonstrated significant long-term improvement in sleep maintenance.[45,46]

To facilitate treatment response, interventions can be adapted to the special needs of older adults. For example, PR can be modified to prevent muscle spasms or arthritic pain by eliminating the muscle tensing (especially for neck and back muscle groups) and having the older adult focus on releasing tension passively.[53] Stimulus-control instructions can be altered for older adults with difficulties ambulating by eliminating the requirement to leave the bedroom during long awakenings.[47]

Most late-life insomnia affects individuals who have comorbid medical conditions, and treatment of the insomnia is omitted while the "primary" medical condition receives full attention.[4] A few recent studies, however, have tested psychological treatments for comorbid late-life insomnia, with promising results (e.g., Rybarczyk et al.[61]).

Only four studies have used polysomnography to objectively measure treatment outcome.[41,45,46,48] These studies suggest that psychological treatments are more effective in improving self-report measures of sleep than polysomnographic measures of sleep.

Very few outcome studies with older adults have included measures of psychological distress, yet a clear relationship exists between poor sleep and psychological distress among older adults.[62] Older adults with insomnia report higher levels of depression and anxiety than older adults without sleep complaints (e.g., Fichten et al.[63]). Future research should examine more closely the success of interventions in alleviating psychological symptoms and improving daytime functioning.

Benefits of Treatment

Psychological treatments for older adults with insomnia offer a high expectancy for relief. These treatments decrease the time it takes to fall asleep, increase total time slept, and improve sleep efficiency, although often, sleep is still not completely normalized. They reduce frequency and duration of nightly awakenings—a finding that is particularly relevant given the prevalence of sleep maintenance insomnia in older adults.

Treated older adults with insomnia also report improved mood and greater self-efficacy in controlling insomnia.[45,48] Psychological treatments present no physical tolerance and dependency risks, and older adults rate psychological interventions as more appropriate and acceptable than pharmacotherapy.[64]

Clinical Course and Prevention

Psychological treatment benefits accumulate gradually in response to treatment visits and home practice. There are typically four to eight visits, usually completed within 1 to 3 months. Occasional booster sessions may help improve long-term gains.

Most insomnia prevention activities are in the realm of health education aimed at decreasing the prevalence of chronic insomnia; at present, the education activities focus on teaching basic facts about normal sleep and sleep hygiene training. *Teaching about normal sleep* helps provide individuals with a foundation for sleeping better, and the knowledge helps shape realistic expectations. Most people receive no formal education about sleep and remain naive about what is normal and abnormal. Incorrect beliefs and unrealistic expectations can increase worry about sleep and may provoke negative sleep habits (e.g., trying too hard to sleep).[65] *Sleep hygiene education* provides research-based advice on the management of sleep.[36,66] The concept of positive sleep hygiene exemplifies the goal of self-management of health. Sleep hygiene recommendations highlight the positive behaviors that promote more reliable and better-quality sleep and point out the negative behaviors that make the occurrence of sleep less reliable and undermine its quality.

Ignorance of basic sleep needs and of aging-related changes in sleep are believed to be contributing factors for some insomnia episodes. Negative sleep hygiene is viewed as a common maintaining factor for chronic insomnia. Available research data, however, have not yet documented a prevention effect from public education efforts, and sleep hygiene as a single treatment has shown inconsistent results[48,56,57] (discussed in Stepanski and Wyatt[67]).

Pitfalls and Controversies

Physicians rarely ask patients about how they sleep, and patients tend not to initiate any discussion of sleep problems. Studies of clinical practice suggest that insomnia most often goes unrecognized by the patient's personal physician and, of course, that means in most instances it is not assessed or treated. Surveys of general practices have found that physicians are often unaware of severe insomnia in their patients. Two studies found that 60% to 64% of severe insomnia cases went unrecognized.[68,69]

Even when physicians identify insomnia and prescribe medication for sleep, there is usually no documented evaluation of sleep. In one study, 88% of the medical charts for patients receiving hypnotic medication contained no reference to sleep in the progress notes.[70]

HYPNOTIC-DEPENDENT INSOMNIA

Chronic use of hypnotic medication can develop HDI, a new disorder characterized by a pattern of tolerance and dependence, and rebound insomnia on discontinuation (see also Chapter 115). This section reviews HDI, with a particular focus on the psychological aspects of dependence and on the benefits of treatment using psychological intervention concurrent with tapered withdrawal.

Epidemiology

Estimating the prevalence of HDI is difficult. Chronic insomnia occurs in 15% to 20% of the population.[30] Although hypnotics are the treatment of choice, not all patients with insomnia are treated with medication, and of those who are, only a small proportion actually develop HDI. Nonetheless, in the absence of data on HDI prevalence, estimates of chronic hypnotic use are the next best available source of information. Approximately 1.5% of adults in the general population[71] and approximately 7.1% of primary care patients report chronic hypnotic use.[29] Rates are generally higher for women and the elderly. Among primary care patients of all ages, 11.4% of women use sleep medication compared with only 8.6% of men.[29] Among older patients (75 years or older), one in five is a consumer of sleep medications.[29]

Pathogenesis

HDI typically develops slowly over time, yet it can develop in as quickly as in 1 week in some cases.[72] Factors influencing the rate of development include half-life, dosage, duration of use, and certain patient characteristics (overall health, other medications). Physical dependence has been documented primarily for benzodiazepines and older hypnotics (e.g., barbiturates), but it may occur with other prescribed and over-the-counter hypnotic medications. Hypnotic medication is recommended only for short-term use.[73] Although most patients intend to use medication for only a few days, some find themselves taking it for much longer as a predictable pattern of tolerance and dependence develops.[74-76] First, tolerance to the initial dosage develops, then insomnia symptoms return, and the patient increases the dosage. Over time, tolerance to the increased dosage develops, insomnia returns, and the dosage is increased again. Attempts to abruptly reduce or stop taking the medication produce withdrawal symptoms (nausea, muscle tension, aches, irritability, restlessness, and nervousness) and a return of insomnia (rebound insomnia and rebound anxiety). Thus, despite diminished therapeutic effectiveness, usage of the hypnotic medication is maintained.

Psychological factors often prolong dependence. *Negative reinforcement* occurs when the resumption of the hypnotic provides rapid relief from withdrawal symptoms. *Anticipation of rebound effects* may discourage withdrawal attempts. A single night of poor sleep can heighten anxiety, reinforcing the belief that sleep medication is necessary. Each failed discontinuation attempt *reduces self-efficacy* and discourages subsequent efforts to quit. Conditioning principles may also play a role. Intermittent or "as needed" administration schedules are recommended to prevent tolerance, but they can promote habitual use. Benzodiazepines can produce *reversed sleep-state misperception,* in which users underestimate the amount of time spent awake while on benzodiazepines and perceive their sleep quality to be better than it is on the basis of sleep electroencephalography. On withdrawal, awareness of sleep difficulties returns and medication is resumed.

Clinical Features

Tolerance and dependence are primary features.[36] Withdrawal symptoms may include rebound insomnia or excessive sleepiness, anxiety, nervousness, and depression. Individuals taking extremely high doses and older adults are at greater risk for more severe withdrawal symptoms, such as seizures and hallucinations.[77]

Diagnosis

The patient typically presents with complaints of poor sleep or excessive daytime sleepiness, despite nearly daily use of a hypnotic medication for at least 3 weeks.[36] Other mental or medical disorders, including other sleep disorders, may be present, but they do not account for the primary symptom.

Treatment

To minimize withdrawal symptoms, gradual tapered withdrawal is generally recommended and typically takes 8 to 12 weeks.[74,78] Two weeks of baseline sleep diary recording is useful for creating a withdrawal plan.[74] Withdrawal often involves dosage reductions of 10% to 25% at 1- to 2-week intervals.[74,77] Once the lowest available dosage is reached, medication-free nights are gradually introduced (1 or 2 nights at first). Finally, medication is stopped completely. If tapered withdrawal fails, DuPont[78] recommended switching to a longer-acting, cross-tolerant medication (e.g., clonazepam) or using medication to suppress the withdrawal symptoms (e.g., carbamazepine). In rare cases, inpatient detoxification may be needed.

Concurrent Psychological Treatment

Psychological treatment either alone[53,79] or combined with tapered withdrawal[80-84] may facilitate medication reduction. In clinical practice settings, Morgan and colleagues[79] found that higher anxiety and a less positive attitude toward symptom control predicted a poor response to psychological treatment for HDI. Morin and colleagues[74] provide an overview of studies examining the efficacy of behavioral interventions in the management of hypnotic discontinuation. The following randomized clinical trials have been performed.

Morin and colleagues[85] recently compared tapered withdrawal, CBT for insomnia, and combined medication withdrawal and CBT in 76 older adults. All three interventions significantly reduced sleep medication usage. However, 85% of participants receiving the combined treatment were medication free at the end of treatment, compared with 48% for tapered withdrawal and 54% for CBT alone. Sleep diary data revealed greater sleep improvements for CBT (alone and combined) than for tapered withdrawal only.

Our laboratory achieved 80% hypnotic medication reduction, modest sleep gains, and minor side effects when testing the results of relaxation[81] and stimulus control.[84] Preliminary data are available on 35 hypnotic-dependent older adults involved in a placebo-controlled clinical trial comparing combined gradual hypnotic withdrawal and psychological treatment (relaxation, stimulus control, and sleep hygiene) to hypnotic withdrawal only and placebo treatment.[80] Despite similar reductions in medication for the three groups (average 84% reduction), self-reported sleep improved only for the combined condition. Polysomnography results revealed no sleep deterioration associated with withdrawal.

Clinical Course and Prevention

Rebound insomnia and other withdrawal symptoms can occur with most hypnotic medications but are more likely to occur after abrupt withdrawal from benzodiazepines with rapid or intermediate elimination rates.[86] Symptoms can appear within 1 or 2 days after discontinuation of short half-life benzodiazepines, but they may not occur until 4 to 10 days after withdrawal from longer half-life benzodiazepines.[87]

Strategies for minimizing the risk of dependence include the following[74]:

1. Minimizing the duration of the hypnotic treatment
2. Education about the psychological factors (described earlier) that can contribute to the development and maintenance of dependence
3. Education about the transient nature of rebound insomnia, and, for those taking benzodiazepines, about reverse sleep-state misperception

Behavioral intervention either alone or initiated with hypnotic treatment may also prove beneficial.

Relapse Prevention after Withdrawal

Morin and colleagues[74] recommend follow-up sessions in addition to encouraging patients to adopt the following strategies:

1. Avoid or prevent situations in which insomnia and hypnotic medication usage are likely to occur.
2. Develop a plan for dealing or coping with an occasional poor night's sleep.
3. Recognize and accept that periodic sleep difficulties are natural and expected. (This can prevent patients from jumping to the conclusion that chronic insomnia has returned.)

Pitfalls and Controversies

The newer nonbenzodiazepine hypnotics, which include zolpidem and zaleplon, and the sedating antidepressants (i.e., trazodone, amitriptyline, and doxepin), have been characterized as highly safe and effective, with little risk of tolerance/dependence. Although scant data support the hypnotic efficacy of the sedating antidepressants, short-term clinical trials with zolpidem[88] and zaleplon[89,90] have typically supported positive expectations. Recently, however, reports of negative effects and side effects have appeared. Both zolpidem and trazodone have produced rebound insomnia on withdrawal[89,91,92] and performance deficits in laboratory tests.[91,92] Zolpidem has also been associated with anxiety, and subjective ratings suggestive of abuse potential.[91] The sedating antidepressants have been associated with a number of negative effects, including physiologic dependence, constipation, cardiac conduction delays, and a higher risk of motor vehicle accidents.[93]

CLINICAL MANAGEMENT RECOMMENDATIONS

Practical, clinical recommendations are available[94] that should help guide the management of these insomnias. Compared with most psychological interventions, treatment of insomnia is relatively short term. A robust treatment course usually involves only 6 to 10 sessions. If drug weaning is required, then the treatment period may be extended, but weekly meetings may not be required to complete tapering. CBT interventions are compatible with each other, and it is common to gather several together in a treatment package. Treatments may be presented concurrently, partially overlapping, or sequentially. We recommend tailoring the package components and their sequence to match the symptom profile of the patient.

Clinical Pearls

When you encounter what appears to be secondary insomnia, proceed on the assumption that it is primary insomnia. You will probably be at least partially correct, and your patients will be grateful.

Physicians should check for sleep problems when they take a history from older adults, and they should offer psychological treatments for late-life insomnia; the treatments are safe and effective.

Women and older adults are particularly susceptible to developing hypnotic-dependent insomnia, a new disorder resulting from chronic use of hypnotic medication. To minimize withdrawal symptoms and to obtain optimal outcomes, tapered withdrawal concurrent with psychological treatment is recommended.

REFERENCES

1. McCrae CS, Lichstein KL: Secondary insomnia: Diagnostic challenges and intervention opportunities. Sleep Med Rev 2001;5: 47-61.
2. Ford DE, Kamerow DB: Epidemiologic study of sleep disturbances and psychiatric disorders: An opportunity for prevention? JAMA 1989;262:1479-1484.
3. Ohayon MM: Prevalence of DSM-IV diagnostic criteria of insomnia: Distinguishing insomnia related to mental disorders from sleep disorders. J Psychiatr Res 1997;31:333-346.
4. Lichstein KL: Secondary insomnia. In Lichstein KL, Morin CM (eds): Treatment of Late-Life Insomnia. Thousand Oaks, Calif, Sage, 2000, pp 297-319.
5. Aldrich MS: Insomnia in neurological diseases. J Psychosom Res 1993;37(Suppl 1):3-11.
6. Moldofsky H: Sleep and pain. Sleep Med Rev 2001;5:387-398.
7. Hu DS, Silberfarb PM: Management of sleep problems in cancer patients. Oncology 1991;59:23-27.
8. Moran MG, Stoudemire A: Sleep disorders in the medically ill patient. J Clin Psychiatry 1992;53(Suppl):29-36.
9. Schneider-Helmert D, Whitehouse I, Kumar A, et al: Insomnia and alpha sleep in chronic non-organic pain as compared to primary insomnia. Neuropsychobiology 2001;43:54-58.
10. Lichstein KL, Durrence HH, Riedel BW, et al: Primary versus secondary insomnia in older adults: Subjective sleep and daytime functioning. Psychol Aging 2001;16:264-271.
11. Smith MT, Perlis ML, Smith MS, et al: Sleep quality and presleep arousal in chronic pain. J Behav Med 2000;23:1-13.
12. Lichstein KL, McCrae CS, Wilson NM: Secondary insomnia: Diagnostic issues, cognitive-behavioral treatment, and future directions. In Perlis ML, Lichstein KL (eds): Treating Sleep Disorders: Principles and Practice of Behavioral Sleep Medicine. New York, Wiley, 2003, pp 286-304.
13. Cannici J, Malcolm R, Peek LA: Treatment of insomnia in cancer patients using muscle relaxation training. J Behav Ther Exp Psychiatry 1983;14:251-256.

14. Currie SR, Wilson KG, Pontefract AJ, et al: Cognitive-behavioral treatment of insomnia secondary to chronic pain. J Consult Clin Psychol 2000;68:407-416.

15. Lichstein KL, Wilson NM, Johnson CT: Psychological treatment of secondary insomnia. Psychol Aging 2000;15:232-240.

16. Katz DA, McHorney CA: Clinical correlates of insomnia in patients with chronic illness. Arch Intern Med 1998;158:1099-1107.

17. Affleck G, Urrows S, Tennen H, et al: Sequential daily relations of sleep pain intensity and attention to pain among women with fibromyalgia. Pain 1996;68:363-368.

18. Morin CM, Kowatch RA, Wade JB: Behavioral management of sleep disturbances secondary to chronic pain. J Behav Ther Exp Psychiatry 1989;20:295-302.

19. Paiva T, Batista A, Martins P, Martins A: The relationship between headaches and sleep disturbances. Headache 1995;35:590-596.

20. Taylor DJ, Lichstein KL, Durrence HH: Insomnia as a health risk factor. Behav Sleep Med 2003;1:227-247.

21. McCrae CS, Lichstein KL: Secondary insomnia: A heuristic model and behavioral approaches to assessment treatment and prevention. Appl Prev Psychol 2001;10:107-123.

22. Marlatt GA, George WH: Relapse prevention and the maintenance of optimal health. In Shumaker SA, Schron EB, Ockene JK, et al (eds): The Handbook of Health Behavior Change, 2nd ed. New York, Springer, 1998, pp 33-58.

23. Meichenbaum D: Cognitive-Behavior Modification: An Integrative Approach. New York, Plenum, 1977.

24. Atkinson JH, Ancoli-Israel S, Slater MA, et al: Subjective sleep disturbance in chronic back pain. Clin J Pain 1988;4:225-232.

25. Pilowsky I, Crettenden I, Townley M: Sleep disturbance in pain clinic patients. Pain 1985;23:27-33.

26. American Psychiatric Association: Diagnostic and Statistical Manual of Mental Disorders, 4th ed. Washington, DC, American Psychiatric Association, 1994.

27. Savard J, Morin CM: Insomnia in the context of cancer: A review of a neglected problem. J Clin Oncol 2001;19:895-908.

28. Lichstein KL, Riedel BW, Means MK: Psychological treatment of late-life insomnia. Annu Rev Gerontol Geriatr 1999;18:74-110.

29. Ohayon MM, Caulet M, Arbus L, et al: Are prescribed medications effective in the treatment of insomnia complaints? J Psychosom Res 1999;47:359-368.

30. Ohayon MM: Epidemiology of insomnia: What we know and what we still need to learn. Sleep Med Rev 2002;6:97-111.

31. WB&A: Sleep in America: 2003. New York, WB&A Market Research, 2003.

32. Mellinger GD, Balter MB, Uhlenhuth EH: Insomnia and its treatment. Arch Gen Psychiatry 1985;42:225-232.

33. Ray WA, Griffin MR, Downey W: Benzodiazepines of long and short elimination half-life and the risk of hip fracture. JAMA 1989;262:3303-3307.

34. Roehrs T, Merlotti L, Zorick F, et al: Sedative, memory, and performance effects of hypnotics. Psychopharmacol 1994;116:130-134.

35. Coleman RM: Diagnosis, treatment and follow-up of about 8,000 sleep/wake disorder patients. In Guilleminault C, Lugaresi E (eds): Sleep/Wake Disorders: Natural History, Epidemiology, and Long-Term Evolution. New York, Raven Press, 1983, pp 87-97.

36. American Sleep Disorders Association: International Classification of Sleep Disorders: Revised. Rochester, Minn, American Sleep Disorders Association, 1997.

37. Sateia MJ, Doghramji K, Hauri PJ, et al: Evaluation of chronic insomnia: An American Academy of Sleep Medicine review. Sleep 2000;23:243-308.

38. Lichstein KL: Clinical Relaxation Strategies. New York, Wiley, 1988.

39. Bootzin RR, Epstein DR: Stimulus control: In Lichstein KL, Morin CM (eds): Treatment of Late-Life Insomnia. Thousand Oaks, Calif, Sage, 2000, pp 167-184.

40. Spielman AJ, Saskin P, Thorpy MJ: Treatment of chronic insomnia by restriction of time in bed. Sleep 1987;10:45-56.

41. Lichstein KL, Riedel BW, Wilson NM, et al: Relaxation and sleep compression for late-life insomnia: A placebo-controlled trial. J Consult Clin Psychol 2001;69:227-239.

42. Morin CM, Savard J, Blais FC: Cognitive Therapy. In Lichstein KL, Morin CM (eds): Treatment of Late-Life Insomnia. Thousand Oaks, Calif, Sage, 2000, pp 207-230.

43. Alperson J, Biglan A: Self-administered treatment of sleep onset insomnia and the importance of age. Behav Ther 1979;10:347-356.

44. Edinger JD, Hoelscher TJ, Marsh GR, et al: A cognitive-behavioral therapy for sleep-maintenance insomnia in older adults. Psychol Aging 1992;7:282-289.

45. Morin CM, Kowatch RA, Barry T, et al: Cognitive-behavior therapy for late-life insomnia. J Consult Clin Psychol 1993;61:137-146.

46. Morin CM, Colecchi C, Stone J, et al: Behavioral and pharmacological therapies for late-life insomnia: A randomized controlled trial. JAMA 1999;281:991-999.

47. Davies R, Lacks P, Storandt M, et al: Countercontrol treatment of sleep-maintenance insomnia in relation to age. Psychol Aging 1986;3:233-238.

48. Engle-Friedman M, Bootzin RR, Hazlewood L, et al: An evaluation of behavioral treatments for insomnia in the older adult. J Clin Psychol 1992;48:77-90.

49. Morin CM, Azrin NH: Behavioral and cognitive treatments of geriatric insomnia. J Consult Clin Psychol 1988;56:748-753.

50. Pallesen S, Nordhus IH, Kvale G, et al: Behavioral treatment of insomnia in older adults: An open clinical trial comparing two interventions. Behav Res Ther 2003;41:31-48.

51. Puder R, Lacks P, Bertelson A, et al: Short-term stimulus control treatment of insomnia in older adults. Behav Ther 1983;14:424-429.

52. Friedman L, Bliwise DL, Yesavage JA, Salom SR: A preliminary study comparing sleep restriction and relaxation treatments for insomnia in older adults. J Gerontol 1991;46:1-8.

53. Lichstein KL, Johnson RS: Relaxation for insomnia and hypnotic medication use in older women. Psychol Aging 1993;8:103-111.

54. Lick JR, Heffler D: Relaxation training and attention placebo in the treatment of severe insomnia. J Consult Clin Psychol 1977;45:153-161.

55. Nicassio P, Bootzin R: A comparison of progressive relaxation and autogenic training as treatments for insomnia. J Abnorm Psychol 1974;83:253-260.

56. Friedman L, Benson K, Noda A, et al: An actigraphic comparison of sleep restriction and sleep hygiene treatments for insomnia in older adults. J Geriatr Psychiatry Neurol 2000;13:17-27.

57. Riedel BW, Lichstein KL, Dwyer WO: Sleep compression and sleep education for older insomniacs: Self-help vs. therapist guidance. Psychol Aging 1995;10:54-63.

58. Morin CM, Culbert JP, Schwartz SM: Nonpharmacological interventions for insomnia: A meta-analysis of treatment efficacy. Am J Psychiatry 1994;151:1172-1180.

59. Brooks JO, Friedman L, Bliwise DL, et al: Use of the wrist actigraph to study insomnia in older adults. Sleep 1993;16:151-155.

60. Chesson AL, Anderson WM, Littner M, et al: Practice parameters for the nonpharmacological treatment of chronic insomnia: An American Academy of Sleep Medicine report. Sleep 1999;22:1128-33.

61. Rybarczyk B, Lopez M, Benson R, et al: Efficacy of two behavioral treatment programs for comorbid geriatric insomnia. Psychol Aging 2002;17:288-298.

62. Bliwise NG: Factors related to sleep quality in healthy elderly women. Psychol Aging 1992;7:83-88.

63. Fichten CS, Creti L, Amsel R, et al: Poor sleepers who do not complain of insomnia: Myths and realities about psychological

and lifestyle characteristics of older good and poor sleepers. J Behav Med 1995;18:189-223.

64. Morin CM, Gaulier B, Barry T, et al: Patients' acceptance of psychological and pharmacological therapies for insomnia. Sleep 1992;15:302-305.

65. Hauri P: The Sleep Disorders, 2nd ed. Kalamazoo, Mich, Upjohn, 1982.

66. Hauri P: Sleep hygiene, relaxation therapy, and cognitive interventions. In Hauri P (ed): Case Studies in Insomnia. New York, Plenum, 1991, pp 65-84.

67. Stepanski EJ, Wyatt JK: Use of sleep hygiene in the treatment of insomnia. Sleep Med Rev 2003;7:215-225.

68. Hohagen F, Rink K, Kappler C, et al: Prevalence and treatment of insomnia in general practice: A longitudinal study. Eur Arch Psychiatry Clin Neurosci. 1993;242:329-36.

69. Schramm E, Hohagen F, Kappler C: Mental comorbidity of chronic insomnia in general practice attenders using DSM-III-R. Acta Psychiatr Scand 1995;91:7-10.

70. Shorr R, Bauwens S: Diagnosis and treatment of outpatient insomnia by psychiatric and non-psychiatric physicians. Am J Med 1992;93:78-82.

71. Ohayon MM, Caulet M, Priest RG, et al: Psychotropic medication consumption patterns in the UK general population. J Clin Epidemiol 1998;51:273-283.

72. Greenblatt DJ, Harmatz JS, Zinny MA, et al: Effect of gradual withdrawal on the rebound sleep disorder after discontinuation of triazolam. N Engl J Med 1987;317:722-728.

73. National Institutes of Health: NIH Consens Statement: The Treatment of Sleep Disorders of Older People, March 26-28, 1990. Sleep 1991;14:169-177.

74. Morin CM, Baillargeon L, Bastien C: Discontinuation of sleep medications. In Lichstein KL, Morin CM (eds): Treatment of Late Life Insomnia. Thousand Oaks, Calif, Sage, 2000, pp 271-296.

75. Barnas C, Whitworth AB, Fleischhacker WW: Are patterns of benzodiazepine use predictable? A follow-up study of benzodiazepine use. Psychopharmacology 1993;111:301-305.

76. Barter G, Cormack M: The long-term use of benzodiazepines: Patients' views, accounts and experiences. Fam Pract 1996;13:491-497.

77. Landry MJ, Smith DE, McDuff DR, Braughman OL 3rd. Benzodiazepine dependence and withdrawal: Identification and medical management. J Am Board Fam Pract 1992;5:167-175.

78. DuPont RL: A physician's guide to discontinuing benzodiazepine therapy. West J Med 1990;152:600-603.

79. Morgan K, Thompson J, Dixon S, et al: Predicting longer-term outcomes following psychological treatment for hypnotic-dependent chronic insomnia. J Psychosom Res 2003;54:21-29.

80. Lichstein KL, McCrae CS, Wilson NM, et al: Treatment of hypnotic dependence in older adults: Pre-post PSG effects. Paper presented at the Associated Professional Sleep Societies, Chicago, Ill, June, 2003.

81. Lichstein KL, Peterson BA, Riedel BW, et al: Relaxation to assist sleep medication withdrawal. Behav Modif 1999;23:379-402.

82. Morin CM, Colecchi CA, Ling WD, et al: Cognitive behavior therapy to facilitate benzodiazepine discontinuation among hypnotic-dependent patients with insomnia. Behavior Therapy 1995;26:733-745.

83. Morin CM, Stone J, McDonald K, et al: Psychological management of insomnia: A clinical replication series with 100 patients. Behav Ther 1994;25:291-309.

84. Riedel BW, Lichstein KL, Peterson BA, et al: A comparison of the efficacy of stimulus control for medicated and non-medicated insomniacs. Behav Modif 1998;22:3-28.

85. Morin CM, Bastien C, Guay B, et al: Randomized clinical trial of supervised tapering and cognitive behavior therapy to facilitate benzodiazepine discontinuation in older adults with chronic insomnia. Am J Psychiatry 2004;161:332-342.

86. Kales A, Soldatos CR, Bixler EO, Kales JD: Rebound insomnia and rebound anxiety: A review. Pharmacology 1983;26:121-137.

87. Gilin JC, Spinweber CL, Johnson, LC: Rebound insomnia: A critical review. J Clin Psychopharmacol 1989;9:161-172.

88. Holm KJ, Goa KL: Zolpidem: An update of its pharmacology, therapeutic efficacy and tolerability in the treatment of insomnia. Drugs 2000;59:865-889.

89. Elie R, Ruther E, Farr I, et al: Sleep latency is shortened during 4 weeks of treatment with zaleplon, a novel nonbenzodiazepine hypnotic. Zaleplon Clinical Study Group. J Clin Psychiatry 1999; 60:536-544.

90. Walsh JK, Vogel GW, Scharf M, et al: A five week, polysomnographic assessment of zaleplon 10 mg for the treatment of primary insomnia. Sleep Med 2000;1:41-49.

91. Rush CR, Baker RW, Wright K: Acute behavioral effects and abuse potential of trazodone, zolpidem and triazolam in humans. Psychopharmacology (Berl) 1999;144:220-233.

92. Troy SM, Lucki I, Unruh M A, et al: Comparison of the effects of zaleplon, zolpidem, and triazolam on memory, learning, and psychomotor performance. J Clin Psychopharmacol 2000; 20:328-337.

93. Buysse DJ, Reynolds CF: Pharmacologic treatment. In Lichstein KL, Morin CM (eds): Treatment of Late-Life Insomnia. Thousand Oaks, Calif, Sage, 2000, pp 231-267.

94. Lichstein KL, Morin CM: Treatment overview. In Lichstein KL, Morin CM (eds): Treatment of Late Life Insomnia. Thousand Oaks, Calif, Sage, 2000, pp 111-124.

Pharmacologic Treatm... of Primary Insomni...

James K. Walsh
Timothy Roehrs
Thomas Roth

ABSTRACT

The benzodiazepine receptor agonists are clearly efficacious in the treatment of insomnia, and they are among the safest central nervous system drugs in common clinical use. Indeed, available data, although limited, suggest a substantial degree of effectiveness in clinical practice. Sufficient variability in pharmacokinetics and receptor selectivity exists among the benzodiazepine receptor agonists to provide the physician with a variety of valuable therapeutic choices. Sedating antidepressants, antihistamines, antipsychotics, and other drugs are also commonly used to promote sleep, despite the absence of adequate efficacy and safety data to allow evidence-based treatment decisions, particularly for the treatment of primary insomnia. Before these drugs are used as a first-line treatment for insomnia, research detailing their efficacy and safety is clearly needed. The changing views of the etiology and morbidities associated with primary insomnia will undoubtedly alter the clinician's approach to pharmacologic management in the future.

A variety of drugs have been shown to possess sedative properties, but a sedative effect does not necessarily translate to hypnotic efficacy. Specifically, it does not provide information about dose-related risk-to-benefit ratios so critical to assessment of therapeutics. Hypnotic efficacy is the capacity of a drug, at a specified dose or dose range, and in the context of controlled research, to improve sleep in people with chronic insomnia or in normal sleepers with a transient disruption to their sleep. Effectiveness of a hypnotic refers to the degree to which insomnia and its morbidity are improved by a drug when utilized in clinical practice or in studies that approximate the typical therapeutic situation. Thus, a hypnotic drug that reduces sleep latency and increases total sleep time may be highly efficacious, but it would be minimally effective if side effects prevent its use in clinical practice. Whether efficacy or effectiveness is of interest, a variety of different measures are available, and conclusions regarding a drug may differ depending on the measure selected.

This chapter reviews what is known about efficacy, effectiveness, and safety for those drugs used to treat insomnia. The classes of drugs and individual agents most commonly used are discussed, including benzodiazepines and nonbenzodiazepines that act at benzodiazepine receptors (together referred to as benzodiazepine receptor agonists [BzRAs]), sedating antidepressants, antihistamines, and antipsychotics.

After the various pharmacologic options are discussed, indications and contraindications for treatment of primary insomnia with hypnotic medication are presented. Finally, implementation and assessment strategies for the pharmacologic treatment of primary insomnia are summarized.

DRUGS COMMONLY USED AS HYPNOTICS

What is known about the efficacy and effectiveness of the drugs most commonly used to treat insomnia varies substantially. Much more is known about drugs with a Food and Drug Administration (FDA) indication for the treatment of insomnia than about "off-label use" of sedating antidepressants and other drugs used as hypnotics. Yet, from 1987 to 1996, the following dramatic changes in the pharmacologic management of insomnia occurred[1]:

1. The use of sedating antidepressants increased 146%.
2. The use of drugs with an FDA indication for the treatment of insomnia decreased 53.7%.
3. The use of "other" sedating drugs (e.g., antihistamines, barbiturates) fell 63.2%.

By 1996, antidepressants were used as frequently as FDA-indicated drugs for the treatment of insomnia. Data from the *Physician Drug and Diagnosis Audit* (Verispan, Yardley, Pa) for 2002 provide an updated estimate of the relative frequency with which various drugs were used to treat insomnia.[2] Antidepressants accounted for 5.268 million occurrences for the treatment of insomnia, compared with 3.442 million for drugs with an insomnia indication, 0.822 million for anxiolytics, 0.815 million for antipsychotics, 0.552 million for anticonvulsants, and 0.220 million for antihistamines. The 16 most commonly identified drugs for the treatment of insomnia in 2002 are shown in Table 63–1. Three of the four drugs with the most insomnia-related occurrences are antidepressants, and only 4 of the top 16 have an FDA indication for insomnia.

To our knowledge, the frequency with which specific medications are used for the treatment of insomnia of different etiologies is unknown; more important, no evidence exists for differential efficacies of sedating drugs for different insomnia etiologies. For example, it is unknown whether antidepressants are, or should be, used more commonly to treat insomnia secondary to depressive disorders than to treat primary insomnia. However, in 1996,[1] fewer than 40% of trazodone occurrences of use for insomnia were concomitant with the use of another antidepressant, and 66.5% were at a dose of

...monly Used Drugs for Insomnia in 2002

	Rank*	FDA Indication(s)	Projected Number of Occurrences (Million)
	1	Depression	2.730
	2	Insomnia	2.074
	3	Depression	0.774
	4	Depression	0.662
	5	Insomnia	0.558
Quetiapine	6	Schizophrenia	0.459
Zaleplon	7	Insomnia	0.405
Clonazepam	8	Seizure and panic disorders	0.394
Hydroxyzine	9	Anxiety; pruritus	0.293
Alprazolam	10	Anxiety and panic disorders	0.287
Lorazepam	11	Anxiety	0.277
Olanzapine	12	Schizophrenia	0.216
Flurazepam	13	Insomnia	0.205
Doxepin	14	Depression	0.199
Cyclobenzaprine	15	Muscle spasm	0.195
Diphenhydramine	16	Allergy; motion sickness; parkinsonism	0.192

*These 16 drugs were identified in the 2002 *Physician Drug and Diagnosis Audit* (Verispan, Yardley, Pa) as having the highest projected number of occurrences of side effects associated with the desired actions of "hypnotic," "promote sleep," or "sedate night."

FDA, U.S. Food and Drug Administration.

100 mg or less (lower than the 150-mg dose recommended as the initial daily dose for depression). In 2002, 84% of trazodone occurrences for treatment of insomnia were doses of 100 mg or less.[2] This information suggests that trazodone is commonly used to treat insomnia regardless of etiology. That is, trazodone and other sedating drugs are being used to provide symptomatic treatment of insomnia in much the way drugs with an indication for insomnia are used.

The majority of investigations characterizing the efficacy and safety of hypnotic drugs were conducted with BzRAs, using either normal volunteers or persons with primary insomnia. The generalizability of those data to other insomnia populations is probably considerable, but it is not well documented. Importantly, much less is known about drugs used to treat insomnia with mechanisms of action other than agonism of the benzodiazepine receptor, despite the frequency of use as discussed previously (see Chapter 37).

BENZODIAZEPINE RECEPTOR AGONISTS

All drugs currently indicated for the treatment of insomnia in the United States are BzRAs, and most experts recommend BzRAs as first-line pharmacologic therapy for insomnia.[3,4] The name of this group of drugs is derived from their recognized mechanism of action (see Chapter 36), which involves occupation of benzodiazepine receptors on the gamma-aminobutyric acid (GABA), type A, receptor complex, resulting in the opening of chloride ion channels and facilitation of GABA inhibition. Some of these drugs (described in Table 63–2) have a benzodiazepine chemical structure (e.g., estazolam, flurazepam, quazepam, temazepam, triazolam) and others do not (zaleplon, zolpidem, eszopiclone). One of the BzRAs under development (indiplon) for which adequate data are available is also included in Table 63–2.

Binding affinities of the benzodiazepines for most GABA, type A, receptor subtypes are similar. On the other hand, the affinities of zolpidem and zaleplon for the receptor subtype with an alpha-1 subunit are much higher than for other subtypes. Because receptors with alpha-1 subunits mediate sedation, amnesia, and some of the anticonvulsant properties, but not anxiolysis or myorelaxation, it is possible that these more selective drugs will have hypnotic effects with fewer side effects.[5] However, this remains to be definitely demonstrated.

The BzRAs are generally recommended as first-line hypnotics for several reasons. All BzRAs have been shown to be efficacious, although there are some differences between drugs, associated with pharmacokinetic properties. Compared with other drug classes, the margin of safety or therapeutic index (i.e., the effective dose relative to lethal dose) is wide.[6] For example, barbiturates have margins of safety on the order of two to four times the effective dose, whereas for BzRAs, the margin of safety can be as great as 100. Abuse of or dependence on BzRAs is infrequent in the therapeutic context, most likely accounted for by the relatively mild reinforcing effects and self-administration patterns. Summaries of the efficacy, effectiveness, and safety characteristics of BzRAs follow. Unless otherwise stated, the summary material refers to recommended dosages of the drugs.

Efficacy and Effectiveness

Measurement of hypnotic efficacy involves polysomnographic (PSG) or patient estimates of induction and maintenance of sleep, or both. Sleep latency (whether PSG or self-report) is the standard sleep induction variable, and the number of awakenings and wake after sleep onset (WASO) are the most common sleep maintenance measures. Total sleep time and sleep efficiency reflect both sleep induction and sleep maintenance properties. Qualitative measures of efficacy are also used, such as morning ratings of sleep quality, sleep depth, or global impression ratings by either an investigator or the patient.

Table 63–2. Characteristics of Benzodiazepine Receptor Agonists for Insomnia

Drug	Chemical Class	Recommended Dose (mg) in Adults; in Older Adults	$t_{1/2}$ (hr)	Receptor Binding
Estazolam	Benzodiazepine	2; 1	8-24	Nonselective
Eszopiclone	Cyclopyrrolone	2, 3; 1	5-7	Nonselective
Flurazepam	Benzodiazepine	30; 15	48-120*	Nonselective
Indiplon	Pyrazolopyrimidine	Under development	1.0-1.5	GABA$_A$ alpha 1
Quazepam	Benzodiazepine	7.5-15; same	48-120*	Nonselective
Temazepam	Benzodiazepine	30; 15	8-20	Nonselective
Triazolam	Benzodiazepine	0.25; 0.125	2-4	Nonselective
Zaleplon	Pyrazolopyrimidine	10; 5	~1.0	GABA$_A$ alpha 1, gamma 3
Zolpidem	Imidazopyridine	10; 5	1.5-2.4	GABA$_A$ alpha 1

The benzodiazepine receptor agonists listed have an FDA indication for treatment of insomnia, or they are currently in phase 3 clinical trials.

*Refers to elimination half-life of active metabolite, desalkylflurazepam.

FDA, U.S. Food and Drug Administration; GABA$_A$, gamma-aminobutyric acid, type A receptor.

The monitoring of motor activity with a wrist-worn sensor (actigraphy) has also been used to evaluate hypnotic efficacy.

Many studies have documented the hypnotic efficacy of BzRAs using patient reports or PSG outcomes, or both.[3,4] A meta-analysis in 1997 concluded that benzodiazepines and zolpidem produce reliable improvements in the sleep of persons with chronic insomnia, although the median duration of the studies included was only 1 week.[7] Other meta-analyses largely concur regarding short-term efficacy. However, the utility of these meta-analyses to assist the clinician is fairly low, because they combine data from multiple drugs with widely different pharmacokinetics (which impacts the outcome variables examined in the meta-analysis). Additionally, two or more doses of a drug may be included in the analysis. It is much more instructive to examine the strengths and weaknesses of individual drugs as opposed to generalizing across all BzRAs, all antidepressants, or other classification of convenience. Here, similarities among BzRAs will be discussed globally, but important differences among drugs will be emphasized.

All of the BzRA hypnotics reduce sleep latency, and most increase total sleep time. The exception is zaleplon, which does not reliably increase total sleep time. The reduction of sleep latency is attributable to a rapid onset of hypnotic effect. Specific sleep maintenance variables, as distinct from total sleep time, have not commonly been reported. Those investigations assessing number of awakenings and/or WASO typically find that the longer the drug's duration of action (i.e., the longer half-life or higher dose), the more likely it is that the drug will show efficacy on these measures. It should be noted that WASO and number of awakenings have not been widely reported or extensively validated as measures of hypnotic efficacy.

Tolerance is defined as a reduction of a drug effect with repeated administration of a constant dose, or the need to increase dose to sustain a specific level of effect. Despite frequent speculations in the medical literature, tolerance to the hypnotic effects of BzRAs does not develop in the vast majority of studies, at least for therapeutic doses and for the periods of time that have been studied. Investigations that are often cited as evidence for tolerance development, such as Mitler et al.,[8]

show gradual improvement in sleep over time in the placebo group, versus a constant effect in the drug group, resulting in loss of statistical significance. Yet the sleep of the active drug groups does not worsen with time on a stable dose of drug. Thus, it cannot be concluded that tolerance has developed, but rather that unspecified changes occur over time with placebo, such as spontaneous remission, regression to the mean (if there are sleep disruption entry criteria), sleep hygiene influences inherent in protocol adherence, Hawthorne effects, and true "placebo" effects.

More than 20 years ago, Oswald and colleagues[9] reported that lormetazepam and nitrazepam, two benzodiazepines, retained their effect by some patient estimates of hypnotic efficacy during 24 weeks of use. More recently, in rigorous PSG studies, zolpidem 10 mg and zaleplon 10 mg (two nonbenzodiazepines) were shown to retain efficacy for 5 weeks of nightly use.[10,11] Unpublished investigations of estazolam 2 mg and triazolam 0.25 mg found sustained efficacy for 10 to 12 weeks of nightly use. A recent landmark study of several hundred patients with primary insomnia showed continued hypnotic efficacy of eszopiclone for 6 months of nightly use.[12] Figure 63–1 illustrates that both subjective sleep latency and WASO are significantly reduced with eszopiclone 3 mg as compared with placebo at each monthly time point. Total sleep time, number of awakenings, and sleep quality were also better than with placebo at each monthly time point.

Efficacy of nonnightly use of zolpidem 10 mg has been investigated for up to 12 weeks.[13,14] In these studies, ratings of sleep latency, total sleep time, number of awakenings, and sleep quality were all improved on nights when zolpidem was taken, as compared with placebo. Additionally, investigator global ratings, which considered both medication nights and nonmedication nights, indicated reduced insomnia severity with zolpidem. Total sleep time data on nights when a pill (either zolpidem or placebo) was taken or not taken during an 8-week study are shown in Figure 63–2. Importantly, an examination of sleep on nights when no drug was taken immediately after a zolpidem night indicated no evidence of rebound insomnia.[13]

Controlled hypnotic effectiveness trials, per se, have not been carried out. However, some reports provide information

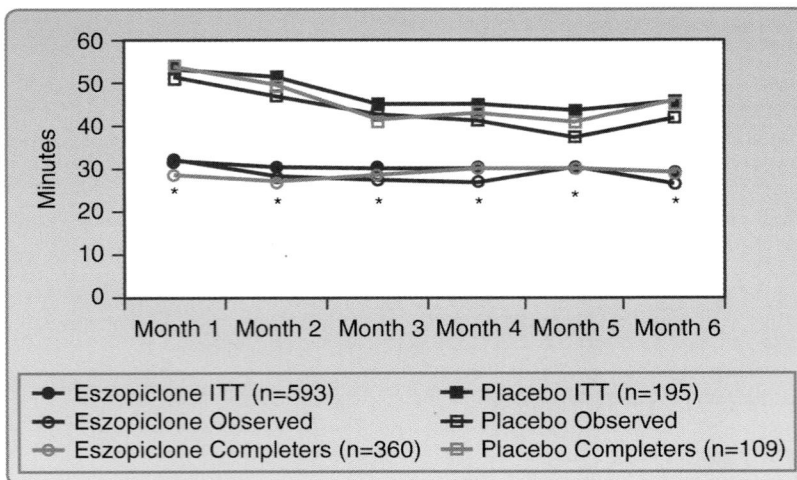

A

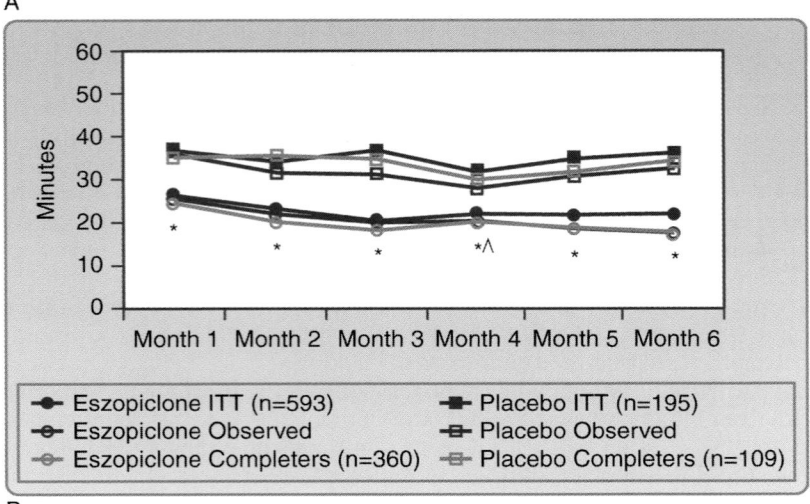

B

Figure 63–1. Results over 6 months of treatment with eszopiclone. Data are shown for the patients included in the intent to treat (ITT), observed case, and completed patient analyses. The nearly identical results obtained with all three analyses provides a high degree of confidence that the long-term efficacy observed cannot be explained by differential drop-out patterns or other factors in the two study groups. **A,** Median sleep latency in minutes. *$P < .005$ for comparison of eszopiclone to placebo for all three analyses. **B,** Median wake after sleep onset in minutes. *$P < .05$ for comparison of eszopiclone to placebo for all three analyses, except ∧ indicates $P = .07$ for the observed case analysis at month 4. (Adapted from Krystal AD, Walsh JK, Laska E, et al: Sustained efficacy of eszopiclone over 6 months of nightly treatment: Results of a randomized, double-blind, placebo-controlled study in adults with chronic insomnia. Sleep 2003;26:793-799.)

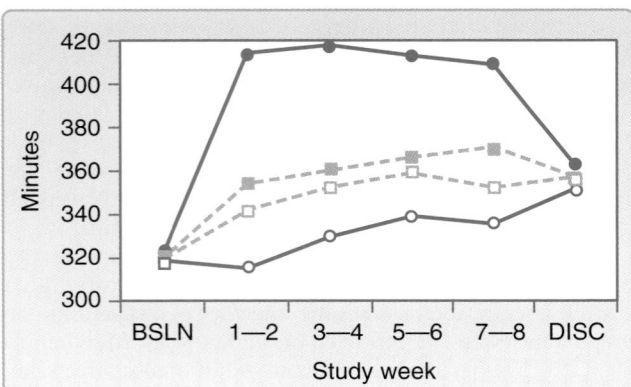

Figure 63–2. Mean subjective total sleep time for (A) zolpidem pill nights *(solid line/solid circles)*, (B) zolpidem no-pill nights *(solid line/open circles)*, (C) placebo pill nights *(dashed line/solid squares)*, and (D) placebo no-pill nights *(dashed line/open squares)* for 8 weeks. $P < .001$ for A versus C and for A versus B, each at study periods 1-2, 3-4, 5-6, and 7-8 weeks. BSLN, baseline (both groups receive placebo, double-blind); DISC, discontinuation week during which both groups received placebo, double-blind. (Adapted from Walsh JK, Roth T, Randazzo AC, et al: Eight weeks of non-nightly use of zolpidem for primary insomnia. Sleep 2000;23:1087-1096.)

on hypnotic use in the general population that may approximate reports of clinical investigations of effectiveness. Using an epidemiologic methodology, Ohayon and colleagues[15] reported that of 532 patients describing chronic insomnia and long-term use of hypnotic medications to help them sleep, 67% rated their sleep quality as improved "a lot," and only 14.4% reported little or no improvement with medication. Balter and Uhlenhuth[16] interviewed individuals who in the past year either reported significant trouble with insomnia or had taken a medication to help them sleep. They found very high satisfaction rates among hypnotic users when asked, "Taking into account both the positive effects on your sleep and daytime functioning and any negative effects you may have experienced, would you take this medication again for the same purpose?" Affirmative responses were received from 84% of those taking triazolam, 82% flurazepam, 74% temazepam, and 61% over-the-counter aids. In summarizing the findings of this intensive interview study, the authors concluded that "the benefits of treatment with prescription hypnotics are substantial and far outweigh the risks as defined in this study." It is important to recognize that in both of these studies, the cited data were obtained from either current users of sleep-promoting medications or those who had used them sometime in the past year. Thus, the generalizability of these findings is unknown.

Long-term open-label studies conducted in outpatient and nursing home settings also provide some information about effectiveness.[17-19] Zolpidem has been evaluated over periods of 6 to 12 months in such studies. In general, patients and physicians report sustained benefit of zolpidem for the duration of the studies, without adverse reactions unique to long-term use. Again, the generalizability of results and the confidence level regarding any conclusions drawn must be tempered by the self-selection of those remaining in these open-label studies.

Daytime Function

Most definitions of insomnia include some form of subjective daytime impairment consequent to the sleep disruption. Theoretically, it should be possible to demonstrate the insomnia-related impairment and a subsequent reduction of impairment with improved sleep. Elimination or reduction of the daytime problem would be another measure of treatment efficacy. Yet few studies have shown objectively documented daytime impairment in primary insomnia patients, and no study of primary insomnia has objectively documented improvement in waking function associated with improvement in sleep.

Related to this issue is the observation that patients with primary insomnia differ from normal subjects in daytime sleepiness/alertness and other measures of physiologic arousal. Rather than showing greater daytime sleepiness, as might be expected given their disturbed sleep and complaints of daytime tiredness, these patients with primary insomnia have longer daytime sleep latencies (as they do at night) than age-matched normal subjects.[20,21] Metabolic rate, heart rate variability, body temperature, and cortisol levels also reflect a hyperarousal trait of patients with primary insomnia, which is hypothesized to lead to disrupted sleep.[21-23] However, in the 6-month eszopiclone study of patients with primary insomnia performed by Krystal et al.,[12] patient reports of daytime alertness, ability to function during the daytime, and physical sense of well-being were all significantly better in the eszopiclone group than in the placebo group.

In contrast to primary insomniac patients, the waking impact of chronic insomnia may differ in other subgroups of insomnia patients. For example, patients with insomnia and periodic limb movement disorder[24] and those with insomnia and rheumatoid arthritis[25] have been shown to have lower than optimal Multiple Sleep Latency Test (MSLT) scores, which improve significantly after 6 nights' treatment with triazolam. A study of older adult patients showed increased daytime alertness on the MSLT resulting from increased sleep time with triazolam treatment.[26] In part, then, the difficulty in finding systematic daytime impairment in chronic insomnia may be the result of differing subgroups of insomniac patients.

Safety

In general, BzRAs are well-tolerated, with few significant safety concerns. For example, adverse reactions recorded in clinical trials or in clinical practice are infrequent and are most commonly rated as mild. For inpatient use in a large academic hospital, the median rate of adverse events, across all hypnotics, was found to be about 1 in every 10,000 doses.[27] Data on the frequency of abuse of hypnotic medications is not available.

However, a study in Switzerland in the early 1980s indicated that abuse of all benzodiazepines (not limited to use as a hypnotic) occurred at the rate of only 2 per 10,000 prescriptions.[28] Specific safety concerns for hypnotics are discussed in the following paragraphs.

RESIDUAL EFFECTS

Many of the side effects associated with BzRAs are mediated by their primary pharmacologic activity, sedation.[29] Residual sedation, which is merely a prolongation of the hypnotic effect of the drug into the daytime, results in adverse reactions such as drowsy feelings, sleepiness, and impairment in psychomotor performance. The likelihood of residual sedation is determined by the duration of drug activity, which in turn is determined by the elimination rate and the dose of the drug. Many studies, using the MSLT and performance assessments, have shown differences in residual effects between short- and long-acting drugs and between different doses of the same drug.

AMNESTIC EFFECTS

Another side effect that is, in part, related to the sedative effects of hypnotics is anterograde amnesia. Anterograde amnesia is memory failure for information presented after consumption of the drug. It is associated with all hypnotics, including all the BzRAs, alcohol, and barbiturates. The extent of amnesia is related to the plasma concentration of the drug. That is, the proximity of information input to peak plasma concentration determines the degree of amnesia, and higher doses, which increase plasma concentration, are associated with both a greater degree of amnesia and a higher prevalence of amnestic events.[30,31] Furthermore, maintaining wakefulness for 10 to 15 minutes after presentation of memory material, rather than allowing a drug-induced rapid sleep onset, attenuates the amnesia.[32]

DISCONTINUATION EFFECTS

The most frequently cited discontinuation effect of BzRAs is rebound insomnia. Sleep is worsened relative to the patient's baseline for 1 to 2 nights after discontinuation of hypnotic use. Rebound insomnia can occur even on discontinuation of short-term hypnotic use[33] and does not increase in severity with the number of repeated nights of use, at least within the time frame of a few weeks of nightly use. Rebound insomnia is more likely to occur after high doses of short- and intermediate-acting BzRAs. It does not occur with long-acting drugs because of the gradual decline in plasma concentration that is inherent to the pharmacology of such drugs. Similarly, it can be minimized with short- and intermediate-acting drugs by gradually tapering the dose over a few nights. Importantly, it usually can be avoided by using the lowest effective dose.

One must differentiate rebound insomnia from recrudescence and from a withdrawal syndrome. Recrudescence is a return of the original symptom at its original severity that does not disappear with time. A withdrawal syndrome is the addition of a new cluster of symptoms (not present prior to treatment), which last several days to weeks rather than 1 or 2 days. Rebound insomnia is the brief (i.e., 1 to 2 nights) exacerbation of the original symptom. It does not reflect the presence of a withdrawal syndrome, which would involve the appearance of new symptoms lasting for more than a night or two.

Also, rebound insomnia does not increase the likelihood of hypnotic self-administration and behavioral dependence.[31] Patient expectancies can also play a role in the experience of rebound insomnia. Discontinuing placebo pills, that is, stopping pill-taking per se, has been found to produce a sleep disturbance.[34]

DEPENDENCE LIABILITY

Dependence on hypnotic medication has continued to be a concern despite minimal evidence to support the concern. Epidemiologic data indicate that the majority of patients use hypnotics for 2 weeks or less.[35,36] A percentage of individuals use them nightly on a chronic basis (i.e., for months or years), with but rare dose escalation.[16] It is unlikely that this pattern of use reflects dependence (i.e., physical or psychological dependence) given the absence of dose escalation and non-therapeutic use of the medications. Although there are reports of physical dependence at therapeutic doses in long-term daytime use of benzodiazepines, no such study of long-term hypnotic use has been done. Daytime studies of the reinforcing effects of these drugs indicate that they have a low behavioral dependence liability.[37] Studies of their behavioral dependence liability in the context of their use as hypnotics have come to a similar conclusion.[34,38] Among individuals, the rate of hypnotic administration varies with the severity of their sleep disturbance; within an individual, rate of administration depends on the degree of sleep disturbance the prior night.[39] Dose escalation in controlled trials (as in the clinical situation) does not occur and daytime use is infrequent.[40] Insomniac patients who do take hypnotic medication during the daytime show the physiologic hyperarousal discussed previously.[40] Hypnotic self-administration in insomniac patients is best explained by therapy-seeking behavior, in that it does not lead to short-term dose escalation, it infrequently generalizes to daytime use (i.e., it does not occur outside the therapeutic context), and the rate of self-administration varies as a function of the severity of the sleep problem.

An area of interest is the potential relationship between benzodiazepine receptor subtype affinity and dependence liability. To the degree that anxiolysis and myorelaxation properties are associated with reinforcing the effects of BzRAs, it is plausible that more selective BzRAs (i.e., those with low affinity for receptors with alpha-2 subunits) may have less dependence liability. However, no data are available to support this hypothesis.

FALLS, COGNITIVE EFFECTS, AND OTHER CONSIDERATIONS FOR OLDER ADULTS

Older adults represent a significant proportion of those using hypnotic medications. Moreover, the therapeutic index for hypnotics in this population is probably narrower than for younger adults because of the increased prevalence (in the former) of medical and neurologic disorders, the common use of concomitant medications (particularly other drugs active on the central nervous system [CNS]), and changes in drug metabolism and excretion.

Those drugs that are primarily metabolized by conjugation are potentially safer for older patients and patients with liver disease. The pharmacokinetics of oxidatively metabolized drugs are altered in these two categories of patients, resulting in increased area under the plasma concentration curve.

For some drugs (e.g., triazolam), this alteration is a consequence of increasing the peak plasma concentration, and for others (e.g., flurazepam), of extending the duration of significant blood levels. The lower recommended dose for most hypnotics when treating older patients is related in part to these kinetic changes.

A number of investigations have demonstrated an increased risk of falls for institutionalized older adults taking benzodiazepines and other psychotropic medications. Results of early studies of community-dwelling older adults are inconsistent,[41-43] but recent large-scale studies suggest elevated risk. Kelly and colleagues[44] found an elevated risk of an injurious fall for seven categories of medications. When controlling for comorbid illness, the elevated risk remained significant only for narcotics, antidepressants, and anticonvulsants. Ensrud et al.[45] reported an elevated fall risk for older women taking antidepressants (both selective serotonin reuptake inhibitors [SSRIs] and tricyclic antidepressants [TCAs]), anticonvulsants, and benzodiazepines, but not narcotics. Data from the same study, however, showed that risk for a fracture was elevated for those taking narcotics and antidepressants but was not affected by use of benzodiazepines and anticonvulsants.[46] Long-acting sedative drugs have been reported to increase risk for falls more than short-acting drugs, but recent data have not borne out this difference.[45] It is important to understand that a variety of CNS-active medications statistically increase fall rates in older adults, and antidepressants often have the highest risks.[47,48]

To our knowledge, no research has attempted to assess fall risk in people specifically taking hypnotics for insomnia. Nor have studies differentiated among BzRAs to determine if receptor selectivity affects fall risk, which would be expected if the degree of myorelaxation impacts falls.

Recently, poor sleep has been identified as a risk factor for falls in older adults. Brassington et al.[49] found that reported sleep problems, but not psychotropic medication use, was an independent risk factor for falls in a large sample of community-dwelling adults aged 64 to 99 years. Future investigations will need to differentiate between sleep disturbance and its treatment in evaluating contributing factors to falls.

Long-term use of benzodiazepines has been reported to be associated with cognitive decline in older adults,[50] although this is certainly not a universal finding.[51] The nature of these investigations (which are predominantly cross-sectional and retrospective) does not allow a firm conclusion regarding causality, because it is extremely difficult to implement proper controls for the aging process, the disease being treated, exposure to other drugs, and other factors. The cognitive changes are often subtle,[52] and the clinical significance of these effects has been questioned.[53] Nevertheless, the possibility that cognitive decline may, at least in part, be attributable to use of hypnotics, or any psychotropic medication, should be kept in mind by the clinician. On the other hand, withholding hypnotic treatment because of the anticipation of cognitive effects does not appear to be warranted on the basis of available information regarding magnitude of risk.

Examination of mortality risk associated with use of medication for sleep frequently demonstrates an elevated risk, the explanation for which is unknown.[54,55] Clearly, these findings merit investigation of the statistical risks. However, a number of factors limit the conclusions that can be drawn from currently available data. First, the epidemiologic nature of the studies (as opposed to controlled experimental trials) prevents any conclusions regarding causality. Second, the exact medications responsible for the elevated mortality risk are not constant from study to study, and, in fact, are often unknown. Data for one study were collected in 1959-1960,[54] when barbiturates were the most commonly used hypnotics; for the second[55] data were collected in 1982, when benzodiazepines were the most commonly used hypnotics. Studies also did not differentiate between prescription and nonprescription drugs. All investigations concluding that an elevated mortality risk exists must include any medication the respondent reports as being taken for sleep, whether a hypnotic or not, and whether the prescribing physician actually intended another indication. The only study that obtained reasonable verification of the actual drugs being taken by respondents found that sedative-hypnotics were not associated with an increased mortality risk. Rather "other drugs" taken for sleep, which in that study were often analgesics, showed a statistically higher mortality risk.[56] Long-term, controlled investigations are needed to clarify whether any medication used to promote sleep increases mortality risk, or whether the statistical risk is explained by the poor health of the users of sleep-promoting drugs, or by other factors.

SEDATING ANTIDEPRESSANTS

According to the *Physician Drug and Diagnosis Audit* database of Verispan (see Table 63–1), trazodone, amitriptyline, and mirtazapine are the three leading sedating antidepressants (SAs) used as hypnotics.[2] It is not clear how much of this use represents treatment of primary insomnia; however, certain data suggest that SA use is not limited to treatment of insomnia with depressive disorders. For example, in 1996, 66.5% of all trazodone drug mentions, regardless of the desired action, were for 100 mg/day or less,[1] whereas the recommended daily dose for the treatment of depression is 150 mg to 400 mg/day. Furthermore, only 38.2% of all trazodone mentions were concomitant with other antidepressant medications. Thus, it seems likely that at least some of the use of SAs as hypnotics is for primary insomnia.

The precise reason for the popularity of SAs in the treatment of insomnia is not clear, and published evidence of efficacy or safety to support this trend is meager. A number of factors probably contribute to the use of SAs as hypnotics: (1) a perception that they are safer than BzRAs, (2) a perception that dependence is less likely, (3) an absence of limitation on recommended duration of use in the package insert (in contrast to all BzRA hypnotics), (4) nonscheduled U.S. Drug Enforcement Administration status (in contrast to all BzRAs), and (5) a view that all or most insomnia is a symptom of depression.

Although the mechanisms of action responsible for the hypnotic properties of BzRAs have been delineated, those of SAs have not. The transmitter systems affected by the various SAs differ. Trazodone antagonizes 5-HT$_{2A}$ (serotonin type 2A), 5-HT$_{2C}$, and alpha$_1$-adrenergic receptors, and it also inhibits 5-HT reuptake.[57,58] Amitriptyline blocks acetylcholine and histamine binding and inhibits the reuptake of norepinephrine and 5-HT.[59-61] Mirtazapine antagonizes alpha$_1$-adrenergic, 5-HT$_{2A}$, 5-HT$_{2C}$, and 5-HT$_3$ receptors, and it is a strong histamine receptor type I (H$_1$) antagonist.[62,63] The antihistaminergic action of amitriptyline and mirtazapine may produce

hypnotic effects, but any hypnotic activity of trazodone would need to be explained through other mechanisms, probably related to 5-HT$_{2A}$, 5-HT$_{2C}$, and alpha$_1$-adrenergic receptors. See Chapter 37 for a more complete discussion of the pharmacology of these drugs.

Efficacy and Effectiveness

Only two studies of the hypnotic efficacy of trazodone in nondepressed insomniac persons have been published, and both have significant methodologic limitations. In a study of nine poor sleepers between 50 and 70 years old (otherwise not characterized), without a parallel placebo group, trazodone 150 mg was taken each night for 3 weeks, and PSG and subjective data were compared with placebo baseline and placebo discontinuation nights.[64] The authors concluded that trazodone improved sleep quality ratings, reduced minutes spent in stage 1, reduced WASO, and increased minutes spent in stage 3/4, but did not increase PSG-determined total sleep time (TST) or shorten PSG sleep latency.

A much larger parallel-group study[65] of well-defined primary insomniac patients compared trazodone 50 mg, zolpidem 10 mg, and placebo during 2 weeks of administration. However, only subjective sleep measures were assessed. Trazodone and zolpidem shortened subjective sleep latency and increased total sleep duration, compared with placebo, although sleep latencies on zolpidem also were shorter than on trazodone. The beneficial effects of trazodone versus placebo occurred only during the first week. In week 2, zolpidem differed from placebo on sleep latency but not on TST results. The findings of this study suggest that trazodone 50 mg may have some short-term hypnotic benefits in primary insomnia, but less so than zolpidem.

A number of studies have assessed the effects of trazodone on the sleep of depressed patients, but they provide little to assist in understanding the drug's hypnotic properties, for several reasons:

1. Determination of the hypnotic characteristics of the drug is confounded by potential antidepressants effects.
2. The results are often contradictory.
3. Most studies have methodologic weaknesses such as having few patients.

The literature on the hypnotic effects of other SAs is equally limited. The TST of persons with primary insomnia tended to increase (but not significantly) with a mean dose of 100 mg of trimipramine taken for approximately 1 month.[66] No data were collected to assess the immediate effects of the drug. Sleep latency and other objective measures were not different in those on placebo. Ratings of sleep quality were reported to be better with trimipramine than placebo. Fifteen persons with primary insomnia were found to have increased TST and sleep quality after 28 nights of treatment with trimipramine (mean dose, 166 ± 48 mg), but the absence of a parallel placebo group, the lack of short-term data, and inadequate washout of other drugs during baseline recordings confound these findings.[67]

Nightly use of doxepin 25 to 50 mg has been evaluated and compared with placebo in persons with primary insomnia.[68] Increased TST, decreased WASO, and enhanced sleep quality were reported with doxepin on nights 1 and 28 of testing, but no differences in sleep latency were documented.

Some researchers have proposed that doxepin may enhance the sleep of persons with primary insomnia via suppression of hypothalamic-pituitary-adrenal axis activity as indexed by nighttime cortisol levels.[69]

Despite the frequent use of amitriptyline and mirtazapine in the treatment of insomnia, no studies of their use in primary insomnia have been published to our knowledge. Furthermore, most studies of these drugs on the sleep of depressed individuals have not included a parallel placebo group. Thus, virtually nothing about their hypnotic efficacy is well established. Conflicting results exist with regard to the ability of amitriptyline to improve the continuity of sleep in depressed persons.[70,71] A pilot study of PSG effects of mirtazapine (15 mg during the first week, 30 mg during the second week) in six patients with major depression, without a parallel placebo group, suggests that sleep latency is decreased and TST increased compared with baseline.[72] A fixed nightly 30-mg dose of mirtazapine for 2 weeks was compared with an escalating dose (15 mg in week 1, 30 mg in week 2) on the self-reported sleep of depressed patients.[63] The authors concluded that the fixed dose was preferred because of greater effects on sleep—specifically, a reduction in sleep latency and an increase in TST; however, the absence of a placebo group does not allow a conclusion to be drawn.

Safety

TCAs and other SAs have more frequent and generally more problematic side effect profiles than BzRAs (see "Falls, Cognitive Effects, and Other Considerations for Older Adults," earlier). In fact, SSRIs have largely supplanted TCAs and other SAs for the treatment of depression because of superior tolerability and safety.[73] The margin between lethal dose and effective dose is much narrower with antidepressants than with BzRAs. The elimination rate of SAs is generally slow, with mean half-lives of about 9 to 30 hours (except for nefazodone, which is 2 to 4 hours), exclusive of any active metabolites. Thus, although residual sedation has not been assessed for these drugs, the pharmacokinetics would indicate that morning carryover is likely and this would negatively impact their overall safety profile.

Unfortunately, most safety data with antidepressants is compiled from studies using antidepressant doses in depressed individuals. The generalizability of this information to the nondepressed person using the lower doses typically administered for insomnia is largely unknown. Two studies of SAs in persons with primary insomnia support the position that SAs used in this context have more frequent and more serious safety concerns than do BzRAs. In an investigation by Hajak et al.,[68] two of four primary insomnia patients who discontinued doxepin treatment had significant adverse events, specifically leukopenia, thrombopenia, and increased liver enzymes. In a direct comparison of lormetazepam and trimipramine in primary insomniac patients,[66] dizziness, dry mouth, headache, and nausea were more frequent, and severe side effects were twice as common, with trimipramine. Mirtazapine is associated with weight gain and increased appetite, as well as high rates of daytime somnolence and dizziness.[74]

Trazodone may be viewed as safe to use as a hypnotic because of the many reports in the 1980s and 1990s that it was safer and caused fewer side effects than did TCAs. However, these studies predate the availability of SSRIs, and comparison of trazodone to SSRIs would probably not be so favorable. Orthostatic hypotension, weakness, and lightheadedness are not uncommon.[75] A number of cases of cardiac conduction abnormalities, hypotension, and other cardiovascular concerns have been reported to be associated with trazodone use by patients with preexisting heart disease.[76-79] Priapism is a rare but potentially serious side effect, even with daily trazodone doses of 100 mg or lower.[80,81] Trazodone 100 to 300 mg does appear to have less performance impairment than BzRAs, as well as fewer subjective effects (which may indicate abuse potential), at least when acutely administered to substance abusers during the daytime.[82]

In sum, use of SAs rather than BzRAs for treatment of insomnia based on overall safety or efficacy profiles is not supported by available information. Known substance abusers are one patient group for whom SAs may have a more favorable benefit-to-risk ratio, as animal models of abuse liability suggest that SAs are less reinforcing than BzRAs.

OTHER DRUGS USED AS HYPNOTICS

As shown in Table 63–1, antipsychotics (quetiapine, olanzapine), antihistamines (hydroxyzine, diphenhydramine), and muscle relaxants (cyclobenzaprine) are not infrequently used for treatment of insomnia. Just as for SAs, the percentage of this use that is directed toward primary insomnia is unknown. Similarly, for most of these drugs little is known about hypnotic efficacy for any patient population. One possible exception is diphenhydramine, for which a small number of studies suggest efficacy at doses of 25 to 50 mg, although the studies lasted only a few days and lacked a parallel placebo group.[83,84] On the other hand, there are two well-designed investigations of the daytime sedating effects of diphenhydramine, given in multiple daytime doses, that clearly show an absence of sedation (i.e., tolerance) by day 3 of administration.[85,86]

For quetiapine and olanzapine, antagonism of H_1 receptors may explain the sedation commonly reported with these drugs, although 5-HT_{2C} antagonism may contribute. Activity at multiple neurotransmitter systems (adrenergic, muscarinic, serotonergic, and dopaminergic) makes these drugs less than ideal for treatment of primary insomnia because of the risk of side effects (e.g., hypotension) and drug interaction related to enzyme induction or inhibition and to multiple neurotransmitter targets. Additionally, olanzapine has a very long duration of action (elimination half-life 20 to 50 hours) and takes several hours to reach peak blood concentrations, neither property characteristic of a good hypnotic. Quetiapine reaches peak plasma levels in about 1.5 hours and has an elimination half-life of approximately 6 hours; thus, morning sedation is likely. The sleep-promoting effects of neither of these antipsychotic medications have been adequately assessed, either in primary or in other forms of insomnia.

INDICATIONS FOR PHARMACOTHERAPY

The 1984 National Institute of Mental Health (NIMH) consensus statement[3] on the use of medications to promote sleep indicated that benzodiazepines (nonbenzodiazepine BzRAs were not available at that time) were the preferred drugs, and that the lowest effective dose should be used for the shortest clinically necessary period of time. Further, pharmacotherapy was acknowledged as an appropriate choice for transient and short-term insomnia (i.e., 4 weeks or less), and use of a short- or an intermediate-acting drug was recommended, unless there was a need for daytime anxiolysis, in which case long-acting drugs might be appropriate. Regarding long-term insomnia, controversy existed over the appropriateness of pharmacotherapy, and the consensus document stated only that "a short trial (less than one month) may also be indicated." The clear position at that time was that hypnotics were not a first-line treatment for chronic insomnia because the insomnia was viewed as a symptom of a medical, psychiatric, or behavioral condition that would remit with treatment of that underlying condition. Nevertheless, long-term use of hypnotics has not been uncommon. Approximately 20% of U.S. users of hypnotic drugs report longest periods of nightly use of 4 months or more.[16]

There continues to be widespread agreement that hypnotics are an appropriate therapy for transient and short-term insomnia. In recent years, a number of advances in our understanding of chronic insomnia, its relation to psychiatric and medical conditions, and the continued development of hypnotic drugs have led many clinicians and investigators to rethink the 1984 consensus statement.[87] In brief, there is considerable evidence that a substantial minority of persons with chronic insomnia have a primary condition without a precipitating psychiatric, medical, or behavioral illness.[88,89] Also, even when insomnia coexists with other medical and psychiatric conditions, the degree of sleep disturbance contributes significantly to overall clinical status. Insomnia is a major risk factor for mood disorders, even a number of years subsequent to the insomnia,[90,91] and there are suggestions that improved sleep may be associated with a more rapid antidepressant response[92] and reduced suicide risk.[93,94] There is also growing evidence that even when underlying conditions are treated, the insomnia does not always remit or even improve significantly.[95] Finally, the already favorable therapeutic margin of hypnotics appears to have improved more with the development of BzRAs with more specific receptor binding profiles.

In recognizing these changes, the NIMH announced it will convene another conference in 2005 to assess current knowledge of insomnia and its treatments. For similar reasons, sleep medicine specialists have begun to clarify the situations in which long-term use of hypnotics would be appropriate.[87,96,97] Although no consensus has yet been reached, the efficacy and safety profile of BzRAs is sufficiently positive that in the absence of dose escalation there appears to be no medical or scientific reason to withdraw or withhold effective long-term therapy from a patient with chronic insomnia. In other words, other than dependence or abuse, there are no contraindications to long-term use of BzRAs for insomnia other than those that apply for short-term use (discussed next).

CONTRAINDICATIONS TO PHARMACOTHERAPY

The primary contraindications to hypnotic therapy are concomitant illnesses, such as sleep apnea, substance abuse disorder, or advanced hepatic disease. All sedative medications have the potential to worsen sleep apnea by blunting arousal from sleep. The dependence liability of BzRAs and other sedative drugs, although low, leads to the conclusion that most patients with a history of alcoholism or drug abuse should not receive BzRAs in outpatient settings without close supervision. Caution is advised for moderate users of alcohol because of additive sedative effects with hypnotics, which narrows the wide margin of safety described earlier. Because most hypnotics undergo hepatic metabolism, advanced liver disease requires the use of a lower dose or avoidance of these medications.

Pharmacotherapy for primary insomnia during pregnancy is also contraindicated; the teratogenic effects of all psychoactive drugs are a matter of concern. People who may be required to awaken and perform duties in the middle of the night should avoid any CNS-depressant drug. All hypnotics have the potential to disrupt alertness and cognitive function for the duration of the sedative activity of the drug, and they may impact motor function.

TREATMENT CONSIDERATIONS

Hypnotic therapy should be considered for primary insomnia when the patient is significantly distressed by the presence or possibility of disturbed sleep, or when the physician judges the sleep disturbance to be deleterious to the patients' safety or health. BzRAs are the recommended hypnotic medications for most patients (the primary exceptions being patients who are substance abusers and patients known to be refractory to BzRAs, for whom SAs could be employed). The specific BzRA should be carefully chosen, considering the pharmacokinetics of the drug and the patient characteristics (e.g., age, concurrent illness). The dose and treatment regimen should be carefully and specifically prescribed, agreed to by the patient, and monitored by the physician. The hypnotic should be taken only at the time and frequency agreed on. The dose should be the lowest clinically indicated dose, and the clinician and patient should jointly determine effectiveness of that dose soon after initiation of treatment (e.g., after 3 to 5 nights). The dose can then be adjusted as appropriate. Patients should generally not be allowed to self-initiate dose adjustment, particularly during the early portion of therapy, as a fluctuating dose makes interpretation of clinical response very difficult.

As suggested earlier, determination of the effectiveness and tolerability of a drug at a specific dose is best accomplished with the patient taking medication every night. The physician should specifically inquire about the aspects of sleep and daytime function that were most problematic for the patient before treatment, rather than relying solely on global statements. A sleep diary can be helpful for comparing pretreatment and posttreatment symptoms. In reasonably healthy persons, one or two monthly visits should be sufficient to identify most potential adverse effects. For older adults or others at increased risk for drug interactions, alterations in drug metabolism, incoordination, or cognitive problems, close follow-up is recommended throughout the period of hypnotic administration. Discontinuation of therapy should be considered if symptoms occur that may be side effects of the medication, to confirm whether they are indeed medication related.

Once a determination of effectiveness and tolerability is made with the patient taking the hypnotic nightly, other administration schedules are possible although not necessary. Hypnotics can be prescribed to be taken every night, on a predetermined intermittent schedule (e.g., every third night), or as needed. There have now been several controlled studies of nonnightly zolpidem use in primary insomnia, all of which indicate that the drug is efficacious on nights that it is taken and that rebound insomnia and other discontinuation phenomena are not significant concerns for the times the drug is not used. Nonnightly schedules were commonly recommended because of the absence of safety data from long-term studies of nightly use, and because of concerns about tolerance and dependence. However, it now seems clear that tolerance does not commonly occur and that dependence is primarily a problem for substance abusers. Moreover, safety concerns with nightly use are generally the same as for short-term use, although the overall risk is affected by the number of exposures. Clearly, after longer-term use, gradual discontinuation, via dose tapering, is best.

There are some theoretical considerations regarding selection of a hypnotic administration schedule. An as-needed prescription may reinforce patients' belief that they are unable to sleep without medication. On the other hand, some patients may benefit from a sense of control over treatment on such a schedule. To the degree that a patient's insomnia may have conditioning features, nightly treatment for a 2- to 3-week period that consistently provides good sleep may decrease the patient's conditioned arousal to the sleep environment, and cognitions regarding the inability to sleep may be extinguished. The intent behind the use of an intermittent schedule is to avoid the possibility of tolerance development in patients being treated chronically. However, as noted earlier, studies have not systematically demonstrated tolerance, physical dependence, or behavioral dependence after chronic treatment of patients with properly diagnosed and treated insomnia. No study has determined whether nightly or intermittent treatment is more likely to have an adverse outcome, and which specific insomnia diagnoses are appropriate and which are inappropriate. Even with a schedule of intermittent treatment, perceptions regarding an inability to sleep may be reinforced.

There are both pharmacologic and behavioral considerations associated with the middle-of-the-night administration of medications. Pharmacologically, it is possible that this protocol will produce daytime residual sedation, as discussed earlier. With the exception of zaleplon, all medications should be taken only when the patient has the opportunity to stay in bed 7 to 8 hours. Zaleplon is an ultra–short-acting drug that has been evaluated in middle-of-the-night dosing protocols (i.e., medication is administered with 5 hours or less of bedtime remaining) and been found to improve sleep in the remaining bedtime without residual effects the next morning.[98,99] If nightly hypnotic use is not appropriate for individual patients, they can be instructed to attempt sleep without medication and, if unsuccessful, to take the drug later, provided there are 4 to 5 hours remaining before they must arise. From a behavioral therapy perspective, middle-of-the-night administration can be thought of as rescue medication. If a particular behavioral treatment fails on a given night, the middle-of-the-night medication serves as a rescue, thereby enabling the patient to avoid frustration with the behavioral treatment. Thus, in cases of sleep maintenance insomnia characterized only by a middle-of-the-night awakening, or in cases of intermittent sleep-onset insomnia, middle-of-the-night administration of an ultra–short-acting medication can be considered.

A LOOK FORWARD

The frequency and significance of changes in the drugs used to treat insomnia over the past few decades are likely to continue in the foreseeable future. The growing view that a chronic disorder of primary insomnia is common and may have significant associated morbidities leads to the need for long-term therapies that not only improve sleep but also reduce consequences and comorbid conditions. Additionally, advances in understanding the neurobiologic mechanisms of sleep–wake state transitions and sleep state stability will provide new neural targets for hypnotic drug development.

Clinical Pearl

Extensive efficacy and safety evidence supports the use of benzodiazepine receptor agonists for the treatment of primary insomnia. Such data for use of other types of medication (e.g., sedating antidepressants) are not currently available. The benzodiazepine receptor agonists demonstrate sufficient variability in pharmacokinetics and receptor selectivity to provide the physician with a variety of therapeutic choices.

REFERENCES

1. Walsh JK, Schweitzer PK: Ten-year trends in the pharmacological treatment of insomnia. Sleep 1999;22:371-375.
2. Compton-McBride S, Schweitzer PK, Walsh JK: Most commonly used drugs to treat insomnia in 2002. Sleep 2004;27(Suppl.): A255.
3. National Institute of Mental Health, Consensus Development Conference: Drugs and insomnia: The use of medications to promote sleep. JAMA 1984;251:2410-2414.
4. American Psychiatric Association Task Force on Benzodiazepine Dependency: Benzodiazepine Dependence, Toxicity, and Abuse. Washington, DC, American Psychiatric Association, 1990.
5. Mohler H, Fritschy JM, Rudolph U: A new benzodiazepine pharmacology. J Pharmacol Exp Ther 2002;300:2-8.
6. Greenblatt DJ, Shader RI: Benzodiazepines in Clinical Practice. New York, Raven Press, 1974.
7. Nowell PD, Mazumdar S, Buysse DJ, et al: Benzodiazepines and zolpidem for chronic insomnia: A meta-analysis of treatment efficacy. JAMA 1997;278:2170-2177.
8. Mitler MM, Seidel WF, Van Den Hoed J, et al: Comparative hypnotic effects of flurazepam, triazolam, and placebo: A long-term simultaneous nighttime and daytime study. J Clin Psychopharmacol 1984;4:2-13.
9. Oswald I, French C, Adam K, et al: Benzodiazepine hypnotics remain effective for 24 weeks. 1982;284:860-863.
10. Scharf MB, Roth T, Vogel GW, et al: A multicenter, placebo-controlled study evaluating zolpidem in the treatment of chronic insomnia. J Clin Psychiatry 1994;55:192-199.
11. Walsh JK, Vogel GW, Scharf M, et al: A five week, polysomnographic assessment of zaleplon 10 mg for the treatment of primary insomnia. Sleep Med 2000;1:41-49.
12. Krystal AD, Walsh JK, Laska E, et al: Sustained efficacy of eszopiclone over 6 months of nightly treatment: Results of a randomized, double-blind, placebo-controlled study in adults with chronic insomnia. Sleep 2003;26:793-799.
13. Walsh JK, Roth T, Randazzo AC, et al: Eight weeks of non-nightly use of zolpidem for primary insomnia. Sleep 2000;23: 1087-1096.

14. Perlis M, McCall WV, Krystal A, et al: Long-term, non-nightly administration of zolpidem in the treatment of patients with primary insomnia. J Clin Psychiat 2004;65:1128-1137.

15. Ohayon MM, Caulet M, Arbus L, et al: Are prescribed medications effective in the treatment of insomnia complaints? J Psychosom Res 1999;47:359-368.

16. Balter MB, Uhlenhuth EH: The beneficial and adverse effects of hypnotics. J Clin Psychiatry 1991;52(Suppl):16-23.

17. Kummer J, Linden J, Eich FX, et al: Long-term polysomnographic efficacy and safety of zolpidem in elderly psychiatric in-patients with insomnia. J Int Med Res 1993;21:171-184.

18. Maarek L, Cramer P, Coquelin JP, et al: The safety and efficacy of zolpidem in insomnia patients: A long-term open study in general practice. J Int Med Res 1991;20:162-170.

19. Schlich D, L'Heritier C, Coquelin JP, et al: Long-term treatment of insomnia with zolpidem: A multicentre general practitioner study of 107 patients. J Int Med Res 1991;19:271-279.

20. Stepanski E, Zorick FJ, Roehrs TA, et al: Daytime alertness in patients with chronic insomnia compared with asymptomatic control subjects. Sleep 1988;11:39-46.

21. Bonnet MH, Arand DL: 24-Hour metabolic rate in insomniacs and normal sleepers. Sleep 1995;18:581-588.

22. Vgontzas AN, Bixler EO, Lin HM, et al: Chronic insomnia is associated with nyctohemeral activation of the hypothalamic-pituitary-adrenal axis: Clinical implications. J Clin Endocrinol Metab 2001;86:3787-3794.

23. Bonnet MH, Arand DL: Heart rate variability in insomniacs and matched normal sleepers. Psychosom Med 1998;60:610-615.

24. Doghramji K, Browman CP, Gaddy JR, et al: Triazolam diminishes daytime sleepiness and sleep fragmentation in patients with periodic leg movements in sleep. J Clin Psychopharmacol 1991;11:284-290.

25. Walsh JK, Muehlbach MJ, Lauter SA, et al: Effects of triazolam on sleep, daytime sleepiness, and morning stiffness in patients with rheumatoid arthritis. J Rheumatol 1996;23:245-252.

26. Roehrs T, Zorick F, Wittig R, et al: Efficacy of a reduced triazolam dose in elderly insomniacs. Neurobiol Aging 1985;6:293-296.

27. Mendelson WB, Thompson C, Franko T: Adverse reactions to sedative/hypnotics: Three years' experience. Sleep 1996;19:702-706.

28. Ladewig D: Abuse of benzodiazepines in western European society: Incidence and prevalence, motives, drug acquisition. Pharmacopsychiatria 1983;16:103-106.

29. Roth T, Roehrs T: Issues in the use of benzodiazepine therapy. J Clin Psychiatry 1992;53:S14-S18.

30. Roth T, Roehrs TA, Stepanski EJ, et al: Hypnotics and behavior. Am J Med 1990;8:43S-46S.

31. Greenblatt D, Harmatz JS, Shapiro L, et al: Sensitivity to triazolam in elderly. N Engl J Med 1991;324:1691-1698.

32. Roehrs T, Zorick F, Sicklesteel J, et al: Effects of hypnotics on memory. J Clin Psychopharmacol 1983;3:310-313.

33. Roehrs T, Vogel G, Roth T: Rebound insomnia: Its determinants and significance. Am J Med 1990;88:39S-42S.

34. Roehrs T, Merlotti L, Zorick F, et al: Rebound insomnia and hypnotic self administration. Psychopharmacology 1992;107:480-484.

35. Mellinger GD, Balter MB, Uhlenhuth EH: Insomnia and its treatment. Arch Gen Psychiatry 1985;42:225-232.

36. Roehrs T, Hollebeek E, Drake C, et al: Substance use for insomnia in Metropolitan Detroit. J Psychosom Res 2002;53:571-576.

37. Griffiths RR, Roache JD: Abuse liability of benzodiazepines: A review of human studies evaluating subjective and/or reinforcing effects. In Smith DE, Wesson DR (eds): The Benzodiazepines: Current Standards for Medical Practice. Hingman, Mass, MTP Press, 1985, pp 209-225.

38. Roehrs T, Pedrosi B, Rosentha L, et al: Hypnotic self administration and dose escalation. Psychopharmacology 1996;127:150-154.

39. Roehrs T, Bonahoom A, Pedrosi B, et al: Disturbed sleep predicts hypnotic self administration. Sleep Med 2002;3:61-66.

40. Roehrs T, Bonahoom A, Pedrosi B, et al: Nighttime versus daytime hypnotic self-administration. Psychopharmacology 2002;161:137-142.

41. Campbell AJ, Borrie MJ, Spears GF: Risk factors for falls in a community based prospective study of people 70 years and older. J Gerontol 1989;44:M112-117.

42. Tinetti ME, Speechley M, Ginter SF: Risk factors for falls among elderly persons living in the community. N Engl J Med 1988;319:1701-1707.

43. Nevitt MC, Cummings SR, Kidd S, et al: Risk factors for recurrent nonsyncopal falls: A prospective study. JAMA 1989;261:2663-2668.

44. Kelly KD, Pickett W, Yiannakoulias N, et al: Medication use and falls in community-dwelling older persons. Age Ageing 2003;32:503-509.

45. Ensrud KE, Blackwell TL, Mangione CM, et al: Central nervous system-active medications and risk for falls in older women. J Am Geriatr Soc 2002;50:1629-1637.

46. Ensrud KE, Blackwell TL, Mangione CM, et al: Central nervous system active medications and risk for fractures in older women. Arch Intern Med 2003;163:949-957.

47. Kallin K, Lundin-Olsson L, Jensen J, et al: Predisposing and precipitating factors for falls among older people in residential care. Public Health 2002;116:263-271.

48. Thapa PB, Gideon P, Cost TW, et al: Antidepressants and the risk of falls among nursing home residents. N Engl J Med 1998;339:875-882.

49. Brassington GS, King AC, Bliwise DL: Sleep problems as a risk factor for falls in a sample of community-dwelling adults aged 64-99 years. J Am Geriatr Soc 2000;48:1234-1240.

50. Paterniti S, Dufouil C, Alperovitch A: Long-term benzodiazepine use and cognitive decline in the elderly: The Epidemiology of Vascular Aging Study. J Clin Psychopharmacol 2002;22:285-293.

51. Allard J, Artero S, Ritchie K: Consumption of psychotropic medication in the elderly: A re-evaluation of its effect on cognitive performance. Int J Geriatr Psychiatry 2003;18:874-878.

52. Curran HV, Collins R, Fletcher S, et al: Older adults and withdrawal from benzodiazepine hypnotics in general practice: Effects on cognitive function, sleep, mood and quality of life. Psychol Med 2003;33:1223-1237.

53. Pat McAndrews M, Weiss RT, Sandor P, et al: Cognitive effects of long-term benzodiazepine use in older adults. Hum Psychopharmacol 2003;18:51-57.

54. Kripke DF, Simons RN, Garfinkel L, et al: Short and long sleep and sleeping pills: Is increased mortality associated? Arch Gen Psychiatry 1979;36:103-116.

55. Kripke DF, Klauber MR, Wingard DL, et al: Mortality hazard associated with prescription hypnotics. Biol Psychiatry 1998;43:687-693.

56. Rumble R, Morgan K: Hypnotics, sleep, and mortality in elderly people. J Am Geriatr Soc 1992;40:787-791.

57. Brogden RN, Heel RC, Speight TM, et al: Trazodone: A review of its pharmacologic properties and therapeutic use in depression and anxiety. Drugs 1981;21:401-429.

58. Jenck F, Moreau JL, Mutel V, et al: Evidence for a role of 5-HT$_{1C}$ receptors in the antiserotonergic properties of some antidepressant drugs. Eur J Pharmacol 1993;231:223-229.

59. Frazer A: Pharmacology of antidepressants. J Clin Psychopharmacol 1997;17(Suppl 1):2S-18S.

60. Preskorn SH: Pharmacokinetics of antidepressants: Why and how they are relevant to treatment. J Clin Psychiatry 1993;54(Suppl):14-34.

61. Richelson E: The pharmacology of antidepressants at the synapse: Focus on newer compounds. J Clin Psychiatry 1994;55(Suppl A):34-39.

62. De Boer T: The pharmacological profile of mirtazapine. J Clin Psychiatry 1996;57(Suppl 4):19-25.

63. Radhakishun FS, van den Bos J, van der Heijden BC, et al: Mirtazapine effects on alertness and sleep in patients as recorded by interactive telecommunication during treatment with different dosing regimens. J Clin Psychopharmacol 2000;20:531-537.

64. Montgomery I, Oswald I, Morgan K, et al: Trazodone enhances sleep in subjective quality but not in objective duration. Br J Clin Pharmacol 1983;16:139-144.

65. Walsh JK, Erman M, Erwin CW, et al: Subjective hypnotic efficacy of trazodone and zolpidem in DSM-III-R primary insomnia. Hum Psychopharmacol 1998;13:191-198.

66. Riemann D, Voderholzer U, Cohrs S, et al: Trimipramine in primary insomnia: Results of a polysomnographic double-blind controlled study. Pharmacopsychiatry 2002;35:165-174.

67. Hohagen F, Montero RF, Weiss E, et al: Treatment of primary insomnia with trimipramine: An alternative to benzodiazepine hypnotics? Eur Arch Psychiatry Clin Neurosci 1994;244:65-72.

68. Hajak G, Rodenbeck A, Voderholzer U, et al: Doxepin in the treatment of primary insomnia: A placebo-controlled, double-blind, polysomnographic study. J Clin Psychiatry 2001;62:453-463.

69. Rodenbeck A, Cohrs S, Jordan W, et al: The sleep-improving effects of doxepin are paralleled by a normalized plasma cortisol secretion in primary insomnia: A placebo-controlled, double-blind, randomized, cross-over study followed by an open treatment over 3 weeks. Psychopharmacology 2003;170:423-428.

70. Gillin JC, Wyatt RJ, Fram D, et al: The relationship between changes in REM sleep and clinical improvement in depressed patients treated with amitriptyline. Psychopharmacol 1978;59:267-272.

71. Hartmann E, Cravens J: The effects of long-term administration of psychotropic drugs on human sleep: III. The effects of amitriptyline. Psychopharmacologia 1973;33:185-202.

72. Winokur A, Sateia MJ, Hayes JB, et al: Acute effects of mirtazapine on sleep continuity and sleep architecture in depressed patients: A pilot study. Biol Psychiatry 2000;48:75-78.

73. Peretti S, Judge R, Hindmarch I: Safety and tolerability considerations: Tricyclic antidepressants vs. selective serotonin reuptake inhibitors. Acta Psychiatr Scand 2000;101(Suppl 403):17-25.

74. Flores BH, Schatzberg AF: Mirtazepine. In Schatzberg A, Nemeroff C (eds): The American Psychiatric Publishing Textbook of Psychopharmacology. Washington, DC, American Psychiatric Publishing, 2004, pp 341-347.

75. Golden RN, Dawkins K, Nicholas L: Trazodone and nefazodone. In Schatzberg A, Nemeroff C (eds): The American Psychiatric Textbook of Psychopharmacology. Washington, DC, American Psychiatric Publishing, 2004, pp 315-325.

76. Rausch JL, Pavlinac DM, Newman PE: Complete heart block following a single dose of trazodone. Am J Psychiatry 1984;141:1472-1473.

77. Irwin M, Spar JE: Reversible cardiac conduction abnormality associated with trazodone administration. Am J Psychiatry 1983;140:945-946.

78. Levenson JL: Prolonged QT interval after trazodone overdose. Am J Psychiatry 1999;156:969-970.

79. Bucknall C, Brooks D, Curry PV, et al: Mianserin and trazodone for cardiac patients with depression. Eur J Clin Pharmacol 1988;33:565-569.

80. Carson CC III, Mino RD: Priapism associated with trazodone therapy. J Urol 1988;139:369-370.

81. Haria M, Fitton A, McTavish D: Trazodone: A review of its pharmacology, therapeutic use in depression and therapeutic potential in other disorders. Drugs Aging 1994;4:331-355.

82. Rush CR, Baker RW, Wright K: Acute behavioral effects and abuse potential of trazodone, zolpidem, and triazolam in humans. Psychopharmacology (Berl) 1999;144:220-233.

83. Kudo Y, Kurihara M: Clinical evaluation of diphenhydramine hydrochloride for the treatment of insomnia in psychiatric patients: A double-blind study. J Clin Pharmacol 1990;30:1041-1048.

84. Rickels K, Morris RJ, Newman H, et al: Diphenhydramine in insomniac family practice patients: A double-blind study. J Clin Pharmacol 1983;23:234-242.

85. Schweitzer PK, Muehlbach MJ, Walsh JK: Sleepiness and performance during three-day administration of cetirizine or diphenhydramine. J Allergy Clin Immunol 1994;94:716-724.

86. Richardson GS, Roehrs TA, Rosenthal L, et al: Tolerance to daytime sedative effects of H1 antihistamines. J Clin Psychopharmacol 2002;22:511-515.

87. Mendelson WB, Roth T, Cassella J, et al: The treatment of chronic insomnia: Drug indications, chronic use and abuse liability. Summary of a 2001 New Clinical Drug Evaluation Unit (NCDEU) meeting symposium. Sleep Med Rev 2004;8:7-17.

88. Ohayon MM: Prevalence of DSM-IV diagnostic criteria of insomnia: Distinguishing insomnia related to mental disorders from sleep disorders. J Psychiat Res 1997;31:333-346.

89. Buysse DJ, Reynolds CR, Kupfer DJ, et al: Clinical diagnoses in 216 insomnia patients using the international classification of sleep disorders (ICSD), DSM-IV and ICD-10 categories: A report from the APA/NIMH DSM-IV field trial. Sleep 1994;17:630-637.

90. Chang PP, Ford DE, Mead LA, et al: Insomnia in young men and subsequent depression: The Johns Hopkins Precursors Study. Am J Epidemiol 1997;146:105-114.

91. Breslau N, Roth T, Rosenthal L, et al: Sleep disturbance and psychiatric disorders: A longitudinal epidemiological study of young adults. Biol Psychiatry 1996;39:411-418.

92. Perlis ML, Giles DE, Buysse DJ, et al: Self-reported sleep disturbance as a prodromal symptom in recurrent depression. J Affect Disord 1997;42:209-212.

93. Agargun MY, Kara H, Solmaz M: Sleep disturbances and suicidal behavior in patients with major depression. J Clin Psychiatr 1997;58:249-251.

94. Hall RC, Platt DE: Suicide risk assessment: A review of risk factors for suicide in 100 patients who made severe suicide attempts. Evaluation of suicide risk in a time of managed care. Psychosomatics 1999;40:18-27.

95. Stark P, Hardison CD: A review of multicenter controlled studies of fluoxetine vs. imipramine and placebo in outpatients with major depressive disorder. J Clin Psychiatry 1985;46:53-58.

96. McCall WV: Pharmacologic treatment of insomnia. In Lee-Chiong TL Jr, Sateia MJ, Carskadon MA (eds): Sleep Medicine. Philadelphia, Hanley & Belfus, 2002, pp 169-176.

97. Roehrs T, Roth T: Hypnotics: An update. Curr Neurol Neurosci Rep 2003;3:181-184.

98. Walsh JK, Pollak CP, Scharf MB, et al: Lack of residual sedation following middle-of-the-night zaleplon administration in sleep maintenance insomnia. Clin Neuropharmacol 2000;23:17-21.

99. Danjou P, Paty I, Fruncillo R, et al: A comparison of the residual effects of zaleplon and zolpidem following administration 5 to 2 hrs before awakening. Br J Clin Pharmacol 1999;48:367-374.

Narcolepsy: Pharmacology, Pathophysiology, and Genetics

Emmanuel Mignot

ABSTRACT

In international classifications, narcolepsy with and without cataplexy are now two distinct diagnostic entries. In almost all cases with cataplexy, and in rare cases without cataplexy, narcolepsy is associated with a deficiency in the hypothalamic neuropeptide hypocretin (Hcrt; or orexin) system. The Hcrt deficiency can be assessed by the demonstration of very low to undetectable Hcrt-1 in the cerebrospinal fluid, a test more specific than the multiple sleep latency test, but recommended only in selected cases. Most cases with cataplexy and fewer cases without cataplexy also carry the human leukocyte antigen (HLA) DQB1*0602, a subtype present in 12% to 38% of control subjects. Both genetic and environmental factors are implicated in the predisposition to the disease. The HLA association suggests a possible autoimmune basis for the Hcrt cell destruction, at least in cases with cataplexy and Hcrt deficiency, but this hypothesis has not been proved. Rare cases of narcolepsy secondary to genetic, tumoral, traumatic, or inflammatory disorders, many of which were shown to affect the hypothalamus or the Hcrt system, have also been reported. Treatments to date are pharmacologically based and do not directly act on the Hcrt system. Our understanding of the pathophysiologic process of narcolepsy has rapidly progressed, thanks to studies in canine and rodent models.

In its original definition, narcolepsy is characterized by "excessive daytime sleepiness that typically is associated with cataplexy and other REM sleep phenomena such as sleep paralysis and hypnagogic hallucinations."[1] Cataplexy, the sudden occurrence of muscle weakness in association with laughing, joking, or anger, has long been considered a pathognomonic symptom.[2-5] A broader definition of narcolepsy includes patients with sleepiness and abnormal rapid eye movement (REM) sleep, such as sleep-onset REM periods during the multiple sleep latency test (MSLT), sleep paralysis, or hypnagogic hallucinations. Disturbed nocturnal sleep is also central to the syndrome.[2-6]

The definition of narcolepsy is being revised in the light of recent scientific discoveries. In most cases with cataplexy and in fewer cases without cataplexy, a deficiency in the neuropeptide hypocretin (Hcrt) system is involved.[7-12] A tight association with the human leukocyte antigen (HLA) DQB1*0602 is also found only in cases with cataplexy.[13,14] An autoimmune mediation of Hcrt cell loss is likely but not established. As a result, in the most recent revision of the International Classification of Sleep Disorders, narcolepsy with and without cataplexy have been separated[1] (Table 64–1).

In this chapter, available information regarding the pathophysiology and pharmacology of narcolepsy is reviewed. The clinical, diagnostic, and therapeutic aspects of the syndrome are discussed in Chapter 65.

PREVALENCE

Prevalence studies for narcolepsy with cataplexy have been performed in multiple ethnic groups and countries. In Finland, 3 subjects with cataplexy and abnormal MSLT results were identified among 11,354 randomly selected subjects, for a prevalence of 0.026%.[15] Similar frequencies (0.013% to 0.067%) were reported in Great Britain, France, Hong Kong, the Czech Republic, and in the United States (see Dauvilliers et al.[6] and Mignot[16] for reviews). A study performed in 1945 in American Navy recruits also identified a prevalence of 0.02% in African Americans.[17] In contrast to these values, narcolepsy-cataplexy may be rare in Israel and more frequent in Japan. Two studies in Japan led to prevalence figures of 0.16% and 0.18%,[18,19] but these studies did not use polysomnography to confirm the diagnosis. In Israel, only a few patients have been identified compared with the large population of subjects with sleep apnea recruited into sleep clinics.[20] This has led to the suggestion that the prevalence of narcolepsy could be as low as 0.002% in Israel.

The prevalence of narcolepsy without cataplexy is more uncertain. In case series, narcolepsy without cataplexy represents 20% to 50% of narcolepsy cases.[13] Patients without cataplexy are, however, probably more likely to be undiagnosed, considering their milder phenotype. Some studies have suggested that 1% to 3% of the adult population may have unexplained sleepiness and multiple sleep-onset REM periods during MSLT testing[21] (also T. Young and E. Mignot, unpublished observations). Other studies have found an even higher prevalence in adolescents or young adults, probably because voluntary chronic sleep deprivation is more common in these populations.[22,23]

Table 64–1. International Classification of Sleep Disorders (ICSD): Definitions and Pathophysiology

Condition	Diagnostic Criteria	Pathophysiology
Narcolepsy with cataplexy	Presence of definite cataplexy (and usually abnormal MSLT results)	90% with low CSF Hcrt-1 and HLA-DQB1*0602
Narcolepsy without cataplexy	MSLT: sleep latency <8 min, ≥2 SOREMPs No or doubtful cataplexy	Unknown, probably heterogeneous, 7–25% with low CSR Hcrt-1, 40% HLA-DQB1*0602
Secondary narcolepsy	As above, but due to other conditions (e.g., neurologic)	With or without Hcrt deficiency; various disorders (see Box 64–1)
Idiopathic hypersomnia	No cataplexy, no SOREMPs during the MSLT	Unknown, probable heterogeneous etiology, with or without prolonged nocturnal sleep

Hcrt, hypocretin; HLA, human leukocyte antigen; MSLT, multiple sleep latency test; SOREMP, sleep-onset rapid eye movement period.

From American Academy of Sleep Medicine: International Classification of Sleep Disorders: Diagnostic and Coding Manual. 2nd ed. Westchester, Ill, American Academy of Sleep Medicine, 2005.

A recent study identified all diagnosed narcoleptic patients in Olmsted County, Minnesota using the medical records linkage system of the Rochester Epidemiology Project.[24] The study identified 0.036% of the population with narcolepsy-cataplexy and 0.021% with narcolepsy without cataplexy, suggesting a significant prevalence for diagnosed cases of narcolepsy without cataplexy.[24]

ANIMAL MODELS

In the last 20 years, narcolepsy research has been facilitated by the existence of a unique animal model, canine narcolepsy. Canine narcolepsy was first reported in the early 1970s in two small breeds by Knecht[25] and Mitler.[26] Early attempts to establish genetic transmission were unsuccessful, suggesting a nongenetic etiology in most cases of canine narcolepsy. In 1975, two narcoleptic Doberman pinschers were reported in a single litter.[27] The breeding of these animals led to the demonstration that narcolepsy was transmitted as a single autosomal recessive gene with full penetrance in this breed. A narcoleptic colony of Dobermans was then established and maintained at Stanford University for more than 20 years. Familial canine narcolepsy was also reported in Labrador retrievers and dachshunds.[27,28] Experiments also indicate that animals heterozygous for the canine narcolepsy gene have subclinical abnormalities such as increased daytime sleepiness. In heterozygous animals, the administration of drugs that increase cholinergic and reduce monoaminergic transmissions (manipulations known to promote REM sleep) has been shown to induce cataplexy at specific developmental stages.[29]

The parallel between human and canine narcolepsy is striking. In MSLT-like procedures, narcoleptic canines have short sleep and REM latencies.[30] Twenty-four-hour recording studies show sleep fragmentation and more daytime sleep than in control animals.[31] Finally, as in human narcolepsy, sudden episodes of muscle weakness akin to cataplexy can be observed in association with strong positive emotions, most typically during the presentation of appetizing food or while at play (Fig. 64–1). These episodes usually last a few seconds and preferentially affect the hind legs, neck, or face. Cataplexy may also escalate to complete muscle paralysis with abolition of tendon reflexes. During these episodes, animals are conscious and able visually to track nearby movement (for video, see http://www.med.stanford.edu/school/Psychiatry/narcolepsy/).

Polygraphic recording indicates a desynchronized, wakelike electroencephalographic pattern at the onset of cataplexy, followed by increased theta activity and genuine REM sleep in long-lasting episodes.[32] A typical picture of narcoleptic canines in the midst of cataplectic attacks is presented in Figure 64–1.

The cause of autosomal recessive canine narcolepsy was identified through positional cloning.[28,33] Three mutations causing complete dysfunction of a receptor for the newly identified neuropeptide system Hcrt (hcrtr2) were identified in Doberman, Labrador, and dachshund pedigrees.[28,33] Sporadic cases of canine narcolepsy were later shown to be associated with low cerebrospinal fluid (CSF) and brain Hcrt levels,[34] as found in human narcolepsy.[7-10]

Several rodent models of narcolepsy are now also available. In one model, Chemelli et al.[35] knocked out the prepro-hypocretin (preproHcrt) gene. The resulting model has fragmented sleep, transitions from wakefulness into REM sleep, and experiences episodes of behavioral arrests akin to cataplexy or sleep-onset paralysis.[35] In another model, a toxic transgene derived from an ataxin-3 human gene mutation was driven by the preproHcrt promoter, resulting in narcoleptic mice lacking Hcrt-containing cells.[36] Rodents lacking either of the two Hcrt receptors, hcrtr1 or hcrtr2, are also available.[37,38] In these

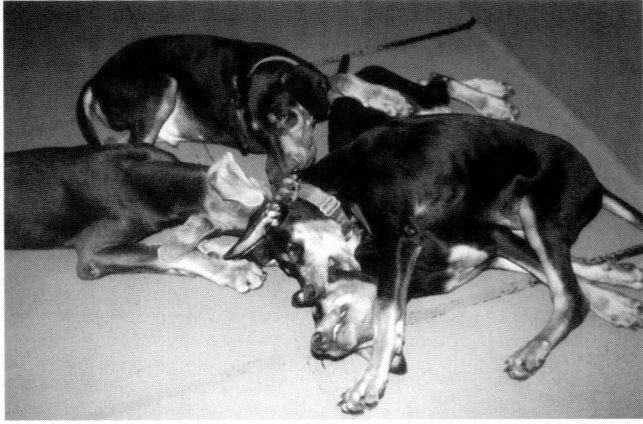

Figure 64–1. Narcoleptic Doberman pinschers in the middle of a cataplectic attack. Note that the eyes are open. Autosomal recessive forms of canine narcolepsy are due to mutations in the hypocretin receptor type 2 gene.[28,33]

models, only hcrtr2 receptor knockout animals experience behavioral arrest episodes similar to cataplexy. Interestingly, however, hcrtr1 knockout animals have fragmented sleep but no behavioral arrest episodes.[38] It is also suggested that hcrtr2 knockout animals are less affected than Hcrt peptide knockout animals, suggesting a role for hcrtr1 in increasing the severity of the phenotype.[37] The rodent models are revolutionizing research in the area. However, it is difficult to differentiate cataplexy from REM sleep onset or sleep paralysis in these models. The link between behavioral arrest and positive emotions is unclear, and pharmacologic characterization has not been performed (see later).

PHARMACOLOGY OF NARCOLEPSY

Adrenergic Uptake Inhibition Mediates the Anticataplectic Effects of Currently Prescribed Antidepressant Medications

In the past, the most commonly prescribed anticataplectic agents were tricyclic antidepressants. More recently, more selective monoaminergic reuptake inhibitors have become available.

Antidepressants have a complex pharmacologic profile that includes monoamine (serotonin, norepinephrine, epinephrine, and dopamine) uptake inhibition, and, for older tricyclic antidepressants, cholinergic, histaminergic, and alpha-adrenergic blocking properties.[30,39,40] In narcoleptic canines, inhibition of adrenergic, but not dopaminergic or serotonergic uptake or other properties mediates therapeutic efficacy for antidepressant compounds.[39,40] This observation fits well with available human pharmacologic data (see Nishino and Mignot[30]; Table 64–2). Protriptyline, desipramine, viloxazine, and atomoxetine, four adrenergic-specific uptake blockers with no effect on serotonin transmission, are effective and potent anticataplectic agents (Table 64–2). In contrast, fluoxetine and other selective serotonin uptake inhibitors are active against cataplexy only at relatively high doses, an effect possibly mediated by the weak adrenergic uptake effects of these compounds and their metabolites.[39,40]

The observation that adrenergic uptake blockers are excellent anticataplectic agents correlates well with their potent inhibitory effects on REM sleep. Adrenergic transmission is reduced during REM sleep (see Chapter 10 in this book for review). The firing rate in the locus coeruleus decreases during cataplexy in narcoleptic canines.[41] Adrenergic uptake

Table 64–2.   Commonly Prescribed Treatments and Their Pharmacologic Properties

Compound	Pharmacologic Properties
Stimulants	
Amphetamine	Increases monoamine release (DA > NE >> 5-HT). Blocks vesicular monoamine storage, monoamine reuptake and MAO at high doses. The D-isomer is more specific for dopaminergic transmission and is a better stimulant compound.
Methamphetamine	More lipophilic than amphetamine, increased central penetration, proportionally fewer peripheral side effects. Because it is an HCl salt and not an SO_4 salt like amphetamine, it contains twice the number of amphetamine molecules per milligram dose.
Methylphenidate	Blocks monoamine uptake at lower dose than amphetamine; slightly less effect on monoamine release; short half-life
Pemoline	Dopamine uptake inhibition; low potency; hepatotoxicity
Selegiline (L-Deprenyl)	MAO B inhibitor; in vivo conversion into amphetamine
Modafinil	Fewer peripheral side effects; mode of action debated
Anticataplectic Compounds	
Venlafaxine	Specific serotonin and adrenergic reuptake blocker (5-HT = NE); very effective but some nausea
Atomoxetine	Specific adrenergic reuptake blocker (NE) normally indicated for attention-deficit/hyperactivity disorder; very effective
Fluoxetine	Specific serotonin uptake blocker (5-HT >> NE = DA). Active metabolite norfluoxetine has more adrenergic effects. High therapeutic doses are often needed.
Protriptyline	Tricyclic antidepressant; monoaminergic uptake blocker (NE > 5-HT > DA); anticholinergic effects
Imipramine	Tricyclic antidepressant; monoaminergic uptake blocker (NE = 5-HT > DA); anticholinergic effects. Desipramine is an active metabolite.
Desipramine	Tricyclic antidepressant; monoaminergic uptake blocker (NE >> 5-HT > DA); anticholinergic effects
Clomipramine	Tricyclic antidepressant; monoaminergic uptake blocker (5-HT > NE >> DA); anticholinergic effects. Desmethyl-clomipramine (NE >> 5-HT > DA) is an active metabolite; no specificity in vivo.
Other	
GHB (sodium oxybate)	May act through gamma-aminobutyric acid B receptors or through specific GHB receptors. Reduces dopamine release.

For details, see references 30, 39, 40, 43, 44, 46, and 98.

DA, dopamine; GHB, gamma-hydroxybutyric acid; 5-HT, 5-hydroxytryptamine (serotonin); MAO, monoamine oxidase; NE, norepinephrine.

blockers might thus increase activity in projection sites involved in REM sleep regulation. The fact that serotonergic uptake blockers, also known to have inhibitory effects on REM sleep, have less or no effect on cataplexy is more surprising. Like adrenergic cells of the locus coeruleus, serotonergic cells of the raphe nuclei dramatically decrease their activity during REM sleep (see Chapter 10). This discrepancy could be explained by a preferential effect of serotonergic projections on REM sleep features other than atonia, for example in the control of eye movements. In this model, adrenergic projections may be more important than serotonergic transmission in the regulation of REM sleep atonia and thus cataplexy.[39] In favor of this hypothesis, a recent experiment has shown that serotonergic activity does not decrease during cataplexy in narcoleptic canines,[42] in contrast to locus coeruleus activity.[41]

Increased Dopaminergic Transmission Mediates the Wake-Promoting Effects of Currently Prescribed Stimulant Compounds

The most commonly prescribed stimulants are amphetamine-like drugs, such as dextroamphetamine, methamphetamine, methylphenidate, pemoline, and the wake-promoting compound modafinil (see Table 64–2). Like tricyclic antidepressant compounds, amphetamine-like drugs are very nonspecific pharmacologically. Their main effect is globally to increase monoaminergic transmission by stimulating monoamine release and blocking monoamine reuptake. Abuse and dose escalation can occur with amphetamine, especially in cases without cataplexy. Less abuse is reported with methylphenidate, and modafinil is not believed to be addictive. Recent studies have demonstrated that the wake-promoting effect of these compounds is secondary to dopamine release stimulation and dopamine reuptake inhibition.[43,44] The mode of action of modafinil is debated, but this compound also selectively inhibits dopamine uptake.[45] All these compounds are ineffective in dopamine transporter knockout mice, suggesting a primary mediation of wake promotion through dopaminergic systems.[44] Compounds selective for dopaminergic transmission have no effect on cataplexy, however, whereas amphetamine-like compounds with combined dopaminergic and adrenergic effects have some anticataplectic properties at high doses.[39,46] Adrenergic effects of amphetamine-like stimulants also correlate with the respective effects of these compounds on normal REM sleep.[30,46] Dopaminergic-specific uptake blockers have little effect on REM sleep compared with adrenergic or serotonergic compounds.[30] The most important effects of dopaminergic uptake blockers are to reduce total sleep time and slow wave sleep.[43] This preferential effect of dopaminergic uptake blockers on non-REM sleep correlates with electrophysiologic data. As opposed to adrenergic or serotonergic neurons, the firing rate of dopaminergic neurons is known to remain relatively constant during REM sleep.[47,48]

Studies in both humans and narcoleptic canines have shown that large doses of stimulants are needed to "normalize" the polysomnogram in narcoleptic subjects. In our narcoleptic Doberman population, amphetamine doses equivalent to 60 mg/day were needed to reduce daytime sleep in our narcoleptic population to control levels.[31] In both control and narcoleptic animals, however, the dose–response curves for modafinil or amphetamine were parallel. This result suggests that there is no difference in sensitivity to stimulants in narcoleptic animals; rather, higher doses are needed in narcoleptic animals because of their extreme baseline sleepiness.[31]

Gamma-Hydroxybutyric Acid/Sodium Oxybate

Gamma-hydroxybutyric (GHB) acid, also called sodium oxybate, is a sedative anesthetic compound known to increase slow wave sleep and, to a lesser extent, REM sleep.[30] Occasional abuse in the context of "rave" parties has been reported, and the prescription of the compound is highly supervised. Because slow wave sleep is associated with growth hormone release, GHB also induces growth hormone release and has been abused by athletes. When administered at night, it consolidates sleep and improves daytime functioning. Because of its short half-life, it must be administered twice a night. Cataplexy and daytime alertness also improve over time, with a full therapeutic effect sometimes produced only after months of treatment and dose adjustments (see Chapter 65).

The mode of action of GHB on sleep and narcolepsy is unclear. GHB has a major effect on dopamine transmission, reducing firing rate and raising brain content of dopamine.[30,49] Other effects on opioid, glutamatergic, and cholinergic transmission have been reported.[49] Specific GHB receptors have been identified, but the compound is also a gamma-aminobutyric acid (GABA) B receptor agonist.[49] Most studies to date suggest that the sedative-hypnotic effect is mediated through $GABA_B$ agonist activity.[49,50] Whether this effect also mediates the anticataplectic effects after long-term administration is unknown. Human or animal studies using other $GABA_B$ agonists, such as high-dose baclofen, would be needed to answer these questions.

Other Known Modulators of Narcolepsy Symptoms

The effects of more than 200 compounds with various modes of action have been examined in human patients and narcoleptic canines (see Nishino and Mignot[30] for review). Almost all the compounds studied are monoaminergic and cholinergic modulators. These systems have been studied more intensively than others because selective pharmacologic probes for these systems are more generally available. With cataplexy being easier to study than sleep in canines, most studies have also focused on cataplexy rather than sleepiness. For cataplexy, the findings were consistent with pharmacologic studies of REM sleep. As is the case for REM sleep, the regulation of cataplexy is modulated positively by cholinergic systems and negatively by monoaminergic tone.[30] Muscarinic M_2 or M_3 receptors mediate the cholinergic effects, whereas monoaminergic effects are mostly modulated by postsynaptic adrenergic $alpha_1$ receptors and presynaptic D_2/D_3 dopaminergic autoreceptors.[30]

A number of studies have shown abnormal cholinergic and monoaminergic receptor density and neurotransmitter levels in human or canine narcolepsy brain and CSF samples.[30,51-63] Local injection studies in selected brain areas of narcoleptic canines have also shown functional relevance for some of these abnormalities.[64-66] Cholinergic hypersensitivity, dopaminergic abnormalities, and decreased histaminergic tone are likely to be critical downstream mediators of the expression of the Hcrt deficiency/narcolepsy symptomatology.[63-66] The cholinergic/monoaminergic imbalances observed in narcolepsy are best illustrated by the finding that in asymptomatic animals heterozygous for the hcrtr2 mutation, a combination of cholinergic agonists with an alpha$_1$-blocker or a D_2/D_3 agonist can trigger cataplexy.[29]

GENETIC ASPECTS OF HUMAN NARCOLEPSY

Familial Aspects of Human Narcolepsy

The familial occurrence of narcolepsy-cataplexy was first reported in 1877 by Westphal.[67] Since then, numerous familial case reports have appeared in the literature. Recent studies have shown that these earlier reports were often confounded by unrecognized obstructive sleep apnea. In more recent studies, the risk for development of narcolepsy-cataplexy in a first-degree relative has been shown to be only 1% to 2% (see Mignot[16] for review). A larger proportion of relatives (4% to 5%) may have isolated daytime sleepiness, when other causes of daytime sleepiness have been excluded.[16] These figures are important to keep in mind because they are helpful in reassuring patients regarding the risk to their children and relatives. A 1% to 2% risk is 10- to 40-fold higher than in the general population, but remains manageable. A 4% to 5% risk for daytime sleepiness is not negligible, but similar values have been reported for excessive daytime sleepiness in the general population independent of narcolepsy.[15,68,69]

Twin Studies and Environmental Factors in Narcolepsy

Twenty monozygotic twin reports are available in literature. Five to seven pairs are discordant for narcolepsy, depending on how strictly concordance is determined.[16,70-72] Most cases of narcolepsy therefore require the influence of environmental factors for the disease to develop. This is also substantiated by the fact that onset is not at birth but typically in adolescence.[6,73] Frequently cited triggering factors are head trauma,[74-76] sudden change in sleep–wake habits,[71,77] or various infections.[78,79] These factors may be involved, but all studies have used a retrospective design, limiting the value of any reported difference. Recent papers have found increased births for narcoleptic patients in March and a decreased frequency in September, suggesting the influence of perinatal factors.[80,81]

Human Narcolepsy, Human Leukocyte Antigen, and the Immune System

The observation that narcolepsy is associated with HLA- (also called major histocompatibility complex, or MHC) DR2 was first reported in Japan in 1983.[82,83] It was quickly confirmed in Europe and North America.[13,14,84-89] This discovery led to the hypothesis that narcolepsy may result from an autoimmune insult to the central nervous system (CNS). The finding of Hcrt cell loss in human narcolepsy[8,9] suggests that the autoimmune process could target this small population of hypothalamic neurons. Attempts at verifying autoimmune mediation have in general been disappointing.[90-93] Human narcolepsy is not associated with striking pathologic changes in the CNS or increased frequency in the occurrence of oligoclonal bands in the CSF.[90-93] Gliosis in human narcolepsy brains has been reported[8,9,94] but remains controversial, as are imaging findings suggesting macroscopic hypothalamic changes.[95-97] Similarly, peripheral immunity does not seem to be altered even around disease onset.[90,91] CD4/CD8 T-lymphocyte populations, various autoantibody levels, erythrocyte sedimentation rate, and C-reactive protein levels are within the normal range and were found not to change up to a year after disease onset. These studies do not exclude the possibility that an autoimmune mechanism will be discovered in the future. Rather, tissue destruction may be difficult to detect because of the small anatomic area involved. In addition, tissue destruction may be short-lasting and confined to the time surrounding disease onset.

Human Leukocyte Antigens DQB1*0602 and DQA1*0102 Are Actual Narcolepsy Susceptibility Genes

Since the initial discovery of the HLA-DR2 association in narcolepsy, HLA testing techniques have changed from serologic, antibody-based technology to molecular typing at the DNA level, resulting in a further layer of complexity for the clinician. The initial narcolepsy marker, DR2, was later defined as DR15 and then DRB1*1501/DRB1*1503. Another gene closely linked with HLA-DR, HLA-DQ, was also found to be associated with narcolepsy. Subtypes of HLA-DQ involved, listed by increased specificity, were DQ1, DQ6, and DQB1*0602. To facilitate the review of this nomenclature, the results are summarized in Figure 64–2 and Table 64–3.

Additional studies across ethnic groups have shown that DQB1*0602 is a better marker for narcolepsy. This is especially important in African Americans, where many patients are DQB1*0602 positive but DR2 negative.[13,14,98,99] Subjects were also found to be DQA1*0102 positive.[13,14,98,99] Novel DNA markers developed in the HLA-DQ region have been tested to map further the narcolepsy susceptibility region within the DQA1-DQB1 interval.[99,100] This segment was entirely sequenced and shown to contain no new genes.[100] In addition, in all narcolepsy susceptibility DR-DQ haplotypes identified, both DQA1*0102 and DQB1*0602 are present,[98,99] thus suggesting that the active DQA1*0102/DQB1*0602 heterodimer is necessary for disease predisposition.[99]

Recent findings in families and in unrelated cases also suggest that most, if not all the DQB1*0602/DQA1*0102 alleles present in the general population predispose equally to narcolepsy. One such finding comes from multiplex families, where several patients are DQB1*0602 positive. In many cases, DQB1*0602 has been inherited from different branches of the family (e.g., in one case from the father and the other case from the mother) and are thus not "identical by descent."[16] It was also recently shown that subjects homozygous for DQB1*0602 are at a twofold to fourfold increased risk for development of narcolepsy compared with DQB1*0602 heterozygous subjects.[14,101]

Finally, risk in DQB1*0602 heterozygous individuals is modulated by the other DQB1 allele. Most notably, risk is increased in DQB1*0602/DQB1*0301 heterozygotes and reduced in DQB1*0602/DQB1*0601 and DQB1*0602/DQB1*0501 heterozygotes.[14] Overall, the data strongly suggest that the HLA-DQ alleles themselves (especially DQB1*0602 and DQA1*0102), and not a yet unknown genetic factor in the region, predispose to narcolepsy.

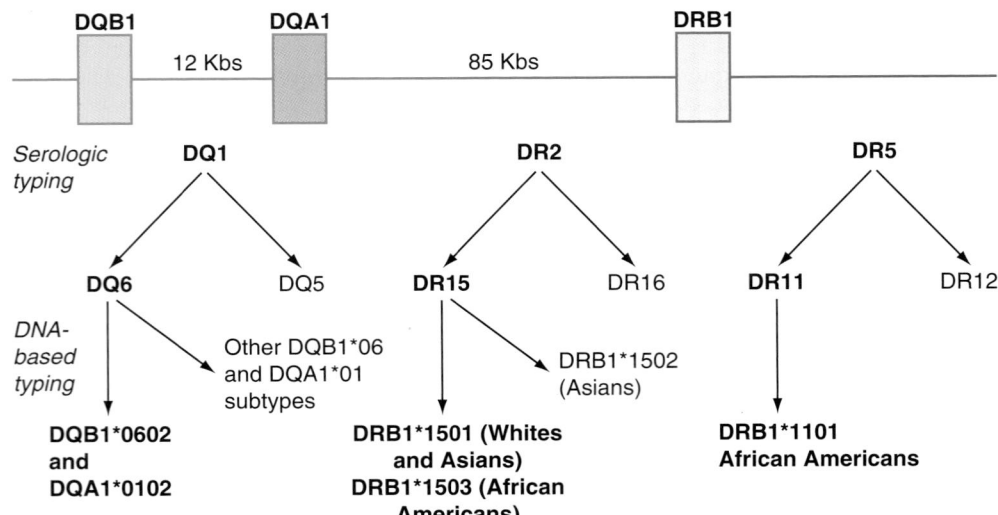

Figure 64–2. Human leukocyte antigen (HLA)-DR and HLA-DQ alleles most typically observed in narcolepsy. The HLA-DR and DQ genes are located very close to each other (85 kb) on chromosome 6p21. These genes encode heterodimeric HLA proteins composed of an α and a β chain. In the DQ locus, both the DQ α and DQ β chains have numerous variable residues and are encoded by two polymorphic genes, DQA1 and DQB1, respectively. Polymorphism at the DR level is mostly encoded by the DRB1 gene, so only this locus is depicted in this figure. At the DR level, DR2 was first split into two subtypes, DR15 and DR16, using serologic typing techniques. DR15 was then identified in DR2 narcoleptic subjects. Molecular subtypes of DR15, DRB1*1501 to DRB1*1514,[158] were further identified at the DRB1 level using DNA sequencing or oligotyping; note that most subtypes except 1501 through 1503 are extremely rare. At the DQ level, all patients were initially found to be DQ1, a very frequent DQ antigen (Table 64–3). DQ1 was then serologically split into DQ5 and DQ6, and all patients were found to be DQ6. Molecular subtypes of DQ6 are identified at the DQB1 level as DQB1*0601 to DQB1*0618 (most subtypes except DQB1*0601, 0602, 0603, 0604, and 0609 are very rare). The DQ6 subtype identified in patients with narcolepsy was found to be DQB1*0602.[13,14,98,99] It is always associated with the DQA1 subtype, DQA1*0102. In whites and Asians, the associated DR2 subtype DRB1*1501 is typically observed with DQB1*0602 (and DQA1*0102) in narcoleptic patients. In African Americans, either DRB1*1503, a DNA-based subtype of DR2, or DRB1*1101, a DNA-based subtype of DR5, is most frequently observed, together with DQB1*0602. Other DRB1 alleles (DRB1*0301, DRB1*0806, DRB1*12022, and DRB1*1602) can be observed together with DQB1*0602, although much more rarely.[13,14,98,99]

Table 64–3. Human Leukocyte Antigen Allele Frequencies in Narcoleptic and Control Subjects across Ethnic Groups

| HLA Marker | Frequency in | | Notes |
	Clear-cut Cataplexy*	Control Subjects†	
HLA-DR2			
Whites	85-100%	26%	Serologic typing (DR15 and DR16 are DR2 subtypes);
African Americans	65-75%	31%	old narcolepsy marker.
Japanese	100%	36%	
HLA-DR15			
Whites	85-100%	23%	Serologic or DNA-based typing; most DR2 antigens are
African Americans	65-75%	29%	DR15 in control subjects and patients; almost
Japanese	100%	35%	equivalent to DR2.
HLA-DRB1*1501			
Whites	85-100%	22%	DNA-based typing; most DR15 antigens are DRB1*1501
African Americans	10-20%	7%	in whites.
Japanese	100%	13%	
HLA-DRB1*1502			
Japanese	2%	22%	DNA-based typing; Asian antigen; two thirds of the DR15
(not associated with narcolepsy)			antigens are DRB1*1502 in Japanese; associated with DQB1*0601 not DQB1*0602.
HLA-DRB1*1503			
African Americans	55-65%	20%	DNA-based typing; African antigen; most DR15 antigens are DRB1*1503 in African Americans.
HLA-DQ1			
Whites	90-100%	67%	
African Americans	>95%	75%	Serologic typing (DQ5 and DQ6 are DQ1 subtypes); very
Japanese	100%	73%	frequent; low specificity; old narcolepsy marker.
HLA-DQB1*0602			
Whites	85-100%	22%	Almost always found with DRB1*1501 in whites
African Americans	90-95%	34%	and Asians.
Japanese	100%	12%	

Table 64–3.   Human Leukocyte Antigen Allele Frequencies in Narcoleptic and Control Subjects across Ethnic Groups—cont'd

HLA Marker	Frequency in Clear-cut Cataplexy*	Control Subjects†	Notes
HLA-DQA1*0102			
Whites	85-100%	36%	More frequent in control subjects than DQB1*0602;
African Americans	90-95%	48%	associated with many DQB1*05 and 06 alleles.
Japanese	100%	26%	
HLA-DQA1*0102/DQB1*0602			
Whites	85-100%	22%	Patients with DQB1*0602 are always DQA1*0102
African Americans	90-95%	33%	positive.
Japanese	100%	12%	

*Narcolepsy values are approximated from references 82-89 and 98-101.

†Control values are population carrier frequencies compiled from composite panels of 333 American white (see references 14, 154 and 98; and courtesy of S. Hsu) and 364 African-American and white control subjects (see references 14, 98, and 154; and courtesy of M. S. Leffell) and 717 Japanese control subjects (courtesy of A. Kimura).

HLA, human leukocyte antigen.

Human Leukocyte Antigen and Narcolepsy in Clinical Practice

The usefulness of HLA typing in clinical practice is limited by several factors. First, the HLA association is very high (more than 90%) only in narcoleptic patients with clear-cut cataplexy.[13] Clear-cut cataplexy is defined as episodes of muscle weakness triggered by laughter, joking, or anger. Muscle weakness episodes triggered by anger, stress, and other negative emotions or physical or sexual activity may not be cataplexy if joking or laughing is not also mentioned as a triggering factor.[4] In patients without cataplexy or with doubtful cataplexy, HLA DQB1*0602 frequency is also increased (40%), but many patients are DQB1*0602 negative.[13] Second, a large number of control individuals (see Table 64–3) have the HLA DQB1*0602 marker without having narcolepsy. Finally, a few rare patients with clear-cut cataplexy do not have the HLA DQB1*0602 marker.[102]

Despite these limitations, HLA typing is probably most useful in atypical cases or in narcolepsy without definite cataplexy. A negative result should lead the clinician to be more cautious in excluding other possible causes of daytime sleepiness, such as abnormal breathing during sleep. Practically, it is always more useful to request HLA-DQ high-resolution typing rather than DR2 or DR15 typing to confirm the diagnosis of narcolepsy. Typical HLA-DR and DQ results are depicted in Table 64–4, together with their interpretation. It is not necessary to test for DQA1*0102 because almost all subjects with DQB1*0602 are also DQA1*0102 positive (see Table 64–3). Most HLA typing laboratories also do not routinely type for DQA1.

Human Leukocyte Antigen DQB1*0602 Negativity

HLA-DQB1*0602–negative subjects with typical and severe cataplexy have been reported, but these subjects are exceptionally rare.[102] An increase in DQB1*0301 in DQB1*0602-negative subjects has been suggested, but needs further substantiation.[14] Most (but not all) of these patients have normal CSF Hcrt-1, suggesting a different pathophysiologic process[10] (Fig. 64–3). Two partially concordant monozygotic twins reported in the literature were DQB1*0602 negative.[16] A number of DQB1*0602-negative families (with normal CSF Hcrt-1) have been reported where narcolepsy and cataplexy seems to be transmitted as a highly penetrant autosomal dominant trait.[10,16] These results emphasize the fact that HLA typing and CSF Hcrt-1 results should be interpreted in conjunction with a careful family history.

HLA-DQB1*0602–negative subjects with cataplexy have also been reported in the context of posttraumatic narcolepsy in the United States.[74-76] This finding would need confirmation in other cultures because the issue could easily be confounded by medicolegal factors in North America.

Genetic Factors Other than Human Leukocyte Antigen

As mentioned previously, genetic factors other than HLA-DQ and DR are likely to be involved in narcolepsy predisposition. The increased risk in first-degree relatives (10-fold in Japanese, 20- to 40-fold in whites) cannot be explained solely by the sharing of HLA subtypes, estimated to explain only a 2- to 3-fold increased risk.[14,16] In addition, the existence of HLA-negative families suggests disease heterogeneity and the possible involvement of other genes. Linkage analysis in HLA-DQB1*0602–positive Japanese families has suggested the existence of a susceptibility gene on 4q13-23.[103] A possible association with tumor necrosis factor-α gene polymorphism (independent of HLA) has been suggested.[104-106] Other results indicate that a polymorphism in the catechol-O-methyltransferase gene, a key enzyme in the degradation of catecholamine, may also modulate disease severity and response to stimulant treatment.[107,108]

As expected from the observation that most cases of human narcolepsy are sporadic and not fully genetic, like in some dogs or mice, an extensive screening study did not identify preprohcrt, hcrtr1, or hcrtr2 mutations in most human narcolepsy cases.[8,109,110] Polymorphisms were observed but were not found to be associated with narcolepsy. Surprisingly, even familial cases of narcolepsy (some of which were HLA-DQB1*0602 negative) did not have any Hcrt gene mutations, suggesting heterogeneity in genetic cases.[8] Rather, only a single case with a signal peptide mutation of the preproHcrt gene was identified.

Table 64–4. **Examples of Human Leukocyte Antigen Typing Results and Their Interpretation**

Clinical Case	HLA Typing*	Interpretation
35-Year-old white man with clear-cut cataplexy	DRB1*1501, DRB1*1101 DQB1*0602, DQB1*0301	Compatible with narcolepsy: DR2+, DQB1*0602+
13-Year-old white boy without cataplexy but SOREMPs	DRB1*1501, DRB1*X† DQB1*0602, DQB1*X	Compatible with narcolepsy: DR2+ homozygous, DQB1*0602+ homozygous
55-Year-old African-American woman with cataplexy	DRB1*1101, DRB1*0401 DQB1*0602, DQB1*0301	Compatible with narcolepsy: DR2–, DQB1*0602+
32-Year-old Japanese man without cataplexy but SOREMPs	DRB1*1502, DRB1*0405 DQB1*0401, DQB1*0601	Not typical for narcolepsy: DR2+ but DRB1*1502 and DQB1*0602–
35-Year-old African-American man without cataplexy but with SOREMPs	DRB1*0302, DRB1*1503 DQB1*0402, DQB1*0602	Compatible with narcolepsy: DR2+, DQB1*0602+
47-Year-old white woman with cataplexy and SOREMPs	DR2+ (insufficient typing resolution)	Compatible with narcolepsy; in whites, almost all DR2+ are DQB1*0602+
25-Year-old white man with possible cataplexy and two SOREMPs	DR1, DR3, DQ1, DQ2 (insufficient typing resolution)	Not typical for narcolepsy. DQ1 has a low specificity. It is also associated with DR1, DR6, and DR10, but DQ1 then is not DQB1*0602.

*HLA typing results may not always be depicted as shown. HLA-DRB1 results do not need to be requested for clinical purposes if HLA-DQB1*0602 results are provided. DRB1 typing results are indicated in this table as a reference to older classifications. HLA-DRB2, DRB3, DRB4, or DRB5 typing results may be reported in addition to HLA-DRB1 typing results, but should be ignored. In subject 2, the subject is "DRB1*X" and "DQB1*X." It is very likely that DRB1*15-DQB1*0602 is present on both chromosomes, thus indicating homozygosity. A theoretically possible alternative explanation would involve undetectable DRB1 and DQB1 alleles on one of the subject's chromosomes (blank). HLA typing in parents of subject 2 would be required to establish homozygosity absolutely. Note that if a patient is homozygous for DQB1*0602, the narcolepsy diagnosis is even more probable; 18-30% of narcoleptic subjects are DQB1*0602 homozygous versus 0-4% in African American and white control subjects.[14,101] In subject 3, one of the HLA haplotypes is most probably DRB1*1101-DQB1*0602 (frequent in African Americans), whereas the other haplotype is DRB1*0401-DQB1*0301 (frequent in all ethnic groups). In whites, DR2 and DQB1*0602 typing is almost equivalent and it is probably unnecessary to retype a patient if he or she has been shown to be DR2 positive using serologic typing techniques (subject 6). Most white subjects with DR2 are also DQB1*0602 positive, but the situation is somewhat different in Asians and African Americans (also see Table 64–3).

†X indicates blank or homozygosity.

HLA, human leukocyte antigen.

This case had an extremely early onset (6 months), severe narcolepsy-cataplexy, DQB1*0602 negativity, and undetectable Hcrtr-1 CSF levels.[8] This important observation indicates that Hcrt system gene mutations can cause narcolepsy in humans, as in animal models. However, Hcrt gene polymorphisms or mutations do not contribute significantly to overall narcolepsy predisposition in the population. Additional studies are thus needed to identify genetic factors predisposing to narcolepsy other than HLA.

HYPOCRETIN DEFICIENCY IN HUMAN NARCOLEPSY

Hypocretin Deficiency in Narcolepsy-Cataplexy

After cloning the canine narcolepsy gene, we found that most sporadic, HLA-DQB1*0602–positive, narcoleptic patients with cataplexy have undetectable Hcrt-1 levels in the CSF (see Fig. 64-3).[7-12,111] Follow-up neuropathologic studies in 10 narcoleptic patients indicated dramatic loss of Hcrt-1, Hcrt-2, and preproHcrt messenger RNA (mRNA) in the brains and hypothalami of narcoleptic patients.[8,9] Figure 64–4 shows a typical loss of Hcrt mRNA in the hypothalamus of a patient with narcolepsy-cataplexy compared with control subjects. As mentioned previously, these subjects have no Hcrt gene mutations[8] and a peripubertal or postpubertal disease onset[73] as opposed to a 6-month onset in the subject with a preproHcrt mutation.[8] Together with the tight HLA association,[13,14] a likely pathophysiologic mechanism in most narcolepsy cases could thus involve an autoimmune alteration of Hcrt-containing cells in the CNS.

The observation that CSF Hcrt-1 levels are decreased in patients with narcolepsy provides a new test to diagnose this disorder. Using a large sample of patients and control subjects, we determined that 110 pg/mL (30% of mean control values) was the most specific and sensitive cut-off value to diagnose narcolepsy.[10] Most samples had undetectable levels (less than 40 pg/mL), whereas a few samples had detectable but very diminished levels (see Fig. 64–3). None of the

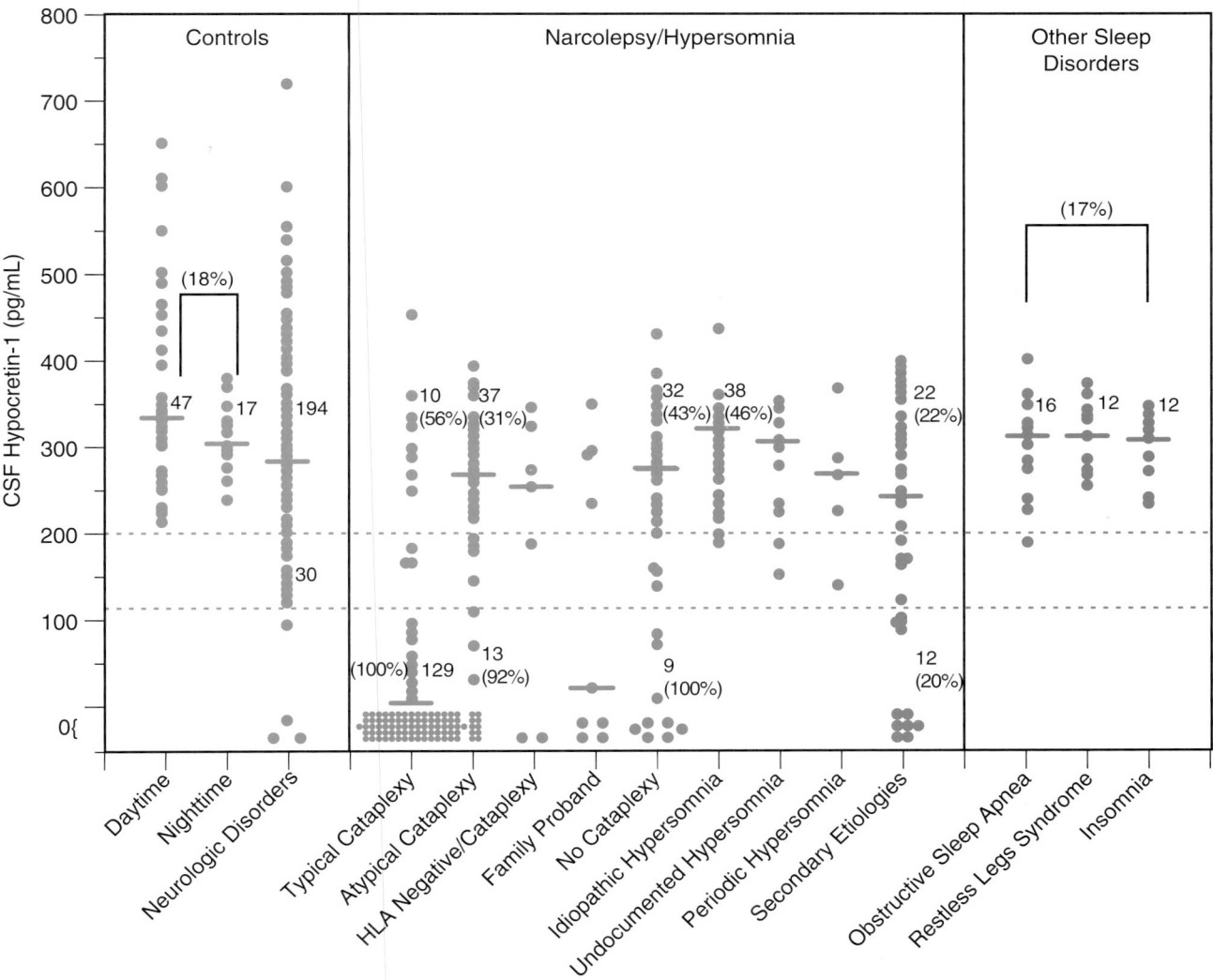

Figure 64–3. Cerebrospinal fluid (CSF) hypocretin-1 (Hcrt-1) concentrations are plotted for individuals across various control and sleep disorders. Each point represents the crude concentration of Hcrt-1 in a single person. The cutoffs for normal (>200 pg/mL) and low (<110 pg/mL) Hcrt-1 concentrations are shown. Also noted is the total number of subjects in each range, and the percentage human leukocyte antigen (HLA)-DQB1*0602 positivity for a given group in a given range is parenthetically noted for certain disorders. Note that control carrier frequencies for DQB1*0602 are 17% to 22% in healthy control subjects and secondary narcolepsy, consistent with control values reported in whites (see Table 64–3). In other patient groups, values are higher, with almost all Hcrt-deficient narcolepsy being HLA DQB1*0602 positive. The median value in each group is shown as a *horizontal bar*. (Updated from previously published data in Mignot E, Lammers GJ, Ripley B, et al.: The role of cerebrospinal fluid hypocretin measurement in the diagnosis of narcolepsy and other hypersomnias. Arch Neurol 2002;59:1553-1562.)

patients with idiopathic hypersomnia, sleep apnea, restless legs syndrome, or insomnia had abnormal Hcrt levels.

Diagnostic Value of Cerebrospinal Fluid Hypocretin-1 Measurements

Using the 110 pg/mL cutoff, CSF Hcrt-1 measurements are especially predictive in patients with definite cataplexy (99% specificity, 87% sensitivity). In these cases, sensitivity and specificity are higher than for the MSLT (Table 64–5). In contrast, CSF Hcrt-1 measurements have a more limited predictive power in cases with atypical or absent cataplexy. Specificity is still extremely high (99%) but sensitivity is low (16%; see Mignot et al.[10]; Fig. 64–3), with most cases having normal levels.[10-12]

This is clearly a dilemma for the clinician because there is more often a need for a definitive diagnosis in these atypical cases.

Possible indications for CSF Hcrt-1 measurements are listed in Table 64–5. The diagnostic value of the CSF Hcrt-1 test needs to be weighed against the trauma associated with obtaining CSF. Lumbar punctures are well known to be safe, but post–lumbar puncture headaches are often observed.[112] The trauma associated with the lumbar puncture must be balanced against the risk of mislabeling a patient with narcolepsy and possibly introducing lifelong treatment. In general, the MSLT is a more useful first step because it is more determinant for the diagnosis and treatment strategies (see Table 64–5). If a lumbar puncture is still required, HLA typing could be useful as a first step because almost all cases of narcolepsy with

Table 64–5.   Advantages and Disadvantages of Selected Diagnostic Procedures for Narcolepsy

Procedures	Advantages	Disadvantages/Limitations	Suggested Indications
MSLT after nocturnal polysomnography* Mean sleep latency <8 min, ≥2 sleep-onset rapid eye movement periods	Identifies concurrent sleep disorders (e.g., sleep-disordered breathing) Safe and painless Measures a physiologic tendency toward sleepiness independent of any biologic cause By definition, positive in cases without cataplexy Available and recognized by insurance companies and other professionals	Cannot be interpreted if sleep was insufficient or disturbed before the MSLT Cannot be conducted in patients on stimulants or antidepressants Has a 15% false-negative rate in narcolepsy-cataplexy False-positive results possible in cases of sleep apnea or sleep deprivation, and in adolescents Not validated in young children Difficult to conduct in very young children and complex cases (i.e., psychiatric cases) Expensive	Most cases, especially if without cataplexy
Cerebrospinal fluid hypocretin-1 measurements Direct assay: <110 pg/mL	Highly specific (99%) and sensitive (87%) in cases with typical cataplexy Biologically based, definitive test for narcolepsy Not sensitive to the presence of psychotropic drugs or of concurrent sleep disorders	High specificity (99%) but low sensitivity (16%) in cases without cataplexy or with atypical cataplexy Painful, long-lasting post–lumbar puncture headache may occur Contraindications (i.e., anticoagulants, high-pressure hydrocephalus) Hypocretin assay not widely available and not standardized Should be interpreted within the clinical context if a severe brain pathologic process is present (e.g., coma, Guillain-Barré syndrome, head trauma) Intermediary values (110-200 pg/mL) of unknown significance	Some cases with possible cataplexy where sleep-disordered breathing or insomnia is severe, making the MSLT difficult to interpret Young children unable to follow MSLT instructions (e.g., younger than 7 years of age) Recent-onset cases with a negative MSLT Patients treated with psychotropic drugs (e.g., antidepressants) unwilling to interrupt treatment Patients with cataplexy in whom narcolepsy is still suspected despite a negative MSLT Individuals unable to afford the cost of an MSLT Individuals with complex associated psychiatric, neurologic, or medical disorders (e.g., secondary narcolepsy) Treatment failures; in need of reevaluation (e.g., patients with cataplexy taking high-dose stimulants without positive response)
HLA-DQ typing Positive for DQB1*0602	Highly sensitive (90%) in cases with cataplexy	Very low specificity; 8-38% of the population is positive Only 40% positive in cases without cataplexy	Very limited interest. Can only assist the diagnosis; should not be used formally to diagnose narcolepsy.

*Other polygraphic tests of possible diagnostic value, such as continuous 24-hour sleep recording studies, are not discussed.

HLA, human leukocyte antigen; MSLT, Multiple Sleep Latency Test.

Narcoleptic Control

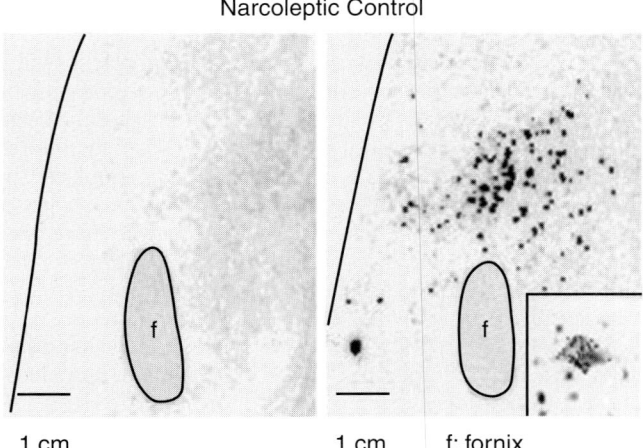

1 cm   1 cm   f; fornix

Figure 64–4. Preprohypocretin messenger RNA staining (in situ hybridization) in a narcoleptic human brain hypothalamus **(A)** contrasted with control **(B).** Each dot in the control represents a hypocretin-producing cell. Note that most of these cells are located close to the fornix area, a white matter tract (f). The dramatic loss of the hypocretin signal is evident in the narcoleptic brain. (From Peyron C, Faraco J, Rogers W, et al.: A mutation in a case of early onset narcolepsy and a generalized absence of hypocretin peptides in human narcoleptic brains. Nat Med 2000;6:991-997.)

low CSF Hcrt-1 levels also are HLA-DQB1*0602 subtype positive[10-12,113]; only three exceptions have been reported (over several hundred patients with low Hcrt-1), including one case where cataplexy was very mild and atypical.[8,10,113] We estimate that the probability of observing low levels of CSF Hcrt-1 in HLA-negative primary narcolepsy cases is far less than 1%.

A rational argument can be made that neither the MSLT nor a CSF Hcrt-1 measurement will affect treatment plans in patients with cataplexy, and therefore such testing may be extraneous in such cases. In fact, the MSLT is not required for the diagnosis of narcolepsy if clear, definite cataplexy is present. However, in many patients presenting with cataplexy, objective data are still recommended. In cases with cataplexy, CSF Hcrt-1 testing may be most helpful when the MSLT is difficult to conduct or interpret (see Table 64–5). In cases without cataplexy, most (but not all) cases with low CSF Hcrt-1 levels have been observed in children in whom cataplexy develops later in the course of the disease.[10,114,115] Therefore, we generally advise that young children with excessive daytime sleepiness but without cataplexy undergo CSF Hcrt-1 testing, as well as cases in which there is a suspicion that cataplexy is present but not clearly reported (Table 64–6).

Although the diagnostic value of low CSF Hcrt-1 (less than 110 pg/mL) has been established, all healthy control values have been shown to be above 200 pg/mL[10] (see Fig. 64–3). In rare cases of narcolepsy and hypersomnia, we have found Hcrt-1 levels between these two values, raising the possibility of partial Hcrt deficiency in these cases.[10] Such values should, however, be cautiously interpreted because in a large series of individuals with various neurologic disorders, we found that up to 15% had CSF Hcrt-1 values within this intermediate range (see Fig. 64–3); most of these cases represented severe brain disease, most notably head trauma, encephalitis, and subarachnoid hemorrhage.[111] Decreased Hcrt-1 levels in these cases may reflect damage to Hcrt transmission, or may be related to changes in CSF flow. Other authors have shown that CSF Hcrt-1 increases with locomotor activity and decreases with treatment with serotonin reuptake inhibitors (but never to near-undetectable, narcolepsy-like levels).[116] Therefore, the finding of Hcrt-1 levels in this intermediate range should alert

Table 64–6.   Cerebrospinal Fluid Hypocretin-1 and Human Leukocyte Antigen Results: Selected Examples

Clinical Case	Cerebrospinal Fluid Hypocretin-1 Level	Notes
8-Year-old boy without cataplexy (onset within 6 mo)	88 pg/mL; HLA+, MSLT+	Diagnostic for narcolepsy, treatment with modafinil, later in association with venlafaxine
17-Year-old boy with rape hallucinations; suspicious and difficult to interview; possible cataplexy	Undetectable (<40 pg/ml); HLA+, refused MSLT	Narcolepsy associated with psychosis, positive effect of venlafaxine
16-Year-old girl with a 5-year history of depression and drug-resistant insomnia; cataplexy on interview	Undetectable (<40 pg/mL); HLA+, MSLT not interpretable	Diagnostic for narcolepsy, now successfully treated with sodium oxybate, modafinil, and atomoxetine
32-Year-old man, post resection of hypothalamic craniopharyngioma, very impaired, possible cataplexy	152 pg/mL ; HLA–, MSLT impossible	Questionable narcolepsy; possibly lesions of other areas; partial effect of stimulants
33-Year-old woman successfully treated with D-amphetamine and fluoxetine; recently moved to the area; no MSLT	Undetectable (<40 pg/mL); HLA+	Diagnostic for narcolepsy, no change in treatment but considering modafinil
15-Year-old girl with sleepiness, no cataplexy	310 pg/mL; HLA+, MSLT+	Narcolepsy without cataplexy; treatment with modafinil

HLA, human leukocyte antigen; HLA+, HLA-DQB1*0602 positive; MSLT, Multiple Sleep Latency Test; MSLT+, mean sleep latency <8 minutes, ≥2 sleep-onset rapid eye movement periods.

the clinician to the possibility of underlying brain disease, which may require additional clinical evaluation, laboratory testing, or imaging. Whether genuine Hcrt deficiency explains abnormal sleep in these neurologic disorders is in need of further investigation (see also next section).

SECONDARY NARCOLEPSY

Von Economo was the first to suggest that narcolepsy may have its origins in the posterior hypothalamus and in some cases a secondary etiology. In his classic study of the encephalitis lethargica pandemic (1916-1923), von Economo recognized three categories of patients: a group with hypersomnia and eye movement abnormalities (somnolent-ophthalmoplegic), a group with insomnia and hyperkinetic movement disorder (sometimes with reversal of the sleep cycle), and a group with parkinsonism (amyostatic-akinetic, often as a residual form).[117,118] Neuropathologic studies revealed involvement of the midbrain periaqueductal gray matter and posterior hypothalamus in the hypersomnolent variant, with frequent extension to the oculomotor nuclei, explaining the oculomotor symptoms. Involvement of the anterior hypothalamus with extension into basal ganglia was observed in the insomnia variant. This led von Economo to speculate that the anterior hypothalamus contained a sleep-promoting area, whereas an area spanning from the posterior wall of the third ventricle to the third nerve was involved in actively promoting wakefulness. The cause of idiopathic narcolepsy, which had been described approximately 50 years earlier,[67] was also speculated to involve this general area.[118]

This hypothesis was further refined by others, who noted that tumors or other lesions located close to the third ventricle were associated with secondary narcolepsy and hypothesized that the posterior hypothalamic region may be the culprit.[117,119] A postulated hypothalamic cause of narcolepsy was widespread until the 1940s, but was then ignored during the psychoanalytic boom, and thereafter replaced by a brainstem hypothesis.[120] Interestingly, only two cases of postencephalitis genuine narcolepsy with cataplexy have been reported.[121,122] In one case, some reversal of symptoms was observed with recovery (whether this was a coincidence or real causality is unknown).

As mentioned, reports of third ventricle lesions (hypothalamus and upper midbrain) in association with narcolepsy (such as tumors) have been described for over 80 years.[117-123] Narcolepsy-like symptoms have also been reported after traumatic brain injury, paramedian thalamic stroke, acute disseminated encephalomyelitis, hypothalamic sarcoidosis, or histiocytosis X, and in association with multiple sclerosis and Parkinson's disease[124-130] (Box 64–1). In some cases, lesions of the hypothalamic Hcrt centers have been clearly identified using magnetic resonance imaging, as in bilateral multiple sclerosis plaques in the hypothalamus, and tumors of the third ventricle.[124-129] Cataplexy may be present in these cases, and CSF Hcrt-1 levels may be either in the narcolepsy range (less than 110 pg/mL) or in the intermediate range[10,124-129] (see Box 64–1). Such intermediate levels may reflect damage to nearby Hcrt projection sites, with sufficient preservation of cell bodies to maintain detectable levels of Hcrt-1. Alternatively (or additionally), other regions, for example, in

---

Box 64–1. Cerebrospinal Fluid Hypocretin-1 Measurements in Secondary Narcolepsy and Hypersomnia*

Secondary Hypersomnia with Low Hypocretin-1 Levels ($\leq$110 pg/mL)

- Acute disseminated encephalomyelitis with sleepiness ($n = 3$)
- Autosomal dominant cerebellar ataxia, deafness, and narcolepsy ($n = 1$)
- Large pituitary adenoma with probable hypothalamic involvement ($n = 1$)
- Late-onset congenital hypoventilation syndrome ($n = 1$)
- Limbic encephalitis ($n = 1$)
- Multiple sclerosis cases with bilateral hypothalamic plaques ($n = 2$)
- Myotonic dystrophy type 1 ($n = 1$)
- Paraneoplastic syndrome with anti Ma2 and sleepiness, possible cataplexy ($n = 4$)
- Post removal of a hypothalamic tumor ($n = 2$); hypothalamic tumor ($n = 1$)
- Prader-Willi syndrome ($n = 1$)
- Steroid-responsive encephalopathy associated with autoimmune thyroiditis ($n = 1$)
- Wernicke encephalopathy with hypothalamic involvement ($n = 1$)
- Whipple's disease with central nervous system involvement ($n = 1$; with hypersomnia)

Secondary Hypersomnia with Intermediate Hypocretin-1 Levels (110-200 pg/mL)

- Limbic encephalitis ($n = 1$)
- Myotonic dystrophy type 1 ($n = 2$)
- Niemann-Pick disease type C with cataplexy ($n = 2$)
- Post diencephalic stroke with hypothalamic and midbrain lesions ($n = 1$)
- Post head trauma ($n = 1$)
- Prader-Willi syndrome ($n = 1$)

Secondary Hypersomnia with Normal Hypocretin-1 Levels (>200 pg/mL)

- Acute disseminated encephalomyelitis with sleepiness ($n = 1$)
- Encephalitis lethargica-like syndrome, post streptococcal ($n = 1$)
- Human immunodeficiency virus encephalopathy with sleepiness ($n = 1$)
- Hypersomnia with depression ($n = 6$)

Box 64–1.   Cerebrospinal Fluid Hypocretin-1 Measurements in Secondary Narcolepsy and Hypersomnia*—cont'd

- Hypersomnia with Parkinson's disease ($n = 3$)
- Multiple sclerosis with hypothalamic involvement ($n = 1$)
- Myotonic dystrophy type 1 ($n = 3$)
- Neurocysticercosis cysts in the hypothalamus and other locations ($n = 1$)
- Niemann-Pick disease type C without cataplexy ($n = 1$)
- Narcolepsy-cataplexy post hypothalamic irradiation ($n = 1$)
- Pontine lesion ($n = 1$)
- Thalamocortical ($n = 1$) and paramedian thalamic ($n = 3$) strokes

Other Pathologies with Intermediate Levels of Hypocretin-1 (No Reported but Possible Sleep Symptoms)[†]

- Traumatic brain injury (numerous cases, probably transitory)
- Various neoplasms of the brain (numerous cases)
- Encephalitis of infectious origin (numerous cases)
- Guillain-Barré syndrome and other inflammatory neuropathies (numerous cases)

Pathologies with Low Levels of Hypocretin-1 (No Reported but Possible Sleep Symptoms)

- Guillain-Barré syndrome ($n = 7$); transitory, unknown significance
- Myxedema coma, no clinical documentation ($n = 1$)
- Post traumatic head injury trauma coma ($n = 1$)

*Cases tested at Stanford University or in centers that used the same standard cerebrospinal fluid (CSF) samples for comparisons are included[124]; measurements in other laboratories cannot be compared.
[†]In another case of Whipple's disease with long-lasting resistant insomnia without hypersomnia, intermediary CSF hypocretin-1 levels were found. This may reflect more complex hypothalamic damage that could include the anterior hypothalamus.
For cases listed in this Box, see references 10, 111, 124-135, and 155-157.

the paramedian thalamus or upper midbrain (as initially proposed by von Economo) may also contribute to the symptomatology, especially sleepiness.

The complex area of genetic or congenital disorders associated with primary central hypersomnolence is also of great interest. Genetic disorders such as Coffin-Lowry syndrome,[131] Möbius syndrome,[132] Norrie's disease,[132] Prader-Willi syndrome,[10] Niemann-Pick disease type C,[10,133,134] and myotonic dystrophy[135] have been reported to be associated with daytime sleepiness or cataplexy-like symptoms. CSF Hcrt-1 has been measured in cases of Niemann-Pick disease type C, a condition where oculomotor symptoms are frequent, and intermediate levels have been found in some cases with cataplexy.[10,133,134] This condition is remarkable because the cataplexy is often triggered by typical emotions (laughing) and partially responsive to anticataplectic treatment. Some diseases are associated with the development of both narcolepsy and sleep-disordered breathing, such as myotonic dystrophy[135] and Prader-Willi syndrome[10]; in such cases, primary hypersomnia should be diagnosed only if excessive daytime sleepiness does not improve after adequate treatment of sleep-disordered breathing. We have explored CSF Hcrt-1 levels in such cases, and have found that some but not all of these patients have very low CSF Hcrt-1 levels (less than 110 pg/mL), suggesting Hcrt deficiency.[10,133] Similarly, in one case of late-onset congenital hypoventilation syndrome, a disorder with reported hypothalamic abnormalities,[136] we found very low CSF Hcrt-1 levels in an individual with otherwise unexplained sleepiness and cataplexy-like episodes.[10] Excellent response to anticataplectic therapy was observed in this case.

Additional studies are needed to expand on these anecdotal reports, to determine whether these changes in CSF Hcrt-1 levels in secondary cases truly represent abnormalities

in their respective cells or their projections, or rather simply represent a nonspecific finding in some secondary etiologies.

TOWARD A NEUROBIOLOGIC MODEL FOR NARCOLEPSY

The role of Hcrt in the regulation of normal sleep is beginning to emerge. In rats and monkeys, Hcrt-1 release is maximal at the end of the active period and minimal at the end of the inactive period.[137,138] These results suggests that Hcrt may be important to promote wakefulness in the evening (in diurnal animals such as humans). In this model, Hcrt would oppose the sleep debt that has accumulated since early morning, allowing a constant level of wakefulness through the day.[138] Additional studies suggest that diurnal fluctuations in Hcrt release are driven both directly by the circadian clock of the suprachiasmatic nucleus and indirectly by the increased sleep debt. Of note, lumbar CSF Hcrt-1 only has limited diurnal fluctuation (10%), suggesting a dampening and delay of brain neurotransmitter changes when reaching the lumbar sack.[116] This finding is important practically because the time of CSF collection has no significant effect for narcolepsy diagnostic purposes.[10,124]

Hcrt neurons project heavily onto monoaminergic cell groups of the locus coeruleus (norepinephrine), ventral tegmental area (dopamine), raphe magnus (serotonin), and tuberomammillary (histamine) neurons. Dopamine and histamine cell groups have one of the highest hcrtr2 receptor densities.[139] Considering the role of hcrtr2 in canine narcolepsy, these projections may be especially important.[140-143] Increased dopamine levels in the amygdala are one of the most consistent neurochemical abnormalities reported in canine narcolepsy.[51,53] Decreased histamine levels are also observed in the brain of narcoleptic canines.[63] In vivo dialysis studies have indicated

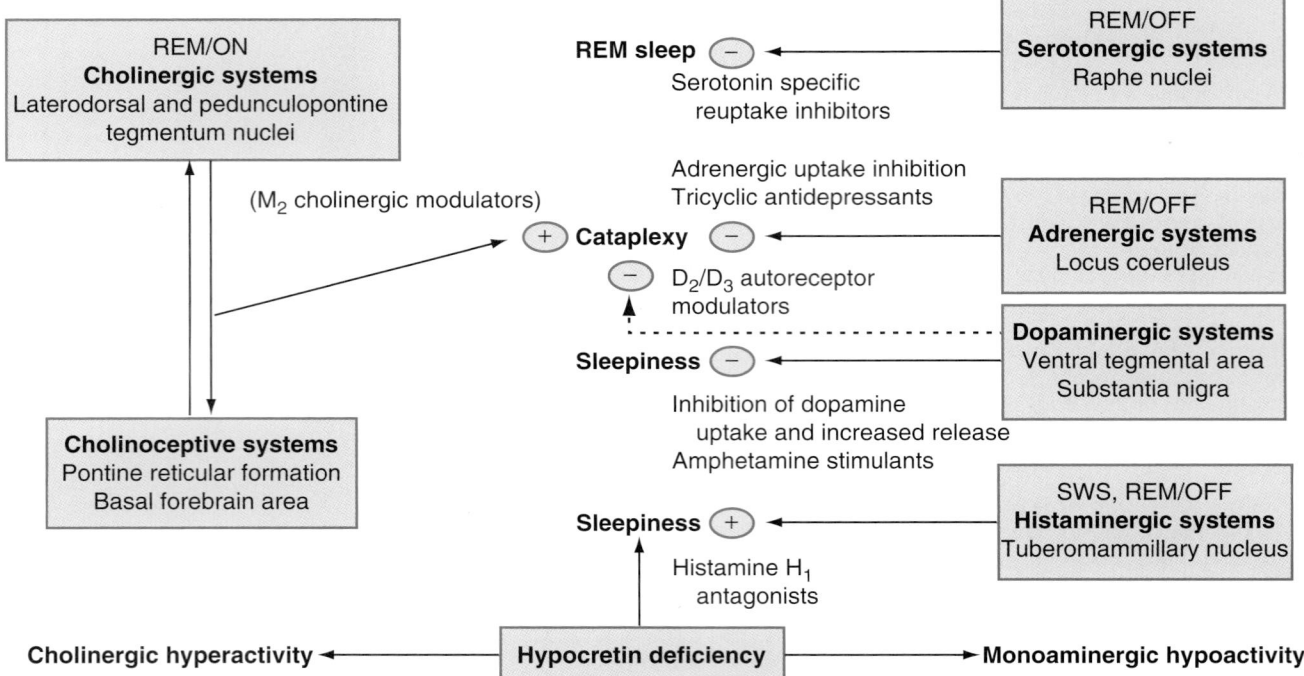

Figure 64–5. Neuropharmacologic and neurochemical control of cataplexy and excessive daytime sleepiness. Narcolepsy in animal models is due to genetic alterations in the hypocretin systems. Note that cataplexy, like rapid eye movement (REM) sleep, is regulated by a balance of activity between adrenergic and cholinergic tone. Anticataplectic antidepressant medications are believed to act primarily by increasing adrenergic tone (adrenergic uptake inhibition). Serotonergic systems are also known to decrease activity during REM sleep, but increasing serotonergic tone with serotonin uptake blockers reduces REM sleep but not cataplexy in narcoleptic dogs. The most commonly prescribed stimulant compounds promote wakefulness by increasing presynaptic dopaminergic transmission (dopamine uptake inhibition or increased dopamine release). Histaminergic systems are likely also to be involved in the expression of daytime sleepiness. Dopaminergic mechanisms may also be involved in the emotional triggering of cataplexy. (For details, see text.)

a critical role for the dopamine mesolimbic and mesocortical system in the regulation of alertness and the triggering of cataplexy by emotions. Histaminergic transmission has long been recognized as a critical wake-promoting neurotransmitter system.[144] Dopamine and histaminergic projections may thus be centrally involved in controlling both cataplexy and alertness. Similar to REM sleep, cataplexy is controlled by pontine cholinergic REM-on cells and aminergic locus REM-off cells.[30] Removing Hcrt excitatory projections to monoamine cell groups could decrease monoaminergic tone and produce a cholinergic-aminergic imbalance consistent with sleepiness and abnormal REM sleep in narcolepsy (Fig. 64–5).

It is also likely that Hcrt is important to the integration of sleep regulation with metabolic status. Narcoleptic patients are slightly more obese[74,145,146] than the general population. Recent results also indicate that Hcrt cells sense glucose, leptin, and ghrelin, responding to metabolic signals, possibly increasing wakefulness when there is a need to search for food during fasting.[147] Hcrt adds another layer of complexity to the understanding of interactions among hypothalamic peptidergic systems in the regulation of appetite, feeding, and metabolism in general.[140]

HYPOCRETIN COMPOUNDS AS POTENTIAL THERAPEUTIC TARGETS

The effects of Hcrt administration on sleep and narcolepsy symptoms have been evaluated.[148,149] Central administration of Hcrt-1, for example in the ventricle of wild-type rodents or normal canines, is strongly wake promoting.[149] The effect is likely to be at least in part mediated by the hcrtr2 receptor because intracerebroventricular Hcrt-1 at the same dose (10 to 30 nmol) has no effects in hcrtr2-mutated narcoleptic canines.[150] Hcrt-2 administration has few if any central effects even in normal animals, most probably because it is biologically unstable and rapidly degraded. The instability may also explain why Hcrt-1 but not Hcrt-2 is detectable in native CSF.[150]

Experiments after intravenous administration of Hcrt-1 have been conducted in hcrtr2-mutated canines and in two Hcrt-deficient narcoleptic dogs. In spite of a previous report,[148] we were unable to detect any significant effect even at extremely high doses in hcrtr2-mutated animals.[149] This result was not surprising, considering the lack of effects after central administration of the same dose in these animals lacking hcrtr2 (see earlier). More interestingly, a possible very slight and brief suppression of cataplexy was observed in a single Hcrt-deficient narcoleptic animal at extremely high doses.[149,151] We also examined the possibility of intrathecal administration by implanting a Medtronic pump with catheterization of the cisterna magna in a single Hcrt-deficient narcoleptic canine.[151] Our hope was that at high dose, some reverse flow would occur back into deeper brain structures, providing therapeutic relief. A positive result would have had therapeutic application because these pumps are frequently used in humans for the treatment of pain or spasticity by intrathecal administration of drug. Disappointingly, however, we did not observe any significant effect on cataplexy,[151] probably because the Hcrt did not diffuse into upper ventricular compartments. Additional studies using intraventricular rather than intracisternal injections are needed to verify that Hcrt-deficient narcoleptic canines are responsive to supplementation.

CONCLUSION

Narcolepsy-cataplexy is most commonly caused by a loss of Hcrt-producing cells in the hypothalamus. Low CSF Hcrt-1 levels can be used to diagnose the condition. The disorder is tightly associated with HLA-DQB1*0602, suggesting that the cause of most of these cases may be an autoimmune destruction of these cells. The Hcrt system sends strong excitatory projections onto monoaminergic cells. The loss of Hcrt creates a cholinergic-monoaminergic imbalance in narcolepsy. Abnormally sensitive cholinergic transmission, together with depressed dopaminergic and histaminergic transmission, are believed to underlie abnormal REM sleep and daytime sleepiness in narcolepsy. Current treatments are symptomatically based and act downstream of the Hcrt abnormality. Presynaptic stimulation of dopaminergic transmission and adrenergic uptake inhibition mediate the wake-promoting and anticataplectic effects of stimulants and antidepressants, respectively. GHB, a sedative compound, may act through $GABA_B$ receptors or specific GHB receptors.

Although most cases of narcolepsy-cataplexy are caused by an Hcrt cell loss, some cases with cataplexy and most cases without cataplexy have normal CSF Hcrt-1 levels. This may reflect either disease heterogeneity or a partial loss of Hcrt neurons without significant CSF Hcrt-1 decrements. A critical area in need of further inquiry is the role of CSF Hcrt-1 testing in predicting therapeutic response to medications already in use to treat narcolepsy.[124] Developing an assay that could

reliably measure Hcrt-1 in plasma may be possible and would also be useful if low levels are observed in narcolepsy.[124]

Whether narcolepsy is an autoimmune disorder is still unclear, but highly suspected. Other possible explanations could involve an infectious agent, with participation of the immune system. Explaining the link between the HLA association and Hcrt deficiency must be a high priority. It may be possible to use CSF Hcrt-1 testing to evaluate the extent of Hcrt cell loss in early stages of the disease (e.g., in children), thus facilitating the development of treatments that may be able to arrest or at least delay disease progression. Similar strategies using immunosuppression have been used in other autoimmune diseases, such as type 1 diabetes mellitus. In one case, 2 months after an abrupt onset, we tried high-dose prednisone, but did not observe significant effects on symptoms and CSF Hcrt-1 levels[152]; however, in this case, very low Hcrt-1 levels were already observed, suggesting the possibility that irreversible damage to cells had already occurred. In another case with recent onset, intravenous immunoglobulin administration was reported to have positive effects, suggesting the need for further studies.[153] We anticipate that in time, patients with narcolepsy will benefit from studies currently underway in sleep medicine as well as other areas of medicine.

Clinical Pearls

Measuring CSF Hcrt-1 is a useful and predictive diagnostic test in patients with cataplexy. The test may be especially useful when the MSLT is difficult to conduct or to interpret, and in complex cases or in young children.

Most cases of narcolepsy are sporadic, so patients diagnosed with narcolepsy should be reassured regarding the low probability of the disorder developing in children or a relative.

HLA typing should never be used to diagnose narcolepsy because it has an extremely low specificity.

When considering treatment for a patient with narcolepsy, it is critical to consider the mode of action of the various compounds available for use. For cataplexy, the most effective pathway to control the symptom may be adrenergic reuptake inhibition, with some additional effect of serotonin reuptake inhibition. GHB most likely acts on GHB and $GABA_B$ receptors; it is effective in cataplexy, disturbed nocturnal sleep, and sleepiness. For sleepiness, most stimulants act by increasing dopaminergic transmission, some by blocking dopamine reuptake, others by stimulating dopamine release. Some stimulants also increase adrenergic release, and thus may participate in the wake-promoting effect. When using stimulants, it is probably best to start with compounds that inhibit dopamine reuptake (modafinil before methylphenidate) and move on to dopamine-releasing agents (amphetamines) only when the other compounds are not effective enough.

REFERENCES

1. American Academy of Sleep Medicine: International Classification of Sleep Disorders: Diagnostic and Coding Manual, 2nd ed. Westchester, Ill, American Academy of Sleep Medicine, 2005.
2. Guilleminault C, Mignot E, Partinen M: Controversies in the diagnosis of narcolepsy. Sleep 1994;17(8 Suppl):S1-S6.
3. Aldrich MS: The clinical spectrum of narcolepsy and idiopathic hypersomnia. Neurology 1996;46:393-401.
4. Anic-Labat S, Guilleminault C, Kraemer HC, et al: Validation of a cataplexy questionnaire in 983 sleep-disorders patients. Sleep 1999;22:77-87.
5. Overeem S, Mignot E, van Dijk JG, Lammers GJ: Narcolepsy: Clinical features, new pathophysiologic insights, and future perspectives. J Clin Neurophysiol 2001;18:78-105.
6. Dauvilliers Y, Billiard M, Montplaisir J: Clinical aspects and pathophysiology of narcolepsy. Clin Neurophysiol 2003;114:2000-2017.
7. Nishino S, Ripley B, Overeem S, et al: Hypocretin (orexin) deficiency in human narcolepsy. Lancet 2000;355:39-40.
8. Peyron C, Faraco J, Rogers W, et al: A mutation in a case of early onset narcolepsy and a generalized absence of hypocretin peptides in human narcoleptic brains. Nat Med 2000;6:991-997.
9. Thannickal TC, Moore RY, Nienhuis R, et al: Reduced number of hypocretin neurons in human narcolepsy. Neuron 2000;27:469-474.
10. Mignot E, Lammers GJ, Ripley B, et al: The role of cerebrospinal fluid hypocretin measurement in the diagnosis of narcolepsy and other hypersomnias. Arch Neurol 2002;59:1553-1562.
11. Kanbayashi T, Inoue Y, Chiba S, et al: CSF hypocretin-1 (orexin-A) concentrations in narcolepsy with and without cataplexy and idiopathic hypersomnia. J Sleep Res 2002;11:91-93.
12. Krahn LE, Pankratz VS, Oliver L, et al: Hypocretin (orexin) levels in cerebrospinal fluid of patients with narcolepsy: Relationship to cataplexy and HLA DQB1*0602 status. Sleep 2002;25:733-736.
13. Mignot E, Hayduk R, Black J, et al: HLA DQB1*0602 is associated with cataplexy in 509 narcoleptic patients. Sleep 1997;20:1012-1020.

14. Mignot E, Lin L, Rogers W, et al: Complex HLA-DR and -DQ interactions confer risk of narcolepsy-cataplexy in three ethnic groups. Am J Hum Genet 2001;68:686-699.

15. Hublin C, Kaprio J, Partinen M, et al: Daytime sleepiness in an adult, Finnish population. J Intern Med 1996;239:417-423.

16. Mignot E: Genetic and familial aspects of narcolepsy. Neurology 1998;50(2 Suppl 1):S16-S22.

17. Solomon P: Narcolepsy in Negroes. Dis Nerv Sys 1945;6:179-183.

18. Tashiro T, Kambayashi T, Hishikawa Y: An Epidemiological Study of Narcolepsy in Japanese. Proceedings of the 4th International Symposium on Narcolepsy; Tokyo, June 16–17, 1994;13.

19. Honda Y: Census of narcolepsy, cataplexy and sleep life among teenagers in Fujisawa City. Sleep Res Online 1979;8:191.

20. Lavie P, Peled R: Narcolepsy is a rare disease in Israel. Sleep 1987;10:608-609.

21. Geisler P, Croeleun F, Tracik F, Zulley J: MSLT: Sleep latency in normals is age and sex related. J Seep Res 1998;7(Suppl 2):99.

22. Bishop C, Rosenthal L, Helmus T, et al: The frequency of multiple sleep onset REM periods among subjects with no excessive daytime sleepiness. Sleep 1996;19:727-730.

23. Carskadon MA, Wolfson A, Acebo C, et al: Adolescent sleep patterns, circadian timing, and sleepiness at a transition to early school days. Sleep 1998;21:271-281.

24. Silber MH, Krahn LE, Olson EJ, Pankratz VS: The epidemiology of narcolepsy in Olmsted County, Minnesota: A population-based study. Sleep 2002;25:197-202.

25. Knecht CD, Oliver JE, Redding R, et al: Narcolepsy in a dog and a cat. J Am Vet Med Assoc 1973;162:1052-1053.

26. Mitler MM, Boysen BG, Campbell L, Dement WC: Narcolepsy-cataplexy in a female dog. Exp Neurol 1974;45:332-340.

27. Baker TL, Foutz AS, McNerney V, et al: Canine model of narcolepsy: Genetic and developmental determinants. Exp Neurol 1982;75:729-742.

28. Hungs M, Fan J, Lin L, et al: Identification and functional analysis of mutations in the hypocretin (orexin) genes of narcoleptic canines. Genome Res 2001;11:531-539.

29. Mignot E, Nishino S, Sharp LH, et al: Heterozygosity at the canarc-1 locus can confer susceptibility for narcolepsy: Induction of cataplexy in heterozygous asymptomatic dogs after administration of a combination of drugs acting on monoaminergic and cholinergic systems. J Neurosci 1993;13:1057-1064.

30. Nishino S, Mignot E: Pharmacological aspects of human and canine narcolepsy. Prog Neurobiol 1997;52:27-78.

31. Shelton J, Nishino S, Vaught J, et al: Comparative effects of modafinil and amphetamine on daytime sleepiness and cataplexy of narcoleptic dogs. Sleep 1995;18:817-826.

32. Kushida CA, Baker TL, Dement WC: Electroencephalographic correlates of cataplectic attacks in narcoleptic canines. Electroencephalogr Clin Neurophysiol 1985;61:61-70.

33. Lin L, Faraco J, Li R, et al: The sleep disorder canine narcolepsy is caused by a mutation in the hypocretin (orexin) receptor 2 gene. Cell 1999;98:365-376.

34. Ripley B, Fujiki N, Okura M, et al: Hypocretin levels in sporadic and familial cases of canine narcolepsy. Neurobiol Dis 2001;8:525-534.

35. Chemelli RM, Willie JT, Sinton CM, et al: Narcolepsy in orexin knockout mice: Molecular genetics of sleep regulation. Cell 1999;98:437-451.

36. Hara J, Beuckmann CT, Nambu T, et al: Genetic ablation of orexin neurons in mice results in narcolepsy, hypophagia, and obesity. Neuron 2001;30:345-354.

37. Willie JT, Chemelli RM, Sinton CM, et al: Distinct narcolepsy syndromes in orexin receptor-2 and orexin null mice: Molecular genetic dissection of non-REM and REM sleep regulatory processes. Neuron 2003;38:715-730.

38. Kisanuki YY, Chemelli RM, Sinton CM, et al: The role of orexin receptor type-1 (OXIR) in the regulation of sleep. Sleep 2000;23(Suppl 2):A91.

39. Mignot E, Renaud A, Nishino S, et al: Canine cataplexy is preferentially controlled by adrenergic mechanisms: Evidence using monoamine selective uptake inhibitors and release enhancers. Psychopharmacology (Berl) 1993;113:76-82.

40. Nishino S, Arrigoni J, Shelton J, et al: Desmethyl metabolites of serotonergic uptake inhibitors are more potent for suppressing canine cataplexy than their parent compounds. Sleep 1993;16:706-712.

41. Wu MF, Gulyani SA, Yau E, et al: Locus coeruleus neurons: Cessation of activity during cataplexy. Neuroscience 1999;91:1389-1399.

42. Wu MF, John J, Boehmer LB, et al: Activity of dorsal raphe cells across the sleep-waking cycle and during cataplexy in narcoleptic dogs. J Physiol (Lond) 2004;554:202-215.

43. Nishino S, Mao J, Sampathkumaran R, Shelton J: Increased dopaminergic transmission mediates the wake-promoting effects of CNS stimulants. Sleep Res Online 1998;1:49-61.

44. Wisor JP, Nishino S, Sora I, et al: Dopaminergic role in stimulant-induced wakefulness. J Neurosci 2001;21:1787-1794.

45. Mignot E, Nishino S, Guilleminault C, Dement WC: Modafinil binds to the dopamine uptake carrier site with low affinity. Sleep 1994;17:436-437.

46. Kanbayashi T, Honda K, Kodama T, et al: Implication of dopaminergic mechanisms in the wake-promoting effects of amphetamine: A study of D- and L-derivatives in canine narcolepsy. Neuroscience 2000;99:651-659.

47. Miller JD, Farber J, Gatz P, et al: Activity of mesencephalic dopamine and non-dopamine neurons across stages of sleep and walking in the rat. Brain Res 1983;273:133-141.

48. Steinfels GF, Heym J, Strecker RE, Jacobs BL: Behavioral correlates of dopaminergic unit activity in freely moving cats. Brain Res 1983;258:217-228.

49. Castelli MP, Ferraro L, Mocci I, et al: Selective gamma-hydroxybutyric acid receptor ligands increase extracellular glutamate in the hippocampus, but fail to activate G protein and to produce the sedative/hypnotic effect of gamma-hydroxybutyric acid. J Neurochem 2003;87:722-732.

50. Queva C, Bremner-Danielsen M, Edlund A, et al: Effects of GABA agonists on body temperature regulation in GABA(B[1])−/− mice. Br J Pharmacol 2003;140:315-322.

51. Baker TL, Dement WC: Canine narcolepsy-cataplexy syndrome: Evidence for an inherited monoaminergic-cholinergic imbalance. In McGinty DJ, Drucker-Colin R, Morrison A, Parmeggiani PL (eds): Brain Mechanisms of Sleep. New York, Raven Press, 1985, pp 199-233.

52. Aldrich MS: The neurobiology of narcolepsy-cataplexy. Prog Neurobiol 1993;41:533-541.

53. Miller JD, Faull KF, Bowersox SS, Dement WC: CNS monoamines and their metabolites in canine narcolepsy: A replication study. Brain Res 1990;509:169-171.

54. Kilduff TS, Bowersox SS, Kaitin KI, et al: Muscarinic cholinergic receptors and the canine model of narcolepsy. Sleep 1986;9:102-106.

55. Kish SJ, Mamelak M, Slimovitch C, et al: Brain neurotransmitter changes in human narcolepsy. Neurology 1992;42:229-234.

56. Aldrich MS, Hollingsworth Z, Penney JB: Dopamine-receptor autoradiography of human narcoleptic brain. Neurology 1992;42:410-415.

57. Aldrich MS, Prokopowicz G, Ockert K, et al: Neurochemical studies of human narcolepsy: Alpha-adrenergic receptor autoradiography of human narcoleptic brain and brainstem. Sleep 1994;17:598-608.

58. Bowersox SS, Kilduff TS, Faull KF, et al: Brain dopamine receptor levels elevated in canine narcolepsy. Brain Res 1987;402:44-48.

59. Khan N, Antonini A, Parkes D, et al: Striatal dopamine D2 receptors in patients with narcolepsy measured with PET and 11C-raclopride. Neurology 1994;44:2102-2104.

60. Rinne JO, Hublin C, Partinen M, et al: Positron emission tomography study of human narcolepsy: No increase in striatal dopamine D2 receptors. Neurology 1995;45:1735-1738.

61. MacFarlane JG, List SJ, Moldofsky H, et al: Dopamine D2 receptors quantified in vivo in human narcolepsy. Biol Psychiatry 1997;41:305-310.

62. Faull KF, Guilleminault C, Berger PA, Barchas JD: Cerebrospinal fluid monoamine metabolites in narcolepsy and hypersomnia. Ann Neurol 1983;13:258-263.

63. Nishino S, Fujiki N, Ripley B, et al: Decreased brain histamine content in hypocretin/orexin receptor-2 mutated narcoleptic dogs. Neurosci Lett 2001;313:125-128.

64. Nishino S, Tafti M, Reid MS, et al: Muscle atonia is triggered by cholinergic stimulation of the basal forebrain: Implication for the pathophysiology of canine narcolepsy. J Neurosci 1995; 15:4806-4814.

65. Reid MS, Nishino S, Tafti M, et al: Neuropharmacological characterization of basal forebrain cholinergic stimulated cataplexy in narcoleptic canines. Exp Neurol 1998;151:89-104.

66. Reid MS, Tafti M, Nishino S, et al: Local administration of dopaminergic drugs into the ventral tegmental area modulates cataplexy in the narcoleptic canine. Brain Res 1996;733: 83-100.

67. Westphal C: Eigenthumliche mit Einschlafen verbundene Anfalle. Arch Psychiatr 1877;7:631-635.

68. Young T, Palta M, Dempsey J, et al: The occurrence of sleep-disordered breathing among middle-aged adults. N Engl J Med 1993;328:1230-1235.

69. D'Alessandro R, Rinaldi R, Cristina E, et al: Prevalence of excessive daytime sleepiness an open epidemiological problem. Sleep 1995;18:389-391.

70. Honda M, Honda Y, Uchida S, et al: Monozygotic twins incompletely concordant for narcolepsy. Biol Psychiatry 2001;49: 943-947.

71. Honda Y: A monozygotic pair completely discordant for narcolepsy, with sleep deprivation as a possible precipitating factor. Sleep Biol Rhythms 2003;1:147-149.

72. Dauvilliers Y, Maret S, Bassetti C, et al: A monozygotic twin pair discordant for narcolepsy and CSF hypocretin-1. Neurology 2004;62:2137.

73. Okun ML, Lin L, Pelin Z, et al: Clinical aspects of narcolepsy-cataplexy across ethnic groups. Sleep 2002;25:27-35.

74. Gill AW: Idiopathic and traumatic narcolepsy. Lancet 1941;1:474.

75. Guilleminault C, Faull KF, Miles L, van den Hoed J: Posttraumatic excessive daytime sleepiness: A review of 20 patients. Neurology 1983;33:1584-1589.

76. Lankford DA, Wellman JJ, O'Hara C: Posttraumatic narcolepsy in mild to moderate closed head injury. Sleep 1994;17(8 Suppl): S25-S28.

77. Orellana C, Villemin E, Tafti M, et al: Life events in the year preceding the onset of narcolepsy. Sleep 1994;17(8 Suppl): S50-S53.

78. Roth B: Narcolepsy and Hypersomnia. Basel, Karger, 1980.

79. Mueller-Eckhardt G, Meier-Ewart K, Schiefer HG: Is there an infectious origin of narcolepsy? Lancet 1990;335:424.

80. Dauvilliers Y, Carlander B, Molinari N, et al: Month of birth as a risk factor for narcolepsy. Sleep 2003;26:663-665.

81. Dahmen N, Tonn P: Season of birth effect in narcolepsy. Neurology 2003;61:1016.

82. Honda Y, Asake A, Tanaka Y, Juji T: Discrimination of narcolepsy by using genetic markers and HLA. Sleep Res 1983; 12:254.

83. Juji T, Satake M, Honda Y, Doi Y: HLA antigens in Japanese patients with narcolepsy: All the patients were DR2 positive. Tissue Antigens 1984;24:316-319.

84. Mueller-Eckhardt G, Meier-Ewert K, Schendel DJ, et al: HLA and narcolepsy in a German population. Tissue Antigens 1986; 28:163-169.

85. Langdon N, Welsh KI, van Dam M, et al: Genetic markers in narcolepsy. Lancet 1984;2:1178-1180.

86. Roth B, Nevsimalova S, Sonka K, et al: A study of the occurrence of HLA DR2 in 124 narcoleptics: Clinical aspects. Schweiz Arch Neurol Psychiatr 1988;139(4):41-51.

87. Sachs C, Moller E: The occurrence of HLA-DR2 in clinically established narcolepsy. Acta Neurol Scand 1987;75:437-439.

88. Billiard M, Seignalet J, Besset A, Cadilhac J: HLA-DR2 and narcolepsy. Sleep 1986;9:149-152.

89. Poirier G, Montplaisir J, Decary F, et al: HLA antigens in narcolepsy and idiopathic central nervous system hypersomnolence. Sleep 1986;9:153-158.

90. Mignot E, Tafti M, Dement WC, Grumet FC: Narcolepsy and immunity. Adv Neuroimmunol 1995;5:23-37.

91. Carlander B, Eliaou JF, Billiard M: Autoimmune hypothesis in narcolepsy. Neurophysiol Clin 1993;23:15-22.

92. Black JL III, Krahn LE, Pankratz VS, Michael S: Search for neuron-specific and nonneuron-specific antibodies in narcoleptic patients with and without HLA DQB1*0602. Sleep 2002;25:719-723.

93. Overeem S, Geleijins K, Garssen MP, et al: Screening for anti-ganglioside antibodies in hypocretin-deficient human narcolepsy. Neurosci Lett 2003;341:13-16.

94. Thannickal TC, Siegel JM, Nienhuis R, Moore RY: Pattern of hypocretin (orexin) soma and axon loss, and gliosis, in human narcolepsy. Brain Pathol 2003;13:340-351.

95. Kaufmann C, Schuld A, Pollmacher T, Auer DP: Reduced cortical gray matter in narcolepsy: Preliminary findings with voxel-based morphometry. Neurology 2002;58:1852-1855.

96. Draganski B, Geisler P, Hajak G, et al: Hypothalamic gray matter changes in narcoleptic patients. Nat Med 2002;8: 1186-1188.

97. Overeem S, Steens SC, Good CD, et al: Voxel-based morphometry in hypocretin-deficient narcolepsy. Sleep 2003;26:44-46.

98. Mignot E, Lin X, Arrigoni J, et al: DQB1*0602 and DQA1*0102 (DQ1) are better markers than DR2 for narcolepsy in Caucasian and black Americans. Sleep 1994;17(8 Suppl):S60-S67.

99. Mignot E, Kimura A, Lattermann A, et al: Extensive HLA class II studies in 58 non-DRB1*15 (DR2) narcoleptic patients with cataplexy. Tissue Antigens 1997;49:329-341.

100. Ellis MC, Hetisimer AH, Ruddy DA, et al: HLA class II haplotype and sequence analysis support a role for DQ in narcolepsy. Immunogenetics 1997;46:410-417.

101. Pelin Z, Guilleminault C, Risch N, et al: HLA-DQB1*0602 homozygosity increases relative risk for narcolepsy but not disease severity in two ethnic groups. U.S. Modafinil in Narcolepsy Multicenter Study Group. Tissue Antigens 1998; 51:96-100.

102. Mignot E, Lin X, Kalil J, et al: DQB1-0602 (DQw1) is not present in most nonDR2 Caucasian narcoleptics. Sleep 1992; 15:415-422.

103. Nakayama J, Miura M, Honda M, et al: Linkage of human narcolepsy with HLA association to chromosome 4p13-q21. Genomics 2000;65:84-86.

104. Hohjoh H, Terada N, Nakayama T, et al: Case-control study with narcoleptic patients and healthy controls who, like the patients, possess both HLA-DRB1*1501 and -DQB1*0602. Tissue Antigens 2001;57:230-235.

105. Kato T, Honda M, Kuwata S, et al: Novel polymorphism in the promoter region of the tumor necrosis factor alpha gene: No association with narcolepsy. Am J Med Genet 1999;88: 301-304.

106. Wieczorek S, Gencik M, Rujescu D, et al: TNFA promoter polymorphisms and narcolepsy. Tissue Antigens 2003;61: 437-442.

107. Dauvilliers Y, Neidhart E, Billiard M, Tafti M. Sexual dimorphism of the catechol-O-methyltransferase gene in narcolepsy is associated with response to modafinil. Pharmacogenom J 2002;2:65-68.

108. Dauvilliers Y, Neidhart E, Lecendreux M, et al: MAO-A and COMT polymorphisms and gene effects in narcolepsy. Mol Psychiatry 2001;6:367-372.

109. Hungs M, Lin L, Okun M, Mignot E: Polymorphisms in the vicinity of the hypocretin/orexin are not associated with human narcolepsy. Neurology 2001;57:1893-1895.

110. Olafsdottir BR, Rye DB, Scammell TE, et al: Polymorphisms in hypocretin/orexin pathway genes and narcolepsy. Neurology 2001;57:1896-1899.

111. Ripley B, Overeem S, Fujiki N, et al: CSF hypocretin/orexin levels in narcolepsy and other neurological conditions. Neurology 2001;57:2253-2258.

112. Evans RW: Complications of lumbar puncture. Neurol Clin 1998;16:83-105.

113. Dalal MA, Schuld A, Pollmacher T: Undetectable CSF level of orexin A (hypocretin-1) in a HLA-DR2 negative patient with narcolepsy-cataplexy. J Sleep Res 2002;11:273.

114. Hecht M, Lin L, Kushida CA, et al: Immunosuppression with prednisone in an 8-year-old boy with an acute onset of hypocretin deficiency/narcolepsy. Sleep 2003;26:809-810.

115. Kubota H, Kanbayashi T, Tanabe Y, et al: Decreased cerebrospinal fluid hypocretin-1 levels near the onset of narcolepsy in 2 prepubertal children. Sleep 2003;26:555-557.

116. Salomon RM, Ripley B, Kennedy JS, et al: Diurnal variation of cerebrospinal fluid hypocretin-1 (orexin-A) levels in control and depressed subjects. Biol Psychiatry 2003;54:96-104.

117. von Economo C: Encephalitis Lethargica: Its Sequelae and Treatment. London, Oxford University Press, 1931.

118. von Economo C: Sleep as a problem of localization. J Nerv Ment Dis 1930;71:249-259.

119. Daniels LE: Narcolepsy. Medicine (Baltimore) 1934;13(1):1-122.

120. Mignot E: A hundred years of narcolepsy research. Arch Ital Biol 2001;139:207-220.

121. Symonds CP: Narcolepsy as a symptom of encephalitis lethargica. Lancet 1926;12:1214-1215.

122. Adie WJ: Idiopathic narcolepsy: A disease sui generis; with remarks on the mechanism of sleep. Brain 1926;49:257-306.

123. Aldrich MS, Naylor MW: Narcolepsy associated with lesions of the diencephalon. Neurology 1989;39:1505-1508.

124. Mignot E, Chen W, Black J: On the value of measuring CSF hypocretin-1 in diagnosing narcolepsy. Sleep 2003;26:646-649.

125. Arii J, Kanbayashi T, Tanabe Y, et al: A hypersomnolent girl with decreased CSF hypocretin level after removal of a hypothalamic tumor. Neurology 2001;56:1775-1776.

126. Dempsey OJ, McGeoch P, De Silva RN, Douglas NJ: Acquired narcolepsy in an acromegalic patient who underwent pituitary irradiation. Neurology 2003;61:537-540.

127. Kato T, Kanbayashi T, Yamamoto K, et al: Hypersomnia and low CSF hypocretin-1 (orexin-A) concentration in a patient with multiple sclerosis showing bilateral hypothalamic lesions. Intern Med 2003;42:743-745.

128. Kubota H, Kanbayashi T, Tanabe Y, et al: A case of acute disseminated encephalomyelitis presenting hypersomnia with decreased hypocretin level in cerebrospinal fluid. J Child Neurol 2002;17:537-539.

129. Scammell TE, Nishino S, Mignot E, Saper CB: Narcolepsy and low CSF orexin (hypocretin) concentration after a diencephalic stroke. Neurology 2001;56:1751-1753.

130. Overeem S, van Hilten JJ, Ripley B, et al: Normal hypocretin-1 levels in Parkinson's disease patients with excessive daytime sleepiness. Neurology 2002;58:498-499.

131. Nelson GB, Hahn JS: Stimulus-induced drop episodes in Coffin-Lowry syndrome. Pediatrics 2003;111:197-202.

132. Parkes JD: Genetic factors in human sleep disorders with special reference to Norrie disease, Prader-Willi syndrome and Moebius syndrome. J Sleep Res 1999;8(Suppl 1):14-22.

133. Kanbayashi T, Abe M, Fujimoto S, et al: Hypocretin deficiency in Niemann-Pick type C with cataplexy. Neuropediatrics 2003;34:52-53.

134. Vankova J, Stepanova I, Jech R, et al: Sleep disturbances and hypocretin deficiency in Niemann-Pick disease type C. Sleep 2003;26:427-430.

135. Martinez-Rodriguez JE, Lin L, Iranzo A, et al: Decreased hypocretin-1 (orexin-A) levels in the cerebrospinal fluid of patients with myotonic dystrophy and excessive daytime sleepiness. Sleep 2003;26:287-290.

136. Katz ES, McGrath S, Marcus CL: Late-onset central hypoventilation with hypothalamic dysfunction: A distinct clinical syndrome. Pediatr Pulmonol 2000;29:62-68.

137. Fujiki N, Yoshida Y, Ripley B, et al: Changes in CSF hypocretin-1 (orexin A) levels in rats across 24 hours and in response to food deprivation. Neuroreport 2001;12:993-997.

138. Zeitzer JM, Buckmaster CL, Parker KJ, et al: Circadian and homeostatic regulation of hypocretin in a primate model: Implications for the consolidation of wakefulness. J Neurosci 2003;23:3555-3560.

139. Marcus JN, Aschkenasi CJ, Lee CE, et al: Differential expression of orexin receptors 1 and 2 in the rat brain. J Comp Neurol 2001;435:6-25.

140. Hungs M, Mignot E: Hypocretin/orexin, sleep and narcolepsy. Bioessays 2001;23:397-408.

141. Taheri S, Zeitzer JM, Mignot E: The role of hypocretins (orexins) in sleep regulation and narcolepsy. Annu Rev Neurosci 2002;25:283-313.

142. Beuckmann CT, Yanagisawa M: Orexins: From neuropeptides to energy homeostasis and sleep/wake regulation. J Mol Med 2002;80:329-342.

143. Mignot E, Taheri S, Nishino S: Sleeping with the hypothalamus: Emerging therapeutic targets for sleep disorders. Nat Neurosci 2002;5(Suppl):1071-1075.

144. Lin JS, Hou Y, Sakai K, Jouvet M: Histaminergic descending inputs to the mesopontine tegmentum and their role in the control of cortical activation and wakefulness in the cat. J Neurosci 1996;16:1523-1537.

145. Schuld A, Hebebrand J, Geller F, Pollmacher T: Increased body-mass index in patients with narcolepsy. Lancet 2000;355:1274-1275.

146. Kok SW, Overeem S, Visscher TL, et al: Hypocretin deficiency in narcoleptic humans is associated with abdominal obesity. Obes Res 2003;11:1147-1154.

147. Yamanaka A, Beuckmann CT, Willie JT, et al: Hypothalamic orexin neurons regulate arousal according to energy balance in mice. Neuron 2003;38:701-713.

148. John J, Wu MF, Siegel JM: Systemic administration of hypocretin-1 reduces cataplexy and normalizes sleep and waking durations in narcoleptic dogs. Sleep Res Online 2000;3:23-28.

149. Nishino S, Fujiki N, Yoshida Y, Mignot E: The effects of hypocretin-1 in hypocretin receptor-2 mutated and hypocretin deficient narcoleptic dogs. Sleep 2003;26(Suppl):A287.

150. Yoshida Y, Fujiki N, Maki RA, et al: Differential kinetics of hypocretins in the cerebrospinal fluid after intracerebroventricular administration in rats. Neurosci Lett 2003;346:182-186.

151. Schatzberg SJ, Barrett J, Cutter K, et al: Case study: Effect of hypocretin replacement therapy in a 3-year-old weimaraner with narcolepsy. J Vet Intern Med 2004;18:586-588.

152. Hecht M, Lin L, Kushida CA, et al: Report of a case of immunosuppression with prednisone in an 8-year-old boy with an acute onset of hypocretin-deficient narcolepsy. Sleep 2003;26:809-810.

153. Lecendreux M, Maret S, Bassetti C, et al: Clinical efficacy of high-dose intravenous immunoglobulins near the onset of narcolepsy in a 10-year-old boy. J Sleep Res 2003;12:1-2.

154. Fernandez-Vina MA, Gao XJ, Moraes ME, et al: Alleles at four HLA class II loci determined by oligonucleotide hybridization and their associations in five ethnic groups. Immunogenetics 1991;34:299-312.

155. Voderholzer U, Riemann D, Gann H, et al: Transient total sleep loss in cerebral Whipple's disease: A longitudinal study. J Sleep Res 2002;11:321-329.

156. Marcus CL, Trescher WH, Halbower AC, Lutz J: Secondary narcolepsy in children with brain tumors. Sleep 2002;25:435-439.

157. Marcus CL, Mignot E: Letter to the editor regarding our previous publication: "Secondary narcolepsy in children with brain tumors," SLEEP 2002;25:435-439. Sleep 2003;26:228.

158. Bodmer JG, Marsh SG, Albert ED, et al: Nomenclature for factors of the HLA system, 1996. Tissue Antigens 1997;49:297-321.

65

Narcolepsy: Diagnosis and Management

Christian Guilleminault

Scott Fromherz

ABSTRACT

Narcolepsy is a syndrome with a prevalence close to 0.04%. It is characterized by abnormal sleep tendencies, including excessive daytime sleepiness, disturbed nocturnal sleep, and manifestations related to rapid eye movement (REM) sleep such as cataplexy (an abrupt drop in muscle tone), sleep paralysis, and hypnopompic more than hypnagogic hallucinations. Its peak age of onset is the second decade. Multiple sleep latency testing after polysomnography shows short sleep latencies and two or more sleep-onset REM sleep periods. The treatment of narcolepsy has improved in recent years, with the newest compounds providing fewer side effects than the classic stimulants (for excessive daytime somnolence) and tricyclic antidepressant medications (for cataplexy). Narcolepsy is a complex syndrome that involves dysfunction in the timing of state changes in wake and sleep. Medications with an alerting effect can help but will never completely control the multifaceted problems associated with this syndrome.

The term *narcolepsy* was first coined by Gélineau[1] in 1880 to designate a pathologic condition characterized by irresistible episodes of sleep of short duration recurring at close intervals. Although Westphal[2] and Fisher[3] had previously published reports of patients with sleepiness and episodic muscle weakness, Gélineau was the first to characterize narcolepsy as a distinct syndrome. He wrote that attacks were sometimes accompanied by falls, or "astasias." Henneberg later referred to these attacks as *cataplexy*.[4] In the 1930s, Daniels[5] emphasized the association of daytime sleepiness, cataplexy, sleep paralysis, and hypnagogic hallucinations. Referring to these symptoms as "the clinical tetrad," Yoss and Daly[6] and Vogel[7] reported nocturnal sleep-onset rapid eye movement (REM) periods in narcoleptic patients, a finding confirmed in the following years.[8-11] Participants in the First International Symposium on Narcolepsy, held in France in 1975, defined the syndrome as follows:

The word "narcolepsy" refers to a syndrome of unknown origin that is characterized by abnormal sleep tendencies, including excessive daytime sleepiness and often disturbed nocturnal sleep and pathological manifestations of REM sleep. The REM sleep abnormalities include sleep onset REM periods and the dissociated REM sleep inhibitory processes, cataplexy and sleep paralysis. Excessive daytime sleepiness, cataplexy, and less often sleep paralysis and hypnagogic hallucinations are the major symptoms of the disease.[12]

The definition strongly emphasizes the dysfunction of REM sleep, but it ignores the notion that genetic factors are frequently involved in the development of narcolepsy. Moreover, although most cases of narcolepsy are idiopathic, secondary causes of narcolepsy have been described.[13]

The discovery of the hypocretin/orexin mutation in narcoleptic Doberman pinschers led to a better understanding of the syndrome and changed, to some degree, our approach to the diagnosis and treatment of disorders of excessive daytime sleepiness (EDS), particularly narcolepsy. Because hypocretins are involved in many hypothalamic functions, narcolepsy may be considered as more than just a disorder of sleep. In addition, it may be considered more as a syndrome of state instability than merely a disorder of dysfunctional REM sleep; patients have the capacity to achieve wakefulness, non-REM, and REM sleep, but are unable to maintain the state. They appear to lack the modulator responsible for maintaining the active sleep state long enough for the normal physiologic "switches" to change the state. Thus, patients with narcolepsy dissociate into the various states of consciousness at inappropriate times. This dissociation is often incomplete, leading to states of consciousness that are a mixture of normal states, such as cataplexy, which represents a combination of the waking state and the paralysis of REM sleep.[14]

CLINICAL FEATURES

The International Classification of Sleep Disorders now includes two entities: narcolepsy with cataplexy and narcolepsy without cataplexy.[15] The classic tetrad for narcolepsy includes EDS, cataplexy, sleep paralysis, and hypnagogic hallucinations. Automatic behaviors and disrupted nighttime sleep also commonly occur. All these symptoms are not present in all patients. Many of the symptoms of narcolepsy can occur in any person who is severely sleep deprived; only cataplexy is unique to narcolepsy.

Sleepiness

Unwanted episodes of sleep recur several times a day—not only under favorable circumstances, such as during monotonous sedentary activity or after a heavy meal, but also in situations in which the patient is fully involved in a task. The duration of the episode may vary from a few minutes, if the patient is in an uncomfortable position, to longer than 1 hour if the patient is reclining. Narcoleptic patients characteristically wake up feeling refreshed, and there is a refractory period of 1 to several hours before the next episode occurs. These relatively short but refreshing naps can help differentiate patients with narcolepsy from patients with idiopathic hypersomnia, who take long, unrefreshing naps.

Apart from sleep episodes, patients may feel abnormally drowsy, resulting in poor performance at work, memory lapses, and even gestural, ambulatory, or speech automatisms. Subjects may complain of chronic tiredness or fatigue while trying to perform despite sleepiness.

Cataplexy

Cataplexy is an abrupt and reversible decrease in or loss of muscle tone, most frequently elicited by emotional responses such as laughter, anger, or surprise, and it may occur in more than two thirds of patients with narcolepsy. It may involve certain muscles or the entire voluntary musculature. Most typically, the jaw sags, the head falls forward, the arms drop to the side, and the knees unlock or buckle.

The severity and extent of cataplectic attacks can vary from a state of absolute powerlessness, which seems to involve the entire voluntary musculature, to a limited involvement of certain muscle groups, or to no more than a fleeting sensation of weakness extending more or less throughout the body. Although the extraocular muscles supposedly are not involved, weakness can occur, and the patient may complain of blurred vision. Complete paralysis of extraocular muscles has never been reported, although the palpebral muscle may be affected. Speech may be impaired and respiration may become irregular during an attack. Long breathing pauses have never been recorded, but short pauses similar to those seen during nocturnal REM sleep in healthy subjects may occur. In a cataplectic attack, there is a complete loss of muscle tone that can lead to total body collapse and the risk of serious injuries such as skull or other bone fractures. Typically, these attacks do not reach that extreme, and may even go unnoticed by nearby individuals. An attack may consist of only a slight buckling of the knees. Patients may perceive this abrupt and short-lasting weakness and simply stop or stand against a wall. Speech may be broken or slurred because of intermittent weakness affecting the arytenoid muscles. As seen during nocturnal REM sleep, the abrupt muscle inhibition is interrupted by sudden bursts of returning muscle tone, which at times even seems enhanced. If the weakness involves only the jaw or speech, the subject may present with wide masticatory movement or an unusual attack of stuttering speech. If it involves the upper limbs, the patient complains of "clumsiness," reporting activity such as dropping cups or plates or spilling liquids when surprised, laughing, and so on.

The short cataplectic attacks are the most common presentation of cataplexy. Because they do not resemble the "classic" full-blown attack of cataplexy, they are often missed by even skilled physicians without the aid of an electromyographic recording. By the same token, however, the skilled physician must be wary not to overdiagnose normal phenomena such as the "rubber knees" that precede the anxiety of public speaking or "rolling on the ground laughing." The duration of each cataplectic attack—whether partial or total—is variable, lasting from a few seconds to 30 minutes, but in most cases 30 seconds to 2 minutes.

Attacks can be elicited by emotion or stress. Laughter and anger seem to be the most common triggers, but the attacks can also be induced by a feeling of elation while listening to music, reading a book, or watching a movie. Cataplexy may be induced merely by remembering a happy or funny situation, and it may rarely occur without clear precipitating acts or emotions, particularly if the patient is sleepy. It often occurs when the patient is telling a joke and frequently occurs when the patient simply anticipates saying something humorous. "Status cataplecticus" is a rare manifestation of cataplexy, characterized by prolonged cataplexy that lasts hours, confining the patient to the bedroom.

The physiology of cataplexy has been partially investigated. Cataplexy is associated with an inhibition of the monosynaptic H-reflex and of the multisynaptic tendon reflexes. H-reflex activity is fully suppressed physiologically only during REM sleep, which emphasizes the relationship between the motor inhibitory component of REM sleep and the sudden atonia and areflexia seen during a cataplectic attack. Muscarinic cholinergic regions of the pontine reticular formation and basal forebrain are sites involved in cataplexy through a multisynaptic descending pathway. An increase in postsynaptic dopamine type 2 (D_2) receptors was observed in the amygdala of narcoleptic dogs with impairment of dopamine release, suggesting that an abnormal cholinergic–dopaminergic interaction could underlie the pathophysiology of narcolepsy.[16]

Sleep Paralysis

This is a terrifying experience that occurs in the narcoleptic patient on falling asleep or on awakening. Patients find themselves suddenly unable to move the limbs, to speak, or even to breathe deeply. This state is frequently accompanied by hallucinations.

During an episode of sleep paralysis, the patient is unable to move the extremities, to speak, or to open the eyes, although he or she is fully aware of the condition and able to recall it completely later. In many episodes of sleep paralysis, but especially the first occurrence, the patient may be prey to extreme anxiety associated with the fear of dying. This anxiety is often greatly intensified by the terrifying hallucinations that may accompany the sleep paralysis. They often interpret the experience as being "scared stiff." With more experience with the phenomenon, however, the patient usually learns that episodes are brief and benign, rarely lasting longer than a few minutes and always ending spontaneously. Sleep paralysis may occur as an independent and isolated phenomenon, and 3% to 5% of the general population may be affected by it.

Hallucinations

Sleep onset, either during daytime sleep episodes or at night, may be unpleasant, with vivid auditory or hypnagogic hallucinations. Similar hallucinations may occur at awakening; these hypnopompic hallucinations may be more characteristic of narcolepsy than the hypnagogic ones. The narcoleptic patient's hypnagogic and hypnopompic hallucinations that accompany sleep paralysis often involve vision. The visual hallucinations usually consist of simple forms (colored circles, parts of objects, and so on) that are constant or changing in size. The image of an animal or a person may present itself abruptly, more often in color. Auditory hallucinations are also common, although other senses are seldom involved. The auditory hallucinations can range from a collection of sounds to an elaborate melody. The patient may also be menaced by threatening sentences or harsh invective. Often hypnopompic hallucinations are perceived as so vividly realistic that the patient acts on them upon awakening. For example, patients with narcolepsy have been known to call 911 about intruders, only to discover after authorities have searched the house that it was all a hallucination. The exact boundary between hypnagogic/hypnopompic hallucinations and dreams is not a clear one. In some cases of unrecognized narcolepsy with daytime hypnagogic/hypnopompic hallucinations, the patient may be mistakenly diagnosed as having a delusional psychosis.[17]

Another common and interesting type of hallucination reported at sleep onset involves elementary cenesthopathic feelings (i.e., experiencing picking, rubbing, or light touching), changes in location of body parts (e.g., arm or leg), or feelings of levitation or extracorporeal experiences (e.g., moving the body in space or floating above the bed) that may be quite elaborate. (For example, the patient may report, "I am above my bed and I can also see my body below"; "I am a few feet up and people jump over my body.") The association of sleep paralysis has led researchers to postulate gamma loop involvement in some of these hallucinations. The abrupt motor inhibition that involves the spinal cord motoneurons may lead to a significant decrease in the feedback of information normally used by the central nervous system (CNS) to gauge the position of the body and the relation of the limb segments to each other.

Sleep Disruption

Night sleep is often interrupted by repeated awakenings and sometimes accompanied by terrifying dreams. Ironically, patients may complain of trouble falling asleep and staying asleep at night, although they may fall asleep repeatedly during the daytime. Rarely, a complaint of insomnia with secondary tiredness is the initial complaint. The sleep disruption may be enhanced by presence of periodic limb movements, which appear to be common in these patients. These movements can be associated with typical episodes of REM behavior disorder.

ONSET OF CLINICAL SYMPTOMS

The first symptoms often develop near the age of puberty; the peak age at which reported symptoms occur is 15 to 25 years, but narcolepsy and other symptoms have been noted as early as 2 years, and at 6 months of age in the case with hypocretin gene mutation.[18] A second, smaller peak of onset has been noted between 35 and 45 years and near menopause in women. There is often a marked delay of over 10 years before diagnosis is made, especially if cataplexy is initially absent.[19]

EDS and irresistible sleep episodes usually occur as the first symptoms, either independently or associated with one or more other symptoms. They are enhanced by high environmental temperature, indoor activity, and idleness. Symptoms may abate with time but never phase out completely. Attacks of cataplexy usually appear in conjunction with abnormal episodes of sleep but may occur as many as 20 years later. They occasionally, but seldom, occur before the abnormal sleep episodes, in which case they are a major source of difficulty in diagnosis. They can vary in frequency from a few episodes during the subject's entire lifetime to one or several episodes per day. Cataplectic attacks have an overall tendency to decrease in frequency with aging.

Hypnagogic/hypnopompic hallucinations and sleep paralysis do not affect all subjects, are often transitory, and occur commonly in the general population.[20] Disturbed nocturnal sleep seldom occurs in the first stages and usually worsens with age.[21] Narcolepsy leads to a variety of complications, such as driving- or machine operation–related accidents; difficulties at work leading to disability, forced retirement, or job dismissal; impotence; and depression.[22]

DIAGNOSTIC PROCEDURES: EVALUATION OF SLEEPINESS

The Stanford Sleepiness Scale,[23] a seven-point scale, was developed to quantify the subjective sleepiness of patients throughout the day, but it is often difficult for patients accurately to rate themselves every 15 to 20 minutes. The Epworth Sleepiness Scale is also used as an index of sleepiness (see Chapter 120).

Several tests have been designed to evaluate sleepiness objectively. Yoss et al.[24] described the electronic pupillogram as a method of measuring decreased levels of sleepiness. Schmidt and Fortin[22] reviewed the advantages and limitations of the electronic pupillogram in arousal disorders. The multiple sleep latency test (MSLT; see Chapter 120) was designed to measure physiologic sleep tendencies in the absence of alerting factors.[25] It consists of five scheduled naps, usually at 10 AM, noon, and 2, 4, and 6 PM, during which the subject is polygraphically monitored in a comfortable, soundproof, dark bedroom, while wearing street clothes. The MSLT records the latency for each nap (time between lights-out and sleep onset), the mean sleep latency, and the presence or absence of REM sleep during any of the naps.[26] On the basis of polygraphic recording, REM sleep that occurs within 15 minutes of sleep onset is considered a sleep-onset REM period.[27] After each 20-minute monitoring period, patients stay awake until the next scheduled nap.

In normal populations, MSLT scores vary with age, and puberty is a critical landmark. Prepubertal children between the ages of 6 and 11 years appear to be hyperalert. In postpubertal subjects, mean MSLT scores under 8 minutes are generally considered to be in the pathologic range; those over 10 minutes are considered to be normal. When the range is between 8 and 10 minutes, age factors interact, so the test must be interpreted with greater care; mean scores of 8 to 10 minutes represent a gray area.[28]

An MSLT performed alone has the same drawbacks as does pupillography—it measures sleepiness regardless of its cause, which may simply be sleep deprivation. The MSLT also ignores repetitive microsleeps that can lead, in borderline cases, to daytime impairment not scored by conventional analysis. To be clinically relevant, the test must be conducted under specific conditions. Subjects must have abstained from medication for a sufficient period (usually 15 days) so that drug interaction is avoided. On the basis of sleep diaries, their sleep–wake schedules are stabilized. On the night preceding the MSLT, the subjects undergo a standard nocturnal polysomnogram. Throughout the total nocturnal sleep period, any sleep-related biologic abnormalities responsible for sleep fragmentation and sleep deprivation are recorded.

The nocturnal polysomnogram may indicate the underlying cause of sleepiness; the MSLT indicates the severity of the problem. Once the nocturnal sleep recording has eliminated specific diseases, the MSLT confirms the diagnosis of narcolepsy with the presence of two or more sleep-onset REM periods.

Browman et al.[29] proposed adding to the MSLT a test for the maintenance of wakefulness. This tests the patient's ability to remain awake in a comfortable sitting position in a dark room for five 20-minute trials given at 10 AM, noon, and 2, 4, and 6 PM. The test may be helpful in specific pharmacologic trials but has proved to be unsatisfactory as a diagnostic procedure.[29] Normally, the test consists of five nap opportunities placed at 2-hour intervals, similar to the MSLT. Each opportunity for sleep lasts 20 minutes, but some studies have claimed that prolonging each test to 30 minutes probably results in improved distinction between a pathologic process and normality.

Another procedure that has been used to document sleepiness is a continuous 24- or 36-hour polysomnogram that provides information about the number, duration, times, and types of daytime sleep episodes. as well as documenting nighttime sleep disruptions. In addition, this long polysomnographic recording may identify the dissociated REM sleep–inhibitory process characterizing cataplexy by showing the elimination of chin and muscle twitches typical of REM sleep in the awake patient. These recordings may be performed using ambulatory equipment.

Broughton et al.[30] proposed using auditory evoked potentials in the evaluation of sleepiness, but this test, which may be helpful in evaluating pharmacologic agents, has not proved sufficiently discriminative to be used as a diagnostic tool.

POSITIVE DIAGNOSIS OF NARCOLEPSY

By consensus the diagnosis of narcolepsy requires a clinical history of sleepiness and a positive MSLT, with a mean sleep latency of less than eight minutes and two or more sleep-onset REM periods.[15] However, there is controversy concerning the criteria needed to confirm narcolepsy in patients with EDS. There is a progressive decrease in the number of sleep-onset REM periods and an increase in the mean sleep latency on the MSLT as a function of age, suggesting that the current criteria used for diagnosis may be too stringent in older patients.[31] Clinicians and researchers in Japan have indicated that their U.S. counterparts have given too much credence to polysomnographic criteria and the presence of two or more sleep-onset REM periods at MSLT.[32] In Japan, a positive history of cataplexy associated with EDS is systematically required for the diagnosis of narcolepsy.[32] Undoubtedly, the presence of cataplexy is pathognomonic of narcolepsy, but it may be difficult to rely on this criterion alone, particularly when cataplexy is partial (i.e., limited to the head and neck or neck and upper arms). Anic-Labat et al.[33] developed a self-administered questionnaire that validated cataplexy in 1000 subjects. Moscovitch et al.[34] also cautioned against the diagnosis of narcolepsy if EDS and two or more sleep-onset REM periods at MSLT are the only positive findings. These authors found that only 84% of the individuals with complaints of EDS and documentation of cataplexy presented with two or more sleep-onset REM periods at MSLT, a replication of findings by Van den Hoed et al.[28] 10 years earlier. They found that all subjects with EDS and cataplexy presented with two or more sleep-onset REM periods at one MSLT if the MSLT was repeated daily for 4 days. Moscovitch et al.[34] recommended that the term *narcolepsy* be used only when EDS and at least a positive history of cataplexy are associated with two or more sleep-onset REM periods. If there is no history of cataplexy, a more descriptive term such as *EDS with several sleep-onset REM periods* could be used, even if other symptoms, such as sleep paralysis or hypnagogic hallucinations, exist.

Genetic testing has been used to aid in the clinical diagnosis of narcolepsy. Mignot et al.[35] showed that 40% of subjects with two or more sleep-onset REM periods were positive for human leukocyte antigen DQB1*0602. However, narcolepsy was clinically suspected in 60% of these cases; thus, genetic testing alone is not sufficient for the diagnosis of narcolepsy. The requirement of a positive history of cataplexy would eliminate subjects in the developing phase of the syndrome, which can take several years. The use of strict criteria will allow better epidemiologic studies to be conducted. Subjects would be classified as narcoleptic only after the presence of EDS and cataplexy had been reported and abnormal daytime alertness

had been confirmed by polysomnographic recording with MSLT. The discovery of the involvement of a second gene in the development of narcolepsy may lead to new diagnostic tests. Hypocretins may one day be measured in the blood of animals and humans. Narcoleptic dogs and mice have mutations that exert an impact directly on the orexin or hypocretin receptor. The discovery of cerebrospinal fluid hypocretins has led to a new diagnostic approach: By performing a lumbar puncture, very low or nonexistent levels of hypocretin can confirm the diagnosis of narcolepsy with cataplexy.[36-39]

PATHOPHYSIOLOGY

Pharmacologic Studies

Because few pharmacologic data are available for human beings, we review pharmacologic studies in canine narcolepsy with cataplexy. This subject is discussed in detail in Chapter 64. In summary, the many pharmacologic investigations performed on the dog suggest that an $alpha_{1b}$ receptor is strongly involved in the control of cataplexy.[40] $Alpha_{1b}$ antagonists drastically worsen cataplexy. Stimulation of $alpha_{1b}$ receptors decreases it, as do noradrenergic reuptake blockers and noradrenergic releasing agents. Other receptors, particularly $alpha_2$ receptors, are also involved in cataplexy, as shown by the effect of several $alpha_2$ antagonists, particularly yohimbine, which completely suppresses cataplexy.[41,42] Central dopamine D_2 agonists significantly suppress cataplexy,[43] whereas most D_2 agonists aggravate it; this suggests an involvement of "presynaptic dopamine receptors" in the regulation of canine cataplexy. However, experimental data suggest that the effect of D_2 compounds on cataplexy is probably mediated by the noradrenergic system.[44,45]

These investigations indicate that a complex loop involving noradrenergic and cholinergic synapses controls the appearance of canine cataplexy. This loop is similar to that suggested by the pharmacologic investigations of REM sleep. The pharmacologic investigations of the narcoleptic dog are even more valuable because they provide information useful to the understanding of REM sleep.[46]

Cerebrospinal Fluid Analysis

Studies in humans with narcolepsy have shown a decrease in dopamine concentration in the cerebrospinal fluid.[47] Studies on narcoleptic dogs performed before and after probenecid administration demonstrated an elevated dopamine turnover with significantly less free homovanillic acid, dihydroxyphenylacetic acid, 3-methoxy-4-hydroxyphenylglycol, and 5-hydroxyindoleacetic acid.[48]

The lower concentration of 5-hydroxyindoleacetic acid in the cerebrospinal fluid of narcoleptic dogs suggests a decreased concentration of the parent amine 5-hydroxytryptamine, a decreased turnover of serotonin in the brain, or both. Similarly, the lower steady-state cerebrospinal fluid concentration of dihydroxyphenylacetic acid and homovanillic acid, as well as the reduced accumulation of dihydroxyphenylacetic acid and homovanillic acid after probenecid, suggests decreased dopamine concentration, decreased turnover, or both. Finally, the lower concentration of 3-methoxy-4-hydroxyphenylglycol after probenecid administration suggests decreased norepinephrine activity.

In most patients with narcolepsy, there is an absence or very low level of hypocretin in the cerebrospinal fluid.[39]

Brain Tissue Analysis

Analyses of both human and animal narcoleptic brain tissue suggest dopaminergic dysfunction. In postmortem human autoradiographic studies, striatal dopamine D_2 receptor binding was increased in narcolepsy, more so than D_1 receptors.[49,50] However, most in vivo studies with single-photon emission computed tomography[51] and positron emission tomography[52] found no increase in striatal D_2 receptor binding in narcolepsy.

Noradrenergic function has also been found to be abnormal. Two different receptor responses can normally be noted, and two different central alpha$_1$ receptors, so-called high-affinity and low-affinity, have been identified.[53] The low-affinity central alpha$_1$ noradrenergic receptors are those involved in canine cataplexy.[40,46]

TREATMENT

In narcolepsy, the goal of all therapeutic approaches is to control the narcoleptic symptoms and allow the patient to have a full family and professional life. Drug prescriptions must take into account possible side effects because narcolepsy is a lifelong illness and patients will have to receive medication for years. Tolerance or addiction may occur with some compounds. In addition, hypertension, abnormal liver function, and psychosis are the most commonly reported complications associated with the long-term use of stimulant medications. The treatment of narcolepsy must balance the maintenance of an active life with the avoidance of side effects and tolerance to medications.[54]

Behavioral Approaches

Part of the difficulty in treating patients with narcolepsy involves the patient's frustration over the delay in diagnosis. In 500 narcoleptic patients surveyed in the United States in the 1980s, the mean time to diagnosis from symptom onset was 15 years. The consequence of this, particularly in a young patient, is the development of reactive depressive symptoms. One of the most important initial treatments is a referral to patient support groups organized by sleep disorders centers, such as the National Sleep Foundation or the Narcolepsy Network. Other support groups exist in most western European countries and in North America. The American Sleep Disorders Association is an integral resource.

Career counseling is also important because patients and their employers must be educated regarding jobs that patients with narcolepsy should avoid, including shift work, on-call schedules, driving and the transportation industry, or any job necessitating continuous attention for long hours without breaks, particularly under monotonous conditions. Some of these difficulties can be overcome if the employer recognizes the importance of short 15- to 20-minute naps every 4 hours during the daytime.

In addition to scheduled naps, other behavioral approaches include a regular sleep–wake schedule, the avoidance of frequent time zone changes, and overall good sleep hygiene (Tables 65–1 and 65–2).

Pharmacologic Treatments

Cataplexy and REM Sleep–Related Symptoms

Investigations have shown that muscle atonia is normally associated with REM sleep; REM-associated muscle atonia occurs at inappropriate times during wakefulness in narcoleptic patients and is responsible for cataplexy. Several neurotransmitter systems have been identified as affecting the inhibitory pathways involving the lower motoneurons, particularly muscarinic cholinergic and noradrenergic systems at the alpha$_{1b}$ and D_2 receptor levels. The best medications are those that target these receptors with the least number of side effects.[55] Tricyclic antidepressants were the first drugs of choice, particularly protriptyline, but the anticholinergic effect led to impotence in more than 40% of male narcoleptic patients.

Table 65–1.   Examples of Initial Treatment Packages (Children)

Prepubertal Children	Pubertal Children
General Measures	
Contact school to alert teachers	Contact school to alert teachers
Nap at lunchtime	Emphasize need for regular nocturnal sleep schedule
Nap at 4 or 5 PM	Try to obtain 9 h of nocturnal sleep
	Nap at lunchtime and 4 or 5 PM
Medication for Sleepiness	
Modafinil 100-200 mg[†]	Modafinil 100-400 mg[†]
Methylphenidate 5 mg (2-4 tablets)	Methylphenidate 5 mg (2-6 tablets*) or 20-mg sustained-release tablet in the morning (on empty stomach)
Medication for Cataplexy[‡]	
Fluoxetine 10-20 mg in the morning	Fluoxetine 10-40 mg in the morning
Venlafaxine 75-150 mg in the morning	Venlafaxine 75-150 mg in the morning
Clomipramine 50 mg at bedtime	

*Usually 10 mg when waking up on an empty stomach, 5 mg around lunchtime, and 5 mg at 3 PM.

[†]Modafinil is started at 100 mg in the morning for 5 days, and a second dose of 100 mg is then added at lunchtime, if needed. This is usually sufficient in prepubertal children. Pubertal children may require a further increase (after 5 days) to an additional 100 mg in the morning and, if still needed later, another 100 mg at noon.

[‡]The use of antidepressants for cataplexy is not approved by the U.S. Food and Drug Administration (FDA). No medications have specifically received approval by the FDA for use in patients with narcolepsy younger than 16 years of age.

Table 65–2. Examples of Initial Treatment Packages (Adults)

General Measures

Avoid shifts in sleep schedule
Avoid heavy meals and alcohol intake
Regular timing of nocturnal sleep: 10:30 PM to 7 AM
Naps: Strategically timed naps, if possible (e.g., 15 min at lunchtime, 15 min at 5:30 PM)

Medication for Sleepiness

The effects of stimulant medications vary widely among patients. The dosing and timing of medications should be individualized to optimize performance. Additional doses, as needed, may be suggested for periods of anticipated sleepiness.
Modafinil 100-200 mg (taken when waking up in the morning) and 100-200 mg at lunchtime, or
Methylphenidate 5 mg (3 or 4 tablets; 10 mg when waking up; 5 mg 30 min before lunch; 5 mg near 3 PM; better action is always obtained if the drug is taken on an empty stomach) or 20 mg SR morning (on empty stomach)

If Persistent Difficulties

Methylphenidate (SR): 20 mg in the morning
5 mg after noon nap
5 mg at 4 PM, or
Modafinil 200 mg in the morning and 200 mg at lunchtime with possible further increase to 300 mg at morning and lunchtime (total daily dosage, 600 mg), or
Add GHB (sodium oxybate) at bedtime: dosage must start low at 1.5 g taken twice while in bed, at bedtime and 2 hours after bedtime; increase to total dosage of 4 to 4.5 g within 3-4 weeks. This is usually an ineffective dose, so keep increasing as indicated on package until 3 g at bedtime and 3 g 2 hours after bedtime. This is a therapeutic dose. Depending on response, dosage can be increased to 9 g total daily dose. Do not increase over 9 g because of risk of side effects during sleep. Effect on cataplexy is seen much faster than effect on sleepiness. Slowly decrease medication taken for sleepiness only when therapeutic dosage has been reached.
Modafinil works best in naive subjects. It should be the drug of first intention in children and adults.

If No Response

Dextroamphetamine sulfate (but will induce rebound hypersomnia)
(Dexedrine Spansule; SR): 15 mg on awakening
5 mg after noon nap
5 mg at 3:30 or 4 PM
(or 15 mg at awakening and 15 mg after noon nap)

Medication for Cataplexy*

Fluoxetine 20-60 mg
Venlafaxine 150-300 mg
GHB (see above)
Clomipramine 75-125 mg, or
Viloxazine 150-200 mg, or
Imipramine 75-125 mg

*Medications may be taken in the evening near bedtime (GHB, clomipramine, imipramine); only in the morning (fluoxetine), or in the morning and at lunchtime (viloxazine, venlafaxine). Tricyclic medications, despite efficacy, should be second-line medications because of side effects The use of antidepressants for cataplexy is not approved by the U.S. Food and Drug Administration (FDA). The only medications specifically approved for use in narcolepsy by the FDA are modafinil and GHB (for cataplexy).

GHB, gamma-hydroxybutyrate; SR, sustained-release tablet.

Most tricyclic antidepressants with significant atropinic side effects are used as a last resort. Similarly, the monoamine oxidase inhibitors are rarely used except for the hybrid selegiline (see later).[56] The newest agent, sodium oxybate (gamma-hydroxybutyrate [GHB]), treats cataplexy through an unknown mechanism that is thought to be related to its consolidation of REM sleep (see later).[57-62] Most medications used for cataplexy have a noradrenergic reuptake blocker action. Viloxazine is available in Europe and is very effective in the treatment of cataplexy. The starting dose is 50 to 100 mg in two divided doses, with a maximum dose of 200 mg/day.[63]

The most commonly used medications are the serotonin reuptake inhibitors that have an active noradrenergic reuptake blocker metabolite; these include clomipramine and its active metabolite desmethyl-clomipramine, fluoxetine and its active metabolite norfluoxetine, and zimeldine and its active metabolite norzimeldine.[64,65] In our experience, we recommend starting with 20 mg fluoxetine in the morning and increasing to 60 to 80 mg/day in two divided doses, or with 50 mg clomipramine at bedtime and increasing to a maximum of 200 mg in two divided doses. The most common dosages are 40 to 60 mg/day of fluoxetine or 100 mg/day of clomipramine. The newer antidepressants have also been found to be effective for cataplexy, sleep paralysis, and hypnagogic/hypnopompic hallucinations. Venlafaxine (75 to 150 mg) has been the most widely used of these new compounds both in adults and in children; it has shown good response and has fewer side effects than the tricyclics, which are now used less often. Atomoxetine (18 to 100 mg once a day or in two divided doses) has been tried in cases of resistant cataplexy after failure of fluoxetine, other serotonin reuptake inhibitors, and venlafaxine. Serotonin, norepinephrine reuptake inhibitors, and selective serotonin reuptake inhibitors, when used during the last trimester of pregnancy, may lead to serious respiratory and feeding side effects in the neonate immediately after birth. Pregnant women may need to be progressively withdrawn from these medications before the third trimester of pregnancy. The withdrawal must be slow to avoid a marked cataplexy rebound that usually occurs on day 3 or 4 and peaks near day 10 after completion of withdrawal.

Common side effects have been well described in previous reports, but there are some side effects that are rarely mentioned that may be more important in narcoleptic patients:

Appearance of periodic limb movement syndrome during sleep. This syndrome is related to the increase in muscle tone induced by these compounds during sleep and may lead to a significant fragmentation of sleep. Levodopa or other dopamine agonists (e.g., pramipexole, pergolide, ropinirole) may be useful.[66,67]

Development of REM behavior disorder, particularly in older subjects. Classically, tricyclic antidepressants and serotonin reuptake inhibitors "decrease" REM sleep. These drugs eliminate or decrease the muscle atonia of REM sleep and dissociate REM sleep (i.e., electroencephalographic patterns of REM sleep without muscle atonia). Although the absence of muscle atonia limits the ability to score this stage as REM sleep using the international rules,[26] the electroencephalographic pattern and dream state of REM persist. Thus, the individual can "act out" his or her dreams. Although REM behavior disorder is a separate sleep disorder, it may occur in narcoleptic patients who already have dysfunction of muscle tone control with cataplexy, and this tendency may be enhanced with anticataplectic drugs. It is unclear if long-term use of anticataplectic drugs may favor this complication.

Rebound of cataplexy and other REM-related symptoms. Abrupt withdrawal of these drugs induces a significant rebound of cataplexy, sleep paralysis, and hypnagogic hallucinations. Patients should be withdrawn from medications slowly; the recommended withdrawal schedule is one dose every 4 days. Even with such a schedule, cataplexy rebound is seen. The problem is related to the disappearance of warning signs and the possibility of abrupt, complete falls that may result in bodily injury. Withdrawal experiments performed at Stanford University with the use of clomipramine showed that rebound was noticeable after 72 hours and peaked at day 10 after withdrawal, and the baseline cataplexy frequency was seen after 15 days. Patients must be warned about this side effect and forbidden from driving during the withdrawal period. When switching medications,

---

Table 65–3.　Narcolepsy Drugs Currently Available

Drug	Usual Dosage* (All Drugs Administered Orally)
Treatment of EDS	
Stimulants[†]	
Modafinil	100-400 mg/day
Methylphenidate	10-60 mg/day
Dextroamphetamine	5-60 mg/day
Methamphetamine	20-25 mg/day
Mazindol	4-8 mg/day (divided dosage)
Sodium oxybate	6-9 g/day (divided in two doses)
Adjunct-effect drugs (i.e., improve EDS if associated with stimulant)[‡]	
Protriptyline	2.5-10 mg/day
Viloxazine[†]	50-200 mg/day
Treatment of Auxiliary Effects (e.g., Cataplexy)	
Gamma-hydroxybutyrate (sodium oxybate)	6-9 g/day (divided in two doses)
Antidepressants[‡] *(without atropinic side effects)*	
Fluoxetine	20-60 mg/day
Venlafaxine	75-300 mg/day
Viloxazine[†]	50-200 mg/day
With atropinic side effects	
Protriptyline	2.5-20 mg/day
Imipramine	25-200 mg/day
Clomipramine	25-200 mg/day
Desipramine	25-200 mg/day

*Occasionally, depending on clinical response, the dose may be outside the usual dosage range.

[†]Most stimulants should be administered in divided doses, commonly in the morning and at lunchtime. This is recommended for amphetamines and modafinil. Methylphenidate has a fast elimination rate; the slow-release (SR) formula may be helpful in the morning (e.g., 20 mg SR). If administered by 5-mg increments, the usual timing of methylphenidate administration is every 3 to 4 hours until 3 PM. Pemoline has been deleted from the list of recommended drugs because of a side effect that may develop years after drug intake.

[‡]The use of antidepressants for cataplexy is not approved by the U.S. Food and Drug Administration (FDA). The only medications specifically approved for use in narcolepsy by the FDA are modafinil and gamma-hydroxybutyrate (sodium oxybate).

EDS, excessive daytime sleepiness.

our experience has been to add the second drug 16 to 24 hours after interruption of the previous medication.[68]

Excessive Daytime Sleepiness

The drugs most widely used to treat EDS (Table 65–3) are the CNS stimulants. Amphetamines were first proposed as a treatment of EDS in narcolepsy by Prinzmetal and Bloomberg in 1935, and the first addiction to amphetamine was reported in 1939.[69] Amphetamines (dextroamphetamines, biamphetamine, methamphetamine), methylphenidate, mazindol, and pemoline had been the most commonly used medications for the treatment of EDS. The introduction of two new agents has given more options to clinicians: modafinil (200 to 600 mg/day) and GHB (6 to 9 g/day). Modafinil is a CNS activating agent that has little or no effect on dopaminergic activity, but it is histaminergic and has highly selective activity in the CNS relative to amphetamines and methylphenidate.[55] GHB is a naturally occurring CNS metabolite that acts as a sedative to consolidate sleep. In addition to its use as an anticataplectic medication, it is also thought to be helpful in the reduction of EDS. Amphetamines and methylphenidate[70-74] are classified as stimulant drugs. Drugs that stimulate norepinephrine release and have dopaminergic activity, such as amphetamines and methylphenidate, have had the greatest impact on sleepiness. The best objective study was reported by Mitler et al.,[65,72] using methamphetamine and evaluating its effect on the MSLT (Fig. 65–1). Compared with dextroamphetamine, methamphetamine accumulates in the CNS and has fewer peripheral side effects. However, our clinical experience does not support this. Our first investigations of narcolepsy and amphetamine treatment were conducted in the 1970s.[54] These studies involved narcoleptic subjects who had received amphetamines for at least 5 years, usually longer than 10 years, and who were receiving more than 80 mg/day

with a maximum dosage of 300 mg/day. All subjects had periods of EDS on a daily basis, and two thirds of the group had hyperexcitation, nervousness, anxiety, and hypertension. Progressive withdrawal of amphetamines in that population led to lowering of blood pressure in all patients but clear worsening of EDS. After a "drug holiday" of 3 to 4 weeks, patients were prescribed stimulant medications at a much lower dose. Subjects had a similar improvement in subjective levels of alertness with fewer side effects.

In adults, methylphenidate and amphetamines at dosages of more than 60 mg/day do not significantly improve EDS without the appearance of long-term side effects, including frequent worsening of the nocturnal sleep disruption. The drug is usually administered in three divided doses with a maximum of 20 mg in the morning, 20 mg at lunchtime, and 20 mg at 3 PM—never later. Therefore, short naps are necessary. The combination of pharmacologic agents and two short naps provides the best daily response to EDS, with no stimulant drug taken after 3 PM. The slow-release form may provide gradual and delayed response during the daytime.

The association between anticataplectic drugs and amphetamine-like medications may enhance the anticataplectic effect of the stimulant medication.[73] Of note, modafinil has no known anticataplectic effects (see later).

Mazindol, an imidazoline, has been helpful in the treatment of EDS in narcolepsy but has not been as clinically effective as the amphetamines.[74] It has been tried at a dosage of 3 to 8 mg/day, with a mean dose of 5 mg mostly taken in the morning. Currently, it is not a commonly used drug.

The two most recently introduced drugs, modafinil and GHB, are the most commonly used agents in newly diagnosed narcoleptic patients.

Modafinil (2-[diphenyl-methyl sulfinyl]acetamide) is a novel stimulant; its mechanism of action is different from that of the amphetamines.[74,75] It acts, at least in part, on the

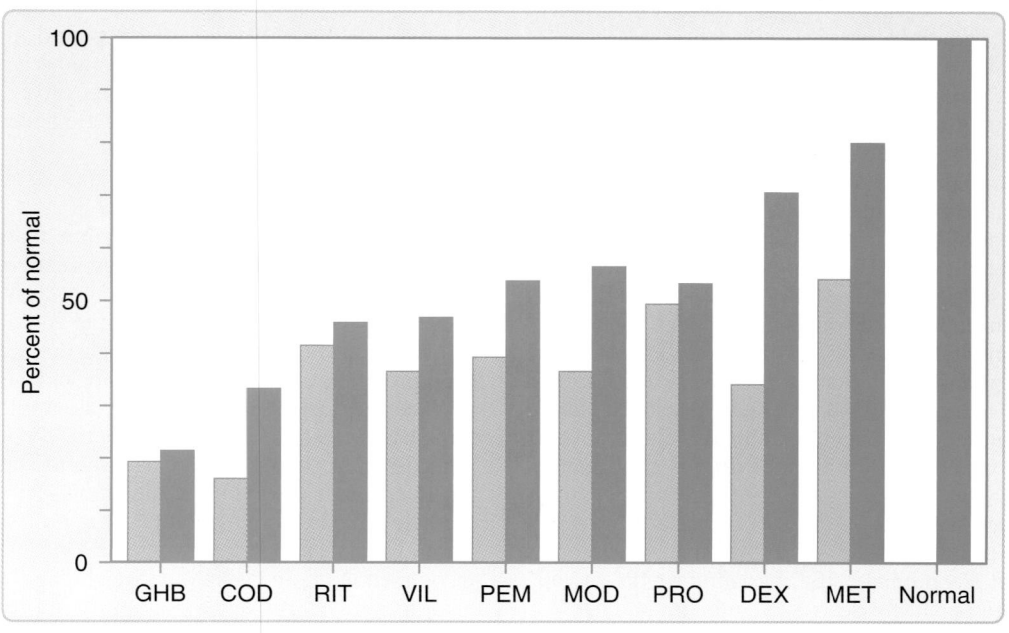

Figure 65–1. Relative efficacy of drugs for treating narcolepsy presented in terms of percentage of normal levels of sleepiness. The lightest shading denotes baseline values. The darkest shading denotes treatment values, or the normal values (extreme right). A comparison between drugs in a blind protocol has not been performed. COD, codeine; DEX, dextroamphetamine; GHB, gamma-hydroxybutyrate; MET, methylphenidate; MOD, modafinil; PEM, pemoline; PRO, protriptyline; RIT, ritanserin; VIL, viloxazine. (From Mitler MM, Hajdukovic R: Relative efficacy of drugs for the treatment of sleepiness in narcolepsy. Sleep 1991;14:218-220.)

histaminergic system. The results from several multicenter studies indicated that modafinil had a significant impact on the objective measures of sleepiness; however, the improvement noted on MSLT was never normalized. This suggests that narcolepsy is a complex disorder in which the mechanisms underlying daytime sleepiness are not yet well understood. Cataplexy and the other REM sleep symptoms are not affected by modafinil. The most important benefit of modafinil concerns its relative lack of side effects. There are no blood pressure side effects; it is not addictive and therefore has a low potential for abuse. Headache is the most common complaint, and this can be reduced by a slow and progressive increase in dosage.[74] Most European studies suggest twice-daily administration, in the morning and at lunchtime. Based on multiple studies (MSLT/Maintenance of Wakefulness Test), this mode of drug intake seems to provide better alertness at the end of the day, but compliance with the noon dose was poorer, particularly in young patients. The most commonly used daily dose in open-label studies has been 400 mg (therapeutic range, 100 to 400 mg/day). Modafinil can be administered concurrently with anticataplectic medications without problems.

Switching patients from a stimulant medication to modafinil may lead to the reappearance of narcoleptic symptoms. Patients who have taken a daily dose of amphetamines of 45 mg or more complain of less control over "sleepiness" than with their prior medications. In our clinical population, after 1 month of daily modafinil intake, 20% of the patients previously treated with amphetamines asked to be switched back to their previous drug. This subjective rating of less control over sleepiness with modafinil occurs despite intake at the upper limits of the recommended dose (commonly 400 to 600 mg daily).

Another problem in the switch from amphetamines to modafinil is the appearance of cataplectic attacks and, more rarely, of sleep paralysis in patients previously well controlled with a combination of stimulants and anticataplectic agents, or by amphetamines alone. Amphetamines have a direct impact on the norepinephrine synapse, thereby helping to control cataplexy and sleep paralysis. Modafinil has none of these activities. With the switch to modafinil, patients who had mild REM sleep–related symptoms controlled by the amphetamine intake may thus experience an abrupt recurrence of these symptoms at the time of the switch of medication, and may need an adjunct compound. In patients already taking an anticataplectic drug simultaneously, an increase in the daily intake of this medication may be needed. The combination of modafinil and venlafaxine (100 mg/day) has provided good results in these specific cases. Modafinil produces the best results in stimulant-naive individuals.

Short-acting methylphenidate may be added as a rescue medication if modafinil's effectiveness is not sustained through the end of the day. GHB (see later) is usually started with modafinil, unless the patient is already taking another alerting drug, in which case the current drug is continued at the same dosage. This is because GHB's effects on sleepiness are slow to appear. After 6 to 9 weeks of taking at least 6 g of GHB (administered in two 3-g doses in bed just at sleep onset and 2 hours after sleep onset), the modafinil or the original alerting agents can be slowly decreased and eliminated.

In declining order, our patients subjectively rate the effectiveness of medications in the treatment of EDS as methylphenidate, pemoline, and then mazindol. Modafinil is probably at the level of effectiveness of methylphenidate. None of the currently available stimulants, including modafinil, has been tested in parallel with a placebo control or in comparison with each other in the narcoleptic population. The first comparative trial is currently ongoing between GHB and modafinil.

Both the stimulant medications and the anticataplectic drugs are hepatically metabolized, so any liver dysfunction will affect both classes of drug. Thus, regular liver function tests are recommended.

The other recent compound is GHB (sodium oxybate).[57-61] It is a naturally occurring metabolite of the human nervous system that is found in the highest concentrations in the hypothalamus and basal ganglia. It was shown to induce a normal sequence of non-REM and REM sleep in normal volunteers lasting 2 to 3 hours at a dose of 30 mg/kg. The first trials on narcoleptic patients were performed in the late 1970s.[60,61] GHB has also been part of multicenter studies in the United States, which has shown long-term efficacy.[61,76] The drug is normally taken at bedtime while the patient is already in bed, to avoid falls. A second dose is taken approximately 2 hours after the first one, again while the patient is in bed. The effective dose has varied from 6 to 9 g, with an increase in total nocturnal sleep time and decrease in sleep paralysis, hypnagogic hallucinations, and nightmares. There is a progressive increase of dose intake over 6 to 8 weeks. The initial dosing is usually too low to have a therapeutic effect, particularly on sleepiness. This progressive effect indicates that the therapeutic effect is an indirect one. All patients subjectively reported progressive improvements in feeling rested on awakening. Overall, a positive effect on cataplexy is reported. The response is gradual, with a significant decrease in the frequency of cataplectic attacks noted. As mentioned previously, this gradual effect means that other alerting agents must initially be given to patients to control sleepiness. If patients wake up in the middle of the night, they may be confused and disoriented, and they may have episodes of enuresis, particularly at high dosages of 6 to 9 g. A transient worsening of cataplexy during the nocturnal period may occur. Nausea may be reported with a high dosage, as well as sluggishness in the early morning. Overall, patients prefer this drug to the anticataplectic drugs because there are fewer side effects.

Treatment in Children

Based on our clinical experience of more than 1000 adults and children with narcolepsy, we recommend modafinil for the treatment of EDS in children with narcolepsy. Modafinil seems to be best when administered morning and noon, but this may be a problem with children, so a single dose in the morning can been prescribed. The drawback of single-dose administration is that the therapeutic effect may not last until late in the day. A 5-mg tablet may be added when the child returns from school, if needed. The drug must not be given too late to avoid inducing sleep-onset insomnia. If modafinil cannot be prescribed, methylphenidate is the second best option; it has a short half-life and is available in a slow-release form.[70,77] In children, the recommended dose is based on weight, and we try to maintain a maximum of 30 mg/day administered as the slow-release form. The drug is given in the morning (15 mg) and at lunchtime (15 mg maximum) in the best case, or as a 20- or 30-mg slow-release preparation in the morning.

Clinical Pearls

Narcolepsy is characterized by the clinical tetrad of excessive daytime sleepiness, cataplexy, sleep paralysis, and hypnagogic/hypnopompic hallucinations, but not all of these must be present for the diagnosis of narcolepsy. The nighttime sleep of a patient with narcolepsy is often disrupted by frequent awakenings.

Patients with narcolepsy typically have two or more sleep-onset REM periods on a multiple sleep latency test (MSLT). The MSLT must be preceded by a nighttime polysomnogram to exclude other, more common causes of daytime sleepiness.

Patients who have narcolepsy with cataplexy usually have absent or very low levels of hypocretin in their spinal fluid.

Cataplexy is defined as a loss of muscle tone, usually triggered by humor or anger. Cataplexy is not associated with a loss of consciousness.

The effectiveness of short naps (15 to 20 minutes) in treating daytime sleepiness should not be underestimated, and this should be made clear to the patient's employer.

GHB (sodium oxybate) has been found to be effective in treating cataplexy without the negative side effects associated with the older tricyclics and the serotonin/norepinephrine reuptake inhibitors.

Modafinil has been found to be effective in treating excessive daytime sleepiness without the negative side effects associated with the older stimulants.

REFERENCES

1. Gélineau J: De la narcolepsie. Gaz Hop (Paris) 1880;53:626-628, 54:635-737.
2. Westphal C: Eigenthümliche mit Einschläfen verbundene Anfälle. Arch Psychiatr 1677;7:631-635.
3. Fisher F: Epileptoide schlafzustände. Arch Psychiatr 1878;8:200-203.
4. Henneberg R: Über genuine Narkolepsie. Neurol Zbl 1916;30:282-290.
5. Daniels L: Narcolepsy. Medicine (Baltimore) 1934;13:1-122.
6. Yoss RE, Daly DD: Criteria for the diagnosis of the narcoleptic syndrome. Proc Staff Meet Mayo Clin 1957;32:320-328.
7. Vogel G: Studies in the psychophysiology of dreams: III. The dream of narcolepsy. Arch Gen Psychiatry 1960;3:421-425.
8. Rechtschaffen A, Wolpert E, Dement WC, et al: Nocturnal sleep of narcoleptics. Electroencephalogr Clin Neurophysiol 1963;15:599-609.
9. Takahashi Y, Jimbo M: Polygraphic study of narcoleptic syndrome with special reference to hypnagogic hallucinations and cataplexy. Folia Psychiatr Neurol Jpn 1963;7(Suppl):343-347.
10. Passouant P, Schwab RS, Cadilhac J, et al: Narcolepsie-cataplexie: Etude du sommeil de nuit et du sommeil de jour. Rev Neurol (Paris) 1964;3:415-426.
11. Hishikawa Y, Kaneko Z: Electroencephalographic study on narcolepsy. Electroencephalogr Clin Neurophysiol 1965;18:249-258.
12. Guilleminault C, Dement WC, Passouant P (eds): Narcolepsy. New York, Spectrum, 1975.
13. Rosen GM, Bendel AE, Neglia JP, et al: Sleep in children with neoplasms of the central nervous system: Case review of 14 children. Pediatrics 2003;112:e46-54.
14. Broughton R, Valley V, Aguirre M, et al: Excessive daytime sleepiness and the pathophysiology of narcolepsy-cataplexy: A laboratory perspective. Sleep 1986;9:205-215.
15. American Academy of Sleep Medicine: International Classification of Sleep Disorders: Diagnostic and Coding Manual, 2nd ed. Westchester, Ill, American Academy of Sleep Medicine, 2005.
16. Guilleminault C, Heinzer R, Mignot E, et al: Investigations into the neurologic basis of narcolepsy. Neurology 1998;50(Suppl 1):S8-S15.
17. Szucs A, Janszky J, Hollo A, et al: Misleading hallucinations in unrecognized narcolepsy. Acta Psychiatr Scand 2003;108:314-316; discussion 316-317.
18. Guilleminault C, Pelayo R: Narcolepsy in prepubertal children. Ann Neurol 1998;43:135-142.
19. Morrish E, King MA, Smith IE, Shneerson JM: Factors associated with a delay in the diagnosis of narcolepsy. Sleep Med 2004;5:37-41.
20. Ohayon MM, Priest RG, Caucet M, et al: Hypnagogic and hypnopompic hallucinations: Pathological phenomenon? Br J Psychiatry 1996;169:459-467.
21. Billiard M, Besset A, Cadilhac J: The clinical and polygraphic development of narcolepsy. In Guilleminault C, Lugaresi E (eds): Sleep/Wake Disorders: Natural History, Epidemiology, and Long Term Evolution. New York, Raven Press, 1983, pp 187-199.
22. Schmidt HS, Fortin LD: Electronic pupillography in disorders of arousal. In Guilleminault C (ed): Sleep and Waking Disorders: Indications and Techniques. Menlo Park, Calif, Addison-Wesley, 1981, pp 127-141.
23. Hoddes E, Dement WC, Zarcone V: The development and use of the Stanford Sleepiness Scale (SSS). Psychophysiology 1972;9:150.
24. Yoss RE, Mayer NJ, Ogle KN: The pupillogram and narcolepsy. Neurology 1969;19:921-928.
25. Carskadon MA, Dement WC: The multiple sleep latency test: What does it measure? Sleep 1982;5:67-72.
26. Rechtschaffen A, Kales AD: A Manual of Standardized Terminology, Techniques and Scoring System for Sleep Stages of Human Subjects. Los Angeles, UCLA Brain Information Service/Brain Research Institute, 1968.
27. Association of Professional Sleep Societies, APSS Guidelines Committee; Carskadon MA, Chairperson: Guidelines for the multiple sleep latency test (MSLT): A standard measure of sleepiness. Sleep 1986;9:519-524.
28. Van den Hoed J, Kraemer H, Guilleminault C, et al: Disorders of excessive daytime somnolence: Polygraphic and clinical data for 100 patients. Sleep 1981;4:23-38.
29. Browman CP, Gujavarty KS, Sampson MG, et al: REM sleep episodes during the maintenance of wakefulness tests in patients with sleep apnea syndrome and patients with narcolepsy. Sleep 1983;6:23-28.
30. Broughton R, Low R, Valley V, et al: Auditory evoked potentials compared to EEG and performance measures of impaired vigilance in narcolepsy-cataplexy. Sleep Res 1981;10:184.
31. Dauvilliers Y, Gosselin A, Paquet J, et al: Effect of age on MSLT results in patients with narcolepsy-cataplexy. Neurology 2004;62:46-50.
32. Honda Y, Juji T (eds): HLA in Narcolepsy. Berlin, Springer-Verlag, 1988.
33. Anic-Labat S, Guilleminault C, Kraemer HC, et al: Validation of a cataplexy questionnaire in 983 sleep-disorders patients. Sleep 1999;22:77-87.
34. Moscovitch A, Partinen M, Patterson N, et al: Cataplexy in differentiation of excessive daytime somnolence. Sleep Res 1991;20:301.
35. Mignot E, Jayduk R, Black J, et al: HLA-DQB1*0602 is associated with narcolepsy in 509 narcoleptic patients. Sleep 1997;20:1012-1020.
36. Lin L, Faraco R, Li R, et al: The sleep disorder canine narcolepsy is caused by a mutation in the hypocretin (orexin) receptor 2 gene. Cell 1999;98:365-376.

37. Chemelli RM, Willie JT, Sinton CM, et al: Narcolepsy in orexin knockout mice: Molecular genetics of sleep regulation. Cell 1999;98:437-451.

38. Peyron C, Tighe DK, van den Pol AN, et al: Neurons containing hypocretin (orexin) project to multiple neuronal systems. J Neurosci 1998;18:9996-10015.

39. Nishino S, Ripley B, Overeem S, et al: Hypocretin (orexin) deficiency in human narcolepsy. Lancet 2000;355:39-40.

40. Mignot E, Guilleminault C, Bowersox S, et al: Effects of alpha-1 adrenoceptor blockade with prazosin in canine narcolepsy. Brain Res 1988;444:184-188.

41. Fruhstorfer B, Mignot E, Bowersox S, et al: Canine narcolepsy is associated with an elevated number of alpha 2 receptors in the locus coeruleus. Brain Res 1989;500:209-214.

42. Nishino S, Haak L, Shepherd H, et al: Effects of central alpha-2 adrenergic compounds on canine narcolepsy, a disorder of rapid eye movement sleep. J Pharmacol Exp Ther 1990;253:1145-1152.

43. Nishino S, Arrigoni J, Valtier D, et al: Dopamine D-2 mechanisms in canine narcolepsy. J Neurosci 1991;11:2666-2671.

44. Langer SZ: Presynaptic regulation of the release of catecholamines. Pharmacol Rev 1981;32:337-362.

45. Laduron PM: Presynaptic heteroreceptors in regulation of neuronal transmission. Biochem Pharmacol 1985;34:467-470.

46. Mignot E, Guilleminault C, Dement WC, et al: Genetically determined animal models of narcolepsy, a disorder of REM sleep. In Driscoll P (ed): Genetically-Defined Animal Models of Neurobehavioral Dysfunction. Cambridge, Mass, Birkhauser, 1992, pp 89-110.

47. Montplaisir J, de Champlain J, Young SN, et al: Narcolepsy and idiopathic hypersomnia: Biogenic amines and related compounds in CSF. Neurology 1982;32:1299-1302.

48. Faull KF, Zeller-DeAmicis LC, Radde L, et al: Biogenic amine concentrations in the brains of normal and narcoleptic canines: Current status. Sleep 1986;9:107-110.

49. Aldrich MS, Hollingsworth Z, Penney JB: Dopamine-receptor autoradiography of human narcoleptic brain. Neurology 1992; 31:503-506.

50. Rinne JP, Hublin C, Partinen M, et al: Striatal dopamine D1 receptors in narcolepsy: A PET study with [^{11}C]NNC756. J Sleep Res 1996;5:262-264.

51. Hublin C, Launes J, Nikkinen P, et al: Dopamine D2 receptors in human narcolepsy: A SPECT study with ^{123}I-IBZM. Acta Neurol Scand 1994;90:186-189.

52. Rinne JO, Hublin C, Partinen M, et al: Positron emission tomography study of human narcolepsy: No increase in striatal dopamine D2 receptors. Neurology 1995;45:1735-1738.

53. Aldrich MS, Prokopowicz G, Ockert K, et al: Neurochemical studies of human narcolepsy: Alpha-adrenergic receptor autoradiography of human narcoleptic brain and brainstem. Sleep 1994;17:598-608.

54. Guilleminault C: Amphetamines and narcolepsy: Use of Stanford database. Sleep 1993;16:199-201.

55. Fry JM: Treatment modalities for narcolepsy. Neurology 1998;50(Suppl 1):S43-S48.

56. Wyatt R, Fram D, Buchbinder R, et al: Treatment of intractable narcolepsy with a monoamine oxidase inhibitor. N Engl J Med 1971;285:987-999.

57. Scharf MB, Brown D, Woods M, et al: The effects and effectiveness of gamma-hydroxybutyrate in patients with narcolepsy. J Clin Psychol 1985;46:222-225.

58. Lammers GJ, Arends J, Declerk AC, et al: Gammahydroxybutyrate and narcolepsy: A double-blind placebo-controlled study. Sleep 1993;16:216-220.

59. Broughton R, Mamelak M: The treatment of narcolepsy-cataplexy with nocturnal gamma hydroxybutyrate. Can J Neurol Sci 1979;5:1-6.

60. Mamelak M, Scharf MB, Woods M: Treatment of narcolepsy with gamma-hydroxybutyrate: A review of clinical and sleep laboratory findings. Sleep 1986;9:285-289.

61. U.S. Xyrem Multicenter Study Group: A randomized, double blind, multicenter trial comparing the effect of 3 doses of orally administered sodium oxybate with placebo for the treatment of narcolepsy. Sleep 2002;25:42-49.

62. Borgen LA, Okerholm RA, Lai A, Scharf MB: The pharmacokinetics of sodium oxybate oral solution following acute and chronic administration to narcoleptic patients. J Clin Pharmacol 2004;44:253-257.

63. Guilleminault C, Mancuso J, Quera Salva MA, et al: Viloxazine hydrochloride in narcolepsy: A preliminary report. Sleep 1986;9:275-279.

64. Langdon N, Bandak S, Shindler J, et al: Fluoxetine in the treatment of cataplexy. Sleep 1986;9:371-372.

65. Mitler MM, Hajdukovic R: Relative efficacy of drugs for the treatment of sleepiness in narcolepsy. Sleep 1991;14:218-220.

66. Bedart MA, Montplaisir J, Godbout R: Effect of L-dopa on periodic movements in sleep in narcoleptics. Eur Neurol 1987;27:35-38.

67. Boivin MA, Montplaisir J, Poirier G: The effect of L-dopa on periodic leg movements and sleep organization in narcolepsy. Clin Neuropharmacol 1989;12:29-37.

68. Parkes JD: Amphetamines and alertness. In: Guilleminault C, Dement WC, Passouant P (eds): Narcolepsy. New York, Spectrum, 1976, pp 643-657.

69. Prinzmetal M, Bloomberg W: The use of benzedrine for treatment of narcolepsy. JAMA 1935;105:2051-2054.

70. Honda Y, Hishikawa Y: Effectiveness of pemoline in narcolepsy. Sleep Res 1970;8:192.

71. U.S. Modafinil in Narcolepsy Study Group: Randomized trial of modafinil for the treatment of pathological somnolence in narcolepsy. Ann Neurol 1998;43:88-97.

72. Mitler M, Erman M, Hajdukovic R: The treatment of excessive somnolence with stimulant drugs. Sleep 1993;16:203-206.

73. Parkes JD, Dahlitz M: Amphetamine prescription. Sleep 1993;16:201-203.

74. Parkes JD, Schacter M: Mazindol in the treatment of narcolepsy. Acta Neurol Scand 1979;60:250-254.

75. Boutrel B, Koob GF: What keeps us awake: The neuropharmacology of stimulants and wakefulness-promoting medications. Sleep 2004;27:1181-1194.

76. U.S. Xyrem Multicenter Study Group: Sodium oxybate demonstrates long-term efficacy for the treatment of cataplexy in patients with narcolepsy. Sleep Med 2004;5:119-123.

77. Yoss RE, Daly DD: Treatment of narcolepsy with Ritalin. Neurology 1959;9:171-173.

66

Idiopathic Hypersomnia

Claudio L. Bassetti

Rafael Pelayo

Christian Guilleminault

ABSTRACT

Idiopathic hypersomnia is a sleep disorder characterized by excessive daytime sleepiness, with episodes of prolonged non-refreshing sleep, a prolonged major sleep episode, and great difficulty waking up either in the morning or at the end of a nap. It is a diagnosis of exclusion with a poorly understood pathophysiology. A broad differential diagnosis needs to be considered. Stimulant medications have been the most common treatment, although the response has been variable.

In the clinical practice of sleep medicine, one of the most frustrating diagnoses to make (and for the patient to receive) is idiopathic hypersomnia. The dissatisfaction stems from diagnostic uncertainty, unclear natural history, and unpredictable response to treatment. This chapter gives an overview of epidemiology, pathogenesis, clinical features, diagnostic workup, treatment, and prognosis of this disorder.

HISTORY

With the clear definition of narcolepsy (see Chapter 65), it became apparent that some patients with hypersomnia suffer from a different disorder. Bedrich Roth was the first in the late 1950s and early 1960s to describe a syndrome characterized by excessive daytime sleepiness (EDS), prolonged sleep and sleep drunkenness, and the absence of "sleep attacks," cataplexy, sleep paralysis, and hallucinations. The terms "independent sleep drunkenness" and "hypersomnia with sleep drunkenness" were initially suggested.[1-4] Features overlapping with narcolepsy were identified from the beginning and led to such labels as "essential narcolepsy," "independent narcolepsy," and "non–rapid eye movement (NREM) sleep narcolepsy."[5,6] Other terms, including "idiopathic central nervous system hypersomnolence" (Diagnostic Classification of Sleep Disorders, 1979), "functional hypersomnia, hypersomnia with automatic behavior,"[7] "harmonious hypersomnia," and "idiopathic hypersomnia" (International Classification of Sleep Disorders, 1990)[8] were also put forward. Idiopathic hypersomnia should not be considered synonymous with hypersomnia of undetermined origin. The term "idiopathic hypersomnia" was indeed used in the medical literature as early as 1829 ("die idiopathische chronische Schlafsucht") for EDS of undetermined origin.

In the absence, until now, of a biological marker for the disorder and the better identification over the last few decades of other potential causes of nonstructural EDS (including subtle forms of sleep disordered breathing), periodic limb movements in sleep, sleep insufficiency, delayed sleep phase syndrome, and hypersomnia associated with psychiatric disorders have raised critical questions about the "true" frequency and clinical picture of idiopathic hypersomnia.[9-11]

EPIDEMIOLOGY

In the absence of systematic studies, the prevalence of idiopathic CNS hypersomnia is unknown. Nosologic uncertainty causes difficulty in determining the epidemiology of the disorder. Recent reports from large sleep centers reported a ratio of idiopathic hypersomnia to narcolepsy of 1:10.[10,11] Hence, the prevalence of idiopathic hypersomnia in the general population may be estimated at around 20 to 50 per million, a figure much lower than the 300 to 600 per million suggested until the early 1980s.[12,13] The age of onset of symptoms varies, but it is frequently between 10 and 30 years. The condition usually develops progressively over several weeks or months. Once established, symptoms are generally stable and long lasting. Spontaneous improvement in EDS may, however, be observed in up to one quarter of patients.[11,14]

PATHOGENESIS

The pathogenesis of idiopathic hypersomnia is unknown. Hypersomnia usually starts insidiously. Occasionally, EDS is first experienced after transient insomnia, abrupt changes in sleep-wake habits, overexertion, general anesthesia, viral illness, or mild head trauma.[11] In about 50% of cases, the disorder has a familial component, and on rare occasions idiopathic hypersomnia and narcolepsy occur in the same family.[10,15] An autosomic dominant mode of inheritance has been discussed, and females may be more affected.[16] In a few series an association with diabetes or obesity was observed.[11,17]

Given the existence of overlapping features between idiopathic hypersomnia and narcolepsy (see later), there has been an interest in potential HLA markers for idiopathic hypersomnia. Despite reports of an increase in HLA DQ1,[11] DR5 and Cw2,[18] and DQ3,[19] and of a decrease of Cw3,[20] no consistent findings have emerged. HLA typing currently does not play a role in the diagnosis of idiopathic hypersomnia.

Cerebrospinal fluid (CSF) analyses in idiopathic hypersomnia have shown normal cell counts, cytology, and protein content. Montplaisir and coworkers found a decrease in dopamine and indoleacetic acid in both patients with idiopathic hypersomnia and with narcolepsy.[21] Faull and colleagues found similar mean concentrations of monoamine metabolites in subjects with narcolepsy or idiopathic hypersomnia and with controls, but—using a principal component analysis—they also found a dysregulation of the dopamine system in narcolepsy and of the norepinephrine system in idiopathic hypersomnia.[22-24]

These metabolic data may support the hypothesis of a primary deficient arousal system in patients with idiopathic hypersomnia. Petitjean and Jouvet observed both hypersomnia and disturbances of monoamine metabolites in the cerebrospinal fluid of cats with a lesion of the ascending noradrenergic pathways.[25]

Disturbances of homeostatic and circadian aspects of sleep-wake regulation have also been suggested in idiopathic hypersomnia. The observations of increased sleep spindle densities during the entire sleep period and decreased slow wave activity in the first two sleep cycles led to the hypothesis of altered NREM sleep homeostasis.[26-28] On the other hand, a disturbed circadian function was hypothesized on the basis of a phase delay found in the rhythm of melatonin and cortisol secretion of patients with idiopathic hypersomnia.[29]

The most recent attempts to understand the pathophysiology of idiopathic hypersomnia relate to the potential role of the hypocretins or orexins. These hypothalamic neuropeptides are involved in the regulation of sleep-wake states. The hypocretin-1 (orexin A) subtype is deficient in about 90% of patients who have narcolepsy with cataplexy.[30-38] However, in narcolepsy without cataplexy, symptomatic narcolepsy, and familial narcolepsy and in narcoleptic twins hypocretin-1 levels may be normal.[17,39-41] Similarly, most studies suggest normal CSF levels of hypocretin-1 in idiopathic hypersomnia.[17,39,40] In the absence of clear cutoffs for normal levels and considering differences in diagnostic criteria, reports of diminished levels of hypocretin-1 and hypocretin-2 must be interpreted with caution.[42,43]

The discovery of biological clock genes and familial circadian disorders allows consideration of possible genetic causes of idiopathic hypersomnia, because mutations or abnormalities of the clock genes may lead to hypersomnia.

CLINICAL FEATURES

Excessive Daytime Sleepiness

Patients complain of a constant and nonimperative excessive daytime sleepiness. The Epworth sleepiness score is typically high (>12-14/24) and does not discriminate patients with narcolepsy and idiopathic hypersomnia. As with narcolepsy, alcohol, exercise, heavy meals, and warm environments can accentuate EDS. Conversely, sleep deprivation is often well tolerated by patients with idiopathic hypersomnia.

Daytime drowsiness leads to naps that are prolonged, interrupted rarely by short awakenings, and frequently unrefreshing. The unrefreshing quality of napping and the sleep drunkenness associated with awakenings (see later) lead patients to fight sleepiness as long as they can. In addition, the work environment may not permit napping.

Subjects who do not nap are particularly prone to episodes of drowsiness and automatic behavior. Episodes of automatic behavior are usually signaled by blank stares. During these episodes, patients act in an unplanned and often inappropriate way; for example, patients have reported finding themselves miles from their homes while driving or performing inappropriate actions such as sprinkling salt on coffee, putting dirty plates in a clothes dryer and turning on the machine, writing incoherent sentences during classes, having loud and

irrelevant bursts of speech, and so on. Amnesia of such occurrences is the rule, although patients are usually aware that they have had one of their "drowsy" episodes when they are later confronted with the results of their automatic behavior.

A few patients with idiopathic hypersomnia occasionally report episodes of irresistible sleep as well as short and refreshing naps.[11] On the other hand, the existence of patients who have narcolepsy with cataplexy and nonimperative EDS, prolonged naps, and nocturnal sleep prove the existence of an overlap between narcolepsy and idiopathic hypersomnia, as suggested also by the occurrence of both conditions in the same family.[9-11,14]

Nocturnal Sleep

Nocturnal sleep is typically subjectively long and undisturbed. A few patients report sleep times of 12 to 19 hours per day on weekends and during holidays. Since most patients do not report improvement of EDS with prolonged sleep, history of extreme sleep times (sleeping more than 12 hours per day) is less frequent than commonly assumed.[11]

In the morning, awakenings are difficult. Sleep "drunkenness" (also called "syndrome d'Elpénor," after the youngest of Odysseus' comrades who was killed in a fall from a roof during an episode of incomplete awakening) was noted in 40% to 60% of patients reported by Roth.[12] These patients are hard to awaken; they can be aggressive and verbally and physically abusive during that twilight state if they are awakened, even at their own request. The patient may be confused and unable to react adequately to external stimuli upon awakening. The "time to get going" (sleep inertia) in the morning may be as long as 2 or 3 hours. Sleep drunkenness can also be noted when patients are awakened from naps.

It should be emphasized that automatic behavior, prolonged sleep episodes, and sleep drunkenness, although very typical for idiopathic hypersomnia, may be seen in a variety of conditions including narcolepsy, hypersomnia associated with psychiatric disorders, and hypersomnia with neurologic disorders.[61]

Associated Features

Depressive symptoms were noted in 15% to 25% of patients in Roth's series and confirmed in later studies.[11,12,15,44,45] Similar figures are found also in patients who have narcolepsy with cataplexy. Mood changes not qualifying for the diagnosis of affective disorder may precede or follow the onset of EDS and evolve independently. The presence of major depression signs are, however, not compatible with the diagnosis of idiopathic hypersomnia (see later).

Sleep paralysis and hallucinations are typical for narcolepsy with cataplexy, but they are not exceptional also in patients with other sleep disorders and even in the healthy population.[9,46,47] It is therefore not surprising that both symptoms may be reported by idiopathic hypersomnia patients, as well, as demonstrated by the only two studies that addressed this issue specifically.[9,11]

Headache is a frequent symptom in patients with EDS. Migraine- and tension-type headaches are reported in about 30% of patients with idiopathic hypersomnia. They may be accompanied by other neurovegetative symptoms such as cold hands and feet; lightheadedness on standing up, orthostatic hypotension; or syncope.[3,11,14,48] The frequency of neurovegetative symptoms is, however, similar in narcolepsy and idiopathic hypersomnia.[14] An increased body mass index has been noted in a few series.[11,17] The overall psychosocial handicap of patients with idiopathic hypersomnia is similar to that of narcoleptics.[49]

DIAGNOSIS

Clinical Criteria

Diagnostic criteria have evolved over time and will no doubt continue to change in the future as our knowledge improves. The International Classification of Sleep Disorders recognizes two types of idiopathic hypersomnia.[50] In one type, idiopathic hypersomnia with long sleep time, the patient typically sleeps more than 10 hours. In idiopathic hypersomnia without long sleep time, the patient typically sleeps more than 6 but less than 10 hours. The minimum diagnostic criteria should include:

- complaint of EDS and prolonged, often unrefreshing naps
- difficulty waking up in the morning or after a nap
- insidious onset prior to age 30
- duration of at least 6 months
- exclusion of conditions that may cause the same symptoms.

This last criterion would typically require sleep studies be performed to rule out other sleep disorders (see later). A recent history of significant head trauma (within 18 months of symptom onset) should not be present.

Given the possibility of circadian disorders manifesting as hypersomnia, the patient should have completed sleep diaries (or actigraphy, see later) for at least 1 to 2 weeks before the polysomnogram. Patients must be set on a regular sleep-wake schedule and must have a minimum of 7 to 8 hours of nocturnal sleep time. Drugs known to affect sleep, sleep latency, and daytime alertness must be carefully evaluated and should be withdrawn for a minimum of 2 weeks before objective polysomnographic testing. It may be helpful to obtain a urine toxicology sample for drug testing at the time of the polysomnogram.

Roth proposed that idiopathic hypersomnia be subdivided into polysymptomatic and monosymptomatic subtypes.[2] The polysymptomatic form, also referred to as the classic form,[11] is characterized by EDS, prolonged nocturnal sleep, and sleep drunkenness. The monosymptomatic form manifests only with EDS. This subdivision or distinction is not currently made in the International Classification of Sleep Disorders.[50] This clinical heterogeneity has led to concerns that idiopathic hypersomnia, and in particular its monosymptomatic variant, is overdiagnosed.[10,11,19,51]

Polysomnographic Criteria

Polysomnographic monitoring of nocturnal sleep is normal in idiopathic hypersomnia except for its prolonged duration and increased amounts of deep (slow wave) NREM sleep (Figure 66–1).[3,11,48] This finding is nonspecific and can be seen also in patients with chronic sleep insufficiency (see later). Amounts of sleep spindles (throughout the sleep period) and of slow wave activity (in the first two sleep cycles) have been reported to be elevated in idiopathic hypersomnia.[26,28] In one study, patients with idiopathic hypersomnia were found to have a higher REM-sleep density than healthy subjects.[52]

Sleep-onset REM episodes are rare, and specific sleep abnormalities such as sleep-disordered breathing (including upper airway resistance syndrome) should be absent. However, the presence of periodic limb movements in patients with EDS—but without restless legs symptoms—does not necessarily preclude the diagnosis of idiopathic hypersomnia.[51,53] In addition, sleep abnormalities may be found in patients in whom the sleep study is performed long after the early onset of the hypersomnia. If upper airway resistance syndrome is suspected, esophageal pressure monitoring or nasal pressure cannula (to measure airflow) should be part of the sleep study.

In a few patients satisfying the clinical criteria for idiopathic hypersomnia, sleep disruption has been described.[11,51]

Multiple Sleep Latency Test Criteria

After the polysomnographic evaluation of nocturnal sleep, a Multiple Sleep Latency Test (MSLT) is usually conducted in a standardized manner the next day. The mean sleep latency score is usually, but not invariably between 5-10 minutes in patients with idiopathic hypersomnia and therefore higher than in narcolepsy (see Fig. 66–1; Figs. 66–2 and 66–3).[11]

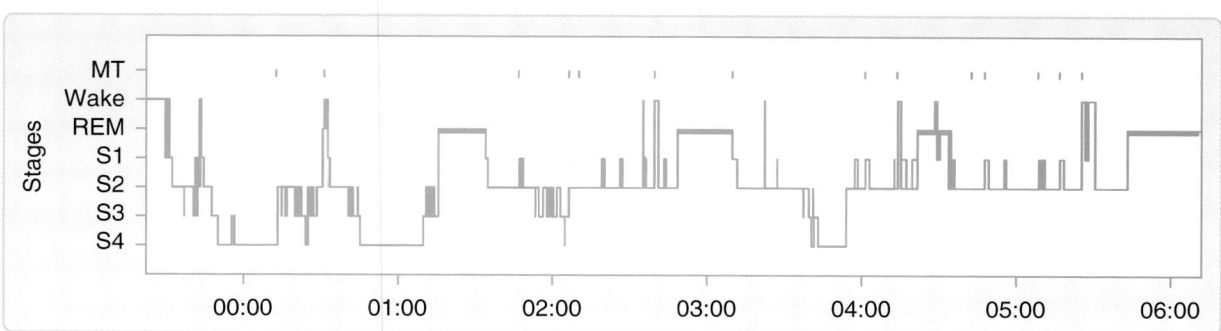

Figure 66–1. A 22-year-old female patient with idiopathic hypersomnia (EDS, prolonged nonrefreshing sleep, sleep drunkenness). Epworth sleepiness score was stable over months at between 17/24 and 18/24. She had frequent hallucinations (while falling asleep or on awakening), no sleep paralysis or cataplexy. Her BMI was 21, and she had a positive family history for EDS. Polysomnography showed sleep efficiency 98%, sleep latency to NREM 2 sleep 10 minutes, slow wave sleep 22% (of sleep period time). No snoring, no apnea, no periodic limb movement in sleep. MSLT: mean sleep latency of 4 minutes, no SOREMP. Actigraphy showed mean time "asleep" (rest/sleep) over 43% of the recording time. Hypocretin-1 in cerebrospinal fluid was normal. Her HLA DQB1*0602 was positive and psychiatric assessment was normal. She experienced no improvement with modafinil up to 300 mg/d. BMI, body mass index; EDS, excessive daytime sleepiness; MSLT, Multiple Sleep Latency Test; MT, movement time; NREM, non–rapid eye movement; SOREMP, sleep-onset rapid eye movement period.

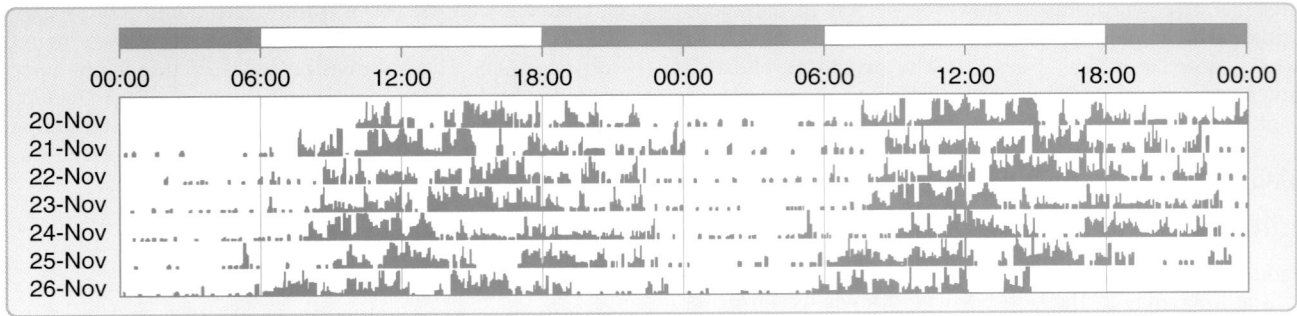

Figure 66–2. A 39-year-old female patient with idiopathic hypersomnia (EDS, prolonged nonrefreshing sleep, sleep drunkenness). Epworth sleepiness score was stable over years between 17/24 and 19/24. No cataplexy, sleep paralysis or hallucinations. The differential diagnosis of hypersomnia associated with psychiatric disorder was discussed in this patient, who had depression in the past. She has a positive family history for EDS (mother of the patient shown in Figure 66–1). Polysomnography showed sleep efficiency 96%, sleep latency to NREM 2 sleep 10 minutes, slow wave sleep 22% (of sleep period time). No snoring, no apnea, no periodic limb movement in sleep. MSLT showed mean sleep latency of 5 minutes, no SOREMP. One-week actigraphy (during holiday) showed mean time "asleep" (rest/sleep) over 50% of the recording time, napping (time "asleep") during the day over a mean of 4 hours. Hypocretin-1 in cerebrospinal fluid was normal. HLA DQB1*0602 was negative. Psychiatric assessment showed signs of dysthymia. She experienced no improvement after mazindol, methylphenidate, modafinil, fluoxetine, or reboxetine. EDS, excessive daytime sleepiness; MSLT, Multiple Sleep Latency Test; NREM, non–rapid eye movement; SOREMP, sleep-onset rapid eye movement period.

A few patients are found to have mean sleep latencies less than 5 minutes or greater than 10 minutes.[11,54,55] Sleep-onset REM periods are rare (4% in a series of 42 patients).[11] Subjective awareness of sleep during naps is higher than in narcoleptics.

The diagnostic value of the MSLT is limited because of the need to wake up the patient from the preceding night's polysomnogram to perform the MSLT. This interferes with the documentation of the prolonged nighttime sleep that is typical in idiopathic hypersomnia. In addition, the standard MSLT protocol of 20-minute nap sessions every 2 hours does not capture the characteristic prolonged daytime sleep episodes. In fact, a few patients with idiopathic hypersomnia may have normal mean sleep latencies on conventional MSLT.

Other Criteria

Some authors have recommended prolonged (24-hour) sleep-wake recordings as a diagnostic tool of idiopathic hypersomnia.[10] This would allow an appreciation of *ad libitum* sleep.

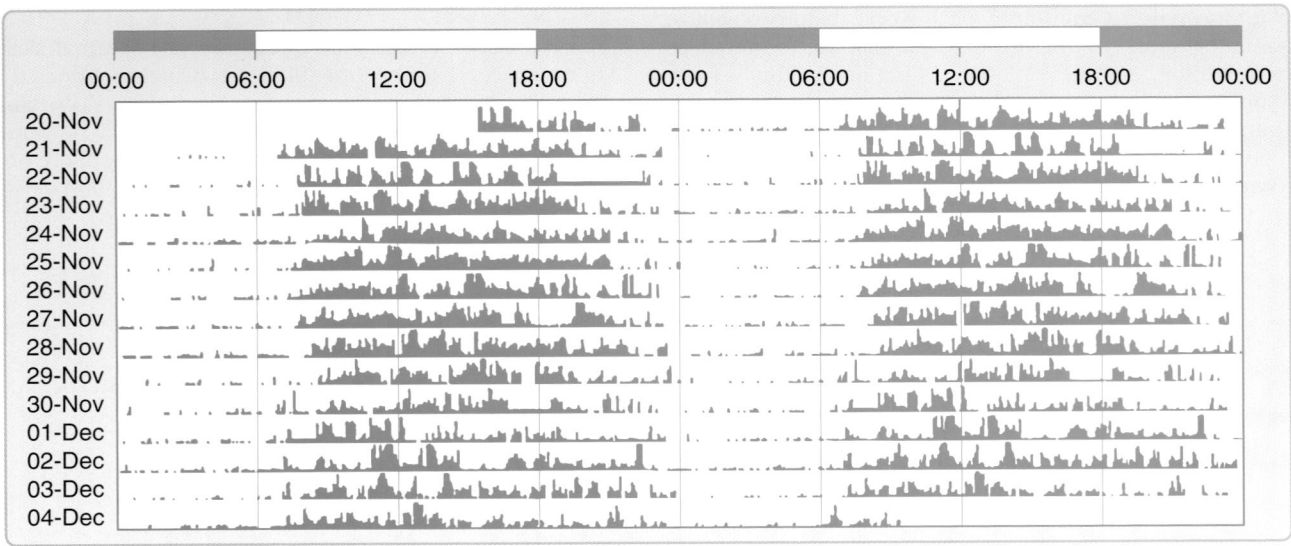

Figure 66–3. A 34-year-old male patient with idiopathic hypersomnia (EDS, prolonged nonrefreshing sleep, sleep drunkenness). Epworth sleepiness score was somewhat variable over years between 14/24 and 19/24. He occasionally had cataplexy-like episodes, sleep paralysis, or hallucinations. His BMI was 20 and he had a negative family history for EDS. Polysomnography showed sleep efficiency 97%, sleep latency to NREM 2 sleep 15 minutes, slow wave sleep 18% (of sleep period time). No snoring, no apnea, no periodic limb movement in sleep. MSLT showed mean sleep latency of 3.5 minutes, no SOREMP. Two-week actigraphy (during working days) showed mean time "asleep" (rest/sleep) over 39% of the recording time, napping (time "asleep") during the day over a mean of 24 hours. Hypocretin-1 in cerebrospinal fluid was normal. HLA DQB1*0602 was positive. Psychiatric assessment was normal. He experienced no improvement after modafinil, methylphenidate, and melatonin. He experienced improvement of EDS with selegilin 30 mg/d. EDS, excessive daytime sleepiness; MSLT, Multiple Sleep Latency Test; NREM, non–rapid eye movement; SOREMP, sleep-onset rapid eye movement period.

Patients with idiopathic hypersomnia have longer and more consolidated nocturnal sleep than do other patients with daytime sleepiness, which a 24-hour recording could demonstrate. In a study of subjects with idiopathic hypersomnia, spontaneous sleep periods of up to 19 hours could be documented.[55] Several 24-hour recordings should be ideally performed to ensure that the patient is saturated with sleep.[48,56]

The counterargument is that the MSLT should be part of the diagnostic workup for idiopathic hypersomnia because it is a diagnosis of exclusion in which narcolepsy without cataplexy is often considered. Performing a standard overnight polysomnogram followed by an MSLT and an additional 24-hour polysomnogram would arguably be ideal, but it would also add considerably to the financial costs of the diagnosis.

In addition, 24-hour polysomnograms have not been standardized. Should these prolonged polysomnograms be performed in an ambulatory or laboratory setting? Should the patient remain in bed or be allowed physical activity? If physical activity is allowed, how much? Finally, prolonged sleep times are not specific for idiopathic hypersomnia and may be observed also in patients with hypersomnia related to neurologic disorders and in depressed patients with EDS who are allowed to sleep *ad libitum*.[57-59]

Instead of an additional 24-hour polysomnogram, ambulatory actigraphy monitoring over several days can also demonstrate the prolonged sleep episodes characteristic of idiopathic hypersomnia (see Figure 66–2).[16,17] However, actigraphy protocols have not been standardized or validated in idiopathic hypersomnia, and the differentiation between sleep and rest while awake ("clinophilia") may be difficult.

Brain magnetic resonance imaging (MRI), HLA-typing, and assessment of CSF hypocretin-1 levels are not useful in the diagnosis of idiopathic hypersomnia, as mentioned before. Differences in melatonin secretion and evoked potential responses (including the P300 wave measure after awakening) have been found between normal subjects, narcoleptics, and idiopathic hypersomnia patients.[16,28,29,60] These findings are, however, of no diagnostic help in a single patient.

DIFFERENTIAL DIAGNOSIS

Narcolepsy with and without Cataplexy

Narcolepsy is a common differential diagnostic consideration, but it is not the most difficult. The presence of EDS with clear-cut (definite) cataplexy, two or more sleep-onset REM periods on the MSLT, and low or undetectable CSF hypocretin-1 levels are diagnostic indications. As pointed out before, some patients fulfilling the current international criteria for idiopathic hypersomnia report a variable EDS associated with irresistible sleep episodes, as well as short and refreshing naps. On the other hand, a few patients who have narcolepsy with cataplexy present with nonimperative EDS, prolonged naps, and prolonged nocturnal sleep.[9,11,61] The narcoleptic syndrome may, in addition, initially manifest as EDS without or with atypical cataplexy, and the positive diagnosis may be in doubt for months or even years. The term *narcolepsy without cataplexy* may be used for this situation.

The presence of sleep-onset REM sleep on polysomnogram or MSLT and the presence of HLA DQB1*0602 help to distinguish narcolepsy from idiopathic hypersomnia. Unfortunately, CSF hypocretin-1 levels have been found to be usually normal in most patients with either narcolepsy without cataplexy or idiopathic hypersomnia.[37,38]

Chronic Sleep Insufficiency and Long Sleepers

A careful history will differentiate patients with idiopathic hypersomnia from those with chronic insufficient nocturnal sleep who have EDS.[62,63] Typically, patients show on questionnaires a difference of 2 to 3 hours between sleep times on weekdays and weekends. Polysomnographic and MSLT findings may be similar to those of patients with idiopathic hypersomnia (see earlier). An actigraphic recording may be helpful if the history is inconclusive. Particularly difficult is the recognition of (relative) sleep insufficiency in long sleepers. It is possible that besides long sleepers, other persons may be more prone to develop hypersomnia in association with sleep insufficiency (Figure 66–4).

Some authors have even suggested that idiopathic hypersomnia may represent an extreme form of a long-sleeper status.[28] However, patients with absolute or relative sleep insufficiency, but usually not those with idiopathic hypersomnia, exhibit a subjective and objective improvement of EDS with prolongation of sleep times or when allowed to sleep *ad libitum*.

Sleep-Disordered Breathing Syndromes

Idiopathic hypersomnia should be distinguished from sleep-disordered breathing syndromes, including the upper airway resistance syndrome.[64-66] Clinically, both men and women complain of isolated EDS and snoring. Examinations of these subjects often reveal a triangular face or a steep mandibular plane, a highly arched palate, a class II malocclusion, and, at times, retroposition of the mandible. All of the patients described have not been obese. Cephalometric radiographs have indicated the presence of a small space behind the base of the tongue (posterior airway space), often near the location of the hyoid bone. The distance between the hyoid bone and the mandibular plane is variable, sometimes small. Several of the nonsnoring women had cervical vertebrae fusions (C3-4, C5-6).

These subjects presented repetitive short ("transient") alpha electroencephalographic arousals lasting 3 to 14 seconds that regularly interrupted the abnormally high inspiratory efforts.[67] Standard polysomnographic recordings of these subjects evoked the diagnosis on the basis of the presence of these repetitive transient arousals, increases in snoring just before the arousal, and an increase in inspiratory time and a decrease in expiratory time, which were determined with the use of well-calibrated sensors. No significant change in SaO_2 was seen, and the respiratory disturbance index was low (less than 5).

If upper airway resistance syndrome is suspected, esophageal pressure monitoring or a nasal pressure cannula should be included in the sleep study. In patients with isolated snoring and idiopathic hypersomnia, a CPAP trial may be warranted. Lack of improvement would support the latter diagnosis.[11,51]

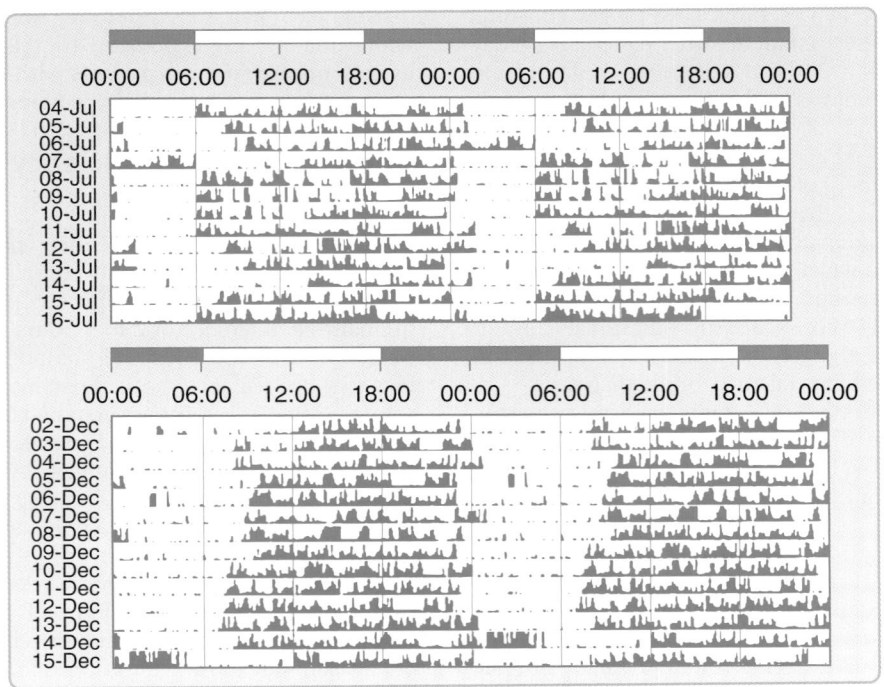

Figure 66–4. A 22-year-old male patient with sleep insufficiency (EDS, sleep drunkenness). Epworth sleepiness score (ESS) was initially 20/24. He occasionally experienced sleep paralysis on awakening but had no cataplexy and no hallucinations. His BMI was 24, and he had a negative family history for EDS. He initially denied sleep insufficiency. The differential diagnosis of hypersomnia associated with psychiatric disorder was discussed for this patient. Polysomnography showed sleep efficiency 90%, sleep latency to NREM 2 sleep 12 minutes, slow wave sleep 7% (of sleep period time). He had no snoring, no apnea, no periodic limb movement in sleep. MSLT showed mean sleep latency of 6 minutes, 3 SOREMP. Two-week actigraphy (during working days) showed irregular sleep-wake rhythms, mean time "asleep" (rest/sleep) over 35% of the recording time. Hypocretin-1 in cerebrospinal fluid was normal and HLA DQB1*0602 was positive. Psychiatric assessment was normal. After sleep extension of >1 h/day (documented by actigraphy, *right inside*) he experienced complete subjective resolution of the EDS and normalization of the ESS (4/24). MSLT showed mean sleep latency of 5 minutes and absence of sleep onset REM periods. EDS, excessive daytime sleepiness; MSLT, Multiple Sleep Latency Test; NREM, non–rapid eye movement; SOREMP, sleep-onset rapid eye movement period.

Hypersomnia Associated with Psychiatric Disorders

Hypersomnia associated with psychiatric disorders (atypical depression, bipolar depression, dysthymia or neurotic depression, neurotic hypersomnia) is not always easy to differentiate from idiopathic hypersomnia. These conditions can share the following symptoms: nonimperative EDS, long nonrefreshing naps, long sleep times, sleep drunkenness or sleep inertia, and depressed mood. The term of atypical or vegetative depression has been used for the association of a major depression with these symptoms.

Particularly difficult is the differential diagnosis between idiopathic hypersomnia and less severe forms of depression (dysthymia, previously called neurotic depression). Polysomnographic findings may be very similar (Fig. 66–5), although patients with hypersomnia associated with psychiatric disorders are generally found to have higher amounts of NREM stage 1 sleep and lower amounts of slow wave sleep.[68] In patients with hypersomnia associated with psychiatric disorders, the MSLT typically shows normal mean sleep latencies. In addition, these patients may spend a large amount of time in bed and acknowledge "resting" more than "sleeping" (clinophilia). Patients with hypersomnia associated with psychiatric disorders may exhibit mean times "asleep" of up to 50% to 60% of the entire actigraphy recording times.[17]

Finally, exacerbation of EDS in winter months, obesity, and improvement of EDS with antidepressants are other typical features of "atypical depression."

Hypersomnia associated with psychiatric disorders may, however, be accompanied also by abnormal MSLT findings (in 36% of cases in the series reported by Billiard et al.[54]) (see Fig. 66–5). Conversely, patients with idiopathic hypersomnia may exhibit normal MSLT findings.[13,17,54,69] In unclear cases, formal psychiatric assessment is needed. Treatment with activating antidepressants (selective serotonin reuptake inhibitors [SSRIs], monoamine oxidase [MAO] inhibitors, noradrenaline reuptake inhibitors [NARIs]) rather than stimulants may be considered in patients in whom a psychiatric disorder as cause of EDS cannot be ruled out with certainty.

Chronic Fatigue Syndrome and Postviral Hypersomnia

Chronic fatigue syndrome is characterized by persistent or relapsing fatigue that does not resolve with sleep or rest. One of the clinical difficulties is that chronic fatigue syndrome is a poorly defined diagnosis, and patients often fail to differentiate between fatigue and desire for sleep and between EDS and need for sleep. The clinical presentation of chronic fatigue is similar to that seen in patients with hypersomnia associated with psychiatric disorders. In addition to fatigue, patients

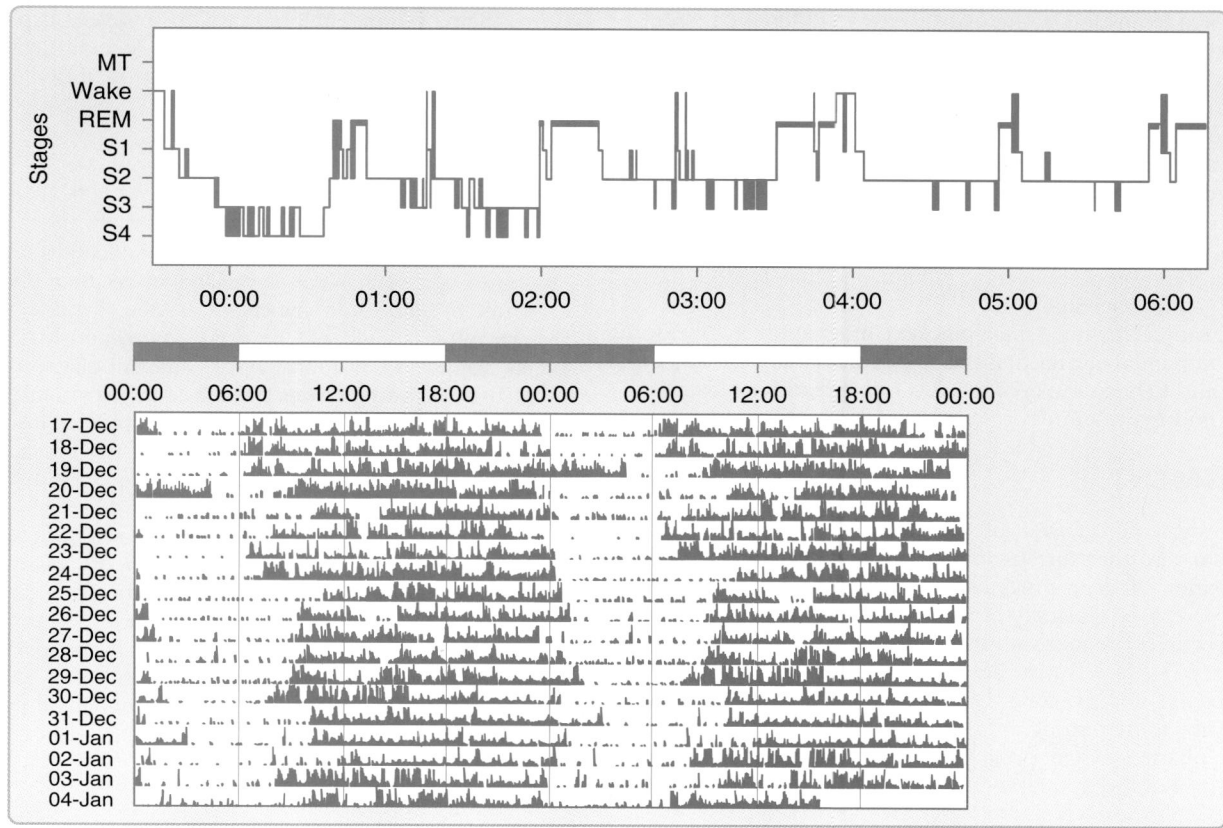

Figure 66–5. A 32-year-old female patient with hypersomnia associated with depression (EDS, prolonged nonrefreshing sleep, mild sleep drunkenness). Epworth sleepiness score (ESS) was 11/24. She had occasional hallucinations on awakening but no cataplexy and no sleep paralysis. Her mood was mildly depressed. Her BMI was 27, and she had a positive family history for EDS and depression. Polysomnography *(top)* shows sleep efficiency 97%, sleep latency to NREM 2 sleep 10 minutes, slow wave sleep 22% (of sleep period time). No snoring, no apnea, no periodic limb movement in sleep. MSLT showed mean sleep latency of 7 minutes, no SOREMP. MWT showed mean sleep latency of 10 minutes, no SOREMP. Actigraphy *(bottom)* showed mean time "asleep" (rest/sleep) over 38% of the recording time. Hypocretin-1 in cerebrospinal fluid was normal. HLA DQB1*0602 was negative. Psychiatric assessment showed depression. She experienced complete subjective resolution of the EDS with citalopram 40 mg/d within one month, normalization of the ESS (2/24), and weight loss (4 kg). EDS, excessive daytime sleepiness; MSLT, Multiple Sleep Latency Test; MWT, Maintenance of Wakefulness Test; MT, movement time; NREM, non–rapid eye movement; SOREMP, sleep-onset rapid eye movement period.

complain of cognitive difficulties, poor mood, anxiety, fever, myalgias, and other symptoms. Polysomnography may show decreased sleep efficiency and recurrent alpha-intrusions, unlike idiopathic hypersomnia. The MSLT is typically normal. A few patients with chronic fatigue syndrome are given a specific sleep diagnosis (sleep apnea, restless legs syndrome, periodic leg movements during sleep) after polysomnographic investigation.[70]

After an acute viral infection (typically mononucleosis or pneumonia) patients may develop a (postviral) syndrome of EDS with features similar to those of chronic fatigue and idiopathic hypersomnia.[71] In some of these patients an encephalitic process or elevated levels of inflammatory cytokines may play a role.[72-74]

Delayed or Advanced Sleep Phase Syndrome

Rarely, EDS during the morning hours in patients with a delayed sleep phase syndrome and EDS during the afternoon hours in patients with advanced sleep phase syndrome may lead to questions regarding the diagnosis, but an appropriate sleep history, sleep logs covering 15 days, and, if needed, actigraphy performed for 1-2 weeks indicate a normal total sleep time but abnormal sleep-onset and wake-up times.

Hypersomnia and Neurologic Disorders

A variety of neurologic disorders including severe head trauma, stroke (particularly at the thalamic or mesencephalic level), parkinsonian syndromes, encephalitis, hypothalamic disorders (tumors, neurosarcoidosis, Whipple's disease), myotonic dystrophy, and communicating hydrocephalus may lead to hypersomnia with prolonged sleep times, sleep drunkenness, nonimperative EDS, and abnormal MSLT findings.[57,58,72,73,75-82] History, clinical findings, and brain imaging are diagnostic tools in these cases.

Other Hypersomnias

Periodic and recurrent hypersomnias, including the Kleine-Levin syndrome and the recurrent hypersomnia associated with the menstrual cycle, occasionally alternating with episodes of hyposomnia, are usually easy to differentiate from idiopathic hypersomnia by history only.[83-88] In some cases periodic hypersomnia may appear after a viral illness.[72,89]

Restless legs syndrome can be associated with EDS.[90,91] Hypersomnia is also a feature of several pediatric syndromes (e.g. Prader-Willy, Niemann-Pick Type C, Möbius', and Norrie's syndromes). Hypophyseal insufficiency, hypothyroidism, and obesity (without sleep disordered breathing) can be associated with apathy, EDS, or hypersomnia.[92,93] Encephalopathies secondary to liver insufficiency, uremia, and hypercapnia may lead to somnolence and EDS.

Medications including beta-blockers, other antihypertensive agents, dopaminergic agents, and antidepressants may lead to fatigue and EDS. Stimulants may over time lead paradoxically to EDS and hypersomnia.[16,94]

TREATMENT

The underlying causes of idiopathic hypersomnia are unknown, and therefore treatment can only be symptomatic. Prolongation of sleep times has been suggested by Roth but has proved to be generally of no help.[11] In fact, restriction of time in bed may be more advantageous. Behavioral approaches and sleep hygiene must be recommended but may have little positive impact alone. Daytime naps are long and most commonly nonrefreshing.

The pharmacologic options for idiopathic hypersomnia have mirrored the developments of treatments of EDS in narcolepsy. Unfortunately the treatment response is often lacking or less robust than in narcolepsy. The list of medications that have been prescribed for patients is extensive and includes tricyclic antidepressants, MAO inhibitors, SSRIs, clonidine, levodopa (isolated or in combination), bromocriptine, selegiline, and amantadine. None of these drugs have fully controlled the symptoms of idiopathic hypersomnia, especially the sleep drunkenness. Historically, the only medications that have brought (often only partial or intermittent) relief have been the stimulants, particularly methylphenidate and amphetamines.

Modafinil (see Chapter 39) has become useful as a first-line treatment for idiopathic hypersomnia.[95] The dose of modafinil is typically started at 100 mg and gradually increased to effectiveness to a maximum of 400 mg. The most common side effect is headache, and this negative effect may be eliminated if there is a progressive dose increase over time. A positive effect has been observed also in children.[96] Recently, Fantini and Montplaisir reported improvement in half of their 10 patients, in whom melatonin (2 mg of slow release at bedtime) was attempted.[51]

Treatment with activating antidepressants (SSRIs and MAO inhibitors) rather than stimulants may be first considered in patients in whom a psychiatric/depressive disorder cannot be ruled out with certainty.

CLINICAL COURSE AND PREVENTION

The overall psychosocial handicap of patients with idiopathic hypersomnia has been found to be similar to that of narcoleptics.[49] At times, the severity of the impairment can place lives in jeopardy (persons with idiopathic hypersomnia have sustained third-degree burns during automatic behavior episodes or have turned on gas furnaces or stoves without lighting them, leading in one case to a severe explosion). In idiopathic hypersomnia, symptoms are generally stable and long lasting; spontaneous improvement in EDS may be observed, however, in up to one quarter of patients.[11,14] No prevention is possible in this disorder.

PITFALLS

Since idiopathic hypersomnia is rare and essentially a diagnosis of exclusion, the main pitfall is making an accurate diagnosis. The terms of idiopathic hypersomnia and hypersomnia of unknown origin should not be used synonymously. Different research groups have historically used different diagnostic criteria, which makes comparisons difficult. This is particularly true of case series that did not exclude mild forms of sleep-disordered breathing (including the upper airway resistance syndrome), sleep insufficiency, and hypersomnia associated with psychiatric disorders.

Careful history, sleep questionnaire, full physical examination, overnight polysomnogram, and MSLT are essential for diagnosis and, more importantly, to rule out other causes of EDS. Demonstration of increased sleep times by prolonged polysomnographic recordings or actigraphy, formal psychiatric testing, CSF hypocretin-1 measurements, and brain MRI may be necessary in unclear cases. Treatment remains difficult in most patients.

Clinical Pearl

The clinician should consider idiopathic hypersomnia in the differential diagnosis of patients with EDS, prolonged nonrefreshing sleep and great difficulty waking up either in the morning or at the end of a nap.

REFERENCES

1. Roth B: Narkolepsie und Hypersomnie. In Roth B (ed): Narkolepsie und Hypersomnie. Berlin: VEB Verlag, 1962.
2. Roth B: Narcolepsy and hypersomnia: Review and classification of 642 personally observed cases. Schweiz Arch Neurol Neurochir Psychiatr 1976;119:31-41.
3. Roth B, Nevsìmalovà S, Rechtschaffen A: Hypersomnia with "sleep drunkeness." Arch Gen Psychiatry 1972;26:456-462.
4. Roth B: Functional hypersomnia. In Guilleminault C, Dement WC, Passouant P (eds): Narcolepsy. Proceedings of the First International Symposium on Narcolepsy. Montpellier, France, Spectrum Publications, 1976, pp 333-349.
5. Dement W, Rechtschaffen A, Gulevich G: The nature of the narcoleptic sleep attack. Neurology 1966;16:18-33.
6. Berti Ceroni G, Coccagna G, Gambi D, Lugaresi E: Considerazioni clinico-poligrafiche sulla narcolessia essenziale "a sonno lento." Sist Nerv 1967;2:81-89.
7. Guilleminault C, Philipps R, Dement WC: A syndrome of hypersomnia with automatic behaviour. Electroencephalogr Clin Neurophysiol 1975;38:408-413.
8. American Sleep Disorders Association: International Classification of Sleep Disorders: Diagnostic and Coding Manual, Revised. Rochester, Minn, American Sleep Disorders Association, 1997.
9. Aldrich M: The clinical spectrum of narcolepsy and idiopathic hypersomnia. Neurology 1996;46:393-401.
10. Billiard M, Dauvilliers Y: Idiopathic hypersomnia. Sleep Med Rev 2001;5:351-360.

11. Bassetti C, Aldrich M: Idiopathic hypersomnia. A study of 42 patients. Brain 1997;120:1423-1435.

12. Roth B: Narcolepsy and hypersomnia. Basel, Karger Libri, 1980.

13. van den Hoed J, Kraemer H, Guilleminault C, et al: Disorders of excessive daytime somnolence: Polygraphic and clinical data for 100 patients. Sleep 1981;4:23-37.

14. Bruck D, Parkes JD: A comparison of idiopathic hypersomnia and narcolepsy-cataplexy using self report measures and sleep diary data. J Neurol Neurosurg Psychiatry 1996;60:576-578.

15. Nevsimalova-Bruhova S, Roth B: Heredofamilial aspects of narcolepsy and hypersomnia. Schweiz Arch Neurol Psychiatr 1972;110:45-54.

16. Nevsimalova S: Differential diagnosis of narcolepsy and other hypersomnias. Vigilia-Sueno 1998;10:S85-S96.

17. Bassetti C, Gugger M, Bischof M, et al: The narcoleptic borderland: A multimodal diagnostic approach including cerebrospinal fluid levels of hypocretin-1 (orexin). Sleep Med 2003;4:7-12.

18. Poirier G, Montplaisir J, Décary F, et al: HLA antigens in narcolepsy and idiopathic central nervous system hypersomnolence. Sleep 1986;9:153-158.

19. Billiard M: Idiopathic hypersomnia. Neurol Clin 1996;14:573-582.

20. Honda Y, Honda M: Idiopathic hypersomnia. Review of literature and clinical experience on 16 Japanese cases. Nippon Rinsho 1998;56:371-375.

21. Montplaisir J, de Champlain J, Young SN, et al: Narcolepsy and idiopathic hypersomnia: Biogenic amines and related compounds in CSF. Neurology 1982;32:1299-1302.

22. Faull KF, Guilleminault C, Berger PA, Barchas JD: Cerebrospinal fluid monoamine metabolites in narcolepsy and hypersomnia. Ann Neurol 1983;13:258-263.

23. Faull KF, Thiemann S, King RJ, Guilleminault C: Monoamine interactions in narcolepsy and hypersomnia: A preliminary report. Sleep 1986;9:246-249.

24. Faull KF, Thiemann S, King RJ, Guilleminault C: Monoamine interactions in narcolepsy and hypersomnia: Reanalysis. Sleep 1989;12:185-186.

25. Petitjean F, Jouvet M: Hypersomnie et augmentation de l'acide 5-hydroxy-indolacétique cérébral par lésion isthmique chez le chat. C R Soc Biol 1970;164:2288-2293.

26. Bove A, Culebras A, Moore JT, Westlake RE: Relationship between sleep spindles and hypersomnia. Sleep 1994;17:449-455.

27. Sforza E, Gaudreau H, Petit D, Montplaisir J: Homeostatic sleep regulation in patients with idiopathic hypersomnia. Clin Neurophysiol 2000;111:277-282.

28. Billiard M, Rondouin G, Espa F, et al: Physiopathologie de l'hypersomnie idiopathique. Rev Neurol (Paris) 2001;157:S101-S106.

29. Nevsimalova S, Blazejova K, Illnerova H, et al: A contribution to pathophysiology of idiopathic hypersomnia. Suppl Clin Neurophysiol 2000;53:366-370.

30. Hublin C, Kaprio J, Partinen M, Koskenvuo M: Limits of self-report in assessing sleep terrors in a population survey. Sleep 1999;22:89-93.

31. Mignot E: Perspectives in narcolepsy and hypocretin (orexin) research. Sleep Med 2000;1:87-90.

32. Nishino N, Ripley B, Overeem S, et al: Hypocretin (orexin) deficiency in human narcolepsy. Lancet 2000;355:39-40.

33. Kilduff TS, Peyron C: The hypocretin/orexin ligand-receptor system: Implications for sleep and sleep disorders. TINS 2000;23:359-365.

34. Caap-Ahlgren M, Dehlin O: Insomnia and depressive symptoms in patients with Parkinson's disease. Relationship to health related quality of life. An interview study of patients living at home. Arch Gerontol Geriatr 2001;32:23-33.

35. Ripley B, Overeem N, Fujiki N, et al: CSF hypocretin/orexin levels in narcolepsy and other neurological conditions. Neurology 2001;57:2253-2258.

36. Bassetti C, Mathis J, Gugger M, et al: Idiopathic hypersomnia and narcolepsy without cataplexy: A multimodal diagnostic approach in 21 patients including cerebrospinal fluid hypocretin levels. Sleep 2001;24:A300.

37. Allen RP, Mignot E, Ripley B, et al: Increased CSF hypocretin-1 (orexin-A) in restless legs syndrome. Neurology 2002;59:639-641.

38. Mignot E, Taheri S, Nishino S: Sleeping with the hypothalamus: Emerging therapeutic targets for sleep disorders. Nature Neurosci 2002;5:1071-1075.

39. Mignot E, Lammers GJ, Ripley B, et al: The role of cerebrospinal fluid hypocretin measurement in the diagnosis of narcolepsy and other hypersomnias. Arch Neurol 2002;59:1553-1562.

40. Dauvilliers Y, Baumann CR, Carlander B, et al: CSF hypocretin-1 levels in narcolepsy, Kleine-Levin syndrome, other hypersomnias and neurological conditions. J Neurol Neurosurg Psychiatry 2003;74:1667-1673.

41. Khatami R, Maret S, Werth E, et al: A monozygotic twin pair concordant for narcolepsy-cataplexy without any detectable abnormality in the hypocretin (orexin) pathway. Lancet 2004;363:1199-1200.

42. Kanbayashi T, Inoue Y, Chiba S, et al: CSF hypocretin-1 (orexin-A) concentrations in narcolepsy with and without cataplexy and idiopathic hypersomnia. J Sleep Res 2002;11:91-93.

43. Ebrahim IO, Sharief KK, De Lacy S, et al: Hypocretin (orexin) deficiency in narcolepsy and primary hypersomnia. J Neurol Neurosurg Psychiatry 2003;74:127-130.

44. Roth B, Nevsimalova S: Depression in narcolepsy and hypersomnia. Schweiz Arch Neurol Psychiatr 1975;116:291-300.

45. Roth B: Idiopathic hypersomnia: A study of 187 personally observed cases. Int J Neurol 1981;15:108-118.

46. Ohayon M, Priest RG, Caulet M, Guilleminault C: Hypnagogic and hypnopompic hallucinations: Pathological phenomena. Br J Psychiatry 1996;169:459-467.

47. Ohayon MM, Zulley J, Guilleminault C, Smirne S: Prevalence and pathologic associations of sleep paralysis in the general population. Neurology 1999;52:1194-1200.

48. Baker TL, Guilleminault C, Nino-Murcia G, Dement WC: Comparative polysomnographic study of narcolepsy and idiopathic central nervous system hypersomnia. Sleep 1986;9:232-242.

49. Broughton R, Nevsimalova S, Roth B: The socio-economic effects of idiopathic hypersomnia-comparison with controls and with compound narcoleptics. In Popoviciu L, Asgian B, Badiu G (eds): Sleep 1978. Basel, Karger, 1980, pp 229-233.

50. American Academy of Sleep Medicine: International Classification of Sleep Disorders: Diagnostic and Coding Manual, 2nd ed. Westchester, Ill, American Academy of Sleep Medicine, 2005.

51. Montplaisir J, Fantini L: Idiopathic hypersomnia: A diagnostic dilemma. Sleep Med Rev 2001;5:361-362.

52. Vankova J, Nevsimalova S, Sonka K, et al: Increased REM density in narcolepsy-cataplexy and the polysymptomatic form of idiopathic hypersomnia. Sleep 2001;15:707-711.

53. Nicolas A, Lespérance P, Montplaisir J: Is excessive daytime sleepiness with periodic leg movements during sleep a specific diagnostic category? Eur Neurol 1998;40:22-26.

54. Billiard M, Dolenc C, Aldaz C, et al: Hypersomnia associated with mood disorders: A new perspective. J Psychosom Res 1994;38(Suppl 1):41-47.

55. Voderholzer U, Backhaus J, Hornyak M, et al: A 19-h spontaneous sleep period in idiopathic central nervous system hypersomnia. J Sleep Res 1998;19:219-223.

56. Montplaisir J, Billiard M, Takahashi S, et al: Twenty-four-hour recording in REM-narcoleptics with special reference to nocturnal sleep disruption. Biol Psychiatry 1978;13:73-89.

57. Ulivelli M, Rossi S, Lombardi C, et al: Polysomnographic characterization of pergolide-induced sleep attacks in idiopathic parkinsonism. Neurology 2002;58:462-465.

58. Bassetti C, Mathis J, Gugger M, et al: Hypersomnia following thalamic stroke. Ann Neurol 1996;39:471-480.

59. Hawkins DR, Taub JM, Van de Castle L: Extended sleep (hypersomnia) in young depressed patients. Am J Psychiatry 1985;142:905-910.

60. Sangal RB, Sangal J: P300 latency: Abnormal in sleep apnea with somnolence and idiopathic hypersomnia but normal in narcolepsy. Clin Electroenceph 1995;26:146-154.

61. Sturzenegger C, Bassetti C: The clinical spectrum of narcolepsy with cataplexy: A reappraisal. J Sleep Res 2004; (in press).

62. Roehrs T, Zorick F, Sicklesteel J, et al: Excessive daytime sleepiness associated with insufficient sleep. Sleep 1983;6:319-325.

63. Roehrs TA, Roth A: Chronic insufficient sleep and its recovery. Sleep Med 2003;4:5-6.

64. Guilleminault C, Stoohs R, Clerk A, et al: A cause of excessive daytime sleepiness: The upper airway resistance syndrome. Chest 1993;104:781-787.

65. Guilleminault C, Stoohs R, Kim YD, et al: Upper airway sleep-disordered breathing in women. Ann Intern Med 1995;122:493-501.

66. Philip P, Stoohs R, Guilleminault C: Sleep fragmentation in normals: A model for sleepiness associated with upper airway resistance syndrome. Sleep 1994;17:242-247.

67. Guilleminault C, Palombini L, Pelayo R, Chervin R: Sleepwalking and sleep terrors in prepubertal children: What triggers them. Pediatrics 2003;111:17-25.

68. Dolenc C, Besset A, Billiard M: Hypersomnia in association with dysthymia in comparison with idiopathic hypersomnia and normal controls. Pflugers Arch 1996;431:R303-R304.

69. Nofzinger EA, Thase ME, Reynolds CF, et al: Hypersomnia in bipolar depression: A comparison with narcolepsy using the multiple sleep latency test. Am J Psychiatry 1991;148:1177-1181.

70. Buchwald D, Pascualy R, Bombardier C, Kith P: Sleep disorders in patients with chronic fatigue. Clin Infect Dis 1994;18:S68-S72.

71. Guilleminault C, Mondini S: Mononucleosis and chronic daytime sleepiness. A long-term follow-up study. Arch Intern Med 1986;146:1333-1335.

72. Merriam AE: Kleine-Levin syndrome following acute viral encephalitis. Biol Psychiatry 1986;21:1301-1304.

73. Castaigne P, Escourolle R: Etude topographique des lésions anatomiques dans les hypersomnies. Revue Neurologique 1967;116:547-584.

74. Vgontzas A, Papanicolaou DA, Bixler EO, et al: Elevation of plasma cytokines in disorders of excessive daytime sleepiness: Role of sleep disturbance and obesity. J Clin Endocrinol Metab 1997;82:1313-1316.

75. Von Economo C: Encephalitis lethargica. Wien Med Wochenschr 1923;73:777-782, 835-838, 1113-1118, 1243-1249, 1334-1338.

76. Lhermitte J, Tournay A: Rapport sur le sommeil normal et pathologique. Rev Neurol (Paris) 1927:751-823.

77. Gordon A: Encéphalite léthargique des centres végétatifs. Syndrome de somnolence périodique avec polyphagie et polydipsie. Rev Neurol (Paris) 1939;71:411-416.

78. Roger H, Roger J: Les hypersomnies. Rev Prat (Paris) 1954;4:1533-1549.

79. Howard RS, Lees AJ: Encephalitis lethargica. A report of four recent cases. Brain 1997;110:19-33.

80. Rubinsztein JS, Rubinsztein DC, Goodburn S, Holland AJ: Apathy and hypersomnia are common features of myotonic dystrophy. J Neurol Neurosurg Psychiatry 1998;64:510-515.

81. Guilleminault C, Faull KF, Miles L, van den Hoed J: Posttraumatic excessive daytime sleepiness: A review of 20 patients. Neurology 1983;33:1584-1589.

82. Laberge L, Begin P, Montplaisir J, Mathieu J: Sleep complaints in patients with myotonic dystrophy. J Sleep Res 2004;13:95-100.

83. Kleine W: Periodische Schlafsucht. Monatschr Psychiatr Neurol 1925;57:285-320.

84. Lhermitte J, Dubois E: Crises d'hypersomnie prolongées rythmées par les règles chez une jeune fille. Rev Neurol (Paris) 1941;73:608-609.

85. Critchley M, Hoffmann HL: The syndrome of periodic somnolence and morbid hunger (Kleine-Levin). BMJ 1942;1:137-139.

86. Critchley M: Periodic hypersomnia and megaphagia in adolescent males. Brain 1962;85:627-656.

87. Bassetti C: Narcolepsy, idiopathic hypersomnia, and periodic hypersomnias. In Culebras A (ed): Sleep disorders and neurological disease. New York, Marcel Dekker, 2000, pp 323-354.

88. Gadoth N, Kesler A, Vainstein G, et al: Clinical and polysomnographic characteristics of 34 patients with Kleine-Levin syndrome. J Sleep Res 2001;10:337-341.

89. Hnayal A, Regli F: Contribution a l'étude clinique des anomalies du sommeil trois cas de "somnolence périodique" (Kleine-Levin). L'encéphale 1967;56:33-44.

90. Bassetti C, Mauerhofer D, Mathis J, et al: Restless legs syndrome: A clinical study of 55 patients. Eur Neurol 2001;45:67-74.

91. Bassetti C, Clavadetscher S, Gugger M, Hess CW: Pergolide-associated "sleep attacks" in a patient with restless legs syndrome. Sleep Med 2002;3:275-277.

92. Vgontzas A, Bixler A, Tan TL, et al: Obesity without sleep apnea is associated with daytime sleepiness. Arch Neurol 1998;158:1333-1337.

93. Aldrich MS, Naylor MW: Narcolepsy associated with lesions of the diencephalon. Neurology 1989;39:1505-1508.

94. Roth T, Roehrs T: Etiologies and sequelae of excessive daytime sleepiness. Clin Ther 1996;18:562-576.

95. Bastuji H, Jouvet M: Successful treatment of idiopathic hypersomnia and narcolepsy with modafinil. Prog Neuro-Psychopharmacol Biol Psychiat 1988;12:695-700.

96. Ivanenko A, Tauman R, Gozal D: Modafinil in the treatment of excessive daytime sleepiness in children. Sleep Med 2003;4:579-582.

67

Parkinsonism

Claudia Trenkwalder

ABSTRACT

Parkinson's disease (PD) and other parkinsonian syndromes are common neurologic diseases, particularly in the elderly. The frequent sleep complaints of patients with PD and the subsequent impaired quality of life in PD and other parkinsonian syndromes have not been sufficiently acknowledged until recently. The sleep disturbance of parkinsonism results from many different factors, some of which are disease specific and others treatment specific. Rapid eye movement (REM) sleep behavior disorder and other motor syndromes during sleep, such as periodic limb movements, tremor, and early morning dystonia, are characteristic features. Daytime sleepiness has recently been investigated and is more a disease-related problem than a treatment-related phenomenon. Respiratory disturbances and sleep apnea should be considered as well. It is necessary to treat sleep symptoms in parkinsonism according to their specific cause. Nocturnal akinesia results mostly from a dopaminergic deficit and should be treated with increased dosages of dopaminergic medication at night, whereas nocturnal REM disorder needs therapy with benzodiazepines, and hallucinations or psychoses require neuroleptic treatments. Respiratory problems may need further polysomnographic diagnosis and specific treatments.

Specific clinical instruments to assess sleep disorders in PD are necessary to guarantee sufficient treatment and to enhance quality of life in PD.

PD is a neurodegenerative disorder with a progressive loss of dopaminergic neurons. It is characterized clinically by akinesia, rigidity, and resting tremor and a positive response to levodopa or the occurrence of levodopa-induced dyskinesias, according to the United Kingdom Brain Bank Criteria.[1] The symptoms start characteristically on one side. When fully developed, the clinical picture is unmistakable. Movements are slow, and reduced facial expressiveness with infrequent blinking and a soft, monotonous voice dominate the picture. The gait is slow and shuffling, with small steps, and the loss of postural reflexes, along with the flexed posture, may lead to a festinating gait with gait initiation problems in the advanced stages of the disease. A coarse resting tremor, mostly unilateral in the beginning, is present when the hands are immobile, but the tremor diminishes or disappears with motion or with complete relaxation, as in stage 1 sleep. Idiopathic PD progresses slowly but inexorably. Walking becomes increasingly difficult because of postural instability and freezing. Descriptions of patients with severe akinesia and feeding tubes have been relegated to medical history since the introduction of levodopa and other dopaminergic medications in the treatment of PD. Death may be associated with the akinetic complications of the disease,

but today patients may live more than 30 years with PD. Complications of falls are mostly hip fractures, which then lead to an immobile, bedridden state. It is important to differentiate PD from other neurodegenerative parkinsonian syndromes such as MSA or PSP.

Similar clinical features occur with secondary parkinsonism, caused by drugs, toxins, infections, and brain lesions. Currently, the most common causes of secondary, mostly intermittent parkinsonism are medications that block dopamine receptors, such as the phenothiazines and butyrophenones. Other causes include manganese intoxication, carbon monoxide poisoning, viral encephalitis, bilateral basal ganglia infarctions, frontal meningiomas, and hypoparathyroidism with basal ganglia calcification. These causes account for a small percentage of parkinsonism cases only and therefore are not discussed in this chapter.

The most common parkinsonian syndromes originate either from vascular parkinsonism or other neurodegenerative diseases, the most common of which is MSA. MSA refers to a group of disorders that cause degeneration of the basal ganglia, substantia nigra, cerebellum, and other brain regions. Consensus criteria have recently defined the clinical spectrum and diagnosis of this disease. The manifestations of these disorders include a parkinsonian syndrome with predominant autonomic failure associated with urinary incontinence or erectile dysfunction and varying combinations of ataxia, eye movement abnormalities, motoneuron degeneration, myoclonus, and dystonia. We distinguish two types of MSA, the striatonigral and the cerebellar types. MSAs are neuropathologically described as synucleinopathies, as opposed to tauopathies. PSP (Steele-Richardson-Olszewski syndrome) belongs to the tauopathies (as does Alzheimer's disease) and is characterized by an akinetic rigid parkinsonian syndrome with the progressive inability to move the eyes voluntarily in the vertical direction, although reflex eye movements are preserved. Pronounced rigidity of the neck and face and early gait disturbance with dizziness and falls are common, and the disorder is not responsive to dopaminergic medications.

Although the major emphasis in this chapter is on PD, much of the discussion also applies to secondary parkinsonism and to the other degenerative disorders associated with parkinsonism.[2]

A variety of neurodegenerative and psychopharmacologic factors can lead to disruption of the normal sleep in patients with parkinsonism. *First,* the neurodegenerative process starts in the lower brainstem areas and follows the six progressive stages described by Braak and collaborators.[3,4] When Lewy bodies, the neuropathologic markers of PD, intrude in the brainstem areas relevant for sleep regulation, the first signs of sleep disruption or disturbance may occur. Rapid eye movement (REM) sleep behavior disorder (RBD) may be a preclinical and premotor sign of PD or a parkinsonian syndrome. Therefore, the observation of early changes in sleep may be of particular importance, especially if neuroprotective agents are available in the future.

Second, the behavioral, respiratory, and motor system phenomena accompanying the disease may produce nocturnal symptoms. *Third*, the medications used as treatment may induce new symptoms, such as nightmares, nocturnal movements, or increased wakefulness. All of these effects on sleep have implications for treatment planning.

HISTORICAL ASPECTS

The clinical features of PD were described by James Parkinson in 1817 in *Essay on the Shaking Palsy*. In addition to his description of daytime symptoms, Parkinson noted that "sleep becomes much disturbed" and that the terminal stage of the disease is associated with "constant sleepiness, with slight delirium, and other marks of extreme exhaustion."[5] Charcot, later in the 19th century, described the impact of severe rigidity and bradykinesia on sleep:

This need of change of position is principally exhibited at night in bed. . . . Half an hour, a quarter of an hour, has scarcely elapsed until they require to be turned again, and if . . . not . . . gratified they give vent to moans, which . . . testify to the intense uneasiness they experience.[6]

The epidemic of encephalitis lethargica in the early 20th century, the major cause of secondary parkinsonism at that time, focused increased attention on the disorder, but despite the writings of Parkinson and Charcot, the sleep problems accompanying parkinsonism received relatively little attention until the 1950s and 1960s, when the first polysomnographic recordings of parkinsonian patients were performed. In the last years, reports of so-called "sleep attacks," mainly consisting of sudden daytime sleepiness, and of concomitant or preceding RBD, have drawn attention to sleep as an important issue for patients with PD. In addition, RBD may develop as a first preclinical sign of PD, and therefore sleep may gain importance for the early diagnosis of PD.

PATHOPHYSIOLOGY

Neuronal depletion and gliosis of pigmented areas of the brainstem are the most striking pathologic features of PD.[7] The loss of dopaminergic input from the substantia nigra leads to a marked reduction in dopamine content of the basal ganglia. The occurrence of parkinsonism in intravenous users of methylphenyltetrahydropyridine (MPTP), a narcotic derivative that is selectively neurotoxic to neurons in the zona compacta of the substantia nigra,[8,9] indicates the importance of these dopamine-containing neurons in the pathogenesis of PD. MPTP is now used in animal models of parkinsonism.

Although the loss of dopaminergic neurons of the substantia nigra is responsible for most of the motor features of PD, other brain abnormalities may account for some of the sleep–wake abnormalities described later in this chapter. Serotonergic neurons originating in the dorsal raphe nuclei are reduced in number, as are noradrenergic neurons originating in the region of the locus coeruleus.[10] Cholinergic neurons of the pedunculopontine nucleus, implicated in the control of REM sleep, are also reduced in number.[11] Because the noradrenergic, serotonergic, and cholinergic systems have all been implicated

in the control and regulation of sleep, abnormalities in these systems may account for some of the sleep disturbance in patients with parkinsonism.

Abnormalities of the mesocorticolimbic dopamine system, as well as the mesostriatal system, are apparent in PD and may contribute to sleep–wake disturbances.[12] Dopamine neurons with cell bodies in the ventral tegmental area of the brainstem project to the cerebral cortex, where the predominant dopamine receptor is the D_1 type.[13] The administration of dopamine D_1 receptor agonists produces electroencephalographic (EEG) desynchronization and behavioral arousal,[14] whereas the administration of antagonists produces sedation,[15] consistent with an arousal function for the ventral tegmental projection neurons. High doses of dopamine D_1 and D_2 receptor agonists, such as apomorphine, reduce total sleep time,[16] although very low doses induce sleep and increase the amount of slow wave sleep. Low doses of apomorphine also induce sleep when injected into the ventral tegmental area, an effect that is blocked by dopamine receptor autoantagonists, suggesting that dopamine D_2 autoreceptors play a role in the mediation of sleep through autoinhibition of the firing rate of ventral tegmental dopaminergic neurons.[17,18] The arousing effects of higher doses of D_2 agonists may be due to effects at postsynaptic receptors. This may also explain the arousal effects that occur when high dosages of dopamine agonists are given during the day.

Dopamine also appears to be involved in the regulation of REM sleep through effects mediated by D_1 and D_2 receptors. Dopamine D_1 receptor antagonists increase the amount and duration of REM sleep, whereas D_1 agonists suppress REM sleep.[17,19] REM sleep is also suppressed by high doses of D_2 agonists.[16] The site of action for the effects of these agents on REM sleep is unknown.

Drugs that enhance activity of dopamine systems, including levodopa (L-dopa), the biochemical precursor of dopamine and norepinephrine, and dopamine agonists such as bromocriptine, pergolide, cabergoline, or nonergoline derivatives such as pramipexole and ropinirole, are frequently used in the treatment of PD. They can also have significant effects on sleep because they predominantly induce wakefulness in higher dosages. In healthy people, L-dopa reduces the amount of REM sleep, an effect that may be due to increased activity of dopamine, norepinephrine, or both. L-Dopa also reduces the amounts of serotonin, tryptophan, and tyrosine in the brain. Consequently, the effects of L-dopa on sleep may be due in part to effects on serotonergic neurons. Dopamine agonists that act directly on dopamine D_2 receptors have little effect on noradrenergic or serotonergic neurons but still alter sleep–wake patterns, presumably through effects on mesocortical dopamine pathways.

Several other aspects of PD also contribute to sleep disturbance (Table 67–1).

EPIDEMIOLOGY

PD is primarily a disease of the elderly: The prevalence increases with age from approximately 0.9% among people 65 to 69 years of age to 5% among people 80 to 84 years of age, with a slight male preponderance.[20] The prevalence is similar worldwide, and the increased proportion of the elderly in industrialized countries will substantially increase the number of patients with PD in the next 10 to 20 years.[21] Only a small percentage of patients, mostly those with the familial forms, experience an onset before the age of 30 years. Sleep problems

Table 67–1.   Contributors to Sleep Disruption in Parkinson's Disease

Cause	Consequence
Neurochemical changes affecting cholinergic and monoaminergic systems	Impaired sleep–wake control; reduced REM sleep
Bradykinesia and rigidity	Reduction in the number of normal body shifts during sleep, leading to discomfort and awakenings; impaired ability to use the bathroom at night
Periodic leg movements, tremor, and medication-induced myoclonus	Arousals
REM sleep behavior disorder	Disrupted REM sleep
Abnormal motor activity affecting respiratory and upper airway muscles	Sleep-disordered breathing
Medication effects	Increased time awake at night, reduced REM sleep
Depression and anxiety	Difficulty falling asleep, early morning awakening
Dementia	Nocturnal confusional episodes

REM, rapid eye movement.

are common in all forms of parkinsonism: In one series of 78 consecutive patients with PD, 67% had difficulties initiating sleep and 88% had difficulty maintaining sleep.[22]

CLINICAL FEATURES

Difficulty falling asleep, difficulty remaining asleep, nocturnal akinesia, and RBD with nocturnal vocalizations and movements are the most common sleep-related complaints. Sleep disturbance tends to increase with disease progression, and daytime drowsiness becomes increasingly common. In recent years, so-called sleep attacks have been described and include sudden sleepiness, mostly related to medication intake. Older patients with on-off phenomena and those with hallucinations are particularly likely to have severe sleep disruption.[23,24] The abnormal sleep features associated with PD include a change of sleep stage patterns, abnormal motor activity, and disturbed breathing.

Sleep–Wake Organization

The most consistent abnormality in PD sleep is sleep fragmentation. Polysomnographic studies have demonstrated increased sleep latency and frequent awakenings, with as much as 30% to 40% of the night spent awake.[25,26] Increased amounts of stage 1 sleep and reduced amounts of stages 3 and 4 sleep and REM sleep are also common, and the duration of REM periods may be reduced, although in milder cases sleep architecture may be normal.[25] Untreated patients with PD show a significant decrease of stages 3 and 4 sleep and increased periodic limb movements.[27]

EEG features of sleep may change; for example, the number of sleep spindles during slow wave sleep is reduced,[26,28] and EEG alpha activity may be prominent during REM sleep.[29,30]

Sleep disturbances are also prominent in other parkinsonian syndromes. In MSA, RBD is even more frequent than in PD,[31] and is an early sign of neurodegeneration. In PSP, poorly formed or absent spindles, increased amounts of slow wave activity during REM sleep, decreased amounts of REM sleep, and insomnia are present; these abnormalities tend to worsen with disease progression.[32] Patients with Shy-Drager syndrome (MSA) may have increased sleep latency and increased numbers of awakenings, along with reductions in REM sleep and stages 3 and 4 sleep.[33]

Motor Activity During Sleep

Although parkinsonian motor symptoms are most prominent during wakefulness, they are not completely abolished during sleep. Both tremor and altered muscle tone occur to varying degrees in the different stages of sleep.

Parkinsonian tremor is predominantly a rest tremor and is reduced by movement and relaxation. Nevertheless, tremor does disappear with the onset of stage 1 sleep, in some cases before alpha EEG activity is entirely gone[34,35] (Fig. 67–1). Furthermore, tremor is rarely present during stages 3 and 4 sleep and is not associated with spindles or K complexes.

Tremor may appear, however, in stages 1 and 2 sleep and with awakenings, arousals, and body movements.[36] Tremor may also appear, with various amplitudes, for a few seconds during sleep stage changes, during bursts of rapid eye movements, and shortly before or after an REM sleep period.[35] In contrast to the quiescence of sleep in healthy persons, increased muscle tone and abnormal simple and complex movements are common and complicate the scoring of polysomnograms in patients with PD. Patterns of simple motor activity during sleep include repeated blinking at the onset of sleep, rapid eye movements during non-REM (NREM) sleep, blepharospasm at the onset of REM sleep, and prolonged tonic contractions of limb extensor or flexor muscles during NREM sleep.[29]

Periodic leg movements in sleep (PLMS) with an index of more than five per hour of sleep (PLMS index greater than 5) occur in up to one third of patients with untreated PD and are even more common in the elderly.[27] PLMS may be associated with arousals.

Symptoms of restless legs syndrome (RLS) are common in patients with PD; however, except in patients with a family history of RLS, they seem to reflect a secondary phenomenon. There is no evidence that RLS symptoms early in life predispose to the subsequent development of PD.[37]

Fragmentary, irregular myoclonic twitches and jerks of the extremities may be recorded, mainly during light NREM sleep.

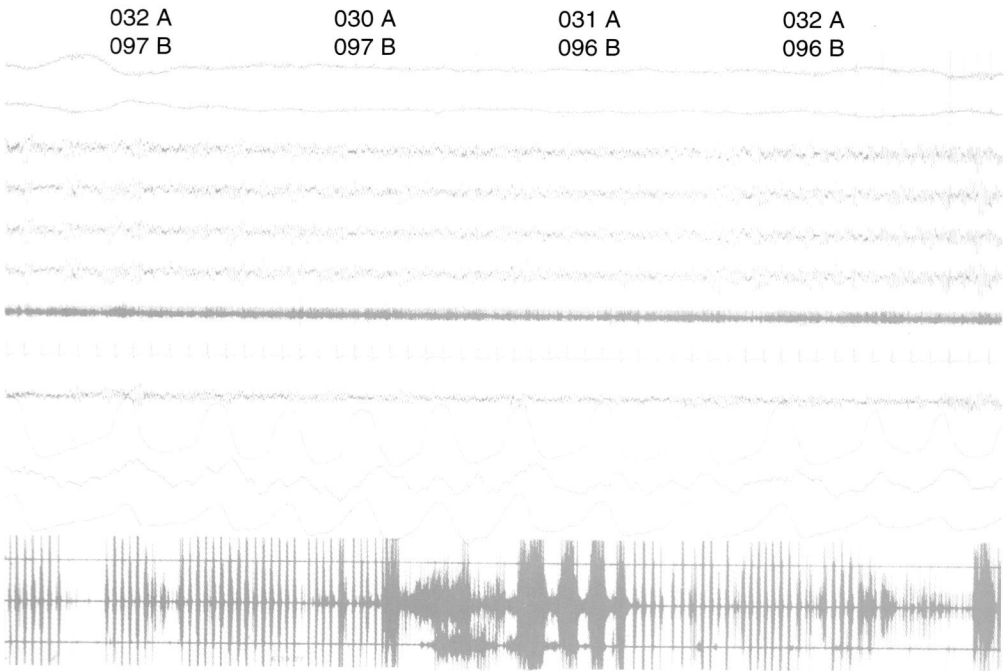

Figure 67–1. Polysomnographic recording of a patient with Parkinson's disease and nocturnal rest tremor of the right leg between wakefulness and stage 1 sleep. The regular unilateral rest tremor is interrupted by bilateral motor activity. Channels, from top down: 1, 2, eye movements; 3-6, electroencephalogram (EEG); 7, chin electromyogram (EMG); 8, ECG; 9, additional EEG; 10-12, respiratory recording with thoracic and abdominal belts; 13, no recording; 14, EMG of right anterior tibialis muscle; 15, EMG of left anterior tibialis muscle.

Repetitive muscle contractions followed by tremor may occur, particularly in the limb primarily affected by the disease, and result in a painful extension of the great toe, finger, or foot as a sign of off-dystonia. Early morning foot dystonia may occur just before waking or soon thereafter and reflects the low concentration of dopamine in the basal ganglia after the last intake of medication at night. It usually starts as a sign of motor response fluctuations 3 to 6 years after initiation of treatment with levodopa. Early morning akinesia and painful off-dystonia are frequent complaints of patients with advanced PD that require adequate nocturnal treatment strategies.[38]

Approximately one third of patients with PD report a "sleep benefit."[39] It is defined as "restoration of mobility on awakening from sleep prior to drug intake."[40] Patients with sleep benefit show a better morning motor function, although no differences in sleep pattern can be detected.[41]

Some patients with familial early-onset PD show marked diurnal variations in rigidity and dystonia, with little rigidity soon after arising but progressively increasing rigidity, tremor, and dysarthria as the day goes on. These symptoms are improved with naps.[42]

Finally, during REM sleep, prolonged elevations of muscle tone may occur, as well as more complex movements, vocalizations, and fully developed RBD. In MSA, RBD is even more frequent than in PD,[31] and is an early sign of neurodegeneration.

REM Sleep Behavior Disorder as an Early Sign of Neurodegeneration

First described by Schenck and collaborators, criteria for RBD are now defined by the American Sleep Disorders Association[43] and include complex behaviors during REM sleep with a loss of skeletal muscle atonia. Mild to harmful body movements are associated with dream mentation and nightmares and disrupt sleep continuity. The underlying cause of RBD is still unknown. RBD most likely reflects dysfunction in the brainstem circuitry and the dorsolateral pontine tegmentum, where REM sleep without atonia can be induced in animal experiments. Recent studies with cohorts of patients with RBD point toward the hypothesis that RBD may represent a preclinical marker of a neurodegenerative process in synucleinopathies such as PD and MSA,[44] and may precede motor symptoms by years.

Comella and coworkers[45] reported a frequency of 15% for clinically diagnosed RBD in patients with PD, whereas Gagnon and coworkers[46] found that one third of an unselected population of patients with PD had RBD when investigated polysomnographically (Fig. 67–2). Only 50% of these patients would have been detected by history only.[46,47] In consecutive patients with MSA, the percentage of clinically diagnosed RBD was 70%, and over 90% if investigated in the sleep laboratory. In 44% of cases, RBD preceded by more than a year the clinical onset of MSA,[48] and polysomnography could differentiate between patients with pure autonomic failure and those developing MSA with autonomic failure.[48] Neuroimaging studies of patients who presented to the sleep clinic with characteristic complaints of RBD revealed a marked reduction of presynaptic dopamine transporter binding, indicating early PD or MSA.[49] RBD seems to be especially frequent in those patients with PD and psychosis or hallucinations,[50] and sometimes is difficult to distinguish by clinical observation at night. Other authors found that sleep disturbances in PD do not occur as early as olfactory deficits, but begin to manifest during the first years of PD.[51]

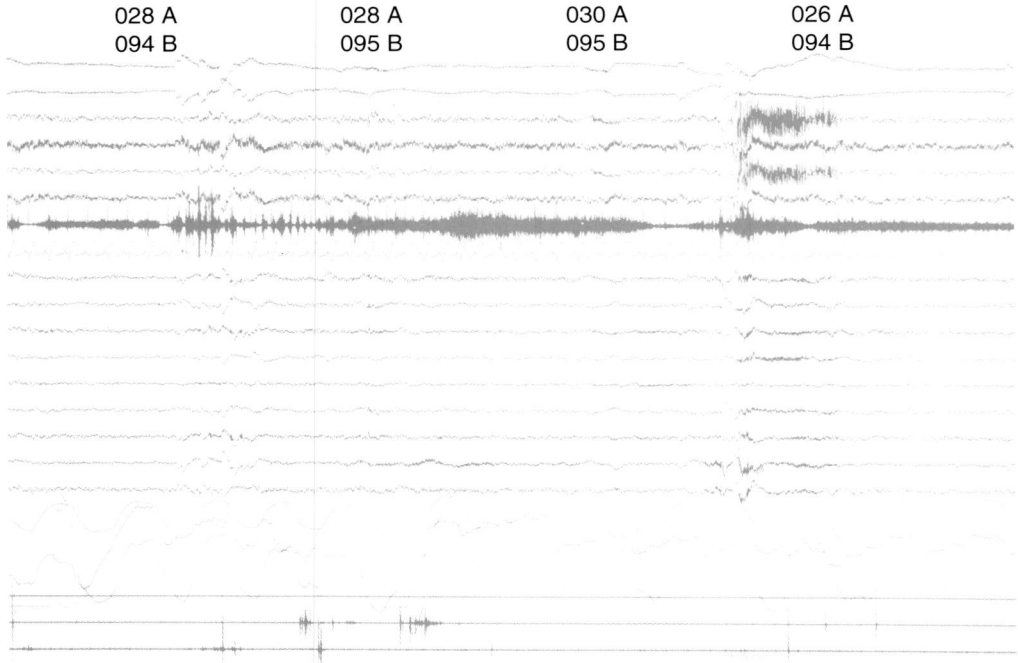

| 028 A | 028 A | 030 A | 026 A |
| 094 B | 095 B | 095 B | 094 B |

Figure 67-2. Polysomnographic recording of a patient with Parkinson's disease with rapid eye movement (REM) sleep behavior disorder. The chin electromyogram (EMG) shows a highly elevated muscle tone, multiple motor activity episodes occur in the recording, and typical muscle twitches are seen in the EMG channels of both legs. Channels, from top down: 1, 2, eye movements showing typical REM sleep pattern; 3-6, electroencephalogram (EEG); 7, chin EMG with increased muscle tone; 8, ECG; 9-17, further EEG channels, showing muscle artifacts of eye movements; 18-20, respiratory recording with thoracic and abdominal belts; 21, no recording; 22, 23, EMG of right and left anterior tibialis muscles.

Respiratory Disorders of Sleep in Parkinsonism

Waking obstructive ventilatory deficits are common in moderate to severe PD and are apparently caused by a combination of upper airway obstruction, probably due at least in part to abnormal tone in upper airway muscles, and respiratory muscle incoordination with decreased effective muscle strength.[52] Although these deficits correlate to some extent with the severity of rigidity and tremor, they do not improve to any great extent with administration of L-dopa. In some patients, upper airway endoscopy has shown intermittent airway closure due to dyskinetic movements of glottic and supraglottic structures caused by either the disease itself or dopaminergic medications.[53]

Although nocturnal respiration is normal in some patients with parkinsonism, other patients show disorganized patterns of respiration with central apneas, obstructive apneas, or episodes of hypoventilation.[54,55] The severity of these respiratory abnormalities tends to be greater in patients with autonomic disturbances.

In some of these patients, daytime respiratory abnormalities include reduced ventilatory responses to hypercapnia and hypoxia.[56,57] Polysomnographic studies have demonstrated obstructive sleep apnea as well as other abnormal breathing patterns, including central sleep apnea, variable-amplitude respirations, and arrhythmic respirations.[58,59] Abnormal vocal cord function, leading to stridor and laryngeal stenosis or obstruction, appears to be a major contributor to abnormal breathing during sleep.[60]

Both hemodynamic and respiratory abnormalities may occur during sleep in patients with Shy-Drager syndrome, including increased systemic arterial pressure during REM and slow wave sleep and sudden phasic swings of blood pressure.[55] The rise of blood pressure during the supine position at night results from the severe autonomic dysregulation in MSA and Shy-Drager syndrome. Obstructive apneas may lead to a reduction in systemic blood pressure in these patients.[61]

Daytime Sleepiness and Sleep Attacks in Parkinson's Disease

Excessive daytime drowsiness, not resulting from respiratory problems in PD, is a well-known phenomenon in patients with PD. Recent studies have described an increased risk for motor vehicle accidents because of sudden sleep onset, so-called sleep attacks.[62] Those episodes were primarily attributed to the intake of non-ergot dopamine agonists, and therefore a variety of studies investigated the effect of dopaminergic drugs on daytime performance and sleepiness in patients with PD. Despite this effort, there are few systematically collected data on the risk of abnormal sleep behavior in patients taking dopaminergic agents compared with other anti-PD medications. Taken together, these studies show conflicting results. One study showed an association of daytime sleepiness with more advanced stages of PD, longer disease duration, and male sex.[63] Other studies could not confirm those results: Higher daily L-dopa dose equivalents were predictors of sleep episodes while driving, whereas sex, age, disease severity, and individual dopaminergic agents were not.[64] Patients with PD preselected for sleepiness, however, did not meet those criteria, and sleepiness did not result from pharmacotherapy or sleep abnormalities but was related to the pathologic process of the disease.[65] Dopaminomimetics may exacerbate sleepiness in a small subset of patients, but the primary pathologic processes appear to be the greatest contributors to the development of daytime sleepiness. These patients may benefit from wake-promoting agents such as bupropion, modafinil, or traditional psychostimulants.[66] An interesting observation is that patients with PD are not as aware of their sleepiness compared with elderly control subjects. Therefore, the patient's history or Epworth Sleepiness Scale (ESS) scores may not be helpful, and only observation or objective measurements of sleepiness such as by polysomnography may solve the question of sleepiness in individual patients with PD.[67]

The most serious issue with daytime sleepiness in PD is the question of whether patients with PD should be allowed to drive and whether there should be special tests for sleepiness. Because the laws differ among countries, it is necessary to advise patients with PD that sudden sleepiness may occur in the course of the disease and may be attributable to specific dopaminergic drugs. Finally, the patients themselves are responsible for their ability to drive, and each must decide individually.

DIAGNOSTIC EVALUATION

A number of factors may contribute to sleep disturbance in parkinsonism, including disease-specific factors, medications, motor activity during sleep, sleep–wake schedule abnormalities, or respiratory disorders (Fig. 67–3). To determine which factors are most important, the clinical history of the patient and that of partners or caregivers, physical examination, and polysomnographic evaluation are used.

Sleep disturbance is rarely the presenting complaint in a patient with previously undiagnosed parkinsonism. More commonly, the diagnosis has been established, and the patient complains of insomnia, daytime sleepiness, or both. The history of the sleep complaint should include all the features the physician would obtain from any patient with a sleep complaint. But it also has to include disease-specific questions about nocturnal akinesia, daytime fatigue in relation to medication intake, and psychiatric symptoms. The use of a disease-specific questionnaire, the Parkinson's Disease Sleep Scale, may be helpful.[68] A careful description from the bed partner is essential to determine the presence and frequency of movements during sleep (and their timing), arousals and awakenings, and periods of daytime sleepiness.

The medication schedule is significant. If dopaminergic medications are not prescribed in the evening, nocturnal rigidity may contribute to the sleep disturbance; on the other hand, excessive evening doses of dopamine agonists may induce sleep-onset insomnia.

Practical Management of Sleep Disorders in Parkinsonism

Some patients with parkinsonism and sleep disturbance require a polysomnogram for diagnosis of the cause of the sleep disorder. Patients who complain about daytime sleepiness with sudden onsets of sleep during the day should be screened for sleep apnea syndrome, and may then require respiratory polysomnography. Patients who present with probable RBD and hallucinations may need a polysomnogram to evaluate better whether both syndromes are relevant,

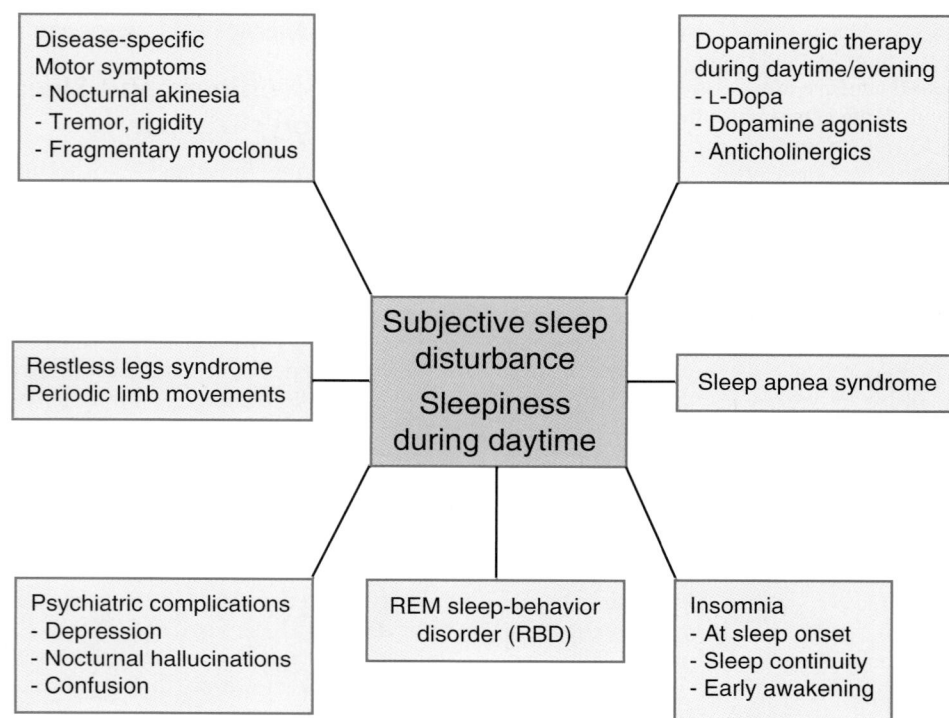

Figure 67–3. Factors contributing to sleep disturbance in parkinsonism.

because the treatment options are different. Simultaneous closed-circuit television monitoring and surface electromyographic monitoring of all four extremities often is helpful if nocturnal myoclonic movements or the RBD is contributing to the sleep disturbance.

If daytime sleepiness is a prominent complaint, a multiple sleep latency test helps to determine its severity and circadian variation. It is usually best to record the patient while he or she is on the usual medication schedule, but if medications appear to be a major factor in the sleep disturbance, definite diagnosis may require 2 or more nights of recording under different treatment regimens.

TREATMENT

The treatment of sleep disturbances in patients with parkinsonism is rarely straightforward because treatment of the disease may affect the sleep disorder. Sleep fragmentation, nocturnal movements and vocalizations, abnormal muscle tone during sleep, and psychiatric syndromes such as depression can all be caused by parkinsonism and by its treatment with dopaminergic agents, such as for psychoses or dyskinesias. The biphasic actions of dopaminergic medications, especially of dopamine agonists, must be kept in mind: Low doses of these medications may promote sleep, whereas high doses during the day and during the evening may lead to increased waking effects, reduction of slow wave sleep, and decreased sleep continuity.[69-71]

Nocturnal Akinesia, Periodic Limb Movements, and Restless Legs Syndrome

In mild cases, nocturnal motor symptoms may disappear with adequate dopaminergic treatment during the day.[72] In other cases, a bedtime dose of a controlled-release formulation containing 200 mg of L-dopa and 50 mg of a decarboxylase inhibitor appears to be particularly useful.[73,74] Trials of several different agents in varying doses are usually warranted if sleep is not improved. Most patients in the advanced stages of PD, however, suffer from severe nocturnal akinesia, which can be treated sufficiently with dopamine agonists (e.g., cabergoline) to improve morning motor problems in particular.[75] PLMS and RLS improve with increased nocturnal dopaminergic stimulation either by L-dopa or dopamine agonists.[75] Factors that may contribute to improved sleep during treatment with dopamine agonists include a reduction of rigidity and bradykinesia with consecutive improvement in nocturnal mobility, reduced numbers of periodic limb movements, disappearance of RLS symptoms, and normalization of sleep muscle activity.[76] Early morning bradykinesia often is also improved. In other patients, fragmentary nocturnal myoclonus and periodic leg movements during NREM sleep develop after L-dopa is taken for extended periods. These complications may be due to medication-induced dysregulation of serotonin activity.[77,78]

REM Sleep Behavior Disorder

RBD may occur in treated or nontreated parkinsonian syndromes and may disturb the patient's sleep by dreams that appear to be "acted out" and therefore disturb sleep continuity. Features of violent or injurious behavior during sleep should be treated for the patient's and bed partner's safety. Because RBD

can easily be treated in most pa[tients with] clonazepam (0.5 to 1 mg), it shou[ld be instituted] early.[79] The occurrence of these [symptoms and] behavior may disrupt the relatio[nship with the] caregiver[45] and be a main reason fo[r . . .]

Insomnia

The first step in the treatment of in[somnia is to identify] psychosocial and behavioral factors [that are contribut]ing to sleep disturbance. Concurrent psychiatric disorders should be addressed. In advanced stages of the disease, the patient's spouse should be encouraged to sleep in a different bed or room; inadequate rest for the spouse or other caregiver may make the patient's sleep disturbance intolerable and lead to institutionalization.

Patients in advanced stages of PD under high doses of dopamine may require further medication for insomnia. In those cases, patients may take low dosages of mirtazapine, which is well tolerated and efficacious, although no studies are available yet.

Insomnia due to dyskinetic nocturnal movements may respond to reduction of the evening dopaminergic dosages. If insomnia is unresponsive to these measures, the judicious use of benzodiazepines, such as triazolam or clonazepam, may be helpful; zolpidem also might be tried for a few days or weeks to normalize the sleep–wake schedule. Although in theory, improved nighttime sleep may lead to reductions in morning tremor and rigidity, in practice, these changes can be hard to assess. Antidepressants with sedating properties, such as amitriptyline (25 to 50 mg) or mirtazapine (15 mg),[80] are frequently helpful for sleep-onset insomnia. The anticholinergic effects of tricyclic antidepressants may have therapeutic benefits for daytime parkinsonian symptoms and depression as well, but they can induce nocturnal delirium in patients with cognitive impairment.

Nocturnal Hallucinations, Psychosis, and Confusion

Unfortunately, when used during the day or in the evening, dopaminergic medications may induce entirely new sleep problems. Vivid dreams, nightmares, and night terrors occur in up to 30% of patients with parkinsonism who are taking L-dopa,[81] especially those with dementia, and may necessitate a reduction in the afternoon or evening doses. For the demented patient with PD, nocturnal confusion and hallucinations often are so disruptive that only low doses of L-dopa can be used, with renunciation of dopamine agonists. In such cases, small doses of clomethiazole or even clozapine (6.25 to 25 mg) at bedtime are sometimes helpful. Nocturnal hallucinations, mostly associated with reduced sleep efficiency and slow wave sleep and altered REM sleep, should be treated with low dosages of clozapine[82] that are slowly increased until a complete remission is achieved. Patients who do not tolerate clozapine may be switched to low-dose quetiapine (12.5 to 50 mg), which is also appropriate for treatment in patients with PD because of its side effect profile.[83,84]

Respiratory Disturbances

The treatment of sleep-related respiratory disturbances in parkinsonism is similar to the treatment of such problems in other patients. A close relation to snoring has been observed

PD with sleepiness, and snoring was the only risk factor for daytime sleepiness in a consecutive ...tion of patients with PD treated with dopaminergic ...ts.[85] In patients with obstructive apneas and hypopneas, ...asal continuous positive airway pressure offers the best chance of success and can be used effectively by most patients with parkinsonism until the advanced stages of the disease are reached. Upper airway surgery may help some patients with redundant palatal or pharyngeal tissue, but the abnormal motor activity of the upper airway remains after surgery. For patients with MSA and severe vocal cord dysfunction, tracheostomy is sometimes necessary.

Appropriate nasal continuous positive airway pressure therapy may improve the condition of a patient with PD substantially, with normalization of nocturnal blood pressure and neuropsychiatric symptoms as well. Daytime fatigue and sudden sleepiness may also result from sleep apnea and should be treated as in nonparkinsonian patients.

Daytime Sleepiness and Sleep Attacks in Parkinson's Disease

Before daytime sleepiness is treated with psychostimulants, respiratory disturbances—especially obstructive sleep apnea syndrome—and pharmacologically induced sleepiness should be excluded, if possible, by polysomnography.[66,85] In nonidiopathic parkinsonian syndromes, the possibility of an encephalitis has been recently discussed in rare cases with somnolence and daytime fatigue.[86] If the degenerative process itself is likely to cause sleepiness or even "sleep attacks," a trial of psychostimulants such as bupropion or modafinil in the morning may be justified.[66] Modafinil is the agent best investigated in patients with PD, and a number of open and some controlled studies are available. Some authors recommend modafinil even if daytime sleepiness is induced by medication.[87] Modafinil (up to 200 mg) given once daily improved subjective daytime sleepiness (measured by ESS scores) significantly in 12 patients with PD with an ESS score greater than 10 who were treated with various dopaminergic agents and did not show any respiratory disturbances.[88] Other authors found that in a small sample, administration of 200 mg/day of modafinil was associated with few side effects and was modestly effective for the treatment of excessive daytime sleepiness in patients with PD.[89] Because long-term studies are still lacking, we cannot predict if these effects remain stable. One should be very cautious in treating patients with PD who are experiencing cognitive decline or psychotic episodes with modafinil because the risk of side effects may be increased.

Clinical Pearl

The clinician should take a careful history of the various sleep problems of a patient with PD and try to distinguish nocturnal akinesia, tremor, respiratory disturbance, off-dystonia, RBD, or psychosis from medication-associated factors and their contribution to the sleep problem. Specific interventions may then be required to increase quality of sleep and reduce daytime sleepiness, thus enhancing quality of life in PD.

REFERENCES

1. Gibb WR, Lees AJ: The relevance of the Lewy body to the pathogenesis of idiopathic Parkinson's disease. J Neurol Neurosurg Psychiatry 1988;51:745-752.
2. Wenning GK, Ben-Shlomo Y, Hughes A, et al: What clinical features are most useful to distinguish definite multiple system atrophy from Parkinson's disease? J Neurol Neurosurg Psychiatry 2000;68:434-440.
3. Braak H, Rüb U, Gai WP, Del Tredici K: Idiopathic Parkinson's disease: Possible routes by which vulnerable neuronal types may be subject to neuroinvasion by an unknown pathogen. J Neural Transm 2003;110:517-536.
4. Del Tredici K, Rüb U, De Vos RA, et al: Where does Parkinson's disease pathology begin in the brain? Neuropathol Exp Neurol 2002;61:413-426.
5. Parkinson J: Essay on the Shaking Palsy. London, Sherwood, Neely, and Jones, 1817, p 17.
6. Charcot JM: Lectures on the diseases of the nervous system [trans. by G. Siegerson]. London, The New Sydenham Society, Lecture V, 1877, p 147.
7. Forno LS: Neuropathology of Parkinson's disease. J Neuropathol Exp Neurol 1996;55:259-272.
8. Langston JW, Forno LS, Rebert CS, et al: Selective nigral toxicity after systemic administration of 1-methyl-4-phenyl-1,2,5, 6-tetrahydropyridine (MPTP) in the squirrel monkey. Brain Res 1984;292:390-394.
9. Burns RS, Chiueh CC, Markey SP, et al: A primate model of parkinsonism: Selective destruction of dopaminergic neurons in the pars compacta of the substantia nigra by N-methy l-4-phenyl-1,2,3,6-tetrahydropyridine. Proc Natl Acad Sci U S A 1983;80:4546-4550.
10. Jellinger K: Pathology of parkinsonism. In Fahn S, Marsden CD, Jenner P, et al (eds): Recent Developments in Parkinson's Disease. New York, Raven Press, 1986, pp 33-66.
11. Zweig RM, Jankel WR, Hedreen JC, et al: The pedunculopontine nucleus in Parkinson's disease. Ann Neurol 1989;26:41-46.
12. Javoy-Agid F, Agid Y: Is the mesocortical dopaminergic system involved in Parkinson's disease? Neurology 1980;30:1326-1330.
13. De Keyser J, Ebinger G, Vauquelin G: Evidence for a widespread dopaminergic innervation of the human cerebral neocortex. Neurosci Lett 1989;104:281-285.
14. Ongini E, Caporali MG, Massotti M: Stimulation of dopamine-D-1 receptors by SKF 38393 induces EEG desynchronization and behavioural arousal. Life Sci 1985;37:2327-2333.
15. Bo P, Ongini E, Giorgetti A, et al: Synchronization of the EEG and sedation induced by neuroleptics depend upon blockade of both D1 and D2 dopamine receptors. Neuropharmacology 1988;27:799.
16. Chianchetti C: Dopamine agonists and sleep in man. In Wauquier A, Gaillard JM, Monti JM, et al (eds): Sleep: Neurotransmitters and Neuromodulators. New York, Raven Press, 1985, pp 121-134.
17. Bagetta G, De Sarro G, Priolo E, et al: Ventral tegmental area site through which dopamine D2-receptor agonists evoke behavioural and electrocortical sleep in rats. Br J Pharmacol 1988; 95:860-866.
18. Svensson K, Alfoldi P, Hajos M, et al: Dopamine autoreceptor antagonists: Effects of sleep-wake activity in the rat. Pharmacol Biochem Behav 1987;26:123-129.
19. Trampus M, Ferri N, Monopoli A, et al: The dopamine D1 receptor is involved in the regulation of REM sleep in the rat. Eur J Pharmacol 1991;194:189-194.
20. de Rijik MC, Tzourio C, Breteler MM, et al: Prevalence of parkinsonism and Parkinson's disease in Europe: The Europarkinson Collaborative Study: European Community Concerted Action on the Epidemiology of Parkinson's Disease. J Neurol Neurosurg Psychiatry 1997;62:10-15.

21. Trenkwalder C, Schwarz J, Gebhard J, et al: Starnberg Trial on Epidemiology of Parkinsonism and Hypertension in the Elderly: Prevalence of Parkinson's disease and related disorders assessed by a door-to-door survey of inhabitants older than 65 years. Arch Neurol 1995;52:1017-1022.

22. Factor SA, McAlarney T, Sanchez-Ramon JR, et al: Sleep disorders and sleep effect in Parkinson's disease. Mov Disord 1990; 4:280-285.

23. Menza MA, Rosen RC: Sleep in Parkinson's disease: The role of depression and anxiety. Psychosomatics 1995;36:262-266.

24. Comella CL, Tanner CM, Ristanovic RK: Polysomnographic sleep measures in Parkinson's disease patients with treatment-induced hallucinations. Ann Neurol 1993;34:710-714.

25. Kales A, Ansel RD, Markham CH, et al: Sleep in patients with Parkinson's disease and normal subjects prior to and following levodopa administration. Clin Pharmacol Ther 1971;12:397-406.

26. Bergonzi P, Chiurulla C, Gambi D, et al: L-Dopa plus dopadecarboxylase inhibitor: Sleep organization in Parkinson's syndrome before and after treatment. Acta Neurol Belg 1975;75:5-10.

27. Wetter TC, Collado-Seidel V, Pollmächer T, et al: Sleep and periodic leg movement patterns in drug-free patients with Parkinson's disease and multiple system atrophy. Sleep 2000;23: 361-367.

28. Friedman A: Sleep pattern in Parkinson's disease. Acta Med Pol 1980;21:193-199.

29. Mouret J: Differences in sleep in patients with Parkinson's disease. Electroencephalogr Clin Neurophysiol 1975;38:653-657.

30. Brunner H, Wetter TC, Hogl B, et al: Microstructure of the non-rapid eye movement sleep electroencephalogram in patients with newly diagnosed Parkinson's disease: Effects of dopaminergic treatment. Mov Disord 2002;17:928-933.

31. Plazzi G, Corsini R, Provini F, et al: REM sleep behaviour disorder in multiple system atrophy. Neurology 1997;48:1094-1097.

32. Aldrich MS, Foster NL, White RF, et al: Sleep abnormalities in progressive supranuclear palsy. Ann Neurol 1989;25:577-581.

33. Martinelli P, Coccagna G, Rizzuto N, et al: Changes in systemic arterial pressure during sleep in Shy-Drager syndrome. Sleep 1981;4:139-146.

34. April RS: Observations on parkinsonian tremor in all-night sleep. Neurology 1966;16:720-724.

35. Stern M, Roffwarg H, Duvoisin R: The parkinsonian tremor in sleep. J Nerv Ment Dis 1968;147:202-210.

36. Fish DR, Sawyers D, Allen PJ, et al: The effect of sleep on the dyskinetic movements of Parkinson's disease, Gilles de la Tourette syndrome, Huntington's disease, and torsion dystonia. Arch Neurol 1991;48:210-214.

37. Ondo WG, Vuong KD, Jankovic J: Exploring the relationship between Parkinson disease and restless legs syndrome. Arch Neurol 2002;59:421-424.

38. Lees AJ, Blackburn NA, Campbell VL: The nighttime problems of Parkinson's disease. Clin Neuropharmacol 1988:11:512-519.

39. Currie LJ, Bennett JP Jr, Harrison MB, et al: Clinical correlates of sleep benefit in Parkinson's disease. Neurology 1997;48: 1115-1117.

40. Bateman DE, Levett K, Marsden CD. Sleep benefit in Parkinson's disease. J Neurol Neurosurg Psychiatry 1999;67:384-385.

41. Hogl BE, Gomez-Arevalo G, Garcia S, et al: A clinical, pharmacologic, and polysomnographic study of sleep benefit in Parkinson's disease. Neurology 1998;50:1332-1339.

42. Yamamura Y, Sobue I, Ando K, et al: Paralysis agitans of early onset with marked diurnal fluctuation of symptoms. Neurology 1973;23:239-244.

43. American Sleep Disorders Association: International Classification of Sleep Disorders, Revised: Diagnostic and Coding Manual. Rochester, Minn, American Sleep Disorders Association, 1997.

44. Olson EJ, Boeve BF, Silber MH: Rapid eye movement sleep behaviour disorder: Demographic, clinical and laboratory findings in 93 cases. Brain 2000;123:331-339.

45. Comella CL, Nardine TM, Diederich NJ, et al: Sleep-related violence, injury, and REM sleep behavior disorder in Parkinson's disease. Neurology 1998;51:526-529.

46. Gagnon JF, Bedard MA, Fantini ML, et al: REM sleep behavior disorder and REM sleep without atonia in Parkinson's disease. Neurology 2002;59:585-589.

47. Eisensehr I, Lindeiner H, Jäger M, et al: REM sleep behavior disorder in sleep-disordered patients with versus without Parkinson's disease: Is there a need for polysomnography? J Neurol Sci 2001;186:7-11.

48. Plazzi G, Cortelli P, Montagna P, et al: REM sleep behaviour disorder differentiates pure autonomic failure from multiple system atrophy with autonomic failure. J Neurol Neurosurg Psychiatry 1998;64:683-685.

49. Eisensehr I, Linke R, Noachtar S, et al: Reduced striatal dopamine transporters in idiopathic rapid eye movement sleep behavior disorder: Comparison with Parkinson's disease and controls. Brain 2000;123:1155-1160.

50. Arnulf I, Bonnet AM, Damier P, et al: Hallucinations, REM sleep, and Parkinson's disease: A medical hypothesis. Neurology 2000;55:281-288.

51. Henderson JM, Lu Y, Wang S, et al: Olfactory deficits and sleep disturbances in Parkinson's disease: A case-control survey. J Neurol Neurosurg Psychiatry 2003;74:956-958.

52. Hovestadt A, Bogaard JM, Meerwaldt JD, et al: Pulmonary function in Parkinson's disease. J Neurol Neurosurg Psychiatry 1989;52: 329-333.

53. Vincken WG, Gauthier SG, Dollfuss RE, et al: Involvement of upper-airway muscles in extrapyramidal disorders: A cause of airflow limitation. N Engl J Med 1984;311:438-442.

54. Hardie RJ, Efthimiou J, Stern GM: Respiration and sleep in Parkinson's disease. J Neurol Neurosurg Psychiatry 1986;49: 1326.

55. Apps MCP, Sheaff PC, Ingram DA, et al: Respiration and sleep in Parkinson's disease. J Neurol Neurosurg Psychiatry 1985;48: 1240-1245.

56. Chokroverty S, Sharp JT, Barron KD: Periodic respiration in erect posture in Shy-Drager syndrome. J Neurol Neurosurg Psychiatry 1978;41:980-986.

57. McNicholas WT, Rutherford R, Grossman R, et al: Abnormal respiratory pattern generation during sleep in patients with autonomic dysfunction. Am Rev Respir Dis 1983;128:429-433.

58. Guilleminault C, Briskin JG, Greenfield MS, et al: The impact of autonomic nervous system dysfunction on breathing during sleep. Sleep 1981;4:263-268.

59. Kenyon GS, Apps MCP, Traub M: Stridor and obstructive sleep apnea in Shy-Drager syndrome treated by laryngofissure and cord lateralization. Laryngoscope 1984;94:1106-1108.

60. Isozaki E, Naito A, Horiguchi S, et al: Early diagnosis and stage classification of vocal cord abductor paralysis in patients with multiple system atrophy. J Neurol Neurosurg Psychiatry 1996;60:399-402.

61. Guilleminault C, Tilkian A, Lehrman K, et al: Sleep apnoea syndrome: States of sleep and autonomic dysfunction. J Neurol Neurosurg Psychiatry 1977;40:718-725.

62. Frucht S, Rogers JD, Greene PE, et al: Falling asleep at the wheel: Motor vehicle mishaps in persons taking pramipexole and ropinirole. Neurology 1999;52:1908-1910.

63. Ondo WG, Dat Vuong K, Khan H, et al: Daytime sleepiness and other sleep disorders in Parkinson's disease. Neurology 2001;57:1392-1396.

64. Brodsky MA, Godbold J, Roth T, et al: Sleepiness in Parkinson's disease: A controlled study. Mov Disord 2003;18:668-672.

65. Arnulf I, Konofal E, Merino-Andreu M, et al: Parkinson's disease and sleepiness: An integral part of PD. Neurology 2002;58:1019-1024.

66. Rye D: Sleepiness and unintended sleep in Parkinson's disease. Curr Treat Options Neurol 2003;5:231-239.

67. Merino-Andreu M, Arnulf I, Konofal E, et al: Unawareness of naps in Parkinson's disease and in disorders with excessive daytime sleepiness. Neurology 2003;60:1553-1554.

68. Chaudhuri KR, Pal S, DiMarco A, et al: The Parkinson's Disease Sleep Scale: A new instrument for assessing sleep and nocturnal disability in Parkinson's disease. J Neurol Neurosurg Psychiatry 2002;73:629-633.

69. Leeman AL, ONeill CJ, Nicholson PW, et al: Parkinson's disease in the elderly: Response to and an optimal spacing of night time dosing with levodopa. Br J Clin Pharmacol 1987;24:637-643.

70. Monti JM, Hawkins M, Jantos H, et al : Biphasic effects of dopamine D-2 receptor agonists on sleep and wakefulness in the rat. Psychopharmacology 1988;95:395-400.

71. Cantor CR, Stern MB: Dopamine agonists and sleep in Parkinson's disease. Neurology 2002;58:S71-S78.

72. Askenasy JJ, Yahr MD: Reversal of sleep disturbance in Parkinson's disease by antiparkinsonian therapy: A preliminary study. Neurology 1985;35:527-532.

73. Jansen EN, Meerwaldtt JD: Madopar HBS in nocturnal symptoms of Parkinson's disease. Adv Neurol 1990;53:527-531.

74. Koller WC, Hutton JT, Tolosa E, et al: Immediate-release and controlled-release carbidopa/levodopa in PD: A 5-year randomized multicenter study. Carbidopa/Levodopa Study Group. Neurology 1999;53:1012-1019.

75. Hogl B, Rothdach A, Wetter TC, et al: The effect of cabergoline on sleep, periodic leg movements in sleep, and early morning motor function in patients with Parkinson's disease. Neuropsychopharmacology 2003;28:1866-1870.

76. Lang AE, Quinn N, Brincat S, et al: Pergolide in late-stage Parkinson disease. Ann Neurol 1982;12:243-247.

77. Klawans HL, Goetz C, Bergen D: Levodopa-induced myoclonus. Arch Neurol 1975;32:331-334.

78. Vardi J, Glaubman H, Rabey J, et al: EEG sleep patterns in Parkinsonian patients treated with bromocriptine and L-dopa: A comparative study. J Neural Transm 1979;45:307-316.

79. Schenck C, Mahowald M: A polysomnographic, neurologic, psychiatric and clinical outcome report on 70 consecutive cases with REM sleep behavior disorder (RBD): Sustained clonazepam efficacy in 89% of 57 treated patients. Cleve Clin J Med 1990;57:10-24.

80. Gordon PH, Pullman SL, Louis ED, et al: Mirtazapine in parkinsonian tremor. Parkinsonism Relat Disord 2002;9:125-126.

81. Scharf B, Moskovitz C, Lupton MD, et al: Dream phenomena induced by chronic levodopa therapy. J Neural Transm 1978;43:143-151.

82. The Parkinson Study Group: Low-dose clozapine for the treatment of drug-induced psychosis in Parkinson's disease. N Engl J Med 1999;340:757-763.

83. Fernandez HH, Friedman JH, Jacques C, et al: Quetiapine for the treatment of drug-induced psychosis in Parkinson's disease. Mov Disord 1999;14:484-487.

84. Reddy S, Factor SA, Molho ES, et al: The effect of quetiapine on psychosis and motor function in parkinsonian patients with and without dementia. Mov Disord 2002;17:676-681.

85. Braga-Neto P, Pereira da Silva-Junior F, Sueli Monte F, et al: Snoring and excessive daytime sleepiness in Parkinson's disease. J Neurol Sci 2004;217:41-45.

86. Dale RC, Church AJ, Surtees RA, et al: Encephalitis lethargica syndrome: 20 new cases and evidence of basal ganglia autoimmunity. Brain 2004;127:21-33.

87. Hauser RA, Wahba MN, Zesiewicz TA, McDowell Anderson W: Modafinil treatment of pramipexole-associated somnolence. Mov Disord 2000;15:1269-1271.

88. Hogl B, Saletu M, Brandauer E, et al: Modafinil for the treatment of daytime sleepiness in Parkinson's disease: A double-blind, randomized, crossover, placebo-controlled polygraphic trial. Sleep 2002;25:905-909.

89. Adler CH, Caviness JN, Hentz JG, et al: Randomized trial of modafinil for treating subjective daytime sleepiness in patients with Parkinson's disease. Mov Disord 2003;18:287-293.

68

Sleep and Stroke

Claudio L. Bassetti

ABSTRACT

Cerebrovascular diseases and sleep disorders are among the most common neurologic problems, and they can occur together by chance alone. In addition, however, each condition can cause the other or can arise from similar predisposing factors. Recent studies have shown that sleep disordered breathing and sleep-wake disorders may have a detrimental effect on neurologic and psychiatric functions and therefore on stroke outcome. In addition, sleep disordered breathing may also increase stroke recurrence and long-term mortality after stroke. The recognition of sleep disordered breathing and sleep-wake disorders represents not only a challenge but also a new therapeutic window in the management of stroke patients.

Over the last 10 years sleep disorders in stroke victims have received increasing attention. The main reasons relate to better recognition of a strong link between sleep disordered breathing and cardio- and cerebrovascular diseases, as well as the high frequency of sleep disorders and sleep architecture changes arising from focal brain damage. This chapter gives an overview of sleep disordered breathing, sleep-wake disturbances (such as hypersomnia and insomnia), sleep architecture changes, and circadian disorders following stroke.

STROKE

Stroke is defined as a focal neurologic deficit of acute onset and vascular origin. Stroke has an incidence of 2 to 18 per 1000 per year and is the most common neurologic disease to warrant hospitalization. Transient ischemic attacks (TIAs), in which neurologic deficits resolve within 24 hours, account for about 20% of acute cerebrovascular events; intracerebral hemorrhage accounts for about 15%. The remaining 65% are ischemic strokes.

Risk factors for stroke include atrial fibrillation, age older than 65 years, arterial hypertension, heart disease, asymptomatic carotid stenosis, history of TIA, alcohol abuse, smoking, diabetes mellitus, and hypercholesterolemia. These factors, however, explain only half the cardiovascular disease risk. Inflammatory markers, infection, homocysteine, and possibly sleep disordered breathing (see later) may represent new risk factors for stroke.[1] According to the criteria of the TOAST (Trial of Acute Stroke Treatment) study, the etiology of stroke can be grouped into five categories: macroangiopathy (large vessel disease), microangiopathy (small vessel disease), cardioembolism, other etiologies (dissection, hypercoagulable states, vasculitis), and unknown origin.[2]

Treatment of acute stroke includes placement of patients in a stroke unit, early recognition of medical complications, and prescription of agents that inhibit platelet aggregation. Fibrinolytic agents can be effective in the first 3 to 6 hours after ischemic stroke. Other treatments under evaluation include neuroprotective agents and endovascular stenting or balloon dilation of stenotic vessels. Surgery may be considered in noncomatose patients with accessible (e.g., cerebellar) hemorrhages.

Primary prevention of stroke includes treatment of risk factors, anticoagulation for atrial fibrillation, and endarterectomy in some patients with significant (70% or greater) carotid stenosis. After an ischemic stroke, prevention of further events often involves aspirin (or clopidogrel), which reduces the relative risk of stroke recurrence by about 20%; statins; and blood-pressure–lowering medications including selective angiotensin I and II blockers.

HISTORY

Changes in sleep and breathing were reported in stroke patients as early as the beginning of the 19th century. In 1818 John Cheyne first described periodic breathing in a patient with cardiac disease and "apoplexy."[3] Hughlings Jackson later recognized that Cheyne-Stokes respiration frequently accompanies bilateral hemispheric stroke. Symptoms of obstructive sleep apnea were first recognized in a patient with intracerebral hemorrhage by Broadbent in 1877.[4] Charles Beevor described the loss of voluntary respiratory control in a patient with pseudobulbar palsy.

Although central apnea in the course of progressive paralysis was described by Weir Mitchell in 1890,[5] failure of automatic respiration during sleep after brainstem stroke was first reported by Ratto in 1955.[6] Hypersomnia following stroke was mentioned by MacNish in 1830,[7] but it was only at the beginning of the 20th century that thalamic and mesencephalic stroke, in particular, were implicated.[8] In 1883 Charcot first reported that a patient lost dream recall after a presumed parietal-occipital stroke.[9] Lhermitte coined the term *peduncular hallucinosis* in 1922 to describe vivid, colorful, dreamlike hallucinations following midbrain stroke.[10] Subsequently abnormalities of sleep spindling in patients with hemispheric stroke and of non–rapid eye movement (NREM) and rapid eye movement (REM) sleep in patients with brainstem stroke were described.[11-13]

SLEEP-DISORDERED BREATHING

Epidemiology

Since the mid-1990s it has been known that about 60% to 70% of all stroke patients exhibit sleep-disordered breathing (SDB) as defined by an apnea-hypopnea index (AHI) of 10 episodes per hour.[14,15] In these as well as subsequent studies, no major differences were found in the frequency of SDB according to topography, subtype (ischemic versus hemorrhagic), and presumed etiology of stroke.[16,17] The prevalence of SDB was found in two studies to be similar also in patients with TIAs and ischemic stroke.[16,17] A recent study found a similarly high frequency of SDB in 86 TIA patients (AHI = 15 in 50%) but no significant differences in frequency or severity of SDB when compared with 86 controls matched for age and sex.[18]

These observations suggest that SDB may precede the onset of stroke in a significant proportion of cases (see also later). This assumption is supported by the results of a recent study in which the presence of *prestroke* cerebrovascular disease and the severity of white matter disease on brain computed tomography (CT) were linked with a more severe *poststroke* SDB.[19]

From the acute to the subacute phase of stroke, SDB tends to improve, but about 50% of patients still exhibit an AHI of 10 per hour three months after the acute event.[17,20,21] Central events probably improve more than obstructive events (Fig. 68–1).[17] One study suggested a better improvement of SDB in hemorrhagic strokes as compared to ischemic strokes.[22]

Pathogenesis

Sleep-Disordered Breathing as a Consequence of Stroke

Although patients at risk for cerebrovascular disease often have SDB before they experience a stroke, some develop the sleep disorder as a consequence of stroke. The observation that recovery from stroke may be accompanied by improvement of SDB gives support to the assumption that obstructive sleep apnea (OSA) is aggravated by stroke or even appears de novo after stroke (see earlier).

A disturbed coordination of upper airway, intercostal, and diaphragm muscles due to brainstem or hemispheric lesions may favor the appearance of OSA.[23] In patients with OSA and rostrolateral medullary lesions, a reduced ventilatory sensitivity to inhaled CO_2 may also play a role.[24]

Cheyne-Stokes breathing (CSB) has been attributed to CO_2 hypersensitivity induced by bilateral supratentorial lesions (see Chapter 81).[25] The presence of bilateral supratentorial or pontine lesions, decreased level of consciousness, and heart failure are crucial for the appearance of CSB during wakefulness.[26,27] Conversely, CSB that occurs only during sleep can be seen also in patients with unilateral lesions of variable topography and without disturbed level of consciousness or clinically overt heart failure.[28] Finally, CSB and OSA may potentiate each other.

Habitual Snoring and Sleep-Disordered Breathing as Risk Factors for Stroke

Whether snoring and SDB cause or contribute to stroke remains a subject of debate. Habitual snoring—that is, snoring that occurs always or almost always—affects 4% to 24% of the adult population, with a maximal prevalence around the age of 50 to 60 years, and it is strongly associated with OSA. Six case-control and three cohort studies have shown that habitual snoring represents an independent risk factor for stroke, with a pooled risk estimate of 1.66 (95% confidence interval [CI], 1.4-2.0).[29] Other studies have suggested that excessive daytime sleepiness and prolonged sleep, which can be symptoms of SDB, may also represent independent risk factors for stroke.[30,31]

Several findings have suggested plausible physiologic mechanisms by which obstructive SDB could cause stroke.

Chronically, habitual snoring and SDB of different degrees of severity are all associated with hypertension, which in turn is an important risk factor for stroke.[32,33] Findings from the Wisconsin sleep cohort have shown that an AHI greater than 15 is independently associated with a threefold increased risk of developing new hypertension within a 4-year period.[34] Furthermore, SDB may cause myocardial infarction, heart failure, and arrhythmias, all of which could also act as intermediate variables in an effect of OSA on risk for stroke.[35]

The immediate consequences of respiratory apneic events include hypoxemia, hypercapnia, arousal from sleep, intrathoracic pressure changes, and sympathetic activation. A series of hemodynamic, neural, metabolic, and inflammatory changes may contribute to diabetes, increased platelet aggregation, decreased fibrinolysis, and increased atherogenesis.[35,36] The observation of an increase in the intima-media thickness of the common carotid artery documented by ultrasound techniques in SDB patients as compared with controls matched for age and vascular risk factors further supports an increased (chronic) atherogenesis in SDB.[37]

Acutely, apneas and hypopneas during sleep may be accompanied by decreased cardiac output, cardiac arrhythmias, systemic hypotension or hypertension, vasodilation due to hypoxia and hypercapnia, and increased intracranial pressure.[38-40] These factors lead to an overall 15% to 20% reduction (in single studies up to 50% reduction) in cerebral blood flow velocities during respiratory events.[39,41,42] Type, duration, and timing of respiratory events may affect hemodynamic consequences. Obstructive apneas of long duration and those that occur during REM sleep may be particularly detrimental.[42-44]

Fluctuations in cerebral blood velocities (and flow) (Fig. 68–2) may be especially harmful because patients with SDB have a diminished vasodilator reserve.[45] Cheyne-Stokes respirations (CSR) and central apneas also can alter cerebral blood flow.[42,46,47] During long apneas, paradoxical embolization caused by right-to-left shunting in patients with patent foramen ovale (PFO) is another potential mechanism of stroke.[48] In view of these observations, it is not surprising that SDB has been associated with the onset of cerebrovascular events at night.[49,50] A direct link between SDB and nocturnal cerebrovascular ischemic events has been suggested for retinal infarcts of embolic origin[51] and in single patients with TIA or minor stroke.[51-53]

A pathogenic role of SDB in vascular disease is further suggested from continuous positive airway pressure (CPAP) treatment studies. A few studies have shown favorable effects of CPAP on mean arterial blood pressure.[54] Pepperell's group reported that therapeutic CPAP reduced mean arterial blood pressure by 2.5 mm Hg, whereas subtherapeutic CPAP levels increased blood pressure by 0.8 mm Hg. Such an effect is expected to be associated with a stroke risk reduction of about 20%. Treatment with CPAP may also favorably influence surrogate markers of vascular disease such as factor VII clotting activity, fibrinogen levels, and platelet activation or aggregation.[55,56]

Clinical Features

Clinical Symptoms

SDB can manifest with a variety of symptoms and signs that are sometimes attributed to the underlying brain damage from stroke. Recent reviews on fatigue after stroke, for example, fail to mention sleep disorders, including SDB, as a possible factor.[57] Nighttime symptoms of SDB include difficulties

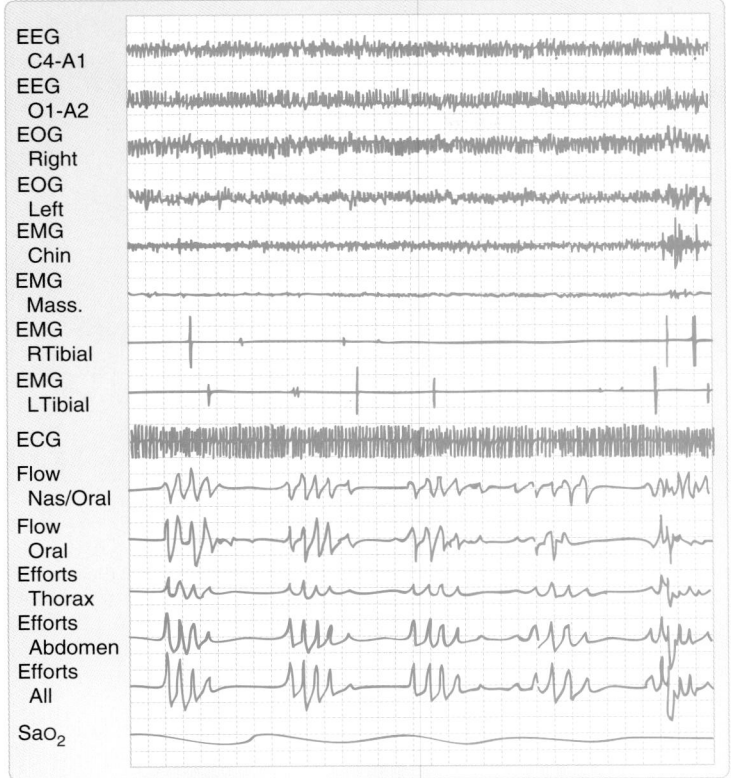

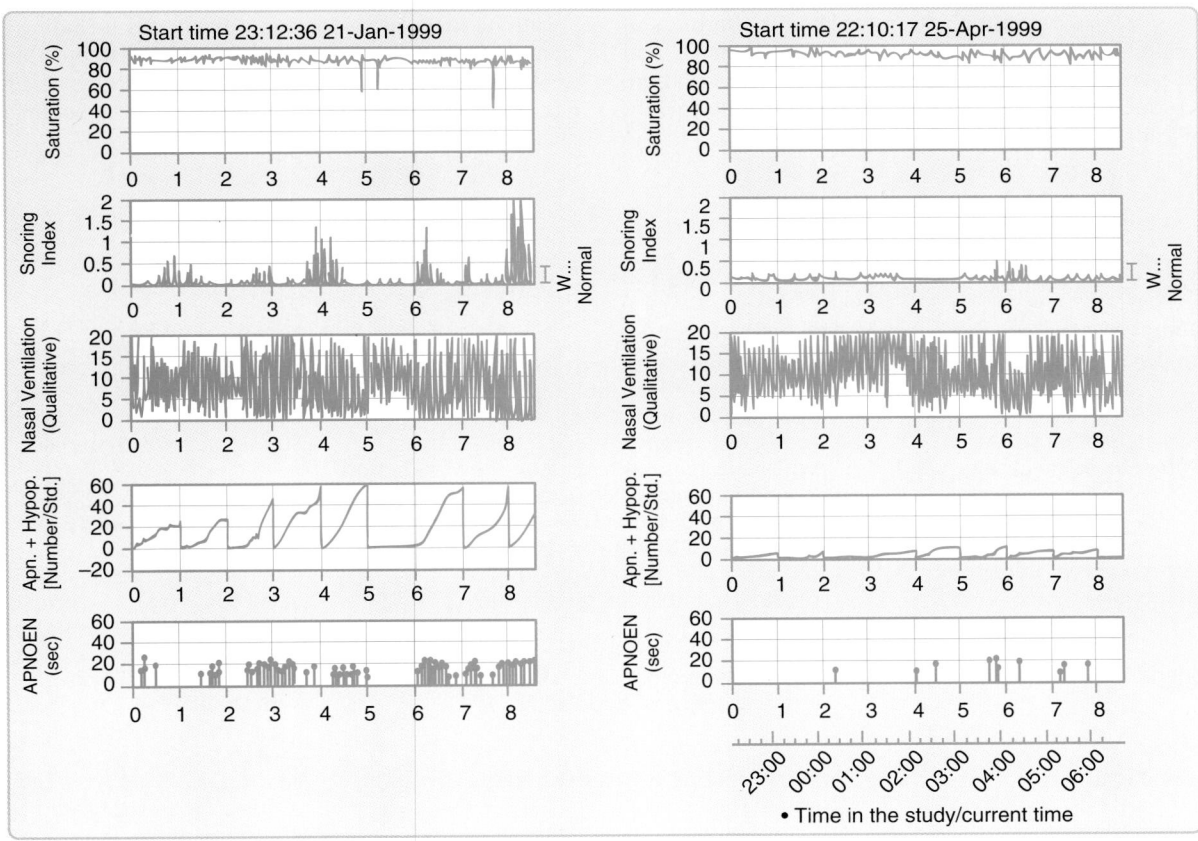

Figure 68–1. Cheyne-Stokes-like breathing (CSB) in acute ischemic stroke. This 68-year-old male patient (BMI = 26) has right thalamo-mesencephalic stroke. Clinically left hemisyndrome, upgaze palsy, dysarthria, mild hypersomnia. No sleep-wake complaints. National Institutes of Health (NIH) Stroke Score = 12. No history of hypertension, no heart failure (ejection fraction on echocardiography = 68%). A sleep study the first night after the stroke event demonstrated severe CSB (AHI = 25). Recording with an "intelligent" continuous positive airway pressure (CPAP) (AutoSet, ResMed, San Diego, Calif) confirmed severe sleep apnea (AHI = 28). A follow-up examination 3 months later demonstrated spontaneous improvement (AHI = 10). EEG, electroencephalogram; ECG, electrocardiogram; EMG, electromyogram; EOG, electrooculogram; SaO_2, oxygen saturation.

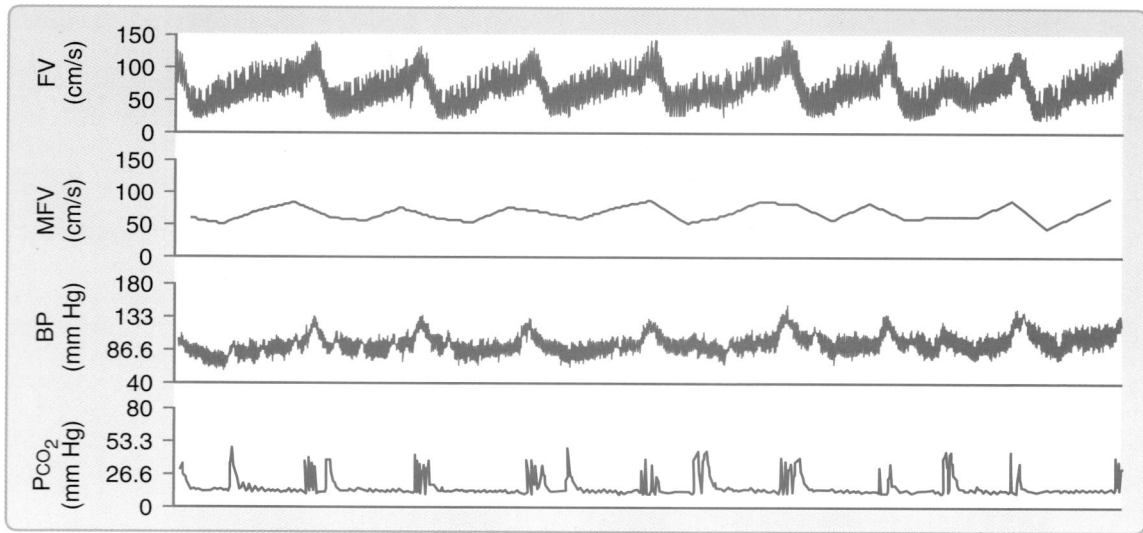

Figure 68–2. Cerebral blood flow velocity and obstructive sleep apnea. Flow velocity (FV) and mean flow velocity (MFV) in the right middle cerebral artery, peripheral blood pressure (BP), and end-expiratory P_{CO_2} in a patient with obstructive sleep apnea. Intervals with low end-expiratory P_{CO_2} show apneic episodes. (From Hajak G, Klingelhöfer J, Schulz-Varszegi M, et al: Sleep apnea syndrome and cerebral hemodynamics. Chest 1996;110:670-679.)

falling asleep (see later); respiratory noises (snoring, stridor); irregular or periodic respiration or apneas; agitated sleep with increased motor activity and frequent awakenings; sudden awakenings with or without choking sensations, shortness of breath, palpitations, and "panic attacks"; orthopnea, and increased sweating. In patients with severe hypoventilation, arousal responses can be suppressed by increasing sleep debt and may lead to death during sleep.

Daytime symptoms of SDB are headaches, fatigue and excessive daytime sleepiness, concentration and memory difficulties, irritability, and depression. Some patients may also exhibit breathing irregularities during wakefulness including dyspnea, apneas, inspiratory breath holding, irregular breathing, rapid shallow breathing (hyperpnea or central hyperventilation), hiccup, and other abnormalities. Table 68–1 summarizes the main breathing abnormalities.

Table 68–1.   Breathing Disturbances and Stroke

Breathing Pattern	Characteristics	Location of Lesions
Obstructive sleep apnea (OSA)	Respiratory events during sleep characterized by a decreased or abolished respiratory flow despite normal respiratory effort	Supra- and infratentorial[16,17]
Central sleep apnea (CSA), Cheyne-Stokes breathing (CSB)	CSA: respiratory events characterized by a similar decrease in respiratory flow and effort CSB: periodic hypopnea or central apnea alternate with hyperpnea in a crescendo-decrescendo ("diamond-form") pattern	Supra- and infratentorial[14,27,62]
Respiratory apraxia, impaired volitional breathing	Impairment of voluntary modulation of breathing amplitude and frequency	Frontal cortex, basal ganglia, capsula interna, ventral pons, ventral medulla, anterior spinal cord[63,64]
Neurogenic hyperventilation	Sustained respiratory rates above 25-30/min in the absence of hypoxemia	Ventro-tegmental pons, bilaterally,[66,68] supratentorial[67] and medial medulla (unilateral)[69]
Apneustic breathing	Erratic variations in breathing frequency and amplitude	Ventro-tegmental pons, infratrigeminal, bilaterally[71]
Ataxic breathing	Erratic variations in breathing frequency and amplitude	Tegmental medulla
Ondine's curse, impaired automatic breathing, central (alveolar) hypoventilation	Impairment or loss of automatic breathing (central apneas and hypoventilation appearing at sleep onset or during sleep)	Tegmental medulla (usually but not invariably bilaterally),[72-75] anterior cervical spinal cord[78]

Obstructive Sleep Apnea

The most common form of SDB in stroke patients is OSA (Figs. 68–3 and 68–4). Occasionally, patients present with coexisting OSA and CSB, with predominance of the first in REM sleep and of the latter in light NREM sleep (see Fig. 68–3).[28,58] Topography and etiology of stroke do not predict OSA in stroke victims,[16,17,28] although first reports suggested an association with brainstem strokes.[59,60]

Cheyne-Stokes Breathing

CSB is a type of periodic breathing in which central apneas and hypopneas are separated by crescendo-decrescendo respiratory patterns. In the first few days after stroke, central sleep apnea or CSB, or both, may be present in up to 30% to 40% of patients (unpublished data; see Fig. 68–1).[17,49] The presence of bilateral strokes, heart failure, and profound disturbances of consciousness, which are traditionally described in stroke patients with CSB, is not always necessary.[28,61] Patients with brainstem stroke can also develop CSB.[27,28,62]

Other Forms of Breathing Disturbance

Unlike OSA and CSB, other breathing abnormalities following *hemispheric strokes* have been less well studied. Such abnormalities include selective impairment of behavioral or volitional respiratory control, with preservation of metabolic control mechanisms. After cerebral stroke, voluntary chest movements are reduced on the paralyzed side.[23,63] Strokes in the frontal cortex, basal ganglia, or capsula interna may cause *respiratory apraxia,* with impairment of voluntary modulation of breathing amplitude and frequency, leaving patients unable to take a deep breath or hold the breath.[63,64]

Several abnormal patterns of breathing, although uncommon, can occur after *brainstem stroke,* especially during sleep or with decreased levels of consciousness. Sustained respiratory rates greater than 25 to 30 per minute in the absence of hypoxemia *(neurogenic hyperventilation)* were originally described in comatose patients as a direct consequence of midbrain or pontine damage.[65,66] Subsequently, neurogenic hyperventilation was also observed in patients with supratentorial and medullary lesions, often in association with

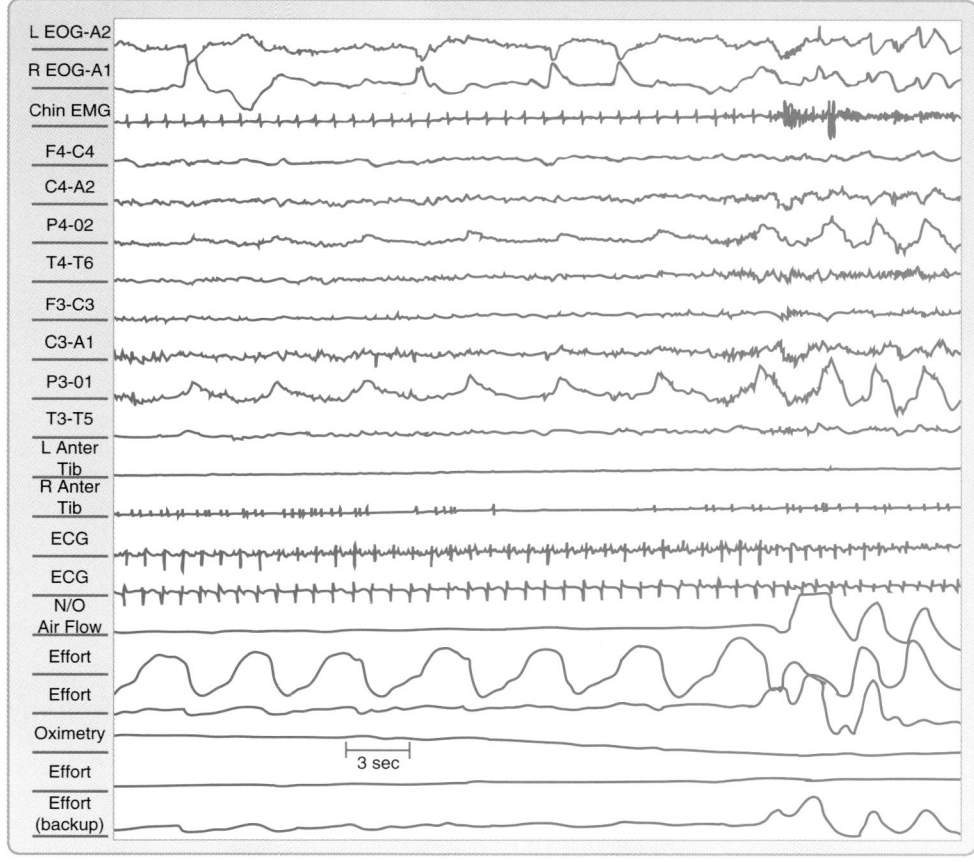

Figure 68–3. Obstructive and central sleep apnea in acute ischemic stroke in a 65-year-old man with right middle cerebral artery stroke following aortocoronary bypass surgery. Before stroke: habitual snoring, no excessive daytime sleepiness. Clinically: severe neurological deficits (Scandinavian Stroke Score of 20/58), no signs of heart failure. Polysomnography (PSG) 48 days after stroke onset: severe sleep apnea with Cheyne-Stokes-like respiration predominantly in light NREM sleep; essentially normal breathing in deep NREM sleep; and obstructive events mainly in rapid eye movement (REM) sleep. Apnea-hypopnea index (AHI) = 104. Sleep-disordered breathing improved (AHI = 2) in a second PSG when continuous positive airway pressure of 8 cm H_2O was applied. ECG, electrocardiogram, EMG, electromyogram; EOG, electrooculogram. (From Bassetti C, Aldrich MS, Quint D: Sleep-disordered breathing in patients with acute supra- and infratentorial stroke. Stroke 1997;28: 1765-1772.)

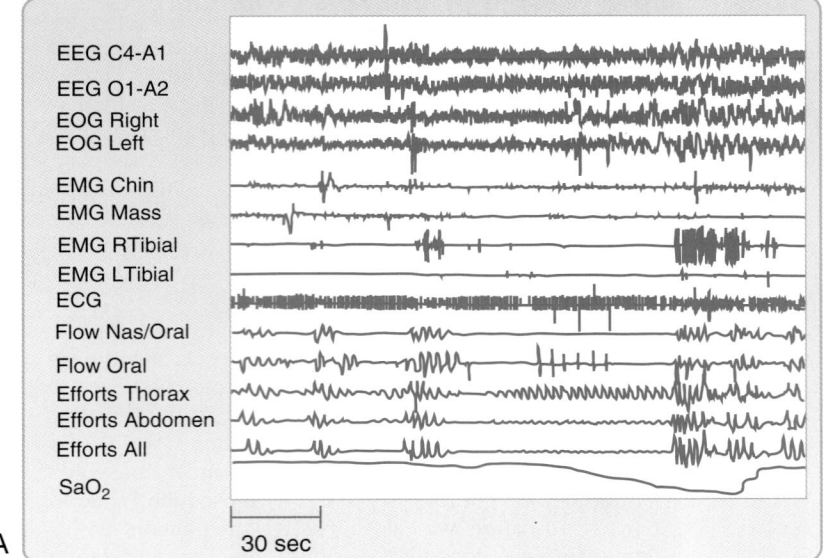

A

30 sec

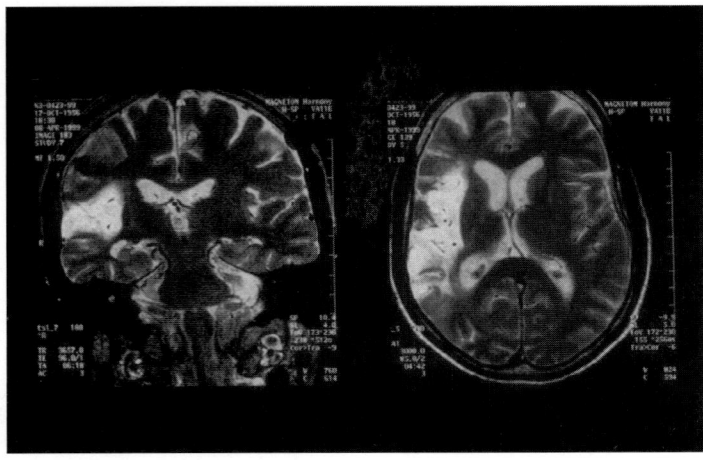

B

Figure 68–4. Obstructive sleep apnea (OSA) and hallucinations in acute ischemic stroke in a 50-year-old male patient (BMI = 28) with right temporo-parietal stroke. Clinically left hemisyndrome, hemianopsia, hemineglect, and anosognosia. Initial National Institutes of Health (NIH) Stroke Score = 8 (progression to hemiplegia in the first hours after admission). Complex visual hallucinations the first 2 days, particularly in the evening hours (two brown snakes and other animals coming though the right window, no insight, duration of several minutes). History of hypertension, hypercholesterolemia, and smoking. No heart failure. A sleep study 3 days after the stroke event demonstrated severe obstructive sleep apnea (AHI = 47). A follow-up examination 2 weeks later demonstrated spontaneous improvement (AHI = 23). EEG, electroencephalogram; ECG, electrocardiogram; EMG, electromyogram; EOG, electrooculogram; Sao₂, oxygen saturation. (MRI pictures courtesy Prof. G. Schroth, Institute of Neuroradiology, University Hospital, Bern, Switzerland.)

pulmonary congestion.[67-69] Neurogenic hyperventilation after stroke usually indicates a poor prognosis.[67,70] Inspiratory breath-holding (*apneustic breathing*), originally described in two patients with bilateral ventrotegmental mediocaudal (infratrigeminal) pontine stroke, is rare and usually secondary to basilar artery occlusion.[71]

Erratic variations in breathing frequency and amplitude (*ataxic* or *Biot's breathing*), and failure of automatic breathing (central sleep apnea or *Ondine's curse*), not uncommonly associated with hiccup, usually imply a lateral medullary stroke, often bilateral.[72-75] Damage to the medullary reticular formation and nucleus ambiguus may be sufficient to cause a loss of automatic breathing, and a lesion that also includes the nucleus tractus solitarius is necessary to cause failure of both automatic and voluntary respiration.[75] Volitional breathing can be impaired by brainstem strokes involving corticobulbar and corticospinal pathways at the pontine and medullary level.[63,64]

Spinal cord stroke can impair both automatic and voluntary breathing control.[76] The topography and extent of the lesion can determine respiratory effects. Anterior spinal artery strokes can affect reticulospinal pathways, located anteriorly in the lateral columns of the first three cervical segments, which are crucial for automatic breathing.[76,77] Failure of automatic breathing

has been described as a complication of anterior spinal cord infarction at the cervical level.[78] In contrast, posterior spinal artery strokes can damage corticospinal pathways in the dorsolateral spinal cord and impair voluntary control of breathing. Strokes that extend up to the C1 level usually cause severe respiratory insufficiency and necessitate ventilatory support.

Clinical Significance

SDB in patients with cerebrovascular disorders may be detrimental even in the absence of a direct causative link between SDB and stroke. In a recent study, SDB detected the first night after brain infarction was found to be associated with early neurologic worsening.[49] Patients with and without stroke progression did not differ with respect to other risk factors, such as body mass index (BMI), arterial hypertension, smoking, diabetes, or hyperlipidemia.

A few studies also suggested a detrimental effect of habitual snoring and SDB on long-term outcome of stroke.[15,79,80] Recent studies have shown that OSA is also linked with length of hospital stay, stroke mortality, and greater functional impairment.[81,82] Furthermore, treatment of SDB has been shown to improve subjective well-being and mood in stroke patients with SDB.[83,84] Based on the blood pressure–lowering effects of CPAP, treatment of SDB could lead to a stroke risk reduction of about 20%.[54]

Diagnosis

The high frequency of SDB, in combination with epidemiologic and physiologic evidence that SDB may be linked pathophysiologically to cerebrovascular disease, suggests that clinicians should investigate the possibility of SDB in all patients who have had a stroke. SDB should be suspected particularly in elderly male patients with a history of habitual snoring or witnessed apnea, multiple cardiovascular risk factors, and stroke onset at night.[16,17,49,50] Stroke topography, etiology, and history of excessive daytime sleepiness are, conversely, poor predictors of SDB in stroke victims.

Objective sleep studies should be considered in patients in whom treatment of SDB is considered as potentially feasible and reasonable (e.g., absence of dementia). Such sleep studies may include pulse oxymetry,[85] portable (ambulatory) respirographies, and "intelligent" CPAP devices (see Fig. 68–1).[50,86] Laboratory polysomnography should be reserved for only a minority of patients.

The optimal timing of sleep studies after stroke or TIA is unknown. Although studies within days of a stroke might be less representative of the baseline condition, treatment of SDB soon after stroke could potentially minimize further damage to injured neural tissue and improve outcome.

Treatment

As a consequence of brain vulnerability to hypoxia and cardiovascular instability, SDB might impede recovery of ischemic but not yet irreversibly damaged brain tissue. Furthermore, SDB can predispose to serious complications, such as aspiration or respiratory arrest, and it can contribute to short-term and long-term morbidity and mortality of stroke patients (see earlier).

Treatment of SDB in stroke patients represents a clinical, technical, and logistic challenge. Treatment strategies should always include prevention and early treatment of secondary complications (e.g. aspiration, respiratory infections, pain) and a cautious use or avoidance of alcohol and sedative-hypnotic drugs, which may all negatively affect breathing control during sleep. Patient positioning in the acute phase may influence oxygen saturation as well.[87]

CPAP is the treatment of choice for OSA. Intelligent CPAP systems can be used for simultaneous detection of upper airway obstructions (see Fig. 68–1) and treatment, which is made possible by automatic titration of CPAP pressure.[86] Compliance with CPAP has been reported by Wessendorf and colleagues to be as high as 70%[84]; however, most other groups reported lower percentages.[20] In our experience, only about 50% of stroke patients with SDB can be treated in the acute phase, and only about half of these patients stay on CPAP long term.[50] Compliance is certainly influenced by the spontaneous improvement of SDB after the acute phase (see earlier) and by the absence of daytime sleepiness in most patients with stroke and SDB.[88] Compliance can be expected to be a problem also in stroke patients with dementia, delirium, aphasia, anosognosia, or pseudobulbar or bulbar palsy.

In patients with central apneas and CSB, improvements of breathing disturbances may be achieved with oxygen.[62]

In addition, a novel method of ventilatory support called "adaptive servoventilation" may also be considered. In a recent study, it was shown that adaptive servoventilation prevented central apneas in stroke patients with heart failure more efficiently than CPAP or oxygen.[84]

Tracheostomy and mechanical ventilation may become necessary in patients with central hypoventilation. Control of central apneas and ataxic breathing usually requires assisted ventilation.

Recently, a few outcome studies have also appeared in patients with stroke and SDB. In a group of patients with stroke and SDB, Wessendorf and coworkers reported an improvement of subjective well-being (analysis of 41 points) and nighttime blood pressure (analysis of 16 points) with CPAP treatment over 10 days.[84] Sandberg and colleagues reported that treatment of SDB is associated with improved ratings for poststroke depression.[83]

SLEEP-WAKE DISTURBANCES

Epidemiology

Sleep-wake disturbances (SWD) are found in at least 20% to 40% of stroke patients. Patients present with increased sleep needs (hypersomnia), excessive daytime sleepiness, or insomnia.[89-92] The ill-defined symptom "fatigue" may be found in an even higher percentage of stroke patients (72% in a series of patients younger than 75 years with mild stroke[92]). Parasomnias and disturbances of time perception ("Zeitgefühl," Fig. 68–5) are observed less often.[93] Sometimes, the transition from wakefulness to sleep and vice versa is

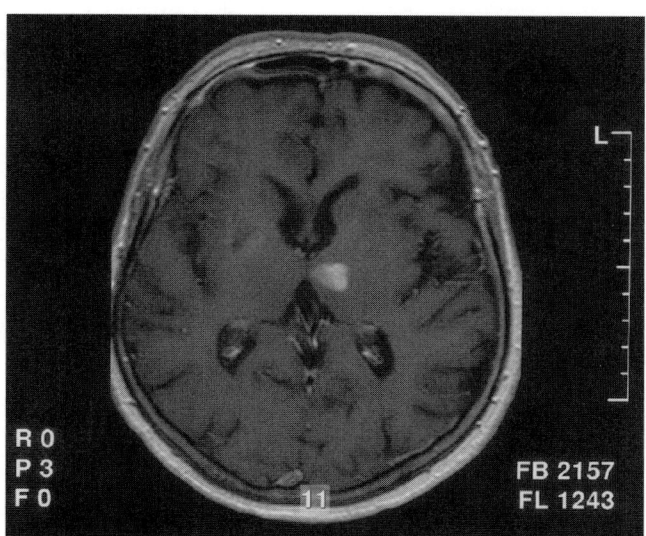

Figure 68–5. Dreamlike hallucinations after unilateral paramedian thalamic stroke in a 62-year-old patient with left paramedian thalamic stroke who presented clinically with confusional state, abulia, anomia, and moderate-severe amnesia, in the absence of major sleep-wake disturbances. In the first few days after hospital admission, recurrent episodes of visual and acoustic hallucinations in the form of human figures (mostly relatives, partial insight), seen on the right side of the visual field, which the patient describes as dreamlike. At 7 months after stroke, the patient had persistent memory problems and reported almost daily episodes of psychic hallucinations ("sensed presence") and a disturbed time perception ("Zeitgefühl"). (MRI picture courtesy Prof. A. Valavanis, Institute of Neuroradiology, University Hospital, Zürich, Switzerland.)

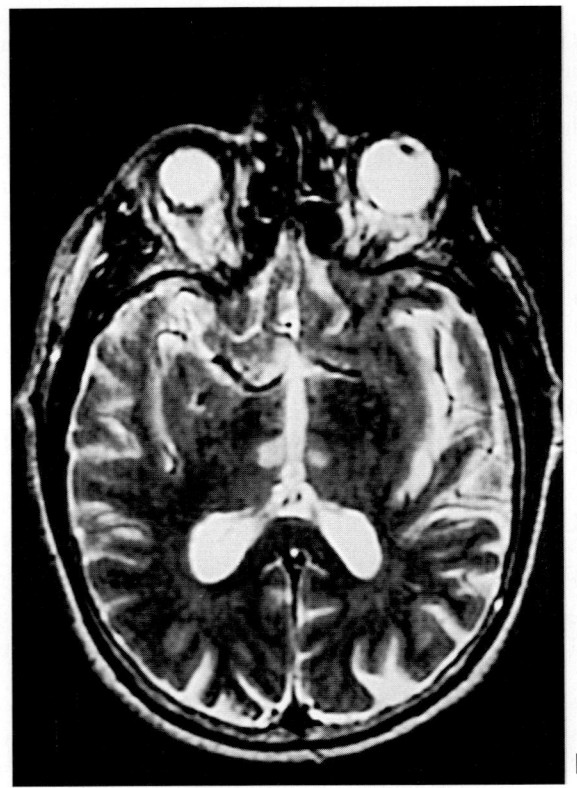

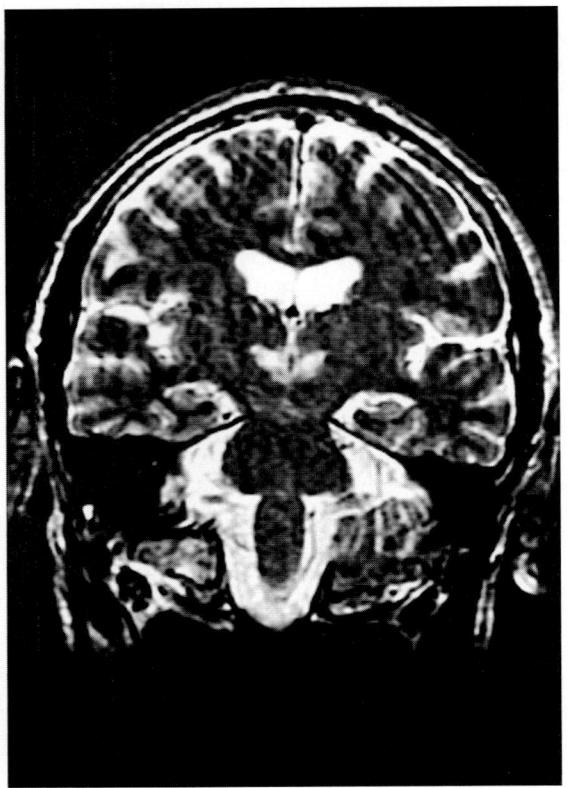

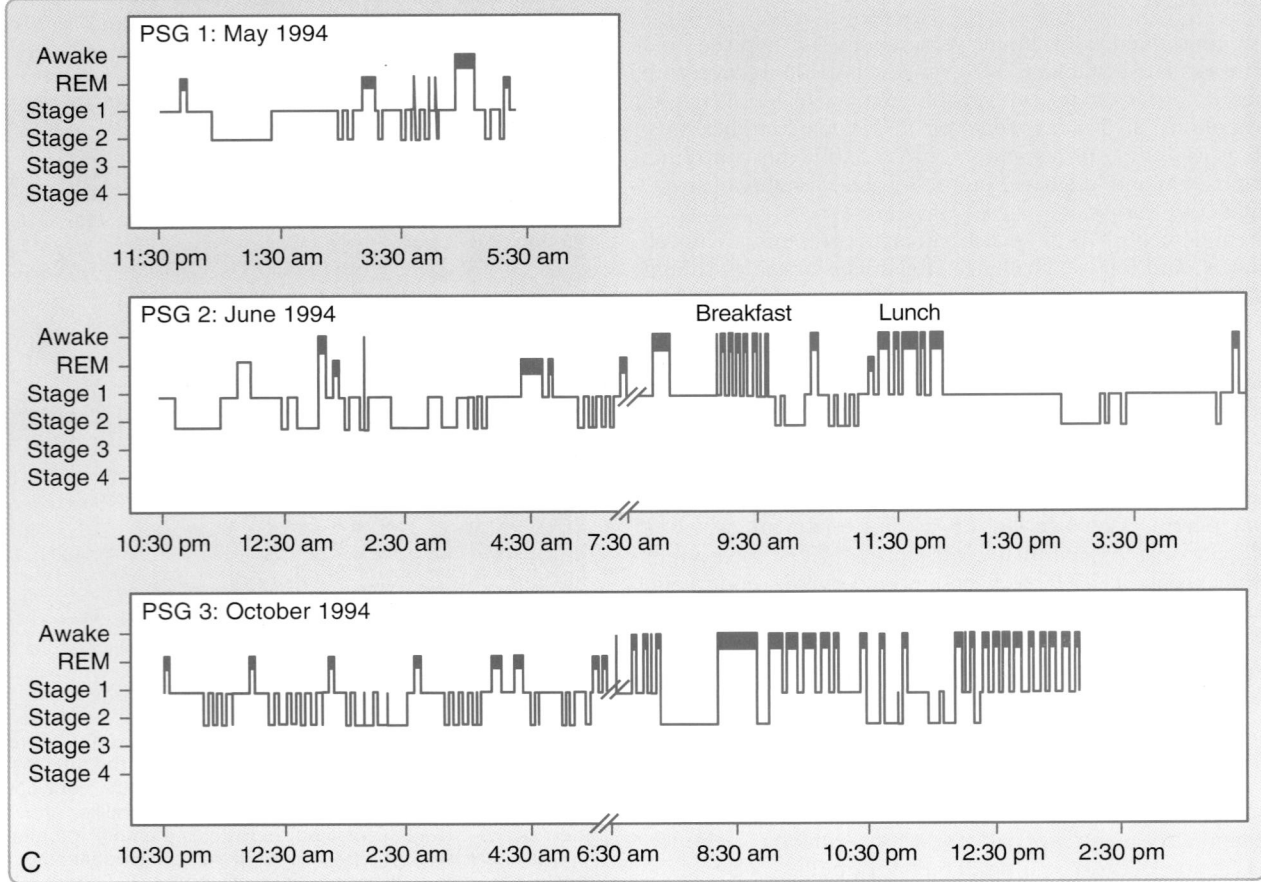

impaired and patients may present with a dream-reality confusion (oneiric state, see Chapter 78).

Pathogenesis

In patients with stroke, SWDs are often of multifactorial origin. In addition to brain damage, environmental factors including noise, light, and intensive medical monitoring may contribute to the development of SWD. Furthermore, SDB, cardiorespiratory disorders, seizures, infections, fever, and drugs may aggravate sleep fragmentation and result in sleep disturbances. Anxiety, depression, and "psychological stress" (difficulties in coping with stroke in general) frequently accompany or complicate stroke and may further contribute to SWD. The importance of these factors is well illustrated by the high occurrence rate of SWD even among intensive care unit (ICU) patients without brain damage.[94,95]

Hypersomnia and Excessive Daytime Sleepiness

A decreased arousal because of lesions involving the ascending reticular activating system (ARAS) is most commonly responsible for poststroke hypersomnia ("passive" hypersomnia). The most severe and persisting forms of "de-arousal" are seen in patients with bilateral lesions of the thalamus, subthalamic or hypothalamic area, tegmental midbrain, and upper pons, where fibers of the ARAS are bundled and can be severely injured even by single small lesions. Such strokes may cause initial coma or, conversely, manic delirium, hyperalertness, and insomnia before hypersomnia evolves. At the thalamomesencephalic level, the dorsomedial nucleus, intralaminar nuclei, centromedian nucleus, and cephalic portions of the ARAS are usually involved. Mental arousal seems to be affected more severely by medial lesions, whereas motor arousal is impaired more strongly by lateral lesions of the ARAS.[95,97]

Other areas in which stroke can occasionally produce hypersomnia include the striatum, tegmental pons, median regions of the medulla, and cerebral hemispheres (Fig. 68–6). Hypersomnia after hemispheric stroke usually implicates large lesions; such lesions occur on the left more than on the right and anteriorly more than posteriorly.[98] In large hemispheric strokes, de-arousal results from disruption of the ARAS in the upper brainstem secondary to vertical (transtentorial) or horizontal displacements of the brain due to brain edema. The occurrence of SWD following cortical or striatal strokes without mass effect[90,97] supports the assumption that the role of these structures is in maintenance of arousal and more generally in sleep-wake regulation.[99,100]

Hypersomnia with increased sleep per 24 hours ("active" hypersomnia) has occasionally been documented polysomnographically in patients with thalamic, mesencephalic, and pontine stroke.[101-103]

In a 23-year-old patient with bilateral diencephalic stroke following surgical removal of a craniopharyngeoma, cerebrospinal fluid (CSF) hypocretin-1 levels were low,[104] suggesting a link between poststroke hypersomnia and deficient hypocretin neurotransmission. However, in two patients with hypersomnia following thalamic and pontine stroke, respectively, we found normal CSF hypocretin-1 levels (unpublished data and Fig. 68–7, respectively).

Fatigue

Fatigue may develop following stroke in association with SWD (hypersomnia, excessive daytime sleepiness, and insomnia), mood and emotional changes, neurologic deficits, and neuropsychological sequelae. A significant overlap exists particularly between poststroke fatigue and poststroke depression. Psychological stress involving inadequate coping with stroke consequences in general probably plays an important role, as suggested by the absence of a correlation between poststroke fatigue and stroke size and site and by a high frequency of fatigue following myocardial infarction (without brain damage).[105] A dysfunction of ARAS and attentional circuits, as suggested also for some forms of poststroke hypersomnia (see earlier), has been postulated for poststroke fatigue.[91]

Insomnia

Mild to moderate insomnia is a frequent, usually nonspecific, often multifactorial complication of acute stroke. Recurrent arousals, sleep discontinuity, and sleep deprivation may result from preexisting disorders (e.g., heart failure, pulmonary disease), SDB, medications, infections and fever, inactivity, environmental disturbances (e.g., patient in ICU), stress, and depression. In a recent study the use of psychotropic agents, anxiety, dementia, preexisting insomnia, and stroke severity were found to be risk factors for poststroke insomnia.[89,106] Insomnia may also be related to brain damage itself, a situation for which the term *agrypnia* has been suggested.[107] Lesions in the dorsal or tegmental brainstem areas, in the paramedian or lateral thalamus, and also subcortically (Fig. 68–8) have been suggested as primary causes of poststroke insomnia.[10,13,108-111] The observation in some of these patients of rapid transitions from insomnia to hypersomnia emphasizes the dual role of such brain areas as thalamus, basal forebrain and pontomesencephalic-medullary junction in sleep-wake regulation.

Clinical Features

Hypersomnia and Excessive Daytime Sleepiness

Hypersomnia is defined clinically as a reduced latency to sleep, increased sleep, or excessive daytime sleepiness. In patients with strokes that affect the reticular formation or the

Figure 68–6. Hypersomnia after bilateral paramedian thalamic stroke in a 60-year-old man with severe hypersomnia (**A** and **B**). Initially sleep-like behavior occured over 19 hours per day. Clinically: upgaze palsy and amnesia. Prolonged polysomnography (PSG) is shown in **C**. PSG 1 shows disruption of nocturnal non–rapid eye movement (NREM) sleep with decreased spindling (automatic sleep spindle counts of 34 per hour on PSG 1 and 116 per hour on PSG 2). PSG 2 shows absent slow wave sleep and PSG 3 shows less severe disruption of rapid eye movement (REM) sleep. The patient was awake during only 30% of daytime hours, remaining for the most part "suspended" in a drowsy state (NREM stage 1 sleep). At 6 months, moderate hypersomnia persisted (sleeplike behavior more than 12 hours per day). Prolonged PSG showed some recovery of nocturnal spindling (162 per hour) and improved REM sleep but continued absence of slow wave sleep. During daytime there was an improvement in wakefulness (54% of time). (From Bassetti C, Mathis J, Gugger M, et al: Hypersomnia following paramedian thalamic stroke. Ann Neurol 1996;39:471-480.)

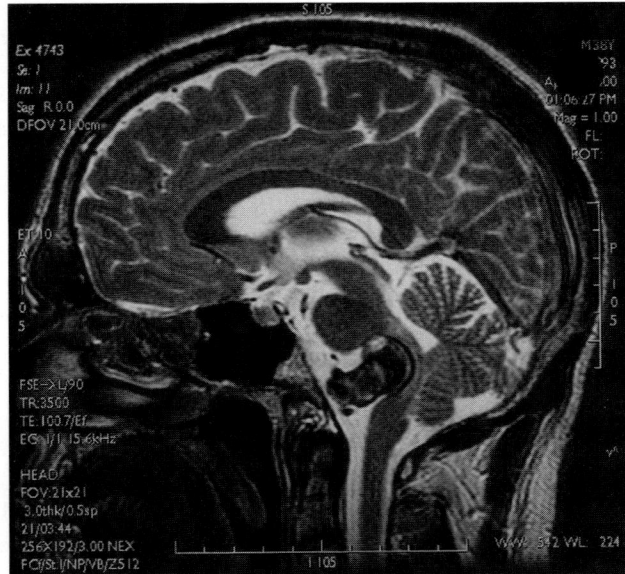

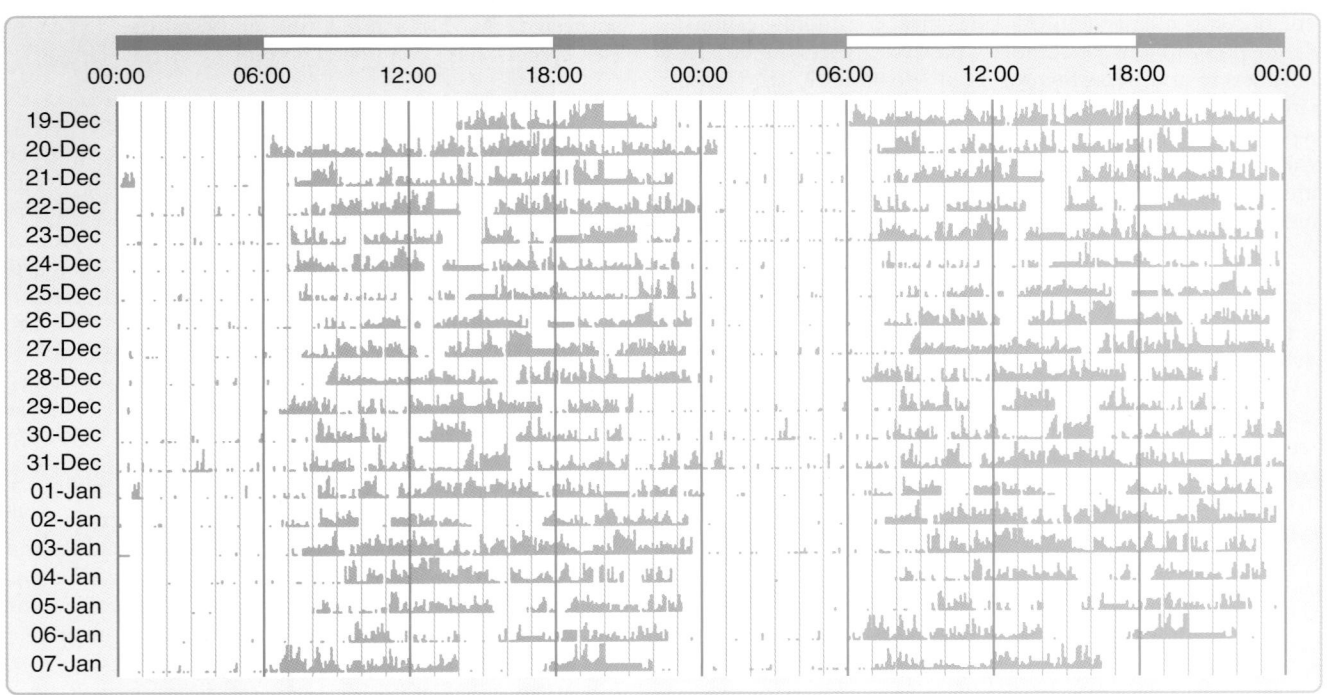

Figure 68–7. Hypersomnia and excessive daytime sleepiness in a 39-year-old male patient with pontomedullary ischemia following subarachnoid hemorrhage and embolization of a giant aneurysm of the basilar artery. Clinically brainstem syndrome with hiccup; left IX, X, and XII palsy; dysarthria; gait ataxia; and mild left hemiparesis. Postintervention severe excessive daytime sleepiness (Epworth sleepiness score = 23/24) and increased sleep needs (12 to 14 hours per day). Polysomnography shows sleep efficiency 97%, slow wave sleep 8% (of total sleep time), no sleep apnea, no periodic limb movements in sleep. Multiple Sleep Latency Test shows mean sleep latency 1 minute, no sleep-onset REM periods. Actigraphy shows time "asleep" (rest or sleep) during 43% of the recording time (2 weeks). Normal cerebrospinal fluid levels of hypocretin-1. Patient refused treatment for his hypersomnia. Jan, January; Dec, December. (From Bassetti C: Sleep and stroke. Semin Neurol [in press]) (MRI picture courtesy Prof. A. Valavanis, Institute of Neuroradiology, University Hospital, Zürich, Switzerland.)

paramedian thalamus, periods of hypersomnia may alternate with periods of insomnia (see earlier). Façon and coworkers described, for example, a 78-year-old patient with a tegmental mesencephalic infarct in whom severe, persistent hypersomnia was accompanied by an inversion of the sleep-wake cycle with nocturnal agitation.[112]

Poststroke hypersomnia, with or without excessive daytime sleepiness, is usually observed in association with thalamic (see Fig. 68–6), mesencephalic, or upper pontine strokes. Less commonly, strokes in the caudate, striatum, lower pons (see Fig. 68–7), medial medulla, and cerebral hemispheres (with or without mass effect, Fig. 68–9) may be complicated by hypersomnia (see earlier). In deep (subcortical) hemispheric and thalamic stroke, hypersomnia may correspond to a presleep behavior, during which patients yawn, stretch, close their eyes, curl up, and assume a normal sleeping

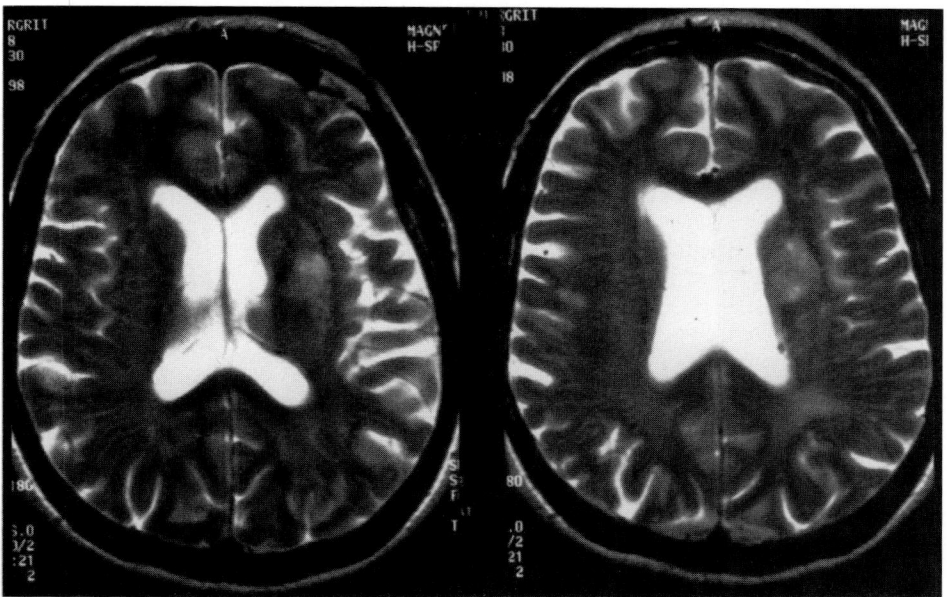

Figure 68–8. Insomnia after subcortical stroke in a 68-year-old female patient with left subcortical hemispheric stroke (corona radiata). Clinically mild right hemisyndrome, National Institutes of Health (NIH) Stroke Score = 6. In the first poststroke week almost complete insomnia and daytime excessive daytime sleepiness (EDS). Two weeks later, recovery from EDS and improvement of insomnia (2 to 3 hours of sleep per night). Normalization of sleep-wake functions after 4 weeks. (MRI picture courtesy Prof. G. Schroth, Institute of Neuroradiology, University Hospital, Bern, Switzerland.)

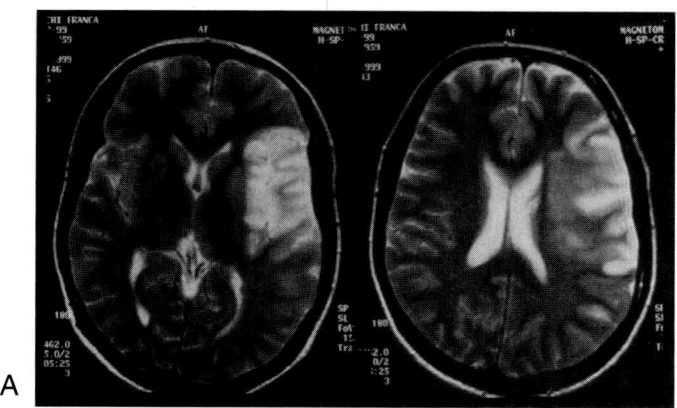

A

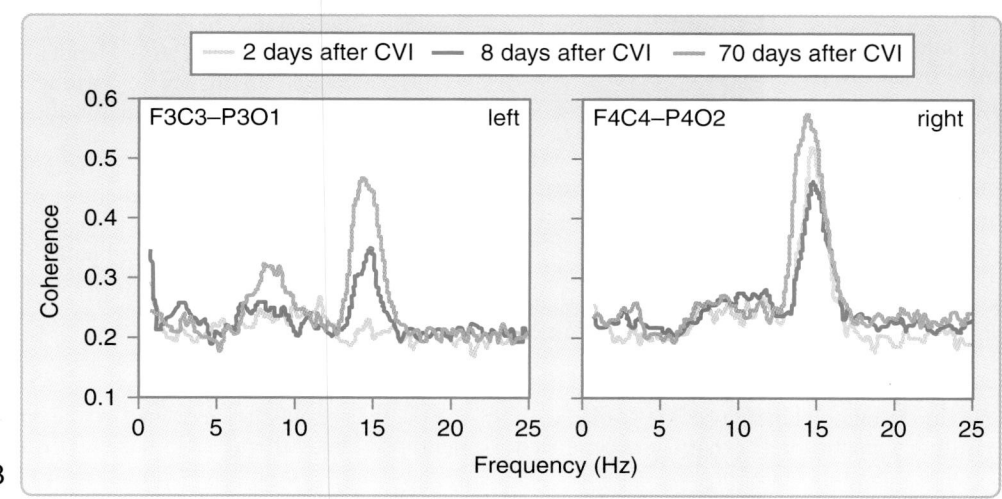

B

Figure 68–9. Hypersomnia and sleep architecture changes after middle cerebral artery stroke in a 39-year-old female patient with aphasia, right hemiparesis, depressed mood, and crying spells. National Institutes of Health (NIH) Stroke Score = 16. In the first 1 to 2 poststroke weeks, increase in sleep needs (12 hours per day as compared with 7 hours per day before stroke). Thereafter, mild excessive daytime sleepiness (Epworth sleepiness score = 12/24). At 12 months patient reported a decrease in sleep needs (10 hours per day). Repeated polysomnographic recordings (days 2, 8, and 70 after stroke) demonstrated a progressive recovery of spindling activity (coherent activity around 12 Hz) over both the affected *(left)* and the nonaffected *(right)* hemisphere. (Recording performed and scored with Dr. P. Achermann, Pharmacology and Toxicology Institute, University of Zürich, Switzerland. MRI pictures courtesy Prof. G. Schroth, Institute of Neuroradiology, University Hospital, Bern, Switzerland.)

posture, while complaining of a constant sleep urge.[113] Some of these patients are able to control this behavior when stimulated or given explicit, active tasks to perform. This presleep behavior may be compulsive in that removal of the patient from bed can result in repeated attempts to lie down and adopt a sleeping posture. However, during what appear to be daytime sleep periods, relatively quick responses to questions or requests suggest wakefulness. For this peculiar lack of autoactivation in the presence of preserved heteroactivation, Laplane suggested the term *athymormia* or "pure psychic akinesia."[114]

In some patients, hypersomnia evolves to extreme apathy with lack of spontaneity and initiative, slowness, poverty of movement, and catalepsy, a condition for which the term *akinetic mutism* was coined. Akinetic mutism, and its less severe form—usually referred to as *abulia*—may persist despite normalization of vigilance or even after appearance of insomnia. Some of these patients are eventually diagnosed to have poststroke fatigue (see later) or poststroke depression.

Hypersomnia with hyperphagia (Kleine-Levin–like syndrome) has been reported after multiple cerebral strokes.[115] In another patient, a narcolepsy-like syndrome with a classic tetrad of symptoms developed after cardiac arrest and pontine stroke despite the absence of the HLA-DR2 haplotype.[116]

Fatigue

A continuum exists between hypersomnia and fatigue, which is defined as a feeling of physical tiredness, exhaustion, and lack of energy accompanied by a strong desire for sleep, with usually normal or (paradoxically decreased) sleep propensity (as assessed, for example, by the Epworth sleepiness score or multiple sleep latency test). Fatigue may be more common in brainstem strokes.[91]

Insomnia

Insomnia is defined by a difficulty in initiating or maintaining sleep, early awakenings, and poor sleep quality. Particularly in patients with subcortical (see Fig. 68–8), thalamic, thalamo-mesencephalic, and large tegmental pontine stroke, insomnia may be accompanied by an inversion of the sleep-wake cycle, with insomnia and agitation during the night and hypersomnia during the day.[108,109,117,118]

In the literature, reports of stroke patients with well-documented insomnia are rare. Van Bogaert and colleagues reported, for example, a patient with pontomesencephalic stroke who presented an almost complete insomnia over more than two months.[108] Freemon and coworkers reported a patient with locked-in syndrome due to pontomesencephalic stroke who presented with polysomnographically confirmed insomnia, which was almost complete for more than one month.[13] Another patient reported by Girard's group had locked-in syndrome due to bilateral basal pontine stroke, with extension to the pontine tegmentum; this patient experienced nearly complete, polysomnographically proven insomnia for as long as 6 months.[109]

Parasomnias

The REM sleep behavior disorder, in which patients are thought to "act out" dreams, occurs because of a loss of physiological REM atonia. Although in most cases the cause of REM sleep behavior disorder is either an unknown or a neurodegenerative process, stroke in the tegmentum of the pons has also been implicated.[119,120]

A reduction in physiologic NREM sleep myoclonus was described in the hemiplegic limbs of a few stroke patients.[121] Periodic leg movements in sleep can increase or decrease after unilateral hemispheric stroke and may persist after spinal stroke.[122,123]

Hallucinations and Altered Dreaming
(See also Chapter 78)

Patients with strokes in the pontomesencephalic or mesencephalic tegmentum and in the paramedian thalamus may experience *peduncular hallucinosis of Lhermitte,* characterized by complex, often colorful, dreamlike visual hallucinations, particularly in the evening and at sleep onset (see Fig. 68–5).[124-127] Peduncular hallucinosis may represent a release of REM-sleep mentation. It can be associated with insomnia, but fortunately it resolves spontaneously in most cases.

The *Charles Bonnet syndrome* generally involves less-complex visual hallucinations that also occur in the setting of diminished arousal.[128] These hallucinations, or "release phenomena," after stroke that involves vision or visual field abnormalities (see Fig. 68–4), may be limited to a hemianopic field.[129-131]

Cessation or reduction of dreaming occurs in the *Charcot-Wilbrand syndrome* and is occasionally limited to alteration of the visual component of the dream (as in the original patient described by Charcot).[9,132] This syndrome can occur in patients with parieto-occipital, occipital, or deep frontal strokes, and the lesions are often bilateral.[133-137] Patients frequently, but not invariably, show deficient revisualization (referred to as *visual irreminiscence),* topographic amnesia, and prosopagnosia.[136] Conversely, REM sleep characteristics may be normal.[138] Hobson recently reported severe insomnia and loss of dreaming following lateral medullary stroke.[111]

Focal (temporal) seizures secondary to stroke can lead to the syndrome of dream-reality confusion or to *recurrent nightmares,* which may be more frequent in right-sided lesions and can be controlled with antiepileptics.[139] Hallucinations as well as increased frequency or vividness of dreaming may occur following stroke, particularly after thalamic, parietal, and occipital stroke.[133,140]

A few patients with severe motor deficits may report the persistence of normal motor functions during dreams for up to several years after stroke. Waking up in the morning may be a source of great distress in these patients. In other patients, motor handicap may, conversely, be incorporated into dreams within a few days of stroke onset.

Clinical Significance

SWDs after stroke are associated with neuropsychological and neuropsychiatric (depression, anxiety) disturbances and have a negative impact on rehabilitation, daily functioning, and quality of life.[89,141] Few studies have, so far, addressed this subject.[103,142]

Diagnosis

The recognition and diagnosis of poststroke SWD occurs primarily on clinical grounds. In stroke patients, the correlation of SWD and sleep EEG is, in fact, often poor.[90,103] In patients with poststroke hypersomnia, sleep EEG may, for example, reveal both a reduction and (less commonly) an increase[143] of NREM sleep or REM sleep, or both. In hypersomnia following thalamic infarcts, sleeplike behavior may be accompanied by a variety of EEG patterns including diffuse low-voltage alpha-beta activity, NREM stage 1 sleep, slow wave activity, and REM sleep.[101,103,144]

Multiple sleep latency testing is also often inadequate for assessment of poststroke SWD.[103] Actigraphy may be helpful to estimate changes in sleep–wake rhythms and sleep and rest needs following stroke (see Fig. 68–7).[145] Neuropsychological and psychiatric assessments should be considered in stroke patients who have SWD that cannot be explained.

Treatment

Hypersomnia and Excessive Daytime Sleepiness

Treatment of poststroke hypersomnia is often ineffective. In individual patients, some improvement has been seen in thalamic and mesencephalic stroke with amphetamines, modafinil, methylphenidate, and dopaminergic agents. In patients with paramedian thalamic stroke, treatment with 20-40 mg bromocriptine may improve apathy and presleep behavior.[113] Improvement of alertness with 200 mg modafinil has been reported in patients with bilateral mesodiencephalic paramedian infarct.[101,110] Treatment of an associated depression with stimulating antidepressants may also improve poststroke hypersomnia. A favorable influence on early post-stroke rehabilitation was reported for both methylphenidate (5-30 mg/day in a 3-week trial) and levodopa (100 mg/day in a 3-week trial), an effect that may at least in part be related to improved alertness in these patients.[146,147]

Insomnia and Parasomnias

Treatment of poststroke insomnia should include placement of patients in private rooms at night, protection from nocturnal noise and light, increased mobilization with exposure to light during the day, and, if necessary, temporary use of hypnotics that are relatively free of cognitive side effects, such as zolpidem or the benzodiazepines. It should be kept in mind, however, that benzodiazepines may not only enhance sedation and neuropsychological deficits in stroke patients but may also lead to the reemergence of other neurologic symptoms.[148]

Treatment of an associated depression with sedative anti-depressants may also improve poststroke insomnia. In a recent study of 51 stroke patients, 60 mg/day mianserin led to a better improvement of insomnia complaints than placebo, even in patients without associated depression.[106] Antidepressants may be preferable for long-term management of poststroke insomnia.

Clonazepam, 0.5 to 2.0 mg, a couple of hours before bed-time is the treatment of first choice in REM sleep behavior disorder. (I usually suggest taking this drug before bedtime because of its slow onset of action.)

SLEEP ARCHITECTURE CHANGES

Abnormalities in sleep macro- and microstructure are common after acute stroke but result only in part from acute brain damage. Changes in sleep architecture depend upon patient and health characteristics present before the stroke (e.g., age, respiratory disturbances), topography and extent of the lesion, associated complications of stroke (e.g., SDB, fever, infections, cardiovascular disturbances, depression, anxiety), drug treatment, and time after stroke onset. Even patients without brain damage who are admitted to an intensive care unit after acute myocardial infarction can have decreased total sleep time, sleep efficiency, REM sleep, and slow wave sleep.[94] Some changes in sleep architecture are more specifically related to brain damage (see later). Examples are persistent alteration of spindling and slow wave sleep in supratentorial stroke and persistent REM sleep abnormalities in infratentorial stroke.

In animal experiments as well as in patients with brain damage, changes in sleep behavior and sleep EEG do not always correlate.[149] In patients with diffuse cortical, thalamic, or pontine stroke, for example, sleep-wake physiological cyclicity in eyelid tone, respiration, temperature, and motor activity may occur despite prominent EEG abnormalities.

Supratentorial Strokes

Reductions in NREM sleep, total sleep time, and sleep efficiency can follow acute supratentorial stroke. Reduction of spin-dling can be ipsilateral[150] or bilateral to unilateral stroke (Fig. 68–10; see Fig. 68–9).[140,151-154] Rarely, spindling and slow wave sleep increase in the acute stage of large middle cerebral artery stroke.[140,155,156] In some such cases, the increase in scored slow wave sleep may reflect a generalized increase in delta activity during both sleep and wakefulness.[143,157] Changes in sleep spindle and slow wave activity usually, but not always, coincide.

Transient reductions in REM sleep can occur in the first days after supratentorial stroke.[140,151] Changes in REM sleep may persist after large hemispheric strokes with poor outcome.[156] Sawtooth waves can be decreased bilaterally in large hemispheric strokes, especially those that involve the right side.[140,151]

Changes in sleep architecture after hemispheric stroke probably do not have high localizing value.[151] Some reports have suggested, however, that right-sided strokes can prefer-entially decrease REM sleep and REM density[158,159] and that left-sided strokes can selectively reduce NREM stage 4 sleep.[158] Cortical blindness has been associated with a reduction of rapid eye movements.[160] Spindling and, to a lesser degree, slow wave activity and K complexes appear to be often (but not invariably) reduced in paramedian thalamic strokes.[101,103,144,161] In severe hypersomnia following paramedian thalamic strokes, prolonged polygraphic recordings can demonstrate an almost continuous state of light NREM stage 1 sleep (see Fig. 68–6), perhaps reflecting inability to make the transition from wakefulness to sleep or to produce full wakefulness.[103] In these patients, REM sleep can occur at night and during the day despite the absence of slow wave sleep.[103]

Like the EEG of wakefulness,[162] the sleep EEG undergoes a reorganization after acute damage, but data on this subject are scarce. Hachinski and colleagues reported that during clin-ical recovery from a large left hemispheric stroke, one patient had progressive deterioration of the sleep EEG on the right side.[140] In patients with paramedian thalamic stroke, recovery from hypersomnia may occur despite the persistence of sig-nificant NREM sleep changes.[101,144] In hemispheric stroke,

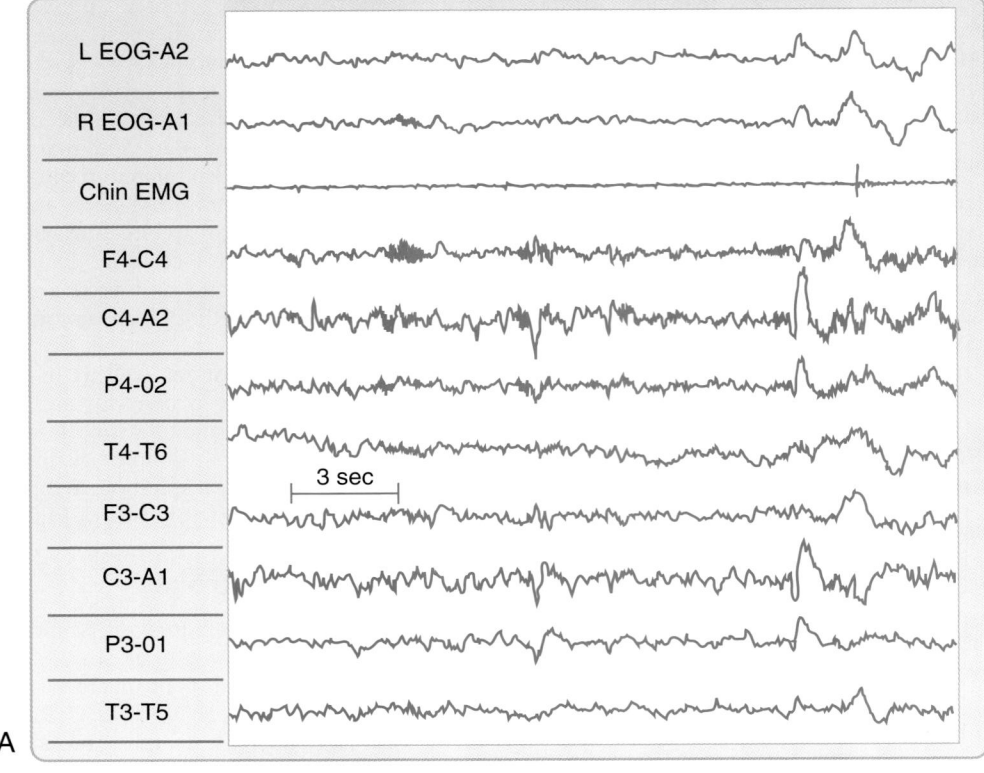

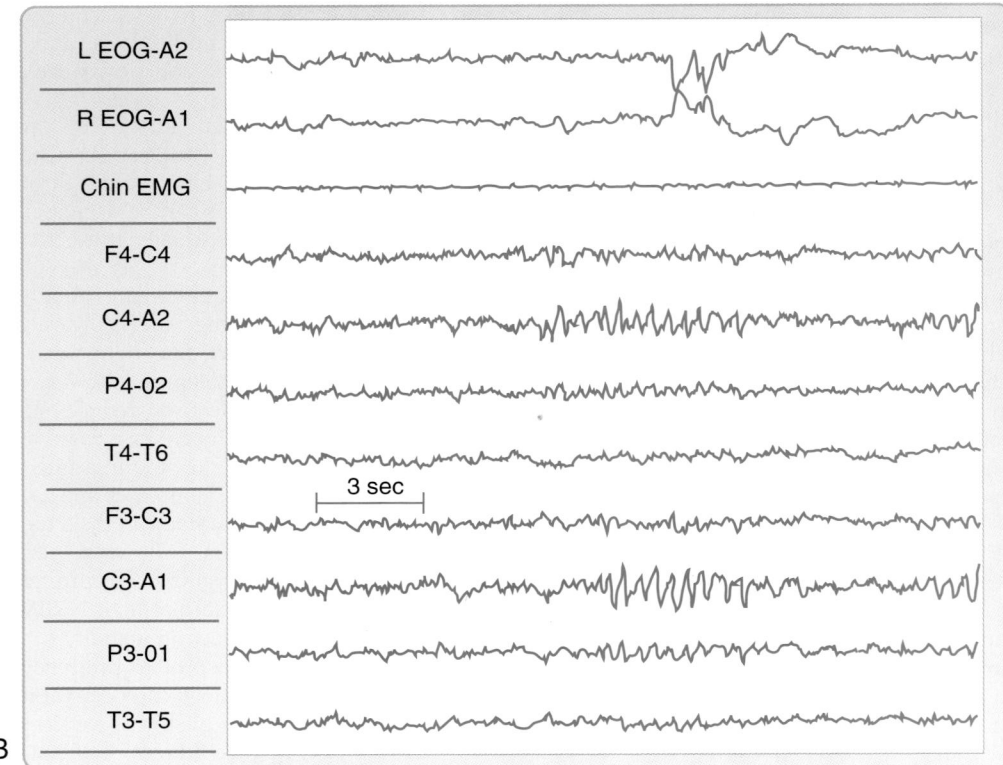

Figure 68–10. Sleep spindles and sawtooth waves after severe middle cerebral artery stroke in a 58-year-old man (Scandinavian Stroke Score of 33/58). Polysomnography 9 days after stroke shows mild obstructive sleep apnea (apnea-hypopnea index = 16). **A,** In NREM sleep, spindling decreased ipsilaterally, with three spindles per hour recorded at C3 and 172 per hour at C4. **B,** In REM sleep, sawtooth waves were symmetrical. EMG, electromyogram; EOG, electrooculogram.

conversely, sleep EEG changes (over the healthy hemisphere) usually recover over time, even in patients with severe strokes (>50 mL in volume).[90]

Infratentorial Strokes

Bilateral, paramedian infarcts in the pontine tegmentum or large bilateral infarcts in the ventrotegmental pons can lead to reduction in NREM and, especially, REM sleep.[102,163-168] Normal sleep EEG features such as sleep spindles, K complexes, and vertex waves may be completely lost.[164,169] Patients usually present clinically with crossed or bilateral sensorimotor deficits, oculomotor disturbances, and, at least initially, disturbances of consciousness. In rare instances, the only focal finding in a patient with severe sleep EEG changes may be a horizontal gaze palsy.[170] Patients with abnormal sleep architecture may complain of insomnia, but isolated REM sleep loss can persist for years without cognitive or behavioral consequences.[166,171]

Bilateral infarction near, but not in, the pontine tegmentum, or infarction of this area only on one side, usually does not alter sleep architecture. Reported examples have included patients with bilateral pontomedullary junction infarcts, bilateral ventral pontine infarcts with locked-in syndrome, and unilateral pontine tegmental infarcts.[169] However, exceptions have also been described: A patient with a hematoma in the left pontine tegmentum had an ipsilateral abnormal EEG during REM sleep despite normal rapid eye movements and muscle atonia,[172] and a patient with a hematoma in the right pontine tegmentum had increased NREM stages 1 and 2 sleep and increased total sleep time in the setting of clinical hypersomnia.[102]

Occasionally, NREM or REM sleep may be altered selectively. Strokes that affect the pontomesencephalic junction tegmentum and the raphe nucleus can lead to a moderate to marked decrease in total sleep time with reduction in NREM sleep but no major changes in REM sleep.[13] Infarctions of the paramedian thalamus and of the lower pons have been associated with absence of slow wave sleep but preservation of REM sleep and appearance of REM at sleep onset.[103,165] In contrast, infarction in the lower pons can cause an almost completely selective decrease in REM sleep.[169] Increased REM sleep has been noted in one patient who had an infarct in the mesencephalic tegmentum and in another with an infarct in the pontomedullary junction.[173] Increased NREM and (to a lesser extent) REM sleep has been reported in patients with mesencephalic stroke.[168]

Clinical Significance

Sleep architecture changes may have prognostic value.[90] Poor sleep efficiency and decreased spindles, K complexes, and slow wave sleep predict poor outcome when found after hemispheric strokes.[11,90,151,153]

CIRCADIAN ASPECTS AND DISTURBANCES

Ischemic stroke, like myocardial infarction and sudden death, occurs most frequently in the morning hours, particularly after awakening, between 6 AM and noon (Fig. 68–11). A meta-analysis of 31 publications reporting the circadian timing of 11,816 strokes found a 49% increase in strokes of all types (ischemic stroke, hemorrhagic stroke, TIA)

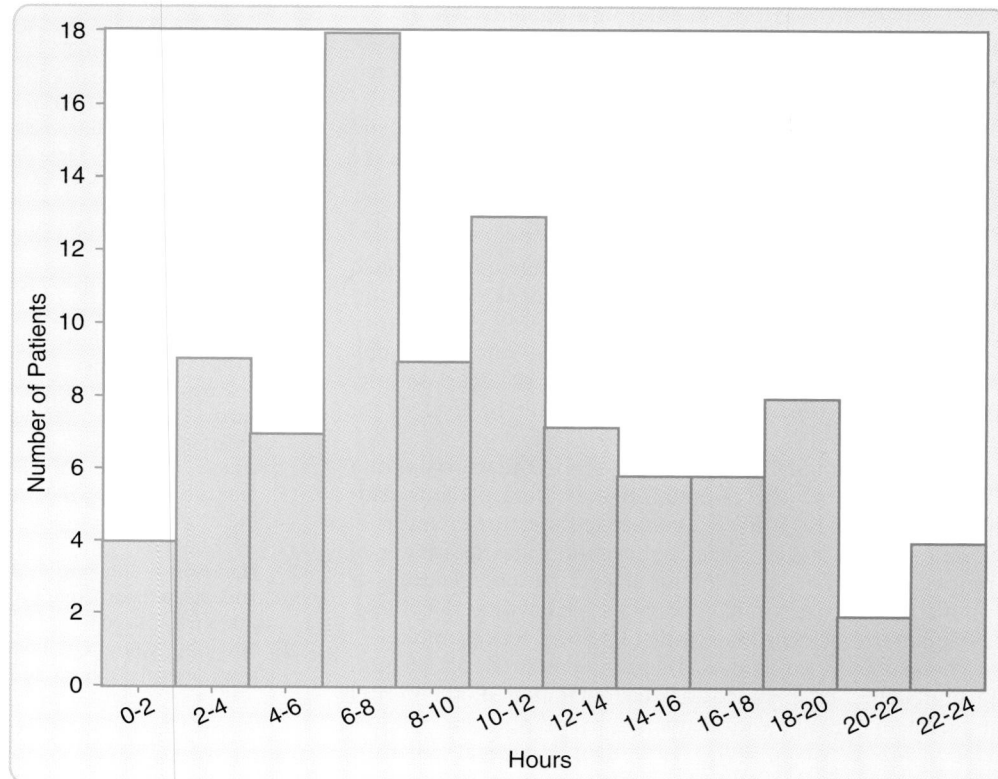

Figure 68–11. Estimated onset time of symptoms in 93 consecutive patients with acute ischemic stroke.

between 6 AM and noon.[174] Lago and colleagues found a higher frequency of strokes on awakening in thrombotic (29%) and lacunar (28%) strokes than in embolic strokes (19%).[175] There was no difference in circadian rhythm between first and recurrent strokes. Possible explanations for this pattern have focused on circadian or postural changes in platelet aggregation, thrombolysis, blood pressure, heart rate, and catecholamine levels that occur after awakening and resumption of physical and mental activities. In addition, the most prolonged REM-sleep period, during which autonomic system instabilities are known to occur,[43,44,176] occurs close to awakening. The highest incidence in the early hours of the morning can be overestimated because of patients who awaken with stroke. Treatment with aspirin does not modify the circadian pattern of stroke onset.[177,178]

Whereas intracerebral and subarachnoid hemorrhages rarely occur at night, 20% to 40% of ischemic strokes occur then.[179] This suggests that sleep may represent a vulnerable phase for a subset of patients with cerebrovascular disease. Two studies have found a significant difference in time of stroke onset between patients with and without sleep apnea.[49,50]

Acute brain infarction—particularly when the right hemisphere and the insula are affected—can disturb normal circadian variation in autonomic functions (e.g., heart rate, blood pressure) and contribute to increased poststroke cardiovascular morbidity.[180-183] Acute stroke also may alter other circadian functions such as sleep-related secretion of growth hormone and melatonin.[155,184]

Actigraphy in a few patients with acute stroke and multi-infarct dementia has shown sleep-wake cycles to be disrupted, shortened, lengthened, or shifted.[103,185] In patients who awaken from coma caused by large hemispheric or brainstem strokes, a polyphasic sleep-wake rhythm often precedes the reappearance of a monophasic rhythm.[96] Alteration of circadian variation in core temperature was documented in a patient with a focal (neoplastic) lesion of the ventral hypothalamus, but never following acute stroke.[186] However, hyperthermia—which may, in some cases, imply diencephalic dysfunction—correlates with stroke severity and represents a bad prognostic sign after acute stroke.[187]

PITFALLS AND CONTROVERSIES

The recognition of sleep-disordered breathing and sleep-wake disturbances in stroke patients requires specific attention to the corresponding symptoms and signs. Ambulatory respirographies, intelligent CPAP machines, and actigraphy are ancillary tests that can be considered in the acute setting. Conventional tests in a sleep laboratory should be reserved for unclear cases.

The etiology of SDB and SWD is often multifactorial. Brain damage per se may be essential in individual patients with specific forms of SDB, SWD, or sleep architecture changes.

Treatment strategies include prevention and treatment of complications of stroke, CPAP for SDB, dopaminergic drugs or stimulants for hypersomnia and excessive daytime sleepiness, and mianserin or benzodiazepine-like drugs for insomnia.

The main controversies relate to the potential role of snoring and SDB as independent risk factors for stroke, the impact of treatment of SDB on stroke incidence and outcome, and the relationship between SWDs (and their treatment) and the neuropsychological and neuropsychiatric outcome of stroke.

Clinical Pearl

Sleep-disordered breathing and sleep-wake disturbances are very common in patients who have ischemic stroke, and recognition of these problems requires a high degree of suspicion. Their treatment represents a new therapeutic window, which has a potential to improve survival, neurologic outcome, and quality of life following stroke. The study of SDB and SWD following focal brain damage may also offer new insights into the brain mechanisms that are responsible for breathing and sleep-wake functions.

REFERENCES

1. Diaz J, Sempere AP: Cerebral ischemia: New risk factors. Cerebrovasc Dis 2004;17(Suppl 1):43-50.
2. Adams HP, Bendixen BH, Kappelle LJ: Classification of subtype of acute ischemic stroke: Definitions for use in a multicenter clinical trial. Stroke 1993;24:35-41.
3. Cheyne J: A case of apoplexy in which the fleshy part of the heart was converted into fat. Dublin Hosp Rep 1818;2:216-218.
4. Broadbent WH: On Cheyne-Stokes respiration in cerebral hemorrhage. Lancet 1877;1:307-309.
5. Mitchell SW: Some disorders of sleep. Am J Med Sci 1890;100:109-127.
6. Goldblatt D: Undine's course. Semin Neurol 1995;15:218-223.
7. Lavie P: The touch of Morpheus: Pre–20th century accounts of sleepy patients. Neurology 1991;41:1841-1844.
8. Claude H, Loyez M: Ramollissement du noyau rouge. Rev Neurol (Paris) 1912;23:40-51.
9. Charcot M: Un cas de suppression brusque et isolée de la vision mentale des signes et des objets (formes et couleurs). Progr Med (Paris) 1883;2:568-571.
10. Lhermitte MJ: Syndrome de la calotte du pédoncule cérébral. Les troubles psycho-sensoriels dans les lésions mésocéphaliques. Rev Neurol (Paris) 1922;29:1359-1365.
11. Cress CH, Gibbs EL: Electroencephalographic asymmetry during sleep. Dis Nerv Syst 1948;9:327-329.
12. Chase TN, Moretti L, Prensky AL: Clinical and electroencephalographic manifestations of vascular lesions of the pons. Neurology 1968;18:357-368.
13. Freemon FR, Salinas-Garcia RF, Ward JW: Sleep patterns in a patient with brainstem infarction involving the raphe nucleus. Electroencephalogr Clin Neurophysiol 1974;36:657-660.
14. Bassetti C, Aldrich M, Chervin R, Quint D: Sleep apnea in the acute phase of TIA and stroke. Neurology 1996;47:1167-1173.
15. Dyken ME, Somers VK, Yamada T, et al: Investigating the relationship between stroke and obstructive sleep apnea. Stroke 1996;27:401-407.
16. Bassetti C, Aldrich M: Sleep apnea in acute cerebrovascular diseases. Final report on 128 patients. Sleep 1999;22:217-223.
17. Parra O, Arboix A, Bechich S, et al: Time course of sleep-related breathing disorders in first-ever stroke or transient ischemic attack. Am J Resp Crit Care Med 2000;161:375-380.
18. McArdle N, Riha RL, Vennelle M, et al: Sleep-disordered breathing as a risk factor for cerebrovascular disease. Stroke 2003;34:2916-2921.
19. Harbison J, Gibson GJ, Birchall D, et al: White matter disease and sleep-disordered breathing after acute stroke. Neurology 2003;61:959-963.
20. Hui DS, Choy DK, Wong LK, et al: Prevalence of sleep-disordered breathing and continuous positive airway pressure compliance: Results in Chinese patients with first-ever ischemic stroke. Chest 2002;122:852-860.
21. Harbison J, Ford GA, James OF, Gibson GJ: Sleep-disordered breathing following acute stroke. Q J Med 2002;95:741-747.

22. Szucs A, Vitrai J, Janszky J, et al: Pathological sleep apnoea frequency remains permanent in ischemic stroke and it is transient in haemorrhagic stroke. Eur Neurol 2002;47:15-19.

23. Urban P, Morgenstern M, Brause K, et al: Distribution and course of cortico-respiratory projections for voluntary activation in man. J Neurol 2002;249:734-744.

24. Morrell MJ, Heywood P, Moosawi SH, et al: Unilateral focal lesions in the rostral medulla influence chemosensitivity and breathing measured during wakefulness, sleep, and exercise. J Neurol Neurosurg Psychiatry 1999;67:637-645.

25. Brown HW, Plum F: The neurologic basis of Cheyne-Stokes respiration. Am J Med 1961;30:849-869.

26. Lee MC, Klassen AC, Resch JA: Respiratory pattern disturbances in ischemic cerebral vascular disease. Stroke 1974;5: 612-616.

27. Lee MC, Klassen AC, Heaney LM, Resch JA: Respiratory rate and pattern disturbances in acute brainstem infarction. Stroke 1976; 7:382-385.

28. Bassetti C, Aldrich MS, Quint D: Sleep-disordered breathing in patients with acute supra- and infratentorial stroke. Stroke 1997; 28:1765-1772.

29. Diehl M, Ragland DR: Habitual snoring as a risk factor for stroke: A meta-analysis. Sleep 2004;(in press).

30. Qreshi AI, Giles WH, Croft JB, Bliwise DL: Habitual sleep patterns and risk for stroke and coronary disease: A 10-year follow-up from NHANES I. Neurology 1997;48:904-910.

31. Davies DP, Rodgers H, Walshaw D, et al: Snoring, daytime sleepiness and stroke: A case-control study of first-ever stroke. J Sleep Res 2003;12:313-318.

32. Brooks D, Horner RL, Kozar L-F, et al: Obstructive sleep apnea as a cause of systemic hypertension. J Clin Invest 1997;99: 106-109.

33. Young T, Peppard P, Palta M, et al: Population-based study of sleep-disordered breathing as a risk factor for hypertension. Arch Intern Med 1997;157:1746-1752.

34. Peppard PE, Young T, Palta M, Skatrud J: Prospective study of the association between sleep-disordered breathing and hypertension. N Engl J Med 2000;342:1378-1384.

35. Shamsuzzaman AS, Gersh BJ, Somers VK: Obstructive sleep apnea. JAMA 2003;290:1906-1914.

36. Wessendorf TE, Thilmann AF, Wang YM, et al: Fibrinogen levels and obstructive sleep apnea in ischemic stroke. Am J Respir Crit Care Med 2000;162:2039-2042.

37. Silvestrini M, Rizzato B, Placidi F, et al: Carotid artery wall thickness in patients with obstructive sleep apnea syndrome. Stroke 2002;33:1782-1785.

38. Jennum P, Borgeson SE: Intracranial pressure and obstructive sleep apnea. Chest 1990;95:279-283.

39. Fischer AQ, Chaudhary BA, Taormina MA, Akhtar B: Intracranial hemodynamics in sleep apnea. Chest 1992;102:1402-1406.

40. Bonsignore MR, Marrone E, Insalaco G, Bonsignore G: The cardiovascular effects of obstructive sleep apnoeas: Analysis of pathogenetic mechanisms. Eur Respir J 1994;7:786-805.

41. Balfors EM, Franklin KA: Impairment of cerebral perfusion during obstructive sleep apneas. Am J Resp Crit Care Med 1994; 150:1587-1591.

42. Netzer N, Werner P, Jochums I, et al: Blood flow of the middle cerebral artery with sleep-disordered breathing. Stroke 1998; 29:87-93.

43. Jung HH, Bassetti C, Hess CW: Near cardiac death following REM-sleep: Polysomnographic report in a patient with sleep apnea and narcolepsy. J Sleep Res 1997;6:57-58.

44. Somers VK, Dyken ME, Clary MP, Abboud FM: Sympathetic neural mechanisms in obstructive sleep apnea. J Clin Invest 1995;96:1897-1904.

45. Diomedi M, Placidi F, Cupini LM, et al: Cerebral hemodynamics changes in sleep apnea and effect of continuous positive airway pressure. Neurology 1998;51:1051-1056.

46. Wardlaw JM: Cheyne-Stokes respiration in patients with acute ischaemic stroke: Observations on middle cerebral artery blood velocity changes using transcranial Doppler ultrasound. Cerebrovasc Dis 1993;3:377-380.

47. Hajak G, Klingelhöfer J, Schulz-Varszegi M, et al: Sleep apnea syndrome and cerebral hemodynamics. Chest 1996;110:670-679.

48. Beelke M, Angeli S, Del Sette M, et al: Obstructive sleep apnea can be provocative for right-to-left shunting through a patent foramen ovale. Sleep 2002;25:856-862.

49. Iranzo A, Santamaria J, Berenguer J, et al: Prevalence and clinical importance of sleep apnea in the first night after cerebral infarction. Neurology 2002;58:911-916.

50. Bassetti C, Milanova M, Gugger M: Sleep disordered breathing and acute stroke: Diagnosis, risk factors, treatment, and longterm outcome (submitted for publication).

51. Bruno A, Biller J, Adams JP, Corbett JJ: Retinal infarction during sleep and wakefulness. Stroke 1990;21:1494-1496.

52. Rivest J, Reiher J: Transient ischemic attacks triggered by symptomatic sleep apneas (abstract). Stroke 1987;18:293.

53. Pressman MR, Schetman WR, Figueroa WG, et al: Transient ischemic attacks and minor stroke during sleep. Stroke 1995; 26:2361-2365.

54. Pepperell JCT, Ramdassingh-Dow S, Crosthwaite N, et al: Ambulatory blood pressure after therapeutic and subtherapeutic nasal continuous positive airway pressure for obstructive sleep apnoea: A randomized parallel trial. Lancet 2001;359: 204-210.

55. Chin K, Ohi M, Kita H, et al: Effects of NCPAP therapy on fibrinogen levels in obstructive sleep apnea syndrome. Am J Resp Crit Care Med 1996;153:1972-1976.

56. Chin K, Kita H, Noguchi T, et al: Improvement of factor VII clotting activity following long-term NCPAP treatment in obstructive sleep apnoea syndrome. Q J Med 1998;91:627-633.

57. van der Werf SP, van den Broek HLP, Anten HWM, Bleijeberg G: Experience of severe fatigue long after stroke and its relation to depressive symptoms and disease characteristics. Eur Neurol 2001;45:28-33.

58. Power WR, Mosko SS, Sassin JF: Sleep-stage dependent Cheyne-Stokes respiration after cerebral infarct: A case study. Neurology 1982;32:763-766.

59. Chaudhary BA, Elguindi A, Kinf DW: Obstructive sleep apnea after lateral medullary syndrome. South Med J 1982;75:65-67.

60. Askenasy JJM, Goldhammer I: Sleep apnea as a feature of bulbar stroke. Stroke 1988;19:637-639.

61. Hermann DM, Kirov P, Gugger M, Bassetti C: Neurogenic Cheyne-Stokes breathing in acute ischemic stroke. Sleep Med 2003;4:S18.

62. Nachtmann A, Siebler M, Rose G, et al: Cheyne-Stokes respiration in ischemic stroke. Neurology 1995;45:820-821.

63. Plum F: Neurological integration of behavioral and metabolic control of breathing. In Porter R (eds): Ciba Foundation Breuer Centenary Symposium: Breathing. London, J and A Churchill, 1970, pp 159-181.

64. Munschauer FE, Mador J, Ahuja A, Jacobs L: Selective paralysis of voluntary but not limbically influenced automatic respiration. Arch Neurol 1991;48:1190-1192.

65. McNealy DE, Plum F: Brainstem dysfunction with supratentorial mass lesions. Arch Neurol 1962;7:10-32.

66. Plum F, Posner JB: The Diagnosis of Stupor and Coma. 3rd ed. Philadelphia, FA Davis, 1980.

67. North JB, Jennett S: Abnormal breathing patterns associated with acute brain damage. Arch Neurol 1974;31:338-344.

68. Siderowf LJ, Balcer LJ, Kenyon LC, et al: Central neurogenic hyperventilation in an awake patient with pontine glioma. Neurology 1996;46:1160-1162.

69. Ducros L, Vahedi K, Similowski T, et al: Uncontrollable high-frequency tachypnea in a case of unilateral medial medullary infarct. Intensive Care Med 2003;29:841-844.

70. Rout MW, Lane DJ, Wollner L: Prognosis in acute cerebrovascular accidents in relation to respiratory pattern and blood gas tensions. BMJ 1971;3:7-9.

71. Plum F, Alvord EC: Apneustic breathing in man. Arch Neurol 1964;10:101-112.

72. Hunziker A, Frick P, Regli F, Rossier PH: Zentralbedingte chronische alveoläre Hypoventilation bei Malazien in der Medulla Oblongata. Beitrag zum Wallenberg-Syndrom. Dtsch Med Wochenschr 1964;89:676-680.

73. Levin BE, Margolis G: Acute failure of automatic respirations secondary to unilateral brainstem infarct. Ann Neurol 1977;1:583-586.

74. Beal MF, Richardson EP, Brandstetter R, et al: Localized brainstem ischemic damage and Ondine's curse after near-drowning. Neurology 1983;33:717-721.

75. Bogousslavsky J, Khurana R, Deruaz JP, et al: Respiratory failure and unilateral caudal brainstem infarction. Ann Neurol 1990;28:668-673.

76. Howard RS, Thorpe J, Barker R, et al: Respiratory insufficiency due to high anterior cervical cord infarction. J Neurol Neurosurg Psychiatry 1998;64:358-361.

77. Newsom-Davis J: Autonomous breathing. Arch Neurol 1974;30:480-483.

78. Manconi M, Mondini S, Fabiani A, et al: Anterior spinal artery syndrome complicated by the Ondine curse. Arch Neurol 2003;60:1787-1790.

79. Spriggs DA, French JM, Murdy JM, et al; Snoring increases the risk of stroke and adversely affects prognosis. Q J Med 1992;303:555-562.

80. Good DC, Henkle JQ, Gelber D, et al: Sleep-disordered breathing and poor functional outcome after stroke. Stroke 1996;27:252-259.

81. Kaneko Y, Hajek V, Zivanovic V, et al: Relationship of sleep apnea to functional capacity and length of hospitalization following stroke. Sleep 2003;26:293-297.

82. Turkington PM, Bamford CR, Wanklyn P, Elliott MW: Prevalence and predictors of upper airway obstruction in the first 24 hours after acute stroke. Stroke 2002;53:2037-2042.

83. Sandberg O, Franklin KA, Bucht G, et al: Nasal continuous positive airway pressure in stroke patients with sleep apnoea: A randomized treatment study. Eur Respir J 2001;18:619-622.

84. Wessendorf TE, Wang YM, Thilmann AF, et al: Treatment of obstructive sleep apnoea with nasal continuous positive airway pressure. Eur Respir J 2001;18:623-629.

85. Roffe C, Sills S, Halim M, et al: Unexpected nocturnal hypoxia in patients with acute stroke. Stroke 2003;34:2641-2645.

86. Disler P, Hansford A, Skelton J, et al: Diagnosis and treatment of obstructive sleep apnea in a stroke rehabilitation unit: A feasibility study. Am J Phys Med Rehabil 2002;81:622-625.

87. Rowat AM, Wardlaw JM, Dennis M, Warlow C: Patient positioning influences oxygen saturation in the acute phase of stroke. Cerebrovasc Dis 2001;12:66-72.

88. Barbé F, Mayoralas LR, Duran J, et al: Treatment with continuous positive airway pressure is not effective in patients with sleep apnea but no daytime sleepiness. Ann Int Med 2001;134:1015-1023.

89. Leppävuori A, Pohjasvaara T, Vataja R, et al: Insomnia in ischemic stroke patients. Cerebrovasc Dis 2002;14:90-97.

90. Vock J, Achermann P, Bischof M, et al: Evolution of sleep and sleep EEG after hemispheric stroke. J Sleep Res 2002;11:331-338.

91. Staub F, Bogousslavksy J: Fatigue after stroke: A major but neglected issue. Cerebrovasc Dis 2001;12:75-81.

92. Carlsson GE, Moller A, Blomstrand C: Consequences of mild stroke in persons <75 years—a 1 year follow-up. Cerebrovasc Dis 2003;16:383-388.

93. Goody W: Disorders of the time sense. In Vinken PJ, Bruyn GW (eds): Handbook of Clinical Neurology. Amsterdam, Elsevier–North Holland,1969, pp 229-250.

94. Broughton R, Baron R: Sleep patterns in the intensive care unit and on the ward after acute myocardial infarction. Electroencephalogr Clin Neurophysiol 1978;45:348-360.

95. Krachmann SL, D'Alonzo GE, Criner GJ: Sleep in the intensive care unit. Chest 1995;107:1713-1720.

96. Passouant P, Cadilhac J, Baldy-Moulinier M: Physio-pathologie des hypersomnies. Rev Neurol (Paris)1967;116:585-629.

97. Castaigne P, Escourolle R: Etude topographique des lésions anatomiques dans les hypersomnies. Rev Neurol (Paris) 1967;116:547-584.

98. Albert ML, Silverberg R, Reches A, Bernam M: Cerebral dominance for consciousness. Arch Neurol 1976;33:453-454.

99. Villablanca JR, Marcus RJ, Olmstead CE: Effect of caudate nuclei or frontal cortex ablations in cats. II. Sleep-wakefulness, EEG, and motor activity. Exp Neurol 1976;53:31-50.

100. Sterman MB, Clemente CD: Forebrain inhibitory mechanisms: Sleep patterns induced by basal forebrain stimulation in the behaving cat. Exp Neurol 1962;6:103-117.

101. Bastuji H, Nighoghossian N, Salord F, et al: Mesodiencephalic infarct with hypersomnia: Sleep recording in two cases. J Sleep Res 1994;3(Suppl 1):16.

102. Arpa J, Rodriguez-Albarino R, Izal E, et al: Hypersomnia after tegmental pontine hematoma: Case report. Neurologia (Spain) 1995;10:140-144.

103. Bassetti C, Mathis J, Gugger M, et al: Hypersomnia following thalamic stroke. Ann Neurol 1996;39:471-480.

104. Scammell TE, Nishino S, Mignot E, Saper CB: Narcolepsy and low CSF orexin (hypocretin) concentration after stroke. Neurology 2001;56:1751-1753.

105. Leegard OF: Diffuse cerebral symptoms in convalescents from cerebral infarction and myocardial infarction. Acta Neurol Scand 1983;67:348-355.

106. Palomäki H, Berg AT, Meririnne E, et al: Complaints of post-stroke insomnia and its treatment with mianserin. Cerebrovasc Dis 2003;15:56-62.

107. Autret A, Henry-Le Bras F, Duvelleroy-Hommet C, et al: Les agrypnies. Neurophysiol Clin 1995;25:360-366.

108. Van Bogaert M: Syndrome de la calotte protubérantielle avec myoclonie localisée et troubles du sommeil. Rev Neurol (Paris) 1926;45:977-988.

109. Girard P, Gerrest F, Tommasi M, Rouves L: Ramollissement géant du pied de la protubérance. Lyon Med 1962;14:877-892.

110. Autret A, Lucas B, Mondon K, et al: Sleep and brain lesions: A critical review of the literature and additional new cases. Neurophysiol Clin 2001;31:356-375.

111. Hobson AJ: Sleep and dream suppression following a lateral medullary infarction: A first-person account. Conscious Cogn 2002;11(3):377-390.

112. Façon E, Steriade M, Wertheim N: Hypersomnie prolongée engendrée par des lésions bilatérale du système activateur médial. Le syndrome thrombotique de la bifurcation du tronc basilaire. Rev Neurol (Paris) 1958;98:117-133.

113. Catsman-Berrevoets CE, Harskamp F: Compulsive pre-sleep behaviour and apathy due to bilateral thalamic stroke. Neurology 1988;38:647-649.

114. Laplane D: La perte d'autoactivation psychique. Rev Neurol (Paris) 1990;146:397-404.

115. Drake ME: Kleine-Levine syndrome after multiple cerebral infarctions. Psychosomatics 1987;28:329-333.

116. Rivera VM, Meyer JS, Hata T, et al: Narcolepsy following cerebral hypoxic ischemia. Ann Neurol 1986;19:505-508.

117. Garrel S, Fau R, Perret J, Chatelain R: Troubles du sommeil dans deux syndromes vasculaires du tronc cérébral dont l'un anatomo-clinique. Rev Neurol (Paris) 1966;115:575-584.

118. Rondot P, Recondo J, Davous P, et al: Infarctus thalamique bilatéral avec mouvements abnormaux et amnésie durable. Rev Neurol (Paris) 1986;142:389-405.

119. Culebras A, Moore JT: Magnetic resonance findings in REM sleep behavior disorder. Neurology 1989;39:1519-1523.

120. Kimura K, Tachibana N, Kohyama J, et al: A discrete pontine ischemic lesion could cause REM sleep behavior disorder. Neurology 2000;55:894-895.

121. Dagnino N, Loeb C, Massazza G, Sacco G: Hypnic physiological myoclonias in man: An EEG-EMG study in normals and neurological patients. European Neurology 1969;2:47-58.

122. Dyken ME, Rodnitzky RL: Periodic, aperiodic, and rhythmic motor disorders of sleep. Neurology 1992;42 (Suppl 6):68-74.

123. Yokota T, Hirose K, Tanabe H, Tsukagoshi H: Sleep-related periodic leg movements (nocturnal myoclonus) due to spinal cord lesion. J Neurol Sci 1991;104:13-18.

124. Van Bogaert L: Syndrome inférieur du noyau rouge, troubles psycho-sensoriels d'origine mésocéphalique. Rev Neurol (Paris) 1924;31:417-423.

125. Van Bogaert L: L'hallucinose pédonculaire. Rev Neurol (Paris) 1927;43:608-617.

126. Geller TJ, Bellur SN: Peduncular hallucinosis: Magnetic resonance imaging confirmation of mesencephalic infarction during life. Ann Neurol 1987;21:602-604.

127. Manford M, Andermann F: Complex visual hallucinations. Brain 1998;121:1819-1840.

128. Teunisse RJ, Cruysberg JR, Hoefnagels WH, et al: Visual hallucinations in psychologically normal people: Charles Bonnet's syndrome. Lancet 1996;347:794-797.

129. Martin R, Bogousslavsky J, Regli F: Striatocapsular infarction and "release" visual hallucinations. Cerebrovasc Dis 1992;2:111-113.

130. Vaphiades MS, Celesia GG, Brigell MG: Positive spontaneous visual phenomena limited to the hemianopic field in lesions of central visual pathways. Neurology 1996;47:408-417.

131. Lepore FE: Spontaneous visual phenomena with visual loss: 104 patients with lesions of retinal and neural afferent pathways. Neurology 1990;40:444-447.

132. Wilbrand H: Ein Fall von Seelenblindheit und Hemianopsie mit Sectionsbefund. Dtsch Z Nervenheilkd 1887;2:361-387.

133. Grünstein AM: Die Erforschung der Träume als eine Methode der topischen Diagnostik bei Grosshirnerkrankungen. Z Gesamte Neurol Psychiatr 1924;93:416-420.

134. Gloning K, Sternbach I: Über das Träumen bei zerebralen Herdläsionen. Wien Z Nervenheilkd 1953;6:302-329.

135. Murri L, Arena R, Siciliano G, et al: Dream recall in patients with focal cerebral lesions. Arch Neurol 1984;41:183-185.

136. Murri L, Massetani R, Siciliano G, et al: Dream recall after sleep interruption in brain-injured patients. Sleep 1985;8:356-362.

137. Solms M: The neuropsychology of dreams. Mahwah, NJ, Lawrence Erlbaum, 1997.

138. Bischof M, Bassetti C: Total dream loss: A distinct neuropsychological dysfunction after bilateral PCA stroke. Ann Neurol 2004;56:583-586.

139. Boller F, Wright D, Cavalieri R, Mitsumoto H: Paroxysmal "nightmares." Neurology 1975;25:1026.

140. Hachinski V, Mamelak M, Norris JW: Clinical recovery and sleep architecture degradation. Can J Neurol Sci 1990;17:332-335.

141. Wyller TB, Holmen J, Laake P, Laake K: Correlates of subjective well-being in stroke patients. Stroke 1998;29:363-367.

142. Ron S, Algom D, Hary D, Cohen M: Time-related changes in the distribution of sleep stages in brain injured patients. Electroencephalogr Clin Neurophysiol 1980;48:432-441.

143. Müller C, Achermann P, Bischof M, et al: Visual and spectral analysis of sleep EEG in acute hemispheric stroke. Eur Neurol 2002;48:164-171.

144. Guilleminault C, Quera-Salva MA, Goldberg MP: Pseudohypersomnia and pre-sleep behaviour with bilateral paramedian thalamic lesions. Brain 1993;116:1549-1563.

145. Bassetti C, Gugger M, Bischof M, et al: The narcoleptic borderland: A multimodal diagnostic approach including cerebrospinal fluid levels of hypocretin-1 (orexin A). Sleep Med 2003;4:7-12.

146. Grade C, Redford B, Chrostowski J, et al: Methylphenidate in early poststroke recovery. A double-blind, placebo controlled study. Arch Phys Med Rehab 1998;79:1047-1050.

147. Scheidtmann K, Fries W, Muller F, Koenig E: Effect of levodopa in combination with physiotherapy on functional recovery after stroke: a prospective, randomized, double-blind study. Lancet 2001;358:787-790.

148. Lazar RM, Fitzsimmons BF, Marshall RS, et al: Reemergence of stroke deficits with midazolam challenge. Stroke 2002;33:283-285.

149. Feldman SM, Waller HJ: Dissociation of electrocortical activation and behavioural arousal. Nature 1962;4861:1320-1322.

150. Greenberg R: Cerebral cortex lesions: The dream process and sleep spindles. Cortex 1966;2:357-366.

151. Bassetti C, Aldrich MS: Sleep electroencephalogram changes in acute hemispheric stroke. Sleep Med 2001;2:185-194.

152. Hachinski VC: Sleep morphology and prognosis in acute cerebrovascular lesions. In Meyer J, Lechner H, Reivich M (eds): Cerebral Vascular Disease. Amsterdam, Excerpta Medica, 1977, pp 69-71.

153. Hachinski VC, Mamelak M, Norris JW: Prognostic value of sleep morphology in cerebral infarction. In Meyer J, Lechner H, Reivich M (eds): Cerebral Vascular Disease. Amsterdam, Excerpta Medica, 1977, pp 287-291.

154. Gottselig J, Bassetti C, Achermann P: Power and coherence of sleep spindle activity following hemispheric stroke. Brain 2002;125:373-385.

155. Culebras A, Miller M: Absence of sleep-related elevation of growth hormone level in patients with stroke. Arch Neurol 1983;40:283-286.

156. Giubilei F, Iannilli M, Vitale A, et al: Sleep patterns in acute ischemic stroke. Acta Neurol Scand 1992;86:567-571.

157. Yokohama E, Nagata K, Hirata Y, et al: Correlation of EEG activities between slow-wave sleep and wakefulness in patients with supratentorial stroke. Brain Topogr 1996;8:269-273.

158. Körner E, Flooh E, Reinhart B, et al: Sleep alterations in ischemic stroke. Eur Neurol 1986;25:104-110.

159. Ribeiro Pinto L, Baptistas Silva A, Tufik S: Rapid eye movements density in patients with stroke (abstract). Sleep Res 1994:076.

160. Appenzeller O, Fischer AP: Disturbances of rapid eye movements during sleep in patients with lesions of the nervous system. Electroencephalogr Clin Neurophysiol 1968;25:29-35.

161. Santamaria J, Pujol M, Orteu N, et al: Unilateral thalamic stroke does not decrease ipsilateral sleep spindles. Sleep 2000;23:333-339.

162. Hirose G, Saeki M, Kosoegawa H, et al: Delta waves in the EEGs of patients with intracerebral hemorrhage. Arch Neurol 1981;38:170-175.

163. Cummings JL, Greenberg R: Sleep patterns in the "locked-in" syndrome. Electroencephalogr Clin Neurophysiol 1977;43:270-271.

164. Autret A, Laffont F, De Toffol B, Cathala HP: A syndrome of REM and non-REM sleep reduction and lateral gaze paresis after medial tegmental pontine stroke. Arch Neurol 1988;45:1236-1242.

165. Tamura K, Karacan I, Williams RL, Meyer JS: Disturbances of the sleep-waking cycle in patients with vascular brain stem lesions. Clin Electroencephalogr 1983;14:35-46.

166. Gironell A, de la Calzada MD, Sagales T, Barraquer-Bordas L: Absence of REM sleep and altered non-REM sleep caused by a hematoma in the pontine tegmentum. J Neurol Neurosurg Psychiatry 1995;59:195-196.

167. Schäfer D, Bianchi O, Greulich W, et al: Störungen von Schlaf und Atmung bei Patienten mit Hirnstammläsionen. Wien Med Wochenschr 1996;146:296-298.

168. Beck U, Kendel K: Polygraphische Nachtsschlafuntersuchugnen bei Patienten mit Hirnstammläsionen. Arch Psychiat Nervenkr 1971;214:331-346.

169. Markand ON, Dyken ML: Sleep abnormalities in patients with brainstem lesions. Neurology 1976;26:769-776.

170. Vallderiola F, Santamaria J, Graus F, Tolosa E: Absence of REM sleep, altered NREM sleep and supranuclear horizontal gaze palsy caused by a lesion of the pontine tegmentum. Sleep 1993;16:184-188.

171. Lavie P, Pratt H, Scharf B, et al: Localized pontine lesion: Nearly total absence of REM sleep. Neurology 1984;34:118-120.

172. Kushida CA, Rye DB, Nummy D: Cortical asymmetry of REM sleep EEG following unilateral pontine hemorrhage. Neurology 1991;41:598-601.

173. Popoviciu L, Asgian B, Corfarici D, et al: Anatomoclinical and polygraphic features in cerebrovascular diseases with disturbances of vigilance. In Tirgu-Mures L, Popoviciu L, Asgia B, et al (eds): Sleep 1978: Fourth European Congress on Sleep Research. New York, Karger, 1980, pp 165-169.

174. Elliott WJ: Circadian variation in the timing of stroke onset: A meta-analysis. Stroke 1998;29:992-996.

175. Lago A, Geffner D, Tembl J, et al: Circadian variation in acute ischemic stroke. A hospital-based study. Stroke 1998;29:1873-1875.

176. Verrier RL, Muller JE, Hobson JA: Sleep, dreams, and sudden death: The case for sleep as an autonomic stress test for the heart. Cardiovascular Research 1996;31:181-211.

177. Marsh EE, Biller J, Adams HP, et al: Circadian variation in onset of acute ischemic stroke. Arch Neurol 1990;47:1178-1180.

178. Bassetti C, Aldrich M: Night time versus daytime transient ischemic attack and ischemic stroke: A prospective study of 110 patients. J Neurol Neurosurg Psychiatry 1999;67:463-467.

179. Wroe SJ, Sandercock P, Bamford J, et al: Diurnal variation in incidence of stroke: Oxfordshire community stroke project. BMJ 1992;304:155-157.

180. Sander D, Klingelhöfer J: Changes of circadian blood pressure patterns and cardiovascular parameters indicate lateralization of sympathetic activation following hemispheric brain infarction. J Neurol 1995;242:313-318.

181. Yoon BW, Morillo CA, Cechetto DF, Hachinski V: Cerebral hemispheric lateralization in cardiac autonomic control. Arch Neurol 1997;54:741-744.

182. Korpelainen JT, Sotaniemi KA, Huikuri HV, Myllylä VV: Circadian rhythm of heart rate variability is reversibly abolished in ischemic stroke. Stroke 1997;28:2150-2154.

183. Dawson SL, Mantelow BN, Robinson TG, et al: Which parameters of beat-to-beat load pressure and variability best predict early outcome after acute ischemic stroke? Stroke 2000;31:463-468.

184. Beloosesky Y, Grinblat J, Laudon M, et al: Melatonin rhythms in stroke patients. Neuroscience Lett 2002;319:103-106.

185. Aharon-Peretz J, Masiah A, Pillar T, et al: Sleep-wake cycles in multi-infarct dementia and dementia of the Alzheimer type. Neurology 1991;41:1616-1619.

186. Schwartz WJ, Busis NA, Hedley-Whyte ET: A discrete lesion of ventral hypothalamus and optic chiasm that disturbed the daily temperature rhythm. J Neurol 1986;233:1-4.

187. Reith J, Jorgensen HS, Pedersen PM, et al: Body temperature in acute stroke: Relations to stroke severity, infarct size, mortality, and outcome. Lancet 1996;347:422-425.

69

Sleep and Neuromuscular Diseases

Charles F. P. George
Christian Guilleminault

ABSTRACT

Neuromuscular disorders are central and peripheral neurologic disorders with impairment of the motor system. The
disability of patients with a neuromuscular disorder worsens
during sleep, and the abnormal sleep and secondary impairment of daytime functions degrade their quality of life. The
nocturnal sleep disruption may be the result of pain and
discomfort related to weakness, rigidity, or spasticity that limit
movements and posture. It may also be related to autonomic
dysfunction (frequently seen in these patients), poor sphincter control, secretion clearance problems, and abnormal
movements and behaviors during sleep. More important,
sleep-related hypoventilation may occur in all patients, and
overlooking this may lead to death. Daytime evaluation will
determine the severity of disability but may not predict the
presence and severity of sleep-related dysfunction. The nonspecific symptoms of fatigue and daytime sleepiness indicate
poor sleep in these patients. Polysomnography is the only test
that can objectively evaluate the severity of sleep-related
dysfunction. By recognizing and treating sleep-related problems, improved survival and better quality of life can be
achieved in this group of patients.

Neuromuscular disorders are central and peripheral neurologic disorders with impairment of the motor system. These
different diseases are secondary to impairments of the motor
unit, formed by lower motor neuron, nerve root, peripheral
nerve, myoneural junction, and muscle. Any classification of
neuromuscular disease may be somewhat arbitrary, and the
astute clinician must keep in mind that the pathologic process
may involve several segments of the nervous system and muscles. For example, myopathies will lead to progressive, peripheral motor and sensory impairment along with autonomic
dysfunction. Conditions such as amyotrophic lateral sclerosis
(ALS) or Creutzfeldt-Jacob disease may progress quickly
toward death, whereas certain chronic polyneuropathies such
as Charcot-Marie-Tooth, or autonomic syndromes such as
familial dysautonomia may have a slower evolution.

Neuromuscular patients are at risk for sleep-related problems. Weakness, rigidity, and spasticity limit movements and
posture changes during sleep, and the limitation leads to discomfort, pain, and disrupted sleep. Difficulty in maintaining
appropriate positions may lead to cramping, abnormal uncontrolled movements, and weakness, which also contribute to
poor sleep. Abnormal sphincter control may induce urinary
and fecal disturbances in the form of nocturia, incomplete
emptying or incontinence, constipation, or painful defecation.

The normal sleep-related changes in respiration (see later)
also put the patient with a neuromuscular disorder at a
specific ventilatory risk by impairing ventilation, which leads
to nocturnal and then diurnal hypoventilation. The slow
progression of ventilatory failure may go undetected for some
time and contribute to increased mortality. Limited attention
is often paid to the impact of sleep in this population, particularly as many clinics may see a very limited number of
patients with neuromuscular disorders. Even in a specialized
neuromuscular clinic, less than 2% of patients are asked
sleep-related questions or had been given a prior sleep
evaluation.[1] Moreover, the common problems (i.e., spasticity,
sphincter dysfunction, pain, abnormal movement, confusional arousal) that lead to sleep fragmentation, insomnia,
parasomnias, daytime tiredness, and sleepiness are rarely
dealt with by the sleep specialist. Thus, a multidisciplinary
approach to treatment is mandatory in these disorders.

EPIDEMIOLOGY AND GENETICS

Each neuromuscular syndrome has its own epidemiology and
its own etiology. For example, ALS affects 0.005% of the U.S.
population, and multiple sclerosis, 0.11%. However, there
are no cumulative prevalence data that include all neuromuscular disorders. Many neurologic disorders, such as Maltase
deficiency myopathy, myotonic dystrophy, Rett syndrome,
or familial dysautonomia, have a clear genetic origin. Other
disorders are secondary to infectious, vascular, malignant, or
degenerative diseases, and the presence or absence of a
genetic component has not been demonstrated.

Despite the number of reports of abnormal sleep and
breathing in patients with neuromuscular diseases, and the
number of studies dealing with the treatment of the concomitant respiratory insufficiency,[2-5] there are almost no studies
that examine the prevalence of sleep-disordered breathing in
these patients. One study from New Mexico[1] attempted to
gather information from its entire clinic population of over
300 patients. (This clinic provides free care, including neurologic, orthopedic, and physical therapy services, and such
access ensures that virtually all patients with neuromuscular
disease from the state will be referred.) Although complete
data are available on only 60 patients (20% of the clinic
population), they demonstrate that sleep and breathing
abnormalities are or may be present in more than 40% of
patients being routinely followed at a neuromuscular diseases
clinic.[1] Such a high prevalence should not be surprising given
the vulnerability of such patients to sleep-related reductions
in muscle tone and overall ventilation.

PATHOPHYSIOLOGY

The diaphragm is the major muscle of respiration during wakefulness and sleep. During non–rapid eye movement (non-REM) sleep, there is an overall reduction in ventilation that is related to sleep state changes in the chemical control of breathing and that is in response to the increased impedance of the respiratory system. However, rib cage activity is maintained, albeit reduced, as is diaphragmatic activity. The importance of the diaphragm is particularly evident during rapid eye movement (REM) sleep. During REM sleep, there is postsynaptic inhibition of somatic motor neurons, which causes further reduction or even complete loss of tone in rib cage and other accessory muscles of respiration, but which leaves the diaphragm relatively unaffected. Thus, the diaphragm is the main muscle of respiration during REM sleep, and any process affecting the diaphragm, whether a myopathy or a process involving its innervation, can be expected to cause significant changes in breathing and oxygenation during this stage of sleep.

In patients with bilateral diaphragmatic paralysis, marked oxygen desaturations can occur in REM sleep.[6-8] The REM sleep–related inhibition of intercostal and accessory muscles leads to profound hypoventilation in this sleep stage, because patients with diaphragmatic paralysis are totally dependent on intercostal and accessory muscles for breathing. As noted previously, this suppression of accessory respiratory muscle tone is a normal concomitant of REM sleep and is seen in normal subjects and in patients with lung diseases.[9-11] Depending on the type of neuromuscular disorder, breathing abnormalities during sleep may be present as central apneas, obstructive apneas, or periods of prolonged hypoventilation.

Sleep disruption with frequent arousals may result in patients with neuromuscular disorders as a result of discomfort in the recumbent position, secretion clearance and sphincter control problems, or increase in upper airway resistance muscle weakness and craniofacial changes. Periods of hypoventilation can also contribute to frequent arousals, reduced sleep time, and sleep deprivation through both ventilatory and arousal responses to changes in oxygen saturation and carbon dioxide levels. Although these changes may be protective to overall ventilation in the short term, over time, ventilatory responses to O_2 and CO_2 become blunted. This leads to worsening hypoventilation, which eventually occurs during both wakefulness and sleep.

CLINICAL FEATURES COMMON TO MOST NEUROMUSCULAR DISORDERS

Nonspecific complaints such as increased tiredness, fatigue, or disrupted nocturnal sleep can be the first manifestations of a slowly evolving neuromuscular disease of adult onset.[1] Such nonspecific complaints may also be the sole indication of a slow progression during sleep. The presence of a neuromuscular condition may bias the clinician toward believing the complaints of tiredness or fatigue are simply part of the neurologic problem, and the impaired sleep mechanisms and sleep-related disturbances may be ignored. Clearance problems of managing saliva or gastric contents can lead to significant drooling, esophageal reflux, or pulmonary congestion from aspiration or retained secretions. Impairment of cough mechanisms may further degrade the ability to clear lung secretions. Autonomic dysfunction may be present in the form of abnormal sensitivity to temperature or to pressure, with discomfort related to sheets and blankets. Cerebral lesions may lead to causalgia with prominence in the evening and early part of the night. Their disease may affect patients psychologically, and its resulting disability may lead to anxiety, depression, and secondary sleep-onset insomnia, as happens with many other chronic illnesses.

Pharmacologic agents that are prescribed to be used in the evening may have alerting effects, whereas others used in the morning may lead to daytime sleepiness. In patients with chronic evolving neuromuscular disorders, many factors may disrupt sleep, worsening daytime functioning and quality of life in general. The added-on sleep problem complicates the already existing neurologic issues.

SPECIFIC NEUROMUSCULAR DISORDERS

Neurodegenerative Diseases

Neurodegenerative diseases are a group of heterogeneous diseases of the central nervous system for which no causal agent has been identified. These include both somatic and autonomic disorders, both of which have direct and indirect effects on sleep. Somatic diseases involve the cortex (e.g., Alzheimer's disease), the basal ganglia or basal ganglia plus syndromes (e.g., Parkinson's disease, progressive supranuclear palsy, Huntington's chorea, torsion dystonia, or Tourette's syndrome), the cerebellum or cerebellum plus syndromes (e.g., spinocerebellar ataxias), or motor neurons (e.g., ALS or motor neuron disease). Autonomic degenerative processes may cause multiple-system atrophy or the Shy-Drager syndrome. Sleep disturbances such as insomnia, hypersomnia, circadian rhythm disturbances, parasomnias, and sleep-disordered breathing may be seen in neurodegenerative disorders. Because these illnesses are more common in older adult patients, the sleep changes occurring with normal aging should also be considered. Still, some of the changes in sleep can also be related to environmental factors (e.g., living in nursing home) or mood disorders.

Although ALS has not been shown to affect the sleep-regulating areas of the brain, it is likely that indirect effects of the disease cause sleep disruption. Periodic limb movements associated with arousals and sleep-disordered breathing contribute to the sleep disruption in some patients with ALS. Respiratory-related sleep disruption is generally not significant until phrenic nerves are involved and the diaphragm becomes paralyzed. In this situation, intensive hypoventilation and oxygen desaturations occur during REM sleep. Almost invariably, these patients ultimately need some form of ventilatory support. However, some patients without any respiratory disturbance or periodic limb movements still have sleep fragmentation, independent of age. This suggests other factors that contribute to disturbed sleep, such as anxiety, depression, pain, choking, excessive secretions, fasciculations and cramps, and the inability to become comfortable or turn oneself freely in bed. Orthopnea, a frequent complaint in ALS, may also contribute to sleep disruption.[12,13]

Spinal Cord Disease

Poliovirus infection targets the nervous system in several ways, producing meningitis and affecting cranial motor nuclei and spinal cord anterior horn cells to cause acute paresis. As a result, there are many possible effects of respiration. Abnormalities in central regulation of breathing in patients with acute and convalescent poliomyelitis were described in 1958 by Plum and Swanson.[14] Subsequently, central, mixed, and obstructive events have been noted.[15] Sleep and breathing abnormalities are seen not only in patients who are on respiratory assistance (rocking beds) during sleep but also before ventilatory assistance is initiated.[16] Sleep abnormalities include decreased sleep efficiency, increased arousal frequency, and varying degrees of apnea and hypopnea. After treatment of these sleep and breathing abnormalities, many symptoms frequently attributed to the postpolio syndrome improve. Thus, although not all symptoms can be explained, daytime symptoms may be explained by poor sleep quality and abnormal respiration during sleep. Inherited metabolic diseases such as subacute necrotizing encephalomyelopathy (Leigh's disease) typically appear in childhood and may be associated with respiratory disturbance. Rarely, this disease may first appear in adulthood, with automatic respiratory failure during sleep.[17]

Poliomyelitis can alter central and peripheral respiratory functions decades after the acute infection, a condition called postpolio syndrome.[18] Muscular atrophy and immobility lead to kyphoscoliosis and potentially more restricted ventilation. The anatomic deformities resulting from poliomyelitis may cause chronic pain and consequent sleep abnormalities. Also, bulbar involvement may affect upper airway muscles. Prolongation of REM latency may result from prolonged recruitment time for damaged neurons in the pontine tegmentum.[19] Whether postpolio syndrome has caused fatigue and weakness or these are the results of disturbed sleep and thus are potentially treatable can be investigated by sleep studies.

Syringomyelia can be associated with central, mixed, and obstructive apneic events. The involvement of the bulbar and high cervical neurons is responsible for the development of hypoventilation and central sleep apnea.[20-22] The syndrome can be associated with other malformations of the base of skull or high cervical junction (platybasia, Chiari malformations[23]) that may also give a variable type of sleep-disordered breathing.

Polyneuropathies

The most common polyneuropathy with sleep-disordered breathing is Charcot-Marie-Tooth syndrome, also called hereditary motor and sensory neuropathy.[24] This is characterized by chronic degeneration of peripheral nerves and roots, resulting in distal muscle atrophy that begins in the feet and legs and later involves the hands. Sleep-disordered breathing can occur in these patients as result of a pharyngeal neuropathy leading to upper airway obstruction (obstructive apnea, upper airway resistance syndrome)[25] or with diaphragmatic dysfunction.[26]

Autonomic neuropathy, particularly when secondary to type 1 diabetes, may be associated with impaired chemosensitivity to carbon dioxide,[27] although these effects on sleep and breathing are not consistent.

Neuromuscular Junction Impairments

Myasthenia gravis is a disorder of the neuromuscular junction characterized by weakness and fatigability of skeletal muscles. Sleep breathing abnormalities can occur as a result of diaphragmatic weakness. Risk factors for the development of sleep-related ventilatory problems in myasthenia gravis patients are age, restrictive pulmonary syndrome, diaphragmatic weakness, and daytime alveolar hypoventilation.[28] Younger patients with a shorter duration of illness are least likely to experience any sleep-related hypoventilation or oxygen desaturation,[29] whereas older patients with moderately increased body mass index, abnormal total lung capacity, and abnormal daytime blood gases are most likely to develop hypopneas or apneas, particularly during REM sleep.[30]

Other neuromuscular disorders that can disturb normal sleep include congenital myasthenic syndromes,[31] botulism, hypermagnesemia, and tick paralysis. Careful history taking is extremely helpful in making the diagnosis in these circumstances. Dyspnea that worsens with activity, morning headache, paroxysmal nocturnal dyspnea, fragmented sleep, and daytime somnolence are among the symptoms that suggest the presence of sleep-disordered breathing in these syndromes.

Muscular Diseases

Myotonic Dystrophy

Myotonic dystrophy (MD) is an autosomal dominant inherited illness; patients present with myotonia and nonmuscular dystrophy. In this illness, there is consistent involvement of facial, masseter, levator palpebrae, sternocleidomastoid, forearm, hand, and pretibial muscles; MD is, in a sense, a distal myopathy. However, pharyngeal and laryngeal muscles may also be involved, as well as respiratory muscles, particularly the diaphragm. Central abnormalities also occur in MD, and these can produce excessive sleepiness via different mechanisms.[32-35] For example, damage in dorsomedial nuclei of the thalamus can lead to a medial thalamic syndrome characterized by apathy, memory loss, and mental deterioration. Loss of 5-hydroxytryptamine (serotonin) neurons of the dorsal raphe nucleus and the superior central nucleus,[35] as well as dysfunction of the hypothalamic hypocretin system,[36] can result in hypersomnia and abnormal results on a multiple sleep latency test (reflecting sleep-onset REM periods) in these patients.[33,36]

Involvement of the respiratory muscles may predispose to breathing and oxygenation changes during sleep. There has been ample evidence for the occurrence of periods of alveolar hypoventilation, predominantly in REM sleep,[37-39] obstructive apneas,[40] and central apneas.[41] However, the development of sleep breathing abnormalities in MD is not simply caused by muscle weakness. When sleep and breathing in patients with MD are compared with those in patients with nonmyotonic respiratory muscle weakness and in control subjects, periods of hypoventilation and apneas (central and obstructive) occurred in those with MD and at higher frequencies than in nonmyotonic patients who had the same degree of muscle weakness (measured by maximal inspiratory and expiratory pressures).[42] This finding adds further evidence that respiratory muscle weakness alone does not account for abnormal breathing in patients with MD. As a result of muscular weakness, development of craniofacial structures in patients with MD is impaired. As a result, they experience more vertical facial growth than normal subjects, have narrower maxillary arches, and deeper palatal depths.[24] These craniofacial changes may contribute to the development of obstructive sleep apnea.

Observations of decreased ventilatory response to hypoxic and hypercapnic stimuli[38,43-46] and extreme sensitivity to sedative drugs have suggested a central origin of the breathing impairments in MD. Whereas response of ventilation to increased carbon dioxide is a standard technique for assessing control of respiration, in patients with MD the respiratory muscles must transduce the chemical stimulus. When these muscles are abnormal, as in MD, it becomes difficult to interpret a reduced ventilatory response. That is, chemoreceptor activity and efferent activity to muscles may be intact, but weak or inefficient respiratory muscles may not permit a normal ventilatory response to a hypoxic stimulus. Measurement of the mouth pressure developed at the beginning of a transiently occluded breath (occlusion pressure, $P_{0.1}$) can also be used as a measure of respiratory center output.[47]

In patients with MD, $P_{0.1}$ may be as high as or higher than that of control subjects at rest and during stimulated breathing, although overall ventilation is lower.[44,48] The finding of high transdiaphragmatic pressure (P_{di}), despite overall lower ventilation, suggests that increased impedance of the respiratory system accounts for incomplete transformation into ventilation of normal or increased respiratory center output. Magnetic stimulation of the cortex, in conjunction with phrenic nerve recordings, can be used to test the corticospinal tract to phrenic motor neuron pathways and is a reliable method for diagnosing and monitoring patients with impaired central respiratory drive.[49] Using transcortical and cervical magnetic stimulation demonstrates that greater than 20% of myotonic patients have impaired central respiratory drive.[50] The finding of neuronal loss in the dorsal central, ventral central, and subtrigeminal medullary nuclei in patients with MD who exhibit alveolar hypoventilation,[51] and the severe neuronal loss and gliosis in the tegmentum of the brainstem[52] also support a central abnormality.

Other Myopathies

Abnormalities in sleep and breathing have been reported in isolated series of patients with various other neuromuscular disorders, such as congenital myopathies (nemaline or congenital fiber-type disproportion myopathy[53-55]) or metabolic myopathies (mitochondrial myopathy [Kearns-Sayre] syndrome,[56-58] acid maltase deficiency).[59-61] In all of these cases, there are various alterations in control of breathing and varied breathing pattern changes, including hypoventilation, obstruction, and central apnea. Severe central sleep apnea and marked oxygen desaturation, particularly during REM sleep, resulting in hypoxia-induced nocturnal seizures, as well as pulmonary hypertension, excessive daytime sleepiness, heart failure, and morning headaches, may be seen in patients with congenital muscular dystrophy,[62] and obstructive sleep apnea has also been described in Thomsen's disease (myotonia congenita).[63]

Myopathies such as Duchenne's muscular dystrophy can cause restrictive lung disease and chest wall deformities.[64] These changes also contribute to ventilatory impairment,

fragmented sleep, frequent arousals and stage changes, hypercapnia and hypoxemia (again, more profound during REM sleep),[65,66] and development of deformities, chronic pain, and discomfort. A special case is maltase deficiency myopathy, in which the rapid, significant diaphragmatic impairment that occurs long before the wasting of other skeletal muscles explains the severity of the sleep-disordered breathing.[67] In fact, the breathing problem during sleep and the secondary daytime tiredness may be the first signs of the myopathy.[68] Although the disease progresses rapidly, the diaphragmatic impairment, with clear evidence of sleep-disordered breathing, remains as a major component of the syndrome.

DIAGNOSTIC EVALUATION

The clinician who evaluates a patient with a neuromuscular disorder has to consider the type of neurologic disorder and the degree of disability seen during wakefulness. During neurologic assessment, the degree of sensory and motor impairment and resulting disability, the associated autonomic defects, the intensity of pain and discomfort, and the impact of the illness on the patient's mood must be assessed. Understanding the patient's interaction with society and family is an important factor for subsequent treatment decisions. A detailed sleep history is required to outline the severity and type of sleep-related problem—for example, the degree and type of nocturnal disruption, sleep-onset insomnia, awakening difficulties, presence or absence of abnormal behavior during sleep (including confusional arousal), nonrestorative sleep, fatigue, and daytime sleepiness. General assessment should also determine the degree of pain and discomfort (particularly in the supine position and during sleep), the presence or absence of sphincter problems and urinary or digestive dysfunction during wake and sleep, and any evidence of autonomic dysfunction already present during wakefulness and suspected during sleep (e.g., orthostatic hypotension, dizziness, lightheadedness when standing up just after awakening, cold hands and feet worsening during the nocturnal period, appearance of skin mottling when supine). The degree of mood impairment caused by illness or sleep disruption should also be characterized.

A number of additional diagnostic tests may supplement the evaluation of sleep in the patient with neuromuscular disease. These include a disability index scale,[1] a sleep disorder questionnaire, and a sleep log or actigraphy (helpful for the investigation of daily rhythms and sleep–wake disturbances during the 24-hour period). The severe respiratory insufficiency questionnaire, a multidimensional health-related quality-of-life instrument, may be used for patients with neuromuscular disorders on assisted ventilation.[69] Routine measures of pulmonary function (spirometry, lung volumes, diffusing capacity) and gas exchange (P_{O_2} and P_{CO_2}) should be performed in all patients at initial presentation. Static lung volume measurements, both upright and after 15 minutes supine, often demonstrate significant changes caused by respiratory muscle weakness, particularly diaphragmatic weakness. A forced expiratory volume in 1 second or forced vital capacity less than 40% of the predicted value, a Pa_{CO_2} greater than 45 mm Hg, and a base excess of 4 mmol/L or greater may indicate that there is a risk for sleep hypoventilation, and it has been suggested that, when these abnormalities are present, polysomnography be done.[70-72]

Overnight polysomnography is the key to a definitive evaluation of sleep and breathing in this patient group. Although it can be done in many settings, including the home, in-laboratory diagnosis allows additional measures such as video monitoring to document any behavioral change (e.g., the presence of confusional arousal), other parasomnias including REM sleep behavior disorder, or anoxic seizure. More importantly, measurement of transcutaneous CO_2 allows continuous tracking of overall ventilation during sleep and can provide a guide for ventilatory assistance during sleep.

TREATMENT OF SLEEP ABNORMALITIES IN PATIENTS WITH NEUROMUSCULAR DISEASE

The greatest advances in the medical treatment of neuromuscular disorders have been for sleep-related abnormalities.[73] The goal is restoration of normal sleep architecture, with subsequent improvement of sleep, daytime function, and quality of life.

Simple measures such as bedding are often overlooked. Many types of beds and mattresses are available with specializations that allow easy position changes, avoidance of skin lesions at pressure points, and segmental inflation and deflation (e.g., air mattresses), thus decreasing the consequences of autonomic dysfunction, cramps, spastic contraction, and rigidity. Great efforts should be made to diminish pain and discomfort of any type. Judicious use of pharmacologic agents in the morning, such as modafinil, 100 to 200 mg, can provide daytime alertness without nocturnal sleep disruption.[74-76] Treatment of abnormal behavior and confusional arousal may necessitate use of sedatives such as benzodiazepines, but such therapy should be considered after careful evaluation of ventilatory function and risk during sleep.

Treatment of abnormal breathing during sleep should be based on polysomnographic findings and should be adjusted with regular follow-up polysomnographic studies.

Various therapies may improve nocturnal hypoventilation or offset the attendant oxygen desaturation. Supplemental oxygen has been used to obviate the REM sleep–related oxygen desaturation in patients with Duchenne's muscular dystrophy. However, little improvement in sleep ensues.[77] Because most of the hypoventilation occurs during REM sleep, pharmacologic manipulation of REM sleep by the use of tricyclic antidepressants is a theoretical option and has been attempted using protriptyline. In a small study of patients with Duchenne's muscular dystrophy, marked improvement in the nocturnal oxygen saturation profile was seen.[78] Similar results of the effectiveness of protriptyline were seen in patients with restrictive lung disease[79]; however, anticholinergic side effects limit the widespread use of such therapy.

Inspiratory muscle training has demonstrated improved waking respiratory failure in one patient with acid maltase deficiency.[60] This patient had abnormal sleep architecture that was unchanged by the muscle training, but there was major improvement in the nocturnal oxygen profile. Muscle weakness can lead to nocturnal hypoventilation and worsening of oxygenation. Repeated nocturnal asphyxia may lead to increased muscle weakness, which begets further oxygen desaturation, and reversal of the hypoxemia may arrest the muscle weakness. Such a case has been reported[80] where nocturnal ventilation ablated nocturnal hypoxemia in a patient with acid maltase deficiency, and muscle weakness did not progress over an 8-year period.

Mechanical ventilation has been a mainstay in supporting ventilation since the days of the poliomyelitis epidemics. Rocking beds, a negative-pressure tank ventilator, and positive-pressure ventilation via tracheostomy have usually been the long-term options. Some patients are still successfully managed with this form of therapy.[2-4] However, all of these options are cumbersome, severely limit the mobility of patients, and, in the case of tracheostomy, may have unwanted complications. Therefore, other forms of assisted ventilation have been developed, including phrenic nerve pacing, cuirass ventilation, nasal continuous positive airway pressure (CPAP), and nasal intermittent positive-pressure ventilation. In contrast to CPAP (in which airway pressures are constant), the bilevel positive airway pressure (BiPAP) system allows different positive pressures on inspiration and expiration. By adjusting the inspiratory pressures to be higher than the expiratory pressures, the BiPAP system emulates a conventional positive-pressure ventilatory device and may be used as a means of enhancing ventilation. This is an effective treatment for a number of neuromuscular diseases[5] and in early stages may be as effective as a conventional ventilator. If, however, this is insufficient, nasal intermittent positive-pressure ventilation with a small ventilator can be used. This last form is rapidly becoming the preferred means of assisting ventilation because of its relative simplicity and because it obviates the need for tracheostomy and its attendant problems. Nasal ventilation has been used predominantly nocturnally for patients with postpoliomyelitis and other neuromuscular disorders,[5,81-88] and it has even been used almost continuously in patients with severe postpoliomyelitis respiratory insufficiency.[85] In almost every case, not only is the nocturnal ventilation normalized but daytime respiratory failure and excessive sleepiness are improved as well. The use of nasal intermittent positive-pressure ventilation can allow a patient to return to work and even travel, something not possible when constrained by reliance on a rocking bed for nocturnal ventilatory support.[16]

THE DECISION TO ASSIST NOCTURNAL VENTILATION

When patients present with disrupted sleep, snoring, excessive daytime sleepiness, and unexplained development of peripheral edema or polycythemia, sleep studies will characterize the breathing disorder, and the decision to assist ventilation is an easy one. For those with obstructive sleep apnea, nasal CPAP or BiPAP is the preferred treatment; patients with predominantly hypoventilation or central apnea and oxygen desaturation should be managed with BiPAP or full nasal ventilation (if tolerated). For a detailed review of noninvasive ventilation, see Chapter 95. However, a change in oxygen saturation (SaO_2) alone is insufficient for deciding whether the patient needs ventilatory assistance. Patients may not be "allowing" themselves to fall asleep, and thus the main abnormality is abnormal sleep structure. In these individuals, the endpoint for successful nasal ventilation is not improvement in SaO_2 but rather improvement in sleep structure.

Only recently is there beginning to emerge a consensus[89] on the management of severe progressive neuromuscular disorders in which respiratory failure plays only a part but other systems are severely affected (e.g., ALS). Issues such as quality of life must be taken into account. Without specific guidance from the literature, each patient must be assessed in detail, and the clinician must bear in mind that nocturnal (and later, 24-hour) ventilation will treat only one (albeit important) aspect of the disorder.

Clinical Pearl

Sleep is a state of vulnerability for patients with neuromuscular disorders, as normal REM sleep–related changes in ventilation are magnified as a result of muscle weakness. Sleep disturbances, in addition to this sleep-disordered breathing, may also be related to spasticity, poor secretion clearance, sphincter dysfunction, inability to turn, pain, and any associated or secondary autonomic dysfunction. All these factors impair sleep and worsen daytime disability.

REFERENCES

1. Labanowski M, Schmidt-Nowara W, Guilleminault C: Sleep and neuromuscular disease: Frequency of sleep-disordered breathing in a neuromuscular disease clinic population. Neurology 1996; 47:1173-1180.
2. Howard RS, Wiles CM, Hirsch NP, et al: Respiratory involvement in primary muscle disorders: Assessment and management. Q J Med 1993;86:175-189.
3. Chalmers RM, Howard RS, Wiles CM, et al: Use of the rocking bed in the treatment of neurogenic respiratory insufficiency. Q J Med 1994;87:423-429.
4. Iber C, Davies SF, Mahowald MW: Nocturnal rocking bed therapy: Improvement in sleep fragmentation in patients with respiratory muscle weakness. Sleep 1989;12:405-412.
5. Guilleminault C, Philip P, Robinson A: Sleep and neuromuscular disease: Bilevel positive airway pressure by nasal mask as a treatment for sleep disordered breathing in patients with neuromuscular disease. J Neurol Neurosurg Psychiatry 1998;65: 225-232.
6. Newsom-Davis J, Goldman M, Loh L, et al: Diaphragm function and alveolar hypoventilation. Q J Med 1975;45:87-100.
7. Kreitzer SM, Feldman NT, Saunders NA, et al: Bilateral diaphragmatic paralysis with hypercapnic respiratory failure. Am J Med 1978;65:89-95.
8. Skatrud J, Iber C, McHugh W, et al: Determinants of hypoventilation during wakefulness and sleep in diaphragmatic paralysis. Am Rev Respir Dis 1980;121:587-593.
9. Muller NL, Francis DW, Gurwitz D, et al: Mechanisms of hemoglobin desaturation during REM sleep in normal subjects and in patients with cystic fibrosis. Am Rev Respir Dis 1980; 121:463-469.
10. Johnson MW, Remmers JE: Accessory muscle activity during sleep in chronic obstructive pulmonary disease. J Appl Physiol 1984;57:1011-1017.
11. Millman BP, Knight H, Kline LR, et al: Changes in compartmental ventilation in association with eye movements during REM sleep. J Appl Physiol 1988;65:1196-1202.
12. Ferguson KA, Strong MJ, Ahmad D, et al: Sleep-disordered breathing in amyotrophic lateral sclerosis. Chest 1996;110: 664-669.
13. David WS, Bundlie SR, Mahdavi Z: Polysomnographic studies in amyotrophic lateral sclerosis. J Neurol Sci 1997;152(Suppl 1): S29-S35.
14. Plum F, Swanson AG: Abnormalities in central regulation of respiration in acute and convalescent poliomyelitis. Arch Neurol Psychiatry 1958;80:267-285.
15. Guilleminault C, Motta J: Sleep apnea syndrome as a long-term sequelae of poliomyelitis. In: Guilleminault C, Dement WC (eds): Sleep Apnea Syndrome. New York, Alan R Liss, 1978, pp 309-315.
16. Steljes DG, Kryger MH, Kirk BW, et al: Sleep in postpolio syndrome. Chest 1990;98:133-140.
17. Cummiskey J, Guilleminault C, Davis R, et al: Automatic respiratory failure: Sleep studies and Leigh's disease. Neurology 1987;37:1876-1878.
18. Burk JB, James AC: Characteristics and management of postpolio syndrome. JAMA 2000;284:412-414.
19. Siegel H, McCutchen C, Dalakas MC, et al: Physiologic events initiating REM sleep in patients with the postpolio syndrome. Neurology 1999;52:516-522.
20. Chokroverty S: Sleep-disordered breathing in neuromuscular disorders: A condition in search of recognition. Muscle Nerve 2001;24:451-455.
21. Kimura K, Tachibana N, Kimura J, Shibasaki H: Sleep-disordered breathing at an early stage of amyotrophic lateral sclerosis. J Neurol Sci 1999;164:37-43.
22. Daube JR: Electrodiagnostic studies in amyotrophic lateral sclerosis and other motor neuron disorders. Muscle Nerve 2000; 23:1488-1502.
23. Lam B, Ryan CF: Arnold-Chiari malformation presenting as sleep apnea syndrome. Sleep Med 2000;1:139-144.
24. Stojkovic T, de Seze J, Dubourg O, et al: Autonomic and respiratory dysfunction in Charcot-Marie-Tooth disease due to Thr124Met mutation in the myelin protein zero gene. Clin Neurophysiol 2003;114:1609-1614.
25. Dematteis M, Pepin JL, Jeanmart M, et al: Charcot-Marie-Tooth disease and sleep apnoea syndrome: A family study. Lancet 2001;357:267-272.
26. Chan CK, Mohsenin V, Loke J, et al: Diaphragmatic dysfunction in siblings with hereditary motor and sensory neuropathy (Charcot-Marie-Tooth disease). Chest 1987;91:567-570.
27. Tantucci C, Bottini P, Fiorani C, Dottorini ML, et al: Cerebrovascular reactivity and hypercapnic respiratory drive in diabetic autonomic neuropathy. J Appl Physiol 2001;90: 889-896.
28. Gajdos P, Quera Salva MA: Respiratory disorders during sleep and myasthenia. Rev Neurol (Paris) 2001;157:S145-147.
29. Manni R, Piccolo G, Sartori I, et al: Breathing during sleep in myasthenia gravis. Ital J Neurol Sci 1995;16:589-594.
30. Quera-Salva MA, Guilleminault C, Chevret S, et al: Breathing disorders during sleep in myasthenia gravis. Ann Neurol 1992; 31:86-92.
31. Iannaccone ST, Mills JK, Harris KM, et al: Congenital myasthenic syndrome with sleep hypoventilation. Muscle Nerve 2000;23: 1129-1132.
32. Phillips MF, Steer HM, Soldan JR, et al: Daytime somnolence in myotonic dystrophy. J Neurol 1999;246:275-282.
33. Gibbs JW 3rd, Ciafaloni E, Radtke RA: Excessive daytime somnolence and increased rapid eye movement pressure in myotonic dystrophy. Sleep 2002;25:672-675.
34. Bourke SC, Gibson GJ: Sleep and breathing in neuromuscular disease. Eur Respir J 2002;19:1194-1201.
35. Ono S, Takahashi K, Jinnai K, et al: Loss of serotonin-containing neurons in the raphe of patients with myotonic dystrophy: A quantitative immunohistochemical study and relation to hypersomnia. Neurology 1998;50:535-538.
36. Martinez-Rodriguez JE, Lin L, Iranzo A, et al: Decreased hypocretin-1 (orexin-A) levels in the cerebrospinal fluid of patients with myotonic dystrophy and excessive daytime sleepiness. Sleep 2003;26:287-290.

37. Kilburn KH, Eagan JT, Sieker HO, et al: Cardiopulmonary insufficiency in myotonic and progressive muscular dystrophy. N Engl J Med 1954;261:1089-1096.

38. Coccagna G, Mantovani M, Parchi C, et al: Alveolar hypoventilation and hypersomnia in myotonic dystrophy. J Neurol Neurosurg Psychiatry 1975;38:977-984.

39. Coccagna G, Martinelli P, Lugaresi E: Sleep and alveolar hypoventilation in myotonic dystrophy. Acta Neurol Belg 1982; 82:185-194.

40. Guilleminault C, Cummiskey J, Motta J, et al: Respiratory and hypodynamics study during wakefulness and sleep in myotonic dystrophy. Sleep 1978;1:19-31.

41. Cirignotta F, Mondini S, Zucconi M, et al: Sleep related breathing impairments in myotonic dystrophy. J Neurol 1987;235: 80-85.

42. Gilmartin JJ, Cooper BG, Griffiths CJ, et al: Breathing during sleep in patients with myotonic dystrophy and non-myotonic respiratory muscle weakness. Q J Med 1991;78:21-31.

43. Serisier DE, Mastaglia FL, Gibson GJ: Respiratory muscle function and ventilatory control: I, in patients with motor neurone disease. II, in patients with myotonic dystrophy. Q J Med 1982; 51:205-226.

44. Begin R, Bureau MA, Lupien L, et al: Pathogenesis of respiratory insufficiency in myotonic dystrophy. Am Rev Respir Dis 1982; 125:312-318.

45. Carroll JE, Zwillich LW, Weil JV: Ventilatory response in myotonic dystrophy. Neurology 1977;27:1125-1128.

46. Gillam PMS, Heaf PJD, Kaufman L, et al: Respiration in dystrophic myotonia. Thorax 1964;19:112-120.

47. Whitelaw WA, Derenne JP, Milic-Emili J: Occlusion pressure as a measure of the respiratory centre output in conscious man. Respir Physiol 1975;23:181-199.

48. Begin P, Mathieu J, Almirall J, et al: Relationship between chronic hypercapnia and inspiratory-muscle weakness in myotonic dystrophy. Am J Respir Crit Care Med 1997;156: 133-139.

49. Zifko UA, Hahn AF, Remtulla H, et al: Central and peripheral respiratory electrophysiological studies in myotonic dystrophy. Brain 1996;119:1911-1922.

50. Zifko U, Remtulla H, Power K, et al: Transcortical and cervical magnetic stimulation with recording of the diaphragm. Muscle Nerve 1996;19:614-620.

51. Ono SF, Kanda F, Takahashi K, et al: Neuronal loss in the medullary reticular formation in myotonic dystrophy: A clinico-pathological study. Neurology 1996;46:A171.

52. Ono S, Kurisaki H, Sakuma A, et al: Myotonic dystrophy with alveolar hypoventilation and hypersomnia: A clinicopathological study. J Neurol Sci 1995;128:225-231.

53. Riley DJ, Santiago RV, Daniele RP, et al: Blunted respiratory drive in congenital myopathy. Am J Med 1977;63:459-466.

54. Maayan C, Springer C, Armen Y, et al: Nemaline myopathy as a cause of sleep hypoventilation. Pediatrics 1986;77:390-395.

55. Wilson DO, Sanders MH, Dauber JH: Abnormal ventilatory chemosensitivity and congenital myopathy. Arch Intern Med 1987;147:1773-1777.

56. Carroll JE, Zwillich C, Weil JV, et al: Depressed ventilatory response in oculocraniosomatic neuromuscular disease. Neurology 1976;26:140-146.

57. Weng TR, Schultz GE, Chang HC, et al: Pulmonary function and ventilatory response to chemical stimuli in familial myopathy. Chest 1985;88:488-495.

58. Kotagal S, Archer CR, Walsh JK, et al: Hypersomnia, bithalamic lesions, and altered sleep architecture in Kearns-Sayre syndrome. Neurology 1985;35:574-577.

59. Bellamy D, Newsom-Davis JM, Mickey BP, et al: A case of primary alveolar hypoventilation associated with mild proximal myopathy. Am Rev Respir Dis 1975;112:867-873.

60. Martin RJ, Sufit RI, Ringel SP, et al: Respiratory improvement by muscle training in adult-onset acid maltase deficiency. Muscle Nerve 1983;6:201-203.

61. Margolis ML, Howlett P, Goldberg R, et al: Obstructive sleep apnea syndrome in acid maltase deficiency. Chest 1994;105: 947-949.

62. Kryger MH, Steljes DG, Yee WC, et al: Central sleep apnea in congenital muscular dystrophy. J Neurol Neurosurg Psychiatry 1991;54:710-712.

63. Striano S, Meo R, Bilo L, et al: Sleep apnea syndrome in Thomsen's disease: A case report. Electroencephalogr Clin Neurophysiol 1983;56:323-325.

64. Gozal D: Pulmonary manifestations of neuromuscular disease with special reference to Duchenne muscular dystrophy and spinal muscular atrophy. Pediatr Pulmonol 2000;29:141-150.

65. American Thoracic Society/European Respiratory Society. ATS/ERS statement on respiratory muscle testing. Am J Respir Crit Care Med 2002;166:518-624.

66. Phillips MF, Smith PE, Carroll N, et al: Nocturnal oxygenation and prognosis in Duchenne muscular dystrophy. Am J Respir Crit Care Med 1999;160:198-202.

67. Mellies U, Ragette R, Schwake C, et al: Sleep-disordered breathing and respiratory failure in acid maltase deficiency. Neurology 2001;57:1290-1295.

68. Guilleminault C, Stoohs RA, Querra-Salva MA: Sleep related obstructive and nonobstructive apneas in neurologic disorders. Neurology 1992;42:S53-S60.

69. Richman DP, Agius MA: Treatment of autoimmune myasthenia gravis. Neurology 2003;61:1652-1661.

70. Hukins CA, Hillman DR: Daytime predictors of sleep hypoventilation in Duchenne muscular dystrophy. Am J Respir Crit Care Med 2000;161:166-170.

71. Ragette R, Mellies U, Schwake C, et al: Patterns and predictors of sleep disordered breathing in primary myopathies. Thorax 2002;57:724-728.

72. Mellies U, Ragette R, Schwake C, et al: Daytime predictors of sleep disordered breathing in children and adolescents with neuromuscular disorders. Neuromuscul Disord 2003;13: 123-128.

73. Bourke SC, Gibson GJ: Sleep and breathing in neuromuscular disease. Eur Respir J 2002;19:1194-1201.

74. MacDonald JR, Hill JD, Tarnopolsky MA: Modafinil reduces excessive somnolence and enhances mood in patients with myotonic dystrophy. Neurology 2002;59:1876-1880.

75. Damian MS, Gerlach A, Schmidt F, et al: Modafinil for excessive daytime sleepiness in myotonic dystrophy. Neurology 2001;56: 794-796.

76. Talbot K, Stradling J, Crosby J, et al: Reduction in excess daytime sleepiness by modafinil in patients with myotonic dystrophy. Neuromuscul Disord 2003;13:357-364.

77. Smith PE, Edwards RH, Calverley PM: Oxygen treatment of sleep hypoxemia in Duchenne muscular dystrophy. Thorax 1989;44:997-1001.

78. Smith PE, Edwards RH, Calverley PM: Protriptyline treatment of sleep hypoxemia in Duchenne muscular dystrophy. Thorax 1989;44:1002-1005.

79. Simons AK, Parker RA, Branthwaite MA: Effects of protriptyline on sleep related disturbance of breathing in restrictive chest wall disease. Thorax 1986;41:586-590.

80. Olsen LG, Hensley MJ, Saunders NA, et al: Sleep breathing and lung disease. In Saunders NA, Sullivan CE (eds): Sleep and Breathing. New York, Marcel Dekker, 1984, pp 517-558.

81. Kerby GR, Mayer LS, Pingleton SK: Nocturnal positive pressure ventilation via nasal mask. Am Rev Respir Dis 1987;135:738-740.

82. Segall D: Noninvasive nasal mask-assisted ventilation in respiratory failure of Duchenne muscular dystrophy. Chest 1988;93: 1298-1300.

83. Ellis ER, Grunstein RR, Chan S, et al: Noninvasive ventilatory support during sleep improves respiratory failure in kyphoscoliosis. Chest 1988;94:811-815.

84. Rodenstein DO, Stanescu DC, Delguste P, et al: Adaptation to intermittent positive pressure ventilation applied through the nose during day and night. Eur Respir J 1989;2:473-478.

85. Bach JR, Alba AS, Shin D: Management alternatives for post-polio respiratory insufficiency: Assisted ventilation by nasal or oral-nasal interface. Am J Phys Med Rehabil 1989;68:264-271.

86. Heckmatt JZ, Loh L, Dubowitz V: Night-time nasal ventilation in neuromuscular disease. Lancet 1990;335:579-581.

87. Barbe F, Quera-Salva MA, deLattre J, et al: Long-term effects of nasal intermittent positive pressure ventilation on pulmonary function and sleep architecture in patients with neuromuscular diseases. Chest 1996;110:1179-1183.

88. Bonekat HW: Noninvasive ventilation in neuromuscular disease. Crit Care Clin 1998;14:775-797.

89. Goldberg A (conference facilitator): Clinical indications for noninvasive positive pressure ventilation in chronic respiratory failure due to restrictive lung disease, COPD, and nocturnal hypoventilation: A consensus conference report. Chest 1999;116:521-534.

Restless Legs Syndrome and Periodic Limb Movements during Sleep

Jacques Montplaisir

Richard P. Allen

Arthur S. Walters

Luigi Ferini-Strambi

ABSTRACT

The restless legs syndrome (RLS) is a neurologic condition characterized by an urge to move, usually associated with paresthesia, that occurs or worsens at rest and is relieved by activity. One of the central characteristics of RLS is the worsening of symptoms in the evening and during the night. Several studies showed that the severity of leg discomfort follows a circadian rhythm, with the maximum occurring after midnight. The symptoms of RLS have a major impact on nocturnal sleep and daytime functioning. Most patients report difficulty falling asleep or waking up shortly after sleep onset with unpleasant leg sensations. They also often experience excessive daytime fatigue and somnolence, probably as a consequence of disrupted nocturnal sleep. Although RLS is usually thought to be a condition of adulthood, it is frequently reported in children, in whom it could be misdiagnosed as growing pains or attention-deficit/hyperactivity disorder. RLS has also been related to several other medical conditions, especially uremia, anemia, and various neuropathies. Several epidemiologic studies showed that the prevalence of RLS symptoms in the white population is probably approximately 10%. There is substantial evidence for a genetic contribution to RLS. Familial aggregation has been well documented, with more than 50% of idiopathic cases reporting a positive family history of RLS. In most pedigrees, it is segregated in an autosomal dominant fashion with a high penetrance rate. Recently, linkage studies revealed the presence of RLS susceptibility genes on chromosomes 12q and 14q. There are major controversies regarding the localization of the neural substrate involved in the pathophysiologic process of RLS. There is increasing evidence for the presence of brain iron deficiency in patients with RLS. As far as treatment is concerned, four categories of medication are commonly prescribed to treat RLS: dopaminergic agents, opioids, anticonvulsants, and benzodiazepines. Because they are more effective and produce fewer adverse effects, dopaminergic agonists are now considered first-line treatment.

DESCRIPTION AND EPIDEMIOLOGY

Sensory and Motor Manifestations

The restless legs syndrome (RLS) has been described for centuries, but it was only in 1945 that it was singled out as a distinct clinical entity and given the name RLS by the Swedish neurologist Carl Ekbom.[1] Patients with RLS report an urge to move associated with dysesthesia when they are at rest.[2] Patients use different terms to describe the dysesthesia. Some say only that the sensations are uncomfortable and unpleasant, whereas others use specific terms such as "creepy-crawly," "jittery," "internal itch," or "shocklike feelings"; up to 50% of patients with RLS describe their sensations as painful. Some people, however, described only an urge to move and are unaware of a sensory component. Although it is called restless *legs* syndrome, the disorder may also involve the arms and other body parts. Michaud et al.[3] showed that almost 50% of patients with RLS have symptoms in the arms. Leg symptoms usually precede arm involvement by several years. The presence of arm paresthesia has been associated with greater severity of the disorder. Involvement of the arms without any involvement of the legs rarely occurs.

The second clinical characteristic of RLS is that the urge to move or the unpleasant leg sensation begins or worsens during periods of rest or inactivity such as lying down or sitting.[2] Typically, patients describe exacerbation of symptoms in situations such as watching television, driving or flying long distances, or attending business meetings. Symptoms also worsen in association with a decrease in central nervous system activity leading to a decrease in alertness. Indeed, several patients report that engaging in intense conversation or playing computer games actually reduces the severity of symptoms.

The urge to move and the unpleasant leg sensations are relieved by activity.[2] Patients use different motor strategies to relieve the discomfort. When symptoms occur, they move their legs vigorously, flexing, stretching, or crossing them one over the other. In severe cases, they may walk around for hours in the evening or during the night to relieve the discomfort. The relief is usually described as beginning immediately or soon after the activity begins, and usually persists as long as the activity continues. In most patients the relief is complete, but patients with severe RLS report that movement does not completely suppress the sensations. When the RLS is so severe that relief with movement does not occur, patients recall that earlier in the course of their disease they were able to obtain relief with movement. In severe cases, symptoms may recur rapidly after the cessation of walking or activity, whereas other patients with less severe disease may remain symptom free for 30 to 60 minutes.

One of the central characteristics of RLS is the worsening of symptoms in the evening or during the night.[2] Several factors may contribute to the worsening of RLS symptoms at that time. One factor is the increase of sleepiness in the evening compared with the daytime. Indeed, it is quite frequent to hear patients with RLS report that their symptoms are worst when they are excessively tired or sleep deprived. Another contributing factor is the decrease of motor activity in the evening compared with the daytime. A third possibility is that the worsening of symptoms is the manifestation of an intrinsic circadian rhythm in RLS symptoms. Recently, three studies used modified constant-routine protocols to investigate the circadian pattern in the occurrence of RLS symptoms.[4-6] Sensory or motor symptoms of RLS were quantified using a method called the *suggested immobilization test* (SIT),[7] which was administered every 2 to 4 hours over 24 to 28 hours. These studies showed that the severity of leg discomfort followed a circadian rhythm, with a maximum occurring after midnight. They also showed that the peak intensity of symptoms occurs on the falling limb of the core body temperature rhythm. Together, these three studies suggest that RLS symptom intensity may be modulated by a circadian factor. In a recent study of seven patients with RLS and seven healthy control subjects,[6] the circadian rhythm of RLS symptoms was significantly correlated with that of subjective vigilance, core body temperature, and salivary melatonin secretion. However, among these variables, the changes in melatonin secretion were the only ones that preceded the increase in sensory or motor symptoms of RLS and could therefore have a causal relationship with the expression of RLS symptoms.

Nocturnal Sleep and Daytime Vigilance

Most patients with RLS also complain of poor sleep. Most patients report difficulty falling asleep because both immobility and circadian factors facilitate the occurrence of RLS symptoms at bedtime. However, some patients fall asleep rapidly but awaken soon thereafter with unpleasant leg sensations that force them to get up and walk around to relieve the discomfort. In a study of 133 patients with RLS, most of the patients (84.7%) frequently experienced difficulty falling asleep at night because of RLS, and 86% reported that symptoms woke them up frequently during the night.[8] Ninety-four percent reported at least one of these two manifestations. Sleep laboratory investigations showed that, as a group, patients with RLS have severe nocturnal sleep disruption compared with normal control subjects (i.e., longer sleep latency and reduced sleep efficiency and total sleep time). A great majority of patients with RLS also experience stereotyped repetitive movements once asleep, a condition known as *periodic limb movements during sleep* (PLMS; for a detailed description of PLMS, see the section on Sleep Laboratory Diagnosis).

Several patients (46.2% of men and 22.2% of women) also reported excessive daytime fatigue or somnolence,[8] probably as a consequence of disrupted nocturnal sleep. On the other hand, it is surprising to find a large number of patients who do not experience fatigue and are fully alert during the day in spite of severe and chronic sleep deprivation. One study has suggested that patients with RLS have an increased level of hypocretin in the central nervous system, which would counteract the effects of poor sleep and sleep deprivation.[9]

Burden of the Illness

Several other problems may result directly from RLS. The incessant bedtime dysesthesia can lead to emotional disturbances in some patients. In severe cases, depression and suicidal thoughts may arise, but RLS should not be confused with the restlessness of anxious patients. RLS may also be responsible for marital difficulties. In several cases of RLS, the main complaint comes from the bed partner; in approximately one third of these cases, couples sleep in separate beds because of the discomfort caused by repetitive leg movements. In a study of 424 patients with RLS, Allen et al.[10] found that patients with RLS have a worse quality of life than the general U.S. population, and that their quality of life is comparable with that of patients with other conditions such as type 2 diabetes mellitus and acute myocardial infarction.

Clinical Course

RLS is thought to be a condition of middle-aged individuals, but there is increasing evidence that RLS may start at an earlier age. Recent studies have shown that familial cases of RLS have an earlier age of onset, typically before the age of 30 years.[11] The intensity of sensory and motor symptoms varies greatly from one case to another; it also fluctuates throughout a patient's life. During some periods, motor symptoms may be present several times a day, whereas at other times they may be totally absent, or nearly so. The sudden remissions, lasting for months or even years, are as difficult to explain as are relapses, which appear without any apparent reason. In severe cases, symptoms are present every night, and in most patients symptom severity increases with advancing age. In women, RLS often appears for the first time during pregnancy, where it was originally associated with a folic acid deficiency.[12] In some cases, RLS is present only during pregnancy, but in several cases in which RLS originally started during pregnancy it eventually became persistent later in life. Positive family history is common in women in whom RLS develops during pregnancy, which suggests that pregnancy facilitates the expression of RLS rather than causes it.

Epidemiology

Based on face-to-face interviews of 500 people, the prevalence of RLS was first estimated by Ekbom to be 5.2% of the population. Subsequently, Lavigne and Montplaisir[13] reported, in a population-based survey of 2019 Canadians, that 15% of individuals reported delayed sleep onset with "restlessness in legs" and 10% reported "unpleasant leg sensations" on awakening from sleep. The percentages were substantially greater for French-speaking than English-speaking Canadians, suggesting a genetic effect. More recently, Phillips and collaborators[14] found that approximately 10% of the adults in Kentucky reported symptoms resembling RLS. In 2000, the National Sleep Foundation[15] conducted a telephone survey in the United States and reported that approximately 15% of adults (18% of women, 11% of men) reported RLS-type feelings of "creeping and crawling, or tingling in the legs a few nights per week." This feeling was reported by 27% of those older than 65 years of age but only by 10% of those between 18 and 29 years of age. More recently, a population-based, direct-interview survey of 369 elderly individuals (65 to 83 years) conducted in Germany reported a prevalence of 9.8%, which was significantly higher for women than for men (13.9% versus 6.1%).[16] Thus, it seems more likely that the true prevalence of RLS is closer to the lower estimates of 5% to 10%, which still makes it the most common movement disorder and among the most common sleep-related disorders.[17]

All the surveys examining the influence of age on RLS found a strong increase in prevalence with age. On the other hand, the surveys differed somewhat regarding findings on sex differences. Neither the Canadian nor the Kentucky survey found significant sex differences (in fact, the prevalence was higher among women in both studies, but the difference was not significant). However, both the U.S. telephone survey and the German study reported notable sex differences, with the prevalence for women being approximately twice that for men. Thus, it seems that this disorder occurs more in the elderly and probably occurs more in women than in men. A recent study looked at the prevalence of RLS in a primary care patient population. This was a prospective, population-based study conducted in a small rural primary care practice with mostly white patients using a validated RLS diagnostic questionnaire. Analyses revealed that 24% of these patients were positive for all four of the essential symptoms required to make the diagnosis of RLS, and 15.3% reported these symptoms at least weekly. In addition, the RLS symptom complex was reported significantly more often by women than by men, and the prevalence of symptoms increased with age until approximately 60 years.[18]

All of the aforementioned epidemiologic studies were performed in adult populations. However, there are some indications that RLS may be quite prevalent among children and adolescents (see section on Restless Legs Syndrome in Childhood).

DIAGNOSIS OF RESTLESS LEGS SYNDROME

Clinical Diagnosis

The diagnosis of RLS is based on the clinical evaluation of the patient. In 1995, a consensus emerged from a large International RLS Study Group (IRLSSG) on the essential criteria for the diagnosis of RLS. This group defined four clinical characteristics of RLS necessary for diagnosis (minimal criteria). These criteria were revised at a recent National Institutes of Health (NIH) RLS workshop[2]; the final formulation of the new RLS diagnostic criteria has been published in *Sleep Medicine*.[2] These criteria are listed in Table 70–1.

These four essential criteria are:

1. An urge to move, usually accompanied or caused by uncomfortable and unpleasant sensations in the legs
2. The urge to move or unpleasant sensations begin or worsen during periods of rest or inactivity such as lying and sitting
3. The urge to move or unpleasant sensations are partially or totally relieved by movement, such as walking or stretching, at least as long as activity continues
4. The urge to move or unpleasant sensations are worse in the evening or night than during the day or occur only in the evening or night

In addition to these essential criteria, there are supportive clinical features that are not essential but can help resolve diagnostic uncertainty. The features include a positive family history of RLS (see the section on Etiology and Pathophysiology) and a positive therapeutic response to dopaminergic medications (see section on Treatment).

Table 70–1.	Diagnostic Criteria Established by the International Restless Legs Syndrome Study Group
Essential features	The patient experiences an urge to move the legs, usually accompanied or caused by uncomfortable and unpleasant sensations in the legs (sometimes the urge to move is present without the uncomfortable sensation, and sometimes the arms or other body parts are involved in addition to the legs). The urge to move or unpleasant sensations begin or worsen during periods of rest or inactivity, such as lying or sitting. The urge to move or unpleasant sensations are partially or totally relieved by movement, such as walking or stretching, at least as long as the activity continues. The urge to move or unpleasant sensations are worse in evening or night than during the day or only occur in the evening or night (when symptoms are very severe, the worsening at night may not be noticeable but must have been previously present).
Nonessential but common features	Family history: The prevalence of RLS among first-degree relatives of people with RLS is three to five times greater than in people without RLS. There is a response to dopaminergic therapy. Patient experiences periodic leg movements during sleep or during wakefulness. Natural clinical course: RLS may begin at any age, but most severely affected patients are in middle to older age—the condition is usually progressive, but a static course or remission may occur. There is sleep disturbance. Medical evaluation/physical examination: No abnormalities in the primary form, but in the secondary form, signs of a peripheral neuropathy or radiculopathy may be present. Iron status should be evaluated because decreased iron stores are a significant potential risk factor that can be treated.

RLS, restless legs syndrome.

Sleep Laboratory Diagnosis

Periodic Limb Movements during Sleep and Periodic Limb Movements while Awake

Originally called *nocturnal myoclonus*, PLMS are best described as rhythmic extensions of the big toe and dorsiflexions of the ankle with occasional flexions of the knee and hip. Methods for recording and scoring PLMS were summarized by Coleman.[19] According to standard criteria, PLMS are scored only if they are part of a series of four or more consecutive movements lasting 0.5 to 5 seconds with an intermovement interval of 4 to 90 seconds. A PLMS index (number of PLMS per hour of sleep) greater than 5 for the entire night of sleep is considered pathologic. The number of PLMS varies from night to night, especially in individuals with less severe sleep complaints. PLMS cluster into episodes, each of which lasts several minutes or even hours. In general, these episodes are more numerous in the first half of the night, but they can also recur throughout the entire sleep period. Diagnostic polysomnography always includes central electroencephalography (EEG), electrooculography, submental electromyography (EMG), and bilateral EMG of the anterior tibialis muscles (Fig. 70–1). Additional EEG and EMG derivations are frequently recorded. The electrographic picture of a single movement can vary from one sustained contraction to a polyclonic burst with a frequency of approximately 5 Hz. PLMS are often associated with EEG signs of arousal. These arousals may be of short duration, insufficient for scoring an epoch of wakefulness, and are therefore termed *EEG arousals* or *microarousals*. In patients with RLS, approximately one third of all PLMS are associated with microarousals. Recently, more attention has been paid to other signs of physiologic activation associated with PLMS. Regardless of the presence of EEG arousals, almost all PLMS are associated with a tachycardia (decreased R-R intervals for 5 to 10 beats) followed by a bradycardia.[20] This autonomic response decreases with age, especially in male patients with RLS.[21]

PLMS were first polygraphically documented in RLS.[22] In fact, most of what is known about PLMS derives from the study of patients with RLS. However, PLMS also occur in a wide range of sleep disorders,[23-25] including narcolepsy,[23] rapid eye movement (REM) sleep behavior disorder,[24] obstructive sleep apnea syndrome,[25] insomnia,[23] and hypersomnia.[26] PLMS were also reported in subjects without any sleep complaint, and although they are rare in young individuals, they are relatively common in the older adult.[27]

When PLMS are seen in patients who complain of primary sleep-onset or sleep-maintenance insomnia or of primary hypersomnia, it is called PLM disorder. The basic assumption is that PLMS are responsible for the nonrestorative sleep and daytime somnolence reported by these patients. Although some studies have suggested that PLMS may be associated with sleep–wake complaints, most authors have concluded that PLMS have little impact on nocturnal sleep or daytime vigilance. In 1980, Coleman and collaborators[26] suggested that there was no evidence that PLMS actually cause insomnia. More recently, several studies conducted in middle-aged or older adults showed a lack of correlation between PLMS and subjective sleep complaints or polysomnographic signs of disrupted sleep.[28] A study of younger insomniac patients with and without PLMS also concluded that PLMS did not appear to be the primary cause of insomnia in these patients.[29] Similarly, in hypersomniac patients with PLMS, there is no indication that PLMS cause sleep disruption resulting in excessive daytime sleepiness.[30] The same conclusion is reached when one considers not only PLMS alone but PLMS associated with arousals.

Although there are major controversies with regard to the functional significance of PLMS, their quantification is a commonly used sleep laboratory diagnostic procedure for RLS. In a recent study of 100 patients with RLS and 50 normal control subjects,[7] 84% of patients showed a PLMS index greater than 5 and 70% an index greater than 10, compared with 36% and 18%, respectively, for the control subjects. Patients also

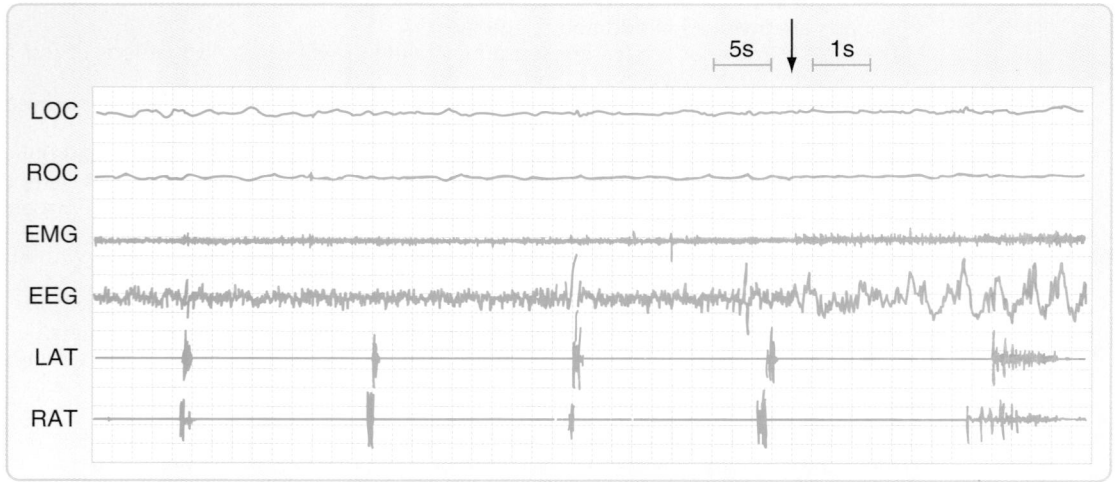

Figure 70–1. Polysomnogram of a patient with restless legs syndrome/periodic leg movements during sleep. *Arrow* points to a change of chart speed from 3 mm/s to 15 mm/s. Left side of the figure shows the periodicity of leg movements, with an interevent interval of 24.5 s; right side of the figure illustrates the arousal reaction accompanying leg movements. LOC, left electrooculogram; ROC, right electrooculogram; EMG, chin electromyogram; EEG, left central electroencephalogram; LAT, left anterior tibialis electromyogram; RAT, right anterior tibialis electromyogram.

showed a greater index of PLMS associated with EEG signs of arousal. In that study, a PLMS index greater than 7 was found to have a sensitivity of 78% and a specificity of 76% in diagnosing RLS. Quantification of PLM while awake (PLMW) was found to be even more sensitive (87%) and specific (80%) for discriminating patients with RLS from normal control subjects. However, these results were obtained in middle-aged individuals; unpublished data show that PLMW are quite common in young, healthy individuals, and this may limit their usefulness in the diagnosis of RLS in younger patients. Almost 50% of patients with RLS also report symptoms in the arms.[8] Polygraphic recordings revealed the presence of periodic arm movements during wakefulness in approximately two thirds of these patients, but only a small number of patients with a complaint of arm paresthesia showed periodic arm movements during sleep (3 of 22, or 13.8%).[31]

Suggested Immobilization Test

The SIT was designed to quantify both sensory and motor manifestations of RLS in wakefulness.[7] During the test, patients remain in bed, reclined at a 45-degree angle with their legs outstretched and eyes open. They are instructed to avoid moving voluntarily for the entire duration of the test, which lasts 1 hour and takes place in the evening before bedtime. Surface EMGs from the right and left anterior tibialis are used to quantify leg movements. In addition, every 5 minutes during the test, the patient has to estimate his or her level of leg discomfort on a 100-mm scale. The descriptors "no discomfort" and "extreme discomfort" are used as the left and right end points of this visual analogue scale. Twelve values are obtained (every 5 minutes for 60 minutes). The mean leg discomfort score (MDS) represents the average value of these 12 measures. Recently, the sensitivity and the specificity of the SIT was tested in 100 patients with RLS and in 50 age-matched normal control subjects. An MDS of 11 was found to discriminate patients with RLS from control subjects with a sensitivity of 82% and a specificity of 84%.

In conclusion, an elevated PLMS index is supportive of the diagnosis of RLS. An elevated index of PLMW at night and a high MDS during the SIT were found to be more sensitive and specific, but these results remain to be confirmed in a large, independent study of patients of different age groups.

Severity Assessments

Recently, the IRLSSG developed a 10-point scale to measure RLS severity (Box 70–1). This scale has been validated[32] by comparing it with independent clinician ratings in a large, multicenter study. This scale is now largely used in clinical trials to assess the outcome of pharmacologic treatments.

Other clinical scales have been used in which severity is scored as mild, moderate, or severe based on global clinical impression or on a specific feature of RLS. For example, the Johns Hopkins RLS Severity scale focuses on the usual time at which the symptoms begin. It is assumed that the time of onset of symptoms indicates the length of time in a day for which the patient is likely to have RLS symptoms.[17] This scale was found to correlate with both PLMS and sleep efficiency. Polygraphic measures of PLMS and PLMW have also been shown to be correlated with subjective RLS severity.[17]

Box 70–1. International Restless Legs Syndrome Study Group Rating Scale

1. Overall, how would you rate the RLS discomfort in your legs or arms?
2. Overall, how would you rate the need to move around because of your RLS symptoms?
3. Overall, how much relief of your RLS arm or leg discomfort do you get from moving around?
4. Overall, how severe is your sleep disturbance from your RLS symptoms?
5. How severe is your tiredness or sleepiness from your RLS symptoms?
6. Overall, how severe is your RLS as a whole?
7. How often do you get RLS symptoms?
8. When you have RLS symptoms, how severe are they on an average day?
9. Overall, how severe is the impact of your RLS symptoms on your ability to carry out your daily affairs, for example carrying out a satisfactory family, home, social, school, or work life?
10. How severe is your mood disturbance from your RLS symptoms—for example, angry, depressed, sad, anxious, or irritable?

Each question (except question 3) has the following multiple choice:
 (4) Very severe, (3) Severe, (2) Moderate, (1) Mild, (0) None (sometimes with a more operational definition in parentheses)
 Question 3: (4) No relief, (3) Slight relief, (2) Moderate relief, (1) Either complete or almost complete relief, (0) No RLS symptoms and therefore question does not apply.

RESTLESS LEGS SYNDROME IN CHILDHOOD

Diagnostic Criteria

Although RLS and PLMS are generally thought to be conditions of adulthood, they have been reported in children.[33] Because children have difficulty verbalizing their symptoms, special criteria for the diagnosis of RLS were established for children at an NIH consensus conference on RLS.[2] For a diagnosis of definite RLS, children must meet all four of the essential diagnostic criteria established for adults, and either (1) the child must be able to describe the leg discomfort in his or her own words; or (2) the child must have two of the three following features: sleep disturbance for age, a PLMS index greater than 5 per hour of sleep, or a biologic parent or sibling with definite RLS. Criteria for probable and possible RLS have also been established.[2]

Prevalence and Relationship to "Growing Pains"

The prevalence of RLS is unknown in childhood, but one study found consistent leg restlessness in 6.1% of 1353 children aged 11 to 13 years over a 3-year period.[34] Retrospective studies of RLS symptoms in two separate series of adults found that 12% to 20% recalled symptom onset before the age of 10 years, and 38.3% to 45% before the age of 20 years.[7,35] In the vast majority of cases, symptoms are mild in childhood and medical attention usually is not sought.

Brenning[36] presented evidence suggesting a close connection between "growing pains" and RLS. First, he showed that adults with RLS-like symptoms are much more likely to have experienced growing pains as children than adults without RLS-like symptoms. Another important observation was that in the parents of children with growing pains, RLS-like features in adulthood occur far more frequently than in control parents. These observations are of potential interest given the familial, presumably autosomal dominant nature of most RLS cases (see section on Genetics).

Relationship to Attention-Deficit/ Hyperactivity Disorder

Much recent literature has focused on the possible relationship between RLS, PLMS, and attention-deficit/hyperactivity disorder (ADHD). In two different series, 26% to 64% of children with ADHD had a PLMS index greater than 5 per hour of sleep.[37,38] In these series, children with both ADHD and a PLMS index greater than 5 per hour of sleep had an increased incidence of both personal and familial history of RLS.[37,38] Not only do children with ADHD have more PLMS, but children with PLMS have more ADHD. Approximately 44% of children with PLMS have been found to have symptoms of ADHD.[39] These data suggest a possible genetic link between RLS/PLMS and ADHD.

In a large, community-based, cross-sectional survey of 866 children, symptoms of ADHD as measured by objective indices were almost twice as likely to occur with symptoms of RLS than would be expected by chance alone.[40] A polysomnographic study of 113 children showed that in children who had a combination of ADHD symptoms, sleep-disordered breathing, and PLMS, only the PLMS showed a linear relationship to ADHD symptoms.[41] However, the linearity was not present in children who had both ADHD and PLMS, but did not have sleep-disordered breathing. Based on these results, Chervin and colleagues have suggested that sleep-disordered breathing acts as a modulator of the more intimate relationship between PLMS and ADHD.[41]

There is evidence that the link between RLS and ADHD may persist into adulthood. Fifty-eight adults with RLS more frequently had symptoms suggestive of ADHD than 59 healthy adult control subjects.[42] A link between ADHD and RLS/PLMS is further suggested by data suggesting that dopaminergic agents improve not only the RLS/PLMS symptoms, but the ADHD symptoms in children with both RLS/PLMS.

SECONDARY RESTLESS LEGS SYNDROME

RLS and PLMS have been related to several other medical conditions, but in only a few cases was the association with RLS well documented.

Uremia

RLS is often associated with uremia, and 15% to 40% of patients undergoing hemodialysis do actually complain of RLS symptomatology, with several of them having very severe RLS.[43-45]

This is dramatic in many patients because hemodialysis requires prolonged periods of immobilization. Several factors may predispose uremic patients to the development of RLS, including anemia and peripheral neuropathy. It is possible that hemodialysis itself plays a role; most data on RLS and kidney failure actually come from patients on hemodialysis. Another interesting observation made in patients with end-stage renal disease is that the presence of RLS relates to an increased mortality rate independent of premature termination of hemodialysis. In one case of uremia, symptoms of RLS were found to resolve after successful kidney transplantation.[46]

Neuropathies

There is some evidence suggesting an association between RLS and peripheral neuropathy, but the extent of this association remains controversial. In 1996, Ondo and Jankovic[47] performed electrophysiologic evaluations (EMG) and nerve conduction velocities in 41 patients with RLS, 15 of which were abnormal (14 neuropathy of mixed types and 1 L5 radiculopathy). Of the 15 neuropathic patients with RLS, only 7 showed clinical signs of neuropathy (decreased vibration in all 7, absent ankle jerks in 6, decreased proprioception in 3, and diminished response to light touch and pinprick in 2). One argument in favor of a causal relationship is the lower prevalence of family history of RLS among those with neuropathic RLS compared with nonneuropathic RLS. Another study,[48] in which a thorough neurologic examination of 22 patients with RLS was performed, found polyneuropathy in 8 of the 22 patients (36%); 5 of the 8 had small-fiber neuropathy based on skin biopsy. The neuropathic cases in this study had an older age of onset and reported sensory symptoms, usually involving pain. In a third study, axonal atrophy was found by sural nerve biopsy performed in eight patients with RLS.[49] All these studies suggest that in a significant number of patients with RLS, neuropathy may be involved. Other studies have questioned the extent of this association between RLS and peripheral neuropathies. RLS was found in only 5.2% of 144 patients presenting with a clinical diagnosis of polyneuropathy,[50] a prevalence not higher than that found in the general population. Similarly, a comparison between 218 patients with RLS and 872 healthy control subjects revealed a low prevalence of neuropathy among patients with RLS, and between-group comparisons showed no difference except for a slightly increased prevalence of neuropathy in female patients with RLS.[51] Similarly, a study of patients with rheumatoid arthritis with and without RLS failed to show a between-group difference for the presence of neuropathy.[52] In summary, it seems that neuropathic RLS may be a secondary form of RLS in some patients, especially those with an older age of onset, sensory symptoms involving pain, and the absence of other affected members in the family.

Anemia

RLS has also been reported in association with iron- and folic acid–deficiency anemia. More recently, iron status was extensively studied and evidence was found that iron deficiency in the central nervous system may be involved in primary RLS even in patients without anemia (see the section on Etiology and Pathophysiology).

Others

RLS was also found in 31% of 135 consecutive patients with fibromyalgia[53] and in 30% of 70 patients with rheumatoid arthritis.[54] RLS has also been reported anecdotally in association with a wide variety of other medical conditions, including diabetes, hypothyroidism and hyperthyroidism, chronic lung disease, leukemia, Isaacs' syndrome, stiff-man syndrome, Huntington's chorea, and amyotrophic lateral sclerosis. However, these associations were found in a limited number of patients. Considering the high prevalence of RLS and PLMS in the general population, these associations should be interpreted with caution. In addition, several substances or medications may induce or worsen RLS or PLMS. These include tricyclic or other antidepressants, lithium carbonate, dopamine D_2 receptor blocking agents, such as classic neuroleptics, as well as caffeine and alcohol.

DIFFERENTIAL DIAGNOSIS

PLMS should be differentiated from other state-dependent motor disorders. Some types of sleep-related "myoclonus" can be observed in normal subjects. So-called hypnic myoclonus or "sleep starts" are observed during the transition from wakefulness to sleep. They consist of short, massive body movements that may also involve the extremities of both sides synchronously but that are devoid of periodicity. Fragmentary myoclonus in the form of phasic REM twitches is normally seen in REM sleep, but it may persist throughout all stages of non-REM sleep in association with several other sleep disorders. Pathologic forms of myoclonus are in general suppressed during sleep, but myoclonic epilepsy is specifically activated by awakenings.

Other conditions can also be misdiagnosed as RLS or PLMS. The "painful legs and moving toes" syndrome[55] is characterized by severe pain in one or both feet, sometimes with a sensation of burning, and associated with repetitive, semicontinuous movements of the toes. However, pain is not necessarily worse at night or relieved by activity. Nocturnal leg cramps are sustained and painful contractions of the leg muscles, mainly the gastrocnemius and the soleus. Such cramping can be precipitated by contraction of these muscles during stretching; it is usually relieved by dorsiflexion of the foot. Although leg cramps can be easily differentiated from RLS clinically, they represent a major confounding factor in epidemiologic studies because patients with nocturnal leg cramps are likely to answer positively to all four diagnostic criteria of RLS listed in Table 70–1. RLS should also be differentiated from neuroleptic-induced akathisia, which is motor restlessness induced by dopamine receptor–blocking antipsychotic agents. Neuroleptic-induced akathisia is not associated with prominent paresthesia, and symptoms are not necessarily worse at night. Inner restlessness rather than leg discomfort is the usual trigger for neuroleptic-induced akathisia. The history of neuroleptic use clarifies the picture. In addition, levodopa (L-dopa) does not suppress akathisia as it does RLS symptoms, and in some cases of parkinsonism, L-dopa may even trigger akathisia. PLMS may occur in neuroleptic-induced akathisia but do not occur in as high a percentage as in RLS.[56]

Vascular conditions such as vascular or neurogenic intermittent claudication are frequent causes of leg pain or discomfort, but unlike RLS, they are relieved by rest with the leg outstretched and worsen during a prolonged upright position or walking.

MEDICAL INVESTIGATION

These observations stress the importance of careful history taking and differential diagnosis. Whenever the diagnosis is doubtful, a polysomnographic recording should be performed. Two consecutive nights of polysomnography are recommended. Because the PLMS index shows night-to-night variability, caution should be exercised in drawing conclusions from single-night studies. Because a significant number of patients with RLS have peripheral neuropathy,[47,48] a careful clinical examination of sensory and motor functions should be performed. EMG and nerve conduction studies should be done if the examination is suggestive of a peripheral neuropathy or radiculopathy. Given the aforementioned associations between RLS and anemia or iron deficiency, iron status should be studied in every patient. Iron deficiency cannot be determined by history and may occur with a normal hemoglobin. Because iron deficiency is usually treatable and because when present it exacerbates or even causes RLS, standard serum tests for ferritin, total iron-binding capacity, and percentage saturation should be considered an essential part of the medical evaluation of RLS. When results are abnormal, further medical evaluation is recommended to determine any possible cause, usually involving blood loss. For example, RLS was found much more commonly in blood donors than in the general population, especially for female donors.[57] Another study reported that the odds ratio of RLS or PLMS was 4.4 times higher for repeat blood donors than for non–repeat blood donors (donated less than five times in lifetime).[58] Repeated blood donation was found to be associated with the induction of RLS due to iron deficiency with or without coexisting anemia.[59]

Although blood loss is usually the cause of iron deficiency, the diet also can be responsible and should be queried. In a recent study on vegan vegetarians, 40% of women younger than 50 years of age were found to be iron deficient.[60]

ETIOLOGY AND PATHOPHYSIOLOGY

Genetics

There is substantial evidence for a genetic contribution to RLS. Several families have been described where members were affected with RLS over a span of three to five generations. Familial aggregation has been well documented, with more than 50% of idiopathic cases reporting a positive family history of RLS.[1,2,8,11,35] In most pedigrees, it segregates in an autosomal dominant fashion, with a high penetrance rate (90% to 100%).[11]

A linkage study revealed the presence of an RLS susceptibility gene on chromosome 12q in one large French-Canadian family (RLS1 locus).[61] In 2003, Bonati et al.[62] excluded the RLS1 locus but reported a new locus on chromosome14q in one large Italian family. This finding was recently confirmed in the French Canadian population.[62a] Genetic heterogeneity was somewhat predictable given the high prevalence of the disease and the reported variability in clinical presentation. Association studies have also looked at candidate genes for RLS. Genes related to dopaminergic transmission (D_1 to D_5 receptors, tyrosine hydroxylase, dopamine-B-hydroxylase) were investigated first, but no association was found.[63]

However, there was some evidence for a genetic association between monoamine oxidase-A and RLS.[64]

Neural Substrates

There are major controversies with regard to the localization of the neural structures involved in the physiopathologic process of RLS. There is some evidence of a peripheral origin of RLS. Although muscle biopsy results were normal in most studies, nerve biopsy revealed the presence of axonal atrophy in a small-fiber sample of patients with RLS.[49] However, there has been no independent replication of this study. As described earlier (see section on Secondary RLS), nerve conduction abnormalities and small-fiber neuropathy were found in a subset of patients with RLS, but these abnormal findings were noted in a small subset of patients with secondary RLS, more frequently in sporadic than in familial RLS and more often in patients with late- rather than early-onset of RLS.

There is most likely a major contribution of the spinal cord to RLS. PLMS and PLMW were also found in several individuals with a spinal cord lesion and even in cases of complete spinal cord transection.[65,66] PLMS were studied by videographic analysis and were found to be similar to the Babinski response,[67] which is found in cortical or spinal cord lesions. More recently, Barra-Jimenez and collaborators studied the flexion reflex of patients with primary RLS by electrically stimulating the plantar nerve.[68] They found a facilitation of the late component of the flexion reflex, indicating hyperexcitability of motoneurons in this condition. They also noted that the late components shared several features with PLMS (similar duration, same muscles involved). Taken together, these studies suggest the presence of a spinal cord generator for the periodic motor manifestations of RLS. This spinal cord generator may be facilitated by the suppression of or a decrease in supraspinal inhibitory inputs.

On the other hand, an additional long latency component of the blink reflex has been reported in some patients with PLMS.[69] This observation, although not found in every patient, could indicate that PLMS is operative at the pontine level or more rostrally. A study using magnetic resonance imaging (MRI) found no anatomic lesion in patients with RLS. However, functional MRI showed that leg-related sensory complaints in RLS were associated with thalamic and cerebellar activation, whereas PLMW were more closely associated with pontine and red nucleus activation. In neither case was any cortical activation found.[70] This result is in agreement with those of back-averaging techniques that found no premovement cortical potentials for PLMS. A study of 18 patients by transcranial magnetic stimulation also supports a subcortical origin of RLS.[71]

Neurotransmitter Dysfunctions

Therapeutic results obtained with opioids and L-dopa have led to some neuropharmacologic hypotheses regarding the physiopathologic process of RLS-PLMS. The therapeutic effects of L-dopa and dopaminergic agonists on RLS and PLMS support the hypothesis that central dopamine may be involved in the pathophysiology of these conditions. Dopamine antagonists usually make RLS symptoms worse and, in one study, precipitated an increase in PLMW in all but one of the patients evaluated.[72] Brain imaging studies have been inconsistent. The only positron emission tomography study with an adequate sample size showed small but significant decreased striatal binding

for raclopride, suggesting either decreased D_2 receptor activity or increased intracellular dopamine, or both.[73] Two of three single-photon emission computed tomography studies comparing patients with RLS with age-matched control subjects failed to find a significant difference,[74,75] whereas one study (the only one performed in early evening) reported a small but statistically significant difference: less binding to D_2 receptors for the patients with RLS.[76] These studies also looked at binding for the dopamine transporter and failed to find any significant difference between patients with RLS and control subjects. In contrast, two 6-[¹⁸F]fluoro-L-dopa (F-DOPA) positron emission tomography studies reported small decreases in binding for patients with RLS. This has been interpreted as indicating a possible presynaptic deficit, but it is known that F-DOPA is somewhat nonspecific, and therefore these results must be considered very cautiously.[73,77] None of these studies, except one, was done during the symptomatic period for RLS. There has been only one cerebrospinal fluid study of a series of patients with RLS compared with control subjects; it failed to find any significant difference for either homovanillic acid or biopterin that was unrelated to age.[78] Overall, aside from the remarkable pharmacologic response to dopaminergic medications, there is scant evidence supporting any significant dopaminergic abnormality in RLS.

The positive pharmacologic response to opioid treatment in RLS and the reversal of that treatment with the opiate receptor blocker naloxone has also been used as an argument in favor of the hypothesis of an endogenous opiate system dysfunction in RLS and PLMS.[79] However, pharmacologic data suggest that the effect of L-dopa is not secondary to the action of dopamine on the opioid system, but rather the reverse. A single-case study showed that blockade of opiate receptors by naloxone does not alter the therapeutic effect of L-dopa, whereas pretreatment with pimozide, a dopamine receptor antagonist, partially blocks the effect of codeine on RLS.[79] Aside from the pharmacologic data, there is no evidence for an opiate system dysfunction in RLS.

Iron

Ekbom was among the first to note that RLS commonly occurs with iron-deficiency anemia.[80] In addition to iron-deficiency anemia, end-stage renal disease, pregnancy, and gastric surgery have been clearly established as causes of secondary RLS. All of these conditions involve iron deficiency. It has been suggested that all conditions that compromise iron status increase the risk of RLS. Treatment of iron-deficiency anemia can completely resolve all RLS symptoms for some patients. Intravenous iron treatment completely resolved all RLS symptoms for 3 to 9 months in 21 of 22 patients in one study.[81] Although the benefits of intravenous iron have not been evaluated in a blinded, placebo-controlled trial, it seems unlikely that the magnitude and duration of these responses could be attributed to a placebo effect. As in adults, RLS has been associated with iron deficiency in adolescents, and treatment of the deficiency resulted in improvement of RLS symptomatology.[82] A very recent study found that serum ferritin levels correlated negatively with ADHD severity in 43 children with ADHD, 44% of whom met the criteria for RLS.[83]

One study of patients with RLS compared with age-matched control subjects showed no significant differences in serum ferritin or iron, but the cerebrospinal fluid ferritin was reduced and transferrin increased, consistent with a central nervous system iron deficiency occurring despite apparently normal peripheral iron status.[84] MRI for regional brain iron content also showed reduced brain iron in the substantia nigra and, to a lesser extent, in the putamen for patients with RLS compared with age-matched control subjects.[85] Autopsy analyses of substantia nigra tissue from patients with RLS compared with age-matched control subjects have revealed a complex pattern of iron-related abnormalities. Iron, H-ferritin, and two primary iron transporters were reduced and transferrin had increased, as expected for an iron-deficiency condition. The transferrin receptor, however, was decreased, contrary to the normal response to iron deficiency.[86] These data suggest that RLS involves an iron deficiency in the substantia nigra that may be associated with an abnormality in the regulation of the transferrin receptor. Thus, the neuromelanin-containing cells of the substantia nigra appear to have a basic iron regulation abnormality in RLS.

Studies of brain iron and RLS consistently found significant abnormalities. These findings, combined with the success of intravenous iron treatments, support the putative concept that a brain iron deficiency causes RLS in many patients. Of interest is the role of iron in dopaminergic transmission in the central nervous system. Iron is an important cofactor for tyrosine hydroxylase, the rate-limiting enzyme in dopamine synthesis, and also plays a major role in the functioning of postsynaptic D_2 receptors.

TREATMENT

Nonpharmacologic

There are no formal studies reporting on the nonpharmacologic strategies used by patients to decrease the urge to move and lessen leg discomfort, but it is important to inform patients to maintain good sleep hygiene to prevent the development of the psychophysiologic insomnia frequently encountered in RLS. Patients should also refrain from drinking alcohol in the evening because alcohol aggravates symptoms in most patients. Massage of the affected parts of the body, taking hot baths or applying something hot or cold, and keeping the mind alert by performing tasks requiring a large amount of concentration have all been reported anecdotally to reduce RLS symptoms. Moderate amounts of exercise have been suggested to help RLS symptoms, although excessive exercise in the evening worsens RLS and further disrupts sleep. Some patients report that they alter their sleep patterns to accommodate their RLS. For instance, they go to bed later at night and remain active during hours when their symptoms make sleep difficult, and some patients with severe RLS may even change their working schedule for that purpose (for review, see Hening et al.[87]).

Pharmacologic

Four categories of medications are commonly prescribed to treat RLS: dopaminergic agents, opioids, anticonvulsants, and benzodiazepines.

Dopaminergic Medications

Levodopa

Dopaminergic medications are now considered the treatment of choice for RLS.[87a] Initially, the emphasis was put on L-dopa. Several open-label studies documented the short-term efficacy of L-dopa given with a dopa-decarboxylase inhibitor, either benserazide or carbidopa. A placebo-controlled study with polysomnography showed that L-dopa administered twice at night produces a significant reduction of RLS symptoms present at bedtime and of PLMS throughout the night.[88] Several studies examined the long-term benefit of L-dopa and found various percentages of persistent efficacy, ranging from 85% after 2 years[89] to 31% after a mean of 31 months.[90] L-Dopa was also found effective in the treatment of RLS in patients with uremia[91] and to reduce PLMS in patients with narcolepsy.

Several adverse effects were reported in patients treated with L-dopa, including nausea, vomiting, tachycardia, orthostatic hypotension, hallucinations, insomnia, and daytime fatigue and sleepiness. Two adverse effects were more specifically studied in patients with RLS treated with L-dopa: morning rebound and RLS augmentation. Morning rebound is characterized by the presence of RLS symptoms occurring de novo as a consequence of evening or nighttime treatment. Similarly, a rebound of PLMS was observed in the last part of the night when L-dopa was administered only at bedtime. In rebound, the reappearance of symptoms is compatible with the timing of withdrawal from medication.

An analogous phenomenon is augmentation. Augmentation is the shifting of symptoms to a period 2 hours or earlier than was the typical period of daily symptoms before pharmacologic intervention. In more severe augmentation, not only do symptoms occur earlier during the day, but the urge to move or unpleasant sensations are extended to previously unaffected body parts, and the duration of the therapeutic effect is shorter than the duration of the initial therapeutic response. Patients may also report an overall increase in intensity of symptoms temporally related to an increase in medication dosage, or a decrease of symptoms related to a decrease in medication dosage. One group found augmentation in 29 of 36(81%) patients treated with L-dopa.[90] Increased severity of RLS and higher dosages of L-dopa were associated with higher risk for development of augmentation. Mild augmentation may be treated by earlier administration of the drug, but in severe cases the medication should be discontinued.

Dopaminergic Agonists

Because they are more effective and produce fewer adverse effects (especially augmentation), dopaminergic agonists are now considered the first-line treatment of RLS. Five agonists have been studied in RLS: bromocriptine, pergolide, cabergoline, pramipexole, and ropinirole. In short-term follow-up studies, the D_2 receptor agonist bromocriptine was found effective in the treatment of RLS and PLMS.[92] However, bromocriptine is frequently associated with severe adverse effects, especially nausea, responsible for withdrawal from bromocriptine shortly after the onset of treatment. Pergolide, another D_2 receptor agonist, was more extensively studied and its efficacy has been well documented in short- and long-term follow-up studies.[93,94] Pergolide was also found superior to L-dopa in alleviating symptoms of RLS. In 28 patients treated for 416 days with pergolide, persistent efficacy was noted in 79% of patients, but adverse effects were noted in 71%, including augmentation in 27% of cases.[94] Cabergoline, a long-acting D_2 receptor agonist, was also used successfully to treat RLS.[95] Like bromocriptine and pergolide, cabergoline is an ergoline derivative drug; agonists of this class are associated with frequent adverse effects, especially nausea and orthostatic hypotension.

It is often necessary to administer domperidone, a peripheral dopamine antagonist, to limit these side effects at least in the early phase of treatment.

Recently, two non–ergoline derivative agonists, pramipexole and ropinirole, were studied for the treatment of RLS. In 1999, pramipexole, a full agonist with high affinity for the D_3 receptor subtype, was studied in a crossover, placebo-controlled study and found to be very effective in treating RLS and suppressing PLMS.[96] Several long-term follow-up studies of patients treated with pramipexole have recently been published.[97,98] These studies showed sustained efficacy of pramipexole in more than 90% of patients. Previous studies have also found augmentation in up to 32% of patients on long-term treatment with pramipexole.[98] Ropinirole, a dopaminergic agonist with a pharmacologic profile similar to that of pramipexole, was also found effective in the treatment of RLS in a placebo-controlled study.[99] Like pramipexole, ropinirole is well tolerated and rarely requires the adjunct use of domperidone. Ropinirole has been approved by the FDA to treat moderate to severe RLS.

Cases of sleepiness associated with sudden onset of sleep were reported in patients with Parkinson's disease treated with pramipexole and ropinirole. Since then, sleepiness was reported in patients with Parkinson's disease treated with several other dopaminergic drugs and in untreated patients with Parkinson's disease (see Chapter 67). In patients with RLS, sleepiness might be seen during treatment with dopamine agonists, but is much less problematic, and no cases of sudden onset of sleep have been reported.[100]

Opioids

The therapeutic effects of opioids were already noted by Ekbom[1] and were recently examined in several open-label and controlled clinical trials. Two are double-blinded, randomized, placebo-controlled trials of oxycodone and propoxyphene using both subjective ratings and polysomnographic measures.[101,101a] Oxycodone administered at a mean daily dose of 15.9 mg both improved subjective ratings and decreased PLMS in 11 patients with RLS, with evidence for decreased arousals and improved sleep efficiency.[101] More recently, a persistent effect of opioids was found in a long-term follow-up study.[102] Open-label trials have also shown the beneficial effect of other opiates, including codeine and methadone.

Opioids are frequently prescribed to patients with severe disease, especially those unresponsive to other treatments. Opioids are also very useful during withdrawal from dopaminergic agents in patients in whom severe augmentation has developed. Although there is little evidence of tolerance or addiction to opioids in the RLS literature, the data are sparse and therefore prescription of opioids should be restricted to patients without a previous history of substance abuse. Opioids should also be used cautiously in patients who snore and are at risk for sleep apnea syndrome.

Anticonvulsants

Anticonvulsants were first studied in the 1980s, beginning with carbamazepine. However, carbamazepine was not found very useful in clinical practice and it is not currently recommended for the treatment of RLS. More recently, studies of anticonvulsants have focused on gabapentin. Several open-label trials and one placebo-controlled study[103] showed subjective improvements with gabapentin at doses of 300 to 2400 mg/day.

Gabapentin produces few adverse effects other than mild daytime somnolence. There have been no comparative studies between gabapentin and dopaminergic agents, but the latter are generally considered more potent. In mild cases or in patients who have experienced adverse effects with dopaminergic medications, gabapentin is a valuable alternative. Because gabapentin is a common treatment of peripheral neuropathy and pain, it has also been recommended for the treatment of neuropathic RLS and in general for patients who use pain as a descriptor for their leg sensations.

Benzodiazepines

Several studies showed that benzodiazepines, including clonazepam, nitrazepam, lorazepam, and temazepam, improve the quality of sleep and reduce PLMS or PLMS associated with arousals in patients with RLS and in patients with both insomnia and PLMS. However, the therapeutic effects of benzodiazepines on subjective ratings of RLS symptoms were either modest or nonsignificant. Therefore, benzodiazepines are mostly used to improve sleep continuity in patients with RLS. Because dopaminergic agents often have a stimulating effect and worsen insomnia, benzodiazepines are often used as an adjunct treatment.

Other Treatments

When the patient's ferritin level is less than 45 to 50 µg/L, oral iron treatment is indicated, usually as supplemental treatment. Oral iron treatment can be ferrous sulfate 325 mg, or its equivalent, with vitamin C 100 to 200 mg taken twice a day, preferably on an empty stomach, depending on how well the iron is tolerated.

Clinical Management of Restless Legs Syndrome

In summary, dopaminergic agonists are now considered the treatment of choice for RLS. Because of their side effects profile, the nonergoline derivatives pramipexole and ropinirole are preferred. One advantage of pramipexole is its longer duration of action. In several patients, RLS occurs sporadically with spontaneous remission lasting weeks or even months. Therefore, the physician should use pharmacologic treatments on an irregular basis or consider a drug holiday when appropriate. Continuous pharmacologic treatment should be considered if patients complain of RLS occurring at least three nights per week. All treatments are symptomatic and do not influence the course of the illness. Therefore, the clinician should carefully assess the therapeutic benefit versus the severity of adverse effects. A therapeutic flowchart appears in Table 70–2. Each drug is presented with its commonly used therapeutic dosage, its most frequent side effects, and the appropriate countermeasures to adopt. Higher doses may be administered in severe cases, but when higher dosage is required, the clinician should carefully assess the presence of augmentation. If augmentation occurs, patients should be switched to another medication. If augmentation occurs with L-dopa, patients should be treated with dopaminergic agonists. If it occurs in the course of treatment with agonists, opioids are usually the best alternative treatment. Because of its pharmacokinetics, cabergoline may also be considered in patients in whom augmentation develops.

Table 70–2. **Flow Chart for the Management of Restless Legs Syndrome**

Steps	Agents	Dosages	Side Effects	Countermeasures
Step 1	DA agonists		Nausea and orthostatic hypotension	Slowly increase dosage *or* use domperidone if available (10-30 mg)
	Pramipexole	0.125-1 mg*	Insomnia	Use small dose of benzodiazepines in association with DA agonists
	Ropinirole	0.25-4 mg*		
	Pergolide	0.1-0.5 mg*	Daytime fatigue and somnolence	Reduce dosage *or* discontinue DA agonists and use levodopa (if severe and persistent)
			Hallucinations	Discontinue DA agonists
			Tolerance	Drug holiday for 2 wk then return to lower dosage
			Augmentation	Use small extra dose during daytime or discontinue DA agonists (if severe and persistent)
Step 2	DA precursors		Same as for DA agonists	See countermeasures for DA agonists (above)
	Levodopa with benserazide or carbidopa	100/25 mg, 200/50 mg,† regular or slow release	Morning rebound or augmentation of restless legs syndrome in early evening	Use small extra dose of levodopa during daytime *or* reduce dosage *or* combine levodopa with DA agonists or benzodiazepines *or* discontinue levodopa (if severe and persistent)
Step 3	Benzodiazepines		Daytime somnolence	Reduce dosage
	Clonazepam	0.5-2 mg*		Drug holiday for 2 wk, then return to lower dosage
	Temazepam	15-30 mg*	Tolerance	
	Nitrazepam	5-10 mg*		
Step 4	Opiates			
	Oxycodone	5-20 mg†	Constipation	Symptomatic treatment
	Codeine	15-120 mg*	Dependency	Drug holiday *or* withdrawal
Step 5	Antiepileptic drugs			
	Carbamazepine	200-400 mg*	Nephrotoxicity	Monitor blood level regularly and adjust dosage
	Gabapentin	100-1800 mg*	Daytime fatigue and somnolence	Reduce dosage

*At bedtime.

†At bedtime and repeated once during the night.

DA, dopamine.

Clinical Pearl

The clinician should keep in mind that RLS is a frequent and underdiagnosed condition with a strong genetic component. Dopaminergic agonists have produced a good therapeutic response in RLS.

REFERENCES

1. Ekbom KA: Restless legs. Acta Med Scand Suppl 1945;158:1-123.
2. Allen R, Picchietti D, Hening WA, et al: Restless legs syndrome: Diagnostic criteria, special considerations, and epidemiology. A report from the restless legs syndrome diagnosis and epidemiology workshop at the National Institutes of Health. Sleep Med 2003;4:101-119.
3. Michaud M, Chabli A, Lavigne G, et al: Arm restlessness in patients with restless legs syndrome. Mov Disord 2000;15:289-293.
4. Trenkwalder C, Hening W, Walters AS, et al: Circadian rhythm of periodic limb movements and sensory symptoms of restless legs syndrome. Mov Disord 1999;14:102-110.
5. Hening WA, Walters AS, Wagner M, et al: Circadian rhythm of motor restlessness and sensory symptoms in the idiopathic restless legs syndrome. Sleep 1999;22:901-912.
6. Michaud M, Dumont M, Selmaoui B, et al: Circadian rhythm of restless legs syndrome symptoms: Relationships with salivary melatonin, core body temperature and subjective vigilance. Ann Neurol 2004;55:372-380.
7. Michaud M, Paquet J, Lavigne G et al: Sleep laboratory diagnosis of restless legs syndrome. Eur Neurol 2002;48:108-113.
8. Montplaisir J, Boucher S, Poirier G, et al: Clinical polysomnographic and genetic characteristics of restless legs syndrome: A study of 133 patients diagnosed with new standard criteria. Mov Disord 1996;12:61-65.
9. Allen RP, Mignot E, Ripley B, et al: Increased CSF hypocretin-1 (orexin-A) in early- versus late-onset restless legs syndrome (RLS): Effects of iron status and amount of activity. Neurology 2002;58(Suppl 3):A514.
10. Allen RP, Bell TJ, Walters A, et al: Impact of restless legs syndrome (RLS) symptoms on the quality of life (QoL) of adult sufferers in the USA. Neurology 2003;60(Suppl 1):A11.
11. Winkelmann J, Muller-Myhsok B, Wittchen HU, et al: Complex segregation analysis of restless legs syndrome provides evidence for an autosomal dominant mode of inheritance in early age at onset families. Ann Neurol 2002;52:297-302.
12. Botez MI, Lambert B: Folate deficiency and restless legs syndrome in pregnancy [letter]. N Engl J Med 1977;297:670.

13. Lavigne G, Montplaisir J: Restless legs syndrome and sleep bruxism: Prevalence and association among Canadians. Sleep 1994;17:739-743.

14. Phillips B, Young T, Finn L, et al: Epidemiology of restless legs symptoms in adults. Arch Intern Med 2000;160:2137-2141.

15. National Sleep Foundation: 2000 Omnibus Sleep in America Poll. 2000. Available at www.sleepfoundation.org/publications/2001poll.html.

16. Rothdach AJ, Trenkwalder C, Haberstock J, et al: Prevalence and risk factors of RLS in an elderly population: The MEMO study. Memory and Morbidity in Augsburg Elderly. Neurology 2000;54:1064-1068.

17. Allen RP, Earley CJ: Restless legs syndrome: A review of clinical and pathophysiologic features. J Clin Neurophysiol 2001;18:128-147.

18. Nichols DA, Allen RP, Grauke JH, et al: Restless legs syndrome symptoms in primary care: A prevalence study. Arch Intern Med 2003;163:2323-2329.

19. Coleman RM: Periodic movements in sleep (nocturnal myoclonus) and restless legs syndrome. In Guilleminault C (ed): Sleeping and Waking Disorders: Indications and Techniques. Menlo Park, Calif, Addison-Wesley, 1982, pp 265-295.

20. Sforza E, Nicolas A, Lavigne G, et al: EEG and cardiac activation during periodic leg movements in sleep: Support for a hierarchy of arousal responses. Neurology 1999;52:786-791.

21. Gosselin N, Lanfranchi P, Michaud M, et al: Age and gender effects on heart rate activation associated with periodic leg movements in patients with restless legs syndrome. Clin Neurophysiol 2003;114:2188-2195.

22. Lugaresi E, Cirignotta F, Coccagna G, et al: Nocturnal myoclonus and restless legs syndrome. Adv Neurol 1986;43:295-307.

23. Montplaisir J, Michaud M, et al: Periodic leg movements are not more prevalent in insomnia or hypersomnia but are specifically associated with sleep disorders involving a dopaminergic impairment. Sleep Med 2000;1:163-167.

24. Fantini L, Michaud M, Gosselin N, et al: Periodic leg movements in REM sleep behavior disorder and related autonomic and EEG activation. Neurology 2002;59:1889-1894.

25. Fry JM, DiPillipo MA, Pressman MR: Periodic leg movements in sleep following treatment of obstructive sleep apnea with nasal continuous positive airway pressure. Chest 1989;96:89-91.

26. Coleman RM, Pollak CP, Weitzman ED: Periodic movements in sleep (nocturnal myoclonus): Relation to sleep disorders. Ann Neurol 1980;8:416-421.

27. Ancoli-Israël S, Kripke DF, Mason W, et al: Sleep apnea and periodic movements in sleep in an aging population. J Gerontol 1985;40:419-425.

28. Karadeniz D, Ondze B, Besset A, et al: Are periodic leg movements during sleep (PLMS) responsible for sleep disruption in insomnia patients? Eur J Neurol 2000;7:331-336.

29. Bastuji H, Garcia-Larrea L: Sleep/wake abnormalities in patients with periodic leg movements during sleep: Factor analysis on data from 24-h ambulatory polygraphy. J Sleep Res 1999;8:217-223.

30. Nicolas A, Lespérance P, Montplaisir J: Is excessive daytime sleepiness with periodic leg movements during sleep a specific diagnostic category? Eur Neurol 1998;40:22-26.

31. Chabli A, Michaud M, Petit D, et al: Periodic arm movements in restless legs syndrome during sleep/wake states. Sleep Res Online 1999;2(Suppl 1):337.

32. The International Restless Legs Syndrome Study Group: Validation of the International Restless Legs Syndrome Study Group rating scale for restless legs syndrome. Sleep Med 2003;4:121-132.

33. Walters AS, Picchietti DL, Ehrenberg BL, Wagner ML: Restless legs syndrome in childhood and adolescence. Pediatr Neurol 1994;11:241-245.

34. Laberge L, Tremblay RE, Vitaro F, et al: Development of parasomnias from childhood to early adolescence. Pediatrics 2000;106:67-74.

35. Walters A, Hickey K, Maltzman J, et al: A questionnaire study of 138 patients with restless legs syndrome: The "Night-Walkers" survey. Neurology 1996;46:92-95.

36. Brenning R: Growing pains. Acta Soc Med Uppsal 1960;65:185-201.

37. Picchietti DL, England SJ, Walters AS, et al: Periodic limb movement disorder and restless legs syndrome in children with attention-deficit hyperactivity disorder. J Child Neurol 1998;13:588-594.

38. Picchietti DL, Underwood DJ, Farris WA, et al: Further studies on periodic limb movement disorder and restless legs syndrome in attention-deficit hyperactivity disorder children. Mov Disord 1999;14:1000-1007.

39. Crabtree VM, Ivanenko A, O'Brien LM, et al: Periodic limb movement disorder of sleep in children. J Sleep Res 2003;12:73-81.

40. Chervin RD, Archbold KH, Dillon JE, et al: Associations between symptoms of inattention, hyperactivity, restless legs, and periodic leg movements. Sleep 2002;25:213-218.

41. Chervin RD, Archbold KH: Hyperactivity and polysomnographic findings in children evaluated for sleep-disordered breathing. Sleep 2001;24:313-320.

42. Wagner ML, Walters AS, Fisher BC, et al: The prevalence of attention deficit hyperactivity disorder and oppositional defiant disorder symptoms in adults is greater in RLS patients than in controls. Neurology 2001;56:A4.

43. Callaghan N: Restless legs syndrome in uremic neuropathy. Neurology 1966;16:359-361.

44. Wetter TC, Stiasny K, Kohnen R, et al: Polysomnographic sleep measures in patients with uremic and idiopathic restless legs syndrome. Mov Disord 1998;13:820-824.

45. Winkelman JW, Chertow GM, Lazarus JM: Restless legs syndrome in end-stage renal disease. Am J Kidney Dis 1996;28:372-378.

46. Yasuda T, Nishimura A, Katsuki Y, et al: Restless legs syndrome treated successfully by kidney transplantation: A case report. Clin Transplant 1986;138:138.

47. Ondo W, Jankovic J: Restless legs syndrome: Clinicoetiologic correlates. Neurology 1996;47:1435-1441.

48. Polydefkis M, Allen RP, Hauer P, et al: Subclinical sensory neuropathy in late-onset restless legs syndrome. Neurology 2000;55:1115-1121.

49. Iannaccone S, Zucconi M, Marchettini P, et al: Evidence of peripheral neuropathy in primary restless legs syndrome. Mov Disord 1995;10:2-9.

50. Rutkove SB, Matheson JK, Logigian EL: Restless legs syndrome in patients with polyneuropathy. Muscle Nerve 1996;19:670-672.

51. Banno K, Delaive K, Wall R, et al: Restless legs syndrome in 218 patients: Associated disorders. Sleep Med 2000;1:221-229.

52. Salih AM, Gray RE, Mills KR, et al: A clinical, serological and neurophysiological study of restless legs syndrome in rheumatoid arthritis. Br J Rheumatol 1994;33:60-63.

53. Yunus MB, Aldag JC: Restless legs syndrome and leg cramps in fibromyalgia syndrome: A controlled study. BMJ 1996;312:1339.

54. Reynolds G, Blake DR, Pall HS, et al: Restless legs syndrome and rheumatoid arthritis. BMJ 1986;292:659-660.

55. Spillane JD, Nathan PW, Kelley RE, et al: Painful legs and moving toes. Brain 1971;94:541-556.

56. Walters AS, Hening WA, Rubinstein M, et al: A clinical and polysomnographic comparison of neuroleptic-induced akathisia and the idiopathic restless legs syndrome. Sleep 1991;14:339-345.

57. Ulberg J, Nystrom B: Restless legs syndrome in blood donors. Sleep Med 2004;5:115-118.

58. Kryger MH, Shepertycky M, Foerster J, et al: Sleep disorders in repeat blood donors. Sleep 2003;26:625-626.

59. Silber MH, Richardson JW: Multiple blood donations associated with iron deficiency in patients with restless legs syndrome. Mayo Clin Proc 2003;78:52-54.

60. Waldmann A, Koschizke JW, Leitzmnn C, et al: Dietary iron intake and iron status of German female vegans: Results of the German Vegan Study. Ann Nutr Metab 2004;48:103-108.

61. Desautels A, Turecki G, Montplaisir J, et al: Identification of a major susceptibility locus for restless legs syndrome on chromosome 12q. Am J Hum Genet 2001;69:1266-1270.

62. Bonati MT, Ferini-Strambi L, Aridon P, et al: Autosomal dominant restless legs syndrome maps on chromosome 14q. Brain 2003;126:1485-1492.

62a. Levchenko A, Montplaisin J-Y, Dubé M-P, et al: The 14q restless legs syndrome locus in the French Canadian population. Ann Neurol 2004;55:887-891.

63. Desautels A, Turecki G, Montplaisir J, et al: Dopaminergic neurotransmission and restless legs syndrome: A genetic association analysis. Neurology 2001;57:1304-1308.

64. Desautels A, Turecki G, Montplaisir J, et al: Evidence for a genetic association between monoamine oxidase A and restless legs syndrome. Neurology 2002;59:215-219.

65. Yokata T, Hirose K, Tanabe H, et al: Sleep-related periodic leg movements (nocturnal myoclonus) due to spinal cord lesions. J Neurol Sci 1991;104:13-18.

66. Dickell MJ, Renfrow SD, Moore PT, et al: Rapid eye movement sleep leg movements in patients with spinal cord injury. Sleep 1994;17:733-738.

67. Smith RC: Relationship of periodic movements in sleep (nocturnal myoclonus) and the Babinski sign. Sleep 1985;8:239-243.

68. Bara-Jimenez W, Aksu M, Graham B, et al: Periodic limb movements in sleep: State-dependent excitability of the spinal flexor reflex. Neurology 2000;54:1609-1616.

69. Briellman RS, Rosler KM, Hess CW: Blink reflex excitability is abnormal in patients with periodic leg movements in sleep. Mov Disord 1996;11:710-714.

70. Bucher SS, Seelos KC, Oertel WH, et al: Cerebral generators involved in the pathogenesis of the restless legs syndrome. Ann Neurol 1997;41:639-645.

71. Tergau F, Wischer S, Paulus W: Motor system excitability in patients with restless legs syndrome. Neurology 2002;52:1060-1063.

72. Winkelmann J, Schadrack J, Wetter TC, et al: Opioid and dopamine antagonist drug challenges in untreated restless legs syndrome patients. Sleep Med 2001;2:57-61.

73. Turjanski N, Lees AJ, Brooks DJ: Striatal dopaminergic function in restless legs syndrome. Neurology 1999;52:932-937.

74. Eisensehr I, Wetter TC, Linke R, et al: Normal IPT and IBZM SPECT in drug-naive and levodopa-treated idiopathic restless legs syndrome. Neurology 2001;57:1307-1309.

75. Tribl GG, Asenbaum S, Klosch G, et al: Normal IPT and IBZM SPECT in drug naive and levodopa-treated idiopathic restless legs syndrome [letter]. Neurology 2002;59:649-650.

76. Michaud M, Soucy JP, Chabli A, et al: SPECT imaging of striatal pre- and postsynaptic dopaminergic status in restless legs syndrome. J Neurol 2002;249:164-170.

77. Ruottinen HM, Partinen M, Hublin C, et al: An FDOPA PET study in patients with periodic limb movement disorder and restless legs syndrome. Neurology 2000;54:502-504.

78. Earley CJ, Hyland K, Allen RP: CSF dopamine, serotonin, and biopterin metabolites in patients with restless legs syndrome. Mov Disord 2001;16:144-149.

79. Montplaisir J, Lorrain D, Godbout R: Restless legs syndrome and periodic leg movements in sleep: The primary role of dopaminergic mechanism. Eur Neurol 1991;31:41-43.

80. Ekbom KA: Restless legs syndrome. Neurology 1960;10, 868-873.

81. Nordlander NB: Therapy in restless legs. Acta Med Scand 1953;145:453-457.

82. Kryger MH, Otake K, Foerster J: Low body stores of iron on restless legs syndrome: A correctable cause of insomnia in adolescents and teenagers. Sleep Med 2002;3:127-132.

83. Konofal E, Lecendreux M, Arnulf I, et al: Restless legs syndrome and serum ferritin levels in ADHD children. Sleep 2003;26: A136-A137.

84. Earley CJ, Connor JR, Beard JL, et al: Abnormalities in CSF concentrations of ferritin and transferrin in restless legs syndrome. Neurology 2000;54:1698-1700.

85. Allen RP, Barker PB, Wehrl F, et al: MRI measurement of brain iron in patients with restless legs syndrome. Neurology 2001;56:263-265.

86. Connor JR, Boyer PJ, Menzies SL, et al: Neuropathological examination suggests impaired brain iron acquisition in restless legs syndrome. Neurology 2003;61:304-309.

87. Hening W, Allen R, Earley C, et al: The treatment of restless legs syndrome and periodic limb movement disorder. Sleep 1999;22:970-999.

87a. Hening WA, Allen RP, Early CJ, et al: An update on the dopaminergic treatment of restless legs syndrome and periodic limb movement disorder. Sleep 2004;27:560-583.

88. Brodeur C, Montplaisir J, Marinier R, et al: Treatment of RLS and PMS with L-dopa: A double-blind controlled study. Neurology 1988;35:1845-1848.

89. Von Scheele, Kempi V: Long-term effect of dopaminergic drugs in restless legs: A 2-year follow-up. Arch Neurol 1990;47:1223-1224.

90. Early CJ, Allen RP: Pergolide and carbidopa/levodopa treatment of the restless legs syndrome and periodic leg movements in sleep in a consecutive series of patients. Sleep 1996;19:801-810.

91. Trenkwalder C, Stiasny K, Pollmächer T, et al: L-dopa therapy of uremic and idiopathic restless legs syndrome: A double-blind, crossover trial. Sleep 1995;18:681-688.

92. Walters A.S, Hening W.A, Chokroverty S, et al: A double-blind randomized crossover trial of bromocriptine and placebo in restless legs syndrome. Ann Neurol 1988;24:455-458.

93. Wetter TC, Stiasny K, Winkelmann J, et al: A randomized controlled study of pergolide in patients with restless legs syndrome. Neurology 1999;52:944-950.

94. Stiasny K, Wetter TC, Winkelmann J, et al: Long-term effects of pergolide in the treatment of restless legs syndrome. Neurology 2001;56:1399-1402.

95. Stiasny K, Robbecke J, Schuler P, et al: Treatment of idiopathic restless legs syndrome (RLS) with the D_2-agonist cabergoline: An open clinical trial. Sleep 2000;23:349-354.

96. Montplaisir J, Nicolas A, Denesle R, et al: Pramipexole alleviates sensory and motor symptoms of restless legs syndrome. Neurology 1998;51:311-312.

97. Silber MH, Girish M, Izurieta R: Pramipexole in the management of restless legs syndrome: An extended study. Sleep 2003;26:819-821.

98. Winkelman JW, Johnston L: Augmentation and tolerance with long-term pramipexole treatment of restless legs syndrome. Sleep Med 2004;5:9-14.

99. Trenkwalder C, Garcia-Borreguero D, Montagna P, et al: Therapy with ropinirole, efficacy and tolerability in RLS-1 Study Group. Ropinirole in the treatment of RLS: Results from the TREAT RLS-1 study, a 12 week, randomized, placebo controlled study in 10 European countries. J Neurol Neurosurg Psychiatry 2004;75:92-97.

100. Stiasny K, Möller JC, Oertel WH: Safety of pramipexole in patients with restless legs syndrome. Neurology 2000;55:1589-1590.

101. Walters AS, Wagner ML, Hening WA, et al: Successful treatment of the idiopathic restless legs syndrome in a randomized double-blind trial of oxycodone versus placebo. Sleep 1993;16:327-332.

101a. Kaplan PW, Allen RP, Buchholz DW, Walters UK: A double-blind, placebo-controlled study of the treatment of periodic limb movements in sleep using carbidopa/levodopa and propoxyphene. Sleep 1993;16:717-723.

102. Walters AS, Winkelmann J, Trenkwalder C, et al: Long-term follow-up on restless legs syndrome patients treated with opioids. Mov Disord 2001;6:1105-1109.

103. Garcia-Barreguero D, Larrosa de la Liave Y, Verger K, et al: Treatment of restless legs syndrome with gabapentin. Neurology 2002;59:1573-1579.

71

Alzheimer's Disease and Other Dementias

Dominique Petit
Jacques Montplaisir
Bradley F. Boeve

ABSTRACT

Abnormalities in sleep are found in a variety of conditions associated with dementia: Alzheimer's disease, progressive supranuclear palsy, Parkinson's disease, dementia with Lewy bodies, vascular dementia, Huntington's disease, Creutzfeldt-Jakob disease, and frontotemporal dementia. The nature of the sleep and electroencephalographic impairment varies in some respects, but a common pattern emerges. Sleep is usually more fragmented, both from more awakenings and a longer duration of time awake; slow wave sleep is decreased; and spindles, K-complexes, and rapid eye movements are less well formed or less numerous, so sleep stages are more difficult to distinguish and rapid eye movement (REM) sleep may be reduced. Quantitative analyses show a slowing of the electroencephalogram during wakefulness and, in Alzheimer's disease, during REM sleep. All these impairments typically worsen with the progression of the disease. Demented patients are also more likely to present with periodic leg movements during sleep, respiratory disturbances, or both. When managing sleep disturbances in patients with dementia, careful assessments of the underlying causes is essential. The clinician should also keep in mind, before prescribing medication to demented patients, that many such agents (especially benzodiazepines) can exacerbate cognitive deficits and obstructive sleep apnea syndrome.

This chapter gives an overview of sleep disturbances, characteristics of sleep architecture and microstructure, and quantitative analyses of the wakefulness and sleep electroencephalogram (EEG) in a variety of conditions associated with dementia: Alzheimer's disease (AD), progressive supranuclear palsy (PSP), Parkinson's disease (PD), dementia with Lewy bodies (DLB), vascular dementia, Huntington's disease, Creutzfeldt-Jakob disease, and frontotemporal dementia (FTD). Some of the goals are (1) to provide useful information for the management and treatment of sleep disorders in individuals suffering from dementia; (2) to understand better the pathophysiologic processes of these conditions; and (3) to develop tools for differential diagnosis.

ALZHEIMER'S DISEASE

AD is a progressive neurodegenerative disorder characterized by progressive decline in memory and other cognitive domains. It is considered the primary cause of irreversible dementia in old age. Diagnostic criteria have been established by the National Institute of Neurological and Communicative Disorders and Stroke–Alzheimer's Disease and Related Disorders Association (NINCDS-ADRDA) Work Group[1] and,

although the sensitivity is good (92%), the specificity is rather low (65%). The accuracy of the diagnosis rests on the clinician's expertise and on the exclusion of other dementias and disorders, including the reversible ones (e.g., folate or vitamin B_{12} deficiency, hypothyroidism).[2] Pathologically, findings include neurofibrillary tangles, neuritic plaques, and neuronal loss.

Most of the literature on sleep disturbances in dementia involves patients clinically diagnosed with AD. However, a significant minority of patients with typical AD clinical features do not have AD when examined postmortem, and instead have one of the non-AD disorders such as DLB, frontotemporal lobar degeneration with or without ubiquitin-positive inclusions, Pick's disease, and so forth. Others have a combination of two or more conditions. The literature on sleep disturbances in dementia has therefore very likely included cases with non-AD disorders, and thus the findings may not be specific for AD. Furthermore, sleep-related issues may be quite different from one disorder to another. This is not the fault of the investigators, but simply reflects the state of the art in dementia diagnosis at that time. We therefore present data and concepts derived from the studies carried out over the past few decades, but ask that readers keep in mind that further research is necessary to define more precisely specific sleep disorder–dementia disorder associations.

Sleep Problems

One of the most noticeable sleep problems of patients with AD is nocturnal agitation or nocturnal wandering, the so-called *sundowning* experienced by the patient.[3] Sundowning refers to agitation or a delirium-like state starting in the evening or at night. In addition to nocturnal agitation, obstructive and central sleep apnea syndromes can contribute to sleep fragmentation. Indeed, obstructive sleep apnea syndrome has been reported to be occurring with a greater prevalence in patients with AD than in the general population.[4] A relationship between AD and apolipoprotein ε (APOE), a lipoprotein made in the liver and brain and involved in cholesterol transport and deposition, was first noted in 1993.[5] It was shown that the risk for development of AD was associated with the APOE4 allele. Recently, an association was found between the APOE4 allele and obstructive sleep apnea.[6]

Polysomnographic Findings

In addition to the presence of sleep problems, sleep architecture is modified in patients with AD. Certain sleep changes seem to be an exaggeration of changes that appear normally with aging. Specifically, patients with AD show an increased number and duration of awakenings and, as a result, an increased percentage of stage 1 sleep. Compared with elderly control subjects, they also show a reduced percentage of slow wave sleep (SWS).[7,8] This is the most consistently reported change in patients with mild to moderate AD, although in some studies the difference has failed to reach significance,[9] probably because patients were in milder stages of the disease. All prior sleep disturbances worsen with increasing severity of AD.[7]

Another change in sleep architecture that suggests accelerated aging in AD is a loss of the specific EEG features of stage 2 sleep. Sleep spindles and K-complexes are poorly formed, of lower amplitude, shorter in duration, and much less numerous.[9,10] With advancing severity of the disease, because of the absence of these characteristic EEG features, it becomes progressively more difficult to separate stage 2 from stage 1 sleep. The proportion of indeterminate non–rapid eye movement (NREM) sleep increases further with the disappearance of the true delta waves of SWS.

Conversely, other sleep changes observed in AD do not suggest accelerated aging. Of particular interest is the percentage of REM sleep, which remains stable in normal aging but which was reduced in patients with AD compared with control subjects, and this as a result of a decrease in mean REM sleep episode duration.[9] Other REM sleep variables, such as REM density, number of REM sleep episodes, and REM sleep latency, are usually unchanged.[8,9,11] In addition, no differences in muscle atonia and phasic electromyographic activity in REM sleep were found compared with age-matched control subjects.[9] In other words, variables pertaining to the initiation of REM sleep and to its characteristic features were unaffected in mild AD. This is probably because these variables are under the control of the mesopontine cholinergic populations, structures that are relatively spared in mild AD. The lower REM sleep percentage, however, could be due to degeneration of the nucleus basalis of Meynert. This nucleus normally exerts an inhibitory influence on the nucleus reticularis of the thalamus,[12] the rhythm generator responsible for NREM sleep.

Quantitative Electroencephalography in Alzheimer's Disease

Wakefulness Electroencephalogram

In AD, waking EEG activity is characterized by greater slowing of the dominant occipital rhythm than is found in the nondemented elderly.[13] There is also an increase in theta and delta activity compared with age-matched control subjects. However, local slowing rarely occurs.[13] Several studies attempted to correlate quantitative waking EEG with clinical severity of AD, with variable results. Some demonstrated that relative theta power separated all four stages of dementia: none, mild, moderate, and severe dementia.[14,15] Some reported that decreases of relative power in alpha and beta bands and increases of power in the delta band were correlated with severity of AD.[16]

REM Sleep Electroencephalogram

EEG slowing was found to be more marked during REM sleep than during wakefulness in patients with AD.[17,18] Using the ratio of slow over fast frequencies from the temporal regions, a correct classification of 90.4% of subjects (sensitivity, 81.5%; specificity, 100%) was obtained for the REM sleep EEG.[18] The best discrimination rate for the waking EEG was only 80.8% (sensitivity, 66.7%; specificity, 96%).[18] Moreover, there was a distinctive topographic pattern of REM sleep EEG slowing in

patients with AD that corresponds with findings from neuroradiologic[19-21] and neuropathologic[22] studies—a pattern not observed for the waking EEG.[23] The quantitative EEG derived from REM sleep (but not from wakefulness) was also correlated with a screening assessment of cognitive functioning in AD (the Mini-Mental State Examination)[24] and with a measure of interhemispheric asymmetry of regional cerebral blood flow.[25] To pinpoint better brain regions presenting significant cortical slowing, significance probability mapping was used in conjunction with a more complete EEG recording.[18] It was confirmed that for REM sleep, EEG slowing was greater in the temporoparietal and frontal regions, whereas for wakefulness EEG slowing was greater for the frontal pole. The discrimination rate obtained with the REM sleep EEG from the temporal region is thus far the best marker of AD using a single measure.

The superiority of the REM sleep EEG over wakefulness EEG may be because the cholinergic basal forebrain, which degenerates early in AD,[26] is likely more crucial for EEG activation during REM sleep than during wakefulness. EEG activation during wakefulness is the result of many convergent neuronal and neurotransmitter systems, many of which (including norepinephrine and histamine) are not active during REM sleep.[27] This leaves mainly the cholinergic nucleus basalis and the glutamatergic thalamocortical system to ensure EEG activation during the latter state. In addition, the importance of the contribution of the cholinergic system to cortical activation in REM sleep may also be due to a relatively enhanced activity in the cholinergic system during that state.[28] Thus, REM sleep EEG might be more useful to detect AD than awake EEG.

PROGRESSIVE SUPRANUCLEAR PALSY

PSP, also called Steele-Richardson-Olszewski syndrome, is characterized by progressive axial rigidity, postural instability, and supranuclear gaze palsy.[29] The dementia syndrome that often evolves in PSP primarily reflects dysfunction in the frontosubcortical neural networks.[29] Because the sleep characteristics of PSP are discussed in Chapter 67, only aspects related to the dementia are reviewed here.

An absence of or drastic reduction in REM sleep is a common finding in patients with PSP.[30-32] A reduction in REM sleep has been generally correlated with a decline in cognitive functioning, which is, in turn, reflected by a slowing of the EEG. One study has quantitatively assessed the EEG from both REM sleep and wakefulness in patients with PSP.[30] For the REM sleep EEG, there were no significant between-group differences in the spectral ratio for any of the 16 regions studied. In awake patients with PSP, a slowing of the EEG (as determined by a spectral ratio) was found mainly for the frontal regions, compared with control subjects.

The frontal EEG slowing during wakefulness is consistent with the results of numerous neuropsychological studies that show deficits to be related to frontal lobe functions.[33,34] The fact that no EEG slowing was found in REM sleep suggests that the slowing observed for wakefulness was not likely due to a cholinergic deficit. This is consistent with findings that normal neocortical and hippocampal choline acetyltransferase activity was found in some patients with PSP.[35] Dopamine levels are, however, severely reduced in the caudate, putamen, and substantia nigra in patients with PSP.[35] A frontal deafferentation from the striatopallidal complex is thought to be responsible for the impairment because there are extensive fiber connections between these nuclei and the prefrontal region.

Indeed, the positive correlations between degree of impairment on frontal tasks and EEG slowing observed in our patients with PSP suggest that both impairments could be at least partially the result of a dopaminergic deficiency.

PARKINSON'S DISEASE

PD is a progressive neurologic disorder characterized by rigidity, resting tremor, bradykinesia, and an impairment of postural reflexes and gait, caused in part by the degeneration of the dopaminergic cells in the substantia nigra.[36] The sleep modifications experienced by patients with PD are discussed in Chapter 67; therefore, only information relevant to the issue of dementia associated with PD is reviewed here.

The incidence of overt dementia in PD is relatively high; in a population-based study of dementia in PD, dementia had developed in approximately 80% of nondemented patients with PD within 8 years.[37] Risk factors include advanced age at onset of motor symptoms, severe motor symptoms (particularly bradykinesia), levodopa-related confusion or hallucinations, presence of speech and axial involvement, presence of depression, and atypical neurologic features, such as modest response to dopaminergic agents or early autonomic dysfunction.[38]

Demented patients with PD often experience hallucinations, but they can also be observed in nondemented patients. One study found that patients with REM sleep anomalies present with more hallucinations than patients without such anomalies.[39] It was proposed that sleep reduction, and particularly REM sleep reduction, would trigger hallucinations by enabling the emergence of REM sleep during wakefulness. Furthermore, hallucinations have been significantly correlated with the presence of REM sleep behavior disorder (RBD) independent of age, sex, disease duration, or Unified Parkinson's Disease Rating Scale score, but related to the amount of dopaminergic medication.[40] RBD is a parasomnia characterized by the loss of normal skeletal muscle atonia and involves complex motor activity occurring specifically during REM sleep in association with dream mentation[41] (for a detailed review, see Chapter 75). There is growing evidence that RBD is an early manifestation of a neurodegenerative disorder, particularly one of the synucleinopathies (e.g., DLB, PD, and multiple system atrophy).[41-43] The incidence of RBD in PD was estimated at 15% with a structured questionnaire,[44] but at 33% using polysomnographic recordings[45]; only half of these had been detected at the clinical interview. The phenomenon of REM sleep without atonia would explain the reduction in REM sleep reported in patients with PD when the sleep staging has been performed according to the standard criteria.[46]

EEG slowing has been frequently reported in PD. Previous studies had shown that approximately one third of patients with PD presented with EEG slowing regardless of the presence of dementia.[40] Even when only nondemented patients with PD were studied, a slowing of the dominant occipital frequency and of the EEG in the temporooccipital and the frontal regions has been found in some patients.[47] A recent study[48] has demonstrated that only nondemented patients with PD who also had RBD showed a slowing of the EEG and of the dominant occipital frequency. A higher theta power was found during wakefulness in frontal, temporal, parietal, and occipital regions in patients with PD and RBD compared with both patients with PD without RBD and control subjects. Moreover, a marked slowing of the dominant occipital frequency was observed only in patients with PD and RBD. The EEG slowing found only in patients with PD and RBD may not be related to an evolutionary stage of PD but rather to the presence of RBD itself. In support of this hypothesis, a higher theta power in frontal, temporal, and occipital regions during wakefulness has also been observed recently in patients with idiopathic RBD without PD.[49] Surprisingly, in light of the fact that the cholinergic basal forebrain is affected by neuronal destruction fairly early in idiopathic PD, no EEG slowing was found in any region in patients with PD and RBD during REM sleep.[48]

Given that the topography of EEG slowing observed in PD with RBD is similar to that of the hypoperfusion and hypometabolism seen in DLB,[50,51] and that many patients with RBD later have DLB,[52,53] there is reason to believe that the presence of RBD in patients with PD may be an early sign of evolution toward DLB. Indeed, some evidence suggests that cortical Lewy body–type degeneration is the main source of dementia in PD.[54] One study reported diffuse cortical Lewy bodies only in demented patients with PD, whereas nondemented patients had only brainstem Lewy bodies.[55] Two other recent studies suggested that α-synuclein–positive cortical (especially frontal) Lewy bodies were associated with cognitive impairment, independent of or more specifically than an AD-type pathologic process.[56,57] However, neurotransmitter abnormalities likely also contribute to cognitive impairment. More studies are necessary to determine the pathologic and neurochemical underpinnings of dementia in PD.

DEMENTIA WITH LEWY BODIES

DLB represents approximately 15% to 20% of cases of dementia in old age.[58] Until recently, it was a much underdiagnosed form of dementia, The core clinical features of DLB are spontaneous parkinsonism, visual hallucinations, and fluctuating cognition or arousal.[59] It is pathologically characterized by the presence of Lewy bodies in limbic or neocortical structures, or both. A questionnaire study showed that patients with DLB had more overall sleep disturbances, more movement disorders while asleep, and more daytime sleepiness than patients with AD.[60] A polysomnographic study[61] of 78 patients with DLB found that 73% of patients had a sleep efficiency below 80%, and half the sample were below 70%. High proportions of these patients also presented pathologic indexes of respiratory disturbances (88%) or of periodic leg movements during sleep (PLMS) with arousal (74%).[61] Moreover, a number of studies or review papers have shown that RBD is a common finding in patients with DLB.[52,53,59] Twelve of 15 cases with RBD plus a neurodegenerative disease had limbic or neocortical Lewy body disease at autopsy (the other 3 having multiple system atrophy), which is indicative of a synucleinopathy.[62] It has even been suggested that the inclusion of RBD in the list of core criteria for DLB would improve the sensitivity and specificity of the diagnosis.[2,53,62,63] As in PD, restless legs syndrome (RLS) is common in DLB.[64] RLS is a condition characterized by an urge to move the legs usually associated with leg paresthesia that occurs predominantly at rest and is worst in the evening and during the night.[65] It is known that RLS is often accompanied by PLMS.[65] RLS and PLMS can play a part in sleep-onset insomnia and nocturnal arousals or awakenings, respectively.

A few quantitative EEG studies have reported a slowing of the awake EEG in DLB, whether expressed as a loss of the alpha rhythm during wakefulness combined with a slowing of both dominant and nondominant rhythms,[66] or as an increase in theta activity,[67,68] which correlates with the degree of dementia.[67]

Frontal intermittent rhythmic delta activity has also been reported.[68] Fluctuating cognition, one of the core features of DLB, was shown to be reflected in cortical activation by the variability of the mean EEG power in patients with DLB compared with both patients with AD and elderly control subjects.[69]

VASCULAR DEMENTIA

The term *vascular dementia* covers a range of problems of various etiologies, and includes the entities known as multiinfarct dementia (MID) and Binswanger's disease. The best-studied form of vascular dementia in sleep medicine is probably MID. An actigraphic study found that patients with MID had a significantly greater disruption of sleep–wake cycles associated with poor sleep quality than patients with AD.[70] There was no correlation, however, between the degree of sleep disruption and the severity of intellectual deterioration. It was reported that sleep apnea syndrome was more strongly associated with MID than with AD.[71] Spectral analysis of the waking EEG of patients with MID revealed a lower dominant occipital frequency,[72,73] a higher theta and slower alpha power, a lower high alpha power, and more numerous delta waves than in control subjects.[72] In addition, in patients with MID, the alpha waves had migrated to more anterior regions. There were no sex differences in the quantitative EEG of patients with MID.[72,73] It was also reported that there was more localized slow wave activity in areas other than the temporal in patients with vascular dementia than in patients with nonvascular dementia.[74]

HUNTINGTON'S DISEASE

Huntington's disease is a well-known autosomal dominant hereditary condition associated with atrophy of basal ganglia structures, especially the caudate nucleus, and characterized by choreic movements and progressive dementia associated with psychotic features.[75] A disturbed sleep pattern has been reported in patients with Huntington's disease. Specifically, they showed a longer sleep latency, a lower sleep efficiency, frequent nocturnal awakenings, and less SWS than age-matched control subjects.[76,77] Contrary to patients with other neurodegenerative diseases, patients with Huntington's disease showed a higher density of sleep spindles compared with healthy control subjects.[77,78] The sleep disturbances correlated with the degree of atrophy of the caudate nucleus and the severity of clinical symptoms.[77] In fact, a study found sleep disturbances only in moderate to severe cases of Huntington's disease, and none in mild cases.[76] Finally, no difference was found in sleep respiratory variables (e.g., apneas, respiratory frequency) between patients with Huntington's disease and healthy control subjects.[79]

On visual inspection, the awake EEG exhibits a gradual slowing and diminution of amplitude as the disease progresses.[80,81] A quantitative analysis of the awake EEG in Huntington's disease revealed that the relative alpha and theta activities were lower than in control subjects and similar to those of patients with AD.[82]

CREUTZFELDT-JAKOB DISEASE

Creutzfeldt-Jakob disease is a prion-related spongiform encephalopathy causing extensive neuronal degeneration and pathologic changes, especially in the cortex, and resulting in myoclonic jerks and rapidly evolving dementia. Sleep apneas, whether central or obstructive, seem prevalent in this condition.[83-85] One PSG study of three patients in the early stage of Creutzfeldt-Jakob disease reported that their sleep patterns were disorganized, with sudden jumps from one sleep stage to the next, very few sleep spindles and K-complexes in stage 2 (which is, however, represented normally but difficult to distinguish from stage 3), an absence of stage 4, and a lower percentage of REM sleep with fewer rapid eye movements.[86]

The awake EEG showed triphasic waves or a slow electrogenesis of low amplitude, suggesting a diffuse cerebral pathologic process.[86] Sleep EEG studies usually report the presence of periodic complexes (also called periodic synchronous discharges or pseudoperiodic discharges) characterized by diffuse slow sharp waves and biphasic or triphasic waves, as early as 1 to 3 months after the onset of symptoms.[83,84,87,88] Two research teams described cyclic changes with periodic complex phases alternating with semirhythmic theta–delta activities.[87,88] Two studies reported that periods of breathing were associated with periodic synchronous discharges, whereas the sleep apneas resulted in a abrupt cessation of these periodic complexes.[84,85] It was suggested that the generator of these periodic discharges might be located in the thalamus or in the upper brainstem.[89]

FRONTOTEMPORAL DEMENTIA

FTD is a category of disorders that includes Pick's disease, corticobasal degeneration, and dementia lacking a distinctive histologic pattern.[2] It is a progressive, degenerative condition characterized by a loss of executive and language abilities and a number of noncognitive symptoms, such as loss of insight, overactivity, lack of social awareness, disinhibition, perseveration, and lack of personal hygiene.[90] In addition, amyotrophic lateral sclerosis also develops in approximately 15% of patients with FTD.[91] On the other hand, concomitant depression is rare.[90] Approximately 5% to 15% of patients with dementia have a disorder in the FTD spectrum. It is thought to be underdiagnosed because, in part, of its similarities with AD, especially later in the progression of the disease. However, unlike AD, FTD initially presents with progressive aphasia and personality changes, whereas memory remains relatively intact. Structural and functional brain imaging showed atrophy, reduced cerebral blood flow, or diminished glucose metabolism in frontal and anterior temporal areas. Pathologic examination revealed neuronal loss in the same regions without plaque formation.

As in AD, FTD is usually accompanied by a disturbance of the activity rhythm and of the sleep–wake rhythm. However, these disturbances manifest differently in the two conditions, supporting the notion that central changes, rather than environmental factors only (such as institutionalization, which often provides insufficient synchronizing signals or zeitgebers), cause the rhythm disturbances. In FTD, the activity rhythm is highly fragmented and phase advanced despite a normal core temperature phase.[92]

Quantitative EEG studies[93,94] first reported normal EEG findings, but more recent studies found some form of EEG slowing in patients with FTD. One study found an increased theta power during both eyes-closed and eyes-open conditions.[95] Another research team reported an increase in both delta and theta power more prominently in anterior regions in a majority of patients.[96] However, 31% had normal EEGs, and most patients had a preserved dominant occipital frequency.[96]

TREATMENT OF SLEEP DISORDERS IN PATIENTS WITH DEMENTIA

One useful approach to address sleep disorders in the demented patient involves considering symptoms within four major categories: (1) insomnia or fragmented sleep; (2) excessive daytime sleepiness; (3) alteration in the sleep–wake circadian rhythm; and (4) excessive motor activity during the night, including RBD, PLMS, and nocturnal agitation or wandering. In addition, one should keep in mind that some of these disturbances could be due to RLS, obstructive sleep apnea syndrome, malnutrition, infections, medication effects (and often polypharmacy), depression, bladder catheterization, fecal impactions, or disturbing environmental factors. Management requires the identification and treatment of the underlying medical or psychiatric disorder. For each of the aforementioned four categories of sleep disorders, we review the appropriate pharmacologic and nonpharmacologic treatment strategies. A summary of selected medications for each problem with suggested dosage and titration schedules also appears in Table 71–1.

Table 71–1. Sleep Disorders and Disturbances in Dementia: Selected Medications with Suggested Dosing Schedules*

Symptom/ Disorder/Behavior	Medication	Initial Dose	Suggested Titrating Schedule	Typical Therapeutic Range
Insomnia	Trazodone	25 mg qhs	Increase in 25-mg increments q3-5d	50-200 mg/night
	Chloral hydrate	500 mg qhs	Increase in 500-mg increments q5-7d	500-1500 mg/night
	Quetiapine	25 mg qhs	Increase in 25-mg increments q3d	25-100 mg/night
	Zolpidem	5 mg qhs	Increase to 10 mg qhs if necessary	5-10 mg/night
Restless legs syndrome	Pramipexole	0.125 mg qhs	Increase in 0.125-mg increments q2-3d	0.25-0.75 mg/night
	Ropinirole	0.25 mg qhs	Increase in 0.25-mg increments q2-3d	0.25-2 mg/night
	Gabapentin	100 mg qhs	Increase in 100-mg increments q2-3d	300-1800 mg/night
Excessive daytime sleepiness	Methylphenidate	2.5 mg qam	Increase in 2.5- to 5-mg increments q3-5d in bid dosing (am and noon)	5 mg qam to 30 mg bid
	Modafinil	100 mg qam	Increase in 100-mg increments q5-7d in bid dosing (am and noon)	100 mg qam to 400 mg/day (400 mg qam or 200 mg bid)
	Amphetamine/ dextroam- phetamine	5 mg qam	Increase in 5-mg increments q7d in qd-bid dosing (am and noon)	5 mg qam; 20 mg bid
REM sleep behavior disorder	Clonazepam	0.25 mg qhs	Increase in 0.25-mg increments q7d	0.25-1.5 mg/night
	Melatonin	3 mg	3-6 mg/night	3-12 mg/night
Psychotic features, behavior dyscontrol, nocturnal agitation, or nocturnal wandering	Donepezil	5 mg qam	Increase to 10 mg qam 4 wk later	5-10 mg qam
	Rivastigmine†	1.5 mg bid	Increase in 1.5-mg increments q4wk in bid dosing (am and hs)	3-6 mg bid
	Galantamine†	4 mg bid	Increase in 4-mg increments q4wk in bid dosing	4-12 mg bid dosing (am and hs)
	Risperidone	0.5 mg qhs	Increase in 0.5-mg increments q7d in bid dosing (am and hs)	0.5 mg qhs to 1.5 mg bid
	Olanzapine	5 mg qhs	Increase in 5-mg increments q7d in bid dosing (am and hs)	5 mg qhs to 10 mg bid
	Clozapine‡	12.5 mg qhs	Increase in 12.5-mg increments q2-3d	12.5-50 mg qhs
	Quetiapine	25 mg qhs	Increase in 25-mg increments q3d	25-100 mg qhs
	Valproic acid‡	125 mg qhs	Increase in 125-mg increments q3-7d in bid to tid dosing	250 mg qhs to 500 mg tid
	Carbamazepine‡	100 mg qhs	Increase in 100-mg increments q3-7d in bid to tid dosing	200 mg qhs to 200 mg tid

*Disclaimer: The choice of which agents to use and which dosing schedules to recommend must be individualized. It is the responsibility of the clinician to consider potential side effects, drug interactions, allergic response, life-threatening reactions (e.g., leukopenia with clozapine), dosing changes due to renal or hepatic dysfunction, and so forth, before administering any drug to any patient, including those listed above. Drs. Petit, Montplaisir, Boeve, their respective institutions, and Elsevier will not be held responsible for any adverse reactions of any kind to any patient regarding the content of this information.

†If insomnia is problematic, second dose can be given no later than evening meal.

‡Requires periodic laboratory monitoring; refer to manufacturer's instructions for laboratory monitoring.

Adapted from Boeve B, Silber M, Ferman T: Current management of sleep disturbances in dementia. Curr Neurol Neurosci Rep 2002;2:169-177.

Insomnia

Patients with dementia are often unable to explain why they are not able to sleep through the night, so caregivers and physicians should carefully investigate the possible sources of the insomnia. Evaluating pain, concomitant medical conditions, and medication effects is essential to treat the patient successfully. For example, both untreated depression and some antidepressant medications (fluoxetine and bupropion) can lead to insomnia. The cholinesterase inhibitors (tacrine, donepezil, rivastigmine, galantamine), which have been shown to improve cognitive and noncognitive symptoms in patients with AD, can also cause insomnia. This problem usually can be avoided if the medication is administered no later than the evening meal, although in some patients the medication must be given no later than lunchtime.

Simple but effective interventions should probably be tried first, such as instituting proper sleep hygiene (e.g., regular schedule, bedtime routine, white noise), limiting caffeine and alcohol intake, and increasing exercise during the day. One study provided empirical evidence that behavioral strategies, which include sleep hygiene instructions, are useful in alleviating sleep problems and nighttime behavioral disturbances in patients with AD.[96a] Before prescribing medication to treat insomnia, the clinician should keep in mind that many such agents (especially benzodiazepines) can exacerbate cognitive deficits and obstructive sleep apnea syndrome, and can induce daytime sleepiness. It has been shown that sedative-hypnotic (and also antipsychotic) use was associated with longer hospital stays in the acute care setting.[97] If no cause is found for the insomnia, trazodone or chloral hydrate can be considered. Melatonin was not found effective in treating insomnia in patients with AD in a multicenter, placebo-controlled trial.[97a]

Restless Legs Syndrome

In some case, insomnia can result from untreated RLS. The exact prevalence of RLS in dementias is not known, but it is a common condition in patients with AD, PD, DLB, FTD, and vascular dementia. Several medications, especially dopaminergic agonists, have been proven efficacious and well tolerated in nondemented individuals with RLS (for review, see Chapter 70). However, no studies have assessed the efficacy and safety of these agents in demented patients. In some patients, dopaminergic agents can cause insomnia because of their stimulating effects or can trigger or exacerbate psychosis.

Excessive Daytime Sleepiness

Excessive sleepiness during the day has been reported mainly in PD. According to Arnulf and collaborators,[98] the daytime sleepiness does not result from poor sleep or from dopaminergic therapy (no correlation found), but is part of PD itself. Personal experience has taught us that sleepiness not resulting another primary sleep problem can also affect patients with AD, DLB, and FTD. In such cases, methylphenidate (at a low dose) or modafinil can be effective in improving alertness without producing undesirable effects.

Obstructive Sleep Apnea Syndrome

Hypersomnolence can also result from obstructive sleep apnea syndrome, a condition frequently associated with degenerative disorders, especially AD. The relationship between sleep apnea syndrome and dementia is complex. On the one hand, it is known that sleep apneas, if left untreated for many years, induce cognitive deficits, some of which are reversible with continuous positive airway pressure (CPAP) therapy.[99] In fact, there have been patients with severe cases of obstructive sleep apnea syndrome who had been diagnosed with dementia and for whom the dementia subsided with CPAP therapy. On the other hand, because of the increase in intracranial pressure and change in perfusion during apneic episodes, cognitive deficits should be associated more with vascular dementia than with AD, for which, however, a much stronger association exists.

Unfortunately, there are no published data on the effects of CPAP therapy on cognitive functioning in patients with a concomitant dementing condition. However, our clinical experience indicates that a small proportion of patients with a dementing illness significantly improve functionally and on psychometric testing with CPAP therapy, that a significant proportion of patients tolerate CPAP and use it nightly, and that even spouses enjoy a more consolidated sleep when their bed partners with dementia are on CPAP therapy.

Disorder of the Sleep–Wake Circadian Rhythm

Several studies have demonstrated a disorder of the sleep–wake rhythm in patients with dementia, especially in DLB, AD, and FTD. In fact, insomnia and excessive daytime sleepiness can be the manifestation of a primary disorder of the circadian rhythm. It has been proposed that degenerative changes in the biological clock, the suprachiasmatic nucleus of the hypothalamus, and in the pineal gland, resulting in a reduced melatonin production, are responsible for the disorganization and flattening of the circadian rhythms.[92,100,101]

Bright-light therapy administered in the evening was found effective in alleviating sleep–wake cycle disturbances in patients with dementia.[102,103] Melatonin can also be helpful for sleep–wake cycle disturbances, as indicated by data from two small samples of patients with dementia.[104,105] In some patients, regular daylight exposure is also effective for day/night reversal problems.

Excessive Motor Activity during the Night

REM Sleep Behavior Disorder

RBD is prevalent in various degenerative conditions, especially in the synucleinopathies (which include PD, DLB, and multiple system atrophy), compared with AD, FTD, and PSP. There is a high interpatient variability in the severity of RBD, but the symptoms in general tend to decrease with the progression of the degenerative disease. It is important to differentiate RDB from nocturnal wandering by taking a careful history. When diagnosis is uncertain and the potential for injury is present, a polysomnographic and video recording is justified. In fact, in a recent study of patients with PD, only half of the polysomnographically confirmed cases of RBD had been detected at the clinical interview.[45]

The first step in the management of RBD is to ensure the safety of the patient, which means removing potentially dangerous objects from the bedroom, perhaps placing a soft mattress on the floor next to the bed, and so forth. Clonazepam, which is the treatment of choice for RBD in nondemented individuals, can potentially worsen some aspects of dementia and can aggravate obstructive sleep apnea. Before prescribing this agent, it is essential to ensure that the patient does not experience obstructive sleep apneas or that CPAP therapy is effective in the apneic patient. Clinical experience shows us that clonazepam was well tolerated and produced few or no cognitive side effects in the vast majority of patients with dementia and concomitant RBD. Pramipexole has been tried in idiopathic RBD and produced modest beneficial results.[106] Melatonin has also been shown to be effective in alleviating RBD symptoms in several patients.[107,108] If depression is also present, treatments other than nefazodone should be considered because this drug increases total REM sleep, contrary to most other antidepressants, and can therefore potentiate RBD.

Periodic Limb Movements during Sleep

The prevalence of PLMS in dementia has not been estimated exactly. However, it is known to be elevated, especially in the synucleinopathies (i.e., PD, DLB, and multiple system atrophy). Without a polysomnographic recording, the severity and clinical significance of PLMS for a given patient are difficult to assess. If they are bothersome to the patient or cause daytime sleepiness as a result of sleep fragmentation, treatment with dopaminergic agonists can be envisaged. Again, dopaminergic agents should be used cautiously, if at all, in patients with psychotic features.

Nocturnal Agitation and Wandering

Apart from the sleep disturbances and EEG abnormalities that have been observed in the various forms of dementia, one of the heavier burdens on families of elderly demented patients and the primary cause of institutionalization is the lack of sleep due to nocturnal agitation or nocturnal wandering, the so-called sundowning experienced by the demented patient.[3] The widely used term *sundowning*, meaning that symptoms are worse in the evening or at night, is ill defined. Because the clinical manifestations of sundowning vary from patient to patient, it might be more appropriate, in order to convey a more meaningful information to health care professionals, caregivers, and researchers, to use descriptive terms such as confusion, delirium, agitation, hallucinations, wandering, pacing, or verbally or physically aggressive behaviors.

Nocturnal agitation could be the result of discomfort (constipation, full bladder, clothing, heat, cold), pain (pressure sores, infection), or environmental interruptions (staff noise, light); hence, verifying the potential sources of discomfort and pain is crucial. As for insomnia management, eliminating alcohol and restricting caffeine intake to the morning may help in alleviating nocturnal agitation. Also, behavioral techniques should be tried before resorting to medication. However, if necessary, atypical neuroleptics (risperidone, olanzapine, clozapine, quetiapine), antiepileptics (carbamazepine, valproic acid), benzodiazepines (clonazepam, lorazepam), as well as trazodone and chloral hydrate can be effective in treating nocturnal agitation (see Table 71–1 for dosages and titration schedules). Cholinesterase inhibitors (donepezil, rivastigmine, galantamine) can significantly ameliorate hallucinations for patients who are frightened or really bothered by them. In these cases, medications with hallucinatory side effects (levodopa, dopamine agonists, anticholinergics, amantadine, selegiline) should be decreased or eliminated.

CONCLUSIONS

Sleep and EEG are customarily impaired in disease associated with dementia. The nature of the impairment varies in some respects, but a common pattern emerges. Sleep is usually more fragmented, from both more awakenings and a longer duration of time awake; SWS is decreased; polygraphic features (spindles, K-complexes, and rapid eye movements) are less well formed and less numerous, so sleep stages are more difficult to distinguish; and REM sleep is often reduced. Moreover, these impairments worsen with the progression of the disease. In addition, demented patients are more likely to present with either PLMS or respiratory disturbances, or both. Although a common general pattern of sleep impairment can be observed in dementia, the study of sleep variables and of the spectral composition of the EEG in different states can provide valuable tools in establishing a diagnosis and in the evaluation of pharmacologic treatment.

> ### Clinical Pearls
>
> *The clinician should keep in mind that, when managing sleep disturbances in patients with dementia, careful assessment of the underlying causes is essential. Nonpharmacologic treatments, along with ensuring that the basic sleep hygiene rules are followed, should be envisaged before considering medication. One should also keep in mind, before prescribing medication to demented patients, that many such agents (especially benzodiazepines) can exacerbate cognitive deficits and obstructive sleep apnea syndrome.*

Acknowledgments

Drs. Petit and Montplaisir are supported by grants from the Canadian Institutes of Health Research. Dr. Boeve is supported by grants AG06786, AG15866, AG16574, and AG17216 from the National Institute on Aging.

REFERENCES

1. McKhann G, Drachman D, Folstein M, et al: Clinical diagnosis of Alzheimer's disease: Report of the NINCDS-ADRDA Work Group under the auspices of Department of Health and Human Services Task Force on Alzheimer's Disease. Neurology 1984;34: 939-944.
2. Knopman DS, Boeve BF, Petersen RC: Essentials of the proper diagnoses of mild cognitive impairment, dementia, and major subtypes of dementia. Mayo Clin Proc 2003;7:1290-1310.
3. Pollak CP, Perlick Linser JP, et al: Sleep problems in the community elderly as predictors of death and nursing home placement. J Commun Health 1990;15:123-135.
4. Bliwise DL: Sleep apnea, APOE4 and Alzheimer's disease: 20 years and counting? J Psychosom Res 2002;53:539-546.
5. Strittmatter WJ, Saunders AM, Schmechel D, et al: Apolipoprotein E: High-avidity binding to β-amyloid and increased frequency of type 4 allele in late-onset familial Alzheimer disease. Proc Natl Acad Sci U S A 1993;90:1977-1981.
6. Kadotani H, Kadotani T, Young T, et al: Association between apolipoprotein E 4 and sleep-disordered breathing in adults. JAMA 2001;285:2888-2890.

7. Prinz PN, Vitaliano PP, Vitiello MV et al: Sleep, EEG and mental function changes in senile dementia of the Alzheimer's type. Neurobiol Aging 1982;3:361-370.

8. Reynolds CF, Kupfer DJ, Taska LS, et al: EEG sleep in elderly depressed, demented, and healthy subjects. Biol Psychiatry 1985;20:431-442.

9. Montplaisir J, Petit D, Lorrain D, et al: Sleep in Alzheimer's disease: Further considerations on the role of brainstem and forebrain cholinergic populations in sleep-wake mechanisms. Sleep 1995;18:145-148.

10. Prinz PN, Peskind ER, Vitaliano PP, et al: Changes in the sleep and waking EEGs of nondemented and demented elderly subjects. J Am Geriatr Soc 1982;30:86-93.

11. Vitiello MV, Bokan JA, Kukull WA, et al: Rapid eye movement sleep measures of Alzheimer's-type dementia patients and optimally healthy aged individuals. Biol Psychiatry 1984;19:721-734.

12. Buzsaki G, Bickford RG, Ponomareff G, et al: Nucleus basalis and thalamic control of neocortical activity in the freely moving rat. J Neurosci 1988;8:4007-4026.

13. Soininen H, Partanen VJ, Helkala E-L, Riekkinen PJ: EEG findings in senile dementia and normal aging. Acta Neurol Scand 1982;65:59-70.

14. Coben LA, Danziger W, Storandt M: A longitudinal EEG study of mild senile dementia of Alzheimer type: Changes at 1 year and at 2.5 years. Electroencephalogr Clin Neurophysiol 1985;61:101-112.

15. Horie T, Koshino Y, Murata T, et al: EEG analysis in patients with senile dementia and Alzheimer's disease. Jpn J Psychiatr Neurol 1990;44:91-98.

16. Primavera A, Novello P, Finocchi C, et al: Correlation between Mini-Mental State Examination and quantitative electroencephalography in senile dementia of Alzheimer type. Neuropsychobiology 1990;23:74-78.

17. Petit D, Montplaisir J, Lorrain D, Gauthier S: Spectral analysis of the rapid eye movement sleep electroencephalogram in right and left temporal regions: A biological marker of Alzheimer's disease. Ann Neurol 1992;32:172-176.

18. Hassania F, Petit D, Nielsen T, et al: Quantitative EEG and statistical mapping of wakefulness and REM sleep in the evaluation of mild to moderate Alzheimer's disease. Eur Neurol 1997;37:219-224.

19. Bonte FJ, Hom J, Weiner MF: Single photon tomography in Alzheimer's disease and the dementias. Semin Nucl Med 1990;20:342-352.

20. Friedland RP, Brun A, Budinger TF: Pathological and positron emission tomographic correlations in Alzheimer's disease. Lancet 1985;19:228.

21. O'Brien JT, Eagger S, Syed GMS, et al: A study of regional cerebral blood flow and cognitive performance in Alzheimer's disease. J Neurol Neurosurg Psychiatry 1992;55:1182-1187.

22. Brun A, Englund E: Brain changes in dementia of Alzheimer's type relevant to new imaging diagnostic methods. Prog Neuropsychopharmacol Biol Psychiatry 1986;10:297-308.

23. Petit D, Lorrain D, Gauthier S, Montplaisir J: Regional spectral analysis of the REM sleep EEG in mild to moderate Alzheimer's disease. Neurobiol Aging 1993;14:141-145.

24. Folstein M, Folstein S, McHugh P: "Mini-Mental State": A practical method for grading the cognitive state of patients for the clinician. J Psychiatr Res 1975;12:189-198.

25. Montplaisir J, Petit D, McNamara D, Gauthier S: Comparisons between SPECT and quantitative EEG measures of cortical impairment in mild to moderate Alzheimer's disease. Eur Neurol 1996;36:197-200.

26. Whitehouse PJ, Price DL, Struble RG, et al: Alzheimer's disease and senile dementia: Loss of neurons in the basal forebrain. Science 1982;215:1237-1239.

27. Hobson JA, McCarley RW, Wyzinshi PW: Sleep cycle oscillation: Reciprocal discharge by two brainstem neuronal groups. Science 1975;189:55-58.

28. Kodama T, Takahashi Y, Honda Y: Enhancement of acetylcholine release during paradoxical sleep in the dorsal tegmental field of the cat brain stem. Neurosci Lett 1990;114:277-282.

29. Litvan I, Agid Y, Calne D, et al: Clinical research criteria for the diagnosis of progressive supranuclear palsy (Steele-Richardson-Olszewski syndrome): Report of the NINDS-SPSP International Workshop. Neurology 1996;47:1-9.

30. Montplaisir J, Petit D, Décary A, et al: Sleep and quantitative EEG in patients with progressive supranuclear palsy. Neurology 1997;49:999-1003.

31. Aldrich MS, Foster NL, White RF, et al: Sleep abnormalities in progressive supranuclear palsy. Neurology 1989;25:577-581.

32. Perret JL, Jouvet M: Etude du sommeil dans la paralysie supranucléaire progressive. Electroencephalogr Clin Neurophysiol 1980;49:323-329.

33. Dubois B, Pillon B, Legault F, et al: Slowing of cognitive processing in progressive supranuclear palsy. Arch Neurol 1988;45:1194-1199.

34. Maher ER, Smith EM, Lees AJ: Cognitive deficits in the Steele-Richardson-Olszewski syndrome (progressive supranuclear palsy). J Neurol Neurosurg Psychiatry 1985;48:1234-1239.

35. Kish SJ, Chang LJ, Mirchandani L, et al: Progressive supranuclear palsy: Relationship between extrapyramidal disturbances, dementia, and brain neurotransmitter markers. Ann Neurol 1985;18:530-536.

36. Hassler RG: Role of the pallidum and its transmitters in the therapy of parkinsonian rigidity and akinesia. Adv Neurol 1984;40:1-14.

37. Aarsland D, Andersen K, Larsen JP, et al: Prevalence and characteristics of dementia in Parkinson disease: An 8-year prospective study. Arch Neurol 2003;60:387-92.

38. Emre M: Dementia associated with Parkinson's disease. Lancet 2003;2:229-237.

39. Comella CL, Ristanovic R, Goetz CG: Parkinson's disease patients with and without REM behavior disorder (RBD): A polysomnographic and clinical comparison. Neurology 1993;43 (Suppl 2):A301.

40. Onofrj M, Thomas A, D'Andreamatteo G, et al: Incidence of RBD and hallucination in patients affected by Parkinson's disease: 8-year follow-up. Neurol Sci 2002;23:S91-S94.

41. Schenck CH, Bundlie SR, Ettinger MG, Mahowald MW: Chronic behavioral disorders of human REM sleep: A new category of parasomnia. Sleep 1986;9:293-308.

42. Boeve, B., Silber M., Ferman T, et al: Association of REM sleep behavior disorder and neurodegenerative disease may reflect an underlying synucleinopathy. Mov Disord 2001;16:622-630.

43. Boeve B, Silber M, Ferman T, et al: REM sleep behavior disorder in Parkinson's disease, dementia with Lewy bodies, and multiple system atrophy. In Bedard M, Agid Y, Chouinard S, et al (eds): Mental and Behavioral Dysfunction in Movement Disorders. Totowa, NJ, Humana Press, 2003, pp 383-397.

44. Comella CL, Nardine TM, Diederich NJ, Stebbins GT: Sleep-related violence, injury, and REM sleep behavior disorder in Parkinson's disease. Neurology 1998;51:526-529.

45. Gagnon JF, Bédard MA, Fantini ML, et al: REM sleep behavior disorder and REM sleep without atonia in Parkinson's disease. Neurology 2002;59:585-589.

46. Rechtschaffen A, Kales A (eds): A Manual of Standardized Terminology, Techniques, and Scoring System for Sleep States Of Human Subjects. U.S. Public Health Service publication no. 204. Washington, DC, U.S. Government Printing Office, 1968.

47. Soikkeli R, Partanen J, Soininen H, et al: Slowing of EEG in Parkinson's disease. Electroencephalogr Clin Neurophysiol 1991;79:159-165.

48. Gagnon JF, Fantini ML, Bédard A, et al: Slowing of EEG in Parkinson's disease without dementia is related to REM sleep behavior disorder. Neurology 2003;60(Suppl 1):A400.

49. Fantini ML, Gagnon J-F, Petit D, et al: Slowing of EEG in idiopathic REM sleep behavior disorder. Ann Neurol 2003;53:774-780.

50. Lobotesis K, Fenwick JD, Phipps A, et al: Occipital hypoperfusion on SPECT in dementia with Lewy bodies but not AD. Neurology 2001;56:643-649.

51. Minoshima S, Foster NL, Sima AA, et al: Alzheimer's disease versus dementia with Lewy bodies: Cerebral metabolic distinction with autopsy confirmation. Ann Neurol 2001;50:358-365.

52. Boeve BF, Silber MH, Ferman TJ, et al: REM sleep behavior disorder and degenerative dementia: An association likely reflecting Lewy body disease. Neurology 1998;51:363-370.

53. Turner RS: Idiopathic rapid eye movement sleep behavior disorder is a harbinger of dementia with Lewy bodies. J Geriatr Psychiatr Neurol 2002;15:195-199.

54. Apaydin H, Ahlskog JE, Parisi JE, et al: Parkinson's disease neuropathology: Later-developing dementia and loss of the levodopa response. Arch Neurol 2002;59:102-112.

55. Kosaka K, Tsuchiya K, Yoshimura M: Lewy body disease with and without dementia: A clinicopathological study of 35 cases. Clin Neuropathol 1988;7:299-305.

56. Mattila PM, Rinne JO, Helenius H, et al: Alpha-synuclein-immunoreactive cortical Lewy bodies are associated with cognitive impairment in Parkinson's disease. Acta Neuropathol 2000; 100:285-290.

57. Hurtig HI, Trojanowski JQ, Galvin J, et al: Alpha-synuclein cortical Lewy bodies correlate with dementia in Parkinson's disease. Neurology 2000;54:1916-1921.

58. Weiner MF: Dementia associated with Lewy bodies. Arch Neurol 1999;56:1441-1442.

59. McKeith IG, Galasko D, Kosaka K, et al: Consensus guidelines for the clinical and pathologic diagnosis of dementia with Lewy bodies (DLB): Report of the Consortium on DLB International Workshop. Neurology 1996;47:1113-1124.

60. Grace JB, Walker MP, McKeith IG: A comparison of sleep profiles in patients with dementia with Lewy bodies and Alzheimer's disease. Int J Geriatr Psychiatry 2000;15:1028-1033.

61. Boeve BF, Ferman TJ, Silber MH, et al: Sleep disturbances in dementia with Lewy bodies involve more than REM sleep behavior disorder. Neurology 2003;60:A79.

62. Boeve BF, Silber MH, Parisi JE, et al: Synucleinopathy pathology and REM sleep behavior disorder plus dementia or parkinsonism Neurology 2003;61:40-45.

63. Ferman TJ, Boeve BF, Smith GE, et al: Dementia with Lewy bodies may present as dementia and REM sleep behavior disorder without parkinsonism or hallucinations. J Int Neuropsychol Soc 2002; 8: 907-914.

64. Boeve BF, Silber MH, Ferman TJ: Current management of sleep disturbances in dementia. Curr Neurol Neurosci Rep 2002;2: 169-177.

65. International Restless Legs Syndrome Study Group, Walters AS (Group organizer and correspondent): Towards a better definition of the restless legs syndrome from the international restless legs syndrome study group. Mov Disord 1995;10:634-642.

66. Briel RCG, McKeith IG, Barker WA, et al: EEG findings in dementia with Lewy bodies and Alzheimer's disease. J Neurol Neurosurg Psychiatry 1999;66:401-403.

67. Barber PA, Varma AR, Lloyd JJ, et al: The electroencephalogram in dementia with Lewy bodies. Acta Neurol Scand 2000; 101:53-56.

68. Calzetti S, Bortone E, Negrotti A, et al: Frontal intermittent rhythmic delta activity (FIRDA) in patients with dementia with Lewy bodies: A diagnostic tool? Neurol Sci 2002;23:S65-S66.

69. Walker MP, Ayre GA, Cummings JL, et al: Quantifying fluctuation in dementia with Lewy bodies, Alzheimer's disease, and vascular dementia. Neurology 2000;54:1616-1624.

70. Aharon-Peretz J, Masiah A, Pillar T, et al: Sleep-wake cycles in multi-infarct dementia and dementia of the Alzheimer type. Neurology 1991;41:1616-1619.

71. Erkinjuntti T, Partinen M, Sulkava R, et al: Sleep apnea in multi-infarct dementia and Alzheimer's disease. Sleep 1987;10:419-425.

72. Sato K, Kamiya S, Okawa M, et al: On the EEG component waves of multi-infarct dementia seniles. Int J Neurosci 1996;86: 95-109.

73. Signorino M, Pucci E, Belardinelli N, et al: EEG spectral analysis in vascular and Alzheimer dementia. Electroencephalogr Clin Neurophysiol 1995;94:313-32.

74. Roberts M, McGeorge AP, Caird FI: Electroencephalography and computerised tomography in vascular and non-vascular dementia in old age. J Neurol Neurosurg Psychiatry 1978;41:903-906.

75. McHugh PR, Folstein MF: Psychiatric syndromes of Huntington's chorea: A clinical and phenomenologic study. In Benson DF, Blumer D (eds): Psychiatric Aspects of Neurologic Disease. New York, Grune and Stratton, 1975, pp 267-285.

76. Hansotia P, Wall R, Berendes J: Sleep disturbances and severity of Huntington's disease. Neurology 1985;35:1672-1674.

77. Wiegand M, Moller AA, Lauer CJ, et al: Nocturnal sleep in Huntington's disease. J Neurol 1991;238:203-208.

78. Emser W, Brenner M, Stober T, Schimrigk K: Changes in nocturnal sleep in Huntington's and Parkinson's disease. J Neurol 1988;235:177-179.

79. Bollen EL, Den Heijer JC, Ponsioen C, et al: Respiration during sleep in Huntington's chorea. J Neurol Sci 1988;84:63-68.

80. Scott DF, Heathfield KWB, Toone B, Margerison JH: The EEG in Huntington's chorea: A clinical and neuropathological study. J Neurol Neurosurg Psychiatry 1972;335:97-102.

81. Sishta SK, Troupe A, Marszalek KS, Kremer LM: Huntington's chorea: An electroencephalographic and psychometric study. Electroencephalogr Clin Neurophysiol 1974;36:387-393.

82. Streletz LJ, Reyes PF, Zalewska M, et al: Computer analysis of EEG activity in dementia of the Alzheimer's type and Huntington's disease. Neurobiol Aging 1990;11:15-20.

83. Kazukawa S, Nakamura I, Endo M, et al: Serial polysomnograms in Creutzfeldt-Jakob disease. Jpn J Psychiatry Neurol 1987;41: 651-661.

84. Mamdani MB, Masdeu J, Ross E, Ohara R: Sleep apnea with unusual changes in Jakob-Creutzfeldt disease. Electroencephalogr Clin Neurophysiol 1983;55:411-416.

85. Kudo Y, Tamaru F, Motomura N, Yamadori A: Disappearance of sleep apnea by tracheal intubation in Creutzfeldt-Jakob disease. Electroencephalogr Clin Neurophysiol 1984;58:226-229.

86. Donnet A, Famarier G, Gambarelli D, et al: Sleep electroencephalogram at the early stage of Creutzfeldt-Jakob disease. Clin Electroencephalogr 1992;23:118-125.

87. Calleja J, Carpizo R, Berciano J, et al: Serial waking-sleep EEGs and evolution of somatosensory potentials in Creutzfeldt-Jakob disease. Electroencephalogr Clin Neurophysiol 1985;60: 504-508.

88. Terzano MG, Parrino L, Pietrini V, et al: Precocious loss of physiological sleep in a case of Creutzfeldt Jakob disease: A serial polygraphic study. Sleep 1995;18:849-858.

89. Szirmai I, Guseo A, Czopf J, Palffy G: Analysis of clinical and electrophysiological findings in Jakob-Creutzfeldt disease. Arch Psychiatr Nervenkr 1976;222:315-323.

90. Diehl J, Kurz A: Frontotemporal dementia: Patient characteristics, cognition, and behaviour. Int J Geriatr Psychiatry 2002;17: 914-918.

91. Vercelletto M, Belliard S, Wiertlewski S, et al: Neuropsychological and scintigraphic aspects of frontotemporal dementia preceding amyotrophic lateral sclerosis. Rev Neurol (Paris) 2003;159:529-542.

92. Harper DG, Stopa EG, McKee AC, et al: Differential circadian rhythm disturbances in men with Alzheimer disease and frontotemporal degeneration. Arch Gen Psychiatry 2001;58: 353-360.

93. Neary D, Snowden JS, Northen B, Goulding P: Dementia of frontal lobe type. J Neurol Neurosurg Psychiatry 1988;51:353-361.

94. Stigsby B, Johannesson G, Ingvar DM: Regional EEG analysis and regional cerebral blood flow in Alzheimer's disease and Pick's disease. Electroencephalogr Clin Neurophysiol 1981;51:537-547.

95. Besthorn C, Sattel H, Hentschel F, et al: Quantitative EEG in frontal lobe dementia. J Neural Transm 1996;47:169-181.

96. Yener GG, Leuchter AF, Jenden D, et al: Quantitative EEG in frontotemporal dementia. Clin Electroencephalogr 1996;27:61-68.

96a. McCurry SM, Logsdon RG, Vitiello MV, Teri L: Treatment of sleep and nighttime disturbances in Alzheimer's disease: A behavioral management approach. Sleep Med 2004;5:373-377.

97. Ray WA, Federspeil CF, Schaffner W: A study of antipsychotic drug use in nursing homes: Epidemiologic evidence suggesting misuse. Am J Public Health 1980;70:485-491.

97a. Singer C, Tractenberg RE, Kaye J, et al: A multicenter, placebo-controlled trial of melatonin for sleep disturbance in Alzheimer's disease. Sleep 2003;26:893-901.

98. Arnulf I, Konofal E, Merino-Andreu M, et al: Parkinson's disease and sleepiness: An integral part of PD. Neurology 2002;58:1019-1024.

99. Montplaisir J, Bédard M-A, Richer F, Rouleau I: Neurobehavioral manifestations in obstructive sleep apnea syndrome before and after treatment with continuous positive airway pressure. Sleep 1992;15:517-519.

100. Mishima K, Tozawa T, Satoh K, et al: Melatonin secretion rhythm disorders in patients with senile dementia of Alzheimer's type with disturbed sleep-waking. Neurobiol Aging 1995;16:765-771.

101. Witting W, Kwa IH, Eikelenboom P, et al: Alterations in the circadian rest-activity rhythm in aging and Alzheimer's disease. Biol Psychiatry 1990;15;27:563-72.

102. Lyketsos C, Lindell Veiel L, Baker A, Steele C: A randomized controlled trial of bright light therapy for agitated behaviors in dementia patients residing in long-term care. Int J Geriatr Psychiatry 1999;14:520-525.

103. Van Someren E, Kessler A, Mirmiran M, Swaab D: Indirect bright light improves circadian rest-activity rhythm disturbances in demented patients. Biol Psychiatry 1997;41:955-963.

104. Singer C, MacArthur A, Hughes R, et al: High dose melatonin and sleep in the elderly. Sleep Res 1995;24A:151.

105. Brusco L, Fainstein I, Marquez M, Cardinali D: Effect of melatonin in selected populations of sleep-disturbed patients. Biol Signals Recept 1999;8:126-131.

106. Fantini ML, Gagnon J-F, Filipini D, Montplaisir J: The effects of pramipexole in REM sleep behavior disorder. Neurology 2003;61;1418-1420.

107. Kunz D, Bes F: Melatonin as a therapy in REM sleep behavior disorder patients: An open-labeled pilot study on the possible influence of melatonin on REM -sleep regulation. Mov Disord 1999;14:507-511.

108. Boeve BF, Silber MH, Ferman TJ: Melatonin for treatment of REM sleep behavior disorder in neurologic disorders: Results in 14 patients. Sleep Med 2003;4:281-284.

72

Epilepsy, Sleep, and Sleep Disorders

Margaret N. Shouse

Mark W. Mahowald

ABSTRACT

Epilepsy is the third most common neurologic disorder after stroke and Alzheimer's disease in the United States. Sleep, sleep disorders, and epilepsy are frequently associated. It is well known that sleep and sleep deprivation increase the incidence of both parasomnias and seizure activity. Conversely, seizure disorders can affect the wake–sleep cycle. Sleep disorders—including parasomnias— may mimic, cause, or even be triggered by epileptic phenomena and vice versa. A high index of suspicion and a full awareness of the broad spectrum of both sleep and epileptic phenomena is instrumental to an accurate diagnosis.

Epilepsy refers to a host of seizure disorders characterized by uncontrolled abnormal brain electrical discharges associated with undesirable motor, verbal, or experiential phenomena.[1,2] These phenomena often occur during sleep.[3] Electroclinical events include *interictal discharges* (IIDs), which are electrographically but not clinically evident, and *ictal events*, which are usually electrographically and clinically evident.

There are many ways of classifying seizure disorders.[1] In spite of considerable diversity in etiologies and in specific ictal/IID characteristics, epileptic seizure manifestations tend to be highly state dependent. Non–rapid eye movement (NREM) sleep is associated with increased incidence and spread of IIDs; clinical accompaniment is most often associated with localization-related epilepsies originating in temporal and frontal lobes.[3-5] Rapid eye movement (REM) sleep is a relatively antiepileptic state in that spread of IID is anatomically localized and clinically evident seizures are usually suppressed.[4,6,7] Arousal from NREM or REM sleep can also provoke or mimic seizures or parasomnias.[8] The facilitation of sleep upon partial seizures depends in part on the location of the epileptic focus.[9] The likelihood that the same basic brain circuitry generates both NREM sleep oscillations and electrical seizures with spike-wave complexes explains the close relationship between seizures and sleep.[10]

With the advent of neurophysiologic monitoring techniques, it has become obvious that state determination is a very complex and dynamic phenomenon involving multiple neural networks, neurotransmitters, neuropeptides, and neurohormones, as well as a myriad of sleep-promoting substances. Given these complexities, it has become clear that the determination of state may be inexact, with components of two or all three states occurring simultaneously or oscillating rapidly. This concept of state dissociation in animals and humans has been extensively reviewed.[11]

These mixed or rapidly oscillating states result in fascinating and perplexing clinical phenomena that may easily be confused with epileptic events; conversely, these sleep disorders may be perfectly imitated by epileptic events. Furthermore, other primary sleep disorders may trigger seizures, and conversely, seizures may trigger abnormal sleep phenomena. Clinically there is substantial overlap among epileptic, sleep, and psychiatric phenomena (Table 72–1).

There are five primary determinants of the quality of nighttime sleep and of daytime alertness: homeostatic (duration of prior wakefulness), circadian (biological clock influence), age, drugs, and central nervous system (CNS) pathology.[12] These factors determine the overall sleep–wake pattern and also play an integral role in epileptic events.

HISTORICAL ASPECTS

In 1965, Gastaut and Broughton[13] reported the clinical and polygraphic characteristics of sleep-related episodic phenomena in human patients. They outlined major symptoms of two major parasomnias, sleepwalking and sleep terrors. Both occur during NREM sleep, usually when the patient emerges from stage 4 NREM sleep. Prior to this study,[13] these parasomnias were associated with seizure disorders. In 1968, Broughton[14] questioned the pathophysiologic mechanisms underlying these paroxysmal (sudden) nocturnal events. Although parasomnias and seizure disorders exhibit common features such as abrupt onset, confusion, disorientation, and retrograde amnesia, Broughton proposed that most if not all of these episodes could be related to a disorder of arousal rather than to epilepsy.

After Broughton's pioneering work, the concept of an arousal disorder generating parasomnias was accepted, but subsequent studies also suggest that arousal disorders can provoke, represent, or be caused by seizure disorders. Certain predisposing factors in NREM sleep seem to increase IID and ictal epileptic events.[3,4] The incidence of arousal-related paroxysms, such as sleep spindles, K-complexes, bursts of slow waves, and ponto-geniculo-occipital (PGO) spikes, is closely associated with the occurrence of generalized or focal spikes, epileptiform spike-and-wave, and polyspike-and-wave in human and animal epilepsy.[15,16] There is also a statistical relationship between the cyclic alternating pattern (CAP) of "fluctuating cortical excitability" with both epilepsy and sleep disorders.[17,18]

EPIDEMIOLOGY

There are no definitive epidemiologic studies on the coincidence of parasomnias and seizure disorders, although available studies suggest that nocturnal seizures rarely represent parasomnias.[13,14,19] Symptoms of parasomnias—such as nightmares, sleep terrors, violent behavior during sleep, sleepwalking,

Table 72–1. Overlap Between Sleep and Epileptic Phenomena

Symptom	Sleep Disorder	Seizure
Normal sleep phenomena	Sleep starts (hypnic jerks) Nightmares	Seizures manifesting as sleep-onset sensorimotor phenomena or nightmares

Hypersomnia	Sleep deprivation
	Idiopathic central nervous system (CNS) hypersomnia
	Narcolepsy
	   Cataplexy
	   Sleep paralysis
	   Hypnagogic hallucinations
	   Automatic behavior
	Recurrent hypersomnia
	   Kleine-Levin
	   Menstruation-related
	Sleep apnea that triggers seizures
		Hypersomnia as a manifestation of having frequent nocturnal seizures resulting in recurrent arousals or hypersomnia as an accompaniment of epilepsy
		Akinetic
		Fugue states
		   Partial complex seizures
		   Subclinical status
		Poriomania
		Recurrent seizures resulting in prolonged periods of "sleepiness"
		
		Seizures resulting in apnea

Insomnia	Medical Psychiatric Psychological Constitutional	Seizures whose sole manifestation is recurrent arousals

Parasomnias	Disorders of arousal: confusional arousals, sleepwalking, sleep terrors, sleepeating
	
	REM sleep behavior disorder (RBD)
	Dreams/nightmares
	Enuresis
	Rhythmic movement disorder
	Periodic limb movement disorder
	Posttraumatic stress disorder
	Cardiopulmonary disorders
	   Cardiac arrhythmias
	   Respiratory dyskinesias
	Gastrointestinal: paroxysmal choking
	Panic disorder
	Psychogenic dissociative disorders
		Mesial frontal, temporal lobe seizures manifesting with complex, bizarre behavior, hypnogenic (nocturnal) paroxysmal dystonia, or autonomic (diencephalic) seizures

Modified from Mahowald MW, Schenck CH: Sleep disorders. In Engel J Jr, Pedley TA (eds): Epilepsy: A Comprehensive Textbook. Philadelphia, Lippincott-Raven, 1997, pp 2705-2715 (with permission).

and REM sleep behavior disorder (RBD)—resemble seizure disorders (notably partial complex seizures), thus warranting comments on reports of incidence, etiology, and clinical course.

The incidence of epilepsy has been studied most often in industrialized countries where overall population percentages are similar; available studies conducted in developing countries indicate a higher prevalence than in industrialized countries. The following statistics reflect well-conducted epidemiologic studies in the United States.[20] The number of patients in the United States with a diagnosis of epilepsy is about 2.5 million, and the cumulative lifetime incidence ranges from 1.3% to 3.1% of the population by the age of 80 years. Epilepsy is the third most common neurologic disorder after stroke and Alzheimer's disease in the United States.

Epilepsies may be classified as generalized (40%), localization related (57%), or unclassified (3%). Localization-related epilepsies may be further subclassified as partial complex (36%), simple partial (14%), and partial unknown (7%).

Localization-related epilepsies, particularly partial complex seizure disorders with tonic-clonic convulsions, are the "prototypical" pure sleep epilepsies; nearly 60% of these patients exhibit convulsions only during sleep.[21,22] Most of these nocturnal seizure disorders are attributed to temporal or frontal lobe foci.[5] Onset can occur at any time, although the average peak age at onset is in adolescence.[21] Electroclinical symptoms tend to persist, and over time ictal events or IID events, or both, are likely to disperse across the sleep–wake cycle.[20-22]

Age at onset of parasomnias such as sleepwalking and sleep terrors is believed to be in childhood. The earlier age at onset of some parasomnias may provide one criterion for differential diagnosis from some nocturnal seizure disorders; however, many epilepsies—such as partial complex seizure disorders—do not remit spontaneously.[20-23] Hereditary factors can be more prevalent in some parasomnias than in partial complex seizure disorders. Still, the most definitive criterion for differential diagnosis is polygraphic evidence of epileptic seizure discharge, and this may be difficult to obtain from surface recordings of patients with deep temporal or frontal lobe foci.[24] It is likely that the rarity of nocturnal seizures manifesting as other parasomnias is more apparent than real—the correct diagnosis having been overlooked for lack of consideration.

PATHOGENESIS

The hypothalamic and brainstem generators of sleep and arousal have diffuse ascending and descending projections[25] that give rise to a number of distinguishing physiologic characteristics called *components*. Components can be tonic (sustained background activity, such as degree of electro-encephalographic [EEG] synchronization and muscle tone) or phasic (periodic transients, such as sleep spindles, K-complexes, and muscle twitches). The association of these tonic and phasic events is important to the integrity of sleep states. Dissociation or abnormality of these components likely contributes to a variety of sleep, arousal, and seizure disorders as well as their interaction.

Direct experimental evidence using dissociative manipulations is best documented with respect to spread of EEG and clinically evident seizures that may coexist with or masquerade as parasomnias.[26] Two state-specific components affecting epilepsy are the degree to which cellular discharge patterns are synchronized and alterations in antigravity muscle tone.[4] NREM sleep and drowsiness differ from alert waking and REM sleep in that EEG activity is synchronized and postural muscle tone is diminished. REM sleep differs from NREM sleep in that EEG activity is desynchronized, and it differs from waking and NREM sleep in that postural muscle tone is absent. REM sleep has sometimes been called "paradoxical sleep"[27] because it is characterized by a "highly active brain in a paralyzed body."[28]

During NREM sleep, virtually every cell in the brain discharges synchronously, and the discharge may even reach paroxysmal levels similar to those in epileptic states.[29] This occurs to a lesser extent in drowsiness. Lasting oscillations of rhythmic burst-pause firing patterns result in concerted synaptic actions. Synchronous synaptic effects, whether excitatory or inhibitory, are likely to augment the magnitude and propagation of postsynaptic responses, including epileptic discharges. During REM sleep and alert waking, cells discharge asynchronously.[30] The divergent synaptic signals associated with asynchronous discharge patterns are less likely to augment the magnitude or propagation of epileptic EEG discharges.

Skeletal muscle tone also varies by sleep or waking state. Antigravity muscle tone is preserved in NREM sleep and waking,[28,31] thus permitting seizure-associated and conceivably parasomnia-associated movement. Profound lower motor neuron inhibition occurs in REM sleep,[28,32] creating virtual paralysis (but sparing the diaphragm to permit continued respiration). Disruption of this important component of REM sleep might underlie RBD and can influence clinically evident motor seizures.

These different EEG and skeletal motor components can be experimentally dissociated, as depicted in Figure 72–1.[6] Figure 72–1A shows normal feline REM sleep. Figure 72–1B shows that NREM sleep–like EEG synchrony during REM sleep can be induced by systemic administration of atropine. Although it is not shown in the figure, atropine also synchronizes the waking EEG. EEG-synchronizing effects are presumably achieved by blocking acetylcholine (ACh) release from cells in the nucleus basalis of the forebrain and pedunculo-pontine-peribrachial nuclei of the brainstem, as these are the critical generators of the asynchronous EEG discharges that occur in waking and to a greater extent in REM sleep.[25,33] Figure 72–1C shows selective loss of postural muscle tone induced by a lesion in the pontine generators of REM sleep atonia.[30] Neural generators are thought to be cholinoceptive and glutaminergic cells in the brainstem atonia regions,[30,34] which hyperpolarize lower motor neurons.[32]

Dissociating these EEG and motor components significantly and differentially influences electrographic and clinical seizure manifestations, as illustrated in Figure 72–2. Figure 72–2A shows the distribution of penicillin-induced spike-wave complexes during intact NREM and REM sleep states. Figure 72–2B shows the effects of atropine administration. The REM sleep EEG is synchronized, and spike-wave discharge rate is comparable with that in NREM sleep. Although it is not shown in the figure, atropine similarly synchronizes the waking EEG in conjunction with an increase in spike-wave discharge rate. Unlike waking and NREM sleep, there is no clinical manifestation during REM sleep, presumably because of the skeletal motor paralysis unique to that state. Figure 72–2C shows that a pontine lesion eliminates REM sleep atonia so that a clinically evident myoclonic seizure occurs in REM sleep.

These results are supported by other experimental and clinical findings indicating that substrates of state-specific components rather than integrity of the state per se can be salient determinants of seizure propagation. Agents that synchronize the EEG, such as cholinergic or noradrenergic antagonists, have proconvulsant effects.[35-37] Conversely, agents that desynchronize the EEG discourage epileptic EEG discharge propagation. Examples are cholinergic and noradrenergic agonists[38-41] as well as beta-carbolines such as abecarnil,[42] which act on central benzodiazepine receptors. Finally, pharmacologic manipulations that induce atonia, such as carbachol infusion into the brainstem, also block clinical motor accompaniment.[40] Consistent observations have been reported in experimental models of primary generalized epilepsy, such as electroconvulsive shock, penicillin epilepsy, and photosensitive epilepsy[6,36,38]; in animal models of localization-related epilepsies, such as limbic system kindling and the cortical alumina cream preparation[40,43]; and in the clinical literature on symptomatic generalized epilepsies such as West's syndrome.[39] Collectively, the findings confirm that cellular discharge patterns and alterations in tone affect electrographic and clinically evident seizure manifestations in diverse epileptic syndromes, including those that mimic parasomnias. There is growing evidence that glial cells play a role in epilepsy.[44,45]

CLINICAL FEATURES

This section discusses various areas of overlap and confusion between sleep disorders and seizures. These areas include normal events, hypersomnia, insomnia, and parasomnias (see Table 72–1).

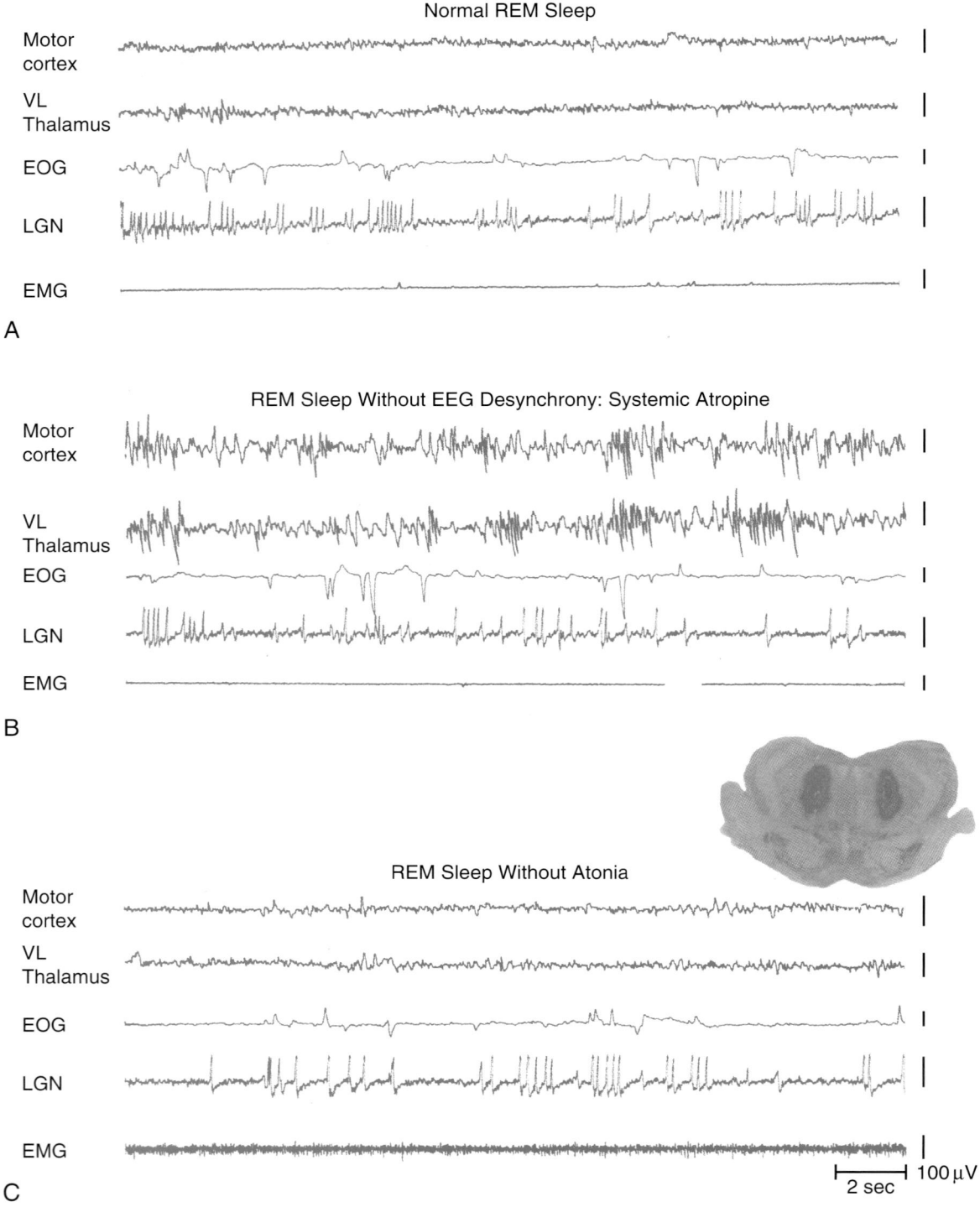

Figure 72–1. The top tracing **(A)** shows normal rapid eye movement (REM) sleep, evidenced by electrogram (EEG) desynchronization and atonia with periodic bursts of phasic events, including REMs and ponto-geniculo-occipital (PGO) spikes. The middle tracing **(B)** shows that systemic atropine selectively abolishes EEG desynchronization. Instead, there is a non–rapid eye movement (NREM) sleep–like EEG with synchronized background and sleep spindles. However, atonia is intact as are eye movements and PGO spikes. Clustering of PGOs is diminished as customarily reported. The bottom tracing **(C)** shows that a pontine lesion selectively eliminates atonia. Note presence of tonic electromyographic (EMG) activity in the bottom channel of this tracing. (From Shouse MN, Siegel JM, Wu FM, et al: Mechanisms of seizure suppression during rapid-eye-movement (REM) sleep in cats. Brain Res 1989;505:271-282.)

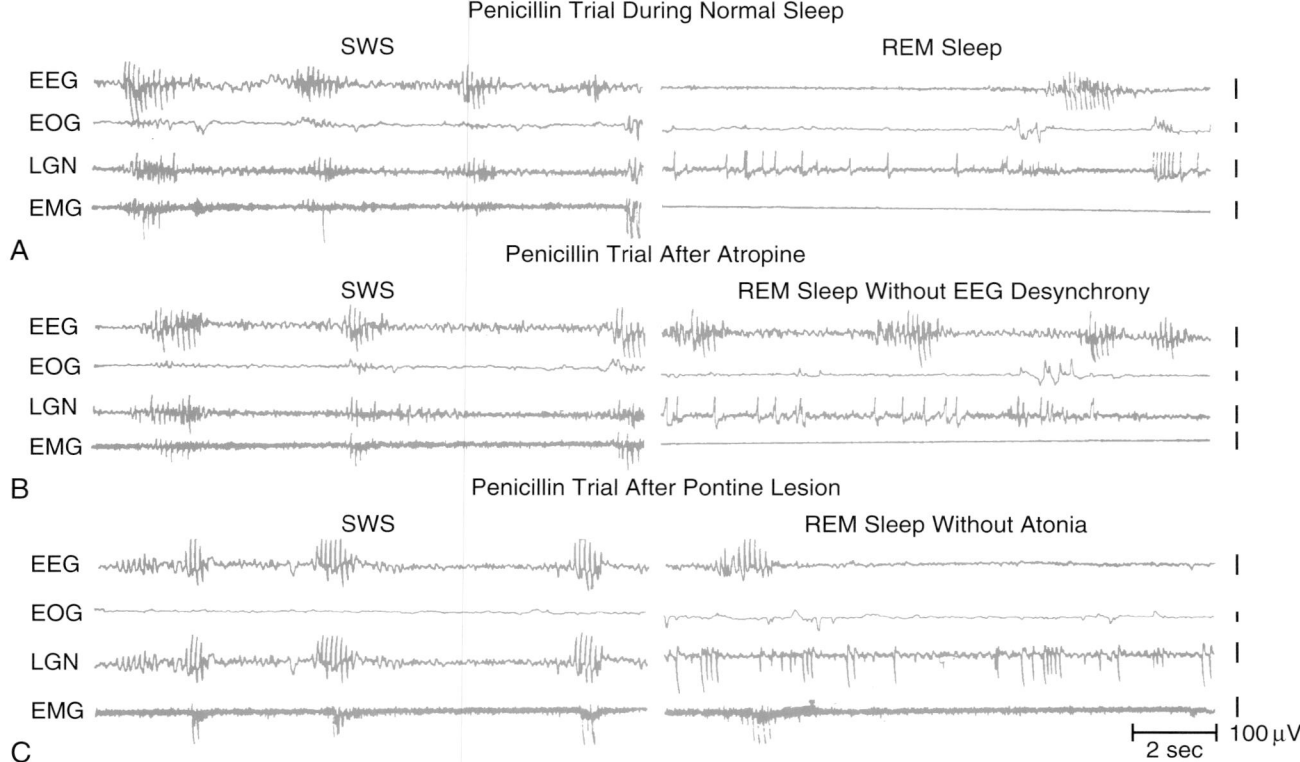

Figure 72–2. Systemic penicillin epilepsy during slow wave sleep (SWS), the equivalent of non–rapid eye movement (NREM) sleep in humans *(left)*, and rapid eye movement (REM) sleep *(right)* before **(A)** and after **(B** and **C)** dissociation of REM-sleep components. Spike-wave paroxysms are visible in the electroencephalogram (EEG) tracing, and myoclonic seizures were associated with electromyographic (EMG) discharges in this cat, as long as lower motor neuron activity is present. (From Shouse MN, Siegel JM, Wu FM, et al: Mechanisms of seizure suppression during rapid-eye-movement [REM] sleep in cats. Brain Res 1989;505:271-282.)

Normal Sleep Phenomena

Sleep Starts

Many healthy people experience sleep starts (hypnic jerks) during the transition from waking to sleep. The most common is the motor sleep start, a sudden jerk of all or part of the body, occasionally awakening the victim or bed partner.[46] Variations include the visual (flashes of light, fragmentary visual hallucinations), auditory (loud bangs, snapping noises), and somesthetic (pain, floating, something flowing through the body) sleep starts, which occur without the body jerk.[47-49] Sleep starts represent a normal (although not understood) physiologic event, and they should not be confused with seizures or other neurologic conditions. It is likely that the "exploding head syndrome" characterized by a sensation of a loud sound like an explosion or a sensation of "bursting" of the head[50] is a variant of a sensory sleep start. Similar phenomena may represent the sole manifestation of a seizure.[51]

Nightmares

Nightmares are frightening dreams that usually awaken the sleeper from REM sleep (see Chapter 77). Unlike disorders of arousal such as sleep terrors (see later), nightmares are not usually associated with prominent motor or vocal behavior or autonomic excitation, and the arousal results in immediate full wakefulness, with memory for the dream sequence of events that caused the awakening.[52] Seizures may manifest as recurrent dreams, nightmares, or disorders of arousal such as sleepwalking and sleep terrors. The diagnosis of seizure-related dreams and nightmares may be overlooked, as the symptom is misinterpreted as a primary sleep phenomenon.[53-56] Autosomal dominant frontal epilepsy may also manifest as recurrent nightmares.[57]

Hypersomnia

Epilepsy

The sole manifestation of nocturnal seizures may be simple arousals—which may or may not be perceived by the patient. If enough arousals occur, the resulting sleep fragmentation will be apparent with symptoms of severe excessive daytime sleepiness (Figure 72–3). These seizure-induced arousals may be associated with very minor motor phenomena.[58]

Some patients with seizures are hypersomnolent during the day—even after discontinuation of antiepileptic medication. Seizure-free preadolescent children with epilepsy are sleepier than healthy controls. In one study, there was no difference in objective sleepiness in children with epilepsy on or off medication, suggesting that antiepileptic drugs do not necessarily cause the daytime sleepiness.[59] Excessive daytime sleepiness in a patient on antiepileptic medications must not summarily be attributed to antiepileptic medication.[60,61]

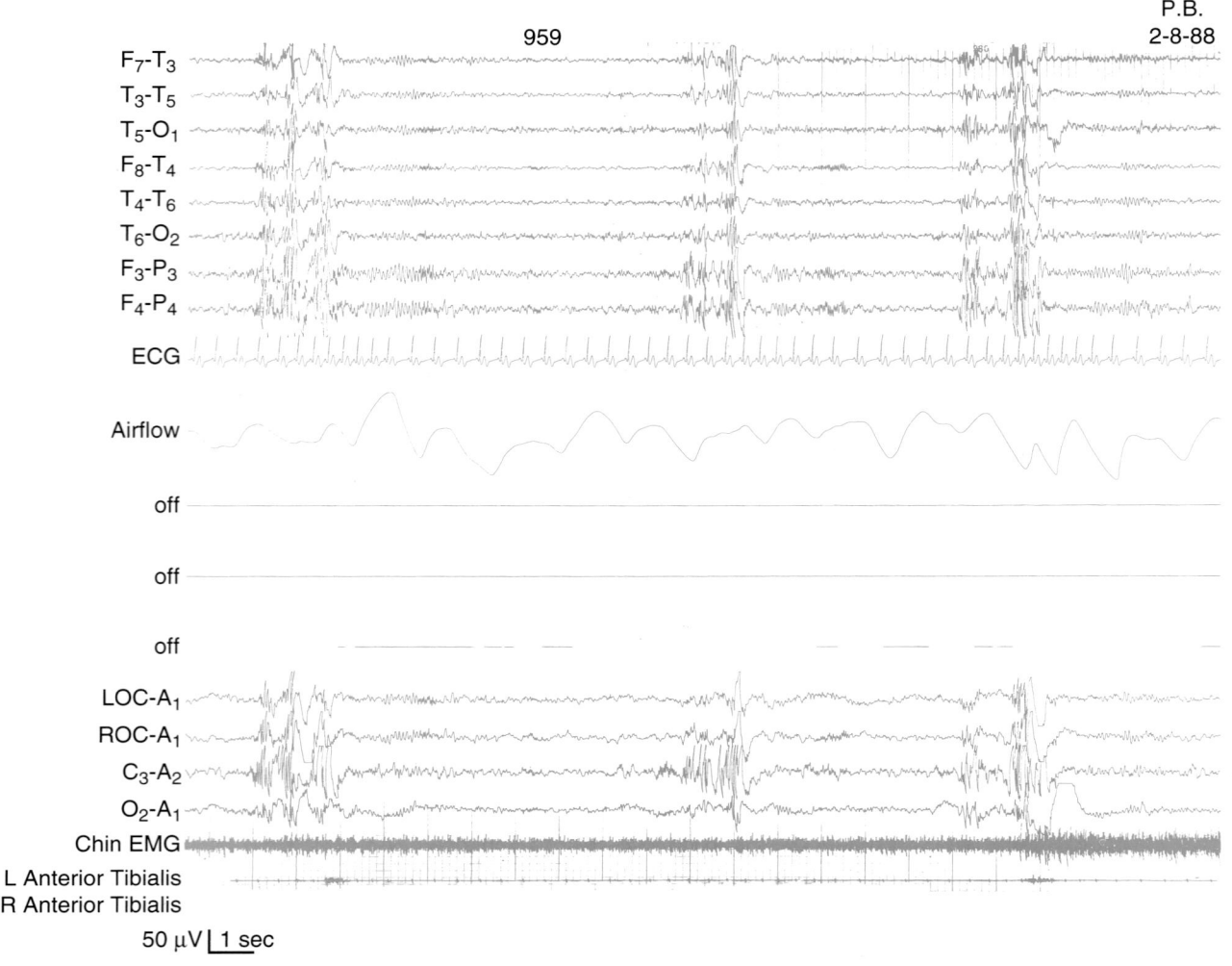

Figure 72–3. Polysomnographic tracing of a child with a history of a "well-controlled" seizure disorder who complained of severe excessive daytime sleepiness. Notice the electroencephalographic (EEG) evidence of arousals, which were the sole manifestation of seizure activity. The seizure-induced arousal index was nearly 100 per hour of sleep—clearly explaining the daytime complaint.

Narcolepsy

Narcolepsy is a genetically determined disorder characterized by excessive daytime sleepiness, cataplexy (the sudden loss of muscle tone triggered by emotionally laden events), sleep paralysis, hypnagogic hallucinations, and automatic behavior during which prolonged, complex activities may be performed without conscious awareness or recall.[62,63] The "spell-like" nature of some sleep attacks, cataplexy, and sleep paralysis may be mistaken for seizures. Conversely, atonic (epileptic negative myoclonus) or inhibitory seizures may mimic cataplexy,[64-70] and the periods of automatic behavior are often misdiagnosed as partial complex seizures, postictal confusion, or priomania.[71,72] The incomplete and waxing and waning nature of cataplexy can imitate tonic-clonic seizure activity.

Periodic Hypersomnia (Kleine-Levin Syndrome)

The Kleine-Levin syndrome is a poorly understood condition characterized by recurrent periods of hypersomnia. The often-cited association with adolescent males and unusual behavior such as hypersexuality and megaphagia have been overrated.[73] Menstruation-related periodic hypersomnia may represent a variant of the Kleine-Levin syndrome.[74] Similar recurrent episodes of hypersomnia may be caused by "ictal sleep" lasting 13 days at 10- to 60-day intervals.[75,76]

Sleep-Disordered Breathing

There is an interesting and important relationship between sleep-disordered breathing and seizures. Nocturnal seizures, probably triggered by periods of hypoxemia, may be the presenting symptom in some individuals with obstructive sleep apnea or sleep-related hypoventilation.[77,78] Furthermore, sleep apnea may exacerbate seizures in patients with epilepsy that is caused by sleep disruption, sleep deprivation, hypoxemia, or decreased cerebral blood flow. Identification and treatment of sleep-disordered breathing in individuals with seizures may improve seizure control.[79,80] Some seizure-like "spells" associated with sleep apnea are actually caused by episodes of cerebral anoxia.[81]

Seizures may also cause periods of apnea, often repetitive, and may closely mimic the conditions of obstructive or central

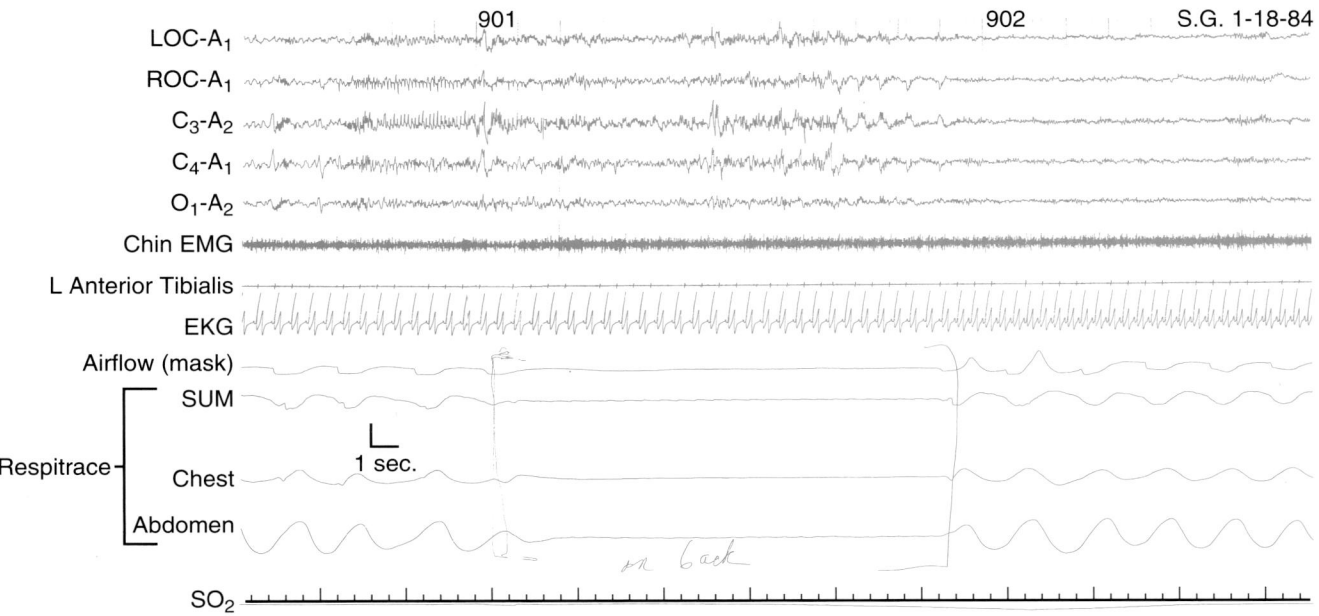

Figure 72–4. Polysomnographic tracing of a 56-year-old man with a long-standing history of well-controlled generalized seizures who developed severe progressive excessive daytime sleepiness. The polysomnogram (PSG) revealed 22 central apneas per hour as the sole manifestation of seizures. Aggressive medical management was unsuccessful. There was marked improvement in his excessive daytime sleepiness following a right frontal lobectomy. (From Mahowald MW, Schenck CH. Sleep disorders. In Engel J Jr, Pedley TA [eds]: Epilepsy: A Comprehensive Textbook. Philadelphia, Lippincott-Raven, 1997, pp 2705-2715.)

sleep apnea.[82-85] Figure 72–4 shows repetitive apneas as the sole manifestation of seizures, and Figure 72–5 shows obstructive sleep apnea inducing electrical seizure activity.

Insomnia

Paroxysmal, otherwise unexplained awakenings may be the sole manifestation of nocturnal seizures and result in the complaint of insomnia.[86-91] Some patients with occasional paroxysmal periodic motor attacks during sleep have very frequent (every 20 to 60 seconds) subclinical arousals causing severe sleep fragmentation.[92] These paroxysmal arousals may be due to deep epileptic foci.[93] The arousal preceding nocturnal seizures may be the initial manifestation of the seizure.[94] Animal studies support the concept of frequent arousals as the manifestation of seizures.[95] This may explain why many patients with epilepsy report frequent, otherwise unexplained nocturnal awakenings.[96]

Parasomnias

Disorders of Arousal

Disorders of arousal are the most common and impressive of the NREM sleep parasomnias, and they may readily be confused with epileptic phenomena (see chapter 74). These occur on a continuum ranging from confusional arousals to sleepwalking to sleep terrors.

Disorders of arousal may difficult to differentiate from nocturnal seizures, and vice versa.[97,98] Preservation of consciousness during seizures may lead to their being confused with disorders of arousal or psychogenic conditions.[99] Crying (dacrystic) or laughing (gelastic) seizures may be misinterpreted as confusional arousals or sleep terrors.[100,101] Both disorders

of arousal and seizures may be related to the menstrual cycle.[102-104]

Arousals of any sort may serve to trigger a disorder of arousal. Therefore, any underlying condition resulting in arousal may cause a disorder of arousal, including sleep apnea, gastroesophageal reflux, or seizures. Thus the clinical event of a sleepwalking or sleep terror episode may, in fact, represent an epiphenomenon of yet a completely different underlying sleep disorder.[19] It is common clinical experience to see an improvement in disorders of arousal following effective treatment of obstructive sleep apnea. Conversely, effective treatment of obstructive sleep apnea with nasal continuous positive airway pressure (CPAP) may result in disorders of arousal, presumably associated with deep NREM-sleep rebound.[105,106] It must be remembered that sleep terrors and seizures may coexist in the same person.[26]

REM Sleep Behavior Disorder

RBD is a recently described condition in which the usual atonia of REM sleep is absent, hypothetically allowing patients to "act out their dreams," often with violent or injurious results (see Chapter 75). RBD is typically a disorder of older men and is frequently misdiagnosed as a nocturnal seizure or psychogenic event. RBD is readily diagnosable by formal sleep studies, which reveal the absence of somatic muscle atonia of REM sleep. RBD responds very well to clonazepam.[107,108] Just as RBD may masquerade as nocturnal seizures, the converse is also true.[109]

Dream and Nightmare Disturbances

As mentioned earlier, dreams (particularly recurrent dreams) or nightmares as the primary manifestation of nocturnal

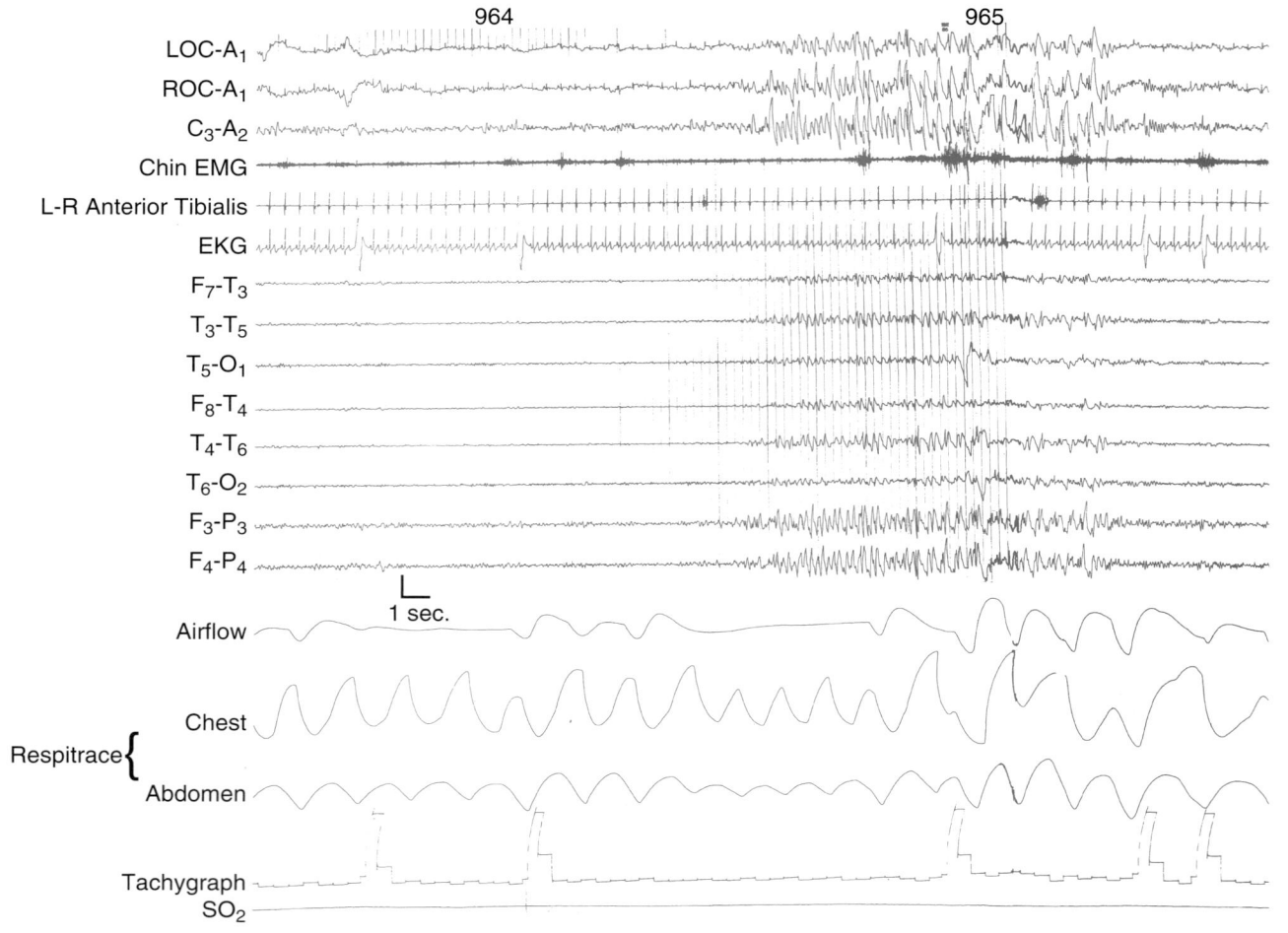

Figure 72–5. Polysomnographic tracing showing electrical seizure activity beginning during an episode of obstructive sleep apnea.

seizures have been well documented. Recurrent dreams as the manifestation of seizures have been well described.[54]

Enuresis

Enuresis was formerly classified as a "disorder of arousal," implying a relationship with NREM or slow wave sleep.[14] However, enuresis may occur during either NREM or REM sleep.[110,111] Enuresis may be the sole manifestation of nocturnal seizures.[19]

Rhythmic Movement Disorder

Rhythmic movement disorder refers to a number of actions characterized by stereotyped movements (rhythmic oscillation of the head or limbs, head-banging, or body-rocking during sleep) seen most frequently in childhood and rarely in adults. Rhythmic movement disorder may occur during any stage of sleep, may be familial, and is not usually associated with underlying psychiatric or psychological conditions.[112] Rarely, rhythmic movement disorder is the sole manifestation of a seizure.[19]

Periodic Limb Movement Disorder

Periodic limb movement disorder (PLMD) is a diagnosis determined by polysomnography. It is characterized by periodic (every 20 to 30 seconds) dorsiflexion of the great toe or

foot or flexion of the entire leg. These movements are not perceived by the patient, and they may be asymptomatic or associated with the complaint of either excessive daytime sleepiness or insomnia.[113,114] When prominent, these movements may be confused with myoclonic seizure activity or may actually represent epileptic phenomena.[115] Propriospinal myoclonus may also be confused with periodic limb movement disorder, and the patient may present with the complaint of insomnia or sleep-related movements that are bothersome to the bed partner.[116,117] Periodic limb movement disorder may be particularly dramatic in patients with underlying renal failure.[118,119]

Posttraumatic Stress Disorder

Posttraumatic stress disorder (PTSD) is often associated with subjective sleep complaints including nightmares and sleep terror–like experiences.[120] It may be confused with nocturnal panic or seizures manifesting solely as arousals with fearful affect.

Seizures

The behavior associated with nocturnal seizures is often bizarre. The seizures thus may masquerade as primary sleep parasomnias, secondary sleep parasomnias, or psychiatric conditions.[121]

The following seizure types are particularly likely to result in diagnostic dilemmas.

CLASSIFIED SEIZURES

Classified seizures occur frequently during sleep.[1] In many people with epilepsy, seizures occur exclusively during sleep, increasing the likelihood of a misdiagnosis of a primary sleep disorder. A conservative estimate is that 10% of patients with epilepsy display seizures exclusively during sleep.[122] One type of seizure that typically occurs predominantly in the sleep period is benign childhood epilepsy with centrotemporal spikes (BECT), also known as benign Rolandic epilepsy. This form of epilepsy is characterized by unilateral somatosensory onset of paresthesias of the tongue, lips, gums, and cheek, with tonic or tonic-clonic movement of the face, lips, tongue, and pharyngeal muscles, and is associated with drooling. The electrical EEG spike discharges are typically activated by sleep (Figure 72–6).[123]

UNUSUAL BEHAVIORAL SEIZURES

Seizures of frontal lobe origin may manifest as bizarre behavior such as running, loud vocalization, or cursing. The extraordinary behavior and the tendency for the behavior to occur during sleep and to cluster in time, promote misdiagnosis (often as a disorder of arousal, RBD, or psychogenic spells).[121,124-128]

Autosomal dominant nocturnal frontal lobe epilepsy (ADNFE) may manifest with predominately or exclusively sleep-related motor behavior,[128,129] as may supplementary sensorimotor seizures.[130] In retrospect, it is probable that many reported unusual nocturnal seizures were due to ADNFE. This condition is characterized by a wide variety of seizure manifestations, previously termed "episodic nocturnal wanderings," and "hypnogenic (nocturnal) paroxysmal dystonia." The seizures often involve hyperkinetic thrashing activity with dystonic posturing, often with vocalization. In addition to the behavioral events, patients with ADNFE may experience innumerable brief arousals from sleep—the sole manifestation of the seizure. The attacks are usually brief and without aura or postictal confusion. The EEG is often obliterated by movement artifact, which makes video-EEG monitoring mandatory.[131,132] ADNFE often responds to carbamazepine.[57] There is evidence that ADNFE represents a channelopathy.[133,134] Nocturnal frontal lobe epilepsy may be particularly difficult to differentiate from disorders of arousal.[98]

Episodic nocturnal wanderings are a manifestation of ADNFE. These wanderings, which respond to anticonvulsants, may be indistinguishable by history from sleepwalking and sleep terrors. The patients ambulate, vocalize, and display

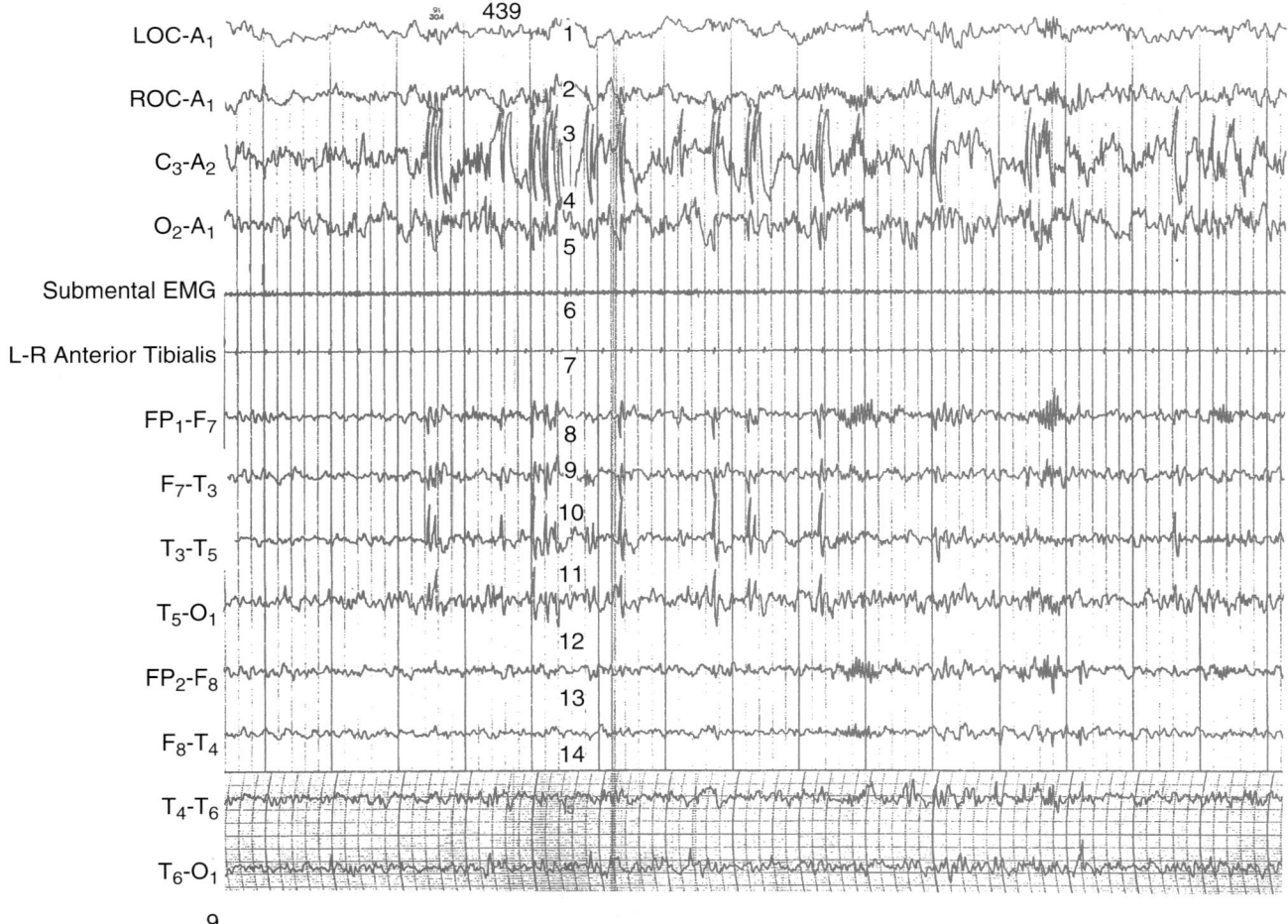

Figure 72–6. Polysomnographic study showing the prominent state-dependent nature of left-sided centromidtemporal spikes, present almost exclusively during non–rapid eye movement (NREM) sleep.

violent behavior during sleep. Not all exhibit waking EEG abnormalities. There is growing evidence that many of these cases represent epileptic phenomena and are actually ambulatory automatisms.[135]

Nocturnal paroxysmal dystonia (NPD) is another manifestation of ADNFE. It is characterized by predominantly or exclusively nocturnal episodes of coarse, occasionally violent, movements of the limbs associated with tonic spasms, often occurring multiple times nightly. Vocalization or laughter may occur. EEGs between events are normal; during events, EEGs display movement artifact, often without clear evidence of electrical seizure activity.[136,137] The cyclic alternating pattern of cortical excitability may play a modulatory role in this condition.[18] It is clear that NPD is a seizure disorder.[138] NPD may be unilateral,[139] and there can be a family history.[140] Nocturnal and diurnal paroxysmal dystonia may exist in the same patient, as can reflex and hypnogenic paroxysmal dystonia. There is considerable overlap among the different clinical categories of paroxysmal dyskinesias.[141] NPD may be posttraumatic[142] and may coexist with panic disorder.[143] Carbamazepine is often very effective in eliminating these spells. Vigilance level–dependent tonic seizures[144] and familial paroxysmal hypnogenic dystonia[140] likely represent variants of this condition.

Pure tonic seizures also likely represent a manifestation of ADNFE with arousal (or paroxysmal polyspike activity with arousal). They appear as insomnia or hypersomnia due to seizure-induced arousals or sleep fragmentation. An interesting subtype of hypnic tonic postural seizures has been described in 10 children, many with a positive family history.[145] This may be a benign epilepsy syndrome similar to benign childhood epilepsy with centrotemporal spikes,[146] childhood epilepsy with occipital paroxysms,[147,148] and primary reading epilepsy.[145]

Autonomic/diencephalic seizures are thought to be rare and could occur with such manifestations as intermittent or paroxysmal apnea,[84,149] stridor,[150] coughing,[151] laryngospasm,[152,153] chest pain and arrhythmias,[154-157] paroxysmal flushing, and localized hyperhidrosis.[158,159] Isolated autonomic symptoms are a well-documented manifestation of seizures and are probably much more common than generally suspected. These simple autonomic seizures are easily confused with other primary or secondary sleep parasomnias or are misattributed to disorders of other organ systems.[160]

Electrical Status Epilepticus of Sleep

Electrical status epilepticus of sleep (ESES) may be detected during a polysomnogram (PSG) performed for other reasons and is characterized by continuous spike and wave activity during NREM sleep.[161] ESES is seen in children who may have a history of seizures or neurologic dysfunction. The prognosis is variable, as ESES can be asymptomatic.[162] ESES may share some features with the Landau-Kleffner syndrome.[163]

Cardiopulmonary Manifestations

CARDIAC ARRHYTHMIAS

Cardiac arrhythmias, including asystole, may be a manifestation of seizures masquerading as nocturnal cardiac abnormalities.[164,165] Conversely, primary cardiac events (e.g., prolonged QT interval) may manifest as seizures.[166] Seizures may manifest as syncope[167] or vice versa.[168]

RESPIRATORY DYSKINESIAS

Peculiar respiratory irregularities may occur or persist during the sleep period. Examples include segmental myoclonus (such as palatal myoclonus[169] or diaphragmatic flutter[170]) and paroxysmal dystonia.[171] Respiratory dyskinesias may also be the manifestation of neuroleptic-induced dyskinesias, which do not always persist during sleep.[172] These dyskinesias should be differentiated from unusual nocturnal seizures that manifest with primarily or exclusively respiratory symptoms.[82]

Gastrointestinal Manifestations

The sole manifestation of nocturnal seizures may be paroxysmal choking.[173]

CASE EXAMPLE

A 3-year-9-month-old girl with tuberous sclerosis was referred for evaluation of progressively severe nocturnal choking and gagging episodes that began at 1½ years of age. There was a remote history of diurnal spells, felt to be seizures, that resolved spontaneously. Aggressive treatment for gastroesophageal reflux had been ineffective. Her father, a nurse anesthetist, was so concerned that she might die during one of these spells that he slept in the same bed with her and kept an intubation tray at her bedside.

A sleep study was requested to evaluate for sleep-disordered breathing, as a tonsillectomy and adenoidectomy were being considered as treatment for these nocturnal choking spells. Because of the possibility of nocturnal seizures, a full seizure montage was employed. Numerous paroxysmal generalized bursts of electrical seizure activity, occasionally associated with coughing or gagging sounds, were present (Figure 72–7). Carbamazepine administered at bedtime resulted in immediate cessation of the nocturnal gagging episodes.

Nocturnal Panic Attacks

Nocturnal panic attacks may occur in patients with diurnal panic or, rarely, may precede the appearance of diurnal panic. In some cases, panic attacks are exclusively nocturnal.[174] The striking similarity of the symptoms of dream anxiety attack, sleep terrors, nocturnal seizures, and nighttime panic urges extreme caution in diagnosis. Obstructive sleep apnea can also cause symptoms of nocturnal panic attacks.[175] The common association of the affect of fear as an accompaniment of nocturnal seizures intensifies their confusion with nocturnal panic attack. It must be remembered that seizures and panic may coexist.[176]

Psychogenic Dissociative States

Complex and potentially injurious behavior, occasionally confined to the sleep period, may be the manifestation of a psychogenic dissociative state. A history of childhood physical or sexual abuse, or both, is virtually always present (but may be difficult to elicit). In this condition, unlike other parasomnias or nocturnal seizures, during EEG monitoring the complex behavior is seen to arise from clear EEG-determined wakefulness.[177] Pseudoseizures may also arise from apparent sleep.[177]

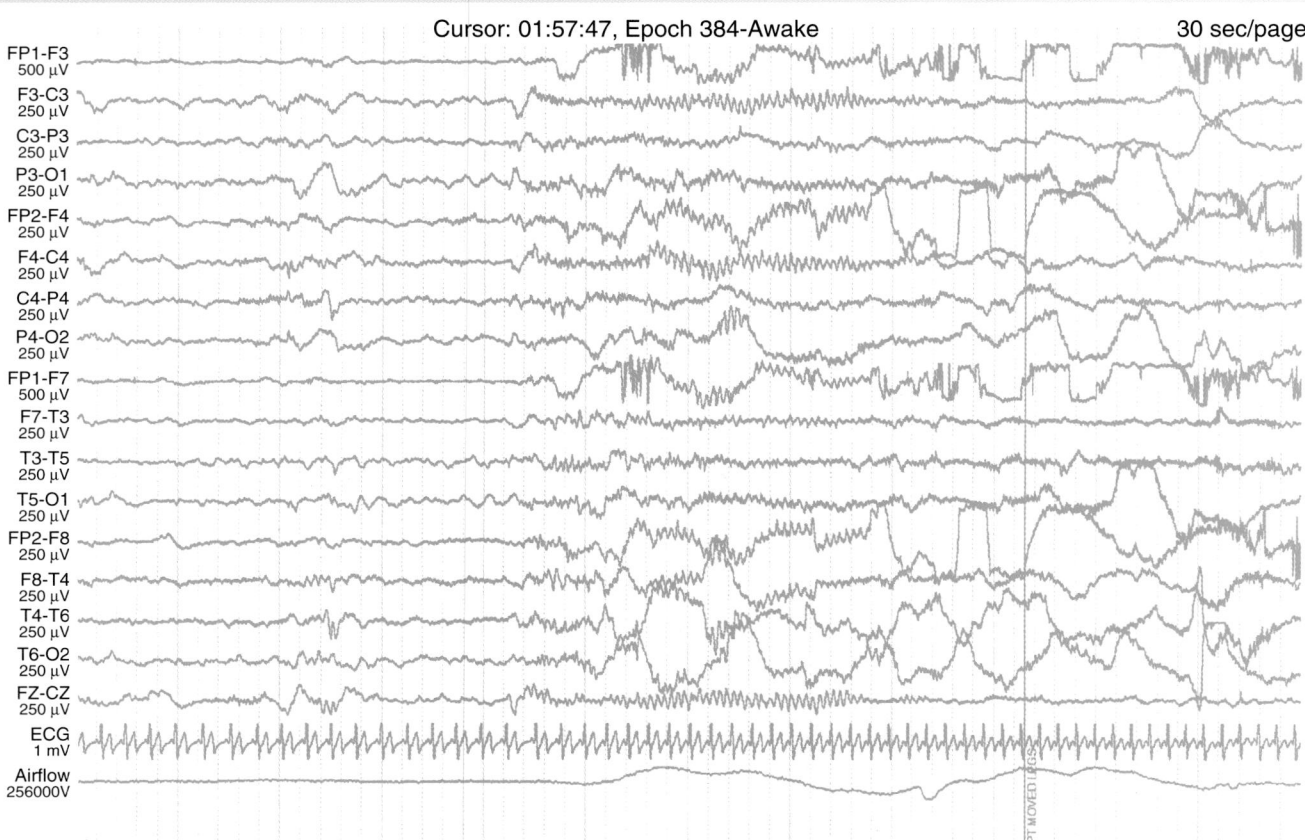

Figure 72–7. Polysomnographic study with a full seizure montage showing generalized paroxysmal rhythmic activity representing electrical seizure activity. This activity was occasionally associated with coughing or gagging and was followed by an arousal.

DIAGNOSTIC EVALUATION

As discussed earlier, clinical differentiation between sleep disorders and epileptic events may often be difficult, if not impossible, because primary or secondary sleep phenomena may perfectly mimic epileptic phenomena and vice versa. Both epileptic and sleep phenomena should be considered in any case of recurrent, stereotyped, and inappropriate unusual sleep-related events.

The decision to investigate unusual nocturnal events depends upon the clinical situation. The most common condition is the disorder of arousal, which is very common (and normal) in the general population. Simple sleepwalking or sleep terrors can readily be diagnosed clinically. Indications for formal evaluation include behavior that is potentially injurious or violent, that causes disruption for other household members, that results in excessive daytime sleepiness, or that displays unusual clinical features.[178]

Clinical differentiation between sleep disorders and epileptic phenomena may be most difficult, and misdiagnosis in both directions is common, particularly in the absence of a history of diurnal spells. Waking and sleep-deprived EEGs may not reveal the diagnosis,[179,180] necessitating all-night polysomnographic study using a full seizure montage, appropriate paper speed, and continuous video recording.[181] Exclusively nocturnal seizures may be uncommon, but they are routinely misdiagnosed and should never be overlooked as the possible etiology in any sleep-related behavior that is recurrent, stereotyped, or inappropriate, regardless of the specific nature of that behavior. Ambulatory EEG monitoring has led to the misdiagnosis of

functional psychiatric disease in a number of our patients who were subsequently demonstrated to have bona fide nocturnal seizures. Erroneous psychogenic branding is reinforced by the bizarre nature of the spells and by the fact that environmental clues may play a role in the context of psychomotor seizures.[182]

Misdiagnosis is common even following formal and appropriate PSG evaluation. Reasons for misdiagnosis include[183]

- Obscuration of the scalp EEG by movement artifact.
- Absence of scalp-EEG manifestation of the seizure activity.
- EEG seizure manifestation appearing to be an arousal pattern.
- Absence of EEG or clinical postictal period.

Extensive polysomnographic monitoring employing a full scalp EEG montage is mandatory. As the clinical events may be infrequent, multiple studies may be necessary to capture an event. Continuous audiovisual monitoring and recording are indicated, and detailed technician observations are invaluable. The difficulties in evaluating unusual sleep-related events emphasize the necessity of extensive, in-person laboratory monitoring with interpretation of all data (clinical, EEG, sleep, video, and technologist-provided information) by personnel experienced in both sleep medicine and epileptology.

TREATMENT

Effective treatment is available for almost all parasomnias, regardless of cause, and is predicated upon an accurate diagnosis. If seizures are responsible for the sleep-wake complaint, treatment is similar to that for other seizure disorders.[184] If a primary sleep disorder (such as narcolepsy, sleep apnea, or other parasomnia) is identified, therapy is dictated by the specific diagnosis. Vagal nerve stimulation for treatment of seizures has been reported to improve daytime alertness[185]; however, vagal nerve stimulation may induce sleep apnea, worsening daytime sleepiness.[186]

CLINICAL COURSE

Few longitudinal studies of nocturnal seizures are available. In some patients the seizures may remit spontaneously, whereas in others the seizures may become diurnal.[187]

PITFALLS AND CONTROVERSIES

Nocturnal seizures are undoubtedly much more common than generally believed. Underdiagnosis is due to the lack of clinical suspicion. The etiologies of many nocturnal paroxysmal events are not clearly defined. Differential diagnosis of epileptic versus nonepileptic manifestations depends primarily on the use of extracranial recordings, although intracranial EEG recordings are sometimes necessary. Specifically, epileptic seizures originating from mesio-orbito-frontal sites often cannot be recorded extracranially, and attacks of uncertain etiology such as sleepwalking, screaming, and complex automatisms may be inaccurately diagnosed as parasomnias. Some evidence also suggests that short-lasting paroxysmal dystonia attacks represent sleep-related frontal lobe seizures.[188] In other cases, parasomnias coexist with limbic epilepsy without an apparent common etiology.

The interface between sleep disorders and epileptic phenomena is vast and compelling, as sleep affects seizures and seizures affect sleep. The myriad of sleep and epileptic phenomena may perfectly counterfeit one another. A high index of suspicion and a full awareness of the broad spectrum of both sleep and epileptic phenomena is instrumental to an accurate diagnosis. A thorough clinical and laboratory evaluation of unusual phenomena that could be either sleep-related or seizure-related usually leads to a specific diagnosis, with important and effective therapeutic implications. Continued close collaboration between clinicians and basic science sleep and epilepsy researchers will undoubtedly lead to important advances in the understanding of both sleep and epilepsy, with vital clinical diagnostic and therapeutic implications.

Clinical Pearl

Nocturnal seizures are routinely misdiagnosed—usually as psychiatric problems or disorders of arousal. Any behavior or experience that is recurrent, stereotyped, and inappropriate may be due to seizures regardless of the nature of the behavior or experience.

Acknowledgment

We thank our technical and nursing staff as well as Paul R. Farber for computer processing and expertise. This work was supported by the Minnesota Regional Sleep Disorders Center and the Hennepin County Medical Center.

REFERENCES

1. Commission Report: Proposal for revised classification of epilepsies and epileptic syndromes. Epilepsia 1989;30:389-399.

2. Drake ME, Pakalnis A, Phillips BB, et al: Sleep and sleep deprived EEG in partial and generalized epilepsy. Acta Neurol Belg 1990;90:11-19.

3. Shouse MN, Martins da Silva A, Sammaritano M: Sleep. In Engel J Jr, Pedley TA (eds): Epilepsy: A Comprehensive Textbook, vol 2. Philadelphia, Lippincott-Raven, 1997, pp 1929-1942.

4. Shouse MN, da Silva AM, Sammaritano M: Circadian rhythm, sleep, and epilepsy. J Clin Neurophysiol 1996;13:32-50.

5. Hauser WA, Kurland LT: The epidemiology of epilepsy in Rochester, MN. Epilepsia 1975;16:1-66.

6. Shouse MN, Siegel JM, Wu FM, et al: Mechanisms of seizure suppression during rapid-eye-movement (REM) sleep in cats. Brain Res 1989;50:271-282.

7. Malow BA, Kushwaha R, Lin X, et al: Relationship of interictal epileptiform discharges to sleep depth in partial epilepsy. EEG Clin Neurophysiol 1997;102:20-26.

8. Mahowald MW, Schenck CH: Sleep disorders. In Engel J Jr, Pedley TA (eds): Epilepsy: A Comprehensive Textbook. Philadelphia, Lippincott-Raven, 1997, pp 2705-2715.

9. Herman ST, Walczak TS, Brazil CW: Distribution of partial seizures during the sleep-wake cycle. Differences by seizure onset site. Neurology 2001;56:1453-1459.

10. Timofeev I, Steriade M: Neocortical seizures: Initiation, development, and cessation. Neuroscience 2004;123:299-336.

11. Mahowald MW, Schenck CH: Evolving concepts of human state dissociation. Arch Ital Biol 2001;139:269-300.

12. Roehrs TA, Carskadon MA, Dement WC, et al: Daytime sleepiness and alertness. In Kryger MH, Roth T, Dement WC (eds): Principles and Practice of Sleep Medicine, 3rd ed. Philadelphia, WB Saunders, 2000, pp 53-71.

13. Gastaut H, Broughton R: A clinical and polygraphic study of episodic phenomena during sleep. Recent Adv Biol Psychiatry 1965;7:197-221.

14. Broughton RJ: Sleep disorders: Disorders of arousal? Science 1968;159:1070-1078.

15. Shouse MN: Physiological basis: How NREM sleep components can promote and REM sleep components can suppress seizure discharge propagation. Clin Neurophysiol 2000;111(Suppl 2):S9-S18.

16. Mendez M, Radtke RA: Interactions between sleep and epilepsy. J Clin Neurophysiol 2001; 18:106-127.

17. Halasz P, Terzano MG, Parrino L: Spike-wave discharge and the microstructure of sleep-wake continuum in idiopathic generalised epilepsy. Neurophysiol Clin 2002;32:38-53.

18. Terzano MG, Monge-Strauss M-F, Mikol F, et al: Cyclic alternating pattern as a provocative factor in nocturnal paroxysmal dystonia. Epilepsia 1997;38:1015-1025.

19. Guilleminault C, Silvestri R: Disorders of arousal and epilepsy during sleep. In Sterman MB, Shouse MN, Passouant PP (eds): Sleep and Epilepsy. New York, Academic Press, 1982, pp 513-531.

20. Hauser WA: Overview: Epidemiology, pathology, and genetics. In Engel J Jr, Pedley TA, (eds): Epilepsy: A Comprehensive Textbook, vol 1. Philadelphia, Lippincott-Raven, 1997, pp 11-14.

21. Janz D: The grand mal epilepsies and the sleeping-waking cycle. Epilepsia 1962;3:69-109.

22. Janz D: Epilepsy and the sleeping-waking cycle. In Vincken PJ, Bruyn GW (eds): Handbook of Clinical Neurology, vol 15. Amsterdam, North Holland, 1974, pp 457-490.

23. Guilleminault C: Parasomnias. In Kryger MH, Roth T, Dement WC (eds): Principles and Practice of Sleep Medicine, 2nd ed. Philadelphia: WB Saunders, 1994, pp 567-601.

24. Sellal F, Hirsch E, Maquet P, et al: Postures et movements anormaux paroxystiques au cours du sommeil: Dystonie paroxystique hypnognique ou epilepsie partielle? Rev Neurol (Paris) 1991;147:121-128.

25. Jones BE: Basic mechanisms of sleep-wake states. In Kryger MH, Roth T, Dement WC (eds): Principles and Practice of Sleep Medicine, 3rd ed. Philadelphia, WB Saunders, 2000, pp 134-154.

26. Tassinari CA, Mancia D, Dalla-Bernardina B, et al: Pavor nocturnus of non-epileptic nature in epileptic children. EEG Clin Neurophysiol 1972;33:603-607.

27. Jouvet M: Recherches sur les structures nerveuses et les mecanismes responsables des differentes phases du sommeil physiologique. Arch Ital Biol 1962;100:125-206.

28. Carskadon MA, Dement WC: Normal human sleep: An overview. In Kryger MH, Roth T, Dement WC (eds): Principles and Practice of Sleep Medicine, 3rd ed. Philadelphia, WB Saunders, 2000, pp 15-25.

29. Steriade M: Impact of network activities on neuronal properties in corticothalamic systems. J Neurophysiol 2001;86:1-39.

30. Siegel J: Brainstem mechanisms generating REM sleep. In Kryger MH, Roth T, Dement WC (eds): Principles and Practice of before Sleep Medicine, 3rd ed. Philadelphia, WB Saunders, 2000, pp 112-133.

31. Rechtschaffen A, Kales A: A Manual of Standardized Terminology: Techniques and Scoring System for Sleep Stages of Human Subjects. Los Angeles, UCLA Brain Information Service/Brain Research Institute, 1968.

32. Chase MH, Morales FR: The control of motoneurons during sleep. In Kryger MH, Roth T, Dement WC (eds): Principles and Practice of Sleep Medicine, 3rd ed. Philadelphia, WB Saunders, 2000, pp 155-168.

33. Baghdoyan HA, Spotts JL, Snyder SG: Simultaneous pontine and basal forebrain microinjections of carbachol suppress REM sleep. J Neuroscience 1993;13:229-242.

34. Lai YY, Siegel JM: Medullary regions mediating atonia. J Neurosci 1988;8: 4790-4796.

35. McIntire DC, Saari M, Pappas BA: Potentiation of amygdala kindling in adult or infant rats by injection of 6-hydroxydopamine. Exp Neurol 1979;63:527-544.

36. Guberman A, Gloor P: Cholinergic drug studies of penicillin epilepsy in the cat. Brain Res 1982;239:203-222.

37. Applegate CD, Burchfield JL, Konkol RJ: Kindling antagonism: Effects of norepinephrine depletion on kindled seizure suppression after concurrent, alternate stimulation in rats. Exp Neurol 1986;94:379-390.

38. Rektor I, Bryere P, Valen A, et al: Physostigmine antagonizes benzodiazepine-induced myoclonus in the baboon, Papio papio. Neurosci Lett 1984;52:91-96.

39. Rektor I, Svejdora M, Silva-Barrat C, et al: Central cholinergic hypofunction in pathophysiology of West's syndrome. In Wolf P, Dam M, Janz D, et al (eds): Advances in Epileptology, vol 16. New York, Raven Press, 1987, pp 139-142.

40. Velasco M, Velasco F: Brain stem regulation of cortical and motor excitability: Effects on experimental and focal motor seizures. In Sterman MB, Shouse MN, Passouant P (eds): Sleep and Epilepsy. New York, Academic Press, 1982, pp 53-61.

41. Corcoran ME: Characteristics of accelerated kindling after depletion of noradrenalin in adult rats. Neuropharmacology 1988; 27:1081-1084.

42. Coenen AM, Stephens DN, Van Luijtelaar EL: Effects of the beta-carboline abecarnil on epileptic activity, EEG, sleep and behavior of rats. Pharmacol Biochem Behav 1992;42: 401-405.

43. Shouse MN, King A, Langer J, et al: Basic mechanisms underlying seizure-prone and seizure-resistant sleep and awakening states in feline kindled and penicillin epilepsy. In Wada JA (ed): Kindling 4. New York, Plenum Press, 1990, pp 313-327.

44. Amzica F: Physiology of sleep and wakefulness as it relates to the physiology of epilepsy. J Clin Neurophysiol 2002;19: 488-503.

45. Amzica F, Massimini M: Glial and neuronal interactions during slow wave and paroxysmal activities in the neocortex. Cereb Cortex 2002;12:1101-1113.

46. Parkes JD: The parasomnias. Lancet 1986;2:1021-1025.

47. Oswald I: Sudden bodily jerks on falling asleep. Brain 1959; 82:92-103.

48. Dagnino N, Loeb C, Massazza G, et al: Hypnic physiological myoclonus in man: An EEG-EMG study in normals and neurological patients. Eur Neurol 1969;2:47-58.

49. Lugaresi E, Coccagna G, Cirignotta F: Phenomena occurring during sleep onset in man. In Popoviciu L, Asgian B, Badiu G (eds): Sleep 1978. Fourth European Congress on Sleep Research, Tirgu-Mures. Basel, Karger, 1980, pp 24-27.

50. Pearce JMS: Exploding head syndrome. Headache 2001;41: 602-603.

51. Walsleben JA, O'Malley EB, Freeman J, et al: Polysomnographic and topographic mapping of EEG in the exploding head syndrome. Sleep Res 1993;22:284.

52. Thorpy MJC, Diagnostic Classification Steering Committee: ICSD—International Classification of Sleep Disorders: Diagnostic and coding manual. Rochester, Minn, American Sleep Disorders Association, 1990.

53. Epstein AW, Hill W: Ictal phenomena during REM sleep of a temporal lobe epileptic. Arch Neurol 1966;15:367-375.

54. Epstein AW: Recurrent dreams. Their relationship to temporal lobe seizures. Arch Gen Psychiatry 1964;10:49-54.

55. Boller F, Wright DG, Cavalieri R, et al: Paroxysmal "nightmares." Neurology 1975;25:1026-1028.

56. Snyder CH: Epileptic equivalents in children. Pediatrics 1958;21:308-318.

57. Scheffer IE, Bhatia KP, Lopes-Cendes I, et al: Autosomal dominant nocturnal frontal lobe epilepsy. A distinctive clinical disorder. Brain 1995;118(Pt 1):61-73.

58. Zucconi M, Oldani A, Ferini-Strambi L, et al: Nocturnal paroxysmal arousals with motor behaviors during sleep: Frontal lobe epilepsy or parasomnia? J Clin Neurophysiol 1997;14:513-522.

59. Palm L, Anderson H, Elmqvist D, et al: Daytime sleep tendency before and after discontinuation of antiepileptic drugs in preadolescent children with epilepsy. Epilepsia 1992;33:687-691.

60. Malow BA, Fromes GA, Aldrich MS: Usefulness of polysomnography in epilepsy patients. Neurology 1997;48:1389-394.

61. Foldvary-Schaefer N: Sleep complaints and epilepsy: The role of seizures, antiepileptic drugs and sleep disorders. J Clin Neurophysiol 2002;19:514-521.

62. Aldrich MS: Narcolepsy. N Engl J Med 1990;323:389-394.

63. Nishino S, Mignot E: Pharmacological aspects of human and canine narcolepsy. Prog Neurobiol 1997;52:27-78.

64. Gambardella A, Reutens DC, Andermann F, et al: Late-onset drop attacks in temporal lobe epilepsy: A reevaluation of the concept of temporal lobe syncope. Neurology 1994; 44:1074-1078.

65. Kanazawa O, Kawai I: Status epilepticus characterized by repetitive asymmetrical atonia: Two cases accompanied by partial seizures. Epilepsia 1990;31:536-543.

66. Guerrini R, Dravet C, Genton P, et al: Epileptic negative myoclonus. Neurology 1993;43:1078-1083.

67. Lee H, Lerner A: Transient inhibitory seizures mimicking crescendo TIAs. Neurology 1990;40:165-166.

68. Andermann F, Tenembaum S: Negative motor phenomena in generalized epilepsies. A study of atonic seizures. In Fahn S, Hallett M, Luders HO, et al (eds): Negative Motor Phenomena, vol 67. Philadelphia, Lippincott-Raven, 1995, pp 9-28.

69. So NK: Atonic phenomena and partial seizures. In Fahn S, Hallett M, Luders HO, et al (eds): Negative Motor Phenomena, vol 67. Philadelphia, Lippincott-Raven, 1995, pp 29-39.

70. Noachtar S, Holthausen H, Luders HO: Epileptic negative myoclonus. Neurology 1997;49:1534-1537.

71. Mayeux R, Alexander MP, Benson DF, et al: Poriomania. Neurology 1979;29:1616-1619.

72. Fagan KJ, Lee SI: Prolonged confusion following convulsions due to generalized nonconvulsive status epilepticus. Neurology 1990;40:1689-1694.

73. Smolik P, Roth B: Kleine-Levin syndrome: Etiopathogenesis and treatment. Acta Univ Carol Med. Monogr 1988;128:5-94 (review).

74. Billiard M, Guilleminault C, Dement WC: A menstruation-linked periodic hypersomnia. Neurology 1975;255:436-443.

75. Mothersill IW, Vogt H, Hilfiker P: Epileptic seizures manifesting as sleep, ictal sleep. Sleep Res 1995;24:410.

76. Wszolek ZK, Groover RV, Klass DW: Seizures presenting as episodic hypersomnolence. Epilepsia 1995;36:108-110.

77. Kryger MH, Steljes DG, Yee W-C, et al: Central sleep apnoea in congenital muscular dystrophy. J Neurol Neurosurg Psychiatry 1991;54:710-712.

78. Barthlen GM, Brown LK, Stacy C: Polysomnographic documentation of seizures in a patient with obstructive sleep apnea syndrome. Neurology 1998;50:309-310.

79. Vaughn BV, D'Cruz OF, Beach J, et al: Improvement of epileptic seizure control with treatment of obstructive sleep apnea. Seizure 1996;5:73-78.

80. Oliveira AJ, Zamagni M, Dolso P, et al: Respiratory disorders during sleep in patients with epilepsy: Effect of ventilatory therapy on EEG interictal epileptiform discharges. Clin Neurophysiol 2000;111(Suppl 2):S141-S145.

81. Cirignotta F, Zucconi M, Mondini S, et al: Cerebral anoxic attacks in sleep apnea syndrome. Sleep 1989;12:400-404.

82. Thach BT: Sleep apnea in infancy and childhood. Med Clin North Am 1985;69:1289-1315.

83. Wantanabe K, Hara K, Hakamada S, et al: Seizures with apnea in children. Pediatrics 1982;70:87-90.

84. Walls TJ, Newman PK, Cumming WJK: Recurrent apnoeic attacks as a manifestation of epilepsy. Postgrad Med J 1981;57:575-576.

85. Monod N, Peirano P, Plouin P, et al: Seizure-induced apnea. Ann N Y Acad Sci 1988;533:411-420.

86. Peled R, Lavie P: Paroxysmal awakenings from sleep associated with excessive daytime somnolence: A form of nocturnal epilepsy. Neurology 1986;36:95-98.

87. Niedermeyer E, Walker AE: Mesio-frontal epilepsy. EEG Clin Neurophysiol 1971;31:104-105.

88. Benner RP, Atkinson R: Generalized paroxysmal fast activity: Electroencephalographic and clinical features. Ann Neurol 1982;11:386-390.

89. Erba G, Cavazzuti V: Pure tonic seizures with arousal. Sleep Res 1981;10:164.

90. Erba G, Ferber R: Sleep disruption by subclinical seizure activity as a cause of increased waking seizures and decreased daytime function. Sleep Res 1983;12:307.

91. Tachibana N, Shinde A, Ikeda A, et al: Supplementary motor area seizure resembling sleep disorder. Sleep 1996;19:811-816.

92. Sforza E, Montagna P, Rinaldi R, et al: Paroxysmal periodic motor attacks during sleep: Clinical and polygraphic features. EEG Clin Neurophysiol 1993;86:161-166.

93. Montagna P, Sforza E, Tinuper F, et al: Paroxysmal arousals during sleep. Neurology 1990;40:1063-1066.

94. Malow BA, Varma NK: Seizures and arousals from sleep—which comes first? Sleep 1995;18:783-786.

95. Shouse MN, Langer J, King A, et al: Paroxysmal microarousals in amygdala-kindled kittens: Could they be subclinical seizures? Epilepsia 1995;36:290-300.

96. Hoeppner JB, Garron DC, Cartwright RD: Self-reported sleep disorder symptoms in epilepsy. Epilepsia 1984;25:434-437.

97. Pedley TA: Differential diagnosis of episodic symptoms. Epilepsia 1983;24(Suppl 1):S31-S44.

98. Zuccconi M, Ferini-Strambi L: NREM parasomnias: Arousal disorders and differentiation from nocturnal frontal lobe epilepsy. Clin Neurophysiol 2000;111(Suppl 2):S129-S135.

99. Ebner A, Dinner DS, Noachtar S, et al: Automatisms with preserved responsiveness: A lateralizing sign in psychomotor seizures. Neurology 1995;45:61-64.

100. Armstrong SC, Watters MR, Pearce JW: A case of nocturnal gelastic epilepsy. Neuropsychiatry, Neuropsychol Behav Neurol 1990;3:213-216.

101. Luciano D, Devinsky O, Perrine K: Crying seizures. Neurology 1993;43:2113-2117.

102. Ichida M, Gomi A, Hiranouchi N, et al: A case of cerebral endometriosis causing catamenial epilepsy. Neurology 1993;43:2708-2709.

103. Newmark ME, Penry JK: Catamenial epilepsy: A review. Epilepsia 1980;21:281-300.

104. Schenck CH, Mahowald MW: Two cases of premenstrual sleep terrors and injurious sleep-walking. J Psychosom Obstet Gynecol 1995;16:79-84.

105. Fietze I, Warmuth R, Witt C, et al: Sleep-related breathing disorder and pavor nocturnus. Sleep Res 1995;24A:301.

106. Millman RP, Kipp GR, Carskadon MA: Sleepwalking precipitated by treatment of sleep apnea with nasal CPAP. Chest 1991;99:750-751.

107. Schenck CH, Bundlie SR, Ettinger MG, et al: Chronic behavioral disorders of human REM sleep: A new category of parasomnia. Sleep 1986;9:293-308.

108. Schenck CH, Mahowald MW: REM sleep behavior disorder: Clinical, developmental, and neuroscience perspectives 16 years after its formal identification in *Sleep*. Sleep 2002;25:120-130.

109. D'Cruz OF, Vaughn BV: Nocturnal seizures mimic REM behavior disorder. Am J Electroneurodiagn Technol 1997;37:258-264.

110. Gillin JC, Rapoport JL, Mikkelsen EJ, et al: EEG sleep patterns in enuresis: A further analysis and comparison with normal controls. Biol Psychiatry 1982;17:947-953.

111. Mikkelsen EJ, Rapoport JL, Nee L, Gruenau C, et al: Childhood enuresis. I. Sleep patterns and psychopathology. Arch Gen Psychiatry 1980;37:1139-1144.

112. Mahowald MW, Thorpy MJ: Non-arousal parasomnias in the child. In Ferber R, Kryger MH (eds): Principles and Practice of Sleep Medicine in the Child. Philadelphia, WB Saunders, 1995, pp 115-123.

113. Montplaisir J, Godbout R, Pelletier G, et al: Restless legs syndrome and periodic limb movements during sleep. In Kryger MH, Roth T, Dement WC (eds): Principles and Practice of Sleep Medicine, 2nd ed. Philadelphia, WB Saunders, 1994, pp 589-597.

114. Mendelson WB: Are periodic leg movements associated with clinical sleep disturbance? Sleep 1996;19:219-223.

115. Lugaresi E, Coccagna G, Mantovani M, et al: The evolution of different types of myoclonus during sleep. A polygraphic study. European Neurology 1970;4:321-331.

116. Plazzi G, Provini F, Ligouri R, et al: Propriospinal myoclonus at the transition from wake to sleep. Sleep Res 1996;26:438.

117. Montagna P, Provini F, Plazzi G, et al: Propriospinal myoclonus upon relaxation and drowsiness: A cause of severe insomnia. Mov Disord 1997;12:66-72.

118. Kimmel PL: Sleep disorders in chronic renal disease. J Nephrol 1989;1:59-65.

119. Pressman MR, Benz RL, Peterson DD: High incidence of sleep disorders in end stage renal disease. Sleep Res 1995;24:417.

120. American Psychiatric Association: Diagnostic and Statistical Manual of Mental Disorders, 4th ed. Washington, DC, American Psychiatric Association, 1994.

121. Stores G, Zaiwalla Z: Misdiagnosis of frontal lobe complex partial seizures in children. Adv Epileptol 1989;17:288-290.

122. Young GB, Blume WT, Wells GA, et al: Differential aspects of sleep epilepsy. Can J Neurol Sci 1985;12:317-320.

123. Lerman P: Benign childhood epilepsy with centrotemporal spikes (BECT). In Engel J, Jr, Pedley TA (eds): Epilepsy: A Comprehensive Textbook. Philadelphia, Lippincott-Raven, 1997, pp 2307-2314.

124. Fusco L, Iani C, Faedda MT, et al: Mesial frontal lobe epilepsy: A clinical entity not sufficiently described. J Epilepsy 1990;3:123-135.

125. Marsh GG: Neuropsychological syndrome in a patient with episodic howling and violent motor behavior. J Neurol Neurosurg Psychiat 1978;41:366-369.

126. Stores G, Zaiwalla Z, Bergel N: Frontal lobe complex partial seizures in children: A form of epilepsy at particular risk of misdiagnosis. Dev Med Child Neurol 1991;33:998-1009.

127. Sussman NM, Jackel RA, Kaplan LR, et al: Bicycling movements as a manifestation of complex partial seizures of temporal lobe origin. Epilepsia 1989;30:527-531.

128. Waterman K, Purves SJ, Kosaka B, et al: An epileptic syndrome caused by mesial frontal lobe seizure foci. Neurology 1987;37:577-582.

129. Hayman M, Scheffer IE, Chinvarun Y, et al: Autosomal dominant nocturnal frontal lobe epilepsy: Demonstration of focal frontal onset and intrafamilial variation. Neurology 1997;49:969-975.

130. King DW, Smith JR: Supplementary sensorimotor area epilepsy in adults. Adv Neurol 1996;70:285-291.

131. Oldani A, Zucconi M, Asselta R, et al: Autosomal dominant nocturnal frontal lobe epilepsy. A video-polysomnographic and genetic appraisal of 40 patients and delineation of the epileptic syndrome. Brain 1998;121:205-223.

132. Oldani A, Zucconi M, Smirne S, et al: The neurophysiological evaluation of nocturnal frontal lobe epilepsy. Seizure 1998;7:317-320.

133. Motamedi GK, Lesser RP: Autosomal dominant nocturnal frontal lobe epilepsy. Adv Neurol 2002;89:463-473.

134. Chang BS, Lowenstein DH: Epilepsy. N Engl J Med 2003;349:1257-1266.

135. Plazzi G, Tinuper P, Montagna P, et al: Epileptic nocturnal wanderings. Neurology 1995;45(Suppl 4):A332.

136. Lugaresi E, Cirignotta F: Hypnogenic paroxysmal dystonia: Epileptic seizure or a new syndrome? Sleep 1981;4:129-138.

137. Hirsch E: Abnormal paroxysmal postures and movements during sleep: Partial epilepsy or paroxysmal hypnogenic dystonia. In Horne J (ed): Sleep '90, Tenth European Congress on Sleep Research, Strasbourg (France). Bochum, Germany, Pontenagle Press, 1990, pp 471-473.

138. Hirsch E, Sellal F, Maton B, et al: Nocturnal paroxysmal dystonia: A clinical form of focal epilepsy. Neurophysiol Clin 1994;24:207-217.

139. Oguni M, Oguni H, Kozasa M, et al: A case with nocturnal paroxysmal unilateral dystonia and interictal right frontal epileptic EEG focus: A lateralized variant of nocturnal paroxysmal dystonia? Brain Dev 1992;14:412-416.

140. Lee BI, Lesser RP, Pippenger CE, et al: Familial paroxysmal hypnogenic dystonia. Neurology 1985;35:1357-1360.

141. Demirkiran M, Jankovic J: Paroxysmal dyskinesias: Clinical features and classification. Ann Neurol 1995;38:571-579.

142. Biary N, Singh B, Bahou Y, et al: Posttraumatic paroxysmal nocturnal hemidystonia. Mov Disord 1994;9:98-99.

143. Stoudemire A, Ninan PT, Wooten V: Hypnogenic paroxysmal dystonia with panic attacks responsive to drug therapy. Psychosomatics 1987;28:280-281.

144. Rajna P, Kundra O, Halasz P: Vigilance level–dependent tonic seizures—epilepsy or sleep disorder? A case report. Epilepsia 1983;24:725-733.

145. Vigevano F, Fusco L: Hypnic tonic postural seizures in healthy children provide evidence for a partial epileptic syndrome of frontal lobe origin. Epilepsia 1993;39:110-119.

146. Holmes GL: Rolandic epilepsy: Clinical and electroencephalographic features. In Degen R, Dreifuss FE (eds): Benign Localized and Generalized Epilepsies of Early Childhood. Amsterdam, Elsevier Science, 1992, pp 29-43.

147. Panayiotopoulos CP: Benign nocturnal childhood occipital epilepsy: A new syndrome with nocturnal seizures, tonic deviation of the eyes, and vomiting. J Child Neurol 1989;4:43-48.

148. Panayiotopoulos CP: Benign childhood epilepsy with occipital paroxysms. In Andermann F, Beaumanoir A, Mira L, et al (eds): Occipital seizures and epilepsy in children. London, John Libbey, 1993, pp 151-164.

149. Sanmarti FX, Estivill E, Campistol J, et al: [Episodes of apnea in an infant: Unusual forms of epileptic seizures]. Rev Electroencephalogr Neurophysiol Clin 1985;14:269-75. French.

150. Maytal J, Resnick TH: Stridor presenting as the sole manifestation of seizures. Ann Neurol 1985;18:414-415.

151. Winans HM: Epileptic equivalents, a cause for somatic symptoms. Am J Med 1949;7:150-152.

152. Ravindran M: Temporal lobe seizure presenting as "laryngospasm." Clin Electroencephalogr 1981;12:139-140.

153. Amir J, Ashkenazi S, Schonfeld T, et al: Laryngospasm as a single manifestation of epilepsy. Arch Dis Child 1983;58:151-153.

154. Devinsky O, Eherenberg B, Barthlen GM, et al: Epilepsy and sleep apnea syndrome. Neurology 1994;44:2060-2064.

155. Kiok MC, Terrence CF, Fromm GH, et al: Sinus arrest in epilepsy. Neurology 1986;36:115-116.

156. Gilchrist JM: Arrhythmogenic seizures: diagnosis by simultaneous EEG/ECG recording. Neurology 1985;35:1503-1506.

157. Hockman CH, Mauch HP, Hoff EC: ECG changes resulting from cerebral stimulation. II. A spectrum of ventricular arrhythmias of sympathetic origin. Am Heart J 1966;71:695-700.

158. Metz SA, Halter JB, Porte DJ, et al: Autonomic epilepsy: clonidine blockade of paroxysmal catecholamine release and flushing. Ann Intern Med 1978;88:189-193.

159. Kuritzky A, Hering R, Goldhammer G, et al: Clonidine treatment in paroxysmal localized hyperhidrosis. Arch Neurol 1984;41:1210-1211.

160. Liporace JD, Sperling MR: Simple autonomic seizures. In Engel J Jr, Pedley TA (eds): Epilepsy: A Comprehensive Textbook. Philadelphia, Lippincott-Raven, 1997, pp 549-555.

161. Kobayashi K, Nishibayashi N, Ohtsuka Y, et al: Epilepsy with electrical status epilepticus during slow sleep and secondary bilateral synchrony. Epilepsia 1994;35:1097-1103.

162. Veggiotti P, Termine C, Granocchio E, et al: Long-term neuropsychological follow-up and nosological considerations in five patients with continuous spikes and waves during slow sleep. Epileptic Disord 2002;4:243-249.

163. Maquet P, Hirsch E, Metz-Lutz MN, et al: Regional cerebral glucose metabolism in children with deterioration of one or more cognitive functions and continuous spike-and-wave discharges during sleep. Brain 1995;118:1497-1520.

164. Rugg-Gunn FJ, Duncan JS, Smith SJM: Epileptic cardiac asystole. J Neurol Neurosurg Psychiatry 2000;68:108-110.

165. Weinstein MD, Albertario C: Cardiac asystole and bradycardia as a manifestation of left temporal lobe complex partial seizure. Ann Intern Med 2000;132:165-166.

166. Pacia SV, Devinsky O, Luciano DJ, et al: The prolonged QT syndrome presenting as epilepsy: A report of two cases and literature review. Neurology 1994;44:1408-1410.

167. Reeves AL, Nollet KE, Klass DW, et al: The ictal bradycardia syndrome. Epilepsia 1996;37:983-987.

168. Bergey GK, Krumholz A, Fleming CP: Complex partial seizure provocation by vasovagal syncope: Video-EEG and intracranial electrode documentation. Epilepsia 1997;38:118-121.

169. Lapresle J: Palatal myoclonus. Adv Neurol 1986;43:265-273.

170. Iliceto G, Thompson BL, Day JC, et al: Diaphragmatic flutter, the moving umbilicus syndrome, and "belly dancer's" dyskinesia. Mov Disord 1990;1:15-22.

171. Sethi KD, Hess DC, Huffnagle VH, et al: Acetazolamide treatment of paroxysmal dystonia in central demyelinating disease. Neurology 1992;42:919-921.

172. Wilcox PG, Bassett A, Jones B, et al: Respiratory dysrhythmias in a patient with tardive dyskinesias. Chest 1994;105:203-207.

173. Brown LW, Fry JM: Paroxysmal nocturnal choking: A newly described manifestation of sleep-related epilepsy. Sleep Res 1988;17:153.

174. Rosenfeld DS, Furman Y: Pure sleep panic: Two case reports and a review of the literature. Sleep 1994;17:462-465.

175. Edlund MJ, McNamara ME, Millman RP: Sleep apnea and panic attacks. Compr Psychiatry 1991;32:130-132.

176. McNamara ME: Absence seizures associated with panic attacks initially misdiagnosed as temporal lobe epilepsy: The importance of prolonged EEG monitoring in diagnosis. J Psychiatry Neurosci 1993;18:46-48.

177. Schenck CS, Milner DM, Hurwitz TD, et al: Dissociative disorders presenting as somnambulism: Polysomnographic, video, and clinical documentation (8 cases). Dissociation 1989; 4:194-204.

178. Mahowald MW, Rosen GM: Parasomnias in children. Pediatrician 1990;17:21-31.

179. Passouant P: Historical views on sleep and epilepsy. In Sterman MB, Shouse MN, Passouant P (eds): Sleep and epilepsy. New York, Academic Press, 1982, pp 1-6.

180. Billiard M, Echenne B, Besset A, et al: All-night polygraphic recordings in the child with suspected epileptic seizures, in spite of normal routine and post-sleep deprivation EEGs. Electroencephalogr Clin Neurophysiol 1981;11:450-460.

181. Aldrich MS, Jahnke B: Diagnostic value of video-EEG polysomnography. Neurology 1991;41:1060-1066.

182. Forster FM, Liske E: Role of environmental clues in temporal lobe epilepsy. Neurology 1963;13:301-305.

183. Mahowald MW, Schenck CH: Parasomnia purgatory—the epileptic/non-epileptic interface. In Rowan AJ, Gates JR (eds): Non-Epileptic Seizures, 2nd ed. Boston, Butterworth-Heinemann, 2000, pp 71-94.

184. Dreifuss FE, Porter RJ: Choice of antiepileptic drugs. In Engel J Jr, Pedley TA (eds): Epilepsy: a Comprehensive Textbook. Philadelphia, Lippincott-Raven, 1997, pp 1233-1236.

185. Rizzo P, Beelke M, De Carli F, et al: Chronic vagus nerve stimulation improves alertness and reduced rapid eye movement sleep in patients affected by refractory epilepsy. Sleep 2003;26:607-611.

186. Holmes MD, Chang M, Kapur V: Sleep apnea and excessive daytime somnolence induced by vagal nerve stimulation. Neurology 2003;61:1126-1129.

187. Park SA, Lee BI, Park SC, et al: Clinical courses of pure sleep epilepsies. Seizure 1998;7:369-377.

188. Montagna P: Nocturnal paroxysmal dystonia and nocturnal wandering. Neurology 1992;42(Suppl 6):61-67.

73

Other Neurological Disorders

Antonio Culebras

ABSTRACT

Sleep may terminate attacks of headache and sleep may trigger or promote headaches. Stage-specific headaches include migraine, cluster headache, chronic paroxysmal hemicrania, and hypnic headache. Stage-specific headaches and the linkage between rapid eye movement (REM) sleep and acute headache attacks point to the influence of circadian sleep rhythms on headaches. Some well-defined sleep disorders are commonly associated with headaches, including sleep apnea, sleep-phase related disorders, and parasomnias. Neurologic conditions with extensive brain damage such as multiple sclerosis, traumatic brain injury, infectious or demyelinating encephalitides, and hereditary neurodegenerative disorders may extensively alter sleep-wake schedules and sleep stages. In some instances, specific sleep disorders, such as narcolepsy in patients with plaques of multiple sclerosis in the hypothalamus or REM sleep behavior disorder in neurodegenerative disorders, afford the opportunity to confirm hypotheses of sleep dysfunction. Clinicians should also keep in mind that upper cervical cord lesions may be associated with obstructive sleep apnea syndrome, and brain tumors may be associated with a variety of sleep disorders.

Sleep is a function of the brain, and brain alterations affect sleep either by defect or excess. Most neurologic conditions that extensively injure brain function, as well as some lesions in such strategic locations as the brainstem, diencephalon, or thalamus, cause sleep abnormalities. There are numerous examples of acute brain injuries causing abrupt changes in sleep patterns or pathologic alterations in sleep. Stroke, head trauma, diffuse encephalopathies, and the encephalitides are just a few examples of such alterations. Chronic diseases with structural alterations of the brain, such as multiple sclerosis or the neurodegenerative disorders, alter sleep; other chronic neurologic disorders not associated with structural brain alterations, such as headache syndromes, show a peculiar but well-established association with sleep anomalies. The clinical study of neurologic disorders and resulting sleep alterations opens up an opportunity to better comprehend sleep and to participate in the alleviation and management of the primary neurologic disorder and of its associated sleep problems.

HEADACHE

There is an intimate relationship between some headache syndromes and sleep.[1] Practitioners and patients have been aware of the peculiar effect of sleep on terminating attacks of headache,[2] and patients have many times complained of being awakened at night or of waking up in the morning with a headache. The discovery of stage-specific headaches and the intriguing linkage between rapid eye movement (REM) sleep and acute headache attacks[3] pointed to the influence that circadian sleep rhythms may have on the advent of headaches. In addition, several well-defined sleep disorders are commonly associated with headaches. These include sleep apnea syndrome and headache on awakening, sleep-phase related headache, and parasomnias and headache.

Epidemiologic studies conducted in headache clinics have noted that 17% of the total headache group reports headaches at night or in the early morning before the final awakening period.[4] Up to 55% of patients in the headache subgroup had a specific sleep disorder identified by polysomnographic monitoring in a sleep center.

Stage-Specific Headaches

Migraine Headaches

Migraine headaches may occur during the night in association with stages 3 and 4 sleep or REM sleep. Fifty-four percent (64% women, 35% men) of patients with narcolepsy report migraine with the full complement of the International Headache Society criteria.[5] Sleep-related migraine attacks are characterized by unilateral throbbing head pain in association with nausea, vomiting, scotomata, visual field defects, photophobia, paresthesias, and even hemiparesis and aphasia. Not all symptoms may be present given the idiosyncratic nature of migraine headaches. Attacks may last for hours to several days. Migraine attacks in children under 8 years of age often resolve after an interval of sleep.[6] Children with migraine may have an increased incidence of disturbed sleep and parasomnias[7] such as somnambulism, night terrors, and enuresis.[8] Prolonged deep sleep is a risk factor for the provocation of sleep terrors and somnambulism, as well as for triggering migraine attacks in susceptible patients at any age.[9]

Although migraine headaches may be provoked by sleep, the most common association is sleep following a migraine attack. The therapeutic effect of sleep[10] in some attacks of migraine may be related to serotonin metabolism, but proof is lacking. The trigeminovascular system, which promotes vasodilation and release of calcitonin gene-related peptide and substance P,[11] has been implicated in the mechanism of migraines because calcitonin gene-related peptide is elevated in the jugular venous blood of migraineurs during the attack.[12]

Serotonin (5-HT) is released from platelets during migraine headaches, and 5-hydroxyindoleacetic acid, the main metabolite of serotonin, is excreted in excess in the urine following a migraine attack.[13] Sumatriptan (an agonist of the 5-HT$_1$ receptor found in cerebral arteries, where it has an inhibitory effect) aborts the migraine headache. Methysergide (antagonist of the 5-HT$_2$ receptor found mainly in temporal arteries, where it has an excitatory effect) also terminates migraines. Thus, serotonin, implicated in mechanisms of non–rapid eye movement (NREM) sleep, is a possible neurotransmitter link between migraine and sleep.

Abnormal patterns of hypothalamic hormone secretion such as decreased nocturnal prolactin peak, increased cortisol concentrations, a delayed nocturnal melatonin peak, and lower melatonin concentrations have been reported in patients with chronic migraine.[14]

Proper sleep hygiene is paramount to aid in the prevention of sleep-related migraine headaches.[15] Bruni and coworkers evaluated the effect of modifying bad sleep habits in 70 migraineurs with poor sleep hygiene. Mean duration and frequency of migraine attacks were significantly reduced when proper sleep hygiene was maintained. Daily administration of preventive therapy should be considered when migraine attacks occur more than twice a month or when they are prolonged and refractory to acute therapy. In women, attacks may cease after menopause.

Cluster Headaches

Cluster headaches occur in 0.4% of men and 0.8% of women.[16] They are characterized by severe unilateral, periorbital, malar and temporal pain with lacrimation, rhinorrhea, nasal engorgement, forehead perspiration, and flushing of the malar area. Attacks are of abrupt onset and termination, generally last 2 hours or less, and recur several times during the 24-hour period, sometimes at the same time each day. Seventy-five percent of cluster headaches occur predominantly at night between 9 PM and 10 AM.[17] Cluster headaches have been linked with REM stage and with sleeping late in the morning, a situation that promotes REM sleep, a possible triggering factor. Spontaneous remissions lasting several months are the norm.

Chronic Paroxysmal Hemicrania

Chronic paroxysmal hemicrania is characterized by attacks of severe pain associated with conjunctival hyperemia, rhinorrhea, and, more rarely, Horner's syndrome. Attacks may appear predominantly at night, usually waking up the patient at the same hour, sometimes in close linkage with REM sleep, leading to the term "REM-sleep locked headache." Chronic paroxysmal hemicrania is considered a variant of cluster headache that features more frequent attacks of pain of shorter duration. It responds quasi-specifically to the therapeutic administration of indomethacin.

Hypnic Headache

Hypnic headache is an idiopathic headache disorder of rare occurrence in older age groups. The mean age of onset is 63 years with a range of 36 to 83.[18] The alternate names—clockwise headache and alarm headache—also attest to its regularity and exclusive occurrence at night. Although it is relatively well known among specialists, this headache syndrome has not yet been included in the classification of the International Headache Society.

Unlike cluster headache and chronic paroxysmal hemicrania, hypnic headache occurs in a diffuse localization in two thirds of patients. Its intensity varies widely, and only one third of patients complain of severe pain. The pain usually lasts longer than 1 hour and generally there is only one attack per night, although more than one attack in a night has also been described. The majority of patients experience the attack during the middle third of the night and report regularity in its occurrence. Less than 10% of patients have associated autonomic symptoms such as lacrimation, nasal congestion, or rhinorrhea, and these are usually mild when they occur.

Results of laboratory tests including magnetic resonance imaging (MRI) of the head, EEG, and Doppler ultrasound have been invariably normal. Polysomnography has shown occurrence of headache attacks during REM sleep in a few but not all patients. Otherwise polysomnograms have been normal. The reports of hypnic headache occurring in REM sleep have led to the speculation that pain structures are activated during REM sleep and to the suggestion that hypnic headache is yet another REM-sleep–related disorder. The appearance of attacks at the same time during the night has led others to suggest a chronobiologic disorder.

The differential diagnosis of hypnic headache, cluster headache, chronic paroxysmal hemicrania, and even nocturnal migraine may be difficult at times. The following characteristics should be helpful to make a diagnosis of hypnic headache: older age group, punctuality of attack occurrence, mild or no autonomic symptoms, diffuse location, duration of 1 hour to a maximum of 2 hours, tendency to appear in relation to dreams, and no symptoms characteristic of migraine such as photophobia, phonophobia, or nausea. Prophylaxis of hypnic headache has been successful with lithium carbonate, flunarizine, indomethacin, and caffeine. The attack itself responds best to the administration of aspirin.

Hemicrania Horologica

Hemicrania horologica, or clock-like hemicrania,[19] is a very rare disorder, with headaches lasting 15 minutes, They occur with clocklike precision every 60 minutes, day and night. Hemicrania horologica differs from chronic paroxysmal hemicrania in the lack of autonomic signs, the clocklike regularity over 24 hours, and the response to nonsteroidal antiinflammatory drugs or indomethacin. Unlike with hypnic headache, attacks also occur during the day.

Exploding Head Syndrome

The exploding head syndrome, originally called "snapping of the brain,"[20] is characterized by the abrupt flashing lights and noises perceived inside the head during the night.[21] The attacks last only seconds and terrify patients despite the absence of pain. The episodes have been shown by polysomnography to appear during any stage of sleep.[22] Generally the exploding head syndrome occurs in persons older than 50 years.

Headache on Awakening

Headache on awakening occurs in half of the patients with sleep apnea syndrome. In at least one study the frequency of headaches was not related to the severity of the syndrome.[23] The headache is generally diffuse and of mild to moderate intensity, with a tendency to disappear as the patient becomes increasingly active. Successful treatment of sleep apnea is associated with significant improvement of the headache in 30% of patients.[24] Prolonged afternoon naps may also be followed by headache.

Headaches on awakening in patients with sleep apnea have been associated with a variety of mechanisms including hypoxemia, hypercapnia, altered cerebral blood flow, and depression. Headaches on awakening may occur with other disorders. These are common in children with brain tumors, but they appear in only 5% of adults with brain tumors. They may also appear in relation to bruxism, systemic hypertension, depression, muscle contraction, alcohol intoxication, and sinus inflammation.

Bruxism, or clenching and grinding of teeth, is a parasomnia that occurs predominantly in stages 1 and 2 of sleep and sometimes in REM sleep, occasionally leading to headache on awakening. The prevalence is 8% in the adult population[25] and somewhat higher in children.[26] It has been related to psychophysiologic stress and iatrogenic interventions, or it may be idiopathic. Both phasic and tonic oromandibular muscle contraction have been observed in bruxism.

Frequent grinding causes abnormal wear of the teeth and occasional fractures of teeth or of tooth restorations; temporomandibular joint disorder and jaw pain are not uncommon when the disorder is chronic and severe. Headaches are presumably caused by temporomandibular joint stress and muscle contraction. Patients with many nocturnal events and associated arousals may complain of fatigue and sleepiness during the ensuing day. Masseter muscle hypertrophy may be observed in patients with chronic sleep bruxism, although daytime bruxism may cause hypertrophy too.

Insomnia and Headache

Insomnia and headache are not uncommonly comorbid conditions. In the postconcussion syndrome, insomnia and headache are prominent symptoms. On the other hand, insomnia and daytime fatigue are frequently reported by patients with chronic headache. Chronic headache sufferers feel more tired (especially the women) and do not sleep as well at night (especially the men).[27] Fibromyalgia occurs in 35.6% of patients with chronic migraine, also known as transformed migraine; this group of patients has a higher incidence of insomnia.[28]

Differential Diagnosis and Diagnostic Workup

Nocturnal migraine, cluster headache, nocturnal paroxysmal hemicrania, and hypnic headache need to be differentiated from other acute severe headaches, such as those associated with intracranial brain tumors, ruptured aneurysm, and meningitis. Patients with intracranial tumors who are awakened at night by headache report improvement on getting out of bed. Headaches on awakening, as observed in sleep apnea patients, are also seen in patients with severe hypertension, depression, intracranial tumor, muscle-contraction headache, alcohol intoxication, and craniofacial sinus disease. Hypnic headache differs from migraine headache, cluster headache, and chronic paroxysmal hemicrania because the pain is commonly diffuse or bilateral and patients are older. Autonomic symptoms are more prominent in cluster headache and chronic paroxysmal hemicrania.

Causes for concern are first or worst-ever headache, associated neurologic symptoms or signs, progressive worsening of headache over days or weeks, intractable nausea or vomiting, fever, lethargy, confusion, and stiff neck. Patients who exhibit causes for concern should have neurologic consultation, neuroimaging studies, and lumbar puncture. Nocturnal polysomnography is indicated for the study of patients suspected of having sleep apnea syndrome or recurrent parasomnias. Videotaping should always be included in the polysomnographic study of parasomnias.

Patients with migraine, cluster headache, and hypnic headache may wake up with an acute attack more frequently during REM sleep than during other stages of sleep, and those with cluster headache and chronic paroxysmal hemicrania may suffer the attack at the same time of the night every night. Attacks of chronic paroxysmal hemicrania may be so closely linked to REM sleep that they have been termed "REM-sleep locked." Bruxism occurs in stage 2 of sleep and less commonly in REM sleep.

Polysomnography has been recommended in patients complaining of early morning and nocturnal headaches.[29] In a study of 25 patients with headache, Paiva and coworkers found 21 patients with disturbed sleep, and in 13 patients the clinical diagnosis had to be reassessed after polysomnography due to the finding of obstructive sleep apnea, periodic limb movements, alpha-delta sleep, and insomnia.

Management

Preventive treatment of migraine, cluster headaches, and chronic paroxysmal hemicrania includes good sleep hygiene, with avoidance of precipitating factors such as sleep deprivation, excessive sleep, stress, trauma, and ingestion of certain idiosyncratic foods including alcohol. Pharmacologic prevention of migraine includes beta-blockers, calcium channel blockers, serotonin receptor antagonists (methysergide, only for use in periods not to exceed 4 weeks), and $5\text{-}HT_2$ antagonists (cyproheptadine and methylergonovine). Prevention may also be achieved with antidepressants that interact with serotonergic receptors such as tricyclics, MAO inhibitors, and selective serotonin reuptake inhibitors (fluoxetine and sertraline); anticonvulsants, particularly in children with abnormal EEG; and nonsteroidal antiinflammatory agents.[30]

Migraine attacks may be aborted with administration of sumatriptan, a $5\text{-}HT_1$ selective agonist, given via subcutaneous injection (6 mg, may repeat after 1 hour, limit 2 injections in 24 hours). Other abortive medications include ergotamine derivatives, acetaminophen, corticosteroids, and nonsteroidal antiinflammatory derivatives. Symptomatic treatment for migraine attacks includes nonsteroidal antiinflammatory derivatives, mixed barbiturate and analgesics, antiemetics (promethazine, 50 mg), and if pain is severe meperidine (50 mg) or codeine sulfate (30 mg).

Cluster headaches may be prevented with ergotamine derivatives at bedtime (1 mg to 3 mg sublingual), amitriptyline (150 mg daily), methysergide (6 mg to 8 mg daily), prednisone (40 mg daily), and lithium carbonate (initial dose 250 mg). Acute attacks are terminated with inhalation of oxygen. Chronic paroxysmal hemicrania responds specifically to indomethacin (50 mg at bedtime or 25 mg 3 times a day). Morning headaches related to sleep apnea syndrome disappear with the successful management of sleep apnea. Hypnic headaches have responded to any of the following regimens at bedtime: coffee; ergotamine tartrate, 0.6 mg;

phenobarbital, 40 mg, with belladona, 0.2 mg; atenolol, 25 mg; aspirin, 325 mg, with caffeine, 40 mg; indomethacin, 25 mg; and flunarazine, 5 mg. Successful prophylaxis with lithium carbonate has also been reported. Reassurance and administration of clomipramine are curative in most instances of exploding head syndrome. Bruxism is treated with stress management, a mouth guard, or an intraoral occlusal splint.[31] For short-term management, diazepam (5 mg) given at bedtime will reduce teeth-grinding. The manifestations of post-concussion syndrome respond in many instances to the administration of tricyclic antidepressants.

HEAD TRAUMA

Severe head trauma, whether open or closed, is characterized by loss of consciousness. Structural lesions ensue following traumatic brain injury; some lesions appear weeks or even months after the event. It is estimated that 500,000 people are hospitalized annually in the United States as a result of head trauma, and 90,000 become permanently disabled, with major medical and social consequences.[32] Severe head trauma disrupts brain functions, including the sleep-wake schedule. Mild head trauma is even more prevalent, affecting close to 1.5 million persons annually,[33] but its sequelae are less predictable and not so well known. When evaluating a patient with a disturbance of the sleep-wake schedule following traumatic brain injury, it is important to determine whether the sleep alteration preceded the injury or appeared following the event.

Traumatic brain injury may cause diffuse or localized brain lesions as well as increased intracranial pressure during the acute stage. Sleep studies of patients with traumatic brain injury have not used uniform measures, and the results have been diverse. The emerging pattern is of major disruption of sleep stages in cases of severe brain injury. Sleep spindles tend to disappear when the lesions are acute and severe,[34] showing a high correlation with the Glasgow outcome scores; recovery of sleep spindles suggests improvement of brain function.

Indeed, in patients with traumatic coma, the occurrence of EEG patterns resembling sleep carries a favorable prognosis. Individual sleep stages are generally less distinct during the acute phase. In the initial phase of recovery while the patient emerges from the coma, hypersomnia is common, with poor recollection of dreams. As the rehabilitation progresses, the organization of sleep stages tends to become normalized. Weeks to months following recovery of consciousness, sleep stages 3 and 4 and REM sleep are decreased along with total sleep time.[35] The early appearance of sleep-wake cycling indicates a better prognosis.

Sleep fragmentation and decreased sleep quality have been reported[36] following minor head injury without loss of consciousness. Surveys performed after mild head injury indicate that insomnia predominates over hypersomnia.[37]

Clinical Manifestations

Sleep-Disordered Breathing

Sleep-disordered breathing (SDB) may be caused by injuries of the brain or cervical cord, and they may be worsened by accompanying injuries in other organs, most prominently the upper airway. In a study of 22 patients with stable spinal cord injury,[38] Short and colleagues found 10 patients with sleep-disordered breathing. The condition has also been observed in studies of patients with posttraumatic quadriplegia.[39,40] Aggravation of sleep-disordered breathing may occur with the administration of sedatives or hypnotics commonly administered to these patients.

Posttraumatic Hypersomnia

Posttraumatic hypersomnia is a common occurrence following significant brain injury. It may appear in patients recovering from posttraumatic coma or in patients whose head trauma was deemed relatively benign and not associated with loss of consciousness. The medico-legal implications are important because patients may lose their job or at the very least complain of deterioration in the quality of life.

In Guilleminault's study of 184 patients with posttraumatic hypersomnia, 103 were involved in litigation.[41] The author divided patients into two groups: group A with premorbid sleep disorder and group B without preceding sleep alteration. Group B was further subdivided into three categories: (1) normal polysomnography with abnormal results on the multiple sleep latency test (MSLT) and an average sleep latency between 6 and 10 minutes; (2) coma, with traumatic brain injury and hydrocephalus; and (3) coma with or without neurologic sequelae followed by a syndrome of subwakefulness independent of depression. In the author's experience, response to treatment is poor in subgroups 1 and 2, whereas subgroup 3 may respond to treatment with amphetamines.

Common complaints of patients with posttraumatic hypersomnolence are, in addition to daytime sleepiness, difficulty performing, inability to work, memory difficulties, speech difficulties, poor concentration, and depressive affect. These patients may complain also of headaches, restless sleep, heavy snoring, leg and body jerks during sleep, night terrors, night sweats, nightmares, and seizures during sleep.

Posttraumatic Narcolepsy

Posttraumatic narcolepsy has been reported in a few cases. Narcolepsy may have preceded the head trauma[42] or the head injury may have served as a triggering factor to unmask premorbid narcolepsy.[43] In light of new knowledge about the etiology of narcolepsy, it is conceivable that severe head trauma may affect the hypothalamic system significantly enough to alter the neurotransmitter hypocretin, either transiently or permanently. It is known that following significant traumatic brain injury there is a decrease in cerebrospinal fluid (CSF) hypocretin levels perhaps nonspecifically as a result of hemodynamic changes.[44]

Narcolepsy-cataplexy developed in a man with acromegaly two weeks following irradiation of the pituitary gland. Since the patient had normal CSF concentrations of hypocretin, the authors suggested that the damage was inflicted to hypocretin receptors rather than to secretors of the neurotransmitter.[45] These observations suggest that symptomatic narcolepsy may be caused by physical damage to the hypocretin system, and it is only a matter of time before posttraumatic hypocretin insufficiency with hypersomnia is reported.[46] Posttraumatic Kleine-Levin syndrome responsive to lithium administration has been reported in two cases.[47]

Circadian Rhythm Disorders

Circadian rhythm disorders have been described following traumatic brain injury. Reversal of the circadian rhythm[48] and resetting of the biological clock in comatose patients following traumatic brain injury have also been reported.[49] Posttraumatic psychiatric and behavioral disorders may lead to sleep-wake alterations, although the premorbid condition needs to be factored in.

Dreaming Disorders

Dreaming may disappear following traumatic brain injury, perhaps related to impairment of visual memory.[50] Paradoxically, studies performed in patients following traumatic brain injury have found no correlation between amount of REM sleep and loss of dreaming.[51] Hallucinations in the recovery phase of traumatic brain injury may reflect the recovery of REM sleep and breakthrough of REM sleep into wakefulness, as a dissociated state.[52]

MULTIPLE SCLEROSIS

The association between multiple sclerosis and sleep disorders is more common than expected by chance. Reports published in the first half of the 20th century cite cases of multiple sclerosis associated with sleep attacks termed "narcolepsy."[53-55] Subsequently, cases of narcolepsy-cataplexy and multiple sclerosis, familial or not, were reported.[56,57] Later reports pointed out that sleep disturbance is relatively common in multiple sclerosis and that a multifactorial etiology that ranges from depression to lesion site[58,59] should be considered.

There is coincidence of genetic susceptibility between multiple sclerosis and narcolepsy. The susceptibility to multiple sclerosis is coded by genes within or close to the human leukocyte antigen DR-DQ subregion.[60] On the other hand, patients with narcolepsy exhibit the highest known association between the human leukocyte antigen DR2 and DQw1 antigens and a disease entity. This has led some authors to postulate a common immunogenetic etiology.[61] Others have postulated that the human leukocyte antigen Dw2 haplotype in patients with multiple sclerosis and narcolepsy extends to the DRB5 locus.[62] Recent publications report hypersomnia in certain multiple sclerosis patients. These patients have lesions seen on MRI that are suggestive of plaques in the hypothalamus, as well as undetectable levels of orexin in spinal fluid.[63]

Clinical Manifestations

Chronic fatigue is common in multiple sclerosis and may confound the interpretation of sleep disturbances. Patients report difficulty falling asleep, restless sleep, nonrestorative sleep, and early morning awakenings more frequently than control subjects.[64] A variety of underlying physical and emotional factors (bladder problems, spasticity, muscle spasms, periodic leg movements, depression, and anxiety) that converge to disturb nocturnal sleep should be considered. Excessive daytime somnolence may be secondary to nocturnal disruption, which is likely amenable to proper management.

In a study of 28 consecutive patients with multiple sclerosis, 54% reported sleep-related problems,[65] including difficulty initiating or maintaining sleep, frequent awakenings due to leg spasms, habitual snoring, and nocturia. Sleep apnea syndrome occurred in two patients, and three showed episodes of nocturnal desaturation. MRI of the brain was abnormal in 20 of 22 cases studied.

Polysomnographic studies of patients with definite multiple sclerosis have shown significantly reduced sleep efficiency and more awakenings during sleep, suggesting a multifactorial etiology of the sleep disorder. In a polysomnographic study of 25 patients with definite multiple sclerosis, sleep efficiency was significantly reduced and awakenings were increased.[66] Periodic leg movements were found in 36% of patients compared with 8% of controls. Central sleep apneas were found in two patients. MRI of the brain showed a greater load of lesions in the cerebellum and brainstem in patients with periodic leg movements.

Management

Fatigue is the most pervasive symptom in multiple sclerosis. Amantadine and modafinil have been suggested for the alleviation of chronic fatigue in these patients.[67,68] Modafinil was assessed in a single-blind study involving 72 patients with multiple sclerosis.[69] The results suggested that 200 mg/day of modafinil significantly improved fatigue and was well tolerated.[69] Some authors have reported a regression of symptoms of sleep disturbance with dexamethasone[70] or prednisolone therapy.[71] Antidepressant medication may be useful for the treatment of sleep disorders in multiple sclerosis and, as in other conditions featuring periodic limb movements, clonazepam may control the movement disorder.

Sleep paralysis in a 40-year-old woman with remitting-progressive multiple sclerosis disappeared with weak electromagnetic field treatments delivered extracerebrally 1 to 2 times per week over a period of 3 weeks.[72] Using this treatment in patients with multiple sclerosis, the same author[73] reported restoration of dream recall in four patients, attenuation of suicidal behavior in three additional patients[74] (which he attributed to improved mental depression), and resolution of partial cataplexy in another patient with chronic progressive multiple sclerosis.[75]

HEREDITARY NEURODEGENERATIVE AND METABOLIC DISORDERS

The occurrence of sleep disorders in this large group of neurologic conditions is limited to case reports and very short series of patients. The list continues to expand with the addition of new reports from the literature.

Neurodegenerative disorders may have predominantly cerebellar dysfunction, as in some forms of olivo-ponto-cerebellar degeneration, extrapyramidal manifestations as in the synucleinopathies, or a combination of cerebellar and sensorimotor signs as in the spino-cerebellar atrophies. Patients with neurodegenerative disorders have many sleep-related complaints including insomnia, hypersomnia, circadian dysrhythmia, abnormal movements, and abnormal behavior in sleep. They are also at risk for the development of sleep apnea syndrome and periodic limb movements in sleep (PLMS). Excessive daytime somnolence secondary to fragmentation of nocturnal sleep caused by sleep apnea, PLMS, or other factors is a common complaint.

The sleep evaluation of patients with a neurodegenerative disorder should include overnight polysomnography followed by a multiple sleep latency test. The objectives are to assess the presence of sleep apnea syndrome, PLMS, and REM sleep without atonia and to measure excessive daytime somnolence. In some cases, the MSLT shows REM sleep in daytime naps with short-onset REM sleep latencies suggestive of narcolepsy. In special circumstances of suspected abnormal motor activity, video recording of nocturnal sleep is desirable. Actigraphy has been used in some laboratories to document motor activity during sleep and waking that may unveil a circadian dysrhythmia.

Management of sleep disorders in patients with neurodegenerative disorders follows the general guidelines. Sedatives and hypnotics should be administered with caution to this group of patients to avoid aggravation of muscle weakness or gait ataxia, not only during daytime hours but also during nocturnal awakenings with ambulation in the dark.

Illustrative Neurodegenerative Disorders

Machado's Disease

Machado's disease[76] is a spinocerebellar ataxia type 3. Increased prevalence of restless legs syndrome and PLMS has also been reported in this condition. The clinical evaluation of patients with spinocerebellar ataxia type 3 should pursue possible presence of sleep apnea syndrome and PLMS. REM sleep behavior disorder (RBD), a condition also prevalent in the synucleinopathies [see Chapter 75], has been reported in association with Machado's disease and may be related to striatal monoaminergic deficit.[77]

Charcot-Marie-Tooth Disease

Charcot-Marie-Tooth disease is a hereditary motor and sensory polyneuropathy characterized by degeneration of peripheral nerves and roots. Patients exhibit distal muscle weakness, atrophy, and sensory impairment. Phrenic neuropathy may cause diaphragmatic dysfunction leading to chronic hypoventilation, particularly in REM sleep.[78] Vocal cord paralysis has also been reported. Patients with Charcot-Marie-Tooth disease have a high incidence of significant sleep apneas, the severity of which is highly correlated with the severity of peripheral neuropathy. Researchers have hypothesized that sleep apneas in Charcot-Marie-Tooth disease are the consequence of pharyngeal neuropathy affecting the function of pharyngeal dilator muscles.[79]

Niemann-Pick Disease

Niemann-Pick disease type C is a rare, autosomal-recessive condition characterized by the accumulation of unesterified cholesterol in many tissues and storage of sphingolipids in liver and brain. Adult patients exhibit ataxia, dystonia, dementia, and vertical supranuclear palsy along with hepatosplenomegaly. Some patients report hypersomnia and cataplexy. Recent investigations have shown reduced CSF levels of hypocretin in this condition, which are likely responsible for sleep abnormalities and cataplexy.[80] Vancova and coworkers suggest that lipid storage abnormalities in Niemann-Pick disease may affect hypocretin-containing cells.

Cataplexy attacks respond to the administration of tricyclic antidepressants.

ACUTE ENCEPHALITIDES

Sleeping sickness is a meningoencephalitis caused by the protozoan Trypanosoma brucei. The parasite is transmitted to humans by the sting of the tsetse fly in Africa, where 20,000 new cases are reported each year. Sleeping sickness begins with a phase of systemic disease, after which the parasite invades the CNS with manifestations of insomnia and daytime hypersomnia, followed by psychomotor retardation. The disease then progresses to extrapyramidal manifestations, ataxia, gait disorder, seizures, coma, and death. Polysomnography reveals sleep onset REM periods shortly after CNS invasion by trypanosomes, then high amplitude slow waves suggestive of a diffuse encephalopathy, with preservation of REM-sleep parameters until the final phases of the disease.[81,81a] CSF analysis has shown increases in cell count, high protein content, and increased immunoglobulin M (IgM) levels.[82] Neuropathologic studies have shown demyelinating lesions in cerebral hemispheres and brainstem.[83]

Acute disseminated encephalomyelitis is an acute inflammatory demyelinating disease of the CNS following viral illness or vaccination. The disorder is probably mediated by immunologic mechanisms. There is a report of hypersomnia in a 5-year-old girl with acute disseminated encephalomyelitis.[84] The CT of the head showed hypodensity lesions involving basal ganglia as well as posterior hypothalamus and brainstem. Following treatment with intravenous dexamethasone, hypersomnia improved and the lesions disappeared. Total sleep time and slow wave sleep were increased, and REM stage was within the normal range in the polysomnographic study during the hypersomnic state. Hypocretin levels in CSF were not assayed.

Transient obstructive sleep apnea has been described in association with presumed viral encephalopathy.[85] Paradoxical respiratory efforts during sleep along with frequent episodes of tachy-bradycardia and asystole led to suspicion of obstructive sleep apnea syndrome, which was documented with portable polysomnography. All apnea events and cardiovascular concomitants resolved with continuous positive airway pressure (CPAP) applications. This case illustrates the occurrence of sleep-related transient respiratory obstructions in diffuse acute encephalopathy that, if undetected, may lead to serious cardiovascular consequences. Similar alterations may occur in acute encephalopathies of different etiologies. Sedating medications commonly administered to patients in the critical care setting may aggravate the sleep apnea syndrome.

BRAIN TUMORS

Brain tumors can disrupt sleep-wake cycles by virtue of their location or indirectly by causing intracranial hypertension or hydrocephalus, or both. Symptomatic narcolepsy has been reported in association with craniopharyngioma compressing the floor of the third ventricle (Fig. 73–1).[86] Symptomatic narcolepsy has also been reported in gliomas and colloid cysts of the third ventricle, as well as in pituitary adenomas and midbrain gliomas.[87] Lower brain stem tumors have been associated with severe hypoventilation and respiratory failure during sleep (Ondine's curse) requiring tracheostomy. Increased intracranial

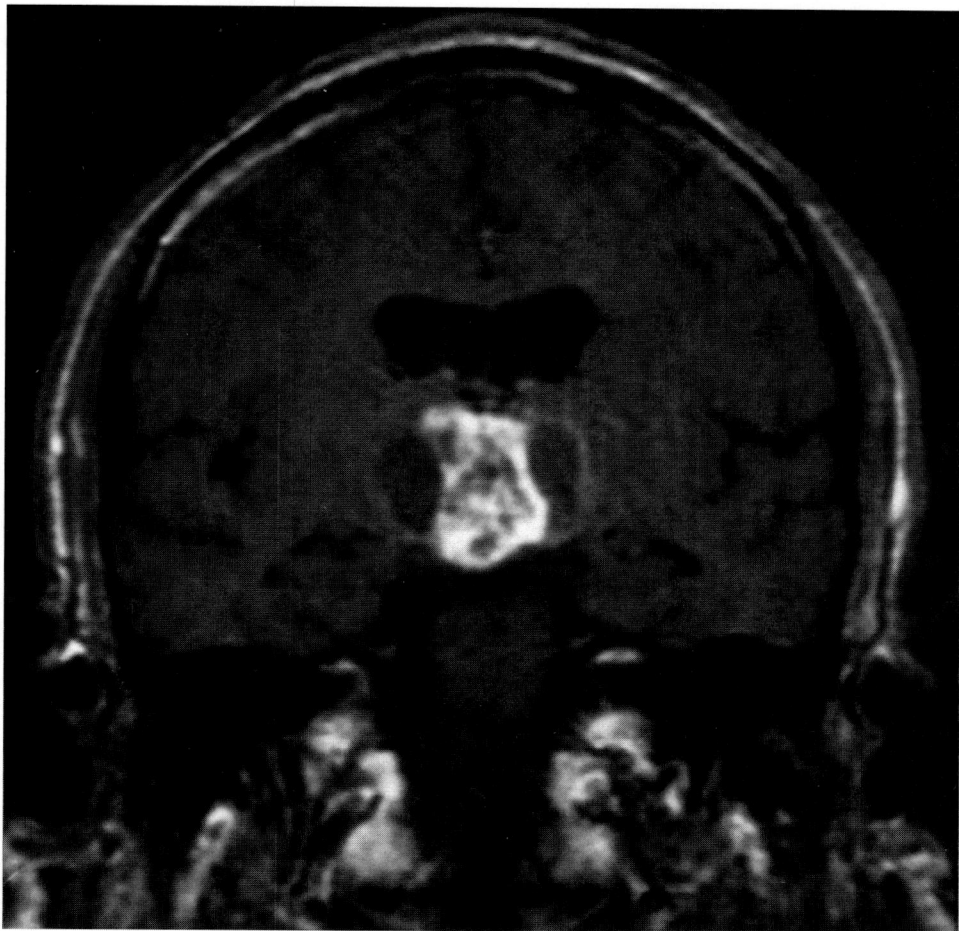

Figure 73–1. CT scan of the head of a 55-year-old man complaining of headaches and excessive daytime somnolence that was initially diagnosed as sleep apnea syndrome. The large cystic mass compressing the diencephalon and floor of the III ventricle was found at operation to be a craniopharyngioma. (Reprinted with permission from Culebras A: Clinical Handbook of Sleep Disorders. Boston, Butterworth-Heinemann, 1996.)

hypertension and obstructive hydrocephalus have been associated with subalertness and lethargy. Sleepiness following hypothalamic injury in the course of resection of an astrocytoma has been reported in association with a low concentration of hypocretin in CSF.[88]

SPINAL CORD DISEASE

Sleep-related ventilatory function depends on the integrity of the spinal cord. In patients with spinal cord lesions, sleep disturbances related to respiratory dysfunction are common. The phrenic nerve controls diaphragmatic motor function. It originates in the phrenic nucleus, which forms the ventral medial cell column of the cervical ventral gray horn, extending from C3 to the caudal part of C5.

The descending respiratory pathway is formed by crossed fibers situated deep in the anterior white column in the vicinity of the anterior horn projecting mainly from the ventral respiratory group in the medulla. High cervical lesions and phrenic nerve damage cause unilateral or bilateral paralysis of the diaphragm, depending on the extent of the cervical cord lesion or on whether one or both phrenic nerves are involved.

The intercostal muscles receive their innervation via descending pathways located dorsal to diaphragmatic pathways in the vicinity of the lateral spinothalamic tract. Voluntary respiration is mediated by fibers in the lateral pyramidal tract, whereas involuntary automatic respiration is mediated by reticulospinal fibers emerging from the brainstem respiratory centers. Spinal motor nuclei situated in segments T1-T11 give origin to intercostal nerves that innervate intercostal muscles.

Accessory respiratory muscles receive innervation from cranial nerve XI and nerves C1-C8. Upper airway muscles involved in nasal, pharyngeal, and laryngeal dilation are innervated by cranial nerves V (m. tensor veli palatine), VII (m. levator alae nasi), X (m. cricothyroid, thyroarytenoid), XII (m. genioglossus, genihyoid, sternohyoid, sternothyroid), and C1-C4 (m. geniohyoid, sternothyroid, sternohyoid). These are unaffected by spinal cord lesions below C5, a lesion compatible with a respirator-free life.

Lesions of the phrenic and intercostal motor neurons in the spinal cord may occur with spinal cord tumors, spinal trauma, spinal surgery (e.g., cervical cordotomy or anterior spinal surgery), and in demyelinating myelitis. Patients with syringomyelia and syringobulbia (fluid-filled cavities in the spinal cord or brainstem, respectively) with dysphonia and dysphagia are particularly prone to severe respiratory disturbances during sleep.[89] In one study of 22 patients with stable spinal cord lesion above T10,[38] 45% had some evidence of obstructive sleep apnea syndrome. Cognitive changes in patients with tetraplegia may be related to sleep apnea syndrome.[90] Although excessive daytime somnolence secondary to sleep-related respiratory dysfunction is the most common symptom, patients with spinal cord diseases may complain of insomnia as a result of immobility, neck pain, and central pain syndrome.

Phrenic nerve damage leads to diaphragmatic paralysis. Unilateral paralysis is asymptomatic, but bilateral paralysis is invariably symptomatic and may be life-threatening. Paresis or weakness with partial diaphragmatic dysfunction may cause sleep-related ventilatory insufficiency. In the supine position, patients complain of profound difficulty breathing because of decreased lung volume and increased respiratory effort as the abdominal contents rise into the thorax. In bilateral severe or acute cases, patients present with nocturnal orthopnea, cyanosis, and fragmented sleep followed by morning headaches, vomiting, and daytime lethargy. Phrenic nerve weakness or paralysis is most prominent in REM sleep when the diaphragm is the only functional respiratory muscle. Upper airway resistance is also higher in REM sleep, contributing to decreased ventilatory efficiency. Patients with weak pharyngeal dilator muscles and a weak diaphragm as a result of a diffuse neuromuscular disorder or bilateral phrenic nerve paralysis exhibit the most serious compromise in REM sleep.[91]

Obstructive sleep apnea syndrome may appear following anterior cervical spine fusion.[92] Guilleminault and coworkers found that placement of anterior cervical plates at the C2-C4 level reduced the size of the upper airway, causing obstructive sleep apnea syndrome. The condition was controlled with positive airway pressure applications.

Restless legs syndrome and PLMS may appear in patients after acute transverse myelitis.[93] Periodic limb movements in sleep have been reported in patients with syringomyelia.[94]

Treatment for sleep-related respiratory dysrhythmias in spinal cord diseases should follow the same general principles as those suggested for neuromuscular disorders. A word of caution comes from a study[95] showing that obese patients who have spinal cord injury and are taking antispasticity medications may have a higher risk for developing snoring and obstructive sleep apnea. The greatest risk appeared in patients taking diazepam or diazepam and baclofen in combination.

> *Clinical Pearls*
>
> *Headaches on awakening, as observed in sleep apnea patients, are also seen in patients with severe hypertension, depression, intracranial tumor, muscle-contraction headache, alcohol intoxication, and craniofacial sinus disease. In headache patients, causes for concern are first or worst-ever headache, associated neurologic symptoms or signs, progressive worsening of headache over days or weeks, intractable nausea or vomiting, fever, lethargy, confusion, and stiff neck.*
>
> *Following significant traumatic brain injury, the early appearance of sleep-wake cycling indicates a better prognosis. The association between multiple sclerosis and sleep disorders is more common than expected by chance. Sleep apnea in patients with Charcot-Marie-Tooth disease may be the consequence of pharyngeal neuropathy affecting the function of pharyngeal dilator muscles.*

REFERENCES

1. Culebras A: Headache Disorders and Sleep. In Culebras A (ed): Sleep Disorders and Neurological Disease, New York, Marcel-Dekker, 2000.
2. Lance JW, Lambert GA, Goadsby PJ, Duckworth JW: Brainstem influences on the cephalic circulation: Experimental data from cat and monkey of relevance to the mechanisms of migraine. Headache 1983;23:258-265.
3. Kayed K, Goadtlibsen OB, Sjaastad O: Chronic paroxysmal hemicrania. IV. "REM sleep locked" nocturnal headache attacks. Sleep 1978;1:91-95.
4. Paiva T, Farinha A, Martins A, et al: Chronic headaches and sleep disorders. Arch Intern Med 1997;157:1701-1705.
5. Dahmen N, Querings K, Grun B, Bierbrauer J: Increased frequency of migraine in narcoleptic patients. Neurology 1999;52:1291-1293.
6. Aaltonen K, Hamalainen ML, Hoppu K: Migraine attacks and sleep in children. Cephalalgia 2000;20:580-584.
7. Bruni O, Fabrizzi P, Ottaviano S: Prevalence of sleep disorders in childhood and adolescence with headache: A case-control study. Cephalalgia 1997;17:492-498.
8. Dexter JD: The relationship between disorders of arousal from sleep and migraine. Headache 1986;26:322.
9. Dalessio DJ: Diagnosing the severe headache. Neurology 1994;44:S6-S12.
10. Dexter JD: Headaches and sleep. Headache 1988;28:671-672.
11. Moskowitz MA, Buzzi MG, Linnik M, Sakas D: Pain mechanisms underlying vascular headaches: Progress report. Rev Neurol 1989;145:181-193.
12. Goadsby PJ, Edvinsson L, Ekman R: Vasoactive peptide release in the extracerebral circulation of humans during migraine headache. Ann Neurol 1990;28:183-187.
13. Sicuteri F, Testi A, Anselmi B: Biomedical investigations in headache: Increase in hydroxyindoleacetic acid excretion during migraine attacks. Int Arch Allergy 1961;19:55-58.
14. Pérez MF, Sánchez del Río M, Seabra ML, et al: Hypothalamic involvement in chronic migraine. J Neurol Neurosurg Psychiatry 2001a;71:747-751.
15. Bruni O, Galli F, Guidetti V: Sleep hygiene and migraine in children and adolescents. Cephalalgia 1999;19:57-59.
16. Kudrow L: Cluster headache: Mechanisms and management. New York, Oxford University Press, 1980.
17. Russell D: Cluster headache: Severity and temporal profile of attacks and patient activity prior to and during attacks. Cephalalgia 1981;1:209-219.
18. Evers S, Goadsby PJ: Hypnic headache. Clinical features, pathophysiology, and treatment. Neurology 2003;60:905-909.
19. Granella F, D'Andrea G: Hemicrania horologica ("clock-like hemicrania"). Neurology 2003;60:1722-1723.
20. Armstrong-Jones R: Snapping of the brain. Lancet 1920;ii:720.
21. Pearce JMS: Clinical features of the exploding head syndrome. J Neurol Neurosurg Psychiatry 1989;52:907-910.
22. Sachs C, Svanborg E: The exploding head syndrome: Polysomnographic recordings and therapeutic suggestions. Sleep 1991;14:263-266.
23. Aldrich MS, Chauncey JB: Are morning headaches part of obstructive sleep apnea syndrome? Arch Intern Med 1990;150:1265-1267.
24. Poceta JS, Dalessio DJ: Identification and treatment of sleep apnea in patients with chronic headache. Headache 1995;35:586-589.
25. Lavigne GJ, Montplaisir JY: Restless legs syndrome and sleep bruxism: Prevalence and association among Canadians. Sleep 1994;17:739.
26. Laberge L, Tremblay RE, Vitaro F, Montplaisir JY: Development of parasomnias from childhood to early adolescence. Pediatrics 2000;106:67.

27. Spierings EL, van Hoof MJ: Fatigue and sleep in chronic headache sufferers: An age- and sex-controlled questionnaire study. Headache 1997;37:549-552.

28. Pérez MF, Young WB, Kaup AO, et al: Fibromyalgia is common in patients with transformed migraine. Neurology 2001b; 57:1326-1328.

29. Paiva T, Batista A, Martins P, Martins A: The relationship between headaches and sleep disturbances. Headache 1995;35:590-596.

30. Baumel B: Migraine: A pharmacologic review with newer options and delivery modalities. Neurology 1994;44:S13-S17.

31. Holmgren K, Sheikholeslam A, Riise C: Effect of full arch maxillary occlusal splint on parafunctional activity during sleep in patients with nocturnal bruxism and signs and symptoms of craniomandibular disorders. J Prosthet Dent 1993;69:293-297.

32. Goldstein M: Traumatic brain injury. Ann Neurol 1990;27:237.

33. Sosin DM, Sniezek JE, Thurman DJ: Incidence of mild and moderate brain injury in the United States Brain Injury 1996;10:47-54.

34. Rae-Grant AD, Barbour PJ, Reed J: Development of a novel EEG rating scale for head injury using dichotomous variables. EEG Clin Neurophysiol 1991;79:349-357.

35. Ron S, Algom D, Hary D, Cohen M: Time-related changes in the distribution of sleep stages in brain-injured patients. Electroencephalogr Clin Neurophysiol 1980;48:432-441.

36. Levin HS, Mattis S, Ruff RM, et al: Neurobehavioral outcome following minor head injury: A three center study. J Neurosurg 1987;66:234-243.

37. Segalowitz SJ, Lawson S: Subtle symptoms associated with self-reported mild head injury. J Learning disabilities 1995;28: 309-319.

38. Short DJ, Stradling JR, Williams SJ: Prevalence of sleep apnea in patients over 40 years of age with spinal cord lesions. J Neurol Neurosurg Psychiatry 1992;55:1032-1036.

39. Cahan C, Gothe B, Decker MJ, et al: Arterial oxygen saturation over time and sleep studies in quadriplegic patients. Paraplegia 1993;31:172-179.

40. Bach JR, Wang TG: Pulmonary function and sleep disordered breathing in patients with traumatic tetraplegia: A longitudinal study. Arch Physical Med Rehabil 1994;75:279-284.

41. Guilleminault C: Post-traumatic hypersomnia. Course 3AS.007. 52nd Annual Meeting of the American Academy of Neurology, San Diego, Calif, 2000.

42. Good JL, Barry E, Fishman PS: Posttraumatic narcolepsy: The complete syndrome with tissue typing. J Neurosurg 1989;71: 765-767.

43. Maccario M, Ruggles KM, Meriewether MW: Post-traumatic narcolepsy. Military Med 1987;152:370-371.

44. Ripley B, Overeem S, Fujiki N, et al: CSF hypocretin/orexin levels in narcolepsy and other neurologic conditions. Neurology 2001;57:2253-2258.

45. Dempsey OJ, McGeoch P, de Silva RN, et al: Acquired narcolepsy in an acromegalic patient who underwent pituitary irradiation. Neurology 2003;61:537-540.

46. Mignot E, Chen W, Black J: On the value of measuring CSF hypocretin-1 in diagnosing narcolepsy. Sleep 2003;26:646-649.

47. Gill RG, Young JPR, Thomas DJ: Kleine-Levin syndrome: Report of two cases with onset of symptoms precipitated by head trauma. Br J Psychiatry 1988;152:410-412.

48. Billiard M, Negri C, Baldy-Moulinier M, et al: Organisations du sommeil chez les sujets attaint d'inconscience post-traumatique chronique. Rev EEG Neurophysiol 1979;9:149-152.

49. Alster J, Pratt H, Feinsod M: Density spectral array, evoked potentials, and temperature rhythms in the evaluation and prognosis of the comatose patient. Brain Injury 1993;7:191-208.

50. Humphrey ME, Zangwill OL: Cessation of dreaming after brain injury. J Neurol Neurosurg Psychiatry 1951;14:322-325.

51. Prigatano GP, Orr WC, Zeiner HK: Sleep and dreaming disturbances in closed head injury patients. J Neurol Neurosurg Psychiatry 1982;45:78-80.

52. Mahowald MW, Woods SR, Schenck CH: Sleeping dreams, waking hallucinations, and the central nervous system. Dreaming 1998;8:89-102.

53. Jacobsohn E: Fall von Narcolepsie. Klin Wochenschr 1926;2:2188.

54. Guillain G, Alajouanine T: La somnolence dans la sclérose en plaques. Les episodes aigus ou subaigus de la sclérose en plaques pouvant simuler l'encéphalite léthargique. Ann Med 1928;24:111-118.

55. Grigioresco D: Contribution a l'étude des troubles du sommeil aux lésions des noyeaux gris centraux dans la sclérose en plaques. Rev Neurol II 1932;27-45.

56. Berg O, Hanley J: Narcolepsy in two cases of multiple sclerosis. Acta Neurol Scand 1963;39:252-257.

57. Ekbom K: Familial multiple sclerosis associated with narcolepsy. Arch Neurol 1966;15:337-344.

58. Leo GJ, Rao M, Bernardin L: Sleep disturbances in multiple sclerosis. Neurology 1991;41:320.

59. Clark CM, Fleming JA, Li D, et al: Sleep disturbance, depression, and lesion site in patients with multiple sclerosis. Arch Neurol 1992;49:641-643.

60. Hillert J, Olerup O: Multiple sclerosis is associated with genes within or close to the HLA-DR-DQ subregion on a normal DR15, DQ6, Dw2 haplotype. Neurology 1993;43:163-168.

61. Younger DS, Pedley TA, Thorpy MJ: Multiple sclerosis and narcolepsy: Possible similar genetic susceptibility. Neurology 1991;41:447-448.

62. Fogdell A, Hillert J, Sachs C, Olerup O: The multiple sclerosis and narcolepsy-associated HLA class II haplotype includes the DRB5*0101 allele. Tissue Antigens 1995;46:333-336.

63. Iseki K, Mezaki T, Oka Y, et al: Hypersomnia in MS. Neurology 2002;59:2006-2007.

64. Saunders J, Whitham R, Schaumann B: Sleep disturbance, fatigue, and depression in multiple sclerosis. Neurology 1991;41:320.

65. Tachibana N, Howard RS, Hirsch NP, et al: Sleep problems in multiple sclerosis. Eur Neurol 1994;34:320-323.

66. Ferini-Strambi L, Filippi M, Martinelli V, et al: Nocturnal sleep study in multiple sclerosis: Correlations with clinical and brain magnetic resonance imaging findings. J Neurol Sci 1994; 125(2):194-197.

67. Zifko UA: Management of fatigue in patients with multiple sclerosis. Drugs 2004;64:1295-1304.

68. Krupp LB, Coyle PK, Doscher C, et al: Fatigue therapy in multiple sclerosis: Results of a double-blind, randomized, parallel trial of amantadine, pemoline, and placebo. Neurology 1995; 45:1956-1961.

69. Rammohan KW, Rosenberg JH, Lynn DJ, et al: Efficacy and safety of modafinil for the treatment of fatigue in multiple sclerosis: A two centre phase study. J Neurol Neurosurg Psychiatry 2002;72:179-183.

70. Schluter B, Aguigah G, Andler W: Hypersomnia in multiple sclerosis. Klin Padiatr 1996;208:103-105.

71. Wang CY, Kawashima H, Takami T, et al: A case of multiple sclerosis with initial symptoms of narcolepsy. Brain Dev 1998; 30:300-306.

72. Sandyk R: Resolution of sleep paralysis by weak electromagnetic fields in a patient with multiple sclerosis. Int J Neurosci 1997;90:145-157.

73. Sandyk R: Weak electromagnetic fields restore dream recall in patients with multiple sclerosis. Int J Neurosci 1995;82: 113-125.

74. Sandyk R: Suicidal behavior is attenuated in patients with multiple sclerosis by treatment with electromagnetic fields. Int J Neurosci 1996a;87:5-15.

75. Sandyk R: Resolution of partial cataplexy in multiple sclerosis by treatment with weak electromagnetic fields. Int J Neurosci 1996b;84:157-164.

76. Syed BH, Rye DB, Singh G: REM sleep behavior disorder and SCA-3 (Machado-Joseph disease). Neurology 2003;60:148.

77. Gilman S, Koeppe RD, Chervin FB, et al: REM sleep behavior disorder is related to striatal monoaminergic deficit in MSA. Neurology 2003;61:29-34.

78. Culebras A: Sleep Disorders and neuromuscular disorders. In: Culebras A (ed): Sleep Disorders and Neurological Disease. New York, Marcel-Dekker, 2000.

79. Dematteis M, Pépin JL, Jeanmart M, et al: Charcot-Marie-Tooth disease and sleep apnoea syndrome: A family study. Lancet 2001;357:267-272.

80. Vankova J, Stepanova I, Jech R, et al: Sleep disturbances and hypocretin deficiency in Niemann-Pick disease type C. Sleep 2003;26:427-430.

81. Schwartz BA, Escande C: Sleeping sickness: Sleep study of a case. Electroencephalogr Clin Neurophysiol 1970;29:83.

81a. Buguet A, Bisser S, Josenando T, et al: Sleep structure: A new diagnostic tool for stage determination in sleeping sickness. Acta Trop 2005;93:107-117.

82. Whittle HC, Greenwood BM, Bidwell DE, et al: IgM and antibody measurements in the diagnosis and management of Gambian trypanosomiasis. Am J Trop Med Hyg 1977;26:1129-1134.

83. Kristensson K, Bentivoglio M: Pathology of trypanosomiasis. In Dumas M, Bouteille B, Bughet A (eds): Progress in Human African Trypanosomiasis, Sleeping Sickness. Paris, Springer, 1999, pp 157-181

84. Kanbayashi T, Goto A, Hishikawa Y, et al: Hypersomnia due to acute disseminated encephalomyelitis in a 5-year old girl. Sleep Medicine 2001;2:347-350.

85. Dyken ME, Yamada T, Berger HA: Transient obstructive sleep apnea and asystole in association with presumed viral encephalopathy. Neurology 2003;60:1692-1694.

86. Culebras A: Psychiatric, medical and neurologic disorders. In Culebras A (ed): Clinical Handbook of Sleep Disorders, Boston, Butterworth-Heinemann, 1996.

87. Aldrich MS, Naylor MW: Narcolepsy associated with lesions of the diencephalons. Neurology 1989;39:1505-1508.

88. Arii J, Kanbayashi T, Tanabe Y, et al: A hypersomnolent girl with decreased CSF hypocretin level after removal of a hypothalamic tumor. Neurology 2001;56:1775-1776.

89. Nogués M, Gene R, Benarroch E, et al: Respiratory disturbances during sleep in syringomyelia and syringobulbia. Neurology 1999;52:1777-1783.

90. Sajkov D, Marshall R, Walker P, et al: Sleep apnea related hypoxia is associated with cognitive disturbances in patients with tetraplegia. Spinal Cord 1998;36:231-239.

91. Culebras A. Sleep and neuromuscular disorders. Neurol Clin 1996;14:791-805.

92. Guilleminault C, Li KK, Philip P, et al: Anterior cervical spine fusion and sleep disordered breathing. Neurology 2003;61:97-99.

93. Brown LK, Heffner JE, Obbens EA: Transverse myelitis associated with restless legs syndrome and periodic movements of sleep responsive to an oral dopaminergic agent but not to intrathecal baclofen. Sleep 2000;23:591-594.

94. Nogués M, Cammarota A, Leiguarda R, et al: Periodic limb movements in syringomyelia and syringobulbia. Move Disord 2000;15:113-119.

95. Ayas NT, Epstein LJ, Lieberman SL, et al: Predictors of loud snoring in persons with spinal cord injury. J Spinal Cord Med 2001;24:30-34.

NREM Sleep–Arousal Parasomnias

Mark W. Mahowald
Michel A. Cramer Bornemann

ABSTRACT

Parasomnias are defined as unpleasant or undesirable behavioral or experiential phenomena that occur predominantly or exclusively during the sleep period. These were initially thought to represent a unitary phenomenon and were often attributed to psychiatric disease. As more parasomnias are being carefully studied both polygraphically and clinically, it is becoming apparent that parasomnias are not a unitary phenomenon but rather are due to a large number of completely different conditions, most of which are diagnosable and treatable. Moreover, most, in fact, are not manifestations of psychiatric disorders and are far more prevalent than previously suspected.

The parasomnias may be conveniently categorized as "primary parasomnias" (disorders of the sleep states per se) and "secondary parasomnias" (organ-system disorders that appear during sleep). The primary sleep parasomnias can be classified according to the sleep state of origin: rapid eye movement (REM) sleep, non–rapid eye movement (NREM) sleep, or miscellaneous (i.e., those not respecting sleep state). The secondary sleep parasomnias can be further classified by the organ system involved (see Table 76–2).

The focus of this chapter is on the NREM sleep–arousal parasomnias, which occur on a broad spectrum and include confusional arousals, sleepwalking, and sleep terrors. The underlying pathophysiology is state dissociation—the brain is partially awake and partially in NREM sleep. The result of this mixed state of being is that the brain is awake enough to perform very complex and often protracted motor or verbal actions, but it is asleep enough not to have conscious awareness of or responsibility for these actions.

There is compelling evidence that extensive reorganization of the central nervous system activity occurs as the brain cycles through the three primary states of being: wakefulness, non–rapid eye movement (NREM) sleep, and rapid eye movement (REM) sleep.[1] The concept that certain parts of the nervous system are active in one state but not in the other two is erroneous. Almost all portions of the nervous system are active across all three states of being, but they are active in a different mode. The *reticular response reversal* phenomenon, in which excitation of the same anatomic site may have opposite effects on motor activity, depending upon the state (wakefulness or REM) during stimulation, is testimony to that fact.[2,3]

Injection of cholinergic drugs into the pontine reticular formation of cats may have dramatically different effects depending upon the state of the animal at the time of injection. If the injection is administered during NREM sleep, then a state identical to naturally occurring REM sleep is induced. However, if the injection is administered during waking, a waking-dissociated state occurs that is characterized by electroencephalographic (EEG) desynchronization and muscle atonia in a cat that appeared to be awake and able to track objects in its visual field.[4] Such a waking-dissociated state is likely the basis for many human parasomnias—both REM and NREM parasomnias.

Parasomnias are clinical phenomena that appear as brain activity becomes reorganized across states; therefore, they are particularly apt to occur during the transition periods from one state to another. In view of the large number of neural networks, neurotransmitters, and other state-determining substances that must be recruited synchronously for full state declaration and considering the frequent transitions among states during the sleep-wake cycle, it is surprising that errors in state declaration do not occur more frequently than they do.[5-7]

The concept that sleep and wakefulness are not invariably mutually exclusive states, and that the various state-determining variables of wakefulness, NREM sleep, and REM sleep may occur simultaneously or oscillate rapidly, is key to understanding the primary sleep parasomnias. The admixture of wakefulness and NREM sleep would explain confusional arousals (sleep-drunkenness), automatic behavior, or microsleeps.[8-11] The tonic and phasic components of REM sleep may become dissociated, intruding or persisting into wakefulness. This dissociation could explain cataplexy, wakeful dreaming, lucid dreaming, and the persistence of motor activity during REM sleep (REM sleep behavior disorder [RBD]).[12]

EPIDEMIOLOGY AND RISK FACTORS

The disorders of arousal are the most impressive and most frequent of the NREM sleep parasomnias. These share common features: They tend to arise from slow wave sleep (stages 3 and 4 of NREM sleep); therefore they usually occur in the first third of the sleep cycle (and rarely during naps). In addition, they are common in childhood, and they usually decrease in frequency with increasing age.[13,14] There is often a family history of disorders of arousal; however, this association has recently been questioned.[15-22] A specific HLA gene (*DQB1*) appears to confer susceptibility to sleepwalking.[23] Importantly, although they most frequently occur during stages 3 and 4 of NREM sleep, disorders of arousal may occur during any stage of NREM sleep, and they may occur late in the sleep period.[24]

Disorders of arousal may be triggered by febrile illness, alcohol, prior sleep deprivation, physical activity, or emotional stress.[25,26] Medication-induced cases have been reported with sedative-hypnotics, neuroleptics, minor tranquilizers, stimulants, and antihistamines, often in combination.[26-29] In some women, disorders of arousal can be exacerbated by pregnancy or menstruation, and in others, disorders of arousal may be alleviated by pregnancy, suggesting hormonal factors.[30-32] Such precipitants should be thought of as triggering events in susceptible individuals, and not as causes.

Numerous other sleep disorders that result in arousals (obstructive sleep apnea,[33] nocturnal seizures, or periodic limb movements) may provoke these disorders. Sleep-disordered breathing is more prevalent in both children and adults with disorders of arousal. One recent study found that sleep fragmentation induced by sleep-disordered breathing is more common in adults with disorders of arousal than in normal subjects.[34,35] The combination of frequent arousals and sleep deprivation seen in these other sleep disorders provide fertile ground for the appearance of disorders of arousal. These cases represent a sleep disorder within a sleep disorder—the clinical event is a disorder of arousal, but the true culprit is a different, unrelated sleep disorder. This would explain the common clinical experience of improvement of disorders of arousal following identification and treatment of obstructive sleep apnea. Conversely, effective treatment of obstructive sleep apnea with nasal continuous positive airway pressure (CPAP) may acutely result in disorders of arousal, which are presumably associated with deep NREM sleep rebound.[36,37]

Persistence of these disorders of arousal beyond childhood or their development in adulthood is often taken as an indication of significant psychopathology.[38,39] Numerous studies have dispelled this myth, indicating that significant psychopathology is usually not present in adults with disorders of arousal.[40-42] One study in children found an association between disorders of arousal and anxiety.[43] These arousals may not be the culmination of ongoing psychologically significant sleep mentation, in that somnambulism can be induced in normal children by standing them up during slow wave sleep[44,45] and sleep terrors can be triggered in susceptible individuals by sounding a buzzer during slow wave sleep.[13,46]

The mechanism of these disorders is not understood, but clearly both genetic[15] and environmental factors contribute. It has been suggested that sleep terrors may be the manifestation of anomalous REM sleep mixed with NREM sleep.[47]

PATHOGENESIS

In addition to the phenomenon of state dissociation, in which two states of being overlap or occur simultaneously, there are likely additional underlying physiologic phenomena that contribute to the appearance of complex motor behavior during sleep. These include locomotor centers, sleep inertia, and sleep state instability.

Locomotor Centers

Locomotor centers are present in multiple sites in the central nervous system and may play a role in the disorders of arousal, which represent motor activity that is dissociated from waking consciousness.[48-51] These areas project to the central pattern generator of the spinal cord, which itself is able to produce complex stepping movements in the absence of supraspinal influence.[52] This accounts for the fact that decorticate experimental and headless barnyard animals can perform very complex, integrated motor acts.[53] A biological substrate is further supported by the similarity between spontaneously occurring sleep terrors in humans and "sham rage" induced in animals.[54-56]

Indeed, human neuropathology may cause similar behavior.[57-61] Dissociation of the locomotor centers from the parent state of NREM sleep would explain the complex motor behavior seen in disorders of arousal. Spontaneous locomotion following decerebration in cats clearly indicates that such centers, if dysfunctional, release motor activity into the sleeping state.[62,63] Single proton emission computed tomography (SPECT) study of a sleepwalker suggested activation of thalamocingulate pathways and persisting deactivation of other thalamocortical arousal systems, resulting in a dissociation between body sleep and mind sleep.[64]

Sleep Inertia

Sleep inertia (also termed *sleep drunkenness*) refers to a period of impaired performance and reduced vigilance following awakening from the regular sleep episode or from a nap. This impairment may be severe, last from minutes to hours, and be accompanied by polygraphically recorded microsleep episodes.[65-68] Support of a gradual disengagement from sleep to wakefulness comes from neurophysiologic studies in animals[69] and cerebral blood-flow studies in humans.[70-72] The persistent reduction, lasting minutes, of the photomyoclonic response upon awakening from NREM sleep is further confirmation of a less-than-immediate transition from sleep to wakefulness.[73] There appears to be great variability among patients in the extent and duration of sleep inertia—both following spontaneous awakening after the major sleep period and following naps. Sleep inertia likely plays a role in the susceptibility to disorders of arousal.[69]

Sleep State Instability

The cyclic alternating pattern (CAP) may also play a role in the disorders of arousal. CAP is a physiologic component of NREM sleep and is functionally correlated with long-lasting arousal oscillations. CAP is a measure of NREM instability with a high level of arousal oscillation.[74] More sophisticated monitoring techniques, such as topographical EEG mapping, suggest that there may be more delta EEG activity prior to the onset of sleep terrors.[75] There is no difference in macrostructural sleep parameters between patients with disorders of arousal and control subjects. However, patients with disorders of arousal have increases in CAP rate, in number of CAP cycles, and in arousals with EEG synchronization.

An increase in sleep instability and in arousal oscillation is a typical microstructural feature of slow wave sleep–related parasomnias and may play a role in triggering abnormal motor episodes during sleep in these patients.[76,77] Microarousals preceded by EEG slow wave synchronization during NREM sleep are more frequent in patients with sleepwalking and sleep terrors than in control subjects. This supports the diagnosis of an arousal disorder in these patients.[76] Some researchers have reported hypersynchronous delta activity on polysomnograms of young adults with sleepwalking,[78] but other researchers have not found this.[79] EEG spectral analysis studies indicate that patients with sleepwalking demonstrate an instability of slow wave sleep, particularly in the early portion of the sleep period.[80-82]

CLINICAL FEATURES

Disorders of arousal occur on a broad continuum ranging from confusional arousals, through somnambulism (sleep walking), to sleep terrors (also termed *pavor nocturnus* and, erroneously, *incubus* or *succubus*). Some take the form of "specialized" behavior (discussed later) such as sleep-related eating and sleep-related sexual activity—without conscious awareness.[83,84]

Confusional Arousals

These are often seen in children and are characterized by movements in bed, occasional thrashing about, or inconsolable crying.[85] "Sleep drunkenness" is probably a variation on this theme.[26] The prevalence of confusional arousals in adults is approximately 4%.[86]

Sleepwalking

Sleepwalking is prevalent in childhood (1% to 17%), peaking at 11 to 12 years of age. It is far more common in adults (nearly 4%) than generally acknowledged.[20,86-88] Sleepwalking may be either calm or agitated, with varying degrees of complexity and duration.

Sleep Terrors

The sleep terror is the most dramatic disorder of arousal. It is frequently initiated by a loud, blood-curdling scream associated with extreme panic, followed by prominent motor activity such as hitting the wall or running around or out of the bedroom—even out of the house—resulting in bodily injury or property damage.

A universal feature is inconsolability. Although the victim appears to be awake, he or she usually misperceives the environment, and attempts at consolation are fruitless and may serve only to prolong or even intensify the confusional state. Some degree of perception may be evident—for example, running for and opening a door or window. Complete amnesia for the activity is typical, but amnesia may be incomplete.[13,14,89]

The intense endogenous arousal and exogenous unarousability constitute a curious paradox. As with sleepwalking, sleep terrors are much more prevalent in adults than generally acknowledged (4% to 5%).[90] Although the episodes are usually benign, the behavior may be violent, resulting in considerable injury to the victim or others or damage to the environment, occasionally with forensic implications.[91,92]

Specialized Forms of Disorders of Arousal

Sleep-Related Eating Disorder

The sleep-related eating disorder likely represents a specialized form of disorder of arousal. It is characterized by frequent episodes of nocturnal eating, generally without full conscious awareness, and is usually not associated with waking eating disorders. This condition often responds to treatment with a combination of dopaminergic and opiate agents. Dexfenfluramine, which is no longer available, was also reported to be effective.[93]

Formal sleep studies are indicated, as sleep-related eating may be the manifestation of other sleep disorders such as restless leg syndrome, periodic limb movements of sleep, or obstructive sleep apnea, all of which predispose to arousal.[83,94-97] Nocturnal binging may be induced by benzodiazepine medication,[98] and sleep-related eating has been associated with zolpidem administration.[99] The sleep-related eating disorder is distinct from the *night-eating syndrome*, which is characterized by morning anorexia, evening hyperphagia (while awake), and insomnia and is associated with hypothalamic-pituitary axis abnormalities.[100-102]

Sleep-Sex

Several researchers have reported inappropriate sexual activities occurring during the sleep state without conscious awareness, presumably the result of a mixture of wakefulness and sleep.[84,103-109] Such activities may result in feelings of guilt or shame or in depression, and they may have medical and legal implications.[110]

CASE EXAMPLE

An 18-year-old white youth who resides in a rural Midwestern farming community is academically doing well as a senior in high school. The patient reluctantly presented to the Sleep Center upon the insistence of his mother, who has had increasing concerns over her only child's safety, particularly at night. According to his parents, since childhood their son has had nocturnal episodes arising within a few hours after sleep onset. Believing that these would resolve as their son grew out of adolescence and into adulthood, the parents were at first not overly concerned and were able to maintain their son's safety by remaining vigilant and subtly intervening when necessary. The patient's nocturnal activities have maintained their almost nightly regularity, but they have developed into occasionally more complex, sustained, and violent actions. The patient has grown to 77 inches tall and a weight of 235 pounds, so it is not surprising that parental interventions to quell their son's suddenly unmanageable nocturnal activities have become problematic for both parties.

The patient states that he has always been completely unaware of these episodes and has no recollection of the events the following morning. The parents are further concerned for their son's safety because he intends to enroll in a college away from home and is looking forward to living in either a dormitory or a high-rise apartment. Without the vigilance of responsible persons in college, the parents fear the worst for their son. Of course the patient, wanting to exert his independence and lacking proper insight into the gravity of his

CASE EXAMPLE—Cont'd

situation, clearly had become antagonistic over his parents' concerns.

The patient's continued lack of awareness in these matters coupled with his sincere denial of any difficulties with either sleep initiation or maintenance made the direct involvement of the patient's parents crucial in attaining a comprehensive history as well as a thorough clinical characterization of the patient's behavior in sleep. According to his mother, since childhood the patient has had "sleep disturbances" almost every night. Typically, these episodes occur within the first two hours after he has gone to bed, and only rarely do they occur in the latter third of the night. The episodes are characterized by somniloquy, somnambulism, and a general "thrashing around in his bed," leaving his bedding in complete disarray. Less frequently, the patient would abruptly wake up the household with fits of "screaming and yelling at the top of his lungs." Despite his parent's efforts at reassurance and solace, the patient remained unreceptive and inconsolable. Just as these "night terrors," as the mother called them, came on suddenly, so too would they would spontaneously abate.

Although the patient's nocturnal activities were unremitting in frequency over recent years, his parents began to discern a trend toward more worrisome physical behavior. These particularly "severe" episodes were punctuated by violent outbursts of punching, hitting, and kicking inflicted upon a foe in the room but unseen to his parents. Never at any time were these combative actions directed toward his parents. Many times over recent years the patient was caught attempting to get out through the front door although he was visibly asleep. On one occasion the mother caught her son just as he was attempting to leave through an upstairs window, having "already completely kicked out the storm window." In the last two years, it has not been uncommon for the patient to sustain bruises and superficial cuts to his extremities as a result of these nocturnal activities. Lastly, the parents note that these "severe" episodes increase in frequency when the patient is staying away from home, such as in a hotel or at summer camp.

Aside from a mild form of delayed sleep-phase syndrome and consequent volitional sleep deprivation supported by three weeks of sleep diaries, the patient has otherwise been absolutely healthy and has not suffered from any medical, neurological, or mental conditions. The patient does not drink alcohol nor does he partake of illicit drugs. The patient does not take any prescription medications, including selective serotonin reuptake inhibitors. The patient does not have a history suggesting sleep-disordered breathing or any other primary sleep disorder. Family history is devoid of any nocturnal behavior suggestive of parasomnias.

Formal nocturnal polysomnography was undertaken using a full seizure montage. The baseline polysomnogram did not reveal any sleep-disordered breathing, nocturnal myoclonus, or periodic limb movements. Sleep architecture was within normal limits and the patient attained a sleep efficiency of 96%. REM stage was attained and observed to have normal atonia. A full seizure montage showed no electrical or clinical seizure activity. Four discrete episodes of spontaneous NREM-related confusional arousals were observed and were associated with complex motor activity (Fig. 74–1) and overt vocalizations. These confusional arousals were not associated with consequent EEG slowing.

As suspected by the clinical history and further supported by the findings on the polysomnogram, the patient's problem was diagnosed as an NREM parasomnia. The patient developed a better understanding of his problem after we replayed his findings on the video monitor. Management strategies included

- *employing proper sleep hygiene and minimizing volitional sleep deprivation;*
- *continuing to refrain from or minimizing alcohol use;*
- *ensuring a supportive environment with appropriate responsible vigilance provided by a team of family and friends;*
- *ensuring safety by, among other measures, attaining housing on the ground level or basement of his chosen residence;*
- *taking a long-acting sedative hypnotic of the benzodiazepine class every night.*

DIAGNOSIS

Isolated, often bizarre, sleep-related activities may be experienced by perfectly healthy people, and most do not warrant further extensive or expensive evaluation. The initial approach to the complaint of unusual sleep-related behavior is to determine whether further evaluation is necessary. The patient should be queried about the exact nature of the events. Because many of these episodes may be associated with partial or complete amnesia, additional descriptive information from a bed partner or other observer may prove invaluable. Home videotapes of the clinical event may be quite helpful. In general, indications for formal evaluation of parasomnias include actions that[1]:

- are potentially violent or injurious
- are extremely disruptive to other household members
- result in the complaint of excessive daytime sleepiness
- are associated with medical, psychiatric, or neurological symptoms or findings

Serious attention should be paid to parasomnia complaints under these circumstances. Formal polysomnographic studies, appropriately performed, provide direct or indirect diagnostic information in the majority of cases. This information is of more than academic interest, as most of these conditions are readily treatable. Emphasis must be placed on the types of studies required; routine polysomnograms performed for unconventional sleep disorders are inadequate. In addition to the physiologic parameters monitored in the standard polysomnogram, there must be an expanded EEG montage and continuous audiovisual monitoring.[78,111] Experienced technologist observation is invaluable. Multiple-night studies may be required to capture an event. Interpretation should be made by a polysomnographer experienced in these disorders. Sleep deprivation prior to formal polysomnographic study may increase the likelihood of capturing an event in the sleep laboratory.[112] Unattended studies have no role in the evaluation of parasomnias.[113]

Differential Diagnosis

Numerous other conditions may perfectly mimic the disorders of arousal. These include obstructive sleep apnea, REM sleep behavior disorder, nocturnal seizures, psychogenic dissociative disorders, or malingering.[114,115] NREM parasomnias may be particularly difficult to differentiate from nocturnal frontal

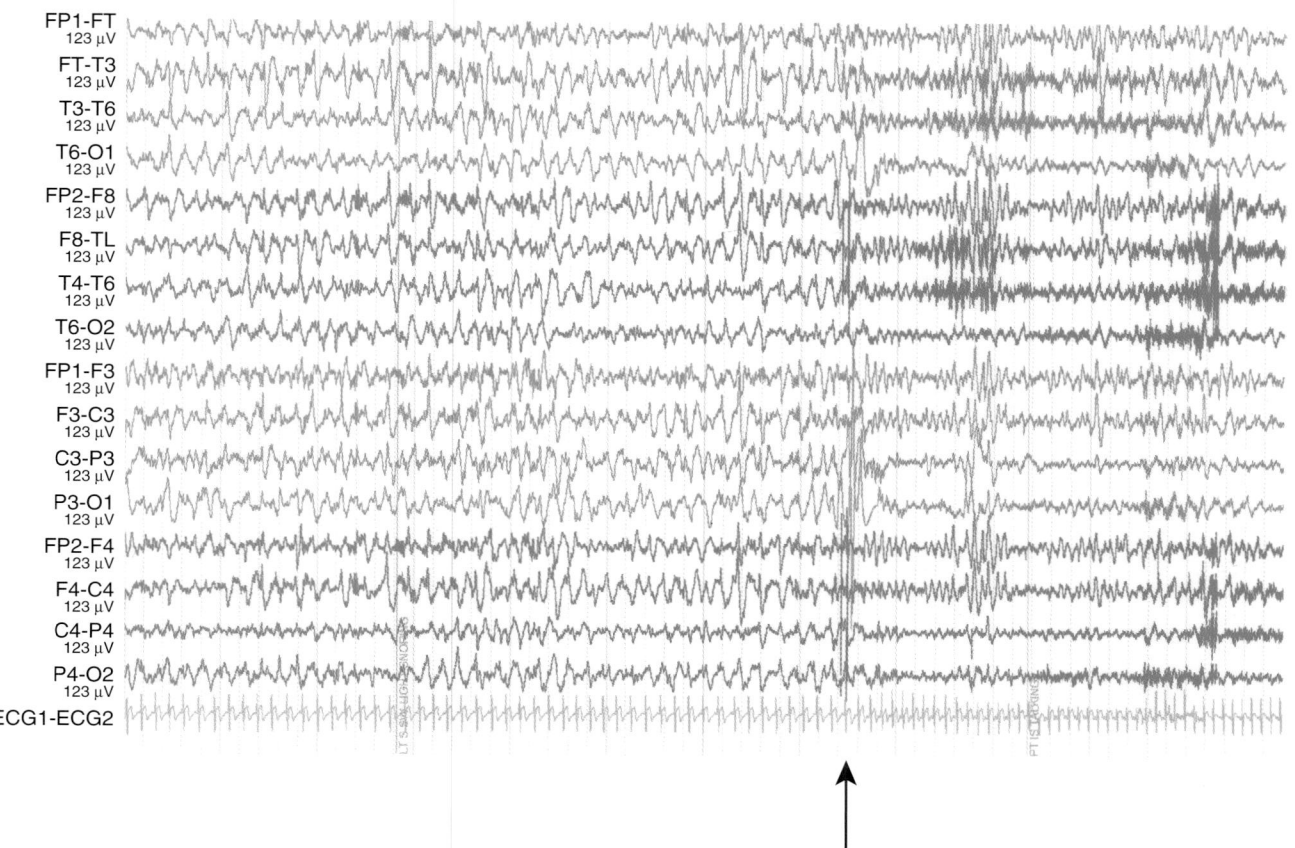

Figure 74–1. Polysomnographic example of disorder of arousal. This is a 1-minute epoch of a full seizure montage of the case presented. Note the precipitous arousal from slow wave sleep *(arrow)* without anticipatory tachycardia. Following the arousal, although the patient is talking and appears to be awake, the EEG shows persistent slowing.

lobe epilepsy.[116] There may be an association with disorders of arousal in children who have migraine headache[117] or Tourette's syndrome.[118,119] In preverbal children, nocturnal cluster headaches may mimic sleep terrors.[120] Obstructive sleep apnea may also manifest as disorders of arousal.[34]

TREATMENT

Given the high prevalence of these disorders in healthy people, formal sleep center evaluation should be confined to those cases in which the activities are potentially injurious or violent, are extremely bothersome to other household members, result in symptoms of excessive daytime sleepiness, or have unusual clinical characteristics. Treatment is often not necessary. Reassurance that they are typically benign, lack psychological significance, and tend to diminish over time is often sufficient. The tricyclic antidepressants and benzodiazepines may be effective, and should be administered if the actions are dangerous to person or property or extremely disruptive to family members.[26]

Paroxetine and trazodone have been reported effective in isolated cases of disorders of arousal.[121,122] Nonpharmacologic treatment such as psychotherapy,[46] progressive relaxation,[123] or hypnosis[124-126] is recommended for long-term management.

Anticipatory awakening has been reported to be effective in treating sleepwalking in children.[127] Avoidance of precipitants such as drugs, alcohol, and sleep deprivation is also important. Administration of dopaminergic agents, opiates, or topiramide has been reportedly effective in the sleep-related eating disorder.[128-130]

CLINICAL COURSE AND PREVENTION

The natural tendency of the disorders of arousal is to diminish with increasing age. However, this pattern is hardly universal, and these conditions may persist into or even begin in adulthood. Identifiable risk factors in a given person, such as sleep deprivation or consumption of alcohol or medication, should be avoided.

PITFALLS AND CONTROVERSIES

The disorders of arousal are extremely prevalent in the normal population, so the decision to treat with pharmacologic or behavioral therapy may be difficult. Certainly if there is a history of potentially violent or injurious behavior, treatment is warranted. Our center has seen patients with a history of very benign and infrequent sleepwalking episodes in childhood present with severely injurious sleep-related episodes as adults.[92]

> *Clinical Pearl*
>
> *Disorders of arousal are very common in both children and adults, and they are not related to significant underlying psychiatric or psychological problems. The behavior may be very complex and protracted. Evaluation and treatment is advised for those individuals whose sleep-related activities are potentially violent or are very disturbing to other family members. Because other parasomnias, particularly the REM sleep behavior disorder and nocturnal seizures, may perfectly mimic disorders of arousal, extensive polysomnographic evaluation by clinicians experienced in these disorders is recommended.*

REFERENCES

1. Mahowald MW, Ettinger MG: Things that go bump in the night—the parasomnias revisited. J Clin Neurophysiol 1990; 7:119-143.
2. Chase MH, Wills N: Brain stem control of maseteric reflex activity during sleep and wakefulness. Exp Neurol 1979;64:118-131.
3. Chase MH: The motor functions of the reticular formation are multifaceted and state-determined. In Hobson JA, Brazier MAB (eds): The Reticular Formation Revisited. New York, Raven Press, 1980, pp 449-472.
4. Lopez-Rodriguez F, Kohlmeier K, Morales FR, Chase MH: State dependency of the effects of microinjection of cholinergic drugs into the nucleus pontalis oralis. Brain Res 1994;649:271-281.
5. Mahowald MW, Schenck CH: Status dissociatus—a perspective on states of being. Sleep 1991;14:69-79.
6. Mahowald MW, Schenck CH: Dissociated states of wakefulness and sleep. Neurology 1992;42:44-52.
7. Mahowald MW, Schenck CH: Evolving concepts of human state dissociation. Arch Ital Biol 2001;139:269-300.
8. Niedermeyer E, Singer HS, Folstein SE, et al: Hypersomnia with simultaneous waking and sleep patterns in the electroencephalogram. J Neurol 1979;221:1-13.
9. Roth B, Nevsimalova S, Rechtschaffen A: Hypersomnia with "sleep drunkenness." Arch Gen Psychiatry 1972;26:456-462.
10. Zorick. FJ, Salis PJ, Roth T, Kramer M: Narcolepsy and automatic behavior: A case report. J Clin Psychiatry 1979;40:194-197.
11. Roth B, Nevsimalova S, Sagova V, et al: Neurological, psychological and polygraphic findings in sleep drunkenness. Schweiz Arch Neurol Neurochir Psychiatr 1981;129:209-222.
12. Mahowald MW, Schenck CH: REM sleep behavior disorder. In Kryger MH, Dement W, Roth T (eds): Principles and Practice of Sleep Medicine, 2nd ed. Philadelphia, Saunders, 1994, pp 574-588.
13. Fisher C, Kahn E, Edwards A, Davis DM: A psychophysiological study of nightmares and night terrors. I. Physiological aspects of the stage 4 night terror. J Nerv Ment Dis 1973;157:75-98.
14. Fisher C, Kahn E, Edwards A, et al: A psychophysiological study of nightmares and night terrors. III. Mental content and recall of stage 4 night terrors. J Nerv Ment Dis 1974;158:174-188.
15. Hori A, Hirose G: Twin studies on parasomnias. Sleep Res 1995; 24A:324.
16. Kales A, Soldatos C, Bixler EO, et al: Hereditary factors in sleepwalking and night terrors. Br J Psychiatry 1980;137:111-118.
17. Abe K, Amatomi M, Oda N: Sleepwalking and recurrent sleeptalking in children of childhood sleepwalkers. Am J Psychiatry 1984;141:800-801.
18. Hallstrom T: Night terrors in adults through three generations. Acta Psychiatry Scand 1972;48:350-352.
19. Bakwin H: Sleep-walking in twins. Lancet 1970;2:446-447.
20. Hublin C, Kaprio J, Partinen M, et al: Prevalence and genetics of sleepwalking: A population-based twin study. Neurology 1997;48:177-181.
21. Hublin C, Kaprio J, Partinen M, Koskenvu M: Parasomnias: Co-occurrence and genetics. Psychiatric Genetics 2001;11:65-70.
22. Hublin C, Kaprio J: Genetic aspects and genetic epidemiology of parasomnias. Sleep Med Rev 2003;7:413-421.
23. Lecendreux M, Bassetti C, Dauvilliers Y, et al: HLA and genetic susceptibility to sleepwalking. Mol Psychiatry 2003;8:114-117.
24. Naylor MW, Aldrich MS: The distribution of confusional arousals across sleep stages and time of night in children and adolescents with sleep terrors. Sleep Res 1991;20:308.
25. Vela Bueno A, Dobladez Blanco B, Vaquero Cajal E: Episodic sleep disorder triggered by fever—a case presentation. Waking Sleeping 1980;4:243-251.
26. Nino-Murcia G, Dement WC: Psychophysiological and pharmacological aspects of somnambulism and night terrors in children. In Meltzer HY (ed): Psychopharmacology: The Third Generation of Progress. New York, Raven Press, 1987, pp 873-879.
27. Warnes H, Osivka S, Montplaisir J: Somnambulistic like behavior induced by lithium-neuroleptic treatment. Sleep Res 1993; 22:287.
28. Mendelson WB: Sleepwalking associated with zolpidem. J Clin Psychopharmacol 1994;14:150.
29. Harazin J, Berigan TR: Zolpidem tartrate and somnambulism. Mil Med 1999;164:669-670.
30. Schenck CH, Mahowald MW: Two cases of premenstrual sleep terrors and injurious sleep-walking. J Psychosom Obstet Gynecol 1995;16:79-84.
31. Snyder S; Unusual case of sleep terror in a pregnant patient. Am J Psychiatry 1986;143:391.
32. Berlin RM; Sleepwalking disorder during pregnancy: A case report. Sleep 1988;11:298-300.
33. Guilleminault C, Silvestri R: Disorders of arousal and epilepsy during sleep. In Sterman MB, Shouse MN, Passouant PP (eds): Sleep and Epilepsy. New York, Academic Press, 1982, pp 513-531.
34. Espa F, Dauvilliers Y, Ondze B, et al: Arousal reactions in sleepwalking and night terrors in adults: The role of respiratory events. Sleep 2002;2:871-875.
35. Guilleminault C, Palombini L, Pelayo R, Chervin RD: Sleepwalking and sleep terrors in prepubertal children: What triggers them? Pediatrics 2003;111:e17-25.
36. Millman RP, Kipp GR, Carskadon MA: Sleepwalking precipitated by treatment of sleep apnea with nasal CPAP. Chest 1991; 99:750-751.
37. Fietze I, Warmuth R, Witt C, Baumann G: Sleep-related breathing disorder and pavor nocturnus. Sleep Res 1995;24A:301.
38. Kales JD, Kales A, Soldatos CR: Night terrors. Clinical characteristics and personality factors. Arch Gen Psychiatry 1980; 47:1413-1417.
39. Soldatos CR, Kales A: Sleep disorders: Research in psychopathology and its practical implications. Acta Psychiatr Scand 1982;65:381-387.
40. Schenck CH, Hurwitz TD, Bundlie SR, Mahowald MW: Sleep-related injury in 100 adult patients: A polysomnographic and clinical report. Am J Psychiatry 1989;146:1166-1173.
41. Guilleminault C, Moscovitch A, Leger D: Forensic sleep medicine: Nocturnal wandering and violence. Sleep 1995;18: 740-748.
42. Llorente MD, Currier MB, Norman S, Mellman TA: Night terrors in adults: Phenomenology and relationship to psychopathology. J Clin Psychiatry 1992;53:392-394.
43. Laberge L, Tremblay RE, Vitaro F, Montplaisir J: Development of parasomnias from childhood to early adolescence. Pediatrics 2000;106:67-74.
44. Broughton RJ: Sleep disorders: Disorders of arousal? Science 1968;159:1070-1078.
45. Kales A, Jacobson A, Paulson MJ, et al: Somnambulism: Psychophysiological correlates. I. All-night EEG studies. Arch Gen Psychiatry 1966;14:586-594.

46. Kales JD, Cadieux RJ, Soldatos CR, Kales A: Psychotherapy with night-terror patients. Am J Psychother 1982;36:399-407.

47. Arkin AM: Night-terrors as anomalous REM sleep component manifestation in slow-wave sleep. Waking Sleeping 1978;2:143-147.

48. Mori SH: Integration of posture and locomotion in acute decerebrate cats and in awake, freely moving cats. Prog Neurobiol 1987;28:161-195.

49. Grillner S, Dubic R: Control of locomotion in vertebrates: Spinal and supraspinal mechanisms. Adv Neurol 1988;47:425-453.

50. Berntson GG, Micco DJ: Organization of brainstem behavioral systems. Brain Res Bull 1976;1:471-483.

51. Mogenson GJ: Limbic-motor integration. Prog Psychobiol Physiol Psychol 1986;12:117-170.

52. Mori S, Nishimura H, Aoki M: Brain stem activation of the spinal stepping generator. In Hobson JA, Brazier MAB (eds): The Reticular Formation Revisited. New York, Raven Press, 1980, pp 241-259.

53. Rossignol S, Dubuc R: Spinal pattern generation. Curr Opin Neurol 1994;4:894-902.

54. Elliott FA. Neuroanatomy and neurology of aggression. Psychiatr Ann 1987;17:385-388.

55. Siegel A, Pott CB: Neural substrates of aggression and flight in the cat. Prog Neurobiol 1988;31:261-283.

56. Bandler R: Brain mechanisms of aggression as revealed by electrical and chemical stimulation: Suggestion of a central role for the midbrain periaqueductal region. Prog Psychobiol Physiol Psychol 1988;13:67-154

57. Kelts KA, Hoehn MM: Hypothalamic atrophy. J Clin Psychiatry 1978;39:357-358.

58. Kelleffer FA, Stern WE: Chronic effects of hypothalamic injury. Arch Neurol 1970;22:419-429.

59. Reeves AG. Hyperphagia, rage, and dementia accompanying a ventromedial hypothalamic neoplasm. Arch Neurol 1969;20:616-624.

60. Haugh RM, Markesbery WR: Hypothalamic astrocytoma. Syndrome of hyperphagia, obesity, and disturbances of behavior and endocrine and autonomic function. Arch Neurol 1983;40:560-563.

61. Sano K, Mayanagi Y: Postermedial hypothalamotomy in the treatment of violent, aggressive behavior. Acta Neurochir (Wien) 1988;44 (Suppl):145-151.

62. Lai YY, Siegel JM: Brainstem-mediated locomotion and myoclonic jerks. I. Neural substrates. Brain Res 1997;745:257-264.

63. Lai YY, Siegel JM. Brainstem-mediated locomotion and myoclonic jerks. II. Pharmacological effects. Brain Res 1997;745:265-270.

64. Bassetti C, Vella S, Donati F, et al: SPECT during sleepwalking. Lancet 2000;356:484-485.

65. Achermann P, Werth E, Dijk D-J, Borbély AA: Time course of sleep inertia after nighttime and daytime sleep episodes. Arch Ital Biol 1995;134:109-119.

66. Dinges DF: Napping patterns and effects in human adults. In Dinges DF, Broughton RJ (eds): Sleeping and Alertness: Chronobiological, Behavioral, and Medical Aspects of Napping. New York, Raven Press, 1989, pp 171-204.

67. Dinges DF: Are you awake? Cognitive performance and reverie during the hypnopompic state. In Bootzin RR, Kihlstrom JF, Schacter DL (eds): Sleep and Cognition. Washington, DC, American Psychological Association, 1990, pp 159-175.

68. Tassi P, Muzet A: Sleep inertia. Sleep Med Rev 2000;4:341-353.

69. Horner RL, Sanford LD, Pack AI, Morrison AR: Activation of a distinct arousal state immediately after spontaneous awakening from sleep. Brain Res 1997;778:127-134.

70. Koboyama T, Hori A, Sato T, et al: Changes in cerebral blood flow velocity in healthy young men during overnight sleep and while awake. EEG Clin Neurophysiol 1997;102:125-131.

71. Balkin TJ, Wesensten NJ, Braun AR, et al: Shaking out the cobwebs: Changes in regional cerebral blood flow (rCBF) across the first 20 minutes of wakefulness. J Sleep Res 1998;21:411A.

72. Balkin TJ, Braun AR, Wesensten NJ, et al: The process of awakening: A PET study of regional brain activity patterns mediating the re-establishment of alertness and consciousness. Brain Res Bulletin 2002;12:2308-2319.

73. Meier-Ewert K, Broughton RJ: Photomyoclonic response of epileptic and non-epileptic subjects during wakefulness, sleep and arousal. EEG Clin Neurophysiol 1967;23:142-151.

74. Terzano MG, Parrino L, Spaggiari MC: The cyclic alternating pattern sequences in the dynamic organization of sleep. EEG Clin Neurophysiol 1988;69:437-447.

75. Zadra AL, Nielsen TA: Topographical EEG mapping in a case of recurrent sleep terrors. Dreaming 1998;8:67-74.

76. Halasz P, Ujszaszi J, Gadoros J: Are microarousals preceded by electroencephalographic slow wave synchronization precursors of confusional awakenings? Sleep 1985;8:231-238.

77. Zuccone M, Oldani A, Ferini-Strambi L, Smirne S: Arousal fluctuations in non–rapid eye movement parasomnias: The role of cyclic alternating pattern as a measure of sleep instability. J Clin Neurophysiol 1995;12:147-154.

78. Blatt I, Peled R, Gadoth N, Lavie P: The value of sleep recording in evaluating somnambulism in young adults. EEG Clin Neurophysiol 1991;78:407-412.

79. Schenck CH, Pareja JA, Patterson AL, Mahowald MW: An analysis of polysomnographic events surrounding 252 slow-wave sleep arousals in 38 adults with injurious sleepwalking and sleep terrors. J Clin Neurophysiol 1998;15:159-166.

80. Gaudreau H, Joncas S, Zadra A, Montplaisir J: Dynamics of slow-wave activity during the NREM sleep of sleepwalkers and control subjects. Sleep 2000;23:755-760.

81. Guilleminault C, Poyares D, Abat F, Palombini L: Sleep and wakefulness in somnambulism. A spectral analysis study. J Psychosom Res 2001;51:411-416.

82. Espa F, Ondze B, Deglise P, et al: Sleep architecture, slow wave activity, and sleep spindles in adult patients with sleepwalking and sleep terrors. Clin Neurophysiol 2000;111:929-939.

83. Schenck CH, Mahowald MW: Review of nocturnal sleep-related eating disorders. Int J Eat Disord 1994;15:343-356.

84. Rosenfeld DS, Elhajjar AJ: Sleepsex: A variant of sleepwalking. Arch Sex Behav 1998;27:269-278.

85. Rosen G, Mahowald MW, Ferber R: Sleepwalking, confusional arousals, and sleep terrors in the child. In Ferber R, Kryger M (eds): Principles and Practice of Sleep Medicine in the Child. Philadelphia, WB Saunders, 1995, pp 99-106.

86. Ohayon M, Guilleminault C, Priest RG: Night terrors, sleepwalking, and confusional arousal in the general population: Their frequency and relationship to other sleep and mental disorders. J Clin Psychiatry 1999;60:268-276.

87. Klackenberg G: Somnambulism in childhood—prevalence, course and behavior correlates. A prospective longitudinal study (6-16 years). Acta Paediatr Scan 1982;71:495-499.

88. Bixler EO, Kales A, Soldatos CR, et al: Prevalence of sleep disorders in the Los Angeles metropolitan area. Am J Psychiatry 1979;136:1257-1262.

89. Kahn E, Fisher C, Edwards A. Night terrors and anxiety dreams. In Ellman SD, Antrobus JS (eds): The Mind in Sleep. Psychology and Psychophysiology, 2nd ed. New York, John Wiley, 1991, pp 437-447.

90. Crisp AH: The sleepwalking/night terrors syndrome in adults. Postgrad Med J 1996;72:599-604.

91. Mahowald MW, Bundlie SR, Hurwitz TD, Schenck CH: Sleep violence—forensic science implications: Polygraphic and video documentation. J Forensic Sci 1990;35:413-432.

92. Mahowald MW, Schenck CH, Goldner M, et al: Parasomnia pseudo-suicide. J Forensic Sci 2003;48:1158-1162.

93. Mancini MC, Aloe F: Nocturnal eating syndrome: A case report with therapeutic response to dexfenfluramine. Sao Paulo Med J 1994;112:569-571.

94. Schenck CH, Hurwitz TD, O'Connor KA, Mahowald MW: Additional categories of sleep-related eating disorders and the current status of treatment. Sleep 1993;16:457-466.

95. Schenck CH, Hurwitz TD, Bundlie SR, Mahowald MW: Sleep-related eating disorders: Polysomnographic correlates of a heterogeneous syndrome distinct from daytime eating disorders. Sleep 1991;14:419-431.

96. Manni R, Ratti MT, Tartara A: Nocturnal eating: Prevalence and features in 120 insomniac referrals. Sleep 1997;20:734-738.

97. Winkelman JW: Clinical and polysomnographic features of sleep-related eating disorder. J Clin Psychiatry 1998;59:14-19.

98. Menkes DB: Triazolam-induced nocturnal bingeing with amnesia. Aust N Z J Psychiatry 1992;26:320-321.

99. Morgenthaler TI, Silber MH: Amnestic sleep-related eating disorder associated with zolpidem. Sleep Med 2002;3:323-327.

100. Birketvedt GS, Florholmen J, Sundsfjord J, et al: Behavioral and neuroendocrine characteristics of the night-eating syndrome. JAMA 1999;282:657-663.

101. Birketvedt GS, Sundsfjord J, Florholmen JR: Hypothalamic-pituitary-adrenal axis in the night eating syndrome. Am J Physiol Endocrinol Metab 2001;282:E366-E369.

102. Stunkard A, Allison KC: Two forms of disordered eating in obesity: Binge eating and night eating. Int J Obes 2003;27:1-12.

103. Wong KE: Masturbation during sleep—a somnambulistic variant? Singapore Med J 1986;27:542-543.

104. Shapiro CM, Fedoroff JP, Trajanovic NN: Sexual behavior in sleep: A newly described parasomnia. Sleep Res 1996;25:367.

105. Hurwitz TD, Mahowald MW, Schenck CH, Schluter JL: Sleep-related sexual abuse of children. Sleep Res 1989;18:246.

106. Buchanan A: Sleepwalking and indecent exposure. Med Sci Law 1991;31:38-40.

107. Fenwick P: Sleep and sexual offending. Med Sci Law 1996;36:122-134.

108. Alves R, Aloe F: Sexual behavior in sleep, sleepwalking and possible REM behavior disorder: A case report (of parasomnia overlap disorder?). Sleep 1998;21(Suppl):64.

109. Shapiro CM, Trajanovic NN, Fedoroff JP: Sexsomnia—a new parasomnia? Can J Psychiatry 2003;48:311-317.

110. Guilleminault C, Moscovitch A, Yuen K, Poyares D: Atypical sexual behavior during sleep. Psychosom Med 2002;64:328-336.

111. Aldrich MS, Jahnke B: Diagnostic value of video-EEG polysomnography. Neurology 1991;41:1060-1066.

112. Joncas S, Zadra A, Paquet J, Montplaisir J: The value of sleep deprivation as a diagnostic tool in adult sleepwalkers. Neurol 2002;58:936-940.

113. Mahowald MW, Schenck CH: Parasomnia purgatory—the epileptic/non-epileptic interface. In Rowan AJ, Gates JR (eds): Non-Epileptic Seizures. Boston, Butterworth-Heinemann, 1993, pp 123-139.

114. Schenck CH, Mahowald MW: REM parasomnias. Neurol Clin 1996;14:697-720.

115. Mahowald MW, Schenck CH: NREM parasomnias. Neurol Clin 1996;14:675-696.

116. Zucconi M, Ferini-Strambi L: NREM parasomnias: Arousal disorders and differentiation from nocturnal frontal lobe epilepsy. Clin Neurophysiol 2000;111(suppl 2):S129-S35.

117. Barabas B, Ferrari M, Matthews WS: Childhood migraine and somnambulism. Neurology 1983;33:948-949.

118. Barabas G, Matthews WS, Ferrari M: Disorders of arousal in Gilles de la Tourette's syndrome. Neurology 1984;34:814-817.

119. Wand RR, Matazow GS, Shady GA, et al: Tourette syndrome: Associated symptoms and most disabling features. Neurosci Biobehav Rev 1993;17:271-275.

120. Isik U, D'Cruz OF: Cluster headaches simulating parasomnias. Ped Neurol 2002;27:227-229.

121. Lillywhite AR, Wilson SJ, Nutt DJ: Successful treatment of night terrors and somnambulism with paroxetine. Br J Psychiatry 1994;164:551-554.

122. Balon R: Sleep terror disorder and insomnia treated with trazodone: A case report. Ann Clin Psychiatry 1994;6:161-163.

123. Kellerman J: Behavioral treatment of night terrors in a child with acute leukemia. J Nerv Ment Dis 1979;167:182-185.

124. Gutnik BD, Reid WH: Adult somnambulism: Two treatment approaches. Nebr Med J 1982;67:309-312.

125. Reid WH, Ahmed I, Levie CA: Treatment of sleepwalking: A controlled study. Am J Psychother 1981;35:27-37.

126. Hurwitz TD, Mahowald MW, Schenck CH, et al: A retrospective outcome study and review of hypnosis as treatment of adults with sleepwalking and sleep terror. J Nerv Ment Dis 1991; 179:228-233.

127. Tobin JD Jr: Treatment of somnambulism with anticipatory awakening. J Pediatr 1993;122:426-427.

128. Schenck CH, Mahowald MW: Combined buproprion-levodopa therapy of nocturnal sleep-related eating and sleep disruption in two adults with chemical dependency (letter). Sleep 2000;23:587-588.

129. Schenck CH, Mahowald MW: Dopaminergic and opiate therapy of nocturnal sleep-related eating disorder associated with sleepwalking or unassociated with another nocturnal disorder. Sleep 2002;45:A249(abstract).

130. Winkelman JW: Treatment of nocturnal eating syndrome and sleep-related eating disorder with topiramate. Sleep Med 2003; 4:243-246.

75

REM Sleep Parasomnias

Mark W. Mahowald

Carlos H. Schenck

ABSTRACT

Parasomnias may be conveniently classified into primary and secondary categories, with the primary category comprising disorders of sleep per se and the secondary category comprising disorders of other organ systems that take advantage of the sleep state to declare themselves (for example, see Chapter 72). The primary parasomnias can be further subcategorized by the state of sleep during which they occur: REM versus NREM. Those primary parasomnias that do not respect sleep state fall into a miscellaneous category.

This chapter focuses on the REM-sleep parasomnias. REM sleep is characterized by numerous physiological variables that usually occur in concert to produce the fully declared REM sleep. The majority of the REM-sleep parasomnias reflect state dissociation, a condition seen when not all of the elements usually composing REM sleep are present, resulting in fascinating clinical phenomena. The most common and best studied REM-sleep parasomnia is the REM sleep behavior disorder (RBD). In patients with RBD, somatic muscle atonia—one of the defining features of REM sleep—is absent, permitting the acting out of dream mentation, often with violent or injurious results. It is overwhelmingly a disorder affecting older men, many of whom will eventually develop neurodegenerative disorders. Increasingly, medications prescribed for psychiatric symptoms (predominantly the selective serotonin reuptake inhibitors) are the cause of RBD. The vast majority of patients with RBD respond to clonazepam. Further study of the REM parasomnias will serve to teach us much about sleep and the function of the central nervous system.

REM SLEEP BEHAVIOR DISORDER

The discovery of rapid eye movement (REM) sleep in 1953 by Aserinsky and Kleitman expanded the states of mammalian being to three: wakefulness, non–rapid eye movement (NREM) sleep and REM sleep. Each of these conditions has its own neuroanatomic, neurophysiologic, neuropharmacologic, and behavioral correlates. Intrusion of components of one state into another may cause severe symptoms in patients.[1,2,214]

In experiments reported in 1965, bilateral lesions of pontine regions adjacent to the locus coeruleus in cats caused absence of the expected atonia associated with REM sleep, allowing the cats to demonstrate prominent motor activities during REM sleep (oneiric behavior).[3] This animal model has been important in further studies demonstrating the similarity between the states of wakefulness and REM sleep[4] and in studies evaluating the state-dependent vulnerability to epileptic activity.[5] In the 1970s, scattered reports of dream-enacting behavior involving humans appeared; the polygraphic and behavioral condition was sometimes referred to as "stage 1-REM with tonic electromyogram."[6-9] Recognition of REM sleep behavior disorder (RBD) as a distinct clinical disorder followed the report in 1986 of a series of adults with RBD.[10] The cat model has recently been extended to the rat.[11,12]

Numerous physiologic phenomena occur during REM sleep[13-26] and fall into two categories: *tonic* (appearing throughout a REM period) and *phasic* (occurring intermittently during a REM period). Tonic elements include electromyographic (EMG) suppression, low voltage desynchronized electroencephalogram (EEG), high arousal threshold, hippocampal theta rhythm, elevated brain temperature, poikilothermia, olfactory bulb activity, and penile tumescence. Phasic elements include rapid eye movements, middle ear muscle activity, tongue movements, somatic muscle-limb twitches, variability of autonomic activity (cardiac and respiratory), and ponto-geniculo-occipital (PGO) spikes. It is not known whether dreaming occurs tonically or phasically during REM sleep.

Whereas the synchronizer (pacemaker) for the sleep-wake cycle appears to reside in the suprachiasmatic nucleus of the hypothalamus,[27,28] the generators or executors of the various REM phenomena, both tonic and phasic, are located in the pons.[17,29,30] It has recently been shown that the identical medullary cells are responsible for both REM atonia and cataplexy.[31]

The tonic and phasic neurophysiologic processes underlying each state can be variously dissociated and recombined across states.[32] For REM sleep, the processes that generally occur in concert may also be seen in dissociated form, both experimentally (e.g., in REM-sleep–deprived animals with PGO spikes occurring in NREM sleep and wakefulness)[33] and in human and animal disease (narcolepsy). In narcolepsy, the best understood dissociated state, the sleep attacks, hypnagogic hallucinations, sleep paralysis, cataplexy, and automatic behavior each represent the intrusion or persistence of one state of being into another (i.e., cataplexy may be the inappropriate isolated intrusion of REM sleep atonia [REM-atonia] into wakefulness, usually induced by an emotionally laden event).[34,35]

Conventional wakefulness is associated with consciousness and muscle tone; REM sleep is associated with dreaming and muscle atonia. Many dissociated conditions involving wakefulness, REM sleep, and NREM sleep are theoretically possible and await discovery or better description (i.e. the disorders of arousal: confusional arousals, sleepwalking, or sleep terrors). If we confine discussion to wakefulness and REM, and if we assume that there must be either consciousness or dreaming and either muscle tone or atonia, and if we recognize that these states can oscillate rapidly, then we see that multiple combinations are possible. The clinical presentation will depend upon the baseline state of wakefulness or REM sleep.

Table 75–1 lists the spectrum of the theoretically possible dissociations in wakefulness and REM sleep. Normal wake and dream states are self-explanatory. Cataplexy, sleep paralysis, and hallucinations are common experiences in narcolepsy.[36] Agrypnia excitata and status dissociatus, discussed below, likely represent extreme examples of state dissociation. The demonstration of willed movements allowing communication during lucid dreaming in REM sleep established the coexistence of dream and conscious mental activity.[37,38]

The counterpart of wakeful automatic behavior that arises during REM sleep constitutes the REM behavior disorder.

Epidemiology and Risk Factors

A recent telephone survey of more than 4900 persons between the ages of 15 and 100 years of age indicated an overall prevalence of violent behavior in general during sleep of 2%, one quarter of which were likely due to RBD, giving an overall prevalence of RBD at 0.5%.[39] Increasingly, RBD is becoming associated with underlying neurologic conditions.

RBD and Extrapyramidal Disease

As more patients with "idiopathic" RBD are carefully followed over time, it is becoming clear that the majority will eventually develop neurodegenerative disorders, most notably the synucleinopathies (Parkinson's disease; multiple system atrophy, including olivopontocerebellar degeneration and the Shy-Drager syndrome; dementia with Lewy body disease). RBD may be the first manifestation of these conditions, and it may precede any other manifestation of the underlying neurodegenerative process by more than 10 years.[40-44] Lai and Siegel have postulated that neuronal degeneration may begin in either the ventral mesopontine junction or the rostroventral midbrain and progress rostrally or caudally. RBD will develop first if the lesion begins in the ventral mesopontine region, but Parkinson's disease will appear first if the lesion begins in the rostroventral midbrain.[45]

Systematic longitudinal study of patients with such neurologic syndromes indicates that RBD and REM sleep without atonia may be far more prevalent than previously suspected. Although the prevalence of RBD in extrapyramidal disease is unknown, subjective reports indicate that 25% of patients with Parkinson's disease exhibit behavior suggestive of RBD or have sleep-related injurious episodes, and polysomnographic studies found RBD in up to 47% of patients with Parkinson's disease who had sleep complaints.[46,47] In one large series of patients with multiple system atrophy (MSA), 90% were found to have REM sleep without atonia and 69% had clinical RBD.[48] In another, nearly half had RBD.[49] The presence of RBD may differentiate pure autonomic failure from MSA with autonomic failure.[50] The finding of incidental Lewy body disease in one patient asymptomatic for Parkinson's disease suggests that this condition may explain idiopathic REM sleep behavior disorder in some older patients.[51] Selegiline may trigger REM sleep behavior disorder in patients with Parkinson's disease and by cholinergic treatment of Alzheimer's disease.[52,53]

RBD and Narcolepsy

There is a higher incidence of RBD in patients with narcolepsy. This association could be expected, because both narcolepsy and RBD are characterized by (state boundary control) abnormalities. The tricyclic antidepressants, selective serotonin reuptake inhibitors (SSRIs), and monoamine oxidase inhibitors, which are used to treat cataplexy, can trigger or exacerbate REM sleep behavior disorder in this population.[54] The demographics of RBD in narcolepsy parallel those of narcolepsy (younger age of onset, and equal sex distribution—unlike the age and sex distribution of spontaneously occurring RBD).

RBD and Other Conditions

Other reported associations include mitochondrial encephalomyopathy, normal pressure hydrocephalus, Tourette's syndrome, Machado-Joseph disease (spinocerebellar ataxia type 3), cerebellopontine angle tumors, group A xeroderma, multiple sclerosis, ischemic or hemorrhagic cerebrovascular

---

Table 75–1. **Spectrum of Dissociated and Transitional States Involving Wakefulness and REM Sleep**

From Wakefulness	Consciousness	Tone	Dream	Atonia	From REM Sleep
Normal waking (ongoing state)	+	+	−	−	Normal waking (normal awakening)
Cataplexy	+	−	−	+	Sleep paralysis
Conscious hallucination	*	+	*	−	Lucid dream with tone
Hypnagogic hallucination (with sleep paralysis)	*	−	*	+	Lucid dream without tone
Conscious delirium (sleep deprivation)	*	†	*	†	Sleep delirium
Automatic behavior (drug withdrawal states)	−	+	+	−	REM sleep behavior disorder (RBD)
Hypnagogic hallucination with intermittent sleep paralysis	−	†	+	†	RBD interruptions
Narcoleptic dream attack with sleep paralysis	−	−	+	+	Normal dream

*Rapidly oscillating shifts in consciousness.
†Rapidly oscillating shifts in muscle tone.
+, present; −, absent.

disease, brainstem neoplasms, autism, and Guillain-Barré syndrome.[55-67]

Pathogenesis

The generalized atonia of REM sleep results from *active inhibition* of motor activity by pontine centers of the peri–locus coeruleus region, which exert an excitatory influence upon the reticularis magnocellularis nucleus of the medulla via the lateral tegmento-reticular tract. The reticularis magnocellularis nucleus, in turn, hyperpolarizes spinal motoneuron postsynaptic membranes via the ventrolateral reticulospinal tract.[68,69] Loss of muscle tone during REM sleep is very complex, and it has been shown to be due to a combination of inactivation of brainstem motor inhibitory systems and inactivation of brainstem facilitory systems.[70,71] Normally the atonia of REM sleep is briefly interrupted by excitatory inputs that produce the rapid eye movements and the muscle jerks and twitches characteristic of REM sleep.[72-74]

Most mammals studied (including humans) exhibit a comparable set of simple REM sleep behavior during early development,[75-82] which may reflect an adaptive maturational delay in central nervous system (CNS) inhibitory capacity with heightened endogenous stimulation.[83-85] The rhesus monkey has less-vigorous REM sleep movements during infancy compared to its juvenile and adult years,[77] which appears to be an exception to the general rule. However, only a small percentage of mammals has been studied during sleep.[86] A recent in utero study of fetal sheep suggests that there is no wakefulness and that all in utero movements represent phasic REM events.[82] For humans, a stable pattern of generalized REM atonia with minimal twitching is achieved during early childhood and persists through adulthood (Table 75–2).[87]

Bilateral pontine tegmental lesions in cats result in a persistent absence of REM atonia associated with prominent motor activity during REM sleep.[3,15,24,69,88-90] That this represents REM sleep rather than waking activity is supported by the presence of other features typical of REM: loss of thermoregulation, the closed nictitating membrane, miotic pupils (despite signs of autonomic activity), and blunted response to stimuli.[22]

Cats receiving pontine tegmental lesions exhibit a range of REM sleep behavior that can appear as soon as the second postlesion day. Loss of REM atonia has been shown to be necessary, but not sufficient, to allow the expression of such REM behavior. The specific site of a pontine lesion determines whether loss of atonia occurs with simple movements or more complex behavior. This suggests that the pontine tegmentum is responsible for two separate mechanisms of skeletal motor inhibition during REM sleep: the atonia system and a system that suppresses phasic brainstem motor pattern generators.[15] A lesion damaging the atonia mechanism would produce only REM sleep with augmented tone (REM without atonia [RWA]), whereas a lesion affecting both mechanisms (tonic and phasic) would also release complex behavior, as listed in Table 75-2, whose stereotypical repertoire is dependent on the precise location of the lesion. Although the classic experimental animal model of RWA involves bilateral peri–locus coeruleus lesions,[3] it is clear that other regions of the central nervous system can affect muscle tone during REM sleep, including the medulla[91] and possibly even the hypothalamus.[30] Recent very relevant animal studies have indicated a co-localization of both the locomotor and atonia systems operating during REM sleep.[92] Given the clear neuroanatomic substrate of a REM behavioral syndrome in cats, "experiments of nature" could be expected, resulting in an analogous disorder in humans. The pathophysiology of RBD in humans may be presumed to be similar to that postulated for experimental cats,[15] namely the loss of REM atonia coupled with enhancement of phasic motor drive.

Neuroimaging studies indicate dopaminergic abnormalities in RBD. Single photon emission computed tomograpy (SPECT) studies have found reduced striatal dopamine transporters,[93,94] and decreased striatal dopaminergic innervation has been reported.[95] Decreased blood flow in the upper portion of the frontal lobe and pons has been reported,[96] as has functional impairment of brainstem neurons.[97] Positron emission tomography (PET) and SPECT studies have revealed decreased nigrostriatal dopaminergic projections in patients with multiple system atrophy and RBD.[98] Decreased blood flow in the upper portion of the frontal lobe and pons has been found in one magnetic resonance imaging (MRI) and SPECT study.[96] Impaired cortical activation as determined by electroencephalographic spectral analysis in patients with idiopathic RBD supports the relationship between RBD and neurodegenerative disorders.[99]

RBD in humans occurs in both an acute and a chronic form. Until recently, most reported cases of *acute* transient RBD fell in the toxic-metabolic category, with the best-studied conditions being the withdrawal states—most commonly involving ethanol.[6] In 1881, Lasegue postulated that dreams and hallucinations may have a common mechanism,[100] and wakeful dreaming has been considered as an etiology for the vivid visual hallucinations associated with delirium tremens.[101-103] Although the theory is controversial, dissociated wakeful-REM phenomena may play a major role in delirium tremens. Japanese investigators in 1975 formally named "Stage 1-REM with tonic EMG" to describe a polygraphic and behavioral condition seen in alcohol and meprobamate withdrawal that appeared to represent REM sleep without atonia.[104] The polygraphic and detailed clinical descriptions of delirium tremens in 1966 by Gross and coworkers[101] resemble those observed in patients with RBD. Comparable patterns have been described with nitrazepam withdrawal and biperiden intoxication.[7,8]

Currently, the most common cause of acute RWA and RBD may be iatrogenic. Medication-induced loss of REM atonia has been carefully documented in patients receiving tricyclic antidepressants,[105-109] monoamine oxidase inhibitors,[110] cholinergic agents,[53,111] and most notably, the serotonin-specific reuptake inhibitors.[112,113] Mirtazapine prescribed for patients with Parkinson's disease may also cause RBD.[114] Excessive caffeine ingestion has also been implicated,[115] as has chocolate ingestion.[116]

The *chronic* form is most often either idiopathic or associated with neurologic disorders. Each basic category of neurologic disease (vascular, neoplastic, toxic-metabolic, infectious, degenerative, traumatic, congenital, and idiopathic) as listed in Table 75-2, could be expected to manifest this disorder. Although RBD has not been reported following infection or trauma, a recent study of persistent hypersomnolence following Epstein-Barr viral infection (infectious mononucleosis and Guillain-Barré syndrome)[117] and a case with absent REM sleep as a sequel to a strategically located pontine shrapnel

Table 75–2. Types of REM Sleep Behavior

REM Sleep Behavior in Mammals		
Developmental (Presumably Most Mammals)[75-82]	**Experimental (Cats)[3,15,24,69,88,89]**	**Pathologic (Animals and Humans)**
Oro-facial behavior and limb jerking are present during late prenatal and early postnatal periods. Atonia then becomes more established and only minimal twitching persists.	Pontine tegmental lesions release stereotypical actions that cluster into 4 categories: a. Unorganized head and limb movements b. Orienting, searching behavior c. Attack behavior d. Locomotion	Spontaneously occurring RBD has been described in household pets (cats and dogs).[126,127]

REM Sleep Behavior Disorder in Humans	
Acute RBD	**Etiology**
Withdrawal	Alcohol[100-103,215] Meprobamate[6] Pentazocine[216] Nitrazepam[8]
Intoxication	Biperidin[7] Tricyclic antidepressants[105-109] Monoamine oxidase inhibitors[110] Caffeine[115]
Chronic RBD	**Etiology**
Toxic-Metabolic	Tricyclic antidepressants[109] Fluoxetine[112] Venlafaxine[113] Selegiline treatment for Parkinson's disease[52] Anticholinergic treatment for Alzheimer's disease[53]
Vascular	Subarachnoid hemorrhage[10] Vasculitis (?)[217] Ischemic[218]
Tumor	Acoustic neuroma[219] Pontine neoplasm[55,125,220]
Infectious, postinfectious	Guillain-Barré syndrome[10]
Degenerative	Amyotrophic lateral sclerosis[221] Anterior-dorsomedial thalamic syndrome Fatal familial insomnia[128] Dementia (including Alzheimer's disease, diffuse Lewy body disease, and corticobasal degeneration)[2,120,140,222-225] Demyelinating disorder[226] Olivo-ponto-cerebellar degeneration[120,227-231] Parkinson's disease[43,154,155,232-234] Progressive supranuclear palsy[40,44,228,229] Shy-Drager syndrome[228,230,235,236] Multiple system atrophy[237-239] Normal pressure hydrocephalus[58]
Traumatic	? (see text)
Developmental, congenital, familial	Developmental, congenital, or familial[125] Narcolepsy[54,240] Tourette's syndrome[59] Group A xeroderma pigmentosum[60] Mitochondrial encephalomyopathy[57]
Idiopathic[10,120,139,241]	(See text)

fragment[118] indicate that these categories will eventually be implicated. Rarely, RBD appears to follow significant psychic trauma[119,120] or to be associated with stress.[121] The phenomenon of stress-related RBD may be explained in part by experience-mediated changes in cortical organization and in synaptic transmission that reflect an impressive plasticity within the central nervous system.[122-124] A familial association has been documented[125] (Figure 75–1A and B) and is occasionally suggested historically during clinical evaluations. Interestingly, spontaneously occurring idiopathic RBD has been reported in dogs and cats.[126,127]

It appears that identifiable structural neuropathology is not necessary for the genesis of RBD. This observation is supported by the concept proposed by a Japanese

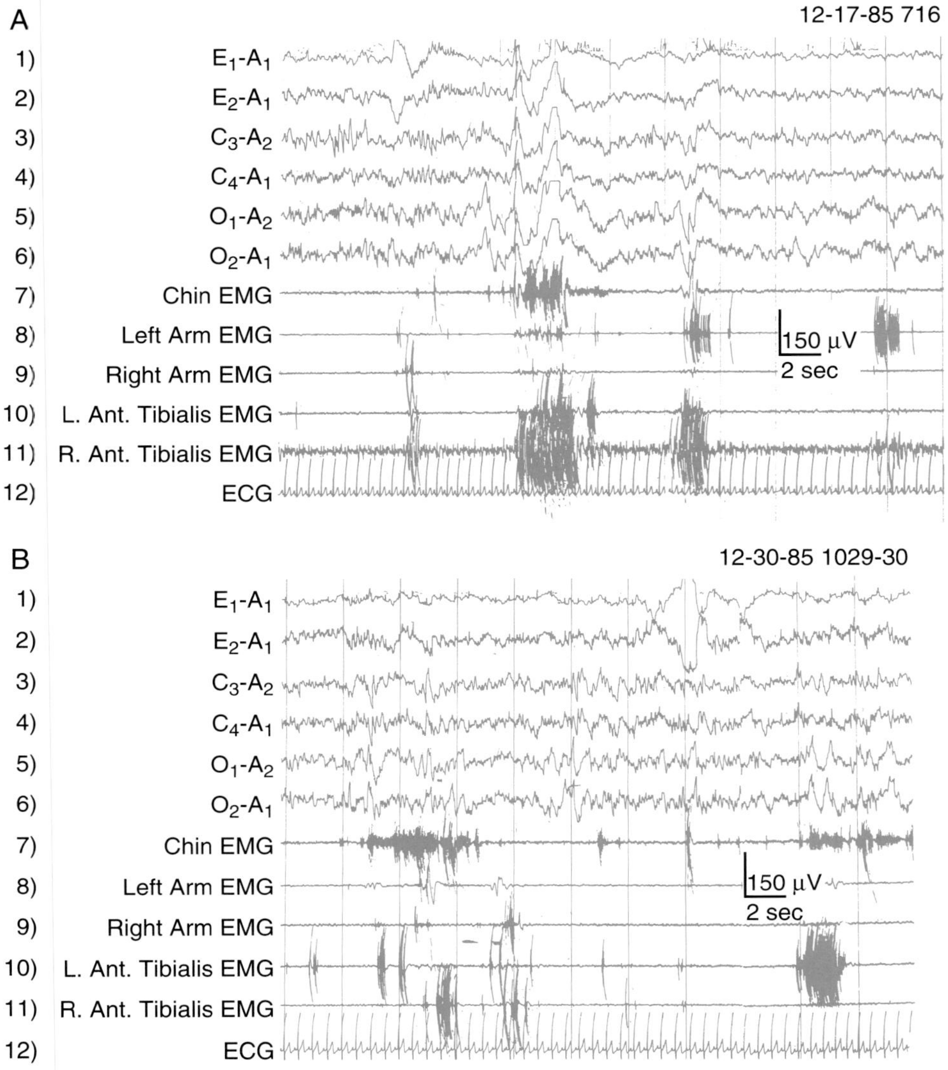

Figure 75-1. Abnormal REM sleep polysomnograms of a 10-year-old girl **(A)** and her 8-year-old brother **(B)**, in which gross body movements accompany bursts of aperiodic chin and limb electromyographic (EMG) twitching (7-11). REM sleep is identified by the presence of rapid eye movements (1-2), an activated electroencephalogram (3-6), and a predominantly atonic chin EMG. These two siblings and their father had demonstrated excessive limb jerking during sleep throughout their lives. For the girl, removal of a brainstem astrocytoma was followed by the onset of nightmares and complex, disruptive sleep behaviors, which persisted for 1 year, when treatment with clonazepam induced prompt control of both dream and motor problems. A, ear; C, central; E, eye; ECG, electrocardiogram; O, occipital; subscripts 1 and 3, left; subscripts 2 and 4, right.

group: "Excited stage 1-REM" (i.e., RBD) was proposed to result from *functional depression* or destruction of the brainstem structures responsible for atonia and *reduced activity* or destruction of brainstem serotonergic and noradrenergic structures, or both, responsible for inhibiting phasic activity.[9] In our group of elderly adults with chronic RBD, we theorize that functional dysregulation associated with the idiopathic subtype may be triggered by subtle but strategic brain changes that do not affect the brainstem primarily. A compromise in descending inhibition to the brainstem may be sufficient to produce RBD, as was strongly suggested in one case of isolated thalamic degeneration[128] and as theoretically discussed in the context of animal experimentation.[129]

Therefore, it appears that the disinhibition ratio of atonic and phasic mechanisms is crucial to the ongoing manifestation of RBD (Figure 75–2), and each mechanism is subject to influences both from within the brainstem and from higher CNS centers. This hypothesis is supported by animal studies that indicate that multiple neural sites may affect REM atonia.[30,91] It has recently been shown that in animals, a colocalization of both the locomotor and atonia systems

operates during REM sleep, indicating that RBD may result from an imbalance in REM-related influence upon these two systems.[92] In fact, RBD behavior can emerge despite maintenance of full submental EMG atonia, suggesting hyperactivation of brainstem locomotor centers without compromise of background atonia.[130,131] Thus, RBD likely may result from either loss of REM atonia or excessive locomotor drive, or both.

The overwhelming male predominance of RBD raises the intriguing question of hormonal influences, as suggested in male-aggression studies in both animals and humans.[132,133] The fact that age-related changes in brain size are more prominent in men may also play a role.[134] The typically late-age onset of RBD suggests an organic brain factor, and it may be a manifestation of the reversal or disintegration of ontogeny of state appearance.[81]

One highly speculative but tantalizing etiologic possibility is that RBD represents a delayed manifestation of REM sleep abnormalities occurring early in development. This explanation invokes the well-documented prolonged effect of pharmacologic manipulation upon developing neural tissues.[135]

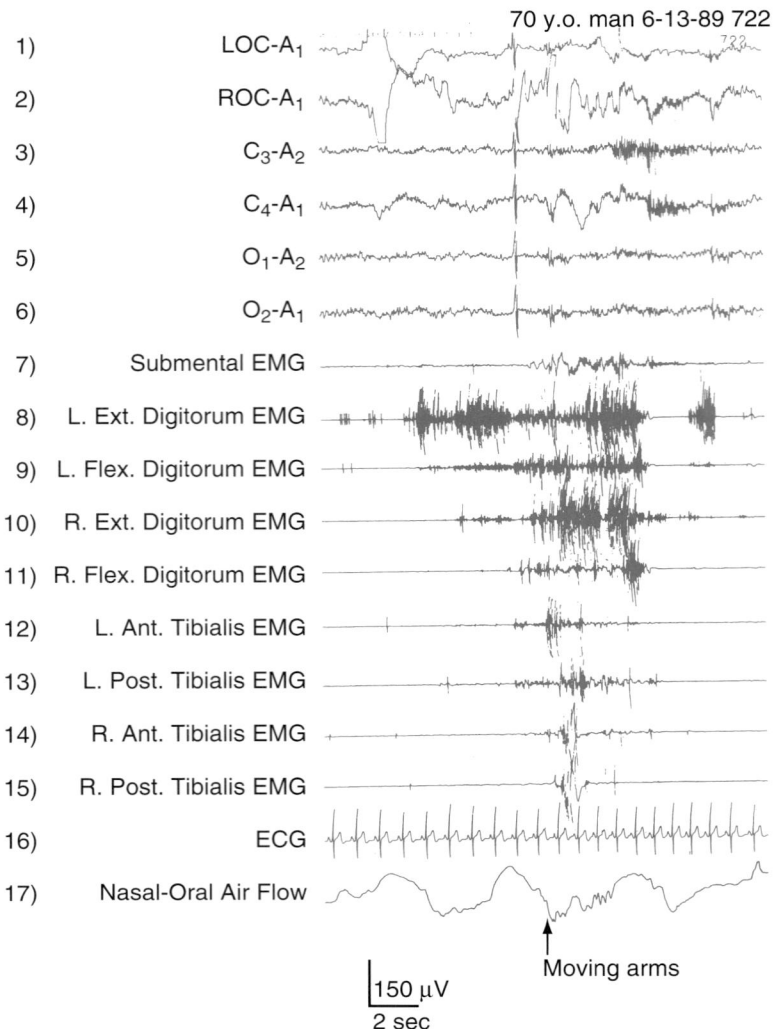

70 y.o. man 6-13-89 722

1) LOC-A₁
2) ROC-A₁
3) C₃-A₂
4) C₄-A₁
5) O₁-A₂
6) O₂-A₁
7) Submental EMG
8) L. Ext. Digitorum EMG
9) L. Flex. Digitorum EMG
10) R. Ext. Digitorum EMG
11) R. Flex. Digitorum EMG
12) L. Ant. Tibialis EMG
13) L. Post. Tibialis EMG
14) R. Ant. Tibialis EMG
15) R. Post. Tibialis EMG
16) ECG
17) Nasal-Oral Air Flow

Moving arms

150 μV
2 sec

Figure 75–2. REM sleep polysomnogram illustrating extensive preservation of submental electromyographic (EMG) atonia *(7)*, despite the emergence of gross arm movements that are noted by the technician and reflected by the prominent twitching in the upper extremity EMGs *(8-11)*. A rapid eye movement *(1-2)* immediately precedes the onset of complex behavior. A, ear; C, central; ECG, electrocardiogram; LOC, left outer canthus; O, occipital; ROC, right outer canthus; subscripts 1 and 3, left; subscripts 2 and 4, right.

In rats, Corner has described an RBD-like PSG pattern persisting into adulthood following clomipramine-induced neonatal REM-sleep suppression.[136] Another etiologic possibility is the possible presence of neuronal-specific antibodies as described in neurological paraneoplastic syndromes and the "stiff-man" syndrome.[137] One study failed to identify anti–locus coeruleus– specific antibodies in patients with RBD.[138] As autopsy material becomes available, direct neuropathologic examination may provide important correlative information. The chronic idiopathic category represents those patients whose RBD is not associated with psychopathology or detectable neuropathology.

CLINICAL FEATURES

The cases reported to date indicate strikingly similar clinical features.[10,120,139] The presenting complaint is that of vigorous sleep activities that usually accompany vivid striking dreams. These activities may result in repeated injury, including ecchymoses, lacerations, and fractures. Some of the self-protection measures taken by the patients (tethering themselves to the bed, using sleeping bags or pillow barricades, or sleeping on a mattress in an empty room) reveal the recurrent and serious nature of these episodes.[139,140] The potential for injury to

self or bed partner raises interesting and difficult forensic medicine issues.[141] RBD may have serious psychological ramifications: One woman with RBD became suicidal because her husband would not share their bed (treatment of her RBD resolved the problem).[142]

Chronic RBD is more common in older men and may be preceded by a lengthy prodrome. In some cases there is a familial predisposition. Since effective and safe treatment is available, precise diagnosis is critical.

It should be noted that RBD and other parasomnias may appear in intensive care units (ICUs). In one series of 20 patients experiencing parasomnias in ICUs, 17 had RBD (3 developed RBD during admission for neurological disorders, 1 was admitted as a consequence of RBD, and 13 displayed preexisting RBD during the course of hospitalization for other medical conditions).[143] Table 75–3 summarizes our experience with RBD and is the basis for discussing the interlocking facets of this clinical disorder.

Case Histories

Four cases illustrate the idiopathic subtype of RBD and describe the main reason for seeking medical attention. Past history and current neurologic and psychiatric evaluations were unremarkable, apart from the findings reported. All four men were known by day to be calm and friendly individuals, and their nocturnal activities were completely out of (waking) character. Clonazepam controlled problematic behavior and abnormal dreams in each.

CASE EXAMPLE 1

A 77-year-old minister presented with a 20-year history of frequent somniloquy and aggressive behavior that occurred during "fighting dreams" of defending himself against assaultive children and adults. Although his wife had sustained repeated blows, she remained in bed to protect him from self-harm. Referral was prompted by an injury to his chest from jumping into a table while dreaming. Despite vigorous sleep movements, he generally awakened feeling refreshed. However, fatigue had recently started to interfere with his busy preaching schedule.

His wife recalled a memorable night when "he said he was flying above some trees and there was a phone sitting out there on the table and it was ringing, so he swooped down to answer the phone and, just as he landed, somebody hit him and when he jumped away, he actually bolted out of the bed and was in the hall, just like that."

Medical history was remarkable for coronary artery bypass surgery three years previously, which was followed by a pronounced depression of consciousness lasting four days and a right-sided hemiplegia that gradually resolved. A mild memory deficit ensued and his preexisting sleep disturbance intensified. Current neurologic examination revealed a memory deficit, mild horizontal nystagmus, modest right-sided cogwheel rigidity, and peripheral neuropathy.

CASE EXAMPLE 2

A 60-year-old surgeon began to punch and kick his wife and jump out of bed during nightmares of being attacked "by criminals, terrorists and monsters who always tried to kill me." Work-related stress was the presumed cause of his sleep disturbance, but the violent behavior intensified despite retirement three years later. He sustained several head lacerations, and his wife once had a severe headache for two days after receiving an accidental blow to the ear. The proper diagnosis was established after 11 years. A prodrome of excessive limb and body jerking during sleep had been present for at least 33 years.

CASE EXAMPLE 3

A 62-year-old industrial plant manager experienced a progressive disorder of "military nightmares" and combative sleep behavior that had begun 10 years previously, after visiting locations where he had fought in World War II. A psychiatrist diagnosed a posttraumatic stress disorder, but treatment was ineffective, and he continued to scream profanities, throw punches, kick, sit up, and jump out of bed while dreaming of being attacked by enemy soldiers. He broke lamps and once kicked a hole in the wall. One dream-incurred head laceration required 10 sutures. He considered his sleep to be sound and had consistent diurnal alertness. He saw four physicians, including two psychiatrists, for this sleep problem before referral to our center. He had a childhood history of sleepwalking. Figure 75–3 illustrates the attempted dream enactments during REM sleep.

CASE EXAMPLE 4

A 57-year-old retired school principal presented with concern over the possibility of injuring his wife. For two years he had inadvertently punched and kicked her during vivid nightmares of protecting himself and family from aggressive people and snakes. Nocturnal arousals were uncommon, and he felt refreshed most mornings. He had developed an adjustment disorder with depressed mood[144] subsequent to a myocardial infarction one year previously, but treatment with desipramine and trazodone failed to control his problematic sleep movements. An MMPI revealed a chronic tendency for somatization. Two brothers reported identical sleep and dream disturbances that had persisted since adolescence. One of them tore the headboard off a bed while dreaming of fighting a bear.

Behavioral Features and Their Bases

The history of dream-enacting behavior occurring at least 90 minutes after sleep onset and as late as the terminal morning awakening strongly suggests an REM-sleep disorder, and in our laboratory nearly all such episodes took place within REM sleep. One rare example of an NREM dream enactment (see Fig. 1 in Schenck et al.[10]) was actually a dissociated state in which an RBD process intruded into the transition from stage 3-4 to stage 2 sleep with rapid eye movements, a vivid dream, and behavioral enactment. This case most likely represents a "parasomnia overlap" state (discussed later under Variations on REM Sleep Behavior Disorder).

Idiopathic RBD is a chronic progressive disorder with increasing complexity, intensity, and frequency of expressed behavior. Although irregular jerking of the limbs may occur nightly, the major movement episodes appear intermittently, with a frequency minimum of once in 2 weeks to a maximum of four times nightly on 10 consecutive nights. Observed somniloquy runs the spectrum from short and garbled to long-winded and clearly articulated speech. Angry speech with shouting, as well as laughter, can emerge. One patient appeared to have a dissociated RBD-lucid dream state in that he could carry on lengthy and coherent conversations with his wife and family while dreaming and incorporate the conversational material into his dreams. The extended prodrome of prominent limb and body movements during sleep in some patients may reflect a developmental failure to fully establish REM sleep atonia, predisposing them to RBD.

Most patients complain of sleep injury but rarely of sleep disruption. They usually are not awakened by their own violent activity but rather by the yelling, often persistent, of their wives.

Two conclusions can be drawn. First, chronic RBD is principally a motor disorder and uncommonly also an arousal disorder. Second, the very high arousal threshold constitutes another physiologic marker of REM sleep, which is known to have the highest threshold for arousal compared to wakefulness or NREM sleep.[18-20] In addition, the autonomic nervous system was generally not activated during episodes of vigorous REM sleep activity, as indicated by Figure 75–3. However, a few patients described episodes of vivid dreaming with behavioral enactment from which they awakened in a terrified state with full subjective autonomic activation. With rare exceptions, the violent nocturnal activities were completely

Table 75–3. Prominent Findings in 70 Consecutive Patients with Polygraphically Documented Chronic REM Sleep Behavior Disorder

Categories	Percentage of Patients	Comments
Sex		
Male	90.0 (63/70)	Mean age at onset (N = 70): 52.6 (± SD 16.1) years; range: 9–73
Female	10.0 (7/70)	Mean age at presentation: 59.3 (± 15.4) years; range:10–77
Prodrome	24.3 (17/70)	Sleeptalking, yelling, limb twitching, and jerking began a mean 22.3 (± 16.8) years before RBD onset; range: 2–48
Chief complaint		
Sleep injury	77.1 (54/70)	Ecchymoses (54); lacerations (24); fractures (5)
Sleep disruption	22.9 (16/70)	
Altered dream process and content	91.4 (64/70)	More vivid, unpleasant, action filled, violent (reported as severe nightmares)
Dream-enacting behaviors	91.4 (64/70)	Talking, laughing, yelling, swearing, gesturing, reaching, grabbing, arm flailing, punching, kicking, sitting, jumping out of bed, crawling, running
Periodic movements of NREM sleep	62.9 (44/70)	Infrequently associated with arousals; involve legs/arms, and occur throughout the entire sleep cycle
Aperiodic movements of NREM sleep	40.0 (28/70)	Infrequently associated with arousals; involve legs/arms, and occur throughout the entire sleep cycle
Elevated percentage of slow-wave (stage 3–4) sleep for age (>58 years)*	84.0 (42/50)	Not associated with prior sleep deprivation; often pronounced: mean percentage for the 42 elevated cases was 25.0 (± 5.8); range: 15–41
Clonazepam treatment efficacy		
Complete	77.2 (44/57)	Rapid control of problem sleep behavior and altered dreams, sustained for up to 7 years
Partial	12.3 (7/57)	
Total	89.5 (51/57)	
Disorders causally associated with RBD[†]		
Central nervous system disorders[‡]	37.5 (24/64)	Degenerative disorders: 11 Dementia (5) Parkinsonism (4) Olivopontocerebellar degeneration (1) Shy-Drager syndrome (1) Narcolepsy: 7 Vascular disorders: 3 Ischemic cerebrovascular disease (2) Subarachnoid hemorrhage (1) Brainstem astrocytoma: 1 Multiple sclerosis: 1 Guillain-Barré syndrome: 1
Psychiatric disorders[§]	9.1 (6/67)	Chronic abstinence states: 3 From ethanol abuse (2) From ethanol/amphetamine abuse (1) Adjustment disorders: 2 (major stressors were divorce and an automobile accident without injury) Combined disorder: 1 (RBD induced by rapid imipramine withdrawal in a patient with chronic major depression)
Endocrinologic disorder	1.4 (1/70)	64-year-old woman abruptly developed RBD after total parathyroidectomy 10 years previously

Adapted from Schenck CH, Mahowald MW. Polysomnographic, neurologic, psychiatric, and clinical outcome report on 70 consecutive cases with the REM sleep behavior disorder (RBD): sustained clonazepam efficacy in 89.5% of 57 treated patients. Cleve Clin J Med. 1990;57:s10–s24.

*Stage 3–4 percentage elevation was defined as greater than 15% of total sleep time. Twenty patients were excluded from analysis who were younger than 58 years old.

[†]The timing of onset and clinical course indicated a causal association with RBD.

[‡]Six patients were excluded from analysis whose neurologic disorders had an indeterminate association with RBD.

[§]Three patients were excluded from analysis whose mood or substance abuse disorders had an indeterminate association with RBD.

RBD, REM sleep behavior disorder.

62 Years 9-11-86

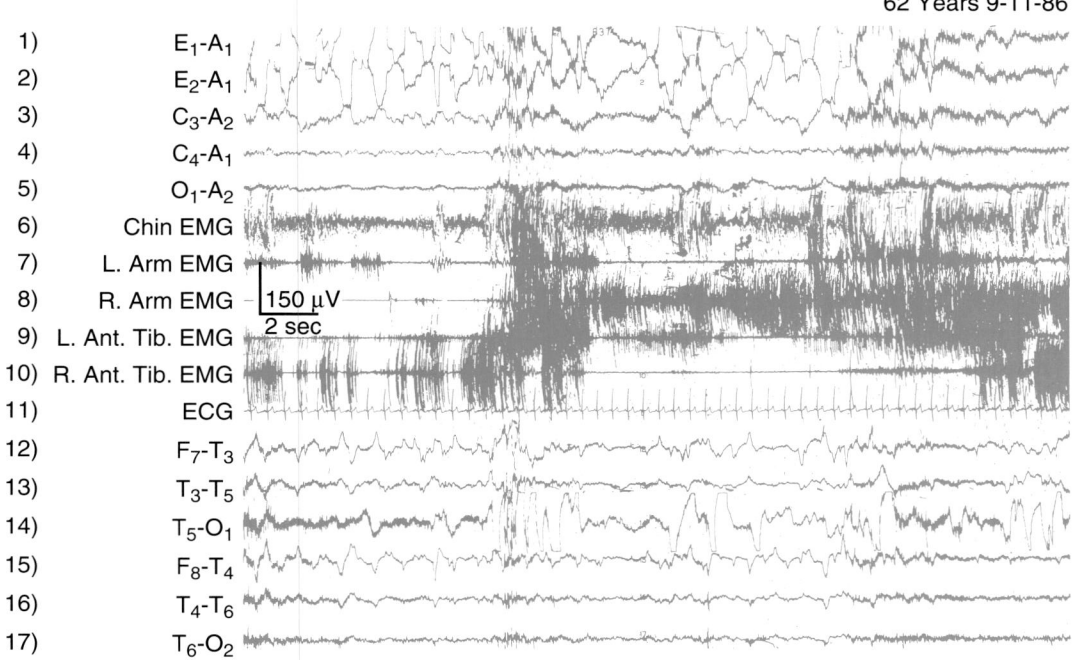

Figure 75–3. Polygraphic correlates of nocturnal dream-enacting behavior. REM sleep contains dense, high-voltage REM activity *(1-2)* and an activated electroencephalogram *(3-5,12-17)*. The electrocardiogram *(11)* has a constant rate of 64 per minute, despite vigorous limb movements, a finding that is consistent with REM sleep and inconsistent with a conventional arousal. Chin electromyographic (EMG) tone is augmented with phasic accentuations *(6)*. Arms *(7-8)* and legs *(9-10)* show aperiodic bursts of intense EMG twitching, which accompany gross behavior noted by the technician. This sequence culminates in a spontaneous awakening, when the man reports a dream of running down a hill in Duluth, Minnesota, and taking shortcuts through backyards, when he suddenly finds himself on a barge that is rocking back and forth. He feels haunted and desperately holds onto anything to prevent falling into the cargo hold, where there are skeletons. He then awakens. A, ear; C, central; E, eye; F, frontal; O, occipital; T, temporal; subscripts 7, 3, 5, and 1, left; subscripts 8, 4, 6, and 2, right.

discordant from the waking personality, supporting the concept that RBD is a state-dependent, neurobehavioral syndrome.

In RBD patients, arousal from sleep to alertness and orientation is usually rapid and accompanied by complete dream recall (very unlike the confusional arousals observed in the disorders of arousal such as sleepwalking or sleep terrors). After awakening, behavior and social interactions are appropriate, militating against an NREM sleep relationship, delirious states, or ictal phenomena but further supporting a REM sleep phenomenon. The activities, although complex and violent, are briefer than those seen in the disorders of arousal. In some persons, the clinical features contain elements of both RBD and disorders of arousal (see Variations on REM Sleep Behavior Disorder). Furthermore, appetitive behaviors (feeding or sexual) have not been seen as a manifestation of RBD in either humans or in the animal model.[15]

REM Behavior Disorder: Both a Dream and a Behavior Disorder

The Hobson and McCarley Activation-Synthesis model of dream formation states that during REM sleep, brainstem generators phasically activate motor, perceptual, affective, cognitive, and amnestic circuits whose information flow is synthesized into dreams by the forebrain.[145,146] This model would theoretically predict the dream changes observed in patients with RBD (see Table 75–3). Intensified activity of these generators or biased activation of particular circuits should induce corresponding changes in dream process and content. We theorize that both of these conditions occur to produce RBD.

As already proposed for pontine-lesioned cats, disinhibition of selective brainstem motor pattern generators accounts for the differential release of stereotypical REM behavior.[15] This same process may produce both the *behavior and dream disorder of RBD*. For example, the generator for violent behavior may become disinhibited and may then coactivate both a descending output to the spinal motor neurons and an ascending output to forebrain dream-synthesizing centers, thus producing the simultaneous movement and dreaming. These two outputs from the same generator may be *isomorphic*, so that command for dream action (fictive movements) is equivalent to command for actual movements,[147] resulting in "acting out of dreams."

In our series of patients with RBD, all who acted violently during REM sleep also had violent dreams. In fact, dream recall was most complete following behavioral enactment. The REM sleep behavior we observed in our patients corresponded to the reported dream mentation.

Most patients repeatedly experienced a "typical RBD nightmare," which consisted of being attacked by animals or unfamiliar people, few of whom were bizarre in appearance. Characteristically, the dreamer would either fight back in self-defense or else attempt to flee. Fear, rather than anger, was the usual accompanying emotion reported. An ironic situation was produced by RBD when a dreaming husband would fight to defend his wife from an aggressor while actually striking her in bed. Her yells would then awaken him to the unfortunate reality of his violent oneiric activity. In these patients, medication suppressed both the vigorous sleep behavior and the abnormal dreaming, which adds further support to the Activation-Synthesis model as described above.

A singular feature of the dream-enacted episodes in this group of patients is that customary dreams are generally not being played out; rather, distinctly altered, stereotypical, repetitive, and "action-packed" dreams are put on display.

Diagnosis

Routine medical history taking should include questions that screen for abnormal sleep movements and altered dreams, especially in older adults, in patients of any age with acute or chronic CNS disorders (particularly those who have neurologic conditions that predispose to RBD such as Parkinson's disease or multiple system atrophy), and in patients receiving psychoactive medications known to trigger RBD. The diagnosis of RBD may be suspected on clinical grounds; however, our experience has shown that polysomnographic confirmation is mandatory. The complaint of sleep-related injurious or violent behavior should be taken very seriously. Reported injuries in our series include lacerations and fractures to patients and bed partners. RBD has also resulted in subdural hematomas and other serious injuries.[148-150]

Detailed polysomnographic data in these patients have been reported elsewhere.[10,120,139] The overall sleep architecture is usually normal, with the expected cycling of NREM and REM sleep. Most of our patients had excessive slow wave sleep for age. Although some of these patients were initially thought to have a seizure disorder causing the movements during sleep, neither EEG electrical nor clinical seizure activity has been detected. The conventional scoring parameters of Rechtschaffen and Kales[87] must be modified to allow for the persistence of EMG tone during epochs that are otherwise clearly REM sleep. These periods are similar to the "stage 1 REM with tonic EMG" described by the Japanese,[9] the "stage 1 REM" seen in delirium tremens,[101] and those recorded in the chronic pontine-lesioned cats.[3,15,24,69,88-90] There is persistence of muscle tone during REM sleep, and it may be strikingly augmented for prolonged periods, occasionally lasting much of the REM sleep cycle. The onset of a REM sleep period is often marked by a sudden increase in chin EMG activity or prominent twitching in conjunction with rapid eye movements.

In addition to the intermittent absence of atonia, there are varying amounts of limb twitching (usually far in excess of that observed in normal REM sleep), gross body movements, and complex, often violent behavior that correlates with reported dream mentation. Interestingly, tachycardia may not accompany these impressive movements. A similar lack of autonomic arousal during REM sleep was observed in a study of delirium tremens.[101] This likely represents paresis of the sympathetic nervous system (inactivation of the locus coeruleus) that is characteristic of REM sleep.[129,151]

A curious feature of the chin EMG and extremity movements seen during the REM period is the variability of involvement and distribution. The chin EMG may be augmented without body movements, or it may be atonic despite flailing extremities, as shown in Figure 75–2. The arms and legs often move independently, necessitating monitoring of all limbs. Some patients demonstrated persistent (over the span of

several years) lateralization of limb EMG activity or also predominant upper or lower extremity movements.

Most all patients displayed prominent aperiodic movements of all extremities in every conceivable combination during all stages of NREM sleep. These aperiodic movements are similar but more intense than the fragmentary myoclonus described by Broughton and coworkers in patients with a wide variety of sleep disorders and occasionally as an incidental observation.[152,153] Most RBD patients also showed conventional periodic movements of sleep usually involving the legs, infrequently associated with arousals. Prolonged periods of aperiodic and periodic movements restricted to the arms were noted occasionally. Figure 75–4A and B and Figure 75–5 exemplify some of these dissociated wake-REM states.

Prominent changes in sleep patterns likely representing variations of RBD have been described in the drug-induced variety of REM sleep without atonia,[106,107] narcolepsy,[54] and Parkinson's disease.[154,155] Our laboratory has studied patients with Parkinson's disease and one each with narcolepsy and advanced olivopontocerebellar degeneration, all with histories highly suggestive of RBD, whose EEG sleep stages were uninterpretable. Their PSG abnormalities consisted of prominent slow and rapid eye movements throughout sleep. These abnormalities were associated with an EEG pattern of generalized slowing, which precluded conventional sleep-stage scoring. Prominent motor activity was present during sleep and reported dreams. Therefore, RBD appears to comprise a spectrum of sleep patterns that ranges from normal to profoundly abnormal. Consequently, the anticipated RBD polysomnographic pattern may be obscured by additional EEG abnormalities associated with the underlying neurologic disorder, necessitating clinical diagnosis.

As predicted by animal experiments, some humans may be expected to display "asymptomatic RBD," that is, RWA without behavioral manifestations. In addition to the patients with narcolepsy and RWA mentioned earlier, our laboratory has seen such cases associated with spinocerebellar degeneration and Parkinson's disease. As already mentioned, commonly prescribed medications such as tricyclic antidepressants and SSRIs may cause RWA or RBD. Figure 75–6 is a dramatic example of venlafaxine-induced RBD in a 9-year-old boy.

Diagnostic Criteria

The minimum diagnostic criteria for RBD we have formulated can be satisfied in either of two ways:

- History of problematic sleep behavior that is
  - harmful or potentially harmful, *or*
  - disruptive of sleep continuity, *or*
  - annoying to self or bed partner, *and*
  - any polysomnographic abnormality listed below.
- No history of problematic sleep behavior *and*
  - any polysomnographic abnormality listed below *and*
  - any videotaped behavioral abnormality listed below.

Polysomnography: At least one of the following during REM sleep:

- excessive augmentation of chin EMG tone
- excessive chin and/or limb EMG twitching, irrespective of chin EMG tone

A

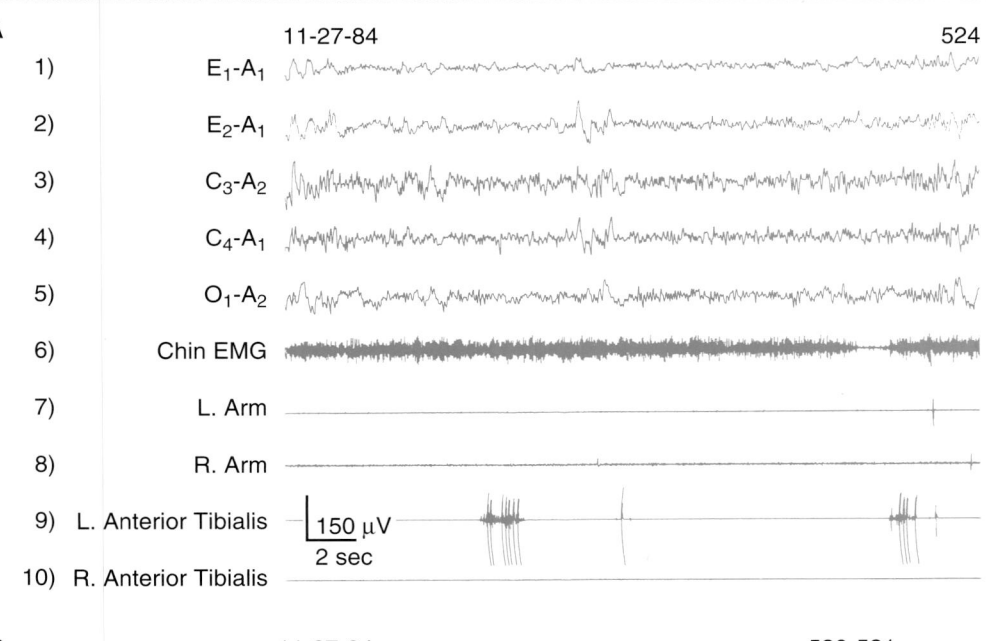

B

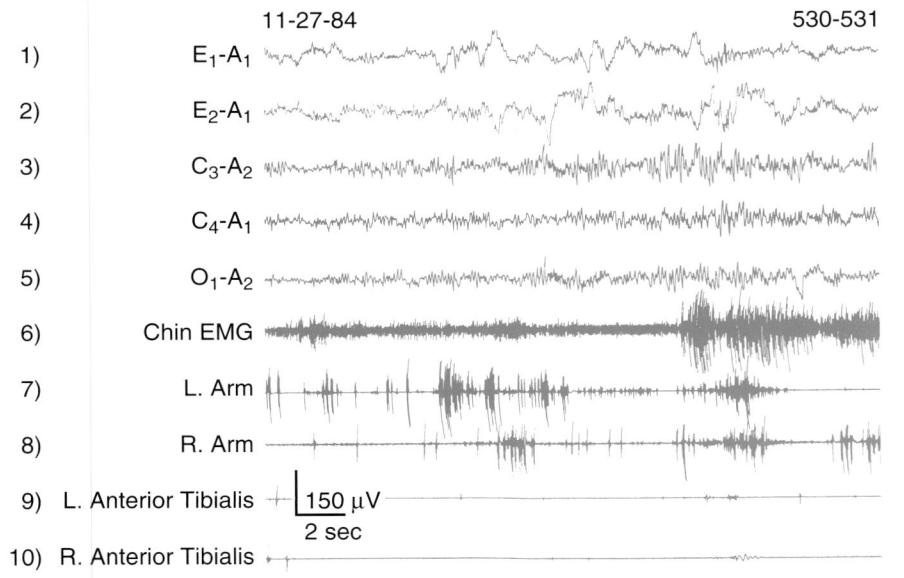

Figure 75–4. Nocturnal polysomnograms that depict contrasting forms of skeletal muscle activity in a 70-year-old man. Eye tracings, 1-2; electroencephalogram, 3-5; electromyogram (EMG) of chin, arms, and legs, 6-10. **A,** Lateralized periodic leg movements appear every 20 to 30 seconds throughout a period of stage 2 NREM sleep. **B,** A different pattern emerges 3 minutes later at the onset of REM sleep, in which both arms have frequent aperiodic movements. REM alpha is present. Chin atonia does not occur in REM sleep but does appear suddenly in NREM sleep just before a leg movement. This man developed a chronic REM sleep behavior disorder at the time of subarachnoid hemorrhage 6 years previously. A, ear; C, central; E, eye; O, occipital; subscripts 1 and 3, left; subscripts 2 and 4, right.

Videotaping of behavior: record at least one of the following during REM sleep:

- excessive limb or body jerking
- complex movements
- vigorous or violent movements

A report of dream changes accompanying the sleep behaviors, such as is listed in Table 75-3, can buttress the history. The determination of what constitutes either excessive EMG augmentation, EMG twitching, or limb jerking requires both meticulous execution of standard recording techniques and an experienced polysomnographer. We recommend that any patient suspected of having RBD undergo a systematic evaluation:

- Review of sleep/wake complaints (from patient and/or bed partner)
- Neurologic and psychiatric examinations

- Sleep laboratory study that includes continuous videotaping of behavior during standard polygraphic monitoring[87] of the electrooculogram (EOG), EEG, EMG (chin, bilateral extensor digitorum, and anterior tibialis muscles), electrocardiogram (ECG), and nasal air flow. A certified technician makes written observations of ongoing actions. The REM density score (REM activity units: 0-8 scale per 1 minute) is determined by a standard technique[156]
- A multiple sleep latency test[157] administered the day following the overnight sleep study.

More extensive neurologic evaluation including multimodal evoked potentials, brain imaging by magnetic resonance imaging (MRI) or computed tomography (CT), or comprehensive neuropsychological testing by methods previously reported,[120] are indicated only if there is a suggestion of neurologic dysfunction by history or neurologic examination.

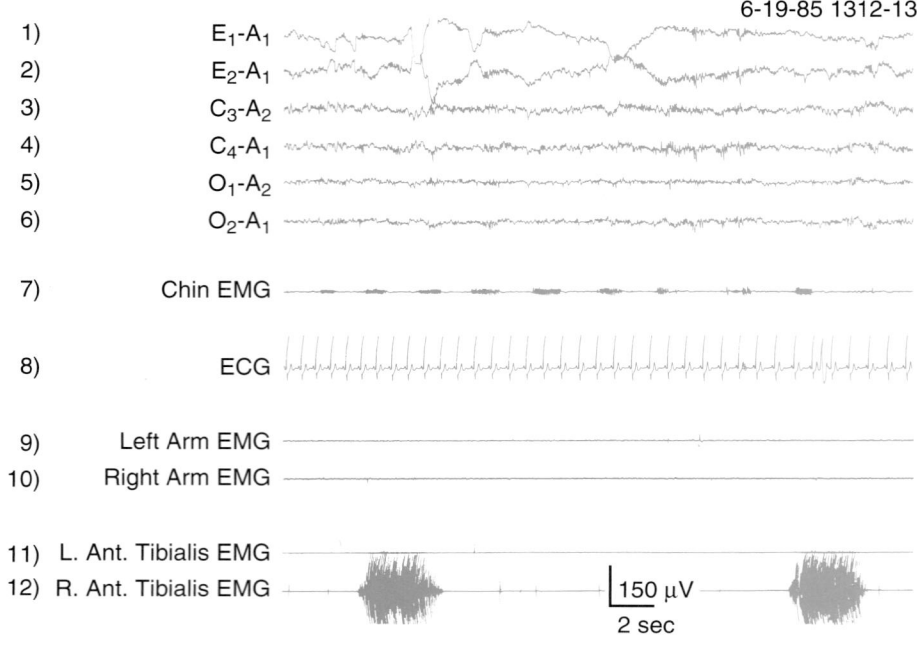

6-19-85 1312-13

1) E_1-A_1
2) E_2-A_1
3) C_3-A_2
4) C_4-A_1
5) O_1-A_2
6) O_2-A_1
7) Chin EMG
8) ECG
9) Left Arm EMG
10) Right Arm EMG
11) L. Ant. Tibialis EMG
12) R. Ant. Tibialis EMG

150 µV
2 sec

Figure 75–5. Nocturnal polysomnogram of a dissociated state in a 58-year-old man with multiple sclerosis. A pathologic process usually confined to NREM sleep—periodic leg movements *(12)*—has intruded into REM sleep, which has typical rapid eye movements *(1-2)* and a desynchronized electroencephalogram *(3-6)*. Chin electromyographic (EMG) atonia alternates every 3 sec with augmented tone *(7)*. A, ear; C, central; E, eye; ECG, electrocardiogram; O, occipital; subscripts 1 and 3, left; subscripts 2 and 4, right.

Differential Diagnosis

RBD can masquerade as many other conditions (Box 75–1). Most conditions in this differential diagnosis represented an initial clinical misdiagnosis in our series, leading to inappropriate and ineffective treatment. The differential diagnosis of these disorders has been extensively reviewed elsewhere.[158] The disorders of arousal, nocturnal seizures, and rhythmic movement disorder are discussed elsewhere in this volume. The clinical event (arousal) may not be primary but rather triggered by an underlying sleep disorder (e.g., apnea leading to arousal leading to sleep terror). Nocturnal behavior induced by obstructive sleep apnea or sleep-related seizures can mimic those of RBD.[159,160]

"Overlap" parasomnias are characterized by a clinical history suggestive of sleepwalking or sleep terrors combined with PSG features of motor disinhibition during both REM and NREM sleep.[161] It is likely that a recent series of somnambulistic-like events in elderly subjects found to have PSG features of RBD represents this phenomenon.[162] Nocturnal panic disorder is poorly understood and requires more study. It is well established that psychogenic dissociative disorders may arise predominantly or exclusively from the sleep period.[163] Finally, our group has seen extremely violent sleep-period behavior believed to represent malingering.[164]

RBD Variations

PARASOMNIA OVERLAP SYNDROME

There is a subgroup of parasomnia patients with both clinical and PSG features of both RBD and disorders of arousal (sleepwalking or sleep terrors). These cases demonstrate motor and behavioral dyscontrol extending across NREM and REM sleep,

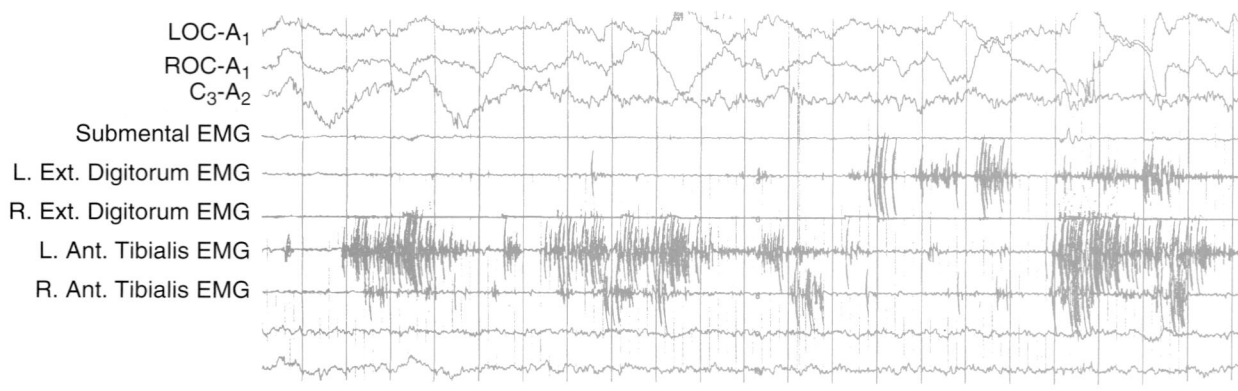

LOC-A_1
ROC-A_1
C_3-A_2
Submental EMG
L. Ext. Digitorum EMG
R. Ext. Digitorum EMG
L. Ant. Tibialis EMG
R. Ant. Tibialis EMG

Venlafaxine-induced RBD in 9 y.o. boy

Figure 75–6. Polysomnogram of a 9-year-old boy who developed REM behavior disorder (RBD) coincident with his being placed on venlafaxine, 550 mg daily. Note the prominent tonic and phasic muscle activity of the extremities during REM sleep. A, ear; C, central; EMG, electromyogram; LOC, left outer canthus; ROC, right outer canthus; subscripts 1 and 3, left; subscript 2, right.

Box 75–1.   RBD-Differential Diagnosis

Disorders of Arousal
Primary

- Confusional Arousals
- Sleepwalking
- Sleep Terrors

Secondary

- Obstructive Sleep Apnea
- Periodic Limb Movement Disorder
- Gastroesophageal Reflux
- Nocturnal Seizures

Parasomnia (Overlap) Syndrome

Nocturnal Seizures

Rhythmic Movement Disorder

Posttraumatic Stress Disorder

Nocturnal Panic Disorder

Psychogenic Dissociative Disorder or Conversion Hysteria

Malingering

and they suggest the possibility of a unifying hypothesis for disorders of arousal and RBD. The primary underlying feature is motor disinhibition during sleep. When motor disinhibition is predominantly during NREM sleep, it manifests as disorders of arousal; when it is predominantly during REM sleep, it manifests as RBD. The parasomnia overlap syndrome occupies an intermediate position, with features of both.[161] One AIDS-related case with prominent brainstem involvement has been identified. The abnormal motor and verbal nocturnal behavior of status dissociatus may respond to treatment with clonazepam.[165,166]

AGRYPNIA EXCITATA

This recently described condition is characterized by generalized overactivity associated with loss of slow wave sleep, mental oneiricism (inability to initiate and maintain sleep, with wakeful dreaming), and marked motor and autonomic sympathetic activation seen in such diverse conditions as delirium tremens, Morvan's fibrillary chorea, and fatal familial insomnia.[167-169] *Oneiric dementia* is likely a related condition.[170]

Agrypnia excitata is similar to "status dissociatus," which may be the most extreme form of RBD and appears to represent the complete breakdown of state-determining boundaries. Clinically, patients with status dissociatus, by observation, appear to be either awake or asleep; however, clinically, their sleep behavior is very atypical, characterized by frequent muscle twitching, vocalization, and reports of dreamlike mentation upon spontaneous or forced awakening. Polygraphically, there are no features of either conventional REM or NREM sleep; rather, there is the simultaneous admixture of elements of wakefulness, REM sleep, and NREM sleep. "Sleep" may be perceived as "normal" and restorative by the patient, despite the nearly continuous motor and verbal actions and absence of polysomnographically defined REM or NREM sleep. Conditions associated with status dissociatus include protracted withdrawal from alcohol abuse, narcolepsy, olivopontocerebellar degeneration, and prior open heart surgery.

The clinical history alone is insufficient to make the diagnosis, which can be established only with extensive PSG evaluation, including employment of a full seizure montage, respiratory recording, monitoring of all extremities, continuous audiovisual documentation, and detailed observations made by experienced technicians. The physical and psychological consequences of an erroneous diagnosis are obvious. The impressive response to treatment emphasizes the importance of a definitive diagnosis.[139,171]

Treatment

Clonazepam is highly effective in the treatment of RBD. The response to clonazepam is impressive both in degree and duration. It is effective in nearly 90% of cases, with little evidence of tolerance or abuse.[139] The majority of our patients and their wives noticed a suppressing effect on problematic sleep behavior and nightmares within the first week, often beginning on the first night. The initial dose was 0.5 mg at bedtime; some cases required a rapid increase to 1.0 mg. Tolerance has been an infrequent and mild problem despite continuous administration for more than 17 years. A hierarchical benefit often occurred: After an initial period (days or months) of marked suppression of sleep motor activity, moderate amounts of limb twitching reemerged along with sleep-talking and more complex behavior. Nevertheless, the medication continued to control the problematic, vigorous activities and the associated nightmares. All instances of drug discontinuation resulted in prompt relapse. Clonazepam may be taken up to two hours before bedtime by those patients complaining of sleep-onset insomnia, prominent limb jerking beginning shortly after sleep onset, or excessive morning sedation.

Consideration of the pathophysiologic mechanisms of RBD leads directly to an examination of clonazepam's beneficial effect. This benzodiazepine has been effective in the control of other motor disorders in various states, such as intention myoclonus,[172] spinal myoclonus,[173] propriospinal myoclonus,[174] rhythmic dystonia,[175] choreiform activity of wakefulness,[176] the motor hyperactivity of bipolar manic states,[177,178] periodic leg movements of NREM sleep,[179-182] and neuroleptic-induced somnambulism.[183] It is also prescribed as an anticonvulsant for infantile spasms and myoclonic epilepsy.[184]

The specific mechanism of action of clonazepam in RBD is unknown, but it likely reflects, in part, its serotonergic property.[185] Disinhibition of REM phasic activity (rapid eye movements and PGO spikes) and hallucinatory behavior were induced in cats by serotonin-depleting drugs and by selective destruction of serotonergic neurons of the brainstem raphe nuclei (reviewed in Hishikawa et al.[9]). Serotonin administration inhibits motor activity in several animal experimental designs.[186-188] Alcohol-dependent mice in withdrawal—a high-risk state for RBD—had a markedly reduced serotonin metabolism.[189] Many of the neurodegenerative conditions associated with RBD involve monoaminergic systems, including the serotonergic raphe nuclei.[9] Although subtle changes in the PSG following effective clinical treatment with clonazepam have been reported,[190] there are no gross changes in sleep stages or in the absence of atonia.[139] The fact that clonazepam causes striking clinical improvement without discernable effect upon the PSG-recorded RWA suggests that it acts preferentially upon the locomotor systems rather than those affecting REM atonia.

Melatonin, often at doses of 3 mg to 12 mg at night, may also be effective.[191-193] Although tricyclic antidepressants may enhance motor activity during REM sleep, they occasionally are effective in treatment of RBD.[194] Desipramine, which has recently been demonstrated to possess a serotonergic effect,[195] induced one temporary and one sustained remission of RBD in our patient sample, but it is less predictably effective than clonazepam.

Pramipexole or levodopa may be effective.[196,197] Carbamazepine has been effective in one case.[198] There have been anecdotal reports of response to gabapentin, monoamine oxidase inhibitors, donepezil, and clonidine.[199,200] Due to the multiplicity of neural networks involved in REM atonia,[15,30,91] it is likely that various medications may be effective in individual cases.

In RBD associated with narcolepsy, the tricyclic antidepressants or monoamine oxidase inhibitors administered for cataplexy may be continued and clonazepam added to the regimen.[54] The treatment of medication-induced or Parkinson's disease–associated RBD is the same as for idiopathic RBD.[43] Pallidotomy has been effective in one case of RBD associated with Parkinson's disease, whereas chronic bilateral subthalamic stimulation was not.[201-203]

The other essential therapeutic intervention concerns environmental safety. Clonazepam is not failsafe: One patient injured himself during a violent dream one year after initiating very satisfactory pharmacotherapy. There was no recurrence during the ensuing five months, even though the dose was not increased. Therefore, potentially dangerous objects should be removed from the bedroom, cushions put around the bed, and perhaps the mattress placed on the floor and windows protected. We anticipate some cases in which drug intolerance or ineffectiveness will lead to discontinuation, requiring maximum environmental safety.

Clinical Course and Prevention

The clinical course will depend upon the etiology. Often, iidiopathic RBD is slowly progressive, as is RBD associated with the synucleinopathies. Interestingly, RBD associated with neurodegenerative disorders may remit spontaneously as the underlying neurodegenerative process progresses. Drug-induced RBD is presumably transient and will improve upon withdrawal of the offending medication. The only known preventable cause of RBD is medication.

Pitfalls and Controversies

Numerous parasomnias can perfectly mimic RBD, mandating formal sleep studies to rule out NREM parasomnias, nocturnal seizures, obstructive sleep apnea, psychogenic dissociative disorders, or malingering.

Perspectives and Implications

A common thread linking RBD and the disorders of arousal is the appearance of motor activity that is dissociated from waking consciousness. In RBD, the motor behavior closely correlates with dream imagery, and in disorders of arousal, it often occurs in the absence of (remembered) mentation. This dissociation of behavior from consciousness may be explained by the presence of locomotor centers (LMCs) from the mesencephalon to the medulla, which are capable of generating complex behavior without cortical input.[204-207] These areas project to the central pattern generator of the spinal cord, which itself is able to produce complex stepping movements in the absence of supraspinal influence.[208] This accounts for the fact that decorticate experimental and barnyard animals are capable of performing very complex, integrated motor acts. It is likely that during NREM sleep the LMCs are not activated, suggesting a release of LMCs during the parent state, just as is seen in the loss of REM atonia. Dissociation of the LMCs from the parent state of REM or NREM sleep would explain the presence of complex motor behavior seen in RBD and disorders of arousal.

RBD is an exciting experiment of nature, extending our understanding of state declaration. Its association with narcolepsy and its clinical similarity to status dissociatus and the parasomnia overlap syndrome expand the concept of state boundary dyscontrol. The identification of yet other state declaration errors, and their induction by or response to specific pharmacologic agents, promises to unveil much about the neuroanatomy, neurophysiology, neurochemistry, and neuropharmacology of waking and sleep. Such experiments of nature underscore the symbiotic relationship between clinical and basic science medicine.

OTHER REM SLEEP PARASOMNIAS

Nightmares

These are discussed by Nielsen in Chapter 77.

REM-Sleep–Related Sinus Arrest

This condition,[209] first described by Guilleminault and colleagues in 1984,[210] is a cardiac rhythm disorder that affects otherwise healthy young adults of either sex. It is characterized by sinus arrest during REM sleep, usually in clusters, with asystoles lasting up to 9 seconds. In one case, vocalizations occurred during periods of REM sleep asystole, with a loud scream and a sensation of being "shocked" (but without chest pain or related symptoms) associated with the longest asystole.[211]

Periods of asystole do not occur during NREM sleep and are not associated with sleep apnea. Some patients experience faintness, light-headedness, and blurred vision during abrupt awakenings, and syncope can occur during ambulation after an awakening. Also, there may be complaints of vague chest pain or tightness, or intermittent palpitations, during the daytime. However, daytime ECG (including Holter monitoring) is usually completely normal, and angiography, when performed, is unremarkable. The underlying pathophysiology, therefore, appears to be autonomic dysfunction. The clinical course is unknown. Complications include loss of consciousness and even cardiac arrest from prolonged asystole. This condition must be considered in cases of sudden, unexplained death during sleep. Treatment is usually not indicated, although prophylactic intervention would include a ventricular-inhibited pacemaker with a low rate limit.

Impaired-Sleep–Related Penile Erections

These are discussed in Chapter 118.

Sleep-Related Painful Erections

This condition[209] is characterized by penile pain with erections that typically occur during REM sleep. Middle-aged or older males are typically affected; they complain of recurrent awakenings with partial or full erections and pain. The cumulative effects of nightly sleep disruption and sleep loss can result in the additional complaints of insomnia, irritability, anxiety, and daytime somnolence. There is usually a history of normal erections during wakefulness. There is little evidence of underlying psychiatric disease, and pathology of the penis is usually not found. Although the course is not well known, it appears that this condition can become more severe over time. No systematic studies of treatment efficacy have been performed, but clozapine, propranolol, or paroxetine may be effective.[212,213]

> *Clinical Pearl*
>
> *The REM sleep behavior disorder is the most common of the REM parasomnias, and it is seen primarily in older men. The presence of RBD in younger individuals, particularly younger female patients, should lead to the suspicion of medication-induced RBD or RBD associated with narcolepsy or a structural central nervous system lesion.*

Acknowledgments

This work was partly supported by a grant from Hennepin Faculty Associates. We acknowledge our ongoing collaboration with Dr. Scott R. Bundlie, Dr. Gerald M. Rosen, and Andrea L. Patterson, RPSGT. We are indebted to Ms. Traci Oletzke for secretarial support and to our dedicated nurses and technologists.

REFERENCES

1. Mahowald MW, Ettinger MG: Things that go bump in the night—the parasomnias revisited. J Clin Neurophysiol 1990;7:119-143.
2. Mahowald MW, Schenck CH: NREM parasomnias. Neurol Clin 1996;14:675-696.
3. Jouvet M, Delorme F: Locus coeruleus et sommeil paradoxal. CR Soc Biol 1965;159:895-899.
4. Morrison AR, Sanford LD, Ball WA, et al: Stimulus-elicited behavior in rapid eye movement sleep without atonia. Behav Neurosci 1995;109:972-979.
5. Shouse MN, Siegel JM, Wu FM, et al: Mechanisms of seizure suppression during rapid-eye-movement (REM) sleep in cats. Brain Res 1989;505:271-282.
6. Tachibana M, Tanaka K, Hishikawa Y, Kaneko Z: A sleep study of acute psychotic states due to alcohol and meprobamate addiction. Adv Sleep Res 1975;2:177-205.
7. Atsumi Y, Kojima T, Matsu'ura M, et al: Polygraphic study of altered consciousness—effect of biperiden on EEG and EOG. Annu Rep Res Psychotrop Drugs 1977;9:171-178 (in Japanese).
8. Sugano T, Suenaga K, Endo S, et al: Withdrawal delirium in a patient with nitrazepam addiction. Jpn J EEG EMG 1980; 8:34-35 (in Japanese).
9. Hishikawa Y, Sugita Y, Iijima S, et al: Mechanisms producing "stage 1-REM" and similar dissociations of REM sleep and their relation to delirium. Adv Neurol Sci (Tokyo) 1981; 25:1129-1147.
10. Schenck CH, Bundlie SR, Ettinger MG, Mahowald MW: Chronic behavioral disorders of human REM sleep: A new category of parasomnia. Sleep 1986;9:293-308.
11. Sanford LD, Cheng CS, Silvestri AJ, et al: Sleep and behavior in rats with pontine lesions producing REM without atonia. Sleep Res Online 2001;4:1-5.
12. Sanford LD, Silvestri AJ, Mann GL, et al: Behavioral release during REM without atonia in rats. Sleep Res Online 1999; 2(suppl 1):76.
13. Aserinski A, Kleitman N: Regularly occurring periods of eye motility, and concomitant phenomena during sleep. Science 1953;118:273-274.
14. Steriade M, Hobson JA: Neuronal activity during the sleep-waking cycle. Prog Neurobiol 1976;6:155-376.
15. Hendricks JC, Morrison AR, Mann GL: Different behaviors during paradoxical sleep without atonia depend upon lesion site. Brain Res 1982;239:81-105.
16. Gaillard J-M: Biochemical pharmacology of paradoxical sleep. Br J Clin Pharmacol 1983;16:205s-230s.
17. Vertes RP: Brainstem control of the events of REM sleep. Prog Neurobiol 1984;22:241-288.
18. Huttenlocher PR: Effects of state of arousal on click responses in the mesencephalic reticular formation. EEG Clin Neurophysiol 1960;12:819-827.
19. Williams HL, Tepas DI, Morlock HC: Evoked responses to clicks and electroencephalographic stages of sleep in man. Science 1962;138:685-686.
20. Hodes R, Suzuki J-I: Comparative thresholds of cortex, vestibular system, and reticular formation in wakefulness, sleep and rapid eye movement periods. EEG Clin Neurophysiol 1965; 18:239-248.
21. Pessah MA, Roffwarg HP: Spontaneous middle ear muscle activity in man: A rapid eye movement sleep phenomenon. Science 1972;178:773-776.
22. Hendricks JC, Bowker RM, Morrison AR: Functional characteristics of cats with pontine lesions during sleep and wakefulness and their usefulness for sleep research. In Koella WP, Levin P (eds): Sleep 1976. Third European Congress Sleep Research, Montpellier, September 1976. Basel, Karger, 1977, pp 207-210.
23. Chokroverty S: Phasic tongue movements in human rapid-eye-movement sleep. Neurology 1980;30:665-668.
24. Jouvet M, Sastre J-P, Sakai K: Toward an etho-ethnology of dreaming. In Karacan I (ed): Psychophysiological Aspects of Sleep. Park Ridge, NJ, Noyes Medical Publishers, 1981.
25. Morrison A: Paradoxical sleep and alert wakefulness: Variations on a theme. In Chase MH, Weitzman ED (eds): Sleep Disorders: Basic and Clinical Research. New York, S. P. Medical and Scientific Books, 1983.
26. Fisher C, Gross J, Zuch J: Cycle of penile erection synchronous with dreaming (REM) sleep: Preliminary report. Arch Gen Psychiatry 1965;12:29-45.
27. Eastman CI, Mistlberger RE, Rechtschaffen A: Suprachiasmatic nuclei lesions eliminate circadian temperature and sleep rhythms in the rat. Physiol Behav 1984;32:357-368.
28. Pickard GE, Turek FW: The suprachiasmatic nuclei: Two circadian clocks? Brain Res 1983;268:201-210.
29. Sakai K: Some anatomical and physiological properties of ponto-mesencephalic tegmental neurons with special reference to the PGO waves and postural atonia during paradoxical sleep in the cat. In Hobson JA, Brazier MAB (eds): The Reticular Formation Revisited. New York, Raven Press, 1980.
30. Morrison AR: Is the pons the site of rapid eye movement sleep generation in normal individuals? Sleep Res 1991;20A:57.
31. Siegel JM, Nienhuis R, Fahringer HM, et al: Neuronal activity in narcolepsy: Identification of cataplexy-related cells in the medial medulla. Science 1991;252:1315-1318.
32. Steriade M, Ropert N, Kitsikis A, Oakson G. Ascending activating neuronal networks in midbrain core and related rostral systems. In Hobson JA, Brazier MAB (eds): The Reticular Formation Revisited. New York, Raven Press, 1980, pp 125-167.

33. Dement WC: The biological role of REM sleep (circa 1968). In Kales A (ed): Sleep Physiology and Pathology. Philadelphia, Lippincott, 1969;245-265.

34. Hishikawa Y, Nan'no H, Tachibana M, et al: The nature of sleep attack and other symptoms of narcolepsy. EEG Clin Neurophysiol 1968;24:1-10.

35. Guilleminault C, Wilson RA, Dement WC: A study on cataplexy. Arch Neurol 1974;31:255-261.

36. Kales A, Cadieux RJ, Soldatos CR, et al: Narcolepsy-cataplexy I. Clinical and electrophysiologic characteristics. Arch Neurol 1982;39:164-168.

37. LaBerge SP, Nagel LE, Dement WC, Zarcone VP: Lucid dreaming verified by volitional communication during REM sleep. Percep Mot Skills 1981;52:727-732.

38. Fenwick P, Schatzman M, Worlsey A, et al: Lucid dreaming: Correspondence between dreamed and actual events in one subject during REM sleep. Biol Psychiatry 1984;18:243-252.

39. Ohayon MM, Caulet M, Priest RG: Violent behavior during sleep. J Clin Psychiatry 1997;58:369-376.

40. Pareja JA, Caminero AB, Masa JF, Dobato JL: A first case of progressive supranuclear palsy and pre-clinical REM sleep behavior disorder presenting as inhibition of speech during wakefulness and somniloquy with phasic muscle twitching during REM sleep. Neurologia 1996;11:304-306.

41. Boeve BF, Silber MH, Ferman JT, et al: Association of REM sleep behavior disorder and neurodegenerative disease may reflect an underlying synucleinopathy. Mov Disord 2001;16: 622-630.

42. Boeve BF, Silber MH, Parisi JE, et al: Synuceinopathy pathology often underlies REM sleep behavior disorder and dementia or parkinsonism. Neurology 2003;61:40-45.

43. Schenck CH, Bundlie SR, Mahowald MW: Delayed emergence of a parkinsonian disorder in 38% of 29 older men initially diagnosed with idiopathic rapid eye movement sleep behavior disorder. Neurology 1996;46:388-393.

44. Montplaisir J, Petit D, Decary A, et al: Sleep and quantitative EEG in patients with progressive supranuclear palsy. Neurology 1997;49:999-1003.

45. Lai YY, Siegel JM: Physiological and anatomical link between Parkinson-like disease and REM sleep behavior disorder. Mol Neurobiol 2003;27:137-152.

46. Comella CL, Nardine TM, Diederich NJ, Stebbins GT: Sleep-related violence, injury, and REM sleep behavior disorder in Parkinson's disease. Neurology 1998;51:526-529.

47. Eisehsehr I, Parrino L, Noachtar S, et al: Sleep in Lennox-Gastaut syndrome: The role of the cyclic alternating pattern (CAP) in the gate control of clinical seizures and generalized polyspikes. Epilepsy Res 2001;46:241-250.

48. Plazzi G, Corsini R, Provini F, et al: REM sleep behavior disorders in multiple system atrophy. Neurology 1997;48:1094-1097.

49. Ghorayeb I, Yekhlef F, Chrysosotome V, et al: Sleep disorders and their determinants in multiple system atrophy. J Neurol Neurosurg Psychiatry 2002;72:798-800.

50. Plazzi G, Cortelli P, Montagna P, et al: REM sleep behavior disorder differentiates pure autonomic failure from multiple system atrophy with autonomic failure. J Neurol Neurosurg Psychiatry 1998;64:683-685.

51. Uchiyama M, Isse K, Tanaka K, et al: Incidental Lewy body disease in a patient with REM sleep behavior disorder. Neurology 1995;45:709-712.

52. Louden MB, Morehead MA, Schmidt HS: Activation by selegiline (Eldepryle) of REM sleep behavior disorder in parkinsonism. W V Med J 1995;91:101.

53. Carlander B, Touchon J, Ondze B, Billiard M: REM sleep behavior disorder induced by cholinergic treatment in Alzheimer's disease. J Sleep Res 1996;5(suppl 1):28.

54. Schenck CH, Mahowald MW: Motor dyscontrol in narcolepsy: Rapid-eye-movement (REM) sleep without atonia and REM sleep behavior disorder. Ann Neurol 1992;32:3-10.

55. Bianchin MM, Ferreira NP, Fernandes LNT, et al: Dissociated sleep components in a patient with a pontomesencephalic astrocytoma. Ann Neurol 1997;42:470 [abstract].

56. Plazzi G, Montagna P: Remitting REM sleep behavior disorder as the initial sign of multiple sclerosis. Sleep Med 2002;3:437-439.

57. Nozawa T, Sato Y, Cho T, Takeuchi T: Polygraphic findings in mitochondrial encephalomyopathy. Sleep Res 1995;24A:403.

58. Uchiyama M, Tanaka K, Isse K, et al: REM sleep behavior disorder in a case with normal pressure hydrocephalus. Jpn J Psychiatry Neurol 1991;45:935-936.

59. Trajanovic NN, Shapiro CM, Sandor P: REM sleep behavior disorder in patients with Tourette's syndrome. Sleep Res 1997;26:524.

60. Kohyama J, Shimohira M, Kondo S, et al: Motor disturbance during REM sleep in group A xeroderma pigmentosum. Acta Neurol Scand 1995;92:91-95.

61. Fukutake T, Shinotoh H, Nishino H, et al: Homozygous Machado-Joseph disease presenting as REM sleep behaviour disorder and prominent psychiatric symptoms. Eur J Neurol 2002;9:97-100.

62. Zambelis T, Paparrigopoulos T, Soldatos CR: REM sleep behavior disorder associated with a neurinoma of the left pontocerebellar angle. J Neurol Neurosurg Psychiatry 2002;72:821-822.

63. Kimura K, Tachibana N, Kohyama J, et al: A discrete pontine ischemic lesion could cause REM sleep behavior disorder. Neurology 2000;55:894-895.

64. Thirumalai SS, Shubin RA, Robinson R: Rapid eye movement sleep behavior disorder in children with autism. J Child Neurol 2002;17:173-178.

65. Friedman JH: Presumed rapid eye movement behavior disorder in Machado-Joseph disease (spinocerebellar ataxia type 3). Mov Disord 2002;17:1350-1353.

66. Syed BH, Rye DB, Singh G: REM sleep behavior disorder and SCA-3 (Machado-Joseph disease). Neurology 2003;60:148.

67. Iranzo A, Munoz E, Santamaria J, et al: REM sleep behavior disorder and vocal cord paralysis in Machado-Joseph disease. Mov Disord 2003;18:1179-1183.

68. Sakai K, Sastre J-P, Kanamori N, Jouvet M: State-specific neurons in the ponto-medullary reticular formation with special reference to the postural atonia during paradoxical sleep in the cat. In Pompeiano O, Ajmone Marsan C (eds): Brain Mechanisms and Perceptual Awareness. New York, Raven Press, 1981, pp 405-429.

69. Webster HW, Frideman L, Jones BE: Modification of paradoxical sleep following transections of the reticular formation at the pontomedullary junction. Sleep 1986;9:1-23.

70. Mileykovskiy BY, Kiyashchenko LI, Kodama T, et al: Activation of pontine medullary motor inhibitory regions reduces discharge in neurons located in the locus coeruleus and the anatomical equivalent of the midbrain locomotor region. J Neurosci 2000;20:8551-8558.

71. Mileykovskiy BY, Kiyashchenko LI, Siegel JM: Cessation of activity in red nucleus neurons during stimulation of medial medulla in decerebrate rats. J Physiol 2002;543:997-1006.

72. Chase MH: The motor functions of the reticular formation are multifaceted and state-determined. In Hobson JA, Brazier MAB (eds): The reticular formation revisited. New York, Raven Press, 1980, pp 449-472.

73. Askenasy JJ, Weitzman ED, Yahr MD: Rapid eye movements—expression of a general muscular phasic event of the REM state. Sleep Res 1983;12:172.

74. Chase MH, Morales FR: Subthreshold excitatory activity and motoneuron discharge during REM periods of active sleep. Science 1983;221:1195-1198.

75. Emde RN, Koenig KL: Neonatal smiling, frowning, and rapid eye movement states II. Sleep-cycle study. J Am Acad Child Psychiatry 1969;8:637-656.

76. Emde RN, Koening KL: Neonatal smiling and rapid eye movement states. J Am Acad Child Psychiatry 1969;8:57-67.

77. Meier GW, Berger RJ: Development of sleep and wakefulness patterns in the infant rhesus monkey. Exp Neurol 1965;12:257-277.

78. Jouvet-Mournier D, Astic L, Lacote D: Ontogenesis of the states of sleep in rat, cat and guinea pig during the first postnatal month. Devel Psychobiol 1970;2:216-239.

79. Luce GG: The development of rhythms: Youth and age. In Luce GG (ed): Biological Rhythms in Psychiatry and Medicine. Washington DC, U.S. Department of Health, Education, and Welfare publication (ADM)78-247, 1970.

80. Corner MA: Maturation of sleep mechanism in the central nervous system. Exp Brain Res 1984;54(Suppl 8):50-66.

81. Corner MA: Ontogeny of brain sleep mechanisms. In McGinty DJ, Drucker-Colin R, Morrison AR, et al (eds): Brain Mechanisms of Sleep. New York, Raven Press, 1985, pp 175-197.

82. Rigatto H, More M, Cates D: Fetal breathing and behavior measured through a double-wall plexiglas window in sheep. J Appl Physiol 1986;61:160-164.

83. Roffwarg HP, Muzzio JN, Dement WC: Ontogenetic development of the human sleep-dream cycle. Science 1966;152:604-619.

84. Corner MA: Spontaneous motor rhythms in early life—phenomenological and neurophysiological aspects. In Corner MA, Baker RE, van de Poll NE, et al (eds): Maturation of the Nervous System, Progress in Brain Research vol 45. Amsterdam, Elsevier, 1978.

85. Denenberg VH, Thoman EB: Evidence for a functional role for active (REM) sleep in infancy. Sleep 1981;4:185-191.

86. Campbell SS, Tobler I: Animal sleep: A review of sleep duration across phylogeny. Neurosci Biobehav Rev 1984;8:269-300.

87. Rechtschaffen A, Kales A: A Manual of Standardized Terminology: Techniques and Scoring System for Sleep Stages of Human Subjects. Los Angeles, UCLA Brain Information Service/Brain Research Institute, 1968.

88. Henly K, Morrison AR: A re-evaluation of the effects of lesions of the pontine tegmentum and locus coeruleus on phenomena of paradoxical sleep in the cat. Acta Neurobiol Exp 1974; 34:215-232.

89. Trulson ME, Jacobs BL, Morrison AR: Raphe unit activity during REM sleep in normal cats and in pontine lesioned cats displaying REM sleep without atonia. Brain Res 1981; 226:75-91.

90. Friedman L, Jones BE: Study of sleep-wakefulness states by computer graphics and cluster analysis before and after lesions of the pontine tegmentum in the cat. EEG Clin Neurophysiol 1984;57:43-56.

91. Lai YY, Siegel JM: Medullary regions mediating atonia. J Neurosci 1988;8:4790-4796.

92. Lai YY, Siegel JM: Muscle tone suppression and stepping produced by stimulation of midbrain and rostral pontine reticular formation. J Neurosci 1990;10:2727-2734.

93. Eisensehr I, Linke R, Noachtar S, et al: Reduced striatal dopamine transporters in idiopathic rapid eye movement sleep behavior disorder. Comparison with Parkinson's disease and controls. Brain 2000;123:1155-1160.

94. Eisensehr I, Linke R, Tatsch K, et al: Increased muscle activity during rapid eye movement sleep correlates with decrease of striatal presynaptic dopamine transporters. IPT and IBZM SPECT imaging in subclinical and clinically manifest idiopathic REM sleep behavior disorder, Parkinson's disease, and controls. Sleep 2003;26:507-512.

95. Albin RL, Koeppe RA, Chervin RD, et al: Decreased striatal dopaminergic innervation in REM sleep behavior disorder. Neurology 2000;55:1410-1412.

96. Shirakawa S-I, Takeuchi N, Uchimura N, et al: Study of image findings in rapid eye movement sleep behavioral disorder. Psychiatry Clin Neurosci 2002;56:291-292.

97. Miyamoto M, Miyamoto T, Kubo J, et al: Brainstem function in rapid eye movement sleep behavior disorder: The evaluation of brainstem function by proton MR spectroscopy (^{1}H-MRS). Psychiatry Clin Neurosci 2000;54:350-351.

98. Gilman S, Koeppe RA, Chervin R, et al: REM sleep behavior disorder is related to striatal monoaminergic deficit in MSA. Neurology 2003;61:29-34.

99. Fantini ML, Gagnon JF, Petit D, et al: Slowing of electroencephalogram in rapid eye movement sleep behavior disorder. Ann Neurol 2003;53:774-780.

100. Lasegue C: Le delire alcoolique n'est pas un delire, mais un reve. Arch Gen Med 1881;88:513-586.

101. Gross MM, Godenough D, Tobin M, et al: Sleep disturbances and hallucinations in the acute alcoholic psychoses. J Nerv Ment Dis 1966;142:493-514.

102. Greenberg R, Pearlman C: Delirium tremens and dreaming. Am J Psychiatry 1967;124:37-46.

103. Hishikawa Y, Sugita Y, Teshima Y, et al: Sleep disorders in alcoholic patients with delirium tremens and transient withdrawal hallucinations—reevaluation of the REM rebound and intrusion theory. In Karacan I (ed): Psychophysiological Aspects of Sleep. Park Ridge, NJ, Noyes Medical Publishers, 1981, pp 109-22.

104. Tachibana M, Tanaka K, Hishikawa Y, Kaneko Z: A sleep study of acute psychotic states due to alcohol and meprobamate addiction. Adv Sleep Res 1975;2:177-205.

105. Passouant P, Cadilhac J, Ribstein M: Les privations de sommeil avec mouvements oculaires par les anti-depresseurs. Rev Neurol 1972;127:173-192.

106. Guilleminault C, Raynal D, Takahashi S, et al: Evaluation of short-term and long-term treatment of the narcolepsy syndrome with clomipramine hydrochloride. Acta Neurol Scand 1976;54:71-87.

107. Besset A: Effect of antidepressants on human sleep. Adv Biosci 1978;21:141-148.

108. Shimizu T, Ookawa M, Iijuma S, et al: Effect of clomipramine on nocturnal sleep of normal human subjects. Ann Rev Pharmacopsychiat Res Found 1985;16:138.

109. Bental E, Lavie P, Sharf B: Severe hypermotility during sleep in treatment of cataplexy with clomipramine. Israel J Med Sci 1979;15:607-609.

110. Akindele MO, Evans JI, Oswald I: Mono-amine oxidase inhibitors, sleep and mood. EEG Clin Neurophysiol 1970;29:47-56.

111. Ross JS, Shua-Haim JR: Aricept-induced nightmares in Alzheimer's disease: 2 case reports. J Am Geriatr Soc 1998;46:119-120.

112. Schenck CH, Mahowald MW, Kim SW, et al: Prominent eye movements during NREM sleep and REM sleep behavior disorder associated with fluoxetine treatment of depression and obsessive-compulsive disorder. Sleep 1992;15:226-235.

113. Schutte S, Doghramji K: REM behavior disorder seen with venlafaxine (Effexor). Sleep Res 1996;25:364.

114. Nash JR, Wilson SJ, Potokar JP, Nutt DJ: Mirtazapine induces REM sleep behavior disorder (RBD) in parkinsonism. Neurology 2003;61:1161.

115. Stolz SE, Aldrich MS: REM sleep behavior disorder associated with caffeine abuse. Sleep Res 1991;20:341.

116. Vorona RD, Ware JC: Exacerbation of REM sleep behavior disorder by chocolate ingestion: A case report. Sleep Med 2002;3:365-367.

117. Guilleminault C, Monini S: Mononucleosis and chronic daytime sleepiness. A long-term follow-up study. Arch Intern Med 1986;146:1333-1335.

118. Lavie P, Pratt H, Sharf B, et al: Localized pontine lesion: Nearly total absence of REM sleep. Neurology 1984;34:118-120.

119. Hefez A, Metz L, Lavie P: Long-term effects of extreme situational stress on sleep and dreaming. Am J Psychiatry 1987;144:344-347.

120. Schenck CH, Bundlie SR, Patterson AL, Mahowald MW: Rapid eye movement sleep behavior disorder. A treatable parasomnia affecting older adults. JAMA 1987;257:1786-1789.

121. Sugita Y, Taniguchi M, Terashima K, et al: A young case of idiopathic REM sleep behavior disorder (RBD) specifically induced by socially stressful conditions. Sleep Res 1991; 20A:394.

122. Cohen LG, Roth BJ, Wassermann EM, et al: Magnetic stimulation of the human cortex, an indicator of reorganization of motor pathways in certain pathological conditions. J Clin Neurophysiol 1991;8:56-65.

123. Kandel ER: Environmental determinants of brain architecture and of behavior: Early experience and learning. In Kandel ER, Schwartz JH (eds): Principles of Neural Science. New York, Elsevier-North Holland, 1981, pp 620-632.

124. Pons TP, Garraghty PE, Ommaya K, et al: Massive cortical reorganization after sensory deafferentation in adult Macaques. Science 1991;252:1857-1860.

125. Schenck CH, Bundlie SR, Smith SA, et al: REM behavior disorder in a 10 year old girl and aperiodic REM and NREM sleep movements in an 8 year old brother. Sleep Res 1986;15:162.

126. Hendricks JC, Lager A, O'Brien D, Morrison AR: Movement disorders during sleep in cats and dogs. J Am Vet Med Assoc 1989;194:686-689.

127. Hendricks JC, Morrison AR, Farnbach GL, et al: Disorder of rapid eye movement sleep in a cat. J Am Vet Med Assoc 1980; 178:55-57.

128. Lugaresi E, Medori R, Montagna P, et al: Fatal familial insomnia and dysautonomia with selective degeneration of thalamic nuclei. N Engl J Med 1986;315:997-1003.

129. Morrison AR, Reiner PB: A dissection of paradoxical sleep. In McGinty DJ, Drucker-Colin R, Morrison A, et al. (eds): Brain Mechanisms of Sleep. New York, Raven Press, 1985.

130. Schenck CH, Duncan E, Hopwood J, et al: The human REM sleep behavior disorder (RBD):quantitative polygraphic and behavioral analysis of 9 cases. Sleep Res 1988;17:14.

131. Lapierre O, Montplaisir J: Polysomnographic features of REM sleep behavior disorder: Development of a scoring method. Neurology 1992;42:1371-1374.

132. Moyer KE: Kinds of aggression and their physiological basis. Comm Behav Biol 1968;2 (part A):65-87.

133. Goldstein M: Brain research and violent behavior. Arch Neurol 1974;30:1-34.

134. Coffey CE, Licke JF, Saxton JA, et al: Sex differences in brain aging. A quantitative magnetic resonance imaging study. Arch Neurol 1998;55:169-179.

135. Corner MA, Ramakers GJA: Spontaneous firing as an epigenetic factor in brain development—physiological consequences of chronic tetrodotoxin and picrotoxin exposure on cultured rat neocortex neurons. Dev Brain Res 1992;65:57-64.

136. Corner MA, Mirmiran M, Bour HLMG, et al: Does rapid eye movement sleep play a role in brain development? Prog Brain Res 1980;53:347-356.

137. Brashear HR, Phillips II LH: Autoantibodies to GABAergic neurons and response to plasmapheresis in stiff-man syndrome. Neurology 1991;41:1588-1592.

138. Schenck CH, Ullevig CM, Mahowald MW, et al: A controlled study of serum anti–locus ceruleus antibodies in REM sleep behavior disorder. Sleep 1997;20:349-351.

139. Schenck CH, Mahowald MW: Polysomnographic, neurologic, psychiatric, and clinical outcome report on 70 consecutive cases with REM sleep behavior disorder (RBD): Sustained clonazepam efficacy in 89.5% of 57 treated patients. Cleve Clin J Med 1990;57(Suppl):S9-S23.

140. Mahowald MW, Schenck CH: REM sleep behavior disorder. In Thorpy MJ (ed): Handbook of Sleep Disorders. New York, Marcel Dekker, 1990, pp 567-593.

141. Mahowald MW, Schenck CH: Parasomnias: Sleepwalking and the law. Sleep Med Rev 2000;4:321-339.

142. Yeh SB, Schenck CH: A case of marital discord and secondary depression with attempted suicide resulting from REM sleep behavior disorder in a 35-year-old woman. Sleep Med 2004; 5:151-154

143. Schenck CH, Mahowald MW: Injurious sleep behavior disorders (parasomnias) affecting patients on intensive care units. Intensive Care Med 1991;17:219-224.

144. American Psychiatric Association: Diagnostic and Statistical Manual of Mental Disorders, 3rd ed. Washington, DC, American Psychiatric Association, 1987.

145. Hobson JA, McCarley RW: The brain as a dream state generator: An activation-synthesis hypothesis of the dream process. Am J Psychiatry 1977;134:1335-1348.

146. McCarley RW, Hobson JA: The form of dreams and the biology of sleep. In Wolman BB (ed): The Handbook of Dreams. New York, Van Nostrand Reinhold, 1979, pp 76-130.

147. McCarley RW: REM dreams, REM sleep and their isomorphisms. In Chase M, Weitzman ED (eds): Sleep Disorders, Basic and Clinical Research. New York, SP Medical and Scientific Books, 1983, pp 363-393.

148. Dyken ME, Lin-Dyken DC, Seaba P, Yamada T: Violent sleep-related behavior leading to subdural hemorrhage. Arch Neurol 1995;52:318-321.

149. Gross PT: REM sleep behavior disorder causing bilateral subdural hematomas. Sleep Res 1992;21:204.

150. Morfis L, Schwartz RS, Cistulli PA: REM sleep behavior disorder; a treatable cause of falls in elderly people. Age Ageing 1997;26:43-44.

151. Siegel JM: Mechanisms of sleep control. J Clin Neurophysiol 1990;7:49-65.

152. Broughton R, Tolentino MA: Fragmentary pathological myoclonus in NREM sleep. EEG Clin Neurophysiol 1984;57: 303-309.

153. Broughton R, Tolentino MA, Krelina M: Excessive fragmentary myoclonus in NREM sleep: A report of 38 cases. EEG Clin Neurophysiol 1985;61:123-133.

154. Mouret J: Differences in sleep in patients with parkinson's disease. EEG Clin Neurophysiol 1975;38:653-657.

155. Askenasy JJM: Sleep patterns in extrapyramidal disorders. Int J Neurol 1981;15:62-76.

156. Taska L, Kupfer D: A system for the quantification of phasic ocular activity during REM sleep. Sleep Watchers 1983; 6:15-17.

157. Carskadon MA, Dement WC, Mitler MM, et al: Guidelines for the multiple sleep latency test (MSLT): A standard measure of sleepiness. Sleep 1986;9:519-524.

158. Mahowald MW, Schenck CH: Parasomnia purgatory—the epileptic/non-epileptic interface. In Rowan AJ, Gates JR (eds): Non-Epileptic Seizures. Boston, Butterworth-Heinemann, 1993, pp 123-139.

159. Nalamalapu U, Goldberg R, DePhillipo M, Fry JM: Behaviors simulating REM behavior disorder in patients with severe obstructive sleep apnea. Sleep Res 1996;25:311.

160. D'Cruz OF, Vaughn BV: Nocturnal seizures mimic REM behavior disorder. Am J Electroneurodiagn Technol 1997;37: 258-264.

161. Schenck CH, Boyd JL, Mahowald MW: A parasomnia overlap disorder involving sleepwalking, sleep terrors, and REM sleep behavior disorder in 33 polysomnographically confirmed cases. Sleep 1997;20:972-981.

162. Tachibana N, Sugita Y, Terashima K, et al: Polysomnographic characteristics of healthy elderly subjects with somnambulism-like behaviors. Biol Psychiatry 1991;30:4-14.

163. Schenck CS, Milner DM, Hurwitz TD, et al: Dissociative disorders presenting as somnambulism: Polysomnographic, video, and clinical documentation (8 cases). Dissociation 1989;4:194-204.

164. Mahowald MW, Schenck CH, Rosen GR, Hurwitz TD: The role of a sleep disorders center in evaluating sleep violence. Arch Neurol 1992;49:604-607.

165. Mahowald MW, Schenck CH: Status dissociatus—a perspective on states of being. Sleep 1991;14:69-79.

166. Mahowald MW, Schenck CH: Dissociated states of wakefulness and sleep. Neurology 1992;42:44-52.

167. Lugaresi E, Provini F: Agrypnia excitata: Clinical features and pathophysiological implications. Sleep Med Rev 2001; 5:313-322.

168. Montagna P, Lugaresi E: Agrypnia excitata: A generalized over-activity syndrome and a useful concept in the neurophysiology of sleep. Clin Neurophysiol 2002;113:552-560.

169. Plazzi G, Montagna P, Meletti S, Lugaresi E: Polysomnographic study of sleeplessness and onericisms in the alcohol withdrawal syndrome. Sleep Med 2002;3:279-282.

170. Cibula JE, Eisenschenk S, Gold M, et al: Progressive dementia and hypersomnolence with dream-enacting behavior. Oneiric dementia. Arch Neurol 2002;59:630-634.

171. Schenck CH, Hurwitz TD, Bundlie SR, Mahowald MW: Sleep-related injury in 100 adult patients: A polysomnographic and clinical report. Am J Psychiatry 1989;146:1166-1173.

172. Goldberg MA, Dorman JD: Intention myoclonus: Successful treatment with clonazepam. Neurology 1976;26:24-26.

173. Hoehn MM, Cherington M: Spinal myoclonus. Neurology 1977;27:942-946.

174. Montagna P, Provini F, Plazzi G, et al: Propriospinal myoclonus upon relaxation and drowsiness: A cause of severe insomnia. Mov Disord 1997;12:66-72.

175. Sunohara N, Mukoyama M, Mano Y, Satoyoshi E: Action-induced rhythmic dystonia: An autopsy case. Neurology 1984;34:321-327.

176. Pieris JB, Boralessa H, Lionel NDW: Clonazepam treatment of choreiform activity. Med J Aust 1976;1:225-227.

177. Chouinard G, Young KN, Annable L: Antimanic effect of clonazepam. Biol Psychiatry 1983;18:451-466.

178. Feinhar JP, Alvarez WH: Use of clonazepam in two cases of acute mania. J Clin Psychiatry 1985;46:29-30.

179. Ohstory MA, Vijayan N: Clonazepam treatment of insomnia due to sleep myoclonus. Arch Neurol 1980;37:119-120.

180. Montplaisir J, Godbout R, Boghen D, et al: Familial restless legs with periodic movements in sleep: Electrophysiologic, biochemical and pharmacologic study. Neurology 1985;35: 130-134.

181. Ohanna N, Peled R, Rubin A-H, et al: Periodic leg movements in sleep: Effect of clonazepam treatment. Neurology 1985; 35:408-411.

182. Mitler MM, Browman CP, Menn SJ, et al: Nocturnal myoclonus: Treatment efficacy of clonazepam and temazepam. Sleep 1986;9:385-392.

183. Goldbloom D, Chouinard G: Clonazepam in the treatment of neuroleptic-induced somnambulism. Am J Psychiatry 1984; 141:1486.

184. Browne TR: Clonazepam. New England J Med 1978;299: 812-818.

185. Chadwick D, Hallet M, Harris R, et al: Clinical, biochemical and physiological features distinguishing myoclonus responsive to 5-hydroxytryptophan, tryptophan with a monoamine oxidase inhibitor and clonazepam. Brain 1977;100:455-487.

186. Green RA, Gillin JC, Wyatt RJ: The inhibitory effect of intraventricular administration of serotonin on spontaneous motor activity of rats. Psychopharmacology 1976;51:81-84.

187. Hollister AS, Breese GR, Kuhn CM, et al: An inhibitory role for brain serotonin-containing systems in the locomotor effects of D-amphetamine. J Pharmacol Exp Ther 1976;198: 12-22.

188. Fleisher LN, Simon JR, Aprison MH: A biochemical-behavioral model for studying serotonergic supersensitivity in brain. J Neurochem 1979;32:1613-1619.

189. Tabakoff B, Hoffman PL: Measures of physical dependence and involvement of serotonin in withdrawal symptomatology. In Gross MM (ed): Alcohol Intoxication and Withdrawal, IIIa. Biological Aspects of Ethanol. New York, Plenum Press, 1977, pp 547-557.

190. Lapierre O, Casademont A, Montplaisir J, et al: Tonic and phasic features of REM sleep behavior disorder. Sleep Res 1991;20:276.

191. Kunz D, Bes F: Effects of exogenous melatonin on periodic limb movment disorder: An open pilot study. Sleep 1999; 22:S162.

192. Boeve BF, Silber MH, Ferman JT: Melatonin for treatment of REM sleep behavior disorder in neurologic disorders: Results in 14 patients. Sleep Med 2003;4:281-284.

193. Takeuchi N, Uchimura N, Hashizume Y, et al: Melatonin therapy for REM sleep behavior disorder. Psychiatry Clin Neurosci 2001;55:267-269.

194. Matsumoto M, Mutoh F, Naoe H, et al: The effects of imipramine on REM sleep behavior disorder in 3 cases. Sleep Res 1991;20A:351.

195. Cowen PJ, Gearey DP, Schacter M, et al: Desipramine treatment in normal subjects. Arch Gen Psychiatry 1986; 43:61-67.

196. Fantini ML, Gagnon J-F, Filipini D, Montplaisir J: The effects of pramipexole in REM sleep behavior disorder. Neurology 2003;61:1418-1420.

197. Tan A, Salgado M, Fahn S: Rapid eye movement sleep behavior disorder preceding Parkinson's disease with therapeutic response to levodopa. Mov Disord 1996;11:214-216.

198. Bamford C: Carbamazepine in REM sleep behavior disorder. Sleep 1993;16:33.

199. Mike ME, Kranz AJ: MAOI suppression of R.B.D. refractory to clonazepam and other agents. Sleep Res 1996;25:63.

200. Ringman JM, Simmons JH: Treatment of REM sleep behavior disorder with donepezil: A report of three cases. Neurology 2000;55:870-871.

201. Rye DB, Dempsay J, Dihenia B, et al: REM-sleep dyscontrol in Parkinson's disease: Case report of effects of elective pallidotomy. Sleep Res 1997;26:591.

202. Iranzo A, Valldeoriola F, Santamaria J, et al: Sleep symptoms and polysomnographic architecture in advanced Parkinson's disease after chronic bilateral subthalamic stimulation. J Neurol Neurosurg Psychiatry 2002;72:661-664.

203. Arnulf I, Bejjani BP, Garma L, et al: Improvement of sleep architecture in PD with subthalamic stimulation. Neurology 2000;55:1732-1734.

204. Mori SH: Integration of posture and locomotion in acute decerebrate cats and in awake, freely moving cats. Prog Neurobiol 1987;28:161-195.

205. Grillner S, Dubic R: Control of locomotion in vertebrates: Spinal and supraspinal mechanisms. Adv Neurol 1988;47: 425-453.

206. Berntson GG, Micco DJ: Organization of brainstem behavioral systems. Brain Res Bull 1976;1:471-483.

207. Mogenson GJ: Limbic-motor integration. Progr Psychobiol Physiol Psychol 1986;12:117-170.

208. Mori S, Nishimura H, Aoki M: Brain stem activation of the spinal stepping generator. In Hobson JA, Brazier MAB (eds): The Reticular Formation Revisited. New York, Raven Press, 1980, pp 241-259.

209. Diagnostic Classification Steering Committee: ICSD: International Classification of Sleep Disorders: Diagnostic and Coding Manual. Rochester, Minn, American Academy of Sleep Medicine, 1990.

210. Guilleminault C, Pool P, Motta J, Gillis AM: Sinus arrest during REM sleep in young adults. N Engl J Med 1984;311: 1106-1110.

211. Rattenborg NC, Lindblom S, Best J, et al: REM sleep-related asystole associated with unusual polysomnographic features: A case history. Sleep Res 1995;24:324.

212. Steiger A, Benkert O: Examination and treatment of sleep-related painful erections—a case report. Arch Sex Behav 1989; 18:263-267.

213. Ferini-Strambi L, Zucconi M, Castronovo V, et al: Sleep-related painful erections: Clinical and polysomnographic findings. Sleep Res 1996;25:241.

214. Schenck CH, Mahowald MW: REM sleep behavior disorder: Clinical, developmental, and neuroscience perspectives 16 years after its formal identification in *Sleep*. Sleep 2002; 25:120-130.

215. Kotorii T, Nakazawa Y, Yokoyama T, et al: The sleep pattern of chronic alcoholics during the alcohol withdrawal period. Folia Psychiat Neurol Jpn 1980;34:89-95.

216. Tanaka K, Kameda H, Sugita Y, Hishikawa Y: A case with pentazocine dependence developing delirium upon withdrawal. Seishin Shinkeigaku Zasshi 1979;81:289-299.

217. Hobson JA: Dreaming sleep attacks and desynchronized sleep enhancement. Arch Gen Psychiatry 1975;32:1421-1424.

218. Culebras A, Moore JT: Magnetic resonance findings in REM sleep behavior disorder. Neurology 1989;39:1519-1523.

219. Isono G, Ishii H, Shibata Y, et al: REM sleep with tonic muscle discharge observed in a patient with acoustic neuroma. Clin Psychiatry 1979;21:1221-1228 (in Japanese).

220. DeBarros-Ferreira M, Chodkiewicz J-P, Lairy GC, Salzarulo P: Disorganized relations of tonic and phasic events of REM sleep in a case of brain-stem tumor. EEG Clin Neurophysiol 1975;38:203-207.

221. Minz M, Autret A, Laffont F, et al: A study on sleep in amyotrophic lateral sclerosis. Biomedicine 1979;30:40-46.

222. Minami R, Harada M: Nocturnal delirium and REM sleep. Clin EEG 1979;21:315-325 (in Japanese).

223. Matsuo R, Iijima S, Sugita Y, et al: Sleep study of aged patients with nocturnal delirium. Jpn J EEG EMG 1980;8:38 (in Japanese).

224. Turner RS, Chervin RD, Frey KA, et al: Probable diffuse Lewy body disease presenting as REM sleep behavior disorder. Neurology 1997;49:523-527.

225. Kimura K, Tachibana N, Aso T, et al: Subclinical REM sleep behavior disorder in a patient with corticobasal degeneration. Sleep 1997;20:891-894.

226. Schenck CH, Slater GE, Sherman RE, et al: Multiple sclerosis and sleep: Survey report and polygraphic detection of REM and NREM motor abnormalities. Sleep Res 1986;15:163.

227. Shimizu T, Tabushi K, Iijima S, et al: Sleep study in patients with OPCA and related diseases. Jpn J EEG EMG 1980;8:38 (in Japanese).

228. Shimizu T, Sugita Y, Iijima S, et al: Sleep study in Shy-Drager syndrome. Clin. Neurol (Japan) 1981;21:218-227.

229. Salva MA, Guilleminault C: Olivopontocerebellar degeneration, abnormal sleep, and REM sleep without atonia. Neurology 1986;36:576-577.

230. Sforza E, Zucconi M, Petronelli R, et al: REM sleep behavioral disorders. Eur Neurol 1988;28:295-300.

231. Tachibana N, Kimura K, Kitajima K, et al: REM sleep without atonia at early stage of sporadic olivopontocerebellar atrophy. J Neurol Sci 1995;132:28-34.

232. April RS: Observations on parkinsonian tremor in all-night sleep. Neurology 1966;16:720-724.

233. Stern M, Roffwarg H, Duvoisin R: The parkinsonian tremor in sleep. J Nerv Men Dis 1968;147:202-210.

234. Boeve BF, Silber MH, Petersen RC, et al: REM sleep behavior disorder and degenerative dementia with or without parkinsonism: A syndrome predictive of Lewy body disease. Neurology 1997;49:a358-359 (abstract).

235. Shimizu T: A polygraphic study of nocturnal sleep in degenerative diseases - a possible mechanism of nocturnal delirium in patients with organic brain conditions. Adv Neurol Sci (Tokyo) 1985;29:154-177.

236. Wright BA, Rosen JR, Buysse DJ, et al: Shy-Drager syndrome presenting as a REM behavior disorder. J Geriatr Psychiatry Neurol 1990;3:110-113.

237. Plazzi G, Corsini R, Provini F, et al: REM sleep behavior disorders in multiple system atrophy. Neurology 1997;48: 1094-1097.

238. Tison F, Wenning GK, Quinn NP, Smith SJM: REM sleep behavior disorder as the presenting symptom of multiple system atrophy. J Neurol Neurosurg Psychiatry 1995;58:379-380.

239. Tachibana N, Kimura K, Kitajima K, et al: REM sleep motor dysfunction in multiple system atrophy. Sleep Res 1995; 24A:415.

240. Mayer G, Meier-Ewert K: Motor dyscontrol in sleep of narcoleptic patients (a lifelong development?). J Sleep Res 1993; 2:143.

241. Ishigooka J, Westendorf F, Oguchi T, et al: Somnambulistic behavior associated with abnormal REM sleep in an elderly woman. Biol Psychiatry 1985;20:1003-1008

76

Other Parasomnias

Mark W. Mahowald

ABSTRACT

Parasomnias may conveniently be divided into two major categories: primary parasomnias, which are due to disorders of sleep per se, and secondary parasomnias, which are due to dysfunction of other organ systems that take advantage of the sleeping state to declare themselves. By far, the primary sleep parasomnias are the most common. They are usually disorders of arousal if from NREM sleep and the REM sleep behavior disorder if from REM sleep. There remains a large group of other parasomnias, many of which are poorly understood, that may cause impressive and distressing behavior arising from the sleep period but that are unrelated to disorders of arousal or RBD. This chapter will discuss these less-common but fascinating phenomena.

NORMAL SLEEP PHENOMENA

Some normal phenomena arising from REM or NREM sleep may be bothersome enough to a patient to seek medical attention.

Sleep Paralysis

Sleep paralysis likely represents the persistence of REM sleep atonia into wakefulness and is extremely common in non-narcoleptics, occurring in more than 33% of the general population. It may be familial, and it is more common in the setting of sleep deprivation and being in the supine position.[1-3] When occurring in isolation, it may lead to erroneous diagnoses such as cardiac disease or seizures or to unwarranted psychiatric diagnoses.[4] Rarely, episodes of periodic paralysis arising from the sleep period may be confused with true sleep paralysis.[5,6] Management is reassurance that this is a normal phenomenon.

Hypnagogic and Hypnopompic Hallucinations

Prominent vivid dream-like mentation may occur at sleep onset, during light NREM sleep, and even during relaxed wakefulness.[7-12] As with sleep paralysis, such sleep onset (hypnagogic) and sleep offset (hypnopompic) hallucinatory phenomena are quite common in the nonnarcoleptic population, and they may be combined with sleep paralysis (often referred to as the "old hag" phenomenon).[13-17] As a matter of fact, the original meaning of the word "nightmare" referred not to the current use of the term (a dream anxiety attack arising from the sleep period) but rather to a combination of sleep paralysis and hypnagogic hallucinations occurring at sleep onset.[18,19] Patients can be reassured that these hallucinations are normal sleep phenomena and not symptoms of psychiatric disease.

Sleep Starts (Hypnic Jerks)

Sleep starts are experienced by many healthy persons during the transition between wake and sleep. The most common is the motor sleep start, a sudden jerk of all or part of the body, occasionally awakening the victim or bed partner. These are so prevalent as to rarely result in neurologic consultation.[20] However, variations on this theme may result in neurologic consultation. These sleep starts include the visual (flashes of light, fragmentary visual hallucinations), auditory (loud bangs, snapping noises) or somesthetic (pain, tingling, floating, something flowing through the body) types. These sensory phenomena may occur without the body jerk.[7,21-24] Explosive tinnitus, characterized by a loud "crashing" or "banging" noise occurring during sleep most likely represents an auditory sleep start.[25]

Sleep starts represent a normal (although not understood) physiologic event, and should not be confused with seizures or other neurologic conditions. Sleep starts may be repetitive and should not be confused with epileptic phenomena.[26,27] Familiarity with nonmotor sleep starts should eliminate unnecessary testing and pharmacologic treatment.[28] It is likely that the exploding head syndrome (see later discussion) is a variant of a sensory sleep start. Management is simply reassurance.

MISCELLANEOUS PRIMARY SLEEP PARASOMNIAS

There remain a number of primary sleep phenomena that are poorly understood and appear not to respect sleep stages. They are listed in Table 76–1.

Sleep-Related Expiratory Groaning (Catathrenia)

Groaning during sleep has been termed "catathrenia."[29] The groans occur intermittently during either REM or NREM sleep and are characterized by prolonged, often very loud, often socially disruptive groaning sounds during expiration. Catathrenia often begins in childhood, but it does not come to medical attention until the individual plans to sleep in a dormitory environment such as in college or the military, or when the patient plans to share a bed with another. It is poorly understood and awaits further definition and therapeutic studies.[30] There is no known effective treatment. There is absolutely no evidence that catathrenia is related to any underlying psychological or psychiatric problems. The fact that continuous positive airway pressure (CPAP) administration eliminated obstructive sleep apnea, but not catathrenia,

Table 76–1.   Sleep Parasomnias

NREM Sleep		REM Sleep		
Normal	**Abnormal**	**Normal**	**Abnormal**	**Miscellaneous**
Sleep starts: Motor Sensory (visual, auditory, somesthetic) Exploding head syndrome Explosive tinnitus	Disorders of arousal: Confusional arousals, sleepwalking, sleep terrors	Sleep paralysis Hypnagogic or hypnopompic hallucinations	REM sleep behavior disorder REM-related painful erections Dream anxiety attacks (nightmares)	Nocturnal groaning (catathrenia) Bruxism Enuresis rhythmic movement disorder Propriospinal myoclonus Somniloquy (sleeptalking)

in one patient with both conditions speaks against static upper airway resistance as an etiology.[31]

Bruxism (Teeth Grinding)

Bruxism is discussed in Chapter 79.

Enuresis

Enuresis was formerly classified as a "disorder of arousal," implying a relationship with slow wave sleep.[32] However, enuresis may occur during either NREM or REM sleep, and the sleep of enuretic children is normal.[33] Enuresis is very frequent in childhood, and it is much more prevalent in adolescence and adulthood than generally appreciated (1% to 2% of 18 year olds and 0.5% of adults).[34,35]

Many etiologies have been suggested, including genetic,[36] behavioral and psychological, bladder size or reactivity abnormalities, lack of vasopressin release during sleep, and delayed development.[37-39] Despite considerable research, the causes of enuresis remain enigmatic.[40] Local urologic abnormalities account for only 2% to 4% of pediatric cases.[41,42] No specific psychopathology has been identified, and there is overwhelming evidence that enuretic children have no more behavioral or psychological problems than nonenuretic children, and that genetic factors are important.[43,44]

Formal urologic evaluation is usually not indicated, and simple reassurance and understanding on the part of both the child and parents are often sufficient. Conditioning with a bell-and-pad device is effective, but it may be transient.[45-47] Psychotherapy is generally ineffective and indicated only if obvious psychopathology is present.[34,40] Tricyclic antidepressants (imipramine or desipramine) are effective and may be employed for short-term treatment, but long-term pharmacologic treatment is to be discouraged. The mechanism of action of the tricyclics is not known, but it appears not to involve peripheral anticholinergic effects.[48] Desmopressin, an intranasally administered vasopressin analogue, has been reported to be of benefit.[49]

Enuresis may be the sole manifestation of nocturnal seizures and may accompany obstructive sleep apnea or other primary sleep disorders.[50] Formal polysomnographic study with a full seizure montage and enuresis detector is indicated in those cases with atypical histories or failure to respond to conventional therapy.

Rhythmic Movement Disorder

Rhythmic movement disorder (RMD), formerly termed *jactatio capitis nocturna,* refers to a group of actions characterized by stereotyped movements (rhythmic oscillation of the head or limbs; head-banging or body-rocking during sleep) seen most frequently in childhood. Its persistence into adulthood is not uncommon.[51,52] It may be familial in some cases. RMD may arise from all stages of sleep, including REM sleep,[53,54] and it may occur in the transition from wake to sleep. Significant injury from repetitive pounding may result.[55]

The etiology of RMD is unknown, and no systematic studies of pharmacologic or behavioral treatment have been reported, although tricyclic antidepressants and benzodiazepines, particularly clonazepam, may be effective.[56-59] Preliminary data suggest that the use of a waterbed may improve the rhythmic behaviors.[60] Hypnosis has been effective in a single case.[61] Posttraumatic cases involving only the foot have been reported.[62] Rarely, RMD may be the sole manifestation of a seizure.[63]

Propriospinal Myoclonus

Propriospinal myoclonus is a spinal-cord–mediated movement disorder that is occasionally associated with acquired spinal cord lesions. Propriospinal myoclonus may be confused with restless leg syndrome or periodic limb movement syndrome, and it may serve to shed light on the pathophysiology of these two sleep disorders.[64] The movements may appear during relaxation, and they may result in severe insomnia, particularly at sleep onset.[65] Clonazepam or anticonvulsant medications may be effective in alleviating these movements.[66] Propriospinal myoclonus may be related to segmental myoclonus, both spinal and palatal.[67-69]

Somniloquy (Sleeptalking)

Sleeptalking is very common in the general population, may have a genetic component,[70-73] and may occur in either REM or NREM sleep.[74,75] Most cases are not associated with serious psychopathology.[71]

SECONDARY SLEEP PARASOMNIAS

The secondary phenomena are those parasomnias representing either abnormal or excessive autonomic or physiologic events arising from specific organ systems and occurring preferentially during the sleep period. These can be approached by addressing the offending organ system. See Table 76–2.

Central Nervous System Parasomnias

Seizures

Nocturnal seizures are an important cause of complex motor behavior arising from the sleep period. They are discussed in Chapter 72.

Table 76–2.   Secondary Sleep Parasomnias

Central Nervous System	Cardiopulmonary	Gastrointestinal	Miscellaneous
Headaches:	Cardiac arrhythmias	Gastroesophageal reflux	Nocturnal muscle cramps
Vascular	Nocturnal angina pectoris	Diffuse esophageal spasm	Nocturnal pruritus
Non-vascular	Nocturnal asthma	Abnormal swallowing	Night sweats
Exploding head syndrome	Respiratory dyskinesias		Nocturnal tongue biting
Hypnic headache	Miscellaneous:		Benign nocturnal alternating
Tinnitus	Sleep hiccup		hemiplegia of childhood
Seizures	Choking		
	Defibrillator shocks		
	Coughing		

Headaches

"VASCULAR" HEADACHES

Although these headaches have historically been referred to as "vascular headaches," there is now overwhelming evidence that the etiology is not vascular but rather is a primary neurologic one.[76] The headache symptoms of cluster headache, chronic paroxysmal hemicrania, and possibly migraines, in some cases, tend to be related to REM sleep, explaining the common report of sleep-related headaches in these conditions.[77-81] The connection with REM sleep explains the worsening of these symptoms following the discontinuation of REM-sleep suppressing agents (which results in a rebound of REM sleep) such as tricyclic antidepressants, monoamine oxidase inhibitors, clonidine, alcohol, and amphetamines.[82-84] Circadian rhythm abnormalities may play a role in cluster headache and chronic paroxysmal hemicrania.[85,86] Episodic paroxysmal hemicrania may respond to calcium channel blockers.[87] Sleep-disordered breathing may serve as a risk factor for headaches in some patients with cluster headaches.[88,89]

NONVASCULAR HEADACHES

Although morning headaches may be more prevalent in people with sleep complaints in general, headaches are not a reliable marker for sleep-disordered breathing.[90-92] However, in some susceptible persons, obstructive sleep apnea may trigger cluster headaches, which are responsive to bilevel positive airway pressure.[88,93] Headaches associated with sleep-disordered breathing are more commonly seen in patients with neuromuscular disease who experience REM-sleep–related hypo ventilation, with hypercapnia-induced migraines arising from the sleep period.

Carbon monoxide poisoning must never be forgotten as a cause of morning headaches.

Exploding Head Syndrome

This syndrome is characterized by the abrupt arousal, usually occurring in the transition from wake to sleep, with the sensation of a loud sound like an explosion or a sensation of "bursting" of the head.[94,95] Most reported cases occur in the twilight state of sleep onset, but polysomnographic recording has documented their occurrence during both wakefulness and well-declared REM sleep.[96,97] These events may represent a variant of sleep starts[98] and are usually benign; however, similar phenomena may represent the sole manifestation of a seizure.[99] Clomipramine or nifedipine may be effective, but they may not be indicated in most cases due to the benign nature of the condition.[96,100]

Hypnic Headache

The hypnic headache syndrome has been described in a number of older patients with regular awakenings from sleep at a consistent time of night (usually between four and six hours after sleep onset), occasionally during a dream. Hypnic headache is a diffuse headache generally lasting 30 to 60 minutes and is associated with nausea but no autonomic symptoms. Although only approximately 50 patients with this syndrome have been reported, it is likely more common than previously thought. The headaches are usually generalized, but they may be unilateral,[101] and they may be protracted.[102] This condition is believed to be a benign sleep-related headache syndrome affecting the elderly. The few cases studied during sleep suggest hypnic headache most frequently arises from REM sleep. It may also represent a circadian-rhythm phenomenon and may respond to lithium, indomethacin, prednisone, flunarizine, gabapentin, acetazolamide, or caffeine administered before bedtime.[103-111] A detailed neurologic history and examination should be performed to rule out focal neurologic conditions such as a posterior fossa meningioma masquerading as hypnic headache.[112]

Tinnitus

Tinnitus may persist during sleep, resulting in sleep complaints in up to 50% of patients.[113-115] The sleep complaints are not associated with mood or emotional distress.[116] Subjective improvement in sleep followed use of an electrical tinnitus suppressor.[117] In another study, nortriptyline decreased depression, functional disability, and loudness of tinnitus, but sleep was not mentioned.[118] This condition is poorly understood and requires more systematic study before any conclusions may be reached. Evidence exists that tinnitus may be centrally mediated.[119] The term "explosive tinnitus" most likely refers to an auditory sleep start.[25] There is no known predictably effective treatment.

Cardiopulmonary Parasomnias

Cardiac Arrhythmias

This topic is covered in Chapter 98.

Nocturnal Angina Pectoris

This topic is covered in Chapter 101.

Nocturnal Asthma

This topic is covered in Chapter 93.

Respiratory Dyskinesias

There are numerous respiratory dyskinesias that may occur or persist during the sleep period. These include segmental myoclonus, such as palatal myoclonus[67,120] or diaphragmatic flutter,[121-123] as well as paroxysmal dystonia.[124] Respiratory dyskinesias may also be the manifestation of neuroleptic-induced dyskinesias, and they may or may not persist during sleep.[125-128] The respiratory dyskenesias should be differentiated from unusual nocturnal seizures that manifest with primarily or exclusively respiratory symptoms.[129-131] Effective treatments remain to be identified.

Sleep Hiccup

Persistent hiccup may continue during all stages of sleep, but its appearance during sleep in persons with chronic hiccup is variable.[132] The frequency diminishes during sleep, more so in REM than NREM sleep. Interestingly, sleep hiccups are rarely associated with arousals.[133,134] No treatment studies are available.

Miscellaneous Cardiopulmonary Parasomnias

Isolated cases of sleep-related dyspnea and choking have been reported. The etiology and treatment are unclear.[30] Paroxysmal choking may be the sole manifestation of nocturnal seizures.[135]

Phantom shocks from implantable cardioverter-defibrillators have been reported. Patients are awakened from a sound sleep with the sensation of having received a defibrillator discharge. These were not associated with dream recall. By observation, there was a motor "jolt" associated with crying out—as though an actual shock had been administered. Review of the counters indicated that no shock had been delivered. These phantom shocks should be verified before medical treatment or device reprogramming is prescribed.[136]

Intractable cough associated with the supine position, presumably due to position-related collapse of the upper airway and responsive to nasal continuous positive airway pressure, has been reported.[137,138]

Gastrointestinal Parasomnias

Numerous gastrointestinal events may result in paroxysmal arousals during sleep, often mimicking disorders of other organ systems.

Gastroesophageal Reflux Disease (GERD)

This topic is covered in Chapter 107.

Diffuse Esophageal Spasm

Nocturnal diffuse esophageal spasm simulates nocturnal cardiac disease, occasionally even resulting in arrhythmias.[139,140] Diagnosis may be made with esophageal manometric monitoring. Treatment includes administration of anticholinergics, nitrates, or calcium antagonists.[141]

Abnormal Swallowing

Abnormal swallowing during sleep may cause arousals induced by coughing, aspiration, or choking. Polysomnographic studies show brief episodes of coughing and gagging.[142] Etiology and treatment are unknown.

Miscellaneous Secondary Parasomnias

Nocturnal Muscle Cramps

The complaint of muscle cramping, frequently nocturnal, is extremely common but poorly understood. The true incidence and etiology are unknown, and there has been no systematic study of nocturnal muscle cramps. A subjective response to quinine sulfate, magnesium, vitamin E, gabapentin, or verapamil has been reported, as has an isolated case responding to transcutaneous nerve stimulation.[143-148]

Nocturnal Pruritus

Patients with a wide variety of dermatologic disorders associated with pruritus may demonstrate recurrent episodes of scratching during sleep, resulting in sleep disruption.[149-151] These scratching episodes occur during all stages of sleep, being most frequent in light NREM, intermediate in REM, and least in slow wave sleep.[152,153] The duration of scratching episodes is the same among the sleep stages.[154] Anecdotal response to lidocaine patches or mirtazapine have been reported.[155,156] Such scratching may interfere with treatment, and it may play a role in factitious dermatoses.[157]

Night Sweats

Night sweats are very common, but tend not to be reported to physicians.[158] Night sweats (unrelated to infectious, endocrine, or malignant conditions) may be associated with a number of unrelated conditions including obstructive sleep apnea,[159] spinal syringomyelia,[160] medications,[158] gastroesophageal reflux,[161] or autonomic seizures.[162] Night sweats may also appear around the time of menopause.[163,164] The degree of sweating during sleep may be impressive, necessitating multiple nightly changes of pajamas and bedding. Benztropine reportedly has been effective in venlafaxine-induced night sweats.[165] There is no known effective treatment of idiopathic recurring night sweats.

Nocturnal Tongue Biting

Tongue biting during sleep has been reported as a manifestation of a number of unrelated conditions, including myoclonic activity, nocturnal seizures, disorders of arousal, or rhythmic movement disorder.[166-171]

Benign Nocturnal Alternating Hemiplegia of Childhood

This presumably rare condition is associated with brief periods of hemiplegia arising from the sleep period, rarely occurring during wakefulness. This condition may resolve spontaneously. There is no known treatment. The mechanism is unknown, but there is a high frequency of migraine in relatives. It may be a channelopathy such as hemiplegic migraine or episodic ataxia type 2.[172]

Functional Disorders

Table 76–3 lists the functional disorders.

Nocturnal Panic Attacks

Sleep-related panic attacks occur in many (30% to 50%) patients with diurnal panic, may precede the appearance of

Table 76-3.	**Functional Disorders**

Nocturnal panic attacks
Posttraumatic stress disorder
Psychogenic dissociative disorder
Malingering, conversion hysteria, Munchausen,
     Munchausen by proxy

diurnal panic, or may be exclusively nocturnal in nature.[173-176] Panic disorder can begin in childhood or adolescence and may masquerade as a wide variety of neurologic syndromes.[177,178] Subjective sleep complaints are common in patients with panic disorder (up to 70%) and include insomnia, nocturnal panic attacks, or fear of going to bed or falling asleep.[179] Formal sleep studies may be unremarkable, with no abnormalities of sleep macrostructure or excessive arousability, but suggest that nocturnal panic is an NREM phenomenon.[180,181] It is easy to understand how nocturnal panic and other sleep disorders characterized by precipitous arousals (particularly sleep apnea or gastroesophageal reflux) may be confused.[182] The striking similarity of the symptoms of dream anxiety attacks, sleep terrors, nocturnal seizures, sleep apnea, and nighttime panic urges caution in diagnosis.[182-188]

Posttraumatic Stress Disorder

This topic is covered in Chapters 46 and 111.

Psychogenic Dissociative States

Complex, potentially injurious behavior, occasionally confined to the sleep period, may be the manifestation of a psychogenic dissociative state.[189] A history of childhood physical or sexual abuse or both is virtually always present (but may be difficult to elicit).[190-192] In this condition (and malingering), unlike other parasomnias, the complex behavior during polysomnographic monitoring is seen to arise from well-developed EEG-determined wakefulness.[193] The term *pseudoparasomnia* has been proposed for this condition.[194]

Malingering, Conversion Hysteria, or Munchausen's Syndrome

Patients with these disorders may present to a sleep specialist with sleep-related stridor, asthma, upper airway obstruction, or sleep-related violent behavior in adults,[195-200] or as sleep apnea (Munchausen by proxy) in children.[201-205] Cyclic hypersomnia has also been reported as a manifestation of a factitious disorder.[206]

Clinical Pearl

The vast majority of parasomnias are due to either disorders of arousal or the REM sleep behavior disorder. There remain a large number of other parasomnias that may be confused with the more common ones. Careful evaluation by history and polysomnographic study usually identifies the true underlying problem. Undoubtedly, as more patients experiencing unusual phenomena arising from the sleep period are evaluated and studied thoroughly, more fascinating parasomnias will be identified, with important therapeutic implications.

REFERENCES

1. Ohayon MM, Zulley J, Guilleminault C, Smirne S: Prevalence and pathologic associations of sleep paralysis in the general population. Neurology 1999;52:1194-1200.
2. Takeuchi T, Fukada K, Sasaki Y: Factors related to the occurrence of isolated sleep paralysis elicited during a multi-phasic sleep-wake schedule. Sleep 2002;25:89-96.
3. Cheyne JA: Situational factors affecting sleep paralysis and associated hallucinations: position and timing effects. J Sleep Res 2002;11:169-177.
4. Herman J, Furman Z, Cantrell G, Peled R: Sleep paralysis: A study in family practice. J R Coll Gen Pract 1988;38:465-467.
5. Celani MF, Bonati ME, Cavalli M: Hypokalemic thyrotoxic periodic paralysis in a Caucasian male with Graves' disease. J Endocrinol Invest 1995;18:228-231.
6. Buzzi G, Mostacci B, Sancisi E, Cirignotta F: Sleep complaints in periodic paralysis: a web survey. Funct Neurol 2001;16: 245-252.
7. Gastaut H, Broughton R: A clinical and polygraphic study of episodic phenomena during sleep. Recent Adv Biol Psychiatry 1967;7:197-221.
8. Foulkes D, Vogel G: Mental activity at sleep onset. J Abnorm Psychol 1965;70:231-243.
9. Vogel G, Foulkes D, Trosman H: Ego functions and dreaming during sleep onset. Arch Gen Psychiatry 1966;14:238-248.
10. Dement WC, Kleitman N: The relation of eye movements during sleep to dream activity: an objective method for the study of dreaming. J Exp Psychol 1957;53:339-346.
11. Rowley JT, Stickgold R, Hobson JA: Eyelid movements and mental activity at sleep onset. Conscious Cogn 1998;7:67-84.
12. Nielsen TA: Mentation during sleep: the NREM/REM distinction. In: Lydic R, Baghdoyan HA (eds): Handbook of Behavioral State Control. Cellular and Molecular Mechanisms. Boca Raton, Fla: CRC Press, 1999, pp 101-128.
13. Liddon SC: Sleep paralysis and hypnagogic hallucinations. Their relationship to the nightmare. Arch Gen Psychiatry 1967; 17:88-96.
14. Ohayon MM, Priest RG, Caulet M, Guilleminault C: Hypnagogic and hypnopompic hallucinations: Pathological phenomena? Br J Psychiatry 1996;169:459-467.
15. Takeuchi T, Miyasita A, Sasaki Y, et al: Isolated sleep paralysis elicited by sleep interruption. Sleep 1992;15:217-225.
16. Takeuchi T, Miyasita A, Inugami M, et al: Laboratory-documented hallucination during sleep-onset REM period in a normal subject. Percept Mot Skills 1994;78:979-985.
17. Ness RC: The old hag phenomenon as sleep paralysis: A biocultural interpretation. Cult Med Psychiatry 1978;2:15-39.
18. Hufford DJ: The terror that comes in the night. Philadelphia, University of Pennsylvania Press, 1982.
19. Mahowald MW, Ettinger MG: Things that go bump in the night—the parasomnias revisited. J Clin Neurophysiol 1990;7: 119-143.
20. Parkes JD: The parasomnias. Lancet 1986;2:1021-1025.
21. Oswald I: Sudden bodily jerks on falling asleep. Brain 1959; 82:92-103.
22. Dagnino N, Loeb C, Massazza G, Sacco G: Hypnic physiological myoclonus in man: An EEG-EMG study in normals and neurological patients. Eur Neurol 1969;2:47-58.
23. Lugaresi E, Coccagna G, Cirignotta F: Phenomena occurring during sleep onset in man. In Popoviciu L, Asgian B, Badiu G (eds): Sleep 1978. Fourth European Congress on Sleep Research, Tirgu-Mures, Romania. Basel: S. Karger, 1980, pp 24-27.
24. Ikeda K, sUrakami K, Isoe K, Nakashima K: Sensory sleep starts. J Neurol Neurosurg Psychiatry 1998;64:690.
25. Teixido MT, Connolly K: Explosive tinnitus: An underrecognized disorder. Otolaryngol Head Neck Surg 1998;118:108-109.
26. Fusco L, Pachatz C, Cusmai R, Vigevano F: Repetitive sleep starts in neurologically impaired children: An unusual non-epileptic manifestation in otherwise epileptic subjects. Epileptic Disord 1999;1:63-67.

27. Kotagal P, Costa M, Wyllie E, Wolgamuth B: Paroxysmal nonepileptic events in children and adolescents. Pediatrics 2002;110:e46.

28. Sander HW, Geisse H, Quinto C, et al: Sensory sleep starts. J Neurol Neurosurg Psychiatry 1998;64:690.

29. Vetrugno R, Provini F, Plazzi G, et al: Catathrenia (nocturnal groaning): A new type of parasomnia. Neurology 2001;56:681-683.

30. DeRoeck J, Van Hoof E, Cluydts R: Sleep-related expiratory groaning: A case report. Sleep Res 1983;12:237.

31. Pevernagie DA, Boon PA, Mariman AN, et al: Vocalization during episodes of prolonged expiration: A parasomnia related to REM sleep. Sleep Med 2001;2:19-30.

32. Broughton RJ: Sleep disorders: Disorders of arousal? Science 1968;159:1070-1078.

33. Bader G, Neveus T, Kruse S, Sillen U: Sleep of primary enuretic children and controls. Sleep 2002;25:579-583.

34. Burke EC, Stikler GB: Enuresis—is it being overtreated? Mayo Clin Proc 1980;55:118-119.

35. Hirasing RA, van Leerdam FJM, Bolk-Bennink L, Janknegt RA: Enuresis nocturnal in adults. Scand J Urol Nephrol 1997;31:533-536.

36. Bakwin H: The genetics of enuresis. In Kolvin I, MacKeith S, Meadow R (eds): Bladder control and enuresis. London, Lavenham Press, 1973.

37. Gillin JC, Rapoport JL, Mikkelsen EJ, et al: EEG sleep patterns in enuresis: A further analysis and comparison with normal controls. Biol Psychiatry 1982;17:947-953.

38. Robert M, Averous M, Besset A, et al: Sleep polygraphic studies using cystomanometry in twenty patients with enuresis. Eur Urol 1993;24:97-102.

39. Butler RJ, Holland P: The three systems a conceptual way of understanding nocturnal enuresis. Scand J Urol Nephrol 2000;34:270-277.

40. Fritz GK, Armbrust, J: Enuresis and encopresis. Psychiatr Clin North Am 1982;5:283-296.

41. Fritz GK, Anders TF: Enuresis: The clinical application of an etiologically based classification system. Child Psychiatry Hum Dev 1979;10:103-113.

42. Hallgren B: Nocturnal enuresis: Etiologic aspects. Acta Pediatr 1958;118(Suppl):66.

43. Lund S: Primary nocturnal enuresis in children. Background and treatment. Scand J Urol Nephrol 1994;156(Suppl):1-48.

44. Hublin C, Kaprio J, Partinen M, Koskenvuo M: Nocturnal enuresis in a nationwide twin cohort. Sleep 1998;21:579-585.

45. Sireling LI, Crisp AH: Sleep and the enuresis alarm device. J R Soc Med 1983;76:131-133.

46. Werry J, Coharssen J: Enuresis: An etiologic and therapeutic study. J Pediatr 1965;67:423-431.

47. Alon US: Nocturnal enuresis. Ped Nephrol 1995;9:94-103.

48. Rapoport JL, Mikkelsen EJ, Zavadil A, et al: Childhood enuresis. II. Psychopathology, tricyclic concentration in plasma, and antidiuretic effect. Arch Gen Psychiatry 1980;37:1146-1152.

49. Neveus T, Bader G, Sullen U: Enuresis, sleep and desmopressin treatment. Acta Paediatr 2002;91:1121-1125.

50. Umlauf MG, Chasens ER: Sleep disordered breathing and nocturnal polyuria: Nocturia and enuresis. Sleep Med Rev 2003;7:403-411.

51. Happe S, Ludemann P, Ringelstein EB: Persistence of rhythmic movement disorder beyond childhood: A videotape demonstration. Mov Disord 2000;15:1296-1297.

52. Kohyama J, Masukura F, Kimura K, Tachibana N: Rhythmic movement disorder: Polysomnographic study and summary of reported cases. Brain Devel 2002;24:33-38.

53. Kempenaers C, Bouillon E, Mendlewicz J: A rhythmic movement disorder in REM sleep: A case report. Sleep 1994;17:274-279.

54. Gagnon P, De Koninck J: Repetitive head movements during REM sleep. Biol Psychiatry 1985;20:176-178.

55. Whyte J, Kavey NB, Gidro-Frank S: A self-destructive variant of jactatio capitis nocturna. J Nerv Ment Dis 1991;179:49-50.

56. Thorpy MJ, Glovinsky PB: Parasomnias. Psychiatr Clin North Am 1987;10:623-639.

57. Manni R, Tartara A: Clonazepam treatment of rhythmic movement disorders. Sleep 1997;20:812.

58. Chisholm T, Morehouse RL: Adult headbanging: sleep studies and treatment. Sleep 1996;19:343-346.

59. Hashizume Y, Yoshijima H, Uchimura N, Maeda H: Case of headbanging that continued to adolescence. Psychiatry Clin Neurosci 2002;56:255-256.

60. Garcia J, Rosen G, Mahowald M: Waterbeds in treatment of rhythmic movement disorders: Experience with two cases. Sleep Res 1996;25:243.

61. Rosenberg C: Elimination of a rhythmic movement disorder with hypnosis—a case report. Sleep 1995;18:608-609.

62. Broughton R: Pathological fragmentary myoclonus, intensified "hypnic jerks" and hypnagogic foot tremor: Three unusual sleep-related movement disorders. In Koella WP, Obal F, Schulz H, et al (eds): Sleep '86. Stuttgart, Gustav Fischer Verlag, 1988, pp 240-243.

63. Guilleminault C, Silvestri R: Disorders of arousal and epilepsy during sleep. In Sterman MB, Shouse MN, Passouant PP (eds): Sleep and Epilepsy. New York, Academic Press, 1982, pp 513-531.

64. Plazzi G, Provini F, Ligouri R, et al: Propriospinal myoclonus at the transition from wake to sleep. Sleep Res 1996;26:438.

65. Vetrugno R, Provini F, Meletti S, et al: Propriospinal myoclonus at the sleep-wake transition: A new type of parasomnia. Sleep 2001;24:835-843.

66. Montagna P, Provini F, Plazzi G, et al: Propriospinal myoclonus upon relaxation and drowsiness: A cause of severe insomnia. Mov Disord 1997;12:66-72.

67. Jankovic J, Pardo R: Segmental myoclonus: clinical and pharmacologic study. Arch Neurol 1986;43:1025-1031.

68. Hoehn MM, Cherington M: Spinal myoclonus. Neurology 1977;27:942-946.

69. Bauleo S, De Mitri P, Coccagna G: Evolution of segmental myoclonus during sleep: Polygraphic study of two cases. Ital J Neurol Sci 1996;17:227-232.

70. Abe K, Shimakawa M: Genetic and developmental aspects of sleeptalking and teeth-grinding. Acta Paedopsychiatr 1966;33:339-344.

71. Hublin C, Kaprio J, Partinen M, Koskenvuo M: Sleeptalking in twins: Epidemiology and psychiatric comorbidity. Behav Genet 1998;28:289-298.

72. Bixler EO, Kales A, Soldatos CR, et al: Prevalence of sleep disorders in the Los Angeles metropolitan area. Am J Psychiatry 1979;136:1257-1262.

73. Reimao RN, Lefevre AB: Prevalence of sleeptalking in childhood. Brain Dev 1980;2:353-357.

74. Arkin AM, Toth MF, Baker J, Hastey JM: The frequency of sleep talking in the laboratory among chronic sleep talkers and good dream recallers. J Nerv Ment Dis 1970;151:369-374.

75. Arkin AM, Toth MG, Baker J, Hastey JM: The degree of concordance between the content of sleep talking and mentation recalled in wakefulness. J Nerv Ment Dis 1970;151:375-393.

76. Welch KM, Cutrer FM, Goadsby PJ: Migraine pathogenesis. Neurology 2003;60(Suppl 2):S9-S14.

77. Dexter JD, Weitzman ED: The relationship of nocturnal headaches to sleep stage patterns. Neurology 1970;20:513-518.

78. Dexter JD, Riley TL: Studies in nocturnal migraine. Headache 1975;15:51-62.

79. Kayed K, Godtlibsen OB, Sjaastad O: Chronic paroxysmal hemicrania. IV. "REM sleep locked" nocturnal headache attacks. Sleep 1978;1:91-95.

80. Pfaffenrath V, Pollmann W, Ruther E: Onset of nocturnal attacks of chronic cluster headache in relation to sleep stages. Acta Neurol. Scand 1986;73:403-407.

81. Sahota PK, Dexter JD: Sleep and headache syndromes: A clinical review. Headache 1990;30:80-84.

82. Kay DC, Blackburn AB, Buckingham JA, Karacan I: Human pharmacology of sleep. In Williams RL, Karacan I (eds): Pharmacology of Sleep. New York, Wiley, 1976, pp 83-210.

83. Jarrott B, Lewis S, Conway EL, et al: The involvement of central alpha adrenoreceptors in the antihypertensive actions of methyldopa and clonidine in the rat. Clin Exp Hypertens 1984;61:387-400.

84. Autret A, Minz M, Beillevaire T, et al: Effect of clonidine on sleep patterns in man. Eur J Clin Pharmacol 1977;12:319-322.

85. Micieli G, Cavallini A, Facchinetti F, et al: Chronic paroxysmal hemicrania: a chronobiological study (case report). Cephalalgia 1989;9:281-286.

86. Bono G, Micieli G, Manzoni GC, et al: Chronobiological basis for the management of periodic headaches. In Rose C (ed): Migraine. Proceedings of the Fifth International Migraine Symposium, London, 1984. Basel, Karger, 1985, pp 206-217.

87. Coria F, Claveria LE, Jimenez-Jimenez FJ, DeSeijas EV: Episodic paroxysmal hemicrania responsive to calcium channel blockers. J Neurol Neurosurg Psychiatry 1992;55:166.

88. Chervin RD, Zallek SN, Lin X, et al: Timing patterns of cluster headaches and association with symptoms of obstructive sleep apnea. Sleep Res Online 2000;3:107-112.

89. Chervin R, Zallek SN, Lin X, et al: Sleep disordered breathing in patients with cluster headache. Neurology 2000;54:2302-2306.

90. Aldrich MS, Chauncey JB: Are morning headaches part of the obstructive sleep apnea syndrome? Arch Intern Med 1990;150:1265-1267.

91. Sand T, Hagen K, Schrader H: Sleep apnoea and chronic headache. Cephalalgia 2003;23:90-95.

92. Goder R, Friege L, Fritzer G, et al: Morning headaches in patients with sleep disorders: A systematic polysomnographic study. Sleep Med 2003;4:385-391.

93. Buckle P, Kerr P, Kryger M: Nocturnal cluster headache associated with sleep apnea. A case report. Sleep 1993;16:487-489.

94. Declerck AC, Arends JB: An exceptional case of parasomnia: The exploding head syndrome. Sleep-Wake Research in the Netherlands 1994;5:41-43.

95. Pearce JMS: Clinical features of the exploding head syndrome. J Neurol Neurosurg Psychiatry 1989;52:907-910.

96. Sachs C, Svanborg E: The exploding head syndrome: Polysomnographic recordings and therapeutic suggestions. Sleep 1991; 14:263-266.

97. Walsleben JA, O'Malley EB, Freeman J, Rapoport DM: Polysomnographic and topographic mapping of EEG in the exploding head syndrome. Sleep Res 1993;22:284.

98. Pearce JMS. Exploding head syndrome. Headache 2001;41:602-603.

99. Fornazzari L, Farcnik K, Smith I, et al: Violent visual hallucinations and aggression in frontal lobe dysfunction: Clinical manifestations of deep orbitofrontal foci. J Neuropsychiatry Clin Neurosci 1992;4:42-44.

100. Jacome DE: Exploding head syndrome and idiopathic stabbing headache relieved by nifedipine. Cephalalgia 2001;21:617-618.

101. Gould JD, Silberstein SD: Unilateral hypnic headache: A case study. Neurology 1997;49:1749-1751.

102. Ghlotto N, Sances G, Di Lorenzo G, et al: Report of eight new cases of hypnic headache and mini-review of the literature. Funct Neurol 2002;17:211-219.

103. Raskin NH: The hypnic headache syndrome. Headache 1988;28:534-536.

104. Newman LC, Lipton RB, Solomon S: The hypnic headache syndrome: A benign headache disorder of the elderly. Neurology 1990;40:1904-1905.

105. Dodick DW, Mosek AC, Campbell JK: The hypnic ("alarm clock") headache syndrome. Cephalalgia 1998;18:152-156.

106. Ivanez V, Soler R, Barreiro P: Hypnic headache syndrome: A case with good response to indomethacin. Cephalalgia 1998;18:225-226.

107. Relja G, Zorzon M, Locatelli L, et al: Hypnic headache: Rapid and long-lasting response to prednisone in two new cases. Cephalalgia 2002;222:157-159.

108. Vieira-Dias M, Esperanca P: Hypnic headache: Report of two cases. Headache 2001;41:726-727.

109. Pinessi I, Rainero I, Cicolin A, et al: Hypnic headache syndrome: Association of the attacks with REM sleep. Cephalalgia 2003;23:150-154.

110. Evers S, Goadsby PJ: Hypnic headache. Clinical features, pathophysiology, and treatment. Neurology 2002;60:905-909.

111. Sibon I, Ghorayeb I, Henry P: Successful treatment of hypnic headache syndrome with acetazolamide. Neurology 2003;61:1157-1158.

112. Peatfield RC, Mendoza ND: Posterior fossa meningioma presenting as hypnic headache. Headache 2003;43:1007-1008.

113. Altster J, Shemesh Z, Ornan M, Attias J: Sleep disturbance associated with chronic tinnitus. Biol Psychiatry 1993;34:84-90.

114. Folmer RL, Griest SE: Tinnitus and insomnia. American J Otolaryngology 2000;21:287-293.

115. Asplund R: Sleepiness and sleep in elderly persons with tinnitus. Arch Gerontol Geriatr 2003;37:139-145.

116. Hallum RS: Correlates of sleep disturbance in chronic distressing tinnitus. Scand Audiol 1996;25:263-266.

117. Matsushima J, Sakai N, Sakajiri M, et al: An experience of the usage of electrical tinnitus suppressor. Artif Organs 1996;20:955-958.

118. Sullivan M, Katon W, Russo J, et al: A randomized trial of nortriptyline for severe chronic tinnitus. Arch Intern Med 1993;153:2251-2259.

119. Plewnia C, Bartels M, Gerloff C: Transient suppression of tinnitus by transcranial magnetic stimulation. Ann Neurol 2002;53:263-266.

120. Lapresle J: Palatal myoclonus. Adv Neurol 1986;43:265-273.

121. Iliceto G, Thompson BL, Day JC: Diaphragmatic flutter, the moving umbilicus syndrome, and "belly dancer's" dyskinesia. Mov Disord 1990;15-22.

122. Phillips JR, Eldridge FL: Respiratory myoclonus (Leeuwenhoek's disease). N Engl J Med 1973;289:1390-1395.

123. Corbett CL: Diaphragmatic flutter. Postgrad Med J 1977;53:399-402.

124. Sethi KD, Hess DC, Huffnagle VH, Adams RJ: Acetazolamide treatment of paroxysmal dystonia in central demyelinating disease. Neurology 1992;42:919-921.

125. Weiner WJ, Goetz CG, Nausieda PA, Klawans HL: Respiratory dyskinesias: Extrapyramidal dysfunction and dyspnea. Ann Intern Med 1978;88:327-331.

126. Kuna ST, Awan R: The irregularly irregular pattern of respiratory dyskinesia. Chest 1986;90:779-781.

127. Wilcox PG, Bassett A, Jones B, Fleetham JA: Respiratory dysrhythmias in patients with tardive dyskinesia. Chest 1994;105:203-207.

128. Rich MW, Radwany SM: Respiratory dyskinesia. An underrecognized phenomenon. Chest 1994;105:1826-1832.

129. Wantanabe K, Hara K, Hakamada S, et al: Seizures with apnea in children. Pediatrics 1982;70:87-90.

130. Thach BT: Sleep apnea in infancy and childhood. Med Clin North Am 1985;69:1289-1315.

131. Walls TJ, Newman PK, Cumming WJK: Recurrent apnoeic attacks as a manifestation of epilepsy. Postgrad Med J 1981;57:575-576.

132. Lanouis S, Bizec JL, Whitelaw WA, et al: Hiccup in adults: An overview. Eur Respir J 1993;6:563-575.

133. Arnulf I, Boisteanu D, Whitelaw WA, et al: Chronic hiccups and sleep. Sleep 1995;19:227-231.

134. Askenasy JJM: Sleep hiccup. Sleep 1988;11:187-194.

135. Brown LW, Fry JM: Paroxysmal nocturnal choking: A newly described manifestation of sleep-related epilepsy. Sleep Res 1988;17:153.

136. Kowey PR, Mainchak RA, Rials SJ: Things that go bang in the night. N Engl J Med 1992;327:1884.

137. Bonnet R, Jorres R, Downey R, et al: Intractable cough associated with the supine body position. Effective therapy with nasal CPAP. Chest 1995;108:581-585.

138. Teng AY, Sullivan CE: Nasal mask continuous positive airway pressure in the treatment of chronic nocturnal cough in a young child. Respirology 1997;2:131-134.

139. Fontan JP, Heldt GP, Heyman MB, et al: Esophageal spasm associated with apnea and bradycardia in an infant. Pediatrics 1984;73:52-55.

140. Bortolotti M, Cirignotta F, Labo G: Atrioventricular block induced by swallowing in a patient with diffuse esophageal spasm. JAMA 1982;248:2297-2299.

141. Traube M, McCallum RW: Primary oesophageal motility disorders. Current therapeutic concepts. Drugs 1985;30:66-77.

142. Guilleminault C, Eldridge FL, Phillips JR, Dement WC: Two occult causes of insomnia and their therapeutic problems. Arch Gen Psychiatry 1976;33:1241-1245.

143. Weiner IH, Weiner HL: Nocturnal leg muscle cramps. JAMA 1980;244:2332-2333.

144. Baltodano N, Gallo BV, Weidler DJ: Verapamil vs quinine in recumbent nocturnal leg cramps in the elderly. Arch Intern Med 1988;148:1969-1970.

145. Mills KR, Newham DJ, Edwards RHT: Severe muscle cramps relieved by transcutaneous nerve stimulation: A case report. J Neurol Neurosurg Psychiatry 1982;45:539-542.

146. Connolly PS, Shirley EA, Wasson JH, Nierenberg DW: Treatment of nocturnal leg cramps. A crossover trial of quinine vs vitamin E. Arch Intern Med 1992;152:1877-1880.

147. Serrao M, Rossi P, Cardinali P, et al: Gabapentin treatment for muscle cramps: An open-label trial. Clinical Neuropharmacol 2000;23:45-49.

148. Kannan N, Sawaya R: Nocturnal leg cramps: Clinically mysterious and painful—but manageable. Geriatrics 2001;56:34-42.

149. Bender BG, Leung SB, Lueng DYM: Actigraphic assessment of sleep disturbance in patients with atopic dermatitis: An objective life quality measure. J Allergy Clin Immunol 2003;111:598-602.

150. Yosipovitch G, Ansari N, Goon A: Clinical characteristics of pruritus in chronic idiopathic urticaria. Br J Dermatol 2002;147:32-36.

151. Stores G, Burrows A, Crawford C: Physiological sleep disturbance in children with atopic dermatitis: a case control study. Pediatr Dermatol 1998;15:264-268.

152. Aoki T, Kushimoto H, Hishikawa Y, Savin JA: Nocturnal scratching and its relationship to the disturbed sleep of itchy subjects. Clin Exp Dermatol 1991;16:268-272.

153. Monti JM, Vignale R, Monti D: Sleep and nighttime pruritus in children with atopic dermatitis. Sleep 1989;12:309-314.

154. Savin JA, Paterson WD, Oswald I, Adam K: Further studies of scratching during sleep. Br J Dermatol 1975;93:297-302.

155. Gabriel GM, Crone CC: Nocturnal pruritus in a cardiac pretransplant patient. Psychosomatics 2001;42:344-346.

156. Sandroni P: Central neuropathic itch: A new treatment option? Neurology 2002;59:778-779.

157. Brodland DG, Staats BA, Peters MS: Factitial leg ulcers associated with an unusual sleep disorder. Arch Dermatol 1989;125:1115-1118.

158. Mold JW, Mathew MK, Shuaib B, DeHaven M: Prevalence of night sweats in primary care patients: An OKPRN and TAFP-Net collaborative study. J Fam Pract 2002;51:452-456.

159. Duhon DR: Night sweats: Two other causes. JAMA 1994;271:1577 (letter).

160. Gordon D: Night sweats: Two other causes. JAMA 1994;271:1577 (letter).

161. Reynolds WA: Are night sweats a sign of esophageal reflux? J Clin Gastroenterol 1989;11:590-591(letter).

162. Solomon GE: Diencephalic autonomic epilepsy caused by a neoplasm. J Pediatr 1973;83:277-280.

163. Woodward S, Freedman RR: The thermoregulatory effects of menopausal hot flashes on sleep. Sleep 1994;17:497-501.

164. Kronenberg F: Menopausal hot flashes: Randomness or rhythmicity. Chaos 1991;1:271-278.

165. Pierre JM, Guze BH: Benztropine for venlafaxine-induced night sweats. J Clin Psychopharmacol 2000;20:269(letter).

166. Johnson LF, Kinsbourne M, Renuart AW: Hereditary chin-trembling with nocturnal myoclonus and tongue-biting in dizygous twins. Dev Med Child Neurol 1971;13:726-729.

167. Vasiknanonte P, Kuasirikul S, Vasiknanonte S: Two faces of nocturnal tongue biting. J Med Assoc Thai 1997;80:500-506.

168. Tuxhorn I, Hoppe M: Parasomnia with rhythmic movements manifesting as nocturnal tongue biting. Neuropediatrics 1993;24:167-168.

169. Edwards JC, Dinner DS, Gordon PH: Violent tongue biting as a parasomnia. Sleep Res 1997;26:358.

170. Aguglia U, Gambardella A, Quattrone A: Sleep-induced masticatory myoclonus: A rare parasomnia associated with insomnia. Sleep 1991;14:80-82.

171. Vetrugno R, Provini F, Plazzi G, et al: Familial nocturnal facio-mandibular myoclonus mimicking sleep bruxism. Neurology 2002;58:644-647.

172. Chaves-Vischer V, Picard F, Andermann E, et al: Benign nocturnal alternating hemiplegia of childhood: Six patients and long-term follow-up. In Brazil CW, Malow BA, Sammaritano M, eds. Sleep and Epilepsy: The Clinical Spectrum. Amsterdam, Eslevier, 2002, pp 283-289.

173. Mellman TA, Uhde TW: Patients with frequent sleep panic: clinical findings and response to medication treatment. J Clin Psychiatry 1990;51:513-516.

174. Rosenfield DS, Furman Y: Pure sleep panic: Two case reports and a review of the literature. Sleep 1994;17:462-465.

175. Craske MG, Rowe MK: Nocturnal panic. Clin Psychol Sci Pract 1997;4:153-174.

176. Craske MG, Kreuger MT: Prevalence of nocturnal panic in a college population. J Anxiety Disord 1990;4:125-139.

177. Herskowitz J: Neurologic presentations of panic disorder in childhood and adolescence. Dev Med Child Neurol 1986;28:617-623.

178. Black B, Robbins DR: Panic disorder in children and adolescents. J Am Acad Child Adolesc Psychiatry 1990;29:36-44.

179. Lepola U, Koponen H, Leinonen E: Sleep in panic disorders. J Psychosom Res 1994;38(Suppl):105-111.

180. Stein MB, Enns MW, Kryger MH: Sleep in nondepressed patients with panic disorder: II. Polysomnographic assessment of sleep architecture and sleep continuity. J Affect Disord 1993;28:1-6.

181. Landry P, Marchand L, Mainguy N, et al: Electroencephalography during sleep of patients with nocturnal panic disorder. J Nerv Ment Dis 2002;190:559-562.

182. Edlund MJ, McNamara ME, Millman RP: Sleep apnea and panic attacks. Compr Psychiatry 1991;32:130-132.

183. Lesser IM, Poland RE, Holcomb C, Rose DE: Electroencephalographic study of nighttime panic attacks. J Nerv Ment Dis 1985;173:744-746.

184. Grunhaus L, Birmaher B: The clinical spectrum of panic attacks. J Clin Psychopharmacol 1985;5:93-99.

185. Hauri P, Friedman M, Ravaris RL, Fisher J: Sleep in agoraphobia with panic attacks. Sleep Res 1985;14:128.

186. Mellman TA, Uhde TW: Sleep panic attacks: new clinical findings and theoretical implications. Am J Psychiatry 1989;146:1204-7.

187. McNamara ME: Absence seizures associated with panic attacks initially misdiagnosed as temporal lobe epilepsy: The importance of prolonged EEG monitoring in diagnosis. J Psychiatry Neurosci 1993;18:46-48.

188. Wall M, Tuchman M, Mielke D: Panic attacks and temporal lobe seizures associated with a right temporal lobe arteriovenous malformation: Case report. J Clin Psychiatry 1985;46:143-145.

189. Agargun MY, Kara H, Ozer OA, et al: Characteristics of patients with nocturnal dissociative disorders. Sleep Hypn 2001;3: 131-134.

190. Chu JA, Dill DL: Dissociative symptoms in relation to childhood physical and sexual abuse. Am J Psychiatry 1990;147: 887-892.

191. Putnam FW, Guroff JJ, Silberman EK, et al: The clinical phenomenology of multiple personality disorder: review of 100 recent cases. J Clin Psychiatry 1986;47:285-293.

192. Agargun MY, Kara H, Ozer OA, et al: Sleep-related violence, dissociative experiences, and childhood traumatic events. Sleep Hypn 2002;4:52-57.

193. Schenck CS, Milner DM, Hurwitz TD, et al: Dissociative disorders presenting as somnambulism: Polysomnographic, video, and clinical documentation (8 cases). Dissociation 1989;4:194-204.

194. Molaie M, Deutsch GK: Psychogenic events presenting as parasomnia. Sleep 1997;20:402-405.

195. Mahowald MW, Schenck CH, Rosen GR, Hurwitz TD: The role of a sleep disorders center in evaluating sleep violence. Arch Neurol 1992;49:604-607.

196. Baker CE, Major E: Munchausen's syndrome. A case presenting as asthma requiring ventilation. Anaesthesia 1994;49: 1050-1051.

197. Elshami AA, Tino G: Coexistent asthma and functional upper airway obstruction. Case reports and review of the literature. Chest 1996;110:1358-1361.

198. Walker FO, Alessi AG, Digre KB, McLean WT: Psychogenic respiratory distress. Arch Neurol 1989;46:196-200.

199. Butani L, O'Connell EJ: Functional respiratory disorders. Ann Allergy Asthma Immunol 1997;79:91-101.

200. Goldman J, Muers M: Vocal cord dysfunction and wheezing. Thorax 1991;46:401-404.

201. Light MJ, Sheridan MS: Munchausen syndrome by proxy and sleep apnea. Clin Pediatr 1990;29:162-168.

202. Griffith JC, Slovik LS: Munchausen by proxy and sleep disorders medicine. Sleep 1989;12:178-183.

203. Skau K, Mouridsen SE: Munchausen syndrome by proxy: A review. Acta Paediatr 1995;84:977-982.

204. Samuels MP, McClaughlin W, Jacobson RR, et al: Fourteen cases of imposed upper airway obstruction. Arch Dis Child 1992;67:162-170.

205. Byard RW, Beal SM: Munchausen syndrome by proxy: Repetitive infantile apnoea and homicide. J Paediatr Child Health 1993;29:77-79.

206. Feldman MD, Russell JL: Factitious cyclic hypersomnia: a new variant of factitious disorder. South Med J 1991;84: 379-381.

77

Nightmares and Other Common Dream Disturbances

Tore A. Nielsen

Antonio Zadra

ABSTRACT

Nightmares and other common disturbances of dreaming involve a perturbation of emotional expression during sleep. Nightmares, the most prevalent dream disturbance, are now recognized to involve disorder in a variety of dysphoric emotions, including especially fear. A genetic basis for nightmares has been demonstrated, and their pathophysiology involves a surprising sympathetic underactivation in many instances. Personality factors, such as nightmare chronicity and distress and coping styles, are mediating determinants of their clinical severity, as are drug and alcohol use. Many treatments have been described, with much support for the effectiveness of short-term cognitive-behavioral interventions such as systematic desensitization and imagery rehearsal. Several related dream disturbances occur at the transitions into or out of sleep and involve dysphoric emotions ranging from malaise to fear to frank terror. These include sleep starts, terrifying hypnagogic hallucinations, sleep paralysis, somniloquy with dream content, false awakenings, and disturbed lucid dreaming. The distinctive nature of these disturbances may be mediated by immediately preceding waking state processes (e.g., consciousness, sensory vividness) that intrude on or carry over into dreaming.

Because most common dreaming disturbances (Table 77–1) involve a perturbation of emotional expression during sleep, their study may help clarify the role of emotion in dream formation, dream function, and sleep mechanisms more generally. Physiologic evidence for emotional activity during rapid eye dreaming (REM) sleep is substantial. Autonomic system variability increases markedly in conjunction with central phasic activation,[1] as seen especially in measures of cardiac function,[2,3] respiration,[4] and skin and muscle sympathetic nerve activity.[5,6] Brain imaging, too, demonstrates increases in metabolic activity in limbic and paralimbic regions during REM sleep activity (see, e.g., Maquet[7] and Braun et al.[8]) similar to that seen during strong emotion in the waking state.[9] These dramatic autonomic fluctuations globally parallel dreamed emotional activity, which is detectable throughout most dreaming when appropriate probes are employed.[10] In fact, most dreamed emotion is negative,[11] primarily fearful,[10] and it may conform to a "surgelike" structure within REM sleep episodes.[12] Many theorists interpret the various peripheral manifestations of phasic ponto-geniculo-occipital activity (see Rechtschaffen[13] for a review) as indicative of dream-related affective activity.[12,14]

Emotional processes during wakefulness are also implicated in dream disturbances. For the most common disturbances, such as nightmares, dreamed emotion becomes unbearably intense and provokes an awakening; this may lead to further distress, which continues to influence waking behavior and mood and may even impair subsequent sleep. Perturbation of dream-related emotion may thus lead to a cycle of sleep disruption and avoidance, insomnia,[15] and psychological distress.[16] This often leads the individual to consult a professional.

However, causal relationships between emotion, dreaming, and other associated symptoms are not well understood. In some disturbances, such as nightmare disorder, emotional disruption may affect primarily sleep-related processes—in which case, dreaming itself might be considered pathologic in some sense (but see also Kramer[17]). However, the widespread belief in dreaming as an emotionally *adaptive* mechanism also leaves room for the possibility that some dream disturbances are adaptive reactions to more basic pathophysiologic factors, rather than signs of pathology per se.

IDIOPATHIC NIGHTMARES

Historical Aspects

The *Diagnostic and Statistical Manual of Mental Disorders, Fourth Edition* (DSM-IV)[18] criteria for Nightmare Disorder (Table 77–2) have not changed substantially since the disorder was previously described as Dream Anxiety Disorder in the DSM-III-R and Dream Anxiety Attack in the DSM-III. The *International Classification of Sleep Disorders, Second Edition* (ICSD-II) criteria for Nightmare Disorder (see Table 77–2) have changed somewhat since the first edition. Some new research on the phenomenology of nightmares has prompted a redefinition of the term *nightmare* in the more recent edition.

The widely accepted definition of a nightmare has long been "a frightening dream that awakens the sleeper," but researchers have come to reevaluate these defining features. Some[19,20] argue that the "awakening" criterion should indeed designate nightmares but that disturbing dreams that do not awaken (i.e., "bad dreams") should nevertheless be considered clinically significant. Whether or not the person awakens presumably reflects a dream's emotional severity, but it is not the only index of severity. First, in patients with various psychosomatic illnesses, even the most macabre and threatening dreams do not necessarily produce awakenings.[21,22] Second, less than one fourth of patients with chronic nightmares report "always" awakening from their nightmares, and these awakenings do not correlate with either nightmare intensity or psychological distress.[20] Third, among subjects with both nightmares and bad dreams, approximately 45% of bad dreams are rated as having an emotional intensity that

Table 77–1. Sleep Disorders in which Disturbed Dreaming is Common

	Code*	Stage	Prevalence	Essential Features
Nightmare Disorder	307.47	REM, 2	Children: 5%-30% Young adults: 2%-5% (see text)	Frightening dreams; awakening
Terrifying Hypnagogic Hallucinations	307.47	Sleep onset	Rare Narcolepsy: 4%-8%	Terrifying sleep onset dreams (now subsumed under Nightmare Disorder)
Sleep Starts, Hypnic Jerks	781.01	Sleep onset	Lifetime: 60%-70% Extreme form: rare	Sudden brief jerks associated with sensory flash, hypnagogic dream, or feeling of falling
Recurrent Isolated Sleep Paralysis	780.56	Sleep onset or offset	Isolated, normals: 1/lifetime in 40%-50% Familial: rare	Paralysis of voluntary muscles; acute anxiety (with or without dreams) is common

*International Classification of Sleep Disorders, Second Edition—Revised from International Classification of Sleep Disorders, Revised: Diagnostic and Coding Manual. Rochester, Minn, American Sleep Disorders Association, 1997.

REM, rapid eye movement (sleep).

equals or exceeds that of the average nightmare.[23] In short, whereas disturbing dreams may frequently awaken a sleeper, awakenings are not the sole or even the best index of the severity of the disorder.

Similarly, researchers have come to define nightmares more inclusively with respect to their emotional tone. This is reflected in the modified ICSD-II definition of nightmares as *disturbing mental experiences* rather than as *frightening dreams* as in the ICSD. Some have argued[20,24] that nightmares can involve any unpleasant emotion, an opinion that is consistent with patients' reports that their nightmares involve intensification of many unpleasant emotions, such as sadness or anger. Nonetheless, fear remains the most frequently reported nightmare emotion.[23]

Table 77–2. Clinical Criteria for Nightmare Disorder

	DSM-IV Diagnostic Criteria for Nightmare Disorder (307.47)	ICSD-II Diagnostic Criteria for Nightmare Disorder (307.47)
Nature of recalled dream	A. Repeated awakenings from the major sleep period or naps with detailed recall of extended and extremely frightening dreams, usually involving threats to survival, security, or self-esteem.	A. Recurrent episodes of awakenings from sleep with recall of intensely disturbing dream mentation, usually involving fear or anxiety but also anger, sadness, disgust and other dysphoric emotions.
Nature of awakening	B. On awakening from the frightening dreams, the person rapidly becomes oriented and alert (in contrast to the confusion and disorientation seen in Sleep Terror Disorder and some forms of epilepsy).	B. Alertness is usually full on awakening, with little confusion or disorientation: recall of sleep mentation is immediate and clear
Nature of distress	C. The dream experience, or the sleep disturbance resulting from the awakening, causes clinically significant distress or impairment in social, occupational, or other important areas of function.	C. Associated features include at least one of the following: • Return to sleep after the episodes is typically delayed and not rapid
Timing	A. The awakenings generally occur during the second half of the sleep period.	• Episodes typically occur in the later half of the habitual sleep period
Differential diagnosis	D. The nightmares do not occur exclusively during the course of another mental disorder (e.g., a delirium, Posttraumatic Stress Disorder) and are not due to the direct physiologic effects of a substance (e.g., a drug of abuse, a medication) or a general medical condition.	*Nightmares are distinguished from several other disorders in a Differential Diagnosis section:* Seizure Disorder, Arousal Disorders (Sleep Terror, Confusional Arousal), REM Sleep Behavior Disorder, Recurrent Isolated Sleep Paralysis, Nocturnal Panic, Posttraumatic Stress Disorder, Acute Stress Disorder

DSM-IV, Diagnostic and Statistical Manual of Mental Disorders, 4th ed.; ICSD-II, International Classification of Sleep Disorders, 2nd ed.; REM, rapid eye movement.

Prevalence and Frequency

Lifetime prevalence in the general population for a nightmare experience is unknown but may well approach 100%. If we consider only attack dreams, which are one of the most common nightmare themes, the lifetime prevalence varies from 67%[25] to 90%.[26] Pursuit, a closely related, highly disturbing theme, has a lifetime prevalence of 92% among women and 85% among men.[26] Age is clearly a mediating factor: children, young adults, and groups of adults and older adults have nightmares "at least sometimes," with a prevalence of 30% to 90%, 40% to 60%, and 60% to 68%, respectively.[27]

Nightmares are both more prevalent and more frequent in childhood. Prevalence increases through the first decade of life and diminishes from adolescence to early adulthood.[28,29] For example, in a clinical context, when nightmare problems were defined as lasting for longer than 3 months, their prevalence was 24% for ages 2 to 5, 41% for ages 6 to 10, and 22% for age 11.[28] Figures of 5% to 30% (for "often or always") and 30% to 90% (for "at least sometimes") have also been reported for children.[27] Two surveys[30,31] indicate that 20% to 30% of 5- to 12-year-old children have at least one nightmare in any 6-month period. There is a large sex difference in the recall ("sometimes" or "often") of bad dreams at age 13 (boys, 25%, versus girls, 40%) and age 16 (20% versus 40%) in the same cohort.[32]

Among adults, prevalence nevertheless is high (8% to 30%) when frequencies of "one or more per month" are considered, as indicated by several studies of college and university students.[20,33-35] When the response choice is "often or always," young adult prevalence is still 2% to 5%, whereas that of adult and older adult samples is only 1% to 2%.[27] Only about 4% of patients spontaneously report a complaint of nightmares to their physicians.[36]

Nightmares are reported more frequently by females than males among adolescents,[32] young adults,[38,39] middle-aged adults,[40,41] and the general population,[42] but not among children,[29,31,43,44] unless, however, estimates are made retrospectively—when the latter have become adults.[41] Our longitudinal study[32] revealed that a marked divergence between boys and girls occurs between 13 and 16 years of age: the proportion of girls responding "often" to a question about nightmare prevalence increases over time (from 2.7% to 4.9%), whereas for boys it decreases (from 2.5% to 0.4%).

Nightmare prevalence may be elevated in clinical populations—for example, 25% of both male chronic alcoholics and female alcohol and drug users report nightmares "every few nights" on the Minnesota Multiphasic Personality Inventory.[45,46] However, other findings of elevated prevalence are difficult to assess because a frequency criterion is not specified—for example, approximately 24% of nonpsychotic patients seen in psychiatric emergency services report nightmares, but with an unknown frequency.[47]

When compared with results from daily home logs, however, retrospective self-reports underestimate current nightmare frequency by a factor of 2.5 in young adults[20,35] and by a factor of over 10 in healthy older adults.[48] In general, a 1-month retrospective estimate is closer to the evidence provided by daily logs than is a 12-month retrospective estimate, so the former is the preferred standard for retrospective assessment. However, as both nightmare prevalence and frequency are seriously underestimated by such instruments, daily logs are the method of choice.

Familial Pattern

Twin-based studies have identified persistent genetic effects on the disposition to nightmares in both childhood, as reported retrospectively by adults, and adulthood,[41] as well as genetic influences on the co-occurrence of nightmares and some other parasomnias, such as sleeptalking, but not others, such as bruxism.[49] In the Finnish nationwide twin cohort study, a substantial genetic basis for nightmares was shown in the proportion of phenotypic variance in trait liability for nightmare prevalence attributable to genetic influences (about 45%).[41]

Pathophysiology

One laboratory study of nightmares[50] indicates moderate arousal—in the form of increased heart and respiration rates—during some nightmare episodes, but unexpectedly low arousal in most others. Although these early findings constitute the principal empirical basis for diagnostic guidelines such as the ICSD and DSM-IV, there are serious problems with the work, such as the inclusion of psychiatric patients and patients with posttraumatic stress disorder (PTSD) in the study sample.

Recordings of heart and respiration rates during nightmare and nonnightmare REM sleep episodes confirmed a moderate level of sympathetic arousal during nightmares.[51] Mean heart rate for nightmare REM sleep was elevated (by about 6 beats per minute) only for the 3 minutes prior to awakening (Fig. 77–1). Most subjects showed heart rate acceleration during nightmare sleep. Mean respiration rate was only marginally higher for the last 3 minutes before awakening, however.

There are changes in cortical activity in the last 2 minutes of nightmare sleep. However, these changes—higher absolute and relative alpha EEG power over primarily right posterior sites—are largely the result of changes occurring immediately before awakening and may reflect the awakening process. Accumulating evidence[52] suggests that dream recall in general is associated with decreases, not increases, in alpha power.

Personality

Although many studies report relationships between nightmare frequency and measures of psychopathology,[16,20,32,37,53] some do not support such a relationship.[24,35] Seemingly weak relationships between nightmares and psychopathology most likely reflect mediating factors, among which three—chronicity of nightmares, nightmare distress, and coping style—have been given some attention.

NIGHTMARE CHRONICITY

Adults with a lifelong history of frequent nightmares make up a subgroup of idiopathic nightmare sufferers who manifest more psychopathologic symptoms than matched controls without nightmares (e.g., higher rates of neuroticism and higher psychopathology scores on the Minnesota Multiphasic Personality Inventory).[54,55] However, Hartmann[56] found that no one measure of psychopathology adequately describes these individuals. He described a general "boundary permeability" personality dimension,[56,57] correlated with nightmare prevalence,[58,59] which at one extreme ("thin boundaries") characterizes lifelong sufferers who are more open, sensitive, and vulnerable to intrusions than "thick boundary" subjects

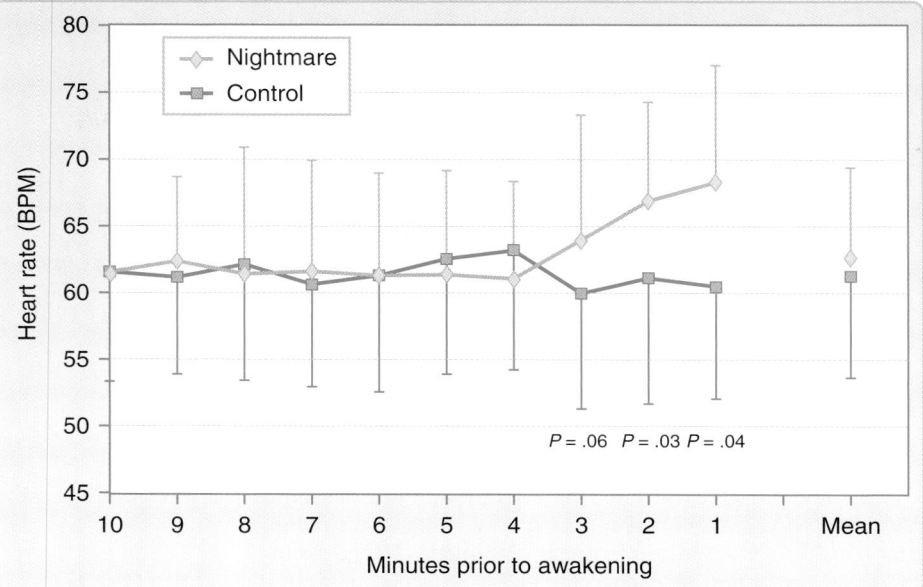

Figure 77–1. Average (± standard error) heart rate 10 minutes prior to awakening in nightmare and nonnightmare rapid eye movement (REM) sleep episodes. Heart rate for nightmare REM sleep was elevated by about 6 beats per minute (BPM) for the 3 minutes prior to awakening, but not earlier than that.

and thus who are more sensitive to events not usually viewed as traumatic.[56]

NIGHTMARE DISTRESS

Nightmare frequency and waking distress over one's nightmares are not equivalent and are only moderately correlated.[16,24,35] Subjects may have only few nightmares (e.g., one per month) yet report high levels of associated distress, or they may report many nightmares (e.g., more than one per week) yet low levels of distress. It is the nightmare distress factor, not necessarily the frequency factor, that is significantly related to psychopathology, especially to measures of anxiety and depression.[16,24] Nightmare distress may be related to more general stress-related factors. For example, whereas both state (stress) and trait personality measures are significantly correlated with nightmare frequency, regression analyses indicate that trait measures do not account for any variance beyond that accounted for by state measures.[53] *Nightmare distress should be evaluated during clinical intake, as it is not among the diagnostic criteria of the DSM-IV or ICSD-II yet it is central to defining nightmares as a clinical problem.*

COPING STYLE

Given the central role of nightmare distress, a person's ability to cope with stress may be critical to whether a clinical problem with nightmares develops. Studies of nightmares that endure for years or even decades after a trauma provide some pertinent findings for coping. College students suffering from nightmares report both a higher rate of childhood traumatic experiences and higher scores on a measure of dissociative coping (i.e., on the Dissociative Experiences Scale) than do students without nightmares.[60] Dysfunctional coping strategies may exacerbate both nightmare distress and chronicity.

Effects of Drugs and Alcohol

Numerous classes of drugs trigger nightmares and bizarre dreams, including catecholaminergic agents, beta-blockers,

some antidepressants, barbiturates, and alcohol. One review[61] suggests that the therapies most often associated with nightmares are sedative/hypnotics, beta-blockers, and amphetamines. Among catecholaminergic agents, reserpine, thioridazine, and levodopa (L-dopa) are all occasionally associated with vivid dreams and nightmares,[62-65] as are beta-blockers such as betaxolol, metoprolol, bisoprolol, and propranolol.[66-70] Among the antidepressants, bupropion leads to more vivid dreams and nightmares than do other antidepressants.[71,72] The selective serotonin reuptake inhibitors paroxetine and fluvoxamine suppress dream recall frequency while simultaneously increasing subjective dream intensity and bizarreness, possibly as a result of serotonergic REM sleep suppression.[73] Bedtime administration of tricyclic and neuroleptic agents leads to a higher recall of frightening dreams than when these are taken in two daily doses,[74,75] even though normal dream recall remains the same. Neuroleptics and tricyclics appear to render dream affect more dysphoric rather than increasing dream recall per se.

Withdrawal from barbiturates is associated with REM sleep rebound, vivid dreaming, and nightmares.[76,77] A hypothesis has been advanced that barbiturate suppression of REM sleep, much like that with alcohol, causes REM sleep rebound after discontinuation of the drug and consequently longer and more vivid dreams.[78] In addition, several case studies have alerted physicians to the nightmarigenic effects of specific substances (Table 77–3).

Sleep and dream disturbances follow alcohol withdrawal. Alcoholic patients report more vivid dreams and nightmares following withdrawal than they do during ingestion; although these are more frequent in the week after withdrawal, they are still present in subsequent weeks. The nightmares and insomnia of withdrawal can lead to resumed drinking in an attempt to normalize sleep. In fact, 29% of a group of 100 alcoholics reported further drinking to alleviate nightmares.[79] This relationship is also of critical importance because of the danger of alcohol self-medication for PTSD[80,81] and for other nightmare-producing disorders.

Table 77–3. Drugs Reported in Case Studies That Increase Frequency of Nightmares

Drug	Function	Reference
Thiothixene	Neuroleptic	Solomon (1983)[134]
Betaxolol	Beta-blocker	Mort (1992)[135]
Carbachol	Cholinergic agent	Mort (1992)[135]
Donepezil	Cholinesterase inhibitor	Ross and Shua-Haim (1998)[136]
Fluoxetine	Antidepressant	Lepkifker et al. (1995),[137] Markowitz (1991)[138]
Naproxen	Nonsteroidal antiinflammatory	Bakht and Miller (1991)[139]
Verapamil	Antimigraine agent	Kumar and Hodges (1988)[140]
Triazolam	Benzodiazepine hypnotic	Forman and Souney (1989),[141] Pagel (1987),[142] Juhl et al. (1984)[143]
Nitrazepam	Benzodiazepine hypnotic	Girwood (1973)[144]
Erythromycin	Antibiotic	Black and Dawson (1988),[145] Williams (1988)[146]

Vivid and macabre dreaming may be central to the delirium tremens (DTs) of acute alcohol withdrawal.[82] Because alcohol suppresses REM sleep, and because percentage of time spent in REM sleep (particularly at sleep onset) is extremely elevated in patients with DTs,[83,84] a theory of DTs hallucinations emphasizing REM sleep rebound and intrusion of dreaming into wakefulness has been proposed.[85] Case studies strongly suggest that hallucinations may continue *uninterrupted* from an ongoing nightmare.[83] Sleep during DTs appears to be a mixture of REM sleep and REM sleep with elevated muscle tone, which distinguishes it from the sleep of alcoholics without DTs.[86] Some, however, have failed to observe this pattern.[87,88] The similarity between sleep in patients with DTs and sleep in patients with REM sleep behavior disorder has also been noted.[89]

The neuropharmacologic basis of drug-induced or withdrawal-associated disturbed dreaming remains unclear. There may be a balance among various neurotransmitter systems such that nightmares are produced by reduced brain norepinephrine and serotonin or by increased dopamine and acetylcholine.[56,73] Dissociation of dream initiation and intensification processes by separate neuromodulatory systems may also be implicated.[73]

Recurrent Dreaming and Nightmares

Repetitive dreams, such as posttraumatic nightmares, depict—with numerous, highly similar versions—an unresolved experience, such as a motor vehicle accident or war trauma. *Recurrent dreams* depict conflicts or stressors metaphorically over time, and they are also primarily unpleasant in nature.[90,91] The most frequent recurrent dreams of adults are pseudonightmarish: being endangered (e.g., chased, threatened with injury), being alone and trapped (e.g., in an elevator), facing natural forces (e.g., volcanic eruptions), losing one's teeth. Dreams with less recurrence—described as *recurrent themes* or *recurrent contents*—extend over long series and are not so clearly associated with psychopathology. However, they may have adaptive functions.[92]

Subjects with recurrent dreams show less successful adaptation on measures of anxiety, depression, personal adjustment, and life-events stress than those without recurrent dreams.[93,94] The maintained cessation of recurrent dreaming may also reflect an upturn in well-being.[94] Further, case studies have described changes in repetitive dream elements toward a progressive pattern as a function of successful psychotherapy.[95]

Treatment

A wide variety of treatments for nightmares have been reported.[19,96] Although psychotherapy aimed at conflict resolution has traditionally been the treatment of choice,[97,98] it lacks empirical support. On the other hand, there is much support for diverse cognitive behavioral interventions that require six or fewer sessions. Systematic desensitization and relaxation techniques, used to condition a relaxation response to anxiety-provoking nightmare contents, have been effective in several case studies and in two controlled studies.[98,99] Imagery rehearsal, which teaches patients to change their remembered nightmares and to rehearse new scenarios, has reduced both nightmare distress and frequency.[100,101] Other treatments with some empirical support are lucid dreaming,[102] eye movement desensitization and reprocessing,[103] and hypnosis.[104]

SLEEP–WAKE TRANSITION DISTURBANCES

Several interrelated dream disturbances occur at the transitions into or out of sleep. These share the attributes of vivid, often intensely real, sensory imagery and disturbing affects such as fear. It may be their close proximity to wakefulness that colors these images with a distinctive reality quality—that is, there may be an interleaving or boundary dissociation of sleep–wake processes at this time. There might be, for example, an intrusion of a real perception into sleep or of a dreamed object or character into wakefulness.[105,106] The nature of the intruding components may well determine the distinctiveness of the transition disturbance, including typical or odd combinations such as a frightening hypnagogic image terminating in a sleep start, or incomprehensible sleeptalking accompanying sleep paralysis.

Sleep Starts

Sleep starts, also known as predormital or hypnic myoclonus or hypnagogic or hypnic jerks, are brief phasic contractions of the muscles of the legs, arms, face, or neck that occur at sleep onset. They are often associated with brief, albeit vivid and impactful, dream events. Perhaps the most common of these events is the illusion of suddenly falling that incites a vigorous and startling jerk. Brief sensory flashes also occur; sometimes they are somatic in nature and somewhat difficult to describe. Complex hypnagogic images may also accompany sleep starts.

Mild starts are a normal—even universal—feature of falling asleep, and a prevalence as high as 60% to 70% has been cited.[107] More extreme starts can engender difficulties in initiating sleep.[108]

Sleep starts bear a striking resemblance to exploding-head syndrome[109] in that the latter also occurs at sleep onset and produces sudden loud auditory sensations and/or bright light flashes. Sounds are described variously as explosions, thunderclaps, clashes of cymbals, doors slamming, electric shocks or explosions, loud snaps, bomblike explosions, and so on.[109] In a sample of 50 patients, 10% reported a simultaneous flash of light, 6% reported a curious sensation as if they had stopped breathing and had to make an "uncomfortable gasp" to start again, and almost all (94%) reported fear, terror, palpitations, or forceful heartbeat as an aftereffect.[109]

It is not known whether chronic sleep starts are primarily a disturbance of motor systems, perhaps akin to periodic limb movements during sleep, or a disturbance of imagery systems, such that intense images provoke the disruptive reflex activity. Electroencephalographic events have been noted to accompany sleep starts,[110] but more systematic studies of sleep starts and the variety of electroencephalographic burst patterns that can accompany drowsiness[111] are needed to clarify this issue.

Terrifying Hypnagogic Hallucinations

Terrifying hypnagogic hallucinations (THHs) are terrifying dreams similar to those in REM sleep. After a sudden awakening at sleep onset, there is prompt recall of frightening content.[107] Sleep-onset REM (SOREM) episodes may be aggravated by factors that predispose to this type of sleep—for example, withdrawal from REM sleep–suppressant medication, chronic sleep deprivation, sleep fragmentation, and narcolepsy. Other sleep and medical disorders may accompany the condition. Content analyses of THHs are lacking, but clinical and anecdotal reports suggest that the themes of attack and aggression found in REM-sleep nightmares are also common. Here, THHs are perhaps more anxiety provoking than most nightmares because of (1) a vivid sense of reality related to their close proximity to wakefulness, and (2) frequently associated feelings of paralysis. These features are illustrated by the following example.

At age 19, a 36-year-old woman, now suffering from PTSD, was abducted and for more than 3 days raped, beaten, burned, and subjected to death threats (Russian roulette) by motorcycle gang members. Although she regularly reexperienced these horrors through flashbacks and nightmares, even worse were the THHs with paralysis occurring as she returned to sleep *after* a nightmare. She felt as though she were awake, aroused, and terrified, yet unable to move; time seemed to be extremely drawn out as she experienced "replays" of her torturous experience in slow motion.[112]

The suffering during such episodes is exacerbated by the individual's simultaneous sense of wakefulness and inability to move or call for help. Furthermore, the intense anxiety may seriously disrupt sleep. For example, recurrent THHs may disrupt sleep onset sufficiently to produce sleep-onset insomnia.[107] Prevalence figures for THHs are not available, but an estimate for patients with narcolepsy is 4% to 8%.[27]

Sleep Paralysis

Physiologic mechanisms of sleep paralysis (SP) have been studied in some detail,[113,114] but the relationship of SP to disturbed dreaming remains unclear. SP is a cardinal symptom of narcolepsy and also occurs among healthy persons. Patients seldom present for symptoms of SP alone, although they may when the frequency of their episodes increases (e.g., to one per day). The clinical disorder of *recurrent isolated sleep paralysis* occurs at sleep onset or on awakening from sleep, whereas "normal" feelings of paralysis or ineffectuality are a common feature of dreaming more generally[14] and, especially, of nightmares.[115] According to some,[116] paralysis feelings render hypnagogic hallucinations threatening or terrifying in nature. Frightening SP episodes have also been referred to as *sleep paralysis nightmares* and their role in the misdiagnosis of hysteria and allegations of abuse described.[117]

Although psychopathology does not seem to be a direct cause of SP,[118] we have found an association between SP with presence imagery and social anxiety.[119] It is also possible that psychopathologic factors influence SP indirectly, by their influence on stress and overwork and subsequent disruptive effects on sleep[118] or by modulating vigilance levels during sleep disruption.[120] Sleep-related life habits, such as poor sleep quality, insufficient sleep, and a proclivity to daytime sleep—all factors that may favor the occurrence of SOREM episodes—are also associated with SP occurrence in nonnarcoleptic populations.[121] In fact, isolated SP episodes have been elicited experimentally by schedules of sleep interruptions that produce SOREM.[120,122]

Another mediating factor may be phase advance or rapid resetting of the circadian clock, as is the case with rapid time-zone change[123] or sleeping in the supine position.[118,124] However, the nature and intensity of imagery generation in both wakefulness and sleep also appears to play a role in the occurrence and frequency of SP. *Imaginativeness*, as indexed by standardized questionnaires, and *vividness of nighttime imagery*, as measured by self-reported frequencies of nightmares/sleep terrors and vividness of dream imagery, are two personality factors found to be *most* predictive of SP occurrence and frequency in a large multivariate study of college students.[118]

SP is typically accompanied by vivid hypnagogic hallucinations. In fact, it is rare to find SP in the absence of other hallucinatory activity. Spanos and coworkers[118] found that only 1.6% (of 387) subjects experienced SP without other attributes. Similarly, of the six experimental SP episodes described by Takeuchi et al.[122] all but one included auditory/visual hallucinations and unpleasant emotions. On the other hand, it is not true that most hypnagogic hallucinations are accompanied by SP. Given this association of SP with hypnagogic hallucinations, it is unclear whether SP is, as some have suggested,[125,126] a *type of perception*—that is, of ongoing REM sleep muscle atonia. Paralysis sensations, much like dreamed emotions and other sensations, *may be at least partially hallucinatory*. This could account for why SP is often reported to be associated with odd feelings of oppression, pressure on the chest and other body parts, even violent choking and beating. It could also explain how paralysis and felt ineffectuality appear routinely and in such variety in dreams and nightmares.[14]

Prevalence

Multiple SP episodes have a low prevalence, occurring "often or always" in only 0% to 1% of young adults and "at least sometimes" in 7% to 8% of young adults.[27] On the other hand, the ICSD[107] cites the lifetime prevalence of SP at 40% to 50%, which is somewhat higher than other estimates. We found rates of 25% to 36% in surveys of three university psychology student groups,[51] which is similar to the value of 26% reported for 208 Japanese undergraduates,[127] of 21% for 1798 Canadian undergraduates,[118] and of 34% for 200 patients with sleep disorders.[51]

Use of a culturally identifiable term for SP, such as *kanashibari* in Japan, can increase the estimate by an additional 8% (to 39%).[127] The latter estimate corresponds well with those drawn from other cultures—for example, 37% of 603 Hong Kong undergraduates report at least one episode of *ghost oppression*, the Chinese equivalent of *kanashibari*.[128] One survey of Newfoundland villagers found as many as 62% admitting to *old hag* attacks.[129]

Somniloquy with Dream Content

Sleeptalking has been observed in all stages of sleep, but especially in non-REM (NREM) sleep stages 2, 3, and 4.[130] Arkin[130] identified various orders of concordance between sleeptalking and later dream reports. For first-order concordances, sleeptalking exactly matches the content in the dream—for example, a subject shouted "No! No!" as she dreamed of shouting these words while seeing her baby fall from the bed. For second-order concordances, a conceptual or emotional link between sleeptalking and the dream is preserved—for example, a patient with nightmares dreamed repeatedly of trying to yell "Burglars!" but in reality called out "Mama!" Absence of concordance is also seen: one study of 28 chronic sleeptalkers found it in 16.7% of REM sleep, 32.9% of stage 2, and 38.5% of stage 3/4 sleep episodes.[130] As with SP, it remains unknown why imagery and behavior are dissociated in this manner.

False Awakening

False awakenings are nowhere classified as pathologic per se, but they are nevertheless dreaming disturbances that can produce anxious reactions. Two types of false awakening have been distinguished, primarily on the basis of the degree of anxious affect associated with them.[106,131] Both types typically depict the person as (falsely) waking up from sleep or, in variations, from a dream, and some confusion ensues while dreaming over whether one is actually awake or asleep. *Type 1* awakenings, the more common type, usually depict realistic instances of the person waking up in the habitual bed followed by, in many cases, depictions of activities such as dressing, eating breakfast, and setting off for work. Some discrepancy in the imagery may fully awaken the person with the surprising realization that it was "just a dream." The dreams are often repetitive, depicting a succession of awakenings or of setting off for work.

Type 2 false awakenings are less pleasant than type 1, in that the apparent awakenings in bed are accompanied by a "stressed, electrified, or tense" atmosphere and feelings of "foreboding or expectancy" that may be "apprehensive or oppressively ominous."[106] There may be hallucinations of ominous or anxiety-provoking sounds, or strange apparitions of persons or monsters. Both type 1 and type 2 false awakening are frequently associated with experiences of separating from the sleeping body (i.e., an out-of-body experience) and

of becoming aware of dreaming while dreaming (i.e., lucid dreaming).[106] False awakenings are clearly not always about a person's own home and bed, because instances have been elicited in laboratory subjects that incorporated the laboratory bed and setting.[132]

Pathologic and Disturbed Lucid Dreaming

Lucid dreaming is occasionally associated with disturbed or pathologic reactions. Typically, lucid dreaming is perceptually vivid—the dreamer often feels awake—with a limited capacity to control the unfolding of some dreamed events. It is often spontaneously triggered within a nightmare and can be used in a therapy context to resolve the distressing contents of recurrent nightmares.[102] However, some have reported diverse negative reactions associated with lucid dreaming, including a type of burnout resulting from too-frequent intentional use of the mental state, mental confusion and quasi-psychotic splits with reality (induced by the overlapping of perceptual and dreamlike mentation), and intense fear associated with the loss of control of the vivid dream contents.[133]

Clinical Pearl

The diagnosis and treatment plan for a great many sleep problems can be enhanced simply by querying patients during the clinical interview as to the nature of their dreams and nightmares and whether they have changed quantitatively or qualitatively since the onset of symptoms.

REFERENCES

1. Parmeggiani PL: The autonomic nervous system in sleep. In Kryger MH, Roth T, Dement WC (eds): Principles and Practice of Sleep Medicine, 2nd ed. Philadelphia, WB Saunders, 1994, pp 194-203.
2. Baharav A, Kotagal S, Gibbons V, et al: Fluctuations in autonomic nervous activity during sleep displayed by power spectrum analysis of heart rate variability. Neurology 1995; 45:1183-1187.
3. Verrier RL, Muller JE, Hobson JA: Sleep, dreams, and sudden death: The case for sleep as an autonomic stress test for the heart. Cardiovasc Res 1996;31:181-211.
4. Orem J: Respiratory neurons and sleep. In Kryger MH, Roth T, Dement WC (eds): Principles and Practice of Sleep Medicine, 2nd ed. Philadelphia, WB Saunders, 1994, pp 177-193.
5. Noll G, Elam M, Kunimoto M, et al: Skin sympathetic nerve activity end-effector function during sleep in humans. Acta Physiol Scand 1994;151:319-329.
6. Takeuchi S, Iwase S, Mano T, et al: Sleep related changes in human muscle and skin sympathetic nerve activities. J Autonom Nerv Syst 1994;47:121-129.
7. Maquet P: Positron emission tomography studies of sleep and sleep disorders. J Neurol 1997;244:S23-S28.
8. Braun AR, Balkin TJ, Wesensten NJ, et al: Dissociated pattern of activity in visual cortices and their projections during human rapid eye movement sleep. Science 1997;279:91-95.
9. Paradiso S, Robinson RG, Andreasen NC, et al: Emotional activation of limbic circuitry in elderly normal subjects in a PET study. Am J Psychiatry 1997;154:384-389.
10. Nielsen TA, Deslauriers D, Baylor GW: Emotions in dream and waking event reports. Dreaming 1991;1:287-300.
11. Hall C, Van de Castle RI: The Content Analysis of Dreams. New York, Appleton-Century-Crofts, 1966.

12. Kramer M: The selective mood regulatory function of dreaming: An update and revision. In Moffitt A, Kramer M, Hoffmann R (eds): The Functions of Dreaming. New York, State University of New York Press, 1993, pp 139-196.

13. Rechtschaffen A: The psychophysiology of mental activity during sleep. In McGuigan FJ, Schoonoer RA (eds): The Psychophysiology of Thinking: Studies of Covert Processes. New York, Academic Press, 1973, pp 153-205.

14. Kuiken D, Sikora S: The impact of dreams on waking thoughts and feelings. In Moffitt A, Kramer M, Hoffmann R (eds): The Functions of Dreaming. New York, State University of New York Press, 1993, pp 419-476.

15. Krakow B, Kellner R, Pathak D, Lambert L: Imagery rehearsal treatment for chronic nightmares. Behav Res Ther 1995;33:837-843.

16. Levin R, Fireman G: Nightmare prevalence, nightmare distress, and self-reported psychological disturbance. Sleep 2002;25:205-212.

17. Kramer M: Nightmares (dream disturbances) in posttraumatic stress disorder: Implication for a theory of dreaming. In Bootzin RR, Kihlstrom JF, Schacter DL (eds): Sleep and Cognition. Washington, DC, American Psychological Association, 1992, pp 190-203.

18. American Psychiatric Association: Diagnostic and Statistical Manual of Mental Disorders, 4th ed (DSM-IV). Washington, DC, American Psychiatric Association, 1994.

19. Halliday G: Direct psychological therapies for nightmares: A review. Clin Psychol Rev 1987;7:501-523.

20. Zadra A, Donderi DC: Nightmares and bad dreams: Their prevalence and relationship to well-being. J Abnorm Psychol 2000;109:273-281.

21. Levitan HL: The significance of certain catastrophic dreams. Psychother Psychosom 1976;27:1-7.

22. Van Bork J: An attempt to clarify a dream-mechanism: Why do people wake up out of an anxiety dream? Int Rev Psychoanal 1982;9:273-277.

23. Zadra A, Donderi DC: Affective content and intensity of nightmares and bad dreams. Sleep 2003;26:A93-A94.

24. Belicki K: Nightmare frequency versus nightmare distress: Relations to psychopathology and cognitive style. J Abnorm Psychol 1992;101:592-597.

25. Harris I: Observations concerning typical anxiety dreams. Psychiatry 1948;11:301-309.

26. Hall CS: The significance of the dream of being attacked. J Pers 1955;24:164-180.

27. Partinen M: Epidemiology of sleep disorders. In Kryger MH, Roth T, Dement WC (eds): Principles and Practice of Sleep Medicine, 2nd ed. Philadelphia, WB Saunders, 1994, pp 437-452.

28. Salzarulo P, Chevalier A: Sleep problems in children and their relationship with early disturbances of the waking-sleeping rhythms. Sleep 1983;6:47-51.

29. Fisher BE, Pauley C, McGuire K: Children's Sleep Behavior Scale: Normative data on 870 children in grades 1 to 6. Percept Motor Skills 1989;68:227-236.

30. Simonds JF, Parraga H: Prevalence of sleep disorders and sleep behaviors in children and adolescents. J Am Acad Child Psychiatry 1982;21:383-388.

31. Vela-Bueno A, Bixler EO, Dobladez-Blanco B, et al: Prevalence of night terrors and nightmares in elementary school children: A pilot study. Res Commun Psychol Psychiatr Behav 1985;10:177-188.

32. Nielsen TA, Laberge L, Paquet J, et al: Development of disturbing dreams during adolescence and their relationship to anxiety symptoms. Sleep 2000;23:727-736.

33. Belicki K, Cuddy MA: Nightmares: Facts, fictions and future directions. In Gackenbach J, Sheikh AA (eds): Dream Images: A Call to Mental Arms. Amityville, NY, Baywood, 1991, pp 99-115.

34. Levin R: Sleep and dreaming characteristics of frequent nightmare subjects in a university population. Dreaming 1994;4:127-137.

35. Wood JM, Bootzin RR: The prevalence of nightmares and their independence from anxiety. J Abnorm Psychol 1990;99:64-68.

36. Bixler EO, Kales A, Soldatos CR: Sleep disorders encountered in medical practice: A national survey of physicians. Behav Med 1979;6:13-21.

37. Chivers L, Blagrove M: Nightmare frequency, personality, and acute psychopathology. Pers Indiv Dif 1999;27:843-851.

38. Coren S: The prevalence of self-reported sleep disturbances in young adults. Int J Neurosci 1994;79:67-73.

39. Tan VL, Hicks RA: Type A-B behavior and nightmare types among college students. Percept Motor Skills 1995;81:15-19.

40. Low JF, Dyster-Aas J, Willebrand M, et al: Chronic nightmares after severe burns: Risk factors and implications for treatment. J Burn Care Rehabil 2003;24:260-267.

41. Hublin C, Kaprio J, Partinen M, Koskenvuo M: Nightmares: Familial aggregation and association with psychiatric disorders in a nationwide twin cohort. Am J Med Genet 1999;88:329-336.

42. Claridge G, Clark K, Davis C: Nightmares, dreams, and schizotypy. Br J Clin Psychol 1997;36:377-386.

43. Muris P, Merckelbach H, Gadet B, et al: Fears, worries, and scary dreams in 4- to 12-year-old children: Their content, developmental pattern, and origins. J Clin Child Psychol 2000;29:43-52.

44. Fisher BE, Wilson AE: Selected sleep disturbances in school children reported by parents: Prevalence, interrelationships, behavioral correlates and parental attributions. Percept Motor Skills 1987;64:1147-1157.

45. Cernovsky ZZ: MMPI and nightmares in male alcoholics. Percept Motor Skills 1985;61:841-842.

46. Cernovsky ZZ: MMPI and nightmare reports in women addicted to alcohol and other drugs. Percept Motor Skills 1986;62:717-718.

47. Brylowski A: Nightmares in crisis: Clinical applications of lucid dreaming techniques. Psychiatr J Univ Ott 1990;15:79-84.

48. Salvio MA, Wood JM, Schwartz J, et al: Nightmare prevalence in the healthy elderly. Psychol Aging 1992;7:324-325.

49. Hublin C, Kaprio J, Partinen M, et al: Parasomnias: Co-occurrence and genetics. Psychiatr Genet 2001;11:65-70.

50. Fisher C, Byrne J, Edwards A, Kahn E: A psychophysiological study of nightmares. J Am Psychoanal Assoc 1970;18:747-782.

51. Nielsen TA, Zadra A: Dreaming disorders. In Kryger M, Roth N, Dement WC (eds): Principles and Practice of Sleep Medicine, 3rd ed. Philadelphia, WB Saunders, 2000, pp 753-772.

52. Esposito MJ, Nielsen TA, Paquette T: Reduced alpha power associated with the recall of mentation from stage 2 and stage REM sleep. Psychophysiology 2004;41:288-297.

53. Schredl M: Effects of state and trait factors on nightmare frequency. Eur Arch Psychiatry Clin Neurosci 2003;253:241-247.

54. Berquier A, Ashton R: Characteristics of the frequent nightmare sufferer. J Abnorm Psychol 1992;101:246-250.

55. Levin R, Raulin ML: Preliminary evidence for the proposed relationship between frequent nightmares and schizotypal symptomatology. J Pers Disord 1991;5:8-14.

56. Hartmann E: The nightmare: The Psychology and the Biology of Terrifying Dreams. New York, Basic Books, 1984.

57. Hartmann E, Elkin R, Garg M: Personality and dreaming: The dreams of people with very thick or very thin boundaries. Dreaming 1991;1:311-324.

58. Hartmann E: Boundaries of dreams, boundaries of dreamers: Thin and thick boundaries as a new personality dimension. Psychiatr J Univ Ott 1989;14:557-560.

59. Levin R, Galin J, Zywiak B: Nightmares, boundaries, and creativity. Dreaming 1991;1:63-74.

60. Agargun MY, Kara H, Ozer OA, et al: Nightmares and dissociative experiences: The key role of childhood traumatic events. Psychiatry Clin Neurosci 2003;57:139-145.

61. Thompson DF, Pierce DR: Drug-induced nightmares (review). Ann Pharmacother 1999;33:93-98.

62. Hartmann E, Cravens J: The effects of long term administration of psychotropic drugs on human sleep: II. The effects of reserpine. Psychopharmacologia 1973;33:169-184.

63. Kales A, Scharf MB, Bixler EO, et al: Sleep laboratory drug evaluation: Thioridazine (Mellaril), a REM enhancing drug. Sleep Res 1974;3:55.

64. Moskovitz C, Moses H, Klawans HL: Levodopa-induced psychosis: A kindling phenomenon. Am J Psychiatry 1978;135:669-675.

65. Sharf B, Moskovitz C, Lupton MD, Klawans HL: Dream phenomena induced by chronic levodopa therapy. J Neural Trans 1978;43:143-151.

66. Bengtsson C, Lennartsson J, Lindquist O, et al: Sleep disturbances, nightmares and other possible central nervous disturbances in a population sample of women, with special reference to those on antihypertensive drugs. Eur J Clin Pharmacol 1980;17:173-177.

67. Cove-Smith JR, Kirk CA: CNS-related side-effects with metoprolol and atenolol. Eur J Pharmacol 1985;28(Suppl):69-72.

68. Davidov ME, Glazer N, Wollam G, et al: Comparison of betaxolol, a new B$_1$-adrenergic antagonist, to propranolol in the treatment of mild to moderate hypertension. Am J Hypertens 1988;1:206S-210S.

69. Henningsen NC, Mattiasson I: Long-term clinical experience with atenolol: A new selective beta-l-blocker with few side effects from the central nervous system. Acta Med Scand 1979;205:61-66.

70. Kuriyama S: Bisoprolol-induced nightmares. J Hum Hypertens 1994;8:730-732.

71. Balon R: Bupropion and nightmares. Am J Psychiatry 1996;153:579-580.

72. Becker RE, Dufresne RL: Perceptual changes with bupropion, a novel antidepressant. Am J Psychiatry 1982;139:1200-1201.

73. Pace-Schott EF, Gersh T, Silvestri R, et al: SSRI treatment suppresses dream recall frequency but increases subjective dream intensity in normal subjects. J Sleep Res 2001;10:129-142.

74. Flemenbaum A: Pavor nocturnus: A complication of single daily tricyclic or neuroleptic dosage. Am J Psychiatry 1976;133:570-572.

75. Strayhorn JM, Nash JL: Frightening dreams and dosage schedule of tricyclic and neuroleptic drugs. J Nerv Ment Dis 1978;166:878-880.

76. Kales A, Bixler EO, Tan TL, et al: Chronic hypnotic use: Ineffectiveness, drug-withdrawal insomnia, and dependence. JAMA 1974;227:513-517.

77. Firth H: Sleeping pills and dream content. Br J Psychiatry 1974;124:547-553.

78. Oswald I, Priest RG: Five weeks to escape the sleeping-pill habit. Br Med J 1965;2:1093-1095.

79. Hershon HI: Alcohol withdrawal symptoms and drinking behavior. J Stud Alcohol 1977;38:953-971.

80. Blake DD, Cook JD, Monaco V, et al: Coping patterns in combat-related PTSD: Alcohol and drug use. Presented at 24th Annual Convention of the Association for Advancement of Behavior Therapy, November, San Francisco, Calif, 1990.

81. Stewart SH: Alcohol abuse in individuals exposed to trauma: A critical review. Psychol Bull 1996;120:83-112.

82. Hishikawa Y, Sugita Y, Teshima T, et al: Sleep disorders in alcoholic patients with delirium tremens and transient withdrawal hallucinations: Reevaluation of the REM rebound and intrusion theory. In Karacan I (ed): Psychophysiological Aspects of Sleep. Park Ridge, NJ, Noyes Medical, 1981, pp 109-122.

83. Gross MM, Goodenough D, Tobin M, et al: Sleep disturbances and hallucinations in the acute alcoholic psychoses. J Nerv Ment Dis 1966;142:493-514.

84. Rowland RH: Sleep onset rapid eye movement periods in neuropsychiatric disorders: Implications for the pathophysiology of psychosis. J Nerv Ment Dis 1997;185:730-738.

85. Feinberg I: Hallucinations, dreaming and REM sleep. In Keup W (ed): Origin and Mechanisms of Hallucinations. New York, Plenum, 1970, pp 125-132.

86. Tachibana M, Tanaka K, Hishikawa Y, et al: A sleep study of acute psychotic states due to alcohol and meprobamate addiction. In Weitzman ED (ed): Advances in Sleep Research, vol 2. New York, Spectrum, 1975, pp 177-205.

87. Wolin SJ, Mello NK: The effects of alcohol on dreams and hallucinations in alcohol addicts. Ann N Y Acad Sci 1973;215:266-302.

88. Allen RP, Wagman A, Faillace LA, et al: Electroencephalographic (EEG) sleep recovery following prolonged alcohol intoxication in alcoholics. J Nerv Ment Dis 1971;153:424-433.

89. Mahowald MW, Schenck CH: REM sleep behavior disorder. In Kryger MH, Roth T, Dement WC (eds): Principles and Practice of Sleep Medicine, 2nd ed. Philadelphia, WB Saunders, 1994, pp 574-588.

90. Cartwright RD: The nature and function of repetitive dreams: A survey and speculation. Psychiatry 1979;42:131-137.

91. Zadra AL: Recurrent dreams: Their relation to life events. In Barrett D (ed): Trauma and Dreams. Cambridge, Mass, Harvard University Press, 1996, pp 231-247.

92. Domhoff GW: The repetition of dreams and dream elements: A possible clue to a function of dreams. In Moffitt A, Kramer M, Hoffmann R (eds): The Functions of Dreaming. New York, State University of New York Press, 1993, pp 293-320.

93. Zadra AL, O'Brien S, Donderi DC: Dream content, dream recurrence and well-being: A replication with a younger sample. J Imag Cogn Pers 1998;17:293-311.

94. Brown RJ, Donderi DC: Dream content and self-reported well-being among recurrent dreamers, past-recurrent dreamers, and nonrecurrent dreamers. J Pers Soc Psychol 1986;50:612-623.

95. Bonime W: The Clinical Use of Dreams. New York, Basic Books, 1962.

96. Coalson B: Nightmare help: Treatment of trauma survivors with PTSD. Psychotherapy 1995;32:381-388.

97. Freud S: The Interpretation of Dreams. New York, Basic Books, 1955.

98. Jones E: On the Nightmare. New York, Liveright, 1951.

99. Miller WR, DiPilato M: Treatment of nightmares via relaxation and desensitization: A controlled evaluation. J Consult Clin Psychol 1983;51:870-877.

100. Germain A, Nielsen TA: Impact of imagery rehearsal treatment on distressing dreams, psychological distress, and sleep parameters in nightmare patients. Behav Sleep Med 2003;1:140-154.

101. Krakow B, Sandoval D, Schrader R, et al: Treatment of chronic nightmares in adjudicated adolescent girls in a residential facility. J Adolesc Health 2001;29:94-100.

102. Zadra AL, Pihl RO: Lucid dreaming as a treatment for recurrent nightmares. Psychother Psychosom 1997;66:50-55.

103. Marquis J: A report on seventy-eight cases treated by eye movement desensitization. J Behav Ther Exp Psychiatry 1991;22:187-192.

104. Kingsbury SJ: Brief hypnotic treatment of repetitive nightmares. Am J Clin Hypn 1993;35:161-169.

105. Mahowald MW, Schenck CH: Dissociated states of wakefulness and sleep. Neurology 1992;42(Suppl 6):44-52.

106. Green C, McCreery C: Lucid Dreaming: The Paradox of Consciousness during Sleep. London, Routledge, 1994.

107. American Sleep Disorders Association: International Classification of Sleep Disorders, Revised: Diagnostic and Coding Manual. Rochester, Minn: American Sleep Disorders Association, 1997.

108. Broughton R: Pathological fragmentary myoclonus, intensified "hypnic jerks" and hypnagogic foot tremor: Three unusual sleep-related movement disorders. In Koella WP, Obal F, Schulz H, et al (eds): Sleep '86. Stuttgart, Germany, Gustav Fischer Verlag, 1988, pp 240-243.

109. Pearce JM: Clinical features of the exploding head syndrome. J Neurol Neurosurg Psychiatry 1989;52:907-910.

110. Oswald I: Sudden bodily jerks on falling asleep. Brain 1959; 82:92-101.

111. Bartel P, Robinson E, Duim W: Burst patterns occurring during drowsiness in clinical EEGs. Am J EEG Technol 1995;283-295.

112. Hudson JI, Manoach DS, Sabo AN, Sternbach SE: Recurrent nightmares in posttraumatic stress disorder: Association with sleep paralysis, hypnopompic hallucinations, and REM sleep. J Nerv Ment Dis 1991;179:572-573.

113. Hishikawa Y, Shimizu T: Physiology of REM sleep, cataplexy, and sleep paralysis. Adv Neurol 1995;67:245-271.

114. Hishikawa Y: Sleep paralysis. In Guilleminault C, Dement WC, Passouant P (eds): Narcolepsy. New York, Spectrum, 1976, pp 97-123.

115. Liddon SC: Sleep paralysis and hypnagogic hallucinations: Their relationship to the nightmare. Arch Gen Psychiatry 1967; 17:88-96.

116. Broughton RJ: Neurology and dreaming. Psychiat J Univ Ott 1982;7:101-110.

117. Powell RA, Nielsen TA: Was Anna O.'s black snake hallucination a sleep paralysis nightmare? Dreams, memories, and trauma. Psychiatry 1998;61:239-241.

118. Spanos NP, DuBreuil C, McNulty SA, et al: The frequency and correlates of sleep paralysis in a university sample. J Res Pers 1995;29:285-305.

119. Simard V, Nielsen TA, Zadra A, et al: Sensed presence as a possible manifestation of social anxiety. Dreaming (submitted). 2004.

120. Takeuchi T, Fukuda K, Sasaki Y, et al: Factors related to the occurrence of isolated sleep paralysis elicited during a multiphasic sleep-wake schedule. Sleep 2002;25:89-96.

121. Takeuchi T, Fukuda K, Yamamoto Y, et al: What kind of sleep-related life style affects the occurrence of sleep paralysis in normal individuals? Sleep Res 1997;26:518.

122. Takeuchi T, Miyasita A, Sasaki Y, et al: Isolated sleep paralysis elicited by sleep interruption. Sleep 1992;15:217-225.

123. Snyder S: Isolated sleep paralysis after rapid time zone change ("jet lag") syndrome. Chronobiologia 1983;10:377-379.

124. Fukuda K, Ogilvie R, Takeuchi T: The prevalence of sleep paralysis among Canadian and Japanese college students. Dreaming 1998;8:59-66.

125. Giaquinto S, Pompeiano O, Somogyi I: Supraspinal inhibitory control of spinal reflexes during natural sleep. Experientia 1963;19:652-653.

126. Hufford DJ: The terror that comes in the night: An experience-centered study of supernatural assault traditions. Philadelphia, University of Pennsylvania Press, 1982.

127. Fukuda K: One explanatory basis for the discrepancy of reported prevalences of sleep paralysis among healthy respondents. Percept Motor Skills 1993;77:803-807.

128. Wing YK, Lee ST, Chen CN: Sleep paralysis in Chinese: Ghost oppression phenomenon in Hong Kong. Sleep 1994;17: 609-613.

129. Ness RC: The Old Hag phenomenon as sleep paralysis: A biocultural interpretation. Cult Med Psychiatry 1978;2:15-39.

130. Arkin AM: Sleep-Talking: Psychology and Psychophysiology. Hillsdale, NJ: Lawrence Erlbaum, 1981.

131. Green CE: Lucid Dreams. Oxford, Institute of Psychophysical Research, 1968.

132. Nielsen TA, Montplaisir J: REM sleep hallucinatory episodes induced by somatic stimulation: A phenomenological report. Tenth Congress of the European Sleep Research Society, Strasbourg, France, May, 1990.

133. Gackenbach J, Bosveld J: Control Your Dreams. New York, Harper & Row, 1989.

134. Solomon K: Thiothixene and bizarre nightmares: An association? J Clin Psychiatry 1983;44:77-78.

135. Mort JR: Nightmare cessation following alteration of ophthalmic administration of a cholinergic and a beta-blocking agent. Ann Pharmacother 1992;26:914-916.

136. Ross JS, Shua-Haim JR: Aricept-induced nightmares in Alzheimer's disease: 2 case reports. J Am Geriatr Soc 1998; 46:119-120.

137. Lepkifker W, Dannon PN, Iancu I, et al: Nightmares related to fluoxetine treatment. Clin Neuropharmacol 1995;18:90-94.

138. Markowitz JC: Fluoxetine and dreaming. J Clin Psychiatry 1991;52:432.

139. Bakht FR, Miller LG: Naproxen-associated nightmares. South Med J 1991;84:1271-1273.

140. Kumar KL, Hodges M: Disturbing dreams with long-acting verapamil. N Engl J Med 1988;318:929-930.

141. Forman JK, Souney PF: Adverse reactions in hospitalized patients receiving triazolam or temazepam. J Geriatr Drug Ther 1989;3:55-66.

142. Pagel JF Jr: Diagnosis and treatment of insomnia. Am Fam Physician 1987;35:191-197.

143. Juhl RP, Daugherty VM, Kroboth PD: Incidence of next-day anterograde amnesia caused by flurazepam hydrochloride and triazolam. Clin Pharm 1984;3:622-625.

144. Girwood RH: Nitrazepam nightmares. BMJ 1973;1:353.

145. Black RJ, Dawson TA: Erythromycin and nightmares. BMJ (Clin Res Ed) 1988;296:1070.

146. Williams NR: Erythromycin: A case of nightmares. BMJ (Clin Res Ed) 1988;296:214.

78

Disturbed Dreaming in Medical Conditions

Tore A. Nielsen

ABSTRACT

Disturbed dreaming has been identified as a common primary or secondary symptom in several medical conditions, in addition to idiopathic nightmares and sleep–wake transition disorders. In these medical conditions, dream disturbances vary along a continuum of dream experience intensity. At the lower extreme of this continuum, dream recall ceases entirely (global cessation of dreaming) or is unusually impoverished in quantity or content (dream impoverishment). Impoverishment affects patients with alexithymia, posttraumatic stress disorder (PTSD), and some brain syndromes. At the higher extreme, dreaming is uncharacteristically excessive, vivid, and emotional (excessive dreaming). Excessive dreaming occurs in patients with epic dreaming, some brain lesions, and withdrawal from some medications. Dreaming may become so intense that it is confused with reality (dream–reality confusion), as is the case with the existential dreams of bereavement, with postpartum infant peril dreams, with intensive care unit delirium dreams, with dreams resulting from limbic lobe damage, and with psychotic dream-related aggression. Intense dreaming may also become rigidly stereotyped in structure (dream stereotypy). Conditions such as rapid eye movement (REM) sleep behavior disorder (RBD) with or without parkinsonism, epilepsy, PTSD reexperiencing dreams, migraine dreams, and prodromal cardiac dreams are affected by dream stereotypy. In many cases, dream disturbances appear to be aberrations of otherwise normal dream qualities, such as intensification, reality-mimesis, or recurrence. Often, sleep fragmentation is implicated in the disturbance, but causal relationships are not yet clear. Although it is primarily REM sleep that is involved, some disturbances are also seen in disorders affecting non-REM sleep. Effective treatments are available for many common disturbances, and other treatments are under development.

In addition to the common dream disturbances of idiopathic nightmares and sleep–wake transition disorders (see Chapter 77), disturbed dreaming has been identified as a common primary or secondary symptom in several other medical conditions (Table 78–1). These disturbances can be organized conveniently along a continuum of varying vividness or intensity of the dream experience. At the lower extreme of this continuum, dream recall ceases entirely or is unusually impoverished in quantity or content. At the higher extreme, it is uncharacteristically excessive, vivid, and emotional, frequently confused with reality or rigidly stereotyped in structure.

GLOBAL CESSATION OF DREAMING

Changes in the recall of dreams and in their global characteristics as a function of neurologic illness have been appreciated

ever since Charcot[1] reported on a patient with complete loss of visual imagery, including loss of visual dreaming.

About a third of patients with neurologic illness queried about *global cessation of dreaming* (GCD) report having ceased dreaming altogether.[2] Parietal lobe involvement is a significant aid to differentiating between patients with and without GCD, as 42% of GCD patients have parietal lesions and an additional 7% have lesions in close proximity to parietal lobe (periparietal). Parietal involvement confirms findings from a previous study.[3] The finding of frontal lobe lesions characterizing some patients (8%) with GCD[2] is consistent with the reduced dream recall seen after frontal lobotomy among schizophrenic patients[4] but not with results from another study.[3] The 43% of GCD cases not linked to parietal or frontal lesions have diffuse and nonlocalizable lesions.[2]

The findings of relatively intact dreaming after right hemispherectomy[5] but extremely impoverished recall after left hemispherectomy[6] support a left-hemisphere lateralization explanation of GCD. Neuropsychological reviews[7,8] also favor a predominant role for *left* hemisphere processes in dream generation more generally.

DREAM IMPOVERISHMENT

Dream impoverishment is a chronic attenuation, but not a total cessation, in the recall, length, vividness, emotionality, or narrative complexity of dream imagery. Impoverished dreaming has been documented above all among psychosomatic patients, particularly those with alexithymia, patients with posttraumatic stress disorder (PTSD) (who also have a high incidence of comorbid alexithymia[9]), and some types of brain syndrome.

Impoverished Dreaming in Alexithymia

Alexithymia refers to a difficulty in verbalizing emotions, literally, to a lack of a lexicon for describing feelings. Early investigations of psychosomatic patients[10,11] linked an alexithymic response style with diminished dream recall and an impoverished imaginal life more generally. An absence of affect in dreams was also frequently noted. Levitan[12] described dreams from many psychosomatic patients with alexithymia in which either the protagonists in the dreams failed to fully perceive their own feelings or their feelings were minimized by attributing them to other characters.

A study[13] of patients with nocturnal asthma—a population with a high incidence of alexithymia[14]—revealed that rapid eye movement (REM) sleep awakenings produced an elevated incidence of dreams with short sentences and impressions of having dreamed but with no specific recall.

Studies have reported evidence of impoverishment in dream sensory and structural features in alexithymia. One study of

Table 78–1. Medical Conditions in which Dreaming Is Disturbed

	Conditions Commonly Affected	Essential Features
Global cessation of dreaming	Charcot-Wilbrand syndrome Frontal lobotomy Parietal lobe lesions	Complete loss of dream recall; often, sudden onset after illness or medical procedure
Dream impoverishment	Alexithymia PTSD Brain syndromes	Reduction in recall, vividness, or complexity of dreaming
Excessive dreaming	Epic dreaming Brain damage Drug withdrawal	Dreaming seems to continue throughout the sleep period; may involve dream vivification, banal or repetitive dream content
Dream–reality confusion	ICU dream delirium Postpartum infant distress Existential dreams Psychotic dream-related aggression	Dream vivification; banal or everyday content may be confused with actual events
Dream stereotypy	RBD/parkinsonism Epilepsy PTSD Migraine Cardiac disease	Frequent recurrence of same dream content; may incorporate features of medical condition (e.g., aura, cardiac symptoms)

Abbreviations: ICU, intensive care unit; PTSD, posttraumatic stress disorder; RBD, REM (rapid eye movement) sleep behavior disorder.

the general Finnish population[15] found that alexithymic subjects reported colorless dreams, and a second[16] found that the dreams of nonclinical alexithymic subjects were less fantastic than those of controls; these groups did not differ on other measures of dream recall and emotion, however.

Sleep studies have not yet identified a consistent pattern of changes that might explain dream impoverishment. In one study,[17] higher alexithymia scores were related to several REM sleep variables: more frequent REM sleep episodes, shorter REM sleep latency, and more stage 1 sleep during and immediately after REM. However, alexithymia was also related to non-REM sleep variables: increased stage 1 and decreased stage 3/4. In a second study,[18] alexithymia scores did not correlate with *any* polysomnographic (PSG) variable or with rapid eye movement density; however, there was an association with shortened REM sleep latency. Finally, a survey study[15] indicated that alexithymia is reliably associated with certain sleep disorders, such as chronic insomnia and parasomnias.

In sum, although converging evidence indicates that dream impoverishment is associated with alexithymia, more research is needed to clarify relationships between alexithymic subcomponents and various attributes of dream recall, dream content, and dream emotion. Sleep measures also require further clarification.

It is also noteworthy that other patterns of disturbed dreaming characterize some alexithymic patients—for example, dreams that are extremely macabre, nightmarish, or lacking in ego and emotional control.[19] A similar manifestation of both impoverished and nightmarish dreams also characterizes patients with PTSD.

Impoverished Dreaming in Posttraumatic Stress Disorder

As unlikely as it might appear from the predominance of nightmares in patients with PTSD (see Chapters 46 and 111),

convergence of evidence suggests that a long-term consequence of PTSD is impoverishment of some features of dreaming. This evidence, as well as findings of sleep changes, have been reviewed concisely.[20,21]

Both home and laboratory studies indicate that patients with PTSD have lower than normal levels of dream recall. Furthermore, the dreams tend to be brief, to deal with trivial daily events, and to be associated with paradoxically high eye-movement densities.[22]

A study of subjects with disturbed dreaming[22] found dream recall only 42% to 54% of the time, compared with 89% to 96% for controls. Similarly, a "well-adjusted" group of 12 patients with PTSD[23] had a significantly lower dream recall rate from REM sleep (33.7%) than groups of either 11 less well-adjusted patients (50.5%) or 10 controls (80%). The well-adjusted patients reported dreams that were less complex and less salient; fewer dreams with anxiety, aggression, and conflict; and higher scores for denial of emotions toward their dreams.

Other studies have not demonstrated reduced dream recall in patients with PTSD[24,25] but at least one has reported, consistent with the previous findings, that laboratory dream recall is *negatively* correlated with trauma severity.[25]

Impoverished dreaming in PTSD remains unexplained, although at least two, very likely interrelated, explanations are feasible. First, the impoverishment may reflect an adaptive response or strategy that reduces overall dream recall and thereby suppresses the occurrence of nightmares.[23] Second, mechanisms responsible for dream impoverishment in alexithymia (see earlier) may also be active in PTSD. There is a high incidence of comorbidity with alexithymia;[9,26] in one study,[27] 85% of patients with PTSD were in the alexithymic range. Hyperarousal and emotional numbing may be common to the etiologies of both conditions. Emotional numbing, which is thought to be equivalent to alexithymia in the PTSD population,[9] is best predicted by the number of hyperarousal symptoms in patients with PTSD.[28] Patients with PTSD may expend so much cognitive, behavioral, and emotional effort managing hyperarousal and reactivity symptoms that they exhaust or deplete their emotional resources including, possibly, a depletion of catecholamines.[29]

Impoverished Dreaming in Brain Syndromes

In chronic brain syndrome, dream recall from REM sleep deteriorates as the illness progresses from mild (57% recall) to severe (35%) to aged and severe (8%).[30] In Korsakoff's psychosis caused by chronic alcohol abuse, near-normal REM sleep time (29.4%) but poor dream recall (3%) is observed.[31] Patients with permanent amnesia for recent events due to mild encephalitis also have impoverished dreaming; the frequency of their reports on awakening from REM sleep (28%) is less than normal (75%), and the report content is simpler, nonsymbolic, and more repetitive, stereotyped, and lacking in emotions and day residues.[32]

EXCESSIVE DREAMING

There are several conditions in which patients complain that their dreams are too abundant, too vivid, or unrelenting. Schenck and Mahowald[33] proposed the term *epic dreaming* to refer to complaints of both excessive dreaming ("dreaming all night long") and daytime fatigue. Apart from a subsequent case study published by our group,[34] this interesting category has not been further elaborated. Patients have the impression that throughout the night they dream about activity that is continuous, trivial, or banal or physical in nature—for example, repetitive housework, endless walking through snow or mud. Intense sensations of acceleration or spinning can also occur. Such dreams occur nightly in 90% of affected patients and 4 nights per week in the remainder.[33] Comorbid nightmares are reported by 70%,[33] although, unlike in nightmares, emotional arousal is strangely absent from epic dreams. Thus, although excessive, epic dreams are paradoxically impoverished in some respects (see earlier). Feelings of fatigue or exhaustion, as well as the recall of endlessly repetitive dreams, may produce distress and lead patients to seek help.

Epic dreaming is more commonly reported by women (85%) than men (15%).[33] PSG evaluation reveals no clinical abnormalities, etiology and pathophysiology remain unknown, and treatments (cognitive, hypnosis, relaxation, medications) have proved largely ineffective.[33] Comparative studies of epic dreams with normal dreams, nightmares, and recurrent dreams might shed light on possible pathophysiologic factors, such as whether the repetitive motor imagery is an amplified form of motor imagery in normal dreaming[35] or whether epic dreams are a type of nightmare stripped of affective intensification.

Other types of excessive dreaming occur in patients with brain lesions[2] and include increases in both the frequency and the vividness of dream imagery.[36,37] Some brain-damaged patients also report more continuous dreaming—that is, dreaming the same content throughout the night, despite intervening episodes of wakefulness.[2,36,37] Neuropsychological evidence points to involvement of the anterior limbic system.

Excessive dreaming may also be induced by withdrawal from certain medications. Excessive, vivid, and early-onset dreaming follows withdrawal from tricyclic antidepressants[38] or short half-life serotonin reuptake inhibitors such as paroxetine or fluvoxamine.[39]

An explanation for excessive dreaming is currently lacking, but it is likely that it, like other dream disorders, is an aberration of one or more characteristics of normal dreaming.

DREAM–REALITY CONFUSIONS

One characteristic of dream intensification is its closer approximation to real sensorimotor, emotional experience (or reality mimesis). This intensified realism is self-evident to anyone in the grips of a vivid nightmare. Heightened reality mimesis during dreaming is also common among patients with sleep paralysis and narcolepsy.[40] Here, dream–reality confusions of varying magnitudes are described for four conditions.

Existential Bereavement Dreams

Kuiken and colleagues[41,42] identified a category of realistic dreams referred to as *existential* dreams that frequently culminate in intensely real endings—often producing awakenings. Such dreams are characterized by a heightened reality mimesis, including distressing emotions (e.g., sadness, despair, guilt), salient bodily feelings (e.g., ineffectuality, paralysis), and failures in goal attainment. Themes frequently involve separation and loss and the appearance of deceased family figures. These features distinguish existential dreams from typical nightmares. Their clinical importance is their appearance during bereavement, which involves a range of distressing emotions other than fear. Bereavement is also characterized by hallucinations and vivid feelings of the presence of the deceased in both dreaming and waking states.[43,44] Existential dreams are common throughout the bereavement period (0 to 5 years after a loss), whereas other dream types are more salient either immediately after (anxiety dreams) or from 3 to 5 years after (transcendent dreams) a loss.[45] A sense of the presence of the deceased also continues throughout bereavement, whereas hallucinations of the deceased diminish over time.[46]

Postpartum Infant Peril Dreams

Postpartum mothers often dream vividly of their infants being either lost or in danger (peril dreams) and may, during these dreams, enact behaviors such as searching, vocalizing, or weeping. A frequent occurrence, what we refer to as BIB (for baby-in-bed) dreams, is that the mother dreams she has lost her infant in the bed and, while asleep, searches anxiously through the covers, weeps, calls out in alarm or touches the spouse thinking that some part of him is the infant.

The prevalence of peril dreams and sleep behaviors is remarkably high.[47] Over 12 postpartum weeks, 77% of women are able to recall the first dream involving their new infant. Of the latter, 73% (50% of total sample) reported at least one peril dream and 63% (44% of total sample) reported associated sleep behaviors. The latter value (44%) is much higher than the number of mothers (28.2%) who reported past or current somnambulism at least "rarely."

The mother's intense emotional and motoric arousal during the dream probably contributes to their appearance. The impact of the dreams is also substantial: 41% of mothers reported continuing anxiety after awakening from them, and

60% reported going to check on the infant. The hallucinated presence of the infant in these dreams suggests possible similarities with mechanisms producing presence imagery in sleep paralysis, narcolepsy, and existential dreams.

Mothers' responses to questioning revealed that peril dreams were predicted by relatively recent, stress-related factors such as difficult pregnancy, sleep disruption, infant–mother bed sharing, and anxiety, whereas sleep behaviors were predicted by sleep disruption and prior psychopathologic factors such as somnambulism, general psychopathology, and attachment disturbance.[47]

Intensive Care Unit Dream Delirium

Nightmarish intensification of dreaming is reported by patients struggling to survive life-threatening conditions in intensive care units (ICUs). The vivid nightmares often convey feelings of extreme horror, dread, or impending mortality, and their content may depict the patients' afflictions, agonizing treatments, isolation, dependency, and the real possibility of death. Few verbatim narratives have been published, but several studies attest to their high prevalence, their alarming nature, and their potentially traumatizing long-term influence on patients.

One assessment[48] of traumatic ICU memories reported by 80 patients with acute respiratory distress syndrome found that nightmares were by far the most frequently remembered "trauma" (i.e., 64% of patients). They were described to be of a "bizarre and extremely terrifying nature" and were far more common than any of the other three types of trauma evaluated: anxiety (41%), pain (40%), and respiratory distress (38%). A follow-up of 52 patients[49] found that nightmares were still the most prevalent traumatic memory (75% versus 46%, 42%, and 42%) and contributed to accurate prediction of future PTSD.

A study of critically ill patients requiring intubation, ventilation, and sedation[50] found that length of stay in the ICU was the best predictor of nightmares. Of the 127 patients who stayed for more than a day, 18.1% reported nightmares and 14.2% hallucinations—many more than the 162 staying less than a day (2.5%, 0.6%). Two thirds of patients premedicated with benzodiazepines later reported postoperative dreams, half of which were nightmares.[51] Several other likely contributing factors included pain, anxiety, noise, and the inability to lie comfortably in bed.[52]

Vivid ICU dreams form part of a larger constellation of psychiatric signs and symptoms that include poor orientation, fluctuating levels of consciousness, paranoid delusions, and hallucinations[53] and that are referred to collectively as ICU psychosis, ICU syndrome, or ICU delirium. Prevalence estimates of the syndrome vary considerably: 13% to 38% in one study,[54] 40% to 57% in another.[55] A recent review[56] of 26 studies found the average incidence to be 37%, with a range of 0% to 74%.

It remains unclear whether or how disturbed sleep contributes to ICU dreams and ICU psychosis more generally.[56] Sleep deprivation and fragmentation are probable contributing factors, as sleep is readily disturbed by illness stress, near-death trauma, excessive noise, night lighting, pain, interruptions from medical or nursing staff, and numerous other variables. Patients who are sleep deprived are more likely to exhibit signs of altered states of consciousness than those who are not.[57]

About a quarter of ICU patients claim that lack of sleep is a problem.[52] Even when optimal sleep conditions are provided, ICU sleep can be poor. For example, in a study[58] of nine surgical patients, sleep time (stage 1 excluded) for the first 2 days was less than 2 hours out of each 24. Stages 3 and 4 and REM sleep were severely or completely suppressed. Because stage 1 sleep accounted for 40% of total sleep time (versus 5% in controls[58]), it is very likely that sleep-onset hypnagogic hallucinations were more frequent and intense and contributed to increased dream and nightmare recall.[59]

Circadian rhythm abnormalities are another possible disruptive factor in ICU psychosis. Delirious patients in general may display a reversal of the circadian cycle, with daytime somnolence and nocturnal restlessness and agitation.[60]

Limbic Lobe Damage

Confusion of dreaming with reality has been described as characteristic of a small subgroup of neurologic patients (10 of 189, or 5.3%).[2] These confusions may be the result of localized anterior limbic lesions, but no one specific pattern of lesions within this region is selectively associated with the symptom. Equal numbers of cases show lesions in medial prefrontal cortex, anterior cingulate gyrus, basal forebrain nuclei, and anteromedial diencephalic nuclei. The most severe cases also involve medial frontal cortex.[2]

Psychotic Dream-Related Aggression

Dream–reality confusion may be at its most extreme among individuals who are either borderline psychotic or in the throes of a psychotic episode. Reports[61-67] of several extreme cases in which violent, psychotic acts were linked to prior dreams raise the possibility of a complete dream–reality *fusion* in some individuals.

In one recent news report,[66] a 53-year-old "deranged" man used knives to attack 10 young children in a church cafeteria: "In my dreams, I heard a voice saying that my wish will be fulfilled and I will live only if I kill many people"; he also told police that he kept hearing the voice even when awake.

Hempel et al.[63] reports five similar cases, two of which involved homicide, and three, violent assaults. All of the individuals were relatively young (27 to 43 years old), four were men, all suffered from paranoid psychosis, and all typically awakened from their dreams in a "very agitated and hostile state" (see p. 611 of Hempel et al.[63]). These authors propose psychotic dream-related aggression as a nosologic category to encompass this phenomenon and to distinguish it from other forms of sleep-related violence such as that seen in severe somnambulism. They and several others (see review[68]) concur that the intensification of dreaming to the point that it is mistaken for reality is a hallmark of psychotic dreaming. During acute psychotic phases, dreams may be lived as real events.[69] Often, realistic dreams anticipate a violent psychotic act itself. In some instances, the dreams even appear to play a direct causal role in the violence (e.g., an authoritative oneiric voice commands a crime) or an indirect role (e.g., the individual reacts to being repeatedly "killed" by others, in dreams, by acting out).[61,63] However, it remains to be determined whether such dreams are, in fact, causally implicated or whether they are simply parallel expressions of a psychotic process that compels its effect independent of sleep state.

DREAM STEREOTYPY

Recurrent dream themes are normal in the general population.[70] Indeed, it might be argued that the predominance of fear in nightmares is the most prevalent stereotyped dream motif. Or, that specific nightmare themes like pursuit, threat, and assault are instances of dream stereotypy, as are the dreams of paralysis and presence seen in sleep paralysis and narcolepsy. However, in the present context, use of the term *dream stereotypy* is restricted to dreams that occur in conjunction with a medical condition and for which their content, structure, or affective quality has become so highly repetitive that patients are distressed. Neurobiologic or psychological features of the associated medical condition may play a role in shaping the precise stereotypical content of such dreams.

REM Sleep Behavior Disorder/ Parkinsonism Assault/Defense Dreams

REM sleep behavior disorder (RBD) is characterized by excessive motor activity during sleep and REM sleep behaviors that may enact the patient's ongoing dreams or nightmares.[71,72] Dream-enacting behaviors were reported by 93%, 87%, and 64% of patients in the three largest series (N = 93, 96, and 52, respectively) reported. PSG recordings indicate that patients do not enact all of the dreams they have in REM sleep. However, partial expression of many dreams is suggested by elevated levels of muscle tone, increased phasic electromyographic activity, and more numerous gross body movements during REM sleep, even in the absence of overt behavior. However, patients do not always recall dream content on awakening from episodes of overt behavior. This may result from factors such as poor recall of dreams among older adults; a lack of salience or memorability of some dreams (e.g., neutral affect, little motor involvement), or the inhibiting effect of sleeping in a laboratory.[73] Nonetheless, most patients do report that since the onset of RBD, their dreams have become more vivid, violent, and action filled and are experienced as nightmares.[74]

Clonazepam not only suppresses the abnormal behaviors of REM sleep but reduces the disturbing dreams associated with them[75,76]; cessation of the medication is followed by a recurrence of both abnormal behaviors and nightmares.[75]

Although a panoply of dream-enacting behaviors has been reported, associated dream themes are largely stereotyped in their structure and emotional content.[77,78] This is shown in Table 78–2, which summarizes examples of dreams for which specific enacting behaviors were identified by the investigator. The most frequent pattern is that of vigorous defense against attack. Of the 17 specific dream instances, the vast majority (82.4%) are of self-defense against assaults by people (58.8%) and animals (23.5%); 11.7% involve sports themes and 5.9% a friendly social gesture. Very similar results are reported for the 37 (of 67) patients with RBD who were able to report dream content to their physicians[79]: most (87%) are again of defense against attacks by either people (57%) or animals (30%).

More rarely, patients have reported recurrent dreams about vestibular activation (e.g., spinning objects and angular motions with acceleration) or instances of atonia intruding into dreamed movements (e.g., suddenly stuck in mud, trapped in deep snow, and falling to the ground and unable to get up).[74] Very similar dream themes were reported by some normal subjects who were administered intense lateralized pressure stimulation during REM sleep,[80] raising the possibility that these types of RBD themes may be shaped by disruption of the sensory–motor balance normally characterizing REM sleep. Sensory–motor imbalance may be induced by lapses in muscle atonia or by disinhibition of patterned motor activity, or by both.[81]

In a similar fashion, stereotypical RBD defense nightmares may also be influenced by sensory–motor imbalance. A defense nightmare may simply be an instance of the most common dream type—pursuit/assault[70]—whose motor engagement and affective intensity has been amplified by sensory–motor imbalance.

It remains unknown to what extent RBD sleep behaviors are, in fact, isomorphic with their associated dream content. Although there is no doubt that reported dreams match associated behaviors in general respects (see Table 78–2), some cases suggest the possibility that dreamed and enacted behaviors may be subtly different. For example, Schenck and Mahowald[74] state that men with RBD often dream about fighting to protect their wives from an attacker but discover on awakening that they are attacking their wives instead. If this "error" is akin to those cases of somnambulistic violence in which, for example, a patient dreams of *removing* an attacker's hands from his wife's neck while he is in fact *throttling* her,[74a] then the possibility of nonisomorphic relationships is feasible. Nonisomorphisms might be explained as being caused by the partial atonia impinging on sleep behaviors leading to modification of the fictive movements associated with them.

The pathophysiology of altered dreaming in RBD may not be limited to the sleeping state. Evidence that patients with RBD suffer from deficits in perceptual–organizational processes[82] suggests a more generalized deficit that is linked to dreaming.[83] RBD patients also suffer from disrupted autonomic function during both sleep and waking,[84] a dysfunction that could well affect the emotional content of dreams.

In sum, the stereotypical nature of RBD dreams may be influenced by consistent pathophysiologic mechanisms that are unique to RBD but that may also affect the waking state. The latter suggestion is further supported by findings of RBD comorbidity with Parkinson's disease, particularly Parkinson's disease with waking or sleep-related hallucinations.

Parkinson's Disease

RBD is now known to presage, often by many years, signs of Parkinson's disease and other synucleinopathic disorders (SNDs) such as dementia with Lewy bodies and multiple system atrophy.[74] About a third (33% to 39%) of patients with Parkinson's disease have RBD, and the proportion is much larger (58% to 64%) when probable cases (i.e., of those people who manifest REM sleep without atonia) are included.[85,86] Vivid dreams, nightmares, and other parasomnias such as nocturnal vocalization and dream enactment are frequent among patients with SND. Presence dreams have also been reported.[87]

Although the precise etiologic overlap between RBD and SND is still unclear, altered dreaming is more prevalent among those patients with SND who hallucinate, and it is possibly also implicated in the genesis of their hallucinations. In one study,[88] 61.3% of hallucinating patients with Parkinson's disease also experienced altered dreaming. In other studies,

Table 78-2. Specific Dreams and Behaviors* of Patients with REM Sleep Behavior Disorder

Author (Year)	Patient Description	Dream Content	Associated Dream-Enacting Behavior
Mahowald and Schenck (2000)[77]	Case 1: 77-year-old man	Flying above some trees, he swoops down to answer a ringing phone on a table. As he lands, someone hits him and he jumps away	Quickly bolted out of the bed into the hallway
	Male, unspecified	Defending wife from an aggressor	Struck wife in bed
Boeve et al. (1998)[112]	Patient 1: 70-year-old man with Lewy body dementia	Running for a touchdown, spikes a football in the end zone	Held wife's head in headlock, moved legs as if running, exclaimed "I'm gonna make that touchdown!" and attempted to throw wife's head down toward foot of the bed
Chiu et al. (1997)[113]	Case 1: 72-year-old woman	Defending herself against an enemy	Grabbed neck of screaming granddaughter and tried to strangle her
		Had won a mahjong game, stood up, and walked away from table	Fell to ground and hit her head
	Case 2: 74-year-old man	Surrounded by snakes, had to roll down a slope to escape	Lying on floor with bruises/lacerations on head and limbs
Morfis et al. (1997)[14]	77-Year-old woman	Standing in a garden, she leaned forward to pat a child on the head	Standing on the bed, fell to the floor and received laceration to forehead
Sforza et al. (1997)[15]	61-Year-old man	Someone wanted to shoot him	Talking and smiling, reaching for or picking up something, tried to sit up in bed screaming and sending someone away
Coy (1996)[116]	45-Year-old man with PTSD	Saw Viet Cong soldiers in the trees outside house, then inside house; chased soldier	Loaded a .22-caliber rifle, checked rooms, tripped over furniture and discharged weapon into his own foot
Chung and Wong (1994)[117]	79-Year-old man	Trying to stop his friends from beating their children	Flailed arms, screamed, moved vigorously
		Being chased by a lion and screaming for help	Screamed aloud during REM sleep
Mahowald and Schenck (1990)[118]	MB: 73-year-old man with Parkinson's disease	In military combat, enemy soldiers above him, aiming their weapons and shooting through a circle made by his arms; clasping his hands down into the ground, he sprang backward rapidly for safety	Flew "over my night table about 4 feet and landed on the floor, cutting my left cheek just below the eye and causing a lengthy nosebleed."
	Figure 7: 69-year-old man	A man had approached him at a party, yanked off his bowtie, threw it in some mud, stomped on it, irritating the patient, who retaliated by throwing punches with his right arm	PSG revealed right arm twitching, chin activation, activation of four limbs, body lifting, and repeated punching of the bedrail with the right arm; banging head on bedrail awakened patient.
Culebras and Moore (1989)[119]	Patient 5: 70-year-old man, treated for diabetes and hypertension	To prevent an alligator from getting into his car, he held its snout with great force	Woke up to wife's shouting as he was "strongly grabbing her arm"
		Threw something at a bear to stop its chasing him	Threw bed covers
Sforza et al. (1988)[120]	Case 1: 62-year-old man with Shy-Drager syndrome	"I was being beaten by someone I had never seen before and I wanted to get away."	Made protective hand and arm movements, leg movements, lifted head and neck with eyes closed as if to avoid or escape something, vocalized, made fearful, pained grimaces
	Case 5: 69-year-old man	"I was dreaming of being caught and tied up by people who were going to beat me and I was terrified."	Moved arms as if to tear someone away, then moved and raised arms and tried to lift legs; after 2 minutes, made sudden body jerks, raised arms in searching and reaching gestures with vocalizations; episode ended in sudden body jerk

*Summary of published instances of dreams by patients with REM sleep behavior disorder (RBD) for which a specific dream-enacting behavior was described as associated.

Abbreviations: PSG, polysomnography; PTSD, posttraumatic stress disorder; REM, rapid eye movement.

the estimates were 59%[89] and 48%.[90] The presence of RBD is associated with the development of hallucinations, even independent of the severity of Parkinson's disease.[91] REM sleep mechanisms may be implicated in both dreams and hallucinations, as there are more REM sleep aberrations (e.g., fragmentation[90] and reduced percentage of time spent in REM sleep) among patients with Parkinson's disease who hallucinate than among those who do not.[92] PSG recordings of patients with Parkinson's disease have demonstrated that hallucinations and delirious episodes can correspond with brief daytime REM sleep episodes.[93] Moreover, sleep fragmentation and daytime dozing occur more frequently in patients with Parkinson's disease than in controls.[89] Hallucinations arising during sleep are also common (e.g., in 22% to 30% of cases[94]).

Although it is also true that drugs commonly used to treat patients with Parkinson's disease and other SNDs, especially dopaminergic agonists such as levodopa, may account for some of the alterations in dreaming,[91] they do not account for the majority of cases.[87,95] The prevalence of altered dreaming after long-term treatment with levodopa is only 31% (27 of 88),[96] and there is no difference in levodopa dosage between those who hallucinate and those who do not.[95]

Epileptic Dream Stereotypy

Case studies[2,97,98] demonstrate stereotypy in the dreams of epilepsy patients in several ways. First, stereotypy is seen when epileptogenic features of seizures (such as auras, phosphenes, or ictal visual, auditory, and olfactory imagery) appear in recurrent nocturnal dreams. Second, it is seen in recurrent dream themes that appear in close proximity to seizures. Third, stereotypy is suggested by recurrent nightmares that precede seizures by substantial intervals.[99]

A laboratory case study has confirmed stereotyped dream content in epilepsy patients.[97] One patient reported in two of three recalled REM sleep dreams (out of 32 awakenings from REM sleep) telling someone else he was dying. A second patient reported that in two of three recalled REM sleep dreams (out of six awakenings) and in one of two end-of-night dreams (stage not specified), she was "on a board" going over water and afraid of falling. These themes were also present in the mental content of their epileptic seizures.

Recurrent dreams *unrelated* to the content of seizures have also been noted,[99] but such relationships are much more difficult to establish given the generally high prevalence of nightmarish typical dream themes in the population[70] and the predominance of fear as an ictal emotion.[100]

Dream stereotypy appears to parallel the discharge pathways active during epileptic seizures; the latter are stereotyped in expression but tend to change spontaneously over time.[101] Right hemisphere temporal structures might be a source of such patterning. A review[2] of 19 published epilepsy cases with recurrent nightmares and for whom localization information was available revealed right hemisphere involvement in 12 (63%), left hemisphere involvement in 2 (11%), and bilateral involvement in 5 (26%). REM sleep anomalies, such as rhythmic temporal epileptiform activity, may also be a source of dream stereotypy.[97]

Patients with temporal lobe epilepsy also display other types of dream disturbance. Dream impoverishment is suggested by the low recall rates (9%, 50%) of the two subjects in the laboratory case studies mentioned earlier[97] and by the fact that, when awakened from REM sleep, they presented dreams with less frequent and less varied emotions. They also have more unpleasant, higher-intensity emotions than do controls,[102] a pattern reminiscent of PTSD (see next paragraphs). These dream disturbances are most likely not a function of medication, because medicated patients describe their dreams as being more vivid than do nonmedicated patients or controls.[102] Type of epileptic focus may play a role: patients with complex partial seizures recall more dreams than those with generalized seizures ($P < .01$), independent of the side of the epileptic focus, the presence of brain lesion, and the presence or absence of seizures on the day of recall.[103]

Reexperiencing Dreams in Posttraumatic Stress Disorder

The reexperiencing of a traumatic event through recurrent nightmares is a widely known feature of patients with PTSD. Patients with PTSD who experienced combat trauma are more likely to state that their nightmares exactly or almost exactly replicate an actual event than are those combat veterans with nightmares but no PTSD diagnosis.[104] To illustrate, one 45-year-old concentration camp survivor reported the same haunting dream (it repeated a traumatic persecution that he had experienced at the age of 6, over 39 years earlier) whether awakening spontaneously from REM or non-REM sleep or being awakened intentionally from REM sleep.[105] PTSD dreams are treated in more detail under "Dream Impoverishment," earlier, and in Chapter 46.

Migraine Dreams

Dream stereotypy is prevalent among headache sufferers—particularly patients with migraine. An early study[106] of patients with migraine proposed criteria for defining three dream patterns that were so consistent as to be useful in diagnosis; these criteria included recurrence, presence of brilliant colors, occurrence at specific times of the patient's life, and particular emotional tones that carry over into waking and, in some cases, carry over as a hallucination. The three patterns defined were horrifying nightmares, nostalgic technicolor, and waking dreams. The latter pattern, in fact, is better described as sleep paralysis attacks, judging by the examples given.

Nightmares of terror were by far the most predominant theme in migraine cases, occurring in 61% of dreams. Other negative affects and themes (frustration, loss, incest, outsized creatures) also occurred. However, these findings are confounded by comorbid PTSD in at least two of the cases (accounting for 11 of the terror and 3 of the negative theme dreams). Negative affect often precedes migraines; migraine dreams contain significantly more anger, misfortune, apprehension, and aggressive interactions.

Prodromal Cardiac Dreams

A form of stereotypy is seen in the recurrent themes of *prodromal* dreams—that is, dreams disturbed by ongoing or occult medical conditions. Such themes may even appear in dreams before any overt symptoms of the condition appear, a phenomenon that has been exploited (and often misunderstood) since the earliest days of medical science.[107] Prodromal dream themes have been proposed for a number of different specific illnesses (e.g., gastrointestinal, pulmonary, gynecologic/obstetric, dental, arthritic).[108]

Studies of nonacute cardiac patients revealed a strong negative relationship between cardiac ejection fraction and dreamed death references (men) and separation references (women).[109] Additional cardiac dream themes can be either direct (e.g., wounds and/or pain or pressure in the arm, heart, chest, or neck), indirect (e.g., clutching or squeezing, references to death, blood, pain), or metaphoric (e.g., explosions) in nature.[108] Patients may present with near-fatal cardiac events following so-called killer dreams, although they had had no warning of a cardiac event (i.e., they had no cardiovascular risk factors).[110] To illustrate, a 23-year-old man awoke with crushing chest pain and had a cardiac arrest 1 hour later; before awakening, he had dreamed that he was murdered along with his father.

TREATMENT CONSIDERATIONS

Because of the emotional, and often bizarre, nature of disturbed dreaming in many medical conditions, a patient's inclination to disclose them to health professionals, and thus the opportunity to provide treatment, is mitigated by various psychological, sociologic, and cultural factors. Expressive difficulties, such as alexithymia, may hinder self-disclosure. Many individuals may consider their dreams to directly or indirectly reflect their state of sanity or mental health and may avoid speaking openly about them. Others attribute a spiritual significance to dreams, believing them to originate in the workings of devils or evil spirits, or to signify a personal rupture with the sacred,[111] and may thus feel guilt, shame, or embarrassment in revealing dreams with taboo or incriminating content. Patients may be more likely to reveal problems with dreaming to sleep specialists because of their professed interest in sleep phenomena. Sensitivity to factors that influence patients' self-disclosures of disturbed dreaming—especially in multicultural settings—may facilitate the accurate diagnosis and treatment of associated sleep disorders.

Successful treatment also depends on proper identification of factors that may perturb sleep and dreaming. Close scrutiny of the medication regimen is important because of the many known and suspected agents that alter sleep and dream quality and whose replacement or dosage change could alleviate symptoms. Similarly, state variables such as stress and anxiety are amenable to short-term interventions that may diminish symptoms rapidly. Evaluation of sleep hygiene is also important to identify behaviors that lead to sleep deprivation and fragmentation, which are known to affect the quality of dreaming. Assessment of personality variables such as alexithymia or depression may also suggest avenues of therapeutic intervention. Many of these factors are amenable to cognitive behavior therapies, which are successful in treating nightmares and other, more common, dream disturbances.

SUMMARY

Dreaming disturbances characterize a variety of medical conditions. These vary along a continuum of intensity from complete cessation of dreaming to total dream–reality confusion. In many cases, these disturbances appear to be aberrations of otherwise normal dream processes, such as recall, intensification, reality mimesis, or recurrence. Often, sleep fragmentation is implicated in the dream disturbance, but causal relationships are not yet clear. Effective treatments are available for many of these disturbances.

> ### Clinical Pearl
>
> *Assessment of changes in dreaming (including impoverishment and intensification) in a variety of sleep disorders and medical conditions may reveal serious comorbid symptoms (1) that negatively affect a patient's recovery and quality of life, (2) that may facilitate diagnosis, and (3) whose prompt treatment may aid long-term prognosis.*

REFERENCES

1. Charcot J-M: Un cas de suppression brusque et isolée de la vision mentale des signes et des objets, (formes et couleurs) [A case of sudden isolated suppression of the mental vision of signs and objects (forms and colors)]. Progrès Médical 1883;11:568-571.
2. Solms M: The Neuropsychology of Dreams. Hillsdale, NJ, Lawrence Erlbaum, 1997.
3. Doricchi F, Violani C: Dream recall in brain-damaged patients: A contribution to the neuropsychology of dreaming through a review of the literature. In Antrobus JS, Bertini M (eds): The Neuropsychology of Sleep and Dreaming. Hillsdale, NJ, Lawrence Erlbaum, 1992, pp 99-129.
4. Jus A, Jus K, Villeneuve A, et al: Studies on dream recall in chronic schizophrenic patients after prefrontal lobotomy. Biol Psychiatry 1973;6:275-293.
5. McCormick L, Nielsen TA, Ptito M, et al: REM sleep dream mentation in right hemispherectomized patients. Neuropsychology 1997;35:695-701.
6. McCormick L, Nielsen T, Ptito M, et al: Case study of REM sleep dream recall after left hemispherectomy. Brain Cogn 1998;37:M15.
7. Greenberg MS, Farah MJ: The laterality of dreaming. Brain Cogn 1986;5:307-321.
8. Antrobus JS: Cortical hemisphere asymmetry and sleep mentation. Psychol Rev 1987;94:359-368.
9. Badura AS: Theoretical and empirical exploration of the similarities between emotional numbing in posttraumatic stress disorder and alexithymia. J Anxiety Disord 2003;17:349-360.
10. Apfel RJ, Sifneos PE: Alexithymia: Concept and measurement. Psychother Psychosom 1979;32:180-190.
11. Sifneos PE: The prevalence of "alexithymic" characteristics in psychosomatic patients. Psychother Psychosom 1973;22:255-262.
12. Levitan HL: The significance of certain dreams reported by psychosomatic patients. Psychother Psychosom 1978;30:137-149.
13. Monday J, Montplaisir J, Malo JL: Dream process in asthmatic subjects with nocturnal attacks. Am J Psychiatry 1987;144:638-640.
14. Feiguine RJ, Johnson FA: Alexithymia and chronic respiratory disease: A review of current research. Psychother Psychosom 1985;43:77-89.
15. Hyyppae MT, Lindholm T, Kronholm E, et al: Functional insomnia in relation to alexithymic features and cortisol hypersecretion in a community sample. Stress Med 1990;6:277-283.
16. Parker JDA, Bauermann TM, Smith CT: Alexithymia and impoverished dream content: Evidence from rapid eye movement sleep awakenings. Psychosom Med 2000;62:486-491.
17. Bazydlo R, Lumley MA, Roehrs T: Alexithymia and polysomnographic measures of sleep in healthy adults. Psychosom Med 2001;63:56-61.
18. De Gennaro L, Ferrara M, Curcio G, et al: Are polysomnographic measures of sleep correlated to alexithymia? A study on laboratory-adapted sleepers. J Psychosom Res 2002;53:1091-1095.
19. Levitan H, Winkler P: Aggressive motifs in the dreams of psychosomatic and psychoneurotic patients. Interfaces 1985;12:11-19.
20. Lavie P: Sleep disturbances in the wake of traumatic events. N Engl J Med 2001;345:1825-1832.

21. Pillar G, Malhotra A, Lavie P: Post-traumatic stress disorder and sleep: What a nightmare! Sleep Med Rev 2000;4:183-200.

22. Kramer M, Schoen LS, Kinney L: Psychological and behavioral features of disturbed dreamers. Psychiat J Univ Ott 1984;9:102-106.

23. Kaminer H, Lavie P: Sleep and dreaming in Holocaust survivors: Dramatic decrease in dream recall in well-adjusted survivors. J Nerv Ment Dis 1991;179:664-669.

24. Dow BM, Kelsoe JR Jr, Gillin JC: Sleep and dreams in Vietnam PTSD and depression. Biol Psychiatry 1996;39:42-50.

25. Lavie P, Katz N, Pillar G, et al: Elevated awaking thresholds during sleep: Characteristics of chronic war-related posttraumatic stress disorder patients. Biol Psychiatry 1998;44:1060-1065.

26. Fukunishi I, Tsuruta T, Hirabayashi N, et al: Association of alexithymic characteristics and posttraumatic stress responses following medical treatment for children with refractory hematological diseases. Psychol Rep 2001;89:527-534.

27. Hyer L, Woods MG, Summers MN, et al: Alexithymia among Vietnam veterans with posttraumatic stress disorder. J Clin Psychiatry 1990;51:243-247.

28. Weems CF, Saltzman KM, Reiss AL, et al: A prospective test of the association between hyperarousal and emotional numbing in youth with a history of traumatic stress. J Clin Child Adolesc Psychol 2003;32:166-171.

29. Litz BT, Schlenger WE, Weathers FW, et al: Predictors of emotional numbing in posttraumatic stress disorder. J Trauma Stress 1997;10:607-618.

30. Kramer M, Roth T, Trinder J: Dreams and dementia: A laboratory exploration of dream recall and dream content in chronic brain syndrome patients, Int J Aging Hum Dev 1975;6:169-178.

31. Greenberg R, Pearlman C, Brooks R, et al: Dreaming and Korsakoff's psychosis. Arch Gen Psychiatry 1968;18:203-209.

32. Torda C: Dreams of subjects with loss of memory for recent events. Psychophysiology 1969;6:358-365.

33. Schenck CH, Mahowald MW: A disorder of epic dreaming with daytime fatigue, usually without polysomnographic abnormalities, that predominantly affects women. Sleep Res 1995;24:137.

34. Zadra AL, Nielsen TA: Epic dreaming: A case report. Sleep Res 1996;25:148.

35. Porte HS, Hobson JA: Physical motion in dreams: One measure of three theories. J Abn Psychol 1996;105:329-335.

36. Whitty CWM, Lewin W: Vivid daydreaming: An unusual form of confusion following anterior cingulectomy. Brain 1957;80:72-76.

37. Lugaresi E, Medori R, Montagna P, et al: Fatal familial insomnia and dysautomania with selective degeneration of thalamic nuclei. N Engl J Med 1986;315:997-1003.

38. Dilsaver SC, Greden JF: Antidepressant withdrawal phenomena. Biol Psychiatry 1984;19:237-256.

39. Belloeuf L, Le Jeunne C, Hugues FC: [Paroxetine withdrawal syndrome.] Ann Med Interne (Paris) 2000;151(Suppl A):A52-A53.

40. Broughton RJ: Neurology and dreaming. Psychiat J Univ Ott 1982;7:101-110.

41. Kuiken D, Sikora S: The impact of dreams on waking thoughts and feelings. In Moffitt A, Kramer M, Hoffmann R (eds): The Functions of Dreaming. New York, State University of New York Press, 1993, pp 419-476.

42. Businck R, Kuiken D: Identifying types of impactful dreams: A replication. Dreaming 1996;6:97-119.

43. Bowlby J: Attachment and Loss: Vol. I. Attachment. London, Hogarth Press, 1969.

44. Parkes CM: Bereavement: Studies of Grief in Adult Life. New York, International Universities Press, 1972.

45. Kuiken D: Euro-North American paths through bereavement. 12th Annual International Conference of the Association for the Study of Dreams, New York, June 20-24, 1995.

46. Grimby A: Bereavement among elderly people: Grief reactions, post-bereavement hallucinations and quality of life. Acta Psychiatr Scand 1993;87:72-80.

47. Nielsen TA, Paquette T: High prevalence of postpartum peril dreams and sleep behaviors. 17th Congress of the European Sleep Research Society, October 5-9, 2004, Prague, Czech Republic, 2004.

48. Schelling G, Stoll C, Haller M, et al: Health-related quality of life and posttraumatic stress disorder in survivors of the acute respiratory distress syndrome. Crit Care Med 1998;26: 651-659.

49. Stoll C, Kapfhammer HP, Rothenhausler HB, et al: Sensitivity and specificity of a screening test to document traumatic experiences and to diagnose post-traumatic stress disorder in ARDS patients after intensive care treatment. Intensive Care Med 1999;25:697-704.

50. Rundshagen I, Schnabel K, Wegner C, et al: Incidence of recall, nightmares, and hallucinations during analgosedation in intensive care. Intensive Care Med 2002;28:38-43.

51. Noble DW, Power I, Spence AA, et al: Sleep and dreams in relation to hospitalization, anaesthesia and surgery: A preliminary analysis of the first 100 patients. In Benno B, Fitch W, Millar K (eds): Memory and Awareness in Anaesthesia. Lisse, The Netherlands, Swets & Zeitlinger, 1990, pp 219-225.

52. Jones J, Hoggart B, Withey J, et al: What the patients say: A study of reactions to an intensive care unit. Intensive Care Med 1979;5:89-92.

53. McGuire BE, Basten CJ, Ryan CJ, et al: Intensive care unit syndrome: A dangerous misnomer. Arch Intern Med 2000;160:906-909.

54. Easton C, MacKenzie F: Sensory-perceptual alterations: delirium in the intensive care unit. Heart Lung 1988;17:229-237.

55. Wilson V: Identification of stressors related to patient's psychological responses to the surgical intensive care unit. Heart Lung 1987;16:267-273.

56. Dyer I: Preventing the ITU syndrome or how not to torture an ICU patient! Part 2. Intensive Crit Care Nurs 1995;11:223-232.

57. Helton MC, Gordon SH, Nunnery SL: The correlation between sleep deprivation and the intensive care unit syndrome. Heart Lung 1980;9:464-468.

58. Aurell J, Elmqvist D: Sleep in the surgical intensive care unit: Continuous polygraphic recording of sleep in nine patients receiving postoperative care. BMJ 1985;290:1029-1032.

59. Jones C, Griffiths RD, Humphris G: Disturbed memory and amnesia related to intensive care. Memory 2000;8:79-94.

60. Henry WD, Mann AM: Diagnosis and treatment of delirium. Can Med Assoc J 1965;93:1156-1166.

61. Felthous AR: Unusual case report: Do violent dreams cause violent acts? Crim Behav Ment Health 1993;3:12-18.

62. Fennig S, Salganik E, Chayat M: Psychotic episodes and nightmares: A case study. J Nerv Ment Dis 1992;180:60.

63. Hempel AG, Felthous AR, Meloy JR: Psychotic dream-related aggression: A critical review and proposal. Aggression Violent Behav 2003;8:599-620.

64. Levin R, Daly RS: Nightmares and psychotic decompensation: A case study. Psychiat Interpers Bio Proc 1998;61:217-222.

65. Martin PA: A psychotic episode following a dream. Psychoanal Q 1958;27:563-567.

66. Associated Press: Man slashes 10 children in Seoul church cafeteria. Montreal Gazette September 5, 2002.

67. Agence France Presse: Il tue trois de ses enfants sur "ordre d'un chat noir." Journal de Montreal 23 Avril, 1995.

68. Capozzi P, de Masi F: The meaning of dreams in the psychotic state: Theoretical considerations and clinical applications. Int J Psychoanal 2001;82:933-952.

69. Racamier P-C: Rêve et psychose: Rêve ou psychose. Rev Fr Psychanal 1976;40:173-193.

70. Nielsen TA, Zadra AL, Simard V, et al: The typical dreams of Canadian university students. Dreaming 2003;13:211-235.

71. Mahowald MW, Schenck CH: REM sleep behavior disorder. In Kryger MH, Roth T, Dement WC (eds): Principles and Practice of Sleep Medicine, 2nd ed. Philadelphia, WB Saunders, 1994, pp 574-588.

72. Schenck CH, Mahowald MW: REM sleep parasomnias. Neurol Clin 1996;14:697-720.

73. Sheldon SH, Jacobson J: REM-sleep motor disorder in children. J Child Neurol 1998;13:257-260.

74. Schenck CH, Mahowald MW: REM sleep behavior disorder: Clinical, developmental, and neuroscience perspectives 16 years after its formal identification in SLEEP. Sleep 2002;25: 120-138.

74a. Nielsen TA, Zadra A: Dreaming disorders. In Kryger M, Roth N, Dement WC (eds): Principles and Practice of Sleep Medicine, 3rd ed. Philadelphia, WB Saunders, pp 753-772.

75. Culebras A: Update on disorders of sleep and the sleep-wake cycle. Psychiatr Clin North Am 1992;15:467-489.

76. Schenck CH, Mahowald MW: Long-term, nightly benzodiazepine treatment of injurious parasomnias and other disorders of disrupted nocturnal sleep in 170 adults. Am J Med 1996;100:333-337.

77. Mahowald MW, Schenck CH: REM sleep parasomnias. In Kryger M, Roth N, Dement WC (eds): Principles and Practice of Sleep Medicine, 3rd ed. Philadelphia, WB Saunders, 2000, pp 724-741.

78. Schenck CH, Bundlie SR, Ettinger MG, et al: Chronic behavioral disorders of human REM sleep: A new category of parasomnia. Sleep 1986;9:293-308.

79. Olson EJ, Boeve BF, Silber MH: Rapid eye movement sleep behaviour disorder: Demographic, clinical and laboratory findings in 93 cases. Brain 2000;123:331-339.

80. Nielsen TA, McGregor DL, Zadra A, et al: Pain in dreams. Sleep 1993;16:490-498.

81. Morrison AR, Mann G, Hendricks J, et al: Release of exploratory behavior in wakefulness by pontine lesions which produce paradoxical sleep without atonia. Anatom Rec 1979;193:628.

82. Ferman TJ, Boeve BF, Smith GE, et al: Dementia with Lewy bodies may present as dementia and REM sleep behavior disorder without parkinsonism or hallucinations. J Int Neuropsychol Soc 2002;8:907-914.

83. Foulkes D: Children's Dreaming and the Development of Consciousness. Cambridge, Mass, Harvard University Press, 1999.

84. Ferini-Strambi L, Zucconi M: REM sleep behavior disorder. Clin Neurophys 2000;111(Suppl 2):S136-S140.

85. Gagnon JF, Bedard MA, Fantini ML, et al: REM sleep behavior disorder and REM sleep without atonia in Parkinson's disease. Neurology 2002;59:585-589.

86. Boeve BF, Silber MH, Ferman TJ, et al: Association of REM sleep behavior disorder and neurodegenerative disease may reflect an underlying synucleinopathy. Mov Disord 2001;16:622-630.

87. Fenelon G, Mahieux F, Huon R, et al: Hallucinations in Parkinson's disease: Prevalence, phenomenology and risk factors. Brain 2000; 123(Pt 4):733-745.

88. Moskovitz C, Moses H, Klawans HL: Levodopa-induced psychosis: A kindling phenomenon. Am J Psychiatry 1978;135: 669-675.

89. Factor SA, McAlarney T, Sanchez-Ramos JR, et al: Sleep disorders and sleep effect in Parkinson's disease. Mov Disord 1990;5:280-285.

90. Pappert EJ, Goetz CG, Niederman FG, et al: Hallucinations, sleep fragmentation, and altered dream phenomena in Parkinson's disease. Mov Disord 1999;14:117-121.

91. Onofrj M, Thomas A, D'Andreamatteo G, et al: Incidence of RBD and hallucination in patients affected by Parkinson's disease: 8-year follow-up. Neurol Sci 2002;23(Suppl 2): S91-S94.

92. Comella CL, Tanner CM, Ristanovic RK: Polysomnographic sleep measures in Parkinson's disease patients with treatment-induced hallucinations, Ann Neurol 1993;34:710-714.

93. Houeto JL, Arnulf I: Psychic disorders and excessive daytime sleepiness. Rev Neurol (Paris) 2002;158:102-107.

94. Askenasy JJ: Sleep disturbances in Parkinsonism. J Neural Transm 2003;110:125-150.

95. Arnulf I, Bonnet AM, Damier P, et al: Hallucinations, REM sleep, and Parkinson's disease: A medical hypothesis. Neurology 2000;55:281-288.

96. Sharf B, Moskovitz C, Lupton MD, et al: Dream phenomena induced by chronic levodopa therapy. J Neural Transm 1978; 43:143-151.

97. Epstein AW: Effect of certain cerebral hemispheric diseases on dreaming. Biol Psychiatry 1979;14:77-93.

98. Reami DO, Silva DF, Albuquerque M, et al: Dreams and epilepsy. Epilepsia 1991;32:51-53.

99. Epstein AW: Recurrent dreams: Their relationship to temporal lobe seizures. Arch Gen Psychiatry 1964;10:25-30.

100. Biraben A, Taussig D, Thomas P, et al: Fear as the main feature of epileptic seizures. J Neurol Neurosurg Psychiatry 2001; 70:186-191.

101. Epstein AW: Dreaming and Other Involuntary Mentation: An Essay in Neuropsychiatry. New York, International Universities Press, 1995.

102. Gruen I, Martinez A, Cruzolloa C, et al: Characteristics of the emotional phenomena in the dreams of patients with temporal lobe epilepsy. Salud Mental 1997;20:8-15.

103. Bonanni E, Cipolli C, Iudice A, et al: Dream recall frequency in epilepsy patients with partial and generalized seizures: A dream diary study. Epilepsia 2002;43:889-895.

104. van der Kolk B, Blitz R, Burr W, et al: Nightmares and trauma: A comparison of nightmares after combat with lifelong nightmares in veterans. Am J Psychiatry 1984;141:187-190.

105. Hefez A, Metz L, Lavie P: Long-term effects of extreme situational stress on sleep and dreaming. Am J Psychiatry 1987;144: 344-347.

106. Lippman CW: Recurrent dreams in migraine: An aid to diagnosis. J Nerv Ment Dis 1954;120:273-276.

107. Gallop D: Aristotle on Sleep and Dreams: A Text and Translation with Introduction, Notes and Glossary. Peterborough, Ontario, Broadview Press, 1990.

108. Garfield P: The Healing Power of Dreams. New York, Simon & Schuster, 1991.

109. Smith RC: Do dreams reflect a biological state? J Nerv Ment Dis 1987;175:201-207.

110. Parmar MS, Luque-Coqui AF: Killer dreams. Can J Cardiol 1998;14:1389-1391.

111. Bulkeley K: Spiritual Dreaming: A Cross-Cultural and Historical Journey. New York, Paulist Press, 1995.

112. Boeve BF, Silber MH, Ferman TJ, et al: REM sleep behavior disorder and degenerative dementia: An association likely reflecting Lewy body disease. Neurology 1998;51:363-370.

113. Chiu HFK, Wing YK, Chung DWS, et al: REM sleep behaviour disorder in the elderly. Int J Geriatr Psychiatry 1997;12: 888-891.

114. Morfis L, Schwartz RS, Cistulli PA: REM sleep behaviour disorder: A treatable cause of falls in elderly people. Age Ageing 1997;26:43-44.

115. Sforza E, Krieger J, Petiau C: REM sleep behavior disorder: Clinical and physiopathological findings. Sleep Med Rev 1997; 1:57-69.

116. Coy JD: To the editor. J Emerg Med 1996;14:760-762.

117. Chung KF, Wong MTH: Rapid eye-movement sleep behavior disorder in a Chinese male (technical note), Aust N Z J Psychiatry 1994;28:144-146.

118. Mahowald MW, Schenck CH: REM-sleep behavior disorder. In Thorpy MJ (ed): Handbook of Sleep Disorders. New York, Marcel Dekker, 1990, pp 567-593.

119. Culebras A, Moore JT: Magnetic resonance findings in REM sleep behavior disorder. Neurology 1989;39:1519-1523.

120. Sforza E, Zucconi M, Petronelli R, et al: REM sleep behavioral disorders. Eur Neurol 1988;28:295-300.

79

Sleep Bruxism

Gilles J. Lavigne

Christiane Manzini

Takafumi Kato

ABSTRACT

Sleep bruxism, characterized by teeth grinding or jaw clenching, causes tooth destruction, headache, orofacial pain, and jaw dysfunction. In the general population, 8% of adults are conscious of teeth grinding sounds during sleep, as are their sleep partners. The causes of sleep bruxism range from psychosocial factors (e.g., life stress, anxiety) to an excessive sleep arousal response. Clinical recognition is based on a current history of teeth grinding or a stiff or painful jaw on awakening; tooth wear is frequently observed but is not a key element in diagnosis, as it may be inaccurate. Final confirmation of current sleep bruxism is made by polygraphic recording of jaw muscle activity, together with, when possible, audio-video signals to rule out frequent but nonspecific orofacial motor manifestations (e.g., myoclonus, tics, swallowing, somniloquy). Techniques for managing sleep bruxism include sleep hygiene improvements, relaxation techniques, oral devices (e.g., occlusal bite splint), and medications (e.g., muscle relaxants).

The first International Classification of Sleep Disorders[1] categorizes sleep bruxism as a parasomnia and the recent one as a sleep-related movement disorder and defines it as "a stereotyped movement disorder characterized by grinding or clenching of the teeth during sleep." Because it is probable that sleep bruxism differs in terms of etiology from daytime parafunctional jaw muscle activity,[2] it should be distinguished from teeth clenching, bracing, or gnashing while awake.[3]

Sleep bruxism frequency is reportedly variable over time[2]; some patients go several nights or even weeks without bruxism/grinding episodes. However, in patients with moderate to severe sleep bruxism, teeth grinding is present every week.[4] Patients with sleep bruxism typically experience either phasic (rhythmic) or tonic (sustained) motor activity in jaw muscles (e.g., the masseter and temporalis) with variable presence of teeth grinding sounds.[2,5] The element of sound is the major reason people seek consultation: teeth grinding sounds disrupt their bed partner's sleep. Other reasons for seeking help are related to tooth wear (Fig. 79–1), orofacial pain or temporal area headaches, and tooth hypersensitivity to cold air, beverages, and food.

Bruxism in the absence of a medical cause is considered to be the primary, or idiopathic, form of the disorder, whereas sleep bruxism associated with a medical condition is the secondary form (Table 79–1 and Box 79–1). The latter is noted after drug intake or withdrawal (e.g., neuroleptics that could induce oral tardive dyskinesia and grinding); this secondary form is classified as iatrogenic. Several orofacial activities are frequently concomitant: grimacing, chewing automatism, or excessive lip and tongue movements such as thrust or protrusion. In this chapter, the term *sleep bruxism* is used to denote tooth oromotor/grinding–related activities occurring during sleep, as reported by the sleep partner or family, regardless of whether it occurs in the primary or secondary (iatrogenic) form.

HISTORICAL ASPECTS

The word bruxism comes from the Greek word *brychein*, meaning "to gnash the teeth." *Bruxism* is defined as teeth grinding usually occurring during sleep, whereas *bruxomania* is the term used for the neurotic habit performed in the daytime. Bruxism is classified as a sleep parasomnia or a sleep-related movement disorder, an orofacial parafunction, a tic, or an automatism.[1,3,6,7] In 1992, the term *brycose* was further suggested for the severe destructive form of bruxism: *brycho* for movement with teeth contact, and *ose* for abnormal exaggerated activity.[8]

Throughout the 20th century, support for different theories regarding the etiology of bruxism has swung like a pendulum; theories range from the role of peripheral dental occlusion[9,10] to a global explanation that includes personality style, the individual's capacity to adapt to life pressures presented by the psychosocial environment, and neurochemical and homeostatic sleep maintenance versus arousal mechanisms associated with activity of the autonomic and motor nervous systems.[2,11-13]

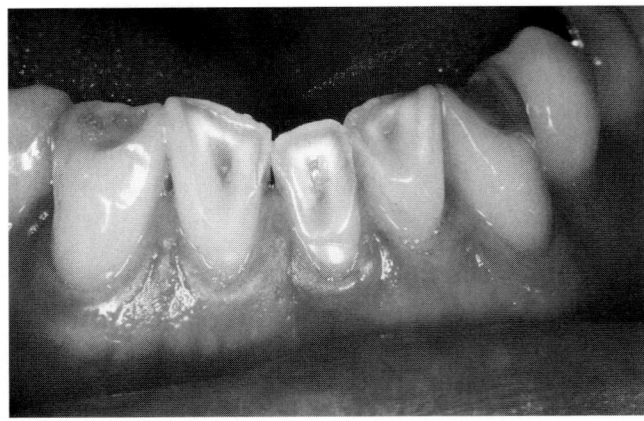

Figure 79–1. Severe attrition (score = 3, see Table 79–2) at lower anterior tooth level, with reduction of crown height (greater than 50%), loss of buccal tooth surface, and secondary dentine reaction at the central area (dental canal). This 55-year-old patient had both protrusive/retrusive and lateral jaw displacements while grinding.

Table 79–1.	Types of Bruxism

1. Awake vs. sleep time
   1.1 Awake time: tooth clenching/tapping, jaw bracing without tooth contact (grinding is rarely noted during the daytime)
   1.2 Sleep time: tooth grinding with phasic (rhythmic) and/or tonic (sustained) or mixed (both types) jaw muscle contractions
2. Primary/idiopathic vs. secondary/iatrogenic forms
   2.1 Primary and/or idiopathic: without known medical or dental causes but could be associated with exacerbating psychosocial factors in some patients
   2.2 Secondary: associated with a medical/psychiatric condition (could also be iatrogenic; see Box 79–1)
   2.3 Iatrogenic: following drug intake or withdrawal

Box 79–1.	Secondary* or Iatrogenic Bruxism

Movement Disorders

- Oral tardive dyskinesia
- Oromandibular dystonia (Meige's syndrome)
- Parkinson's disease
- Tics: simple (grunting) and complex (Tourette's disease)
- Huntingdon's disease
- Hemifacial spasm

Sleep-Related Disorders

- Restless legs syndrome or periodic limb movements during sleep (limb myoclonus)
- Sleep fragmentary myoclonus: oromandibular, facial, lingual
- Apnea or snoring
- Rapid eye movement sleep behavior disorder
- Epilepsy (not observed yet in our sleep bruxism sample)
- Sleep terrors or confusional awakening

Neurologic or Psychiatric Disorders

- Cerebellar hemorrhage or infarct
- Olivopontocerebellar atrophy and Shy-Drager syndrome
- Coma
- Neurologic complication related to Whipple's disease
- Mental health problems such as dementia, depression, mental retardation

Chemical Substances and Medications Related to Secondary Bruxism

- Iatrogenic bruxism (risk for initiation or exacerbation)

Chemical Substances with Abuse Potential

- Alcohol
- Nicotine (smoking)
- Caffeine
- Cocaine
- MDMA (3,4-methylenedioxymethamphetamine [ecstasy])

Medications

- Amphetamines: methylphenidate (Ritalin, for attention-deficit/hyperactivity disorder)
- Antidopaminergic drugs: haloperidol (Haldol)
- Antipsychotic drugs: haloperidol, lithium (e.g., Lithane), chlorpromazine (Thorazine)
- Antidepressive drugs (selective serotonin reuptake inhibitors): fluoxetine (Prozac), sertraline (Zoloft), citalopram (Celexa)
- Cardioactive: calcium blockers (flunarizine [Sibelium, Cinnarizine]), antiarrhythmic drugs (flecainide [Tambocor])

*Includes teeth grinding and/or bruxism-like (not necessarily sleep-related) orofacial motor activities associated with medical conditions and some drugs or chemicals, as reported in the literature.[2,7,18,21,22,29,56,61,64,80,87,93,108,112]

EPIDEMIOLOGY AND RISK FACTORS

Most studies and surveys reporting the prevalence (the number of positive cases at a given time) of sleep bruxism are based on self-reports of clenching during the daytime, or both clenching and grinding during sleep. As yet, no longitudinal study using biologic recordings has been conducted to estimate sleep bruxism fluctuation or its persistence in a given individual with respect to age. Moreover, many patients with sleep bruxism are not aware of grinding if they sleep alone or with a "deep sleep" partner. The overall prevalence of daytime clenching is approximately 20% of the adult population, with more women reporting their awareness of clenching than men.[14,15] According to parental reports, the incidence of sleep grinding in children is between 14% and 20% in children younger than 11 years of age. Concomitant oral activity such as nail biting (onychophagia) is also noted in 9% to 28% of those reporting sleep bruxism, and thumb sucking is seen in 21% of children and snoring found in 14%.[16,17] In adults, the prevalence of grinding drops with age, from 13% in those 18 to 29 years old, to 3% in those 60 years and older, with a mean of 8%.[18] No further sex differences have been noted. Caution is necessary in interpreting these numbers, however, because reduced incidence with age can result from an inaccurate estimate resulting from the high prevalence of denture users in the older population (e.g., greater than 40% in some geographic areas).

Several concomitant risk factors have been linked to sleep bruxism. Psychological factors such as anxiety, competitiveness, and stress have been associated with sleep bruxism exacerbation, but some findings remain controversial.[19,20] Restless legs syndrome is associated with sleep bruxism, but in only 10% of the population. Although survey results showed sleep apnea to be a risk factor, laboratory recordings were less supportive.[21,22] Smoking and caffeine and alcohol consumption are risk factors (significant odds ratio),[21,23] although it remains to be determined whether the variance could be explained by the physiologic influences of nicotine or the perception of smoking as an oral habit. Another variable is the concomitant finding of orofacial pain or joint sound or lock at the temporomandibular level; patients with sleep bruxism are three to four times more at risk for pain and

jaw limitation.[15,24] For example, we found that one third of patients with severe sleep bruxism reported moderate pain in the morning, which was associated with a lower frequency of sleep bruxism episodes per hour of sleep than in matched controls.[24,25] The prevalence of grinding noted in an institutionalized mentally retarded population is similar to the figure reported in the general population.[18,26] Consequently, mental retardation could not be considered as a strong risk factor or as a major factor in the etiopathophysiology of sleep bruxism. Use of several medications or recreational drugs is a risk factor for sleep bruxism (see Box 79–1).

PATHOPHYSIOLOGY

No single mechanism or theory explains sleep bruxism pathophysiology. Rather, this motor activity is more likely to be the product of biologic and psychosocial influences in a given individual. Bruxism probably results from a series of influences that do not obey a mechanistic model or the logic of an algorithm.

RHYTHMIC MASTICATORY MUSCLE ACTIVITY DURING SLEEP IN ASYMPTOMATIC SLEEPERS

Research involving the recording of masseter electromyographic (EMG) activity to assess rhythmic masticatory motor activity (RMMA) in the jaw-closer muscles found that about 60% of "normal" sleepers exhibited RMMA (three masseter muscle bursts or contractions within an episode, and this in the absence of teeth grinding) during sleep.[27] In patients with somnambulism and sleep terrors, the term *chewing automatism* was used to describe the slow rhythmic masticatory activity.[28] This term was later used in the identification of the orofacial activities noticed with the rapid eye movement (REM) behavior disorders.[29] Phasic oromotor activity is associated with RMMA, and in sleep bruxism it is probably an extreme manifestation of an ongoing or natural activity during sleep.

STRESS AND PSYCHOSOCIAL INFLUENCES

As recently as 1949, bruxism was associated with anxiety and hyperactivity by several authors, despite the fact that the Minnesota Multiphasic Personality Inventory and the Cornell Medical Index gave different or confounding outcomes.[30,31] Rigorous evidence is lacking, however, to support the notion that sleep bruxism is an anxiety-related disorder.[19,21] Consequently, the common belief among patients and clinicians that stress triggers sleep bruxism needs to be reconsidered. Patients with sleep bruxism seem to be more task oriented as a result of their personality and coping style, as opposed to being in a pathologic stress or anxiety-related pattern.

FINDINGS IN SLEEP

Studies comparing patients with sleep bruxism and control subjects[5,32-34] have shown that the former demonstrate normal sleep organization and macrostructure. Their sleep latency, total sleep time, percentage of time spent in the various sleep stages, and number of awakenings are within normal limits. They also report a normal amount of time spent awake during the sleep period, and they demonstrate sleep efficiency that falls within the usual range of good sleepers (greater than 90%). Thus, they do not complain about sleeping poorly.[33] Interestingly, and like episodes of sleep apnea in patients with that disorder, most sleep bruxism episodes (74%) were observed in the supine position.[35]

Sleep bruxism episodes are most frequently (greater than 80% of the time) scored in sleep stages 1 and 2,[33,34,36] although the literature is confusing on this point. It was first reported that sleep bruxism occurs mainly in REM sleep, but later the authors retracted this statement because of a methodologic

error in scoring.[38] A high incidence of "destructive" sleep bruxism, scored from electroencephalographic (EEG) artifacts, was also previously reported in REM sleep[39] in patients suffering from depression, and this probably represented secondary sleep bruxism. However, one study reported that some patients with severe sleep bruxism (who were older than those in most published studies) had 20% less REM sleep than would be expected from the literature[40]; these interesting data need to be reproduced in a controlled study. In young sleep bruxism subjects we observed that approximately 5% to 10% of sleep bruxism occurred in REM.[41]

Recent studies do not support the idea that sleep bruxism triggers sleep arousal but rather that sleep bruxism is concomitant or secondary to cyclic alteration in sleep patterns. During sleep, every 20 to 60 seconds, a cyclic electroencephalographic–electrocardiographic–electromyographic (EEG-ECG-EMG) activation was observed and called the cyclic alternating pattern (CAP). Interestingly, between 60% and 88% of sleep bruxism episodes were observed in association with these CAPs, which may act as a reset for physiologic functions in relation to sleep environment or endogenous factors.[34,42] The association between sleep bruxism and CAP is supported by recent findings showing that more than 50% of sleep bruxism episodes occur in clusters (within 100 seconds), and that approximately 15% to 20% occur in the transition from deep sleep (stage 3/4) to REM sleep.[34,43] These findings are also consistent with the observation that sleep bruxism is preceded by alpha EEG activity and is associated with a tachycardia.[36,44-48]

We have also noticed that RMMA or sleep bruxism episodes occurred after physiologic events. In the minute preceding RMMA or sleep bruxism episodes, there is a slight change in autonomic-cardiac sympathetic (increased) and parasympathetic (decreased) balance; then at minus 4 seconds, there is a rise in EEG alpha and delta activity, followed by a tachycardia initiated one heartbeat before the onset of jaw-opener muscle activity, and about 800 msec later, the jaw-closer muscle contractions start.[47,49] These findings support the concept that sleep bruxism is secondary to exaggerated transient motor and autonomic nervous system activation in relation to microarousals. Also, young and otherwise healthy patients with sleep bruxism show a normal rate of microarousals (less than 14 per hour of sleep).[36,50] To further challenge the mechanism involved in the initiation of sudden RMMA or sleep bruxism/teeth grinding in sleep, we developed an experimental model that could trigger arousals during sleep without inducing awakenings. The application of a brief vibrotactile stimulation induced frequent sleep arousals that were followed by RMMA in all patients with sleep bruxism, with teeth grinding occurring in 86% of trials.[51] We suggest that sleep bruxism/teeth grinding is one of the events occurring along the sequence of physiologic activations associated with microarousals (Fig. 79–2).[13,47]

The role of cortical EEG activity in the genesis of sleep bruxism has also been studied. There is an increase in alpha and delta activity in the cascade of physiologic activations associated with microarousals.[47] EEG K-complexes were not reported to be more frequent in the 60 seconds before sleep bruxism episodes, and, overall, patients with sleep bruxism had 40% fewer K-complex events than matched normals.[52] This finding is contrary to previous reports based on studies made in the absence of comparison with normal sleepers.[5,45]

SEQUENCE IN SLEEP BRUXISM

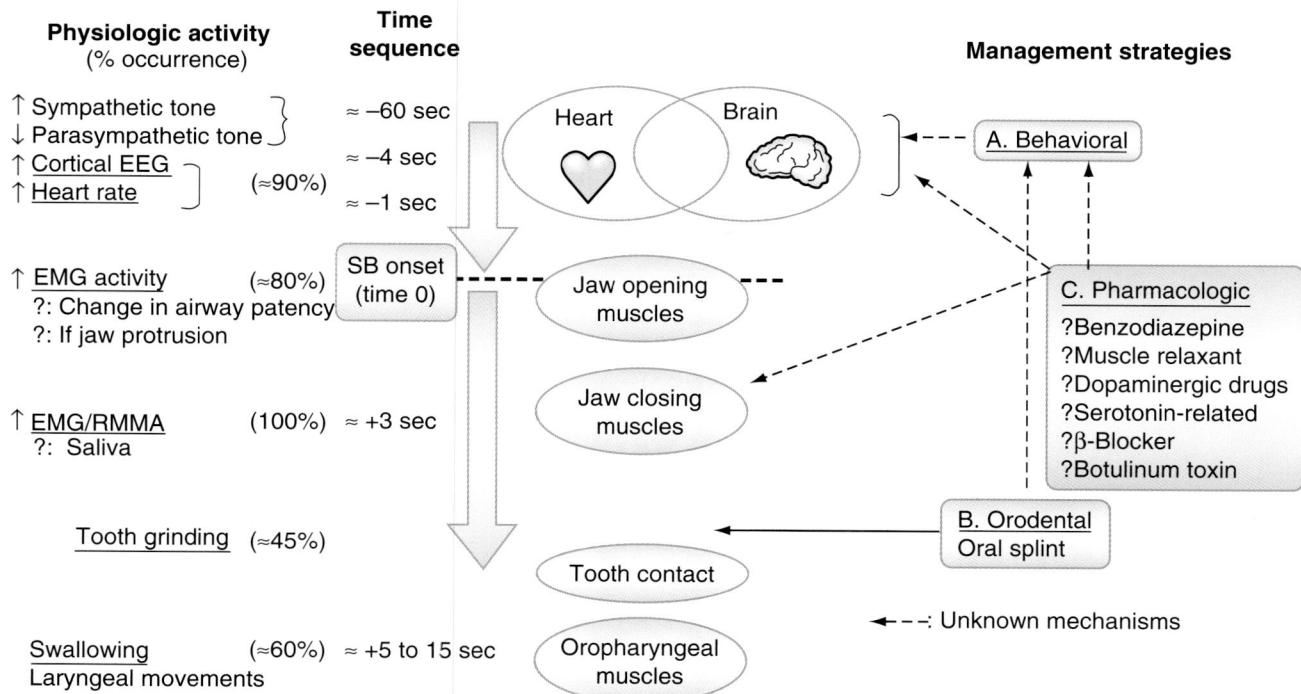

Figure 79–2. Physiologic sequence in the appearance of sleep bruxism or rhythmic masticatory motor activity (RMMA), and management strategies. EEG, electroencephalography; EMG, electromyography; SB, sleep bruxism.

This finding was at first surprising, because K-complexes are frequent in patients with periodic limb movements during sleep (PLMS); however, unlike patients with restless legs syndrome, our patients with sleep bruxism are good sleepers.

OROMOTOR EXCITABILITY

There is little experimental evidence to support a role for the motor system as a primary factor in the genesis of sleep bruxism. At best, some very indirect information from animal physiologic studies may help us understand how the motor system is comodulated during sleep.[13] For humans, as for animals, it has been suggested that fluctuations in the activity of the reticular motor area in relation to sleep onset and maintenance could be associated with brief periodic motor excitation.[53,54]

CATECHOLAMINES AND NEUROCHEMISTRY

An early report on Parkinson's disease linking the use of levodopa (L-dopa) to teeth grinding provided initial support for the suggestion that grinding may be related to dopaminergic, brain-related neurotransmitters.[2,45,55] Teeth grinding was also reported for some schizophrenic patients treated with neuroleptic drugs, as a manifestation of oromandibular tardive dyskinesia.[56] From these reports, the association of dopamine (DA) with sleep bruxism pathophysiology was somewhat weak. These patients already had altered nigrostriatal neurons due to disease or medication.[55,56]

Some recent evidence suggests that catecholamines, such as DA and noradrenaline, may have a role in sleep bruxism pathophysiology. A controlled polysomnographic study of patients with sleep bruxism with the catecholamine precursor L-dopa revealed a modest reduction in sleep bruxism frequency in comparison to placebo.[57] The use of a dopaminergic modest agonist, bromocriptine, in a double-blind control design (using domperidone, a peripheral DA blocker, to prevent side effects such as nausea or vomiting) failed to show either reduction in sleep bruxism motor episodes or a change in DA striatal binding.[58] The role of DA has also been challenged in a nuclear medicine brain imaging study. The total binding of DA by the ligand at the nigrostriatal level was similar to that in controls.[59]

The other catecholamine-related medication reported to reduce sleep bruxism and teeth grinding is propranolol, a beta-blocker. In an open polysomnographic study, propranolol was reported to reduce sleep bruxism motor activity in one subject with severe sleep bruxism but without any medical disorder.[60] In another study, the same medication was also associated with a reduction in daytime teeth grinding in two neuroleptic-treated patients presenting with abnormal orofacial movements.[61] However, a recently completed controlled study done in young patients with sleep bruxism revealed that propranolol was not deleterious to their sleep and neither reduced teeth grinding nor influenced the frequency and duration of jaw muscle contraction.[62] Also, when interpreting studies using specific pharmacologic agents in sleep bruxism, it should be noted that other neurotransmitters (e.g., serotonin, cholecystokinin, gamma-aminobutyric acid) and drugs (e.g., selective serotonin reuptake inhibitors, DA antagonists, calcium channel inhibitors) exacerbate teeth grinding and rhythmic movement modulation[12,63,64] (see Box 79–1).

GENETICS AND FAMILIAL PREDISPOSITION

As yet, no genetic markers have been found for sleep bruxism transmission. It is, however, interesting that between 21% and 50% of patients with sleep bruxism have a direct family member who ground teeth in childhood.[16,65] Furthermore, studies made of monozygotic and dizygotic twins showed that sleep bruxism was more frequently observed in monozygotic twins.[66,67] A concomitant finding in a recent Finnish study revealed that childhood sleep bruxism persisted in a large number of adults (greater than 86.9%).[67] On the other hand, a recent twin study did not find any genetic correlation with sleep bruxism.[68] Thus, the pattern of inheritance for sleep bruxism is unknown and the role and influences of familial and environmental factors remain to be assessed.[67]

POSSIBLE ROLE OF LOCAL FACTORS SUCH AS DENTAL OCCLUSION

In the 1960s, findings from physiologic EMG recordings made during the daytime[69] suggested that tooth occlusal or morphologic interferences were responsible for teeth grinding. Although this concept of a peripheral cause for sleep bruxism is still reported in literature, it is controversial.[9-11,70-72] On the basis of noncontrolled evidences, tooth contact is not a dominant activity in a 24-hour cycle; it has been estimated to occur for approximately 17.5 minutes per 24 hours.[73] Moreover, during sleep, oromotor sleep bruxism–related muscle activity is present for approximately 8 minutes (about 2% of sleep time) over a 7- to 8-hour sleep period and does not always occur with tooth contact; grinding sounds are reported in approximately 44% of sleep bruxism/RMMA episodes.[5,35] The debate over the role of dental occlusion in sleep bruxism is beyond the scope of this chapter; a recent review has described peripheral sensory influences on sleep bruxism.[72]

REDUCED SALIVARY FLOW, AIRWAY PATENCY, AND JAW MOTOR ACTIVITY DURING SLEEP

Another question is whether the lower salivary flow during sleep increases the risk for tooth wear.[74,75] It appears that no sleep data directly support this premise. The low salivary flow observed during sleep may be related to low swallowing frequency: between 2.1 and 9.1 swallowing movements per hour are observed in sleep, compared with 25 per hour during daytime.[76] From data retrieved from a recent analysis of laryngeal swallowing movements observed in controls and in sleep bruxism subjects, it was hypothesized that RMMA could be associated with an increase in salivary flow during sleep to lubricate the oroesophageal tissues.[35,74] Lack of saliva, a natural orodental lubricant, may then cause a dramatic breakdown of tooth structure in patients with sleep bruxism. Consequently, specific clinical management could be planned for oral dryness in sleep.[74] However, it remains to be understood why some frequent teeth grinders show little tooth wear; it may be that a better quality and volume of saliva lubrication or a stronger tooth enamel (e.g., density) explains such observations.

Sleep breathing disorders (e.g., sleep apnea) have recently been associated with sleep bruxism. Results from a large-population survey suggested that self-reports of sleep apnea were two to three times higher in subjects also aware of teeth grinding.[21] However, no correlation was found between sleep apnea and masseter muscle activation when polysomnographic variables were analyzed.[22] As sleep is usually associated with a jaw opening–retrude position, a tongue muscle relaxation (e.g., the genioglossus), and a reduction of airway patency, it remains to be investigated whether RMMA-related sleep arousal assists in the recovery of airway patency or whether this is just a concomitant and typical motor response associated with sleep arousal.[13,77-79]

CLINICAL FEATURES

Clinicians can diagnose sleep bruxism in their patients using the following clinical features as a guide[1-3] (Box 79–2):

1. Teeth grinding or tapping sounds noticed by the patient's sleep partner or a family member
2. Complaints of jaw muscle discomfort, fatigue, or stiffness, and occasional headaches (e.g., temporalis muscles)
3. The presence of tooth wear (see Table 79–2 and Fig. 79–1)
4. Tooth sensitivity to hot or cold (one tooth or several teeth)
5. Muscle hypertrophy

Box 79–2. **Clinical Features of Bruxism**

Reported by Patients

During Sleep

- Teeth grinding sounds, usually noticed by another person
- Possible teeth tapping/oromandibular myoclonus

On Awakening during Sleep or at Morning

- Tooth wear or "chipping" at incisal border
- Muscle hypertrophy affecting aesthetics
- Jaw muscle discomfort (fatigue or tension), with or without pain
- Temporal muscle headache or tenderness
- Stiff jaw, reduced mobility, or difficulty in biting food at breakfast
- Exacerbation by life pressure/stress
- Teeth hypersensitive to cold food, liquid, or air (sometimes to heat)
- Frequent tooth restoration failure (e.g., filling, bridge)

Observed by Clinicians

- Tooth wear or fracture (see Fig. 79–1), shiny spots on filling
- Masseter muscle hypertrophy on voluntary jaw clenching (less important at temporalis level)
- Muscle (masseter, temporalis, pterygoid, sternocleidal [at mastoid insertion]) or temporomandibular joint tenderness or pain on digital palpation
- Tongue indentation
- Tense personality or hypervigilant patient (subjective appreciation)
- Polygraphic observation of jaw muscle activity with audible teeth grinding sounds

Others

- Exacerbation of periodontal disease (a controversial issue)
- Reduction in salivary flow, or xerostomia
- Lip or cheek biting
- Burning tongue, with concomitant oral habits

Table 79–2.	**Ordinal Scale of Tooth Wear**

Score	Wear Condition
0	No wear or presence of facets (shiny spots on tooth)
1	Visible wear restricted to enamel or chipped incisal ridge or cuspid tips
2	Visible wear with dentin exposure and loss of $\leq 1/3$ of clinical crown
3	Loss of $> 1/3$ but $< 2/3$ of clinical crown
4	Loss $\geq 2/3$ of clinical crown

Procedure to assess tooth wear: Dry the tooth with air or cotton and use a dental mirror.

An index of wear could be calculated from the cumulative scores of all the teeth evaluated divided by the number of teeth. However, a concurrent assessment should be made of the validity of the relationship between the wear and sleep bruxism.

From refs. 84 and 85.

6. Temporomandibular joint (TMJ) sound (clicking) or jaw lock (e.g., reduction of opening amplitude)
7. Tongue indentation

Teeth grinding or tapping sounds have to be objectively distinguished from confounding oral sounds during sleep such as snoring, throat grunting, tongue clicking, or TMJ sounds with jaw movements.[80,81] The presence of muscle or TMJ tenderness, or pain, is usually confirmed by digital palpation. Use of a visual analogue scale (e.g., 0 to 100 mm with no pain, and worst pain at both extremes) or numerical scale (0 to 10) can be used to score the patient's subjective reports. Approximately one patient in five with sleep bruxism will complain of pain on awakening and occasionally during sleep. By contrast, patients with diurnal clenching will mainly report pain toward the end of the afternoon and in the evening.[24,25]

The presence of tooth wear (see Fig. 79–1) represents a challenge for clinical recognition of current sleep bruxism. Attrition caused by bruxism differs from attrition resulting from dental work (e.g., crown, bridge or denture, tooth equilibration with a dental bur) or trauma (e.g., pipe, sports injury, abrasive dust in working milieu) or from erosion due to chemical causes (e.g., lemon sucking or gastroesophageal reflux or vomiting [e.g., bulimia]). Tooth wear may be exacerbated by craniodental morphology, which changes with aging. Clinicians need to be aware that observations at the time of examination may have no link with current muscle activity, because teeth grinding frequency fluctuates over time.[2,4,82] Wear can also be localized to one tooth, a few teeth, or a full segment (e.g., the lower incisors). The wear pattern can be seen within normal movement range or in an eccentric jaw position. Finally, although 100% of those with bruxism show tooth wear, so do 40% of those who are asymptomatic.[83] Thus, tooth wear alone cannot be relied on for a definite diagnosis of sleep bruxism, and the other factors mentioned must be taken into consideration. Moreover, tooth sensitivity to temperature stimulations (e.g., cold liquid or air) is also reported after sleep periods with teeth clenching, grinding, or tapping.

Another clinical feature used to recognize sleep bruxism is the presence of masseter muscle hypertrophy. This is easily seen when the subject is voluntarily clenching the teeth together: a unilateral or bilateral mass will protrude on the side of the face below the zygomatic arch. On relaxation, this mass disappears. This condition needs to be differentiated from swelling resulting from periodontal abscess or the trauma of wisdom tooth extraction; parotid gland tumor, or the blockage of the parotid salivary duct by a calculus; or sustained contraction of the masseter muscle that constricts the salivary flow. This last problem is named the parotid–masseter syndrome.[2]

DIAGNOSTIC EVALUATION

Clinical

Clinical diagnosis of sleep bruxism is based on the patient's history and orofacial examination. The presence of tooth wear (see Fig. 79–1) can be scored (see Table 79–2) from criteria derived from the literature.[82,84,85] To assess tooth wear, dry the tooth with air or cotton and use a dental mirror with a light source. Tooth wear can be monitored over time by taking dental arch impressions and visually analyzing wear patterns using casts or models. For research purposes, scanning electron microscopy or computerized laser analysis could be used. Another technique monitors wear intensity using intraoral appliances (e.g., the Bruxscore Plate).[86] The validity of this measure for assessment of sleep bruxism frequency is, however, questionable, because Bruxscore Plate data do not correlate strongly with ongoing sleep bruxism muscle activity as monitored with ambulatory EMG units.[86] Moreover, the presence of an oral appliance can influence ongoing EMG activity (causing either an increase or a decrease).[87,88]

The diagnosis of muscle hypertrophy is made by considering the patient's age and dentofacial morphology, having ruled out any unusual condition (see earlier) or swelling caused by infection in the salivary gland. The patient is then asked to clench the teeth, which induces a protruding mass at the masseter muscle level (rarely, the temporalis). Using the fingers, a positive score is given if the contracted muscle volume increases at least twofold. For research purposes, sliding rules or ultrasonography measures can also be used, although they have not yet been validated for sleep bruxism diagnosis.[89]

In addition, we suggest that the following be noted in the patient file:

1. Tooth wear location and severity (see Table 79–2)
2. The presence or absence of masseter muscle hypertrophy
3. Report of sensitive teeth, pain, or tenderness on digital palpation of muscles and the TMJ
4. Maximum jaw displacement (use the space between both upper and lower central incisors as a reference point)
5. The presence or absence of joint sounds (e.g., TMJ clicking or grating) using finger palpation

Ambulatory Monitoring and Sleep Laboratory Recording

The monitoring of sleep bruxism motor activity is also possible using other techniques, but their use is recommended only for those with severe teeth grinding or in the presence of other sleep disorders (e.g., apnea, epilepsia), or in a clinical trial. First, audio-video home recordings (home camera with black light in room) can help to estimate sound frequency and jaw displacement. However, in the absence of polygraphy, it can be very difficult to distinguish the sounds of snoring, throat grunting, teeth tapping, TMJ clicking, teeth grinding, and jaw movements such as swallowing, rumination, typical chewing-like movements, smiling, and orofacial myoclonia.[80]

Second, ambulatory EMG recordings can be used to monitor sleep bruxism at home. Some systems allow only one channel to be used to monitor masseteric EMG (surface) activity during sleep.[87,90] Full ambulatory multichannel (EEG, EMG, ECG, respiration, movement) recorders, with a very good quality EMG signal, are also currently available (e.g., Biosaca, Sweden; Embla, Iceland). Although the use of ambulatory recordings allows patients to be monitored in the home environment, they have some limitations. In the absence of audio and video recordings, it is difficult to assess precisely the specificity of EMG activity over the large spectrum of orofacial activities that occur during sleep, such as swallowing, coughing, grunting, sighs, yawning, sleep talking, and smiling.[80,91] Moreover, up to 40% of all orofacial activities scored during sleep (polygraphic and audio-video recordings) may not be specific to sleep bruxism.[33]

Despite these limitations, ambulatory recordings are a valuable complement to sleep laboratory recordings because they allow low-cost monitoring over several nights in the patient's natural environment. The suggested sleep bruxism scoring algorithm for ambulatory recordings needs further validation along with laboratory polysomnography (Table 79–3).[90,92]

In the sleep laboratory (a highly controlled but decidedly less natural milieu), recording the following biologic signals frequently completes the diagnosis of sleep bruxism (Fig. 79–3):

1. Two EEG readings (C3A2, O2A1)
2. Right and left electrooculograms
3. EMGs (surface) from both jaw masseter (right and left; in single or jump channel) and temporalis (optional; to improve scoring) muscles for sleep bruxism, scoring of chin and suprahyoid muscles for standard sleep hypotonia in REM sleep, and of the anterior tibialis to rule out PLMS
4. Nasal air flow, respiratory effort (via chest belt), and microphone recording for sleep apnea and snoring assessments
5. Audio-video recordings to identify and quantify jaw and orofacial activities (zoom on face)

These recordings should be made in a temperature-controlled room where light (use black lights for video) and sound are minimal. Before sleep, subjects should swallow, cough, open the jaw vertically and laterally, as well as clench and tap the teeth to help score and assess EMG signal recognition pattern. All-night data are recorded with a computer at a minimum acquisition speed of 128 Hz[33] and analyzed according to the standard Rechtschaffen and Kales criteria described in Chapter 116. Computer screen segments of 20 or 30 seconds can be used. The EMG sleep bruxism episodes of at least 10% to 20% of the maximum voluntary contraction while awake are scored in parallel with audio-video signals. Three types of sleep bruxism events are identified[5,33,39] (see Table 79–3): phasic, tonic, or mixed, according to criteria derived from the literature. If bursts of less than 0.25 second are noticed in the temporalis or masseter muscles, they are scored as myoclonic events and are separated from bruxism.[80,93] We found that 10% of those who were clinically diagnosed with sleep bruxism had this activity during sleep. Because repetitive myoclonus can be confused with epileptic spikes, these patients were recorded for a third night using a full EEG

Table 79–3. Criteria for Diagnosis of Sleep Bruxism (SB)

Ambulatory Criteria	
EMG (RMS) level	>10% of maximum (voluntary clench while awake)
EMG periodicity	<5 sec between events
EMG duration	>3 sec (minimum >0.25 sec to rule out myoclonus)
Heart rate change	>5% change in beats per minute with an EMG event
Minimum acquisition	16.7 Hz or 0.05 sec frequency for EMG or time resolution
Sleep Laboratory Criteria	
Mean SB EMG potential	>10% or 20% of the maximal clench while awake (masseter muscles)
SB episodes types are scored as	
1. Phasic (rhythmic)	More than three EMG bursts, separated by two interburst pauses, in masseter or temporalis muscle; each burst lasts >0.25 sec and <2.0 sec
2. Tonic (sustained)	One EMG burst, lasting >2.0 sec
3. Mixed	Both phasic and tonic types
Minimum acquisition	128 Hz frequency
Diagnostic Cutoff Criteria	
Sensitivity, >72%; specificity, >94%	Bruxism episodes/hr > 4 Bruxism bursts/hr > 25 At least one episode of grinding per sleep period

Data are expressed as number of SB episodes/hr of sleep, number of SB bursts (contractions)/hr of sleep, number of SB episodes/night, duration of SB EMG activity/hr of sleep.

RMS, root mean square (here, of masseter muscle).

Ambulatory criteria from refs. 90 and 92; sleep laboratory criteria from refs. 5, 27, 33, 37, and 39.

montage; no such neurologic events were found in any of our patients with oromandibular myoclonus.

The frequency of sleep bruxism bursts (single EMG events) is quantified in episodes per night and per hour of sleep, with or without the presence of grinding sounds or leg movement. Another index of sleep bruxism duration per hour of sleep has also recently been proposed: total duration of sleep bruxism episodes divided by total sleep time.[94] Through training, individuals can achieve a strong reliability in scoring the frequencies of events, and a moderate capacity to discriminate episode types (i.e., phasic, tonic, or mixed).[33] Again, it is strongly suggested that the audio-video signal be used in parallel with a polygraphic recording to differentiate sleep bruxism episodes occurring with snoring, swallowing, major body movement, somniloquy, and so forth.

Other Diagnostic Features

Using the cutoff criteria described in Table 79–3 to establish a sleep diagnosis, bruxism can be correctly predicted in 83.3%

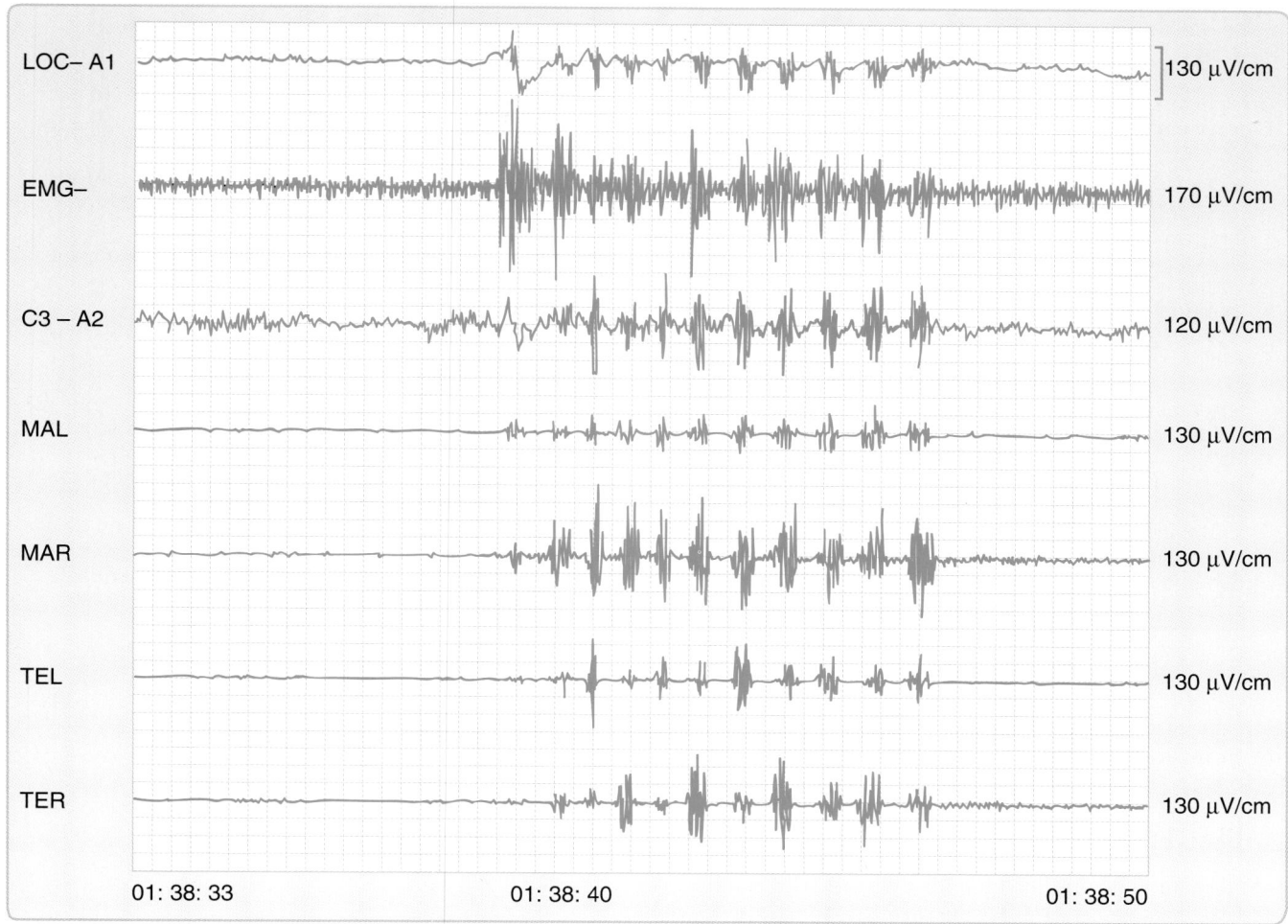

Figure 79–3. Polygraphic traces of one rhythmic sleep bruxism episode. The three upper traces, which are the electrooculogram (EOG) of the left eye (LOC–A1), submental electromyogram (EMG), and electroencephalography (EEG) at C3–A2, all show the rhythmic pattern with movement artifacts in both EOG and EEG. The left (L) and right (R) masseter (MA) and temporalis (TE) muscle activity is associated with 11 phasic (rhythmic) bursts. In this patient, the level of muscle activity was elevated, and co-contraction between closer (MA and TE) and submental opener muscles is noted.

of patients with sleep bruxism, and asymptomatic status can be confirmed in 81.3% of controls.[33] The clinical use of these research cutoffs needs further validation in a larger population. Even when the first night was used simply for habituation, approximately 10% of subjects with sleep bruxism invited to the sleep laboratory did not have a full first night of sleep (i.e., they had several awakenings with no habituation to sleep laboratory conditions, or they refused to appear for the experimental second night). When using polygraphy to evaluate patients with severe sleep bruxism, it is important to rule out other sleep disorders (such as apnea, PLMS, epilepsy, and REM sleep behavior disorder) and other activities (see Boxes 79–1 and 79–3). In a retrospective analysis of patients with sleep bruxism, lasting 2 months to 7.5 years (with 3- to 8-night recordings), we estimated that the time-to-time variability of RMMA/sleep bruxism index per hour of sleep was 25.3%, whereas the number of episodes of teeth grinding was 53%.[4]

Other sleep architecture variables, such as sleep duration and efficiency, number of awakenings and arousal movements, and sleep stage distribution, do not usually differ between patients with primary sleep bruxism and asymptomatic controls.[5,12,32-34] However, the most significant sleep-related variables characterizing sleep bruxism are the following:

1. Up to three times more EMG bruxism episodes occur per hour of sleep.[12,32-34]
2. Most sleep bruxism episodes can usually be scored in light-sleep stages (60% to 85% in stages 1 and 2)[5,12,32-34] rather than in REM sleep.[39,40]
3. More sleep bruxism episodes can be noted when subjects sleep on their backs.[35,95]

No obvious differences were noted in the frequency of PLMS.[33,36,96] At the EEG level, most sleep bruxism episodes can be observed in relationship to the active phase of the CAP,[34,42] and the presence of K-complexes is two to three times less frequent than in matched asymptomatic subjects. Some EEG alpha wave intrusions may also be noted before sleep bruxism episodes, but the specificity of this observation needs further validation in a controlled study.[36] Finally, an autonomic response is noticeable with sleep bruxism episodes

---

Box 79-3. **Differential Diagnosis of Sleep Bruxism**

Information from Electromyography (EMG) or Electroencephalography (EEG)

- Natural, ongoing rhythmic masticatory muscle activity or chewing automatism
- Clenching associated with muscle spasm or drug intake (e.g., cocaine, Ecstasy)
- Orofacial or cervical myoclonia, dystonia (Meige's syndrome), or tardive dyskinesia
- Abnormal swallowing pattern
- Orofacial movements with sighs, somniloquy, smiling, swallowing, coughing
- Epileptic activity (frontal EEG electrode position over temporalis muscle could give rise to artifact)

Sounds

- Teeth grinding (oral tardive dyskinesia, Meige's syndrome, Parkinson's disease, or other neurologic condition)
- Sounds such as snoring, throat grunting, temporomandibular joint sound (click), somniloquy, sighing (EMG and audio-video recordings help to discriminate)

Box 79-4. **Palliative Management of Sleep Bruxism**

Behavioral (None Supported by Strong Evidence)

- Explanation of causes or exacerbation factors of sleep bruxism
- Reversing the habit of clenching teeth or bracing the jaw during daytime in reaction to life pressures (e.g., by abdominal breathing)
- Lifestyle and sleep hygiene and relaxation, autohypnosis, winding down before sleep
- Biofeedback
- Physical therapy and training (relaxation, breathing)
- Psychology (stress/life pressure management)

Orodental

- Mouth guard (soft, short term) for tooth protection (−)*
- Bite splint (hard, need control visits) for tooth protection (+), but risk of aggravating sleep apnea in patients with respiratory disturbance in sleep
- Splint with vibration or electrical lip stimulation device (new) (+)
- Anterior tooth device (e.g., Nociceptive Trigeminal Inhibition [NTI], Sved appliance); lack of controlled study (?)
- Dental occlusion (but controversy over tooth equilibration and orthodontic bite corrections) (?)

Pharmacologic (Short-Term Use in Clinic for Acute or Severe Condition)

Sedative and Muscle Relaxant Properties

- Diazepam (+/cr), clonazepam (?), lorazepam (?)
- Methocarbamol (+), cyclobenzaprine (?)
- Buspirone (+/cr)

Serotonin Related

- Tryptophan (0)
- Amitriptyline (0)
- Venlafaxine (+/cr)
- Trazodone (?)

Dopaminergic Related

- L-dopa (+)
- Bromocriptine (0)
- Pergolide (?)
- Pramipexole (?)
- Gamma-hydroxybutyrate (+/cr)

Cardioactive

- Propranolol (+ and − for teeth grinding)
- Clonidine (+)/risk hypotension

Other

- Botulinum toxin (?/no controlled study for sleep bruxism)
- Continuous positive airway pressure or oral device for sleep apnea (mandibular advancement device); under study in our laboratory

*Levels of evidence: (+), positive evidence of sleep bruxism reduction; (−), evidence of sleep bruxism exacerbation; (0), no effect; (?), evidence questionable or unknown; (cr), mostly based on case reports.

Evidence related to orodental management from refs 71, 72, 81, 100, 101, 103, and 104; evidence related to pharmacologic management from refs 7, 64, and 81.

(as is the case for body movements during sleep) and acceleration in heart rate precedes or is concomitant with sleep bruxism.[12,36,47,48]

MANAGEMENT

As yet, there is no specific cure for bruxism. The clinician's role is to manage sleep bruxism, with the primary goals of preventing damage to the orofacial structures and reducing sensory complaints. Current interventions are oriented toward behavioral, orodental, and pharmacologic strategies, but controlled studies confirming the efficacy of these strategies are still required.[11,47,64] Some of the following recommendations directly address the patient's awareness of the disorder and management of life stress and anxiety (Boxes 79–4 and 79–5, and see Fig. 79–2).

Behavioral strategies should begin with a short and comprehensive explanation of bruxism to the patient, including its definition, causes, and consequences. Next, the clinician should give instructions on sleep hygiene (see Chapter 61). The psychological and behavioral management strategies for sleep bruxism have been of major interest for years.[30,97] No persistent or clear effects have been obtained with strategies aimed at relaxation and tension reduction or exercise,[30,97,98] but several patients have reported a sensation of well-being. One study reported a reduction in both EMG activity and grinding frequency after hypnotherapy.[99] However, no control therapy was used. The use of biofeedback, with loud sounds, is also reported to reduce sleep bruxism EMG activity, but this effect may not last over time without the regular use of the device.[91,97]

Occlusal appliances such as a mouth guard or stabilization bite splint can protect the orofacial structures from damage. The soft mouth guard is usually recommended for use only on a short-term basis because degradation can occur rapidly. The hard occlusal stabilization splint, covering a full dental

Box 79–5.   Other Modalities for Management of Sleep Bruxism

For Children and Teenagers

- Behavioral management
- Soft mouth guard for teenagers (replace frequently as bones grow) (see Box 79–4)
- Control for presence of oropharyngeal obstruction (tonsillar mass)

For Hypersensitive Teeth Secondary to Bruxism

- Local application of 0.4% stannous fluoride gel (e.g., Gel Kam) to protect teeth; can be applied in mouth guard or splint

For Dry Mouth (Xerostomia), Which Could Increase Tooth Wear

- Have a medical evaluation to rule out primary condition (e.g., diabetes, Sjögren's syndrome).
- Avoid coffee, tea, colas, and smoking in the evening.
- At bedtime, rinse mouth with water mixed with olive oil to lubricate oral tissues, and use a water spray in room.
- On every nighttime awakening, sip water.
- Sialagogue drugs (e.g., anetholtrithione [Sialor] or pilocarpine [Salagen]) may help but efficacy is unknown; as yet, there is no controlled clinical trial related to sleep xerostomia.

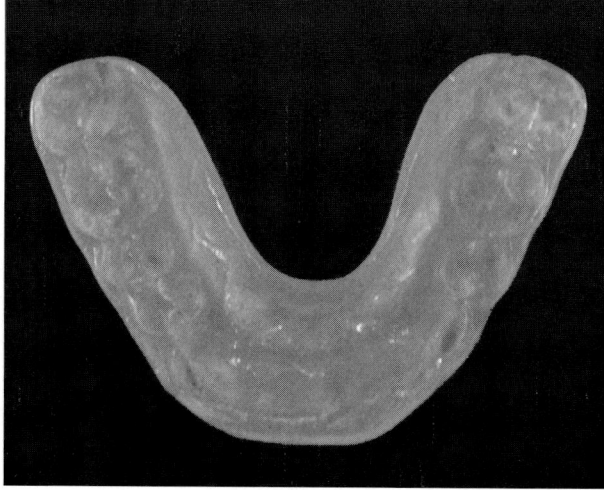

A

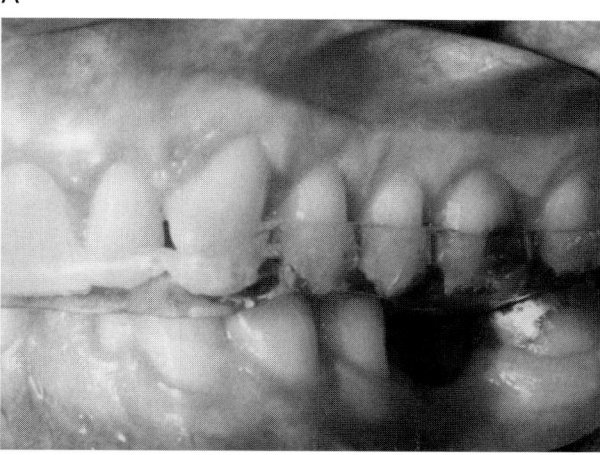

B

Figure 79–4. A, An oral appliance (bite splint) made of hard acrylic to protect upper teeth from wear associated with grinding. **B,** A similar appliance in the mouth.

arch (Fig. 79–4), is particularly useful (e.g., for tooth protection) for patients who are frequent and severe grinders or clenchers.[11] However, not every patient finds relief with these orthopedic treatments. In a crossover controlled polygraphic study comparing full maxillary tooth coverage and a palatal splint without tooth coverage, we observed a 40% to 50% reduction in the number of sleep bruxism/RMMA teeth grinding episodes, but no further difference was observed between the two oral devices.[100] Moreover, use of a maxillary occlusal splint is not recommended in patients with sleep apnea because it may aggravate respiratory disturbances.[101] Patient compliance with these oral devices is low over time, and splints may therefore be considered as "crutches" or "bumpers" that prevent tissue damage or influence oral habits.[102]

Other oral devices are used with patients with sleep bruxism. The mandibular advancement devices (using full maxillary and mandibular tooth coverage devices) that allow horizontal and vertical freedom for rhythmic jaw movements seem to be well tolerated in patients with concomitant sleep bruxism and sleep apnea, although failure (breaking parts) of the device is not uncommon (see Chapter 91). Various types of anterior bite block are also available, but their efficacy and safety in the management of sleep bruxism is yet to be proven in a polygraphic controlled study. Last, three new and very original devices have been proposed: one delivers an electric shock, another a vibration, and the third a bad taste when there is excessive tooth contact with the device.[103-105]

Tooth equilibration, to reduce occlusal interference, has also been suggested as a treatment for sleep bruxism.[9,69] Although the efficacy of such therapy for bruxism is controversial,[11,71,72] it is sometimes appropriate after major dental restoration (e.g., crown and bridge work) or orthodontic treatment, to restore oral comfort.

Pharmacologic management is indicated on a short-term basis only (see Box 79–4).[64] Clinicians report that centrally acting drugs in the benzodiazepine group and muscle relaxants reduce bruxism-related motor activity. To our knowledge, only diazepam and methocarbamol have been tested in open study design.[2,7,81] These medications are usually prescribed at bedtime, and patients must be informed of possible side effects (e.g., no driving in the morning, because of potential drowsiness).

Antidepressants such as tricyclics have also been used for the management of sleep bruxism.[64] Two controlled studies using ambulatory EMG failed to support the efficacy of a small dose of amitriptyline in sleep bruxism management.[106,107] The associated xerostomia, frequently reported in the first few weeks, can be managed (see Box 79–5). The use of *selective serotonin reuptake inhibitors* such as fluoxetine, sertraline, and citalopram has been reported to induce clenching or grinding. Finally, as recently reviewed, the use of L-tryptophan (a serotonin precursor) in sleep bruxism management has been reported to have no effect, and the use of a weight control medication related to serotonin, fenfluramine (Ponderal), has been noted to exacerbate grinding.[64] Therefore, caution is suggested before using serotonin-related medication in patients with sleep bruxism.

The literature on the safe use of *dopamine*-related medications is inconclusive.[64] Patients with chronic antidopaminergic drug exposure (e.g., haloperidol, a dopaminergic antagonist) exhibited iatrogenic grinding similar to that associated with oral tardive dyskinesia, and a similar effect was seen with L-dopa (a dopaminergic precursor) in a patient already suffering from Parkinson's disease.[55,61] A recent study demonstrated that acutely administered L-dopa modestly reduced bruxism activity in otherwise healthy patients with sleep bruxism, whereas bromocriptine had no effect.[57,58] To avoid waking the patient for the second administration of L-dopa in the middle of the night, a sustained slow-release drug (e.g., Sinemet CR [levodopa/carbidopa]) could be prescribed. So far, too few studies have been performed on dopaminergic regimens (e.g., L-dopa) to consider these in the long-term management of sleep bruxism. It also remains to be demonstrated whether, as in the case of PLMS (see Chapter 70), a pharmacologic rebound will induce a rebound of sleep bruxism activity later in the night or during the next day.

Another pharmacologic avenue for sleep bruxism management is the use of a *beta-adrenergic antagonist*, such as propranolol. Two recent case studies reported a reduction of sleep bruxism in one patient without any medical history[60] and in two patients in whom iatrogenic sleep bruxism was noted secondary to antipsychotic (dopaminergic antagonist) medication.[61] A recently controlled study done in our laboratory with young patients with sleep bruxism, using placebo or long-action propranolol (120 mg), resulted in no net reduction of sleep bruxism, and the medication had no effect on sleep variables.[62]

Botulinum toxin is frequently used in the management of cervicofacial dystonia and was recently suggested for control of masseter muscle hypertrophy.[109,110] At this time, no controlled studies with polygraphic recordings have demonstrated that the toxin has long-term efficacy and safety for sleep bruxism. Moreover, it has been reported that the botulinum toxin is carried to the central nervous system, and it is not known whether this explains its effects or whether it signifies a potential risk for the patient.[111]

In Box 79–5, further advice is given for the management of sleep bruxism: (1) in children and teenagers, (2) in patients of all ages who have sleep bruxism and secondarily hypersensitive teeth, and (3) for the occasional dry mouth and xerostomia brought on by stress and the influence of hormones, age, and drug use (e.g., tricyclic antidepressant, benzodiazepine).

PITFALLS AND CONTROVERSIES

The presence of tooth wear alone is not sufficient to diagnose sleep bruxism, as the tooth wear may have occurred years ago. At a clinical examination, a current report of teeth grinding by the patient's sleep partner is the most reliable clinical indicator of ongoing sleep bruxism. Polysomnographic recording, including EMG of the jaw muscles, is not mandatory except if the patient presents with a concomitant sleep disorder (e.g., apnea, sleep epilepsy, or teeth tapping) or if a clinical trial is planned. In this case, the specificity of polygraphy is greatly improved through the use of audio and video recordings to compare with RMMA and to exclude teeth grinding sounds caused by concomitant orofacial activities during sleep, such as sleeptalking, teeth tapping, snoring, TMJ sounds, or grunting.

Current studies on the pathophysiology of sleep bruxism suggest that RMMA and teeth grinding are secondary to ongoing sleep microarousals. The role of dental occlusion (i.e., interferences between tooth microcontacts) and of dopaminergic substances are less significant in the genesis of sleep bruxism than was originally thought. However, we do not know enough about the role of familial and genetically transmitted factors.

Because of the absence of controlled studies, the management of sleep bruxism in children is not evidence based. For adults, most pharmacologic treatments have not been submitted to the quality assessment of randomized clinical trials with quantitative outcomes; for example, the use of cardioactive agents to manage sleep bruxism needs more study, with regard to both efficacy and safety, before recommendations can be made (e.g., effect of clonidine). In patients with sleep apnea, bite splints that protect teeth from wear are not recommended.

Clinical Pearl

In the management of sleep bruxism, the sleep medicine clinician should distinguish primary sleep bruxism from secondary sleep bruxism related to sleep or medical disorders (e.g., arousal-related disorders such as sleep apnea, tics such as grunting, teeth tapping and/or sleep-related epilepsy, medication-related tardive dyskinesia, cerebral infarct). Dental splints reduce tooth damage and teeth grinding sounds but are not recommended for use by patients with sleep apnea. Medications, such as muscle relaxants and anxiolytics, are indicated for more severe cases. In children, cognitive behavior approaches and the use of a soft mouth guard for those with severe grinding is an option, but in the absence of further evidence, clinicians should be prudent and closely monitor the evolution of signs and symptoms, controlling for respiratory disturbances.

Acknowledgments

The sleep bruxism studies done by the authors were made possible by the support of the Canadian Institutes of Health Research and the Fonds de Recherché en Santé du Québec. Our thanks to Clare Lord and Alice Peterson for editing text, and to Francine Bélanger and Carmen Remo for manuscript preparation.

REFERENCES

1. Thorpy MJ: International Classification of Sleep Disorders: Diagnostic and Coding Manual, Revised. Lawrence, Kan, Allen Press, 1997.
2. Rugh JD, Harlan J: Nocturnal bruxism and temporomandibular disorders. Adv Neurol 1988;49:329-341.
3. Okeson JP: Orofacial Pain Guidelines for Assessment, Diagnosis, and Management. Chicago, Quintessence, 1996.
4. Lavigne GJ, Guitard F, Rompré PH, et al: Variability in sleep bruxism activity over time. J Sleep Res 2001;103:237-244.
5. Reding GR, Zepelin H, Robinson JE Jr, et al: Nocturnal teeth-grinding: All-night psychophysiologic studies. J Dent Res 1968; 47:786-797.
6. Adams RD, Victor M: Principles of Neurology. New York, McGraw Hill, 1993.

7. Kato T, Blanchet PJ, Montplaisir JY, et al: Sleep bruxism and other disorders with orofacial activity during sleep. In Chokroverty S, Hening WA, Walters A (eds): Sleep and Movement Disorders, Philadelphia, Butterworth Heinemann 2003, pp 273-285.

8. Rozencweig D: Bruxisme et parafonctions: Maladies expressives. Meeting summary of College National Occlusodontologie, France. 1992;9:95-100.

9. Yustin D, Neff P, Rieger MR, Hurst T: Characterization of 86 bruxing patients and long term study of their management with occlusal devices and other forms of therapy. J Orofac Pain 1993;7:54-60.

10. Kobayashi Y: Management of bruxism. J Orofac Pain 1996; 10:173-174.

11. Okeson JP: Management of Temporomandibular Disorders and Occlusion, 5th ed. St. Louis, Mosby, 2003.

12. Sjöholm T: Sleep bruxism: Pathophysiology, diagnosis, and treatment [thesis]. Turku, Finland, University of Turku, 1995.

13. Lavigne GJ, Kato T, Kolta A, et al: Neurobiological mechanisms involved in sleep bruxism. Crit Rev Oral Biol Med 2003;14: 30-46.

14. Glaros AG: Incidence of diurnal and nocturnal bruxism. J Prosthet Dent 1981;45:545-549.

15. Goulet JP, Lund JP, Montplaisir J, et al: Daily clenching, nocturnal bruxism, and stress and their association with TMD symptoms. J Orofac Pain 1993;7:89.

16. Abe K, Shimakawa M: Genetic and developmental aspects of sleeptalking and teeth-grinding. Acta Paedopsychiatr 1966; 33:339-344.

17. Laberge L, Tremblay RE, Vitaro F, et al: Development of parasomnias from childhood to early adolescence. Pediatrics 2000; 106:67-74.

18. Lavigne GJ, Montplaisir J: Restless legs syndrome and sleep bruxism: Prevalence and association among Canadians. Sleep 1994;17:739-743.

19. Pierce CJ, Chrisman K, Bennett ME, et al: Stress, anticipatory stress, and psychologic measures related to sleep bruxism. J Orofac Pain 1995;9:51-56.

20. Major M, Rompré PH, Guitard F, et al: A controlled daytime challenge of motor performance and vigilance in sleep bruxers. J Dent Res 1999;78:1754-1762.

21. Ohayon MM, Li KK, Guilleminault C: Risk factors for sleep bruxism in the general population. Chest 2001;119:53-61.

22. Sjöholm TT, Lowe AA, Miyamoto K, et al: Sleep bruxism in patients with sleep-disordered breathing. Arch Oral Biol 2000; 45:889-896.

23. Lavigne GJ, Lobbezoo F, Rompré PH, et al: Cigarette smoking as a risk factor or an exacerbating factor for restless legs syndrome and sleep bruxism. Sleep 1997;20:290-293.

24. Dao TTT, Lund JP, Lavigne GJ: Comparison of pain and quality of life in bruxers and patients with myofascial pain of the masticatory muscles. J Orofac Pain 1994;8:350-356.

25. Lavigne GJ, Rompré PH, Montplaisir J, et al: Motor activity in sleep bruxism with concomitant jaw muscle pain. Eur J Oral Sci 1997;105:92-95.

26. Richmond G, Rugh JD, Dolfi R, et al: Survey of bruxism in an institutionalized mentally retarded population. Am J Ment Defic 1984;88:418-421.

27. Lavigne GJ, Rompré PH, Poirier G, et al: Rhythmic masticatory muscle activity during sleep in humans. J Sleep Res 2001;80:443-448.

28. Halász P, Ujszaszi J, Gadoros J: Are microarousals preceded by electroencephalographic slow wave synchronization precursors of confusional awakenings? Sleep 1985;8:231-238.

29. Sforza E, Zucconi M, Petronelli R, et al: REM sleep behavioral disorders. Eur Neurol 1988;28:295-300.

30. Glaros AG, Rao SM: Bruxism: A critical review. Psychol Bull 1977;84:767-781.

31. Harness DM, Peltier B: Comparison of MMPI scores with self-report of sleep disturbance and bruxism in the facial pain population. Cranio 1992;10:70-74.

32. Sjöholm T, Lehtinen I, Helenius H: Masseter muscle activity in diagnosed sleep bruxists compared with non-symptomatic controls. J Sleep Res 1995;4:48-55.

33. Lavigne GJ, Rompré PH, Montplaisir J: Sleep bruxism: Validity of clinical research diagnostic criteria in a controlled polysomnographic study. J Dent Res 1996;75:546-552.

34. Macaluso GM, Guerra P, Di Giovanni G, et al: Sleep bruxism is a disorder related to periodic arousals during sleep. J Dent Res 1998;77:565-573.

35. Miyawaki S, Lavigne GJ, Mayer P, et al: Association between sleep bruxism, swallowing-related laryngeal movement, and sleep positions. Sleep 2003;26:461-465.

36. Bader GG, Kampe T, Tagdae T, et al: Descriptive physiological data on a sleep bruxism population. Sleep 1997;20:982-990.

37. Tosun T, Karabuda C, Cuhadaroglu C: Evaluation of sleep bruxism by polysomnographic analysis in patients with dental implants. Int J Oral Maxillofac Implants 2003;18:286-292.

38. Reding GR, Zepelin H, Robinson JE Jr, et al: Sleep pattern of bruxism: A revision [abstract]. Associated Professional Sleep Societies Meeting, 1967;4:396.

39. Ware JC, Rugh JD: Destructive bruxism: Sleep stage relationship. Sleep 1988;11:172-181.

40. Boutros NN, Montgomery MT, Nishioka G, et al: The effects of severe bruxism on sleep architecture: A preliminary report. Clin Electroencephalogr 1993;24:59-62.

41. Saber M, Guitard F, Rompré PH, et al: Distribution of rhythmic masticatory muscle activity across sleep stages and association with sleep stage shifts. J Dent Res 2002;81:A297.

42. Zucconi M, Oldani A, Ferini-Strambi L, et al: Arousal fluctuations in non-rapid eye movement parasomnias: The role of cyclic alternating pattern as a measure of sleep instability. Clin Neurophysiol 1995;12:147-154.

43. Saber M, Kato T, Rompré PH, et al: Correlation between slow wave activity, rhythmic masticatory muscle activity/bruxism and micro-arousals across sleep cycles. Sleep 2003;26:A320-321.

44. Tani K, Yoshii N, Yoshino I, et al: Electroencephalographic study of parasomnia: Sleep-talking, enuresis and bruxism. Physiol Behav 1966;1:241-243.

45. Satoh T, Harada Y: Electrophysiological study on tooth-grinding during sleep. Electroenceph Clin Neurophysiol 1973;35: 267-275.

46. Sjöholm T, Piha SJ, Lehtinen I: Cardiovascular autonomic control is disturbed in nocturnal teethgrinders. Clin Physiol 1995;15:349-354.

47. Kato T, Rompré PH, Montplaisir JY, et al: Sleep bruxism: An oromotor activity secondary to microarousal. J Dent Res 2001;80:1940-1944.

48. Okura K, Makano M, Bando E, et al: Analysis of biological signals during sleep associated bruxism. J Jpn Soc Stomatognath Funct 1996;3:83-93.

49. Huynh N, Kato T, de Champlain J, et al: Sleep bruxism is associated with a higher sympathetic and a lower parasympathetic tone before the onset of masticatory muscle activation. Sleep 2003;26:A320.

50. Boselli M, Parrino L, Smerieri A, et al: Effect of age on EEG arousals in normal sleep. Sleep 1998;21:351-357.

51. Kato T, Montplaisir JY, Guitard F, et al: Evidence that experimentally-induced sleep bruxism is a consequence of transient arousal. J Dent Res 2003;82:284-288.

52. Lavigne GJ, Rompré PH, Guitard F, et al: Lower number of K-complexes and K-alphas in sleep bruxism: A controlled quantitative study. Clin Neurophysiol 2002;113:686-693.

53. Chase MH, Morales FR: The controls of motoneurons during sleep. In Kryger MH, Roth T, Dement WC (eds): Principles and

Practice of Sleep Medicine, 2nd ed. Philadelphia, WB Saunders, 1994, pp 163-175.

54. Gottesmann C: Introduction to the neurophysiological study of sleep: central regulation of skeletal and ocular activities. Arch Ital Biol 1997;135:279-314.

55. Magee KR: Bruxism related to levodopa therapy. J Am Dent Assoc 1970;214:147.

56. Micheli F, Pardal MF, Gatto M, et al: Bruxism secondary to chronic antidopaminergic drug exposure. Clin Neuropharmacol 1993;16:315-323.

57. Lobbezoo F, Lavigne GJ, Tanguay R, et al: The effect of catecholamine precursor L-dopa on sleep bruxism: A controlled clinical trial. Mov Disord 1997;12:73-78.

58. Lavigne GJ, Soucy J-P, Lobbezoo F, et al: Double blind, crossover, placebo-controlled trial with bromocriptine in patients with sleep bruxism. Clin Neuropharmacol 2001;4:145-149.

59. Lobbezoo F, Soucy JP, Montplaisir J, Lavigne GJ: Striatal D2 receptor binding in sleep bruxism: A controlled study with iodine-123-iodobenzamide and single photon emission computed tomography. J Dent Res 1996;75:1804-1810.

60. Sjöholm T, Lehtinen I, Piha SJ: The effect of propranolol on sleep bruxism: Hypothetical considerations based on a case study. Clin Auton Res 1996;6:37-40.

61. Amir I, Hermesh H, Gavish A: Bruxism secondary to antipsychotic drug exposure: A positive response to propranolol. Clin Neuropharmacol 1997;20:86-89.

62. Huynh N, Guitard F, Manzini C, et al: Lack of effect of propranolol on sleep bruxism: A controlled double-blind study (abstract). Sleep 2004;27:A286.

63. Nakamura Y, Katakura N: Generation of masticatory rhythm in the brainstem. Neurosci Res 1995;23:1-19.

64. Winocur E, Gavish A, Voikovitch M, et al: Drugs and bruxism: A critical review. J Orofac Pain 2003;17:99-111.

65. Kuch EV, Till MJ, Messer LB: Bruxing and non-bruxing children: A comparison of their personality traits. Pediatr Dent 1979;1:182-187.

66. Lindqvist B: Bruxism in twins. Acta Odontol Scand 1974;32:177-187.

67. Hublin C, Kaprio J, Partinen M, et al: Sleep bruxism based on self-report in a nationwide twin cohort. J Sleep Res 1998;7:61-67.

68. Michalowicz BS, Pihlstrom BL, Hodges JS, et al: No heritability of temporomandibular joint signs and symptoms. J Dent Res 2000;79:1573-1578.

69. Ramfjord SP, Mich AA: Bruxism: A clinical and electromyographic study. J Am Dent Assoc 1961;62:35-58.

70. LeResche L, Truelove EL, Dworkin SF: Temporomandibular disorders: A survey of dentists' knowledge and beliefs. J Am Dent Assoc 1993;124:90-106.

71. Tsukiyama Y, Baba K, Clark GT: An evidence-based assessment of occlusal adjustment as a treatment for temporomandibular disorders. J Prosthet Dent 2001;86:57-66.

72. Kato T, Thie NMR, Huynh N, et al: Topical review: Sleep bruxism and the role of peripheral sensory influences. J Orofac Pain 2003;17:191-213.

73. Graf H: Bruxism. Dent Clin North Am 1969;13:659-665.

74. Thie NM, Kato T, Bader G, et al: The significance of saliva during sleep and the relevance of oromotor movements. Sleep Med Rev 2002;6:213-227.

75. Schneyer LH, Pigman W, Hanahan L, et al: Rate of flow of human parotid, sublingual, and submaxillary secretions during sleep. J Dent Res 1956;35:109-114.

76. Lichter I, Muir RC: The pattern of swallowing during sleep. Electroencephalogr Clin Neurophysiol 1975;38:427-432.

77. Miyamoto K, Ozbek MM, Lowe AA, et al: Mandibular posture during sleep in patients with obstructive sleep apnoea. Arch Oral Biol 1999;44:657-664.

78. Shea SA, Edwards JK, White DP: Effect of wake-sleep transitions and rapid eye movement sleep on pharyngeal muscle response to negative pressure in humans. J Physiol 1999; 520:897-908.

79. Trudo FJ, Gefter WB, Welch KC, et al: State-related changes in upper airway caliber and surrounding soft-tissue structures in normal subjects. Am J Respir Crit Care Med 1998;158: 1259-1270.

80. Velly-Miguel AM, Montplaisir J, Rompré PH, et al: Bruxism and other orofacial movements during sleep. J Craniomandib Disord 1992;6:71-81.

81. Kato T, Thie N, Montplaisir J, et al: Bruxism and orofacial movements during sleep. Dent Clin North Am 2001;45:657-684.

82. Seligman DA, Pullinger AG: The degree to which dental attrition in modern society is a function of age and of canine contact. J Orofac Pain 1995;9:266-275.

83. Menapace SE, Rinchuse DJ, Zullo T, et al: The dentofacial morphology of bruxers versus non-bruxers. Angle Orthod 1994;64:43-52.

84. Johansson A, Haraldson T, Omar R, et al: A system for assessing the severity and progression of occlusal wear. J Oral Rehabil 1993;20:125-131.

85. Lobbezoo F, Naeije M: Bruxism is mainly regulated centrally, not peripherally. J Oral Rehabil 2001;28:1085-1091.

86. Pierce CJ, Gale EN: Methodological considerations concerning the use of bruxcore plates to evaluate nocturnal bruxism. J Dent Res 1989;68:1110-1114.

87. Clark GT, Beemsterboer PL, Solberg WK, et al: Nocturnal electromyographic evaluation of myofascial pain dysfunction in patients undergoing occlusal splint therapy. J Am Dent Assoc 1979;99:607-611.

88. Okeson JP: The effects of hard and soft occlusal splints on nocturnal bruxism. J Am Dent Assoc 1987;114:788-791.

89. Bakke M, Thomsen CE, Vilmann A, et al: Ultrasonographic assessment of the swelling of the human masseter muscle after static and dynamic activity. Arch Oral Biol 1996;41:133-140.

90. Gallo LM, Lavigne GJ, Rompré PH: Reliability of scoring EMG orofacial events: Polysomnography compared ambulatory recordings. J Sleep Res 1997;6:259-263.

91. Hudzinski LG, Walters PJ: Use of a portable electromyogram integrator and biofeedback unit in the treatment of chronic nocturnal bruxism. J Prosthet Dent 1987;58:698-701.

92. Ikeda T, Nishigawa K, Kondo K, et al: Criteria for the detection of sleep-associated bruxism in humans. J Orofac Pain 1996;10:270-282.

93. Kato T, Montplaisir J, Blanchet P, et al: Idiopathic myoclonus in the oromandibular region during sleep: A possible source of confusion in sleep bruxism diagnosis. Mov Disord 1999;14:865-871.

94. Lobbezoo F, Huddleston Slater JJ: Variation in masticatory muscle activity during subsequent, submaximal clenching efforts. J Oral Rehabil 2002;29:504-509.

95. Okeson JP, Phillips BA, Berry DTR, et al: Nocturnal bruxing events in healthy geriatric subjects. J Oral Rehabil 1990;17:411-418.

96. Okeson JP, Phillips BA, Berry DTR, et al: Nocturnal bruxing events in subjects with sleep-disordered breathing and control subjects. J Craniomandib Disord 1991;5:258-264.

97. Pierce CJ, Gale EN: A comparison of different treatments for nocturnal bruxism. J Dent Res 1988;67:597-601.

98. Moss RA, Hammer D, Adams HE, et al: A more efficient biofeedback procedure for the treatment of nocturnal bruxism. J Oral Rehabil 1982;9:125-131.

99. Clarke JH, Reynolds PJ: Suggestive hypnotherapy for nocturnal bruxism: A pilot study. Am J Clin Hypn 1991;33:248-253.

100. Dube C, Rompre PH, Manzini C, et al: Quantitative polygraphic controlled study on efficacy and safety of oral splint devices in tooth-grinding subjects. J Dent Res 2004;83:398-403.

101. Gagnon Y, Mayer P, Morisson F, et al: Aggravation of respiratory disturbances by the use of an occlusal splint in apneic patients: A pilot study. Int J Prosthodont 2004;17:151-157.

102. Dao TTT, Lavigne GJ: Oral splints: The crutches for temporomandibular disorders and bruxism? Crit Rev Oral Biol Med 1998;9:345-361.

103. Watanabe T, Baba K, Yamagata K, et al: A vibratory stimulation-based inhibition system for nocturnal bruxism: A clinical report. J Prosthet Dent 2001;85:233-235.

104. Nishigawa K, Kondo K, Takeuchi H, et al: Contingent electrical lip stimulation for sleep bruxism: A pilot study. J Prosthet Dent 2003;89:412-417.

105. Nissani M: Can taste aversion prevent bruxism? Appl Psychophysiol Biofeedback 2000;25:43-54.

106. Mohamed SE, Christensen LV, Penchas J: A randomized double-blind clinical trial of the effect of Amitriptyline on nocturnal masseteric motor activity (sleep bruxism). Cranio 1997;15:326-332.

107. Raigrodski A, Christensen L, Mohamed S, Gardiner DM: The effect of four-week administration of amitriptyline on sleep bruxism. A double-blind crossover clinical study. Cranio 2001;19:21-25.

108. Longstaff M: Do β-blockers pose an unacceptable risk to patients with obstructive sleep apnea (OSA)? Sleep 1997;20:920.

109. Tan EK, Jankovic J: Treating severe bruxism with botulinum toxin. J Am Dent Assoc 2000;131:211-217.

110. Smyth AG: Botulinum toxin treatment of bilateral masseteric hypertrophy. Br J Oral Maxillofac Surg 1994;32:29-33.

111. Filippi GM, Errico P, Santarelli R, et al: Botulinum A toxin effects on rat jaw muscle spindles. Acta Otolaryngol 1993;113:400-404.

112. Weiner WJ, Lang AE: Movement Disorders: A Comprehensive Study. Mt. Kisco, NY, Futura, 1989.

80

Violent Parasomnias: Forensic Medicine Issues

Mark W. Mahowald

Carlos H. Schenck

In all of us, even in good men,
there is a lawless, wild-beast nature
which peers out in sleep.

PLATO—THE REPUBLIC

Acts done by a person asleep cannot be criminal,
there being no consciousness.

P. J. FITZGERALD[1]

ABSTRACT

Increasingly, sleep medicine practitioners are asked to render opinions regarding legal issues pertaining to violent or injurious behaviors purported to have arisen from sleep. Such acts, if having arisen from sleep without conscious awareness, would constitute an *automatism*. Automatic behaviors (or automatisms) resulting in illegal acts have been described in many different medical, neurologic, and psychiatric conditions. Medical and psychiatric automatisms arising from wakefulness are reasonably well understood. Recent advances in sleep medicine have made it apparent that some complex behaviors, occasionally violent or injurious with forensic science implications, are exquisitely state dependent, meaning that they arise exclusively, or predominately, from the sleep period. Violent behaviors arising from the sleep period are more common than previously thought, being reported by 2% of the adult population. The medical and the legal concepts of automatisms differ greatly.

SLEEP-RELATED VIOLENCE

State-Dependent Violence

The concept that sleep is simply the passive absence of wakefulness is no longer tenable. Not only is sleep an active rather than a passive process but it is now clear that sleep is composed of two completely different states: non–rapid eye movement (NREM) sleep, and rapid eye movement (REM) sleep. Therefore, our lives are spent in three entirely different states of being—wakefulness, REM sleep, and NREM sleep. Recent studies have indicated that bizarre behavioral syndromes can, and do, result from the incomplete declaration or the rapid oscillation of these states.[3,4] Although the automatic behaviors of some "mixed states" are relatively benign (e.g., shoplifting in narcolepsy),[5] others may be associated with very violent or injurious behaviors.

The fact that violent or injurious behaviors may arise in the absence of conscious wakefulness and without conscious

> **CASE STUDY**
>
> *This 24-year-old man enjoyed a stellar college academic and athletic record and had no history of psychiatric disease, of drug or substance abuse, or of any sleep disorder, and he had absolutely no prior history of interpersonal violence. In December 1993, he was living in Japan, working as a teacher, and was very sleep deprived prior to returning to the United States. On his return, he went to a friend's house. He estimates that he had received no more than 15 hours of sleep in the preceding 4 days. He drank one and a half beers and took one hit of marijuana. He was noticed to be acting "peculiar." He got out of the car and saw a policeman approaching. He told his friends it was "OK," as he knew the officer (not true).*
>
> *He sat down in the police car. The officer drove him to where his friends were waiting. Each got out of the car and they met behind the car. He then viciously attacked the officer, fracturing his jaw and knocking him unconscious. Another officer arrived. He was finally subdued by a number of people. According to his friends, his behavior was extremely inappropriate, irrational, and completely out of character for him.*
>
> *He had no recollection of any of the event from riding in the car until he "came to" in a hospital. He does remember "dreamlike" images. He stated, "I thought I was in hell." He remembers being held down by a number of arms, but he could not identify bodies or faces. He thinks he thought he was in hell because of the burning sensation on his face. In retrospect, he thought this may have been fragmentary imagery of being held down by the policemen and of having been sprayed in the face with Mace. Extensive psychiatric and chemical dependency evaluations performed after the incident were unrevealing.*
>
> *Based on reports from his friends and the police, and on his fragmentary memories, he never denied having committed the violent act. He was charged with a felony. If convicted on the basis of an "insane" automatism, his plans of developing a business in Japan would be destroyed, as he would not be allowed to leave the United States. He wished to have his behavior declared a "noninsane" automatism, which would have very different legal consequences.*

awareness raises the crucial question of how such complex behavior can occur. Extensive animal experimental studies provide preliminary answers. The widely held view that the brainstem and other, more primitive neural structures primarily participate in elemental/vegetative rather than behavioral activities is inaccurate. Overwhelming amounts of data document that highly complex emotional and motor behaviors can originate from these more primitive structures, without involvement of higher neural structures such as the cortex.[6,7]

Sleep-Related Disorders Associated with Violence

Violent sleep-related behaviors have been recently reviewed in the context of automatic behavior in general.[8] There are well-documented cases of (1) somnambulistic homicide, filicide, attempted homicide, and suicide, (2) murders and other crimes with sleep drunkenness (confusional arousals), and (3) sleep terrors/sleepwalking with potential violence/injury. A wide variety of disorders may result in sleep-related violence.[2,3,9] Conditions associated with violence related to sleep period are listed in Table 80–1. These fall into two major categories: neurologic and psychiatric.

NEUROLOGIC CONDITIONS ASSOCIATED WITH VIOLENT BEHAVIORS

Extrapolating from animal experimental data to the human condition, it has been shown that structural lesions at multiple levels of the nervous system may result in wakeful violence.[10-13] Animal studies provide insights to violent behaviors in disorders of arousal, REM behavioral disorder (RBD), and sleep-related seizures.

Table 80–1.	**Conditions Associated with Automatic Behavior**

Organic Neurologic Disorders

A. Vascular
  1. Transient global amnesia (including migraine)
B. Mass lesions
  1. Increased intracranial pressure
  2. Deep midline structural lesions
C. Toxic/metabolic
  1. Endocrine
  2. Hypoxia/carbon monoxide poisoning
  3. Drugs/alcohol (intoxication/withdrawal)
  4. Thiamine deficiency (Wernicke-Korsakoff syndrome)
D. Infectious (limbic encephalitis)
E. Central nervous system (CNS) trauma
F. Seizures
G. Sleep disorders
  1. Disorders of arousal (confusional arousals [sleep drunkenness], sleepwalking, sleep terrors)
  2. Rapid eye movement (REM) sleep behavior disorder
  3. Nocturnal seizures
  4. Automatic behavior
     a. Narcolepsy and idiopathic CNS hypersomnia
     b. Sleep apnea
     c. Sleep deprivation (including jet-lag)
  5. Hypnagogic hallucinations

Psychogenic Disorders

A. Dissociative states (may arise exclusively from sleep)
  1. Fugues
  2. Multiple personality disorder
  3. Psychogenic amnesia
B. Posttraumatic stress disorder
C. Malingering
D. Munchausen by proxy

Disorders of Arousal (Confusional Arousals, Sleepwalking/Sleep Terrors)

The disorders of arousal comprise a spectrum ranging from confusional arousals (sleep drunkenness) to sleepwalking to sleep terrors[14,15] (see Chapter 74). Although there is usually amnesia for the event,[16,17] vivid dreamlike mentation may occasionally be experienced and reported.[18] Contrary to popular opinion, these disorders may actually begin in adulthood, and they are most often not associated with psychopathology.[18,19] Recent population surveys indicate that the disorders of arousal are quite prevalent in the adult population, being reported by 3% to 4% of all adults and occurring weekly in 0.4%.[20]

Febrile illness, alcohol, prior sleep deprivation, and emotional stress may trigger disorders of arousal in susceptible individuals.[21-23] Sleep deprivation is known to result in confusion, disorientation, and hallucinatory phenomena.[24-29] Medications such as sedatives/hypnotics, neuroleptics, minor tranquilizers, stimulants, and antihistamines, often in combination with each other or with alcohol, may also play a role.[30-32] Many of the reported medicolegal cases of sleepwalking-related violence involved alcohol consumption in an individual prone to experience spontaneous disorders of arousal.

Confusional arousals, the mildest form of disorder of arousal, occur during the transition between sleep and wakefulness and represent a disturbance of cognition and attention despite the motor behavior of wakefulness, resulting in complex behavior without conscious awareness.[33-35] These may be potentiated by prior sleep deprivation or the ingestion of alcohol or sedatives/hypnotics before sleep onset.[36] These episodes of automatic behavior occur in the setting of chronic sleep deprivation or other conditions associated with state admixture (shoplifting has been reported during a period of automatic behavior in a narcoleptic).[5,37,38]

Pathophysiology of Disorders of Arousal

The behavioral similarities between the documented disorder of arousal-related violence in humans and sham rage as seen in the hypothalamic savage syndrome are striking.[39] Although it has been assumed that the sham rage animal models are awake, there is some suggestion that similar models are behaviorally awake and yet (partially) physiologically asleep, with apparent hallucinatory behavior (possibly representing REM sleep dreaming) occurring during wakefulness, and dissociated from other REM state markers.[40]

The neural bases of aggression and rage in the cat have been recently reviewed, indicating that there is clearly an anatomic basis for some forms of violent behavior.[41] The prosencephalic system may serve to control and elaborate, rather than initiate, behaviors originating from deeper structures.[42] In confusional arousals in humans, which can result in confusion or aggression, there is clear electroencephalographic evidence of rapid oscillations between wakefulness and sleep.[35,43] It may be that such behaviors occurring in states other than wakefulness are the expression of motor/affective activity generated by lower structures—unmonitored and unmodified by the cortex.

Some very important factors are beyond the scope of this chapter: (1) the known effect of genetics on violence, and

(2) the well-demonstrated effects of environmental and social factors on the structure and function of the nervous system.[44] (In one study of 31 individuals awaiting trial or sentencing for murder, none was neurologically or psychiatrically normal.[11]) The plasticity of the nervous system in response to environmental influences is greater than previously thought.[45,46] Psychobiologic and sociocultural factors are undoubtedly operant in both wakeful and sleep-related violence.[47,48]

Treatment of the disorders of arousal include both pharmacologic (benzodiazepine and tricyclic antidepressant) and behavioral (hypnosis) approaches.[49]

Various associations exist between obstructive sleep apnea and confusional arousals. Patients suffering from obstructive sleep apnea may experience frequent arousals, which may serve to trigger arousal-induced precipitous motor activity.[50] Therefore, the observed clinical behavior—a confusional arousal—is actually the result of another underlying primary sleep disorder—obstructive sleep apnea. This is another example of why overnight polysomnographic (PSG) studies with extensive physiologic monitoring are mandatory in the evaluation of problematic motor parasomnias. Disorders of arousal may also be precipitated by inadequate or incomplete treatment of sleep apnea with nasal continuous positive airway pressure.[51,52]

Disorders of Arousal and Human Violence

The commonly held belief that disorders of arousal are always benign is erroneous: the accompanying behaviors may be violent, resulting in considerable self-harm, injury to others, or damage to the environment.[3,18] Apparently criminal acts without conscious awareness that occur during sleep drunkenness (formerly termed somnolentia) are not a recently described condition: dramatic cases were described in a classic book on sleep, well over a century ago. The author's conclusion regarding sleep drunkenness was, "It is a natural phenomenon, to which all are liable" (p. 315).[53]

Sleepwalking resulting in injury to self or others has been termed Elpenor's syndrome, after an incident in Book 10 of Homer's *Odyssey*. A youth named Elpenor became intoxicated and fell asleep on the roof of a house. He was suddenly awakened by the noise of others preparing to leave the island of Aeoli, and he ran off the rooftop rather than taking the staircase, sustaining a fatal cervical fracture.

Not only is sleep a very active process but the generators or effectors of many components of both REM and NREM sleep reside in the brainstem and other lower centers. Therefore, it is not surprising that, during sleep, prominent motoric and affective behaviors do occur. Specific incidents have included:

1. Somnambulistic homicide, attempted homicide, filicide[30,54-70]
2. Murders and other crimes with sleep drunkenness,[22] including sleep apnea[23] and narcolepsy[5]
3. Suicide, or fear of committing suicide[9,69,71-74]
4. Sleep terrors/sleepwalking with potential violence/injury[75-78] (may be drug induced[30,79,80])
5. Inappropriate sexual behaviors during the sleep state, presumably the results of and admixture of wakefulness and sleep[80a-80g]

Violent sleep-related behaviors can also result in posttraumatic stress in a spouse.[81]

Some very dramatic cases have been tried using the confusional arousal defense. In one, the *Parks* case in Canada, the defendant drove 23 kilometers, killed his mother-in-law, and attempted to kill his father-in-law. Somnambulism was the legal defense, and he was acquitted.[82] In another case, in Butler, Pennsylvania, a confusional arousal attributed to underlying obstructive sleep apnea was offered as a criminal defense for a man who fatally shot his wife during his usual sleeping hours. He was found guilty.[83]

Accidental death resulting from self-injury incurred during sleepwalking may be erroneously attributed to suicide.[9,74]

REM Sleep Behavior Disorder

RBD represents an experiment of nature, predicted in 1965 by animal experiments[84] and recently identified in humans[85] (see Chapter 75). Normally during REM sleep, there is active paralysis of all somatic muscles (sparing the diaphragm and eye movement muscles). In RBD, there is an absence of REM sleep atonia, which permits the acting out of dreams, often with dramatic and violent or injurious behaviors. The oneiric (dream) behavior demonstrated by cats with bilateral peri–locus ceruleus lesions and by humans with spontaneously occurring RBD clearly arises from and continues to occur *during* REM sleep.[84-86] These oneiric behaviors displayed by patients with RBD are often misdiagnosed as manifestations of a seizure or psychiatric disorder. RBD is often associated with underlying neurologic disorders.[87] The overwhelming male predominance (90%) of RBD[88] raises interesting questions about the relationship of sexual hormones to aggression and violence.[89,90] The violent and injurious nature of RBD behaviors has been extensively reviewed elsewhere.[80,88,91-93] Treatment with clonazepam is highly effective.[87]

Recently, a parasomnia overlap syndrome, which contains both clinical and PSG features of both disorders of arousal and RBD, has been described.[94] Other sleep disorders such as disorders of arousal, underlying sleep apnea, and nocturnal seizures may perfectly simulate RBD, again underscoring the necessity for thorough PSG evaluation of these cases.[95,96]

Nocturnal Seizures

The association between seizures and violence has long been debated. It is plain that, on occasion, seizures may result in violent, injurious, or murderous behaviors.[3,97] Frantic, elaborate, and complex nocturnal motor activity may result from seizures originating in the orbital, mesial, or prefrontal region.[98-103] Episodic nocturnal wanderings, a condition that is clinically indistinguishable from other forms of sleep-related motor activity (such as complex sleepwalking) but that is responsive to anticonvulsant therapy, has also been described.[104-106] Aggression and violence may be seen preictally, ictally, and postictally. Postictal wanderings may result in confused or violent behaviors.[107,108] Some postictal violence is induced or perpetuated by the good intentions of bystanders trying to calm the patient after a seizure.[109] A fascinating postictal aggression syndrome has been described: the aggressive behaviors begin hours to days after the confusional postictal period and may last for hours to several days. Interestingly, as with many other violent states, this is a male phenomenon.[110]

As mentioned earlier, other sleep disorders such as obstructive sleep apnea or RBD may masquerade as nocturnal seizures.[96,111-113]

Compelling Hypnagogic Hallucinations

Recurrent, sexually oriented hypnagogic hallucinations experienced by patients with narcolepsy may be so vivid and convincing to the victim that they may support false accusations.[114]

Sleeptalking

Sleeptalking has also been addressed by the legal system.[115] It is interesting to speculate whether utterances made during sleep are admissible in court.

PSYCHIATRIC CONDITIONS

Psychogenic Dissociative States

Waking dissociative states may result in violence.[116] Dissociative disorders may arise exclusively or predominately from the sleep period.[117,118] Virtually all patients with nocturnal dissociative disorders evaluated at our center were victims of repeated physical and/or sexual abuse, beginning in childhood.[118]

Posttraumatic Stress Disorder

Dissociative states and injury related to nightmare behaviors have been reported in association with posttraumatic stress disorder.[119,120] The limbic psychotic trigger reaction, in which motiveless and unplanned homicidal acts occur, is speculated to represent partial limbic seizures which are "kindled" by highly individualized and specific trigger stimuli, reviving past repetitive stress.[121] If the speculation is correct, this is an example of environmentally induced changes in brain function.

Malingering

Although uncommon, malingering must also be considered in cases of apparent sleep-related violence. Our center has seen a young man who developed progressively violent behaviors, apparently arising from sleep, directed exclusively at his wife. This behavior included beating her and chasing her with a hammer. Following exhaustive neurologic, psychiatric, and PSG evaluation, it was determined that this behavior represented malingering. It was suspected that he was attempting to have the sleep center legitimize his behaviors, should his wife be murdered during one of these episodes.

Munchausen Syndrome by Proxy

In Munchausen syndrome by proxy, a child is reported to have apparently medically serious symptoms, which, in fact, are induced by an adult, usually a caregiver, often a parent. The use of surreptitious video monitoring in sleep disorder centers during sleep (with the parent present) has documented the true etiology for reported sleep apnea and other unusual nocturnal spells.[122-129]

MEDICOLEGAL EVALUATION

Automatisms and the Law

Actus non facit reum nisi mens sit rea—"the deed does not make a man guilty unless his mind is guilty."[130]

In the United States and the United Kingdom, a criminal act (*actus rea*), in order to be criminal, must be paired with a culpable mental state (*mens rea*), meaning a knowing intent to commit a crime. The legal definition of automatism is based on this doctrine. A recent book is devoted to the various forensic aspects of sleep medicine.[131]

Most of the conditions mentioned thus far that have resulted in violent or injurious behaviors are termed automatisms. Automatism is difficult to define.[132-134] Fenwick has proposed the following definition:[130] "An automatism is an involuntary piece of behavior over which an individual has no control. The behavior is usually inappropriate to the circumstances, and may be out of character for the individual. It can be complex, coordinated, and apparently purposeful and directed, though lacking in judgment. Afterwards the individual may have no recollection or only partial and confused memory for his actions. In organic automatisms there must be some disturbance of brain function sufficient to give rise to the above features."

Although the medical concept of automatism (i.e., complex behavior in the absence of conscious awareness or volitional intent) is relatively straightforward, the judicial concept is quite different. Legally, there are two forms of automatism: sane and insane. The *sane* automatism results from an external or extrinsic factor, the *insane* from an internal or endogenous cause. This choice results in two very different consequences for the accused: commitment to a mental hospital for an indefinite period of time if deemed insane, or acquittal without any mandated medical consultation or follow-up if deemed sane. For example, a criminal act resulting from altered behavior due to hypoglycemia induced by injection of too much insulin would be a sane automatism, whereas the same act resulting from hypoglycemia caused by an insulinoma would be an insane automatism. By this unscientific paradigm, criminal behavior associated with epilepsy is, by definition, an insane automatism.[132,135] In the United States, the approach to automatism varies from state to state.[136]

The current legal system unfortunately must consider a sleep-related violence case strictly in terms of choosing between insane or noninsane automatism, without any stipulated deterrent concerning a recurrence of sleepwalking with criminal charges that was induced by a recurrence of the high-risk behavior. If sleepwalking is deemed an insane automatism, then a significant percentage of the general population is legally insane. Clearly, dialogue between the medical and legal professions regarding this important area would be helpful to both and to those arrested during automatisms.[137]

One reasonable approach to dealing with these automatisms from a legal standpoint would be to add a category of acquittal that allowed for innocence based on lack of guilt consequent to set diagnoses—that is, specific illnesses that could be categorized by a group of subspecialty clinicians in consultation with the legal profession.[138]

Another suggestion has been a two-stage trial, which would first establish who committed the act, and then deal separately with the issue of culpability. The first part would be held before a jury, and the second in front of a judge with medical advisors present.[134]

One fortunate (and unexplained) fact is that nocturnal sleep-related violence is hardly ever a recurrent phenomenon.[139] Rarely, recurrence is reported, and possibly it should be termed a noninsane automatism. Thorough evaluation and effective treatment are mandatory before the patient can be regarded as no longer a menace to society.[140] In some cases, clear precipitating events can be identified, and these must be avoided if the individual is to be exonerated of legal culpability. These concepts have led to the proposal of two new forensic categories: (1) parasomnia with continuing danger as a non-insane automatism, and (2) intermittent, state-dependent continuing danger.[140-142]

The Role of the Sleep Medicine Specialist

With the increasing identification of causes, manifestations, and consequences of sleep-related violence comes an opportunity for neurologists and sleep medicine professionals to educate the public and practicing clinicians about the occurrence and nature of such behaviors, and about their successful treatment. More important, the onus is on the sleep medicine professional to educate and assist the legal profession in cases of sleep-related violence that result in forensic medicine issues. This often presents ethical problems, as most expert witnesses are retained by either the defense or the prosecution, leading to a tendency for them to become a partisan for one side or the other. Historically, this has been fertile ground for the appearance of "junk science" in the courtroom,[143] from Bendectin to triazolam to breast implants. Junk science leads to junk justice, and to altered standards of care,[144] and recommendations have been made to minimize its occurrence.

The judicial system is increasingly paying more attention to the process of authentic science and may move to accept only valid scientific evidence.[145,146] In the 1920s, in an attempt to reduce incompetence on the part of expert witnesses, the *Frey* rule was issued. *Frey* allowed experts into court only if their testimony was based on evidence that was "generally accepted" as valid among other scientists in their field. In 1975, the Federal Rules of Evidence were codified and made no mention of *Frey*, and the standards for expert testimony all but disappeared.[143] In 1993, the *Daubert* decision (after the Bendectin debacle) made it the judge's responsibility to determine the legitimacy of scientific evidence before admitting it.[147] The gatekeeping power (and responsibility) of judges to exclude evidence based on subjective belief or unsupported speculation was further elevated by the Supreme Court in the *General Electric Co. et al. v. Joiner* (No. 96-188) decision.

Forensic Sleep Medicine Expert as Impartial Friend of the Court (Amicus Curiae)

One infrequently used tactic that could improve scientific testimony is to use a court-appointed impartial expert.[143] When approached to testify, the expert could encourage this practice by volunteering to serve as a court-appointed expert, rather than being paid by either the prosecution or the defense. Other proposals include the development of a section in scientific journals dedicated to expert witness testimony extracted from public documents, with requests for opinions and consensus statements from appropriate specialists, and the development of a library of circulating expert testimony, which could be used to discredit irresponsible (i.e., paid professional) witnesses.[143] Good science is not determined by

the credentials of the expert witness but rather by scientific consensus.[144]

Prior to accepting a case, the sleep professional should become familiar with this most important issue. A good starting point is a highly informative book, *Galileo's Revenge: Junk Science in the Courtroom*.[143] Many professional societies are calling for, and some have developed guidelines for, expert witness qualifications and testimony.[148-150] Similarly, the American Sleep Disorders Association and the American Academy of Neurology have adopted their own guidelines, which include the following[151,152]:

A. Expert witness qualifications
1. Must have a current, valid, unrestricted license
2. Must be a Diplomat of the American Board of Sleep Medicine
3. Must be familiar with the clinical practice of sleep medicine and should have been actively involved in clinical practice at the time of the event

B. Guidelines for expert testimony
1. Must be impartial: Ultimate test for accuracy and impartiality is a willingness to prepare testimony that could be presented unchanged for use by either the plaintiff or the defendant.
2. Fees should relate to time and effort and not be contingent upon the outcome of the claim. Fees should not exceed 20% of the practitioner's annual income.
3. Practitioner should be willing to submit the testimony for peer review.
4. To establish consistency, the expert witness should make records from previous expert witness testimonies available to the attorneys and expert witnesses of both parties.
5. The expert witness must not become a partisan or advocate in the legal proceedings.

Familiarization with these guidelines may be helpful, and expert witnesses from both sides should be held to the same standards.[153]

Clinical and Laboratory Evaluation of Waking and Sleep-Related Violence

The history of complex, violent, or potentially injurious motor behavior arising from the sleep period should suggest the possibility of one of the conditions mentioned earlier. Our experience with over 200 adults involved in sleep-related injury or violence has repeatedly indicated that clinical differentiation between RBD, disorders of arousal, sleep apnea, and sleep-related psychogenic dissociative states and other psychiatric conditions is often impossible without a PSG study.[154] It is likely that violence arising from the sleep period is more frequent than previously assumed.[155]

The legal implications of automatic behavior have been debated in both the medical and legal literature.[1,156-159] As with nonsleep automatisms, the identification of a specific underlying organic or psychiatric sleep-plus-violence condition does not establish causality for any given deed. Two questions accompany each case of reportedly sleep-related violence: (1) is it possible for behavior this complex to have arisen in a mixed state of wakefulness and sleep without conscious awareness or responsibility for the act? and (2) is that what happened at the time of the incident? The answer to the first is often yes. The second can never be determined with surety, as "the thief has fled in the night."

To assist in the determination of the putative role of an underlying sleep disorder in a specific violent act, we have proposed guidelines, modified from Bonkalo[22] (sleepwalking), Walker[160] (epilepsy), and Glasgow[161] (automatism in general), and formulated from our clinical experience[3]:

1. There should be reason (by history or formal sleep laboratory evaluation) to suspect a bona fide sleep disorder. Similar episodes, with benign or morbid outcome, should have occurred previously. (It must be remembered that disorders of arousal *may begin* in adulthood.)
2. The duration of the action is usually brief (minutes).
3. The behavior is usually abrupt, immediate, impulsive, and senseless—without apparent motivation. Although ostensibly purposeful, it is completely inappropriate to the total situation, out of (waking) character for the individual, and without evidence of premeditation.
4. The victim is someone who merely happened to be present, and who may have been the stimulus for the arousal.
5. Immediately after return of consciousness, there is perplexity or horror, without attempt to escape, conceal, or cover up the action. There is evidence of lack of awareness on the part of the individual during the event.
6. There is usually some degree of amnesia for the event; however, this amnesia need not be complete.
7. In the case of sleep terrors, sleepwalking, or sleep drunkenness, the act may conform to one of the following:
   a. It may occur on awakening (rarely immediately on falling asleep), and usually at least 1 hour after sleep onset.
   b. It may occur upon attempts to awaken the subject.
   c. It may have been potentiated by alcohol ingestion, sedative or hypnotic administration, or prior sleep deprivation.

Most of these conditions are diagnosable and most are treatable. Clinical evaluation should include a complete review of sleep/wake complaints from both the victim and bed partner (if available). This should be followed by thorough examinations: general physical, neurologic, and psychiatric. The diagnosis may be only suspected clinically. Extensive PSG study including scalp electroencephalography, electromyographic monitoring of all four extremities, and continuous audiovisual recording is mandatory for correct diagnosis in atypical cases.[50,105,162-168] Establishing the diagnosis of nocturnal seizures may be particularly difficult (see Chapter 72).

The proposition that sleep disorders may be a legitimate defense in cases of violence arising from the sleep period has been met with immense skepticism.[139] For credibility, evaluations of such complex cases are best performed in experienced sleep disorders centers with interpretation by a veteran clinical polysomnographer. Because of the complex nature of many of these disorders, a multidisciplinary approach is highly recommended.[154,169]

SUMMARY AND FUTURE DIRECTIONS

It is abundantly clear that violence may occur during any one of the three states of being. That which occurs during REM or NREM sleep may have occurred without conscious awareness and may be caused by one of a number of completely different disorders. Violent behavior during sleep may result in events that have forensic science implications. The apparent suicide (e.g., a leap to death from a second-story window) or assault or murder (e.g., molestation, strangulation, stabbing, shooting) may be the unintentional, nonculpable but catastrophic result of disorders of arousal, sleep-related seizures, RBD, or psychogenic dissociative states. The majority of these conditions are diagnosable and, more important, are treatable. The social and legal implications are obvious.

The field of sleep medicine must pursue further productive study, and request adequate funding to objectively study the following important questions: What is the true prevalence of these disorders? How are they best and most accurately diagnosed? What would make the prodromes, which are usually present, be taken seriously? Why is there male predominance in many? How can they best be treated or, better yet, prevented? Are social stressors truly more prevalent in this population? What is the best way to deal with forensic science issues? What is to be done with the offender? What is the likelihood of recurrence? Is such behavior a sane or an insane automatism?[68] How can the potential victim be protected?

More research, both basic science and clinical, is urgently needed to further identify and elaborate on the components of both waking and sleep-related violence, with particular emphasis on neurobiologic, neuroplastic, genetic, and socioenvironmental factors.[11,12,47] The study of violence and aggression will be greatly enhanced by close cooperation among clinicians, basic science researchers, and social scientists.

Clinical Pearl

Homicide, suicide, and inappropriate sexual behavior can occur in the context of sleep-related confusional arousals, without conscious awareness or responsibility on the part of the perpetrator. These behaviors may have important forensic medicine implications. Sleep medicine clinicians involved in such cases should be aware of the differing medical and legal concepts of automatisms, and they should closely follow the guidelines for expert testimony developed by a number of professional organizations.

REFERENCES

1. Fitzgerald PJ: Voluntary and involuntary acts. In Guest AG (ed): Oxford Essays in Jurisprudence. New York, Oxford University Press, 1961, pp 1-28.
2. Ohayon MM, Caulet M, Priest RG: Violent behavior during sleep. J Clin Psychiatry 1997;58:369-376.
3. Mahowald MW, Bundlie SR, Hurwitz TD, Schenck CH: Sleep violence—Forensic science implications: Polygraphic and video documentation. J Forensic Sci 1990;35:413-432.
4. Mahowald MW, Schenck CH: Dissociated states of wakefulness and sleep. Neurology 1992;42:44-52.
5. Zorick FJ, Salis PJ, Roth T, Kramer M: Narcolepsy and automatic behavior: A case report. J Clin Psychiatry 1979;40:194-197.
6. Grillner S, Dubic R: Control of locomotion in vertebrates: Spinal and supraspinal mechanisms. Adv Neurol 1988;47:425-453.
7. Bandler R: Brain mechanisms of aggression as revealed by electrical and chemical stimulation: Suggestion of a central role for the midbrain periaqueductal region. Prog Psychobiol Physiol Psychol 1988;13:67-154.
8. Mahowald MW, Schenck CH: Parasomnias: Sleepwalking and the law. Sleep Med Rev 2000;4:321-339.

9. Mahowald MW, Schenck CH, Goldner M, et al: Parasomnia pseudo-suicide. J Forensic Sci 2003;48:1158-1162.

10. Weiger WA, Bear DM: An approach to the neurology of aggression. J Psychiatr Res 1988;22:85-98.

11. Blake PY, Pincus JH, Buckner C: Neurologic abnormalities in murderers. Neurology 1995;45:1641-1647.

12. Elliott FA: Violence: The neurologic contribution—An overview. Arch Neurol 1992;49:595-603.

13. Greene AF, Lynch TF, Decker B, Coles CJ: A psychobiological theoretical characterization of interpersonal violence offenders. Aggress Violent Behav 1997;2:273-284.

14. Mahowald MW, Schenck CH: Parasomnia purgatory: The epileptic/non-epileptic interface. In Rowan AJ, Gates JR (eds): Non-Epileptic Seizures. Boston, Butterworth-Heinemann, 1993, pp 123-139.

15. Mahowald MW, Ettinger MG: Things that go bump in the night: The parasomnias revisited. J Clin Neurophysiol 1990;7:119-143.

16. Fisher C, Kahn E, Edwards A, et al: A psychophysiological study of nightmares and night terrors: III. Mental content and recall of stage 4 night terrors. J Nerv Ment Dis 1974;158:174-188.

17. Thorpy MJC, Diagnostic Classification Steering Committee. ICSD—International Classification of Sleep Disorders: Diagnostic and Coding Manual. Rochester, Minn, American Sleep Disorders Association, 1990.

18. Schenck CH, Hurwitz TD, Bundlie SR, Mahowald MW: Sleep-related injury in 100 adult patients: A polysomnographic and clinical report. Am J Psychiatry 1989;146:1166-1173.

19. Hartmann E, Greenwald D, Brune P: Night-terrors–sleep walking: Personality characteristics. Sleep Res 1982;11:121.

20. Hublin C, Kaprio J, Partinen M, et al: Prevalence and genetics of sleepwalking: A population-based twin study. Neurology 1997; 48:177-181.

21. Vela Bueno A, Blanco BD, Cajal FV: Episodic sleep disorder triggered by fever: A case presentation. Waking Sleeping 1980;4: 243-251.

22. Bonkalo A: Impulsive acts and confusional states during incomplete arousal from sleep: Criminological and forensic implications. Psychiatric Q 1974;48:400-409.

23. Raschka LB: Sleep and violence. Can J Psychiatry 1984;29: 132-134.

24. Nielsen TA, Dumont M, Montplaisir J: A 20-h recovery sleep after prolonged sleep restriction: Some effects of competing in a world record-setting cinemarathon. J Sleep Res 1995;4:78-85.

25. Williams HL, Morris GO, Lubin A: Illusions, hallucinations and sleep loss. In West L (ed): Hallucinations. New York, Grune and Stratton, 1962, pp 158-165.

26. Shurley JT: Hallucinations in sensory deprivation and sleep loss. In West L (ed): Hallucinations. New York, Grune and Stratton, 1962, pp 87-91.

27. Babkoff H, Sing HC, Thorne DR, et al: Perceptual distortions and hallucinations reported during the course of sleep deprivation. Percept Motor Skills 1989;68:787-798.

28. Brauchi JT, West LJ: Sleep deprivation. JAMA 1959;171:1-14.

29. Belenky GL: Unusual visual experiences reported by subjects in the British army study of sustained operations, Exercise Early Call. Mil Med 1979;144:695-696.

30. Luchins DJ, Sherwood PM, Gillin JC, et al: Filicide during psychotropic-induced somnambulism: A case report. Am J Psychiatry 1978;135:1404-1405.

31. Huapaya LVM: Seven cases of somnambulism induced by drugs. Am J Psychiatry 1979;136:985-986.

32. Charney DS, Kales A, Soldatos CR, Nelson JC: Somnambulistic-like episodes secondary to combined lithium-neuroleptic treatment. Br J Psychiatry 1979;135:418-424.

33. Lipowski ZJ: Delirium (acute confusional state). JAMA 1987; 258:1789-1792.

34. Guilleminault C, Billiard M, Montplaisir J, Dement WC: Altered states of consciousness in disorders of daytime sleepiness. J Neurol Sci 1975;26:377-393.

35. Roth B, Nevsimalova S, Sagova V, et al: Neurological, psychological and polygraphic findings in sleep drunkenness. Arch Suisses Neurol Neurochir Psychiatr 1981;129:209-222.

36. Roth B, Nevsimalova S, Rechtschaffen A: Hypersomnia with "sleep drunkenness." Arch Gen Psychol 1972;26:456-462.

37. Mahowald MW, Schenck CH: REM sleep behavior disorder. In Kryger MH, Dement W, Roth T (eds): Principles and Practice of Sleep Medicine, 2nd ed. Philadelphia, Saunders, 1994, pp 574-588.

38. Parkes JD: Sleep and Its Disorders. Philadelphia, WB Saunders, 1985.

39. Glusman M: The hypothalamic "savage" syndrome. Res Publ Assoc Res Nerv Ment Dis 1974;52:52-92.

40. Kitsikis A, Steriade M: Immediate behavioral effects of kainic acid injections into the midbrain reticular core. Behav Brain Res 1981;3:361-380.

41. Siegel A, Shaikh MB: The neural bases of aggression and rage in the cat. Aggress Violent Behav 1997;2:241-271.

42. Berntson GG, Micco DJ: Organization of brainstem behavioral systems. Brain Res Bull 1976;1:471-483.

43. Guilleminault C, Phillips R, Dement WC: A syndrome of hypersomnia with automatic behavior. Electroencephalogr Clin Neurophysiol 1975;38:403-413.

44. Valzelli L: Psychobiology of Aggression and Violence. New York, Raven Press, 1981.

45. Pons TP, Garraghty PE, Ommaya K, et al: Massive cortical reorganization after sensory deafferentation in adult Macaques. Science 1991;252:1857-1860.

46. Edelman GM: Neural Darwinism. New York, Basic Books, 1987.

47. Greene AF, Lynch TF, Decker B, Coles CL: A psychobiological theoretical characterization of interpersonal violence offenders. Aggress Violent Behav 1997;2:273-284.

48. Golden CJ, Jackson ML, Peterson-Rohne A, Gontkovsky ST: Neuropsychological correlates of violence and aggression: A review of the clinical literature. Aggress Violent Behav 1996;1:3-25.

49. Mahowald MW, Schenck CH: NREM parasomnias. Neurol Clin 1996;14:675-696.

50. Guilleminault C, Silvestri R: Disorders of arousal and epilepsy during sleep. In Sterman MB, Shouse MN, Passouant PP (eds): Sleep and Epilepsy. New York, Academic Press, 1982, pp 513-31.

51. Millman RP, Kipp GR, Carskadon MA: Sleepwalking precipitated by treatment of sleep apnea with nasal CPAP. Chest 1991;99:750-751.

52. Pressman MR, Meyer TJ, Kendrick-Mohamed J, et al: Night terrors in an adult precipitated by sleep apnea. Sleep 1995;18:773-775.

53. Hammond WA: Sleep and Its Derangements. Philadelphia, JB Lippincott, 1869.

54. Hopwood JS, Snell HK: Amnesia in relation to crime. J Ment Sci 1933;79:27-41.

55. Tarsh MJ: On serious violence during sleep-walking. Br J Psychiatry 1986;148:476.

56. Bartholomew AA: On serious violence during sleep-walking. Br J Psychiatry 1986;148:476-477.

57. Sleepwalking and guilt (editorial). Br Med J 1970;2:186.

58. Oswald I, Evans J: On serious violence during sleepwalking. Br J Psychiatry 1985;147:688-691.

59. Morris N: Somnambulistic homicide: Ghosts, spiders, and North Koreans. Res Judicatae 1951;5:29-33.

60. Fenwick P: Murdering while asleep. Br Med J 1986;293:574-575.

61. Podolsky E: Somnambulistic homicide. Dis Nerv Syst 1959;20: 534-536.

62. Podolsky E: Somnambulistic homicide. Med Sci Law 1961;1: 260-265.

63. Yellowlees D: Homicide by a somnambulist. J Ment Sci 1878;24: 451-458.

64. Howard C, D'Orban PT: Violence in sleep: Medico-legal issues and two case reports. Psychol Med 1987;17:915-925.

65. Schatzman M: To sleep, perchance to kill. New Sci 1986;26:60-62.

66. Lochel M: Sleepwalking in children and adolescents: Medical history, child psychiatric and electro-encephalographic aspects. Acta Paedopsychiatrica 1989;52:112-120.

67. Ovuga EBL: Murder during sleepwalking. East Afr Med J 1992;69:533-534.

68. Brooks AD: Law, Psychiatry and the Mental Health System. Boston, Little, Brown, 1974.

69. Bornstein S, Guegen B, Hache E: [Elpenor's syndrome or somnambulistic murder?] Ann Med Psychol (Paris) 1996;154: 195-201.

70. Hamer BA, Payne A: Sleep automatism: Clinical study in forensic nursing. Perspect Psychiatr Care 1993;29:7-11.

71. Kleitman N: Sleep and Wakefulness. Chicago, University of Chicago Press, 1963.

72. Chuaqui C: Suicide and abnormalities of consciousness. Can Psychiatr Assoc J 1975;20:25-28.

73. Lauerma H: Fear of suicide during sleepwalking. Psychiatry 1996;59:206-211.

74. Shatkin JP, Feinfield K, Strober M: The misinterpretation of a non-REM sleep parasomnia as suicidal behavior in an adolescent. Sleep Breath 2002;6:175-179.

75. Hartmann E: Two case reports: Night terrors with sleepwalking—A potentially lethal disorder. J Nerv Ment Dis 1983; 171: 503-505.

76. Rauch PK, Stern TA: Life-threatening injuries resulting from sleepwalking and night terrors. Psychosomatics 1986;27:62-64.

77. Ferber R, Boyle MP: Injury associated with sleepwalking and sleep terrors in children. Sleep Res 1984;13:141.

78. Chin CN: Sleep walking in adults: Two case reports. Med J Malaysia 1987;42:132-133.

79. Scott AIF: Attempted strangulation during phenothiazine-induced sleep-walking and night terrors. Br J Psychiatry 1988; 153:692-694.

80. Schenck CH, Mahowald MW: Injurious sleep behavior disorders (parasomnias) affecting patients on intensive care units. Intensive Care Med 1991;17:219-224.

80a. Buchanan A: Sleepwalking and indecent exposure. Med Sci Law 1991;31:38-40.

80b. Fenwick P: Sleep and sexual offending. Med Sci Law 1996; 36;122-134.

80c. Hurwitz TD, Mahowald MW, Schenck CH, Schulter JL: Sleep-related sexual abuse of children. Sleep Res 1989;18:246.

80d. Rosenfeld DS, Elhajjar AJ: Sleepsex: A variant of sleepwalking. Arch Sex Behav 1998;27:269-278.

80e. Shapiro CM, Fedoroff JP, Trajanovic NN: Sexual behavior in sleep: A newly described parasomnia. Sleep Res 1996;25:367.

80f. Shapiro CM, Trajanovic NN, Fedoroff JP: Sexsomnia – a new parasomnia? Can J Psychiatry 2003;48:311-317.

80g. Wong KE: Masturbation during sleep – a somnambulistic variant? Singapore Med J 1986;27:542-543.

81. Baran AS, Richert AC, Goldberg R, Fry JM: Posttraumatic stress disorder in the spouse of a patient with sleep terrors. Sleep Med 2003;4:73-75.

82. Broughton R, Billings R, Cartwright R, et al: Homicidal somnambulism: A case report. Sleep 1994;17:253-264.

83. Nofzinger EA, Wettstein RM: Homicidal behavior and sleep apnea: A case report and medicolegal discussion. Sleep 1995; 18:776-782.

84. Jouvet M, Delorme F: Locus coeruleus et sommeil paradoxal. CR Séances Soc Biol Fil 1965;159:895-899.

85. Schenck CH, Bundlie SR, Ettinger MG, Mahowald MW: Chronic behavioral disorders of human REM sleep: A new category of parasomnia. Sleep 1986;9:293-308.

86. Hendricks JC, Morrison AR, Mann GL: Different behaviors during paradoxical sleep without atonia depend upon lesion site. Brain Res 1982;239:81-105.

87. Schenck CH, Mahowald MW: REM sleep behavior disorder: Clinical, developmental, and neuroscience perspectives 16 years after its formal identification in Sleep. Sleep 2002;25:120-130.

88. Schenck CH, Hurwitz TD, Mahowald MW: REM sleep behavior disorder: A report on a series of 96 consecutive cases and a review of the literature. J Sleep Res 1993;2:224-231.

89. Goldstein M: Brain research and violent behavior. Arch Neurol 1974;30:1-34.

90. Moyer KE: Kinds of aggression and their physiological basis. Commun Behav Biol 1968;2:65-87.

91. Dyken ME, Lin-Dyken DC, Seaba P, Yamada T: Violent sleep-related behavior leading to subdural hemorrhage. Arch Neurol 1995;52:318-321.

92. Gross PT: REM sleep behavior disorder causing bilateral subdural hematomas. Sleep Res 1992;21:204.

93. Morfis L, Schwartz RS, Cistulli PA: REM sleep behavior disorder: A treatable cause of falls in the elderly. Age Ageing 1997;26: 43-44.

94. Schenck CH, Boyd JL, Mahowald MW: A parasomnia overlap disorder involving sleepwalking, sleep terrors, and REM sleep behavior disorder in 33 polysomnographically confirmed cases. Sleep 1997;20:972-981.

95. Nalamalapu U, Goldberg R, DePhillipo M, Fry JM: Behaviors simulating REM behavior disorder in patients with severe obstructive sleep apnea. Sleep Res 1996;25:311.

96. D'Cruz OF, Vaughn BV: Nocturnal seizures mimic REM behavior disorder. Am J Electroneurodiagn Technol 1997;37:258-264.

97. Hindler CG: Epilepsy and violence. Br J Psychiatry 1989;155: 246-249.

98. Collins RC, Carnes KM, Price JL: Prefrontal-limbic epilepsy: Experimental functional anatomy. J Clin Neurophysiol 1988; 5:105-117.

99. Quesney LF, Krieger C, Leitner C, et al: Frontal lobe epilepsy: Clinical and electrographic presentation. In Porter RJ, Mattson RH, Ward AAJ, et al. (eds): Advances in Epileptology: XVth Epilepsy International Symposium. New York, Raven Press, 1984, pp 503-508.

100. Ludwig B, Ajmone Marsan B, Strauss E, Wada JA: Cerebral seizures of probable orbitofrontal origin. Epilepsia 1987;16:141-158.

101. Waterman K, Purves SJ, Kosaka B, et al: An epileptic syndrome caused by mesial frontal lobe seizure foci. Neurology 1987;37:577-582.

102. Tharp B: Orbital frontal seizures: An unique electroencephalographic and clinical syndrome. Epilepsia 1972;13:627-642.

103. Williamson PD, Spencer SS: Clinical and EEG features of complex partial seizures of extratemporal origin. Epilepsia 1986;27(Suppl 2):s46-s63.

104. Maselli RA, Rosenberg RS, Spire JP: Episodic nocturnal wanderings in non-epileptic young patients. Sleep 1988;11: 156-161.

105. Pedley TA, Guilleminault C: Episodic nocturnal wanderings responsive to anticonvulsant drug therapy. Ann Neurol 1977;2:30-35.

106. Plazzi G, Tinuper P, Montagna P, et al: Epileptic nocturnal wanderings. Neurology 1995;45(Suppl 4):A332.

107. Mayeux R, Alexander MP, Benson DF, et al: Poriomania. Neurology 1979;29:1616-1619.

108. Borum R, Appelbaum KL: Epilepsy, aggression, and criminal responsibility. Psychiatr Serv 1996;47:762-763.

109. Fenwick P: The nature and management of aggression in epilepsy. J Neuropsychiatry 1989;1:418-425.

110. Gerard ME, Spitz MC, Towbin JA, Shantz D: Subacute postictal aggression. Neurology 1998;50:384-388.

111. Houdart R, Mamo H, Tomkiewicz H: La forme epileptogene du syndrome de Pickwick. Rev Neurol 1960;103:466-468.

112. Kryger M, Quesney LF, Holder D, et al: The sleep deprivation syndrome of the obese patient. Am J Med 1974;56:531-539.

113. Guilleminault C: Natural history, cardiac impact and long-term follow-up of sleep apnea syndrome. In Guillemiault C, Lugaresi E (eds): Sleep/Wake Disorders: Natural History, Epidemiology, and Long-term Evolution. New York, Raven Press, 1983, pp 107-125.

114. Hays P: False but sincere accusations of sexual assault made by narcoleptic patients. Medico-Legal Bull 1992;60:265-271.

115. *Regina v. Warner*. Ontario Reports Feb. 17, 1995:136-157.

116. McCaldon RJ: Automatism. Can Med Assoc J 1964;91:914-920.

117. Fleming J: Dissociative episodes presenting as somnambulism. Sleep Res 1987;16:263.

118. Schenck CS, Milner DM, Hurwitz TD, et al: Dissociative disorders presenting as somnambulism: Polysomnographic, video, and clinical documentation (8 cases). Dissociation 1989; 4:194-204.

119. Coy JD: Letter to Editor. J Emerg Med 1996;14:760-762.

120. Bisson JI: Automatism and post-traumatic stress disorder. Br J Psychiatry 1993;163:830-832.

121. Pontius AA: Homicide linked to moderate repetitive stresses kindling limbic seizures in 14 cases of limbic psychotic trigger reaction. Aggress Violent Behav 1997;2:125-141.

122. Rosenberg DA: Web of deceit: A literature review of Munchausen syndrome by proxy. Child Abuse Neglect 1987; 11:547-563.

123. Light MJ, Sheridan MS: Munchausen syndrome by proxy and sleep apnea. Clin Pediatr 1990;29:162-168.

124. Griffith JC, Slovik LS: Munchausen by proxy and sleep disorders medicine. Sleep 1989;12:178-183.

125. Byard RW, Beal SM: Munchausen syndrome by proxy: Repetitive infantile apnoea and homicide. J Paediatr Child Health 1993;29:77-79.

126. Samuels MP, McClaughlin W, Jacobson RR, et al: Fourteen cases of imposed upper airway obstruction. Arch Dis Child 1992;67:162-170.

127. Mydlo JH, Maccia RJ, Kanter JL: Munchausen's syndrome: A medico-legal dilemma. Med Sci Law 1997;37:198-201.

128. Bryk M, Siegel PT: My mother caused my illness: The story of a survivor of Munchausen by proxy syndrome. Pediatrics 1997; 100:1-7.

129. Skau K, Mouridsen SE: Munchausen syndrome by proxy: A review. Acta Paediatr 1995;84:977-982.

130. Fenwick P: Sleep and sexual offending. Med Sci Law 1996;36: 122-134.

131. Shapiro C, McCall Smith A: Forensic Aspects of Sleep. Chichester, England, John Wiley & Sons, 1997:208.

132. Fenwick P: Automatism. In Bluglass R, Bowden P (eds): Principles and Practice of Forensic Psychiatry. Edinburgh, Churchill Livingstone, 1990, pp 271-285.

133. Jang D, Coles EM: The evolution and definition of the concept of "automatism" in Canadian case law. Med Law 1995;14:221-238.

134. Fenwick P: Automatism, medicine, and the law. Psychol Med Monogr Suppl 1990;17:1-27.

135. Fenwick P: Epilepsy, automatism, and the English law. Med Law 1997;16:349-358.

136. McCall Smith A, Shapiro CM: Sleep disorders and the criminal law. In Shapiro C, McCall Smith A (eds): Forensic Aspects of Sleep. Chichester, England, John Wiley & Sons, 1997, pp 29-64.

137. Thomas TN: Sleepwalking disorder and mens rea: A review and case report. J Forensic Sci 1997;42:17-24.

138. Beran RG: Automatisms: The current legal position related to clinical practice and medicolegal interpretation. Clin Exp Neurol 1992;29:81-91.

139. Guilleminault C, Moscovitch A, Leger D: Forensic sleep medicine: Nocturnal wandering and violence. Sleep 1995;18:740-748.

140. Schenck CH, Mahowald MW: A polysomnographically documented case of adult somnambulism with long-distance automobile driving with frequent nocturnal violence: Parasomnia with continuing danger as a noninsane automatism. Sleep 1995;18:765-772.

141. Schenck CH, Mahowald MW: An analysis of a recent criminal trial involving sexual misconduct with a child, alcohol abuse, and a successful sleepwalking defense: Arguments supporting two proposed new forensic categories. Med Sci Law 1998;38: 147-152.

142. Schenck CH, Mahowald MW: Sleepwalking and indecent exposure (letter). Med Sci Law 1992;32:86-87.

143. Huber PW: Galileo's Revenge: Junk Science in the Courtroom. New York, Basic Books, 1991.

144. Weintraub MI: Expert witness testimony: A time for self-regulation? Neurology 1995;45:855-858.

145. Loevinger L: Science as evidence. Jurimetrics J 1995;153:153-190.

146. Foster KR, Bernstein DE, Huber PW: Phantom Risk: Scientific Inference and the Law. Cambridge, Mass, MIT Press, 1993.

147. Re: *Daubert et al v Merril Dow Pharmaceuticals* 92-102. June 28, 1993. 113 SCt 2768 (1993).

148. Committee on Medical Liability: Guidelines for expert witness testimony. Pediatrics 1989;83:312-313.

149. Anonymous: Guidelines for the physician expert witness: American College of Physicians. Ann Intern Med 1990;113:789.

150. Bone R, Rosenow E: ACCP guidelines for an expert witness. Chest 1990;98:1006.

151. American Sleep Disorders Association: ASDA Guidelines for expert witness qualifications and testimony. APSS Newsletter 1993;8:23.

152. American Academy of Neurology: Qualifications and guidelines for the physician expert witness (newsletter). Neurology 1989;39:9A.

153. Mahowald MW, Schenck CH: Complex motor behavior arising during the sleep period: Forensic science implications. Sleep 1995;18:724-727.

154. Mahowald MW, Schenck CH, Rosen GR, Hurwitz TD: The role of a sleep disorders center in evaluating sleep violence. Arch Neurol 1992;49:604-607.

155. Broughton RJ, Shimizu T: Sleep-related violence: A medical and forensic challenge. Sleep 1995;18:727-730.

156. Whitlock FA: Criminal Responsibility and Mental Illness. London, Butterworth, 1963.

157. Prevezer S: Automatism and involuntary conduct. Criminal Law Rev 1958:361-367.

158. Williams G: Criminal Law. London, Stevens and Sons, 1961.

159. Shroder O, Mather NJ: Forensic psychiatry. In Camps FE (ed): Gradwohl's Legal Medicine. Chicago, John Wright & Sons, 1976, p 505.

160. Walker EA: Murder or epilepsy? J Nerv Ment Dis 1961;133: 430-437.

161. Glasgow GL: The anatomy of automatism. N Z Med J 1965;64: 491-495.

162. Soldatos CR, Vela-Bueno A, Bixler EO, et al: Sleepwalking and night terrors in adulthood: Clinical and EEG findings. Clin Electroencephalogr 1980;11:136-139.

163. Halbreich U, Assael M: Electroencephalogram with sphenoidal needles in sleepwalkers. Psychiatr Clin 1978;11:213-218.

164. Popoviciu L, Szabo L, Corfariu O, et al: A study of the relationships of certain pavor nocturnus (PN) attacks with nocturnal epilepsy. In Popoviciu L, Asgian B, Badiu G (eds): Sleep 1978. Fourth European congress on sleep research. Tirgu-Mures. Basel, Karger, 1980, pp 599-605.

165. Dervent A, Karacan I, Ware JC, Williams RL: Somnambulism: A case report. Sleep Res 1978;7:220.

166. Amir N, Navon P, Silverberg-Shalev R: Interictal electroencephalography in night terrors and somnambulism. Isr J Med Sci 1985;21:22-26.

167. Broughton R: Childhood sleepwalking, sleep terrors, and enuresis nocturna: Their pathophysiology and differentiation from nocturnal epileptic seizures. In Popoviciu L, Badiu G (eds): Sleep 1978. Fourth European congress on sleep research. Tirgu-Mures. Basel, Karger, 1980, pp 103-122.

168. Mahowald MW, Schenck CS: Parasomnia purgatory: The epileptic/non-epileptic interface. In Rowan AJ, Gates JR (eds): Non-Epileptic Seizures. Boston, Butterworth-Heinemann, 1993, pp 123-139.

169. Aldrich MS, Jahnke B: Diagnostic value of video-EEG polysomnography. Neurology 1991;41:1060-1066.

170. Mahowald MW, Schenck CH: Violent parasomnias: Forensic medicine issues. In Kryger MH, Roth T, Dement WC (eds): Principles and Practice of Sleep Medicine, 3rd ed. Philadelphia, WB Saunders, 2000, pp 786-795.

Central Sleep Apnea

David P. White

ABSTRACT

Central sleep apnea is a disorder characterized by recurrent episodes of apnea during sleep resulting from temporary loss of ventilatory effort. Such apneas generally result from the strong dependence of ventilation during sleep on the metabolic control system and, in particular, arterial P_{CO_2}. Thus, they occur during the wake–sleep transition, when waking P_{CO_2} may be below sleeping levels and therefore nonstimulatory to ventilatory effort (sleep onset apneas), when the gain of the ventilatory control system is high (idiopathic central sleep apnea), when high gain is combined with prolonged circulation time (Cheyne-Stokes respiration), or when P_{CO_2} control mechanisms are defective (hypercapnic respiratory failure). Regardless of the cause, central apneas are often associated with arousal from sleep, which can lead to difficulty sustaining sleep and daytime somnolence. This reflects the symptoms with which these patients may present. The prevalences of most disorders that are associated with central sleep apnea have been minimally studied, although most are believed to be relatively uncommon. Cheyne-Stokes respiration may be an exception, as a high prevalence has been observed in patients with congestive heart failure. Diagnosis of central sleep apnea generally requires a full-night polysomnographic evaluation, ideally including measurement of esophageal pressure. However, use of chest–abdominal wall motion as a marker of respiratory effort would be unlikely to lead to an incorrect diagnosis. Treatment of central sleep apnea must be directed, as much as possible, toward the underlying cause. Idiopathic central sleep apnea frequently responds to oxygen or acetazolamide, whereas Cheyne-Stokes respiration (associated with congestive heart failure) is best managed with continuous positive airway pressure, which regularizes the respiratory pattern as cardiac function improves. Hypercapnic respiratory failure, on the other hand, often requires noninvasive nocturnal ventilation. Thus, the cause of the disordered breathing must be clarified to optimize management.

Cessation of breathing during sleep can result from obstruction of the upper airway (obstructive apnea), loss of ventilatory effort (central apnea), or a combination of the two. The term *central sleep apnea* is used to describe both the pattern of an individual event and the clinical disorder characterized by repeated episodes of apnea during sleep resulting from the temporary loss of ventilatory effort.[1] A central apnea is conventionally defined as a period of at least 10 seconds without airflow, during which no ventilatory effort is evident. This condition differs from the obstructive or mixed apnea by the absence of upper airway obstruction and subsequent ventilatory attempts against an occluded airway (Fig. 81–1). Although this chapter is concerned with central sleep apnea, central and obstructive events are rarely seen in isolation. The vast majority of patients with central apneas also have some obstructive events. This observation suggests that the mechanisms responsible for the different types of apnea must overlap, and research indicates this is likely to be the case.

The muscles of the upper airway (the genioglossus and others) behave as respiratory muscles,[2] dilating or stiffening the pharynx on inspiration. If a decrease or loss of activity occurs in both upper airway muscles and the diaphragm,[3] one of several consequences seems likely:

1. The decrement in motor tone of the pharyngeal dilator muscles could lead to upper airway occlusion, with subsequent obstructed ventilatory efforts when diaphragmatic inspiratory activity resumes (a mixed apnea).
2. This loss of pharyngeal muscle activity could yield upper airway collapse, but pharyngeal and diaphragmatic muscles resume activation simultaneously, giving the appearance of a central apnea when airway obstruction was actually present during the apnea.
3. If loss of upper airway muscle activity does not lead to pharyngeal obstruction, a pure central apnea will very likely be seen, with no activation of the diaphragm.

The propensity of the upper airway to collapse may therefore be important in determining whether central or obstructive apnea results when cycling output to respiratory muscles occurs during sleep.

After tracheostomy for obstructive sleep apnea, many patients develop central apnea, which generally resolves over a period of months.[4] This may also occur when continuous positive airway pressure (CPAP) is initiated to alleviate upper airway obstruction. In addition, it has been observed that the treatment of central apneas with either a respiratory stimulant (e.g., acetazolamide[5]) or diaphragmatic pacing[6] can result in obstructive events. Finally, studies report objective evidence of

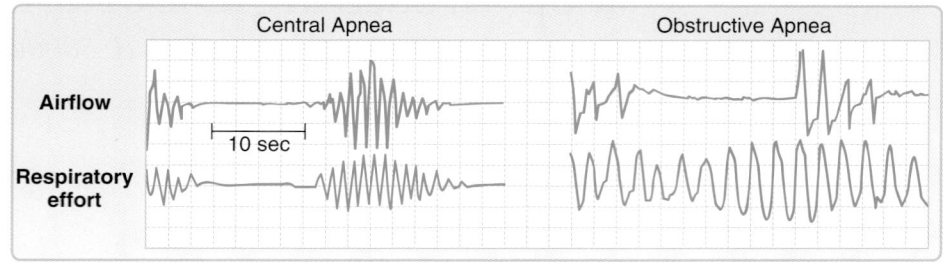

Figure 81–1. The relation between airflow and respiratory effort is demonstrated in both central and obstructive apnea. During a central apnea, there is cessation of airflow for at least 10 seconds with no associated ventilatory effort. An obstructive apnea is defined as a similar cessation of airflow but with continued respiratory effort.

pharyngeal airway narrowing during purely central apneas. These observations imply some commonality in the pathophysiology of the various types of apnea, so it is not surprising that central and obstructive apneas are frequently seen in the same individual.

Patients with predominantly central sleep apnea constitute fewer than 10% of apneic individuals in most sleep laboratory populations,[1,7] with studies suggesting only about 4%.[8,9] As a result, only a small number of studies with more than a few such patients have been reported, which makes knowledge of this disorder scant. Most of this chapter provides a discussion of patients with central sleep apnea who breathe normally during the day; however, any patient with hypoventilation during wakefulness will almost certainly have hypoventilation with central apneas at night.

It should be recognized from the beginning that a central pause in breathing may result from a variety of physiologic or pathophysiologic events. The term *central sleep apnea* reflects several breathing patterns, all of which include pauses in inspiratory effort; it does not represent a single entity or result from a single cause. Examples include Cheyne-Stokes respiration, periodic breathing at altitude, and the idiopathic central sleep apnea observed at sea level. Each has a different pathogenesis but is manifested by central apneas during sleep. To understand central sleep apnea, the normal mechanisms controlling ventilation awake and asleep and pathologic influences on these mechanisms must be understood. All possible causes of central apnea must be considered in caring for patients with this disorder.

PATHOPHYSIOLOGY

Because central apneas are defined as pauses in breathing without ventilatory effort, a complete loss of electromyographic activity of the respiratory muscles during such an apnea would be expected, and this has been demonstrated.[3] After the apnea, there is a resumption of normal ventilatory muscle activity. This finding implies that the neuronal output to the respiratory muscles ceases during central apnea and returns at the end of the ventilatory pause. Central apneas therefore represent a loss of inspiratory drive. Although the cause of central apnea in many patients remains obscure, investigation into the control of breathing during sleep and the association of central apneas with certain disease processes has pointed to a number of possible mechanisms, all of which are characterized by instability of respiratory control.

Control of Breathing

Ventilation is controlled by a number of processes that have been generally grouped under three headings (see Chapter 18).[10] The first is the automatic or metabolic control system, consisting of the chemoreceptors (carotid body for hypoxia and carotid body plus medullary chemoreceptor for hypercapnia), vagally mediated intrapulmonary receptors, and numerous brainstem mechanisms that both process the information from these peripheral receptors and control the pattern of breathing. This metabolic system keeps ventilation regular and ensures that the quantity of ventilation occurring at any time is well matched to metabolic and homeostatic requirements. The second such system is called the "behavioral" control system. It seems clear that the activities of normal life, such as talking and eating, can influence ventilation and are thought of as behavioral or volitional influences. The origin of this neural input to respiration is probably in the forebrain. The third ventilatory control process in awake humans and animals is referred to as the "wakefulness" stimulus, with increased ventilation being inherent to the waking state.[10] Although the mechanisms responsible for this effect of wakefulness on ventilation are poorly defined, it has been proposed that it either results from the influence of the descending arousal systems on respiratory pattern generators in the brainstem or it is a product of tonic input from nonrespiratory sensory mechanisms such as sight or hearing on the respiratory control system.[11,12] The important point is that during wakefulness, ventilation is controlled by both the metabolic and the behavior systems, including possibly this wakefulness stimulus. Ventilation is likely to persist during wakefulness even with the complete absence of metabolic mechanisms.

During sleep, particularly non–rapid eye movement (NREM) sleep, breathing is controlled almost solely by the metabolic control system, with ventilation being tightly linked to afferent input from chemoreceptors and vagal intrapulmonary receptors.[13] This observation was demonstrated in dogs by blocking the input from each of these receptors and monitoring the change in ventilatory pattern (Fig. 81–2). These interventions produced a marked slowing of ventilatory frequency, with long apneic periods. Although this has not been compellingly demonstrated in humans, there is evidence suggesting that a similar control system is present. Oxygen administration, which reduces the hypoxic stimulus to breathing, has been shown to decrease ventilation during sleep and to initially prolong apneas in some individuals in whom such

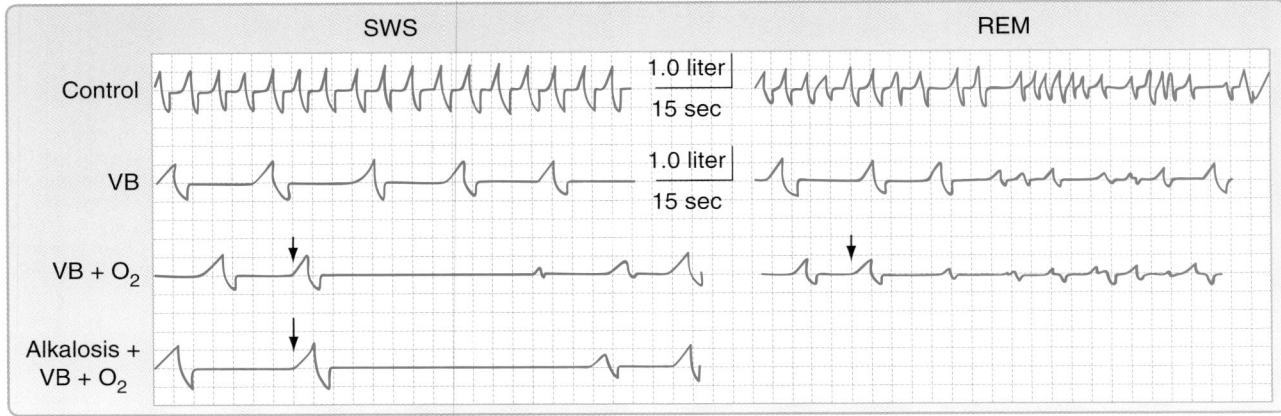

Figure 81–2. Recorder tracing from the dog, showing effects of decreased respiratory afferent stimulation during slow wave sleep (SWS) and rapid eye movement (REM) sleep. Tracings show inspired and expired volumes. Note change in volume calibration for all records during vagal blockage (VB). VB + O_2, one breath of 100% oxygen inspired (*at arrow*) during vagal blockage; Alkalosis + VB + O_2, one breath of 100% oxygen inspired (*at arrow*) during vagal blockage and chronic metabolic alkalosis. (From Guilleminault C, Dement W [eds]: Sleep Apnea Syndromes. New York, Alan R Liss, 1978, p 58.)

events were already present. In addition, hypocapnic alkalosis, which reduces the hypercapnic ventilatory drive, has been shown to produce central apneas in otherwise normal men.[14,15] This combination of studies indicates the importance of both the hypoxic and the hypercapnic influences on breathing during sleep. The implication is that maintenance of neuronal output to the respiratory muscles during sleep may be critically dependent on incoming stimuli, such as those from chemoreceptors.

Considerable investigation has been directed at determining the influence of sleep itself on chemoreceptor activity.[16,17] Although this is still controversial, the majority of the available information suggests that ventilatory responses to both hypoxia and hypercapnia are reduced somewhat during NREM sleep and fall further during rapid eye movement (REM) sleep.[16,17] However, several studies indicate that the decrement during NREM sleep is very likely a product of diminished resistive load compensation (reduced defense of ventilation in the presence of the normal, physiologic increase in upper airway resistance associated with NREM sleep) rather than a true loss of chemosensitivity.[18] Most investigators believe that chemoresponsiveness is reasonably well maintained during sleep, particularly NREM sleep, and is probably important in maintaining rhythmic ventilation during sleep.

Arterial Carbon Dioxide Tension (Pco_2) and Breathing during Sleep

The important role of arterial Pco_2 in the maintenance of normal rhythmic ventilation during sleep has been known for years and was outlined by Cherniack.[19] Within the usual physiologic range, there is a linear relationship between increasing Pco_2 and ventilation, with only a small rise above the resting Pco_2 level being required to increase ventilation (Fig. 81–3). The hypoxic drive, described by the arterial oxygen tension (Pao_2)–ventilation relationship, on the other hand, is a hyperbolic response, with little change in ventilation occurring despite fairly large fluctuations in Po_2 around the normal range (see Fig. 81–3). This arrangement yields a

stable ventilatory control system for several reasons. Pco_2 is arguably the dominant ventilatory stimulus during sleep, and as stated, the relationship between Pco_2 and ventilation is linear. In addition, there are relatively large stores of carbon dioxide in the body, so that large increases in ventilation are necessary to produce changes in Pco_2, especially in the central nervous system, where such changes are detected. As a result, a "damped" and stable feedback system exists. On the other hand, the hypoxic response is neither linear nor damped because oxygen stores in the body (lungs and blood) are small. Changes in Po_2 in the normal range, however, have little influence on ventilation. Thus, any process disturbing this arrangement could make ventilatory control unstable, yielding apnea or cycling breathing. The validity of these observations has been confirmed by a number of investigators.

In his classic studies, Bülow[20] showed that "periodic breathing" during sleep was related to Pco_2 in an important way. He observed that apnea or pronounced hypoventilation occurred "only when the preceding Pco_2 was relatively low," which suggests that a reduced Pco_2 during sleep may decrease the drive to breathe to the point of apnea. Other studies have confirmed the prominent role played by Pco_2 in the maintenance of rhythmic breathing during sleep. Skatrud and Dempsey[14,21] showed that passive, positive-pressure hyperventilation of sleeping subjects yielded apnea by reducing Pco_2 only 3 to 6 mm Hg below the sleeping value (Fig. 81–4). The actual Pco_2 level associated with apnea was often only 1 to 2 mm Hg below the awake value as Pco_2 rose from wakefulness to sleep. Each individual had an "apnea threshold," a Pco_2 level below which apnea was commonly seen. It seemed, therefore, that the waking Pco_2 level was at or near this apnea threshold, such that waking Pco_2 levels may be inadequate to stimulate ventilation during sleep. It was also demonstrated that the periodic breathing during sleep that is frequently seen with prolonged hypoxia could be abolished by elevating the Pco_2 above the predetermined "apnea threshold." This finding suggests that the hypocapnia induced by hypoxia, not hypoxia itself, is the pivotal element in this periodic breathing. The authors[15] concluded "that effective ventilatory rhythmogenesis

HYPERCAPNIC RESPONSE   HYPOXIC RESPONSE

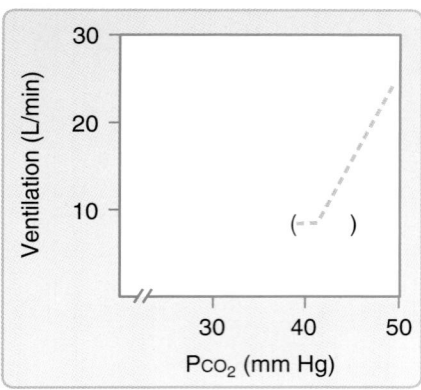 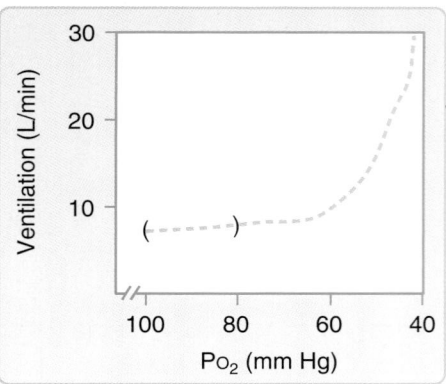

Figure 81–3. Schematic representation of normal hypercapnic and hypoxic ventilatory responses. *Parentheses* enclose normal ranges for P_{CO_2} and P_{O_2}. Little change from the resting P_{CO_2} value is necessary to stimulate ventilation, whereas ventilation is minimally affected by alteration of P_{O_2} in the normal range.

in the absence of stimuli associated with wakefulness is critically dependent on chemoreceptor stimulation secondary to P_{CO_2}-[H⁺]." It should be noted that subsequent studies by this same investigative group now suggest that increased tidal volume (vagal mechanisms) may also be a primary mechanism inhibiting respiration after a series of large breaths.[22] However, the concept of hyperventilation ultimately leading to an inhibition of respiration with central apnea (whether secondary to hypocapnia or vagal mechanisms) remains intact and is likely to be an important one in understanding the pathogenesis of central sleep apnea.

These findings have important implications in the pathogenesis of the central sleep apnea or periodic breathing that is observed at increased altitude, which is discussed in more detail in Chapter 20. It has long been known that humans acutely exposed to high altitude have periodic breathing during sleep with central apnea. The previously described studies suggest that this apnea is a product of the hypocapnia induced by hypoxia (hyperventilation) and not of the hypoxia itself. Whether hypoxia is a further destabilizing influence on ventilation, as

suggested by Cherniack, remains unresolved. It seems that increasing the influence of the hypoxic drive (a hyperbolic, undamped response) might amplify breathing dysrhythmias, but further investigations are necessary to document this.

Ventilatory Control Stability

These mechanisms are all seemingly designed to maintain ventilatory stability during wakefulness and sleep, thus avoiding large swings in respiratory pattern and arterial blood gases. However, abnormalities in the various components of this ventilatory control system can lead to instability in respiration. This can best be understood by introducing the concept of "loop gain," an engineering term describing the gain of a system controlled by multiple feedback loops.[23] Although greatly simplified, as shown in Figure 81–5, loop gain in the ventilatory control system is primarily influenced by three variables:

- *Plant gain:* The efficiency by which CO_2 is removed from the body by the lung apparatus (parenchyma and respiratory muscles)

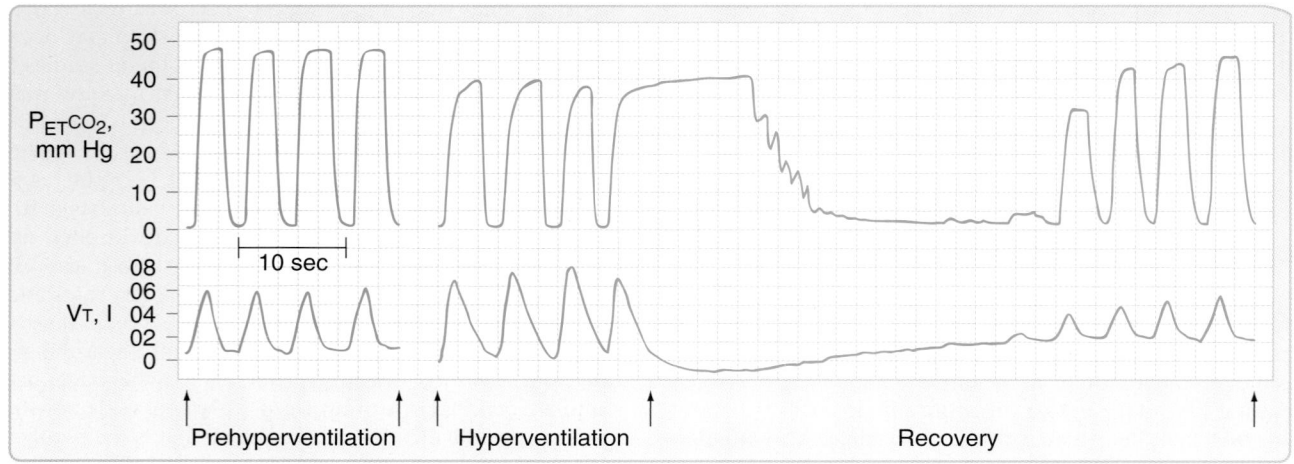

Figure 81–4. Posthyperventilation apnea after 3 minutes of passive, positive-pressure hyperventilation during non–rapid eye movement sleep. Oxygen saturation was 100% in prehyperventilation, hyperventilation, and recovery periods. Small tidal volume (V_t) on first breath after apnea resulted in a poor end-tidal P_{CO_2} sample that was not representative of the alveolar partial pressure of carbon dioxide during or at the end of the apneic episode. $P_{ET}CO_2$, end-tidal P_{CO_2}. (From Skatrud J, Dempsey J: Interaction of sleep state and chemical stimuli in sustaining rhythmic ventilation. J Appl Physiol 1983;55:813-822.)

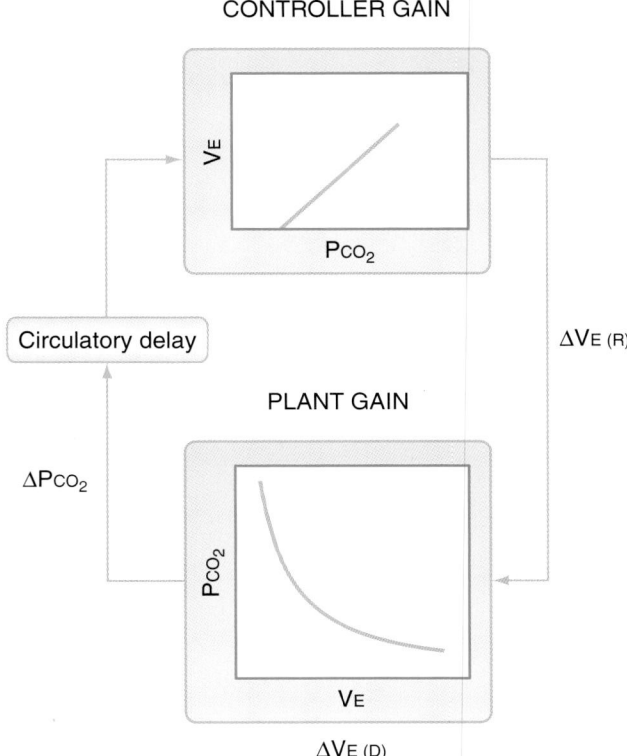

CONTROLLER GAIN

PLANT GAIN

Circulatory delay

$\Delta V_{E(R)}$

ΔP_{CO_2}

$\Delta V_{E(D)}$

Figure 81–5. The major components of loop gain. Plant gain indicates the ability of the lung apparatus to eliminate CO_2. Controller gain is the responsiveness of the respiratory system to increasing P_{CO_2}. Circulatory delay is the delay between blood gas changes in the lung and the arrival of the new blood gas at the medullary chemoreceptor. $V_{E(D)}$ is the ventilatory disturbance and $V_{E(R)}$ is the response to the disturbance.

- *Controller gain:* The responsiveness of the ventilatory control system, primarily to changes in P_{CO_2} but also, to a lesser extent, P_{O_2}
- *Circulation time:* The interval between changes in blood gases in the lung and the arrival of the new blood gases at the CO_2 sensor in the brainstem (influenced primarily by cardiac output)

Although loop gain can be quantified in a number of ways, it can most easily be thought of as the ratio of the ventilatory response to a disturbance to the disturbance itself (i.e., {response to disturbance/disturbance}). As shown in Figure 81–6, a stable ventilatory control system has a small to moderate response to a disturbance (e.g., an apnea), and ventilation quickly decays back to the normal pattern. Thus, a low loop gain (less than 1 and generally less than 0.5) yields stable respiration. On the other hand, a very high loop gain (greater than 1), as shown in Figure 81–6, leads to a waxing and waning of ventilation because the response to the respiratory disturbance is always greater than or equal to the disturbance. Thus ventilation can never stabilize. A high loop gain is generally the product of high controller gain (increased hypercapnic responsiveness) and a prolonged circulation time (low cardiac output), although high plant gain (rapid CO_2 elimination) may play a role. This context can be used in understanding the various causes of central sleep apnea.[24]

Central Apnea Caused by Ventilatory Control Instability

Sleep Onset Central Apneas

It should be evident that ventilation is remarkably dependent on the metabolic control system during sleep and that the primary stimulus to ventilation during sleep is arterial P_{CO_2}. Several circumstances could therefore lead to central apneas during sleep. First, if the P_{CO_2} drops below a certain level, the *apnea threshold*,[21] breathing is likely to become dysrhythmic. This drop may in part explain the dysrhythmic breathing frequently seen at sleep onset. As an individual changes from wakefulness to stage 1 or stage 2 sleep, the P_{CO_2} level that was adequate to stimulate ventilation during wakefulness may be inadequate to do so during sleep (i.e., the P_{CO_2} is below the apnea threshold), and an apnea occurs. During the apnea, P_{CO_2} rises until it is above this apnea threshold and ventilation resumes. This resumption of ventilation may arouse the individual, and the process repeats itself when the individual falls back to sleep. Once a stable sleep stage is reached, ventilation should become regular under metabolic control. Therefore, any process that leads to frequent sleep–wake transitions over the course of the night (such as insomnia) may increase the number of central apneas. In addition, it should be clear that nonrepetitive central apneas in the sleep–wake transition are probably normal events.

Hypercapnic Respiratory Failure

With loss of wakefulness, ventilation becomes completely dependent on metabolic control mechanisms. In individuals with deficient ventilatory control (i.e., low or absent hypoxic/hypercapnic responsiveness), breathing during wakefulness may be maintained by behavioral or wakeful stimuli. However, during sleep, when these wakeful mechanisms are no longer operative, there may be little residual drive to ventilation because metabolic mechanisms are defective.

Thus, the slope of the ventilatory response to hypercapnia (frequently measured during wakefulness) is an important variable in defining loop gain and the subsequent development of central apneas during sleep. In patients with markedly diminished or absent chemosensitivity, in whom hypercapnia is commonly encountered during wakefulness, loop gain would be quite low and cycling central apneas during sleep unexpected. This is generally the case, as these patients most often demonstrate hypoventilation during sleep, particularly during REM sleep, with few central apneas. However, when carbon dioxide sensitivity is very low or absent, there may be little to no stimulus to ventilation during sleep, and central apneas can occur although they are not common: patients with disorders such as central alveolar hypoventilation (Ondine's curse)[25] and the obesity–hypoventilation (pickwickian) syndrome would fall into this group.[26] These individuals have virtually no measurable chemosensitivity during wakefulness and tend to hypoventilate during the day. When these patients are asleep, this hypoventilation becomes worse, with further hypoxia and carbon dioxide retention. Apneas, both central and obstructive, can occur, although cycling, recurrent central apneas would be uncommon.

NORMAL LOOP GAIN

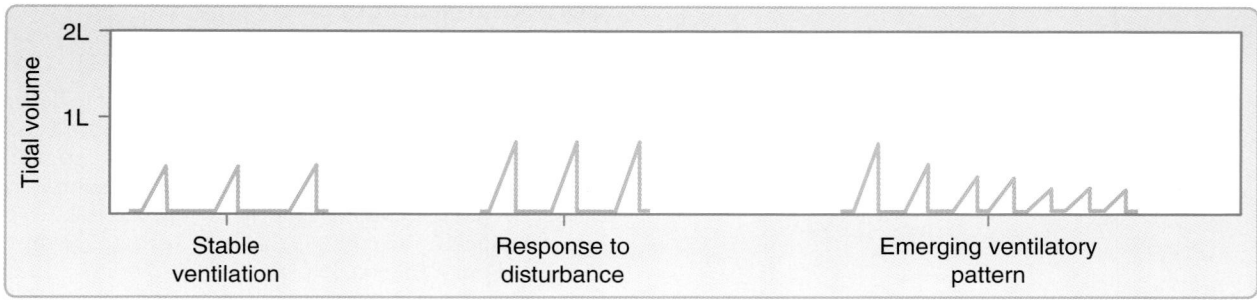

HIGH LOOP GAIN

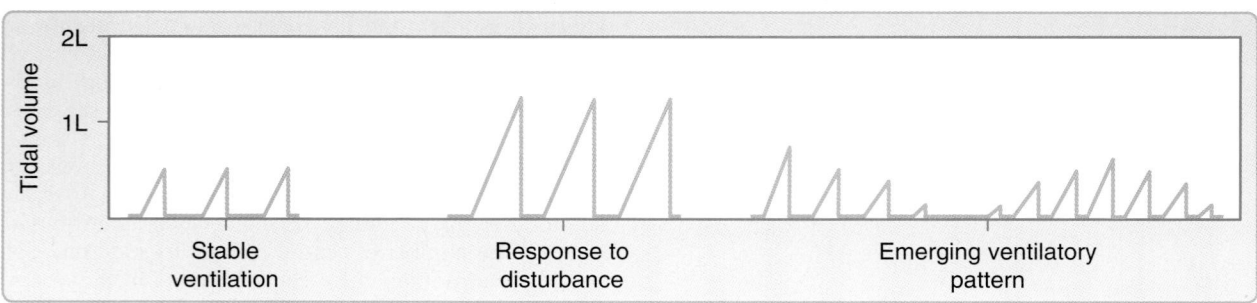

Figure 81–6. Ventilatory response to a disturbance in an individual with a normal and in an individual with a high loop gain. In the normal loop gain situation, the disturbance yields a moderate increase in ventilation, which decays back to normal relatively quickly. With a high loop gain, there is a larger response to the disturbance, and a cycling unstable ventilatory pattern emerges from the disturbance.

Idiopathic Central Sleep Apnea

Increased hypercapnic sensitivity may also be associated with problems during sleep. Bradley et al.,[27] observed two distinct groups of patients with central apneas. One had a low hypercapnic ventilatory response (0.6 ± 0.2 L/min/mm Hg) and hypercapnia during wakefulness. In contrast, the other group, patients with idiopathic central sleep apnea, tended to have a high hypercapnic response (2.9 ± 0.4 L/min/mm Hg) and low arterial P_{CO_2} levels during wakefulness. In this latter group of patients, it was postulated that the unusually steep hypercapnic response led to a high loop gain with respiratory instability, yielding a waxing and waning of ventilation. Such cycling ventilation probably results from the marked increments in ventilation that occur with relatively modest increments in P_{CO_2}.

Bradley et al.[27] subsequently validated these concepts by documenting that indeed most apneas in patients with idiopathic central sleep apnea are associated with arousal-induced hyperventilation and subsequent hypocapnia.[28] This reinforces the importance of P_{CO_2} as a potent stimulus to breathing during sleep. These investigators also observed that patients with central apnea have lower waking and sleeping P_{CO_2} levels in conjunction with higher hypercapnic ventilatory responsiveness compared with normal control subjects.[29] As a result of the lower awake P_{CO_2}, these patients are breathing closer to their P_{CO_2} apnea threshold during sleep. In addition, Grunstein et al.[30] reported a higher incidence of central apnea in patients with acromegaly, noting that the patients with central apnea had quite high ventilatory responsiveness to rising CO_2. Thus, a high waking hypercapnic response is the most consistent finding in patients with idiopathic central sleep apnea and is quite likely the primary cause of the high loop gain.

These mechanisms of the pathogenesis of idiopathic central sleep apnea provide a viable explanation for the disorder. However, careful examination of the actual respiratory pattern suggests other mechanisms must be involved as well. A pure cycling of chemoreceptor (P_{CO_2})-mediated respiratory output would yield a gradual waxing and waning of ventilation, with an apnea or hypopnea at the nadir as is seen in Cheyne-Stokes respiration (see later). In idiopathic central sleep apnea, the respiratory pauses are terminated with an abrupt, large breath, not with a gradual increment in ventilation. Although the explanation for this has not been fully elucidated, this pattern strongly suggests that the mechanisms involved in respiratory switching (expiration to inspiration) are affected by this disorder.[24] The long expiratory pause that characterizes these central apneas seems to be a failure of the expiratory-to-inspiratory switch, which may be influenced by not only the chemoreceptors but other mechanisms as well (lung volume, chest wall mechanoreceptors, blood pressure). How these inputs individually contribute to this cycling respiratory pattern is unclear. However, the respiratory pattern of central sleep apnea clearly suggests a different mechanism from that of Cheyne-Stokes breathing.

Cheyne-Stokes Respiration

It has long been recognized that congestive heart failure is associated with Cheyne-Stokes respiration during wakefulness and sleep (see Chapter 102). This breathing pattern is characterized by a crescendo–decrescendo ventilatory pattern with a central apnea or hypopnea at the nadir (Fig. 81–7). As stated earlier, this is quite different from the more abrupt onset and offset of idiopathic central apnea. This breathing pattern is almost entirely a product of ventilatory control system instability (high loop gain) resulting from both a prolonged circulation time and increased ventilatory responsiveness to rising P_{CO_2}.[31] It has been demonstrated in anesthetized animals that lengthening a normal circulation time can induce Cheyne-Stokes respiration.[32] Such an increased circulation time produces unstable ventilation due to the delay that occurs between mechanical changes in respiration (hyperpnea or hypopnea) and receptor stimulation resulting from changes in arterial blood gases. Thus, ventilation can wax and wane, with actual apneas occurring at the nadir of this cycle. It has been argued that this is not the mechanism of Cheyne-Stokes respiration seen with congestive heart failure, because a several-fold increase in circulation time is necessary to produce such breathing dysrhythmias in animals.[33] This is probably a greater change than commonly occurs with heart failure. However, when a moderately prolonged circulation time is combined with an increased ventilatory responsiveness to rising P_{CO_2}, Cheyne-Stokes respiration will emerge.[34] Thus, both conditions (increased hypercapnic responsiveness and prolonged circulation time) are required for Cheyne-Stokes respiration. This probably explains why heart failure severity alone does not account for the presence or absence of Cheyne-Stokes breathing.

Whether apneas in patients with congestive heart failure are central or obstructive may depend on the characteristics of the individual's upper airway (size, collapsibility), with obstructive events potentially resulting from decreased upper airway muscle tone at the nadir of the respiratory cycle in an individual with a susceptible airway. However, most such events are likely to be central in nature.

Cheyne-Stokes respiration has been reported in patients with neurologic disease as well, primarily cerebrovascular disorders[35]; however, the actual ventilatory pattern in these patients has been less well characterized than in patients with congestive heart failure, and the mechanisms remain less well understood.

Upper Airway Causes of Central Apnea

Nasal Obstruction

It is generally acknowledged that the common cold is associated with sleep disturbance; the reason for this, however, has remained obscure. It has been demonstrated that nasal obstruction can affect breathing pattern during sleep, with both central and obstructive apneas being reported.[36] A number of investigators have observed sleep-disordered breathing (central and obstructive apneas, as well as hypopneas) in individuals with nasal obstruction, whether occurring naturally, as in allergic rhinitis[37] or deviated nasal septum,[38] or produced artificially.[36] The etiology of these events remains unresolved,

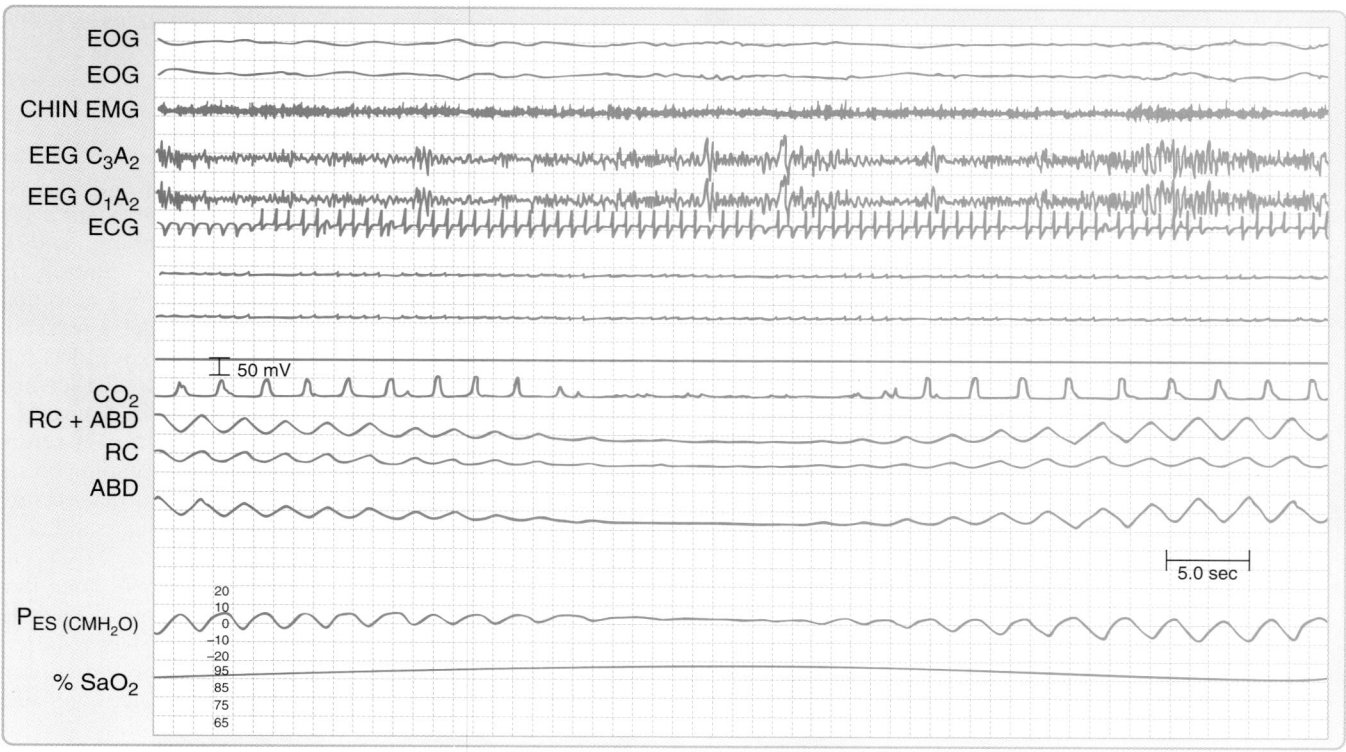

Figure 81–7. Representative tracing in stage 2 non–rapid eye movement sleep, showing central apnea at the nadir of a Cheyne-Stokes respiration event. Note the gradual decrease and eventual disappearance of esophageal pressure (P_{ES}), abdominal movement (ABD), rib cage movement (RC), and RC + ABD excursions during the central apneic portion of the event, followed by a smooth increase in these tracings. EEG, electroencephalogram; ECG, electrocardiogram; EMG, electromyogram; EOG, electrooculogram. (From Dowdell WT, Javaheri S, McGinnis W: Cheyne-Stokes respiration presenting as sleep apnea syndrome. Am Rev Respir Dis 1990;141:874.)

although several explanations seem possible. A number of studies suggest that airflow can be detected by receptors in the nose and that these receptor mechanisms may influence respiration.[39] If this is the case, then loss of such input due to obstruction of air flow could alter the respiratory pattern. The other possible explanation relates to the simple loss of the nose as a breathing route. Humans may be more obligate nasal breathers during sleep than was previously appreciated, and the transition to the oral route could prove to be difficult. In addition, the increased negative airway pressures that must be generated to breathe through a partially occluded nasal passage tend to collapse the pharynx during sleep, yielding obstructive apneas. As a result, both central and obstructive events may result from nasal disease, although obstructive events are probably more common.

Upper Airway Receptors (Nonnasal)

There are also data suggesting that other (nonnasal) pharyngeal airway reflexes may initiate apneas. Davies et al.[40] observed that apneas in infants occurred frequently after the instillation of small boluses of water or warm saline into the oropharynx. They believe this to be a protective reflex. More relevant to adults, Issa and Sullivan[41] reported that pharyngeal airway collapse during sleep may initiate reflexes inhibiting respiration, thus yielding central apneas. In eight patients with predominantly central sleep apnea, they noted that (1) central apneas occurred more frequently when in the supine posture, a position likely to produce pharyngeal collapse during sleep; (2) oropharyngeal anesthesia abolished central apneas in two patients; and (3) high levels of nasal CPAP eliminated all apneas, including central ones. This final observation has been confirmed.[42] Thus, pharyngeal obstruction may inhibit respiration, yielding central apnea, a concept supported by data from studies in animals.[43] This should be kept in mind in evaluating the obese, snoring patient in whom predominantly central apneas are observed in the sleep laboratory. Such patients may respond to therapies aimed at relieving upper airway obstruction.

Neurologic Disorders and Central Sleep Apnea

As stated, ventilation during sleep is highly dependent on the metabolic control system. As a result, any neurologic disorder affecting this system could influence the ventilatory pattern while the individual is asleep, possibly leading to central sleep apnea. Various neurologic processes have been implicated in the development of central sleep apnea. Patients with autonomic dysfunction,[44] such as the Shy-Drager syndrome, familial dysautonomia, or diabetes mellitus, frequently have apneas that are generally of central origin, although obstructive events are also reported. These patients have also been noted to have erratic breathing during sleep even when central apneas are not obvious.

Because the brainstem is the primary source of both ventilatory pattern generation and the processing of respiratory afferent input from chemoreceptors and intrapulmonary receptors, any disease process affecting this area could influence ventilation during sleep. Damage to the brainstem, particularly the medullary area, may lead to hypoventilation during wakefulness but more commonly affects ventilation during sleep early in the disease. An example is poliomyelitis, a disease well known to damage medullary neurons.[45] In the early stages of the postpolio syndrome, respiration during wakefulness is normal, although short central apneas or mild hypoventilation may occur during sleep. With progression of this process (which may take decades), ventilation during sleep becomes progressively more abnormal, with longer, more frequent apneas, and with greater hypoventilation as hypoventilation during wakefulness may become apparent. Finally, some patients may actually require ventilatory support during sleep and wakefulness if the disease progresses that far. Other processes, such as tumor,[46] infarction,[47] hemorrhage, or encephalitis,[48] can damage the medullary area, leading to breathing dysrhythmias during sleep, with central apneas being a prominent feature.

In addition, if the neural pathways from these medullary respiratory neurons to the motoneurons of the ventilatory muscles are interrupted (without damage to the brainstem itself), the metabolic control of breathing may be affected. This interruption is not an uncommon event after cervical cordotomy,[49] with central apnea being described after this procedure.

Finally, chronic neuromuscular diseases, such as muscular dystrophy or myasthenia gravis, may lead to waking alveolar hypoventilation with further hypoventilation during sleep. This may occasionally be associated with central apneas, although hypoventilation is the more prominent disorder. In fact, as with most patients with postpolio syndrome, ventilation during sleep in patients with respiratory muscle disease frequently deteriorates well before waking ventilation is affected. The treatment of the nocturnal hypoventilation with noninvasive nasal ventilation may delay frank waking respiratory failure.

EPIDEMIOLOGY

If abnormal nocturnal breathing is to be understood and recognized, it is important to determine how commonly central apneas occur in normal individuals (see Chapter 19). The reported frequency of disordered breathing, and in particular the individual patterns, varies depending on the population studied, the methods used for apnea detection, and the threshold used to define abnormalities.[50] Carskadon and Dement[51] found that 37.5% of all subjects over the age of 62 had apneas or hypopneas, and that most of the time, "when determinations were possible, apneas were primarily of central type." Other studies report an incidence of central sleep apnea of between 12% and 66%,[52-55] depending on the population investigated. Lugaresi et al.[56] stated that "central apneas lasting 5-15 sec may appear during light and REM sleep" in normal subjects.

With these limitations in mind, a frequency of more than five central apneas per hour of sleep is generally considered abnormal. Although most research-based studies require a greater frequency of events for inclusion, a recent report from the American Academy of Sleep Medicine defined idiopathic central sleep apnea syndrome as the presence of five or more central apneas per hour of sleep in patients with an arterial P_{CO_2} of less than 45 mm Hg who are either excessively sleepy during the day or have frequent nocturnal arousals or awakenings.[57] This same report defined the Cheyne-Stokes respiration syndrome as the presence of at least three consecutive respiratory cycles, with a crescendo–decrescendo pattern and a cycle length near 60 seconds, in a patient with either congestive heart failure or cerebrovascular disease. In addition, these patients must have either five or more central apneas or hypopneas per hour of sleep or 10 consecutive minutes of crescendo–decrescendo breathing.[57] Thus, a standard now exists for defining these syndromes.

In the four studies that specifically considered patients with symptomatic idiopathic central sleep apnea, no consistent epidemiologic trends emerge. Guilleminault et al.,[1] White et al.,[58] and Bradley et al.[27] reported a strong male predominance; Roehrs et al.[7] observed central apneas more commonly in women. No explanation can be offered for this discrepancy. All studies, however, noted this disorder to occur most commonly in middle-aged to older adult individuals, although a few younger patients have been reported.

In the case of Cheyne-Stokes respiration, a number of reports suggest that patients with congestive heart failure, without obvious breathing abnormalities during the day, may have periodic breathing during sleep.[59,60] One study suggests that 45% of patients with congestive heart failure (left ventricular ejection fraction of less than 40%) have more than 20 central apneas plus hypopneas per hour of sleep.[61] Thus, Cheyne-Stokes respiration during sleep in patients with congestive heart failure is likely to be quite common.

CLINICAL FEATURES AND CONSEQUENCES

Idiopathic Central Sleep Apnea

The clinical presentation of patients with central sleep apnea varies dramatically depending on the cause of the apnea (Table 81–1). Patients with alveolar hypoventilation (waking hypercapnia) due to a number of possible causes (see "Pathophysiology," earlier) make up a small percentage of patients with central apnea and generally present with symptoms suggestive of respiratory failure,[27,62] including cor pulmonale, peripheral edema, and polycythemia. Restless sleep and daytime sleepiness are also commonly reported in these patients. On the other hand, nonhypoventilating (normocapnic) patients with idiopathic central sleep apnea have no symptoms of respiratory failure; these patients have a symptom complex that may be similar to that of the patient with obstructive apnea, although differences do exist.[1,7,58]

On the basis of several studies[1,27,58] and personal experience, it seems that individuals with pure idiopathic central sleep apnea less commonly complain of daytime hypersomnolence than do patients with obstructive sleep apnea, although such daytime sleepiness has been commonly

described in patients with central apnea.[27] As the proportion of obstructive or mixed events increases in these patients (still with predominantly central apnea), hypersomnolence may become more frequent. The primary complaint of many patients with central apnea tends to be insomnia, restless sleep, or frequent awakenings during the night. Such awakenings may be accompanied by gasping for air or shortness of breath. Patients with these central apneas also tend to have a normal body habitus, unlike the characteristically obese patient with obstructive apnea. As a result, patients with central sleep apnea as a group may be clinically distinguishable from those with obstructive apnea, although separation of the two disorders by history alone is often difficult (see Table 81–1).

The frequency and duration of central apneas required to produce the clinical symptoms described are difficult to determine from the available literature.[1,7,27,58,63] The actual number of apneas, either central or obstructive, necessary to yield insomnia, hypersomnolence, or hemodynamic sequelae is quite variable between patients, although recent data primarily addressing patients with obstructive apnea suggest that hypertension and other adverse cardiovascular sequelae may occur in patients with quite mild sleep apnea.[64] Despite this limited information, as stated, five central events per hour of sleep is considered the upper limit of normal. Although this number is somewhat arbitrary, we must await new information before a more meaningful figure can be chosen.

As expected, arterial oxygen desaturation occurs with central apneas. The degree to which the saturation falls during a given apnea is likely to be related to the saturation (or P_{O_2}) at the time ventilation ceased, the duration of the apnea, and the lung volume at which the apnea occurred.[65] Whether ventilatory effort is occurring (obstructive apnea) or not (central apnea) may also have a minor effect on the rate of desaturation.[66] Patients with obstructive apnea generally seem to reach a lower arterial oxygen saturation during an apnea than do individuals with central events; this is probably a product of longer apnea duration, reduced lung volume (lower in patients with obstructive apnea due to obesity), and the presence of ventilatory efforts in the patient with obstructive apnea.

The hemodynamic consequences of central apneas have been poorly investigated. Early studies by Schroeder et al.[67] reported that pulmonary artery pressures increased from 26/16 mm Hg during wakefulness to 41/26 mm Hg during central apneic episodes. A study by Podszus et al.[68] reported virtually no change in pulmonary artery pressure during central apneas or the central component of mixed apneas despite considerable arterial oxygen desaturation; however, it seems highly probable that any elevation in pulmonary pressure associated with central apnea will result from hypoxemia and

Table 81–1. Clinical Characteristics of Patients with Sleep Apnea

Central		Obstructive
Hypercapnic	**Nonhypercapnic**	
Respiratory failure	Daytime sleepiness	Daytime sleepiness
Cor pulmonale	Insomnia (restless sleep)	Prominent snoring
Polycythemia	Mild and intermittent snoring	Witnessed apneas/gasping
Daytime sleepiness	Awakenings (± choking, shortness of breath)	Commonly obese
Snoring	Normal body habitus	

hypercapnia, with the hypoventilating patient with central apnea demonstrating more severe pressure elevations. There are few data addressing the impact of central apnea on systemic pressures, but Schroeder et al.[67] reported systemic arterial pressures to increase from 155/84 to 188/117 mm Hg during central apneas in a small number of patients. In addition, White et al.[69] reported very similar increases in both systemic and pulmonary artery pressures during and after central and obstructive apneas in an anesthetized baboon model.

That dysrhythmic breathing can disrupt normal sleep architecture is well known; however, little information is available that specifically addresses central sleep apnea in this role. White et al.[58] reported an improvement in sleep efficiency and a trend toward more time in deeper (stages 3 and 4) and REM sleep after the treatment of central sleep apnea, which suggests that sleep was disrupted by the apneas. In fact, the six patients reported in that study had a mean of 209 apnea-associated awakenings and arousals during 1 night before therapy. Roehrs et al.[7] also found a reduction in what is generally considered a normal percentage of stage 3 or 4 sleep and an increase in stage 1 or 2 sleep in a group of patients with about 50% central apneas. The results of these studies suggest that the frequent arousals and awakenings generally associated with the hypercapnia after an apnea can lead to disruption of the normal distribution of sleep stages.

Cheyne-Stokes Respiration

Considerable data also indicate important adverse consequences from Cheyne-Stokes respiration (see Chapter 102). These studies indicate that the hyperpneic phase of this cycling ventilation leads to frequent arousals and poor sleep quality. In addition, several studies have reported reduced survival rates in individuals with left ventricular failure and Cheyne-Stokes respiration[70,71] compared with patients with heart failure who breathed rhythmically. At least two studies specifically associated central apneas during sleep with decreased survival rates in these patients.[70,71] This may be a product of the increased hypoxia and catecholamines[72] found in patients with Cheyne-Stokes respiration. Thus, this nocturnal respiratory pattern has serious potential health consequences.

DIAGNOSTIC EVALUATION

The diagnosis of central sleep apnea generally requires a full night's recording of standard polysomnographic variables with a particular focus on respiratory effort. To prove that an apnea is indeed central, it must be documented that there is no respiratory effort throughout the event.[57] This is most effectively and consistently accomplished with an esophageal balloon or catheter recording intrathoracic pressure swings reflective of ventilatory effort.[73,74] Therefore, in the research setting, esophageal pressure should be measured to definitively document apnea type. Recognizing the difficulty in using an esophageal balloon and its infrequent use in clinical practice, other strategies have been used. Most evidence suggests that respiratory inductive plethysmography (RIP), calibrated or uncalibrated, can adequately assess respiratory effort.[57,73,75] If there is a complete absence of thoracoabdominal motion (RIP or strain gauges) throughout an apnea, this strongly suggests the event is central in origin. Although recent evidence suggests that chest–abdominal wall motion as a measure of effort may overestimate the frequency of central apnea, rarely will

the patient be misclassified with the use of this methodology.[73] A third method of assessing effort would be the use of diaphragmatic electromyelography,[57] although this is frequently difficult to obtain and therefore cannot always be relied on. Finally, classic teaching has suggested that pulse wave artifacts in the oronasal flow signal indicate a patent airway and, therefore, a central apnea. However, the study by Morrell et al.[76] indicates that this approach cannot be relied on.

Distinguishing central from obstructive hypopneas is extraordinarily difficult and cannot be reliably accomplished with standard monitoring techniques. As a result, central apneas, not hypopneas, must be documented to make a definitive diagnosis of central sleep apnea.

As stated, five central apneas per hour of sleep is considered the upper limit of normal, and a greater frequency implies an abnormal state. In a patient with both central and obstructive events, it is frequently difficult to discern the primary abnormality. As a result, no definitive event percentage can be provided that will always indicate a central process. For research purposes, generally 75% to 85% of events must be central for patient inclusion,[27-29] although occasionally a lower percentage has been used.[7] Because obstructive apneas are considerably more common and diagnostic methodologies tend to overestimate the frequency of central apneas,[73,75] the use of 80% central events as a threshold seems reasonable. This value can be adjusted up or down as the clinical scenario dictates, but, in general, a high percentage of central apneas should be present before the disorder is considered central as opposed to obstructive on the basis of the prevalences of the two disorders.

To diagnose Cheyne-Stokes respiration, an esophageal balloon again represents the gold standard, but a crescendo–decrescendo pattern of breathing as detected by chest wall–abdominal motion (RIP[57,77]) is likely to be adequate (see Fig. 81–7). As stated earlier, this respiratory pattern commonly has a cycle length of about 60 seconds, with 10 minutes of continuous crescendo–decrescendo breathing often being required to document its existence.

TREATMENT

Patients with Alveolar Hypoventilation and Central Sleep Apnea

Because there are few large series of patients with central sleep apnea, investigation into treatment has been somewhat limited. Two general types of therapeutic approaches have emerged depending on the cause of the central apnea. For the hypercapnic patient with alveolar hypoventilation during wakefulness and worsening hypoventilation during sleep with occasional central apneas, nocturnal ventilation is the most appropriate approach. Initially, such ventilation was accomplished only with tracheostomy with a mechanical respirator, diaphragmatic pacing, or negative-pressure (cuirass) ventilators.[74,78,79] Newer studies indicate that nocturnal ventilation can be accomplished satisfactorily with a nasal mask and a pressure-cycled ventilator,[80-82] so the ease of administration of nocturnal ventilation has improved substantially, as has patient acceptance. As stated, most individuals in whom these techniques have been used have some form of central alveolar hypoventilation or respiratory nerve/muscle disease with severe nocturnal hypoxia and hypercapnia (see Chapter 95).

Idiopathic Central Sleep Apnea

For the individual with insomnia, restless sleep, waking hypersomnolence, and mild-to-moderate nocturnal hypoxemia, all secondary to central sleep apnea, a number of therapeutic options are available. First, if any of the previously described conditions known to be associated with central apnea are present (e.g., nasal obstruction, pharyngeal collapse), the abnormality should be treated aggressively and the central apnea reassessed. Second, the literature suggests that these central apneas may resolve spontaneously in about 20% of patients. As a result, if the symptoms are not debilitating or other therapies fail, it may be appropriate to follow some patients with central apnea. Third, if the problem persists or if no known predisposing abnormality can be found, several pharmacologic approaches can be attempted. Acetazolamide, a carbonic anhydrase inhibitor known to produce a metabolic acidosis and probably a shift in the P_{CO_2} apnea threshold to a lower value, has been used to treat central sleep apnea.[58] In a series of six patients, acetazolamide (250 mg four times daily) was shown to reduce central apnea substantially in all participants when used over a short period (1 to 2 weeks). Long-term use of this medication was assessed in only two individuals and was successful in one and unsuccessful in the other. However, a study[8] of 14 patients with central apnea suggests that acetazolamide may lead to a more sustained improvement in apnea frequency and symptoms (primarily hypersomnolence). Of note, subsequent discontinuation of acetazolamide did not lead to an immediate return of symptoms or events.[9] On the other hand, several studies have reported the development of obstructive apneas after acetazolamide administration in patients previously demonstrated to have central events.[5] The explanation for this remains obscure but may relate to the respiratory stimulating activity of acetazolamide in an individual with a collapsing airway during sleep. When little ventilatory effort is present, the apneas appear central. However, when respiration is stimulated, obstructive events develop. Clearly, follow-up sleep studies are necessary in patients being treated with acetazolamide, particularly if symptoms persist.

Isolated reports of the use of other medications, such as theophylline, naloxone, and medroxyprogesterone acetate, imply that these drugs have little efficacy in the treatment of central apnea.[1] Clomipramine (a tricyclic antidepressant), on the other hand, was found to be successful in several patients in whom it was tried.[1] Theophylline improved apnea in a patient with a damaged brainstem.[83] None of these drugs has been studied systematically, so firm recommendations regarding their use cannot be made.

Nasal CPAP has been shown to be an effective therapy for some patients with central sleep apnea.[41,42] These patients probably fall into several groups. First, as stated previously, pharyngeal airway collapse or closure during sleep may initiate a reflex inhibition of ventilation in some patients and therefore a central apnea. With nasal CPAP, airway closure is prevented, and such apneas abolished. In obese, snoring patients in whom predominantly central apneas are observed, nasal CPAP may be an effective form of therapy. Second, an abstract suggests that CPAP may also be a viable form of therapy in idiopathic central sleep apnea.[84] This efficacy was attributed primarily to a CPAP-induced increase in arterial P_{CO_2}. As a result, P_{CO_2} was kept above the apnea threshold.

Thus, some patients with central apnea may respond to CPAP, although the final role of this therapeutic modality in central apnea must await further investigation.

A number of studies suggest that oxygen may be a useful method of treating central sleep apnea. Martin et al.[85] observed that central apneas were completely abolished with oxygen administration in two patients during a short-nap study. McNicholas et al.[86] found a considerable reduction in the number of central apneas present in a patient with central alveolar hypoventilation after oxygen therapy was begun. Finally, a study evaluating the effects of low-flow oxygen in nine obese patients with a large component of central apneas reported a considerable reduction in these central events.[87] However, the frequency of obstructive apneas was somewhat increased. Although the mechanism by which oxygen administration reduces central apneas has not yet been established, two explanations seem possible. One relates to the potential destabilizing influence of the hypoxic ventilatory response on respiratory control. As at altitude, an individual with hypoxia will hyperventilate, yielding hypocapnia and alkalosis. As previously stated, hypocapnia may inhibit respiration during sleep. Thus, cycling ventilation may develop, with central apneas occurring at the nadir of this periodic breathing. With the administration of oxygen, the hypoxic influence on ventilation may be reduced and breathing regularized. The other possible explanation relates to the fact that hypoxia can be a ventilatory depressant. If respiration is depressed by hypoxia, then central apneas may occur. Oxygen administration in this situation could reduce apneas. Regardless of the mechanism, low-flow oxygen may be an effective treatment for central sleep apnea.

When attempting to treat a patient with predominantly central sleep apnea, it must be remembered that both central and obstructive apneas are commonly seen in the same individual. In these patients, it is frequently difficult to determine whether the primary cause of the apnea is of central origin or relates to upper airway obstruction, or both. Therefore, in patients who have central apnea with a large component of obstructive events, treatment of the airway obstruction via one of the currently available methods may have beneficial effects on both types of apnea.

Cheyne-Stokes Respiration

The treatment of Cheyne-Stokes respiration requires special comment because it has been the subject of a number of studies (see also Chapter 102). First, as stated, the heart failure (if present) should be treated as aggressively as possible. Optimal medical treatment, however, abolishes the sleep apnea in only a minority of patients who had originally presented with acute left ventricular failure.[88] Second, should this fail, a number of additional options are available. Nocturnal oxygen administration has been shown to reduce apnea frequency and improve symptoms in several studies of congestive heart failure and Cheyne-Stokes respiration.[89-91] Several medications have also demonstrated some efficacy; these include theophylline[92] and possibly hypnotic agents.[93,94] Finally, CPAP has been shown both to improve cardiac function in patients with Cheyne-Stokes respiration when used chronically and to substantially reduce apnea frequency yielding improved sleep quality.[95,96] CPAP in those patients may improve cardiac function in a number of ways, but it works primarily by reducing transmural pressure. Over time, this leads to an increased ejection fraction, reduced circulation time, and, as a result, more stable respiration.[96] Cycling ventilation is reduced or eliminated, yielding fewer arousals, less hypoxemia, and improved sleep. Thus CPAP should be considered the optimal therapy in patients with Cheyne-Stokes respiration secondary to heart failure. Of note, there has been an effort to develop positive pressure devices that immediately eliminate Cheyne-Stokes respiration rather than requiring several weeks to achieve this result as is often the case with CPAP.[97] The concept is that these devices may improve compliance because the patient should feel better immediately. How such devices will ultimately fit into the therapeutic options for Cheyne-Stokes respiration is unclear at this time.

SUMMARY

A logical approach to the treatment of central sleep apnea in the symptomatic patient, when it is certain that the apneas are of central origin, would be to first rule out treatable causes; these include nasal obstruction, pharyngeal collapse, congestive heart failure, and, certainly, alveolar hypoventilation. If present, the condition should be corrected. If no such problem is found, the therapeutic approach must be individualized to the patient. First, if the patient is obese and snoring or has heart failure, nasal CPAP may be an appropriate first choice. Second, if the patient is hypoxemic during central apneas or the apneas have a clearly periodic nature, then nocturnally administered oxygen may be most appropriate. Finally, if none of these conditions exists, then acetazolamide (at 250 mg four times daily) or possibly hypnotics should be considered.

> ### Clinical Pearls
>
> *Central sleep apnea is a condition characterized by ventilatory control system instability, most often with increased responsiveness to hypercapnia leading to this instability.*
>
> *Ventilation during sleep, particularly NREM sleep, is primarily driven by arterial P_{CO_2}. Therefore, any event or condition leading to reduced P_{CO_2} can precipitate central apneas.*
>
> *The treatment of central sleep apnea must be individualized to the cause of the ventilatory instability. Idiopathic central sleep apnea often responds to oxygen or acetazolamide, whereas Cheyne-Stokes respiration is best treated with continuous positive airway pressure.*
>
> *In the obese patient who snores and has substantial central sleep apnea on polysomnography, upper airway obstruction responsive to CPAP is the most likely diagnosis.*

REFERENCES

1. Guilleminault C, van den Hoed J, Mitler M: Clinical overview of the sleep apnea syndromes. In Guilleminault C, Dement W (eds): Sleep Apnea Syndromes. New York, Alan R Liss, 1978, pp 1-11.
2. Onal E, Lopata M, O'Connor T: Genioglossal and diaphragmatic EMG responses to CO_2 rebreathing in humans. J Appl Physiol 1981;50:1052-1055.
3. Onal E, Lopata M, O'Connor T: Pathogenesis of apnea in hypersomnia-sleep apnea syndrome. Am Rev Respir Dis 1982;125:167-174.
4. Fletcher EC: Recurrence of sleep apnea syndrome following tracheostomy: A shift from obstructive to central apnea. Chest 1989;95:205-209.
5. Sharp J, Druz W, D'Souza V, et al: Effect of metabolic acidosis upon sleep apnea. Chest 1985;87:619-624.
6. Hyland R, Hutcheon M, Perl A, et al: Upper airway occlusion induced by diaphragm pacing for primary alveolar hypoventilation: Implications for the pathogenesis of obstructive sleep apnea. Am Rev Respir Dis 1981;124:180-185.
7. Roehrs T, Conway W, Wittig R, et al: Sleep complaints in patients with sleep-related respiratory disturbances. Am Rev Respir Dis 1985;132:520-523.
8. DeBacker WA, Verbraecken J, Willeman M, et al: Central apnea index decreases after prolonged treatment with acetazolamide. Am J Respir Crit Care Med 1995;151:87-91.
9. DeBacker WA: Central sleep apnoea, pathogenesis and treatment: An overview and perspective. Eur Respir J 1995;8:1372-1383.
10. Phillipson EA: Control of breathing during sleep. Am Rev Respir Dis 1978;118:909-939.
11. Orem J, Lydic R, Norris P: Experimental control of diaphragm and laryngeal abductor muscles by brain stem arousal systems. Respir Physiol 1979;38:203-221.
12. Sears TA, Newsom-Davis J: The control of respiratory muscles during voluntary breathing. Ann N Y Acad Sci 1968;155:183.
13. Sullivan C, Kozar L, Murphy E, et al: Primary role of respiratory afferents in sustaining breathing rhythm. J Appl Physiol 1978;45:11-17.
14. Berssenbrugge A, Dempsey J, Skatrud J: Hypoxic versus hypocapnic effects on periodic breathing during sleep. In West J, Lahiri S (eds): High Altitude and Man, Clinical Physiology Series. Bethesda, Md, American Physiological Society, 1984, pp 115-127.
15. Skatrud J, Dempsey J: Interaction of sleep state and chemical stimuli in sustaining rhythmic ventilation. J Appl Physiol 1983;55:813-822.
16. Berthon-Jones M, Sullivan C: Ventilatory and arousal responses to hypoxia in sleeping humans. Am Rev Respir Dis 1982;125:632-639.
17. Douglas N, White D, Pickett C, et al: Hypercapnic ventilatory response in sleeping adults. Am Rev Respir Dis 1982;126:758-762.
18. White DP: Occlusion pressure and ventilation during sleep in normal humans. J Appl Physiol 1986;61:1279-1287.
19. Cherniack N: Sleep apnea and its causes. J Clin Invest 1984;73:1501-1506.
20. Bülow K: Respiration and wakefulness in man. Acta Physiol Scand 1963;53(Suppl 209):1-110.
21. Dempsey JA, Skatrud JB: A sleep induced apneic threshold and its consequences. Am Rev Respir Dis 1986;133:1163-1170.
22. Chow CM, Xi L, Smith CA, et al: A volume-dependent apnea threshold during NREM sleep in the dog. J Appl Physiol 1994;76:2315-2325.
23. Meza S, Giannouli E, Younes M: Control of breathing during sleep assessed by proportional assist ventilation. J Appl Physiol 1998;84:3-12.
24. Younes M: The physiologic basis of central apnea and periodic breathing. Curr Pulmonol 1989;10:265-326.
25. Mellins R, Balfour H, Turino G, et al: Failure of autonomic control of ventilation (Ondine's curse). Medicine 1970;49:487-504.
26. Tassinari C, Dalla Bernardina B, Cirignotta F, et al: Apnoeic periods and the respiratory related arousal patterns during sleep in the pickwickian syndrome. Bull Physiopathol Respir 1972;8:1087-1102.
27. Bradley TD, McNicholas WT, Rutherford R, et al: Clinical and physiological heterogeneity of the central sleep apnea syndrome. Am Rev Respir Dis 1986;134:217-221.
28. Xie A, Wong B, Phillipson EA, et al: Interaction of hyperventilation and arousal in the pathogenesis of idiopathic central sleep apnea. Am J Respir Crit Care Med 1994;150:489-495.

29. Xie A, Rutherford R, Rankin F, et al: Hypocapnia and increased ventilatory responsiveness in patients with idiopathic central sleep apnea. Am J Respir Crit Care Med 1995;152:1950-1955.

30. Grunstein RR, Ho KY, Berthon-Jones M, et al: Central sleep apnea is associated with increased ventilatory responses to carbon dioxide and hypersecretion of growth hormone in patients with acromegaly. Am J Respir Crit Care Med 1994; 150:496-502.

31. Javaheri S: A mechanism of central sleep apnea in patients with heart failure. N Engl J Med 1999;341:949-954.

32. Lange R, Hecht H: The mechanism of Cheyne-Stokes respiration. J Clin Invest 1962;41:42-52.

33. Guyton A, Crowell J, Moore J: Basic oscillating mechanism of Cheyne-Stokes breathing. Am J Physiol 1979;187:185-200.

34. Wilcox I, McNamara SG, Dodd MJ, et al: Ventilatory control in patients with sleep apnoea and left ventricular dysfunction: Comparison of obstructive and central sleep apnoea. Eur Respir J 1998;11:7-13.

35. Nachtmann A, Siebler M, Rose G, et al: Cheyne-Stoke respiration in ischemic stroke. Neurology 1995;45:820-821.

36. Suratt PM, Turner BL, Withoit SC: Effect of intranasal obstruction on breathing during sleep. Chest 1986;90:324-329.

37. McNicholas W, Tarlo S, Cole P, et al: Obstructive apneas during sleep in patients with seasonal allergic rhinitis. Am Rev Respir Dis 1982;126:625-628.

38. Heimer D, Scharf S, Lieberman A, et al: Sleep apnea syndrome treated by repair of deviated nasal septum. Chest 1983;84: 184-185.

39. Ramos J: On the integration of respiratory movements: III. The fifth nerve afferents. Acta Physiol Lat Am 1960;10:104-113.

40. Davies AM, Koenig JC, Thach BT: Upper airway chemoreflex responses to saline and water in preterm infants. J Appl Physiol 1988;64:1412-1420.

41. Issa F, Sullivan C: Reversal of central sleep apnea using nasal CPAP. Chest 1986;90:165-171.

42. Hoffstein V, Slutsky AS: Central sleep apnea reversed by continuous positive airway pressure. Am Rev Respir Dis 1987;135: 1210-1212.

43. Mathew OP, Farber JP: Effect of upper airway negative pressure on respiratory timing. Respir Physiol 1983;54:259-268.

44. McNicholas W, Rutherford R, Grossman R, et al: Abnormal respiratory pattern generation during sleep in patients with autonomic dysfunction. Am Rev Respir Dis 1983;128: 429-433.

45. Plum F, Swanson AG: Abnormalities in central regulation of respiration in acute and convalescent poliomyelitis. Arch Neurol Psychiatr 1958;80:267-285.

46. Devereaux M, Keane J, Davis R: Autonomic respiratory failure. Arch Neurol 1973;29:46-52.

47. Levin B, Margolis G: Acute failure of autonomic respirations secondary to unilateral brainstem infarct. Ann Neurol 1977;1: 583-586.

48. White D, Miller F, Erickson R: Sleep apnea and nocturnal hypoventilation following Western equine encephalitis. Am Rev Respir Dis 1983;127:132-133.

49. Krieger A, Rosomoff H: Sleep induced apnea: A respiratory and autonomic dysfunction syndrome following bilateral percutaneous cervical cordotomy. J Neurosurg 1974;39:168-180.

50. Ancoli-Israel S: Epidemiology of sleep disorders. Clin Geriatr Med 1989;5:347-362.

51. Carskadon M, Dement W: Respiration during sleep in the aged human. J Gerontol 1981;36:420-425.

52. Bixler E, Kales A, Soldatos C, et al: Sleep apneic activity in a normal population. Res Commun Chem Pathol Pharmacol 1982;36:141-152.

53. Block A, Boysen P, Wayne J, et al: Sleep apnea, hypopnea, and oxygen desaturation in normal subjects. N Engl J Med 1979; 300:513-517.

54. Block A, Wynne J, Boysen P: Sleep-disordered breathing and nocturnal oxygen desaturation in postmenopausal women. Am J Med 1980;69:75-79.

55. Webb P: Periodic breathing during sleep. J Appl Physiol 1974;37:899-903.

56. Lugaresi E, Coccagna G, Cirignotta F, et al: Breathing during sleep in normal and pathological conditions. Adv Exp Med Biol 1978;99:35-45.

57. American Academy of Sleep Medicine Task Force: Sleep-related breathing disorders in adults: Recommendations for syndrome definitions and measurement technique in clinical research. Sleep 1999;22:667-689.

58. White D, Zwillich C, Pickett C, et al: Central sleep apnea: Improvement with acetazolamide therapy. Arch Intern Med 1982;142:1816-1819.

59. Javaheri S, Parker T, Liming J, et al: Sleep apnea in 81 ambulatory male patients with stable heart failure. Circulation 1998;97: 2154-2159.

60. Sin DD, Fitzgerald F, Parker J, et al: Risk factors for central and obstructive sleep apnea in 450 men and women with congestive heart failure. Am J Respir Crit Care Med 1999;160: 1101-1106.

61. Javaheri S, Parker TJ, Wexler L, et al: Occult sleep-disordered breathing in stable congestive heart failure. Ann Intern Med 1995;122:487-492.

62. Bradley TD, Phillipson EA: Central sleep apnea. Clin Chest Med 1992;13:493-505.

63. Guilleminault C, Tilkian A, Dement W: The sleep apnea syndromes. Annu Rev Med 1976;27:465-484.

64. Shahar E, Whitney CW, Redline S, et al: Sleep disordered breathing and cardiovascular disease: Cross-sectional results of the Sleep Heart Health Study. Am J Respir Crit Care Med 2001; 163:19-25.

65. Findley LJ, Ries AL, Tisi GM, et al: Hypoxemia during apnea in normal subjects: Mechanisms and impact of lung volume. J Appl Physiol 1983;55:1777-1783.

66. Fletcher EC: The rate of fall of arterial oxyhemoglobin saturation on obstructive sleep apnea. Chest 1989;96:717-722.

67. Schroeder J, Motta J, Guilleminault C: Hemodynamic studies in sleep apnea. In Guilleminault C, Dement W (eds): Sleep Apnea Syndromes. New York, Alan R Liss, 1978, pp 177-196.

68. Podszus T, Peter JH, Renke A, et al: Pulmonary artery pressure during central sleep apnea. Sleep Res 1988;17:236.

69. White SG, Fletcher EC, Miller CC: Acute systemic blood pressure elevation in obstructive and nonobstructive breath hold in primates. J Appl Physiol 1995;79:324-330.

70. Hanly P, Zuberi-Khakhar NS: Increased mortality associated with Cheyne-Stokes respiration in patients with congestive heart failure. Am J Respir Crit Care Med 1996;153:272-276.

71. Lanfranchi PA, Braghiroli A, Bosimini E, et al: Prognostic value of nocturnal Cheyne-Stokes respiration in chronic heart failure. Circulation 1999;99:1435-1440.

72. Naughton M, Benard D, Liu P, et al: Effects of nasal CPAP on sympathetic activity in patients with heart failures and central sleep apnea. Am J Respir Crit Care Med 1995;152:473-479.

73. Boudewyns A, Willemen M, Wagemans M, et al: Assessment of respiratory effort by means of strain gauge and esophageal pressure swings: A comparative study. Sleep 1997; 20:168-170.

74. Glenn W, Phelps M, Gersten L: Diaphragm pacing in the management of central alveolar hypoventilation. In Guilleminault C, Dement W (eds): Sleep Apnea Syndromes. New York, Alan R Liss, 1978, pp 333-345.

75. Staats BA, Bonekat HW, Harris CD, et al: Chest wall motion in sleep apnea. Am Rev Respir Dis 1984;130:59-63.

76. Morrell MJ, Badr S, Harms CA, et al: The assessment of upper airway patency during apnea using cardiogenic oscillations in the airflow signal. Sleep 1995;18:651-658.

77. Dowdell WT, Javahari S, McGinnis W: Cheyne-Stokes respiration presenting as sleep apnea syndrome. Am Rev Respir Dis 1990; 141:871-879.

78. Coleman M, Boros S, Huseby T, et al: Congenital central hypoventilation syndrome. Am Rev Respir Dis 1979;119: 901-902.

79. Godfrey C, Man M, Jones R, et al: Primary alveolar hypoventilation managed by negative-pressure ventilators. Chest 1979;76: 219-221.

80. Guilleminault C, Stoohs R, Schnieder H, et al: Central alveolar hypoventilation and sleep: Treatment by intermittent positive-pressure ventilation through nasal mask in an adult. Chest 1989;96:1210-1212.

81. Make BJ, Hill NS, Goldberg AI, et al: Mechanical ventilation beyond the intensive care unit: Report of a consensus conference of the American College of Chest Physicians. Chest 1998; 113(Suppl):2895-3445.

82. Shneerson JM, Simonds AK: Noninvasive ventilation for chest wall and neuromuscular disorders. Eur Respir J 2002;20: 480-487.

83. Raetzo MA, Junod AF, Kryger MH: Effect of aminophylline and relief from hypoxia on central sleep apnea due to medullary damage. Bull Eur Physiopathol Respir 1987;23:171-175.

84. Rutherford R, Popkin J, Phillipson EA, et al: Effect of CPAP on Cheyne-Stokes respiration and idiopathic central sleep apnea. Am Rev Respir Dis 1991;143(Suppl):A197.

85. Martin R, Sanders M, Gray B, et al: Acute and long-term ventilatory effects of hypoxia in the adult sleep apnea syndrome. Am Rev Respir Dis 1982;125:175-180.

86. McNicholas W, Carter J, Rutherford R, et al: Beneficial effect of oxygen in primary alveolar hypoventilation with central sleep apnea. Am Rev Respir Dis 1982;125:773-775.

87. Gold AV, Bleecker ER, Smith PL: A shift from central and mixed sleep apnea to obstructive apnea resulting from low-flow oxygen. Am Rev Respir Dis 1985;132:220-223.

88. Tremel F, Pepin J, Veale D, et al: High prevalence and persistence of sleep apnoea in patients referred for acute left ventricular failure and medically treated over 2 months. Eur Heart J 1999;20:1201-1209.

89. Franklin KA, Eriksson P, Sahlin C, et al: Reversal of central sleep apnea with oxygen. Chest 1997;111:163-169.

90. Hanly PJ, Millar TW, Steljes DG, et al: The effect of oxygen on respiration and sleep in patients with congestive heart failure. Ann Intern Med 1989;111:777-782.

91. Krachman SL, D'Alonzo GE, Berger TJ, et al: Comparison of oxygen therapy with nasal continuous positive airway pressure on Cheyne-Stokes respiration during sleep in congestive heart failure. Chest 1999;116:1550-1557.

92. Javaheri S, Parker TJ, Wexler L, et al: Effects of theophylline on sleep disordered breathing in stable heart failure: A prospective, double-blind, placebo controlled, crossover study. N Engl J Med 1996;335:562-567.

93. Biberdorf DJ, Steens R, Millar TW, et al: Benzodiazepines in congestive heart failure: Effects of temazepam on arousability and Cheyne-Stokes respiration. Sleep 1993;16:529-538.

94. Bonnet MH, Dexter JR, Arand DL: The effect of triazolam on arousal and respiration in central sleep apnea patients. Sleep 1990;13:31-41.

95. Naughton MT, Liu PP, Bernard DC et al: Treatment of congestive heart failure and Cheyne-Stokes respiration during sleep by continuous positive airway pressure. Am J Respir Crit Care Med 1995;151:92-97.

96. Sin D, Logan A, Fitzgerald F, et al: Effects of continuous positive airway pressure on cardiovascular outcomes in heart failure patients with and without Cheyne-Stokes respiration. Circulation 2000;102:61-66.

97. Teschler H, Dohring J, Wang YM, Berthon-Jones M: Adaptive pressure support servo-ventilation: A novel treatment for Cheyne-Stokes respiration in heart failure. Am J Respir Crit Care Med 2001;164:614-619.

Anatomy and Physiology of Upper Airway Obstruction

Richard J. Schwab

Samuel T. Kuna

John E. Remmers

ABSTRACT

The upper airway is a very complex structure, and the pathogenesis of pharyngeal airway closure in patients with obstructive sleep apne a is not fully understood. However, sophisticated physiologic and imaging studies have significantly advanced our understanding of the anatomic risk factors for obstructive sleep apnea and illuminated the biomechanical mechanisms by which therapeutic interventions for this disorder—such as continuous positive airway pressure, weight loss, oral appliances, and surgery—increase upper airway caliber. Pharyngeal airway patency is maintained by two counteracting forces: the activity of the upper airway muscles, which dilate and stiffen the airway, and negative intraluminal pressure. However, this balance can be disturbed by abnormalities in upper airway anatomy and neural control. Patients with obstructive sleep apnea have been shown to have a narrowed, more collapsible pharyngeal airway. Sleep-related reduction in upper airway dilating muscle activity can lead to greater negative intraluminal pharyngeal pressure, which leads in turn to further narrowing and complete closure of the airway.

Although obstructive sleep apnea is a major public health problem affecting a significant portion of the population (see Chapter 52), the pathogenesis of this disorder is not well understood. However, studies examining the upper airway with sophisticated imaging and physiologic techniques have started to provide important insights into the pathogenesis of sleep apnea and the efficacy of different treatment options, including continuous positive airway pressure (CPAP), weight loss, oral appliances, and surgery. In addition, physiologic studies have generated new information about the dynamic and state-dependent changes in the biomechanical behavior of the upper airway in patients with sleep apnea.

This chapter reviews the anatomy and physiology of upper airway obstruction in patients with obstructive sleep apnea. We review normal upper airway anatomy, static and dynamic properties of the normal upper airway, and upper airway pharyngeal muscle activation. We also examine differences in soft tissue and craniofacial structures between healthy subjects and patients with apnea and the factors leading to these differences, as well as dynamic physiologic changes in upper airway structures in patients with sleep apnea and obstruction of the pharynx during sleep. Finally, we discuss mechanisms by which the therapeutic interventions for sleep apnea increase upper airway caliber and a model for upper airway closure in patients with sleep-disordered breathing.

UPPER AIRWAY FUNCTION

The upper airway technically includes the extrathoracic trachea, larynx, pharynx, and nose. The pharyngeal airway is bounded cranially by the nasopharynx and caudally by the larynx. This chapter will focus on the pharyngeal airway because it is the site of upper airway closure or narrowing during sleep.

The upper airway is a very complicated multipurpose passage transmitting air, liquid, and solids. It is a common pathway for digestion, phonation, and respiration. Structures surrounding the pharyngeal airway close the airway during deglutition, and they valve and shape the airway during phonation. Because the pharynx is a conduit for airflow connecting the nose with the larynx, pharyngeal patency is critical. With the exception of the two ends of the respiratory airway tract (the nares and the small intrapulmonary airways), the pharynx is the only collapsible segment of the respiratory tract.

Normally, the pharynx remains open at all times, except during momentary closures associated with swallowing, regurgitation, eructation, and speech. Pharyngeal patency during wakefulness is, in large part, attributable to continual neuromuscular control by the higher nervous system, which coordinates the need for a patent airway with the need for swallowing and phonation in such a way that the airway closes only briefly in coordination with respiratory movements of the thoracic pump.

The sleep state is associated with a decrease in motor output to pharyngeal muscles. When this occurs against the background of upper airway anatomic abnormalities, severe narrowing or closure of the pharyngeal airway can occur.

NORMAL UPPER AIRWAY ANATOMY

The upper airway is separated into three regions: the nasopharynx, which is defined from the nasal turbinates to the hard palate; the oropharynx, subdivided into the retropalatal region (defined from the hard palate to the caudal margin of the soft palate) and the retroglossal region (defined from the caudal margin of the soft palate to the base of the epiglottis); and the hypopharynx, which is defined from the base of the tongue to the larynx (Fig. 82–1). The majority of patients with obstructive sleep apnea manifest upper airway closure or narrowing during sleep in the retropalatal and retroglossal regions.[1-3]

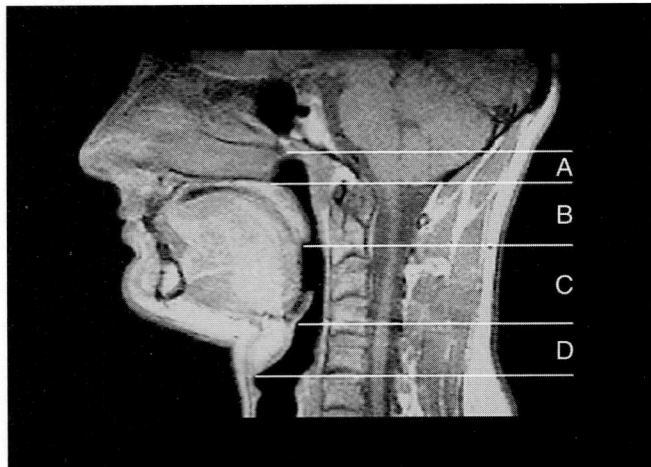

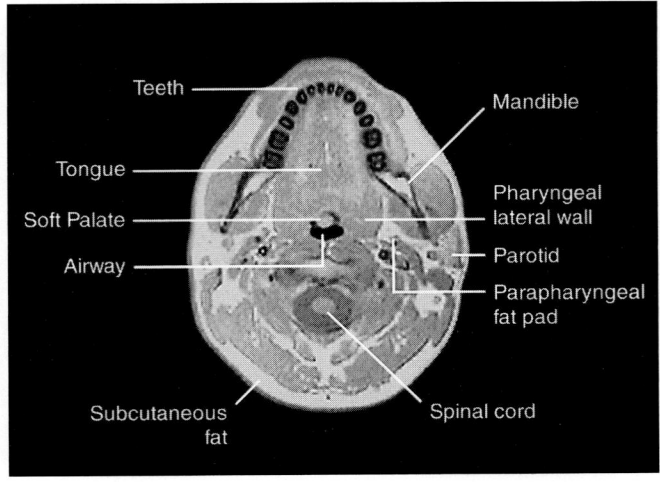

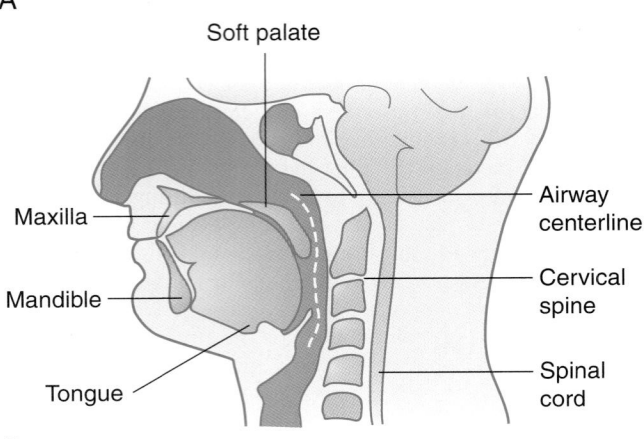

Figure 82–1. **A,** Midsagittal magnetic resonance (MR) image in a normal subject showing the four upper airway regions: A is the nasopharynx, which is defined from the nasal turbinates to the hard palate; B is the retropalatal oropharynx, which extends from the hard palate to the caudal margin of the soft palate; C is the retroglossal region, which extends from the caudal margin of the soft palate to the base of the epiglottis; and D is the hypopharynx, which is defined from the base of the tongue to the larynx. **B,** Diagram demonstrating important midsagittal upper airway, soft tissue, and bony structures.

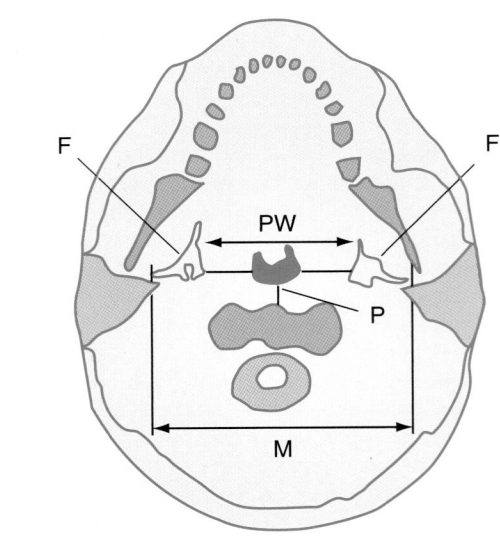

Figure 82–2. **A,** Axial magnetic resonance (MR) image in a normal subject in the retropalatal region. The tongue, soft palate, parapharyngeal fat pads (fat is white on an MR image), lateral parapharyngeal walls (muscles between the airway and lateral parapharyngeal fat pads), and mandibular rami can all be visualized on this axial MRI. **B,** Diagram demonstrating important soft tissue and craniofacial structures on an axial MR image in the retropalatal region. F, distance between the parapharyngeal fat pads; M, distance between the mandibular rami; P, posterior airway wall thickness; PW, lateral pharyngeal wall thickness.

To understand airway closure in patients with obstructive sleep apnea, we need to understand how pharyngeal wall structures determine airway size, or, to put it another way, examine the doughnut as well as the hole in the doughnut. The anterior wall of the oropharynx is formed primarily by the soft palate and tongue, whereas the posterior wall of the oropharynx primarily comprises the superior, middle, and inferior constrictor muscles. The lateral oropharyngeal walls are formed by several different structures including oropharyngeal muscles (hyoglossus, styloglossus, stylohyoid, stylopharyngeus, palatoglossus, palatopharyngeus, and the pharyngeal constrictors [superior, middle, and inferior]), lymphoid tissue (palatine tonsils), and adipose tissue (parapharyngeal fat pads). The mandibular rami bound all the structures that form the lateral pharyngeal walls (Figs. 82–2 and 82–3).

STATIC AND DYNAMIC PROPERTIES OF THE NORMAL PHARYNGEAL AIRWAY

To understand why the pharyngeal airway collapses during sleep in patients with obstructive sleep apnea, one must first understand the static and dynamic properties of the upper airway under normal conditions. The mechanical behavior of the upper airway under passive conditions—that is, when neuromuscular influences have been suppressed[4-7]—can best be described in terms of the relationship between cross-sectional airway area (A) and transmural pressure (P_{tm}).

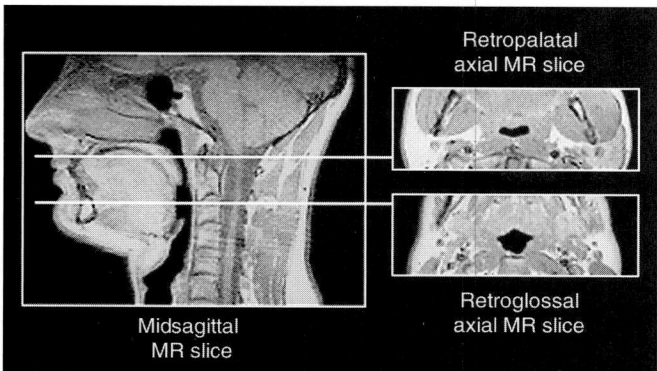

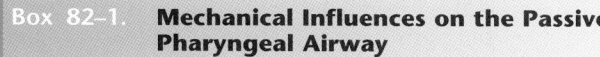

Figure 82–3. Midsagittal magnetic resonance (MR) image in a normal subject, depicting the midretropalatal and midretroglossal regions.

As depicted in Figure 82–4A, transmural pressure is the difference between intraluminal pressure (P_l) and tissue pressure (P_{ti}): $P_{tm} = P_l - P_{ti}$. An increase in transmural pressure, caused either by more positive intraluminal pressure or more negative tissue pressure, distends and enlarges the airway area; conversely, a decrease in transmural pressure, caused either by more negative intraluminal pressure or more positive tissue pressure, narrows the airway.

The overall behavior at a particular region of the passive pharynx is revealed in a plot of transmural pressure against intraluminal cross-sectional area, as depicted in Figure 82–4B. Such a plot is referred to as the "tube law" and describes the dependence of cross-sectional area on transmural pressure. The transmural pressure at which area reaches zero is referred to as closing pressure (P_{close}), and the area at which the curve plateaus is the maximal area. The slope of the line at any point in the relationship ($\Delta A/\Delta P_{tm}$) is referred to as the effective compliance of that particular region of the airway.

Box 82–1.	**Mechanical Influences on the Passive Pharyngeal Airway**

Static Factors

Surface adhesive forces
Neck and jaw posture
Tracheal tug
Gravity

Dynamic Factors

Upstream resistance within the nasal airway and pharynx
Bernoulli effect
Dynamic compliance

A number of mechanical influences (Box 82–1) impinge on the upper airway to cause it to be fully open, narrowed, or closed. These factors can be classified as static or dynamic influences, and they interact with the tube law of the pharynx to determine, at any time, the cross-sectional area of various segments of the upper airway.

Static Factors Influencing Behavior of the Normal Pharyngeal Airway

Surface Adhesive Forces

Clinical observations, as well as studies in anesthetized animals, indicate that surface adhesive forces between opposed luminal surfaces may contribute to airway patency and closure. During nasal breathing with the mouth closed, surface adhesive forces help maintain the soft palate in apposition to the base of the tongue and promote contact of the tongue with the mucosa of the fixed-space oral cavity. Mouth opening potentially destabilizes the airway by freeing the mucosal

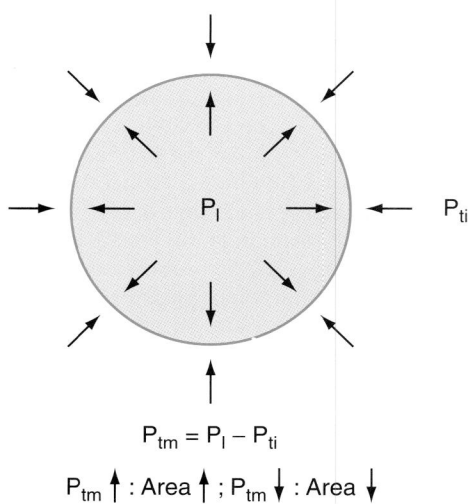

$$P_{tm} = P_l - P_{ti}$$

$$P_{tm} \uparrow : \text{Area} \uparrow ; P_{tm} \downarrow : \text{Area} \downarrow$$

A

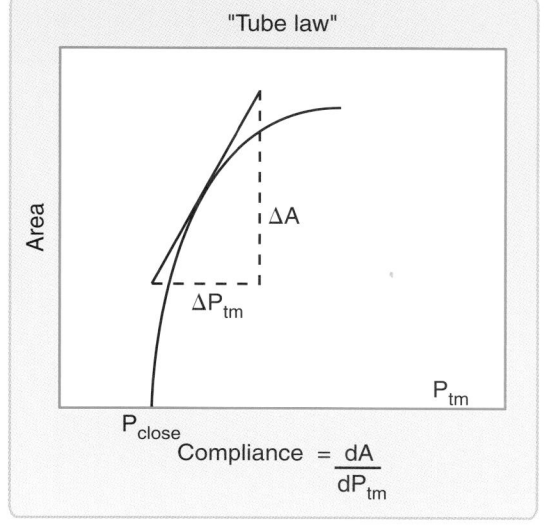

B

Figure 82–4. The concept of transmural pressure (P_{tm}) and a "tube law" of the pharynx are schematized. **A,** P_{tm} is defined as intraluminal pressure (P_l) minus surrounding tissue pressure (P_{ti}). **B,** An increase in P_{tm} results in an increase in the cross-sectional area (A) in accordance with a tube law of the pharynx. The slope of the tube law represents compliance of the pharynx. P_{close}, closing pressure; P_{ti}, tissue pressure.

attachments of the tongue and soft palate and allowing the now freely moving structures to move posteriorly and compromise the pharyngeal airway. Surface adhesive forces may also make restoration of airway patency more difficult and may explain why the pressure needed to open an already closed airway (opening pressure) is greater than the closing pressure.[5,8]

Neck and Jaw Posture

A number of studies indicate that neck flexion tends to close the airway and neck extension acts to open it.[9,10] Whether the action is principally in the oropharynx or hypopharynx has not been documented, but it is likely that retropalatal and retroglossal regions of the upper airway are narrowed as the neck is flexed.

Jaw posture has also been documented to influence the size of the upper airway. Opening the jaw slightly may actually increase the size of the pharynx by providing more room in the oral cavity for the tongue. This may be particularly important if the tongue is large relative to the oral cavity. However, progressive opening of the jaw leads to posterior movement of the genu of the mandible—that is, the genu moves closer to the posterior pharyngeal wall because the mandibular condyle of the temporomandibular joint is considerably rostral to the plane of the mandible (Fig. 82–5). This posterior movement of the genu of the mandible with mouth opening causes the tongue and hyoid apparatus to move posteriorly and thereby narrow the pharynx.

Tracheal Tug

Increases in lung volume are thought to increase pharyngeal cross-sectional area, reduce closing pressure, and stiffen the upper airway.[11-14] This action is probably exerted through axial

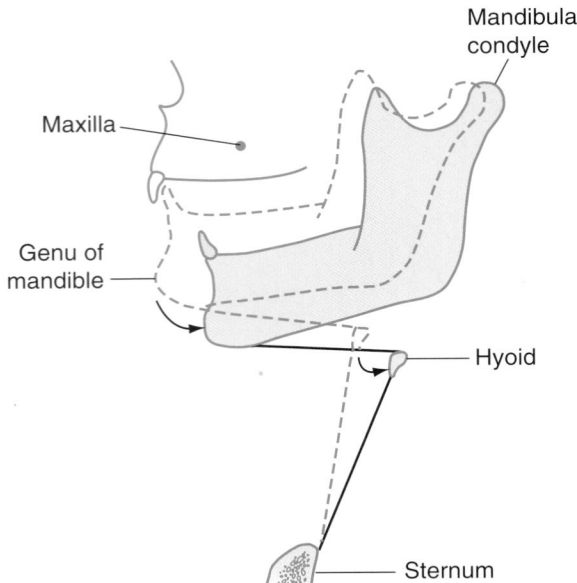

Figure 82–5. Mouth opening causes a posterior and caudal displacement of the genu of the mandible, as well as the floating hyoid bone, through the many hyomandibular attachments. As a result, the anterior pharyngeal wall structures such as the tongue and epiglottis move in a posterior direction, decreasing pharyngeal airway size. Neck flexion would have a similar effect on the hyoid, tongue, and epiglottis even without a change in the relationship between the mandible and the maxilla.

forces in the trachea—a so-called tracheal tug. Increasing lung volume causes a caudal displacement of the intrathoracic trachea that, in turn, exerts caudally directed forces on the pharynx. The resulting passive axial tension in the pharyngeal wall tends to open the pharynx.

Gravity

Gravity is thought to have an important influence on pharyngeal airway patency, and it is common for patients with obstructive sleep apnea to have a higher apnea-hypopnea index in the supine than in the nonsupine position. When the patient is supine, gravity can narrow the pharyngeal airway by pulling the tongue and soft palate in a posterior direction.

Dynamic Properties of the Normal Pharyngeal Airway

A model of the upper airway under dynamic conditions that has been advanced and effectively employed is derived from an analogy of the upper airway to a Starling resistor.[15,16] In essence, *Starling resistor* is a term used to describe a highly collapsible tube having infinite compliance at one transmural pressure and low compliance at a higher or lower transmural pressure. The tube is completely closed at one luminal pressure and completely open at a higher luminal pressure. The luminal pressure at which the airway shifts from fully open to fully closed (i.e., the point of infinite compliance) is determined by the extramural pressure and is referred to as the critical pressure (P_{crit}).

Factors Influencing the Dynamic Properties of the Passive Pharyngeal Airway

Upstream Resistance within the Nasal Airway

Airflow is generated through the nose owing to a pressure drop between the nasal inlet and the nasopharynx. This driving pressure for airflow is generated by a reduction in nasopharyngeal pressure secondary to active contraction of the diaphragm and other inspiratory pump muscles.

The nose has a relatively high resistance and turbulent flow. The resistance is enhanced in situations where the nasal airway is narrowed by mucosal congestion. Accordingly, the increase in nasal resistance that occurs during inspiration is alinear relative to inspiratory airflow such that greater inspiratory airflow leads to disproportionately more negative nasopharyngeal intraluminal pressure.

Nasopharyngeal pressure is, effectively, the equivalent of intraluminal pressure for the pharynx if the resistance within the pharynx is relatively low. All other factors being equal, increases in nasal resistance will produce a greater negative pharyngeal intraluminal pressure and reduced pharyngeal cross-sectional area. The extent to which the lumen narrows depends on regional airway compliance, that is, the relative compliance of each segment.

Upstream Resistance within the Pharynx

As is the case with nasal resistance, a high resistance within the pharynx is associated with a decrease in intraluminal pressure at more caudal (more downstream) segments during inspiration.

In other words, a narrowing at the retropalatal region is associated with a further decline in intraluminal pressure during inspiration at sites caudal to the retropalatal region, thereby increasing the tendency for closure in the retroglossal region and hypopharynx.

Bernoulli Effect

Two physical phenomena cause a reduction in intraluminal pressure as gas flows through a tube: loss of energy and the Bernoulli effect. Energy is lost by work done in overcoming flow-resistance aspects of the airway; the Bernoulli effect is the conversion of energy from static to kinetic caused by an increase in the velocity of airflow when the lumen size decreases. The first phenomenon relates to upstream resistance to airflow. Whenever gas flows through a resistance, potential energy is dissipated in overcoming friction; consequently, intraluminal pressure decreases. The second phenomenon relates to acceleration of gas as it flows through a narrowed segment of a tube. Both phenomena contribute to decreasing pharyngeal intraluminal pressure during inspiration; therefore, both tend to narrow the pharynx during inspiration.

To generate an inspiratory flow through the high-resistance air passage presented by the nose, pharyngeal pressure must fall below pressure at the nares. Nasal resistance contributes to the development of negative intraluminal pressure in the absence of inspiratory flow limitation. However, once inspiratory flow limitation is present, the relatively rigid nasal passage does not contribute to further pressure drop across the collapsible airway segment. By contrast, progressive narrowing of the pharyngeal upstream segment would produce progressively more negative intraluminal pressures caudal to the site of narrowing, regardless of inspiratory flow limitation, because of increased viscous energy losses in the narrowed region.

If the cross-sectional area of the pharyngeal lumen decreases in some regions, the velocity of airflow will be elevated in these regions. This increase in airflow velocity implies an increase in kinetic energy of the airstream and, hence, a decrease in lateral wall pressure. This reduction in lateral wall pressure allows further narrowing of the tube according to the tube law of the pharynx.

Dynamic Compliance

During inspiration, the decrease in intraluminal pressure at any point in the upper airway interacts with the dynamic compliance of that segment of the upper airway.[17] If intraluminal pressure at the beginning of inspiration is a value that lies on the steep portion of the pressure-area relationship, the upper airway narrows as intraluminal pressure decreases during inspiration. The degree to which pharyngeal cross-sectional area decreases depends on the dynamic compliance of the upper airway.

This mechanical property also influences the likelihood of yet further airway collapse. Specifically, narrowing during inspiration due to a decrease in intraluminal pressure might decrease the area significantly, which in turn increases the velocity of gas flowing through that segment. The velocity increase causes further reductions in intraluminal pressure because of the conversion of static to kinetic energy with decreased lateral wall (or distending) pressure. Such a decline in luminal pressure tends to further decrease airway area. This sequence of events describes dynamic narrowing of the upper airway, which is typically observed under normal conditions if the pharyngeal muscles are relatively hypotonic.

ACTIVATION OF THE UPPER AIRWAY PHARYNGEAL MUSCLES

Many of the 20 or more skeletal muscles surrounding the pharyngeal airway, including the medial pterygoid, tensor palatini, genioglossus, geniohyoid, and sternohyoid, receive phasic activation during inspiration and tend to promote a patent pharyngeal lumen by dilating the airway and stiffening the airway walls.[18] As shown in Figure 82–6A,B, the pharyngeal muscles have complex anatomic relationships. These muscles can be classified into muscles regulating the position of the soft palate, tongue, hyoid apparatus, and posterolateral pharyngeal walls.

Contraction of specific muscles within these groups can have antagonistic effects on the pharyngeal airway. For example, contraction of the palatal muscle levator palatini, along with the superior pharyngeal constrictor, closes the retropalatal airway; contraction of other palatal muscles, the palatopharyngeus and glossopharyngeus, opens the airway in the retropalatal region.[19] Similarly, the extrinsic tongue muscles include tongue protrudors (genioglossus and geniohyoid) and retractors (hyoglossus and styloglossus).

Pharyngeal muscles can have different effects when activated in concert than when activated individually. Coactivation of the hyoid muscles is a particularly good example of this phenomenon (see Fig. 82–6).[20] The hyoid bone in humans, unlike that in other mammals, does not articulate with any other bony or cartilaginous structure. The position of the relatively compliant ventral pharyngeal wall is, therefore, determined by the numerous muscle attachments to this floating bony structure.

Muscles inserting on the hyoid include the geniohyoid and genioglossus. Contraction of these muscles pulls the hyoid in a rostral and anterior direction. Strap muscles originating from the sternum (sternohyoid) and thyroid cartilage (thyrohyoid) also insert on the hyoid and pull it in a caudal direction. With simultaneous contraction of all four muscles, the resultant force vector acting on the hyoid is directed caudally and anteriorly. This combined effect moves the anterior pharyngeal wall outward and promotes upper airway patency. Evidence also indicates that simultaneous activation of the antagonstic protrudor and retractor tongue muscles, as occurs under hypercapnic and hypoxic conditions, has a synergistic effect in promoting upper airway patency.[21,22]

The action of any upper airway muscle depends not only on whether other muscles are simultaneously active but also on precise anatomic arrangements at the time of activation. For instance, mouth opening decreases the length of the genioglossus and geniohyoid muscles, and hence the force developed by a particular level of efferent neural activity is lessened. Similarly, neck flexion changes the position of the hyoid bone. This alters the anatomic relationships of a variety of muscles acting on the hyoid, shifting the resultant vector of their forces in a more caudal direction.

Other evidence suggests that a particular pharyngeal muscle may have different mechanical effects on the airway depending on the size of the airway at the time of muscle activation.[23,24] The ability of a given muscle to produce different mechanical effects may be due to changes in muscle fiber orientation, with concomitant changes in airway size and shape.

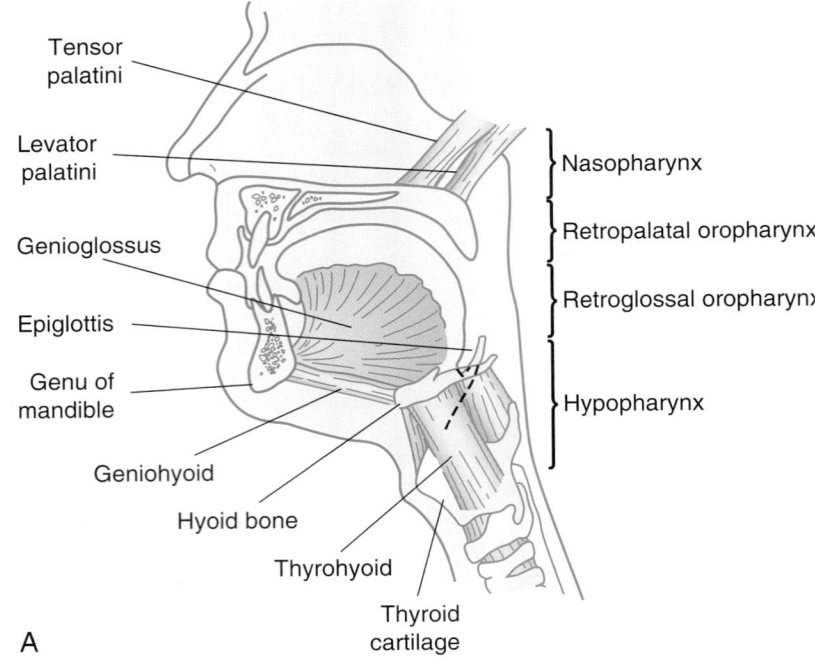

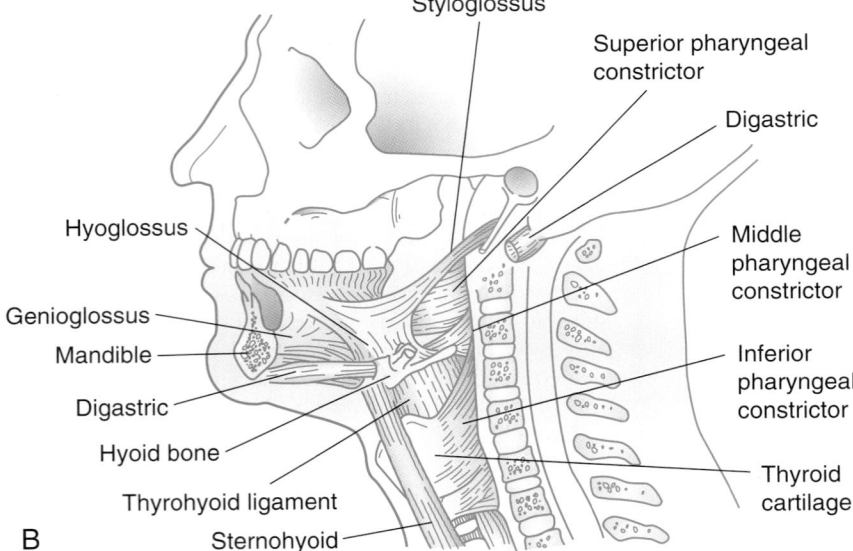

Figure 82–6. A, Schematic diagram of upper airway anatomy. The tensor palatini moves the soft palate ventrally. The genioglossus acts to displace the tongue ventrally. Coactivation of the muscles in the anterior pharyngeal wall such as the geniohyoid and sternohyoid (not shown) act on the hyoid bone to move it ventrally. **B,** Schematic diagram of upper airway muscles. Among the many upper airway muscles attaching to the floating hyoid bone are the genioglossus, geniohyoid (not shown), hyoglossus, middle pharyngeal constrictor, sternohyoid, and digastric.

In addition, the timing of muscle activation relative to the phase of respiration may play a role in determining the mechanical effects of such activation.[25]

The differing mechanical effects of the pharyngeal muscles, depending on airway conditions at the time of activation, may help explain how pharyngeal muscles can play a role in such disparate functions as respiration, deglutition, and phonation. Rather than a separate set of muscles performing one particular function, activation of a given muscle can have diametrically different mechanical effects on the airway, depending on what other muscles are simultaneously active and on precise anatomic arrangements at the time of activation.

Factors Modulating Pharyngeal Muscle Activation

Activation of pharyngeal muscles can alter the mechanical characteristics of the upper airway. The effect of pharyngeal dilator muscle activation on the tube law of the pharynx is shown in Figure 82–7. Under active conditions, the pressure-area relationship is shifted upward and to the left. At any given transmural pressure, muscle activation increases area and stiffens the airway; that is, it decreases effective compliance.

The effect of muscle activation on the tube law is quantified by the term P_{mus}, the effective pressure exerted by muscle

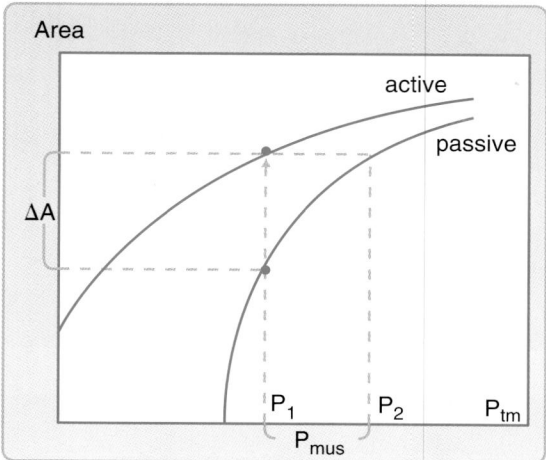

Figure 82–7. Airway area under passive conditions (i.e., no muscle activation) can be increased by a rise in transmural pressure (P_{tm}). Such a change occurs with the application of a positive intraluminal pressure, such as with nasal continuous positive airway pressure (CPAP). Contraction of pharyngeal dilators shifts the passive curve up and to the left. The muscle contraction increases P_{tm}, and ($P_2 - P_1$) now represents P_{mus} (muscle pressure).

activation, which is equivalent to the change in transmural pressure required to yield the equivalent change in area on the passive curve (see Fig. 82–7). Under certain conditions, pharyngeal dilating muscles generally display inspiratory bursting activity together with tonic expiratory activity. Alcohol, sleep deprivation, anesthesia, and sedative-hypnotics suppress respiratory-related pharyngeal muscle activation.[26] Additional factors that modulate respiratory-related activity of

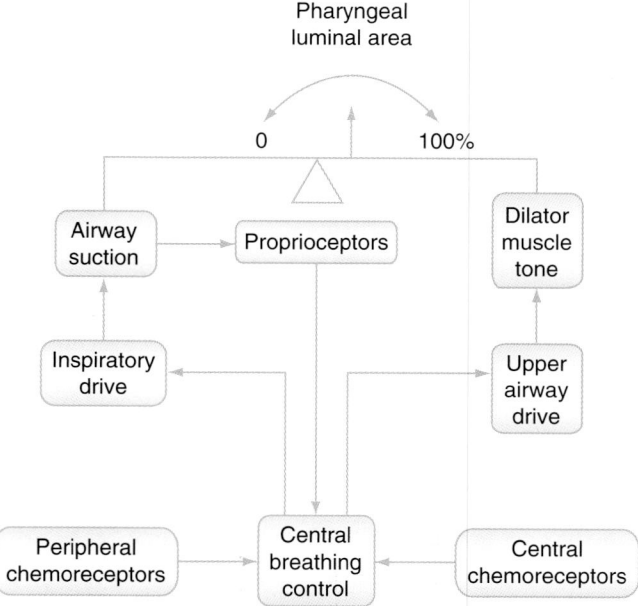

Figure 82–8. Balance of forces that sustain upper airway patency. The two major forces are airway suction pressure and upper airway muscle tone that dilates and stiffens the airway. These in turn are influenced by other factors.

pharyngeal airway motor neurons include changes in state, proprioceptive feedback, and chemical drive (Fig. 82–8).

Changes in State

Perhaps the most convincing evidence demonstrating the overall importance of changes in state on the neuromuscular maintenance of airway patency is that obstructive sleep apnea is a sleep disorder. Modification of neuromuscular factors by sleep is a normal phenomenon; this fact can be inferred from measurements of supraglottic resistance in healthy persons— that is, resistance from the nares to the region above the glottis. With sleep onset, this resistance rises from the low values (e.g., 1 to 2 cm H_2O/L/sec) to high values (e.g., 5 to 10 cm H_2O/L/sec).[27,28] Supraglottic airway resistance is abnormally high in patients with obstructive sleep apnea while they are awake, and the resistance rises significantly with sleep onset, reaching infinity with complete airway closure.[27,29]

These observations in healthy persons, snorers, and patients with obstructive sleep apnea indicate that a reversible change in upper airway caliber occurs with a shift in neural state. Such behavior is explained by a change in neural output to upper airway muscles, which causes a decrease in P_{mus} at one or more sites within the pharyngeal airway. Electromyographic (EMG) recordings of pharyngeal muscles, such as the genioglossus and tensor palatini, confirm this decrease in pharyngeal muscle activity during the transition from wakefulness to sleep.[28,30] An even more pronounced reduction in motor output to pharyngeal muscles occurs in rapid eye movement (REM) sleep, particularly in phasic REM.[31,32] Although there is compelling evidence that sleep compromises the neural output to pharyngeal dilator muscles, the corresponding effects on inspiratory pump muscles are much less convincing.

Proprioceptive Stimuli

Proprioceptive feedback from thoracic and upper airway receptors can modulate the motor output to pharyngeal muscles. During non–rapid eye movement (NREM) sleep and general anesthesia in animals, withdrawal of vagally mediated phasic volume feedback by tracheal occlusion during inspiration results in an immediate large augmentation in motor output to many upper airway and chest wall inspiratory pump muscles.[33-35] Neurally mediated upper airway muscle activation also occurs with introduction of subatmospheric pressure into an isolated, sealed upper airway in spontaneously breathing tracheotomized animals.[36,37] Because topical anesthesia of the upper airway inactivates the response, the upper airway receptors mediating this reflex activation are believed to be located superficially in the airway wall.[37,38] The majority of upper airway respiratory-related afferents appear to be located in the upper trachea and larynx and are carried in the internal branch of the superior laryngeal nerve. Proprioceptive information from the upper airway is also transmitted in the glossopharyngeal and trigeminal nerves.[37,39]

Both intrathoracic and upper airway proprioceptive information may also reduce motor output to the thoracic inspiratory muscles, thereby increasing intraluminal pressure below the site of airway obstruction.[40] The reflex effects elicited in animals on upper airway and respiratory pump muscles could represent a powerful defense mechanism for the maintenance of upper airway patency during sleep. Presumably, neural reflex activation of pharyngeal muscles by upper airway and thoracic receptors are initiated by upper airway obstruction and tend to compensate for airway obstruction by dilating and stiffening the pharynx.

Chemical Stimuli

Respiratory-related pharyngeal muscle activity, which can be absent during quiet breathing, usually appears under hypercapnic or hypoxic conditions.[41,42] These EMG differences are only significant as they relate to their mechanical effects. These electromechanical relationships are largely unexplored, but it appears unlikely that changes in electrical output to upper airway or thoracic pump muscles have a direct, linear relationship to the resulting mechanical changes in the pharyngeal airway.

Upper airway and phrenic motor neurons also differ in their response to hypocapnia. Upper airway motor neurons appear to have a higher CO_2 threshold for activation than respiratory pump muscles. With passive hyperventilation in a tracheotomized, vagotomized, anesthetized animal, phasic upper airway motor neuron activity disappears prior to phrenic activity. When the CO_2 level is then allowed to rise, phasic activity first reappears in the phrenic nerve. Thus, cyclic changes in arterial CO_2 around the CO_2 threshold for activation of upper airway motor neuron activity could lead to an imbalance of forces acting on the pharyngeal airway and favor closure.

DIFFERENCES IN STATIC UPPER AIRWAY ANATOMY IN PATIENTS WITH SLEEP APNEA

Most studies have shown that the upper airway is smaller in patients with sleep apnea compared with normal subjects.[1,43-48] The airway narrowing found in these studies is primarily in the retropalatal region.[43,49,50] Why is the upper airway smaller in patients with sleep apnea? The reduction in the size of the apneic upper airway compared with the normal airway must be secondary to enlargement of the surrounding soft tissues and to reductions in or changes to the craniofacial structures.[46,47]

Studies using cephalometrics have demonstrated reductions in mandibular body length (retrognathia), inferiorly positioned hyoid bone, and retroposition of the maxilla in patients with sleep apnea compared with normal subjects.[51-54] Reduction in mandibular body length, in particular, has been shown to be an important risk factor for obstructive sleep apnea.[55] In addition to craniofacial differences, enlargement of the upper airway soft tissue structures (tongue, lateral pharyngeal walls, soft palate, parapharyngeal fat pads) has also been demonstrated in patients with sleep apnea compared with normal subjects.[46,47]

Imaging studies with computed tomography (CT) or magnetic resonance (MR) imaging have demonstrated decreased cross-sectional area and increased dimensions of the soft palate, tongue, parapharyngeal fat pads, and lateral pharyngeal walls in patients with sleep apnea.[2,43,48,56-58] Figure 82–9A (a midsagittal MR image) demonstrates narrowing of the upper airway and elongation of the soft palate and tongue in an apneic patient compared with a normal subject. Figure 82–9B (an axial MR image in the retropalatal region) demonstrates lateral airway narrowing in a patient with sleep apnea compared with a normal subject.

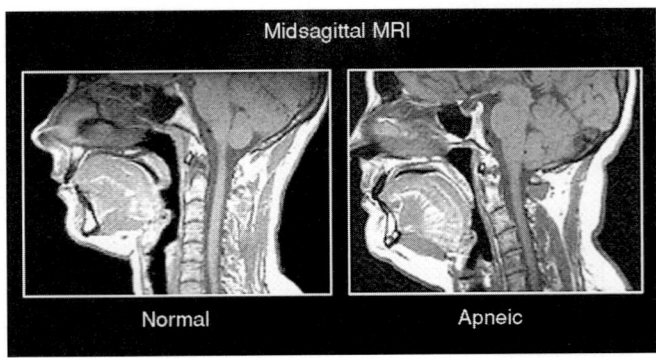

A

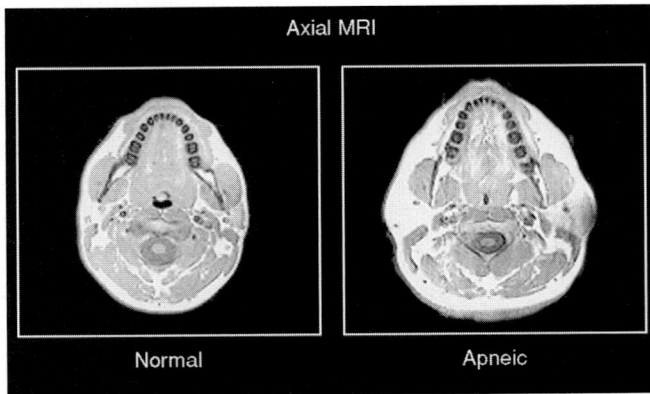

B

Figure 82–9. A, Midsagittal magnetic resonance (MR) image of a normal subject *(left)* and a patient with sleep apnea *(right)*. The upper airway is smaller and the soft palate is longer in the patient with sleep apnea. The amount of subcutaneous fat (white area at the back of the neck) is greater in the apneic than in the normal subject. **B,** Axial MR image in the retropalatal region of a normal subject *(left)* and a patient with sleep apnea *(right)*. The upper airway is smaller (primarily narrowed in the lateral dimension) in the patient with sleep apnea.

Recently, a case-control study demonstrated that the volume of the upper airway soft tissue structures (tongue, lateral pharyngeal walls, soft palate, parapharyngeal fat pads; Fig. 82–10) was significantly greater in apneic patients than normal ones.[46] The volume of the lateral pharyngeal walls, tongue, and total soft tissue surrounding the upper airway remained significantly larger in apneic patients than in normal persons after covariate adjustments for sex, age, ethnicity, craniofacial size, and fat surrounding the upper airway. Moreover, this study demonstrated that increased volume of the lateral pharyngeal walls, tongue, and total upper airway soft tissue significantly increased the risk for sleep apnea even after the covariate adjustments.[46]

Causes of Upper Airway Soft Tissue Enlargement

Why are the upper airway soft tissue structures enlarged in patients with sleep apnea? Although there is not a specific answer to this question, there are several possible mechanisms explaining the etiology of the enlargement of the upper airway soft tissue structures in apneic persons, including edema secondary to negative pressure from airway closure or trauma, weight gain, muscle injury, gender, and genetic factors.

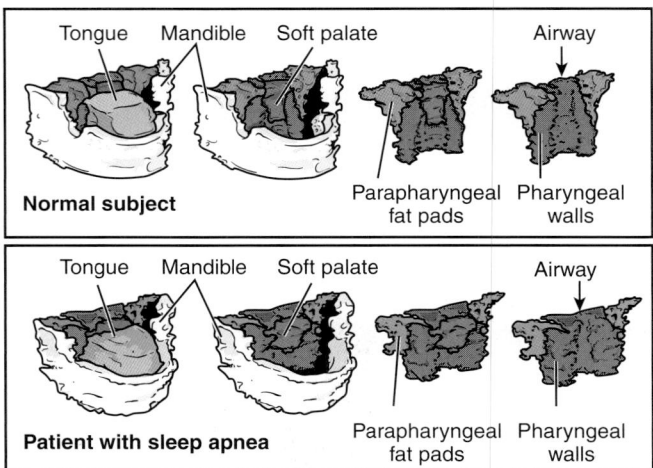

Tongue   Mandible   Soft palate   Airway

Normal subject

Parapharyngeal   Pharyngeal
fat pads   walls

Tongue   Mandible   Soft palate   Airway

Patient with sleep apnea

Parapharyngeal   Pharyngeal
fat pads   walls

Figure 82–10. Volumetric reconstruction of axial magnetic resonance (MR) images in a normal subject and a patient with sleep apnea. The mandible is depicted in white, the tongue in light blue, the soft palate in dark blue, the lateral parapharyngeal fat pads in medium blue, and the lateral/posterior pharyngeal walls in gray. Both subjects had an elevated body mass index (32.5 kg/m²). The normal subject has a larger airway than the patient with sleep apnea. The tongue, soft palate, and lateral pharyngeal walls of the patient with sleep apnea are all larger than in the normal subject.

Edema

Negative pressure during airway closure or trauma from repeated apneic events may cause edema in the soft tissue structures surrounding the upper airway. This edema could increase the size of these soft tissue structures. The soft palate is especially at risk for the development of edema because it can be tugged caudally and traumatized during apneas. CPAP is thought to reduce upper airway edema.[56] Quantitative MR mapping has indicated that there is more edema or fat, or both, in the genioglossus muscles of apneic persons than in normal ones.[59,60] Histologic studies have also shown that patients with sleep apnea have increased edema in the uvula compared with normal persons.[61]

Obesity and Weight Gain

Obesity is known to be an important risk factor for obstructive sleep apnea.[62,63] Although the relationship between obesity and sleep apnea is not well understood, it appears that obesity decreases pharyngeal airway size and increases airway collapsibility. Increased neck size, a better surrogate of upper airway fat distribution than body mass index (BMI), has been demonstrated to be an excellent predictor of sleep apnea.[63,64] It is thought that the increased neck size in obese patients with obstructive sleep apnea is related to fat deposition in the neck.[1,43,65-68]

Upper airway imaging studies have demonstrated increased adipose tissue surrounding the airway (primarily enlargement of the lateral parapharyngeal fat pads—see Figs. 82–2, 82–9B, and 82–10) in obese patients with sleep apnea.[1,43,65-68] These studies suggest that obesity increases fat deposition in the lateral pharyngeal fat pads, which, in turn, has been hypothesized to compress the lateral walls and reduce upper airway size.[1,43,65-68] Fat deposition within the tongue or soft palate may also be important in increasing the size of the soft tissue structures and reducing the caliber of the upper airway. Fat has been shown to be deposited in the uvula of patients with sleep apnea, which supports the hypothesis that fat deposited outside of the parapharyngeal fat pads may be important in the pathogenesis of sleep apnea.[69,70]

It has also been argued that the total amount of fat surrounding the upper airway may be a more important contributor to sleep apnea than fat localized in a particular anatomic site. Shelton and coworkers[67] have hypothesized that fat deposition in the space bounded by the mandibular rami increases tissue pressure, which in turn would lead to airway narrowing.

In addition to direct deposition of fat, weight gain may also alter the muscle tissue surrounding the upper airway. Weight gain not only increases adipose tissue but also has been shown to increase muscle mass.[71,72] Approximately 25% of the increased weight in obese patients is secondary to fat-free tissue[72,73]; it has been shown that patients with sleep apnea have a larger percentage of muscle in the uvula than normal subjects do.[69,74] These data suggest that weight gain may predispose to obstructive sleep apnea by increasing the size of the muscular soft tissue structures (tongue, soft palate, lateral pharyngeal walls) surrounding the upper airway in addition to the direct deposition of fat in the parapharyngeal fat pads. This hypothesis is supported by data in obese nonapneic women that show that weight loss decreases the volume of the lateral pharyngeal walls and parapharyngeal fat pads (Fig. 82–11A,B).[75]

Other explanations for the relationship between obesity and sleep apnea include changes in upper airway compliance and alterations in the biomechanical relationships of the upper airway muscles.[76] Thus, although obesity has been shown to be an important risk factor for sleep apnea, the specific effect of weight gain on the upper airway soft tissue structures is not entirely understood.

Muscle Injury

Researchers have also hypothesized that patients with obstructive sleep apnea have a primary myopathy that contributes to the enlargement of the upper airway soft tissue structures.[77] Several studies have shown an increase in type II fast-twitch fibers in the genioglossus muscle of apneic persons.[74,78,79] Type II fibers are more likely to fatigue than type I fibers, so the upper airway muscles in patients with sleep apnea would be more susceptible to fatigue than those in nonapneic subjects.

The remodeling of the upper airway muscles in patients with sleep apnea may be a primary or secondary phenomenon; in other words, it might be a consequence rather than the cause of apneas. Carrera and coworkers[78] studied the structure and function of the genioglossus in apneic subjects and nonapneic subjects and demonstrated that the myopathy is a secondary phenomenon. These investigators found increased type II fibers in the genioglossus muscle of apneic subjects; however, the changes in the genioglossus muscle were reversed with CPAP.

Gender

Gender may also have an important effect on the size of the upper airway soft tissue structures. Several studies have

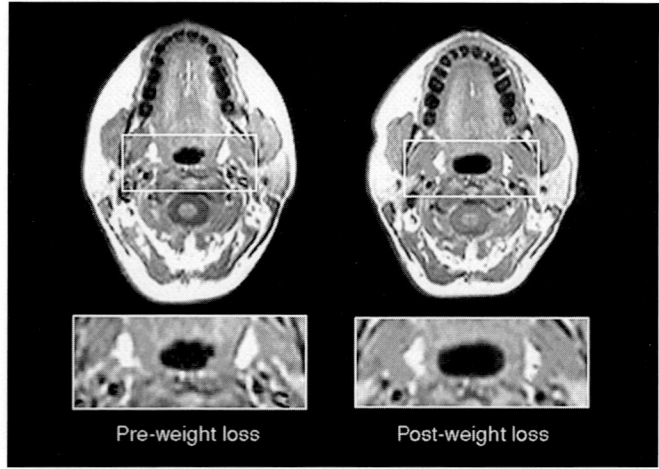

A

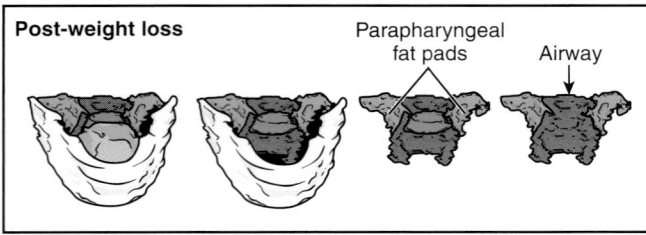

B

Figure 82–11. **A,** Axial magnetic resonance images of a normal subject, before and after weight loss in the retropalatal region. Airway area and lateral airway dimensions increase with weight loss. The thickness of lateral pharyngeal walls and the size of the parapharyngeal fat pads decrease with weight loss. **B,** Volumetric reconstructions of the upper airway soft tissues (soft palate [dark blue], the tongue [light blue], the lateral pharyngeal walls [gray], parapharyngeal fat pads [medium blue]), and craniofacial (mandible [white]) before and after weight loss in a normal subject. The size of the upper airway increases with weight loss. The lateral pharyngeal walls and the parapharyngeal fat pads demonstrated the largest reductions in size with weight loss. Mandibular volume did not change with weight loss.

demonstrated that upper airway size is smaller in women than in men.[80,81] In addition, studies have shown that neck size is smaller in women than in men[82] so the size of the upper airway soft tissue structures (tongue, soft palate, lateral pharyngeal walls, lateral parapharyngeal fat pads) are hypothetically also smaller in women than men. Moreover, fat distribution is different in women than in men.[83,84] In men, fat is deposited primarily in the upper body and trunk, whereas in women it is deposited primarily in the lower body and extremities.[83,84] These gender-related differences in overall fat distribution suggest that the size of the lateral parapharyngeal fat pads may be greater in men than in women.

Two studies have used MR imaging to examine gender-related differences in upper airway soft tissue structures in normal subjects.[85,86] Both studies showed that the tongue size, soft palate size, and total soft tissue were greater in normal men than in women.[85,86] Whittle and colleagues[85] demonstrated that the total volume of soft tissues and the size of both the tongue and soft palate were larger in men than in women. Malhotra and coworkers[86] demonstrated that airway length, soft palate size, and tongue size were greater in men than women. Surprisingly, neither study found significant differences in the size of the lateral pharyngeal fat pads in the normal men and women.[85,86] These data suggest that gender may not have a significant effect on the amount of visceral (parapharygneal fat pads) neck fat but may have an important effect on the size of the other upper airway soft tissue structures.

Genetic Factors

Although some researchers hypothesize that genetic factors play an important role in determining the size of the upper airway soft tissue structures, few data support this hypothesis. Family aggregation of craniofacial anatomy (reduction in posterior airway space, increase in mandible-to-hyoid distance, inferior hyoid placement) has been shown in patients with sleep apnea.[82,87] The data from these studies suggest that elements of craniofacial structure are likely inherited in apneic patients, but studies examining the heritability of the upper airway soft tissue structures (tongue, soft palate, lateral pharyngeal walls, lateral parapharyngeal fat pads) have not yet been performed. Macroglossia has been shown to be a risk factor for sleep apnea in patients with trisomy 21,[88] but otherwise the effect of genetic factors on the size of upper airway soft tissue structures has not been well studied. Nonetheless it seems plausible that the size of the tongue, soft palate, and lateral pharyngeal walls is at least partially genetically mediated.

DYNAMIC PHYSIOLOGIC CHANGES IN UPPER AIRWAY STRUCTURES

Although we have gained important insights into the anatomic risk factors for sleep apnea with static studies of the upper airway, examination of the dynamic behavior of the upper airway is also necessary to completely understand the pathogenesis of sleep-disordered breathing. CT, MR imaging, and nasopharyngoscopy have been used to examine dynamic changes in upper airway caliber and the surrounding soft tissue structures during the respiratory cycle.[48,89-93] Electron beam CT has been used to demonstrate that upper airway size changes during four distinct phases of the respiratory cycle in normal subjects and patients with sleep apnea (Fig. 82–12).[45,49]

In early inspiration (phase 1, see Fig. 82–12) there is a small increase in upper airway size, but during most of inspiration (phase 2, see Fig. 82–12) upper airway caliber remains relatively constant. The finding that upper airway caliber is relatively constant in inspiration during wakefulness suggests a balance between the action of the upper airway dilator muscles to increase airway size and negative intraluminal pressure to decrease airway size. In early expiration, upper airway caliber increases (phase 3, see Fig. 82–12) secondary to positive intraluminal pressure (the upper airway dilator muscles are not active during expiration). Upper airway caliber was largest in early expiration.[45,49] At the end of expiration (phase 4, see Fig. 82–12) there is a large reduction in upper airway caliber.

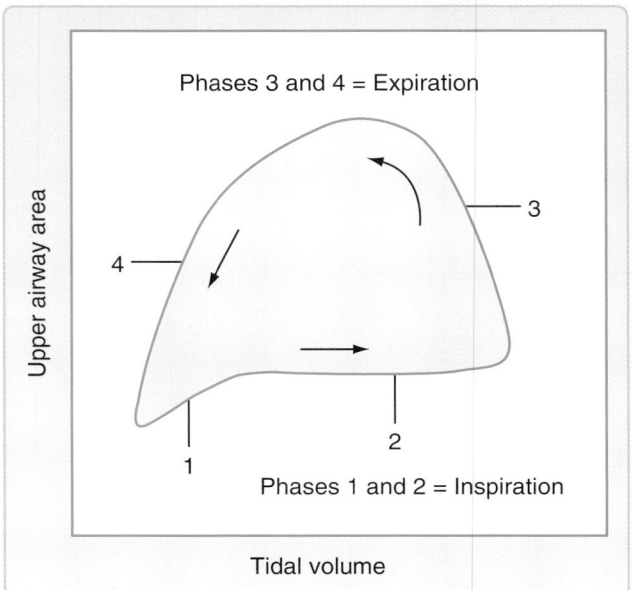

Figure 82–12. Diagram of the changes in upper airway area as a function of tidal volume during the respiratory cycle. Airway caliber is relatively constant in inspiration (phases 1 and 2), whereas airway size increases in early expiration (phase 3) and decreases in late expiration (phase 4).

Researchers have hypothesized that the end of expiration is a vulnerable time for upper airway narrowing or collapse because the upper airway is no longer kept open by the phasic action of the upper airway dilator muscles (phases 1 and 2, during inspiration) or positive intraluminal pressure (phase 3, early expiration).[45,49] In these investigations, upper airway caliber was smallest at the end of expiration.[45,49] This finding may have important implications with regard to the timing of sleep-induced upper airway closure.

Apneic events during sleep are thought to occur during inspiration secondary to negative intraluminal pressure generated by contraction of the chest wall.[94] However, studies examining airway resistance have demonstrated that airway closure in patients with sleep apnea can occur during both expiration and inspiration.[95,96] Studies using nasopharyngoscopy have also shown that airway closure during sleep occurs during expiration and that subatmospheric intraluminal pressure was not required for pharyngeal closure.[43,97] These data indicate that the upper airway is vulnerable to collapse at the end of expiration in addition to collapse during inspiration.

OBSTRUCTION OF THE PHARYNX DURING SLEEP

Periodic and Nonperiodic Obstruction of the Pharynx during Sleep

A typical polygraphic recording from a patient displaying periodic pharyngeal occlusion during sleep is shown in Figure 82–13A. Periods during which airflow is absent are interspersed with somewhat briefer periods during which airflow is present. During the periods of pharyngeal occlusion, arterial oxygen saturation progressively drops, and the magnitude

of respiratory fluctuations in the esophageal pressure recording progressively increases. The apneic episodes terminate with an arousal that is associated with a large burst of submental EMG activity.

Narrowing of the pharyngeal lumen can also produce nonperiodic obstruction characterized by a relatively stable elevated respiratory resistance associated with sustained arterial oxygen desaturation and repetitive, large inspiratory efforts associated with chin muscle activation (see Fig. 82–13B).[98,99] As is the case with periodic occlusion, the location of the airway narrowing can be identified as the pharynx by measurement of airflow and supraglottic pressure, which may reveal upper airway resistance exceeding 75 cm H_2O/L/sec.

This tracing also provides insight into a consequence of a collapsible pharyngeal tube–inspiratory flow limitation. Note that despite a progressively larger driving pressure (as reflected by abnormally negative esophageal pressure) during an inspiratory effort, airflow remains constant, indicating increasing resistance during inspiration, presumably resulting from the progressive reduction of the pharyngeal lumen.

Site and Patterns of Pharyngeal Obstruction

The retropalatal region is the most common primary site of airway narrowing or closure during sleep in patients with obstructive sleep apnea, although upper airway narrowing can also occur in the retroglossal region.[1,3,19,48,100-102] However, most patients with obstructive sleep apnea have more than one site of narrowing.[101] The retropalatal region usually collapses in a sphincter-like fashion, which is characterized by movement of both the anterior and lateral walls rather than the more rigid posterior wall.[103] Studies examining state-dependent changes in the upper airway also demonstrate that airway narrowing during sleep occurs in both the lateral and anterior-posterior dimensions (Fig. 82–14).[1,3,91,97,100]

EFFECT OF TREATMENT ON UPPER AIRWAY CALIBER

In the following sections we will review data on the effect of weight loss, CPAP, oral appliances, and surgery on upper airway size and the surrounding soft tissue and craniofacial structure.

Weight Loss

Weight loss (see Chapter 88) on the order of 5% to 10% has been shown in several investigations to improve obstructive sleep apnea and decrease the collapsibility of the airway.[61,76,104,105] However, it is not entirely clear how weight loss decreases the severity of obstructive sleep apnea or alters the size or configuration of the upper airway soft tissue structures (soft palate, tongue, parapharyngeal fat pads, lateral pharyngeal walls). Weight loss probably decreases the volume of the parapharyngeal fat pads, which, in turn, could increase the size of the upper airway.

Continuous Positive Airway Pressure

Although CPAP (see Chapter 89) suppresses upper airway muscle activity, it increases airway caliber by establishing a positive transmural pressure along the entire pharyngeal airway, functioning as a pneumatic splint.[44,106,107] Initially it

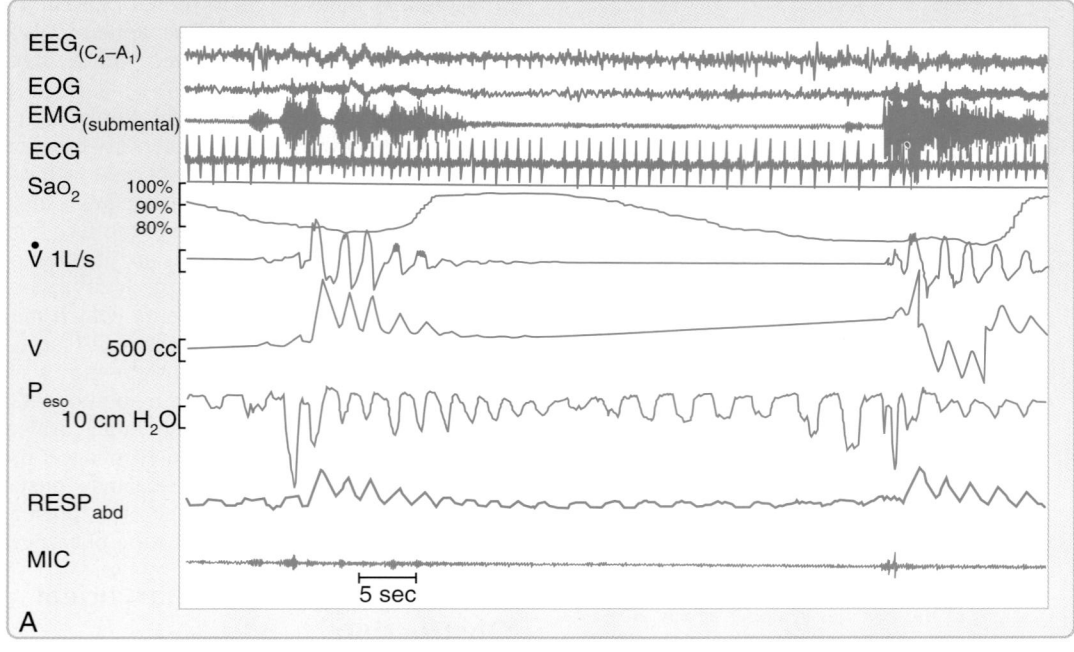

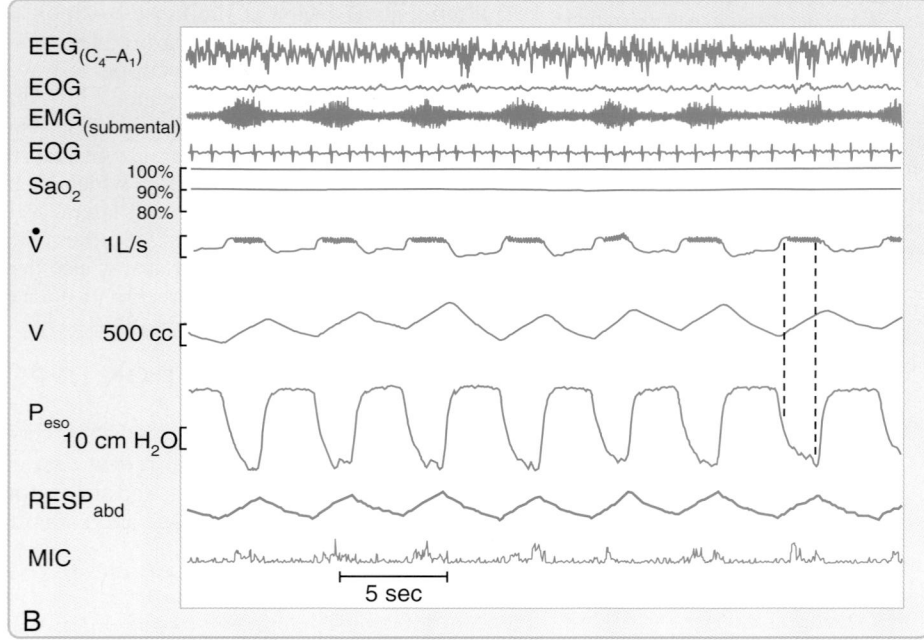

Figure 82–13. A, A typical tracing from a patient with severe obstructive sleep apnea. Bioelectric measurements *(top three channels)* indicate that the patient is in light sleep between periods of arousals associated with activation of submental electromyogram (EMG). Arterial oxygen saturation (Sao₂) decreases periodically and increases after onset of airflow (V̇). Esophageal pressure (P_eso) and abdominal motion (RESP_abd) show continuous respiratory efforts. **B,** A typical tracing derived from a patient with obstructive sleep hypopnea. A submental electromyogram indicates rhythmic bursts of pharyngeal inspiratory muscles. Sao₂ reveals stable mild hypoxemia. Airflow demonstrates flow limitation during inspiration. Despite a progressively larger driving pressure during an inspiratory effort *(time between dashed vertical lines),* flow remains constant, which indicates increasing resistance during inspiration, presumably resulting from progressive narrowing of the pharyngeal lumen. The thickened tracing at this time results from high-frequency oscillation in airflow caused by snoring. EEG, electroencephalogram; ECG, electrocardiogram; EOG, electrooculogram; MIC, microphone; V, volume.

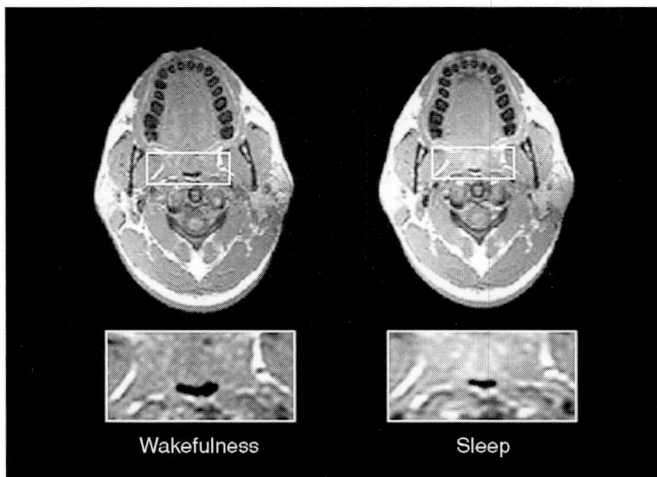

Figure 82–14. Magnetic resonance image in the retropalatal region of a normal subject during wakefulness and sleep. Airway area is smaller during sleep in this normal subject. The state-dependent change in airway caliber is a result of decreases in the lateral and anterior-posterior airway dimensions. Thickening of the lateral pharyngeal walls is demonstrated during sleep.

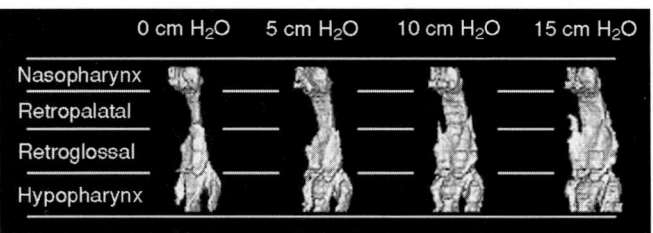

A

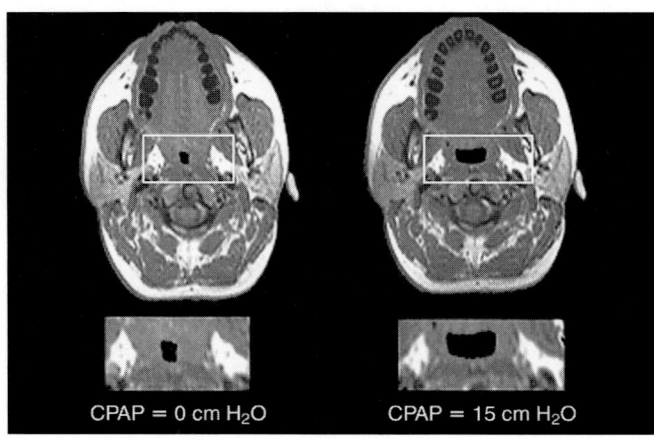

B

Figure 82–15. A, Volumetric reconstruction of the upper airway with progressively greater continuous positive airway pressure (CPAP) (0 to 15 cm H_2O) settings in a normal subject. There are significant increases in upper airway volume in the retropalatal and retroglossal regions with higher levels of CPAP. **B,** Axial magnetic resonance image in a normal subject at two levels of CPAP (0 and 15 cm H_2O) in the retropalatal region. Airway area is significantly greater at 15 cm H_2O. The airway enlargement is predominantly in the lateral dimension. Airway enlargement with CPAP results in thinning of the lateral pharyngeal walls, although the parapharyngeal fat pads are not displaced.

was thought that CPAP increased the caliber of the upper airway by anteriorly displacing the tongue and soft palate. However, CT and MR imaging studies have shown that the dilation of the upper airway with CPAP is greater in the lateral dimension than in the anterior-posterior dimension.[2,44] If the tongue and soft palate had been displaced anteriorly with CPAP, the increase in airway dimensions should have been in the anterior-posterior, not the lateral, direction. Progressive increases in CPAP (up to 15 cm H_2O) not only increased airway caliber in the lateral dimension but also significantly increased airway volume (three-fold) and airway area in the retropalatal and retroglossal regions (Fig. 82–15A,B).

Oral Appliances

Oral mandibular advancement devices (see Chapter 91) are also used to treat patients with obstructive sleep apnea.[108,109] These devices have been shown to increase the posterior airway space.[108,110-112] However, the specific biomechanical mechanisms that explain the increase in airway caliber with these devices are not well understood. Furthermore there is no gold standard oral appliance, and each of them (more than 50 appliances are available) may have a different mechanism of action.

Mandibular repositioning devices hypothetically increase airway size more in the retroglossal than in the retropalatal region because these devices advance the mandible and pull the tongue forward.[113,114] However, recent studies have shown that mandibular repositioning devices increase airway size in the retropalatal as well as the retroglossal region.[110,114] The increase in retropalatal airway area was predominantly in the lateral dimension,[114] suggesting that the mechanism of action of oral appliances may be more complex than simply pulling the tongue and soft palate forward.

Upper Airway Surgery

Uvulopalatopharyngoplasty (UPPP) is the most common surgical procedure (see Chapter 90) for patients with sleep

apnea.[115,116] In UPPP the tonsils (if present), uvula, distal margin of the soft palate, and any excessive pharyngeal tissue are removed. The success rate of UPPP is partially dependent on the site of airway closure.[19,50,56] Patients with retropalatal obstruction have better results after UPPP than those with retroglossal obstruction.[19,50,56] Unfortunately the success rate in patients undergoing UPPP surgery is only 50%, which is an unacceptably high failure rate. More favorable results with UPPP have been demonstrated if the surgery reduces the critical closing pressure.[117]

Thus far, the biomechanical changes in the upper airway soft tissue structures that underlie the efficacy, or lack of efficacy, of UPPP have not been identified.[2,59,118] Nonetheless, preliminary studies with MR imaging have demonstrated that in patients who have undergone UPPP, the airway remains small in the nonresected portion of the soft palate, whereas the airway enlarges in the resected portion of the soft palate (Fig. 82–16A,B).[119] CT studies have also demonstrated increased width of the soft palate after UPPP.[108] Persistent upper airway narrowing in the nonresected portion of the soft palate after UPPP may explain why UPPP has not been more successful in treating patients with obstructive sleep apnea.[2,59,118,119]

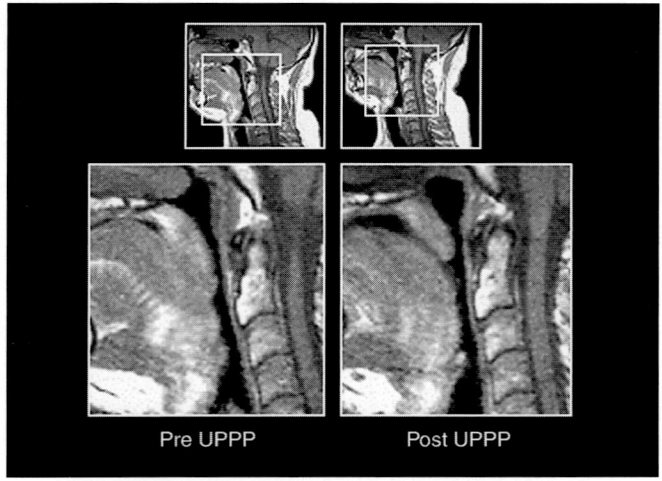

Pre UPPP Post UPPP

A

Uvula

Pre UPPP Post UPPP

B

Figure 82–16. **A,** Midsagittal magnetic resonance (MR) image in a patient with sleep apnea before and after a uvulopalatopharyngoplasty (UPPP). The uvula is shorter after the UPPP. However, the airway remains narrow in the region where the soft palate is not resected. **B,** Axial MR image before and after UPPP in the region where the uvula was resected. Airway caliber increases substantially after the UPPP in this region of the airway.

INTERACTION OF ANATOMIC AND NEUROLOGIC FACTORS: A SCHEMATIC MODEL

The overall balance of airway pressure and P_{mus} generated by upper airway muscles for subjects with normal anatomy and patients with sleep apnea is depicted in Figure 82–17, where a seesaw shows the balance between luminal pressure and pharyngeal P_{mus} and the angle of equilibrium indicates the pharyngeal luminal area. The position of the fulcrum is determined by the anatomy of the upper airway. In awake normal subjects (see Fig. 82–17A), equal values of negative luminal pressure and P_{mus} result in a widely dilated upper airway area because the anatomy of the upper airway favors patency—that is, the fulcrum is to the left of center. In contrast, an anatomic abnormality in patients with obstructive sleep apnea moves the pivot position of the balance to the right of center (see Fig. 82–17B). This means that even in the presence of increased upper airway muscle activity and normal intraluminal airway pressure (as may be present during wakefulness), the pharyngeal airway is still smaller than normal.

The effect of sleep on these equilibriums under normal conditions and in obstructive sleep apnea is shown in Figure 82–17C and D. In a normal subject, sleep is associated with a decrease in pharyngeal luminal area because of a sleep-induced decrease in upper airway muscle activity and a persistence of subatmospheric luminal pressure during inspiration. This means that the upper airway narrows during sleep compared to wakefulness but does not narrow severely. However, the patient with obstructive sleep apnea sustains a severe narrowing and closure on falling asleep, because sleep-induced loss of upper airway activity occurs against the background of an anatomic impairment and the airway narrows more significantly.

Although there is no doubt that sleep induces a decrease in pharyngeal muscle activity in normal subjects and in patients with sleep apnea, the more fundamental question regarding the pathogenesis of obstructive sleep apnea is whether this decrease in motor output constitutes a key abnormality or whether it occurs against the background of an abnormally narrow passive pharynx, which constitutes the principal pathogenic alteration. Specifically, is the sleep-related decrease in pharyngeal neural activity in patients with obstructive sleep apnea greater than in normal people? One can hypothesize that a sleep-induced reduction in pharyngeal muscle activity is the primary abnormality of obstructive sleep apnea or, alternatively, that a structural abnormality of the pharynx is the principal pathogenic factor, with the sleep-related decrement in pharyngeal dilator muscle activity playing a permissive role in the development of upper airway closure in patients with obstructive sleep apnea. The former can be referred to as the *neural hypothesis* of the pathogenesis of airway occlusion, and the latter can be referred to as the *anatomic hypothesis*.

Neural Hypothesis

Does a sleep-related neuromuscular abnormality contribute to obstructive sleep apnea? There is no evidence at present to indicate the existence of a primary neural abnormality in patients with obstructive sleep apnea, but this may simply reflect our inability to quantify and compare changes from wakefulness to sleep across populations of obstructive sleep apnea patients and normal subjects. Because there is no possibility that anatomic factors can change immediately upon going to sleep, one is driven to the conclusion that essential neuromuscular influences dilating the pharyngeal airway are compromised at sleep onset.

Studies of awake patients with obstructive sleep apnea reveal that the supraglottic resistance is elevated[27] and that the pharyngeal airway lumen is somewhat narrowed.[11,120] These alterations are apparent despite neural compensations that effectively increase the activity of the genioglossus muscle during wakefulness in patients to a level that is higher than that seen in normal subjects.[121,122] This indicates that neuromuscular factors during wakefulness play an important compensatory or protective role in increasing P_{mus} of the pharyngeal muscles by shifting the pressure-area relationship of the pharynx, as shown in Figure 82–8. Loss of pharyngeal muscle activity at sleep onset decreases P_{mus} and thereby changes the tube law relationship. This induces pharyngeal narrowing, which becomes more severe as intraluminal pressure falls during inspiration. Whether the level of neuromuscular

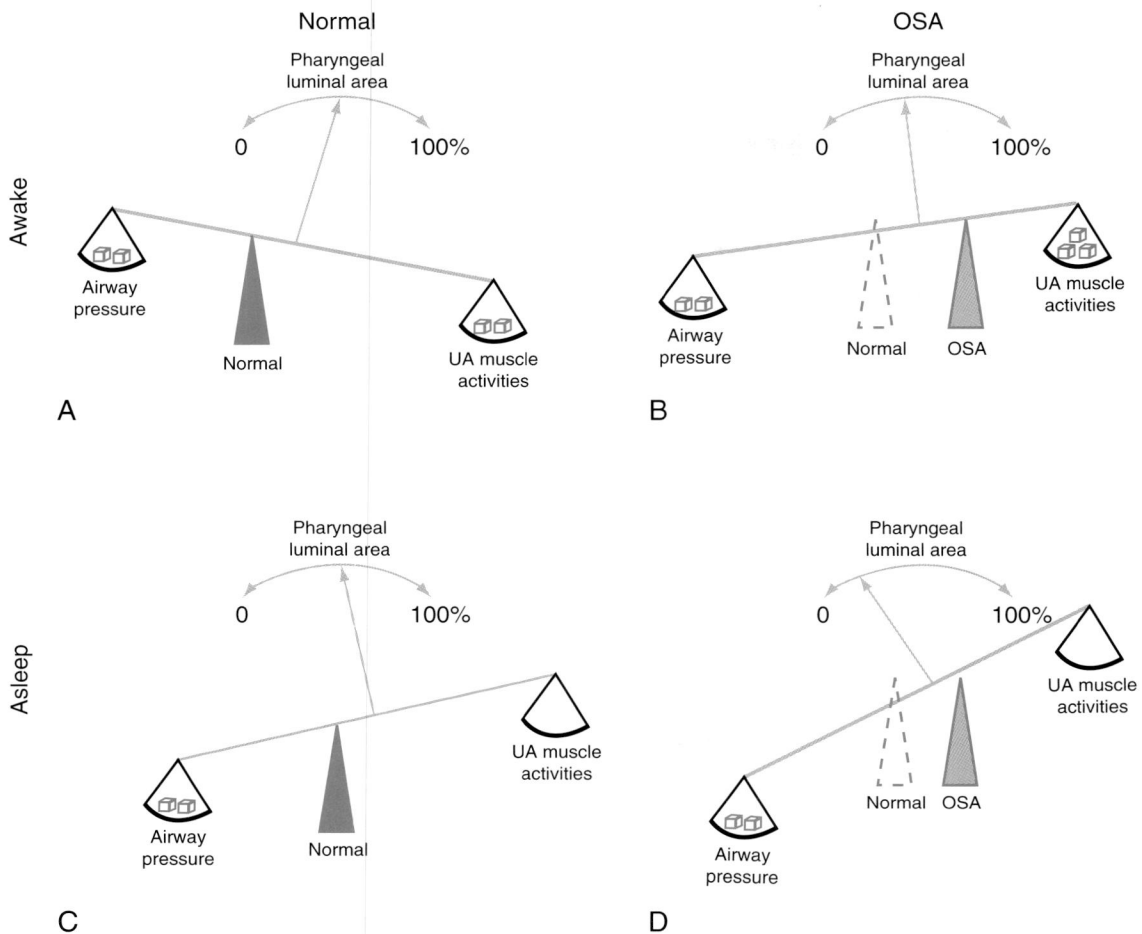

Figure 82–17. Schematic model explaining pharyngeal airway patency, showing upper airway (UA) muscle activities and airway pressure on either side of a fulcrum that represents the intrinsic mechanical properties of the passive upper airway (i.e., upper airway anatomy). The fulcrum of sleep apneic subjects (**B** and **D**) is suggested to be to the right side of normal subjects (**A** and **C**). OSA, obstructive sleep apnea. (From Isono S, Remmers JE, Tanaka A, et al: Anatomy of pharynx in patients with obstructive sleep apnea and in normal subjects. J Appl Physiol. 1997;82: 1319-1326.)

activation during sleep in obstructive sleep apnea patients is abnormally reduced as a reflection of a primary abnormality or whether it reflects a normal sleep-related loss of function remains a question at issue.

Even if there is no fundamental abnormality of upper airway muscle activation during sleep in patients with obstructive sleep apnea, it is possible that such a reduction may occur secondarily as a result of the disease process. Evidence implicates the nervous system as a secondary contributor in the pathogenesis of obstructive sleep apnea. These findings reveal a compromise in the response of the genioglossus to increases in the hypercapnic stimulus in normal subjects following sleep deprivation.[123] The sleep fragmentation associated with obstructive sleep apnea might produce a similar reduction in motor output to pharyngeal muscles, thereby further reducing P_{mus} during sleep and exacerbating the disorder.

Anatomic Hypothesis

As detailed throughout this chapter, there is now strong evidence supporting the anatomic hypothesis. This evidence

principally takes the form of observations that obstructive sleep apnea is associated with enlargement of the tongue, lateral pharyngeal walls, tonsils, and total soft tissue as well as with obesity and craniofacial abnormalities.[46,77] Sleep apnea improves with weight loss, tonsillectomy, or correction of the craniofacial abnormalities, indicating that these abnormalities play a role in initiating or perpetuating the disorder.

Isono and colleagues[124] have supplied more direct evidence, showing that patients with sleep-disordered breathing had a higher closing pressure than did normal subjects. These results provide additional evidence for the anatomic hypothesis, indicating that independent of neuromuscular factors, structural abnormalities contribute importantly to the pathogenesis of sleep-disordered breathing.

In addition, Schwab and coworkers[46] recently demonstrated that the volume of the tongue, lateral pharyngeal walls, and total soft tissue were larger in apneic subjects than in normal subjects and that volumetric enlargement of these structures significantly increased the risk for obstructive sleep apnea. Thus, abnormalities in upper airway anatomy are clearly important in the pathogenesis of sleep apnea.

Clinical Pearls

Enlargement of the upper airway soft tissue structures or abnormality of skeletal structures are important risk factors for obstructive sleep apnea. In obstructive sleep apnea, the location of upper airway closure is usually in the oropharynx (either retropalatal or retroglossal regions), and there are often multiple sites of pharyngeal airway closure in these patients with sleep apnea. Pharyngeal airway patency is maintained by a balance between the action of the upper airway dilator muscles and negative intraluminal pressure. Abnormal upper airway anatomy and possible abnormal neural control during sleep can lead to pharyngeal airway collapse in patients with obstructive sleep apnea.

REFERENCES

1. Horner RL, Shea SA, McIvor J, Guz A: Pharyngeal size and shape during wakefulness and sleep in patients with obstructive sleep apnoea. Q J Med 1989;72:719-735.
2. Schwab RJ, Goldberg AN: Upper airway assessment: Radiographic and other imaging techniques. Otolaryngol Clin North Am 1998;31:931-968.
3. Suto Y, Matsuo T, Kato T, et al: Evaluation of the pharyngeal airway in patients with sleep apnea: Value of ultrafast MR imaging. AJR Am J Roentgenol 1993;160:311-314.
4. Isono S, Morrison DL, Launois SH, et al: Static mechanics of the velopharynx of patients with obstructive sleep apnea. J Appl Physiol 1993;75:148-154.
5. Issa FG, Sullivan CE: Upper airway closing pressures in snorers. J Appl Physiol 1984;57:528-535.
6. Issa FG, Sullivan CE: Upper airway closing pressures in obstructive sleep apnea. J Appl Physiol 1984;57:520-527.
7. Strohl KP, Redline S: Nasal CPAP therapy, upper airway muscle activation, and obstructive sleep apnea. Am Rev Respir Dis 1986;134:555-558.
8. Roberts JL, Reed WR, Mathew OP, et al: Assessment of pharyngeal airway stability in normal and micrognathic infants. J Appl Physiol 1985;58:290-299.
9. Safar P, Escarraga LA, Chang F: Upper airway obstruction in the unconscious patient. J Appl Physiol 1959;14:760-764.
10. Morikawa S, Safar P, DeCarlo J: Influence of head-jaw position upon upper airway patency. Anesthesiology 1981;22:265-270.
11. Hoffstein V, Zamel N, Phillipson EA: Lung volume dependence of pharyngeal cross-sectional area in patients with obstructive sleep apnea. Am Rev Respir Dis 1984;130:175-178.
12. Rowley JA, Permutt S, Willey S, et al: Effect of tracheal and tongue displacement on upper ariway airflow dynamics. J Appl Physiol 1996;80:2171-2178.
13. Thut DC, Schwartz AR, Roach D, et al: Tracheal and neck position influence upper airway airflow dynamics by altering airway length. J Appl Physiol 1993;75:2084-2090.
14. Van de Graaff WB: Thoracic influence on upper airway patency. J Appl Physiol 1988;65:2124-2131.
15. Smith PL, Wise RA, Gold AR, et al: Upper airway pressure-flow relationships in obstructive sleep apnea. J Appl Physiol 1988;64:789-795.
16. Schwartz AR, Smith PL, Wise RA, et al: Induction of upper airway occlusion in sleeping individuals with subatmospheric nasal pressure. J Appl Physiol 1988;64:535-542.
17. Isono S, Feroah TR, Hajduk EA, et al: Interaction of cross-sectional area, driving pressure, and airflow of passive velopharynx. J Appl Physiol 1997;83:851-859.
18. Series F: Upper airway muscles awake and asleep. Sleep Med Rev 2002;6:229-242.
19. Launois SH, Feroah TR, Campbell WN, et al: Site of pharyngeal narrowing predicts outcome of surgery for obstructive sleep apnea. Am Rev Respir Dis 1993;147:182-189.
20. Van de Graaff WB, Gottfried SB, Mitra J, et al: Respiratory function of the hyoid muscles and hyoid arch. J Appl Physiol 1984;57:197-204.
21. Fregosi RF, Fuller DD: Respiratory-related control of extrinsic tongue muscle activity. Respir Physiol 1997;110:295-306.
22. Fuller DD, Mateika JH, Fregosi RF: Co-activation of tongue protrudor and retractor muscles during chemotherapy stimulation in the rat. J Physiol (Lond) 1998;507:265-276.
23. Kuna ST, Vanoye CR: Mechanical effects of pharyngeal constrictor activation on pharyngeal airway function. J Appl Physiol 1999;86:411-417.
24. Kuna ST, Brennick MJ: Effects of pharyngeal muscle activation on airway pressure-area relationships. Am J Respir Crit Care Med 2002;166:972-977.
25. Hudgel DW, Harasick T: Fluctuation in timing of upper airway and chest wall inspiratory muscle activity in obstructive sleep apnea. J Appl Physiol 1990;69:443-450.
26. Ayappa I, Rapoport DM: The upper airway in sleep: Physiology of the pharynx. Sleep Med Rev 2003;7:9-33.
27. Anch AM, Remmers JE, Bunce H: Supraglottic airway resistance in normal subjects and patients with occlusive sleep apnea. J Appl Physiol 1982;53:1158-1163.
28. Tangel DJ, Mezzanotte WS, White DP: The influence of sleep on tensor palatini EMG and upper airway resistance in normal subjects. J Appl Physiol 1991;70:2574-2581.
29. Anch AM, Remmers JE, Sauerland EK, deGroot WJ: Oropharyngeal patency during waking and sleep in the pickwickian syndrome: Electromyographic activity of the tensor veli palatini. Electromyogr Clin Neurophysiol 1981;21:317-330.
30. Tangel DJ, Mezzanotte WS, Sandberg EJ, White DP: Influences of NREM sleep on the activity of tonic versus inspiratory phasic muscles in normal men. J Appl Physiol 1992;73:1058-1066.
31. Pack AI: Changes in respiratory motor activity during rapid eye movement sleep. In Dempsey JA, Pack AI (eds): Regulation of Breathing. New York, Marcel Dekker, 1995, pp 983-1010.
32. Wiegand L, Zwillich CW, Wiegand D, White DP: Changes in upper airway muscle activation and ventilation during phasic REM sleep in normal men. J Appl Physiol 1991;71:488-497.
33. Kuna ST: Inhibition of inspiratory upper airway motoneuron activity by phasic feedback. J Appl Physiol 1986;60:1373-1379.
34. van Lunteren E, Strohl KP, Parker DM, et al: Phasic volume-related feedback on upper airway muscle activity. J Appl Physiol 1984;56:730-736.
35. van Lunteren E, Van de Graaff WB, Parker DM, et al: Nasal and laryngeal reflex responses to negative upper airway pressure. J Appl Physiol 1984;56:746-752.
36. Mathew OP: Upper airway negative-pressure effects on respiratory activity of upper airway muscles. J Appl Physiol 1984;56:500-505.
37. Mathew OP, Abu-Osba YK, Thach BT: Influence of upper airway pressure changes on genioglossus muscle respiratory activity. J Appl Physiol 1982;52:438-444.
38. Horner RL, Innes JA, Holden HB, Guz A: Afferent pathways for pharyngeal dilator reflex to negative pressure in man: A study using upper airway anesthesia. J Physiol (Lond) 1991;436:31-44.
39. Hwang JC, St. John WM, Bartlett D Jr: Respiratory-related hypoglossal nerve activity: Influence of anesthetics. J Appl Physiol 1983;55:785-792.
40. Thach BT, Schefft GL, Pickens DL, Menon AP: Influence of upper airway negative pressure reflex on response to airway occlusion in sleeping infants. J Appl Physiol 1989;67:749-755.
41. Onal E, Lopata M, O'Connor T: Diaphragmatic and genioglossal electromyogram responses to isocapnic hypoxia in humans. Am Rev Respir Dis 1981;124:215-217.
42. Weiner D, Mitra J, Salamone J, Cherniack NS: Effect of chemical stimuli on nerves supplying upper airway muscles. J Appl Physiol 1982;52:530-536.
43. Schwab RJ, Gupta KB, Gefter WB, et al: Upper airway and soft tissue anatomy in normal subjects and patients with

sleep-disordered breathing. Significance of the lateral pharyngeal walls. Am J Respir Crit Care Med 1995;152(5 Pt 1):1673-1689.

44. Kuna ST, Bedi DG, Ryckman C: Effect of nasal airway positive pressure on upper airway size and configuration. Am Rev Respir Dis 1988;138:969-975.

45. Schwab RJ, Gefter WB, Pack AI, Hoffman EA: Dynamic imaging of the upper airway during respiration in normal subjects. J Appl Physiol 1993;74:1504-1514.

46. Schwab RJ, Pasirstein M, Pierson R, et al: Identification of upper airway anatomic risk factors for obstructive sleep apnea with volumetric MRI. Am J Respir Crit Care Med 2003;168:522-530.

47. Schwab RJ: Pro: Sleep apnea is an anatomic disorder. Am J Respir Crit Care Med 2003;168:270-271; discussion 273.

48. Ciscar MA, Juan G, Martinez V, et al: Magnetic resonance imaging of the pharynx in OSA patients and healthy subjects. Eur Respir J 2001;17:79-86.

49. Schwab RJ, Gefter WB, Hoffman EA, et al: Dynamic upper airway imaging during awake respiration in normal subjects and patients with sleep disordered breathing. Am Rev Respir Dis 1993;148:1385-1400.

50. Shepard JW, Jr., Thawley SE: Evaluation of the upper airway by computerized tomography in patients undergoing uvulopalato-pharyngoplasty for obstructive sleep apnea. Am Rev Respir Dis 1989;140:711-716.

51. Bacon WH, Turlot JC, Krieger J, Stierle JL: Cephalometric evaluation of pharyngeal obstructive factors in patients with sleep apnea syndrome. Angle Orthod 1990;60:115-122.

52. deBerry-Borowiecki B, Kukwa A, Blanks RH: Cephalometric analysis for diagnosis and treatment of obstructive sleep apnea. Laryngoscope 1988;98:226-234.

53. Lowe AA, Fleetham JA, Adachi S, Ryan CF: Cephalometric and computed tomographic predictors of obstructive sleep apnea severity. Am J Orthod Dentofacial Orthop 1995;107:589-595.

54. Pracharktam N, Hans MG, Strohl KP, Redline S: Upright and supine cephalometric evaluation of obstructive sleep apnea syndrome and snoring subjects. Angle Orthod 1994;64:63-73.

55. Miles PG, Vig PS, Weyant RJ, et al: Craniofacial structure and obstructive sleep apnea syndrome—a qualitative analysis and meta-analysis of the literature. Am J Orthod Dentofacial Orthop 1996;109:163-172.

56. Ryan CF, Lowe AA, Li D, Fleetham JA: Three-dimensional upper airway computed tomography in obstructive sleep apnea. A prospective study in patients treated by uvulopalatopharyngo-plasty. Am Rev Respir Dis 1991;144:428-432.

57. Caballero P, Alvarez-Sala R, Garcia-Rio F, et al: CT in the evaluation of the upper airway in healthy subjects and in patients with obstructive sleep apnea syndrome. Chest 1998;11:111-116.

58. Do KL, Ferreyra H, Healy JF, Davidson TM: Does tongue size differ between patients with and without sleep-disordered breathing? Laryngoscope 2000;110:1552-1555.

59. Schwab RJ: Upper airway imaging. Clin Chest Med 1998;19:33-54.

60. Schotland HM, Insko EK, Schwab RJ: Quantitative magnetic resonance imaging demonstrates alterations of the lingual musculature in obstructive sleep apnea. Sleep 1999;22:605-613.

61. Schwartz AR, Gold AR, Schubert N, et al: Effect of weight loss on upper airway collapsibility in obstructive sleep apnea. Am Rev Respir Dis 1991;144(3 Pt 1):494-498.

62. Bliwise DL, Feldman DE, Bliwise NG, et al: Risk factors for sleep disordered breathing in heterogeneous geriatric populations. J Am Geriatr Soc 1987;35:132-141.

63. Young T, Palta M, Dempsey J, et al: The occurrence of sleep-disordered breathing among middle-aged adults. N Engl J Med 1993;328:1230-1235.

64. Davies RJ, Ali NJ, Stradling JR: Neck circumference and other clinical features in the diagnosis of the obstructive sleep apnoea syndrome. Thorax 1992;47:101-105.

65. Horner RL, Mohiaddin RH, Lowell DG, et al: Sites and sizes of fat deposits around the pharynx in obese patients with obstructive

sleep apnoea and weight matched controls. Eur Respir J 1989;2:613-622.

66. Mortimore IL, Marshall I, Wraith PK, et al: Neck and total body fat deposition in nonobese and obese patients with sleep apnea compared with that in control subjects. Am J Respir Crit Care Med 1998;157:280-283.

67. Shelton KE, Gay SB, Hollowell DE, et al: Mandible enclosure of upper airway and weight in obstructive sleep apnea. Am Rev Respir Dis 1993;148:195-200.

68. Shelton KE, Woodson H, Gay S, Suratt PM: Pharyngeal fat in obstructive sleep apnea. Am Rev Respir Dis 1993;148:462-466.

69. Stauffer JL, Buick MK, Bixler EO, et al: Morphology of the uvula in obstructive sleep apnea. Am Rev Respir Dis 1989;140:724-728.

70. Zohar Y, Sabo R, Strauss M, et al: Oropharyngeal fatty infiltration in obstructive sleep apnea patients: A histologic study. Ann Otol Rhinol Laryngol 1998;107:170-174.

71. Hill JO, Sparling PB, Shields TW, Heller PA: Effects of exercise and food restriction on body composition and metabolic rate in obese women. Am J Clin Nutr 1987;46:622-630.

72. Wadden TA, Foster GD, Letizia KA, Mullen JL: Long-term effects of dieting on resting metabolic rate in obese outpatients. JAMA 1990;264:707-711.

73. Foster GD, Wadden TA, Mullen JL, et al: Resting energy expenditure, body composition, and excess weight in the obese. Metabolism 1988;37:467-472.

74. Series F, Cote C, Simoneau JA, et al: Physiologic, metabolic, and muscle fiber type characteristics of musculus uvulae in sleep apnea hypopnea syndrome and in snorers. J Clin Invest 1995;95:20-25.

75. Welch KC, Foster GD, Ritter CT, et al: A novel volumetric magnetic resonance imaging paradigm to study upper airway anatomy. Sleep 2002;25:532-542.

76. Strobel RJ, Rosen RC: Obesity and weight loss in obstructive sleep apnea: A critical review. Sleep 1996;19:104-115.

77. Schwab RJ: Imaging for the snoring and sleep apnea patient. Dent Clin North Am 2001;45:759-796.

78. Carrera M, Barbe F, Sauleda J, et al: Patients with obstructive sleep apnea exhibit genioglossus dysfunction that is normalized after treatment with continuous positive airway pressure. Am J Respir Crit Care Med 1999;159:1960-1966.

79. Friberg D, Ansved T, Borg K, et al: Histological indications of a progressive snorer's disease in an upper airway muscle. Am J Respir Crit Care Med 1998;157:586-593.

80. Brooks LJ, Strohl KP: Size and mechanical properties of the pharynx in healthy men and women. Am Rev Respir Dis 1992;146:1394-1397.

81. Brown IG, Zamel N, Hoffstein V: Pharyngeal cross-sectional area in normal men and women. J Appl Physiol 1986;61:890-895.

82. Guilleminault C, Partinen M, Hollman K, et al: Familial aggregates in obstructive sleep apnea syndrome. Chest 1995;107:1545-1551.

83. Legato MJ: Gender-specific aspects of obesity. Int J Fertil Womens Med 1997;42:184-197.

84. Millman RP, Carlisle CC, McGarvey ST, et al: Body fat distribution and sleep apnea severity in women. Chest 1995;107: 362-366.

85. Whittle AT, Marshall I, Mortimore IL, et al: Neck soft tissue and fat distribution: Comparison between normal men and women by magnetic resonance imaging. Thorax 1999;54:323-328.

86. Malhotra A, Huang Y, Fogel RB, et al: The male predisposition to pharyngeal collapse: Importance of airway length. Am J Respir Crit Care Med 2002;166:1388-1395.

87. Mathur R, Douglas NJ: Family studies in patients with the sleep apnea-hypopnea syndrome. Ann Intern Med 1995;122:174-178.

88. Marcus CL, Keens TG, Bautista DB, et al: Obstructive sleep apnea in children with Down syndrome. Pediatrics 1991;88: 132-139.

89. Burger CD, Stanson AW, Daniels BK, et al: Fast-CT evaluation of the effect of lung volume on upper airway size and function in normal men. Am Rev Respir Dis 1992;146:335-339.

90. Burger CD, Stanson AW, Daniels BK, et al: Fast-computed tomographic evaluation of the effect of route of breathing on upper airway size and function in normal men. Chest 1993; 103:1032-1037.

91. Morrell MJ, Arabi Y, Zahn B, Badr MS: Progressive retropalatal narrowing preceding obstructive apnea. Am J Respir Crit Care Med 1998;158:1974-1981.

92. Shepard JW Jr, Stanson AW, Sheedy PF, Westbrook PR: Fast-CT evaluation of the upper airway during wakefulness in patients with obstructive sleep apnea. In Suratt PM (ed): Proceedings of the First International Symposium on Sleep and Respiration. New York, Alan R. Liss, 1990, pp 273-282.

93. Welch KC, Ritter CT, Gefter WB, Schwab RJ: Dynamic respiratory related upper airway imaging during wakefulness in normal subjects and patients with sleep disordered breathing using MRI. Am J Respir Crit Care Med 1998;157:A54.

94. Suratt PM, Wilhoit SC, Cooper K: Induction of airway collapse with subatmospheric pressure in awake patients with sleep apnea. J Appl Physiol 1984;57:140-146.

95. Sanders MH, Moore SE: Inspiratory and expiratory partitioning of airway resistance during sleep in patients with sleep apnea. Am Rev Respir Dis 1983;127:554-558.

96. Sanders MH, Kern N: Obstructive sleep apnea treated by independently adjusted inspiratory and expiratory positive airway pressures via nasal mask. Physiologic and clinical implications. Chest 1990;98:317-324.

97. Badr MS, Toiber F, Skatrud JB, Dempsey J: Pharyngeal narrowing/occlusion during central sleep apnea. J Appl Physiol 1995; 78:1806-1815.

98. Skatrud JB, Dempsey JA: Airway resistance and respiratory muscle function in snorers during NREM sleep. J Appl Physiol 1985;59:328-335.

99. Stoohs R, Guilleminault C: Snoring during NREM sleep: Respiratory timing, esophageal pressure and EEG arousal. Respir Physiol 1991;85:151-167.

100. Trudo FJ, Gefter WB, Welch KC, et al: State-related changes in upper airway caliber and surrounding soft-tissue structures in normal subjects. Am J Respir Crit Care Med 1998;158:1259-1270.

101. Morrison DL, Launois SH, Isono S, et al: Pharyngeal narrowing and closing pressures in patients with obstructive sleep apnea. Am Rev Respir Dis 1993;148:606-611.

102. Hudgel DW: Palate and hypopharynx—sites of inspiratory narrowing of the upper airway during sleep. Am Rev Respir Dis 1988;138:1542-1547.

103. Weitzman ED, Pollak CP, Borowiecki B, et al: The hypersomnia-sleep apnea syndrome: Site and mechanism of upper airway obstruction. In Guilleminault C, Dement WD (eds): Sleep Apnea Syndromes. New York, Alan R. Liss, 1978, pp 235-248.

104. Smith PL, Gold AR, Meyers DA, et al: Weight loss in mildly to moderately obese patients with obstructive sleep apnea. Ann Intern Med 1985;103(Pt 1):850-855.

105. Wittels EH, Thompson S: Obstructive sleep apnea and obesity. Otolaryngol Clin North Am 1990;23:751-760.

106. Collop NA, Block AJ, Hellard D: The effect of nightly nasal CPAP treatment on underlying obstructive sleep apnea and pharyngeal size. Chest 1991;99:855-860.

107. Ryan CF, Lowe AA, Li D, Fleetham JA: Magnetic resonance imaging of the upper airway in obstructive sleep apnea before and after chronic nasal continuous positive airway pressure therapy. Am Rev Respir Dis 1991;144:939-944.

108. Schmidt-Nowara W, Lowe A, Wiegand L, et al: Oral appliances for the treatment of snoring and obstructive sleep apnea: A review. Sleep 1995;18:501-510.

109. Strollo PJ Jr, Rogers RM: Obstructive sleep apnea. N Engl J Med 1996;334:99-104.

110. Liu Y, Zeng X, Fu M, Huang X, Lowe AA: Effects of a mandibular repositioner on obstructive sleep apnea. Am J Orthod Dentofacial Orthop 2000;118:248-256.

111. Schmidt-Nowara WW, Meade TE, Hays MB: Treatment of snoring and obstructive sleep apnea with a dental orthosis. Chest 1991;99:1378-1385.

112. Bonham PE, Currier GF, Orr WC, et al: The effect of a modified functional appliance on obstructive sleep apnea. Am J Orthod Dentofacial Orthop 1988;94:384-392.

113. Bennett LS, Davies RJ, Stradling JR: Oral appliances for the management of snoring and obstructive sleep apnoea. Thorax 1998;53(Suppl 2):S58-S64.

114. Ryan CF, Love LL, Peat D, et al: Mandibular advancement oral appliance therapy for obstructive sleep apnoea: Effect on awake calibre of the velopharynx. Thorax 1999;54:972-977.

115. Schwab RJ, Goldberg AN, Pack AI: Sleep apnea syndromes. In Fishman AP (ed): Pulmonary Diseases and Disorders, 3rd ed. New York, McGraw-Hill, 1998, pp 1617-1637.

116. Sher AE, Schechtman KB, Piccirillo JF: The efficacy of surgical modifications of the upper airway in adults with obstructive sleep apnea syndrome. Sleep 1996;19:156-177.

117. Schwartz AR, Schubert N, Rothman W, et al: Effect of uvulopalatopharyngoplasty on upper airway collapsibility in obstructive sleep apnea. Am Rev Respir Dis 1992;145:527-532.

118. Langin T, Pepin JL, Pendlebury S, et al: Upper airway changes in snorers and mild sleep apnea sufferers after uvulopalatopharyngoplasty (UPPP). Chest 1998;113:1595-1603.

119. Welch KC, Goldberg AN, Trudo FJ, et al: Upper airway anatomic changes with magnetic resonance imaging in uvulopalatopharyngoplasty patients. Am J Respir Crit Care Med 1997;155:A938.

120. Suratt PM, Dee P, Atkinson RL, et al: Fluoroscopic and computed tomographic features of the pharyngeal airway in obstructive sleep apnea. Am Rev Respir Dis 1983;127:487-492.

121. Mezzanotte WS, Tangel DJ, White DP: Waking genioglossal EMG in sleep apnea patients versus normal controls (a neuromuscular compensatory mechanism). J Clin Invest 1992;89: 1571-1579.

122. Suratt PM, McTier RF, Wilhoit SC: Upper airway muscle activation is augmented in patients with obstructive sleep apnea compared with that in normal subjects. Am Rev Respir Dis 1988;137:889-894.

123. Leiter JC, Knuth SL, Bartlett D Jr: The effect of sleep deprivation on activity of the genioglossus muscle in man. Am Rev Respir Dis 1985;132:1242-1245.

124. Isono S, Remmers JE, Tanaka A, et al: Anatomy of pharynx in patients with obstructive sleep apnea and in normal subjects. J Appl Physiol 1997;82:1319-1326.

83

Snoring and Upper Airway Resistance

Victor Hoffstein

ABSTRACT

Snoring is common, occurring in about 40% of the adult population, although the prevalence varies greatly between studies because of the highly subjective nature of this symptom. Snoring originates in the pharynx when normal physiologic changes in pharyngeal mechanics during sleep become superimposed on underlying pharyngeal abnormalities present during wakefulness. Upper airway narrowing implies increased work of breathing, which may lead to arousals from sleep, resulting in sleep fragmentation, unrefreshing sleep, and daytime neurocognitive dysfunction. This constellation of findings is termed the upper airway resistance syndrome (UARS), and nocturnal polysomnography is required for the diagnosis. The main clinical significance of snoring is that it is a marker of UARS and obstructive sleep apnea. To date, there is no evidence of a causal relationship between snoring and hypertension, coronary artery disease, or cerebrovascular disease. The best way to treat snoring is to modify the risk factors, including obesity and alcohol ingestion; body position training (if applicable in a particular case) is beneficial. If these treatments are not possible or effective, oral appliances and continuous positive airway pressure are the noninvasive treatments of choice. Other treatment modalities including nasal lubricants, other over-the-counter remedies, and nasal dilators, have not been proven effective, although they may improve snoring in individual patients. Pharyngeal surgery (uvulopalatopharyngoplasty, laser-assisted palatoplasty, radiofrequency ablation, and various modifications thereof) has not achieved a high rate of application. However, when carried out by surgeons experienced in treating sleep disordered breathing, these procedures may be effective in some individuals; consequently, surgical assessment of nonapneic snorers is certainly warranted.

Snoring is the most common complaint precipitating a referral to a sleep laboratory. Increased awareness of sleep apnea has resulted in a concern on the part of some snorers that they may have this disorder. Others simply wish to do something about the objectionable noise that disturbs bed partners and others in the sleep environment, and to avoid the social embarrassment caused by snoring (e.g., during travel, while sharing a hotel room, during camping trips).

Prior to the 1970s, snoring was thought to be simply a nuisance. For example, the author of the first authoritative book dealing with sleep[1] concluded that "snoring is harmless to the sleeper, but can be very annoying to others who may be awake at the time, or have been aroused by the loud noises." Beginning in the 1970s, concomitant with the recognition of sleep apnea syndrome, snoring assumed a new importance. It was realized that snoring is almost invariably a symptom of obstructive sleep apnea and in fact may be a precursor to this disorder.[2] Because sleep apnea syndrome was found to be associated with daytime tiredness, sleepiness, poor memory, decreased ability to concentrate, and adverse vascular events such as increased risk of hypertension, strokes, and heart attacks, the question arose as to whether nonapneic snoring might have the same health consequences. Early studies[3] indicated that snoring may be an independent risk factor for hypertension, and that even trivial snoring might be the first step in the continuum, termed *heavy snorer's disease,*[2] eventually leading to full-blown sleep apnea syndrome. Although this orderly progression from normal breathing to snoring and then on to sleep apnea is an attractive and plausible hypothesis, there is no convincing evidence that this is the case. In fact, more than 40% of habitual snorers reported resolution rather than worsening of their snoring when asked about it 10 years later.[4]

In the 1990s, snoring was linked to another possible adverse health effect when it was demonstrated[5] that elevated upper airway resistance during sleep (which occurs during snoring) may lead to arousals and sleep fragmentation. The term *upper airway resistance syndrome* (UARS) was coined to describe tired and sleepy nonapneic patients, many of whom are heavy snorers. There is continuing debate over whether this entity constitutes a separate disease, whether it is part of the spectrum of sleep-disordered breathing, and whether there is a relationship between the severity of sleep-disordered breathing and adverse health effects. One consequence of this debate is a shift in the attitude of some clinicians toward objectively investigating complaints related to snoring, with more liberal use of nocturnal polysomnography in habitual snorers.

This chapter is a review of the pathophysiology, clinical features, diagnostic evaluation, and management of snoring. As much as possible, the discussion and recommendations are based on evidence obtained from studies of nonapneic snorers. Such evidence is not always available, because most investigations have not clearly differentiated apneic from nonapneic snorers in the study populations. Many studies are also limited by the lack of nonsnoring controls, which further complicates the attribution of pathology to snoring alone.

DEFINITIONS

The *Random House Dictionary of the English Language* defines snoring as "breathing during sleep with hoarse or harsh sounds as caused by the vibration of the soft palate." The *New Webster's Dictionary* gives an almost identical definition, with the sole qualifier that the harsh breathing is "through the open mouth and the nose when asleep." Both definitions imply something about the pathogenesis—namely, that snoring is produced by the vibrating soft tissues. Page 195 of the

International Classification of Sleep Disorders manual defines *primary snoring* (ICSD 780.53-1) as "loud upper airway breathing sounds in sleep, without episodes of apnea or hypoventilation."[6] No matter which definition of snoring is adopted, it is essential to remember that snoring is a subjective impression on the part of the listener. The subjectivity with which patients and bed partners characterize snoring is a difficult issue that must be taken into account when analyzing, interpreting, and applying the results of investigations dealing with snoring.

PATHOPHYSIOLOGY AND MEASUREMENT OF SNORING

Snoring is a sound produced by the vibrating structures of the upper airway. It is not caused by a local abnormality within the airway (e.g., the soft palate or uvula). Endoscopic observation of the upper airway in snoring patients during natural or induced sleep demonstrates that any membranous part of the upper airway that lacks cartilaginous support may vibrate. This includes the soft palate, uvula, faucial pillars, pharyngeal walls, and the rest of the upper airway, almost to the level of the vocal cords. It is this diffuse, rather than local, involvement of the upper airway that makes successful treatment of snoring difficult, particularly when techniques directed only to a local modification of the airway segment are employed.

Several theoretical models of the human upper airway have been developed[7-9] (see Chapter 82). These models include the effects of airway wall compliance, gas density, and airway dimensions on the pressure–flow relationships. They predict that, depending on pharyngeal mechanical properties of the pharynx, the walls of the upper airway may be stable (normal breathing), may exhibit vibration or fluttering (snoring), or may narrow or collapse completely (obstructive hypopnea or apnea, respectively). Some predictions have been verified experimentally. For example, it is well known that alcohol ingestion, which reduces pharyngeal dilator muscle tone and increases airway wall compliance (making the pharynx more "floppy"), promotes snoring. On the other hand, breathing lower-density gas mixtures (e.g., helium plus oxygen) reduces snoring because airflow is less turbulent, the pressure–flow relationship in the pharynx is altered favorably, and the wall vibrations are reduced or completely eliminated.

Snoring is usually an inspiratory sound, but it may also be present during expiration. It occurs in all sleep stages, although it may be more common in stages 2, 3, and 4. The sound of snoring can be analyzed (by spectral analysis) to determine its frequency components. The *power spectrum* describes how much power is contributed by each constituent frequency component. Because snoring may be generated at several sites along the airway, sometimes at multiple sites simultaneously, the power spectrum of snoring is wide, encompassing a range of frequencies up to 10,000 Hz. The spectral characteristics of snoring sounds are influenced by the route of breathing, sleep stage, whether the sleep is natural or induced, posture, weight, airway wall mass and elasticity, and other factors affecting the upper airway. To what extent each factor is responsible for the power spectrum of snoring sound is not known; our current state of knowledge does not allow us to work backward—that is, to use the measured power spectrum of snoring sound to determine the segment of the airway most responsible for producing the sound.

Clearly, such information would be diagnostically and therapeutically useful. To be able to measure, analyze, and quantify snoring would allow us to determine the site of sound generation and to study the relationship between snoring and adverse health outcomes. The effects of treatments could be evaluated in a more objective and consistent fashion.

Several different techniques for measuring and quantifying snoring have been described.[10] Unlike apneas, there is no uniformly accepted way to conduct this measurement. A standard method to measure the mechanics of snoring, which would include mechanical calibration of the microphone against a known sound source, standardized positioning of the microphone relative to the upper airway, and a biologic calibration, is needed. Until such a method is developed, a combination of objective sound measurements and subjective assessment using currently available questionnaires should be used to characterize snoring. Because recorded sound must be perceived by a listener to be identified as snoring rather than simply background noise (e.g., heavy breathing, wheezing, or other noises), it is necessary to define physical cutoffs for amplitude and frequency to separate snores from other noises.

EPIDEMIOLOGY AND PREVALENCE OF SNORING

It is recognized that snoring is common, but estimates of its prevalence in different populations vary widely (Table 83–1). The prevalence of snoring ranges from 5% to 86% in men, and from 2% to 57% in women. To a large degree, these differences depend on the methods used. Snoring, being a perception of the listener, may be reported differently depending on who answers the question (the snorer or the bed partner), how the question is phrased, and whether the bed partner is present during the interview. In addition, snoring (or absence thereof) assessed during sleep in the sleep laboratory may not be representative of that which occurs during sleep at home. In one study, 15% of self-confessed snorers did not snore at all when studied in the sleep laboratory. On the other hand, 15% of those who said they never snore actually snored for at least 50% of the night. Overall, correlation between self-reported and measured snoring is poor. On the basis of the more rigorous studies conducted in the United States, the prevalence of snoring in the adult population is between 30% and 40%.

Male predominance, observed in all epidemiologic studies, remains unexplained. Sex differences in the prevalence of sleep apnea and its symptoms have received much attention in the last several years. Possible contributing factors (summarized in a recent review[11]) include differences in perception of snoring between men and women, differences in hormonal factors, and differences in pharyngeal anatomy and function.

The apparent reduction in snoring with age, observed in some studies, is probably related to several factors, such as the loss of a bed partner, altered perception of snoring, survival bias, or methodologic problems.

Finally, clinical observations suggest that genetic factors (see Chapter 84), including factors such as obesity, play a role in snoring. The family history of patients presenting to the sleep clinic because of snoring and suspected sleep apnea frequently includes at least one other family member (parent or sibling) with a similar problem. Although the evidence is in its early stages, it justifies inquiring about the family history of

Table 83–1. Prevalence of Snoring*

Study	Country	N	Prevalence (%) Men	Prevalence (%) Women
Lugaresi et al. (1980)[3]	Italy	5713	40	28
Norton 1983	Canada	279	86	57
Mondini 1983	Italy	1898	24	14
Koskenvuo 1985	Finland	7511	9	4
Norton 1985	Canada	2001	71	51
Stradling 1990	United Kingdom	890	10	—
Wiggins 1990	United States	360	34	18
Bliwise 1991	United States	1409	40	15
Young 1993	United States	1255	44	28
Bearpark 1995	Australia	294	10	—
Olson 1995	Australia	441	52 (both genders)	
Janson 1995	Sweden, Iceland, Belgium	2202	5	2-3
Marin 1997	Spain	1222	64	36
Ohayon 1997	United Kingdom	4972	48	34
Stoohs 1998	United States	289	6-32	—
Neven 1998	Netherlands	2182	39	20
Ng 1998	Singapore	2298	7 (both genders)	
Keenan 1998	Canada	437	27	—
Hui 1999	Hong Kong	1910	26 (both genders; students)	
Ferini-Strambi 1999	Italy	750	—	20
Zamarron 1999	Spain	1414	40 (both genders)	
Zielinski 1999	Poland	1186	48	27
Kayukawa 2000	Japan	6445	16	7
Ip 2001	Hong Kong	773	23	—
Duran 2001	Spain	2148	46	25
Kim 2001	Korea	640	35 (both genders)	
Teculescu 2001	France	299	32	—
Bednarek 2001	Poland	1186	78	59
Hui 2002	Hong Kong	216	37 (both genders; bus drivers)	
Young 2002	United States	5615	34 (both genders; habitual snorers only)	
Larsson 2003	Sweden	4648	18	7
Tishler 2003	United States	754	42 (both genders)	
Shin 2003	Korea	3871	12.4 (boys)	8.5 (girls)
Udwadia 2004	India	658	26	—
Ip 2004	Hong Kong	854	—	15
Liu 2004	Taiwan	1252	57	37
Ersu 2004	Turkey	2147	9 (boys)	6 (girls)

*References for the studies in the table are at the end of the reference list in alphabetical order by author.

snoring in all patients who are being assessed for sleep-related breathing disorders.

HEALTH EFFECTS OF SNORING

Is snoring associated with adverse health outcomes? Isolated studies suggest that snoring may be a risk factor for some common medical conditions (e.g., type II diabetes, headaches). However, because snoring is common, it is possible that the relationship is simply coincidental rather than causal, and evidence for a causal linkage between snoring and these disorders is weak. The two most common adverse health effects that are believed to be causally linked to snoring are daytime dysfunction and cardiovascular disease.

Snoring and Upper Airway Resistance Syndrome

The most interesting and controversial development in the debate regarding health effects of snoring is the description of the upper airway resistance syndrome (UARS) by Guilleminault et al.[5] to characterize tired and sleepy patients whose polysomnography reveals fragmented sleep without sleep apnea. Although snoring is not a prerequisite for this syndrome, the presence of snoring implies an elevated upper airway resistance. This is why, in current clinical practice, the term UARS is used to diagnose tired and sleepy snorers whose polysomnography shows nonapneic sleep fragmentation.

Is UARS a distinct entity or simply a mild form of sleep apnea syndrome?[12,13] The current view is that UARS represents an intermediate point on the continuum of sleep-disordered breathing, between nonsnoring, nonapneic, asymptomatic subjects at one end and tired sleepy snorers with severe sleep apnea at the other end. Changes in pharyngeal mechanics mirror this clinical continuum: pharyngeal properties in patients with UARS are intermediate between those with sleep apnea and normal nonapneic controls.[14] In the International Classification of Sleep Disorders, UARS is not listed as a separate entity but as an alternate name for "obstructive sleep apnea, adult."[14a]

The debate regarding the existence of UARS helped to direct attention to respiratory events other than apneas and hypopneas that fragment sleep and may therefore lead to daytime symptoms. During these events, the inspiratory flow is reduced, although not enough to satisfy the definition of hypopnea.[15] In addition, as the respiratory effort increases, so does the upper airway resistance, and as a result the flow remains constant—that is, limited. These episodes of flow limitation are frequently terminated by an arousal, called respiratory effort–related arousal,[16] after which there is reduction in upper airway resistance and resumption of stable airflow and pressure.

Sleep fragmentation resulting from the respiratory effort–related arousals may lead to the same adverse consequences as conventional apneas and hypopneas. The *respiratory disturbance index* (RDI) describes all of the abnormal respiratory events during sleep—apneas, hypopneas, and episodes of airflow limitation. The importance of respiratory effort–related arousals in the pathogenesis of UARS has been emphasized by a task force of the American Academy of Sleep Medicine (AASM).[17]

Nonapneic snoring is not synonymous with UARS. Although snoring implies elevated upper airway resistance, it does not automatically imply sleep fragmentation. Termination of snoring is not always associated with arousals, at least when a conventional definition of arousals is used. However, there is evidence that nonapneic snoring *is* associated with daytime dysfunction. Nonsnorers with an RDI of less than 15 participating in the Sleep Heart Health Study[18] scored 6.7 on the Epworth Sleepiness Scale, compared with 8.9 in nightly snorers with the same RDI. Self-confessed snorers who complained of excessive sleepiness had approximately twice the risk of having an occupational accident during the following 10 years compared to nonsleepy snorers or sleepy nonsnorers[19]; however, sleep apnea was not ruled out in that population. There appears to be a direct relationship between neuropsychiatric deficits and severity of sleep-disordered breathing, implying that even those with an apnea-hypopnea index (AHI) of less than 10 can be at risk for daytime dysfunction.

The most compelling argument in favor of UARS would be demonstration that elimination of snoring (e.g., by continuous positive airway pressure [CPAP]) decreases arousals and reduces symptoms, but this contention cannot be fully supported at this time. Such evidence would support a causal relationship between snoring and daytime dysfunction, and when present in clinical circumstances, would establish the diagnosis of UARS in individual patients. However, most nonapneic snorers tolerate CPAP poorly and their compliance with treatment is low. When these patients are seen in follow-up, side effects of CPAP assume such a prominent role that it is difficult for the treating physician to decide whether the treatment was beneficial but poorly tolerated, or whether it was of no benefit at all. Objective measures of daytime function are also difficult to quantify. Recent randomized controlled trials[20,21] of CPAP versus placebo in patients with mild sleep apnea (mean AHI of 13), which can almost be considered UARS, showed that CPAP improved snoring and some subjective symptoms but failed to improve multiple sleep latency test scores, Epworth Sleepiness Scale scores, and scores on other questionnaires dealing with daytime function. Patients with UARS seem to perceive their symptoms differently from those with obstructive sleep apnea syndrome (OSAS): they have more functional somatic complaints (insomnia, headaches, irritable bowel, bruxism) than patients with sleep apnea.[22] Whether increased upper airway resistance during sleep and/or snoring is responsible for these complaints has not been investigated.

Given the evidence to date, UARS should be accepted as different from sleep apnea syndrome as currently defined, and the diagnosis of UARS should be considered in nonapneic (AHI less than 10) snorers with daytime symptoms and sleep fragmentation (arousal index greater than 10).

Because the AHI, pharyngeal mechanics, and clinical presentation form a continuum from UARS to OSAS, perhaps this continuum should be extended by defining the sleep-disordered breathing syndrome (SDBS), which would include asymptomatic nonapneic snorers, UARS, and OSAS.

Snoring and Cardiovascular Disease

Lugaresi and colleagues[23] raised the possibility that snoring and cardiovascular disease are related when they demonstrated that episodes of snoring are associated with acute simultaneous elevations of blood pressure. In addition, some snorers do not exhibit the normal reduction of blood pressure during sleep. Thus, it is possible that transient nocturnal abnormalities in blood pressure control may carry over into wakefulness and lead to hypertension. However, this hypothesis is still unproven.

Several studies appearing since the start of the new millennium have examined the relationship between sleep-disordered breathing and blood pressure. Although none of them specifically address the issue of snoring and hypertension, they all include nonapneic subjects (AHI less than 10) and some provide information about snoring status. One study[24] of 1741 community dwellers, all of whom had nocturnal polysomnography and measurements of blood pressure, found that nonapneic snoring was weakly but independently associated with hypertension—the odds ratio was 1.6 (confidence interval, 1.09-2.20).

Two large studies address the issue of sleep-disordered breathing and hypertension—the Sleep Heart Health Study[25] and the Wisconsin Sleep Cohort Study.[26] The former is a cross-sectional study involving over 6000 participants, and the latter is a longitudinal study of over 700 participants followed for 4 years. Differences in study design, sample size, ethnic mix, age, recording of snoring, and definition of hypopnea make it difficult to compare the results. In the Sleep Heart Health Study, no significant association between self-reported snoring and hypertension was found. In the Wisconsin Sleep Cohort Study, participants with an AHI of less than 5 at baseline had an approximately 40% chance of developing hypertension after 4 years; however, snoring status of these subjects either at baseline or at follow-up was not given. The evidence to date is insufficient to conclude that snoring is a risk factor for hypertension.

What is the relationship between nonapneic snoring and cardiovascular or cerebrovascular disease? The evidence here is even weaker than for hypertension. Several epidemiologic and case-control studies indicate that odds ratios for cardiovascular and cerebrovascular events are higher in snorers than in nonsnorers. However, all of them suffer from a number of limitations, which necessitate a cautious interpretation of the results.

The limitations include absence of sleep study data, lack of proper study groups (nonapneic snorers versus nonapneic nonsnorers), inadequate treatment of the confounders, and selection bias. The Sleep Heart Health Study, designed to overcome some of the these limitations, probably does not support the association between snoring and cardiovascular disease. Although there was no separate analysis for snoring, the data for nonapneic subjects (AHI less than 11) reveal no significantly higher risk of cardiovascular disease (odds ratio, 1.24; 95% confidence interval, 0.97-1.59).[27]

Some authors suggest that the association between snoring and cardiovascular disease has been confirmed,[28] but others caution against this conclusion.[29] At this time, it would be incorrect to assume the existence of a positive independent association between snoring and vascular disease.

CLINICAL FEATURES AND DIAGNOSTIC ASSESSMENT

Snoring is a symptom. The purposes of obtaining the history of and performing a physical examination on a snorer are to determine the likelihood of sleep apnea, identify the presence of risk factors associated with snoring, identify anatomic or functional abnormalities whose correction may improve or abolish snoring, and give advice regarding treatment. Which laboratory tests to perform is, to some extent, directed by the findings obtained. The major decision in all patients is whether to perform nocturnal polysomnography.

History

The history is best obtained in the presence of the bed partner, because the snorer is not aware of snoring. The visit to the physician is usually instigated by the bed partner, who can help to determine whether snoring is positional, whether it occurs nightly, and whether it is associated with breathing pauses. In obtaining the history from the bed partner, the clinician should be cognizant that some bed partners may be particularly sensitive to noise and find it difficult to fall asleep even when exposed to normal breathing sounds. Others may have an ulterior motive—to not sleep with the patient—and use snoring as an excuse to accomplish this goal. Consequently, the clinician must inquire whether other bed partners, family members, or friends who have shared a room with the patient or observed the patient during sleep have also complained about loud and disruptive snoring.

Studies of snoring have identified a number of risk factors (e.g., overweight, alcohol, allergies, nasal obstruction, muscle relaxants, smoking), but only overweight, alcohol, and perhaps nasal obstruction (e.g., during allergy season) have been shown to be causally related to snoring. If snoring has appeared recently or changed for the worse, it is important to determine whether there was a change in any of these risk factors.

Therapeutic decision making can be guided by the nature and severity of the patient's complaints. The interviewer should assess the individual's daytime function and quality of life. Does the snorer wake up feeling refreshed? Is he or she tired or excessively sleepy during the day? Is performance at work adequate? Are there difficulties with memory, ability to concentrate, and the performance of routine tasks? Several questionnaires that are employed in assessing patients with sleep apnea (e.g., the Epworth Sleepiness Scale) are also useful for determining daytime function in snorers. Particularly if there is evidence of daytime dysfunction, the adequacy of sleep hygiene should be explored to establish whether sleep restriction could account for the patient's symptoms.

Systemic diseases leading to snoring (and usually to sleep apnea) by virtue of altering upper airway anatomy or function are rare but should not be overlooked. Examples include hypothyroidism and acromegaly. A routine search for them by biochemical tests of hormone levels is not indicated, and testing should be guided by the clinical circumstances. Several uncommon congenital conditions affect pharyngeal area and collapsibility, such as achondroplasia, dwarfism, fusion of cervical vertebrae (e.g., Klippel-Feil anomaly), and other neck deformities. These are apparent during the physical examination.

The history should reveal previous surgery or trauma to the upper airways at any site between the nose and the larynx, because the local airway area or compliance may have been affected in such a way as to lead to snoring.

Physical Examination

The physical examination should document the presence of general or regional obesity (by body mass index [BMI], neck circumference), hypertension, and local anatomic abnormalities of the upper airway such as nasal polyps and enlarged tonsils or adenoids. It is also useful observe whether the pharynx is small and crowded, whether the tongue is large, and whether the uvula is inflamed, bulky, or simply long, hardly lifting off the base of the tongue during phonation. Positive findings probably do not have therapeutic implications, but they are useful for confirming long-standing snoring, and they increase suspicion of sleep apnea. Examination, including fiberoptic nasopharyngoscopy, of the upper airway by an otolaryngologist should be routine for all habitual snorers seeking medical attention. The results are useful for visualizing the anatomic structures and the amount of redundant tissue present, and for making a subjective judgment about the patient's suitability as a surgical candidate. Simulating snoring or performing Müller's maneuver during endoscopic examination is not useful for determining the site of obstruction and predicting surgical success. Opinions vary in this regard, however.

Laboratory Investigations

The two main investigations to be considered are assessment of the upper airway and nocturnal polysomnography.

Upper airway assessment can be carried out during sleep or during wakefulness. The latter is usually done using various imaging techniques—x-ray cephalometry, computed tomography, or magnetic resonance imaging. The results, however, are neither predictive of snoring nor helpful in selecting surgical candidates, so these techniques are not indicated for the assessment of snorers. Only patients who might undergo maxillofacial surgery (a rare occurrence for treatment of nonapneic snoring) should have radiographic imaging of the airway. On the other hand, upper airway assessment during sleep, either by direct observation using a nasopharyngoscope or by measuring the pressures along the upper airway, may indeed be of value, as it can be used to localize the anatomic site of obstruction, help to diagnose UARS, and select optimal surgical candidates. However, there are other, less invasive ways to diagnose UARS. Furthermore, as snoring is a result of a diffuse rather than a localized abnormality of the upper airway, identification of the site of partial collapse of the airway does not improve surgical outcome.[30] Consequently, outside of particular research protocols, such measurements cannot be recommended for therapeutic decisions in nonapneic snorers.

Should polysomnography be performed in all snorers? Snorers with any symptoms—unrefreshing sleep, daytime sleepiness, fatigue—should be evaluated with this modality in the sleep laboratory to establish or exclude diagnoses including OSAS and UARS. Snorers who are planning to have surgery should be evaluated with polysomnography for diagnostic purposes as well as to establish their baseline status, which is useful when assessing the surgical outcome (in some cases, patients report feeling worse after surgery; see Chapter 90). When sleep apnea is confirmed by polysomnography, a trial of CPAP prior to surgery can be discussed.

A more difficult decision is whether *asymptomatic* snorers should have full-night polysomnography. In the past, it was thought that this was not necessary in this group of patients, because their chance of having sleep apnea was small. However, evolution of our knowledge regarding sleep-disordered breathing and its consequences led to a shift in this paradigm for the following reasons. First, many patients with sleep apnea tend to underestimate their symptoms. Second, several epidemiologic studies have pointed out a high prevalence of unsuspected sleep apnea in snorers. For example, among community-dwelling adult participants of the Sleep Heart Health Study,[27] loud habitual snorers had a fourfold higher risk of having AHI of 15 or greater. Our own sleep clinic data indicate that almost 30% of patients referred because of habitual snoring without any other symptoms of sleep apnea have an AHI of greater than 10. Third, clinical prediction rules for sleep apnea may facilitate prioritization of patients for polysomnography, but they do not possess sufficient accuracy to predict snorers with sleep apnea.[31] Fourth, if sleep-disordered breathing represents a continuum of upper airway dysfunction during sleep, and if we accept that there is a relationship between AHI and adverse health outcomes, UARS and sleep apnea should be identified as early as possible so that corrective measures can be instituted. For all of these reasons, it is prudent to carry out sleep monitoring in all habitual snorers referred to sleep disorders clinics. This monitoring must include careful examination of the tracings for arousals and episodes of flow limitation. Therefore, it is best performed in the sleep laboratory rather than at home, where reliance on unattended monitoring, limited equipment, and inability to deal with temporary malfunctions or other unexpected problems may result in an unsatisfactory study.

TREATMENT

Treatment of snoring is generally similar to that of sleep apnea. The first decision is whether nonapneic snorers should be treated at all. This requires individual consideration in each case. Clearly, some patients were referred to the sleep clinic only because of their (or their bed partner's) fear of sleep apnea, and they require no treatment. They should be advised that they do not have this disorder, told about the risk factors (generally obesity and alcohol ingestion), informed about the symptoms of UARS and sleep apnea, and advised to return if such symptoms develop.

Snorers with unrefreshing sleep (even in the absence of polysomnographically confirmed UARS), snorers with cardiovascular disease, and those whose snoring interferes with their bed partner's sleep or causes embarrassment should all be provided with an appropriate therapeutic trial.

Once treatment is initiated, it is imperative to assess the outcome of the intervention. Superficially, this appears simple. There is a subjective method, based on responses to specific questions, and an objective method, based on measurement of snoring. However, subjective assessment must be used with caution because snoring is a symptom perceived by the listener and not by the snorer; improvement or lack thereof after intervention is best decided by the person who voiced the initial complaint, which is seldom done. Objective methods are also problematic because, as previously discussed, measurements of snoring lack standardized techniques and data analysis protocols. In addition, there is no compelling evidence that measured sound agrees with the listener's perception of the snoring. Given these methodologic problems, the important issue is not which method to use but to make certain that the same assessment tool is used before and after treatment.

Treatment options for all sleep-related breathing disorders (sleep apnea, nonapneic asymptomatic snoring, and UARS) fall into four general categories—lifestyle modification, surgery, oral appliances, and CPAP. When the results of polysomnography are known, these approaches should be discussed with the patient and the most applicable option selected.

Figure 83–1 describes the sequence of treatment decisions, beginning with identification and correction of risk factors and followed by use of an oral appliance, use of CPAP, and finally surgery. This approach should be followed in obese snorers without obvious anatomic abnormality of the upper airway. Treatment should be individualized on the basis of the clinical circumstances and patient preferences. For example, patients shown to have tonsillar hypertrophy, large adenoids, or significant septal deviation should be referred for surgical assessment early, after being informed about CPAP and oral appliances. Some may wish to try one of these latter options and should be encouraged to do so. Those who are considering surgery should be advised not to expect complete elimination of snoring, and that even if snoring is initially reduced or even eliminated by surgery, there is no guarantee that this favorable result will persist. Patients should be advised to discuss specific issues (e.g., surgical techniques, side effects, recovery time, pain control, morbidity, mortality) with the surgeon.

After patients have been informed about the approach options, they invariably ask for a recommendation. Noninvasive treatments must be recommended first. Although financial and health insurance considerations may influence the course of treatment, they should not cloud proper medical advice, which must be based on the available evidence.

Medical Treatment

It is clinically observed that *weight loss* improves, and sometimes cures, snoring, but studies confirming this hypothesis in nonapneic snorers are lacking. In patients with sleep apnea, almost all studies demonstrate marked improvement in snoring and sleep apnea with weight loss. In a study of 123 patients 1 year after bariatric surgery (which reduced average

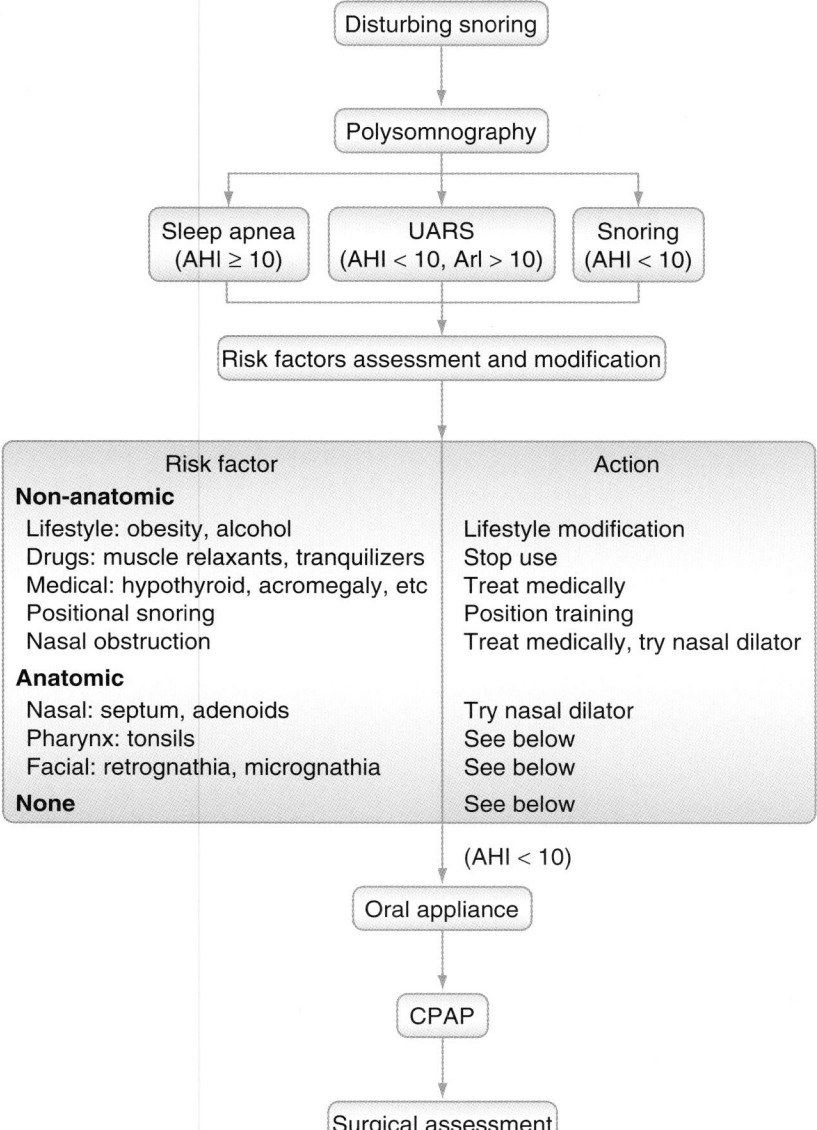

Figure 83–1. Algorithm for treatment of snoring.

BMI from 46 kg/m² to 35 kg/m²), the percentage of habitual snorers dropped from 82% to 14%.[32]

In general, it is not possible to predict the amount of weight loss required to abolish snoring in an individual, but sometimes as little as 3 kg is sufficient. Obesity, even when defined in a very liberal fashion as BMI greater than 30 kg/m², is very common among snorers; therefore, weight reduction should be the first recommendation given to all snorers, regardless of whether they have sleep apnea and whether other treatment methods are contemplated.

A second recommendation is *avoidance of alcohol*. It is clinically observed, and well known to bed partners of snorers, that alcohol ingested prior to going to bed worsens snoring. However, there are no sleep laboratory measurements to confirm this; in fact, in one study, snoring intensity was measured before and after alcohol ingestion and no significant difference was found.[33] What *has* been shown is that, depending on the blood alcohol level, nonapneic snorers develop increased

upper airway resistance during sleep, increased pharyngeal collapsibility, reduction in nocturnal oxygen saturation, and increased AHI.[34,35] The deleterious effect of alcohol on breathing during sleep is directly related to the timing of alcohol ingestion, the amount ingested, and the individual's metabolism, and the effect may be evident for up to 5 hours after ingestion. Snorers who drink alcoholic beverages should be cautioned not to ingest alcohol within 2 to 5 hours of going to bed.

Medical therapy of sleep apnea is discussed in Chapter 88. No medication consistently cures or improves snoring in all snorers. Preparations that have been tried include protriptyline, nasal lubricants, nasal decongestants, and nasal steroids. Nasal decongestants and intranasal steroids are probably the most common drugs used to reduce snoring in patients with chronic nasal problems. Almost all studies in community[36] and clinic populations indicate that nasal congestion and measured nasal resistance correlate with snoring; furthermore, nasal resistance decreases significantly with decongestants and intranasal steroids. However, no objective evidence supports their beneficial effect on snoring.[37]

Members of the Clinical Practice Review Committee of the AASM recently reviewed the use of nasal lubricants (and other nonprescription pharmacologic products) regarding their usefulness in the treatment of snoring; they found the existing data inconclusive and could not make a definitive recommendation.[38] However, because a short trial (4 weeks) of intranasal steroid is generally quite safe, and because it is not possible to predict who will respond, it is reasonable to offer it to nonapneic snorers with nasal symptoms. The patients must be informed about the low chance of success and the possible risks. Adequate follow-up must be arranged to assess the efficacy of treatment and to determine whether it should be continued.

Some medications, such as sedatives and muscle relaxants, may worsen snoring in some patients, and it is a good general measure to advise snorers to abstain from taking these drugs.

Positional training can sometimes be recommended. Snoring is generally position dependent, being worse in supine position. Bed partners of snorers, when disturbed by loud snoring, frequently comment that kicking the snorer forces a change in position that stops the snoring, although only temporarily. Sleep laboratory investigations indicate that snoring and apneas are position dependent in up to 50% of patients. A recent retrospective review of snoring in 21 nonapneic patients showed significant reduction in the snoring index and sound intensity with a change from supine to lateral position.[39] Although other factors (e.g., obesity and sleep stage) may modulate positional effect on snoring, this is a benign intervention, and all snorers should be advised to learn to avoid sleeping in the supine position.

Nasal dilators were introduced almost 15 years ago. Although internal and external nasal dilators met with initial enthusiasm, studies[40,41] that measured snoring objectively have not supported that approval. Recent randomized controlled trials of nasal dilators found either no change in recorded snoring at all[42] or only minor, partial benefits.[43,44]

Having reviewed the literature dealing with nasal dilators, the Clinical Practice Review Committee of the AASM concluded that these devices may be useful to treat nonapneic snoring,[38] although they acknowledged that robust data supporting this conclusion is missing. Despite the lack of objective data, clinical experience shows that there are some patients whose bed partners report subjective improvement in snoring with nasal dilation. Given the rather low cost and benign nature of this treatment, there is no harm in recommending it as a therapeutic trial for nonapneic snorers. They will quickly determine for themselves whether it is beneficial.

Oral appliances, patented in the late 19th century for treatment of snoring, were at first relatively neglected because of their discomfort. More recently, however, there has been considerable progress in the design, material, manufacturing techniques, and the ability to customize the appliance to an individual patient. They have become the treatment of choice in idiopathic, nonapneic snorers and patients with UARS—in preference to CPAP (which is more successful but poorly tolerated by these patients) or surgery (the results of which have been disappointing). Different types of appliances, their mechanism of action, their side effects, patient suitability for this treatment, and the results of recent placebo-controlled studies have been recently reviewed[45,46] and are also discussed in Chapter 91. A summary of data involving almost 500 patients indicates 40% to 50% objective improvement in the measured number of snores per hour of sleep and a 70% to 100% subjective rate of satisfaction; 50% to 75% of patients continued to use their appliance 12 to 60 months later.

Surgical

Surgery is an attractive alternative to treatment of nonapneic snoring for several reasons. It offers the possibility of a quick fix without the necessity of lifestyle modification or the wearing of an appliance. Also, some patients respond beneficially to surgery. Finally, it is generally safe and patients are willing to undergo a procedure even if the chance of success is no more than 50%.

Surgical procedures used to treat nonapneic snoring, like those for sleep apnea, involve operations on the nose, the mouth, and the jaw (although the latter is generally reserved for patients with sleep apnea). These are described in Chapter 90. Surgical tools include scalpel, laser, and microwaves. Determining success rates is difficult because almost all of the studies suffer from various shortcomings, such as inconsistent endpoint assessment, short follow-up time, differences in surgical techniques, selection bias, lack of preoperative and postoperative sleep studies, and differences in snoring assessments. Overall, however, surgical results for treatment of idiopathic snoring (i.e., unassociated with clinically recognizable upper airway pathology) have been disappointing. The following paragraphs summarize the results of recent studies (generally published after the year 2000) that included any (subjective or objective) assessment of snoring.

Nasal Surgery

Nasal obstruction promotes snoring by increasing negative intrathoracic pressure during sleep; this leads to a reduction in the pharyngeal cross-sectional area, pharyngeal collapse, turbulent flow, and vibration of pharyngeal structures. The Wisconsin Sleep Cohort Study[39] indicates that nocturnal nasal congestion is strongly associated with habitual snoring, with an odds ratio of about 3.0. However, despite the existence of this association between nasal obstruction and sleep-disordered breathing, there is no evidence that this association is causal—that is, that relief of nasal obstruction consistently improves or eliminates snoring. There is very good evidence that surgical correction of nasal obstruction (e.g., nasal polypectomy, or septoplasty, or turbinate reduction) reduces nasal resistance and improves nasal breathing, but only a minority of patients report reduction in snoring.[47]

Pharyngeal Surgery

UVULOPALATOPHARYNGOPLASTY

Uvulopalatopharyngoplasty (UPPP) was described in the early 1980s and quickly became the surgical treatment of choice for apneic and nonapneic snorers. Review of the surgical results up to 1999 indicates that the success rates of UPPP for treatment of snoring are highly variable and may reach up to 90%.[48] More recent studies, with longer follow-up, show that subjective improvement in snoring, as assessed 2 to 5 years after surgery, ranges from 18% to 65% and is highest within 6 months after surgery, dropping off by at least 50% with longer follow-up.[49]

It is not possible to predict the success of UPPP from preoperative assessment of the airway either during wakefulness or during sleep, because snoring is a consequence of diffuse and dynamic, rather than localized and static, abnormality of the upper airway. In general, younger, thinner (BMI less than 30 kg/m²), nonapneic snorers have a better success rate than the older and more obese ones. Those with large tonsils have a better success rate than idiopathic snorers. A bulky and inflamed uvula, frequently seen in habitual heavy snorers, is more likely a consequence of snoring than the cause, and is not an indication for surgery.

The patient should be informed that UPPP will not result in complete abolition of snoring, but it may lower the sound intensity and change the spectral frequency (i.e., the pitch) of the sound, making it less objectionable to the bed partner. Side effects of UPPP for treatment of snoring are the same as for treatment of sleep apnea (see Chapter 90).

LASER-ASSISTED UVULOPALATOPLASTY

Laser-assisted uvulopalatoplasty (LAUP) was launched in 1990 as an alternative to UPPP. It is an office procedure done under local anesthesia, which can be performed several times (generally three times) at 1- to 3-week intervals to achieve the desired effect. Less tissue is resected than during UPPP. The efficacy of this procedure for treatment of snoring is not higher than for UPPP, and the main reason for selecting this procedure is to avoid general anesthetic.

There are two randomized trials of LAUP for treatment of snoring. In the first trial[50] (LAUP vs. no treatment) the authors studied 45 patients with mild sleep apnea (AHI < 27). After 8 months' follow-up, 48% of operated patients reported improvement in snoring, versus none in the untreated group. In the second study,[50a] which was a randomized, placebo-controlled trial of LAUP versus sham surgery in 25 patients with AHI < 20, no difference in subjective impression or objective measurements of snoring were found at 3 months follow-up.

The Standards of Practice Committee of the AASM critically reviewed the results published up to September 2000 and concluded that "long-term effectiveness of LAUP on treatment of snoring has not been convincingly established" (p. 605 of Littner et al.[51]). The committee pointed out marked variability between individual studies, undoubtedly due to differences in assessment of snoring, length of follow-up, sample size, and drop-out rate, for example, which resulted in rates of improvement in snoring that varied between 43% and 90%. Since that report, several more studies of the effect of LAUP on mild obstructive sleep apnea (and snoring) were published[50,52]; the results are substantially the same—snoring improves in 22% to 92% of patients, depending on the length of follow-up. Although within the first month, up to 90% of patients may be satisfied with the effect of surgery, by 18 to 24 months only about 50% are satisfied, and by 70 to 75 months this rate drops to only 20%.[53] In the 3 years that have passed since the report of the Standards of Practice Committee of the AASM,[51] no new data have emerged to justify a less cautious approach than that recommended in 2001.

RADIOFREQUENCY ABLATION

Radiofrequency ablation (RFA) is a new outpatient procedure pioneered in 1998 by Powell and colleagues.[54] It is based on delivering thermal (radiofrequency) energy to the pharyngeal tissues—palate, tonsils, uvula, and base of the tongue. The tissues are heated and ablated, causing volume reduction and stiffening of the pharynx, thus making the walls less susceptible to vibration and collapse.

The initial results were encouraging. They showed a reduction in subjective snoring score from 8.3 (out of 10) to 1.9 within 2 to 3 months after the procedure; the score increased to 3.8 with longer follow-up (14 months).[56] Between 1998 and 2003, over 20 studies involving over 700 patients were published. Most were prospective case series. Almost all the patients in these studies had preoperative and most had postoperative polysomnography. Snoring was seldom measured objectively but was assessed subjectively by the patient (or bed partner) on a scale from 0 (minimal or absent) to 10 (maximal or most severe). Average follow-up time was only 8 months, with a maximum of 16 months. Within the limitations of the studies (no placebo control, inconsistent preoperative and postoperative measurements of respiration, selection bias), the results indicate an approximately 53% reduction in the snoring scores, with satisfaction rates ranging from 0% to 90%. Objective measurements of snoring, when available, generally showed minimal or no improvement, sometimes despite subjective satisfaction, once again emphasizing the very subjective nature of self- or bed partner–reported snoring.

Recently, Woodson et al.[56] conducted a randomized, placebo-controlled trial of RFA versus CPAP. The placebo group had sham surgery—the probes were inserted but no energy was delivered. Follow-up time was short—approximately 3 to 4 weeks. Although the sample included patients with an AHI of less than 10, no separate analysis for this group of patients was carried out. There was no significant difference between the placebo and surgical groups in the symptoms of nocturnal obstruction and related events (SNORE25) questionnaire, although there was a significant improvement in the post-treatment score compared with the pretreatment one. There are few studies that compare RFA with LAUP and UPPP, but RFA does not appear to be any more successful than the other surgical procedures.

RFA is still too new to determine its ultimate efficacy in treatment of snoring. A recent review of RFA[57] concluded that according to the published data the procedure leads to a significant reduction in subjective snoring. However, the authors pointed out that this conclusion remains unconfirmed by controlled clinical trials.

Other Surgical Procedures

Some of the other surgical procedures that modify the upper airway, such as tracheostomy, genioglossal advancement, hyoid myotomy, and maxillomandibular osteotomy, are used exclusively in the context of sleep apnea; they have not been applied specifically to treat nonapneic snoring. Tonsillectomy, however, has been used to treat snoring and sleep apnea. In the rare adult who has tonsillar hypertrophy that is bilateral, severe, and associated with sleep apnea, it is successful in reducing snoring and apnea.[58] Other procedures, such as diathermy palatoplasty, injection snoreplasty, and lateral pharyngoplasty, have been used in isolated case series to treat snoring and apnea, but the utility of these procedures cannot be evaluated; although surgical details are different, these procedures share many features with the more standard procedures described earlier.

SUMMARY

Snoring is common in the general population. It occurs when normal sleep-induced physiologic changes in pharyngeal properties are superimposed on underlying pharyngeal pathology; the latter may be anatomic (large tonsils or adenoids), or it may be caused by obesity or the ingestion of alcohol or medications. When certain critical conditions in the flow rate, cross-sectional area of the pharynx, gas density, and collapsibility of pharyngeal walls are met during breathing, the airway begins to narrow and pharyngeal walls start to flutter, producing the snoring sound. In about 5% to 10% of snorers, this pharyngeal narrowing proceeds to complete occlusion, leading to OSAS. In others (the precise incidence is unknown), the increase in airway resistance is only sufficient to augment significantly the work of breathing and cause brief arousals from sleep, which leads to sleep fragmentation and UARS. Some snorers progress to sleep apnea if they gain weight, drink alcohol in the evening, or develop systemic disease such as hypothyroidism or acromegaly.

The most important clinical significance of snoring is that it serves as a marker of UARS or OSAS. Much has been written about snoring as a risk factor for hypertension or cardiovascular or cerebrovascular disease. All of these conditions are common, and it is not surprising that they coexist in the same patient. However, at present there is no unequivocal evidence for a definite association or a causal relationship between snoring and vascular disease.

Treatment of nonapneic snoring begins with identification and correction of risk factors (including surgical risk factors, if applicable), proceeding to noninvasive methods, of which oral appliances and nasal CPAP have the highest chances of success, and then to surgical assessment.

Clinical Pearl

Snoring is caused by diffuse vibrations of pharyngeal walls. It implies increased upper airway resistance during sleep. Snorers who complain of unrefreshing sleep and poor daytime functioning warrant investigations to rule out upper airway resistance syndrome or sleep apnea. Although many snorers may have coexisting hypertension, neither causality nor independent association between snoring and vascular disease has been confirmed.

REFERENCES

1. Kleitman N: Sleep and Wakefulness. Chicago, University of Chicago Press, 1963, pp 48-52.
2. Lugaresi E, Mondini S, Zucconi M, et al: Staging of heavy snorers' disease: A proposal. Bull Eur Physiopathol Respir 1983;19:590-594.
3. Lugaresi E, Cirignotta F, Piana G: Some epidemiological data on snoring and cardiocirculatory disturbances. Sleep 1980;3:221-224.
4. Lindberg E, Taube A, Janson C, et al: A 10-year follow-up of snoring in men. Chest 1998;114:1048-1055.
5. Guilleminault C, Stoohs R, Clerk A, et al: A cause of excessive daytime sleepiness: The upper airway resistance syndrome. Chest 1993;104:781-787.
6. Diagnostic Classification Steering Committee: International Classification of Sleep Disorders: Diagnostic and Coding Manual. Rochester, Minn, American Sleep Disorders Association, 1990, p 195.
7. Gavriely N, Jensen O: Theory and measurement of snores. J Appl Physiol 1993;74:2828-2837.
8. Aittokallio T, Gyllenberg M, Polo O: A model of snorer's upper airway. Math Biosci 2001;170:79-90.
9. Huang L, Williams JE: Neuromechanical interaction in human snoring and upper airway obstruction. J Appl Physiol 1999;86:1759-1763.
10. Dalmasso F, Prota R: Snoring: Analysis, measurement, clinical implications, and applications. Eur Respir J 1996;9:146-159.
11. Kapsimalis F, Kryger MH: Gender and obstructive sleep apnea syndrome: Part I. Clinical features. Sleep 2002;25:409-416.
12. Guilleminault C, Chowdhuri S: Upper airway resistance syndrome is a distinct syndrome. Am J Respir Crit Care Med 2000;161:1412-1413.
13. Douglas NJ: Upper airway resistance syndrome is not a distinct syndrome. Am J Respir Crit Care Med 2000;161:1413-1415.
14. Gold AR, Marcus CL, Dipalo F. Gold MS: Upper airway collapsibility during sleep in upper airway resistance syndrome. Chest 2002;121:1531-1540.
14a. American Academy of Sleep Medicine. International Classification of Sleep Disorders: Diagnostic and Coding Manual, 2nd edition. Westchesler, IL: American Academy of Sleep Medicine, 2005.
15. Meoli AL, Casey KR, Clark RW, et al: Hypopnea in sleep-disordered breathing in adults. Sleep 2001;24:469-470.
16. Ayappa I, Norman RG, Krieger AC, et al: Non-invasive detection of respiratory effort-related arousals (RERAs) by a nasal cannula/pressure transducer system. Sleep 2000;23:763-771.
17. American Academy of Sleep Medicine: Sleep-related breathing disorders in adults: Recommendations for syndrome definition and measurement techniques in clinical research. Report of the American Academy of Sleep Medicine Task Force. Sleep 1999;22:667-689.
18. Gottlieb DJ, Yao Q, Redline S, et al, for the Sleep Heart Health Study Research Group: Does snoring predict sleepiness independently of apnea and hypopnea frequency? Am J Respir Crit Care Med 2000;162:1512-1517.
19. Lindberg E, Carter N, Gislason T, Janson T: Role of snoring and daytime sleepiness in occupational accidents. Am J Respir Crit Care Med 2001;164:2031-2035.
20. Engleman HM, Kingshott RN, Wraith PK, et al: Randomized placebo-controlled crossover trial of continuous positive airway pressure for mild sleep apnea/hypopnea syndrome. Am J Respir Crit Care Med 1999;159:461-467.
21. Barnes M, Houston D, Worsnop CJ, et al: A randomized controlled trial of continuous positive airway pressure in mild obstructive sleep apnea. Am J Respir Crit Care Med 2002;165:773-780.
22. Gold AR, Dipalo F, Gold MS, O'Hearn D: The symptoms and signs of upper airway resistance syndrome: A link to functional somatic syndromes. Chest 2003;123:87-95.
23. Lugaresi E, Coccagna G, Farnetti P, et al: Snoring. Electroencephalogr Clin Neurol 1975;39:59-64.
24. Bixler EO, Vgontzas AN, Lin HM, et al: Association of hypertension and sleep-disordered breathing. Arch Intern Med 2000;160:2289-2295.
25. Nieto FJ, Young TB, Lind BK, et al, for the Sleep Heart Health Study: Association of sleep-disordered breathing, sleep apnea, and hypertension in a large community-based study. JAMA 2000;283:1829-1836.
26. Peppard PE, Young T, Palta M, Skatrud J: Prospective study of the association between sleep-disordered breathing and hypertension. N Engl J Med 2000;342:1378-1384.
27. Shahar E, Whitney CW, Redline S, et al., for the Sleep Heart Health Study Research Group. Sleep-disordered breathing and cardiovascular disease: Cross-sectional results of the Sleep Heart Health Study. Am J Respir Crit Care Med 2001;163:19-25.

28. Roux F, D'Ambrosio C, Mohsenin V: Sleep-related breathing disorders and cardiovascular disease. Am J Med 2000;108:396-402.

29. Dart RA, Gregoire JR, Gutterman DD, Woolf SH: The association of hypertension of and secondary cardiovascular disease with sleep-disordered breathing. Chest 2003;123:244-260.

30. El Badawey MR, McKee G, Heggie N, et al: Predictive value of sleep nasendoscopy in the management of habitual snorers. Ann Otol Rhinol Laryngol 2003;112:40-44.

31. Tsai WH, Remmers JE, Brant R, et al: A decision rule for diagnostic testing in obstructive sleep apnea. Am J Respir Crit Care Med 2003;167:1427-1432.

32. Dixon JB, Schachter LM, O'Brien PE: Sleep disturbance and obesity: changes following surgically induced weight loss. Arch Intern Med 2001;161:102-106.

33. Scanlan MF, Roebuck T, Little PJ, et al: Effect of moderate alcohol upon obstructive sleep apnea. Eur Respir J 2000;16:909-913.

34. Issa FG, Sullivan CE: Alcohol, snoring and sleep apnea. J Neurol Neurosurg Psychiatry 1982;45;353-359.

35. Mitler MM, Dawson A, Henriksen SJ, et al: Bedtime ethanol increases resistance of upper airways and produces sleep apneas in asymptomatic snorers. Alcohol Clin Exp Res 1988;12:801-805.

36. Young T, Finn L, Palta M: Chronic nasal congestion at night is a risk factor for snoring in a population-based cohort study. Arch Intern Med 2001;161:1514-1519.

37. Kiely JL, Nolan P, McNicholas WT: Intranasal corticosteroid therapy for obstructive sleep apnea in patients with co-existing rhinitis. Thorax 2004;59:50-55.

38. Meoli AM, Rosen CL, Kristo D, et al: Nonprescription treatments of snoring or obstructive seep apnea: An evaluation of products with limited scientific evidence. Sleep 2003;26:619-624.

39. Nakano H, Ikeda T, Hayashi M, et al: Effects of body position on snoring in apneic and nonapneic snorers. Sleep 2003;26:169-172.

40. Liistro G, Rombaux P, Dury M, et al: Effects of Breathe Right on snoring: A polysomnographic study. Respir Med 1998;92:1076-1078.

41. Schönhofer B, Franklin KA, Brünig H, et al: Effect of nasal valve dilation on obstructive sleep apnea. Chest 2000;118:587-590.

42. Djupesland PG, Skatvedt O, Borgersen K: Dichotomous physiological effects of nocturnal external nasal dilation in heavy snorers: The answer to a rhinologic controversy? Am J Rhinol 2001;15:95-103.

43. Pevernagie D, Hamans E, Van Cauwenberge P, Pauwels R: External nasal dilation reduces snoring in chronic rhinitis patients: A randomized controlled trial. Eur Respir J 2000; 15: 996-1000.

44. Bahammam AS, Tate R, Manfreda J, Kryger MH: Upper airway resistance syndrome: Effect of nasal dilation, sleep stage, and sleep position. Sleep 1999;22:592-598.

45. Mohsenin N, Mostofi MT, Mohsenin V: The role of oral appliances in treating obstructive sleep apnea. J Am Dent Assoc 2003;134:442-449.

46. Ferguson KA: The role of oral appliance therapy in the treatment of obstructive sleep apnea. Clin Chest Med 2003;24:355-364.

47. Friedman M, Tanyeri H, Lim JW, et al: Effect of improved nasal breathing on obstructive sleep apnea. Otolaryngol Head Neck Surg 2000;122:71-74.

48. Coleman J, Rathfoot C: Oropharyngeal surgery in the management of upper airway obstruction during sleep. Otolaryngol Clin North Am 1999;32:263-276.

49. Hessel NS, de Vries N: Results of uvulopalatopharyngoplasty after diagnostic workup with polysomnography and sleep endoscopy: A report of 136 patients. Eur Arch Otorhinolaryngol 2003;260:91-95.

50. Ferguson KA, Heighway K, Ruby RRF: A randomized trial of laser-assisted uvulopalatoplasty in the treatment of mild obstructive sleep apnea. Am J Respir Crit Care Med 2003:167:15-19.

50a. Larrosa F, Hernandez L, Morello A, et al: Laser-assisted uvulopalatoplasty for snoring: Does it meet the expectations? Eur Respir J 2004;24:66-70.

51. Littner M, Kushida CA, Hartse K, et al: Practice parameters for the use of laser-assisted uvulopalatoplasty: An update for 2000. Sleep 2001;24:603-608.

52. Kyrmizakis DE, Chimona TS, Papadakis CE, et al: Laser-assisted uvulopalatoplasty for the treatment of snoring and mild obstructive sleep apnea syndrome. J Otolaryngol 2003;32:172-179.

53. Sharp HR, Mitchell DB: Long-term results of laser-assisted uvulopalatoplasty for snoring. J Laryngol Otol 2001;115:897-900.

54. Powell NB, Riley RW, Troell RJ, et al: Radiofrequency volumetric tissue reduction of the palate in subjects with sleep-disordered breathing. Chest 1998;113:1163-1174.

55. Li KK, Powell NB, Riley RW, et al: Radiofrequency volumetric reduction of the palate: An extended follow-up study. Otolaryngol Head Neck Surg 2000;122:410-414.

56. Woodson BT, Steward DL, Weaver EM, Javaheri S: A randomized trial of temperature-controlled radiofrequency, continuous positive airway pressure, and placebo for obstructive sleep apnea syndrome. Otolaryngol Head Neck Surg 2003;128:848-861.

57. Stuck BA, Maurer JT, Hein G, et al: Radiofrequency surgery of the soft palate in the treatment of snoring. Sleep 2004;27:551-555.

58. Verse T, Kroker B, Pirsig W, Brosch S: Tonsillectomy as a treatment of obstructive sleep apnea in adults with tonsillar hypertrophy. Laryngoscope 2000;110:1556-1559.

REFERENCES FOR STUDIES IN TABLE 83–1

Bearpark H, Elliott L, Grunstein R, et al: Snoring and sleep apnea: A population study in Australian men. Am J Respir Crit Care Med 1995;151:1459-1465.

Bednarek M, Polakowska M, Kurjata P, et al: Snoring and excessive daytime somnolence and risk of cardiovascular diseases. Pol Arch Med Wewn 2001;105:11-17.

Bliwise DL, Nekich JC, Dement WC: Relative validity of self-reported snoring as a symptom of sleep apnea in a sleep clinic population. Chest 1991;99:600-608.

Duran J, Esnaola S, Rubio R, Iztueta A: Obstructive sleep apnea-hypopnea and related clinical features in a population-based sample of subjects aged 30 to 70 yr. Am J Respir Crit Care Med 2001;163(Pt 1):685-689.

Ersu R, Arman AR, Save D, et al: Prevalence of snoring and symptoms of sleep-disordered breathing in primary school children in Istanbul. Chest 2004;126:19-24.

Ferini-Strambi L, Zucconi M, Castronovo V, et al: Snoring and sleep apnea: A population study in Italian women. Sleep 1999;22:859-864.

Hui DS, Chan JK, Ho AS, et al: Prevalence of snoring and sleep disordered breathing in a student population. Chest 1999 Dec;116(6):1530-1536.

Hui DS, Chan JK, Ko FW, et al: Prevalence of snoring and sleep-disordered breathing in a group of commercial bus drivers in Hong Kong. Intern Med J 2002;32:149-157.

Ip MS, Lam B, Tang LC, et al: A community study of sleep-disordered breathing in middle-aged Chinese women in Hong Kong: Prevalence and gender differences. Chest 2004;125:127-134.

Ip MS, Lauder IJ, Tsang KW, et al: A community study of sleep-disordered breathing in middle-aged Chinese men in Hong Kong. Chest 2001;119:62-69.

Janson C, Gislason T, De Backer W, et al: Daytime sleepiness, snoring, and gastro-oesophageal reflux amongst adults in three European countries. J Intern Med 1995;237:277-285.

Kayukawa Y, Shirakawa S, Hayakawa T, et al: Habitual snoring in an outpatient population in Japan. Psychiatry Clin Neurosci 2000;54:385-391.

Keenan SP, Ferguson KA, Chen-Yeung M, Fleetham J: Prevalence of sleep disordered breathing in a population of Canadian grainworkers. Can Respir J 1998;3:184-190.

Kim JS, Song WH, Shin C, et al: The prevalence and awareness of hypertension and the relationship between hypertension and snoring in the Korean population. Korean J Intern Med 2001; 16:62-68.

Koskenvuo M, Kaprio J, Partinen M, et al: Snoring as a risk factor for hypertension and angina pectoris. Lancet 1985;1:893-895.

Larsson G-L, Lindberg A, Franklin KA, Lundbäck B: Gender differences in symptoms related to sleep apnea in a general population and in relation to referral to sleep clinic. Chest 2003;124: 204-211.

Liu SA, Liu CY: Prevalence of snoring in Taichung area: An epidemiological study. J Clin Med Assoc 2004;67:32-36.

Lugaresi E, Cirignotta F, Piana G: Some epidemiological data on snoring and cardiocirculatory disturbances. Sleep 1980;3:221-224.

Marin JM, Gascon JM, Carrizo S, Gispert J: Prevalence of sleep apnoea syndrome in the Spanish adult population. Int J Epidemiol 1997;26:381-386.

Mondini S, Zucconi M, Cirignotta F, et al: Snoring as a risk factor for cardiac and circulatory problems: An epidemiological study. In Guilleminault C, Lugaresi E (eds): Sleep/wake Disorders: Natural History, Epidemiology and Long-term Evolution. New York, Raven Press, 1983, pp 99-105.

Neven AK, Middelkoop HA, Kemp B, et al: The prevalence of clinically significant sleep apnoea syndrome in The Netherlands. Thorax 1998;53:638-642.

Ng TP, Scow A, Tan WC: Prevalence of snoring and sleep breathing-related disorders in Chinese, Malay and Indian adults in Singapore. Eur Respir J 1998;12:198-203.

Norton PG, Dunn EV. Snoring as a risk factor for disease: An epidemiological survey. Br Med J 1985;231:630-632.

Norton PG, Dunn EV, Haight JS: Snoring in adults: Some epidemiological aspects. Can Med Assoc J 1983;128:674-675.

Ohayon MM, Guilleminault C, Priest RG, Caulet M: Snoring and breathing pauses during sleep: Telephone interview survey of a United Kingdom population sample. Br Med J 1997;314: 860-863.

Olson LG, King MT, Hensley MJ, Saunders NA: A community study of snoring and sleep-disordered breathing: Prevalence. Am J Respir Crit Care Med 1995;152:711-714.

Shin C, Joo S, Kim J, Kim T. Prevalence and correlates of habitual snoring in high school students. Chest 2003;124:1709-715.

Stoohs RA, Blum HC, Haselhorst M, et al: Normative data on snoring: A comparison between younger and older adults. Eur Respir J 1998 Feb;11(2):451-457.

Stradling JR, Crosby JH: Relation between systemic hypertension and sleep hypoxemia and snoring: Analysis in 748 men drawn from general practice. Br Med J 1990;300:75-78.

Teculescu D, Hannhart B, Cornette A, et al: Prevalence of habitual snoring in a sample of French males. Role of "minor" nose-throat abnormalities. Respiration 2001;68:365-370.

Tishler PV, Larkin EK, Schluchter MD, Redline S: Incidence of sleep-disordered breathing in an urban adult population: The relative importance of risk factors in the development of sleep-disordered breathing. JAMA 2003;289:2230-2237.

Udwadia ZF, Doshi AV, Lonkar SG, Singh CI: Prevalence of sleep-disordered breathing and sleep apnea in middle-aged urban Indian men. Am J Respir Crit Care Med 2004;169:168-173.

Wiggins CL, Schmidt-Nowara WW, Coultas DB, Samet JM: Comparison of self- and spouse reports of snoring and other symptoms associated with sleep apnea syndrome. Sleep 1990;13:245-252.

Young T, Palta M, Dempsey J, et al: The occurrence of sleep-disordered breathing among middle-aged adults. N Engl J Med 1993;328:1230-1235.

Young T, Shahar E, Nieto FJ, et al: Predictors of sleep-disordered breathing in community-dwelling adults: The Sleep Heart Health Study. Arch Intern Med 2002;162:893-900.

Zamarron C, Gude F, Otero Y, et al: Prevalence of sleep disordered breathing and sleep apnea in 50- to 70-year-old individuals; a survey. Respiration 1999;66:317-322.

Zielinski J, Zgierska A, Polakowska M, et al: Snoring and excessive daytime somnolence among Polish middle-aged adults. Eur Respir J 1999;14:946-950.

84

Genetics of Obstructive Sleep Apnea

Susan Redline

ABSTRACT

Obstructive sleep apnea (OSA) is substantially influenced by familial and probably genetic factors. Studies of the familial aggregation of OSA have included reports of families with multiple affected members, twin and cohort studies, studies of OSA prevalence among relatives of affected probands, and quantification of the familial aggregation of OSA by comparing the prevalence of OSA among relatives of affected probands with that in control samples.

There is clear evidence that a positive family history of OSA is an important risk factor for an elevated apnea-hypopnea index (AHI) and associated symptoms such as snoring, daytime sleepiness, and apneas. Studies of families sampled from diverse populations have consistently shown familial aggregation of OSA, AHI level, and symptoms of OSA. Familial aggregation has been observed in studies of both children and adults and in samples that have included both obese and nonobese subjects, with recurrent risks varying from 1.6 to more than 8.0. Overall heritability estimates for the AHI are .30 to .40. Segregation analysis of the AHI has further defined the likely mode of inheritance and provides estimates for the magnitude of genetic influences.

These analyses suggest that a recessive or codominant gene may explain 17% to 35% of the variance in the trait. Preliminary linkage studies have identified several areas where biologically plausible candidate genes are located, including candidates for metabolic syndrome and obesity. Future research to study candidate gene areas in more detail and to replicate preliminary findings in other populations will be required. If novel genetic determinants of OSA can be identified, important new insights into OSA pathophysiology, and ultimately treatment, could result.

Astute clinicians have long observed that their patients with obstructive sleep apnea (OSA) often have relatives—parents, siblings, and children—who have similar symptoms or a diagnosis of OSA, or both. Related family members with OSA often share similar anthropomorphic or craniofacial characteristics. In some instances, family resemblances appear strongest for weight and weight distribution (e.g., increased central adiposity); in others, family similarities are noted for jaw size and position (micro- or retrognathia) or face and head shape.

Genetic studies of OSA have generally lagged behind those of other common chronic cardiorespiratory conditions such as asthma and coronary artery disease; however, in the last decade these anecdotal observations have been supplemented by growing data that have quantified the role of genetics in OSA. Genetic studies have quantified the heritability of OSA, described potential modes of transmission, and identified suggestive or biologically plausible candidate genes.

Modern advances in both genetic and genomic methods, as well as in our understanding of the physiologic underpinnings of OSA and its associated comorbidities, indicate that OSA is strongly heritable. This realization has spurred growing international work aimed at gene discovery. Although much of this work is still in its infancy, the evidence to date provides insights into the genetics of OSA, and these insights potentially have broad implications for understanding other complex diseases associated with OSA, such as the metabolic syndrome and some cardiovascular diseases.

In this chapter, both general and specific approaches for investigating the genetic basis of OSA are reviewed, and those candidate genes and intermediate traits that are likely important in determining the expression and severity of the syndrome are described. The latter knowledge may eventually help elucidate physiologically specific approaches for treating (and possibly preventing) OSA and its common comorbidities.

DEFINITION OF THE OSA PHENOTYPE

As is the case with many other complex disorders, there is no standardized phenotypic definition of OSA. Clinically, OSA is recognized as a *syndrome* that is defined by the occurrence of repetitive episodes of complete or partial upper airway obstruction during sleep; these episodes usually occur in association with loud snoring and daytime sleepiness.[1] However, operationally, there is much variability in how specific respiratory events are identified, what threshold level for increased numbers of events is considered pathologic, and which other clinical and polysomnographic data are considered necessary for characterizing disease status.[2,3]

Most family and genetic studies of OSA have used the apnea-hypopnea index (AHI, often used synonymously in the literature with "respiratory disturbance index," RDI), to define phenotype. The advantages of using the AHI include its relative simplicity, generally high night-to-night reproducibility,[4] and widespread clinical use. In addition, it is often used clinically to identify cases and to justify third-party reimbursement for treatment, and it is often followed as a key outcome in OSA treatment studies. Because the AHI has been shown to be moderately correlated with other indices of OSA severity, such as nighttime oxygen desaturation and sleep fragmentation,[3] it may provide information about several correlated traits that are important in disease expression. All genetic studies of OSA that use the AHI as the outcome variable have demonstrated significant familial aggregation,[5-7] suggesting that this measure captures useful information for quantifying genetic associations.

Combining polysomnographic data with other information, including symptoms, signs, and outcome data, to derive a multidimensional phenotype is one approach for producing a more comprehensive description. In the Cleveland Family Study, multivariate models provided improved classification of people into more homogeneous strata. Specifically, a stronger relationship between familial risk and OSA was observed when OSA was defined by an AHI level greater than15 plus reported daytime sleepiness than when disease was defined by AHI level alone.[8] Additional power may be gained in future genetic studies of OSA that use multidimensional phenotypes.

As part of this effort, the polysomnographic variables that best identify specific phenotypes must be clarified. For example, alternatives to the AHI, such as indices of flow limitation during sleep or spectral analysis of sleep architecture, may prove to be superior markers for genetic studies. However, a phenotype must be feasible for use in the large numbers of subjects that are needed for genetic epidemiologic studies of complex traits.[9] The choice of phenotype will be influenced by the cost, degree of invasiveness, degree of participant burden, and applicability across the spectrum of age and body mass index (BMI), as well as by its accuracy and reliability.

INTERMEDIATE PHENOTYPES

OSA is a complex syndrome that is defined using clinically and physiologically relevant terms; identifying genes that determine "intermediate" phenotypes that are on a causal pathway leading to OSA is one way to study it. Such intermediate traits may be more closely associated with specific gene products and may be less influenced by environmental modification than more complex phenotypes.

In OSA, a number of risk factors probably interact to increase propensity for repetitive upper airway collapse that occurs with sleep. In a given individual, the relevant attributes may be determined by anatomic and neuromuscular factors that influence upper airway size and function. Recognized risk factors are obesity, male gender,[10] small upper airway size,[11,12] ventilatory control mechanisms,[13-15] and possibly elements of sleep and circadian rhythm control.[16,17] These factors are probably influenced substantially by genetic elements.

There may be at least four[18] primary intermediate pathogenic pathways through which genes might act to increase susceptibility to OSA[18]: obesity and related metabolic syndrome phenotypes, craniofacial and upper airway morphometry, control of ventilation, and control of sleep and circadian rhythm.[19,20] These are discussed in more detail later (see "Candidate Gene [Association] and Genetic Linkage Studies"). The limitation of this approach is that the genes so identified may not be sufficient to describe the clinically important phenotype, which may only occur in the context of other genetic and environmental factors. Specifically, susceptibility genes for intermediate traits associated with OSA may not be equivalent to the susceptibility genes for OSA.

Obesity and Body Fat Distribution

Obesity increases risk of OSA approximately 10- to 14-fold, and the most marked effects are observed in middle age.[21] Central body fat distribution appears especially important. It is unclear whether this is because of the mechanical effects of central adiposity on lung mechanics and ventilation or upper airway size, or both,[22] or because visceral fat is metabolically active. Both central obesity and OSA are associated with hypertension, type 2 diabetes, and hyperlipidemia.[23-26] Thus, the association of central obesity and OSA may indicate a specific phenotype based on a gene or set of genes influencing

adipocyte biology, ventilatory control, chemoreflexes, or craniofacial morphology.

Obesity, like OSA, is strongly heritable, with heritability estimates for obesity-associated phenotypes such as BMI, skinfold thickness, regional body fat distribution, fat mass, and leptin levels between 40% and 70%.[27-31] Several mutations affecting genes that influence appetite regulation, thermogenesis, and other metabolic functions have been implicated in rare forms of human obesity. Animal models suggest that more than 85 quantitative trait loci potentially influence weight and body fat distribution, and most of these loci individually explain less than 4% of the phenotypic variation. To date, researchers have not identified large single or oligogenic effects that account for a sizable fraction of the variance in obesity levels in the population.

Analyses of obesity as an intermediate OSA trait require careful consideration of the potential causal relationships between obesity and OSA. Causal modeling, performed using data from the Cleveland Family Study, indicates complex relationships between indices of obesity (BMI and neck circumference) and AHI. These analyses showed that AHI and body mass index (BMI) are closely associated. The narrow-sense heritability [$h(2)_N$, the proportion of the variance of the trait attributable to the additive effects of genes] of BMI was 52.8%. After considering the additive genetic variance attributable to AHI, the $h(2)_N$ was modestly reduced to 42.9%, suggesting that BMI and AHI are related by both shared and unshared genetic pathways.[7] Continued application of sophisticated statistical methods is needed to better determine the genetic causal pathways that underlie the complex relationships between obesity and OSA.

Craniofacial Morphology

Craniofacial morphology, which affects both bony and soft tissues, is thought to predispose to OSA by reducing upper airway patency. Structural features that have been described in patients with OSA using techniques such as cephalometry include reduction of the anterior-posterior dimension of the cranial base, a reduced nasion-sella-basion angle, reduction of the size of the posterior and superior airway spaces, inferior displacement of the hyoid, elongation of the soft palate, macroglossia, hypertrophy of adenoids and tonsils, increased vertical facial dimension with a disproportionate increase in the lower facial height, and mandibular retrognathia or micrognathia.[11] A brachycephalic head form, measured by anthropometry, is often found in association with reduced upper airway dimensions. This head form is associated with a small but significant increased risk of OSA in whites,[32] and it also identifies families at risk for both OSA and sudden infant death.[33] In African Americans, this head form is uncommon and does not appear to increase risk of OSA.[32]

Acoustic reflectometry, which is a noninvasive technique for assessing airway cross-sectional area as a function of airway distance, has identified associations of OSA with mean and minimal airway cross-sectional areas.[34] Because this technique is relatively simple and portable, it may be particularly suitable in large-scale genetic epidemiologic studies. Magnetic resonance imaging has been used to precisely characterize anatomy in terms of muscle, fat, and bone contributions. Such studies have shown that the lateral pharyngeal wall and tongue are larger in OSA patients compared with matched controls.[35] Preliminary data from family studies indicate that these characteristics are also highly heritable.

Twin and family studies have consistently suggested a genetic basis for craniofacial morphology. Heritability estimates from twin studies of cephalometric data have ranged from 60% to 90%.[36,37] Micrognathia can be found in a number of genetic syndromes, suggesting that normal human craniofacial growth may be influenced by a number of genes, perhaps with specific dosage requirements. There are at least 50 syndromes in which congenital malformations of mandibular and maxillary structure occur, many of which also are associated with respiratory impairment and upper airway obstruction. These include Pierre Robin syndrome and Treacher Collins syndrome.[38] Identifying the genetic bases for these disorders may provide valuable insights into the pathogenetic basis of OSA.

Inherited abnormalities of craniofacial structure appear to explain at least some of the familial aggregation of OSA. Relatives of OSA probands have been shown to have decreased total pharyngeal volumes and glottic cross-sectional areas, retropositioned maxillae and mandibles, and longer soft palates compared with relatives of controls.[39] In another study population, relatives of patients with OSA were shown by cephalometry to have a more retropositioned mandible and smaller posterior superior airway space as compared to normative data.[40] In the Cleveland Family Study, both hard tissue (e.g., head form, intermaxillary length) and soft tissue (e.g., soft palate length, tongue volume) factors predicted the AHI level in white families. In black families, soft tissue factors also predicted AHI levels, but hard tissue anatomic features appeared to be only weakly associated with OSA.[32,41] These data support the importance of structural features in increasing susceptibility to OSA, but they also suggest that the anatomic underpinnings and the genes for upper airway anatomy may differ among ethnic groups.

Ventilatory Control Patterns

Upper airway patency is dynamically influenced by many complex processes linked with the control of both chest wall and upper airway neuromuscular function. Potentially inherited abnormalities of ventilatory control may predispose to obstructive or central sleep apnea by affecting ventilation during sleep and promoting upper airway collapsibility. This might occur by preferential reduction in the level of activation of upper airway muscles as compared with chest wall muscles.[42]

Altered ventilatory drive also may cause apnea by promoting ventilatory control instability and, subsequently, periodic breathing.[43] Recently, Tankersley and associates suggested that OSA may occur when ventilatory responses are inadequate to overcome physical obstruction of the upper airway, and they proposed measurement of the inspiratory "duty cycle" (the ratio of inspiratory time to tidal ventilation) as an intermediate trait that varies in the population and provides information on susceptibility to OSA.[44]

An inherited basis for ventilatory responsiveness to hypoxemia or hypercapnia has been suggested by familial studies of several respiratory diseases. Abnormalities in hypoxic or hypercapnic ventilatory responsiveness have been described in the first-degree relatives of probands with unexplained respiratory failure,[45,46] chronic obstructive pulmonary disease,[47-49] and asthma.[50] A genetic basis for ventilatory chemoresponsiveness has been suggested by several twin studies.[51-53]

Population differences in ventilatory patterns and hypoxic sensitivity have been identified for populations that have adapted to living at high altitude.[53,54] Heritability estimates for oxygen saturation or chemoresponsiveness to oxygen saturation levels range from approximately 30% to 75%, suggesting a substantial contribution of inheritance to this trait.[53,54]

A potential role for inherited impairments of ventilatory control in influencing susceptibility to OSA has been suggested by several studies of carefully characterized families.[14,15,55] These studies have demonstrated blunted hypoxic responses and impairment in load compensation in the families of OSA patients compared with controls. Thus, the familial aggregation of OSA may in some instances be based on inherited abnormalities in ventilatory control, perhaps related to chemoregulation or load compensation.

Control of Sleep and Circadian Rhythm

Given the impact of sleep-wake state on respiratory motor neuron activation, insights into the susceptibility of upper airway muscles to collapse during sleep may require delineation of the genetics of sleep-wake control. Remarkable advances in our understanding of narcolepsy have provided important information on genes that may control sleep-wake regulation. Experimental studies in both dogs and rodents have implicated deficiencies in the orexins (hypocretins; two polypeptides that are ligands for two G protein–coupled receptors in the brain) in causing the phenotypic abnormalities in sleep regulation that characterize narcolepsy (cataplexy, rapid eye movement [REM]-onset sleep, and hypersomnolence).[56-58]

One can speculate that abnormalities in orexin genes, or genes coding for their receptors, could be relevant to studies of OSA because of the potential impact of these neuropeptides on arousal and muscle tone, both of which influence the behavior of respiratory systems or because of the close proximity of these neurons to central respiratory control centers, with potential interactions between arousal and respiratory centers. Orexins have also been shown to play a role in energy homeostasis and the regulation of feeding.[59]

In addition to considering the impact of genetic abnormalities on processes that regulate sleep-wake state, it may be useful to consider how respiratory motor neuron control may be influenced by genetic processes that determine circadian clocks, which are known to drive important metabolic and behavioral rhythms. Studies of *Drosophila* and mouse models have identified a number of genes that influence periodicity and persistence of circadian rhythms.[60,61] A family has been reported with a marked phase advance of their clock.[17] The relevance of these findings to OSA is unclear. However, genetic variations in regulation of sleep-wake rhythm may be factors that influence the expression of OSA (e.g., ability to compensate or show sleepiness in response to recurrent apneas and sleep disruption).

Familial Aggregation of OSA

Significant familial aggregation of AHI, or of symptoms of OSA, has been observed in studies from the United States, Finland, Denmark, the United Kingdom, Israel, and Iceland.[39,40,59,62-66] Studies have used a variety of designs, including cohorts, small and large pedigrees, twins, and case-control studies; they have included adults and children; and they have employed varying approaches for assessing phenotype. Despite study design and population differences, all studies have consistently shown familial aggregation of the AHI level and symptoms of OSA in both children and adults and in obese and nonobese subjects.[39,55,64,65,67-71] These studies have provided clear evidence that a positive family history of OSA is an important risk factor for an elevated AHI and for associated symptoms such as snoring, daytime sleepiness, and apneas. However, the estimated magnitude of effects has varied greatly.

Four large twin studies have shown that concordance rates for snoring, a cardinal symptom of OSA, were significantly higher in monozygotic twins than in dizygotic twins.[62,72-74] A recent study of adult male twins showed significant genetic correlations for daytime sleepiness as well as snoring, and models were consistent with common genes underlying both symptoms.[73] Carmelli's group recently extended their research, establishing significant heritability for objectively measured AHI levels in this twin population.[75] A large Danish cohort study[63] showed that the age, BMI, and comorbidity-adjusted risk of snoring was increased threefold when one first-degree relative was a snorer, and it increased fourfold when both parents were snorers.

The prevalence of objectively measured OSA among first-degree relatives of OSA probands has been reported to vary from 22% to 84%.[39,40,65,66,70] Among the studies that included controls, the odds ratio, which relates the odds of a person with OSA in a family with affected relatives to that for someone without an affected relative, has varied from 2 to 46.[39,40,65] Pedigree studies from both the United States and Iceland have shown consistent associations; the overall recurrent risk for OSA in a family member of an affected proband is approximately 2,[65,71] which is lower than that reported from case control studies. Heritability estimates for the AHI from both pedigree[7] and twin[75] studies are approximately 35% to 40%. Similar parent-offspring ($r = .21$, $P = .002$) and sib-sib correlations ($r = .21$, $P = .003$)[65] have been observed, and they are greater than spouse-spouse correlations.[65]

OSA has been described as occurring more commonly as a multiplex (affecting at least two members) than a simplex (occurring in a single family member) disorder. Further evidence for a genetic basis for OSA is derived from the observation that the odds of sleep apnea syndrome, defined as AHI >15 and self-reported daytime sleepiness, increases with increasing numbers of affected relatives. Table 84-1 shows the odds for sleep apnea syndrome given one, two, or three affected

relatives with these findings, as compared with OSA patients who have no affected relatives, adjusted for age, gender, ethnicity, and BMI.[65]

These results support the utility of ascertaining family history as part of the evaluation of the patient for OSA. Information on snoring, apneas, and sleepiness among first-degree relatives can be used to refine the likelihood of OSA in any given patient. However, perhaps more importantly, such information can be used to make it easier to diagnose cases by identifying the need for other family members to seek sleep evaluations.

GENETIC ANALYSES

Segregation Analysis

Segregation analysis is an approach whereby statistical models that make alternative assumptions about the underlying mode of inheritance and the impact of environmental factors on a given trait are compared in an attempt to identify the model that best explains the underlying distribution of traits. These analyses are particularly useful in identifying potential patterns of inheritance.

In the Tucson Epidemiologic Survey, segregation analyses of self-reported snoring in 584 pedigrees suggested a major gene effect; however, evidence for the connection weakened after adjustments were made for obesity and gender.[75] Segregation analysis was applied to a sample of whites (177 families, 1202 members) and African Americans (123 families, 709 members) in the Cleveland Family Study. The data suggest that the observed distribution of the AHI is consistent with the segregation of major genetic factors within both sets of families,[6] although the results suggested possible ethnic differences in the mode of inheritance.

In whites, analysis suggested recessive Mendelian inheritance of the AHI, which accounts for 21% to 27% of the variance and an additional 8% to 9% of the variation caused by other familial factors, either environmental or polygenic. In African Americans, the BMI-adjusted and age-adjusted AHI gave evidence of segregation of a codominant gene with an allele frequency of 0.14 that accounts for 35% of the total variance of this trait. Adjustment of the AHI for BMI weakened the findings in the whites and strengthened them in the African Americans. These results provide support for an underlying genetic basis for OSA in African Americans independent of the contribution of BMI. The analyses in whites suggested that a major gene for OSA might be closely related to genes for obesity.

Table 84–1.	**Familial Correlations for Apnea-Hypopnea Index**				
	Partially Adjusted*			**BMI-Adjusted†**	
Relationship	**Familial Correlation Coefficient**	**P Value**		**Familial Correlation Coefficient**	**P Value**
Parent-offspring	.21	.002		.17	.017
Sib-sib	.21	.003		.18	.008

BMI, body mass index.

*Adjusted for age, age^2, ethnic group, and gender.

†Adjusted for BMI, age, age^2, ethnic group, and gender.

From Redline S, Tishler PV, Tosteson TD, et al: The familial aggregation of obstructive sleep apnea. Am J Respir Crit Care Med 1995;151:682-687.

Causal Pathway Modeling

As discussed earlier, OSA is closely associated with a number of intermediate phenotypes, and it is likely to result from dysregulation involving several interacting biologic systems. Although these factors are closely related, it is uncertain to what extent associations reflect the action of shared genetic determinants. Informed genetic analysis—models that appropriately specify relationships among the covariates (such as BMI) associated with OSA—will not be possible until the basic mechanisms and interactions underlying these pathophysiologic factors are understood.

Causal pathway modeling has been applied to the Cleveland Family data to dissect the genetic etiology of OSA and associated traits by investigating the sharing or nonsharing of the genetic and nongenetic determinants of correlated phenotypes. Evidence of shared additive genetic determinants would suggest that the close association of these traits with OSA and with each other is at least partially the result of shared genetic factors. Evidence of unshared additive genetic determinants suggests the existence of multiple, distinct genetic pathways modulating genetic susceptibility to OSA.

The relationships among AHI- and OSA-associated traits—BMI, neck circumference, and high-density lipoprotein (HDL) cholesterol levels—suggest that the patterns of association are different among white and African American families and that the pathogenetic mechanisms leading to OSA are complex and involve a number of genetically distinct pathways.[76] Only 19% to 30% of the additive genetic variance for BMI and AHI overlapped, suggesting that there are both shared and unshared genetic factors underlying susceptibility to OSA and obesity.

Candidate Genes and Biochemical Markers

Genes that influence obesity and body fat distribution, craniofacial morphology, ventilatory control, and the sleep-wake state may be relevant in determining the OSA phenotype. In rodents, numerous genes have been identified that influence the expression or regulation of proteins or receptors that could be relevant in the pathogenesis of OSA. Most studies of inbred strains and back-crosses have suggested strong genetic

regulation of obesity,[77,78] ventilatory control,[79] and craniofacial morphometry.[80] Candidate genes for intermediate OSA phenotypes are summarized in Table 84–2.

Obesity and Body Fat Distribution

The genetics of obesity has been the subject of several detailed reviews.[27,78,81] Numerous cross-breeding experiments in animal models of obesity have been undertaken, suggesting that more than 85 potential quantitative trait loci may regulate body weight or body fat.[78] However, only a few humans appear to have genetic mutations in homologous genes.

Recent interest has been directed at elucidating genes that regulate the expression of a range of proteins involved in the hypothalamic-pituitary-adrenal-thyroid axis. Through complex positive- and negative-feedback loops, including signaling from fat, muscle, liver, and the gastrointestinal tract, these proteins affect appetite, nutrient turnover, and thermogenesis (see Table 84–2). Some genes may have effects that vary by sex, age, and subphenotypes and that are differentially influenced by environmental factors.

Of potential interest in regard to OSA are genes associated with leptin, a protein with a number of pleiotropic effects relevant to the OSA phenotype. Leptin-deficient mice are markedly obese, as are the very rare human cases with leptin deficiency.[82] However, the majority of obese humans, including patients with OSA,[83] have increased leptin levels, suggesting that human obesity and OSA are associated with leptin resistance. One target for leptin is pro-opiomelanocortin (POMC), a precursor protein in the hypothalamus for several other proteins involved in weight homeostasis, including alpha-melanocyte–stimulating hormone.[84] Humans with POMC mutations are obese.[85] Results of the first published genome-wide linkage analysis for the AHI shows suggestive linkage to an area on chromosome 2, near the POMC gene.[7]

Ventilatory Control

Mouse models have been used to identify genes potentially important in the control of ventilation, including genes that determine respiratory timing, frequency, awake ventilation, chemosensitivity, and load responses. Clear strain differences have been observed for many of these phenotypes, with evidence

Trait	Candidate Genes*
Obesity	Leptin, pro-opiomelanocortin, melanocyte-stimulating hormone, melanocortin 4-receptor, neuropeptidase Y, insulin-like growth factor, glucokinase, adenosine deaminase, tumor necrosis factor-α, glucose regulatory protein, agouti signaling protein, β3-adrenergic receptor, carboxypeptidase E, insulin signaling protein, resistin, ghrelin, adiponectin, gamma-aminobutyric acid transporter, orexin
Ventilatory control	RET proto-oncogene, *PHOX2B, HOX IIL2, KROX-20*, receptor tyrosine kinase, neurotrophic growth factors (brain-derived, glia-derived neurotrophic factors, neurotrophic factor-4, platelet-derived growth factors), neuronal synthase, acetylcholine receptor, dopaminergic receptor, substance P, glutamyl transpeptidase, endothelin-1, endothelin-3, leptin, *KROX-20, en-1, gsh-2*, orexin
Craniofacial and airway structure	Class I homeobox genes, growth hormone receptors, growth factor receptors, retinoic acid, endothelin-1, collagen types I and II, tumor necrosis factor-α

Table 84–2.   Candidate Genes for Intermediate Phenotypes for Obstructive Sleep Apnea

*Includes related proteins and receptors.

of quantitative trait loci near plausible candidate genes.[79,86-89] Knockout and transgenic mice also have helped identify the role of specific proteins and receptors in ventilatory responses.

Generally, genetic determinants of ventilatory control have focused on genes that influence respiratory chemoreception, neuromuscular transmission, and neural integration. Broadly, these include genes that influence the segmentation of the brainstem during development (*HOX* genes, *Krox20*), influence autonomic nervous system development (*HOX* genes, *RET* proto-oncogene), and influence the growth and survival of glomus cells of the carotid body and other peripheral chemoreceptors and neurotrophic factors, as well as neurotransmitters involved in afferent or efferent pathways linked to the central or peripheral controllers of respiration (e.g., substance P, dopaminergic and acetylcholine receptors, neuronal nitrous oxide synthase).

Homeobox genes are transcription factors characterized by a highly conserved DNA binding homeodomain; they play a critical role in brain development, including development of centers of cardiorespiratory control. In mice, targeted deletion of several genes critical for hindbrain development, especially of the medullary respiratory centers and nucleus tractus solitarius, such as zinc finger protein Krox-20, HOXIIL2, and Gsn-2, results in phenotypes characterized by frequent apneas, respiratory failure, and abnormal respiratory patterns.[90-92]

Heterozygous and homozygous *RET* (a proto-oncogene involved in embryonic neural crest development) knockout mice, which survive only briefly, demonstrate reductions in hypercapnic ventilatory responsiveness.[93] One homeobox gene, *PHOX2B*, expressed in the peripheral and central autonomic nervous system tissue, was mutated in 18 of 29 humans with congenital central hypoventilation syndrome,[94] suggesting a critical role for this gene in the normal patterning of ventilation.

In a knockout mouse model, loss of brain-derived neurotrophic factor (BDNF) resulted in reduced survival of neurons in the nodose-petrosal ganglion.[95] Other data have implicated other neurotropic factors in the survival and growth of cells that mediate chemoreception.[96,97]

Endothelin-1 (ET-1) is a potent vasoactive peptide expressed in the central and peripheral nervous system as well as the lung and other organs and is highly expressed embryonically in the pharyngeal arch. Mutant mice deficient in ET-1 have impaired ventilatory responses to both hypoxia and hypercapnia.[98] Hypoxia-related ventilation appears to be mediated by *S*-nitrosothiols at the nucleus tractus solitarius. Deficiencies in these and related signaling molecules are thought to contribute to abnormal hypoxic responses.[99]

In summary, these studies emphasize the complexity of the respiratory control system, and they indicate that a number of genes important in different regulatory functions might influence ventilatory phenotypes potentially relevant to OSA.

Craniofacial Structure

Mouse models have suggested that a number of different genes may influence craniofacial development. Craniofacial abnormalities, including retrognathia and micrognathia, have been described in mice deficient in the growth and differentiating factor transforming growth factor-β2,[100] in mice deficient for the retinoic acid receptor-αγ,[101] and in mice with collagen gene mutations (types II and XI).[102] Further understanding of

homeobox genes and genes controlling growth factors may contribute to our clarifying the origins of craniofacial dysmorphisms found in OSA.

Pleiotropic Effects: Proteins with Multiple Effects Relevant to OSA

A number of the candidate genes for intermediate phenotypes (e.g., leptin, ET-1, orexins) may affect the expression of several other OSA-related traits, for example, obesity,[103] ventilation,[28,104,105] sleep architecture,[106,107] lung structure,[108] and craniofacial structure. For example, a number of candidate genes for obesity (e.g., leptin, adenosine deaminase, and melanocortin-4 receptor) are expressed in a variety of tissues and brain sites important for regulating breathing.

Candidate Gene (Association) and Genetic Linkage Studies

Researchers have begun to investigate the molecular genetics of OSA using two general approaches: candidate gene approaches (association studies) and whole genome screens followed by positional cloning attempts. Most candidate gene approaches compare the frequency of specific polymorphisms of interest in groups with and without OSA. Genetic linkage studies, in contrast, examine the cosegregation of a disease locus and a marker locus among family members. Typically, the strength of genetic associations is expressed as a LOD score (the log-odds summarizing the probability of receiving alleles at two loci). A LOD score of 3.0 or more usually is considered strong evidence for linkage, while a LOD score of less than −2.0 is interpreted as evidence against linkage.

Association Studies

ANGIOTENSIN-CONVERTING ENZYME

Several types of experimental and anthropologic studies indicate that an insertion polymorphism in the angiotensin I–converting enzyme (ACE) gene, which results in reduced serum and tissue ACE activity, is more frequent in persons with greater endurance and better adaptation to high altitude, suggesting a relationship between this gene and ventilatory regulation.[109,110] The relationship of this ACE polymorphism to ventilatory control pattern is an area of active investigation. A preliminary study from China, which reported an association between a polymorphism in the ACE gene and severity of OSA, suggests the potential importance of this gene in moderating expression of OSA, possibly by effects on hypoxic arousal.[5]

APOLIPOPROTEIN E

An allele of the apolipoprotein E gene (ε4) that has been previously associated with increased risk for both cardiovascular disease and Alzheimer's disease[111] has been shown to be associated with an elevated AHI level in two cohort studies[112,113] of predominantly white populations. However, this finding was not replicated in two other studies, including a study of an older Japanese American cohort.[114,115]

Linkage Analyses

A whole genome screen for OSA and associated phenotypes was recently completed in a subset of African American and white families selected from the Cleveland Family Study.[116] Multipoint model-free variance component linkage analysis was performed for the quantitative phenotype AHI. In the white families, candidate regions on chromosomes 1p, 2p, 12p, and 19p gave suggestive evidence for linkage to AHI. The highest LOD scores were 1.64 on chromosome 2 (2p16), 1.43 on chromosome 12 (12p13), and 1.40 on chromosome 19 (19q13). In the African American families, a candidate region on chromosome 8 gave suggestive evidence for linkage to AHI.

Several biologically plausible candidate genes are located within the most promising chromosome regions in these analyses. The chromosome 2p region contains acid phosphatase 1, apoprotein B precursor, POMC, and the alpha-2B-adrenergic receptor. Although the linkage associations were only suggestive, they pointed to plausible candidate genes for OSA that have also been implicated in genetic studies of obesity, where BMI, percentage of body fat, and serum leptin levels were examined as relevant phenotypes.

Special Challenges in Studying the Genetics of OSA

As described earlier, the AHI has been the most common measure used in genetic studies of OSA. However, it is not clear that this is the trait that has the highest degree of heritability or whether it provides an index of disease severity that is consistent across the population. As a "count," it may not provide maximal information regarding severity of individual events (duration, associated hypoxemia, arousal) and event characteristics (e.g., extent of pleural pressure swings).

The AHI may be conceptualized as a category that includes a variety of event patterns (e.g., obstructive, central, mixed, periodic, or Cheyne-Stokes respiration), each of which may occur in different age or disease contexts and reflect different genetic influences. For example, central events and Cheyne-Stokes respiration may occur in association with underlying heart failure or central nervous system disease, both of which may increase with aging. An overall AHI in an older population may represent somewhat different physiologic perturbations than one derived in a younger population.

Genetic determinants also may distinguish persons with a predominance of central events, in whom neural mechanisms may play a potentially greater role than do factors that more directly influence airway collapsibility. Certain genetic influences may affect predominantly the duration rather than the number of respiratory events. For example, preliminary association studies suggest that duration of apneas, possibly a surrogate for arousability or other ventilatory traits, may vary according to ACE polymorphisms,[5] which may prove to be an important genetic determinant of susceptibility to severe OSA. More comprehensive physiologic data may better capture features that define clearer and more specific phenotypes.

The AHI as a trait-defining variable also presents special statistical challenges in genetic studies. Analyses of quantitative trait loci usually provide the greater statistical power in genetic analyses than analyses of binary traits (e.g., present or absent). These analyses are very sensitive to normality assumptions. However, the AHI follows an extremely skewed distribution that even extensive statistical transformations often do not fully normalize. Additionally, these distributions may vary by sex, with different mean values as well as variances for males and females.[6]

These statistical challenges have required some studies to use specialized statistical transformations applied to each sex separately.[6] Additionally, in the general population, AHI strongly correlates with BMI.[6] Initial linkage studies, statistical analyses examining the cosegregation of alleles, suggest that there are both common and independent genetic determinants for the AHI and BMI.[7] Thus, strategies where the AHI is statistically adjusted for BMI may not be appropriate for identifying genes that causally affect both traits. On the other hand, analyses that do not account for BMI have limited interpretability regarding the specificity for OSA of any observed genetic associations.

Challenges also arise in association studies, where it is necessary to define specific thresholds for classifying disease status. The absolute threshold values that distinguish disease subgroups are very sensitive to the specific application of polysomnographic measurement techniques,[9] and they may also vary according to the age and other characteristics of the population. Because the AHI has a strong age dependency, with marked increases with advancing age and in women after menopause, a single threshold disease-defining value may not be appropriate across the age span.

SUMMARY

Despite the challenges in studying an inherently complex trait, there is growing evidence from clinical and epidemiologic studies that genetic factors influence the expression of OSA. The overall magnitude of effect that may be attributable to specific genes requires further definition. Differences in phenotype definition and sampling have hindered comparisons between studies. However, the largest pedigree and twin studies consistently estimate heritability for the AHI to be between 35% and 40%, with recurrent risk factors of approximately 2.

The recurrence of OSA in families suggests a multifactorial etiology. Although innumerable potential candidate genes for OSA and related phenotypes exist, segregation analysis suggests that a small number of genes likely account for approximately 20% of the variance in the trait. Investigating the genetic etiology of OSA offers a means of better understanding its pathogenesis, with the goal of improving preventive strategies, diagnostic tools, and therapies.

Molecular studies of OSA itself are in their infancy, but initial promising findings suggest potentially important genetic mechanisms. Animal models have been developed in parallel with human studies to assist in identifying OSA-susceptibility genes. The successful integration of information from human and animal studies should lead to the mapping of genes for traits that substantially influence the expression of OSA.

Clinical Pearl

A positive family history of OSA (or of related symptoms) is useful in identifying patients at increased risk for the disorder. Craniofacial abnormalities and obesity may each have a genetic basis and are risk factors for sleep apnea. Clinicians should ask about apnea symptoms in family members. Children and siblings of patients with craniofacial abnormalities may have similar abnormalities that may be amenable to treatment.

REFERENCES

1. Guilleminault C: Obstructive sleep apnea: The clinical syndrome and historical perspective. Med Clin N America 1985;69:1187-1203.
2. Flemons WW, Buysse D, Redline S, et al: Sleep-related breathing disorders in adults: Recommendations for syndrome definition and measurement techniques in clinical research: The report of an American Academy of Sleep Medicine Task Force. Sleep 1999; 22:533-570.
3. Gould GA, Whyte KF, Rhind GB, et al: The sleep hypopnea syndrome. Am Rev Respir Dis 1988;137:895-898.
4. Quan SF, Griswold ME, Iber C, et al: Short-term variability of respiration and sleep during unattended nonlaboratory polysomnography—The Sleep Heart Health Study. Sleep 2002; 25:843-849.
5. Xiao Y, Huang X, Qiu C, et al: Angiotensin 1 converting enzyme gene polymorphism in Chinese patients with obstructive sleep apnea syndrome. Chin Med J 1999;112:701-704.
6. Buxbaum SG, Elston RC, Tishler PV, Redline S: Genetics of the apnea hypopnea index in Caucasians and African Americans: I. Segregation analysis. Genet Epidemiol 2002;22:243-53.
7. Palmer LJ, Buxbaum SG, Larkin E, et al: A whole-genome scan for obstructive sleep apnea and obesity. Am J Hum Genet 2003; 72:340-50.
8. Redline S, Tishler PV: Familial influences on sleep apnea. In Saunders NA (ed): Sleep and Breathing, 2nd ed. New York, Marcel Dekker, 1994, pp 363-377.
9. Redline S, Sanders MH, Lind BK, et al: Methods for obtaining and analyzing unattended polysomnography data for a multi-center study. Sleep 1998;21:759-767.
10. Strohl KP, Redline S: Recognition of obstructive sleep apnea. Am J Respir Crit Care Med 1996;154:279-289.
11. Lowe AA, Ozbek MM, Miyamoto K, et al: Cephalometric and demographic characteristics of obstructive sleep apnea: An evaluation with partial least squares analysis. Angle Orthod 1997;67:143-153.
12. Pracharktam N, Nelson S, Hans MG, et al: Cephalometric assessment in obstructive sleep apnea. Am J Orthod Dentofacial Orthop 1996;109:410-419.
13. Lavie P, Rubin AE: Effects of nasal occlusion on respiration in sleep: Evidence of inheritability of sleep apnea prognosis. Acta Otolaryngol 1984;97:127-130.
14. Pillar G, Schnall RP, Peled NIR, et al: Impaired respiratory response to resistive loading during sleep in healthy offspring of patients with obstructive sleep apnea. Am J Respir Crit Care Med 1997;155:1602-1608.
15. Redline S, Leitner J, Arnold J, et al: Ventilatory-control abnormalities in familial sleep apnea. Am J Respir Crit Care Med 1997;156:155-60.
16. Heath AC, Kendler KS, Eaves LJ, Martin N: Evidence for genetic influences on sleep disturbance and sleep pattern in twins. Sleep 1990;13:318-335.
17. Jones CR, Campbell SS, Zone SE, et al: Familial advanced sleep-phase syndrome: A short-period circadian rhythm variant in humans. Nat Med 1999;5:1062-1065.
18. Palmer LJ, Redline S: Genomic approaches to understanding obstructive sleep apnea. Respir Physiol Neurobiol 2003; 135:187-205.
19. Redline S, Young T: Epidemiology and natural history of obstructive sleep apnea. Ear Nose Throat J 1993;72:20-21, 24-26.
20. Redline SR, Tishler PV: The genetics of sleep apnea. Sleep Med Rev 2000;4:583-602.
21. Redline S: Age-related differences in sleep apnea: Generalizability of finding in older populations. In Kuna S (ed): Sleep and Respiration in Aging Adults. New York, Elsevier, 1991, pp 189-194.
22. Horner RL, Mohiaddin RH, Lowell DG, et al: Sites and sizes of fat deposits around the pharynx in obese patients with obstructive sleep apnea and weight matched controls. Eur Respir J 1989;2:613-622.
23. Ferrannini E, De Fronzo RA: The association of hypertension, diabetes, and obesity: A review. J Nephrol 1989;1:3-15.
24. Katsumada K, Okada T, Miyao M, Katsumata Y: High incidence of sleep apnea syndrome in a male diabetic population. Diab Res Clin Prac 1991;13:45-52.
25. Strohl KP, Novak RD, Singer W, et al: Insulin levels, blood pressure and sleep apnea. Sleep 1994;17:614-618.
26. Strohl KP: Diabetes and sleep apnea. Sleep 1996;19:225-228.
27. Comuzzie AG, Allison DB: The search for human obesity genes. Science 1998;280:1374-1377.
28. Bray G, Bouchard C: Genetics of human obesity: Research directions. FASEB J 1997;11:937-945.
29. Arner P: Obesity—a genetic disease of adipose tissue? Br J Nutr 2000 83(Suppl 1):S9-S16.
30. Barsh GS, Farooqi IS, O'Rahilly S: Genetics of body-weight regulation. Nature 2000;404:644-51.
31. Chagnon YC, Perusse L, Weisnagel SJ, et al: The human obesity gene map: The 1999 update. Obes Res 2000;8:89-117.
32. Cakirer B, Hans MG, Graham G, et al: The relationship between craniofacial morphology and obstructive sleep apnea in whites and in African-Americans. Am J Respir Crit Care Med 2001;163: 947-950.
33. Tishler PV, Redline S, Ferrette V, et al: The association of sudden unexpected infant death with obstructive sleep apnea. Am J Respir Crit Care Med 1996;153:1857-1863.
34. Monahan KJ, Larkin EK, Rosen CL, et al: Utility of noninvasive pharyngometry in epidemiologic studies of childhood sleep-disordered breathing. Am J Respir Crit Care Med 2002;165: 1499-1503.
35. Schwab RJ, Pasirstein M, Pierson R, et al: Identification of upper airway anatomic risk factors for obstructive sleep apnea with volumetric magnetic resonance imaging. Am J Respir Crit Care Med 2003;168:522-530.
36. Arya R, Duggirala R, Comuzzie AG, et al: Heritability of anthropometric phenotypes in caste populations in Visakhapatnam, India. Hum Biol 2002;74:325-344.
37. Osborne RH, De George FV: Genetic Basis of Morphologic Variation: An Evaluation and Application of the Twin Study Method. Cambridge, Mass: Harvard University Press, 1959.
38. McKusick V: Mendelian Inheritance in Man. Baltimore: Johns Hopkins University Press, 1992.
39. Mathur R, Douglas NJ: Family studies in patients with the sleep apnea-hypopnea syndrome. Ann Intern Med 1995;122:174-178.
40. Guilleminault C, Partinen M, Hollman K, et al: Familial aggregates in obstructive sleep apnea syndrome. Chest 1995;107:1545-1551.
41. Redline S, Tishler PV, Hans MG, et al: Racial differences in sleep-disordered breathing in African-Americans and Caucasians. Am J Respir Crit Care Med 1997;155:186-192.
42. Strohl KP, Cherniack NS, Gothe B: Physiologic basis of therapy for sleep apnea. Am Rev Respir Dis 1986;134:791-802.
43. Cherniack NS: Respiratory dysrhythmias during sleep. N Engl J Med 1981;305:325-330.
44. Tankersley CG: Genetic aspects of breathing: On interactions between hypercapnia and hypoxia. Respir Physiol Neurobiol 2003;135:167-178.
45. Martin RJ, Ballard RD, Hudgel DW, Hill PL: The effects of weight and chemosensitivity on respiratory sleep abnormalities: A family study. Int J Obes 1986;10:283-292.
46. Moore GC, Zwillich CW, Battaglia JD, et al: Respiratory failure associated with familial depression of ventilatory response to hypoxia and hypercapnia. N Engl J Med 1976;295:861-865.
47. Fleetham JA, Arnup ME, Anthonisen NR: Familial aspects of ventilatory control in patients with chronic obstructive pulmonary disease. Am Rev Respir Dis 1984;129:3-7.
48. Kawakami Y, Irie T, Shida A, Yoshikawa T: Familial factors affecting arterial blood gas values and respiratory chemosensitivity in chronic obstructive pulmonary disease. Am Rev Respir Dis 1982;125:420-425.

49. Mountain R, Zwillich C, Weil J: Hypoventilation in obstructive lung disease: The role of familial factors. N Engl J Med 1978; 298:521-525.

50. Hudgel DW, Weil JV: Asthma associated with decreased hypoxic ventilatory drive: A family study. Ann Intern Med 1974;80: 622-625.

51. Collins DD, Scoggin CH, Zwillich CW, Weil JV: Hereditary aspects of decreased hypoxic response. J Clin Invest 1978;62: 105-110.

52. Kawakami Y, Yamamoto H, Yoshikawa T, Shida A: Chemical and behavioral control of breathing in adult twins. Am Rev Respir Dis 1984;129:703-707.

53. Thomas DA, Swaminathan S, Beardsmore CS, et al: Comparison of peripheral chemoreceptor responses in monozygotic and dizygotic twin infants. Am Rev Respir Dis 1993;148:1605-1609.

54. Beall C, Strohl K, Blangero J, et al: Quantitative genetic analysis of arterial oxygen saturation in Tibetan highlanders. Hum Biol 1997;69:597-604.

55. el Bayadi S, Millman RP, Tishler PV, et al: A family study of sleep apnea. Anatomic and physiologic interactions. Chest 1990;98: 554-559.

56. Chemelli RM, Willie JT, Sinton CM, et al: Narcolepsy in orexin knockout mice: Molecular genetics of sleep regulation. Cell 1999;98:437-451.

57. Nishino S, Mignot E: Pharmacological aspects of human and canine narcolepsy. Prog Neurobiol 1997;52:27-78.

58. Nishino S, Ripley B, Overcom S, et al: Hypocretin (orexin) deficiency in human narcolepsy. Lancet 2000;355:39-40.

59. Smart D, Haynes AC, Williams G, Arch JR: Orexins and the treatment of obesity. Eur J Pharmacol. 2002;440:199-212.

60. Gekakis N, Staknis D, Nguyen HB, et al: Role of the CLOCK protein in the mammalian circadian mechanism. Science 1998; 280:1564-1568.

61. Hao H, Allen DL, Hardin PE: A circadian enhancer mediates PER-dependent mRNA cycling in *Drosophila melanogaster*. Mol Cell Biol 1997;17:3687-3693.

62. Kaprio J, Koskenvuo M, Partinen M, Telakivi I: A twin study of snoring (abstract). Sleep Res 1988;17:365.

63. Jennum P, Hein HO, Suadicani P, et al: Snoring, family history, and genetic markers in men: The Copenhagen Male Study. Chest 1995;107:1289-1293.

64. Redline S, Tosteson T, Tishler PV, et al: Studies in the genetics of obstructive sleep apnea. Familial aggregation of symptoms associated with sleep-related breathing disturbances. Am Rev Respir Dis 1992;145:440-444.

65. Redline S, Tishler PV, Tosteson TD, et al: The familial aggregation of obstructive sleep apnea. Am J Respir Crit Care Med 1995; 151:682-687.

66. Pillar G, Lavie P: Assessment of the role of inheritance in sleep apnea syndrome. Am J Respir Crit Care Med 1995;151:688-691.

67. Strohl KP, Saunders NA, Feldman NT, Hallett M: Obstructive sleep apnea in family members. N Engl J Med 1978;299:969-973.

68. Wittig RM, Zorick FJ, Roehrs TA, et al: Familial childhood sleep apnea. Henry Ford Hosp Med J 1988;36:13-15.

69. Manon-Espaillat R, Gothe B, Adams N, et al: Familial "sleep apnea plus" syndrome. Report of a family. Neurology 1988;38: 190-193.

70. Douglas NJ, Luke M, Mathur R: Is the sleep apnoea/hypopnoea syndrome inherited? Thorax 1993;48:719-721.

71. Gislason T, Johannsson JH, Haraldsson A, et al: Familial predisposition and cosegregation analysis of adult obstructive sleep apnea and the sudden infant death syndrome. Am J Respir Crit Care Med 2002;166:833-838.

72. Ferini-Strambi L, Calori G, Oldani A, et al: Snoring in twins. Respir Med 1995;89:337-340.

73. Carmelli D, Bliwise DL, Swan GE, Reed T: Genetic factors in self-reported snoring and excessive daytime sleepiness: A twin study. Am J Respir Crit Care Med 2001;164:949-952.

74. Carmelli D, Colrain IM, Swan GE, Bliwise DL: Genetic and environmental influences in sleep disordered breathing in older male twins. Sleep 2004;27:917-922.

75. Holberg CJ, Natrajan S, Cline MG, Quan SF: Familial aggregation and segregation analysis of snoring and symptoms of obstructive sleep apnea. Sleep Breath 2000;4:21-30.

76. Redline S, Palmer LJ, Elston RC: Genetics of obstructive sleep apnea and related phenotypes. Am J Respir Cell Biol 2004; 2(supp):51-81.

77. Tschop M, Heiman ML: Rodent obesity models: An overview. Exp Clin Endocrinol Diabetes 2001;109:307-319.

78. Rankinen T, Perusse L, Weisnagel SJ, et al: The human obesity gene map: The 2001 update. Obes Res 2002;10:196-243.

79. Strohl K, Thomas A, St. Jean P, et al: Estimates of heritability for ventilatory traits from a rat intercross. Am J Respir Crit Care 1997;155:A444.

80. Wilkie AO, Morriss-Kay GM: Genetics of craniofacial development and malformation. Nat Rev Genet 2001;2:458-468.

81. Commuzzie AG, Hixson JE, Almasy L, et al: A major quantitative trait locus determining serum leptin levels and fat mass is located on human chromosome 2. Nat Genet 1997;15:273-276.

82. Montague CT, Farooqi IS, Whitehead JP, et al: Congenital leptin deficiency is associated with early-onset obesity in humans. Nature 1997;387:903-908.

83. Patel SR, Palmer LJ, Larkin EK, et al: Obstructive sleep apnea and diurnal leptin rhythm. Sleep 2004;15:235-239.

84. Wardlaw SL: Obesity as a neuroendocrine disease: Lessons to be learned from proopiomelanocortin and melanocortin receptor mutations in mice and men. J Clin Endocrinol Metab 2001;86: 1442-1446.

85. Challis BG, Pritchard LE, Creemers JW, et al: A missense mutation disrupting a dibasic prohormone processing site in pro-opiomelanocortin (POMC) increases susceptibility to early-onset obesity through a novel molecular mechanism. Hum Mol Genet 2002;11:1997-2004.

86. Tankersley CG, DiSilvestre DA, Jedlicka AE, et al: Differential inspiratory timing is genetically linked to mouse chromosome 3. J Appl Physiol 1998;85:360-365.

87. Tankersley CG, Fitzgerald RS, Levitt RC, et al: Genetic control of differential baseline breathing pattern. J Appl Physiol 1997; 82:874-881.

88. Strohl KP, Thomas AJ, St. Jean P, et al: Ventilation and metabolism among rat strains. J Appl Physiol 1997;82:317-323.

89. Tankersley CG, Fitzgerald RS, Mitzner WA, Kleeberger SR: Hypercapnic ventilatory responses in mice differentially susceptible to acute ozone exposure. J Appl Physiol 1993;75: 2613-2619.

90. Shirasawa S, Arata A, Onimaru H, et al: Rnx deficiency results in congenital central hypoventilation. Nat Genet 2000;24: 287-290.

91. Szucsik JC, Witte DP, Li H, et al: Altered forebrain and hindbrain development in mice mutant for the Gsh-2 homeobox gene. Dev Biol 1997;191:230-242.

92. Jacquin TD, Borday V, Schneider-Maunoury S, et al: Reorganization of pontine rhythmogenic neuronal networks in Krox-20 knockout mice. Neuron 1996;17:747-758.

93. Burton MD, Kawashima A, Brayer JA, et al: RET proto-oncogene is important for the development of respiratory CO_2 sensitivity. J Auton Nerv Syst 1997;63:137-143.

94. Amiel J, Laudier B, Attie-Bitach T, et al: Polyalanine expansion and frameshift mutations of the paired-like homeobox gene PHOX2B in congenital central hypoventilation syndrome. Nat Genet 2003;33:459-461.

95. Erickson JT, Conover JC, Borday V, et al: Mice lacking brain-derived neurotrophic factor exhibit visceral sensory neuron losses distinct from mice lacking NT4 and display a severe developmental deficit in control of breathing. J Neurosci 1996; 16:5361-5371.

96. Katz DM, Balkowiec A: New insights into the ontogeny of breathing from genetically engineered mice. Curr Opin Pul Med 1997;3:433-439.

97. Durbec P, Marcos-Gutierrez CV, Kilkenny C, et al: GDNF signalling through the Ret receptor tyrosine kinase. Nature 1996;381:789-793.

98. Kurihara Y, Kurihara H, Suzuki H, et al: Elevated blood pressure and craniofacial abnormalities in mice deficient in endothelin-1. Nature 1994;368:703-710.

99. Lipton SA: Physiology: Nitric oxide and respiration. Nature 2001;413:118-119.

100. Sanford LP, Ormsby I, Gittenberger-de Groot AC, et al: TGF beta–2 knockout mice have multiple developmental defects that are non-overlapping with other TGF beta knockout phenotypes. Development 1997;124:2659-2670.

101. Lohnes D, Mark M, Mendelsohn C, et al: Function of the retinoic acid receptors (RARs) during development. (I) Craniofacial and skeletal abnormalities in RAR double mutants. Development 1994;120:2723-2748.

102. Marks SC, Jr, Odgren PR, Popoff SN, Wurtz T: Sutures, growth plates and the craniofacial base—experimental studies in the toothless (tl-osteopetrotic) rat. Ann Acad Med Singapore 1999; 28:650-654.

103. Wiesner G, Vaz M, Collier G, et al: Leptin is released from the human brain: Influence of adiposity and gender. J Clin Endocrinol Metab 1999;84:2270-2274.

104. O'Donnell CP, Schaub CD, Haines AS, et al: Leptin prevents respiratory depression in obesity. Am J Respir Crit Care Med 1999;159:1477-1484.

105. Kuwaki T, Cao W-H, Kurihara Y, et al: Impaired ventilatory responses to hypoxia and hypercapnia in mutant mice deficient in endothelin-1. Am J Physiol 1996;270: R1279-R1286.

106. Sinton CM, Fitch TE, Gershenfeld HK: The effects of leptin on REM sleep and slow wave delta in rats are reversed by food deprivation. J Sleep Res 1999;8:197-203.

107. Franken P, Chollet D, Tafti M: The homeostatic regulation of sleep need is under genetic control. J Neurosci 2001;21: 2610-2621.

108. Tsuchiya T, Shimizu H, Horie T, Mori M: Expression of leptin receptors in lung: Leptin as a growth factor. Eur J Pharmacol 1999;365:273-279.

109. Woods DR, Montgomery HE: Angiotensin-converting enzyme and genetics at high altitude. High Alt Med Biol 2001;2:201-210.

110. Qadar Pasha MA, Khan AP, Kumar R, et al: Angiotensin converting enzyme insertion allele in relation to high altitude adaptation. Ann Hum Genet 2001;65:531-536.

111. Ordovas JM, Schaefer EJ: Genetic determinants of plasma lipid response to dietary intervention: The role of the APOA1/C3/A4 gene cluster and the APOE gene. Br J Nutr 2000;83(Suppl 1): S127-S136.

112. Kadotani H, Kadotani T, Young T, et al: Association between apolipoprotein E e4 and sleep-disordered breathing in adults. JAMA 2001;285:2888-2890.

113. Gottlieb DJ, DeStefano AI, Foley DJ, et al: A POE e4 is associated with obstructive sleep apnea/hypopnea: The Sleep Heart Health Study. Neurology 2004;63:664-668.

114. Saarelainen S, Lehtimaki T, Kallonen R, et al: No relation between apolipoprotein E alleles and obstructive sleep apnea. Clin Genet 1998;53:147-148.

115. Foley DJ, Masaki K, White L, Redline S: Relationship between apolipoprotein E epsilon4 and sleep-disordered breathing at different ages. JAMA 2001;286:1447-1448.

116. Palmer LJ, Buxbaum SG, Larkin EK, et al: A genome-wide search for quantitative trait loci underlying obstructive sleep apnea. Am J Respir Crit Care Med 2002;165:A419.

85

Cognition and Performance in Patients with Obstructive Sleep Apnea

Terri E. Weaver

Charles F. P. George

ABSTRACT

Patients with obstructive sleep apnea demonstrate variable degrees of cognitive and performance deficits. The impact of the cognitive and performance deficits is more easily identified in those with more severe disease (higher apnea-hypopnea index, greater hypoxemia). Deficits are found in cognitive processing, sustained attention, executive functioning, and quality of life; findings regarding memory are mixed. The mechanisms leading to such deficits and the relative contribution of sleep disruption, hypoxemia, and daytime sleepiness remain unclear.

Treatment of obstructive sleep apnea with continuous positive airway pressure results in consistent improvement in cognition and performance, although the magnitude of improvement is variable. The role of continuous positive airway pressure as first-line therapy in mild obstructive sleep apnea is currently unknown; long-term effectiveness with regard to cognitive and performance deficits needs further study.

Practically speaking, the health care provider must be aware of the patient's potential for cognitive and performance deficits and routinely ask about performance at work, ability to concentrate and maintain attention, irritability, and difficulties performing everyday tasks. It is the practitioner's obligation to inform the patient of the risks associated with such deficits, protecting the public through appropriate action until the patient is successfully treated.

Untreated obstructive sleep apnea (OSA) has an adverse impact on the patient 24 hours a day. Sleep is chronically disturbed, and daytime functioning is impaired by slowed thought processes, forgetfulness, retarded responses, and inability to concentrate. The cognitive and performance deficits experienced by patients with OSA are associated with decreased work performance,[1] increased accidents,[2-8] and diminished quality of life.[9-14] Proposed mechanisms for these neurobehavioral deficits have stemmed from the physiologic hallmarks of OSA—hypoxemia related to episodic collapse of the upper airway and fragmented sleep attributed to the accompanying arousals. These deficits constitute a threat to the patient and to the well-being of others, which presents legal challenges to practitioners. Whether a patient should be denied the right to drive or work because of this risk is a matter of professional debate and legislative consideration.

This chapter describes the cognitive and performance deficits in patients with OSA, considers the scope of this problem, and proposes etiologic mechanisms, methods of assessment, and response to treatment. The legal ramifications of impaired functioning and practitioner liability are also addressed. As respiratory disturbance index (RDI) and apnea-hypopnea index (AHI) are often used interchangeably in the literature, the term used in the cited literature will be the term applied in the chapter.

EPIDEMIOLOGY

The percentage of persons who experience OSA symptoms remains unknown. It has been estimated that approximately 80% of OSA patients complain of both excessive daytime sleepiness and cognitive impairments, and half report personality changes.[15] Traffic- and work-related accidents represent surrogate indicators of neurobehavioral performance deficits.

Four percent of a randomly selected population sample aged 18 to 84 years identified themselves as habitual sleepy drivers, defined as fear of falling asleep while driving at least one of every three times at the wheel.[16] The presence of abnormal breathing events during sleep was an independent risk factor for auto crashes in the habitually sleepy drivers. Based on driving records, 34% of OSA patients had at least one accident in the 5 years preceding diagnosis, compared with 26% of age- and sex-matched controls.[6,7]

DEFINITION, ASSESSMENT, AND IMPACT

To understand the cognitive and neurobehavioral performance deficits that might affect patients with OSA, it is instructive to approach these phenomena from a categorical perspective. The effects of sleep loss on performance includes changes in cognitive performance, difficulty with working memory, slowing of response across the duration of the task (sustained attention), declines in the best effort or fastest response, lapses (acts of omission), and false responses (acts of commission).[14] False responses (responding when no stimulus is presented, lack of behavior inhibition), problems with working memory and contextual memory, problems with cognitive processing (analysis and synthesis), deficits in the pattern of responses (set shifting), and self-regulation of affect and arousal, which are also associated with OSA, are components of executive functioning.[17] Table 85–1 presents a description of the performance deficits and commonly used assessment techniques in OSA. Further information regarding the neurobehavioral tests may be found in Lezak's *Neuropsychological Assessment*.[18]

The impact of OSA on cognitive processing, memory, sustained attention, and executive and motor functioning is summarized in Figure 85–1, which portrays the effect of OSA compared with normal performance. This difference can be

Table 85–1. Definitions and Assessment of Cognitive and Neurobehavioral Deficits Associated with Obstructive Sleep Apnea

Concept	Behavior	Measures Commonly Used to Assess Deficit in Obstructive Sleep Apnea

Cognitive processing	Decreased ability to digest information:
	  slowing on task
	  increased errors
	  decline in total number correct and/or completed per unit time
		"Self-paced" tasks of short duration (1-5 min)—arithmetic calculations, communication, concept attainment:
		  Paced Auditory Serial Addition task (PASAT)
		  Trailmaking A and B (sequencing numbers [A] or letters and numbers [B])
		  Category Test (six sets of items organized around different principles, with a seventh set comprising previously shown items)
		  Digit Symbol Substitution Test (supplying matching symbol given the corresponding number)
		  Digit Backward (stating verbally provided numbers in reverse order)
		  Letter Cancellation (cancellation of target alphabets from presentation of randomized alphabets)

Memory	Decreased ability to register, store, retain, and retrieve information	Short-term memory—timed tasks of up to 10 min that require free recall of words, numbers, paragraph, or figure:
		  Probed, Recall Memory Task (words)
		  Digit Span Forward (numbers)
		  Weschler Memory Scale Story Task (paragraph)
		  Rey Auditory-Verbal Learning Test (figure)
		Long-term memory: presenting the subject with lists of items that are longer than the 7-item memory capacity:
		  California Verbal Learning Test
		  Procedural memory: gradual acquisition and the maintenance of motor skills and procedures:
		  Mirror Tracing Task
		  Rotary Pursuit Task

Sustained attention or vigilance	Inability to maintain attention over time:
	  slowing of response time (time on task)
	  increased errors
	  reduction in the fastest optimal response times
	  periods of delayed responses or nonresponses (lapses)
	  response to stimuli when none are presented (false responses)
		Short-duration tasks of <30 min:
		  Psychomotor Vigilance Task (PVT)
		  Four-Choice Reaction Time Test
		  Steer Clear
		  Continuous Performance Tests

Divided attention	Inability to respond to more than one task or stimulus, such as with driving	Divided Attention Driving Test (DADT): mimics vigilant-related behavior essential to driving:
		  Tracking (the ability to stay within the driving lane)
		  Visual search (looking for and avoiding obstacles, traffic lights, etc.)

Executive functioning	Problems with manipulating and processing information
	Inadequate planning and execution of plans
	Disorganization: poor judgment, decision making
	Inflexible: emotional lability
	Impulsivity
	Difficulty maintaining motivation
		Volition component or intentional behavior:
		  Assessed by asking the patient's preferences, what they like to do, or what makes them angry
		Planning component:
		  Porteus Maze Test
		  Tower Tests—Tower of London, Tower of Toronto, Tower of Hanoi
		  Wisconsin Card Sorting Test
		Purposive action:
		  Tinkertoy Test
		Effective performance:
		  Random Generation Task

Adapted from Dinges D: Probing the limits of functional capability: The effects of sleep loss on short-duration tasks. In Broughton R, Ogilvie R (eds): Sleep, Arousal, and Performance. Boston, Birkhauser, 1992, pp 177-188.

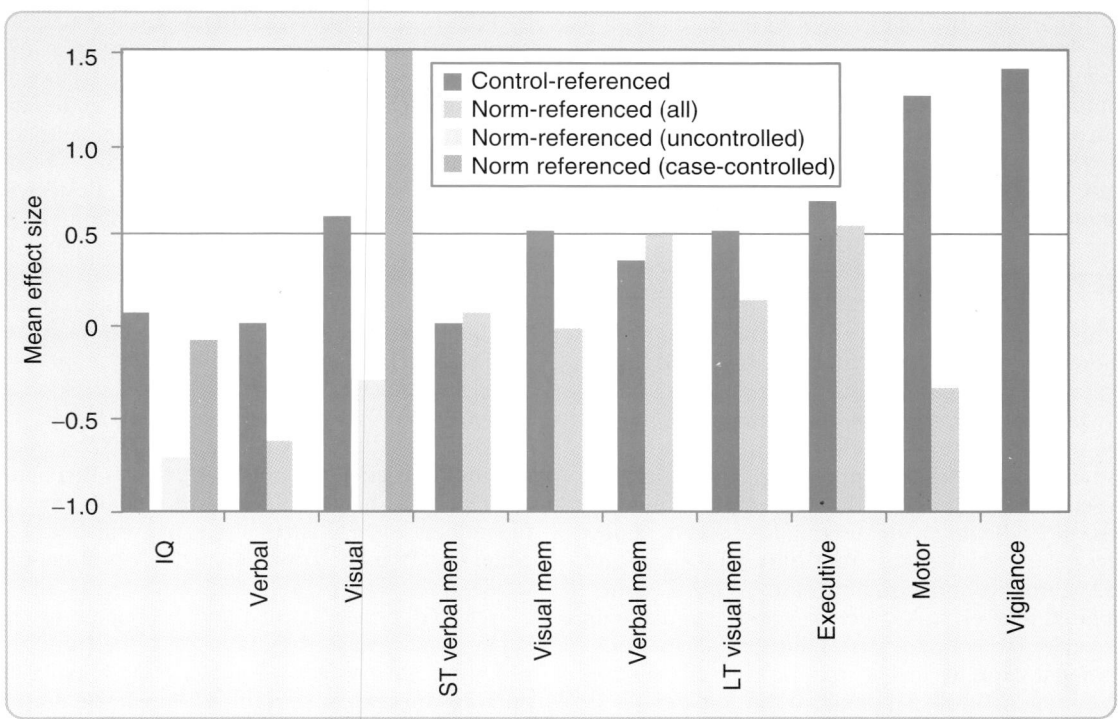

Figure 85–1. Summary of mean effect sizes across domains and data sets. Positive values indicate deficits relative to healthy adults, and negative values indicate strengths relative to healthy adults. The data set for moderate intelligence and visual functioning is split into case-controlled and uncontrolled samples for those domains where study design (case-controlled versus uncontrolled) moderated the data. The line at 0.5 indicates clinically important effect size. IQ, intelligence quotient; LT mem, long-term memory; ST mem, short-term memory. (From Beebe DW, Groesz L, Wells C, et al: The neuropsychological effects of obstructive sleep apnea: A meta-analysis of norm-referenced and case-controlled data. Sleep 2003;26:298-307, p 302.)

quantified in terms of an effect size or differences expressed in terms of standard deviations. An effect size of 0.2 (differences being 0.2 standard deviations) is considered to be small and clinically nonsignificant, 0.5 is moderate and clinically meaningful, and 0.8 is large.[19]

COGNITIVE PROCESSING

There is considerable evidence of impairment in cognitive processing in studies employing clinic-based samples, although the sample sizes in these investigations have typically been small, and few provided power analyses.[20-24] Compared with historical controls, OSA patients have impaired cognitive processing.[20] OSA patients had more difficulty with cognitive challenges than age-matched and education-matched healthy controls.[21,22,24] However, the evidence provided by larger population-based studies is less compelling than that generated from the clinic-based samples, reflecting the selection bias of more-impaired persons referred for evaluation.[25-27]

Subjects with milder OSA (AHI 10 to 30) did not have deficits in cognitive processing compared with normal controls (AHI < 5), which suggests ability to compensate in less severe disease.[23] However, the level of objectively and subjectively measured daytime sleepiness of the patients was the same as the controls,[23] which was not the case in studies of patients with more-severe OSA.[21,24] In this light, several studies found robust differences in cognitive processing in moderate to severe OSA patients (AHI > 15) compared with normal controls.[21,24]

MEMORY

Memory has been defined as the ability to register, store, retain, and retrieve information.[28] The psychological processes involved in memory include registration, short-term memory, rehearsal, long-term memory, and retrieval.[18]

Registration, or sensory memory, is the first recognition of a stimulus and serves as evidence of consciousness. Registered information is either processed as short-term memory or quickly decays.[18] Evidence of impaired registration pertinent to OSA is decreased alertness. Short-term, or working, memory involves a limited-capacity "holding unit" for storage of up to seven bits of information and operates in conjunction with an executive system to hold and internalize information to direct behavior.[18] When these components of memory malfunction, new information is immediately lost and there is a reduction in memory span.[18] Thus, short-term memory maintains information for immediate use.[28] Repetitive mental processes, or rehearsal, increase the likelihood that the memory trace will endure or be maintained.[18] Reduced learning efficiency and loss of new information occurs when there are deficits in rehearsal.[18]

Long-term information storage involves the process of consolidation, or organizing information based on meaning.[18] Neuropsychological deficits resulting from the inability to store information for the long term result in the inability to learn, retain, or execute skills or functions.[18] Finally, retrieval involves recall of information; spontaneous recall is lost when there is a deficit in this process.[18] Procedural memory is the gradual acquisition and the maintenance of motor skills and procedures.[28]

Studies comparing memory function of OSA patients with those of controls have provided inconsistent results.[24,29-31] Differences in samples—clinic versus population-based, level of disease severity, and the use of normal controls versus norm-referenced comparisons—may account for the lack of clarity in the literature regarding this issue.

SUSTAINED ATTENTION

Attention is the composite of different capacities or processes that reflect how stimuli are received and processed.[18] It can be sustained or tonic, as in the case of vigilance; or it can be phasic, in which attention shifts to changing stimuli.[18] *Concentration* refers to focused or selective attention to home in on important stimuli while suppressing other stimuli.[18] Sometimes used interchangeably with concentration, *sustained attention* is the most salient faculty used in assessment of day-time sleepiness, and it is likely the root cause of a significant source of OSA morbidity and mortality: motor vehicle crashes.

With increased time on task, a person's ability to maintain attention becomes more taxed, producing uneven performance.[32] Attentional capacity has a limit, so that engaging in one task requiring controlled attention can interfere with another task requiring the same processing requirements.[18] Divided attention is the ability to respond to more than one task or to different stimuli, and it is sensitive to situations of reduced attentional capacity.[18]

OSA patients initially perform as well as normal controls during short-duration tasks (e.g., 10 minutes), but performance instability occurs over the duration of the task, causing increasing response time, lapses or failure to respond, and responses without prior stimuli (acts of commission) (Fig. 85–2).[32,33] The magnitude of the impact of OSA on sustained-attention tasks is illustrated by effect sizes ranging from 0.2 to 3.0, indicating deviation from performance by normal individuals

by 0.25 to 3 standard deviations.[31] The smallest impact was reported in large community-based subjects with lower levels of disease severity, with the highest effect documented in clinic-based subjects, who suffer higher levels of disease severity. In the clinic-based subjects, the average impairment reflected a large effect size (mean RDI = 36), which decreases to a more moderate effect size when sample size is considered.[31]

The effect of OSA on sustained attention can be illustrated using a meaningful example: Performance on the Psychomotor Vigilance Task (PVT) was measured in OSA patients and compared with normal controls who ingested alcohol to incrementally raise their blood alcohol level from zero to a mean of 0.80 g/210 L of breath.[34] Differences in performance were noted immediately on the first trial at a blood alcohol level higher than 0.057 g/210 L, a level that would limit driving a commercial vehicle in California.[34] On subsequent trials, the maximum reaction time of OSA patients was poorer than that at a blood alcohol level (0.08 g/dL) that defines driving under the influence in California.[34] The performance of a 47-year-old patient with mild to moderate OSA was comparable to or worse than that of a healthy nonsleepy, alcohol-impaired 27-year-old subject who would be unable to legally drive a commercial vehicle in most states in the United States.[34]

Drivers do not always notice their impairment and continue to drive while sleepy.[35] OSA patients are 6 to 10 times more likely to have an accident than healthy controls and twice as likely to have an accident than controls in the past 3 years.[35] Patients with more severe disease (AHI > 40) contribute most to this elevated risk.[7] Human error, chiefly inattention, was indicated as a cause in 40% of traffic accidents in the state of Indiana.[36] On driving simulators, patients with sleep apnea hit more obstacles, have increased error in tracking and visual search, have increased response time, and drive more times out of bounds (Fig. 85–3).[33] In a sophisticated driving simulator, untreated OSA patients compared with healthy controls had increased off-road events, slower brake-reaction time, and increased lateral-position deviation.[36]

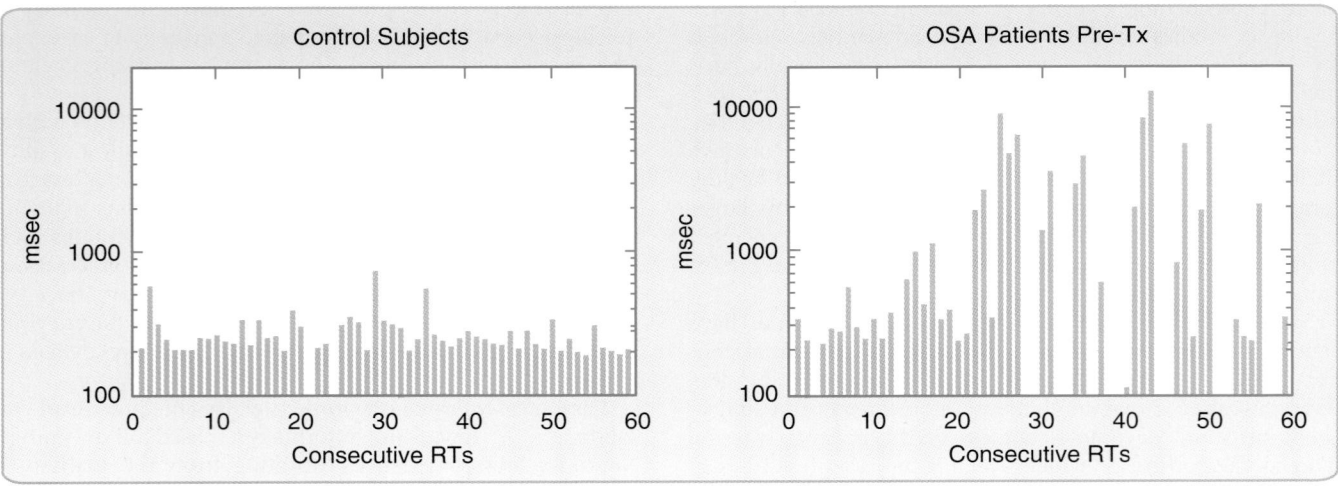

Figure 85–2. Comparison of performance of normal controls and sleep apnea patients on the Psychomotor Vigilance Task. Sleep apnea patients demonstrate increased reaction time, indicated by the bars, and lapses in response, indicated by the blank spaces. OSA, obstructive sleep apnea; RT, reaction time; Tx, treatment. (From Chugh D, Dinges D: Mechanisms of sleepiness. In Pack A [ed]: Pathogenesis, Diagnosis, and Treatment of Sleep Apnea. New York, Marcel Dekker, 2002, p 273.)

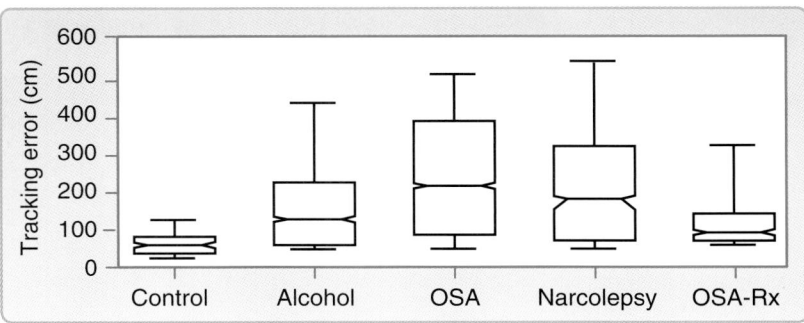

Figure 85–3. Summary of tracking errors by different groups on the Divided Attention Driving Task. OSA, obstructive sleep apnea; OSA-Rx, treated obstructive sleep apnea. (From George CF: Vigilance impairment: Assessment by driving simulators. Sleep 2000;23 (Suppl 4):S115-S118, p S116.)

EXECUTIVE FUNCTIONS

In assessment of cognitive functions, the researcher asks what the person knows or can do; in evaluation of executive functions, the researcher asks how or whether the person goes about accomplishing a task.[18] Executive functions are those facilities that produce purposive, independent, self-serving behavior and represent frontal lobe functioning.[18] Even with considerable loss in cognitive functioning, if the executive functioning is preserved, the person can be independent and productive.[18]

However, the reverse is not true: The loss of executive functions renders the person incapable of performing self-care, working independently, or maintaining normal social relationships even though cognitive functioning remains intact.[18] There may also be emotional lability, increased irritability, or impulsivity. The person with impaired executive function lacks motivation, is unable to initiate activity, and has problems planning and carrying out activities that require goal-directed behavior.[18]

Inconsistencies in the literature regarding the impact of OSA on memory may be explained by executive function deficits and the associated impact on organization and retrieval but not long-term storage.[29,37] Deficiencies in executive functioning in conjunction with difficulties with concentration, sustained attention, cognitive processing, and memory may contribute to the decrements in functional status that have been reported in OSA patients, although this link has not been systematically studied.[10,13,38-44]

Performances related to executive functions may be the performance parameter that is most affected by sleep apnea.[17] Studies comparing the performance of patients with that of normal controls or norm-referenced data suggest that OSA has a moderate to large impact on executive functioning. The deviation in executive functions from normal performance evaluated with a community-acquired sample of patients with more mild disease[23,25] show an effect that is not clinically important; this is not the case with clinic-based samples, where the effect is moderate to large.[31] Impairments identified in the sleep apnea population include problems with verbal fluency, planning, sequential thinking, and constructional ability.[40]

QUALITY OF LIFE

Measuring the impact of illness on the patient's ability to conduct everyday tasks and fulfill roles from the patient's perspective is a key component in outcome management and the evaluation of treatment efficacy. Quality of life, health-related quality of life, and functional status are distinct concepts, but they have been used to describe the effect of illness on everyday life.[10] The term *quality of life* encompasses such attributes as standard of living, economic status, life satisfaction, housing quality, health, and job satisfaction; *health-related quality of life* comprises only those domains considered to be affected by illness.[10] *Functional status,* a component of quality of life, is multidimensional and defines the ability to carry out activities and tasks necessary to fulfill current life roles.[10]

Measures of quality of life are categorized as either generic or disease-specific. Generic measures assess a wide variety of activities and domains and are designed for heterogeneous populations, which is useful for cross-illness comparisons (Table 85–2).[10] Compared with generic measures, disease-specific measures provide more depth regarding the aspects of daily functioning most likely to be affected by the illness or symptom of interest.[10] Disease-specific measures that have been designed for use in assessing the impact of OSA include the Functional Outcomes of Sleep Questionnaire (FOSQ), Calgary Sleep Apnea Quality of Life Instrument (SAQLI), and OSA Patient Oriented Severity Index.[10]

As disease-specific measures of quality of life have recently been developed, the majority of research evaluating quality of life in untreated OSA has employed generic measures, such as the Medical Outcomes Study Short Form 36 (SF36). Large, community-acquired samples indicate that OSA affects quality of life and has an impact similar to that experienced by those with other chronic disorders of moderate severity.[45] Even patients with mild OSA appear to have difficulties carrying out their daily activities, although whether there is a linear relationship with degree of sleep disordered breathing is uncertain.[44-46] However, several studies indicate that those with more severe disease experience the greatest deficits, with an odds ratio of approximately 1.5 times those with less severe disease.[46] One study of older black volunteers showed that the association between AHI and general physical and mental functioning reflected the escalation in AHI from 1 to 15, but no greater deficit was documented beyond that level, suggesting a threshold effect.[45]

Studies using clinical samples employing norm-referenced data or normal controls for comparison have demonstrated impaired quality of life in OSA patients on both generic and disease-specific measures.[10,47] Studies using disease-specific questionnaires demonstrated a greater array of affected tasks and roles than generic measures did.[10] Patients reported problems in aspects of daily living beyond vigilance-related

Table 85–2. Comparison of Domains Addressed by Quality of Life Instruments

Domain	WHO QOL-BREF*	Sickness Impact Profile (SIP)	Functional Limitations Profile (FIP)	Medical Outcome Study Short Form 36 (SF36)	Nottingham Health Profile (NHP)	EuroQoL Questionnaire
Physical functioning	×	×	×	×	×	×
Mental health	×	×	×	×	×	×
Psychological distress		×	×	×	×	×
Psychological well-being				×		
Role functioning		×	×	×		
Social functioning	×	×	×	×	×	
Health perceptions				×		
Pain				×	×	×
Vitality				×	×	
Mobility/travel		×	×			×
Sleep		×	×		×	
Cognitive functioning		×	×			
Eating		×	×			
Recreation and hobbies		×	×			
Communication		×	×			
Environment	×					
Home management		×	×			

*Measure developed by the World Health Organization.

From Weaver TE: Outcome measurement in sleep medicine practice and research. Part 1: Assessment of symptoms, subjective and objective daytime sleepiness, health-related quality of life and functional status. Sleep Med Rev 2001;5:103-128.

activities, which indicates the pervasive effect of OSA.[10] For example, OSA patients had greater deficits than normal controls by up to two standard deviations in all subscales of the FOSQ, reflecting the domains of general productivity, vigilance, activity level, social outcome, and sexual relationships.[47]

Although several studies have suggested a linear relationship between severity of OSA and components of quality of life, prediction of impaired daily functioning is not consistently found.[40] For example, a dose relationship between scores on SF36, the generic instrument, with OSA severity (controlling for age, body mass index [BMI], and other pertinent factors) was documented in one community-based study, but only for the vitality/energy subscale when desaturation was included in the definition of disease severity.[44,46] Self-reported sleepiness has been reported to reflect daytime sleepiness, but the relationship is dependent on consideration of other critical factors such as chronic illness, BMI, and age.[37,44,48] Evaluations of dysfunction in OSA using disease-specific quality of life instruments have not supported a statistically significant relationship between quality of life and severity of OSA,[49] but they have indicated a more robust link with self-reported daytime sleepiness.[10,49]

ETIOLOGY AND MECHANISMS

Researchers have speculated for some time that the cognitive and performance deficits associated with OSA are related to two etiologies: fragmented sleep and nocturnal hypoxemia.[17] The relationship between the respiratory disturbance index and cognitive and neurobehavior deficits have been either weak or not statistically reliable.[26,31,40,50] Although sleep disruption and nocturnal hypoxemia have been linked to cognitive

and neurobehavior dysfunction, their relative contributions remain unclear.[17]

The prefrontal model has been proposed as a conceptual framework for the relationship between sleep disruption and nocturnal hypoxemia and primarily frontal deficits (cognitive and neurobehavioral dysfunction) (Fig. 85–4).[17] This model posits that the sleep disruption, intermittent hypoxemia, and intermittent hypercarbia experienced by OSA patients alters the normal restorative process that occurs during sleep. This alteration generates cellular and biochemical stresses that result in disruption of functional homeostasis and altered neuronal and glial viability within certain brain regions, primarily the prefrontal regions of the brain cortex.[17] Investigations of animal models of sleep apnea have demonstrated poor maze learning and increased neuron apoptosis in specific regions of the hippocampus and overlying cortical region.[17]

These physiologic alterations destabilize the executive system, which causes behavioral disturbance in inhibition, maintenance of performance, self-regulation of affect and arousal, working memory, analysis and synthesis, and contextual memory.[17] Alterations in the executive system can adversely affect cognitive abilities, resulting in the types of maladaptive behavior depicted in Figure 85–4.[17] The impairments associated with sleep disorders produce inefficient performance and *not* the inability to perform.[17] When a debilitated system, such as those required for memory or divided attention, attempts to perform, other systems are recruited. However, their contributions are suboptimal because they themselves are impaired. This may account for the increased activations of the prefrontal cortex under conditions of sleep deprivation documented by functional magnetic resonance imaging.[17]

OSA AND PREFRONTAL FUNCTIONING

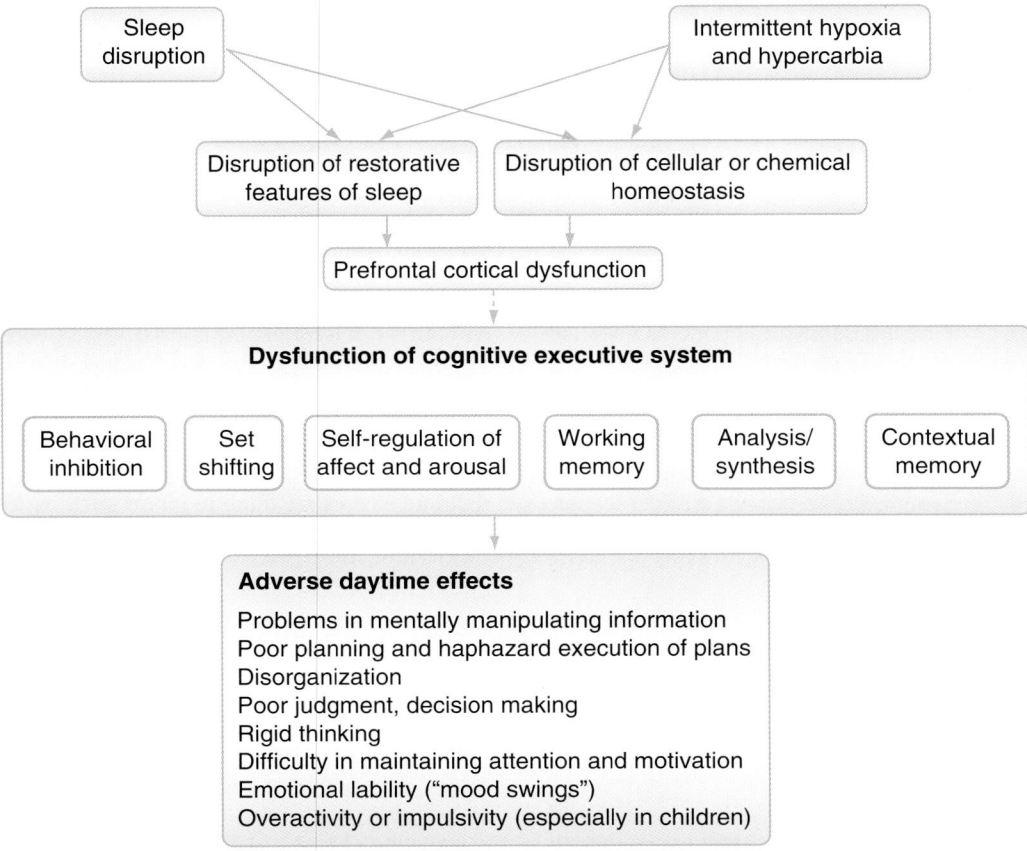

Figure 85–4. The proposed prefrontal model. In this model, OSA-related sleep disruption and intermittent hypoxemia and hypercarbia alter the efficacy of restorative processes occurring during sleep and disrupt the functional homeostasis and neuronal and glial viability within particular brain regions, particularly the prefrontal regions of the brain cortex. (From Beebe DW, Gozal D: Obstructive sleep apnea and the prefrontal cortex: Towards a comprehensive model linking nocturnal upper airway obstruction to daytime cognitive and behavioral deficits. J Sleep Res 2002;11:1-16, p 3.)

Studies examining the relationships among sleep, respiratory variables, hypoxemia, and cognitive and neurobehavioral functioning have not produced conclusive findings.[40,51] Studies have shown that hypoxemia is linked to attention, executive function, perceptual speed, organization and motor speed, memory, and verbal fluency.[40,51] Other studies have supported the relationship between sleep disruption and executive function.[40,51]

A comparison of cognitive and neurobehavioral functioning in patients with chronic obstructive pulmonary disease (who also suffer from hypoxemia) and patients with OSA showed that OSA patients were similarly impaired.[20] Both types of patients showed problems with cognitive processing and memory, indicating the role of hypoxemia. However, sleep apnea patients demonstrated more dysfunction on tests of sustained attention that were sensitive to sleepiness.[20] Other studies have suggested that sleepiness plays an important role in cognitive and neurobehavioral performance.[20]

These (and other[31]) findings suggest that the small to moderate deficits in cognitive processing and large impairments in objective sleepiness indicate that sleepiness and decrements in performance share a common biologic substrate.[31] For example, in rodent models of long-term intermittent hypoxemia,

the observed increased sleepiness is related to oxidative injuries to the wake-promoting regions of the forebrain.[52]

Using factor analysis and by comparing the relative contributions of sleep disturbance, hypoxemia, and sleep quality, others have attempted to more directly isolate the mechanisms that produce cognitive and neurobehavioral deficits.[50] In this study, executive functioning was not related to these three variables, but it was more strongly related to subjective sleepiness.

EFFECT OF TREATMENT

Evaluating the evidence of the effectiveness of treatment on the cognitive and performance impairments exhibited by OSA patients is challenging because of differences in adherence to treatment, length of treatment, type of controls, and placebos employed.

In uncontrolled studies, continuous positive airway pressure (CPAP) treatment had a moderate to large effect on cognitive processing, memory, sustained attention, and executive functions.[22] However, there is evidence of persistent cognitive and neurobehavioral deficits despite treatment; these are attributed to permanent hypoxia-related insults.[53,54] Compared with baseline values, CPAP treatment produced moderate to large changes in cognitive and neurobehavioral performance.[31] These gains are not evident when treatment outcomes are compared with placebo.[31]

Although a meta-analysis of the efficacy of CPAP treatment evaluated in studies employing tablet placebos have demonstrated the positive impact of this treatment on cognitive and neurobehavioral performance,[31] the evidence is less convincing when sham-CPAP was employed as the placebo.[55,56] Treatment duration may affect clinical outcomes.[57]

The majority of controlled clinical trials evaluating the efficacy of CPAP treatment have predominantly involved patients who have moderate to severe OSA, and the few studies examining the utility of CPAP treatment involved patients who have mild OSA.[58] Compared to conservative therapy, the only improvement in aspects of quality of life after 8 weeks of CPAP treatment was in vitality.[58] The variable results in these studies may reflect the fact that with milder disease severity there is less cognitive impairment and, thus, less potential for gains following therapy.[59-61] Sample size, especially where the effect of treatment may be more blunted (such as in patients with milder disease), may also contribute to inconsistencies across outcomes and studies.

Improvements in cognitive and neurobehavioral performance might also be a function of baseline level of daytime sleepiness. Controlled studies that have examined treatment response in patients who do not present with daytime sleepiness but who have mild[58] or severe[62] pathology have not found CPAP superior to conservative therapy[58] or sham-CPAP[62] across outcomes.

Several studies have explored the impact of CPAP treatment on cognitive and neurobehavioral outcomes compared with other forms of treatment. Compared with nasal oxygen therapy, CPAP treatment produces equivalent positive benefits for enhanced sustained attention and memory, but CPAP therapy yields greater gains for cognitive processing in mild OSA.[63] CPAP treatment and surgery appear to have equipoise compared with conservative therapy with respect to cognitive and neurobehavioral function. Positional therapy has no greater effect than CPAP treatment on cognitive performance or general health, with the exception of improved energy levels associated only with CPAP treatment.[64] Two months of CPAP treatment compared with 2 months of treatment with a mandibular repositioning device demonstrated higher quality of life measured with disease-specific and generic measures, but it showed no difference in cognitive and neurobehavioral performance.[65] The magnitude of these differences was moderate, but it was larger for those in the sample with mild disease.[65]

MEDICAL AND LEGAL ASPECTS OF COGNITIVE AND PERFORMANCE DEFICITS

The majority of accidental injuries or death can be explained by human error. Because sleepiness increases periods of inattention, it is not surprising that sleepiness has been linked to accidents both on the road and in occupational settings.[6,66-68] The courts have long recognized civil liability claims and defense for injury caused by loss of consciousness or diminished alertness. More recently, sleep-related civil liability issues have increased in frequency and complexity, and determining fitness to drive has been problematic for sleep clinicians, particularly in view of the varied laws and jurisdictions.

Clearly, a motor vehicle operator has an obligation to drive safely in order to avoid foreseeable harm to others. However, the courts often agree that the driver is not criminally negligent when falling asleep while driving unless it appears that he or she continued to drive in reckless disregard of warning symptoms. Table 85–3 illustrates the legal consequence of cases of fall-asleep motor vehicle accidents. A recent and notable exception is in New Jersey, where the state senate enacted "Maggie's Law" on June 23, 2003. Falling asleep at the wheel and fatigued driving now count as recklessness under the existing vehicular homicide law (NJS 2C:11-5). This legislation is the first bill in the United States to specifically address the issue of driving while fatigued, where "fatigue" is defined as being without sleep for a period in excess of 24 consecutive hours.

As a result, physicians who believe that a patient is unfit to drive because of sleepiness should inform the patient of this opinion. Those patients who continue to drive and who are believed to be a public health risk should be reported by the physician to the authorities in jurisdictions where they are required to do so. Failure to report such patients can result in personal liability for clinicians.

In the 1990s, two Ontario Court of Appeal judgments found physicians liable because they had failed to report potentially unfit medical patients to the motor vehicle licensing authorities, and the patients subsequently had traumatic car accidents.[69,70] The courts emphasized the importance of the physicians' statutory reporting duty to the public. This duty superseded the physicians' private duty with regard to confidentiality and the dictates of the therapeutic relationship. The courts' interpretation was a departure from earlier case law. In addition, the courts were unmoved by the physicians' explanations for their failure to report. It was immaterial that the physicians deemed the medical conditions to be temporary or that they trusted their patients to comply with their medication regimen and instructions against driving.

It is therefore important for physicians to fulfill their statutory duties in a diligent yet sensible manner, reporting those patients whom they believe have a medical condition that might reasonably make it dangerous to drive, especially where there is a mandatory reporting system.

The data for sleep apnea are numerous and consistent: As a group, OSA patients' risk of motor vehicle collisions is increased two to fourfold. Still, not all patients have accidents, and as many as two thirds may never have a collision.[4] Identifying those at greatest risk is still not clear from the available literature, thereby complicating decision making from a medical and legal perspective.

Accordingly, physicians must work to ensure that patients understand the balance between physician's duty of care to the patient and their statutory duty under the law. They should educate patients about the increased risk of sleepy driving in sleep apnea, pointing out the patient's civil responsibilities that accompany the privilege of having a driver's license. Further, by instructing patients in proper sleep hygiene and effective countermeasures to sleepy driving (rest stops, caffeine, napping), physicians begin to modify the risks of drowsy driving.

Although it may be argued that mandatory reporting of drivers with sleep apnea will discourage many sleepy drivers from being evaluated for OSA, data supporting this argument are lacking. There are data, however, supporting the concept that effective treatment of sleep apnea will reduce collision risk to normal.[4,71]

Table 85–3.   Case Details of Fall-Asleep Motor Vehicle Accidents

Case (Diagnosis)	Overnight Sleep Study	MSLT or MWT	Accident Outcome	Legal Outcome	Remained Licensed?
A (OSA and PLMD)	With CPAP: AI, 30; AHI, 10; PLMI, 20	MWT20, 4.75 min	2 vehicles, 1 fatality, 2 others injured	No-billed	Yes
B (OSA and UARS)	AI, 41; AHI, 10	MSLT, 9.4 min	2 vehicles, 1 fatality, 2 others injured	No-billed	Yes
C (sleep deprivation)	AHI, 2.4; AHI, 1	MWT40, 40 min	4 vehicles, 5 fatalities, several others injured	Acquitted	Yes; later withdrawn by RTA and then contested in court
D (OSA)	AHI, 30	MWT40, 11 min	6 vehicles, 2 fatalities, 12 others injured	Found guilty, jailed	Yes
E (idiopathic hypersomnolence)	AHI, 0.4	MWT20, 8 min	5 vehicles, 1 fatality, 2 others injured	Pleaded guilty	Yes
F (OSA)	AHI, 23	MSLT, 5.5 min	3 vehicles, 2 fatalities	Pleaded guilty, jailed	Yes
G (OSA)	AHI, 17	Not performed	2 vehicles, 1 fatality	Found guilty, jailed	Yes; later withdrawn by judge

AHI, apnea-hypopnea index; AI, arousal index; CPAP, continuous positive airway pressure; MSLT, multiple sleep latency test; MWT, Maintenance of Wakefulness Test; MWT20, MWT 20-minute protocol; MWT40, MWT 40-minute protocol, OSA, obstructive sleep apnea; PLMD, periodic limb movement disorder; PLMI, periodic limb movement index; RTA, Roads and Traffic Authority; UARS, upper-airway resistance syndrome.

Normal values: AHI, 0-5 per hour; AI, 0-10 per hour; MWT20 (sleep onset defined as the first occurrence of one epoch of any stage of sleep in 20 minute protocol), 11-20 minutes; MWT40 (sleep onset defined as three consecutive epochs of stage 1 sleep or any single epoch of another sleep stage in 40 minute protocol), 19-40 minutes; MSLT, 10-20 minutes; PLMI, 0-5 per hour.

From Rajaratnam SM: Legal issues in accidents caused by sleepiness. J Hum Ergol (Tokyo) 2001;30:107-111.

Therefore, where mandatory reporting is in place, treating patients at the same time as notifying the motor vehicle authorities can discharge the clinician's statutory duty while still maintaining the patient's ability to drive and earn a living. This strategy assumes appropriate access to care, which regrettably is not yet universal.[72] In situations where there is no mandatory reporting, and in cases where ongoing sleepiness is a major concern, physicians must balance the personal risk of litigation for disclosing private medical information without consent against public safety.

SUMMARY

Patients with OSA demonstrate variable degrees of cognitive and performance deficits. Evidence of these impairments is greater in studies using control-referenced compared with norm-referenced samples. There also seems to be stronger evidence in those studies using clinic-based instead of community-based samples, which reflects the increased disease severity in clinic-based samples. Thus, the impact of the cognitive and performance deficits is more easily identified in those with more severe disease. Indeed, those with more severe disease display deficits in cognitive processing, sustained attention, executive functioning, and quality of life, with mixed findings regarding memory.

The mechanistic processes that lead to such deficits remain unclear with respect to the relative contribution of sleep disruption, hypoxemia, and daytime sleepiness. The potential role of obesity, hypertension, diabetes, and cardiovascular disease in the etiology of these deficits is relatively unknown. Uncontrolled studies present a convincing picture of the positive impact of CPAP therapy. However, the benefit of this treatment is less persuasive in controlled trials, particularly those employing a sham-CPAP placebo. The role of CPAP as first-line therapy in patients with mild OSA remains undetermined, and long-term effectiveness with regard to cognitive and performance deficits needs further exploration.

Despite the need for more evidence regarding cognitive and performance deficits in community-acquired samples in sham-CPAP–controlled studies, there is sufficient documentation to suggest that untreated and nonadherent patients are at risk for traffic- and occupation-related accidents. Legislation such as Maggie's Law will increase public awareness of the hazard of driving sleepy. However, it is also the duty of the health care provider to assess the patient for cognitive and performance deficits by asking about performance at work, ability to concentrate, ability to maintain attention, irritability, and difficulties performing everyday tasks. It is the practitioner's obligation to inform the patient of the risks associated with such deficits, protecting the public through appropriate action until the patient is successfully treated.

Clinical Pearl

Sleep fragmentation and hypoxemia due to sleep apnea commonly influence cognitive ability and daytime performance. Awareness of these impairments and prompt treatment will reduce burden of illness on the patient, reduce public risk, and minimize the physician's medical and legal risk.

REFERENCES

1. Ulfberg J, Carter N, Talback M, et al: Excessive daytime sleepiness at work and subjective work performance in the general population and among heavy snorers and patients with obstructive sleep apnea. Chest 1996;110:659-663.
2. Krieger J, Meslier N, Lebrun T, et al: Accidents in obstructive sleep apnea patients treated with nasal continuous positive airway pressure: A prospective study. The Working Group ANTADIR, Paris, and CRESGE, Lille, France. Association Nationale de Traitement a Domicile des Insuffisants Respiratoires. Chest 1997;112:1561-1566.
3. Hakkanen J, Summala H: Sleepiness at work among commercial truck drivers. Sleep 2000;23:49-57.
4. George CF: Reduction in motor vehicle collisions following treatment of sleep apnoea with nasal CPAP. Thorax 2001;56:508-512.
5. Horstmann S, Hess C, Bassetti C, et al: Sleepiness-related accidents in sleep apnea patients. Sleep 2000;23:383-389.
6. Teran-Santos J, Jimenez-Gomez A, Cordero-Guevara J: The association between sleep apnea and the risk of traffic accidents. Cooperative Group Burgos-Santander. N Engl J Med 1999;340:847-851.
7. George CF, Smiley A: Sleep apnea and automobile crashes. Sleep 1999;22:790-795.
8. Barbé F, Pericás J, Muñoz A, et al: Automobile accidents in patients with sleep apnea syndrome: An epidemiological and mechanistic study. Am J Respir Crit Care Med 1998;158:18-22.
9. Veale D, Poussin G, Benes F, et al: Identification of quality of life concerns of patients with obstructive sleep apnoea at the time of initiation of continuous positive airway pressure: A discourse analysis. Qual Life Res 2002;11:389-399.
10. Weaver TE: Outcome measurement in sleep medicine practice and research. Part 1: Assessment of symptoms, subjective and objective daytime sleepiness, health-related quality of life and functional status. Sleep Med Rev 2001;5:103-128.
11. Kingshott R, Vennelle M, Hoy C, et al: Predictors of improvements in daytime function outcomes with CPAP therapy. Am J Respir Crit Care Med 2000;161:866-871.
12. Jenkinson C, Stradling J, Petersen S, et al: Comparison of three measures of quality of life outcome in the evaluation of continuous positive airways pressure therapy for sleep apnoea. J Sleep Res 1997;6:199-204.
13. Jenkinson C, Davies RJO, Mullins R, et al: Comparison of therapeutic and subtherapeutic nasal continuous positive airway pressure for obstructive sleep apnoea: A randomised prospective parallel trial. Lancet 1999;353:2100-2105.
14. Dinges D: Probing the limits of functional capability: The effects of sleep loss on short-duration tasks. In Broughton R, Ogilvie R (eds): Sleep, Arousal, and Performance. Boston, Birkhauser, 1992, pp 177-188.
15. Guilleminault C, Hoed JVD, Mitler M, et al: Clinical overview of the sleep apnea syndromes. In Guilleminault C, Dement W (eds): Sleep Apnea Syndromes. New York, Allan R Liss, 1978, pp 1-12.
16. Masa JF, Rubio M, Findley LJ, et al: Habitually sleepy drivers have a high frequency of automobile crashes associated with respiratory disorders during sleep. Am J Respir Crit Care Med 2000;162:1407-1412.
17. Beebe DW, Gozal D: Obstructive sleep apnea and the prefrontal cortex: Towards a comprehensive model linking nocturnal upper airway obstruction to daytime cognitive and behavioral deficits. J Sleep Res 2002;11:1-16.
18. Lezak M: Neuropsychological Assessment. New York, Oxford University Press, 1995.
19. Cohen J: Statistical Power Analysis for the Behavioral Sciences. Hillsdale, NJ, Lawrence Erlbaum Associates, 1988.
20. Roehrs T, Merrion M, Pedrosi B, et al: Neuropsychological function in obstructive sleep apnea syndrome (OSAS) compared to chronic obstructive pulmonary disease (COPD). Sleep 1995;18:382-388.
21. Bedard MA, Montplaisir J, Malo J, et al: Persistent neuropsychological deficits and vigilance impairment in sleep apnea syndrome after treatment with continuous positive airways pressure (CPAP). J Clin Exp Neuropsychol 1993;15:330-341.
22. Naegele B, Thouvard V, Pepin JL, et al: Deficits of cognitive executive functions in patients with sleep apnea syndrome. Sleep 1995;18:43-52.
23. Redline S, Strauss ME, Adams N, et al: Neuropsychological function in mild sleep-disordered breathing. Sleep 1997;20:160-167.
24. Rouleau I, Decary A, Chicoine AJ, et al: Procedural skill learning in obstructive sleep apnea syndrome. Sleep 2002;25:401-411.
25. Kim HC, Young T, Matthews CG, et al: Sleep-disordered breathing and neuropsychological deficits. A population-based study. Am J Respir Crit Care Med 1997;156:1813-1819.
26. Boland LL, Shahar E, Iber C, et al: Measures of cognitive function in persons with varying degrees of sleep-disordered breathing: The Sleep Heart Health Study. J Sleep Res 2002;11:265-272.
27. Jennum P, Sjol A: Self-assessed cognitive function in snorers and sleep apneics. An epidemiological study of 1,504 females and males aged 30-60 years: The Dan-MONICA II Study. Eur Neurol 1994;34:204-208.
28. Decary A, Rouleau I, Montplaisir J, et al: Cognitive deficits associated with sleep apnea syndrome: A proposed neuropsychological test battery. Sleep 2000;23:369-381.
29. Beebe DW, Groesz L, Wells C, et al: The neuropsychological effects of obstructive sleep apnea: A meta-analysis of norm-referenced and case-controlled data. Sleep 2003;26:298-307.
30. Bedard MA, Montplaisir J, Richer F, et al: Obstructive sleep apnea syndrome: Pathogenesis of neuropsychological deficits. J Clin Exp Neuropsychol 1991;13:950-964.
31. Engleman HM, Kingshott RN, Martin SE, et al: Cognitive function in the sleep apnea/hypopnea syndrome (SAHS). Sleep 2000;23(Suppl 4):S102-S108.
32. Chugh D, Dinges D: Mechanisms of sleepiness. In Pack A (ed): Pathogenesis, Diagnosis, and Treatment of Sleep Apnea. New York, Marcel Dekker, 2002; pp 265-285.
33. Weaver TE: Outcome measurement in sleep medicine practice and research. Part 2: Assessment of neurobehavioral performance and mood. Sleep Med Rev 2001;5:223-236.
34. Powell NB, Riley RW, Schechtman KB, et al: A comparative model: Reaction time performance in sleep-disordered breathing versus alcohol-impaired controls. Laryngoscope 1999;109:1648-1654.
35. George CF: Driving simulators in clinical practice. Sleep Med Rev 2003;7:311-320.
36. George CF: Vigilance impairment: Assessment by driving simulators. Sleep 2000;23(Suppl 4):S115-S118.
37. Bennett LS, Barbour C, Langford B, et al: Health status in obstructive sleep apnea: Relationship with sleep fragmentation and daytine sleepiness, and effects of continuous positive airway pressure treatment. Am J Resp Crit Care Med 1999;159:1884-1890.
38. Gall R, Isaac L, Kryger M, et al: Quality of life in mild obstructive sleep apnea. Sleep 1993;16:S59-S61.
39. Jenkinson C, Stradling J, Petersen S, et al: How should we evaluate health status? A comparison of three methods in patients presenting with obstructive sleep apnoea. Qual Life Res 1998;7:95-100.
40. Sateia MJ: Neuropsychological impairment and quality of life in obstructive sleep apnea. Clin Chest Med 2003;24:249-259.
41. Rosen CL, Palermo TM, Larkin EK, et al: Health-related quality of life and sleep-disordered breathing in children. Sleep 2002;25:657-666.
42. Flemons WW, Reimer MA: Development of a disease-specific health-related quality of life questionnaire for sleep apnea. Am J Respir Crit Care Med 1998;158:494-503.

43. Akashiba T, Kawahara S, Akahoshi T, et al: Relationship between quality of life and mood or depression in patients with severe obstructive sleep apnea syndrome. Chest 2002;122:861-865.

44. Baldwin CM, Griffith KA, Nieto FJ, et al: The association of sleep-disordered breathing and sleep symptoms with quality of life in the Sleep Heart Health Study. Sleep 2001;24:96-105.

45. Young T, Peppard PE, Gottlieb DJ, et al: Epidemiology of obstructive sleep apnea: A population health perspective. Am J Respir Crit Care Med 2002;165:1217-1239.

46. Finn L, Young T, Palta M, et al: Sleep-disordered breathing and self-reported general health status in the Wisconsin Sleep Cohort Study. Sleep 1998;21:701-706.

47. Engleman H, Joffe D: Neuropsychological function in obstructive sleep apnoea. Sleep Med Rev 1999;3:59-78.

48. Briones B, Adams N, Strauss M, et al: Relationship between sleepiness and general health status. Sleep 1996;19:583-588.

49. Flemons WW, Reimer MA: Measurement properties of the Calgary Sleep Apnea Quality of Life Index. Am J Respir Crit Care Med 2002;165:159-164.

50. Naismith S, Winter V, Gotsopoulos H, et al: Neurobehavioral functioning in obstructive sleep apnea: Differential effects of sleep quality, hypoxemia and subjective sleepiness. J Clin Exp Neuropsychol 2004;26:43-54.

51. Smith IE, Shneerson JM: Is the SF 36 sensitive to sleep disruption? A study in subjects with sleep apnoea. J Sleep Res 1995;4:183-188.

52. Veasey SC, Davis CW, Fenik P, et al: Long-term intermittent hypoxia in mice: Protracted hypersomnolence with oxidative injury to sleep-wake brain regions. Sleep 2004;27:194-201.

53. Valencia-Flores M, Bliwise DL, Guilleminault C, et al: Cognitive function in patients with sleep apnea after acute nocturnal nasal continuous positive airway pressure (CPAP) treatment: Sleepiness and hypoxemia effects. J Clin Exp Neuropsychol 1996;18:197-210.

54. Kotterba S, Rasche K, Widdig W, et al: Neuropsychological investigations and event-related potentials in obstructive sleep apnea syndrome before and during CPAP-therapy. J Neurol Sci 1998;159:45-50.

55. Henke KG, Grady JJ, Kuna ST, et al: Effect of nasal continuous positive airway pressure on neuropsychological function in sleep apnea-hypopnea syndrome. A randomized, placebo-controlled trial. Am J Respir Crit Care Med 2001;163:911-917.

56. Bardwell WA, Ancoli-Israel S, Berry CC, et al: Neuropsychological effects of one-week continuous positive airway pressure treatment in patients with obstructive sleep apnea: A placebo-controlled study. Psychosom Med 2001;63:579-584.

57. McMahon JP, Foresman BH, Chisholm RC, et al: The influence of CPAP on the neurobehavioral performance of patients with obstructive sleep apnea hypopnea syndrome: A systematic review. WMJ 2003;102:36-43.

58. Redline S, Adams N, Strauss ME, et al: Improvement of mild sleep-disordered breathing with CPAP compared with conservative therapy. Am J Resp Crit Care Med 1998;157:858-865.

59. Engleman HM, Kingshott RN, Wraith PK, et al: Randomized placebo-controlled crossover trial of continuous positive airway pressure for mild sleep apnea/hypopnea syndrome. Am J Respir Crit Care Med 1999;159:461-467.

60. Barnes M, Houston D, Worsnop CJ, et al: A randomized controlled trial of continuous positive airway pressure in mild obstructive sleep apnea. Am J Respir Crit Care Med 2002;165: 773-780.

61. Engleman HM, Martin SE, Deary IJ, et al: Effect of CPAP therapy on daytime function in patients with mild sleep apnoea/hypopnoea syndrome. Thorax 1997;52:114-119.

62. Barbé F, Mayoralas LR, Duran J, et al: Treatment with continuous positive airway pressure is not effective in patients with sleep apnea but no daytime sleepiness. A randomized, controlled trial. Ann Intern Med 2001;134:1015-1023.

63. Phillips BA, Schmitt FA, Berry DT, et al: Treatment of obstructive sleep apnea. A preliminary report comparing nasal CPAP to nasal oxygen in patients with mild OSA. Chest 1990;98:325-330.

64. Jokic R, Klimaszewski A, Crossley M, et al: Positional treatment vs continuous positive airway pressure in patients with positional obstructive sleep apnea syndrome. Chest 1999;115:771-781.

65. Engleman HM, McDonald JP, Graham D, et al: Randomized crossover trial of two treatments for sleep apnea/hypopnea syndrome: Continuous positive airway pressure and mandibular repositioning splint. Am J Respir Crit Care Med 2002;166: 855-859.

66. Lindberg E, Carter N, Gislason T, et al: Role of snoring and daytime sleepiness in occupational accidents. Am J Respir Crit Care Med 2001;164:2031-2035.

67. George CF, Nickerson PW, Hanly PJ, et al: Sleep apnoea patients have more automobile accidents. Lancet 1987;2:447.

68. Findley LJ, Unverzagt ME, Suratt PM, et al: Automobile accidents involving patients with obstructive sleep apnea. Am Rev Respir Dis 1988;138:337-340.

69. Spillane v. Wasserman (1992) 13 CCLT (2d) 267 (GD), [1998] OJ No. 2470 (CA).

70. Toms v. Foster [1994] OJ No. 1413 (CA).

71. Findley L, Smith C, Hooper J, et al: Treatment with nasal CPAP decreases automobile accidents in patients with sleep apnea. Am J Respir Crit Care Med 2000;161:857-859.

72. Flemons WW, Douglas NJ, Kuna ST, et al: Access to diagnosis and treatment of patients with suspected sleep apnea. Am J Respir Crit Care Med 2004;169:668-672.

86

Sleep Apnea and Metabolic Dysfunction

Naresh M. Punjabi

Brock A. Beamer

ABSTRACT

The dramatic increase in the prevalence of obesity worldwide is posing a substantial public health problem in both developed and developing countries. Clinical sequelae of obesity are numerous and include conditions such as hypertension, type 2 diabetes mellitus, and sleep apnea. It is also well established that obesity is a leading cause of glucose intolerance and insulin resistance that, in turn, can lead to cardiovascular disease.

There has been increasing recognition that sleep apnea may also predispose to impaired glucose metabolism. Experimental and observational data from human studies support the notion that sleep apnea and its associated physiologic consequences of intermittent hypoxemia and recurrent arousals are associated with glucose intolerance and insulin resistance. Data from animal studies also show that hypoxia can promote insulin resistance.

Increase in sympathetic activity, alteration in hypothalamic-pituitary-adrenal function, and a predisposition to a proinflammatory state have been implicated in the putative causal pathway between sleep apnea and metabolic dysfunction. Elevated levels of interleukin-6, tumor necrosis factor-α, and leptin—factors known to increase the predisposition to metabolic dysfunction—are found in patients with sleep apnea.

Although the effect of continuous positive pressure therapy on glucose homeostasis is a topic of intense investigation, emerging data demonstrates improvement in metabolic function with therapy. Whether sleep apnea is a precursor of glucose intolerance, insulin resistance, or diabetes independent of obesity or whether sleep apnea represents another component of the metabolic syndrome remains to be determined. Regardless of the directionality of associations, understanding the relationship between sleep apnea and metabolic function has implications for both clinicians and the research community.

It is becoming increasingly evident that normal sleep has a vital role in glucose homeostasis. Recent data suggest that even partial sleep loss can induce glucose intolerance. Extensive research on the relationship between sleep and endocrine function has demonstrated that disturbances in the normal sleep-wake cycle can disrupt the activity of the corticotropic, thyrotropic, and somatotropic axes.

Sleep apnea is a chronic and prevalent condition that is associated with disruption of sleep continuity and intermittent hypoxemia, engendering a number of adverse health-related consequences. Over the past decade, there has been a growing body of evidence suggesting that sleep apnea may be independently, and perhaps causally, associated with altered glucose metabolism and the development of type 2 diabetes mellitus.

Based on epidemiologic data from several population-based studies that have used polysomnography, approximately 5% of the general population may have moderate to severe sleep apnea.[1] Factors that increase the risk for sleep apnea include male gender,[2-5] age,[5-7] ethnicity,[8] and obesity.[9-12] Most, if not all, cross-sectional surveys of clinic and population samples show that obesity and in particular visceral adiposity are the strongest risk factors for sleep apnea.[9-15]

Defining the exact prevalence of type 2 diabetes in the general population is fraught with some of the same challenges as defining the prevalence of sleep apnea, including inconsistencies in disease definition and methodological differences in quantifying the severity and diversity of the study samples. Methods for ascertaining abnormalities of glucose metabolism and the classification of hyperglycemic states have varied significantly across studies and provided a wide range of prevalence estimates.

Data from the Third National Health and Nutrition Examination Survey indicate that 5.1% of adults have physician-diagnosed diabetes; an additional 2.7% have a fasting glucose higher than 126 mg/dL but remain undiagnosed.[16] Because obesity and visceral adiposity are risk factors for type 2 diabetes mellitus,[17] it is not surprising to find that sleep apnea and type 2 diabetes mellitus frequently coexist. The primary focus of this chapter is to describe the current evidence for this relationship, examine the relative importance of intermittent hypoxemia and sleep fragmentation, and describe candidate mechanisms in the putative causal pathway.

DEFINITIONS

Before discussing the link between sleep apnea and impaired glucose metabolism, it is appropriate to provide brief definitions of glucose intolerance, insulin resistance, and diabetes mellitus and to summarize the methods currently used for assessing these hyperglycemic states.

The American Diabetes Association (ADA) guidelines divide diabetes mellitus into four distinct clinical and pathophysiologic types.[18] The ADA has outlined the criteria for defining diabetes mellitus and other categories of hyperglycemia (Table 86–1). The consensus statement[19] requires that testing be performed on two separate occasions and recommends fasting glucose as the principal means for establishing the diagnosis of diabetes mellitus.

Type 1 diabetes mellitus (formerly known as insulin-dependent diabetes mellitus) results from cell-mediated autoimmune destruction of the pancreatic β-cells. It usually occurs in young, nonobese persons and accounts for approximately 7% of those with a diagnosis of diabetes mellitus.[20] Type 2 diabetes mellitus (formerly known as non–insulin dependent diabetes mellitus) is a state of insulin resistance that is accompanied by

Table 86–1. Criteria for Diagnosing Diabetes Mellitus and Other Categories of Hyperglycemia

Hyperglycemia	Test	Glucose Concentration mg/dL	(mmol/L)
Diabetes mellitus	Fasting glucose	≥126	(7.0)
	2-hour post-glucose load	≥200	(11.1)
Impaired glucose tolerance	Fasting glucose (if measured)	<126	(7.0)
	2-hour post-glucose load	140-199	(7.8-11.0)
Impaired fasting glucose	Fasting glucose	100-125	(6.1-6.9)

inadequate compensatory response in insulin secretion. It usually occurs among middle-aged obese adults and accounts for more than 85% of individuals with diagnosed diabetes mellitus.

Gestational diabetes mellitus is the occurrence of glucose intolerance during pregnancy. Gestational diabetes complicates approximately 4% of the pregnancies in the United States, resulting in 135,000 cases annually.[21] Other secondary types of diabetes mellitus can result from genetic defects of the β-cell function and insulin action (e.g., leprechaunism), other endocrinopathies (e.g., Cushing's syndrome), and pancreas destruction by specific drugs and toxins. The ADA also provides definitions for two other hyperglycemic states, including impaired glucose tolerance and impaired fasting glucose. Both of these hyperglycemic states are known risk factors for type 2 diabetes and are independently associated with increased cardiovascular risk.[22,23]

Studies relating sleep apnea to glucose metabolism have employed fasting glucose values and results of the oral glucose tolerance test as the primary outcomes. Several studies have also incorporated other measures of insulin sensitivity as the dependent variable. The gold standard technique for assessing insulin sensitivity is the hyperinsulinemic euglycemic clamp.[24] With this method, exogenous insulin is administered at a rate designed to maintain a stable level of hyperinsulinemia while exogenous glucose is infused to maintain the serum glucose concentration at normal fasting levels. At steady state, the exogenous glucose infusion rate represents the amount of glucose uptake by the tissues and provides a measure of insulin sensitivity.

Because the hyperinsulinemic clamp method may not be practical in field studies, several alternative and simpler measures of insulin sensitivity are available. Fasting and postglucose challenge levels of serum insulin are widely used as surrogate measures for insulin sensitivity. The product of fasting insulin and glucose levels[25] and the ratio of these measures[26] have been used as proxies for insulin sensitivity. Finally, the insulin suppression test and the intravenous glucose tolerance test provide alternative measures of insulin sensitivity.[27]

SLEEP APNEA AND DIABETES MELLITUS: A BIDIRECTIONAL ASSOCIATION

Diabetes Mellitus as a Cause of Sleep Apnea

Most of the earlier studies examining the association between sleep apnea and type 2 diabetes provided simple descriptions of breathing abnormalities during sleep in diabetic patients. Although these studies included small case-based samples and could not segregate cause and effect, a uniform observation emerged suggesting that diabetic patients with autonomic neuropathy were more likely to manifest obstructive or central sleep apnea, or both, than those without autonomic neuropathy.[28-33] Given that normal breathing during sleep is dependent on central respiratory motor control and upper airway patency, a major implication of these earlier reports is that central and obstructive sleep apnea might be consequences of autonomic dysfunction.

More recently, data from the Sleep Heart Health Study has provided compelling evidence for an independent relationship between sleep apnea and type 2 diabetes.[34] In a large cohort of community-dwelling individuals without cardiovascular disease, diabetic subjects exhibited a higher frequency of obstructive and central respiratory events during sleep than nondiabetic subjects. Differences between the two groups, however, dissipated after adjustment for age, sex, race, and obesity. Nevertheless, diabetic subjects were more likely to manifest periodic breathing during sleep compared with their nondiabetic counterparts.

Animal studies that have examined the effects of diabetes on respiratory function provide further support for the hypothesis that patients with type 2 diabetes have increased susceptibility to sleep apnea. Experimentally induced diabetes mellitus in animal models[35,36] can depress baseline ventilatory function and diminish reflex responses to hypoxia and hypercapnia—factors that can promote breathing abnormalities during sleep. Human studies that have characterized the pathophysiologic consequences of autonomic dysfunction also show that with underlying neuropathy, diabetic patients have increased central and decreased peripheral chemosensitivity to carbon dioxide.[37] Because excessive responsiveness of the respiratory centers to carbon dioxide can promote periodic breathing, there is good biologic plausibility for a causal link between type 2 diabetes and sleep apnea. However, further studies are needed to clarify the role of autonomic neuropathy in abnormalities of upper airway collapsibility and control of breathing during sleep.

Sleep Apnea as a Cause of Diabetes Mellitus

In addition to the possibility that complications of type 2 diabetes may contribute to breathing disturbances during sleep, a growing body of literature suggests that sleep apnea may independently contribute to the incidence of type 2

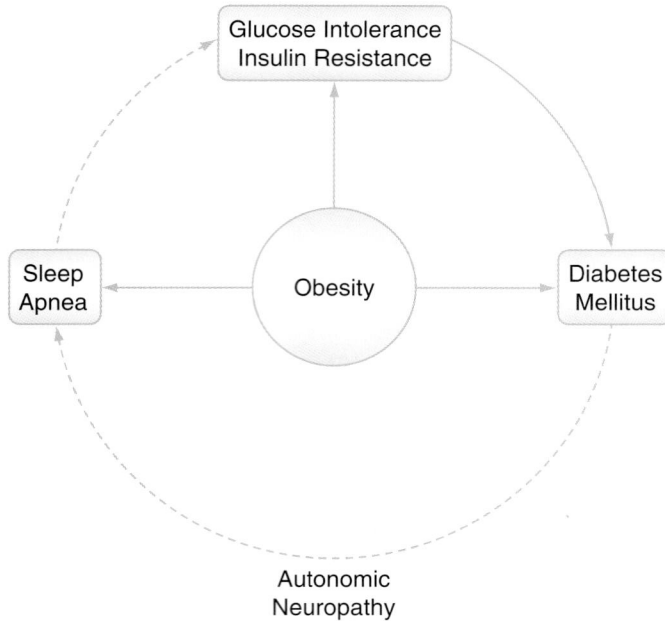

Figure 86–1. Sleep apnea and diabetes mellitus.

diabetes (Fig. 86–1). Given that the two disorders share several common risk factors, separating a causal from a noncausal association is challenging.

Perhaps the best evidence for a causal link is found in two recent cohort studies that assessed the association between sleep apnea symptoms and the development of type 2 diabetes.[38,39] In the first study, habitual snoring in 2668 Swedish men was associated with a higher incidence of self-reported diabetes over a 10-year period.[38] Obesity and habitual snoring were noted to be additive in their associated risks for type 2 diabetes. Despite the large sample size and long-term follow-up, a major weakness of that study was that self-reports were used to assess diabetes and sleep apnea status.

The potential misclassification due to self-reports was subsequently addressed by data from the Nurses' Health Study,[39] in which type 2 diabetes was diagnosed as the presence of any of the following conditions: classical symptoms (e.g., excessive thirst, polyuria, weight loss, hunger), with a fasting glucose greater than 140 mg/dL or a random glucose greater than 200 mg/dL; no symptoms but two elevated plasma glucose levels on different occasions; or treatment with insulin or oral hypoglycemic medications. In a sample of 69,852 women with longitudinal data over a 10-year period, the relative risk for diabetes mellitus comparing regular snorers to nonsnorers was 2.03 (95% confidence interval, 1.71-2.40). The higher incidence of type 2 diabetes in snoring women was independent of age, body mass index, smoking, physical activity, family history of diabetes, and number of hours of sleep. As with the Swedish study, a major weakness in the Nurses' Health Study was the use of snoring as a surrogate for sleep apnea.

Although these two studies provide compelling evidence for an independent and perhaps causal association between snoring and type 2 diabetes, prospective data from population-based studies that include objective measures of sleep apnea are unavailable. Thus, it remains to be determined whether sleep apnea mediates the observed association between snoring and the occurrence of type 2 diabetes.

SLEEP APNEA, GLUCOSE INTOLERANCE, AND INSULIN RESISTANCE

Studies relating sleep apnea to altered glucose metabolism have been categorized into three major groups. The first group consists of studies on the association between symptoms of sleep apnea (e.g., snoring) and glucose metabolism.[38-42] The second group consists of studies that have used objective measures of sleep and breathing and correlated these indices with abnormalities in glucose metabolism.[43-56] The third group consists of studies on the effects of continuous positive airway pressure (CPAP) therapy on glucose metabolism. Although studies from the first group provide longitudinal data[38,39] and support a causal association between snoring and glucose metabolism, a major deficiency is the lack of polysomnographic data. Thus, the underlying mechanisms linking snoring to metabolic disturbance cannot be delineated.

Physiologic insight into the causal pathways among snoring, sleep apnea, and metabolic impairment can be found in studies that have used polysomnography to characterize nocturnal oxyhemoglobin saturation and sleep architecture.[43-56] Early investigations using oximetry in conjunction with cardiorespiratory monitoring or full-montage polysomnography did not demonstrate an independent association between sleep apnea and glucose metabolism. The lack of a significant association may have been due to the small sample sizes with insufficient statistical power.

Subsequently, several groups with larger study samples have shown that regardless of the outcome (i.e., fasting glucose or insulin levels, oral glucose tolerance test, or insulin sensitivity), an independent association does exist between sleep apnea and altered glucose metabolism. In these studies, severity of sleep-related hypoxemia has been a consistent correlate of glucose intolerance or insulin resistance, suggesting that the metabolic effects of sleep apnea are perhaps mediated through oxyhemoglobin desaturation associated with the occurrence of apneas and hypopneas. Data from the Sleep Heart Health Study[56] also show that in addition to the degree of nocturnal oxygen levels, the frequency of nocturnal arousals is independently correlated with the degree of insulin resistance.

Support for a causal association between sleep apnea and glucose metabolism is also evident in studies that have examined the effects of CPAP on metabolic function. If sleep apnea precedes glucose intolerance and insulin resistance, then CPAP should mitigate the metabolic disturbance. Although results in a number of initial studies were equivocal on the effects of CPAP,[45,48,57-63] emerging data from several laboratories have shown a beneficial effect of CPAP on glucose metabolism.[59,64]

In the largest study to date,[64] improvement in insulin sensitivity, as assessed by the hyperinsulinemic euglycemic clamp, was observed over a three-month period after initiating CPAP. Interestingly, insulin sensitivity increased within two days of therapy, with further improvements occurring at the three-month follow-up. As expected, obesity was an important modifier of the treatment effect: Nonobese patients experienced a rapid improvement in insulin sensitivity compared with obese patients. Despite the favorable effects of CPAP on insulin sensitivity, several questions remain, including the role of compliance with therapy, defining responsive and non-responsive subgroups, and quantifying the long-term benefits of improved metabolic function on cardiovascular outcomes in sleep apnea.

Mechanisms

Currently, the mechanisms underlying the predisposition to glucose intolerance, insulin resistance, and type 2 diabetes in sleep apnea are not known. The following sections review the available evidence on hypoxia and sleep fragmentation as the primary etiologic factors and candidate mechanisms that may explain the observed associations.

Effects of Hypoxia on Glucose Metabolism

Literature from animal and human studies indicates that hypoxia can have detrimental effects on insulin sensitivity. Using the hyperinsulinemic euglycemic clamp in healthy young men, a 50% decrease in insulin sensitivity was observed within two days after rapid passive ascent from sea level to an altitude of 4559 meters.[65] The decrease in insulin sensitivity with altitude hypoxia was associated with an increase in cortisol and norepinephrine concentrations. However, with prolonged exposure to hypoxic conditions, the acute metabolic derangements improved.

Subsequently, similar findings were also reported in a sample of healthy women who were subjected to high-altitude conditions in a hypobaric chamber (~4300 meters). Relative to normoxic conditions, 16 hours of hypobaric hypoxia was associated with a 61% decrease in insulin sensitivity.[66] As noted with the experiment at high altitude, hypobaric hypoxia increased sympathetic activity with elevations in circulating levels of epinephrine and norepinephrine.

Experimental studies in newborn calves[67] and rats[68,69] also show that exposure to continuous hypoxia can increase serum insulin levels with as little as two hours of exposure.

Taken together, these studies suggest that continuous hypoxia may be an important risk factor for altered glucose metabolism in sleep apnea. However, the physiologic consequences of chronic sustained hypoxia may significantly differ from the consequences of intermittent hypoxemia in sleep apnea. Currently, the adverse effects of intermittent hypoxemia on glucose metabolism are relatively unexplored.

In an animal model of intermittent hypoxia, short-term (5 days) and long-term (12 weeks) alterations in glucose metabolism were examined in strains of lean and genetically obese leptin-deficient mice.[70] With short-term exposure, intermittent hypoxia was associated with improved glucose tolerance in the lean and leptin-deficient obese mice. Although insulin levels remained unchanged in the lean mice at 5 days, serum leptin levels increased. In the obese leptin-deficient mice, however, insulin levels increased with short-term exposure to intermittent hypoxia.

The improvement in glucose tolerance in the two strains with acute hypoxic exposure is most likely due to the increase in the insulin-sensitizing effects of leptin in lean mice, whereas the improvement in obese leptin-deficient mice is due to the increase in insulin secretion. With long-term or chronic exposure to intermittent hypoxia, obese mice manifest a time-dependent increase in insulin levels and demonstrate worsening glucose tolerance. These data suggest that, at least in the presence of obesity, intermittent hypoxemia may be a potential causative factor for metabolic dysfunction.

Effects of Sleep Disruption on Glucose Metabolism

Glucose metabolism depends on a complex interaction among insulin secretion, insulin sensitivity, and glucose effectiveness.[71] Insulin sensitivity is the ability of insulin to accelerate the uptake of glucose by the peripheral tissues. Glucose effectiveness quantifies the ability of glucose to normalize its own concentration. Thus, glucose effectiveness represents glucose uptake by peripheral tissues that is independent of insulin-receptor function.

Using the intravenous glucose tolerance test to measure glucose tolerance, insulin sensitivity, and glucose effectiveness in a well-designed pre-post study, experimental sleep restriction to 4 hours per night for 6 nights led to glucose intolerance in healthy men.[72] Results from the intravenous glucose tolerance test revealed that insulin sensitivity was preserved and glucose effectiveness decreased by 30%. The decrease in glucose effectiveness with sleep restriction was on the same order of magnitude as that observed between patients with type 2 diabetes and normoglycemic subjects.

Although the physiologic relevance of glucose effectiveness in the pathogenesis of type 2 diabetes mellitus is controversial, several investigators have argued that reduced glucose effectiveness may also be an important determinant of metabolic dysfunction. Because apnea-related sleep fragmentation can cause secondary sleep debt, it would be reasonable to speculate that disruption of sleep continuity in sleep apnea may also contribute to metabolic dysfunction. Results from the Sleep Heart Health Study indicate that after adjusting for a number of confounders including total sleep time, the frequency of arousals at night does correlate with insulin resistance.

Despite the wealth of emerging data, the current state of the art with regard to the effects of sleep fragmentation on metabolic function is limited, and further research is under way in several laboratories to separate the independent effects of sleep fragmentation from intermittent hypoxemia.

Intermediate Pathways

If intermittent hypoxia and sleep fragmentation promote metabolic dysfunction in sleep apnea, then what are the underlying mechanisms that might mediate their effects? Candidate pathways that might be responsible include the sympathetic nervous system, the hypothalamic-pituitary-adrenal axis, and adipocyte-derived inflammatory mediators including interleukin-6 (IL-6), tumor necrosis factor-α (TNF-α), and leptin. Figure 86–2 shows these candidate pathways, which are discussed in the following sections.

The Sympathetic Nervous System

Untreated patients with sleep apnea manifest elevated sympathetic tone during wakefulness and sleep that decreases with CPAP therapy.[73] Sympathetic stimulation can influence glucose homeostasis by increasing muscle glycogenolysis and hepatic glucose output.[74] In addition, a number of studies have shown that adipose tissue is innervated with sympathetic nerve fibers[75] and that stimulation of sympathetic nerve

endings promotes lipolysis and the release of free fatty acids, which can induce peripheral insulin resistance.[76] It is therefore plausible that heightened sympathetic activity represents one process linking sleep apnea to altered glucose regulation.

The Hypothalamic-Pituitary-Adrenal Axis

Predisposition to glucose dysregulation in sleep apnea patients may also occur through the effects of sleep apnea on the hypothalamic-pituitary-adrenal axis. Experimentally induced partial or total sleep deprivation increases plasma cortisol levels by 37% and 45%, respectively, on the following evening at a time when the circadian variation of the hypothalamic-pituitary-adrenal axis is at its nadir.[77] The increase in evening cortisol can have marked effects on glucose levels, serum insulin concentrations, and insulin secretion. Although the paradigm of sleep disruption in sleep apnea is different from that of sleep loss, serum cortisol levels may also be abnormal in patients with sleep apnea.[78]

Experimental work in animals[79,80] also shows that hypoxia and hypercapnia can stimulate production of glucagon and glucocorticoids from the pancreas and adrenals, respectively. Glucocorticoids oppose insulin action on peripheral glucose uptake, enhance gluconeogenesis in the liver,[81] and thereby

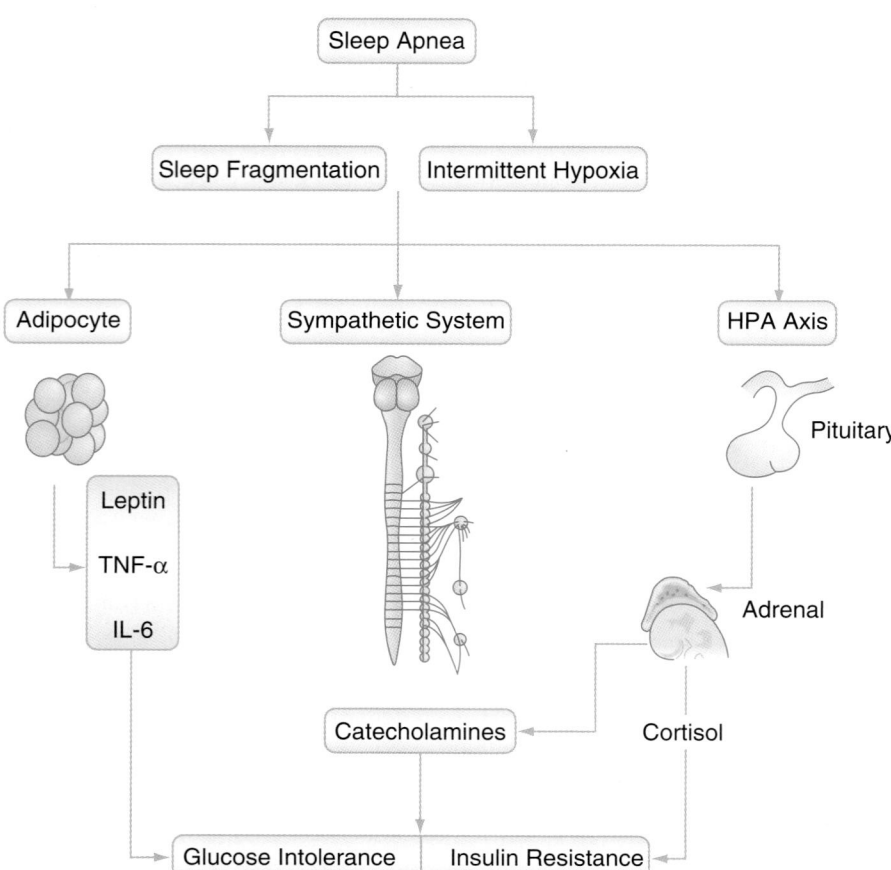

Figure 86–2. Intermediate pathways linking sleep apnea, glucose intolerance, and insulin resistance.

lead to insulin resistance and glucose intolerance. Finally, glucocorticoids can stimulate adipocytes to secrete leptin,[82] which may be directly involved in the pathogenesis of type 2 diabetes mellitus.

Adipocyte-Derived Inflammatory Mediators

Cyclic hypoxia may also lead to glucose intolerance and insulin resistance by promoting the release of several adipocyte-derived factors including IL-6, TNF-α, and leptin.

IL-6 is an inflammatory mediator that is released, in part, by subcutaneous adipose tissue. Serum levels of IL-6 correlate with indices of insulin resistance,[83,84] and higher levels are associated with an increased risk for type 2 diabetes mellitus.[85] Although very little is known about the IL-6 response to intermittent hypoxia, a few studies have shown that circulating levels of IL-6 increase with altitude hypoxia.[86,87] Furthermore, cross-sectional clinic-based studies have shown that patients with sleep apnea manifest elevated circulating levels of IL-6.[49,88] Although these studies did not rigorously address the confounding effects of obesity, one month of CPAP therapy decreased IL-6 levels,[89] suggesting that sleep apnea might independently increase IL-6, possibly through the effects of intermittent hypoxemia or sleep fragmentation.

Recent data also indicate that TNF-α has an important role in the development of insulin resistance. TNF-α is a cytokine mediator that contributes to insulin resistance by antagonizing insulin action. Animal studies that target disruption of the TNF-α gene suggest that the gene also regulates plasma triglyceride levels and body fat.[90] Although mice that have homozygous null mutations at the TNF-α or TNF-receptor loci become obese, they appear protected from developing obesity-related insulin resistance.[91] Finally, insulin-sensitizing thiazolidinediones decrease TNF-α release and antagonize TNF-α–induced inhibition of insulin signaling.[92] While the effects of sleep apnea on TNF-α require further exploration, observational studies of relatively limited sample size demonstrated higher TNF-α levels in patients with sleep apnea compared with control subjects.[49,88] Interestingly, a recent preliminary placebo-controlled, double-blind study on etanercept, a TNF-α antagonist, showed no significant change in glucose or insulin levels in a small sample of eight patients with sleep apnea.[92a] Clearly, further work is needed to delineate whether sleep apnea can alter TNF-α levels and whether these changes are responsible for metabolic dysfunction.

Leptin is the third factor implicated in the pathogenesis of sleep apnea–related metabolic disturbance. It is widely accepted that leptin, an adipocyte-derived factor, acts on the hypothalamus to control food intake and energy expenditure. Leptin also decreases insulin secretion from the pancreatic β-cell in response to the amount of body fat stores. Insulin, on the other hand, stimulates leptin biosynthesis and secretion from adipose tissue. Thus, a feedback loop between adipose tissue and the pancreas is established that regulates glucose homeostasis according to the needs that are determined by adipose mass.

In animal models of obesity and most obese patients, leptin levels are generally higher and the effects of leptin are blunted. Leptin resistance[93] would lead to the dysregulation of the feedback loop and promote hyperinsulinemia, which then sets the stage for the development of hyperglycemia and type 2 diabetes mellitus.

Although the effect of hypoxia on leptin levels remains a topic of intense investigation, in vitro studies demonstrate that hypoxia can increase leptin promoter activity and leptin secretion in the cultured adipocytes.[94] Studies in patients with sleep apnea also show elevated leptin levels that decrease with effective treatment.[48,95-100] The improvement in leptin with CPAP therapy is independent of changes in body weight, suggesting that sleep apnea is associated with elevated leptin levels and that a leptin resistance in sleep apnea may predispose to alterations of glucose metabolism.

CONCLUSION

The natural history and pathogenesis of type 2 diabetes consists of several elements, including dietary, genetic, and environmental factors. The evidence reviewed here suggests that sleep apnea may also contribute to the risk for developing glucose intolerance, insulin resistance, and type 2 diabetes. Defining the underlying relationships between sleep apnea and altered glucose metabolism would add to the current understanding of whether sleep apnea represents yet another component of the metabolic syndrome, which is characterized by central obesity, hyperinsulinemia, insulin resistance, hyperlipidemia, hypertension, and a proinflammatory state.

It is well established that the metabolic syndrome is a significant risk factor for coronary heart disease and accounts for more than half the population-attributable risk for type 2 diabetes. Thus, delineating the role of sleep apnea as a component or a risk factor for metabolic syndrome has major implications from a clinical and public health perspective. Clearly, there are several major gaps in our knowledge of the interrelationship between glucose metabolism and sleep apnea. Further research is needed to provide confirming evidence for a causal link between sleep apnea and glucose metabolism, delineate the role of intermittent hypoxemia and sleep fragmentation, determine effect modification by other factors including age and obesity, and establish whether treatment with CPAP therapy can reverse the associated abnormalities and curtail cardiovascular risk.

> *Clinical Pearl*
>
> *Sleep apnea is associated with glucose intolerance and insulin resistance and may predispose to the development of type 2 diabetes mellitus independent of obesity. Intermittent hypoxemia and recurrent arousals related to apneas and hypopneas may mediate the metabolic disturbance in sleep apnea.*

REFERENCES

1. Young T, Peppard PE, Gottlieb DJ: Epidemiology of obstructive sleep apnea: A population health perspective. Am J Respir Crit Care Med 2002;165:1217-1239.
2. Young T, Palta M, Dempsey J, et al: The occurrence of sleep-disordered breathing among middle-aged adults. N Engl J Med 1993;328:1230-1235.
3. Redline S, Kump K, Tishler PV, et al: Gender differences in sleep disordered breathing in a community-based sample. Am J Respir Crit Care Med 1994;149:722-726.
4. Bixler EO, Vgontzas AN, Lin HM, et al: Prevalence of sleep-disordered breathing in women: Effects of gender. Am J Respir Crit Care Med 2001;163:608-613.

5. Young T, Shahar E, Nieto FJ, et al: Predictors of sleep-disordered breathing in community-dwelling adults: The Sleep Heart Health Study. Arch Intern Med 2002;162:893-900.

6. Bixler EO, Vgontzas AN, Ten Have T, et al: Effects of age on sleep apnea in men: I. Prevalence and severity. Am J Respir Crit Care Med 1998;157:144-148.

7. Duran J, Esnaola S, Rubio R, Iztueta A: Obstructive sleep apnea-hypopnea and related clinical features in a population-based sample of subjects aged 30 to 70 yr. Am J Respir Crit Care Med 2001;163:685-689.

8. Redline S, Tishler PV, Hans MG, et al: Racial differences in sleep-disordered breathing in African-Americans and Caucasians. Am J Respir Crit Care Med 1997;155:186-192.

9. Olson LG, King MT, Hensley MJ, Saunders NA: A community study of snoring and sleep-disordered breathing. Prevalence. Am J Respir Crit Care Med 1995;152:711-716.

10. Shinohara E, Kihara S, Yamashita S, et al: Visceral fat accumulation as an important risk factor for obstructive sleep apnoea syndrome in obese subjects. J Intern Med 1997;241:11-18.

11. Ferini-Strambi L, Zucconi M, Castronovo V, et al: Snoring and sleep apnea: A population study in Italian women. Sleep 1999;22:859-864.

12. Newman AB, Nieto FJ, Guidry U, et al: Relation of sleep-disordered breathing to cardiovascular disease risk factors: The Sleep Heart Health Study. Am J Epidemiol 2001;154:50-59.

13. Hoffstein V, Mateika S: Differences in abdominal and neck circumferences in patients with and without obstructive sleep apnoea. Eur Respir J 1992;5:377-381.

14. Grunstein R, Wilcox I, Yang TS, et al: Snoring and sleep apnoea in men: Association with central obesity and hypertension. Int J Obes Relat Metab Disord 1993;17:533-540.

15. Jennum P, Sjol A: Snoring, sleep apnoea and cardiovascular risk factors: The MONICA II Study. Int J Epidemiol 1993;22:439-444.

16. Harris MI, Flegal KM, Cowie CC, et al: Prevalence of diabetes, impaired fasting glucose, and impaired glucose tolerance in U.S. adults. The Third National Health and Nutrition Examination Survey, 1988-1994. Diabetes Care 1998;21:518-524.

17. Rewers M, Hamman RF: Risk factors for non-insulin dependent diabetes mellitus. In National Diabetes Group: Diabetes in America, 2nd ed. Washington, DC, US Government Printing Office, 1995, pp 179-220. PDF available at http://diabetes.niddk.nih.gov/dm/pubs/america/

18. American Diabetes Association: Diagnosis and classification of diabetes mellitus. Diabetes Care 2004;27(Suppl 1):S5-S10.

19. American Diabetes Association: Screening for type 2 diabetes. Diabetes Care 2004;27(Suppl 1):S11-S14.

20. Harris MI: Classification, diagnostic criteria, and screening for diabetes. In National Diabetes Group: Diabetes in America, 2 ed. Washington, DC, US Government Printing Office, 1995, pp 15-36. PDF available at http://diabetes.niddk.nih.gov/dm/pubs/america/

21. Engelgau MM, Herman WH, Smith PJ, et al: The epidemiology of diabetes and pregnancy in the U.S., 1988. Diabetes Care 1995;18:1029-1033.

22. DECODE Study Group: Glucose tolerance and mortality: Comparison of WHO and American Diabetes Association diagnostic criteria. The DECODE study group. European Diabetes Epidemiology Group. Diabetes Epidemiology: Collaborative analysis Of Diagnostic criteria in Europe. Lancet 1999;354:617-621.

23. Coutinho M, Gerstein HC, Wang Y, Yusuf S: The relationship between glucose and incident cardiovascular events. A meta-regression analysis of published data from 20 studies of 95,783 individuals followed for 12.4 years. Diabetes Care 1999;22:233-240.

24. DeFronzo RA, Tobin JD, Andres R: Glucose clamp technique: A method for quantifying insulin secretion and resistance. Am J Physiol 1979;237:E214-E223.

25. Matthews DR, Hosker JP, Rudenski AS, et al: Homeostasis model assessment: Insulin resistance and beta-cell function from fasting plasma glucose and insulin concentrations in man. Diabetologia 1985;28:412-419.

26. Caro JF: Insulin resistance in obese and nonobese man. J Clin Endocrinol Metab 1991;73:691-695.

27. Bergman RN, Finegood DT, Ader M: Assessment of insulin sensitivity in vivo. Endocr Rev 1985;6:45-86.

28. Guilleminault C, Briskin JG, Greenfield MS, Silvestri R: The impact of autonomic nervous system dysfunction on breathing during sleep. Sleep 1981;4:263-278.

29. Rees PJ, Prior JG, Cochrane GM, Clark TJ: Sleep apnoea in diabetic patients with autonomic neuropathy. J R Soc Med 1981;74:192-195.

30. Catterall JR, Calverley PM, Ewing DJ, et al: Breathing, sleep, and diabetic autonomic neuropathy. Diabetes 1984;33:1025-1027.

31. Mondini S, Guilleminault C: Abnormal breathing patterns during sleep in diabetes. Ann Neurol 1985;17:391-395.

32. Neumann C, Martinez D, Schmid H: Nocturnal oxygen desaturation in diabetic patients with severe autonomic neuropathy. Diabetes Res Clin Pract 1995;28:97-102.

33. Ficker JH, Dertinger SH, Siegfried W, et al: Obstructive sleep apnoea and diabetes mellitus: The role of cardiovascular autonomic neuropathy. Eur Respir J 1998;11:14-19.

34. Resnick HE, Redline S, Shahar E, et al: Diabetes and sleep disturbances: Findings from the Sleep Heart Health Study. Diabetes Care 2003;26:702-709.

35. Hein MS, Schlenker EH, Patel KP: Altered control of ventilation in streptozotocin-induced diabetic rats. Proc Soc Exp Biol Med 1994;207:213-219.

36. Polotsky VY, Wilson JA, Haines AS, et al: The impact of insulin-dependent diabetes on ventilatory control in the mouse. Am J Respir Crit Care Med 2001;163:624-632.

37. Bottini P, Dottorini ML, Cristina CM, et al: Sleep-disordered breathing in nonobese diabetic subjects with autonomic neuropathy. Eur Respir J 2003;22:654-660.

38. Elmasry A, Janson C, Lindberg E, et al: The role of habitual snoring and obesity in the development of diabetes: A 10-year follow-up study in a male population. J Intern Med 2000;248:13-20.

39. Al Delaimy WK, Manson JE, Willett WC, et al: Snoring as a risk factor for type II diabetes mellitus: A prospective study. Am J Epidemiol 2002;155:387-393.

40. Enright PL, Newman AB, Wahl PW, et al: Prevalence and correlates of snoring and observed apneas in 5,201 older adults. Sleep 1996;19:531-538.

41. Grunstein RR, Stenlof K, Hedner J, Sjostrom L: Impact of obstructive sleep apnea and sleepiness on metabolic and cardiovascular risk factors in the Swedish Obese Subjects (SOS) Study. Int J Obes Relat Metab Disord 1995;19:410-418.

42. Jennum P, Schultz-Larsen K, Christensen N: Snoring, sympathetic activity and cardiovascular risk factors in a 70 year old population. Eur J Epidemiol 1993;9:477-482.

43. Levinson PD, McGarvey ST, Carlisle CC, et al: Adiposity and cardiovascular risk factors in men with obstructive sleep apnea. Chest 1993;103:1336-1342.

44. Tiihonen M, Partinen M, Narvanen S: The severity of obstructive sleep apnoea is associated with insulin resistance. J Sleep Res 1993;2:56-61.

45. Davies RJ, Turner R, Crosby J, Stradling JR: Plasma insulin and lipid levels in untreated obstructive sleep apnoea and snoring: Their comparison with matched controls and response to treatment. J Sleep Res 1994;3:180-185.

46. Strohl KP, Novak RD, Singer W, et al: Insulin levels, blood pressure and sleep apnea. Sleep 1994;17:614-618.

47. Stoohs RA, Facchini F, Guilleminault C: Insulin resistance and sleep-disordered breathing in healthy humans. Am J Respir Crit Care Med 1996;154:170-174.

48. Ip MS, Lam KS, Ho C, et al: Serum leptin and vascular risk factors in obstructive sleep apnea. Chest 2000;118:580-586.

49. Vgontzas AN, Papanicolaou DA, Bixler EO, et al: Sleep apnea and daytime sleepiness and fatigue: Relation to visceral obesity, insulin resistance, and hypercytokinemia. J Clin Endocrinol Metab 2000;85:1151-1158.

50. Elmasry A, Lindberg E, Berne C, et al: Sleep-disordered breathing and glucose metabolism in hypertensive men: A population-based study. J Intern Med 2001;249:153-161.

51. De La Eva RC, Baur LA, Donaghue KC, Waters KA: Metabolic correlates with obstructive sleep apnea in obese subjects. J Pediatr 2002;140:654-659.

52. Ip MS, Lam B, Ng MM, et al: Obstructive sleep apnea is independently associated with insulin resistance. Am J Respir Crit Care Med 2002;165:670-676.

53. Manzella D, Parillo M, Razzino T, et al: Soluble leptin receptor and insulin resistance as determinant of sleep apnea. Int J Obes Relat Metab Disord 2002;26:370-375.

54. Punjabi NM, Sorkin JD, Katzel LI, et al: Sleep-disordered breathing and insulin resistance in middle-aged and overweight men. Am J Respir Crit Care Med 2002;165:677-682.

55. Coughlin SR, Mawdsley L, Mugarza JA, et al: Obstructive sleep apnoea is independently associated with an increased prevalence of metabolic syndrome. Eur Heart J 2004;25:735-741.

56. Punjabi NM, Shahar E, Redline S, et al: Sleep-disordered breathing, glucose intolerance, and insulin resistance: The Sleep Heart Health Study. Am J Epidemiol 2004;160(6):521-530.

57. Saini J, Krieger J, Brandenberger G, et al: Continuous positive airway pressure treatment. Effects on growth hormone, insulin and glucose profiles in obstructive sleep apnea patients. Horm Metab Res 1993;25:375-381.

58. Stoohs RA, Facchini FS, Philip P, et al: Selected cardiovascular risk factors in patients with obstructive sleep apnea: Effect of nasal continuous positive airway pressure (n-CPAP). Sleep 1993;16:S141-S142.

59. Brooks B, Cistulli PA, Borkman M, et al: Obstructive sleep apnea in obese noninsulin-dependent diabetic patients: Effect of continuous positive airway pressure treatment on insulin responsiveness. J Clin Endocrinol Metab 1994;79:1681-1685.

60. Cooper BG, White JE, Ashworth LA, et al: Hormonal and metabolic profiles in subjects with obstructive sleep apnea syndrome and the acute effects of nasal continuous positive airway pressure (CPAP) treatment. Sleep 1995;18:172-179.

61. Saarelainen S, Lahtela J, Kallonen E: Effect of nasal CPAP treatment on insulin sensitivity and plasma leptin. J Sleep Res 1997;6:146-147.

62. Chin K, Shimizu K, Nakamura T, et al: Changes in intra-abdominal visceral fat and serum leptin levels in patients with obstructive sleep apnea syndrome following nasal continuous positive airway pressure therapy. Circulation 1999;100:706-712.

63. Smurra M, Philip P, Taillard J, et al: CPAP treatment does not affect glucose-insulin metabolism in sleep apneic patients. Sleep Med 2001;2:207-213.

64. Harsch IA, Schahin SP, Radespiel-Troger M, et al: Continuous positive airway pressure treatment rapidly improves insulin sensitivity in patients with obstructive sleep apnea syndrome. Am J Respir Crit Care Med 2003;169:156-162.

65. Larsen JJ, Hansen JM, Olsen NV, et al: The effect of altitude hypoxia on glucose homeostasis in men. J Physiol (Lond) 1997;504(Pt 1):241-249.

66. Braun B, Rock PB, Zamudio S, et al: Women at altitude: Short-term exposure to hypoxia and/or alpha(1)-adrenergic blockade reduces insulin sensitivity. J Appl Physiol 2001;91:623-631.

67. Cheng N, Cai W, Jiang M, Wu S: Effect of hypoxia on blood glucose, hormones, and insulin receptor functions in newborn calves. Pediatr Res 1997;41:852-856.

68. Raff H, Bruder ED, Jankowski BM: The effect of hypoxia on plasma leptin and insulin in newborn and juvenile rats. Endocrine 1999;11:37-39.

69. Raff H, Bruder ED, Jankowski BM, Colman RJ: Effect of neonatal hypoxia on leptin, insulin, growth hormone and body composition in the rat. Horm Metab Res 2001;33:151-155.

70. Polotsky VY, Li J, Punjabi NM, et al: Intermittent hypoxia increases insulin resistance in genetically obese mice. J Physiol 2003;552:253-264.

71. Bergman RN, Phillips LS, Cobelli C: Physiologic evaluation of factors controlling glucose tolerance in man: Measurement of insulin sensitivity and beta-cell glucose sensitivity from the response to intravenous glucose. J Clin Invest 1981;68:1456-1467.

72. Spiegel K, Leproult R, Van Cauter E: Impact of sleep debt on metabolic and endocrine function. Lancet 1999;354:1435-1439.

73. Narkiewicz K, Somers VK: Sympathetic nerve activity in obstructive sleep apnoea. Acta Physiol Scand 2003;177:385-390.

74. Nonogaki K: New insights into sympathetic regulation of glucose and fat metabolism. Diabetologia 2000;43:533-549.

75. Bartness TJ, Bamshad M: Innervation of mammalian white adipose tissue: Implications for the regulation of total body fat. Am J Physiol 1998;275:R1399-R1411.

76. Boden G: Free fatty acids, insulin resistance, and type 2 diabetes mellitus. Proc Assoc Am Physicians 1999;111:241-248.

77. Leproult R, Copinschi G, Buxton O, Van Cauter E: Sleep loss results in an elevation of cortisol levels the next evening. Sleep 1997;20:865-870.

78. Bratel T, Wennlund A, Carlstrom K: Pituitary reactivity, androgens and catecholamines in obstructive sleep apnoea. Effects of continuous positive airway pressure treatment (CPAP). Respir Med 1999;93:1-7.

79. Bloom SR, Edwards AV, Hardy RN, Silver M: Adrenal and pancreatic endocrine responses to hypoxia in the conscious calf. J Physiol 1976;261:271-283.

80. Bloom SR, Edwards AV, Hardy RN: Adrenal and pancreatic endocrine responses to hypoxia and hypercapnia in the calf. J Physiol 1977;269:131-154.

81. Andrews RC, Walker BR: Glucocorticoids and insulin resistance: Old hormones, new targets. Clin Sci (Lond) 1999;96: 513-523.

82. Leal-Cerro A, Soto A, Martinez MA, et al: Influence of cortisol status on leptin secretion. Pituitary 2001;4:111-116.

83. Kern PA, Ranganathan S, Li C, Wood L, Ranganathan G: Adipose tissue tumor necrosis factor and interleukin-6 expression in human obesity and insulin resistance. Am J Physiol Endocrinol Metab 2001;280:E745-E751.

84. Fernandez-Real JM, Vayreda M, Richart C, et al: Circulating interleukin 6 levels, blood pressure, and insulin sensitivity in apparently healthy men and women. J Clin Endocrinol Metab 2001;86:1154-1159.

85. Pradhan AD, Manson JE, Rifai N, et al: C-reactive protein, interleukin 6, and risk of developing type 2 diabetes mellitus. JAMA. 2001;286:327-334.

86. Klausen T, Olsen NV, Poulsen TD, et al: Hypoxemia increases serum interleukin-6 in humans. Eur J Appl Physiol Occup Physiol 1997;76:480-482.

87. Hartmann G, Tschop M, Fischer R, et al: High altitude increases circulating interleukin-6, interleukin-1 receptor antagonist and C-reactive protein. Cytokine 2000;12:246-252.

88. Liu H, Liu J, Xiong S, et al: The change of interleukin-6 and tumor necrosis factor in patients with obstructive sleep apnea syndrome. J Tongji Med Univ 2000;20:200-202.

89. Yokoe T, Minoguchi K, Matsuo H, et al: Elevated levels of C-reactive protein and interleukin-6 in patients with obstructive sleep apnea syndrome are decreased by nasal continuous positive airway pressure. Circulation 2003;107:1129-1134.

90. Ventre J, Doebber T, Wu M, et al: Targeted disruption of the tumor necrosis factor-alpha gene: metabolic consequences in obese and nonobese mice. Diabetes 1997;46:1526-1531.

91. Uysal KT, Wiesbrock SM, Marino MW, Hotamisligil GS: Protection from obesity-induced insulin resistance in mice lacking TNF-alpha function. Nature 1997;389:610-614.

92. Peraldi P, Xu M, Spiegelman BM: Thiazolidinediones block tumor necrosis factor-alpha-induced inhibition of insulin signaling. J Clin Invest 1997;100:1863-1869.

92a. Vgontzas AN, Zoumakis E, Lin HM, et al: Marked decrease in sleepiness in patients with sleep apnea by etanercept, a tumor necrosis factor-alpha antagonist. J Clin Endocrinol Metab 2004;89(9):4409-4413.

93. Ceddia RB, Koistinen HA, Zierath JR, Sweeney G: Analysis of paradoxical observations on the association between leptin and insulin resistance. FASEB J 2002;16:1163-1176.

94. Grosfeld A, Zilberfarb V, Turban S, et al: Hypoxia increases leptin expression in human PAZ6 adipose cells. Diabetologia 2002;45:527-530.

95. Chin K, Shimizu K, Nakamura T, et al: Changes in intra-abdominal visceral fat and serum leptin levels in patients with obstructive sleep apnea syndrome following nasal continuous positive airway pressure therapy. Circulation 1999;100:706-712.

96. Phillips BG, Kato M, Narkiewicz K, et al: Increases in leptin levels, sympathetic drive, and weight gain in obstructive sleep apnea. Am J Physiol Heart Circ Physiol 2000;279:H234-H237.

97. Shimizu K, Chin K, Nakamura T, et al: Plasma leptin levels and cardiac sympathetic function in patients with obstructive sleep apnoea-hypopnoea syndrome. Thorax 2002;57:429-434.

98. Chin K, Nakamura T, Takahashi K, et al: Effects of obstructive sleep apnea syndrome on serum aminotransferase levels in obese patients. Am J Med 2003;114:370-376.

99. Ozturk L, Unal M, Tamer L, Celikoglu F: The association of the severity of obstructive sleep apnea with plasma leptin levels. Arch Otolaryngol Head Neck Surg 2003;129:538-540.

100. Sanner BM, Kollhosser P, Buechner N, et al: Influence of treatment on leptin levels in patients with obstructive sleep apnoea. Eur Respir J 2004;23:601-604.

87

Clinical Features and Evaluation of Obstructive Sleep Apnea–Hypopnea Syndrome and Upper Airway Resistance Syndrome

Christian Guilleminault

Ali Bassiri

ABSTRACT

Sleep disordered breathing (SDB) includes obstructive sleep apnea–hypopnea syndrome (OSAHS) and upper airway resistance syndrome (UARS). Obesity and craniofacial dysmorphism are major risk factors for these syndromes. Polysomnography distinguishes UARS from OSAHS, with the former characterized by the absence of obstructive apneas, a respiratory disturbance index of fewer than five events per hour, and a lack of oxygen desaturation. Typical daytime symptoms of OSAHS patients include daytime sleepiness, afternoon drowsiness, forgetfulness, impaired concentration and attention, personality changes, and morning headaches. UARS patients may have more symptoms associated with functional somatic syndromes, with more daytime fatigue than sleepiness, myalgias (sometimes similar to those reported by fibromyalgia patients), migraine-like headaches, and postural hypotension and dizziness. Nocturnal signs and symptoms of SDB may variably include snoring, snorting, observed apneas, restless sleep, sweating during sleep, nocturia, bruxism, and nocturnal gastroesophageal reflux. Insomnia, disrupted sleep, sleepwalking, sleep terrors, and confusional arousals are more commonly expressed by UARS subjects. The validity of separating OSAHS and UARS into different syndromes is controversial. The important issue is to be aware that in the appropriate clinical context, a symptomatic patient who does not fulfill the diagnostic criteria for OSAHS may have UARS.

Obstructive sleep apnea–hypopnea syndrome (OSAHS) and the related upper airway resistance syndrome (UARS) are becoming increasingly recognized as leading causes of daytime sleepiness. Collectively they are referred to as sleep-disordered breathing (SDB). Obesity and certain craniofacial features are notable predisposing factors for SDB, and a thorough clinical evaluation can strongly suggest the diagnosis. A definite diagnosis, however, requires the integration of clinical evaluation and an overnight sleep study. Obstructive sleep apnea is characterized by episodes of complete or partial pharyngeal obstruction during sleep. It is a polysomnographic finding. When apneas and hypopneas occur with a specified frequency during sleep and in conjunction with symptoms such as daytime somnolence, the term *obstructive sleep apnea–hypopnea syndrome* (OSAHS) is applied.[1] In this chapter we review the clinical features and the pathophysiology of OSAHS and discuss the current thoughts regarding UARS.

EPIDEMIOLOGY

Obstructive sleep apnea was first recognized during polysomnographic monitoring of severely obese patients with the pickwickian syndrome.[2] Epidemiologic studies based on general population or community-based cohorts between 30 and 60 years of age estimate that 2% to 5% of the population are affected by OSAHS.[3-9] It should be noted that these figures mainly apply to whites. The incidence may vary in other ethnic groups.

CLINICAL SYMPTOMS

The most common symptoms or observations made by a bed partner of an OSAHS patient are snoring, excessive daytime sleepiness, nocturnal snorting and gasping, and witnessed apneas.[10] Nocturnal symptoms tend to be more specific for OSAHS than are the daytime symptoms, which are usually the result of abnormal sleep regardless of the cause.

NIGHTTIME SYMPTOMS

Almost all OSAHS patients and many UARS patients snore. Snoring can be extremely loud. A characteristic pattern in OSAHS is that of loud snoring or brief gasps that alternate with episodes of silence typically lasting 20 to 30 seconds.[10,11] The complaint of snoring often precedes the complaint of daytime sleepiness, and the intensity increases with weight gain and bedtime alcohol intake. Snoring is not uncommonly a factor in marital discord; in one study, 46% of the patients slept in separate bedrooms from their partners.[10]

Pregnancy is associated with an increase in snoring due to the upward displacement of the diaphragm and nasopharyngeal edema. Although up to 30% of pregnant women snore, overt OSAHS is uncommon.[12-16]

An interview of the bed partner as well as the patient often provides notable diagnostic insights. Apneic episodes are reported by about 75% of bed partners.[17] The cessation of breathing can cause considerable anxiety, and many bed partners shake the patient for the fear that breathing may not resume. Respiratory movements can usually be observed during these periods of obstructive apneas. Apneic episodes are usually terminated by gasps, chokes, snorts, vocalizations, or brief awakenings. Bed partners report a sudden cessation of snoring followed by a loud snort and a resumption of snoring. Although some patients awaken with a sensation of having stopped breathing, most are unaware of the apneas.

Rarely, particularly in the elderly, is there awareness of frequent awakenings, and these persons may present with a complaint of insomnia and unrefreshing sleep.

About half of OSAHS patients report restless sleep (tossing and turning) and diaphoresis, usually in the neck and upper chest area.[18,19] These symptoms are probably related to increased breathing efforts during periods of upper airway obstruction. Bed partners readily attest to excessive body movements because these can at times be violent. Patients without bed partners usually notice disheveled bed sheets in the morning.

A sensation of choking or dyspnea that interrupts sleep is reported by 18% to 31% of patients.[10,18,19] During episodes of upper airway obstruction, progressively more vigorous inspiratory efforts lead to more negative intrathoracic pressure swings, with an increase in venous return. This may increase the pulmonary capillary wedge pressure and contribute to the sensation of dyspnea.[20] Because nocturnal dyspnea may also occur in patients with congestive heart failure (paroxysmal nocturnal dyspnea), it is important to inquire about other typical symptoms to distinguish heart failure from OSAHS.[21] However, it is not unusual for the two disorders to coexist (see Chapter 102). In our experience, nocturnal dyspnea from OSAHS usually resolves quickly on awakening, whereas the paroxysmal nocturnal dyspnea that is characteristic of congestive heart failure patients takes much longer to resolve.

Esophageal reflux is another frequently observed symptom among patients with OSAHS. Increased breathing efforts during periods of apnea and hypopnea increase intraabdominal pressures while making the intrathoracic pressures more negative. Reflux results when an increased gradient between intra-abdominal and intrathoracic pressures favors the movement of gastric contents cephalad into the esophagus. Patients report awakening with heartburn. In one case, reflux led to laryngospasm.[22]

Nocturia is a relatively common symptom in OSAHS.[17] In our experience, 28% of patients report four to seven nightly trips to the bathroom.[23] Rarely, an adult patient complains of enuresis. Increased intra-abdominal pressure, confusion associated with arousals, and increased secretion of atrial natriuretic peptide[24] have been proposed contributors to nocturia.

About 74% of patients report dry mouth and the need to drink water either in the morning or during the night.[10] Drooling occurs in 36%.[10] These symptoms are most likely the result of mouth breathing, commonly seen in patients with OSAHS. OSAHS is also commonly associated with nocturnal bruxism.[25]

DAYTIME SYMPTOMS

Daytime sleepiness or fatigue is the most common complaint of patients with OSAHS.[10,17,18] Sleepiness may be subtle (such as midafternoon drowsiness during a group meeting or an occasional nap), severe (such as falling asleep while eating or talking), or catastrophic (such as falling asleep while driving). In general, it is not normal to feel sleepy immediately after a meal or while watching television. Such drowsiness usually indicates some degree of sleep deprivation or fragmentation, and OSAHS may be the underlying factor.

It is essential to inquire about sleepiness during machine and motor vehicle operation, not only because of the increased risk of accidents[26-28] but also because the safety of innocent bystanders is involved. The evidence of functional impairment in these regards may be subtle. Some drivers recall an occasional honk from the car behind alerting them to the changing of the traffic light. Others routinely roll down the windows or drink coffee to stay awake. Others report having fallen asleep while driving. Some pathologically sleepy patients deny any problems with driving, fearing restrictions on their licenses.

Patients may report clumsiness in tasks requiring dexterity, concentration, attention, memory, or judgment. Such difficulties may be so severe that job performance or even the ability to maintain employment is affected. Such intellectual impairment can be detected on neuropsychological testing.[29] Personality changes, such as aggressiveness, irritability, anxiety, or depression, may also be observed. Treatment with nasal continuous positive airway pressure (CPAP) has been shown to improve some of the symptoms such as depression and fatigue.[30] In our experience, a third of the patients also report decreased libido or impotence, which also tends to improve with treatment.

Morning or nocturnal headaches are reported in about half of the patients and often are described as dull and generalized.[10] They usually last 1 to 2 hours and may prompt the ingestion of analgesics. A study from a headache clinic found OSAHS to be the main cause of nocturnal or morning headaches.[31] None of these patients had been previously investigated for OSAHS. Other sleep disorders, such as periodic limb movements, also caused headaches; hence, patients with morning headaches[31] should be asked about sleep habits and symptoms.

Any one person will probably not report all symptoms. There also is a notable lack of specificity for most of these symptoms, and many overlap with other disorders such as depression or hypothyroidism.[32,33] In most patients with depression, the presence of daytime sleepiness should prompt a sleep study to rule out coexisting OSAHS. With respect to thyroid function, one study detected hypothyroidism in 3 of 103 patients (2.9%) with OSAHS versus 1 of 135 control subjects (0.7%).[34] The difference was not significant. The authors concluded that routine thyroid function testing is not indicated in the absence of signs or symptoms of hypothyroidism, although an exception may be made for high-risk groups such as women over the age of 60 years.

UPPER AIRWAY RESISTANCE SYNDROME

Although most of the symptoms of OSAHS overlap with UARS, some important differences have been noted in recent studies. In our experience, chronic insomnia tends to be much more common in patients with UARS than in those with OSAHS. Many UARS patients report nocturnal awakenings and find it difficult to return to sleep. In younger subjects, parasomnias are more frequently reported.[35,36] The most common parasomnia is sleepwalking with or without sleep terrors and associated confusional arousal. The treatment of UARS usually eliminates these parasomnias.

Patients with UARS are more likely to complain of daytime fatigue than sleepiness. About half of UARS patients complain of symptoms of cold hands and feet and about a third have lightheadedness upon standing or bending abruptly. This latter complaint may be related to the observation that systolic blood pressure less than 105 mm Hg and usually below 90 mm Hg is more frequently associated with UARS[37] than with OSAHS, which is commonly associated with hypertension.[38]

Finally, somatic functional complaints such as muscle pain, fainting (occasionally precipitated by emotions), or nonspecific somatic complaints are commonly seen in UARS and may be misinterpreted as chronic fatigue syndrome or fibromyalgia or, in the occasional case, may prompt a referral to psychiatry.[39] As further studies are conducted on UARS, its relation to OSAHS will become clearer. For now it may be helpful to keep in mind that the treatment options available for UARS are closely related to the ones for OSAHS.

RISK FACTORS

The presence of certain risk factors can strengthen a clinical suspicion of OSAHS. The strongest risk factors for OSAHS are obesity and age greater than 65 years.[40-46] The body mass index (BMI, weight in kg/height in m²) is commonly used to define and quantify obesity (see Table 94–1, Chapter 94). In one study, a BMI of at least 25 kg/m² had a sensitivity of 93% and a specificity of 74% for OSAHS.[46] Though obesity is common in patients with OSAHS, an increased BMI is uncommon in UARS patients.

There is currently speculation regarding the association between OSAHS and android-type obesity (fat deposition predominantly in the neck and abdomen, in contradistinction to gynecoid-type obesity, fat deposition in hips and legs), which is commonly associated with the Metabolic Syndrome or Syndrome X. In this context, male gender represents another risk factor for OSAHS. In community-based studies, the male-to-female ratio for OSAHS is 2-3:1, whereas in clinic-based studies the ratio is increased to 10-90:1.[40] The risk in women increases with obesity and postmenopausal status.[47-50] This ratio may not be applicable to UARS patients where, in our experience, the ratio is closer to 1:1.

A positive family history increases the risk of sleep disordered breathing (SDB) by twofold to fourfold.[51-53] First-degree relatives of OSAHS patients have a 21% to 84% chance of having SDB compared with 10% to 12% of the control subjects.[51-53] This genetic predisposition is likely to be expressed through craniofacial anatomy that predisposes to OSAHS, although the genetic predisposition for obesity has also been considered as a potential hereditable pathway to OSAHS.

The craniofacial features that augment risk for OSAHS include a high and narrow hard palate, an elongated soft palate, small chin, and an abnormal overjet (i.e. distance between upper and lower incisors, a dental pattern indicative of abnormal growth pattern of the maxilla, maxilla and mandible, or mandible) and may be passed on from parent to child. There is indication that these anatomical features may become more pronounced as the child grows, if the growth period is punctuated by repetitive bouts of allergies and upper respiratory tract infections and development of mouth breathing. Mouth breathing may contribute to enlargement of the tonsils, a common finding in childhood OSAHS.[54]

Several studies have shown that SDB is exacerbated by alcohol ingestion, especially around bedtime.[55-57] Alcohol ingestion reduces the activity of the genioglossus muscle and other dilator muscles that are involved in maintaining the patency of the upper airway. Decreased genioglossal activity can predispose to upper airway collapse and apneas.

Additional potential risk factors include race (African Americans, Mexican Americans, Pacific Islanders, and East Asians[58-61]) and disorders with craniofacial abnormalities such as Marfan's disease, Down's syndrome, the Pierre-Robin syndrome and other congenital craniofacial anomalies.[62-64] Isolated studies have implicated tobacco use[65] and low vital capacity as independent risk factors for SDB[66]; however, there is currently insufficient data to include them as part of the accepted risk factors for OSAHS.

Finally, sleep disordered breathing may be aggravated by certain factors such as sedatives, sleep deprivation, and supine posture.[67-69] Respiratory allergies and nasal congestion may also aggravate snoring and SDB. In addition, lesions of the autonomic nervous system (type 1 diabetes, chronic uremia, dysautonomia)[70,71] that impair sensory input and delay adjustment to abnormal airway narrowing and its consequences can worsen or even lead to OSAHS. All of these factors should be identified during the initial clinical evaluation.

The patency of the upper airway is related to the balance between negative transpharyngeal pressure developed during inspiration and a counteracting dilating force due to the contraction of the upper airway dilating muscles. The reflexes involved in this activity are mediated at least in part through receptors embedded in the pharyngeal mucosa. Signs of local nerve lesions have been demonstrated in the pharynx in patients with OSAHS. Presence of a local polyneuropathy[72-77] has been well demonstrated using electrophysiology, histology, electron microscopy, histochemistry, and evoked potentials responses. However, a systematic search for local neurologic lesions (local polyneuropathies[72-77]) in the upper airway is not part of the systematic examination of patients with SDB, despite good demonstration of their existence. The authors who support dissociation between an upper airway resistance syndrome and OSAHS base the difference in part on clinical presentation and in part on the presence or absence of decreased local sensory input due to these local lesions.[72-78] More effort should be made to evaluate them in a systematic fashion, as it may have an impact on therapeutic indications, particularly soft palate surgery.

CLINICAL EXAMINATION

As with any other patient, a complete physical examination is required to assess a patient suspected of having OSAHS. Special attention, however, must be given to the evaluation of body habitus and the upper airway.

Obesity and Neck Circumference

Measurement of height and weight and the calculation of BMI, as well as the measurement of neck circumference, should be obtained in every patient. Neck circumference has been reported to correlate better with presence of obstructive apnea than body mass index does, and circumference greater than 40 cm should lead to questions related to presence of SDB.

Katz and colleagues[79] reported that the mean neck circumference (measured at the superior border of the cricothyroid membrane, with the patient in the upright position) was 43.7 cm (±4.5 cm) (mean (SD) in patients with OSAHS and 39.6 cm (±4.5 cm) in patients without OSAHS ($P = .0001$). Another study found a correlation between neck circumference and the severity of OSAHS.[80] In their morphometric model of OSAHS, Kushida et al.[81] observed that neck circumference at and above a threshold of 40 cm is associated with a sensitivity of 61% and a specificity of 93% for OSAHS, regardless of the patient's gender.

Upper Airway

The purpose of the upper airway examination is to identify structures or abnormalities that potentially narrow the airway and increase its resistance during sleep. Some clinical indices suggesting presence of OSAHS are based on measurement of anatomic structures limiting the upper airway.[82] This examination is also important to support therapeutic suggestions, and it may indicate the need to add specific treatment, such as septoplasty or radiofrequency treatment of inferior nasal turbinates, to a prescription of nasal CPAP. The patient should preferably be examined in both the seated and supine positions because the latter may provide a relatively better reflection of the anatomy during sleep, and it frequently aggravates snoring and OSAHS. The examination is the same in patients suspected of OSAHS or UARS.

The presence of retrognathia and dental overjet (a forward extrusion of the upper incisors beyond the lower incisors) should be identified. Teeth are inserted in maxilla and mandible, and analysis of their relative positions helps classify a subject with a prognathic, orthognathic, or retrognathic mandible. The retrognathic mandible carries the risk of narrow upper airway behind the base of the tongue. The craniofacial dysmorphism that predisposes to OSAHS can result from delayed growth of the maxilla or mandible, or both, narrowing the caliber of the upper airway and producing retrognathia.[82]

Dental malocclusion and overlapping teeth are indicators of small oral cavity leading to tongue malposition, and dislocation of the temporomandibular joint during mouth opening may also contribute to an airway predisposed to collapse. Questioning about dental history during the teenage years and early 20s, and examination of teeth, can bring further information. In a general population study, OSAHS has been found to be the most common association with bruxism, and signs of dental clenching and grinding can be noted. Early in life, extraction of wisdom teeth is mostly due to impaction related to a small maxilla or mandible—again, a risk factor for narrow upper airway.

The oropharynx should be examined for the presence of macroglossia, another cause of narrow upper airway and partial airway occlusion. A visual estimate of the space between the back of the tongue and the posterior pharyngeal wall should be made, because the retroglossal area is a common site of airway obstruction during sleep. The distinction between real macroglossia and small oral cavity with relative macroglossia (in reality normal tongue size) can be difficult.

The uvula and soft palate are assessed for size, length, and height. These soft tissues represent the anterior limit of the upper airway. A small airway diameter increases suspicion that the airway is more susceptible to collapse during sleep. The soft palate examination must always be coupled with an evaluation of the hard palate (Fig. 87–1) because the positions of both are influenced by development of the maxilla early in life, and any abnormality suggests a narrow oropharynx with, again, increased risk of narrowing or collapse during sleep.

Edema or erythema of the uvula may indicate repetitive vibration trauma from snoring. A low-lying soft palate and uvula are

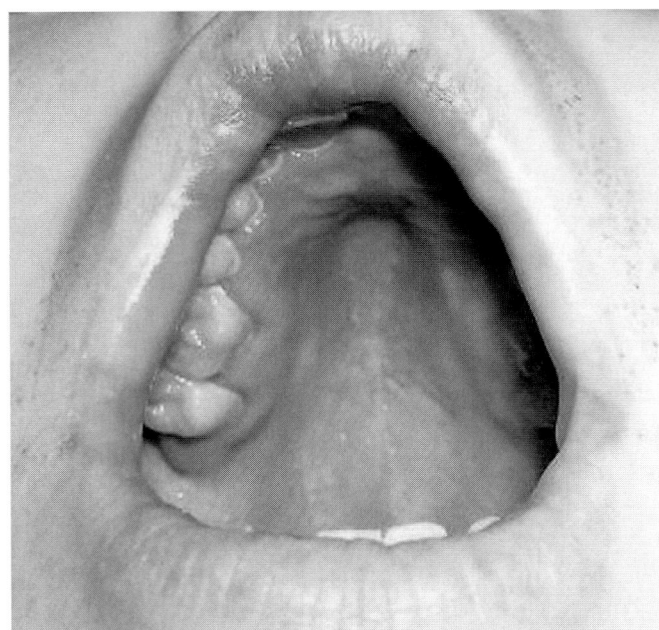

Figure 87–1. Photograph of high arched palate.

commonly seen in patients with OSAHS, and the retropalatal area can be a site of occlusion in these patients. Accurate visualization of this area, however, may require endoscopy, which is usually carried out by an otolaryngologist. Tonsillar hypertrophy and the size of the tonsillar pillars (occasionally referred to as "redundant tissue") should be noted. Enlarged tonsils are a far more important source of obstruction in children than in adults, though occasionally one sees the adult in whom enlarged, "kissing" tonsils cause significant airway narrowing and OSAHS.

Clinical scales have been useful for standardizing oropharyngeal clinical evaluation. The most commonly used is the Mallampati scale.[83] When it was initially described, subjects were asked to open their mouth wide and to protrude their tongue forward. A modified technique is performed with the mouth open and without protusion of the tongue.[84] In both cases, the oropharynx is visually assessed and the respective positions of the soft palate, the tip of the uvula, the lateral pillars, and the tongue are noted. The degree of oropharyngeal crowding is assigned a score between 1 and 4, with "1" reflecting an unobstructed, wide oropharynx with uvula clearly above the tongue, "2" indicating visible pillars and part of the inferior segment of the uvula, "3" marking a much more limited visualization of the oropharynx with the base of the uvula barely visible, and "4" indicating a very crowded oropharynx with only the hard palate visible because the uvula is entirely masked by the tongue. Scores of 3 and 4 have been associated with difficult intubation and usually imply an abnormally small oropharynx. Tonsils are also graded. Often a scale from 0 to 4 is used, with 0 indicating complete absence of the tonsils and 4 indicating "kissing" tonsils that completely obstruct the oropharynx.

Finally, one should inspect the nose for aspect and collapsibility of nasal valves, size and asymmetry of nares (Fig. 87–2), septal deviation, evidence of trauma, or enlarged inferior nasal turbinates that may lead to nasal obstruction and high nasal resistance. Although the nasal obstruction

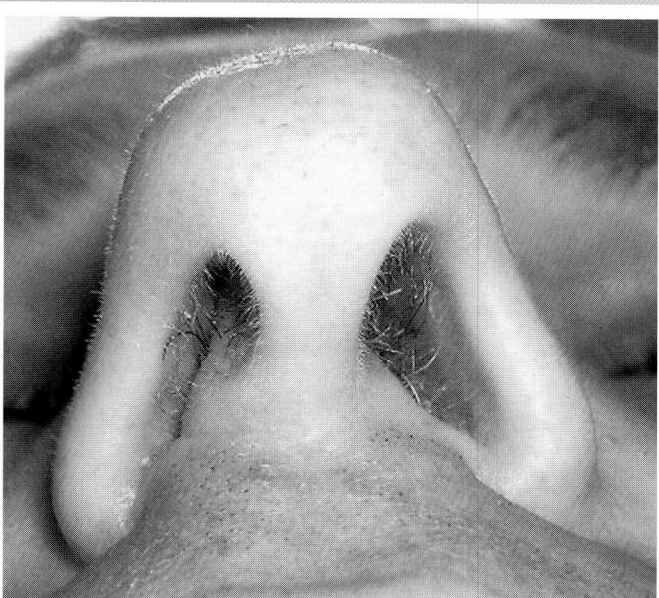

Figure 87–2. Abnormal nasal anatomy in a patient with upper airway resistance syndrome. Note the deviation of the septum, the asymmetrical size of the nares, and the collapse of the nasal external valves.

alone is rarely the sole cause of OSAHS, it may nevertheless contribute to increased airway resistance (abnormal nasal resistance plays a major role in mouth breathing in children, with a secondary impact on craniofacial growth) and may be a more significant factor in patients with UARS.[85]

Kushida and colleagues[81] described four measurements that characterize the narrow airway: palatal height, maxillary intermolar distance, mandibular intermolar distance, and overjet. Use of scales such as the abovementioned Mallampati scale[83] (developed to assess the likelihood of difficult airway intubation) has been described to help predict the likelihood of OSAHS. In general, the more difficult the airway is to intubate, the greater the likelihood is of OSAHS.

Whether one chooses to use a scale or not, routine visual examination of the upper airway in patients with and without SDB will quickly familiarize the examiner with the typical appearance of the narrow upper airway. An example of a narrowed airway is given in Figure 87–1 where one observes a high, narrow palate and an overjet. Figure 87–2 shows the abnormal nose of a patient with UARS.

Gender

In 1995 Guilleminault and coworkers[86] characterized women as the "forgotten gender" during the early descriptions of OSAHS. This was well demonstrated by Kapsimalis and Kryger in 2002.[87] The lack of recognition of the syndrome in adults and the large discrepancies in ratio of the syndrome reported between men and women ranging between 5 and 90 to 1 was not scrutinized for a long time, despite the acknowledgment of a similar proportion of boys and girls among children with SDB.

In the 1980s, the rare reports on OSAHS in women emphasized obesity and the fact that women were much more overweight than men for similar respiratory disturbance index (RDI),[42,48,49] a fact confirmed by Young's group[5] in the Wisconsin Sleep Cohort study. But a clear bias was demonstrated: In 1995,

a case-control study of 334 women with SDB reported a significant difference (mean, 9.7 years) in the duration of symptoms associated with SDB and appropriate referral and diagnosis in women between 30 and 60 years of age, compared to similar-age men.[86] This difference disappeared when BMI was greater than 30 kg/m^2.

Two elements emerged in the early 1990s: recognition of SDB in women occurred when obesity was present,[86] whereas normal-weight women were not only usually ignored, but when the diagnosis of SDB was considered, the clinical presentation and polysomnographic findings[88] usually led to denial of the problem. In their very large cohort, Young and colleagues[5] showed that women with an apnea-hypopnea index (AHI) >15 events/hour have snoring, snorting, daytime sleepiness, and breathing pauses similar to those of men with the same degree of apnea severity. Several authors[86-89] have indicated that many women have symptoms of UARS and an AHI < 5. The discrepancy between recognizing SDB in women in the clinical setting and recognizing it in large cohorts or the general population is most probably linked to lack of recognition of the specific symptomatology with which patients present and the recording of a low AHI or presence of UARS polygraphic patterns that are not given proper pathological significance.

Women complain more of insomnia, fatigue, tiredness, morning headache, muscle pain mimicking fibromyalgia, and anxiety, which Gold and coworkers called "functional somatic symptoms."[39] When comparing men and women seen for SDB in a clinical setting, Shepertycky and colleagues[90] found that women had a significantly higher incidence of depression (odds ratio (OR) = 4.6), history of thyroid disease (OR=5.6), and history of asthma or allergy (OR=1.9). Guilleminault and colleagues[86] noted a significantly greater degree of social isolation and depression in women with SDB; premenopausal women had increased reports of amenorrhea and dysmenorrhea. Thus, women often have a different clinical presentation than men.

Predictive Value of Clinical Examination

Hoffstein and Szalai studied 594 patients referred to their sleep laboratory and reported that clinical impression alone is insufficient to identify patients with OSAHS.[17] Subjective impression had a sensitivity of 60% and a specificity of 63%. The positive predictive value for snoring was 49%, bed partner's observation of apnea was 56%, and nocturnal choking was 44%. Physical examination of the pharynx revealed that 54% of the patients had an abnormal pharynx (bulky or long uvula that failed to elevate from the base of the tongue during phonation, large tonsils, or small and narrow pharyngeal orifice). In contrast, 35% of the patients without OSAHS had an abnormal pharynx. The authors concluded that history and physical examination (including blood pressure and BMI) can predict OSAHS in only about 50% of patients. Definitive diagnosis of OSAHS and of UARS therefore requires a sleep study.

DEFINITIONS (See also Chapter 117)

Apnea is defined as the complete cessation of airflow for a minimum of 10 seconds regardless of whether or not there is associated oxygen desaturation[91] or sleep fragmentation (electroencephalographically defined arousal), although they are usually present. The definition of *hypopnea* has not been universally accepted, but it is common to use a 30% or greater reduction in airflow associated with at least a 3% to 4% drop in oxygen saturation or an EEG alpha wave arousal.[91]

Certain patients with daytime symptoms similar to that described by OSAHS patients display a pattern of increased inspiratory effort leading to sleep disruption in the absence of currently defined apneas and hypopneas.[92] It is believed that these disruptions result in significant daytime symptoms such as excessive fatigue or sleepiness. These patterns can be detected by esophageal manometry (the gold standard) or the newer nasal cannula pressure transducers.[93,94] Esophageal manometry is the measurement of esophageal pressure (P_{es}) and provides a reflection of intrathoracic pressure fluctuations associated with breathing efforts. The greater the respiratory effort, the greater the swings in intrathoracic pressure, and hence the greater the oscillations in P_{es}. Normally, the most negative P_{es} value generated during inspiration (measured from the end of expiration to the most negative pressure during inspiration) varies between −2 to −3 cm H_2O in a small woman to −8 to −9 cm H_2O in a healthy large man.[95]

Three patterns of increased respiratory effort are recognized by P_{es} measurements. P_{es} *crescendo*[86] is a progressive breath-by-breath increase in P_{es} terminating either in an alpha wave or a mixture of alpha- and beta-wave EEG arousal or in a burst of delta wave activation.[96] The alpha-wave or alpha- and beta-wave burst is also referred to as a *respiratory effort–related arousal* (RERA).[1] Activation is a subcortical event and at present can only be recognized on the EEG by a sudden burst of delta waves, or a K-complex. These patterns can be part of a cyclical alternating pattern[97] and are not usually associated with a drop in oxygen saturation. *Sustained continuous effort* is a relatively stable but persistent increase in P_{es} over time (several epochs) terminated with EEG patterns similar to P_{es} crescendos. P_{es} *reversal* is an abrupt drop in P_{es} after a sequence of variable respiration efforts, independent of the EEG pattern seen (Figs. 87–3, 87–4, 87–5).[95]

Nasal cannula–pressure transducer systems (see Chapter 117), which are being used increasingly in sleep laboratories, allow one to detect increased respiratory effort by its effects on the inspiratory airflow wave contour.[93,94] Normally, inspiration produces an airflow waveform with a rounded peak. Increased respiratory efforts produce a plateau or a flattening of this peak, or an abrupt decrease immediately after an initial peak. Obstructive sleep apnea has historically been quantified by the AHI (the average number of apneas and hypopneas per hour of sleep). OSAHS is diagnosed when the patient has clinical symptoms, the most common being excessive sleepiness

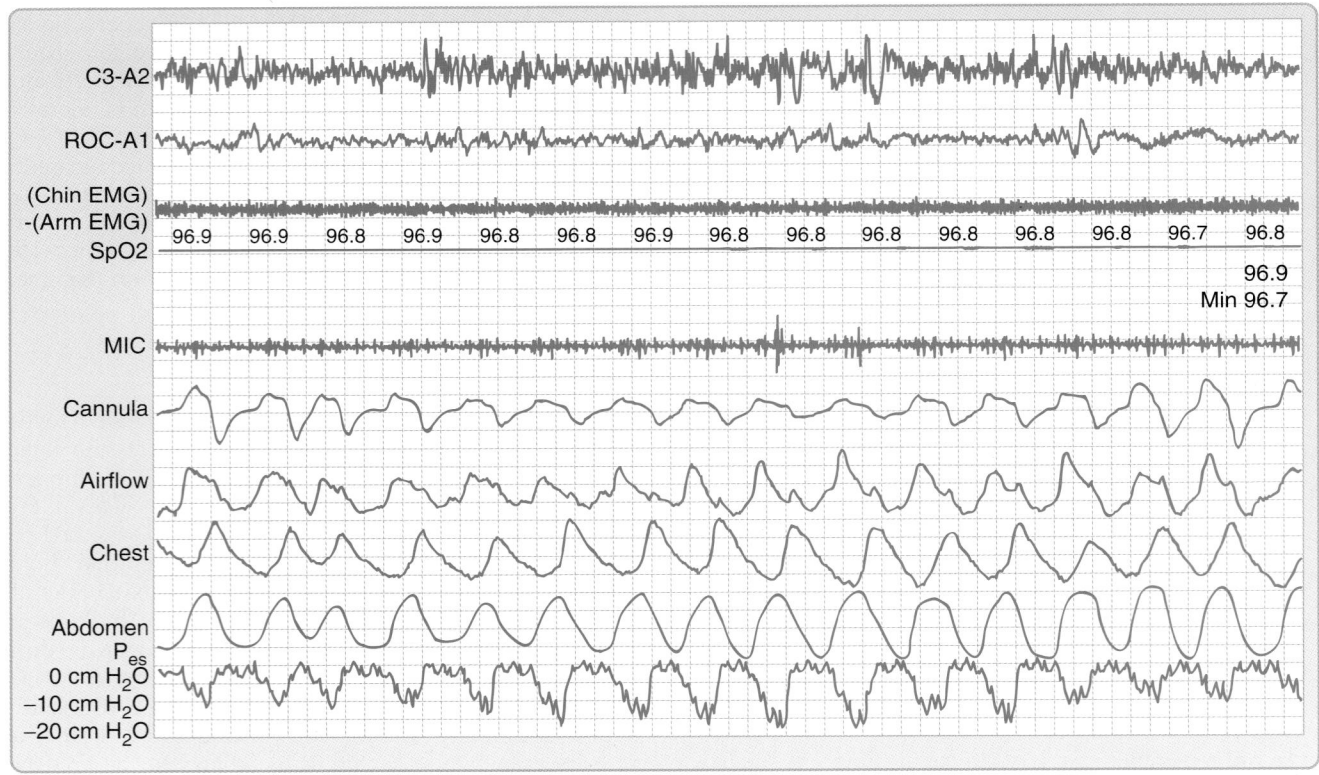

Figure 87–3. Example of a snorer with progressive worsening of the "flattening" of the nasal cannula–pressure transducer recording *(channel 6 from top)*. Simultaneously there is a progressive increase in respiratory effort as indicated by the more and more negative peak end inspiratory esophageal pressure (P_{es}) recording *(channel 10 from top)*. The progressive increase in effort gives a "crescendo" pattern to the tracing of P_{es}. At the end of the sequence there is a clear electroencephalogram (EEG) arousal indicated by the changes in EEG frequencies *(channel 1 from top)*. This is associated with a return of respiratory efforts to a less important amount, translated by a reduction of the negative deflection of P_{es} *(channel 10 from top)*, called a "P_{es} reversal." The nasal cannula-pressure transducer shows also a disappearance of the reduction in nasal flow *(channel 6 from top)*. Note that the subject snores and has a clear flow of air through the mouth *("airflow" channel 7)*. Normally humans are nose breathers; mouth breathing is abnormal and requires a larger amount of effort than nose breathing. The recording lasts 60 seconds. Note that no oxygen saturation change is seen and SaO_2 is greater than 95%. Channel labeling from top to bottom: EEG with monopolar derivation, right eye lead (electrooculogram), chin EMG (electromyogram), microphone to record snoring, nasal cannula to record pressure fluctuations at the nose to reflect airflow, chest breathing movement, abdominal movement, and esophageal pressure.

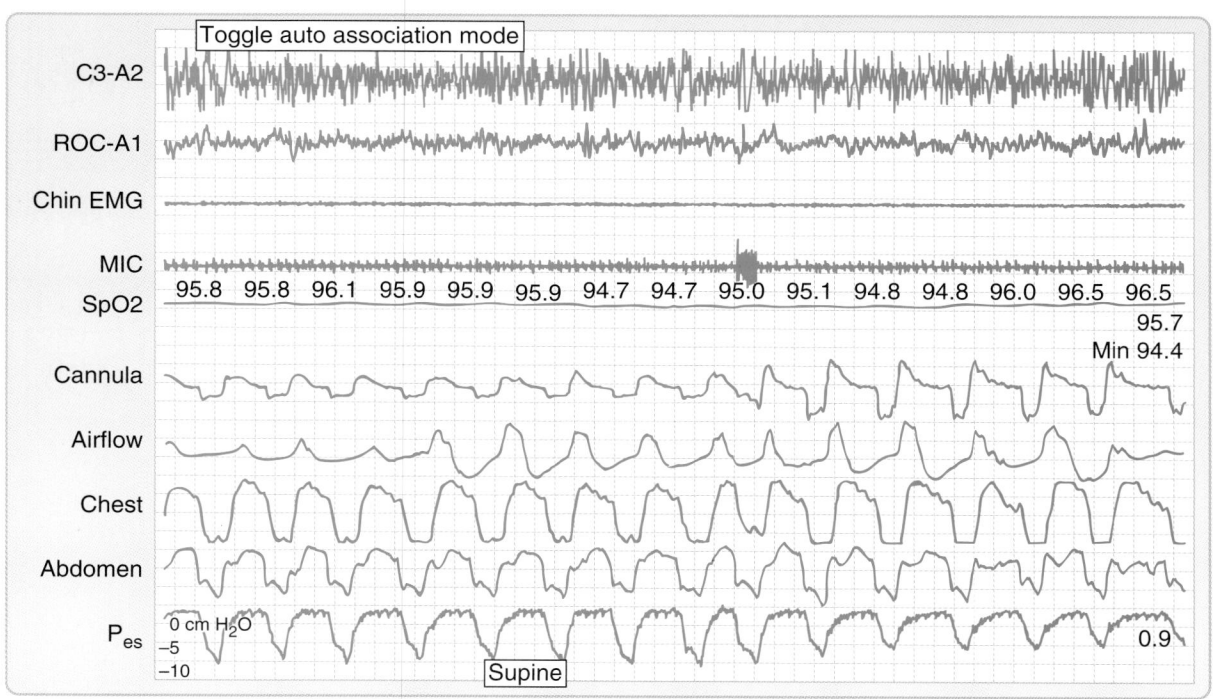

Figure 87–4. Continuous flow limitation indicated by nasal cannula–pressure transducer recording *(channel 6 from top)* but not reaching the criterion for "hypopnea" (i.e., decrease of flow by 30% from prior unobstructed recording) and leading to continuous increased effort (indicated by esophageal pressure [P_{es}] recording) *(bottom channel)* in an intermittent snorer with complaint of insomnia and fatigue. Note that the P_{es} reaches 15 cm H_2O at peak end inspiration with each breath; there is no "crescendo" pattern but a continuous maintenance of the same amount of effort during the first part of the segment. When the patient has normal breathing in other parts of the recording, the P_{es} oscillates to a peak negative inspiratory P_{es} of –3 to –4 cm H_2O. This is the normal respiratory effort during sleep for this individual. Note that there is minimal Sao_2 change (1%) in this 60-second segment *(channel 5 from top)*. In the last third of the recording *(right)* there is a short respiratory noise, not preceded by any prior snoring (microphone channel 4 from top) and an abrupt decrease in effort indicated by a less negative peak P_{es} (P_{es} reversal). The nasal cannula, channel 6 from top, indicates a better nasal flow. Visual scoring of sleep performed at slower speed (30-second epoch) does not show presence of an electroencephalogram (EEG) arousal of 3 seconds or longer, but a high-amplitude slow wave is noted concomitant with the P_{es} reversal. Channel labeling from top to bottom: EEG with monopolar derivation, right eye lead (electrooculogram), chin EMG (electromyogram), microphone to record snoring, nasal cannula to record pressure fluctuations at the nose to reflect airflow, chest movement, abdominal movement, and esophageal pressure.

in conjunction with an AHI greater than 5 per hour. With the recognition of the other patterns of increased ventilatory effort, a new index was needed. Hence the respiratory disturbance index (RDI) was introduced, and it is slowly replacing the AHI as a more inclusive method of describing SDB.

Respiratory Disturbance Index versus Apnea-Hypopnea Index in Diagnosis

The RDI is the number of apneas plus hypopneas plus RERAs and other respiratory events per hour of sleep. Some authors have used RDI as an equivalent of AHI, which it is not. Using the RDI, OSAHS is diagnosed by an RDI greater than 5 per hour and symptoms of daytime sleepiness.

This switch from an AHI to an RDI has been somewhat confusing; it is difficult in the literature to always assess what abnormal breathing event has really been measured. Proper application of the RDI parameter requires using more sensitive sensors to measure limitation of airflow.

An unresolved issue is the definition of a hypopnea. Currently, there is no clear consensus in this regard. It has been suggested that any flow limitation is a hypopnea, but no data exist to demonstrate the validity of the claim; the duration of the disturbance of flow necessary to define a "hypopnea" is also unclear. The seminal work that led to selection of a

10-second duration criterion for "apnea" (i.e. longer than 2 breaths in healthy 25- to 45-year-old men) was performed more than 30 years ago, and it considered oxygen saturation or sleep EEG changes. It is now recognized that visually scored alpha EEG arousal may not present a full indication of the sleep disturbance.[8] Also it was known from arterial blood sampling and blood gas measurements that changes in Pao_2 may not be reflected in a drop of oxygen saturation of 3% to 4%. The type of oximeter used, the sampling rate of the equipment, the location on the body of the sensor, skin pigmentation, autonomic nervous system activation, and the degree of peripheral vasoconstriction may also influence oximeter reading. Only in prepubertal children have efforts been made to assess rules for scoring SDB by comparison with clinical outcome and in the context of interscorer reliability and sleep disturbance unseen by visual scoring.[98-100] In light of these considerations, the type of sensor used, the type of event scored, and what is included behind the terms AHI and RDI should be systematically expressed in any medical report.

UARS has traditionally been diagnosed when the AHI is less than 5, but the simultaneously calculated RDI is often, but not necessarily, greater than 5 per hour of sleep, the difference in the indices being due to RERAs and other respiratory events. Hence, these other events are considered the diagnostic hallmark of UARS.[92] With the RDI beginning to

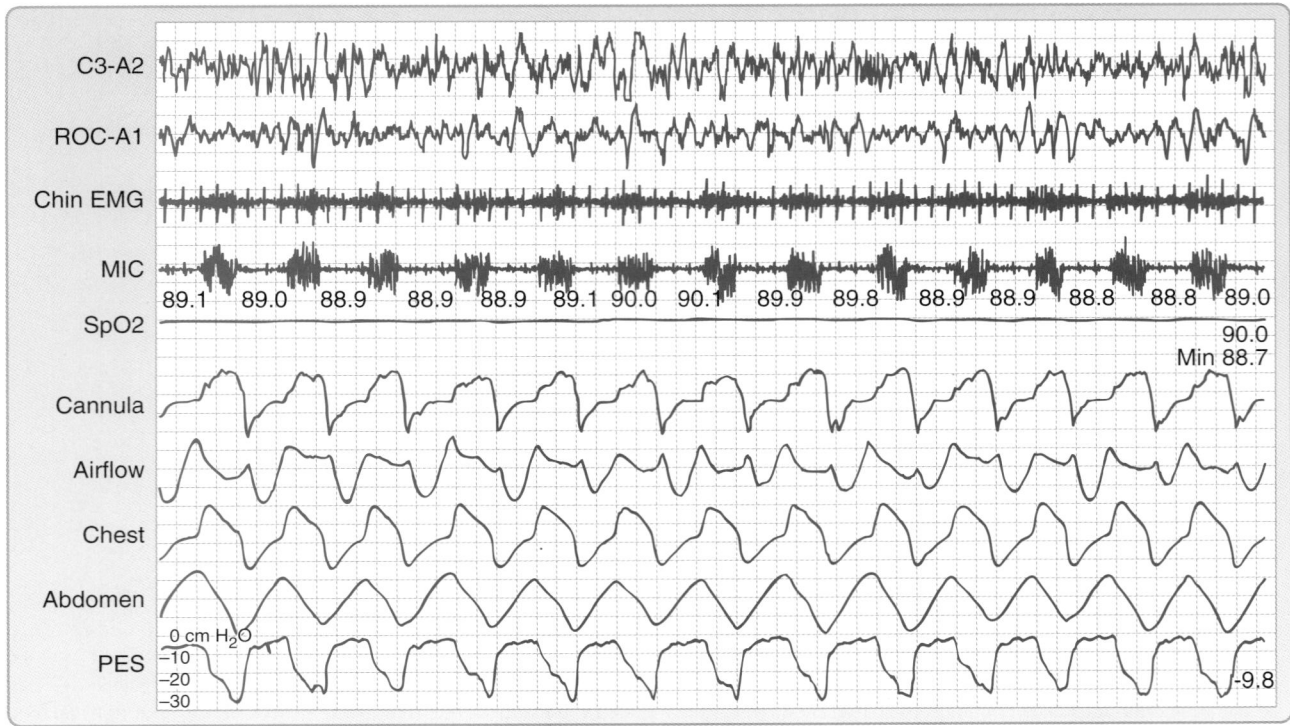

Figure 87–5. Example of a "continuous sustained effort." This recording is from a man with continuous snoring and, as in the patients in Figures 87–3 and 87–4, absence of apneas. With normal breathing respiratory effort measured by esophageal pressure, recording is a maximum of 9 cm H_2O. As can be seen with obstructed breathing, the patient presents a mild change in the nasal cannula–pressure transducer curve *(channel 6 from top)*, but the respiratory effort is greatly increased as demonstrated by the peak end inspiratory pressure (P_{es}) *(channel 10 from top)*. There is maintenance of the same amount of effort during the entire sequence of increased respiratory effort. The sequence lasted 3 minutes 46 seconds. There is no indication of change of electroencephalogram (EEG) in the 60 seconds presented here and thereafter. The termination of the sequence was indicated by a burst of delta waves. Channel labeling from top to bottom: EEG with monopolar derivation, right eye lead (electrooculogram), chin EMG (electromyogram), microphone to record snoring, nasal cannula to record pressure fluctuations at the nose to reflect airflow, chest movement, abdominal movement, and esophageal pressure.

replace the AHI, and a greater number of events being scored, more and more patients who were previously considered "chronic snorers" now have a diagnosis of OSAHS. This change now raises the question of how one diagnoses UARS. In light of recent studies showing that UARS has peculiar features that differ from OSAHS,[37,39,78,92,101] establishing the criteria for its diagnosis has become more significant. Again, clinical symptoms are associated with a polysomnographic pattern: No instances of apnea are seen and oxygen saturation is above 92% at termination of the abnormal breathing event. The abnormal breathing events usually do not meet the criteria for hypopnea as currently defined, with a duration of 10 seconds and a drop in nasal flow of 30% or more, but they are associated with the presence of well-defined cyclical alternating patterns,[97] EEG activation,[98] or alpha EEG arousal.[1]

SUMMARY

Complete assessment of the symptoms and signs, followed by a polysomnogram, is necessary for evaluating the patient with SDB. As more physicians become familiar with the clinical presentation of OSAHS and UARS, the number of diagnoses of this disorder will increase. Further studies are required to clarify the nature and the significance of the upper airway resistance syndrome. As the link between SDB and a variety of medical and psychiatric diseases becomes more secure, referrals to sleep specialists will undoubtedly increase. Furthermore, the

public is becoming increasingly aware of the importance of sleep to well being. These are exciting times in the field of sleep medicine, and the role of the sleep specialist is likely to become much more prominent in the future.

Clinical Pearls

A full assessment of the symptoms and signs followed by a polysomnogram is necessary in the evaluation of the patient with suspected SDB. Obesity and certain craniofacial features are notable predisposing factors for SDB, and a thorough clinical evaluation can strongly suggest the diagnosis. A positive family history increases the risk of SDB by twofold to fourfold. This genetic predisposition is likely to be expressed through craniofacial anatomy that predisposes to OSAHS, although the genetic predisposition for obesity has also been considered a potential heritable pathway to OSAHS.

REFERENCES

1. American Academy of Sleep Medicine: Sleep related breathing disorders in adults: Recommendations for syndrome definition and measurement techniques in clinical research. Sleep 1999; 22: 667-689.
2. Gastaut H, Tassinari CA, Duron B: Polygraphic study of the episodic diurnal and nocturnal (hypnic and respiratory) manifestations of the Pickwick syndrome. Brain Res 1965;2:167-186.

3. Bresnitz EA, Goldberg R, Kosinski RM: Epidemiology of obstructive sleep apnea. Epidemiol Rev 1994;16:210-227.

4. Olson LG, King MT, Hensley MJ, et al: A community study of snoring and sleep-disordered breathing: Prevalence. Am J Respir Crit Care Med 1995;152:711-716.

5. Kripke DF, Ancoli-Israel S, Klauber MR, et al: Prevalence of sleep-disordered breathing in ages 40-64 years: A population-based survey. Sleep 1997;20:65-76.

6. Young T, Palta M, Dempsey J, et al: The occurrence of sleep-disordered breathing among middle-aged adults. N Engl J Med 1993;328:1230-1235.

7. Ohayon MM, Guilleminault C, Priest RG, et al: Snoring and breathing pauses during sleep: Telephone interview survey of a United Kingdom population sample. BMJ 1997;314:860-863.

8. Ip MS, Lam B, Laudwe IJ, et al: A community study of sleep disordered breathing in middle-aged Chinese men in Hong Kong. Chest 2001;119:69-79.

9. Gislason T, Benedikisdottir B, Bjornsson JK, et al: Snoring, hypertension and sleep apnea syndrome. An epidemiologic survey of middle-aged women. Chest 1993;103:1147-1151.

10. Kales A, Cadieux RJ, Bixler EO, et al: Severe obstructive sleep apnea. I: Onset, clinical course, and characteristics. J Chron Dis 1985;38:419-425.

11. Guilleminault C, Tilkian A, Dement WC: The sleep apnea syndromes. Ann Rev Med 1976;27:465-484.

12. Feinsilver SH, Hertz G: Respiration during sleep in pregnancy. Clin Chest Med 1992;13:637-644.

13. Charbonneau M, Falcone T, Cosio MG, et al: Obstructive sleep apnea during pregnancy. Am Rev Respir Dis 1991;144:461-463.

14. Loube DI, Poceta JS, Morales MC, et al: Self-reported snoring during pregnancy: Association with fetal outcome. Chest 1996;109:885-889.

15. Franklin KA, Holmgren PA, Jonsson F, et al: Snoring, pregnancy-induced hypertension, and growth retardation of the fetus. Chest 2000;117:137-141.

16. Guilleminault C, Querra-Salva MA, Chowdhury S, Poyares D: Normal pregnancy, daytime sleeping, snoring, and blood pressure. Sleep Med 2000:289-297.

17. Hoffstein V, Szalai JP: Predictive value of clinical features in diagnosing obstructive sleep apnea. Sleep 1993;16:118-122.

18. Maislin G, Pack AI, Kribbs NB, et al: A survey screen for prediction of apnea. Sleep 1995;18:158-166.

19. Coverdale SGM, Read DJC, Woolcock AJ, et al: The importance of suspecting sleep apnea as a common cause of excessive daytime sleepiness: Further experience from the diagnosis and management of 19 patients. Aust N Z J Med 1980;10:284-288.

20. Buda AJ, Schroeder JS, Guilleminault C: Abnormalities of pulmonary artery wedge pressure in sleep-induced apnea. Int J Cardiol 1981;1:67-74.

21. Yamashiro Y, Kryger MH: Review: Sleep in heart failure. Sleep 1993;16:513-523.

22. Guilleminault C, Miles L: Differential diagnosis of obstructive apnea syndrome: The abnormal esophageal reflux and laryngospasm during sleep (abstract). Sleep Res 1980;16:410.

23. Hajduk IA, Strollo PJ Jr, Jasani RR, et al: Prevalence and prediction of nocturia in obstructive sleep apnea–hypopnea syndrome— a retrospective study. Sleep 2003;26;61-64.

24. Krieger J, Laks L, Wilcox I, et al: Atrial natriuretic peptide release during sleep in patients with obstructive sleep apnoea before and during treatment with nasal continuous positive airway pressure. Clin Sci 1989;77:407-411.

25. Ohayon MM, Li KK, Guilleminault C: Risk factors for sleep bruxism in the general population. Chest 2001;119:53-61.

26. George CF, Nickerson PW, Hanly PJ, et al: Sleep apnoea patients have more automobile accidents. Lancet 1987;2:447.

27. Findley LJ, Unverzadt M, Suratt P: Automobile accidents in patients with obstructive sleep apnea. Am Rev Respir Dis 1988;138:337-340.

28. Gonsalves MA, Paiva T, Ramos E, Guilleminault C: Obstructive sleep apnea syndrome, sleepiness and quality of life. Chest 2004;125:2091-2096.

29. Greenberg GD, Watson RK, Deptula D: Neuropsychological dysfunction in sleep apnea. Sleep 1987;10:254.

30. Derderian SS, Bridenbaugh RH, Rajagopal KR: Neuropsychologic symptoms in obstructive sleep apnea improve after treatment with nasal continuous positive airway pressure. Chest 1988;94:1023-1027.

31. Paiva T, Farinha A, Martins A, Guilleminault C: Chronic headaches and sleep disorders. Arch Intern Med 1997;157:1701-1705.

32. Skjodt NM, Atkar R, Easton PA: Screening for hypothyroidism in sleep apnea. Am J Respir Crit Care Med 1999;160:732-735.

33. Winkelman JW, Goldman H, Piscatelli N, et al: Are thyroid function tests necessary in patients with suspected sleep apnea? Sleep 1996;19:790-793.

34. Rajagopal KR, Abbrecht PH, Derderian SS: Obstructive sleep apnea in hypothyroidism. Ann Intern Med 1984;101:471-474.

35. Guilleminault C, Palombini L, Pelayo R, Chervin RD: Sleepwalking and night terrors in prepubertal children: what triggers them? Pediatrics 2003;111:17-25.

36. Guilleminault C, Kirisoglu C, da Rosa A, et al: Continuous NREM sleep instability in sleep walking and treatment of the underlying cause. J Sleep Res (abstract) 2004;13(suppl 1):281.

37. Guilleminault C, Faul JL, Stoohs R: Sleep disordered breathing and hypotension. Am J Respir Crit Care Med 2001;164:1242-1247.

38. Peppard PE, Young T, Palta M, et al: Prospective study of the association between sleep disordered breathing and hypertension. N Engl J Med 2000;342:1378-1384.

39. Gold AR, Dipalo F, Gold MS, O'Hearn D: Symptoms and signs of upper airway resistance syndrome: A link to the functional somatic syndromes. Chest 2003;123:87-95.

40. Strohl KP, Redline S: Recognition of obstructive sleep apnea. Am J Respir Crit Care Med 1996;154:279-289.

41. Levinson PD, McGarvey ST, Carlisle CC, et al: Adiposity and cardiovascular risk factors in men with obstructive sleep apnea. Chest 1993;103:1336-1342.

42. Rajala RM, Partinen M, Sane T, et al: Obstructive sleep apnea in morbidly obese patients. J Intern Med 1991;230:125-129.

43. Phillips B, Cook Y, Schmitt F, et al: Sleep apnea: Prevalence of risk factors in the general population. South Med J 1989;82:1090-1092.

44. Bloom JW, Kaltenborn WT, Quan SF: Risk factors in the general population for snoring: Importance of cigarette smoking and obesity. Chest 1988;93:678-683.

45. Dealberto M-J, Ferber C, Garma L, et al: Factors related to sleep apnea syndrome in sleep clinic patients. Chest 1994;105:1753-1758.

46. Grunstein R, Wilcox I, Yang T, et al: Snoring and sleep apnoea in men: Association with central obesity and hypertension. Int J Obes 1993;17:533-540.

47. Wilhoit SC, Suratt PM: Obstructive sleep apnea in premenopausal women: A comparison with men and with post-menopausal women. Chest 1987;91:654-658.

48. Leech JA, Onal E, Dulberg C, et al: A comparison of men and women with occlusive sleep apnea syndrome. Chest 1988;94:983-988.

49. Guilleminault C, Quera-Salva A, Partinen M, et al: Women and the obstructive sleep apnea syndrome. Chest 1988;93:104-109.

50. Richmond RM, Elliot LM, Burns CM, et al: The prevalence of obstructive sleep apnoea in an obese female population. Int J Obes 1994;18:173-177.

51. Redline S, Tishler PV, Williamson J, et al: The familial aggregates of sleep apnea. Am J Respir Crit Care Med 1995;151:682-687.

52. Pillar G, Lavie P: Assessment of the role of inheritance in sleep apnea syndrome. Am J Respir Crit Care Med 1995;151:688-691.

53. Guilleminault C, Partinen M, Hollman K, et al: Familial aggregates in obstructive sleep apnea syndrome. Chest 1995;107:1545-1551.

54. Behlfelt K: Enlarged tonsils and the effect of tonsillectomy. characteristics of the dentition and facial skeleton. Posture of the head, hyoid bone and tongue. Mode of breathing. Swed Dent J 1990;72(Suppl):1-35.

55. Taasan VC, Block AJ, Boysen PG, et al: Alcohol increases sleep apnea and oxygen desaturation in asymptomatic men. Am J Med 1981;71:240-245.

56. Krol RC, Knuth SL, Bartlett D Jr: Selective reduction of genioglossal muscle activity by alcohol in normal human subjects. Am Rev Respir Dis 1984;129:247-250.

57. Scrima L, Broudy M, Nay KN, et al: Increased severity of obstructive sleep apnea after bedtime alcohol ingestion: Diagnostic potential and proposed mechanism of action. Sleep 1982;5:318-328.

58. Redline S, Hans M, Pracharktam N, et al: Differences in the age distribution and risk factors for sleep-disordered breathing in blacks and whites. Am J Respir Crit Care Med 1994;149:577.

59. Schmid-Nowara WW, Coultas D, Wiggins C, et al: Snoring in a Hispanic-American population: Risk factors and association with hypertension and other morbidity. Arch Intern Med 1990;150:597-601.

60. Grunstein RR, Lawrence S, Spies JM, et al: Snoring in paradise: the Western Samoa Sleep Survey. Eur Respir J 1989;2(S5):4015.

61. Li KK, Powell NB, Riley RW, Guilleminault C: Obstructive sleep apnea syndrome: A comparison between Far-East Asian and white men. Laryngoscope 2000;110:1689-1693.

62. Cistulli P, Sullivan CE: Sleep apnea in Marfan's syndrome. Am Rev Respir Dis 1993;147:645-648.

63. Telekavi T, Partinen M, Salmi T, et al: Nocturnal periodic breathing in adults with Down syndrome. J Ment Defic Res 1987;31:31-39.

64. Resta O, Barbaro MP, Giliberti T, et al: Sleep related breathing disorders in adults with Down syndrome. Down Syndr Res Pract 2003;8:115-119.

65. Wetter D, Young T, Bidwall T, et al: Smoking as a risk factor for sleep disordered breathing. Arch Intern Med 1994;154: 2219-2224.

66. Bliwise DL, Bliwise NG, Partinen M, et al: Sleep apnea and mortality in an aged cohort. Am J Public Health 1988;78:544-547.

67. Roth T, Roehrs T, Zorick F, et al: Pharmacological effects of sedative-hypnotics, narcotic analgesics, and alcohol during sleep. Med Clin North Am 1985;69:1281-1288.

68. Mendelson WB, Garnett D, Gillin JC: Flurazepam-induced sleep apnea syndrome in a patient with insomnia and mild sleep-related respiratory changes. J Nerv Ment Dis 1981;169:261-264.

69. Dolly FR, Block AJ: Effects of flurazepam on sleep-disordered breathing and nocturnal oxygen desaturation in asymptomatic subjects. Am J Med 1982;73:239-243.

70. Mondini S, Guilleminault C: Abnormal breathing patterns during sleep in diabetes. Ann Neurol 1985;17:391-395.

71. Resnick HE, Redline S, Shahar E, et al: Diabetes and sleep disturbances: Findings from the Sleep Heart Study. Diabetes Care 2003;26:702-709.

72. Edstrom L, Larson H, Larson L: Neurogenic effects on the palato pharyngeal muscle in patients with obstructive sleep apnea: A muscle biopsy study. J Neurol Neurosurg Psychiatr 1992;55:916-920.

73. Friberg D, Answed T, Borg K, et al: Histological indications of a progressive snorer disease in upper airway muscle. Am J Respir Crit Care Med 1998;157:586-593.

74. Friberg D, Gazelius B, Holfelt T, et al: Abnormal afferent nerve endings in the soft palatal mucosa of sleep apneics and habitual snorers. Regul Pept 1997;71:29-36.

75. Kimoff JR, Sforza E, Champagne V, et al: Upper airway sensation in snoring and obstructive sleep apnea. Am J Respir Crit Care Med 2001;164:250-255.

76. Petrof BJ, Hendricks JC, Pack AI: Does upper airway muscle injury trigger a vicious cycle in obstructive sleep apnea? A hypothesis. Sleep 1996;19:465-471.

77. Affifi L, Guilleminault C, Colrain I: Sleep and respiratory stimulus specific dampening of cortical responsiveness in OSAS. Respir Physiol Neurobiol 2003;136:221-234.

78. Guilleminault C, Li K, Chen NH, Poyares D: Two point palatal discrimination in upper airway resistance syndrome, OSAS and normal controls. Chest 2002;122:866-870.

79. Katz I, Stradling J, Slutsky AS, et al: Do patients with obstructive sleep apnea have thick necks? Am Rev Respir Dis 1990;141:1228-1231.

80. Davies RJO, Stradling JR: The relationship between neck circumference, radiographic pharyngeal anatomy, and the obstructive sleep apnoea syndrome. Eur Respir J 1990;3:509-514.

81. Kushida CA, Efron B, Guilleminault C: A predictive morphometric model for the obstructive sleep apnea syndrome. Ann Intern Med 1997;127:581-587.

82. Jamieson A, Guilleminault C, Partinen M, et al: Obstructive sleep apnea patients have craniomandibular abnormalities. Sleep 1986;9:469-477.

83. Mallampati SR, Gugino LD, Ga SP, et al: A clinical sign to predict difficult tracheal intubation: A prospective study. Can Anesth Soc J 1985;32:429-434.

84. Friedman M, Tanyeri H, La Rosa M, et al: Clinical predictors of obstructive sleep apnea. Laryngoscope 1999;109:1901-1907.

85. Guilleminault C, Kim YD, Stoohs RA: Upper airway resistance syndrome. Oral Maxillofac Surg Clin North Am 1995;7:397-406.

86. Guilleminault C, Stoohs R, Kim YD, et al: Upper airway sleep disordered breathing in women. Ann Intern Med 1995;122: 493-501.

87. Kapsimalis F, Kryger MH: Gender and obstructive sleep apnea syndrome, part 1: Clinical features. Sleep 2002;25:412-419.

88. Guilleminault C, Stoohs R, Clerk A, et al: Excessive daytime somnolence in women with abnormal respiratory effort during sleep. Sleep 1993;16:S137-S138.

89. Mohsenin V: Gender differences in the expression of sleep disordered breathing: Role of upper airway dimensions. Chest 2001;120:1442-1447.

90. Shepertycky MR, Banno K, Kryger MH: Differences between men and women in the clinical presentation of patients diagnosed with obstructive sleep apnea syndrome. Sleep 2005;28:309-314.

91. Butkov N: Atlas of Clinical Polysomnography. Vol II. Ashland, Ore, Synapse Media, 1996, pp 184-189.

92. Guilleminault C, Stoohs R, Clerk AC, et al: A cause of excessive daytime sleepiness: the upper airway resistance syndrome. Chest 1993;104:781-787.

93. Ayap I, Norman RG, Krieger AC, et al: Noninvasive detection of respiratory effort-related arousals (RERAs) by a nasal cannula/pressure transducer system. Sleep 2000;23:763-771.

94. Hosselet JJ, Norman RG, Ayappa I, Rapoport D: Detection of flow limitation with nasal cannula/pressure transducer system. Am J Respir Crit Care Med 1998;157:1461-1467.

95. Guilleminault C, Poyares D, Palombini L, et al: Variability of respiratory effort in relationship with sleep stages in normal controls and upper airway resistance syndrome patients. Sleep Med 2001;2:397-406.

96. Black J, Guilleminault C, Colrain I, Carillo O: Upper airway resistance syndrome: Central EEG power and changes in breathing effort. Am J Respir Crit Care Med 2000;162:406-411.

97. Terzano MG, Parrino L, Sherieri A, et al: Atlas, rules and recording techniques for the scoring of the cyclical alternating pattern (CAP) in human sleep. Sleep Med 2001;2:537-554.

98. Guilleminault C, Li K, Khramtsov A, et al: Breathing patterns in pre-pubertal children with sleep disordered breathing. Arch Pediatr Adolesc Med 2004;158:153-161.

99. Chervin RD, Burns JW, Subotic NS, et al: Correlates of respiratory cycle-related EEG changes in children with sleep disordered breathing. Sleep 2004;27:116-122.

100. Wong TK, Galster P, Lau C, et al: Reliability of scoring arousal in children. Sleep 2004 in press.

101. Guilleminault C, Kim YD, Chowdhuri S, et al: Sleep and daytime sleepiness in upper airway resistance syndrome compared to obstructive sleep apnea syndrome. Eur Respir J 2001;17:838-847.

88

Medical Therapy for Obstructive Sleep Apnea–Hypopnea Syndrome

Patrick J. Strollo, Jr.

Charles W. Atwood, Jr.

Mark H. Sanders

ABSTRACT

Although measures that physically increase the size of the upper airway (continuous positive airway pressure [CPAP], oral appliances, and surgery) are usually used as primary treatment in patients with obstructive sleep apnea–hypopnea syndrome, other medical interventions play a role in management. Among these is weight loss (either by dietary modification or surgery), which, when successful, might ameliorate or completely reverse obstructive sleep apnea in obese patients. Because alcohol and some drugs such as hypnotic sedatives and opiates may worsen episodes of apnea, such drugs should be avoided. Neither drugs that may stimulate breathing, such as progestational agents and methylxanthines, nor medications used in an attempt to increase upper airway patency (e.g., antidepressants) have been demonstrated to be efficacious. Estrogen–progesterone combinations may be effective in selected menopausal patients with sleep apnea, but not as sole treatment. The role of such therapy in postmenopausal women has not been studied in clinical trials, and it is not known whether the potential benefits in this group of patients outweigh the risks. Modafinil, a wake-promoting medication, may play a role in treating residual sleepiness in patients compliant with CPAP therapy. Oxygen has not been shown to be efficacious as a primary treatment of obstructive sleep apnea, but it may have a role in patients with obstructive sleep apnea who demonstrate severe hypoxemia during sleep but who do not tolerate any other therapy. Oxygen should be used cautiously in this setting because it may prolong episodes of apnea.

The principal medical therapy for the obstructive sleep apnea–hypopnea syndrome (OSAHS) remains positive pressure administered through a mask (see Chapter 89). Oral appliances can be useful in selected patients who cannot tolerate continuous positive airway pressure (CPAP; see Chapter 91). Other medical options may be important as adjuncts to these treatment options or as therapeutic interventions alone if the patient cannot accept or tolerate CPAP or oral appliance therapy as a primary treatment. The focus of this chapter is to review these options in detail.

BEHAVIORAL INTERVENTIONS

Good medical care mandates a thorough look at the patient's lifestyle and how it may complicate the underlying medical problem. This is particularly true in the patient with OSAHS.

There are a number of lifestyle considerations that place the patient at increased risk. Modification of these behaviors can have a favorable impact on risk. These behavioral risks are dealt with in separate sections for clarity. It should be kept in mind that multiple interventions may be appropriate in a given patient.

Weight Loss

The adverse effect of obesity on upper airway function is in part mediated through a direct mechanical influence on upper airway geometry. Studies in animals have indicated that upper airway resistance is influenced by mass loading of the anterior neck, which may simulate the clinical scenario of excessive adipose tissue deposits in this area.[1] Further support for a significant pathophysiologic role of cervical obesity is provided by the observation that changes in pressure surrounding the neck are transmitted to the airway lumen and that cyclic pressure fluctuations in the pharyngeal fat pad coincide with intrapharyngeal pressure fluctuations.[2,3] These data also support the relevance of the observation that patients with OSAHS have "thick" necks[4] and that increased neck circumference is a predictive factor for OSAHS.[5-7] Furthermore, velopharyngeal collapsibility increases with increasing neck circumference, at least in awake patients with OSAHS.[8]

The presence of intrapharyngeal fat deposition may also be of pathophysiologic significance. Several groups of investigators have observed increased intrapharyngeal adipose tissue or increased lateral fat pad size on magnetic resonance imaging of patients with OSAHS.[9,10] The significance of a space-occupying intrapharyngeal mass on pharyngeal function has been demonstrated in an animal model with increased upper airway resistance that is related to the magnitude of inflation of a balloon catheter in the region of the upper airway lateral fat pad.[3,11]

It has been well documented that either medical or surgical weight reduction can have a substantial ameliorative impact on this disorder.[12-16] In a prospective cohort study examining the association between weight change and the severity of sleep-disordered breathing, Young et al. demonstrated that a 10% weight loss predicted a 26% reduction in the apnea-hypopnea index (Fig. 88–1). Smith and colleagues reported that a relatively modest weight loss may provide a significant benefit for some individuals.[13]

Although it is clear that there remains a population of nonobese patients with OSAHS and that there are some

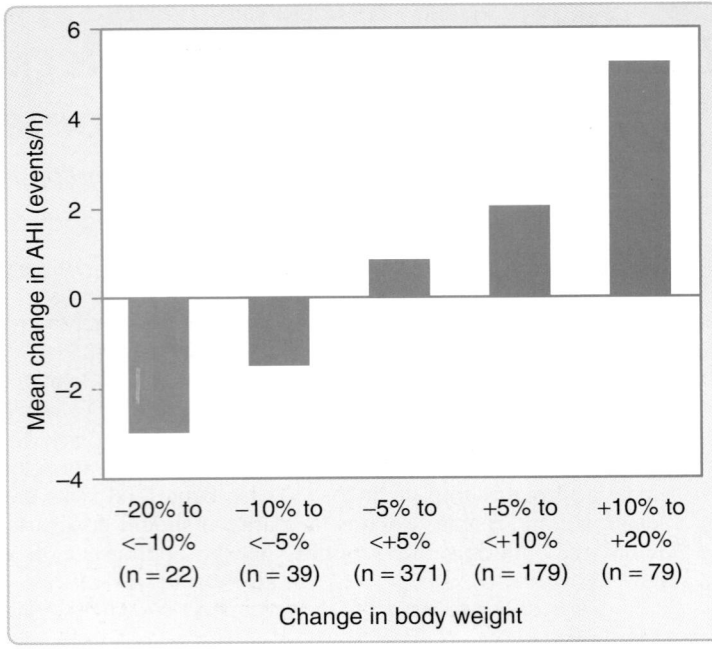

Figure 88–1. The effect of the change in body weight on the mean change in the apnea-hypopnea index (AHI) over a 4-year period. (Redrawn from Peppard PE, Young T, Palta M, et al: Longitudinal study of moderate weight change and sleep-disordered breathing. JAMA 2000;284:3015-3021.)

patients who do not obtain benefit from weight reduction,[13,14] obese patients should always be encouraged to lose weight. A multidisciplinary team approach to weight reduction, encompassing lifestyle and dietary modification as well as pharmacologic and surgical options, may optimize clinical results.[17] Not only will this have a beneficial impact on overall health, it has a high likelihood of reducing the severity of upper airway dysfunction during sleep. Conceivably, the "nonresponders" reflect those who have not lost sufficient weight or have coexistent craniofacial abnormalities. Because of the poor long-term success rate with weight loss in this group, bariatric surgery is being done more frequently in the treatment of these patients, with sometimes excellent results.[18] In fact, most patients referred for bariatric surgery, regardless of whether apnea is suspected, are found to have sleep apnea, and it has been suggested that all patients referred for bariatric surgery should have preoperative polysomnography.[19,20] Patients with sleep apnea may have a higher complication rate with such surgery.[21,22]

Smoking Cessation

Tobacco use is known to have a detrimental effect on sleep. Cigarette users have more difficulty initiating and maintaining sleep and experience increased daytime sleepiness as well.[23] Although there are a variety of possible explanations for this, including the impact of nicotine withdrawal, it is conceivable that one mechanism is an association between smoking and sleep-disordered breathing. Smokers have an odds ratio that is fourfold to fivefold greater than that of never-smokers for having at least moderate sleep-disordered breathing.[24] Heavy smokers are at greatest risk. Cigarette smoking may contribute to upper airway dysfunction during sleep by eliciting mucosal edema and increased upper airway resistance. It is obvious that tobacco use should be discouraged on the basis of its adverse multisystem effects.

The observation that nicotine administered as gum reduces apnea frequency over the first several hours of sleep[25] is of conceptual if not practical interest. The short duration of action of this mode of delivery precludes effective therapeutic application of nicotine gum for OSAHS. Additional studies have subsequently demonstrated that there was no clinically significant reduction in disordered breathing event frequency after application of transdermal nicotine patches, which have an extended duration of delivery. Apnea duration and snoring intensity were reduced, although the magnitude of the latter was insufficient to be therapeutically useful. Adverse effects were observed in conjunction with the transdermal patch, including reduced total sleep time, sleep efficiency, and rapid eye movement (REM) sleep.[26] Other side effects, including gastrointestinal complaints, lightheadedness, and tremor, were also reported.

Sleep Hygiene and Sleep Deprivation

We live in a sleep-deprived society.[27] In addition to the intuitively obvious adverse impact of sleep deprivation on performance, several lines of evidence suggest that absolute deprivation, as well as repetitive sleep disruption, may also predispose to or worsen existing OSAHS. Sleep deprivation is associated with blunted hypoxic and hypercapnic ventilatory chemoresponsiveness during wakefulness,[28,29] and may prolong apneas and hypopneas with consequently greater oxyhemoglobin desaturation by depressing the arousal response.[30,31] Sériès et al. have reported that upper airway collapsibility increased after sleep fragmentation but not after short-term sleep deprivation.[32]

Patients should be encouraged to maintain good sleep hygiene, although this advice is often unheeded because of social and financial pressures. It may be useful to remind them that to do otherwise may have an adverse impact on their sleep-disordered breathing and contribute to a vicious cycle in which insufficient or fragmented sleep promotes OSAHS, which in turn promotes poor-quality sleep.

Body Position

A bed partner's prompting to move to the lateral recumbent position constitutes one of the oldest interventions for snoring and OSAHS. In many patients, the frequency of sleep-disordered breathing events is substantially greater during sleep in the supine position than in the lateral recumbent position.[33-35] Sleeping in the supine position may increase the probability of upper airway occlusion because of the effect of gravity on the tongue, which tends to relapse posteriorly and come into apposition with the posterior pharyngeal wall. If the mass of soft tissue in the anterior cervical region enhances the propensity for upper airway dysfunction,[1,4] it is reasonable to speculate that this factor interacts with body position to compromise upper airway patency during sleep.

Body position dependency is inversely related to the degree of obesity,[36] with a greater likelihood that more obese patients will have OSAHS regardless of position. It should not be assumed that a patient with normal body weight has position-dependent OSAHS.[36] The presence or absence of obesity is not an invariable predictor of supine position–dependent sleep-disordered breathing. It has been suggested that there is no effect of body position specifically during REM sleep.[35] Position-related alterations in overall apnea frequency are present primarily during non-REM (NREM) sleep. There is no body position effect on apnea duration, suggesting that the arousal mechanism is influenced by sleep stage but not by body position.

Sleeping with the head and trunk elevated at a 30- to 60-degree angle to the horizontal has a favorable impact on OSAHS.[37,38] Upper airway closing pressure (the magnitude of negative pressure when applied to the airway that results in occlusion) is more negative (indicating greater stability) in the 30-degree head-elevated position than in the supine and lateral recumbent positions during NREM sleep.[38] Opening pressure (the magnitude of nasal CPAP that eliminates apnea, hypopneas, and oxyhemoglobin desaturation) is less in the head-elevated position than in the supine position, but not significantly different from the lateral recumbent position. These data suggest that 30-degree head elevation may be more effective in stabilizing the upper airway than sleeping in the lateral recumbent position, but that head elevation may not reduce the required magnitude of CPAP relative to lateral recumbency.

The data are sufficiently suggestive that body position influences upper airway patency during sleep in some patients to warrant specific questioning of the patient and bed partner regarding position dependence of sleep-disordered breathing. It is prudent to objectively evaluate sleep and breathing in this context. If there is sufficient control of OSAHS, as well as maintenance of acceptable oxygenation and sleep continuity in the lateral recumbent position during REM and NREM sleep, therapeutic management of body position during sleep may be considered. The "sleep ball" or similar technique to facilitate maintenance of the lateral recumbent position during sleep may be used. This technique entails sewing a pocket into the back of the patient's sleeping garment and placing an object such as one or more tennis balls in this pocket. Alternatively, the objects may be placed in a sock, which is safety-pinned to the back of the sleeping garment.

Over time, the patient may become trained to sleep in the lateral recumbent position, without the need for a physical reminder. The clinician must also recognize the practical issues involved with prescribing a head-elevated position because this may require a wedge on which the patient may sleep (cumbersome with regard to sharing a bed) or a specialized and potentially costly bed.

In addition to affecting OSAHS frequency, body position may influence "central" apnea. We have seen several patients with supine body position–dependent mixed and central apneas. Issa et al.[39] also remarked on the presence of supine position–dependent central apnea in patients with predominantly obstructive apnea. It has been postulated that occlusion of the upper airway in the supine position is an important element in the pathogenesis of these central apneas. Sanders and colleagues[40] suggested that upper airway obstruction during exhalation could result in prolonged, low-level expiratory airflow, which is usually below the threshold for detection by usual recording techniques, thereby simulating true central apnea. Several additional reports using video-endoscopy have demonstrated the presence of upper airway occlusion during otherwise central apneas.[41,42] Issa et al.[39] postulated that supine position–dependent (gravity-related) apposition of the pharyngeal walls precipitates central apnea through reflex inhibition of ventilation. The tendency for improvement of these central apneas by nasal CPAP[39,40,43] or, in some cases, by maintaining the lateral recumbent body position supports a pathophysiologic role of upper airway obstruction in these events.

In summary, manipulation of body position to promote sleeping in the lateral recumbent posture or with a 30- to 60-degree head elevation may lead to clinically significant improvement of OSAHS in an undefined proportion of patients. It is important to analyze each patient's historical and polysomnographic data with this in mind. The potential impact of variation in body position should be considered when critically evaluating published reports describing the effects of other therapeutic interventions for OSAHS. The effect of variations in head, neck, and shoulder position on upper airway patency during sleep remains to be fully investigated.

Alcohol

Bed partners and housemates are probably the first to recognize the association between alcohol consumption and upper airway dysfunction during sleep. It is clear that alcohol evokes obstructive apnea in individuals who otherwise only snore and increases the apnea frequency in patients with preexisting OSAHS.[44-46] In addition to increasing the frequency of sleep-disordered breathing events, alcohol consumption increases the duration of these events.[47,48]

Alcohol may also have a particularly adverse impact on daytime alertness in patients with OSAHS. The hypnotic effect of this agent is enhanced in the presence of underlying sleepiness. Alcohol consumption superimposed on sleepiness, as in sleep deprivation, is associated with worse driving simulator test performance compared with sleep deprivation and placebo.[49] It would be expected that alcohol would have a notably greater detrimental impact on daytime alertness in patients with OSAHS who have increased basal sleepiness.

The key message is that individuals with OSAHS, treated or untreated, would be best served by abstinence from alcohol.

Although this is prudent advice, not all patients will follow this directive. If a patient is unwilling to abstain completely, he or she should be told to limit the alcohol intake to small quantity, and not to consume alcohol for a time before bedtime that is sufficient to permit the blood alcohol level to fall to nil. There is inconsistency in the literature regarding the impact of alcohol on the magnitude of the positive-pressure prescription[50-52]; patients who are unlikely to alter their alcohol consumption should have a therapeutic trial under usual lifestyle conditions. Therapy needs to be proven successful despite the presence of exogenous as well as endogenous influences on the pathophysiologic processes. This includes not only alcohol consumption, but other factors, such as body position during sleep (some individuals may be able to sleep only in the supine position) or unavoidable need for treatment with pharmacologic agents that may adversely effect upper airway stability during sleep (e.g., benzodiazepines).

Sedatives

Although the effect of every individual benzodiazepine on breathing during sleep has not been evaluated, flurazepam has been the subject of several investigations. This agent may worsen OSAHS in some individuals who otherwise have minimal sleep-disordered breathing.[53-55] Reports addressing the impact of benzodiazepine on breathing during sleep in otherwise healthy subjects provide inconsistent results.[55,56]

There have been a limited number of studies examining the impact of benzodiazepines other than flurazepam and diazepam. In a group of patients with mild insomnia and sleep apnea (respiratory disturbance index [RDI]: 8.8 ± 5.3 [mean ± standard error]), 15 to 30 mg of temazepam did not significantly increase the RDI or alter the degree of oxyhemoglobin desaturation compared with placebo.[57] In a group of patients with mild chronic obstructive pulmonary disease, no significant increase in the group average RDI was observed after 0.25 mg of triazolam.[58] The investigators were careful to note that individual patients met their criteria for worsened sleep-disordered breathing after administration of this agent.[58]

Because of the small populations evaluated in published investigations, as well as the conflicting results of these studies, the safety of benzodiazepine administration to patients with OSAHS remains uncertain and the issue continues to be debated.[59] In usual hypnotic doses, benzodiazepines may not present a substantial risk for evoking OSAHS in some otherwise normal individuals. In view of the inconclusive data regarding the margin of safety, it is prudent to avoid this class of agents in patients who have been diagnosed with OSAHS and those with risk factors for this disorder.

Narcotics and Anesthetics

There have been anecdotal reports of clinically significant upper airway obstruction developing after administration of intravenous narcotics.[60-62] Healthy subjects failed to demonstrate a change in breathing during sleep after *oral* administration of hydromorphone hydrochloride, in 2- and 4-mg doses.[63] It may not be valid to extrapolate these results to the administration of higher doses of narcotics or giving them to patients who have, or are at risk for upper airway dysfunction during sleep. It is prudent to withhold, or at least minimize narcotics given to patients with OSAHS or those with risk factors for this disorder. There are instances when humane medical

practice requires analgesia, such as in the postoperative setting or during some procedures (e.g., bronchoscopy or colonoscopy). If nonnarcotic or nonventilatory depressant agents cannot provide adequate pain control, and if the risk is deemed clinically acceptable, minimal doses of narcotics should be administered with careful monitoring. An experienced airway management team should be available to reestablish upper airway patency emergently if the need arises. Patients who are already on nasal CPAP for OSAHS should use this therapy in the postoperative/periprocedure period. They may have increased pressure requirements in the presence of narcotics and after general anesthesia. The latter can also promote upper airway instability by selectively reducing the innervation to the upper airway dilator muscles.[64] If patients have not previously required aggressive intervention for OSAHS, nasal CPAP therapy at appropriate levels, empirically determined if necessary, should be considered until there is no longer a need for drugs with the potential to destabilize the upper airway.

Barbiturates

There have been no systematic assessments of the impact of barbiturates on upper airway function during sleep. Like alcohol, this class of agents selectively reduces the neural output through the hypoglossal nerve, reduces the tone of the upper airway dilator muscles, and predisposes to upper airway occlusion during sleep.[65,66] It is prudent to avoid barbiturates in patients who are predisposed to, or are known to have sleep-disordered breathing.

ENDOCRINE CONSIDERATIONS

Hypothyroidism

The physiologic relationship between thyroid function and sleep-disordered breathing is addressed in Chapter 105. Although the magnitude of the clinical association between hypothyroidism and OSAHS is not clear, there are considerable data in support of the former condition reflecting a risk factor for the latter.[67-70]

Patients with OSAHS may benefit from thyroid replacement therapy with a reduction of apnea frequency.[69] On the basis of the data suggesting that this therapy improves upper airway function during sleep, clinicians should consider the possibility of hypothyroidism adversely affecting OSAHS. Hypothyroid patients (and their bed partners) should be specifically interviewed and examined to detect factors that raise the probability that OSAHS is present.

Although OSAHS may be reduced after initiation of thyroid replacement therapy, the degree of improvement may be insufficient to obviate the need for additional treatment.[69,71] It is important to repeat an objective assessment of breathing during sleep after restoration of the euthyroid state. Grunstein et al.[71] made the important observation that thyroid replacement therapy in patients with untreated OSAHS may precipitate cardiac complications attributable to ischemia in the setting of augmented metabolism and persistent nocturnal hypoxemia. For this reason, as well as the benefit of more rapid relief of OSAHS, the authors suggested treatment with nasal CPAP during thyroid replacement therapy. This recommendation could be extrapolated to include successful oral appliance therapy. This strategy appears prudent until objective reassessment is performed when the patient is clinically and chemically euthyroid and further management decisions can be made based on the additional data.

The utility of screening unselected patients with OSAHS for hypothyroidism is controversial. Winkelman and coworkers[72] have reported a similar prevalence of chemical hypothyroidism in patients with OSAHS and individuals without OSAHS. These authors concluded that routine screening for thyroid dysfunction is not indicated in patients with OSAHS unless there are corroborating signs and symptoms. Concomitant hypothyroidism should be explored in patients with OSAHS on adequate therapy, who continue to report symptoms of fatigue and daytime sleepiness.

Estrogen and Progesterone

The effect of gender on OSAHS has been well defined, indicating a male-to-female ratio of 2:1 or 3:1.[73] The postmenopausal state increases the risk of OSAHS.[74,75] The exact mechanisms that confer this risk are incompletely understood, but appear to be in part due to estrogen and progesterone levels.[76] Recent reports have demonstrated that hormonal replacement therapy (HRT) has a favorable effect on the OSAHS.[74,75]

The current data indicate that HRT affects a number of organ systems, both favorably and unfavorably. The Heart and Estrogen/Progestin Replacement Study II (HERS II) and Women's Health Initiative (WHI) failed to demonstrate a favorable effect of HRT on cardiovascular risk.[77] In HERS II, there was a twofold risk of venous thromboembolism and a 50% increase in the rate of gallbladder disease that required surgery.[78] The estrogen/progestin arm of the WHI study was prematurely halted after 5.2 years of follow-up because of an increased risk of invasive breast cancer.[79] A recent U.S. Preventative Services Task Force scientific review concluded that HRT was not advisable in postmenopausal women for prevention of chronic conditions.[80]

Although a favorable effect of HRT on OSAHS has been demonstrated in postmenopausal women, the additional risks cited previously outweigh the potential benefit. Further research

may define subsets of patients and dosing regimens that are safe and effective. It is unlikely that this intervention would be robust enough to preclude the use of positive pressure in severe OSAHS.[76]

PHARMACOLOGIC INTERVENTIONS

Oxygen

In addition to sleep fragmentation, many of the clinically and physiologically evident consequences of OSAHS are attributable to nocturnal hypoxemia. Prevention of hypoxemia is a worthwhile therapeutic goal in patients with OSAHS. Several older studies reported that administration of supplemental oxygen to patients with OSAHS may significantly increase apnea duration with associated hypercapnia and respiratory acidosis.[81-83] Martin et al.[83] observed an initial prolongation of apnea duration in a group of eucapnic patients with OSAHS in conjunction with a significant reduction in apnea frequency. There was no change in the mean apnea duration after 30 minutes of oxygen administration compared with a period of room air breathing. This resulted in decreased apnea time and maintenance of satisfactory oxyhemoglobin saturation over the study period (Fig. 88–2). The bradycardia that accompanied apnea was eliminated by supplemental oxygen administration. Gold and coworkers[84] subsequently reported that supplemental oxygen administration was associated with a statistically, but probably not clinically significant reduction of apnea frequency, particularly during NREM sleep, as well as improved oxyhemoglobin saturation. Apnea duration increased slightly by an average of 4 to 7 seconds across the study group. There was no improvement in subjective or objective measures of daytime sleepiness during the period of nocturnal oxygen supplementation.

The evidence suggests that, in and of itself, providing supplemental oxygen during sleep is not sufficiently effective in reducing apnea frequency and increasing daytime alertness to stand alone as therapy for most patients. There may be a population of individuals who are asymptomatic with regard to the consequences of sleep fragmentation (i.e., hypersomnolence) or

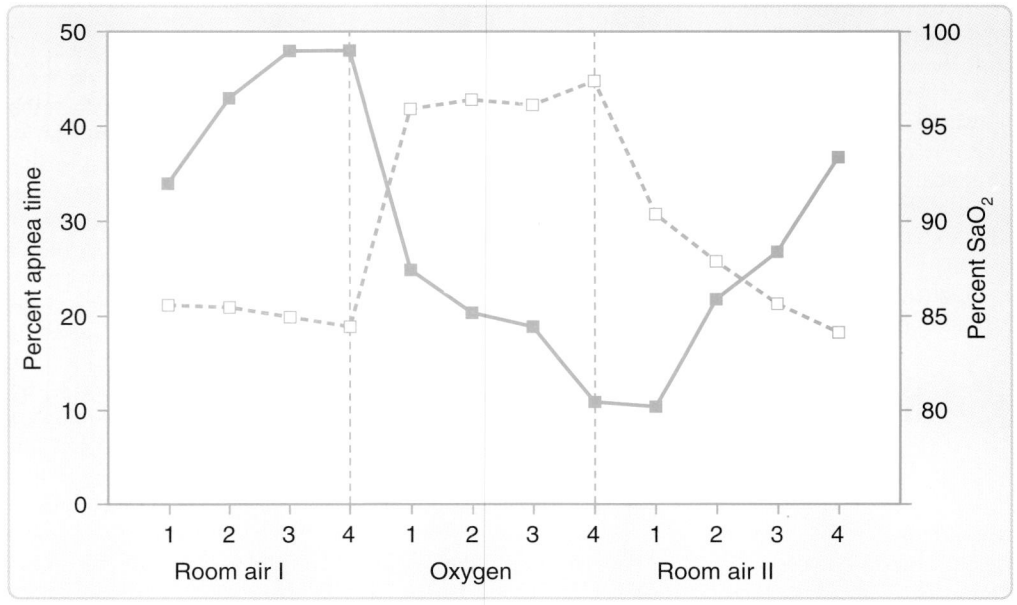

Figure 88–2. Mean percent apnea time for eight patients (*closed squares, solid line*) and the average nadir of oxyhemoglobin saturation per apnea (*open squares, dashed line*) for each 7.5-minute interval during the three study conditions (Room Air I, Oxygen, Room Air II). (Redrawn from Martin RJ, et al: Acute and long-term ventilatory effects of hyperoxia in the adult sleep apnea syndrome. Am Rev Respir Dis 1982;125:175-180.)

have a minimal frequency of OSAHS events, but who experience unacceptable oxyhemoglobin desaturation during sleep. In these patients, increasing nocturnal oxyhemoglobin saturation may be the major if not the only therapeutic goal.[85] The degree and duration of oxyhemoglobin desaturation that is ultimately harmful remains to be determined.[86] Patients with coronary artery disease or cerebrovascular disease and only a marginally elevated frequency of abnormal breathing events during sleep, with unacceptable oxyhemoglobin desaturation during those events, might benefit from supplemental oxygen.[87,88] Outcome studies are clearly needed to determine at what level of desaturation there is cost–benefit justification for providing oxygen therapy. Consideration should be given to performing initial trials of oxygen therapy during attended monitoring. This may be particularly important in patients with concomitant hypercapnia during wakefulness.[89] Such monitoring is also necessary to determine the flow of supplemental oxygen required for maintenance of acceptable oxyhemoglobin saturation.

In addition to providing sole therapy in selected patients with OSAHS, oxygen may be a useful adjunct to positive airway pressure (CPAP or bilevel positive pressure).[90] Patients with OSAHS who are sufficiently hypoxemic or borderline hypoxemic during wakefulness to warrant supplemental oxygen therapy usually meet the criteria for this therapy during sleep, even if positive airway pressure treatment maintains upper airway patency.[91] It should be determined if persistent desaturation on CPAP is related to hypoventilation resulting from the high mechanical impedance to expiration or increased dead space–tidal volume ratio that may be associated with this modality.[92] Bilevel positive pressure may permit sufficient reduction of expiratory pressure to avoid significant hypoventilation and desaturation and obviate the need for supplemental oxygen.

Transtracheal Oxygen Delivery

Several studies have described the impact of transtracheal oxygen administration to patients with OSAHS.[93,94] The data are too limited to provide substantive insight into the clinical utility of this mode of oxygen delivery, or to determine if it provides meaningful benefit over less invasive methods of oxygen delivery. If the transtracheal route of oxygen delivery is effective and superior to nasal cannulae in reducing OSAHS, it could be the result of stimulation of flow- or temperature-sensitive receptors in the upper airway. Large, well-designed studies are necessary to evaluate the role of this intervention. The frequency and severity of complications resulting from transtracheal oxygen therapy in a predominantly obese patient population have not been well characterized. Availability of this information is essential before this therapeutic modality could be accepted. At present, transtracheal oxygen should be considered investigational in the treatment of patients with OSAHS.

Psychotrophic Agents (Anxiolytics and Hypnotics)

Protriptyline

The tricyclic antidepressant protriptyline may reduce OSAHS by reducing the duration of REM sleep[95] and by increasing the tone of the upper airway dilator muscles[96] with increased hypoglossal and recurrent laryngeal nerve activity. Protriptyline may alter the distribution of obstructive apneas and hypopneas, with a decreased frequency of the former and increased frequency of the latter.[97] The clinical significance of converting obstructive apneas to hypopneas is not clear because both may result in arousals, autonomic nervous system activation, and potentially deleterious cardiovascular impact. Although protriptyline administration may result in a statistically significant reduction in sleep-disordered breathing events in study populations, breathing and oxygenation during sleep generally remain abnormal.[98]

Patients with OSAHS receiving protriptyline report subjective improvement in daytime sleepiness despite a persistently elevated arousal frequency.[95] This has led to speculation that this agent has specific "alerting" properties, over and above any effect on breathing. This has clinical relevance in that changes in symptoms after initiation of protriptyline therapy cannot be used as a reflection of physiologic changes in breathing during sleep, and objective assessment is required to evaluate therapeutic impact.

Protriptyline has a number of side effects, primarily related to its anticholinergic properties, that further limit its utility.[95,99] Side effects vary in severity and may limit use. They include dry mouth, urinary hesitancy, constipation, confusion, and ataxia. No significant cardiac dysrhythmias were observed at the dosages used (up to 30 mg daily).

Because of its lack of clinically significant therapeutic impact and potentially troublesome side effects, protriptyline is not considered to be a standard intervention in the treatment of OSAHS.

Serotonin Uptake Inhibitors

Several studies have suggested that serotonin may mediate both upper airway dilator muscle and diaphragm activity.[98,100] It has been further postulated that the reduction in upper airway dilator muscle tone, particularly during REM sleep, is due to withdrawal of serotonin-related excitatory input to the hypoglossal motor neurons.[101] If these postulates are true, it could have substantial implications for the treatment of patients with OSAHS.

Buspirone is a clinically available anxiolytic agent, the mechanism of action of which is believed to be at least partly mediated through serotonin receptors in the central nervous system.[102,103] Several animal studies have suggested that administration of buspirone augments ventilation during wakefulness and sleep and enhances ventilatory responsiveness to carbon dioxide.[102,103] In addition, the apneic threshold for carbon dioxide is reduced by an average of 3.7 mm Hg.

These data suggest that as a class of agents, serotonin agonists may have a therapeutic role in OSAHS. Although in theory, buspirone has characteristics that may provide therapeutic benefit in OSAHS, there are insufficient data on which to base judgments regarding its safety or efficacy. Other serotonin agonists have been evaluated to limited degrees. After administration of 20 mg/day of fluoxetine, one study found a statistically significant reduction in the apnea plus hypopnea frequency, from 57 ± 9 to 34 ± 6 (mean $\pm$ SE), although there was wide intersubject variability and there was no significant impact on the arousal frequency.[98] Fluoxetine increased sleep latency independent of its effect on sleep-disordered breathing, and reduced the percentage of REM sleep. Although these results are disappointing, knowledge regarding the relationship between the serotoninergic system, sleep, and breathing is continuing to evolve. There is reason to be hopeful that further knowledge of the relevant receptors will result in more effective interventions.[104,105]

A discussion of OSAHS therapy using serotonin-related agents would be incomplete without mention and caution with regard to L-tryptophan. Several studies were published in the 1980s that reported the impact of L-tryptophan in the treatment of OSAHS.[106] The evidence for consistent, clinically significant amelioration of OSAHS was at best arguable. It was subsequently observed that L-tryptophan has an unacceptable safety profile and should not be used because of its association with development of the eosinophilia-myalgia syndrome.[107]

Use of Medications to Promote Wakefulness

There are a number of potential reasons why a patient with OSAHS, who is thought to be on adequate treatment to reverse upper airway dysfunction and maintain acceptable oxyhemoglobin saturation as well as sleep continuity, may still complain of disturbing diurnal sleepiness or lack of alertness. Mean sleep latency improves during CPAP therapy, but in many cases does not return to clearly normal values.[108] The clinician must consider the possibility of noncompliance with a volitional treatment regimen (e.g., CPAP, oral appliances, body position modification), an inadequate prescription (e.g., CPAP level or mandibular advancement), changing external factors (e.g., weight gain, medications, sleep hygiene, shift work, other medical/psychiatric disorders), or a nonpulmonary sleep–wake disorder, to name a few. Even after these issues have been addressed, some patients remain unacceptably and perhaps dangerously sleepy or inattentive.

Recent animal data have demonstrated that long-term intermittent hypoxia (LTIH) can result in oxidative injury to the sleep–wake regions of the brain.[109] After the withdrawal of LTIH, objective sleepiness persisted, supporting the notion that sleepiness associated with sleep apnea may not be completely reversible.

Historically, amphetamines have been the class of agents used as stimulants. Unfortunately, this group of drugs has considerable potential for harmful cardiovascular consequences as well as adverse psychiatric and sleep effects. Modafinil is an agent that is thought to be a central alpha$_1$-adrenergic agonist with possible dopaminergic properties.[110] Limited studies have suggested that modafinil increases daytime alertness and vigilance and memory performance without significant side effects in patients without and with OSAHS.[110,111] There was no change in the apnea-hypopnea index or the nadir of oxyhemoglobin saturation on modafinil in patients with OSAHS.

Modafinil has recently been approved by the U.S. Food and Drug Administration for the treatment of residual sleepiness in OSAHS adequately treated with positive pressure by mask. Pack et al.[112] have shown in a 4-week, randomized, double-blinded, placebo-controlled, parallel-group study that there was significant improvement in daytime sleepiness on modafinil compared with placebo in patients with OSAHS who were objectively adherent to CPAP therapy. There was no decrease in CPAP use in the modafinil versus the placebo group at the 4-week end point. In a subsequent 12-week open-label study involving 125 patients, improvements in

subjective daytime sleepiness and sleep-related functional status were maintained.[113] There was a statistically significant decrease in CPAP use from 6.3 ± 1.3 hours per night at baseline to 5.9 ± 1.4 hours per night at the 12-week point, suggesting that modafinil may adversely affect adherence to CPAP. The most common side effects were headache (28%), anxiety (16%), and nervousness (14%).

Prescription of stimulants without a diagnostic evaluation risks masking important persistent and significant sleep-related pathologic processes that may have a negative impact on the quality and duration of the patient's life, independent of the issue of daytime sleepiness.[87,88,114-118] Careful follow-up with objective assessment of adherence to positive-pressure therapy should be pursued in patients treated with stimulants.

MECHANICAL THERAPY

Nasal Dilators

Elevated nasal resistance may promote upper airway closure during sleep.[119,120] Although the therapeutic benefit remains somewhat controversial, approximately 10% of patients with snoring and apnea have been reported to improve after administration of mucosal vasoconstrictors.[121] A variety of devices have recently become available that mechanically dilate the anterior nasal valve to reduce nasal airway resistance and putatively decrease the propensity toward OSAHS.

In one of the few studies to assess objectively the impact of nasal dilation on sleep, breathing, and oxygenation, Hoijer et al.[122] assessed the impact of an external nasal dilator in 10 snorers, 7 of whom had an apnea index in excess of 5. Although the average apnea index fell from 18 to 6.4 and the minimum oxyhemoglobin saturation also improved while asleep with the nasal dilator, the saturation remained severely reduced in those individuals with more severe baseline desaturation. Snoring intensity was reduced, although there was no subjective effect of the nasal dilator on arousal frequency or daytime sleepiness after 10 nights of use. Neither the hypopnea index nor objectively measured arousal frequency were reported in this study, and it is possible that neither the apnea-hypopnea index nor arousal index was favorably affected by the nasal dilator. It is also noteworthy that only four patients expressed a desire to continue to use the nasal dilator. In contrast, Hoffstein et al.[123] concluded that dilation of the anterior nasal valve using an external dilator has no impact on sleep-disordered breathing, nadir of desaturation, and mean oxyhemoglobin saturation, although a reduction in snoring intensity was noted. As the authors indicated, it is possible that their results may have been biased by the absence of a randomized treatment order. This possibility is highlighted by the fact that there was a greater percentage of REM sleep during the period in which the nasal dilator was applied and the recognition that OSAHS severity may worsen as the night progresses.

Using an intranasally applied dilator, Scharf et al.[124] reported that a significant proportion of 20 participants had improved Stanford Sleepiness Scale scores, morning concentration, and subjective quality of sleep, as well as reduced sleepiness on awakening and number of awakenings. Using a numeric scale, there was no difference in subjective sleep depth, refreshing quality of sleep, morning sleepiness, sleep quality, number of awakenings, and other subjective parameters. A significant number of bed partners reported decreased snoring loudness but no change in snoring regularity. Unfortunately, there was no objective assessment of sleep and breathing, either at study entry or with the nasal dilator. In another study, cyclic alternating pattern sequences in nonapneic snorers were reduced during use of an intranasally applied dilator, suggesting improved sleep continuity.[125]

The existing literature suggests that these devices may offer some benefit for selected patients, but most studies have notable deficiencies. It is evident that more objective, controlled, and well-designed studies must be done before any conclusions can be reached regarding the utility of nasal dilators for OSAHS.

Nasopharyngeal Airway

Although the concept of nasopharyngeal intubation to maintain upper airway patency during sleep was originally reported in the literature in the 1970s,[126] there have been relatively few reports describing its use.[127,128]

Nasopharyngeal intubation has limited therapeutic utility. A substantial proportion of patients do not tolerate this intervention and, of those who do, only approximately two thirds may have a clinically significant improvement in sleep-disordered breathing as defined by a reduction in disordered breathing event frequency of 65%, or an apnea index less than 5 *and* an apnea-hypopnea index less than 10.[128] Some of these patients continued to experience notable oxyhemoglobin desaturation, and there was no major improvement in sleep quality and architecture. Thus, the limited available data suggest that there is substantial patient intolerance of this form of therapy and many of the apparent "responders" still have a noteworthy degree of sleep-disordered breathing as well as persistently abnormal sleep quality and architecture. In selected patients, especially those in whom other, usually more successful noninvasive therapies have failed, a trial of this modality may be considered. Alternating nostrils in which the nasopharyngeal airway is placed, in conjunction with adequate lubrication (avoiding substances that may cause lipoid pneumonia), may improve acceptance.

Upper Airway Stimulation

Phasic activity of the upper airway dilators during inspiration is increased during wakefulness in patients with OSAHS compared with control subjects.[129] This is consistent with ongoing physiologic compensation for compromised upper airway patency. This compensatory augmentation may be diminished during sleep and, consequently, upper airway dilator muscle tone becomes insufficient to overcome those factors promoting airway occlusion. It is reasonable to speculate that external augmentation of upper airway dilator muscle activity will enhance luminal patency during periods when these occlusive forces are operative and natural compensatory mechanisms are reduced.

Attempts to stimulate the upper airway dilator muscles using transcutaneous submental or transhyoid electrodes as well as intraoral electrodes have met with either disappointing results or concern regarding the possible impact of unintentional patient arousal.[130] In contrast, promising results have been obtained using direct intramuscular genioglossal or hypoglossal stimulation. Unilateral electrical stimulation of those branches of the hypoglossal nerve supplying the genioglossus muscle reduces (i.e., makes more negative) the

upper airway critical closing pressure or increases maximal inspiratory airflow in feline and canine models.[131,132] Schwartz et al.[133] applied direct electrical stimulation to the genioglossus muscle in several patients with OSAHS. The electrical stimulus is triggered by the development of negative intrapharyngeal or esophageal pressure, consistent with the onset of inspiration. In a small number of patients, this reduced the number of inspiratory flow-limited breaths by approximately 50%, as well as the apnea-hypopnea index. Electrical stimulation did not appear to induce arousal because there was no change in the electroencephalogram immediately after the stimulus train compared with the period immediately before application of the stimulus, nor was there a difference in the heart rate across the periods before, during, or after stimulation. In a small group of patients with OSAHS with inspiratory airflow limitation, unilateral hypoglossal nerve stimulation using electrodes applied directly either to the main hypoglossal nerve trunk or specifically to those branches innervating the genioglossus muscle increased maximal inspiratory airflow.[134,135] Stimulation significantly improved the apnea-hypopnea index and the oxyhemoglobin desaturations (Figs. 88–3 and 88–4).

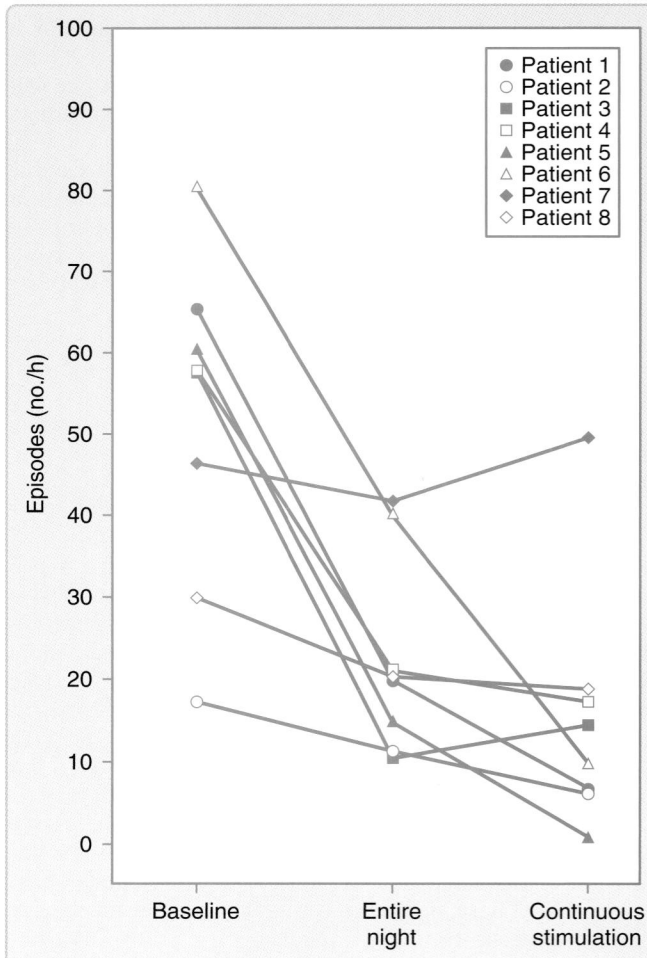

Figure 88–3. Non–rapid eye movement sleep apnea-hypopnea indexes at baseline versus mean data (months 1, 3, and 6) for the entire night versus mean data (months 1, 3, and 6) for continuous stimulation. (Redrawn from Schwartz AR, et al: Therapeutic electrical stimulation of the hypoglossal nerve in obstructive sleep apnea. Arch Otolaryngol Head Neck Surg 2001;127:1216-1223.)

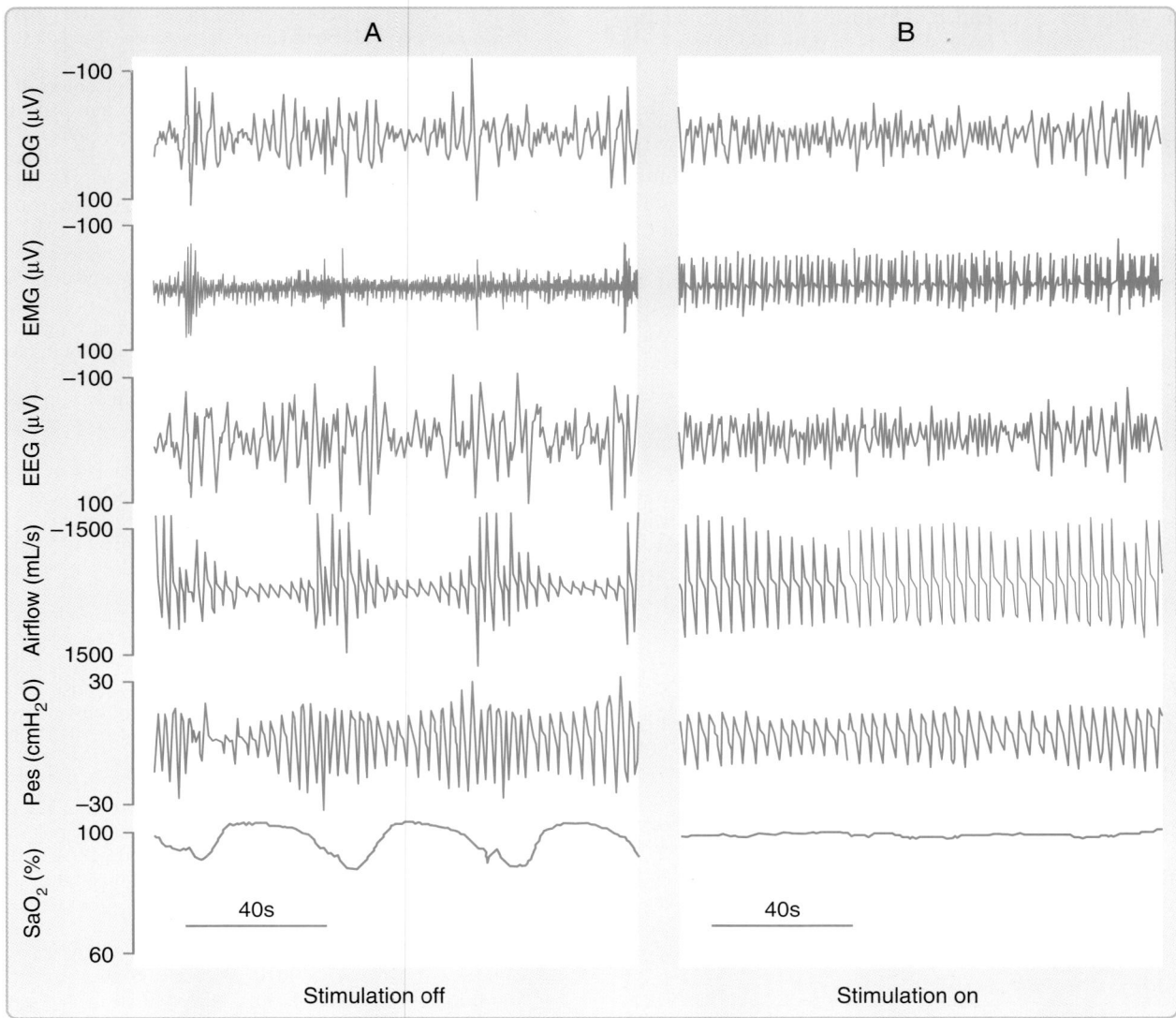

Figure 88–4. A, Breathing pattern during non–rapid eye movement (NREM) sleep with hypoglossal stimulation off. **B,** Breathing pattern during NREM sleep with hypoglossal stimulation on. EOG, electrooculogram; EMG, electromyogram; EEG, C3–A2 electroencephalogram; P_{es}, esophageal pressure; SaO_2, oxyhemoglobin saturation. (Redrawn from Schwartz AR, et al: Therapeutic electrical stimulation of the hypoglossal nerve in obstructive sleep apnea. Arch Otolaryngol Head Neck Surg 2001;127:1216-1223.)

A trend toward deeper stages of NREM sleep was observed. Only three of eight patients remained free from stimulator malfunction at 6 months.

The results of hypoglossal nerve stimulation are encouraging but require confirmation in larger studies. The data suggesting that stimulation does not precipitate arousal are of particular importance, but whether this remains the case in patients after the initial treatment period and reduction of sleep pressure requires confirmation. The limited available data suggest that electrical stimulation improves, but may not eliminate OSAHS. If the impact of this intervention is incomplete, it may be related to the unilateral stimulation technique (one would be reluctant to implant bilateral electrodes owing to concern regarding potential bilateral nerve trauma), the importance of other, unstimulated upper airway muscles, or factors related to upper airway lateral wall instability. A durable and reliable system is needed.[131] Technical issues related to

electrode breakage and malfunction need to be solved before considering hypoglossal nerve stimulation as alternative therapy to positive pressure. Electrical stimulation techniques reflect one of the most exciting new prospects in the treatment of patients with OSAHS.

PITFALLS AND CONTROVERSIES

The chronic care of the patient with OSAHS frequently includes medical interventions other than positive pressure applied by mask or oral appliance therapy. Behavioral interventions involving avoidance of sleep deprivation, fitness, smoking cessation, and reduction of alcohol consumption should be pursued, when appropriate, in all patients. Lifestyle interventions can clearly augment overall management of OSAHS. Recent data have demonstrated that adequate treatment with CPAP does not result in weight loss. Specific therapy addressing weight loss must be provided.[17] Instituting behavioral change is difficult. Avoiding discussions regarding lifestyle change ensures lack of success.

HRT can have a favorable impact on OSAHS, although the effect is modest.[76] The current evidence indicates that the benefit of chronic HRT for the purpose of improving OSAHS is outweighed by the potential risk of other medical complications.[80,136,137] It is unknown whether alternate preparations or dosing regimens will favorably modify these significant medical risks.

Recent experiments using a murine model support the notion that residual daytime sleepiness may persist despite adequate control of sleep-disordered breathing.[109] Wake-promoting agents have been shown to improve daytime sleepiness in patients adequately treated with CPAP.[112] There may be a temptation to treat sleepiness in patients with OSAHS who lack adequate adherence to positive pressure or refuse CPAP or bilevel therapy.[138,139] The long-term impact on other important physiologic consequences (i.e., cardiovascular risk and the metabolic syndrome) of treatment with wake-promoting agents is unknown, and their use may mask a symptom that could motivate the patient to adhere to positive-pressure therapy.

Clinical Pearls

Treatment of OSAHS in elderly patients can be challenging. If the patient is intolerant of positive-pressure therapy, treatment options are frequently limited. Oral appliance therapy may be compromised by the lack an adequate number of teeth. One possible approach is to combine oxygen by nasal cannula with head of bed elevation.[37,38,140] Although somewhat expensive, head of bed elevation with a hospital bed is usually well tolerated. Oxygen by nasal cannula is frequently easier to accept than positive pressure by mask. Objective assessment of the response to therapy is advisable.

Acknowledgment

Supported in part by National Heart, Lung, and Blood Institute Training Grant #5T32HL07563-07.

References

1. Koenig JS, Thach BT: Effects of mass loading on the upper airway. J Appl Physiol 1988;64:2294-2299.
2. Wolin AD, Strohl KP, Acree BN, Fouke JM: Responses to negative pressure surrounding the neck in anesthetized animals. J Appl Physiol 1990;68:154-160.
3. Winter WC, Gampper T, Gay SB, Suratt PM: Lateral pharyngeal fat pad pressure during breathing. Sleep 1996;19:S178-S179.
4. Katz I, Stradling J, Slutsky AS, et al: Do patients with obstructive sleep apnea have thick necks? Am Rev Respir Dis 1990;141:1228-1231.
5. Davies RJO, Stradling JR: The relationship between neck circumference, radiographic pharyngeal anatomy, and obstructive sleep apnoea syndrome. Eur Respir J 1990;3:509-514.
6. Hoffstein V, Mateika S: Differences in abdominal and neck circumferences in patients with and without obstructive sleep apnoea. Eur Respir J 1992;5:377-381.
7. Hoffstein V, Mateika S: Predicting nasal continuous positive airway pressure. Am J Respir Crit Care Med 1994;150:486-488.
8. Ryan CF, Love LL: Mechanical properties of the velopharynx in obese patients with obstructive sleep apnea. Am J Respir Crit Care Med 1996;154:806-812.
9. Schwab RJ, Gupta KB, Hoffman EA, et al: Differences in upper airway soft tissue anatomy in normal subjects and patients with sleep-disordered breathing. Am Rev Respir Dis 1993;147:A947.
10. Schwab RJ: Diagnostic imaging in the diagnostic evaluation of the upper airway. In Rose B, Weinberger S (eds): UpToDate in Pulmonary and Critical Care Medicine. New York, American Thoracic Society, 1997.
11. Winter WC, Gampper T, Gay SB, Suratt PM: Enlargement of the lateral pharyngeal fat pad space in pigs increases upper airway resistance. J Appl Physiol 1995;79:726-731.
12. Harman EM, Wynne JW, Block AJ: The effect of weight loss on sleep-disordered breathing and oxygen desaturation in morbidly obese men. Chest 1982;82:291-294.
13. Smith PL, Gold AR, Meyers DA, et al: Weight loss in mildly to moderately obese patients with obstructive sleep apnea. Ann Intern Med 1983; 103:850-855.
14. Suratt PM, McTier RF, Findley LJ, et al: Changes in breathing and the pharynx after weight loss in obstructive sleep apnea. Chest 1987;92:631-637.
15. Schwartz AR, Gold AR, Schubert N, et al: Effect of weight loss on upper airway collapsibility in obstructive sleep apnea. Am Rev Respir Dis 1991;144:494-498.
16. Sugarman HJ, Fairman RP, Sood RK: Long-term effects of gastric surgery for treating respiratory insufficiency of obesity. Am J Clin Nutr 1992;55: 597S-601S.
17. Kajaste S, Brander PE, Telakivi T, et al: A cognitive-behavioral weight reduction program in the treatment of obstructive sleep apnea syndrome with or without initial nasal CPAP: A randomized study. Sleep Med 2004;5:125-131.
18. Buchwald H, Avidor Y, Braunwald, E, et al: Bariatric surgery: A systematic review and meta-analysis. JAMA 2004;292:1724-1737.
19. O'Keeffe T, Patterson EJ: Evidence supporting routine polysomnography before bariatric surgery. Obes Surg 2004;14: 23-26.
20. Frey WC, Pilcher J: Obstructive sleep-related breathing disorders in patients evaluated for bariatric surgery. Obes Surg 2003; 13:676-683.
21. Fernandez AZ Jr, DeMaria EJ, Tichansky DS, et al: Experience with over 3,000 open and laparoscopic bariatric procedures: Multivariate analysis of factors related to leak and resultant mortality. Surg Endosc 2004;18:193-197.
22. Perugini RA, Mason R, Czerniach DR, et al: Predictors of complication and suboptimal weight loss after laparoscopic Roux-en-Y gastric bypass: A series of 188 patients. Arch Surg 2003; 138:541-545.
23. Phillips B, Danner F: Cigarette smoking and sleep disturbance. Arch Intern Med 1995;155:734-737.
24. Wetter DW, et al: Smoking as a risk factor for sleep-disordered breathing. Arch Intern Med 1994;154:2219-2224.
25. Gothe B, Strohl KP, Cherniack NS: Nicotine: A different approach to treatment of obstructive sleep apnea. Chest 1985;87:11-17.
26. Davila DG, Hurt RD, Offord KP, et al: Acute effects of transdermal nicotine on sleep architecture, snoring, and sleep-disordered breathing in nonsmokers. Am J Respir Crit Care Med 1994; 150:469-474.
27. Bonnet MH, Arand DL: We are chronically sleep deprived. Sleep 1995;18:908-911.
28. Schiffman PL, Trontell MC, Mazar MF, Edelman NH: Sleep deprivation decreases ventilatory response to CO_2 but not load compensation. Chest 1983;84: 695-698.
29. White DP, Douglas NJ, Pickett CK, et al: Sleep deprivation and the control of ventilation. Am Rev Respir Dis 1983;128: 984-986.
30. Guilleminault C, Rosekind M: The arousal threshold: Sleep deprivation, sleep fragmentation, and obstructive sleep apnea syndrome. Bull Eur Pathophysiol Respir 1981;17:341-349.

31. Bowes G, Woolf GM, Sullivan CE, Phillipson EA: Effect of sleep fragmentation on ventilatory and arousal responses of sleeping dogs to respiratory stimuli. Am Rev Respir Dis 1980;122:899-908.

32. Sériès F, Cormier Y, La Forge J, Desmeules M: Mechanisms of the effectiveness of continuous positive airway pressure in obstructive sleep apnea. Sleep 1992; 15:S47-S49.

33. Cartwright RD, Lloyd S, Lilie J, Kravitz H: Sleep position training as treatment for sleep apnea syndrome: A preliminary study. Sleep 1985;8:87-94.

34. Phillips BA, Okeson J, Paesani D, Gilmore R: Effect of sleep position on sleep apnea and parafunctional activity. Chest 1986;90:424-429.

35. George CF, Millar TW, Kryger MH: Sleep apnea and body position during sleep. Sleep 1988;11:90-99.

36. Cartwright RD: Effect of sleep position on sleep apnea severity. Sleep 1984;7:110-114.

37. McEvoy RD, Sharp DJ, Thornton AT: The effects of posture on obstructive sleep apnea. Am Rev Respir Dis 1986;133:662-666.

38. Neill AM, Angus SM, Sajkov D, McEvoy RD: Effects of sleep posture on upper airway stability in patients with obstructive sleep apnea. Am J Respir Crit Care Med 1997;155:199-204.

39. Issa FG, Sullivan CE: Reversal of central sleep apnea using nasal CPAP. Chest 1986;90:165-171.

40. Sanders MH, Rogers RM, Pennock BE: Prolonged expiratory phase in sleep apnea: A unifying hypothesis. Am Rev Respir Dis 1985;131:401-408.

41. Badr MS, Toiber F, Skatrud JB, Dempsey J: Pharyngeal narrowing/occlusion during central sleep apnea. J Appl Physiol 1995;78:1806-1815.

42. Morrell MJ, et al: The assessment of upper airway patency during apnea using cardiogenic oscillations in the airflow signal. Sleep 1995;18:651-658.

43. Sanders MH: Nasal CPAP effect on patterns of sleep apnea. Chest 1984;86:839-844.

44. Issa FG, Sullivan CE: Alcohol, snoring and sleep apnea. J Neurol Neurosurg Psychiatry 1982;45:353-359.

45. Scrima L, Broudy M, Nay KN, Cohn MA: Increased severity of obstructive sleep apnea after bedtime alcohol ingestion: Diagnostic potential and proposed mechanism of action. Sleep 1982;5:318-328.

46. Taasan VC, Block AJ, Boysen PG, Wynne JW: Alcohol increases sleep apnea and oxygen desaturation in asymptomatic men. Am J Med 1981;71:240-245.

47. Gleeson K, Zwillich CW, White DP: The influence of increasing ventilatory effort on arousal from sleep. Am Rev Respir Dis 1990;142:295-300.

48. Berry RB, Bonnet MH, Light RW: Effect of ethanol on the arousal response to airway occlusion during sleep in normal subjects. Am Rev Respir Dis 1992;145:445-452.

49. Roehrs T, Beare D, Zorick F, Roth T: Sleepiness and ethanol effects on simulated driving. Alcohol Clin Exp Res 1994;18:154-158.

50. Berry RT, Desa MM, Light RW: Effect of ethanol on the efficacy of nasal continuous positive airway pressure as a treatment of obstructive sleep apnea. Chest 1991;99:339-343.

51. Mitler MM, Dawson A, Henriksen SJ, et al: Bedtime ethanol increases resistance of upper airways and produces sleep apneas in asymptomatic snorers. Alcohol Clin Exp Res 1988;12:801-805.

52. Teschler H, Berthon-Jones M, Wessendorf T, et al: Influence of moderate alcohol consumption on obstructive sleep apnoea with and without AutoSet™ nasal CPAP therapy. Eur Respir J 1996;9:2371-2377.

53. Dolly FR, Block AJ: Effect of flurazepam on sleep-disordered breathing and nocturnal desaturation in asymptomatic subjects. Am J Med 1982;73:239-243.

54. Mendelson WB, Garnett D, Gillin JC: Flurazepam-induced sleep apnea syndrome in a patient with insomnia and mild sleep-related respiratory changes. J Nerv Ment Dis 1981;160:261-264.

55. Guilleminault C, Silvestri R, Mondini S, Coburn S: Aging and sleep apnea: Action of benzodiazepine, acetazolamide, alcohol and sleep deprivation in a healthy elderly group. J Gerontol 1984;39:655-661.

56. Guilleminault C, Cummiskey J, Silvestri R: Benzodiazepines and respiration during sleep. In Usdin E, Skolnick P, Tallman JF, et al. (eds): Pharmacology of Benzodiazepines, pp 229-236. London, Macmillan, 1982.

57. Camacho ME, Morin CM: The effect of temazepam on respiration in elderly insomniacs with mild sleep apnea. Sleep 1995;18:644-645.

58. Steens RD, et al: Effects of zolpidem and triazolam on sleep and respiration in mild to moderate chronic obstructive pulmonary disease. Sleep 1993;16:318-326.

59. Hanly P, Powles P: Hypnotics should never be used in patients with sleep apnea. J Psychosom Res 1993;37(Suppl 1):59-65.

60. Rafferty TD, Ruskis A, Sasaki C, Gee JB: Perioperative considerations in the management of tracheostomy for the obstructive sleep apnea patient. Br J Anaesth 1980;52:619-621.

61. Cately DM, Thornton C, Jordan C, et al: Pronounced episodic oxygen desaturation in the postoperative period: Its association with ventilatory pattern and analgesic regimen. Anesthesiology 1985;63:20-28.

62. Boushra NN: Anesthetic management of patients with sleep apnea syndrome. Can J Anaesth 1996;43:599-616.

63. Robinson RW, Zwillich CW, Bixler EO, et al: Effects of oral narcotics on sleep-disordered breathing in healthy adults. Chest 1987;91:197-203.

64. Nishino T, Shirahata M, Yonezawa T, Honda Y: Comparison of changes in the hypoglossal and phrenic nerve activity in response to increasing depth of anesthesia in cats. Anesthesiology 1984;60:19-24.

65. Brouillette RT, Thach BT: A neuromuscular mechanism maintaining extrathoracic airway patency. J Appl Physiol 1979;46:772-779.

66. Drummond GB: Influence of thiopentone on upper airway muscles. Br J Anaesth 1989;63:212-221.

67. Skatrud J, Iber C, Ewart R, et al: Disordered breathing during sleep in hypothyroidism. Am Rev Respir Dis 1981;124:325-329.

68. Orr WC, Males JL, Imes NK: Myxedema and obstructive sleep apnea. Am J Med 1981;70:1061-1066.

69. Rajagopal KR, Abbrecht PH, Derderian SS, et al: Obstructive sleep apnea in hypothyroidism. Ann Intern Med 1984;101:491-494.

70. Pelttari L, Rauhala E, Polo O, et al: Upper airway obstruction in hypothyroidism. J Intern Med 1995;236:177-181.

71. Grunstein RR, Sullivan CE: Sleep apnea and hypothyroidism: Mechanisms and management. Am J Med 1988;85:775-779.

72. Winkelman JW, Goldman H, Piscatelli N, et al: Are thyroid function tests necessary in patients with suspected sleep apnea? Sleep 1996;19:790-793.

73. Jordan AS, McEvoy RD: Gender differences in sleep apnea: Epidemiology, clinical presentation and pathogenic mechanisms [see comment]. Sleep Med Rev 2003;7:377-389.

74. Bixler EO, Vgontzas AN, Lin HM, et al: Prevalence of sleep-disordered breathing in women: Effects of gender [see comment]. Am J Respir Crit Care Med 2001;163:608-613.

75. Shahar E, Redline S, Young T, et al: Hormone replacement therapy and sleep-disordered breathing [see comment]. Am J Respir Crit Care Med 2003;167:1186-1192.

76. White DP: The hormone replacement dilemma for the pulmonologist [comment]. Am J Respir Crit Care Med 2003;167:1165-1166.

77. Paoletti R, Wenger NK: Review of the International Position Paper on Women's Health and Menopause: A comprehensive approach. Circulation 2003;107:1336-1339.

78. Grady D, Herrington D, Bittner V, et al: Cardiovascular disease outcomes during 6.8 years of hormone therapy: Heart and Estrogen/progestin Replacement Study follow-up (HERS II). JAMA 2002;288:49-57.

79. Rossouw JE, Anderson GL, Prentice RL, et al: Risks and benefits of estrogen plus progestin in healthy postmenopausal women: principal results From the Women's Health Initiative randomized controlled trial. JAMA 2002;288:321-333.

80. Nelson HD, Humphrey LL, Nygren P, et al: Postmenopausal hormone replacement therapy: Scientific review. JAMA 2002; 288:872-881.

81. Motta J, Guilleminault C: Effects of oxygen administration in sleep-induced apneas. In Guilleminault C, Dement WC (eds): Sleep Apnea Syndromes, pp 137-144. New York, Alan R. Liss, 1978.

82. Kimoff RJ, Cheong TH, Olha AE, et al: Mechanisms of apnea termination in obstructive sleep apnea: Role of chemoreceptor and mechanoreceptor stimuli. Am J Respir Crit Care Med 1994;149:707-714.

83. Martin RJ, Sanders MH, Gray BA, Pennock BE: Acute and long-term ventilatory effects of hyperoxia in the adult sleep apnea syndrome. Am Rev Respir Dis 1982;125:175-180.

84. Gold AR, Schwartz AR, Bleecker ER, Smith PL: The effect of chronic nocturnal oxygen administration upon sleep apnea. Am Rev Respir Dis 1986;134:925-929.

85. Strollo PJ Jr: Indications for treatment of obstructive sleep apnea in adults. Clin Chest Med 2003;24:307-313.

86. Sanders MH, Rogers RM: Sleep apnea: When does better become benefit? Chest 1985;88:320-321.

87. Hanly P, Sasson Z, Zuberi N, Lunn K: ST-segment depression during sleep in obstructive sleep apnea. Am J Cardiol 1993; 71:1341-1345.

88. Franklin KA, Nilsson JB, Sahlin C, Naslund U: Sleep apnoea and nocturnal angina. Lancet 1995;345:1085-1087.

89. Krieger J, Weitzenblum E, Monassier JP, et al: Dangerous hypoxaemia during continuous positive airway pressure treatment of obstructive sleep apnoea. Lancet 1983;2:1429-1430.

90. Sanders MH, Kern N: Obstructive sleep apnea treated by independently adjusted inspiratory and expiratory positive airway pressures via nasal mask: Physiologic and clinical implications. Chest 1990;98:317-324.

91. Piper AJ, Sullivan CE: Effects of short-term NIPPV in the treatment of patients with severe obstructive sleep apnea and hypercapnia. Chest 1994;105:434-440.

92. Martin T, Sanders M, Atwood C: Correlation between changes in $PaCO_2$ and CPAP in obstructive sleep apnea (OSA) patients. Am Rev Respir Dis 1993;147:A681.

93. Chauncey JB, Aldrich MS: Preliminary findings in the treatment of obstructive sleep apnea with transtracheal oxygen. Sleep 1990;13:167-174.

94. Farney RJ, Walker JM, Elmer JC, et al: Transtracheal oxygen, nasal CPAP and nasal oxygen in five patients with obstructive sleep apnea. Chest 1992;101:1228-1235.

95. Brownell LG, West P, Sweatman P, et al: Protriptyline in obstructive sleep apnea: A double blind trial. N Engl J Med 1982;307: 1037-1042.

96. Bonora M, St. John WM, Bledsoe TA: Differential elevation by protriptyline and depression by diazepam of upper airway respiratory muscle activity. Am Rev Respir Dis 1985;131:41-45.

97. Smith PL, Haponik EF, Allen RP, Bleecker ER: The effects of protriptyline in sleep-disordered breathing. Am Rev Respir Dis 1983;127:8-13.

98. Hanzel DA, Proia NG, Hudgel DW: Response of obstructive sleep apnea to fluoxetine and protriptyline. Chest 1991;100: 416-421.

99. Conway WA, Zorick F, Piccione P, Roth T: Protriptyline in the treatment of sleep apnoea. Thorax 1982;37:49-53.

100. Richmonds C, Hudgel DW: Hypoglossal and phrenic motoneuron responses to serotoninergic active agents in rats. Respir Physiol 1996;106:153-160.

101. Veasy SC, Panckeri KA, Hofman EA, et al: The effects of serotonin antagonists in an animal model of sleep-disordered breathing. Am J Respir Crit Care Med 1996;153:776-786.

102. Mendelson WB, Martin JV, Rapoport DM: Effects of buspirone on sleep and respiration. Am Rev Respir Dis 1990;141: 1527-1530.

103. Garner SJ, Eldridge FL, Wagner PG, Dowell T: Buspirone, an anxiolytic drug that stimulates respiration. Am Rev Respir Dis 1989;139:946-950.

104. Horner RL: The neuropharmacology of upper airway motor control in the awake and asleep states: Implications for obstructive sleep apnoea. Respir Res 2001;2:286-294.

105. Veasey SC: Pharmacotherapies for obstructive sleep apnea: How close are we? Curr Opin Pulm Med 2001;7:399-403.

106. Schmidt HS: Combined L-tryptophan and protriptyline in the treatment of obstructive sleep apnea. Sleep Res 1985; 14:209.

107. Hertzman PA, Blevins WL, Mayer J, et al: Association of the eosinophilia-myalgia syndrome with the ingestion of tryptophan. N Engl J Med 1990;322:869-873.

108. Engleman HM, Martin SE, Deary IJ, Douglas NJ: Effect of continuous positive airway pressure treatment on daytime function in sleep apnoea/hypopnoea syndrome. Lancet 1994;343: 572-575.

109. Veasey SC, Davis CW, Fenik P, et al: Long-term intermittent hypoxia in mice: Protracted hypersomnolence with oxidative injury to sleep-wake brain regions. Sleep 2004;27:194-201.

110. Lyons TJ, French J: Modafinil: The unique properties of a new stimulant. Aviat Space Environ Med 1991;62:432-435.

111. Arnulf I, et al: Modafinil in obstructive sleep apnea-hypopnea syndrome: A pilot study in 6 patients. Respiration 1997;64: 159-161.

112. Pack AI, Black JE, Schwartz JR, Matheson JK: Modafinil as adjunct therapy for daytime sleepiness in obstructive sleep apnea. Am J Respir Crit Care Med 2001;164:1675-1681.

113. Schwartz JR, Hirshkowitz M, Erman MK, Schmidt-Nowara W: Modafinil as adjunct therapy for daytime sleepiness in obstructive sleep apnea: A 12-week, open-label study. Chest 2003;124:2192-2199.

114. Bradley TD, Rutherford R, Grossman RF, et al: Role of daytime hypoxemia in the pathogenesis of right heart failure in the obstructive sleep apnea syndrome. Am Rev Respir Dis 1985;131:835-839.

115. Fletcher EC: The relationship between systemic hypertension and obstructive sleep apnea: Facts and theory. Am J Med 1995; 98:118-128.

116. Guilleminault C, Connolly S, Winkle RA: Cardiac arrhythmia and conduction disturbances during sleep in 400 patients with sleep apnea syndrome. Am J Cardiol 1983;52:490-494.

117. Hla KM, Young TB, Bidwell T, et al: Sleep apnea and hypertension. Ann Intern Med 1994;120:382-388.

118. Zwillich C, Devlin T, White D, et al: Bradycardia during sleep apnea: Characteristics and mechanism. J Clin Invest 1982;69: 1286-1292.

119. Suratt PM, Turner BL, Wilhoit SC: Effect of intranasal obstruction on breathing during sleep. Chest 1986;90:324-329.

120. Lavie P, Fischel N, Zomer J, Eliaschar I: The effects of partial and complete mechanical occlusion of the nasal passages on sleep architecture and breathing during sleep. Acta Otolaryngol 1983;95:161-166.

121. Fairbanks DNF, Fairbanks DW: Obstructive sleep apnea: Therapeutic alternatives. Am J Otolaryngol 1992;13:265-270.

122. Hoijer U, Ejnell H, Hedner J, et al: The effects of nasal dilation on snoring and obstructive sleep apnea. Arch Otolaryngol Head Neck Surg 1992;118:281-284.

123. Hoffstein V, Mateika S, Metes A: Effect of nasal dilation on snoring and apneas during different stages of sleep. Sleep 1993;16:360-365.

124. Scharf MB, Brannen DE, McDonnold M: A subjective evaluation of a nasal dilator on sleep and snoring. Ear Nose Throat J 1994;73:395-401.

125. Scharf MB, McDonnold MD, Zaretsky NT, et al: Cyclic alternating pattern sequences in non-apneic snorers with and without nasal dilation. Ear Nose Throat J 1996;75:617-619.

126. Kravath RE, Pollack CP, Borowiecki B: Hypoventilation during sleep in children who have lymphoid airway obstruction treated by nasopharyngeal tube and tonsillectomy and adenoidectomy. Pediatrics 1977;59:865-871.

127. Afzelius L-E, Elmqvist D, Hougaard K, et al: Sleep apnea syndrome: An alternative treatment to tracheostomy. Laryngoscope 1981;91:285-291.

128. Nahmias JS, Karetzky MS: Treatment of the obstructive sleep apnea syndrome using a nasopharyngeal tube. Chest 1988;94: 1142-1147.

129. Mezzanotte WS, Tangel DJ, White DP: Influence of sleep onset on upper airway muscle activity in apnea patients versus normal controls. Am J Respir Crit Care Med 1996;153:1880-1887.

130. Guilleminault C, Powell N, Bowman B, Stoohs R: The effect of electrical stimulation on obstructive sleep apnea. Chest 1995;107:67-73.

131. Goding GS, Eisele DW, Testerman R, et al: Relief of upper airway obstruction with hypoglossal nerve stimulation in the canine. Laryngoscope 1998;108:162-169.

132. Schwartz AR, Thut DC, Russ B, et al: Effect of electrical stimulation of the hypoglossal nerve on airflow mechanics in the isolated upper airway. Am Rev Respir Dis 1993;147:1144-1150.

133. Schwartz AR, Eisele DW, Hari A, et al: Electrical stimulation of the lingual musculature in obstructive sleep apnea. J Appl Physiol 1996;81:643-652.

134. Schwartz AR, Bennett ML, Smith PL, et al: Therapeutic electrical stimulation of the hypoglossal nerve in obstructive sleep apnea. Arch Otolaryngol Head Neck Surg 2001;127: 1216-1223.

135. Eisele DW, Smith PL, Alam DS, Schwartz AR: Direct hypoglossal nerve stimulation in obstructive sleep apnea. Arch Otolaryngol Head Neck Surg 1997;123:57-61.

136. Nelson HD: Assessing benefits and harms of hormone replacement therapy: Clinical applications. JAMA 2002;288: 882-884.

137. Miller J, Chan BK, Nelson HD: Postmenopausal estrogen replacement and risk for venous thromboembolism: A systematic review and meta-analysis for the U.S. Preventive Services Task Force. Ann Intern Med 2002;136:680-690.

138. Black J: Pro: Modafinil has a role in management of sleep apnea. Am J Respir Crit Care Med 2003;167:105-106; discussion 108.

139. Pollak CP: Con: Modafinil has no role in management of sleep apnea. Am J Respir Crit Care Med 2003;167:106-107; discussion 107-108.

140. Landsberg R, Friedman M, Ascher-Landsberg J: Treatment of hypoxemia in obstructive sleep apnea. Am J Rhinol 2001; 15:311-313.

Continuous Positive Airway Pressure Treatment for Obstructive Sleep Apnea–Hypopnea Syndrome

Ronald Grunstein

ABSTRACT

Nasal continuous positive airway pressure (CPAP) is the treatment of choice for moderate to severe obstructive sleep apnea–hypopnea syndrome. At an appropriately set pressure, CPAP is almost always effective for this syndrome. The main limitations to CPAP usage are lack of patient acceptance and lack of tolerance of treatment. Newer modalities of CPAP, such as autotitrating CPAP, have been advocated to avoid complex sleep laboratory investigation and to maximize CPAP usage. More research is required before this viewpoint can be fully supported.

Nasally applied continuous positive airway pressure (CPAP) is now the established treatment for obstructive sleep apnea–hypopnea syndrome (OSAHS) and for some forms of central apnea. Studies have provided information on different aspects of the usage, compliance, and efficacy of CPAP therapy. In this chapter, these data are summarized, with an emphasis on the practical use of CPAP therapy in clinical management of patients with OSAHS.

Nasal CPAP therapy for sleep apnea was first described in 1981,[1] but it was not until about 1985 that it began to be recognized as a realistic form of long-term therapy in other centers. Although patients needed to use an adhesive to attach the mask, the prompt relief of sleepiness led to an increasing number of users. By 1985, over 100 patients were using this therapy on a regular basis.[2] Subsequently, technical improvements were made in the design of the masks and pressure delivery systems. Over the past 10 years, the evidence supporting the use of CPAP has improved both in quantity and quality, driven by the demands of government funding authorities and health maintenance organizations and by the availability of industry sponsorship with the increasing commercial success of the CPAP equipment.[3]

Nevertheless, studies to assess and validate a mechanical device such as CPAP are more difficult to design than the studies required for pharmaceutical registration or approval. Performing true double-blind, randomized, controlled trials of CPAP treatment or variants is problematic. "Sham CPAP" by its nature has less efficacy on unavoidably observable variables such as snoring and apnea, with consequent frustration of efforts to blind the study participants. It is also quite difficult to effectively blind a CPAP therapist or doctor involved in such studies compared with pharmaceutical trials involving placebo medications. The most recent phase in CPAP development has been the advent of automatically titrating CPAP devices, which have major implications for the delivery of health care to patients with sleep apnea, and for the traditional relationship between sleep laboratory and patient. It is important to ensure that use of all new devices for routine CPAP treatment is driven by evidence, not by marketing.

Currently, nasal CPAP is the gold standard of treatment for moderate to severe OSAHS. However, many patients do not use it, or they use it irregularly. Comparative, intention-to-treat trials involving all degrees of severity of OSAHS are needed to delineate treatment pathways. These studies, which will focus on comparative treatments and how to obtain better acceptance of and compliance with CPAP, will form the next phase in the development of this treatment. A viable pharmacologic therapy for sleep apnea[4] does not appear to be in the foreseeable future.

NASAL CONTINUOUS POSITIVE AIRWAY PRESSURE

Mode of Action

The original experiments with CPAP followed from the concept that closure of the oropharynx results from an imbalance of the forces[5] that normally keep the upper airway open (see Chapter 82). In the first description of CPAP use for treatment of OSAHS in 1981,[1] it was suggested that nasal CPAP acts as a pneumatic splint to prevent collapse of the pharyngeal airway, and that it does this by elevating the pressure in the oropharyngeal airway and reversing the transmural pressure gradient across the pharyngeal airway (Fig. 89–1). This notion

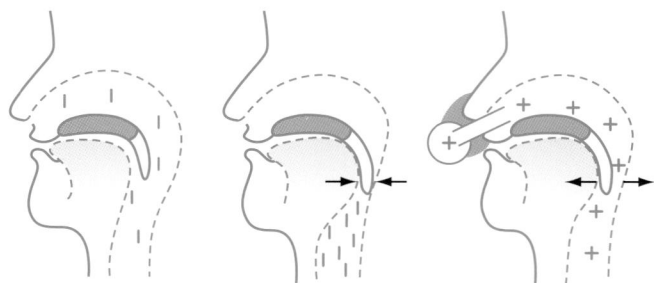

Figure 89–1. Mechanism of upper airway occlusion and its prevention by nasal continuous positive airway pressure (CPAP). When the patient is awake *(left)*, muscle tone prevents collapse of the upper airway during inspiration. During sleep, the tongue and soft palate are sucked against the posterior oropharyngeal wall *(middle)*. CPAP with low pressure provides a pneumatic splint and keeps the upper airway open *(right)*. (Adapted from Sullivan CE, Issa FG, Bethon-Jones M, et al: Reversal of obstructive sleep apnea by continuous positive airway pressure applied through the nares. Lancet 1981;1:862-865.)

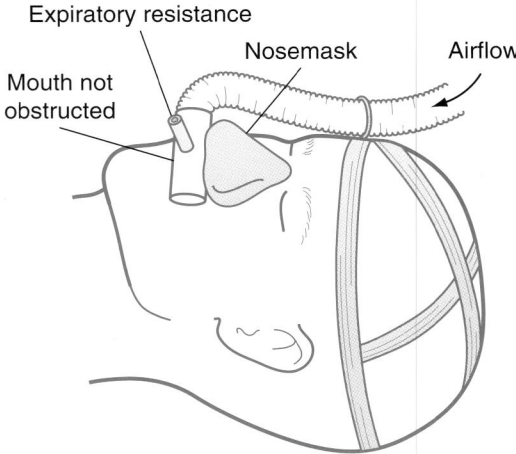

Figure 89–2. Diagram of method of applying continuous positive airway pressure by nose mask. (From Sullivan CE, Issa FG, Berthon-Jones M, et al: Home treatment of obstructive sleep apnea with continuous positive airway pressure applied through a nosemask. Bull Eur Physiopathol Respir 1984;20:49-54.)

has been confirmed by a number of studies that either demonstrated the "pneumatic splint" by endoscopic or other imaging or showed that CPAP does *not* increase upper airway muscle activity by reflex mechanisms.[6] Detailed magnetic resonance imaging has confirmed that CPAP increases airway volume and airway area and reduces lateral pharyngeal wall thickness and the upper airway edema that result from chronic vibration and occlusion of the airway.[7]

The apparatus providing the pressure at the nasal airway must have the capacity to maintain any given pressure during inspiration (Fig. 89–2). The simplest CPAP systems involve an air blower with sufficient pressure-flow characteristics to provide CPAP via a fixed resistive leak in the system (typically adjacent to the mask).

CPAP and Central Apnea

Regardless of the mechanism, nasal CPAP has been documented to be effective in eliminating both mixed and obstructive apneas.[8] Some central apneas, particularly those observed in patients with predominantly obstructive events, are also eliminated by nasal CPAP (Fig. 89–3).[8] Clearly, some central apneas are associated with increased upper airway resistance and it could be argued that it is better to consider apnea classification as being CPAP responsive or CPAP nonresponsive. CPAP is also effective in central apneas associated with cardiac failure (see later).

PRACTICAL ASPECTS OF TREATMENT

Currently, most patients commence CPAP under supervision, usually in a hospital-based sleep laboratory. The purposes of the supervision are to ensure that the patient is appropriately educated about the therapy, to determine the adequacy of CPAP through the night, and to evaluate immediate acceptance or problems with the therapy. Economic pressures within health systems, however, are challenging this approach and moving in the direction of less intensive staffing or even home commencement of CPAP.

Regardless of the location or method of CPAP titration, there is a need for proper patient assessment (to determine, e.g., whether the patient has awake respiratory failure or marked hypoxemia in sleep), and this requires specific physician training and experience. There is no evidence for the safety and efficacy of CPAP titration outside of a medically supervised process.[9] Current evidence supports the use of trained technologists to provide patient education, technical aspects of titration, and follow-up. However, recent data from small patient groups has challenged the notion of close medical supervision, and this should become a major research focus.[10] The dominant determinants of CPAP usage are patient understanding of the therapy, its impact on symptoms, and close professional support, regardless of mask type, CPAP manufacturer, and mode of delivery.

The First Night

Sleeping with a nose mask and feeling the pressure sensation of CPAP, although not necessarily uncomfortable, are novel experiences for the patient. Physician explanation, video programs, and mask acclimation sessions prior to beginning

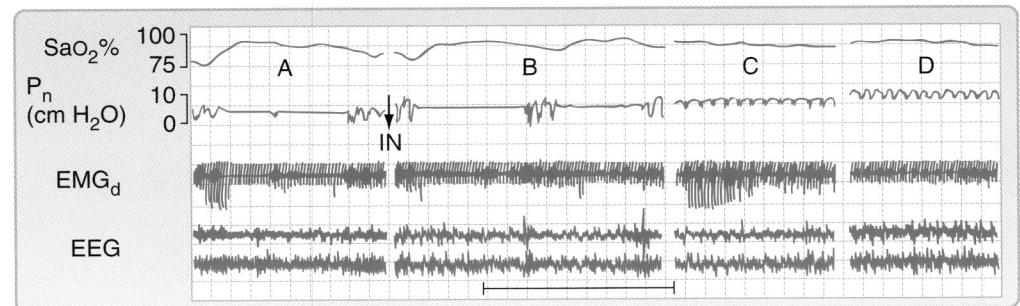

Figure 89–3. Polygraphic records demonstrating prevention of central sleep apnea by continuous positive airway pressure (CPAP) applied through the nose. **A,** Note the presence of central apnea at a nasal CPAP of 2 cm H_2O. **B,** Elevation of nasal CPAP to 6.6 cm H_2O changes the apnea from a central to a mixed type. Further increase of nasal CPAP to 10 cm H_2O (not shown) leads to a change in the apnea pattern from a mixed to an obstructive apnea. **C,** Loud, continuous snoring occurs when the nasal CPAP is elevated to 11.5 cm H_2O. **D,** Finally, at a nasal CPAP of 14.5 cm H_2O, the patient breathes with an open airway. EEG, electroencephalogram; EMG_d, diaphragm electromyogram; IN, inspiration; P_n, nasal pressure; SaO_2, arterial oxyhemoglobin saturation (scale, 100% to 75%); time scale is in seconds. Patient is in the supine position. (Adapted from Issa FG, Sullivan CE: Reversal of central sleep apnea using nasal CPAP. Chest 1986;90:165-171.)

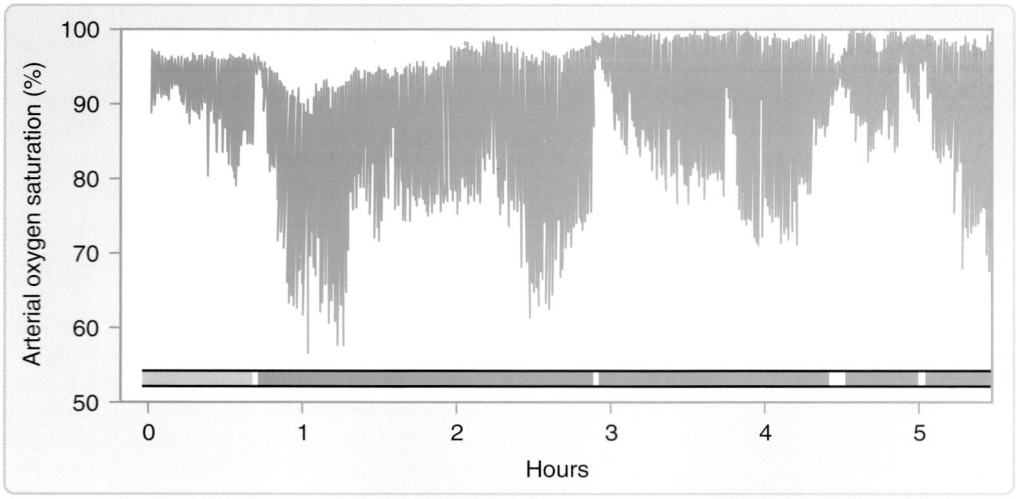

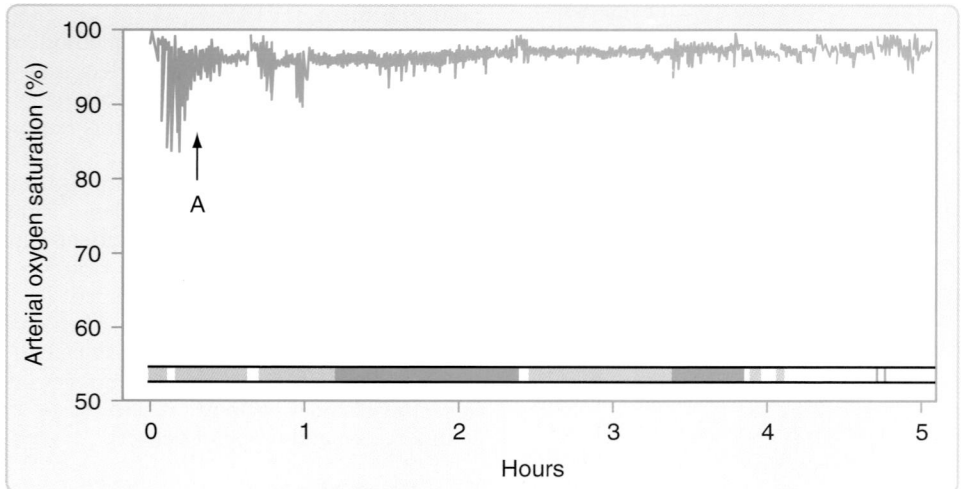

Figure 89–4. All-night recordings of arterial hemoglobin saturation in one of the earliest patients to use home continuous positive airway pressure (CPAP). **Top,** Control night. **Bottom,** CPAP trial night. *Light blue bar,* non–rapid eye movement (NREM) sleep; *dark blue bar,* rapid eye movement (REM) sleep; *open bar,* awake. A CPAP of 7 cm H_2O was applied at *arrow A* and continued for the rest of the night. (Adapted from Sullivan CE, Issa FG, Berthon-Jones M, et al: Reversal of obstructive sleep apnea by continuous positive airway pressure applied through the nares. Lancet 1981;1:862-865.)

CPAP are routine in many centers. Education about CPAP reduces patient anxiety and improves acceptance. Current evidence provides support for the benefit of more intensive patient education in CPAP usage.[9]

On the first night of treatment, it is important to ensure that the pressure level that is identified as being most therapeutically effective is sufficient to prevent not only apnea and oxyhemoglobin desaturation but also respiratory-related arousals in all sleep stages and in all postures of sleep (Fig. 89–4). *Thus, simple apnea prevention is not the endpoint of CPAP titration.* It must be ensured that the airflow pressure tracing is normal and not "chopped off," to avoid residual partial airway obstruction (Fig. 89–5).[3] It is important to correct this flow limitation, as it may indicate residual upper airway obstruction, potentially causing arousal.[11] Studies have emphasized the importance of proper airflow measurement in CPAP titration using pressure-flow transducers rather than

thermistors or other more indirect airflow measures.[12] Proper airflow measurement can help determine the optimal pressure level by providing insights regarding the etiology of arousals—for example, whether they are related to respiratory events (respiratory-related arousals) and whether increasing pressure has a beneficial effect on sleep continuity. Although acute (1-night) studies suggest that flow limitation correction may be the preferred endpoint of CPAP titration, long-term data are sparse.[13]

When the correct pressure level is reached and the airway is open, sleep should no longer be fragmented by repetitive arousals, but there is often "rebound" slow wave and rapid eye movement (REM) sleep (Fig. 89–6).[14] This rebound phase of recovery from severe sleep fragmentation lasts about a week; the duration and intensity of these rebound sleep episodes decrease quickly after the first night of treatment.[14] However, the improvement in sleep architecture is usually

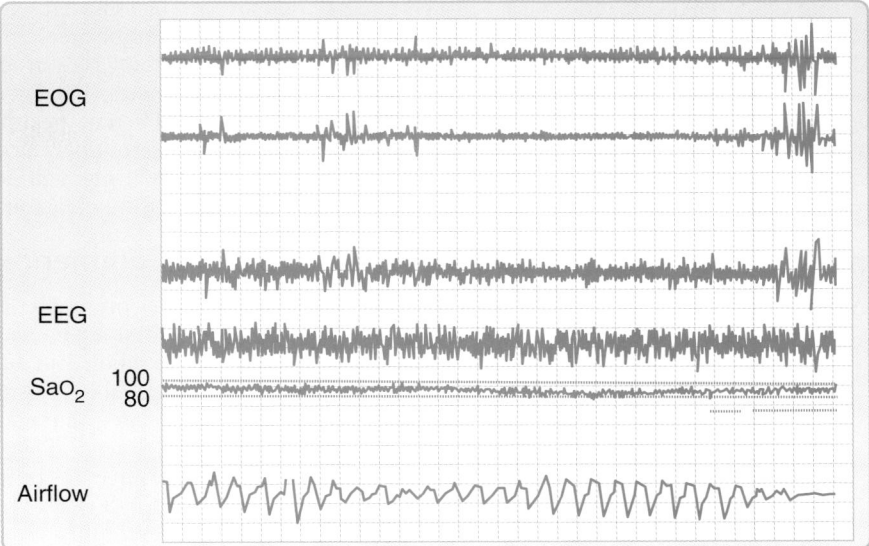

Figure 89–5. Two-minute tracing of rapid eye movement (REM) sleep in a patient exhibiting persisting upper airway flow limitation. The second part of the flow tracing demonstrates "chopped-off" airflow.

immediate and can be used as a sign of an effective pressure level. Continued frequent arousals may indicate that a critical level of upper airway resistance persists, especially if associated with flow limitation. Continued snoring is another sign of inadequate CPAP pressure.

Other data demonstrate that hysteresis exists in the relationship between CPAP and upper airway resistance. In other words, to eliminate inspiratory flow limitation, higher pressures are required during upward titration of CPAP than with downward titration from higher pressures.[15] This means that patients with OSAHS may actually normalize their breathing during sleep at a lower pressure level if manual or automatic titration involves both upward titration till airflow is sinusoidal in shape and downward titration till obstructed events recur. This may be an important concept in patients with complications of CPAP caused by higher pressure levels, such as mask or mouth leak, or when an autotitrating CPAP

(auto-CPAP) does not allow for this up-and-down titration approach.

Considering the length of time CPAP has been used to treat patients with sleep apnea, the published data on the variability in CPAP pressure with posture or sleep stage are surprisingly limited. Some evidence exists for higher pressure requirements with the supine posture[16] and in REM sleep.[17]

It appears that a pressure level accurately set on one night is generally effective on subsequent nights.[18] Early work and clinical experience suggested that this was the case, but the use of auto-CPAP technology in the home has provided the research to support this view.[19] For patients who respond immediately to CPAP but then report continued daytime sleepiness on home treatment, it may be appropriate to empirically increase CPAP pressure, assuming that the laboratory study underestimated the pressure requirement. However, this has not been specifically studied. Other factors may have

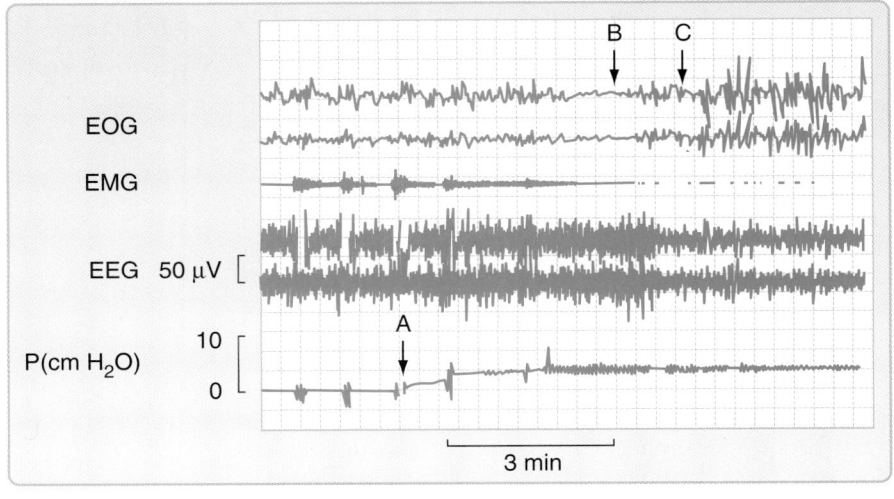

Figure 89–6. Recordings demonstrating the rapid onset of rapid eye movement (REM) sleep soon after obstructive apnea was prevented by nasal continuous positive airway pressure (CPAP). Note that the onset of each episode of obstructive apnea *(left side)* is accompanied by fadeout on the electromyogram (EMG). Apneas were prevented when nasal CPAP was increased *(arrow A)*. Note the fadeout of postural EMG activity *(arrow B)* preceding the changes in electroencephalogram (EEG) and electrooculogram (EOG) characteristic of REM sleep *(arrow C)*. P, nasal airway pressure. (From Sullivan CE, Issa FG, Berthon-Jones M, et al: Pathophysiology of sleep apnea. In Saunders NA, Sullivan CE [eds]: Sleep and Breathing. New York, Marcel Dekker, 1984, pp 299-364.)

an impact on the therapeutic efficacy of a given CPAP pressure in the home. Weight gain may lead to a need for a higher CPAP setting.[20] Heavy (but not moderate) alcohol consumption may affect CPAP pressure, presumably because alcohol depresses upper airway neuromuscular tone.[21] Nasal congestion or a different posture in the home may also lead to different pressure requirements, but this has not been well researched.

Treatment of Decompensated Patients with Cardiorespiratory Failure

Patients with carbon dioxide retention, heart failure, and extreme nocturnal hypoxemia (i.e., an arterial oxyhemoglobin saturation [SaO_2] of 50% or less) require close supervision when commencing CPAP. Such patients may have confusion at night, from delirium due to their blood gas derangement, that may be exacerbated by someone trying to attach a mask to their face. The nurse or technician must be aware that the patient may try to pull the mask off repeatedly throughout the night. After the first few nights, these patients typically settle down and sleep with the CPAP unit without the need for intensive nursing.

Previously, the therapy choice for these patients was intubation or urgent tracheostomy. Intubation may still be the appropriate option; however, in trained hands, nasally applied CPAP or noninvasive ventilation (see Chapter 95) will readily control the breathing disturbance during sleep. Many of these patients have both upper airway obstruction and hypoventilation, and nasal CPAP may not be adequate to normalize gas exchange.[22] Increasingly, the clinical approach in these patients is to employ bilevel positive airway pressure therapy. Auto-CPAP approaches are inappropriate in such patients. When possible, hospitalization would be the most reasonable approach in management of patients with severe CO_2 retention due to a hypoventilation syndrome or chronic lung disease until studies showing the safety of ambulatory approaches are available.

CPAP on the Night Sleep Apnea Is Diagnosed?—The Split-Night Study

It has been suggested that CPAP treatment can be initiated on the same night the diagnosis is established.[23,24] However, in these studies, patient selection was not randomized: "split-night" studies (with the first part of the night used for diagnosis and the second part for treatment) tended to be performed in patients with more severe disease who had been waiting a shorter time for CPAP titration. Other studies[31] have identified a subset of patients for whom a split-night study provided insufficient time for CPAP titration to achieve a satisfactory prescription. Patients with milder degrees of sleep-disordered breathing (i.e., with an apnea-hypopnea index less than 20) in whom the titration was initiated later in the night (because prolonged monitoring was required to establish a diagnosis) were more likely to have unsuccessful split-night titrations.

CPAP titration can potentially be accomplished during the day.[26] In this study, both daytime and nocturnal CPAP titration studies yielded sufficient amounts of REM and non-REM sleep to help determine CPAP settings. The diurnal and nocturnal CPAP titrations resulted in comparable therapeutic pressures, resolution of sleep-disordered breathing, and 1-week compliance. Split-night or day studies may appear attractive from a short-term, economic point of view in the United States, but data in larger numbers of unselected patients in different health systems are required before this approach is routinely accepted. It is possible that a combination of split-night titration and subsequent home autotitration may be an adequate strategy, but as yet this is speculative.

Commencement of CPAP at Home?

Theoretically, it may be economically advantageous to start CPAP at home and avoid a formal polysomnographic CPAP titration, but outcome studies showing true cost utility are not available. Current reviews and guidelines do not advocate home commencement of CPAP, particularly using autotitrating devices.[27] This is a controversial area, as it implies a major change in practice in sleep centers. One study observed poorer CPAP compliance in patients assessed only with respiratory monitoring[28] but this is not a universal finding.[29] Other workers have found reasonable utility with unattended in-hospital CPAP titration in patients with mild to moderate disease but not with severe OSAHS.[30] Other studies have suggested that equations can be determined that would allow an empirical pressure level to be set, potentially preventing the need for any investigation of CPAP efficacy.[31] Recent data in a small group of patients support this empirical method of home CPAP titration instead of laboratory initiation.[10] Again, long-term outcome data are lacking. The ongoing studies in several countries should provide clearer evidence-based guidelines for initiating CPAP.

PROBLEMS AND SIDE EFFECTS

Side effects reported by the patient are usually, but not exclusively, related to pressure or airflow or the mask–nose interface (Table 89–1). Side effects are important for CPAP usage, because patients who complain of side effects use CPAP less frequently than those without side effects.[32] A nonspecific sense of claustrophobia may be reported by patients, but this often involves either mask/interface problems, nasal congestion, or exhalation difficulties. Dangerous complications

Table 89–1. Side Effects of Nasal Continuous Positive Airway Pressure

Type of Problem	Side Effect
Nasal	Rhinorrhea
	Nasal congestion, oronasal dryness
	Epistaxis
Mask	Skin abrasion/rash
	Conjunctivitis from air leak
Flow-related	Chest discomfort
	Aerophagy
	Sinus discomfort
	Claustrophobia
	Difficulty exhaling
	Pneumothorax (very rare)
	Pneumoencephaly (very rare)
Noise	—
Partner intolerance	—
Inconvenience	—

of nasal CPAP therapy (e.g., pulmonary barotrauma, pneumocephalus, increased intraocular pressure, tympanic membrane rupture, massive epistaxis, and subcutaneous emphysema after facial trauma) are extremely rare and represent isolated case reports in the literature.[33] Caution should be used when implementing CPAP therapy after neurosurgery or facial surgery. Irritating side effects such as aerophagy and musculoskeletal chest discomfort (presumably related to increased lung volumes) have also been reported.[33]

Nasal Congestion

Nasal congestion is a common side effect of CPAP therapy.[33] Although most patients experience initial self-limiting nasal congestion, at least 10% complain of persistent nasal stuffiness to some degree after 6 months of therapy.[34] There appear to be many reasons for nasal symptoms. CPAP may provoke pressure-sensitive mucosal receptors, leading to vasodilation and mucus production. In some patients, it may unmask allergic rhinitis by restoring the nasal route of breathing after years of mouth breathing. In others, fixed nasal obstruction with polyps or a deviated septum may produce symptoms. Mouth leaks also cause increased nasal resistance, probably by exposing the nasal mucosa to higher flows and reduced relative humidity.[35]

Treatment of nasal congestion depends on the cause. Mouth leak may be minimized by ensuring that the correct CPAP pressure is used. Sometimes, it may be necessary to use a chin strap. These are often uncomfortable and acclimation to this device is often necessary. Heated, rather than cold, pass-over humidification is best suited to increase the relative humidity and may be used to treat nasal congestion.[35,36] Nasal congestion can be treated with antihistamines, topical steroids, or topical saline sprays, and humidification of the circuit will improve nasal dryness. Intranasal ipratropium bromide can be helpful in abating CPAP-induced rhinorrhea.

Patients with persistent symptoms of nasal congestion or those with obvious nasal obstruction should have nasopharyngoscopy performed and may require corrective surgery for an obstructive lesion such as a polyp, marked mucosal thickening, or deviated septum. There is some limited evidence of benefit in improving CPAP compliance.[37] Oral masks may also be of value in managing patients with nasal side effects.[38]

The Interface

Initially, masks were custom made, but in the mid-1980s, new forms of plastic self-sealing masks became more convenient to use. Mask technology has improved greatly, and this is important as mask comfort remains a pivotal influence on CPAP acceptance and compliance. Poorly fitting masks permit air leakage, and the resultant drop in pressure leads to persistent OSAHS and sleep fragmentation. The leak is usually the source of considerable discomfort; if it is directed toward the eye, it may cause conjunctivitis.[39] A potential problem with a poorly fitting mask is the development of bruising or even ulceration of the bridge of the nose.

Few studies compare different mask types despite the constant availability of new designs. Anecdotally, the newer generation of mask types appears to be associated with fewer mask-fit problems. Nevertheless, certain patients become claustrophobic when using nasal CPAP with any mask. Changing the interface prescription from a nasal mask to the less confining nasal prongs or "pillows" may correct that problem.

However, nasal prongs may cause irritation in the nares, and long-term use data are needed. Newer interfaces are constantly being developed to address mask problems, but for some patients, particularly younger patients with mild disease, aesthetic problems with CPAP, regardless of interface, preclude this treatment modality.

An infrequent but difficult problem is the patient who has no upper front teeth. The upper teeth provide the rigid structure against which the lower part of the mask can be pulled. If there is no dentition, the mask simply rolls around the top gums into the mouth, with loss of an adequate seal. The problem may be rectified by providing a denture[40] or possibly an oronasal mask.

Pressure Level and Airflow

Although the air pressure created by the CPAP apparatus is frequently mentioned as a problem, there is no convincing evidence that it actually impairs compliance (see "Autotitrating CPAP," later). Some patients complain of initial increased resistance to exhalation or the sensation of too much pressure in the nose. For these patients, a CPAP unit with a ramp feature may be worth considering. The ramp allows the pressure to increase to the optimal CPAP pressure gradually over a set time interval (usually 5 to 30 minutes). No studies have been performed to show that a ramp feature improves acceptance or compliance with CPAP; however, an interesting case of "ramp abuse" has been reported, in which continuous application of the ramp function by the patient led to undertreatment of sleep apnea.[41]

Alternatively, a bilevel positive airway pressure system, in which inspiratory positive airway pressure and expiratory positive airway pressure can be adjusted independently, may be used, as this approach lowers mean airway pressure and resistance to expiration. Again, it is not clear whether these approaches will improve compliance. Limited data indicate that use of bilevel devices does not affect the number of hours of use of positive pressure in patients with OSAHS. However, the same study showed a higher dropout rate.[42] It is the impression of some clinicians that bilevel pressure is more acceptable to patients with lung or chest wall diseases who also have OSAHS, but this has not been studied systematically. For such patients, CPAP may result in hyperinflation and a sensation of breathlessness, and they may complain of difficulty breathing out. More recently, a novel type of CPAP with modification of the expiratory pressure–time profile has become available, but there is no evidence of increased patient compliance using this modality.[43]

Patients occasionally find the air generated by the CPAP unit too warm or too cold. If moving the machine from the floor to a bedside table, heating the bedroom, or placing tubing under the blankets does not correct the problem, incorporating a heated humidifier into the circuit may help. Bed partners may also experience cold air on their bodies from the expiratory port of the device. Another complaint, also usually from the bed partner, is that the CPAP machine generates too much noise. Removing the machine from the bedside or placing it in a closet may remedy the problem. Extra tubing may be needed, and it is important to recheck pressures if nonstandard tubing is used. Noise or a changing level of noise may be a problem in some auto-CPAP devices because of the nature of their motors.

Comparison with Other Treatments

Compared with other treatments, one of the great advantages of nasal CPAP is that it is immediately and demonstrably effective in relieving OSAHS.[1,44] Another is that it can be offered on a trial basis and withdrawn if not tolerated, in contrast to surgical options. This is particularly important in milder cases of OSAHS, or where the contribution of OSAHS to the patient's symptomatology is unclear. A few studies have attempted to compare CPAP with other treatments for OSAHS using formal protocols. The conclusion of most of these studies is that CPAP is the appropriate therapy for patients with moderate to severe sleep apnea.[53-56]

COMPLIANCE

General Issues

Compliance is a term that, in medical use, refers to a patient-administered pharmacologic therapy. The word evolved in the context of clinical drug trials and implied one of the following: (1) adherence of patients to medical advice and prescriptions, (2) adherence of investigators to a protocol and related administrative responsibilities, and (3) adherence of sponsors to regulatory and other legal responsibilities.[47] In terms of mechanical therapies, compliance may be interpreted in different ways (see later). More accurate compliance measurements are possible with devices such as CPAP than with medications.

At least 40% to 50% of patients do not use oral medications and inhalers as prescribed. For example, despite efforts to enhance compliance, over 70% of patients with chronic obstructive lung disease in a clinical trial did not comply with their prescribed drug treatment. Moreover, 15% of the patients deliberately "dump" their medications in an effort to appear to be following the physician's orders.[48] In general, compliance is not associated with age, sex, educational level, economic status, or personality, or with the characteristics of a disease, including diagnosis or severity or frequency of symptoms. In general, physicians cannot predict which of their patients will be compliant. Therefore, it appears that compliance is not easily associated with any factor that might be used in everyday practice to make predictions about patients' behavior.[49]

Several factors are associated with improved compliance.[49] These include simplicity of the regimen, family support, the patient's perception that the disease is serious, a belief that the proposed therapy will be effective, patient understanding of the rationale of treatment, provision of accurate details of the treatment planned, and a close patient–clinician relationship, including close clinician supervision of therapy.

Compliance and CPAP

In assessing the long-term results of CPAP, a variety of words have been used to describe the patient–CPAP interaction. To a large extent, these terms describe different measures. *Acceptance* and *tolerance* are subjective terms used in early studies. More recent studies measure CPAP *usage* or *compliance* utilizing time meters or more sophisticated devices that measure both run-time and pressure delivery. True *efficacy* studies have yet to be performed, as they would need to measure total sleep time over a set period and compare this with CPAP usage and the actual number of respiratory events not prevented by CPAP. Nevertheless, when looking at all the CPAP usage data currently available, compliance with CPAP devices compares favorably with medication use. Terms that have been suggested to describe CPAP usage[3] are listed in Table 89–2. The criteria set for the terms may vary: for example, good compliance for one group may be 6 hours of CPAP, 6 nights per week, whereas for others, such criteria may be too strict.

Several factors can affect CPAP compliance, including machine cost, technical advances in equipment, and prescriber motivation. In some countries, machines are provided free of cost, whereas in others, the cost may vary between $1000 and $3000. This may lead to variable acceptance and prescription of the therapy. In addition, there have been rapid changes in CPAP technology. Current machines are quieter, with apparently more comfortable masks, and with a ramp facility to slowly increase the pressure over the first period of sleep. Many older CPAP usage studies employed equipment that has been replaced by newer devices, and compliance data need to be continually updated to verify whether these technical changes actually influence CPAP use or are merely cosmetic marketing ploys. This situation is analogous to clinical trials of new medications within the same drug class—for example, comparative studies of beta-blockers.

Unlike for inhalers,[48] CPAP "dumping" is not a major factor. If a CPAP mask is taken off the face, there is detectable drop in pressure. Thus, if patients simply switch on their machine and leave the mask on the floor, there is a major discrepancy between "machine-on" time and "mask-on-face" time. This is not the case, as simultaneous studies of CPAP use and pressure delivery at the mask revealed a high correlation between usage and compliance.[50]

Table 89–2.	**Suggested Terminology for Patient Interaction with Continuous Positive Airway Pressure (CPAP)**
Term	**Definition**
Acceptance	Patient meets selection criteria for CPAP treatment *and* actually proceeds to have CPAP pressure level determined
Prescription	Patient accepts CPAP *and* commences home treatment
Adherence	Patient is prescribed CPAP and *reports* continuing use of CPAP
Tolerance	Patient *reports* ability to use CPAP without side effects (term used interchangeably with *adherence*)
Usage	Patient's CPAP machine is *switched on* more than an arbitrary period of time
Compliance	Patient *uses* CPAP machine *and it delivers* a preset level (i.e., the mask is likely to be on the patient's face)

Dosage studies are not available for CPAP. Do patients have to use CPAP every night to receive beneficial therapeutic effects? Mean CPAP use of less than 4 hours per night produces a demonstrable reduction in sleepiness.[51] Another study showed that 1 night off CPAP in compliant CPAP users led to a recurrence in daytime sleepiness.[52] Early studies[53] sought a biomarker of CPAP efficacy and usage akin to glycosylated hemoglobin as a biomarker of diabetic control, but none has been developed. However, these studies have not simultaneously measured the biologic endpoint and objectively measured CPAP usage. At this stage, all criteria set for CPAP usage or nonusage or compliance or noncompliance[50,51] are essentially arbitrary.

However, even partial-night CPAP use can lead to measurable clinical improvement. Some sleep apnea patients use CPAP for only part of the night because they derive a satisfactory degree of symptomatic benefit from that limited application.[54] This may reflect interindividual variation in function with sleep loss or fragmentation, as some patients report that they require less sleep to function at a reasonable level during wakefulness.[55] However, given the evidence that shortened sleep hours are associated with significant performance deficit (see Chapter 6), patients should be warned about the risk of persisting alertness problems with limited hours of CPAP use. Newer-generation CPAP devices that allow monitoring of more precise patterns of use and efficacy will give us insight into the minimal duration of CPAP use that is needed to maintain normal daytime neurobehavioral function and, possibly, to modify the vascular consequences of sleep apnea.

Studies of CPAP Usage

The paragraphs below use the terminology suggested in Table 89–2 to discuss the data on interactions between patients and CPAP.

Patient Acceptance of CPAP

Limited data are available on patient acceptance of CPAP, as most studies discuss patient data only from the night of CPAP pressure determination or later. Studies suggest that 70% of patients offered a CPAP trial night accepted it.[56] It is unknown how many people with moderate to severe obstructive sleep apnea avoid even consultation, or seek referral to surgeons or dentists because they will not accept the concept of CPAP.

Patient Agreement to Prescription of Home CPAP

The percentage of patients who refuse CPAP after an in-hospital trial ranges from 58% to 80%.[57] CPAP purchase rates after CPAP titration with polysomnography are over 50%, based on a calculation comparing new CPAP machine sales (provided by manufacturers) with national insurance data on multiple sleep study frequency.[58] In other words, over 50% of patients completing a sleep laboratory trial ultimately purchase a CPAP machine or have one purchased for them by the health system.

Long-Term Use of CPAP

Covert objective monitoring of nasal CPAP has demonstrated that compliance is substantially lower than that seen in studies where compliance is reported on the basis of subjective patient data.[50] The covert objective monitoring revealed that only 46% of patients used nasal CPAP equal to or greater than

4 hours for 70% of the observed nights. Compliance at 1 month predicted compliance at 3 months.[50,59] Other studies have generally confirmed this degree of usage.

Follow-up studies of CPAP cohorts are biased by the same factors that affect clinical trials of pharmaceuticals. Patient populations are often highly selected for lack of comorbidity, intellectual capacity, geographic access, and health consciousness—all factors that may affect compliance in the real world. Larger, more open studies from a variety of sleep clinics[60] would provide better information on true CPAP compliance.

Baseline Indicators That Influence CPAP Usage

Several studies have confirmed that severity of symptoms has a major impact on continuing usage of CPAP—that is, patients with good objective usage or reported adherence were sleepier at baseline.[33,50,60-62] Although daytime sleepiness as measured by the multiple sleep latency test (MSLT) improves after CPAP treatment,[51] baseline MSLT scores do not appear to predict CPAP compliance. It is controversial whether degree of improvement in MSLT scores can predict compliance.[50,61] It is possible that in patients with sleep apnea, the Maintenance of Wakefulness Test may be a better predictor of CPAP use, but this is untested. Sleep fragmentation measured by an electroencephalographic neural network analysis or movement events on video recordings is reasonably correlated with CPAP compliance.[63] Improved compliance has also been linked to the higher degree of improvement in sleep efficiency and quality between diagnostic and treatment studies.[64] Other factors that may be related to reduced usage include previous palatal surgery and fewer years of education. Surprisingly, considering potential discomfort and potential mask leak, having a higher pressure level has not had a negative impact on compliance.[5,9,10,33] In fact, it may be associated with better compliance, although these data could be confounded by more marked symptoms in patients requiring higher pressures.[60] We do not really know whether strategies to lower pressure levels will improve compliance in poor-compliance users experiencing mask or mouth leak.

Motivation Supplied by Clinician

Surely, the greater the positive reinforcement given to patients, the more likely it is that the patient will use CPAP as prescribed. Various studies have shown the value of patient education, but it is unclear how much education and support is necessary to improve compliance.[9,10,65]

Management of CPAP Failure

What constitutes CPAP failure is a subjective issue, and practice varies from center to center in the absence of hard data addressing the diverse health consequences of varying degrees of sleep apnea. CPAP failure has been defined as the "use of CPAP for less than 4 hours per night on 70% of the nights and/or lack of symptomatic improvement."[50] This figure equates to 2.7 hours of use per night, but it was essentially an arbitrary figure based on the authors' expert clinical opinion.[50] Some clinicians have adopted a policy of reclaiming loaned CPAP machines if use is less than 2 hours per night.[60] Sometimes patients use CPAP effectively but for only part of their total sleep time. This may represent CPAP failure, depending on the endpoint of therapy.[66,67]

A cause should be identified when there is CPAP failure. Some common side effects and potential solutions have been mentioned. Ear, nose, and throat assessment may be appropriate in looking for any structural reasons to explain CPAP failure. Other considerations include misdiagnosis and coexisting causes of sleepiness.[67]

HEALTH OUTCOMES AND NASAL CPAP

Over the past decade, a number of randomized controlled trials have demonstrated that CPAP is effective in improving neurobehavioral outcomes such as daytime sleepiness or blood pressure in patients with moderate to severe OSAHS.[62,69,70] However, the evidence is less clear in patients with more severe disease who do not report sleepiness[61] and in patients with mild disease.[71] A detailed discussion of the treatment effect on neurocognition and performance in obstructive sleep apnea is provided in Chapter 85.

Researchers have employed either an oral placebo or a sham (or subtherapeutic) CPAP as a control arm in randomized controlled trials examining the effects of CPAP. There is no perfect placebo for CPAP, and each approach has limitations and difficulties in blinding. For example, a patient on sham CPAP may be told by the bed partner that the snoring persists. However, existing studies have clearly defined a role for CPAP in moderate to severe symptomatic obstructive sleep apnea. The treatment for the asymptomatic patient with milder disease remains controversial.[71]

CPAP and Cardiac Failure

Sleep apnea is common in patients with cardiac failure (see Chapter 102).[72] A number of studies have reported the presence of central sleep apnea in patients with ventricular dysfunction. Central apnea appears to be an adverse prognostic factor in such patients.[73] OSAHS is also prevalent in patients with cardiac failure.[74] It has been suggested that OSAHS may cause or exacerbate ventricular dysfunction by a number of mechanisms. These include increasing left ventricular afterload through the combined effects of elevations in systemic blood pressure and the generation of exaggerated negative intrathoracic pressure, and by activating the sympathetic nervous system through the influence of hypoxia and arousals from sleep.[74] Use of nasal CPAP for 1 month[75] and 3 months[76] in patients with OSAHS and cardiac failure leads to improvement in left ventricular function. A number of studies, including some with a randomized controlled design, have demonstrated improvement in various endpoints, including reduced mitral regurgitant fraction, atrial natriuretic factor secretion, inspiratory muscle strength, reduced left ventricular afterload, increasing P_{CO_2} (toward normal), and decreasing norepinephrine concentrations with CPAP treatment in patients with cardiac failure and central sleep apnea.[73] Ongoing research is aimed at determining the optimal type of device and the influence of CPAP on patient survival.[76a,77]

AUTOTITRATING CPAP: DEVELOPMENT AND RATIONALE

The aims of auto-CPAP devices are to simultaneously detect and prevent upper airway obstruction using the lowest possible pressure level across the night.[78] If pressure requirements vary with changes in upper airway resistance (nasal obstruction, alcohol or sedative use), then an auto-CPAP machine would, in theory, adjust to these changes, unlike a fixed-pressure machine. An overnight tracing from one such device is shown in Figure 89–7. Economic benefits could also accrue if auto-CPAP reduced technician time, eliminated in-hospital polysomnography for CPAP titration, or reduced clinic visits of patients with CPAP compliance problems.

Accuracy of Auto-CPAP Devices

Recent research studies in selected patients have generally shown that auto-CPAP provides pressures that are similar to those of fixed-pressure CPAP machines. However, there is often great variability in study methodology,[27,79] with some patients initially undergoing manual titration in the laboratory *before* home use of auto-CPAP. For in-laboratory studies comparing technician-determined and autotitrated pressures, the technician and machine should be trying to achieve the same titration outcomes. Also, it may be inappropriate to depend on a flow signal provided by the auto-CPAP device itself; for research and comparative purposes, independent verification should be obtained. Finally, data obtained in the sleep laboratory with technician supervision cannot be extrapolated to unattended CPAP titration at home, where correction of a leak or mask adjustment is not possible.

Compliance and Usage with Autotitrating CPAP Devices

One of the main reasons for developing auto-CPAP was to decrease average pressure levels and improve compliance. However, a recent meta-analysis of randomized trials comparing auto-CPAP with fixed-pressure CPAP concluded that there were no differences in hours of use and other outcomes, despite a mean decrease in overnight pressure of 2 cm H_2O.[80]

Thus, auto-CPAP does not appear to significantly influence compliance. There is no evidence that the availability of auto-CPAP has led to a dramatic increase in hours of CPAP use by patients or to an increase of acceptance of this therapy in patients refusing fixed-pressure CPAP. Given the current costs of auto-CPAP devices, there is no rationale, at this stage, for their use as the standard initial home device, replacing the cheaper, fixed-pressure CPAP.[80] Even if the pressure level required to treat sleep apnea decreases over time in compliant patients, such changes in pressure are usually small. It is not clear what the advantage of lowering pressure would be in patients who are, presumably, successfully established on therapy. Auto-CPAP may have a role in replacing in-hospital titration of CPAP, but this needs to be tested in large studies that evaluate cost versus utility, that look at a wide range of unselected patients, and that compare in-hospital titration with empirical home treatment.[29,80,81]

Problems with Autotitrating CPAP

Potential problems with auto-CPAP include overcompensation for mask or mouth leaks, with resultant unnecessarily high pressures (Fig. 89–8). This could lead to a worsening air leak. Other potential problems include undertreatment because of slow responses to airway obstruction or even to the presence of central apnea or hypoventilation (Fig. 89–9), which may not be detected if flow limitation is the only

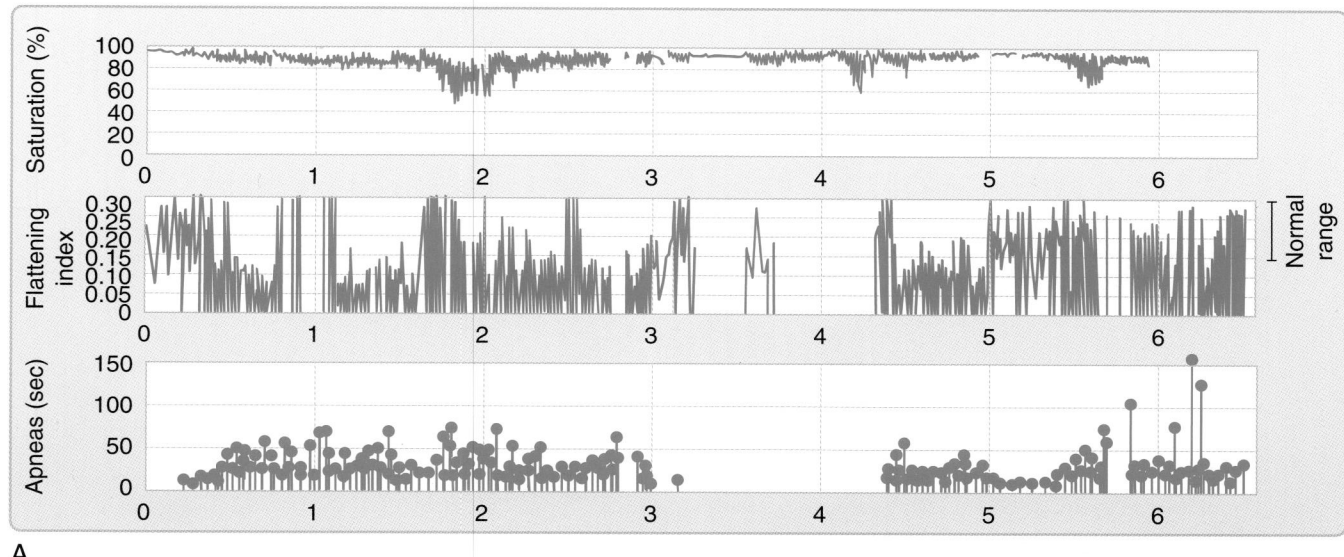

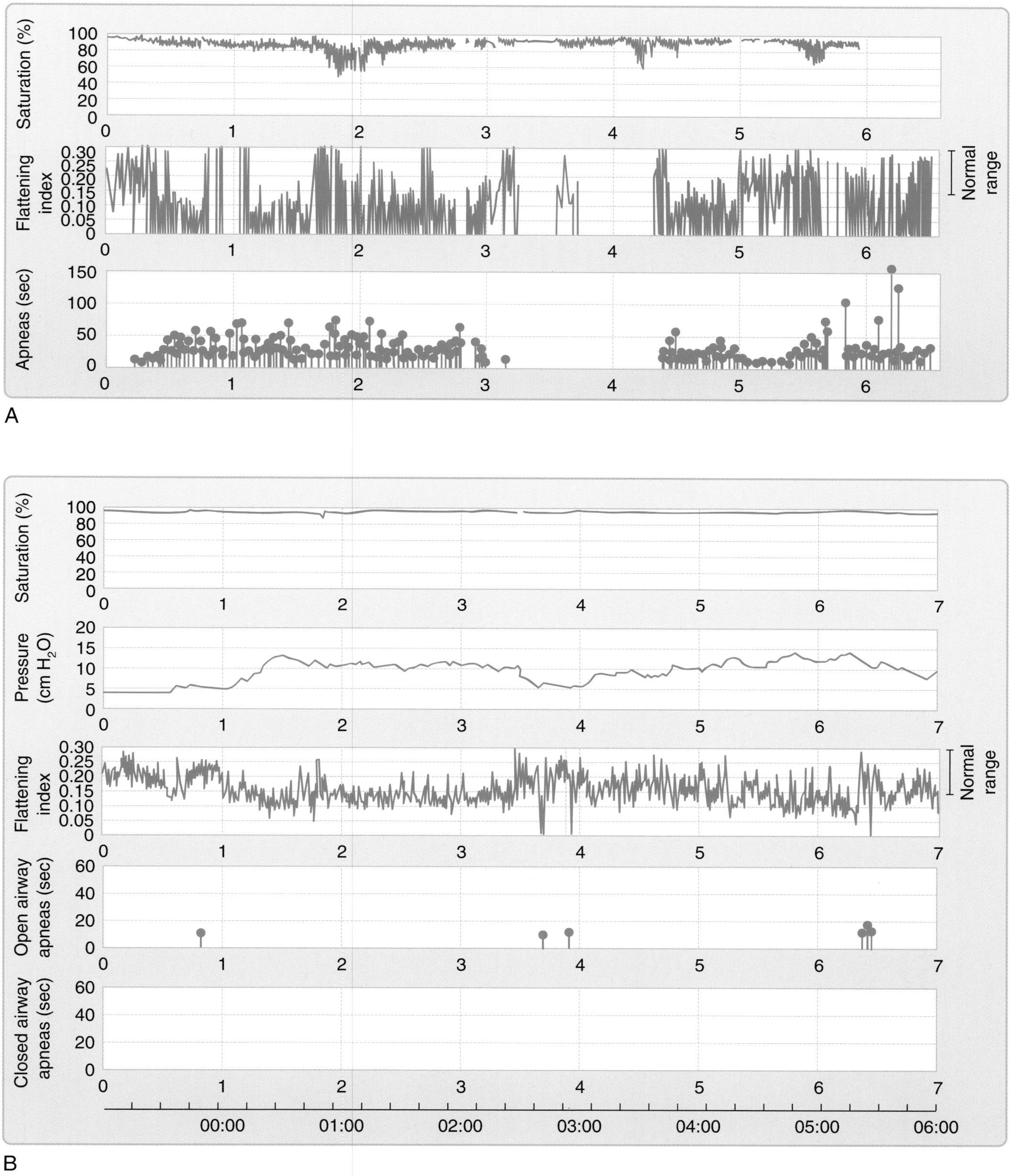

Figure 89–7. Autotitrating continuous positive airway pressure (auto-CPAP) tracing of a patient with severe obstructive sleep apnea before (**A**) and during (**B**) nasal CPAP treatment. In **B,** CPAP level varies automatically to prevent flow limitation (denoted by an arbitrary index based on flattening of the shape of the inspiratory flow curve) and apneas.

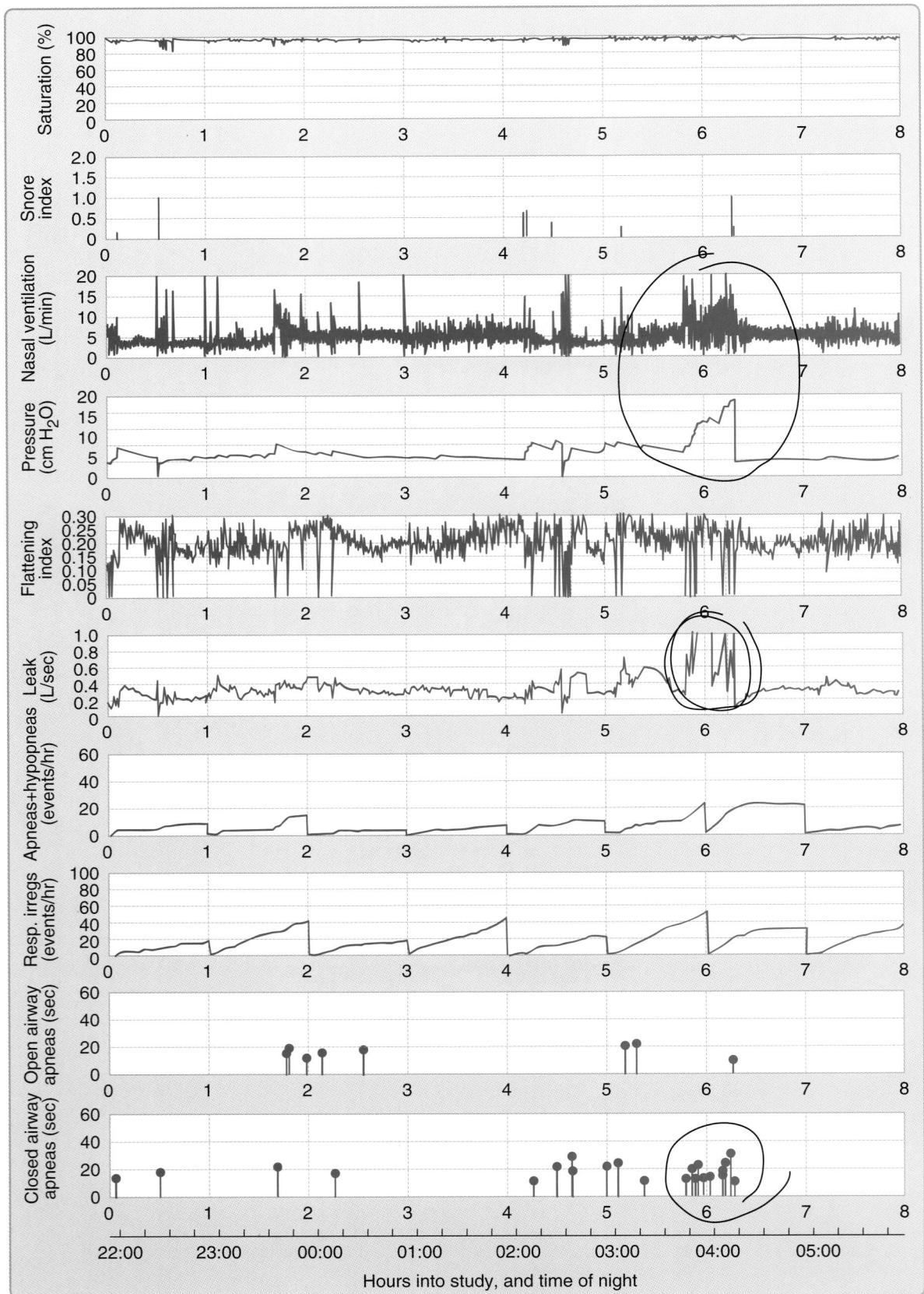

Figure 89–8. Autotitrating continuous positive airway pressure (auto-CPAP) tracing from one device demonstrating persisting apneas with constant increase in pressure in the presence of a mask leak *(roughly circled areas)*. The pressure rises over a 22-minute period from 6 cm to nearly 20 cm, eventually resulting in the patient's attempting to pull the mask off and a drop in pressure.

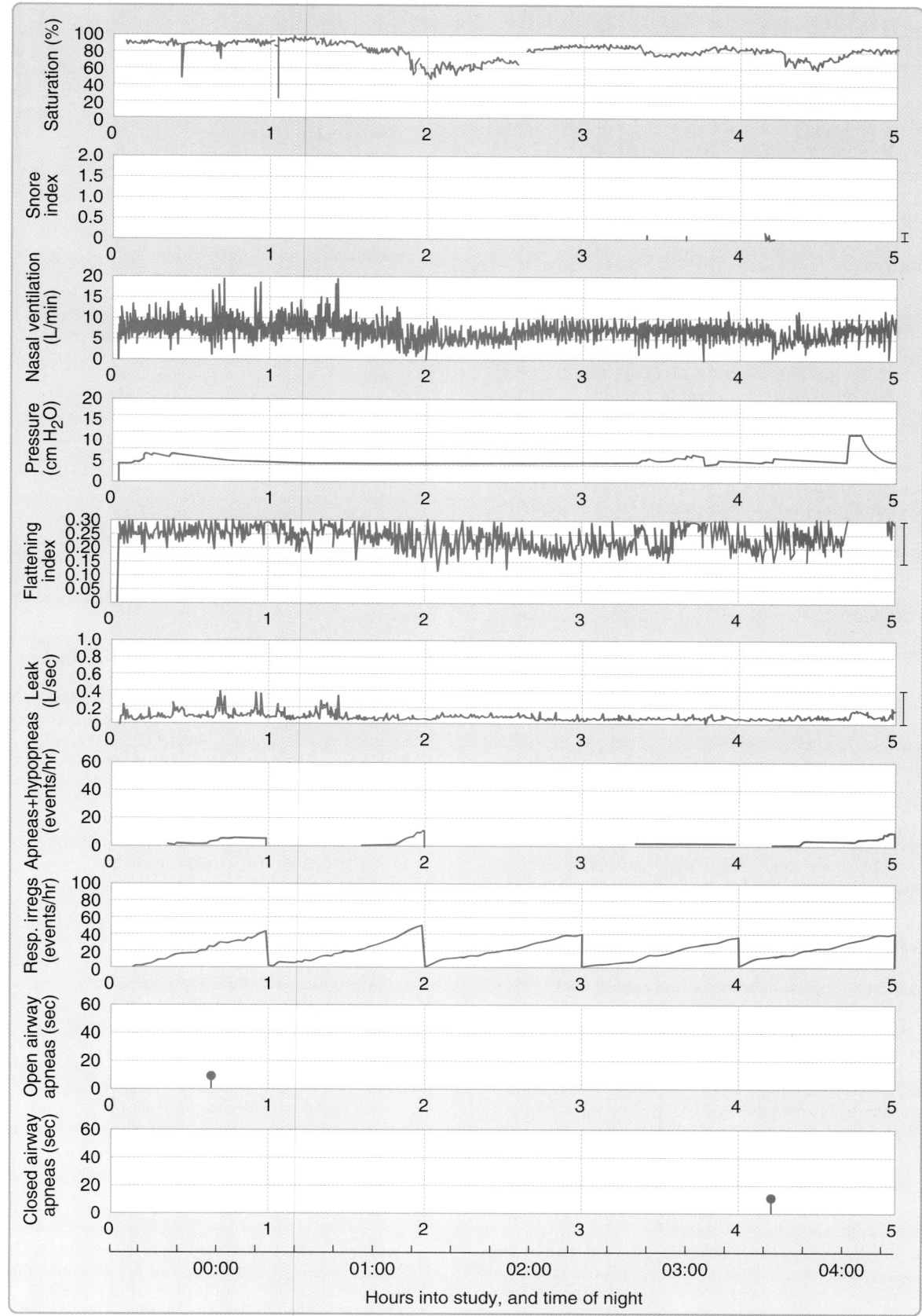

Figure 89–9. Patient with long-standing sleep apnea and obesity. There is evidence of marked reduction in arterial oxyhemoglobin saturation (SaO₂) during sleep. There is no increase in continuous positive airway pressure (CPAP) with auto-CPAP, presumably because no upper airway obstruction, flow limitation, or snoring is detected.

end point used by the device's diagnostic algorithm. Auto-CPAP does not appear to easily correct the flow limitation caused by acute nasal congestion, and it may have difficulty treating patients in whom central apneas appear after adequate correction of obstructive events. Other work has shown mask leaks to be a significant problem in auto-CPAP as well as in manual titration.[27] They may lead to overshoots in pressure level, compromising sleep structure.[17] Finally, it is important to recognize that data from studies investigating one type of autotitrating machine cannot be extrapolated to other autotitrating devices.[27]

> ### Clinical Pearl
>
> Nasal CPAP is the standard form of treatment for patients with moderate to severe symptomatic OSAHS or forms of central sleep apnea that respond to CPAP. Correction of flow limitation appears to be the most practical and effective endpoint for pressure titration. Severe side effects are rare, but nasal and mask problems may limit compliance. Compliance varies from 40% to 80%, depending on the study, and is probably influenced by the degree to which education and support are provided to the patient. Randomized controlled studies have provided an evidence-based rationale for CPAP treatment.

Acknowledgment

Supported by a Practitioner Fellowship from the National Health and Medical Research Council of Australia.

References

1. Sullivan CE, Issa FG, Berthon-Jones M, et al: Reversal of obstructive sleep apnea by continuous positive airway pressure applied through the nares. Lancet 1981;1:862-865.
2. Grunstein RR, Dodd MJ, Costas L, et al: Home nasal CPAP for sleep apnea: Acceptance of home therapy and its usefulness. Aust N Z J Med 1986;16:635.
3. Grunstein RR: Sleep-related breathing disorders: 5. nasal continuous positive airway pressure treatment for obstructive sleep apnoea. Thorax 1995;50:1106-1113.
4. Grunstein RR, Hedner J, Grote L: Therapy of sleep apnea. Drugs 2001;61:237-251.
5. Remmers JE, De Groot WJ, Sauerland EK, et al: Pathogenesis of upper airway occlusion during sleep. J Appl Physiol 1978;44:931-938.
6. Strohl KP, Redline S: Nasal CPAP therapy, upper air-way muscle activation and obstructive sleep apnea. Am Rev Respir Dis 1986;134:555-558.
7. Schwab RJ, Pack AI, Gupta KB, et al: Upper airway and soft tissue structural changes induced by CPAP in normal subjects. Am J Respir Crit Care Med 1996;154:1106-1116.
8. Issa FG, Sullivan CE: Reversal of central sleep apnea using nasal CPAP. Chest 1986;90:165-171.
9. Zozula R, Rosen R: Compliance with continuous positive airway pressure therapy: Assessing and improving treatment outcomes. Curr Opin Pulm Med 2001;7:391-398.
10. Fitzpatrick MF, Alloway CED, Wakeford TM, et al: Can patients with obstructive sleep apnea titrate their own continuous positive airway pressure? Am J Respir Crit Care Med 2003;167:716-722.
11. Montserrat JM, Ballester E, Olivi H, et al: Time-course of stepwise CPAP titration: Behavior of respiratory and neurological variables. Am J Respir Crit Care Med 1995;152:1854-1859.
12. Hosselet JJ, Norman RG, Ayappa I, et al: Detection of flow limitation with a nasal cannula/pressure transducer system. Am J Respir Crit Care Med 1998;157:1461-1467.
13. Meurice JC, Paquereau J, Denjean A, et al: Influence of correction of flow limitation on continuous positive airway pressure efficiency in sleep apnoea/hypopnoea syndrome. Eur Respir J 1998;11:1121-1127.
14. Issa FG, Sullivan CE: The immediate effects of nasal continuous positive airway pressure treatment on sleep pattern in patients with obstructive sleep apnea syndrome. Electroencephalogr Clin Neurophysiol 1986;63:10-17.
15. Condos R, Norman RG, Krishnasamy I, et al: Flow limitation as a noninvasive assessment of residual upper-airway resistance during continuous positive airway pressure therapy of obstructive sleep apnea. Am J Respir Crit Care Med 1994;150:475-480.
16. Pevernagie DA, Shepard JW Jr: Relations between sleep stage, posture and effective nasal CPAP levels in OSAHS. Sleep 1992;15:162-167.
17. Marrone O, Insalaco G, Bonsignore MR, et al: Sleep structure correlates of continuous positive airway pressure variations during application of an autotitrating continuous positive airway pressure machine in patients with obstructive sleep apnea syndrome. Chest 2002;121:759-767.
18. Jokic R, Klimaszewski A, Sridhar G, et al: Continuous positive airway pressure requirement during the first month of treatment in patients with severe obstructive sleep apnea. Chest 1998;114:1061-1069.
19. Willson G, Grunstein RR, Doyle J, et al: Domiciliary use of autoset nasal continuous positive airway pressure (nCPAP): Feasibility, efficacy and night to night variability. Sleep Res 1996;25:210.
20. Miljeteigh H, Hoffstein V: Continuous positive airway pressure for treatment of obstructive sleep apnea. Am Rev Respir Dis 1993;147:1526-1530.
21. Berry RB, Desa MM, Light RW: Effect of ethanol on the efficacy of nasal continuous positive airway pressure as a treatment for obstructive sleep apnea. Chest 1991;99:339-343.
22. Becker HF, Piper AJ, Flynn WE, et al: Breathing during sleep in patients with nocturnal desaturation. Am J Respir Crit Care Med 1999;159:112-118.
23. Sanders MH, Kern NB, Costantino JP, et al: Adequacy of prescribing positive airway pressure therapy by mask for sleep apnea on the basis of a partial-night trial. Am Rev Respir Dis 1993;147:1169-1174.
24. McArdle N, Grove A, Devereux G, et al: Split-night versus full-night studies for sleep apnoea/hypopnoea syndrome. Eur Respir J 2000;15:670-675.
25. Yamashiro Y, Kryger MH: CPAP titration for sleep apnea using a split-night protocol. Chest 1995;107:62-66.
26. Rosenthal L, Nykamp K, Guido P, et al: Daytime CPAP titration: A viable alternative for patients with severe obstructive sleep apnea. Chest 1998;114:1056-1060.
27. Littner M, Hirshkowitz M, Davila D, et al, Standards of Practice Committee of the American Academy of Sleep Medicine: Practice parameters for the use of auto-titrating continuous positive airway pressure devices for titrating pressures and treating adult patients with obstructive sleep apnea syndrome. An American Academy of Sleep Medicine report. Sleep 2002;25:143-147.
28. Krieger J, Sforza E, Petiau C, et al: Simplified diagnostic procedure for obstructive sleep apnoea syndrome: Lower subsequent compliance with CPAP. Eur Respir J 1998;12:776-779.
29. White DP, Gibb TJ: Evaluation of the Healthdyne NightWatch system to titrate CPAP in the home. Sleep 1998;21:198-204.
30. Juhasz J, Schillen J, Urbigkeit A, et al: Unattended continuous positive airway pressure titration: Clinical relevance and cardiorespiratory hazards of the method. Am J Respir Crit Care Med 1996;154:359-365.

31. Hoffstein V, Mateika S: Predicting nasal continuous positive airway pressure. Am J Respir Crit Care Med 1994;150:486-488.

32. Engleman HM, Asgari-Jirhandeh N, McLeod AL, et al: Self-reported use of CPAP and benefits of CPAP therapy: A patient survey. Chest 1996;109:1470-1476.

33. Strollo PJ Jr, Sanders MH, Atwood CW: Positive pressure therapy. Clin Chest Med 1998;19:55-68.

34. Pepin JL, Leger P, Veale D, et al: Side effects of nasal continuous positive airway pressure in sleep apnea syndrome: Study of 193 patients in two French sleep centers. Chest 1995;107:375-381.

35. Richards GN, Cistulli PA, Unger RG, et al: Mouth leak with nasal continuous positive airway pressure increases nasal airway resistance. Am J Respir Crit Care Med 1996;154:182-186.

36. Martins de Araujo MT, Vieira SB, Vasquez EC, et al: Heated humidification or face mask to prevent upper airway dryness during continuous positive airway pressure therapy. Chest 2000;117:142-147.

37. Friedman M, Tanyeri H, Lim JW, et al: Effect of improved nasal breathing on obstructive sleep apnea. Otolaryngol Head Neck Surg 2000;122:71-74.

38. Beecroft J, Zanon S, Lukic D, Hanly P: Oral continuous positive airway pressure for sleep apnea: Effectiveness, patient preference, and adherence. Chest 2003;124:2200-2208.

39. Stauffer JL, Fayter NA, McClure BJ: Conjunctivitis from nasal CPAP apparatus. Chest 1984;86:802.

40. Bucca C, Carossa S, Pivetti S, et al: Edentulism and worsening of obstructive sleep apnoea. Lancet 1999;353:121-122.

41. Pressman MR, Peterson DD, Meyer TJ, et al: Ramp abuse: A novel form of patient noncompliance to administration of nasal continuous positive airway pressure for treatment of obstructive sleep apnea. Am J Respir Crit Care Med 1995;151:1632-1634.

42. Reeves-Hoche MK, Hudgel DW, Meck R, et al: Continuous versus bilevel positive airway pressure for obstructive sleep apnea. Am J Respir Crit Care Med 1995;151:443-449.

43. Gay PC, Herold DL, Olson EJ: A randomized, double-blind clinical trial comparing continuous positive airway pressure with a novel bilevel pressure system for treatment of obstructive sleep apnea syndrome. Sleep 2003;26:864-869.

44. Lojander J, Maasilta P, Partinen M, et al: Nasal-CPAP, surgery, and conservative management for treatment of obstructive sleep apnea syndrome: A randomized study. Chest 1996;110:114-119.

45. Engleman HM, McDonald JP, Graham D, et al: Randomized crossover trial of two treatments for sleep apnea/hypopnea syndrome: Continuous positive airway pressure and mandibular repositioning splint. Am J Respir Crit Care Med 2002;166:855-859.

46. Woodson BT, Steward DL, Weaver EM, et al: A randomized trial of temperature-controlled radiofrequency, continuous positive airway pressure, and placebo for obstructive sleep apnea syndrome. Otolaryngol Head Neck Surg 2003;128:848-861.

47. Spilker B: Guide to Clinical Trials. New York, Raven Press, 1991.

48. Rand CS, Wise RA, Nides N, et al: Medication adherence in a clinical trial. Am Rev Respir Dis 1992;146:1559-1564.

49. Haynes RB, Taylor DW, Sackett DL: Compliance in Health. Baltimore, Johns Hopkins University Press, 1979.

50. Kribbs NB, Pack AI, Kline LR, et al: Objective measurement of patterns of nasal CPAP use by patients with obstructive sleep apnea. Am Rev Respir Dis 1993;147:887-895.

51. Engleman HM, Martin SE, Deary IJ, et al: Effect of continuous positive airway pressure treatment on daytime function in sleep apnoea/hypopnoea syndrome. Lancet 1994;343:572-575.

52. Kribbs NB, Pack AI, Kline LR, et al: Effects of one night without nasal CPAP treatment on sleep and sleepiness in patients with obstructive sleep apnea. Am Rev Respir Dis 1993;147:1162-1168.

53. Grunstein RR, Handelsman DJ, Lawrence S, et al: Neuroendocrine dysfunction in sleep apnea: reversal by nasal continuous positive airways pressure. J Clin Endocrinol Metab 1989;68:352-358.

54. Hers V, Liistro G, Dury M, et al: Residual effect of nCPAP applied for part of the night in patients with obstructive sleep apnoea. Eur Respir J 1997;10:973-976.

55. Van Dongen HP, Maislin G, Dinges DF: Dealing with inter-individual differences in the temporal dynamics of fatigue and performance: Importance and techniques. Aviat Space Environ Med 2004;75(Suppl 3):A147-154.

56. Rauscher H, Popp W, Wanke T, et al: Acceptance of CPAP therapy for sleep apnea. Chest 1991;100:1019-1023.

57. Meurice JC, Dore P, Paquereau J, et al: Predictive factors of long term compliance with nasal continuous positive airway pressure treatment in sleep apnea syndrome. Chest 1994;105:429-433.

58. Grunstein R: Investigation and treatment of sleep apnea in Australia 1991-95. Am J Respir Crit Care Med 1997;155:A133.

59. Weaver TE, Kribbs NB, Pack AI, et al: Night-to-night variability in CPAP use over the first three months of treatment. Sleep 1997;20:278-283.

60. McArdle N, Devereux G, Heidarnejad H, et al: Long-term use of CPAP therapy for sleep apnea/hypopnea syndrome. Am J Respir Crit Care Med 1999;159:1108-1114.

61. Barbe F, Mayoralas LR, Duran J, et al: Treatment with continuous positive airway pressure is not effective in patients with sleep apnea but no daytime sleepiness: A randomized, controlled trial. Ann Intern Med 2001;134:1015-1023.

62. Patel SR, White DP, Malhotra A, et al: Continuous positive airway pressure therapy for treating sleepiness in a diverse population with obstructive sleep apnea: Results of a meta-analysis. Arch Intern Med 2003;163:565-571.

63. Bennett LS, Langford BA, Stradling JR, et al: Sleep fragmentation indices as predictors of daytime sleepiness and nCPAP response in obstructive sleep apnea. Am J Respir Crit Care Med 1998;158:778-786.

64. Drake CL, Day R, Hudgel D, et al: Sleep during titration predicts continuous positive airway pressure compliance. Sleep 2003;26:308-311.

65. Hoy CJ, Vennelle M, Kingshott RN, et al: Can intensive support improve continuous positive airway pressure use in patients with the sleep apnea/hypopnea syndrome? Am J Respir Crit Care Med 1999;159:1096-1100.

66. Grote L, Hedner J, Grunstein R, Kraiczi H: Therapy with nCPAP: Incomplete elimination of sleep related breathing disorder. Eur Respir J 2000;16:921-927.

67. Stepnowsky CJ Jr, Moore PJ: Nasal CPAP treatment for obstructive sleep apnea: Developing a new perspective on dosing strategies and compliance. J Psychosom Res 2003;54:599-605.

68. Pack AI, Black JE, Schwartz JR, Matheson JK: Modafinil as adjunct therapy for daytime sleepiness in obstructive sleep apnea. Am J Respir Crit Care Med 2001;164:1675-1681.

69. White J, Cates C, Wright J: Continuous positive airways pressure for obstructive sleep apnoea. Cochrane Database Syst Rev 2002;(2):CD001106.

70. Pepperell JC, Ramdassingh-Dow S, Crosthwaite N, et al: Ambulatory blood pressure after therapeutic and subtherapeutic nasal continuous positive airway pressure for obstructive sleep apnoea: A randomised parallel trial. Lancet 2002;359:204-210.

71. Barnes M, Houston D, Worsnop CJ, et al: A randomized controlled trial of continuous positive airway pressure in mild obstructive sleep apnea. Am J Respir Crit Care Med 2002;165:773-780.

72. Javaheri S, Parker TJ, Liming JD, et al: Sleep apnea in 81 ambulatory male patients with stable heart failure: Types and their prevalences, consequences, and presentations. Circulation 1998;97:2154-2159.

73. Bradley TD, Floras JS: Sleep apnea and heart failure: Part II. Central sleep apnea. Circulation 2003;107:1822-1826.

74. Bradley TD, Floras JS: Sleep apnea and heart failure: Part I. Obstructive sleep apnea. Circulation 2003;107:1671-1678.

75. Kaneko Y, Floras JS, Usui K, et al: Cardiovascular effects of continuous positive airway pressure in patients with heart failure and obstructive sleep apnea. N Engl J Med 2003;348:1233-1241.

76. Mansfield DR, Gollogly NC, Kaye DM, et al: Controlled trial of continuous positive airway pressure in obstructive sleep apnea and heart failure. Am J Respir Crit Care Med 2004;169: 361-366.

76a. Topfer V, El-Sebai M, Wessendorf TE, et al: Adaptive servoventilation: Effect on Cheyne-Stokes respiration and on quality of life. Pneumologie 2004;58:28-32.

77. Bradley TD, Logan AG, Floras JS, CANPAP Investigators: Rationale and design of the Canadian Continuous Positive Airway Pressure Trial for Congestive Heart Failure Patients with Central Sleep Apnea—CANPAP. Can J Cardiol 2001;17:677-684.

78. Berthon-Jones M: Feasibility of a self-setting CPAP machine. Sleep 1993;16:S120-121.

79. Roux FJ, Hilbert J: Continuous positive airway pressure: new generations. Clin Chest Med 2003;24:315-342.

80. Ayas NT, Patel SR, Malhotra A, et al: Auto-titrating versus standard continuous positive airway pressure for the treatment of obstructive sleep apnea: Results of a meta-analysis. Sleep 2004;27:249-253.

81. Kuna ST: Can continuous positive airway pressure be self-titrated? Am J Respir Crit Care Med 2003;167:674-675.

82. Lafond C, Sériès F: Influence of nasal obstruction on auto-CPAP behaviour in the treatment of obstructive sleep apnea/hypopnea syndrome. Thorax 1998;53:780-783.

Surgical Management of Sleep-Disordered Breathing

Nelson B. Powell

Robert W. Riley

Christian Guilleminault

ABSTRACT

Obstructive sleep-disordered breathing (SDB) is defined by partial or total collapse of the upper airway during sleep. This disorder should be potentially amenable to a surgical solution. Initially, the only treatment available for patients with obstructive SDB was a tracheotomy that bypassed the obstruction and resulted in a 100% cure. However, this was not readily accepted by most patients. With increased understanding of the varied upper airway presentations seen in SDB, surgical methods other than tracheotomy were developed to successfully clear the upper airway during sleep by making the airway bigger without creating adverse effects. The three major anatomic regions of potential collapse during sleep in SDB are the nose, palate, and tongue base. Each region can be surgically reconstructed on its own or in combinations as necessary. Surgical techniques are currently available that may be applied to each region of the obstructed airway. Soft tissue can be repositioned or removed, and in some cases the jaws may be repositioned forward to expand the posterior airway space and improve nocturnal breathing. A commitment must be made by the surgeon to clearly advise the patient of all possible treatments, protocols, medical alternatives, and risks. Implementation and completion of the necessary airway reconstruction in a systematic, phased protocol should result in outcomes that are equivalent to those of medical management.

Obstructive sleep-disordered breathing (SDB) is a collective term that encompasses snoring, upper airway resistance syndrome (UARS), obstructive sleep apnea syndrome, and obstructive sleep apnea–hypopnea syndrome (OSAHS). Obstructive SDB is thought to be caused by partial or complete obstruction of the upper airway during sleep, combined with some yet unidentified central nervous system imbalance.[1] This nocturnal disordered breathing results in sleep fragmentation and subsequent excessive daytime sleepiness (EDS).

Patients with the pickwickian syndrome[2] were some of the first to undergo surgery for an anatomic narrowing or blockage of the upper airway during sleep. This early surgical intervention was a tracheotomy, which, although it did not address the anatomic collapse, successfully bypassed the obstruction.

The causes leading to obstructive SDB are multifactorial, but generally they entail a negative influence on the delicate balance necessary to maintain upper airway patency during sleep. Ideally, surgical approaches strive to intervene at identified levels of obstruction. Medical approaches, including risk modification (manipulation of body position during sleep, avoidance of alcohol and sedating medications, weight loss), continuous positive airway pressure (CPAP), or bi-level positive airway pressure devices are usually the first avenues of treatment (see Chapters 88 and 89). Patients who are unable or unwilling to comply with medical management may be surgical candidates.

RATIONALE AND INDICATIONS FOR SURGICAL TREATMENT OF SDB

Rationale

The rationale for surgical intervention, as for any intervention in patients with objectively documented SDB, is to improve the quality of life, reduce the risk for medical morbidity, and potentially enhance longevity. This rationale should take into consideration the behavioral and pathophysiologic derangements caused by nocturnal upper airway obstructions. The derangements are associated with adversely altered quality of life secondary to arousals, fragmented sleep, and subsequent EDS. The pathophysiologic manifestations of SDB commonly affect the cardiovascular, pulmonary, neurologic, and gastrointestinal systems. Two examples of the enhancement by SDB (specifically hypoxia) of biologic processes that promote cardiovascular and central nervous system morbidity were recently reported by Dyugovskaya et al.[3] (increased monocyte adhesion to endothelial cells) and Macey et al.[4] (gray matter loss).

Surgical Indications

Surgical indications are listed in Box 90–1. For patients whose average number of apneas plus hypopneas per hour of sleep (i.e., respiratory disturbance index [RDI]), is less than 20, and whose associated EDS interferes with daily functioning, surgery may be appropriate. In some cases, a trial of CPAP may indicate the need for surgery, and scores on the Multiple Sleep Latency Test (MSLT) or the Maintenance of Wakefulness Test (MWT) are helpful in assessing prior medical treatment outcome. In addition, these tests may demonstrate a link (or lack thereof) between SBD and clinical symptoms and signs, thereby facilitating therapeutic decision making. For example, if a patient's symptoms do not improve during a CPAP trial despite alleviation of SDB, it is unlikely that surgery will be beneficial, and an alternative etiology for the symptoms should be sought.

Relative contraindications to surgery are listed in Box 90–2.

Sleep-Disordered Breathing: Surgical Indications

- Excessive daytime sleepiness (EDS)
- Respiratory disturbance index (RDI) >20*
- Oxygen desaturation <90%
- Arrhythmia or hypertension
- Esophageal pressure more negative than −10 cm H_2O
- Anatomic airway abnormalities
- Failure of medical management

*Or an RDI <20 with severe EDS. Like the apnea-hypopnea index, the RDI usually reflects the average number of apneas plus hypopneas per hour of sleep.

Box 90–2. **Relative Contraindications for Surgery**

- Morbid obesity
- Severe pulmonary disease
- Unstable cardiovascular status
- Psychological instability
- Alcohol or drug abuse
- Older age
- Unrealistic expectation of outcome

MEDICAL AND SURGICAL EVALUATION

Patients with SDB usually present with EDS and other symptoms (see Chapters 81, 83, and 85). Because EDS has numerous other causes, such as narcolepsy, insomnia, and sleep deprivation, the workup should include a complete medical and sleep history, with a head and neck evaluation, to assess health and detect comorbid medical conditions. The pretreatment evaluation should include nocturnal polysomnography (PSG). A radiographic cephalometric analysis, along with fiberoptic nasopharyngoscopy, is helpful in evaluating skeletal anatomy and the airway. No single test or procedure should be relied on to make a definitive surgical treatment plan. A systematic medical and surgical review should determine the type of sleep disorder, establish parameters of severity, identify comorbidity factors, identify probable sites of upper airway obstruction, decide if treatment is emergent or elective, and assess the risk-to-benefit ratio of surgery.

Although the exact etiology of SDB is not well understood, the areas producing anatomic obstruction are usually, but not always, well defined.[5–8] SDB can thus be viewed as a surgically responsive problem caused by the presence of areas of disproportionate anatomy and diffuse upper airway collapse (nose, palate and pharyngeal wall, and base of tongue). A systematic approach and application of a surgical protocol will yield improved clinical outcomes.

Clinical Evaluation

Routine vital signs, neck circumference, body habitus, and facial skeletal pattern should be documented. A detailed head and neck examination should rule out pathology and then highlight the three major anatomic regions of potential upper airway obstruction: nose, palate (oropharynx), and base of

tongue (hypopharynx). The boundaries of these regions are as follows:

- Nose: includes the septum, turbinates, and nasal valve
- Palate (oropharynx): extends superiorly to the hard palate and inferiorly to the hyoid bone, and includes tonsils
- Base of tongue (hypopharynx): extends from the plane of the hyoid bone inferiorly to the cricoid cartilage below; does not include the larynx; is bounded anteriorly by the tongue base, posteriorly by the pharyngeal wall, and laterally by the lateral pharyngeal wall

The nasal examination should be performed while the patient is breathing quietly and during deep inspiration. This allows assessment of alar support and nasal valve function during dynamic breathing. Nasal septal deflection, turbinate enlargement, webs, polyps, or masses are potentially important in the patient with SDB. The oral cavity should be examined by assessing dental health, class of occlusion (I, II, or III), and the character of the oral mucous membranes and tongue. Examination of the pharynx includes evaluating the length of the soft palate, any lateral pharyngeal redundancy, and the size of the tonsils.

The facial skeletal portion of the examination involves evaluating the positions of the upper and lower jaws and their relationship to each other. The size of the tongue is evaluated relative to the space available. A laryngeal examination is essential on all patients because there may be laryngeal dysfunction secondary to webs, cysts, tumors, or vocal cord paralysis. The anatomy of the epiglottis can be important, especially if it is omega shaped (folded). The presence of "floppy" redundant supraglottic mucosa and tissue should not be overlooked. Cephalometric radiographs assist in the overall evaluation of the soft tissue and bony configuration. Other valuable upper airway imaging methods include magnetic resonance imaging (MRI) and volumetric computed tomography.[9,10] However, because of cost and time, these methods are usually reserved for investigational studies. Fujita[11] proposed a classification of obstructive regions in the upper airway that is useful in planning therapy and for standardization of scientific reporting (Table 90–1).

Fiberoptic Nasopharyngolaryngoscopy

A flexible fiberoptic scope can be used to evaluate the nasal airway, pharynx, hypopharynx, and larynx. Müller's maneuver (inspiratory effort against an occluded mouthpiece, with nose clips in place but with the patient keeping the glottis open), which exposes the pharynx to negative intraluminal pressures in an attempt to identify areas of potential obstruction and

Table 90–1. **Fujita Classification of Obstructive Regions**

Type I	Palate (normal base of tongue)
Type II	Palate and base of tongue
Type III	Base of tongue (normal palate)

From Fujita S: Pharyngeal surgery for obstructive sleep apnea and snoring. In Fairbanks D, Fujita S, Ikematsu T, et al: Snoring and Obstructive Sleep Apnea. New York, Raven Press, 1987, pp 101-128.

thus more accurately predict the likelihood of success of selected surgical procedures, has been evaluated by Sher et al.[12]

Radiographic Evaluation

The cephalometric radiograph is the simplest and most practical upper airway imaging technique. It is a lateral radiographic view of the head that details bone and soft tissue landmarks (Fig. 90–1). Although this technique has limitations, the image provides reliable presurgical and postsurgical data on soft tissue and skeletal relationships, length of soft palate, posterior airway space, and hyoid position. The use of cephalometric radiographs and the anthropomorphic measurements (except SNA and SNB) seen in Figure 90–1 were first described in 1983 by Riley et al.[13] Additional evaluations showed a statistically significant correlation of this two-dimensional cephalometric study with three-dimensional volumetric computed tomographic scans.[14] This correlation gave added confidence to using cephalometric evaluations to assess upper airway abnormalities in SDB, especially at the posterior airway space. It has been a reliable and relatively inexpensive diagnostic tool. The cephalometric evaluation is limited in that the patient is evaluated while awake and seated, and because it is not a dynamic study obtained during sleep. This technique cannot be relied on alone to determine the most appropriate surgical intervention.

Approach to Surgical Treatment

A systematic approach to the surgical management of patients with SDB is essential for quality care (Box 90–3). Because the

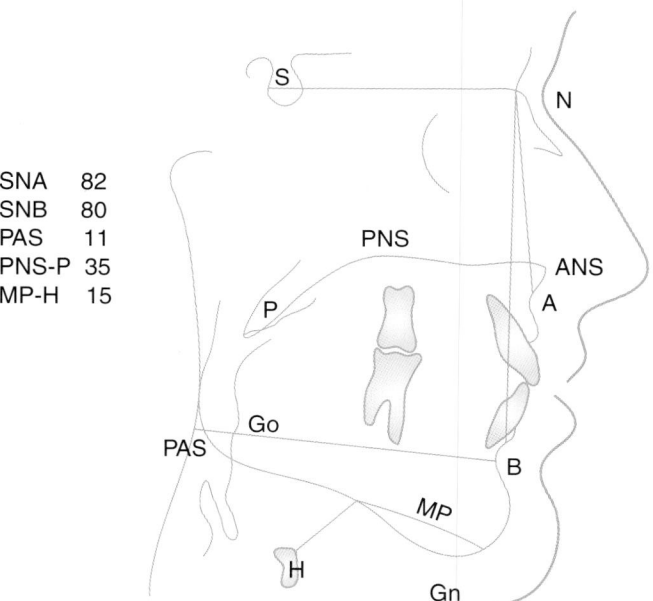

SNA	82
SNB	80
PAS	11
PNS-P	35
MP-H	15

Figure 90–1. Cephalometric analysis used for evaluation of patients with sleep-disordered breathing. SNA = 82° (SD ± 2), maxilla to cranial base; SNB = 80° (SD ± 2), mandible to cranial base; PAS = 11 mm (SD ± 1), posterior airway space; PNS-P = 37 mm (SD ± 3), length of soft palate; MP-H = 15.4 mm (SD ± 3), distance of hyoid from inferior mandible. MP-H, distance between mandibular plane and hyoid; PNS-P, distance between posterior nasal spine and point B; SNA, angle from sella to nasion to point A; SNB, angle from sella to nasion to point B. (From Riley RW, Powell NB, Guilleminault C: Obstructive sleep apnea syndrome: A surgical protocol for dynamic upper airway reconstruction. J Oral Maxillofac Surg 1993;51:742-747.)

Box 90–3.   Philosophy of Surgical Treatment

Goal
- Treat to cure.

Methods
- Careful and systematic plan of management
- Obstructions in the entire upper airway are treated (i.e., upper airway reconstruction [UAR]).
- Full disclosure of options and risks
- Staged surgical management
- Follow-up of all treatments

---

potential exists for upper airway narrowing at multiple sites in a given SDB patient, it may be necessary for surgical intervention to address more than one anatomic site. Failures will result if the objective is not complete upper airway reconstruction.

Although SDB is considered a surgical problem related to anatomic obstruction, medical management is usually considered first in formulating the surgical treatment philosophy. Medical management primarily uses risk factor reduction and either CPAP or a bi-level positive airway pressure device. Weight loss was recognized over 20 years ago as an important treatment. Although the ability of patients with SDB to control weight has been limited, a resurgence of interest in obesity may yield new methods of control. The merit of weight loss in obese patients with SDB is well documented. For example, Peppard et al.[15] recently reported that weight gain in SDB, even as minor as 10% (relative to stable weight), can result in an approximate increase in a patient's apnea–hypopnea index of 32%. In some morbidly obese patients with SDB, bariatric surgery is indicated. Sleep medicine surgeons may be asked to participate in the care of such patients who have attempted but failed medical therapy. The following phased protocol has proved, over time, to be effective and safe for controlling upper airway collapse in patients with SDB.

TWO-PHASE SURGICAL PROTOCOL

The Powell-Riley surgical protocol is a two-phase procedure that directs surgical treatment toward the specific regions of obstruction during sleep. Its benefits are listed in Box 90–4. Phase I of the surgical intervention includes nasal reconstruction, uvulopalatopharyngoplasty (UPPP), and a limited mandibular osteotomy with genioglossus advancement–hyoid myotomy and suspension (GAHMS). We are currently evaluating the use of radiofrequency (RF) technology using

---

Box 90–4.   Rationales for Powell-Riley Stanford University Phased Surgical Protocol

- Decreases risk of overoperating
- Treats conservatively because outcomes are difficult to predict
- Decreases hospital stay
- Limits postoperative risk
- Causes less trauma and pain
- Better accepted by most patients
- Improves cure rates in phase II

> **Box 90–5.** **Powell-Riley Protocol for Upper Airway Reconstruction**
>
> **Phase I**
> - Nasal reconstruction
> - Pharynx (uvulopalatopharyngoplasty [UPPP] with or without tonsillectomy)
> - Hypopharynx (genioglossus advancement–hyoid myotomy and suspension [GAHMS])
> - Possible use of radiofrequency (RF) technique
> - Reevaluation at 4 to 6 months
>
> **Phase II (When Phase I Treatment Is Insufficient)**
> - Maxillary and mandibular advancement (MMO)
> - *Alternative:* Surgical or RF tongue reduction

temperature-controlled RF (TCRF) in combination with GAHMS to be applied in phase I. The protocol sequence for addressing nasal, oropharyngeal, and hypopharyngeal obstruction during sleep is presented in Box 90–5. A patient needing intervention at any of these three anatomic levels should complete phase I surgery, in a sequence that would least jeopardize the upper airway during recovery, before moving on to phase II. This sequence should not interfere with the patient's ability to use CPAP after surgery. Phase II represents skeletal reconstruction and consists of bi-maxillary advancement, commonly referred to as maxillary and mandibular osteotomy (MMO). Combining phase I and phase II in one surgical procedure is discouraged because of an increased possibility of postoperative edema and upper airway compromise. In addition, both phases may not be necessary.

All possible medical and surgical options should be reviewed with the patient and the family well in advance, with the rationale for each clearly explained. Furthermore, it is mandatory that the patients be medically and psychologically stable, and that they wish to undergo the surgical procedure with knowledge of the potential risks, benefits, and likelihoods of success and failure.

Because surgical outcomes can vary, all patients must be reevaluated after each intervention. This minimizes the possibility of unnecessary additional surgery and readily identifies those who require further attention. To determine the outcome, each patient who has undergone phase I surgery is reevaluated by PSG and reassessed clinically after a 4- to 6-month healing period. Patients who have persistent SDB following phase I surgery become candidates for phase II (i.e., MMO). In conjunction with each surgical phase, weight management is encouraged as an essential part of the protocol.

In 1988, concern about postoperative upper airway compromise secondary to surgery prompted us to investigate perioperative CPAP. Our findings led to the establishment of a CPAP surgical strategy.[16] All patients are encouraged to use CPAP, and those who have an RDI of greater than 40 and an oxyhemoglobin desaturation (SaO_2) of less than 80% are required to use CPAP for at least 2 weeks before surgery, unless they cannot tolerate the device. Patients are also maintained on CPAP immediately after extubation and are encouraged to remain on this therapy during sleep until 2 weeks before the 4- to 6-month postoperative PSG reevaluation. Patients with severe sleep apnea (i.e., an RDI greater than 60, an SaO_2 of less than 70%, and significant comorbidities such

as severe hypertension, cardiac sequela, or morbid obesity with body mass index [BMI] of 35) who are intolerant of nasal CPAP should be considered for temporary or permanent tracheotomy.

Every treatment protocol has exceptions. In many instances, local resources, experience, and expertise dictate the type of surgical therapy a patient may receive. Some procedures require surgeons with multidisciplinary training, and none may be available in the patient's community. In such cases, surgical treatment must be left to the choice of the surgeon and the patient. Fortunately, myriad diagnostic and surgical procedures (see later) are available that can minimize risks and complications.

Definition of Phase I

Three regions of the upper airway are evaluated for treatment as directed by the systematic workup. For each region, only the most conservative surgery is used, and treatment at that level is considered only if it is the location of significant obstruction during sleep. Phase I surgery address the following susceptible regions:

Nasal region: Phase I procedures may correct nasal obstruction depending on the anatomic deformity (septum, turbinates, or nasal valve deformities).

Pharyngeal region: Phase I procedures improve pharyngeal airway space (UPPP or the equivalent, with tonsillectomy if present).

Hypopharyngeal region: Phase I procedures may place tension on the tongue base to help resist prolapse during sleep (genioglossus advancement [with or without hyoid myotomy and suspension]). Reduction techniques use laser midline glossectomy and lingualplasty, partial glossectomy, or TCRF technology.

Four to 6 months after phase I is completed (sufficient time for healing, weight stabilization, and neurologic equilibration), the patient undergoes a PSG, a new sleep assessment, and a clinical examination to assess clinical outcomes.[17] Patients who are incompletely treated or unchanged could advance to phase II.

Definition of Phase II

Phase II reflects skeletal midface advancement, or MMO. If the protocol has been followed, the only region that is as yet incompletely treated is the hypopharynx (i.e., the base of the tongue). Tracheotomy or nasal CPAP may be considered for tongue base control instead of MMO. Other techniques that are used less often but may be considered include laser midline glossectomy and lingualplasty, partial glossectomy, and TCRF technology. Except for TCRF, these procedures are seldom used by our center for phase II reconstruction.

Clinical Outcome: Responder

Previous reporting methods defined responders as those who were 50% improved according to the apnea or apnea-hypopnea index. However, most clinicians and researchers no longer consider this definition valid. A more stringent surgical goal combines specific PSG parameters with quality-of-life issues, and the outcome should compare favorably with the results of medical management (CPAP or bi-level positive airway pressure).

Box 90–6. Criteria for Responders to Powell-Riley Surgical Protocol

A patient is a responder (or a cure) if items 1 through 4, or items 4 and 5 are accomplished.

1. Respiratory disturbance index (RDI) <20, or a reduction to 50% (or better) of the preoperative RDI*
2. Oxygen saturation >90%
3. Normalization of sleep architecture
4. Resolution of excessive daytime sleepiness (EDS)
5. Response equivalent to continuous positive airway pressure (CPAP) on full-night titration

*If the RDI was 22 then the postoperative RDI would need to be 11 to qualify as a responder.

Box 90–8. Nasal Reconstruction

Rationale
- The nasal passage is an integral part of the upper airway.
- Any obstruction causes increased airway resistance.
- Rotation of the mandible with mouth breathing and prolapse of tongue into the posterior airway space

Internal and External Indications
- Deviated septum
- Enlarged turbinates
- Nasal valve or alar collapse
- External nasal deformities

Our criteria for designating a responder are presented in Box 90–6.

Surgical Procedures for SDB

Contemporary surgical techniques and a new technology are listed in Box 90–7.

Tracheotomy: Airway Bypass Surgery

Rationale: Tracheotomy provides immediate resolution of upper airway obstruction during sleep.

Indications: Tracheotomy should be employed when an emergent airway is necessary, or where there is neither the specialized equipment nor the surgical expertise to offer an alternative procedure. It may be indicated in selected patients with obesity (BMI, 30), morbid obesity (BMI, 40 kg/m^2), severe hypoxemia (Sao_2 less than or equal to 70%), serious arrhythmia or dysrhythmia, or uncontrolled hypertension. When edema resulting from surgery to alleviate upper airway obstruction may compromise the airway, or when CPAP is not tolerated by the patient, tracheotomy is an option. It is usually, but not always, poorly tolerated or accepted, especially in light of the successful use of nasal CPAP for severe SDB.[16] In the majority of cases, tracheotomy has taken a second position to CPAP in the treatment of SDB.

Techniques: Temporary or permanent tracheotomy may be employed to maintain the airway.

Box 90–7. Surgical Techniques

Contemporary Techniques
- Tracheotomy
- Nasal reconstruction
- Uvulopalatopharyngoplasty (UPPP)
- Tongue reduction (surgical)
- Genioglossus advancement–hyoid myotomy and suspension (GAHMS)
- Bi-maxillary advancement, or maxillary and mandibular osteotomy (MMO)

New Technology
- Temperature-controlled radiofrequency (turbinates, palate, tongue)

Clinical outcomes: Tracheotomy may be considered to ensure airway protection in patients with severe SDB and especially in those who are morbidly obese. In the absence of other confounding conditions (e.g., altered control of breathing physiology), tracheotomy can usually be expected to provide alleviation of SDB with 100% certainty.

Nasal Reconstruction (Phase I)

Rationale: A patent nasal airway establishes physiologic breathing and may minimize mouth breathing (Box 90–8). When the mouth is opened, the lower jaw rotates down and back, allowing the tongue to be repositioned into the posterior airway space. In some patients, improvement of the nasal airway may also improve CPAP tolerance or compliance.[18]

Indications: Nasal reconstruction is used for symptomatic nasal airway blockage caused by bony, cartilaginous, or hypertrophied tissues that interfere with nasal breathing during sleep.

Techniques: Septal or bony intranasal reconstruction, alar valve or alar rim reconstruction, and turbinectomy are variably applied in nasal reconstruction.

Clinical outcomes: The ease and high success rate of nasal reconstruction in improving nasal airway patency makes this procedure a very valuable technique for those with nasal obstruction and SDB. However, by itself, nasal reconstruction is less likely to have a significant impact on moderate or severe SDB than palatal or tongue base surgery. However, it is still an essential part of the upper airway and should not be ignored in the overall treatment of SDB. Correction of any defects at this level minimizes mouth breathing and decreases negative-pressure breathing during sleep.

Pharyngeal Reconstruction: Uvulopalatopharyngoplasty (Phase I)

In 1964, Ikematsu[19] proposed UPPP in Japan for the treatment of habitual snoring. Fujita[20] brought this technique to the United States as a procedure to treat not only snoring but also SDB.

Rationale: The palatal and lateral pharyngeal tissues have been found to be the most compliant of the upper airway, and documentation of collapse at this level in SDB is well established[21-23] (Box 90–9).

Indications: Pharyngeal reconstruction can be used to improve a long soft palate, a narrow inlet to the nasopharynx, hypertrophic tonsils, and a redundant lateral pharyngeal mucosa.

Box 90–9.   **Uvulopalatopharyngoplasty**

Rationales
- Opens the pharyngeal airway
- Excellent technique for this level

Indications
- Long floppy soft palate
- Enlarged tonsils
- Redundant lateral pharyngeal wall

This level of obstruction is classified as Fujita type I (see Table 90–1).

Techniques: Many surgical methods, including traditional UPPP and many variations of it, can be used to adapt the pharyngeal region[24] (Fig. 90–2). Transpalatal advancements, surgical flaps, lasers, and radiofrequency have also been used.[25-28]

Clinical outcomes: Results vary with the experience of the surgeon, the patients' anatomy, the severity of the SDB, and the technique selected. The removal, shrinking, or repositioning of the tissue blockage at this level is essential to the improvement of SDB, and the contemporary techniques are excellent in accomplishing this goal. However, these procedures have not maintained widespread popularity over the years because of the pain and discomfort after surgery and because cure rates have been so variable. Although most UPPP techniques do clear the pharyngeal level of obstruction, the procedure itself has often been associated with failure, partly because of unrecognized tongue base (hypopharyngeal) obstruction. In patients who have been carefully selected for upper airway reconstruction and whose site of primary obstruction is at the oropharyngeal level (Fujita type I), the cure rate can be very favorable.

In 1996, the American Sleep Disorders Association sponsored a meta-analysis of the surgical literature for the treatment of obstructive sleep apnea syndrome.[29] This review covered the previous 29 years of surgical therapy. UPPP was found to have approximately an overall 40% success rate for correcting obstructive sleep apnea syndrome. UPPP has seldom been credited with curing moderate or severe SDB. Although there is often an improvement in SDB after UPPP, the degree of improvement is frequently insufficient to define surgical success. We suggest that UPPP is probably overused as an *isolated* procedure by those who have failed to identify other existing obstructive sites.

UVULOPALATAL FLAP: AN ALTERNATE PROCEDURE FOR PHARYNGEAL RECONSTRUCTION

Rationale and indications: The rationale and indications for the uvulopalatal flap (UPF) are the same as for UPPP, except that the UPF is contraindicated when the palate and uvula are excessively long and bulky. We developed the UPF as a modification of the UPPP.[26] The goal was to reduce the risk of nasopharyngeal incompetence by using a potentially reversible flap that could be taken down in the early postoperative period. Additionally, it was found that because there were no sutures along the free edge of the palate, there was less postoperative pain than with the traditional UPPP or laser technique.

Technique: The technique is demonstrated in Figure 90–3.

Clinical outcomes: In a study of 80 patients examined in a prospective, nonrandomized, consecutive manner, there were no statistically significant differences between the UPPP group and the UPF group in the preoperative and postoperative variables including BMI, RDI, lowest oxygen desaturation during sleep, and subjective snoring scale. There were no significant complications in the UPF group. Using a visual analogue scale to assess pain, there was significantly less pain in the UPF group than in the UPPP group. Patients with long soft palates and uvulas, or with thick palates and uvulas, are not good candidates for this technique. Creating a flap with this much tissue bulk can create an abnormal thickness to the palate and diminish or eliminate favorable outcomes.

LASER-ASSISTED UVULOPALATOPLASTY

Rationale and indications: The rationale and indications for laser-assisted uvulopalatoplasty (LAUP) are the same as for a traditional UPPP. LAUP, an office-based surgical procedure,

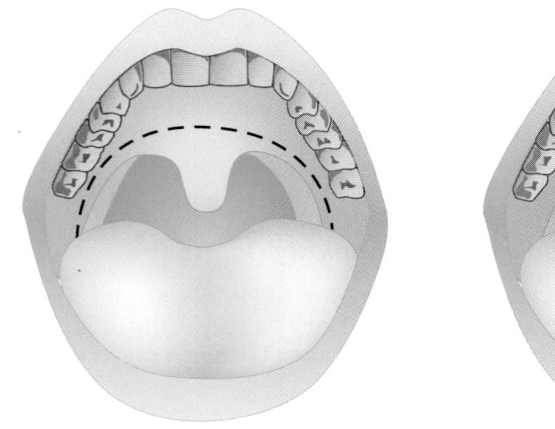 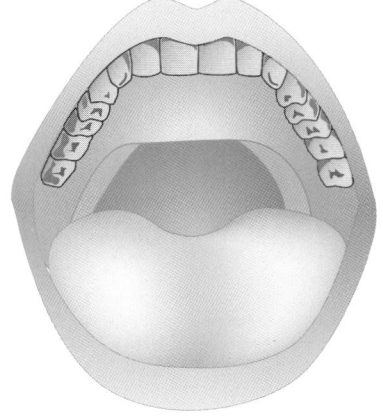 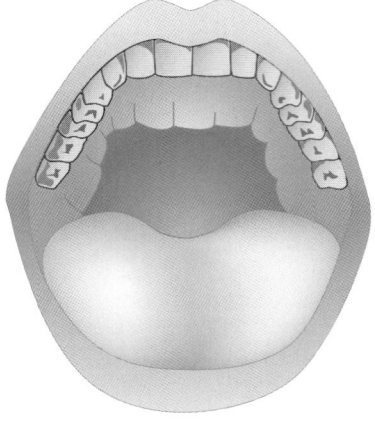

A   B   C

Figure 90–2. Uvulopalatopharyngoplasty technique. **A,** Redundant soft palate and tonsillar pillar mucosa are outlined. **B,** Tonsils, tonsillar pillar mucosa, and posterior soft palate have been excised. The extent of soft palate excision is determined by placing traction on the uvula and noting the position of the mucosal crease. **C,** Mucosal flaps of the lateral pharyngeal wall and nasal palatal muscle are advanced to the anterior pillar and oral mucosa of the soft palate. The wound is closed with 3-0 Vicryl braided suture. (From Troell RJ, Strom CG: Surgical therapy for snoring. Fed Practitioner 1997;14:29-52.)

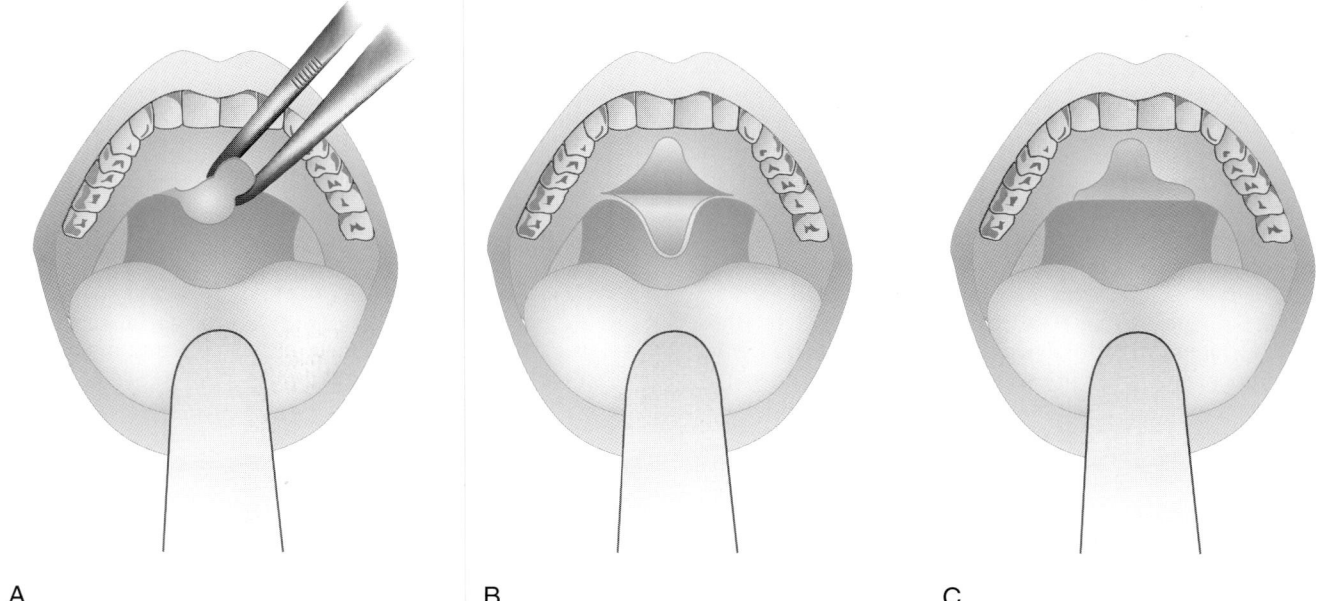

Figure 90–3. Reversible uvulopalatal flap technique (UPF). **A,** Uvula reflected to identify mucosal crease of muscular sling. **B,** Knife removes mucosa on proposed flap site. **C,** Wound is closed with a half-buried suture of 3-0 Vicryl braided suture at the tip of the uvula and simple interrupted sutures along the mucosal closure. (From Troell RJ, Strom CG: Surgical therapy for snoring. Fed Practitioner 1997;14:29-52.)

was introduced in 1990 as a new approach for the treatment of snoring.

Technique: This technique progressively shortens and tightens the uvula and palate through a series of carbon dioxide laser incisions and vaporizations. Most of the uvula is amputated, and the soft palate is incised by vertical trenches up to the muscular sling, 1 to 2 cm lateral to the uvula. Additionally, mucosal or tonsillar pillar tissue is vaporized as needed (Fig. 90–4).

Clinical outcomes: Most early studies evaluating the efficacy of LAUP for snoring and SDB were flawed by methodologic discrepancies or statistical inadequacies such as ill-defined criteria for response and lack of adequate follow-up. A more recent study by Walker et al.[27] is far more reliable and demonstrates that positive outcomes are possible with a 48% success rate (a postoperative RDI of less than 10). However, 21% of patients had worsening of SDB, 15% had no significant change, and 36% still had a postoperative RDI of greater than 20.

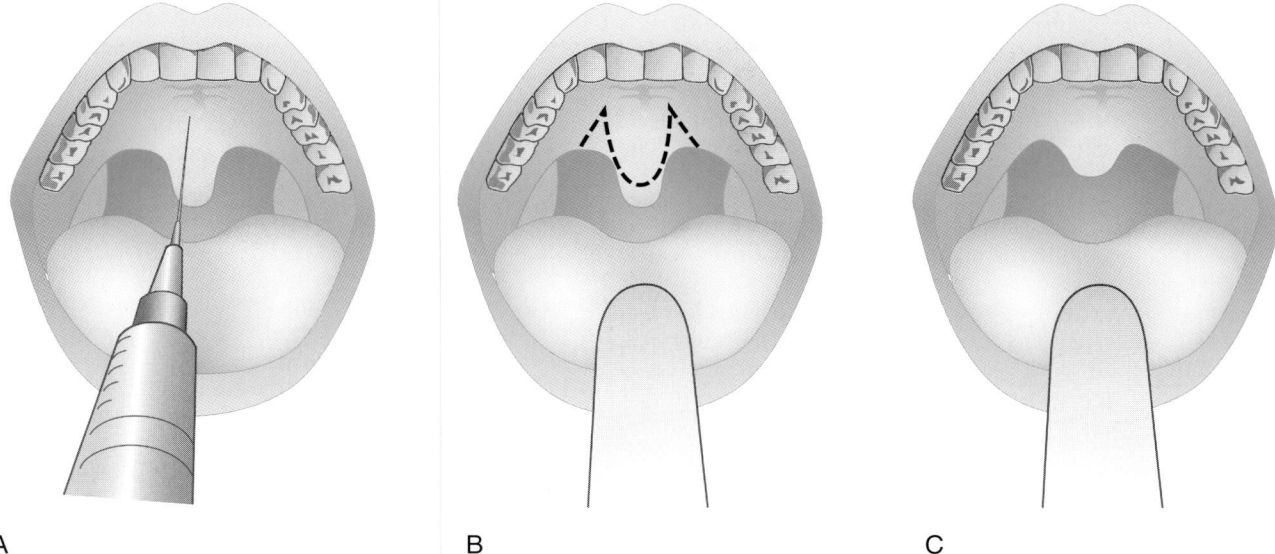

Figure 90–4. Laser-assisted uvulopalatoplasty technique (LAUP). **A,** Local anesthetic injected. **B,** The CO_2 laser is used to excise vertical trenches in the soft palate on either aspect of the uvula up to the muscular sling; 30% to 90% of the uvula is amputated or vaporized. **C,** The postoperative result necessitates 4 to 5 weeks for complete healing. (From Troell RJ, Strom CG: Surgical therapy for snoring. Fed Practitioner 1997;14:29-52.)

There is concern about the safety of performing upper airway surgery, including LAUP, on an ambulatory basis, especially with respect to edema secondary to surgical trauma in the early postoperative period.

Terris et al.[30] evaluated LAUP using MRI and PSG in patients with a mean preoperative RDI of 11.3 and a mean overnight, lowest oxyhemoglobin saturation (LSAT) of 87.7%. After LAUP they described a doubling of the RDI, a fourfold increase in the apnea index, stable oxygen saturation, and a decrease in the cross-sectional area at the palate level of as much as 48% at 72 hours. They concluded that patients with mild SDB (RDI less than 20, SaO_2 greater than 85%) may be offered LAUP, but those with moderate to severe SDB should be counseled about other, more prudent surgical options such as UPPP, UPF, or hypopharyngeal reconstructive techniques. The application of LAUP is waning, mostly because of pain problems and the controversy concerning efficacy and potential risks.[31]

Hypopharyngeal Region: Base of Tongue Obstruction (Phase I)

The hypopharynx may be bypassed by tracheotomy, or the hypopharyngeal region can be addressed by making more room for the tongue or by reducing the tongue size. The midportion of the tongue base can be removed with laser midline glossectomy and lingualplasty, partial glossectomy, or shrinkage by RF techniques. The more contemporary approaches utilize repositioning of the genioglossus attachment and hyoid (GAHMS), and skeletal advancements (MMO).

MANDIBULAR OSTEOTOMY: GENIOGLOSSUS ADVANCEMENT–HYOID MYOTOMY AND SUSPENSION

The GAHMS procedure is referred to as phase I of the Powell-Riley protocol, which includes genioglossus advancement, with or without hyoid myotomy and suspension. The surgery is limited in that the jaw and teeth are not moved; only the genial tubercle and hyoid complex are advanced. These advancements place tension on the tongue musculature (genioglossus and geniohyoid) and thereby limit the posterior displacement during sleep. No additional room for the tongue is created. This is in contrast to mandibular advancement or MMO (phase II), which not only places further tension on the genioglossus (after phase I) but also creates more physical space for the tongue. (The hyoid myotomy and suspension will be described later.)

Rationale: The rationale of the GAHMS procedure is to minimize the posterior displacement of the tongue into the posterior airway space during sleep (Box 90–10). The genioglossus muscle is attached to the lingual surface of the mandible at the geniotubercle and also to the hyoid complex just above the larynx. Movement forward of either or both of these anatomic structures will stabilize the tongue base along with the associated pharyngeal dilatators. Forward movement of the mandible or isolated geniotubercle advancement will, in most cases, improve the posterior airway space, as in the typical "jaw thrust" used in cardiopulmonary resuscitation to establish an emergency airway.

Indications: Indications for the GAHMS procedure include the general indications for surgery with additional findings of clinical tongue base obstruction.

Technique: Detailed knowledge of the preoperative anatomy is essential to the surgeon in planning the procedure. A radiographic analysis should include a lateral cephalometric

---

> **Box 90–10. Genioglossus Advancement–Hyoid Myotomy and Suspension (GAHMS)**
>
> **Rationales**
> - Places genioglossus under tension
> - Fixes major dilators of pharynx
> - Does not gain additional room for tongue
>
> **Indications**
> - Documented base of tongue obstruction
> - Failure of medical management
> - Severe sleep-disordered breathing in patients who, because of the severity of the disorder and their excess weight, are being prepared for maxillary and mandibular osteotomy (MMO) in a stepped sequence using the phased protocol
> - Applied in phase I or II

radiograph and a panoramic dental radiograph. The Panorex depicts the course of the inferior alveolar nerve canal and the location of the mental foramen. It further shows the root length of the mandibular canines and central incisor teeth and potential pathologic processes (e.g., periodontal disease, cyst, and tumor). The health of the periodontal structures and root length can be assessed and measured from this film and will help limit inadvertent damage to the dentition or bone during surgery. Surgery may be performed under general anesthesia or intravenous sedation. The technique creates less surgical trauma by advancing only the genioglossus muscle with the genial tubercle, thus maintaining the inferior mandibular border. This should reduce postoperative morbidity, as it minimizes fractures and bleeding. The technique is illustrated in Figure 90–5.

Clinical outcomes: Our first attempt to move the geniotubercle forward for SDB was presented as a single case report in 1984.[32] As measured by PSG, the RDI decreased from 60 to 45, and the lowest oxyhemoglobin saturation (LSAT) increased from 66% to 83% at the third postoperative month. However, this was accomplished using a modified horizontal mandibular sliding osteotomy. Although there was modest improvement, the technique was insufficient, in this case, to improve tongue base obstruction. We abandoned the technique after further tries and in 1986 developed a completely new osteotomy for geniotubercle advancement.[33,34] In 1993, in 239 patients who completed phase I and underwent preoperative and postoperative PSG, the responder or cure rate ranged from 42% to 77%, depending on the severity of the disorder.[35] Overall, the mean responder rate was 61%. To better view the outcomes, the results were stratified as to severity (Table 90–2). Outcome results reported by our center and by other centers in the United States and abroad vary from a 23% to a 69% response rate. In many cases, techniques were modified and definitions for control were not the same. However, for the most part, the overall outcomes were similar to those achieved at our center. A chronologic summary of the genioglossus advancement with and without hyoid myotomy and suspension is seen in Table 90–3.[33-43]

HYOID MYOTOMY AND SUSPENSION

Rationale: The rationale for including hyoid myotomy and suspension in the treatment of base of tongue obstruction is that

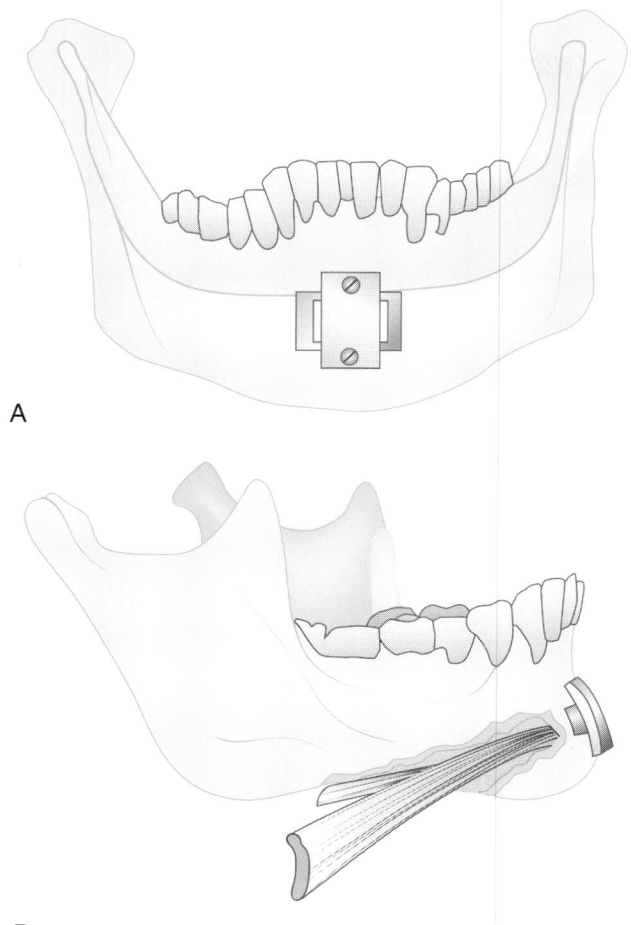

A

B

Figure 90–5. Limited mandibular osteotomy with genioglossus advancement procedure (GA). A rectangular window of symphyseal bone consisting of the geniotubercle is advanced anteriorly, rotated to allow bony overlap, and immobilized with a titanium screw. **A,** Anterior view. **B,** Lateral view. (From Troell RJ, Powell NB, Riley RW: Hypopharyngeal airway surgery for obstructive sleep apnea syndrome. Semin Respir Crit Care Med 1998;19:175-183.)

Table 90–2. Phase I Surgical Protocol: Results from 239 Patients

Sleep-Disordered Breathing		Patient Successes/ Total Patients	Success Rate (%)
Mild	(RDI <20) (LSAT >85)	20/26	77
Moderate	(RDI 20-40) (LSAT >80)	45/58	78
Moderate to severe	(RDI 40-60) (LSAT >70)	36/51	71
Severe	(RDI >60) (LSAT <70)	44/104	42

LSAT, lowest oxyhemoglobin saturation; RDI, respiratory disturbance index.

From Riley RW, Powell NB, Guilleminault C: Obstructive sleep apnea syndrome: A review of 306 consecutively treated surgical patients. Otolaryngol Head Neck Surg 1993;108: 117-125.

Table 90–3. Genioglossus Advancement–Hyoid Myotomy and Suspension (GAHMS): Clinical Outcomes

Date	Authors (ref.)	N	Responders* (%)
Index Case			
1986	Riley et al. (33)	5	RDI, 73 to 20; SaO₂, 43% to 77%
Subsequent Studies			
1989	Riley et al. (34)	55	67
1993	Riley et al. (35)	239	61
1994	Johnson and Chin (36)	9	69
1996	Ramirez and Loube (37)	12	53
1998	Yoa et al. (38)	23	68
1999	Lee et al. (39)	35	69
2000	Wagner et al. (40)	21	25
2001	Bettega et al. (41)	44	23
2002	Vilaseca et al. (42)	20	35
2003	Neruntarat (43)	31	70

*Responder rates varied, in part because the criteria used by the individual investigators to define success varied, and in part because technique variations and deletion of steps were common.

anatomically, the hyoid complex is an integral part of the hypopharynx, both statically and dynamically. Van de Graaff et al.[44] reported that in dogs, the hyoid complex helps to maintain the upper airway space. Forward movement of the complex improves the posterior airway space. We evaluated lateral cephalometric radiographs of patients with SDB who were receiving CPAP treatment at their preset therapeutic pressure level, and we observed an improved opening at the vallecular and tongue base level, which is also seen after a hyoid myotomy and suspension. Numerous reports have supported the concept that surgical intervention at the hyoid level improves the posterior airway space.[45,46]

Indications: Hyoid myotomy and suspension is an adjunctive procedure to the genioglossus advancement.

Two parameters that need to be considered are the linear distances from the inferior mandibular plane to the hyoid bone and the posterior airway space. Distances between the inferior mandibular plane and the hyoid of greater than 15 mm suggest a backward rotation of the tongue with resultant narrowing of the posterior airway space. Abnormal distance between the mandibular plane and the hyoid may reflect an enlarged tongue or a skeletal abnormality in the mandibular plane angle, either of which can result in a posteriorly based tongue or a narrow posterior airway space. In these cases, caution is recommended, because the vector of pull is so far below the tongue base that anterior repositioning could rotate the tongue base backward and result in an undesirable narrowing of the posterior airway space. The use of just the mandibular plane and the hyoid measurement is not recommended in decision making, and each patient must be evaluated individually for this confound.

The hyoid myotomy and suspension is part of phase I treatment, but it is not always included at the same time as the genioglossus advancement. In patients with severe SDB (RDI greater than 40, SaO₂ less than 80% to 85%, BMI greater than 30), we generally combine the genioglossus advancement only

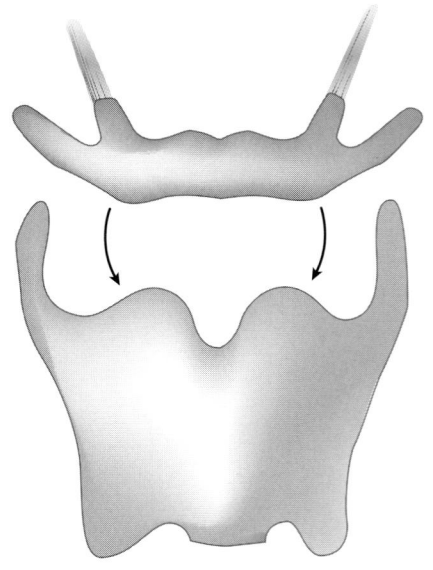

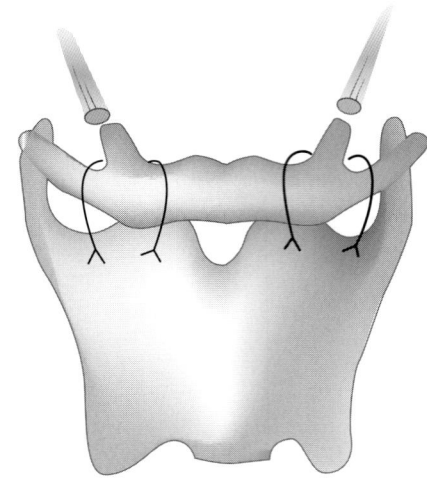

Figure 90–6. Modified hyoid myotomy and suspension procedure (HMS). The hyoid bone is isolated; the inferior body is dissected clean, and the majority of the suprahyoid musculature remains intact. The hyoid is advanced over the thyroid lamina and immobilized with sutures placed through the superior aspect of the thyroid cartilage. (From Troell RJ, Powell NB, Riley RW: Hypopharyngeal airway surgery for obstructive sleep apnea syndrome. Semin Respir Crit Care Med 1998;19: 175-183.)

with the UPPP. The additional insult to the infrahyoid region when the hyoid myotomy and suspension is included was found to be very difficult for many of these patients to tolerate. When evaluating patients after UPPP and genioglossus advancement, we have also found that the posterior airway space in some members of this group was sufficiently improved to obviate the need for a hyoid procedure.

Technique: Although the original description of the hyoid suspension technique involved suspending the hyoid to the anterior mandible with fascia lata,[33] the technique has been modified by suspending the hyoid to the thyroid cartilage. This modification was designed to decrease the risk of posterior rotation of the tongue (as described earlier) and to lessen the extent of surgery (i.e., less dissection, no grafting)[47] (Figure 90–6). We are investigating the use of the hyoid myotomy and suspension combined with ventral and base of tongue TCRF. This approach may decrease the need for phase II intervention, although multiple treatments of TCRF would be necessary.[48]

Clinical outcomes: Fifteen consecutively treated subjects were assessed before and after hyoid myotomy and suspension surgery (isolated hyoid myotomy and suspension to the laryngeal cartilage) with full PSG and sleepiness evaluations. All patients had previously undergone either UPPP plus genioglossus advancement (n = 11), UPPP only (n = 1), or genioglossus advancement only (n = 3), with incomplete treatment results. Before hyoid surgery, the mean RDI was 46.9 and the LSAT was 81% (BMI, 29.6 kg/m²; mean age, 51.8 years). After hyoid myotomy and suspension surgery, the mean RDI was 21.3 and the LSAT was 85% with no significant change in BMI. Twelve of the 15 (75%) had correction of their EDS and improvement of their SDB.[47] We do not consider this technique a primary therapy, but we do use it as an adjunctive addition to treating tongue base obstruction.

Maxillary Mandibular Osteotomy (Phase II)

The first reports of mandibular skeletal surgery for SDB came from Kuo et al.[49] in 1979 (n = 3) and Bear and Priest[50] in 1980

(n = 1). They reported subjective improvement, but there was no objective PSG data to support outcomes. We presented an additional mandibular advancement for severe SDB in 1983[51] in a somnolent 31-year-old, morbidly obese man with an RDI of 52 and an LSAT of 44%. After mandibular advancement surgery (with unchanged weight), his RDI was 21.4, with an LSAT of 73% and an improved EDS.

Rationale: This phase II surgery is specifically for the treatment of hypopharyngeal (base of the tongue) obstruction (Box 90–11). Mandibular, or maxillary and mandibular, advancement helps to clear hypopharyngeal obstruction. The reverse of mandibular advancement is a mandibular setback, which is used for the correction of a mandibular prognathism. This procedure has the potential to produce SDB in some patients by narrowing the posterior airway space.[52]

Indications: With few exceptions, patients enter phase II surgical management after they have undergone phase I and are found incompletely treated due to continued base of tongue obstruction. Some authors have advocated MMO as the first intervention, or only for patients with significant craniofacial disorders (e.g., maxillomandibular deficiency). The utilization of MMO as the primary treatment modality is

---

Box 90–11.   Bi-maxillary Surgery in Patients with Sleep-Disordered Breathing

Rationales

- Moves mid-face forward (palate, maxilla, and mandible)
- Increases posterior airway space
- Provides more tension than genioglossus advancement–hyoid myotomy and suspension (GAHMS)
- Increases room for the tongue

Indications

- Documented base of tongue obstruction
- Recommended when remaining upper airway has been maximally treated

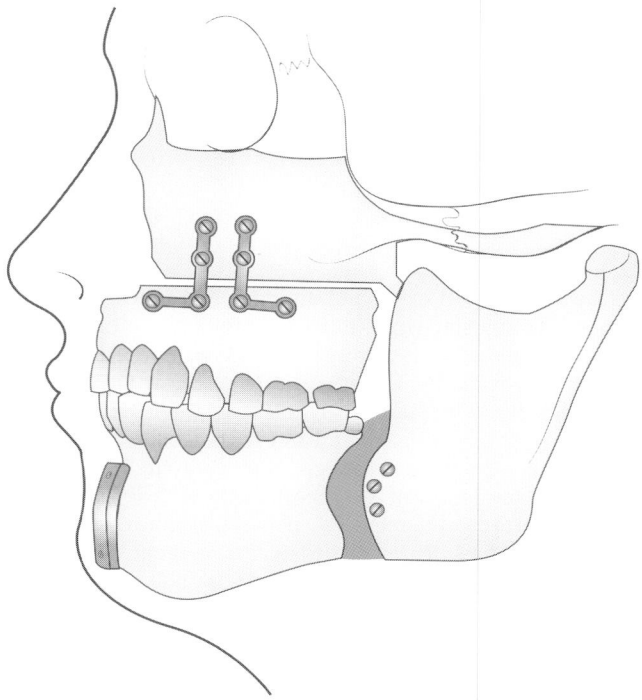

Figure 90–7. Maxillomandibular advancement osteotomy procedure (MMO). Lefort I maxillary osteotomy with rigid plate fixation and a bilateral sagittal split mandibular osteotomy with bicortical screw fixation. The advancement is at least 10 mm. A previous genioglossus advancement is shown. (From Troell RJ, Powell NB, Riley RW: Hypopharyngeal airway surgery for obstructive sleep apnea syndrome. Semin Respir Crit Care Med 1998;19:175-183.)

generally not advocated by our center because of the acceptable control rates achieved for many patients with the less invasive phase I surgery.

Technique: The maxillomandibular advancement procedure creates further tension and physical room for the tongue, thus expanding the posterior airway space. Achieving such clearance, especially for long-term improvement, usually necessitates an advancement of 10 to 15 mm of the maxilla and mandible (Figs. 90–7 and 90–8).

Clinical outcomes: In 1989, we reported on 25 patients who underwent MMO for SDB. The mean RDI preoperatively was 67.8, the LSAT was 65.9%, and the number of SaO_2 events below 90% was 276. Postoperatively, the mean RDI was 9.3, the LSAT was 87.2%, and the number of SaO_2 events below 90% was 12.6.[53] The cure rate for these 25 patients, as well as for a subsequent larger group ($n = 91$), was greater than 90%.[35] Long-term follow-up of a group of our patients who underwent MMO ($n = 40$) at a mean of 50.7 months (range, 12 to 146 months) showed 36 of 40 (90%) with long-term control.[54] In 1990, we reported[55] on 30 consecutive patients who underwent maxillofacial surgery and who had previously been users of nasal CPAP. There were no statistical differences between the preoperative PSG parameters and the same PSG findings after surgical intervention. Studies by other centers using MMO (bi-maxillary surgery) for the treatment of SDB are combined with our reports and are listed in chronologic order in Table 90–4.[35,41,53,56-58]

Adverse Effects of Phases I and II

As seen at our center, adverse effects associated with the genioglossus advancement and hyoid suspension, although minimal, may include infection (less than 2%), need for root

Figure 90–8. This patient has undergone phase I and phase II upper airway reconstruction (UAR). Note the improvement of the posterior airway space (PAS).

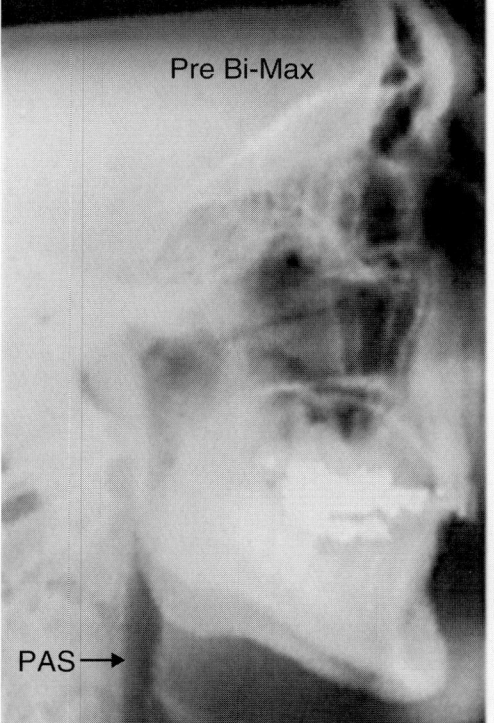

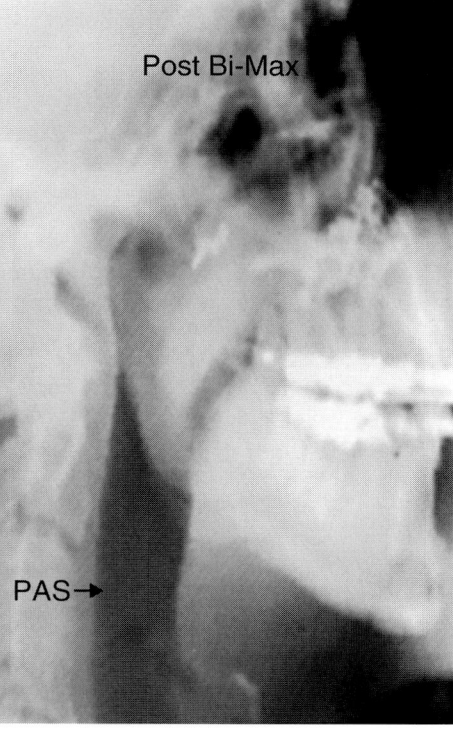

Table 90–4. Bi-maxillary Advancement*: Clinical Outcomes

Date	Authors (ref.)	N	Cure or Responder Rate (%)
1989	Riley et al. (53)	25	>90
1989	Waite et al. (56)	23	65
1993	Riley et al. (35)	91	>90
1997	Hochban et al. (57)	38	>95
1999	Prinsell (58)	50	100
2002	Bettega et al. (41)	20	75

*Often referred to as maxillary and mandibular osteotomy (MMO).

canal therapy (less than 1%), permanent tooth anesthesia (less than 6%), seroma (less than 2%), mandibular fracture (0%), and aspiration (0%). Maxillomandibular advancement osteotomy may have similar adverse consequences. We have experienced no significant episodes of bleeding or infection. Paresthesias or anesthesia of the lip or chin area seldom lasts more than 6 to 12 months, if it occurs at all. There has been some skeletal relapse, with 15% of the patients developing a malocclusion. The severity is limited and it is not unusual to see minor dental interferences that may require occlusal equilibration or orthodontic follow-up. On very rare occasions, a revision surgical procedure may be necessary.

TREATMENT ALTERNATIVES FOR TONGUE BASE OBSTRUCTION

Thus far, we have focused on our experience and that of others over the past 20 years in the surgical management of SDB. Several alternative methodologies are also relevant. Previously used therapies such as laser midline glossectomy and lingualplasty or partial glossectomy are now seldom used because of their inherent invasiveness. In addition, there is the relatively noninvasive alternative of TCRF for control of upper airway obstruction.

Laser Midline Glossectomy and Lingualplasty

The removal of the center part of the tongue base using a laser evaporation technique was described by Woodson and Fugita along with lingualplasty.[59] This procedure was an alternative to skeletal surgery and their results were equivalent or slightly better to our phase I GAHMS surgery.

Clinical outcomes: Woodson and Fugita reported a 77% responder rate in their series using criteria of an RDI of less than or equal to 20 and at least a 50% decrease in the RDI. At times, a protective tracheotomy and an extended hospital stay were required. In addition, postoperative bleeding was experienced (25%). Regardless of these drawbacks, the use of the laser for tongue reduction was very innovative.

Surgical Tongue Resection

Tongue reduction surgery (in various configurations) has been used in the past to treat macroglossia such as is seen in patients with Down syndrome. Its use in SDB has been limited because of morbidity. In 1992, two centers in Norway reported tongue reduction procedures in a series that combined a modified UPPP with base of tongue resection.[60-62] Objective data was limited. However, the procedures were aggressive for this period (1987-1992).

Clinical outcomes: In 1997, Mickelson and Rosenthal[63] published their experience in 12 patients who had surgical midline glossectomy combined with an epiglottidectomy for obstructive sleep apnea syndrome. Three patients (25%) responded to treatment using as a criterion an RDI of below 20 for cure or responder rate.

Chabolle et al.[64] described an extra oral incision through the neck (transpharyngeal exposure) for tongue base reduction in patients with severe SDB. A hyoidepiglottoplasty (suspension of the hyoid with sutures to the anterior inferior mandible) was included with the tongue base resection. Chabolle's group reported a greater than 80% success rate in this study using a postoperative RDI of less than 20 events per hour and a reduction of the preoperative RDI of greater than 50%. Unfortunately, most of these procedures have not caught on, because the patients tend to be reluctant to have this type of tongue surgery, and because not all surgeons have the desire or skill to undertake this form of management.

New Technology: Temperature-Controlled Radiofrequency

The advent of RF tissue ablation and subsequent reduction has been studied extensively in many medical and surgical specialties. RF has been employed for precise tissue ablation in conditions affecting vital organs such as the central nervous system, where accurate ablation of the abnormal tissue is mandatory and excess ablation is dangerous. In cardiology, RF is used for ablation of aberrant pathways in Wolfe-Parkinson-White syndrome.[65] Additionally, it is used in the treatment of patients with symptomatic benign prostatic hyperplasia with excellent efficacy through transurethral needle ablation.[66] Until recently, however, it had not been used in the delicate tissues of the upper airway. The advantages of RF over electrocautery and laser energy surgery reside in its precision in ablating tissues and in the ease of control of operation. With RF, the temperatures of the targeted tissue remain within a range of 60° C to 90° C, thus limiting heat dissipation and damage to adjacent tissue. Electrocautery and laser temperatures are significantly higher (750° C to 900° C), which results in significant heat propagation beyond the therapeutic need. The lower RF temperatures allow a more accurate, minimally invasive, and less morbid procedure without compromising treatment efficacy.

Animal Model

We investigated the application of TCRF technology in a series of prospective studies to treat the soft tissues of the upper airway. The goal of these investigations was to evaluate the feasibility, efficacy, and safety of TCRF for the purpose of later determining its clinical applications in SDB. The initial studies were performed in a porcine model (tongue) to establish parameters of TCRF energy to the tongue base (later studies were performed in humans [palate, nose, and tongue]). The investigation used histologic and volumetric analyses to establish tissue response, healing, and outcomes. RF energy was delivered by a custom-fabricated needle electrode with two thermocouples energized by a TCRF generator.[67]

Clinical outcomes: Histologic assessments done serially over time (1 hour through 3 weeks) showed a well-circumscribed lesion with a healing progression, similar to that of a healing myocardial infarction, and no peripheral damage to nerves. Volumetric analysis documented a very mild initial edematous response (6%), which promptly tapered and resolved at 24 to 48 hours. Ten days after TCRF, there was a 23% volume reduction documented using implanted micro-ultrasonic crystals that transmitted data to a special software program for three-dimensional analyses of volumetric changes.

Human TCRF Studies

TREATMENT OF THE PALATE

Subsequent to the animal studies, TCRF technology was applied to the human palate.[28] This prospective nonrandomized investigation was structured to evaluate pain, swallowing, speech, edematous response, tissue shrinkage, sleep, snoring, and safety after RF treatment to the palate in 22 subjects with snoring or UARS. PSG, radiographic imaging, and infrared thermography, along with questionnaires and visual analogue scales, were used to evaluate the effects of TCRF treatment to the palate. RF was delivered to the submucosa of the palate with a custom-fabricated electrode. Reduction of snoring scores determined the endpoint of the study.

Clinical outcomes: Neither speech nor swallowing was adversely affected. Pain was of short duration (1 to 5 days) and was controlled with acetaminophen. There were no infections. Although there was edema at 24 to 48 hours, there was no clinical airway compromise. PSG data showed improvement in esophageal pressure measurements in terms of the mean nadir and the 95th percentile nadir ($P = .031$ and $P = .001$, respectively), as well as in terms of the mean sleep efficiency index ($P = .002$). Radiographic imaging showed longitudinal shrinkage of the mid palate with a mean of 5.5 ± 3.7 mm ($P < .0001$). Subjective snoring scores fell by a mean of 77% (8.3 ± 1.8 to 1.9 ± 1.7; $P = .0001$), accompanied by improved mean scores on the Epworth Sleepiness Scale (8.5 ± 4.4 to 5.2 ± 3.3; $P = .0001$).

TREATMENT OF THE TURBINATES

TCRF to treat hypertrophied turbinates was studied in subjects with nasal obstruction as is commonly seen in SDB, especially in patients on nasal CPAP.[68] In a nonrandomized prospective study, 22 consecutive patients with nasal obstruction and associated inferior turbinate hypertrophy, refractory to medical therapy, were evaluated for TCRF. Clinical examinations, patient questionnaires, and visual analogue scales were utilized to assess treatment outcomes.

Clinical outcomes: No adverse effects, such as bleeding, crusting, dryness, infection, adhesion, or a worsening of obstruction, were encountered. Mild edema was noted in all patients, but it was of short duration (24 to 48 hours) and did not interfere with nightly use of CPAP. Posttreatment discomfort was well controlled with acetaminophen. Visual analogue scales of pain, degree and frequency of obstruction, snoring, and patient satisfaction were used as outcome measures. At 8 weeks after treatment, subjective nasal breathing improved in 21 of 22 patients, with a 58.5% reduction in severity and a 56.5% decrease in the frequency of nasal obstruction.

TREATMENT OF THE TONGUE

Eighteen patients with SDB entered and completed the study investigating the feasibility, safety, and efficacy of TCRF applied to the tongue base.[69] An RF electrode delivered energy to the subsurface tongue base using only local anesthetic. TCRF treatments at 4-week intervals were given for a mean total energy of 8490 joules per patient. PSG, quantitative speech and swallowing studies, questionnaires, and visual analogue scales were used to assess outcomes. MRI of the upper airway (posterior airway space and tongue) was performed prior to TCRF treatment, at 48 to 72 hours after treatment, and again at the end of the treatment protocol (12 weeks after the last treatment). These studies assessed the edematous response to treatment as well as tongue volume changes.

Clinical outcomes: The mean pretreatment RDI was 39.6, with a mean LSAT of 81.9%. The mean posttreatment RDI was 17.8, with a mean SaO_2 nadir of 88.3%. Weight increased slightly; speech and swallowing did not change. Questionnaires and visual analogue scale scores showed improvement in study variables. Tongue volume was reduced by a mean of 17%. Oral hydrocodone controlled pain for 3 to 4 days on an as-needed basis. The one infection seen resolved promptly with incision, drainage, and antibiotics. Long-term follow-up showed some relapse but persistent improvement.[70]

Summary of Temperature-Controlled Radiofrequency

TCRF treatment at the *nasal level* has shown a positive treatment effect for turbinate hypertrophy, especially in patients who are struggling with this problem during use of CPAP. This was reported in a prospective, randomized, double-blind, placebo-controlled study on TCRF turbinate reduction and CPAP usage.[18] Additional studies support the use of RF technology in turbinate hypertrophy.[71-75]

TCRF treatment at the *pharyngeal level* also showed positive results when used for simple snoring.[76-80] TCRF use in the palate for primary treatment of SDB obstruction is probably limited because of the mass of excess tissue usually encountered. However, Blumen et al.[81] reported on 29 patients with mild to moderate SDB who were treated with TCRF for soft palate obstruction. The mean RDI decreased significantly, from 19.1 (range, 10 to 30) to 9.8 events per hour of sleep, with a nonsignificant LSAT of 85.3% to 86.4%. EDS, snoring, and PSG results were remarkably improved.

TCRF treatment at the *hypopharyngeal level* for tongue base obstruction should be done on a case-by-case basis, as the treatment outcomes vary because of the multifactorial findings typical of SDB. A few of these factors include age, health, weight, tongue size, skeletal deficiency, other areas of obstruction, and severity of SDB. Our center and others have reported on the application of RF to the tongue, and, although outcomes vary, encouraging results have been noted.[67,69,70,82-85] We consider tongue base treatment with TCRF to be adjunctive in nature and not usually a primary procedure. Occasional confounding problems with the use of TCRF in SDB include the multiple visits required to safely deliver RF energy. When increased TCRF energy is delivered to reduce the number of treatments, the benefit of the minimal invasiveness of the therapy is defeated. Treatment provided as a single-dose method may result in complications and is less likely to be successful due to the biophysics of energy delivery. Appropriate patient

Table 90–5. Papers on Radiofrequency Technology to Treat Upper Airway Obstruction

Studies (n)	Year	Tongue	Palate	Turbinates	Tonsils	Other	Subjects (n)
1*	1997	1	—	—	—	—	19 (porcine)
2	1998	—	1	1	—	—	44
10	1999	1	4	3	—	2	218
12	2000	2	7	2	—	1	258
15	2001	2	4	3	3	3	413
15	2002	2	8	1	1	3	345
Total Number of Papers							
55	—	8	24	10	4	9	—
Total Number of Human Subjects†							
—	—	187	793	222	76	105	1278

*Index study.

†Some subjects received treatment at more than one location.

Studies performed in 11 countries (United States, France, Norway, Sweden, Finland, Germany, Turkey, Korea, Saudi Arabia, Brazil, and Belgium) and published in peer-reviewed journals.

selection is essential. Furthermore, there is a learning curve for the surgeon, which may not be recognized because of the simplicity of the technique. Finally, after treatment, airway protection protocols must be carefully followed, as the edematous response varies widely between individuals. As the surgeon becomes more familiar with the technology, the limits of the technique, and thus its efficacy and safety, can be improved.

The effort in evaluating RF thus far has been remarkable. From the first report in 1997 through the end of 2002, 55 papers were published in peer-reviewed journals on animal models and humans for the treatment of upper airway obstruction using RF (Table 90–5). This technology has a promising future in the treatment of SDB as long as it is approached with patience and used cautiously.

RISK MANAGEMENT

Although rare, life-threatening complications have been associated with sleep apnea surgery. Fairbanks,[86] on the basis of a national survey, reported 16 fatalities and seven near fatalities from UPPP in the early postoperative period. Respiratory obstruction, secondary to pharmacologic sedation and surgical edema, was the most frequently cited cause. Several authors have cautioned against the use of narcotics in patients with SDB undergoing upper airway or other surgery.[87-90]

In an earlier study, we observed that nasal CPAP protected postoperative patients with SDB from airway obstruction and hypoxemia and could be used in some cases to avoid tracheotomy.[16] Subsequently, we adopted the use of nasal CPAP as a standard whenever possible for all patients undergoing surgery for SDB, and we developed a risk management surgical protocol for patients with SDB. This protocol is frequently updated to provide ongoing improvements in patient safety.

An outcomes review of the risk management protocol was performed on 182 consecutively treated patients with SDB undergoing 210 surgical procedures in 1995.[91] Data examined included the patient's age, sex, weight (BMI), facial skeletal development, coexisting medical problems, complications with anesthetic induction and extubation, postoperative vital signs, medication requirements for all postoperative days, days in the intensive care unit, and total length of hospital stay. The review concluded that patients undergoing surgical reconstruction of the airway for SDB often have coexisting

Box 90–12. Risk Management Protocol

1. Patients with a respiratory disturbance index (RDI) >40 and lowest oxyhemoglobin saturation (LSAT) <80 begin using nasal continuous positive airway pressure (CPAP) at least 2 weeks before surgery and continue with it postoperatively until polysomnography is performed (at 4 to 6 months) to document outcome.

2. Surgeons are present for anesthetic induction and intubation. For potentially difficult airways, a fiberoptic intubation is performed with the patient awake.

3. Patients are extubated when awake in the operating room immediately after surgery.

4. A patient undergoing multiple procedures (e.g., uvulopalatopharyngoplasty and maxillofacial surgery), or a single procedure when there are significant coexisting medical problems (e.g., hypertension, coronary artery disease), is monitored in the intensive care unit (ICU) for the 1st day after surgery and then in the surgical ward. The patient is monitored by oximetry throughout the hospital stay.

5. Patients with nasal CPAP must continue to use CPAP during all periods of sleep after surgery. All other patients are maintained on humidified oxygen (35%) via face tent.

6. Analgesia consists of intravenous morphine sulfate or meperidine HCl in the ICU. IV narcotics are administered by a nurse in small, graduated doses while the respiratory rate is monitored. All nurses caring for patients with sleep-disordered breathing (SDB) are educated about the mechanisms of SDB and the use of narcotics in this population. Patient-controlled analgesia (PCA pump) is not recommended. Intramuscular meperidine HCl and oxycodone elixir are used in the surgical ward. Oral hydrocodone or codeine and acetaminophen are used after discharge.

7. Requirements for discharge include adequate oral intake of fluids, satisfactory pain control, stable or resolving surgical edema, and the use of nasal CPAP if the patient can tolerate it. A fiberoptic nasopharyngoscopy is done on each patient at the bedside to assess the status of the airway prior to discharge. This procedure can reveal significant potential (but asymptomatic at this time) airway compromise that may contribute to an airway problem after discharge.

medical problems (cardiovascular disease being the most significant) that can complicate therapy. A risk management protocol is seen in Box 90–12.

Clinical Pearl

Sleep-disordered breathing is primarily caused by an anatomic collapse of the upper airway during sleep and hence is a surgical problem. Surgical procedures have been developed over the years to manage and control SDB. Not all of these procedures have equivalent outcomes, but there are combinations that offer the same control of SDB as medical management.

REFERENCES

1. Schwab R: Pro: Sleep apnea is an anatomic disorder. Am J Respir Crit Care Med 2003;168:270-273.
2. Kuhlo W, Doll E, Franck MD: Erfolgreiche Behandlung eines Pickwick Syndroms durch eine Dauertrachekanuele. Dtsch Med Wochenschr 1969;94:1286-1290.
3. Dyugovskaya L, Lavie P, Lavie L: Increased adhesion molecules expression and production of reactive oxygen species in leukocytes of sleep apnea patients. Am J Respir Crit Care Med 2002; 165:934-939.
4. Macey P, Henderson L, Macey K, et al: Brain morphology associated with obstructive sleep apnea. Am J Respir Crit Care Med 2002;166:1382-1387.
5. Shepard J, Gefter W, Guilleminault C, et al: Evaluation of the upper airway in patients with obstructive sleep apnea. Sleep 1991;14:361-371.
6. Riley R, Guilleminault C, Powell NB, et al: Palatopharyngoplasty failure, cephalometric roentgenograms, and obstructive sleep apnea. Otolaryngol Head Neck Surg 1985;93:240-244.
7. Rivlin J, Hoffstein V, Kalbfleisch J, et al: Upper airway morphology in patients with idiopathic obstructive sleep apnea. Am Rev Respir Dis 1984;129:355-360.
8. Remmers JE, DeGrott WJ, Sauerland EK, et al: Pathogenesis of upper airway occlusion during sleep. J Appl Physiol 1978;44: 931-938.
9. Schwab RJ, Pasirstein M, Pierson R, et al: Identification of upper airway anatomic risk factors for obstructive sleep apnea with volumetric MRI. Am J Respir Crit Care Med 2003;168:522-530.
10. Shepard JW, Stanson AW, Sheedy PF, et al: Fast-CT evaluation of the upper airway during wakefulness in patients with obstructive sleep apnea. Prog Clin Biol Res 1990;345:273-279.
11. Fujita S: Pharyngeal surgery for obstructive sleep apnea and snoring. In Fairbanks D, Fujita S, Ikematsu T, et al: Snoring and Obstructive Sleep Apnea. New York, Raven Press, 1987, pp 101-128.
12. Sher AE, Thorpy MJ, Shrintzen RJ, et al: Predictive value of Muller maneuver in selection of patient for uvulopalatopharyngoplasty. Laryngoscope 1985;95:1483-1487.
13. Riley R, Guilleminault C, Herran J, Powell N: Cephalometric analyses and flow volume loops in obstructive sleep apnea patients. Sleep 1983;6:304-307.
14. Riley R, Powell N, Guilleminault C: Cephalometric roentgenograms and computerized tomographic scans in obstructive sleep apnea. Sleep 1986;9:514-515.
15. Peppard P, Young T, Palta M, et al: Longitudinal study of moderate weight change and sleep-disordered breathing. JAMA 2000;284:3015-3021.
16. Powell N, Riley R, Guilleminault C: Obstructive sleep apnea, continuous positive airway pressure, and surgery. Otolaryngol Head Neck Surg 1988;99:362-369.

17. Guilleminault C, Mondini S: Need for multi-diagnostic approaches before considering treatment in obstructive sleep apnea. Bull Eur Physiopathol Respir 1983;19:583-589.
18. Powell N, Zonato A, Weaver E, et al: Radiofrequency treatment of turbinate hypertrophy in subjects using continuous positive airway pressure: A randomized, double-blind, placebo-controlled clinical pilot trial. Laryngoscope 2001;111:1783-1790.
19. Ikematsu T: Study of snoring, 4th report: Therapy [in Japanese]. Jpn Otorhinolaryngol 1964;64:434-435.
20. Fujita S, Conway W, Zorick F, et al: Surgical correction of anatomic abnormalities in obstructive sleep apnea syndrome: Uvulopalatopharyngoplasty. Otolaryngol Head Neck Surg 1981;89:923-934.
21. Rojewski TE, Schuller DE, Clark RW, et al: Videoendoscopic determination of the mechanism of obstruction in obstructive sleep apnea. Otolaryngol Head Neck Surg 1984;92:127-131.
22. Rivlin J, Hoffstein V, Kalbfleisch J, et al: Upper airway morphology in patients with idiopathic obstructive sleep apnea. Am Rev Respir Dis 1984;129:355-360.
23. Remmers JE, DeGrott WJ, Sauerland EK, et al: Pathogenesis of upper airway occlusion during sleep. J Appl Physiol 1978;44: 931-938.
24. Fairbanks D: Operative techniques of uvulopalatopharyngoplasty. Otolaryngol Head Neck Surg 1991;2:104-106.
25. Woodson BT, Toohill RJ: Transpalatal advancement pharyngoplasty for obstructive sleep apnea. Laryngoscope 1993;103: 269-276.
26. Powell NB, Riley RW, Guilleminault C, et al: A reversible uvulopalatal flap for snoring and obstructive sleep. Sleep 1996;19: 593-599.
27. Walker RP, Grigg-Damberger MM, Gopalsami C, et al: Laser-assisted uvulopalatoplasty for snoring and obstructive sleep apnea: Results in 170 patients. Laryngoscope 1995;105: 938-943.
28. Powell NB, Riley RW, Troell RJ, et al: Radiofrequency volumetric tissue reduction of the palate in subjects with sleep-disordered breathing. Chest 1998;113:1163-1174.
29. Sher A, Schechtman K, Piccirillo J: An American Sleep Disorders Association review: The efficacy of surgical modifications of the upper airway in adults with obstructive sleep apnea syndrome. Sleep 1996;19:156-177.
30. Terris DJ, Clerk AA, Norbash AM, et al: Characterization of post-operative edema following laser-assisted uvulopalatoplasty using MRI and polysomnography: Implication for the outpatient treatment of obstructive sleep apnea syndrome. Laryngoscope 1996; 106:124-128.
31. Finkelstein Y, Stein G, Ophir D, et al: Laser-assisted uvulopalatoplasty for the management of obstructive sleep apnea. Arch Otolaryngol Head Neck Surg 2002;128:429-434.
32. Riley R, Guilleminault C, Powell N, et al: Mandibular osteotomy and hyoid bone advancement for obstructive sleep apnea: A case report. Sleep 1984;7:79-82.
33. Riley R, Powell N, Guilleminault C: Inferior sagittal osteotomy of the mandible with hyoid myotomy-suspension: A new procedure for obstructive sleep apnea. Otolaryngol Head Neck Surg 1986;94:589-593.
34. Riley RW, Powell NB, Guilleminault C: Inferior mandibular osteotomy and hyoid myotomy suspension for obstructive sleep apnea: A review of 55 patients. J Oral Maxillofac Surg 1989; 47:159-164.
35. Riley RW, Powell NB, Guilleminault C: Obstructive sleep apnea syndrome: A review of 306 consecutively treated surgical patients. Otolaryngol Head Neck Surg 1993;108:117-125.
36. Johnson, NT, Chinn J: Uvulopalatopharyngoplasty and inferior sagittal mandibular osteotomy with genioglossus advancement for treatment of obstructive sleep apnea. Chest 1994;105:278.
37. Ramirez SG, Loube DI: Inferior sagittal osteotomy with hyoid bone suspension for obese patients with sleep apnea. Arch Otolaryngol Head Neck Surg 1996;122:953.

38. Yoa M, Utley D, Terris D: Cephalometric parameters after multi-level pharyngeal surgery for patients with obstructive sleep apnea. Laryngoscope 1998;108:789-795.

39. Lee N, Givens C, Wilson J, et al: Staged surgical treatment of obstructive sleep apnea syndrome: A review of 35 patients. J Oral Maxillofac Surg 1999;57:382-385.

40. Wagner I, Coiffier T, Sequert C, et al: Surgical treatment of severe sleep apnea syndrome by maxillomandibular advancing or mental transposition. Ann Otolaryngol Chir Cervicofac 2000;117:137-146.

41. Bettega G, Pépin J, Veale D, et al: Obstructive sleep apnea syndrome: Fifty-one consecutive patients treated by maxillofacial surgery. Am J Crit Care Med 2000;162:641-649.

42. Vilaseca I, Morello A, Montserrat J, et al: Usefulness of uvulopalatopharyngoplasty with genioglossus and hyoid advancement in the treatment of obstructive sleep apnea. Arch Otolaryngol Head Neck Surg 2002;128:435-440.

43. Neruntarat C: Genioglossus advancement and hyoid myotomy under local anesthesia. Otolaryngol Head Neck Surg 2003;129:85-91.

44. Van de Graaff W, Gottfried S, Mitra J, et al: Respiratory function of hyoid muscles and hyoid arch. J Appl Physiol 1984;57:197-204.

45. Kaya N: Sectioning the hyoid bone as a therapeutic approach for obstructive sleep apnea. Sleep 1984;7:77-78.

46. Patton TJ, Thawley SE, Water RC, et al: Expansion hyoid-plasty: A potential surgical procedure designed for selected patients with obstructive sleep apnea syndrome—Experimental canine results. Laryngoscope 1983;93:1387-1396.

47. Riley RW, Powell NB, Guilleminault C: Obstructive sleep apnea and the hyoid: A revised surgical procedure. Otolaryngol Head Neck Surg 1994;111:717-721.

48. Riley R, Powell N, Li K, et al: An adjunctive method of radiofrequency volumetric tissue reduction of the tongue for OSAS. Otolaryngol Head Neck Surg 2003;129:37-42.

49. Kuo PC, West RA, Bloomquist DS, et al: The effect of mandibular osteotomy in three patients with hypersomnia and sleep apnea. Oral Surg Oral Med Oral Pathol 1979;48:385-392.

50. Bear SE, Priest JH: Sleep apnea syndrome: Correction with surgical advancement of the mandible. J Oral Surg 1980;38:543-549.

51. Powell N, Guilleminault C, Riley R, et al: Mandibular advancement and obstructive sleep apnea syndrome. Bull Eur Physiopathol Respir 1983;19:607-610.

52. Guilleminault C, Riley R, Powell N: Sleep apnea in normal subjects following mandibular osteotomy with retrusion. Chest 1985;88:776-778.

53. Riley R, Powell N, Guilleminault C: Maxillofacial surgery and obstructive sleep apnea: A review of 80 patients. Otolaryngol Head Neck Surg 1989;101:353-361.

54. Riley R, Powell N, Li K, et al: Surgery and obstructive sleep apnea: Long-term clinical outcomes. Otolaryngol Head Neck Surg 2000;122:415-421.

55. Riley R, Powell N, Guilleminault C: Maxillofacial surgery and nasal CPAP: A comparison of treatment for obstructive sleep apnea syndrome. Chest 1990;98:1421-1425.

56. Waite PD, Wooten V, Lachner J, et al: Maxillomandibular advancement surgery in 23 patients with obstructive sleep apnea syndrome. J Oral Maxillofac Surg 1989;47:1256.

57. Hochban W, Conradt R, Brandenburg U, et al: Surgical maxillofacial treatment of obstructive sleep apnea. Plast Reconstr Surg 1995;99:619.

58. Prinsell J: Maxillomandibular advancement surgery in a site-specific treatment approach for obstructive sleep apnea in 50 consecutive patients. Chest 1999;116:1519-1529.

59. Woodson BT, Fujita S: Clinical experience with lingualplasty as part of the treatment of severe obstructive sleep apnea. Otolaryngol Head Neck Surg 1992;107:40.

60. Djupesland G, Lyberg T, Krogstad O: Cephalometric analysis and surgical treatment of patients with obstructive sleep apnea syndrome. Acta Otolaryngol 1987;103:551-557.

61. Miljeteig H, Tvinnereim M: Uvulopalatopharyngoplasty (UPPGP) in the treatment of the obstructive sleep apnea syndrome. Acta Otolaryngol 1992;492(Suppl):86-89.

62. Faye-Lund H, Djupesland G, Lyberg T: Glossopexia: Evaluation of a new surgical method for treating obstructive sleep apnea syndrome. Acta Otolaryngol 1992;492(Suppl):46-49.

63. Mickleson S, Rosenthal L: Midline glossectomy and epiglottidectomy for obstructive sleep apnea syndrome. Laryngoscope 1997;107:614-619.

64. Chabolle F, Wagner I, Blumen MB, et al: Tongue base reduction with hyoepiglottoplasty: A treatment for severe obstructive sleep apnea. Laryngoscope 1999;1109:1273-1280.

65. Jackman WM, Wang XZ, Friday KJ, et al: Catheter ablation of accessory atrioventricular pathways (Wolff-Parkinson-White syndrome) by radiofrequency current. N Engl J Med 1991;324:1605-1611.

66. Issa M, Oesterling J: Transurethral needle ablation (TUNA): An overview of radiofrequency thermal therapy for the treatment of benign prostatic hyperplasia. Curr Opin Urol 1996;6:20-27.

67. Powell NB, Riley RW, Troell RJ, et al: Radiofrequency volumetric reduction of the tongue: A porcine pilot study for the treatment of obstructive sleep apnea syndrome. Chest 1997;111:1348-1355.

68. Li K, Powell N, Riley R, et al: Radiofrequency volumetric tissue reduction for treatment of turbinate hypertrophy: A pilot study. Otolaryngol Head Neck Surg 1998;119:569-573.

69. Powell N, Riley R, Guilleminault C: Radiofrequency tongue base reduction in sleep-disordered breathing: A pilot study. Otolaryngol Head Neck Surg 1999;120:656-664.

70. Li K, Powell N, Riley R, et al: Temperature-controlled radiofrequency tongue base reduction for sleep-disordered breathing: Long-term outcomes. Otolaryngol Head Neck Surg 2002;127:230-234.

71. Coste A, Yona L, Blumen M, et al: Radiofrequency is a safe and effective treatment of turbinate hypertrophy. Laryngoscope 2001;111:894-899.

72. Smith T, Correa A, Kuo T, et al: Radiofrequency tissue ablation of the inferior turbinates using a thermocouple feedback electrode. Laryngoscope 1999;109:1760-1765.

73. Utley D, Goode R, Hakim I: Radiofrequency energy tissue ablation for the treatment of nasal obstruction secondary to turbinate hypertrophy. Laryngoscope 1999;109:683-686.

74. Rhee C, Kim D, Won T, et al: Changes of nasal function after temperature-controlled radiofrequency tissue volume reduction for the turbinate. Laryngoscope 2001;111:153-158.

75. Seeger J, Zenev E, Gundlach P, et al: Bipolar radiofrequency-induced thermotherapy of turbinate hypertrophy: Pilot study and 20 months' follow-up. Laryngoscope 2003;113:130-135.

76. Back L, Tervahartiala P, Piilonen A, et al: Bipolar radiofrequency thermal ablation of the soft palate in habitual snorers without significant desaturations assessed by magnetic resonance imaging. Am J Respir Crit Care Med 2002;166:865-871.

77. Wedman J, Miljeteig H: Treatment of simple snoring using radio waves for ablation of uvula and soft palate: A day-case surgery procedure. Laryngoscope 2002;112:1256-1259.

78. Johnson J, Pollack G, Wagner R: Transoral radiofrequency treatment of snoring. Otolaryngol Head Neck Surg 2002;127:235-237.

79. Attal P, Popot B, Le Pajolec C, et al: Short term evaluation of a new treatment method for primary snoring: Radiofrequency energy. Ann Otolaryngol Chir Cervicofac 2000;117:259-265.

80. Blumen M, Dahan S, Wagner I, et al: Radiofrequency versus LAUP for the treatment of snoring. Otolaryngol Head Neck Surg 2002;126:67-73.

81. Blumen M, Dahan S, Fleury B, et al: Radiofrequency ablation for the treatment of mild to moderate obstructive sleep apnea. Laryngoscope 2002;112:2086-2092.

82. Woodson B, Nelson L, Mickelson S, et al: A multi-institutional study of radiofrequency volumetric tissue reduction for OSAS. Otolaryngol Head Neck Surg 2001;125:303-311.

83. Stuck B, Maurer J, Hormann K: Tongue base reduction with radiofrequency tissue ablation: Preliminary results after two treatment sessions. Sleep Breath 2000;4:155-162.

84. Nelson L: Combined temperature-controlled radiofrequency tongue reduction and UPPP in apnea surgery. Ear Nose Throat J 2001;80:640-644.

85. Stuck B, Maurer J, Verse T, et al: Tongue base reduction with temperature-controlled radiofrequency volumetric tissue reduction for treatment of obstructive sleep apnea syndrome. Acta Otolaryngol 2002;122:531-536.

86. Fairbanks D: Uvulopalatopharyngoplasty complications and avoidance strategies. Otolaryngol Head Neck Surg 1990;102: 239-245.

87. Esclamado RM, Glenn MG, McCulloch TM, et al: Perioperative complications and risk factors in the surgical treatment of obstructive sleep apnea syndrome. Laryngoscope 1989;99: 1125-1129.

88. Gabrielczyk MR: Acute airway obstruction after uvulopalatopharyngoplasty for obstructive sleep apnea syndrome. Anesthesiology 1988;69:941-943.

89. Kravath RE, Pollak CP, Borowiecki B, et al: Obstructive sleep apnea and death associated with surgical correction of velopharyngeal incompetence. J Pediatr 1980;96:645-648.

90. den Herder C, Schmeck J, Appelboom DJ, et al: Risks of general anaesthesia in people with obstructive sleep apnoea. BMJ 2004; 329:955-959.

91. Riley RW, Powell NB, Guilleminault C, et al: Obstructive sleep apnea surgery: Risk management and complications. Otolaryngol Head Neck Surg 1997;117:648-652.

Oral Appliances for Sleep-Disordered Breathing

Kathleen A. Ferguson

Alan A. Lowe

ABSTRACT

Oral appliances (OAs) are an established treatment option for snoring and mild obstructive sleep apnea (OSA). OA therapy is a simple, reversible approach to treatment. OAs appear to work as a result of an increase in airway space, the provision of a stable anterior position of the mandible, advancement of the tongue or soft palate, and possibly a change in upper airway muscle activity. Recent randomized, controlled trials of OA therapy have shown a good level of effectiveness in patients with mild to moderate OSA and effectiveness in some patients with more severe OSA. In most of the studies comparing OAs with continuous positive airway pressure (CPAP), patients exhibited a preference for the OA even though CPAP lowered the apnea-hypopnea index more effectively. With evidence of effectiveness from randomized, controlled trials, it is now reasonable to expand the indications for first-line therapy with an OA to the treatment of patients with moderate OSA.

Most patients report improvements in sleep quality and excessive daytime sleepiness with OA therapy, and these devices are generally well tolerated. Short-term side effects are usually minor and are related to excessive salivation, jaw and tooth discomfort, and occasionally joint discomfort. These symptoms usually improve over time. Significant temporomandibular joint (TMJ) complications are rare, but occlusal changes are more common than previously thought.

OA therapy is a unique opportunity for dentists and physicians to work together to select the ideal patients for this form of treatment. Each plays a crucial role in providing the patient with optimal care. With collaboration and good communication between the dentist and the sleep clinician, many patients with snoring or OSA can be treated effectively with OAs.

Oral appliances (OAs) are an established treatment option for simple snoring and mild obstructive sleep apnea (OSA). There are two main appliance types in common clinical use—devices that advance the tongue and devices that advance the mandible during sleep. In 1995, the American Academy of Sleep Medicine published guidelines about the use of OA therapy in the treatment of OSA.[1] These guidelines stated that OAs are indicated as first-line therapy in patients with simple snoring and mild OSA and second-line therapy for moderate to severe OSA when other therapies have failed. At the time the guidelines were published, the available studies were uncontrolled, small, mostly retrospective case series. Since then, many prospective studies have been published, including randomized, controlled clinical trials with comparisons with continuous positive airway pressure (CPAP), other appliances, surgery, and placebo.[2-17] With evidence of effectiveness from randomized, controlled trials, it is now reasonable to expand the indications for first-line therapy with an OA to the treatment of patients with moderate OSA.

This chapter reviews the available data about the mechanism of action and the evidence for using OA therapy. The role of the physician and dentist is discussed. It also reviews indications for, side effects and complications of, and predictors of outcome of OA therapy.

MECHANISM OF ACTION

Current evidence suggests that the pathogenesis of OSA involves a combination of reduced upper airway size and altered upper airway muscle activity. OAs may improve upper airway patency during sleep by enlarging the upper airway or by decreasing upper airway collapsibility (e.g., improving upper airway muscle tone). The effects of OAs on upper airway size vary between studies, and these differences are likely due to the different imaging techniques used, the study methods (i.e., evaluation during wakefulness versus during sleep), differences with regard to the subject's body position (i.e., supine versus upright), and different types of appliances and degrees of protrusion. Most imaging studies suggest that OAs have a direct effect on mandibular posture and thereby increase airway size. The effects on upper airway size are summarized in Table 91–1. Effects on upper airway muscles have been less well studied.

Mandibular repositioning appliances (MRA) cover the upper and lower teeth and hold the mandible in a forward position. An example of the effect of an MRA on airway size is illustrated in Figure 91–1. Tongue-advancing appliances hold the tongue in a forward position without mandibular advancement. Some tongue-advancing appliances like the tongue-retaining device (TRD) hold the tongue forward in a bulb using suction (Fig. 91–2).

Simple anterior movement of the tongue or mandible during wakefulness can increase cross-sectional airway size at all levels in subjects with and without OSA.[18] Passive mandibular advancement during general anesthesia (done by a jaw thrust maneuver) stabilizes the upper airway by increasing airway size in both the retropalatal and retroglossal area and by reducing upper airway closing pressure (the level of intraluminal pressure at which closure occurs).[19] Mandibular advancement with an MRA reduces closing pressure (e.g., makes it more negative) and therefore decreases upper airway collapsibility.[20]

Effects of Mandibular and Tongue Advancement on Upper Airway Muscle Tone

TRDs affect genioglossus muscle activity in patients with OSA (awake or asleep),[21,22] but effects of the TRD on other upper

Table 91–1. **Effect of Mandibular Repositioning Appliances on Upper Airway Size**

Imaging Modality	Image Obtained	Body Position	Dimension	Effect	References
Lateral cephalometry	Awake	Upright	Posterior airway space	Increased	29,67
	Awake	Upright	Posterior airway space	Unchanged	68
	Awake	Upright	Retropalatal airway space	Increased	69
	Awake	Upright	Tongue posture	Flattened	69,70
	Awake	Upright	Oropharynx size	Increased	70
	Awake	Upright	Hypopharynx size	Increased	71
	Awake	Supine	Velopharynx size	Increased	72
			Oropharynx size	Unchanged	
	Awake	Supine	Sagittal cross-sectional area of the pharynx	Increased	60
	Awake	Upright	Mandibular plane to hyoid distance	Decreased	67,69,70
	Awake	Supine	Mandibular plane to hyoid distance	Decreased	60
Computed tomography	Awake	Supine	Pharyngeal cross-sectional airway size	Increased	73
Magnetic resonance imaging	Asleep	Supine	Velopharynx size	Increased	67
	Awake	Supine	Oropharynx size	Increased	74
			Hypopharynx size	Increased	
Videoendoscopy	Awake	Supine	Velopharynx size	Increased	75

airway muscles have not been evaluated. A TRD worn during sleep reduced the apnea-hypopnea index (AHI),[22] and when the TRD was worn without tongue advancement (no bulb), the AHI decreased and peak genioglossus activity, measured just before airway opening, increased. The mechanism for this effect and its significance is not certain, but increased genioglossus tone may contribute to upper airway reopening.

A study using an MRA found that upper airway muscle tone increased with an MRA except in the post-apnea period, when genioglossus tone was lower.[23] Another study also found augmentation of genioglossus tone with mandibular advancement.[24] These studies suggest that activation of the upper airway muscles by an MRA may contribute to airway patency. In a more recent, placebo-controlled trial the presence

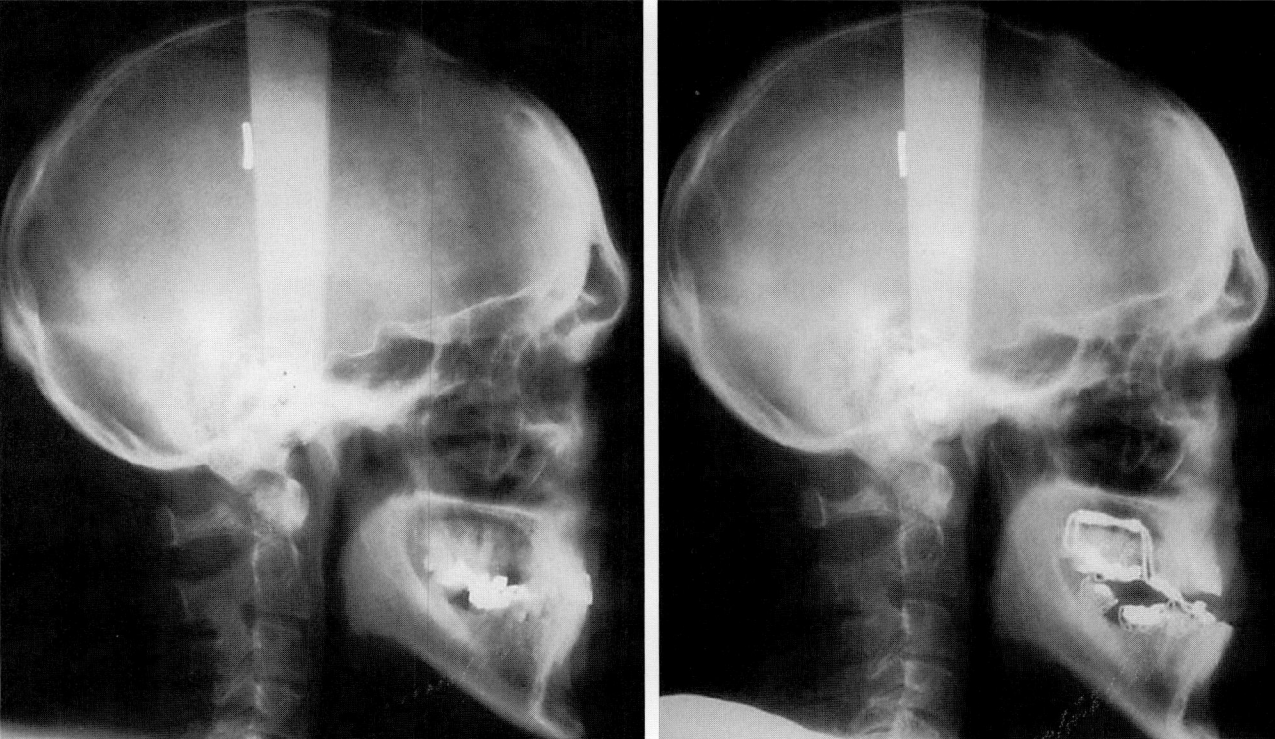

Figure 91–1. Lateral cephalograms of a patient pretreatment (*left*) and while wearing a Klearway mandibular repositioning appliance (*right*).

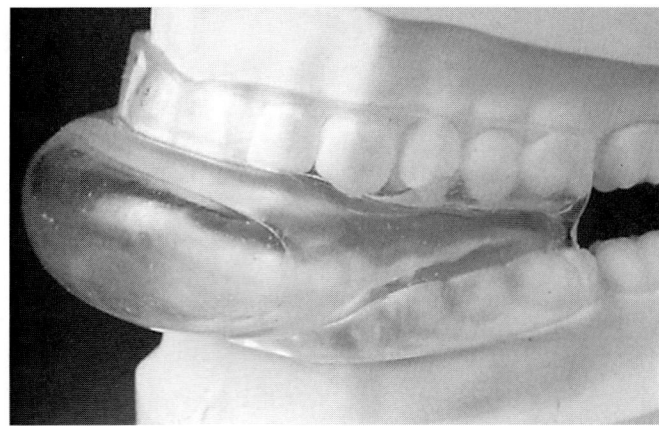

Figure 91–2. A tongue-retaining device. (Photograph courtesy of Dr. Alan Lowe, University of British Columbia, Vancouver, British Columbia, Canada.)

of an intraoral device that did not advance the mandible had no impact on the AHI or on oxygen levels.[7] This study suggests that effects on upper airway tone are insufficient to reduce apnea and that mandibular advancement is required for the appliance to improve OSA.

CLINICAL PROTOCOL FOR ORAL APPLIANCE THERAPY

Successful OA therapy requires that a physician and dentist work together to manage the patient optimally. OSA and snoring are medical conditions treated with a dental therapy. Guidelines from the American Academy of Sleep Medicine[1] recommend a protocol for the management of OA therapy in the treatment of snoring and OSA and define the roles of the physician and dentist in the provision of this therapy.

Pretreatment Assessment

Before treating either snoring or OSA with an OA, an assessment by a sleep clinician is required. The sleep clinician must determine if the patient is a good medical candidate for OA therapy. An overnight diagnostic assessment in accordance with local practice is conducted before OA therapy. If treatment with an OA is medically indicated, the clinician provides the dentist with a written referral and a copy of the diagnostic report. The sleep clinician can do a preliminary screen for dental suitability for oral appliance therapy by asking the patient if he or she wears dentures, is missing teeth, or has a history of periodontal disease or TMJ problems.

The dentist determines whether or not the patient is a good dental candidate for an MRA. The evaluation includes a medical and dental history and a complete intraoral examination. This includes a soft tissue, periodontal, TMJ, and occlusal assessment. The occlusion is assessed and the teeth and restorations are examined. The dentist determines if the patient has sufficient number of healthy teeth (usually eight teeth in the upper and in the lower jaw) to wear an MRA (the device is held in place by the teeth). The patient should have the ability to protrude the mandible forward more than 5 mm in order to achieve a therapeutic result. Full upper and lower dentures likely preclude the use of an MRA, but some edentulous

patients may respond to a TRD. Dental records are obtained and may include dental radiographs and a panoramic or full-mouth survey. Some practitioners obtain a cephalogram. The dentist obtains informed consent about the risks and benefits of OA therapy. A discussion about potential long-term side effects and complications should take place as part of the informed consent process.

Moderate to severe TMJ problems, bruxism, an inadequate protrusive range, and advanced periodontal disease are all relative contraindications to MRA use. Thirty-four of 100 patients consecutively assessed by oral and maxillofacial surgeons were found to have contraindications to therapy and 16% to have dental issues that would require close follow-up.[25] Not all TMJ problems are contraindications to MRA therapy—mild problems may be lessened by a forward jaw position. TRDs do not necessarily require teeth and do not require mandibular protrusion. Patients who are claustrophobic with CPAP may also be claustrophobic with an appliance.

Appliance Selection and Management

Types of Oral Appliances

The dentist determines the most appropriate type of appliance to use. There are two main appliance groups in common clinical use—tongue-repositioning devices and MRAs (see Figs. 91–2 through 91–6). The dentist chooses which type of appliance to use. Tongue-repositioning devices, such as the TRD, are often used in patients with large tongues, an inadequate protrusive range, or insufficient teeth to use an MRA. Information about OAs that have received 510k market clearance from the U.S. Food and Drug Administration for the treatment of snoring or OSA is available at the Academy of Dental Sleep Medicine website (http://www.dentalsleepmed.org/fda.htm). Soft palate lifters are used rarely for snoring or OSA. Because this device is poorly tolerated and is ineffective in the treatment of snoring[16] and OSA,[26] it is not discussed.

Appliance Selection, Fabrication, Insertion, and Management

An appliance may be "off the shelf" or be custom, may provide partial or full occlusal coverage, may be made of soft or hard materials, and may be rigid or allow jaw movement. Some appliances are made of temperature-sensitive acrylic (Fig. 91–3). These appliances become pliable in hot water and when they cool to mouth temperature they firmly grip the teeth and are very retentive. Bruxism is common in patients with OSA[27] and may be a contraindication to MRA therapy. Patients who experience jaw discomfort after wearing a rigid MRA may benefit from using an appliance that allows lateral and vertical jaw movement. A small amount of movement may improve comfort for patients with bruxism who use an MRA. Plaster models are obtained as appropriate for the specific OA. Boil-and-bite appliances are fit to the patient in the office. Custom appliances may be fabricated by the dentist or by the dental laboratory.

Appliances may be nonadjustable and worn in one position or be partly adjustable (more than one possible preset position). Newer appliances tend to be fully adjustable. This allows the mandible to be incrementally advanced to obtain the therapeutic position. The initial position is usually set between 50% and 75% of maximum mandibular protrusion.

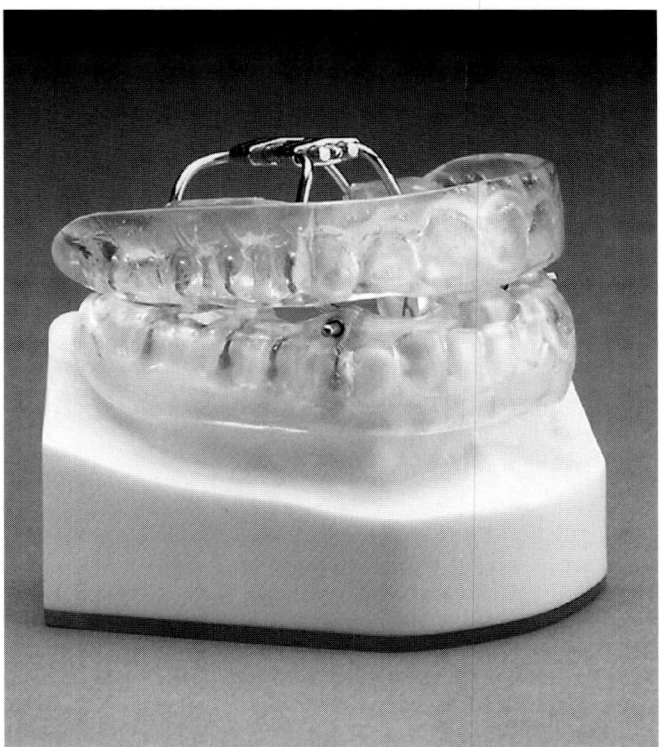

Figure 91–3. The Klearway adjustable oral appliance. (Courtesy of Great Lakes Orthodontics, Ltd., Tonawanda, NY.)

Patients tolerate the initial amount of protrusion differently and sometimes need to start at less than 50% of maximum. Appliances with a single jaw position can usually be remade if the initial position is too far forward and uncomfortable or if it is not forward enough to provide benefit.

A typical titration protocol would consist of gradual forward adjustments of the MRA to a position associated with relief of snoring and other symptoms but without significant side effects. Patients vary considerably in the speed of advancement during titration of an MRA and in how far forward they can comfortably go in terms of the amount of protrusion achieved. Gradual forward titration of the mandible by the patient without remaking the MRA each time is an advantage of adjustable MRAs. If an optimal position is not obtained (e.g., persistent snoring), the MRA is set at the maximum forward position that does not produce significant side effects.

TRDs are custom made for the patient. The patient advances the tongue into the bulb while squeezing the bulb to create negative suction. The patient experiments with the amount of forward positioning of the tongue that is required to decrease snoring and symptoms. Denture adhesive powder may be placed into the bulb to enhance retention of the tongue during sleep.

The dentist teaches the patient how to use the appliance, to care for it, to adjust it (if that is a feature of the design), and what side effects and complications to look for. The appliance may need repairs, modification, further advancement, or even redesign or replacement with a different device if side effects develop or if there is an inadequate subjective or objective improvement. Patient compliance should be monitored at each visit. Once a satisfactory improvement in symptoms has

taken place, the patient is referred back to the attending physician for a clinical assessment or repeat overnight assessment. Medical follow-up is necessary to evaluate treatment response and to assess for recurrence of OSA. It is recommended that follow-up overnight studies be performed to verify the improvement in apnea, oxygenation, and sleep fragmentation by the OA.[1] This recommendation is supported by the evidence that some patients have an increase in AHI with OA treatment.[3,4,28-30] Regular follow-up visits are continued as long as the patient is using OA therapy. The dentist monitors device usage, symptoms, side effects, complications, and the degree of advancement at follow-up visits. The dentist monitors effectiveness, fit, and comfort, as well as TMJ, occlusal, and dental status at all follow-up visits.

OVERVIEW OF ORAL APPLIANCE EFFECTIVENESS

A comprehensive review of OA therapy was published in 1995,[31] along with practice parameters for their use.[1] The literature at that time consisted of case reports and retrospective and prospective case series. The authors pooled the results for the TRDs and MRAs of different designs. Seventy percent of the 304 subjects had a reduction in AHI by at least 50% from baseline. Fifty-one percent had a post-treatment AHI of less than 10, but as much as 40% of subjects had a post-treatment AHI of greater than 20. Snoring was reported improved in most patients. Since 1995, many prospective studies have been published, including randomized and controlled trials. In the more recent prospective case series of OA therapy, 54% to 84% of patients had a reduction in AHI by at least 50%,[30,32-35] and 51% to 82% of patients had a post-treatment AHI of less than 10.[32-37]

Mandibular Repositioning Appliances

Seventeen controlled clinical studies have been published on OA therapy and OSA or snoring. There are six crossover studies comparing MRAs with CPAP (five randomized,[2,3,10,12,13] one nonrandomized[38]); five randomized studies comparing two different MRAs or appliance designs;[4,6,8,11,15] and three randomized, placebo-controlled trials.[7,9,14] There is one randomized study comparing an MRA with uvulopalatopharyngoplasty (UPPP),[5] with additional data in three subsequent manuscripts.[39-41] Two randomized studies in snoring have been published—one comparing three appliances[16] and one comparing an MRA with placebo.[17]

Randomized, Crossover Studies of Oral Appliances with Continuous Positive Airway Pressure

The first randomized, controlled, crossover study of OA therapy was published in 1996.[2] The investigators compared the efficacy, side effects, compliance, and preference between an MRA (fixed position, boil-and-bite [SnoreGuard]) and CPAP in patients with mild to moderate OSA (AHI 15 to 40). Treatment success for the MRA was 48% (reduction in AHI to 10 or less with relief of symptoms) and for CPAP was 62%. The AHI was lower with CPAP than with the MRA. The MRA was well tolerated, with fewer side effects than CPAP, but some patients (24%) were unable or unwilling to use the MRA because of poor retention (ability to keep the OA in place in the oral cavity) or discomfort. The MRA was effective in reducing snoring in most patients and in reducing daytime sleepiness. Side effects were more common and the patients were less satisfied with CPAP. The authors concluded that a simple fixed-position appliance was an effective treatment in some patients with mild to moderate OSA and was associated with fewer side effects and greater patient satisfaction than CPAP. A second randomized, crossover study evaluated a partly adjustable custom appliance.[3] This MRA was successful (AHI of 10 or less and relief of symptoms) in treating 55% of patients. Sleep quality was improved more by CPAP and CPAP was more effective at reducing the AHI. Daytime sleepiness was equally improved by the two treatments.

Another randomized, crossover study of an intraoral sleep apnea device (a type of MRA) versus CPAP was conducted in patients with mild to moderate OSA (AHI between 5 and 30).[10] The MRA was arbitrarily set at two thirds of maximum mandibular protrusion and was not further adjusted during the study. After 6 weeks of therapy, CPAP was more effective at improving snoring, the AHI, and oxygenation. This MRA was not particularly effective at reducing the AHI (baseline AHI 17.5 ± 7.7 to 13.8 ± 11.1 at 6 weeks, P = not significant), although patients reported greater ease of use and higher compliance with the MRA. Subjective sleepiness was improved equally with both treatments. Overall, only 30% of patients (6 of 20) had an AHI of less than 10 with the MRA. The relatively low level of efficacy of this MRA may be related to the lack of titration of the appliance during the study.

Another randomized, crossover study of CPAP and OA in patients with OSA (AHI 11 to 43) and at least two OSA symptoms was published.[13] The patients were selected for the presence of sleepiness. The study included objective measures of sleepiness and assessments of quality of life and performance. The appliance was set at roughly 80% of maximum mandibular protrusion. The two appliances chosen for the study were fixed-position appliances. CPAP was more effective than the MRA for improving AHI and subjective ratings of daytime function even in the patients with milder OSA. There were no differences between the treatments in the effect on objective measures of sleepiness or cognition, or patient preference. Patients who preferred CPAP therapy had a higher body mass index and greater daytime impairment. The researchers concluded that CPAP would be the preferred first-line therapy in patients with OSA who have significant functional impairment and sleepiness even if they had mild OSA (defined by a lower AHI). The lower level of effectiveness of OA therapy in this study may be related to the selected appliance (single position, not state of the art) being compared with state-of-the-art CPAP therapy and the lack of titration of the MRA during the study.

A randomized, crossover trial of an MRA and CPAP therapy in 24 patients with mild to moderate OSA was published in 2002.[12] Two types of appliances were used—a single-piece device and a two-part appliance. Both appliances were set at approximately 75% of maximal protrusion but could be advanced further if needed. The AHI decreased from 22.2 to 8 with the MRA and to 3.1 with CPAP. Sleepiness as measured by the Epworth Sleepiness Scale (ESS) score was improved by both treatments (P < .001). Sixteen of the 23 patients (70%) who completed MRA therapy (22 completed CPAP therapy) had an AHI of less than 10.

SUMMARY

In these five published randomized, crossover studies of MRA therapy compared with CPAP in the treatment of OSA, CPAP was more effective in reducing snoring, improving oxygenation, and decreasing the AHI. In three of the five studies, they were equally effective in relieving excessive daytime sleepiness.[2,3,10] The MRA was the form of therapy preferred by patients in most studies.

Randomized, Controlled Studies of Two Appliances or Two Designs

Five studies have compared different MRAs or MRA designs. One study evaluated a fixed-position appliance (SnoreGuard) and a modified device in 24 patients with mild OSA.[4] The device that protruded the mandible (device A) was more effective in reducing the AHI than the device that minimally opened the vertical dimension without mandibular protrusion (device B). Some patients had an increase in AHI using device A or device B. A randomized, controlled, crossover study of the Herbst (Fig. 91–4) and the Monobloc appliance (Fig. 91–5) has been published.[6] The AHI was less than 10 in 75% of patients with the Monobloc and in 67% of patients with the Herbst. Both devices reduced sleepiness and snoring, but patients preferred the Monobloc.

One randomized, crossover study specifically evaluated the effect of vertical opening on the efficacy of an MRA.[8] The splint was constructed with 4 mm of interincisal opening or 14 mm of opening. Twenty-three patients wore each MRA for 2 weeks in random order. Both MRAs had similar efficacy

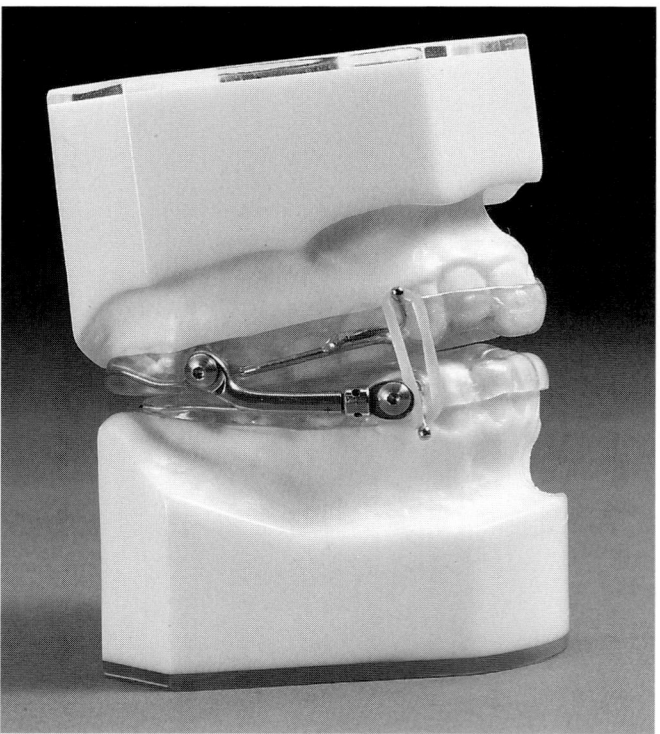

Figure 91–4. An adjustable Herbst appliance. (Courtesy of Great Lakes Orthodontics, Ltd., Tonawanda, NY.)

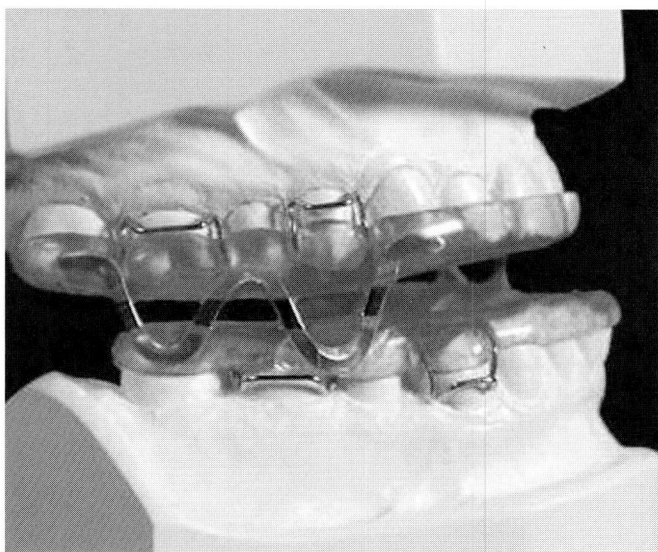

Figure 91–5. The Monobloc appliance. (Courtesy of Dr. Konrad Bloch, University of Zurich, Zurich, Switzerland.)

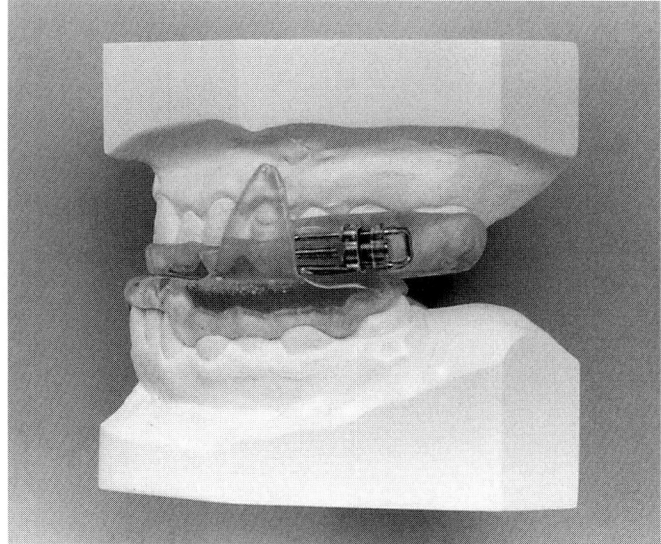

Figure 91–6. The mandibular advancement splint. (From Gotsopoulos H, Chen C, Qian J, Cistulli PA: Oral appliance therapy improves symptoms in obstructive sleep apnea: A randomized, controlled trial. Am J Respir Crit Care Med 2002;166:743-748.)

in reducing the AHI. Both MRAs improved snoring and sleepiness, but there was a trend to more jaw discomfort with the greater incisal opening. Overall, the patients preferred the appliance with less incisal opening for treatment. In this short-term study, increasing the vertical opening did not have an impact on efficacy, but there is concern that with long-term use it could increase side effects.

Another randomized, crossover study of two distinct MRAs for the treatment of mild OSA in 26 patients was published in 2002.[11] The appliances differed in materials, the amount of vertical opening, and the type of retention. Both were set at approximately 75% of maximum protrusion. Both MRAs improved symptoms like snoring, sleepiness, and sleep quality. The MRA made of hard material with more vertical opening had more side effects and was less effective at improving OSA. Another study evaluated two different amounts of mandibular protrusion, 75% or 50%, with an MRA in 86 men with severe OSA.[15] There were no more side effects with further protrusion. The MRA set at 75% reduced the AHI to less than 10 in 52% of patients, whereas the MRA set at 50% reduced the AHI to less than 10 in 31% of patients ($P = .04$).

SUMMARY

Different MRAs have different levels of effectiveness at reducing the AHI. There may be differences in terms of side effects, comfort, and preference. These differences may be related to design features of the appliance such as amount of vertical opening and the amount of protrusion.

Randomized, Placebo-Controlled Studies

The first randomized, placebo-controlled, crossover trial of an MRA (Fig. 91–6) for the treatment of OSA was published in 2001.[7] The authors studied 28 patients who wore an MRA that was incrementally advanced until symptoms resolved or maximum tolerated protrusion was obtained. Patients were randomly assigned to treatment with the placebo (lower plate

of the appliance only) or with the MRA. A partial response was defined as symptomatic improvement with an AHI reduced by at least 50% but greater than 5 at outcome, and a complete response was defined as a resolution of symptoms and an AHI of less than 5. The MRA resulted in a partial response in 15 patients (62.5%) and a complete response in 9 (37.5%). Seventy-one percent had an AHI of less than 10 with the MRA. The placebo device had no impact on AHI or on oxygen saturation. The MRA improved snoring, sleep structure, oxygenation, and daytime symptoms. There were few important side effects and no complications.

Another randomized, placebo-controlled, crossover study evaluated the effect of an MRA on subjective and objective sleepiness in 73 subjects.[9] Sixty-two subjects (85%) had moderate to severe OSA (AHI of 15 or more) and 38 (52%) reported sleepiness (ESS score greater than 10). The MRA was set at roughly 80% of maximum protrusion. The MRA improved snoring and reduced the AHI by 52%, with 63% having a complete or partial response (as defined for the study discussed previously). The MRA reduced the ESS score and increased the mean sleep latency compared with placebo.

A further randomized, crossover study compared an MRA set at 75% maximum protrusion with a placebo maxillary splint.[14] The MRA decreased the AHI, but there was a small increase in AHI with the placebo. Six of the 18 patients had a reduction in AHI to less than 10 with the MRA. Subjects reported a high level of compliance.

SUMMARY

Placebo-controlled trials of OA therapy consistently demonstrate that devices that advance the mandible are effective at lowering the AHI. In general, the active devices improve symptoms better than the placebo, but not always. Most of these studies are small, and larger placebo-controlled trials might find more improvement in subjective outcomes.

Randomized Study Comparing a Mandibular Repositioning Appliance with Uvulopalatopharyngoplasty

There is one randomized study of UPPP versus an MRA in patients with mild to moderate OSA.[5] The MRA was set at 50% of maximum protrusion and the surgical group had a conventional UPPP. Similar numbers of patients withdrew before treatment from both groups, but additional patients withdrew from the MRA group during the 1-year treatment period. The MRA was more effective at lowering the AHI (AHI of less than 10 in 78% with the MRA versus 51% with UPPP). The treatments were equally effective at improving subjective sleepiness. MRA side effects were described as minor and infrequent in a later publication, with no significant occlusal changes.[39] After 4 years, 10% of patients with UPPP had persistent swallowing complaints.[41] Quality-of-life scores improved in both treatment groups at 1 year.[40] Although the MRA reduced the AHI by more than UPPP, there was no difference in vitality and sleep scores between the treatments. Contentment scores were higher in the UPPP group. After 4 years of treatment, five patients in the MRA group had stopped using the device.[41] Some patients in the UPPP group had begun using an MRA because of persisting OSA.

Randomized, Prospective Studies of Snoring

There have been two randomized studies of OA for snoring. One study evaluated three different appliances in a crossover design.[16] The appliance that advanced the mandible improved snoring in four of five patients. Another study found that an MRA was effective at reducing the frequency and loudness of snoring compared with the placebo (upper plate of the appliance).[17]

Summary of Randomized, Prospective Studies

In summary, MRAs are an effective treatment option for many patients with OSA, including some patients with more severe OSA (higher AHI). They improve snoring and daytime symptoms, reduce the AHI, and improve oxygenation during sleep. They are not as effective as CPAP in reducing the AHI or snoring or at improving oxygenation. In some studies they are not as effective in reducing symptoms of sleepiness as CPAP, but in other studies they were. Overall, CPAP is more effective than an MRA and is considered first-line therapy in patients with more severe symptoms and in patients with more severe OSA, particularly if there is significant impairment of oxygenation.

Tongue-Advancing Appliances

Tongue-repositioning devices include the TRD, which is the best studied of these devices (see Fig. 91–2). The TRD is a custom-made, soft acrylic appliance that covers the upper and lower teeth and has an anterior bulb. It uses negative suction pressure to hold the tongue in a forward position inside the bulb. For those patients with limited nasal breathing, the TRD may be modified by the addition of lateral airway tubes that permit mouth breathing. The TRD appliance may be particularly useful in patients who have a relatively large tongue, poor dentition, or a poor protrusive range. Side effects include tongue soreness and excessive salivation, and some patients have difficulty using the TRD for the entire night.

In 1982, Cartwright and Samelson reported their initial experience with the TRD in 20 patients.[42] Fourteen of the 20 patients had undergone polysomnography before and with the TRD. There was a reduction in AHI of approximately 50% even though patients wore the TRD only half the night. Cartwright reported a second uncontrolled study of the TRD in 16 patients.[28] Treatment success in this study was defined as a reduction in apnea index (AI) to the normal range (0 to 6) or a 50% reduction in AI. Sixty-nine percent were successfully treated by the TRD by these criteria. The TRD was more effective in patients who were less severely overweight and in patients with positional apnea (apnea that is more severe in the supine position). Sleep architecture was improved with the TRD. When obesity, age, and the position ratio were used in a discriminant function analysis, these three variables predicted TRD success (as defined by an AI of less than 6 or a 50% reduction in AI) correctly for 13 (81%) of the patients. In a subsequent case series comparing treatments for positional OSA, the success rate with the TRD was reported as 80% for the reduction of the AHI to less than 10.[43]

Other tongue-advancing appliances have also been developed. A tongue-stabilizing device was assessed in a pilot study of six patients.[44] This device is based on the bulb component of the TRD and because it does not cover the dentition, it is an "off-the-shelf" product. The tongue-stabilizing device reduced snoring significantly, but the reduction in AHI (from 26 ± 17 to 15 ± 13; $P = .06$) was not significant.

SIDE EFFECTS AND COMPLICATIONS

Several studies have been published that have evaluated long-term side effects and complications from OA therapy. Pantin and others assessed 132 of 191 (69%) patients consecutively treated with an MRA during a 5-year period and performed a dental examination on 106 patients.[45] Ten patients had stopped using the MRA because of minor dental side effects. Occlusal changes were seen in 14%, and in two cases they recommended the patient stop treatment. Marklund and colleagues investigated side effects of a soft and a hard acrylic MRA in 75 patients who reported using the device more than 50% of nights for approximately 2.5 years.[46] Overbite and overjet decreased and three patients reported a permanent occlusal change. Hard acrylic appliances and larger amounts of protrusion were associated with more occlusal changes. Fritsch and colleagues evaluated 22 patients who had used either a Monobloc or a Herbst MRA for the treatment of OSA.[47] Common side effects included mucosal dryness (86%), tooth discomfort (59%), excessive salivation (55%), and jaw pain (41%), but they were described as minor. Long-term appliance use was associated with small orthodontic changes—decreased overjet and overbite, retroclined maxillary incisors, and slight anterior movement of the first mandibular molars. Patients reported that symptoms due to these changes usually resolved after a few minutes in the morning. Other long-term studies that have carefully evaluated the patient's dental status have confirmed the presence of small orthodontic changes[48,49] and indicate that the changes may be progressive with time.[50]

Overall, there is a degree of occlusal change in patients with long-term MRA use and these changes need to be monitored and addressed when they arise. Usually, the changes are minor and reversible when treatment is discontinued. Rarely, the occlusal changes are permanent.[51] Patients need to be informed of the potential for occlusal change when they embark on OA therapy. TMJ problems in patients without pre-existing joint problems are very uncommon, and long-term use does not seem to predispose to joint dysfunction.[52,53]

Occasionally, an OA can worsen apnea severity.[3,4,28-30] In one recent trial, 4 of 28 subjects (14%) had an increase in AHI with the appliance.[30] The reason for this increase could not be determined from a review of the patient data.

PREDICTORS OF TREATMENT OUTCOME

Although many studies have examined variables that may be associated with treatment outcome, most studies have been underpowered to find relationships between outcome and these variables. Clinical variables and upper airway characteristics associated with good treatment outcome are summarized in Box 91–1. In general, a younger, thinner patient with positional OSA (AHI higher when supine) and an overall lower AHI is the preferred candidate for OA therapy. One study found that heavier patients responded better to MRA treatment than thinner patients.[10] Marklund and colleagues reviewed 630 patients treated with MRAs and found that women had greater success with the device than men.[54] They also found that weight gain in treated male patients and nasal obstruction symptoms in female patients decreased treatment success. Some studies have demonstrated reasonably good success rates in patients with more severe OSA.[7,26,30,34,55,56]

Published studies have used a variety of imaging techniques to assess the upper airway and the factors associated with treatment response. Upper airway features associated with a good response are summarized in Box 91–1. It has been suggested that a more micrognathic or retrognathic mandible is associated with improved treatment response,[57] but other studies have suggested that a normal mandibular length and less overjet is associated with a better outcome.[58] A hypopharyngeal site of obstruction may be associated with improved treatment outcome,[59] but many patients with velopharyngeal closure still get a good result.[30] Increased hypopharyngeal size and middle airway space (airway width at the tip of the soft palate) with the MRA were associated with a good response in one study of 16 patients using supine cephalography.[60]

TREATMENT COMPLIANCE

In recent studies, 76% to 90% of patients have reported regular use of the MRA.[35,61] In two of the studies comparing OAs with CPAP, compliance was measured by patient reports.[2,3] There was no difference in reported nightly use between the treatments (roughly 60% for all treatment arms). Until objective compliance monitors are available for OAs, compliance rates will be uncertain given the unreliability of self-report. One preliminary study using a built-in compliance monitor embedded in the device[55] found that patients were using the MRA an average of 6.8 hours per night (range, 5.6 to 7.5).

INDICATIONS FOR ORAL APPLIANCE THERAPY

Prospective, controlled trials of OA therapy have shown a good level of effectiveness in patients with mild to moderate OSA and effectiveness in some patients with more severe OSA. In most of the studies comparing OAs with CPAP, patients exhibited a strong preference for the OA even though CPAP lowered the AHI more effectively. There may be difficulties implementing CPAP therapy in patients who have previously had UPPP,[62] but OAs may be effective in this group.[33] There are case reports detailing the successful use of an OA in the treatment of upper airway resistance syndrome,[63,64] with improvements in objective daytime sleepiness.[65]

OAs are usually not indicated as first-line therapy for severe OSA or severe sleepiness, or in patients who have very abnormal oxygen levels during sleep. CPAP therapy can be titrated in 1 night, but it can take weeks to months to optimize protrusion of an MRA. Two published studies have assessed overnight titration of an MRA to determine the therapeutic position and efficacy.[56,66] This is a promising approach that may allow identification of patients in whom an OA might be effective. Overnight titration might allow patients with more severe OSA to be treated without delay.

SUMMARY

OA therapy is a simple, reversible approach to treatment. Patients require alternatives to surgery and CPAP and the usefulness of OA therapy is no longer in question. Randomized, controlled clinical trials have shown them to be an effective treatment option for many patients, particularly in patients with less severe OSA. They are indicated in patients who have failed other treatments even if they have severe OSA. OAs appear to work as a result of an increase in airway space, the provision of a stable anterior position of the mandible, advancement of the tongue or soft palate, and possibly by a change in upper airway muscle activity.

Although MRAs are not as effective as CPAP therapy, they work in most patients to relieve symptoms and apnea and are well tolerated by most patients. Most patients report improvements in sleep quality and excessive daytime sleepiness. Short-term side effects are usually minor and are related to excessive salivation, jaw and tooth discomfort, and occasionally joint discomfort. These symptoms usually improve over time.

Box 91–1.   Predictors of Treatment Outcome

Clinical Variables

- Younger age[10,60,76]
- Lower body mass index[28,76]
- Smaller neck circumference[7]
- Positional obstructive sleep apnea (OSA): apnea-hypopnea index (AHI) higher when supine[28,54,77]
- Lower AHI (not a consistent predictor)[7,29,30,38,54,76]
- Increased amount of protrusion by appliance[11,15,53,78]

Variables from Upper Airway Imaging

- Smaller or narrow oropharynx[60,70,76]
- Smaller overjet[76]
- Normal mandible length[58]
- Shorter mandibular plane to hyoid distance[68]
- Shorter soft palate length[68]
- Normal or reduced lower facial height[58]
- Small soft palate and tongue[58]
- Increased retropalatal airway space[7]

Significant TMJ complications are rare, but occlusal changes are more common than previously thought.

OA therapy is a unique opportunity for dentists and physicians to work together to select the ideal patients for this form of treatment. Each plays a crucial role in providing the patient with optimal care. With collaboration and good communication between the dentist and the sleep clinician, many patients with snoring or OSA can be treated effectively with OAs.

FUTURE DIRECTIONS

Future studies are needed to compare the effectiveness of different types of appliances and different design features (e.g., the amount of vertical opening). The precise indications, complication rates, and reasons for treatment failure need to be determined for each OA if it is going to be used in clinical practice. Ongoing refinements of appliance design may eventually lead to improved outcomes. Only when the mechanisms of action are fully understood can more effective appliances be developed. On the horizon for the field of OA therapy are the introduction of a compliance monitor that will allow an objective determination of appliance use, and more rapid overnight titration approaches for implementing OA therapy quickly.

> *Clinical Pearls*
>
> *OAs are not as effective as CPAP for the treatment of patients with OSA. In particular, they work less well in patients with significant hypoxemia or morbid obesity. They are most effective in younger, thinner patients with milder OSA. Randomized, controlled clinical trials have indicated that OAs may be used as first-line therapy for the treatment of mild to moderate OSA. However, OAs are not the preferred treatment for patients with severe sleepiness because of the time it may take to achieve the final therapeutic position.*

REFERENCES

1. Standards of Practice Committee of the American Sleep Disorders Association: Practice parameters for the treatment of snoring and obstructive sleep apnea with oral appliances. Sleep 1995;18:511-513.
2. Ferguson KA, Ono T, Lowe AA, et al: A randomized crossover study of an oral appliance vs nasal-continuous positive airway pressure in the treatment of mild-moderate obstructive sleep apnea. Chest 1996;109:1269-1275.
3. Ferguson KA, Ono T, Lowe AA, et al: A short term controlled trial of an adjustable oral appliance for the treatment of mild to moderate obstructive sleep apnoea. Thorax 1997;52:362-368.
4. Hans MG, Nelson S, Luks VG, et al: Comparison of two dental devices for treatment of obstructive sleep apnea syndrome (OSAS). Am J Orthod Dentofacial Orthop 1997;111:562-570.
5. Wilhelmsson B, Tegelberg Å, Walker-Engström ML, et al: A prospective randomized study of a dental appliance compared with uvulopalatopharyngoplasty in the treatment of obstructive sleep apnoea. Acta Otolaryngol 1999;119:503-509.
6. Bloch KE, Iseli A, Zhang JN, et al: A randomized, controlled crossover trial of two oral appliances for sleep apnea treatment. Am J Respir Crit Care Med 2000;162:246-251.
7. Mehta A, Qian J, Petocz P, et al: A randomized, controlled study of a mandibular advancement splint for obstructive sleep apnea. Am J Respir Crit Care Med 2001;163:1457-1461.
8. Pitsis AJ, Darendeliler MA, Gotsopoulos H, et al: Effect of vertical dimension on efficacy of oral appliance therapy in obstructive sleep apnea. Am J Respir Crit Care Med 2002; 166:860-864.
9. Gotsopoulos H, Chen C, Qian J, et al: Oral appliance therapy improves symptoms in obstructive sleep apnea: A randomized, controlled trial. Am J Respir Crit Care Med 2002;166:743-748.
10. Randerath WJ, Heise M, Hinz R, et al: An individually adjustable oral appliance vs continuous positive airway pressure in mild-to-moderate obstructive sleep apnea syndrome. Chest 2002;122: 569-575.
11. Rose E, Staats R, Virchow C, et al: A comparative study of two mandibular advancement appliances for the treatment of obstructive sleep apnoea. Eur J Orthod 2002;24:191-198.
12. Tan YK, L'Estrange PR, Luo YM, et al: Mandibular advancement splints and continuous positive airway pressure in patients with obstructive sleep apnoea: A randomized cross-over trial. Eur J Orthod 2002;24:239-249.
13. Engleman HM, McDonald JP, Graham D, et al: Randomized crossover trial of two treatments for sleep apnea/hypopnea syndrome: Continuous positive airway pressure and mandibular repositioning splint. Am J Respir Crit Care Med 2002;166: 855-859.
14. Johnston CD, Gleadhill IC, Cinnamond MJ, et al: Mandibular advancement appliances and obstructive sleep apnoea: A randomized clinical trial. Eur J Orthod 2002;24:251-262.
15. Walker-Engström ML, Ringqvist I, Vestling O, et al: A prospective randomized study comparing two different degrees of mandibular advancement with a dental appliance in treatment of severe obstructive sleep apnea. Sleep Breath 2003;7:119-130.
16. Marklund M, Franklin KA: Dental appliances in the treatment of snoring: A comparison between an activator, a soft-palate lifter, and a mouth-shield. Swed Dent J 1996;20:183-188.
17. Johnston CD, Gleadhill IC, Cinnamond MJ, et al: Oral appliances for the management of severe snoring: A randomized controlled trial. Eur J Orthod 2001;23:127-134.
18. Ferguson KA, Love LL, Ryan CF: Effect of mandibular and tongue protrusion on upper airway size. Am J Respir Crit Care Med 1997;155:1748-1754.
19. Isono S, Tanaka A, Sho Y, et al: Advancement of the mandible improves velopharyngeal airway patency. J Appl Physiol 1995;79:2132-2138.
20. Ng AT, Gotsopoulos H, Qian J, et al: Effect of oral appliance therapy on upper airway collapsibility in obstructive sleep apnea. Am J Respir Crit Care Med 2003;168:238-241.
21. Ono T, Lowe AA, Ferguson KA, et al: The effect of the tongue retaining device on awake genioglossus muscle activity in patients with obstructive sleep apnea. Am J Orthod Dentofacial Orthop 1996;110:28-35.
22. Ono T, Lowe AA, Ferguson KA, et al: A tongue retaining device and sleep-state genioglossus muscle activity in patients with obstructive sleep apnea. Angle Orthodontist 1996;66:273-280.
23. Yoshida K: Effect of a prosthetic appliance for treatment of sleep apnea syndrome on masticatory and tongue muscle activity. J Prosthet Dent 1998;79:537-544.
24. Tsuiki S, Ono T, Kuroda T: Mandibular advancement modulates respiratory-related genioglossus electromyographic activity. Sleep Breath 2000;4:53-58.
25. Petit FX, Pépin JL, Bettega G, et al: Mandibular advancement devices: rate of contraindications in 100 consecutive obstructive sleep apnea patients. Am J Respir Crit Care Med 2002;166: 274-278.
26. Barthlen GM, Brown LK, Wiland MR, et al: Comparison of three oral appliances for treatment of severe obstructive sleep apnea syndrome. Sleep Med 2000;1:299-305.
27. Sjöholm TT, Lowe AA, Miyamoto K, et al: Sleep bruxism in patients with sleep-disordered breathing. Arch Oral Biol 2000;45:889-896.

28. Cartwright RD: Predicting response to the tongue retaining device for sleep apnea syndrome. Arch Otolaryngol 1985;111: 385-388.

29. Schmidt-Nowara WW, Meade TE, Hays MB: Treatment of snoring and obstructive sleep apnea with a dental orthosis. Chest 1991;99:1378-1385.

30. Henke KG, Frantz DE, Kuna ST: An oral elastic mandibular advancement device for obstructive sleep apnea. Am J Respir Crit Care Med 2000;161:420-425.

31. Schmidt-Nowara W, Lowe A, Wiegand L, et al: Oral appliances for the treatment of snoring and obstructive sleep apnea: A review. Sleep 1995;18:501-510.

32. Cohen R: Obstructive sleep apnea: Oral appliance therapy and severity of condition. Oral Surg Oral Med Oral Pathol Oral Radiol Endod 1998;85:388-392.

33. Millman RP, Rosenberg CL, Carlisle CC, et al: The efficacy of oral appliances in the treatment of persistent sleep apnea after uvulopalatopharyngoplasty. Chest 1998;113:992-996.

34. Pancer J, Al-Faifi S, Al-Faifi M, et al: Evaluation of variable mandibular advancement appliance for treatment of snoring and sleep apnea. Chest 1999;116:1511-1518.

35. Yoshida K: Effects of a mandibular advancement device for the treatment of sleep apnea syndrome and snoring on respiratory function and sleep quality. Cranio 2000;18:98-105.

36. Menn SJ, Loube DI, Morgan TD, et al: The mandibular repositioning device: Role in the treatment of obstructive sleep apnea. Sleep 1996;19:794-800.

37. Marklund M, Sahlin C, Stenlund H, et al: Mandibular advancement device in patients with obstructive sleep apnea: Long-term effects on apnea and sleep. Chest 2001;120:162-169.

38. Clark GT, Blumenfeld I, Yoffe N, et al: A crossover study comparing the efficacy of continuous positive airway pressure with anterior mandibular positioning devices on patients with obstructive sleep apnea. Chest 1996;109:1477-1483.

39. Tegelberg Å, Wilhelmsson B, Walker-Engström ML, et al: Effects and adverse events of a dental appliance for treatment of obstructive sleep apnoea. Swed Dent J 1999;23:117-126.

40. Walker-Engström ML, Wilhelmsson B, Tegelberg Å, et al: Quality of life assessment of treatment with dental appliance or UPPP in patients with mild to moderate obstructive sleep apnoea: A prospective randomized 1-year follow-up study. J Sleep Res 2000;9:303-308.

41. Walker-Engström ML, Tegelberg Å, Wilhelmsson B, et al: 4-year follow-up of treatment with dental appliance or uvulopalatopharyngoplasty in patients with obstructive sleep apnea: A randomized study. Chest 2002;121:739-746.

42. Cartwright RD, Samelson CF: The effects of a nonsurgical treatment for obstructive sleep apnea. JAMA 1982;248: 705-709.

43. Cartwright R, Ristanovic R, Diaz F, et al: A comparative study of treatments for positional sleep apnea. Sleep 1991;14:546-552.

44. Kingshott RN, Jones DR, Taylor DR, et al: The efficacy of a novel tongue-stabilizing device on polysomnographic variables in sleep-disordered breathing: A pilot study. Sleep Breath 2002; 6:69-76.

45. Pantin CC, Hillman DR, Tennant M: Dental side effects of an oral device to treat snoring and obstructive sleep apnea. Sleep 1999;22:237-240.

46. Marklund M, Franklin KA, Persson M: Orthodontic side-effects of mandibular advancement devices during treatment of snoring and sleep apnoea. Eur J Orthod 2001;23:135-144.

47. Fritsch KM, Iseli A, Russi EW, et al: Side effects of mandibular advancement devices for sleep apnea treatment. Am J Respir Crit Care Med 2001;164:813-818.

48. Fransson AM, Tegelberg Å, Svenson BA, et al: Influence of mandibular protruding device on airway passages and dentofacial characteristics in obstructive sleep apnea and snoring. Am J Orthod Dentofacial Orthop 2002;122:371-379.

49. Rose EC, Staats R, Virchow C Jr, et al: Occlusal and skeletal effects of an oral appliance in the treatment of obstructive sleep apnea. Chest 2002;122:871-877.

50. Robertson CJ: Dental and skeletal changes associated with long-term mandibular advancement. Sleep 2001;24:531-537.

51. Panula K, Keski-Nisula K: Irreversible alteration in occlusion caused by a mandibular advancement appliance: an unexpected complication of sleep apnea treatment. Int J Adult Orthod Orthognath Surg 2000;15:192-196.

52. Bondemark L, Lindman R: Craniomandibular status and function in patients with habitual snoring and obstructive sleep apnoea after nocturnal treatment with a mandibular advancement splint: A 2-year follow-up. Eur J Orthod 2000;22:53-60.

53. de Almeida FR, Bittencourt LR, de Almeida CI, et al: Effects of mandibular posture on obstructive sleep apnea severity and the temporomandibular joint in patients fitted with an oral appliance. Sleep 2002;25:507-513.

54. Marklund M, Stenlund H, Franklin KA: Mandibular advancement devices in 630 men and women with obstructive sleep apnea and snoring. Chest 2004;125:1270-1278.

55. Lowe AA, Sjoholm TT, Ryan CF, et al: Treatment, airway and compliance effects of a titratable oral appliance. Sleep 2000;23:S172-178.

56. Pételle B, Vincent G, Gagnadoux F, et al: One-night mandibular advancement titration for obstructive sleep apnea syndrome: A pilot study. Am J Respir Crit Care Med 2002;165:1150-1153.

57. Yoshida K: Prosthetic therapy for sleep apnea syndrome. J Prosthet Dent 1994;72:296-302.

58. L'Estrange PR, Battagel JM, Harkness B, et al: A method of studying adaptive changes of the oropharynx to variation in mandibular position in patients with obstructive sleep apnoea. J Oral Rehabil 1996;23:699-711.

59. Fransson AM, Isacsson G, Leissner LC, et al: Treatment of snoring and obstructive sleep apnea with a mandibular protruding device: An open-label study. Sleep Breath 2001;5:23-33.

60. Liu Y, Park YC, Lowe AA, et al: Supine cephalometric analyses of an adjustable oral appliance used in the treatment of obstructive sleep apnea. Sleep Breath 2000;4:59-66.

61. Johal A, Battagel JM: An investigation into the changes in airway dimension and the efficacy of mandibular advancement appliances in subjects with obstructive sleep apnoea. Br J Orthod 1999;26:205-210.

62. Mortimore IL, Bradley PA, Murray JA, et al: Uvulopalato pharyngoplasty may compromise nasal CPAP therapy in sleep apnea syndrome. Am J Respir Crit Care Med 1996;154:1759-1762.

63. Loube DI, Andrada T, Shanmagum N, et al: Successful treatment of upper airway resistance syndrome with an oral appliance. Sleep Breath 1998;2:98-101.

64. Guerrero M, Lepler L, Kristo D: The upper airway resistance syndrome masquerading as nocturnal asthma and successfully treated with an oral appliance. Sleep Breath 2001;5:93-96.

65. Rose E, Frucht S, Sobanski T, et al: Improvement in daytime sleepiness by the use of an oral appliance in a patient with upper airway resistance syndrome. Sleep Breath 2000;4:85-87.

66. Raphaelson MA, Alpher EJ, Bakker KW, et al: Oral appliance therapy for obstructive sleep apnea syndrome: progressive mandibular advancement during polysomnography. Cranio 1998;16:44-50.

67. Ishida M, Inoue Y, Suto Y, et al: Mechanism of action and therapeutic indication of prosthetic mandibular advancement in obstructive sleep apnea syndrome. Psychiatry Clin Neurosci 1998;52:227-229.

68. Eveloff SE, Rosenberg CL, Carlisle CC, et al: Efficacy of a Herbst mandibular advancement device in obstructive sleep apnea. Am J Respir Crit Care Med 1994;149:905-909.

69. Liu Y, Zeng X, Fu M, et al: Effects of a mandibular repositioner on obstructive sleep apnea. Am J Orthod Dentofacial Orthop 2000;118:248-256.

70. Mayer G, Meier-Ewert K: Cephalometric predictors for orthopaedic mandibular advancement in obstructive sleep apnoea. Eur J Orthod 1995;17:35-43.

71. Bernhold M, Bondemark L: A magnetic appliance for treatment of snoring patients with and without obstructive sleep apnea. Am J Orthod Dentofacial Orthop 1998;113:144-155.

72. Tsuiki S, Hiyama S, Ono T, et al: Effects of a titratable oral appliance on supine airway size in awake non-apneic individuals. Sleep 2001;24:554-560.

73. Gale DJ, Sawyer RH, Woodcock A, et al: Do oral appliances enlarge the airway in patients with obstructive sleep apnoea? A prospective computerized tomographic study. Eur J Orthod 2000;22:159-168.

74. Gao XM, Zeng XL, Fu MK, et al: Magnetic resonance imaging of the upper airway in obstructive sleep apnea before and after oral appliance therapy. Chin J Dent Res 1999;2:27-35.

75. Ryan CF, Love LL, Peat D, et al: Mandibular advancement oral appliance therapy for obstructive sleep apnoea: Effect on awake calibre of the velopharynx. Thorax 1999;54:972-977.

76. Liu Y, Lowe AA, Fleetham JA, et al: Cephalometric and physiologic predictors of the efficacy of an adjustable oral appliance for treating obstructive sleep apnea. Am J Orthod Dentofacial Orthop 2001;120:639-647.

77. Yoshida K: Influence of sleep posture on response to oral appliance therapy for sleep apnea syndrome. Sleep 2001;24:538-544.

78. Marklund M, Franklin KA, Sahlin C, et al: The effect of a mandibular advancement device on apneas and sleep in patients with obstructive sleep apnea. Chest 1998;113:707-713.

Management of Obstructive Sleep Apnea–Hypopnea Syndrome: Overview

Barbara Phillips

Meir H. Kryger

ABSTRACT

Sleep-disordered breathing (SDB) is a spectrum, and boundaries between pathologic and normal are still not precisely defined. The reported prevalence of sleep apnea is rising, driven by the increasing recognition of people who have the disorder and by the increasing ubiquity of risk factors, notably obesity and aging, which enhance the incidence of SDB; perhaps 5% of the population of the developed world has significant sleep-disordered breathing. Although the prototypical patient with sleep apnea is a middle-aged, obese man, is has become clear that neither obesity nor male sex is a necessary feature. Tools to monitor breathing during sleep and definitions for describing and stratifying SDB are becoming more precise and standardized, although they remain imperfect. The clinical importance of a disorder may be judged by the prevalence and severity of its outcomes. In this regard, strong associations between SDB and important sequelae, notably cardiovascular disease, automobile accidents, cognitive impairment, and derangements in the endocrine system, have become evident. Home ("ambulatory") multivariable testing, screening oximetry, and clinical algorithms will probably gain in importance as diagnostic tools because of the notable burden engendered by the large numbers of patients requiring evaluation for SDB and the growing recognition of the seriousness of this problem. Continuous positive airway pressure remains the treatment of choice, but behavioral change should be part of the overall management.

Sleep-related breathing disorders are common, are present in all age groups, and can result in significant morbidity and mortality. Eighty percent of patients presenting to sleep disorders centers have sleep-disordered breathing (SDB) as the primary diagnosis. The term *sleep-disordered breathing* has been used synonymously with the term *obstructive sleep apnea syndrome* (OSAS), which has been supplanted by the term *obstructive sleep apnea–hypopnea syndrome* (OSAHS). In this chapter, these terms will be used interchangeably. SDB is a spectrum (Fig. 92–1), and it is not yet clear where to draw the line between normal and pathologic.

Intermittent snoring is the mildest form of SDB, and it is often considered to be a benign nuisance (see Chapter 83). However, some evidence suggests that even "simple" snoring may have significant consequences. The most severe form of SDB is the obesity–hypoventilation syndrome (formerly called the pickwickian syndrome), which is associated with severe morbidity and very high mortality. Between these two extremes are disorders of gradually increasing impact on morbidity and mortality: persistent snoring, upper airway resistance syndrome, and obstructive sleep apnea syndrome.

This chapter presents an overview of the identification and management of patients with SDB. Details of diagnosis, clinical features, pathophysiology and treatment are presented in Chapters 81 to 91.

EPIDEMIOLOGY AND RISK FACTORS

Prevalence in the General Population

The Wisconsin Sleep Cohort Study reported that 4% of men and 2% of women in a middle-aged cohort (ages 30 to 60 years) had obstructive sleep apnea, as defined by an apnea-hypopnea index (AHI: the average number of apneas plus hypopneas per hour of sleep) of greater than 5 associated with daytime hypersomnolence.[1] In this cohort, 44% of men and 28% of women were habitual snorers. Since this report in 1993, the general population has become heavier and older. The risk for significant SDB rises both with body mass index (BMI: weight in kilograms per height in meters squared)[2] and with age.[3] It is difficult to identify a precise prevalence for sleep apnea for two reasons: risk factors in the general population are increasing, and the diagnostic criteria continue to change. However, the Sleep Heart Health Study (SHHS)

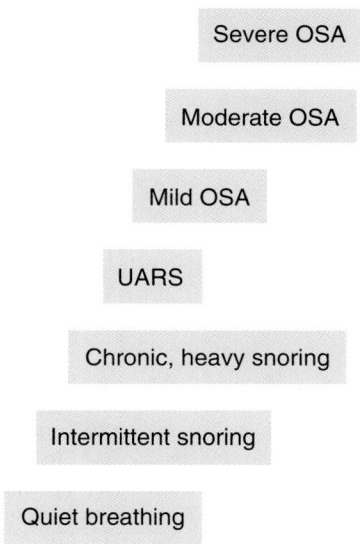

Figure 92–1. The spectrum of sleep-disordered breathing.

reported that 22% of 1824 people had a respiratory disturbance index (RDI, which in the context of this research was the same as the AHI) of greater than 15 events per hour, which most practitioners would consider to be significant sleep apnea.[4] On the basis of an exhaustive review of currently available data, it has been estimated that 5% of adults in developed countries have OSAHS with sleepiness, and an unknown percentage have SDB without overt sleepiness.[5]

The Cleveland Family Study of 285 individuals without significant sleep apnea at baseline reported that the incidence of developing SDB (as defined by an AHI greater than five events per hour) is about 7% per year, and the incidence of developing an AHI of greater than 15 events per hour is about 2% per year.[6] In addition to establishing the first incidence data for SDB, this study confirmed that with aging, male sex and BMI lose importance as risk factors for obstructive sleep apnea.[3,6] After menopause, the incidence of SDB rises in women, and the prevalence difference between the sexes is essentially the same.[7]

Genetic Influences

SDB is seen more commonly in patients with a family history of SDB. In one study, 41% of the offspring of 45 randomly selected patients with OSAHS had an AHI of greater than 5, and 13.3% had an AHI of greater than 20.[8] Other large family studies have reported a much higher prevalence of OSAHS among offspring of family members with OSAS when compared to the general population[5] (see Chapter 81). Ethnicity also appears to play a role in the development of SDB. African-American, Asian, and Hispanic individuals are at increased risk for sleep apnea, even controlling for other important risk factors.[2,5,9,10]

Associated Medical Disorders

Although it was recognized long ago that heart failure may result in repetitive central apneas (Cheyne-Stokes breathing), it is now clear that OSAHS may result in congestive heart failure, so sleep-related breathing disorders should be suspected in all cases of heart failure.[11] Hypothyroidism is more prevalent in those with sleep apnea than in those without, and it may contribute to the development of SDB by several mechanisms, including obesity, increased tongue size, and reduced respiratory drive.[5,12] Nasal obstruction and rhinitis are also associated with increased snoring and SDB.[13] Enlarged tonsils and adenoids may cause sleep apnea, particularly in children. SDB should be strongly suspected in syndromes that affect airway caliber such as trisomy 21, achondroplasia, Arnold-Chiari malformation, mucopolysaccharidoses, and Klippel-Feil, Pierre Robin, Alpert's, Treacher Collins, and Marfan's syndromes.[5]

Behavioral Factors

Alcohol and sedative medications decrease upper airway neuromuscular drive, predisposing to recurrent upper airway collapse.[5,14] Tobacco smoke causes an increase in nasal and pharyngeal irritation, resulting in narrowing of the upper airway. Obstructive sleep apnea (OSA) has been shown to be more prevalent in current smokers than in nonsmokers or ex-smokers.[5,15]

PATHOGENESIS

Epidemiologic and genetic studies indicate that the inheritance of OSAS is likely to be multigenic, and its development depends on environmental as well as genetic factors (see Chapter 84). A reduced airspace behind the uvula or tongue base results in increased inspiratory airflow resistance. Obesity increases the work of breathing, causing abnormally high levels of negative pressure against the narrowed upper airway. This causes edema by suction, which is exacerbated by trauma of snoring. If there is nasal obstruction (polyps, septal deviation), then increased *upstream* airway resistance increases the effects of the increased *downstream* negative pressure (intrathoracic vacuum). Retrognathia, which results in posterior displacement of the tongue, also leads to posterior airway narrowing and may increase the risk for SDB. For more on the pathophysiology of sleep-disordered breathing, see Chapter 82.

CLINICAL FEATURES

History

Snoring

"Heavy" snoring is the most common symptom in patients with SDB (Box 92–1). About 50% of men and 25% of women snore, but somewhat fewer than that have sleep apnea, so snoring alone is clearly not diagnostic. Snoring accompanied by apnea, snorting, gasping, and choking during sleep is predictive of OSAS.[16-18] Witnessed apneas are more predictive of SDB than are self-reported episodes of waking up gasping for breath, which may be a symptom of other diseases such as congestive heart failure, gastroesophageal reflux disease, nocturnal asthma, and panic disorder.

Sleepiness

Although excessive daytime sleepiness has many possible etiologies, this complaint should increase the suspicion for OSAHS. Subjective sleepiness can be assessed by the Epworth Sleepiness Scale (see Chapters 49, 120), which has been validated in clinical studies and correlates very roughly with objective measures

---

Box 92–1. **Symptoms and Signs of Sleep-Disordered Breathing**

Symptoms
- Snoring
- Witnessed apneas
- Gasping for breath during sleep
- Sleepiness
- Enuresis, nocturia
- Mood, memory, or learning problems
- Impotence
- Recent weight gain
- Morning headache
- Dry mouth or dry throat in the morning

Signs
- Obesity
- Hypertension
- Crowded oropharynx
- Retrognathia

of sleepiness.[19] Patients both underreport and overreport their sleepiness,[19a] so querying members of their household is also useful. An Epworth Sleepiness Scale score greater than 10 suggests significant daytime sleepiness, but this is not specific for OSAS. Sleepiness can be objectively measured with a multiple sleep latency test or with the Maintenance of Wakefulness Test, but these tests are rarely indicated in the evaluation of individuals with SDB. Patients who report falling asleep while driving should be evaluated for sleep disorders, including SDB. Because of the threat posed to the patient and others by this symptom, clinicians should have a low threshold for evaluation of patients who report this problem.

Other Symptoms

Nocturia,[20] impotence,[21] attention deficits, cognitive impairment (see Chapter 85), morning headache, dry or sore throat in the morning, and problems with vision[22-24] are other symptoms that may be associated with OSAHS. Recent weight gain is an almost invariable finding, and it may be both the cause and the consequence of sleep disordered breathing (see Chapter 86).

Gender and Symptoms

Female patients with OSAHS are much more likely than male patients to present with insomnia, and they are less likely to present with a history of observed apnea. Women with OSAHS are much more likely than men to have been diagnosed with a mood disorder and previous hypothyroidism.[25] Alcohol and caffeine have been found to be used more by male than by female patients.

PHYSICAL FINDINGS

The physical finding that is most predictive of OSAS is central obesity. A BMI greater than 28 kg/m^2 in both men and women reflects a risk factor and should increase the suspicion for OSAS. Approximately 40% of individuals with a BMI greater than 40 and 50% of those with a BMI greater than 50 have significant SDB,[2] although premenopausal women are generally much heavier than their male counterparts, and both obesity and sex become less important risk factors for sleep apnea after age 50.[5] Measures of central obesity such as neck size are very useful in predicting the presence of OSAS. Men with a neck circumference greater than 17 in (43 cm) and women with a neck circumference greater than 16 in (41 cm) are very likely to have OSAS confirmed by overnight polysomnography.[17,26,27]

Nasal obstruction from any cause appears to be a risk factor for SDB including snoring.[28] A narrow posterior oropharynx, deviated nasal septum, retrognathia, and other craniofacial abnormalities which result in airway narrowing are frequently seen in patients with sleep apnea. Several diagnostic schemes are based on intraoral measurements, notably a narrowed posterior oropharynx.[18,28,29]

Measurement of systemic arterial blood pressure is, of course, a standard part of the physical examination. It is therefore noteworthy that several large epidemiologic studies have demonstrated that OSAHS is a risk factor for hypertension[30-32] in a "dose-dependent" way. Analysis of data obtained from 6132 subjects in the SHHS revealed an odds ratio for hypertension of 1.37 (95% confidence interval, 1.03-1.83), comparing the highest category of AHI (greater than 30 per hour)

with the lowest (less than 1.5 per hour).[30] As many as 83% of patients with drug-resistant hypertension have sleep apnea.[33]

DIAGNOSIS

Polysomnography

The gold standard for the diagnosis of OSAHS remains overnight polysomnography (PSG) (Fig. 92–2). A nocturnal PSG includes recordings of airflow, ventilatory effort, oxygen saturation, and body position, and electrocardiography, electromyography, and electroencephalography. In standard, laboratory-based polysomnography, a technician is present to monitor the patient for the entire study. A single overnight study is generally sufficient to diagnose OSAHS. In many instances, the level of SDB is severe enough that the diagnosis of OSAHS can be established early in the study. In this event, a split-night study may be performed, in which the second half of the study is used to titrate treatment (positive airway pressure) for OSAHS.

Definitions

The *apnea-hypopnea index* is the most commonly used criterion to establish the diagnosis of OSAS and to quantify its severity. The AHI is defined as the total number of apneas plus hypopneas divided by the hours of sleep (Box 92–2) in a single night's study. Obstructive apneas and hypopneas are characterized by an absence or a reduction of airflow, respectively, despite continued ventilatory efforts. Some authors have suggested that the presence of continuous positive airway pressure (CPAP) responsiveness might add additional precision to the diagnosis.[34] In central apneas and hypopneas, ventilatory effort is absent or reduced during the period of apnea or reduced airflow.

Recently, a consensus for defining apneas and hypopneas has been achieved, largely as a result of the *Sleep Heart Health Study*. The SHHS is a longitudinal follow-up of more than 6000 individuals who were enrolled in ongoing studies of cardiovascular disease, including in-home polysomnography.[35] In this study (which is limited to middle-aged and older adults), apneas were identified by absence of airflow for greater than 10 seconds, and hypopneas were defined by a reduction of airflow (to 30% of baseline for apneas, and to 70% of baseline for hypopneas) for greater than 10 seconds. In the SHHS, the definitions of both apneas and hypopneas require an oxygen desaturation of 4% or more, and they do not include any measure of sleep disturbance or arousal.[35-37] These criteria were adopted largely because they are both predictive of cardiovascular sequelae[37] and very reproducible.[35,36]

The definition of apnea proposed by the American Academy of Sleep Medicine (AASM)[38] and by the Centers for Medicare and Medicaid Services[39] (CMS; see "Indications," later) do not require oxygen desaturation (although the definition of hypopnea does). The definition of hypopnea published by the AASM prior to recognition of these events[40] called for a 3% or more oxygen desaturation.

Diagnostic Criteria for Obstructive Sleep Apnea–Hypopnea Syndrome

According to the AASM, OSAHS exists when a patient has five or more obstructed breathing events per hour of sleep, with an appropriate clinical presentation (Box 92–3).[38]

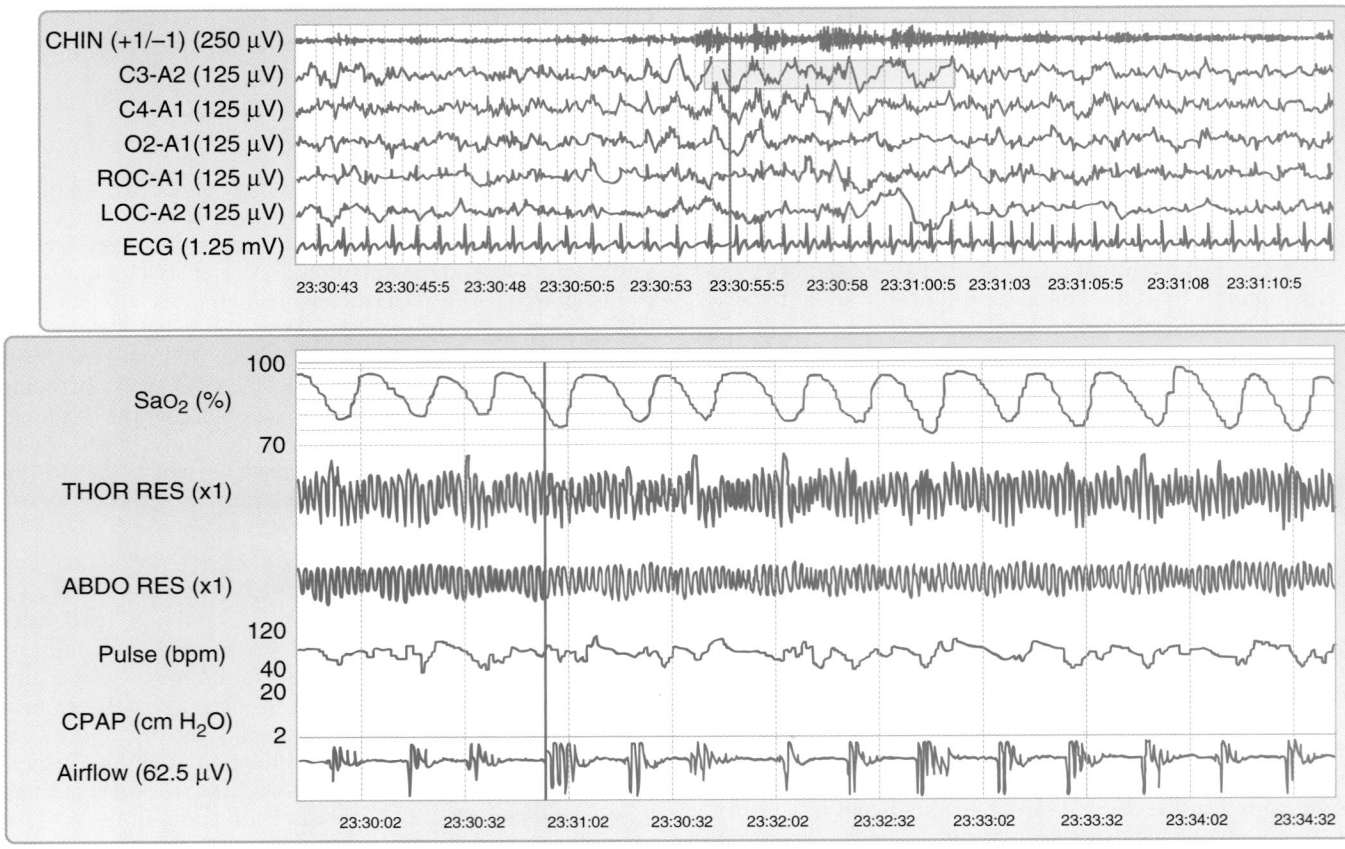

Figure 92–2. Polysomnogram from a patient with severe obstructive sleep apnea syndrome. The top seven channels represent about 30 seconds of data and show the electrocardiogram (ECG) and information used to stage sleep. The top channel is chin electromyography. The next three channels are used for electroencephalography (EEG), the next two for eye movements, and the seventh is the ECG. The bottom six channels represent about 5 minutes of data and show the information used to document apnea type. The channels from top to bottom are oxyhemoglobin saturation (SaO2), thoracic movement, abdominal movement, pulse rate, CPAP pressure, and nasal airflow. The 14 apneic episodes in this segment are associated with efforts to breathe, as seen in the chest wall and abdomen channels, but note the intermittent cessation of airflow in the bottom channel. The *vertical dark blue line* in each segment corresponds to an identical moment in time. Notice that resumption of breathing occurs right after an arousal on EEG *(light blue box)*. Also note the marked variability in pulse rate. CPAP, continuous positive airway pressure.

Although there is now some consistency in the definitions of SDB, considerable variation continues to exist in recording techniques for measures of airflow and respiratory effort (see Chapter 117).[38,40] The innate inaccuracy and variability of current measurement techniques have almost certainly resulted in varying sensitivities for detection of SDB events.

Diagnostic Criteria for Upper Airway Resistance Syndrome

A probable consequence of the lack of standardized definitions and measurement techniques for SDB is the confusion and controversy surrounding the upper airway resistance syndrome (UARS).[41] Patients with UARS have increased inspiratory efforts with frequent arousals but without overt apneas. This fragmented sleep results in increased subjective and objective daytime sleepiness. In the original description of UARS, increased respiratory effort was identified by esophageal pressure nadirs more negative than one standard deviation below the mean, followed by transient electroencephalography arousals. A recent AASM panel defined a respiratory effort–related arousal event as "a sequence of breaths characterized by increasing respiratory effort leading to an arousal from sleep, but which does not meet criteria for an apnea or hypopnea."[38]

Techniques currently used to detect UARS in sleep laboratories vary greatly in clinical practice, but few clinical centers actually define and measure UARS as it was originally defined. Since there is no clear standard of diagnosis for this condition, it is probably both underdiagnosed and overdiagnosed (see Chapter 83).

Other Diagnostic Approaches

Prediction Formulae

Because individual features from the history and physical diagnosis are nondiagnostic, several groups have suggested the use of prediction formulae based on combinations of findings.[16-18,27] Among the most useful of such findings are history of witnessed apneas, male sex, BMI, and neck circumference. The Berlin Questionnaire,[17] which is widely used, focuses on a limited set of known risk factors for sleep apnea. It includes questions about snoring, daytime sleepiness, and high blood pressure, as well as age, weight, height, sex, and neck circumference (see Chapter 50).

Box 92–2. Definitions

Apnea and hypopnea: Decrease in airflow or chest wall movement to an amplitude smaller than approximately 25% (apnea) or 70% (hypopnea) of baseline. These events must last at least 10 seconds. They are associated with oxyhemoglobin desaturation of 4% or greater compared with baseline.[35,36]

Apnea-hypopnea index (AHI): Apneas plus hypopneas per total sleep time (in hours).

Respiratory effort–related arousal (RERA): A sequence of breaths characterized by increasing respiratory effort and leading to an arousal from sleep, but not meeting the criteria for an apnea or a hypopnea. These events must fulfill both of the following criteria: a pattern of progressively more negative esophageal pressure, which is terminated by a sudden change in pressure to a less negative level and an arousal. The event lasts 10 seconds or longer.[38]

Upper airway resistance syndrome (UARS): A clinical syndrome of sleepiness resulting from RERAs.[39]

Respiratory disturbance index (RDI): AHI, more or less (may include RERAs).

Sleep-disordered breathing (SDB): An ill-defined term used to encompass nonspecified respiratory disturbances during sleep; may include snoring, asymptomatic apneas, and full-blown sleep apnea.

These formulae and questionnaires can be used to help determine which patients are likely to benefit from further evaluation and diagnostic testing. Specific oropharyngeal measurements are also highly predictive.[18,29] Investigators of prediction formulae typically analyze the ability of the proposed formula to predict a given AHI. However, the AHI is a poor standard. A more clinically relevant outcome for prediction formulae might be a positive response to CPAP treatment.[34] In general, these formulae perform well when applied to individuals with a high likelihood of severe SDB; but this is when such formalized algorithms are least needed

---

Box 92–3. Diagnostic Criteria for the Obstructive Sleep Apnea–Hypopnea Syndrome

The individual must fulfill criterion A or B, plus criterion C

A. Excessive daytime sleepiness that is not better explained by other factors

B. Two or more of the following (not better explained by other factors)
1. Choking or gasping during sleep
2. Recurrent awakenings from sleep
3. Unrefreshing sleep
4. Daytime fatigue
5. Impaired concentration

C. Overnight monitoring demonstrating five or more obstructed breathing events per hour during sleep; events may include any combination of obstructive apneas/hypopneas or respiratory effort–related arousals

Adapted from American Academy of Sleep Medicine Task Force: Sleep-related breathing disorders in adults: Recommendations for syndrome definition and measurement techniques in clinical research. Sleep 1999;22:667-689.

---

by the clinician. Prediction formulae probably do have a place in the expedited diagnosis and/or triage of patients with severe sleep apnea.

Ambulatory Monitoring and Oximetry

AMBULATORY MULTICHANNEL STUDIES

Controversy exists about where sleep studies are best done and about the role of screening in general.[42,43] The studies that are available in a community reflect both scientific validity (see Chapter 50) and the likelihood of being reimbursed, as well as the data required to start the patient on treatment. Ambulatory monitors, which measure as many channels as laboratory PSG does, have been available for some time. Proponents of home testing point to the benefits of increased accessibility, enhanced patient convenience, reduced cost, and better sleep in the familiar environment. Opponents point out that titrations cannot be done, equipment problems cannot be corrected, non-OSAHS disorders cannot be detected, and patient compliance might somehow be worsened. Autotitrating CPAP performs at least as well as in-laboratory titrated CPAP (see later and Chapter 89). The SHHS, using rigid protocols and a centralized PSG reading laboratory, has demonstrated that home monitoring can produce reliable data with acceptable rates of data loss.[35] The two nonapneic sleep disorders most likely to be identified by laboratory PSG are narcolepsy, which cannot be diagnosed by overnight study alone, and periodic limb movements during sleep. Periodic limb movements are extremely common in sleep disorders,[44] often unassociated with sleepiness in the nonapneic patient,[44] and are likely to be a marker of SDB anyway.[45] A comparison of laboratory PSG and titration with home diagnosis and autotitration found no difference in CPAP compliance between groups, although the home testing group was evaluated more quickly and less expensively.[46]

OXIMETRY

Oximetry results are the basis for the current definitions of SDB, in that oxygen desaturations of varying degrees are included or required criteria for measures of SDB, notably hypopneas.[36-40] Oximetry has better inter-rater reliability, and it is a better predictor of the response to CPAP treatment than is the AHI.[47,48] In general, patients with significant sleep apnea have a greater fluctuation in oxygen saturation (and heart rate) than do those without. However, thinner, younger patients without lung disease can have significant breathing and sleep disturbance without remarkable oxygen desaturation. Furthermore, patients with underlying lung disease may have oxygen desaturation without OSA. Thus, oximetry is neither sensitive nor specific for SDB. Several studies have investigated it as a screening or diagnostic tool for sleep apnea, but their conclusions often conflict. In general, like prediction models, oximetry performs best with more severely affected patients.

Other Diagnostic Tools

Several other tools have been developed to aid in the evaluation of SDB. Among them are measures of movement such as actigraphy[49] and static charge–sensitive bed assessment.[50] Also being developed, are measures of heart rate variability and pulse pressure, Holter monitoring, and measures of sympathetic nervous system tone.[51-53]

> **Box 92–4.   Consequences of Untreated Sleep Apnea**
>
> - Impaired cognitive function
> - Impaired quality of life
> - Daytime sleepiness
> - Increased risk of automobile accidents
> - Increased health care costs
> - Hypertension
> - Cardiovascular disease
> - Worsened glucose tolerance
> - Increased mortality rates
> - Impotence

> **Box 92–5.   CMS Indications for CPAP Reimbursement to Patients with Obstructive Sleep Apnea**
>
> Continuous positive airway pressure (CPAP) therapy is covered for adults who have sleep-disordered breathing and the following symptoms or disorders:
>
> - AHI > 15, OR
> - AHI > 5 with any of the following:
>   - Hypertension
>   - Stroke
>   - Sleepiness
>   - Ischemic heart disease
>   - Insomnia
>   - Mood disorders
>
> AHI, apnea-hypopnea index; CMS, Centers for Medicare and Medicaid Services.
>
> Information obtained from Centers for Medicare and Medicaid Services. http://www.cms.hhs.gov/manuals/pm_trans/R150CIM.pdf.

CLINICAL COURSE AND PREVENTION

Several large studies controlling for obesity and for other confounders have established that SDB is a clear-cut risk factor for hypertension,[30,32,54] car crashes,[55,56] neurocognitive dysfunction,[57,58] and cardiovascular disease,[37,59,60] including strokes. Other likely but less well established sequelae include impotence,[21] depression,[61] glucose intolerance,[62,63] reduced quality of life,[4,64] and increased health care costs[65] (see Chapters 85-87) (Box 92–4).

Substantial progression of SDB can occur over relatively short time periods.[6,66] In the Wisconsin Sleep Cohort, the overall mean AHI increased by 2.6 events per hour of sleep in 8 years. Both snoring and obesity appear to be predictors of progression.

A report in 1997 estimated that 93% of women and 82% of men with moderate to severe SDB had not been clinically diagnosed.[67] At this point, the need for aggressive diagnosis and treatment of severe, symptomatic SDB is widely recognized. The next frontier is likely to be an understanding of the risks and natural progression associated with milder levels of SDB. This will necessarily involve developing more precise tools and definitions for its identification. At present, even "simple" snoring is associated with some of the risks known to result from unequivocal sleep apnea (see Chapter 83).[68,69] This is likely to be because the tools that we use to assess both breathing disturbances during sleep and their sequelae are very imprecise. Although some data on cardiovascular morbidity are emerging from the SHHS,[36] much more needs to be known about the consequences of "mild" SDB. Because of the burden of illness associated with this disorder, and because the risk of vehicular crashes makes it a public health problem, increasing efforts toward effective diagnosis and cure are appropriate.

TREATMENT

Indications

Patients meeting the AASM criteria for the diagnosis of OSAHS should be treated. In different communities, governments and insurance companies may impose their own criteria. The published criteria of the CMS are similar to those of the AASM. The CMS reimburses for CPAP treatment for patients with an AHI greater than 15, or with an AHI greater than 5 and concurrent hypertension, stroke, sleepiness, ischemic heart disease, or mood disorders[39] (Box 92–5).

General Measures

Behavior change has a major role in causing and in the treatment of sleep apnea. Weight loss can be curative, and even modest weight loss (10%) can relieve mild SDB.[70] The relationship between weight, sleep, and appetite is complex, probably mediated in part by leptin, cortisol, insulin, and metabolic rate (see Chapter 86). Patients newly diagnosed with obstructive sleep apnea have a greater increase in weight in the year prior to diagnosis than do their weight-matched controls, and patients who comply with CPAP treatment tend to gain weight.[70] All obese patients with SDB should be counseled about weight loss. Unfortunately, weight loss takes time, and only a minority of patients can maintain weight loss. In the long run, simple advice about caloric intake and output may be most effective. The two pharmacologic approaches that are still available in the United States have respectable long-term (2-year) weight loss results of 8% to 10%. Recently, a commercially available program (Weight Watchers) has been shown to promote and maintain weight loss more effectively than a self-help approach.[71]

Some patients with sleep apnea have chronic rhinitis. Intranasal corticosteroid therapy may improve their apnea severity, but not necessarily their snoring or sleep quality.[72]

Although the data are inconsistent, cigarette smoking has been implicated as a risk factor for snoring and for sleep apnea, as well as for chronic obstructive pulmonary disease (COPD).[4,14] In addition, nicotine disrupts sleep. In general, smokers have more sleep disturbances than nonsmokers.[73] Smoking cessation advice should be routine in the management of all patients who smoke.

Muscle relaxants, including alcohol and sleeping pills, can make apneas longer by reducing airway tone and by increasing the arousal threshold. Moderate drinking has been clearly shown to exacerbate OSAHS and should be discouraged.[5,74]

A subset of patients (usually thinner, older, and with milder disease) may have position-dependent apnea. In these individuals, sleeping on the side may totally eliminate SDB. Unfortunately, the state of the art of "position training" is still a tennis ball in a pocket in the back of a T-shirt. Most clinicians are uncomfortable treating a condition known to have serious cardiovascular and public health consequences with this technique.

Continuous Positive Airway Pressure

The first line of treatment for OSAHS is CPAP (see Chapter 89). Typically applied in the range of 5 to 15 cm H_2O through a nasal or oronasal mask, CPAP splints open the entire airway (from nares to alveoli), increases functional residual capacity, may increase pharyngeal dilator activity, and reduces afterload on the heart. CPAP is often titrated in a sleep laboratory, with mask fitting and CPAP adjustment done in the second half of the night after the diagnosis of sleep apnea is established. Diagnosing SDB and titrating CPAP in a single-night study, or split night testing, is currently the standard approach. The CMS (formerly known as the Health Care Financing Administration) requires that the patient get at least 2 hours of sleep in the untreated state before the titration is begun. CPAP is begun at 3 to 5 cm H_2O, and it is gradually increased until all measures of SDB, including snoring and arousals, are eliminated. Most people end up on CPAP pressures of 8 to 14 cm H_2O. CPAP requirements vary with airway resistance, and they tend to be higher in more obese patients, in rapid eye movement sleep, in the supine position, and when alcohol or other muscle relaxants have been consumed. For this reason, achieving a perfect CPAP pressure in a single night's (or a half night's) titration is more difficult than it sounds.

Autotitrating CPAP machines are now available.[75-77] These devices infer airflow reduction by sensing vibration of upper airway tissues or by measures of airflow, and they deliver flow (and thus pressure) to eliminate the vibration or reduced inspiratory airflow. They use different algorithms to accomplish this, and probably all are not equally effective.[78] However, they have been validated in both laboratory and home studies. Currently, no guidelines exist about how to remedy an inadequate attempt at CPAP titration on a split-night study. Autotitrating CPAP may be a cost-effective alternative to laboratory titration for many of these patients. However, for patients who have severe oxygen desaturation or sleep disruption, problems with mask leaks or open-mouthed sleep, hypoventilation, or possible central apnea, laboratory titration with a technician in attendance may be the solution.

Compliance with CPAP (somewhat arbitrarily defined as use for 4 or more hours on 5 or more nights a week) remains the most difficult part of CPAP treatment. Probably only about 50% to 60% of patients comply with CPAP.[79-81] Humidification of inspired air (warm better than cold, but cold better than nothing) and education have been shown to improve CPAP compliance.[82,83] Autotitrating CPAP may have better rates of compliance and results in reduced overall pressure. Bilevel pressure has not been shown to improve compliance compared with "straight" CPAP in a head-to-head trial. Mask fit and type, nasal steroids, and decongestants are believed by many clinicians to enhance CPAP use, but there is no convincing evidence that they do so, with the possible exception of the use of one kind of nasal pillow.

Complications of CPAP treatment are relatively minor and include epistaxis, ulcer, rashes or irritation on the bridge of the nose, rhinorrhea, chest or sinus discomfort, claustrophobia, nasal congestion, and conjunctivitis. Most of these can be addressed with good mask fit and humidification.

CPAP has been shown to reverse many of the sequelae of OSAHS, including mortality,[84] automobile accidents,[56,85] hypertension and other cardiovascular diseases,[59,60,86,87] cognitive impairment,[46,88,89] sleepiness,[89,90] increased health care costs,[65] impaired quality of life,[91] depression,[61] and impotence.[21] Most studies documenting improved outcomes with CPAP treatment have shown benefit with an intention-to-treat model. In other words, if the patient accepts CPAP, benefit occurs even in the absence of well-documented compliance.

Surgery

A variety of surgical approaches have been applied to SDB, including tracheostomy, uvulopalatopharyngoplasty (UPPP), laser-assisted uvulopalatopharyngoplasty (LAUP), septoplasty, oromaxillofacial surgery, and radiofrequency volumetric tissue reduction (also known as somnoplasty). In addition, bariatric surgery has been applied to morbid obesity in patients with sleep apnea. Chapter 88 addresses surgical treatment of sleep apnea in detail.

In general, surgical approaches to the treatment of SDB have been poorly evaluated. Long-term follow-up and measures of effects on automobile accidents, quality of life, blood pressure, cognitive performance, and health care costs are minimal.[92,93]

Uvulopalatopharyngoplasty

UPPP is the most commonly performed and best studied of the surgical procedures used to treat sleep apnea. In a meta-analysis of 37 papers including over 500 patients, Sher noted that the mean decrease in apnea index is 55%, with a mean decrease in RDI of 38%.[92] Unfortunately, reducing the RDI by about one third rarely results in a cure. Surgical success is defined in this meta-analysis (as in many papers in the surgical literature) by some ratio of preoperative to postoperative RDI *plus* a postoperative RDI or apnea index of 10 to 20 events per hour of sleep. Because cardiac and neurocognitive effects may involve RDIs of even as low as five events per hour of sleep, designating these kinds of responses as a success is questionable.[37,94] Even accepting these definitions, UPPP has a success rate of approximately 50%, and it appears to be even less effective in more severely affected, heavier patients.[95] In particular, outcomes are poorer for those with a BMI greater than 30, or with a lowest SaO_2 below 88%. Relapse also occurs in as many as half in that fraction who get an initial response, usually (but not always) related to weight gain.[92] Complications of UPPP appear to be velopharyngeal insufficiency in up to 2%, postoperative bleeding in about 1%, nasopharyngeal stenosis (1%), voice change (1%), perioperative upper airway obstruction (0.3%), and death (0.2%). Sher also reported that many papers do not comment on the presence of complications at all.

Laser-Assisted Uvulopalatopharyngoplasty

LAUP has a surgically defined success rate of 0% to 48% for OSAHS,[92] depending on the criteria used. Sher notes that most case series report preoperative and postoperative results in only a fraction of those who had the procedure. In addition, very few long-term results or data about complications are available. Importantly, LAUP has been associated with an acute exacerbation of SDB.[96] Because LAUP has typically been done as an outpatient procedure, it could actually pose a risk to patients. At present, many surgeons believe that LAUP is an operation appropriate for snoring only.[92]

Radiofrequency Volumetric Tissue Reduction

Radiofrequency volumetric tissue reduction (RFVTR) has been applied to the palate, tongue base, and nasal septum. Originally reported as a treatment for SDB,[97] this procedure appears to be safer and less painful than LAUP. Follow-up data for RFVTR of both palate and tongue suggest that the initial response is generally not what would be considered a cure by most sleep specialists, and that relapse is a significant problem. This procedure is now used primarily for snoring rather than for significant OSAHS.[92]

Oromaxillofacial Surgery

Maxillomandibular advancement (MMA) may be of benefit[98] to carefully selected (nonobese) patients who cannot or will not accept CPAP and who are willing to accept the risk of a procedure whose short-term efficacy appears modest and whose long-term efficacy and consequences are unknown.

Combination Surgical Treatment

There are a variety of combination surgical procedures, typically including some combination of genioglossal advancement, hyoid myotomy and suspension, UPPP, and RFVTR (see Chapter 90). Studies evaluating these procedures typically include 10 or fewer patients; they often offer a loose definition of success and provide no long-term follow-up.

Tracheostomy

Tracheostomy remains the gold standard approach to severe sleep apnea in those who are CPAP intolerant and face an immediate life-threatening risk. Early resolution of sleep apnea occurs promptly in 83%, and central apneas slowly resolve in the remainder. Sleepiness resolves in 82% and hypertension resolves in 40% of those who undergo tracheostomy.[92] At a mean follow-up of 8 years, tracheostomy was uniformly successful in 79 patients who had severe obstructive sleep apnea.[99] Of those patients, 16 had decannulation, but five needed CPAP, three had UPPP, two achieved weight loss, and three were lost to follow-up. Immediate complications of tracheostomy included one perioperative myocardial infarction and one tracheal–innominate fistula.

Bariatric Surgery

Of the several types of weight-reduction surgeries, gastric bypass done laparoscopically is probably the treatment of choice as it results in greater weight loss, better weight loss maintenance, and fewer complications. Overall, perioperative morbidity and mortality are 10% and less than 1%, respectively. Incisional hernias, wound infections, and vitamin deficiencies may result in the long run. In several studies to date, gastric bypass surgery appears to be very effective in the treatment of OSAHS caused by obesity.[100]

Oral Appliances

Oral appliances are indicated for patients who have mild SDB or are CPAP intolerant. The appliances have beneficial effects on snoring, sleepiness, and mild SDB.[101,102] Patients consistently prefer oral appliance over CPAP therapy.[101] Furthermore, oral appliances are more effective than UPPP in both the long and the short term.[102] Although complications of oral appliance therapy are uncommon, possibly a third of patients have a contraindication to this therapy, such as insufficient teeth, periodontal problems, or temporomandibular joint disorder (see Chapter 91).[103]

COMMON CLINICAL PROBLEMS ENCOUNTERED IN MANAGING PATIENTS WITH OSAHS

Negative Sleep Studies

When the results of an overnight study are normal, significant SDB is unlikely but cannot be completely excluded. Factors that may contribute to a false-negative sleep study include the following:

1. Poor-quality sleep during the study (particularly, absence of rapid eye movement sleep)
2. Sleeping on one's side during the study instead of the usual supine sleeping position (sleep apnea tends to be most severe in the supine position)
3. Omitting one's usual alcohol or sedative agent on the night of the study
4. Insensitive (or, more accurately, overly sensitive) monitors of airflow or respiratory effort, which allow subtle decrements in airflow or marked increases in respiratory effort to go undetected[104]

As originally described, UARS occurs in patients with clinical symptoms suggestive of sleep apnea but with negative sleep studies.[41] Overreliance on the AHI also probably results in undertreatment of patients who would benefit from CPAP. The AHI does not take into account the duration of SDB events, the degree of oxygen desaturation or sleep disruption, or associated cardiac arrhythmias. A significant number of symptomatic patients would almost certainly benefit from treatment even though they have sleep study findings that do not meet reimbursement criteria for treatment.

CPAP Compliance

Second to weight loss, CPAP compliance remains the most significant therapeutic challenge, even though some work suggests that the benefits of CPAP are directly related to the average duration of nightly use.[86,59,93] Patients who do not accept or comply with CPAP need written and verbal discussion of the risks of untreated sleep apnea, emphasizing automobile accidents and cardiovascular risk, as these are the best documented consequences of untreated SDB. For medicolegal purposes, this discussion should be documented in the medical record. Such patients also deserve a frank discussion of alternative treatments, including surgery and oral appliances. They should always have the option of using CPAP even when another treatment was selected first. Documentation should note that the patient was told that neither surgery nor oral appliances have been shown to be as effective as CPAP in alleviating the consequences of sleep apnea.

Driving Risk

SDB increases the risk of motor vehicle accidents. Doctors should familiarize themselves with local laws concerning sleepiness and driving. Estimates of increased risk range from 2 to 7 times that in the nonaffected population.[105] Identifying those at greatest risk is more art than science; a prior history of automobile accidents or near misses and an elevated score on the Epworth Sleepiness Scale may help to predict those at greatest risk. Some recent evidence reveals that driving simulator technology may discriminate apneic drivers from control drivers, and it may be able to identify those with apnea who are at lesser risk for automobile crashes. Both driving simulator data and real-life experience have demonstrated that driving capabilities return quickly (within days) to baseline when patients with sleep apnea are treated with nasal CPAP.[106,107] The prevention of driving accidents in patients with sleep apnea appears cost effective and may reduce fatalities.[108] Both education of the patient with sleep apnea about sleepy driving and objective documentation of treatment efficacy are important in reducing the likelihood of accidents.

Vorona and Ware recommend the following approach to reduce the risk of accidents for patients with SDB:[105]

1. Educate patients with OSAS about the increased risk of sleepy driving. Inform them that sleep-related accidents are disproportionately severe. Provide access to written materials on sleep apnea and driving.
2. Ask patients with OSAS about a previous history of sleepy driving and any history of motor vehicle accidents. Pay particular attention to patients with a history of previous sleepy accidents and those who drive professionally.
3. Instruct patients in proper sleep hygiene and encourage them to obtain adequate hours of sleep.
4. Encourage caffeine and use of rest stops as effective countermeasures to sleepy driving. Napping has also been shown to counteract sleepiness in driving activities.
5. Order time-of-use meters on CPAP units for objective documentation of patient compliance.
6. Use PSG to document efficacy of treatment for those undergoing other treatments such as surgery or an oral appliance. Patients who drive professionally may benefit from a driving simulator. This test appears more effective for stratifying those most likely to avoid accidents. In the absence of a driving simulator, another measure of alertness (a multiple sleep latency test or the Multiple Wakefulness Test) may be used, although data supporting their utility are inconclusive.
7. Discourage driving for those patients not complying with therapy and believed to be at risk for motor vehicle accidents. Those patients continuing to drive and believed to be a public health risk should be reported by the physician to the authorities if state statutes allow. Although some might propose obligatory reporting to the state of all with sleep apnea, caution is urged. Recent work by Findley[109] suggests that this might reduce the likelihood that patients will seek medical attention.

Inadequate Response: When to Restudy

Repeat testing is usually not routine for several reasons. Most sleep laboratories are overbooked with patients who have not yet been diagnosed, sleep studies are expensive and inconvenient, and insurance often does not cover repeat testing. However, for some patients a repeat test can be very helpful. Among them are patients who have a nondiagnostic first study

(see earlier), who are still sleepy on adequate CPAP, who gain or lose significant amounts of weight, or who undergo surgery or fabrication of an oral appliance to treat their SDB. Patients who remain sleepy on treatment or whose sleepiness and other symptoms recur after an initial good clinical response may benefit from reassessment.

The Patient Who Remains Sleepy on CPAP Treatment

Sleepiness after initiation of CPAP treatment is common and takes two forms: the patient who has an initial excellent response to treatment and subsequently becomes sleepy again, and the patient who has never had an improvement in sleepiness despite CPAP use. The prevalence of this problem is unknown, but several studies have documented that the mean level of sleepiness does not return to normal in individuals treated with CPAP.[110,111] Box 92–6 lists the likely causes of sleepiness after CPAP treatment is initiated. The first step in evaluating such patients should probably be to obtain some measure of compliance, typically accomplished by a meter or a card on the CPAP machine. Although acceptable compliance is often suggested to be 4 or 5 hours of CPAP use, optimal CPAP use for individual patients is not known. Evaluation of the patient for another sleep disorder, particularly shift work sleep disorder, may clarify the issue. Medications and their effects on nocturnal sleep and daytime alertness should be investigated.

Two groups[110,112] have investigated the use of modafinil in carefully selected, CPAP-compliant patients who were still objectively and subjectively sleepy. Each study found improvement in some measure of sleepiness with 400 mg of modafinil a day. Whether and when to use this approach for patients with SDB who are still sleepy is likely to remain controversial. Objective measurements of CPAP compliance and of sleepiness would seem to be minimal prerequisites to such treatment.

Managing OSAHS in Special Patient Groups

The Patient Who Has Both Chronic Obstructive Pulmonary Disease and OSAHS

The term *overlap syndrome* was coined to refer to patients who have both COPD and OSAHS[113] (see Chapter 93). Data from the SHHS suggest that although there is no association between generally mild COPD and sleep apnea–hypopnea, oxygen desaturation is greater in individuals who have both conditions than in those who have either condition alone.[114]

Box 92–6. **Potential Causes of Sleepiness despite CPAP Treatment**

- Noncompliance
- Inadequate total sleep time (e.g., self-imposed sleep restriction)
- Medication effects
- A coexisting sleep disorder
- Depression
- Permanent brain damage from untreated sleep-disordered breathing

CPAP, continuous positive airway pressure.

CPAP is an effective treatment for the SDB in these patients and may reduce cardiovascular risk. It often appears remarkably effective in reversing the hypoxemia that is associated as well. Unfortunately, CPAP compliance in smokers and in individuals who have COPD appears to be lower than in nonsmokers or in those who do not have COPD.[79]

Some patients with COPD (and other lung diseases) have difficulty tolerating CPAP, or they remain hypoxemic on CPAP pressures that are high enough to eliminate the episodes of apnea. It is possible that bilevel pressure, with or without a set rate, may be of benefit in these situations. Supplemental oxygen can be added to the CPAP circuit to normalize oxygenation. Very little is known about the likelihood of carbon dioxide retention in this situation or its effects.

Smoking cessation is imperative for these patients. Not only do ex-smokers appear to have a normalized risk for sleep apnea compared with active smokers,[15] but also smokers in general sleep more poorly than do nonsmokers.[73] Optimal medical management of these patients includes, in addition to CPAP, inhaled bronchodilators and perhaps inhaled antiinflammatory agents to minimize the effects of cough and wheezing on sleep structure.

Management of Sleep Apnea in the Perioperative Patient

The scientific data about optimal perioperative management of patients known or suspected to have SDB are limited. According to a statement by the Clinical Practice Committee of the AASM and a recent review,[115,116] critical issues in preventing perioperative mishaps in patients with OSAHS include having a high degree of clinical suspicion, controlling the airway throughout the perioperative period, using medications very judiciously, and employing appropriate monitoring. Orthopedic patients appear to be at particularly increased risk. Further research is clearly needed to define the magnitude of risk and optimal perioperative care.

Management of Sleep Apnea in the Critically Ill Patient

Patients with sleep apnea have increased health care costs because of cardiovascular risk and other comorbid conditions such as obesity, diabetes, and hypertension.[65] It is to be expected, then, that they arrive frequently to the intensive care unit (ICU). For patients with known sleep apnea, an attempt to treat with CPAP or bilevel pressure may be of benefit. However, many patients with diagnosed sleep apnea arrive in the ICU because they have been unwilling or unable to use the CPAP machine. Furthermore, coughing, vomiting, nasogastric tubes, procedures, and patient discomfort may result in intermittent CPAP use. For critically ill patients, intermittent airway patency is a great deal less than optimal. Intubation may be the most definitive and effective initial course for the critically ill patient with sleep apnea who has respiratory distress. In patients with known sleep apnea who arrive in the ICU because of inability to use CPAP, tracheostomy is a long-term solution that may prevent another hospitalization. All the caveats of care that are applicable to perioperative patients apply to those in the ICU.

For management of OSAHS in the pregnant woman, see Chapter 109, and in the patient with heart failure, see Chapter 102.

Clinical Pearl

Sleep apnea is a common condition with significant cardiac, metabolic, and cognitive consequences. Although there is clearly a genetic predisposition, lifestyle factors are important and modifiable risk factors. Witnessed apneas, heavy snoring, daytime sleepiness, obesity, and hypertension are the classic symptoms and signs of sleep-disordered breathing. CPAP is clearly the most effective treatment, and achieving compliance with this treatment remains an important clinical challenge.

REFERENCES

1. Young T, Palta M, Dempsey J, et al: The occurrence of sleep-disordered breathing among middle-aged adults. N Engl J Med 1993;328:1230-1235.
2. Kripke DF, Ancoli-Israel S, Klauber MR, et al: Prevalence of sleep-disordered breathing in ages 40-64 years: A population-based survey. Sleep 1997;20:65-76.
3. Young T, Shahar E, Nieto FJ, and the Sleep Heart Health Study Research Group: Predictors of sleep-disordered breathing in community-dwelling adults: The Sleep Heart Health Study. Arch Intern Med 2002;162:893-900.
4. Gottlieb DJ, Whitney CW, Bonekat WH, et al: Relation of sleepiness to respiratory disturbance index: The Sleep Heart Health Study. Am J Respir Crit Care Med 1999;159:502-507.
5. Young T, Peppard PE, Gottlieb DJ: Epidemiology of obstructive sleep apnea. Am J Respir Crit Care Med 2002;165:1217-1239.
6. Tischler PV, Larkin EK, Schluchter MD, Redline S: Incidence of sleep-disordered breathing in an urban adult population: The relative importance of risk factors in the development of sleep-disordered breathing. JAMA 2003;289:2230-2237.
7. Young T, Finn L, Austin D, Peterson A: Menopausal status and sleep-disordered breathing in the Wisconsin Sleep Cohort Study. Am J Respir Crit Care Med 2003;167:1181-1185.
8. Pillar G, Lavie P: Assessment of the role of inheritance in sleep apnea syndrome. Am J Resp Crit Care Med 1995;151:688-691.
9. Redline S, Tishler PV, Hans MG, et al: Racial differences in sleep-disordered breathing in African-Americans and Caucasians. Am J Respir Crit Care Med 1997;155:186-192.
10. Ip MS, Tsan WT, Lam WK, Oam B: Obstructive sleep apnea syndrome: An experience in Chinese adults in Hong Kong. Chin Med J 1998;111:257-260.
11. Lanfranchi PA, Somers VK: Sleep-disordered breathing in heart failure: Characteristics and implications. Respir Physiol Neurobiol 2003;136:153-165.
12. Skjodt NM, Atkar R, Easton PA: Screening for hypothyroidism in sleep apnea. Am J Respir Crit Care Med 1999;160:732-735.
13. Watanabe T, Isono S, Tanaka A, et al: Contribution of body habitus and craniofacial characteristics to segmental closing pressures of the passive pharynx in patients with sleep-disordered breathing. Am J Respir Crit Care Med 2002;165:260-265.
14. Scanlan MF, Roebuck T, Little PJ, et al: Effect of moderate alcohol upon obstructive sleep apnoea. Eur Respir J 2000;16:909-913.
15. Wetter DW, Young TB, Bidwell TR, et al: Smoking as a risk factor for sleep-disordered breathing Arch Intern Med 1994;154:2219-2224.
16. Maislin G, Pack AI, Kribbs NB, et al: A survey screen for prediction of apnea. Sleep 1995;18:158-166.
17. Netzer NC, Stoohs RA, Netzer CM, et al: Using the Berlin Questionnaire to identify patients at risk for the sleep apnea syndrome. Ann Intern Med 1999;131:485-491.
18. Tsai WH, Remmers JE, Brant R, et al: A decision rule for diagnostic testing in obstructive sleep apnea. Am J Respir Crit Care Med 2003;167:1427-1432.

19. Johns MW: A new method for measuring daytime sleepiness: The Epworth sleepiness scale. Sleep 1991;14:540-545.

19a. Chin K, Fukuhara S, Takahashi K, et al: Response to shift in perception of sleepiness in obstructive sleep apnea-hypopnea syndrome before and after treatment with nasal CPAP. Sleep 2004;27:490-493.

20. Hajduk IA, Strollo PJ Jr, Jasani RR, et al: Prevalence and predictors of nocturia in obstructive sleep apnea-hypopnea syndrome: A retrospective study. Sleep 2003;26:61-64.

21. Karacan I, Karatas M: Erectile dysfunction in sleep apnea and response to CPAP. J Sex Marital Ther 1995;21:239-247.

22. Mojon DS, Hedges TR 3rd, Ehrenberg B, et al: Association between sleep apnea syndrome and nonarteritic anterior ischemic optic neuropathy. Arch Ophthalmol 2002;120: 601-605.

23. Purvin VA, Kawasaki A, Yee RD: Papilledema and obstructive sleep apnea syndrome. Arch Ophthalmol 2000;118:1626-1630.

24. Mojon DS, Hess CW, Goldblum D, et al: High prevalence of glaucoma in patients with sleep apnea syndrome. Ophthalmology 1999;106:1009-1012.

25. Shepertycky MR, Banno K, Kryger MH: Differences between men and women in the clinical presentation of patients diagnosed with obstructive sleep apnea syndrome. Sleep 2005;28:309-314.

26. Viner S, Szalai JP, Hoffstein V: Are history and physical examination a good screening test for sleep apnea? Ann Intern Med 1991;115:356-359.

27. Davies RJ, Ali NJ, Stradling JR: Neck circumference and other clinical features in the diagnosis of the obstructive sleep apnoea syndrome. Thorax 1992;47:101-105.

28. Young T, Finn L, Palta M: Chronic nasal congestion at night is a risk factor for snoring in a population-based cohort study. Arch Intern Med 2001 25;161:1514-1519.

29. Kushida CA, Efron B, Guilleminault C: A predictive morphometric model for the obstructive sleep apnea syndrome. Ann Intern Med 1997;127:581-587.

30. Nieto FJ, Young TB, Lind BK, et al: Association of sleep-disordered breathing, sleep apnea, and hypertension in a large community-based study. JAMA 2000;283:1829-1836.

31. Grote L, Ploch T, Heitmann J, et al: Sleep-related breathing disorder is an independent risk factor for systemic hypertension. Am J Respir Crit Care Med 1999;160:1875-1882.

32. Peppard PE, Young T, Palta M, Skatrud J: Prospective study of the association between sleep-disordered breathing and hypertension. N Engl J Med 2000;342:1378-1384.

33. Logan AG, Perlikowski SM, Mente A, et al: High prevalence of unrecognized sleep apnoea in drug-resistant hypertension. J Hypertens 2001;19:2271-2277.

34. Stradling JR, Davies RJ: Sleep: 1. Obstructive sleep apnoea/hypopnoea syndrome—Definitions, epidemiology, and natural history. Thorax 2004;59:73-78.

35. Kapur VK, Rapoport DM, Sanders MH, et al: Rates of sensor loss in unattended home polysomnography: The influence of age, gender, obesity, and sleep-disordered breathing. Sleep 2000; 23:682-688.

36. Whitney CW, Gottlieb DJ, Redline S, et al: Reliability of scoring respiratory disturbance indices and sleep staging. Sleep 1998;21:749-757.

37. Shahar E, Whitney CW, Redline S, et al: Sleep-disordered breathing and cardiovascular disease: Cross-sectional results of the Sleep Heart Health Study. Am J Respir Crit Care Med 2001;163:19-25.

38. American Academy of Sleep Medicine Task Force: Sleep-related breathing disorders in adults: Recommendations for syndrome definition and measurement techniques in clinical research. Sleep 1999;22:667-689.

39. Centers for Medicare & Medicaid Services: Available at http://www.cms.hhs.gov/manuals/pm_trans/R150CIM.pdf.

40. Meoli AL, Casey KR, Clark RW, and the Clinical Practice Review Committee of the American Academy of Sleep Medicine: Hypopnea in sleep-disordered breathing in adults. Sleep 2001; 24:469-470.

41. Guilleminault C, Stoohs R, Clerk A, et al: A Cause of excessive daytime sleepiness. Chest 1993;104:781-787.

42. Douglas NJ: Home diagnosis of the obstructive sleep apnoea/hypopnea syndrome. Sleep Med Rev 2003;7:53-59.

43. ASDA Standards of Practice: Practice parameters for the use of portable recording in the assessment of obstructive sleep apnea. Sleep 1994;17:372-377.

44. Chervin RD: Periodic leg movements and sleepiness in patients evaluated for sleep-disordered breathing. Am J Respir Crit Care Med 2001;164:1454-1458.

45. Exar EN, Collop NA: The association of upper airway resistance with periodic limb movements. Sleep 2001;24:188-192.

46. Whittle AT, Finch SP, Mortimore IL, et al: Use of home sleep studies for diagnosis of the sleep apnoea/hypopnoea syndrome. Thorax 1997;52:1068-1073.

47. Kingshott RN, Vennelle M, Hoy CJ, et al: Predictors of improvements in daytime function outcomes with CPAP therapy. Am J Respir Crit Care Med 2000;161;866-871.

48. Bennett LS, Langford BA, Stradling JR, Davies RJ: Sleep fragmentation indices as predictors of daytime sleepiness and nCPAP response in obstructive sleep apnea. Am J Respir Crit Care Med 1998;158:778-786.

49. Elbaz M, Roue GM, Lofaso F, Quera Salva MA: Utility of actigraphy in the diagnosis of obstructive sleep apnea. Sleep 2002; 25:527-531.

50. Lojander J, Salmi T, Maasilta P: Reproducibility of oximetry with a static charge-sensitive bed in evaluation of obstructive sleep apnoea. Clin Physiol 1998;18:225-233.

51. Grote L, Zou D, Kraiczi H, Hedner J: Finger plethysmography: A method for monitoring finger blood flow during sleep-disordered breathing. Respir Physiol Neurobiol 2003;136: 141-152.

52. Stein PK, Duntley SP, Domitrovich PP, et al: A simple method to identify sleep apnea using Holter recordings. J Cardiovasc Electrophysiol 2003;14:467-473.

53. Bar A, Pillar G, Dvir I, et al: Evaluation of a portable device based on peripheral arterial tone for unattended home sleep studies. Chest. 2003;123:695-703.

54. Lenfant C, Chobanian AV, Jones DW, Roccella EJ, and the Joint National Committee on the Prevention, Detection, Evaluation, and Treatment of High Blood Pressure: Seventh report of the Committee (JNC 7): Resetting the hypertension sails. Hypertension 2003;41:1178-1179; Epub 2003 May 19.

55. Barbe F, Pericas J, Munoz A, et al: Automobile accidents in patients with sleep apnea syndrome. An epidemiological and mechanistic study. Am J Respir Crit Care Med 1998;158:18-22.

56. Hack M, Davies RJ, Mullins R, et al: Randomised prospective parallel trial of therapeutic versus subtherapeutic nasal continuous positive airway pressure on simulated steering performance inpatients with obstructive sleep apnoea. Thorax 2000;55:224-231.

57. Fulda S, Schulz H: Cognitive dysfunction in sleep disorders. Sleep Med Rev 2001;5:423-445.

58. Redline S, Strauss M, Adams N, et al: Neuropsychological function in mild sleep-disordered breathing. Sleep 1997;20:160-167.

59. Kaneko Y, Floras JS, Usui K, et al: Cardiovascular effects of continuous positive airway pressure in patients with heart failure and obstructive sleep apnea. N Engl J Med 2003;348:1233-1241.

60. Peker Y, Hedner J, Norum J, et al: Increased incidence of cardiovascular disease in middle-aged men with obstructive sleep apnea: A 7-year follow-up. Am J Respir Crit Care Med 2002; 166:159-165.

61. Means MK, Lichstein KL, Edinger JD, et al: Changes in depressive symptoms after continuous positive airway pressure treatment for obstructive sleep apnea. Sleep Breath 2003;7:31-42.

62. Punjabi N, Sorkin J, Katzel L, et al: Sleep-disordered breathing and insulin resistance in middle-aged and overweight men. Am J Respir Crit Care Med 2002;165:677-682.

63. Ip M, Lam B, Ng M, et al: Obstructive sleep apnea is independently associated with insulin resistance. Am J Respir Crit Care Med 2002;165:670-676.

64. Baldwin CM, Griffith KA, Nieto FJ, et al: The association of sleep-disordered breathing and sleep symptoms with quality of life in the Sleep Heart Health Study. Sleep 2001;24:96-105.

65. Bahammam A, Delaive K, Ronald J, et al: Health care utilization in males with obstructive sleep apnea syndrome two years after diagnosis and treatment. Sleep 1999;22:740-747.

66. Redline S, Larkin E, Schluchter M, et al: Incidence of sleep disordered breathing in a population-based sample. Sleep 2001; 24:511.

67. Young T, Evans L, Finn L, Palta M: Estimation of the clinically diagnosed proportion of sleep apnea syndrome in middle-aged men and women. Sleep 1997;20:705-706.

68. Lindberg E, Janson C, Gislason T, et al: Snoring and hypertension: A 10 year follow-up. Eur Respir J 1998;11:884-889.

69. Al-Delaimy W, Manson J, Willett W, et al: Snoring as a risk factor for type 2 diabetes mellitus: A prospective study. Am J Epidemiol 2002;155:387-393.

70. Peppard PE, Young T, Palta M, et al: Longitudinal study of moderate weight change and sleep-disordered breathing. JAMA 2000;284:3015-3021.

71. Foster GD: Principles and practices in the management of obesity. Am J Respir Crit Care Med 2003;168:274-280.

72. Kiely JL, Nolan P, McNicholas WT: Intranasal corticosteroid therapy for obstructive sleep apnoea in patients with co-existing rhinitis. Thorax 2004;59:50-55.

73. Phillips BA, Danner FJ: Cigarette smoking and sleep disturbance. Arch Intern Med 1995;155:734-737.

74. Scanlan MF, Roebuck T, Little PJ, et al: Effect of moderate alcohol upon obstructive sleep apnoea. Eur Respir J 2000;16:909-913.

75. Littner M, Hirshkowitz M, Davila D, et al: Practice parameters for the use of auto-titrating continuous positive airway pressure devices for titrating pressures and treating adult patients with obstructive sleep apnea syndrome. Sleep 2002;25:143-147.

76. Randerath W, Schraeder O, Galetke W, et al: Autoadjusting CPAP therapy based on impedance efficacy, compliance and acceptance. Am J Crit Care Med 2001;163:652-657.

77. Massie CA, McArdle N, Hart RW, et al: Comparison between automatic and fixed positive airway pressure in the home. Am J Respir Crit Care Med 2003;167:20-23.

78. Farre R, Montserrat JM, Rigau J, et al: Response of automatic continuous positive airway pressure devices to different sleep breathing patterns: A bench study. Am J Respir Crit Care Med 2002;166:469-473.

79. Kribbs NB, Pack AI, Kline LR, et al: Objective measurement of patterns of nasal CPAP use by patients with obstructive sleep apnea. Am Rev Respir Dis 1993;147:887-895.

80. Janson C, Noges E, Svedberg-Brandt S, Lindberg E: What characterized patients who are unable to tolerate continuous positive airway pressure (CPAP) treatment? Respir Med 2000; 94:145-149.

81. McArdle N, Devereux G, Heidarnejad H, et al: Long-term use of CPAP therapy for sleep apnea/hypopnea syndrome. Am J Respir Crit Care Med 1999;159:1108-1114.

82. Weist G, Lehnert G, Bruck WM, et al: A heated humidifier reduced airway dryness during continuous positive airway pressure therapy. Respir Med 1999;93:211-226.

83. Massie CA, Hart RW, Richards GN: The effects of humidification on nasal symptoms and compliance in sleep apnea patients using continuous positive airway pressure. Chest 1999;116:403-409.

84. He J, Kryger MH, Zorick FJ, et al: Mortality and apnea index in obstructive sleep apnea: Experience in 385 male patients. Chest 1988;94:9-14.

85. Wright J, Johns R, Watt I, et al: The health effects of obstructive sleep apnoea and the effectiveness of treatment with continuous positive airway pressure: A systematic review of the research evidence. BMJ 1997;314:851-860.

86. Pepperell JCT, Ramdassingh-Dow S, Crosthwaite N, et al: Ambulatory blood pressure after therapeutic and subtherapeutic nasal continuous positive airway pressure for obstructive sleep apnoea: A randomised parallel trial. Lancet 2002; 359:204-214.

87. Becker HF, Jerrentrup A, Ploch T, et al: Effect of nasal continuous positive airway pressure treatment on blood pressure in patients with obstructive sleep apnea. Circulation 2003; 107:68-73.

88. Bardwell WA, Ancoli-Israel S, Berry CC, Dimsdale J: Neuropsychological effects of one-week continuous positive airway pressure treatment in patients with obstructive sleep apnea: A placebo-controlled study. Psychosom Med 2001; 63:579-584.

89. Redline S, Adams N, Strauss ME, et al: Improvement of mild sleep-disordered breathing with CPAP compared with conservative therapy. Am J Respir Crit Care Med 1998;157:858-865.

90. Jenkinson C, Davies RJ, Mullins R, Stradling JR: Comparison of therapeutic and subtherapeutic nasal continuous positive airway pressure for obstructive sleep apnoea: A randomised prospective parallel trial. Lancet 1999;353:2100-2105.

91. Engleman HM, Martin SE, Deary IJ, Douglas NJ: Effect of continuous positive airway pressure treatment on daytime function in sleep apnoea/hypopnoea syndrome. Lancet 1994;343:572-575.

92. Sher AE: Upper airway surgery for obstructive sleep apnea. Sleep Med Rev 2002;6:195-212.

93. Weaver T, Maislin G, Venditti L, et al: CPAP dose duration for effective outcome response. Am J Respir Crit Care Med 2003; 167:A324.

94. Engleman HM, Kingshott RN, Wraith PK, et al: Randomized placebo-controlled crossover trial of continuous positive airway pressure for mild sleep apnea/hypopnea syndrome. Am J Respir Crit Care Med 1999;159:461-467.

95. Walker R, Grigg-Damberger MM, Gopalsami C, et al: Laser-assisted uvulopalatoplasty for snoring and obstructive sleep apnea: results in 170 patients. Laryngoscope 1995;105: 938-943.

96. Finkelstein Y, Stein G, Ophir D, et al: Laser-assisted uvulopalatoplasty for the management of obstructive sleep apnea: Myths and facts. Arch Otolaryngol Head Neck Surg 2002;128: 429-434.

97. Powell NB, Riley RW, Troell RJ, et al: Radiofrequency volumetric reduction of the palate in subjects with sleep-disordered breathing. Chest 1998;113:1163-1174.

98. Prinsell JR: Maxillomandibular advancement surgery for obstructive sleep apnea syndrome. J Am Dent Assoc 2002;133: 1489-1497.

99. Thatcher GW, Maisel RH: The long-term evaluation of tracheostomy in the management of severe obstructive sleep apnea. Laryngoscope 2003;113:201-204.

100. Buchwald H, Avidor Y, Braunwald E, et al: Bariatric surgery: A systematic review and meta-analysis. JAMA 2004;292: 1724-1737.

101. Schmidt-Nowara W: Recent developments in oral appliance therapy of sleep disordered breathing. Sleep Breath 1999;3: 103-106.

102. Walker-Engstrom ML, Tegelberg A, Wilhelmsson B, Ringqvist I: 4-year follow up of treatment with dental appliance or uvulopalatopharyngoplasty in patients with obstructive sleep apnea: A randomized study. Chest 2002;121:739-746.

103. Petit FX, Pepin JL, Bettega G, et al: Mandibular advancement devices: Rate of contraindications in 100 consecutive obstructive sleep apnea patients. Am J Respir Crit Care Med 2002; 166:274-278.

104. Hosselet JJ, Norman RG, Ayappa I, Rapoport DM: Detection of flow limitation with a nasal cannula/pressure transducer system. Am J Respir Crit Care Med 1998;157:1461-1467.

105. Vorona RD, Ware JC: Sleep disordered breathing and driving risk. Curr Opin Pulm Med 2002;8:506-510.

106. George CF: Reduction in motor vehicle collisions following treatment of sleep apnoea with nasal CPAP. Thorax 2001;56:508-512.

107. Turkington PM, Sircar M, Saralaya D, Elliott MW: Time course of changes in driving simulator performance with and without treatment in patients with sleep apnoea hypopnoea syndrome. Thorax 2004;59:56-59.

108. Sassani A, Findley LJ, Kryger M, et al: Reducing motor vehicle collisions, costs, and fatalities by treating obstructive sleep apnea syndrome. Sleep 2004;27:453-458.

109. Findley L: The threat of mandatory reporting to a driver's license agency discourages sleepy drivers from being evaluated for sleep apnea. Sleep 2002;25:A224.

110. Pack AI, Black JE, Schwartz JR, Matheson JK: Modafinil as adjunct therapy for daytime sleepiness in obstructive sleep apnea. Am J Respir Crit Care Med 2001;164:1675-1681.

111. Lamphere J, Roehrs T, Wittig R, et al: Recovery of alertness after CPAP in apnea. Chest 1989;96:1364-1367.

112. Kingshott RN, Vennelle M, Coleman EL, et al: Randomized, double-blind, placebo-controlled crossover trial of modafinil in the treatment of residual excessive daytime sleepiness in the sleep apnea/hypopnea syndrome. Am J Respir Crit Care Med 2001;163:918-923.

113. Chaout A, Weitzenblum E, Kreiger J, et al: Association of chronic obstructive pulmonary disease and sleep apnea syndrome. Am J Respir Crit Care Med 1995;151:82-86.

114. Sanders MH, Newman AB, Haggerty CL, et al: Sleep and sleep-disordered breathing in adults with predominantly mild obstructive airway disease. Am J Respir Crit Care Med 2003;167:7-14.

115. Clinical Practice Review Committee, American Academy of Sleep Medicine: Upper airway management of the adult patient with obstructive sleep apnea in the perioperative period: Avoiding complications. Sleep 2003;26:1060-1065.

116. den Herder C, Schmeck J, Appelboom DJ, et al: Risks of general anaesthesia in people with obstructive sleep apnoea. BMJ 2004;329:955-959.

93

Asthma and Chronic Obstructive Pulmonary Disease

Neil J. Douglas

ABSTRACT

Patients with asthma are often troubled by nocturnal cough, wheeze, and breathlessness. This results from sleep-related nocturnal narrowing of the lower airways. The main mechanism is probably alteration in neural control of airway caliber during sleep. Usually nocturnal asthma is inconvenient and unpleasant, but occasionally it can be life-threatening. The new development of nocturnal symptoms is an indicator of deteriorating asthma control, and it is an indication for intensifying therapy. Treatment is by optimizing inhaled steroids and beta-agonists, often with the addition of long-acting inhaled beta-agonists.

Patients with chronic obstructive pulmonary disease experience oxyhemoglobin desaturation during sleep, especially during rapid eye movement sleep. This is caused by normal physiologic hypoventilation during sleep, but nevertheless it may have deleterious cardiovascular and hematologic effects. The need for treatment depends on daytime levels of arterial oxygen tension, and there is no evidence that overnight polysomnography is helpful in the management of such patients unless there is a clinical suspicion for obstructive sleep apnea–hypopnea syndrome. The treatments of choice are oxygen therapy, or oxygen plus nocturnal noninvasive intermittent positive-pressure ventilation.

NOCTURNAL ASTHMA

Asthma, a disease characterized by variable bronchoconstriction, occurs in about 5% of the population. The bronchoconstriction is, at least initially, totally reversible with therapy. Besides spasm of bronchial smooth muscle, other causes of the airflow obstruction are viscous bronchial secretions and inflammation and swelling of the mucosa and submucosa. There is no evidence that asthma is more common in obese subjects.

The airways of asthmatic patients are hyperresponsive: bronchoconstriction may follow exposure to allergens (pollen, animal dander) or nonallergenic stimuli (viral infections, cold, fumes). In many patients, asthma is worse at night or in the early morning, causing cough, wheeze, or breathlessness. These symptoms reflect overnight bronchoconstriction, which occurs in over two thirds of asthmatic patients.[1]

Although the cause of nocturnal bronchospasm remains uncertain, its management is improving with advances in medications. The observation that many asthmatic patients wheeze at night is not new. In 1698, Dr. (later Sir) John Floyer, himself asthmatic, wrote: "I have observed the fit always to happen after sleep in the night. . . . At first waking, about one or two of the clock in the night, the fit of asthma more evidently begins, the

breath is very slow . . . the diaphragm seems stiff and tied. . . . It is not without much difficulty moved downwards."[2] Despite the clarity of this description, over 2 centuries passed before nocturnal asthma received much further attention.

The forced expiratory volume in 1 second (FEV_1) and peak flow rates fall overnight in patients with asthma,[3] the fall being over 50% in some patients. Patients with such overnight bronchoconstriction have been called "morning dippers" (Fig. 93–1).[4] In asthmatics recovering from exacerbations, about one third have bronchoconstriction during the night, and another third have bronchoconstriction before sleep and continue to have it overnight.[1] Thus, two thirds of such patients have their lowest flow rates between 10 PM, and 8 AM with a mean amplitude of variation of peak flow rates of 29%.[1]

Circadian Rhythm of Airway Caliber

Most unaffected people also have circadian changes in airway caliber with mild nocturnal bronchoconstriction.[5] The largest series comparing circadian changes in peak flow in healthy subjects and unstable asthmatic patients[5] shows that the changes in flow rate are synchronous in asthmatic and healthy subjects, whereas the amplitude of the peak flow rate changes is far greater in asthmatic patients (50%) than in healthy subjects (8%). Thus, nocturnal bronchoconstriction in asthma appears to be an exaggeration of the normal circadian changes in airway caliber. Asthmatic patients are hyperreactive to constrictor stimuli; thus, nocturnal bronchoconstriction in asthmatic patients is probably an expression of hyperresponsiveness

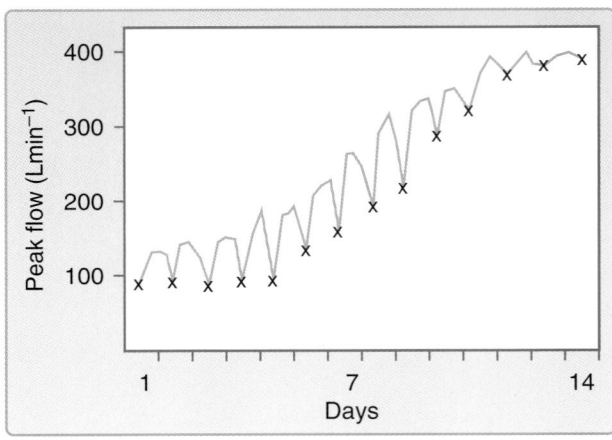

Figure 93–1. Peak flow rate over a 2-week period in a 62-year-old nonallergic asthmatic woman. The flow rate on waking is indicated with a *cross*. There is marked "morning dipping." (From Douglas NJ: Asthma at night. Clin Chest Med 1985;6:663-674.)

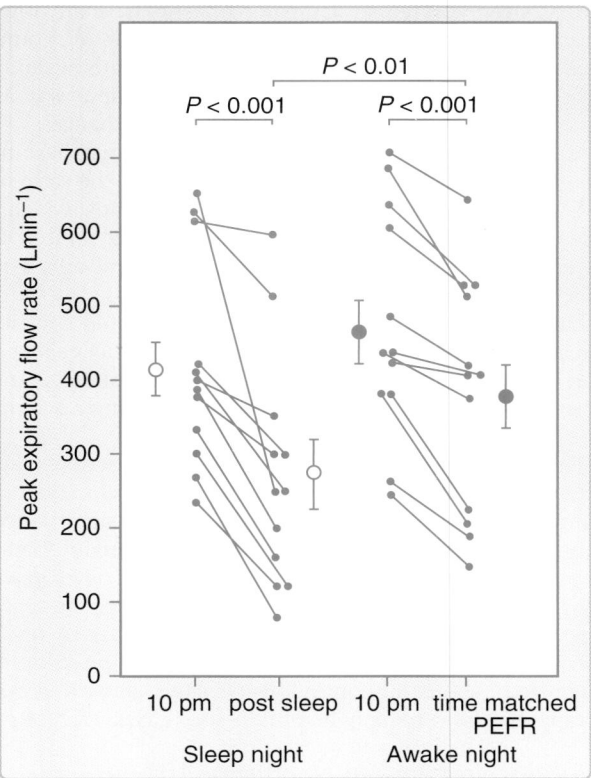

Figure 93–2. Peak expiratory flow rate (PEFR) at night and in the morning on both the asleep and the awake nights. All patients developed bronchoconstriction on both nights, but although the 10 PM peak flow rates were not significantly different, morning peak flow was higher after the awake night. Data are presented as mean ± SEM. (From Catterall JR, Rhind GB, Stewart IC, et al: Effect of sleep deprivation on overnight bronchoconstriction in nocturnal asthma. Thorax 1986;41:676-680.)

to the factors that produce mild nocturnal bronchoconstriction in healthy subjects.

Synchronization of Circadian Rhythm

As with other circadian rhythms, the major synchronizing factor is sleep. Overnight sleep deprivation reduces, but does not abolish, nocturnal airway narrowing (Fig. 93–2).[6,7] In asthmatic shift workers, sleep time determines the timing of nocturnal airway narrowing,[8] with rapid inversion of airway caliber changes with inversion of the sleep pattern. That some overnight airway narrowing persists even if patients are kept awake all night could be the result of a lag between altered sleep times and readjustment of circadian rhythms.

Pathogenesis of Nocturnal Airway Narrowing

Factors that have been suggested but seem unlikely to be primary causes of nocturnal airway narrowing include the sleeping posture, interruption of bronchodilator or other treatment, and allergens in bedding.

Posture is not a major factor because patients who lie in bed throughout the 24-hour period continue to exhibit overnight bronchoconstriction,[3] and lying down does not produce sustained bronchoconstriction.[9] The treatment interval is not critical; regular spacing of treatments throughout the 24 hours does not abolish nocturnal bronchospasm,[4] and nocturnal wheeze is a presenting complaint of many untreated asthmatic patients.

Allergens

It is unlikely that allergens in bedding are prime causes of nocturnal asthma, because avoidance of such allergens does not abolish nocturnal airway narrowing.[10] In addition, overnight bronchoconstriction occurs in both allergic and nonallergic asthmatic patients,[1] and in healthy people.[5] Allergic factors can, however, produce nocturnal wheeze; experimental allergen inhalation can cause bronchoconstriction on subsequent nights[11] and scrupulous exclusion of allergens can reduce circadian changes in peak flow rates and in the frequency and severity of asthmatic attacks.[12]

These findings suggest that allergic reactions—and particularly, perhaps, late or delayed allergic reactions—are important in the development of nocturnal wheeze in some patients. There is a close relationship between the extent of nocturnal airway narrowing and the degree of airway twitchiness or bronchial reactivity.[13] It seems likely that such allergen exposure increases bronchial reactivity in predisposed patients and thus may result in nocturnal bronchoconstriction.

Airway Cooling

Cold, dry air causes bronchoconstriction in asthmatic patients. It had been suggested that nocturnal asthma might be caused either by breathing cooler air at night or by bronchial wall cooling as a result of the overnight decrease in body core temperature. However, overnight bronchoconstriction persists in healthy subjects when temperature and humidity are kept constant throughout the 24-hour day.[14] Nevertheless, it has been reported that breathing warm, humid air (36° C to 37° C, 100% saturation) overnight, compared with breathing room air (23° C, 17% to 24% saturation) overnight, abolished nocturnal bronchoconstriction in six of seven asthmatic patients.[15] It is not clear how well the patients slept when breathing the warm, humid air. If it kept them awake, this could explain the lack of bronchoconstriction.

Gastroesophageal Reflux

There seems to be a high incidence of gastroesophageal reflux (GER) in people with asthma, especially in those with nocturnal wheeze,[16] and the GER may be clinically "silent." There is no convincing evidence that spontaneous GER causes nocturnal bronchoconstriction.[17] Gastric acid suppression with the proton pump inhibitor omeprazole produced a small improvement in nocturnal but not daytime asthma symptoms.[16] There was a minor deterioration in lung function in the overall study population.[16]

Mucociliary Clearance

Mucociliary clearance is impaired during sleep, and the accumulation of mucus in the airways could contribute to nocturnal airway narrowing. However, this accumulation seems unlikely to be a major factor in nocturnal wheeze, as bronchodilators are rapidly effective.

Bronchial Hyperreactivity

Bronchial responsiveness to inhaled histamine and allergens increases throughout the night.[18] However, the airways are narrower at this time, and thus the increased response could reflect greater initial bronchomotor tone at night rather than any change in mucosal permeability or receptor or neuromuscular function. A skin prick test for allergens and histamine shows marked circadian variation: maximal effects are in the late evening, and a minimum is reached by early morning.[19] Thus, there may be circadian variations in reactivity, although the changes in sensitivity to skin tests are about 8 hours ahead of the circadian changes in airway reactivity.

Is Nocturnal Wheeze Related to Sleep Stage?

Several groups have recorded electroencephalograms (EEGs) of sleeping asthmatic patients and have noted the stage the patients were in when they awoke with attacks of asthma. An early study suggestion that patients awoke more frequently from rapid eye movement (REM) sleep than would be expected by chance has not been confirmed, asthmatic attacks being randomly distributed throughout the stages of sleep in proportion to the amount of time spent in each sleep stage[20] (Fig. 93–3).

Esophageal pressure measurements suggest that pulmonary resistance does not differ between sleep stages.[7] It thus appears unlikely that there is any difference in the degree of airway narrowing between sleep stages.

Breathing Patterns during Sleep

Ventilation in asthmatic patients, like that in normal subjects,[21] decreases from wakefulness to sleep, becoming lower during non-REM (NREM) sleep than during wakefulness, and lowest

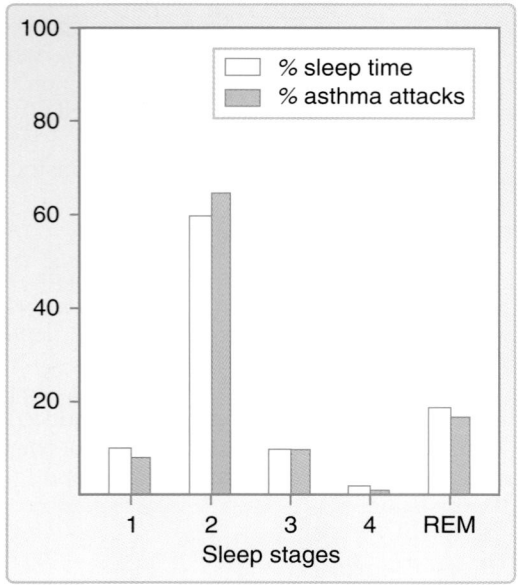

Figure 93–3. Comparison of percentage of night spent in each sleep stage with percentage of asthmatic awakenings from that stage. The asthmatic attack frequency was proportional to the frequency of each sleep stage. (Redrawn from Kales A, Beall GN, Bajor GF, et al: Sleep studies in asthmatic adults: Relationship of attacks to sleep stage and time of night. J Allergy 1968;41:164-173.)

in REM sleep.[22] Whether asthmatic patients have any breathing pattern abnormality during sleep is unclear. We found a small, but significant, increase in irregular breathing in asthmatic patients, caused almost entirely by more apneas in asthmatic patients,[23] but others found no such changes.[22] The increased number of apneas that we observed may have been the result of the study having been performed in the early summer, when the patients may have had mild rhinitis, which has been shown to increase apneas. In addition, the apneas were few and brief and were not associated with significant hypoxemia; thus, their clinical significance is dubious.

Lung volume falls during sleep, and this could contribute to increasing resistance to airflow because airway caliber will drop as lung volume decreases. However, this is not a major cause of sleep-related airway narrowing, although it may be contributory.[24]

There is some evidence that distal lung function may be preferentially impaired at night in patients with nocturnal asthma.[25] However, neither the cause nor the significance of this observation is clear. Some nocturnal asthmatic patients who snore or have obstructive sleep apnea may develop worsening of their asthma, perhaps as a reflex response to their upper airway vibration. This appears to be a relatively uncommon cause of nocturnal asthma, but it is important that it be recognized, as nasal continuous positive airway pressure therapy may be extremely helpful in such cases[26] (Fig. 93–4).

Relationship between Nocturnal Asthma and Obesity

There has been speculation that asthma is directly related to obesity and thus might be more common in patients with the obstructive sleep apnea–hypopnea syndrome. However there is no convincing evidence of an association between asthma and obesity.[27]

Causes of Nocturnal Airway Narrowing: Conclusions

Nocturnal asthma is largely a sleep-synchronized circadian rhythm in airway caliber. The following paragraphs describe how this results in airway narrowing.

Mechanisms and Effector Systems for Nocturnal Airway Narrowing

Autonomic Function

Bronchial muscle receives efferent innervation from the parasympathetic system via the vagus nerve, but there is no evidence of direct sympathetic innervation to the muscle in humans. However, there are sympathetic nerves to the airway, and some probably terminate on the vagal ganglia in the bronchial wall. Circulating (or inhaled) catecholamines probably cause bronchodilation by acting directly on bronchial smooth muscle. In addition, a third component of the autonomic nervous system—the nonadrenergic, noncholinergic (NANC) bronchodilating system—passes in the vagus nerve and produces bronchodilation.

PARASYMPATHETIC NERVOUS SYSTEM

Parasympathetic tone tends to be increased at night. Studies using cholinergic blockade[28,29] indicate that an increase in

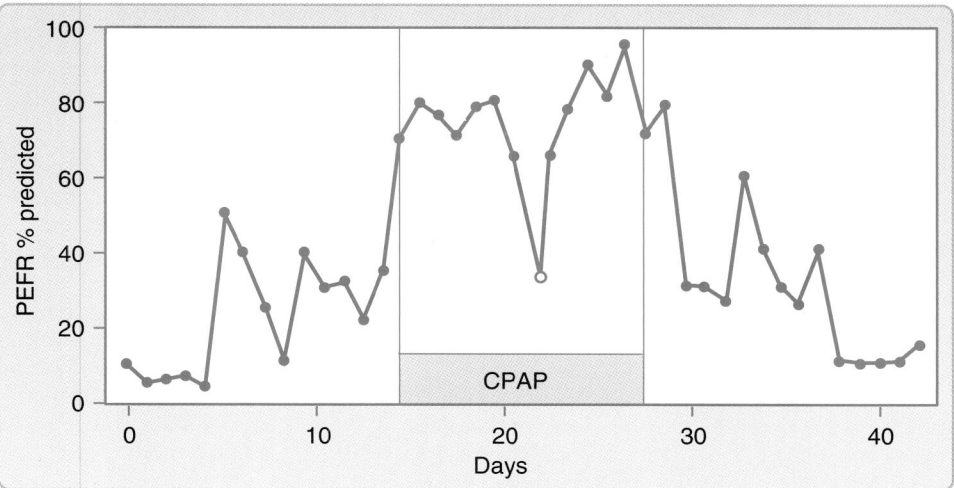

Figure 93–4. Peak expiratory flow rate (PEFR), as percentage predicted, at 3 AM in a snoring asthmatic patient measured during a control period, during a period of nocturnal continuous positive airway pressure (CPAP) therapy, and during a subsequent period after CPAP withdrawal. The *open circle* during the CPAP period represents a single night when the CPAP period was withdrawn. (Redrawn from Chan CS, Woolcock AJ, Sullivan CE: Nocturnal asthma: Role of snoring and obstructive sleep apnea. Am Rev Respir Dis 1988;137:1502-1504.)

airway parasympathetic tone contributes significantly to the development of nocturnal asthma.[29] However, increased vagal tone does not account for all the nocturnal airway narrowing.[29]

SYMPATHETIC NERVOUS SYSTEM

No studies have been performed on the intrinsic sympathetic tone in nocturnal asthma. The bronchodilator response to infused epinephrine is unchanged at night[30]; thus, circadian changes in beta-adrenergic receptor sensitivity cannot explain nocturnal asthma.

NONADRENERGIC, NONCHOLINERGIC NERVOUS SYSTEM

The other autonomic nervous system affecting the airway is the NANC bronchodilating system. The precise role of this nervous system and the neurotransmitters involved are still unclear. However, there is evidence that the activity of the NANC bronchodilating system is impaired in the early morning,[31] and this may contribute to tipping the balance of airway caliber toward the development of overnight bronchoconstriction.

Circadian Variation of Hormones

CORTISOL

Nocturnal breathlessness in asthmatic patients is most marked when the urinary excretion of 17-hydroxycorticosteroid is at its nadir and peak flow rates parallel changes in the levels of circulating steroids.[1] This relationship is not causal: overnight falls in peak flow rate remain unchanged if plasma levels of 11-hydroxycorticosteroids are kept constant by infusion of hydrocortisone. In addition, therapy with large doses of steroids does not abolish morning dipping.[3] Thus, it seems that circadian changes in circulating cortisol levels are not important in the pathogenesis of nocturnal bronchoconstriction.

CATECHOLAMINES AND OTHER MEDIATORS

Circulating catecholamine levels show diurnal changes, with a nocturnal nadir. Urinary catecholamine excretion falls to a minimum coincident with the lowest peak flow rates in some patients.[32] However, catechol infusion does not abolish nocturnal airway narrowing.[33]

Airway Inflammation

Despite considerable recent interest, there is conflicting evidence whether there are consistent changes in airway inflammatory cell populations or mediators in nocturnal asthma.[34-41] Increased inflammatory cells in bronchoalveolar lavage specimens at 4:00 AM have been found in some[36,37] but not all[34,40,42] studies. Bronchial biopsies at 4:00 AM showed no change in cell populations.[36,40] Furthermore, there is no evidence of any causal relationship between changes in inflammatory cell numbers and nocturnal airway narrowing.[36,40,42] One study has suggested a correlation between the FEV_1 at 4:00 AM and CD4+ cells in alveolar tissue,[35] but no causative role has been established. Increases in bronchoalveolar lavage cytokines, eosinophil cationic protein,[36] and interleukin-1-beta[41] have been found in some studies. There is no evidence of increased expression of vascular adhesion molecules at 4:00 AM in patients with nocturnal asthma.[38] This confusing situation could be summarized by stating that some inconsistent changes in inflammatory markers have been found overnight in the lungs of patients with nocturnal asthma, but their relevance is not yet clear.

Summary

Airway narrowing at night is a normal physiologic phenomenon, more obvious in asthmatic patients because their airways are already narrower by day. The major cause is a sleep-synchronized circadian rhythm probably effected largely by changes in the autonomic tone to the airways, with increased parasympathetic bronchoconstrictor tone and decreased NANC bronchodilator function in the early morning.

Clinical Features

Nocturnal wheezing causes inconvenience and disturbed sleep and probably also hypoxemia and death.

Sleep Disturbance

The major complaints of patients with nocturnal wheeze are that their sleep is interrupted and that they feel tired in the daytime. This sleep disruption, which has been confirmed by EEG studies,[20,43] probably results in the impairment in daytime cognitive function in patients with nocturnal asthma in comparison with age- and education-matched healthy subjects.[43] There was no evidence that this impairment in cognitive function resulted from drug therapy.[43] Indeed, treatment of nocturnal asthma has been reported to improve cognitive function, but this improvement could have been the result of increased familiarity with the tests used to assess neurocognition.[44] Nevertheless, the potential damage to daytime cognitive function and to work and school performance caused by nocturnal sleep disruption underlines the importance of intensifying therapy in patients with nocturnal asthma.

Hypoxemia

Patients with nocturnal asthma can undoubtedly become hypoxemic during the night, but the hypoxemia is rarely severe: in stable asthmatic patients studied at sea level, the lowest saturation is normally in the range of 85% to 95%. However, no large studies have been performed in unstable patients with nocturnal asthma, and these patients may become more hypoxemic.

Nocturnal Asthmatic Attacks

Asthmatic patients present with attacks more frequently by night than by day, both to their family physician and to the emergency department. In addition to the adverse medical impact of these events, this timing significantly impairs the quality of life of all concerned.

Death

Fortunately, deaths from asthma are uncommon, but there are more asthmatic deaths per hour at night than by day.[45] When subdivided according to place of death, there was an excess nocturnal rate for the 146 deaths that occurred at home ($P < .05$). The same trend was seen for the 73 deaths occurring in hospital ($.15 > P > .10$). The death rate is, of course, higher at night than by day in the general population, but the average increase between midnight and 8:00 AM is only 5%, in contrast to the 28% increase observed in asthmatic patients.[45]

Excess nocturnal mortality could be caused by many factors, including the failure of sleeping subjects to be rapidly awakened by hypoxia,[46] hypercapnia,[47] or increased airflow resistance[48] (with resultant delays in treatment), reticence to summon family or medical help at night, and delay in the arrival of medical assistance. Eight of 10 ventilatory arrests in asthmatic patients in hospital occurred in the early morning,[49] suggesting that the unavailability of medical assistance is not a major factor. One of the most important causes of nocturnal death seems to be nocturnal bronchospasm. The two asthmatic patients who died at night during a prospective study were both morning dippers,[50] which suggests that nocturnal bronchoconstriction can be life-threatening. Thus, the morning dip pattern of asthma should be sought and recognized as potentially dangerous when it is marked in unstable asthmatic patients.

Diagnosis

Nocturnal asthma comprises a combination of related symptoms—nocturnal wheeze, cough, and breathlessness—associated with a greater than 10% fall in overnight peak airflow rate. Peak flow rates should be measured in triplicate,

and the highest value taken, at least three times a day for at least 2 weeks. An overnight fall in peak flow rate that is consistently greater than 15% is strong evidence of nocturnal asthma.

Treatment

Nocturnal bronchoconstriction is a sign of inadequate control of asthma, and the new development of nocturnal wheeze in a patient must be regarded as a dangerous sign requiring monitoring and urgent treatment. Nocturnal wheeze often responds to increasing conventional daytime maintenance treatment with either prophylactic agents or bronchodilators, and recent evidence indicates that inhaled steroids may help overnight airway narrowing within 12 hours.[51] Only when optimal daytime control does not abolish nocturnal symptoms should additional treatment be directed at nocturnal wheeze.

Inhalation of bronchodilators immediately before sleep, repeated whenever the patient is awakened by wheeze, is the initial treatment of choice; side effects are few. However, conventional inhaled beta$_2$ agonists last only around 4 hours, and most people sleep for longer than that. Inhaled ipratropium and tiotropium last longer, but this increased duration has proved disappointing in clinical practice.

For those in whom these treatments are insufficient, long-acting bronchodilators—either inhaled or oral—should be used. Salmeterol is a beta$_2$ agonist that lasts more than 12 hours after inhalation. Salmeterol improves symptoms, overnight peak flow rates, and sleep quality[52] and also quality of life[53] in patients with nocturnal asthma (Fig. 93–5). Formoterol, another long-acting inhaled agent, has been shown to improve overnight lung function.[54]

In terms of oral bronchodilators, there appears to be little difference, from the bronchodilation point of view, between oral theophyllines[55] and oral beta$_2$ agonists.[56] Both can

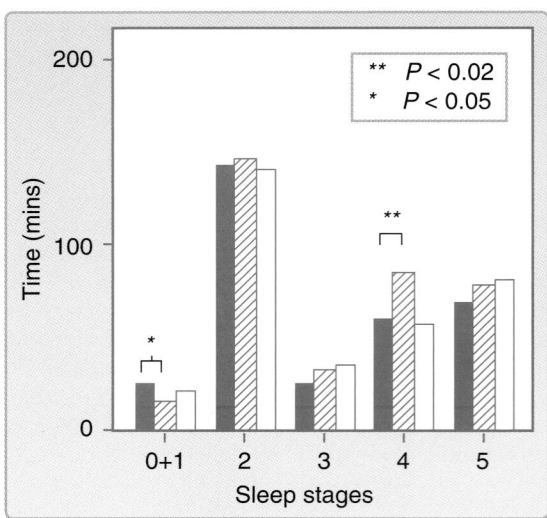

Figure 93–5. Mean (SE) time spent in each sleep stage by 18 asthmatic patients receiving placebo *(solid bar)* or salmeterol, 50 µg *(hatched bar)* or 100 µg *(open bar)* twice daily. (Redrawn from Fitzpatrick MF, Mackay T, Driver H, et al: Salmeterol in nocturnal asthma: A double blind, placebo controlled trial of a long acting inhaled beta$_2$ agonist. Br Med J 1990;301:1365-1368.)

markedly reduce nocturnal symptoms, and the choice is largely determined by whether the patient develops side effects. These agents can often be taken effectively once a day immediately before going to bed, thus reducing daytime side effects.[55] Theophylline absorption tends to be lower at night than in the morning. This is not caused by diurnal variations in theophylline absorption or disposition but probably results from differences between nocturnal and morning gastric content, physical activity, and posture. However, it is important to be aware of this difference, because larger dosages can be given at night. It has been reported that oral theophylline disturbs sleep, as judged by the EEG in patients with nocturnal asthma, despite improving nocturnal symptoms and overnight changes in airflow rates.[57] However, there was no evidence of sleep disturbance in a medium-term study of healthy subjects being treated with theophylline.[58]

Relatively few studies have compared long-acting inhaled beta$_2$ agonists with other agents in the management of nocturnal asthma.[59,60] One such study showed no major difference in efficacy between salmeterol and oral theophylline, although there were marginal benefits in favor of salmeterol in terms of frequency of arousals from sleep and improved quality of life.[59] Another study showed that salmeterol compared with theophylline resulted in less deterioration in nighttime lung function and improvement in subjective sleep quality.[60] Salmeterol was superior to oral slow-release terbutaline in terms of the number of nights free of awakenings, morning peak flow rates, and assessment of clinical efficacy.[61] Salmeterol 50 µg twice daily was similar in efficacy to fluticasone 250 µg twice daily in improving nocturnal asthma.[62] Inhaled long-acting bronchodilators are now more often prescribed than oral long-acting bronchodilators, as side effects are fewer.

The role of proton pump inhibitors remains unclear.[16] However, this is a rational treatment to try in patients with symptomatic gastroesophageal reflux or others who respond poorly to standard measures.

Patients who do not respond to these measures will require oral steroid therapy. A very small minority will need further immunosuppression—for example, with methotrexate, which can improve symptoms and FEV$_1$.

In the small minority of asthmatic patients whose nocturnal airway narrowing relates to their snoring or obstructive apneas, weight loss (if appropriate) and continuous positive airway pressure therapy should be tried.[26] In my experience, such therapy does not often improve nocturnal asthma.

Conclusions

Although there have been advances in our understanding of both pathophysiology and therapeutics, overnight wheeze remains a problem for many patients with the common condition of asthma. Overnight wheeze is caused by a circadian rhythm in airway caliber that is at least partially controlled by neural factors. Development of long-acting inhaled bronchodilators has simplified the management of these symptoms.

CHRONIC OBSTRUCTIVE PULMONARY DISEASE

Chronic obstructive pulmonary disease (COPD) is an umbrella term describing a disease state characterized by airflow limitation that is not fully reversible. The airflow limitation is usually both progressive and associated with an abnormal inflammatory response of the lungs to noxious particles or gases.[62a] Patients with COPD become more hypoxemic during sleep than when awake—even more hypoxemic than during exercise.[63] They become slightly more hypoxemic as they fall into NREM sleep, and much more hypoxemic in REM sleep, when oxygen saturation may fall to extremely low levels,[64] especially in those whose oxygenation is poor even before sleep (Fig. 93–6). This sleep-related hypoxemia affects the cardiovascular and hematologic systems and is thus of clinical significance.

Pathogenesis of Hypoxemia during Sleep in Patients with COPD

Many factors have been proposed as causes of hypoxemia during sleep in patients with COPD, including hypoventilation, a decrease in functional residual capacity, and ventilation–perfusion mismatch.

Hypoventilation

Minute ventilation decreases during all sleep stages compared with wakefulness in both healthy subjects[21] and patients with COPD.[65] The reduction in ventilation from wakefulness to NREM sleep is small, but during REM sleep, there is intermittent marked hypoventilation.[21,65] This hypoventilation in healthy subjects is most severe during periods of frequent eye movements,[66] when tidal volume falls substantially.

The typical REM sleep–related desaturation in patients with COPD is accompanied by hypoventilation and not by apneas[67,68] (Fig. 93–7). The breathing pattern during REM sleep is similar in patients with COPD and healthy subjects.[67] Alveolar ventilation in healthy subjects is about 40% lower during bursts of eye movements in REM sleep than during wakefulness. Measurements made in patients with COPD sleeping with 4 cm H$_2$O continuous positive airway pressure are compatible with these estimates.[65] Because patients with COPD have increased physiologic dead space, the rapid shallow breathing during bursts of eye movements in REM sleep would be expected to produce an even greater decrease in alveolar ventilation than occurs in healthy subjects. This contributes significantly to their REM sleep–related hypoxemia, and could account for all the hypoxemia observed in REM sleep in patients with COPD.[69]

Many factors contribute to hypoventilation during sleep. In NREM sleep, ventilation falls in healthy subjects despite an increase in respiratory effort as measured by occlusion pressure.[70] It is likely that this hypoventilation in NREM sleep is in part the result of increased upper airway resistance.[71] Furthermore, the ventilatory response to added respiratory resistance is impaired during NREM sleep,[72] which allows hypoventilation to occur. There also may be loss of the "wakefulness drive to breathing," which contributes to hypoventilation during NREM sleep,[46] and there may be an effect from the fall in basal metabolic rate during sleep.[73]

The marked intermittent hypoventilation during REM sleep seems unlikely to be caused by further increases in upper airway resistance, because overall airway resistance is no greater in REM sleep than in NREM sleep, at least in healthy subjects.[71] Furthermore, although few measurements have been made, it appears that the ventilatory response to inspiratory

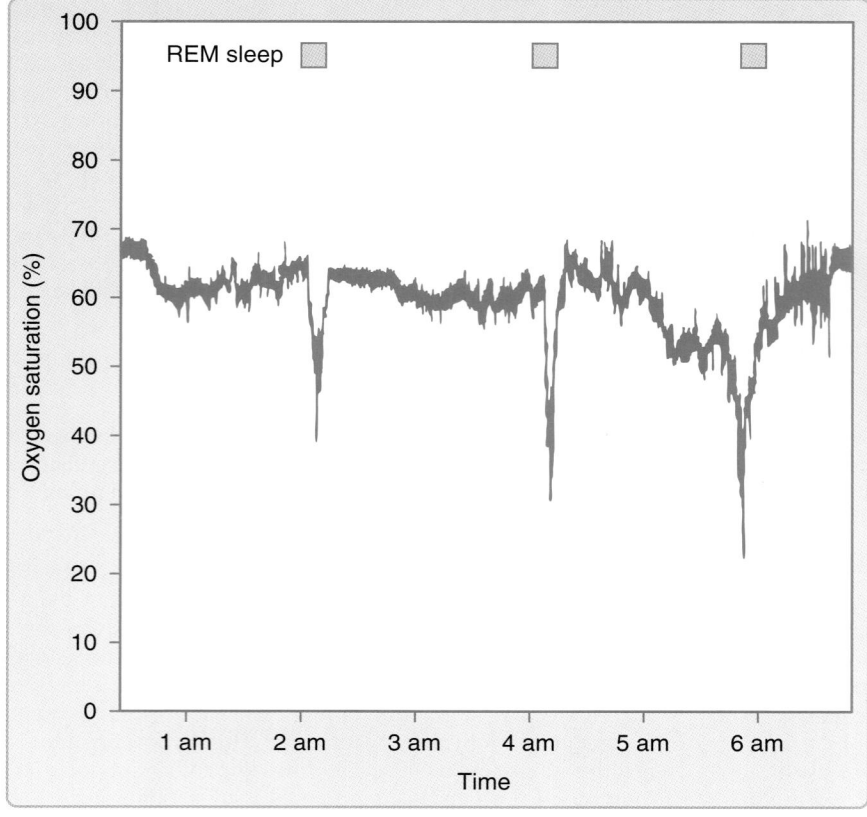

Figure 93–6. Overnight oxygen saturation in a patient with chronic obstructive pulmonary disease. *Shaded areas* represent REM sleep during which marked oxygen desaturation occurs.

resistance is similar in NREM and in REM sleep.[72] During REM sleep, there is altered brainstem function with phasic activity of respiratory neurons, and diminution in central respiratory output may be a major factor in producing REM sleep–related hypoventilation. During REM sleep, there is hypotonia of postural muscles, including the intercostal muscles, so that the rib cage contributes less to ventilation.[74] This further decreases ventilation during REM sleep in hyperinflated patients with COPD, in whom the flattened diaphragm pulls in the flaccid lower chest wall, with resultant highly inefficient ventilation. This may explain why patients with COPD become more hypoxemic during sleep than

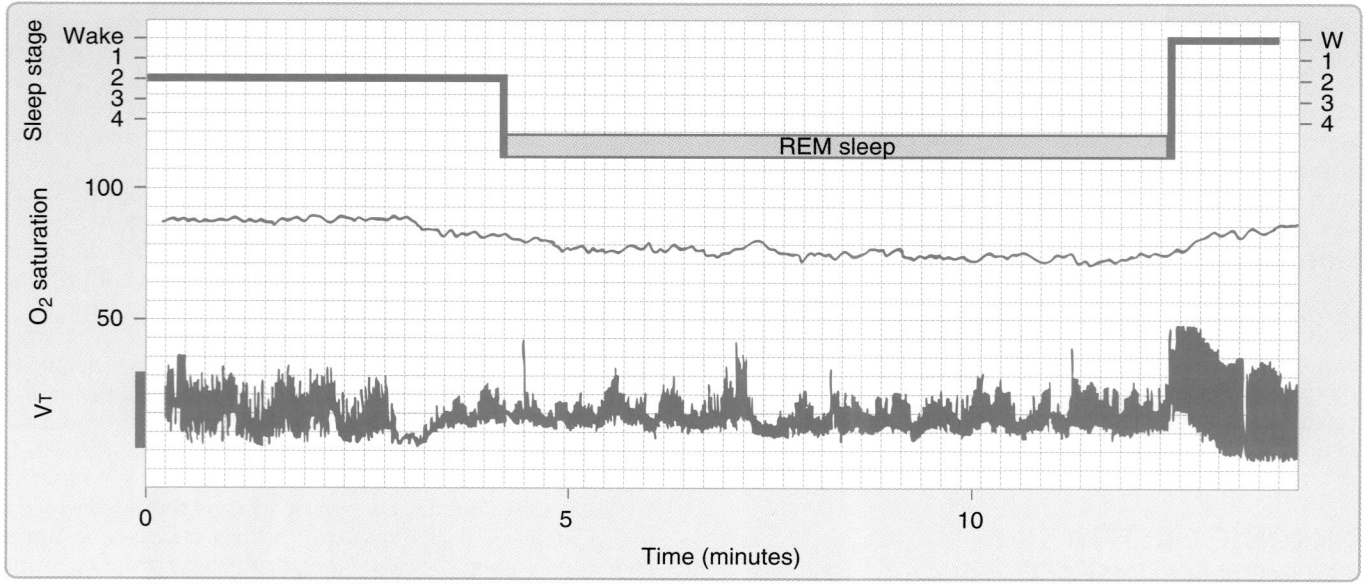

Figure 93–7. Tidal volume (V_T), O_2 saturation, and sleep stage in a patient with chronic obstructive pulmonary disease illustrated in the drop in O_2 saturation and irregular hyperventilation during REM sleep. (Redrawn from Fletcher EC, Gray BA, Levin DC: Nonapneic mechanisms of arterial oxygen desaturation during rapid-eye movement sleep. J Appl Physiol 1983;54:632-639.)

patients with pulmonary fibrosis.[75] In addition, the postural hypotonia of REM sleep involves not only the intercostal muscles but also the accessory muscles of respiration,[76] which may be important in maintaining adequate ventilation in patients with COPD.

The hypoventilation of REM sleep is accompanied by a marked diminution of both the hypoxic[46] and hypercapnic[47] ventilatory responses. The normal defense mechanisms of the body to the resulting hypoxemia and hypercapnia are diminished.

Decrease in Functional Residual Capacity

Functional residual capacity decreases during REM sleep in healthy subjects.[71] However, body plethysmographic studies indicate that functional residual capacity does not change during sleep in patients with COPD, although these data were gathered in only five patients.[77]

Ventilation–Perfusion Mismatch

It is inevitable that additional ventilation–perfusion mismatch occurs in patients with COPD during the marked hypoventilation of REM sleep. This is supported by evidence that cardiac output is maintained during these episodes of hypoventilation, which indicates changes in global ventilation–perfusion match.[78] Unfortunately, technology does not allow assessment of the importance of ventilation–perfusion match relative to the other mechanisms involved. Techniques for quantifying ventilation–perfusion mismatch are reliant on a steady state of both ventilation and metabolism; certainly, the former does not occur during REM sleep, in which ventilation is extremely variable.[78] This negates many of the arguments previously advanced for the importance of ventilation–perfusion mismatch. For example, it has been suggested that the greater decrease in alveolar PO_2 compared with the rise in arterial PCO_2 indicates the importance of ventilation–perfusion changes during REM sleep in patients with COPD. However, because the body's storage capacity for carbon dioxide is much larger than that for oxygen, the transient episodes of hypoventilation that occur during REM sleep produce much greater decreases in PO_2 than rises in PCO_2, which is exactly what has been observed.[78]

COPD Combined with Obstructive Sleep Apnea–Hypopnea Syndrome

Both COPD and obstructive sleep apnea–hypopnea syndrome (OSAHS) are common. These two conditions coexist in some patients, although the prevalence of OSAHS in patients with COPD seems to be no greater than the prevalence of OSAHS[79,80] in the unaffected population. In a small minority of patients with COPD, perhaps about 2%,[80] nocturnal hypoxemia results from obstructive apneas or hypopneas, in addition to REM sleep–related hypoventilation. Viewing this in a different way, one study suggested that 10% of patients with OSAHS may have some degree of coexisting COPD.[81] In patients with both conditions, the pattern of nocturnal desaturation is different: frequent desaturation results in a broad-band saturation trace rather than the relatively clearly defined "spike" of desaturation typically found in REM sleep (see Fig. 93–6). Hypercapnic patients with COPD may have narrower upper airways when awake, predisposing them to OSAHS.[82]

Summary

Hypoventilation is the major cause of hypoxemia during REM sleep in patients with COPD. There may be additional contributions from ventilation–perfusion mismatch and a decrease in functional residual capacity. In a small minority of patients with COPD, there may also be coexisting OSAHS.

Clinical Consequences of Sleep Hypoxemia

Hypoxemia during sleep in patients with COPD has significant cardiovascular and neurophysiologic effects, may have hematologic consequences, and may contribute to the incidence of nocturnal death.

Cardiac Dysrhythmias

Patients with COPD have more ventricular ectopic beats during sleep. Although in most patients there is no direct relationship between ventricular ectopic frequency and oxygen saturation,[83] in a minority of the most hypoxic patients a significant relationship can be found between ventricular ectopic frequency and nocturnal oxygen saturation.

Hemodynamics

Pulmonary arterial pressure rises as oxygen saturation falls during REM sleep. Coccagna and Lugaresi[84] observed in 12 patients with COPD that mean pulmonary arterial pressure rose from 37 to 55 mm Hg during REM sleep, as the average arterial oxygen tension fell from 56 to 43 mm Hg. Boysen et al.[85] observed an inverse correlation between oxygenation and mean pulmonary arterial pressure, and although individual values varied widely, on average a 1% fall in oxygen saturation led to a 1-mm Hg rise in mean pulmonary arterial pressure. The clinical significance of these transient episodes of pulmonary arterial pressure elevation is unknown; however, in rats, intermittent hypoxemia induced by breathing 12% oxygen for as little as 2 hours each day for 4 weeks significantly elevated right ventricular mass, even when individual episodes of hypoxia were as short as 30 minutes.[86] It thus seems probable that the intermittent REM sleep hypoxemia in patients with COPD has similar effects on the human myocardium.

Polycythemia

Intermittent hypoxemia in rats results in an elevation of red cell mass[86]; the nocturnal desaturation in patients with COPD might also stimulate erythropoiesis. Morning erythropoietin levels are raised in some patients with COPD.[87]

A study examined red cell mass and pulmonary hemodynamics in 36 patients with COPD who experienced nocturnal desaturation to a nadir of 85% or lower (with more than 5 minutes spent below 90% saturation), and compared them to these variables in 30 patients who did not reach such a desaturation.[88] Those with nocturnal desaturation had significantly higher daytime pulmonary arterial pressures and red cell mass than those without. Although these differences could have resulted from the nocturnal events, those who achieved nocturnal desaturation also had significantly poorer daytime oxygenation levels, which could account for the hemodynamic and hematologic differences.

Nocturnal erythropoietin rises only in those patients with COPD whose oxygen saturations fall below 60% at night.[87] This suggests that a relatively minor degree of nocturnal desaturation may be of little hematologic consequence.

Sleep Quality

Both subjective and objective[89] assessments indicate that patients with COPD sleep poorly compared with healthy subjects. Although arousals and sleep fragmentation are common during episodes of desaturation,[89] the extent of sleep disruption is at least as great in relatively normoxic patients with COPD. Despite these reports of poor sleep, there is no objective evidence of daytime sleepiness as assessed by a multiple sleep latency test in patients with COPD.[90]

Consequences of COPD Combined with OSAHS

Patients with both COPD and OSAHS are more likely to develop pulmonary hypertension, right-sided heart failure, and carbon dioxide retention than are patients with OSAHS alone.[91] Indeed, these complications develop earlier in patients with both COPD and OSAHS than in patients with COPD alone. Certainly, many patients with both COPD and OSAHS who have these complications have relatively good lung function. This seems likely to be because they have two causes for nocturnal hypoxemia, resulting in more severe nocturnal hypoxemia than would have occurred if they had only one such condition.

Prediction of Nocturnal Oxygenation

Oxygenation during wakefulness in patients with COPD is a major predictor of the mean and lowest levels of oxygenation during sleep and also of the extent of desaturation during sleep.[80] Because the hypoxemic complications of pulmonary hypertension and polycythemia relate to the patient's absolute arterial oxygenation rather than to the change in saturation, the more important relationship is the one between absolute levels of nocturnal oxygenation and measurements that can be taken during wakefulness. Several different equations relating these variables have been derived, but their clinical significance is limited because the scatter around the regression lines is wide,[80] especially for the more severely hypoxemic patients (Fig. 93–8). Regression relationships show that the extent of nocturnal hypoxemia relates not only to daytime oxygenation but also to daytime arterial carbon dioxide tension and to the duration of REM sleep.[80]

Clinical Value of Sleep Studies in Chronic Obstructive Pulmonary Disease

Studies of breathing and oxygenation during sleep in patients with COPD could be of clinical relevance by (1) detecting unsuspected cases of OSAHS, (2) detecting which patients had clinically important excess nocturnal hypoxemia, (3) guiding which patients might benefit from nocturnal oxygen therapy, and (4) determining the optimal inspired oxygen concentration for nocturnal oxygen therapy. The last two roles are discussed under "Treatment of Nocturnal Hypoxemia in Chronic Obstructive Pulmonary Disease," later.

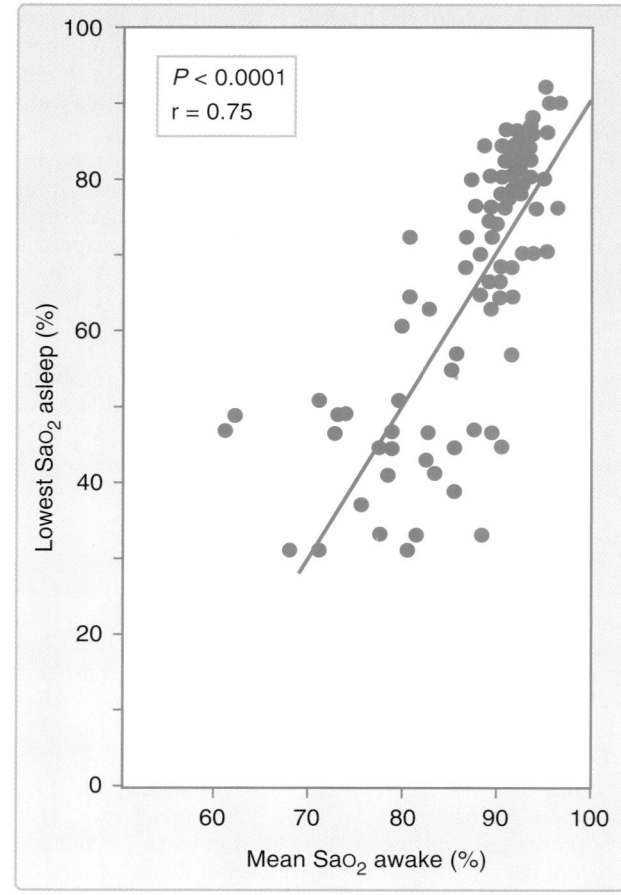

Figure 93–8. Relationship between mean oxygen saturation (SaO_2) awake and lowest oxygen saturation during sleep in 97 patients with chronic obstructive pulmonary disease. (Redrawn from Connaughton JJ, Catterall JR, Elton RA, et al: Do sleep studies contribute to the management of patients with severe chronic obstructive pulmonary disease? Am Rev Respir Dis 1988;138:341-345.)

There is no evidence that the prevalence of OSAHS is increased in patients with COPD,[67,79] but large population studies are lacking. When OSAHS and COPD coexist, the typical symptoms of OSAHS are present, and it appears that sleep studies do not yield unsuspected cases of OSAHS.[80] Thus, all patients with COPD should be questioned about the occurrence of symptoms of OSAHS, and, if major symptoms are elicited, polysomnography should be performed.

Oxygenation during sleep can be predicted on the basis of awake arterial blood gas tensions.[80] These predictions leave considerable unexplained residual variance, but it is unclear whether this is of clinical significance. Measurement of the extent of nocturnal hypoxemia in such patients has been held to be a useful guide for treatment. To clarify the clinical importance of this variability in the extent of nocturnal hypoxemia, Connaughton et al.[80] studied the relationship between nocturnal oxygen saturation and survival in 97 patients with severe COPD, with follow-up to a median of 70 months. Both the mean nocturnal oxygen saturation and the lowest nocturnal oxygen saturation were significantly related to survival: the lower the nocturnal oxygenation, the worse the prognosis was. However, neither nocturnal measure significantly improved the prediction of survival that could be obtained from the easier and cheaper measurements of vital capacity or oxygen saturation when awake.[80]

These data[80] were also analyzed to determine the significance of the scatter around the regression relation between measurements of oxygen saturation and Pa_{CO_2} when awake and oxygen saturation during sleep. The patients were divided into those who had excess nocturnal hypoxemia, defined as those whose oxygen saturation during sleep was lower than that predicted on the basis of their awake oxygen saturation and arterial P_{CO_2}, and those who became less hypoxemic than predicted at night. There was no difference in survival rates at a median of 70 months between those with excess nocturnal hypoxemia and those who became less hypoxemic at night than might be predicted on the basis of the awake oxygenation and Pa_{CO_2} (Fig. 93–9). Thus, measurement of nocturnal oxygenation does not yield useful prognostic information in addition to that obtained during wakefulness. Another study in a group of patients with daytime arterial oxygen tensions of 56 to 69 mm Hg found no significant relationship between the magnitude of nocturnal hypoxemia and the development of pulmonary hypertension or the worsening of arterial blood gas tensions.[92] This, again, suggests that the contribution of the additional hypoxemia during sleep to overall daytime pulmonary arterial pressure is relatively small.

There seems to be no clinical advantage, therefore, to performing routine polysomnography in patients with COPD, although undoubtedly many research areas require clarification by this technique. I believe that clinical polysomnography is indicated in patients with COPD only if OSAHS is suspected (i.e., symptoms of OSAHS are developing) or in patients with hypoxemic complications (e.g., cor pulmonale and polycythemia) and with a daytime arterial oxygen tension of greater than 60 mm Hg. There is no evidence that recording overnight oxygenation in patients with COPD provides evidence that helps management or predicts prognosis.[80,92]

Treatment of Nocturnal Hypoxemia in Chronic Obstructive Pulmonary Disease

Oxygen Therapy

Not surprisingly, nocturnal oxygen therapy improves oxygenation during sleep in patients with COPD.[64] Some nocturnal desaturation still occurs, particularly during REM sleep, but the hypoxemia is not so profound. A few patients report morning headaches due to carbon dioxide retention as a result of nocturnal oxygen therapy. This may be a particular problem in patients with coexisting OSAHS,[93] and it is as an indication for polysomnography.

The patients who become most severely hypoxemic at night are those with daytime hypoxemia.[80] Long-term domiciliary oxygen therapy remains the only treatment shown by controlled clinical trials to prolong life in such patients. Because the period of oxygen administration almost always includes the night, it is possible that some of the benefit of oxygen therapy is due to preventing nocturnal hypoxemia.

Long-term domiciliary oxygen therapy is based on data obtained when oxygen treatment depended solely on measurement of arterial blood gas tensions when the patient was awake. There is at present no proven role for studies of breathing and oxygenation during sleep to aid selection of patients for nocturnal oxygen therapy. Studies of patients with daytime arterial tensions of greater than 55 mm Hg but with nocturnal desaturation reported that nocturnal oxygen therapy did not improve patient survival rates.[94] The only patients for whom I suggest that polysomnography be performed in relation to oxygen therapy in COPD are those who develop morning headaches with oxygen therapy, because this may indicate coexisting OSAHS.

Almitrine

The use of almitrine can raise arterial oxygen tension in patients with COPD. In a randomized double-blind study, 50 mg of almitrine twice daily for 2 weeks improved oxygenation during sleep in patients with COPD.[95] The role, if any, of almitrine in patients with COPD is not yet clear, as this medication was not found to be effective in long-term treatment.[96] The reported side effects include clinical and laboratory evidence consistent with peripheral neuropathy. Other, inconsistently reported effects include dyspnea, weight loss, and increased pulmonary artery pressure.

Protriptyline

The results of a nonrandomized, nonblinded trial[97] suggested that protriptyline may improve daytime arterial oxygen and carbon dioxide tensions in patients with COPD, but side effects were common, causing cessation of therapy within 10 weeks in 4 of 14 patients. The acceptability of long-term protriptyline and its effect on survival remain to be assessed.

Medroxyprogesterone Acetate

Despite suggestions that medroxyprogesterone acetate might be beneficial, in a double-blind, placebo-controlled trial,

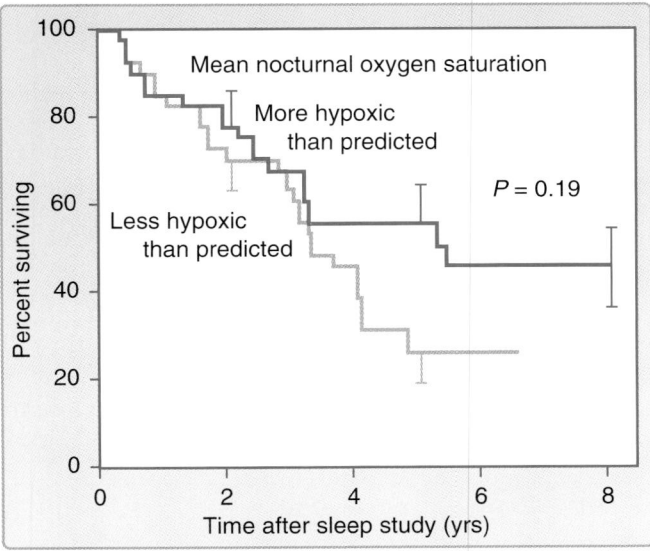

Figure 93–9. Survival curves for patients who are more hypoxic than predicted from their awake oxygen saturation and carbon dioxide level, compared with those who are less hypoxic than predicted. There was no significant difference in the survival curves of the two groups. (Redrawn from Connaughton JJ, Catterall JR, Elton RA, et al: Do sleep studies contribute to the management of patients with severe chronic obstructive pulmonary disease? Am Rev Respir Dis 1988;138:341-345.)

Dolly and Block[98] found no significant change in the lowest oxygen saturation during sleep in 19 patients with COPD who were taking medroxyprogesterone acetate. In addition, medroxyprogesterone acetate may cause troublesome side effects, including impotence. The clinical role of the drug appears to be limited.

Theophylline

The use of oral theophylline may improve overnight oxygen saturation and transcutaneous carbon dioxide levels.[99] However, the benefits are limited and often outweighed by the side effects.

Beta Agonists and Anticholinergic Bronchodilators

The use of oral sustained-release salbutamol had no effect on sleep, oxygenation, or morning FEV_1 in 14 patients with moderately severe COPD.[100] In a placebo-controlled, randomized, double-blind trial involving 36 patients, ipratropium bromide improved oxygenation and sleep quality.[101]

Noninvasive Intermittent Positive-Pressure Ventilation

Nocturnal nasal intermittent positive-pressure ventilation (NIPPV) via a nasal mask or a face mask was developed for use in patients with chest wall or neuromuscular disorders. Some patients with COPD find this technique acceptable, and it has a theoretical advantage over long-term oxygen therapy of reducing, rather than raising, $PaCO_2$. In patients who can tolerate NIPPV, improvements in arterial blood gas tensions and sleep may be achieved, but nocturnal oxygenation is improved more with nocturnal oxygen therapy than with NIPPV alone.[102] Simultaneous NIPPV and nocturnal oxygen therapy produced greater improvements in $PaCO_2$ and quality of life than did oxygen therapy alone in randomized controlled trials.[103,104] A more-detailed review of NIPPV is given in Chapter 95.

Treatment of COPD Combined with OSAHS

There are remarkably few data indicating how to treat patients who have both COPD and OSAHS. A nonrandomized study found that daytime arterial blood gas tensions (Fig. 93–10) and pulmonary arterial pressures in patients with both conditions improved when they were adequately treated for OSAHS but not when they received domiciliary oxygen therapy in the absence of adequate therapy for OSAHS.[105] It is important to recognize coexisting OSAHS in such patients and to treat it appropriately, usually with continuous positive airway pressure therapy. In some who are markedly hypoxemic during both day and night, despite continuous positive airway pressure, supplemental oxygen may have to be added to the continuous positive airway pressure line. In such patients, NIPPV administered via a nasal mask may be a viable alternative.

Treatment of Insomnia in Patients with COPD

Many patients with COPD receive hypnotics when they complain of sleep disturbance. Hypnotics should not be used in hypercapnic patients, lest ventilatory responses be further inhibited and acute or chronic respiratory failure precipitated. In normocapnic patients with COPD, benzodiazepines have

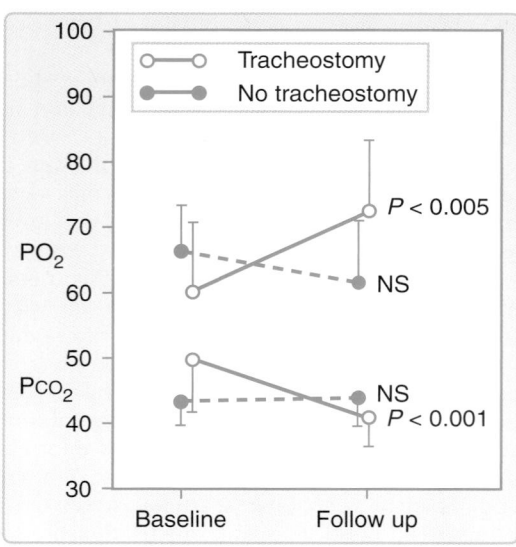

Figure 93–10. Arterial oxygen (PO_2) and carbon dioxide (PCO_2) tensions (in mm Hg) in patients with both chronic obstructive pulmonary disease and sleep apnea at baseline and subsequent follow-up. *Open circles* indicate those who were treated with tracheostomy, and *closed circles* indicate those who were treated by other techniques, which largely consisted of long-term oxygen therapy. The *P* values indicate significant improvements in arterial blood gas tensions in the patients treated with tracheostomy. (Redrawn from Fletcher EC, Schaaf JW, Miller J, et al: Long-term cardiopulmonary sequelae in patients with sleep apnea and chronic lung disease. Am Rev Respir Dis 1987;135: 525-533.)

been found to increase sleep duration in some[106,107] but not all[108] studies, but the frequency and severity of nocturnal hypoxemia may increase.[106] The imidazopyridines and pyrazolopyrimidines may be safer,[109-111] but more data are needed to prove this. Thus at present, hypnotics should only be used with great care in COPD, even in normocapnic patients.

Conclusions

Patients with COPD become hypoxemic during sleep, particularly during episodes of dense eye movements in REM sleep. The measurement of nocturnal hypoxemia and breathing pattern in individual patients does not provide prognostic information that significantly adds to the more simple measurements of oxygenation and lung function during wakefulness. In a small minority of patients with COPD, OSAHS coexists, and any patient with COPD and a history suggestive of OSAHS should undergo full polysomnography. Those found to have OSAHS should be aggressively treated. Domiciliary oxygen therapy is the treatment of choice for patients with COPD who are hypoxemic in the day and night, but the roles of respiratory stimulants and of IPPV via a nasal mask may grow.

Clinical Pearls

Nocturnal asthma should always be suspected in any patient presenting with nocturnal cough, wheeze, or breathlessness and should be confirmed by demonstration of circadian variation in peak flow rates.

Patients with chronic obstructive pulmonary disease become hypoxemic during sleep, and this is one of the main causes of a fall in oxygen saturation in hospitalized patients.

REFERENCES

1. Connolly CK: Diurnal rhythms in airway obstruction. Br J Dis Chest 1979;73:357-366.
2. Floyer J: A Treatise on the Asthma. Printed for Richard Wilkin at the King's-Head in St. Paul's Church-Yard, London, 1698.
3. Clark TJ, Hetzel MR: Diurnal variation of asthma. Br J Dis Chest 1977;71:87-92.
4. Turner-Warwick M: On observing patterns of airflow obstruction in chronic asthma. Br J Dis Chest 1977;71:73-86.
5. Hetzel MR, Clark TJ: Comparison of normal and asthmatic circadian rhythms in peak expiratory flow rate. Thorax 1980;35:732-738.
6. Catterall JR, Rhind GB, Stewart IC, et al: Effect of sleep deprivation on overnight bronchoconstriction in nocturnal asthma. Thorax 1986;41:676-680.
7. Ballard RD, Saathoff MC, Patel DK, et al: Effect of sleep on nocturnal bronchoconstriction and ventilatory patterns in asthmatics. J Appl Physiol 1989;67:243-249.
8. Hetzel MR, Clark TJ: Does sleep cause nocturnal asthma? Thorax 1979;34:749-754.
9. Whyte KF, Douglas NJ: Posture and nocturnal asthma. Thorax 1989;44:579-581.
10. Woodcock A, Forster L, Matthews E, et al: Control of exposure to mite allergen and allergen-impermeable bed covers for adults with asthma. N Engl J Med 2003;349:225-236.
11. Davies RJ, Green M, Schofield NM: Recurrent nocturnal asthma after exposure to grain dust. Am Rev Respir Dis 1976;114:1011-1019.
12. Platts-Mills TA, Tovey ER, Mitchell EB, et al: Reduction of bronchial hyperreactivity during prolonged allergen avoidance. Lancet 1982;2:675-678.
13. Ryan G, Latimer KM, Dolovich J, Hargreave FE: Bronchial responsiveness to histamine: Relationship to diurnal variation of peak flow rate, improvement after bronchodilator, and airway calibre. Thorax 1982;37:423-429.
14. Kerr HD: Diurnal variation of respiratory function independent of air quality: Experience with an environmentally controlled exposure chamber for human subjects. Arch Environ Health 1973;26:144-152.
15. Chen WY, Chai H: Airway cooling and nocturnal asthma. Chest 1982;81:675-680.
16. Kiljander TO, Salomaa ER, Hietanen EK, Terho EO: Gastroesophageal reflux in asthmatics: A double-blind, placebo-controlled crossover study with omeprazole. Chest 1999;116:1257-1264.
17. Nagel RA, Brown P, Perks WH, et al: Ambulatory pH monitoring of gastro-oesophageal reflux in "morning dipper" asthmatics. BMJ 1988;297:1371-1373.
18. Gervais P, Reinberg A, Gervais C, et al: Twenty-four-hour rhythm in the bronchial hyperreactivity to house dust in asthmatics. J Allergy Clin Immunol 1977;59:207-213.
19. Smolensky MH, Reinberg A, Queng JT: The chronobiology and chronopharmacology of allergy. Ann Allergy 1981;47:234-252.
20. Kales A, Beall GN, Bajor GF, et al: Sleep studies in asthmatic adults: Relationship of attacks to sleep stage and time of night. J Allergy 1968;41:164-173.
21. Douglas NJ, White DP, Pickett CK, et al: Respiration during sleep in normal man. Thorax 1982;37:840-844.
22. Tabachnik E, Muller NL, Levison H, Bryan AC: Chest wall mechanics and pattern of breathing during sleep in asthmatic adolescents. Am Rev Respir Dis 1981;124:269-273.
23. Catterall JR, Douglas NJ, Calverley PM, et al: Irregular breathing and hypoxaemia during sleep in chronic stable asthma. Lancet 1982;1:301-304.
24. Ballard RD, Irvin CG, Martin RJ, et al: Influence of sleep on lung volume in asthmatic patients and normal subjects. J Appl Physiol 1990;68:2034-2041.
25. Kraft M, Pak J, Martin RJ, et al: Distal lung dysfunction at night in nocturnal asthma. Am J Respir Crit Care Med 2001;163:1551-1556.
26. Chan CS, Woolcock AJ, Sullivan CE: Nocturnal asthma: Role of snoring and obstructive sleep apnea. Am Rev Respir Dis 1988;137:1502-1504.
27. Chinn S: Asthma and obesity: Where are we now? Thorax 2003;58:1008-1010.
28. Catterall JR, Rhind GB, Whyte KF, et al: Is nocturnal asthma caused by changes in airway cholinergic activity? Thorax 1988;43:720-724.
29. Morrison JF, Pearson SB, Dean HG: Parasympathetic nervous system in nocturnal asthma. Br Med J (Clin Res Ed) 1988;296:1427-1429.
30. Barnes P, FitzGerald G, Brown M, Dollery C: Nocturnal asthma and changes in circulating epinephrine, histamine, and cortisol. N Engl J Med 1980;303:263-267.
31. Mackay TW, Hulks G, Douglas NJ: Non-adrenergic, non-cholinergic function in the human airway. Respir Med 1998;92:461-466.
32. Soutar CA, Carruthers M, Pickering CA: Nocturnal asthma and urinary adrenaline and noradrenaline excretion. Thorax 1977;32:677-683.
33. Morrison JF, Teale C, Pearson SB, et al: Adrenaline and nocturnal asthma. BMJ 1990;301:473-476.
34. Jarjour NN, Busse WW, Calhoun WJ: Enhanced production of oxygen radicals in nocturnal asthma. Am Rev Respir Dis 1992;146:905-911.
35. Kraft M, Martin RJ, Wilson S, et al: Lymphocyte and eosinophil influx into alveolar tissue in nocturnal asthma. Am J Respir Crit Care Med 1999;159:228-234.
36. Mackay TW, Wallace WA, Howie SE, et al: Role of inflammation in nocturnal asthma. Thorax 1994;49:257-262.
37. Martin RJ, Cicutto LC, Smith HR, et al: Airways inflammation in nocturnal asthma. Am Rev Respir Dis 1991;143:351-357.
38. ten Hacken NH, Postma DS, Bosma F, et al: Vascular adhesion molecules in nocturnal asthma: A possible role for VCAM-1 in ongoing airway wall inflammation. Clin Exp Allergy 1998;28:1518-1525.
39. Kraft M, Striz I, Georges G, et al: Expression of epithelial markers in nocturnal asthma. J Allergy Clin Immunol 1998;102:376-381.
40. ten Hacken NH, Timens W, Smith M, et al: Increased peak expiratory flow variation in asthma: Severe persistent increase but not nocturnal worsening of airway inflammation. Eur Respir J 1998;12:546-550.
41. Jarjour NN, Busse WW: Cytokines in bronchoalveolar lavage fluid of patients with nocturnal asthma. Am J Respir Crit Care Med 1995;152:1474-1477.
42. Oosterhoff Y, Kauffman HF, Rutgers B, et al: Inflammatory cell number and mediators in bronchoalveolar lavage fluid and peripheral blood in subjects with asthma with increased nocturnal airways narrowing. J Allergy Clin Immunol 1995;96:219-229.
43. Fitzpatrick MF, Engleman H, Whyte KF, et al: Morbidity in nocturnal asthma: Sleep quality and daytime cognitive performance. Thorax 1991;46:569-573.
44. Weersink EJ, van Zomeren EH, Koeter GH, Postma DS: Treatment of nocturnal airway obstruction improves daytime cognitive performance in asthmatics. Am J Respir Crit Care Med 1997;156:1144-1150.
45. Douglas NJ: Asthma at night. Clin Chest Med 1985;6:663-674.
46. Douglas NJ, White DP, Weil JV, et al: Hypoxic ventilatory response decreases during sleep in normal men. Am Rev Respir Dis 1982;125:286-289.
47. Douglas NJ, White DP, Weil JV, et al: Hypercapnic ventilatory response in sleeping adults. Am Rev Respir Dis 1982;126:758-762.

48. Gugger M, Molloy J, Gould GA, et al: Ventilatory and arousal responses to added inspiratory resistance during sleep. Am Rev Respir Dis 1989;140:1301-1307.

49. Hetzel MR, Clark TJ, Branthwaite MA: Asthma: Analysis of sudden deaths and ventilatory arrests in hospital. BMJ 1977; 1:808-811.

50. Bateman JR, Clarke SW: Sudden death in asthma. Thorax 1979; 34:40-44.

51. Frezza G, Terra-Filho J, Martinez JA, Vianna EO: Rapid effect of inhaled steroids on nocturnal worsening of asthma. Thorax 2003;58:632-633.

52. Fitzpatrick MF, Mackay T, Driver H, Douglas NJ: Salmeterol in nocturnal asthma: A double blind, placebo controlled trial of a long acting inhaled beta 2 agonist. BMJ 1990;301:1365-1368.

53. Lockey RF, DuBuske LM, Friedman B, et al: Nocturnal asthma: Effect of salmeterol on quality of life and clinical outcomes. Chest 1999;115:666-673.

54. Maesen FP, Smeets JJ, Gubbelmans HL, Zweers PG: Formoterol in the treatment of nocturnal asthma. Chest 1990;98:866-870.

55. Barnes PJ, Greening AP, Neville L, et al: Single-dose slow-release aminophylline at night prevents nocturnal asthma. Lancet 1982; 1:299-301.

56. Crompton GK, Ayres JG, Basran G, et al: Comparison of oral bambuterol and inhaled salmeterol in patients with symptomatic asthma and using inhaled corticosteroids. Am J Respir Crit Care Med 1999;159:824-828.

57. Rhind GB, Connaughton JJ, McFie J, et al: Sustained release choline theophyllinate in nocturnal asthma. Br Med J (Clin Res Ed) 1985;291:1605-1607.

58. Fitzpatrick MF, Engleman HM, Boellert F, et al: Effect of therapeutic theophylline levels on the sleep quality and daytime cognitive performance of normal subjects. Am Rev Respir Dis 1992;145:1355-1358.

59. Selby C, Engleman HM, Fitzpatrick MF, et al: Inhaled salmeterol or oral theophylline in nocturnal asthma? Am J Respir Crit Care Med 1997;155:104-108.

60. Wiegand L, Mende CN, Zaidel G, et al: Salmeterol vs theophylline: Sleep and efficacy outcomes in patients with nocturnal asthma. Chest 1999;115:1525-1532.

61. Brambilla C, Chastang C, Georges D, Bertin L: Salmeterol compared with slow-release terbutaline in nocturnal asthma: A multicenter, randomized, double-blind, double-dummy, sequential clinical trial. French Multicenter Study Group. Allergy 1994;49:421-426.

62. Weersink EJ, Douma RR, Postma DS, Koeter GH: Fluticasone propionate, salmeterol xinafoate, and their combination in the treatment of nocturnal asthma. Am J Respir Crit Care Med 1997;155:1241-1246.

62a. Global Initiative for Obstructive Lung Disease. http://www.goldcopd.com.

63. Mulloy E, McNicholas WT: Ventilation and gas exchange during sleep and exercise in severe COPD. Chest 1996;109:387-394.

64. Douglas NJ, Calverley PM, Leggett RJ, et al. Transient hypoxaemia during sleep in chronic bronchitis and emphysema. Lancet 1979;1:1-4.

65. Becker HF, Piper AJ, Flynn WE, et al: Breathing during sleep in patients with nocturnal desaturation. Am J Respir Crit Care Med 1999;159:112-118.

66. Gould GA, Gugger M, Molloy J, et al: Breathing pattern and eye movement density during REM sleep in humans. Am Rev Respir Dis 1988;138:874-877.

67. Catterall JR, Douglas NJ, Calverley PM, et al: Transient hypoxemia during sleep in chronic obstructive pulmonary disease is not a sleep apnea syndrome. Am Rev Respir Dis 1983;128: 24-29.

68. George CF, West P, Kryger MH: Oxygenation and breathing pattern during phasic and tonic REM in patients with chronic obstructive pulmonary disease. Sleep 1987;10:234-243.

69. Catterall JR, Calverley PM, MacNee W, et al: Mechanism of transient nocturnal hypoxemia in hypoxic chronic bronchitis and emphysema. J Appl Physiol 1985;59:1698-1703.

70. White DP: Occlusion pressure and ventilation during sleep in normal humans. J Appl Physiol 1986;61:1279-1287.

71. Hudgel DW, Martin RJ, Johnson B, Hill P: Mechanics of the respiratory system and breathing pattern during sleep in normal humans. J Appl Physiol 1984;56:133-137.

72. Wiegand L, Zwillich CW, White DP: Sleep and the ventilatory response to resistive loading in normal men. J Appl Physiol 1988;64:1186-1195.

73. White DP, Weil JV, Zwillich CW: Metabolic rate and breathing during sleep. J Appl Physiol 1985;59:384-391.

74. White JE, Drinnan MJ, Smithson AJ, et al: Respiratory muscle activity during rapid eye movement (REM) sleep in patients with chronic obstructive pulmonary disease. Thorax 1995;50:376-382.

75. Midgren B: Oxygen desaturation during sleep as a function of the underlying respiratory disease. Am Rev Respir Dis 1990;141: 43-46.

76. Johnson MW, Remmers JE: Accessory muscle activity during sleep in chronic obstructive pulmonary disease. J Appl Physiol 1984;57:1011-1017.

77. Ballard RD, Clover CW, Suh BY: Influence of sleep on respiratory function in emphysema. Am J Respir Crit Care Med 1995;151: 945-951.

78. Catterall JR, Calverley PM, MacNee W, et al: Mechanism of transient nocturnal hypoxemia in hypoxic chronic bronchitis and emphysema. J Appl Physiol 1985;59:1698-1703.

79. Sanders MH, Newman AB, Haggerty CL, et al: Sleep and sleep-disordered breathing in adults with predominantly mild obstructive airway disease. Am J Respir Crit Care Med 2003;167:7-14.

80. Connaughton JJ, Catterall JR, Elton RA, et al: Do sleep studies contribute to the management of patients with severe chronic obstructive pulmonary disease? Am Rev Respir Dis 1988;138: 341-344.

81. Chaouat A, Weitzenblum E, Krieger J, et al: Association of chronic obstructive pulmonary disease and sleep apnea syndrome. Am J Respir Crit Care Med 1995;151:82-86.

82. Chan CS, Bye PT, Woolcock AJ, Sullivan CE: Eucapnia and hypercapnia in patients with chronic airflow limitation: The role of the upper airway. Am Rev Respir Dis 1990;141:861-865.

83. Shepard JW Jr, Garrison MW, Grither DA: Relationship of ventricular ectopy to nocturnal oxygen desaturation in patients with chronic obstructive pulmonary disease. Am J Med 1985; 78:28-34.

84. Coccagna G, Lugaresi E: Arterial blood gases and pulmonary and systemic arterial pressure during sleep in chronic obstructive pulmonary disease. Sleep 1978;1:117-124.

85. Boysen PG, Block AJ, Wynne JW, et al: Nocturnal pulmonary hypertension in patients with chronic obstructive pulmonary disease. Chest 1979;76:536-542.

86. Moore-Gillon JC, Cameron IR: Right ventricular hypertrophy and polycythaemia in rats after intermittent exposure to hypoxia. Clin Sci (Lond) 1985;69:595-599.

87. Fitzpatrick MF, Mackay T, Whyte KF, et al: Nocturnal desaturation and serum erythropoietin: A study in patients with chronic obstructive pulmonary disease and in normal subjects. Clin Sci (Lond) 1993;84:319-324.

88. Fletcher EC, Luckett RA, Miller T, et al: Pulmonary vascular hemodynamics in chronic lung disease patients with and without oxyhemoglobin desaturation during sleep. Chest 1989; 95:757-764.

89. Fleetham J, West P, Mezon B, et al: Sleep, arousals, and oxygen desaturation in chronic obstructive pulmonary disease: The effect of oxygen therapy. Am Rev Respir Dis 1982;126:429-433.

90. Orr WC, Shamma-Othman Z, Levin D, et al: Persistent hypoxemia and excessive daytime sleepiness in chronic obstructive pulmonary disease (COPD). Chest 1990;97:583-585.

91. Bradley TD, Rutherford R, Grossman RF, et al: Role of daytime hypoxemia in the pathogenesis of right heart failure in the obstructive sleep apnea syndrome. Am Rev Respir Dis 1985; 131:835-839.

92. Chaouat A, Weitzenblum E, Kessler R, et al: Outcome of COPD patients with mild daytime hypoxaemia with or without sleep-related oxygen desaturation. Eur Respir J 2001;17: 848-855.

93. Goldstein RS, Ramcharan V, Bowes G, et al: Effect of supplemental nocturnal oxygen on gas exchange in patients with severe obstructive lung disease. N Engl J Med 1984;310: 425-429.

94. Chaouat A, Weitzenblum E, Kessler R, et al: A randomized trial of nocturnal oxygen therapy in chronic obstructive pulmonary disease patients. Eur Respir J 1999;14:1002-1008.

95. Connaughton JJ, Douglas NJ, Morgan AD, et al: Almitrine improves oxygenation when both awake and asleep in patients with hypoxia and carbon dioxide retention caused by chronic bronchitis and emphysema. Am Rev Respir Dis 1985;132: 206-210.

96. Saas-Torres J, Domingo C, Moron A, et al: Long-term effects of almitrine bismesylate in COPD patients with chronic hypoxaemia. Respir Med 2003;97:599-605.

97. Series F, Cormier Y: Effects of protriptyline on diurnal and nocturnal oxygenation in patients with chronic obstructive pulmonary disease. Ann Intern Med 1990;113:507-511.

98. Dolly FR, Block AJ: Medroxyprogesterone acetate and COPD: Effect on breathing and oxygenation in sleeping and awake patients. Chest 1983;84:394-398.

99. Mulloy E, McNicholas WT: Theophylline improves gas exchange during rest, exercise, and sleep in severe chronic obstructive pulmonary disease. Am Rev Respir Dis 1993;148: 1030-1036.

100. Veale D, Cooper BG, Griffiths CJ, et al: The effect of controlled-release salbutamol on sleep and nocturnal oxygenation in patients with asthma and chronic obstructive pulmonary disease. Respir Med 1994;88:121-124.

101. Martin RJ, Bartelson BL, Smith P, et al: Effect of ipratropium bromide treatment on oxygen saturation and sleep quality in COPD. Chest 1999;115:1338-1345.

102. Lin CC: Comparison between nocturnal nasal positive pressure ventilation combined with oxygen therapy and oxygen monotherapy in patients with severe COPD. Am J Respir Crit Care Med 1996;154:353-358.

103. Clini E, Sturani C, Rossi A, et al: The Italian multicentre study on noninvasive ventilation in chronic obstructive pulmonary disease patients. Eur Respir J 2002;20:529-538.

104. Meecham Jones DJ, Paul EA, Jones PW, Wedzicha JA: Nasal pressure support ventilation plus oxygen compared with oxygen therapy alone in hypercapnic COPD. Am J Respir Crit Care Med 1995;152:538-544.

105. Fletcher EC, Schaaf JW, Miller J, Fletcher JG: Long-term cardiopulmonary sequelae in patients with sleep apnea and chronic lung disease. Am Rev Respir Dis 1987;135:525-533.

106. Block AJ, Dolly FR, Slayton PC: Does flurazepam ingestion affect breathing and oxygenation during sleep in patients with chronic obstructive lung disease? Am Rev Respir Dis 1984;129: 230-233.

107. Midgren B, Hansson L, Skeidsvoll H, et al: The effects of nitrazepam and flunitrazepam on oxygen desaturation during sleep in stable hypoxemic nonhypercapnic COPD. Chest 1989; 95:765-768.

108. Cummiskey J, Guilleminault C, Rio GD, et al: The effects of flurazepam on sleep studies in patients with chronic obstructive pulmonary disease. Chest 1983;84:143-147.

109. Girault C, Muir JF, Mihaltan F, et al: Effects of repeated administration of zolpidem on sleep, diurnal and nocturnal respiratory function, vigilance, and physical performance in patients with COPD. Chest 1996;110:1203-1211.

110. George CF, Bayliff CD: Management of insomnia in patients with chronic obstructive pulmonary disease. Drugs 2003;63: 379-387.

111. Kutty K: Sleep and chronic obstructive pulmonary disease. Curr Opin Pulm Med 2004;10:104-112.

94

Restrictive Lung Disorders

Meir H. Kryger

ABSTRACT

Disorders of structures surrounding the lungs, the most common being obesity and kyphoscoliosis, commonly result in breathing problems during sleep and consequent daytime symptoms. The most severe cases result in hypoventilation and cardiorespiratory failure. Obesity most often leads to upper airway obstruction, which may lead to obstructive sleep apnea–hypopnea syndrome and the obesity–hypoventilation syndrome. The obesity is managed with weight loss, whereas treatment of the sleep-related breathing problem is usually with continuous positive airway pressure or bilevel positive pressure. Kyphoscoliosis that results in hypoventilation is usually treated with bilevel positive pressure or positive-pressure ventilation employing a volume-cycled ventilator. Diffuse diseases of the lungs causing restriction have many causes, the most common being idiopathic pulmonary fibrosis. Stimulation of pulmonary receptors results in a rapid, shallow breathing pattern and hyperventilation. Sleep apnea is uncommon in this group. Daytime symptoms such as dyspnea dominate. The most common treatment of sleep hypoxemia in these cases is the administration of oxygen.

Lung volume is determined by two opposing forces: (1) the elasticity of the lung, which tends to reduce lung volume, and (2) the normal outward recoil of the thoracic cage and the activity of the inspiratory muscles. "Resting" lung volume (the volume at the end of a normal exhalation) is determined solely by the balance between the elasticity of the lung and the normal outward recoil properties of the chest wall. Restriction of lung expansion may thus be the result of disorders of the lungs (intrapulmonary restriction) or disorders of structures surrounding the lungs, such as the skeletal and soft tissue components of the chest wall (extrapulmonary restriction).

The physiologic consequences of these two types of restriction are different and result in different effects on respiratory control. In general, intrapulmonary restriction is characterized by stimulation of pulmonary vagal receptors with resultant tachypnea and hyperventilation. Patients with extrapulmonary restriction may exhibit blunted ventilatory chemosensitivity and hypoventilation. On the basis of differences during the awake state, one would expect these two groups to behave differently during sleep. Lung restriction is most commonly seen in five conditions: obesity, kyphoscoliosis, interstitial lung disease, neuromuscular diseases, and pregnancy. Sleep disorders in pregnancy are reviewed in detail in Chapter 109, and neuromuscular diseases are reviewed in Chapter 69.

OBESITY

Epidemiology and Risk Factors

Obesity is the excessive accumulation of fat and the resulting generalized increase in body mass. The most common clinical measure of adult obesity is the body mass index (BMI).[1,2] The combination of BMI and waist circumference can be used as a gauge of disease risk (Table 94–1).

There is a worldwide epidemic of obesity.[1,3] Among adults in the United States, about 19.9% of men and 24.9% of women have a BMI of greater than 30,[4] and the rate is similar in other developed countries.[5] In just the decade ending with 2000, the prevalence of BMIs greater than 40 tripled.[6] Obesity has been linked to an increased mortality from a variety of diseases including cancer.[7-9] It has been reported that 30% of people with a BMI of greater than 30, and 50% of people with a BMI of greater than 40, have obstructive sleep apnea.[10]

Obesity is associated with increased morbidity from arterial hypertension, diabetes mellitus, and degenerative joint disease,

Table 94–1. NIH Obesity Classification and Disease Risk

NIH Classification	Body Mass Index[†]	Obesity Class	Disease Risk*	
			Normal Waist Circumference	Increased Waist Circumference[‡]
Normal	18.5-24.9	—	—	—
Overweight	25-29.9	—	Increased	High
Obesity class I	30-34.9	I	High	Very high
Obesity class II	35-39.9	II	Very high	Very high
Extreme obesity	≥40	III	Extremely high	Extremely high

*Risk for type 2 diabetes, hypertension, and cardiovascular disease.
[†]BMI ≥ 30 is classified as obese.
[‡]Waist circumference increased: for men, >102 cm (>40 inches); for women, >88 cm (>35 inches).
Adapted from Table ES-4 of National Institutes of Health (NIH): Clinical Guidelines for the Identification, Evaluation, and Treatment of Overweight and Obesity in Adults. Bethesda, Md, National Institutes of Health, 1998; available at http://www.nhlbi.nih.gov/guidelines/obesity/ob_gdlns.pdf.

and it is a component of the metabolic syndrome. Metabolic syndrome is a constellation of findings whose features include obesity, insulin resistance, hypertension, and dyslipidemia (see Chapter 86). Some investigators have suggested that obstructive sleep apnea–hypopnea syndrome (OSAHS) is a component of the metabolic syndrome.[11] Patients with the metabolic syndrome have about three times the risk of death from coronary heart disease as those without.[12] The metabolic syndrome is estimated to affect 25% of the adult population.[13]

The distribution of fat is important. Epidemiologic studies show that central obesity (increased abdominal fat) is associated with increased cholesterol, blood pressure, and blood glucose, and with an increased incidence of cardiovascular disease and an increased death rate.[2]

Pathogenesis

Obese patients have compromised respiratory function while awake and seated. Their ventilatory function may become worse on assuming the supine position and may worsen further during sleep.

Awake Ventilation in Obesity

Obese people have increased metabolic demands, and this is reflected by an increased oxygen uptake ($\dot{V}O_2$) and a higher carbon dioxide production ($\dot{V}CO_2$). Thus, to maintain normal arterial blood gas tensions PaO_2 and $PaCO_2$, they must maintain an elevated level of alveolar ventilation. The work of breathing is increased in obesity, mainly because of the increased stiffness (reduced compliance) and inertance of the thoracic cage, which results from the accumulation of adipose tissue in and around the ribs, abdomen, and diaphragm.

In obese patients, the mass loading of the chest wall by adipose tissue reduces the tendency to recoil outward. Thus, resting lung volume (measured as functional residual capacity [FRC]) is reduced in these patients, and thus the oxygen stores in their lungs are reduced. During expiration, when lung volume falls below a certain level, airways at the lung bases begin to close. Perfusion may continue to lung units having closed (and therefore poorly ventilated) airways, which results in mismatching of ventilation and perfusion ($\dot{V}/\dot{Q}$) and causes hypoxemia.

Obesity and the Supine Position

In the supine position, the hydrostatic force of the abdomen is applied through the diaphragm to the lungs. In addition, the chest wall of obese people is stiffer in the supine than in the upright position. Thus, FRC is lower in the supine position, which exacerbates the hypoxemia caused, in part, by breathing at lung volumes below the closing volume. In addition, there is a further increase in the work of breathing during sleep, related to increases in upper airway resistance. This would be the case even in the absence of obstructive apnea given the normal increase in airway resistance that normally accompanies sleep.

Breathing during Sleep in Obesity

Obese patients with and without the obesity–hypoventilation syndrome (see later), may demonstrate the following breathing abnormalities during sleep.

HEAVY SNORING WITH NO DEMONSTRABLE APNEA OR HYPOPNEA

Some patients may have severe snoring without having hypoxemia. When such patients have increased respiratory effort–related arousals during sleep, and excessive daytime sleepiness, their symptoms fit the criteria for upper airway resistance syndrome.[14]

HYPOXEMIA WITH NO DEMONSTRABLE APNEA OR HYPOPNEA

Hypoxemia without demonstrable apnea or hypopnea is most likely related to the low lung volumes seen in the supine position. Some obese patients may have an oxyhemoglobin saturation (SaO_2) in the range of 90% to 94% during non–rapid eye movement (NREM) sleep, with further reductions during rapid eye movement (REM) sleep. The lack of overt apneas in these patients may reflect normal drives to breathe and an absence of upper airway obstruction.

PERIODIC HYPOXEMIA WITHOUT APNEAS

Swings in SaO_2 may be present without overt apneas. In some cases, these may be related to periodic changes in ventilation or to incomplete upper airway occlusion—the sleep hypopnea syndrome. Such patients may have the same sequelae as do those with apnea, including multiple arousals, cyclic hypoxemia, sleepiness, and right-sided heart failure.[15] Many laboratories no longer differentiate sleep hypopnea syndrome from OSAHS. Periodic hypoxemia without apneas may represent a transition between upper airway resistance syndrome, in which there are no discrete hypopneas or apneas, and OSAHS characterized by overt apneic or hypopneic events.

SLEEP APNEA AND HYPOVENTILATION

Although many obese patients develop repetitive sleep apneas, some do not. Increased weight alone is not sufficient to cause sleep apnea. About half of adults with a BMI exceeding 40 can be expected not to have sleep apnea.[10] It is likely that the distribution of fat with an associated anatomic predisposition to upper airway obstruction is a key element in the genesis of sleep apnea. Increased compliance of the walls of the upper airway may also be present, making it more collapsible (see Chapter 82). Obese sleepy patients fall into two distinct groups: those without hypoventilation while awake (most of whom have OSAHS), and those having hypoventilation while both awake and asleep. Patients in the latter group have reduced chemical (i.e., hypoxic and hypercapnic) drives to breathe. They have obesity–hypoventilation syndrome, also called the pickwickian syndrome (see later). Obstructive sleep apnea–hypopnea syndrome is discussed in greater detail in Chapters 84 to 92.

Clinical Features

The clinical presentation of people with obesity reflects obesity-related comorbidities that can also affect sleep. For example, they might present with diabetes, cardiovascular disease, joint diseases, and sleep breathing disorders. Many patients have combinations of symptoms related to several of these conditions. The features related to sleep breathing disorders in obese patients with OSAHS are reviewed in Chapter 87.

Diagnosis

Obesity is most commonly quantified by using the BMI (see Table 94–1). Other measures of adiposity include waist circumference, waist-to-hip ratio, and neck circumference. Epidemiologic studies suggest that waist circumference is a better marker of abdominal visceral fat content than the waist-to-hip ratio, and that it is the most practical measurement for abdominal fat.[2] Computed tomography and magnetic resonance imaging are more accurate in quantifying visceral fat, but they are not clinically practical.[2] Large neck size in both male and female snorers is highly predictive of obstructive sleep apnea. Men with a neck circumference of 17 inches (43 cm) or more and women with a neck circumference of 16 inches (40.6 cm) or more are at higher risk for having obstructive sleep apnea, but an even better predictor of apnea severity is the ratio of neck size to height.[16]

Treatment

Achieving and maintaining normal weight is a challenge, and the strategies for treating obesity are beyond the scope of this chapter (see Chapter 88). However, many approaches to weight loss have been studied, and an algorithm developed by the National Institutes of Health (NIH) is presented in Figure 94–1. The comprehensive recommendations in Table 94–2 are from a systematic review by the NIH, and the reader is encouraged to download them from the website given in the table.[2] No randomized clinical trials of the efficacy of weight loss methods have been reported for obese subjects with sleep breathing disorders,[17] although many studies have reported improvement of breathing during sleep after weight loss. There has been an increase in the use of bariatric surgery in morbidly obese sleep apnea patients.[17a]

OBESITY–HYPOVENTILATION SYNDROME (PICKWICKIAN SYNDROME)

Classification, Epidemiology, and Risk Factors

Originally, obesity–hypoventilation syndrome (OHS) was the diagnosis used for obese patients who had hypoventilation while awake,[18] and there is still some controversy about the name.[19] Hypoventilation in the awake state is present in about 10% of sleepy obese patients.[20] About half of sleep apnea patients with a BMI exceeding 40 can be expected to have awake hypoventilation.[21] The disorder is classified as sleep-related non-obstructive alveolar hypoventilation, secondary to neuromuscular and chest wall disorders in the International Classification of Sleep Disorders when hypercapnia is present and BMI ≥ 35.[21a] Women make up a high proportion of OHS patients; in several reports, they make up more than half of all cases.[22-25] The high prevalence in women may reflect the fact that morbid obesity is more common in women than in men.

Pathogenesis

The chemical drives to breathe—both hypoxic and hypercapnic—have been found to be reduced in OHS.[26] Respiratory mechanics and weight do not adequately explain why relatively few obese patients develop hypoventilation while awake and the majority do not. Indeed, hypoventilation may occur with only mildly impaired ventilatory function.[27] Control of ventilation plays a role. If the limiting factor were simply the stiffness of the respiratory system, these patients should demonstrate increased muscle work compared with obese patients without hypoventilation while awake,[28] but they do not.

The hypoventilation causes hypoxemia. This promotes the production of red blood cells (erythrocytosis),[27] which is followed by pulmonary vasoconstriction leading to pulmonary arterial hypertension,[29] which may in turn cause right heart failure (cor pulmonale), systemic venous hypertension, and peripheral edema.

The hormone leptin, produced by fat cells and thought to reduce appetite, may also act in the nervous system to increase ventilation (see Chapter 86). It has been suggested that the hypercapnic respiratory failure in OHS may be due to an acquired central resistance to the effect of the high levels of leptin.[30]

Clinical Features

The classic clinical features of patients with OHS are obesity, excessive daytime sleepiness, a plethoric complexion, cyanosis, and evidence of right heart failure including peripheral edema. Surprisingly, despite obvious hypoxemia, the patients may not complain of dyspnea. The latter finding is found in patients with depressed drives to breathe.

Diagnosis

Diagnostic criteria for sleep hypoventilation syndromes have been published[31] and can be applied to OHS patients. The patient with OHS has BMI ≥ 35 and awake hypoventilation (confirmed by an elevated $PaCO_2$) and one or more features of chronic hypoventilation (cor pulmonale, pulmonary hypertension, erythrocytosis), and an overnight sleep study that documents either an increase in PCO_2 of more than 10 mm Hg or an oxygen desaturation not explained by apnea or hypopnea. Patients may demonstrate a spectrum of findings: episodes of obstruction, hypoventilation, or sustained obstructive hypoventilation due to partial upper airway obstruction.[25] Clinicians should make sure that the patient does not have hypothyroidism, which in severe cases may lead to hypoventilation and mimic OHS.

Treatment

The approaches to treating OHS include weight loss, continuous positive airway pressure (CPAP) or bilevel positive airway pressure (PAP), and ventilatory stimulation with progestational agents. Ventilatory chemoresponsiveness may normalize with weight loss and may result in clinical improvement.[18] Ventilatory assistance with CPAP may be effective in some cases, whereas others may require bilevel PAP.[22,32] Because these patients are often medically unstable, CPAP or bilevel PAP titration should be done in an experienced laboratory, not in an ambulatory or unattended setting. The patients sometimes require oxygen to be added to the CPAP or bilevel PAP systems.

Progesterone increases the chemical drive to breathe without altering lung mechanics. That reduced drive plays a role in many of the features of OHS is shown by the sometimes dramatic improvement when these patients are treated with progestational agents (e.g., medroxyprogesterone acetate [MPA]).[33,34] Few patients with classic OHS have been reported as having been treated with MPA.[34] We have used MPA, 30 to 60 mg daily as a single dose, and documented the effect with arterial blood gas values: a clinical response (a drop in $PaCO_2$), if one is going

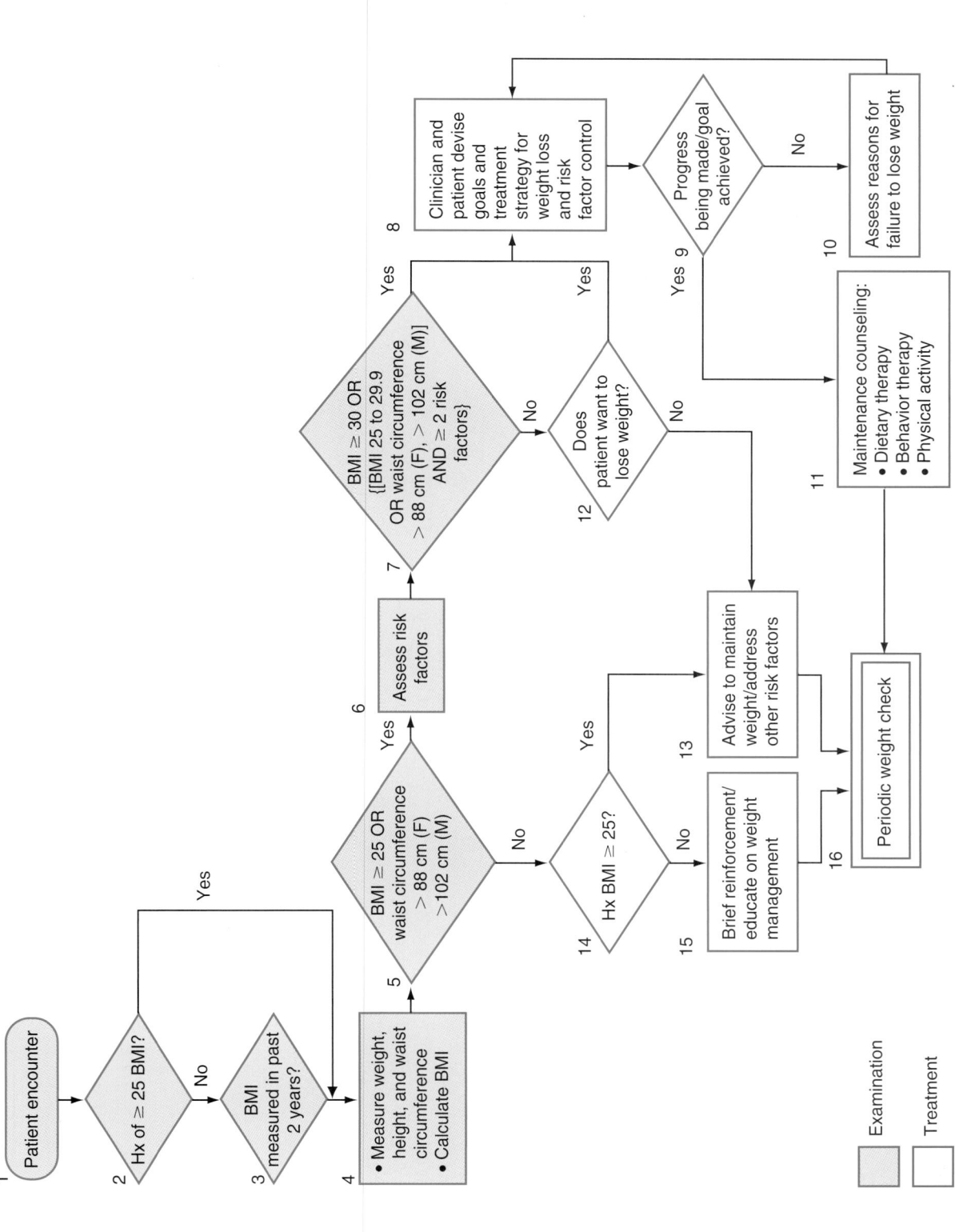

1 Patient encounter

2 Hx of ≥ 25 BMI?
— Yes
— No

3 BMI measured in past 2 years?

4 • Measure weight, height, and waist circumference
• Calculate BMI

5 BMI ≥ 25 OR waist circumference > 88 cm (F) >102 cm (M)
— Yes
— No

6 Assess risk factors
— Yes

7 BMI ≥ 30 OR {[BMI 25 to 29.9 OR waist circumference > 88 cm (F), > 102 cm (M)] AND ≥ 2 risk factors}
— Yes
— No

8 Clinician and patient devise goals and treatment strategy for weight loss and risk factor control

9 Progress being made/goal achieved?
— Yes
— No

10 Assess reasons for failure to lose weight

11 Maintenance counseling:
• Dietary therapy
• Behavior therapy
• Physical activity

12 Does patient want to lose weight?
— Yes
— No

13 Advise to maintain weight/address other risk factors

14 Hx BMI ≥ 25?
— Yes
— No

15 Brief reinforcement/educate on weight management

16 Periodic weight check

Examination
Treatment

* This algorithm applies only to the assessment for overweight and obesity and subsequent decisions based on that assessment. It does not include any initial overall assessment for cardiovascular risk factors or diseases that are indicated.

Figure 94–1. Obesity treatment algorithm. (From National Institutes of Health: Clinical Guidelines for the Identification, Evaluation, Treatment of Overweight and Obesity in Adults. Bethesda, Md, National Institutes of Health, 1998; available at http://www.nhlbi.nih/gov/guidelines/obesity/ob_gdlns.pdf.) BMI, body mass index; F, female; M, male.

Table 94–2. Treatment Modalities and Their Efficacy in Obesity

1. Dietary Therapy

- Low-calorie diets are recommended for weight loss in overweight and obese persons. Evidence Category A.
- Reducing fat as part of a low-calorie diet is a practical way to reduce calories. Evidence Category A.
- Reducing dietary fat alone without reducing calories is not sufficient for weight loss. However, reducing dietary fat, along with reducing dietary carbohydrates, can facilitate caloric reduction. Evidence Category A.
- A diet that is individually planned to help create a deficit of 500 to 1,000 kcal/day should be an integral part of any program aimed at achieving a weight loss of 1 to 2 lb/week. Evidence Category A.

2. Physical Activity

- Physical activity is recommended as part of a comprehensive weight loss therapy and weight maintenance program because it modestly contributes to weight loss (Evidence Category A), may decrease abdominal fat (Evidence Category B), and may help with maintenance of weight loss (Evidence Category C).
- Initially, moderate levels of physical activity for 30-45 minutes, 3-5 days per week should be encouraged. Adults should set a long-term goal to accumulate at least 30 minutes or more of moderate intensity physical activity on most, and preferably all, days of the week. Evidence Category B.
- The combination of a reduced calorie diet and increased physical activity is recommended since it produces weight loss, decreases abdominal fat, and increases cardiorespiratory fitness. Evidence Category A.

3. Behavior Therapy

- Behavior therapy is a useful adjunct when incorporated into treatment for weight loss and weight maintenance. Evidence Category B.
- Practitioners need to assess the patient's motivation to enter weight loss therapy; assess the readiness of the patient to implement the plan and then take appropriate steps to motivate the patient for treatment. Evidence Category D.
- Behavior therapy strategies to promote diet and physical activity should be used routinely, as they are helpful in achieving weight loss and weight maintenance. Evidence Category B.

4. Combined Therapy

- Weight loss and weight maintenance therapy should employ the combination of low-calorie diet, increased physical activity, and behavior therapy. Evidence Category A.

5. Pharmacotherapy

- Weight loss drugs approved by the FDA may be used as part of a comprehensive weight loss program including diet and physical activity for patients with a BMI of ≥30 with no concomitant obesity-related risk factors or diseases, and for patients with a BMI of ≥27 with concomitant obesity-related risk factors of diseases. Drugs should never be used without concomitant lifestyle modification. Continual assessment of drug therapy for efficacy and safety is necessary. If the drug is efficacious in helping the patient lose and/or maintain weight loss and there are no serious adverse effects, it can be continued. If not, it should be discontinued. Evidence Category B.

6. Weight Loss Surgery

- Weight loss surgery is an option in carefully selected patients with *clinically severe obesity* (BMI ≥40 or ≥35 with comorbid conditions) when less invasive methods of weight loss have failed and the patient is at high risk for obesity-associated morbidity or mortality. Evidence Category B.

From National Institutes of Health: Clinical Guidelines for the Identification, Evaluation, and Treatment of Overweight and Obesity in Adults. Bethesda, Md, National Institutes of Health, 1998; http://www.nhlbi.nih.gov/guidelines/obesity/ob_gdlns.pdf.

to occur, is usually apparent within 24 hours. Pulse therapy using MPA has been suggested as helpful in postmenopausal women with OHS.[35] Whether MPA is clinically useful long term is unclear. One might use MPA for patients with OHS who have an inadequate response to CPAP or bilevel PAP therapy.

KYPHOSCOLIOSIS

Epidemiology and Risk Factors

Scoliosis refers to a lateral curvature of the spine, whereas kyphosis refers to anteroposterior curvature of the spine. Kyphoscoliosis, a combination of the two, causing significant thoracic cage deformity, is usually idiopathic in origin (80% of cases) but may be a consequence of many diseases, including paralytic poliomyelitis, neurofibromatosis, Pott's disease, ankylosing spondylitis, Marfan's syndrome, and the mucopolysaccharidoses. Chest wall deformity is more common in females than males. Very severe kyphoscoliosis occurs in about 1 person in 10,000.[36]

Pathogenesis

Depending on the cause and degree of spinal curvature, kyphoscoliosis can produce respiratory failure at ages ranging from adolescence to late adulthood.[37] Scoliosis by itself is insufficient to cause respiratory failure. About 100 degrees of curvature is present in kyphoscoliosis patients with respiratory failure; in most of the studies reporting on sleep in kyphoscoliosis, the spinal deformity has been of this magnitude.[38-40]

Lung Mechanics

Between episodes of acute respiratory failure, these patients have the rapid, shallow breathing pattern of a marked restrictive defect. This breathing pattern is adopted because it is associated with a reduced work of breathing in the context of the stiff chest wall associated with kyphoscoliosis. In addition, the ventilatory muscles, abnormally positioned because of the chest wall deformity, are inefficient. This also promotes the development of a breathing pattern that will operate with the greatest efficiency. There is an important tradeoff engendered by a rapid, shallow breathing pattern, because it is associated with relatively increased ventilation of the anatomic dead space (the larger, more central airways that do not participate in gas exchange) with a smaller percentage of the inspired tidal volume getting to the alveoli. The deformity also causes an abnormal distribution of inspired air, with consequent atelectasis and ventilation and perfusion ($\dot{V}/\dot{Q}$) mismatching. The small tidal volumes also probably promote airway closure and thus perpetuate the atelectasis.

Another factor that may play a role is the low FRC. Patients with a low FRC have reduced oxygen stores in the lungs. If such a patient becomes apneic, oxygen uptake from the lungs into the pulmonary circulation will continue with abnormally rapid depletion of oxygen stores, thus causing a precipitous fall in alveolar P_{O_2}.

Control of Breathing

Control of ventilation in kyphoscoliosis may be abnormal for two reasons. First, if the kyphoscoliosis was caused by poliomyelitis, the defect in respiratory drive may be secondary to involvement of the respiratory control system in the medulla, or it may be the result of weakness of the respiratory muscles.

Second, the blunting of drive may be acquired—it may be related to the enormous mechanical load, as may occur with obesity. Respiratory failure may first occur in patients with postpoliomyelitic kyphoscoliosis 20 to 30 years after their acute infection and recovery. The ventilatory response to hypercapnia may be markedly reduced.[37,41] This blunting of hypercapnic drive may result from mechanical impairment (chest wall deformity, ventilatory muscle weakness) alone. However, when hypercapnia is present, peak ventilation remains well below the patient's maximal voluntary minute ventilation, which suggests a primary defect in ventilatory drive. Hypoxic ventilatory drive may also be blunted in some patients.

Clinical Features

Although, in some cases, hypoventilation during wakefulness is chronic, in most patients it appears to be episodically precipitated by infections and less frequently by pulmonary emboli or respiratory depressant agents, such as hypnotics or opiates. Patients with chronic hypoventilation have the sequelae of chronic hypoxemia, polycythemia, pulmonary hypertension, and cor pulmonale. Interestingly, even when these patients are hypoxic and hypercapnic, they may not have the sensation of dyspnea.

Sleep

Patients may complain of excessive daytime sleepiness and disrupted nocturnal sleep.[38] Some patients have severe nocturnal or morning headaches, probably caused by carbon dioxide retention during sleep. Both hypercapnia and hypoxia are known to increase cerebral blood flow by vasodilation, which is the likely mechanism by which these headaches occur. Sleep studies show that sleep in these patients is "lighter," with an increase in stage 1 and a reduction in stage 2 sleep.[39]

Sleep Breathing Patterns and Gas Exchange

Kyphoscoliosis patients may have a Cheyne-Stokes respiration pattern (i.e., a periodic breathing pattern with or without apneas; see Chapter 81), severe central apneas, or hypoventilation (primarily during REM sleep),[39] and obstructive apneas.[38] Apnea duration is substantially greater in REM sleep than in NREM sleep. The cause of the REM apneas is unclear, but they may be linked to REM sleep–related loss of tone in the intercostal and accessory muscles of respiration. The hypoventilation of sleep results in an elevation of the Pa_{CO_2}, there being a positive correlation between the awake Pa_{CO_2} and the nocturnal rise in Pa_{CO_2}[42,43]; that is, the greater the degree of hypercapnia during wakefulness, the greater are the increases in Pa_{CO_2} during sleep.

The Sa_{O_2} is much lower in REM sleep than in NREM sleep, and the lowest Sa_{O_2} of the night was less than 60% in most reported cases.[38-40,44] Patients with cor pulmonale have the most severe drops in Sa_{O_2}.[39] In one report, elevated hematocrit, hypoxemia during the awake state, and cor pulmonale were present in two of the five patients with severe oxygen desaturation.[39] It is interesting that the degree of impairment of lung function did not seem to correlate with desaturation during sleep.

The patient's sex may play a role in the development of sleep breathing abnormalities in kyphoscoliosis. In one report, all the patients were men.[38] In the other, the only two patients with severe desaturation were men; the two women who had the most impaired lung function demonstrated little desaturation during sleep.[39] However, I have encountered several women with kyphoscoliosis secondary to poliomyelitis who had severe breathing abnormalities during sleep.

Daytime Sequelae

In one report, four patients with severe kyphoscoliosis and a previous history of poliomyelitis had hypercapnic respiratory failure during wakefulness that seemed related to abnormalities in sleep.[45] When these patients were mechanically ventilated at night, the daytime hypoventilation resolved. This finding suggests that one of two mechanisms may be involved in producing spillover hypoventilation. One is respiratory muscle fatigue. These patients must generate high pleural pressures to maintain tidal volume in the presence of altered mechanics. The respiratory muscles, which may be abnormal in the first place, may fatigue during the night.[46] The other possible mechanism causing hypoxemia is a progressive loss of lung volume during sleep. It is believed that low tidal volume breathing with no or few sighs promotes airway closure and microatelectasis.

Diagnosis

Kyphoscoliosis is easily diagnosed by physical examination, and the impact on physiology is documented by lung function testing and arterial blood gases. In the most severe cases, sleep symptoms (nocturnal or morning headaches, sleepiness) and cardiorespiratory failure are common. Comprehensive diagnostic polysomnography followed by titration on bilevel pressure support or mechanical ventilation using a nasal mask (or, in some cases, other noninvasive interfaces) are indicated in patients with significant headaches, sleepiness, or cardiorespiratory failure.

Treatment

Untreated patients with kyphoscoliosis, respiratory failure, and cor pulmonale have a poor prognosis. Tracheostomy alone, which was used in the past in an attempt to reduce anatomic dead space, is probably not indicated unless severe obstructive apnea is documented. The use of tracheostomy does not result in consistent improvement in respiratory failure.[45,47]

The uncontrolled administration of CPAP in patients with kyphoscoliosis but without obstructive apnea may have detrimental effects. Because of the extreme stiffness of the chest wall, increasing FRC may result in the patient's having to generate great pressure to breathe in. Patients with kyphoscoliosis have developed acute respiratory failure with the institution of CPAP.

Nasal ventilation using either a home ventilator or a bilevel PAP device can also be expected to be effective, and excellent long-term results have been reported[47-49] (see Chapters 89 and 95). With such treatment, one can expect a reduction in nocturnal carbon dioxide levels and improvement in daytime somnolence and the sensation of dyspnea.[48] In one report, if patients did not have coexisting obstructive apnea, the inspiratory pressure used was the highest that was tolerated by the patient, and the expiratory pressure was 2 to 4 cm H_2O.[48] If the patients had obstructive apnea, the expiratory pressure value was the previously determined effective CPAP level, and the inspiratory pressure level was increased until oxygen desaturations were eliminated. If bilevel PAP is stopped when the patient has shown clinical improvement, there is a return of daytime sleepiness, morning headaches, dyspnea, and a loss of energy within a week.[49]

When ventilation is not possible with these noninvasive modalities, a tracheostomy may become necessary. Tracheostomy and chronic nighttime ventilation with high inflation pressures

resulted in dramatic improvements in $PaCO_2$ and in PaO_2 during wakefulness, and in a normalization of hematocrit.[45]

Medications in the Nonventilated Patient

Although breathing oxygen-enriched gas mixtures is known to increase waking values of $PaCO_2$ in patients with kyphoscoliosis who are already hypercapnic, it is not known whether the benefit of increased PaO_2 offsets the rise in $PaCO_2$.[37] I have seen several hypercapnic patients with kyphoscoliosis who became comatose with oxygen administration. Thus, the sensorium and $PaCO_2$ should be monitored closely until the patient is stable. It has been shown that although oxygen administration increases SaO_2 during sleep in these patients, dyspnea, morning headache, and sleepiness are not systematically improved, in contrast to the improvement seen in patients with these symptoms who have received ventilatory support.[50]

Because the most severe oxygen desaturations occur in REM sleep, suppression of REM sleep may theoretically be of benefit. Protriptyline, a nonsedating tricyclic antidepressant, was evaluated in eight patients with chest wall restriction.[40] A dose of 10 to 20 mg at bedtime reduced REM sleep by about 50%. Oxygenation was significantly improved while the patients were asleep and awake. Hypercapnia was also improved during sleep. Anticholinergic side effects were not a severe problem in this report; however, seven of the eight patients were women, who are less likely than are men to develop urinary hesitancy. There are no published systematic trials of respiratory stimulants such as progesterone or acetazolamide in kyphoscoliosis. In the absence of adequate trials, no medications can be recommended as treatment of hypoventilation in kyphoscoliosis.

INTERSTITIAL LUNG DISEASE

Epidemiology and Risk Factors

The accumulation of abnormal cells, tissues, or fluid in the interstitial space of the lung alters the mechanical properties of the lung, making it substantially stiffer and increasing its recoil, which reduces lung volume. Although diffuse interstitial lung disease (ILD) can be caused by over a hundred diseases, the disorders most commonly responsible are idiopathic pulmonary fibrosis[50a] (also called interstitial pneumonitis or cryptogenic fibrosing alveolitis), sarcoidosis, occupational dust exposures, malignancy, and reaction to drugs.[51]

Pathogenesis

Patients with ILD have a rapid, shallow breathing pattern thought to be related to lung vagal stimulation by a pathologic process in the lungs. The resultant level of ventilation is usually excessive for the level of carbon dioxide production, which causes hypocapnia to occur.[52]

Clinical Features

During the awake state, patients with ILD have dyspnea, which may become quite severe with exercise. Nonproductive cough is another common symptom.

Sleep

Patients with ILD have very disrupted sleep, with more arousals, sleep-stage changes, and sleep fragmentation than normal subjects.[53,54] The multiple arousals could be related to coughing or to chemical stimuli. Patients with an SaO_2 of less than 90% had more disrupted sleep than did those with an

SaO_2 above 90%. Sleep stages were also redistributed, with a marked increase in stage 1 and a reduction in REM sleep.

Sleep Breathing Patterns and Gas Exchange

Hypoxemia during sleep is common in these patients and may result in an impaired quality of life.[51a] In studies of SaO_2 during sleep, three patterns of oxygen desaturation have been reported in patients with ILD.[52] In the first and most common pattern, oxygen desaturation occurred primarily during REM sleep and seemed to be related to episodic hypoventilation. The lower the baseline SaO_2, the greater the fall in SaO_2 from awake to REM sleep.[55] In the second pattern, there were sustained falls in SaO_2 during both REM sleep and NREM sleep. The third group of patients consisted of those who snored, some of whom had the classic OSAS. Although a low incidence of apnea and hypopnea was present in one series, it was found that patients with interstitial lung disease with an SaO_2 of less than 90% had drops in SaO_2 when they snored.[54] Profound hypoxemic episodes tend to be brief and rare, and the maximal fall in SaO_2 is similar to that seen during maximal exercise.[56] Because the hypoxemic episodes may be brief, the mean sleep SaO_2 may fall only slightly from awake values.[56] At moderate altitude, patients with ILD have a low baseline SaO_2.[57]

Breathing frequency tends to remain high but may decrease during sleep. Transcutaneous PCO_2 may stay the same as at awake levels,[58] or it may increase as it does in normal subjects.[43] Hypoventilation does not seem to occur.[43,55] Thus, although many reflexes are inhibited by the sleep state, those that maintain the rapid breathing pattern remain during sleep. Apnea frequency is low in these patients, perhaps reflecting a high drive to breathe. Control of breathing does appear to be important in maintaining ventilation in interstitial fibrosis; patients with lower hypercapnic ventilatory responses have greater falls in SaO_2 during sleep.[55] Obstructive sleep apnea has been described in patients with disorders that may cause interstitial lung diseases, including rheumatoid arthritis[59] and sarcoidosis.[60]

Diagnosis

Several methods are used to determine the impact of ILD on physiology (lung function tests and exercise oximetry) and to diagnose it (chest radiograph, computerized tomography, and lung biopsy). Daytime symptoms, especially dyspnea, can be quite severe, so in general these patients are not referred to a sleep laboratory, and therapy is geared toward attempts to reverse the lung disease and toward the use of oxygen based on exercise oximetry.

Treatment

In view of the high drive to breathe and the low incidence of apnea, it is unlikely that nocturnal oxygen therapy would cause either significant apneas or hypoventilation. There are no randomized clinical trials examining the use of oxygen in patients with ILD.[61] In the absence of any literature dealing with indications for nocturnal oxygen therapy in this group, it seems prudent to start with the criteria of the Nocturnal Oxygen Therapy Trial Group.[62] One would use supplemental oxygen if awake PaO_2 is less than 55 mm Hg, or if it is less than 60 mm Hg in the presence of hypoxemic complications (polycythemia or peripheral edema). However, because many of these patients desaturate rapidly with minimal exercise, criteria for home oxygen therapy should be more liberal, and many centers use exercise oximetry as a guide in determining the need for home oxygen. Some patients may need oxygen therapy only with exercise. Respiratory stimulants probably do not have a role in interstitial lung disease because respiratory drive is usually already high. At moderately high altitude, oxygen administration improved SaO_2 and decreased heart rate and breathing frequency, but it had little effect on sleep efficiency or arousal rate.[57]

> ### Clinical Pearls
>
> Patients with extrapulmonary lung restriction may develop severe hypoventilation during sleep, with resultant cardiorespiratory failure. Treatment with bilevel positive airway pressure or mechanical ventilation can result in improved clinical status and even resolution of daytime hypoventilation. Patients with intrapulmonary restriction generally hyperventilate, and sleep apnea is uncommon.

References

1. World Health Organization: Obesity: Preventing and managing the global epidemic—Report of a WHO consultation on obesity. Geneva, World Health Organization, 1998, pp 1-276.
2. National Institutes of Health: Clinical Guidelines for the Identification, Evaluation, and Treatment of Overweight and Obesity in Adults. Bethesda, Md, National Institutes of Health, 1998; available at http://www.nhlbi.nih.gov/guidelines/obesity/ob_gdlns.pdf.
3. York DA, Rossner S, Caterson I, et al: American Heart Association. Prevention Conference VII: Obesity, a worldwide epidemic related to heart disease and stroke: Group I: worldwide demographics of obesity. Circulation 2004;110(18):e463-470.
4. Flegal K, Carroll M, Kuczmarski R, Johnson C: Overweight and obesity in the United States: Prevalence and trends, 1960-1994. Int J Obes Relat Metab Disord 1998;22:39-47.
5. Birmingham CL, Muller JL, Palepu A, et al: The cost of obesity in Canada. CMAJ 1999;160:483-488.
6. Freedman DS, Khan LK, Serdula MK, et al: Trends and correlates of class 3 obesity in the United states from 1990 through 2000. JAMA 2002;288:1758-1761.
7. Fontaine KR, Redden DT, Wang C, et al: Years of life lost due to obesity. JAMA 2003;289:187-193.
8. Peeters A, Barendregt JJ, Willekens F, et al: Obesity in adulthood and its consequences for life expectancy: A life-table analysis. Ann Intern Med 2003;138:24-32.
9. Calle EE, Rodriguez C, Walker-Thurmond K, Thun MJ: Overweight, obesity, and mortality from cancer in a prospectively studied cohort of U.S. adults. N Engl J Med 2003;348:1625-1638.
10. Resta O, Foschino-Barbaro MP, Legari G, et al: Sleep-related breathing disorders, loud snoring and excessive daytime sleepiness in obese subjects. Int J Obes Relat Metab Disord 2001;25:669-675.
11. Coughlin S, Calverley P, Wilding J: Sleep disordered breathing: A new component of syndrome x? Obes Rev 2001;2:267-274.
12. Lakka H-M, Laaksonen DE, Laaka TA, et al: The metabolic syndrome and total and cardiovascular disease mortality in middle aged males. JAMA 2002;288:2709-2716.
13. Ford ES: Prevalence of the metabolic syndrome in US populations. Endocrinol Metab Clin North Am 2004;33:333-350.
14. Exar EN, Collop NA: The upper airway resistance syndrome. Chest 1999;115:1127-1139.
15. Gould G, Whyte KF, Rhind GB, et al: The sleep hypopnea syndrome. Am Rev Respir Dis 1988;137:895-898.
16. Dancey DR, Hanly PJ, Soong C, et al: Gender differences in sleep apnea: The role of neck circumference. Chest 2003;123:1544-1550.
17. Shneerson J, Wright NJ: Lifestyle modification for obstructive sleep apnoea. Cochrane Database Syst Rev 2001;(1):CD002875.
17a. Buchwald H, Avidor Y, Braunwald E, et al: Bariatric surgery:A systematic review and meta-analysis. JAMA 2004;292:1724-1737.

18. Burwell CS, Robin ED, Whaley RD, et al: Extreme obesity associated with alveolar hypoventilation: A pickwickian syndrome. Am J Med 1956;21:811-818.

19. Bandyopadhyay T: Obesity-hypoventilation syndrome: The name game continues. Chest 2004;125:352.

20. Kessler R, Chaouat A, Weitzenblum E, et al: Pulmonary hypertension in the obstructive sleep apnea syndrome: Prevalence, causes and therapeutic consequences. Eur Respir J 1996;9:787-794.

21. Laaban JP, Orvoen-Frija E, Cassuto D, et al: Mechanisms of diurnal hypercapnia in sleep apnea syndromes associated with morbid obesity. Presse Med 1996;25:12-16.

21a. American Academy of Sleep Medicine. International Classification of Sleep Disorders: Diagnostic and Coding Manual, 2nd ed. Westchester, IL: American Academy of Sleep Medicine, 2005.

22. Berg G, Delaive K, Manfreda J, et al: The use of health-care resources in obesity-hypoventilation syndrome. Chest 2001;120:377-383.

23. MacGregor MI, Block AJ, Ball WC: Serious complications and sudden death in the Pickwickian syndrome. Hopkins Med J 1970;126:279-295.

24. Miller A, Granada M: In-hospital mortality in the pickwickian syndrome. Am J Med 1974;56:144-150.

25. Berger KI, Ayappa I, Chatr-Amontri B, et al: Obesity hypoventilation syndrome as a spectrum of respiratory disturbances during sleep. Chest 2001;120:1231-1238.

26. Zwillich CW, Sutton FO, Pierson DJ, et al: Decreased hypoxic ventilatory drive in the obesity-hypoventilation syndrome. Am J Med 1975;59:343-347.

27. Brzecka A, Zukowska H, Werynska B: Chronic alveolar hypoventilation in obstructive sleep apnea syndrome. Pol Merkuriusz Lek 1996;1:8-10.

28. Lourenco RV: Diaphragm activity in obesity. J Clin Invest 1969;48:1609-1614.

29. Ahmed Q, Chung-Park M, Tomashefski JF Jr: Cardiopulmonary pathology in patients with sleep apnea/obesity hypoventilation syndrome. Hum Pathol 1997;28:264-269.

30. Phipps PR, Starritt E, Caterson I, Grunstein RR: Association of serum leptin with hypoventilation in human obesity. Thorax 2002;57:75-76.

31. American Academy of Sleep Medicine: Sleep-related breathing disorders in adults: Recommendations for syndrome definition and measurement techniques in clinical research. Sleep 1999;22:667-689.

32. Resta O, Guido P, Picca V, et al: Prescription of nCPAP and nBIPAP in obstructive sleep apnoea syndrome: Italian experience in 105 subjects—A prospective two centre study. Respir Med 1998;92:820-827.

33. Lyons HH, Huang CT: Therapeutic use of progesterone in alveolar hypoventilation associated with obesity. Am J Med 1968;44:881-888.

34. Hudgel DW, Thanakitcharu S: Pharmacologic treatment of sleep-disordered breathing. Am J Respir Crit Care Med 1998;158:691-699.

35. Saaresranta T, Polo-Kantola P, Irjala K, et al: Respiratory insufficiency in postmenopausal women: Sustained improvement with short-term medroxyprogesterone acetate. Chest 1999;115:1581-1587.

36. Simonds AK: Scoliosis and kyphoscoliosis. In Albert R, Spiro S, Jett J (eds): Comprehensive Respiratory Medicine. London, Mosby, 2001, 71.1-71.4.

37. Bergofsky EH, Turinto GM, Fishman AP: Cardiorespiratory failure in kyphoscoliosis. Medicine (Baltimore) 1959;38:263.

38. Guilleminault C, Kurland G, Winkle R, et al: Severe kyphoscoliosis, breathing, and sleep: The "Quasimodo" syndrome during sleep. Chest 1981;79:6.

39. Mezon BL, West P, Israels J, et al: Sleep breathing abnormalities in kyphoscoliosis. Am Rev Respir Dis 1980;122:617.

40. Simonds AK, Parker RA, Branthwaite MA: Effects of protriptyline on sleep-related disturbances of breathing in restrictive chest wall disease. Thorax 1986;41:586-590.

41. Kafer ER: Respiratory function in paralytic scoliosis. Am Rev Respir Dis 1974;110:450.

42. Sawicka EH, Branthwaite MA: Respiration during sleep in kyphoscoliosis. Thorax 1987;42:801-808.

43. Midgren B, Hansson L: Changes in transcutaneous PCO2 with sleep in normal subjects and in patients with chronic respiratory diseases. Eur J Respir Dis 1987;71:388-394.

44. Midgren B: Oxygen desaturation during sleep as a function of the underlying respiratory disease. Am Rev Respir Dis 1990;141:43-46.

45. Hoeppner VH, Cockcroft DW, Dosman JA, et al: Night-time ventilation improves respiratory failure in secondary kyphoscoliosis. Am Rev Respir Dis 1984;129:240.

46. Levine S, Henson D, Levy S: Respiratory muscle rest therapy. Clin Chest Med 1988;9:297-309.

47. Bruderman I, Stein M: Physiologic evaluation and treatment of kyphoscoliotic patients. Ann Intern Med 1961;55:94.

48. Fuschillo S, De Felice A, Gaudiosi C, et al: Nocturnal mechanical ventilation improves exercise capacity in kyphoscoliotic patients with respiratory impairment. Monaldi Arch Chest Dis 2003;59:281-286.

49. Hill NS, Eveloff SE, Carlisle CC, et al: Efficacy of nocturnal nasal ventilation in patients with restrictive thoracic disease. Am Rev Respir Dis 1992;145:365-371.

50. Masa JF: Noninvasive positive pressure ventilation and not oxygen may prevent overt ventilatory failure in patients with chest wall disease. Chest 1997;112:207-213.

50a. Khalil N, O'Connor R: Idiopathic pulmonary fibrosis: Current understanding of the pathogenesis and the status of treatment. CMAJ 2004;17:153-160.

51. Warren CPW: Lung restriction. In Kryger M (ed): Introduction to Respiratory Medicine. New York, Churchill Livingstone, 1990, pp 45-73.

51a. Clark M, Cooper B, Singh S, et al: A survey of nocturnal hypoxaemia and health related quality of life in patients with cryptogenic fibrosing alveolitis. Thorax 2001;56:482-486.

52. Lourenco RV, Turino GM, Davidson LA, et al: The regulation of ventilation in diffuse pulmonary fibrosis. Am J Med 1965;38:199-216.

53. Bye PT, Issa F, Berthon-Jones M, et al: Studies of oxygenation during sleep in patients with interstitial lung disease. Am Rev Respir Dis 1984;129:27-32.

54. Perez-Padilla R, West P, Lertzman M, et al: Breathing during sleep in patients with interstitial lung disease. Am Rev Respir Dis 1985;132:224-229.

55. Tatsumi K, Kimuar H, Kunitomo F, et al: Arterial oxygen desaturation during sleep in interstitial pulmonary disease: Correlation with chemical control of breathing during wakefulness. Chest 1989;95:962-967.

56. Midgren B, Hansson L, Eriksson L, et al: Oxygen desaturation during sleep and exercise in patients with interstitial lung disease. Thorax 1987;42:353-356.

57. Vazquez JC, Perez-Padilla R: Effect of oxygen on sleep and breathing in patients with interstitial lung disease at moderate altitude. Respiration 2001;68:584-589.

58. Shea SA, Winning AJ, McKenzie E, et al: Does the abnormal pattern of breathing in patients with interstitial lung disease persist in deep, non-rapid eye movement sleep? Am Rev Respir Dis 1989;139:653-658.

59. Offers E, Herbort C, Dumke K, et al: Complicated course of rheumatoid arthritis with pulmonary involvement, myocardial fibrosis and sleep apnea syndrome. Pneumologie 1996;50:906-911.

60. Turner GA, Lower EE, Corser BC, et al: Sleep apnea in sarcoidosis. Sarcoidosis Vasc Diffuse Lung Dis 1997;14:61-64.

61. Crockett AJ, Cranston JM, Antic N: Domiciliary oxygen for interstitial lung disease. Cochrane Database Syst Rev 2001;(3):CD002883.

62. Nocturnal Oxygen Therapy Trial Group: Continuous or nocturnal oxygen therapy in hypoxemic chronic obstructive lung disease. Ann Intern Med 1980;93:391-398.

95

Noninvasive Ventilation for Chronic Respiratory Failure

Dominique Robert

Patrick Leger

ABSTRACT

Early experience with long-term mechanical ventilation using tracheostomy or negative-pressure ventilation in the home revealed that even those patients with essentially no ventilatory function could be continuously supported, and individuals who retained partial ventilatory function could do well with intermittent (e.g., during sleep) ventilatory assistance. Since it was recognized that noninvasive ventilation with a nasal mask often obviates or postpones the need for a tracheostomy, this alternative has become available for an increasing number of patients, who now benefit from long-term ventilation.

Patients with all categories of chronic respiratory diseases resulting in alveolar hypoventilation may benefit from chronic, noninvasive ventilatory assistance, but individuals with neuromuscular or chest wall disorders exhibit the best results and the longest extension of life, although clear evidence is still lacking in patients with chronic obstructive pulmonary disease. Careful choice and adjustment of masks and ventilator settings are key elements of clinical success. Both volume- and pressure-preset modes provide good results, but pressure preset modes, which provide better leak compensation, are better suited for noninvasive ventilation. For patients such as those with advanced neuromuscular disorders, who need diurnal as well as nocturnal ventilatory assistance, noninvasive ventilation can be applied with a mouthpiece interface during wakefulness. However, when the need for ventilatory assistance is long term and quite continuous, tracheostomy may still be the best choice for ventilation, despite its invasiveness.

The first patients to receive long-term mechanical ventilatory assistance were those with sequelae of poliomyelitis or Duchenne's muscular dystrophy (DMD). Either noninvasive ventilation (negative-pressure body ventilators or positive pressure via a mouthpiece, or both) or invasive ventilation (via tracheotomy) was employed.[1-6] Early experience revealed that even those patients with essentially no ventilatory function could be continuously supported, and individuals who retained partial ventilatory function could do well with intermittent ventilatory assistance (e.g., during sleep).[3,4,7] It is now recognized that continuous positive airway pressure and intermittent positive-pressure ventilation can be comfortably and noninvasively delivered through a nasal mask.[6,8-10] In light of its successful application, the use of noninvasive positive-pressure ventilation (NPPV) for long-term mechanical ventilatory assistance has increased substantially, both in patients with restrictive disorders due to neuromuscular or chest wall disorders and, to a somewhat lesser degree, in patients with lung parenchymal disorders such as chronic obstructive pulmonary disease (COPD). This chapter will address the treatment of patients, other than those with obstructive sleep apnea, who require NPPV during sleep to achieve physiologic and clinical improvement while asleep as well as during wakefulness. This chapter will also contrast treatment with NPPV and treatment with negative-pressure modalities. The use of positive airway pressure to treat patients with obstructive sleep apnea is reviewed in Chapter 89.

NOCTURNAL NASAL NONINVASIVE POSITIVE-PRESSURE VENTILATION

Diseases

The principal diseases that may be successfully addressed using NPPV therapy are kyphoscoliosis, sequelae of tuberculosis, spinal muscular atrophy, acid maltase deficit, DMD, myotonic myopathy, amyotrophic lateral sclerosis, chronic obstructive pulmonary disease, bronchiectasis, cystic fibrosis, idiopathic hypoventilation, and obesity–hypoventilation syndrome (Table 95–1). If these diseases become severe enough, all of them may cause sufficient alveolar hypoventilation to impair the quality of life or to be life-threatening. In deciding whether to initiate nocturnal NPPV therapy, the primary considerations are as follows:

1. The relative contributions of chest wall abnormalities, ventilatory muscle weakness or inefficiency, and pulmonary parenchymal pathology to hypoventilation.
2. The natural history of the disease process, so that the likelihood of evolution from nocturnal-only NPPV to diurnal ventilatory assistance can be anticipated.
3. The associated comorbidities that may dominate the prognosis.

Clinical Severity

When deciding whether to initiate nocturnal NPPV, the first step is to identify the clinical symptoms or physiologic markers of hypoventilation and to determine the severity of disease. The clinical symptoms of hypoventilation (Box 95–1) must be carefully evaluated, because even when modest, they indicate disease severity and can affect the prognosis. Hypoventilation is defined by an abnormally elevated arterial carbon dioxide tension ($PaCO_2$) and high serum bicarbonate levels with an associated reduction of arterial oxygen tension (PaO_2). Although the values above which NPPV is definitely indicated

Table 95–1. Representative Disorders for Which Benefit May Be Obtained from NPPV Therapy: Classified by Clinical Category and Pulmonary Functional Test Profile

- Extra-Pulmonary Restrictive Disorders
  ↓ VC, ↓ FEV_1, ↔ FEV_1/VC, ↓ RV, ↓ TLC*

  Chest Wall Disorders
  Kyphoscoliosis
  Sequelae of thoracoplasty for tuberculosis

  Neuromuscular Disorders
  Spinal muscular atrophy
  Acid maltase deficit
  Myotonic myopathy
  Amyotrophic lateral sclerosis

- Obstructive Lung Diseases
  ↔ or ↓ VC, ↓ FEV_1, ↓ FEV_1/VC, ↑ RV, ↑ TLC*

  Chronic obstructive pulmonary disease (COPD)
  Bronchiectasis
  Cystic fibrosis

- Abnormal Central Ventilatory Control but Normal Lung Function: Normal Pulmonary Function Tests

  Idiopathic hypoventilation
  Obesity–hypoventilation syndrome (may also be considered a form of extra-pulmonary restriction)

*Symbols indicate actual compared to theoretical values: ↓ or ↑, decrease or increase; ↔, normal.

FEV_1: forced expiratory volume in 1 second; RV, residual volume; TLC, total lung capacity; VC, vital capacity.

Table 95–2. Severity of Hypoventilation Based on Clinical Signs and Blood Gases

Severity	Clinical Signs*	Diurnal Hypoventilation†	Nocturnal Hypoventilation‡
Severe	Yes	Yes	Yes
Moderate	Yes	No	Yes
Mild	No	No	Yes
No	No	No	No

*Symptoms of chronic ventilatory failure (see Box 95–1).

†PaO_2 under 65 and $PaCO_2$ above 50 to 55 mm Hg.

‡Proven with at least an overnight SpO_2, possibly with an associated CO_2 recording (transcutaneous or end-tidal capnography).

In patients with mild or moderate underlying disease (e.g., a neuromuscular disorder in the absence of hypoventilation, or hypercapnia during wakefulness), a sleep study is required to document nocturnal hypoventilation. Nocturnal hypoventilation may occur in all sleep stages, but when it occurs exclusively in rapid eye movement (REM) sleep, a trial of NPPV is justified. Pulmonary function tests help define and quantify the ventilatory aspects of respiratory disease, but they have poor predictive values for chronic, sleep-related hypoventilation, the management of which requires expertise in sleep medicine and experience with NPPV.

Indications for Nocturnal NPPV

The decision to use NPPV reflects a balance of three issues:

- The disease process and its natural rate of progression.
- The severity at the time of the decision making.
- The patient's willingness to undertake the therapy (the willingness is mandatory).

In clinical practice, NPPV is initiated either electively or in the context of acute ventilatory failure. In the latter circumstance, the long-term use of NPPV should be reevaluated during follow-up, because the indications for NPPV may change as the clinical condition stabilizes.[11] Indications for NPPV are listed in Table 95–3. NPPV is indicated in patients with restrictive disorders (including only chest wall and neuromuscular disorders but not lung disorders such as fibrosis) in the presence of clinical symptoms attributable to either diurnal or nocturnal hypoventilation.[12-14] With increasing ventilator dependency, the daily duration of NPPV may be progressively extended from sleep time alone to throughout the 24-hour day.[15] Alternatively, a tracheostomy may be performed to facilitate ventilatory assistance.[4,16,17] On the other hand, in patients with COPD, even if symptoms are essentially the same, the evidence does not support the unequivocal utility of NPPV. Observed cohorts treated with NPPV plus supplemental oxygen (O_2) did not experience improved survival. This was confirmed in two relatively large, randomized, controlled trials, which have not shown substantial benefits.[18,19] Nevertheless, this question remains open, as other parameters (secondary to survival), such as quality of life or hospitalization days, may have improved.[18-20] Presently, we discuss NPPV as an option in patients with symptoms of hypoventilation, or hypoventilation contributing to hypoxemia and recurrence

have not been established, many clinicians consider treating a patient who has an awake $PaCO_2$ of greater than 50 to 55 mm Hg and a PaO_2 of less than 65 mm Hg. NPPV may be considered for any of the three degrees of severity presented in Table 95–2.

Chronic daytime hypoventilation indicates a very low respiratory reserve. It should be considered an unstable state with increased susceptibility to life-threatening acute ventilatory failure, which may be triggered by otherwise trivial additional factors. Sleep-related hypoventilation is invariably present, and it probably preceded diurnal hypoventilation. A primary reason for overnight polysomnography (PSG) in patients with diurnal hypoventilation is to rule out obstructive or central apnea.

Box 95–1. Clinical Features of Alveolar Hypoventilation

- Shortness of breath during activities of daily living in the absence of paralysis
- Orthopnea in patients with disordered diaphragmatic dysfunction
- Poor sleep quality: insomnia, nightmares, frequent arousals
- Nocturnal or early morning headaches
- Daytime fatigue and sleepiness, loss of energy
- Decrease in intellectual performance
- Loss of appetite and weight loss
- Appearance of recurrent complications: respiratory infections
- Cor pulmonale

Table 95–3.   Typical Indications for Nocturnal NPPV According to Disease Process and Severity

Disease	Clinical Signs* + Diurnal Hypoventilation†	Clinical Signs + Nocturnal Hypoventilation‡	Nocturnal Hypoventilation Only	Neither Clinical Signs nor Hypoventilation	Maintenance on Nocturnal NPPV, if Indicated (yr)
Scoliosis	Yes	Yes	Perhaps	No	>10-20
Tuberculosis	Yes	Yes	No	No	10
Neuromuscular (slow)	Yes	Yes	No	No	10-15
Neuromuscular (intermediate)	Yes	Yes	No	No	5
Neuromuscular (severe)	Yes	Yes	No	No	0-5
Chronic obstructive pulmonary disease	Perhaps	No	No	No	1-5
Bronchiectasis, cystic fibrosis	Yes	Perhaps	No	No	1-5
Obesity–hypoventilation	Yes	Yes	Perhaps	No	>10-20

*Symptoms of chronic ventilatory failure (see Box 95–1).

†Pao_2 under 65 and $Paco_2$ above 50 to 55 mm Hg.

‡Proven by at least overnight Spo_2, possibly with an associated CO_2 recording (transcutaneous or end-tidal capnography).

of acute/subacute ventilatory failure, provided that long-term oxygen therapy has already been optimally adjusted.

In cases of isolated sleep hypoventilation (i.e., in the absence of clinical symptoms and diurnal hypercapnia), NPPV may be indicated only in diseases known to rapidly worsen (typically, amyotrophic lateral sclerosis). Otherwise, reinforced follow-up is recommended to avoid missing the appearance of clinical symptoms.

The data are limited regarding use of NPPV as prophylaxis against acute ventilatory failure or to increase survival in patients who do not have chronic ventilatory failure. However, one study, although frequently criticized on methodologic grounds, reported that there was no benefit of such use in patients with muscular dystrophy.[21,22]

Patients Needing Continuous Assistance with NPPV

With time, many patients, particularly those with progressive neuromuscular disease, require ventilatory assistance during wakefulness as well as during sleep. At this point, the clinician must reconsider the suitability of NPPV. It is evident that an interface such as a nasal mask, which functions well during sleep, is generally inappropriate during wakefulness. Thus, when diurnal *and* nocturnal NPPV ventilation are needed, the interface may vary with the time of day—for example, a nasal interface can be used at night and a mouthpiece during the day (Fig. 95–1). Such application has been reported by different teams in stable neuromuscular patients, such as those with sequelae of poliomyelitis, high-level spinal cord injury, or DMD.[5,15,23] Nevertheless, some clinicians prefer creation of a tracheostomy when 24-hour or nearly 24-hour ventilatory assistance is required, often because it ensures access to the airway and facilitates secretion removal.[4,12,24] Continuation of NPPV assumes that the medical team, patient, family, and caregivers have a good understanding of assisted cough and secretion removal techniques. However, this clinical issue may be problematic under the best of circumstances when providing NPPV. It is difficult to determine whether and beyond what time a patient is better or more safely ventilated by tracheostomy or NPPV. In our experience, patients with DMD

who were using NPPV for 16 to 20 hours a day and subsequently convert to ventilatory assistance via a tracheostomy demonstrate weight gain and psychological improvement. This may be because during the daytime, these patients now consistently receive ventilatory assistance via the tracheostomy, releasing them from the obligation to repeatedly access the mouthpiece for few assisted breaths.

The most difficult situations involve patients with motor neuron disease, which usually devastates all muscle function within a few years of diagnosis. NPPV or tracheostomy may prolong life despite further muscle loss, with the result that 50% of the patients achieve a locked-in state or a state of minimal communication.[17,25-27] This debate will probably continue, and ultimately the decision to convert to tracheostomy

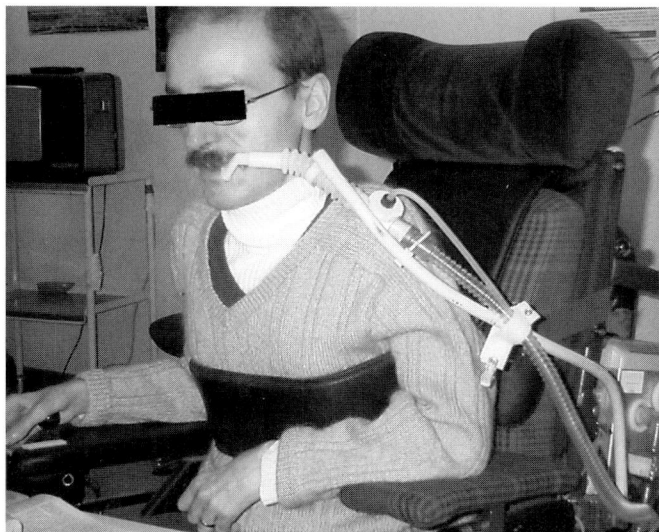

Figure 95–1. This patient requiring continuous ventilatory assistance is using only noninvasive ventilation. He uses a nasal mask during sleep and a mouthpiece during the day. The mouthpiece is positioned close to his mouth. He alternates between receiving insufflations from the ventilator (on the back of the wheelchair) and breathing spontaneously.

is highly dependent on the philosophy and capabilities of the clinical team, as well as on the preferences of the patient and the family. It is essential that discussion of such issues be started early in the patient's clinical course, well before a decision becomes imminently imperative, and that an expert team in the field of long-term mechanical ventilatory assistance be involved.

Contraindications

The only major contraindications to NPPV are in those patients with upper airway dysfunction who are prone to swallowing difficulties and aspiration (particularly frequent in patients with amyotrophic lateral sclerosis), or in patients with neurologic disorders that render them insufficiently cooperative. In patients with a chronically obstructed airway, the inability to clear secretions despite assisted cough techniques may also be a contraindication to NPPV.

Positive versus Negative Pressure for Noninvasive Ventilation

Negative-pressure ventilators function by alternatively applying subatmospheric (negative) and atmospheric (zero) pressures around the thorax and the abdomen. The result is negative intrathoracic pressure that simulates spontaneous inspiration, with resultant airflow into the airway and lungs. Three categories of negative-pressure ventilators are available.[28] With the typical iron lung, the entire body (except the head) is exposed to negative pressure. Both the chest cuirass (a rigid shell) and wraptype systems (a nylon poncho surrounding a semicylindrical, tentlike support over the chest) are enclosures that allow application of negative pressure to the thorax only. Efficacy in generating tidal volume is related to the body surface area that is exposed to negative pressure, and it is therefore greater with the iron lung than with the cuirass or the poncho type of negative-pressure ventilators.

Negative-pressure ventilation was successfully and predominantly used for long-term mechanical ventilatory assistance until the mid 1980s.[3,5,7,15] Currently, negative pressure is applied in a limited number of cases, primarily in patients with neuromuscular diseases. Since the late 1980s, reported applications of negative-pressure ventilatory assistance were limited to short-term or physiologic studies and to one long-term study of patients with chest wall diseases.[22,29-32] There is presently little interest in long-term mechanical ventilatory assistance using negative-pressure devices, probably because their efficacy is lower than that of NPPV in providing ventilatory support to patients with altered pulmonary or chest wall mechanics and to those who have comorbid obstructive sleep apnea–hypopnea (OSAH). In addition, negative-pressure ventilation may precipitate OSAH.[33,34] From a patient-use perspective, negative-pressure modalities are cumbersome and relatively impractical. In this regard, the literature suggests that, particularly in patients with non-neuromuscular diseases, long-term compliance with negative-pressure ventilation is poor because of discomfort.[22,31]

TECHNICAL CONSIDERATIONS

Methods of NPPV

Interfaces

The need to select an appropriate and properly fitted interface cannot be overemphasized. Its impact on the quality of ventilation, sleep, patient comfort, tolerance, and compliance with therapy is significant. A variety of interfaces are used,[35] and Table 95–4 summarizes their advantages, disadvantages, and indications.

Table 95–4. Interfaces: Advantages, Disadvantages, and Indications

Interface	Advantages	Disadvantages	Indications
Nasal mask	Physiologic Natural humidification Can speak and expectorate	Damage to nasal bridge Mouth leaks	First interface to use
Commercially made	Large choice Easy to size	—	First choice
Custom-made	Large contact area with face limits skin damage	Time consuming Risk of nares compression in case of an overtightened internal space of the mask	Second choice More indicated for volume- than pressure-preset ventilation
Mouthpiece (commercially available lip seal or customized)	Better control of leaks	Cannot expectorate or talk Aerophagia Initial hypersalivation Dental pain Orthodontic problem Nasal leaks No physiologic humidification	Nasal obstruction Massive oral air leaks Intermittent daytime ventilation
Oronasal mask (commercially available or customized)	Control of oral air leaks	Less choice available for long-term use Difficult to size Claustrophobia Dead space Facial skin necrosis	Nocturnal use Massive air leaks

Nasal Interfaces

Many nasal interfaces are commercially available, and these are frequently the first option offered to the patient. Some suggestions for their use include the following:

1. Follow the manufacturer's suggestions for proper sizing.
2. Use the smallest mask size that encompasses the nose without pinching the nares.
3. Use forehead supports.
4. To avoid air leaks, avoid overtightening the head straps; maintain a very low tolerance for air leaks.
5. Check the skin regularly and intervene if signs of a pressure sore develop by using mask or skin barriers, or alternate different types of interfaces (e.g., masks versus prongs), or both.

Custom-made nasal masks are an option for patients who present unusual challenges, although some teams use them routinely.[12,36] Usually, such masks are directly molded on the face with formable material, such as silicone paste or thermoplastic, that will not lose its shape. Creating this mask requires specific skill and regular practice. When tidal volume preset modes of ventilation are used, custom nasal interfaces have been found to limit leaks and dead space more effectively than commercially available nasal masks.[37]

Nasal pillows or prongs can help when a nasal bridge sore develops, or when a nasal mask is considered too obtrusive. Some patients with limited arm movement have also found these interfaces to be easier to put on and remove.

Oronasal (Full-Face) Masks

When mouth leaks are significant and prevent adequate ventilatory support, a full-face or oronasal mask may be indicated. Oronasal mask ventilation is used extensively during acute respiratory failure[38]: some clinicians estimate that as many as 30% to 40% of their patients receiving chronic ventilatory assistance use this type of interface.[39,40] As with nasal masks, proper sizing minimizes leaks and increases tolerance. Oronasal masks can add significant dead space, and ventilator settings need to be adjusted accordingly.[41] Oronasal interfaces should incorporate a safety valve to permit entrainment of fresh air in case of ventilator failure. When employing an oronasal interface, the clinician must also consider the risk associated with vomiting and aspiration in the mask. Patients should be counseled regarding this risk and advised to contact their physician should circumstances predispose to such events.

Oral Interfaces during Sleep

Some clinicians have demonstrated success using an oral interface (e.g., a mouthpiece) to apply noninvasive ventilation in patients with postpoliomyelitis.[6] The oral interface may be either a commercial model or one that is custom-made. The main reasons to use it are to avoid major mouth leaks during nasal ventilation and to achieve ventilation when the patient has nasal obstruction. The major drawbacks include swallowing difficulties and inability to speak. With the development of better full-face masks, nocturnal mouthpiece ventilation is rarely used by most teams.

Daytime Use of an Oral Interface

The primary indication for an oral interface is a need for daytime ventilation. The daytime oral interface is an excellent adjunct to nocturnal ventilation in patients who are unable to maintain acceptable diurnal arterial blood gases on nocturnal ventilation alone. Especially for patients with neuromuscular problems, the mouthpiece can be positioned close to the mouth, where it may be intermittently captured to take a few assisted breaths from the ventilator and then released. Thus, the patient needing ventilatory assistance night and day may use a combination of interfaces.

Ventilator and Settings

Ventilators use one of two basic methods to deliver, assist, or augment tidal volume: volume-preset and pressure-preset. With volume-preset, the ventilator always delivers the tidal volume, which is set by the clinician, regardless of the patient's pulmonary system mechanics (compliance, resistance, and active inspiration). However, leaks in the system (including, e.g., at the skin–mask interface, or mouth leaks when using a nasal interface) reduce the volume received by the patient.

In contrast, with pressure-preset, changes in pulmonary mechanics directly influence the flow and the delivered tidal volume; within limits, depending on the type of ventilator, there is some compensation for leaks. The beginning and end of inspiration are either initiated by the ventilator or occur in response to the patient's effort to breathe.

Three ventilator modes are used:

- *Control mode:* The ventilator starts and ends inspiration specifically and uniquely, according to the settings prescribed by the clinician.
- *Assist–control mode:* The delivery of inspiratory flow/volume is initiated either by the patient's effort or according to programmed settings prescribed by the clinician (e.g., if the patient does not initiate a breath within a specified time interval).
- *Assist or spontaneous mode:* The patient's effort starts and ends the inspiration.

Assist mode is possible only with pressure-preset. Modern home ventilators may deliver all three modes of ventilation.[42]

Besides the classic circuitry including two valves (on the inspiratory and expiratory limbs of the ventilator circuit), bilevel ventilators, which alternately close and open, are simpler and therefore lend themselves to home mechanical ventilation.[43] Inspiratory and expiratory pressures are alternately established in a single circuit that incorporates an intentional, calibrated leak located close to the patient or even on the mask. The theoretical drawback of such a circuit is the risk of a variable CO_2 rebreathing. The amount of rebreathing is decreased by using positive expiratory pressure (at least 2 to 4 cm H_2O).[44,45] Table 95–5 compares volume- and pressure-preset ventilators. Depending on the ventilator, the modes and refined settings usually applied in the intensive care unit are also available for home ventilation. Besides the basic options (the control, assist-control, and spontaneous modes), home mechanical ventilators may permit setting inspiratory time (fixed, minimal, or maximal), initial rate (slope) of inspiratory airflow, backup ventilation, and even closed-loop mode (volume-assured pressure support, or proportional assist ventilation). Some ventilators may analyze ventilation in an ongoing manner, keep it in an internal memory, and provide the data for further assessment. The general objective is to provide many possible settings and thus to have enough tools and

Table 95–5. Advantages and Disadvantages of Preset Ventilators for Home Ventilation

	Volume-Preset	Pressure-Preset
Advantages	Tidal volume (V_T) always delivered Internal batteries	Comfort Responsive to patient demand Positive end-expiratory pressure Leak compensation V_T variable
Disadvantages	Decrease of V_T in presence of leaks No compensation for leaks Poor response to patient demand Desynchronization	Decrease of V_T when resistance increases Failure to maintain pressure and to cycle with massive leaks Variability of forced inspiratory oxygen
First choice	For neuromuscular patients when battery is convenient	In chronic obstructive pulmonary disease In chest wall disorder or tuberculosis
Second choice	Failure of pressure-preset	Failure of volume-preset

flexibility to optimize patient–machine synchronization. Although this concept is attractive, sufficient studies have not been performed to document or refute the advantages of such complexity in the context of home ventilation.

Choice of Ventilator

Few studies have compared volume- and pressure-preset ventilators. Their short-term results show no major differences in the correction of hypoventilation in patients with neuromuscular and chest-wall–restrictive disorders or COPD.[46,47] Nevertheless, it was shown that in 10 of 28 patients with restrictive disorders who were adequately ventilated with volume-preset mode and who were then ventilated with pressure-preset mode, significant worsening occurred after 4 weeks. These 10 patients were converted back to volume-preset ventilators, and after 4 months all were improved.[48] On the other hand, in another study, patients were found to have some improvement in arterial blood gases when they switched from volume- to pressure-preset ventilation.[49] Clearly, some patients respond better than others to pressure-preset ventilation.

Many clinicians prefer the pressure-preset ventilator in assist mode, considering it to offer the better synchronization for the majority of patients. However, batteries are unavailable for bilevel ventilators, and this limits the mobility of patients with neuromuscular disorders who have hypoventilation during wakefulness. It is thus important to remain flexible, trying alternative approaches if problems occur with one type of ventilator. In a retrospective study of 211 patients with different diseases, survival and probability of continuing to use NPPV do not differ in the context of using a volume- or pressure-preset ventilator.[50]

Initiation and Settings of NPPV

The goals of NPPV include provision of patient comfort, synchrony with the ventilator, improvement of sleep, and improvement in arterial blood gases on and off ventilation. The first selection and adjustment of the ventilator settings should be done while the patient is awake, as this ensures physiologic adequacy and patient comfort for at least 1 or 2 hours. One study found that clinical observation was as efficient as the use of physiologic measurements (including esophageal pressure) for setting the ventilator parameters.[51]

Next, the clinician should judge adequacy when the patient is sleeping, during a nap and/or nocturnal use. Ideally, expiratory tidal volume, airway pressure, and arterial blood gas measurements are made. However, the difficulty and the resources required for frequent arterial blood sampling have led most clinicians to assess efficacy by monitoring oxyhemoglobin saturation (SpO_2), transcutaneous carbon dioxide tension ($PtcCO_2$), or end-tidal CO_2 tension ($PetCO_2$); rib cage and abdomen excursion; and sleep staging.[52] When resources are not available to perform these detailed recordings, it is recommended that at least the SpO_2 be recorded, and anything else that is possible. In addition, data related to patient tolerance, comfort, and changes in sleep quality and well-being should be obtained. If $PtcCO_2$ is employed as a measure of alveolar ventilation, it should be validated against $PaCO_2$ (measured in arterial blood). Reduction of awake $PaCO_2$ after several nights confirms the efficacy of NPPV. Evidence of a good tolerance and a decrease in $PaCO_2$ will confirm that the settings are adequate. If the results are not satisfactory, alterations must be made to the settings, and their effects checked again. In most cases, success is seen in a few days.

If assist pressure-preset ventilation is used, 10 cm H_2O of inspiratory pressure support is a suggested starting point. If necessary, the pressure level is progressively increased to achieve evidence of improvement. Pressure support higher than 20 cm H_2O is rarely necessary and is frequently not well tolerated. In patients with COPD, the addition of positive end-expiratory pressure (PEEP) should improve patient triggering when intrinsic PEEP exists, but no long-term study has proved its clinical usefulness.[53,54] Depending on the ventilator capabilities and on observations of the compatibility of the patient and the ventilator, more subtle settings concerning triggers, initial flow, and inspiratory time limit can be tried. A backup frequency that is set close to the spontaneous frequency of the patient during sleep is a reasonable substitute for inspiratory trigger failure.

When a volume-preset ventilator is employed, the initial settings may be established by adjusting the frequency of ventilator-delivered breaths so that it approximates the patient's spontaneous breathing frequency during sleep, an inspiratory time or total breathing cycle time of between 0.33 and 0.5, and a tidal volume of around 10 mL/kg.

Supplemental oxygen (O_2) should be added into the ventilator circuit for those patients who have lung parenchymal disease (e.g., COPD) and require oxygen while awake. In the absence of parenchymal disease, it is only after trying to optimize all technical parameters that residual desaturation may justify adding more O_2 into the ventilator circuit, provided there is maintenance of an acceptable $PaCO_2$ (or an appropriately valid surrogate) during sleep.[55]

When Should Patients Use NPPV?

Nasal ventilation is used mainly at night for physiologic and practical reasons, but it should also be encouraged during daytime naps. However, it has been shown that in the short term, awake ventilatory support provides results that are very similar to 8 consecutive hours during the night.[56]

FOLLOW-UP

Clinical follow-up should be conducted and daytime arterial blood gases checked once or twice a year. When possible, the same parameters that were measured when NPPV was initiated should be recorded while the patient is asleep and on NPPV. Whenever there are indications of unsatisfactory results (e.g., recurrence of clinical symptoms or hypoventilation indicated by arterial blood gases), inadequate NPPV must be suspected, and an objective evaluation during sleep must be undertaken. At the very least, nocturnal oximetry must be done. When NPPV is determined to be suboptimal, a change in ventilator modality or setting may be indicated. Increasing the total duration of NPPV use per day should also be considered, particularly when the underlying disease has progressed. Masks have to be checked and changed or adapted as needed.

MANAGEMENT OF COMPLICATIONS

Air Leaks during NPPV

All patients using NPPV during sleep experience leaks to some degree. The major potential adverse effects of such leaks are reduced efficiency of ventilation and sleep fragmentation.[57-60] A variety of measures have been suggested to address this problem, and their effectiveness must be confirmed during a sleep recording. They include the use of preset-pressure ventilation, prevention of neck flexion, having the patient assume a semirecumbent position, discouraging the mouth from opening and preventing the fall of the mandible by use of a chin strap or a cervical collar, and decreasing the peak inspiratory pressure. If upper airway obstruction is documented or suspected, judicious addition of PEEP, preferably during a polysomnographic recording, may be tried.

Nasal Dryness, Congestion, Rhinitis

Nasal dryness, congestion, and rhinitis are addressed in Chapter 89. In our experience, humidification during NPPV is usually not necessary, but for some patients, nasal and mouth dryness (usually related to leaks) can increase nasal airway resistance and be a source of discomfort.[61] A pass-over or heated humidifier can be used in this situation and also for patients with high sputum production (bronchiectasis, cystic fibrosis). Heat or moisture exchangers are not well suited for dealing with leaks, because the "dry" flow from the ventilator is greater than the "dampened" flow returning from the patient because of the usual air leaks.

Aerophagia

Aerophagia, or swallowing of air, is frequently reported by patients on NPPV, but it is rarely intolerable.[62] Aerophagia usually depends on the level of inspiratory pressure and is more commonly seen when using volume-preset or mouthpiece ventilation. The incidence decreases considerably if the peak inspiratory pressure is kept below 25 cm H_2O pressure.

OUTCOMES OF NOCTURNAL NPPV

Effects of NPPV during Ventilatory Assistance

During ventilatory assistance, gas exchange is improved, as reflected by improvements in overnight SpO_2 and $PtcCO_2$.[13,16,20,40,48,63-65] Nevertheless, significant episodes of transient hypoventilation may persist, and they appear to be related to mouth leaks.[57-60]

Total sleep duration increases slightly during NPPV, regardless of etiology.[16,66-71] Among five series studying patients with COPD, three showed increases and two showed decreases in sleep duration. The two series that studied patients with restrictive disorders showed increases in sleep duration. Sleep efficiency was similar, from 70% ± 9% to 73% ± 11%, in patients with COPD and restrictive disorders, respectively.[16,18,20,72] No significant changes were reported in percentage of non-REM sleep, REM sleep, or arousals in patients with any disorders.[13,58,69,70] Thus, NPPV improves nocturnal hypoventilation, but improvement in sleep *quality* is inconsistent.

Effects of NPPV on Daytime Respiratory Function during Spontaneous Breathing

The following data relate to patients who use nocturnal NPPV but are able to breathe spontaneously (e.g., without ventilatory assistance) for at least 8 hours during the day. Comparison of arterial blood gases during wakefulness before and after NPPV are summarized in Table 95–6. In contrast to improvements seen in patients with restrictive disorders, it appears that in patients with COPD, there is little or no improvement in diurnal arterial blood gases with NPPV. Comparison of maximal inspiratory pressure and vital capacity reveals some improvement in patients with restrictive disorders (Table 95–7). Five controlled, randomized trials with patients who had COPD demonstrated no treatment effect on forced expiratory volume in 1 second (FEV_1), forced vital capacity, maximal inspiratory pressure, PaO_2, or $PaCO_2$.[16,18-20,72] Only the 6-minute walking test and maximal expiratory pressure show a trend to improvement.

Three hypotheses have been proposed to explain the improvements in diurnal arterial blood gases during spontaneous breathing after initiation of NPPV during sleep in patients with restrictive disorders. These hypotheses involve improved respiratory muscle strength, resetting of the chemoreceptors, and decrease of the ventilatory load.

The first hypothesis is based on the idea that ventilatory assistance rests the respiratory muscles, thus reversing fatigue. The change of the ventilatory pattern in spontaneous breathing, characterized by lower frequency and higher tidal volume, that is observed in some patients using nocturnal

Table 95–6. Blood Gas Compositions during Spontaneous Breathing in Response to Noninvasive Mechanical Ventilation

Disease and Mode of Ventilatory Support	Patients/Studies	Arterial Blood Gases (mm Hg)			
		Pao_2		$Paco_2$	
		Baseline	Change	Baseline	Change
Chronic obstructive pulmonary disease, using noninvasive positive-pressure ventilation (NPPV)	314/16*	56 ± 16	5 ± 5	54 ± 7	-3 ± 4
Kyphoscoliosis, tuberculosis, using NPPV	543/16†	54 ± 9	10 ± 5	54 ± 5	-13 ± 10
Neuromuscular disorders, using NPPV or negative pressure ventilation	179/14‡	65 ± 7	13 ± 6	57 ± 3	-10 ± 5

*References: 12, 14, 16, 18-20, 40, 50, 68, 70, 84-90.

†References: 13, 36, 48, 50, 56, 57, 60, 66, 75, 83, 84, 88, 91-94.

‡References: 3, 14, 28, 50, 64, 95-101.

NPPV means that muscles could develop more force per breath, thus favoring this hypothesis.[48]

The second hypothesis suggests that in response to chronic hypercapnia, the respiratory centers change their set point, which perpetuates the hypoventilation, rather than trying to generate nonsustainable ventilatory muscle effort.[73-76] The third hypothesis suggests that an improvment of respiratory chest wall compliance during spontaneous breathing reduces the ventilatory load and increases the efficiency of the muscles. One study has shown transitory improvement of dynamic compliance in kyphoscoliosis after hyperinflation.[77] However, the generally modest improvement of forced vital capacity often associated with increased maximal inspiratory pressure does not favor the hypothesis of changes of respiratory mechanics.

Even if the mechanisms that explain the efficacy of nocturnal assisted ventilation are unknown, it is evident that improvement is more or less related to the normalization, or at least the improvement, of alveolar ventilation.[20] The minimal mandatory duration of assistance is unknown.[56]

In general, it is likely that in addition to its reducing the burden of breathing in patients with chest wall or neuromuscular diseases, NPPV favorably impacts ventilatory mechanics or muscle function during spontaneous breathing, despite intrinsic neuromuscular abnormality. In patients with COPD, two studies that aimed to put respiratory muscles at rest with negative-pressure ventilators have not shown improvements.[22,31] This could be explained by the relatively low impairment of respiratory muscles in such diseases.

Effects on Hospitalization

The home care system in France allows precise tabulation of the days that patients spend in hospital. Comparison between the year before and the first and second year after beginning nocturnal NPPV reveals a significant reduction in the number of days of hospitalization: 34 days versus 6 during the first year after and 5 during the second year after for patients with scoliosis, 31 days versus 10 and 9 for the sequelae of tuberculosis, and 18 versus 7 and 2 for patients with DMD. In contrast, the number of hospital days for patients with COPD decreased significantly only during the first year on NPPV (49 days versus 17 and 25).[12] This reflects the modest long-term effect of NPPV in patients with COPD. In the two controlled prospective trials on patients with COPD, hospitalizations were not significantly decreased with NPPV.[18,19] For patients with bronchiectasis, there was no statistical change in the number of hospital days after initiation of NPPV.[12,78]

Effect on Quality of Life

Besides the fact that staying at home rather than in hospital can affect the quality of life in some ways, specific measurements have been made. The Medical Outcomes Study 36-Item Short-Form Health Status Survey (SF36) quantifies numerous physical and mental domains.[79] In a cross-sectional study, performed during NPPV on a group of 78 patients with COPD and 57 patients with scoliosis, their physical components and mental components scored at 30% and 70%, respectively, of

Table 95–7. Ventilatory Responses to Noninvasive Positive-Pressure Ventilation

Disease	Vital Capacity (mL)			Maximal Inspiratory Pressure (cm H_2O)		
	Patient/ Study	Base	Change	Patient/ Study	Base	Change
Chronic obstructive pulmonary disease	35/3*	1980 ± 228	$+57 \pm 143$	52/4‡	-48 ± 2	-1 ± 11
Kyphoscoliosis, tuberculosis	178/6†	1097 ± 219	110 ± 98	112/6§	-39 ± 6	-14 ± 10

*References: 16, 20, 90.

†References: 56, 57, 91, 93, 94.

‡References: 16, 68, 87, 89.

§References: 13, 16, 48, 56, 66, 68, 87, 89, 91, 94.

Table 95–8.   Long-Term Outcomes of Patients on Noninvasive Positive-Pressure Ventilation (NPPV)

Authors	Patients (Number/ Mean Age)	NPPV Continuation (%) at 5 Years	NPPV Withdrawal*	Tracheostomy	Death
Scoliosis					
Simonds and Elliott[14]	47/49	79	1 (2%)	Tech NA[†]	7 (9%)
Leger et al.[83]	105/57	73	7 (7%)	5 (5%)	15 (14%)
Janssens et al.[50]	19/60	71	2 (10%)	0 (0%)	3 (16%)
Tuberculosis					
Simonds and Elliott[14]	20/61	94	0	Tech NA	1 (5%)
Leger et al.[83]	80/64	68	1 (1%)	11(14%)	17 (21%)
Janssens et al.[50]	23/75	40	0 (0%)	1 (4%)	11 (48%)
Poliomyelitis					
Simonds and Elliott[14]	30/51	100	0 (0%)	Tech NA	0
Janssens et al.[50]	12/67	40	0 (0%)	1 (8%)	5 (42%)
Duchenne's Disease					
Leger et al.[83]	16/21	47	0	7 (44%)	2 (13%)
Simonds et al.[82]	23/20	73	0	Tech NA	5 (22%)
Chronic Obstructive Pulmonary Disease					
Simonds and Elliott[14]	33/57	43	5 (15%)	Tech NA	6 (19%)
Leger et al.[83]	50/63	31	4 (8%)*	12 (24%)	15 (30%)
Sivasothy et al.[40]	26/66	68	0 (0%)	Tech NA	6 (23%)
Janssens et al.[50]	58/63	28	4 (7%)	0 (0%)	23 (40%)
Bronchiectasis					
Simonds and Elliott[14]	13/41	< 20	0	Tech NA	7 (54%)
Leger et al.[83]	25/55	62	0	2 (8%)	6 (24%)
Benhamou et al.[65]	14/64	29	0	Tech NA	10 (71%)

*Lung transplantations not included in the withdrawn patients.
[†]Technique not available in this study.

those in the normal population. Patients with scoliosis, according to mental component scores, do better than patients with COPD.[80] In a longitudinal study of 45 patients with thoracic or neuromuscular diseases surveyed 18 months before and then during NPPV,[81] patients with thoracic disorders experienced a significant and durable improvement, whereas patients with neuromuscular disorders had relatively little improvement. Two controlled trials on patients with COPD have demonstrated some improvement.[19,20]

Withdrawal from Therapy versus Continuation, and Survival

For patients on NPPV, outcomes can be divided into continuation (i.e., the use of NPPV continues) and noncontinuation, a broader category that includes death, tracheostomy, and withdrawal (defined as stopping NPPV for reasons other than death, tracheostomy, or lung transplantation). Among the studies of long-term NPPV use, interpretation is confounded by the absence of control groups and of correlation with age. Table 95–8 reviews several series with a 5-year follow-up.[12,14,40,50,82] Overall, continued use of therapy beyond 5 years is greater than 70% for patients with chest wall disorders and less than 70% for patients with DMD, COPD, and bronchiectasis. Differences in continuation between series involving patients with tuberculosis, poliomyelitis, DMD, and

COPD are probably related to different medical practices and patient age when starting NPPV.[50,83] On the other hand, differences in continued use in patients with bronchiectasis are related to survival and probably to age.[14,65,83] Comparison of survival between patients initially treated with NPPV and those initially treated with tracheostomy show that they are in the same range.[4] Finally, in patients with COPD, the results with NPPV are approximately the same as those obtained with long-term O_2 therapy,[18,19] except that one observational study reported better survival.[40] This result is probably related to patient selection.

CONCLUSION

Chronic ventilatory support using NPPV improves and stabilizes the clinical course of many patients with chronic ventilatory failure. The results appear to be better in patients with restrictive disorders than in COPD. Among the neuromuscular disorders, results are better in the more slowly progressive ones. In restrictive disorders, the benefit of NPPV is reflected by the improvements in survival, blood gas composition, and clinical stability. Because of its relative simplicity and its noninvasive nature, NPPV permits long-term mechanical ventilation to be an acceptable option for patients who would not have been treated if tracheostomy were the only alternative. In this way, nocturnal NPPV represents progress.

Clinical Pearl

Noninvasive positive-pressure ventilation using nasal interfaces and portable ventilators is now the treatment of choice for patients with chronic alveolar hypoventilation due to neuromuscular or chest wall diseases. Many of these patients experience improved blood gas measurements during wakefulness after initiation of ventilatory assistance during sleep. Quality of life and survival are also improved. For those patients with alveolar hypoventilation due to underlying COPD, uniform benefit from noninvasive mechanical ventilation has not been documented, and it remains to be determined which subgroups may eventually benefit from these techniques.

REFERENCES

1. Bertoye A, Garin JP, Vincent P, et al: Le retour à domicile des insuffisants respiratoires chroniques appareillés. Lyon Med 1965; 38:389-410.
2. Wiers PW, Le Coultre R, Dallinga OT, et al: Cuirass respirator treatment of chronic respiratory failure in scoliotic patients. Thorax 1977;32:221-228.
3. Curran FJ: Night ventilation by body respirators for patients in chronic respiratory failure due to late stage Duchenne muscular dystrophy. Arch Phys Med Rehabil 1981;62:270-274.
4. Robert D, Gerard M, Leger P, et al: Permanent mechanical ventilation at home via a tracheotomy in chronic respiratory insufficiency. Rev Fr Mal Respir 1983;11:923-936.
5. Splaingard ML, Frates RC Jr, Harrison GM, et al: Home positive-pressure ventilation: Twenty years' experience. Chest 1983;84:376-382.
6. Bach JR, Alba A, Mosher R, et al: Intermittent positive pressure ventilation via nasal access in the management of respiratory insufficiency. Chest 1987;92:168-170.
7. Garay SM, Turino GM, Goldring RM: Sustained reversal of chronic hypercapnia in patients with alveolar hypoventilation syndromes: Long-term maintenance with noninvasive nocturnal mechanical ventilation. Am J Med 1981;70:269-274.
8. Sullivan CE, Issa FG, Berthon-Jones M, et al: Reversal of obstructive sleep apnea by continuous positive airway pressure applied the nares. Lancet 1981;1:862-865.
9. Ellis ER, Bye PT, Bruderer JW, et al: Treatment of respiratory failure during sleep in patients with neuromuscular disease: Positive-pressure ventilation through a nose mask. Am Rev Respir Dis 1987;135:148-152.
10. Leger P, Jennequin J, Gerard M, et al: Home positive pressure ventilation via nasal mask for patients with neuromusculoskeletal disorders. Eur Respir J Suppl 1989;7:640s-644s.
11. De Miguel Diez J, De Lucas Ramos P, Perez Parra JJ, et al: Analysis of withdrawal from noninvasive mechanical ventilation in patients with obesity-hypoventilation syndrome: Medium term results. Arch Bronconeumol 2003;39:292-297.
12. Leger P, Bedicam JM, Cornette A, et al: Nasal intermittent positive pressure ventilation: Long-term follow-up in patients with severe chronic respiratory insufficiency. Chest 1994;105:100-105.
13. Masa JF, Celli BR, Riesco JA, et al: Noninvasive positive pressure ventilation and not oxygen may prevent overt ventilatory failure in patients with chest wall diseases. Chest 1997;112:207-213.
14. Simonds AK, Elliott MW: Outcome of domiciliary nasal intermittent positive pressure ventilation in restrictive and obstructive disorders. Thorax 1995;50:604-609.
15. Curran FJ, Colbert AP: Ventilator management in Duchenne muscular dystrophy and postpoliomyelitis syndrome: Twelve years' experience. Arch Phys Med Rehabil 1989;70:180-185.
16. Strumpf DA, Millman RP, Carlisle CC, et al: Nocturnal positive-pressure ventilation via nasal mask in patients with severe chronic obstructive pulmonary disease. Am Rev Respir Dis 1991;144:1234-1239.
17. Polkey MI, Lyall RA, Davidson AC, et al: Ethical and clinical issues in the use of home non-invasive mechanical ventilation for the palliation of breathlessness in motor neurone disease. Thorax 1999;54:367-371.
18. Casanova C, Celli BR, Tost L, et al: Long-term controlled trial of nocturnal nasal positive pressure ventilation in patients with severe COPD. Chest 2000;118:1582-1590.
19. Clini E, Sturani C, Rossi A, et al: The Italian multicentre study on noninvasive ventilation in chronic obstructive pulmonary disease patients. Eur Respir J 2002;20:529-538.
20. Meecham Jones DJ, Paul EA, Jones PW, et al: Nasal pressure support ventilation plus oxygen compared with oxygen therapy alone in hypercapnic COPD. Am J Respir Crit Care Med 1995;152:538-544.
21. Raphael JC, Chevret S, Chastang C, et al: Randomised trial of preventive nasal ventilation in Duchenne muscular dystrophy. French Multicentre Cooperative Group on Home Mechanical Ventilation Assistance in Duchenne de Boulogne Muscular Dystrophy. Lancet 1994;343:1600-1604.
22. Celli B, Lee H, Criner G, et al: Controlled trial of external negative pressure ventilation in patients with severe chronic airflow obstruction. Am Rev Respir Dis 1989;140:1251-1256.
23. Bach JR, Alba AS, Saporito LR: Intermittent positive pressure ventilation via the mouth as an alternative to tracheostomy for 257 ventilator users. Chest 1993;103:174-182.
24. Robert D, Willig TN, Paulus J, et al: Long-term nasal ventilation in neuromuscular disorders: Report of a consensus conference. Eur Respir J 1993;6:599-606.
25. Kleopa KA, Sherman M, Neal B, et al: Bipap improves survival and rate of pulmonary function decline in patients with ALS. J Neurol Sci 1999;164:82-88.
26. Bach JR, Baird JS, Plosky D, et al: Spinal muscular atrophy type 1: Management and outcomes. Pediatr Pulmonol 2002;34:16-22.
27. Hayashi H, Oppenheimer E: ALS patients on TPPV: Totally locked-in state, neurologic findings and clinical implications. Neurology 2003;61:135-137.
28. Hill NS: Clinical applications of body ventilators. Chest 1986;90:897-905.
29. Goldstein RS, Molotiu N, Skrastins R, et al: Assisting ventilation in respiratory failure by negative pressure ventilation and by rocking bed. Chest 1987;92:470-474.
30. Kinnear W, Petch M, Taylor G, et al: Assisted ventilation using cuirass respirators. Eur Respir J 1988;1:198-203.
31. Shapiro SH, Ernst P, Gray-Donald K, et al: Effect of negative pressure ventilation in severe chronic obstructive pulmonary disease [see comments]. Lancet 1992;340:1425-1429.
32. Jackson M, Kinnear W, King M, et al: The effects of five years of nocturnal cuirass-assisted ventilation in chest wall disease. Eur Respir J 1993;6:630-635.
33. Levy RD, Cosio MG, Gibbons L, et al: Induction of sleep apnea with negative pressure ventilation in patients with chronic obstructive lung disease. Thorax 1992;47:612-615.
34. Hill NS, Redline S, Carskadon MA, et al: Sleep-disordered breathing in patients with Duchenne muscular dystrophy using negative pressure ventilators. Chest 1992;102:1656-1662.
35. Bach JR, Sortor SM, Saporito LR: Interfaces for non-invasive intermittent positive pressure ventilatory support in North America. Eur Respir Rev 1993;3:254-259.
36. Leger P, Jennequin J, Gerard M, et al: Nocturnal mechanical ventilation in intermittent positive pressure at home by nasal route in chronic restrictive respiratory insufficiency: An effective substitute for tracheotomy [letter]. Presse Med 1988;17:874.

37. Tsuboi T: Noninvasive positive pressure ventilation in patients with COPD. Nippon Rinsho 1999;57:2074-2082.

38. Meduri GU, Conoscenti CC, Menashe P, et al: Noninvasive face mask ventilation in patients with acute respiratory failure. Chest 1989;95:865-870.

39. Criner GJ, Travaline JM, Brennan KJ, et al: Efficacy of a new full face mask for noninvasive positive pressure ventilation. Chest 1994;106:1109-1115.

40. Sivasothy P, Smith IE, Shneerson JM: Mask intermittent positive pressure ventilation in chronic hypercapnic respiratory failure due to chronic obstructive pulmonary disease. Eur Respir J 1998;11:34-40.

41. Schettino GP, Chatmongkolchart S, Hess DR, et al: Position of exhalation port and mask design affect CO_2 rebreathing during noninvasive positive pressure ventilation. Crit Care Med 2003;31:2178-2182.

42. Lofaso F, Brochard L, Hang T, et al: Home versus intensive care pressure support devices: Experimental and clinical comparison. Am J Respir Crit Care Med 1996;153:1591-1599.

43. Strumpf DA, Carlisle CC, Millman RP, et al: An evaluation of the respironics BiPAP Bi-Level CPAP device for delivery of assisted ventilation. Respiratory Care 1990;35:415-422.

44. Ferguson GT, Gilmartin M: CO_2 rebreathing during BiPAP ventilatory assistance. Am J Respir Crit Care Med 1995;151:1126-1135.

45. Lofaso F, Brochard L, Touchard D, et al: Evaluation of carbon dioxide rebreathing during pressure support ventilation with airway management system (BiPAP) devices. Chest 1995;108:772-778.

46. Meecham Jones DJ, Wedzichia JA: Comparison of pressure and volume preset nasal ventilator systems in stable chronic respiratory failure. Eur Respir J 1993;6:1060-1064.

47. Restrick LJ, Fox NC, Braid G, et al: Comparison of nasal pressure support ventilation with nasal intermittent positive pressure ventilation in patients with nocturnal hypoventilation. Eur Respir J 1993;6:364-370.

48. Schonhofer B, Sonneborn M, Haidl P, et al: Comparison of two different modes for noninvasive mechanical ventilation in chronic respiratory failure: Volume versus pressure controlled device. Eur Respir J 1997;10:184-191.

49. Smith IE, Laroche CM, Jamieson SA, et al: Kyphosis secondary to tuberculosis osteomyelitis as a cause of ventilatory failure: Clinical features, mechanisms, and management. Chest 1996;110:1105-1110.

50. Janssens JP, Derivaz S, Breitenstein E, et al: Changing patterns in long-term noninvasive ventilation: A 7-year prospective study in the Geneva Lake area. Chest 2003;123:67-79.

51. Vitacca M, Nava S, Confalonieri M, et al: The appropriate setting of noninvasive pressure support ventilation in stable COPD patients. Chest 2000;118:1286-1293.

52. Gonzalez MM, Parreira VF, Rodenstein DO, et al: Non-invasive ventilation and sleep, effects of hypocapnic hyperventilation on the response to hypoxia in normal subjects receiving intermittent positive-pressure ventilation. Sleep Med Rev 2002;6:29-44.

53. Nava S, Ambrosino N, Rubini F, et al: Effect of nasal pressure support ventilation and external PEEP on diaphragmatic activity in patients with severe stable COPD. Chest 1993;103:143-150.

54. Appendini L, Patessio A, Zanaboni S, et al: Physiologic effects of positive end expiratory pressure and mask pressure support during exacerbation of chronic obstructive pulmonary disease. Am J Respir Crit Care Med 1994;149:1069-1076.

55. Thys F, Liistro G, Dozin O, et al: Determinants of Fi,O2 with oxygen supplementation during noninvasive two-level positive pressure ventilation. Eur Respir J 2002;19:653-657.

56. Schonhofer B, Geibel M, Sonneborn M, et al: Daytime mechanical ventilation in chronic respiratory insufficiency. Eur Respir J 1997;10:2840-2846.

57. Bach JR, Robert D, Leger P, et al: Sleep fragmentation in kyphoscoliotic individuals with alveolar hypoventilation treated by NIPPV. Chest 1995;107:1552-1558.

58. Meyer TJ, Pressman MR, Benditt J, et al: Air leaking through the mouth during nocturnal nasal ventilation: Effect on sleep quality. Sleep 1997;20:561-569.

59. Teschler H, Stampa J, Ragette R, et al: Effect of mouth leak on effectiveness of nasal bilevel ventilatory assistance and sleep architecture. Eur Respir J 1999;14:1251-1257.

60. Gonzalez J, Sharshar T, Hart N, et al: Air leaks during mechanical ventilation as a cause of persistent hypercapnia in neuromuscular disorders. Intensive Care Med 2003;29:596-602.

61. Richards GN, Cistulli PA, Ungar RG, et al: Mouth leak with nasal continuous positive airway pressure increases nasal airway resistance. Am J Respir Crit Care Med 1996;154:182-186.

62. Hill NS: Complications of noninvasive ventilation. Respir Care 2000;45:480-481.

63. Elliott MW: Noninvasive ventilation in chronic ventilatory failure due to chronic obstructive pulmonary disease. Eur Respir J 2002;20:511-514.

64. Barbé F, Quera-Salva MA, de Lattre J, et al: Long-term effects of nasal intermittent positive-pressure ventilation on pulmonary function and sleep architecture in patients with neuromuscular diseases. Chest 1996;110:1179-1183.

65. Benhamou D, Muir JF, Raspaud C, et al: Long-term efficiency of home nasal mask ventilation in patients with diffuse bronchiectasis and severe chronic respiratory failure. Chest 1997;112:1259-1266.

66. Goldstein RS, De Rosie JA, Avendano MA, et al: Influence of noninvasive positive pressure ventilation on inspiratory muscles. Chest 1991;99:408-415.

67. Barbe F, Quera-Salva MA, McCann C, et al: Sleep-related respiratory disturbances in patients with Duchenne muscular dystrophy. Eur Respir J 1994;7:1403-1408.

68. Lin CC. Comparison between nocturnal nasal positive pressure ventilation combined with oxygen therapy and oxygen monotherapy in patients with severe COPD. Am j Respir Crit Care Med 1996;154:353-358.

69. Gozal D. Nocturnal ventilatory support in patients with cystic fibrosis: Comparison with supplemental oxygen. Eur Respir J 1997;10:1999-2003.

70. Krachman SL, Quaranta AJ, Berger TJ, et al: Effects of noninvasive positive pressure ventilation on gas exchange and sleep in COPD patients. Chest 1997;112:623-628.

71. Jones SE, Packham S, Hebden M, et al: Domiciliary nocturnal intermittent positive pressure ventilation in patients with respiratory failure due to severe COPD: Long-term follow up and effect on survival. Thorax 1998;53:495-498.

72. Gay PC, Hubmayr RD, Stroetz RW: Efficacy of nocturnal nasal ventilation in stable, severe chronic obstructive pulmonary disease during a 3-month controlled trial. Mayo Clin Proc 1996;71:533-542.

73. Elliott MW, Mulvey DA, Moxham J, et al: Domiciliary nocturnal nasal intermittent positive pressure ventilation in COPD: Mechanisms underlying changes in arterial blood gas tensions. Eur Respir J 1991;4:1044-1052.

74. Fernandez E, Weinert P, Meltzer E, et al: Sustained improvement in gas exchange after negative pressure ventilation for 8 hours per day on 2 successive days in chronic airflow limitation. Am Rev Respir Dis 1991;144:390-394.

75. Hill NS, Eveloff SE, Carlisle C, et al: Efficacy of nocturnal nasal ventilation in patients with restrictive thoracic disease. Am Rev Respir Dis 1992;145:365-371.

76. Annane D, Chevrolet JC, Chevret S, et al: Nocturnal mechanical ventilation for chronic hypoventilation in patients with neuromuscular and chest wall disorders. Cochrane Database Syst Rev 2000;(2):CD001941.

77. Bergowsky EH: State of the art: Respiratory failure in disorders of the thoracic cage. Am Rev Respir J 1979;119:643-669.

78. Gacouin A, Desrues B, Lena H, et al: Long-term nasal intermittent positive pressure ventilation (NIPPV) in sixteen consecutive patients with bronchiectasis: A retrospective study. Eur Respir J 1996;9:1246-1250.

79. Ware JE, Kosinski M, Gandek B, et al: The factor structure of the SF-36 Health Survey in 10 countries: Results from the IQOLA Project. International Quality of Life Assessment. J Clin Epidemiol 1998;51:1159-1165.

80. Windisch W, Freidel K, Schucher B, et al: Evaluation of health-related quality of life using the MOS 36-Item Short-Form Health Status Survey in patients receiving noninvasive positive pressure ventilation. Intensive Care Med 2003;29:615-621.

81. Domenech-Clar R, Nauffal-Manzur D, Perpina-Tordera M, et al: Home mechanical ventilation for restrictive thoracic diseases: Effects on patient quality-of-life and hospitalizations. Respir Med 2003;97:1320-1327.

82. Simonds AK, Muntoni F, Heather S, et al: Impact of nasal ventilation on survival in hypercapnic Duchenne muscular dystrophy. Thorax 1998;53:949-952.

83. Leger P, Petitjean T, Langevin B, et al: Long term effects of nocturnal nasal positive pressure ventilation at home. Paris, Arnette-Blackwell, 1995.

84. Carroll N, Branthwaite M: Control of nocturnal hypoventilation by nasal intermittent positive ventilation. Thorax 1988;43:349-353.

85. Elliott MW, Simonds AK, Carroll MP, et al: Domiciliary nocturnal nasal intermittent positive pressure ventilation in hypercapnic respiratory failure due to chronic obstructive lung disease: Effects on sleep and quality of life. Thorax 1992;47:342-348.

86. Lin MC, Huang CC, Lan RS, et al: Home mechanical ventilation: investigation of 34 cases in Taiwan. Chang Keng I Hsueh 1996;19:42-49.

87. Renston JP, DiMarco AF, Supinski GS: Respiratory muscle rest using nasal BiPAP ventilation in patients with stable severe COPD. Chest 1994;105:1053-1060.

88. Laier-Groeneveld G, Hüttemenn U, Criée CP: Nasal inspiratory positive pressure ventilation. Eur Respir Rev 1992;2:389-397.

89. Clini E, Vitacca M, Foglio K, et al: Long-term home care programmes may reduce hospital admissions in COPD with chronic hypercapnia. Eur Respir J 1996;9:1605-1610.

90. Perrin C, El Far Y, Vandenbos F, et al: Domiciliary nasal intermittent positive pressure ventilation in severe COPD: Effects on lung function and quality of life. Eur Respir J 1997;10:2835-2839.

91. Ellis ER, Grunstein RR, Chan S, et al: Noninvasive ventilatory support during sleep improves respiratory failure in kyphoscoliosis. Chest 1988;94:811-815.

92. Waldhorn RE: Nocturnal nasal intermittent positive pressure ventilation with bi-level positive airway pressure (BiPAP) in respiratory failure. Chest 1992;101:516-521.

93. Leger P, Robert D, Langevin B, et al: Indications of home mechanical ventilation in patients with chest wall deformities due to idiopathic kyphoscoliosis or sequelae of tuberculosis. Eur Respir Rev 1992;2:362-368.

94. Jackson M, Smith I, King M, et al: Long term non-invasive domiciliary assisted ventilation for respiratory failure following thoracoplasty. Thorax 1994;49:915-919.

95. Ellis ER, McCauley B, Mellis C, et al: Treatment of alveolar hypoventilation in a six-year-old girl with intermittent positive pressure ventilation through a nose mask. Am Rev Respir Dis 1987;136:188-191.

96. Kinnear W, Hockley S, Harvey J, et al: The effects of one year of nocturnal cuirass-assisted ventilation in chest wall disease. Eur Respir J 1988;1:204-208.

97. Heckmatt JZ, Loh L, Dubowitz V: Night-time nasal ventilation in neuromuscular disease. Lancet 1990;335:579-582.

98. Piper AJ, Sullivan CE: Effects of long term nocturnal nasal ventilation on spontaneous breathing during sleep in neuromuscular and chest wall disorders. Eur Respir J 1996;9:1515-1522.

99. Vianello A, Bevilacqua M, Salvador V, et al: Long-term nasal intermittent positive pressure ventilation in advanced Duchenne's muscular dystrophy. Chest 1994;105:445-448.

100. Sawicka EH, Loh L, Branthwaite MA: Domiciliary ventilatory support: An analysis of outcome. Thorax 1988;43:31-35.

101. Nugent AM, Lyons JD, Gleadhill IC, et al: Home ventilation in Northern Ireland. Ulster Med J 1996;65:47-50.

Cardiovascular Disorders **13**
Shahrokh Javaheri

96

Sleep and Cardiovascular Disease: Present and Future

Shahrokh Javaheri

ABSTRACT

Cardiovascular disorders are very common, affecting 23% of the population. They are associated with excess morbidity and mortality, and huge economic costs. One of the most significant recent developments in the field has been the recognition that sleep disorders such as sleep apnea can cause or worsen cardiovascular disease and, conversely, that cardiovascular disease can cause sleep disorders.

CARDIOVASCULAR DISEASE

Cardiovascular disorders are highly prevalent and are associated with excessive morbidity and mortality, and huge economic costs[1] (Table 96–1). Approximately 23% of the U.S. population (one in five men or women) have some form of cardiovascular disease. Hypertension alone, a disorder that has been proven to be caused by obstructive sleep apnea (see Chapter 100), affects 50 million Americans. Many of these patients may be erroneously diagnosed as having essential hypertension. Congestive heart failure and stroke, disorders frequently associated with both central and obstructive sleep apnea, are also highly prevalent, each affecting approximately 5 million Americans (see Table 96–1).

In 2001, cardiovascular disorders accounted for approximately 931,000 deaths, which is 38.5% of all deaths in the United States. In fact, since 1900, cardiovascular disease has been the number one killer every year except 1918. In 2004, the annual cost for cardiovascular diseases was estimated to be 368 billion U.S. dollars and for congestive heart failure, approximately 29 billion dollars (see Table 96–1).

Since polysomnography became a common tool and sleep apnea was recognized as a medical disorder, perhaps the most important development in this field has been the recognition of the association of sleep apnea, both obstructive and central, with cardiovascular disorders[2–7] (Fig. 96–1, Table 96–2).

Table 96–1. Prevalence, Mortality, and Economic Burden of Cardiovascular and Cerebrovascular Disorders in the United States

Population Group	Prevalence 2001	Mortality 2001	Hospital Discharge 2001	Cost (U.S. Dollars) 2004
Total	64 Million (23%)	930,000 (39% of all deaths in United States)	6 Million	368 Billion
Age 65 yr or older	25 Million (40% of 64 million)			
Women	33 Million (22.4%)	502,200 (54%)	3 Million (50%)	
Men	31 Million (21.5%)	390,600 (46%)	3 Million (50%)	
Hypertension	50 Million			55.5 Billion
Coronary heart disease	13 Million			133 Billion
Myocardial infarction	7.5 Million			
Angina	6.5 Million			
Congestive heart failure	5 Million	266,200*	1 Million	29 Billion
Stroke	4.8 Million	164,000	1 Million	54 Billion

*Total mentioned mortality.

Data from American Heart Association: Heart Disease and Stroke Statistics—2004 Update. Dallas, American Heart Association, 2004.

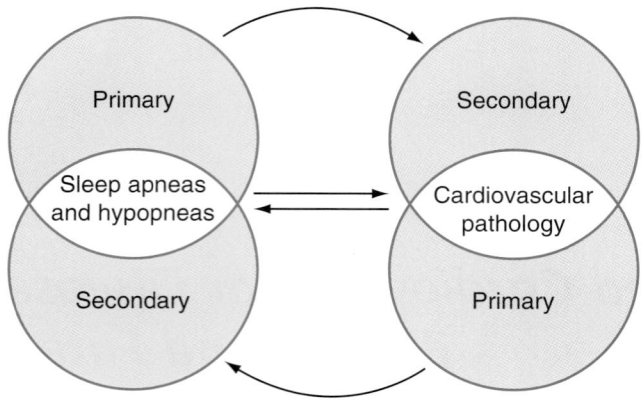

Figure 96–1. The relationship between obstructive sleep apnea (a primary sleep disorder), which secondarily could result in cardiovascular diseases, and a primary cardiovascular disease, specifically congestive heart failure, which secondarily could result in sleep-related breathing disorders.

SLEEP APNEA

There has been an explosion of basic science and physiologic studies both in experimental animals and in humans, as well as epidemiologic and clinical studies that support the bidirectional linking of sleep apnea to a variety of cardiovascular disorders[2-7] (see Fig. 96–1 and Table 96–2; see Chapters 99 through 102). Although much more research is to be done in this area, it is interesting to note that cor pulmonale was recognized as a feature of pickwickian syndrome before it became known that the underlying pathologic process of cor pulmonale is a sleep disorder.

Obstructive sleep apnea is associated with a number of biochemical and cellular abnormalities. Obstructive apnea results in neurohormonal activation, release of inflammatory mediators such as cytokines and C-reactive protein, increased expression of adhesion molecules, resulting in attachment of white blood cells to endothelial cells and their transmigration, and oxidative stress (see Chapter 99). Perhaps through increased production of reactive oxygen species,[8] a number of transcription factors are activated, increasing the expression of redox-sensitive genes and resulting in the production of vasoactive and inflammatory proteins. These reactions

Table 96–2.	Potential Cardiovascular and Cerebrovascular Complications of Obstructive Sleep Apnea

Cardiovascular diseases
  Hypertension
    Systemic
    Pulmonary (cor pulmonale)
  Heart failure
  Arrhythmias
  Coronary artery disease
Cerebrovascular diseases
  Stroke; transient ischemic attack
  Neuropsychological dysfunction
  Dementia

underlie the pathologic processes involved in endothelial dysfunction syndrome, atherosclerosis, hypertension, stroke, heart failure, and coronary artery disease (Fig. 96–2).

Because of the aforementioned abnormalities, and along with cyclic changes in blood pressure resulting in wall stress, changes in coronary and cerebral blood flow, and diminished oxygen delivery, obstructive sleep apnea could play a causative role or contribute to the development of atherosclerosis (see Fig. 96–2). In this context, treatment of obstructive sleep apnea with nasal continuous positive airway pressure (CPAP) devices results in reversal of a number of biochemical abnormalities, indicating a cause-and-effect relationship (see Chapter 99). Furthermore, preliminary studies also demonstrate that in patients with obstructive sleep apnea, treatment with CPAP results in a reduction in systemic and pulmonary hypertension[4,9,10] (see Chapter 100). I therefore hope that long-term treatment of obstructive sleep apnea will be reflected in the prevention of cardiovascular and cerebrovascular diseases.

With regard to systemic hypertension, studies show a significant drop in blood pressure with even short-term use of CPAP. The most beneficial therapeutic effects are observed in severe obstructive sleep apnea and in those patients who are compliant with CPAP[9,10] (see Chapter 100). Importantly, it has been shown that even small reductions in blood pressure over the long term significantly decrease the incidence of cerebrovascular and cardiovascular diseases.[11] In prospective studies of 420,000 patients, with a mean follow-up of 10 years, drops in diastolic blood pressure of 5, 7.5, and 10 mm Hg were respectively associated with at least 34%, 46%, and 56% less stroke and at least 21%, 29%, and 37% less coronary heart disease.[11] Therefore, in patients with obstructive sleep apnea, even a small drop in blood pressure, which could be maintained with long-term use of CPAP, is clinically meaningful. Further, treatment of obstructive sleep apnea with CPAP may afford additional protection against vascular disorders because obstructive sleep apnea may contribute to cardiovascular and cerebrovascular disease by a variety of mechanisms in addition to hypertension (see Fig. 96–2).

METABOLIC SYNDROME

With the emergence of metabolic syndrome (see Chapter 86), a precursor of incident cerebrovascular and cardiovascular diseases, a new epidemic is evolving.[12-14] This syndrome grows hand in hand with obesity, and is characterized by hypertension, hyperglycemia, insulin resistance, hyperinsulinemia, and hypertriglyceridemia. Metabolic syndrome is a proinflammatory and prothrombotic condition with increased concentrations of serum high-sensitivity C-reactive protein, fibrinogen, and von Willebrand factor, and increased platelet aggregation. Metabolic syndrome is highly prevalent, affecting 24% of all adults.[14] However, its prevalence progressively increases with age, reaching approximately 45% in those 60 years of age or older.[14] Because metabolic syndrome is a precursor of cerebrovascular and cardiovascular disorders, its early recognition and targeted therapy have been emphasized by different medical societies.[13-15] However, obstructive sleep apnea also accompanies obesity, and it shares a large number of biochemical abnormalities that are markers of metabolic syndrome (see Chapter 86). As an example, through sympathetic stimulation, obstructive sleep apnea contributes to insulin resistance and hypertension. Therefore, metabolic

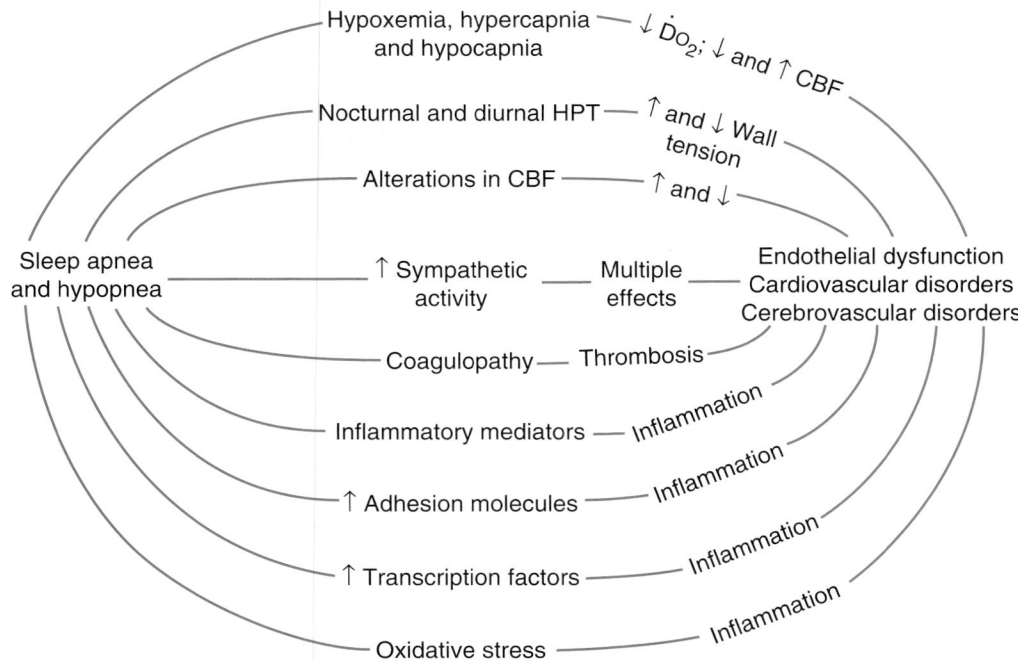

Figure 96–2. The mechanisms by which sleep apnea may result in endothelial dysfunction and cerebrovascular and cardiovascular disorders. CBF, coronary/cerebral blood flow; $\dot{D}_{O_2}$, oxygen delivery; HPT, hypertension; ↑, increase; ↓, decrease. (Adapted from Javaheri S: Heart failure and sleep apnea: Emphasis on practical therapeutic options. Clin Chest Med 2003;24:207-222.)

syndrome, obesity, and obstructive sleep apnea together are components of a vicious cycle. In concert with emphasis on early recognition of metabolic syndrome,[13-15] early recognition of obstructive sleep apnea as a companion of metabolic syndrome also needs to be emphasized, particularly because treatment of obstructive sleep apnea with CPAP has been shown to reverse some of the aforementioned abnormalities (see Chapter 86) associated with metabolic syndrome. Therefore, I also hope that longitudinal studies will be conducted to determine whether early recognition and treatment of obstructive sleep apnea as a companion of metabolic syndrome will have a preventive effect on cerebrovascular and cardiovascular diseases.

SLEEP IN HEART FAILURE

Another major development in the field is the rediscovery of central sleep apnea and Cheyne-Stokes respiration in congestive heart failure with systolic dysfunction[17] (see Chapter 102), although the discovery of this disorder dates back to John Hunter,[16,17] 37 years before John Cheyne's description in 1818.[18] There has been an explosion of physiologic and clinical research studies in this field[17] (see Chapter 102). Many studies show that both central and obstructive sleep apnea are common in patients with congestive heart failure, and preliminary studies have shown that treatment of sleep apnea improves the surrogates of mortality in heart failure.

IMPACT

For two major reasons, the recognition of the association of sleep-related breathing disorders and cardiovascular diseases is important. First, as noted previously (see Table 96–1),

cardiovascular disorders pose a great burden to patients and society. Second, recent studies show that treatment of obstructive and central sleep apnea results in improvement in the cardiovascular disorder.

I expect that future studies will demonstrate that treatment of sleep apnea increases survival and health-related quality of life of patients with various cardiovascular disorders. I expect this because therapeutic interventions to treat obstructive and central sleep apnea have resulted in improvement in the associated biochemical abnormalities (surrogates of morbidity and mortality) and the cardiovascular disease.

Because of the importance of the relation of sleep-related breathing disorders, both obstructive and central sleep apnea, with cardiovascular disorders, this edition of *Principles and Practice of Sleep Medicine* is the first to devote a series of chapters to cardiovascular diseases and sleep. In Chapters 97 and 98, a number of cardiovascular disorders related to sleep but unrelated to sleep apnea are reviewed. In Chapter 97, emphasis is placed on nocturnal myocardial ischemia and infarction, and in Chapter 98 on arrhythmias as they relate to changes in autonomic nervous system and sleep stages. The remaining chapters are devoted to obstructive and central sleep apnea and their relationship to cardiovascular diseases.

Much more research remains to be done in this field. I particularly hope that therapeutic studies will show that treatment of obstructive sleep apnea may reduce the morbidity and mortality of cardiovascular and cerebrovascular disorders. Similarly, prospective therapeutic studies will determine whether treatment of sleep apnea, both central and obstructive, will influence the natural history of left ventricular dysfunction in systolic and diastolic heart failure. I must emphasize that there have been no systematic studies in diastolic heart failure, which is the most common form of left ventricular heart failure in the older population, in whom sleep apnea is also common. And there is ample pathophysiologic evidence that the consequences of sleep apnea can cause left ventricular diastolic dysfunction.

Clinical Pearls

Cardiovascular disorders are highly prevalent and associated with excess morbidity and mortality and huge economic costs.

Sleep-related breathing disorders are common in patients with cardiovascular disorders and may either play a causative role or contribute to the progression of the cardiovascular pathologic process.

Preliminary studies of treatment of sleep apnea in heart failure have been promising.

REFERENCES

1. American Heart Association: Heart Disease and Stroke Statistics—2004 Update. Dallas, American Heart Association, 2004.
2. Peppard PE, Young T, Palta M, Skatrud J: Prospective study of the association between sleep-disordered breathing and hypertension. N Engl J Med 2000;342:1378-1384.
3. Nieto FJ, Young TB, Lind BK, et al: Association of sleep-disordered breathing, sleep apnea, and hypertension in a large community-based study. JAMA 2000;283:1829-1836.
4. Marrone O, Bonsignore MR: Pulmonary hemodynamics in obstructive sleep apnea. Sleep Med Rev 2002;6:175-193.
5. Guilleminault C, Connolly SJ, Winkle RA: Cardiac arrhythmia and conduction disturbances during sleep in 400 patients with sleep apnea syndrome. Am J Cardiol 1983;52:490-494.
6. Koehler U, Fus E, Grimm W, et al: Heart block in patients with obstructive sleep apnoea: Pathogenetic factors and effects of treatment. Eur Respir J 1998;11:434-439.
7. Javaheri S: Sleep-related breathing disorders in heart failure. In Mann DL (ed): Heart Failure: A Companion to Braunwald's Heart Disease. Philadelphia, WB Saunders, 2004, pp 471-487.
8. Lavie L: Obstructive sleep apnoea syndrome: An oxidative stress disorder. Sleep Med Rev 2003;7:35-51.
9. Becker HF, Jerrentrup A, Ploch T, et al: Effect of nasal continuous positive airway pressure treatment on blood pressure in patients with obstructive sleep apnea. Circulation 2003;107:68-73.
10. Pepperell JC, Randassingh-Dow S, Crosthwaite N, et al: Ambulatory blood pressure after therapeutic and subtherapeutic nasal continuous positive airway pressure for obstructive sleep apnoea: A randomized parallel trial. Lancet 2002;359:204-210.
11. MacMahon S, Peto R, Culter J, et al: Epidemiology: Blood pressure, stroke, and coronary artery disease: Part 1. Prolonged differences in blood pressures: Prospective observational studies corrected for the regression dilution bias. Lancet 1990;335:765-774.
12. Ninomiya JK, L'Italien G, Criqui MH, et al: Association of the metabolic syndrome with history of myocardial infarction and stroke in Third National Health and Nutrition Examination Survey. Circulation 2004;109:42-45.
13. Deedwania PC: Metabolic syndrome and vascular disease: Is nature or nurture leading to new epidemic of cardiovascular disease? Circulation 2004;109:2-4.
14. Ford ESF, Giles WH, Dietz WH: Prevalence of the metabolic syndrome among US adults: findings from the Third National Health and Nutrition Examination Survey. JAMA 2002;287:356-359.
15. Grundy SM, Hansen B, Smith SC: Clinical management of metabolic syndrome: Report of the American Heart Association/National Heart, Lung, and Blood Institute/American Diabetes Association Conference on Scientific Issues Related to Management. Circulation 2004;109:551-556.
16. Ward M: Periodic respiration: A short historical note. Ann R Coll Surg Engl 1973;52:330-334.
17. Allen R, Truk JL, Muricy R: The Case Books of John Hunter, FRS. New York, Parthenon, 1993.
18. Cheyne J: A case of apoplexy, in which the fleshy part of the heart was converted into fat. Dublin Hosp Rep Commun 1818;2:216-223.

97

Sleep-Related Cardiac Risk

Richard L. Verrier
Murray A. Mittleman

ABSTRACT

The brain, in subserving its needs for periodic reexcitation during rapid eye movement (REM) sleep and dreaming, imposes significant demands on the heart by inducing bursts in sympathetic nerve activity, which reaches levels higher than during wakefulness. In patients with cardiac disease, such neural activity may compromise coronary artery blood flow, as metabolic demand outstrips supply, and may trigger sympathetically mediated life-threatening arrhythmias in response to functional myocardial ischemia. An additional challenge is presented by non-REM sleep, when hypotension may lead to malperfusion of the heart and brain as a result of a lowered blood pressure gradient through stenosed vessels. Impairment of ventilation by sleep-related breathing disorders, including obstructive sleep apnea and central sleep apnea, which afflict millions of Americans, can generate reductions in arterial oxygen saturation and other pathophysiologic sequelae. Obstructive sleep apnea has been strongly implicated, when severe, in the etiology of hypertension, myocardial ischemia, arrhythmias, myocardial infarction, and sudden death in individuals with coexisting ischemic heart disease. Similarly, central sleep apnea has been associated with a variety of atrial and ventricular arrhythmias. Atrial fibrillation may be triggered by autonomic or respiratory disturbances during sleep in certain patient populations. Medications that cross the blood–brain barrier may alter sleep structure and provoke nightmares with severe cardiac autonomic discharge.

In healthy individuals, sleep is usually salutary and restorative. Ironically, during sleep in patients with respiratory or heart disease, the brain can precipitate breathing disorders, myocardial ischemia, arrhythmias, and even death. Our observation that 20% of myocardial infarctions (MIs) and 15% of sudden deaths occur during the period from midnight to 6:00 AM projects to an estimated 250,000 nocturnal MIs and 38,000 nocturnal sudden deaths annually in the U.S. population.[1] The latter figure is equivalent to 87% of the number of U.S. fatalities due to automobile accidents and is more than 2.5 fold the number of U.S. deaths due to human immunodeficiency virus infection. Thus, sleep is not a protected state. Furthermore, the nonuniform distribution of deaths and MIs during the night is consonant with provocation by pathophysiologic triggers. The two main factors implicated in nocturnal cardiac events are sleep state–dependent surges in autonomic activity[2] and depression of respiratory control mechanisms,[3] which affect a vulnerable cardiac substrate. Precise characterization of their interaction in precipitating nocturnal cardiac events is, however, incomplete. Although sudden death during sleep can be presumed to be painless, in many cases it is premature because it occurs in infants and adolescents and in adults with ischemic heart disease, for whom the median age is 59 years. Populations at elevated risk for nocturnal cardiorespiratory events include a number of large patient groups (Table 97–1).

An insidious component of the problem of nocturnal risk results from the fact that many people are unaware of their respiratory or cardiac distress at night and therefore take no corrective action. Thus, sleep presents unique autonomic, hemodynamic, and respiratory challenges to the diseased myocardium that cannot be monitored by daytime diagnostic tests. The importance of nocturnal monitoring of patients with cardiac disease extends beyond identifying sleep state–dependent triggers of cardiac events because nighttime myocardial ischemia, arrhythmias, autonomic activity, and respiratory disturbances carry predictive value for daytime events (Box 97–1).

In this chapter we discuss the pathophysiologic mechanisms responsible for sleep-related cardiac morbidity and mortality. For a review of mechanisms and treatment of nocturnal arrhythmias, see Chapter 98.

AUTONOMIC ACTIVITY AND CIRCULATORY FUNCTION DURING SLEEP

The generalized decrease in mean heart rate and arterial blood pressure at the onset of sleep and throughout non–rapid eye movement (NREM) sleep, which occupies 80% of sleep time, has prompted the assumption that sleep is a period of relative autonomic inactivity. NREM sleep, the initial stage, is characterized by marked stability of autonomic regulation with a high degree of parasympathetic neural tone and prominent respiratory sinus arrhythmia.[2,4] Baroreceptor gain is high and contributes to the stability of arterial blood pressure and to overall cardiovascular homeostasis.[5-8] Muscle sympathetic nerve activity is stable, falls with the transition from awake to NREM sleep, and decreases progressively with depth of sleep,[2,9,10] reaching half the awake value during stage 4.[2] Short-lasting increases in muscle sympathetic nerve activity, heart rate, and arterial blood pressure accompany the appearance of high-amplitude K complexes during stage 2.[2,9,10] Heart rate accelerations may even precede the electroencephalographic arousals of stage 2 and REM sleep.[11] During transitions from NREM to REM sleep, bursts of vagus nerve activity may result in pauses in heart rhythm and frank asystole. Transitions between REM and NREM sleep elicit posture shifts that are associated with varying degrees of autonomic activation and attendant changes in heart rate and arterial blood pressure.[12,13] These shifts in body position increase in frequency as individuals age and sleep becomes fragmented.

Table 97–1. **Patient Groups at Potentially Increased Risk for Nocturnal Cardiac Events**

Indication (U.S. Patients/Year)	Possible Mechanism
Angina, myocardial infarction, arrhythmias, ischemia, or cardiac arrest at night	The nocturnal pattern suggests a sleep state–dependent autonomic trigger or respiratory distress; 20% of myocardial infarctions (~250,000 cases/yr) and 15% of sudden deaths (~38,000 cases/yr) occur between midnight and 6:00 AM.
Unstable angina, Prinzmetal's angina	Nondemand ischemia and angina peak between midnight and 6:00 AM.
Acute MI (1.5 million)	Disturbances in sleep, respiration, and autonomic balance may be factors in nocturnal arrhythmogenesis. Nocturnal onset of MI is more frequent in older and sicker patients and carries a higher risk of congestive heart failure.
Spousal or family report of highly irregular breathing, excessive snoring, or apnea in patients with coronary disease (5–10 million patients with apnea)	Patients with hypertension or atrial or ventricular arrhythmias should be screened for the presence of sleep apnea.
Long QT syndrome	The profound cycle-length changes associated with sleep may trigger pause-dependent torsades de pointes in these patients.
Near-miss or siblings of victims of sudden infant death syndrome	Sudden infant death commonly occurs during sleep with characteristic cardiorespiratory symptoms.
Asians with warning signs of SUNDS	SUNDS is a sleep-related phenomenon in which night terrors may play a role.
Atrial fibrillation (2.5 million)	Twenty-nine percent of episodes occur between midnight and 6:00 AM. Respiratory and autonomic mechanisms are suspected.
Patients on cardiac medications (13.5 million patients with cardiovascular disease)	Beta-blockers and calcium channel blockers that cross the blood–brain barrier may increase nighttime risk because poor sleep and violent dreams may be triggered. Medications that increase the QT interval may conduce to pause-dependent torsades de pointes during the profound cycle-length changes of sleep. Because arterial blood pressure is decreased during non–rapid eye movement sleep, additional lowering by antihypertensive agents may introduce a risk of ischemia and infarction due to lowered coronary perfusion.

MI, myocardial infarction; SUNDS, sudden unexplained nocturnal death syndrome.

Autonomic nervous system activity is dramatically altered when REM sleep is initiated (Fig. 97–1). REM sleep is marked by profound muscle sympathetic nerve activation, in terms of both frequency and amplitude,[2,9,10] which attains levels significantly higher than in wakefulness.[2] Sympathetic nerve activity is concentrated in short, irregular periods that are most striking when accompanied by intense eye movements.[2] These bursts trigger intermittent increases in heart rate and arterial blood pressure to levels similar to those in wakefulness, with increased variability.[2,5,6,9-11] Significant surges and pauses in heart rate during REM sleep have been described in several species, including humans.[9-11] Cardiac efferent vagal tone and baroreceptor regulation[7] are generally suppressed during REM sleep, and breathing patterns may become highly irregular and may lead, in susceptible individuals, to oxygen desaturation. Thus, while subserving the neurochemical functions of the brain, REM sleep can disrupt cardiorespiratory homeostasis. The brain's increased excitability during REM sleep can also trigger major surges in sympathetic nerve activity to the skeletal muscular beds, accompanied by muscular twitching,[2] which interrupts the generalized skeletal atonia of REM.[12,14] The peripheral autonomic status characterized by

muscle sympathetic nerve recording is compatible with reduced neuronal activity in the brainstem and other regions of the brain[15] and reduced cerebral blood flow[16] during NREM sleep and, during REM sleep, with increased brain activity in several discrete regions to levels above waking values.[16,17]

The decline in autonomic activity during sleep is also evident in peroneal muscle sympathetic nerve activity[2,9,10] and peripheral levels of epinephrine and norepinephrine, and mirrors the generalized sleep-induced decline in heart rate and arterial blood pressure.[18,19] A nocturnal nadir in plasma catecholamines is evident at 1 hour after sleep onset.[19] Plasma cortisol is also depressed during sleep; increased levels are initiated at 5:00 AM.[20]

In the absence of readily achieved, direct measures of cardiac-bound nerve activity, analysis of heart rate variability (HRV) has emerged as a widely accepted method for measuring cardiac sympathetic versus parasympathetic neural dominance.[21] High-frequency (HF) HRV is a general indicator of cardiac parasympathetic tone and includes the effects of respiration. The low- to high-frequency ratio (LF/HF) is widely accepted as an approximation of cardiac-bound sympathetic nerve activity, as validated by studies involving beta-adrenergic

Box 97–1. Predictive Value of Nocturnal Cardiorespiratory Status

- Because parasympathetic nerve activity is elevated during sleep in healthy individuals, lack of circadian pattern of heart rate variability and baroreflex sensitivity may be readily monitored for increased risk of cardiac events.
- Nondemand nocturnal ischemic episodes may disclose a critical underlying coronary lesion, coronary vasospasm, or transient coronary artery stenosis.
- In elderly subjects, nighttime multifocal ventricular ectopic activity predicts increased mortality from cardiac causes independently of clinically evident cardiac diseases.
- Sleep apnea, which may be screened by heart rate variability analysis, conduces to hypertension, ischemia, and atrial and ventricular arrhythmias, and is a risk factor for lethal daytime cardiac events, including myocardial infarction.
- Cheyne-Stokes respiration accelerates deterioration in cardiac function in patients with heart failure; the apnea-hypopnea index predicts poor prognoses in these patients.
- Hypertensive patients with less than a 10% nocturnal decline in blood pressure are at increased risk of total and cardiovascular mortality and all cardiovascular end points, myocardial ischemia, frequent or complex ventricular arrhythmias, cerebrovascular insult, and increased organ damage, including cardiac hypertrophy.
- Nocturnal hypertension is a marker of left ventricular filling impairment.

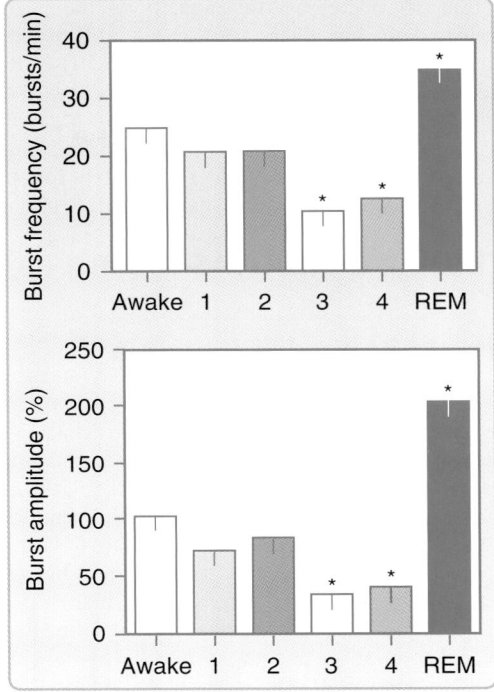

Figure 97–1. Sympathetic burst frequency and amplitude during wakefulness, non–rapid eye movement (NREM) sleep (eight subjects), and REM sleep (six subjects). Sympathetic activity was significantly lower during stages 3 and 4 (*$P < .001$). During REM sleep, sympathetic activity increased significantly ($P < .001$). Values are means ± standard error of the mean. (From Somers VK, Dyken ME, Mark AL, et al: Sympathetic nerve activity during sleep in normal subjects. N Engl J Med 1993;328:303-307. Copyright © 1993 Massachusetts Medical Society. All rights reserved.)

receptor blockers.[21] Decreased HRV, indicating a decline in parasympathetic nerve activity, is an established indicator of risk for sudden cardiac death after MI.[21] HRV analysis reveals a generalized increase in vagus nerve activity and a decrease in cardiac sympathetic nerve activity across the sleep period,[22,23] probably reflecting the dominance of total sleep time by NREM sleep. HRV studies using 5-minute intervals provide results consistent with muscle nerve recording, indicating increased HF and decreased LF (or parasympathetic nerve dominance) in NREM sleep, but decreased HF and increased LF (or predominant sympathetic nerve activity) in REM sleep and during wakefulness.[11] In healthy individuals, the increase in HRV measures of cardiac sympathetic nerve activity at onset of REM sleep is initiated before[11,23] the transition from NREM sleep as classically defined from the polysomnographic record.

The typical circadian pattern of decreased nocturnal cardiac sympathetic nerve activity as described by heart rate and HRV studies is altered in patients with coronary artery disease,[24,25] MI,[22,26,27] and diabetes,[28,29] suggesting either increased nocturnal cardiac sympathetic nerve activity or decreased parasympathetic nerve activity compared with healthy subjects. The HF component has been observed to decrease approximately 10 minutes before onset of nocturnal myocardial ischemia.[25] In unmedicated patients with a recent MI, the LF/HF ratio was significantly increased during both REM and NREM sleep, in contrast to healthy subjects, in whom this ratio during REM sleep is similar to awake levels and higher than during NREM sleep[22] (Fig. 97–2). The conclusions were

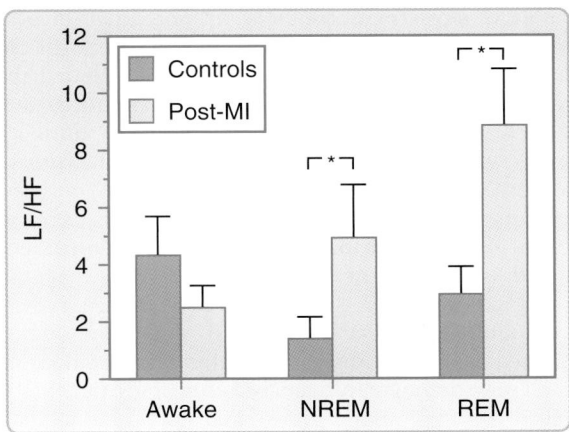

Figure 97–2. Bar graphs indicating low- to high-frequency ratio (LF/HF) of heart rate variability during the awake state (left), during non–rapid eye movement (NREM) sleep (middle), and during REM sleep (right) in healthy subjects and in post–myocardial infarction (MI) patients (*$P < .01$ when comparing control subjects vs. post-MI patients). Values are means ± standard error of mean. (From Vanoli E, Adamson PB, Ba-Lin, et al: Heart rate variability during specific sleep stages: A comparison of healthy subjects with patients after myocardial infarction. Circulation 1995;91:1918–1922.)

reached that MI decreases the capacity of the vagus nerve to be activated during sleep, resulting in unbridled cardiac sympathetic nerve activity,[22] and that loss of rise in the HF component is characteristic of patients post-MI with residual myocardial ischemia.[27]

These sleep state–dependent profiles of autonomic activity have significant potential to affect coronary function and cardiac electrical stability in patients with ischemic heart disease.

NOCTURNAL CARDIOVASCULAR EVENTS

Nocturnal Myocardial Ischemia and Angina

Accurate assessment and treatment of nocturnal angina has been a subject of concern for over two centuries. Heberden in 1768 described angina that "will often oblige [the patients] to rise up out of their bed every night for many months altogether."[30] John Hunter, the well-known 18th-century surgeon, reported chest pains that "seized him in his sleep so as to awaken him."[31] As early as 1923, MacWilliam[32] postulated that the mechanisms of nocturnal ventricular fibrillation and angina were stimulation of sympathetic nerves and increased arterial blood pressure. He described "reflex excitations, dreams, nightmares, etc., sometimes accompanied by extensive rises of arterial blood pressure (hitherto not recognized), increased heart action, changes in respiration, and various reflex effects" and noted "the suddenness of development of the functional disturbances in arterial blood pressure, heart action, etc., in the dreaming state." He documented greater stress on the circulatory system during dreaming than during wakefulness, with arterial blood pressures reaching 200 mm Hg. In the middle of the last century, the renowned cardiologists Paul Dudley White[30] and Samuel Levine[33] remarked on the frequency of MI and angina in sleep and suggested an association with dreams.

Ischemic activity is an important prognostic marker in patients with cardiac disease, and characteristics of both REM and NREM sleep may conduce to nocturnal myocardial ischemia and angina. The few studies in patients with cardiac disease that have used sleep staging have concluded that in the absence of significant depression of left ventricular function, nocturnal ischemic events occur primarily during REM sleep,[34,35] which is characterized by increased sympathetic nerve activity, metabolic demands, and heart rate surges. In patients with stable coronary artery disease, myocardial ischemia is largely attributable to bouts of sympathetically mediated surges in heart rate and resultant metabolic demands in flow-limited, stenotic coronary arteries.[4,13,25,26,35-41] Nowlin and coworkers[35] attributed nocturnal angina to heightened blood pressure after performing detailed, multisession polysomnographic analysis of four patients with advanced coronary artery disease and nocturnal angina pectoris and established that attacks of nocturnal angina occurred predominantly during REM sleep (32 of 39 recordings) and were associated with heart rate acceleration. Dream content, in patients who could describe it, included awareness of chest pain and involved strenuous physical activity or emotions of fear, anger, or frustration.

That nocturnal myocardial ischemia is generated by mechanisms in addition to sympathetic nerve activity and unsatisfied metabolic demands is indicated by the finding that nighttime ischemic events remain, although they are less frequent, in patients receiving beta-adrenergic receptor blockade therapy, the primary therapy that effectively reduces the overall incidence of and suppresses the morning peak in cardiac events by containing sympathetic nerve activity and demand-related myocardial ischemia.[37,41,42] The main factors that may contribute to non–demand-related myocardial ischemia during NREM sleep are decreased coronary perfusion pressure as the result of hypotension[4,41,43,44] and increased coronary vasomotor tone.[37,43] These influences decrease the metabolic threshold for induction of nocturnal myocardial ischemia, which has a nadir between 1:00 AM and 3:00 AM.[13,36,43,45] During these hours in patients with stable coronary disease, Benhorin and colleagues[43] observed that myocardial ischemia can be provoked at heart rates of 83 beats per minute (bpm), in contrast to 96 bpm during midday, and that its incidence was not affected by beta-adrenergic receptor blockade. Patel et al.[42] noted that nocturnal myocardial ischemia is attended by heart rate elevations of 6 bpm or less in patients with unstable angina receiving beta-adrenergic receptor blocking agents. Mancia[4] hypothesized that the hypotension of NREM sleep is a major contributor to nocturnal myocardial ischemia and MI because it "reduces the volume and velocity of blood flow, favoring the development of thrombi and embolic and ischemic phenomena before and after arousal." It has also been postulated that myocardial ischemia provoked by transient thrombus formation[46,47] is attributable to the nocturnal nadir in endogenous fibrinolytic activity,[46-48] as well as peaks in serum levels of plasminogen activator inhibitor[46-48] and tissue plasminogen activator antigen,[48] increasing blood viscosity or hypercoagulability at night, and free-radical generation.[49]

Nondemand nocturnal myocardial ischemia is prevalent in patients with more severe coronary disease,[13,41,45,50] acute coronary syndromes,[42,51] diabetes,[52] and Prinzmetal's angina,[13,48,53] patient populations with significant endothelial dysfunction. Indeed, it has been concluded that nondemand nocturnal ischemic episodes disclose a critical underlying coronary lesion, coronary vasospasm, or transient coronary artery stenosis.[42] Patel and colleagues[42] documented a nocturnal peak in ischemic events in their study of 256 hospitalized patients with the acute coronary syndromes of unstable angina and non–Q-wave MI (Fig. 97–3). Electrocardiograms were recorded within hours after patients' admission for chest pain to the coronary care unit for new-onset angina, sudden acceleration of previously stable angina, or angina within 1 month of MI. In hospital, they received optimal medical therapy aimed at containing demand-related myocardial ischemia. It is important to note, however, that the peak in out-of-hospital onset of the syndromes followed the usual circadian pattern, as reported by Cannon and coworkers[54] in the Thrombosis in Myocardial Infarction (TIMI) III study of 3318 patients. By contrast, in patients with longstanding diabetes or with documented autonomic nervous system dysfunction, there is no nocturnal decrease in myocardial ischemia or onset of acute MI.[52]

Patients with Prinzmetal's variant angina, in whom REM sleep is associated with coronary vasospasm, experience no nighttime trough in the incidence of nocturnal myocardial ischemia,[41,53] which is both demand related and non-demand related.[13,53] Masuda et al.[48] discovered that the nocturnal peak

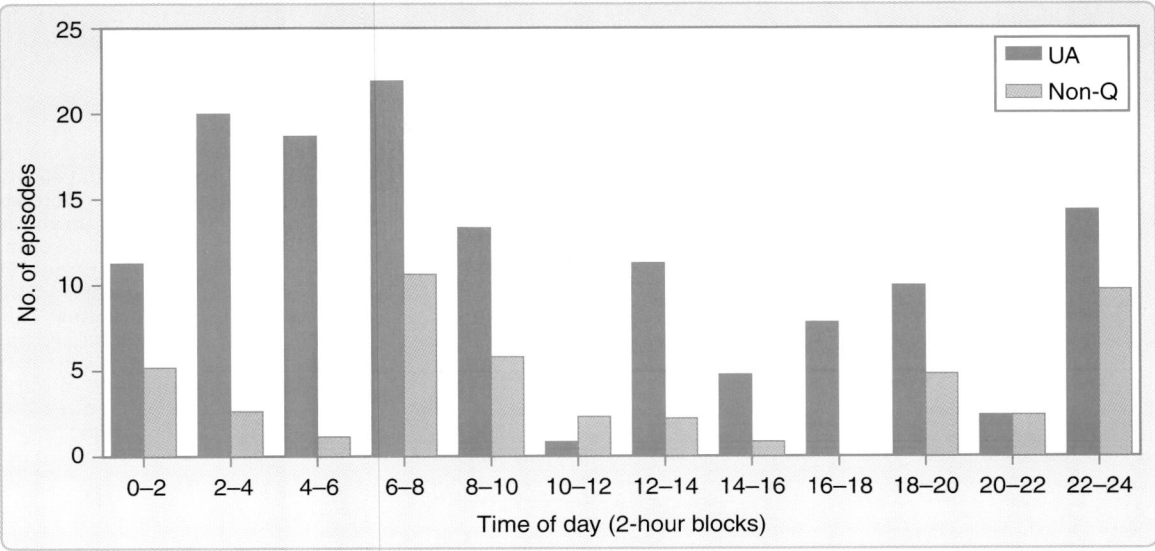

Figure 97–3. The circadian variation of ischemic activity based on 2-hr time blocks for the in-hospital study population. There is a single peak of ischemic activity at night between 10:00 PM and 8:00 AM, and no morning peak in ischemia activity is apparent. More than 64% of episodes occurred during this period (P < .001 compared with daytime). The circadian distribution of ischemic episodes in unstable angina (UA) and non–Q-wave myocardial infarction (Non-Q) is similar to the overall pattern of ischemic activity. (From Patel DJ, Knight CJ, Holdright DR, et al: Pathophysiology of transient myocardial ischemia in acute coronary syndromes: Characterization by continuous ST-segment monitoring. Circulation 1997;95:1185-1192.)

in ischemic activity in these patients coincided with a nadir in fibrinolytic activity.

Treatment of sleep apnea is capable of ameliorating angina in some patients.[55] However, impaired breathing and oxygen desaturation are not prerequisites of nocturnal ischemic episodes in patients with coronary disease. Myocardial ischemia need not be concomitant with decreased oxygen saturation,[56] and recorded episodes of myocardial ischemia[56] or oxygen desaturation[57] were not necessarily accompanied by apnea.

Demand-related ischemic episodes can be effectively contained by beta-adrenergic receptor blockade,[40,42] but antihypertensive treatment does not reduce the nocturnal incidence of non–demand-related myocardial ischemia.[58] The use of vasodilators to treat nondemand episodes due to endothelial dysfunction is the subject of debate.[40] The incidence of nocturnal ischemic activity in patients with unstable angina and non–Q-wave MI who were receiving optimal medical therapy suggests that current approaches to management do not adequately address the factors involved.[42] The lack of sleep staging and arterial blood pressure monitoring in patients with nocturnal myocardial ischemia leaves unidentified any contribution by autonomic and hemodynamic activity dictated by sleep states. Such monitoring would also disclose the prevalence of the established proischemic influences of nocturnal arousal and rising from bed.[24,59]

Post–Myocardial Infarction Patients

During the first weeks after MI, sleep is significantly disturbed,[44,60] and nocturnal oxygen desaturation, especially in patients with impaired left ventricular function, may be

generalized or episodic and directly provoke tachycardia, ventricular premature beats, and ST segment changes[60-64] (Fig. 97–4). Both the duration and number of nighttime ischemic events are increased, consonant with increased cardiac sympathetic nerve activity[26,42,65,66] or decreased parasympathetic nerve activity[22] (see Fig. 97–2), particularly in patients with residual myocardial ischemia.[27] Nocturnal levels of norepinephrine are increased and nocturnal secretion of melatonin, an endogenous hormone that suppresses sympathetic nerve activity, is impaired.[67] These symptoms become normal over time so that within the first 6 months, ventricular tachycardia during sleep is relatively rare and is characteristic of patients whose heart rates in sleep had averaged greater than 80 bpm at the time of the crisis.[62] If the nighttime heart rate remains high, averaging over 90 bpm, the risk of fatal events is increased.

The most detailed study to date of sleep in post-MI patients was performed in 1978 by Broughton and Baron,[44] who reported on the sleep and cardiovascular condition of 12 patients, aged 33 to 70 years, after severe MI, first during their stay in the intensive care unit and then in the hospital ward. They noted a "marked disturbance of nocturnal sleep patterns … characterized by high amounts of wakefulness, stage 1, and number of awakenings, and REM density and low amounts of REM sleep, shorter REM periods with prolonged REM latencies. Sleep efficiency was substantially reduced."[44] All of these sleep quality parameters improved in parallel with time after MI until on day 9 the only remaining abnormal feature was a high content of NREM sleep stages 3 and 4. REM density peaked on postinfarction nights 3 and 4 and NREM sleep on night 4. On subsequent hospital visits after discharge, the patients described terrifying dreams, suggesting

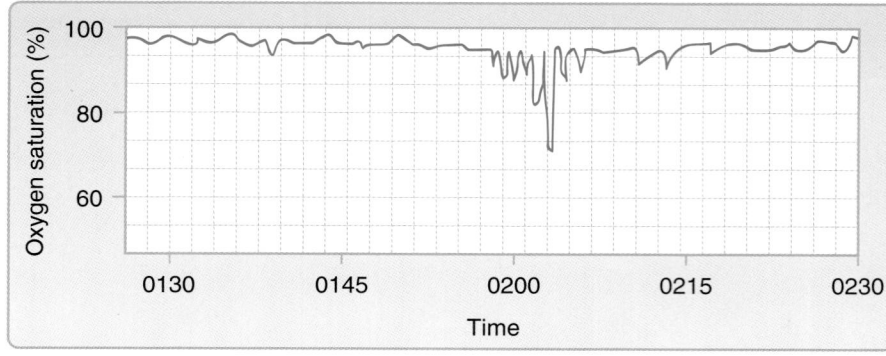

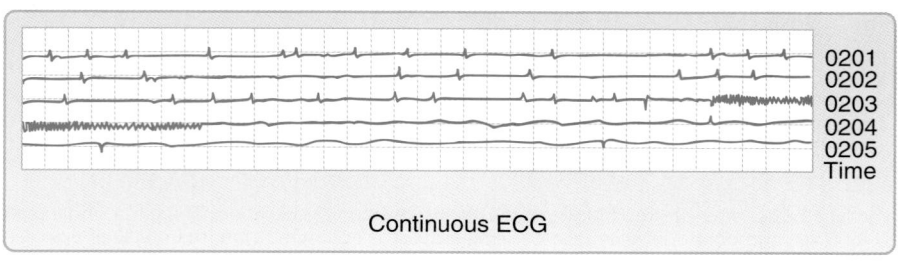

Continuous ECG

Figure 97–4. Importance of monitoring nocturnal oxygen saturation in patients who have sustained a myocardial infarction. Nonsustained ventricular tachycardia (lower panel) and hypoxemia measured by pulse oximetry (upper panel) occurred simultaneously in a patient on the third night after infarction. The patient died on the following day of cardiogenic shock. ECG, electrocardiogram. (From Galatius-Jensen S, Hansen J, Rasmussen V, et al: Nocturnal hypoxemia after myocardial infarction: Association with nocturnal myocardial ischaemia and arrhythmias. Br Heart J 1994; 72:23-30.)

that REM suppression was followed by REM rebound more than 2 weeks after the crisis. Importantly, Broughton and Baron observed that NREM sleep provoked nocturnal angina and awakening. They postulated that the hypotension associated with NREM sleep resulted in a diminution in perfusion pressure of the major coronary and collateral vessels supplying the mechanically compromised myocardium. The decreased heart rates typical of NREM sleep, however, were not observed, and heart rates were higher in NREM sleep than in wakefulness on half the nights recorded, indicating enhanced cardiac sympathetic nerve activity even in NREM sleep. In half of the cases, the electrocardiogram amplitude decreased during anginal attacks. T-wave alternans, a marker of vulnerability to lethal arrhythmias in post-MI patients,[68] appeared in the electrocardiogram of one of these patients during angina in NREM sleep.

Nocturnal Myocardial Infarction

Although only 20% of MIs occur between midnight and 6:00 AM, their nonuniform distribution implicates pathophysiologic triggers.[1] The dynamic perturbations in autonomic nervous system activity both independent of and in conjunction with apnea[69] are likely to constitute important triggers of MI at night. REM-induced surges in sympathetic nerve activity have the potential to provoke tachycardia and hypertension, alterations that carry the potential for inducing MI secondary to coronary artery plaque rupture as well as to inappropriate decreases in the myocardial oxygen supply–demand relationship or alpha-adrenergically mediated coronary vasoconstriction.[70]

Alternatively, in a starkly opposite manner, the hypotension of slow wave sleep may lead to malperfusion of the myocardium due to reduced coronary perfusion pressure through stenotic vessel segments. Several investigators[42,71-73] have attributed nocturnal MI and myocardial ischemia to the relative hypotension of NREM sleep, which "reduces the volume and velocity of blood flow, favoring the development of thrombi and embolic and ischemic phenomena before and

after arousal."[4] Mancia[4] therefore advocated avoiding drugs that enhance the hypotension of NREM sleep and prescribing antihypertensive medications only for daytime therapy. He echoed the argument of Floras,[58] who observed that antihypertensive treatment did not reduce the incidence of nocturnal MI and myocardial ischemia. Further evidence of the risk of hypotension-induced infarction has been provided by Kleiman and colleagues,[72] who reported that the incidence of subendocardial MI clustered at 2:00 AM to 4:00 AM, simultaneously with the nadir in arterial blood pressure. Other factors known to contribute to MI are operative during sleep, including increased ventricular diastolic pressures and volumes due to the fluid shifts resulting from assuming a supine posture, unfavorable alterations in the balance of fibrinolytic and thrombotic factors,[46-49] and chronic or episodic oxygen desaturation.[44,60-64] It is unknown which of these factors contributed in the case report of onset of nocturnal angina and transmural MI[74] in which myocardial ischemia–induced T-wave alternans, a marker of risk for lethal tachyarrhythmias,[68] was recorded during sleep (Fig. 97–5). Alternans, evident in the precordial leads, disappeared as the myocardial ischemia and pain resolved.

Specific patient groups experience an increased incidence of nighttime MIs, particularly in those with poor ventricular function,[75] advanced age,[75] or diabetes.[76-78] The risk for development of congestive heart failure is higher for nighttime than daytime MIs,[79] potentially because of either the pathologic process or a delay in obtaining high-quality care.

Hypertension

Hypertensive patients whose nighttime arterial blood pressure declines less than 10% from day to night (called "nondippers") are at increased risk of total and cardiovascular mortality, as well as all cardiovascular end points,[80] frequent or complex ventricular arrhythmias,[81] myocardial ischemia,[82] cerebrovascular insult,[83,84] and increased organ damage,[83] including cardiac hypertrophy.[85] The absence of a nocturnal decline in

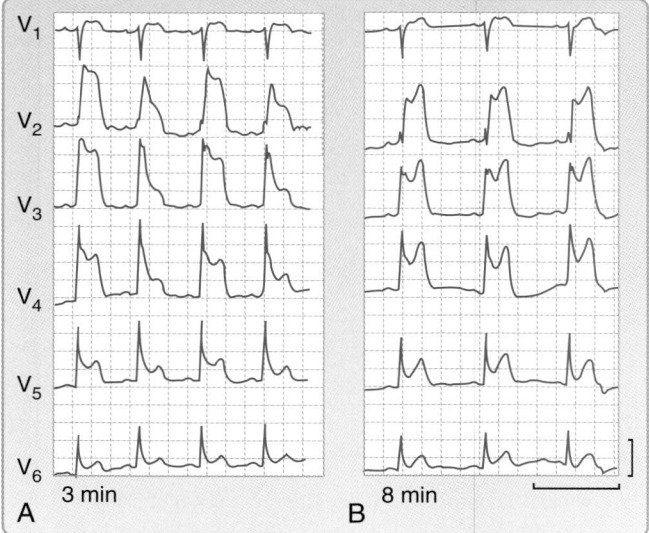

Figure 97–5. **A,** Alternation in precordial leads V_2 to V_5 at 3 min after onset of nocturnal angina during transmural myocardial infarction. **B,** Eight minutes after beginning of pain, alternation has disappeared. (From Cinca J, Janse MJ, Moréna H, et al: Mechanism and time course of the early electrical changes during acute coronary artery occlusion: An attempt to correlate the early ECG changes in man to the cellular electrophysiology in the pig. Chest 1980; 77:499-505.)

blood pressure may be an important marker of complications among patients with type 1 diabetes[86] or may be reflected in the significant incidence of death at 2:00 to 4:00 AM in hypertensive women reported by Mitler and colleagues[87] (Fig. 97–6). Pickering and James[88] argued that the pathologic basis for this increased risk is the challenge of a higher average 24-hour arterial blood pressure. An alternative explanation may be that a high average nocturnal diastolic arterial blood pressure is a powerful marker of left ventricular filling impairment, itself a strong indicator of cardiovascular risk.[89] Faulty baroreceptor activation may account for the fact that arterial blood pressure during sleep remains significantly elevated in these hypertensive patients, who typically show evidence of central hypersympathetic nerve activity with an increased number of microarousals, reduced length and depth of NREM sleep, and a shortened REM latency. Blunted endothelium-dependent vasodilation is also implicated.[90]

Elderly Patients

Elderly individuals' reports of daytime sleepiness, suggesting poor quality of sleep, are associated with mortality, cardiovascular morbidity and mortality, MI, and congestive heart failure, particularly in women.[91] Depression, poor health, daytime angina, a limited activity level,[92] and cardiac arrhythmias[93] may accompany disturbed sleep in elderly individuals. Initiating a moderately intense exercise program significantly improves sleep quality[94] and autonomic status[95] in formerly sedentary older people. Nocturnal myocardial ischemia is not uncommon in older patients with vascular disease who experience regular episodes of oxygen desaturation and increased heart rate.[96] Conflicting evidence has been presented of increased risk for nighttime compared with daytime MI and sudden cardiac death in the elderly.[73,76,97] Impaired baroreceptor sensitivity,[98] a measure of the capacity for reflex vagus nerve activation,[7] and increased LF power of HRV[99] are evident at night in susceptible elderly patients. Given this autonomic background, it is not surprising that nighttime multifocal activity in elderly patients is a predictor of cardiac mortality.

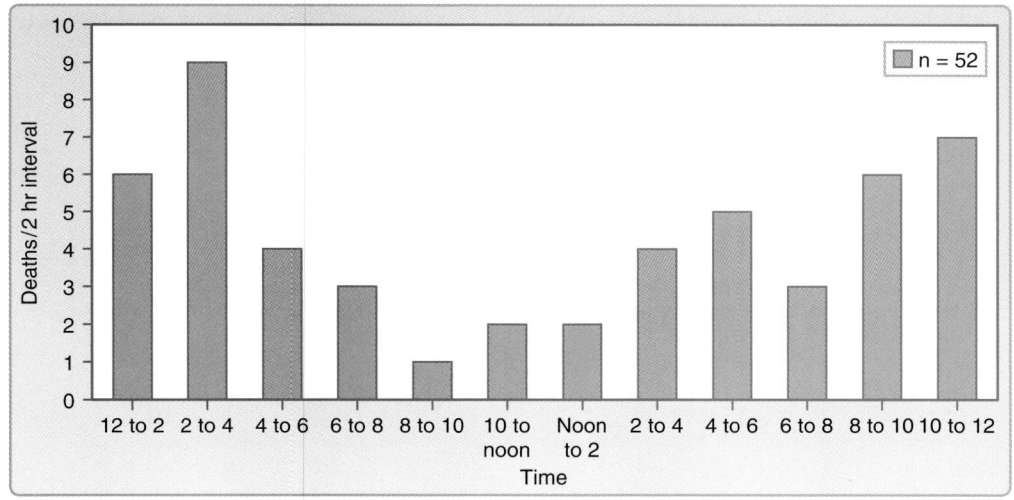

FEMALE DEATHS FROM HYPERTENSIVE DISEASE

Figure 97–6. The temporal distribution of female deaths attributed to hypertensive disease peaked at 2:00 to 4:00 AM. The temporal concentration was statistically significant ($P < .01$). Data were derived from a 4600-person (>8%) sample of deaths due to disease in New York City in 1979. (Reprinted from Mitler MM, Hajdukovic RM, Shafor R, et al: When people die: Cause of death versus time of death, *American Journal of Medicine*, 82:266-274, Copyright 1987, with permission from Excerpta Medica Inc.)

Clinical Pearls

Sleep exerts a major impact on the health of the patient with cardiac disease, through both direct cardiovascular influences and through sleep-disordered breathing.[100] In a sense, the diseased heart and lungs are unwitting victims of the needs of the sleeping brain, which commands dramatic alterations in autonomic and respiratory activity. A sizeable population experiences cardiac events during sleep, with identifiable high-risk groups (see Table 97–1). Sleep also presents unusual opportunities to monitor the patient with cardiac disease because there is growing appreciation of the fact that nighttime heart rate, blood pressure, myocardial ischemia, arrhythmias, and respiratory disturbances carry predictive value for daytime events (see Box 97–1). Daytime tests cannot substitute for nighttime monitoring of the patient with cardiac disease because exercise treadmill testing and daytime ambulatory monitoring cannot replicate the autonomic, hemodynamic, or respiratory challenges that uniquely accompany sleep. Improved identification of the precise triggers of nocturnal cardiac events may be anticipated when technologies are integrated for monitoring sleep state, respiration, and cardiovascular variables.

Acknowledgments

Supported by grant ES 08129 from the National Institute of Environmental Health, National Institutes of Health, Bethesda, Maryland. The authors thank Sandra Verrier for her editorial contributions.

REFERENCES

1. Lavery CE, Mittleman MA, Cohen MC, et al: Nonuniform nighttime distribution of acute cardiac events: A possible effect of sleep states. Circulation 1997;5:3321-3327.
2. Somers VK, Dyken ME, Mark AL, et al: Sympathetic nerve activity during sleep in normal subjects. N Engl J Med 1993;328:303-307.
3. Young T, Palta M, Dempsey J, et al: The occurrence of sleep-disordered breathing among middle-aged adults. N Engl J Med 1993;328:1230-1235.
4. Mancia G: Autonomic modulation of the cardiovascular system during sleep. N Engl J Med 1993;328:347-349.
5. Coccagna G, Mantovani M, Brignani F, et al: Laboratory note: Arterial pressure changes during spontaneous sleep in man. Electroencephalogr Clin Neurophysiol 1971;31:277-281.
6. Snyder F, Hobson JA, Morrison DF, et al: Changes in respiration, heart rate, and systolic blood pressure in human sleep. J Appl Physiol 1964;19:417-422.
7. Smyth HS, Sleight P, Pickering GW: Reflex regulation of arterial pressure during sleep in man: A quantitative method of assessing baroreflex sensitivity. Circ Res 1969;24:109-121.
8. Conway J, Boon N, Jones JV, et al: Involvement of the baroreceptor reflexes in the changes in blood pressure with sleep and mental arousal. Hypertension 1983;5:746-748.
9. Hornyak M, Cejnar M, Elam M, et al: Sympathetic muscle nerve activity during sleep in man. Brain 1991;114:1281-1295.
10. Okada H, Iwase S, Mano T, et al: Changes in muscle sympathetic nerve activity during sleep in humans. Neurology 1991;41:1961-1966.
11. Bonnet MH, Arand DL: Heart rate variability: Sleep stage, time of night, and arousal influences. Electroencephalogr Clin Neurophysiol 1997;102:390-396.
12. Hobson JA, Spagna T, Malenka R: Ethology of sleep studied with time-lapse photography: postural immobility and sleep-cycle phase in humans. Science 1979;201:1251-1253.
13. Quyyumi AA, Efthimiou J, Quyyumi A, et al: Nocturnal angina: precipitating factors in patients with coronary artery disease and those with variant angina. Br Heart J 1986;56:346-352.
14. Khatri IM, Freis ED: Hemodynamic changes during sleep. J Appl Physiol 1967;22:867-873.
15. Siegel JM: Mechanisms of sleep control. J Clin Neurophysiol 1990;7:49-65.
16. Townsend RE, Prinz PN, Obrist WD: Human cerebral blood flow during sleep and waking. J Appl Physiol 1973;35:620-625.
17. Maquet P, Peters J, Aerts J, et al: Functional neuroanatomy of human rapid-eye-movement sleep and dreaming. Nature 1996;383:163-166.
18. Dodt C, Breckling U, Derad I, et al: Plasma epinephrine and norepinephrine concentrations of healthy humans associated with nighttime sleep and morning arousal. Hypertension 1997;30:71-76.
19. Irwin M, Thompson J, Miller C, et al: Effects of sleep and sleep deprivation on catecholamine and interleukin-2 levels in humans: clinical implications. J Clin Endocrinol Metab 1999;84:1979-1985.
20. Weitzman ED, Fukushima D, Nogeire C, et al: Twenty-four hour pattern of the episodic secretion of cortisol in normal subjects. J Clin Endocrinol Metab 1971;33:14-22.
21. Task Force of the European Society of Cardiology and the North American Society of Pacing and Electrophysiology: Heart rate variability: Standards of measurement, physiological interpretation and clinical use. Circulation 1996;93:1043-1065.
22. Vanoli E, Adamson PB, Ba-Lin, et al: Heart rate variability during specific sleep stages: A comparison of healthy subjects with patients after myocardial infarction. Circulation 1995;91:1918-1922.
23. Otzenberger H, Simon C, Gronfier C, et al: Temporal relationship between dynamic heart rate variability and electroencephalographic activity during sleep in man. Neurosci Lett 1997;229:173-176.
24. Huikuri HV, Niemela MJ, Ojala S, et al: Circadian rhythms of frequency domain measures of heart rate variability in healthy subjects and patients with coronary artery disease: Effects of arousal and upright posture. Circulation 1994;90:121-126.
25. Vardas PE, Kochiadakis GE, Manios EG, et al: Spectral analysis of heart rate variability before and during episodes of nocturnal ischaemia in patients with extensive coronary artery disease. Eur Heart J 1996;17:388-393.
26. Marchant B, Stevenson R, Vaishnav S, et al: Influence of the autonomic nervous system on circadian patterns of myocardial ischaemia: Comparison of stable angina with the early post-infarction period. Br Heart J 1994;71:329-333.
27. Cerati D, Nador F, Maestri R, et al: Influence of residual ischaemia on heart rate variability after myocardial infarction. Eur Heart J 1997;18:78-83.
28. Bernardi L, Ricordi L, Lazzari P, et al: Impaired circadian modulation of sympathovagal activity in diabetes: A possible explanation for altered temporal onset of cardiovascular disease. Circulation 1992;86:1443-1452.
29. Aronson D, Weinrauch LA, D'Elia JA, et al: Circadian patterns of heart rate variability, fibrinolytic activity, and hemostatic factors in type I diabetes mellitus with cardiac autonomic neuropathy. Am J Cardiol 1999;84:449-453.
30. White PD: Heart Disease, 3rd ed. New York, Macmillan, 1944, p 87.
31. Home E: Life of John Hunter. In Major RH (ed): Classic Descriptions of Disease, 4th ed. Springfield, Ill, Charles C Thomas, 1955, p 423.
32. Mac William JA: Blood pressure and heart action in sleep and dreams: Their relation to haemorrhages, angina, and sudden death. BMJ 1923;22:1196-2000.

33. Levine S: Clinical Heart Disease. Philadelphia, WB Saunders, 1951, p 816.

34. Kales A, Kales JD: Evaluation, diagnosis, and treatment of clinical conditions related to sleep. JAMA 1970;213:2229-2232.

35. Nowlin JB, Troyer WG Jr, Collins WS, et al: The association of nocturnal angina pectoris with dreaming. Ann Intern Med 1965;63:1040-1046.

36. Quyyumi AA, Wright CA, Mockus LJ, et al: Mechanisms of nocturnal angina pectoris: Importance of increased myocardial oxygen demand in patients with severe coronary artery disease. Lancet 1984;1:1207-1209.

37. Mulcahy D, Cunningham D, Crean P, et al: Circadian variation of total ischaemic burden and its alteration with anti-anginal agents. Lancet 1988;1:755-759.

38. Deedwania PC, Nelson JR: Pathophysiology of silent myocardial ischemia during daily life: Hemodynamic evaluation by simultaneous electrocardiographic and blood pressure monitoring. Circulation 1990;92:1296-1304.

39. Behar S, Reicher-Reiss H, Goldbourt U, et al: Circadian variation in pain onset in unstable angina pectoris. Am J Cardiol 1991;67:91-93.

40. Deedwania PC: Increased demand versus reduced supply and the circadian variations in ambulatory myocardial ischemia: Therapeutic implications [editorial]. Circulation 1993;98:328-331.

41. Andrews TC, Fenton T, Toyosaki N, et al., for the Angina and Silent Ischemia Study Group (ASIS): Subsets of ambulatory myocardial ischemia based on heart rate activity: Circadian distribution and response to anti-ischemic medication. Circulation 1993;98:92-100.

42. Patel DJ, Knight CJ, Holdright DR, et al: Pathophysiology of transient myocardial ischemia in acute coronary syndromes: Characterization by continuous ST-segment monitoring. Circulation 1997;95:1185-1192.

43. Benhorin J, Banai S, Moriel M, et al: Circadian variations in ischemic threshold and their relation to the occurrence of ischemic episodes. Circulation 1993;97:808-814.

44. Broughton R, Baron R: Sleep patterns in the intensive care unit and on the ward after acute myocardial infarction. Electroencephalogr Clin Neurophysiol 1978;45:348-360.

45. Figueras J, Cinca J, Balda F, et al: Resting angina with fixed coronary artery stenosis: Nocturnal decline in ischemic threshold. Circulation 1986;74:1248-1254.

46. Andreotti F, Davies GJ, Hackett DR, et al: Major circadian fluctuations in fibrinolytic factors and possible relevance to time of onset of myocardial infarction, sudden cardiac death, and stroke. Am J Cardiol 1988;62:635-637.

47. Bridges AB, McLaren M, Scott NA, et al: Circadian variation of tissue plasminogen activator and its inhibitor, von Willebrand factor antigen, and prostacyclin stimulating factor in men with ischemic heart disease. Br Heart J 1993;69:121-124.

48. Masuda T, Ogawa H, Miyao Y, et al: Circadian variation in fibrinolytic activity in patients with variant angina. Br Heart J 1994;71:156-161.

49. Bridges AB, Scott NA, McNeill GP, et al: Circadian variation in white blood cell aggregation and free radical indices in men with ischaemic heart disease. Eur Heart J 1992;13:1632-1636.

50. Selwyn AP, Fox K, Eves M, et al: Myocardial ischaemia in patients with frequent angina pectoris. BMJ 1978;2:1594-1596.

51. Langer AL, Freeman MR, Armstrong PW: ST-segment shift in unstable angina: pathophysiology and association with coronary anatomy and hospital outcome. J Am Coll Cardiol 1989;13:1495-1502.

52. Zarich S, Waxman S, Freeman RT, et al: Effect of autonomic nervous system dysfunction on the circadian pattern of myocardial ischemia in diabetes mellitus. J Am Coll Cardiol 1994;24:956-962.

53. Araki H, Koiwaya Y, Nakagaki O, et al: Diurnal distribution of ST-segment elevation and related arrhythmias in patients with variant angina: A study by ambulatory ECG monitoring. Circulation 1983;67:995-1000.

54. Cannon CP, McCabe CH, Stone PH, et al: Circadian variation in the onset of unstable angina and non-Q-wave acute myocardial infarction (the TIMI III Registry and TIMI IIIB). Am J Cardiol 1997;79:253-258.

55. Franklin KA, Nilsson JB, Sahlin C, et al: Sleep apnea and nocturnal angina. Lancet 1995;345:1085-1087.

56. Keyl C, Lemberger P, Rodig G, et al: Hypoxaemia and myocardial ischaemia on the night before coronary bypass surgery. Br J Anaesth 1994;73:157-161.

57. Pollock JS, Kenny GN: Effect of lorazepam on oxygen saturation before cardiac surgery. Br J Anaesth 1993;70:219-220.

58. Floras JS: Antihypertensive treatment, myocardial infarction, and nocturnal myocardial ischaemia. Lancet 1988;2:994-996.

59. Parker JD, Testa MA, Jimenez AH, et al: Morning increase in ambulatory ischemia in patients with stable coronary artery disease: Importance of physical activity and increased cardiac demand. Circulation 1994;99:604-614.

60. Galatius-Jensen S, Hansen J, Rasmussen V, et al: Nocturnal hypoxemia after myocardial infarction: Association with nocturnal myocardial ischaemia and arrhythmias. Br Heart J 1994;72:23-30.

61. Spudge DD, Seires SF, Maron BJ, et al: Prevalence of arrhythmias during 24-hour Holter electrocardiographic monitoring and exercise testing in patients with obstructive and nonobstructive hypertrophic cardiomyopathy. Circulation 1979;59:866-875.

62. Møller M, Lyager Nielsen B, Fabricius J: Paroxysmal VT during repeated 24-hr ambulatory electrographic monitoring of post-MI patients. Br Heart J 1980;43:447-453.

63. Davies SW, John LM, Wedzicha JA, et al: Overnight studies in severe chronic left heart failure: arrhythmias and oxygen desaturation. Br Heart J 1991;65:77-83.

64. Cripps T, Rocker G, Stradling J: Nocturnal hypoxia and arrhythmias in patients with impaired left ventricular function. Br Heart J 1992;68:382-386.

65. Mickley H, Pless P, Nielsen JR, et al: Circadian variation of transient myocardial ischemia in the early out-of-hospital period after first acute myocardial infarction. Am J Cardiol 1991;67:927-932.

66. Casolo GC, Stroder P, Signorini C, et al: Heart rate variability during the acute phase of myocardial infarction. Circulation 1992;95:2073-2079.

67. Brugger P, Marktl W, Herold M: Impaired nocturnal secretion of melatonin in coronary heart disease. Lancet 1995;345:1408.

68. Verrier RL, Nearing BD, LaRovere MT, et al: Ambulatory ECG-based tracking of T-wave alternans in post-myocardial infarction patients to assess risk of cardiac arrest or arrhythmic death. J Cardiovasc Electrophysiol 2003;14:705-711.

69. Hung J, Whitford EG, Parsons RW, et al: Association of sleep apnoea with myocardial infarction in men. Lancet 1990;336:261-264.

70. Peters RW, Zoble RG, Liebson PR, et al: Identification of a secondary peak in myocardial infarction onset 11 to 12 hours after awakening: The Cardiac Arrhythmia Suppression Trial (CAST) experience. J Am Coll Cardiol 1993;22:998-1003.

71. Gibson RS, Boden WE, Theroux P, et al: Diltiazem and reinfarction in patients with non-Q-wave myocardial infarction: Results of a double-blind, randomized, multicenter trial. N Engl J Med 1986;315:423-429.

72. Kleiman NS, Schechtman KB, Young PM, et al., and the Diltiazem Reinfarction Study Investigators: Lack of diurnal variation in the onset of non-Q-wave infarction. Circulation 1990;91:548-555.

73. Hansen O, Johannsson BW, Gullberg B: Circadian distribution of onset of acute myocardial infarction in subgroups from analysis of 10,791 patients treated in a single center. Am J Cardiol 1992;69:1003-1008.

74. Cinca J, Janse MJ, Moréna H, et al: Mechanism and time course of the early electrical changes during acute coronary artery occlusion: An attempt to correlate the early ECG changes in man to the cellular electrophysiology in the pig. Chest 1980;77:499-505.

75. Peters RW, Zoble RG, Brooks MM: Onset of acute myocardial infarction during sleep. Clin Cardiol 2002;25:237-241.

76. Hjalmarson A, Gilpin EA, Nicod P, et al: Differing circadian patterns of symptom onset in subgroups of patients with acute myocardial infarction. Circulation 1989;90:267-275.

77. Fava S, Azzopardi J, Muscat HA, et al: Absence of circadian variation in the onset of acute myocardial infarction in diabetic subjects. Br Heart J 1995;74:370-372.

78. Rana JS, Mukamal KJ, Morgan JP, et al: Circadian variation in the onset of myocardial infarction: effect of duration of diabetes. Diabetes 2003;52:1464-1468.

79. Mukamal KJ, Muller JA, Maclure M, et al: Increased risk of congestive heart failure among infarctions with nighttime onset. Am Heart J 2000;140:439-442.

80. Staessen JA, Thijs L, Fagard R, et al: Predicting cardiovascular risk using conventional vs ambulatory blood pressure in older patients with systolic hypertension: Systolic Hypertension in Europe Trial Investigators. JAMA 1999;282:539-546.

81. Schillaci G, Verdecchia P, Borgioni C, et al: Association between persistent pressure overload and ventricular arrhythmias in essential hypertension. Hypertension 1996;28:284-289.

82. Pierdomenico SD, Bucci A, Costantini F, et al: Circadian blood pressure changes and myocardial ischemia in hypertensive patients with coronary artery disease. J Am Coll Cardiol 1998;31:1627-1634.

83. Verdecchia P, Schillaci G, Gatteschi C, et al: Blunted nocturnal fall in blood pressure in hypertensive women with future cardiovascular morbid events. Circulation 1993;98:986-992.

84. Kario K, Matsuo T, Kobayashi H, et al: Nocturnal fall of blood pressure and silent cerebrovascular damage in elderly hypertensive patients: Advanced silent cerebrovascular damage in extreme dippers. Hypertension 1997;27:130-135.

85. Verdecchia P, Schillaci G, Guerrieri M, et al: Circadian blood pressure changes and left ventricular hypertrophy in essential hypertension. Circulation 1990;91:523-536.

86. Lurbe E, Redon J, Kesani A, et al: Increase in nocturnal blood pressure and progression to microalbuminuria in type 1 diabetes. N Engl J Med 2002;347:797-805.

87. Mitler MM, Hajdukovic RM, Shafor R, et al: When people die: Cause of death versus time of death. Am J Med 1987;82:266-274.

88. Pickering TG, James GD: Determinants and consequences of the diurnal rhythm of blood pressure. Am J Hypertens 1993;6:166S-169S.

89. Galderisi M, Petrocelli A, Alfieri A, et al: Impact of ambulatory blood pressure on left ventricular diastolic dysfunction in uncomplicated arterial systemic hypertension. Am J Cardiol 1996;77:597-601.

90. Higashi Y, Nakagawa K, Kimura M, et al: Circadian variation of blood pressure and endothelial function in patients with essential hypertension: A comparison of dippers and nondippers. J Am Coll Cardiol 2002;40:2039-2043.

91. Newman AB, Spiekerman CF, Enright P, et al: Daytime sleepiness predicts mortality and cardiovascular disease in older adults: The Cardiovascular Health Study Research Group. J Am Geriatr Soc 2000;48:115-123.

92. Newman AB, Enright PL, Manolio TA, et al: Sleep disturbance, psychosocial correlates, and cardiovascular disease in 5201 older adults: The Cardiovascular Health Study. J Am Geriatr Soc 1997;45:1-7.

93. Asplund R: Sleep and cardiac disease amongst elderly people. J Intern Med 1994;236:65-71.

94. King AC, Oman RF, Brassington GS, et al: Moderate-intensity exercise and self-rated quality of sleep in older adults: A randomized controlled trial. JAMA 1997;277:32-37.

95. Stein PK, Ehsani AA, Domitrovich PP, et al: Effect of exercise training on heart rate variability in healthy older adults. Am Heart J 1999;138:567-576.

96. Goldman MD, Reeder MK, Muir AD, et al: Repetitive nocturnal arterial oxygen desaturation and silent myocardial ischemia in patients presenting for vascular surgery. J Am Geriatr Soc 1993;41:703-709.

97. Aronow WS, Ahn C: Circadian variation of primary cardiac arrest or sudden cardiac death in patients aged 62 to 100 years (mean 82). Am J Cardiol 1993;71:1455-1456.

98. Parati G, Frattola A, Di Rienzo M, et al: Effects of aging on 24-h dynamic baroreceptor control of heart rate in ambulant subjects. Am J Physiol 1995;268:H1606-1612.

99. Yamasaki Y, Kodama M, Matsuhisa M, et al: Diurnal heart rate variability in healthy subjects: Effects of aging and sex difference. Am J Physiol 1996;271:H303-310.

100. Quan SF, Gersh B: Cardiovascular consequences of sleep-disordered breathing: Past, present and future. Report of a Workshop from the National Center on Sleep Disorders Research and the National Heart, Lung, and Blood Institute. Circulation 2004;109:951-957.

98

Cardiac Arrhythmogenesis during Sleep: Mechanisms, Diagnosis, and Therapy

Richard L. Verrier

Mark E. Josephson

ABSTRACT

The pronounced sleep state–dependent changes in autonomic nervous system activity and respiration can provoke both atrial and ventricular arrhythmias in patients with cardiovascular disease. Mortality is most common during sleep in the distinct syndromes of sudden infant death, sudden unexplained nocturnal death, and the Brugada syndrome, each of which has been linked to genetic abnormalities. Because the etiology of nocturnal arrhythmias is multifactorial, their management necessitates a comprehensive approach and consideration of a host of cardiovascular and respiratory factors. Treatment must be tailored to contain neurally induced arrhythmias while avoiding exacerbation of the hypotension of non–rapid eye movement sleep. The proarrhythmic potential of class III antiarrhythmic agents (potassium channel blockers) for patients with significant heart rate pauses and the sleep-disrupting effect of medications must be considered.

Cardiac arrhythmias are prevalent in the 13.5 million Americans with heart disease, with potentially severe consequences. Approximately 15% of lethal ventricular arrhythmias occur during sleep, and most atrial arrhythmias in patients younger than 61 years old have their onset at nighttime. Lack of streamlined technology for concurrent monitoring of sleep state, electrocardiogram, and respiration continues to hamper diagnosis and evaluation of therapy of these arrhythmias. In this chapter we review the current state of knowledge regarding epidemiology, risk factors, pathogenesis, and treatment options for each nocturnal arrhythmia type.

VENTRICULAR ARRHYTHMIAS

Malignant ventricular arrhythmias are usually suppressed during sleep, as is evidenced by the nocturnal trough in incidence of myocardial infarction, sudden cardiac death, implantable cardioverter-defibrillator discharge, myocardial ischemic events, and arrhythmias in patients with ischemic heart disease[1,2] (Fig. 98–1). This decrement coincides with lessened metabolic demands during non–rapid eye movement (NREM) sleep, which occupies approximately 80% of sleep time. However, sleep is not entirely free of risk because the nocturnal incidence of sudden cardiac death, which is attributable to ventricular fibrillation, has been calculated at approximately 15%,[3] or 38,000 cases annually in the United States alone. Moreover, the nonuniformity of the nighttime distribution of these events[3] suggests physiologic triggering that may be amenable to monitoring for improved diagnosis and therapy.

Surges in cardiac sympathetic nerve activity during REM sleep have been implicated in nocturnal ventricular arrhythmias[4] and myocardial ischemia.[5-7] The specific mechanisms of REM-induced cardiac events include direct effects on electrophysiologic status or indirect consequences of heart rate and arterial blood pressure accelerations, which may disrupt plaques and lead to intraarterial platelet aggregates, releasing proarrhythmic constituents such as thromboxane A_2.[8] Myocardial ischemia or other changes in cardiac substrate and mechanical function due to disease,[9] infarction,[10] or ageing[11] can amplify nocturnal electrical instability. Sleep apnea has been found to trigger nighttime ventricular tachycardia in patients with cardiac disease after myocardial infarction[10] or in those with heart failure[9] as a result of surges in arterial blood pressure and sympathetic nerve activity provoked by severe oxygen desaturation. Frequent or complex arrhythmias are also characteristic of hypertensive patients in whom the typical nocturnal trough in blood pressure is not observed.[12] The nocturnal increase in QT interval dispersion among survivors of sudden cardiac death[13] provides evidence of increased vulnerability to cardiac arrhythmias at night.

REM-related nocturnal arrhythmogenesis may have a significant affective component. REM sleep dreams, which may be vivid, bizarre, and emotionally intense, commonly generate the emotions of anger and fear. Because these emotions have been linked in wakefulness to the onset of myocardial infarction and sudden death,[14] it is reasonable to hypothesize that when these affective states are evoked during dreaming, they may trigger lethal events. This possibility is illustrated by a case report of recurrence of ventricular fibrillation in a 39-year-old man with normal coronary arteries and cardiac function while sleeping. A subsequent sleep study determined that ventricular premature beats were substantially increased during REM and that dreams at the same hour that fibrillation had occurred were emotionally charged.[15]

In some cases, arrhythmia frequency may be enhanced during NREM sleep, when latent automatic foci are exposed by the generalized reduction in heart rate after withdrawal of overdrive suppression, or when hypotension exacerbates impaired coronary perfusion.

Therapy

In most cases, an electrically unstable substrate underlies the propensity to develop nocturnal ventricular arrhythmias, and treatment is similar to that for daytime arrhythmias.

SUDDEN CARDIAC DEATH
(n = 2,203)

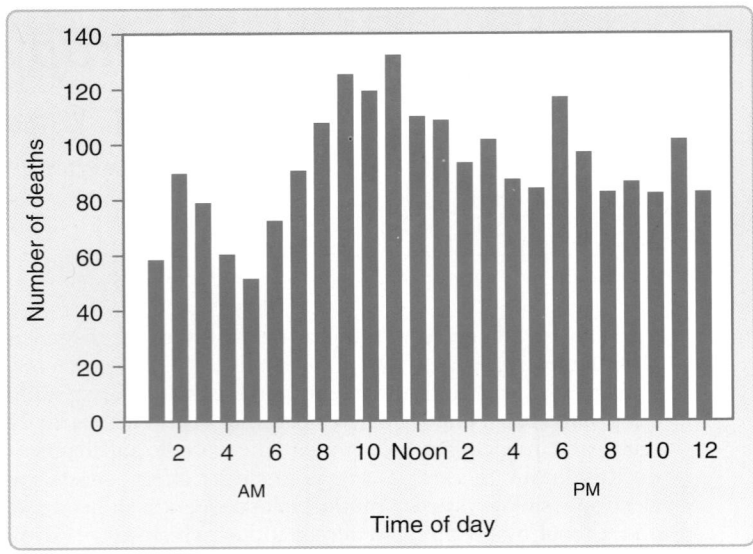

Figure 98–1. Time of day of out-of-hospital sudden cardiac death (<1 hr from onset of symptoms to death) for 2203 persons dying in Massachusetts in 1983. A significant circadian rhythm is present (*P* < .001) with a morning peak between 7 and 11 AM and a secondary peak between 5 and 6 PM. (From Muller JE, Ludmer PL, Willich SN, et al: Circadian variation in the frequency of sudden cardiac death. Circulation 1987;75:131-138.)

If surges in sympathetic nerve activity, which typically occur during REM sleep and dreaming, are suspected, beta-adrenergic receptor blockade therapy may prove helpful, with careful attention to avoiding medications that disrupt sleep.[16]

In treating hypertensive patients, it is important to appreciate Mancia's[17] suggestion that pharmacologic therapy that exacerbates the hypotensive effect of NREM sleep may introduce the potential risk of thrombosis and embolism in patients with stenotic lesions in the heart or brain. Floras[18] determined that the nocturnal incidence of myocardial infarction was not diminished in patients treated with antihypertensive agents and suggested that the agents induced nocturnal hypotension. Thus, special attention should be given to the hemodynamic effects of antihypertensive drugs and vasodilators to avoid precipitating cardiac events by inducing profound hypotension. The importance of ruling out "white coat" hypertension is underscored because more than 30% of individuals with elevated blood pressure readings in the physician's office or hospital prove to be normotensive during daily life as documented by ambulatory blood pressure monitoring.[19]

The nighttime onset of ventricular arrhythmias may also indicate provocation by disturbed breathing, which can be treated by continuous positive airway pressure (CPAP).

NOCTURNAL ASYSTOLE AND QT INTERVAL PROLONGATION

In individuals who are young[20,21] or physically fit, such as athletes[22,23] and heavy laborers,[24] sinus pauses of less than 2 seconds,[25] prolonged atrioventricular (AV) conduction,

Wenckebach AV block, and bradycardia are well documented and are attributed to effects of increased parasympathetic activity on AV node conduction.[26] More extreme cases were observed by Guilleminault and colleagues,[27] who reported periods of sinus arrest of up to 9 seconds during REM sleep in young adults with apparently normal cardiac function. It was concluded that the nocturnal asystoles were the result of exaggerated, if not abnormally elevated, vagal tone because muscarinic receptor blockers significantly reduced the duration of the nocturnal asystoles but did not prevent them. No further therapeutic intervention was warranted.

However, in patients with cardiac disease, who number 13.5 million in the United States alone, especially those taking class III antiarrhythmic drugs (potassium channel blocking agents), nocturnal asystolic events can set the stage for ventricular arrhythmias. Such prolongation of cycle length can facilitate the development of early afterdepolarizations and the lethal arrhythmia torsade de pointes. In patients with damaged endothelium due to coronary atherosclerosis, the acetylcholine released by surges in vagus nerve activity could result in vasoconstriction rather than vasodilation owing to impaired release of endothelium-derived relaxing factor.[28]

Nocturnal heart rate pauses may be particularly arrhythmogenic in a subset of patients with the long QT syndrome who have mutations on the sodium channel, voltage-gated, type V, alpha gene (SCN5A).[29] The lethal arrhythmias occur almost exclusively at rest or during sleep, when the QT interval is typically prolonged[30] (see section on Sudden Infant Death Syndrome, later).

Therapy

Ascertaining whether patients exhibit nocturnal heart rate pauses is important in treating individuals for whom class III antiarrhythmic drugs (potassium channel blockers) are the primary option.

ATRIAL FIBRILLATION

In the 2.5 million U.S. patients with atrial fibrillation, which has serious consequences in terms of increased morbidity and mortality,[31] it is likely that 10% to 25% of the arrhythmias are facilitated by vagal influences. Several investigators have reported nocturnal peaks in onset of paroxysmal atrial fibrillation.[32-34] A significant midnight to 2:00 AM peak in atrial fibrillation onset and a higher average nocturnal incidence were documented by Rostagno and colleagues in their review of records from 10 years of responses by mobile coronary care units staffed by cardiologists in Florence, Italy.[32] This arrhythmia was also found to exhibit a peak in frequency of onset at midnight in a Japanese population 60 years of age or younger. The maximum duration of the arrhythmia (77 ± 27 minutes per episode) was also greatest between midnight and 6:00 AM[33] (Fig. 98–2). This has been termed *vagally mediated atrial fibrillation*. Other investigators characterized a 4:00 to 5:00 AM peak in onset of paroxysmal atrial fibrillation that was refractory to antiarrhythmic drugs in a 3-month study of 67 patients with implantable cardioverters.[34] The 514 recorded episodes with an atrial rate of greater than 220 beats per minute lasted more than 1 minute before termination by pacing or spontaneous reversion. A potential contribution of sympathetic nerve activity is implicated by the timing of these bouts of atrial fibrillation, which occurred during a period of sleep when REM typically emerges. However, this potential of REM sleep to trigger the arrhythmia was not discussed.

Few records exist of concurrent monitoring of sleep stage and nocturnal onset of atrial fibrillation. Available evidence indicates that nocturnal atrial fibrillation is provoked during periods of intense vagus nerve activity, as indicated by heart rate variability studies,[35,36] and the presence of bradycardia,[37] in individuals with structurally normal hearts. Enhanced adrenergic activity may interact in a complex manner with changes in vagal tone to affect atrial refractoriness and dispersion of repolarization and alter intraatrial conduction, thus increasing the propensity to develop this arrhythmia.[31,37] The high level of vagus nerve tone maintained during slow wave sleep has the capacity to exacerbate atrial fibrillation in patients whose atria are particularly prone to the arrhythmogenic influence of acetylcholine.[31]

Risk of atrial fibrillation is doubled if breathing during sleep is disordered[38] because apnea can provoke nocturnal hypoxemia, sympathetic nerve activity, and hemodynamic stress. Obstructive apnea–induced surges in blood pressure distend atrial chambers and can activate stretch receptors.

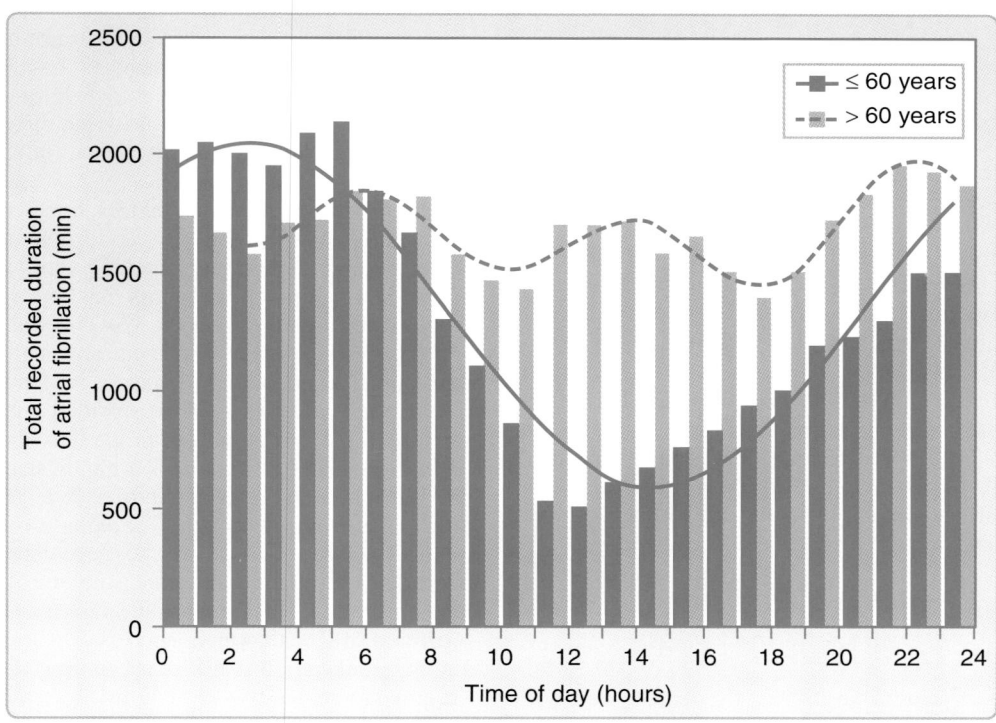

Figure 98–2. Hourly total duration of paroxysmal atrial fibrillation in younger (≤60 yr of age; *dark blue bars*) and older patients (*light blue bars*). The single harmonic fit of the data in the younger patients is shown by the *unbroken line*. The triple harmonic fit in the older patients is shown by the *broken line*. A prominent monophasic circadian rhythm is present in younger patients, in contrast to a toneless triphasic rhythm in older patients. (From: Yamashita T, Murakawa Y, Hayami N, et al: Relation between aging and circadian variation of paroxysmal atrial fibrillation. Am J Cardiol 1998;82:1364-1367.)

Therapy

Medical therapy is similar to that for patients whose arrhythmias occur during the day, including therapy to control rate or terminate the arrhythmia pharmacologically or with an atrial cardioverter-defibrillator. In addition, individuals with nocturnal onset of atrial fibrillation should be monitored for the presence of sleep-disordered breathing, which can be effectively treated by CPAP.[39] No additional information or instruction has been provided with reference to therapy of atrial fibrillation with nocturnal rather than daytime onset.

IMPACT OF RESPIRATORY CHALLENGES

Obstructive and central sleep apnea are common disorders, affecting millions of Americans. Obstructive sleep apnea is a risk factor for development of hypertension[40-42] and myocardial infarction.[43] In patients with cardiovascular disease, apneic episodes and oxygen desaturation are highly conducive to bradyarrhythmias,[44,45] sinus arrest,[46] asystole,[47] and supraventricular[26,27,38,39] and ventricular[9,10] arrhythmias. Importantly, the segment of the population at greatest risk for cardiovascular disease, namely unfit individuals from the sixth decade of life, is also at elevated risk for sleep apnea. A graded positive cross-sectional association between sleep-disordered breathing and prevalent cardiac disease has been demonstrated in a large, multicity community-based study.[48] Central sleep apnea is also common in patients with systolic heart failure and is associated with a number of atrial and ventricular arrhythmias (see Chapter 102).

Therapy

The facts that risk factors for cardiac disease and sleep apnea overlap, that myocardial infarction and sudden cardiac death may be unheralded by prodromes, and that the presence of cardiovascular disease is frequently underdiagnosed provide a rationale for investigating whether apnea may be provoking nocturnal arrhythmias in individual patients.

Screening for obstructive sleep apnea and treatment by CPAP may eliminate unwarranted pacemaker implantation for nocturnal bradyarrhythmias[44] and sinus arrest and heart block.[46] CPAP minimizes or eliminates apnea-provoked atrial[39] and ventricular[9,44,45] arrhythmias, improves fibrinogen levels[49] and insulin responsiveness,[50,51] lessens myocardial ischemia,[52] and reduces apnea-induced elevations in arterial[53] and pulmonary[54] blood pressure and sympathetic nerve activity.[53,55] Similarly, treatment of central sleep apnea in heart failure may decrease nocturnal ventricular arrhythmias.[9]

SUDDEN INFANT DEATH SYNDROME

Sudden infant death syndrome (SIDS), the leading cause of mortality in infants between 1 week and 1 year of age, occurs during sleep.[56] The definition of the syndrome is a "diagnosis of exclusion"; that is, it includes all causes that "remain unexplained after a thorough case investigation, including performance of a complete autopsy, examination of the death scene, and review of the clinical history."[56] Thus, SIDS, which took a toll of 2234 infants in 2001 in the United States[57] or 8.1% of infant deaths, may be attributable to a variety of etiologies that challenge the developing cardiorespiratory system. The fatal event in SIDS victims is characterized by hypotension and bradycardia[58] and appears to be attributable to a deficit in the normal reflex coordination of heart rate, arterial blood pressure, and respiration during sleep.[59] This failure to respond to cardiorespiratory challenges during sleep may result from a binding deficit in the arcuate nucleus of SIDS infants,[59] because muscarinic cholinergic activity in this structure at the ventricular medullary surface is postulated to be involved in cardiorespiratory control. Heart rates in infants who later died of SIDS are generally higher and exhibit a reduced range, suggesting altered autonomic control.[60] Autonomic instability has also been documented in NREM sleep in infants with aborted SIDS events.[61]

Repolarization abnormalities have also been observed. Recent evidence from a 19-year, prospective, multicenter observational study of more than 33,000 infants determined that significant prolongation (35 msec or more) of the QT interval characterized the 24 (0.07%) infants who died of SIDS within the first year of life.[62] These results suggest that SIDS may be attributed to a genetic defect that produces a developmental abnormality in cardiac sympathetic innervation and alters repolarization to increase the risk of ventricular arrhythmia. Nocturnal demise is frequent among infants and children with the long QT syndrome genotype linked to chromosome 3 (LQT3). A defect in the sodium channel gene SCN5A is responsible for the arrhythmias and reduced heart rates. The genetic locus of the defect and the length of the QT interval are independent predictors of risk.[63] T-wave alternans, an electrocardiographic indicator of heightened vulnerability to sudden cardiac death,[64] has been reported in infants who became SIDS victims[65,66] or were successfully treated with pacing[67] or beta-blockade therapy.[68,69] The latter therapy diminished T-wave alternans, indicating antiarrhythmic efficacy.

Among environmental influences, the increased risk of SIDS during the winter season is well documented[70,71] and is not related to bronchiolitis.[72] A genetic susceptibility that may interact with environmental factors has been implicated by a 5.8-fold increase in recurrence of SIDS within families.[73] Tishler and colleagues[74] reported a significant incidence of deficits in ventilatory responses to hypoxia in families with apnea. Conflicting evidence has been provided regarding the relative increase in risk attributable to prone (face-down) sleeping.[75-79]

Passive cigarette smoking is a highly significant modifiable risk factor in SIDS. A reduction of 61% in the number of SIDS deaths has been projected if smoking were eliminated from infants' environments.[74-77,80] A dose-dependent effect has been demonstrated.[75] Maternal smoking during gestation is also implicated.[80-82] Established SIDS risk factors of preterm birth and low birth weight increased risk more than 15-fold among smokers[82] but not at all among nonsmokers. Illegal drug use increases risk of SIDS by more than fourfold.[80] The mechanisms may include impairment in chemoreceptor responsiveness due to decreased sensitivity to carbon dioxide in infants of substance-abusing mothers.[83] The increase in SIDS due to passive smoking may be attributable to nicotine's adverse effect on chemoreceptor activation of respiration,[84] dulling the response to hypoxia.[85] Nicotine and its meta-bolites have been found at autopsy in the pericardial fluid of SIDS infants.[86,87] Epicardial nicotine is associated with hypopnea[88] and affects the sinoatrial node and epicardial neural fibers to induce hypotension and bradycardia,[89,90] the documented symptomatology of the final event in SIDS infants.[58]

Therapy

This profile suggests some straightforward opportunities for intervention, including placing infants in a supine (face-up) position for sleeping and avoidance of maternal smoking during gestation and passive smoking during infancy. Theoretically, sodium channel blockade[29] or cardiac pac-ing[29,67] might be useful in treating infants diagnosed with the long QT3 syndrome, but prospective studies are required. Beta-blockade is the current treatment of choice.[29,68,69] Assessment of vulnerability to arrhythmias by monitoring for QT interval prolongation has been suggested by a prospective study[62] and for T-wave alternans by multiple clinical reports.[65-69]

THE BRUGADA SYNDROME AND SUDDEN UNEXPLAINED NOCTURNAL DEATH

The striking phenomenon of sudden death during sleep has been reported in Western adults diagnosed with the Brugada syndrome, which strikes men almost exclusively, and in young, apparently healthy Southeast Asian men with the sudden unexplained nocturnal death syndrome (SUNDS). The latter syndrome is named *lai-tai* ("sleep death") in Laos, *pokkuri* ("sudden and unexpected death") in Japan, and *bangungut* ("to rise and moan in sleep") in the Philippines. These syndromes probably represent the same disorder, which is characterized by right precordial ST segment elevation.[91,92]

The Brugada syndrome is considered responsible for 4% to 12% of all sudden cardiac deaths and for approximately 20% of deaths in patients with structurally normal hearts.[91] The electrocardiographic abnormality is estimated to be present in approximately 5 per 10,000 inhabitants, and, apart from accidents, in geographic regions where it is widespread, this inherited syndrome is the leading cause of death of men younger than 50 years of age. A single sodium channel muta-tion in the SCN5A gene has been identified in an eight-generation kindred with a high incidence of nocturnal sudden cardiac death, QT interval prolongation, and Brugada-like electrocardiogram. Genetic defects in the sodium channel are also associated with progressive conduction system disease. Bradycardia is the dominant arrhythmia. Wichter and colleagues[93] suggested presynaptic sympathetic cardiac dysfunction based on abnormal ^{123}I-MIBG uptake, with bradycardia-dependent QT prolongation, intrinsic sinus node dysfunction, conduction abnormalities, and absence of ventricular ectopy.

In the United States, 117 SUNDS deaths have been regis-tered among male Southeast Asian immigrants or their descen-dants since 1981, with 12 of the most recent 13 cases documented as occurring during sleep.[94] Autopsies of SUNDS cases have established that cardiovascular disease is absent, but, in some instances, that conduction pathways are develop-mentally abnormal.[92] Companions have reported that the immediate symptoms are onset of agonal respirations during sleep along with vocalization, violent motor activity, nonarous-ability, rapid, irregular deep breathing, perspiration, heart rate surges, and severe autonomic discharge. Several victims revived by vigorous massage reported sensations of airway obstruction, chest discomfort or pressure, and numb and weak limbs. When these symptoms recurred within weeks to months, they culminated in death.[95] Three victims who had been resuscitated from ventricular fibrillation then experienced recurring fibrillation in hospital during sleep accompanied by similar moaning vocalizations. In these three patients, there was no evidence of atherosclerosis or structural abnormalities and no sleep apnea, but creatine kinase levels were markedly elevated and potassium was depressed. Vagal tone is lower in SUNDS survivors compared with healthy individuals, particu-larly at night.[96]

Therapy

Development of effective therapy for these syndromes has been particularly challenging. Currently, implantation of cardioverter-defibrillators appears to be the most effective approach in patients with Brugada syndrome[91] or SUNDS.[92]

SLEEP-DISRUPTING EFFECTS OF CARDIAC MEDICATIONS

Several important medications that are widely prescribed for patients with cardiac disease, including antihypertensive agents, beta-blockers that cross the blood–brain barrier, have the potential to disrupt sleep[16] (Fig. 98–3). In particular, the lipophilic beta-blockers (pindolol, propranolol, and metopro-lol) increase the total number of awakenings and total wake-fulness compared with placebo and with the nonlipophilic atenolol.[16] Penetration of the blood–brain barrier occurs with prolonged therapy, when these distinctions may become less apparent. In addition, pindolol, which has intrinsic sympath-omimetic activity, increases REM latency and, as a result, decreases REM sleep time.[16] Sleep disruption may provoke daytime fatigue and lethargy, symptoms widely reported by patients taking beta-blockers that may prompt discontin-uation of the medication or noncompliance. It has been postulated that the mechanism of sleep disruption by beta-blocking agents is their well-known tendency to deplete endogenous melatonin,[97] a key sleep-regulating hormone that modulates sympathetic nerve activity. An additional important side effect of these beta-blockers[16] is their poten-tial to provoke nightmares. Despite these effects, it is the lipophilic beta-blockers (propranolol, metoprolol, carvedilol) that have been shown to reduce the risk of sudden cardiac death. Sleep disturbance has also been documented in conjunction with the widely used antiarrhythmic agent amio-darone.[98,99] Neurologic side effects were attributed to amio-darone in 20% to 40% of patients.[99] Optimum antiarrhythmic management with this agent to minimize side effects dictates prescription of lower dosages and close patient monitoring and follow-up.[99]

SLEEP CONTINUITY

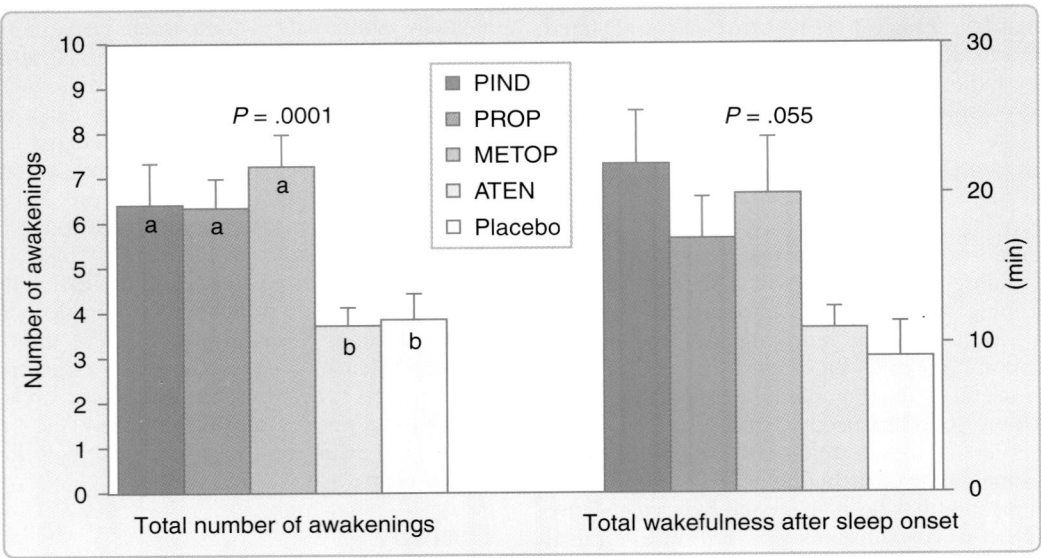

Figure 98–3. Polysomnographic measures of sleep continuity in 30 healthy male subjects during 1 night after 1 week of treatment with beta-blockers or placebo. Lipophilic beta-blockers pindolol (PIND), propranolol (PROP), and metoprolol (METOP) significantly disturbed sleep, as indicated by the number of awakenings, which was significantly reduced with nonlipophilic atenolol (ATEN). Bars with the same letters (a or b) are not significantly different. Values are reported as means ± standard error of the mean. (From Kostis JB, Rosen RC: Central nervous system effects of beta-adrenergic-blocking drugs: The role of ancillary properties. Circulation 1987;75:204-212.)

Clinical Pearl

Diagnosing and treating patients with nocturnal arrhythmias have been hampered by a paucity of information about concurrent autonomic nervous system activity, cardiac electrical instability, and breathing disturbances. It is now possible to assess autonomic nervous system activity with noninvasive markers such as heart rate variability, a measure of autonomic nervous system tone, and heart rate turbulence, an indicator of baroreceptor function based on the pattern of heart rhythm recovery after a ventricular premature beat.[100] Simultaneous measurement of these indicators, along with clinical history and analysis of cardiac electrical instability with QT interval dispersion[13] or T-wave alternans,[64] promises to provide valuable information regarding vulnerability to nocturnal arrhythmias and potential provocation by the autonomic nervous system. Because nighttime arrhythmias may be triggered by apnea, concurrent monitoring of oxygen saturation and respiratory patterns will provide essential information.

Acknowledgments

Supported by grant ES 08129 from the National Institute of Environmental Health, National Institutes of Health, Bethesda, Maryland. The authors thank Sandra Verrier for her editorial contributions.

REFERENCES

1. Muller JE, Ludmer PL, Willich SN, et al: Circadian variation in the frequency of sudden cardiac death. Circulation 1987; 75:131-138.

2. Andrews TC, Fenton T, Toyosaki N, et al for the Angina and Silent Ischemia Study Group (ASIS): Subsets of ambulatory myocardial ischemia based on heart rate activity: Circadian distribution and response to anti-ischemic medication. Circulation 1993;98: 92-100.

3. Lavery CE, Mittleman MA, Cohen MC, et al: Nonuniform nighttime distribution of acute cardiac events: A possible effect of sleep states. Circulation 1997;5:3321-3327.

4. Smith R, Johnson L, Rothfeld D, et al: Sleep and cardiac arrhythmias. Arch Intern Med 1972;130:751-753.

5. Kales A, Kales JD: Evaluation, diagnosis, and treatment of clinical conditions related to sleep. JAMA 1970;213:2229-2232.

6. Nowlin JB, Troyer WG Jr, Collins WS, et al: The association of nocturnal angina pectoris with dreaming. Ann Intern Med 1965; 63:1040-1046.

7. King MJ, Zir LM, Kaltman AJ, et al: Variant angina associated with angiographically demonstrated coronary artery spasm and REM sleep. Am J Med Sci 1973;265:419-422.

8. Curtis MJ, Pugsley MK, Walker MJ: Endogenous chemical mediators of ventricular arrhythmias in ischaemic heart disease. Cardiovasc Res 1993;27:703-719.

9. Javaheri S: Effects of continuous positive airway pressure on sleep apnea and ventricular irritability in patients with heart failure. Circulation 2000;101:392-397.

10. Galatius-Jensen S, Hansen J, Rasmussen V, et al: Nocturnal hypoxemia after myocardial infarction: Association with nocturnal myocardial ischaemia and arrhythmias. Br Heart J 1994; 72:23-30.

11. Asplund R: Sleep and cardiac disease amongst elderly people. J Intern Med 1994;236:65-71.

12. Schillaci G, Verdecchia P, Borgioni C, et al: Association between persistent pressure overload and ventricular arrhythmias in essential hypertension. Hypertension 1996;28:284-289.

13. Molnar J, Rosenthal JE, Weiss JS, et al: QT interval dispersion in healthy subjects and survivors of sudden cardiac death: Circadian variation in a 24-hour assessment. Am J Cardiol 1997; 79:1190-1193.

14. Mittleman MA, Maclure M, Sherwood JB, et al: Triggering of acute myocardial infarction onset by episodes of anger: Determinants of Myocardial Infarction Onset Study Investigators. Circulation 1995;92:1720-1725.

15. Lown B, Temte JV, Reich P, et al: Basis for recurring ventricular fibrillation in the absence of coronary heart disease and its management. N Engl J Med 1976;294:623-629.

16. Kostis JB, Rosen RC: Central nervous system effects of beta-adrenergic blocking drugs: The role of ancillary properties. Circulation 1987;75:204-212.

17. Mancia G: Autonomic modulation of the cardiovascular system during sleep. N Engl J Med 1993;328:347-349.

18. Floras JS: Antihypertensive treatment, myocardial infarction, and nocturnal myocardial ischaemia. Lancet 1988;2:994-996.

19. Myers MG, Reeves RA: White coat effect in treated hypertensive patients: Sex differences. J Hum Hypertens 1995;9:729-733.

20. Brodsky M, Wu D, Denes P, et al: Arrhythmias documented by 24-hour continuous electrocardiographic monitoring in 50 male medical students without apparent heart disease. Am J Cardiol 1977;39:390-395.

21. Sobotka PA, Mayer JH, Bauernfeind RA, et al: Arrhythmias documented by 24-hour continuous ambulatory electrocardiographic monitoring in young women without apparent heart disease. Am Heart J 1981;101:753-759.

22. Viitasalo MT, Kala R, Eisalo A: Ambulatory electrocardiographic recording in endurance athletes. Br Heart J 1982;47:213-220.

23. Ector H, Bourgois J, Verlinden M, et al: Bradycardia, ventricular pauses, syncope, and sports. Lancet 1984;2:591-594.

24. Bortkiewicz A, Palczynski C, Makowiec-Dabrowska T, et al: Cardiac arrhythmia in women performing heavy physical work. Int J Occup Med Environ Health 1995;9:23-31.

25. Bjerregaard P: Mean 24 hour heart rate, minimal heart rate and pauses in healthy subjects 40-79 years of age. Eur Heart J 1983;4:44-51.

26. Otsuka K, Ichimaru Y, Yanaga T: Studies of arrhythmias by 24-hour polygraphic recordings: Relationship between atrio-ventricular block and sleep states. Am Heart J 1983;105:934-940.

27. Guilleminault CP, Pool P, Motta J, et al: Sinus arrest during REM sleep in young adults. N Engl J Med 1984;311:1006-1010.

28. Ludmer PL, Selwyn AP, Shook TL, et al: Paradoxical vasoconstriction induced by acetylcholine in atherosclerotic coronary arteries. N Engl J Med 1986;315:1046-1051.

29. Schwartz PJ, Priori SG, Spazzolini C, et al: Genotype-phenotype correlation in the long-QT syndrome: Gene-specific triggers for life-threatening arrhythmias. Circulation 2001;103:89-95.

30. Molnar J, Zhang F, Weiss J, et al: Diurnal pattern of QTc interval: how long is prolonged? Possible relation to circadian triggers of cardiovascular events. J Am Coll Cardiol 1996;27:76-83.

31. Josephson ME: Atrial flutter and fibrillation. In Josephson ME (ed): Clinical Cardiac Electrophysiology Techniques and Interpretations. Philadelphia, Lea & Febiger, 2002.

32. Rostagno C, Taddei T, Paladini B, et al: The onset of symptomatic atrial fibrillation and paroxysmal supraventricular tachycardia is characterized by different circadian rhythms. Am J Cardiol 1993;71:453-455.

33. Yamashita T, Murakawa Y, Hayami N, et al: Relation between aging and circadian variation of paroxysmal atrial fibrillation. Am J Cardiol 1998;82:1364-1367.

34. Gillis AM, Connolly SJ, Dubuc M, et al: Circadian variation of paroxysmal atrial fibrillation. Am J Cardiol 2001;87:794-798.

35. Andresen D, Bruggemann T: Heart rate variability preceding onset of atrial fibrillation. J Cardiovasc Electrophysiol 1998;9(8 Suppl):S26-S29.

36. Herweg B, Dalal P, Nagy B, et al: Power spectral analysis of heart period variability of preceding sinus rhythm before initiation of paroxysmal atrial fibrillation. Am J Cardiol 1998;82:869-874.

37. Allessie M: Reentrant mechanisms underlying atrial fibrillation. In Zipes DP, Jalife J (eds): Cardiac Electrophysiology: From Cell to Bedside. Philadelphia, WB Saunders, 1995.

38. Kanagala R, Murali NS, Friedman PA, et al: Obstructive sleep apnea and the recurrence of atrial fibrillation. Circulation 2003;107:2589-2594.

39. Haffajee CI, Chaudhry GM, Casavant D, et al: Efficacy and tolerability of automatic nighttime atrial fibrillation shocks in patients with permanent internal atrial defibrillators. Am J Cardiol 2002;89:875-878.

40. Carlson JT, Hedner JA, Ejnell H, et al: High prevalence of hypertension in sleep apnea patients independent of obesity. Am J Respir Crit Care Med 1994;150:72-77.

41. Hla KM, Young TB, Bidwell T, et al: Sleep apnea and hypertension: A population-based study. Ann Intern Med 1994;120:382-388.

42. Young T, Peppard P, Palta M, et al: Population-based study of sleep-disordered breathing as a risk factor for hypertension. Arch Intern Med 1997;157:1746-1762.

43. Hung J, Whitford EG, Parsons RW, et al: Association of sleep apnoea with myocardial infarction in men. Lancet 1990;336:261-264.

44. Stegman SS, Burroughs JM, Henthorn RW: Asymptomatic bradyarrhythmias as a marker for sleep apnea: Appropriate recognition and treatment may reduce the need for pacemaker therapy. Pacing Clin Electrophysiol 1996;19:899-904.

45. Grimm W, Koehler U, Fus E, et al: Outcome of patients with sleep apnea-associated severe bradyarrhythmias after continuous positive airway pressure therapy. Am J Cardiol 2000;86:688-692.

46. Becker H, Brandenburg U, Peter JH, et al: Reversal of sinus arrest and atrioventricular conduction block in patients with sleep apnea during nasal continuous positive airway pressure. Am J Respir Crit Care Med 1995;151:215-218.

47. Grimm W, Hoffman J, Menz V, et al: Electrophysiologic evaluation of sinus node function and atrioventricular conduction in patients with prolonged ventricular asystole during obstructive sleep apnea. Am J Cardiol 1996;77:1310-1314.

48. Shahar E, Whitney CW, Redline S, et al: Sleep-disordered breathing and cardiovascular disease: Cross-sectional results of the Sleep Heart Health Study. Am J Respir Crit Care Med 2001;163:19-25.

49. Chin K, Ohi M, Kita H, et al: Effects of NCPAP therapy on fibrinogen levels in obstructive sleep apnea syndrome. Am J Respir Crit Care Med 1996;153:1972-1976.

50. Brooks B, Cistulli PA, Borkman M, et al: Obstructive sleep apnea in obese non-insulin-dependent diabetic patients: Effect of continuous positive airway pressure treatment on insulin responsiveness. J Clin Endocrinol Metab 1994;79:1681-1685.

51. Ip MS, Lam B, Ng MM, et al: Obstructive sleep apnea is independently associated with insulin resistance. Am J Respir Crit Care Med 2002;165:670-676.

52. Peled N, Abinader EG, Pillar G, et al: Nocturnal ischemic events in patients with obstructive sleep apnea syndrome and ischemic heart disease: Effects of continuous positive air pressure treatment. J Am Coll Cardiol 1999;34:1744-1749.

53. Somers VK, Dyken ME, Clary MP, et al: Sympathetic neural mechanisms in obstructive sleep apnea. J Clin Invest 1995;96:1897-1904.

54. Sajkov D, Wang T, Saunders NA, et al: Continuous positive airway pressure treatment improves pulmonary hemodynamics in patients with obstructive sleep apnea. Am J Respir Crit Care Med 2002;165:152-158.

55. Narkiewicz K, Kato M, Phillips BG, et al: Nocturnal continuous positive airway pressure decreases daytime sympathetic traffic in obstructive sleep apnea. Circulation 1999;100:2332-2335.

56. Centers for Disease Control and Prevention: Sudden infant death syndrome—United States, 1983–1994. MMWR Morb Mortal Wkly Rep 1996;45:859-863.

57. National Center for Health Statistics: Deaths: Final data for 2001. National Vital Statistics Report 2003;52. Available at http://www.cdc.gov/nchs/data/nvsr/nvsr52/nvsr52_03.pdf.

58. Meny RF, Carroll JL, Carbone MT, et al: Cardiorespiratory recordings from infants dying suddenly and unexpectedly at home. Pediatrics 1994;93:43-49.

59. Kinney HC, Filiano JJ, Sleeper LA, et al: Decreased muscarinic receptor binding in the arcuate nucleus in sudden infant death syndrome. Science 1995;269:1446-1450.

60. Schechtman VL, Harper RK, Harper RM: Aberrant temporal patterning of slow-wave sleep in siblings of SIDS victims. Electroencephalogr Clin Neurophysiol 1995;94:95-102.

61. Pincus SM, Cummins TR, Haddad GG: Heart rate control in normal and aborted-SIDS infants. Am J Physiol 1993;264:R638-R646.

62. Schwartz PJ, Stramba-Badiale M, Segantini A, et al: Prolongation of the QT interval and the sudden infant death syndrome. N Engl J Med 1998;338:1709-1714.

63. Priori SG, Schwartz PJ, Napolitano C, et al: Risk stratification in the long-QT syndrome. N Engl J Med 2003;348:1866-1874.

64. Verrier RL, Nearing BD, LaRovere MT, et al: Ambulatory ECG-based tracking of T-wave alternans in post-myocardial infarction patients to assess risk of cardiac arrest or arrhythmic death. J Cardiovasc Electrophysiol 2003;14:705-711.

65. Smith TA, Mason JM, Bell JS, et al: Sleep apnea and QT interval prolongation: A particularly lethal combination. Am Heart J 1979;97:505-507.

66. Weintraub RG, Gow RM, Wilkinson JL: The congenital long QT syndromes in childhood. J Am Coll Cardiol 1990;16:674-680.

67. Tanel RE, Triedman JK, Walsh EP, et al: High-rate atrial pacing as an innovative bridging therapy in a neonate with congenital long QT syndrome. J Cardiovasc Electrophysiol 1997;8:812-817.

68. Mache CJ, Beitzke A, Haidvogl M, et al: Perinatal manifestations of idiopathic long QT syndrome. Pediatr Cardiol 1996;17:118-121.

69. Bosi G, Cappato R, Priori SG, et al: Complex electrocardiographic findings in a neonate with long QT syndrome. Ital Heart J 2002;3:605-607.

70. Haglund B, Cnattingius S, Otterblad-Olausson P: Sudden infant death syndrome in Sweden, 1983-1990: Season at death, age at death, and maternal smoking. Am J Epidemiol 1995;142:619-624.

71. Douglas AS, Allan TM, Helms PJ: Seasonality and the sudden infant death syndrome during 1987-9 and 1991-3 in Australia and Britain. BMJ 1996;312:1381-1383.

72. Gupta R, Helms PJ, Jolliffe IT, et al: Seasonal variation in sudden infant death syndrome and bronchiolitis: A common mechanism? Am J Respir Crit Care Med 1996;154:431-435.

73. Oyen N, Skjaerven R, Irgens LM: Population-based recurrence risk of sudden infant death syndrome compared with other infant and fetal deaths. Am J Epidemiol 1996;144:300-305.

74. Tishler PV, Redline S, Ferrette V, et al: The association of sudden unexpected infant death with obstructive sleep apnea. Am J Respir Crit Care Med 1996;153:1857-1863.

75. Dwyer T, Ponsonby AL, Blizzard L, et al: The contribution of changes in the prevalence of prone sleeping position to the decline in sudden infant death syndrome in Tasmania. JAMA 1995;273:783-789.

76. Klonoff-Cohen HS, Edelstein SL: A case-control study of routine and death scene sleep position and sudden infant death syndrome in Southern California. JAMA 1995;273:790-794.

77. Klonoff-Cohen HS, Edelstein SL, Lefkowitz ES, et al: The effect of passive smoking and tobacco exposure through breast milk on sudden infant death syndrome. JAMA 1995;273:795-798.

78. Fleming PJ, Blair PS, Bacon C, et al: Environment of infants during sleep and risk of the sudden infant death syndrome: Results of 1993-1995 case-control study for confidential inquiry into stillbirths and deaths in infancy. Confidential Enquiry into Stillbirths and Deaths Regional Coordinators and Researchers. BMJ 1996;313:191-195.

79. Brooke H, Gibson A, Tappin D, et al: Case-control study of sudden infant death syndrome in Scotland, 1992-5. BMJ 1997;314:1516-1520.

80. Blair PS, Fleming PJ, Bensley D, et al: Smoking and the sudden infant death syndrome: Results from 1993-5 case-control study for confidential inquiry into stillbirths and deaths in infancy. Confidential Enquiry into Stillbirths and Deaths Regional Coordinators and Researchers. BMJ 1996;313:195-198.

81. MacDorman MF, Cnattingius S, Hoffman HJ, et al: Sudden infant death syndrome and smoking in the United States and Sweden. Am J Epidemiol 1997;146:249-257.

82. Schellscheidt J, Oyen N, Jorch G: Interactions between maternal smoking and other prenatal risk factors for sudden infant death syndrome (SIDS). Acta Paediatr 1997;96:857-863.

83. Wingkun JG, Knisely JS, Schnoll SH, et al: Decreased carbon dioxide sensitivity in infants of substance-abusing mothers. Pediatrics 1995;95:864-867.

84. Slotkin TA, Lappi SE, McCook EC, et al: Loss of neonatal hypoxia tolerance after prenatal nicotine exposure: Implications for sudden infant death syndrome. Brain Res Bull 1995;38:69-75.

85. Cutz E, Ma TK, Perrin DG, et al: Peripheral chemoreceptors in congenital central hypoventilation syndrome. Am J Respir Crit Care Med 1997;155:358-363.

86. Milerad J, Majs J, Gidlund E: Nicotine and cotinine levels in pericardial fluid in victims of SIDS. Acta Pediatr 1994;93:59-62.

87. Rajs J, Rasten-Almqvist P, Falck G, et al: Sudden infant death syndrome: postmortem findings of nicotine and cotinine in pericardial fluid of infants in relation to morphological changes and position at death. Pediatr Pathol Lab Med 1997;17:83-97.

88. Evans RG, Ludbrook J, Michalicek J: Use of nicotine, bradykinin and veratridine to elicit cardiovascular chemoreflexes in unanesthetized rabbits. Clin Exp Pharmacol Physiol 1991;18:245-254.

89. Staszewska-Barczak J: Prostanoids and cardiac reflexes of sympathetic and vagal origin. Am J Cardiol 1983;52:36A-45A.

90. Barber MJ, Mueller TM, Davies BG, et al: Phenol topically applied to canine left ventricular epicardium interrupts sympathetic but not vagal afferents. Circ Res 1984;55:532-544.

91. Antzelevitch C, Brugada P, Brugada J, et al: Brugada syndrome: A decade of progress. Circ Res 2002;91:1114-1118.

92. Nademanee K, Veerakul G, Mower M, et al: Defibrillator Versus Beta-Blockers For Unexplained Death in Thailand (DEBUT): A randomized clinical trial. Circulation 2003;107:2221-2226.

93. Wichter T, Matheja P, Eckardt L, et al: Cardiac autonomic dysfunction in Brugada syndrome. Circulation 2002;105:702-706.

94. National Center for Health Statistics: Update: Sudden unexplained death syndrome among Southeast Asian refugees—United States. MMWR Morb Mortal Wkly Rep 1988;37:568-570. Available at http://www.cdc.gov/mmwr/preview/mmwrhtml/00001278.htm.

95. Munger RG: Sudden death in sleep of Laotian-Hmong refugees in Thailand: A case-control study. Am J Public Health 1987;77:1187-1190.

96. Krittayaphong R, Veerakul G, Bhuripanyo K, et al: Heart rate variability in patients with sudden unexpected cardiac arrest in Thailand. Am J Cardiol 2003;91:77-81.

97. Garrick NA, Tamarkin L, Taylor PL, et al: Light and propranolol suppress the nocturnal elevation of serotonin in the cerebrospinal fluid of rhesus monkeys. Science 1983;221:474-476.

98. Bucknall CA, Keeton BR, Curry PV, et al: Intravenous and oral amiodarone for arrhythmias in children. Br Heart J 1986;56:278-284.

99. Hilleman D, Miller MA, Parker R, et al: Optimal management of amiodarone therapy: Efficacy and side effects. Pharmacotherapy 1998;18:138S-145S.

100. Schmidt G, Malik M, Barthel P, et al: Heart-rate turbulence after ventricular premature beats as a predictor of mortality after acute myocardial infarction. Lancet 1999;353:1390-1396.

Cardiovascular Effects of Sleep-Related Breathing Disorders

Virend K. Somers

Shahrokh Javaheri

ABSTRACT

The cycle of apnea–recovery causes (1) hypoxemia–reoxygenation, (2) hypercapnia–hypocapnia, (3) changes in intrathoracic pressure, and arousals. These consequences of sleep apnea, both obstructive and central apnea, adversely affect cardiovascular function. The cardiovascular effects of sleep apnea may be mediated by redox-sensitive gene activation, altered autonomic nervous system activity, oxidative stress, and release of inflammatory mediators. Pathophysiologic consequences of sleep apnea elicit acute and chronic cardiovascular changes.

Hemodynamic changes have been most studied in obstructive sleep apnea. Studies in humans document that exposure to obstructive sleep apnea elicits acute hemodynamic changes. Chronic exposure results in left ventricular systolic and diastolic dysfunction. A limited number of studies have shown that treatment of obstructive sleep apnea with nasal continuous positive airway pressure devices or tracheostomy can result in reversal of left ventricular dysfunction and arrhythmias.

Periodic breathing is characterized by cyclic changes in tidal breathing with intervening episodes of obstructive or central apnea or hypopnea. These disordered breathing events result in three basic pathophysiologic consequences: (1) intermittent arterial blood gas abnormalities characterized by hypoxemia–reoxygenation and hypercapnia–hypocapnia; (2) arousals and shift to light sleep stages; and (3) large negative swings in intrathoracic pressure[1-3] (Fig. 99–1). These pathophysiologic consequences of apnea and hypopnea, both obstructive and central, adversely affect cardiovascular function, acutely and chronically.

ARTERIAL BLOOD GAS ABNORMALITIES AND THEIR CONSEQUENCES

Periodic breathing consists of cyclic changes in breathing pattern that include episodes of apnea and hypopnea, resulting in hypoxemia and hypercapnia. After apnea and hypopnea, hyperpnea ensues, resulting in reoxygenation and hypocapnia. The alterations in blood gases affect the cardiovascular system in different ways.

Hypoxemia–Reoxygenation

Hypoxemia has direct (decreased myocardial oxygen delivery) and indirect (activation of sympathetic nervous system, promotion of endothelial cell dysfunction, and pulmonary arteriolar vasoconstriction) cardiovascular effects. Hypoxemia with reoxygenation may be analogous to ischemia–reperfusion, and reoxygenation may cause additional damage through further production of free radical species. Biochemical injury due to hypoxemia–reoxygenation has considerable relevance to sleep apnea–hypopnea, where intermittent and profound alterations in the partial pressure of oxygen (PO_2) may occur many times during sleep.

Direct Effects of Hypoxia on Myocardium

Decreased myocardial oxygen delivery may result in an imbalance between myocardial oxygen consumption and demand, resulting in myocardial hypoxia, particularly if there is already coronary artery disease. Potential clinical consequences include nocturnal angina, myocardial infarction, and arrhythmias. Hypoxia may also impair myocardial contractility and cause diastolic dysfunction.[4,5]

Hypoxemia–Reoxygenation and Coronary Endothelial Dysfunction

Coronary vessel endothelial cells play a central role in vasoregulation, coagulation, and inflammation.[6,7] Blood flow and coagulation are modulated by production and release of vasoactive substances that include vasodilators and platelet deaggregators (e.g., nitric oxide, prostacyclin), and vasoconstrictors and platelet aggregators (e.g., endothelin and thromboxane). The balance between vasoregulatory agents is important in regulating coronary blood flow and coagulation status in both health and disease.

Through activation of certain transcription factors such as hypoxia-inducible factor-1 and nuclear factor-κB,[8,9] hypoxia increases the expression of a number of genes such as those encoding endothelin-1, a potent vasoconstrictor with proinflammatory properties, vascular endothelial growth factor, and platelet-derived growth factor. In contrast, hypoxia suppresses the transcriptional rate of endothelial nitric oxide synthase,[10] resulting in decreased production of nitric oxide, which is vasodilatory and has antimitogenic properties. Hypoxia enhances expression of adhesion molecules and promotes leukocyte rolling and endothelial adherence.[11] Hypoxia is also involved in induction of endothelial and myocyte apoptosis.[12]

Some of the aforementioned adverse effects of sustained hypoxia have also been observed with intermittent hypoxia (i.e., hypoxia–reoxygenation).[13-23] In this context, intermittent hypoxia has been proposed to be more deleterious than sustained hypoxia.[18,19] Reoxygenation through delivery of

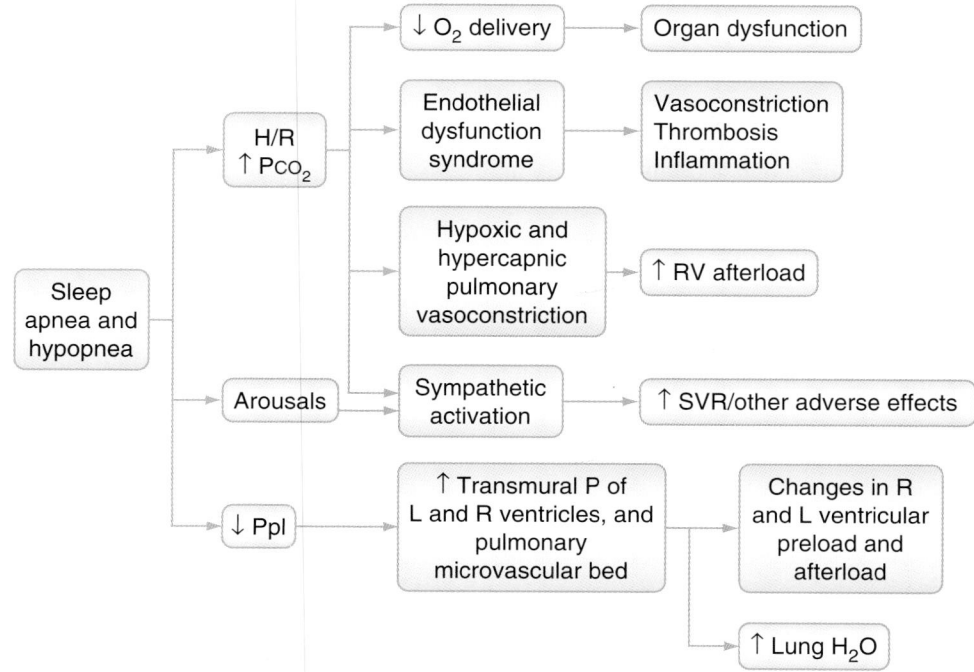

Figure 99–1. Pathophysiologic consequences of sleep apnea and hypopnea. Pleural pressure (Ppl) is a surrogate of the pressure surrounding the heart and other vascular structures. H/R, hypoxia–reoxygenation; ↑, increased; ↓, decreased; RV, right ventricular; SVR, systemic vascular resistance; R, right; L, left; P, pressure. (Adapted from Javaheri S: Sleep-related breathing disorders in heart failure. In Mann DL (ed): Heart Failure: A Companion to Braunwald's Heart Disease. Philadelphia, Saunders, 2003, p 478.)

oxygen molecules provides a substrate for additional production of oxygen radicals and may contribute to oxidative stress.

The pathophysiologic consequences of hypoxemia–reoxygenation could lead to vascular inflammation and remodeling, similar to atherosclerosis.[6,23] Endothelial dysfunction has been demonstrated in a number of cardiovascular disorders, including hypertension, myocardial infarction, and stroke. Interestingly, these disorders have been also associated with obstructive sleep apnea (OSA). It is therefore conceivable that endothelial dysfunction due to sleep-related breathing disorders may contribute to worsening of atherosclerosis, atherothrombosis, and left ventricular dysfunction.[1,24]

The inflammatory and neurohormonal (see later) consequences of altered blood gas chemistry have been best studied in patients with OSA. OSA has been shown to be associated with increased sympathetic activity, high concentrations of endothelin, adhesion molecules, and inflammatory cytokines, activation of white blood cells, oxidative stress, and hypercoagulopathy.[1,22,24-39] These biochemical alterations may be reversed with use of nasal continuous positive airway pressure (CPAP) to treat OSA. However, such systematic studies are lacking in central sleep apnea, with the exception of studies showing increased overnight and morning sympathetic activity in patients with heart failure with central sleep apnea compared with those without central sleep apnea[40] (for details, see Chapter 102).

Hypoxemia–Hypercapnia and the Autonomic Nervous System

Sleep apneas and hypopneas, both obstructive and central (Figs. 99–2 and 99–3), increase sympathetic activity through complex mechanisms. Hypoxemia stimulates the peripheral arterial chemoreceptors in the carotid bodies, triggering reflex increases in sympathetic activity.[41,42] Hypercapnia acts primarily on the central chemoreceptors located in the region of the brainstem, also increasing sympathetic activity.

Both hypoxemia and hypercapnia increase ventilation, which, perhaps acting though the thoracic afferents, buffers the increases in sympathetic drive during hypoxemia, and to a lesser extent during hypercapnia.[41,42] Thus, when hypoxemia or hypercapnia occurs during apnea, the absence of ventilatory inhibition results in a potentiation of sympathetic activation and consequent vasoconstriction and blood pressure surges. In this context, and especially when there are potentiated chemoreflex responses to hypoxemia–hypercapnia,[43,44] the sympathetic and pressor responses to hypoxemia–hypercapnia, particularly in the absence of inhibitory effects of breathing, are marked.

Alveolar Hypoxia–Hypercapnia and Pulmonary Arteriolar Vasoconstriction

Alveolar hypoxia, in part through release of endothelin, and hypercapnia cause pulmonary arteriolar vasoconstriction and hypertension, which could adversely affect right ventricular function (see Chapter 100).

Hypocapnia

Episodes of hyperpnea after apneas and hypopneas result in hypocapnia. Hypocapnia may impair myocardial oxygen delivery and uptake by coronary artery vasoconstriction[45] and shifting of the oxygen–hemoglobin dissociation curve to the left. Hypocapnia may also contribute to arrhythmogenesis.

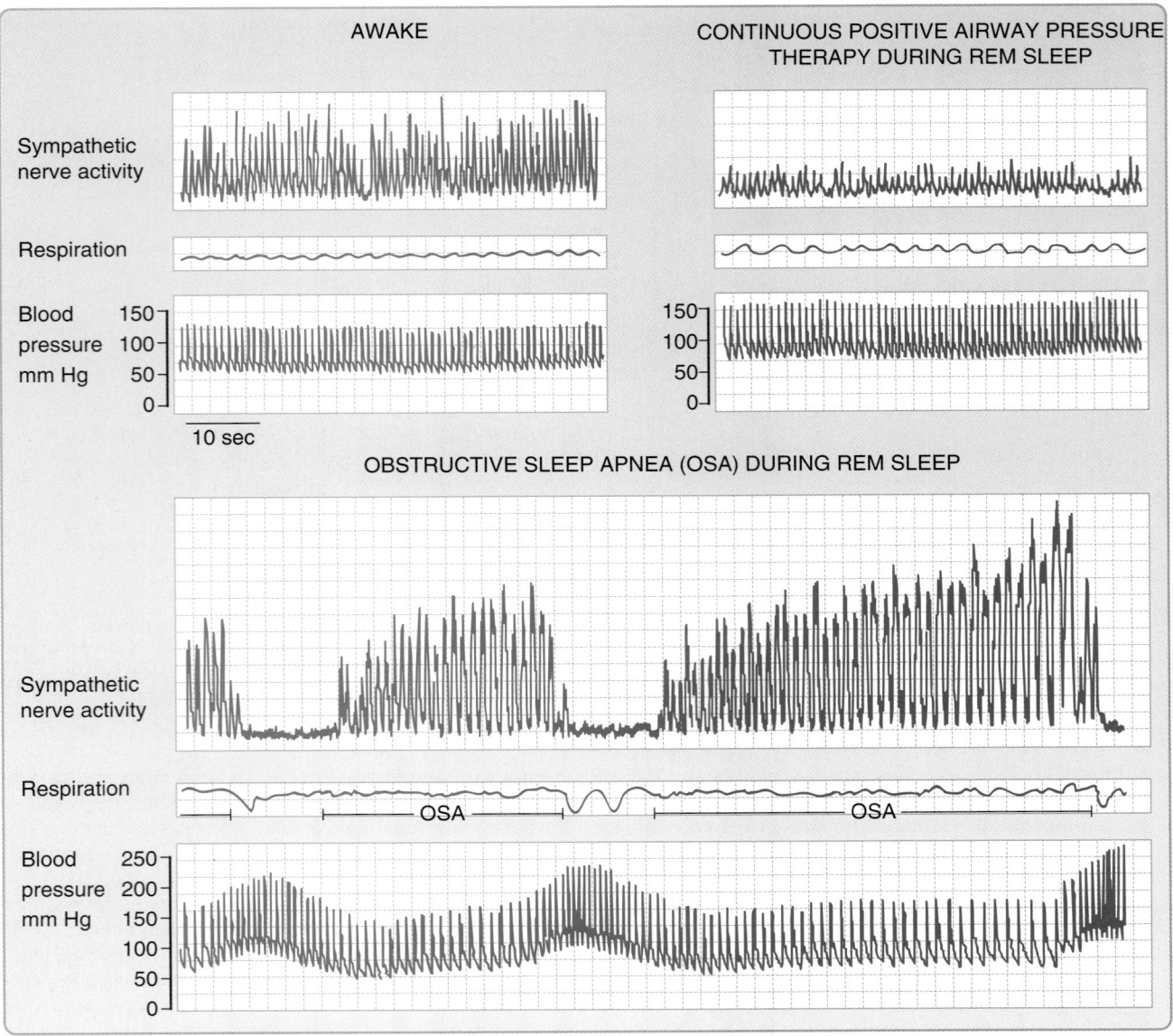

Figure 99–2. Recordings of sympathetic nerve activity, intraarterial blood pressure, and breathing in a normotensive patient with obstructive sleep apnea (OSA) during resting normoxic wakefulness (*top left panel*). The patient was free of any other overt cardiovascular disease and on no medications. Note the high levels of sympathetic nerve traffic even in the absence of apneic events. During rapid eye movement (REM) sleep (*lower panel*), the repetitive hypoxemia and hypercapnia elicit chemoreflex-mediated sympathetic activation and vasoconstriction. At the end of apneas, with increases in cardiac output and severe vasoconstriction, intraarterial blood pressure can reach levels from 130/60 mm Hg during wakefulness to a peak of 220/130 mm Hg during apneas. At the end of apneas, there also is abrupt inhibition of sympathetic traffic because of the increase in blood pressure acting through the baroreflexes and the sympathetic inhibitory effects of the thoracic afferents. After treatment of OSA with continuous positive airway pressure (*top right panel*), there is a marked reduction in sympathetic traffic and in blood pressure. (From Somers VK, Dyken ME, Clary MP, et al: Sympathetic neural mechanisms in obstructive sleep apnea. J Clin Invest 1995;96:1897-1904.)

AROUSALS, SHIFT TO LIGHT SLEEP STAGES, AND THE AUTONOMIC NERVOUS SYSTEM

Compared with wakefulness, the balance of activity of sympathetic and parasympathetic nervous system reverses in normal sleep.[46,47] Normally, there is a progressive reduction in sympathetic nerve traffic, heart rate, and blood pressure during the deepening stages of non–rapid eye movement sleep, such that sympathetic activity, heart rate, and blood pressure in stage 4 sleep are substantially lower than during

supine resting wakefulness.[46,47] During phasic rapid eye movement (REM) sleep, there is an abrupt increase in sympathetic activity, resulting in intermittent and brief surges in blood pressure and heart rate. On average, blood pressure and heart rate during REM sleep are similar to levels recorded during wakefulness. Thus, during normal sleep, there is a well-regulated pattern of alteration in autonomic and hemodynamic measures, modulated by changes in sleep stage. These organized responses to normal sleep are completely disrupted in patients with sleep-related breathing disorders, both obstructive and central sleep apnea. Sleep architecture is dramatically

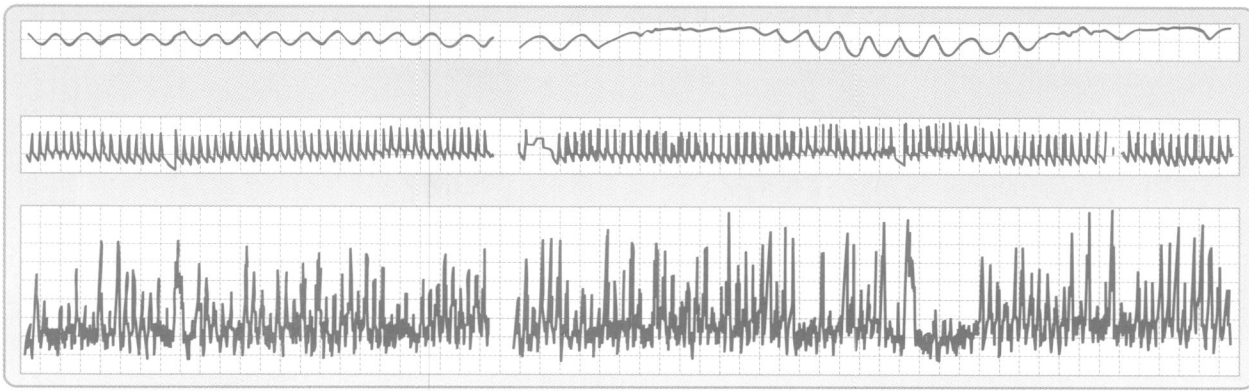

Figure 99–3. Recordings of breathing (*top*), beat-by-beat blood pressure (*middle*), and muscle sympathetic nerve activity (MSNA; *bottom*) in a patient with severe congestive heart failure, during normal breathing on the *left* and during Cheyne-Stokes breathing on the *right*. Oxygen saturation was 94% during normal breathing and oscillated between 97% and 90% during Cheyne-Stokes breathing. MSNA total burst amplitude increased from 1533 arbitrary units per minute during normal breathing to 1759 arbitrary units per minute during Cheyne-Stokes breathing. Mean blood pressure was 70 mm Hg during normal breathing and peaked at 82 mm Hg during the hyperventilation that followed central apnea. Patients with heart failure have high levels of sympathetic drive even during normal breathing. During central apneas, there is a modest but significant further increase in sympathetic activity.

altered in patients with OSA–hypopnea, and also in patients with heart failure and central sleep apnea. There is a shift to light sleep stages. Most important, however, apneas and hypopneas commonly result in arousals that are also associated with an increase in sympathetic activity and a decrease in parasympathetic activity,[47,48] increasing blood pressure and heart rate. In OSA, arousals occur at the end of the apnea and result in patency of the upper airway and resumption of breathing. In patients with central sleep apnea and a Cheyne-Stokes respiration pattern, arousals occur at the peak of hyperventilation, further disrupting sleep quality.

In addition to arousals, sleep-related breathing disorders may increase sympathetic activity by hypoxemia, hypercapnia, and changes in ventilation, as noted previously.

There are multiple adverse cardiac consequences of sympathetic activation. These include increased systemic vascular resistance and left ventricular afterload, venoconstriction with increased right ventricular preload, increased myocardial contractility, hypertrophy, tachycardia, and arrhythmias. Furthermore, increased myocardial norepinephrine may cause myocyte toxicity and apoptosis.[49,50]

Central sleep apnea and OSA increase sympathetic activity as measured by either microneurography or blood and urinary norepinephrine levels.[51-56] Treatment of obstructive[54-56] and central sleep apnea[52,57] decreases sympathetic activity, with important implications. First, with regard to central sleep apnea in heart failure, increased sympathetic activity is associated with poor survival; therefore, a reduction in sympathetic activity should have favorable prognostic implications. OSA causes nocturnal increases in sympathetic activity and blood pressure, which carry over into the daytime. OSA is a known cause of hypertension, and blood pressure decreases relatively quickly with effective treatment of OSA with CPAP (see Chapter 100).

In summary, pathophysiologic consequences of sleep-related breathing disorders, such as increased periods of wakefulness (interruption insomnia), arousals, hypoxemia, and hypercapnia, collectively contribute to increased sympathetic activity.

EXAGGERATED NEGATIVE INTRATHORACIC PRESSURE AND ITS CONSEQUENCES

Large negative intrathoracic pressures are generated during episodes of obstructive apnea. In central sleep apnea, relatively large negative pressure deflections occur during hyperpnea, particularly in the face of less compliant (stiff) lungs (due to heart failure). However, pleural pressure changes are usually more pronounced in obstructive than in central sleep apnea.

There are a large number of studies addressing the cardiovascular consequences of both negative and positive pressure deflections affecting right and left ventricular function.[58,59] Negative intrathoracic pressure increases the transmural pressure (pressure inside minus pressure outside; Fig. 99–4) of the intrathoracic vascular structures, including aorta, pulmonary vascular bed, and ventricles.

According to Laplace's law, increased transmural myocardial pressure increases wall tension and myocardial oxygen consumption. Furthermore, negative intrathoracic perivascular pressure could increase extravascular lung water by favoring fluid transudation across the pulmonary microvascular bed and by diminishing lymph outflow from the lung.[60] This may account in part for cases of flash pulmonary edema reported in OSA, and sleep apnea may contribute to excess lung water and pulmonary edema in congestive heart failure. In addition, decreased intrathoracic pressure increases venous inflow, resulting in increased right ventricular diastolic size, which in turn may decrease left ventricular compliance and volume, a phenomenon called *ventricular interdependence*. Application of nasal CPAP to treat sleep apnea, both obstructive and central, reduces transmural pressure by two mechanisms. First, and most important, it decreases or eliminates apneas, desaturation, and arousals, which collectively increase sympathetic activity and result in cyclic surges in arterial blood pressure. Second, nasal CPAP not only attenuates steep surges in intrathoracic pressure, it actually increases the pleural pressure, thus decreasing transmural pressures across intrathoracic structures (see Fig. 99–4).

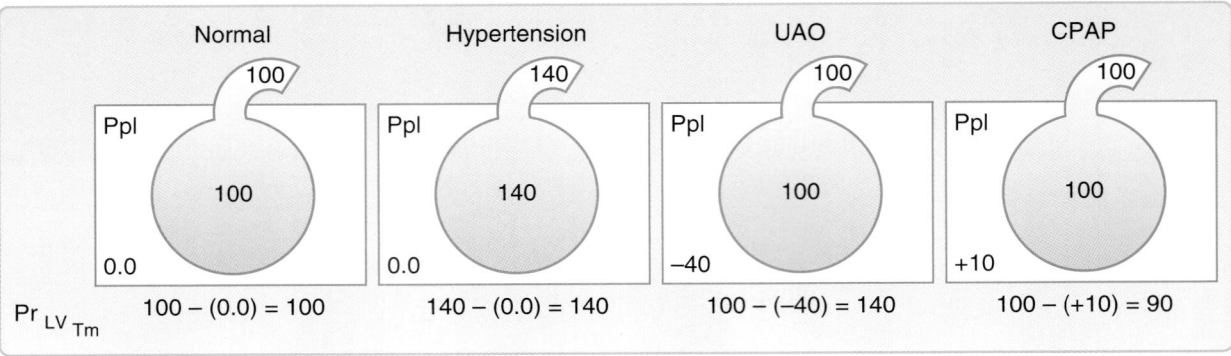

Figure 99–4. Transmural (Tm) pressure (Pr) of the left ventricle (LV) during systole. Because of an obstructive apnea (UAO, upper airway occlusion), a negative pleural pressure (Ppl) of –40 mm Hg is generated. This increases left ventricular transmural pressure from 100 to 140 mm Hg, which is equivalent to an increase in systolic aortic blood pressure from 100 to 140 mm Hg. Note the reduction in left ventricular transmural pressure with application of nasal continuous positive airway pressure (CPAP). (Adapted from Javaheri S: Sleep-related breathing disorders in heart failure. In Mann DL (ed): Heart Failure: A Companion to Braunwald's Heart Disease. Philadelphia, Saunders, 2003, p 480.)

ACUTE HEMODYNAMIC EFFECTS OF SLEEP APNEA

The circulatory responses to individual apneas and hypopneas are governed by the interaction of stresses and physiologic consequences described previously.[61,62] Hemodynamic changes are related to development of hypoxemia, hypercapnia, presence or absence of breathing, changes in intrathoracic pressure, and the consequent mechanical effects.

Hemodynamic changes have been best studied in human OSA.[61,63,64] The evolution of a cycle of apnea–recovery is complex and represents an unsteady hemodynamic state. For these reasons, hemodynamic changes occur during the course of an apnea, and these changes are different from those occurring during the immediate or late postapnea periods. During recovery, arousals and ventilation further affect hemodynamics. Cyclic changes in heart rate and systemic and pulmonary arterial blood pressure paralleling periodic breathing occur commonly.[61,63-66] In some patients, there is a very clear and progressive bradycardia toward the end of apnea, with abrupt development of tachycardia with resumption of breathing, because of the vagolytic effects of lung inflation and arousals. This manifests as a pattern of repetitive bradycardias/tachycardias during sleep, which may be evident on Holter monitoring and may signify the presence of OSA. In experimental sleep apnea, decreases in heart rate are more severe during central than obstructive apnea, reflecting lack of activation of thoracic afferents.[62]

The bradycardias may be especially severe,[65,66] and are elicited because of activation of the diving reflex by the combination of hypoxemia and apnea. Episodes of up to 10 seconds or more of sinus arrest may occur because of the chemoreflex-mediated vagal activation. The consequent absence of perfusion, because of asystole, may have implications for patients with preexisting severe cerebral or cardiac ischemia.

At the termination of obstructive apneas, there are surges in blood pressure. This cyclic change in blood pressure is one of the most consistent hemodynamic findings in OSA. Multiple mechanisms are involved. During apnea, the increased hypoxemia and hypercapnia, acting through the chemoreflexes, progressively elicit sympathetic activation and vasoconstriction.[53] With resumption of breathing, because of the inspiratory increase in right ventricular filling, stroke volume may increase. Vagolytic effects of inspiration result in tachycardia. The increased stroke volume and heart rate result in an increased cardiac output entering a vasoconstricted peripheral circulation, with consequent acute increases in blood pressure.[53] However, just after termination of an obstructive apnea, there is abrupt inhibition of sympathetic activity to the peripheral blood vessels, in part because the deep breathing inhibits sympathetic activity through thoracic afferents, and in part because of baroreflex inhibition of sympathetic activity secondary to the postapneic blood pressure surge. Nevertheless, despite the interruption in sympathetic nerve traffic, vasoconstriction persists for several seconds after termination of the sympathetic nerve discharge because of the kinetics of norepinephrine uptake, release, and washout at the neurovascular junction.

Another consistent finding is a mild reduction in stroke volume during obstructive apnea, which has been documented using noninvasive techniques for measuring beat-to-beat cardiac output.[61] This is probably due to a decrease in left ventricular preload and an increase in afterload. Changes in stroke volume after termination of the apnea depend on where in the recovery cycle it is being measured.[61]

OBSTRUCTIVE SLEEP APNEA, LEFT VENTRICULAR DYSFUNCTION, AND HEART FAILURE

The relation between central sleep apnea and heart failure is discussed in Chapter 102. In this section, we review OSA as a cause of heart failure.

Obstructive Sleep Apnea and Systolic Heart Failure

In a canine model mimicking severe OSA,[67] within a 1- to 3-month period of exposure to apneas during sleep, left ventricular systolic dysfunction developed. Left ventricular ejection fraction, measured during the daytime, decreased significantly because of an increase in left ventricular systolic volume.

In humans, there are two kinds of studies relating left ventricular systolic dysfunction and OSA: first, studies in which patients with OSA have been assessed for the presence of left ventricular dysfunction,[68-71] and second, studies in patients with established left ventricular systolic dysfunction who have been assessed to determine the prevalence of OSA.[72,73] In some studies,[74-76] changes in left ventricular ejection fraction in response to treatment of OSA have been also described.

Results of studies assessing left ventricular systolic function in OSA patients are conflicting.[68-70] However, in the two studies[69,70] in which technetium-99m was used to assess left ventricular systolic function, OSA was associated with left ventricular systolic dysfunction. Use of radionuclide ventriculography to assess left ventricular function is important because in obese subjects, echocardiography, which has been used in some studies, may be associated with technical difficulties.

Alchanatis et al.[69] studied 29 patients with severe OSA (apnea-hypopnea index [AHI] greater than 15/hour; mean AHI, 54/hour; lowest arterial oxygen saturation, 62%) and 12 control subjects (AHI, 9/hour; lowest saturation, 92%). The subjects were without known cardiovascular disease. The mean left ventricular ejection fraction was significantly lower in patients with OSA compared with the control group (53% versus 61%; P <.003). Six months after treatment with CPAP, left ventricular ejection fraction increased significantly to 56% (P <.001). Left ventricular diastolic dysfunction also improved significantly (see later).

In a large study[70] of 169 patients with OSA (AHI greater than 10/hour; mean AHI, 47/hour), 13 subjects (8%) had left ventricular systolic dysfunction (range, 32% to 50%). Left ventricular systolic dysfunction was not due to ischemic disease as evidenced by echocardiography and dipyridamole stress testing. In seven patients who were treated for OSA (six with CPAP and one with upper airway surgery), 1 year after therapy, mean left ventricular ejection increased significantly from 44% to 63%.[70]

In the cross-sectional analysis of over 6000 patients enrolled in the Sleep Health Heart Study,[71] the presence of OSA increased the likelihood of having a history of heart failure by an odds ratio of 2.5. Furthermore, there was a significant dose-dependent correlation between AHI and the prevalence of heart failure.

In studies of patients with established left ventricular systolic dysfunction undergoing polysomnography (reviewed in Chapter 102), the prevalence of OSA, defined as an AHI of at least 15/hour, ranged from 5% to 32%. This wide range is not particularly surprising. The prevalence depends on a number of factors, including the number of obese patients with heart failure enrolled in each study and the different polysomnographic criteria used by various investigators for diagnosis of OSA.

In a prospective study[72] of 81 patients with known systolic dysfunction and in whom no question was asked regarding snoring or other symptoms associated with OSA, 11% had OSA with a mean AHI of 36/hour and a lowest arterial oxygen saturation of 72%. In a retrospective study[73] of 450 patients with systolic dysfunction who were referred for a sleep study because of loud snoring and other symptoms of sleep apnea, 32% had OSA. From the aforementioned studies, however, it cannot be determined whether OSA preceded heart failure. Yet, as is discussed later, treatment of OSA with nasal CPAP increases left ventricular ejection fraction, indicating that OSA contributes to worsening of left ventricular systolic dysfunction.

The mechanisms by which OSA may impair left ventricular systolic function are multiple. Hypoxemia plays a critical role, both by impairing myocardial contractility and through a host of neurohormonal mechanisms. In addition, increases in left ventricular wall stress and transmural pressure occur because of additive effects of the excess negative juxtacardiac pressure (during obstructive apneas) and development of hypertension.

Two studies involving a small number of patients report that treatment of OSA with CPAP improves left ventricular systolic function.[69,70] In one study,[69] ejection fraction increased significantly from 53% to 56% after 6 months of therapy, and in the other from 44% to 63% after 1 year.[70] On the other hand, two randomized studies of subjects with known heart failure and left ventricular systolic dysfunction report that use of CPAP to treat OSA significantly increased left ventricular ejection fraction within 1 to 3 months[75,76] (Fig. 99–5). This finding has important implications because in systolic heart failure, ejection fraction predicts survival.

Obstructive Sleep Apnea and Diastolic Heart Failure

Isolated left ventricular diastolic heart failure with relative preservation of left ventricular systolic function is the most common form of heart failure in elderly subjects. The pathophysiologic consequences of this form of heart failure relate to a hypertrophied, noncompliant left ventricle, shifting the pressure–volume curve upward and to the left. Therefore, for a given left ventricular volume, left ventricular end-diastolic pressure increases, resulting in elevated left atrial and pulmonary capillary pressure, and pulmonary congestion and edema.

As noted previously, hemodynamic studies[63,64] of patients with OSA have documented that pulmonary capillary pressure increases during the course of an obstructive apnea, indicating development of diastolic dysfunction. During obstructive apnea, left ventricular transmural wall tension increases because of an increase in aortic blood pressure and a simultaneous decrease in juxtacardiac pressure. Furthermore, hypoxemia may impair left ventricular relaxation, further impairing diastolic function.[77] Repeated exposure to nocturnal hypertension and hypoxemia, and consequent development of OSA-induced systemic hypertension and increased left ventricular mass, may also contribute to left ventricular diastolic dysfunction.

Some studies, but not all, show that OSA is associated with an increase in left ventricular mass.[78-81] An early study[78] reported that OSA may cause left ventricular hypertrophy even in the absence of daytime systemic hypertension. This finding was later supported by another study[79] comparing patients with OSA (AHI greater than 20/hour) with those without OSA (AHI less than 20/hour).

In the largest study,[81] consisting of 533 subjects referred to a sleep laboratory, patients with OSA (n = 353; AHI greater than 5/hour) had a significantly greater left ventricular mass than patients without OSA (n = 180; AHI less than 5/hour). In multiple regression analysis, left ventricular mass correlated with body mass index, age, and hypertension, but not with AHI or desaturation. This is not surprising because if OSA causes an increase in left ventricular mass, hypertension may well be the main mechanism for this effect. Nevertheless, the multiple comorbidities associated with OSA make any clear

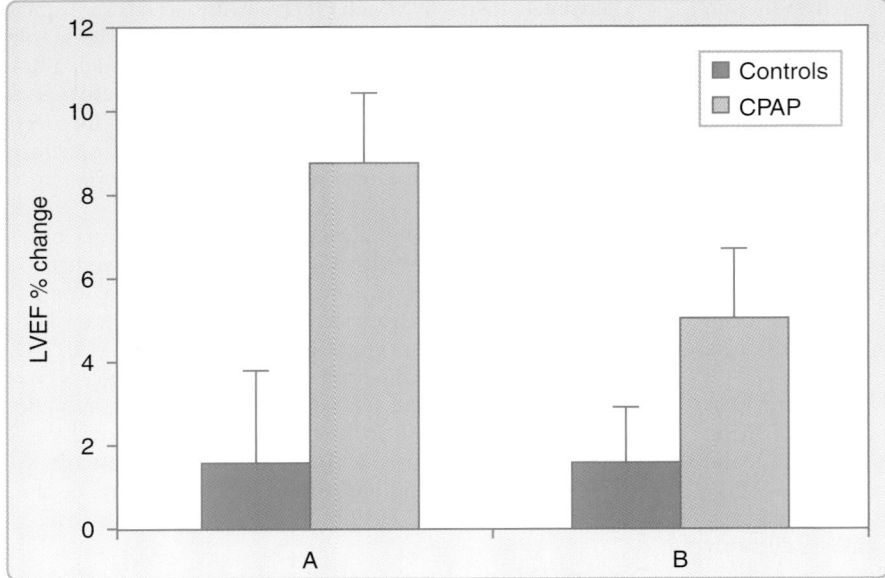

Figure 99–5. Data from two randomized studies of treatment of obstructive sleep apnea in heart failure showing increases in left ventricular ejection fraction (LVEF) in untreated control subjects compared with patients treated with continuous positive airway pressure (CPAP) for 1 month (**A**) to 3 months (**B**). (**A** adapted from Kaneko Y, Floras JS, Usui K, et al: Cardiovascular effects of continuous positive airway pressure in patients with heart failure and obstructive sleep apnea. N Engl J Med 2003;348:1233-1241; **B** adapted from Mansfield DR, Gollogly NC, Kaye DM, et al: Controlled trial of continuous positive airway pressure in obstructive sleep apnea and heart failure. Am J Respir Crit Care Med 2004; 169:361-366.)

cause–effect relationship between OSA and left ventricular hypertrophy difficult to quantify definitively.

Although the prevalence of sleep apnea in patients with systolic heart failure has been systematically studied,[72,73] the prevalence and the impact of OSA in diastolic heart failure need to be determined. In one study[82] of 20 patients with diastolic heart failure, approximately half of the patients had sleep apnea. As noted earlier, isolated diastolic heart failure is highly prevalent in elderly subjects. Furthermore, elderly subjects have a high prevalence of OSA. It is speculated that OSA could be the cause of diastolic heart failure, or the presence of OSA could contribute to the worsening of left ventricular diastolic dysfunction. In this regard, a preliminary study reports that treatment of OSA improves left ventricular diastolic dysfunction,[69] an observation similar to the improvement seen in systolic function when patients with heart failure and OSA are treated with CPAP[74-76] (see Fig. 99–5).

ARRHYTHMIAS IN OBSTRUCTIVE SLEEP APNEA

Obstructive Sleep Apnea Predisposing to an Arrhythmogenic Substrate

Repetitive nocturnal apneas elicit severe derangements in cardiovascular homeostasis. Hypoxemia, hypercapnia, acidosis, adrenergic activation, increased afterload, and rapid fluctuations in cardiac wall stress would reasonably be expected to be conducive to tachycardia–brachycardia oscillations and atrial and ventricular arrhythmias (Figs. 99–6 and 99–7). A variety of atrioventricular arrhythmias, including complete heart block and ventricular asystole during sleep, have been observed in patients with OSA[83-85] and have been eliminated by either tracheostomy or use of nasal CPAP.[83,84] Profound OSA-induced arrhythmias can occur in the absence of any major structural abnormalities in the conduction system.[85]

Although the normal heart would be less likely to manifest malignant arrhythmias in the setting of severe obstructive apnea, the ischemic, hypertrophied, or failing heart would be more susceptible.[86] Nevertheless, activation of the diving reflex[66,87,88] during apneas can elicit often severe brady-arrhythmias, even in the setting of a normal myocardium and normal cardiac electrophysiologic function.

Tachycardia–Bradycardia Oscillations

Patients undergoing Holter monitoring may be noted to have repetitive cyclic episodes of tachycardias and bradycardias during the night.[89,90] These cyclic fluctuations may be attributable to obstructive apneas, although this cannot be confirmed because standard Holter monitoring does not incorporate simultaneous measurements of either breathing pattern or oxygen saturation.

These oscillations in cardiac rate are for the most part explained by changes in cardiac autonomic drive related to breathing pattern. During the course of apnea, incremental hypoxemia elicits the diving reflex so that bradycardia becomes progressively more marked. With termination of apnea, hyperpnea occurs with consequent activation of thoracic afferents, which is vagolytic.[91] Thus, with resumption of breathing, abrupt lung inflation interrupts vagal drive to the heart, resulting in rapid-onset tachycardia. Furthermore, increased cardiac-bound sympathetic drive and withdrawal of parasympathetic activity due to arousals should also contribute to the tachycardia seen with termination of obstructive apnea. It is interesting that tachycardia persists even though blood pressure increases strikingly with termination of apnea. The vagolytic effects of inspiration and the arousal-associated changes in the autonomic nervous system not only interrupt the chemoreflex-mediated cardiac vagal drive, but blunt the expected cardiac vagal drive that would occur secondary to baroreflex activation by the postapnea surge in blood pressure.

Because of the repetitive nature of nocturnal apneas, Holter or other electrocardiographic monitoring at night manifests as a tachycardia–bradycardia pattern. This cardiac rate oscillation is less apparent in patients with autonomic dysfunction,

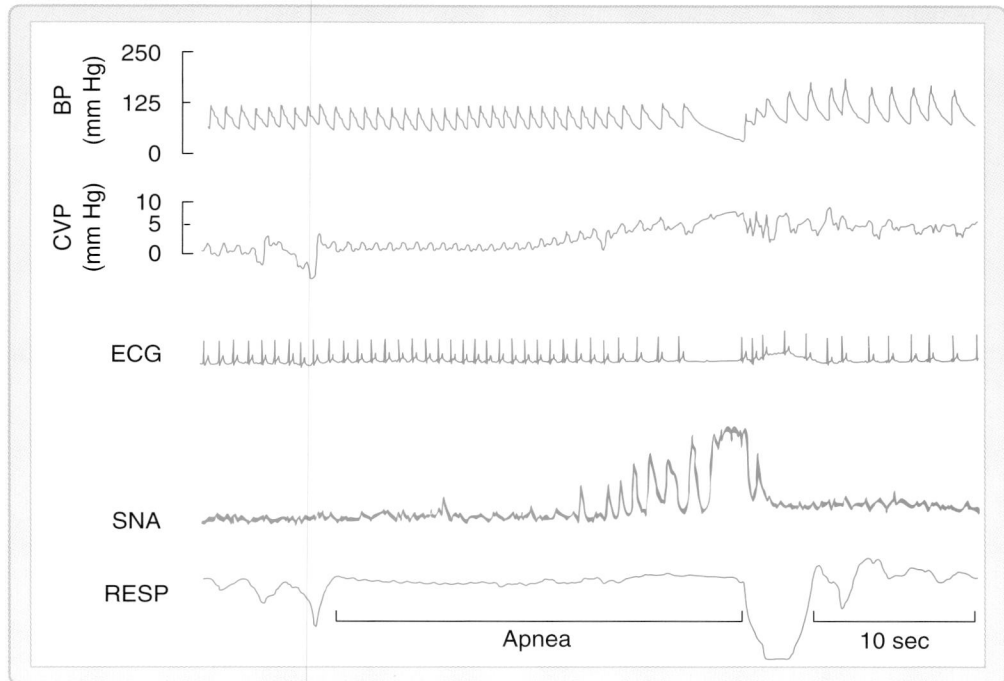

Figure 99–6. Recordings of intraarterial blood pressure (BP), central venous pressure (CVP), electrocardiogram (ECG), sympathetic nerve activity (SNA), and respiratory patterns (RESP) in a healthy subject during voluntary end-expiratory apnea. During apnea there is a progressive increase in the RR interval on the ECG with eventual sinus pause and atrioventricular block. Accompanying this is increased sympathetic activity. The simultaneous sympathetic activation to peripheral blood vessels and vagal activation of the heart is characteristic of the diving reflex. Note the rapid increase in heart rate and sympathetic inhibition during resumption of breathing. This occurs in part because thoracic afferents activated by inspiration inhibit both sympathetic traffic and vagal cardiac drive. (From Somers VK, Dyken MK, Mark AL, et al: Parasympathetic hyperresponsiveness and bradyarrhythmias during apnea in hypertension. Clin Auton Res 1992;2: 171-176.)

such as patients with long-standing diabetes, or cardiac transplant recipients with denervated hearts. Although the changes in cardiac rate are predominantly reflex mediated, breathing-related changes in cardiac filling, as well as rapid changes in cardiac transmural pressures due to the Mueller maneuver, also modulate heart rate by variations in stretch of cardiac conduction tissue.

Bradyarrhythmias

The primary response to hypoxia is bradycardia.[87,88] When hypoxia is accompanied by the action of breathing, the bradycardic response is masked because of inhibition of cardiac vagal drive by ventilation.[66] The sympathetic response to hypoxemia, although evident to some extent during breathing,

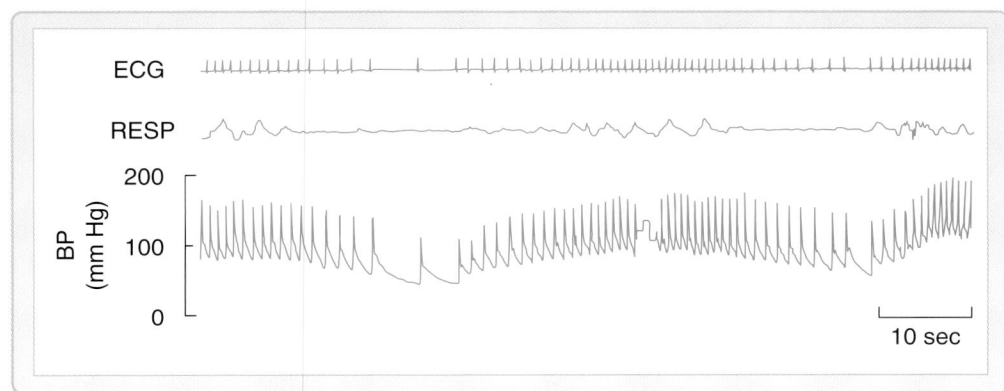

Figure 99–7. A patient with sleep apnea manifesting prolonged and profound bradyarrhythmias with absence of either atrial or ventricular contraction. The beat-by-beat blood pressure (BP) recording confirms the absence of any perfusion during the bradycardia. ECG, electrocardiogram; RESP, respiratory pattern. (From Somers VK, Dyken MK, Mark AL, et al: Parasympathetic hyperresponsiveness and bradyarrhythmias during apnea in hypertension. Clin Auton Res 1992;2:171-176.)

is also attenuated by ventilation and is therefore potentiated during apnea.[92,93] Patients with OSA may be particularly susceptible to hypoxia-induced bradyarrhythmias because their peripheral chemoreflex is heightened, so that even during voluntary apneas, hypoxemia elicits greater bradycardia than is seen in closely matched control subjects.[94] The arterial baroreflexes serve as an important buffer to diminish chemoreflex gain.[95] Impaired baroreflex sensitivity, such as is seen in hypertension[96] and heart failure,[97] may be associated with further increased chemoreflex drive. Thus, patients with hypertension or heart failure who have OSA may manifest even greater sympathetic, and perhaps bradycardic, responses to obstructive apneas.

Profound bradyarrhythmias may have important consequences, particularly in patients with underlying cardiovascular disease. As an example, in the absence of recognition of OSA as a potential cause of the bradyarrhythmia, patients may receive pacemaker implantation, even though their cardiac conduction system may be completely normal and the bradyarrhythmias could be abolished by effective treatment with CPAP.[83,84,98] Second, prolonged episodes of asystole result in absence of perfusion (see Fig. 99–7). Absence of perfusion in the setting of apnea-induced hypoxemia, occurring repetitively through the night, may have important implications for ischemic damage to end organs in which there may already be preexisting circulatory compromise.

Ventricular Arrhythmias

There is an extensive literature on sleep apnea inducing nocturnal angina and cardiac ischemia evidenced by ST segment depression.[99,100] Thus, there is a potential contribution of OSA to ventricular arrhythmias through ventricular ectopy during profound bradycardia, as well as polymorphic ventricular tachycardia due to cardiac hypoxia/ischemia. These episodes occur primarily with severe desaturation,[83,84] are more common in patients with coronary heart disease,[86] and are virtually eliminated with treatment.[83,84,98] The prevalence of these arrhythmias is low in patients without premorbid cardiorespiratory disease or severe desaturation.[101]

Atrial Fibrillation

In patients cardioverted for atrial fibrillation, those with polysomnographically proven OSA who were not receiving effective CPAP treatment had a 12-month recurrence rate of 82%, compared with a 42% recurrence rate in patients with OSA receiving effective CPAP.[102] In patients cardioverted for atrial fibrillation in whom no sleep study had been done, the recurrence rate was 53%. This risk for recurrence in the patients with atrial fibrillation without a previous sleep study suggests that undiagnosed OSA may be present in a large proportion of patients with atrial fibrillation. In addition, in the untreated patients with OSA, those experiencing a recurrence of atrial fibrillation had more severe nocturnal hypoxemia than those without a recurrence. Furthermore, the increased recurrence in patients with untreated OSA could not be explained by factors such as antiarrhythmic medication, body mass index, hypertension, cardiac function, or atrial size.

Mooe et al.[103] observed that after coronary artery bypass surgery, patients with OSA were more likely to experience postoperative atrial fibrillation. However, it is not clear whether this was explained by other variables in the patients with OSA.

There are many reasons why OSA may be conducive to atrial fibrillation. Hypoxemia, pressor surges, and sympathetic activation are all potential mechanisms leading to atrial fibrillation. High levels of C-reactive protein may also independently predict the development of atrial fibrillation.[104] Patients with OSA have increased C-reactive protein.[105] Furthermore, abrupt and dramatic changes in intrathoracic negative pressures may especially affect the atria, with their relatively thin walls compared with the ventricles. Increased pressure gradients with consequent increased atrial wall stretch, occurring repetitively through the night, may be expected to induce mechanical and electrical changes also conducive to atrial fibrillation. Indeed, about 50% of patients presenting for cardioversion have a high risk for sleep apnea, compared with 30% of patients from a general cardiology clinic.[106]

SUMMARY

Sleep-related breathing disorders affect cardiovascular function in a variety of ways. OSA and central sleep apnea act through multiple mechanisms to elicit acute circulatory responses, which have implications for the development of chronic vascular and cardiac dysfunction. The acute responses to apnea are mediated in large part by the effects of apnea on blood gas chemistry, which exerts important cardiovascular effects directly on the myocardium and blood vessels, and also acts through reflex mechanisms. Acute neural, circulatory, endothelial, inflammatory, and other responses to repetitive nocturnal hypoxemia and hypercapnia may act to induce long-term damage to the myocardium and to the coronary and other vascular beds. With the development of functional and structural cardiovascular disease, the consequences of acute apneas are magnified. For example, severe hypoxemia in the setting of sleep apnea is more easily tolerated by an overtly healthy cardiovascular system compared with one where myocardial ischemia or left ventricular dysfunction is present, with consequent diminished cardiovascular reserve. Small, short-term studies have suggested that effective prevention of recurrent apneas may favorably affect surrogates of cardiovascular disease outcome, such as sympathetic activity, blood pressure, and left ventricular ejection fraction.

Clinical Pearls

Apnea–recovery cycles result in three basic abnormalities: alterations in blood gases, arousals, and changes in intrathoracic pressure.

Hypoxemia–reoxygenation has deleterious effects on the cardiovascular system. This activates redox-sensitive genes, resulting in synthesis of vasoconstrictor and inflammatory mediators; increases sympathetic activity; and causes oxidative stress. These alterations have been best studied in OSA.

Untreated OSA may increase the risk of recurrence of atrial fibrillation after cardioversion.

Sleep apnea can induce severe bradyarrhythmias, including prolonged periods of asystole and heart block, even in the setting of a normal myocardium and cardiac electrophysiologic function.

OSA should be considered in patients who have ST segment depression or angina occurring primarily at night. Heart failure may be significantly linked to the presence of either central sleep apnea or OSA.

REFERENCES

1. Javaheri S: Sleep related breathing disorders in heart failure. In Mann DL (ed): Heart Failure: A Companion to Braunwald's Heart Disease. Philadelphia, WB Saunders, 2003, pp 471-487.
2. Leung RST, Bradley TD: Sleep apnea and cardiovascular disease. Am J Respir Crit Care Med 2001;164:2147-2165.
3. Javaheri S: Central sleep apnea-hypopnea syndrome in heart failure: Prevalence, impact and treatment. Sleep 1996;19:S229-S231.
4. Cargill JI, Kiely DG, Lipworth BJ: Adverse effects of hypoxemia on diastolic filling in humans. Clin Sci 1995;89:165-169.
5. Kusuoka H, Weisfeildt ML, Zweier JL, et al: Mechanism of early contractile failure during hypoxia in intact ferret heart: Evidence for modulation of maximal Ca^{2+}-activated force by inorganic phosphate. Circ Res 1986;59:270-282.
6. Mombouli JV, Vanhoutte PM: Endothelial dysfunction: from physiology to therapy. J Mol Cell Cardiol 1999;31:61-74.
7. Faller DV: Endothelial cell responses to hypoxic stress. Clin Exp Pharmacol Physiol 1999;26:74-84.
8. Yu AY, Shimoda LA, Iyer NV, et al: Impaired physiological responses to chronic hypoxia in mice partially deficient for hypoxia-inducible factor 1α. J Clin Invest 1999;103:691-696.
9. Koong AC, Chen EY, Giaccia AJ: Hypoxia causes the activation of nuclear factor kB through the phosphorylation of IκBα on tyrosine residues. Cancer Res 1994;54:1425-1430.
10. Phelan MW, Faller DV: Hypoxia decreases constitutive nitric oxide synthase transcript and protein in cultured endothelial cells. J Cell Physiol 1996;167:469-476.
11. Gonzalez NC, Wood JG: Leukocyte-endothelial interactions in environmental hypoxia. Adv Exp Med Biol 2001;502:39-60.
12. Aoki M, Nata T, Morishita R, et al: Endothelial apoptosis induced by oxidative stress through activation of NF-kB: Antiapoptotic effect of antioxidant agents on endothelial cells. Hypertension 2001;38:48-55.
13. Kanagy NL, Walker BR, Nelin LD: Role of endothelin in intermittent hypoxia-induced hypertension. Hypertension 2001;37:511-515.
14. Adhikary G, Kline D, Yuan G, et al: Gene regulation during intermittent hypoxia: Evidence for the involvement of reactive oxygen species. Adv Exp Med Biol 2001;499:297-302.
15. Ichikawa H, Flores S, Kvietys PR, et al: Molecular mechanisms of anoxia/reoxygenation-induced neutrophil adherence to cultured endothelial cells. Circ Res 1997;81:922-931.
16. Samarasinghe DA, Tapner M, Farrell GC: Role of oxidative stress in hypoxia-reoxygenation injury to cultured rat hepatic sinusoidal endothelial cells. Hepatology 2000;31:1600-1605.
17. Willam C, Schindler R, Frei U, et al: Increases in oxygen tension stimulate expression of ICAM-1 and VCAM-1 on human endothelial cells. Am J Physiol 1999;276:H2044-H2052.
18. Prabhakar NR: Physiological and genomic consequences of intermittent hypoxia. Invited review: Oxygen sensing during intermittent hypoxia: cellular and molecular mechanisms. J Appl Physiol 2001;90:1986.
19. Prabhakar NR: Sleep Apneas: An oxidative stress? Am J Respir Crit Care Med 2002;165:859-860.
20. Gozal D, Daniel JM, Dohanich GP: Behavioral and anatomical correlates of chronic episodic hypoxia during sleep in the rat. J Neurosci 2001;21:2442-2450.
21. Row BW, Liu R, Xu W, et al: Intermittent hypoxia is associated with oxidative stress and spatial learning deficits in the rat. Am J Respir Crit Care Med 2003;167:1548-1553.
22. Lavie L: Obstructive sleep apnoea syndrome: An oxidative stress disorder. Sleep Med Rev 2003;7:35-51.
23. Biegelsen ES, Loscalzo J: Endothelial function and atherosclerosis. Coron Artery Dis 1999;10:241-256.
24. Javaheri S: Heart failure and sleep apnea: Emphasis on practical therapeutic options. Clin Chest Med 2003;24:207-222.
25. Hedner J, Darpo B, Ejnell H, et al: Reduction in sympathetic activity after long-term CPAP treatment in sleep apnoea: Cardiovascular implications. Eur Respir J 1995;8:222-229.

26. Narkiewicz K, Kato M, Phillips BG, et al: Nocturnal continuous positive airway pressure decreases daytime sympathetic traffic in obstructive sleep apnea. Circulation 1999;100;2332-2335.
27. Schulz R, Schmidt D, Blum A, et al: Decreased plasma levels of nitric oxide derivatives in obstructive sleep apnoea: Response to CPAP therapy. Thorax 2000;55:1046-1051.
28. Ip MSM, Lam B, Chan LY, et al: Circulating nitric oxide is suppressed in obstructive sleep apnea and is reversed by nasal continuous positive airway pressure. Am J Respir Crit Care Med 2000;162:2166-2171.
29. Kato M, Roberts-Thompson P, Phillips BG, et al: Impairment of endothelium-dependent vasodilation of resistance vessels in patients with obstructive sleep apnea. Circulation 2001;102:2607-2610.
30. Miyasaka M, Ohi M: Effects of nasal continuous positive airway pressure on soluble cell adhesion molecules in patients with obstructive sleep apnea syndrome. Am J Med 2000;109:562-567.
31. Schulz R, Mahmoudi S, Hattar K, et al: Enhanced release of superoxide from polymorphonuclear neutrophils in obstructive sleep apnea. Am J Respir Crit Care Med 2000;162:566-570.
32. Phillips BG, Narkiewicz K, Pesek CA, et al: Effects of obstructive sleep apnea on endothelin-1 and blood pressure. J Hypertens 1999;17:61-66.
33. Chin K, Ohi M, Kita H, et al: Effects of NCPAP therapy on fibrinogen level in obstructive sleep apnea syndrome. Am J Respir Crit Care Med 1996;153:1972-1976.
34. Bobinsky G, Miller M, Ault K, et al: Spontaneous platelet activation and aggregation during obstructive sleep apnea and its response to therapy with nasal continuous positive airway pressure. Chest 1995;108:625-630.
35. Sanner BM, Konermann M, Tepel M, et al: Platelet function in patients with obstructive sleep apnoea syndrome. Eur Respir J 2000;16:648-652.
36. Yokoe T, Minoguchi K, Matsuo H, et al: Elevated levels of C-reactive protein and interleukin-6 in patients with obstructive sleep apnea syndrome are decreased by nasal continuous positive airway pressure. Circulation 2003;1129-1134.
37. Carpagnano GE, Kharitonov SA, Resta O, et al: 8-Isoprostane, a marker of oxidative stress, is increased in exhaled breath condensate of patients with obstructive sleep apnea after night and is reduced by continuous positive airway pressure therapy. Chest 2003;124:1386-1392.
38. Dyugovskaya L, Lavie P, Lavie L: Phenotypic and functional characterization of γδ T cells in sleep apnea. Am J Respir Crit Care Med 2003;168:242-249.
39. Christou K, Markoulis N, Moulas AN, et al: Reactive oxygen metabolites (ROMs) as an index of oxidative stress in obstructive sleep apnea patients. Sleep Breath 2003;7:105-109.
40. Naughton MT, Bernard DC, Liu PP, et al: Effects of nasal CPAP on sympathetic activity in patients with heart failure and central sleep apnea. Am J Respir Crit Care Med 1995;152:473-479.
41. Somers VK, Zavala DC, Mark AL, Abboud FM: Contrasting effects of hypoxia and hypercapnia on ventilation and sympathetic activity in humans. J Appl Physiol 1989;67:2101-2106.
42. Somers VK, Zavala DC, Mark AL, et al: Influence of ventilation and hypocapnia on sympathetic nerve responses to hypoxia in normal humans. J Appl Physiol 1989;67:2095-2100.
43. Narkiewicz K, van de Borne P, Pesek C, et al: Selective potentiation of peripheral chemoreceptor sensitivity in obstructive sleep apnea. Circulation 1999;99:1183-1189.
44. Javaheri S: A mechanism of central sleep apnea in patients with heart failure. N Engl J Med 1999;341:949-954.
45. Nakao K, Ohgushi M, Yoshimura M, et al: Hyperventilation as a specific test for diagnosis of coronary artery spasm. Am J Cardiol 1997;80:545-549.
46. Mancia G: Autonomic modulation of the cardiovascular system during sleep. N Engl J Med 1993;238:347-349.

47. Somers VK, Dyken ME, Mark AL, et al: Sympathetic-nerve activity during sleep in normal subjects. N Engl J Med 1993; 328:303-307.

48. Horner RL, Brooks D, Kozar LF, et al: Immediate effects of arousal from sleep on cardiac autonomic outflow in the absence of breathing in dogs. J Appl Physiol 1995;79:151-162.

49. Mann DL, Kent RL, Parsons B, et al: Adrenergic effects on the biology of the adult mammalian cardiocyte. Circulation 1992;85:790-804.

50. Communal C, Singh K, Pimental DR, et al: Norepinephrine stimulates apoptosis in adult rat ventricular myocytes by activation of the β-adrenergic pathway. Circulation 1998;98:1329-1334.

51. Van de Borne P, Oren R, Abouassaly C, et al: Effect of Cheyne-Stokes respiration on muscle sympathetic nerve activity in severe congestive heart failure secondary to ischemic or idiopathic dilated cardiomyopathy. Am J Cardiol 1998;81:432-436.

52. Naughton MT, Benard DC, Liu PP, et al: Effects of nasal CPAP on sympathetic activity in patients with heart failure and central sleep apnea. Am J Respir Crit Care Med 1995;152:473-479.

53. Somers VK, Dyken ME, Clary MP, et al: Sympathetic neural mechanisms in obstructive sleep apnea. J Clin Invest 1995;96:1897-1904.

54. Fletcher EC, Miller J, Schaaf JW, et al: Urinary catecholamines before and after tracheostomy in patients with obstructive sleep apnea and hypertension. Sleep 1987;10:35-44.

55. Waravdekar NV, Sinoway LI, Zwillich CW, et al: Influence of treatment on muscle sympathetic nerve activity in sleep apnea. Am J Respir Crit Care Med 1996;153:1333-1338.

56. Narkiewicz K, Kato M, Phillips BG, et al: Nocturnal continuous positive airway pressure decreases daytime sympathetic traffic in obstructive sleep apnea. Circulation 1999;100:2332-2335.

57. Staniforth AD, Kinneart WJM, Hetmanski DJ, et al: Effect of oxygen on sleep quality, cognitive function and sympathetic activity in patients with chronic heart failure and Cheyne-Stokes respiration. Eur Heart J 1998;19:922-928.

58. Buda AJ, Pinsky MR, Ingels NB, et al: Effect of intrathoracic pressure on left ventricular performance. N Engl J Med 1979; 301:453-459.

59. Brinker JA, Weiss JL, Lappe DL, et al: Leftward septal displacement during right ventricular loading in man. Circulation 1980;61:626-632.

60. Fletcher EC, Proctor M, Yu J, et al: Pulmonary edema develops after recurrent obstructive apneas. Am J Respir Crit Care Med 1999;160:1688-1696.

61. Weiss JW, Remsburg S, Garpestad E, et al: Hemodynamic consequences of obstructive sleep apnea. Sleep 1996;19:388-397.

62. Tarasiuk A, Scharf SM: Cardiovascular effects of periodic obstructive and central apneas in dogs. Am J Respir Crit Care Med 1994;150:83-89.

63. Tilkian AG, Guilleminault C, Schroeder JS, et al: Hemodynamics in sleep-induced apnea: Studies during wakefulness and sleep. Ann Intern Med 1976;85:714-719.

64. Buda AJ, Schroeder JS, Guilleminault C: Abnormalities of pulmonary artery wedge pressures in sleep-induced apnea. J Cardiol 1981;1:67-74.

65. Guilleminault C, Connolly S, Winkle R, et al: Cyclical variation of the heart rate in sleep apnoea syndrome: Mechanisms, and usefulness of 24 h electrocardiography as a screening technique. Lancet 1984;1:126-131.

66. Somers VK, Dyken MK, Mark AL, et al: Parasympathetic hyper-responsiveness and bradyarrhythmias during apnea in hypertension. Clin Auton Res 1992;2:171-176.

67. Parker JD, Brooks D, Kozar LF: Acute and chronic effects of airway obstruction on canine left ventricular performance. Am J Respir Crit Care Med 1999;160:1888-1896.

68. Hanly P, Sasson Z, Zuberi N, et al: Ventricular function in snorers and patients with obstructive sleep apnea. Chest 1992;102:100-105.

69. Alchanatis M, Tourkohoriti G, Kosmas EN, et al: Evidence of left ventricular dysfunction in patients with obstructive sleep apnoea syndrome. Eur Respir J 2002;20:1239-1245.

70. Laaban JP, Fascal-Sebaoun S, Bloch E, et al: Left ventricular systolic dysfunction in patients with obstructive sleep apnea syndrome. Chest 2002;122:1133-1138.

71. Shahar E, Whitney CW, Redline S, et al: Sleep-disordered breathing and cardiovascular disease: Cross-sectional results of the Sleep Heart Health study. Am J Respir Crit Care Med 2001; 163:19-25.

72. Javaheri S, Parker TJ, Liming JD, et al: Sleep apnea in 81 ambulatory male patients with stable heart failure: Types and their prevalences, consequences and presentations. Circulation 1998;97:2154-2159.

73. Sin DD, Fitzgerald F, Parker JD, et al: Risk factors for central and obstructive sleep apnea in 450 men and women with congestive heart failure. Am J Respir Crit Care Med 1999;160:1101.

74. Malone S, Liu PP, Holloway R, et al: Obstructive sleep apnea in patients with dilated cardiomyopathy: Effects of continuous positive airway pressure. Lancet 1991;338:1480.

75. Kaneko Y, Floras JS, Usui K, et al: Cardiovascular effects of continuous positive airway pressure in patients with heart failure and obstructive sleep apnea. N Engl J Med 2003;348:1233-1241.

76. Mansfield DR, Gollogly NC, Kaye DM, et al: Controlled trial of continuous positive airway pressure in obstructive sleep apnea and heart failure. Am J Respir Crit Care Med 2004;169:361-366.

77. Cargill JI, Keily DG, Liworth BJ: Adverse effects of hypoxemia on diastolic filling in humans. Clin Sci 1995;89:165.

78. Hender J, Enjell H, Caidahl K: Left ventricular hypertrophy independently of hypertension in patients with obstructive sleep apnea. J Hypertens 1990;8:941-946.

79. Noda A, Okada T, Yasuma F, et al: Cardiac hypertrophy in obstructive sleep apnea syndrome. Chest 1995;107:1538-1544.

80. Davis RJ, Crosby J, Prothero A, et al: Ambulatory blood pressure and left ventricular hypertrophy in subjects with untreated obstructive sleep apnea and snoring, compared with matched control subjects and their response to treatment. Clin Sci 1994; 86:417-424.

81. Niroumand M, Kuperstein R, Sasson Z, et al: Impact of obstructive sleep apnea on left ventricular mass and diastolic function. Am J Respir Crit Care Med 2001;163:1632-1636.

82. Chan J, Sanderson J, Chan W, et al: Prevalence of sleep-disordered breathing in diastolic heart failure. Chest 1997;111: 1488-1493.

83. Guilleminault C, Connolly SJ, Winkle RA: Cardiac arrhythmia and conduction disturbances during sleep in 400 patients with sleep apnea syndrome. Am J Cardiol 1983;52:490-494.

84. Koehler U, Fus E, Grimm W, et al: Heart block in patients with obstructive sleep apnoea: Pathogenetic factors and effects of treatment. Eur Respir J 1998;11:434-439.

85. Grimm W, Hoffmann J, Menz V, et al: Electrophysiologic evaluation of sinus node function and atrioventricular conduction in patients with prolonged ventricular asystole during obstructive sleep apnea. Am J Cardiol 1996;77:1310-1314.

86. Koehler U, Glaremin DT, Junkermann H, et al: Nocturnal myocardial ischemia and cardiac arrhythmia in patients with sleep apnea with and without coronary heart disease. Klin Wochenschr 1991;69:474-482.

87. de Burgh Daly M, Elsner R, Angel-James JE: Cardiorespiratory control by carotid chemoreceptors during experimental dives in the seal. Am J Physiol 1977;232:H508-H516.

88. de Burgh Daly M, Angell-James J, Elsner R: Role of carotid-body chemoreceptors and their reflex interactions in bradycardia and cardiac arrest. Lancet 1997;1:764-767.

89. Roche F, Gaspoz J-M, Court-Fortune I, et al: Screening of obstructive sleep apnea syndrome by heart rate variability analysis. Circulation 1999;100:1411-1415.

90. Stein PK, Domitrovich PP: Detecting OSAHS from patterns seen on heart-rate tachograms. Comput Cardiol 2000;27:271-274.

91. Anrep GV, Pascual W, Rossler R: Respiratory variations of the heart rate: II. The central mechanism of the respiratory arrhythmia and the interrelations between the central and reflex mechanisms. Proc R Soc Lond Ser B 1936;119:218-230.

92. Somers VK, Zavala DC, Mark AL, et al: Contrasting effects of hypoxia and hypercapnia on ventilation and sympathetic activity in humans. J Appl Physiol 1989;67:2101-2106.

93. Somers VK, Zavala DC, Mark AL, et al: Influence of ventilation and hypocapnia on sympathetic nerve responses to hypoxia in normal humans. J Appl Physiol 1989;67:2095-2210.

94. Narkiewicz K, van de Borne P, Pesek C, et al: Selective potentiation of peripheral chemoreceptor sensitivity in obstructive sleep apnea. Circulation 1999;99:1183-1189.

95. Somers VK, Mark AL, Abboud FM: Interaction of baroreceptor and chemoreceptor reflex control of sympathetic nerve activity in normal humans. J Clin Invest 1991;87:1953-1957.

96. Bristow J, Honour A, Pickering G, et al: Diminished baroreflex sensitivity in high blood pressure. Circulation 1969;39:48-54.

97. Zucker I: Baro and cardiac reflex abnormalities in chronic heart failure. In Zucker I, Gilmore J (eds): Reflex Control of the Circulation. Boca Raton, Fla, CRC Press, 1991, pp 849-873.

98. Stegman SS, Burroughs JM, Henthorn RW: Asymptomatic bradyarrhythmias as a marker for sleep apnea: Appropriate recognition and treatment may reduce the need for pacemaker therapy. Pacing Clin Electrophysiol 1996;19:899-904.

99. Hanly P, Sasson Z, Zuberi N, et al: ST-segment depression during sleep in obstructive sleep apnea. Am J Cardiol 1993;71:1341-1345.

100. Peled N, Abinader EG, Pillar G, et al: Nocturnal ischemic events in patients with obstructive sleep apnea syndrome and ischemic heart disease: effects of continuous positive air pressure treatment. J Am Coll Cardiol 1999;34:1744-1749.

101. Flemons WW, Remmers JE, Gillis AM: Sleep apnea and cardiac arrhythmias: Is there a relationship? Am Rev Respir Dis 1993;148:618-621.

102. Kanagala R, Murali N, Friedman P, et al: Obstructive sleep apnea and the recurrence of atrial fibrillation. Circulation 2003;107:2589-2594.

103. Mooe T, Gullsby S, Rabben T, Eriksson P: Sleep-disordered breathing: A novel predictor of atrial fibrillation after coronary artery bypass surgery. Coron Artery Dis 1996;7:475-478.

104. Chung MK, Martin DO, Sprecher D, et al: C-reactive protein elevation in patients with atrial arrhythmias: Inflammatory mechanisms and persistence of atrial fibrillation. Circulation 2001;104:2886-2891.

105. Shamsuzzaman ASM, Winnicki M, Wolk R, et al: An independent association between plasma leptin and C-reactive protein in healthy humans. Circulation 2004;109:2181-2185.

106. Gami AS, Pressman G, Caples SM, et al: Association of atrial fibrillation and obstructive sleep apnea. Circulation 2004;110:364-367.

Systemic and Pulmonary Hypertension in Obstructive Sleep Apnea

Terry Young

Shahrokh Javaheri

ABSTRACT

Findings from investigations based on diverse populations and different study designs have consistently supported a role for obstructive sleep apnea (OSA) in systemic and pulmonary hypertension. Both cross-sectional and prospective population-based epidemiology studies have shown that persons with polysomnographically indicated OSA (15 or more apnea or hypopnea events per hour of sleep) have 2 to 3 times the odds of having systemic hypertension or developing new systemic hypertension compared with persons who do not have OSA. The associations are not explained by confounding factors such as increased body mass index or age. Some studies suggest that the link between OSA and hypertension is stronger with younger age and lower BMI. A dose-dependent association for OSA and hypertension is seen in the mild to moderate OSA range, but the association appears to plateau with more-severe OSA.

In both population and clinical studies with ambulatory blood pressure monitoring, mean systolic and diastolic blood pressures are higher in OSA groups compared with controls. The associations are seen during both sleep and wake, and there is some evidence that the relationship of OSA and blood pressure is strongest during sleep and early morning. Pulmonary arterial hypertension (PAH), ranging from mild to severe, is prevalent in patients with OSA. Mild PAH may occur in OSA patients without daytime hypoxemia or chronic obstructive pulmonary disease (COPD), but these comorbidities are more common in severe OSA.

Although definitive randomized clinical trials have not been completed, most studies of both systemic and pulmonary arterial blood pressures before and after continuous positive airway pressure (CPAP) have shown decreases in blood pressure. Intervention trials have generally shown modest reductions in systemic blood pressure with CPAP use (2 to 10 mm Hg), and the largest effects are seen in effectively treated severe OSA. Importantly, such small changes in blood pressure, if maintained, significantly decrease the incidence of cerebrovascular and cardiovascular disease. Decreases of up to 12 mm Hg in pulmonary artery pressures have been reported after several months of CPAP treatment.

Several early studies[1-3] using intraarterial and Swan-Ganz catheters to measure systemic blood pressure and central hemodynamics documented acute cyclic changes in systemic and pulmonary arterial blood pressures that parallel episodes of obstructive sleep apnea (OSA). Only recently, however, have convincing data emerged from hypothesis-testing studies of the causal role of OSA in chronic hypertension and other cardiovascular conditions. Evidence from basic and physiologic studies showing biologic plausibility (see Chapter 99), and evidence from observational and interventional studies, support the hypothesis that nightly exposure to repeated episodes of OSA is associated with elevated daytime systemic and pulmonary arterial blood pressure.

The potential importance of OSA in cardiovascular disease is gaining recognition beyond the field of sleep research. In the Seventh Report of the Joint National Committee on Prevention, Detection, Evaluation, and Treatment of High Blood Pressure, OSA is recognized as an identifiable cause of hypertension.[4] Similarly, the World Health Organization has recognized OSA as a cause of secondary pulmonary arterial hypertension.[5]

Although an accurate estimate of the fraction of systemic hypertension that can be *causally* attributed to OSA is lacking and data on OSA and pulmonary hypertension are sparse, it is clear that clinical recognition of the high prevalence of systemic and pulmonary hypertension in people with OSA,[6,7] as well as the high occurrence of OSA in hypertensive patients,[8-10] is imperative. The aim of this chapter is to present the epidemiologic data in support of a role of OSA in systemic and pulmonary hypertension and to describe the clinical issues in identification and treatment of patients with OSA and hypertension.

SYSTEMIC HYPERTENSION

Epidemiologic Evidence for a Role of OSA in Systemic Hypertension

The early observations of hypertension in sleep apnea patients stimulated several cross-sectional clinic- and community-based studies that attempted to determine whether there was an association of OSA and hypertension not explained by excess body weight or other factors common to both OSA and hypertension (see also Chapter 52).[7] Results were mixed, but many of the studies had some methodologic shortcomings such as inadequate sample size, flawed comparison groups, measurement error, or limited statistical analysis.[11,12] Since then, findings from both population and clinical studies have shed important new light on this association.

OSA and Hypertension Defined by Blood Pressure Cutpoints

Reports from several well-designed epidemiology studies have consistently shown statistically significant associations of polysomnographically determined OSA and hypertension, defined by blood pressure thresholds or use of antihypertensive medication, independent of age, gender, and body habitus measures.[13,14]

The strongest epidemiologic evidence for a causal association comes from longitudinal analyses of data from the ongoing Wisconsin Sleep Cohort Study of middle-aged state employees, reported by Peppard and colleagues.[15,16] OSA status, indicated by the frequency of apnea and hypopnea events and resting blood pressure obtained during an overnight protocol, was available for 709 men and women who had been followed for at least 4 years. The incidence of new hypertension, defined as systolic blood pressure at least 140 mm Hg, diastolic blood pressure at least 90 mm Hg, or use of antihypertensive medication at follow-up, was significantly dependent on baseline level of OSA.

Using categories based on the apnea-hypopnea index (AHI, number of apnea and hypopnea events per hour of sleep), the 4-year incidence of hypertension was 9.7%, 17.1%, 31.5%, and 32.1% for baseline AHI categories of 0, 1 to 5, 5 to 15, and greater than 15, respectively. After adjustment for confounding factors, a dose-response association persisted: Relative to study participants without OSA, the likelihood of developing new hypertension over 4 years was two-fold greater for those with AHI of 5 to 15 and three-fold greater for those with AHI greater than 15 at baseline, compared with participants without OSA at baseline (i.e., AHI < 1). As would be expected with the use of more powerful longitudinal analyses, these odds ratios are consistent with, but they are somewhat higher and more precise than, those reported from earlier cross-sectional analyses of baseline data on the entire cohort (N = 1060).[17]

Cross-sectional analyses of baseline data from three other cohorts, with measurements, definitions, and statistical models to adjust for confounding similar to those used in the Wisconsin Sleep Cohort Study, have also shown OSA to be a statistically significant risk factor for hypertension (Table 100–1 and Fig. 100–1). Nieto and colleagues[18] analyzed OSA measured with in-home polysomnography and blood pressure collected in the multicenter Sleep Heart Health Study of 6132 men and women, ages 40 to 97 years. Although the magnitude of odds ratios for hypertension with AHI categories was lower than that found in the other cohorts, a significant dose-response trend was found, with odds ratios for hypertension ranging from 1.1 (AHI 1.5 to 4.9 versus AHI < 1.5) to 1.37 (AHI ≥ 30 versus AHI < 1.5).

Results reported by Bixler and colleagues[19] from the Pennsylvania cohort of 1741 men and women ages 20 to 100 years revealed considerably higher odds ratios for hypertension of 6.9 for AHI at least 15 versus AHI of 0, and 2.3 for AHI of 0.1 to 14.9 versus AHI of 0. Duran's group[20] studied 555 men and women from Vitoria-Gasteiz, Spain, with polysomnography, selected as a subsample from a larger household census sample. Adjusted odds ratios did not show a dose-response trend, but they suggested an overall twofold risk of hypertension for AHI greater than 0 versus AHI of 0.

Collectively, the relationship of OSA and hypertension has been assessed with state of the art measurements of 9488 men and women from the general population, and results have been consistent. Confidence in the validity of the findings is increased as a result of the care taken by investigators to evaluate the effects of methodologic limitations. In all studies, potential confounding factors and optimal ways to account for their influence were carefully considered. With the exception of the Sleep Heart Health Study, the studies were based on probability samples and participation bias was assessed and found to be minimal. Researchers ensured that statistical model assumptions were met, and some investigators conducted

Table 100–1.   Association of Polysomnographically Determined Sleep Disordered Breathing and Hypertension in Four Population Studies

		Odds Ratio* for Hypertension† (95% Confidence Interval)				
			AHI Category			
Study Design	N	<1.0‡	1-4.9	5.0-14.9	≥15	≥30
Wisconsin Sleep Cohort Study,[15] state employees, ages 30 to 65 years,[16] prospective 4-8 years follow-up	709	1.0	1.2 (1.1, 1.8)	2.0 (1.3, 3.2)	2.9 (1.5, 5.6)	—
Sleep Heart Health Study,[18] multicenter, ages 40 to 97 years, cross-sectional	6132	1.0	1.1 (0.9, 1.3)	1.2 (1.0, 1.4)	1.3 (1.9, 1.6)	1.4 (1.0, 1.8)
Southern Pennsylvania,[19] population sample via random-digit dialing, ages 20 to 100 years, cross-sectional	1741	1.0	—	2.3§ (1.4, 3.6)	6.9§ (2.0, 26.4)	—
Vitoria-Gasteiz, Spain,[20] random census sample, ages 30 to 70 years, cross-sectional	552	1.0	2.5 (1.1, 5.8)	1.3 (0.5, 4.1)	2.3 (0.9, 5.7)	—

*Odds ratios are all adjusted for age, sex, BMI, neck circumference, alcohol intake, and cigarette smoking. Additional adjustments are made for baseline hypertension and waist circumference in the Wisconsin study, for ethnicity and waist-to-hip ratio in the Sleep Heart Health Study, and for ethnicity, menopause, and hormone replacement therapy in the Southern Pennsylvania study.

†Defined by systolic blood pressure ≥140, diastolic blood pressure ≥90, or use of antihypertensive medication.

‡Reference category for odds ratio.

§Estimated at the mean age and BMI of the sample.

AHI, apnea-hypopnea index.

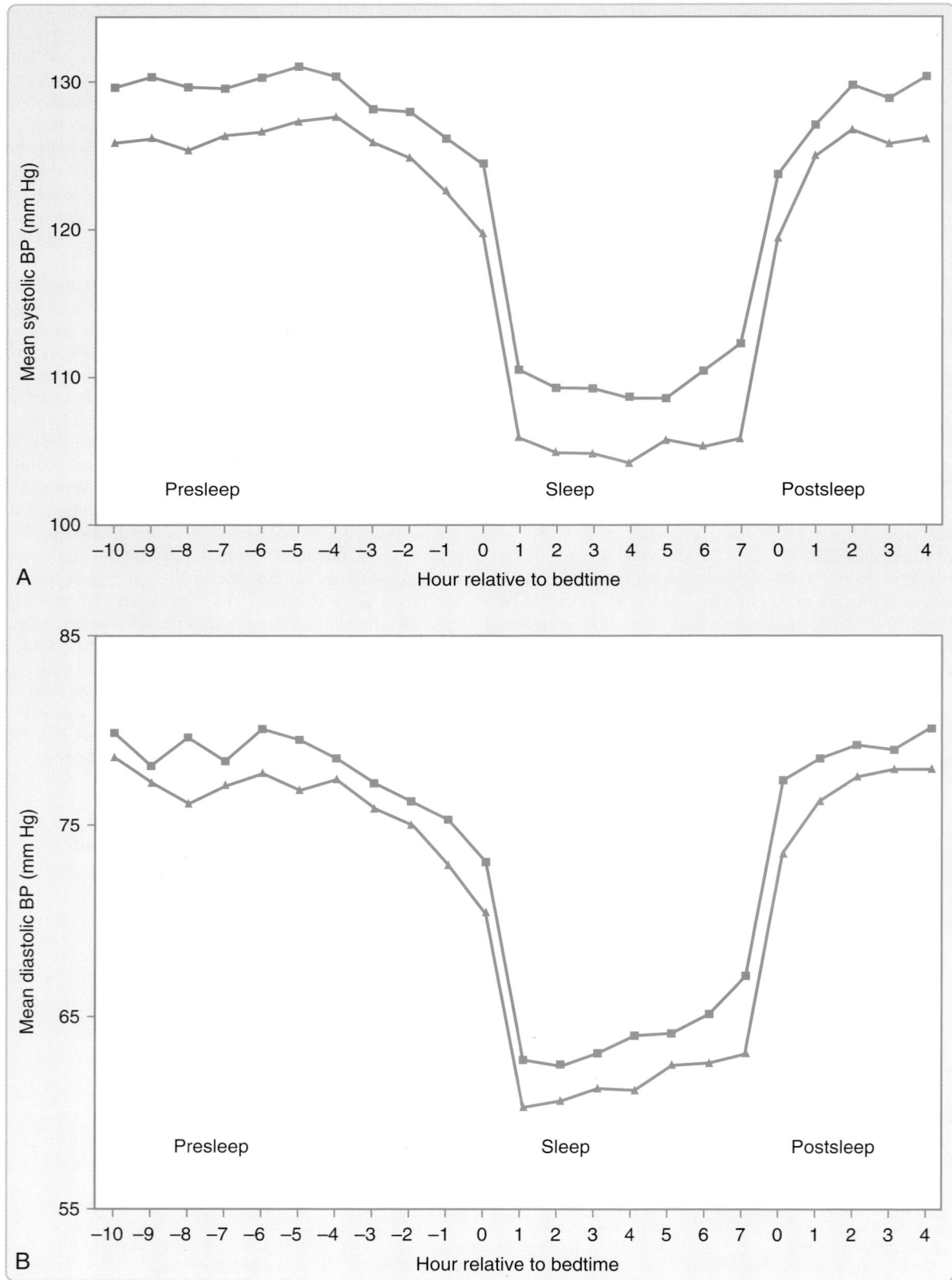

Figure 100–1. Ambulatory blood pressure during presleep, sleep, and postsleep by apnea-hypopnea index (AHI) category (the line with triangles shows AHI < 5, number of patients = 537; the line with squares shows AHI ≥ 5, number of patients = 231); Wisconsin Sleep Cohort Study. **A** shows systolic blood pressure and **B** shows diastolic blood pressure. Mean blood pressure values are adjusted for age, sex, and body mass index.

sensitivity analyses and simulations to investigate measurement error.[15,21] If the epidemiology findings do reflect a causal relationship, as is suggested by the prospective data, a harder look must be taken at the importance of preventing OSA or at treating even mild OSA, discussed more fully below.

In three of the population studies, despite a dose-response association of AHI categories with cutpoints up to 15 or 30 and hypertension, the odds of hypertension do not appear to increase further past this level of moderate OSA severity. It is possible that such a threshold exists, but methodologic limitations may account for this. This feature may reflect a survival bias against persons with high OSA and cardiovascular disease, greater measurement error at higher AHI levels, or study power limitations from the relatively small number of persons with very severe OSA in the general population.

Data from a clinic-based study in Marburg (N = 1087), with a severity distribution skewed toward higher AHI values (88 patients with AHI > 40), however, show similar odds ratios (OR) for hypertension with AHI categories of 5 to 20 (OR = 1.8), 20 to 40 (OR = 1.8) and greater than 40 (OR = 1.9).[22] Although the odds ratio for the category of AHI greater than 40 was higher when hypertension was defined by higher cutpoints of 160/95 mm Hg, the confidence intervals for all the categories were overlapping.

A substantial number of patients with higher AHI were included in a study of 2677 sleep clinic patients in Toronto,[23] where 363 patients had AHI values greater than 50. The proportion of patients with hypertension did increase with AHI category, but these data were not adjusted for confounding factors. However, a small dose-response relationship was suggested by results from a regression model using AHI as a continuous variable: An increase in systolic pressure of 1.0 mm Hg and increase in diastolic pressure of 0.7 mm Hg was seen for increments of 10 AHI units, adjusted for confounding factors. The authors did not mention whether quadratic or other terms to test for a departure from linearity or a plateau effect were investigated in the regression modeling, so the possibility of a plateau in risk of elevated blood pressure or hypertension cannot be ruled out.

A threshold for hypertension in OSA also may exist because the presence of pathophysiologic consequences of severe OSA, such as nocturia and heart failure, could lessen hypertension. In regard to heart failure, severe OSA has been associated with left ventricular systolic dysfunction[24]; in the Sleep Health Heart Study, there was a dose-dependent relation between AHI and prevalence of heart failure.[25] If left ventricular systolic dysfunction occurs as OSA becomes more severe, adequate left ventricular stroke volume may not be maintained to sustain a high blood pressure.

Furthermore, biologically, the mechanisms mediating hypertension in OSA may be threshold dependent and become saturated at a certain level of AHI. In this regard, in a two-arm study[26] of therapeutic and subtherapeutic CPAP in OSA, there were no changes in systemic arterial blood pressure from baseline in the subtherapeutic CPAP trial arm despite a decrease in average AHI from 65 to 33 per hour. These results are consistent with a threshold effect for AHI in mediating existing systemic hypertension, although conclusive evidence for or against a stronger risk of developing new hypertension with severe OSA requires further longitudinal data.

OSA and Hypertension in Population Subgroups

Some findings on whether the association of OSA and hypertension varies in strength by gender, ethnicity, age, and body mass index have emerged. Although the odds ratios for hypertension with OSA were slightly smaller for women compared with men in the report from the Sleep Heart Health Study,[18] no other study has reported a gender effect, which suggests that the risk of hypertension with OSA is no less significant in women, relative to men. This message is particularly important given the past underdiagnosis and treatment of OSA in women and the possibility that less-aggressive evaluation and treatment of OSA in women may lead to a survival disadvantage in women with OSA.[27]

Few studies have included sufficient population diversity to determine if the association of OSA and hypertension varies by ethnicity. Findings from the Sleep Heart Health Study, with a sample of approximately 10% African American and 12% American Indian, have not shown a significantly higher or lower risk of hypertension with OSA in these groups compared with the risk in whites.[18] No interaction of OSA with ethnicity was found in the Pennsylvania cohort.[19]

Cross-sectional regression analyses of two of the cohort studies with age ranges that include sufficient older people have suggested a negative interaction of age and AHI with respect to hypertension. Bixler and coworkers found that odds ratios for hypertension and AHI of 30 or greater versus AHI of 0 exponentially decreased as age increased; there was essentially no risk of hypertension associated with OSA for those 70 years and older.[19] Similar findings were reported by Nieto's group: After stratifying the Sleep Heart Health Study sample with a cutpoint of age 65 years, the odds ratio for hypertension with AHI greater than 30 versus AHI less than 1.5 was lower and not statistically significant for ages 65 years and older (OR = 1.23), compared with ages 40 to 65 years (OR = 1.64).[18]

Hass and colleagues[28] pursued the Sleep Heart Health Study findings further by considering whether an association of OSA and hypertension was being diluted by the high prevalence of isolated systolic hypertension inherent in the older age group. Isolated systolic hypertension, the most common form of hypertension in older people, is the result of an age-related loss of arterial compliance, manifested clinically by a widened pulse pressure. The definition of hypertension used in the previous study of Sleep Heart Health Study and other cohort studies has not discriminated essential hypertension from isolated systolic hypertension; both types are captured in the commonly used definition of systolic pressure at least 140 mm Hg or diastolic pressure at least 90 mm Hg or use of antihypertensive drugs.

In the Hass group's study, after distinguishing the two forms of hypertension in the Sleep Heart Health Study, OSA was not found to be associated with isolated systolic hypertension, regardless of age, as expected. However, even after exclusion of subjects with isolated systolic hypertension, the association of OSA and hypertension did not increase in the older age group. Some investigators have posited that a different form of OSA, with more events of central rather than obstructive origin, is manifested in older age,[29] but Hass's group also reported that excluding people with central sleep apnea from the Sleep Heart Health Study analysis did not explain the age effect.

Although it is possible that OSA is truly less likely to be associated with hypertension in older people, methodologic difficulties arising from high comorbidity and survival bias are inherent in studying health effects of OSA in older populations and could cause a spurious age effect. Cross-sectional studies are particularly vulnerable to these problems; longitudinal studies following people from middle to older age are essential to accurately determine the hypertension risk in older people with OSA. Clinical practice should not be influenced by the notion that health risks of OSA in older people are lower until there are conclusive data.

The magnitude of the OSA-hypertension link did not vary by BMI categories in the Sleep Heart Health Study, but BMI was a significant modifier in studies by Young and coworkers[17] and Bixler and coworkers.[19] The odds ratio for hypertension and OSA increased in magnitude with decreasing BMI, indicating that in leaner people, those with OSA compared to those without may be at particularly high risk for hypertension. This finding has clinical implications, particularly in primary care, where sleep apnea is not likely to be suspected in nonobese patients, even in the presence of symptoms.

OSA and Diurnal Blood Pressure

Hypertension defined by chronic elevated daytime pressure is generally considered to be the outcome of interest, but it is not clear what specific features of elevated blood pressure are important. OSA-related nocturnal perturbations include repeated spiking of pressures that exceed hypertension cut-points (blood pressure load) and elevated average nighttime blood pressure, as well as a carry-over effect resulting in elevated daytime blood pressure. Early studies of hemodynamics in OSA involved invasive blood pressure monitoring; more recent studies of circadian patterns of blood pressure rely on ambulatory monitors that sample blood pressure at 15- to 30-minute intervals with arm cuff inflation-based methods.

Most studies with ambulatory blood pressure monitoring have been conducted on sleep apnea patients. A Marburg study of 93 OSA patients[30] showed the number of oxygen desaturation events per hour of presumed sleep was linearly related to both daytime and nighttime systolic and diastolic blood pressure, and it was related most strongly to nighttime pressures. In Great Britain, Davies and colleagues[31] performed ambulatory blood pressure studies on 45 pairs of sleep apnea patients and community controls matched to the patients on age, BMI, and treated hypertension. Sleep apnea patients had significantly higher diastolic pressures during the day and night, higher systolic pressures during the night, and a notably smaller nocturnal dip.

Nocturnal blood pressure relative to daytime pressure has been of special interest, as studies have shown that the lack of the normal nighttime decline (nondipping) in blood pressure, usually considered to be a nighttime drop of at least 10% of the daytime pressure, is related to adverse cardiovascular outcomes independent of hypertension.[32] Some findings from relatively small clinic-based samples do suggest that patients with OSA have a smaller nocturnal decline in blood pressure, but strong evidence for a clear, significant risk of nondipping is lacking.[30,31,33-36,37]

Data from population studies with polysomnography and nocturnal blood pressure measures are sparse. In a preliminary study of 147 Wisconsin Sleep Cohort Study subjects,[38]

OSA was associated with elevated blood pressure from 24-hour ambulatory monitoring. Average systolic and diastolic blood pressures during wake and sleep, and systolic blood pressure load during wake and sleep, were all statistically significantly higher in the participants with AHI greater than 5. Findings from an update on a much larger cohort sample (N = 768) are shown in Figure 100–2: Blood pressures, adjusted for confounding factors, were higher at every hour before, during, and after sleep for those with AHI greater than 5 versus AHI less than 5.

Collectively, the ambulatory blood pressure studies do support an association of OSA in elevated blood pressure during both the nighttime and daytime, and some studies suggest that the effect is greatest during nighttime. These findings are particularly important because elevated ambulatory blood pressure has been shown to predict cardiovascular events independently of office-measured blood pressure and other cardiovascular risk factors.[39]

Upper Airway Resistance and Snoring as Predictors of Hypertension

Controversy about whether there is a hypertension risk associated with upper airway resistance or snoring in the absence of frank apnea and hypopnea events has been ongoing for many years.[40-43,45] Several surveys of diverse populations have been conducted, with comparisons of hypertension prevalence in nonsnorers and snorers, a category that encompasses the full range of OSA from simple snoring to severe apnea.[46,47] In the prospective study conducted on the large Nurses Heath Study sample (N = 73,231), self-reported snorers compared to nonsnorers had twice the odds of hypertension.[46]

It is possible that only those snorers with OSA explain the snoring-hypertension association. However, in two cohort

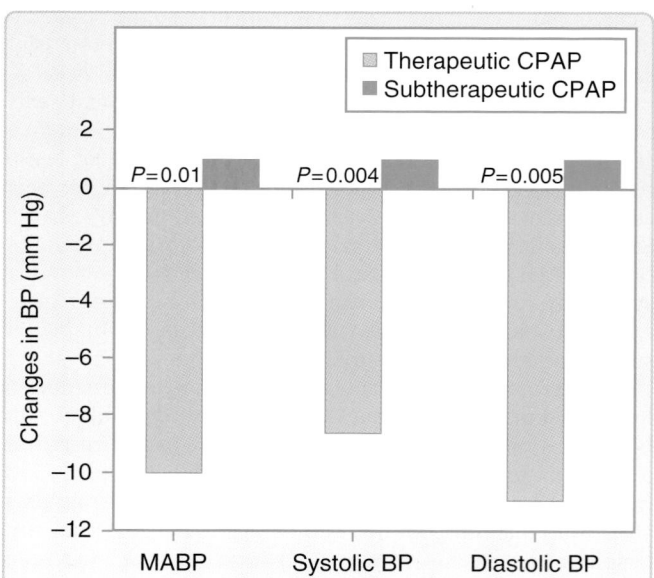

Figure 100–2. Treatment with therapeutic continuous positive airway pressure (CPAP) decreased systemic blood pressure, whereas use of subtherapeutic CPAP failed to decrease blood pressure. (From Becker HF, Jerrentrup A, Ploch T, et al: Effect of nasal continuous positive airway pressure treatment on blood pressure in patients with obstructive sleep apnea. Circulation 2003;107:68-73.)

studies, after exclusion of subjects with OSA using polysomnographic data, small odds ratios were still seen for simple snoring and hypertension.[19,47] In addition, upper airway resistance syndrome, where frank apneic events are not present, has been linked with hypertension.[48] The prevalence of simple snoring is high, and thus understanding what role, if any, snoring has in hypertension is an important question.

Blood Pressure Changes after CPAP Treatment of OSA

Studies of the effect of CPAP on blood pressure have evolved from clinical observations of treated patients to sophisticated randomized, double-blind trials, with sham-CPAP as the control condition and objectively measured compliance. Information from these studies is important to the more basic question of whether OSA has a causal role in elevated blood pressure and adverse circadian patterns as intermediates for cardiovascular disease. Clinical trial results, in general, support a contribution of OSA to elevated blood pressure.

A significant lowering of blood pressure with CPAP was reported by Pepperell and coworkers[49] in a study of 118 OSA patients with an average oxygen desaturation index (ODI) of 37 per hour, randomized to CPAP or subtherapeutic CPAP (pressure about 1 cm H_2O) for 4 weeks. Ambulatory blood pressure data showed mean blood pressure drops of 2.4 mm Hg during sleep and 3.4 mm Hg during wake in the CPAP group, and an increase of 0.8 for the control group. The largest CPAP effect was seen in patients with the most severe OSA (ODI > 33/hour, decrease in blood pressure of 5.1 mm Hg) and in those being treated with antihypertensive drugs. Furthermore, in patients who used therapeutic CPAP for longer than 5 hours average per night, mean blood pressure fell by about 5 mm Hg, compared with no change in blood pressure in those who used CPAP for less than 5 hours. As will be discussed later, the small changes in blood pressure, if long-term, have important implications in preventing cerebrovascular and cardiovascular incidents.

The largest effect of CPAP was reported by Becker and colleagues,[26] in a double-blind 9-week trial, completed by 32 of 60 eligible sleep clinic patients. Full night polysomnography, continuous noninvasive blood pressure monitoring (Portapress, FMS, Amsterdam), and a relatively long-term follow-up provided the most detailed look at the effects of CPAP on OSA and 24-hour blood pressure profile. There were no changes in medications or body weight during the 9-week trial. In the therapeutic CPAP group, AHI decreased from 63 per hour to 3 per hour. In the subtherapeutic CPAP group, AHI decreased from 65 per hour to 33 per hr. Compliance with CPAP was monitored and averaged about 5.5 hours per night in both groups. In the therapeutic CPAP group, there was a decrease of approximately 10 mm Hg in systolic and diastolic blood pressure, during both day and night. Even though the subtherapeutic group had a 50% reduction in AHI, there was no change in blood pressure. In general these results are consistent with those reported by Pepperell's group,[49] indicating that use of CPAP in severe OSA decreases blood pressure. Both studies stress the need for effective treatment of OSA.

With a different study design, Hla and coworkers[50] investigated the effect of 3 weeks of CPAP on blood pressure in hypertensive subjects with and without OSA to control for effects that CPAP might have on blood pressure independent of an effect from elimination of apnea and hypopnea events. Newly diagnosed unmedicated hypertensive men from primary care settings were assessed for OSA by laboratory polysomnography to identify 14 men with AHI greater than 5 (mean AHI = 25) and 10 men with AHI less than 5 (mean AHI = 1).

The OSA group received therapeutic CPAP, and the non-OSA group received CPAP at a pressure of 5 cm H_2O for 3 weeks. Ambulatory blood pressure monitoring was done pre-CPAP, on the last night and day of CPAP, and post-CPAP. Nocturnal blood pressure in the OSA group dropped significantly with CPAP (−10.3 mm Hg systolic, −4.5 mm Hg diastolic) but was essentially unchanged with CPAP in the no-OSA group. There was a greater but statistically nonsignificant difference in blood pressure drop in the OSA versus non-OSA group in daytime blood pressure (−2.4 mm Hg systolic, −0.6 mm Hg diastolic).

Most interesting, in the OSA group, the blood pressure–lowering effect persisted during the night post CPAP and was of magnitude similar to the lowering seen during the night with CPAP. The explanation for a carry-over blood pressure effect to the post-CPAP night, but only a small effect on daytime pressure, is not clear; the short-term improvements in upper airway caliber such as reduced edema, or a short persistence in the positive effects of CPAP on intermediate consequences of apnea and hypopnea events, such as vascular responsiveness and sympathetic activity, may account for this observation. Although interpretations are very limited by the small sample, these results suggest that there are important hemodynamic effects of the apnea and hypopnea events beyond the acute spikes in blood pressure in the pathway to elevated blood pressure.

Clinical Relevance of a Role of OSA in Hypertension

In contrast to the state of evidence 10 years ago, findings in support of a role of OSA in the development of hypertension would be difficult to dismiss as spurious. Translating the findings described above to clinical settings, however, poses new challenges. These findings, as well as new guidelines on hypertension detection and treatment, support case-finding for OSA in patients with hypertension in primary care settings; but what is the next step? While it is clear that diagnosis and treatment of a patient with hypertension and symptomatic OSA is a priority, a critical and much-debated question is the course of action that should be taken if a hypertensive patient has mild OSA without daytime symptoms of sleepiness.

Is treatment of mild, asymptomatic OSA warranted on the basis of potential cardiovascular consequences? Arguments against treatment point to lack of conclusive data: Any effect of CPAP on blood pressure is too small to be of clinical significance and thus would not replace use of antihypertensive drugs for controlling blood pressure.[51] In addition, data showing that CPAP does not improve daytime functioning, including cognitive function and objective sleepiness in patients without subjective sleepiness, leads to skepticism that such patients would be compliant with CPAP use.[52]

Alternatively, there are arguments for considering CPAP treatment in patients with mild, asymptomatic OSA and coexisting hypertension.[53,54] Worsening of mild sleep apnea over time is likely, and cardiovascular consequences that might be attributable to severe OSA could be prevented.[54] Some data suggest that CPAP treatment of patients with OSA and drug-resistant hypertension may be of benefit in lowering blood pressure.[55] Furthermore, little is known about the interaction of OSA and hypertension in cardiovascular morbidity and mortality. Given the acute negative cardiovascular effects of apnea and hypopnea events, it is plausible that OSA worsens existing hypertension and speeds progression to cardiovascular disease. It is possible that eliminating the disordered breathing would improve overall cardiovascular prognosis; research on this is clearly warranted.

Clinicians increasingly recognize the markers of OSA, such as snoring, and are becoming more aware of the OSA-hypertension association. Consequently, referrals of patients with mild, asymptomatic OSA will increase and heighten the dilemma of whom to treat in the face of limited medical resources. Further understanding of the costs and benefits of OSA treatment in preventing the incidence and progression of hypertension and other cardiovascular diseases is needed before this problem can be satisfactorily addressed.

Meanwhile, clinicians taking care of OSA patients on CPAP should underscore the importance of full compliance as well as adequate control of disordered breathing events with CPAP, as evidenced by studies showing the importance of these two variables to lower blood pressure.[26,49] In this regard, it must be emphasized that long-term small changes in blood pressure have major preventive effects. In prospective studies of 420,000 persons, a decrease of 5 mm Hg in diastolic blood pressure lessened the incidence of stroke and coronary heart disease by approximately 34% and 21%, respectively, and there was a dose-dependent reduction in blood pressure and incident cardiovascular diseases.[56] Therefore, in patients with OSA, long-term compliance with CPAP may be effective in preventing adverse cerebrovascular and cardiovascular diseases.

PULMONARY ARTERIAL HYPERTENSION

Obstructive Sleep Apnea as a Cause of Pulmonary Arterial Hypertension

In 1998, the second World Health Organization conference on pulmonary arterial hypertension (PAH)[5] recognized sleep disordered breathing as a secondary cause of PAH. PAH may be defined as an elevation in the mean pulmonary artery pressure to at least 20 mm Hg at rest or to at least 30 mm Hg during exercise. In patients with OSA, the prevalence of PAH varies from about 15% to 70%.[61] PAH is usually mild, although it could also be severe, resulting in cor pulmonale, a feature of pickwickian syndrome (hypercapnic OSA syndrome).

An early study[1] in 12 patients with OSA who had undergone right heart catherization showed cyclic changes in pulmonary artery pressure coinciding with episodes of OSA. Marked degree of hypoxemia and hypercapnia was associated with these hemodynamic abnormalities. In some of these patients, systolic pulmonary artery pressure exceeded 60 mm Hg. During wakefulness, four patients had mild PAH, and mean pressure ranged from 20 to 22 mm Hg. One of these 4 patients had an elevated pulmonary capillary wedge pressure of 16 mm Hg. With exercise most of the patients developed PAH with mean pulmonary artery pressure about 30 mm Hg.

In some of these patients, the wedge pressure increased with exercise, unmasking left ventricular diastolic dysfunction. This study indicated that OSA impaired the physiologic processes that normally operate to enable pulmonary circulation and left ventricular function to maintain pulmonary artery pressure close to normal in the face of increases in cardiac output.

Since the study of Tilkian and colleagues,[1] many studies have demonstrated that PAH is relatively common in patients with OSA.[57] Box 100–1 summarizes three large studies in which full night polysomnography and right heart catheterization, the gold standard for diagnosis of OSA and PAH, were performed. In a French study[58] involving 220 consecutive patients with AHI greater than 20, 37 patients (17%) had resting mean pulmonary artery pressure of at least 20 mm Hg (range 20 to 44 mm Hg). Patients with PAH had more severe OSA, a higher $PaCO_2$, a higher body mass index, and a lower PaO_2 than patients without PAH. Furthermore, patients with PAH had higher prevalence of both obstructive and restrictive pulmonary defects. $PaCO_2$ and FEV_1 were the two major predictors of PAH.

In an Australian study[59] of 100 consecutive patients with an AHI of 20 or more, 42% had PAH, with the mean pulmonary artery pressure ranging from about 20 to 52 mm Hg. In this study $PaCO_2$, PaO_2, and FEV_1 accounted for about 33% of variability in pulmonary artery pressure. Six patients with PAH had normal PaO_2.

In a German study[60] of 92 consecutive patients with AHI greater than 10, and using COPD as an exclusion criterion,

---

Box 100–1.	**Pulmonary Arterial Hypertension in Obstructive Sleep Apnea**

Chaouat et al[58]

- 220 consecutive French patients with AHI > 20/hr
- 17% had mean PAP > 20 mm Hg
- Patients with PAH had more severe OSA, higher $PaCO_2$ and BMI, lower PaO_2, and more obstructive and restrictive defect
- $PaCO_2$ and FEV_1 were independent predictors of PAH

Laks et al[59]

- 100 consecutive Australian patients with AHI > 20/hr
- 42% had mean PAP > 20 mm Hg; range, 20 to 52 mm Hg
- $PaCO_2$, PaO_2, and FEV_1 accounted for 33% of variability in PAH
- 6 patients with PAH had normal PaO_2

Sanner et al[60]

- 92 consecutive German patients with OSA and AHI > 10/hr; range, 10-100/hr
- COPD was an exclusion criterion
- 20% had mild PAH; range, 20 to 25 mm Hg
- 8 patients had increased PCWP; all had systemic hypertension
- PCWP and time <90% saturation were independent predictors of PAH

AHI, apnea-hypopnea index; BMI, body mass index; COPD, chronic obstructive pulmonary disease; PAP, pulmonary artery pressure; PCWP, pulmonary capillary wedge pressure.

20% had mild PAH with a mean pulmonary artery pressure of 20 to 25 mm Hg. Eight patients had increased pulmonary capillary wedge pressure, and all of these patients had systemic hypertension that was presumably causing left ventricular diastolic dysfunction. Pulmonary capillary wedge pressure and time spent below saturation of 90% were the independent variables predicting PAH.

Presence of PAH in patients with OSA but without COPD has been also confirmed in another French study.[61] COPD was defined as an FEV_1 of less than 70% predicted and FEV_1/FVC ratio of less than 60% predicted. In this study, which involved 44 patients, 12 patients (27%) had precapillary PAH. The authors reported that mean pulmonary artery pressure was positively correlated with body mass index and negatively correlated with PaO_2. Patients with PAH had significantly lower values for FVC and FEV_1. The mechanisms by which body mass index positively correlated with PAH could have been multifactorial and related to restrictive lung defect and hypoxemia.

In conclusion, mild PAH is common in patients with OSA and may occur in the absence of COPD as well as daytime hypoxemia. However, severe OSA, severe hypoxemia, and obstructive or restrictive lung defects are more commonly associated with PAH.

Mechanisms of Pulmonary Arterial Hypertension

Multiple mechanisms mediate nocturnal rises in pulmonary artery pressure. These include alterations in blood gases, cardiac output, lung volume, intrathoracic pressure, compliance of pulmonary circulation, and left ventricular diastolic dysfunction.

Diurnal PAH could be precapillary, capillary, or postcapillary, in part depending on comorbid disorders that may contribute to development of PAH in OSA (Box 100–2). Postcapillary PAH could be due to left ventricular hypertrophy and diastolic dysfunction caused by diurnal systemic hypertension. However, left ventricular hypertrophy could be present in OSA even in the absence of daytime systemic hypertension,[62] presumably because of nocturnal cyclic changes in systemic artery blood pressure and hypoxemia during sleep.[63]

Box 100–2.	**Mechanisms of Pulmonary Arterial Hypertension in Obstructive Sleep Apnea**

Precapillary PAH

Hypoxemia
Hypercapnia
Changes in intrathoracic pressure
Endothelial dysfunction or remodeling

Capillary PAH

Loss of vascular surface area due to a cormorbid disorder, such as in COPD

Postcapillary PAH

LVH and diastolic dysfunction

COPD, chronic obstructive pulmonary disease; LVH, left ventricular hypertrophy; PAH, pulmonary arterial hypertension.

In the presence of a hypertrophied, noncompliant left ventricle, end-diastolic pressure increases, resulting in an increase in pulmonary capillary and pulmonary artery systolic and diastolic pressures (postcapillary PAH). Left ventricular diastolic dysfunction may become unmasked when cardiac output increases. This may account for high prevalence of PAH with exercise in patients with OSA.[57,64]

Loss of vascular surface area, as may occur in COPD, is an important cause of capillary PAH, and may significantly contribute to PAH in patients with OSA. Several studies[58,59,65] have shown that COPD and a low FEV_1 are predictors of PAH in patients with OSA. COPD could also contribute to PAH by way of hypoxemia and hypercapnia resulting in precapillary PAH (see below).

Finally, an important mechanism contributing to or mediating PAH in OSA is the presence of factors that cause constriction of pulmonary arterioles, which leads to precapillary PAH. The best-known stimulus is alveolar hypoxia, and hypoxemia is an independent predictor of PAH in OSA (see Box 100–1). However, hypercapnia and changes in intrathoracic pressure could also increase pulmonary arterial blood pressure.

The molecular mechanisms of PAH are complex and multifactorial.[66] Both acquired and genetic factors are involved. Disordered endothelial cell function, in part caused by hypoxia, and manifested biochemically in an imbalance between concentrations of local vasodilators (e.g., NO and prostacyclins) and vasoconstrictors (e.g., endothelin-1, thromboxane, and serotonin), as occurs in endothelial dysfunction syndrome, mediates development of PAH.[66] It is also conceivable that if OSA is longstanding, pulmonary vascular remodeling similar to that in COPD could occur, as a number of mediators such as vascular endothelial growth factor are proliferative and angiogenic.

Even though cyclic PAH occurs regularly with episodes of apnea during sleep, it is not clear why only some patients with OSA develop diurnal PAH. The same is true for systemic hypertension. Genetic predisposition, however, may confer an increased risk for the occurrence of PAH in some patients. In families with inherited PAH, mutations in the gene for bone morphogenetic protein receptor type 2 (BMPR2) have been reported.[67]

Most recently,[68] aberrant production of angiopoietin-1 was observed in a variety of disorders with acquired PAH, including thromboembolic disease, scleroderma, and mitral regurgitation. The expression of angiopoietin-1 messenger RNA and the protein itself were unregulated in the lungs of these patients, and it correlated directly with the severity of the disease. Angiopoietin-1 is an angiogenic factor that recruits smooth muscle cells to the endothelial vascular network during the embrogenic stage. However, after development is completed, angiopoietin-1 is expressed only minimally in normal human lung. In contrast, in patients with the various forms of acquired PAH, the level of angiopoietin-1 is increased.[68] Although the mechanisms leading to upregulation of angiopoietin-1 are unclear, it is conceivable that its upregulation could mediate PAH in some patients with OSA.

In summary, the consequence of OSA on pulmonary circulation may vary from those of cyclic nocturnal PAH, which occurs in virtually all patients, to daytime PAH, right ventricular dysfunction, and eventually cor pulmonale, a feature of pickwickian syndrome. However, even in the absence of cor pulmonale, which is the manifestation of longstanding severe PAH, presence of PAH increases right ventricular afterload and myocardial oxygen consumption. If PAH develops as a result of increases in cardiac output, for example with exercise, it may cause dyspnea and exercise intolerance.

Treatment

Since mechanisms of PAH in OSA are multifactorial (see Box 100–2), the behavioral response of pulmonary circulation to therapy of OSA probably depends on several factors. For example, if loss of vascular surface area (capillary PAH) due to presence of COPD or other comorbid pulmonary disorders is contributing to PAH in OSA, this component is irreversible. Similarly, if remodeling of the pulmonary vascular bed has occurred, longstanding effective therapy is necessary to effect any reversal. Therefore, if CPAP is used to treat OSA, long-term compliance with therapy is critical and needs to be confirmed by covert monitoring. Large, long-term systematic studies considering these important factors are necessary to determine effects of treatment of OSA on pulmonary circulation. Lack of such considerations may lead to serious underestimation of effects.

There is no doubt that effective treatment of OSA eliminates nocturnal PAH. Motta and coworkers[69] studied 6 patients with severe OSA (apnea index 60 to 80 per hour) before and after tracheostomy. After tracheostomy, the mean pulmonary artery pressure decreased significantly from 45 ± 4 mm Hg (SEM) to 22 ± 2 mm Hg.

Alchanatis and colleagues[70] used Doppler echocardiography to estimate pulmonary artery pressure before and after 6 months of effective treatment with CPAP in 29 patients with OSA and without COPD. In six patients who had mild PAH, the mean pulmonary artery pressure decreased significantly from about 26 mm Hg to 20 mm Hg 6 months after treatment with CPAP. In the study by Sforza and colleagues,[71] 8 patients had mild PAH (mean = 23 ± 1 mm Hg $\pm$ SEM). After treatment with CPAP for a year, the mean pulmonary artery pressure

was $21(\pm 1)$ mm Hg. For such a small change to be statistically significant, a large sample of patients is imperative.

Sajkov's group,[72] using Doppler echocardiography, studied pulmonary hemodynamics in 20 patients with OSA (average AHI = 49) before and 4 months after treatment with CPAP. In this study, CPAP compliance was objectively monitored and the average was 5 hours per night. Patients had normal lung function. Five patients who had mild PAH (range 20 to 32 mm Hg) showed the most dramatic decrease in the pulmonary artery pressure, all decreasing below 20 mm Hg, after 4 months of effective treatment with CPAP. In a subject who was not compliant with CPAP, there was no change in pulmonary artery pressure. Although this was a single observation, this finding and those reported for systemic hypertension strongly indicate that effective use of CPAP is necessary to lower systemic and pulmonary artery pressures.

REFERENCES

1. Tilkian AG, Guilleminault C, Schroeder JS, et al: Hemodynamics in sleep-induced apnea. Studies during wakefulness and sleep. Ann Intern Med 1976;85:714-719.
2. Coccagna G, Mantovani M, Brignani F, et al: Continuous recording of the pulmonary and systemic arterial pressure during sleep in syndromes of hypersomnia with periodic breathing. Bull Physiopathol Respir 1972;8:1159-1172.
3. Podszus T, Mayer J, Penzel T, et al: Nocturnal hemodynamics in patients with sleep apnea. Eur J Respir Dis Suppl 1986;146: 435-442.
4. Chobanian AV, Bakris GL, Black HR, et al: The Seventh Report of the Joint National Committee on Prevention, Detection, Evaluation, and Treatment of High Blood Pressure: The JNC 7 report. JAMA 2003;289:2560-2572.
5. Rich S (ed): Primary pulmonary hypertension: Executive summary from the World Symposium on Primary Pulmonary Hypertension. Geneva, World Health Organization, 1998.
6. Carlson JT, Hedner JA, Ejnell H, et al: High prevalence of hypertension in sleep apnea patients independent of obesity. Am J Respir Crit Care Med 1994;150:72-77.
7. Levinson PD, Millman RP: Causes and consequences of blood pressure alterations in obstructive sleep apnea. Arch Intern Med 1991;151:455-462.
8. Warley AR, Mitchell JH, Stradling JR: Prevalence of nocturnal hypoxaemia amongst men with mild to moderate hypertension. Q J Med 1988;68:637-644.
9. Fletcher EC, DeBehnke RD, Lovoi MS, et al: Undiagnosed sleep apnea in patients with essential hypertension. Ann Intern Med 1985;103:190-195.
10. Lavie P, Ben-Yosef R, Rubin AE: Prevalence of sleep apnea syndrome among patients with essential hypertension. Am Heart J 1984; 108:373-376.
11. Stradling J: Sleep apnea and the misuse of evidence-based medicine. Lancet 1997;349:201-202.
12. Wright J, Johns R, Watt I, et al: Health effects of obstructive sleep apnoea and the effectiveness of continous positive airways pressure: A systematic review of the research evidence. BMJ 1997; 314:851-860.
13. Young T, Peppard PE, Gottlieb DJ: Epidemiology of obstructive sleep apnea: A population health perspective. Am J Respir Crit Care Med 2002;165:1217-1239.
14. Pepperell JC, Davies RJ, Stradling JR: Systemic hypertension and obstructive sleep apnoea. Sleep Med Rev 2002;6:157-173.
15. Peppard PE, Young T, Palta M, Skatrud J: Prospective study of the association between sleep-disordered breathing and hypertension. N Engl J Med 2000;342:1378-1384.
16. Peppard PE, Young T: Sleep-disordered breathing and hypertension. Reply. N Engl J Med 2000;343:967.

Clinical Pearls

Recent evidence from several well-designed epidemiology studies supports a causal role of OSA in systemic hypertension independent of BMI, measures of fat distribution, age, gender, and other possible confounding factors.

Effective treatment of OSA with CPAP has been shown to lower systemic blood pressure. These studies have been performed in patients with severe OSA.

Even small decrements in blood pressure, maintained for the long term, have been shown to significantly lessen the incidence of cerebrovascular and cardiovascular diseases. Thus, the potential lowering of blood pressure from CPAP treatment holds promise for decreasing cerebrovascular or cardiovascular disease. However, adequate control of OSA and compliance with CPAP, particularly in patients with severe OSA, are critical.

Obstructive sleep apnea is a cause of secondary pulmonary arterial hypertension, and this has been recognized by international health organizations. Pulmonary arterial hypertension may decrease with use of CPAP to treat OSA.

17. Young T, Peppard P, Palta M, et al: Population-based study of sleep-disordered breathing as a risk factor for hypertension. Arch Intern Med 1997;157:1746-1752.

18. Nieto FJ, Young TB, Lind BK, et al: Association of sleep-disordered breathing, sleep apnea, and hypertension in a large community-based study. JAMA 2000;283:1829-1836.

19. Bixler EO, Vgontzas AN, Lin HM, et al: Association of hypertension and sleep-disordered breathing. Arch Intern Med 2000; 160:2289-2295.

20. Duran J, Esnaola S, Rubio R, et al: Obstructive sleep apnea-hypopnea and related clinical features in a population-based sample of subjects aged 30 to 70 yr. Am J Respir Crit Care Med 2001;163:685-689.

21. Young T, Peppard P: Epidemiological evidence for an association of sleep-disordered breathing with hypertension and cardiovascular disease. In Bradley TFJ (ed): Sleep Apnea: Implications in Cardiovascular and Cerebrovascular Disease. New York, Marcel Dekker, 2000.

22. Grote L, Ploch T, Heitmann J, et al: Sleep-related breathing disorder is an independent risk factor for systemic hypertension. Am J Respir Crit Care Med 1999;160:1875-1882.

23. Lavie P, Herer P, Hoffstein V: Obstructive sleep apnoea syndrome as a risk factor for hypertension: population study. BMJ 2000; 320:479-482.

24. Laaban JP, Pascal-Sebaoun S, Bloch E, et al: Left ventricular systolic dysfunction in patients with obstructive sleep apnea syndrome. Chest 2002;122:1133-1138.

25. Shahar E, Whitney CW, Redline S, et al: Sleep disordered breathing and cardiovascular disease: Cross-sectional results of the Sleep Heart Health Study. Am J Resp Crit Care Med 2001;163:19-25.

26. Becker HF, Jerrentrup A, Ploch T, et al: Effect of nasal continuous positive airway pressure treatment on blood pressure in patients with obstructive sleep apnea. Circulation 2003;107:68-73.

27. Young T, Finn L: Epidemiological insights into the public health burden of sleep disordered breathing: Sex differences in survival among sleep clinic patients. Thorax 1998;53:S16-S19.

28. Hass D: Sleep disordered breathing: The importance of discriminating between essential hypertension and isolated systolic hypertension [abstract]. Am Heart J 2003.

29. Bixler E, Vgontzas A, Have T, et al: Effects of age on sleep apnea in men. Am J Respir Crit Care Med 1998;157:144-148.

30. Pankow W, Nabe B, Lies A, et al: Influence of sleep apnea on 24-hour blood pressure. Chest 1997;112:1253-1258.

31. Davies CW, Crosby JH, Mullins RL, et al: Case-control study of 24 hour ambulatory blood pressure in patients with obstructive sleep apnoea and normal matched control subjects. Thorax 2000;55:736-740.

32. Verdecchia P, Schillaci G, Borgioni C, et al: Altered circadian blood pressure profile and prognosis. Blood Press Monit 1997; 2:347-352.

33. Wilcox I, Grunstein RR, Collins FL, et al: Circadian rhythm of blood pressure in patients with obstructive sleep apnea. Blood Press 1992;1:219-222.

34. Noda A, Okada T, Hayashi H, et al: 24-hour ambulatory blood pressure variability in obstructive sleep apnea syndrome. Chest 1993;103:1343-1347.

35. Nabe B, Lies A, Pankow W, et al: Determinants of circadian blood pressure rhythm and blood pressure variability in obstructive sleep apnoea. J Sleep Res 1995;4:97-101.

36. Suzuki M, Guilleminault C, Otsuka K, Shiomi T: Blood pressure "dipping" and "non-dipping" in obstructive sleep apnea syndrome patients. Sleep 1996;19:382-387.

37. Portaluppi F, Provini F, Cortelli P, et al: Undiagnosed sleep-disordered breathing among male nondippers with essential hypertension. J Hypertens 1997;15:1227-1233.

38. Hla KM, Young TB, Bidwell T, et al: Sleep apnea and hypertension. A population-based study. Ann Intern Med 1994;120: 382-388.

39. Clement DL, De Buyzere ML, De Bacquer DA, et al: Prognostic value of ambulatory blood-pressure recordings in patients with treated hypertension. N Eng J Med 2003;348:2407-2415.

40. Hoffstein V: Is snoring dangerous to your health? Sleep 1996; 19:506-516.

41. Hoffstein V: Blood pressure, snoring, obesity, and nocturnal hypoxaemia. Lancet 1994;344:643-645.

42. Dart RA, Gregoire JR, Gutterman DD, et al: The association of hypertension and secondary cardiovascular disease with sleep-disordered breathing. Chest 2003;123:244-260.

43. Jeong DU, Dimsdale JE: Sleep apnea and essential hypertension: a critical review of the epidemiological evidence for co-morbidity. Clin Exp Hypertens A 1989;11:1301-1323.

44. Gislason T, Benediktsdottir B, Bjornsson JK, et al: Snoring, hypertension, and the sleep apnea syndrome. An epidemiologic survey of middle-aged women. Chest 1993;103:1147-1151.

45. Lugaresi E, Plazzi G: Heavy snorer disease: From snoring to the sleep apnea syndrome—an overview. Respiration 1997;64:11-14.

46. Hu FB, Willett WC, Colditz GA, et al: Prospective study of snoring and risk of hypertension in women. Am J Epidemiol 1999; 150:806-816.

47. Young T, Finn L, Hla KM, et al: Snoring as part of a dose-response relationship between sleep-disordered breathing and blood pressure. Sleep 1996;19:S202-S205.

48. Guilleminault C, Stoohs R, Shiomi T, et al: Upper airway resistance syndrome, nocturnal blood pressure monitoring, and borderline hypertension. Chest 1996;109:901-908.

49. Pepperell JC, Ramdassingh-Dow S, Crosthwaite N, et al: Ambulatory blood pressure after therapeutic and subtherapeutic nasal continuous positive airway pressure for obstructive sleep apnoea: A randomised parallel trial. Lancet 2002;359:204-210.

50. Hla KM, Skatrud JB, Finn L, et al: The effect of correction of sleep-disordered breathing on BP in untreated hypertension. Chest 2002;122:1125-1132.

51. Montserrat JM, Barbe F, Rodenstein DO: Should all sleep apnoea patients be treated? Sleep Med Rev 2002;6:7-14; discussion 15-16.

52. Barbe F, Mayoralas LR, Duran J, et al: Treatment with continuous positive airway pressure is not effective in patients with sleep apnea but no daytime sleepiness. A randomized, controlled trial. Ann Intern Med 2001;134:1015-1023.

53. Levy P, Pepin JL, McNicholas WT: Should all sleep apnoea patients be treated? Yes. Sleep Med Rev 2002;6:17-26; discussion 27.

54. Pack AI, Maislin G: Who should get treated for sleep apnea? Ann Intern Med 2001;134:1065-1067.

55. Logan AG, Tkacova R, Perlikowski SM, et al: Refractory hypertension and sleep apnoea: Effect of CPAP on blood pressure and baroreflex. Eur Respir J 2003;21:241-247.

56. MacMahon S, Peto R, Cutler J, et al: Epidemiology: Blood pressure, stroke, and coronary heart disease; Part 1, prolonged difference in blood pressure: prospective observational studies corrected for the regression dilution bias. Lancet 1990;335: 765-774.

57. Marrone O, Bonsignore MR: Pulmonary hemodynamics in obstructive sleep apnoea. Sleep Med Rev 2002;6:175-193.

58. Chaouat A, Weitzenblum E, Krieger J, et al: Pulmonary hemodynamics in the obstructive sleep apnea syndrome. Chest 1996; 109:380-386.

59. Laks L, Lehrhaft B, Grunstein RR, et al: Pulmonary hypertension in obstructive sleep apnea. Eur Respir J 1995;8:537-541.

60. Sanner BM, Doberauer C, Konermann M, et al: Pulmonary hypertension in patients with obstructive sleep apnea syndrome. Arch Intern Med 1997;157:2483-2487.

61. Bady E, Achkar A, Pascal S, et al: Pulmonary arterial hypertension in patients with sleep apnea syndrome. Thorax 2000;55: 934-939.

62. Hedner J, Enjell H, Caidahl K: Left ventricular hypetrophy independently of hypertension in patients with obstructive sleep apnea. J Hypertens 1990;8:941-946.

63. Cargill JI, Kiely DG, Lipworth BJ: Adverse effects of hypoxemia on diastolic filling in humans. Clin Sci 1995;89:165-169.

64. Podszus T, Bauer W, Mayer J, et al: Sleep apnea and pulmonary hypertension. Klin Wochenschr 1986;64:131-134.

65. Bradley TD, Rutherford R, Grossman RF, et al: Role of daytime hypoxemia in the pathogenesis of right heart failure in the obstructive sleep apnea syndrome. Am Rev Respir Dis 1985; 131:835-839.

66. Budhiraja R, Tuder RM, Hassoun PM: Endothelial dysfunction in pulmonary hypertension. Circulation 2004;109:159-165.

67. Deng Z, Morse JH, Slager SL, et al: Familial primary pulmonary hypertension (gene *ppH1*) is caused by mutations in the bone morphogenetic protein receptor-II gene. Am J Hum Genet 2000; 67:737-744.

68. Du L, Sullivan CC, Chu D, et al: Signaling molecules in nonfamilial pulmonary hypertension. N Engl J Med 2003;348:500-509.

69. Motta J, Guilleminault C, Schroeder JS, et al: Tracheostomy and hemodynamic changes in sleep-induced apnea. Ann Int Med 1978;89:454-458.

70. Alchanatis M, Tourkohoriti G, Kakouros S, et al: Daytime pulmonary hypertension in patients with obstructive sleep apnea. Respiration 2001;68:566-572.

71. Sforza E, Krieger J, Weitzenblum E, et al: Long-term effects of treatment with nasal continuous positive airway pressure on daytime lung function and pulmonary hemodynamics in patients with obstructive sleep apnea. Am Rev Respir Dis 1990;141: 866-870.

72. Sajkov D, Wang T, Saunders NA, et al: Continuous positive airway pressure treatment improves pulmonary hemodynamics in patients with obstructive sleep apnea. Am J Respir Crit Care Med 2002;165:152-158.

Coronary Artery Disease and Obstructive Sleep Apnea

Jan Hedner

Karl A. Franklin

Yüksel Peker

ABSTRACT

Recurrent apneas during sleep lead to a sequence of events that, independently or in concert with other recognized risk factors, are likely to have harmful effects on vascular structure and function. The epidemiologic support for a causal relationship between obstructive sleep apnea (OSA) and coronary artery disease (CAD) is rapidly increasing but is not yet fully confirmed. This relationship is stronger in clinical cohorts compared with the general population, which suggests that comorbid OSA in obese, hypertensive, smoking, and hyperlipidemic subjects may provide an additive or synergistic risk factor for development of CAD. OSA-related phenomena including hypoxemia, reoxygenation, and recurrent vascular wall stress may induce coronary artery disease, and the events may by themselves aggravate already existing compromised coronary artery flow reserve.

Patients with CAD, including nocturnal angina, should therefore be considered for sleep recording because elimination of apneas by nasal continuous positive airway pressure (CPAP) during sleep has been shown to reduce angina attacks and nocturnal myocardial ischemia. The long-term tentative causal association between OSA and CAD is supported by experimental data suggesting endothelial dysfunction, acceleration of vascular inflammation, and development of atherosclerotic disease as a result of the breathing disorder. Increased recognition of the adverse impact of OSA on vascular disease may open a perspective of new primary and secondary prevention models for CAD that involve identification and elimination of the sleep and breathing disorder.

Epidemiologic data suggest that obstructive sleep apnea (OSA) is overrepresented in patients with coronary artery disease (CAD). Conversely, evidence suggests that the clinical course of CAD is initiated or accelerated by the presence of the breathing disorder. A rapidly evolving field of experimental data suggests that OSA, by phenomena such as hypoxemia and reoxygenation, may trigger a sequence of events involved in the development of atherosclerotic disease.

Vascular disease and CAD development is influenced by a number of genotypic and phenotypic risk factors, several of which have been associated with OSA. Sleep apneic events induce a state of increased csardiac oxygen demand but are also frequently associated with low oxygen reserve due to lack of ventilation. Nocturnal angina can therefore be triggered by sleep apneas in patients with CAD. There is growing evidence that elimination of sleep apnea can benefit patients with OSA at risk of CAD in the immediate and long term. This chapter reviews the evidence of an association between these two conditions.

EPIDEMIOLOGY

The risk of experiencing angina pectoris or an acute coronary syndrome such as unstable angina, acute myocardial infarction (MI), or sudden cardiac death appears to be increased during the late hours of sleep or in the hours after awakening.[1] Researchers have speculated that this circadian distribution in part is explained by obstructive breathing. The epidemiologic support for a causal relationship between OSA and CAD is rapidly increasing but not yet fully confirmed.

In general, there is a stronger relationship between OSA and CAD in clinical cohorts compared with the general population because clinical cohort studies are particularly influenced by comorbidity and confounding factors including obesity, hypertension, smoking, and hyperlipidemia. In this perspective, OSA may provide an additive or synergistic risk factor for development of CAD. This chapter reviews evidence of a relationship between OSA and CAD in the general population as well as in populations with either OSA or CAD or both.

Prevalence of OSA and CAD in the General Population

Snoring, a common symptom of OSA, is associated with an up to fivefold risk increase for MI.[2,3] It has been claimed that snoring is a relatively insensitive measure of sleep-disordered breathing. However, the strength of these data is that snoring is an accessible symptom in large-scale studies, permitting appropriate adjustment for confounding risk factors. Snoring per se is a hard-to-quantify and observer-dependent phenomenon, but intrathoracic pressure changes typical of snoring may play an important role in the pathogenesis of CAD. This speculation is supported by a smaller-scale community study of 441 subjects[4] with sleep recordings showing an increased prevalence of CAD in nonapneic snorers (12%) compared with nonsnorers (7%), and there was a further increase (20%) in apneic snorers (crude odds ratio for CAD for apneic snorers versus nonsnorers, 3.5; 95% confidence interval, 1.2 to 10.0).

The largest study to date addressing OSA and CAD is the Sleep Heart Health Study.[5] The investigators performed a cross-sectional analysis of 6132 subjects undergoing unattended polysomnography (PSG). There was a modest but significant risk increase (peaking at an odds ratio of 1.42) for self-reported cardiovascular disease, but not specifically CAD, across the quartiles. The weak association in this prevalence study may be explained by a proportionally high age and a low median apnea-hypopnea index (AHI) in this population.

Prevalence of CAD in OSA

Clinical studies of CAD in sleep clinic cohorts generally involve OSA patients with daytime symptoms. Consequently, compared with studies in the general population, these studies selectively deal with symptomatic patients, those likely to suffer from more-severe sleep apnea, and potentially also patients with more obesity and other cardiovascular comorbidities. Available data in this area are to a large extent based on uncontrolled studies. For instance, in a sleep clinic cohort of 386 subjects,[6] CAD was present in almost one fourth of OSA subjects, and the percentage of patients with CAD was high among those with moderate to severe OSA.

Simultaneous PSG and electrocardiographic (ECG) recordings demonstrated that episodes of nocturnal ischemia were more common in OSA patients with CAD and mainly so during REM sleep, during episodes of high apnea activity as well as during sustained hypoxemia.[7] Moreover, ST-segment depression on ECG was not uncommon during sleep in OSA patients without a history of CAD, and these changes were eliminated by CPAP[8] Studies using invasive measures that were angiographically identified were able to verify CAD in more than 20% of investigated subjects with OSA,[9] and an even higher prevalence (68%) was reported in a slightly larger study of unselected OSA patients.[10] Collectively these data suggest proportionally high prevalence of CAD in sleep clinic cohorts.

Prevalence of OSA in CAD

Sleep disordered breathing appears to be common in patients with CAD. An early small study[11] demonstrated obstructive sleep apnea or central sleep apnea (CSA) with Cheyne-Stokes respiration (CSR) in more than 75% of subjects with CAD. A subsequent Australian case-control study that investigated middle-aged male survivors of acute MI and age-matched controls[12] provided the first clinic-based epidemiologic evidence of an increased prevalence of OSA in CAD patients. OSA (AHI = 5) was found in approximately one third of the patients compared with only 4% of controls and constituted

an independent predictor of MI after adjustment for traditional risk factors.

A larger case-control study[13] provided a similar OSA prevalence (approximately 30%), whereas the prevalence in the control group was 20%. In this population, an AHI of 20 was associated with a history of MI (odds ratio, 2.0). Finally, in a tightly matched Swedish case-control study of 62 patients, OSA provided an independent odds ratio of 3.1 for CAD.[14]

The OSA and CAD association may also be influenced by gender. In patients with angiographically verified CAD, AHI greater than 10 was almost twice as common in men[15] but three times more common in women[16] younger than 70 years and compared with age-matched controls.

The possibility that OSA may trigger episodes of nocturnal angina in patients with disabling CAD was addressed in an interventional study.[17] OSA was found in 9 of 10 investigated CAD patients with nocturnal angina, and episodes of ischemia were reversed after CPAP treatment. A subsequent larger cross-sectional study found signs of silent nocturnal myocardial ischemia in 31% of 226 CAD patients[18] but failed to demonstrate a general and immediate temporal relationship between sleep-disordered breathing events and episodes of myocardial ischemia. However, a direct association could be documented in a small subgroup of patients and, in general, episodes of silent ischemia appeared to be more frequent in those with more-severe sleep disordered breathing.

In summary, OSA is common in patients with MI, but mean AHI is relatively mild in most published reports (Table 101–1). Moreover, the prevalence of OSA is higher in patients with MI than in those with angina pectoris. This finding may be explained by occurrence of Cheyne-Stokes respiration as a result of reduced ejection fraction.[18] Nocturnal angina may be associated with severe OSA in CAD patients. Available studies on the OSA prevalence in the CAD population (see Table 101–1) include 518 patients, and approximately one third of those had an AHI exceeding 10.

Incidence of CAD in Longitudinal Studies

Incidence of CAD has been investigated in three large studies with focus on snoring habits. In a Finnish cohort of 4388 men aged 40 to 69 years, snoring provided a 1.9-fold increased risk of CAD during a 3-year follow-up.[22] The association was somewhat weakened after CAD risk-factor adjustment. A subsequent

Table 101–1. **Prevalence of Sleep Apnea* in Patients with Coronary Artery Disease**

Author	Publication Year	N	Sex	AHI > 10	Controls
De Olazabal[11]	1982	17	Male	76%	
Andreas[19]	1996	50	Male, female	50%	
Mooe[15]	1996	142	Male	37%	yes
Mooe[16]	1996	102	Female	30%	yes
Koehler[7]	1996	74	Male	35%	
Peker[14]	1999	62	Male, female	31%	yes
Moruzzi[20]	1999	22	Male, female	9%	
Sanner[21]	2001	49	Male, female	27%	
Total		518		37%	

*AHI > 10.

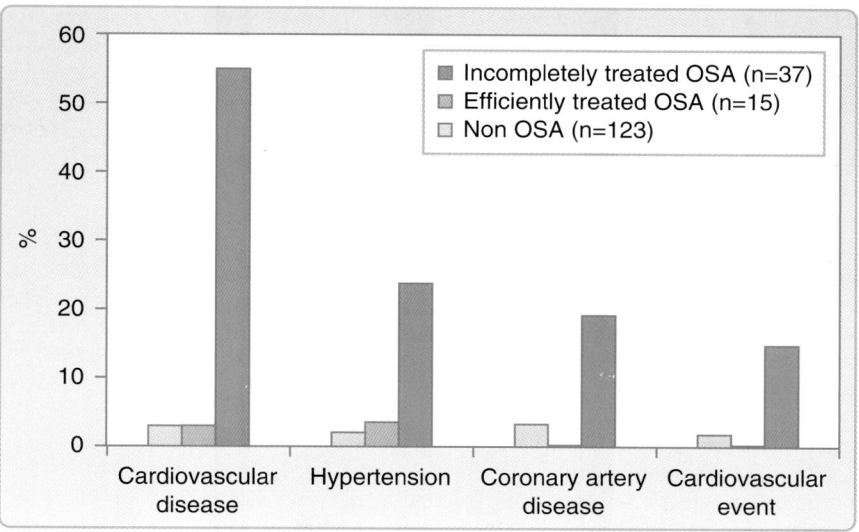

Figure 101–1. Incidence of cardiovascular disease during a 7-year follow-up in middle-aged men otherwise healthy at baseline. Fraction of individuals with incidence of cardiovascular disease, hypertension, coronary artery disease (CAD), and cardiovascular event (stroke, myocardial infarction [MI], or cardiovascular death). Depicted are data from patients without OSA (non OSA) as well as from those incompletely or efficiently treated for their sleep and breathing disorder. (Reprinted from Peker Y, Hedner J, Norum J, et al: Increased incidence of cardiovascular disease in middle-aged men with obstructive sleep apnea: A seven-year follow-up. Am J Respir Crit Care 2002;166:159-165.)

smaller prospective study[23] in 400 subjects suggested that snoring worsened the prognosis of patients with already-known risk factors for cardiovascular disease but did not constitute an independent or predictive risk factor in itself. A large Danish prospective investigation on self-reported snoring habits in middle-aged men[24] failed to identify an increased incidence of CAD, although a trend was seen in the younger half of the cohort.

These data are supported by a well-controlled 4-year prospective Spanish study,[25] which showed a tripled risk for acute MI in snorers compared with nonsnorers. Moreover, a large follow-up study[26] showed an almost tripled risk of cardiovascular death when the symptom of daytime sleepiness was added to snoring. The association was stronger in men younger than 60 years.

As already mentioned, it is likely that snoring only provides an unspecific measure of OSA. These studies are likely to contain variable contribution of patients with OSA, and it remains unknown if any specific aspect of snoring such as profound negative intrathoracic pressures may be involved in CAD development.

Incident CAD data from the longitudinal analysis of the Sleep Heart Health Study are not yet available. A smaller retrospective sleep laboratory cohort study reported incident CAD in almost a quarter of untreated OSA patients during a 7-year follow-up period.[27] The corresponding number in treated sleep apnea patients and nonapneic snorers were 4% and 6%, respectively. Moreover, more than 50% of a normotensive cohort not treated for OSA developed at least one cardiovascular disease during the 7-year follow-up (Fig. 101–1). New cases with CAD were also found among those maintaining normotension.[28] These findings suggest that development of CAD may be in part independent of diurnal systemic hypertension induced by OSA.

PATHOGENESIS

Obstructive sleep apnea is associated with considerable immediate hemodynamic change (see Chapter 99). During the cycle of the apneic event there is increased work of breathing, considerable negative intrathoracic pressure, recurrent hypoxia and reoxygenation, and fluctuating autonomic activity (see Chapter 99). Heart rate and blood pressure also fluctuate considerably across the cycle, but the absolute contribution of these changes to development of cardiovascular disease is unknown. Increased oxygen demand and reduced oxygen supply (i.e., hypoxemia) following sleep disordered breathing may trigger an attack of angina pectoris in patients with CAD who already have reduced coronary flow reserve.[11,17,19]

Another study reported signs of apnea-induced ischemia predominantly during REM sleep,[7] a finding that may be explained by the frequently more prolonged and severe apneic events that commonly occur in this sleep stage. OSA is also associated with long-term alteration of cardiac structure, hemodynamic reflex function, and vascular structure or function. The disorder leads to immediate and sustained sympathetic activation.[29] Baroreceptor and chemoreceptor responsiveness is altered,[30] and vascular reactivity in terms of responsiveness to hypoxemia or vasoconstrictors appears to be elevated.[31] A series of recent studies demonstrated that vascular endothelial function, expressed in terms of nitric oxide vascular dilating capacity, appears to be reduced in OSA.[32] Changes are specific to OSA in the sense that they are reversed by CPAP (see Chapter 99).[33]

The mechanisms responsible for endothelial cell damage and dysfunction are not entirely understood. However, recent investigations have shown that oxidative stress, potentially as a result of hypoxia and reperfusion, is enhanced in OSA.[34] Oxidative stress results in compromised nitric oxide bioavailability and leads to an activation of redox-sensitive gene expression. Ensuing steps in this chain of events include increased expression of adhesion molecules by an activated endothelium and leukocytes, which finally leads to acceleration of vascular inflammation and atherosclerotic disease.

This hypothesis (see Chapter 96, Fig. 96–2)[35] is supported by data from OSA patients demonstrating increased free radical production,[34] increased plasma-lipid peroxidation, increased adenosine and uric acid levels,[35] and increased levels of redox-sensitive gene expression products including vascular endothelial growth factor[36] and inflammatory cytokines.[37] Moreover, circulating levels of adhesion molecules[38] as well as adhesion molecule–dependent monocyte-to-endothelial cell avidity appears to be increased in OSA.[39] Finally, sleep apnea appears to provide an additive stimulus for adhesion molecule expression in patients with CAD.[40]

The tentative association between OSA and CAD is therefore supported by experimental data suggesting endothelial dysfunction, acceleration of vascular inflammation, and development of atherosclerotic disease as a result of the breathing disorder. Atherosclerotic plaque formation may jeopardize coronary flow reserve and generate symptoms of nocturnal angina during periods of increased flow demand. Such episodes occur repeatedly in sleep apnea, and they are associated with hypoxemia that further enhances the vulnerability for ischemia.

On the other hand, the majority of heart attacks (i.e., acute MI or sudden cardiac death) stem from sudden rupture of less-obtrusive plaques, which triggers thrombus formation in coronary vessels.[41] Several studies suggest that the risk of experiencing acute MI peaks in the early hours after awakening from sleep (see Chapter 97).[1] Therefore, OSA may contribute to the vascular changes of CAD, and it is also possible that sleep disordered breathing influences the circadian acute coronary event distribution. OSA may lead to a disproportionate number of events that occur during or soon after the sleeping period.

Although there is scientific support for a considerable impact of OSA on vascular structure and function, it is likely that development of CAD and other forms of vascular disease is determined by multiple genotypic and phenotypic factors. The absolute role of OSA in this concerted influence should evidently be better clarified. However, with the increasing recognition of OSA as an independent, additive, or even synergistic risk factor for CAD, we are facing a need for early identification of high-risk persons and a consensus on well-defined treatment strategies in such patients.

CLINICAL COURSE AND PREVENTION

Early recognition and treatment of OSA may be beneficial in terms of CAD prevention. A retrospective analysis of a sleep laboratory cohort followed over 7 years found a reduction (relative risk, 0.29; confidence interval, 0.10 to 0.82) of incident CAD in effectively treated OSA compared with ineffectively treated or untreated patients.[27] Conversely, in a group of CAD patients followed for 5 years, mortality was higher in those with comorbid OSA (38%) compared with those with no OSA (9%).[42] Although the higher mortality in part was explained by the presence of other traditional risk factors, there was an independent influence by the breathing disorder. Another study followed 408 patients with stable angina and angiographically verified CAD during 5 years after sleep apnea recordings. The risk for a cerebrovascular event including stroke and transient ischemic attack was tripled in CAD patients with concomitant OSA (AHI > 10).[43]

Patients with CAD and nocturnal angina should be considered for sleep recording, because nasal CPAP reduces angina attacks and nocturnal myocardial ischemia.[17] In the study of 10 severely disabled patients with a history of frequent nocturnal angina, 9 had sleep apnea. Treatment with CPAP reduced episodes of nocturnal ischemia. There is no evidence to suggest that medication used for treatment of CAD affects the severity of the breathing disorder. A double-blind crossover study of nitrates in OSA patients with or without CAD found lower oxygen saturation during apnea-associated ischemic episodes than during ischemia not associated with apnea (77.3% vs. 93.1%), and nitrate administration did not reduce the number of ischemic episodes associated with apnea.[44]

Clinical Pearls

Recurrent apneas during sleep lead to a sequence of events that independently or in concert with other recognized risk factors are likely to have harmful effects on vascular structure and function.

Not only may phenomena such as hypoxemia, reoxygenation, and recurrent vascular wall stress induce coronary artery disease (CAD), but also the events in themselves may aggravate already existing compromised coronary artery flow reserve.

The adverse health effects of OSA in terms of CAD development, progression, and proneness to complications are likely to depend on genotypic and phenotypic factors. Markers or predictors for identification of high-risk persons in this context are still lacking.

Approximately one third of patients with CAD have OSA defined according to conventional criteria. A large fraction of these patients do not exhibit daytime sleepiness. Compliance with CPAP treatment in nonsleepy OSA patients is low, and there are no data on CPAP compliance for OSA patients with CAD.

Recognition of the adverse impact of OSA on vascular disease will open a perspective of new primary and secondary prevention models for CAD that involve identifying and eliminating the sleep and breathing disorder.

REFERENCES

1. Muller JE, Tofler GH, Stone PH: Circadian variation and triggers of onset of acute cardiovascular disease. Circulation 1989;79:733-743.
2. D'Alessandro R, Magelli C, Gamberini G, et al: Snoring every night as a risk factor for myocardial infarction: A case-control study. BMJ 1990;300:1557-1558.
3. Koskenvuo M, Kaprio J, Telakivi T, et al: Snoring as a risk factor for ischaemic heart disease and stroke in men. BMJ 1987;294:16-19.
4. Olson LG, King MT, Hensley MJ, Saunders NA: A community study of snoring and sleep-disordered breathing. Health outcomes. Am J Respir Crit Care Med 1995;152:717-720.
5. Shahar E, Whitney CW, Redline S, et al: Sleep-disordered breathing and cardiovascular disease: Cross-sectional results of the Sleep Heart Health Study. Am J Respir Crit Care Med 2001;163:19-25.
6. Maekawa M, Shiomi T, Usui K, et al: Prevalence of ischemic heart disease among patients with sleep apnea syndrome. Psychiatry Clin Neurosci 1998;52:219-220.
7. Koehler U, Dubler H, Glaremin T, et al: Nocturnal myocardial ischemia and cardiac arrhythmia in patients with sleep apnea with and without coronary heart disease. Klin Wochenschr 1991;69: 474-482.
8. Hanly P, Sasson Z, Zuberi N, Lunn K: ST-segment depression during sleep in obstructive sleep apnea. Am J Card 1993;71:1341-1345.
9. Akasaka K, Akiba Y, Ishii Y, et al: Association between sleep apnea syndrome and coronary artery disease. Nippon Kyobu Shikkan Gakkai Zasshi 1997;35:16-21.

10. Bauer T, Ewig S, Schafer H, et al: Heart rate variability in patients with sleep-related breathing disorders. Cardiology 1996;87: 492-496.

11. De Olazabel JR, Miller MJ, Cook WR, Mithoefer JC: Disordered breathing and hypoxia during sleep in coronary artery disease. Chest 1982;82:548-552.

12. Hung J, Whitford EG, Parsons RW, Hillman DR: Association of sleep apnoea with myocardial infarction in men. Lancet 1990;336:261-264.

13. Schafer H, Koehler U, Ewig S, et al: Obstructive sleep apnea as a risk marker in coronary artery disease. Cardiology 1999;92: 79-84.

14. Peker Y, Kraiczi H, Hedner J, et al: An independent association between obstructive sleep apnoea and coronary artery disease. Eur Respir J 1999;14:179-184.

15. Mooe T, Rabben T, Wiklund U, et al: Sleep-disordered breathing in men with coronary artery disease. Chest 1996;109:659-663.

16. Mooe T, Rabben T, Wiklund U, et al: Sleep-disordered breathing in women: Occurrence and association with coronary artery disease. Am J Med 1996;101:251-256.

17. Franklin KA, Nilsson JB, Sahlin C, Näslund U: Sleep apnea and nocturnal angina. Lancet 1995;345:1085-1087.

18. Mooe T, Franklin KA, Wiklund U, et al: Sleep-disordered breathing in patients with coronary artery disease. Chest 2000;117: 1597-1602.

19. Andreas S, Schulz R, Werner GS, Kreuzer H: Prevalence of obstructive sleep apnoea in patients with coronary artery disease. Coron Artery Dis 1996;7:541-545.

20. Moruzzi P, Sarzi-Braga S, Rossi M, Contini M: Sleep apnoea in ischaemic heart disease: Differences between acute and chronic coronary syndromes. Heart 1999;82:343-347.

21. Sanner BM, Konermann M, Doberauer C, et al: Sleep-disordered breathing in patients referred for angina evaluation—association with left ventricular dysfunction. Clin Cardiol 2001;24:146-150.

22. Koskenvuo M, Kaprio J, Telakivi T, et al: Snoring as a risk factor for ischaemic heart disease and stroke in men. BMJ 1987;294: 16-19.

23. Zaninelli A, Fariello R, Boni E, et al: Snoring and risk of cardiovascular disease. Int J Cardiol 1991;32:347-352.

24. Jennum P, Hein HO, Suadicani P, Gyntelberg F: Risk of ischemic heart disease in self-reported snorers. A prospective study of 2,937 men aged 54 to 74 years: The Copenhagen male study. Chest 1995;108:138-142.

25. Zamarron C, Gude F, Otero Otero Y, Rodriguez-Suarez JR: Snoring and myocardial infarction: A 4-year follow-up study. Respir Med 1999;93:108-112.

26. Lindberg E, Janson C, Svärdsudd K, et al: Increased mortality among sleepy snorers: A prospective population based study. Thorax 1998;53:631-637.

27. Peker Y, Norum J, Hedner J, Carlson J: Increased incidence of coronary artery disease in obstructive sleep apnoea: A seven-year follow-up. Eur Respir J 2001;18(Suppl 33):518S. (abstract).

28. Peker Y, Hedner J, Norum J, et al: Increased incidence of cardiovascular disease in middle-aged men with obstructive sleep apnea: A seven-year follow-up. Am J Respir Crit Care 2002;166: 159-165.

29. Hedner J, Ejnell H, Sellgren J, et al: Is high and fluctuating muscle nerve sympathetic activity in the sleep apnoea syndrome of pathogenetic importance for the development of hypertension? J Hypertension 1988;6(suppl 4):529-531.

30. Parati G, Di Rienzo M, Bonsignore MR, et al: Autonomic cardiac regulation in obstructive sleep apnoea syndrome: Evidence from spontaneous baroreflex analysis during sleep. J Hypertension 1997;15(12 Pt 2):1621-1626.

31. Kraiczi H, Hedner J, Peker Y, Carlson J: Increased vasoconstrictor sensitivity in obstructive sleep apnoea. J Appl Physiol 2000; 89:493-498.

32. Carlson JT, Rangemark C, Hedner JA: Attenuated endothelium-dependent vascular relaxation in patients with sleep apnoea. J Hypertension 1996;14:577-584.

33. Narkiewicz K, Somers VK: Sympathetic nerve activity in obstructive sleep apnoea. Acta Physiol Scand 2003;177:385-390.

34. Schulz R, Mahmoudi S, Hattar K, et al: Enhanced release of superoxide from polymorphonuclear neutrophils in obstructive sleep apnea. Impact of continuous positive airway pressure therapy. Am J Respir Crit Care Med 2000;162:566-570.

35. Lavie L: Obstructive sleep apnoea syndrome—an oxidative stress disorder. Sleep Med Rev 2003;7:35-51.

36. Lavie L, Kraiczi H, Hefetz A, et al: Plasma vascular endothelial growth factor in sleep apnea syndrome: effects of nasal continuous positive air pressure treatment. Am J Respir Crit Care Med 2002;165:1624-1628.

37. Yokoe T, Minoguchi K, Matsuo H, et al: Elevated levels of C-reactive protein and interleukin-6 in patients with obstructive sleep apnea syndrome are decreased by nasal continuous positive airway pressure. Circulation 2003;107:1129-1134.

38. Ohga E, Tomita T, Wada H, et al: Effects of obstructive sleep apnea on circulating ICAM-1, IL-8, and MCP-1. J Appl Physiol 2003;94:179-184.

39. Dyugovskaya L, Lavie P, Lavie L: Phenotypic and functional characterization of blood γδ T cells in sleep apnea. Am J Respir Crit Care Med 2003;168:242-249.

40. El-Solh AA, Mador MJ, Sikka P, et al: Adhesion molecules in patients with coronary artery disease and moderate-to-severe obstructive sleep apnea. Chest 2002;121:1541-1547.

41. Libby P: Atherosclerosis: The new view. Sci Am 2002;286:46-55.

42. Peker Y, Hedner J, Kraiczi H, Löth S: Respiratory disturbance Index: An independent predictor of mortality in coronary artery disease. Am J Respir Crit Care Med 2000;162:81-86.

43. Mooe T, Franklin KA, Holmström K, et al: Sleep-disordered breathing and coronary artery disease: Long-term prognosis. Am J Respir Crit Care Med 2001;164:1910-1913.

44. Schafer H, Koehler U, Ploch T, Peter JH: Sleep-related myocardial ischemia and sleep structure in patients with obstructive sleep apnea and coronary heart disease. Chest 1997;111:387-393.

Heart Failure

Shahrokh Javaheri

ABSTRACT

Heart failure is a common disorder that has a significant economic impact and is associated with excess morbidity and mortality. Because of increased average life span and improved therapy for hypertension and ischemic coronary artery disease, the incidence and prevalence of heart failure will continue to rise into the 21st century.

One factor that may contribute to the progressively declining course of heart failure is the occurrence of periodic breathing, with repetitive episodes of apnea, hypopnea, and hyperpnea. Episodes of apnea, hypopnea, and hyperpnea cause sleep disruption, arousals, hypoxemia and reoxygenation, hypercapnia and hypocapnia, and changes in intrathoracic pressure. These pathophysiologic consequences of sleep-related breathing disorders have deleterious effects on the cardiovascular system, and they may be most pronounced in the setting of established heart failure and coronary artery disease. Diagnosis and treatment of sleep-related breathing disorders may therefore improve morbidity and mortality of patients with heart failure.

Heart failure has been known for more than two centuries to be associated with abnormal breathing patterns. John Cheyne and William Stokes have been credited for visual description of a unique pattern of breathing in heart failure known as Cheyne-Stokes breathing.[1,2] However, 37 years earlier, John Hunter,[3,4] a British physician, was the first to actually describe this breathing pattern, which is characterized by gradual crescendo-decrescendo changes in tidal volume, commonly with an intervening central apnea (Fig. 81–1).[5-9]

Periodic breathing is a pattern of breathing characterized by cyclic fluctuations in the amplitude of tidal volume.[10] It consists of recurring cycles of apnea or hypopnea, or both, followed by hyperpnea. The apneas and hypopneas may be obstructive (i.e., due to upper airway occlusion) or central in nature.[10] Obstructive sleep apnea–hypopnea is the most common form of periodic breathing in persons without heart failure. However, in patients with heart failure, both obstructive and central periodic breathing occur, although central sleep apnea–hypopnea is predominant.

Cheyne-Stokes breathing is a form of periodic breathing that occurs in systolic heart failure and has a long cycle time.[11] This is an important feature of Cheyne-Stokes breathing and reflects the prolonged circulation time that is a pathologic feature of systolic heart failure. Cheyne-Stokes breathing is a subjective description and is not readily quantifiable. For these reasons, the term *central sleep apnea* is preferable, and it also avoids misrepresentation, since the credit for the discovery of Cheyne-Stokes breathing has not been given to the original discoverer.

Cheyne-Stokes breathing observed in awake heart failure patients has been considered a rare entity and potentially an indicator of terminal prognosis. However, like obstructive apnea, central apnea occurs primarily during sleep, and recent polysomnographic studies have reported a high prevalence of this disorder in patients with heart failure.[8,9,12-14] This finding is important, because the consequences of sleep-related breathing disorders such as hypoxemia may affect the natural history of heart failure. Therefore, treatment of sleep apnea could potentially improve morbidity and mortality of patients with heart failure.

EPIDEMIOLOGY OF HEART FAILURE AND SLEEP-RELATED BREATHING DISORDERS

Epidemiology of Heart Failure

Heart failure is approaching epidemic proportions and has become a major public health problem.[15] It is the only cardiovascular disorder with increasing incidence and prevalence, causing excessive morbidity and mortality. It is estimated that heart failure may contribute directly or indirectly to 266,400 deaths each year. The death rate increases progressively with advanced symptomatology, approaching 30% to 40% annually in patients with heart failure in New York Heart Association class IV. It is the largest single Medicare expenditure because it is the leading cause of hospitalization for patients older than age 65 years. Not surprisingly, therefore, the economic impact of heart failure is also huge, with an estimated cost of $29 billion in 2004 (see Chapter 96, Table 96–1).[15]

Left ventricular myocardial failure is the most common cause of heart failure in adults, and it could be predominantly diastolic in nature or manifested by combined systolic and diastolic dysfunction. The underlying pathology in diastolic heart failure is a stiff, noncompliant left ventricle with preserved systolic function. The principal hallmark of diastolic dysfunction, therefore, is an elevation in left ventricular end-diastolic pressure and consequently in pulmonary capillary pressure, resulting in pulmonary congestion, pulmonary edema, and shortness of breath (backward failure). In contrast, the hallmark of the left ventricular systolic dysfunction is a depressed ejection fraction, which is commonly associated with an increase in left ventricular end-diastolic and systolic volumes. The symptoms, which are due to both diminished cardiac output and the concomitant diastolic dysfunction, include fatigue, shortness of breath, and exercise intolerance.

It is estimated that 1.5% to 2% of the United States population has heart failure.[15] Heart failure is a disorder of elderly persons, and its prevalence increases to approximately 6% to 10% in those older than 65 years. Heart failure is the only cardiovascular disease with increasing incidence and prevalence.

In this regard, it is estimated that 20 million people may have asymptomatic cardiac dysfunction, and with time, these persons are likely to become symptomatic. Because of increased average life span and improved therapy of ischemic coronary artery disease and hypertension, which are risk factors for heart failure, it is predicted that incidence and prevalence of heart failure will continue to rise in the 21st century.

Sleep Apnea in Systolic Heart Failure

The prevalence of sleep-related breathing disorders has been systematically studied in patients with systolic heart failure.[5,16] These studies[9,12-14,17-21] show that about 40% to 80% of such patients have an apnea-hypopnea index (AHI) of 15 events per hour (Table 102–1). High prevalence rates have been reported in subjects who have systolic heart failure and are awaiting transplantation,[17] those with valve disease,[18] and those with an implanted cardiac defibrillator.[19]

The largest prospective study in systolic heart failure[9] involved 81 ambulatory male subjects with stable, treated heart failure. Using an AHI of 15 per hour or greater as the threshold, 41 subjects (51% of all patients) had moderate to severe sleep apnea–hypopnea, with an average AHI of 44. In comparison, a population study of subjects without heart failure[22] showed that 9% of working men and women age 30 to 60 years had an AHI greater than 15. An AHI of 5 or greater has been used to define presence of a significant number of disordered breathing events in obstructive sleep apnea–hypopnea syndrome.[22] Therefore, with a much higher prevalence of sleep apnea (see Table 102–1) observed in patients with heart failure than in the general population, systolic heart failure should be the leading risk factor for sleep apnea in the general population.

Studies have reported that 5% to 32% of patients with systolic heart failure have predominantly obstructive sleep apnea, and 30% to 60% have central sleep apnea (see Table 102–1). The major reasons for differences in the prevalence rates are the criteria used to define hypopnea, the accuracy of classification of disordered breathing events (obstructive versus central, particularly in regard to hypopneas), the criteria used to define predominant obstructive versus central sleep apnea, the number of obese heart failure patients enrolled, the level of arterial P_{CO_2}, and the severity of left ventricular systolic dysfunction.

Obesity is an important risk factor for development of obstructive sleep apnea in patients with heart failure,[9,12] as it is for patients without heart failure.[22] Subjects with systolic heart failure and obstructive sleep apnea are significantly heavier, snore habitually, and have a higher systemic arterial blood pressure than subjects with central sleep apnea.[9,12]

Sleep Apnea in Isolated Diastolic Heart Failure

Little is known about prevalence of sleep-related breathing disorders and their impact in patients with isolated diastolic heart failure.[23] Yet both disorders are prevalent in the older population, and the major consequences of sleep-related breathing disorders such as sympathetic activation, nocturnal hypertension, and hypoxemia could impair left ventricular diastolic function. It is, therefore, conceivable that sleep-related breathing disorders are a cause of diastolic dysfunction or contribute to its progression. Epidemiologic and therapeutic studies are needed to define the relation of these two disorders, particularly in the older population, and the impact of treatment of sleep apnea on the natural history of isolated diastolic heart failure.

GENDER AND SLEEP-RELATED BREATHING DISORDERS IN SYSTOLIC HEART FAILURE

In the general population, the prevalence of obstructive sleep apnea is significantly higher in men than in women.[22,24] This also holds true for central sleep apnea in systolic heart failure. Combining the results of several studies of patients with systolic heart failure,[12-14,17,18] 40% of the male patients and 18% of the female patients have central sleep apnea (Fig. 102–1). A similar trend was found for obstructive sleep apnea.

The reasons for a low prevalence of obstructive and central sleep apnea in women are not well understood, but female hormones may play an important role. The results of population studies of subjects without heart failure (reviewed by Young et al.[24]) suggest that menopause may be a risk factor for obstructive sleep apnea and that the risk is probably reduced by hormone replacement therapy. In women with congestive

Table 102–1. Prevalence of Sleep-Related Breathing Disorders in Patients with Systolic Heart Failure

Study Site (Reference)	N	Sex (M/F)	LVEF (%)	AHI ≥ 10 (%)	AHI ≥ 15/h (%)	CSA with AHI ≥ 15 (%)	OSA with AHI ≥ 15 (%)
Cincinnati*[9]	81	81/0	25	57	51	40	11
Grenoble*[14]	34	28/6	300	—	82	62	20
Veruno*†[21]	66	58/8	23	76	—	—	6
Créteil*[17]	20	17/3	<25	45	45	40	5
Melbourne*[13]	75	61/14	<40	59	43	32	11
Toronto‡[12]	450	382/68	27	72	61	29	32

*Prospective

†In this study electroencephalography was not recorded.

‡Retrospective

—, not available or not reported.

AHI, apnea-hypopnea index; CSA, central sleep apnea; F, female; LVEF, left ventricular ejection fraction; M, male; OSA, obstructive sleep apnea.

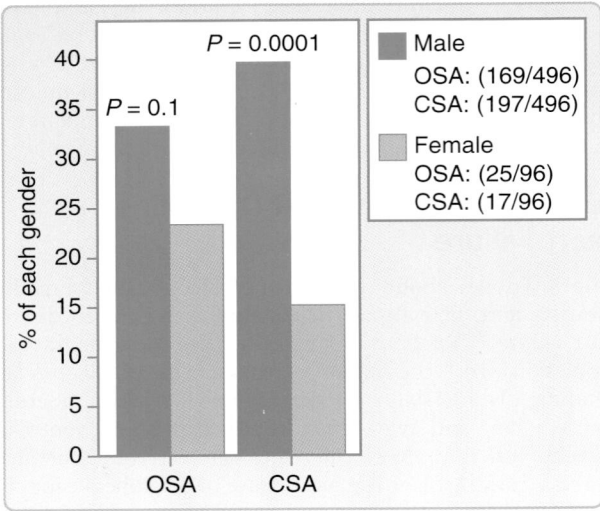

Figure 102–1. Prevalence of obstructive sleep apnea (OSA) and central sleep apnea (CSA) in men and women with systolic heart failure. The prevalence of CSA is much lower in women than in men. A similar trend is found in OSA, though it is not statistically significant. (From Javaheri S: Sleep related breathing disorders in heart failure. In Mann DL [ed]: Heart Failure: A Companion to Braunwald's Heart Disease. Philadelphia, WB Saunders, 2004, pp 471-487.)

heart failure and systolic dysfunction, risk of central sleep apnea was six times higher in those age 60 years or older when compared with those younger than 60 years.[12] A similar difference was also reported for obstructive sleep apnea–hypopnea before and after age 60 years.[12]

Progesterone is a known respiratory stimulant, and its effects on the respiratory system may in part explain the lower prevalence of central and obstructive sleep apnea in menstruating women. Progesterone increases ventilation[25] and the tone of the dilator muscles of the upper airway.[26] Furthermore, premenopausal women have a significantly lower apneic threshold than men.[27] This should decrease the probability of developing central apnea during sleep in female subjects (see Mechanisms of Central Sleep Apnea).

MECHANISMS OF SLEEP-RELATED BREATHING DISORDERS IN HEART FAILURE

Mechanisms of Central Sleep Apnea

The mechanisms of periodic breathing and central sleep apnea in heart failure are complex and multifactorial[5,28-31] (see Chapter 81). In heart failure, alterations occur in various components of the negative feedback system controlling breathing that increase the likelihood of developing periodic breathing, both during sleep and wakefulness. In addition, there are specific sleep-related mechanisms that explain the genesis of central sleep apnea and the reason periodic breathing becomes so prevalent during sleep. Mathematical models of the negative feedback system predict that increased arterial circulation time (which delays the transfer of information regarding changes in P_{O_2} and P_{CO_2}) from pulmonary capillary blood to the chemoreceptors, enhanced gain of the chemoreceptors, and enhanced plant gain (decreased functional residual capacity) collectively increase the likelihood of periodic breathing.[5,29,30]

Delay in transfer of information plays a fundamental role in destabilization of a negative feedback system.[5,29-31] It has the potential to convert a negative feedback system to a positive feedback system. In heart failure, arterial circulation time may be increased for a variety of reasons including dilation of cardiac chambers, increased pulmonary blood volume, and decreased cardiac output. However, patients with systolic heart failure invariably have increased circulation time. Therefore, although increased circulation time is necessary to develop periodic breathing, it does not explain why only some heart failure patients have periodic breathing.

The second factor that increases the likelihood of occurrence of periodic breathing (and also central apnea during sleep), is the gain of the chemoreceptors.[25] In persons with increased sensitivity to carbon dioxide (or hypoxia), the chemoreceptors elicit a large ventilatory response whenever the partial pressure of carbon dioxide rises (or P_{O_2} decreases). The consequent intense hyperventilation, by driving the P_{CO_2} below the apneic threshold, results in central apnea. Due to central apnea, P_{CO_2} rises (and P_{O_2} falls) and the cycles of hyperventilation and hypoventilation or central apnea are maintained.[25] Differences in the gain of the chemoreceptors among patients with heart failure may in part explain why only some patients develop periodic breathing and central sleep apnea.[28]

The third factor that may contribute to the development of periodic breathing in heart failure is decreased functional residual capacity, which results in underdamping.[5,29,31] This means that for a given change in ventilation (e.g., a pause in breathing), changes in the controlled variables—namely P_{O_2} and P_{CO_2}—will be augmented. In turn, the augmented changes in P_{O_2} and P_{CO_2} result in a pronounced compensatory ventilatory response, and overcompensation tends to destabilize breathing. Patients with heart failure may have decreased functional residual capacity for a variety of reasons, including pleural effusion, cardiomegaly, and decreased compliance of the respiratory system. Functional residual capacity may decrease further in the supine position, facilitating development of periodic breathing in this position.

The aforementioned mechanisms underlying periodic breathing are present both during sleep and wakefulness. However, in the supine position and during sleep, changes such as reduction in functional residual capacity, metabolic rate, and cardiac output occur that will further increase the likelihood of developing periodic breathing during sleep beyond that observed during wakefulness. Meanwhile, like obstructive apnea, central apnea usually occurs during sleep or when a subject is dozing. The genesis of central sleep apnea during sleep relates specifically to the removal of the non-chemical drive of wakefulness on breathing and to the unmasking of the apneic threshold, the level of P_{CO_2} below which rhythmic breathing ceases.[32-34] The difference between the two P_{CO_2} set points—the prevailing P_{CO_2} minus the P_{CO_2} at the apneic threshold—is a critical factor for occurrence of central sleep apnea. The smaller this difference, the greater the likelihood of occurrence of apnea (see later).

Normally, with the onset of sleep, ventilation decreases and P_{CO_2} increases. As long as the prevailing P_{CO_2} is above the apneic threshold, rhythmic breathing continues.[35-36] However, in some patients with heart failure, the awake prevailing P_{CO_2} does not significantly rise during sleep.[34,37] Therefore, because of the proximity of the prevailing P_{CO_2} to the apneic threshold, the likelihood of developing central apnea increases during sleep.

The reason for the lack of normally observed rise in PCO_2 in some patients with heart failure is not clear. It could be due to the lack of normally observed sleep-induced decrease in ventilation. Conceivably, because of increased venous return in the supine position, and in the presence of a stiff left ventricle, pulmonary capillary pressure could rise. This results in an increase in respiratory rate and ventilation, preventing the normally observed rise in PCO_2.

Several studies[38-40] have shown that subjects with heart failure and low arterial PCO_2 have a high probability of developing central apnea during sleep. Predictive value of a low arterial PCO_2 (<35 mm Hg) is about 80%.[40] However, although an awake low arterial PCO_2 is highly predictive of central sleep apnea, it is *not* a prerequisite. Many patients with heart failure and central sleep apnea have a normal awake $PaCO_2$.[40,41] What is important is the proximity of the apneic threshold to the arterial PCO_2.

Mechanisms of Obstructive Sleep Apnea

Another profound effect of sleep on breathing relates to the neuromuscular control of the upper airway dilator muscles. Periodic breathing due to systolic heart failure may particularly predispose the susceptible subjects to develop upper-airway occlusion during the nadir of the ventilatory cycles of periodic breathing.[7]

Obesity, which causes narrowing of the upper airway, is a major risk factor for obstructive sleep apnea in the general population.[22,24] This is also true in subjects with heart failure.[5,9,12]

Increased venous congestion and pressure due to right heart failure also may diminish upper airway size[42] and theoretically facilitate upper airway occlusion. Venous congestion of the upper airway may be worse in the supine (than in the erect) position. Decreased upper airway size due to both venous congestion and obesity may predispose patients with heart failure to develop upper airway occlusion during the nadir of the ventilatory cycles of periodic breathing,[7] when the tone of the dilator muscles of the upper airway decreases the most.[43]

PATHOLOGIC CONSEQUENCES AND PROGNOSTIC SIGNIFICANCE OF SLEEP-RELATED BREATHING DISORDERS IN HEART FAILURE

There are three major adverse consequences of obstructive and central sleep apneas and hypopneas.[5] These include intermittent arterial blood gas abnormalities characterized by hypoxemia-reoxygenation and hypercapnia-hypocapnia, excessive arousals and shift to light sleep stages, and large negative swings in intrathoracic pressure (for details see Chapter 92, Fig. 92–2). The pathophysiologic consequences of obstructive and central sleep apneas and hypopneas adversely affect various cardiovascular functions and are potentially most detrimental in the presence of established coronary artery disease and left ventricular systolic and diastolic dysfunction.[5]

In patients with established coronary artery disease, obstructive sleep apnea is an independent prognostic factor for recurrent cardiovascular disorders and survival.[44,45] In patients with systolic heart failure, presence of obstructive sleep apnea is associated with a reduction in left ventricular ejection fraction, which is reversed by treating sleep apnea with nasal continuous positive airway pressure (CPAP).[46,47] This is important, because left ventricular ejection fraction is a predictor of survival in patients with systolic heart failure.

In regard to central sleep apnea, several studies (Table 102–2) have suggested that presence of central sleep apnea decreases survival of patients with systolic heart failure.[19,21,48-52] In one study,[53] a similar trend was reported, but the difference in mortality was not significant. Although these studies may be criticized for a number of reasons,[16] they collectively suggest a trend toward increased mortality of heart failure patients who have periodic breathing and central sleep apnea. Furthermore, treatment of central sleep apnea decreases sympathetic activity, increases left ventricular ejection fraction, and may improve survival.[5,51]

Table 102–2. Survival in Patients with Heart Failure and without (Group I) or with (Group II) Central Sleep Apnea

Author (ref)	No. of Patients I	No. of Patients II	Age (years) I	Age (years) II	LVEF (%) I	LVEF (%) II	AHI (no./h) I	AHI (no./h) II	Death (%) I	Death (%) II	Follow up (mo)
Findley[48]	9	6	56	68	34 (N = 6)	28 (N = 3)	1	30*	33	100*	6
Hanly[49]	7	9	63	61	24	22	6	41*	14	78*	36-54
Andreas[53]	16	20	48	59*	22	20	6	39*	6	20	11-53
Lanfranchi[21]	44	18	58	56	24	20*	<30	≥30*	14	59*	28
Fries[19]	24	9	65	65	37	32	<10	32	13	44*	24
Sin[51]	37	29	58	60	23	20	7	39	32	48*	60

*$P < 0.05$

AHI, apnea-hypopnea index; LVEF, left ventricular ejection fraction.

These studies show that periodic breathing and central sleep apnea are risk factors for increased mortality in subjects with systolic heart failure.

CLINICAL PRESENTATION OF OBSTRUCTIVE AND CENTRAL SLEEP APNEA IN HEART FAILURE

Sleep-onset insomnia and sleep-maintenance insomnia are common complaints in heart failure patients. Orthopnea and paroxysmal dyspnea may be especially troubling in those with severe failure. It is often difficult to clinically suspect sleep apnea in heart failure because most patients deny excessive sleepiness. We have found that prevalence of sleepiness is similar in heart failure patients with sleep apnea to that of those without.[9]

Furthermore, symptoms of sleep apnea and heart failure are overlapping. These symptoms include sleep maintenance insomnia, nocturia, waking up with shortness of breath or gasping, waking up unrested, and daytime fatigue. The overlapping of symptoms of heart failure with those of sleep apnea undoubtedly contributes to the underdiagnosis of sleep-related breathing disorders in heart failure. Central sleep apnea in particular is most difficult to diagnose,[8] since obesity and habitual snoring, which are the two hallmarks of obstructive sleep apnea in the general population and in patients with heart failure, are commonly absent in heart failure patients with central sleep apnea.[8,9]

INDICATIONS FOR POLYSOMNOGRAPHY IN HEART FAILURE

As noted above, patients with heart failure and sleep apnea do not generally present with symptoms that distinguish them from heart failure patients without sleep apnea. Furthermore, because heart failure is common, it is not possible to perform sleep studies on all heart failure patients. However, there are a number of clinical and laboratory findings that, when present in patients with heart failure, should increase clinical suspicion for sleep apnea. These markers are different from obstructive and central sleep apnea.

Risk factors for obstructive sleep apnea–hypopnea in patients with heart failure are similar to those without heart failure. These include obesity, increased neck size, habitual snoring, and hypertension. These risk factors and others such as witnessed apnea, waking up unrested, and excessive daytime sleepiness, when present, should increase suspicion for the presence of obstructive sleep apnea.

Nocturnal angina—substernal chest pain that awakens the patient—should increase suspicion for sleep apnea in general population and subjects with coronary heart disease and heart failure.

Paroxysmal nocturnal dyspnea characteristically awakens the patient with shortness of breath, which is relieved with resumption of an erect position. However, this symptom may be a perception of shortness of breath occurring during the hyperpneic phase of periodic breathing, suggesting presence of sleep apnea.

Restless sleep, maintenance insomnia, and leg movements may reflect periodic arousals and movements following apneas and hypopneas. Periodic limb movement, however, is also commonly found in patients with systolic heart failure.[54]

Patients with heart failure and *progressive ventricular systolic or diastolic dysfunction* or patients who remain in New York Heart Association classes III or IV despite intensive medical therapy should have a diagnostic sleep study.

In patients with a *cardioverter or defibrillator*, prevalence of central sleep apnea is high and it is associated with increased mortality.[19] Such patients should have polysomnography and may benefit from appropriate therapy of sleep-related breathing disorders.

The prevalence of sleep-related breathing disorders is high in *patients awaiting cardiac transplantation.*[17] The waiting period for transplantation is long, and a large number of patients succumb to consequences of heart failure while awaiting. It is conceivable that survival of these pretransplant subjects may improve if their sleep-related breathing disorders are treated. If so, the chance of receiving cardiac transplantation may increase.

As noted earlier, several studies[38-40] have shown that heart failure patients with *low arterial* P_{CO_2} have high prevalence of central sleep apnea. The predictive value of low P_{CO_2} (<35 mm Hg) is about 80%.[40] It must be emphasized, however, that many patients with heart failure have central sleep apnea without daytime hypocapnia.[40,41]

Several studies have shown that heart failure patients with sleep apnea have a higher prevalence of *atrioventricular arrhythmias*, especially atrial fibrillation[9,12,55] and ventricular arrhythmias.[9,56,57] Presence of these arrhythmias should increase suspicion for presence of central sleep apnea.

TREATMENT OF SLEEP-RELATED BREATHING DISORDERS IN HEART FAILURE

Depending on the nature of sleep apnea, there are different therapeutic options to treat obstructive and central sleep apnea.

Obstructive Sleep Apnea

In general, treatment of obstructive sleep apnea–hypopnea in heart failure is similar to that in the absence of heart failure, although there are some differences (Box 102–1).

Box 102–1. **Treatment of Obstructive Sleep Apnea in Heart Failure**

- Optimization of cardiopulmonary function
  - to eliminate or improve periodic breathing
  - to decrease right atrial and central venous pressure upper airway congestion/edema, which may increase upper airway size
  - to improve functional residual capacity, which may increase upper airway size as lung volume increases
- Weight loss
- Nasal positive airway pressure mechanical devices
  - Continuous positive airway pressure (CPAP)
  - Bilevel positive airway pressure (BiPAP) (Chapter 89)
- Supplemental nocturnal nasal oxygen to minimize desaturation and to decrease periodic breathing
- Upper airway procedures
  - Oral appliances (Chapter 91)
  - Uvulopalatopharyngoplasty (Chapter 90)
  - Laser surgery (Chapter 90)
  - Radiofrequency volume reduction (Chapter 90)

Optimization of Cardiopulmonary Function

Optimal treatment of heart failure by improving periodic breathing and central apneas may decrease the likelihood of developing upper airway occlusion. Upper airway occlusion may occur at the nadir of the ventilatory cycle of periodic breathing,[43] and in some patients with heart failure, the first few breaths following central apneas are obstructed.[7] Furthermore, in biventricular heart failure, elevated right atrial and central venous pressure may result in pharyngeal congestion and edema, so using therapeutic measures to decrease venous pressure and upper airway narrowing[42] is advisable. Finally, optimal treatment of heart failure to increase lung volumes may also increase upper airway size, which is dependent on lung volume.

Weight Loss

In the general population, weight reduction improves obstructive sleep apnea. Since many patients with heart failure and obstructive sleep apnea are also obese,[9,12] weight loss should be advised.

Nasal Positive Airway Pressure Devices

Nasal mechanical devices have been most successfully used to treat obstructive sleep apnea in the general population and in patients with heart failure.[46,47,58] These devices are the treatment of choice. First-night application of nasal CPAP results in a significant decrease in disordered breathing, arterial oxyhemoglobin desaturation, and arousals.[58] Short-term use of CPAP in patients with heart failure and obstructive sleep apnea improves left ventricular ejection fraction, blood pressure, and ventricular systolic volume.[46,47] For CPAP-noncompliant subjects who complain of a high expiratory pressure, bilevel mechanical devices should be tried.

Supplemental Nasal Oxygen

For subjects with heart failure who cannot tolerate mechanical devices, oxygen is an alternative for treating obstructive sleep apnea. The rationale for use of nocturnal supplemental nasal oxygen is to improve both hypoxemia and periodic breathing. Minimizing desaturation and hypoxemia-reoxygenation may have important therapeutic implications. Furthermore, as noted earlier, improvement in periodic breathing may decrease in obstructive disordered breathing events that occur at the nadir of ventilation.[7,43]

Upper Airway Procedures

Oral appliances are used and upper airway surgical procedures are performed for treatment of obstructive sleep apnea in the general population, but there are no data in patients with heart failure.

Central Sleep Apnea

Figure 102–2 depicts our present approach to treatment of this disorder in heart failure.

Optimization of Cardiopulmonary Function

Intensive therapy of heart failure with diuretics, angiotensin converting enzyme inhibitors, and beta-blockers improves and may even eliminate periodic breathing.[5] With therapy, hypocapnic patients may become eucapnic. The mechanism may be related to the elimination of tachypnea due to a decrease in pulmonary capillary congestion and pressure, which decrease J receptor stimulation. Furthermore, with therapy, arterial circulation time decreases (as stroke volume increases and cardiopulmonary blood volume decreases), and functional residual capacity may increase (due to a decrease in cardiac size, pleural effusion, and intra- and extravascular lung water). These changes contribute to stabilization of breathing.

Beta-blockers, by increasing stroke volume and decreasing pulmonary capillary pressure, should be particularly helpful in improving periodic breathing in systolic heart failure. An additional beneficial effect of beta-blockers may relate to their counterbalancing of nocturnal cardiac sympathetic hyperactivity due to repetitive arousals and desaturation. The reduction in cardiac sympathetic activity may have contributed to

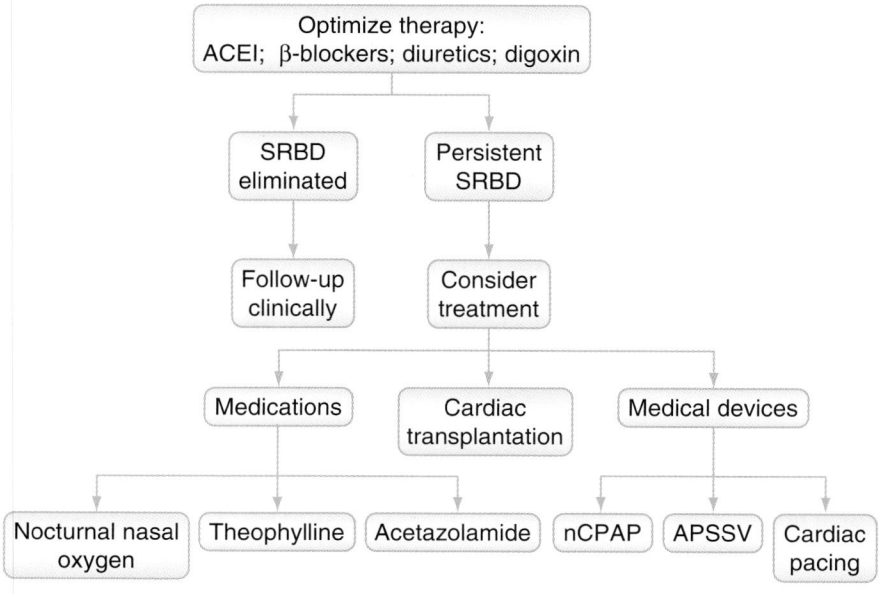

Figure 102–2. Treatment of central sleep apnea in systolic heart failure. ACEI, angiotensin converting enzyme inhibitor; APSSV, adaptive pressure support servoventilation; nCPAP, nasal continuous positive airway pressure; SRBD, sleep-related breathing disorders. (Adapted from Javaheri S: Sleep-related breathing disorders in heart failure. In Mann DL (ed): Heart Failure: A Companion to Braunwald's Heart Disease. Philadelphia, Saunders, 2004, p 482.)

improved survival in trials of beta-blockers in patients with heart failure. One particular side effect of beta-blockers, however, relates to their effect on melatonin. Melatonin, a sleep-promoting chemical, is secreted via the cyclic adenosine monophosphate (cAMP)-mediated beta-blockers signal transduction system. Beta-blockers, except carvedilol, by inhibiting this process, decrease melatonin secretion.[59,60]

After optimizing cardiopulmonary function, if periodic breathing persists, several approaches are possible (see Fig. 102–2).

Cardiac Transplantation

Preliminary studies (reviewed in Javaheri[5]) suggest that after cardiac transplantation, central sleep apnea is virtually eliminated. However, with time a large number (about 36%) of cardiac transplant recipients develop obstructive sleep apnea.[61] This is because of weight gain, which is most probably due to the use of corticosteroids.

Medical Devices

A number of studies (reviewed in Javaheri[5]) have reported on the use of nasal positive airway pressure devices, and one study has reported the use of an atrial pacing device to treat central sleep apnea.

NASAL POSITIVE AIRWAY PRESSURE DEVICES

Several devices, including continuous positive airway pressure, bilevel pressure, and adaptive pressure support servoventilation (APSSV), have been used to treat central sleep apnea in patients with systolic heart failure.[5,62]

One-night use of CPAP has been shown to eliminate central sleep apnea in 43% of the subjects with systolic heart failure.[58] Typically, these CPAP-responsive patients had mild to moderate central sleep apnea, and the average AHI decreased from 36 to 4, with elimination of desaturation. An important observation was that the number of premature ventricular contractions, couplets, and ventricular tachycardias decreased. This effect was presumed to be due to decreased sympathetic activity because arousals decreased and saturation improved. Heart failure patients with severe central sleep apnea (57% of the patients) did not respond to CPAP, and use of CPAP had no significant effect on ventricular irritability in these patients.[58]

Chronic trials (1 to 3 months) of nasal CPAP devices in subjects with heart failure show reduced AHI, improved desaturation, decreased plasma and urinary norepinephrine, and increased left ventricular ejection fraction (reviewed in Javaheri[5,62] and Naughton et al.[63]). Since sudden death (presumably caused by ventricular arrhythmias) and pump failure are the two major causes of death in heart failure patients, long-term use of CPAP by decreasing ventricular arrhythmias[58] and improving ejection fraction[63] may increase survival of patients with systolic heart failure and central sleep apnea.[51]

Caution, however, should be exercised with use of nasal CPAP.[5,62] Because of increased intrathoracic pressure, cardiac output may decrease, resulting in hypotension.[64] If coronary blood flow decreases, particularly in patients with coronary artery disease, CPAP may result in myocardial ischemia and arrhythmias. Furthermore, negative studies have been reported[65-67] and reviewed,[5,62] and subjects with severe central sleep apnea may not respond to CPAP.[58] Long-term compliance with CPAP in heart failure is not known and could be low. Successful use of CPAP in subjects with central sleep apnea requires teamwork and a referral to a sleep center familiar with heart failure and sleep disorders.

Therapeutic mechanisms of nasal CPAP are multifunctional. They may relate to an increase in PCO_2, which presumably may increase the differences between the prevailing and the apneic threshold PCO_2. They may improve stroke volume by decreasing left ventricular afterload, which decreases arterial circulation time; they may increase functional residual capacity, which decreases underdamping; and they may open the upper airway, as in some patients with central sleep apnea upper airway closure (see Javaheri[5,62] for review).

APSSV provides varying amounts of ventilatory support during different phases of periodic breathing.[62a] The support is minimal during the hyperpneic phase of periodic breathing and maximal during periods of diminished breathing and central apnea. In an acute (one-night) study[68] of 14 subjects with systolic heart failure and central sleep apnea, the APSSV device decreased the AHI more than oxygen, CPAP, and bilevel devices did. The APSSV device may be particularly helpful in those heart failure patients who have severe central sleep apnea and who may be noncompliant or nonresponsive[63] to CPAP devices.

CARDIAC PACING

In 15 subjects with predominantly mild to moderate central sleep apnea, some of whom had mild left ventricular systolic dysfunction, atrial overdrive pacing improved periodic breathing.[69] These subjects had permanent atrial-synchronized ventricular pacemakers placed for symptomatic sinus bradycardia. Atrial overdrive (average 72 beats per minute versus spontaneous 57 beats per minute) moderately but significantly decreased the AHI from 28 to 11, improved arterial oxyhemoglobin desaturation, and decreased arousals. The mechanisms remain unclear and the study needs to be confirmed. However, if cardiac pacing improves central sleep apnea, biventricular pacing[70] may be therapeutically more effective than atrial pacing overdrive.

Medications

OXYGEN

Systematic studies in patients with systolic heart failure[5,71-75] have shown that nocturnal therapy with supplemental nasal oxygen improves central sleep apnea (Fig. 102–3). Oxygen therapy may also decrease arousals and improve the hypnogram by shifting sleep structure to deep sleep stages. In addition, randomized, placebo-controlled, double-blind studies have shown that short-term (1 to 4 weeks) administration of nocturnal supplemental nasal oxygen improves maximum exercise capacity[74] and decreases overnight urinary norepinephrine excretion.[75]

Supplemental administration of nasal oxygen may decrease periodic breathing by several mechanisms.[5,71] These include a small rise in PCO_2, which presumably may increase the difference between the prevailing PCO_2 and the PCO_2 at the apneic threshold; reduction in ventilatory response to carbon dioxide and perhaps to hypoxemia; and an increase in body stores (e.g., lung contents) of oxygen, which increases damping. Prospective, placebo-controlled long-term studies, however, are necessary[71] to determine if nocturnal oxygen therapy has the potential to decrease morbidity and mortality of patients with systolic heart failure.

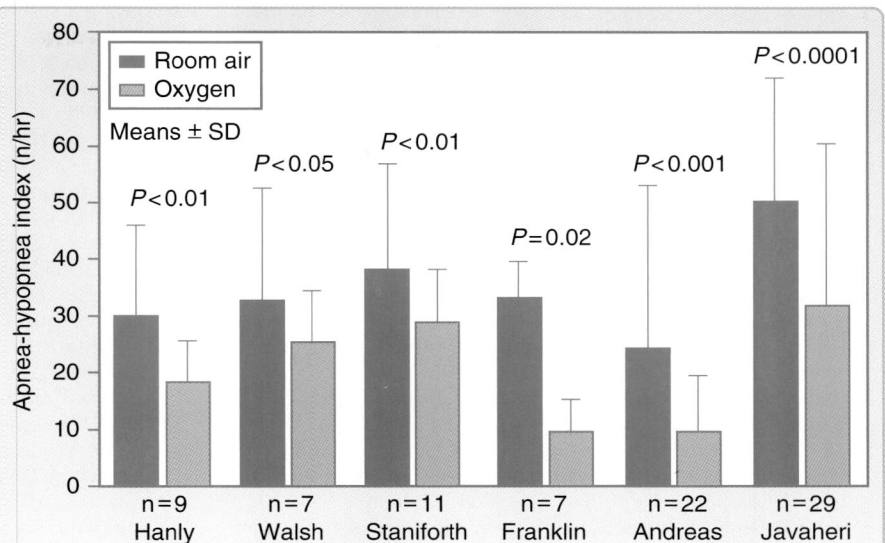

Figure 102–3. Effects of supplemental nasal oxygen on apnea-hypopnea index in patients with systolic heart failure.

THEOPHYLLINE

Open and blind studies[7,76] have shown the efficacy of theophylline in the treatment of central sleep apnea in heart failure (reviewed in Javaheri et al.[76]). In a double blind, randomized, placebo-controlled crossover study[76] of 15 patients with treated, stable systolic heart failure, oral theophylline at therapeutic plasma concentration (11 µg/mL, range 7 to 15 µg/mL), decreased the AHI by about 50% and improved arterial oxyhemoglobin saturation.[76]

Mechanisms of action of theophylline in improving central apnea remain unclear.[76] At therapeutic serum concentrations, theophylline competes with adenosine at some of its receptor sites. In the central nervous system, adenosine is a respiratory depressant and theophylline stimulates respiration by competing with adenosine. Conceivably, therefore, an increase in ventilation by theophylline could decrease central apnea during sleep. Theophylline does not increase ventilatory response to CO_2.

Potential arrhythmogenic effects and phosphodiesterase inhibition are common concerns with long-term use of theophylline in patients with heart failure. Therefore, further controlled studies are necessary to ensure its safety. If theophylline is used to treat central sleep apnea, frequent and careful follow-ups are necessary.

ACETAZOLAMIDE

By inhibiting carbonic anhydrase in red blood cells, kidney, and choroid plexus, acetazolamide causes acidosis in the blood and cerebrospinal fluid[77-79] and stimulates breathing. For this reason, acetazolamide has been used to treat idiopathic central sleep apnea and periodic breathing at high altitude.[80-81] Acetazolamide should be therapeutically effective in treatment of central sleep apnea in heart failure, but no systematic studies are available.

BENZODIAZEPINES

Benzodiazepines, by decreasing arousals, may decrease central sleep apnea. However, a placebo-controlled, double-blind study[82] showed a reduction in arousals but failed to show any improvement in central sleep apnea in patients with systolic heart failure. Although benzodiazepines do not increase the number of central apneas, their use may increase the likelihood of developing obstructive apneas in some heart failure patients.

Clinical Pearls

Heart failure is a highly prevalent disorder. Because of increased average life span and improved therapy of ischemic coronary artery disease and hypertension, the prevalence of heart failure will continue to rise in the 21st century.

Sleep-related breathing disorders may contribute to the progressively declining course of heart failure in some patients.

Periodic breathing is characterized by apnea, hypopnea, and hyperpnea, which cause sleep disruption, arousals, hypoxemia-reoxygenation, hypercapnia-hypocapnia, and changes in intrathoracic pressure. All of these adversely affect sleep and cardiovascular function.

Treatment of sleep-related breathing disorders may improve morbidity and mortality of patients with heart failure.

REFERENCES

1. Cheyne J: A case of apoplexy, in which the fleshy part of the heart was converted into fat. Dublin Hospital Reports and Communications 1818;2:216-223.
2. Stokes W: Observations on some cases of permanently slow pulse. Dublin Quarterly Journal of Medical Sciences 1846;2: 73-85.
3. Ward M: Periodic respiration. A short historical note. Ann R Coll Surg Engl 1973;52:330-334.
4. Allen R, Truk JL, Muricy R: The Case Books of John Hunter, FRS. New York, Parthenon, 1993.
5. Javaheri S: Sleep related breathing disorders in heart failure. In Mann DL (ed): Heart Failure: A Companion to Braunwald's Heart Disease. Philadelphia, WB Saunders, 2004, pp 471-487.

6. Hanly PJ, Millar TW, Steljes DG, et al: Respiration and abnormal sleep in patients with congestive heart failure. Chest 1989;96: 480-488.

7. Dowdell WT, Javaheri S, McGinnis W: Cheyne-Stokes respiration presenting as sleep apnea syndrome. Clinical and polysomnographic features. Am Rev Respir Dis 1990;141:871-879.

8. Javaheri S, Parker TJ, Wexler L, et al: Occult sleep-disordered breathing in stable congestive heart failure. Ann Intern Med 1995;122:487-492. Erratum, Ann Intern Med 1995;123:77.

9. Javaheri S, Parker TJ, Liming JD, et al: Sleep apnea in 81 ambulatory male patients with stable heart failure: Types and their prevalences, consequences, and presentations. Circulation 1998;97:2154-2159.

10. Cherniack NS: Apnea and periodic breathing during sleep. N Engl J Med 1999;341:985-987.

11. Millar TW, Hanly PJ, Hunt B, et al: The entrainment of low frequency breathing periodicity. Chest 1990;98:1143-1148.

12. Sin DD, Fitzgerald F, Parker JD, et al: Risk factors for central and obstructive sleep apnea in 450 men and women with congestive heart failure. Am J Respir Crit Care Med 1999;160:1101-1106.

13. Solin P, Bergin P, Richardson M, et al: Influence of pulmonary capillary wedge pressure on central apnea in heart failure. Circulation 1999;99:1574-1579.

14. Tremel F, Pépin J-L, Veale D, et al: High prevalence and persistence of sleep apnoea in patients referred for acute left ventricular failure and medically treated over 2 months. Eur Heart J 1999;20:1201-1209.

15. American Heart Association: Heart Disease and Stroke Statistics—2004 Update. Dallas, American Heart Association, 2004.

16. Javaheri S: Prevalence and prognostic significance of sleep apnea in heart failure. In Bradley TD, Floras JS (eds): Sleep Apnea. Implications in Cardiovascular and Cerebrovascular Disease. New York, Marcel Dekker, 2000, pp 415-433.

17. Lofaso F, Verschueren P, Rande JL, et al: Prevalence of sleep-disordered breathing in patients on a heart transplant waiting list. Chest 1994;106:1689-1694.

18. Yasuma F, Nomura H, Hayashi H, et al: Breathing abnormalities during sleep in patients with chronic heart failure. Jpn Circ J 1989;53:1506-1510.

19. Fries R, Bauer D, Heisel A, et al: Clinical significance of sleep-related breathing disorders in patients with implantable cardioverter defibrillators. Pace 1999;22:223-227.

20. Staniforth AD, Kinnear WJ, Starling R, et al: Nocturnal desaturation in patients with stable heart failure. Heart 1998; 79:394-399.

21. Lanfranchi PA, Braghiroli A, Bosimini E, et al: Prognostic value of nocturnal Cheyne-Stokes respiration in chronic heart failure. Circulation 1999;99:1435-1440.

22. Young T, Palta M, Dempsey J, et al: The occurrence of sleep-disordered breathing among middle-aged adults. N Engl J Med 1993;328:1230-1235.

23. Chan J, Sanderson J, Chan W, et al: Prevalence of sleep-disordered breathing in diastolic heart failure. Chest 1997;111: 1488-1493.

24. Young T, Peppard PE, Gottlieb DJ: Epidemiology of obstructive sleep apnea. Am J Respir Crit Care Med 2002;165:1217-1239.

25. Javaheri S, Guerra LF: Effects of domperidone and medroxyprogesterone acetate on ventilation in man. Respir Physiol 1990;81:359-370.

26. St. John WM, Bartlett D Jr., Knuth KV, et al: Differential depression of hypoglossal nerve activity by alcohol. Protection by pretreatment with medroxyprogesterone acetate. Am Rev Respir Dis 1986;133:46-48.

27. Zhou XS, Shahabuddin S, Zahn BR, et al: Effect of gender on the development of hypocapnic apnea/hypopnea during NREM sleep. J Appl Physiol 2000;89:192-199.

28. Javaheri S: A mechanism of central sleep apnea in patients with heart failure. N Eng J Med 1999;341:949-954.

29. Cherniack NS, Longobardo GS: Cheyne-Stokes breathing: An instability in physiologic control. N Eng J Med 1973;288: 952-957.

30. Khoo MCK: Theoretical models of periodic breathing in sleep apnea. In Bradley TD, Floras JS (eds): Sleep Apnea: Implications in Cardiovascular and Cerebrovascular Disease. New York, Marcel Dekker, 2000, pp 335-384.

31. Guyton AC, Crowell JW, Moore JW: Basic oscillating mechanisms of Cheyne-Stokes breathing. Am J Physiol 1956;187:395-398.

32. Dempsey JA, Skatrud JB: A sleep-induced apneic threshold and its consequences. Am Rev Respir Dis 1986;133:1163-1170.

33. Nakayama H, Smith CA, Rodman JR, et al: Effect of ventilatory drive on CO_2 sensitivity below eupnea during sleep. Am J Critical Care Med 2002;165:1251-1259.

34. Xie A, Skatrud JB, Puleo DS, et al: Apnea-hypopnea threshold for CO_2 in patients with congestive heart failure. Am J Respir Crit Care Med 2002;165:1245-1250.

35. Skatrud JB, Dempsey JA: Interaction of sleep state and chemical stimuli in sustaining rhythmic ventilation. J Appl Physiol 1983; 55:813-822.

36. Dempsey JA, Skatrud JB: Fundamental effects of sleep state on breathing. Cur Pulmonol 1988;9:267-304.

37. Tkacova R, Hall ML, Luie PP, et al: Left ventricular volume in patients with heart failure and Cheyne-Stokes respiration during sleep. Am J Respir Crit Care Med 1997;156:1549-1555.

38. Hanly P, Zuberi N, Gray R: Pathogenesis of Cheyne-Stokes respiration in patients with congestive heart failure, Relationship to arterial P_{CO_2}.Chest 1993;104:1079-1084.

39. Naughton M, Bernard D, Tam A, et al: Role of hyperventilation in the pathogenesis of central sleep apneas in patients with congestive heart failure. Am Rev Respir Dis 1993;148:330-338.

40. Javaheri S, Corbett WS: Association of low $PaCO_2$ with central sleep apnea and ventricular arrhythmias in ambulatory patients with stable heart failure. Ann Intern Med 1998;128:204-207.

41. Javaheri S: Central sleep apnea and heart failure. Circulation 2000;342:293-294.

42. Shepard JW Jr, Pevernagie DA, Stanson AW, et al: Effects of changes in central venous pressure on upper airway size in patients with obstructive sleep apnea. Am J Respir Crit Care Med 1996;153:250-254.

43. Hudgel D, Chapman KR, Faulks C, Hendricks C: Changes in inspiratory muscle electrical activity and upper airway resistance during periodic breathing induced by hypoxia during sleep. Am Rev Respir Dis 1987;135:899-906.

44. Mooe T, Franklin KA, Holmstrom K, et al: Sleep-disordered breathing and coronary artery disease: Long-term prognosis. Am J Respir Crit Care Med 2001;164:1910-1913.

45. Peker Y, Hedner J, Kraiczi H, et al: Respiratory disturbance index: An independent predictor of mortality in coronary artery disease. Am J Respir Crit Care Med 2000;162:81-86.

46. Kaneko Y, Floras JS, Usui K, et al: Cardiovascular effects of continuous positive airway pressure in patients with heart failure and obstructive sleep apnea. N Engl J Med 2003;248:1233-1241.

47. Mansfield DR, Gollogly C, Kaye DM: Controlled trail of continuous positive airway pressure in obstructive sleep apnea and heart failure. Am J Respir Crit Care Med 2004;169:361-366.

48. Findley LJ, Zwillich CW, Ancoli-Israel S, et al: Cheyne-Stokes breathing during sleep in patients with left ventricular heart failure. South Med J 1985;78:11-15.

49. Hanly P, Zuberi-Khokhar N: Increased mortality associated with Cheyne-Stokes respiration in patients with congestive heart failure. Am J Respir Crit Care Med 1996;153:272-276.

50. Ancoli-Israel S, DuHamel ER, Stepnowsky C, et al: The relationship between congestive heart failure, sleep apnea and mortality in older men. Chest 2003;124:1400-1405.

51. Sin DD, Logan AG, Fitzgerald FS, et al: Effects of continuous positive airway pressure on cardiovascular outcomes in heart failure patients with and without Cheyne-Stokes respiration. Circulation 2000;102:61-66.

52. Leite JJ, Mansur AJ, de Freitas HFG, et al: Periodic breathing during incremental exercise predicts mortality in patients with chronic heart failure evaluated for cardiac transplantation. J Am Coll Cardiol 2003;41:2175-2181.

53. Andreas S, Hagenah G, Möller C, et al: Cheyne-Stokes respiration and prognosis in congestive heart failure. Am J Cardiol 1996;78:1260-1264.

54. Hanly PJ, Zuberi-Khokhar N: Periodic limb movements during sleep in patients with congestive heart failure. Chest 1996;109:1497-1502.

55. Blackshear JL, Kaplan J, Thompson RC, et al: Nocturnal dyspnea and atrial fibrillation predict Cheyne-Stokes respirations in patients with congestive heart failure. Arch Inter Med 1995;155:1297-1302.

56. Cripps T, Rocker G, Strading J: Nocturnal hypoxia and arrhythmias in patients with impaired left ventricular function. Br Heart J 1992;68:382-386.

57. Lanfranchi PA, Somers VK, Braghiroli A, et al: Central sleep apnea in left ventricular dysfunction: Prevalence and implications for arrhythmic risk. Circulation 2003;107:727-732.

58. Javaheri S: Effects of continuous positive airway pressure on sleep apnea and ventricular irritability in patients with heart failure. Circulation 2000;101:392-397.

59. Arendt J, Bojkowski C, Franey C, et al: Immunoassay of 6-hydroxymelatonin sulfate in human plasma and urine: Abolition of urinary 24-hour rhythm with atenolol. J Clin Endocrinol Metab 1985;60:1166-1173.

60. Stoschizky K, Sakotnik A, Lercher P, et al: Influence of beta-blockers on melatonin release. Eur J Clin Pharmacol 1999;55:111-115.

61. Javaheri S, Abraham W, Brown C, et al: Prevalence of obstructive sleep apnea and periodic limb movement in 45 subjects with heart transplantation. Eur Heart J 2004;25:260-266.

62. Javaheri S: Heart failure and sleep apnea: emphasis on practical therapeutic options. Clin Chest Med 2003;24:207-222.

62a. Topfer V, El-Sebai M, Wessendorf TE, et al: Adaptive servoventilation: Effect on Cheyne-Stokes-Respiration and on quality of life. Pneumologie 2004;58:28-32.

63. Naughton MT, Bernard DC, Liu PP, et al: Effects of nasal CPAP on sympathetic activity in patients with heart failure and central sleep apnea. Am J Respir Crit Care Med 1995;152:473-479.

64. Keily JL, Deegan P, Buckley A, et al: Efficacy of nasal continuous positive airway pressure therapy in chronic heart failure: Importance of underlying cardiac rhythm. Thorax 1998;53:956-962.

65. Guilleminault C, Clerk A, Labanowski M, et al: Cardiac Failure and benzodiazepines. Sleep 1993;16:524-528.

66. Davies RJ, Harrington KJ, Ormerod OJ et al: Nasal continuous positive airway pressure in chronic heart failure with sleep-disordered breathing. Am Rev Respir Dis 1993;147:630-634.

67. Buckle P, Millar T, Kryger M: The effects of short-term nasal CPAP on Cheyne-Stokes respiration in congestive heart failure. Chest 1992;102:31-35.

68. Teschler H, Döhring J, Wang YM, et al: Adaptive pressure support servo-ventilation. Am J Respir Crit Care Med 2001;64:614-619.

69. Garrigue S, Bordier P, Jaïs P, et al: Benefit of atrial pacing in sleep apnea syndrome. N Engl Med 2002;346:404-412.

70. Abraham WT, Hayes DL: Cardiac resynchronization therapy for heart failure. Circulation 2004;108:2596-2603.

71. Javaheri S: Pembrey's Dream: The time has come for a long-term trial of nocturnal supplemental nasal oxygen to treat central sleep apnea in congestive heart failure. Chest 2003;123:322-325.

72. Hanly PF, Millar TW, Steljes DG, et al: The effect of oxygen on respiration and sleep in patients with congestive heart failure. Ann Intern Med 1989;111:777-782.

73. Javaheri S, Ahmed M, Parker TJ, with technical assistance of Brown CR: Effects of nasal O_2 on sleep-related disordered breathing in ambulatory patients with stable heart failure. Sleep 1999;22:1101-1106.

74. Andreas S, Clemens C, Sandholzer H, et al: Improvement of exercise capacity with treatment of Cheyne-Stokes respiration in patients with congestive heart failure. J Am Coll Cardiol 1996;27:1486-1490.

75. Staniforth AD, Kinnear WJ, Starling R, et al: Effect of oxygen on sleep quality, cognitive function and sympathetic activity in patients with chronic heart failure and Cheyne-Stokes respiration. Eur Heart J 1998;19:922-928.

76. Javaheri S, Parker TJ, Wexler L, et al: Effect of theophylline on sleep-disordered breathing in heart failure. N Engl J Med 1996;335:562-567.

77. Javaheri S, Kennealy J, Runck CD, et al: Cerebrospinal fluid ions in metabolic acidosis in dogs: Effects of acetazolamide. J Appl Physiol 1986;61:633-639.

78. Javaheri S, Weyne J, Demeester G, et al: Effects of acetazolamide on ionic composition of cisternal fluid during acute respiratory acidosis. J Appl Physiol 1984;57:92-97.

79. Javaheri S: Effects of acetazolamide on cerebrospinal fluid ions in metabolic alkalosis in dogs. J Appl Physiol 1987;62:1582-1588.

80. White DP, Zwillich CW, Pickett CK, et al: Central sleep apnea. Arch Intern Med 1982;142:1816-1819.

81. DeBacker WA, Verbraecken J, Willeman M, et al: Central apnea index decreases after prolonged treatment with acetazolamide. Am J Respir Crit Care Med 1995;151:87-91.

82. Biberdorf DJ, Steens R, Millar TW, et al: Benzodiazepines in congestive heart failure: Effects of temazepam on arousability and Cheyne-Stokes respiration. Sleep 1993;16:529-538.

Sleep and Fatigue in Cancer Patients

Sonia Ancoli-Israel

ABSTRACT

The study of sleep and fatigue in cancer is fairly new. Little is known about the cause or the mechanisms of the sleep disruption or the fatigue experienced by these patients. Evidence is accumulating that sleep is often disturbed probably secondary to a variety of factors. Fatigue is described as a major complaint in patients with cancer before treatment, while undergoing chemotherapy or radiation therapy, and after the completion of therapy.

The relationship, if any, between fatigue and the quality or quantity of sleep or between fatigue and the sleep-wake circadian rhythm is unknown. One hypothesis is that some of the cancer-related fatigue may be related to disturbed sleep or to disturbed sleep-wake rhythms. Different dimensions of fatigue (physical, attentional and cognitive, emotional or affective) are likely to be associated in some way with disrupted sleep and desynchronized sleep-wake rhythms. In cancer patients, as in other medically ill patients, disturbed sleep may be important not only to the expression of fatigue but also to the patients' quality of life, to their tolerance of treatment, and to the development of mood disorders, particularly clinical depression.

Disruptions in circadian rhythms themselves affect sleep quality as well as disrupting many other physiological mechanisms that pertain to fatigue. Lack of entrainment to the day-night cycle and not keeping regular hours can lead to feelings of grogginess, similar to the feeling of jet lag.

The degree of sleep disruption found in patients with cancer is not trivial. Objectively recorded sleep and biological rhythms have not been well investigated in patients with cancer, but since it appears that most may in fact not be getting a good night's sleep, the goal of future research should be to better characterize the sleep disruption and to find new treatment approaches to improve sleep in this population.

Fatigue is described as a major complaint in patients with cancer, before treatment, while undergoing chemotherapy or radiation therapy, and after the completion of therapy.[1-4a] Sleep disruption is also a common complaint in cancer patients,[5-7] and the poor sleep likely contributes to decreased quality of life.[1,8,9] Little is known about the relationship between fatigue and the quality or quantity of sleep or between fatigue and the sleep-wake circadian rhythm cycle. In fact, few studies have examined the circadian rhythms of cancer patients.[10-13] This chapter reviews the evidence on cancer-related sleep disruption, as well as the possible contribution of poor sleep and desynchronized circadian rhythms to cancer-related fatigue.

EPIDEMIOLOGY AND RISK FACTORS

Sleep Disruption

Nature of Sleep Disruption

There have been no large-scale epidemiologic studies of sleep disturbance in patients with cancer, but the prevalence of sleep complaints has been studied in small samples with a few different methodologies. Most of the early studies used questionnaires to examine self-reports of sleep disturbances. Two of the earliest studies examined subjective reports of sleep but never questioned the severity of the sleep disturbance.[14,15] Their results confirmed that patients complained of difficulty falling asleep, difficulty staying asleep, frequent awakening, and difficulty falling back to sleep both before[16] and during treatment.[17,18]

In an extensive sleep-related telephone survey of 150 patients with either breast or lung cancer in different stages of treatment and undergoing various types of treatment, 44% reported a sleep problem in the previous month.[18] Similar to other patients with insomnia,[19] only 17% of them communicated the problem to their physician. In a second survey, 45% reported having had a sleep problem in the previous month, and half of those rated the sleep problem moderate, severe, or intolerable. Ninety percent reported awakening during the night as the most frequent problem, 85% complained of not getting enough sleep, 75% complained of difficulty falling back to sleep, and 39% reported napping.

Another way to gather information about sleep disturbance is by extrapolating that information from data on sedative-hypnotic use.[5] In a group of more than 1500 cancer patients, hypnotics were the most frequent form of psychotropic prescription and accounted for 48% of total prescriptions. The indication for the hypnotic prescription was poor sleep in 85% of the cases, but it was only 14% for "medical procedure," 1% for "nausea/vomiting," 1% for "psychological distress," none for "pain," and none for "other." These results were later replicated,[20] with 44% of prescriptions in more than 200 consecutive cancer clinic patients being for hypnotic medications. The interpretation of this large number of prescriptions for hypnotics was that sleeping difficulties were a major problem in cancer patients.

In a large questionnaire study of more than 900 patients with different types of cancer, the most prevalent complaints were fatigue (44%), leg restlessness (41%), insomnia (31%), and excessive sleepiness (28%).[21] The greatest number of problems was in the lung cancer patients, although breast cancer patients also had a high prevalence of complaints of insomnia and fatigue. Recent treatment was also associated with excessive fatigue and hypersomnolence.

Another survey showed that 61% of the cancer patients had significant sleep deficits, but there was no difference in sleep complaints between the cancer patients and patients with medical conditions other than cancer.[22] The patients with breast cancer reported a mean time to sleep onset of 21 minutes and a mean sleep duration of 6.9 hours. Almost half of the group had a sleep efficiency below 85%, and the sleep problems predicted deficits in quality of life. In addition, those patients receiving therapy tended to have more sleep disturbances than those not receiving treatment. Many of the patients attributed their poor sleep to pain, nocturia, feeling too hot, coughing, or snoring loudly.

In another study of patients with metastatic breast cancer, 63% reported sleeping difficulties. Depression was significantly associated with both difficulty falling asleep and increased awakening during the night, and pain was associated with difficultly falling asleep.[23] In one of the largest survey studies to date, in a sample of almost 1500 women, women who reported more pain, depression, and sleep complaints also reported more fatigue, and pain, depression, and fatigue were all positively correlated with sleep complaints.[24]

There have also been a few objective studies using either polysomnography or actigraphy. Full polysomnography was used to examine the sleep of patients with breast cancer, patients with lung cancer, patients with insomnia, and healthy volunteers. Of the four groups, the insomnia patients had the shortest total sleep time; the lung cancer patients had the longest sleep onset latency, lowest sleep efficiency, and greatest wake time during the night. There were no differences in stress levels or emotional state between the cancer patients and the healthy volunteers. There also was no difference in reported total sleep time between the cancer patients and the others; however, when compared with the insomnia patients, the cancer patients did not underestimate total sleep time or overestimate wake time during the night.[7]

Cancer patients also have a higher prevalence of periodic limb movements in sleep (PLMS) than insomnia patients or healthy volunteers, but no difference in the amount of sleep disordered breathing has been found.[7] In ongoing research in our own laboratory, the prevalence of PLMS in women with breast cancer who have completed chemotherapy was 36%. This high preponderance of PLMS may help explain some of the sleep disturbance found in this population.

Actigraphy to Characterize Sleep Disruption

Actigraphy, a noninvasive, continuous ambulatory measure of sleep and circadian rhythms,[25] has also been used to characterize the sleep and rhythms of patients with cancer.[12,13,26,27]

Daytime inactivity and nighttime restlessness were associated with higher subjective ratings of cancer-related fatigue.[13,28] Women with breast cancer who were undergoing adjuvant chemotherapy reported more fatigue during treatment, and less fatigue at chemotherapy cycle midpoints, in a roller coaster pattern.

Activity levels were negatively correlated with reports of fatigue: those with more fatigue showed less activity. Activity levels were reduced during the three treatment sessions compared with the cycle midpoints, thus showing the reverse roller coaster pattern, and changing simultaneously with fatigue scores, albeit in the opposite direction. Patients tended to have more nighttime restlessness at treatment times compared to cycle midpoints when higher activity during the day prevailed and there were fewer nighttime awakenings.[13,28]

In another study, wrist actigraphy was used to examine sleep in patients who had bone metastases and were undergoing radiation therapy. As therapy progressed, sleep efficiency declined. However, it was the frequent need to urinate, rather than pain intensity, that was reported to be the main cause of awakenings at night.[11] Similar to previous findings,[13,28] sleep was fragmented and not consolidated, being broken up with periods of wakefulness.

The periods in which the greatest fatigue was experienced were periods of diminished dichotomization of the sleep-wake schedule: periods with less activity during the day and more awakenings during the night. Fatigue was associated with periods of greater inactivity rather than resulting from increased activity. Instead of activity occurring during the day and rest at night, there was a polyphasic rhythm that suggested diminished daytime activity and increased numbers of daytime naps. Few other studies have examined napping behavior in this population, so little is known about whether taking naps reduces fatigue or increases it.[11]

It has also been shown that the contrast between daytime and nighttime activity in patients with metastatic colon and rectal cancer is smaller than that of healthy individuals.[26] Five days of actigraphy recordings confirmed that the patients had altered rest-activity cycles, with more interpatient variability and less differentiation between night and day. Whether or not cancer patients have altered rest-activity circadian patterns due to their diagnosis or due to a vicious circle of fatigue and inactivity remains to be established.[29]

In our own laboratory, women with breast cancer have worn actigraphs for 72 consecutive hours before and during chemotherapy. In almost 60 women studied before the start of chemotherapy, the mean total sleep time was 6 hours, with only 76% of the night spent asleep. Each sleep bout was approximately 32 minutes long, and each wake bout was approximately 6 minutes long. On average, the women napped for about 1 hour a day. After the start of chemotherapy, the percentage of sleep at night decreased, with sleep bouts getting shorter and wake bouts getting longer. In addition, naptime increased to almost two hours.

Fatigue

There are multiple definitions of fatigue,[30] including a decrease in strength and performance, tiredness, weakness, lack of energy, lethargy, depression, difficulty with concentration, lack of motivation, and sleepiness.[3,30] Fatigue is one of the most frequent and disturbing complaints of patients with cancer.[1,2]

More than 75% of patients who undergo chemotherapy or radiation therapy report feeling weak and tired.[3,4] It has been reported that 76% of patients receiving chemotherapy report fatigue at least once per week; 18% identify it as the most significant problem during treatment,[31] interfering with daily life, reducing quality of life,[1,8,9] and being one of the key reasons for discontinuing treatment.[3]

In the study described earlier from our laboratory, the amount of fatigue reported increased during treatment, with 66% of the women reporting at least some fatigue before treatment and 84% reporting it during treatment. Additionally, the percentage of women reporting extreme fatigue doubled from approximately 5% before treatment to approximately 10% during treatment.

PATHOGENESIS

Pathogenesis of Sleep Disruption

Patients with cancer may complain of insomnia, hypersomnia, or both, but the pathogenesis of this sleep disruption can be quite varied. Most of the research conducted on sleep and cancer has been in patients with either breast or lung cancer. Although these studies agree that patients experience difficulties with sleep,[7,32,33,33a] they are less clear about the cause of this sleep disruption. Chemotherapy or radiation therapy may be some of the problem, as both are known to disrupt sleep. Hot flashes may cause insomnia in breast cancer survivors.[33b] In one survey of sleep quality in patients with different types of cancer undergoing different types of treatment, cancer patients generally reported worse overall sleep quality and consequently more daytime dysfunction than controls with no cancer.[17] In addition, commonly administered analgesics, such as opioids, are also known to disrupt sleep.[34]

The amount of insomnia in cancer patients can be as high as the amount of insomnia found in depressed patients.[35] Therefore, clinicians should not overlook the possibility that poor sleep in cancer patients may indicate some depression.[36] Many studies have suggested that the sleep disruption is secondary to pain and psychological distress.[6] It is not yet known to what extent these may affect sleep or whether the pain, for example, is a primary cause of the sleep disruption or whether the medications used to treat the pain are causing the sleep disruption. In fact, there are surprisingly few studies supporting the notion that pain in cancer leads to disrupted sleep.

In a study examining the relationship between pain and sleep disruption, patients with breast cancer, patients with lung cancer, patients with insomnia (but no cancer), and healthy controls were questioned, and whereas those with breast cancer reported pain prior to bedtime, neither their poor sleep nor that of the patients with lung cancer was associated with reports of pain.[7] In the study of patients with bone metastases,[11] ratings of fatigue and pain were collected in the morning and evening. Although ratings of pain were fairly consistent throughout the 48-hour recording period, fatigue ratings were higher in the evening and lower in the morning, suggesting that the fatigue was independent of the pain.

Along the same lines, patients with breast cancer who had not yet begun treatment completed questionnaires on sleep quality, fatigue, and distress. Insomnia was the most frequent symptom, reported by 88% of the sample, and was correlated with high levels of distress and anxiety.[16] However, contrary to the belief that disturbed sleep prior to treatment is attributable to the increased stress and anxiety found with a recent diagnosis of a life-threatening illness, insomnia and fatigue were rated high even in those patients who rated themselves low on anxiety.

Pain has often been thought to be the cause of sleep disruption, not only in patients with cancer[37] but also in patients with a multitude of other medical conditions.[38] The results of these studies suggest, however, that the sleep problems in patients with cancer may be independent of these psychological and physiologic factors. One hypothesis is that pain may be the initial cause of the frequent awakenings, but psychological distress is what prevents the patient from falling back to sleep.[18] A second hypothesis is that whereas sleep leads to recovery and repair of tissue and may offer a temporary cessation of the psychological awareness of pain, poor sleep leads to difficulty managing pain.[38] In this way, a cycle of pain and poor sleep may become self-perpetuating.

Pathogenesis of Fatigue

Fatigue is believed to be caused by physical factors, such as cachexia; weight loss; biochemical, hematologic, and endocrine abnormalities[39,40]; psychological factors, such as depression[4,41-43]; and social factors (Fig. 103–1).[39,44] There has been no overwhelming evidence to suggest a causal relationship between nutritional status and fatigue in cancer patients.[41,42]

Biochemical abnormalities, such as anemia, are known to be present in patients with cancer and to cause fatigue, yet one study examining the incremental effect of increasing hemoglobin on quality of life found that improving the anemia only improved quality of life to a point beyond which there was no further improvement.[45] Hemoglobin levels are only moderately related to fatigue and quality of life.[46] Few studies have examined the relationship between endocrine abnormalities and fatigue[39] or between biochemical abnormalities and fatigue[41] in cancer patients.

One survey showed a relationship between reports of fatigue and of depression, and between reports of menopausal symptoms and of sleep quality and sleeping during the day,

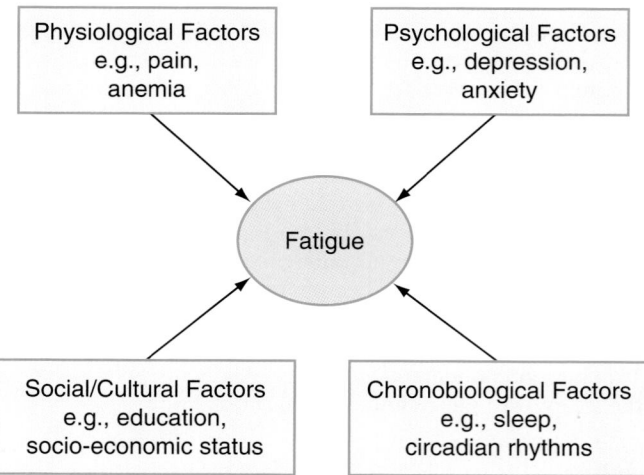

Figure 103–1. Diagrammatic representation of possible factors affecting fatigue. (Reprinted from Ancoli-Israel, S, Moore PJ, Jones V: The relationship between fatigue and sleep in cancer patients: A review. Eur J Cancer Care (Engl) 2001;10:245-255.)

but no causal relationships were determined.[43] It has been shown that the fatigue experienced by patients with cancer is different from that experienced by patients with depression but that sleep disturbance is a significant predictor of severe fatigue in these patients.[47]

Few studies to date have followed cancer patients over time, but some evidence suggests that the amount of fatigue varies before, during, and after treatment.[8,48-50] In addition, several studies have suggested that fatigue can continue for months after the completion of therapy.[41,51-54] When women with breast cancer were followed for 1 year after the completion of their chemotherapy and compared with women who had no history of breast cancer, patients reported more severe fatigue, poorer quality of life secondary to their fatigue, and more severe symptoms of menopause.[43]

TREATMENT

The complaints of sleep disturbances and fatigue are often overlooked and rarely treated, aside from occasional use of sedative-hypnotics or sedating antidepressants.[22] Some researchers have recommended sleep hygiene.[55]

A major problem is that the etiology of these complaints is not fully understood. For example, although treatments may be available for different symptoms of fatigue (e.g., depression, pain, anemia, metabolic abnormalities), there are no known treatments for the full syndrome of fatigue.[56] Corticosteroids have been used to treat fatigue in patients with advanced cancer, but because of potential complications, their use has been limited.[56] Several other clinical trials have primarily examined outcome interventions such as support groups, relaxation, and psychotherapy, all which showed improvement, but none targeted fatigue per se.[57-59] Several other studies have examined novel treatment approaches for sleep, but no one treatment was effective for all of the complaints.

DIFFERENTIAL DIAGNOSIS: IS IT SLEEPINESS, FATIGUE, OR SOMETHING ELSE?

The clinician needs to try to determine the cause of a patient's symptoms, recognizing that the words used by the patient to describe the symptoms may be vague (see Chapter 104). Is the symptom related to *sleepiness* (the patient may describe unintended episodes of falling asleep in the daytime or have an elevated Epworth sleepiness score), or to *fatigue* (complaints of muscle weakness or of lack of energy but without sleepiness)? Patients may also have symptoms attributable to specific effects of cancer or its treatment. When the patient has complaints related to one or more of these realms, the complaints sometimes become very difficult to manage.

Sleepiness or Insomnia

Sleep disorders resulting in daytime sleepiness should be treated specifically if possible. If a patient has restless legs syndrome, the clinician should make sure that the patient is not iron deficient, as commonly occurs in gastrointestinal carcinomas. If the patient has developed movement disorders secondary to a chemotherapeutic agent, then a trial of a dopaminergic agent to treat the movements could be tried. If a patient has developed obstructive sleep apnea, for example,

secondary to enlarged lymph nodes in the pharynx as might occur with lymphoma or with nasopharyngeal carcinoma, then specific treatment directed at these areas could be initiated. If the patient has developed clinical depression, then therapy of the mood disorder might help the sleep disorder.

Fatigue

Fatigue, weakness, and loss of energy are all hallmarks of cancer. Although the pathophysiology is as yet poorly understood, the clinician should try to determine if the fatigue is caused in part by a correctable factor such as electrolyte imbalance (this might occur in a patient on chemotherapy with severe nausea or vomiting), an underlying infection, or an undiagnosed metabolic disorder such as thyroid disease or diabetes mellitus. The latter may develop as a result of some therapy, for example large doses of corticosteroid.

Physical activity often improves fatigue.[60] Going for a self-paced walk three or four times per week often results in lower ratings of fatigue as well as lower ratings of anxiety, depression, and difficulty sleeping. The benefit of the mild exercise program may be successful for a variety of reasons, including that mild exercise synchronizes the rest-activity rhythms.

A second benefit of taking walks would be the increased exposure to bright light, which may promote greater daytime alertness. Patients who report more fatigue tend to be exposed to less light. Although the cause of fatigue and light exposure in breast cancer patients is not confirmed, there may be a negative feedback loop in which less light exposure desynchronizes the patients circadian rhythms, which then causes or increases fatigue, leading further to less light exposure.[61]

Direct Effect of Cancer

If the cancer is causing pain that is disturbing sleep, the pain must be treated. Hypoxemia caused by spread of cancer to the lung, or the development of lung fibrosis in response to chemotherapy or radiation therapy, may require treatment, because patients with hypoxemia are known to have disturbed sleep.

When sleep complaints are due to the stress associated with cancer, mindfulness-based stress reduction intervention has been shown to improve daily sleep quality measures.[62] Therapy that includes stimulus control, relaxation, sleep education, setting aside a worry time, and cognitive restructuring has been shown to consolidate sleep; improvement is typically seen in number of awakenings, time awake, sleep efficiency and sleep quality ratings, decreased fatigue, and enhanced ability to perform tasks.[63] A combination of relaxation, stimulus control, and sleep restriction in women with breast cancer has been shown to improve sleep and wake patterns.[64]

Nonspecific Treatment

In the end, the clinician, having corrected as much as is clinically feasible, might prescribe hypnotics (see Chapter 63) to improve a patient's sleep. Recently, drugs such as modafinil have been used at low doses and found to be effective in some patients who have fatigue caused by cancer.

Chronotherapy for Cancer

Chronotherapy is a relatively new method of treatment that is based on the premise that administering medications at

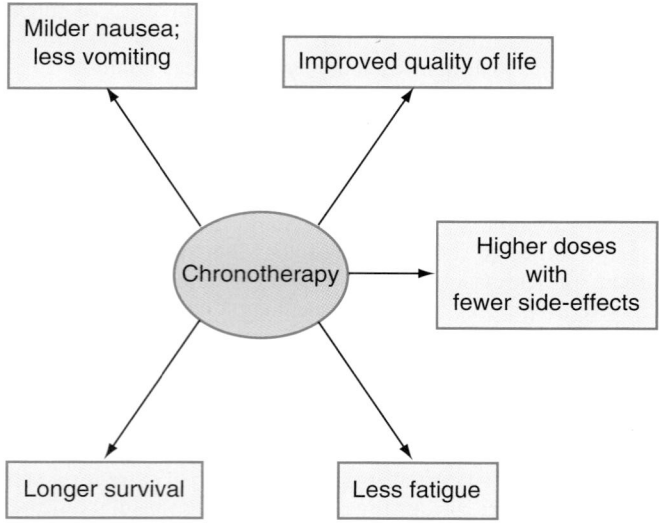

Figure 103–2. Diagrammatic representation of the effects of chronotherapy. (Reprinted from Ancoli-Israel S, Moore PJ, Jones V: The relationship between fatigue and sleep in cancer patients: A review. Eur J Cancer Care (Engl) 2001;10:245-255.)

different times of the circadian cycle will minimize side effects and maximize therapeutic effects (Fig. 103–2). Clinical trials have documented that both toxicity and antitumor activity of cancer drugs are time dependent.[65,66] Studies in mice and rats have shown that the tolerability of 30 different drugs for cancer varied by as much as 50% depending on the time of administration in relation to the circadian rhythm, and the dose could be increased at certain times without increasing side effects.[65]

Circadian influences on a variety of measures in tumor cells and in healthy tissues in cancer have been studied by administering drugs at different times of the day and night. Results suggested that the same dose of an anticancer drug became lethally toxic only when administered at certain times of day, whereas at other times of day, a 10-fold increase in dose was tolerated.[10,67]

In certain types of cancer, rest-activity rhythms deteriorate in some patients with advanced disease, but it is unknown whether these patients are less responsive to the external environmental time cues or whether the round-the-clock-care and continuous low lighting results in the loss of meaningful time cues. In some patients, there are indications that the tumor itself shows signs of abnormal circadian rhythmicity.[29] Patients with marked activity rhythms (i.e., greater activity out of bed than in bed) have been shown to have better quality of life, less reported fatigue, and most importantly, a fivefold higher survival at two-year follow-up, than those with less-synchronized rhythms. The authors concluded that the rest-activity cycle can be used to determine prognosis for cancer patients' survival and tumor response.[68]

The rhythm of the immune system of cancer patients has also been examined to determine if timing of medications might affect outcome.[69-71] Chronobiologic infusion of floxuridine has been shown to result in low toxicity and a long period of stable disease in 12% of patients.[70] When administration of cytostatics in the evening was compared with administration in the morning in testicular and ovarian cancer patients, the response rate was the same for both times of day; however, there were fewer hematologic and renal side effects, milder nausea, and less vomiting in those receiving the chemotherapy in the evening.[71]

Along similar lines, it has been shown that adjusted administration of chemotherapy (oxaliplatin, fluorouracil, and folinic acid) that coincided with relevant circadian rhythms (i.e., chronotherapy) was significantly less toxic and more effective than a constant rate of infusion.[72] There was a positive response in 51% of those on chronotherapy compared with only 29% in the constant infusion group. In addition, chronotherapy reduced fivefold the rate of mucosal toxicity and halved the functional impairment from peripheral sensory neuropathy. In addition to reduced toxicity, other benefits included improved quality of life and fewer days of hospitalization.[73]

The effect of chronotherapy on quality of life was compared with traditional therapy in patients with metastatic cancer. Those undergoing chronotherapy showed better psychosocial adaptation (including better social relations, less feeling of loss of independence, less anxiety, less depression, and less somatic discomfort) than patients receiving traditional therapy.[74]

PITFALLS AND CONTROVERSIES

The degree of sleep disruption found in patients with cancer is not trivial. Disruptions in circadian rhythms themselves affect sleep quality as well as disrupting many other physiologic mechanisms that pertain to fatigue. Lack of entrainment to the day-night cycle and not keeping regular hours can lead to feelings of grogginess, similar to the feelings of jet lag.

The area of sleep and fatigue in cancer is a fairly new one. Little is known about the cause or the mechanisms of the sleep disruption or of the fatigue.[75] New survey methodologies, particularly validated questionnaires designed specifically for the study of fatigue in cancer, will help the research move forward.[29] Although the number of research studies in the last few years has increased, much still remains unknown about the cause, consequences, or cures of sleeping difficulties in patients with cancer.

> *Clinical Pearl*
> *Fatigue is the most common and most distressing complaint of patients with cancer.*

Acknowledgments

This work was supported by NCI CA85264, NIA AG08415, Rebecca and John Moores, UCSD Cancer Center, the Department of Veterans Affairs VISN-22 Mental Illness Research, Education and Clinical Center (MIRECC); and the Research Service of the Veterans Affairs San Diego Healthcare System.

This chapter is dedicated to the memory of Dr. J. Christian Gillin, dear friend and colleague, who died of cancer and was fatigued, but never let it get to him. He was an inspiration and role model to us all.

References

1. Richardson A: Fatigue in cancer patients: A review of the literature. Eur J Cancer Care 1995;4:20-32.
2. Stein KD, Martin SC, Hann DM, Jacobsen PB: A multidimensional measure of fatigue for use with cancer patients. Cancer Pract 1998;6:143-152.

3. Winningham ML, Nail LM, Burke MB, et al: Fatigue and the cancer experience: The state of the knowledge. Oncol Nurs Forum 1994;21:23-36.

4. Smets EM, Garssen B, Cull A, de Haes JC: Application of the multidimensional fatigue inventory in cancer patients receiving radiotherapy. Br J Cancer 1996;73:241-245.

4a. Lee K, Cho M, Miaskowski C, Dodd M: Impaired sleep and rhythms in persons with cancer. Sleep Medicine Reviews 2004;8:199-212.

5. Derogatis LR, Feldstein M, Morrow G, et al: A survey of psychotropic drug prescriptions in an oncology population. Cancer 1979;44:1919-1929.

6. Hu D, Silberfarb PM: Management of sleep problems in cancer patients. Oncology 1991;5:23-27.

7. Silberfarb PM, Hauri PJ, Oxman TE, Schnurr PP: Assessment of sleep in patients with lung cancer and breast cancer. J Clin Oncol 1993;11:997-1004.

8. Visser MR, Smets EM: Fatigue, depression and quality of life in cancer patients: How are they related? Support Care Cancer 1998;6:101-108.

9. Stromborg MF, Wright P: Ambulatory cancer patients' perception of the physical and psychosocial changes in their lives since the diagnosis of cancer. Cancer Nurs 1984;7:117-130.

10. Mormont MC, Levi F: Circadian system alterations during cancer processes: A review. Int J Cancer 1997;70:241-247.

11. Miaskowski C, Lee KA: Pain, fatigue and sleep disturbances in oncology outpatients receiving radiation therapy for bone metastasis: A pilot study. J Pain Symptom Manage 1999;17: 320-332.

12. Morrow G, Tian L, Roscoe J, et al: The relationship between circadian rhythm and fatigue in breast cancer patients [abstract]. Ann Behav Med 2000;22:S188.

13. Berger AM: Patterns of fatigue and activity and rest during adjuvant breast cancer chemotherapy. Oncol Nurs Forum 1998; 25:51-62.

14. Beszterczey A, Lipowski ZJ: Insomnia in cancer patients. Can Med Assoc J 1977;116:355.

15. Kaye J, Kaye K, Madow L: Sleep patterns in patients with cancer and patients with cardiac disease. J Psychol 1983;114:107-113.

16. Cimprich B: Pretreatment symptom distress in women newly diagnosed with breast cancer. Cancer Nurs 1999;22:185-194.

17. Owen DC, Parker KP, McGuire DB: Comparison of subjective sleep quality in patients with cancer and healthy subjects. Oncol Nurs Forum 1999;26:1649-1651.

18. Engstrom CA, Strohl RA, Rose L, et al: Sleep alterations in cancer patients. Cancer Nurs 1999;22:143-148.

19. Ancoli-Israel S, Roth T: Characteristics of insomnia in the United States: Results of the 1991 National Sleep Foundation Survey. I. Sleep 1999;22(Suppl 2):S347-S353.

20. Stiefel FC, Kornblith AB, Holland JC: Changes in the prescription patterns of psychotropic drugs over a 10-year period. Cancer 1990;65:1048-1053.

21. Davidson JR, MacLean AW, Brundage MD, Schulze K: Sleep disturbance in cancer patients. Soc Sci Med 2002;54:1309-1321.

22. Fortner BV, Stepanski EJ, Wang SC, et al: Sleep and quality of life in breast cancer patients. J Pain Symptom Manage 2002;24: 471-480.

23. Koopman C, Nouriani B, Erickson V, et al: Sleep disturbances in women with metastatic breast cancer. Breast J 2002;8:362-370.

24. Profant J: Fatigue and Sleep Complaints in Women Treated for Breast Cancer [dissertation]. San Diego, San Diego State University and University of California at San Diego, 2003.

25. Ancoli-Israel S, Cole R, Alessi CA, et al: The role of actigraphy in the study of sleep and circadian rhythms. Sleep 2003;26: 342-392.

26. Mormont MC, De Prins J, Levi F: Assessment of activity rhythms by wrist actigraphy: Preliminary results in 30 patients with colorectal cancer. Biol Rhythm Res 1995;6:423.

27. Brown AC, Smolensky MH, D'Alonzo GE, Redman DP: Actigraphy: A means of assessing circadian patterns in human activity. Chronobiol Int 1990;7:125-133.

28. Berger AM, Farr L: The influence of daytime inactivity and nighttime restlessness on cancer-related fatigue. Oncol Nurs Forum 1999;26:1663-1671.

29. Ancoli-Israel S, Schnierow B, Kelsoe J, Fink R: A pedigree of one family with delayed sleep phase syndrome. Chronobiol Int 2001;18:831-841.

30. Glaus A: Fatigue in Patients with Cancer: Analysis and Assessment. Berlin, Springer-Verlag, 1998.

31. Curt G, Breitbart W, Cella DF, et al: Impact of cancer-related fatigue on the lives of patients [abstract]. Proceedings of the American Society of Clinical Oncology 1999;18:573a.

32. Knobf MT: Physical and psychological distress associated with adjuvant chemotherapy in women with breast cancer. J Clin Oncol 1986;4:678-684.

33. Berglund G, Bolund C, Fornander T, et al: Late effects of adjuvant chemotherapy and postoperative radiotherapy on quality of life among breast cancer patients. Cancer 1991;27: 1075-1081.

33a. Savard J, Simard S, Hervouet S, et al: Insomnia in men treated with radical prostatectomy for prostate cancer. Psychooncology 2004:Jun 14 [Epub ahead of print].

33b. Savard J, Davidson JR, Ivers H, et al: The association between nocturnal hot flashes and sleep in breast cancer survivors. J Pain Symptom Manage 2004;27:513-522.

34. Moore P, Dimsdale JE: Opioids, sleep, and cancer-related fatigue. Med Hypotheses 2002;58:77-82.

35. Holland JC, Plumb M: A comparative study of depressive symptoms in patients with advanced cancer. Proc Am Assoc Cancer Res 1977;18:201.

36. McDaniel JS, Musselman DL, Porter MR, et al: Depression in patients with cancer: Diagnosis, biology and treatment. Arch Gen Psychiat 1995;52:89-99.

37. Strang P, Qvarner H: Cancer-related pain and its influence on quality of life. Anticancer Res 1990;10:109-112.

38. Lewin DS, Dahl RE: Importance of sleep in the management of pediatric pain. J Devel Behav Pediatr 1999;20:244-252.

39. Stone P, Richards M, Hardy J: Fatigue in patients with cancer. Eur J Cancer Care 1998;34:1670-1676.

40. Morrow GR, Andrews PL, Hickok JT, et al: Fatigue associated with cancer and its treatment. Support Care Cancer 2002;10: 389-398.

41. Bruera E, Brenneis C, Michaud M, et al: Association between asthenia and nutritional status, lean body mass, anemia, psychological status, and tumor mass in patients with advanced breast cancer. J Pain Symptom Manage 1989;4:59-63.

42. Morant R, Stiefel F, Berchtold W, et al: Preliminary results of a study assessing asthenia and related psychological and biological phenomena in patients with advanced cancer. Support Care Cancer 1993;1:101-107.

43. Broeckel J, Jacobsen PB, Horton J, et al: Characteristics and correlates of fatigue after adjuvant chemotherapy for breast cancer. J Cinical Oncol 1998;16:1689-1696.

44. Ancoli-Israel S, Moore PJ, Jones V: The relationship between fatigue and sleep in cancer patients: A review. Eur J Cancer Care (Engl) 2001;10:245-255.

45. Cleeland C, Demetri G, Glaspy J, et al: Identifying hemoglobin level for optimal quality of life: Results of an incremental analysis [abstract]. Proceedings of the American Society of Clinical Oncology 1999;18:574a.

46. Holzner B, Kemmler G, Greil R, et al: The impact of hemoglobin levels on fatigue and quality of life in cancer patients. Ann Oncol 2002;13:965-973.

47. Anderson KO, Getto CJ, Mendoza TR, et al: Fatigue and sleep disturbance in patients with cancer, patients with clinical depression, and community-dwelling adults. J Pain Symptom Manage 2003;25:307-318.

48. Haes J, Raategever J, Van der Berg M, et al: Evaluation of the quality of life of patients with advanced ovarian cancer treated with combination chemotherapy. In Aaronson N, Beckmann J (eds): Quality of Life of Cancer Patients. New York, Raven Press, 1987, pp 215-226.

49. Greenberg DB, Sawicka J, Eisenthal S, Ross D: Fatigue syndrome due to localized radiation. J Pain Symptom Manage 1992;7:38-45.

50. Greenberg DB, Gray JL, Mannix CM, et al: Treatment-related fatigue and serum interleukin-1 levels in patients during external beam irradiation for prostate cancer. J Pain Symptom Manage 1993;8:196-200.

51. Dow KH, Ferrell BR, Leigh S, et al: An evaluation of the quality of life among long-term survivors of breast cancer. Breast Cancer Res Treat 1996;39:261-273.

52. Ferrell BR, Grant M, Funk B, et al: Quality of life in breast cancer. Cancer Pract 1996;4:331-340.

53. Ganz P, Coscarelli A, Fred C, et al: Breast cancer survivors: Psychosocial concerns and quality of life. Breast Cancer Res Treat 1996;38:183-199.

54. Goldstein D, Scott E, Bennett B, et al: Post malignancy fatigue syndrome—results of long term follow-up in a cross-sectional study in women following adjuvant treatment for breast cancer [abstract]. Proceedings of the American Society of Clinical Oncology Annual Meeting 2000;19:623a.

55. Older H, Winningham ML: Select psychiatric and psychological considerations. In Winningham ML, Barton Burke M (eds): Fatigue in Cancer: A Multidimensional Approach. London, Jones and Bartlett Publishers, 2000, pp 217-218.

56. Berger AM: Treating fatigue in cancer patients. Oncologist 2003;8(Suppl 1):10-14.

57. Spiegel D, Bloom JR, Yalom I: Group support for patients with metastatic cancer. A randomized outcome study. Arch Gen Psychiat 1981;38:527-533.

58. Forester B, Kornfeld DS, Fleiss JL: Psychotherapy during radiotherapy: Effects on emotional and physical distress. Am J Psychiatry 1985;142:22-27.

59. Decker TW, Cline-Elsen J, Gallagher M: Relaxation therapy as an adjunct in radiation oncology. J Clin Psychol 1992;48:388-393.

60. Mock V, Hassey D, Meares CJ, et al: Effects of exercise on fatigue, physical functioning and emotional distress during radiation therapy for breast cancer. Oncol Nurs Forum 1997;24:991-1000.

61. Liu LQ, Johnson SS, Jones V, et al: The relationship between fatigue and light exposure in breast cancer [abstract]. Sleep 2003;26:A356.

62. Shapiro SL, Bootzin RR, Figueredo AJ, et al: The efficacy of mindfulness-based stress reduction in the treatment of sleep disturbance in women with breast cancer: An exploratory study. J Psychosom Res 2003;54:85-91.

63. Davidson JR, Waisberg JL, Brundage MD, Maclean A: Nonpharmacologic group treatment of insomnia: A preliminary study with cancer survivors. Psychooncology 2001;10:389-397.

64. Berger AM, VonEssen S, Kuhn BR, et al: Adherence, sleep, and fatigue outcomes after adjuvant breast cancer chemotherapy: Results of a feasibility intervention study. Oncol Nurs Forum 2003;30:513-522.

65. Levi F: Chronopharmacology and chronotherapy of cancers. Pathol Biol (Paris) 1996;44:631-644.

66. Hrushesky WJ, Martynowicz M, Markiewicz M, et al: Chronotherapy of cancer—a major drug-delivery challenge. Advan Drug Delivery Rev 1992;9:1-83.

67. Mormont MC, Boughattas NA, Levi F: Mechanisms of circadian rhythms in the toxicity and the efficacy of anti-cancer drugs: Relevance for the development of new analogs. In Lemmer B (ed): Chronopharmacology: Cellular and Biochemical Interactions. New York, Marcel Dekker, 1989, pp 395-437.

68. Mormont MC, Waterhouse J, Bleuzen P, et al: Marked 24-h rest/activity rhythms are associated with better quality of life, better response and longer survival in patients with metastatic colorectal cancer and good performance status. Clin Cancer Res 2000;6:3038-3045.

69. Levi F, Bourin P, Depres-Brummer P, Adam R: Chronobiology of the immune system: Implication for the delivery of therapeutic agents. Clin Immunother 1994;2:53-64.

70. Aveta P, Terrone C, Neira D, et al: Chemotherapy with FUDR in the management of metastatic renal cell carcinoma. Ann Urol (Paris) 1997;31:159-163.

71. Zuchowska-Vogelgesang B, Pernal J, Zemelka T: Toxicity and efficacy of chemotherapy dependent on circadian time of cytostatic drug administration. Przegl Lek 1996;53:870-873.

72. Levi F, Zidani R, Misset JL: Randomised multicentre trial of chronotherapy with oxaliplatin, fluorouracil, and folinic acid in metastatic colorectal cancer. Lancet 1997;350:681-686.

73. Wood PA, Hrushesky WJ: Circadian rhythms and cancer chemotherapy. Criti Rev Eukaryot Gene Expr 1996;6:299-343.

74. Bertolini R, Focan C, Bartholome F, Baro V: Comparative psychological aspects of two different types of chemotherapeutic administration (chronotherapy vs. traditional chemotherapy) on quality of life of cancer patients at advanced stage. In Vivo 1995;9:583-587.

75. Ahlberg K, Ekman T, Gaston-Johansson F, Mock V: Assessment and management of cancer-related fatigue in adults. Lancet 2003;362:640-650.

Fibromyalgia and Chronic Fatigue Syndromes

Harvey Moldofsky
James G. MacFarlane

ABSTRACT

The diagnosis and the management of patients with fibromyalgia syndrome and chronic fatigue syndrome are complex. These patients present with persistent tiredness or physical fatigue, accompanied by unrefreshing sleep and generalized muscular pain but in the absence of a specific medical disease or a primary psychiatric disorder. Tiredness is a complaint that commonly brings patients to their physicians. Because of the various meanings that have come to be applied to the symptom, the chronically tired patient is a challenge for the physician to diagnose and manage. An understanding of what the patient means by *tired* is essential for the physician to determine the investigations that can aid in diagnosis and management.

A key component of these syndromes is unrefreshing sleep. The first step is to determine the contributing factors. The multiple sleep latency test permits differentiation between tiredness characterized by physical exhaustion and tiredness that results from uncontrollable sleepiness. Overnight polysomnography may be important to rule out comorbid sleep disorders, such as sleep apnea, restless legs syndrome, or periodic leg movements during sleep. The sleep electroencephalogram (EEG) may reveal nonperiodic arousals in association with movement arousals or sleep fragmentation. Periodic EEG arousals or a continuous alpha-EEG arousal pattern may correlate with reports of unrefreshing sleep.

Nonspecific treatments include behavioral approaches to improve sleep hygiene, such as aerobic fitness and eating habits that help to regularize potential disturbances in circadian sleep–wake rhythms. Although helpful in initiating and maintaining sleep and thus in reducing daytime tiredness, traditional hypnotic agents do not provide restorative sleep or reduce pain. Tricyclic drugs (e.g., amitriptyline, cyclobenzaprine) may improve sleep quality but do not reduce pain in the long term. No systematic studies have shown that treating restless legs syndrome, periodic leg movements during sleep, or sleep apnea improves the unrefreshing sleep, fatigue, and pain of patients with fibromyalgia syndrome and chronic fatigue syndrome.

Chronic fatigue syndrome (CFS) and fibromyalgia syndrome (FMS) are chronic clinical conditions characterized by a variety of nonspecific somatic complaints. The two most prominent complaints for both are intractable fatigue and unrefreshing sleep. In FMS, prominent diffuse musculoskeletal discomfort is the differentiating symptom. However, in terms of demographics and general clinical features, these two conditions cannot be clearly distinguished. That is, the prevalent symptoms of each disorder are present in the other.[1]

Sleep disturbance is the common complaint that has kept these conditions within the purview of sleep disorders medicine. The combination of perceived sleep disturbance and chronic fatigue often prompts referrals to a sleep disorders clinic. It is then up to the sleep disorders specialist to decide whether there is evidence for a primary sleep disorder that could explain the daytime impairment. The subjective experience of feeling "tired" is most often the focal point of the clinical evaluation. The term is commonly used to describe an unpleasant and ill-defined subjective experience, troublesome enough to bring people to their physicians. What each patient means by this complaint must be defined, because *tired* has several attributions.[2]

"Tiredness" may imply any of the following descriptive categories:

1. *Central fatigue:* The person describes mental exhaustion with impairment in concentration or thinking that occurs as the result of intellectually demanding activities. The person may be unmotivated, bored, disinterested, or fed up with a particular task. If the lack of motivation is affecting all aspects of the personality, the complaint of tiredness may be a mask for abulia, which characterizes a negative symptom of chronic schizophrenia, or the presence of a degenerative brain disease (e.g., Alzheimer's, Huntington's, or Parkinson's disease). Tiredness is often used in the context of a mood disorder, in which the additional symptoms of sadness, irritability, guilt, and poor self-image may indicate a major depressive disorder. Other psychiatric disorders that have tiredness as a symptom may include general anxiety disorder, dysthymic disorder, and somatoform disorder, including neurasthenia.

2. *Physical fatigue:* A sense of overall physical exhaustion or depletion of energy as the result of physical effort can occur with or without any medical disease. Such chronic diseases as cancer; neuroendocrine, metabolic, infectious, or rheumatic diseases; and chronic painful diseases all have an adverse effect on energy. Various drugs, radiation, and immunosuppressants may induce profound physical exhaustion. On the other hand, where there is no evidence for a primary medical disease or psychiatric disorder and the fatigue is accompanied by unrefreshing sleep, such patients may be diagnosed with CFS or FMS. Physical fatigue may be more specific in conditions of muscular weakness such as neuromotor diseases: amyotrophic lateral sclerosis, postpolio syndrome, or myasthenia gravis.

3. *Sleepiness:* The person feels an urge to return to sleep, in the absence of central or physical fatigue. This person may actually avoid the sedentary situations preferred by those with FMS and CFS, because to be inactive is to increase the propensity for falling asleep. Whereas fatigue may be

relieved or reduced to some extent by rest or withdrawal from mental activities, sleepiness is relieved only by sleep.

The literature provides further semiotic confusion when the word *fatigue* is used to describe operational impairment in task performance (e.g., driver fatigue) or sleepiness. Because of the language confusion in the medical literature and the various meanings intended by patients, the clinician must carefully interpret what each patient means or risk prescribing unnecessary and expensive diagnostic procedures or inappropriate treatments.

Other chapters in this volume address the diagnostic features and management of those sleep disorders in which tiredness is a synonym for sleepiness; furthermore, the evaluation of the medical and psychiatric conditions that result in tiredness are outside the scope of this chapter. This chapter will focus on the assessment and management of those chronically tired patients who complain of unrefreshing sleep or chronic mental and physical fatigue in the absence of physical or laboratory evidence for a primary medical disease or behavioral evidence for a primary psychiatric disorder. Often, when generalized and ill-defined musculoskeletal pain and tenderness in specific anatomic regions accompany the fatigue, these people acquire descriptive labels such as *chronic fatigue syndrome*[3] or *fibromyalgia syndrome*.[4]

EPIDEMIOLOGY

Epidemiologic studies reveal that 23% of the adult population in the United States report having experienced the symptom of persistent fatigue sometime during their life.[5] A cross-national epidemiologic study of primary care physicians shows that unexplained substantial fatigue occurring for more than 1 month affects approximately 8% of patients, with a range from 12% to 15% in Berlin, Santiago, and Manchester to a low prevalence of between 2% and 4% in Ibadan, Verona, Shanghai, Seattle, and Bangalore.[1] Within these variable prevalence clusters of patients with unexplained fatigue lie smaller groups of overlapping primary diagnoses, which include CFS and FMS. In the United States and Japan, between 0.4% and 1.5% of people are affected with CFS (i.e., these patients complain of persistent fatigue for more than 6 months).[6,7] FMS affects approximately 2% of the population (more than 80% of them women), and debilitating fatigue affects between 76% and 81% of these patients.[4,8] Because of the similarities of the symptoms, there is considerable overlap between the diagnoses of CFS and FMS, which are also comorbid with such regional pain syndromes as temporomandibular joint disorder, irritable bowel syndrome, migraine, and tension headaches.[9]

PATHOGENESIS

There are no known specific causes for CFS and FMS. Various hypotheses, including genetics; infectious agents; neurotransmitter, neuroendocrine, neuroimmune, and autonomic disturbances; and psychological stress factors have been proposed for the etiology of these disorders. The fatigue and bodily hypersensitivity are thought to be the result of disturbances in central nervous system functions.[10] In particular, the myalgia and tender points in specific anatomic regions have been associated with unrefreshing sleep. The poor quality of sleep is related to the number of tender points in patients with fibromyalgia but not to psychological factors.[11] The importance

of disturbances in sleep physiology for the symptoms of these patients has been shown in four types of experiments:

1. Experimental disruption of slow wave sleep with noise in healthy subjects artificially induces both musculoskeletal pain and fatigue symptoms.[12-14] One of these studies failed to show significant differences in tender point threshold after sleep disruption. Procedural differences, including the absence of an adaptation night, may have accounted for this discrepancy. Another study showed altered pain thresholds, but there was no associated increase in alpha-EEG activity.[14] However, alpha-EEG activity was quantified by computer-generated frequency analysis rather than visual scoring techniques.

2. Experimental pain induction during sleep by infusion of 6% hypertonic saline resulted in increased sleep disturbance, with the appearance of increased alpha- and reduced delta-EEG sleep.[15]

3. Experimental sleep deprivation of 40 hours' duration was shown to reduce pain thresholds, which returned to baseline values specifically after slow wave sleep recovery.[16]

4. Sleep disruption was quantified in patients with a clear diagnosis of fibromyalgia. Various studies have shown protracted sleep latencies,[17,18] a reduced sleep efficiency index,[16,19] a reduction of slow wave sleep and rapid eye movement (REM) sleep,[17-20] increased motor activity during sleep, generalized restlessness,[17-19,21-25] and an increase in alpha-EEG activity during non-REM sleep.[12,18,20,26-29] The alpha-EEG non-REM sleep anomaly is the most extensively studied correlate of nonrestorative sleep, especially as it applies to CFS and FMS. However, it is not specific to these conditions, and some studies have reported a low sensitivity.[30]

One report of electrocardiographic analyses of patients with FMS found that sympathetic activity increases overnight, although sympathetic activity usually declines during sleep.[31] This finding is consistent with the autonomic disturbances, which have symptoms that include faintness, unsteadiness, palpitations, paresthesias, and blurring of vision. Another preliminary report examined heart rate variability and did not confirm autonomic nervous system dysregulation during sleep in patients with FMS.[32]

Some studies have shown changes in autonomic, neuroendocrine, and immune functions of the body related to the circadian sleep–wake cycle, and alterations in neurotransmitter functions that affect substance P, catecholamine, serotonin, and neuroendocrine metabolism.[10,33] However, many of these changes may be confounded by disturbances in sleep physiology, pain, psychological distress, and physical deconditioning.[34] Although no specific neuroendocrine, cytokine, or neuroimmune dysfunctions have been directly related to FMS, the abnormalities that have been reported provide further evidence for the importance of disturbances in the sleeping/waking brain in the pathogenesis of the syndrome.[10,33,35-41]

CLINICAL FEATURES

The clinical criteria for CFS are shown in Box 104–1, and those for FMS are shown in Box 104–2.

The American College of Rheumatology criteria emphasize pain and tenderness (Fig. 104–1) for the diagnosis of FMS, but this may actually limit sensitivity and specificity.[42] An evaluation for FMS should investigate complaints of chronic fatigue,

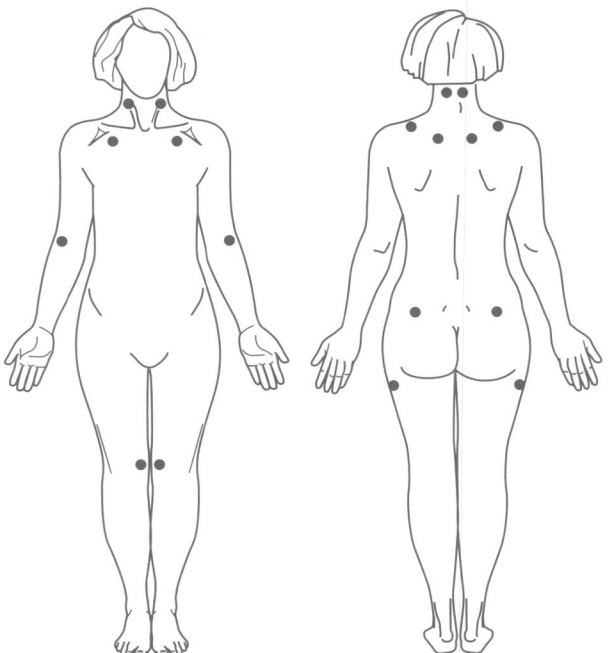

Figure 104–1. Anatomic distribution of 18 tender points in fibromyalgia syndrome.

unrefreshing sleep, cognitive difficulties, and psychological distress. Whereas fatigue, postexertional malaise, and impairment in cognitive functioning are the focus of attention in CFS, unrefreshing sleep, chronic muscular pain, and tenderness also prevail. These symptoms may follow a viral illness or a physical or psychological traumatic event (e.g., an automobile whiplash injury or a work-related soft tissue injury), or they may appear for no apparent reason. FMS may occur in the context of potentially disabling arthritic disease (e.g., rheumatoid arthritis) or connective tissue disease (e.g., systemic lupus erythematosus), human immunodeficiency virus infection, or Lyme disease.

In patients with either CFS or FMS, the quality of sleep is usually impaired. More than 80% of patients with chronic fatigue describe significant impairment in their sleep quality.[43] Patients commonly complain of light or superficial sleep, describing sensitivity to noise or inability to turn off thinking during sleep, so their sleep is unrefreshing. Their mental fatigue results in word lapses, word confusions, and problems in multitasking, so they are slower in performing such tasks. However, they do not make more errors than unaffected individuals.[44] Their sensory sensitivities may include lowered intolerance to noise, noxious smells or strong perfumes, and bright light. In addition to external sensory hypersensitivities, they may describe internal sensitivities (e.g., intolerance to certain foods and symptoms of irritable bowel syndrome or irritable bladder).

The fatigue that characterizes FMS and CFS shows a diurnal variation that is different from that of the sleepiness. On morning awakening from light and unrefreshing sleep, patients with CFS and FMS rate their pain and fatigue as high. Depending on the severity of the symptoms, they may improve during the interval between 1000 hours and 1500 hours, but this is followed by a feeling of exhaustion and increased pain during the latter part of the afternoon and evening. Typically, the patients feel no better when they awaken than when they went to sleep, or they have more aching, stiffness, and fatigue in the morning, which is indicative of their sleep being nonrestorative.[45]

In contrast, in those medical conditions characterized by muscular weakness, the motor tiredness increases coincident with physical activity over the course of the day, and it improves with rest. The tiredness associated with major depressive disorder is greater on awakening (when the depression is more severe) than in the evening (when both mood and tiredness improve). In dysthymic disorder, the tiredness increases progressively over the course of the day.[46] Sleepiness as the result of sleep restriction or disruption leaves the person feeling drowsy in the morning and again in the mid-afternoon. However, there is reduced late afternoon and early evening sleepiness as a result of circadian variation in alertness. In narcolepsy, the sleepiness is prevalent throughout the day.

DIAGNOSES

Although the diagnoses of CFS and FMS are based on clinical criteria, sleep physiologic analyses may provide an added dimension of understanding and a rationale for treatment. Neuropsychiatric assessment may be required to determine whether there is a brain or peripheral neuromotor disease that could explain the fatigue and weakness, or a whether there is a primary psychiatric disorder (e.g., major depressive disorder, general anxiety disorder, dysthymia, or somatoform pain disorder). Psychosocial concerns, such as current stressors and interpersonal, economic, insurance, and medicolegal problems, need to be assessed as part of the overall management strategy.

CLINICAL ASSESSMENT

Specific enquiry about the quality of sleep (e.g., whether sleep is light and unrefreshing) is essential. Sleep–wake habits can be assessed with the aid of a sleep diary. Attention should be directed to potential agents that could interfere with sleep—for example, excessive use of caffeine, alcohol, nicotine, and certain classes of drugs. Some patients may have loud snoring and interruptions of breathing, which could indicate sleep apnea.[47-49] Others may describe dysesthesia and uncontrollable leg movements in the evening and restlessness or kicking during sleep, which characterize restless legs syndrome and involuntary periodic limb movements (PLM) disorder.[50,51] Tiredness as the result of excessive daytime sleepiness should be differentiated from physical and central fatigue. Routine laboratory tests help to exclude a primary medical disease. The routine use of expensive tests (e.g., imaging studies) is not required. However, patients with FMS or CFS may have concomitant rheumatic or connective tissue disease that requires careful medical diagnostic appraisal. Furthermore, because unrefreshing sleep, fatigue, and cognitive impairment are often accompanied by anxiety or depression, assessment of psychological disturbances is required as part of an overall plan of management.

Sleep–Wake Diary

A self-monitored sleep–wake diary helps to clarify behaviors (e.g., excessive use of stimulants, alcohol, sedatives, hypnotics, or consumption of street drugs) that may contribute to the tiredness. This simple, inexpensive tool may save costly and unrewarding investigative procedures. Moreover, the diary can assist in reeducation to correct the faulty habits and poor sleep hygiene that contribute to the complaint of tiredness.

Clinical Rating Scales for Various Attributes of Tiredness

Self-Rating Scales

Tiredness that is a symptom of depression is included in the Beck Depression Inventory.[52] Fatigue scales that provide information about various aspects of fatigue include the following:

1. The *Multidimensional Fatigue Inventory* (MFI-20)[53] is a 20-item, five-point Likert scale questionnaire that comprises five subscales, which include general fatigue, physical fatigue, reduced activity, reduced motivation, and mental fatigue.
2. The *fatigue scale* by Chalder and colleagues[54] has 11 items; it measures fatigue intensity and separates mental from physical fatigue.
3. The *fatigue severity scale*[55] includes nine items that provide a measure of fatigue severity. This simple scale was originally standardized on patients with fatigue related to multiple sclerosis and systemic lupus erythematosus.

These fatigue instruments, however, do not evaluate or exclude sleepiness. Sleepiness scales are commonly used in sleep research and clinical sleep laboratories. These include:

1. The *Stanford Sleepiness Scale* measures sleepiness at the time of the test. This instrument was originally developed for narcolepsy and comprises seven categories, ranging from "1," indicating alert and wide awake, to "7," indicating almost asleep.[56]
2. The *Epworth Sleepiness Scale*, which measures an ongoing tendency for sleepiness, inquires about the chance of dozing in eight different situations.[57] The chance of dozing is ranked from "0," meaning never, to "3," meaning there is a high chance of dozing. These passive situations include sitting and reading or watching television, sitting inactive in a public place (such as a theater or a meeting, or as a passenger in a car), lying down to rest in the afternoon, sitting and talking to someone, sitting quietly after lunch without alcohol, and finally sitting in a car that is stopped for a few minutes in traffic. The sum of the responses gives a global score from 0 to 24, and higher ratings are related to pathologic sleepiness. Interestingly, the Epworth Sleepiness Scale does not include a question regarding irresistible daytime sleepiness.

Qualitative and Quantitative Self-Rating Scales of Sleep

In addition to a subscale rating of subjective sleep quality, the Pittsburgh Sleep Quality Index questionnaire provides subscale measures of sleep latency, sleep duration, and habitual sleep efficiency. Some components relate to sleep disturbances, use of sleeping medication, and daytime dysfunction. The sum of the scores for these seven components yields one global score that is a composite of sleep quality and quantity.[58]

In the Sleep Assessment Questionnaire (SAQ), a 17-item, four-point Likert scale, nonrestorative sleep is a specific sleep factor. Five other factors are insomnia/hypersomnia, restless leg/motility, sleep schedule, excessive daytime sleeping, and sleep apnea. Importantly, this instrument has been validated against data (e.g., the alpha EEG sleep disorder in patients with FMS and CFS) obtained from polysomnography. The SAQ shows favorable sensitivity and specificity as a simple screening instrument for nonrestorative sleep disorders and other sleep pathologies. It has been found to be useful in screening for sleep pathologies in an epidemiologic study of a chronically fatigued population.[59]

The Karolinska Sleep Diary[60] consists of seven self-rated items on a five-point Likert scale. It yields two factors: (1) the sleep quality index, which assesses the sleep quality, ease of falling asleep, and maintenance and calmness of sleep, and (2) a second factor that assesses the sufficiency of sleep, the ease of awakening, and achievement of a refreshed feeling. The amount of slow wave sleep and degree of sleep efficiency were found to be predictors for the sleep quality index.

Performance Tasks

The difficulty with self-rating estimates of fatigue is that they are not necessarily related to the observed behavior. Therefore, performance tasks of vigilance are employed, especially if daytime sleepiness (e.g., resulting from sleep deprivation or a primary sleep disorder) is being assessed. This psychomotor vigilance task involves a 10-minute computerized assessment battery that is sensitive to the effects of sleep loss and circadian rhythmicity and is devoid of practice effects.[61,62] Efforts are underway to objectively measure performance in specific tasks (e.g., driving a car or truck).[63,64] Motor vehicle accidents are a common outcome of driver fatigue, in which there are inattention or lapses in alertness as symptoms of sleepiness.[65]

Many of these assessment tools are too cumbersome for routine use in the sleep disorders clinic. The most practical tools are (1) the sleep–wake diary to assess scheduling and behavioral factors that may be compounding existing symptoms, (2) the Beck Depression Inventory to rule out comorbid depression, and (3) the SAQ or other screening questionnaires to rule out comorbid sleep disorders.

Polysomnography

When the diagnosis is uncertain or a primary sleep disorder is suspected, overnight polysomnography can provide objective evidence for the unrefreshing sleep and a rationale for treatment of the underlying sleep disorder. These sleep disorders include the alpha EEG sleep disorder, which is often associated with poor quality or light and unrefreshing sleep.[66] Initially, this sleep disorder was termed alpha-delta sleep, and it was described in a heterogeneous group of psychiatric patients with somatic malaise and fatigue.[67] Subsequently, alpha EEG sleep was found in stages 2, 3, and 4 non-REM sleep in adults and children with FMS[12,68-72] and in some patients with CFS or unexplained chronic fatigue.[73,74]

The alpha EEG anomaly is not specific to CFS and FMS. Other disorders in which alpha EEG sleep, nonrestorative sleep, and pain and fatigue symptoms may occur include rheumatoid arthritis[75-77] and systemic lupus erythematosus.[68] Furthermore, it may be found in patients with psychophysiologic insomnia and unrefreshing sleep and fatigue,[78] in some patients with various primary sleep disorders (e.g., PLM disorder, non–24-hour sleep–wake syndrome, sleep apnea, and narcolepsy), and occasionally in normal people.[79-83] Studies examining the sensitivity of the alpha EEG intrusion as a marker for FMS and CFS have been equivocal. Also, the relative presence of the alpha EEG anomaly is not always correlated with symptom severity.[30] Unfortunately, variations in methodology, including frequency analysis techniques and inclusion and exclusion criteria, hamper valid comparisons between many studies. Still, this common but as yet unexplained EEG finding provides an opportunity for additional research into the mechanisms of disease. More recent studies have attempted to clarify the exact nature of the alpha EEG anomaly and its permutations. Frequency analyses show that there is a progressive decline in the alpha EEG through the night. Detailed EEG frequency analyses differentiate three types of alpha EEG sleep:

1. Tonic alpha EEG sleep occurs throughout sleep stages 2, 3, and 4, where global rating of alpha intrusion is 3–5 (i.e., greater than 40% prevalence of the alpha frequency).[12]
2. Phasic alpha EEG sleep, in which the alpha frequency coincides with stages 3 and 4 sleep (alpha-delta sleep), has maximal frontal alpha power localized symmetrically in the left and right anterior cingulum.[68]
3. Periodic K-alpha and periodic polyphasic EEG burst activity (K-alpha/polyphasic burst variety of cyclical alternating pattern) is recorded when four or more consecutive K-complexes, immediately followed by alpha EEG activity

of 0.5- to 5.0-second duration, or four or more polyphasic bursts occur in a sequence of approximately 20- to 40-second intervals. A rapid frequency, with an index of greater than 15 per hour of sleep, is associated with unrefreshing sleep, fatigue, and muscle symptoms.[84] Additional EEG details are found in the Appendix (later).

Other sleep disorders, such as restless legs syndrome and sleep-related PLM disorder, occur in about 20% of patients with FMS, and 5% of patients with FMS have significant obstructive sleep apnea.[85]

The Multiple Sleep Latency Test aids in the differentiation of types of tiredness. For some patients, physical and mental fatigue fails to lead to rapid onset of sleep in daytime naps, whereas others have excessive daytime sleepiness and difficulty remaining alert that interferes with concentration. This test is especially important in those patients who, in addition to having FMS or CFS, have hypersomnolence[86] or even narcolepsy.[87,88]

TREATMENT

Despite clinical criteria for recognizing these fatigue and pain syndromes, there is no satisfactory effective treatment for improving sleep quality, fatigue, and debilitating somatic symptoms. Treatment is either nonspecific (e.g., improving sleep habits) or it employs medications that aim to relieve symptoms or aspects of the sleep disorder.

Nonspecific Treatment Methods

Overall sleep hygiene and nonspecific methods provide a suitable background regimen that is helpful for regularizing and facilitating sleep.[89] Based on the principle that there is a dysregulation of the sleep and the rhythms of the body, the management involves regularizing the patient's behavioral and physiologic functions. The psychological methods for improving circadian sleep–wake behavior are central to any cognitive behavior therapy approach in the management of FMS. Sleep hygiene enables regulation of the circadian rhythm of sleep–wakefulness when the pattern is disorganized because of faulty sleep habits.

Two of the most common faulty habits, variable bedtimes and inadequate nocturnal sleep time, result in disorganization of circadian rhythms and sleep deprivation with sleepiness and fatigue. Efforts should be directed to stabilize the regulatory functions of sleep by going to bed and awakening at suitable times to ensure adequate duration of sleep. Establishing a regular daily routine not only includes meeting the sleep requirements of the body but also requires a regular schedule of nutritious meals and a suitable exercise program. The exercise program should involve a gentle, graded aerobic fitness routine during the part of the day when there is least fatigue and pain—commonly between 10 AM and 3 PM. Vigorous physical activities should be avoided before bedtime, because their stimulating effects interfere with sleep. Patients who are sensitive to the stimulating effects of caffeine and alcohol should avoid their use.

In attending to the sleep environment, the aim is to reduce any psychological or environmental disturbances that are disruptive to sleep. Other behavioral methods, such as hypnosis and biofeedback treatments, that reduce psychological distress are helpful in modulating symptoms. Hypnotherapy results in improvements in muscle pain, fatigue, and sleep disturbance.[90]

Electromyographic biofeedback therapy helps to improve pain, tender points, and stiffness on awakening in the morning.[91]

Physical methods, which include massage and acupuncture, provide temporary improvement.[92] Ultrasound and interferential current treatment decrease unrefreshing sleep, fatigue, pain, tender points, and tenderness while increasing slow wave sleep and decreasing the percentage of stage 1 sleep.[93] A gentle daily cardiovascular fitness training may improve sleep and symptoms of fibromyalgia.[94]

Specific Treatment Methods

Sleep-Promoting Agents

Medications intended to improve sleep appear to help in some patients but have not been demonstrated to provide lasting benefit for pain. Tricyclic antidepressant agents, which facilitate central nervous system serotonin metabolism, may have favorable effects on sleep for up to 2 or 3 months (e.g., cyclobenzaprine) or 5 months (e.g., amitriptyline).[95,96] However, sleep EEG studies show that neither cyclobenzaprine nor amitriptyline reduces the alpha EEG sleep disorder.[30,97] Selective serotonin reuptake inhibitors (e.g., fluoxetine) provide no consistent benefits.[98,99] Agents that increase slow wave sleep and reduce the alpha EEG sleep may benefit both the quality of sleep and the pain and fatigue symptoms of FMS.

Traditional sedatives and hypnotic benzodiazepines alone do not provide any specific benefit. Nonbenzodiazepine hypnotic drugs (such as zopiclone[100] and zolpidem[101]) improve subjective sleep and daytime tiredness but do not modify alpha EEG sleep or benefit pain symptoms. Over-the-counter sedatives such as antihistamines and herbal agents (e.g., valerian) have not been systematically assessed. L-Tryptophan facilitates sleep, but there is no effect on alpha EEG sleep, pain, or mood symptoms in patients with FMS.[102] However, 5-hydroxytryptophan, a direct precursor of brain serotonin, tends to improve pain and sleep quality,[103] although its effect on the sleep physiology of patients with FMS is unknown. Although chlorpromazine has been shown to decrease pain and improve sleep physiology by reducing the alpha EEG sleep and increasing slow wave sleep, the risk for long-term adverse effects does not make this a desirable drug.[102] Agents that have been classified as anticonvulsants (e.g., gabapentin, pregabalin, carbamazepine) have sedative properties and antinociceptive effects but have not been systematically assessed in terms of sleep physiology. Sodium oxybate improves sleep quality and symptoms of FMS while reducing alpha and increasing delta sleep.[104] These findings require further, large-scale confirmation. Further research should help provide a better understanding of CFS and FMS and pave the way for devising and testing specific molecules that would help to improve sleep quality and illnesses where fatigue problems prevail.

An important consideration when employing any medication for the management of symptoms related to FMS or CFS is that these patients are very often exquisitely sensitive to pharmacologic agents and are thus likely to report troublesome side effects. It is not uncommon for them to derive a therapeutic benefit from a fraction of the recommended adult starting dose. Such a minimal dose will, in turn, minimize side effects.

Sleep-Related Neuroendocrine Substances

No consistent abnormalities have been reported in the secretion of melatonin in patients with either CFS or FMS, nor has its administration been found to be useful in controlled studies.[34] Furthermore, the use of morning bright-light treatment, which tends to modify the timing of the nocturnal secretion of melatonin and is helpful in seasonal affective disorder, does not benefit sleep, pain, or mood symptoms in patients with FMS.[105] On the other hand, growth hormone, which is found to be reduced in patients with FMS, improves its symptoms,[37] but its high cost and the need for daily injections make its use impractical.

Management of Primary Sleep Disorders

For patients with other primary sleep disorders (e.g., restless legs syndrome, PLM disorder, or sleep apnea), some specific remedial measures have been demonstrated to provide relief, and these should be considered. Unfortunately, as yet there are no systematic studies of their benefits for the pain and fatigue symptoms in patients with FMS.[89]

PITFALLS AND CONTROVERSIES

Despite the existence of clinical criteria for the diagnoses of CFS and FMS, the subjective nature of these nonspecific pain and fatigue disorders may become confounded by the psychological distress. This may be especially apparent in patients who are involved with insurance and medicolegal matters related to disability claims. Their need to provide proof of disability and the symptoms of distress may magnify the sleep, fatigue, and pain symptoms and result in controversy about whether symptoms are indications of medical illnesses or are illness behavior.

Also, the symptoms are not specific. Similar symptoms of fatigue, pain, and unrefreshing sleep appear with other diagnostic labels that have emerged in various medical specialties to address unexplained symptoms—for example, Gulf War syndrome, multiple chemical sensitivity syndrome, and sick building syndrome (in the fields of allergy, clinical immunology) and chronic pain in somatoform disorder (in psychiatry). These fatigue, pain, and sleep symptoms also occur with other difficult-to-diagnose illnesses, such as irritable bowel syndrome, temporomandibular joint pain syndrome, interstitial cystitis, migraine, chronic headache, and atypical chest pain.[106] Furthermore, FMS is not distinctive; the same symptoms may accompany rheumatic or connective tissue disease (e.g., osteoarthritis, rheumatoid arthritis), systemic lupus erythematosus, Lyme disease, endocrine disorder, and myxedema,[107,108] and in patients with psychiatric illness such as major depression, general anxiety disorder, and posttraumatic stress disorder.[109]

Given the lack of specificity of symptoms, it is understandable that abnormalities in sleep physiology (e.g., alpha EEG sleep disorder) also lack diagnostic reliability. Contributing to this are the various techniques used to quantify the EEG frequencies (e.g., computer-based spectral analysis, visual scoring techniques). Furthermore, not all researchers adhere to conventional Rechtschaffen and Kales methodology. Attention has been directed to specific stages of sleep and obtaining consensus on observer rating of transient EEG arousals. Others have been interested in examining periodic or continuous EEG physiologic anomalies within these stages of sleep. Indeed, Rechtschaffen and Kales, in Figure 38 of their sleep scoring manual, illustrate an "epoch of unambiguous stage 4" of normal sleep that actually features the alpha-delta EEG sleep anomaly.[110] The clinical observer ratings of MacLean and colleagues[111] and the cyclical alternating pattern methodology of Terzano et al.[112] should help advance the field of enquiry of EEG sleep physiology.[84]

CLINICAL COURSE AND PREVENTION

Long-term outcome studies indicate that patients with CFS rarely return to the premorbid levels of energy. Similarly, the prognosis for patients with CFS remains poor because current treatments are limited and equivocal in efficacy, and symptoms may persist over extended periods of time. There are no known measures to prevent CFS and FMS.

Clinical Pearl

An accurate diagnosis of CFS and FMS must begin with a clear definition of the most common symptomatic descriptor, "feeling tired." Furthermore, this must be differentiated from excessive daytime sleepiness, and comorbid sleep disorders must be ruled out. Given the multidisciplinary nature of sleep disorders medicine, this differentiation may only be possible within the realm of the sleep disorders clinic. Even though treatment for these syndromes is limited, diagnosis remains essential, as validation for the patient is often the critical first step toward self-management and rehabilitation.

CHAPTER 104 APPENDIX: TECHNICAL CONSIDERATIONS AND SCORING CRITERIA

Alpha EEG: Recording Techniques and Scoring Rules

The quantification of non-REM alpha EEG has traditionally depended on visual scoring. Records are collected and scored using standard Rechtschaffen and Kales criteria.[110] In addition to the central leads, it is preferable to include occipital (Oz) and frontal (Fz) leads. Sensitivity should be set at 50 μV/cm. Alpha EEG activity is assessed from the EEG channel with the most prominent alpha activity.

The alpha frequency (7 to 12 Hz) is identified during non-REM stages 2, and/or 3 and 4 sleep with a minimum peak-to-peak amplitude of 5 μV. This alpha frequency is approximately 2 Hz slower in sleep than in wake, and more prominent in the frontal lobes. Observer ratings may use a single global rating or serial epoch ratings for more detailed analysis. The global ratings for prevalence during non-REM sleep range from 1 (0% to 20%), 2 (21% to 40%), 3 (41% to 60%), 4 (61% to 80%), to 5 (81% to 100%).[111] (Figure 104–2 shows an alpha rating of 1 in stage 2 sleep; Figure 104–3 shows an alpha rating of 5 in stage 2 sleep).

Periodic EEG Phenomena: Recording Techniques and Scoring Rules.

Cyclic alternating pattern (CAP) had been traditionally measured using a bipolar 10-lead EEG. This is not practical for most sleep laboratories. Bipolar montages using C3-A2, C4-A1, plus Oz and Fz referred to A1 or A2 are suboptimal but adequate for detection.

Previous CAP studies have described the quantification of CAP in terms of CAP rates. The CAP rate is defined as the temporal sum of all CAP sequences, and it is expressed as a percentage ratio of CAP time to total sleep time. The higher the CAP rate, the poorer is the sleep quality.[113] Unfortunately, this concept deviates from the standard nomenclature of PSG, which generally relies on indices rather than on ratios. Other studies specifically examining the relationship between periodic EEG phenomena during sleep and symptoms of nonrestorative sleep have used an index of greater than 15 per hour of sleep as the cutoff for clinical significance.[84]

Some studies have described variations in CAP in terms of both amplitude and rate. These events have been described as follows:

1. *Periodic K-alpha EEG bursts*[84]: Characterized by a K-complex (i.e., an EEG waveform of approximately 0.5 seconds' duration, consisting of a well-delineated negative component, followed by a positive deflection), immediately followed by 0.5 to 5.0

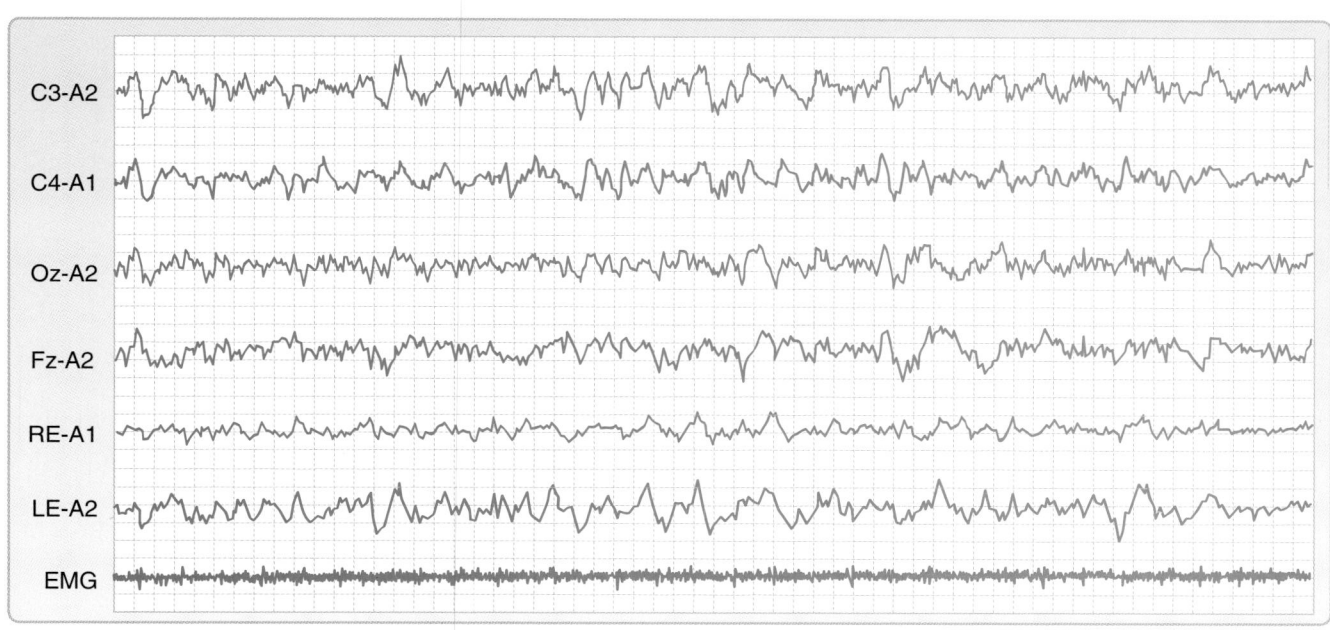

Figure 104–2. Example of alpha rating of 1 in stage 2 sleep.

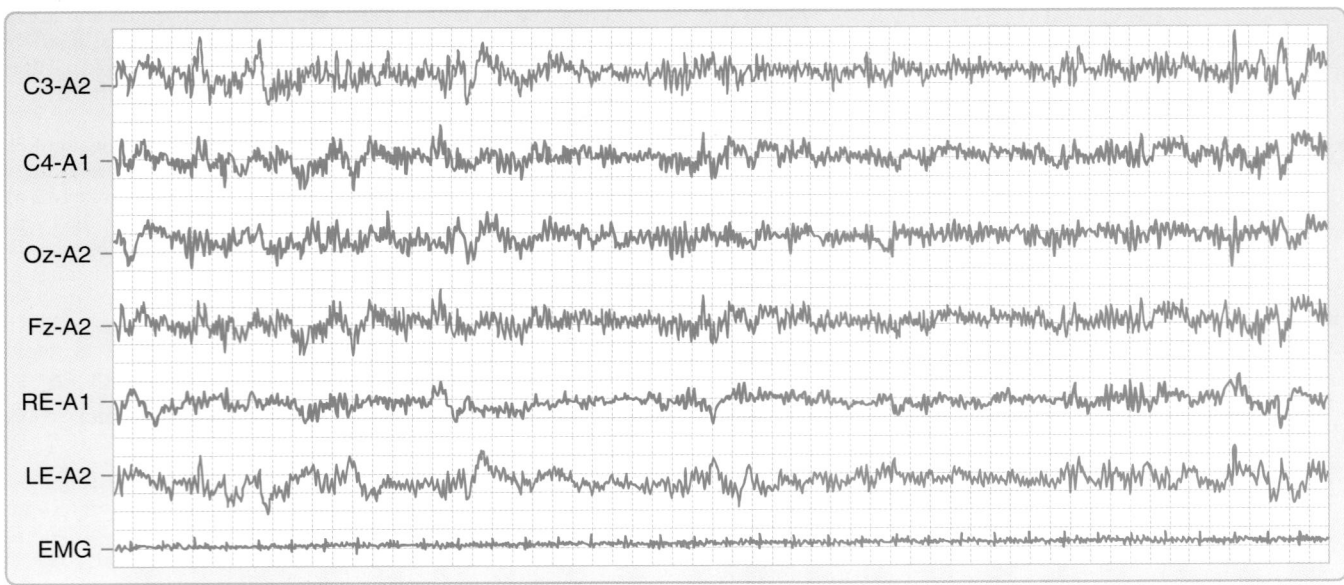

Figure 104–3. Example of an alpha rating of 5 in stage 2 sleep.

seconds of alpha EEG activity. Periodic K-alpha is scored when four or more consecutive K-alpha sequences occur within a periodicity range of 5 to 120 seconds. If a submental EMG burst immediately follows the K-alpha, this event is tagged as both a K-alpha event and a spontaneous arousal (Fig. 104–4).

2. *Periodic polyphasic EEG bursts* (PPBs)[114]: Characterized by periodic clusters of high-amplitude delta waves, with overlapping alpha, beta, and occasional theta activity. PPBs usually contain 3 to 12 delta peaks but may contain more than 20 delta peaks. They occur most often in stages 2 and 3. If a submental EMG burst immediately follows the PPB, this event is tagged as a PPB and a spontaneous arousal. Figures 104–5 and 104–6 show a 19-lead bipolar montage at 30 seconds and at 60 seconds. Note that the key features of K-alpha and PPBs are more easily identified from the frontal leads.

Strict amplitude criteria have yet to be established. Normal phase-A CAP requires a 30% increase over background EEG activity.

Abnormal phase-A CAP variants generally show a 100% to 500% increase over background.

Other Techniques

A preliminary study has used low-resolution electromagnetic tomography (LORETA) to determine cortical spatiotemporal genesis of the abnormal phase-A CAP EEG anomaly in patients with fibromyalgia and nonrestorative sleep.[115] This technique allows determination of current density and source localization across the entire EEG frequency band using a minimum 19-lead bipolar montage. Abnormal increases in current density occurred during phase-A of the CAP event and were in the delta, theta, and alpha bands. The current density increase was more than 4000% in some frequency bands, as compared with the average 300% increase noted in normal phase-A CAP. Maximal increases for delta and theta occurred in the medial frontal gyrus, and in the middle temporal gyrus for the alpha band. These findings further

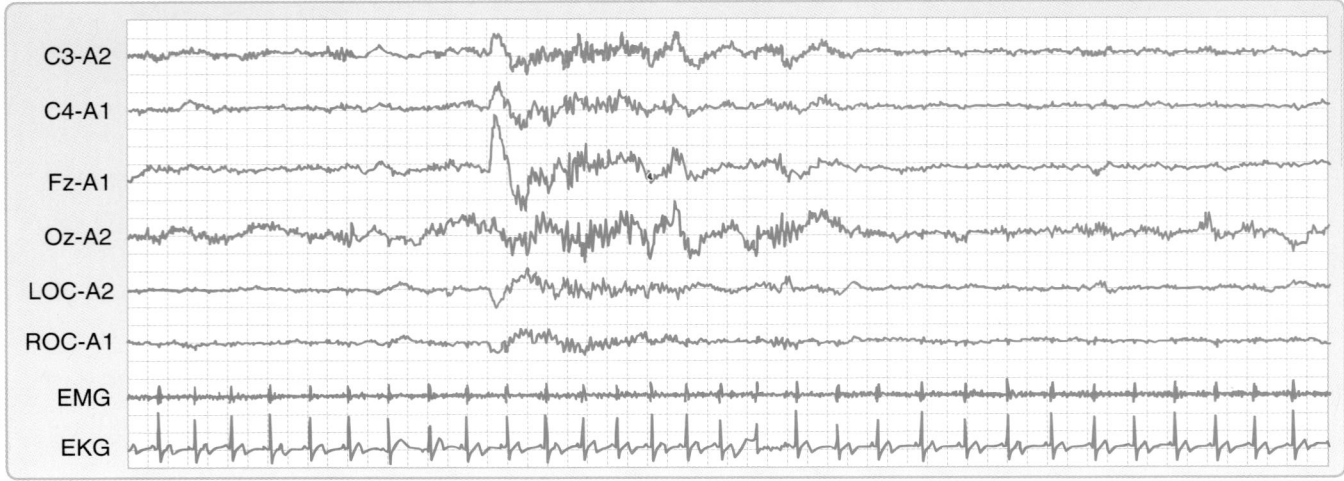

Figure 104–4. This event is tagged as a K-alpha event.

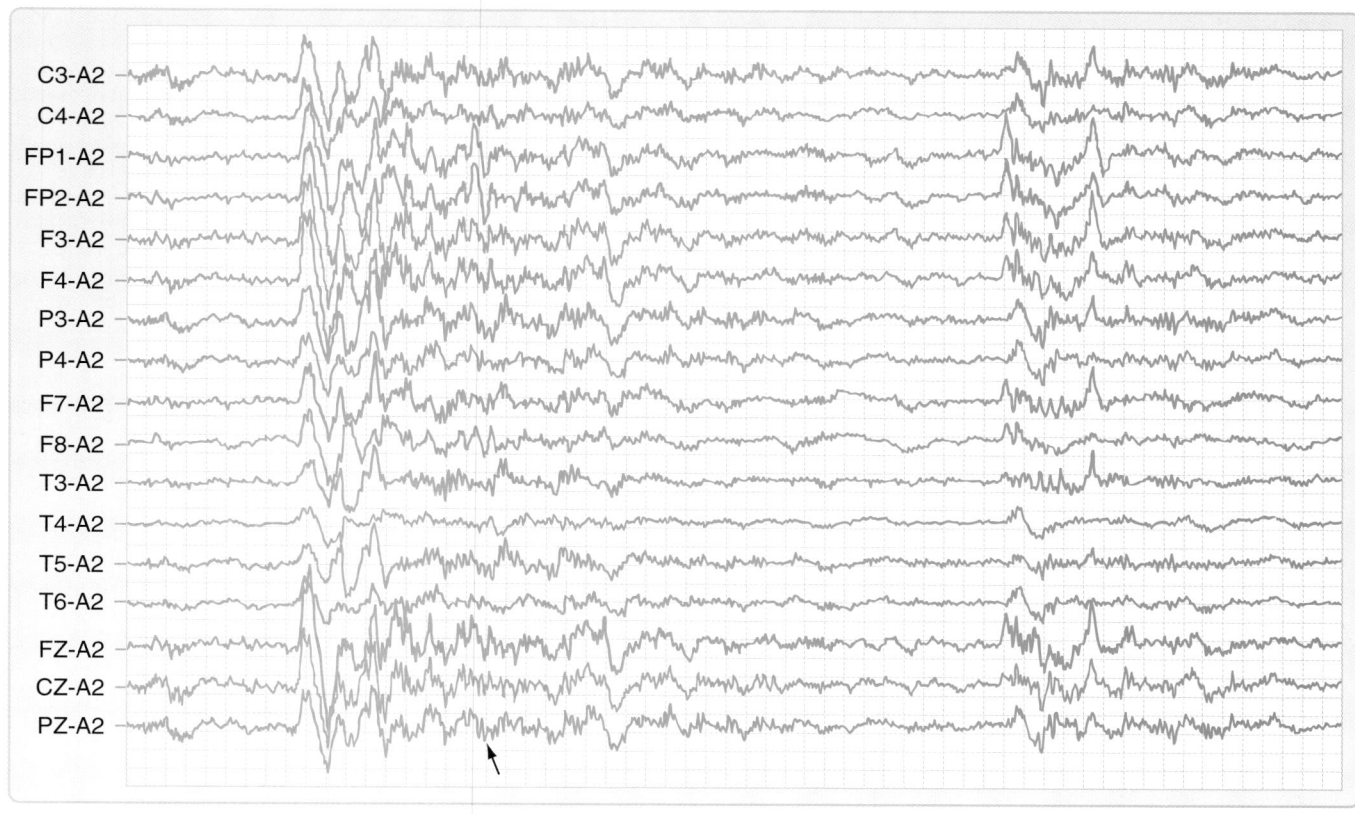

Figure 104–5. A 19-lead bipolar montage with an epoch length of 30 seconds. The key features of K-alpha and periodic polyphasic EEG bursts are more easily identified from the frontal leads.

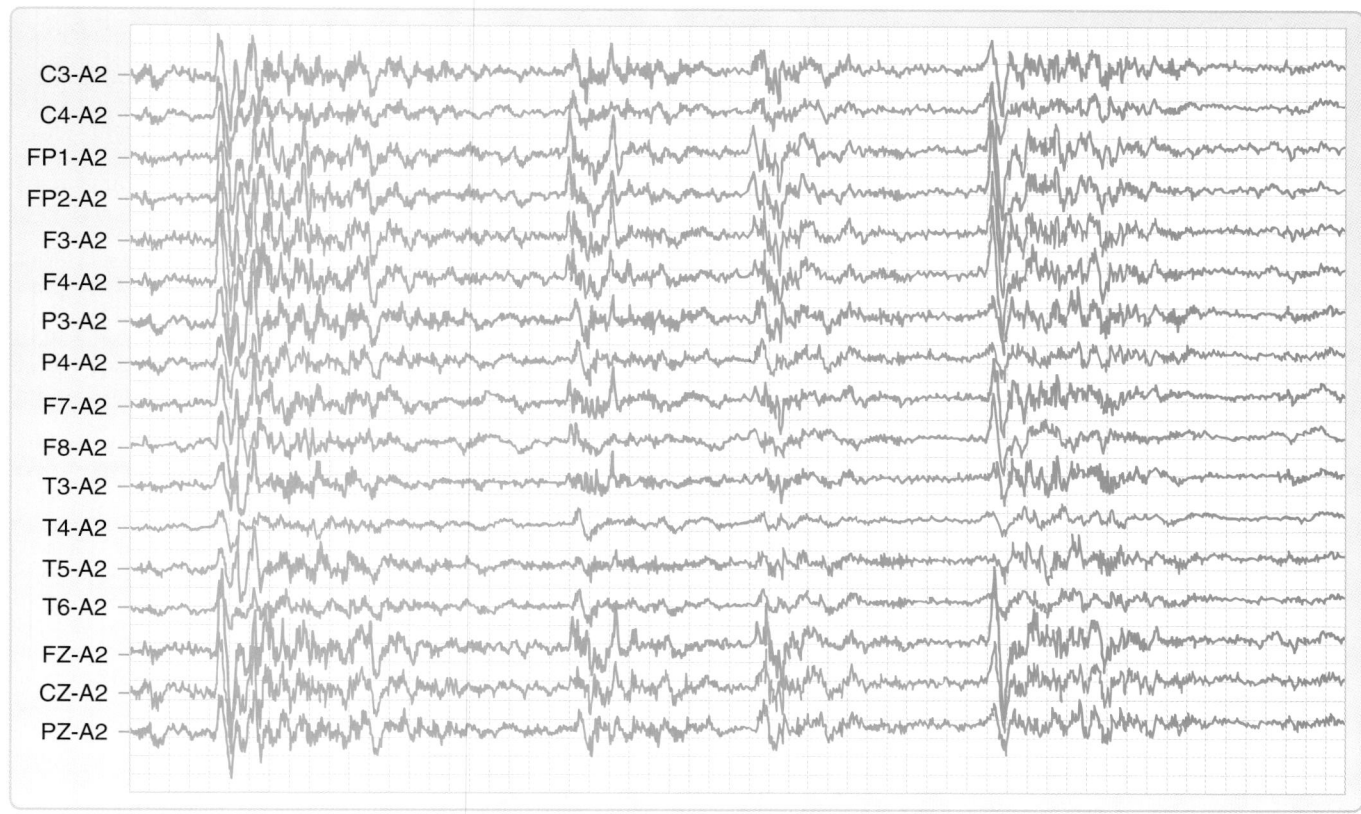

Figure 104–6. A 19-lead bipolar montage with an epoch length of 60 seconds.

demonstrate the importance of including frontal EEG measurements (i.e., Fz) as part of the standard PSG montage.

REFERENCES

1. Skapinakis P, Lewis G, Mavreas V: Cross-cultural differences in the epidemiology of unexplained fatigue syndromes in primary care. Br J Psych 2003;182:205-209.
2. Lindberg A (ed): Oxford American Thesaurus of Current English. New York, Oxford University Press, 1999.
3. Fukuda K, Straus SE, Hickie I, et al: The chronic fatigue syndrome: A comprehensive approach to its definition and study. International Chronic Fatigue Syndrome Study Group. Ann Intern Med 1994;121:953-959.
4. Wolfe F, Smythe HA, Yunus MB, et al: American College of Rheumatology 1990 criteria for the classification of fibromyalgia. Report of the Multicenter Criteria Committee. Arthritis Rheum 1990;33:160-172.
5. Price RK, North CS, Wessely S, et al: Estimating the prevalence of chronic fatigue syndrome and associated symptoms in the community. Public Health Rep 1992;107:514-522.
6. Jason LA, Richman JA, Rademaker AW, et al: A community-based study of chronic fatigue syndrome. Arch Intern Med 1999;159:2129-2137.
7. Kawakami N, Iwata N, Fujihara S, et al: Prevalence of chronic fatigue syndrome in a community population in Japan. Tohoku J Exp Med 1998;186:33-41.
8. Wolfe F, Hawley DJ, Wilson K: The prevalence and meaning of fatigue in rheumatic disease. J Rheumatol 1996;23:1407-1417.
9. Aaron LA, Burke MM, Buchwald D: Overlapping conditions among patients with chronic fatigue syndrome, fibromyalgia, and temporomandibular disorder. Arch Intern Med 2000;24; 160:221-227.
10. Pillemer SR, Bradley LA, Crofford LJ, et al: The neuroscience and endocrinology of fibromyalgia. Conference summary. Arthritis Rheum 1991;34:15-21.
11. Yunus MB, Ahles TA, Aldag JC, et al: The relationship of the clinical features with psychological status in primary fibromyalgia. Arthritis Rheum 1991;34:15-21.
12. Moldofsky H, Scarisbrick P, England R, et al: Musculoskeletal symptoms and non-REM sleep disturbance in patients with "fibrositis syndrome" and healthy subjects. Psychosomat Med 1975;37:341-351.
13. Older SA, Battafarano DF, Danning CL, et al: The effects of delta wave sleep interruption on pain thresholds and fibromyalgia-like symptoms in healthy subjects: Correlations with insulin-like growth factor I. J Rheumatol 1998;25:1180-1186.
14. Lentz MJ, Landis CA, Rothermel J, et al: Effects of selective slow wave sleep disruption on musculoskeletal pain and fatigue in middle aged women. J Rheumatol 1999;26:1586-1592.
15. Drewes AM, Nielson KD, Arendt-Nielson L, et al: The effect of cutaneous and deep pain on the electroencephalogram during sleep: An experimental study. Sleep 1997;20:632-640.
16. Onen SH, Alloui A, Gross A, et al: The effects of total sleep deprivation selective sleep interruption and sleep recovery on pain tolerance thresholds in healthy subjects. J Sleep Res 2001; 10:35-42.
17. Horne JA, Shackell BS: Alpha-like EEG activity in non-REM sleep and the fibromyalgia (fibrositis) syndrome. Electroencephalogr Clin Neurophysiol 1991;79:271-276.
18. Branco J, Atalaia A, Paiva T: Sleep cycles and alpha-delta sleep in fibromyalgia syndrome. J Rheumatol 1994;21:1113-1117.
19. Touchon J, Besset A, Billiard M, et al: Fibrositis syndrome: Polysomnographic and psychological aspects. In Koella WP, Obál F, Schulz H, et al. (eds): SLEEP '86: New York, Gustav Fischer Verlag, 1988, pp 445-447.
20. Drewes AM, Nielsen KD, Taagholt SJ, et al: Sleep intensity in fibromyalgia: Focus on the microstructure of the sleep process. Br J Rheumatol 1995;34:629-635.
21. Shaver JL, Lentz M, Landis CA, et al: Sleep, psychological distress, and stress arousal in women with fibromyalgia, Res Nurs Health 1997;20:247-257.
22. Wittig RM, Zorick FJ, Blumer D, et al: Disturbed sleep in patients complaining of chronic pain. J Nerv Ment Dis 1982;70:429-431.
23. Molony RR, MacPeek DM, Schiffman PL, et al: Sleep, sleep apnea, and fibromyalgia syndrome. J Rheumatol 1986;13:797-800.
24. Clauw D, Blank C, Hiltz R, et al: Polysomnography in fibromyalgia patients (abstract). Arthritis Rheum 1994;37(Suppl 9):S348.
25. Staedt J, Windt H, Hajaki G, et al: Cluster arousal analysis in chronic pain-disturbed sleep. J Sleep Res 1993;2:134-137.
26. Roizenblatt S, Tufik S, Goldenberg J, et al: Juvenile fibromyalgia: Clinical and polysomnographic aspects. J Rheumatol 1977;24: 579-585.
27. Drewes AM, Gade J, Nielsen KD, et al: Clustering of sleep electroencaphalopathic patterns in patients with the fibromyalgia syndrome. Br J Rheumatol 1995;34:1151-1140.
28. Perlis ML, Giles DE, Bootzin RR, et al: Alpha sleep and information processing, perception of sleep, pain and arousability in fibromyalgia. Int J Neurosci 1997;89:265-280.
29. Ware JC, Russell IJ, Campos E: Alpha intrusions into the sleep of depression and fibromyalgia syndrome (fibrositis) patients (abstract). Sleep Res 1986;15:210.
30. Carette S, Oakson G, Guimont C, et al: Sleep electroencephalography and the clinical response to amitriptyline in patients with fibromyalgia. Arthritis Rheum 1995;38:1211-1217.
31. Martinez-Lavin M, Hermosillo AG, Rosas M, et al: Circadian studies of autonomic nervous balance in patients with fibromyalgia: A heart rate variability analysis. Arthritis Rheum 1998;41:1966-1971.
32. McMillan DE, Landis CA, Lentz MJ, et al: Heart rate variability during sleep in women with fibromyalgia. Sleep 2004;27:A724.
33. Landis CA, Lentz MJ, Rothermel J, et al: Decreased nocturnal levels of prolactin and growth hormone in women with fibromyalgia. J Clin Endocrinol Metab 2001;86:1672-1678.
34. Geenen R, Jacobs JW, Bijlsma JW: Evaluation and management of endocrine dysfunction in fibromyalgia. Rheum Dis Clin North Am 2002;28:389-404.
35. Bennett RM, Clark SC, Campbell SM, et al: Low levels of somatomedin C in patients with the fibromyalgia syndrome: A possible link between sleep and muscle pain. Arthritis Rheum 1992;35:1113-1116.
36. Paiva ES, Deodhar A, Jones KD, et al: Impaired growth hormone secretion in fibromyalgia patients: Evidence for augmented hypothalamic somatostatin. Arthritis Rheum 2002;46:440-450.
37. Bennett RM, Clark SC, Walczyk J: A randomized, double-blind, placebo-controlled study of growth hormone in the treatment of fibromyalgia. Am J Med 1998;104:227-231.
38. Demitrack MA, Crofford LJ: Evidence for and pathophysiologic implications of the hypothalamic-pituitary-adrenal axis dysregulation in fibromyalgia and chronic fatigue syndrome. Ann N Y Acad Sci 1998;840:684-697.
39. Adler GK, Kinsley BT, Hurwitz S, et al: Reduced hypothalamic-pituitary-adrenal and sympathoadrenal responses to hypoglycemia in women with fibromyalgia syndrome. Am J Med 1999;106: 534-543.
40. Klerman EB, Goldenberg DL, Brown EN, et al: Circadian rhythms of women with fibromyalgia. J Clin Endocrin Metab 2001;86:1034-1039.
41. Moldofsky H, Lue FA, Dickstein J, et al: Disordered circadian sleep-wake neuroendocrine and immune functions in chronic fatigue syndrome. Presented at the bi-annual research conference of the American Association for Chronic Fatigue Syndrome. Cambridge, Mass, October 10-11, 1998.
42. Schochat T, Raspe H: Elements of fibromyalgia in an open population. Rheumatology 2003;42:829-835.
43. Unger ER, Nisenbaum R, Moldofsky H, et al. Sleep assessment in a population-based study of chronic fatigue syndrome. BMC Neurol 2004;19:4-6.

44. Coté KA, Moldofsky H: Sleep, daytime symptoms, and cognitive performance in patients with fibromyalgia. J Rheumatol 1997; 24:2014-2023.

45. Moldofsky H: Sleep and pain. Sleep Med Rev 2001;5: 387-398.

46. Moldofsky H: The contribution of sleep medicine to the assessment of the tired patient. Can J Psychiatry 2000;45:51-55.

47. Carette S, Oakson G, Guimont C, et al: Sleep EEG and clinical response to amitriptyline in patients with fibromyalgia. Arthritis Rheum 1995;38:1211-1217.

48. May KP, West SG, Baker MR, et al: Sleep apnea in male patients with fibromyalgia syndrome. Am J Med 1993;94:505-508.

49. Alvarez Lario B, Alonso Valdivielso JL, Alegre Lopez J, et al: Fibromyalgia syndrome: Overnight falls in arterial oxygen saturation. Am J Med 1996;101:54-60.

50. Yunus MB, Aldag JC: Restless legs syndrome and leg cramps in fibromyalgia: Controlled study. BMJ 1996;312:1339.

51. Tayag-Kier CE, Keenan GF, Scalzi LV, et al: Sleep and periodic limb movements in sleep in juvenile fibromyalgia. Pediatrics 2000;106:E70.

52. Beck AT, Ward CH, Mendelson M, et al: An inventory for measuring depression. Arch Gen Psychiatry 1961;4:561-567.

53. Smets EM, Garssen B, Bonke B, et al: The Multidimensional Fatigue Inventory (MFI): Psychometric qualities of an instrument to assess fatigue. J Psychosomat Res 1995;39:315-325.

54. Chalder T, Berelowitz G, Pawlikowska T, et al: Development of a fatigue scale. J Psychosomat Med 1993;37:147-153.

55. Krupp LB, LaRocca NG, Muir-Nash J, et al: The fatigue severity scale: Application to patients with multiple sclerosis and systemic lupus erythematosus. Arch Neurol 1989;46:1121-1123.

56. Hoddes E, Zarcone V, Smythe H, et al: Quantification of sleepiness: A new approach. Psychophysiology 1973;10:431-436.

57. John MW: A new method for measuring daytime sleepiness: The Epworth Sleepiness Scale. Sleep 1991;14:540-545.

58. Buysse DJ, Reynolds CF 3rd, Monk TH, et al: The Pittsburgh Sleep Quality Index: A new instrument for psychiatric practice and research. Psychiatr Res 1989;28:193-213.

59. Unger ER, Nisenbaum R, Moldofsky H, et al: Sleep assessment in a population-based study of chronic fatigue syndrome. BMC Neurol 2004;4:6.

60. Keklund G, Akerstedt T: Objective components of individual differences in subjective sleep quality. J Sleep Res 1997;6:217-220.

61. Dinges DF, Powell JW: Microcomputer analyses of performance on a portable simple visual RT task during sustained operations. Behav Res Meth Instr Comp 1985;17:652-655.

62. Van Dongen HP, Dinges DF: Investigating the interaction between the homeostatic and circadian processes of sleep-wake regulation for the prediction of waking neurobehavioural performance. J Sleep Res 2003;12:181-187

63. Horne JA, Reyner LA: Sleep related vehicle accidents. BMJ 1995; 310:565-567.

64. Mitler MM, Miller JC, Lipsitz JJ, et al: The sleep of long-haul drivers. N Engl J Med 1997;337:755-761.

65. Aldrich MS: Automobile accidents in patients with sleep disorders. Sleep 1989;12:487-494.

66. Benca R, Moldofsky H, Ancoli Israel S: Special considerations in insomnia diagnosis and management: Depressed, elderly, and chronic pain populations. J Clin Psychiatry 2004;65(Suppl 8): 26-35.

67. Hauri P, Hawkins D: Alpha delta sleep. Electroencephalogr Clin Neurophysiol 1973;34:233-237.

68. Anch AM, Lue FA, MacLean AW, et al: Sleep physiology and psychological aspects of the fibrositis (fibromyalgia) syndrome. Can J Psychol 1991;45:178-184.

69. Branco J, Atalaia A, Paiva T: Sleep cycles and alpha-delta sleep in fibromyalgia syndrome. J Rheumatol 1994;21:1113-1117.

70. Drewes AM, Nielsen KD, Taagholt SJ, et al: Sleep intensity in fibromyalgia: Focus on the microstructure of the sleep process. Br J Rheumatol 1995;34:629-635.

71. Roizenblatt S, Tufik S, Goldenberg J, et al: Juvenile fibromyalgia: Clinical and polysomnographic aspects. J Rheumatol 1997;24: 579-585.

72. Roizenblatt S, Moldofsky H, Benedito-Silva AA, et al: Alpha sleep characteristics in fibromyalgia. Arthritis Rheum 2001;44:222-230.

73. Whelton CL, Salit I, Moldofsky H: Sleep, Epstein-Barr virus infection, musculoskeletal pain, and depressive symptoms in chronic fatigue syndrome. J Rheumatol 1992;19:939-943.

74. Manu P, Lane TJ, Matthews Castriotta RJ, et al: Alpha-delta sleep in patients with a chief complaint of chronic fatigue. South Med J 1994;87:465-470.

75. Moldofsky H, Lue FA, Smythe HA: Alpha EEG and morning symptoms in rheumatoid arthritis. J Rheumatol 1983;10:373-379.

76. Drewes AM, Svendsen L, Taagholt SJ, et al: Sleep in rheumatoid arthritis: A comparison with healthy subjects and studies of sleep/wake interactions. Br J Rheumatol 1998;37:71-81.

77. Mahowald MW, Mahowald ML, Bundlie SR, et al: Sleep fragmentation in rheumatoid arthritis. Arthritis Rheum 1989;32:974-978.

78. Schneider-Helmert D, Kumar A: Sleep, its subjective perception and daytime performance in insomniacs with a pattern of alpha sleep. Biol Psychiatry 1995;37:99-105.

79. Saskin P, Moldofsky H, Lue FA: Periodic movements in sleep and sleep-wake complaint. Sleep 1985;8:318-324.

80. Honda M, Koga E, Ishikawa T, et al: Alpha-delta sleep in a case of non-24 h sleep-wake syndrome: Quantitative electroencephalogram analysis of alpha and delta band waves. Psychiatry Clin Neurosci 1997;51:387-392.

81. Pivik RT, Harman KA: Reconceptualization of EEG alpha activity during sleep: All alpha activity is not equal. J Sleep Res 1995; 4:131-137.

82. Scheuler W, Kubicki S, Marquardt J, et al: The sleep pattern-quantitative analysis and functional aspects. In Koella WP, Obál F, Schulz H, et al (eds): Sleep '86. New York, Gustav Fischer Verlag, 1988, pp 284-286.

83. Connemann BJ, Mann K, Pascual-Marki RD, Roschke J: Limbic activity in slow wave sleep in a healthy subject with alpha-delta sleep. Psychiatry Res 2001;107:165-171.

84. MacFarlane JG, Shahal B, Moldofsky H: Periodic K-alpha sleep EEG activity and periodic leg movements during sleep: Comparisons of clinical features and sleep parameters. Sleep 1996;19:200-204.

85. Moldofsky H, Cesta A, Mously C, et al: Prevalence of sleep disorders in fibromyalgia. Sleep 2002;25(Suppl):A501.

86. Sarzi-Puttini P, Rizzi M, Andreoli A, et al: Hypersomnolence in fibromyalgia syndrome. Clin Exp Rheumatol 2002;20:69-72.

87. Disdier P, Genton P, Harle JR, et al: Fibromyalgia and narcolepsy. J Rheumatol 1993;20:888-889.

88. Disdier P, Genton P, Bolla G, et al: Clinical screening for narcolepsy/cataplexy in patients with fibromyalgia. Clin Rheumatol 1994;13:132-134.

89. Moldofsky H: Management of sleep disorders in fibromyalgia. Rheum Dis Clin North Am 2002;28:353-365.

90. Haanen HC, Hoenderdos HT, Van Romunde LK, et al: Controlled trial of hypnotherapy in the treatment of refractory fibromyalgia. J Rheumatol 1991;18:72-75.

91. Ferraccioli G, Ghirelli L, Scita F, et al: EMG biofeedback training in fibromyalgia syndrome. J Rheumatol 1987;14:820-825.

92. Deluze C, Bosia L, Zirbs A, et al: Electroacupuncture in fibromyalgia: Results of a controlled trial. BMJ 1992;305:1249-1252.

93. Almeida TF, Roizenblatt S, Benedito-Silva AA, et al: The effect of combined therapy (ultrasound and interferential current) on pain and sleep in fibromyalgia. Pain 2003;104:665-672.

94. Burckhardt CS, Mannerkorpi K, Hedenberg L, et al: A randomized, controlled clinical trial of education and physical training for women with fibromyalgia. J Rheumatol 1994;21:714-720.

95. Bennett RM, Gatter RA, Campbell SM, et al: A comparison of cyclobenzaprine and placebo in the management of fibrositis: A double blind controlled study. Arthritis Rheum 1988;3: 1535-1542.

96. Carette S, Bell MV, Reynolds WJ, et al: Comparison of amitriptyline, cyclobenzaprine and placebo in the treatment of fibromyalgia: A randomized double blind clinical trial. Arthritis Rheum 1994; 37:32-40.

97. Reynolds WJ, Moldofsky H, Saskin P, et al: The effects of cyclobenzaprine on sleep physiology and symptoms in patients with fibromyalgia. J Rheumatol 1991;18:452-454.

98. Goldenberg D, Mayskiy M, Mossey C, et al: A randomized, double-blind crossover trial of fluoxetine and amitriptyline in the treatment of fibromyalgia. Arthritis Rheum 1996;39: 1852-1859.

99. Wolfe F, Cathey MA, Hawley DJ: A double blind placebo controlled trial of fluoxetine in fibromyalgia. Scand J Rheumatol 1994;23:255-259.

100. Drewes AM, Andreasen A, Jennum P, et al: Zopiclone in the treatment of sleep abnormalities in fibromyalgia. Scand J Rheumatol 1991;20:288-293.

101. Moldofsky H, Lue FA, Mously C, et al: The effect of zolpidem in patients with fibromyalgia: A dose ranging, double blind, placebo controlled, modified crossover study. J Rheumatol 1966; 23:529-533.

102. Moldofsky H, Lue FA: The relationship of alpha and delta EEG frequencies to pain and mood in "fibrositis" patients treated with chlorpromazine and L-tryptophan. Electroencephalogr Clin Neurophysiol 1980;50:71-80.

103. Caruso I, Sarzi Puttini P, Cazzola M, et al: Double-blind study of 5-hydroxytryptophan versus placebo in the treatment of primary fibromyalgia syndrome. J Int Med Res 1990;18: 201-209.

104. Scharf MB, Baumann M, Berkowitz DV: The effects of sodium oxybate on clinical symptoms and sleep patterns in patients with fibromyalgia. J Rheumatol 2003;30:1070-1074.

105. Pearl SJ, Lue F, MacLean AW, et al: The effects of bright light treatment on the symptoms of fibromyalgia. J Rheumatol 1996; 23:896-902.

106. Silver DS, Wallace DJ: The management of fibromyalgia-associated syndromes. Rheum Dis Clin North Am 2002;28:405-417.

107. Golding DN: Hypothyroidism presenting with musculoskeletal symptoms. Ann Rheum Dis 1970;29:10-14.

108. Bland JH, Frymoyer JW: Rheumatic syndromes of myxedema. N Engl J Med 1970;282:1171-1174.

109. Yunus MA: Comprehensive medical evaluation of patients with fibromyalgia. Rheum Dis Clin North Am 2003;28:201-217.

110. Rechtschaffen A, Kales A (eds): A Manual of Standardized Terminology, Techniques and Scoring System for Sleep Stages of Human Subjects. Washington, DC, Public Health Service, U.S. Government Printing Office, 1968.

111. MacLean AW, Lue FA, Moldofsky H: The reliability of visual scoring of alpha EEG sleep. Sleep 1995;18:565-569.

112. Terzano MG, Parino L, Sherieri A, et al: Consensus report: Atlas, rules, and recording techniques for the scoring of cyclic alternating pattern (CAP) in human sleep. Sleep Med 2002;3: 187-199.

113. Terzano MG, Paino L, Fioti G, et al: Modifications of sleep structure induced by increasing levels of acoustic perturbation in normal subjects. Electroencephalogr Clin Neurophysiol 1990: 76:29-38.

114. MacFarlane JG, Ball BA, MacLean AW, Moldofsky H: Sleep and symptoms in patients with periodic polyphasic EEG burst activity vs periodic leg movements during sleep. Sleep Res 1997:26:420.

115. MacFarlane JG, Doidge M, Twining L, et al: Source localization of abnormal cyclic alternating pattern in fibromyalgia patients with non-restorative sleep. Sleep 2004;27:A283.

105

Endocrine Disorders

Ronald Grunstein

ABSTRACT

Sleep disorders, particularly sleep apnea, are common in many endocrine conditions. Most patients with acromegaly have some degree of sleep apnea with an unusually high prevalence of central sleep apnea. Androgens appear to exacerbate sleep apnea, whereas there is some evidence of a protective effect of female sex steroids on upper airway obstruction during sleep. It is controversial whether hypothyroidism is a risk factor for sleep breathing disorders. Finally, sleep apnea is associated with endocrine disorders linked to obesity such as diabetes. Some evidence exists supporting a role of sleep disorders in the pathogenesis of metabolic disturbances associated with obesity.

There are many diverse associations between human endocrine function and sleep. Importantly, neuroendocrine and metabolic physiology is often influenced by behavioral states of sleep and wakefulness (see Chapter 22). Extensive research in this area has flourished owing to the development of better assays of endocrine function, paralleling the growth of human sleep research stimulated by the availability of polysomnography. Endocrine rhythms have often been labeled either sleep related (when the predominant change in fluctuation is nocturnal) or circadian (when the rhythm appears to be regulated by an internal clock rather than periodic changes in the external environment). The predominant influences are intrinsic circadian rhythmicity and sleep, which interact to varying degrees to produce the characteristic 24-hour rhythm of each hormone. Conversely, aberrations of normal endocrine function may influence sleep or alter state-affected parameters such as breathing or the electroencephalogram (EEG). This chapter concentrates on these changes, limiting discussion to particular endocrine disorders in adults and children.

ACROMEGALY AND OTHER GROWTH HORMONE DISORDERS

Acromegaly is a condition of growth hormone (GH) excess in adults characterized by the insidious development of coarsening of facial features, bony proliferation, and soft tissue swelling.[1] It is usually secondary to a GH-producing pituitary adenoma, which may be either a microadenoma or macroadenoma. Rarely, the GH excess commences before puberty and closure of the epiphyses and then the condition is termed *gigantism*. It occurs with equal frequency in both sexes, with a prevalence of 50 to 70 cases per million. The clinical features may be due to the local effects of an expanding pituitary mass in addition to the effects of excess GH secretion, which include disordered somatic cell growth and insulin resistance.

The mortality rate of untreated or partially treated acromegaly is approximately double the expected rate in healthy subjects matched for age.[2] Acromegaly was first described as a clinical entity by Marie in 1876. Ten years later, Roxburgh and Collis[3] described daytime sleepiness and Chappell and Booth[4] observed upper airway obstruction as features of acromegaly, but the association between sleep apnea and acromegaly was described only 90 years later.[5]

Epidemiology and Risk Factors

Sleep-disordered breathing is extremely common in acromegaly. Studies have shown that at least 60% of unselected patients with acromegaly have sleep apnea[6] (Fig. 105–1). Almost all patients with acromegaly in this series were noted to have heavy snoring. A number of prevalence studies using limited nocturnal respiratory monitoring have also shown a very high prevalence of sleep breathing disorders in acromegaly.[7,8] In keeping with typical sleep apnea epidemiology, abnormal breathing during sleep in acromegaly is associated with increasing age. However, obesity has less influence on the prevalence of sleep apnea in acromegaly.[6-8] Increases in body mass index in acromegaly may be due to increased muscle mass rather than the increased body fat typically seen in obesity.[1]

Pathogenesis

Although it would appear logical that sleep apnea in acromegaly is secondary to macroglossia causing narrowing of the hypopharynx, the exact etiology is unclear.[6] Endoscopic studies of the upper airway have indicated little posterior movement of the tongue,[7] whereas other studies using cephalometry have produced divergent findings when examining craniofacial anatomy in patients with acromegaly both with and without sleep apnea.[9]

Patients with acromegaly have a high rate of central apnea, with up to 34% of the total group of patients with sleep apnea in one study.[6,10] Others,[11] using full sleep studies, reported that two of their three patients with sleep apnea and acromegaly had predominantly or exclusively central apnea. A waxing-and-waning central apnea pattern of breathing on static charge–sensitive bed studies has also been reported as more common in acromegaly as opposed to typical upper airway obstruction.[7]

The high prevalence of central apnea in acromegaly suggests that abnormalities of central respiratory control are involved. This has been supported by the finding that patients with central sleep apnea had significantly lower awake arterial carbon dioxide levels and increased ventilatory responsiveness[12] than those with obstructive sleep apnea (OSA)[6,12] (Fig. 105–2). Central apnea occurs in association with a wide range of disorders and many potential mechanisms have been

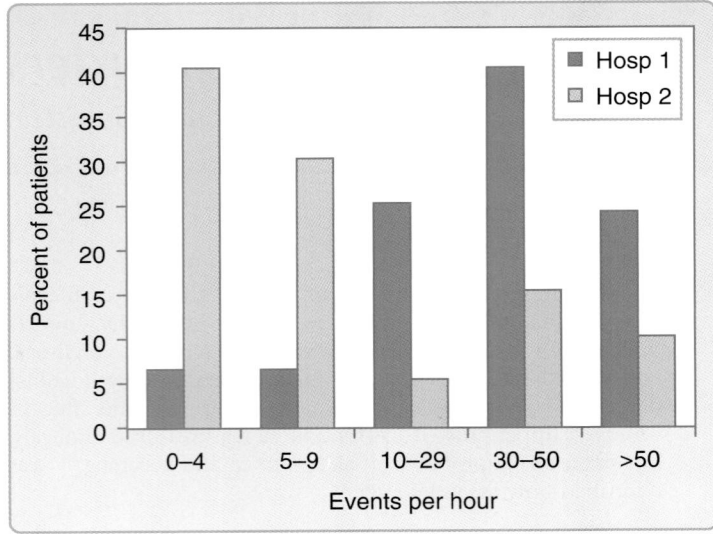

Figure 105–1. Prevalence of sleep apnea in acromegaly in two cohorts in Sydney, Australia. In hospital 1, which has a sleep laboratory, almost all patients with acromegaly have sleep apnea. In hospital 2, a regional endocrine center without sleep investigation facilities, 60% of patients have sleep apnea (defined by respiratory disturbance index > 5).

described, including disordered central respiratory control.[12] The precise cause in acromegaly is unclear, but there are a number of hypotheses, including alterations in central somatostatin pathways disinhibiting respiratory control.[12] Other mechanisms include an effect of GH on central respiratory control, either directly or by altering metabolic rate, inducing central apnea. This is supported by the correlation between GH hypersecretion and the prevalence of central apnea.[6,12] Apparent central apneas have been observed in beagles exposed to medroxyprogesterone, which in turn increases GH secretion and causes an acromegaly-like condition.[12]

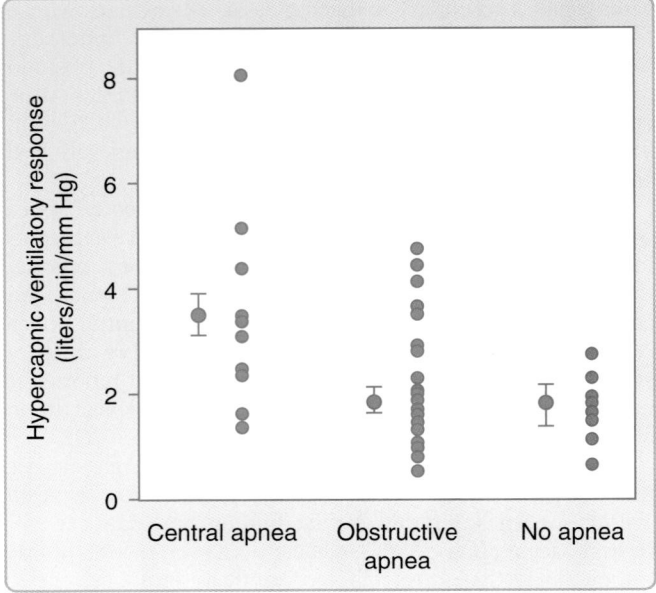

Figure 105–2. Ventilatory responses to hypercapnia in patients with acromegaly. Patients with predominantly central sleep apnea have increased ventilatory responses.

Disease Activity in Acromegaly and Sleep Apnea

In view of the morbidity and mortality of acromegaly, it is important to define active and inactive (cured) disease. High circulating insulin-like growth factor-1 (IGF-1) and GH levels reflect increased GH production and therefore disease activity. Studies describing "cure" after pituitary surgery often use inadequate criteria of disease inactivity.[1] True cure involves observing a physiologic 24-hour GH secretion, normal IGF-1 levels, and normal GH responses to glucose. Even in patients with acromegaly and normal IGF-1 and GH profiles, GH secretory patterns are still different from those of healthy subjects.[10]

Most studies have observed persisting sleep apnea despite treatment of acromegaly by pituitary surgery. However, no correlation has been found between disease activity and sleep apnea severity,[6] and in the same study, no significant differences in mean GH and IGF-1 levels in patients with and without sleep apnea were observed. In this study,[6] 23 patients had detailed 24-hour GH secretory profiles and 16 had sleep apnea (2 predominantly central and 14 predominantly obstructive). In this subgroup with more extensive GH measurements, no significant differences in mean GH and GH pulsatility were found between patients with and without sleep apnea. In contrast, lower GH levels have been reported in some patients with milder sleep apnea.[8] Studies using octreotide, a somatostatin analogue, have shown powerful GH reduction with a parallel decrease in apnea severity.[10] However, even in this study, there was no relationship between the decrease in apnea and the decrease in GH levels.[10]

At present, it is not known what proportion of patients with both sleep apnea and acromegaly will have complete resolution of their sleep apnea after cure of acromegaly. This will require careful prospective studies accurately monitoring the true cure of acromegaly. However, it is clear that sleep apnea does occur in cured acromegaly.[6,10] The combination of inactive acromegaly and sleep apnea may occur for a number of reasons. First, sleep apnea is a common disorder and may be coincident to acromegaly in patients with other risk factors for sleep apnea. Second, it may take a long time after normalization of GH secretion for the effects of acromegaly to resolve or there may be permanent effects on upper airway function or sleep breathing regulation.

Although there appears to be no relationship between disease activity and severity of sleep apnea, patients with central sleep apnea have much higher IGF-1 and fasting GH levels compared with patients with OSA.[6,12]

Morbidity and Mortality of Acromegaly and Sleep Apnea

The adverse health risks of both acromegaly and sleep apnea are well established. Both disorders are associated with an increased risk of hypertension.[1] In acromegaly, the blood pressure level is sometimes reduced by successful transsphenoidal surgery. One postulated mechanism for hypertension in acromegaly is sodium and water retention secondary to GH overproduction.[1]

Sleep apnea and hypertension may be closely linked. In one study,[6] over 50% of patients with both acromegaly and sleep apnea had hypertension, but all patients with acromegaly who did not have sleep apnea were normotensive. Patients who were hypertensive had significantly higher respiratory disturbance indices and a greater degree of sleep hypoxemia than those who were normotensive. Mean 24-hour GH and IGF-1 levels and the degree of obesity were not significantly different in those with hypertension compared with those without hypertension. Using multiple regression analysis, both the respiratory disturbance index and age were found to be independent predictors of hypertension.[6]

Examination of the causes of death in patients with acromegaly at four London hospitals has found an excess of deaths due to cardiovascular and respiratory causes.[2] In this report, the authors commented that "The excess of deaths due to respiratory disease was an unexpected finding for which there was no obvious explanation." This finding was inexplicable because there is no apparent excess of chronic lung disease in acromegaly. Lung function is usually normal or supernormal. With our new understanding of the high prevalence of sleep apnea in acromegaly, it is likely that this is the mechanism of the deaths attributed at that time to respiratory disease. Another potential link is sleep apnea and upper airway obstruction complicating anesthesia in these patients.[13]

Does Acromegaly Cause Nonrespiratory Sleep Disorders?

Somnolence has long been recognized as part of the clinical spectrum of acromegaly. Early descriptions of sleepiness in patients with acromegaly suggested a link with narcolepsy.[14] However, subsequent data support the view that the dominant sleep disorder caused by acromegaly is sleep apnea. A direct effect of increased GH in promoting sleep and sleepiness has been suggested.[15] Alternatively, sleepiness in the absence of sleep apnea may be due to the effects of radiation therapy.[16] Given the close proximity of the sleep-regulating centers in the hypothalamus to sites of irradiation for acromegaly, it may be worth reviewing previously reported cases of narcolepsy in acromegaly.[14]

Growth Hormone Deficiency

Adults with sleep apnea appear to have relative GH deficiency, which is reversible by nasal continuous positive airway pressure (CPAP)[17,18] (Fig. 105–3). This deficiency in untreated patients is likely related to abnormal sleep structure (see Chapter 22) and hypoxemia during sleep. In individuals with primary GH deficiency, a reduction in power in delta sleep has been observed.[19] There are few data on GH-inducing sleep apnea in hypopituitary patients. There is one report[20] of the development of sleep apnea in four children (two obstructive, two mixed) after GH administration.

SEX HORMONE DISORDERS

Male Hormonal Disorders

Since the early 1980s, there have a number of reports describing the development of sleep apnea in both sexes after testosterone therapy.[21-23] These cases certainly suggest that testosterone may be important in the regulation of breathing during sleep and in the pathogenesis of sleep apnea. Testosterone also was reported to exacerbate sleep apnea in a 13-year-old boy, associated with an increase in upper airway collapsibility during sleep.[24]

Other studies have examined the sleep breathing effects of exogenous testosterone on hypogonadal patients using before-and-after observational designs.[25,26] These studies show an overall increase in sleep apnea in these patients, but clinically

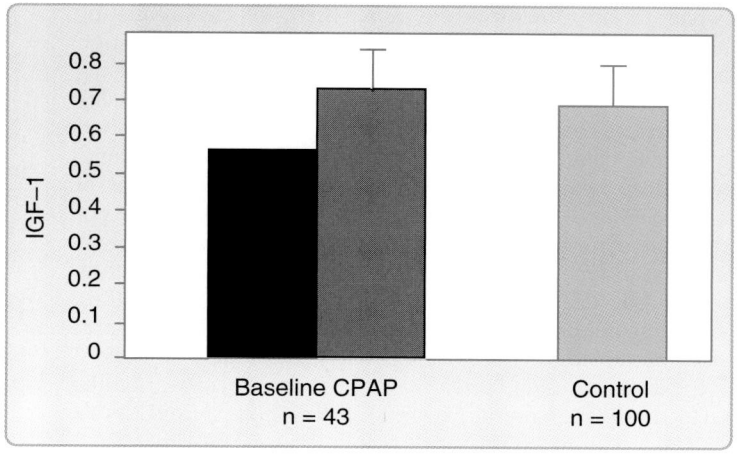

Figure 105–3. Insulin-like growth factor-1 (IGF-1) levels in sleep apnea in 43 men before (*black bar*) and 3 months after (*gray bar*) nasal continuous positive airway pressure (CPAP) therapy. IGF-1 levels increased to levels similar to those observed in a control group (*blue bar*) of 100 hospital volunteers (mean age, 40 years).

significant increases occurred in a minority of patients. Recently, a placebo-controlled, double-blinded trial of high-dose testosterone in otherwise healthy elderly men has shown that testosterone worsens coexisting undiagnosed sleep apnea and shortens total sleep time.[27] Despite this effect on sleep and breathing, there were no observed effects on driving task performance and cognitive tests. The clinical message from these studies is that patients commencing on androgen replacement should be questioned closely for sleep apnea symptomatology and monitored during the course of their therapy to check if such symptoms develop. The possibility of more extensive use of testosterone therapy in eugonadal men for contraception or for "andropause" will likely bring testosterone-induced apnea into clinical practice. Simple device-based methods for sleep apnea "screening" may also need to be used in such patients.

Testosterone also influences sleep architecture. In a study of pharmacologically induced hypogonadism,[28] with and without gonadal steroid replacement, hypogonadal male patients had reduced 24-hour prolactin (PRL) levels and percentage of stage 4 sleep in the hypogonadal state compared with testosterone replacement. Melatonin secretion is increased in male patients with gonadotropin-releasing hormone deficiency and in low-testosterone, hypergonadotropic, hypogonadal patients.[29] However there are no data on the prevalence of sleep disturbance in these patients. The observation of reduced total sleep time without worsening alertness on task with high-dose testosterone therapy is intriguing in this context.[27] Recent data demonstrating lower testosterone levels in those with sleep disturbances and shift work sleep disorder[30] indicate that the topic of sex steroids and sleep is an area worthy of more extensive research.

Low testosterone levels have been reported in men with sleep apnea.[17,31] In the largest study,[17] hormone level suppression by sleep apnea was independent of age, degree of obesity, and presence of awake hypoxemia and hypercapnia. Testosterone levels increase with treatment of sleep apnea using nasal CPAP or even successful uvulopalatopharyngoplasty.[17,31] These androgen abnormalities in sleep apnea (decreased sex hormone–binding globulin [SHBG] and free and total testosterone) are qualitatively as well as quantitatively distinct from those reported in aging (increased SHBG, decreased free and total testosterone) and obesity (decreased SHBG and total testosterone, normal free testosterone). Importantly, despite the fall in plasma free and total testosterone levels, there was no increase in basal plasma gonadotropin (luteinizing hormone [LH], follicle-stimulating hormone) levels. These findings, together with the retention of pituitary sensitivity to exogenous gonadotropin-releasing hormone in sleep apnea,[32] point to a hypothalamic abnormality as the cause of the fall in testosterone levels. This is supported by recent data indicating impaired LH secretion in patients with sleep apnea[33] and partial correction with 9 months of nasal CPAP treatment.[34] The potential causes of this hypothalamic abnormality are essentially similar to those involved in reduced GH secretion. Testosterone levels are significantly reduced by sleep deprivation and fragmentation.[35] Therefore, sleep fragmentation in sleep apnea may lead to disruption of sleep-entrained rhythms in LH and testosterone secretion. Hypoxemia in sleep apnea may be involved because, unlike GH, there are several reports of low sex steroid levels in patients with chronic airflow limitation.[14] In other large studies,[14] the apparent effects of awake hypoxemia and impaired lung function were entirely accounted for by sleep hypoxemia. It is possible that the sexual dysfunction reported in sleep apnea may be mediated by the sex hormone changes seen in sleep-disordered breathing. The low testosterone levels may also interact with low IGF-1 levels and impair anabolism. Androgens may exacerbate sleep apnea, and it is possible that the fall in androgen levels may be part of an adaptive homeostatic mechanism to reduce sleep-disordered breathing. However, androgen-lowering therapy with the nonsteroidal androgen antagonist flutamide did not alter sleep-disordered breathing or awake ventilatory drive.[36]

Female Sex Hormones and Sleep

Studies about the impact of the menstrual cycle and use of oral contraceptives on sleep parameters are limited by sample size and design. Sleep disruption during pregnancy and postpartum is well recognized and menopause is associated with insomnia due to several factors, including hot flashes, mood disorders, and increased sleep-disordered breathing (see Chapters 108 through 110). Longitudinal studies of sleep during the postpartum period and large-scale investigation of the effect of hormone replacement therapy on sleep and breathing are needed.[37]

Recent epidemiologic studies have confirmed an increase in prevalence of sleep-disordered breathing among postmenopausal women.[38] Other work has suggested that hormone replacement therapy is associated with a lower risk of sleep apnea in postmenopausal women.[39] Experimental studies have also shown that testosterone administration in women increases breathing instability during sleep, a finding that is relevant for sleep apnea considering the increased androgen-to-estrogen balance postmenopause.[40] However, despite these studies, definitive data showing a benefit for female sex hormones in women with sleep apnea are lacking. Although progesterone levels fall after menopause and progestogens have been shown to stimulate ventilation during the luteal phase of the menstrual cycle, in pregnancy, in healthy male subjects, and in conditions of alveolar hypoventilation, there is no consistent therapeutic effect of progestogens in sleep apnea.[41,42] Similarly, there is no obvious benefit seen in other studies directly examining the role of female sex hormone therapy on breathing during sleep.[41,42] Again, definitive, double-blinded, placebo-controlled trials are lacking.

Increasing central obesity develops with the estrogen deficiency of menopause.[43] This is likely to be the main factor in the increased prevalence of sleep apnea in the postmenopause state. Obesity occurs in approximately 50% of hyperandrogenic anovulatory women, some of whom also have type 2 diabetes mellitus. This is typically associated with the polycystic ovary syndrome (PCOS). There are two studies indicating that PCOS is strongly associated with the presence of sleep apnea and, in turn, that sleep apnea in PCOS is strongly associated with the degree of androgen excess and increased central fat.[44,45]

Prolactinoma

Short-term administration of PRL and even long-term hyperprolactinemia in animals increases rapid eye movement (REM) sleep.[46] In one study,[47] sleep in drug-free patients with prolactinoma (mean PRL levels, 1450 ± 1810 ng/mL; range, 146 to 5106 ng/mL) was compared with that of matched control subjects. The patients had secondary hypogonadism but no other endocrine abnormalities. They spent more time in slow wave sleep (SWS) than the control subjects. REM sleep variables did not differ between the groups. It appears that chronic excessive enhancement of PRL levels exerts different influences on the sleep EEG in humans compared with the enhanced REM sleep produced by hyperprolactinemia in rats. These findings are in accordance with reports of good sleep quality in patients with prolactinoma. Sleep apnea is also associated with reduced PRL secretory pulse frequency.[48]

THYROID

Hypothyroidism and Sleep Apnea

Apneic breathing in myxedema was first reported in 1964.[49] Although myxedema coma is now rare, in retrospect many cases were probably due to severe sleepiness and obtundation secondary to severe sleep apnea, coupled with the hypercapnic respiratory failure of sleep apnea. Several mechanisms have been suggested to explain the association between sleep apnea and hypothyroidism. These include reduced upper airway patency due to myxedematous infiltration of tissues, impaired function of upper airway muscles, and reduced central drive to upper airway muscles.[50]

Several studies have questioned the strength of the association between sleep apnea and hypothyroidism. In a study of 20 hypothyroid patients,[51] all reported snoring, but only 2 patients had moderate to severe OSA and 3 had mild OSA. Another study[52] compared 26 patients with hypothyroidism with 188 euthyroid control subjects. Fifty percent of the hypothyroid patients and 29.3% of the control subjects had at least some episodes of partial or complete upper airway obstruction. Severe obstruction with episodes of repetitive apnea was present in 7.7% of the patients and in 1.5% of the control subjects. However, this association was largely explained by coexisting obesity and male sex. It has also been claimed that routine thyroid function testing in sleep apnea is not cost-effective[53] except in certain high-risk groups such as elderly women. Several large studies have been completed with conflicting conclusions on the strength of the association between sleep apnea and hypothyroidism and whether all patients with OSA should be screened for this disorder.[53,54] It is likely that the prevalence of the association in sleep apnea cohorts is too low, and further case-control studies in larger cohorts of patients with sleep apnea are needed. There are no large, prospective studies investigating the prevalence of sleep apnea in patients with hypothyroidism. It has been asserted that the prevalence of sleep apnea in this group is high.[55]

The effect of adequate thyroid hormone replacement on sleep apnea in hypothyroidism has been variable. An early case report[56] described three obese patients with myxedema and sleep apnea and reported cure of sleep apnea when they became euthyroid. Other case reports[51] either describe similar cures or no significant reduction in apnea index for both obese and nonobese patients. The mean apnea index fell from 99.5 to less than 20 in the six obese patients without weight change, and in all patients there was an associated decrease in apnea duration. The three nonobese patients reduced their apnea indices to less than 5 after achieving euthyroid status. In contrast, in another study of 10 patients,[50] only 2 of them had a complete resolution of their sleep apnea when they became euthyroid. Five patients had moderate improvement in their sleep apnea, although they continued to require nasal CPAP, whereas three patients had an increase in their apnea frequency.

The failure of sleep apnea to resolve after thyroxine treatment supports the view of a chance rather than causal association. An alternative explanation may be that hypothyroidism induces long-term changes in upper airway mechanics[57] or breathing control that do not resolve immediately after a euthyroid state is achieved. However, in two sleep apnea case-control studies, past hypothyroidism did not appear to be a risk factor for sleep apnea.[53,54]

A number of studies have suggested a link between sleep apnea and cardiovascular complications in the initial stages of thyroid hormone replacement therapy. It is well recognized that rapid restoration of the euthyroid state in hypothyroid patients may entail significant cardiovascular morbidity and mortality.[50] This is particularly so in the elderly or those with preexisting cardiovascular disease. In one report, one male patient had extremely long apneas lasting over 2 minutes, yet the oxyhemoglobin saturation fell only to 64%.[51] It is likely that his low metabolic rate and oxygen consumption (reduced to 50% of normal) contributed to his ability to maintain such saturation levels despite long apneas. After commencing thyroxine treatment, the increase in basal metabolic rate and oxygen consumption may be more rapid than clearance of abnormal myxedematous mucoprotein from the upper airway and normalization of depressed ventilatory responses. Long apneas may then be associated with lower oxyhemoglobin saturation as the oxygen consumption rate increases, therefore posing a potential risk of dangerous hypoxemia for a patient with compromised coronary blood supply. In the same study,[51] two female patients had cardiac complications after commencing thyroxine before a sleep study and the use of nasal CPAP therapy. One had a myocardial infarction with residual nocturnal angina after her thyroxine dosage was increased. Her nocturnal angina resolved after nasal CPAP was commenced. Another had nocturnal ventricular arrhythmias and unstable angina after thyroxine was commenced. Both complications resolved with CPAP therapy. In a case report,[58] extreme bradycardia and hypotension complicating sleep apnea were seen in a patient with myxedema successfully managed with nasal CPAP before commencing thyroxine. Others[56] have described a myxedematous patient with OSA and cardiac arrhythmias who had a tracheotomy performed, resolving both the OSA and the arrhythmias. It would seem appropriate to institute thyroid hormone replacement cautiously in patients with hypothyroidism, sleep apnea, and probable cardiovascular disease.

Sleep Quality in Hypothyroidism

Sleepiness has long been observed as a symptom in hypothyroidism. Although sleep apnea may be one cause, a primary central effect on sleep is also possible in some patients. A marked reduction in SWS has been seen in patients with hypothyroidism, which is reversible with treatment.[59] In congenital hypothyroidism, increased movement in sleep and reduced REM sleep have been noted.[60]

Hyperthyroidism and Sleep

A number of studies have shown an association between hyperthyroidism and sleep disturbance. This is not surprising in view of theoretical links between increased metabolic rates and insomnia.[61] Hyperthyroid patients complain of insomnia and have consequent impairment in mood.[62] However, these changes are not obvious in asymptomatic hyperthyroidism detected on random testing.[63] In addition, definitive controlled studies of sleep in hyperthyroid patients are lacking.

DISORDERED CORTICOSTEROID SECRETION AND SLEEP

Patients with corticosteroid excess secondary to Cushing's disease are characterized by truncal obesity, hypertension, and depression. In the only published data, approximately one third of patients appear to have sleep apnea.[64] Patients with Cushing's disease who do not have sleep apnea exhibit poorer sleep continuity, shortened REM latency, and increased first REM period density compared with normal subjects.[65] Other workers have suggested that, apart from insufficient inhibition of hypothalamic-pituitary-adrenal secretory activity during early sleep, patients with Cushing's disease have reduced SWS.[66] Interestingly, reduced SWS occurs in Addison's disease,[67] suggesting that normal cortisol secretion is needed for maintenance of SWS.

DIABETES AND CENTRAL OBESITY

No specific sleep architecture abnormalities are associated with diabetes. Even hypoglycemic episodes during sleep are not apparently associated with EEG evidence of arousal.[68] Periodic movements in sleep may be more common in diabetes (see Chapter 70), and sleep may be disrupted in those with painful neuropathy.[69] Sleep apnea is common in diabetes and even more common in diabetic patients with autonomic neuropathy.[70,71] The fundamental link between diabetes and sleep apnea is through a coassociation with obesity.[70,72]

Central obesity is often a more crucial determinant of morbidity and mortality than total adiposity.[73] Centrally obese individuals have increased risk of cardiovascular and cerebrovascular disease, diabetes, hypertension, hyperlipidemia, hyperuricemia, and insulin resistance relative to peripherally obese individuals—the so-called metabolic syndrome. Central obesity is the most common metabolic abnormality in sleep apnea.[72,74] The health risks of obesity and sleep apnea are similar and data are complicated by mutually confounding variables.[72] Multivariate analyses of data or CPAP intervention studies suggest that both sleep apnea and central obesity are additive in the pathogenesis of obesity-related morbidity.

Central obesity is a powerful epidemiologic predictor of sleep apnea,[72,74] and weight reduction may lead to marked improvement in sleep apnea severity. However, there are certainly less data addressing the reverse possibility—that sleep apnea may promote the development of obesity.[18] Unfortunately, no long-term longitudinal studies examining the developmental relationship between upper airway obstruction and obesity exist. It is tempting to think that chronic intermittent hypoxia and sleep fragmentation over years in sleep apnea can lead to changes in central control of energy regulation, appetite control, feeding, and metabolism, which would promote weight gain and thus worsen sleep apnea further. Moreover, if this is the case, could this vicious circle be broken by successful CPAP therapy? Or are there clear interindividual differences in underlying hypothalamic function leading to divergent responses in energy balance in patients with sleep apnea?

During sleep, energy expenditure (EE) typically falls relative to the awake basal state.[61] In severe sleep apnea, sleep EE appears to increase during apneic sleep and falls with CPAP therapy[75] (Fig. 105–4). This would seem to be paradoxical; such EE changes would favor weight loss before CPAP and weight gain after CPAP. However, the 24-hour EE may be

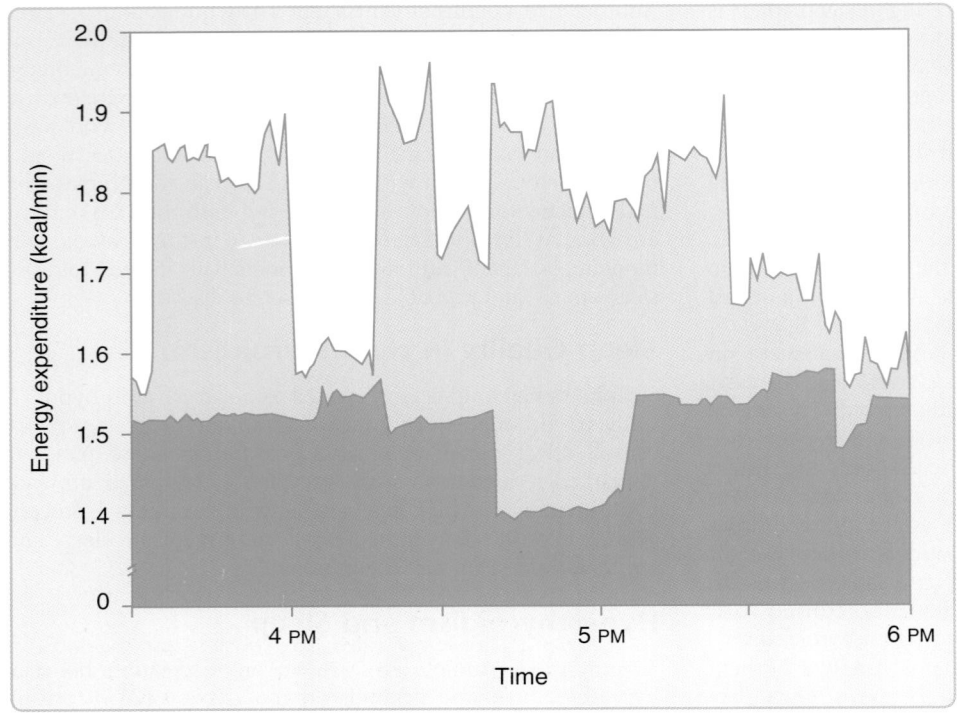

Figure 105–4. Sleep energy expenditure (SEE) curve for a subject (age 26 years, body mass index 40 kg/m²) with severe obstructive sleep apnea before treatment with nasal continuous positive airway pressure (CPAP; *top curve*) and reduction in SEE with CPAP therapy (*bottom curve*). (Adapted from Stenlöf K, Grunstein RR, Hedner J, et al: Energy expenditure in obstructive sleep apnea: Effects of treatment with continuous positive airway pressure. Am J Physiol 1996;271: E1036-E1043.)

different in untreated sleep apnea, with reduced spontaneous physical activity (fidgeting, routine physical activities) due to fatigue and sleepiness producing a net decrease in EE, despite increased EE in sleep due to respiratory effort and sleep fragmentation. Other intriguing data suggest that patients with sleep apnea may have altered serotonergic sensitivity in the hypothalamus. In one study[76] the cortisol response to L-5-hydroxytryptophan, a serotonin precursor, was elevated relative to control nonapneic subjects and was not readily explained by changes in weight. Subsequent data have shown that treatment with nasal CPAP reverses the elevated cortisol response to serotonergic stimulation.[77] These investigators have speculated that the exaggerated cortisol responses in sleep apnea indicate supersensitivity of postsynaptic serotonergic receptors in the hypothalamus caused by a serotonergic-"deficient" state induced by sleep apnea. Certainly, short periods of sleep deprivation in human beings and animals produce evidence of increased serotonin turnover[78]; whether chronic sleep fragmentation and hypoxemia in sleep apnea produce serotonin depletion in the hypothalamus and other regions is entirely speculative. Another potential factor that may promote obesity is leptin resistance. Leptin is a fat-regulating mediator produced widely in the body, especially by fat cells. Central resistance to leptin is not uncommon in obesity and has been observed in sleep apnea.[79]

There are parallel findings of a serotonin-deficient state in central obesity.[80] A cluster of disorders is associated with central obesity,[80] including abnormalities of the hypothalamic–pituitary–end-organ axis (low GH and testosterone, high cortisol), a "defeat" reaction to stress with psychosocial disability, and carbohydrate craving promoted by a low serotonergic state. Specific serotonergic agonists have been used as treatments in central obesity. The observed low testosterone and GH in sleep apnea also occur in central obesity. In central obesity, recombinant GH appears to reduce central body fat.[81] Perhaps, restoration of GH secretion during sleep with nasal CPAP in sleep apnea may have similar effects.[17,18] In this context, it also has been shown that nasal CPAP reduces visceral fat deposits even without change in body mass index in patients with sleep apnea.[82]

Central obesity is associated with hyperinsulinemia and insulin resistance.[73,79,80] The exact link between obesity, sleep apnea, and insulin resistance is unclear (see Chapter 86). Certainly, some data also point to increased insulin levels in sleep apnea independent of weight and central obesity.[83,84] Nasal CPAP also improves insulin sensitivity in type 2 diabetes mellitus.[70] However, in community cohorts, any relationship between sleep apnea and insulin resistance appears to be mediated by obesity.[85] Recent CPAP intervention data suggest that sleep apnea aggravates insulin resistance in moderately overweight patients, whereas the effect is less clear in the more obese.[86] Another direction of research linking OSA with the pathogenesis of the health risks of obesity is work showing an overproduction of certain cytokines and the formation of a "pro-inflammatory state in OSA."[87] These changes favor the development of increased vascular risk, insulin resistance, and metabolic syndrome. Other data linking shortened sleep with propensity to diabetes and OSA[84] are intriguing in the context of the current epidemic of diabetes and obesity. How the endocrine effects of shortened sleep relate to the effects of OSA on the endocrine system is clearly a potential area for future research. In summary, diabetes and central obesity, in

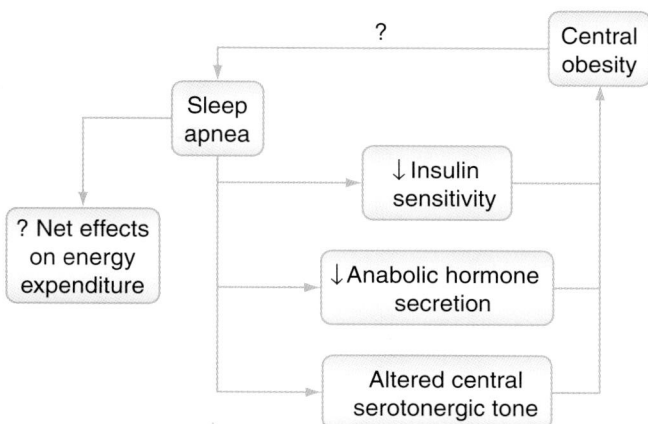

Figure 105–5. Factors involved in the relationship between central obesity and sleep apnea. Sleep apnea is linked with reduced insulin sensitivity and secretion of anabolic hormones, which would favor development of central obesity. The observed changes in serotonergic "tone" in sleep apnea would also theoretically promote the obese state. Although continuous positive airway pressure treatment of sleep apnea reduces energy expenditure, the net effects of sleep apnea on energy expenditure are unknown.

particular, are closely linked to sleep breathing disorders. A schema of the association between sleep apnea and central obesity is outlined in Figure 105–5.

> *Clinical Pearl*
>
> *It is important to consider the potential development of sleep apnea in any patient with an endocrine disorder or who is receiving certain hormonal therapies.*

Acknowledgments

Supported by a Practitioner Fellowship from the National Health and Medical Research Council of Australia.

References

1. Melmed S: Acromegaly. N Engl J Med 1990;322:966-977.
2. Wright AD, Hill DM, Lowy C, et al: Mortality in acromegaly. QJM 1970;39:1-16.
3. Roxburgh F, Collis AJ: Notes on a case of acromegaly. BMJ 1886; 2:63-65.
4. Chappell WF, Booth JA: A case of acromegaly with laryngeal symptoms and pharyngeal symptoms. J Laryngol Otol 1886;1: 142-150.
5. Laroche C, Festal G, Poenaru S, et al: Une observation de respiration périodique chez une acromégalie. Ann Med Intern 1976;127: 381-385.
6. Grunstein RR, Ho KY, Sullivan CE: Acromegaly and sleep apnea. Ann Intern Med 1991;115:527-532.
7. Pelttari L, Polo O, Rauhala E, et al: Nocturnal breathing abnormalities in acromegaly after adenomectomy. Clin Endocrinol (Oxf) 1995;43:175-182.
8. Rosenow F, Reuter S, Deuss U, et al: Sleep apnoea in treated acromegaly: Relative frequency and predisposing factors. Clin Endocrinol (Oxf) 1996;45:563-569.
9. Dostalova S, Sonka K, Smahel Z, et al: Craniofacial abnormalities and their relevance for sleep apnoea syndrome aetiopathogenesis in acromegaly. Eur J Endocrinol 2001;144:491-497.

10. Grunstein RR, Ho KY, Sullivan CE: Effect of octreotide on sleep apnoea in acromegaly. Ann Intern Med 1994;121:478-483.

11. Perks WH, Horrocks PM, Cooper RA, et al: Sleep apnea in acromegaly. BMJ 1980;280:894.

12. Grunstein RR, Ho KY, Berthon-Jones M, et al: Central sleep apnea is associated with increased ventilatory response to carbon dioxide and hypersecretion of growth hormone in patients with acromegaly. Am J Respir Crit Care Med 1994;150:496-502.

13. Bengtsson BA, Eden S, Ernst I, et al: Epidemiology and long term survival in acromegaly. Acta Med Scand 1988;223:327-335.

14. Barnes AJ, Pallis C, Joplin GF: Acromegaly and narcolepsy. Lancet 1979;2:332-333.

15. Astrom C, Christensen L, Gjerris F, et al: Sleep in acromegaly before and after treatment with adenomectomy. Neuroendocrinology 1991;53:328-331.

16. Faithfull S: Patients' experiences following cranial radiotherapy: A study of the somnolence syndrome. J Adv Nurs 1991;16:939-946.

17. Grunstein RR, Handelsman DJ, Lawrence S, et al: Neuroendocrine dysfunction in sleep apnea: reversal by nasal continuous positive airway pressure. J Clin Endocrinol Metab 1989;68:352-358.

18. Grunstein RR: Metabolic aspects of sleep apnea. Sleep 1996;19(Suppl):S218-S220.

19. Astrom C, Jochumsen PL: Decrease in delta sleep in growth hormone deficiency assessed by a new power spectrum analysis. Sleep 1989;12:508-515.

20. Gerard JM, Garibaldi L, Myers SE, et al: Sleep apnea in patients receiving growth hormone. Clin Pediatr 1997;36:321-326.

21. Sandblom RE, Matsumoto AM, Schoene RB, et al: Obstructive sleep apnea induced by testosterone administration. N Engl J Med 1983;308:506-510.

22. Johnson MW, Arch AM, Remmers JE: Induction of the obstructive sleep apnea syndrome in a woman by exogenous androgen administration. Am Rev Respir Dis 1984;129:1023.

23. Dexter DD, Dovre EJ: Obstructive sleep apnea due to endogenous testosterone production in a woman. Mayo Clin Proc 1998;73:246-248.

24. Cistulli PA, Grunstein RR, Sullivan CE: Effect of testosterone administration on upper airway collapsibility during sleep. Am J Respir Crit Care Med 1994;149:530-532.

25. Matsumoto AM, Sandblom RE, Schoene RB, et al: Testosterone replacement in hypogonadal males: Effects on obstructive sleep apnea, respiratory drives and sleep. Clin Endocrinol (Oxf) 1985; 22:713-717.

26. Schneider BK, Pickett CK, Zwillich CW, et al: Influence of testosterone on breathing during sleep. J Appl Physiol 1986;61:618-624.

27. Liu PY, Yee B, Wishart SM, et al: The short-term effects of high-dose testosterone on sleep, breathing, and function in older men. J Clin Endocrinol Metab 2003;88:3605-3613.

28. Leibenluft E, Schmidt PJ, Turner EH, et al: Effects of leuprolide-induced hypogonadism and testosterone replacement on sleep, melatonin, and prolactin secretion in men. J Clin Endocrinol Metab 1997;82:3203-3207.

29. Luboshitzky R, Wagner O, Lavi S, et al: Abnormal melatonin secretion in male patients with hypogonadism. J Mol Neurosci 1996;7:91-98.

30. Axelsson J, Akerstedt T, Kecklund G, et al: Hormonal changes in satisfied and dissatisfied shift workers across a shift cycle. J Appl Physiol 2003;95:2099-2105.

31. Santamaria JD, Prior JC, Fleetham JA: Reversible reproductive dysfunction in men with obstructive sleep apnea. Clin Endocrinol (Oxf) 1988;28:461-470.

32. Stewart DA, Grunstein RR, Sullivan CE, et al: Neuroendocrine changes in sleep apnea are not related to a pituitary defect. Sleep Res 1989;18:308.

33. Luboshitzky R, Aviv A, Hefetz A, et al: Decreased pituitary-gonadal secretion in men with obstructive sleep apnea. J Clin Endocrinol Metab 2002;87:3394-3398.

34. Luboshitzky R, Lavie L, Shen-Orr Z, Lavie P: Pituitary-gonadal function in men with obstructive sleep apnea: The effect of continuous positive airways pressure treatment. Neuroendocrinol Lett 2003;24:463-467.

35. Akerstedt T, Palmblad J, de la Torre B, et al: Adrenocortical and gonadal steroids during sleep deprivation. Sleep 1980;3:23-30.

36. Stewart DA, Grunstein RR, Berthon-Jones M, et al: Androgen blockade does not affect sleep-disordered breathing or chemosensitivity in men with obstructive sleep apnea. Am Rev Respir Dis 1992;146:1389-1393.

37. Moline ML, Broch L, Zak R, Gross V: Sleep in women across the life cycle from adulthood through menopause. Sleep Med Rev 2003;7:155-177.

38. Young T, Finn L, Austin D, Peterson A: Menopausal status and sleep-disordered breathing in the Wisconsin Sleep Cohort Study. Am J Respir Crit Care Med 2003;167:1181-1185.

39. Shahar E, Redline S, Young T, et al: Hormone replacement therapy and sleep-disordered breathing. Am J Respir Crit Care Med 2003;167:1186-1192.

40. Zhou XS, Rowley JA, Demirovic F, et al: Effect of testosterone on the apneic threshold in women during NREM sleep. J Appl Physiol 2003;94(1):101-107.

41. Cistulli PA, Barnes DJ, Grunstein RR, et al: Effect of short-term hormone replacement in the treatment of obstructive sleep apnoea in postmenopausal women. Thorax 1994;49:699-702.

42. Saaresranta T, Polo O: Sleep-disordered breathing and hormones. Eur Respir J 2003;22:161-172.

43. Carr MC: The emergence of the metabolic syndrome with menopause. J Clin Endocrinol Metab 2003;88:2404-2411.

44. Fogel RB, Malhotra A, Pillar G, et al: Increased prevalence of obstructive sleep apnea syndrome in obese women with polycystic ovary syndrome. J Clin Endocrinol Metab 2001;86:1175-1180.

45. Vgontzas AN, Legro RS, Bixler EO, et al: Polycystic ovary syndrome is associated with obstructive sleep apnea and daytime sleepiness: Role of insulin resistance. J Clin Endocrinol Metab 2001;86:517-520.

46. Obal F Jr, Kacsoh B, Bredow S, et al: Sleep in rats rendered chronically hyperprolactinemic with anterior pituitary grafts. Brain Res 1997;25;755:130-136.

47. Frieboes RM, Murck H, Stalla GK, et al: Enhanced slow wave sleep in patients with prolactinoma. J Clin Endocrinol Metab 1998;83:2706-2710.

48. Spiegel K, Follenius M, Krieger J, et al: Prolactin secretion during sleep in obstructive sleep apnoea patients. J Sleep Res 1995;4:56-62.

49. Massumi RA, Winnacker JL: Severe depression of the respiratory center in myxedema. Am J Med 1964;36:876-882.

50. Grunstein RR, Sullivan CE: Hypothyroidism and sleep apnea: Mechanisms and management. Am J Med 1988;85:775-779.

51. Lin CC, Tsan KW, Chen PJ: The relationship between sleep apnea syndrome and hypothyroidism. Chest 1992;102:1663-1667.

52. Pelttari L, Rauhala E, Polo O, et al: Upper airway obstruction in hypothyroidism. J Intern Med 1994;236:177-181.

53. Kapur VK, Koepsell TD, deMaube J, et al: Association of hypothyroidism and obstructive sleep apnea. Am J Respir Crit Care Med 1998;158:1379-1383.

54. Sjokdt NM, Aktar R, Easton PA: Screening for hypothyroidism in sleep apnea. Am J Respir Crit Care Med 1999;160:732-735.

55. Rajagopal KR, Abbrecht PH, Derderian SS, et al: Obstructive sleep apnea in hypothyroidism. Ann Intern Med 1984;101:471-474.

56. Orr WC, Males JL, Imes NK: Myxedema and obstructive sleep apnea. Am J Med 1981;70:1061-1066.

57. Petrof BJ, Kelly AM, Rubinstein NA, et al: Effect of hypothyroidism on myosin heavy chain expression in rat pharyngeal dilator muscles. J Appl Physiol 1992;73:179-187.

58. Abouganem D, Taylor AL, Donna E, et al: Extreme bradycardia during sleep apnea caused by myxedema. Arch Intern Med 1987;147:1497-1499.

59. Ruiz-Primo E, Jurado JL, Solis H, et al: Polysomnographic effects of thyroid hormones in primary myxedema. Electroencephalogr Clin Neurophysiol 1982;53:559-564.

60. Hayashi M, Araki S, Kohyama J, et al: Sleep development in children with congenital and acquired hypothyroidism. Brain Dev 1997;19:43-49.

61. Bonnet MH, Berry RB, Arand DL: Metabolism during normal, fragmented and recovery sleep. J Appl Physiol 1991;71: 1112-1118.

62. Huang YR, Wang GH: Study on quality of sleep and mental health in patients with hyperthyroidism. Chung Hua Hu Li Tsa Chih 1997;32:435-439.

63. Schlote B, Schaaf L, Schmidt R, et al: Mental and physical state in subclinical hyperthyroidism: Investigations in a normal working population. Biol Psychiatry 1992;32:48-56.

64. Shipley JE, Schteingart DE, Tandon R, et al: Sleep architecture and sleep apnea in patients with Cushing's disease. Sleep 1992; 15:514-518.

65. Shipley JE, Schteingart DE, Tandon R, et al: EEG sleep in Cushing's disease and Cushing's syndrome: Comparison with patients with major depressive disorder. Biol Psychiatry 1992; 32:146-155.

66. Born J, Fehm HL: Hypothalamus-pituitary-adrenal activity during human sleep: A coordinating role for the limbic hippocampal system. Exp Clin Endocrinol Diabetes 1998;106:153-163.

67. Gillin JC, Jacobs LS, Snyder F, et al: Effects of decreased adrenal corticosteroids: Changes in sleep in normal subjects and patients with adrenal cortical insufficiency. Electroencephalogr Clin Neurophysiol 1974;36:283-289.

68. Porter PA, Byrne G, Stick S, et al: Nocturnal hypoglycaemia and sleep disturbances in young teenagers with insulin dependent diabetes mellitus. Arch Dis Child 1996;75:120-123.

69. Backonja M, Beydoun A, Edwards KR, et al: Gabapentin for the symptomatic treatment of painful neuropathy in patients with diabetes mellitus: A randomized controlled trial. JAMA 1998; 280:1831-1836.

70. Brooks B, Cistulli PA, Borkman M, et al: Effect of nasal continuous positive airway pressure treatment on insulin sensitivity in patients with type II diabetes and obstructive sleep apnea. J Clin Endocrinol Metab 1994;79:1681-1685.

71. Ficker JH, Dertinger SH, Siegfried W, et al: Obstructive sleep apnoea and diabetes mellitus: The role of cardiovascular autonomic neuropathy. Eur Respir J 1998;11:14-19.

72. Grunstein RR, Wilcox I, Yang TS, et al: Snoring and sleep apnoea in men: Association with central obesity and hypertension. Int J Obes 1993;17:533-540.

73. Bjorntorp P: Obesity. Lancet 1997;350:423-426.

74. Grunstein RR, Stenlöf K, Hedner J, et al: Impact of self reported sleep apnea symptoms on psycho-social performance in the Swedish Obese Subjects (SOS) Study. Sleep 1995;18:635-643.

75. Stenlöf K, Grunstein RR, Hedner J, et al: Energy expenditure in obstructive sleep apnea: Effects of treatment with continuous positive airway pressure. Am J Physiol 1996;271:E1036-E1043.

76. Hudgel DW, Gordon EA, Meltzer HY: Abnormal serotonergic stimulation of cortisol production in obstructive sleep apnea. Am J Respir Crit Care Med 1995;152:186-192.

77. Hudgel DW, Gordon EA: Serotonin-induced cortisol release in CPAP-treated obstructive sleep apnea patients. Chest 1997;111: 632-638.

78. Heiser P, Dickhaus B, Opper C, et al: Platelet serotonin and interleukin-1 beta after sleep deprivation and recovery sleep in humans. J Neural Transm 1997;104:1049-1058.

79. Harsch IA, Konturek PC, Koebnick C, et al: Leptin and ghrelin levels in patients with obstructive sleep apnoea: Effect of CPAP treatment. Eur Respir J 2003;22:251-257.

80. Bjorntorp P: Neuroendocrine abnormalities in human obesity. Metabolism 1995;44(Suppl 2):38-41.

81. Johannsson G, Marin P, Lonn L, et al: Growth hormone treatment of abdominally obese men reduces abdominal fat mass, improves glucose and lipoprotein metabolism, and reduces diastolic blood pressure. J Clin Endocrinol Metab 1997;82: 727-734.

82. Chin K, Shimizu K, Nakamura T, et al: Changes in intra-abdominal visceral fat and serum leptin levels in patients with obstructive sleep apnea following nasal continuous positive airway pressure. Circulation 1999;100:706-712.

83. Grunstein RR, Stenlöf K, Hedner J, et al: Impact of obstructive sleep apnea and sleepiness on metabolic and cardiovascular risk factors in the Swedish Obese Subjects (SOS) Study. Int J Obes 1995:151:410-418.

84. Tasali E, Van Cauter E: Sleep-disordered breathing and the current epidemic of obesity: Consequence or contributing factor? Am J Respir Crit Care Med 2002;165:562-563.

85. Stoohs RA, Facchini F, Guilleminault C: Insulin resistance and sleep-disordered breathing in healthy humans. Am J Respir Crit Care Med 1996;154:170-174.

86. Harsch IA, Pour Schahin S, Radespiel-Troger M, et al: CPAP treatment rapidly improves insulin sensitivity in patients with OSAS. Am J Respir Crit Care Med 2004;169:156-162.

87. Vgontzas AN, Bixler EO, Chrousos GP: Metabolic disturbances in obesity versus sleep apnoea: The importance of visceral obesity and insulin resistance. J Intern Med 2003;254:32-44.

106

Pain and Sleep

Gilles J. Lavigne
Diana McMillan
Marco Zucconi

ABSTRACT

Pain is an acute or chronic condition associated with a sensory and emotional experience reported to interfere with sleep. The impact of acute pain on sleep (e.g., delay in sleep onset, sleep awakening, poor sleep quality, low restorative effectiveness) is usually short term and reversible. However, the presence of chronic pain can be associated with a vicious cycle pattern: A day with intense pain may be followed by a night of poor sleep quality, and a night of poor sleep may increase pain the next day. Chronic pain is reported by approximately 11% of the adult population, and two thirds of them complain of poor sleep quality. Coexistent conditions such as anxiety, depression, insomnia, apnea, periodic limb movements during sleep (PLMS), aging, and use of medications (e.g., cardioactive, morphine) are among risk factors for poor sleep in the presence of pain such as arthritis, fibromyalgia, previous traumatic nerve injury, and neuropathic or cancer pain. The interaction between pain and poor sleep could be explained by sleep fragmentation (arousal, sleep stage shift), lower percentage of slow wave activity during sleep, and/or sympathetic overactivity (e.g., high cardiac heart beat variability). Most patients with chronic pain report daytime fatigue and sleepiness, reduced cognitive functioning (e.g., memory), and poorer quality of life.

A clinical interview and polygraphic recording are needed to rule out poor sleep hygiene, insomnia, PLMS, apnea, and altered circadian rhythm. Cognitive and behavioral management is recognized to be useful, and medications that improve sleep and reduce pain are indicated, although some may alter sleep quality (e.g., morphine, nonsteroidal antiinflammatory drugs). The role of the sleep clinician is to recognize that pain interferes with sleep quality, educate patients about sleep hygiene and poor sleep habits, guide the patient to cognitive and behavioral or physical therapies, and review and prescribe analgesic and sleep-promoting medications.

A majority (50% to 90%) of patients with chronic pain report poor-quality sleep. This chapter provides a better understanding of the mechanisms associated with poor sleep in the presence of pain, and a guide to sleep management for the pain patient. At present, there are no evidence-based guidelines for such problems. Pain of various origins and causes is associated with poor sleep quality. Pain can cause sleep fragmentation and gave rise to reports of unrefreshing sleep in relation to several clinical pain conditions, including restless legs syndrome/periodic limb movements during sleep (PLMS), headaches with or without apnea, irritable bowel, gastric ulcer, visceral distention (bladder or intestinal), cancer pain, musculoskeletal pain (neck or back pain, limb pain, fibromyalgia), neuropathic pain, dental and orofacial pain, spinal cord damage, sensory dysfunction, and burn or trauma.

As defined by the International Association for the Study of Pain,[1] pain is an "unpleasant sensory and emotional experience associated with actual or potential tissue damage or described in terms of such damage." The emotional dimension is concomitant with both acute pain (e.g., postoperative) and chronic pain (e.g., arthritic pain, herpetic neuralgia, diabetic neuropathy). In the presence of acute pain, such as a toothache, relief is predictable with appropriate dental care, and the consequences for quality of life and health are usually short term. When pain becomes chronic, that is if it lasts more than several weeks or months, the patient may report poor quality of life and poor daytime performance at work or familial tasks. For some patients, day-to-day life with intense pain is so unbearable that a suicide attempt is possible if the distress associated with suffering is not managed. The sudden reappearance of a pain episode can be a sign of the recurrence of a potentially fatal disease (e.g., cancer pain), and its potential effects on patient well-being, anxiety, and sleep quality are obvious.

Interest in the interaction of pain and sleep emerges from the basic sciences literature of the 1960s, which described the processing of tactile-cutaneous sensory inputs at the level of the brainstem mesencephalic-reticular formation and the trigeminal sensory nucleus during wakefulness and sleep.[2,3] Clinical interest began in the late 1960s with a series of publications suggesting that patients with chronic pain could demonstrate disturbed sleep homeostasis. At that time, the emerging concept of electroencephalographic (EEG) instability—referred to as "alpha intrusions" during non–rapid eye movement (NREM) deep sleep—was associated with somatic pain.[4,5]

It is commonly accepted that pain is a protective response, involving several neuronal mechanisms, from cellular activity (e.g., gene expression, ionic channel and receptor activation) to integrated behavior such as the "fight-or-fight" reaction with the activation of several limbic structures such as the hypothalamus, amygdala, cingulate, and frontal cortical areas.[6-8] Chronic pain may also be considered as a disorder of the nervous system; when it is persistent, there are either reversible or permanent changes associated with neuronal plasticity or modifications at cellular or network levels. Pain is associated either with direct nerve activation (e.g., trigeminal neuralgia), inflammation (e.g., arthritis), changes in nerve environment (e.g., neuropathic pain), or changes at the cortical sensory representation areas (enlargement of the sensory cortical territory, a reverberating loop that potentiates sensory nonpain inputs to a frequency that is interpreted as pain). In summary, with most somatic pain there is a usual sequence of activation from nociception to pain perception that involves the following: (1) activation of nerve endings; (2) transmission through sensory A delta and C sensory fibers; (3) first relay at spinal cord neurons; (4) second relay at thalamic levels and interactions with brainstem cells; (5) cortical neuronal network activation; and (6) the final reaction to pain, such as withdrawal or escape behaviors with or without emotional reactions such as tearing, crying, or anxiety.

Visceral pain behaves differently from most somatic pain. In the presence of visceral pain (e.g., irritable bowel syndrome), it is thought that the sensation is diffuse and poorly localized.[9] When visceral nociceptors are activated, they tend to react to innocuous and noxious stimuli without further discrimination. As such, the tissue sensory ending and its brain localization become oversolicited (i.e., hypersensitive), which can result in allodynia (i.e., nonpain stimulation such as touch is described by the patient as a pain sensation).

Interestingly, pain perception can be attenuated by the activation of brain descending influences that are either localized on specific neurons or diffuse; the net result is a better tolerance of pain. Such mechanisms are linked to brain-derived opioid, serotonin, and norepinephrine neurochemicals and other substances acting at the spinal cord or brainstem levels.

EPIDEMIOLOGY, RELATIONSHIP BETWEEN PAIN AND SLEEP, AND RISK FACTORS

The prevalence of chronic pain in the adult population is estimated to be 11%, but figures as high as 29% have been reported depending on the specificity of the questions asked to the general population.[10,11] Between 50% and 90% of patients with chronic pain report complaints of poor sleep in relation to their pain conditions, which include arthritis, cervical pain, fibromyalgia, facial joint and muscle pain (temporomandibular pain), and low back pain.[12-19] Other medical conditions with concomitant pain that are also reported to interfere with sleep quality are headaches, irritable bowel syndrome, spinal cord injury, and metastatic breast cancer.[4,20-24] Among the risk factors that contribute to perpetuation of poor

sleep is chronic pain, with an adjusted odds ratio of approximately 1.5 (i.e., 44% of patients with chronic pain report insomnia versus 19% for subjects without pain).[4,25] Prospective and quantitative studies will help to quantify and validate the nature of the interaction between pain and sleep. The influence of concomitant conditions such as anxiety, fatigue, mood disturbance, depression, and poor physical fitness are further described in the next paragraph in relation to the vicious cycle interaction between pain and sleep.

In addition to the supporting epidemiologic data,[25a] the causal relationship between pain and sleep needs to be reproduced experimentally, a criterion that is described in the section on Pathogenesis. Clinically, it can be shown that a linear relation exists between pain and sleep. As described in Figure 106–1, pain can precede the poor sleep complaints, or vice versa. With acute pain, the poor sleep complaints do not usually continue after pain resolution. However, the initial linear sequence (i.e., pain precedes poor sleep) can be transformed into a vicious circle pattern when pain lasts too long (i.e., a day with intense pain is followed by a night with poor sleep quality, and a night with poor sleep by more pain the next day). The linear relation was reported by 53% to 89% of patients with various musculoskeletal types of pain.[14,15,17] The vicious cycle is reported for patients with chronic pain such as fibromyalgia or severe skin burns.[26-28]

Sleep and pain interactions are influenced by multiple factors. Much of the preceding data are derived from surveys done with general populations or with patient cohorts, where pain intensity and sleep quality reports are subjective, and up to 30% of the interaction between pain and sleep can be explained by the presence of concomitant fatigue, depression/mood alteration, poor physical condition, and anxiety.[17,19,21,28-31] Sex and aging are also concomitant variables. Chronic pain is more frequently reported by women, at approximately double the rate in men. With age, pain becomes more prevalent (25% to 50% in patients older than 55 years of age) and lasts longer, although older patients seem to cope better with pain and tend to be more stoic.[11,32-34] Insomnia complaints are also partly related to lower scores on physical, emotional, bodily pain, and vitality domains when the Short-Form Health Survey (SF 36) is administered to older patients. This suggests a more complex interaction between aging, pain, and poor sleep complaints.[35]

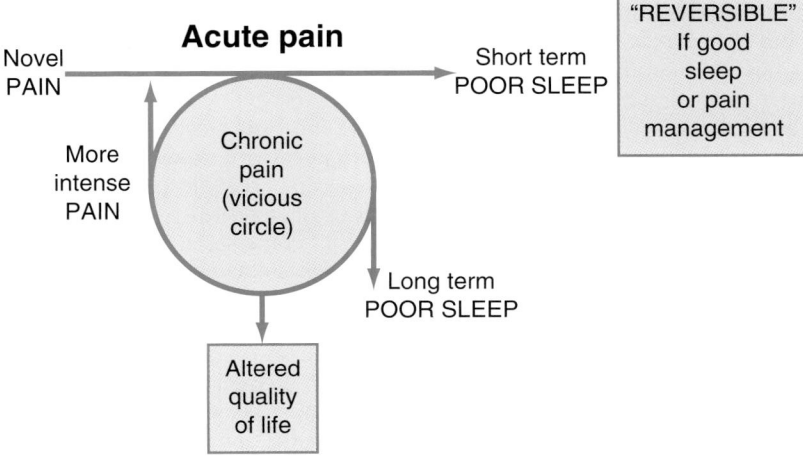

Figure 106–1. Linear (acute pain) and vicious circle (chronic pain) relationship.

PATHOGENESIS

The interaction between pain and poor sleep could be explained by sleep fragmentation (arousal, sleep stage shift), lower percentage of slow wave sleep (SWS; stages 3 and 4 or deep or restorative sleep), and/or sympathetic overactivity (e.g., high cardiac heart beat variability) during sleep. Indeed, most patients with chronic pain report daytime fatigue and sleepiness, reduced cognitive function (e.g., memory impairment), and poor quality of life. So far, no clear and simple mechanism explains the pathophysiology of the interaction between pain and poor sleep quality, or the presence of the vicious cycle pattern found in several patients with chronic pain (see Fig. 106–1). Pain perception and modulation are altered in relation to sleep state. In general, sensory information is filtered during sleep, but relevant inputs threatening body homeostasis may trigger a rapid return of consciousness, with the patient reporting pain upon awakening.

Neurobiologic Basis of Sensory–Pain Perception in Sleep

Recent animal studies have confirmed that in the presence of brief sensory or pain stimulations during sleep, the spinoreticular and trigeminothalamic tract neurons (part of the ascending sensory–pain pathways) behave as a gate control mechanism to trigger or inhibit an awakening response. Such activity is not homogeneous across sleep stages (quiet NREM or active REM sleep) and seems to depend on brainstem raphe magnus cell activity (serotonergic or not).[36-38] Moreover, the latency of the pain-related sensorimotor reflex, the tail flick, is a sensitive method to assess spinal nociception. Compared with wakefulness, the reflex latency in cats is increased threefold in NREM and fivefold in REM sleep.[39] The spinal tail withdrawal reflex seems to be under the influence of cholinergic neurons located in the medial pontine reticular formation. In the presence of chronic pain, arthritic rats show a loss of the typical sleep and wake pattern, with an increased number of sleep periods.[40] Based on animal findings, it is now accepted that a sleeping brain is not completely isolated from the external milieu, and that neuronal sensory-motor networks related to vigilance and body protection remain active in sleep.[37,41]

In humans, the perception of pain during sleep depends on the type of sensory stimulation. Differing stimuli—brief sensory nerve, mid-duration thermal, or long chemical or mechanical stimulations—produce very different outcomes, from spinal reflex to integrated cortical response and autonomic sleep arousal–awakening, all the way up to conscious awareness of stimulation. The spinal nociceptive reflex is a short-loop spinal reflex triggered by intense and brief electrical stimulation of the sural nerve area. Compared with wakefulness, the latency of this reflex is longer in deep NREM sleep and REM sleep, with its threshold significantly increased by 60% in NREM and by 200% in REM sleep.[42] In contrast, laser stimulations (approximately 60 milliseconds) sufficient to evoke a brief negative and positive cortical potential during the waking state do not produce any observable cortical response during sleep stage 2.[43]

However, mid-duration (6- to 12-second) thermal pain stimulations, causing a pain sensation with an intensity of 6 on a 10-point scale during wakefulness, triggered clear cortical microarousals with approximately 50% of stimulations in stage 2 sleep and responses with only approximately 30% of stimulations in SWS (stages 3 and 4) or REM sleep. These data indicate that the nociceptive temperature threshold is higher in SWS and REM sleep.[44] Another pain model infuses hypertonic saline (5%) in muscle to evoke during wakefulness a pain intensity of 3 of 10 for more than 70 seconds. Using this model, where experimental pain mimics a muscle cramp, clear awakening responses are produced with a similar response rate across sleep stage; interestingly, most patients remembered a pain experience during their sleep, in contrast to the thermal stimulation experiments described previously.[45,46] This experimental model is closer to what patients report (i.e., being awakened by pain at various times during sleep); but again, very few data are available to demonstrate how ongoing sleep is interrupted by clinical pain.

Circadian Variation in Pain Perception

In healthy subjects, most studies suggest that pain perception to experimental thermal stimulation, chemical infusion, or mechanical pressure does not show variation over a 24-hour period or between evening and morning measurements when data are controlled for mood state and sex.[44,47-50] However, pain perception in patients with chronic pain is variable with daytime symptoms. For example, patients with arthritis report that pain is worst in the morning with body motion. Those with muscle-related pain, including headaches, report higher pain intensity in the afternoon and evening, whereas pain from torticollis is completely relieved by sleep.[13,51-53]

Cognitive Impairment, Sleep Deprivation, and Pain Perception

Regardless of cause, sleep fragmentation is associated with a subsequent increase in sleepiness and fatigue and a decrease in cognitive and motor performance. Effects of pain on sleep and cognition may therefore be nonspecific and mediated simply by the degree to which pain causes sleep fragmentation.[4,54]

Recent studies suggest that memory and attention are impaired in patients with chronic musculoskeletal pain and fibromyalgia.[55-57] More studies are needed to clarify the cognitive changes associated with chronic pain and poor sleep, taking into consideration the impact of sleep fragmentation and of concomitant anxiety, mood dysfunction, fatigue, and the like. Development or validation of more naturalistic tests related to real-life working or driving performance may provide new information on the cognitive deficit related to the interaction of pain and sleep or secondary to medication prescribed in its management.[58,59] Moreover, all sleep stages seem to be necessary for memory consolidation, and a nap of minimum 60- to 90-minute duration offers similar advantages.[60,61] In studying the interaction of pain and sleep, it is important to control for both napping and sleep continuity in the assessment of poor sleep quality in patients with chronic pain in whom daytime napping habits are unknown.[54]

Some short-term studies tested the impact of acute sleep deprivation on pain perception. Sleep stage 4 (or SWS) deprivation by sound induces more muscle tenderness and lower pain thresholds (mechanical pressure) on awakening in healthy subjects and patients with fibromyalgia. However, these findings must be interpreted in light of concomitant physical tiredness and fatigue.[62,63] Moreover, no increase in alpha EEG intrusions was observed when an automated measure of the EEG power was done.[63] In addition, the original findings of an increase in muscle tenderness and lower pain threshold on awakening were not reproduced in the healthy subjects without pain.[64] Finally, selectively depriving healthy subjects of SWS, REM sleep, or total sleep duration revealed interesting information on pain perception and its interaction with sleep.[65] The mechanical pain threshold is significantly decreased (8%) only by total sleep deprivation, whereas the thermal pain threshold is unchanged by any of the sleep stage interruptions. After sleep recovery, the mechanical pain threshold is increased by 15%, suggesting that SWS recovery induces an analgesic effect. Obviously, sleep deprivation studies need to be controlled for the complex interactions between fatigue and lower mental and sensory processing of pain sensations involving both emotional and sensory dimensions. In addition, sleep deprivation is an extreme manipulation of sleep fragmentation that is not highly representative of sleep complaints in patients with chronic pain. At present, there is little evidence that patients with chronic pain suffer long periods of wakefulness during sleep, although insomnia is not uncommon.[4]

Aging, Pain Perception, and Dysfunctional Endogenous Analgesia

With age, pain perception is altered but, paradoxically, older patients are reported to cope better with the consequences of chronic pain than middle-aged subjects.[66-68] Pain sensitivity is lower and the pain threshold higher probably because of age-related changes in tissues (e.g., reduced thickness, changes in microcirculation). In addition, there is lower cerebral discrimination of sensory information (processing at spinal cord or cortical levels), but with a paradoxically lower endogenous pain modulatory activity (described as *diffuse nociceptive inhibitory control* [DNIC]).[67,69] The DNIC system is an upper brain function that reduces pain perception in the whole body through the activation of neurochemicals (e.g., opioids) in distant body areas, in a nonselective distribution (i.e., a diffuse general reduction in pain threshold is found). As demonstrated by experimental manipulations, DNIC activation is apparently dysfunctional in patients with fibromyalgia.[70,71] This is further supported by the evidence that in the presence of generalized pain, such as in patients with fibromyalgia, an abnormal sensitization (e.g., generalized body pain) and abnormal temporal summation of pain are dominant.[72] So far, there is no evidence to support that the DNIC system is dysfunctional in patients with pain and poor sleep complaints.

Alpha Electroencephalogram Intrusions, Phasic Arousal, and Autonomic Activity

So-called alpha EEG intrusions were found in several sleep studies in patients with fibromyalgia, but more recent controlled and quantitative scoring failed to support the notion that alpha EEG intrusions were pain or fibromyalgia specific.[21,71,73-77] The current trend is to reassess such findings in the setting of mood alterations and sleep respiratory and movement events (e.g., apnea, PLMS) and to reconcile them with the fact that patients with pain have arousals in clusters or in a sequence of phasic events, also termed the *cyclic alternating pattern.*[4,18,78,78a]

Finally, a recent study has demonstrated that the usual reduction in heart rate variability during sleep of healthy subjects is absent in insomniac patients and patients with fibromyalgia.[79,80] If such findings can be confirmed in patients with pain without mood alteration or respiratory-motor sleep disorders, this would add support to the notion that complaints of poor sleep in chronic pain are due to sleep instability, associated with maintenance of sympathetic activation and nonrestorative function. Obviously, this hypothesis needs more study.

Neurochemistry in the Interaction of Pain and Sleep

As briefly described previously, there is indirect evidence that pain modulatory systems may be altered in the context of chronic pain and poor sleep. Animal findings suggest that serotonergic and nonserotonergic brainstem neurons modify alertness in relation to so-called raphe magnus "off" cells, which prevent arousal from external sensory stimulations such as pain.[38] Surprisingly, almost no evidence links the "alertness" or vigilance network (i.e., ascending reticular activating system) to changes in cholinergic, dopaminergic, gamma-aminobutyric acid–ergic, or adrenergic neuronal reticular and hypothalamic activity in relation to alterations in sleep homeostasis in the presence of chronic pain.[39,81] Moreover, it is unknown whether hypocretin (orexin) gene activity—with its role in alertness—or *Clock* gene expression—with its circadian rhythm regulatory role—is altered in the presence of chronic pain with secondary sleep alterations.[82]

In patients with fibromyalgia, substance P has been found in higher concentration in the cerebrospinal fluid. Because generalized hyperalgesia is also found in these patients, it is possible that several other classic pain-facilitating agents, receptors, or ionic channels are activated in the presence of chronic pain (e.g., glutamate, N-methyl-D-aspartate, serotonin, neurokinins).[6,8,72,73] Special interest has been devoted to growth hormone because its release is associated with SWS. However, there is limited evidence to support an alteration in serum levels of insulin-like growth factor or somatomedin C in patients with fibromyalgia or other pain; furthermore, this suggestion is not supported by experimental sleep deprivation challenge.[64,83-86] Clearly, there is a paucity of evidence supporting a relationship between chronic pain, poor sleep, and altered neurochemistry. Moreover, the role of other changes associated with chronic pain, such as generalized hyperexcitability and low inhibition from upper brain centers such as the DNIC, needs to be investigated in parallel.

CLINICAL FEATURES

Most of the sleep-related variables described in Box 106–1 and associated with pain and poor sleep are not pain specific because they may also be found with several sleep disorders such as sleep apnea, PLMS, or insomnia. During the day, patients with pain commonly complain of unrefreshing sleep, fatigue, headache, sleepiness while driving, or anxiety with occasional anger at fulfilling home or work tasks. The reports of more intense pain during the day after a night with poor

> **Box 106–1.** **Selected Sleep-Related Symptoms and Findings in the Presence of Pain***
>
> **Bedtime Symptoms**
> - Delay in sleep onset
> - Anxiety, rumination
> - Intense fatigue and more intense pain
>
> **Sleep Time Findings**
> - Lower sleep efficacy (<90%)
> - Longer percentage sleep time in stage 1, with less in stages 3 and 4
> - Numerous sleep stage shifts (stages 3 and 4 toward stages 2 or 1)
> - Fragmentation of sleep continuity (increase in number of microarousals, awakenings, sleep stage shifts, respiratory events, movement intrusions)
> - Alpha electroencephalographic intrusions in stages 3 and 4 with or without elevated phasic arousals (cyclic alternating pattern)
> - Absence of reduction in heart rate variability in sleep (cardiac sympathetic overactivation)
> - Nightmares, periodic leg movements, apnea, sweating, heart palpitations
> - Wake time in sleep with pain (e.g., neck, lower back, visceral, tooth)
>
> **Wake Time Symptoms**
> - Unrefreshing sleep sensation, fatigue, headache, and the like
> - Sleepiness if driving
> - Anxiety and anger over fulfilling daytime requirements at home or work
>
> *Most are not pain specific.

sleep or the sensation of unrefreshing sleep when the pain was intense during the day or night before are good indicators of a circular relationship between pain and sleep quality/efficacy (see Fig. 106–1). As pointed out by others, estimating such variables in a clinical setting requires skill and time—for example, what type of fatigue is reported, that associated with intense physical work, or with monotony due to lack of stimulation or motivation? The location of the pain, how long it lasts, and its impact on sleep and daytime function are all related issues.[76]

At bedtime, reports of delayed sleep onset (more than 20 to 30 minutes) with anxiety or rumination related to daytime stressful events, intense fatigue that prevents the behavioral relaxation/wind-down process, and persistence of intense pain are all key elements that help us in the selection of sleep hygiene advice or choice of treatment (Table 106–1). During sleep, complaints of sudden awakenings with pain (e.g., neck, lower back, visceral, tooth) are strong indicators of pain as an intruder. If the patient cannot resume sleep, it stands to reason that pain triggers secondary insomnia, and management should be planned accordingly.

DIAGNOSIS

Clinical

When evaluating a patient complaining of both pain and sleep problems, the first task is to identify the possible risk factors.

These are many and can be related to concomitant anxiety, mood alteration, pain, alcohol or drug abuse, poor life style, lack of physical activities, long delay in sleep onset or awakening during sleep time, snoring, poor quality of the sleep environment, and so forth.

Pain intensity and related emotional feelings may be assessed using several available self-report scales. In the investigation of the interaction between pain and sleep, patient diaries are clinically valuable in identifying bad habits and customizing management of each patient. Whether completed on paper or hand-held computer, such diaries can highlight pain intensity and interference with sleep and napping, as well as the sleep time–awakening temporal pattern. Each tool has limitations, and selection depends on the goal—whether evaluating, for example, clinical patients or research subjects, children or adults, or patients on psychoactive medication.[21,87,88] For pain assessments, the McGill Pain Questionnaire provides detailed information but takes a long time to complete and interpret. Other questionnaires are also available, including body map drawings, category scales (no pain, mild, moderate, or severe pain), visual analogue scales (10-cm line with the "no pain" at one extreme and the "most intense pain" at the other), verbal graphic ratings on a scale (words below the 10-cm scale), and numeric scales (0 for no pain to 10 for maximum pain).[87,88] The last is a popular tool in emergency room or clinical settings because the rating score is given verbally and noted in the patient file with little time expenditure. In children, a set of face drawings (smile for no pain up to tears and sad face for intense pain) is useful.

For muscle and joint pain, manual palpation using the fingers or pressure devices can localize tender, pain-related spots. These are well-known techniques that correlate well with patient verbal pain reports. For assessing nerve damage or neuropathy, many modalities are used, including the brush, pin and needle, von Frey hairs of various sizes, two-point/touch discrimination, as well as ice, heat, and vibration. Unfortunately the validity and reliability of these tools have not been fully demonstrated. Pain threshold (subject detects a sensory stimulus as being painful 50% of the time) and tolerance (maximum pain a subject can accept) assessments with electrical, thermal, chemical, or mechanical modalities are excellent research tools but are complicated to use and time-consuming in a clinical sleep laboratory.[42,44,45] Moreover, some of the most common outcome variables in pain and sleep investigations are reflex threshold and latency; changes in rate of sleep arousal and awakening as scored with EEG, electromyography, and electrocardiography; and morning subject reports of being aware of stimulus perception during sleep. A laser-evoked cortical potential is not a sensitive method to assess pain perception and related sensory processing during sleep because no cortical response is observed. This is probably due to the short duration (milliseconds) of laser stimulation or the sleep-related filtering of sensory information.[43] Distention of a rectal balloon is commonly used in the clinic to assess the visceral pain threshold, but to our knowledge this has never been done during sleep. Brain imaging has revealed very important information regarding pain perception and modulation, but it also is not currently used in assessing clinical pain perception, and it is methodologically difficult to perform during sleep.[89]

Patients with sleep complaints are frequently evaluated with visual analogue or numeric scales to assess pain (as described

Table 106–1.   Management Algorithm for Presence of Concomitant Pain and Sleep Problems*

Step 1 Detection of a primary sleep disorder	Examples: insomnia, sleep-disordered breathing, primary snoring, periodic leg movements during sleep, headache-bruxism, daytime fatigue/sleepiness
Step 2 Sleep hygiene overview	Evaluation of: Sleep environment (e.g., dark, cool, and quiet bedroom) Wake–sleep cycle (e.g., consistent bedtime and morning awakening) Lifestyle habits (e.g., intense exercise, smoking, or alcohol at night) Presence of nonsleeping infant, snoring or tooth-grinding sleep partner
Step 3 Behavioral–cognitive strategies and physical management	Establish regular routines for evening relaxation, avoid "bringing work home" and intense/troubling evening discussions, develop a short nap schedule if possible during daytime (≤20 min) Moist heat application (10-20 min) or ice massage (5 min) Physical manipulations: massage-fascia therapy, physical therapy (osteopathy, manipulation, chiropractic); transcutaneous electrical nerve stimulation (TENS)

Step 4
Pharmacologic interventions†
	Short term:
	Analgesic either alone or combined with a muscle relaxant in the evening:
	Ibuprofen, aspirin, or acetaminophen
	Acetaminophen with chlorzoxazone
	Methocarbamol with acetaminophen, aspirin, or ibuprofen
	
	Mild condition:
	A. Muscle relaxant/sedative (in evening to reduce morning dizziness):
	   Low-dose cyclobenzaprine (½ or full 10-mg tablet)
	   Clonazepam (lowest dose available, short term because of risk of dependence) ± analgesic such as acetaminophen, ibuprofen, or aspirin in the evening
	B. Sleep facilitator:
	   Triazolam
	   Temazepam
	   Zopiclone
	   Zolpidem
	   Zaleplon (ideal for patients with sleep apnea; very short acting, useful for mid- or late-night wakefulness/insomnia)
	   Low-dose gabapentin (low dose at bedtime)
	
	More severe/persistent cases (physician consult recommended):
	Low-dose amitriptyline (lowest dose at first in increasing doses if required in the evening; daytime sedation frequent) or mortriptyline
	Trazodone
	Nefazodone
	Gabapentin, codeine + morphine; morphine could cause poor sleep quality by reduction of slow-wave sleep duration
	Anesthetic nerve block, surgical implantation of brain stimulator, surgical nerve debridement (vertebra)

Other products with unknown efficacy on comorbid pain and sleep conditions	Natural products such as valerian, lavender Glucosamine sulfate for osteoarthritis Muscle relaxants such as carisoprodol or tizanidine *Plus*: Antihistamines, local anesthetics (lidocaine patches), or topical agents (capsaicin)

*No recognized guidelines are available at this time. The evidence level is low (few blinded, prospective, large, controlled studies) for most treatments because of the paucity of specific pain and sleep studies.

†For steps 3 and 4, combined strategies could be considered, but only on a case-by-case basis. Caution for step 4: Because of daytime sleepiness and dizziness with most of these medications, it is recommended that patients avoid driving (e.g., in the morning if residual sleepiness is present) and that they take care with use of any potentially hazardous tool or decision-making process. Although popular in the clinic, some medications have not been specifically approved by governing bodies or agencies for pain or sleep management (e.g., gabapentin, clonazepam).

Modified from Brousseau M, Manzini C, Thie NMR, et al: Understanding and managing the interaction between sleep and pain: An update for the dentist. J Can Dent Assoc 2003;69:440-445.

previously), sleep quality, and fatigue. However, several other questionnaires have been selected for specific assessments, including (1) for health and mood, the Beck Anxiety–Depression Inventory, the SF 36, the Symptom Checklist-90, the Sickness Impact Scale, and the Impact of Event Scale; (2) for pain, the McGill Pain Questionnaire and the Multidimensional Pain Inventory; and (3) for sleep, the Pittsburgh Sleep Quality Index and a dream inventory.[15,17,19,30,31,35,90] Future directions include developing scales to assess daytime consequences of poor sleep in relation to pain. Recent studies suggested that memory and attention are impaired in patients with chronic musculoskeletal pain and fibromyalgia.[55-57] More studies are needed to clarify the cognitive changes associated with chronic pain and poor sleep, taking into consideration such factors as concomitant anxiety, mood dysfunction, and the like; tests related to real-life working or driving performance may provide new information on the cognitive deficits related to the interaction of pain and sleep or secondary to the medication prescribed in the management of pain.[58,59]

Sleep Recordings

Both ambulatory (actigraphy) and sleep laboratory (polygraphy) recordings are done to assess patients with pain and sleep complaints. Although data collected with these ambulatory devices should be interpreted with caution, they are powerful population-based tools for longer-term study.[16,21,76,91] The standard polygraphic techniques include EEG, electrocardiographic, electromyographic, and electrooculographic recordings plus video to rule out movement disorders (PLMS), and respiratory sensors to rule out respiratory disorders (apnea). Currently, dedicated software allows unbiased, rapid, and powerful quantitative (spectral) analysis of EEG and heart rate variability.[74,79]

In the absence of other sleep disorders, the most common sleep abnormalities found in patients with chronic pain are listed in Box 106–1. In more detail, these nonspecific findings are as follows:

Lower sleep efficacy (below 90%): In a recent analysis done in our laboratory with healthy subjects matched to patients with a medical and sleep diagnosis of insomnia, PLMS, fibromyalgia, or somatic pain, we noted that the patients with pain had a sleep efficiency of only 77.6% compared with scores of 81.1%, between 84.5 and 88.1%, and 91.3% in insomniac patients, patients with PLMS, patients with fibromyalgia, and healthy subjects, respectively.[92] Similar findings are reported for patients with irritable bowel syndrome, fibromyalgia, rheumatoid arthritis, and back pain (75% to 86%) compared with subjects without pain.[12,16,77,91,93]

Longer percentage of sleep time in stage 1 with less in stages 3 and 4: The stage 1 sleep duration is reported to be shorter in patients with fibromyalgia and longer in patients with irritable bowel syndrome than in healthy subjects in some but not all studies. Differences in patient selection and concomitant psychobehavioral changes could account for these findings. Conflicting results for stage 3 and 4 sleep duration may also be seen.[12,16,18,74,91]

Numerous sleep stage shifts (stages 3 and 4 toward stages 2 or 1): Surprisingly, there are very few data on this sleep variable. In our comparative study with healthy subjects and

patients with fibromyalgia and pain, we found no difference, but there were significantly more shifts in patients with irritable bowel syndrome.[91]

Fragmentation of sleep continuity assessed by an increase in the number of microarousals, awakenings, respiratory disturbances, and movement intrusions: This seems to be a stronger group of variables because most studies show an increase in the microarousal and awakening index or absolute number, but again a lack of standard scoring criteria prevents us from drawing any firm conclusions. Some found no difference in microarousal index for patients with back pain and those with fibromyalgia,[18,78] although an increase in the global arousal–awakening index is also reported in the literature.[16,91,93] For the microarousal index, again depending on the scoring criteria selected, an index below 15 per hour of sleep in young adults and below 30 per hour in older persons is considered acceptable, although the impact of sleep fragmentation needs careful investigation because chronic long-term sleep disruption may alter several physiologic functions.[54,94] The presence of respiratory disturbances (e.g., apnea syndrome) in patients with fibromyalgia does not explain the poor sleep, but it remains to be seen whether brief hypopnea–apnea influences sleep fragmentation in the general pain population.[16,76] The intrusion of body movement is also frequent in patients with fibromyalgia and rheumatoid arthritis,[12,93] and although the association with PLMS is not very clear, we found significantly more PLMS in patients with pain and those with fibromyalgia than in healthy subjects (approximately 10 versus 1.7 per hour of sleep, respectively).[16,77,92]

Alpha EEG intrusions in stages 3 and 4 sleep with or without elevated phasic arousal (cyclic alternating pattern): So-called alpha EEG intrusions were found in several sleep studies in patients with fibromyalgia, but more recent controlled and quantitative scoring failed to support such a strong association.[21,74-77] The current trend is to reassess such findings with corrections for mood alterations and sleep respiratory and movement events (e.g., apnea, PLMS) and to reconcile them with the fact that patients with pain experience arousals in clusters or in a sequence of phasic events (i.e., cyclic alternating pattern), as described previously in the section on Pathogenesis.[4,18,78,78a]

Absence of reduction in heart rate variability in sleep, suggesting cardiac sympathetic overactivation during sleep: Finally, recent observations in insomniac patients and patients with fibromyalgia showed that sleep in these subjects lacked the usual reduction in heart rate variability.[79,80] If these findings can be confirmed in patients with pain without mood alteration or respiratory-motor sleep disorders, it may support patient complaints of poor sleep due to sleep instability associated with maintenance of sympathetic activation and nonrestorative function. The significance of this variable in the interaction of pain and sleep deserves more study.

TREATMENT

First, it should be emphasized that no consensus has been reached regarding guidelines or principles in managing the interaction of pain and sleep, as has been done for acute and cancer pain.[95] Several suggestions have been made in the literature, and the current section is based on a few recent reviews.[16,20,21,96] To mitigate the deleterious effects of pain on sleep, most of the management focus is directed at alleviating nighttime complaints by reducing pain and related anxiety. The prevention of sleep disturbance (e.g., reduction of noise to prevent excessive sleep fragmentation as indicated by the presence of microarousals, awakenings, and stage shifts) may also be as effective as the treatment of nighttime pain for patients with chronic pain. In the absence of comprehensive studies to support one or the other management strategy, targeting either pain relief or sleep quality is appropriate. For most of these patients, the treatment is selected on a subjective basis without instrumental or objective measures of sleep. However, polysomnographic assessment of sleep structure is usually reserved for patients complaining of severe pain, of nighttime disturbances (e.g., movement, respiratory perturbation), and of daytime sleepiness or fatigue. As a management algorithm, we suggest the following steps, as outlined in Table 106–1: (1) detection of the pain and sleep condition with differential diagnosis; (2) sleep hygiene instruction; (3) when possible, behavioral–cognitive strategies and physical management; and (4) medications for pain relief and sleep improvement.

Consumption of analgesics is very frequent in these patients. Although most analgesic medications (nonsteroidal antiinflammatory drugs [NSAIDs], opioids) are taken during the day, very little is known about the potential risk for sleep architecture disruption or the best timing or circadian "window" for maximal medication efficacy. Patients with pain are commonly reported to have an increased consumption of hypnotics compared with the otherwise healthy population (3 to 14 times higher). Moreover, in many cases, combination therapy of analgesics with hypnotics or antidepressives (amitriptyline, trazodone) is necessary. Again, very little is known about the carryover of analgesic, hypnotic, and antidepressive medication effects to daytime functioning (work performance, memory, risk of transportation or work accidents).

CLINICAL COURSE AND PREVENTION

In the presence of poorly managed acute pain, the risk for the development of chronic pain is ever present. However, not every patient is at risk for persistent pain. In the presence of acute pain, most sleep complaints are rapidly reversible when the pain is resolved. Whether chronic pain will ensue depends on a number of factors. These include socioeconomic factors (e.g., secondary benefit, depression, anxiety) and genetic makeup, which might predispose to poor healing and subsequent changes at either the sensory nerve or brain/hemispheric level—and which is why prompt pain management is beneficial. The long waiting lists in pain clinics and the lack of efficient medications for some chronic pain (e.g., neuropathic pain), coupled with the complexity of the interaction between sleep and pain, all contribute to perpetuating the pain and poor sleep "vicious circle." As described previously, chronic pain tends to interfere with sleep architecture and initiates the vicious circle (see Fig. 106–1) between chronic pain, poor sleep, and low quality of life. The success rate of most pain and sleep management approaches described in Table 106–1 is unknown, and so far no consensus has been reached on guidelines or principles that clinicians may use as a resource.

PITFALLS AND CONTROVERSIES

The most common pitfall for clinicians is to fasten exclusively on alpha EEG intrusions to explain the influence of pain on sleep. Recent evidence suggests that alpha EEG intrusions are nonspecific to pain, and instead represent the sleep fragmentation process consisting of phasic and recurrent arousals during sleep, referred to as the *cyclic alternating pattern*.[4,18,76-78,78a] The influence of other physiologic activities, such as sympathetic cardiac activation during sleep, needs to be further investigated in patients with chronic pain and complaints of poor sleep quality and insomnia, and more efficient management strategies developed.[54,79,80,92,97]

The other pitfall is the potentially harmful influence of analgesics (e.g., NSAIDs, morphine) on sleep architectures (e.g., awakenings, reduction in SWS and REM sleep). This paradoxical effect needs further investigation. Moreover, the carryover of several medications, such as opioid analgesics and antidepressants, on next-day functioning needs to be estimated objectively in relation to cognitive function and vigilance, such as during driving or attending classes. Again, in the absence of evidence-based algorithms or guides in the choice of medication, clinicians must select their management strategy based on the experience of so-called experts.

Clinical Pearl

In the management of poor sleep complaints associated with pain, the sleep medicine clinician should recognize the presence of concomitant sleep disorders and related causes (e.g., insomnia, sleep apnea, PLMS). It should be clear to the clinician that the influence of acute pain on sleep is usually brief and reversible. In patients reporting chronic pain, sleep can be disturbed to the point that comprehensive management is required, including review of sleep hygiene, cognitive and behavioral approaches, and use of analgesic and hypnotic medications or antidepressant drugs in more persistent cases.

REFERENCES

1. Merskey H, Bogduk N: Classification of Chronic Pain. Seattle, IASP Press, 1994.
2. Pompeiano O, Swett JE: Actions of graded cutaneous and muscular afferent volleys on brain stem units in the decerebrate, cerebellectomized cat. Arch Ital Biol 1963;101:552-583.
3. Hernandez-Peon R, O'Flaherty JJ, Mazzuchelli-O'Flaherty AL: Modifications of tactile evoked potentials at the spinal trigeminal sensory nucleus during wakefulness and sleep. Exp Neurol 1965;13:40-57.
4. Moldofsky H: Sleep and pain: Clinical review. Sleep Med Rev 2001;5:387-398.
5. Hauri P, Hawkins DR: Alpha-delta sleep. Electroencephalogr Clin Neurophysiol 1973;34:233-237.
6. Woolf CJ, Salter MW: Neuronal plasticity: increasing the gain in pain. Science 2000;288:1765-1768.
7. Price DD: Psychological and neural mechanisms of the affective dimension of pain. Science 2000;288:1769-1772.
8. Julius D, Basbaum AI: Molecular mechanisms of nociception. Nature 2001;413:203-210.
9. Cervero F, Laird JM: Visceral pain. Lancet 1999;353:2145-2148.
10. Harstall C, Ospina M: How prevalent is chronic pain? Pain Clin Updates 2003;11:1-4.

11. Moulin DE, Clark AJ, Speechley M, et al: Chronic pain in Canada: Prevalence, treatment, impact and the role of opioid analgesia. Pain Res Manage 2002;7:179-184.

12. Atkinson JH, Ancoli-Israel S, Slater MA, et al: Subjective sleep disturbance in chronic back pain. Clin J Pain 1988;4:225-232.

13. Dao TTT, Lavigne GJ, Charbonneau A, et al: The efficacy of oral splints in the treatment of myofascial pain of the jaw muscles: A controlled clinical trial. Pain 1994;56:85-94.

14. Morin CM, Gibson D, Wade J: Self-reported sleep and mood disturbance in chronic pain patients. Clin J Pain 1998;14:311-314.

15. Smith MT, Perlis ML, Smith MS, et al: Sleep quality and presleep arousal in chronic pain. J Behav Med 2000;23:1-13.

16. Dauvilliers Y, Touchon J: Le sommeil du fibromyalgique: Revue des données cliniques et polygraphiques. Neurophysiol Clin 2001;31:18-33.

17. Riley III JL, Benson MB, Gremillion HA, et al: Sleep disturbances in orofacial pain patients: Pain-related or emotional distress? J Craniomandib Pract 2001;19:106-113.

18. Roizenblatt S, Moldofsky H, Benedito-Silva AA, et al: Alpha sleep characteristics in fibromyalgia. Arthritis Rheum 2001;44:222-230.

19. McCracken LM, Iverson GL: Disrupted sleep patterns and daily functioning in patients with chronic pain. Pain Res Manage 2002;7:75-79.

20. Cohen M, Menefee LA, Doghramji K, et al: Sleep in chronic pain: Problems and treatments. Int Rev Psychiatry 2000;12: 115-126.

21. Menefee LA, Cohen M, Anderson WR, et al: Sleep disturbance and nonmalignant chronic pain: A comprehensive review of the literature. Pain Med 2000;1:156-172.

22. Widerstrom-Noga EG, Felipe-Cuervo E, Yezierski RP: Chronic pain after spinal injury: Interference with sleep and daily activities. Arch Phys Med Rehabil 2001;82:1571-1577.

23. Rains JC, Penzien DB: Chronic headache and sleep disturbance. Curr Pain Headache Rep 2002;6:498-504.

24. Koopman C, Nouriani B, Erickson V, et al: Sleep disturbances in women with metastatic breast cancer. Breast J 2002;6:362-370.

25. Sutton DA, Moldofsky H, Badley EM: Insomnia and health problems in Canadians. Sleep 2001;24:665-670.

25a. Ohayon MM: Relationship between chronic painful physical condition and insomnia. J Psychiatr Res 2005;39:151-159.

26. Affleck G, Urrows S, Tennen H, et al: Sequential daily relations of sleep, pain intensity, and attention to pain among women with fibromyalgia. Pain 1996;68:363-368.

27. Raymond I, Nielsen TA, Lavigne GJ, et al: Quality of sleep and its daily relationship to pain intensity in hospitalized adult burn patients. Pain 2001;92:381-388.

28. Nicassio PM, Moxham EG, Schuman CE, et al: The contribution of pain, reported sleep quality, and depressive symptoms to fatigue in fibromyalgia. Pain 2002;100:271-279.

29. Smith RP, Veale D, Pepin JL, et al: Obstructive sleep apnoea and the autonomic nervous system. Sleep Med Rev 1998;2:69-92.

30. Sayar K, Arikan M, Yontem T: Sleep quality in chronic pain patients. Can J Psychiatry 2002;47:844-848.

31. Yatani H, Studts J, Cordova M, et al: Comparison of sleep quality and clinical and psychologic characteristics in patients with temporomandibular disorders. J Orofac Pain 2002;16:221-228.

32. Cook AJ, Chastain DC: The classification of patients with chronic pain: Age and sex differences. Pain Res Manage 2001;6:142-151.

33. Scudds RJ, Ostbye T: Pain and pain-related interference with function in older Canadians: The Canadian Study of Health and Aging. Disabil Rehabil 2001;15:654-664.

34. Ohayon MM, Schatzberg AF: Using chronic pain to predict depressive morbidity in the general population. Arch Gen Psychiatry 2003;60:39-47.

35. Schubert CR, Cruickshanks KJ, Dalton DS, et al: Prevalence of sleep problems and quality of life in an older population. Sleep 2002;25:889-893.

36. Cairns BE, McErlane SA, Fragoso MC, et al: Spontaneous discharge and peripherally evoked orofacial responses of trigemino-thalamic tract neurons during wakefulness and sleep. J Neurosci 1996;16:8149-8159.

37. Soja PJ, Pang W, Taepavarapruk N, et al: Spontaneous spike activity of spinoreticular tract neurons during sleep and wakefulness. Sleep 2001;24:18-25.

38. Foo H, Mason P: Brainstem modulation of pain during sleep and waking. Sleep Med Rev 2003;7:145-154.

39. Kshatri AM, Baghdoyan HA, Lydic R: Cholinomimetics, but not morphine, increase antinociceptive behavior from pontine reticular regions regulating rapid-eye movement sleep. Sleep 1998;21:677-685.

40. Landis CA, Robinson CR, Levine JD: Sleep fragmentation in the arthritic rat. Pain 1988;34:93-99.

41. Velluti RA, Pena JL, Pedemonte M: Reciprocal actions between sensory signals and sleep. Biol Signals Recept 2000;9:297-308.

42. Sandrini G, Milanov I, Rossi B, et al: Effects of sleep on spinal nociceptive reflexes in humans. Sleep 2001;24:13-17.

43. Beydoun A, Morrow TJ, Shen J, et al: Variability of laser-evoked potentials: attention, arousal and lateralized differences. Electroencephalogr Clin Neurophysiol 1993;88:173-181.

44. Lavigne GJ, Zucconi M, Castronovo C, et al: Sleep arousal response to experimental thermal stimulation during sleep in human subjects free of pain and sleep problems. Pain 2000; 84:283-290.

45. Drewes AM, Nielsen KM, Arendt-Nielsen L, et al: The effect of cutaneous and deep pain on the electroencephalogram during sleep: An experimental study. Sleep 1997;20:623-640.

46. Lavigne G, Brousseau M, Kato T, et al: Experimental pain perception remains equally active over all sleep stages. Pain 2004;110:646-655.

47. Rogers EJ, Vilkin B: Diurnal variation in sensory and pain thresholds correlated with mood states. J Clin Psychiatry 1978; 39:431-438.

48. Strian F, Lautenbacher S, Galfe G, et al: Diurnal variations in pain perception and thermal sensitivity. Pain 1989;36:125-131.

49. Koltyn KF, Focht BC, Ancker JM, et al: Experimentally induced pain perception in men and women in the morning and evening. Int J Neurosci 1999;98:1-11.

50. Bentley AJ, Newton S, Zio CD: Sensitivity of sleep stages to painful thermal stimuli. J Sleep Res 2003;12:143-147.

51. Bellamy N, Sothern RB, Campbell J, et al: Circadian rhythm in pain, stiffness, and manual dexterity in rheumatoid arthritis: Relation between discomfort and disability. Ann Rheum Dis 1991;50:243-248.

52. Reilly PA, Littlejohn GO: Diurnal variation in the symptoms and signs of the fibromyalgia syndrome (FS). J Musculoskeletal Pain 1993;1:237-243.

53. Lobbezoo F, Thu Thon M, Montplaisir J, et al: Relationship between sleep, neck muscle activity, and pain in cervical dystonia. Can J Neurol Sci 1996;23:285-290.

54. Bonnet MH, Arand DL: Clinical effects of sleep fragmentation versus sleep deprivation. Sleep Med Rev 2003;7:297-310.

55. Kewman DG, Vaishampayan N, Zald D, et al: Cognitive impairment in musculoskeletal pain patients. Int J Psychiatry Med 1991;21:253-262.

56. Landro NI, Stiles TC, Sletvold H: Memory functioning in patients with primary fibromyalgia and major depression and healthy controls. J Psychosom Res 1997;42:297-306.

57. Côté KA, Moldofsky H: Sleep, daytime symptoms, and cognitive performance in patients with fibromyalgia. J Rheumatol 1997; 24:2014-2023.

58. George CFP: Driving simulators in clinical practice. Sleep Med Rev 2003;7:311-320.

59. Chapman S: The effects of opioids on driving ability in patients with chronic pain. APS Bull 2001;11:5-9.

60. Stickgold R, James LT, Hobson JA: Visual discrimination learning requires sleep after training. Nat Neurosci 2000;3:1237-1238.

61. Mednick S, Nakayama K, Stickgold R: Sleep dependent learning: a nap is as good as a night. Nat Neurosci 2003;6:697-698.

62. Moldofsky H, Scarisbrick P: Induction of neurasthenic musculoskeletal pain syndrome by selective sleep stage deprivation. Psychosom Med 1976;38:35-44.

63. Lentz MJ, Landis CA, Rothermel J, et al: Effects of selective slow wave sleep disruption on musculoskeletal pain and fatigue in middle aged women. J Rheumatol 1999;26:1586-1592.

64. Older SA, Battafarano DF, Danning CL, et al: The effects of delta wave sleep interruption on pain thresholds and fibromyalgia like symptoms in healthy subjects: Correlations with insulin like growth factor I. J Rheumatol 1998;25:1180-1186.

65. Onen AH, Alloui A, Gross A, et al: The effects of total sleep deprivation, selective sleep interruption and sleep recovery on pain tolerance thresholds in healthy subjects. J Sleep Res 2001;10: 35-42.

66. Kaasalainen S, Molly W: Pain and aging. Geriatr Today 2004;4:32-37.

67. Farrell MJ: Pain and aging. Am Pain Soc Bull 2000;10:1, 8-11.

68. Riley JL, Wade JB, Robinson ME, et al: The stages of pain processing across the adult lifespan. J Pain 2000;1:162-170.

69. Edwards RR, Fillingim RB: Effects of age on temporal summation and habituation of thermal pain: Clinical relevance in healthy older and younger adults. J Pain 2001;2:307-317.

70. Lautenbacher S, Rollman GB: Possible deficiencies of pain modulation in fibromyalgia. Clin J Pain 1997;13:189-196.

71. Bennett RM: Emerging concepts in the neurobiology of chronic pain: Evidence of abnormal sensory processing in fibromyalgia. Mayo Clin Proc 1999;74:385-398.

72. Staud R, Vierck CJ, Cannon RL, et al: Abnormal sensitization and temporal summation of second pain (wind-up) in patients with fibromyalgia syndrome. Pain 2001;91:165-175.

73. Pillemer SR, Bradley LA, Crofford LJ, et al: The neuroscience and endocrinology of fibromyalgia. Arthritis Rheum 1997;40:1928-1939.

74. Carette S, Oakson G, Guimont C, et al: Sleep electroencephalography and the clinical response to amitriptyline in patients with fibromyalgia. Arthritis Rheum 1995;38:1211-1217.

75. Drewes AM: Pain and sleep disturbances with special reference to fibromyalgia and rheumatoid arthritis. Rheumatology 1999;38:1035-1044.

76. Mahowald ML, Mahowald MW: Nighttime sleep and daytime functioning (sleepiness and fatigue) in less well-defined chronic rheumatic diseases with particular reference to the "alpha-delta NREM sleep anomaly." Sleep Med 2000;1:195-207.

77. Rains JC, Penzien DB: Sleep and chronic pain challenges to the α-EEG sleep pattern as a pain specific sleep anomaly. J Psychosom Res 2003;54:77-83.

78. Staedt J, Windt H, Hajak G, et al: Cluster arousal analysis in chronic pain-disturbed sleep. J Sleep Res 1993;2:134-137.

78a. Rizzi M, Sarzi-Puttini P, Atzeni F, et al: Cyclic alternating pattern: A new marker of sleep alteration in patients with fibromyalgia? J Rheumatol 2004;31:1193-1199.

79. Bonnet MH, Arand DL: Heart rate variability in insomniacs and matched normal sleepers. Psychosom Med 1998;60:610-615.

80. Martinez-Lavin M, Hermosillo AG, Rosas M, et al: Circadian studies of autonomic nervous balance in patients with fibromyalgia: a heart rate variability analysis. Arthritis Rheum 1998;41:1966-1971.

81. Mignot E, Taheri S, Nishino S: Sleeping with the hypothalamus: Emerging therapeutic targets for sleep disorders. Nat Neurosci 2002;5(Suppl):1071-1075.

82. Taheri S, Mignot E: The genetics of sleep disorders. Lancet Neurol 2002;1:242-250.

83. Gronfier C, Luthringer R, Follenius M, et al: A quantitative evaluation of the relationships between growth hormone secretion and delta wave electroencephalographic activity during normal sleep and after enrichment in delta waves. Sleep 1996;19:817-824.

84. Van Cauter E, Leproult R, Plat L: Age-related changes in slow wave sleep and REM sleep and relationship with growth hormone and cortisol levels in healthy men. JAMA 2000;287:861-868.

85. Bennett JS, Gossett KA, McCarthy MP, et al: Effects of ketamine hydrochloride on serum biochemical and hematologic variables in rhesus monkeys (*Macaca mulatta*). Vet Clin Pathol 1992;21:15-18.

86. Bagge E, Bengtsson BA, Carlsson L, et al: Low growth hormone secretion in patients with fibromyalgia: A preliminary report on 10 patients and 10 controls. J Rheumatol 1998;25:145-148.

87. Turk DC, Melzack R: Handbook of Pain Assessment. New York, Guilford Press, 2001.

88. McDowell I, Newell C: Measuring Health: A Guide to Rating Scales and Questionnaires, 2nd ed. New York, Oxford University Press, 1996.

89. Casey KL, Bushnell MC: Pain Imaging, vol 18. Seattle, IASP Press, 2000.

90. Raymond I, Nielsen T, Lavigne GJ: Incorporation of pain in dreams of hospitalized burn victims. Sleep 2002;7:765-770.

91. Rotem AY, Sperber AD, Krugliak P, et al: Polysomnographic and actigraphic evidence of sleep fragmentation in patients with irritable bowel syndrome. Sleep 2003;26:747-752.

92. Okura K, Rompré S, Manzini C, et al: Sleep duration and quality in chronic pain patients in comparison to the sleep of fibromyalgia, insomnia, RLS and control subjects [abstract]. Sleep 2004;27:A329-A330.

93. Mahowald MW, Mahowald SR, Bundlie SR, et al: Sleep fragmentation in rheumatoid arthritis. Arthritis Rheum 1989;32:974-983.

94. Boselli M, Parrino L, Smerieri A, et al: Effect of age on EEG arousals in normal sleep. Sleep 1998;21:351-357.

95. Miaskowski C, Cleary J, Burney R, et al: Guideline for the Management of Cancer Pain in Adults and Children. American Pain Society, Glenview, IL, 2003.

96. Brousseau M, Manzini C, Thie NMR, et al: Understanding and managing the interaction between sleep and pain: An update for the dentist. J Can Dent Assoc 2003b;69:440-445.

97. Brousseau M, Mayer P, Lavigne G: Physiologie et manipulations expérimentales des interrelations entre la douleur et le sommeil. Doul Analg 2003;2:79-87.

107

Gastrointestinal Disorders

William C. Orr

ABSTRACT

Alterations in physiologic functioning have been shown to be critically important in the development of a variety of disease states, particularly those related to respiratory disorders, such as sleep apnea. It is becoming increasingly clear that alterations in gastrointestinal functioning during sleep also play an important role in the pathophysiology of various gastrointestinal disorders. Alterations in gastrointestinal functioning during sleep can often manifest themselves in terms of symptoms, most notably the epigastric pain that awakens patients from sleep who have duodenal ulcer disease. Sleep disturbance has also been described as a common occurrence in patients with gastroesophageal reflux disease (GERD) and irritable bowel syndrome (IBS). Although *Helicobacter pylori* has been shown to be important in the pathogenesis of duodenal ulcer disease, suppression of nocturnal acid secretion remains an important element in healing duodenal ulcers. Alterations in typical responses to acid mucosal contact during sleep have also been shown to be important in the development of the esophageal and extraesophageal complications of acid reflux disease. In addition, the pattern of esophageal acid contact during waking and sleeping is quite different and also contributes to the development of these complications. Sleep is associated with fewer episodes of acid reflux, but a much more prolonged interval of esophageal acid contact. Suppression of nocturnal acid secretion therefore also remains a mainstay in the treatment of GERD. Sleep-related acid reflux also appears to relate importantly to the various respiratory complications of GERD. Although our understanding of the relationship between sleep and altered intestinal motility is evolving, it appears clear that patients with IBS do manifest alterations in intestinal motility and visceral perception, and these may be related to alterations in autonomic functioning during sleep.

This chapter reviews how sleep alters the manifestation or pathogenesis of gastrointestinal and related disorders. The chapter focuses on adults, and only research that has appeared in peer-reviewed journals is included, unless a specific abstract is mentioned to focus on a particularly interesting or promising area of work. In instances where there are numerous articles that convey similar results, only a few of the articles that best represent the consensus of data in the area are presented. In general, case reports and case series are not included.

NOCTURNAL GASTROINTESTINAL SYMPTOMS

The manifestation of gastrointestinal symptoms during sleep is quite familiar to the practicing gastroenterologist. Perhaps the most obvious and common example is the occurrence of epigastric pain characteristically awakening the patient from sleep in the early morning hours. This pattern of awakening from sleep is quite predictable by the patient and can help significantly in establishing a diagnosis of duodenal ulcer disease. Patients may also have awakenings from sleep with symptoms that ostensibly are not related to gastrointestinal disorders. For example, individuals may complain of sleep disruption secondary to awakening from sleep with chest pain, heartburn, or regurgitation into the throat. Asthmatic patients may awaken from sleep by the exacerbation of bronchial asthma secondary to gastroesophageal reflux (GER). Numerous studies suggest that respiratory symptoms secondary to GER are common, and these symptoms are noted often secondary to sleep-related GER.[1]

Other symptoms encountered by the practicing gastroenterologist that may occur during the day but whose occurrence during sleep adds a disconcerting dimension to the symptom include nocturnal diarrhea, fecal incontinence, chest pain, or the respiratory disorders noted previously. Although a denial of symptoms thought to be related to gastrointestinal problems such as GER does not necessarily preclude the occurrence of the sleep-related abnormalities, a positive symptom history enhances the probability of the existence of a nocturnal gastrointestinal disorder, as may be the case in patients with functional bowel disorders such as irritable bowel syndrome (IBS) or functional dyspepsia.

NOCTURNAL ACID SECRETION IN DUODENAL ULCER DISEASE

Patients with duodenal ulcer disease maintain a circadian pattern of gastric acid secretion, and the levels of secretion are enhanced.[2] The peak of basal acid secretion occurs at approximately midnight, with minimal acid secretion occurring during the day in the absence of food ingestion. In addition, as reviewed in Chapter 23, there does not appear to be any relation between the stages of sleep and gastric acid secretion. However, patients with duodenal ulcer disease demonstrate a failure to inhibit acid during the first 2 hours of sleep.[3] Multicenter trials with bedtime administration of histamine type 2 (H_2) receptor antagonists have documented the efficacy of healing duodenal ulcers through nocturnal acid suppression.[4,5] These studies uniformly documented that duodenal ulcer healing rates were at least as good with a once-a-day, bedtime dose of these potent acid-suppressing compounds as with the more conventional multiple daily dosing regimens. When looking at published data on nocturnal dosing of H_2 receptor antagonists in more than 12,000 patients with duodenal ulcer disease, nocturnal dosing clearly shows an advantage over multiple daily doses.[6] Taken together, these data strongly support the notion that nocturnal acid suppression alone is sufficient to heal a duodenal ulcer.

Other studies in patients with refractory duodenal ulcer suggest that nocturnal acid suppression is not only sufficient but necessary for duodenal ulcer healing. Reduction in nocturnal acid secretion through parietal cell vagotomy produced an enhanced healing rate in patients who were unresponsive to conventional cimetidine treatment.[7] When treated with conventional H_2 blockers, only patients with a substantial suppression of nocturnal acid secretion demonstrate ulcer healing, whereas patients whose ulcer again failed to heal maintained a nocturnal peak in gastric acid secretion.[8] A subsequent study found that in persons who have had a parietal cell vagotomy, nocturnal acid secretion was significantly greater in those who experienced ulcer recurrence than in those who did not.[9] Further support for the important role of nocturnal acid secretion in the pathogenesis of duodenal ulcer disease comes from data showing that the maintenance of a modest degree of nocturnal acid suppression effectively prevents the recurrence of duodenal ulcer disease.[10-12] These studies compared the use of 150 mg ranitidine at bedtime with 400 mg cimetidine at bedtime and found ranitidine to be superior in the prevention of ulcer recurrence. This finding is most likely due to the increased potency of ranitidine and its enhanced effectiveness in producing nocturnal acid suppression.

Therapeutic Considerations

The data reviewed concerning ulcer healing and the prevention of ulcer relapse strongly suggest that suppression of nocturnal gastric acid secretion is an important element in ulcer pathogenesis and healing. This observation does not imply that the numerous other factors (such as *Helicobacter pylori*) that have been implicated in the pathogenesis of duodenal ulcer disease are not equally important; it simply strongly affirms that nocturnal acid secretion appears to be an important element in ulcer formation. Even though the pathogenesis of duodenal ulcer disease is complex, these data appear to make it clear that ulcer healing will not occur, or will be severely retarded, without effective nocturnal acid suppression.

GASTROESOPHAGEAL REFLUX DURING SLEEP

GER, particularly with its familiar symptom of heartburn, is recognized as a common phenomenon. Most healthy people experience occasional bouts of heartburn. Approximately 7% of the otherwise healthy population experiences heartburn nearly every day.[13] Furthermore, the majority of patients with frequent heartburn complain of nighttime GER symptoms, and a substantial proportion (more than 50%) of these patients report that their symptoms disrupt their sleep and affect their daytime functioning.[14-16] Many patients who present to a physician with a complaint of heartburn can be readily treated with simple alterations in lifestyle, such as the avoidance of certain provocative foods and the use of antacid therapy, although there are no data specifically on the utility of these measures in treating sleep-related symptoms.[16] The familiarity of this symptom and its rapid response in most instances to relatively simple therapeutic measures belie the severity and potential complications of this disease process. As reviewed in the following, the complications of GER appear to be the result of recurrent episodes of sleep-related GER.

GER events do occur during sleep, but appear to occur most commonly during brief arousals from sleep.[16a] Two studies have been published that were remarkably similar in their results in that reflux events occurred much more frequently in patients with diagnosed gastroesophageal reflux disease (GERD), and relatively infrequently in healthy volunteers.[17,18] Most of the reflux events in both studies did occur in association with polygraphically determined brief arousal responses.

Attention has been focused on the importance of different patterns of GER associated with waking and sleeping.[19] These patterns were documented in studies involving 24-hour monitoring of the distal esophageal pH. GER is identified when the pH falls below 4 for a period of more than 30 seconds, and the reflux episode is arbitrarily terminated when the pH reaches 4 or 5. This landmark study described two different patterns of reflux.[19] Reflux in the upright position occurs most often postprandially and usually consists of two or three reflux episodes that are rapidly cleared (2 to 3 minutes). Reflux in the supine position is usually associated with sleep and with more prolonged clearance time.

These studies documented highly significant increases in acid–mucosa contact time in patients with esophagitis, and these differences were most impressive when the supine position or sleep interval was considered; that is, there was a greater difference between patients and control subjects in the supine position as opposed to the upright position. Even though acid–mucosa contact time may be equivalent in the upright and supine positions, the prolonged acid clearance times associated with sleep appeared to result in greater damage to the esophageal mucosa.[20] In another study, the patterns of GER, as determined by 24-hour esophageal pH monitoring, and the endoscopic evaluation of the esophageal mucosa were correlated.[21] Patients were identified as primarily *upright* (waking) *refluxers*, *supine* (sleep) *refluxers*, and *combined refluxers*, those whose reflux was evident throughout the 24-hour day. The severity of endoscopic change according to three grades of esophagitis was determined. Grade 1 esophagitis was defined simply as distal erythema and friability; grade 2 esophagitis was defined when mucosal erosions were noted; and grade 3 esophagitis involved more severe ulcerations and strictures. The data indicated that an increasing incidence of nocturnal acid exposure was associated with more severe esophageal mucosal damage. An additional study compared the results of 24-hour esophageal pH monitoring in patients who had either normal findings on endoscopy or erosive esophagitis.[22] The results of this study showed that total acid exposure time and the number of reflux episodes requiring longer than 5 minutes to clear were found most reliably to discriminate these two groups of patients. Furthermore, it was noted that 50% of the patients with reflux symptoms had normal results on 24-hour pH monitoring and that 29% of the patients with erosive esophagitis also had normal pH studies. The most effective variable in distinguishing the two groups of patients was the number of episodes requiring longer than 5 minutes to clear (to pH 4). These findings have been extended using 24-hour pH monitoring in a group of symptomatic patients with heartburn and normal endoscopic results and a group of patients with severe complications of GER, including erosive esophagitis, stricture, and Barrett's esophagus.[23] The results show that the best discriminator between the two groups is the number of episodes of prolonged acid clearance (longer than 5 minutes) in the supine position. These episodes appear to be more likely to occur during sleep, confirming the notion that prolonged acid clearance is an important determinant in the development of esophagitis. Other studies have not been as positive in supporting nocturnal GER as an important factor in the pathogenesis of reflux esophagitis, and have suggested that postprandial acid exposure was the best predictor of the severity of esophagitis.[24]

ESOPHAGEAL ACID CLEARANCE DURING SLEEP

As previously noted, acid clearance during sleep seems to be an important contributing factor in the development of reflux esophagitis. The process of acid clearance takes place in two phases: an initial phase, termed *volume clearance*, and a second phase, termed *acid neutralization*.[25] The vast majority of the volume of refluxed material is cleared from the esophagus quite rapidly by the first two or three swallows. There remains a coating of acid on the esophageal mucosa, which keeps the esophageal pH well below 4. Subsequent swallows serve to deliver saliva to the distal esophagus, and, with its potent buffering capacity, the distal esophageal pH is returned to its normal level (5.5 to 6.5). A subsequent study confirmed these findings in that acid clearance was found to be independent of the swallowing rate but significantly altered by an anticholinergic drug that inhibits salivation.[26]

Both swallowing frequency and salivation have been shown to be markedly depressed during sleep; as a result, one would hypothesize a prolongation of acid clearance during sleep.[27,28] Swallowing occurs sporadically during sleep, and there are long periods (longer than 30 minutes) without swallowing.[27] Overall, the rate of swallowing during sleep is approximately six swallows per hour, and the swallows usually occur in association with a movement arousal. The highest frequency of these events is in stages 1 and 2 and rapid eye movement (REM) sleep.[27] A marked reduction in swallows associated with esophageal acid infusion during sleep has also been demonstrated.[29] Studies have focused specifically on the issue of the parameters of esophageal acid clearance during sleep. A model that incorporated the clearance of infused acid (15.0/mL 0.1 N HCl) during sleep was used in these studies. As opposed simply to analyzing spontaneous GER, this approach allowed the infusion of acid into the distal esophagus during specific periods of documented sleep (REM versus non-REM [NREM]), and it allowed the precise timing of infusions such that the amount of sleep before each infusion could be relatively well controlled. This model also permitted a precise comparison of acid clearance during waking and during sleep under well-controlled conditions.

The initial study in this series involved a comparison of acid clearance during sleep in healthy volunteers and patients with mild to moderate esophagitis.[29] The results revealed that sleep infusions in both groups were associated with a statistically significant prolongation of acid clearance time. In minutes, the absolute clearance time was nearly doubled in both groups. However, there was no significant difference between the clearance times in the patients and in the control subjects. The latter finding is believed to be a somewhat academic point because, as noted previously, healthy persons rarely have reflux during sleep, whereas it is somewhat more common in patients with esophagitis. In addition, it was clear from the polysomnographic observations that clearance was invariably associated with an arousal from sleep, and if this did not occur, there was a marked prolongation in acid clearance time. To evaluate this notion more precisely, clearance intervals which had more or less than 50% of waking during the clearance interval were compared. The clearance trials that involved more than 50% of waking had significantly faster clearance times. These data led to the conclusion that both arousal responses and waking are important elements in the response to an acidic distal esophagus.

To evaluate the motor functioning of the esophagus during sleep and the associated arousals from sleep, a subsequent study was performed using a specially designed esophageal probe (Konigsberg Instruments, Inc., Los Angeles, California) to monitor not only distal esophageal pH but esophageal peristalsis.[30] This study also confirmed the importance of arousal responses in the efficient clearance of acid from the distal esophagus. The test was performed on healthy volunteers who had a negative acid perfusion test; that is, they did not show any sensitivity to acid dripped in the distal esophagus and could not distinguish acid from water in the esophagus. However, the determination of arousal responses to these two different substances infused during sleep revealed that the acid infusions produced a significantly greater number of arousal responses. In addition, an exponential relation was described between the percentage of waking during the acid clearance interval and the acid clearance time; that is, the greater the amount of waking during the acid clearance interval, the faster the clearance time. Again, this finding substantiates those from the previous study of patients with esophagitis. This study did not document any difference between peristaltic parameters during sleep and during waking.

To test more definitively the hypothesis that complications of GER are associated with prolonged acid clearance, a group of 13 patients with Barrett's esophagus was studied.[31] Barrett's esophagus is a condition believed to be related to chronic, severe GER, which results in the replacement of normal esophageal squamous epithelium with gastric columnar epithelium. The results of this study proved to be quite surprising in that the patients with Barrett's esophagus were shown to have significantly faster acid clearance during sleep and waking compared with the control subjects. These data were, however, quite compatible with previous results in documenting the importance of arousal responses in the clearance process. The patients with Barrett's esophagus showed both a higher frequency of arousal responses and a shorter latency to the first swallow than did the control subjects.

Further illustrating the importance of these parameters in differentiating the patients with Barrett's esophagus from the control subjects is the fact that they could not be distinguished on the basis of any parameters associated with esophageal motor functioning, such as the amplitude of the peristaltic contraction or the esophageal transit time. It is especially notable in this study that there were a remarkable number of episodes of spontaneous GER in the group with Barrett's esophagus compared with the control subjects. These data led to the conclusion that the severe esophagitis in the patients with Barrett's esophagus is acquired through repeated episodes of spontaneous GER during sleep, which are associated with a prolongation of the acid clearance time (even though this was demonstrated to be faster than in normal control subjects, the acid clearance still is substantially longer than that occurring during waking).

Therapeutic Considerations

GER appears to be affected by sleeping position; in particular, sleeping in the left lateral position significantly reduced the incidence of GER.[32] The results of previously cited studies suggest that the pattern of GER during waking and sleep is important in that sleep-related reflux produces a prolongation of acid clearance.[22,23] Additional documentation of the importance of this pattern of the prolongation of acid clearance comes from studies that have shown that the back-diffusion of hydrogen ions in the esophagus is directly related to the duration of acid–mucosa contact time.[33] Further evidence for the importance of nocturnal GER comes from a clinical study that documented individuals with symptoms of nocturnal heartburn, as well as dysphagia and chest pain, were much more likely to have demonstrable esophageal disease.[34]

These results, as well as those described in the cited studies, tend to substantiate the time-honored clinical approach to persistent reflux, which is the suggestion that the patient sleep with the head of the bed elevated.[34a] This clinical axiom had survived for decades with little in the way of objective documentation of its therapeutic effect. Subsequent testing using intraesophageal pH monitoring during sleep has confirmed that sleeping with the head of the bed elevated produced a 67% improvement in the acid clearance time, although the frequency of reflux episodes remains unchanged.[35] The use of a cholinergic drug (bethanechol) that produces an elevation in lower esophageal sphincter pressure and increases esophageal peristaltic efficiency resulted in a decrease in both reflux frequency (30%) and acid clearance time (53%). Another clinical axiom, avoidance of late evening meals, has also been directly tested.[36] Reflux events during monitored sleep were not increased by a late evening provocative meal in patients with symptomatic GER disease. However, an over-the-counter dose (75 mg) of ranitidine at bedtime was effective in significantly reducing reflux events during sleep.

The use of H_2 receptor antagonists to suppress gastric acid secretion has been shown to be effective in the relief of heartburn.[37,38] One study using 24-hour ambulatory esophageal pH assessments in patients with symptomatic heartburn and documented GER demonstrated that increasing doses (40 mg at bedtime, 20 mg twice daily, and 40 mg twice daily) of an H_2 receptor antagonist (famotidine) produced increasing reductions in daytime and total acid–mucosa contact.[39] The three dosing regimens were equally effective in reducing nocturnal acid contact time. Thus, in contrast to duodenal ulcer disease, it does not appear that bedtime-only dosing is adequate to treat GER. However, these data suggest that GER can be adequately controlled through effective gastric acid suppression. Powerful acid suppression is the most common treatment for GERD, and long-acting proton pump inhibitors (PPIs) have been shown to be effective in suppressing GER during both daytime and at night, as well as providing effective remission of symptoms of nighttime heartburn.[40] Two PPIs appear to have a slight advantage regarding nighttime suppression of acid secretion or intragastric pH. Esomeprazole has advantages with regard to the time the intragastric pH is below 4.0, and pantoprazole has a more prolonged area under the curve for blood levels (see Cohen et al.[40] for review). No direct comparisons are available regarding how the various PPIs compare in the suppression of nighttime GER and symptom control. The "breakthrough" of acid suppression has been described

as a drop in the intragastric pH that occurs during the sleeping interval with PPI treatment.[41] It has been suggested that adding an H_2 receptor blocker at bedtime can control this phenomenon.[42] There are data, however, that cast considerable doubt on the clinical relevance of this phenomenon. Studies have shown that the addition of an H_2 blocker at bedtime does not alter the occurrence of nighttime GER.[43]

Sleep-related GER and heartburn symptoms are both significantly decreased with Nissen fundoplication.[40] Subjective and objective sleep measures are also improved after surgery. More specifically, there was a very small, but significant increase (approximately 5%) in NREM sleep, whereas there were more robust improvements in difficulty falling asleep, sleep quality, and daytime sleepiness. There are data to suggest that the administration of nasal continuous positive airway pressure (CPAP) to patients who are being treated for obstructive sleep apnea (OSA) had the additional therapeutic benefit of reducing GER during sleep and consequent esophageal acid–mucosa contact time.[41] Similar improvement was reported in patients with GER without apnea.[42] In fact, patients with sleep apnea have a high incidence of GER,[43,44] although there is little relation between severity of sleep apnea and GER, or between apneic events and reflux events. Similar results have been reported in other studies, but an overall increase in reflux events and acid clearance time was noted despite the absence of a clear relationship between obstructive apneic events and reflux events.[45] The question remains as to what is the pathogenesis of increased sleep-related GER in patients with OSA. They clearly share some risk factors, such as obesity, alcohol consumption, and perhaps hiatal hernia, but based on some clinical and physiologic data, obesity alone would not appear to be an adequate explanation for this relationship. An association between obesity and symptoms of OSA, but no relationship between obesity and reflux symptoms, was noted in a study that addressed this issue.[46] On the other hand, another questionnaire study showed a significant reduction in nighttime heartburn symptoms after CPAP treatment, and those with higher CPAP levels had a greater reduction in symptoms of nighttime heartburn.[47] Another study that evaluated reflux symptoms (i.e. heartburn, acid regurgitation) in patients with a diagnosis of OSA found that there was no difference in reflux symptoms between those with the diagnosis of OSA and those designated as "simple snorers."[48] Furthermore, no relationship was found between the severity of OSA and reflux symptoms. However, this investigation did not specifically address nighttime GER symptoms. In addition, the incidence of reflux symptoms did not appear to be greater than that noted in some general population surveys in one of these studies.[48] An interesting physiologic study addressed the issue of the relationship between GER and OSA by identifying individuals with significant OSA and GER, and treating them with acid suppression with a PPI.[49] In this study, it was noted that after treatment with the PPI for 1 month, there was a significant reduction in complete obstructive events, although the overall respiratory disturbance index only showed a strong trend toward a reduction after treatment ($P < .06$).

On the basis of these data, it would appear that the incidence of nighttime heartburn is elevated in patients with OSA at a rate (62% in one study) that is similar to that in patients with frequent heartburn complaints.[14,47] Furthermore, the frequency shows a very significant decline with CPAP treatment.

This coincides well with other physiologic studies that have clearly shown a significant decline in esophageal acid–mucosa contact time with CPAP treatment.[41,42] The mechanism by which CPAP reduces esophageal acid contact time remains controversial, but an interesting study from this same group has suggested that some residual lower esophageal sphincter pressure (>10 mm Hg) may be necessary for nasal CPAP to affect nocturnal reflux.[50]

Of considerable interest is the fact that studies have documented that commonly consumed sedating drugs such as benzodiazepines and alcohol have been shown to prolong acid clearance during sleep.[51,52] One study has shown that alcohol consumption approximately 3 hours before sleep resulted in marked prolongation of the clearance of spontaneous episodes of GER.[51] In another investigation of the effect of the administration of commonly used hypnotic drugs, a decrease in the arousal latency and a prolongation in the acid clearance time were shown with triazolam.[52]

To summarize, these studies on acid clearance during sleep lend increasing support to the idea that sleep is a time of considerable risk for patients with reflux esophagitis and that intact afferent arousal mechanisms are important in allowing normal acid clearance from the distal esophagus. Furthermore, commonly ingested sedating compounds such as hypnotic drugs and alcohol appear to result in a prolongation of acid clearance time, which might make otherwise benign GER a more clinically significant event.

PULMONARY COMPLICATIONS OF SLEEP-RELATED GASTROESOPHAGEAL REFLUX

In an important epidemiologic study, it was noted that in a random population study, individuals who reported GER symptoms once or twice per week were significantly more likely to report symptoms of sleep-disordered breathing, and subjects with a combination of asthma and GER had a higher prevalence of nocturnal cough and sleep-related symptoms.[53] It was concluded that the occurrence of nocturnal GER is strongly associated with both asthma and respiratory symptoms, as well as symptoms of OSA syndrome. In another report from the same data set, these investigators noted that symptoms of nocturnal GER were associated with daytime sleepiness with an odds ratio of 2.6, and with daytime tiredness/fatigue with an odds ratio of 4.5.[54] In addition, in a study that addressed symptoms of GER in older adults, a complaint of insomnia was independently associated with symptoms suggestive of GERD.[55]

Nocturnal wheezing in persons with asthma and chronic nocturnal cough are pulmonary symptoms that have been linked to the occurrence of GER.[1,56-57a] The GER may be clinically "silent," and treatment of the GER may reduce nocturnal asthma symptoms.[57] In fact, a much greater incidence of nocturnal symptoms was identified in asthmatic patients who were subsequently found to have GER.[58] In the same study, symptoms such as night cough, nocturnal wheezing, shortness of breath, and other upper gastrointestinal complaints, especially when positionally induced, were significantly more common in asthmatic patients with GER than in those without reflux. One study has demonstrated that 47% of patients with chronic bronchitis have GER, and that the most striking

abnormality in these patients was a significant impairment of acid clearance.[59] Results of the studies reviewed strongly suggest that prolonged acid clearance is most likely to occur during sleep. Furthermore, an abnormal degree of GER is substantially more common in a group of unselected asthmatic patients than in control subjects.[60] Cuttitta et al.[1] concluded that GER duration may determine the severity of nocturnal bronchoconstriction in asthmatic patients with GER. In an interesting study that supports the important role of sleep, infraglottic resistance in asthmatic subjects has been shown to increase significantly during sleep.[61] Another investigation has provided data on esophageal function in another group of patients with lung dysfunction (i.e., chronic obstructive pulmonary disease).[62] In this study, patients with chronic obstructive pulmonary disease failed to show any reflex bronchial constriction to esophageal acid infusion, and their nocturnal and diurnal acid exposure times were completely normal on 24-hour pH monitoring. Thus, with regard to the relation between pulmonary functioning and reflux during sleep, it appears that there is something unique to the asthmatic patient.

Only rarely does acute or chronic inflammatory lung disease develop as the direct consequence of GER. In an editorial concerning respiratory symptoms in patients with GER, Orringer[63] commented, "Far more commonly than is generally appreciated, however, gastroesophageal reflux triggers a variety of respiratory symptoms in the absence of actual aspiration of gastric contents into the tracheal bronchial tree." He points out that because GER-related symptoms usually occur in the supine position during sleep and are usually resolved by assuming the upright position, symptoms such as shortness of breath may be confused with paroxysmal nocturnal dyspnea. Although it is clear that there are pulmonary symptoms that suggest nocturnal GER in their pathogenesis, daytime symptoms suggesting GER are not as consistently obvious. In a study of patients with esophageal pH and symptoms indicative of pulmonary aspiration, only approximately half of the patients had significant symptoms of heartburn.[64] The common symptoms associated with GER are not necessarily reliable indicators of the physiologic presence of GER, particularly in patients with chronic pulmonary symptomatology.

Of considerable interest is the fact that there are a number of parameters of GER that are believed to be related to the likelihood of pulmonary aspiration and subsequent damage to the lung parenchyma; two of these are volume refluxed and pH of the refluxant. Questions concerning esophageal responsiveness to these critical stimuli during sleep were addressed subsequent to a previous study from our laboratory that suggested arousals to esophageal acid stimulation were enhanced during sleep.[30] It was shown that in healthy, asymptomatic volunteers with a negative acid perfusion test (no distinction between acid and water infused into the esophagus), acid provoked a marked increase in arousal responses during sleep. This suggested that esophageal responsivity was altered during sleep and that the enhanced arousal responses and shortened latency to swallowing were endogenous mechanisms designed to protect the trachea and bronchial tree from the aspiration of esophageal contents. Another parameter of importance may be the degree of proximal acid migration in the esophagus. It has been shown in cats that tracheal stimulation with minute amounts of acid produces a markedly greater bronchoconstrictive response than occurs with much larger volumes placed in the distal esophagus.[65] In addition, proximal esophageal acid contact acts as a strong arousal stimulus in infants.[66]

These study results are compatible with the notion that responses to a noxious and potentially dangerous stimulus such as acid are altered or amplified under circumstances of increased risk, (i.e., decreased level of consciousness such as the sleeping state). This hypothesis was tested by investigating the effect of parameters that would produce an increased risk of pulmonary aspiration. As noted, two of these parameters are volume and pH. An increasing volume of reflux into the esophagus would be considered a greater risk for pulmonary aspiration, and it would be hypothesized that larger volumes would produce more prompt and vigorous responses. To test this hypothesis, three different volumes of 0.1 N HCl were infused into the distal esophagus during waking and sleep.[67] The data revealed that acid clearance was more rapid for the higher volumes; during waking, the latency to the first swallow was not noted to be significantly different, but subsequent to acid infusion during sleep, the latency clearly progressively decreased with increasing volume. Similarly, the latency to the arousal from sleep was significantly reduced with increasing volume.

In a follow-up study, as a further test of the hypothesis of differential esophageal acid sensitivity during sleep, the effect of different pH levels infused with constant volume was studied.[68] It has been well established, for example, that aspiration of fluid into the lungs at a relatively high pH (above 3) does not produce any significant damage to the lungs.[69] However, considerable damage and, in some instances, death can occur with the aspiration of more acidic gastric contents. When acid (0.1 N HCl) is infused into the esophagus at a constant volume (15 mL) but with varying pH (1.2, 3, or 5), esophageal acid sensitivity is enhanced during sleep compared with during the waking state.[68] Arousal latency, for example, was shown to be significantly decreased with an infusion of the lowest pH compared with the highest pH, and the latency to the first swallow was significantly decreased with pH 1.2 compared with 5. No differences were noted with infusions in the waking state. Data from these two experiments are quite consistent with the notion that the esophagus responds differentially during sleep to stimuli that would be considered to produce an increased risk of esophageal injury or pulmonary aspiration.

Published observations that acid in the distal esophagus can induce a reflex bronchoconstriction, presumably leading to pulmonary symptoms, have markedly changed the views on the medical significance of the relation between GER and pulmonary symptoms. If the latter occur only in the presence of true aspiration of gastric contents, obviously the significance of this complication diminishes substantially because it is well known that this is a relatively rare phenomenon. In 15 asthmatic patients, all of whom had a positive acid perfusion test (i.e., reproduction of typical substernal pyrosis with acid infusion into the esophagus), acid alone in the distal esophagus produced an increase in pulmonary resistance.[70] In a subsequent, better-controlled study,[71] the same investigators noted that the increased pulmonary resistance and decreased air flow occurred only in patients with a positive acid perfusion test. In both of these studies, symptoms were relieved with antacid ingestion, further substantiating the notion that the pulmonary changes were reflexly induced by the presence of acid in the distal esophagus.

Obviously, GER can occur during waking or sleep; therefore, symptom induction by this mechanism would be expected to occur both during the daytime and at night. In our experience, symptom provocation in most people with esophagitis may take 5 minutes or longer with the acid perfusion test, so one might extrapolate from this that the esophagus must be perfused for a period of several minutes before symptoms occur. From the results of previous studies, it is suspected that this would most commonly occur with nocturnal GER.

A clinical study has documented a significant resolution of nocturnal symptoms only in those asthmatic patients treated with an H_2 receptor antagonist (cimetidine).[72] There also was significant improvement in reflux symptoms in 14 of the 18 patients studied. In another group of asthmatic patients with predominantly nocturnal wheezing, respiratory symptoms significantly abated with treatment for GER with 150 mg of ranitidine twice daily.[73] The authors specifically commented in their discussion that GER should be considered in the pathogenesis of asthma symptoms, particularly in persons with nocturnal wheezing. These data lend additional support to the notion that the adequate treatment of reflux symptoms can substantially improve asthmatic symptoms. Although the presence of the clinical symptoms of GER in patients with pulmonary disease is notable, as emphasized previously, the presence of GER as a contributing factor to the pulmonary disease cannot be ruled out on the basis of an absence of symptoms of GER. This was again emphasized in a study that documented the presence of "silent" physiologic reflux in a group of asthmatic patients who had no reflux symptoms.[74]

In an excellent review, it has been pointed out that the relationship among small airway disease, GER, and symptoms can be difficult to document historically because small airway resistance due to bronchial asthma can intensify at night without accompanying symptom exacerbation.[75] It seems clear, however, that regardless of the mechanism, empirical therapy can determine this relation by resolving pulmonary symptoms through a reduction in nocturnal GER.

The physiologic and clinical data noted earlier suggest a relation between asthmatic symptoms, particularly nocturnal wheezing, and a reflex bronchoconstriction caused by GER. Despite the numerous studies noted, controversy remains, and any parsimonious explanation of these phenomena must account for some significant negative data. For example, in an excellent study, patients with nocturnal wheezing were studied at night with the use of respiratory and polysomnographic monitoring.[76] These data showed no relation between spontaneous GER and pulmonary resistance measures, nor was there any relation with the exogenous infusion of acid. Similarly, in another study in patients with chronic obstructive pulmonary disease and varying degrees of reversible lung disease, acidification of the distal esophagus did not produce any notable change in respiratory resistance or conductance. Furthermore, these patients did not exhibit any alterations in daytime or nocturnal GER as noted with 24-hour pH monitoring.

Further documentation of the relation between nocturnal pulmonary symptoms and nocturnal aspiration of gastric contents comes from a study that used a scintiscanning technique that involved the instillation of a radionuclide into the stomach before sleep and a lung scan the next morning to identify any radioactivity.[77] Positive scans were documented in three of six patients suspected of having nocturnal pulmonary aspiration. In the patients with positive scans, the investigators also documented the presence of prolonged episodes of reflux during sleep. It is of interest that a similar study documented a positive lung scan in 45% of healthy persons who had a radionuclide placed in the posterior pharynx during sleep.[78] These data suggest that subtle pulmonary aspiration occurs in healthy persons during sleep. It is particularly interesting that depressed consciousness markedly enhanced the rate of positive lung scans in this study and that of the healthy persons who were studied, those who reported multiple awakenings (arousals) during sleep uniformly had negative scans. These data suggest that arousals from sleep, as emphasized earlier, are important elements in the response to acid in the upper airway.

Similar techniques have been applied to asthmatic patients with nocturnal wheezing. No evidence of pulmonary aspiration was found in this patient population, suggesting that either the technique itself may lack adequate sensitivity or that pulmonary aspiration is relatively uncommon in asthmatic persons with nocturnal symptoms. Although the actual aspiration of gastric contents into the lungs may be uncommon,[79] there are numerous studies suggesting that the aspiration of gastric contents is not necessary to produce symptoms. It has been suggested that a reflex gradient exists from the distal esophagus to the posterior pharyngeal airway and results in increasing intensity of reflex bronchoconstriction when acid is introduced in these areas.[65] Although there have been some studies suggesting that proximal esophageal acid exposure can produce symptoms such as chronic cough, there are no definitive studies related to the occurrence of these symptoms and their relation to polysomnographically monitored sleep and esophageal acid exposure. Of interest, however, is a study that suggests that sleep itself may predispose to the proximal migration of acidic fluid in the distal esophagus.[80] In this study, 1 mL of infused volume into the distal esophagus revealed no evidence of proximal migration in the waking state; however, during sleep, 40% of the healthy volunteers studied showed evidence of proximal migration. An increase in the volume to 3 mL led to a substantial increase in the percentage of subjects showing proximal migration (80%).

INTESTINAL MOTILITY

Because of the technological and practical difficulties in monitoring intestinal activity, there is limited information on intestinal motility during sleeping and waking in patient populations of interest. However, some data have been gradually appearing in the medical literature. In one study of patients with IBS, 24-hour ambulatory monitoring of small intestinal motility showed that nocturnal motor patterns could not differentiate the patient group from the control subjects, and it was noted that there was a marked prolongation in phase II of the migrating motor complex (MMC; see Chapter 23 for definition) in the waking state in patients with IBS.[81] The notable lack of motility activity during sleep suggests that the changes in motor functioning noted are primarily the result of reactions to various "stressful" events occurring in the waking state.

In another study that examined the effects of alcohol on the MMC, it was noted that alcohol reduces phase II of the MMC during sleep (although the authors did not polysomnographically monitor sleep).[82] The authors noted that the actual contractions during phase II were enhanced, and they interpreted this to suggest that these findings were more related to the central effects of alcohol than to the local effects. They pointed out that much of the alcohol would be metabolized by the time the actual effects on the amplitude were noted.

However, a subsequent study showing a marked increase in REM sleep in patients with IBS lends additional support to the speculation that this syndrome has a central nervous system pathogenesis.[83] The observation that REM sleep was enhanced in patients with IBS has prompted a number of investigations into sleep and functional bowel disorders to include IBS and functional dyspepsia. Using subjective reports of sleep quality, it has been documented that the exacerbations of IBS symptoms and poor sleep show a strong correlation.[84] The problems of a subjective study without physiologic measurement of sleep are obvious: The occurrence of waking symptomatology may unduly influence the perception of the previous night's sleep, and without polysomnographic documentation of sleep, this influence cannot be discounted.[85] In a study in patients with nonulcer dyspepsia (characterized by epigastric postprandial bloating, nausea, or early satiety), two thirds of 65 patients with nonulcer dyspepsia complained of general sleep disturbances suggestive of nonrestorative sleep (i.e., numerous wakenings after sleep onset, morning awakenings without feeling rested).[86] These were significantly more common than noted in control subjects, and 65% of those complaining of sleep disturbance attributed their sleep problem to their abdominal symptoms. Ten patients were also studied for a 24-hour period with intestinal manometric monitoring, and a change in the rhythmicity of the MMC was found in the functional dyspeptic patients characterized by a significant decrease in the number of MMCs during the nocturnal recording interval. In a subsequent study, a marked increase in sleep complaints was noted in patients with functional bowel disorders (i.e., IBS and functional dyspepsia) compared with healthy control subjects.[87] In addition, the dyspeptic patients had more complaints of sleep disturbance, perhaps because of more intense abdominal pain.

Several studies have documented increased sleep complaints in patients with IBS.[88-90] In all of these studies, full polysomnography was conducted. One study found no difference in any of the sleep measures reported between patients with IBS and healthy subjects,[88] whereas the other did show a significant prolongation of REM sleep.[89] However, in one study, the investigators noted a number of significant polysomnographic differences in the patients with IBS compared with control groups, including decreased slow wave sleep, increased arousal responses, and increased waking after sleep onset. Further research with larger sample sizes and stratification by IBS diagnostic subtype may help elucidate and resolve these discrepancies. The original study that noted the enhancement of REM sleep in patients with IBS reported on only six individuals who had a single night of sleep subsequent to small bowel intubation for monitoring of intestinal motility.[82] With a small number of subjects and no attempt to adapt individuals to the laboratory setting (even though a control group was used), there is a high probability that these results were spurious. A subsequent study attempted to replicate this study while at the same time noninvasively monitoring a gastrointestinal measure so that more natural sleep could be obtained.[91] Nine patients with IBS and nine control subjects were studied with full polysomnographic monitoring and gastric electrical activity monitored by the surface electrogastrogram. In this study, a statistically significant increase in REM sleep was documented in the patients with IBS, but the absolute level of REM sleep was not nearly in the range reported in the previous study.[82] In addition, specific electrogastrographic changes were found to be associated with sleep in healthy subjects that were not noted in patients with IBS. Healthy volunteers showed a significant decrease in the spectral amplitude of the electrogastrographic three-cycle-per-minute rhythm during NREM sleep compared with waking. During REM sleep, however, the amplitude was significantly increased to levels approaching those in the waking state. The patients with IBS failed significantly to modulate the amplitude of the dominant frequency of the gastric electrical rhythm during any of these states of consciousness. The lack of modulation of the dominant frequency of the electrogastrographic amplitude during sleep in patients with IBS raises the possibility that other autonomic abnormalities may be unmasked by further study of physiologic functioning during sleep.

In a subsequent study it was noted that patients with IBS who had dyspeptic symptoms in addition to classic symptoms of abdominal pain and cramping did not exhibit the increase in sympathetic dominance in REM sleep that was noted only in the patients with abdominal cramping alone as part of their IBS symptomatology.[92] In a series of published studies, none has replicated the finding of an increase in REM sleep in patients with IBS.[80,92,93]

Collectively, these results from various sleep investigations in patients with functional bowel disorders suggest not only that there are sleep disturbances noted in this patient population but that the sleep disturbances may contribute to altered gastrointestinal functioning. Certainly, these studies confirm the notion that there are central nervous system alterations in patients with functional bowel disorders and that these alterations are perhaps uniquely identified during sleep. Future studies on sleep in patients with functional bowel disorders will undoubtedly provide additional understanding of the pathophysiology of the brain–gut axis and its alterations during sleep.

Colonic motility has been monitored for 24 hours in healthy volunteers and in patients with chronic constipation.[94] Although there was a decrease in the number and duration of mass movements in the patients with chronic constipation, as well as a circadian pattern of decrease in mass movements during the night, no significant difference was noted between patients and control subjects with regard to the circadian pattern itself. In a similar study, the motor activity of the distal colon, rectum, and anal canal was monitored over a 24-hour interval in patients with slow-transit constipation.[95] These patients were compared with 10 healthy control subjects. The patients with slow-transit constipation were noted to have impaired responses to feeding as well as reduced colonic contractile activity on awakening from sleep in the morning.

Another interesting observation concerning alterations in anorectal functioning during sleep concerns a study in which the authors monitored rectal motor activity during sleep in patients who had undergone ileoanal anastomosis.[96] The investigators noted that decreases in anal resting pressure coupled with marked minute-to-minute variations in pressure during sleep occurred in control subjects and in patients and, when particularly profound, led to nocturnal fecal incontinence in some patients.

CONCLUSIONS

It appears that there is an important relation between sleep and the development of various acid peptic diseases, such as duodenal ulcer disease and GERD. The pathogenesis and treatment of these disorders relate in large measure to the control of acid secretion during sleep. The suppression of nocturnal acid secretion appears to be an essential element in the healing of duodenal ulcers, and the occurrence of nocturnal GER is an unquestionably important aspect of the development of serious complications of this disorder. Continuous monitoring of the distal esophageal pH to document nocturnal GER is emerging as an important and useful diagnostic tool. The respiratory complications of GER also appear to be associated with sleep-related GER. In addition, prolonged monitoring of small and large bowel motility appears to be a promising tool in further understanding the pathogenesis of various gastrointestinal diseases and how these diseases may be altered by sleep. Functional bowel disorders, as well as GER, appear to be associated with an increased incidence of sleep complaints, and autonomic dysfunction specifically noted during REM sleep appears to characterize a subset of patients diagnosed with IBS. An awareness of these sleep-related phenomena is becoming an important element in the practice of state-of-the-art gastroenterology, and future research will undoubtedly further substantiate the important role of sleep in the pathogenesis of gastrointestinal disease.

> *Clinical Pearl*
>
> *Suppression of nocturnal acid secretion is an important element in healing duodenal ulcers and remains a mainstay in the treatment of GERD. This in turn can reduce the pulmonary complications of GERD.*

References

1. Cuttitta G, Cibella F, Visconti A, et al: Spontaneous gastroesophageal reflux and airway patency during the night in adult asthmatics. Am J Respir Crit Care Med 2000;161:177-181.
2. Feldman M, Richardson CT: Total 24-hour gastric acid secretion in patients with duodenal ulcer: Comparison with normal subjects and effects of cimetidine and parietal cell vagotomy. Gastroenterology 1986;90:540-544.
3. Orr WC, Hall WH, Stahl ML, et al: Sleep patterns and gastric acid secretion in duodenal ulcer disease. Arch Intern Med 1976;136:655-660.
4. Kildebo S, Aronsen O, Bernersen B, et al: Cimetidine, 800 mg at night, in the treatment of duodenal ulcers. Scand J Gastroenterol 1985;20:1147-1150.
5. Colin-Jones DG, Ireland A, Gear P, et al: Reducing overnight secretion of acid to heal duodenal ulcers: Comparison of standard divided dose of ranitidine with a single dose administered at night. Am J Med 1984;77:116-122.
6. Howden CW, Jones DB, Hunt RH: Nocturnal doses of H$_2$ receptor antagonists for duodenal ulcer. Lancet 1985;1:647-648.
7. Gledhill T, Buck M, Paul A, et al: Comparison of the effects of proximal gastric vagotomy, cimetidine, and placebo on nocturnal intragastric acidity and acid secretion in patients with cimetidine resistant duodenal ulcer. Br J Surg 1983;70:704-706.
8. Galmiche JP, Tranvouez JL, Denis P, et al: L'enregistrement nocturne du pH gastrique permet-il de prévoir la réponse thérapeutique des ulc: Ageres duodenaux sév; ageres traites par la ranitidine? Gastroenterol Clin Biol 1985;9:583-589.

9. Gotthard R, Strom M, Sjodahl R, et al: 24-Hour study of gastric acidity and bile acid concentration after parietal cell vagotomy. Scand J Gastroenterol 1986;21:503-508.

10. Gough KR, Bardhan KD, Crowe JP, et al: Ranitidine and cimetidine in prevention of duodenal ulcer relapse. Lancet 1984;2:659-662.

11. Silvis SE: Final report on the United States multicenter trial comparing ranitidine to cimetidine as maintenance therapy following healing of duodenal ulcer. J Clin Gastroenterol 1985; 7:482-487.

12. Santana IA, Sharma BK, Pounder RE, et al: 24-Hour intragastric acidity during maintenance treatment with ranitidine. BMJ 1984;289:1420.

13. Nebel OT, Fornes MF, Castell DO: Symptomatic gastro-esophageal reflux: Incidence and precipitating factors. Am J Dig Dis 1976;21:953-956.

14. Shaker R, Castell DO, Schoenfeld PS, et al: Nighttime heart-burn is an under-appreciated clinical problem that impacts sleep and daytime function: The results of a Gallup survey conducted on behalf of the American Gastroenterological Association. Am J Gastroenterol 2003;98:1487-1493.

15. Farup C, Kleinman L, Sloan S, et al: The impact of nocturnal symptoms associated with gastroesophageal reflux disease on health-related quality of life. Arch Intern Med 2001;151:45-52.

15a. Shaker R, Brunton S, Elfant A, et al: Impact of night-time reflux on lifestyle–unrecognized issues in reflux disease. Aliment Pharmacol Ther 2004;9 (Dec 20 Suppl):3-13.

16. Orr WC: Lifestyle measures for the treatment of gastro-esophageal reflux disease. In Bayless TM, Diehl AM (eds): Advanced Therapy in Gastroenterology and Liver Disease. Hamilton, Ontario, BC Decker, 2005.

16a. Orr WC, Heading R, Johnson LF, et al: Sleep and its relationship to gastro-oesophageal reflux. Aliment Pharmacol Ther 2004;9 (Dec 20 Suppl):39-46.

17. Freidin N, Fisher MJ, Taylor W, et al: Sleep and nocturnal acid reflux in normal subjects and patients with reflux oesophagitis. Gut 1991;32:1275-1279.

18. Penzel T, Becker HR, Brandenburg U, et al: Arousal in patients with gastro-esophageal reflux and sleep apnea. Eur Respir J 1999;14:1266-1270.

19. Johnson LF, DeMeester TR: Twenty-four hour pH monitoring of the distal esophagus. Am J Gastroenterol 1974;62:325-332.

20. DeMeester TR, Johnson LF, Guy JJ, et al: Patterns of gastro-esophageal reflux in health and disease. Ann Surg 1976;184:459-470.

21. Johnson LF, DeMeester TR, Haggitt RC: Esophageal epithelial response to gastroesophageal reflux: A quantitative study. Am J Dig Dis 1978;23:498-509.

22. Schlesinger PK, Honahue PE, Schmid B, et al: Limitations of 24-hour intraesophageal pH monitoring in the hospital setting. Gastroenterology 1985;89:797-804.

23. Orr WC, Allen ML, Robinson M: The pattern of nocturnal and diurnal esophageal acid exposure in the pathogenesis of erosive mucosal damage. Am J Gastroenterol 1994;89:509-512.

24. De Caestecker, Blackwell JH, Brown J, et al: When is acid reflux most damaging to the esophagus [abstract]? Gastroenterology 1985;88:1360.

25. Helm JF, Dodds WJ, Hogan WJ, et al: Acid neutralizing capacity of human saliva. Gastroenterology 1982;83:69-74.

26. Allen ML, Orr WC, Woodruff DM, et al: The effects of swallowing frequency and transdermal scopolamine on esophageal acid clearance. Am J Gastroenterol 1985;80:669-672.

27. Lichter J, Muir RC: The pattern of swallowing during sleep. Electroencephalogr Clin Neurophysiol 1975;38:427-432.

28. Schneyer LH, Pigman W, Hanahan L, et al: Rate of flow of human parotid, sublingual, and submaxillary secretions during sleep. J Dent Res 1956;35:109-114.

29. Orr WC, Johnson LF, Robinson MG: The effect of sleep on swallowing, esophageal peristalsis, and acid clearance. Gastroenterology 1984;86:814-819.

30. Orr WC, Robinson MG, Johnson LF: Acid clearing during sleep in the pathogenesis of reflux esophagitis. Dig Dis Sci 1981;26:423-427.

31. Orr WC, Lackey C, Robinson MG, et al: Acid clearance and reflux during sleep in Barrett's esophagus. Gastroenterology 1983;84:1265.

32. Khoury R, Camacho-Lobato L, Katz P, et al: Influence of spontaneous sleep positions on nighttime recumbent reflux in patients with gastroesophageal reflux disease. Am J Gastroenterol 1999; 94:2069-2073.

33. Johnson LF, Harmon JW: Experimental esophagitis in a rabbit model: Clinical relevance. J Clin Gastroenterol 1986;8(Suppl 1): 26-44.

34. Andersen LI, Madsen PV, Dalgaard P, et al: Validity of clinical symptoms in benign esophageal disease, assessed by questionnaire. Acta Med Scand 1987;221:171-177.

34a. McGuigan JE, Belafsky PC, Fromer L, et al: Diagnosis and management of night-time reflux. Aliment Pharmacol Ther 2004;9 (Dec 20 Suppl):57-72.

35. Johnson LF, DeMeester TR: Evaluation of the head of the bed, bethanechol, and antacid foam tablets on gastroesophageal reflux. Dig Dis Sci 1981;26:673-680.

36. Orr WC, Harnish MJ: Sleep-related gastro-oesophageal reflux: Provocation with a late evening meal and treatment with acid suppression. Aliment Pharmacol Ther 1998;12:1033-1038.

37. Behar J, Brand DL, Brown FC, et al: Cimetidine in the treatment of symptomatic gastroesophageal reflux: A double-blind controlled trial. Gastroenterology 1978;74:441-448.

38. Sontag S, Glaxo GERD Research Group: Ranitidine therapy for gastroesophageal reflux disease: Results of a large double-blind trial. Arch Intern Med 1987;147:1485-1491.

39. Orr WC, Robinson MG, Humphries T: Dose response effect of famotidine on patterns of gastroesophageal reflux. Aliment Pharmacol Ther 1988;2:229-235.

40. Cohen JA, Arain A, Harris PA, et al: Surgical trial investigating nocturnal gastroesophageal reflux and sleep (STINGERS). Surg Endosc 2003;17:394-400.

41. Kerr P, Shoenut P, Millar T, et al: Nasal CPAP reduces gastroesophageal reflux in obstructive sleep apnea syndrome. Chest 1992;101:1539-1544.

42. Kerr P, Shoenut JP, Steens RD, et al: Nasal CPAP: A new treatment for nocturnal gastroesophageal reflux. J Clin Gastroenterol 1993; 17:276-280.

43. Graf KI, Karaus M, Heinemann S, et al: Gastroesophageal reflux in patients with sleep apnea syndrome. Z Gastroenterol 1995; 33:689-693.

44. Tardif C, Denis P, Verdure-Poussin A, et al: Gastro-oesophageien pendant le sommeil chez l'obese. Neurophysiol Clin 1988; 18:323-332.

45. Ing AJ, Ngu MC, Breslin AB: Obstructive sleep apnea and gastroesophageal reflux. Am J Med 2000;108(Suppl 4a):120S-125S.

46. Suganuma N, Shigedo Y, Adachi H, et al: Association of gastroesophageal reflux disease with weight gain and apnea, and their disturbance on sleep. Psychiatry Clin Neurosci 2001;55: 255-256.

47. Green BT, Broughton WA, O'Connor JB: Marked improvement in nocturnal gastroesophageal reflux in a large cohort of patients with obstructive sleep apnea treated with continuous positive airway pressure. Arch Intern Med 2003;163:41-45.

48. Valipour A, Makker H, Hardy R, et al: Symptomatic gastroesophageal reflux in subjects with a breathing sleep disorder. Chest 2002;121:1748-1753.

49. Senior BA, Khan M, Schwimmer C, et al: Gastroesophageal reflux and obstructive sleep apnea. Laryngoscope 2001;111:2144-2146.

50. Shoenut JP, Kerr P, Micflikier AB, et al: The effect of nasal CPAP on nocturnal reflux in patients with aperistaltic esophagus. Chest 1994;106:738-741.

51. Vitale GC, Cheadle WG, Patel B, et al: The effect of alcohol on nocturnal gastroesophageal reflux. JAMA 1987;258:2077-2079.

52. Orr WC, Robinson MG, Rundell OH: The effect of hypnotic drugs on acid clearance during sleep. Gastroenterology 1985; 88:1526.

53. Gisalson T, Janson C, Vermeire P, et al: Respiratory symptoms and nocturnal gastroesophageal reflux. Chest 2002;121:158-163.

54. Janson C, Gislason T, DeBacker W, et al: Daytime sleepiness, snoring and gastro-oesophageal reflux amongst young adults in three European countries. J Intern Med 1995;237:277-285.

55. Raiha I, Impivaara O, Seppala M, et al: Determinants of symptoms suggestive of gastroesophageal reflux disease in the elderly. Scand J Gastroenterol 1993;28:1011-1014.

56. Field SK: Gastroesophageal reflux and asthma: Are they related? J Asthma 1999;36:631-644.

57. Kiljander TO, Salomaa ER, Hietanen EK, et al: Gastroesophageal reflux in asthmatics: A double-blind, placebo-controlled crossover study with omeprazole. Chest 1999;116:1257-1264.

57a. Fass R, Achem SR, Harding S, et al: Supra-oesophageal manifestations of gastro-oesophageal reflux disease and the role of night-time gastro-oesophageal reflux. Aliment Pharmacol Ther 2004;9 (Dec 20 Suppl):26-38.

58. Perrin-Foyalle M, Bell A, Kofman J, et al: Asthma and gastro-esophageal reflux: Results of a survey of over 250 cases. Poumon Coeur 1980;36:225-230.

59. David P, Denis P, Nouvet G, et al: Lung function and gastro-esophageal reflux during chronic bronchitis. Bull Eur Physiopathol Respir 1982;18:81-86.

60. Sontag SJ, O'Connell S, Khandelwal S, et al: Most asthmatics have gastroesophageal reflux with or without bronchodilator therapy. Gastroenterology 1990;99:613-620.

61. Ballard RD, Saathoff MC, Patel DK, et al: The effect of sleep on nocturnal bronchoconstriction and ventilatory patterns in asthmatics. J Appl Physiol 1989;67:243-249.

62. Orr WC, Shamma-Othman Z, Allen M, et al: Esophageal function and gastroesophageal reflux during sleep and waking in patients with chronic obstructive pulmonary disease. Chest 1992;101:1521-1525.

63. Orringer MB: Respiratory symptoms and esophageal reflux. Chest 1979;76:618-619.

64. Pelligrini CA, DeMeester TR, Johnson LF, et al: Gastroesophageal reflux and pulmonary aspiration: incidence, functional abnormality, and results of surgical therapy. Surgery 1979;86:110-119.

65. Tuchman DN, Boyle JT, Pack AI, et al: Comparison of airway responses following tracheal or esophageal acidification in the cat. Gastroenterology 1984;87:872-881.

66. Kahn A, Rebuffate E, Sottiaux M, et al: Arousals induced by proximal esophageal reflux in infants. Sleep 1991;14:39-42.

67. Orr WC, Robinson MG, Johnson LF: The effect of esophageal acid volume on arousals from sleep and acid clearance. Chest 1991;99:351-355.

68. Orr WC, Johnson LF: Responses to different levels of esophageal acidification during waking and sleep. Dig Dis Sci 1998;43:241-245.

69. Terry PB, Fuller SD: Pulmonary consequences of aspiration. Dysphagia 1989;3:179-183.

70. Mansfield LE, Stein MR: Gastroesophageal reflux and asthma: A possible reflex mechanism. Ann Allergy 1978;41:224-226.

71. Spaulding HS, Mansfield LE, Stein MR, et al: Further investigation of the association between gastroesophageal reflux and bronchoconstriction. J Allergy Clin Immunol 1982;69:516-521.

72. Goodall RJ, Earis JE, Cooper DN, et al: Relationship between asthma and gastro-oesophageal reflux. Thorax 1981;36:116-121.

73. Harper PC, Bergner A, Kaye MD: Antireflux treatment for asthma: Improvement in patients with associated gastroesophageal reflux. Arch Intern Med 1987;147:56-60.

74. Berquist WE, Rachelefsky GS, Rawshan N, et al: Quantitative gastroesophageal reflux and pulmonary function in asthmatic children and normal adults receiving placebo, theophylline, and metaproterenol sulfate therapy. J Allergy Clin Immunol 1984;73: 253-258.

75. Murphy JR, Johnson LF: Sleep and the respiratory complications of gastroesophageal reflux. Pract Gastroenterol 1993;17: 16-29.

76. Tan WC, Martin RJ, Pandey R, et al: Effects of spontaneous and simulated gastroesophageal reflux on sleeping asthmatics. Am Rev Respir Dis 1990;141:1394-1399.

77. Chernow B, Johnson LF, Janowitz WR, et al: Pulmonary aspiration as a consequence of gastroesophageal reflux: A diagnostic approach. Dig Dis Sci 1979;24:839-844.

78. Huxley EJ, Viroslav J, Gray WR, et al: Pharyngeal aspiration in normal adults with depressed consciousness. Am J Med 1978; 64:564-568.

79. Ghaed N, Stein MR: Assessment of a technique for scintigraphic monitoring of pulmonary aspiration of gastric contents in asthmatics with gastroesophageal reflux. Ann Allergy 1979;42: 306-308.

80. Orr WC, Elsenbruch S, Harnish MJ: Autonomic regulation of cardiac function during sleep in patients with irritable bowel syndrome. Am J Gastroenterol 2000;98:2865-2871.

81. Kellow JE, Gill RG, Wingate DL: Prolonged ambulant recordings of small bowel motility demonstrate abnormalities in the irritable bowel syndrome. Gastroenterology 1990;98:1208-1218.

82. Charles F, Evans DF, Castillo FD, et al: Daytime indigestion of alcohol alters nighttime jejunal motility in man. Dig Dis Sci 1994;39:51-58.

83. Kumar D, Thompson PD, Wingate DL, et al: Abnormal REM sleep in the irritable bowel syndrome. Gastroenterology 1992; 103:12-17.

84. Goldsmith G, Levin JS: Effect of sleep quality on symptoms of irritable bowel syndrome. Dig Dis Sci 1993;38:1809-1814.

85. Wingate D: An association between poor sleep quality and the severity of IBS symptoms [letter]. Dig Dis Sci 1994;39: 2350-2351.

86. David D, Mertz H, Fefer L, et al: Sleep and duodenal motor activity in patients with severe non-ulcer dyspepsia. Gut 1994; 35:916-925.

87. Fass R, Fullerton S, Tung S, et al: Sleep disturbances in clinic patients with functional bowel disorders. Am J Gastroenterol 2000;95:1195-2000.

88. Heitkemper M, Charman AB, Shaver J, et al: Self-report and polysomnographic measures of sleep in women with irritable bowel syndrome. Nurs Res 1998;47:270-277.

89. Elsenbruch S, Harnish MJ, Orr WC: Subjective and objective sleep quality in irritable bowel syndrome. Am J Gastroenterol 1999;94:2447-2452.

90. Rotem AY, Sperber AD, Krugliak P, et al: Polysomnographic and actigraphic evidence of sleep fragmentation in patients with irritable bowel syndrome. Sleep 2003;26:747-752.

91. Orr WC, Crowell MD, Lin B, et al: Sleep and gastric function in irritable bowel syndrome: Derailing the brain-gut axis. Gut 1997;41:390-393.

92. Thompson JJ, Elsenbruch S, Harnish MJ, et al: Autonomic functioning during REM sleep differentiates IBS symptom subgroups. Am J Gastroenterol 2002;97:3147-3153.

93. Elsenbruch S, Thompson JJ, Harnish MJ, et al: Behavioral and physiological sleep characteristics in women with irritable bowel syndrome. Am J Gastroenterol 2002;97:2306-2314.

94. Bassotti G, Gaburri M, Imbimbo BP, et al: Alimentary tract and pancreas: Colonic mass movements in idiopathic chronic constipation. Gut 1988;29:1173-1179.

95. Ferrara A, Pemberton JH, Hanson RB: Motor responses of the sigmoid, rectum and anal canal in health and in patients with slow transit constipation (STC). Gastroenterology 1991;100:A441.

96. Orkin BA, Soper NJ, Kelly KA, et al: Influence of sleep on anal sphincter pressure in health and after ileal pouch-anal anastomosis. Dis Colon Rectum 1992;35:137-144.

The Menstrual Cycle and Circadian Rhythms

Roseanne Armitage

Fiona C. Baker

Barbara L. Parry

ABSTRACT

Despite compelling evidence of sexual dimorphism in brain structure, function, and regulation, there have been few systematic studies of sex differences in sleep and circadian rhythms. This chapter reviews sex differences and hormonal influences on sleep, circadian rhythms, and health-related issues pertaining to women's sleep. The focus is first on sex differences in sleep and circadian rhythms from childhood throughout the early adult years, with the conclusion that the most dramatic sex differences are evident in age-related changes in sleep architecture and regulation. The second focus is on sleep and circadian rhythms as influenced by the menstrual cycle and alterations in ovarian hormones. The monthly fluctuations in menstrual cycle hormones can affect circadian temperature rhythms and sleep architecture as well as subjective sleep. During women's premenstrual phase, from ovulation to onset of menses, circadian amplitudes are dampened, rapid eye movement sleep is likely to be altered, and women report disturbed sleep and poorer sleep quality. The last focus is on common health problems in young women of reproductive age, and the associated sleep disturbances. Depression, a mental health problem more common in women than in men, is associated with changes in sleep architecture. One of the most common physical causes of infertility in young women is polycystic ovaries, which entail excess androgen production and estrogen insufficiency. Sleep-disordered breathing is prevalent in women with polycystic ovaries, regardless of body weight. Implications for women's health and well-being during their reproductive years are discussed in terms of these common clinical conditions.

SEX DIFFERENCES IN SLEEP FROM CHILDHOOD TO ADULTHOOD

There is extensive evidence of sexual dimorphism in brain structure, function, and regulation in studies ranging from fruit flies to humans (Table 108–1). Circadian clock genes,[1] growth hormone,[2] respiratory control,[3] stress response and hypothalamic-pituitary-adrenal axis,[4] density of hypothalamic nuclei,[5] and sex hormone receptors in the suprachiasmatic nucleus (SCN),[5] to name but a few, are all sexually dimorphic and have strong implications for sex differences in sleep and circadian rhythm regulation. Despite this evidence, however, sleep and circadian rhythm research has lagged behind in the study of sex differences in either animals or humans.[6-8a] The following paragraphs review the findings on sex differences in sleep and circadian rhythms from childhood to early adulthood, focusing on studies of healthy individuals.

Infancy

It remains controversial whether the development of sleep states and circadian rhythms is sex dependent. Only a few studies have noted statistical differences between boys and girls, and others have failed to find sex differences in sleep consolidation or architecture.[9,10] Only a few studies have examined the structure of sleep by quantitative or computerized electroencephalographic (EEG) analysis in infants, and none of them have evaluated potential differences with regard to sex.[11-14] Thus, these paragraphs focus on sleep architecture in infants based on observational scoring schemas.

At an early age, infant boys may have less total sleep and more frequent awakenings than infant girls[15,16] (although one study reported more wakefulness in girls[17]). Two studies have also found less non–rapid eye movement (REM) sleep in young boys, particularly in the first few months of life.[15,18] Interestingly, Bach et al.[15] have interpreted these sex differences to reflect greater adaptive capability and maturation of the central nervous system in infant girls. This suggestion was based on increased variability in response to a thermal challenge among male infants compared with a longer duration of non-REM sleep in female infants. Although the suggestion is provocative, such a conclusion would require an assessment of age-related changes in the development of the sleep–wake cycle. Ironically, one study did include sex-by-age interactions in healthy infants, and there was less non-REM sleep in girls older than 3 months.[17] Thus, if non-REM sleep is an index of central nervous system maturation, there is conflicting data on whether development is precocious in boys or girls.

Table 108–1.   Sex Differences Relevant to Sleep and Rhythms

Compared Aspect	Species	Reference Number
By Neuroanatomic Location		
Hypothalamus		
Preoptic area		
3-8 times larger in males	Rats	5
2 times larger in men	Humans	5
Bed nucleus of stria terminalis		
40 times larger in men	Humans	5
Suprachiasmatic nuclei		
Vasopressin-containing neurons	Humans	5
Greater in men under 40 years old		
Greater in women over 40 years old		
More axiospinal synapses in males	Rats	5
More androgen receptors in men	Humans	5
More estrogen receptors in women		
Volume greater in males	Gerbils	5
Brainstem		
Respiratory nuclei		
Serotonin levels higher in females	Rats	3
By Function		
Growth hormone		
higher in women	Humans	2
Epinephrine		
lower in women	Humans	2
Adrenocorticotropic hormone secretion		
Greater in males	Rats	4
Men > follicular women	Humans	4
Luteal women > follicular women	Humans	
Corticosterone secretion		
Greater in males	Rats	4
Clock Genes		
Cycle (BMALI)	Fruit flies	1
Reduced response to "sleep" deprivation in males		
Enhanced response in females		

Cornwell[17] also contrasted age and sex differences in healthy infants and those at high risk for sudden infant death syndrome and found greater sex differences in the high-risk group, with a maturational lag in boys. The prevalence of sudden infant death syndrome is higher in infant boys than in infant girls, and it has been suggested that circadian factors may play a key role in the pathogenesis of the syndrome.[18] Specifically, developmental lags in (1) the establishment of circadian rhythms in temperature regulation and (2) in sleep–wake differentiation have been suggested as risk factors for sudden ventilatory events.[19,20] Taken together, these findings suggest that delayed development of circadian rhythms early in infancy may contribute to differential risk for disease in boys and girls. The data on sleep and circadian rhythms in early onset depression also support this view.[21]

Childhood

A fairly large body of literature (from prior to 1960) on sex and sleep suggests few differences between boys and girls until after 8 years of age. According to a review by Kleitman,[22] there was some disagreement among the studies, but most indicated longer sleep durations in girls. In children between 3 and 5 years of age, Williams and colleagues[23] reported longer sleep

time, longer REM sleep, and more stage 2 sleep in boys than in girls. Among 6- to 9-year-olds, only the latency to the first slow wave sleep (SWS; delta sleep, stage 3/4) period differed between boys and girls, with a longer latency among girls. Sex differences were not evident in older children. However, these early studies included very small sample sizes, typically with 10 to 12 children in each sex and age group. As few of these early studies involved quantitative EEG frequency analyses in children,[24,25] they are excluded from more recent work discussed next.

Recent research has identified sex differences in children's sleep, but findings have not been consistent across all studies. For example, the laboratory-based sleep studies from Carskadon's group,[26-28] conducted over the past 25 years, fail to show significant sex differences in sleep parameters when children are matched by stage of pubertal development. Similarly, a questionnaire-based study found no significant sex effect for time spent in bed, for feeling the need for more sleep, or for time to become alert on awakening; however, the authors did not evaluate potential differences as they relate to both age and sex, nor did they control for pubertal status.[29] By contrast, a later study of Dutch children,[30] based on sleep diary data, indicated a significantly earlier bedtime and more time in bed for girls. These authors also reported significant sex differences in control of aggression at school, and in relationships between control of aggression and sleep variables. Thus, the relationship between sleep and psychological dimensions of health and behavior appears to be strongly influenced by sex.

In assessing only those children with sleep problems, it does appear that the nature of the difficulty and perhaps its severity are sex dependent.[31] Boys had a greater likelihood of awakening prior to 5:00 AM and of having excessive daytime sleepiness. Boys were also more likely to exhibit parasomnias such as head banging. Girls, on the other hand, were three times more likely to sleep with their parents than their male counterparts.

Actigraphy data have also been useful in exploring sex differences in sleep in the home environment. In a study[32] of children in the 2nd, 4th, and 6th grades, girls appeared to sleep longer than boys. Although both boys and girls showed the expected decline in total sleep time with increasing age, the decrease in sleep time appeared to be most dramatic in girls between 4th and 6th grade. These findings support laboratory-based reports of sex differences for time in bed and amount of stage 2 and stage 4 sleep in children between 10 and 17 years of age.[33] Boys had more stage 4 sleep and less stage 2 sleep than girls, but girls spent less time in bed. When these sex differences were evaluated in comparison with a group of men and women, significant sex-by-group interactions were also evident. A larger age-related decline in stage 4 sleep occurs in boys than in girls, in line with accepted sex differences noted in prior studies.[23]

Other researchers have failed to find significant sex effects on sleep, but they generally included very small samples of boys and girls or did not directly assess sex differences.[34-36] Moreover, most studies do not present sleep data separately for each sex,[11,29,35,37-39] and thus the discrepant findings can not be easily synthesized through meta-analyses of published studies.

Additional studies relevant to sex differences in children's sleep are mostly in the context of differentiating healthy children from those with psychiatric disorders. These studies[40-42] found that, although most sleep architecture measures did not differ statistically between healthy boys and girls of 8 to 12 years of age, there was a tendency toward shorter REM onset latency in girls (100.9 minutes) than in boys (134.5 minutes). Girls also had significantly lower delta amplitudes in their first non-REM period than boys.[42]

In summary, only a few studies have examined potential sex differences in children using EEG sleep measures. Although they may have controlled for age, very few used adequate indicators of pubertal status. The majority of studies indicate few reliable differences between healthy boys and girls prior to puberty. As discussed later, and as is evident in the sleep changes from infancy to childhood, the most consistent sex differences are evident in age-related changes in sleep (Table 108–2).

Adolescence

The majority of sleep studies in adolescents also fail to consider potential differences according to sex. One study[7] reported no sex differences in the amount of time boys and girls took to fall asleep, but girls reported an earlier awake time during the school week, with a greater propensity to fall asleep while riding on the bus or in the car on the way home from school. It was suggested that the greater consumption of caffeinated beverages by boys may have contributed to the increased rate of girls falling asleep on the way home from school. Although there were no sex differences in bedtimes or overall amount of sleep on weekdays or weekends, boys were significantly more likely to report earlier wake times on weekends.

Several survey studies have reported significant sex differences on a number of sleep measures.[43,44] Boys had a later bedtime and rise time on weekends, and on school days as well in one study.[43] Compared with girls, the boys also slept less and had a greater tendency to nap, particularly in older adolescence.[43] Regardless of age, however, daytime sleepiness was more prevalent in girls than in boys, supporting earlier findings.[7] Several studies have also noted that complaints about difficulty falling asleep at bedtime were more common among girls.[44-47]

In a large-scale laboratory study of children, adolescent boys and girls showed equivalent sleep architecture, but differences between child and adolescent boys were more dramatic than differences between child and adolescent girls.[42] Adolescent boys had more stage 1 sleep than younger boys, whereas younger and older girls did not differ. Similarly, the age differences in the amount of REM sleep, wake time, and total sleep time were also significantly influenced by sex.

Table 108–2.	**Gender Differences in Sleep**	
Life Stage	**Compared Aspect**	**Reference Number**
Infancy	Less sleep and more awakenings in boys	15, 16, 18
Childhood	Longer sleep length in girls	22, 30, 32, 33
	Earlier bedtime in girls	30
	More severe sleep problems in boys	31
Adolescence	Longer sleep time in girls	7, 43, 44
	Earlier wake-up time in girls	7, 43
	More sleepiness in girls	7, 43
	More awakenings in boys	42
Adults	More stage 1 in men	48
	More slow wave sleep in women	42
	More awakenings in men	48, 50
	Subjective sleep worse in women	51-53
Most consistent finding	Greater age-related sleep changes in males	23, 40-42, 48-50, 59

Adolescent girls had more REM sleep than younger girls, whereas adolescent boys had less REM sleep than younger boys. Adolescent boys had more wake time than younger boys, an effect that was opposite to that observed in girls. In addition, the shorter REM onset latency and reduced total sleep time from younger to older children were more dramatic in boys than in girls. Compared to younger children, there were lower amounts of SWS in adolescents regardless of sex. Thus, not only were the age-related changes in sleep more dramatic in boys, they were often in the opposite direction from those observed in girls.

These findings are in general agreement with those of Acebo and colleagues,[33] who also identified more dramatic age-related sleep changes in boys than in girls, and are consistent with the several reports on infants and children discussed earlier. However, updating their prior studies of sleep in children, Carskadon and Acebo[28] suggest that there are few consistent sex differences once age and maturation (usually assessed with Tanner criteria for stage of puberty) are factored into the analysis. Because it is well documented that girls reach maturity before boys, it is essential that developmental maturity be considered in research studies. There are too few normative studies at this point to determine whether quantitative EEG sleep measures or circadian rhythms differ between boys and girls at similar stages of puberty. Nevertheless, not only do sex differences in sleep and biologic rhythms persist into adulthood but they are also generally greater than those observed in childhood and adolescence.

Adults

Several early studies reported more disturbed sleep in men than in women across the lifespan, with lower sleep efficiency, more stage 1 sleep, and more awakenings in men, but they were largely restricted to later adulthood.[23] These studies also suggested that women lost less SWS across their lifespan. Recent studies also suggest more disturbed, lighter sleep in men than in women, particularly among older individuals.[48] A meta-analysis of published work confirmed that the greatest age-related changes in sleep occur in men,[49] findings further supported by actigraphy data.[50] Interestingly, polysomnographic (PSG) and actigraphic measures indicate worse sleep in men, whereas it is women who report worse subjective sleep, particularly after age 40.[51-53]

The findings in younger adults may be more equivocal and may also depend on the methods used to quantify sleep. For example, studies using quantitative EEG frequency analysis have reported sex difference in sleep spindles[54] and slow wave delta activity in non-REM sleep, and men typically show lower delta amplitude than women.[40,41] Yet these studies did not always control for menstrual cycle phase or oral contraceptive use.[55-57] One study that did control for these two variables found no significant differences in sleep architecture between young women and men, although the naturally cycling women tended to have more SWS.[58] Nevertheless, most studies suggest that the age-related decrease in delta activity may also be sex dependent,[40,41,59] echoing the changes from childhood to adolescence. In contrast, one recent study presented a different view and documented higher power in delta, theta, alpha, and sigma frequency bands in women than in men between 20 and 60 years of age.[60]

None of these studies have demonstrated a differential time course of delta activity (presumed to reflect the basic homeostatic sleep drive), providing little evidence that sleep regulation differs between men and women.[40,41,56,57] As discussed later, however, sex differences may be more evident under challenge conditions.

It has been argued that sex differences in sleep regulation are quite subtle in healthy young individuals, but that they may become more prevalent under challenge conditions such as sleep deprivation, environmental or pharmacologic stressors, or in diseases associated with immune or hypothalamic-pituitary-adrenal axis abnormalities, such as major depressive disorder.[61] This argument is based on findings of a greater delta response to sleep deprivation in healthy young women,[62] sex differences during sleep that are two to five times greater in depressed patients than in healthy individuals,[40,41] and sexual dimorphism in neuroendocrine and neurotransmitter function.[63] There may be greater biologic flexibility and adaptation among women, as reflected in a greater response to a challenge condition. However, Rhodes and Rubin[63] and Van Cauter et al.[64] have hypothesized that women should be less responsive to a challenge in order to preserve sleep, neuroendocrine function, and circadian phase and amplitude. A similar position is held by Kirschbaum et al.[4] Although these viewpoints may appear inconsistent, modulating or dampening the response to a neuroendocrine challenge may reflect a better adaptive response and a greater effort to preserve homeostasis. However, it must be noted that ovarian hormones, either endogenous levels that fluctuate with phase of the menstrual cycle or exogenous levels associated with oral contraceptive use or hormone replacement therapy, can have dramatic effects on stress response.[4] Regardless, both positions provide strong support for sex differences in sleep and neuroendocrine function.

Sex differences in secretion of hormones from the hypothalamus have also been reported. Compared with men, women have a greater amplitude in their circadian secretion pattern of prolactin, a hormone known to be sleep dependent.[65] Diurnal growth hormone concentrations are substantially higher in young women than in men,[2] and the sex difference in growth hormone secretion is independent of gonadal steroids.[66] In older adults between 60 and 73 years of age, growth hormone secretion and the secretory pattern of cortisol secretion become more disorganized and chaotic in women than in men.[64] Plasma cortisol levels appear to be lower in women but increase with age, whereas age-related changes in men are significantly smaller.[64] As observed in studies of children and adolescents, the effects of aging on circadian rhythms for hormone secretion may also be sex dependent.[67-69]

Finally, recent work has also demonstrated sex differences in the neuroanatomy of the suprachiasmatic nucleus and other hypothalamic structures in both humans and animals.[5] Taken together with clinical and laboratory data on sleep and circadian rhythms, these findings provide a strong neurophysiologic and neuroanatomic basis for sex differences and may also be relevant to sex differences in risk factors for neurologic and psychiatric disease. Although the evidence for sex differences is strongest in adulthood, an increasing number of studies suggest a differential maturation time course in males and females that may influence circadian rhythms and sleep–wake cycles. The roots of the divergent maturational influences may be evident very early in human development. Further longitudinal studies are necessary, however, to determine the time period at which these sex differences emerge and how they are shaped by maturation of sex steroids, neuro-endocrine function, gene transcription factors, and environment.

THE MENSTRUAL CYCLE AND EFFECTS OF OVARIAN HORMONES ON SLEEP AND CIRCADIAN RHYTHMS

Female reproductive hormones, specifically estrogen and progesterone, not only regulate reproductive tissue function during the menstrual cycle, but through their secondary actions in the central nervous system, these hormones also influence other physiologic processes, such as sleep and circadian rhythms.

Conventionally, in a normal menstrual cycle of 28 days, day 1 is identified as the first day of bleeding (menses). Ovulation occurs around day 14, dividing the cycle into two phases: a preovulatory follicular phase and a postovulatory luteal phase[70] (Fig. 108–1). Under the control of the hypothalamic–anterior pituitary axis, ovarian follicles grow during the follicular phase, with an associated rise in plasma estradiol. Circulating estradiol levels peak just before ovulation, triggering a surge in luteinizing hormone (LH) secretion from the anterior pituitary.

Ovulation occurs 12 to 16 hours later, around day 14. In the luteal phase, progesterone dominates, being secreted from the ruptured dominant follicle (corpus luteum), together with estradiol. Approximately 14 days after ovulation, if there is no implantation of a fertilized ovum, hormone levels drop precipitously, heralding the onset of menstruation. Ovulatory cycles are typically between 25 and 35 days.

Circadian Rhythms during the Menstrual Cycle

In women, circadian rhythms for hormone secretion, body temperature, and sleep–wake activity are superimposed on the menstrual cycle rhythm. The interaction between the menstrual cycle and circadian rhythms in young women has been studied to a limited extent and mostly in relation to body temperature. The circadian rhythm of body temperature differs with menstrual cycle phase. Women with ovulatory menstrual cycles show an increase in average daily body temperature of approximately 0.3° to 0.4° C after ovulation (luteal phase), due to the thermogenic action of progesterone secreted from the corpus luteum.[58,71-74] With the exception of two studies,[58,75]

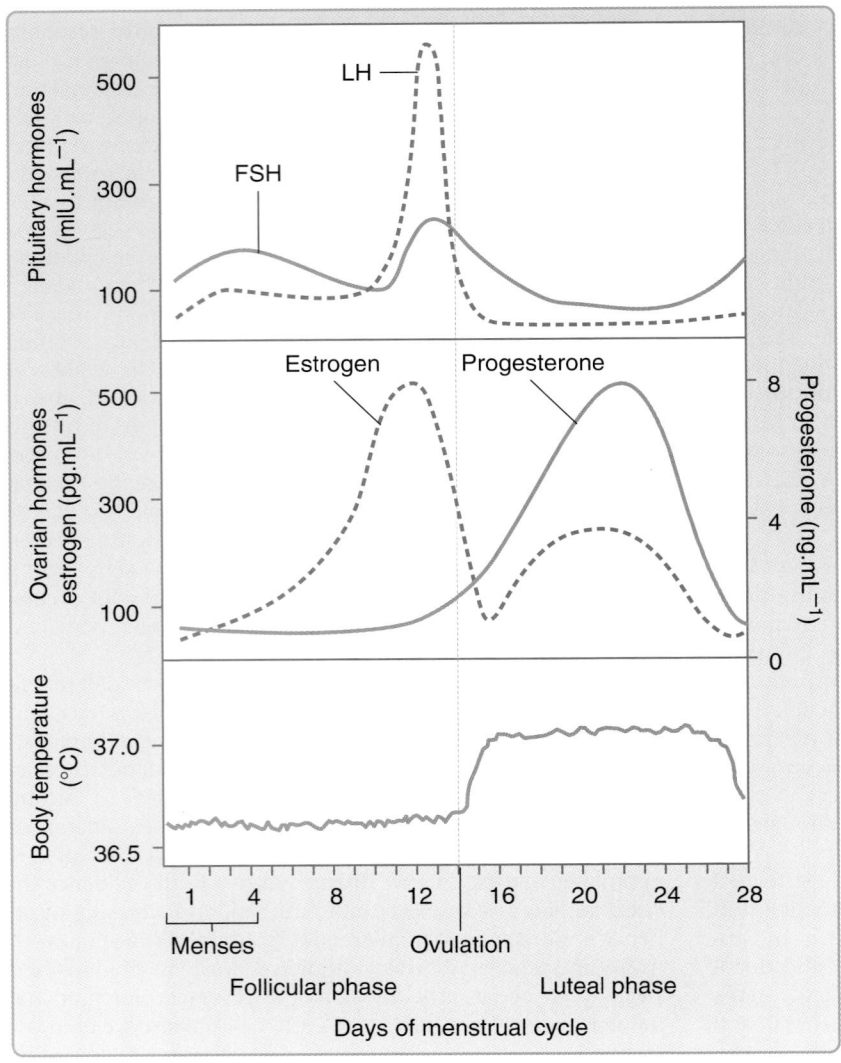

Figure 108–1. Mean daily plasma concentrations of estradiol, progesterone, follicle-stimulating hormone (FSH) and luteinizing hormone (LH), and basal body temperature throughout a "typical" 28-day ovulatory menstrual cycle. (Adapted from Pocock G, Richards CD: Human Physiology: The Basis of Medicine. New York, Oxford University Press, 1999, p 450.)

most studies[71-74,76] have found that the nocturnal decline in body temperature is blunted, reducing the circadian amplitude in the luteal phase compared with the follicular phase. Amplitude of the circadian body temperature rhythm is negatively related to the progesterone-to-estradiol ratio.[72]

Most researchers have not found a change in the time of the minimum (nadir) or maximum (acrophase) temperature associated with menstrual phase, although there are some conflicting reports in the literature.[72] There also is no difference in melatonin onset or offset, duration, or acrophase of the melatonin rhythm between the follicular and luteal phases of the menstrual cycle in young women, on the basis of studies that used either a constant routine protocol[75] or a multiple nap, ultradian routine.[76] However, the amplitude of the melatonin rhythm may become blunted in the luteal phase compared with the follicular phase.[76] With similar dampening of amplitudes for cortisol, thyroid-stimulating hormone, and body temperature, these findings suggest that amplitude of the endogenous oscillator of the circadian pacemaker is blunted after exposure to ovulatory hormones.[76] Indeed, the presence of progesterone and estrogen receptors in the suprachiasmatic nuclei of the hypothalamus[5] suggests the possibility that progesterone and estrogen may influence circadian rhythmicity directly. Studies are still needed in larger groups of women and with more frequent sampling during the menstrual cycle to firmly establish menstrual cycle effects on circadian rhythmicity of temperature and hormone release.

Shift Work and Menstrual Rhythms

Limited research shows that altered circadian rhythms—by shift-work schedules, for example—affect reproductive function in women. Female shift workers have more menstrual cycle irregularities, painful menstruation (dysmenorrhea), and longer menstrual cycles than non–shift workers.[77-79] Also, shift-work nurses who report changes in menstrual function, compared with those who do not, report significantly more sleep disturbances, symptoms of shift-work intolerance, and longer sleep onset latencies, suggesting an association between sleep disturbances and menstrual irregularities.[79] Reproductive health problems associated with shift work could be caused by increased stress as well as disrupted rhythms in secretion of hormones, particularly LH and follicle-stimulating hormone, that directly influence ovarian hormone secretion.[79]

Sleep Complaints during the Menstrual Cycle

Female reproductive hormones, particularly the ovarian hormones progesterone and estrogen, influence sleep, and some of the most important findings are discussed here.[8,80-82] Women (age 18 to 35) report more sleep disturbances during the premenstrual week and during the first few days of menstruation than at other times. A poll conducted by the National Sleep Foundation[52] found that 71% of 514 menstruating women in the United States reported that their sleep was affected by menstrual symptoms, such as bloating and tender breasts, on an average of 2.5 days every month. In menstruating women, subjective sleep disturbances are most evident in the late luteal phase compared with the mid-follicular phase, regardless of whether these women report premenstrual symptoms.[83,84] Studies that have investigated sleep objectively with EEG measures have found variable menstrual cycle phase

effects on sleep that do not always corroborate findings from subjective sleep studies. One reason for the inconclusive findings in objective sleep studies is the daunting methodologic challenges facing the researcher when studying sleep during the menstrual cycle in young women.[85,86] Factors that need to be considered include the presence and timing of ovulation, the identification of menstruation-associated disorders, sampling times during the menstrual cycle, and sample size. Individual studies have generally been performed on a small number of women (less than 10) and at selected phases of the menstrual cycle.[87]

Sleep EEG Changes across the Menstrual Cycle

The main findings from PSG sleep studies using EEG in young women who are at different phases of the menstrual cycle are summarized in Table 108–3. Contrary to subjective sleep assessments, most studies have found that sleep onset latency (time from "lights out" to stage 1 or stage 2 sleep) and sleep efficiency remain stable at different phases of the menstrual cycle in young women. Studies have found variable effects of menstrual cycle phase on SWS.[88,89] Baker and colleagues[90] increased statistical power by combining data from 20 women with normal menstrual cycles from three different studies and found no difference in sleep onset latency, SWS latency, or amount of SWS or stage 2 sleep between the mid-follicular and mid-luteal phases of the menstrual cycle.

Discrete recordings during the menstrual cycle may not detect variations in sleep that occur as a function of the continuous nature of the menstrual cycle. The only over-the-cycle study of sleep included nine healthy young women with normal ovulatory menstrual cycles who spent every other night in the laboratory throughout one ovulatory menstrual cycle, and neither the time course of SWS nor slow wave delta activity changed across the menstrual cycle.[91] Interestingly, EEG activity in the 14.25- to 15.0-Hz band, which corresponds to the upper frequency range of sleep spindles, was increased during the luteal phase compared with other phases of the menstrual cycle,[91] an effect also reported by others.[92] The increased spindle frequency activity is reminiscent of the effects of the progesterone metabolite allopregnanolone on the EEG in rats,[93] and it may represent an interaction between endogenous progesterone metabolites and gamma-aminobutyric acid-A ($GABA_A$) membrane receptors in the luteal phase.[91] Benzodiazepines and barbiturates also exert their sedative effects by binding to the $GABA_A$ receptor, but probably at a different site from that to which progesterone metabolites bind.[94,95]

SWS and sleep continuity are often considered markers of sleep homeostasis.[96] Taken together, findings of no change in sleep onset latency, overall sleep efficiency, wakefulness after sleep onset, or SWS support the conclusion that sleep homeostasis is maintained across the menstrual cycle in young healthy women.

REM sleep, however, is influenced by the menstrual cycle (see Table 108–3). Women have a shorter REM onset latency and a small decrease in the amount of REM sleep in the luteal phase compared with the follicular phase.[90,91,97] Women with ovulatory cycles also have a shorter REM onset latency in the luteal phase than women with anovulatory cycles.[98] In the absence of ovulation, women do not secrete sufficient ovarian hormones or increase their core body temperature and thus do not experience a true luteal phase in the 2 weeks prior to menses.

Variation in REM sleep during the menstrual cycle may be related to altered circadian processes. During the luteal phase of the menstrual cycle, higher core temperature or the dampened amplitude of the temperature rhythm may lower the threshold for earlier REM sleep onset.[97] However, REM sleep was inhibited by experimentally induced increases in body temperature,[99] ovariectomized female rats had more REM sleep than intact rats,[100] and cycling rats had less REM sleep in the presence of progesterone.[101]

In conclusion, sleep is remarkably stable across the normal menstrual cycle, despite the large changes in hormone milieu. There are, however, some changes in sleep, most notably an increase in spindle frequency activity and a small decrease in REM sleep in the luteal phase compared with the follicular phase. It is therefore essential for researchers to consider menstrual cycle phase in sleep studies that include young women. Menstrual cycle–related changes in sleep may manifest more in older women and in women with menstrual cycle–associated pain or mood changes, as discussed in the following paragraph.

Sleep in Women with Menstrual Cycle Disorders

A small proportion of women experience drastic changes in sleep behavior associated with their menstrual cycles, such as severe hypersomnia or a premenstrual night or two of insomnia[81,83] to the extent that they are classified as having a sleep disorder.[102] Other women who suffer from a menstrual cycle–associated disorder also may experience more marked changes in sleep during the menstrual cycle than do women without any menstrual complaints.

Polycystic Ovary Syndrome

Polycystic ovary syndrome (PCOS) is one of the most common reproductive endocrine disorders, occurring in approximately

Table 108–3.	Polysomnographic Sleep Studies in Women across the Menstrual Cycle		
Menstrual Cycle Status (Number of Women)	**Protocol**	**Luteal Phase Compared with Follicular Phase**	**Reference (Chronological)**
Presumed ovulatory (7, of whom 3 were psychiatric patients)	1 night/wk for 3 mo	↑ REM (trend) with large variance	Hartmann (1966)[110]
Presumed ovulatory (3)	2 nights each phase for 3 menstrual cycles: premenstrual (late luteal), menses, early follicular	↑ Variability stage 3 onset latency ↑ SWS premenstrually	Henderson et al. (1970)[128]
Ovulatory (3) Amenorrhea (3)	Just before/after menses Estrogen peak Night after ovulation High progesterone	TST and SWS varied, but not correlated with hormone levels	Billiard and Passouant (1972)[88]
Presumed ovulatory (3) Possible PMS (1)	8 nights in one menstrual cycle	No menstrual phase effect **PMS vs controls:** ↓ SWS and ↑ stage 2	Cluydts and Visser (1980)[111]
Ovulatory (8) Moderate PMS (8)	2 nights/wk in one menstrual cycle Early and late follicular Early and late luteal	↓ Stage 3 (trend) and ↑ WASO trend late luteal phase **PMS vs controls:** ↑ Stage 2 and ↓ REM	Parry et al. (1989)[113]
Ovulatory (6) PMS (7) On OC (3)	2 nights in each phase: Follicular (days 3-10)* Luteal (3-12 days after ovulation)	↓ REM onset latency **PMS vs controls:** ↑ Stage 2 and ↓ SWS	Lee et al. (1990)[97]
Ovulatory, based on body temperature (7)	Every 3rd night for one menstrual cycle	↓ SWS	Ito et al. (1993)[89]
Ovulatory (5)	3 nights/wk for one menstrual cycle	↑ Spindle frequency 3 days before menstruation	Ishizuka et al. (1994)[92]
Ovulatory (9)	Every other night for one menstrual cycle	↑ Stage 2 and spindle frequency ↓ REM (trend)	Driver et al. (1996)[91]
Ovulatory (6) PMS (3)	Follicular (day 8) Periovulation (day 15) Late luteal (day 25)	No menstrual phase or PMS effect	Chuong et al. (1997)[112]
Ovulatory (8) Dysmenorrhea (10)	1 night in each phase: Follicular (days 7-10) Luteal (5 or 6 days after ovulation) Menstruation (day 1)	↓ REM **Dysmenorrheics vs controls:** ↓ Sleep efficiency (menstruation) ↓ REM (all phases)	Baker et al. (1999)[119]

Continued

Table 108-3.   Polysomnographic Sleep Studies in Women across the Menstrual Cycle—Cont'd

Menstrual Cycle Status (Number of Women)	Protocol	Luteal Phase Compared with Follicular Phase	Reference (Chronological)
Ovulatory (9) PMDD (14)	1 baseline night each phase: Follicular (days 6-10) Late luteal (2-4 days before menstruation)	↓ REM ↑ REM latency ↑ Stage 1 **PMDD vs controls:** No significant differences	Parry et al. (1999)[117]
Ovulatory (22) Anovulatory (12)	2 nights at home each phase: Follicular (days 4-10) Luteal (days 16-25)	↓ REM both groups **Anovulatory vs ovulatory:** ↑ Wake and ↑ REM latency	Lee et al. (2000)[98]
Ovulatory (8)	48 ten-min naps during a 26-hr ultra-short sleep–wake schedule: Follicular (days 5-8) Late luteal (3-5 days before menstruation)	↑ SWS-containing naps	Shibui et al. (2000)[76]
Ovulatory (8) On OCs (8) Men (8)	1 night each phase: Mid-follicular (days 7-10) Mid-luteal (5-6 days after ovulation)	Women with ovulatory cycles: ↓ Stage 3 latency ↓ REM (trend)	Baker et al. (2001)[58]
Ovulatory (9) On OCs (10)	1 night each phase: Mid-follicular (days 7-10) Mid-luteal (5-6 days after ovulation)	Women with ovulatory cycles: ↑ SWS (trend)	Baker et al. (2001)[122]
Ovulatory (16, including 8 women with dysmenorrhea)	1 night each phase: Mid-follicular (days 7-10) Mid-luteal (5-6 days after ovulation)	↓ REM ↑ SWS **Dysmenorrheics vs controls:** No significant differences	Baker et al. (2002)[120]

*Day 1 is defined as the first day of menstruation.

OCs, oral contraceptives; PMS, premenstrual syndrome; PMDD, premenstrual dysphoric disorder; REM, rapid eye movement sleep; SWS, slow wave sleep (delta deep sleep, stages 3/4); TST, total sleep time; WASO, wake after sleep onset.

Modified from Driver HS, Baker FC: Menstrual factors in sleep. Sleep Med Rev 1998;2:213-229.

4% of women of childbearing age.[103] The theca cell hyperplasia evident in PCOS results in excessive ovarian androgen production, and follicle-stimulating hormone becomes suppressed while LH pulses become faster and of higher amplitude throughout the menstrual cycle.[104] The high androgen secretion in women with PCOS predisposes them to insulin resistance. Furthermore, obesity occurs in approximately 50% of cases.[105] The combination of obesity, excess androgen production, and insulin resistance places women with PCOS at increased risk for sleep-disordered breathing (SDB) as well as hypertension and cardiovascular disease. Indeed, women with PCOS were found to be 30 times more likely to suffer from SDB than controls.[106] Obesity is an important risk factor for SDB, but even when compared with healthy age- and weight-matched controls, women with PCOS are more likely to have SDB during their reproductive years[106,107] and are more likely to report excessive daytime sleepiness (80%) than healthy women (27%), even after controlling for body weight.[107] PCOS can be a useful model for understanding common mechanisms involved in SDB, insulin and glucose metabolism, and risks of cardiovascular disease in a young female population.

Sleep and Circadian Rhythm Alterations in Women with Major Depression

Depressive disorders during the menstrual cycle are referred to as premenstrual dysphoric disorder (PMDD) in the Diagnostic and Statistical Manual of Mental Disorders (DSM).[108] A large-scale study[109] found that women with premenstrual depression reported more hypersomnia than insomnia. The earliest PSG study was done in four healthy women and three inpatients with depression or schizophrenia taking multiple medications, including oral contraceptives, Dexedrine, and Prolixin.[110] They were studied once a week across three menstrual cycles; REM sleep (minutes and percent) was increased in the premenstrual period and correlated with severity of "premenstrual tension" symptoms.

More recent controlled studies have found other differences in sleep EEG measures between asymptomatic and symptomatic women (see Table 108–3).[111-114] Women who met DSM criteria for premenstrual depression had a higher percentage of stage 2 sleep and less REM sleep than controls, whereas SWS and number of awakenings varied with phase of the menstrual cycle.[113] During the luteal phase, symptomatic women also tend to have an earlier nadir and blunted amplitude in their core body temperature rhythm that improves after sleep deprivation.[114] They also have low melatonin levels and a shorter duration of melatonin secretion during the night in the luteal phase of their menstrual cycle.[114] Parry et al.[114] also found that women with premenstrual dysphoric disorder (PMDD) have more resistance to circadian phase shifting in response to bright light therapy.[115]

For women with PMDD, sleep deprivation during the symptomatic luteal menstrual cycle phase may be therapeutic. Eight of 10 women responded to sleep deprivation in one study and maintained improved mood after a night of recovery sleep.[116] In responders, subsequent late-night sleep deprivation was more effective than early-night deprivation. In a follow-up study, mood continued to improve after recovery sleep, but late-night deprivation did not have a greater benefit than early-night deprivation.[116] Although there were no group differences in sleep EEG measures during baseline follicular or luteal phases, both those with PMDD and controls had longer REM onset latencies and less REM sleep in their luteal phase than in their follicular phase. Women with PMDD had better sleep quality and improved mood during recovery nights compared with controls. REM sleep measures were also normalized in association with clinical improvement in women who responded to the sleep deprivation therapy.[117]

Primary Dysmenorrhea

Primary dysmenorrhea is painful menstruation in the absence of visible pelvic pathology, and it occurs in as many as 50% of young women.[118] The painful menstrual cramps experienced every month reduce productivity and work quality, and disrupt personal and family lives.[118] Unlike women with PMDD, women with dysmenorrhea do not necessarily experience physical or emotional symptoms premenstrually. One study has investigated the effect of dysmenorrheic pain using sleep PSG.[119] Women with primary dysmenorrhea had a lower sleep efficiency (because of increased time spent awake, movement activity, and stage 1 light sleep) and a poorer subjective sleep quality when they were suffering from menstrual pain compared with the pain-free phases of the menstrual cycle, and compared with women without menstrual pain.

Improvements in sleep, possibly with the aid of analgesics to alleviate the pain, may positively impact mood and productivity in these women. Interestingly, the women with dysmenorrhea also showed signs of altered sleep and temperature in the mid-luteal phase before the onset of pain; these women had reduced REM sleep and raised nocturnal body temperatures compared with women with normal menstrual cycles,[119] although this finding was not replicated in a subsequent study.[120] Primary dysmenorrhea not only may be a disorder of menstruation but may manifest itself at pain-free phases of the menstrual cycle.

Oral Contraceptives, Body Temperature, and Sleep

Many women control their menstrual cycles artificially using oral contraceptives. Oral contraceptives are combined formulations of a low-dose progestin and a synthetic estrogen and, unlike other commonly prescribed drugs, they are taken by healthy women for long periods of time.[121] Oral contraceptives suppress endogenous reproductive hormones and therefore prevent ovulation so that women taking these preparations do not have normal cycles. Women taking oral contraceptives are often used as control subjects in physiology studies because their reproductive hormone status is stable. However, oral contraceptives themselves influence body temperature and sleep.

Women taking oral contraceptives containing estrogen and a progestin have elevated rectal temperatures and raised circadian body temperature profiles, with temperature minimums occurring at a similar time as in ovulating women in the luteal phase.[58,71,75,122] Surprisingly, during the 7-day placebo period of the oral contraceptive pack, 24-hour body temperatures remain elevated,[122] suggesting that continuous use of synthetic reproductive steroids may have long-term influences on thermoregulation. Oral contraceptives also may influence melatonin levels, although findings are inconsistent.[75,123-126] In one study involving a constant routine procedure, researchers found no significant differences in melatonin levels between naturally cycling women and women taking oral contraceptives, although there was a trend in this small sample for increased melatonin levels in the latter part of the night in women taking oral contraceptives.[75]

Sleep is altered by oral contraceptives. Consistently, studies have found that women taking oral contraceptives have less SWS than do women with natural menstrual cycles.[58,122,127,128] Stage 2 sleep is significantly increased in women while taking active oral contraceptives compared with the placebo pills, and compared with naturally cycling women in both menstrual cycle phases.[122] Other sleep effects reported in oral contraceptive users include a shorter REM onset latency,[97,127] a shorter sleep onset latency, and more REM sleep[127] than in women with natural menstrual cycles. Exogenous steroid hormones therefore appear to influence sleep differently from endogenous progesterone and estrogen. These differences may be a consequence of the greater potency of synthetic steroids[129] as well as the sustained sex steroid hormone concentrations in women taking oral contraceptives as opposed to the cyclical variations that occur in reproductive hormones over the natural menstrual cycle.[122]

Clinical Pearls

There is strong evidence for neurophysiologic and neuroanatomic sex differences in sleep, particularly with maturation. The finding of progesterone and estrogen receptors in the hypothalamus suggests that these hormones may influence circadian rhythmicity and sleep patterns directly. They may also affect immune function.[130] Sex differences in sleep and rhythms may be risk factors for neurologic, immunologic, and psychiatric disease, and the relationship between sleep and psychological health and behavior appears to be strongly influenced by sex. Women are likely to experience a decrease in sleep quality before and during menstruation compared with other phases of their menstrual cycle, and compared with ovulating women, those taking oral contraceptives have less SWS, the deep stages of sleep thought to be restful and restorative.

References

1. Hendricks JC, Lu S, Kume K, et al: Gender dimorphism in the role of cycle (BMAL1) in rest, rest regulation, and longevity in *Drosophila melanogaster*. J Biol Rhythms 2003;18:12-25.

2. Engstrom BE, Karlsson A, Wide L: Gender differences in diurnal growth hormone and epinephrine values in young adults during ambulation. Clin Chem 1999;45:1235-1239.

3. Behan M, Zabka AG, Mitchell GS: Age and gender effects on serotonin-dependent plasticity in respiratory motor control. Respir Physiol Neurobiol 2002;131:65-77.

4. Kirschbaum C, Kudielka BM, Gaab J, et al: Impact of gender, menstrual cycle phase, and oral contraceptives on the activity of the hypothalamus-pituitary-adrenal axis. Psychosom Med 1999;61:154-162.

5. Swaab DF, Chung WCJ, Kruijver FPM, et al: Sex differences in the hypothalamus in the different stages of human life. Neurobiol Aging 2003;24:S1-S16.

6. Fang J, Fishbein W: Sex differences in paradoxical sleep: Influences of estrus cycle and ovariectomy. Brain Res 1996;734:275-285.

7. Lee KA, McEnany G, Weekes D: Gender differences in sleep patterns for early adolescents. J Adolesc Health 1999;24:16-20.

8. Manber R, Armitage R: Sex steroids and sleep: A review. Sleep 1999;22:540-555 [errata, 2000;23:145-149].

8a. Dzaja A, Arber S, Hislop J, et al: Women's sleep in health and disease. J Psychiatr Res 2005;39:55-76.

9. Anders TF, Kenner M: Developmental course of nighttime sleep-wake patterns in full-term and premature infants during the first year of life. Sleep 1985;8:173-192.

10. Jacklin CN, Snow ME, Gahart M, et al: Sleep pattern development from 6 through 33 months. J Pediatr Psychol 1980;5:295-303.

11. Bes F, Schulz H, Navelet Y, et al: The distribution of slow-wave sleep across the night: A comparison for infants, children, and adults. Sleep 1991;14:5-12.

12. Bes F, Fagioli I, Peirano P, et al: Trends in electroencephalographic synchronization across nonrapid eye movement sleep in infants. Sleep 1994;17:323-328.

13. Eiselt M, Schendel M, Witte H, et al: Quantitative analysis of discontinuous EEG in premature and full-term newborns during quiet sleep. Electroencephalogr Clin Neurophysiol 1997;103:528-534.

14. Witte H, Putsche P, Eiselt M, et al: Analysis of the interrelations between a low-frequency and a high-frequency signal component in human neonatal EEG during quiet sleep. Neurosci Lett 1997;236:175-179.

15. Bach V, Telliez F, Leke A, et al: Gender-related sleep differences in neonates in thermoneutral and cool environments. J Sleep Res 2000;9:249-254.

16. Moss HA, Robson KS: The relation between the amount of time infants spend at various states and the development of visual behavior. Child Devel 1970;41:509-517.

17. Cornwell AC: Sex differences in the maturation of sleep/wake patterns in high risk for SIDS infants. Neuropedia 1993;24:8-14.

18. Hoppenbrouwers T, Hodgman J, Arakawa K, et al: Polysomnographic sleep and waking states are similar in subsequent siblings of SIDS and control infants during the first six months of life. Sleep 1989;12:265-276.

19. Rivkees SA: Mechanisms and clinical significance of circadian rhythms in children. Curr Opin Pediatr 2001;74:160-171.

20. McGraw K, Hoffmann R, Harker C, et al: The development of circadian rhythms in a human infant. Sleep 1999;22:303-310.

21. Armitage R, Hoffmann R, Emslie G, et al: Rest-activity cycles in childhood and adolescent depression. J Am Acad Child Adolesc Psychiatry 2004;43:761-769.

22. Kleitman N: Sleep and Wakefulness, Chicago, University of Chicago Press, 1963.

23. Williams R, Karacan I, Hursch C: Electroencephalography of Human Sleep: Clinical Applications. New York, Wiley, 1974.

24. Coble PA, Reynolds CF III, Kupfer DJ, et al: Electroencephalographic sleep of healthy children: Part II. Findings using automated delta and REM sleep measurement methods. Sleep 1987;10:551-562.

25. Ferri R, Pettinato S, Alicata F, et al: Correlation dimension of EEG slow-wave activity during sleep in children and young adults, Electroencephalogr Clin Neurophysiol 1998;106:424-428.

26. Carskadon MA, Harvey K, Duke P, et al: Pubertal changes in daytime sleepiness. Sleep 1980;25:453-460.

27. Carskadon MA, Orav EJ, Dement WC: Evolution of sleep and daytime sleepiness in adolescents. In Guilleminault C, Lugaresi E (eds): Sleep/Wake Disorders: Natural History, Epidemiology, and Long-Term Evolution. New York, Raven Press, 1983, pp 201-216.

28. Carskadon MA, Acebo C: Regulation of sleepiness in adolescents: Update, insights and speculation. Sleep 2002;25:606-614.

29. Strauch I, Meier B: Sleep need in adolescents: A longitudinal approach. Sleep 1988;11:378-386.

30. Meijer AM, Habekothé HT, Van den Wittenboer GLH: Time in bed, quality of sleep and school functioning of children. J Sleep Res 2000;9:145-153.

31. Quine L: Sleep problems in primary school children: Comparison between mainstream and special school children. Child Care Health Dev 2001;27:201-221.

32. Sadeh A, Raviv A, Gruber R: Sleep patterns and sleep disruptions in school-age children. Dev Psychol 2000;36:291-301.

33. Acebo C, Millman RP, Rosenberg C, et al: Sleep, breathing and cephalometrics in older children and young adults: Part I. Normative values. Chest 1996;109:664-672.

34. Bader G, Neveus T, Kruse S, et al: Sleep of primary enuretic children and controls. Sleep 2002;25:579-583.

35. Palm L, Elmqvist D, Blennow D: Automatic versus visual EEG sleep staging in preadolescent children. Sleep 1989;12:150-156.

36. Villa MP, Piro S, Dotta A, et al: Validation of automated sleep analysis in normal children. Eur Respir J 1998;11:458-461.

37. Park YM, Matsumoto K, Shinkoda H, et al: Age and gender difference in habitual sleep-wake rhythm. Psychiatry Clin Neurosci 2001;55:201-202.

38. Sadeh A, Gruber R, Raviv A: Sleep, neurobehavioral functioning, and behavior problems in school-age children. Child Dev 2002;73:405-417.

39. Thorleifsdottir B, Bjornsson JK, Benediktsdottir B, et al: Sleep and sleep habits from childhood to young adulthood over a 10-year period. J Psychosom Res 2002;53:529-537.

40. Armitage R, Hoffmann R, Fitch T, et al: Temporal characteristics of delta activity during NREM sleep in depressed outpatients and healthy adults: group and sex effects. Sleep 2000;23:607-617.

41. Armitage R, Hoffmann R, Trivedi M, et al: Slow-wave activity in NREM sleep: Sex and age effects in depressed outpatients and healthy controls. Psychiatry Res 2000;95:201-213.

42. Lewis K, Hoffmann R, Emslie G, et al: REM sleep architecture in depressed children and adolescents. Sleep 2003;26(Suppl):A128.

43. Giannotti F, Cortesi F, Sebastiani T, et al: Circadian preference, sleep and daytime behaviour in adolescence. J Sleep Res 2002;11:191-199.

44. Laberge L, Petit D, Simard C, et al: Development of sleep patterns in early adolescence. J Sleep Res 2001;10:59-67.

45. Choquet M, Tesson F, Stevenot A: Les adolescents et leur sommeil: Approche epidemiologique. Neuropsychiatrie Enfant Adolescent 1988;36:399-410.

46. Kirmil-Gray K, Eagleston JR, Gibson E, et al: Sleep disturbance in adolescents: Sleep quality, sleep habits, beliefs about sleep and daytime functioning. J Youth Adolesc 1984;13:375-384.

47. Price VA, Coates TJ, Thoresen CE, et al: Prevalence and correlates of poor sleep among adolescents. Am J Dis Child 1978;132:583-586.

48. Bixler EO, Kales A, Jacoby JA, et al: Nocturnal sleep and wakefulness: Effects of age and sex in normal sleepers. Int J Neurosci 1984;23:33-42.

49. Rediehs MH, Reis JS, Creason NS: Sleep in old age: Focus on gender differences. Sleep 1990;13:410-424.

50. Sakakibara S, Kohsaka M, Kobayashi R, et al: Gender differences in self-evaluated sleep quality and activity of middle-aged and aged subjects. Psychiatry Clin Neurosci 1998;52:184-186.

51. Middelkoop HA, Smilde-van den Doel DA, Neven AK, et al: Subjective sleep characteristics of 1,485 males and females aged 50-90: effects of sex and age, and factors related to self-evaluated quality of sleep. J Gerontol A Biol Sci Med Sci 1996; 51A:M108-115.

52. National Sleep Foundation: The National Sleep Foundation's 1998 Women and Sleep Poll. Washington, DC, The National Sleep Foundation, 1998.

53. Reyner A, Horne JA: Gender- and age-related differences in sleep determined by home-recorded sleep logs and actimetry from 400 adults. Sleep 1995;18:127-134.

54. Huupponen E, Himanen SL, Varri A, et al: A study on gender and age differences in sleep spindles. Neuropsychobiology 2002;45:99-105.

55. Armitage R, Roffwarg HP: Distribution of period-analyzed delta activity during sleep. Sleep 1992;15:556-561.

56. Dijk DJ, Beersma DG, Bloem GM: Sex differences in the sleep EEG of young adults: Visual scoring and spectral analysis. Sleep 1989;12:500-507.

57. Mourtazaev MS, Kemp B, Zwinderman AH, et al: Age and gender affect different characteristics of slow waves in the sleep EEG. Sleep 1995;18:557-564.

58. Baker FC, Waner JI, Vieira EF, et al: Sleep and 24-hour body temperatures: A comparison in young men, naturally cycling women, and in women taking hormonal contraceptives. J Physiol 2001;530:565-574.

59. Ehlers CL, Kupfer DJ: Slow-wave sleep: Do young adult men and women age differently? J Sleep Res 1997;6:211-215.

60. Carrier J, Land S, Buysse DJ, et al: The effects of age and gender on sleep EEG power spectral density in the middle years of life (ages 20-60 years old). Psychophysiology 2001;38:232-242.

61. Armitage R, Hoffmann R: Sleep EEG, depression and gender. Sleep Med Rev 2001;5:237-246.

62. Armitage R, Smith C, Thompson S, et al: Sex differences in slow-wave activity in response to sleep deprivation. Sleep Res Online 2001;4:33-41.

63. Rhodes ME, Rubin RT: Functional sex differences ("sexual diergism") of central nervous system cholinergic systems, vasopressin, and hypothalamic-pituitary-adrenal axis activity in mammals: A selective review. Brain Res Rev 1999;30:135-152.

64. Van Cauter E, Leproult R, Kupfer DJ: Effects of gender and age on the levels and circadian rhythmicity of plasma cortisol. J Clin Endocrinol Metab 1996;81:2468-2473.

65. Waldstreicher J, Duffy JF, Brown EN, et al: Gender differences in the temporal organization of prolactin (PRL) secretion: Evidence for a sleep-independent circadian rhythm of circulating PRL levels—A clinical research center study. J Clin Endocrinol Metab 1996;81:1483-1487.

66. Schmidt PJ, Raju J, Danaceau MA, et al: The effects of gender and gonadal steroids on the neuroendocrine and temperature response to m-chlorophenylpiperazine in leuprolide-induced hypogonadism in women and men. Neuropsychopharmacology 2002;27:800-812.

67. Campbell SS, Gillin JC, Kripke DF, et al: Gender differences in the circadian temperature rhythms of healthy elderly subjects: Relationships to sleep quality. Sleep 1989;12:529-536.

68. Moe KE, Prinz PN, Vitiello MV, et al: Healthy elderly women and men have different entrained circadian temperature rhythms. J Am Geriatr Soc 1991;39:383-387.

69. Wever RA: Sex differences in human circadian rhythms: Intrinsic periods and sleep fractions. Experientia 1984;40:1226-1234.

70. Pocock G, Richards CD: Human Physiology: The Basis of Medicine. New York, Oxford University Press, 1999, p 450.

71. Lee KA: Circadian temperature rhythms in relation to menstrual cycle phase. J Biol Rhythm 1988;3:255-263.

72. Cagnacci A, Arangino S, Tuveri F, et al: Regulation of the 24h body temperature rhythm of women in the luteal phase: Role of gonadal steroids and prostaglandins. Chronobiol Int 2002; 19:721-730.

73. Kattapong K, Fogg L, Eastman C: Effect of gender, menstrual cycle phase and hormonal contraceptive use on circadian body temperature rhythms. Chronobiol Int 1995;12:257-266.

74. Coyne MD, Kesick CM, Doherty TJ, et al: Circadian rhythm changes in core temperature over the menstrual cycle: Method for noninvasive monitoring. Am J Physiol Regul Integr Comp Physiol 2000;279:R1316-1320.

75. Wright KP, Badia P: Effects of menstrual cycle phase and oral contraceptives on alertness, cognitive performance, and circadian rhythms during sleep deprivation. Behav Brain Res 1999;103:185-194.

76. Shibui K, Uchiyama M, Okawa M, et al: Diurnal fluctuation of sleep propensity and hormonal secretion across the menstrual cycle. Biol Psychiatry 2000;48:1062-1068.

77. Lee KA: Prevalence of perimenstrual symptoms in employed women. Women's Health 1991;17:17-32.

78. Messing K, Saurel-Cubizolles MJ, Bourgine M, Kaminski M: Menstrual-cycle characteristics and work conditions of workers in poultry slaughterhouses and canneries. Scand J Work Environ Health 1992;18:302-309.

79. Labyak S, Lava S, Turek F, Zee P: Effects of shiftwork on sleep and menstrual function in nurses. Health Care Women Int 2002;23:703-714.

80. Driver HS, Baker FC: Menstrual factors in sleep. Sleep Med Rev 1998;2:213-229.

81. Moline ML, Broch L, Zak R, Gross V: Sleep in women across the life cycle from adulthood through menopause. Sleep Med Rev 2003;7:55-177.

82. Shaver JLF: Women and sleep. Nurs Clin North Am 2002; 37:707-718.

83. Manber R, Bootzin RR: Sleep and the menstrual cycle. Health Psychol 1997;6:209-214.

84. Baker FC, Driver HS: Self-reported sleep across the menstrual cycle in young, healthy women. J Psychosom Res 2004;56:239-243.

85. Metcalf M: Incidence of ovulation from the menarche to the menopause: Observations of 622 New Zealand women. N Z Med J 1983;96:645-648.

86. Leibenluft E, Fiero PL, Rubinow DR: Effects of the menstrual cycle on dependent variables in mood disorder research. Arch Gen Psychiatry 1994;51:761-781.

87. Gardner K, Sanders D: Premenstrual syndrome. In McPherson A, Waller D (eds): Women's Health, 4th ed. New York, Oxford University Press, 1997, pp 280-302.

88. Billiard M, Passouant P: Sleep study in women. In Sleep: Physiology, Biochemistry, Psychology, Pharmacology and Clinical Implications (First European Congress on Sleep Research). Basel, Karger, 1972, pp 395-399.

89. Ito M, Kohsaka M, Fukuda N, et al: Effects of menstrual cycle on plasma melatonin level and sleep characteristics. Jpn J Psychiatry Neurol 1993;47:478-479.

90. Baker FC, Mitchell D, Driver HS: Sleep in the follicular and luteal phases of the menstrual cycle. Actas Fisiología 2001;7:154.

91. Driver HS, Dijk DJ, Werth E, et al: Menstrual cycle effects on sleep EEG in young healthy women. J Clin Endocrinol Metab 1996;81:728-735.

92. Ishizuka Y, Pollak CP, Shirakawa S, et al: Sleep spindle frequency changes across the menstrual cycle. J Sleep Res 1994;3:26-29.

93. Damianisch K, Rupprecht R, Lancel M: The influence of sub-chronic administration of the neurosteroid allopregnanolone on sleep in the rat. Neuropsychopharmacology 2001;25:576-584.

94. Lancel M: Role of GABA$_A$ receptors in the regulation of sleep: Initial sleep responses to peripherally administered modulators and agonists. Sleep 1999;22:33-42.

95. Concas A, Follesa P, Barbaccia ML, et al: Physiological modulation of GABA$_A$ receptor plasticity by progesterone metabolites. Eur J Pharmacol 1999;375:225-235.

96. Dijk DJ, Cajochen C, Tobler I, Borbély AA: Sleep extension in humans: Sleep stages, EEG power spectra and body temperature. Sleep 1991;14:294-306.

97. Lee KA, Shaver JF, Giblin EC, Woods WF: Sleep patterns related to menstrual cycle phase and premenstrual affective symptoms. Sleep 1990;13:403-439.

98. Lee KA, McEnany G, Zaffke ME: REM sleep and mood state in childbearing women: Sleepy or weepy? Sleep 2000;23:877-885.

99. Baker FC, Selsick H, Driver HS, et al: Different nocturnal body temperatures and sleep with forced-air warming in men and in women taking hormonal contraceptives. J Sleep Res 1998;7:175-181.

100. Li H, Satinoff E: Body temperature and sleep in intact and ovariectomized female rats. Am J Physiol 1996;271:R1753-1758.

101. Schwierin B, Borbély A, Tobler I: Sleep homeostasis in the female rat during the estrous cycle. Brain Res 1998;811:96-104.

102. Diagnostic Classification Steering Committee, Thorpy MJ (Chairman): The International Classification of Sleep Disorders: Diagnostic and coding manual. Rochester, Minn, American Sleep Disorders Association, 1990.

103. Guzick DS: Polycystic ovary syndrome. Obstet Gynecol 2004;103:181-193.

104. Waldstreicher J: Hyperfunction of the hypothalamic-pituitary axis in women with polycystic ovarian disease: Indirect evidence for partial gonadotroph desensitization. J Clin Endocrinol Metab 1988;66:165-172.

105. Dunaif A: Insulin resistance and the polycystic ovary syndrome: Mechanism and implications for pathogenesis. Endocr Rev 1997;18:774-800.

106. Vgontas NA, Legro RS, Bixler EO, et al: Polycystic ovary syndrome is associated with obstructive sleep apnea and daytime sleepiness: Role of insulin resistance. J Clin Endocrin Metab 2001;86:517-520.

107. Gopal M, Duntley S, Uhles M, Attarian H: The role of obesity in the increased prevalence of obstructive sleep apnea syndrome in patients with polycystic ovarian syndrome. Sleep Med 2002;3:401-404.

108. American Psychiatric Association: Diagnostic and Statistical Manual for Mental Disorders, 4th ed. Washington, DC, American Psychiatric Press, 1994.

109. Halbreich U, Endicott J, Nee J: Premenstrual depressive changes: Value of differentiation. Arch Gen Psychiatry 1983;40:535-542.

110. Hartmann E: Dreaming sleep (the D-state) and the menstrual cycle. J Nervous Mental Dis 1966;143:406-416.

111. Cluydts R, Visser P: Mood and sleep: I. Effects of the menstrual cycle. Waking Sleeping 1980;4:193-197.

112. Chuong CJ, Kim SR, Taskin O, Karacan I: Sleep pattern changes in menstrual cycles of women with premenstrual syndrome: A preliminary study. Am J Obstet Gynecol 1997;177:554-558.

113. Parry BL, Mendelson WB, Duncan WC, et al: Longitudinal sleep EEG, temperature and activity measurements across the menstrual cycle in patients with premenstrual depression and in age-matched controls. Psychiatry Res 1989;30:285-303.

114. Parry BL, LeVeau B, Mostofi N, et al: Temperature circadian rhythms during the menstrual cycle and sleep deprivation in premenstrual dysphoric disorder and normal comparison subjects. J Biol Rhythms 1997;12:34-46.

115. Parry BL, Udell C, Elliott JA, et al: Blunted phase-shift responses to morning bright light in premenstrual dysphoric disorder. J Biol Rhythms 1997;12:443-456.

116. Parry BL, Cover H, Mostofi N, et al: Early versus late partial sleep deprivation in patients with premenstrual dysphoric disorder and normal comparison subjects. Am J Psychiatry 1995;152:404-412.

117. Parry BL, Mostofi N, LeVeau B: Sleep EEG studies during early and late partial sleep deprivation in premenstrual dysphoric disorder and normal control subjects. Psychiatry Res 1999;85:127-143.

118. Dawood MY: Dysmenorrhea. Clin Obstet Gynecol 1990;33:168-178.

119. Baker FC, Driver HS, Paiker J, Mitchell D: High nocturnal body temperatures and disturbed sleep in women with primary dysmenorrhea. Am J Physiol 1999;277:E1013-1021.

120. Baker FC, Rogers G, Paiker J, et al: Acetaminophen does not affect 24-hour body temperature nor sleep in the luteal phase of the menstrual cycle in young women. J Appl Physiol 2002;92:1684-1691.

121. Cerel-Suhl SL, Yeager BF: Update on oral contraceptive pills. Am Fam Physician 1999;60:2073-2084.

122. Baker FC, Mitchell D, Driver HS: Oral contraceptives alter sleep and raise body temperature in young women. Pflügers Arch 2001;442:729-737.

123. Brun J, Claustrat B, David M: Urinary melatonin, LH, oestradiol, progesterone excretion during the menstrual cycle or in women taking oral contraceptives. Acta Endocrinol 1987;116:145-149.

124. Delfs TM, Baars S, Fock C, et al: Sex steroids do not alter melatonin secretion in the human. Hum Reprod 1994;9:49-54.

125. Reinberg AE, Touitou Y, Soudant E, et al: Oral contraceptives alter circadian rhythm parameters of cortisol, melatonin, blood pressure, heart rate, skin blood flow, transepidermal water loss, and skin amino acids of healthy young women. Chronobiol Int 1996;13:199-211.

126. Webley GE, Leidenberger F: The circadian pattern of melatonin and its positive relationship with progesterone in women. J Clin Endocrinol Metab 1986;63:323-328.

127. Burdick RS, Hoffmann R, Armitage R: Short note: Oral contraceptives and sleep in depressed and healthy women. Sleep 2002;25:347-349.

128. Henderson A, Nemes G, Gordon NB, Roos L: The sleep of regularly menstruating women and of women taking an oral contraceptive. Psychophysiology 1970;7:337.

129. Rogers SM, Baker MA: Thermoregulation during exercise in women who are taking hormonal contraceptives. Eur J Appl Physiol 1997;75:34-38.

130. Moldofsky H, Lue FA, Shahal B, et al: Diurnal sleep/wake-related immune functions during the menstrual cycle of healthy young women. J Sleep Res 1995;4:150-159.

109

Pregnancy and the Postpartum Period

Amy R. Wolfson

Kathryn A. Lee

ABSTRACT

Pregnancy and the postpartum period are times in a woman's life when sleep patterns are greatly disturbed. Hormonal changes in the first trimester, the large fetus and anxiety about labor and delivery during the third trimester, and a newborn with unpredictable sleep patterns in the postpartum period contribute to her poor sleep. The incidence and types of sleep disorders during the perinatal period remain unknown, but any complaint of excessive sleepiness and fatigue should be pursued and evaluated by health care providers because of potential harm to the fetus or newborn.

Many women experience considerable daytime sleepiness and fatigue as a result of disrupted sleep as they transition through their pregnancies into the first few postpartum months. Additionally, some women develop specific sleep disorders such as restless legs syndrome (RLS), sleep apnea, and insomnia during pregnancy, and others may develop postpartum depression. Complaints of heartburn and leg cramps increase during pregnancy and need to be taken seriously because of the potential for severe sleep deprivation for the mother if heartburn progresses to severe nocturnal esophageal reflux, or if leg cramps are undifferentiated from severe RLS. Evaluation of sleep disorders and depression should be a part of routine antepartum and postpartum assessments. Occurrence of sleep apnea and RLS has been associated with adverse pregnancy outcomes; therefore, particular attention should be given to complaints of leg movements, to overweight women who become obese during pregnancy, and to those who develop complications of pregnancy such as preeclampsia.

Pharmacologic options for sleep disorders and disturbances should be viewed with caution during pregnancy and during lactation, not only because of the risk to fetal and newborn development but also particularly in relationship to the dosage of hypnotics and anesthetics with their potentiating effects on the high endogenous levels of progesterone during pregnancy. During the first prenatal visit, health care providers should stress the importance of adequate uninterrupted sleep and provide anticipatory guidance regarding fatigue and sleepiness to women as early in the pregnancy as possible, and they should continue to do so throughout the postpartum months. Childbirth educators should also address the importance of adequate sleep during the postpartum period.

Sleep disruption has been discussed among pregnant and postpartum women themselves for centuries. Yet, it was not until the late 1960s that researchers began to describe specific alterations in sleep patterns during pregnancy and after birth. Although it is a challenge for researchers to study sleep during pregnancy, sleep becomes much more difficult to study during postpartum recovery and the first few months after birth. Although study designs and measures may differ (e.g., sleep laboratory studies, home monitoring, self-report questionnaires, actigraphy, observations, and clinical interviews), sleep during pregnancy has been a focused area of research during the last decade, and consistent results are summarized in this chapter. However, sleep disturbance during the postpartum period and its effects on maternal role functioning and maternal–infant interactions are not well understood. Confounding factors such as type of delivery, type of infant feeding, infant temperament, return-to-work issues, and availability of nighttime support from the father of the baby or from other members of the family can all have an impact on quality and quantity of sleep in new mothers, especially until the infant begins to sleep through the night.

In this chapter, we discuss the sleep changes that occur during pregnancy. The impact of childbirth on sleep, and sleep patterns during the early months of motherhood are discussed. Common sleep disorders during pregnancy are reviewed, and the use of medications for sleep during pregnancy and lactation are discussed. Conclusions are presented within the context of sleep and circadian rhythm disturbances for childbearing women, and the implications for maternal role functioning and maternal–infant interaction are discussed.

PHYSIOLOGIC CHANGES DURING PREGNANCY AND THE POSTPARTUM PERIOD

Increasing levels of placental hormones over the course of pregnancy influence sleep both directly and indirectly, and the abrupt drop in these hormone levels after the birth of the placenta may affect a new mother's sleep as much as the 24-hour care she provides for her newborn. During the first 12 weeks of pregnancy, many hormonal changes promote implantation and gestation, and the increases in secretion of placental estrogen, progesterone, and prolactin are dramatic.[1,2] Early on, increased progesterone levels may be soporific, and feelings of sleepiness or fatigue may be a woman's first symptom of pregnancy. The experience of first-trimester nausea and urinary frequency can influence sleep, but it is not until the growing uterus begins to press on a woman's bladder and her breasts enlarge and become tender that sleep becomes much more fragmented. Late in the third trimester, the high level of progesterone and the elevated diaphragm contribute to an increased rate of breathing and complaints of feeling short of breath. In addition, the enlarged uterus pressing on the bladder reduces bladder capacity and increases urinary frequency. As a result of the growing fetus, the intestines and esophageal

Table 109–1.   Sleep Changes Typical during Pregnancy and Postpartum

First Trimester	Second Trimester	Third Trimester	Postpartum
High levels of progesterone from placenta (20-30 ng/mL)	Progesterone levels rise, but more slowly (50-100 ng/mL)	Progesterone levels peak (300-400 ng/mL)	No progesterone No estrogen Prolactin levels fluctuate with lactation
More difficulty sleeping through the night due to increased urinary frequency	Sleep less disrupted by urinary frequency More daytime energy	Sleep disturbances due to leg cramps, heartburn, nasal congestion, and increased need to urinate	Sleep disrupted due to infant care and feeding Sleep more disrupted for first-time mothers than for experienced mothers Breast-feeding mothers awake longer during the night than formula-feeding mothers
Daytime sleepiness Daytime fatigue	Snoring may begin Risk of sleep apnea Risk of hypertension	Increased daytime sleepiness Increased fatigue Difficulty with sleeping positions	Increased daytime sleepiness More opportunity to nap if not employed outside the home
Morning or evening nausea		Discomfort due to irregular uterine contractions, shortness of breath, and breast tenderness	Risk of postpartum depression
Tend to sleep more than prior to pregnancy	More wake time during the night	More wake time during the night Possible RLS and PLM	Tendency to sleep later into the morning hours Issues of co-sleeping and bed sharing emerge
Less SWS	Less SWS	Less SWS	Increased SWS

PLM, periodic leg movements; RLS, restless legs syndrome; SWS, slow wave sleep.

sphincter are displaced, causing esophageal reflux and complaints of heartburn. Leg cramps also become a frequent occurrence. The first pregnancy experience has more of an impact on a woman's postpartum sleep than subsequent pregnancies[3] (Table 109–1).

SLEEP DURING PREGNANCY

Karacan and colleagues[4] conducted one of the first clinical studies of sleep during pregnancy and compared seven women during the last month of pregnancy to age-matched nonpregnant women. The two groups spent about the same amount of time in bed trying to sleep, but the pregnant women had less total sleep. Although pregnant women frequently report sleep complaints to their obstetrician, it has been only in the last decade that studies of sleep during pregnancy have been more systematic and with larger samples of women.

Pregnancy affects a woman's sleep both physiologically and psychologically.[4a] Women report that sleep is interrupted during the first trimester by nausea, vomiting, backaches, and the increased need to urinate.[5] In the second trimester, women also report that they are awakened by fetal movements and heartburn; however, they frequently note that their sleep is improved from the first trimester and that they have more energy during the day. During the third trimester, sleep is disrupted because of urinary frequency, backaches, shortness of breath, and leg cramps.[5,6] The uterus itself may begin to contract, but in a disorganized manner (Braxton-Hicks contractions) until such time as true labor begins with forceful contractions

that are regularly spaced and signify the onset of labor. Although these reasons for disturbed sleep disappear with the birth of the infant, they are replaced with maternal caregiving activities and the newborn's schedule of frequent feedings that can be as often as every 2 to 3 hours around the clock.

Polysomnographic studies indicate more wake after sleep onset as pregnancy progresses, resulting in lower sleep efficiency compared with nonpregnant women.[4,7-13] Sleep architecture is also altered during pregnancy, but study results conflict because of small samples. The amount of time spent in rapid eye movement (REM) sleep either remains the same or decreases slightly as the pregnancy progresses, but this may depend on whether REM sleep is reported as an absolute number of minutes or as a percentage of total sleep time.[13-16] Changes in amount of REM sleep, latency to the first REM sleep period, and amount of slow wave sleep (SWS) are unclear.[17-19]

First Trimester (Months 1 to 3)

Although there are individual differences in women's pregnancies, the majority of women report more fatigue, daytime sleepiness, and night awakenings during their first trimester.[8] Sleep begins to change as early as the tenth week of gestation. Progesterone's soporific and sedating effect potentiates any central nervous system depressant medication such as anesthetics or analgesics, its thermogenic effect results in increased body temperature, and its inhibitory effect on smooth muscle acts on the urinary tract to cause frequent urination.

Second Trimester (Months 4 to 6)

Many women report that they are relieved to move into the second trimester, as sleep improves at night and they report more daytime energy.[8] As women transition into the second trimester, progesterone levels continue to rise, but more slowly. The growing fetus begins to move above the bladder, and many women no longer need to urinate as frequently. Both subjective and objective sleep parameters are better during this trimester, but about 30% report onset of snoring that did not exist prior to pregnancy[5,6,18]; snoring is an indication of increased congestion in the nasal passages resulting from estrogen's effects on vascular tissue. As discussed later, pregnant women who snore may be at risk of preeclampsia (pregnancy-induced hypertension) and sleep apnea syndrome. Further changes in SWS and REM sleep architecture during the second trimester may also occur, but results are not consistent in these small samples.[4,8-16]

Third Trimester (Months 7 to 9)

The quality of sleep in the last trimester is worse than during the first two trimesters.[20,21] Women report sleep problems and feel physically uncomfortable. Leg cramps increase from about 20% during the first trimester to 75% in the third trimester.[22,23] Many women also describe longer sleep onset latencies, more awakenings, less total sleep, and increasing levels of morning sleepiness over the course of the third trimester.[5,6] In one study, women were particularly bothered in the last few weeks of pregnancy by not being able to find a comfortable position for sleep (70%), by waking up frequently to use the bathroom (nearly 85%), by feeling too hot or perspiring (nearly 45%), and by their baby's movements (nearly 40%).[5] Carpal tunnel pain, heartburn, and bad dreams also occur,[6] and up to 20% of pregnant women develop restless legs syndrome during their third trimester[23,24] (see "Leg Cramps, Periodic Limb Movements, and Restless Legs Syndrome," later section).

Overall, both cross-sectional and longitudinal studies conclude that pregnant women have more awake time during the night as a result of the many symptoms and physical changes that occur over the 9 months of gestation. In contrast, changes in sleep architecture seem to be minimal. REM sleep, however, either remains unchanged or diminishes slightly from the first trimester to the third trimester, and changes in the amount of SWS remain inconclusive.[17-19] More studies, however, document less SWS over the course of pregnancy.[3,4,8,11-13] It appears that more frequent or longer wake episodes during the sleep period have little effect on REM sleep but result in less SWS and total sleep time.[7-16]

CIRCADIAN RHYTHMS AND PREGNANCY

Several hormones have a circadian rhythm that may change over the course of pregnancy and affect sleep architecture.[18] The hormones include growth hormone, prolactin, melatonin, cortisol, thyroid-stimulating hormone, and placental hormones (progesterone, estriol).[1] As mentioned earlier, estrogen and progesterone progressively increase during pregnancy and are thought to be responsible for the increase in the basal levels of prolactin that rapidly increase between 25 weeks gestation and term. Estrogen is known to decrease REM sleep, but the placental form of estrogen (estriol) is much weaker than the ovarian source.[1] Progesterone, on the other hand, has a sedating effect in both men and women when exogenously administered, and it appears to increase non-REM sleep,[25,26] but the circadian rhythms of both estrogen and progesterone have not been described in pregnant women. Prolactin secretion associated with meals and sleep is similar in pregnant and in nonpregnant women[27] (see also Chapter 22), but the basal level rapidly declines during active labor and peaks again for up to 6 hours after vaginal delivery. This dramatic fluctuation in prolactin is not seen in elective cesarean births.[28-30]

Cortisol concentrations continue to peak in the early morning hours, but the half-life of cortisol is prolonged during pregnancy and levels increase twofold in late pregnancy and fourfold during labor.[31] Pregnant women who report sleeping poorly in the third trimester may have lower cortisol-to-melatonin ratios than good sleepers because of a lower early morning cortisol peak and a higher concentration of melatonin.[32] Although less studied in humans, melatonin secretion does not seem to change over the course of pregnancy or during labor and delivery.[18,33] Additionally, uterine activity peaks at night along with peaks in oxytocin secretion and may explain the increased incidence of labor and delivery during the evening and night.[18,31-34]

LABOR AND DELIVERY

Sleep quality diminishes as women approach labor,[4,35] yet very little research has been done to examine the effect of sleep disturbance on labor and delivery outcomes. Common clinical practice has involved administration of morphine sulfate to women in the early and nonprogressing latent phase of labor to induce sleep and reduce uterine contractions by reducing epinephrine levels,[36] and the laboring patient typically awakens from the sleep period with more regular and active labor contractions.

As mentioned earlier, prolactin secretion is affected by the type of delivery. During active labor, there is a precipitous drop in blood levels of prolactin, beginning about 4 hours prior to birth, that reaches a nadir about 2 hours before delivery. At delivery, there is a dramatic spike in prolactin levels that lasts for 4 to 6 hours, at which time levels return to their normal circadian secretory pattern.[30] Infants who are delivered by elective cesarean birth, rather than emergency cesarean or vaginal delivery, have a significantly lower prolactin level in their umbilical venous plasma.[37] After an emergency cesarean delivery, women fail to experience the rise in prolactin levels typically seen about 30 minutes after the onset of breastfeeding during the first few postpartum days.[38]

There appears to be no relationship between sleep quality and quantity and any adverse birth outcomes.[18,35] For the most part, maternal sleep efficiency is poor on the first night after delivery but begins to improve over the following days.[4,39] Being in labor during the night may be related to depressed mood during the first week after delivery[40] (see "Postpartum Depression," later).

SLEEP DURING POSTPARTUM RECOVERY

Postpartum recovery is generally defined as the first 6 months after delivery. It is interesting that maternity leave for employed women is typically only 6 weeks, whereas in actuality, most women would say that the postpartum period continues from birth until the infant is sleeping through the night with predictable day and night sleeping patterns.[41] In the early postpartum days, there is a rapid decline in all placental hormones, and 35% to 80% of women experience postpartum distress or blues approximately 3 to 5 days after birth. For most women, the blues are confined to the first 2 weeks after childbirth, but a major episode of postpartum depression can occur at any time during the first 6 months after childbirth.[41] About 20% of women develop depression in the postpartum period, a prevalence that is similar to that of women at other stages of life (see "Postpartum Depression," later).

Both self-report and actigraphy studies have demonstrated that nearly 30% of mothers have disturbed sleep after the birth of their baby and that they experience more nighttime awakenings because of disruptions during the initial postpartum weeks (2 to 4 weeks) in comparison to the end of pregnancy and later postpartum months.[5,13,15,42-44] Although total sleep time may change little over this period, a mother's sleep is far more disrupted and less efficient during these early postpartum weeks than at other points in her life. Women seem to compensate for their sleep disruptions by spending more time napping and sleeping later in the morning during the first postpartum month.[5,13,44,45] Compared with early in postpartum recovery, awake and arise times occur earlier at 3 to 4 postpartum months and at 12 to 15 postpartum months,[5] presumably because women are returning to work.

Researchers have also examined changes in fatigue and lack of energy from pregnancy into the postpartum period, as well as through the year after delivery, through self-report and physiologic measures such as progesterone levels, thyroid functioning, and iron or other nutrient deficiencies.[8,46-48] On the basis of these studies, nulliparas and multiparas do not differ significantly in their perception of fatigue. However, 3 to 6 weeks after delivery is especially fatiguing for first-time mothers, and fatigue levels remain high at 3 postpartum months compared with prepregnancy reports.[8,47-50] Postpartum fatigue is associated with reduced sleep time, low hemoglobin, and low levels of ferritin.[8] When these measures are taken together, researchers conclude that the level of progesterone is unrelated to fatigue and that social factors, such as employment and family responsibilities, influence perception of fatigue during the postpartum period.[8,50]

A small number of studies have described sleep architecture in the postpartum period. It appears that mothers, regardless of the number of children, have a significant increase in SWS and less stage 1 and stage 2 sleep (light sleep) at 1 postpartum month.[3,8-13,18] This may be caused in part by the action of prolactin (see the following section).

Breast-Feeding and Formula Feeding

Self-reported sleep disturbance and perception of fatigue are unrelated to type of infant feeding, whereas wrist actigraphy measures document more wake time during the night in women who are exclusively breast-feeding at 3 to 4 weeks after the birth.[45,51,52] During the first 2 weeks after birth, REM sleep is stable for women who are breast-feeding, but it gradually decreases for women who are not lactating.[15]

For lactating women, basal levels of prolactin are high and there is a burst of prolactin secretion at the onset of each breast-feeding event, regardless of when sleep occurs, but the bursts seem to be of a higher magnitude in the evening compared with morning.[53] Both basal levels and bursts diminish to prepregnancy levels by about 3 postpartum months. The effect of lactation on sleep patterns of mothers and infants has not been a focus of research, but Blyton and coworkers[54] studied women in their home environment with portable polysomnography, and the lactating women had less stage 1 and stage 2 light sleep, fewer arousals, and more SWS, especially in the second half of the night, compared with nonlactating postpartum women. There was no difference in the amount of REM sleep or total sleep time between the two groups.[54] Within 24 hours of weaning, prolactin levels return to low basal levels and to the circadian sleep-associated patterns found in healthy adults.[55]

Bed Sharing and Co-Sleeping

Although few studies have examined the relationship between bed sharing and mothers' sleep–wake patterns, parent–infant bed sharing and co-sleeping have become increasingly common during the postpartum period.[56-60] The proportion of bed-sharing infants rose from 5.5% in 1993-1994 to 12.8% in 1999-2000.[60] Bed sharing is defined as an infant sleeping in the same bed with the caregiver, whereas co-sleeping means that the infant sleeps in the same room as, and in close proximity to, a parent or caregiver, but does not necessarily occupy the same bed. Some studies suggest that bed sharing reduces the risk of sudden infant death syndrome because the bed-sharing infant has more arousals due to the mother's body heat, sounds, oxygen and carbon dioxide exchange, smells, movement, and touch.[57] It has been postulated that infants are at risk for dying from sudden infant death syndrome because of their immature neurologic systems and difficulty arousing from sleep to breathe.[57] However, greater risks for bed-sharing infants may be posed by the presence of pillows, comforters, soft surfaces, and multiple bodies, particularly obese adults.[56]

Bed-sharing mothers report disrupted, inefficient sleep. In a polysomnographic study, Mosko and colleagues[56] demonstrated that bed sharing had no effect on REM sleep, but that it increased the number of arousals and modestly reduced SWS, and that it increased stage 1 and stage 2 light sleep in breast-feeding women. Bed sharing is not necessarily associated with breast-feeding practices or with household crowding.[59] Because the trend for infant bed sharing is on the rise and may be more commonly practiced among low-income women,[59,60] the impact of bed sharing or co-sleeping on the sleep–wake patterns of the new mother and father, as well as on the infant's sleep, requires further investigation.

PREGNANCY AND POSTPARTUM HEALTH PROBLEMS ASSOCIATED WITH DISTURBED SLEEP

Several sleep disorders, such as sleep-disordered breathing, periodic limb movements, esophageal reflux, or restless legs syndrome, can be triggered or worsened by pregnancy.[17-19] Although the timing, symptoms, and occurrence of these sleep disorders may vary, they are most prevalent during the third trimester. Pharmacologic treatment for sleep problems during pregnancy and during lactation is of great concern because of potential effects on fetal development and on the

Table 109–2. Drug Use Related to Sleep during Pregnancy and Lactation*

Class B† Low Risk	Class C Some Risk	Class D High Risk
Hypnotics		
Diphenhydramine Zolpidem	Clonazepam Zaleplon	Alcohol (ethanol) Alprazolam Diazepam Lorazepam Midazolam Secobarbital
Antidepressants		
Sertraline	Fluoxetine Paroxetine Trazodone Venlafaxine	Amitriptyline Imipramine
Dopaminergics		
—	Carbamazepine Carbidopa Levodopa	—
Opioids		
Meperidine Oxymorphone	Codeine Morphine	—
Stimulants		
Caffeine Pemoline	Dextroamphetamine Methamphetamine Mazindol Modafinil	—

*Dosages should begin with half of the lowest recommended dosage due to increased sensitivity; lactating women should consider alternatives to breastfeeding due to unknown long-term effects on newborn growth and neurodevelopment.

†Classes:
  Class A: Fetal harm is remote. There are no class A drugs in any category listed.
  Class B: There is no risk seen in animal studies, but human studies not done, or risk in animals is documented but no risk to fetus in controlled human studies.
  Class C: Animal studies document teratogenic effects, but no studies done in women.
  Class D: Risk to fetus is present, but use in pregnancy may outweigh risk of serious danger or disease to mother.
  Class X: Studies demonstrate high risk for fetal abnormalities and drug is contraindicated for pregnant women. Class X hypnotic drugs include flurazepam, temazepam, and triazolam.

Adapted from Briggs GG, Freeman RK, Yaffe SJ (eds): Drugs in Pregnancy and Lactation. Philadelphia, Lippincott Williams & Wilkins, 2002.

newborn's growth and development. Table 109–2 contains a summary of common sleep-related medications and their ratings for potential harm to the fetus or newborn.[61]

Pregnancy-Induced Hypertension (Preeclampsia)

Pregnancy-induced hypertension (PIH), also known as preeclampsia or toxemia of pregnancy, is a disorder that occurs in about 5% to 10% of pregnancies.[62] First-time pregnancies, long intervals between pregnancies (over 10 years),

multiple pregnancies (twins or more), women younger than 20 or older than 35 years, or women who are overweight or have a history of hypertension, kidney disease, or diabetes are all at risk for PIH.[63] PIH is characterized by high blood pressure that has a flat circadian rhythm, without the nocturnal dip associated with sleep,[62] and proteinuria thought to be pathologically induced by an autoimmune maternal inflammatory response in the uterine spiral arteries.[64] Cytokines, plasma lipoproteins, and fatty acids are all elevated in PIH.[64] Symptoms include excessive edema, severe headaches, dizziness and nausea, blurred or double vision, and sleepiness.[62] Preeclampsia can progress to a life-threatening condition called eclampsia, which includes seizures and risk of coma and death of the mother and infant, or to the life-threatening HELLP syndrome characterized by hemolysis (H), elevated liver enzymes (EL), and low platelets (LP). To prevent seizures, drug therapy focuses on controlling the hypertension, but the only definitive treatment is the delivery of the fetus and placenta.

A small number of studies have investigated the effects of PIH on sleep.[62,63] PIH is associated with an increased incidence of periodic limb movements as well as significantly narrowed upper airways and limited airflow during sleep, most likely the result of mucosal and pharyngeal edema.[63,64] Women with PIH have significantly larger neck circumference than healthy pregnant women, and in one study 75% of women with PIH reported that they snored, compared with 28% of healthy pregnant women.[63] Because PIH is associated with restricted airflow and hypertension, frequent arousals from sleep are noted and, as a result, continuous positive airway pressure (CPAP) may improve sleep, reduce daytime sleepiness, and lower blood pressure and levels of uric acid in women with PIH.[62] Although CPAP did not change the time spent in SWS or REM sleep,[62] it may extend gestation closer to full term and, unlike antihypertensive medications, CPAP does not appear to adversely affect the mother or fetus.

Snoring and Sleep-Disordered Breathing

During the normal course of pregnancy, increased respiratory rate is common because of the effects of progesterone, and shortness of breath is a common complaint during the third trimester, particularly when functional residual capacity is maximally reduced by about 20% before the fetus descends into the pelvis. Gas exchange is even more compromised in the supine position, and women often find it more comfortable to sleep in a sitting position for complaints of heartburn as well as dyspnea. Despite the potential for compromised pulmonary function, oxygen saturation levels remain stable during sleep in nonobese women. This is probably a result of the increased ventilatory drive effects of progesterone and the overall increase in minute ventilation.[65-67] Because these changes in lung function during normal pregnancy result in a state of respiratory alkalosis, with a higher pH of 7.44 at rest, there is a greater risk of hypoxemia and compromised oxygen delivery to the fetus, even during a very brief apneic event, if uterine blood flow is restricted by placental insufficiency or by positioning on the back and allowing the gravid uterus to compress the vena cava (supine hypotensive syndrome, or Posiero effect).

It is also during pregnancy when about 15% to 20% of women report a new onset of snoring, whereas fewer than 5%

report snoring prior to pregnancy.[67-69] The sound synonymous with snoring results from a blocked airway as a result of narrowed passages, and most likely is caused by the increased fluid volume during pregnancy and the effects of estrogen on vascular tissue, which result in congested nasal passages.[66]

In one recent retrospective survey, snoring was associated with higher blood pressure, and 10% of the pregnant snorers developed PIH compared with only 4% of nonsnoring women.[67] Infants born to the snoring mothers also had lower Apgar scores as well as higher risk of intrauterine growth retardation (7.1% versus 2.6%), but these findings have not been replicated in prospective studies.[68,69]

Although the changes in lung function during pregnancy can mimic a state of obesity, the overall distribution of adipose tissue is somewhat different in pregnancy, and the presence of high levels of progesterone may be protective against sleep-disordered breathing. Obese women who become pregnant, however, are at greater risk of sleep apnea. When obese women were compared with nonobese women at about 12 weeks and 30 weeks of gestation, the obese group had a lower level of progesterone level and more snoring.[70] Sleep-disordered breathing during early pregnancy was common in the obese group, and by 30 weeks' gestation, 50% of their sleep time was spent snoring, primarily during REM sleep. Only one of the 11 obese women developed PIH with mild obstructive sleep apnea, and one mother with oxygen saturation of less than 90% during 6% of her sleep time delivered a newborn who was small for gestational age, but all other infants were delivered without complications. At 30 weeks' gestation, both obese and nonobese pregnant women had about 30 minutes less total sleep time and more wakefulness during the night than they had at 12 weeks, but REM and SWS were not adversely affected.[70]

Studies have shown that overweight women who become pregnant, women who gain excessive weight, and women who report snoring during pregnancy should be evaluated for sleep-disordered breathing, because the hypoxic events associated with apnea may result in intrauterine growth retardation or other neonatal complications.[67,68,71] External nasal dilation may be effective in women who snore without apneic events,[72] but nasal CPAP (see Chapter 89) appears to have no adverse effects on the mother or fetus and is effective in treating sleep-disordered breathing during pregnancy.[73]

Leg Cramps and Restless Legs Syndrome

Over the course of pregnancy, about one in three women consistently reports episodes of jerkiness of the extremities while falling asleep, a rate that does not differ from prepregnancy or the postpartum period. However, those who experience awakenings during the night from leg cramps increase from a low of 8% to 10% before and after pregnancy to a rate of 12% to 21% during the first trimester, 49% to 57% during the second trimester, and 73% to 75% in the third trimester.[22,23]

Restless Legs Syndrome (RLS) (see Chapter 70) is rare in healthy young adult women. Because of its association with iron deficiency anemia, however, between 15% and 25% of women develop RLS during pregnancy.[23,24,74] Although the RLS symptoms typically reverse after delivery, it can be "torture" when added to all of the other discomforts and difficulty sleeping in the third trimester. The women most at risk are those with low folate levels or low ferritin and hemoglobin prior to conception. Even when taking vitamin and iron supplementation, fetal growth and red blood cell formation require so much folate and iron substrate that, beginning in the second trimester, levels of hemoglobin, ferritin, and vitamin B_{12} start to fall regardless of adequate dietary measures. Those who develop RLS, however, have lower folate levels even prior to pregnancy and are consistently lower throughout gestation than those who do not develop RLS.[23]

Women who received multivitamins with folate and iron during pregnancy did not develop RLS at the same rate as those who took only multivitamins with iron.[75] Most women who receive early prenatal care are counseled to begin taking prenatal vitamins with iron and folic acid early in their pregnancy to prevent fetal neural tube defects. Women should also be assessed early in pregnancy for risk of RLS. RLS is a reversible syndrome in pregnancy and is typically limited to the third trimester.

During the third trimester, when sleep is more disrupted and there is less total sleep time, pregnant women with RLS also experience a longer sleep onset latency, longer REM sleep onset latency, and more depressed mood than those without RLS.[23] Therefore, intervention is important even if the RLS is time limited. The standard medications for RLS that include dopaminergics or opioids, with potential risk to the fetus (see Table 109-2), should be avoided, and preventative measures should begin with encouraging folate-enriched breads and cereals at the first prenatal visit.

Postpartum Depression

Up to 50% to 60% of all new mothers experience a postpartum blues during the first 2 postpartum weeks. The blues manifest as excessive and unpredictable crying episodes and sadness during a time that should be quite joyful. At some point during the first 3 to 6 months after delivery, between 10% and 15% of new mothers experience diagnosable postpartum depression.[76,77] Symptoms of postpartum depression are similar to depression experienced at other times of life (see Chapter 112), but they also include difficulty sleeping when the baby sleeps and worrying about hurting the baby.[76] Various mechanisms for postpartum depression have been proposed, including the dramatic drop in progesterone and estrogen levels during the first few postpartum days,[77] poor supportive relationships, overly high expectations of the baby and motherhood, type of delivery, unexpected difficulties with labor and delivery or postpartum infant care, and a sudden shift in attention from the mother to the baby. However, these contextual variables have not been shown to be directly related to postpartum depression.[76,77]

One additional contextual variable that seems obvious but has previously been overlooked is sleep deprivation and disrupted sleep–wake cycles. Sleep deprivation is likely to contribute to postpartum mood changes.[4,11-16,51] Being in labor during the night and a prior history of sleep disruption at the end of pregnancy may result in a higher incidence of postpartum blues.[5,40] Specifically, one study reported that new mothers had increased dysphoric mood during the first postpartum week, but this significant effect was eliminated when the effect of "time awake" was controlled for in the analysis.[43] The frequency of night awakenings, rather than a change in hormone levels, was related to negative mood at 1 postpartum month, and REM sleep onset latency was significantly shorter (less than 60 minutes) for the postpartum women who reported higher levels of depressed mood.[14]

Moreover, mothers who develop elevated depressive symptoms at 2 to 4 postpartum weeks have significantly different sleep schedules at the end of their pregnancies compared with nondepressed mothers.[5] On average, mothers who developed postpartum depressive symptoms reported later rise times, longer naps, and more total sleep at the end of their pregnancies. Postpartum mothers' increased time awake during the night and poor sleep quality were strongly associated with increased negative daytime mood, or blues, particularly in the first 4 weeks after delivery.[5,15,37,51] Lee and colleagues[14] compared sleep patterns for women with positive postpartum affect at 1 postpartum month to women with negative postpartum affect. The positive mood group had stable sleep times from the last trimester to 1 postpartum month, whereas the negative mood group reported that they slept 80 minutes less at 1 postpartum month.[14]

Although Wolfson and coworkers[5] did not examine the data in this fashion, the women with clinically significant depressed mood at 2 to 4 postpartum weeks reported more changes in their sleep (e.g., decreased total sleep from the end of pregnancy to early postpartum weeks) than the nondepressed women. Future studies need to examine the impact of changes in sleep patterns from pregnancy to the early postpartum weeks on the possible development of postpartum depression.

Postpartum depression can have an impact on maternal–infant bonding as well as marital satisfaction and infant development.[78] A few women go on to develop postpartum psychosis, of which insomnia is one of the most frequent symptoms.[76-80] Although women with a history of mental illness are at increased risk for postpartum depression or postpartum psychosis, Coble and colleagues[11] followed women until their eighth postpartum month and found no differences in sleep architecture between those with a history of mental health problems and controls, and no woman in their study developed postpartum depression.

Women with major depression during pregnancy or the postpartum period were found to have more REM sleep than women without a pregnancy-related depressive episode,[81] suggesting a greater sleep-related risk for depression. However, in women with a history of mood disorder, less REM sleep was noted early in pregnancy and persisted even at 8 postpartum months in one study,[11] and REM sleep was not different during pregnancy or postpartum compared with matched controls.[82]

Because of the risks of antidepressant drug therapy to the fetus and to the newborn during breast-feeding (see Table 109–2), health care providers are hesitant to prescribe medications, and some women refuse pharmacologic therapy or have intolerable side effects that include sedation, disrupted sleep, or insomnia.[76,76a] For postpartum women, it is recommended that any drug therapy should start with half of the lowest recommended level and be increased slowly in small increments.[76] If drug therapy is not a reasonable option, REM sleep deprivation or light therapy may be useful to consider (see Chapters 112 and 121). Women with postpartum depression who were allowed to sleep only from 2100 to 0100 hours and kept awake during the second half of the night responded more favorably to this sleep deprivation therapy than women allowed to sleep from 0300 to 0700 hours.[82,83] Light treatment, or phototherapy, may be effective for depressive episodes during pregnancy, but there may be side effects such as nausea, premature birth, or a high rate of cesarean births,[84] and, as with any drug use in pregnancy, caution is warranted. During postpartum depressive episodes, light treatment may be effective if administered over weeks rather than days.[85]

Clinical Pearls

The cause of excessive sleepiness and fatigue in a pregnant woman should be determined because of potential harm to the fetus or newborn. Some pregnant women develop specific sleep disorders such as RLS, sleep apnea, or insomnia, and others may develop postpartum depression. Occurrence of sleep apnea or RLS has been associated with adverse pregnancy outcomes; therefore, particular attention should be given to complaints of leg movements, to overweight women who become obese during pregnancy, and to those who develop complications of pregnancy such as preeclampsia.

REFERENCES

1. Carsten ME: Endocrinology of pregnancy and parturition. In Hacker NF, Moore JG (eds): Essentials of Obstetrics and Gynecology. Philadelphia, WB Saunders, 1998, pp 76-84.
2. Sahota PK, Jain SS, Dhand R: Sleep disorders in pregnancy. Curr Opin Pulm Med 2003;9:477-483.
3. Lee KA, Zaffke ME, McEnany G: Parity and sleep patterns during and after pregnancy. Obstet Gynecol 2000;95:14-18.
4. Karacan I, Heine W, Agnew HW, et al: Characteristics of sleep patterns during late pregnancy and the postpartum periods. Am J Obstet Gynecol 1968;101:579-585.
4a. Dzaja A, Arber S, Hislop J, et al: Women's sleep in health and disease. J Psychiatr Res 2005;39:55-76.
5. Wolfson AR, Crowley S, Anwer U, et al: Changes in sleep patterns and depressive symptoms in first-time mothers: Last trimester to one-year postpartum. Behav Sleep Med 2003;1:54-67.
6. Baratte-Beebe KR, Lee K: Sources of midsleep awakenings in childbearing women. Clin Nurs Res 1999;8:386-397.
7. Hertz G, Fast A, Feinsilver SH, et al: Sleep in normal late pregnancy. Sleep 1992;15:246-251.
8. Lee KA, Zaffke ME: Longitudinal changes in fatigue and energy during pregnancy and the postpartum period. J Obstet Gynecol Neonatal Nurs 1999;28:183-191.
9. Brunner DP, Munch M, Biedermann K, et al: Changes in sleep and sleep electroencephalogram during pregnancy. Sleep 1994;17:576-582.
10. Driver HS, Shapiro CM: A longitudinal study of sleep stages in young women during pregnancy and postpartum. Sleep 1992;15:449-453.
11. Coble PA, Reynolds CF, Kupfer DJ, et al: Childbearing in women with and without a history of affective disorder: II. Electroencephalographic sleep. Compr Psychiatry 1994;35:215-224.
12. Karacan I, Williams RL, Hursch CJ, et al: Some implications of the sleep patterns of pregnancy for postpartum emotional disturbances. Br J Psychol 1969;115:929-935.
13. Nishihara K, Horiuchi S: Changes in sleep patterns of young women from late pregnancy to postpartum: Relationships to their infants' movements. Percept Mot Skills 1998;87:1043-1056.
14. Lee KA, McEnany G, Zaffke ME: REM sleep and mood state in childbearing women: Sleepy or weepy? Sleep 2000;23:877-884.
15. Petre-Quadens O, De Lee C: Sleep-cycle alterations during pregnancy, postpartum and the menstrual cycle. In Ferin M,

Halberg F, Richart RM, et al. (eds): Biorhythms and Human Reproduction. New York, John Wiley, 1974, 335-351.

16. Schorr SJ, Chawla A, Devidas M, et al: Sleep patterns in pregnancy: A longitudinal study of polysomnography recordings during pregnancy. J Perinatol 1998;6:427-430.

17. Lee K: Alterations in sleep during pregnancy and postpartum. Sleep Med Rev 1998;2:231-242.

18. Santiago JR, Nolledo MS, Kinzler W, et al: Sleep and sleep disorders in pregnancy. Ann Intern Med 2001;134:396-408.

19. Moline ML, Broch L, Zak R, et al: Sleep in women across the life cycle from adulthood through menopause. Sleep Med Rev 2003; 7:155-177.

20. Hedman C, Pohjasvaara T, Tolonen U, et al: Effects of pregnancy on mothers' sleep. Sleep Med 2002;3:37-42.

21. National Sleep Foundation: Women and Sleep Poll. Washington, DC, National Sleep Foundation, 1998.

22. Gupta MA, Schork NJ, Gay C: Nocturnal leg cramps in pregnancy: A prospective study of clinical features. Sleep Res 1992;21:294.

23. Lee KA, Zaffke ME, Baratte-Beebe K: Restless legs syndrome and sleep disturbance during pregnancy: The role of folate and iron. J Womens Health Gend Based Med 2001;10:335-341.

24. Goodman JDS, Brodie C, Ayida GA: Restless legs syndrome in pregnancy. BMJ 1998;297:1101-1102.

25. Little BC, Matta RJ, Zahn TP: Physiological and psychological effects of progesterone in man. J Nerv Ment Dis 1974;159: 256-262.

26. Friess E, Tagaya H, Trachsel L, et al: Progesterone-induced changes in sleep in male subjects. Am J Physiol 1997;272:885-891.

27. Spiegel K, Luthringer R, Follenius M, et al: Temporal relationship between prolactin secretion and slow-wave electroencephalic activity during sleep. Sleep 1995;18:543-548.

28. Quigley ME, Ishizuka B, Ropert JF, Yen SSC: The food-entrained prolactin and cortisol release in late pregnancy and prolactinoma patients. J Clin Endocrinol Metab 1982;54:1109-1112.

29. Boyar RM, Finkelstein JW, Kapen S, Hellman L: Twenty-four hour prolactin secretion pattern during pregnancy. J Clin Endocrinol Metab 1975;40:1117-1120.

30. Rigg LA, Yen SSC: Multiphasic prolactin secretion during parturition in human subjects. Am J Obstet Gynecol 1977;128: 215-218.

31. Cousins L, Rigg L, Hollingsworth D, et al: Qualitative and quantitative assessment of the circadian rhythm of cortisol in pregnancy. Am J Obstet Gynecol 1983;145:411-416.

32. Suziki S, Greenwood KM, Armstrong SM, et al: Melatonin and hormonal changes in disturbed sleep during late pregnancy. J Pineal Res 1993;15:191-198.

33. Kivela A, Kauppila A, Leppaluoto J, et al: Serum and amniotic fluid melatonin during human labor. J Clin Endocrinol Metab 1989;69:1065-1068.

34. Seron-Ferre M, Ducsay CA, Valenzuela GJ: Circadian rhythms during pregnancy. Endocr Rev 1993;14:594-609.

35. Evans ML, Dick MJ, Clark AS: Sleep during the week before labor: Relationships to labor outcomes. Clin Nurs Res 1995;4: 238-252.

36. Conklin KA: Obstetric analgesia and anesthesia. In Hacker NF, Moore JG (eds): Essentials of Obstetrics and Gynecology. Philadelphia, WB Saunders, 1998, 169-170.

37. Heasman L, Spencer JAD, Symonds ME: Plasma prolactin concentrations after caesarean section or vaginal delivery. Arch Dis Child Fetal Neonatal Ed 1997;77;F237-238.

38. Nissen E, Uvnas-Moberg K, Svensson K, et al: Different patterns of oxytocin, prolactin but not cortisol release during breastfeeding in women delivered by caesarean section or by the vaginal route. Early Hum Dev 1996;5:103-118.

39. Zaffke ME, Lee KA: Sleep architecture in a postpartum sample: A comparative analysis. Sleep Res 1992;21:327.

40. Wilke G, Shapiro CM: Sleep deprivation and the postnatal blues. J Psychosom Res 1992;36:309-316.

41. Wolfson AR: The Woman's Book of Sleep: A Complete Resource Guide. Oakland, Calif, New Harbinger, 2001.

42. O'Hara MW, Zekoski EM, Philipps LH: Controlled perspective study of postpartum mood disorders: Comparison of childbearing and nonchildbearing women. J Abnorm Psychol 1990;99:3-15.

43. Salazaro P: Long lasting disturbances in women after childbirth. J Reprod Infant Psychol 1987;5:245-246.

44. Swain AM, O'Hara MW, Starr KR, et al: A prospective study of sleep, mood, and cognitive function in postpartum and non-postpartum women. Obstet Gynecol 1997;90:381-386.

45. Gay CL, Lee KA, Lee S: Sleep patterns and fatigue in new mothers and fathers. Biol Res Nurs 2004;5:311-318.

46. Kang MJ, Matsumoto K, Shinkoda H, et al: Longitudinal study of sleep-wake behaviors of mothers from pre-partum to post-partum using actigraph and sleep logs. Psychiatry Clin Neurosci 2002;56:251-252.

47. Reeves N, Potempa K, Gallo A: Fatigue in early pregnancy: An exploratory study. J Nurse Midwifery 1991;36:303-309.

48. Elek SM, Hudson DB, Fleck MO: Expectant parents' experience with fatigue and sleep during pregnancy. Birth 1997;24:49-54.

49. Gjerdinger DK, Froberg DG, Chaloner KM, et al: Changes in women's physical health during the first postpartum year. Arch Fam Med 1993;2:277-283.

50. Troy NW: A comparison of fatigue and energy levels at 6 weeks and 14 to 19 months postpartum. Clin Nurs Res 1999;8:135-152.

51. Quillan SI: Infant and mother sleep patterns during 4th post-partum week. Issues Compr Pediatr Nurs 1997;20:115-123.

52. Wambach KA: Maternal fatigue in breastfeeding primiparae during the first 9 weeks postpartum. J Hum Lact 1998;14:219-229.

53. Noel GL, Suh HK, Frantz AG: Prolactin release during nursing and breast stimulation in postpartum and nonpostpartum patients. J Clin Endocrinol Metab 1974;38:413-423.

54. Blyton DM, Sullivan CE, Edwards N: Lactation is associated with an increase in slow-wave sleep in women. J Sleep Res 2002; 11:297-303.

55. Uvnas-Moberg K, Widstrom AM, Werner S, et al: Oxytocin and prolactin levels in breast-feeding women: Correlation with milk yield and duration of breast-feeding. Acta Obstet Gynecol Scand 1990;69:301-306.

56. Mosko S, Richard C, McKenna J: Maternal sleep and arousals during bedsharing with infants. Sleep 1997;20:142-150.

57. McKenna J, Mosko S, Richard C, et al: Experimental studies of infant-parent co-sleeping: Mutual physiological and behavioral influences and their relevance to SIDS (sudden infant death syndrome). Early Hum Dev 1994;38:187-201.

58. Okami P, Weisner T, Olmstead R: Outcome correlates of parent-child bedsharing: An eighteen-year longitudinal study. J Dev Behav Pediatr 2002;4:244-253.

59. Brenner RA, Simons-Morton BG, Bhaskar B, et al: Infant-parent bed sharing in an inner-city population. Arch Pediatr Adolesc Med 2003;157:33-39.

60. Willinger M, Ko C, Hoffman HJ, et al: Trends in infant bed sharing in the United States, 1993-2000. Arch Pediatr Adolesc Med 2003;157:43-49.

61. Briggs GG, Freeman RK, Yaffe SJ (eds): Drugs in Pregnancy and Lactation. Philadelphia, Lippincott Williams & Wilkins, 2002.

62. Edwards N, Blyton DM, Kirjavainen T, et al: Nasal continuous positive airway pressure reduces sleep-induced blood pressure increments in preeclampsia. Am J Respir Crit Care Med 2000; 162:252-257.

63. Izci B, Riha RL, Martin SE, et al: The upper airway in pregnancy and pre-eclampsia. Am J Respir Crit Care Med 2002;167:137-140.

64. Taylor RN, Roberts JM: Endothelial cell dysfunction. In Linhheimer MD, Roberts JM (eds): Chesley's hypertension disorders in pregnancy. Stamford, Conn, Appleton & Lange, 1999, pp 395-429.

65. Ekholm EM, Polo O, Rauhala ER, et al: Sleep quality in preeclampsia. Am J Obstet Gynecol 1992;167:1262-1266.

66. Edwards N, Middleton PG, Blyton DM, Sullivan CE: Sleep disordered breathing and pregnancy. Thorax 2002;57: 555-558.

67. Franklin KA, Holmgren PA, Jönsson F, et al: Snoring, pregnancy-induced hypertension, and growth retardation of the fetus. Chest 2000;117:137-141.

68. Loube DI, Poceta JS, Morales MC, et al: Self-reported snoring in pregnancy: Association with fetal outcome. Chest 1996;109: 885-889.

69. Guilleminault C, Querra-Salva M, Chowdhuri S, Poyares D: Normal pregnancy, daytime sleeping, snoring and blood pressure. Sleep Med 2000;1:289-297.

70. Maasilta P, Bachour A, Teramo K, et al: Sleep-related disordered breathing during pregnancy in obese women. Chest 2000;120: 1448-1454.

71. Schutte S, Del Conte A, Doghramji K, et al: Snoring during pregnancy and its impact on fetal outcome. Sleep Res 1994; 23:325.

72. Turnbull GL, Rundell OH, Rayburn WF, et al: Managing pregnancy-related nocturnal nasal congestion: The external nasal dilator. J Reprod Med 1996;41:897-902.

73. Guilleminault C, Kreutzer M, Chang JL: Pregnancy, sleep disordered breathing and treatment with nasal continuous positive airway pressure. Sleep Med 2004;5:43-51.

74. McParland P, Pearce JM: Restless legs syndrome in pregnancy: Case reports. Clin Exp Obstet Gynecol 1990;17:5-6.

75. Botez MI, Lambert B: Folate deficiency and restless legs syndrome in pregnancy (Letter). N Engl J Med 1977;297:670.

76. Wisner KL, Parry BL, Piontek CM: Postpartum depression. N Engl J Med 2002;347:194-199.

76a. Dennis CL, Stewart DE: Treatment of postpartum depression, part 1: A critical review of biological interventions. J Clin Psychiatry 2004;65:1242-1251.

77. Bloch M, Schmidt PJ, Danaceau M, et al: Effects of gonadal steroids in women with a history of postpartum depression. Am J Psychiatry 2000;157:924-930.

78. Weinberg MK, Tronick EZ: Emotional characteristics of infants associated with maternal depression and anxiety. Pediatrics 1998;102(Suppl E):1298-1304.

79. Sharma V, Mazmanian D: Sleep loss and postpartum psychosis. Bipolar Disord 2003;5:98-105.

80. Rohde A, Marneros A: Postpartum psychoses: Onset and long-term course. Psychopathology 1993;26:203-209.

81. Frank E, Kupfer DJ, Jacob M, et al: Pregnancy-related affective episodes among women with recurrent depression. Am J Psychiatry 1987;144:288-293.

82. Parry BL, Sorenson DL, Meliska CJ, et al: Hormonal basis of mood and postpartum disorders. Curr Sci 2003;3:230-235.

83. Parry BL, Curran ML, Stuenkel CA, et al: Can critically timed sleep deprivation be useful in pregnancy and postpartum depressions? J Affect Disord 2000;60:201-212.

84. Oren DA, Wisner KL, Spinelli M, et al: An open trial of morning light therapy for treatment of antepartum depression. Am J Psychiatry 2002;159:666-669.

85. Corral M, Kuan A, Kostaras D: Bright light therapy's effect on postpartum depression. Am J Psychiatry 2000;157:303-304.

110

Menopause

Karen E. Moe

ABSTRACT

Menopause is a normal event in a woman's life. It is the physiologic centerpiece of a major developmental stage in the normal aging process. Most women now live long enough to become menopausal. In 1998, there were more than 477 million postmenopausal women in the world; approximately 40 million live in the United States, and numbers are expected to increase with time because of longer life expectancy.

There is accumulating evidence that the hormonal and other biologic changes that comprise menopause may have health consequences for some women that extend beyond the classic reproductive tissues and functions. In particular, changes in sleep are commonly experienced during and after menopause. Insomnia and fatigue are among the most frequent health complaints of perimenopausal women, including those who are not seeking treatment for menopausal symptoms. This chapter discusses several clinical conditions commonly associated with menopause that may contribute to sleep disruption in midlife and older women. Hormone replacement therapy has been the treatment of choice for menopausal hot flashes and night sweats, and the effect of these therapies on sleep has been the focus of considerable research.

Sleep-disordered breathing is also more prevalent in women after menopause. This may be strongly related to other menopause-related changes, particularly the increased prevalence of obesity. Depression, thyroid disease, and cancer are also more common after menopause. This chapter provides an overview of menopause and discusses these common clinical conditions and their impact on women's sleep.

PHASES OF THE MENOPAUSAL TRANSITION

Menopause is the anchor point of a woman's transition to midlife and, because menstrual cycles can be irregular for many reasons, menopause can be declared only after 12 months of amenorrhea. Menopause occurs at a mean of 51.4 years of age for Western women, but the range can be as wide as 40 to 58 years of age. For many years, menopause was considered to be simply a consequence of the depletion of ovarian follicles (the primary source of estrogen and progesterone). However, it is now clear that transitional processes and events begin several years before menopause itself, and continue for several years after menopause. This perimenopausal developmental transition in a woman's life is a dynamic process that consists of a series of complex and interactive changes in the endocrine system and central nervous system.[1,2]

A menopause terminology and staging system has been developed to provide a consistent way of describing this transition in midlife women[3] (Fig. 110–1). The *early menopausal transition stage* is characterized by elevated follicle-stimulating hormone (FSH) and a variable cycle length (more than 7 days deviation from normal). FSH levels increase in response to the absence of estrogen and progesterone that would normally provide negative feedback to the hypothalamus to inhibit FSH secretion. The *late menopausal transition stage* is characterized by two or more skipped menstrual cycles and an interval of amenorrhea (at least 60 days) as well as elevated FSH levels. The postmenopausal period is also divided into stages. The *early postmenopause stage* is defined as 5 years since the final menstrual period, and is subdivided into two segments: (1) the first 12 months after the final menstrual period, and (2) the next 4 years. The *late menopause stage* begins with year 6 after the final menstrual period and continues through the remaining life span.

Menopause is a universal phenomenon, but the timing of these stages and associated signs and symptoms vary considerably from woman to woman. The age at which menopause occurs is strongly influenced by several factors: smoking, adiposity, race/ethnicity, and reproductive variables such as age at menarche, duration of breastfeeding, and oral contraceptive use. The vasomotor signs and symptoms associated with menopause, such as hot flashes and night sweats, also vary to such a great extent that they are not specified as one of the staging criteria[3] for ascertaining phases of menopause (see Fig. 110–1). The perimenopausal transition and postmenopausal experience for an individual woman arise from a complex interaction of biologic, cultural, psychological, and environmental factors. The timing and duration of this midlife transition cannot be easily predicted.

NORMAL SLEEP PATTERNS DURING MENOPAUSE

Disturbed sleep and daytime fatigue are among the most frequent complaints of women during the menopausal transition.[4,5] Population survey studies of menopause show that sleep problems are more common in perimenopausal and postmenopausal women compared with premenopausal women. The prevalence of sleep disturbance varies widely from study to study, but most report increases of 50% to 100% for perimenopausal and postmenopausal women compared with premenopausal women. For example, Kuh and colleagues[6] found that 40% of premenopausal women reported trouble sleeping, compared with 50% and 63% of perimenopausal and postmenopausal women. The large Wisconsin Sleep Cohort Study found that perimenopausal and postmenopausal women were twice as likely to be dissatisfied with their sleep than premenopausal women.[7] The most common menopausal sleep complaint is difficulty falling asleep, but significant increases in self-reported nighttime awakenings and daytime drowsiness have also been described.[7,8]

Stages:	−5	−4	−3	−2	−1	0 (FMP)	+1	+2
Terminology:	Reproductive			Menopausal transition			Postmenopause	
	Early	Peak	Late	Early	Late*		Early*	Late
				Perimenopause				
Duration of stage:	variable			variable		(a) 1 yr	(b) 4 yrs	until demise
Menstrual cycles:	variable to regular	regular		variable cycle length (> 7 days different from normal)	≥ 2 skipped cycles and an interval of amenorrhea (≥ 60 days)	Amen × 12 mos	none	
Endocrine:	normal FSH		↑ FSH	↑ FSH			↑ FSH	

*Stages most likely to be characterized by vasomotor symptoms   ↑ = elevated

Figure 110–1. Stages of normal reproductive aging in women. The final menstrual period (FMP) is the time in a woman's life when she has missed 12 consecutive menstrual periods (amenorrhea) (a) and is considered early postmenopausal for the next 4 years (b) before becoming late postmenopausal for the duration of her life. Before permanent cessation of menstrual cycles, women vary in the duration of their cycles during the stage known as perimenopause. Follicle-stimulating hormone (FSH) is elevated throughout early and late perimenopause because of a lack of adequate levels of ovarian hormones to inhibit secretion of FSH from the hypothalamus. Note that the reproductive stages most likely to see hot flashes and night sweats are late perimenopause and early postmenopause, with wide and unpredictable variations in duration of these stages of normal reproductive aging. (Adapted from Soules MR, Sherman S, Parrott E, et al: Executive summary: Stages of Reproductive Aging Workshop [STRAW]. Fertil Steril 2001;76:874-878.)

These findings persist even in studies that control for confounding factors such as depression and age.[4-9]

Despite the frequency of insomnia and fatigue complaints by menopausal women, very few studies have used objective techniques such as polysomnography or actigraphy to assess sleep before, during, and after menopause. An actigraphic study of 15 perimenopausal women and 13 age-matched premenopausal women found that perimenopausal women experienced significantly greater sleep disruption, as indicated by longer and more frequent arousals during the night.[10] Their sleep disruption was consistent with self-reported sleep quality. The perimenopausal women were significantly more dissatisfied with their overall sleep quality because of more spontaneous awakenings during the night, daytime drowsiness, and a feeling of needing extra sleep. However, studies using polysomnography to measure sleep quality have not supported a prominent general effect of menopause.[7,11,12] Shaver and colleagues[11] reported a nonsignificant trend toward increased sleep fragmentation in perimenopausal and postmenopausal women, but no difference in total sleep time, slow wave or rapid eye movement (REM) sleep, or sleep latency compared with premenopausal control subjects. Investigators for the two largest studies of menopause and sleep[7,13] found that their midlife subjects perceived poor sleep quality concurrently with objective measures showing no detectable decline in sleep quality.

In short, the subjective experience of menopause-related insomnia is well documented, but it is not concordant with the limited data from standard objective sleep measures. This "mismatch" has been called *sleep state misperception*, and it is not unique to menopausal women.[14,15] The cause of this discrepancy is unknown. One possibility is that polysomnography may not be a sensitive measure for some important element of sleep quality that is reflected in subjective ratings.[16] Quantitative analysis of the sleep electroencephalogram (i.e., power spectral analysis of specific waveforms and frequency bands, such as delta waves) is likely to be a powerful source of additional information about sleep quality that would address this question.[16] Another possibility is that the impact of menopause on objective sleep measures is heterogeneous, that is, there may be a subgroup of women whose objectively measured sleep quality shows a menopause-related decline. This would not be surprising, given the heterogeneity of women's experiences with hot flash symptoms. Also, cultural attitudes and expectations about menopause can influence women's experiences and may affect perception of sleep quality.[17]

One prominent theory of reproductive aging is that menopause results from the aging of multiple pacemakers in the brain and the ovaries that control and coordinate a variety of circadian and other rhythms.[2] The suprachiasmatic nuclei of the hypothalamus are a primary source of these endogenous rhythms and their synchrony. The sleep–wake cycle is the most visible human circadian rhythm, and it is profoundly influenced by the suprachiasmatic nuclei and by other circadian rhythms, particularly the rhythms of body temperature and melatonin secretion. Numerous studies have shown estrogen's impact on circadian rhythms in female mammals.[18] These data suggest that the circadian control of sleep might be changed or compromised with menopause. However, this hypothesis is purely speculative at present. No studies have attempted to distinguish menopause effects on circadian rhythm from the well-known effects of aging per se.

Aging is associated with a decline in sleep quality.[19,20] Although investigators studying midlife women (40 to 60 years of age) usually consider menopausal status when describing women's health and experiences, the significant effect of age is often ignored. That is, some sleep effects ascribed to menopause may in fact be due to aging. One approach to this issue is to control the confounding factor of age with statistical techniques (e.g., using age as a covariate).[7] Another approach is to report experiences and symptoms for specific narrow age ranges in midlife, such that the specific contributions of age and menopause can be identified.[4] These techniques may not be entirely successful because there is little overlap between ages of premenopausal and postmenopausal women. In short, sleep disturbance in some midlife women may be related to conditions associated with aging (e.g., thyroid dysfunction, depression) rather than menopause.

COMMON CLINICAL CONDITIONS IN MIDLIFE WOMEN

Hot Flashes and Night Sweats

It has long been suspected that at least some of the self-reported sleep disturbance associated with menopause is secondary to vasomotor symptoms of hot flashes and night sweats. A hot flash (often called a hot flush, or a "night sweat" when it occurs during the night) is a sudden, transient, and recurrent subjective sensation of moderate to intense heat that usually begins in the upper body. It is primarily a thermoregulatory phenomenon,[21] with all the characteristics of a heat dissipation response: (1) peripheral vasodilation, which causes increased heat loss; and (2) increased sweating, which causes evaporative cooling. There is tremendous individual variability in hot flashes. A hot flash typically lasts 3 to 5 minutes, but can be more than 20 minutes in some women. The subjective intensity of the flash can also vary widely, ranging from severely disruptive to mild. Some women have hot flashes 20 or more times each day, whereas others report only 1 or 2 per week.

The etiology of hot flashes is unknown.[22] Although they are generally associated with menopause, hot flashes are also associated with androgen-suppressive hormone treatment in men with prostate cancer, and the use of selective estrogen receptor modulators such as tamoxifen for treatment of estrogen-sensitive breast cancer. Surgical menopause, smoking, and physical inactivity increase the likelihood of hot flashes.[23,24] The prevalence of hot flashes also varies by racial/ethnic groups. In the recent Study of Women's Health Across the Nation (SWAN) with 15,000 participants, approximately 39% of African-American women experienced hot flashes, compared with 26% of Hispanic women and 24% of white women. Asian Americans had the lowest prevalence: 16% for Chinese-American women and 12% for Japanese-American women.[23] It is not clear whether differences in the experience of hot flashes are the result of differences in lifestyle stressors, diet, or cultural factors, or unidentified biologic factors.[17]

Hot flashes are associated with reduced self-reported sleep quality.[25,26] This relationship has been confirmed in a variety of study designs, ethnic groups, and nationalities. However, little is known about how hot flashes affect objectively measured sleep quality. Only two studies have used polysomnography and a concurrent objective measure of hot flashes to compare the sleep of women with and without hot flashes. Both showed that hot flashes disrupt sleep, as indicated by more nocturnal awakenings, lower sleep efficiency, and more sleep stage changes.[27,28] Erlik and colleagues also assessed the effect of each nocturnal hot flash on sleep in 9 menopausal women; of the 47 objectively measured hot flashes, 45 were associated with a waking episode.[28]

Some research suggests that hot flashes are unrelated to polysomnographic sleep quality.[7] Most of these studies relied on self-reports of hot flashes, often for nights other than the polysomnography nights. This is problematic because women are not always aware of hot flashes that occur during sleep. The concordance between self-reported and objectively identified hot flashes (i.e., measured changes in galvanic skin resistance) is extremely high during daytime hours, but drops significantly during bedtime hours. In one study, postmenopausal women were provisionally enrolled in a "no hot flash" group based on self-reports. Subsequent objective monitoring revealed that half of them were having nocturnal hot flashes.[29]

Collectively, existing research indicates that hot flashes and night sweats can cause significant sleep disruption, especially awakenings during the night. However, some important questions remain unanswered. Most of the research in this area is based on women's perceptions of their sleep when they are having hot flashes. Consequently, little is known about how hot flashes affect particular types of sleep (such as REM or slow wave sleep), whether hot flashes are more likely to occur during particular sleep stages, or whether hot flashes sometimes cause sleep to become "lighter" and less restful but do not result in an outright awakening. Data from large population studies suggest that some women continue to have hot flashes for many years, even decades, after menopause.[30] Hot flashes are not always labeled as "hot flashes" by older postmenopausal women because of their previous association with menopausal transition. Rather, they may describe their vasomotor symptoms in terms of waking up during the night "feeling too warm" and feeling the need to throw off the bedcovers. The effect of chronic hot flashes on the sleep of older women is unknown. Finally, not all women who have menopause-related sleep problems also complain of hot flashes.[31] This suggests that there are other reasons why menopause may be associated with sleep disturbance.

Sleep disruption associated with hot flashes may be treated in several ways. Hormone replacement therapy (HRT) has historically been the standard treatment. Although HRT is still recommended for the short-term alleviation of vasomotor symptoms in women who do not have a history of breast cancer or stroke, patients and health care providers are increasingly reluctant to pursue this option because of health risks. Many other options are available.[32] Antidepressants that inhibit serotonin reuptake (selective serotonin reuptake inhibitors [SSRIs]; e.g., paroxetine)[33] and gabapentin[34] have been used with some success. Complementary or alternative therapies may help,[32,35] although data on their effectiveness have been decidedly mixed. Clinical trials are underway to assess the efficacy of acupuncture, yoga, phytoestrogens such as soy and red clover, and herbal treatments such as dong quai and black cohosh. Appropriate changes to the sleeping environment and bedclothes may be helpful because a warm ambient temperature or elevated body core temperature increases the likelihood of hot flashes.

Effects of Hormone Replacement Therapy on Sleep

Estrogen and progesterone levels fluctuate dramatically during the perimenopause and ultimately decline to very low postmenopausal levels.[1] Consequently, estrogen therapy (ET) or HRT was commonly prescribed for midlife and older women on a long-term basis in an effort to counter hormone deficiency and protect against osteoporosis, heart disease, and Alzheimer's dementia. However, the Women's Health Initiative results abruptly reversed this practice. This national clinical trial showed that use of a common HRT regimen for 1 to 7 years significantly increased the risk of breast cancer, stroke, heart disease, and vascular dementia.[36] Women are now being advised to use HRT for only a short time to provide relief from hot flashes and other symptoms during the menopausal transition.

Because many women do continue to use exogenous ET or HRT to counter the changes in their endogenous hormone levels and thereby obtain short-term relief of menopausal symptoms, it is important to understand the effects of these hormone therapies on sleep. Moreover, the effects of ET/HRT can be considered a clue to mechanisms for how menopause-related hormone changes may influence the sleep of midlife and older women. If these hormonal changes contribute directly or indirectly to menopause-related sleep disturbance, then ET or HRT should improve sleep.

ET or HRT is currently the most effective treatment for hot flashes.[37] Dozens of epidemiologic studies and small clinical trials have shown that ET/HRT reduces hot flashes and concurrently improves *self-reported* sleep quality. The size of this effect varies from a significant but clinically small effect[38] in some studies to other studies that document alleviation of hot flashes as highly predictive of improvements in sleep.[31] Polysomnography studies have generally replicated these findings. In women who were experiencing frequent hot flashes, ET decreased the number[28,39] and duration[39] of nighttime awakenings, increased REM sleep,[39-41] and shortened latency to sleep onset.[40] However, in studies where many or all of the women had only mild or infrequent hot flashes, neither ET[42] nor HRT[43] had an effect on polysomnographic recorded sleep stages. With one exception,[39] these polysomnography studies were based on small groups of 4 to 16 women. The presence or frequency of hot flashes may also explain the failure of a large cross-sectional epidemiologic study to find differences in the polysomnographic sleep of women using HRT compared with women who were not.[7] If hot flashes are not measured concurrently with polysomnography, if data on general hot flash frequency or severity are not reported, or if asymptomatic women do not opt to take HRT and symptomatic women selectively use HRT to alleviate hot flashes, no differences in sleep would be detected between the two groups.

Progesterone

Virtually nothing is known about how menopausal changes in endogenous progesterone levels affect sleep. Progesterone given by itself can have acute effects of sleepiness similar to sedative-hypnotic medications. A high clinical dose (300 mg) of micronized progesterone given orally 1.5 hours before bedtime significantly shorted the latency to REM sleep and increased the amount of non-REM sleep in a small group of young men.[44] There are also numerous clinical reports and anecdotes about sleepiness side effects of progesterone, particularly daytime drowsiness that occurs in a significant percentage of women after taking progesterone in the morning as part of HRT.[45] Clinically, women on HRT are often advised to take their progesterone in the evening because of this daytime drowsiness phenomenon.[45]

There may be significant differences among progestins in their impact on sleep. Montplaisir and colleagues[46] found that conjugated equine estrogens (Premarin) plus micronized progesterone significantly improved the sleep of postmenopausal women, whereas the same estrogens plus the synthetic medroxyprogesterone acetate had no effect. This is consistent with emerging evidence that there are significant differences between progestins in the multitude of their nonendometrial biologic effects.[47] For example, unlike medroxyprogesterone acetate, micronized progesterone is metabolized to potent neurosteroids such as allopregnanolone and pregnanolone. These neurosteroids interact with the same brain gamma-aminobutyric acid type A receptor as sedative-hypnotic medications, and they are soporific.[48]

In sum, a clear picture has not yet emerged about the effects of ET or HRT on the sleep of midlife and older women independent of the presence or absence of vasomotor symptoms such as hot flashes. Also, there is a discrepancy between effects of HRT on subjective experience of sleep and polysomnographic measures of sleep. Finally, the few clinical trials using polysomnography involved small numbers of subjects. Given the current lack of knowledge and the sobering results of the Women's Health Initiative study, it is clearly inappropriate at present to suggest ET or HRT as a treatment for menopause-related insomnia except when that sleep disturbance is clearly due to frequent and severe hot flashes.

Hormone Withdrawal

Because of the results from the Women's Health Initiative study, many women have abruptly discontinued HRT. The number of prescriptions written for HRT declined by 66% during the 6-month period soon after results were published.[49] The sleep effects of withdrawal from ET or HRT are unknown. Two recent studies have shown that abrupt estrogen withdrawal can result in significant hot flashes,[50,51] suggesting that there might be sleep consequences to ET or HRT discontinuation.

Stress Reactivity

One way in which menopausal hormone changes could influence sleep is through changes in stress reactivity. Stress can disrupt sleep; mild psychological distress or stressors such as daily "hassles" can increase arousal, waking, and the subjective experience of sleep disturbance.[52] Several studies suggest that a low estrogen level during and after menopause is associated with enhanced cardiovascular and hormonal responses to stress,[53] whereas ET reduces stress reactivity to psychological stress in postmenopausal women.[54] Moe and colleagues[55] showed more directly how the relationship between stress reactivity and estrogen levels might affect sleep in postmenopausal women who underwent frequent remote nocturnal blood sampling (a mild stressor) during one night of a sleep study. Those not on ET had significantly more disrupted sleep from this mild blood sampling stressor than women on ET. They had less total sleep time, more time awake during the night, more episodes of awakenings, a longer latency to the onset of sleep, and less slow wave sleep.

Apnea, Obesity, and Hypertension

Obesity, hypertension, and sleep-disordered breathing (SDB) are strongly associated with each other[56] (see Chapter 87). All three are common clinical conditions in postmenopausal women, and considerable research suggests that menopause contributes to these conditions. The well-documented gender gap in prevalence of SDB[57] begins to narrow with menopause. Bixler and colleagues[58] found a female/male ratio of 1:3.3 for clinically defined apnea in their sample of 1741 men and women aged 20 to 100 years; this ratio fell to 1:1.44 for postmenopausal women when matched with men by age and body mass index (BMI).

Sleep-Disordered Breathing

Menopause has long been described as a risk factor for SDB.[59] Previous studies yielded inconsistent or unconvincing results because of small sample sizes, menopausal status defined by age rather than menstrual history or hormonal assay,[12,60] or lack of controls for age, adiposity, and sleep clinic referral bias. However, two large and well-designed population studies now provide strong support for the hypothesis that menopause increases the risk of SDB.[58,61]

In the first study, Bixler and colleagues performed polysomnography on 1000 women drawn from a random telephone survey.[58] The postmenopausal women had a significantly higher prevalence of SDB compared with the premenopausal women. The prevalence of mild SDB (defined as an apnea-hypopnea index [AHI] between 0 and 15, together with a self-report of moderate or severe snoring) was 3.2% for premenopausal women but 9.7% for postmenopausal women who were not using HRT. The prevalence of more severe SDB (AHI of at least 15) was 0.6% for premenopausal women versus 2.7% for postmenopausal women not using HRT. SDB prevalence remained significantly higher for postmenopausal women even after adjusting for known risk factors of age and BMI.

In the other study, Young and colleagues examined polysomnographic data collected on 589 middle-aged women participating in the longitudinal Wisconsin Sleep Cohort Study.[61] The detailed attention paid to menopausal staging in this study allowed the investigators to determine SDB prevalence and odds ratios for premenopause as well as perimenopause and postmenopause. Postmenopausal women were 2.6 times more likely than premenopausal women to have SDB (defined as AHI of at least 5), and 3.5 times more likely to have more severe SDB (AHI of at least 15). The odds of having SDB were not significantly higher for perimenopausal women compared with premenopausal women. However, the data did suggest that the risk for SDB increases throughout the menopausal transition. When women were stratified on years since last menstrual period, there was a significant linear trend toward increased risk for AHI of at least 5 with increasing postmenopause duration up to 5 years. One additional strength of this study was the careful use of multivariate models to adjust for several known risk factors for SDB, particularly age, BMI, smoking, and alcohol use. Despite the inclusion of these potent risk factors in the analyses, menopausal status remained a strong and significant independent risk factor for SDB.[61]

The mechanism by which menopause increases the risk of SDB is not yet clear. One possibility is the menopause-related decline in levels of endogenous estrogen or progesterone.[59] This hypothesis grew from early work showing that progesterone increases ventilatory drive.[62] Although several studies have examined the effects of progesterone on ventilation in general, on oxygen saturation, or on measures of apnea, only a few have included female subjects. Postmenopausal women with SDB had improved nocturnal ventilation with exogenous progesterone administration, but no change in the number of apneas or hypopneas.[63] In healthy postmenopausal women, progesterone improved resting ventilation and hypoxic ventilatory response[64] and decreased the number of apneas and hypopneas.[59] HRT may improve OSAS in postmenopausal women.[64a]

Menopause and Obesity

Menopause and the postmenopausal years are characterized by some weight gain. Contrary to widely held belief, this increased weight is likely associated with normal aging and with a reduction in physical activity, rather than menopause per se.[65] Regardless of etiology, excessive weight is a significant problem for perimenopausal and postmenopausal women in the United States. Over 37% of midlife women (40 to 59 years of age) are considered obese, as defined by a BMI of 30 or more.[66] Excess weight is a similar problem for older women (60 to 74 years of age), with more than 35% considered obese.[66] Increased adiposity is a primary risk factor for SDB (see Chapter 87). The prevalence and severity of SDB in general are highly and positively correlated with excess weight.[67]

Hypertension

The prevalence of hypertension in women rises sharply with onset of menopause. The etiology of this phenomenon is complex and still under investigation, but two factors strongly associated with hypertension are obesity and SDB, conditions common in perimenopausal and postmenopausal women. The National Health and Nutrition Examination Survey III (NHANES III) documented a strong association between hypertension and BMI in women.[68] For midlife women (40 to 59 years of age), the prevalence of hypertension was approximately 10% when BMI was less than 25, but rose to 39% when BMI was 30 or more. For older women (60 to 79 years of age), 52% with a BMI less than 25 had hypertension, but over 72% had hypertension if BMI was 30 or more. A panel recently convened by the American College of Chest Physicians[69] confirmed the strong association of SDB and hypertension. In sum, midlife women are at increased risk of hypertension and SDB by virtue of their increased risk of obesity.

Metabolic Syndrome

The strong association of SDB with obesity, visceral adiposity, and hypertension has led to the suggestion that sleep apnea is a manifestation of the metabolic syndrome[70] (see Chapter 86). The metabolic syndrome is a constellation of closely related symptoms (visceral adiposity, hypertension, insulin resistance, elevated glucose, dyslipidemia) that together convey substantially increased risk of cardiovascular disease.[71] Visceral adiposity is first and foremost among these symptoms, and it is thought by many to be the major determinant of the metabolic syndrome. These features of the metabolic syndrome become much more common in women as they transition from premenopause to postmenopause.[71] Regardless of whether there is any weight gain, the menopausal transition is associated with a decrease in lean body mass and an increase in body fat composition. Also, there is a preferential increase in the intraabdominal or visceral deposition of fat relative to other areas. This effect is independent of age and total body adiposity.[71] It may be due to menopause-related hormone changes because HRT decreases the shift to visceral adiposity.[72] Visceral fat correlates especially strongly with SDB, and is believed by some to be the principal culprit leading to SDB.[70] Thus, the increased adiposity and visceral fat accumulation associated with menopause places women at increased risk for SDB.

Collectively, these data suggest that midlife and older women may be doubly at risk for SDB compared with younger women because of possibly decreased ventilatory drive resulting from lower estrogen/progesterone and because of increased visceral adiposity. Hypertension and obesity together in midlife women should be considered high risk factors for SDB and other serious health problems, including cardiovascular disease and type 2 diabetes.

HRT may have some beneficial effects on respiration and visceral adiposity. In epidemiologic population studies, HRT has been associated with a lower prevalence of sleep apnea in postmenopausal women.[7,58] This relationship was confirmed in the Sleep Heart Health Study[73] even after controlling for well-documented differences (e.g., education level, body weight, health awareness) between women who choose to use HRT and those who do not. Most small clinical trials of HRT are consistent with these results, suggesting that HRT has some efficacy in alleviating SDB.[74] However, it is premature to conclude that HRT is an effective or desirable treatment for SDB in women. No large clinical trial has been conducted. The wide variability in response to HRT among individual patients suggests that, if these hormones affect SDB, they do so through a specific unidentified mechanism that is not common to all cases of SDB. Also, there are significant and serious health risks associated with using HRT. If it is eventually determined that low endogenous hormone levels play a role in SDB, the relative risks and benefits of HRT compared with other treatment options (e.g., nasal continuous positive airway pressure or surgery; see Chapters 89 and 90) will require thorough consideration for each individual woman. Also, weight loss and exercise (specifically to reduce adiposity) should be strongly considered for any SDB treatment plan.

Depression

Several longitudinal studies have found that depressive symptoms increase in the transition from premenopause to perimenopause and then begin to decrease in the years after menopause.[75,76] Although these studies controlled for age and other known predictors of depression, it remains unclear whether depression is a menopausal symptom per se.[77]

Depression in general has a significant negative impact on sleep (see Chapter 112), and this is true of depression during menopause. Perimenopausal women have more mood alterations as well as longer and more numerous nocturnal awakenings than premenopausal women.[10] Also, perimenopausal and postmenopausal women with major depression have been shown to have reduced sleep efficiency and less delta-wave sleep than nondepressed women of similar menopausal status.[78]

HRT has reduced symptoms of depression and anxiety in perimenopausal and postmenopausal women in some but not all studies,[79] leading to the hypothesis that a low estrogen or progesterone level can increase the risk for mood disorders. Moreover, there is a strong relationship between hot flash severity and depression in menopausal women.[76,78] Results from a large HRT clinical trial that examined depression, vasomotor symptoms, and fatigue in 2763 postmenopausal women revealed that effects of HRT on these symptoms depended on the presence or absence of hot flashes.[80] Women with hot flashes assigned to HRT had fewer depressive symptoms and less fatigue after treatment than those assigned to placebo. However, another study has shown that, even after ET, menopausal women with major depression continue to have a longer duration of awakenings.[78]

Hysterectomy

Hysterectomy is the second most common surgery for women in the United States, with approximately 633,000 hysterectomies performed each year.[81] The average age at hysterectomy is 40 to 45 years; approximately 37% of women in the United States have had a hysterectomy by 60 years of age. At least 50% of these patients also undergo concurrent bilateral oophorectomy (removal of both ovaries). In these women there is an abrupt onset of menopause known as "surgical" menopause.

Disturbed sleep and fatigue are common postoperative symptoms after hysterectomy.[82] In addition, women who undergo surgical menopause are more likely to experience hot flashes than women who experience natural menopause. Moreover, the hot flashes that follow surgical menopause are more severe and continue longer than hot flashes after natural menopause.[83] Significant depression or anxiety may also occur subsequent to hysterectomy to confound sleep complaints.[82]

These findings suggest that women undergoing hysterectomy may be more vulnerable to sleep disruption beyond the immediate postoperative period. Insomnia, daytime sleepiness, and fatigue should be explored and reviewed in the context of these biologic and psychological factors so that appropriate treatment strategies can be devised. These may include pharmacologic therapies (antidepressants, short-term sedative-hypnotics, short-term HRT) or nonpharmacologic approaches such as good sleep hygiene and behavioral-cognitive therapies directed at insomnia or depression.

Cancer

With age, women are more likely to have cancer of the breast, lung, colon, ovary, gallbladder, or thyroid gland. During midlife, women 40 to 59 years of age, for example, have a 1:11 probability for development of an invasive cancer.[84] Persons with cancer commonly experience sleep disturbance.[85] As discussed in Chapter 103, the etiology of cancer-related sleep disruption is often complex,[86-88] with multiple factors that are likely to precipitate sleep problems. These include pain and discomfort, physical effects of the cancer itself, depression and anxiety, and side effects of chemotherapy or radiation treatments (e.g., nausea, vomiting, diarrhea, urinary frequency). In addition to the sleep-disrupting factors commonly experienced by most patients with cancer, women with breast cancer are likely to experience hot flashes.[88] Hot flashes are a side effect of chemotherapy-induced ovarian disruption and they also occur with the use of adjuvant hormone therapy. Women with estrogen receptor–positive tumors are treated with the anti-estrogen tamoxifen citrate or aromatase inhibitors (anastrozole, letrozole, exemestane) to prevent endogenous estrogens from stimulating the growth of residual tumors or micrometastases. More than 50% of tamoxifen users experience hot flashes, and the hot flashes associated with the use of these agents are usually more frequent and more severe than hot flashes associated with natural menopause.[89] Because standard treatment with adjuvant hormone therapy typically lasts for 5 years, breast cancer survivors are subjected to significant hot flashes and sleep disruption for a considerable period. Although HRT is not indicated for treatment of hot flashes in women with cancer,[90] antidepressants (SSRIs such as venlafaxine) and gabapentin have been used with some success.[89]

Thyroid Dysfunction

The prevalence of thyroid disease, particularly hypothyroidism, increases with age and is far higher in women than men. For midlife women living in iodine-replete areas, the prevalence of impaired thyroid function (i.e., thyroid-stimulating hormone [TSH] values outside the euthyroid range) is 9.6%.[91] Of these, the majority (6.2%) have elevated TSH, indicating clinical or subclinical hypothyroidism. Because hypothyroidism is typically characterized by tiredness and fatigue, such complaints by perimenopausal and postmenopausal women should be clinically evaluated in light of a TSH level.

Women with hypothyroidism may be more likely than euthyroid women to have SDB (see Chapter 105), suggesting that hypothyroidism may also be a risk factor for SDB.[92] Midlife and older women with hypothyroidism should also be screened for clinical signs and symptoms indicative of SDB.

SUMMARY

Menopause as an area of women's health is a rapidly growing field of clinical practice and research.[93] Sleep disruption is one of the most common symptoms reported by midlife and older women, so there is great interest in understanding how menopause affects sleep and how to treat menopausal sleep complaints. Despite major gaps in research on this issue, some clear diagnostic and therapeutic implications are emerging.

One of the most important considerations is the interrelationship between menopausal status and aging. There is a tendency to assume a cause-and-effect relationship between menopause and symptoms whose prevalence is linked to menopause. In particular, symptoms tend to be attributed to the hormonal changes that occur as part of menopause. This focus on menopause may obscure the presence and contribution of age-related factors to sleep complaints. Several common concomitants of aging make midlife women more vulnerable to sleep problems, independent of menopause. These include weight gain, reduced physical activity, changes in physiologic stress reactivity, and increased risk of several diseases and chronic conditions that affect sleep (e.g., thyroid dysfunction, cancer, surgical menopause, arthritis). Although a woman of menopausal age may attribute the appearance of sleep disturbance to the onset of menopause or "hormone problems," the symptoms and their treatment should be viewed in the wider context of aging as well. One important example of this is the increased risk of SDB in midlife and older women. Fatigue or sleep complaints combined with hypertension and excessive weight should prompt consideration of snoring and SDB in a clinical evaluation. Likewise, sleep disturbance in a woman younger than the expected age for menopause may be due to a premature and unexpected perimenopausal transition, and an FSH level should be obtained to evaluate stage of menopause as a possible explanation for her fatigue or sleep complaints.

The subjective experience of menopause-related insomnia is well documented. However, the limited research using polysomnography to investigate this phenomenon has not yet identified features of sleep architecture that correspond to these self-reports of poor sleep quality. Thus, polysomnography may not be of much value in assessing older women's sleep complaints, except in specific cases when clinical signs and symptoms suggest SDB. Instead, it may be more useful to concentrate on a careful clinical interview and assessment that thoroughly explores menopause-related issues (e.g., hot flashes), aging-related vulnerabilities (e.g., thyroid dysfunction, depression, widowhood, chronic musculoskeletal pain), lifestyle (physical activity, stress, and coping strategies), sleep environment (exposure to light, noise, or violence) and sleep hygiene practices, as well as her expectations of menopause, sleep, and aging.

Hot flashes have long been recognized as a possible disruptive influence on sleep during the menopausal transition. Some women are more likely to experience disruptive hot flashes; the possibility that hot flashes are contributing to insomnia should definitely be explored in women who have undergone surgical menopause or breast cancer treatment, or who have abruptly discontinued HRT. Also, hot flashes are popularly assumed to end within a few years after the last menstrual period. However, data from several large studies show that a significant number of postmenopausal women continue to have hot flashes for many years, even decades, after menopause. This possibility should be kept in mind while exploring insomnia complaints with older women, particularly when accompanied by descriptions of waking up during the night and feeling too warm. Although HRT remains the single most effective treatment for hot flashes, women and their health care providers are now more reluctant to support its use because of significant health risks. Even women with severe hot flashes may be reluctant to consider HRT, and many women have discontinued their long-term HRT. A growing number of alternatives to HRT have been identified as successful for at least some women. These include the SSRI class of antidepressants, clonidine, gabapentin, herbal remedies, and lifestyle modifications (e.g., exercise, stress reduction, smoking cessation, and weight loss programs).

PITFALLS AND CONTROVERSIES

One important challenge for midlife women's health research is to determine whether changes in sleep and other dimensions of health that occur during and after menopause are directly attributable to menopause rather than to aging. This is methodologically difficult, and will require creative research designs and analytic methods. Another challenge arises from data suggesting that there may be racial/ethnic differences in menopausal experiences. For example, the prevalence of hot flashes is higher among African-American women and lower among Asian-American women, compared with other groups.[23] The nature and implications of these differences have not been adequately explored, and the possible role of cultural differences and expectations has been underinvestigated.

There are several unanswered questions about HRT. These include the sleep consequences of discontinuing long-term HRT, and determining whether there are any sleep-related conditions for which HRT is appropriate. Clearly there is a need for alternative treatments for hot flashes and related insomnia. Determining the etiology of hot flashes would help identify possible alternatives.

Perhaps the most important need is for additional research on the links between obesity, hypertension, and SDB in perimenopausal and postmenopausal women. Older women have an elevated risk of SDB as well as obesity and hypertension. Because SDB is more commonly found in men, most research on mechanisms and treatments has focused on men, with very little representation of women in the study samples. There may be significant sex differences in the etiology, expression, and effective treatment modalities for SDB in relation to menopausal status, regardless of age and body weight.

Clinical Pearls

Midlife women may assume that hormonal changes associated with menopausal transition are responsible for any symptoms they experience, and this assumption may obscure other, more likely causes such as weight gain, reduced physical activity, stress, thyroid dysfunction, cancer, or chronic illness. Postmenopausal women are at increased risk of SDB, and fatigue or sleep complaints combined with hypertension and excessive weight should prompt consideration of snoring and SDB in a clinical evaluation. Women in their fifth decade and younger than the expected age for menopause could have premature menopause, and an FSH level should be obtained to evaluate stage of menopause as a possible explanation for their fatigue or sleep complaint.

REFERENCES

1. Santoro N, Brown JR, Adel T, et al: Characterization of reproductive hormonal dynamics in the perimenopause. J Clin Endocrinol Metab 1996;81:1495-1501.
2. Wise PM, Krajnak KM, Kashon ML: Menopause: the aging of multiple pacemakers. Science 1996;273:67-70.
3. Soules MR, Sherman S, Parrott E, et al: Executive summary: Stages of Reproductive Aging Workshop (STRAW). Fertil Steril 2001;76:874-878.
4. Lee KA, Taylor DL: Is there a generic midlife woman? The health and symptom experience of midlife women. Menopause 1996;3:154-164.
5. Owens JF, Mathews KA: Sleep disturbance in healthy middle-aged women. Maturitas 1998;30:41-50.
6. Kuh DL, Wadsworth M, Hardy R: Women's health in midlife: The influence of the menopause, social factors and health in earlier life. Br J Obstet Gynaecol 1997;104:923-933.
7. Young T, Rabago D, Zgierska A, et al: Objective and subjective sleep quality in premenopausal, perimenopausal, and postmenopausal women in the Wisconsin Sleep Cohort Study. Sleep 2003;26:667-672.
8. Ballinger CB: Psychiatric morbidity and the menopause: Clinical features. BMJ 1976;1:1183-1185.
9. Kravitz HM, Ganz PA, Bromberger J, et al: Sleep difficulty in women at midlife: A community survey of sleep and the menopausal transition. Menopause 2003;10:19-28.
10. Baker A, Simpson S, Dawson D: Sleep disruption and mood changes associated with menopause. J Psychosom Res 1997;43:359-369.
11. Shaver J, Giblin E, Lentz M, et al: Sleep patterns and stability in perimenopausal women. Sleep 1988;11:556-561.
12. Sharkey KM, Bearpark HM, Acebo C, et al: Effects of menopausal status on sleep in midlife women. Behav Sleep Med 2003;1:69-80.
13. Shaver JLF, Giblin E, Paulsen V: Sleep quality subtypes in midlife women. Sleep 1991;14:18-23.
14. Carskadon MA, Dement WC, Mitler MM, et al: Self-reports versus sleep laboratory findings in 122 drug-free subjects with complaints of chronic insomnia. Am J Psychiatry 1976;133:1382-1388.
15. Vitiello MV, Larsen LH, Moe KE: Age-related sleep change: Gender and estrogen effects on the subjective-objective sleep quality relationships of healthy, noncomplaining older men and women. J Psychosom Res 2004;56:503-510.
16. Polo O: Sleep in postmenopausal women: better sleep for less satisfaction. Sleep 2003;29:652-653.
17. Lock M, Kaufert P: Menopause, local biologies, and cultures of aging. Am J Biol 2001;13:494-504.
18. Leibenluft E: Do gonadal steroids regulate circadian rhythms in humans? J Affect Disord 1993;29:175-181.
19. Vitiello MV: Sleep disorders and aging. Curr Opin Psychiatry 1996;9:284-289.
20. Middelkoop HA, Smilde van den Doel DA, Neven AK, et al: Subjective sleep characteristics of 1,485 males and females aged 50-93: Effects of sex and age, and factors related to self-evaluated quality of sleep. J Gerontol A Biol Sci Med Sci 1996;51A:M108-M115.
21. Freedman RR: Physiology of hot flashes. Am J Hum Biol 2001;13:453-464.
22. Kronenberg F: Hot flashes: Phenomenology, quality of life, and search for treatment options. Exp Gerontol 1994;29:319-336.
23. Avis NE, Stellato R, Crawford S, et al: Is there a menopausal syndrome? Menopausal status and symptoms across racial/ethnic groups. Soc Med 2001;52:345-356.
24. Whiteman MK, Staropoli CA, Benedict JC, et al: Risk factors for hot flashes in midlife women. J Womens Health 2003;12:459-472.
25. Polo-Kantola P, Erkkola R, Irjala K, et al: Climacteric symptoms and sleep quality. Obstet Gynecol 1999;94:219-224.
26. Hollander LE, Freeman EW, Sammel MD, et al: Sleep quality, estradiol levels, and behavioral factors in late reproductive age women. Obstet Gynecol 2001;98:391-397.
27. Woodward S, Freedman RR: The thermoregulatory effects of menopausal hot flashes on sleep. Sleep 1994;17:497-501.
28. Erlik Y, Tataryn IV, Meldrum DR, et al: Association of waking episodes with menopausal flushes. JAMA 1981;245:1741-1744.
29. Freedman RR, Roehrs TA: Menopausal sleep disturbance. Sleep 2003;26(Suppl):A161.
30. Barnabei VM, Grady D, Stovall DW, et al: Menopausal symptoms in older women and the effects of treatment with hormone therapy. Obstet Gynecol 2002;100:1209-1218.
31. Polo-Kantola P, Erkkola R, Helenius H, et al: When does estrogen replacement therapy improve sleep quality? Am J Obstet Gynecol 1998;178:1002-1009.
32. North American Menopause Society: Treatment of menopause-associated vasomotor symptoms: Position statement of The North American Menopause Society. Menopause 2004;11:11-33.
33. Stearns V, Beebe KL, Iyengar M, et al: Paroxetine controlled release in the treatment of menopausal hot flashes: A randomized controlled trial. JAMA 2003;289:2827-2834.
34. Guttuso T, Kurlan R, McDermott MP, et al: Gabapentin's effects on hot flashes in postmenopausal women: A randomized controlled trial. Obstet Gynecol 2003;101:337-345.
35. Newton KM, Buist DSM, Keenan NL, et al: Use of alternative therapies for menopause symptoms: Results of a population-based survey. Obstet Gynecol 2002;100:18-25.

36. Writing Group for the Women's Health Initiative: Risks and benefits of estrogen plus progestin in healthy postmenopausal women: Principal results from the Women's Health Initiative randomized controlled trial. JAMA 2002;288:2819-2825.

37. MacLennan A, Lester S, Moore V: Oral estrogen replacement therapy versus placebo for hot flushes: A systematic review. Climacteric 2001;4:58-74.

38. Hays J, Ockene JK, Brunner RL, et al: Effects of estrogen plus progestin on health-related quality of life. N Engl J Med 2003; 348:1839-1854.

39. Thomson J, Oswald I: Effect of oestrogen on the sleep, mood, and anxiety of menopausal women. BMJ 1977;2:1317-1319.

40. Schiff I, Regenstein Q, Tulchensky D, et al: Effects of estrogens on sleep and psychological state of hypogonadal women. JAMA 1979;242:2405-2407.

41. Scharf MB, McDannold MD, Stover R, et al: Effects of estrogen replacement therapy on rates of cyclic alternating patterns and hot-flush events during sleep in postmenopausal women: A pilot study. Clin Ther 1997;19:304-311.

42. Polo-Kantola P, Erkkola R, Irjala K, et al: Effect of short-term trans-dermal estrogen replacement therapy on sleep: A randomized, double-blind crossover trial in postmenopausal women. Fertil Steril 1999;71:873-880.

43. Purdie DW, Empson JAC, Crichton C, et al: Hormone replacement therapy, sleep quality and psychological well-being. Br J Obstet Gynaecol 1995;102:735-739.

44. Friess E, Tagaya H, Trachsel L, et al: Progesterone-induced changes in sleep in male subjects. Am J Physiol 1997;272: E885-E891.

45. de Lignieres B: Oral micronized progesterone. Clin Ther 1999; 21:41-60.

46. Montplaisir J, Lorrain J, Denesle R, Petit D: Sleep in menopause: differential effects of two forms of hormone replacement therapy. Menopause 2001;8:10-16.

47. Schindler AE: Differential effects of progestins. Maturitas 2003; 46(Suppl 1):S3-S5.

48. Schulz H, Jobert M, Gee KW, et al: Soporific effect of the neuro-steroid pregnanolone in relation to the substance's plasma level: A pilot study. Neuropsychobiology 1996;34:106-112.

49. Hersh AL, Stefanick ML, Stafford RS: National use of post-menopausal hormone therapy: Annual trends and response to recent evidence. JAMA 2004;291:47-53.

50. Simon JA, Mack CJ: Counseling patients who elect to discontinue hormone therapy. Int J Fertil Womens Med 2003;48:111-116.

51. Grady D, Ettinger B, Tosteson ANA, et al: Predictors of difficulty when discontinuing postmenopausal hormone therapy. Obstet Gynecol 2003;102:1233-1239.

52. Shaver JLF, Johnston SK, Lentz MJ, et al: Stress exposure, psychological distress, and physiological stress activation in midlife women with insomnia. Psychosom Med 2002;64:793-802.

53. Saab PG, Matthews KA, Stoney CM, et al: Premenopausal women and postmenopausal women differ in their cardiovascular and neuroendocrine response to behavioral stressors. Psychophysiology 1989;26:270-280.

54. Lindheim SR, Legro RS, Berstein L, et al: Behavioral stress responses in premenopausal and postmenopausal women and the effects of estrogen. Am J Obstet Gynecol 1992;167: 1831-1836.

55. Moe KE, Larsen LH, Vitiello MV, et al: Estrogen replacement therapy moderates the sleep disruption associated with nocturnal blood sampling. Sleep 2001;24:886-894.

56. Wolk R, Shamsuzzaman ASM, Somers VK: Obesity, sleep apnea, and hypertension. Hypertension 2003;42:1067-1074.

57. Kapsimalis F, Kryger MH: Gender and obstructive sleep apnea syndrome: Part 1. Clinical features. Sleep 2002;25:412-419.

58. Bixler EO, Vgontzas AN, Lin H-M, et al: Prevalence of sleep-disordered breathing in women. Am J Respir Crit Care Med 2001;163:608-613.

59. Block AJ, Wynne JW, Boysen PG: Sleep-disordered breathing and nocturnal oxygen desaturation in postmenopausal women. Am J Med 1980;69:75-79.

60. Dancy DR, Hanly PJ, Soong C, et al: Impact of menopause on the prevalence and severity of sleep apnea. Chest 2001;120: 151-155.

61. Young T, Finn L, Austin D, et al: Menopausal status and sleep-disordered breathing in the Wisconsin Sleep Cohort Study. Am J Respir Crit Care Med 2003;167:1181-1185.

62. Skatrud JB, Dempsey JA, Kaiser DG: Ventilatory response to medroxyprogesterone acetate in normal subjects: Time course and mechanism. J Appl Physiol 1978;44:939-944.

63. Saaresranta T, Polo-Kantola P, Rauhala E, et al: Medroxy-progesterone in postmenopausal females with partial upper airway obstruction during sleep. Eur Respir J 2001;18: 989-995.

64a. Wesstrom J, Ulfberg J, Nilsson S: Sleep apnea and hormone replacement therapy: A pilot study and a literature review. Acta Obstet Gynecol Scand 2005;84:54-57.

64. Regensteiner JG, Woodward WD, Hagerman DDH, et al: Combined effects of female hormones and metabolic rate on ventilatory drives in women. J Appl Physiol 1989;66:808-813.

65. MacDonald HM, New SA, Campbell MK, et al: Longitudinal changes in weight in perimenopausal and early post-menopausal women: Effects of dietary energy intake, energy expenditure, dietary calcium intake and hormone replacement therapy. Int J Obes 2003;27:669-676.

66. Flegal KM, Carroll MD, Ogden CL, et al: Prevalence and trends in obesity among US adults, 1999-2000. JAMA 2002;288: 1723-1727.

67. Young T, Peppard PE, Gottlieb DJ: Epidemiology of obstructive sleep apnea. Am J Respir Crit Care Med 2002;165:1217-1239.

68. Brown CD, Higgins M, Donato KA, et al: Body mass index and the prevalence of hypertension and dyslipidemia. Obes Res 2000;8:605-619.

69. Dart RA, Gregoire JR, Gutterman DD, et al: The association of hypertension and secondary cardiovascular disease with sleep-disordered breathing. Chest 2003;123:244-260.

70. Vgontzas AN, Bixler EO, Chrousos GP: Metabolic disturbances in obesity versus sleep apnoea: The importance of visceral obesity and insulin resistance. J Intern Med 2003;254:32-44.

71. Carr MC: The emergence of the metabolic syndrome with menopause. J Clin Endocrinol Metab 2003;88:2404-2411.

72. Reubinoff BE, Wurtman J, Rojanski L, et al: Effects of hormone replacement therapy on weight, body composition, fat distribution, and foot intake in early postmenopausal women: A prospective study. Fertil Steril 1995;64:963-968.

73. Shahar E, Redline S, Young T, et al: Hormone replacement therapy and sleep-disordered breathing. Am J Respir Crit Care Med 2003;167:1186-1192.

74. Manber R, Kuo TF, Cataldo N, et al: The effects of hormone replacement therapy on sleep-disordered breathing in postmenopausal women: A pilot study. Sleep 2003;2:163-168.

75. Maartens LWF, Knottnerus JA, Pop VJ: Menopausal transition and increased depressive symptomatology: A community based prospective study. Maturitas 2002;42:195-200.

76. Freeman EW, Sammel MD, Li L, et al: Hormones and menopausal status as predictors of depression in women in transition to menopause. Arch Gen Psychiatry 2004;61:62-70.

77. Woods NF, Mariella A, Mitchell ES: Patterns of depressed mood across the menopausal transition: Approaches to studying patterns in longitudinal data. Acta Obstet Gynecol Scand 2002;81:623-632.

78. Parry BL, Meliska CJ, Basavaraj N, et al: Menopause: Neuro-endocrine changes and hormone replacement therapy. J Am Med Womens Assoc 2004;59:135-145.

79. Birkhauser M: Depression, menopause and estrogens: Is there a correlation? Maturitas 2002;41(Suppl 1):S3-S8.

80. Hlatky MA, Boothroyd D, Vittinghoff E, et al: Quality-of-life and depressive symptoms in postmenopausal women after receiving hormone therapy. JAMA 2002;287:591-597.

81. Hall MJ, Owings, MF: National Hospital Discharge Survey: Advance Data from Vital and Health Statistics. DHHS publication no. 2002-1250.Washington, DC, National Center for Health Statistics, 2002.

82. Kim KH, Lee KA: Symptom experience in women after hysterectomy. J Obstet Gynecol Neonatal Nurs 2001;30:472-480.

83. Stadberg E, Mattson LA, Milsom I: Factors associated with climacteric symptoms and the use of hormone replacement therapy. Acta Obstet Gynecol Scand 2000;79:286-292.

84. Feuer EJ, Wun LM: DEVCAN: Probability of Developing or Dying of Cancer [software]. Version 4.2. Bethesda, MD, National Cancer Institute, 2002.

85. Lee K, Cho M, Miaskowski C, et al: Impaired sleep and rhythms in persons with cancer. Sleep Med Rev 2004;8:199-212.

86. Savard J, Morin CM: Insomnia in the context of cancer: A review of a neglected problem. J Clin Oncol 2001;19:895-908.

87. Davidson JR, MacLean AW, Brundage MD, et al: Sleep disturbance in cancer patients. Soc Sci Med 2002;54:1309-1321.

88. Carpenter JS, Andrykowski MA, Cordova M, et al: Hot flashes in postmenopausal women treated for breast cancer: Prevalence, severity, correlates, management, and relation to quality of life. Cancer 1998;82:1682-1691.

89. Hoda D, Perez DG, Loprinzi CL: Hot flashes in breast cancer survivors. Breast J 2003;9:431-438.

90. Holmberg L, Anderson H, HABITS Steering and Data Monitoring Committees: HABITS (Hormonal Replacement Therapy After Breast Cancer—Is It Safe?), a randomised comparison: Trial stopped. Lancet 2004;363:453-455.

91. Sowers MF, Luborsky J, Perdue C, et al: Thyroid stimulating hormone (TSH) concentrations and menopausal status in women at the mid-life: SWAN. Clin Endocrinol 2003;58: 340-347.

92. Mickelson SA, Lian T, Rosenthal L: Thyroid testing and thyroid hormone replacement in patients with sleep disordered breathing. Ear Nose Throat J 1999;78:768-775.

93. Dzaja A, Arber S, Hislop J, et al: Women's sleep in health and disease. J Psychiatr Res 2005;39:55-76.

Anxiety Disorders

Murray B. Stein
Thomas A. Mellman

ABSTRACT

Anxiety disorders are frequently associated with complaints of disturbed sleep. This chapter provides a review of the diagnostic criteria, sleep features, and treatment of sleep-related problems in patients with panic disorder, generalized anxiety disorder (GAD), social phobia, obsessive-compulsive disorder (OCD), and posttraumatic stress disorder (PTSD). Subjective sleep complaints are most prominent in patients with PTSD, panic disorder, and GAD, and must be understood in the context of depressive disorders that are commonly comorbid. Abrupt nocturnal awakenings are not uncommonly encountered in anxiety disorders such as panic disorder and PTSD, where they are thought to be non–rapid eye movement (NREM) and REM sleep–related phenomena, respectively. Treatments that target sleep can improve outcomes in patients with anxiety disorders.

Anxiety disorders are among the most common of mental disorders, affecting more than 10% of persons in the general population in a 1-year period, and even more during a lifetime. A large, cross-national epidemiologic survey conducted in the early 1990s, the National Comorbidity Survey (NCS), found that 24.9% of adults in the age group 15 to 54 years had a lifetime anxiety disorder diagnosis.[1] In a large European survey of over 14,000 persons in the general population, approximately 1 in 4 respondents with insomnia had a current diagnosis of mental disorders and 25.6% had a psychiatric history. In that study, whereas insomnia antedated (more than 40%) or started in tandem (more than 22%) with mood disorder symptoms among respondents with depressive disorders, when anxiety disorders were involved, insomnia appeared mostly concurrently with (more than 38%) or after (more than 34%) the anxiety disorder.[2] Thus, from an epidemiologic perspective, anxiety disorder onset often heralds the onset of sleep problems, suggesting that a sizable portion of the burden of insomnia in the general population is associated with—and perhaps even etiologically attributable to—anxiety disorders.

Anxiety disorders are also frequently seen in patients presenting to their primary care physicians for general medical care, where complaints of sleep problems are often prominent.[3] Sleep disturbances are included among the diagnostic features of two of the six categories for anxiety disorders in the *Diagnostic and Statistical Manual of Mental Disorders*, 4th edition (DSM-IV; PTSD and GAD) and are commonly associated with others although not incorporated into the diagnostic criteria, per se (e.g., panic disorder). Treatments for sleep problems and those targeting worry, tension, and other manifestations of anxiety often use similar approaches (e.g., relaxation, cognitive or behavioral techniques, benzodiazepine medications). Thus, from a clinical perspective, it is important to consider the diagnosis and treatment of anxiety disorders when caring for a patient with prominent sleep complaints. The converse is equally true: Attention to sleep problems is integral to the quality management of patients with anxiety disorders.

There are also theoretical links between anxiety and sleep disorders. Sleep is a necessary and restorative state of diminished cortical arousal. Anxiety and fear states manifest with heightened cortical and peripheral arousal. Increased arousal is also implicated when sleep initiation or maintenance are disturbed. Thus, insights into mechanisms of arousal regulation would be applicable as well to anxiety and sleep disorders (and their overlapping features). Whereas sleep has been extensively studied in depressive disorders, the polysomnographic (PSG) study of anxiety disorders is less well developed. PSG studies of anxiety disorders provide information regarding measurable objective disturbances in sleep initiation, maintenance, and structure, as well as the presence of a primary sleep pathologic process. Such studies are the primary focus of the material reviewed in this chapter. Sleep disturbance does not seem related to specific phobias, and this subject has been little studied, so it is not included here. In the cases of panic disorder and PTSD, an additional focus relates to the core paroxysmal events that can manifest in relation to sleep (e.g., panic attacks, nightmares). In addition to reviewing PSG studies in the anxiety disorders, this chapter reviews current pathophysiologic concepts for sleep disturbances in the anxiety disorders, and reviews the types of treatments (and their outcomes) that target or indirectly influence sleep in these conditions.

*Deceased.

PANIC DISORDER

Epidemiology and Clinical Features

Panic disorder has a 12-month general population prevalence of 1% to 2%, is more common in women than men, and has a typical age of onset in late teens or early twenties (although it can start earlier in life).[4] It is sufficiently unusual for panic attacks to begin in later life that their de novo occurrence in this context should spur a search for underlying medical (e.g., thyroid disease) or iatrogenic (e.g., prescription drug interactions) causes.[5,6] The characteristic feature of panic disorder is recurrent, unexpected *panic attacks* (Box 111–1), which are acute episodes of severe anxiety associated with a wide array of somatic symptoms, such as chest pain, heart palpitations, tachycardia, psychosensory disturbances (i.e., changes in sound or light intensity, alterations in the perception of time, depersonalization or derealization), gastrointestinal discomfort, and lightheadedness. Classic panic attacks reach peak severity within 10 minutes and are typically brief, lasting only seconds to minutes in most cases. Panic attacks can occur during sleep; in this chapter, the terms *nocturnal panic* and *sleep panic* are synonymous and refer to the same phenomenon.

Panic disorder is diagnosed when an individual experiences *recurrent* unexpected panic attacks. Some individuals may experience infrequent panic attacks for years without conspicuous changes in their health. More often, however, panic attacks are complicated by anticipatory anxiety (i.e., apprehension about future attacks) or worry about possible underlying medical disorders (e.g., heart disease). Such concerns, if lasting for 1 month or longer after the panic attack or attacks, justify the diagnosis of panic disorder. Alternatively, behavioral change (e.g., frequent visits to the emergency department; avoidance of places where attacks have occurred in the past) subsequent to the attacks also justifies this diagnosis. Patients also may become frightened of places or situations in which unexpected panic attacks have occurred. The actual avoidance

---

Box 111–1. DSM-IV Criteria for Panic Attack

A discrete period of intense fear or discomfort, in which four (or more) of the following symptoms developed abruptly and reached a peak within 10 minutes:

- Palpitations, pounding heart, or accelerated heart rate
- Sweating
- Trembling or shaking
- Sensations of shortness of breath or smothering
- Feeling of choking
- Chest pain or discomfort
- Nausea or abdominal distress
- Feeling dizzy, unsteady, lightheaded, or faint
- Derealization (feelings of unreality) or depersonalization (being detached from oneself)
- Fear of losing control or going crazy
- Fear of dying
- Paresthesias (numbness or tingling sensations)
- Chills or hot flashes

DSM-IV, Diagnostic and Statistical Manual of Mental Disorders, 4th edition.

Reprinted with permission from the American Psychiatric Association: Diagnostic and Statistical Manual of Mental Disorders, 4th ed. Washington, DC, American Psychiatric Press, 1994. Copyright 1994 American Psychiatric Association.

Box 111–2. Criteria for Agoraphobia*

A. Anxiety about being in places or situations from which escape might be difficult (or embarrassing) or in which help may not be available in the event of having an unexpected or situationally predisposed panic attack or panic-like symptoms. Agoraphobic fears typically involve characteristic clusters of situations that include being outside the home alone, being in a crowd or standing in a line, being on a bridge, and traveling in a bus, train, or automobile.

Note: Consider the diagnosis of *Specific phobia* if the avoidance is limited to one or only a few specific situations, or *Social phobia* if the avoidance is limited to social situations.

B. The situations are avoided (e.g., travel is restricted) or else are endured with marked distress or with anxiety about having a panic attack or panic-like symptoms or require the presence of a companion.

C. The anxiety or phobic avoidance is not better accounted for by another mental disorder, such as *Social phobia* (e.g., avoidance limited to social situations because of fear of embarrassment), *Specific phobia* (e.g., avoidance limited to a single situation, like elevators), *Obsessive-compulsive disorder* (e.g., avoidance of dirt in someone with an obsession about contamination), *Posttraumatic stress disorder* (e.g., avoidance of stimuli associated with a severe stressor), or *Separation anxiety* disorder (e.g., avoidance of leaving home or relatives).

*Agoraphobia is not a DSM-IV disorder that can be coded. Code the specific disorder in which the agoraphobia occurs (e.g., *Panic disorder with agoraphobia* or *Agoraphobia without history of panic disorder*).

DSM-IV, Diagnostic and Statistical Manual of Mental Disorders, 4th edition.

---

of places (e.g., bridges, tunnels, airplanes) or situations (e.g., driving, shopping, traveling) in which unexpected panic attacks or panic-like symptoms have occurred in the past is referred to as *agoraphobia* (Box 111–2). Depending on the absence or presence of agoraphobia, respectively, patients are given a diagnosis of panic disorder *without* or *with* agoraphobia (Boxes 111–3 and 111–4). Agoraphobia may also occur independently of panic disorder, although this is thought to be relatively rare. In such circumstances, agoraphobia (i.e., fear and avoidance of particular situations owing to fear of incapacitation or embarrassment) may be a complication of illness (and the repercussions thereof) such as vertigo or other forms of physical incapacity.

Sleep Features

Surveys document increased complaints of insomnia in patients with panic disorder compared with nonanxious comparison subjects.[7,8] Most PSG studies have found decreased sleep efficiency and sleep duration with panic disorder,[9-11] although some studies have not found such disturbances.[12] Panic disorder and depressive illness are so frequently comorbid[13] that it is difficult to interpret the sleep findings without taking this fact into consideration. In this context, it may be interpreted that much of the associated sleep disturbance is a function of depressive illness that is commonly comorbid with panic disorder. Another possibility is that depression may

Box 111–3. DSM-IV Criteria for Panic Disorder without Agoraphobia

A. Both 1 and 2:
  1. Recurrent unexpected panic attacks
  2. At least one of the attacks has been followed by 1 month (or more) of one (or more) of the following:
     a. Persistent concern about having additional attacks
     b. Worry about the implications of the attack or its consequences (e.g., losing control, having a heart attack, "going crazy")
     c. A significant change in behavior related to the attacks

B. The absence of agoraphobia

C. The panic attacks are not due to the direct physiological effects of a substance (e.g., a drug of abuse, a medication) or a general medical condition (e.g., hyperthyroidism)

D. The panic attacks are not better accounted for by another mental disorder such as *Social phobia* (e.g., occurring on exposure to feared social situations), *Specific phobia* (e.g., on exposure to a specific phobic situation), *Obsessive-compulsive disorder* (e.g., on exposure to dirt in someone with an obsession about contamination), *Posttraumatic stress disorder* (e.g., in response to stimuli associated with severe stressor), or *Separation anxiety* (e.g., in response to being away from home or close relatives).

DSM-IV, Diagnostic and Statistical Manual of Mental Disorders, 4th edition.

Reprinted with permission from the American Psychiatric Association: Diagnostic and Statistical Manual of Mental Disorders, 4th ed. Washington, DC, American Psychiatric Press, 1994. Copyright 1994 American Psychiatric Association.

serve as a marker of a more severe variant of panic disorder. Although it has been suggested that nocturnal panic may itself be a marker of more severe panic disorder, this has not consistently been found across studies.[14] Greater motor activity during sleep as evidenced by increased epochs of movement time has also been reported with panic disorder, with additional evidence that patients may move *less* on the nights where they subsequently experience sleep panic attacks.[15]

Several surveys and studies of populations with panic disorder have documented the occurrence of panic attacks emerging from sleep as a not uncommon feature of the disorder. The presence of sleep panic attacks may delineate a subgroup of patients with panic disorder with early difficulties with anxiety, and comorbid mood and anxiety disorders as adults.[16]

Box 111–4. DSM-IV Criteria for Panic Disorder with Agoraphobia

A. Meets the criteria for *Panic disorder*

B. Meets the criteria for *Agoraphobia*

DSM-IV, Diagnostic and Statistical Manual of Mental Disorders, 4th edition.

Reprinted with permission from the American Psychiatric Association: Diagnostic and Statistical Manual of Mental Disorders, 4th ed. Washington, DC, American Psychiatric Press, 1994. Copyright 1994 American Psychiatric Association.

In a study that used ambulatory monitoring, 18% of panic attacks were found to occur during sleep hours[17] and approximately one half of patients with panic disorder report experiencing sleep panic attacks at some point during the course of their illness.[7,18] These episodes are often described as being awakened abruptly from sleep, usually with physical symptoms such as shortness of breath that also characterize the individual's panic attacks in awake states. Sleep panic attack episodes appear to be non–rapid eye movement (NREM) sleep phenomena because they have been observed to be preceded by either stage 2 or stage 3 sleep[9]; additional research will be necessary to confirm this stage specificity of sleep panic. This observation does, nonetheless, suggest a possible relationship between diminishing arousal during NREM sleep (i.e., transition into early slow wave sleep) and the onset of sleep panic attacks.

The apparently paradoxical triggering of panic from states of diminished arousal may have implications for our understanding of the pathophysiology of panic disorder. It has been suggested that the occurrence of panic attacks during NREM sleep implicates a more endogenous, physiologic (rather than cognitive or attributional) mechanism for triggering anxiety. Specific mechanisms that have been proposed include sensitivity to subtle increases in blood carbon dioxide levels,[19] irregular breathing during slow wave sleep,[20] and abnormalities in autonomic activity.[9,10] It has been reported that patients with panic disorder have greater cardiac and respiratory reactivity to sodium lactate than healthy comparison subjects during sleep, when the influence of cognitive factors is minimal or absent.[21] Another research group, using pentagastrin to elicit panic attacks during sleep, found that intravenous administration of this drug during stage 2 to 3 sleep resulted in abrupt awakenings, consistent with the notion that panic attacks can occur in the absence of elevated arousal.[22] It has also been reported, using caffeine administration during sleep, that the more fully elaborated panic attacks were preceded by a period of lighter sleep before awakening, providing support for a mixture of physiologic and cognitive influences on sleep panic.[23] In fact, a strong case can be made that the emergence of panic attacks from sleep is consistent with cognitive-behavioral models that view panic attacks as being the result of fearful and catastrophic beliefs about the experience of the attacks themselves,[24] and that a differential physiology for nocturnal panic need not be posited.[25]

CASE STUDY: SLEEP PANIC

Ms. R. is a 28-year-old woman with a 2- to 3-month history of onset of episodes during sleep where she awakes abruptly with a feeling of fear and shortness of breath. She is also aware of tachycardia at the time of awakening. She otherwise feels intensely alert, with no sense of confusion and no dream recall, on awakening. She and her significant other deny somnambulism. After experiencing an episode, she typically gets out of bed, and has great difficulty going back to sleep. She also reported increasing worries and avoidance about going to sleep.

The patient reports that she has been experiencing somewhat similar attacks during the daytime on an occasional basis since the age of 17 years. She reports having experienced these episodes—which feature shortness of breath,

Continued

tremulousness, tachycardia, and dizziness—on multiple occasions (i.e., several times weekly) from 17 to 20 years of age; during this period, she sought care in the emergency department and had multiple medical tests conducted to rule out a seizure disorder or a vestibular disorder. The attacks eventually waned, although she admits to experiencing lesser forms of these attacks once or twice monthly from age 20 years through to the time of her presentation. She states that she had learned that these attacks were bothersome but not dangerous, and she was able to function well despite their continued occurrence during this period. Because the pattern of attacks has now changed to occur during sleep, she is concerned that her belief about their innocuous nature might be mistaken. She also admits to an increase in work-related stresses concurrent with the onset of the nocturnal attacks. She is not depressed, and denies suicidal ideation. She also denies substance abuse or excessive caffeine use.

Although Ms. R. was thin and had no obvious physical risk factors for sleep apnea, an ambulatory sleep-breathing evaluation was conducted that revealed no evidence of obstructive apnea. Thyroid-stimulating hormone level was normal.

In light of the clear history of daytime panic attacks in the past, despite their relative infrequency in recent years, a probable diagnosis of panic disorder was applied. Ms. R. was given a choice of participating in a course of cognitive-behavioral therapy directed toward the panic disorder, or starting on an antianxiety medication that would be intended to block the occurrence of the attacks. Citing time constraints that would make it difficult for her to begin cognitive-behavioral therapy, she opted for treatment with a selective serotonin reuptake inhibitor (SSRI)—a pharmacologic treatment with a good evidence base for its efficacy in the treatment of panic disorder (although data supporting the efficacy of any treatment specifically for nocturnal panic are sorely lacking).[26]

Treatment

The aim of drug treatment is to block panic attacks (waking and nocturnal panic attacks) and to eliminate secondary fears and avoidance behaviors (e.g., sleep phobias). The removal of exogenous (e.g., caffeine) factors or the correction of maladaptive behaviors (e.g., sleep deprivation) that often exacerbate panic disorder should also be an integral part of the treatment program. If a thorough medical assessment has not recently been performed, this should be conducted (including, routinely, thyroid-stimulating hormone measurement to rule out most thyroid problems) before proceeding with antipanic treatments.

Historically, tricyclic antidepressants (e.g., imipramine) and monoamine oxidase inhibitors (e.g., phenelzine) were mainstays in the treatment of panic disorder. For reasons of tolerability, these have been largely supplanted by the selective serotonin reuptake inhibitors (SSRIs; e.g., fluoxetine, sertraline, paroxetine, and controlled-release paroxetine are currently indicated by the U.S. Food and Drug Administration [FDA] for this purpose), which have been found to be effective in the treatment of panic disorder (with or without agoraphobia). High-potency benzodiazepines (alprazolam, extended-release alprazolam, and clonazepam are currently indicated by the FDA for this purpose) have also been widely used to treat panic disorder (with or without agoraphobia). Some medications (e.g., propranolol, buspirone) used often in the management of other

forms of anxiety have been shown to be *ineffective* in the treatment of panic disorder. Cognitive-behavioral techniques are also valuable in the prevention of panic attacks and in the treatment of avoidance behaviors, and have the benefit of yielding long-lasting effects.[27] Preliminary observations support that sleep panic attacks are responsive to antidepressant/ antipanic medications.[28] There is otherwise little information to guide the specific treatment of patients with panic disorder who have nocturnal panic attacks; this remains an area ripe for further research. In the absence of empirical data in this regard, it is recommended that patients with sleep panic attacks be treated with an antipanic agent or with cognitive-behavioral therapy and be instructed on the implementation of good sleep hygiene measures (see Chapter 61).

GENERALIZED ANXIETY DISORDER

Epidemiology and Clinical Features

GAD is typified by chronic anxiety and excessive, pervasive worry (Box 111–5). In community surveys, the 12-month prevalence of GAD is approximately 3%, with lifetime rates being somewhat higher (approximately 5%).[29] As is the case for all of the anxiety disorders, with the exception of OCD, the prevalence is higher in women than in men, with GAD showing an approximate 2:1 female-to-male ratio. The natural course of GAD can be characterized as chronic with few complete remissions, a waxing and waning course of symptoms, and the occurrence of substantial depressive comorbidity.

GAD, it might be argued, has been poorly named. This has led to a tendency to consider it a "generic" form of anxiety, and to make the diagnosis inappropriately and pervasively. Many anxiety (and depressive) disorders are characterized by chronic anxiety and tension; these features alone are therefore insufficient to make this diagnosis. It is the presence of extensive and uncontrollable worry—about multiple factors, such as work, health (where GAD merges with hypochondriasis), and family—that defines GAD. Patients with GAD often present to their primary care practitioner, where somatic complaints (e.g., headache, back pain, chronic gastrointestinal distress) may predominate.

Sleep Features

Sleep disturbance, further defined as difficulty initiating or maintaining sleep, or sleep that is restless and unsatisfying, is one of the six features (a total of three of which are needed to establish the diagnosis) associated with chronic worry in the DSM-IV criteria for GAD. Two of the other features, fatigue and irritability, can be considered consequences of sleep loss. The core cognitive feature of GAD, "excessive worry (apprehensive expectation)," is commonly implicated in the genesis and maintenance of insomnia problems, in that patients often report their worry as most uncontrollable and bothersome at bedtime, interfering with their ability to fall asleep.

The PSG sleep of insomniac patients with GAD has been compared with that of healthy control subjects in a handful of studies, with a synthesis of the findings published.[30] In this synthesis, it is concluded that, compared with healthy control subjects, patients with GAD have increased sleep latency, increased wake time after sleep onset, and reduced total sleep time and lower sleep efficiency.[30] The sleep architecture

---

Box 111–5. DSM-IV Criteria for Generalized Anxiety Disorder

A. Excessive anxiety and worry (apprehensive expectation) occur more days than not for at least 6 months, about a number of events or activities (such as work or school performance).

B. The person finds it difficult to control the worry.

C. The anxiety and worry are associated with three (or more) of the following six symptoms (with at least some symptoms present for more days than not for the past 6 months).
   Note: Only one item is required in children.
   1. Restlessness or feeling keyed up or on edge
   2. Being easily fatigued
   3. Difficulty concentrating or mind going blank
   4. Irritability
   5. Muscle tension
   6. Sleep disturbance (difficulty falling or staying asleep, or restless, unsatisfying sleep)

D. The focus of the anxiety and worry is not confined to features of an axis 1 disorder and the anxiety or worry is not about having a panic attack (as in *Panic disorder*), being embarrassed in public (as in *Social phobia*), being contaminated (as in *Obsessive-compulsive disorder*), gaining weight (as in *Anorexia nervosa*), having multiple physical complaints (as in *Somatization disorder*), or having multiple illness (as in *Hypochondriasis*); and the anxiety and worry do not occur exclusively during *Posttraumatic stress disorder*.

E. The anxiety, worry, or physical symptoms cause clinically significant distress or impairment in social, occupational, or other important areas of functioning.

F. The disturbance is not due to the direct physiological effects of a substance (e.g., a drug of abuse, a medication) or a general medical condition (e.g., hyperthyroidism) and does not occur exclusively during a mood disorder, psychotic disorder, or pervasive development disorder.

DSM-IV, Diagnostic and Statistical Manual of Mental Disorders, 4th edition.

Reprinted with permission from the American Psychiatric Association: Diagnostic and Statistical Manual of Mental Disorders, 4th ed. Washington, DC, American Psychiatric Press, 1994. Copyright 1994 American Psychiatric Association.

---

findings in GAD are unremarkable, and the conclusion is that GAD is characterized by a nonspecific sleep-onset and sleep-maintenance insomnia that compromises sleep quality. Notably, these studies provide evidence that GAD can be differentiated from major depression: The classic reduction in REM latency seen in endogenous major depression is usually *not* seen in nondepressed patients with GAD.[31-33] However, given that most patients with GAD, particularly those encountered in general medical settings, also suffer from major depression, it should be expected that more classic depression-related sleep problems (e.g., early morning awakening) also will be seen. It is doubtful that differentiation of GAD from other anxiety or depressive disorders can be made on the basis of differences in sleep symptoms or PSG findings.

Treatment

Benzodiazepines (e.g., alprazolam, clonazepam) are used extensively in the management of GAD, although strong evidence from double-blinded, placebo-controlled studies indicates that certain classes of antidepressants such as the SSRIs[34] and the dual reuptake inhibitors (also known as norepinephrine and serotonin reuptake inhibitors [NSRIs], e.g., venlafaxine extended-release)[34a] are also efficacious.[34b] Antihistamines may also be helpful for treating core GAD symptoms,[35] although their role in the treatment of insomnia remains controversial. Tricyclic antidepressants are also effective, although their use has largely been supplanted by that of the SSRIs and NSRIs. Treatment for this chronic condition is, not surprisingly, frequently prolonged (i.e., several years). Although tolerance to the hypnotic effects of benzodiazepines is commonly encountered, the available evidence suggests that the antianxiety effects of these compounds persist indefinitely in most cases and are not associated with dosage escalation in the long term.[36] Clinical experience suggests that improvement in insomnia parallels the overall benefits associated with benzodiazepine treatment; however, the relation of insomnia to treatment outcome requires double-blinded, placebo-controlled studies. A substantial advantage of antidepressants over benzodiazepines is the fact that the former treat comorbid depression, whereas the latter do not. New treatments on the horizon for GAD include the medication pregabalin,[37] which may be especially useful for sleep complaints associated with GAD.

Cognitive-behavioral treatments for GAD have also been shown to be highly effective.[38] Such treatments have been shown to have specific beneficial effects on insomnia in patients with GAD.[38a] In older adults, where benzodiazepines may be relatively contraindicated because of concerns about adverse effects (e.g., falls leading to fractures), psychosocial treatments may be particularly appealing.[39] The potential efficiency of integrating psychotherapeutic interventions that target excessive generalized worries, and worries about sleep, warrants exploration.

SOCIAL PHOBIA

Epidemiology and Clinical Features

The term *social anxiety disorder* is synonymous with *social phobia*, and the two terms can be used interchangeably. According to the DSM-IV,[40] social phobia consists of "a marked and persistent fear of one or more social or performance situations in

Box 111–6. DSM-IV Criteria for Social Phobia

A. A marked and persistent fear of one or more social or performance situations in which the person is exposed to unfamiliar people or to possible scrutiny by others. The individual fears that he or she will act in a way (or show anxiety symptoms) that will be humiliating or embarrassing. **Note:** In children, there must be evidence of the capacity for age-appropriate social relationships with familiar people and the anxiety must occur in peer settings, not just in interactions with adults.

B. Exposure to the feared social situation almost invariably provokes anxiety, which may take the form of a situationally bound or situationally predisposed panic attack. **Note:** In children, the anxiety may be expressed by crying, tantrums, freezing, or shrinking from social situations with unfamiliar people.

C. The person recognizes that the fear is excessive or unreasonable. **Note:** In children, this feature may be absent.

D. The feared social or performance situations are avoided or are endured with intense anxiety or distress.

E. The avoidance, anxious anticipation, or distress in the feared social or performance situation(s) interferes significantly with the person's normal routine, occupational (academic) functioning, or social activities or relationships or there is marked distress about having the phobia.

F. In individuals younger than 18 years, the duration is at least 6 months.

G. The fear or avoidance is not due to the direct physiological effects of a substance (e.g., a drug of abuse, a medication) or a general medical condition and is not better accounted for by another mental disorder (e.g., *Panic disorder with* or *without agoraphobia, Separation anxiety disorder, Body dysmorphic disorder, Pervasive developmental disorder,* or *Schizoid personality disorder*).

H. If a general medical condition or another mental disorder is present, the fear in Criterion A is unrelated to it, e.g., the fear is not of stuttering, trembling in Parkinson's disease, or exhibiting abnormal eating behavior in anorexia nervosa or bulimia nervosa.

Specify whether *Generalized:* if the fears include most social situations (also consider the additional diagnosis of *Avoidant personality disorder*).

DSM-IV, Diagnostic and Statistical Manual of Mental Disorders, 4th edition.

Reprinted with permission from the American Psychiatric Association: Diagnostic and Statistical Manual of Mental Disorders, 4th ed. Washington, DC, American Psychiatric Press, 1994. Copyright 1994 American Psychiatric Association.

which the person is exposed to unfamiliar people or to possible scrutiny by others. The individual fears that he or she will act in a way (or show anxiety symptoms) that will be humiliating or embarrassing..." (p. 411) (Box 111–6).

When individuals with social phobia are faced with a situation where they might be scrutinized by others, they experience extreme anxiety. This anxiety can take the form of a panic attack, marked by extreme discomfort, physical symptoms like heart racing and skipped heartbeats, shaking, sweating, blushing, and other symptoms. What differentiates panic attacks seen in social phobia from those seen in panic disorder is that the former are not experienced as unexpected or spontaneous; rather, the individual is acutely aware that his or her anxiety relates to concerns about scrutiny and embarrassment. In other cases, the symptoms may be milder, but last longer. This is often the case when the social anxiety occurs in anticipation of a social situation, such as when someone might worry for days or weeks ahead of time about having to attend a dinner party. Blushing and sweating are symptoms that are often of special concern to the patient with social phobia. In fact, any overt sign of discomfort (tremors in voice, motor tics) that might be visualized by another person is distressing to the social phobic patient. One of these symptoms ("I sweat too much"; "I have the shakes") might be the chief and exclusive complaint of the social phobic patient when seeking treatment from his or her family physician. A careful history, however, will uncover a wider array of complaints typical of the patient with social phobia. It is also important to be aware that although public speaking may be endorsed as a prominent

source of anxiety, further inquiry often reveals social fears and avoidance in many more socially "routine" situations such as speaking to small groups, interacting with authority figures, and relating to peers. In situations where social fears and avoidance are pervasive, a diagnosis of *generalized social phobia* is applied. The generalized type of social phobia is more likely to be associated with disability, and with depressive or substance abuse comorbidity, than the nongeneralized type (e.g., public speaking fears only).

Another aspect of social phobia, in addition to the anxiety experience itself, is the tendency to *avoid*. Many individuals with social phobia avoid the situations that make them anxious, if they are able to do so. Often, though, they are unable to avoid the situation or they are able to resist the temptation do so. In such cases, they endure the situations with intense anxiety or distress. The anxiety symptoms and the avoidance, which may be pervasive, can significantly interfere with daily functioning and reduce quality of life.[41]

Many patients with social phobia report that they always have been "shy"; onset of the disorder is in early childhood (i.e., it has "always been there") in approximately half of cases, whereas in the other half it appears to develop de novo in adolescence among those without a background of pathologic shyness. Social phobia affects slightly more women than men, although men more commonly present to mental health treatment settings for its treatment. Social phobia is often associated with panic disorder or major depression. Alcohol and drug abuse may develop as a complication of social phobia, particularly in men.

CASE STUDY: GENERALIZED SOCIAL PHOBIA

Mr. W is a 54-year-old high school English teacher. He has never been married, nor has he been in a long-term relationship. He comes to us for treatment of what he calls his "debilitating shyness." He reports a lifelong history of social anxiety and discomfort, peaking in severity in his early twenties. At that time, he used alcohol in excess ("to feel more comfortable around others ... it seemed like the thing to do") to the point that his grades suffered and he dropped out of college. After several years of unemployment and ongoing drinking, he joined Alcoholics Anonymous (AA) and returned to school to complete his degree. He has subsequently been gainfully employed as a teacher, but has had virtually no romantic social life or even close friendships despite a strong expressed desire for these. Mr. W states that he feels inadequate around his peers at work, seldom makes eye contact with them, and even less frequently engages them in conversation. When he pushes himself to interact, he reports intense tachycardia, sweating, and "trouble keeping my thoughts straight."

Mr. W does not complain spontaneously of sleep problems, although these are readily elicited. He reports experiencing intermittent problems with initial insomnia. His trouble falling asleep occurs exclusively in relation to certain situations, such as knowing that he will need to attend a staff meeting later in the week. In anticipation of these situations, he lies awake in bed and worries about what he is going to say, how others are going to perceive him, and whether he will make a fool of himself. When such situations are not on the immediate horizon, he sleeps well. He has available an old prescription for a benzodiazepine hypnotic (lorazepam) that he uses when his sleep problems mount over several consecutive nights, but he uses it sparingly for fear of becoming dependent on it.

Treatment was started with an SSRI (sertraline) at a dose of 50 mg at bedtime with instructions to the patient that this would be increased in weekly 50-mg increments to a usual therapeutic dose of 100 to 200 mg/day. The patient phoned his physician after 3 nights of taking the sertraline, reporting that he was waking up after a few hours of sleep, feeling nervous and unable to fall back asleep. He also reported having very vivid dreams, although these were not disturbing to him. His physician suggested he cut back to 25 mg of sertraline daily, and switch to a morning dosing. When seen at the next visit, the patient reported tolerating the medicine well with the change in dose and timing, and the dose was gradually increased to 125 mg/day (in 25-mg weekly increments), all taken during the daytime. After 4 weeks of treatment at 125 mg sertraline per day, the patient reported marked improvement in his level of "self-consciousness." He was encouraged to "test out" the medication effect by participating in social situations that usually made him nervous. Seen 1 month later, the patient reported that he felt much more comfortable in these situations, and intended to practice even more in future weeks and months to improve his confidence.

Sleep Features

Complaints of insomnia are not uncommon in patients with social phobia if the clinician specifically elicits them, although it is rare for a patient with social phobia to present with sleep disturbances as his or her chief complaint. The one study that specifically focused on subjective sleep in patients with social phobia found reports of poorer sleep quality, longer sleep latency, and more frequent sleep disturbance and daytime dysfunction compared with control subjects.[42] The results of PSG are largely normal in social phobia, with sleep latency and sleep efficiency being similar in patients with social phobia and in healthy control subjects; REM latency, REM distribution, and REM density are also normal in social phobia.[43]

Sleep problems in social phobia may, in some cases, be attributable to comorbid depressive illness. Secondary sleep problems may also develop in patients who abuse alcohol. Prominent sleep complaints in social phobia should, in fact, prompt a further exploration as to etiology, including taking a thorough substance abuse history.

Treatment

There is a solid evidence base for the management of social phobia with either pharmacotherapy or cognitive-behavioral therapy. Five classes of medications are effective in the treatment of social phobia: high-potency benzodiazepines (i.e., alprazolam, clonazepam), monoamine oxidase inhibitor antidepressants (i.e., phenelzine, tranylcypromine), SSRIs (paroxetine and sertraline have FDA indications for the treatment of social phobia), NSRIs (venlafaxine extended-release has FDA indication for the treatment of social phobia), and, in certain cases, beta-blockers (e.g., atenolol, propranolol).[26] Clinical experience suggests that some patients with nongeneralized social phobias (e.g., public speaking or limited to other performance situations such as playing a musical instrument in public) may respond to beta-blockers on an as-needed basis, whereas the more generalized, pervasive form of social phobia requires regular dosing with either a benzodiazepine or one of the aforementioned antidepressants. Group cognitive-behavioral therapy for social phobia and, to a lesser extent in terms of strength of evidence, individual therapy are also effective in the treatment of social anxiety disorder, and their duration of effects is longer than that for medication treatments.[44] A combination of psychosocial and drug therapies may be necessary to achieve an optimal response, although research demonstrating the utility of such combinations is still lacking. The impact of successful social anxiety disorder treatment on sleep symptoms has not been ascertained.

OBSESSIVE-COMPULSIVE DISORDER

Epidemiology and Clinical Features

Lifetime prevalence of OCD is approximately 2% to 3%, with the 12-month prevalence in the range of 0.5% to 1.0%. The disorder is approximately equally distributed among men and women in adulthood, although in childhood a predominance of boys is apparent (where it is often comorbid with attention-deficit/hyperactivity disorder). The age of onset is adolescence or early adulthood, although it can begin in childhood, where it often assumes a more malignant course than when it starts later in life. Up to one in five patients with OCD has comorbid tic disorders.

The key signs and symptoms of OCD are obsession or compulsions. Obsessions are thoughts or ideas recognized by the patient as being irrational or foolish. A common example of an obsession is the belief that objects are contaminated with germs, which will lead to illness. An individual with OCD will be able to say that, logically, this makes little sense because other people do not seem to be falling ill at remarkable rates. Yet, despite the ability to "reality test" in this way, the patient cannot rid himself or herself of the obsessions. Obsessions can also take the form of impulses (e.g., a mother's impulse to strangle her baby), which are experienced by the individual as horrific and repulsive.

Compulsions are repetitive but deliberate behaviors performed by the patient in response to a particular obsession (Box 111–7). These are distinguished from tics, which are not purposeful, although they may share with compulsions the ability to suppress them temporarily. The compulsions are performed in a predictable fashion according to specific rules in an attempt to lessen, neutralize, or ward off distressing obsessions. In the example of the patient with fears about germ contamination, the corresponding compulsion commonly consists of avoidance of touching "contaminated" surfaces and the need to wash repeatedly if contact is made. As with obsessions, almost all individuals recognize the illogical nature of their compulsions and, as a result, actively resist the urge to act. Other examples of classic compulsions include repeating (words, or repeated touching or tapping) or checking (the stove to be sure that it is turned off; the door to be sure that it is locked).

Sleep Features

Neither the core syndromal manifestations nor prominent associated features of OCD include sleep disturbances.

An early study that used PSG did find evidence for impaired sleep maintenance, as well as reduced latency to REM sleep in a group with OCD; a majority of these cases were reported to feature histories of abnormal sleep patterns.[45] Two more recent PSG studies of patients with OCD have not replicated these findings and have concluded sleep patterns of patients with OCD are essentially normal.[46,47] Some patients with OCD have problems with sleep. In such cases, the sleep problem is either related to their comorbid depressive illness, or to the obsessions and compulsions themselves (e.g., need to check the alarms and stove repetitively before going to bed).

Treatment

Treatment is targeted toward the management of obsessions or compulsions, and the treatment of comorbid depressive symptoms. Pharmacologic treatment for OCD consists of the administration of antidepressant drugs that block synaptic reuptake of serotonin; these include a tricyclic antidepressant, clomipramine, and the SSRIs (e.g., fluoxetine, fluvoxamine, sertraline, paroxetine). Drug therapy should be continued for a prolonged period (several years) and, in some cases, indefinitely, because the available data suggest that patients' symptoms will return within several months after medications are stopped. Specialized behavioral (or cognitive-behavioral) treatments are

---

Box 111–7. DSM-IV Criteria for Obsessive-Compulsive Disorder

A. Either obsessions or compulsions:

Obsessions

1. Recurrent and persistent thoughts, impulses, or images that are experienced, at some time during the disturbance, as intrusive and inappropriate and that cause marked anxiety or distress.
2. The thoughts, impulses, or images are not simply excessive worries about real-life problems.
3. The person attempts to ignore or suppress such thoughts, impulses, or images or to neutralize them with some other thought or action.
4. The person recognizes that the obsessional thoughts, impulses, or images are a product of his or her own mind (not imposed from without as in thought insertion).

Compulsions

1. Repetitive behaviors (e.g., hand washing, ordering, checking) or mental acts (e.g., praying, counting, repeating words silently) that the person feels driven to perform in response to an obsession, or according to rules that must be applied rigidly.
2. The behaviors or mental acts are aimed at preventing or reducing distress or preventing some dreaded event or situation; however, these behaviors or mental acts either are not connected in a realistic way with what they are designed to neutralize or prevent or are clearly excessive.

B. At some point during the course of the disorder, the person has recognized that the obsessions or compulsions are excessive or unreasonable. **Note:** This does not apply to children.

C. The obsessions or compulsions cause marked distress, are time consuming (take more than 1 hour a day), or significantly interfere with the person's normal routine, occupational (or academic) functioning, or usual social activities or relationships.

D. If another axis 1 disorder is present, the content of the obsessions or compulsions is not restricted to it (e.g., preoccupation with food in the presence of an eating disorder, hair pulling in the presence of trichotillomania, concern with appearance in the presence of body dysmorphic disorder, preoccupation with drugs in the presence of a substance use disorder, preoccupation with having a serious illness in the presence of hypochondriasis, preoccupation with sexual urges in the presence of a paraphilia, or guilty ruminations in the presence of major depressive disorder).

E. The disturbance is not due to the direct physiological effects of a substance (e.g., a drug of abuse, a medication) or a general medical condition.

DSM-IV, Diagnostic and Statistical Manual of Mental Disorders, 4th edition.

Reprinted with permission from the American Psychiatric Association: Diagnostic and Statistical Manual of Mental Disorders, 4th ed. Washington, DC, American Psychiatric Press, 1994. Copyright 1994 American Psychiatric Association.

also useful in treating OCD, although some patients find it too difficult to engage in these treatments and may require considerable encouragement (or concomitant pharmacotherapy) to do so. Available data strongly suggest that providing behavior therapy while the patient is taking medication may delay or prevent relapse when medication is discontinued. In extreme cases, patients with severe, disabling, and treatment-refractory (i.e., unresponsive to several good pharmacotherapy trials and at least one good trial of behavior therapy) OCD may be considered for psychosurgery (i.e., cingulotomy or limbic leukotomy).[48]

POSTTRAUMATIC STRESS DISORDER

Epidemiology and Clinical Features

This disorder is characterized by the recurrent, unwanted reexperiencing of a previous traumatic event. The trauma is one that would be experienced by almost anyone as profoundly disturbing, usually falling in the category of an event that was life-threatening (e.g., violent attack with physical injury; sexual assault; serious motor vehicle collision) or profoundly and abruptly life-altering (e.g., sudden death of a loved one from accidental or unanticipated medical causes). Traumatic experiences that yield PTSD, such as repeated episodes of military combat or domestic violence (i.e., intimate partner abuse), frequently are not single events. After exposure to severe traumatic experiences, it is the norm for individuals to experience brief (lasting several days) periods of anxiety, recurrent thinking about the event, and insomnia. In cases where these symptoms persist more than a few days and cause functional impairment, accompanied by prominent feelings of unreality or memory problems (i.e., dissociative symptoms), a diagnosis of *acute stress disorder* may be applied. In most such cases, the symptoms wane over the ensuing weeks, but when they do *not* (which is the pattern in 10% to 30% of cases, depending on the nature and severity of the traumatic event) and the symptoms interfere with functioning or cause great distress, a diagnosis of PTSD may be applied. To qualify for a PTSD diagnosis, characteristic symptoms must be noted in three domains: (1) reexperiencing symptoms (e.g., nightmares or daytime intrusive thoughts or images, including flashbacks); (2) avoidance symptoms (e.g., avoidance of reminders of the trauma); and (3) hyperarousal symptoms (e.g., insomnia or increased startle response; Box 111–8).

Lifetime prevalence of PTSD is reported to be as high as 7% to 8%, with a 12-month prevalence in the range of 2% to 3%. PTSD is approximately twice as prevalent in women as men in the general population. Common sources of PTSD in men are military combat, and in women, intimate partner violence and violent injury (often associated with sexual assault). Like many of the other anxiety disorders, PTSD is often encountered comorbid with major depression, both in general population samples as well as in clinical settings. More than any of the other anxiety disorders, sleep complaints in almost any context should warrant inclusion of PTSD in the differential diagnosis.

Sleep complaints are myriad and often severe in patients with PTSD.[49] Patients sometimes report not having slept well for decades, with these reports corroborated by their bed partners. Extreme hypervigilance (sometimes bordering on paranoia, but evidently linked to habits learned during combat experiences) may take the form of a combat veteran with PTSD spending several hours each evening "patrolling" the perimeter of his home to ensure that it is protected from intruders. Nightmares, often (although not always) accompanied by vivid recall and, according to companions' reports, extreme motoric activity, are commonplace. It is not uncommon to encounter patients who have tried numerous over-the-counter and prescription medications to help with their sleep, to no avail. Many patients also have alcohol abuse problems, which can complicate the clinical picture and make determination of the nature of the sleep disorder even more difficult. In some cases, other risk factors for disorders of sleep initiation and maintenance—such as obstructive sleep apnea—are present, making an informed evaluation by a sleep expert (with a particular focus on possible sleep-disordered breathing) of considerable value.

Sleep Features

The diagnostic criteria for PTSD prominently feature two types of sleep complaints: nightmares (which are viewed as reexperiencing phenomena) and insomnia (i.e., impairment in initiating and maintaining sleep). A survey of male Vietnam veterans with PTSD confirms that insomnia complaints are very common symptoms of PTSD, although nightmares are more specific manifestations of the disorder.[50] In a Canadian community survey, PTSD was frequently (approximately 70% of cases) associated with violent or injurious behaviors during sleep, sleep paralysis, sleep talking, and hypnagogic and hypnopompic hallucinations[51]; these rates seem very high and need to be replicated, but they do point to the usefulness of a thorough sleep assessment in conjunction with diagnostic assessment of PTSD and other trauma-related disorders. Clinical and survey data further suggest that sleep manifestations of heightened arousal in PTSD include excessive motor activity and awakenings with somatic anxiety symptoms.[52] Understanding the relationship between sleep problems and functional disability in PTSD will be particularly important because there are indications that somatic symptoms associated with PTSD are mediated by the severity of sleep disturbance.[53]

In a study conducted 6 to 8 months after a natural disaster (Hurricane Andrew in Florida), subjects with PTSD did demonstrate some tendencies toward impaired sleep continuity.[54] In patients injured in motor vehicle collisions, sleep complaints at 1 month postinjury predict subsequent PTSD development at 12 months postinjury.[55] Almost all of the initial PSG studies of subjects with PTSD have featured male combat veterans during a chronic phase of the disorder. In these studies, findings are mixed with respect to the presence of impaired sleep initiation and maintenance. Several studies reported reduced sleep time or efficiency or increased awakenings in the patients with PTSD,[52,56] whereas in other studies measures of sleep maintenance did not differ between patients with PTSD and control subjects.[57-59] There are two published studies that corroborate the complaint of excessive motor activity by documenting frequent limb or gross body movement during sleep,[52,60] whereas other studies show reduced movement time during sleep in patients with PTSD.[61] Several studies in patients with PTSD (including men with military combat–related PTSD and women with sexual trauma–related PTSD) have found many patients to have evidence of sleep-disordered breathing.[62] Although not yet widely replicated in other laboratories, the likelihood that PTSD may frequently be associated with sleep-disordered breathing and might, taken a step

Box 111–8. DSM-IV Criteria for Posttraumatic Stress Disorder

A. The person has been exposed to a traumatic event in which both of the following were present.
1. The person experienced, witnessed, or was confronted with an event or events that involved actual or threatened death or serious injury, or a threat to the physical integrity of self or others.
2. The person's response involved intense fear, helplessness, or horror. **Note:** In children, this may be expressed instead by disorganized or agitated behavior.

B. The traumatic event is persistently reexperienced in one (or more) of the following ways:
1. Recurrent and intrusive distressing recollections of the event, including images, thoughts, perceptions. **Note:** In young children, repetitive play may occur in which themes or aspects of the trauma are expressed.
2. Recurrent distressing dreams of the event. **Note:** In children, there may be frightening dreams without recognizable content.
3. Acting or feeling as if the traumatic event were recurring (includes a sense of reliving the experience, illusions, hallucinations, and dissociative flashback episodes, including those that occur on awakening or when intoxicated).
4. Intense psychological distress at exposure to internal or external cues that symbolize or resemble an aspect of the traumatic event.
5. Physiological reactivity on exposure to internal or external cues that symbolize or resemble an aspect of the traumatic event.

C. Persistent avoidance of stimuli associated with the trauma and numbing of general responsiveness (not present before the trauma), as indicated by three (or more) of the following:
1. Efforts to avoid thoughts, feelings, or conversations associated with the trauma
2. Efforts to avoid activities, places, or people that arouse recollections of the trauma
3. Inability to recall an important aspect of the trauma
4. Markedly diminished interest or participation in significant activities
5. Feeling of detachment or estrangement from others
6. Restricted range of affect (e.g., unable to have loving feelings)
7. Sense of foreshortened future (e.g., does not expect to have a career, marriage, children, or a normal life span)

D. Persistent symptoms of increased arousal (not present before the trauma), as indicated by two (or more) of the following:
1. Difficulty falling or staying asleep
2. Irritability or outbursts of anger
3. Difficulty concentrating
4. Hypervigilance
5. Exaggerated startle response

E. Duration of the disturbance (symptoms in criteria B, C, and D) is longer than 1 month.

F. The disturbance causes clinically significant distress or impairment in social, occupational, or other important areas of functioning.

Specify if
- **Acute:** Duration of symptoms is less than 3 months
- **Chronic:** Duration of symptoms is 3 months or longer

Specify if
- **With delayed onset:** Onset of symptoms is at least 6 months after the stressor.

DSM-IV, Diagnostic and Statistical Manual of Mental Disorders, 4th edition.

Reprinted with permission from the American Psychiatric Association: Diagnostic and Statistical Manual of Mental Disorders, 4th ed. Washington, DC, American Psychiatric Press, 1994. Copyright 1994 American Psychiatric Association.

further, be amenable to treatments that target the breathing abnormality (e.g., continuous positive airway pressure) is a very promising avenue for future research.

The prominence of nightmares in PTSD and the strong association of the REM state and dream mentation has focused interest on REM sleep variables. PTSD nightmares most typically arise from REM sleep.[52,58] Abnormalities in the timing or amount of REM sleep in PTSD have not been consistently found. Two studies of combat veterans with chronic PTSD have reported increases in the frequency of eye movements in REM sleep periods (REM density).[58,63] Increased phasic muscle activation during REM sleep with PTSD has also been reported.[64] Symptomatic awakenings with and without dream recall were found to have been preceded more commonly by REM than other sleep stages,[52] suggesting greater arousal during REM sleep and the possibility of REM sleep sometimes being disrupted with chronic PTSD.

In addition, there is some evidence to suggest a relationship between REM sleep activity in the acute aftermath of trauma and the subsequent development of PTSD. In a study of 21 physically injured subjects admitted to hospital who had at least one night of PSG recording within a month of injury, development of PTSD symptoms was associated with a shorter average duration of REM sleep before a stage change, and more periods of REM sleep.[65] More recently, in a subsequent report from a subset of this sample, digitized electrocardiographic recordings were extracted from early and late REM and preceding NREM sleep periods, and the ratio of low- to high-frequency spectral densities was calculated as an index of sympathetic activation.[66] Low-frequency/high-frequency ratios were higher during the REM sleep of the 9 subjects who were positive for PTSD symptoms, compared with the 10 subjects who were PTSD negative. Taken together, these studies suggest that the development of PTSD symptoms after traumatic injury is associated with a more fragmented pattern of REM sleep and, moreover, that increased noradrenergic activity during REM sleep may contribute to the development of PTSD. These hypotheses deserve to be further explored because they may suggest avenues for pharmacologic intervention to prevent the development of PTSD in persons exposed to traumatic events.

Most recently, in the largest PSG study of PTSD conducted to date, investigators conducted sleep studies for 2 consecutive nights with a subset of a representative cohort of young adult community residents followed for 10 years for exposure to trauma and PTSD.[67] Of 439 eligible subjects, 292 (66.5%) participated, including 71 with lifetime PTSD. On standard measures of sleep disturbance, no differences were detected between subjects with PTSD and control subjects, regardless of history of trauma or major depression in the control subjects. Persons with PTSD had higher rates of brief arousals from REM sleep. The investigators concluded that they found no objective evidence for clinically relevant sleep disturbances in PTSD. The increased number of brief arousals from REM sleep that was detected was hypothesized to represent amplified perceptions of these arousals in persons with PTSD. This study calls into question the universality of objective PSG-detectable sleep disturbances in patients with PTSD. It raises the possibility that the presence of sleep disturbance in PTSD may be a prevailing factor in determining treatment-seeking and disability in PTSD, such that patient samples are enriched for sleep disturbance. If this is true, then our efforts to ameliorate sleep disturbance in PTSD should be further intensified.

Treatment

As noted previously, thorough assessment of sleep complaints is integral to the overall management of PTSD. Although the absolute rates of sleep disturbances such as obstructive sleep apnea or parasomnias in patients with PTSD remain to be determined, clinical experience suggests that these are not uncommonly encountered in this clinical population and should be seriously considered in most cases. This may require, in select cases where the suspicion is high, referral to a sleep physician for assessment. Patients with PTSD are also likely to have comorbid mental disorders such as major depression and other anxiety disorders such as panic disorder. Treatment therefore needs to encompass these clinical entities, as well as comorbid alcohol or other substance abuse or dependence, which are also frequently encountered in patients with PTSD.

There is a strong and growing evidence base for particular pharmacologic and psychological treatments for PTSD. Pharmacologic treatments with proven efficacy in the treatment of PTSD include the SSRIs (sertraline and paroxetine are approved by the FDA for this indication) and, to a lesser extent in terms of strength of evidence, tricyclic antidepressants and monoamine oxidase inhibitors.[26,68] Novel and promising treatments for PTSD that may have a particular beneficial impact on sleep include the alpha$_1$-adrenergic receptor antagonist, prazosin,[69] anticonvulsants such as tiagabine,[70] and the adjunctive (or monotherapeutic) use of atypical antipsychotics (e.g., olanzapine, risperidone, or quetiapine).[71]

More than in any of the other anxiety disorders (with the possible exception of OCD, where behavioral therapy is very important), the use of evidence-based psychotherapy is critical either as a primary or adjunctive treatment for PTSD.[72] There is accumulating evidence that psychosocial treatments that focus on sleep aspects of PTSD such as nightmares may have strong therapeutic effects across the full spectrum of PTSD symptoms.[73-75]

PITFALLS AND CONTROVERSIES

The anxiety disorders are often, but not always, associated with disturbances in initiating and maintaining sleep. But when comorbid conditions such as major depression are present—which is frequently the case in many of the anxiety disorders—then sleep problems may be accentuated and take on the features of the predominating mood disorder. The frequent comorbidity of mood and anxiety disorders makes it very difficult, in fact, to paint a particular sleep symptomatic or PSG portrait of the anxiety disorders. Moreover, it could be argued that because comorbid anxiety disorders have been so rarely accounted for in studies of major depression that their presence could contribute to some of the variability in PSG findings seen in major depression.

Patients with GAD may have significant reductions in total sleep time and sleep efficiency. Clinical experience suggests these disturbances, when present, are tightly linked to pathologic worry, and improvement in insomnia closely parallels the successful amelioration of core anxiety symptoms.

PTSD and, to a lesser extent, panic disorder, are frequently characterized by recurrent frightening arousals from sleep. Sleep complaints are so prevalent in PTSD that it could be argued that every assessment of sleep disturbance should include the taking of a thorough history of traumatic events. Available evidence suggests that the predominating sleep pathologic process in PTSD relates to REM sleep, whereas that in nocturnal panic relates to NREM sleep. But reports of high rates of obstructive sleep apnea and parasomnias in PTSD suggest that a more complex etiology for sleep disturbance may exist in individual patients with this disorder. Reports of a high prevalence of sleep breathing disturbances in PTSD are controversial, and remain to be widely replicated and differentiated from a high base rate of sleep-related breathing disorders that might otherwise be seen in patients with PTSD (e.g., when male combat veterans in their sixth decade, with comorbid obesity and other medical problems, are studied). It has recently been suggested that PTSD and panic disorder seem to converge on several sleep-related parameters, namely, sleep quality, presence of episodic parasomnias, and movement time, whereas they diverge in the particular phenomenologic nature of episodic parasomnias, namely, nightmares or nocturnal panic attacks.[75] As suggested by the authors of that report, further investigations focusing on sleep disturbances in PTSD and panic disorder have the potential to further our understanding of the biology of these disorders.

As this research advances, it will be important that sleep studies include representative samples of persons with the disorders of interest, so that our vantage point is not constrained to the most severe, treatment-seeking patients.

Many evidence-based pharmacologic and psychosocial treatments for anxiety disorders improve sleep as part of their spectrum of therapeutic effects, but this is not always the case. In some instances, preferred medications with good evidence of efficacy for anxiety disorders (e.g., SSRIs) may actually worsen sleep while they ameliorate daytime and phobic anxiety. What is a clinician to do in such cases? Here, there is little in the way of guidance to be found in the published literature. There seems to be great interindividual variability in the impact of SSRIs on sleep, such that it may make sense to switch to a different SSRI in the hope that sleep problems are ameliorated. But it may also be the case that direct therapeutic benefits on anxiety are so substantial that the patient (and the clinician) is reluctant to make a switch. In such cases, or when switching between antidepressants does not improve the insomnia, therapeutic trials of adjunctive sleep aids (e.g., benzodiazepines, low-dose atypical antipsychotics) may be considered on an individualized basis. This is an area where further research is sorely needed.

Clinical Pearls

Effective treatment of anxiety disorders includes the assessment and management of sleep symptoms. Clinical experience suggests that education and encouragement about basic sleep hygiene measures can be helpful as an adjunct to treatment in nearly all cases. In some cases, such as panic disorder, where individuals appear to be especially sensitive to caffeine, education about limiting caffeine intake can be of primary therapeutic benefit.

If sleep disturbances persist after the successful treatment of the primary anxiety disorder (and are not an obvious iatrogenic result of treatment, as described previously), the clinician should reevaluate the patient for other possible medical or sleep disorders. In the case of PTSD, where there is reason to suspect that comorbid medical problems and sleep disorders (e.g., obstructive sleep apnea) may be particularly common, a high index of suspicion should be maintained and a thorough medical and sleep evaluation may be considered early in the course of assessment and treatment.

REFERENCES

1. Kessler RC, McGonagle KA, Zhao S, et al: Lifetime and 12-month prevalence of psychiatric disorders in the United States: Results from the National Comorbidity Survey. Arch Gen Psychiatry 1994;51:8-19.
2. Ohayon MM, Roth T: Place of chronic insomnia in the course of depressive and anxiety disorders. J Psychiatr Res 2003;37:9-15.
3. Stein MB: Attending to anxiety disorders in primary care. J Clin Psychiatry 2003;64(Suppl 15):35-39.
4. Sheikh JI, Leskin GA, Klein DF: Gender differences in panic disorder: Findings from the National Comorbidity Survey. Am J Psychiatry 2002;159:55-58.
5. Lang AJ, Stein MB: Anxiety disorders: How to recognize and treat the medical symptoms of emotional illness. Geriatrics 2001;56:24-34.
6. Sheikh JI, Swales PJ, Carlson EB, et al: Aging and panic disorder: Phenomenology, comorbidity, and risk factors. Am J Geriatr Psychiatry 2004;12:102-109.
7. Mellman TA, Uhde TW: Sleep panic attacks: New clinical findings and theoretical implications. Am J Psychiatry 1989;146:1204-1207.
8. Stein MB, Chartier MJ, Walker JR: Sleep in nondepressed patients with panic disorder: I. Systematic assessment of subjective sleep quality and sleep disturbance. Sleep 1993;16:724-726.
9. Mellman TA, Uhde TW: Electroencephalographic sleep in panic disorder: A focus on sleep-related panic attacks. Arch Gen Psychiatry 1989;46:178-184.
10. Sloan EP, Natarajan M, Baker B, et al: Nocturnal and daytime panic attacks: Comparison of sleep architecture, heart rate variability, and response to sodium lactate challenge. Biol Psychiatry 1999;45:1313-1320.
11. Arriaga F, Paiva T, Matos-Pires A, et al: The sleep of non-depressed patients with panic disorder: A comparison with normal controls. Acta Psychiatr Scand 1996;93:191-194.
12. Stein MB, Enns MW, Kryger MH: Sleep in nondepressed patients with panic disorder: II. Polysomnographic assessment of sleep architecture and sleep continuity. J Affect Disord 1993;28:1-6.
13. Roy-Byrne PP, Stang P, Wittchen H-U, et al: Lifetime panic-depression comorbidity in the National Comorbidity Survey: Association with symptoms, impairment, course and help-seeking. Br J Psychiatry 2000;176:229-235.
14. Craske MG, Lang AJ, Mystkowski JL, et al: Does nocturnal panic represent a more severe form of panic disorder? J Nerv Ment Dis 2002;190:611-618.
15. Brown TM, Uhde TW: Sleep panic attacks: A micro-movement analysis. Depress Anxiety 2003;18:214-220.
16. Labbate LA, Pollack MH, Otto MW, et al: Sleep panic attacks: An association with childhood anxiety and adult psychopathology. Biol Psychiatry 1994;36:57-60.
17. Taylor CB, Sheikh J, Agras WS, et al: Ambulatory heart rate changes in patients with panic attacks. Am J Psychiatry 1986;143:478-482.
18. Barlow DH, Brown TA, Craske MG: Definitions of panic attacks and panic disorder in the DSM-IV: Implications for research. J Abnorm Psychol 1994;103:553-564.
19. Klein DF: False suffocation alarms, spontaneous panics and related conditions: An integrative hypothesis. Arch Gen Psychiatry 1993;50:306-317.
20. Stein MB, Millar TW, Larsen DK, et al: Irregular breathing during sleep in patients with panic disorder. Am J Psychiatry 1995;152:1168-1173.
21. Koenigsberg HW, Pollak CP, Fine J, et al: Cardiac and respiratory activity in panic disorder: Effects of sleep and sleep lactate infusions. Am J Psychiatry 1994;151:1148-1152.
22. Geraci M, Anderson TS, Slate-Cothren S, et al: Pentagastrin-induced sleep panic attacks: Panic in the absence of elevated baseline arousal. Biol Psychiatry 2002;52:1183-1189.
23. Koenigsberg HW, Pollak CP, Ferro D: Can panic be induced in deep sleep? Examining the necessity of cognitive processing for panic. Depress Anxiety 1998;8:126-130.
24. Craske MG, Freed S: Expectations about arousal and nocturnal panic. J Abnorm Psychol 1995;104:567-575.
25. Craske MG, Lang AJ, Rowe M, et al: Presleep attributions about arousal during sleep: Nocturnal panic. J Abnorm Psychol 2002;111:53-62.
26. Sareen J, Stein MB: Pharmacotherapy for anxiety disorders in the new millennium. Psychiatr Clin North Am 2000;7:173-186.
27. Barlow DH, Gorman JM, Shear MK, et al: Cognitive-behavioral therapy, imipramine, or their combination for panic disorder: A randomized controlled trial. JAMA 2000;283:2529-2536.
28. Mellman TA, Uhde TW: Patients with frequent sleep panic: Clinical findings and response to medication treatment. J Clin Psychiatry 1990;51:513-516.

29. Wittchen H-U, Zhao S, Kessler RC, et al: DSM-III-R generalized anxiety disorder in the National Comorbidity Survey. Arch Gen Psychiatry 1994;51:355-364.

30. Monti JM, Monti D: Sleep disturbance in generalized anxiety disorder and its treatment. Sleep Med Rev 2000;4:263-276.

31. Saletu-Zyhlarz G, Saletu B, Anderer P, et al: Nonorganic insomnia in generalized anxiety disorder: 1. Controlled studies on sleep, awakening and daytime vigilance utilizing polysomnography and EEG mapping. Neuropsychobiology 1997;36:117-129.

32. Arriaga F, Paiva T: Clinical and EEG sleep changes in primary dysthymia and generalized anxiety: A comparison with normal controls. Neuropsychobiology 1990;24:109-114.

33. Papadimitriou GN, Kerkhofs M, Kempenaers C, et al: EEG sleep studies in patients with generalized anxiety disorder. Psychiatry Res 1988;26:183-190.

34. Davidson JR, Bose A, Korotzer A, et al: Escitalopram in the treatment of generalized anxiety disorder: Double-blind, placebo controlled, flexible dose study. Depress Anxiety 2004;19:234-240.

34a. Gelenberg AJ, Lydiard RB, Rudolph RL, et al: Efficacy of venlafaxine extended-release capsules in nondepressed outpatients with generalized anxiety disorder: A 6-month randomized controlled trial. JAMA 2000;283:3082-3088.

34b. Fricchione G: Clinical practice. Generalized anxiety disorder. N Engl J Med 2004;351:675-682.

35. Llorca PM, Spadone C, Sol O, et al: Efficacy and safety of hydroxyzine in the treatment of generalized anxiety disorder: A 3-month double-blind study. J Clin Psychiatry 2002;63:1020-1027.

36. Soumerai SB, Simoni-Wastila L, Singer C, et al: Lack of relationship between long-term use of benzodiazepines and escalation to high dosages. Psychiatr Serv 2003;54:1006-1011.

37. Pande AC, Crockatt JG, Feltner DE, et al: Pregabalin in generalized anxiety disorder: A placebo-controlled trial. Am J Psychiatry 2003;160:533-540.

38. Dugas MJ, Ladouceur R, Leger E, et al: Group cognitive-behavioral therapy for generalized anxiety disorder: Treatment outcome and long-term follow-up. J Consult Clin Psychol 2003;71:821-825.

38a. Belanger L, Morin CM, Langlois F, et al: Insomnia and generalized anxiety disorder: Effects of cognitive behavior therapy for GAD on insomnia symptoms. J Anxiety Disord 2004;18:561-571.

39. Wetherell JL, Gatz M, Craske MG: Treatment of generalized anxiety disorder in older adults. J Consult Clin Psychol 2003;71:31-40.

40. American Psychiatric Association: Diagnostic and Statistical Manual of Mental Disorders, 4th ed. Washington, DC, American Psychiatric Press, 1994.

41. Stein MB, Kean Y: Disability and quality of life in social phobia. Am J Psychiatry 2000;157:1606-1613.

42. Stein MB, Kroft CDL, Walker JR: Sleep impairment in patients with social phobia. Psychiatry Res 1993;49:251-256.

43. Brown TM, Black B, Uhde TW: The sleep architecture of social phobia. Biol Psychiatry 1994;35:420-421.

44. Heimberg RG, Liebowitz MR, Hope DA, et al: Cognitive behavioral group therapy vs phenelzine therapy for social phobia. Arch Gen Psychiatry 1998;55:1133-1141.

45. Insel TR, Gillin JC, Moore A, et al: The sleep of patients with obsessive-compulsive disorder. Arch Gen Psychiatry 1982;39:1372-1377.

46. Hohagen F, Lis S, Krieger S, et al: Sleep EEG of patients with obsessive-compulsive disorder. Eur Arch Psychiatry Clin Neurosci 1994;243:273-278.

47. Robinson D, Walsleben J, Pollack S, et al: Nocturnal polysomnography in obsessive-compulsive disorder. Psychiatry Res 1998;80:257-263.

48. Dougherty DD, Baer L, Cosgrove GR, et al: Prospective long-term follow-up of 44 patients who received cingulotomy for treatment-refractory obsessive-compulsive disorder. Am J Psychiatry 2002;159:269-275.

49. Lavie P: Sleep disturbances in the wake of traumatic events. N Engl J Med 2001;345:1825-1832.

50. Neylan TC, Marmar CR, Metzler TJ, et al: Sleep disturbances in the Vietnam generation: Findings from a nationally representative sample of male Vietnam veterans. Am J Psychiatry 1998;155:929-933.

51. Ohayon MM, Shapiro CM: Sleep disturbances and psychiatric disorders associated with posttraumatic stress disorder in the general population. Compr Psychiatry 2000;41:469-478.

52. Mellman TA, Kulick-Bell R, Ashlock LE, et al: Sleep events among veterans with combat-related posttraumatic stress disorder. Am J Psychiatry 1995;152:110-115.

53. Mohr D, Vedantham K, Neylan T, et al: The mediating effects of sleep in the relationship between traumatic stress and health symptoms in urban police officers. Psychosom Med 2003;65:485-489.

54. Mellman TA, David D, Kulick-Bell R, et al: Sleep disturbance and its relationship to psychiatric morbidity after Hurricane Andrew. Am J Psychiatry 1995;152:1659-1663.

55. Koren D, Arnon I, Lavie P, et al: Sleep complaints as early predictors of posttraumatic stress disorder: A 1-year prospective study of injured survivors of motor vehicle accidents. Am J Psychiatry 2002;159:855-857.

56. Dow BM, Kelsoe JR Jr, Gillin JC: Sleep and dreams in Vietnam PTSD and depression. Biol Psychiatry 1996;39:42-50.

57. Dagan Y, Lavie P, Bleich A: Elevated awakening thresholds in sleep stage 3-4 in war-related post-traumatic stress disorder. Biol Psychiatry 1991;30:618-622.

58. Ross RJ, Ball WA, Dinges DF, et al: Rapid eye movement sleep disturbance in posttraumatic stress disorder. Biol Psychiatry 1994;35:195-202.

59. Hurwitz TD, Mahowald MW, Kuskowski M, et al: Polysomnographic sleep is not clinically impaired in Vietnam combat veterans with chronic posttraumatic stress disorder. Biol Psychiatry 1998;44:1066-1073.

60. Brown TM, Boudewyns PA: Periodic limb movements of sleep in combat veterans with posttraumatic stress disorder. J Trauma Stress 1996;9:129-136.

61. Woodward SH, Leskin GA, Sheikh JI: Movement during sleep: Associations with posttraumatic stress disorder, nightmares, and comorbid panic disorder. Sleep 2002;25:681-688.

62. Krakow B, Melendrez D, Warner TD, et al: To breathe, perchance to sleep: Sleep-disordered breathing and chronic insomnia among trauma survivors. Sleep Breath 2002;6:189-202.

63. Mellman TA, Nolan B, Hebding J, et al: A polysomnographic comparison of veterans with combat-related PTSD, depressed men, and non-ill controls. Sleep 1997;20:46-51.

64. Ross RJ, Ball WA, Dinges DF, et al: Motor dysfunction during sleep in posttraumatic stress disorder. Sleep 1994;17:723-732.

65. Mellman TA, Bustamante V, Fins AI, et al: REM sleep and the early development of posttraumatic stress disorder. Am J Psychiatry 2002;159:1696-1701.

66. Mellman TA, Knorr BR, Pigeon WR, et al: Heart rate variability during sleep and the early development of posttraumatic stress disorder. Biol Psychiatry 2004;55:953-956.

67. Breslau N, Roth T, Burduvali E, et al: Sleep in lifetime posttraumatic stress disorder: A community-based polysomnographic study. Arch Gen Psychiatry 2004;61:508-516.

68. Stein MB: A 46-year-old man with anxiety and nightmares after a motor vehicle collision. JAMA 2002;288:1513-1522.

69. Raskind MA, Peskind ER, Kanter ED, et al: Reduction of nightmares and other PTSD symptoms in combat veterans by prazosin: A placebo-controlled study. Am J Psychiatry 2003;160:371-373.

70. Taylor FB: Tiagabine for posttraumatic stress disorder: A case series of 7 women. J Clin Psychiatry 2003;64:1421-1425.

71. Stein MB, Kline NA, Matloff JL: Adjunctive olanzapine for SSRI-resistant combat-related posttraumatic stress disorder: A double-blind, placebo-controlled study. Am J Psychiatry 2002;159: 1777-1779.

72. Ballenger JC, Davidson JR, Lecrubier Y, et al: Consensus statement on posttraumatic stress disorder from the International Consensus Group on Depression and Anxiety. J Clin Psychiatry 2000;61(Suppl 5):60-66.

73. Krakow B, Johnston L, Melendrez D, et al: An open-label trial of evidence-based cognitive behavior therapy for nightmares and insomnia in crime victims with PTSD. Am J Psychiatry 2001;158:2043-2047.

74. Krakow B, Hollifield M, Johnston L, et al: Imagery rehearsal therapy for chronic nightmares in sexual assault survivors with posttraumatic stress disorder. JAMA 2001;286:537-545.

75. Sheikh JI, Woodward SH, Leskin GA: Sleep in post-traumatic stress disorder and panic: Convergence and divergence. Depress Anxiety 2003;18:187-197.

Mood Disorders

Ruth M. Benca

ABSTRACT

Mood disorders, including major depressive disorder and bipolar disorder, are commonly associated with sleep disturbance, and sleep problems are part of the diagnostic criteria for these disorders. Although subjective complaints of insomnia are most common, hypersomnolence is sometimes reported during periods of depression as well. Polysomnographic studies of depressed patients have consistently revealed abnormalities in sleep architecture compared with control subjects, including disrupted sleep continuity, loss of slow wave sleep (SWS), and reduced latency to rapid eye movement sleep onset. Both subjective and objective sleep abnormalities may persist even during periods of clinical remission from mood disorders, making sleep disturbance a chronic problem for many patients with a history of depression. Not only is insomnia common in patients with mood disorders, it is predictive of individuals at higher risk for the development of depression. Depression thus must be assessed in any patient with a sleep complaint, and sleep problems often require specific and potentially chronic treatment in individuals with mood disorders.

It is difficult to underestimate the medical importance of mood disorders. Not only are these disorders prevalent, but their associated disability is among the highest reported for any disease. The World Health Organization recently reported in its *Global Burden of Disease* study that in industrialized countries, disability due to major depression was second only to that due to ischemic heart disease.[1]

Disturbed sleep is characteristic of patients with mood disorders, and changes in sleep patterns are among the clinical diagnostic criteria for these illnesses. Over the past 50 years, sleep has been studied more extensively in patients with depression than with any other psychiatric disorder. Not only do depressive patients show significantly elevated rates of insomnia and other sleep disturbances, they exhibit robust and relatively specific changes in sleep architecture that may relate to the underlying neurobiology of depression. This chapter provides an overview of the clinical features and epidemiology of mood disorders and discusses current views of neurobiologic mechanisms and their relationship to sleep changes in mood disorders. It also discusses the treatment of mood disorders and associated sleep problems, including effects of antidepressant and mood-stabilizing medications on sleep.

DIAGNOSIS

Mood disorders are subclassified into depressive disorders and bipolar disorders.[2] Depressive disorders include major depressive disorder or unipolar depression, diagnosed in people who have experienced one or more major depressive episodes. Diagnostic criteria for a major depressive episode are listed in Box 112–1. At least five symptoms must be present for the same 2-week period, and at least one symptom must be either depressed mood or loss of interest or pleasure. Other symptoms of major depressive episodes include insomnia or hypersomnia, weight gain or loss, increased or decreased psychomotor activity, decreased energy, poor concentration, feelings of worthlessness or guilt, or suicidal thoughts. Suicidal ideation is common in more severe depression, and up to 15% of patients with a history of severe depressive episodes ultimately commit suicide. Individuals who are chronically depressed for at least 2 years but do not meet full criteria for major depression during that period are classified as dysthymic.

Bipolar disorder is diagnosed in patients who have experienced at least one manic or mixed episode; most patients have had depressive episodes as well. Manic episodes are described in Box 112–2 and are characterized by elevated or irritable mood. Other symptoms may include decreased sleep (usually perceived as decreased need for sleep), grandiosity, rapid thought and speech, psychomotor agitation, distractibility, or hedonistic indulgences such as shopping sprees, drinking, or sexual activity. Mixed episodes occur when patients meet criteria for both a manic episode and a major depressive episode nearly every day for a 1-week period. During a hypomanic episode, the mood disturbance and some of the associated symptoms are present but are not as severe as in a full manic episode. Patients who experience one or more manic or mixed episodes are classified as having bipolar I disorder, whereas those with at least one major depressive episode and at least one hypomanic episode are classified as having bipolar II disorder. Individuals with cyclothymia have alternating episodes of hypomania and depressed mood.

Major depressive episodes may be categorized with one of several specifiers. Melancholic features include either loss of pleasure in all, or almost all, activities or a lack of improvement in mood in response to normally pleasurable stimuli. Patients with melancholic features also may complain of early morning awakening and diurnal variation in mood, with depression worse in the morning. Depressed patients with atypical features, in contrast, show significant mood reactivity to positive events. They characteristically show significant weight gain and hypersomnia during periods of depression. Patients with catatonic features have psychomotor disturbances that may range from excessive, purposeless motor activity to catalepsy, stupor, or mutism. In bipolar disorder, occurrence of major depressive episodes may show a seasonal pattern, most typically with onset of depression in the fall to winter. Remissions from depression, or even episodes of hypomania or mania, may also be seasonal, with a peak in the spring and possibly in the fall as well. Episodes of major depression or mania may also present with psychotic features. Overall, no specific biologic marker has been identified for

Box 112–1. **DSM-IV Criteria for Major Depressive Episode**

A. Five (or more) of the following symptoms have been present during the same 2-week period and represent a change from previous functioning; at least one of the symptoms is either (1) depressed mood or (2) loss of interest or pleasure.
Note: Do not include symptoms that are clearly due to a general medical condition, or mood-incongruent delusions or hallucinations.

   1. Depressed mood most of the day, nearly every day, as indicated by either subjective report (e.g., feels sad or empty) or observation made by others (e.g., appears tearful). **Note:** In children and adolescents, can be irritable mood.
   2. Markedly diminished interest or pleasure in all, or almost all, activities most of the day, nearly every day (as indicated by either subjective account or observation made by others)
   3. Significant weight loss when not dieting or weight gain (e.g., a change of more than 5% of body weight in a month), or decrease or increase in appetite nearly every day. **Note:** In children, consider failure to make expected weight gains.
   4. Insomnia or hypersomnia nearly every day
   5. Psychomotor agitation or retardation nearly every day (observable by others, not merely subjective feelings of restlessness or being slowed down)
   6. Fatigue or loss of energy nearly every day
   7. Feelings of worthlessness or excessive or inappropriate guilt (which may be delusional) nearly every day (not merely self-reproach or guilt about being sick)
   8. Diminished ability to think or concentrate, or indecisiveness, nearly every day (either by subjective account or as observed by others)
   9. Recurrent thoughts of death (not just fear of dying), recurrent suicidal ideation without a specific plan, or a suicide attempt or a specific plan for committing suicide

B. The symptoms do not meet criteria for a Mixed Episode.

C. The symptoms cause clinically significant distress or impairment in social, occupational, or other important areas of functioning.

D. The symptoms are not due to the direct physiological effects of a substance (e.g., a drug of abuse, a medication) or a general medical condition (e.g., hypothyroidism).

E. The symptoms are not better accounted for by Bereavement, i.e., after the loss of a loved one, the symptoms persist for longer than 2 months or are characterized by marked functional impairment, morbid preoccupation with worthlessness, suicidal ideation, psychotic symptoms, or psychomotor retardation.

DSM-IV, *Diagnostic and Statistical Manual of Mental Disorders*, 4th edition.

Reprinted with permission from the American Psychiatric Association: Diagnostic and Statistical Manual of Mental Disorders, 4th ed. Washington, DC, American Psychiatric Press, 1994. Copyright 1994 American Psychiatric Association.

Box 112–2. **DSM-IV Criteria for Manic Episode**

A. A distinct period of abnormally and persistently elevated, expansive, or irritable mood, lasting at least 1 week (or any duration if hospitalization is necessary).

B. During the period of mood disturbance, three (or more) of the following symptoms have persisted (four if the mood is only irritable) and have been present to a significant degree:

   1. Inflated self-esteem or grandiosity
   2. Decreased need for sleep (e.g., feels rested after only 3 hours of sleep)
   3. More talkative than usual or pressure to keep talking
   4. Flight of ideas or subjective experience that thoughts are racing
   5. Distractibility (i.e., attention too easily drawn to unimportant or irrelevant external stimuli)
   6. Increase in goal-directed activity (either socially, at work or school, or sexually) or psychomotor agitation
   7. Excessive involvement in pleasurable activities that have a high potential for painful consequences (e.g., engaging in unrestrained buying sprees, sexual indiscretion, or foolish business investments)

C. The symptoms do not meet criteria for a Mixed Episode.

D. The mood disturbance is sufficiently severe to cause marked impairment in occupational functioning or in usual social activities or relationships with others, or to necessitate hospitalization to prevent harm to self or others, or there are psychotic features.

E. The symptoms are not due to the direct physiological effects of a substance (e.g., a drug of abuse, a medication, or other treatment) or a general medical condition (e.g., hyperthyroidism).

Note: Manic-like episodes that are clearly caused by somatic antidepressant treatment (e.g., medication, electroconvulsive therapy, light therapy) should not count toward a diagnosis of Bipolar I Disorder.

DSM-IV, *Diagnostic and Statistical Manual of Mental Disorders*, 4th edition.

Reprinted with permission from the American Psychiatric Association: Diagnostic and Statistical Manual of Mental Disorders, 4th ed. Washington, DC, American Psychiatric Press, 1994. Copyright 1994 American Psychiatric Association.

these subtypes, although certain subgroups tend to show evidence of more significant biologic disturbances, such as sleep abnormalities. In both bipolar and major depressive disorders, sleep disturbances are more severe during acute episodes of illness, but may persist during periods of partial or complete remission.

EPIDEMIOLOGY AND RISK FACTORS

Major depression is a common disorder and is reported to have a lifetime prevalence of up to 5% to 12% in men and 10% to 25% in women.[3] The reason for increased rates of major depressive episodes in women is unclear, but may include hormonal factors as well as differences in psychosocial stressors. Given the strong associations between insomnia and mood disorders, discussed later, it is likely that the increased rates of insomnia in women are related to their increased rates of depression.

In contrast to major depression, bipolar I disorder affects only approximately 1% of the population and shows no sexual predilection. The prevalence of bipolar II disorder has also been estimated to be approximately 1% of the population, but the incidence could in fact be higher; many patients with bipolar II disorder may be diagnosed with major depression because hypomanic episodes may be clinically more difficult to detect. Bipolar II disorder, like major depression, is also more common in women. Interestingly, bipolar disorder may occur at higher rates in creative individuals such as writers, and among those in higher socioeconomic groups.

Major depressive disorder tends to appear in the fourth to fifth decade of life and most patients experience their first episode between the ages of 20 and 50 years, whereas bipolar disorder appears somewhat earlier, usually during the third decade of life. Both disorders can appear at any point in the life span, however, and both are being diagnosed at increasing rates in children and adolescents. Although the reasons for the earlier ages of onset of illness are unknown, they may include increased rates of substance abuse and greater psychosocial stressors in our society.

Most episodes of depression or mania last less than 6 months, and patients tend to recover between acute episodes. As the overall duration of illness increases, individual episodes may occur more frequently and last longer. There is increasing evidence that repeated episodes of mood disorders may lead to an overall worse prognosis, with greater number and severity of episodes and poorer interepisode recovery, suggesting that chronic treatment may be beneficial for patients with recurrent illness.

A variety of factors have been associated with an increased risk for mood disorders, including chronic pain or illness, increasing numbers of somatic symptoms, lack of psychosocial supports, a history of alcohol or substance abuse, and recent stressors. Mood disorders also occur with increased frequency in first-degree relatives of affected individuals. Although almost half of the risk for depression may be due to genetic factors,[4] specific genes for depression have not yet been identified, probably because depression may be a heterogeneous disorder with multiple genes potentially involved. As discussed later in this chapter, sleep disturbance—including insomnia or hypersomnia—is one of the most highly predictive symptoms of individuals at risk of having or acquiring a mood disorder.

PATHOGENESIS

Despite the devastating impact of mood disorders, relatively little is known about their etiology or pathophysiology. It has long been hypothesized that abnormalities in central nervous system monoaminergic systems are responsible, specifically deficiencies in noradrenergic, serotonergic, or dopaminergic neurotransmission. This theory is supported by the demonstration of abnormal levels of biogenic amines and their metabolites, and by the fact that most effective antidepressant treatments, including tricyclic antidepressants, monoamine oxidase inhibitors, electroconvulsive therapy, and the newer antidepressants, all regulate intrasynaptic concentrations of monoamines. Conversely, treatment with antihypertensive medications, which are known to deplete monoamines, has been shown to precipitate depressive symptoms. Antidepressants may also precipitate mania in susceptible individuals, which supports the theory that mania may be related to increased monoaminergic activity.

Although considerable research has focused on monoaminergic abnormalities, these investigations have done little to elucidate the pathogenesis of mood disorders. A common phenomenon in pharmacologic treatment for mood disorders involves a considerable lag time between the onset of drug therapy and clinical effect, suggesting a role for neuroadaptive responses in the mode of action of these treatments. Clinical and preclinical studies have suggested that signaling pathways involved in regulating cell survival and cell death might be the long-term targets for the actions of both mood stabilizers and antidepressants. This evidence has led many in the clinical neuroscience field to embrace the notion that impairments of neuroplasticity and cellular resilience might underlie the pathophysiology of mood disorders.[5,6]

Recent studies using a variety of structural and functional brain imaging techniques have suggested that mood disorders are associated with abnormalities in specific brain regions that are known to be involved in emotional regulation (reviewed in Soares and Mann,[7] Davidson et al.,[8] and Nestler et al.[9]). Abnormalities in prefrontal cortex have been documented most consistently in patients with major depression and bipolar disorder; they include decreased volume and reduced blood flow and metabolism, as well as a shift in activation patterns, with bilateral decrements or relative right-sided activation of prefrontal cortex. Other structures involved in regulation of mood and emotion are abnormal in depressive patients, with reports of increased activation in anterior cingulate cortex and decreased volume of the hippocampus; the amygdala, in contrast, tends to show increased activation in depressive patients, during both wakefulness and sleep. Interestingly, the amygdala is normally most activated during rapid eye movement (REM) sleep and many depressive patients show increased REM sleep volume and reduced latency to REM sleep onset, as described later.

In addition to these structural and functional abnormalities, it has been increasingly recognized that the hypothalamic-pituitary-adrenal (HPA) axis is overactivated in depression, with increased secretion of both corticotropin-releasing hormone (CRH) and cortisol (reviewed in Nestler et al.[9]). It has been postulated that cortisol hypersecretion may be responsible for damage to hippocampal neurons, which in turn decrease their inhibition of HPA axis activity. Other potential mechanisms for depression include decrements in neurotrophin production, leading to decreased neurogenesis and loss of hippocampal neurons. Although it is not yet known which of these observed abnormalities is responsible for depression, clearly most of the systems involved in mood regulation also appear to be involved in the regulation of sleep and wakefulness (see Chapter 11), suggesting that dysfunction in particular brain regions may lead to both mood and sleep abnormalities. Possible mechanisms accounting for sleep changes in depression are discussed later.

CLINICAL FEATURES

Subjective Sleep Complaints

Most patients with major depression complain of insomnia. Specific features may include difficulty falling asleep, frequent nocturnal awakenings, early morning awakening, nonrestorative sleep, decreased total sleep, and disturbing dreams. In addition, depressed patients frequently report increased daytime fatigue, and they may attempt to compensate with daytime napping, although they do not consistently show evidence of increased daytime sleepiness.[10,11]

Most patients with bipolar disorder also report insomnia while depressed, but a significant percentage of patients with bipolar depression report symptoms of hypersomnia, with extended nocturnal sleep periods, difficulty awakening, and excessive daytime sleepiness.[12] Similarly, patients with seasonal affective disorder (described in Box 112–3), who have episodes of major depression occurring only during the winter months, may also complain of excessive fatigue or sleepiness. During manic periods, however, patients usually report significantly reduced amounts of total sleep, often with a subjective sense of a decreased need for sleep.

Episodes of depression and mania are often preceded by several weeks of subjectively reported increases in sleep disturbance, and prodromal insomnia may be even more common in mania than depression.[13,14] In many cases, switches into manic episodes are preceded or even precipitated by periods of sleeplessness. Although sleep disturbance frequently worsens during acute episodes of illness, sleep may not normalize even during periods of clinical remission from mood disorders. Several studies have demonstrated that insomnia often persists in treated depressive patients, and may be one of the most troublesome and chronic symptoms despite resolution of the depressive episode.[15]

Association of Sleep Disturbance and Mood Disorders

Epidemiologic studies have demonstrated strong associations between sleep disturbance and depression. In the general adult population, 14% to 20% of individuals with significant complaints of insomnia and approximately 10% of those with hypersomnia showed evidence of major depression, whereas rates of depression were less than 1% in those without sleep complaints.[16,17] An assessment of the lifetime prevalence of sleep disturbance and psychiatric disorders in young adults also found greatly increased rates of major depression in individuals with sleep complaints (31.1% for those with insomnia, 25.3% for those with hypersomnia, and 54.3% for those with both insomnia and hypersomnia) compared with individuals with no sleep complaints (2.7%).[18]

The association between insomnia and depression may be even greater in clinical samples. A study of patients presenting to general medical clinics found that the symptoms of sleep disturbance and fatigue had the greatest positive predictive values (61% and 69%, respectively) for significant depressive symptoms.[19] Studies of diagnostic patterns in sleep disorder centers have found that the most common primary diagnosis for patients presenting with a complaint of insomnia is a psychiatric illness, particularly depression. In a multicenter study of patients evaluated by clinical interview and polysomnography, a diagnosis of insomnia related to psychiatric disorders was made in 35% of cases, and half of those had mood disorders.[20] Over half of the insomniac and medical/psychiatric patients evaluated by clinical interview in sleep disorder centers were diagnosed with sleep disorder associated with mood disorder, according to the International Classification of Sleep Disorders diagnosis.[21] In children seen in general pediatrics clinics, insomnia and daytime fatigue were strongly correlated with elevated scores on the Child Behavior Checklist, and insomnia was particularly associated with symptoms of depression, anxiety, and attentional problems.[22]

It has historically been assumed that mood disorders cause changes in sleep patterns. Possible explanations for sleep

---

Box 112–3.   DSM-IV Criteria for Seasonal Pattern Specifier

A. There has been a regular temporal relationship between the onset of Major Depressive Episodes in Bipolar I or Bipolar II Disorder or Major Depressive Disorder, Recurrent, and a particular time of the year (e.g., regular appearance of the Major Depressive Episode in the fall or winter).
   Note: Do not include cases in which there is an obvious effect of seasonal-related psychosocial stressors (e.g., regularly being unemployed every winter).

B. Full remissions (or a change from depression to mania or hypomania) also occur at a characteristic time of the year (e.g., depression disappears in the spring).

C. In the last 2 years, two Major Depressive Episodes have occurred that demonstrate the temporal seasonal relationships defined in Criteria A and B, and no nonseasonal Major Depressive Episodes have occurred during that same period.

D. Seasonal Major Depressive Episodes (as described above) substantially outnumber the nonseasonal Major Depressive Episodes that may have occurred over the individual's lifetime.

DSM-IV, *Diagnostic and Statistical Manual of Mental Disorders*, 4th edition.

Reprinted with permission from the American Psychiatric Association: Diagnostic and Statistical Manual of Mental Disorders, 4th ed. Washington, DC, American Psychiatric Press, 1994. Copyright 1994 American Psychiatric Association.

disturbance include the increased anxiety and arousal experienced by most patients with mood disorders, abnormalities in circadian rhythms, and the fact that neurobiologic systems involved in mood and behavior may also mediate sleep. Sleep disturbances, however, may also affect mood disorders, and increasing amounts of epidemiologic data support this contention. Insomnia often precedes the onset of a first episode of major depression, but is even more common before episodes of recurrent depression[23]; in contrast, insomnia was more likely to occur subsequently to the onset of anxiety disorders.

In a prospective study, subjects who reported insomnia at both an initial interview and a 1-year follow-up interview were more likely to have developed a new major depression (odds ratio, 39.8) than were individuals whose insomnia had resolved by the second interview (odds ratio, 1.6).[17] In a subsequent study using a similar two-wave longitudinal design, Breslau et al. found that a history of sleep disturbance in the baseline interview was associated with an increased risk for new onset of major depression, anxiety disorders, substance abuse disorders, and nicotine dependence.[18] The association appeared to be strongest between sleep disturbance and major depression, even when depression was defined on criterion symptoms other than sleep disturbance.

A long-term prospective study found that men who reported insomnia or difficulty sleeping under stress while in medical school showed significantly increased relative risks (2.0 and 1.8, respectively) for development of major depression during a median follow-up period of 34 years.[24] In a meta-analysis of prospective studies on risk factors for depression among community-dwelling elderly individuals, 57% of the risk for depression was attributable to insomnia, and insomnia was second only to recent bereavement in predicting depression.[25] Symptoms of depression and reduced self-esteem were more likely to develop in children who reported decreased amounts of sleep.[26] These data suggest that insomnia is predictive of depression across the life span and may even contribute to the development of mood disorders.

Polysomnographic Findings

Major depression has been studied polysomnographically more than any other psychiatric disorder, and most patients have shown objective sleep disturbances (reviewed in Benca et al.[27]). Sleep abnormalities in depression have been grouped into three general categories[28]:

1. *Sleep continuity disturbances.* Depressed patients showed prolonged sleep latency, increased wakefulness during sleep, and early morning awakening, which results in sleep fragmentation and decreased sleep efficiency.

2. *SWS deficits.* Patients with depression have decreased amounts of SWS, both as a proportion of total sleep as well as minutes spent in SWS during the night. Computer analyses have shown that SWS loss is most significant during the first non-REM (NREM) period, and that depressive patients appeared to have reduced delta wave power and delta wave counts across the night.[29] Abnormalities in SWS distribution have also been observed, with a decrease in slow wave activity in the first NREM period relative to the second NREM period.[30] In addition to SWS loss, depressive patients show elevations in fast-frequency electroencephalographic (EEG) patterns and decreased interhemispheric coherence between beta and theta rhythms, and decreased intrahemispheric coherence between beta and delta rhythms, even in the absence of differences in sleep stage amounts.[31] Armitage and colleagues have also reported that slow wave activity abnormalities may be more robust in men than in women.[32]

3. *REM sleep abnormalities.* A number of changes in REM sleep parameters have been reported, with the most robust finding that REM sleep latency (period of time from sleep onset to REM sleep onset) is significantly reduced in depression. Other reported abnormalities in the REM sleep of patients with depression include prolonged duration of the first REM sleep period and increased rate of rapid eye movements (increased REM density) during REM sleep. Increased percentage of REM sleep has also been observed. Common sleep complaints and polysomnographic abnormalities are listed in Table 112–1.

Although the polysomnographic features listed earlier have been documented most extensively in patients with major depression, studies of manic subjects have reported similar findings. In contrast, dysthymic subjects tended to show sleep

---

Table 112–1.   Sleep Abnormalities in Depression

Subjective Complaints	Polygraphic Findings
Insomnia, including	Sleep continuity disturbances
Difficulty falling asleep	Prolonged sleep latency
Increased awakening at night	Increased wake time during sleep
Early morning awakening	Increased early morning wake time
Decreased amounts of sleep	Decreased total sleep time
Less "deep" sleep	SWS deficits
	Decreased SWS amount
	Decreased SWS percentage of total sleep
Disturbing dreams	REM sleep abnormalities
	Reduced REM sleep latency
	Prolongation of the first REM sleep period
	Increased REM activity (total number of eye movements during the night)
	Increased REM density (REM activity/total REM sleep time)
	Increased REM sleep percentage of total sleep

REM, rapid eye movement; SWS, slow wave sleep.

patterns comparable with those of healthy control subjects. Hypersomniac patients with bipolar depression did not show reduced REM sleep latency consistently, and although they complained of daytime sleepiness, their sleep latency, as measured on the multiple sleep latency test, was relatively normal.[33]

Various attempts have been made to correlate sleep abnormalities with specific symptoms, duration, or global severity of illness. Significant sleep disturbances were not seen in depressed patients who did not meet criteria for major depression and in individuals with depressed mood but not a mood disorder[34]; this finding suggested that a depressed mood alone does not produce the polysomnographic abnormalities of depression. Giles et al.[35] have shown that the symptoms of terminal insomnia, decreased appetite, anhedonia, and unreactive mood were more strongly associated with reduced REM sleep latency in patients with endogenous depression. A recent multivariate analysis of sleep variables and depressive symptoms found that a constellation of 15 depressive symptoms, including depressed mood, weight loss, decreased libido, disturbed sleep, anxiety, and self-blame, were correlated with 9 sleep variables, particularly decreased delta activity, increased stage 1 sleep percentage of total sleep, and increased REM activity.[36] These findings suggest that the relationship between sleep abnormalities and depression is based on associations between a number of core depressive symptoms and predominantly NREM sleep abnormalities.

There is evidence to suggest that duration of the depressive episode may correlate with the degree of observed sleep abnormalities. In studies of middle-aged patients, REM sleep abnormalities were more pronounced during the early phase of a recurrent episode of depression compared with a more chronic phase of a previous episode.[37] A study of elderly subjects found that both REM and NREM sleep abnormalities were more severe in patients during the early phase of a depressive episode compared with patients who had been depressed for longer periods of time.[38] These findings suggest that more significant REM sleep abnormalities may be associated with an earlier phase of the depressive episode or recurrence.

The presence of sleep disturbance does not necessarily indicate that a patient is acutely ill at the time of study. Several studies have reported sleep parameters in patients in remission as well as during episodes of illness. Some sleep abnormalities may be more severe in acute versus remitted phases, including increased REM density and reduced sleep efficiency.[39] However, reduced REM sleep latency and decreased SWS can persist for prolonged periods in otherwise asymptomatic individuals. Thus, sleep disturbances—particularly reduced REM sleep latency and SWS abnormalities—may be trait markers for some patients with mood disorders rather than simply indications of an acute state of illness. The persistence of sleep abnormalities in the absence of clinical illness has been interpreted in two ways: (1) Sleep disturbance may indicate a biologic susceptibility for depression and predate the illness, or (2) sleep changes may be caused by depression and persist much longer than other affective symptoms.[28]

The hypothesis of reduced REM sleep latency as a trait rather than a state marker is further supported by data from family studies. First-degree relatives with major depression tend to show concordance in REM sleep latency measures.[40] Furthermore, first-degree relatives of probands with major depression and short REM sleep latency are themselves more likely to show reduced REM sleep latency and SWS deficits, even without a personal history of a mood disorder.[41] Another study compared non–psychiatrically ill subjects who had at least one first-degree relative with a mood disorder (high-risk probands) with healthy subjects without any family history of psychiatric illness (normal probands). Although their affected first-degree relatives were not characterized polysomnographically, the high-risk probands showed increased phasic REM sleep and reduced SWS compared with the normal probands.[42] These data suggest familial transmission of polysomnographic features of sleep associated with depression. Ongoing longitudinal studies will determine whether the sleep abnormalities confer increased risk for development of mood disorders.

Age strongly affects the relationship between sleep patterns and mood disorders. An analysis of age and sex effects in people with depression showed that REM sleep latency, SWS amount, and sleep efficiency declined with age, and that SWS amounts were greater in women than men.[43] Younger groups with depression were generally indistinguishable from control subjects in most sleep parameters.[27] The interaction of depression and age on sleep parameters suggests that depression may accelerate the effects of aging on sleep. This is probably not the case because some sleep parameters that change with age do not show increased effects of depression. For example, elderly patients with depression do not tend to have significant reductions in SWS compared with control subjects; the absence of a difference may result from both groups having very little SWS by that time. The duration of the first REM sleep period, sleep latency, and other sleep-continuity measures also do not show evidence of depression-age interactions.[27] In summary, although adult groups of patients are more easily distinguished from control subjects, the effects of age on sleep in depression cannot yet be explained easily.

Mechanisms for Sleep Changes in Mood Disorders

Attempts have been made to explain the mechanisms for sleep changes in mood disorders as well as correlate them with other biologic abnormalities in depression. A number of hypotheses have been advanced, and include those discussed in the following sections.

Cholinergic–Aminergic Imbalance

Considerable evidence suggests that REM sleep is promoted by cholinergic activation in the medial pontine reticular formation and inhibited by aminergic (serotonergic and noradrenergic) activation[44] (see Chapter 10). Thus, either enhanced cholinergic neurotransmission or diminished aminergic neurotransmission could account for the short REM sleep latency and elevated REM density and, possibly, for the reduced total sleep time and sleep efficiency of depression. Increased cholinergic activation may also suppress SWS; animal studies have demonstrated that pontine reticular formation neurons inhibit delta wave production by thalamocortical neurons.[45] Furthermore, these same changes might account for the HPA axis activation of depression.[46,47] This interpretation of the sleep and neuroendocrine abnormalities of depression would also be consistent with the cholinergic–aminergic imbalance hypothesis of affective disorders originally proposed by Janowsky et al.[48] Cholinergic, muscarinic receptor supersensitivity has been proposed to play an important role in the pathophysiology of depression, particularly the associated changes in sleep.[49] Healthy volunteers treated with scopolamine, a muscarinic antagonist, for 3 days and studied during a period of withdrawal showed many of the sleep changes typical of depression, including short REM sleep latency, elevated REM sleep density, and shortened sleep.[49,50] Consistent with the cholinergic supersensitivity hypothesis, depressed patients, compared with control subjects, show faster REM sleep induction with the muscarinic agonists arecoline[51] and RS-86[52] and more frequent awakening with infusions of physostigmine (an anticholinesterase).[53] Increased sensitivity to cholinergic REM sleep induction, like short REM sleep latency, may also be a marker for depression because concordance has been demonstrated in twin and family studies.[54]

The Two-Process Model of Sleep Regulation: Deficiency of Process S

Borbély[55] proposed that sleep is regulated by the interaction of two processes: a homeostatic, sleep-inducing process (process S), which rises exponentially during wakefulness and declines exponentially during sleep; and a circadian process (process C), which reflects an internal clock that governs circadian propensity for sleep (see Chapter 33). He has suggested that process S is deficient in patients with depression.[56] Process S is considered to be an inhibitor of REM sleep; therefore, the less SWS (which reflects process S), the shorter the REM sleep latency, the longer the first REM sleep period, and the higher the REM sleep density. Because process S is inferred from the time course of delta activity (or, more technically, EEG power density in the low-frequency range) across the night, this hypothesis reflects the reduction of SWS in depression. When compared with healthy control subjects, depressed patients show a reduction of both the integrated EEG power density and the average delta count (delta waves/minute).[29,57] The hypothesis may also explain the antidepressant effect of total and partial sleep deprivation because process S increases with sleep deprivation.

Increased REM Sleep Pressure

Related to the observations that REM sleep latency is reduced and REM sleep proportion is increased in depressive patients, Vogel and colleagues have postulated that depression may be caused by excessive amounts of REM sleep and the resulting decrease in REM sleep pressure.[58] According to this view, the sleep deprivation therapies work by suppressing REM sleep and thus increasing REM sleep pressure. In addition, most antidepressant medications suppress REM sleep for prolonged periods, a point that Vogel et al. have used to support their hypothesis. Further evidence for a relationship between increased REM sleep pressure and antidepressant response is suggested by the positive correlations between clinical response and either REM sleep suppression early in the course of treatment with tricyclics or REM sleep rebound after cessation of REM sleep deprivation or tricyclic administration.[59,60] The fact that a number of effective medications (e.g., bupropion, nefazodone, and trazodone) do not reduce REM sleep, however, suggests that REM sleep suppression is not necessary for an antidepressant response.

Circadian Phase Advance

The phase-advance hypothesis suggests that the circadian oscillator controlling REM sleep, temperature, and cortisol is phase-advanced in depressed patients. That is, when a depressed patient retires at midnight, the NREM–REM sleep cycles are similar to the NREM–REM sleep cycles of a normal person beginning much later in the night. Wehr and Wirz-Justice[61] proposed the internal phase coincidence model to explain REM sleep abnormalities in depression. They hypothesized that REM sleep is phase-advanced relative to the sleep–wake cycle in depressive patients, and that depression results from awakening at sensitive circadian phases. Studies in healthy subjects have confirmed that an acute phase delay in bedtime results in REM sleep changes similar to those seen in depression.[62]

The phase-advance hypothesis would account for the short REM sleep latency and, possibly, the increased length and duration of the first REM sleep period. However, it is not clear that short REM sleep latency at night invariably means phase advance of the REM sleep circadian system. For example, Kupfer et al.[63] reported that REM sleep latency during daytime naps was correlated with REM sleep latency at night. Schulz and Tetzlaff[64] also reported that REM sleep latency was short in depressed patients after awakenings at night. Thus, the available data suggest that REM sleep latency is short whenever sleep occurs in depressed patients. Furthermore, other studies have suggested that REM sleep does not appear to be phase-advanced when measured relative to "clock" time (i.e., REM sleep appeared to occur at the same time of night, but earlier relative to sleep onset).[65] The data on circadian temperature rhythms do not show a consistent phase advance in depressed patients but suggest instead that, if anything, the nocturnal temperature of depressed patients is elevated,[66] whereas the amplitude of the circadian temperature rhythm is reduced.[67,68] Other studies have demonstrated a possible phase advance of the temperature curve, including earlier appearances of maximal and minimal body temperatures.[69] Although cortisol rhythm may show a phase advance in depression,[70] the effect is relatively small and has not been found consistently. One possible explanation for these findings is that circadian rhythms are "flat" (i.e., have reduced amplitude) in depression. Although phase advance of bedtime has been shown to have antidepressant effects and has been proposed to support the phase-advance hypothesis,[71] not all studies have been able to confirm the antidepressant effects of phase advance.[72]

Hypothalamic-Pituitary-Adrenal Axis Dysregulation

Many patients with depression show dysregulation of their HPA axis, characterized by excessive CRH and cortisol secretion; they also show a lack of cortisol suppression in response to challenge with dexamethasone.[9] One question that has been addressed is whether people with depression who fail to reduce cortisol secretion in response to the dexamethasone suppression test are the same people who exhibit short REM sleep latency. Although the two groups (dexamethasone suppression test nonsuppressors and those with short REM sleep latency) are not identical, the two parameters tend to be correlated.[73]

It is possible that increased activity of the HPA axis could contribute to sleep changes in depression because people with depression tend to secrete excessive daily amounts of cortisol, and cortisol hypersecretors tend to have reduced REM sleep latency.[74] CRH is known to increase arousal, disrupt sleep, and possibly contribute to reduced REM sleep latency (reviewed in Steiger[75]). Elevated CRH levels in the brain may also contribute to other symptoms of depression, and HPA axis activity normalizes in treated depressive patients in association with clinical improvement.[76]

Primary Sleep Disorders and Mood Disorders

There may also be an increased association between primary sleep disorders and mood disorders. For example, patients with sleep apnea or narcolepsy appear to have elevated levels of anxiety, depression, and substance abuse. A recent general population study has demonstrated that approximately one in five individuals with sleep apnea has major depressive disorder, and vice versa.[77] Patients with restless legs syndrome or periodic limb movements showed elevated depressive symptomatology.[78] Conversely, as described later, antidepressants may precipitate or exacerbate movement disorders in sleep. Patients with mood disorders and sleep disturbance thus should be screened for primary sleep disorders.

TREATMENT

Treatment of Sleep Disturbance in Patients with Mood Disorders

The diagnosis of a mood disorder is often complicated by the failure of the patient to recognize the nature of the illness. Patients with mood disorders may present to primary care physicians or sleep clinics with complaints of insomnia or fatigue alone. People with depression often try to deny the presence of an emotional disturbance and attribute their symptoms of low energy, poor concentration, lack of motivation, and loss of interest to sleep loss. Because of the strong association between mood disorders and insomnia suggested in recent surveys of the general population, as discussed previously, any patient presenting with sleep complaints must be screened for depression. Recognition of major depression is important for determining appropriate treatment and must include careful assessment of possible suicide risk, given the high rate of suicide in this patient group. Obviously, patients with suicidal ideation should not be given potentially lethal amounts of hypnotics or antidepressants.

In screening patients for depression, it is important for the clinician to establish rapport and create a permissive and supportive atmosphere for the patient to discuss any psychological symptoms. It is frequently necessary to ask about depressed mood and anhedonia in several ways before a patient will admit to these symptoms. Some examples of the kinds of questions that can be used for this purpose are listed in Box 112–4. Patients who have either depressed mood or loss of interest or pleasure in activities for at least a 2-week period should be questioned about the additional symptoms listed in Box 112–1 to make the diagnosis of a major depressive episode.

Mood disorders and the accompanying sleep disturbances may be treated with medication, psychotherapy, or a combination of both. Patients meeting criteria for major depression with moderate to severe symptoms usually are treated with

---

Box 112–4. Examples of Questions to Elicit Primary Symptoms of Depression

Depressed mood:

- How has your mood been recently?
- Have you been feeling down/depressed/sad/blue lately?
- Has your sleep problem affected your mood?

Loss of interest or pleasure:

- Has your ability to enjoy things changed?
- Has your interest in things decreased?
- Are you less motivated to do things that are normally enjoyable for you?

---

medication (Table 112–2). Slightly over one half of all depressed patients improve regardless of the choice of drug. Individuals with the melancholic type of depression, including diurnal variation in mood, loss of interest or pleasure, lack of mood reactivity to environmental stimuli, early morning awakening, and weight loss, have a significantly greater response rate to somatic therapies. The tricyclic antidepressants and most of the newer agents are roughly equivalent in terms of overall clinical efficacy, although individual patients may respond preferentially to particular drugs. The initial choice of antidepressant is therefore often made on the basis of side effect profile or the physician's experience with the drug; patients with agitated depression and severe insomnia might be started on a more sedating antidepressant, for example. Pharmacologic treatments for mood disorders all have significant effects on sleep, including both the tendency to normalize sleep patterns by treating the underlying illness as well as direct effects on sleep.

Selective serotonin reuptake inhibitors (SSRIs) are currently the most widely prescribed class of drugs for depression in the United States. Along with some of the other newer agents (e.g., bupropion, mirtazapine, and venlafaxine), they have become first-line agents because of their safety and improved side effect profiles compared with the older tricyclics and monoamine oxidase inhibitors (MAOIs). SSRIs, bupropion, and venlafaxine can cause significant sleep disruption and worsen insomnia in some patients, however.[79-81] In contrast, trazodone, nefazodone, and mirtazapine are sedating and may improve sleep initiation and maintenance.

Although use of tricyclic antidepressants has diminished because of the associated side effects and greater toxicity, these drugs may be effective in patients who fail to improve with SSRIs or other, newer antidepressants. Most tricyclics are quite sedating, and therefore may be helpful to depressed patients with insomnia; they continue to be used for treatment of migraine headaches and other chronic pain conditions. Low doses of tricyclics such as amitriptyline have commonly been prescribed for insomnia, although there are no controlled studies for use of tricyclics as hypnotics in the absence of significant depression.

MAOIs are sometimes used, albeit rarely, in patients who fail to improve with other agents or in those with atypical features (hypersomnia, increased appetite) or a significant component of anxiety. The drawback to using these agents is the danger of hypertensive crisis if used in combination with sympathomimetic drugs or with foods containing tyramine.

Table 112–2. Treatment of Major Depression

Medication	Usual Dosage Range	Pharmacologic Mechanism	Side Effects	Effects on Sleep
Heterocyclics				
Amitriptyline (Elavil)	75-150 mg	Inhibit serotonin and norepinephrine reuptake	Anticholinergic effects (drugs listed in decreasing order of severity): blurred vision, dry mouth, urinary retention, orthostatic hypotension, flushing, tachycardia, confusion, others	Sedation (drugs listed in decreasing order; clomipramine desipramine, and protriptyline may be nonsedating or activating)
Imipramine (Tofranil)	100-300 mg			
Doxepin (Sinequan)	75-300 mg	Anticholinergic		
Nortriptyline (Pamelor)	50-150 mg	Antihistaminergic		
Clomipramine (Anafranil)	100-250 mg			REM sleep suppression
Desipramine (Norpramin)	75-200 mg		Other side effects include liver toxicity, lowering of seizure threshold, sweating, weight gain	Increased stage 2 sleep
Protriptyline (Vivactil)	15-60 mg			
Monoamine Oxidase Inhibitors				
Phenelzine (Nardil)	45-90 mg	Inhibit monoamine oxidase, increasing norepinephrine, serotonin, and dopamine	Hypertensive crisis in combination with tyramine-containing foods or sympathomimetics	Insomnia
Isocarboxazid (Marplan)	10-30 mg			Potent REM sleep suppression
Tranylcypromine (Parnate)	30-60 mg		Anticholinergic effects Dizziness, agitation, liver toxicity Weight gain	
Selective Serotonin Reuptake Inhibitors (SSRIs)				
Fluoxetine (Prozac)	20-60 mg	Inhibits serotonin reuptake	Gastrointestinal disturbances	Insomnia
Paroxetine (Paxil)	20-60 mg		Sexual dysfunction	REM sleep suppression
Sertraline (Zoloft)	50-200 mg		Anxiety, agitation Possible increased risk for suicide	Increased eye movements in non-REM sleep
Other Antidepressants				
Trazodone (Desyrel)	150-600 mg	Inhibits serotonin reuptake Blocks alpha₁ adrenoreceptors Serotonin-2A receptor antagonist	Few anticholinergic effects Nausea, dizziness, dry mouth Priapism	Sedation
Nefazodone (Serzone)	200-300 mg	Inhibits serotonin and norepinephrine reuptake Serotonin-2A receptor antagonist	Nausea, dizziness, dry mouth Hepatic failure Priapism	Sedation
Bupropion (Wellbutrin)	100-450 mg	Inhibits norepinephrine and dopamine reuptake	Gastrointestinal upset Lowering of seizure threshold	Insomnia
Venlafaxine (Effexor)	75-375 mg	Inhibits serotonin, norepinephrine, and dopamine reuptake	Anxiety Anorexia Hypertension Possible increased risk for suicide	Insomnia REM sleep suppression
Mirtazapine (Remeron)	15-45 mg	Alpha₂ receptor antagonist Serotonin-2 and -3 receptor antagonist Antihistaminergic	Increased appetite, weight gain Dizziness	Sedation REM sleep suppression

REM, rapid eye movement.

Severely depressed patients, including those with psychotic features or strong suicidal intent, may require a course of electroconvulsive therapy treatments. Antipsychotics are also used in combination with antidepressants in delusional or psychotic patients, or those who are treatment resistant to antidepressants alone. Many of the newer, atypical antipsychotics (e.g., risperidone, olanzapine, and quetiapine) are used to enhance antidepressant responses to SSRIs or as mood stabilizers in bipolar patients because of their antimanic properties (see Chapter 113 for further discussion of atypical antipsychotic agents). Commonly used antidepressants and their dose ranges and side effects are listed in Table 112–2.

Many antidepressant medications have REM sleep–suppressing effects, which has led to the theory that some antidepressants work by causing selective REM sleep deprivation.[58] MAOIs are the most potent suppressors of REM sleep, and they may virtually eliminate REM sleep for prolonged periods of treatment.[82] Tricyclics, SSRIs, and venlafaxine also reduce REM sleep amounts and prolong REM sleep latency.[80,81,83] Electroconvulsive therapy has also been reported to prolong REM sleep latency but has little effect on REM sleep amount.[84] Not surprisingly, abrupt cessation of REM sleep–suppressing antidepressants is associated with REM sleep rebound, with accompanying symptoms of bizarre, intense, or frightening dreams and sleep fragmentation.

Some of the newer antidepressants, however, do not suppress REM sleep, suggesting that REM sleep suppression is not necessary for clinical efficacy. Trazodone and nefazodone are relatively sedating drugs with no consistent effects on REM sleep patterns. Bupropion, a more activating agent, has even been reported to cause increases in REM sleep in some cases.[85]

Antidepressants may also show a variety of other effects on sleep. Some patients complain of "hangover" effects from the more sedating or anticholinergic agents, such as trazodone, nefazodone, mirtazapine, and tricyclics. Fluoxetine and other SSRIs have been associated with frequent eye movements in NREM sleep, which may persist for prolonged periods after cessation of treatment; the clinical significance of this effect is unknown.[86] Tricyclic antidepressants and SSRIs have been implicated in precipitating or exacerbating restless legs/ periodic leg movements, and may thus exacerbate symptoms of insomnia or daytime fatigue by this mechanism in some patients.[87,88] REM sleep behavior disorder also has been reported after administration of various REM sleep–suppressing antidepressants.[86,89]

Patients with bipolar disorders usually require the use of mood stabilizers (Table 112–3). Lithium carbonate is the treatment of choice for most manic patients, although antipsychotics may also be required during the acute phase of a manic episode. The anticonvulsants carbamazepine, oxcarbazepine, sodium valproate, and topiramate also have been found to be effective treatments for some patients with bipolar disorders that cannot be controlled with lithium, and may be used alone or in combination with lithium. The efficacy of both lithium and the anticonvulsants depends on achieving adequate plasma drug levels. Mood-stabilizing agents have more potent antimanic than antidepressant effects, and depressed patients with bipolar disorders may require antidepressant medication in addition; one exception to this rule is lamotrigine, an anticonvulsant that appears to be effective in treating bipolar depression and prolonging time to recurrence of mania, but does not seem to have significant antimanic properties.

Lithium carbonate may prolong REM sleep latency and suppress REM sleep time.[90] In manic patients, it has been shown to increase SWS amounts as well. Lithium and the mood-stabilizing anticonvulsants can lead to increased daytime sleepiness, particularly at higher plasma levels. Lithium has also been reported to induce restless legs syndrome.[91]

In treating patients with mood disorders and prominent sleep disturbances, it is important to focus on both the

Table 112–3.   Treatment of Mania

Medication	Usual Dosage Range	Side Effects	Effects on Sleep
Lithium carbonate	600-1800 mg/day Plasma level: 0.7-1.5 mEq/L	Increased white blood cell count Polyuria, polydypsia Diabetes insipidus Decreased thyroid function Weight gain Gastrointestinal upset Tremor	Sedation Increased total sleep May increase slow wave sleep, decrease rapid eye movement sleep
Carbamazepine	800-1200 mg/day Plasma level: 4-12 µg/mL	Bone marrow suppression (rare) Liver toxicity Rashes	Sedation
Sodium valproate	30-60 mg/kg/day Plasma level: 50-100 µg/mL	Gastrointestinal upset Liver toxicity Tremor Weight gain Rashes	Mild sedation No significant effects on sleep
Lamotrigine*	100-400 mg/day	Rash Stevens-Johnson Syndrome	Minimal effects on sleep architecture Mild sedation

*Not directly antimanic; more useful for bipolar depression but may prevent recurrence of mania.

psychiatric illness as well as the sleep complaint. As the acute illness resolves, the sleep problem may improve, although it may not resolve completely. In mild to moderate cases of depression or hypomania, insomnia can be an important target symptom and a gauge of treatment efficacy. The degree of sleep disturbance is not always linked with the clinical course of a mood disturbance, however. For example, fluoxetine was found to be equally as effective as nefazodone in ameliorating depression, but significantly more disruptive of sleep.[92,93] Furthermore, insomnia may be exacerbated directly by activation antidepressants or stimulants, and psychotropic medications can produce sleep disturbance indirectly by exacerbating or precipitating sleep disorders (e.g., antidepressant-induced restless legs syndrome/periodic leg movements during sleep, or sleep apnea worsened by weight gain from lithium, antipsychotics, or some antidepressants).

The choice of a specific drug regimen should be influenced by the patient's sleep complaint. Patients with agitated depression or mania and total insomnia may initially require a hypnotic or sedating antipsychotic medication if psychosis is present or insomnia is severe and refractory to other agents. It may be particularly important to treat insomnia in mania because sleep loss is a trigger for manic episodes in some patients. For depressed patients with insomnia, more highly sedating antidepressants can be administered in a single dose at bedtime. Although the mood stabilizers (e.g., lithium carbonate, carbamazepine, sodium valproate, or lamotrigine) usually need to be given in divided doses throughout the day to maintain adequate plasma levels, they also tend to be sedating, and a larger proportion of medication may be given at bedtime. If antipsychotic medications are indicated, they should also be given at bedtime to obtain maximal benefit from their sleep-inducing effects.

When treating sleep disorders associated with depression, it is usually necessary to administer antidepressant medications in full therapeutic dosages. Low doses of antidepressants are commonly prescribed for a variety of sleep disorders, including insomnia, narcolepsy, and some parasomnias, but they may not be effective for treatment of the insomnia that accompanies major depression. An adequate clinical trial of an antidepressant usually requires a minimum of 3 weeks at a therapeutic dose (see Table 112–2).

Insomnia occurring in patients treated with activating antidepressants (e.g., SSRIs or bupropion), or which persists in spite of treatment with other antidepressants or mood stabilizers, may require additional pharmacotherapy. Trazodone has been shown to be effective as a hypnotic in patients with insomnia and depression,[94,95] and is frequently combined with other antidepressants to improve sleep.[96] Hypnotics can usually be safely combined with antidepressants, although care should be taken when combining drugs that are metabolized by the cytochrome P-450 system, such as the SSRIs, nefazodone, benzodiazepines (alprazolam, clonazepam, diazepam, and triazolam), and zolpidem.

Patients with mood disorders and chronic sleep disturbances often manifest a superimposed component of psychophysiologic insomnia and can benefit from behavioral therapies. Patients with significant insomnia should be instructed in the basic aspects of sleep hygiene, and behavioral techniques such as relaxation of stimulus control may be useful for some patients as well (see Chapters 61 and 62). The use of stimulants should be discouraged. Likewise, alcohol

use must be avoided for its negative effects on both sleep and affective illnesses. For patients with significant hypersomnia, sleep restriction (i.e., limiting the number of hours in bed) as well as stimulant medications may be indicated.

For patients with winter depression and hypersomnia, bright light therapy has been shown to be effective, either alone or in combination with antidepressant medication. Light therapy and its use in treating depression is reviewed in detail in Chapter 121. Patients with severe fatigue or hypersomnia may also benefit from adjunctive use of stimulant medications.

Finally, for patients with mood disorders and significant insomnia or hypersomnia that does not respond to appropriate pharmacotherapy of the underlying illness, it is important to consider the possibility of a concomitant primary sleep disorder. For example, patients with narcolepsy or sleep apnea have higher rates of depression; both sleep disorders are associated with nocturnal sleep disruption, daytime fatigue, and hypersomnia, or impaired daytime concentration, all of which may be confused with the "vegetative" symptoms of depression.

Clinical Application of Sleep Studies

Sleep studies have potential utility in psychiatry, both for diagnosis and treatment evaluation. Although a specific psychiatric diagnosis cannot be made solely on the basis of standard polysomnographic data, sleep studies can sometimes answer specific questions. For example, reduced REM sleep latency may suggest a concomitant diagnosis of depression in patients with significant anxiety complaints or dementia. Although sleep complaints in most patients with mood disorders are usually related to the underlying psychiatric illness, in some cases a sleep study may help in diagnosis of an occult primary sleep disorder. Both sleep apnea and periodic limb movements can disrupt nocturnal sleep and lead to fatigue and poor concentration during the day, which are also symptoms of depression. In depressed patients whose sleep complaints continue in spite of aggressive treatment and resolution of depressed mood, a sleep study should be considered for further evaluation. In some cases, medications also may be responsible for precipitating or exacerbating sleep disorders (i.e., tricyclic antidepressants and periodic leg movements, benzodiazepines and sleep apnea).

The potential prognostic utility of sleep studies in mood disorders has not yet been fully realized. It is possible that specific sleep abnormalities may be predictive of treatment response. For example, patients with reduced REM sleep latency may be more likely to respond to antidepressant medication than those with normal REM sleep latency.[97] A multicenter study comparing response to fluoxetine versus placebo, however, found no difference in response rates in patients with short versus normal REM sleep latencies.[98] In one study of depressed inpatients, response to amitriptyline was related to more severe initial depression rating and less baseline stage 4 sleep.[99] However, another study found no correlations between sleep variables and response to cognitive therapy.[100]

Alternatively, medication-induced changes in sleep patterns may be correlated with antidepressant effects. For patients with depression and reduced REM sleep latencies, it has been shown that the REM sleep–suppressing effects of an antidepressant medication predicted clinical efficacy.[101] The amount of REM sleep suppression during the first night of treatment

| | | |

Box 112–5. Clinical Conditions in Which Reduced REM Sleep Latency Has Been Reported

- Psychiatric disorders
  - Mood disorders
  - Borderline personality disorder
  - Eating disorders
  - Anxiety disorders
  - Alcoholism
  - Schizophrenia
- Narcolepsy
- After cessation of treatment with rapid eye movement sleep–suppressing drugs
  - Benzodiazepines
  - Antidepressants
- During alcohol withdrawal
- During recovery sleep after sleep deprivation

with tricyclic antidepressants was correlated with eventual antidepressant response in several studies,[60,101] although prolongation of REM sleep latency alone was less consistent in predicting treatment response. Increased amounts of REM sleep rebound after abrupt discontinuation of amitriptyline were also indicative of clinical response to the drug[101]; in this case, the amount of rebound may have reflected the amount of prior deprivation. Given the cost and inconvenience of performing sleep studies in laboratory situations, however, it is unlikely that multinight sleep studies will be performed to assess antidepressant treatment efficacy using current technology.

Sleep variables may also be helpful in identifying individuals susceptible to development of affective illnesses or relapses. Kupfer et al.[102] have shown that a decreased delta sleep ratio (average delta wave counts in the first versus second NREM periods) correlated with an increased risk of relapse. New-onset depression was more likely to develop in healthy adolescents with increased phasic REM sleep and a trend for shorter REM sleep latency than in subjects with normal sleep patterns.[103] Short REM sleep latency also appeared to be correlated with earlier recurrence of illness.[104] If reduced REM sleep latency or other sleep abnormalities indicate a susceptibility to depression, it might be useful to consider whether individuals with subjective sleep complaints and short REM sleep latency should be treated prophylactically with antidepressants.

In interpreting sleep studies in clinical settings, it is important to bear in mind that reduced REM sleep latency can be present in a variety of conditions other than mood disorders. As mentioned previously, short REM sleep latency has been reported in some groups of patients with schizophrenia, borderline personality, eating disorders, and alcoholism. Early appearance of REM sleep, of course, is also characteristic of narcolepsy. Short REM sleep latency and REM sleep rebound commonly occur in patients who have been withdrawn recently from antidepressant medications, benzodiazepines, or alcohol. After sleep deprivation, REM sleep latency reductions may occur during recovery sleep, although usually not during the first night. Common causes of reduced REM sleep latency are listed in Box 112–5.

Treatment of Mood Disorders with Sleep Deprivation

A variety of sleep manipulations have been shown to have antidepressant effects, although they have not come into widespread clinical use. They include selective deprivation of REM sleep, partial and total sleep deprivation, and, possibly, phase advance of the sleep period relative to clock time.[105,106] A single night of sleep deprivation usually shows antidepressant effects, with response rates of 50% or greater. Antidepressant effects peak by the afternoon after a night of total sleep loss.[107] Patients with endogenous depression and a more pronounced diurnal pattern of illness have better responses to sleep deprivation. A study of depressed adolescents suggested that more severely ill patients may have a greater benefit from sleep deprivation than mildly depressed subjects, who showed no significant effects of sleep deprivation on mood[108]; remitted patients and healthy control subjects reported worsening of mood after sleep deprivation, consistent with other reports.[109] The major drawback to total sleep deprivation as a therapy for depression, however, has been the immediate reversibility of the antidepressant effects by recovery sleep, including short naps, not to mention the problems associated with sleep deprivation itself (e.g., increased sleepiness). Chronic REM sleep deprivation also improved depressive symptomatology.[58] However, unlike total sleep deprivation, the antidepressant effects took several weeks to appear and were not immediately reversed after recovery sleep.

Antidepressant effects have been produced by partial sleep deprivation, particularly when performed during the latter half of the night, which proportionately reduces REM sleep more than NREM sleep.[110] Like total sleep deprivation, partial deprivation was immediately effective and had comparable response rates.[111] It has been suggested that sleep during the early morning hours is more "depressogenic"[61] and that the antidepressant effect of sleep deprivation accrues from avoiding sleep during this period. Antidepressant effects of total sleep deprivation may be prolonged if sleep is phase-advanced during the period immediately after a night of sleep deprivation.[112] Sleep phase advance may also potentiate effects of antidepressant medications.[113] Intermittent partial sleep deprivation administered 1 or more nights per week may also be useful as a prophylactic or adjunctive treatment for depression.

The mood-elevating effects of sleep deprivation have been most dramatically demonstrated by reports that sleep deprivation triggered manic episodes in some patients with bipolar depression.[114] Furthermore, manic episodes are often immediately preceded by periods of sleeplessness, suggesting that decreased sleep may contribute to mania.[115,116]

Although the mechanism for the antidepressant effects of sleep deprivation is not known, functional neuroimaging studies suggest that they are correlated with effects on limbic structures. Increased rates of glucose metabolism[117] and blood flow[118,119] in the amygdala and cingulate have been reported in depressed subjects who respond to sleep deprivation. Normalization of activity in these limbic structures was associated with a decrease in depression.[117]

CLINICAL COURSE AND PREVENTION

Mood disorders tend to be remitting and relapsing disorders with long courses, although there are some patients who may experience only a single episode. Depressive episodes last for an average of 6 to 12 months without treatment, whereas manic episodes may last approximately 3 months. Treatment reduces episode length, but should be continued for at least 6 months to a year after remission because the risk of relapse is greater during this time. Increasingly, it is recognized that repeated episodes of mood disorders contribute to a poor prognosis, emphasizing the importance of early and effective treatment. Patients with multiple episodes of illness probably require chronic medication treatment to prevent or minimize recurrence. The course of bipolar disorder is characterized by a decreased interval between episodes as the number of episodes increases; patients with four or more episodes per year are considered rapid cyclers. Patients with bipolar disorder usually begin with an episode of major depression; a minority of patients may experience only manic episodes. Bipolar disorder is more likely to be recurrent than major depression; at least 90% of bipolar patients have multiple episodes. Overall, bipolar patients have a worse prognosis than those with major depressive disorder; over one third have a chronically progressive course.

After treatment with pharmacotherapy or psychotherapy, approximately one third of depressed patients recover fully, one third have partial remissions, and one third do not respond significantly to treatment. All patients, including those considered to be in remission, may continue to experience residual symptoms of depression. Sleep disturbance is one of the more common residual symptoms and has been estimated to occur in up to 44% of patients in remission from major depression.[120] In addition, insomnia is one of the most predictive symptoms heralding the onset of an episode of mania or depression, as discussed earlier in this chapter. Thus, it is not surprising that patients with mood disorders often suffer from chronic sleep problems.

PITFALLS AND CONTROVERSIES

Clinical Utility of Polysomnography

The potential diagnostic utility of polysomnography in mood disorders depends on the specificity and sensitivity of the sleep abnormalities. Although most patients with mood disorders show significant sleep abnormalities on EEG testing compared with healthy control subjects, so do other psychiatric patients.[27]

Most studies have assessed sensitivity and specificity of either REM sleep latency alone or combinations of sleep parameters for distinguishing mood disorder patients from healthy control subjects. Short REM sleep latency alone has shown sensitivities of up to 70% and even higher degrees of specificity in identifying depressed patients.[40,121] However, one of the problems in attempting to define cut-off values for REM sleep latency has been the lack of a standardized definition for REM sleep latency. Different definitions (yielding different calculated values of REM sleep latency) show varying degrees of sensitivity and specificity for depression.[122,123] REM density (number of eye movements divided by REM sleep time) has been shown to distinguish people with depression from controls,[124,125] but it is also a parameter without a uniformly accepted definition.

The fact that REM sleep latency reductions can be found in patients with psychiatric disorders other than primary major depression has led to the speculation that the presence of short REM sleep latency may signify the presence of a concomitant depressive illness. Alternatively, it may indicate common biologic factors in different disorders. Short REM sleep latency has been reported occasionally in panic disorder, posttraumatic stress disorder, eating disorders, alcoholism, schizophrenia, and schizoaffective disorder.[27] All of these disorders can be accompanied by depression, but decreased REM sleep latency could not be accounted for by coexisting depression in all studies. Clearly, reduced REM sleep latency may be seen in patients with secondary depression, but it is not yet known whether reduced REM sleep latency is a specific indicator of past or current depression.

Despite the lack of an ideal theory, there is considerable evidence to suggest that sleep is biologically linked to mood disorders. Perhaps the most basic question is whether a causal link exists between sleep and depression, regardless of the specific mechanism involved. For example, does depression cause sleep abnormalities? This is probably not the case because many people with depression, particularly younger patients, fail to exhibit short REM sleep latency, reduced SWS, or sleep disruption. Also, depression-like sleep patterns are seen during remission and in first-degree relatives without depression. Alternatively, does the abnormal sleep pattern specifically lead to an increased susceptibility to depression, as suggested by some of the longitudinal and family studies? Indirect evidence suggests that changes in sleep are correlated with improvement in mood disorders; patients whose sleep improved more rapidly also showed a more rapid improvement in depression or mania.[13,126,127] On the other hand, narcoleptic patients with short REM sleep latency are not invariably depressed, and inducing "depressive" sleep patterns in healthy subjects with cholinergic agents does not cause depression. A third possibility is that separate biologic processes can lead to the clinical syndrome of depression and the characteristic sleep abnormalities. Whether the psychiatric illness, the sleep disturbance, or both are expressed may depend on other biologic factors. Continued study of sleep in mood disorders and the psychiatric disorders in general will elucidate neuropharmacologic and genetic mechanisms involved in sleep regulation and psychiatric illnesses. An understanding of the sleep abnormalities and sleep disorders commonly found in patients with mood disorders can lead to more effective clinical management of this large patient population.

Clinical Pearl

Because of the strong association between sleep disturbance and mood disorders, all patients with sleep complaints should be screened for mood disorders. Sleep may not normalize with resolution of mood disorders, and many patients with mood disorder may require specific and chronic treatment of their sleep problems.

REFERENCES

1. Murray CJ, Lopez AD: The Global Burden of Disease. Geneva: World Health Organization, 1996.
2. American Psychiatric Association: Diagnostic and Statistical Manual of Mental Disorders, 4th ed. Washington, DC, American Psychiatric Press, 1994.

3. Boyd JH, Weissman MM: Epidemiology of affective disorders: A reexamination and future directions [review]. Arch Gen Psychiatry 1981;38:1039-1046.

4. Fava M, Kendler KS: Major depressive disorder. Neuron 2000; 28:335-341.

5. Manji HK, Moore GJ, Rajkowska G, et al: Neuroplasticity and cellular resilience in mood disorders. Mol Psychiatry 2000; 5:578-593.

6. Manji HK, Quiroz JA, Sporn J, et al: Enhancing neuronal plasticity and cellular resilience to develop novel, improved therapeutics for difficult-to-treat depression. Biol Psychiatry 2003; 53:707-742.

7. Soares JC, Mann JJ: The anatomy of mood disorders: Review of structural neuroimaging studies. Biol Psychiatry 1997;41:86-106.

8. Davidson RJ, Pizzagalli D, Nitschke JB, et al: Depression: perspectives from affective neuroscience. Annu Rev Psychol 2002; 53:545-574.

9. Nestler EJ, Barrot M, DiLeone RJ, et al: Neurobiology of depression. Neuron 2002;34:13-25.

10. Billiard M, Dolenc L, Aldaz C, et al: Hypersomnia associated with mood disorders: A new perspective. J Psychosom Res 1994;38(Suppl 1):41-47.

11. Reynolds CF III, Coble PA, Kupfer DJ, et al: Application of the multiple sleep latency test in disorders of excessive sleepiness. Electroencephalogr Clin Neurophysiol 1982;53:443-452.

12. Detre TP, Himmelhoch JM, Swartzburg M, et al: Hypersomnia and manic-depressive disease. Am J Psychiatry 1972;128:1303-1305.

13. Perlis ML, Giles DE, Buysse DJ, et al: Self-reported sleep disturbance as a prodromal symptom in recurrent depression. J Affect Disord 1997;42:209-212.

14. Jackson A, Cavanagh J, Scott J: A systematic review of manic and depressive prodromes. J Affect Disord 2003;74:209-217.

15. Tranter R, O'Donovan C, Chandarana P, et al: Prevalence and outcome of partial remission in depression. J Psychiatry Neurosci 2002;27:241-247.

16. Mellinger GD, Balter MB, Uhlenhuth EH: Insomnia and its treatment: Prevalence and correlates. Arch Gen Psychiatry 1985; 42:225-232.

17. Ford DE, Kamerow DB: Epidemiologic study of sleep disturbance and psychiatric disorders: An opportunity for prevention?. JAMA 1989;262:1479-1484.

18. Breslau N, Roth T, Rosenthal L, et al: Sleep disturbance and psychiatric disorders: A longitudinal epidemiological study of young adults. Biol Psychiatry 1996;39:411-418.

19. Gerber PD, Barrett JE, Barrett JA, et al: The relationship of presenting physical complaints to depressive symptoms in primary care. J Gen Intern Med 1992;7:170-173.

20. Coleman RM, Roffwarg HP, Kennedy SJ, et al: Sleep-wake disorders based on a polysomnographic diagnosis: A national cooperative study. JAMA 1982;247:997-1003.

21. Buysse DJ, Reynolds CF III, Kupfer DJ, et al: Clinical diagnoses in 216 insomnia patients using the International Classification of Sleep Disorders (ICSD), DSM-IV and ICD-10 categories: A report from the APA/NIMH DSM-IV Field Trial. Sleep 1994;17:630-637.

22. Stein MA, Mendelsohn J, Obermeyer WH, et al: Sleep and behavior problems in school-aged children. Pediatrics 2001;107:E60.

23. Ohayon MM, Roth T: Place of chronic insomnia in the course of depressive and anxiety disorders. J Psychiatr Res 2003;37:9-15.

24. Chang PP, Ford DE, Mead LA, et al: Insomnia in young men and subsequent depression: The Johns Hopkins Precursors Study. Am J Epidemiol 1997;146:105-114.

25. Cole MG, Dendukuri N: Risk factors for depression among elderly community subjects: A systematic review and meta-analysis. Am J Psychiatry 2003;160:1147-1156.

26. Fredriksen K, Rhodes J, Reddy R, et al: Sleepless in Chicago: Tracking the effects of adolescent sleep loss during the middle school years. Child Dev 2004;75:84-95.

27. Benca RM, Obermeyer WH, Thisted RA, et al: Sleep and psychiatric disorders: A meta-analysis. Arch Gen Psychiatry 1992;49:651-668.

28. Reynolds CF III, Kupfer DJ: Sleep research in affective illness: State of the art circa 1987. Sleep 1987;10:199-215.

29. Borbély AA, Tobler I, Loepfe M, et al: All-night spectral analysis of the sleep EEG in untreated depressives and normal controls. Psychiatry Res 1984;12:27-33.

30. Kupfer DJ, Reynolds CF III, Ulrich RF, et al: Comparison of automated REM and slow-wave sleep analysis in young and middle-aged depressed subjects. Biol Psychiatry 1986;21:189-200.

31. Armitage R, Hoffmann RF, Rush AJ: Biological rhythm disturbance in depression: Temporal coherence of ultradian sleep EEG rhythms. Psychol Med 1999;29:1435-1448.

32. Armitage R, Hoffmann R, Trivedi M, et al: Slow-wave activity in NREM sleep: Sex and age effects in depressed outpatients and healthy controls. Psychiatry Res 2000;95:201-213.

33. Nofzinger EA, Thase ME, Reynolds CF III, et al: Hypersomnia in bipolar depression: A comparison with narcolepsy using the multiple sleep latency test. Am J Psychiatry 1991;148:1177-1181.

34. Cohen DB: Dysphoric affect and REM sleep. J Abnorm Psychol 1979;88:73-77.

35. Giles DE, Roffwarg HP, Schlesser MA, et al: Which endogenous depressive symptoms relate to REM latency reduction? Biol Psychiatry 1986;21:473-482.

36. Perlis M, Giles D, Buysse D, et al: Which depressive symptoms are related to which sleep electroencephalographic variables? Biol Psychiatry 1997;42:904-913.

37. Kupfer DJ, Ehlers CL, Frank E, et al: EEG sleep profiles and recurrent depression. Biol Psychiatry 1991;30:641-655.

38. Dew MA, Reynolds CF III, Buysse DJ, et al: Electroencephalographic sleep profiles during depression: Effects of episode duration and other clinical and psychosocial factors in older adults. Arch Gen Psychiatry 1996;53:148-156.

39. Thase ME, Fasiczka AL, Berman SR, et al: Electroencephalographic sleep profiles before and after cognitive behavior therapy of depression. Arch Gen Psychiatry 1998;55:138-144.

40. Giles DE, Roffwarg HP, Rush AJ: A cross sectional study of the effects of depression on REM latency. Biol Psychiatry 1990;28:697-704.

41. Giles DE, Kupfer DJ, Rush AJ, et al: Controlled comparison of electrophysiological sleep in families of probands with unipolar depression. Am J Psychiatry 1998;155:192-199.

42. Lauer CJ, Schreiber W, Holsboer F, et al: In quest of identifying vulnerability markers for psychiatric disorders by all-night polysomnography. Arch Gen Psychiatry 1995;52:145-153.

43. Reynolds CF III, Kupfer DJ, Thase ME, et al: Sleep, gender and depression: An analysis of gender effects on the electroencephalographic sleep of 302 depressed outpatients. Biol Psychiatry 1990; 28:673-684.

44. Pace-Schott EF, Hobson JA: The neurobiology of sleep: genetics, cellular physiology and subcortical networks. Nat Rev Neurosci 2002;3:591-605.

45. Steriade M, Curro Dossi RC, Nunez A: Network modulation of a slow intrinsic oscillation of cat thalamocortical neurons implicated in sleep delta waves: Cortically induced synchronization and brainstem cholinergic suppression. J Neurosci 1991;11:3200-3217.

46. Risch SC, Janowsky DS, Mott MA, et al: Central and peripheral cholinesterase inhibition: Effects on anterior pituitary and sympathomimetic function. Psychoneuroendocrinology 1986; 11:221-230.

47. Berger M, Doerr P, von Zerssen D: Physostigmine influence on DST results. Am J Psychiatry 1982;141:469-470.

48. Janowsky DS, Davis JM, El-Yousef MK, et al: A cholinergic-adrenergic hypothesis of mania and depression. Lancet 1972; 2:632-635.

49. Gillin JC, Sitaram N, Duncan WC: Muscarinic supersensitivity: A possible model for the sleep disturbance of primary depression. Psychiatry Res 1979;1:17-22.

50. Sagales T, Erill S, Domino EF: Effects of repeated doses of scopolamine on the electroencephalographic stages of sleep in normal volunteers. Clin Pharmacol Ther 1975;18:727-732.

51. Gillin JC, Sutton L, Ruiz C, et al: The cholinergic rapid eye movement induction test with arecoline in depression. Arch Gen Psychiatry 1991;48:264-270.

52. Berger M, Hochli D, Zulley J, et al: Cholinomimetic drug RS 86, REM sleep, and depression. Lancet 1985;1:1385-1386.

53. Berger M, Lund RD, Bronisch T, et al: REM latency in neurotic and endogenous depression and cholinergic REM induction test. Psychiatry Res 1983;10:113-123.

54. Sitaram N, Dube S, Keshavan M, et al: The association of supersensitive cholinergic REM-induction and affective illness within pedigrees. J Psychiatr Res 1987;21:487-497.

55. Borbély AA: A two process model of sleep regulation. Hum Neurobiol 1982;1:195-204.

56. Borbély AA, Wirz-Justice A: Sleep, sleep deprivation and depression: A hypothesis derived from a model of sleep regulation. Hum Neurobiol 1982;1:205-210.

57. Kupfer DJ, Ulrich RF, Coble PA, et al: Application of automated REM and slow wave sleep analysis: II. Testing the assumption of the two-process model of sleep regulation in normal and depressed subjects. Psychiatry Res 1984;13:335-343.

58. Vogel GW, Buffenstein A, Minter K, et al: Drug effects on REM sleep and on endogenous depression. Neurosci Biobehav Rev 1990;14:49-63.

59. Vogel GW, Vogel F, McAbee RS, et al: Improvement of depression by REM sleep deprivation: New findings and a theory. Arch Gen Psychiatry 1980;37:247-253.

60. Kupfer DJ, Spiker DG, Coble PA, et al: Sleep and treatment prediction in endogenous depression. Am J Psychiatry 1981;138:429-434.

61. Wehr TA, Wirz-Justice A: Internal coincidence model for sleep deprivation and depression. In Koella WP (ed): Sleep 1980. Basel, Karger, 1981, pp 26-33.

62. David MM, MacLean AW, Knowles JB, et al: Rapid eye movement latency and mood following a delay of bedtime in healthy subjects: Do the effects mimic changes in depressive illness? Acta Psychiatr Scand 1991;84:33-39.

63. Kupfer DJ, Gillin JC, Coble PA, et al: REM sleep, naps, and depression. Psychiatry Res 1981;5:195-203.

64. Schulz H, Tetzlaff W: Distribution of REM latencies after sleep interruption in depressive patients and control subjects. Biol Psychiatry 1982;17:1367-1376.

65. Buysse DJ, Jarrett DB, Miewald JM, et al: Minute-by-minute analysis of REM sleep timing in major depression. Biol Psychiatry 1990;28:911-925.

66. Avery DH, Wildschiodtz G, Smallwood RG, et al: REM latency and core temperature relationships in primary depression. Acta Psychiatr Scand 1986;74:269-280.

67. Avery DH, Wildschiodtz G, Rafaelsen O: REM latency and temperature in affective disorder before and after treatment. Biol Psychiatry 1982;17:463-470.

68. Tsujimoto T, Yamada N, Shimoda K, et al: Circadian rhythms in depression: Part II. Circadian rhythms in inpatients with various mental disorders. J Affect Disord 1990;18:199-210.

69. Wehr TA, Muscettola G, Goodwin FK: Urinary 3-methoxy-4-hydroxyphenylglycol circadian rhythm: Early timing (phase advance) in manic-depressives compared with normal subjects. Arch Gen Psychiatry 1980;37:257-263.

70. Halbreich U, Asnis GM, Shindledecker R, et al: Cortisol secretion in endogenous depression: I. Basal plasma levels. Arch Gen Psychiatry 1985;42:904-908.

71. Riemann D, Hohagen F, König A, et al: Advanced vs. normal sleep timing: Effects on depressed mood after response to sleep deprivation in patients with a major depressive disorder. J Affect Disord 1996;37.2-3:121-128.

72. Elsenga S, Van den Hoofdakker RH: Clinical effects of several sleep-wake manipulations on endogenous depression, Sleep Res 1983;12:326.

73. Kerkhofs M, Missa J-N, Mendlewicz J: Sleep electroencephalographic measures in primary major depressive disorder: Distinction between DST suppressor and nonsuppressor patients. Biol Psychiatry 1986;21:225-228.

74. Asnis GM, Halbreich U, Sachar EJ, et al: Plasma cortisol secretion and REM period latency in adult endogenous depression. Am J Psychiatry 1983;140:750-753.

75. Steiger A: Sleep and the hypothalamo-pituitary-adrenocortical system. Sleep Med Rev 2002;6:125-138.

76. Arborelius L, Owens MJ, Plotsky PM, et al: The role of corticotropin-releasing factor in depression and anxiety disorders. J Endocrinol 1999;160:1-12.

77. Ohayon MM: The effects of breathing-related sleep disorders on mood disturbances in the general population. J Clin Psychiatry 2003;64:1195-1200; quiz, 1274-1196.

78. Saletu B, Anderer P, Saletu M, et al: EEG mapping, psychometric, and polysomnographic studies in restless legs syndrome (RLS) and periodic limb movement disorder (PLMD) patients as compared with normal controls. Sleep Med 2002;3(Suppl):S35-S42.

79. Armitage R, Emslie G, Rintelmann J: The effect of fluoxetine on sleep EEG in childhood depression: A preliminary report. Neuropsychopharmacology 1997;17:241-245.

80. Staner L, Kerkhofs M, Detroux D, et al: Acute, subchronic and withdrawal sleep EEG changes during treatment with paroxetine and amitriptyline: A double-blind randomized trial in major depression. Sleep 1995;18:470-477.

81. Luthringer R, Toussaint M, Schaltenbrand N, et al: A double-blind, placebo-controlled evaluation of the effects of orally administered venlafaxine on sleep in inpatients with major depression. Psychopharmacol Bull 1996;32:637-646.

82. Wyatt RJ, Fram DH, Kupfer DJ, et al: Total prolonged drug-induced REM sleep suppression in anxious-depressed patients. Arch Gen Psychiatry 1971;24:145-155.

83. Kupfer DJ, Spiker DG, Rossi A, et al: Nortriptyline and EEG sleep in depressed patients. Biol Psychiatry 1982;17:535-546.

84. Grunhaus L, Tiongco D, Pande A, et al: Monitoring of antidepressant response to ECT with polysomnographic recordings and dexamethasone suppression test. Psychiatry Res 1988;24:177-185.

85. Nofzinger EA, Reynolds CF III, Thase ME, et al: REM sleep enhancement by bupropion in depressed men. Am J Psychiatry 1995;152:274-276.

86. Schenck CH, Mahowald MW, Kim SW, et al: Prominent eye movements during NREM sleep and REM sleep behavior disorder associated with fluoxetine treatment of depression and obsessive-compulsive disorder. Sleep 1992;15:226-235.

87. Salin-Pascual RJ, Galicia-Polo L, Drucker-Colin R: Sleep changes after 4 consecutive days of venlafaxine administration in normal volunteers. J Clin Psychiatry 1997;58:348-350.

88. Bakshi R: Fluoxetine and restless legs syndrome. J Neurol Sci 1996;142:151-152.

89. Schenck CH, Mahowald MW: Motor dyscontrol in narcolepsy: Rapid-eye-movement (REM) sleep without atonia and REM sleep behavior disorder. Ann Neurol 1992;32:3-10.

90. Kupfer DJ, Reynolds CF III, Weiss BL, et al: Lithium carbonate and sleep in affective disorders: Further considerations. Arch Gen Psychiatry 1974;30:79-84.

91. Terao T, Terao M, Yoshimura R, et al: Restless legs syndrome induced by lithium. Biol Psychiatry 1991;30:1167-1170.

92. Gillin JC, Rapaport M, Erman MK, et al: A comparison of nefazodone and fluoxetine on mood and on objective, subjective, and clinician-rated measures of sleep in depressed patients: A double-blind, 8-week clinical trial [published erratum appears in J Clin Psychiatry 1997;58:275]. J Clin Psychiatry 1997;58:185-192.

93. Rush AJ, Armitage R, Gillin JC, et al: Comparative effects of nefazodone and fluoxetine on sleep in outpatients with major depressive disorder. Biol Psychiatry 1998;44.1:3-14.

94. Parrino L, Spaggiari MC, Boselli M, et al: Clinical and polysomnographic effects of trazodone CR in chronic insomnia associated with dysthymia. Psychopharmacology 1994;116:389-395.

95. Scharf MB, Sachais BA: Sleep laboratory evaluation of the effects and efficacy of trazodone in depressed insomniac patients. J Clin Psychiatry 1990;51(Suppl):13-17.

96. Kaynak H, Kaynak D, Gozukirmizi E, et al: The effects of trazodone on sleep in patients treated with stimulant antidepressants. Sleep Med 2004;5:15-20.

97. Rush AJ, Giles DE, Jarrett RB, et al: Reduced REM latency predicts response to tricyclic medication in depressed outpatients. Biol Psychiatry 1989;26:61-72.

98. Heiligenstein JH, Faries DE, Rush AJ, et al: Latency to rapid eye movement sleep as a predictor of treatment response to fluoxetine and placebo in nonpsychotic depressed outpatients. Psychiatry Res 1994;52:327-339.

99. Mendlewicz J, Kempenaers C, de Maertelaer V: Sleep EEG and amitriptyline treatment in depressed inpatients. Biol Psychiatry 1991;30:691-702.

100. Jarrett RB, Rush AJ, Khatami M, et al: Does the pretreatment polysomnogram predict response to cognitive therapy in depressed outpatients? A preliminary report. Psychiatry Res 1990;33:285-299.

101. Gillin JC, Wyatt RJ, Fram DH, et al: The relationship between changes in REM sleep and clinical improvement in depressed patients treated with amitriptyline. Psychopharmacology 1978;59:267-272.

102. Kupfer DJ, Frank E, McEachran AB, et al: Delta sleep ratio: A biological correlate of early recurrence in unipolar affective disorder. Arch Gen Psychiatry 1990;47:1100-1105.

103. Rao U, Dahl RE, Ryan ND, et al: The relationship between longitudinal clinical course and sleep and cortisol changes in adolescent depression. Biol Psychiatry 1996;40:474-484.

104. Giles DE, Jarrett RB, Roffwarg HP, et al: Reduced rapid eye movement latency: A predictor of recurrence in depression. Neuropharmacology 1987;1:33-39.

105. Ringel BL, Szuba MP: Potential mechanisms of the sleep therapies for depression. Depress Anxiety 2001;14:29-36.

106. Giedke H, Schwarzler F: Therapeutic use of sleep deprivation in depression. Sleep Med Rev 2002;6:361-377.

107. Wu JC, Bunney WE: The biological basis of an antidepressant response to sleep deprivation and relapse: Review and hypothesis. Am J Psychiatry 1990;147:14-21.

108. Naylor MW, King CA, Lindsay KA, et al: Sleep deprivation in depressed adolescents and psychiatric controls. J Am Acad Child Adolesc Psychiatry 1993;32:753-759.

109. Pilcher JJ, Huffcutt AI: Effects of sleep deprivation on performance: A meta-analysis. Sleep 1996;19:318-326.

110. Sack DA, Duncan W, Rosenthal NE, et al: The timing and duration of sleep in partial sleep deprivation therapy of depression. Acta Psychiatr Scand 1988;77:219-224.

111. Szuba MP, Baxter LRJ, Fairbanks LA, et al: Effects of partial sleep deprivation on the diurnal variation of mood and motor activity in major depression. Biol Psychiatry 1991;30:817-829.

112. Berger M, Vollmann J, Hohagen F, et al: Sleep deprivation combined with consecutive sleep phase advance as a fast-acting therapy in depression: An open pilot trial in medicated and unmedicated patients. Am J Psychiatry 1997;154:870-872.

113. Sack DA, Nurnberger J, Rosenthal NE, et al: Potentiation of antidepressant medications by phase advance of the sleep-wake cycle. Am J Psychiatry 1985;142:606-608.

114. Wehr TA: Sleep-loss as a possible mediator of diverse causes of mania. Br J Psychiatry 1991;159:576-578.

115. Wehr TA, Sack DA, Rosenthal NE: Sleep reduction as a final common pathway in the genesis of mania. Am J Psychiatry 1987;144:201-204.

116. Leibenluft E, Albert PS, Rosenthal NE, et al: Relationship between sleep and mood in patients with rapid-cycling bipolar disorder. Psychiatry Res 1996;63:161-168.

117. Wu JC, Gillin JC, Buchsbaum MS, et al: Effect of sleep deprivation on brain metabolism of depressed patients. Am J Psychiatry 1992;149:538-543.

118. Ebert D, Feistel H, Barocka A: Effects of sleep deprivation on the limbic system and the frontal lobes in affective disorders: a study with Tc-99m-HMPAO SPECT. Psychiatry Res 1991;40:247-251.

119. Ebert D, Feistel H, Kaschka W, et al: Single photon emission computerized tomography assessment of cerebral dopamine D2 receptor blockade in depression before and after sleep deprivation: Preliminary results. Biol Psychiatry 1994;35:880-885.

120. Nierenberg AA, Wright EC: Evolution of remission as the new standard in the treatment of depression. J Clin Psychiatry 1999;60(Suppl 22):7-11.

121. Somoza E, Mossman D: Optimizing REM latency as a diagnostic test for depression using receiver operating characteristic analysis and information theory. Biol Psychiatry 1989;27:990-1006.

122. Knowles JB, MacLean AW, Cairns J: Definitions of REM latency: Some comparisons with particular reference to depression. Biol Psychiatry 1982;17:993-1002.

123. Reynolds CF III, Shaw DH, Newton TF, et al: EEG sleep in outpatients with generalized anxiety: A preliminary comparison with depressed outpatients. Psychiatry Res 1983;8:81-89.

124. King D, Akiskal HS, Lemmi H, et al: REM density in the differential diagnosis of psychiatric from medical-neurologic disorders: A replication. Psychiatry Res 1981;5:267-276.

125. Lauer CJ, Garcia D, Pollmacher T, et al: All-night EEG sleep in anxiety disorders and major depression. In Horne J (ed): Sleep '90. Bochum, Germany, Pontenagel Press, 1991.

126. Fava GA, Grandi S, Canestrari R, et al: Prodromal symptoms in primary major depressive disorder. J Affect Disord 1990;19:149-152.

127. Nowlin-Finch NL, Altshuler LL, Szuba MP, et al: Rapid resolution of first episodes of mania: Sleep related? J Clin Psychiatry 1994;55:26-29.

113

Schizophrenia

Kathleen L. Benson
Vincent P. Zarcone, Jr.

ABSTRACT

Schizophrenia is perhaps the most devastating neuropsychiatric illness. Worldwide, the prevalence rate is approximately 1%. Although the etiology remains unknown, schizophrenia is considered a neurodevelopmental disorder involving the interplay of susceptibility genes and environmental factors. There is a wide range of pathologic findings, but there is no specific laboratory abnormality. Consequently, schizophrenia is a clinical diagnosis and the defining symptom is thought disorder or cognitive impairment.

Sleep patterns in schizophrenic patients can be markedly disturbed. In times of severe psychotic agitation, schizophrenic patients may experience a profound insomnia or total sleeplessness. They may also develop sleep–wake reversals with a preference for sleeping during the day. Severe insomnia is one of the prodromal symptoms associated with psychotic relapse. Clinically stable, medicated patients with schizophrenia may also experience sleep disturbance, particularly early and middle insomnia. Many polysomnographic abnormalities have been identified, but none is diagnostic of schizophrenia. Such abnormalities can include poor sleep efficiency, slow wave sleep deficits, and short rapid eye movement sleep latencies. The most consistently observed sleep abnormality is early insomnia or difficulty attaining a state of persistent sleep.

Although a minority of schizophrenic patients have a full recovery after an initial psychotic episode, the majority are in long-term treatment with antipsychotic (AP) medications. These agents are classified as first-generation (traditional) APs or second-generation (atypical) APs. They differ in their receptor binding profiles, clinical outcome, and range of side effects. Relative to the atypical APs, the traditional APs are associated with more extrapyramidal side effects as well as tardive dyskinesia (TD). Several of the atypical APs are associated with significant weight gain as well as abnormal glucose regulation.

Broadly speaking, most APs augment total sleep and improve sleep continuity. Some atypicals, like olanzapine and risperidone, may also increase slow wave sleep. Schizophrenic patients also suffer from a range of intrinsic and extrinsic dyssomnias, including inadequate sleep hygiene, irregular sleep–wake patterns, obstructive sleep apnea syndrome, restless legs syndrome, and periodic limb movements during sleep. The second-generation APs include agents that can induce or augment sleep-disordered breathing, restless legs syndrome, or periodic limb movements during sleep. Sleep disorder specialists should make every effort to treat schizophrenic patients with dyssomnias in the same manner as they do other referrals. Also, sleep disorder specialists should educate mental health care providers about the possible emergence of sleep disorders associated with AP treatment.

More than a hundred years ago, Jackson[1] and Wundt[2] reflected on the similarities between dreaming and psychosis. In dreaming sleep, hallucinations, perceptual distortions, bizarre thinking, and temporary delusions are intimately mixed with more normal thought and perceptual processes. In 1953, when Aserinsky and Kleitman[3] discovered rapid eye movement (REM) sleep and its associated dream reports, not only did they usher in the modern era of sleep research, but also many of the seminal studies of schizophrenia. Both Dement[4] and Rechtschaffen and colleagues[5] explored the hypothesis that REM sleep abnormalities (or the intrusion of the dream state into waking) might explain schizophrenia. These first polysomnographic (PSG) studies of sleep in schizophrenic patients found no gross abnormalities of REM sleep, nor any intrusion of REM sleep into wakefulness, but, in the ensuing years, other significant sleep abnormalities came to be documented.

This chapter reviews those findings, but it is important to remember that the studies of the sleep of schizophrenic patients have more than historical significance. Schizophrenia is associated with immense human and economic cost. It is also associated with severe insomnia, particularly during episodes of psychotic exacerbation.

This chapter provides an overview of the clinical features of schizophrenia, as well as associated risk factors and neuropathology. It also describes the sleep abnormalities characteristic of schizophrenia and their neurobiologic correlates. Finally, we address the issues surrounding antipsychotic (AP) medications and their side effects, particularly those associated with the development of comorbid dyssomnias.

EPIDEMIOLOGY AND RISK FACTORS

Because of cultural differences, as well as differences in methodology and diagnostic criteria, prevalence rates for schizophrenia derived from U.S. and international studies vary widely. Tsuang et al.[6] found that the prevalence of schizophrenia ranged from 0.6 to 17 cases per 1000. As a general trend, most of these studies suggested a prevalence rate of 5 cases per 1000.[6] Lifetime prevalence, which in part corrects for age of onset, was approximately 1% worldwide.[6] Annual new case appearance, or incidence, was estimated to be 0.35 cases per 1000 population.[6] Schizophrenia is equally common in both sexes. Although the age of onset is usually in the second decade of life, the disorder seems to begin earlier in male than in female patients.

Although the etiology of schizophrenia remains unknown, there are several factors associated with an increased likelihood for development of schizophrenia. First and foremost, a genetic predisposition greatly elevates the risk for development of schizophrenia. Family, twin, and adoption studies provided strong evidence that schizophrenia is highly heritable. The prevailing genetic model of the etiology of schizophrenia envisions multiple susceptibility genes, each of small effect, no one gene being necessary or sufficient for the development of the disease.[7] Multiple susceptibility genes interacting with one another, and with environmental factors, suggest that multiple forms of schizophrenia might exist. Because the concordance rate for monozygotic twins only approaches 50%, genetic makeup alone is not sufficient for the development of schizophrenia, and nongenetic or sporadic forms of the disorder should also exist.

Among the environmental factors that could play a role in the development of schizophrenia are obstetric complications and viral infection.[6] Obstetric complications could include premature birth, low birth weight, trauma, and poor oxygenation. Obstetric complications are neither necessary nor sufficient causes of schizophrenia but, rather, they could trigger schizophrenia in those genetically predisposed. Seasonality in the births of schizophrenic patients suggests that a viral infection during fetal development might also activate the disorder. Schizophrenic patients are more likely to be born in late winter or in spring months, when the developing fetus has an increased risk of exposure to maternal viral infections. Some conceptualize that schizophrenia is an autoimmune disease potentially triggered by maternal antibodies to viral infection.[8] In conclusion, a better understanding of both genetic and environmental

risk factors and their interaction should open a window on the etiology and pathophysiology of the disease.

THE DIAGNOSIS OF SCHIZOPHRENIA

The term *schizophrenia* derives from Bleuler's description of the splitting or disintegration of normal thought processes.[9] His belief that cognitive impairment or "thought disorder" is the fundamental defining symptom of schizophrenia shaped the course of diagnostic criteria developed during the 20th century, particularly with their emphasis on manifest symptoms rather than course of illness. Current criteria for the diagnosis of schizophrenia are defined in the *Diagnostic and Statistical Manual of Mental Disorders*, 4th edition[10] (DSM-IV; Box 113–1).

As reviewed by Black and Andreasen,[11] schizophrenia is a clinical diagnosis because there are no specific laboratory abnormalities diagnostic of the disorder. It is also, in large part, a diagnosis of exclusion, eliminating psychotic disturbances attributable to a variety of medical, psychiatric, and substance abuse disorders. The number and diversity of symptoms also complicates the clinical presentation.

To simplify the task of the clinician, Criterion A[10] (see Box 113–1) has been organized into two main categories, namely, positive and negative symptoms. According to DSM-IV, "positive symptoms appear to reflect an excess or distortion of normal

---

Box 113–1. DSM-IV Diagnostic Criteria for Schizophrenia

A. *Characteristic symptoms:* Two (or more) of the following, each present for a significant portion of time during a 1-month period (or less if successfully treated):

1. Delusions
2. Hallucinations
3. Disorganized speech (e.g., frequent derailment or incoherence)
4. Grossly disorganized or catatonic behavior
5. Negative symptoms (i.e., affective flattening, alogia, or avolition)

Note: Only one Criterion A symptom is required if delusions are bizarre or hallucinations consist of a voice keeping up a running commentary on the person's behavior or thoughts, or two or more voices conversing with each other.

B. *Social/occupational dysfunction:* For a significant portion of the time since the onset of the disturbance, one or more major areas of functioning such as work, interpersonal relations, or self-care are markedly below the level achieved prior to the onset (or when the onset is in childhood or adolescence, failure to achieve expected level of interpersonal, academic, or occupational achievement).

C. *Duration:* Continuous signs of the disturbance persist for at least 6 months. This 6-month period must include at least 1 month of symptoms (or less if successfully treated) that meet Criterion A (i.e., active-phase symptoms) and may include periods of prodromal or residual symptoms. During these prodromal or residual periods, the signs of the disturbance may be manifested by only negative symptoms or two or more symptoms listed in Criterion A presented in an attenuated form (e.g., odd beliefs, unusual perceptual experiences).

D. *Schizoaffective and Mood Disorder exclusion:* Schizoaffective Disorder and Mood Disorder with Psychotic Features have been ruled out because either (1) no Major Depressive, Manic, or Mixed Episodes have occurred concurrently with the active-phase symptoms; or (2) if mood episodes have occurred during active-phase symptoms, their total duration has been brief relative to the duration of the active and residual periods.

E. *Substance/general medical condition exclusion:* The disturbance is not due to the direct physiological effects of a substance (e.g., a drug of abuse, a medication) or a general medical condition.

F. *Relationship to a Pervasive Developmental Disorder:* If there is a history of Autistic Disorder or another Pervasive Developmental Disorder, the additional diagnosis of schizophrenia is made only if prominent delusions or hallucinations are also present for at least a month (or less if successfully treated).

DSM-IV, Diagnostic and Statistical Manual of Mental Disorders, 4th edition.

functions, whereas the negative symptoms appear to reflect a diminution or loss of normal functions." Positive symptoms can be further subdivided into a "psychotic dimension" that includes hallucinations and delusions and a disorganization dimension that includes disorganized speech and behavior. Negative symptoms include affective flattening, avolition, and poverty of speech. Criterion B[10] (see Box 113–1) reflects a marked deterioration in occupational and social functioning.

Finally, the sleep abnormalities found in schizophrenia lack diagnostic specificity. Consequently, they do not reliably differentiate schizophrenia from other psychiatric disorders. *It is unlikely, therefore, that a sleep clinic will be asked to apply PSG to diagnose schizophrenia.* However, the sleep clinic could help differentiate schizophrenia from narcolepsy, which can present with a strong hallucinatory component.[12]

PATHOGENESIS

The etiology of schizophrenia is poorly understood, but accumulating evidence has revealed a wide range of brain abnormalities.[6,11] Brain structural abnormalities have been found in postmortem studies as well as in in vivo imaging using computed tomography (CT) and magnetic resonance imaging technology. Regarding the latter, structural dysmorphologies have included enlarged lateral and third ventricles, loss of total gray matter, frontal, and temporal lobe volume, as well as a reduction in total brain size. These findings seem to be present at the onset of illness and cannot be attributed to progressive degeneration; however, most findings are nonspecific, having been observed in other psychiatric disorders. Functional imaging studies utilizing positron emission tomography or regional cerebral blood flow have observed decreased metabolism in the frontal cortex (hypofrontality), as well as left hemisphere dysfunction.

Abnormalities of neurotransmitter systems have also been extensively investigated. For many years, the prevailing theory of schizophrenia has centered on the dopamine (DA) system. The DA hypothesis of schizophrenia derived from two observations. First, the potency of standard AP medication correlates with the amount of DA (D_2) receptor blockade. Second, drugs such as amphetamines, which enhance DA activity, can cause psychosis or exacerbate schizophrenic symptoms. The DA hypothesis holds that psychotic symptoms such as hallucinations and delusions are associated with hyperactivity of the DA mesolimbic system. In a similar vein, both serotonin (5-hydroxytryptamine [5-HT]) and norepinephrine have been associated with the pathophysiology of schizophrenia because the potency of the newest generation of APs has been linked to 5-HT and alpha-adrenergic receptor blockade. Finally, the role of the neurotransmitter glutamate in the pathophysiology of schizophrenia is gaining greater credence in part because several of the recently identified schizophrenia susceptibility genes target glutamatergic transmission.[7,13]

The range of these findings may reflect both genetic and environmental effects as well as the clinical heterogeneity of schizophrenia. Because no discrete pathologic abnormality has emerged as an etiologic factor, schizophrenia could be an abnormality of neuronal connectivity[14] or of integrative neuronal circuits.[15] Neither of these theories is inconsistent with the broader and prevailing view that schizophrenia is a neurodevelopmental disorder.[16] Although abnormal events may occur early in development (prenatal or perinatal), maturational abnormalities may present during the second decade of life[17] or even into middle age.[18]

CLINICAL FEATURES

Subjective Complaints

As Bleuler[9] pointed out over 90 years ago, "In schizophrenia, sleep is habitually disturbed." With the onset of psychotic symptoms, and with each subsequent relapse, sleep can be markedly impaired. The sleep of schizophrenic patients who are in a state of psychotic agitation is characterized by prolonged periods of total sleeplessness. In times of less severe psychotic agitation, sleep is often characterized by a pronounced insomnia—long sleep-onset latencies, reduced total sleep time (TST), and sleep fragmented by bouts of waking. There is a fairly frequent reversal of sleep and wake so that the patient sleeps in the daylight hours, preferring to do so because it relieves him or her of some of the responsibility and anxiety of interacting with other people. Schizophrenic patients can also experience profoundly disturbing hypnagogic hallucinations. Many also suffer from nightmares. Although there are no systematic studies, anecdotal clinical reports indicate that alcohol and substance abuse can both disturb sleep and cause the patient to relapse. Even among clinically stable, medicated patients with schizophrenia, subjectively experienced sleep disturbance is common, particularly early and middle insomnia.[19]

Polysomnographic Features

Total Sleep, Sleep Maintenance, and Sleep Continuity

The sleep of schizophrenic patients is characterized by poor sleep efficiency (SE).[20-29] Often this takes the form of a reduction in TST as well as early, middle, and late insomnia. The most consistently reported abnormality shown in empirical studies of sleep patterns in schizophrenia is early insomnia or difficulty reaching a state of persistent sleep. Typically, sleep latency (SL) in healthy control subjects ranges from 10 to 20 minutes; in contrast, SL in schizophrenic patients typically exceeds 30 minutes, and is often in the 50- to 100-minute range. Severe insomnia is one of the prodromal symptoms associated with psychotic decompensation or relapse after AP discontinuation.[30-32]

Abnormalities of REM Sleep Time and REM Sleep Phasic Events

Despite early speculation regarding potential REM sleep abnormalities in schizophrenia, studies comparing schizophrenic patients with healthy control subjects have consistently shown that REM sleep time is neither systematically augmented nor reduced.[20,21] In schizophrenic patients, a cross-sectional study found little difference in REM sleep time between seven hallucinating patients and four nonhallucinating patients.[33] And in a longitudinal study of acutely disturbed patients with schizophrenia, REM sleep did not appear to be abnormally shortened in the waxing phase of the psychosis.[34]

REM phasic events have also been studied, particularly REM sleep eye movements. Because the number of eye movements in REM sleep depends, in part, on the availability of background stage REM sleep time, measures of eye movement density correct for this confounding effect. Eye movement density is typically computed as the ratio of eye movement frequency to stage REM sleep minutes. Visual scoring of REM sleep eye movement activity found no difference in eye movement density between schizophrenic patients and control subjects.[27-29,35] Furthermore, use of an automated eye movement detection system[36] yielded the same conclusion, but extended the observation to finding no difference in eye movement density between schizophrenic patients, nonpsychiatric control subjects, and patients with major depressive disorder.

REM Sleep Latency

Many studies of nocturnal sleep in schizophrenia have observed that the latency to the onset of the first REM sleep period (REML) is less than normal. Since 1965, several studies[22-28,35,37-39] have compared the REML of unmedicated schizophrenic patients with that of nonpsychiatric control subjects. Half[22,25,26,37-39] reported significant between-group differences, with the schizophrenic patients demonstrating abnormally short REML. Even among those studies finding no between-group differences, a bimodal distribution of REML values in schizophrenic patients has been observed, suggesting that there are subgroups of schizophrenic patients with sleep-onset REM periods.[24,27,35,40]

Abnormalities of Non-REM Sleep

Although short REML in schizophrenia is a common observation, there is lack of agreement about the underlying mechanism. Short REML could represent an active, or primary alteration of REM sleep mechanisms. Alternatively, as suggested by Feinberg et al.,[41] a slow wave sleep (SWS) deficit in the first non-REM (NREM) period could permit the passive advance or early onset of the first REM period. SWS deficits are frequently, but not consistently, observed in PSG recordings of schizophrenic patients. In visually scored PSG, SWS is reported as the summation of sleep stages 3 and 4, with stage 4 sleep having the greater incidence of underlying slow wave activity. In the Feinberg et al. study,[41] schizophrenic patients and control subjects did not differ in the amount of stage 3 sleep, but schizophrenic patients had significantly less stage 4 sleep. A complete absence of stage 4 sleep has been reported in a sizable proportion of patients with schizophrenia.[42] In the intervening decades, some[22,28,43] but not all[24-27] studies have observed stage 4 or SWS deficits in schizophrenic patients relative to nonpsychiatric control subjects. Although some research has suggested that prior exposure to, or withdrawal from, APs might explain these inconsistencies,[27] other factors come into play such as the insensitivity of visual scoring to the incidence and amplitude of slow wave (0 to 3 Hz) activity underlying SWS. Those studies[23,28,39] using computer processing of electroencephalograms (EEGs; Fourier analysis, period and amplitude analysis) have confirmed the degradation of sleep-related slow wave activity in schizophrenic patients relative to nonpsychiatric control subjects. For example, significant differences in slow wave amplitude between schizophrenic patients and nonpsychiatric control subjects (schizophrenic patients less than control subjects) have been observed despite comparable amounts of visually scored SWS.[29]

SWS deficits, whether scored visually or measured digitally, raise concern about the integrity of homeostatic regulatory mechanisms in schizophrenia. In healthy subjects, SWS increases in proportion to the amount of prior waking, and this homeostatic or dynamic response may serve a restorative role in the central nervous system. In healthy subjects, this homeostatic drive is clearly demonstrated by a rebound in SWS or slow wave activity after the naturalistic probe of total sleep deprivation (TSD). On an idealized daily basis, the homeostatic drive builds up during 16 hours of daytime waking and is dissipated by nocturnal slow wave activity, which declines across successive NREM sleep cycles. Few studies have looked at potential homeostatic dysregulation in schizophrenia. Luby and Caldwell[44] found no homeostatic recovery of SWS in schizophrenic patients after 85 hours of TSD. More recently, both visual and computer scoring of slow wave activity[45] was examined after 1 night of TSD. Recovery sleep revealed decreases in SL and stage 1, as well as increases in TST and stages 2 and 3. Stage 4 sleep could not be visually scored either on the baseline or recovery night, but period and amplitude analysis of EEG slow wave activity revealed a significant (although modest) recovery night increase in slow-wave incidence and amplitude relative to baseline. Therefore, it would appear that the homeostatic drive in schizophrenia is diminished but intact. In support of this conclusion, it has been shown that on an intranight basis, the time course of slow-wave activity dissipation over all NREM sleep cycles is normal in schizophrenic patients.[29]

Correlation with Clinical Symptoms

Having reviewed the sleep abnormalities associated with schizophrenia, we now turn to how these abnormalities relate to clinical presentation. Global symptom severity has been associated with increased waking, reduced REM sleep time, SWS deficits, and short REML.[24,25,46] Positive symptoms are one component of global severity. Depending on the clinical instrument, positive symptoms may include ratings of unusual thought content, conceptual disorganization, delusions, and hallucinatory behavior. Positive symptoms correlate with increased REM sleep eye movement density,[35,36] short REML,[25,27,47] reduced SE,[48] and prolonged SL.[49]

Negative symptoms are another component of global severity and have also been linked to short REML[25,40] as well as SWS deficits.[23,50-53] More recently, cognitive dysfunction in schizophrenia has correlated with SWS deficits.[54] Although attempts to link short REML in schizophrenia to depression have been unsuccessful,[25,27] enhanced REM sleep time and REM sleep eye movement activity in schizophrenia have been associated with suicidality.[55,56] Finally, longitudinal outcome studies have observed that a poor clinical and psychosocial outcome is associated with both short REML[40,57] and SWS deficits.[58]

Broadly viewed, these studies do not produce a necessarily consistent picture, perhaps because of different rating scales and clinical instruments, different algorithms to quantify sleep parameters, small sample sizes, differences in medication status and history, and patient heterogeneity. These studies relied almost exclusively on a cross-sectional design and demonstrate a need for within-patient longitudinal assessment of sleep patterns across changing clinical states. However, a tentative synthesis of studies to date might suggest that insomnia and REM sleep eye movement augmentation are associated with psychosis, positive symptoms, and emotionality, whereas SWS deficits are related to negative symptoms and cognitive dysfunction.

Correlation with Other Biologic Systems

Although the pathophysiology of the sleep abnormalities found in schizophrenia is unknown, several neurobiologic correlates have been observed and theoretical models have been suggested.

Structural and Functional Neuroimaging

On a theoretical level, SWS deficits have been associated with microstructure brain abnormalities. Feinberg[17] has proposed that schizophrenia is a neurodevelopmental disorder arising from a malfunction in the normal maturational process of synaptic elimination during the second decade of life; excess synaptic pruning would result in less capability for synchronous EEG slow wave activity and a resultant SWS deficit.

Empirically, SWS deficits in schizophrenia have been investigated using brain imaging technology. A significant negative correlation between stage 4 sleep and CT measures of ventricular–brain ratio has been reported.[50] Although follow-up studies[59] do not concur, all measures of SWS correlated inversely with ventricular system volume in schizophrenia when ventricular volume was corrected for normal variation in age and head size.[60] Furthermore, SWS deficits have been associated with decreased brain anabolic processes using functional neuroimaging (i.e., phosphorus-31 magnetic resonance spectroscopy).[51]

Research studies have also noted a relationship between brain anatomic features and abnormalities of SE, another robust characteristic of the sleep disturbance found in schizophrenia. Studies have found a negative correlation between the size of the third ventricle and both TST[50] and sleep maintenance.[61] Finally, CT imaging of ventricular–brain ratio correlated with measures of awakening in drug-naive schizophrenic patients.[27] Taken together, these studies suggest that certain sleep abnormalities in schizophrenia may have underlying brain neuroanatomic concomitants contributing to a stable or traitlike presentation.

Neurochemical Abnormalities

Dopamine

Although DA dysfunction has assumed a prominent role in the pathophysiology of schizophrenia, there has been little study of the relationship of sleep abnormalities in schizophrenia to the DA system. Although such studies warrant attention, they are likely to be confounded by long-term exposure to the DA antagonist properties of AP medication. For example, patients with longer AP exposure as well as TD have more abnormalities of REM sleep time and REML during medication-free sleep recordings than do schizophrenic patients with a briefer history of AP exposure without TD.[46]

Acetylcholine

Our understanding of how cholinergic mechanisms might be involved in the sleep abnormalities of schizophrenia is limited and derives, in large part, from extrapolations of the study of cholinergic mechanisms in affective illness. The Cholinergic REM Induction Test (CRIT)[62] has been used to advance the hypothesis that short REML in depressive patients reflects cholinergic supersensitivity. Because short REML is also present in schizophrenic patients, they too have undergone testing with the CRIT and responded similarly to patients with mood disorder, suggesting that short REML in schizophrenic patients also involves cholinergic mechanisms.[63] Independent of sleep abnormalities, a link between cholinergic hyperactivity and schizophrenia has been proposed as part of a comprehensive model of cholinergic–dopaminergic interaction in schizophrenia.[64]

Serotonin

For decades, research studies have noted that 5-HT plays a key role in sleep regulation. SWS deficits in schizophrenia have been associated with a 5-HT mechanism in a study reporting a positive correlation between cerebrospinal fluid (CSF) levels of the 5-HT metabolite, 5-hydroxyindole acetic acid, and SWS time in unmedicated patients with schizophrenia.[65] Many of the novel or atypical APs like olanzapine and risperidone act in part through 5-HT receptor blockade.

Norepinephrine

As reported earlier in this chapter, severe insomnia is one of the prodromal symptoms associated with psychotic decompensation and relapse.[30] This study also noted that increased CSF levels of norepinephrine and its metabolite, 3-methoxy-4-hydroxyphenylglycol, accompanied this relapse-related insomnia.

Hypocretin

Hypocretin (orexin) deficiency[66] has been observed in human narcolepsy, a sleep disorder associated with excessive daytime sleepiness. Because severe insomnia is characteristic of schizophrenia and because hypocretin excites midbrain DA neurons, it was hypothesized that hypocretin levels might be abnormally elevated in schizophrenic patients. No difference in CSF hypocretin levels was found between schizophrenic patients and nonpsychiatric control subjects; however, in the patients with schizophrenia, CSF hypocretin was correlated with SL, suggesting a relationship between hypocretin and hyperarousal in schizophrenia.[67]

TREATMENT

Antipsychotic Medication

It is unlikely that a sleep specialist will treat an emergent schizophrenic psychosis, either at onset or at relapse. Instead, this situation is typically encountered in a hospital emergency department or inpatient psychiatric facility where treatment involves administration of APs (e.g., haloperidol or ziprasidone) and tranquilizers until the patient is sedated or markedly less psychotic. However, rapid tranquilization with barbiturates might induce significant apneic events in susceptible patients and must be carefully monitored. Because of the high prevalence of dyssomnias in schizophrenia, it is more likely that the sleep disorder specialist will be asked to diagnose and treat symptomatically stable schizophrenic patients on maintenance doses of APs such as those shown in Table 113–1.

APs differ in their chemical design and have differential effects on DA, 5-HT, alpha-adrenergic, cholinergic, and histaminic receptors and their various subtypes.[68,69] Although most therapeutic effects are mainly achieved through receptor blockade, APs may also act as partial agonists and reuptake blockers. The differential receptor binding profile of these

Table 113–1.	Commonly Used Antipsychotic Medications	
Antipsychotic Medications	**Usual Adult Daily Maintenance Dose (mg)**
Typical or Traditional Antipsychotics	
Chlorpromazine (Thorazine)	50-400
Fluphenazine (Prolixin)	1-15
Haloperidol (Haldol)	1-15
Perphenazine (Trilafon)	8-24
Thioridazine (Mellaril)	50-400
Thiothixene (Navane)	6-30
Trifluoperazine (Stelazine)	4-30
Atypical or Novel Antipsychotics	
Aripiprazole (Abilify)	10-30
Clozapine (Clozaril)	200-600
Olanzapine (Zyprexa)	5-20
Quetiapine (Seroquel)	150-750
Risperidone (Risperdal)	2-8
Ziprasidone (Geodon)	80-160

agents has been associated with different side effect profiles and clinical outcome.

First-Generation, Traditional, or Typical Antipsychotics

Historically, the therapeutic efficacy of the first generation of APs has been attributed to their affinity for the D_2 postsynaptic receptor. However, the benefits associated with the traditional APs do not accrue without cost; these APs bind to D_2 receptors in the striatum, resulting in extrapyramidal side effects (EPS) such as akathisia, dystonia, and parkinsonism. Effects are dose dependent and may occur to some degree in 50% to 75% of patients. A more damaging side effect associated with DA blockade is TD; this is a potentially irreversible side effect occurring in approximately 20% of schizophrenic patients receiving typical APs. The traditional APs are also associated to varying degrees with cholinergic side effects, sedation, changes in both blood pressure and myocardial conduction, sexual dysfunction, and weight gain. Also, a relatively rare but potentially lethal side effect associated with hyperthermia is the neuroleptic malignant syndrome.

Some of the side effects associated with the typical APs correlate with the range of potency per milligram. For example, low-milligram, high-potency APs such as haloperidol and fluphenazine strongly antagonize DA receptors and tend to have prominent EPS but fewer adverse anticholinergic and blood pressure effects. In contrast, high-milligram, low-potency agents such as chlorpromazine and thioridazine have a weaker affinity for DA receptors and less risk of EPS but produce more sedation, hypotension, and anticholinergic effects.

Second-Generation, Novel, or Atypical Antipsychotics

Several factors played a role in motivating the development of the second-generation APs. From the perspective of outcome, up to 30% of patients with chronic schizophrenia have a poor or inadequate response to traditional APs. Furthermore, although traditional APs have demonstrated success in

ameliorating positive symptoms, they have been less successful in treating negative symptoms such as avolition. Finally, the side effects associated with the use of the traditional APs, particularly EPS and TD, were a source of noncompliance and difficult management issues. Clozapine was the first of the second-generation APs to demonstrate good clinical efficacy with no EPS. The atypical APs now include five other agents listed in Table 113–1. Although they demonstrate unique receptor binding profiles and other pharmacologic features, as a group, they are characterized by weaker affinity for the D_2 receptor (relative to traditional APs), and strong affinity for 5-HT$_2$ receptors.[69] The atypical APs are now considered first-line treatment for schizophrenia. Relative to the traditional APs, they offer better compliance and less hospitalization.

However, the atypical APs are not the panacea once envisioned.[70] Only clozapine has clearly demonstrated effectiveness in treatment-refractory schizophrenia, and none of the atypical APs has proven strongly effective against negative symptoms. And like the traditional APs, the atypical APs are not without adverse side effects. Although the incidence of TD remains low with atypical APs, acute EPS may occur with both olanzapine and risperidone. Clozapine is associated with increased risk of agranulocytosis and of seizures at higher doses. Finally, the atypical APs are associated with increased morbidity owing to weight gain, dyslipidemias, impaired glucose regulation, and type 2 diabetes mellitus. Weight gain may be particularly striking and puts the patient at increased risk for development of sleep-related breathing disorders and other obesity-related morbidities. Abnormalities of glucose regulation may occur independent of weight gain.

Antipsychotics, Sedation, and Sleep Patterns

Among the traditional APs, sedation is a side effect associated with high-milligram, low-potency agents such as chlorpromazine and thioridazine. In contrast, the low-milligram, high-potency agents such as fluphenazine, haloperidol, and thiothixene have lower sedation rates. Of the novel or atypical APs, clozapine and olanzapine are the most sedating, and risperidone the least. The remaining atypical agents have intermediate rates of sedation. The relationship of sedation rates to AP receptor binding profiles remains largely speculative.

Broadly speaking, traditional APs alter sleep architecture by improving sleep maintenance. Studies have noted an augmentation of TST and SE as well as reductions in SL and waking.[71-76] With less consistency, the traditional APs have been associated with increased REML,[71-75] increased REM sleep time,[73,74] and increased REM eye movement density.[71,74,76] In one study, chlorpromazine was associated with increased SWS time.[71]

With regard to the effect of atypical APs on sleep patterns in schizophrenic patients, clozapine has been the most widely studied. Clozapine has been shown to have strong consolidating effects on sleep; these effects include increased TST, SE, and stage 2 sleep, and decreased SL and wake time after sleep onset.[76,77,78] Relative to a medication-free baseline, a significant decline in SWS and stage 4 sleep was observed in schizophrenic patients treated with clozapine.[77] In a direct comparison of clozapine with traditional APs, it was reported that clozapine caused greater consolidation of NREM sleep, that is, more stage 2 and less stage 1 sleep.[76]

Olanzapine has also been shown to be a sleep-promoting agent in schizophrenia. Relative to a medication-free baseline, olanzapine increased TST, stage 2 sleep, and eye movement density and decreased both wake and stage 1 sleep.[79] There was also a twofold to threefold increase in SWS. Finally, a direct comparison of risperidone and haloperidol reported that, with one exception, there were no differences in sleep patterns between the risperidone- and haloperidol-treated patients; the exception was a significant enhancement of SWS time in the risperidone-treated patients with schizophrenia.[80]

In summary, the acute administration of atypical APs promotes sleep maintenance and enhances stage 2 sleep and REM eye movement density. They appear to have no effect on REM sleep. They may increase SWS (olanzapine and risperidone) or decrease SWS (clozapine). Finally, although typical and atypical APs show PSG-measured improvements in sleep maintenance, the atypical agents (e.g., risperidone) may also be associated with subjectively reported superior sleep quality and morning alertness.[81] Finally, one might speculate that the PSG-measured improvements in sleep reported in these studies are secondary to, or byproducts of, clinical improvement. This conclusion is hard to reconcile with the fact that sleep improvement occurs during acute or short-term AP administration, whereas therapeutic effects lag behind (by days or weeks) the initiation of medication. Instead, the positive effect of APs on sleep maintenance and structure may contribute to their efficacy and their tolerance.

Adjunct Medications

Judicious intermittent use of benzodiazepine tranquilizers and hypnotics may be important, but sleep-related breathing disorders should be ruled out before chronic use. Benzodiazepines should also be avoided if patients have a history of alcoholism or alcohol abuse. In addition, patients with schizoaffective disorder and those with impulse control problems are often treated with mood stabilizers such as valproate. This usually has a continuing beneficial effect on sleep.

Comorbid Sleep Disorders

Although a primary sleep disturbance is characteristic of schizophrenia, schizophrenic patients can also suffer from a variety of intrinsic and extrinsic dyssomnias, including inadequate sleep hygiene, sleep disorders associated with the abuse of, or withdrawal from, alcohol and psychoactive drugs, obstructive sleep apnea syndrome (OSAS), restless legs syndrome (RLS), periodic limb movements during sleep (PLMS), and irregular sleep–wake patterns. Whenever possible, schizophrenic patients with dyssomnias must be approached in the same manner as any other patient referred to the sleep disorders specialist.

The patient with schizophrenia is a good candidate for sleep hygiene counseling. Lacking daytime structure and wanting to isolate themselves socially to avoid painful interactions with other people, many schizophrenic patients develop bad habits in relation to sleep initiation and sleep maintenance, including sleep reversals and polyphasic sleep patterns; this situation is sometimes complicated by heavy self-prescribed administration of alcohol or other psychoactive drugs such as cocaine. Because many schizophrenic patients are followed over the long term in day hospitals and outpatient clinics, the opportunity exists for sleep disorder clinics to educate mental health care providers so that they might incorporate sleep hygiene counseling into their programs.

The prevalence of OSAS among schizophrenic patients is unknown. Among schizophrenic patients not referred to a sleep clinic for suspected OSAS, reported estimates include the following: 17%,[82] 19%,[83] and 48%.[84] These studies varied in terms of sample size, age, sex, inpatient/outpatient status, APs, and measurement instrument (oximetry, ambulatory apnea monitor, and PSG). In contrast, among schizophrenic patients referred for a sleep clinic evaluation for a suspected sleep disorder, over 46% had a respiratory disturbance index greater than 10 events/hour; the mean respiratory disturbance index was 64.8 events/hour.[85] In this study, the most powerful predictor of OSAS was obesity. Obesity is widespread among patients with schizophrenia. Historically, weight gain has been associated with APs, but, as discussed previously, weight gain secondary to the use of the atypical APs has become a very serious morbidity issue. A recent case study reported on the development of moderate to severe OSAS in one patient treated with clozapine and a second patient treated with risperidone; the former was associated with a 40-lb weight gain and the latter with a 65-lb weight gain.[86] Because daytime somnolence in AP-treated schizophrenic patients is not uncommon, the possibility of OSAS must be seriously considered for patients who are obese by history or who have undergone weight gain secondary to atypical APs. Depending on the level of symptomatology, many schizophrenic patients with sleep-disordered breathing can be effectively treated with nasal continuous positive airway pressure and demonstrate relatively good compliance.

The prevalence rates for RLS and PLMS in schizophrenia are also unknown. Because RLS and PLMS respond to DA agonists, DA deficiency has been linked to their pathophysiology.[87] Likewise, D_2 receptor blockade has been correlated with AP efficacy and, as noted previously, the prevailing theory has been that DA hyperactivity might underlie the pathophysiology of schizophrenia.[6] As previously discussed, the traditional APs, with their strong affinity for the D_2 receptor, have a long history of associated movement disorders. Unfortunately, no data are available on the naturally occurring prevalence rates of RLS and PLMS in AP-naive schizophrenic patients in relationship to the general population.

It would also be useful to know, from a clinical perspective, if APs can induce or augment RLS or PLMS because they diminish DA neurotransmission. On this point some data are available. PLMS rates of 13%[82] and 14%[84] have been reported, respectively, in patients AP-free for 2 or more weeks and in currently AP-treated patients. In patients with AP-associated movement disorders, PLMS were observed in 5 of 9 residual schizophrenic patients with akathisia[88] and 10 of 10 elderly schizophrenic patients (7 with TD) who were in long-term AP treatment.[89] Finally, two case reports have been published linking the atypical APs to the development of RLS. In the first case, RLS and clinically significant PLMS developed in a patient after 6 weeks treatment with olanzapine; he was switched to clozapine, with resolution of both RLS and PLMS.[90] In the second case, RLS and PLMS were induced by risperidone but resolved on switching to quetiapine.[91] Finally, akathisia is one of the prominent side effects of APs and is characterized by intense motor restlessness and pacing. It too can lead to significant sleep disruption and relapse, but can be differentiated from RLS by history and clinical presentation. Akathisia is often treated with propranolol.

For many schizophrenic patients, the new generation of APs surpasses the old in terms of clinical efficacy and risk of persistent EPS such as TD, but these patients may be at even greater risk for the development of significant sleep disorders such as sleep-related breathing disorders, RLS, and PLMS. In addition to the medical morbidity associated with these disorders, the impact of untreated sleep disorders may augment the fragility of underlying sleep processes in schizophrenia, with potentially adverse effects on treatment compliance and clinical outcome.

CLINICAL COURSE AND PREVENTION

In the prevailing pathophysiologic model, schizophrenia is viewed as a neurodevelopmental disorder with onset typically (but not always) in late adolescence. The onset may be abrupt or insidious—that is, beginning with a prodromal phase characterized by subtle changes in behavior, mild thought disorder, and social withdrawal. The prodromal phase is followed by an active phase marked by positive psychotic symptoms such as hallucinations and delusions. This phase may wax and wane but some degree of psychoticism usually persists during the waning or residual phase. Positive symptomatology (relapse or acute exacerbation) may recur episodically. Finally, over the course of the illness, positive psychotic symptoms may gradually decline; in contrast, negative symptoms such as affective flattening and avolition increase with the progression of the disease.

For approximately 50% of patients, the onset of the illness is both progressive and insidious; for the remainder, the onset is acute with little or no prodromal syndrome. Also, for approximately 50% of patients, the course of the illness is continuous; for others the course is marked by episodic flareups. The likelihood of relapse has been associated with stressful life events, a critical and hostile family environment, and drug abuse.

If outcome is defined as the absence of psychotic symptoms and normal levels of social functioning, long-term follow-up studies suggest that 20% to 30% of patients may have a full recovery. Another 20% to 30% of patients have a mild outcome and recover to levels where they can function occupationally and socially. Approximately 50% continue to show moderate to severe dysfunction requiring numerous outpatient interventions or rehospitalization with each relapse. Perhaps approximately one fifth requires long-term institutionalization. Although the atypical APs may lower the number of hospitalizations, AP treatment does not fundamentally alter these outcomes. Finally, a better outcome has been associated with acute onset, episodic course, female sex, and lack of family history of schizophrenia.

The course of illness in schizophrenia can be characterized by dysphoria or depressive episodes, particularly early in the course of illness. Relative to other major psychiatric disorders, schizophrenic patients tend to marry less frequently, are more likely found in an institutional setting, and have poorer occupational functioning. Schizophrenic patients also have a higher mortality rate owing to suicide as well as physical illness. In summary, schizophrenia is possibly the most devastating of all psychiatric illnesses. We can neither cure this disorder nor prevent its occurrence. And most patients, after an early onset, can anticipate lifelong mental disability as well as social and economic marginalization.

PITFALLS AND CONTROVERSIES

One of the ongoing controversies concerns the issue of diagnostic specificity. Although a range of sleep abnormalities is observed in schizophrenia, these abnormalities lack diagnostic specificity. Long sleep-onset latencies and other sleep maintenance abnormalities found in schizophrenia are also observed in primary insomnia as well as in psychotic depression. Sleep-onset REM periods and SWS deficits are also observed in depressive illness. Certain schizophrenic patients appear to have normal amounts of SWS, which may reflect some dimension of the heterogeneity of the samples studied. However, other patients with schizophrenia are severely affected, having no visually scored minutes of stage 4 sleep. This observation raises a secondary issue. What role do SWS deficits in schizophrenia have in clinical presentation and outcome? The homeostatic property of SWS suggests some central nervous system restorative function with potential neuropsychiatric consequences, and, if so, are SWS deficits in schizophrenia associated with greater cognitive impairment and thought disorder, and do those schizophrenic patients with less SWS impairment face a better clinical outcome? Finally, do agents that augment SWS, such as certain atypical APs (olanzapine and risperidone), exert a greater likelihood of positive clinical outcome?

Clinical Pearl

Schizophrenia is associated with insomnia, often severe. Because insomnia is a prodromal sign of relapse, outpatient clinics should always query schizophrenic patients about changes in their sleep patterns. This query should also address the possible emergence of sleep disorders associated with AP treatment.

REFERENCES

1. Jackson JH: In Taylor J, Holmes G, Walshe FMR (eds): Selected Writings of John Hughlings Jackson, vol 2. New York, Basic Books, 1958, p 412.
2. Wundt W: Outlines of Psychology: Scholarly Publications, East St. Clair Shores, MI, 1897.
3. Aserinsky E, Kleitman N: Regularly occurring periods of eye motility, and concomitant phenomena, during sleep. Science 1953;118:273-274.
4. Dement W: Dream recall and eye movements during sleep in schizophrenics and normals. J Nerv Ment Dis 1955;122:263-269.
5. Rechtschaffen A, Schulsinger F, Mednick S: Schizophrenia and physiological indices of dreaming. Arch Gen Psychiatry 1964; 10:89-93.
6. Tsuang MT, Faraone SV, Green AI: Schizophrenia and other psychotic disorders. In Nicholi AM (ed): The Harvard Guide to Psychiatry, 3rd ed. Cambridge, Mass, Belknap Press of Harvard University Press, 1999, pp 240-280.
7. Harrison PJ, Own MJ: Genes for schizophrenia? Recent findings and their pathophysiological implications. Lancet 2003;361:417-419.
8. Wright P, Gill M, Murray RM: Schizophrenia: Genetics and the maternal immune response to viral infection. Am J Med Genet 1993;48:40-46.
9. Bleuler E: Dementia Praecox, or the Group of Schizophrenias. New York, International University Press, 1950, pp 168-169.
10. American Psychiatric Association: Diagnostic and Statistical Manual of Mental Disorders, 4th ed. Washington, DC, American Psychiatric Press, 1994, pp 273-290.
11. Black DW, Andreasen NC: Schizophrenia, schizophreniform disorder, and delusional (paranoid) disorders. In Hales RE, Yudofsky SC, Talbott JA (eds): Textbook of Psychiatry, 3rd ed. Washington, DC, American Psychiatric Press, 1999, pp 425-477.
12. Douglass AB: Narcolepsy: Differential diagnosis or etiology in some cases of bipolar disorder and schizophrenia? CNS Spectrums 2003;8:120-126.

13. Goff DC, Coyle JT: The emerging role of glutamate in the pathophysiology and treatment of schizophrenia. Am J Psychiatry 2001;158:1367-1377.

14. Davis KL, Stewart DG, Friedman JI, et al: White matter changes in schizophrenia: Evidence for myelin-related dysfunction. Arch Gen Psychiatry 2003;60:443-456.

15. Feinberg I, Guazzelli M: Schizophrenia: A disorder of the corollary discharge systems that integrate the motor systems of thought with the sensory systems of consciousness. Br J Psychiatry 1999; 174:196-204.

16. Lewis DA, Levitt P: Schizophrenia as a disorder of neurodevelopment. Annu Rev Neurosci 2002;25:409-432.

17. Feinberg I: Schizophrenia: Caused by a fault in programmed synaptic elimination during adolescence? J Psychiatr Res 1983; 17:319-334.

18. Bartzokis G: Schizophrenia: Breakdown in the well-regulated lifelong process of brain development and maturation. Neuropsychopharmacology 2002;27:672-683.

19. Haffmans PM, Hoencamp E, Knegtering HJ, et al: Sleep disturbance in schizophrenia. Br J Psychiatry 1994;165:697-698.

20. Benca RM, Obermeyer WH, Thisted RA, et al: Sleep and psychiatric disorders: A meta-analysis. Arch Gen Psychiatry 1992;49:651-668.

21. Chouinard S, Poulin J, Stip E, et al: Sleep in untreated patients with schizophrenia: A meta-analysis. Schizophr Bull (submitted).

22. Zarcone VP, Benson KL, Berger PA: Abnormal rapid eye movement latencies in schizophrenia. Arch Gen Psychiatry 1987;44:45-48.

23. Ganguli R, Reynolds CF, Kupfer DJ: EEG sleep in young, never medicated, schizophrenic patients: A comparison with delusional and nondelusional depressives and with healthy controls. Arch Gen Psychiatry 1987;44:36-45.

24. Kempenaers C, Kerkhofs M, Linkowski P, et al: Sleep EEG variables in young schizophrenic and depressive patients. Biol Psychiatry 1988;24:833-838.

25. Tandon R, Shipley JE, Taylor S, et al: Electroencephalographic sleep abnormalities in schizophrenia. Arch Gen Psychiatry 1992;49:185-194.

26. Hudson JI, Lipinski JF, Keck PE, et al: Polysomnographic characteristics of schizophrenia in comparison with mania and depression. Biol Psychiatry 1993;34:191-193.

27. Lauer CJ, Schreiber W, Pollmächer T, et al: Sleep in schizophrenia: A polysomnographic study on drug-naive patients. Neuropsychopharmacology 1997;16:51-60.

28. Keshavan MS, Reynolds CF, Miewald JM, et al: Delta sleep deficits in schizophrenia. Arch Gen Psychiatry 1998;55:443-448.

29. Hoffman R, Hendrickse W, Rush AJ, et al: Slow-wave activity during non-REM sleep in men with schizophrenia and major depressive disorders. Psychiatry Res 2000;95:215-225.

30. Van Kammen DP, van Kammen WB, Peters JL, et al: CSF MHPG, sleep and psychosis in schizophrenia. Clin Neuropharmacol 1986;9(Suppl 4):575-577.

31. Dencker SJ, Malm U, Lepp M: Schizophrenic relapse after drug withdrawal is predictable. Acta Psychiatr Scand 1986;73:181-185.

32. Chemerinski E, Ho B, Flaum M, et al: Insomnia as a predictor for symptom worsening following antipsychotic withdrawal in schizophrenia. Compr Psychiatry 2002;43:393-396.

33. Koresko R, Snyder F, Feinberg I: "Dream time" in hallucinating and non-hallucinating schizophrenic patients. Nature 1963;199: 1118-1119.

34. Kupfer DJ, Wyatt RJ, Scott J, et al: Sleep disturbance in acute schizophrenic patients. Am J Psychiatry 1970;126:1213-1223.

35. Feinberg I, Koresko RL, Gottlieb F: Further observations on electrophysiological sleep patterns in schizophrenia. Compr Psychiatry 1965;6:21-24.

36. Benson KL, Zarcone VP: REM sleep eye movement activity in schizophrenia and depression. Arch Gen Psychiatry 1993;50: 474-482.

37. Jus K, Bouchard M, Jus AK, et al: Sleep EEG studies in untreated long-term schizophrenic patients. Arch Gen Psychiatry 1973;29: 386-390.

38. Stern M, Fram D, Wyatt R, et al: All night sleep studies of acute schizophrenics. Arch Gen Psychiatry 1969;20:470-477.

39. Hiatt JF, Floyd TC, Katz PH, et al: Further evidence of abnormal NREM sleep in schizophrenia. Arch Gen Psychiatry 1985;42: 797-802.

40. Taylor SF, Tandon R, Shipley JE, et al: Sleep onset REM periods in schizophrenic patients. Biol Psychiatry 1991;30:205-209.

41. Feinberg I, Braum N, Koresko RL, et al: Stage 4 sleep in schizophrenia. Arch Gen Psychiatry 1969;21:262-266.

42. Caldwell DF, Domino EF: Electroencephalographic and eye movement patterns during sleep in chronic schizophrenic patients. Electroencephalogr Clin Neurophysiol 1967;22:414-420.

43. Traub AC: Sleep stage deficits in chronic schizophrenia. Psychol Rep 1972;31:815-820.

44. Luby ED, Caldwell DF: Sleep deprivation and EEG slow wave activity in chronic schizophrenia. Arch Gen Psychiatry 1967;17: 361-364.

45. Benson KL, Lim KO, Zarcone VP: The effect of total sleep deprivation on slow wave activity and clinical symptoms in schizophrenia. Sleep Res 1995;24:382.

46. Thaker GK, Wagman AMI, Tamminga CA: Sleep polygraphy in schizophrenia: Methodological issues. Biol Psychiatry 1990;28: 240-246.

47. Howland RH: Sleep-onset rapid eye movement periods in neuropsychiatric disorders: Implications for the pathophysiology of psychosis. J Nerv Ment Dis 1997;185:730-738.

48. Neylan TC, van Kammen DP, Kelley ME, et al: Sleep in schizophrenic patients on and off haloperidol therapy. Arch Gen Psychiatry 1992;49:643-649.

49. Zarcone VP, Benson KL: BPRS symptom factors and sleep variables in schizophrenia. Psychiatry Res 1997;66:111-120.

50. Van Kammen DP, van Kammen WM, Peters J, et al: Decreased slow-wave sleep and enlarged lateral ventricles in schizophrenia. Neuropsychopharmacology 1988;1:265-271.

51. Keshavan MS, Pettegrew JW, Reynolds CF, et al: Biological correlates of slow wave sleep deficits in functional psychoses: ^{31}P-magnetic resonance spectroscopy. Psychiatry Res 1995;57:91-100.

52. Keshavan MS, Miewald J, Haas G, et al: Slow-wave sleep and symptomatology in schizophrenia and related psychotic disorders. J Psychiatr Res 1995;29:303-314.

53. Kato M, Kajimura N, Okuma T, et al: Association between delta waves during sleep and negative symptoms in schizophrenia. Neuropsychobiology 1999;39:165-172.

54. Yang CK, Winkelman J, Yoo SY: The clinical significance of sleep EEG abnormalities in chronic schizophrenia. Unpublished data, 2003.

55. Keshavan MS, Reynolds CF, Montrose D, et al: Sleep and suicidality in psychotic patients. Acta Psychiatr Scand 1994;89:122-125.

56. Lewis CF, Tandon R, Shipley JE, et al: Biological predictors of suicidality in schizophrenia. Acta Psychiatr Scand 1996;94: 416-420.

57. Goldman M, Tandon R, DeQuardo JR, et al: Biological predictors of 1-year outcome in schizophrenia in males and females. Schizophr Res 1996;21:65-73.

58. Keshavan MS, Reynolds CF III, Miewald J, et al: Slow-wave sleep deficits and outcome in schizophrenia and schizoaffective disorder. Acta Psychiatr Scand 1995;91:289-292.

59. Lauer CJ, Krieg J-C: Slow-wave sleep and ventricular size: A comparative study in schizophrenia and major depression. Biol Psychiatry 1998;44:121-128.

60. Benson KL, Sullivan EV, Lim KO, et al: Slow wave sleep and CT measures of brain morphology in schizophrenia. Psychiatry Res 1996;60:125-134.

61. Keshavan MS, Reynolds CF, Ganguli R, et al: Electroencephalographic sleep and cerebral morphology in functional psychosis: A preliminary study with computed tomography. Psychiatry Res 1991;39:293-301.

62. Gillin JC, Sitaram N, Nurnberger JI, et al: The cholinergic REM induction test. Psychopharmacol Bull 1983;19:668-670.

63. Riemann D, Hohagen F, Krieger S, et al: Cholinergic REM induction test: Muscarinic supersensitivity underlies polysomnographic findings in both depression and schizophrenia. J Psychiatr Res 1994;28:195-210.

64. Tandon R, Greden JF: Cholinergic hyperactivity and negative schizophrenia symptoms. Arch Gen Psychiatry 1989;46:745-753.

65. Benson KL, Faull KF, Zarcone VP: Evidence for the role of serotonin in the regulation of slow wave sleep in schizophrenia. Sleep 1991;14:133-139.

66. Nishino S, Ripley B, Overeem S, et al: Hypocretin (orexin) deficiency in human narcolepsy. Lancet 2000;355:39-40.

67. Nishino S, Ripley B, Mignot E, et al: CSF Hypocretin-1 levels in schizophrenia and controls: Relationship to sleep architecture. Psychiatry Res 2002;110:1-7.

68. Bymaster FP, Calligaro DO, Falcone JF, et al: Radioreceptor binding profile of the atypical antipsychotic olanzapine. Neuropsychopharmacology 1996;14:87-96.

69. Meltzer HY, Li Z, Kaneda Y, Ichikawa J: Serotonin receptors: Their key role in drugs to treat schizophrenia. Prog Neuropsychopharmacol Biol Psychiatry 2003;27:1159-1172.

70. Bridler R, Umbricht D: Atypical antipsychotics in the treatment of schizophrenia. Swiss Med Wkly 2003,133:63-76.

71. Kaplan J, Dawson S, Vaughan T, et al: Effect of prolonged chlorpromazine administration on the sleep of chronic schizophrenics. Arch Gen Psychiatry 1974;31:62-66.

72. Taylor SF, Tandon R, Shipley JE, et al: Effect of neuroleptic treatment on polysomnographic measures in schizophrenia. Biol Psychiatry 1991;30:904-912.

73. Nofzinger EA, van Kammen DP, Gilbertson MW, et al: Electroencephalographic sleep in clinically stable schizophrenic patients: Two-weeks versus six-weeks neuroleptic free. Biol Psychiatry 1993;33:829-835.

74. Keshavan MS, Reynolds CF, Miewald JM, et al: A longitudinal study of EEG sleep in schizophrenia. Psychiatry Res 1996;59:203-211.

75. Maixner S, Tandon R, Eiser A, et al: Effects of antipsychotic treatment on polysomnographic measures in schizophrenia: A replication and extension. Am J Psychiatry 1998;155:1600-1602.

76. Wetter TC, Lauer CJ, Gillich G, et al: The electroencephalographic sleep pattern in schizophrenic patients treated with clozapine or classical antipsychotic drugs. J Psychiatr Res 1996;30:411-419.

77. Hinze-Selch D, Mullington J, Orth A, et al: Effects of clozapine on sleep: A longitudinal study. Biol Psychiatry 1997;42:260-266.

78. Lee JH, Woo JI, Meltzer HY: Effects of clozapine on sleep measures and sleep-associated changes in growth hormone and cortisol in patients with schizophrenia. Psychiatry Res 2001;103:157-166.

79. Salin-Pascual RJ, Herrera-Estrella M, Galicia-Polo L, et al: Olanzapine acute administration in schizophrenic patients increases delta sleep and sleep efficiency. Biol Psychiatry 1999;46:141-143.

80. Yamashita H, Morinobu S, Yamawaki S, et al: Effect of risperidone on sleep in schizophrenia: A comparison with haloperidol. Psychiatry Res 2002;109:137-142.

81. Dursun SM, Patel JK, Burke JG, et al: Effects of typical antipsychotic drugs and risperidone on the quality of sleep in patients with schizophrenia: A pilot study. J Psychiatry Neurosci 1999;24:333-337.

82. Benson KL, Zarcone VP: Sleep abnormalities in schizophrenia and other psychotic disorders. Rev Psychiatry 1994;13:677-705.

83. Takahashi KI, Shimizu T, Sugita T, et al: Prevalence of sleep-related respiratory disorders in 101 schizophrenic patients. Psychiatry Clin Neurosci 1998;52:229-231.

84. Ancoli-Israel S, Martin J, Jones DW, et al: Sleep disordered breathing and periodic limb movements in sleep in older patients with schizophrenia. Biol Psychiatry 1999;45:1426-1432.

85. Winkelman JW: Schizophrenia, obesity, and obstructive sleep apnea. J Clin Psychiatry 2001;62:8-11.

86. Wirshing DA, Pierre JM, Wirshing WC: Sleep apnea associated with antipsychotic-induced obesity. J Clin Psychiatry 2002;63:369-370.

87. Allen RP, Earley CJ: Restless legs syndrome: A review of clinical and pathophysiologic features. J Clin Neurophysiol 2001;18:128-147.

88. Walters AS, Hening W, Rubinstein M, et al: A clinical and polysomnographic comparison of neuroleptic-induced akathisia and the idiopathic restless legs syndrome. Sleep 1991;14:339-345.

89. Steadt J, Dewes D, Danos P, et al: Can chronic neuroleptic treatment promote sleep disturbances in elderly schizophrenic patients? Int J Geriatr Psychiatry 2000;15:170-176.

90. Kraus T, Schuld A, Pollmächer T: Periodic leg movements in sleep and restless legs syndrome probably caused by olanzapine. J Clin Psychopharmacol 1999;19:487-479.

91. Wetter TC, Brunner J, Bronisch T: Restless legs syndrome probably induced by risperidone treatment. Pharmacopsychiatry 2002;35:109-111.

114

Sleep and Eating Disorders

Ruth M. Benca
Carlos H. Schenck

ABSTRACT

It is increasingly recognized that sleep and feeding, perhaps the two behaviors most critical for survival, are interrelated. Patients with eating disorders show sleep abnormalities in comparisons with normal subjects, and starvation and overeating can influence sleep patterns. Individuals with anorexia nervosa tend to have insomnia, with sleep electroencephalographic findings of reduced sleep efficiency and decreased total sleep amounts. Patients with bulimia nervosa do not consistently show objective sleep abnormalities, although they may report episodes of hypersomnolence after eating binges. A specific sleep and eating parasomnia that has been described, sleep-related eating disorder (SRED), consists of involuntary eating episodes that occur during partial arousals from sleep.

The eating disorders anorexia nervosa and bulimia nervosa are most prevalent during adolescence and young adulthood, respectively—an age range in which sleep tends to be least disturbed by psychiatric illness. Nevertheless, sleep problems are not uncommon in patients with anorexia nervosa or bulimia nervosa, and objective sleep abnormalities have been documented, particularly in patients with anorexia nervosa. Initially, sleep electroencephalographic studies were performed in patients with eating disorders to determine whether they showed sleep abnormalities similar to patients with mood disorders. In addition, the effects of feeding patterns and nutrition on sleep have been studied. More recently, eating disorders specific to the sleep period have been described, ranging from nocturnal eating syndrome to SRED. The recent discovery of peptides that affect both feeding and sleep will, it is hoped, lead to a better understanding of the mechanisms underlying these disorders. This chapter reviews the sleep changes associated with eating disorders, the relationship between nutritional status and sleep, and SRED.

PRIMARY EATING DISORDERS AND SLEEP

Diagnosis, Epidemiology, and Risk Factors

Anorexia nervosa and bulimia nervosa are classified as eating disorders and both are characterized by abnormalities in eating behavior as a result of fear of losing control and being overweight (Box 114–1). The pursuit of thinness in anorexia nervosa leads to severe pathologic weight loss and malnutrition, whereas in bulimia nervosa bouts of binge eating often followed by vomiting result in sometimes unpredictable metabolic and endocrine changes, with large weight fluctuations

within the normal range of body weight. After eating binges, patients with bulimia attempt to prevent weight gain by vomiting, using diuretics or laxatives, restricting food intake, or exercising excessively. Hormonal and metabolic disturbances are regularly associated with anorexia nervosa; their presence and severity are largely functions of the weight loss and nutritional deficiencies.[1]

Anorexia nervosa and bulimia nervosa occur almost exclusively in women, with female-to-male ratios of 20:1 for anorexia nervosa and 20:5 for bulimia nervosa. Anorexia nervosa typically occurs in early or middle adolescence, whereas bulimia nervosa often has its onset in middle to late adolescence or early adulthood. Bulimia nervosa is 5 to 10 times more common than anorexia nervosa.

Eating disorders are unusual in patients older than 40 years of age, and then they usually reflect a chronic condition. The current mortality rate for anorexia nervosa is approximately 5% to 7%, from either the disease itself or suicide. Suicidal ideation may occur at an increased rate in bulimia nervosa as well; the overall mortality rate is unknown, but lower than in anorexia nervosa, and most often the result of metabolic or physiologic disturbances secondary to vomiting.

There is an increased incidence of major depression in patients with bulimia nervosa, which has led to the speculation that the two categories of mood and eating disorders may be related biologically.[2] Although like people with major depressive disorder,[3] those with anorexia and bulimia may show abnormally elevated cortisol secretion both at baseline[4,5] and after administration of dexamethasone,[6-9] profound underweight has been shown to account for these changes in anorexia nervosa, and intermittent caloric restriction contributes to these changes in bulimia nervosa.[10,11] A further biologic link between eating disorders and depressive disorders is suggested by the fact that antidepressant drugs have been shown to be effective in the treatment of bulimia nervosa.[12,13] In addition, patients with bipolar depression may present with hyperphagia, often accompanied by hypersomnia (see Chapter 112). All patients with significant eating abnormalities and sleep disturbance should, therefore, be evaluated for mood disorders.

Clinical Features

Insomnia and decreased amounts of sleep are common, as long as weight is subnormal.[14] However, patients with anorexia nervosa rarely if ever complain of insomnia. Quite to the contrary, individuals with anorexia nervosa tend to use the time gained by their reduced need for sleep for activities and exercise. People with bulimia nervosa frequently binge into or throughout the night and tend to fall asleep after midnight, often sleeping through the morning hours. Increased amounts of sleep may occur after eating binges.

Box 114–1. DSM-IV Criteria for Eating Disorders

Anorexia Nervosa

A. Refusal to maintain body weight at or above a minimally normal weight for age and height (e.g., weight loss leading to maintenance of body weight less than 85% of that expected; or failure to make expected weight gain during period of growth, leading to body weight less than 85% of that expected).

B. Intense fear of gaining weight or becoming fat, even though underweight.

C. Disturbance in the way in which one's body weight or shape is experienced, undue influence of body weight or shape on self-evaluation, or denial of the seriousness of the current low body weight.

D. In postmenarcheal females, amenorrhea, i.e., the absence of at least three consecutive menstrual cycles. (A woman is considered to have amenorrhea if her periods occur only following hormone, e.g., estrogen, administration.)

Bulimia Nervosa

A. Recurrent episodes of binge eating. An episode of binge eating is characterized by both of the following:

  1. Eating, in a discrete period of time (e.g., within any 2-hour period), an amount of food that is definitely larger than most people would eat during a similar period of time and under similar circumstances
  2. A sense of lack of control over eating during the episode (e.g., a feeling that one cannot stop eating or control what or how much one is eating)

B. Recurrent inappropriate compensatory behavior in order to prevent weight gain, such as self-induced vomiting; misuse of laxatives, diuretics, enemas, or other medications; fasting; or excessive exercise.

C. The binge eating and inappropriate compensatory behaviors both occur, on average, at least twice a week for 3 months.

D. Self-evaluation is unduly influenced by body shape and weight.

The disturbance does not occur exclusively during episodes of anorexia nervosa.

DSM-IV, Diagnostic and Statistical Manual of Mental Disorders, 4th edition.

Reprinted with permission from the American Psychiatric Association: Diagnostic and Statistical Manual of Mental Disorders, 4th ed. Washington, DC, American Psychiatric Press, 1994. Copyright 1994 American Psychiatric Association.

Patients with bulimia nervosa anecdotally report sleep-walking and binge eating, occasionally even shopping for food during the night after having fallen asleep, with partial recollection of the episode. Sometimes the only evidence of the behavior is the presence of store receipts or partially eaten food the next morning. Guirguis reported a case of a 32-year-old woman who went on uncontrollable nightly eating binges in a dreamlike state.[15] Gupta found one third of 32 patients with bulimia nervosa to have experienced sleep-related eating; this behavior was reported to be similar to that in other parasomnias in that patients often did not awaken completely while eating, nor did they have recall of the behavior the next morning.[16] A majority of the subjects reported sleepwalking as children; episodes of sleeptalking and recurrent bruxism were reported less frequently. Parasomnias have not been described in restricting anorexia nervosa. Clinical experience and published reports suggest that parasomnias deserve to be investigated more systematically in bulimia nervosa or in conditions associated with binge eating (see "Sleep-Related Eating Disorder," later in this chapter).

Polysomnographic Findings

Polysomnographic studies have been performed on patients with eating disorders to define the associated changes in sleep architecture and to determine whether eating disorders and major depression share biologic markers. As discussed in Chapter 112, sleep in depression is characterized by sleep continuity disruption, decreased slow wave sleep (SWS) amounts, and rapid eye movement (REM) sleep abnormalities consistent with increased REM sleep drive. A number of studies have been performed on patients with anorexia nervosa, bulimia nervosa, and mixed eating disorders. In general, patients with bulimia nervosa are not easily distinguishable from age-matched control subjects.[17-21] Patients with anorexia nervosa have been found to have significant decrements in sleep efficiency, total sleep time, or SWS amounts.[18-23] Reduced REM sleep latency, the sleep abnormality most specific for depression, was reported in several studies.[22,24,25] Paradoxically, REM density was reduced compared with control subjects in two studies.[4,22]

The failure to demonstrate consistent sleep abnormalities in patients with eating disorders does not necessarily imply that they do not share common features with those having depression. In four studies,[18,23,25,26] age-matched groups with major depression were included, and these groups with depression generally failed to show robust differences compared with control subjects. Only one depressed group exhibited reduced REM sleep latency,[25] three groups had disturbed sleep continuity,[17,23,25] and two groups showed increased REM density,[25,26] but no other sleep abnormality was reported in these young patients. Eating disorder groups were significantly different from these groups with depression in their decrease in REM density[17,26] and an increase in nocturnal awakenings.[23]

Because some individuals with eating disorders showed reduced REM sleep latency, investigators have questioned whether short REM sleep latency in a patient with an eating disorder might signify the presence of concurrent depressive symptoms or a concomitant affective disorder. Indeed, Katz et al. found a significant negative correlation between Hamilton depression ratings and REM sleep latency in patients with eating disorders.[24] A study by Walsh et al. failed to find a similar association between Hamilton scores and REM sleep latency; however, they did find that subgroups of patients with eating disorders who also qualified for a diagnosis of major depression tended to have shorter REM sleep latency than those without major depression.[21] On the other hand, two studies have failed to document reduced REM sleep latency in patients with eating disorders and depressive illness,[20,26] although one study reported increased REM density in patients with depressive disorder and eating disorders.[20]

To assess further the similarities in sleep between patients with eating disorders and those with mood disorders, polysomnographic findings from studies of patients with eating disorders were compared with those of groups of patients with affective disorders and healthy control subjects of comparable ages using meta-analysis,[27] a statistical technique for combining data from different studies. Depending on whether eating disorder groups were compared with their own control subjects or with a larger pool of age-matched control subjects, they showed tendencies toward decreased total sleep and sleep efficiency and reduced REM sleep latency. Compared with those with affective disorders, they seemed to show less significant disruption of sleep continuity, and REM sleep latency was indistinguishable (in controlled studies) or prolonged (for all studies combined). Of interest was the fact that although REM sleep latency was not reduced in the studies of patients with eating disorders compared with their own matched control subjects in the meta-analysis, REM sleep latency appeared to be significantly reduced compared with a larger pool of control data in the same age group. This discrepancy could be explained by the somewhat shorter-than-average REM sleep latencies reported for control groups in the few studies of eating disorders. Because of the lack of robust findings in patients with eating disorders in the age groups tested, it is generally not possible to use sleep markers to distinguish them reliably from healthy subjects or those with depression. Thus, the issue as to whether REM sleep latency is reduced in eating disorders, or whether short REM sleep latency in patients with an eating disorder represents a component of major depressive illness, has yet to be resolved.

Correlation of Sleep Findings with Other Markers

The cholinergic REM induction test has been performed to assess the possibility of abnormal cholinergic regulation of REM sleep in eating disorders. People with depressive disorders tend to show abnormally rapid appearance of REM sleep in response to cholinomimetic agents (see Chapter 112). In tests of the responses of patients with anorexia nervosa to the cholinergic REM sleep induction test (RIT), Sitaram et al. found that most patients with both anorexia nervosa and major depression showed more rapid REM sleep induction in response to arecoline.[28] However, in later studies by Lauer et al., no differences in patients with anorexia nervosa were demonstrated compared with control subjects.[18,26] Although an age-matched group with depression showed more rapid REM sleep onset after the RIT,[26] normal RIT responses were observed in patients with anorexia nervosa, including those with concomitant major depression.

A single study of cortisol responses and sleep in non-depressed bulimic patients found that although the group showed elevated baseline and post–dexamethasone suppression test cortisol levels, REM sleep latency values were not reduced on average.[4] Furthermore, no significant correlation was found between reduced REM sleep latency and dexa-methasone suppression test nonsuppression. Overall, these findings do not unequivocally support the hypothesis that sleep patterns and other neurobiologic markers are similar in eating disorders and mood disorders.

Clinical Factors Influencing Sleep

Although sleep studies have not reliably distinguished eating disorder groups from either control subjects or groups of depressed patients, this does not necessarily mean that sleep is unaffected in patients with eating disorders. The major problem with most recent studies on sleep in eating disorders has been the failure to consider those factors that specifically affect sleep patterns in these patients, including age, sex, weight loss, and nutritional status.

AGE

One explanation for the failure to find many significant abnormalities in either eating disorder or depressive groups is that the groups studied may have been too young to exhibit the full spectrum of sleep abnormalities; in all cases, mean group ages were between 20 and 30 years. As discussed in Chapter 112, age has profound effects on sleep in depression. Younger patient groups often fail to show the characteristic sleep abnormalities. The lack of studies of patient groups with mean ages over 30 years makes it difficult to determine whether patients with eating disorders have sleep abnormalities in common with those with depression, and difficult to define the effects of age on sleep in eating disorders. On the other hand, the early age at onset, especially for anorexia nervosa, suggests that if patients older than 30 years of age are being studied, either they have been chronically ill for many years and thus would represent selective treatment-resistant cases, or, if their symptoms have developed in their late twenties, they would be considered atypical cases. Thus, it may not be possible to explore the effects of age on sleep in patients with eating disorders, nor may the potential "depressive" effects of eating disorders on sleep become fully expressed, if most treatment-responsive patients have long had remission by the age at which sleep abnormalities become most pronounced.

SEX

The effect of sex on sleep in eating disorders is impossible to determine, because too few patients studied were male. A previous study of the effects of sex on sleep in depression has shown that SWS amounts declined less significantly with age in women than in men, although other parameters did not appear to be affected.[29]

WEIGHT LOSS

In addition to possible effects of depression on sleep in eating disorders, the degree of weight loss may strongly influence sleep patterns. Some of the first data on the effects of starvation on sleep were obtained from animal studies. Food deprivation caused severe insomnia and significantly increased activity in rats.[30,31] Early clinical studies suggested that weight loss was responsible for insomnia during acute starvation and strongly associated with insomnia in populations with psychiatric illness, whereas hypersomnia was more commonly found during periods of significant weight gain.[14,32] Several studies have been performed to assess the effects of weight gain on sleep in anorexia nervosa. During periods of severely reduced weight, patients with anorexia nervosa reported insomnia and reduced amounts of total sleep; after treatment and significant weight gain, patients reported increased amounts of sleep and decreased wakefulness during sleep hours.[14] Similar results were obtained in polysomnographic studies of patients with anorexia nervosa, with significant increases in total sleep, SWS, and REM sleep amounts after weight gain.[33,34] In other studies, Levy et al. have found significant positive correlations between percentage of ideal body weight (IBW) and SWS amount in one study,[19] and between percentage of IBW and total sleep time and sleep efficiency in another.[20] Others have failed to confirm significant relationships between percentage of IBW and sleep parameters in patients with eating disorders.[18,26] Possible explanations for these discrepancies include independent effects of drug treatment and psychotherapy in some of the earlier studies, and differences in correlations performed within individual patients over time versus cross-sectional studies of patients.

NUTRITIONAL STATUS AND NEUROENDOCRINE FACTORS

The eating habits of patients with anorexia nervosa vary so markedly that the only common denominator is profoundly reduced caloric intake, usually between 400 to 800 kcal/day. However, the composition of the food differs widely, from consumption of only apricot juice for weeks or months to lettuce and rice cakes or boiled eggs and tea. On the other hand, for patients with bulimia nervosa, the amount of calories consumed during one binge can fluctuate from a few hundred to several thousand, depending on binge frequency, and can amount to a maximum of 10,000 to 30,000 kcal/day. Some patients with bulimia prefer high-fat foods such as ice cream, chocolate cake, bread and butter, whereas others may binge on meat or bread. Similarly, vomiting may occur immediately after a binge or at variable intervals thereafter, resulting in considerable differences in absorption. Thus, to determine whether nutritional factors influence sleep, it is necessary to obtain detailed dietary records or to stabilize the patient's condition on a controlled diet under supervision.

Virtually none of the recent studies of sleep in eating disorders reported the eating behavior, body weight changes, or caloric intake during the week preceding sleep studies; any of these factors may influence sleep patterns. Acute fasting in humans, rats, and birds has been shown to increase SWS amounts.[35-39] With prolonged starvation resulting in increased protein catabolism, waking time increased, and both SWS and REM sleep amounts were significantly reduced.[36,38] Conversely, ingestion of food may lead to sleepiness. Animal studies have shown that fat-containing food in the gastrointestinal tract causes drowsiness.[40]

A number of recent studies have assessed the effects of eating on sleepiness in healthy human subjects. A high-calorie, high-carbohydrate noontime meal led to a prolonged duration of postprandial sleep in a group of healthy men.[41] Orr et al. found that solid but not liquid meals led to decreased sleep latencies, but could not detect a difference in the soporific effects of high-fat versus high-carbohydrate meals.[42] Similarly, both high-fat/low-carbohydrate and low-fat/high-carbohydrate meals increased sleepiness and reduced sleep latency in another study by Wells and colleagues.[43] A previous study by the same authors found subjective sleepiness increased by both types of meals, but more so by high fat content.[44]

It is not clear whether increased sleep after feeding is caused by specific food substances, the increased metabolic rate after eating, or endogenous peptides released in response to food. The sleep-promoting effects of the gastrointestinal peptide cholecystokinin (CCK), released in response to food intake, have been assessed in several studies. Direct administration of CCK to rats has been shown to have sleep-inducing effects in some studies,[45-47] and CCK caused drowsiness in humans.[48] Other studies, however, have failed to confirm hypnotic effects of CCK.[49-51] Healthy subjects who had ingested high-fat/low-carbohydrate meals had higher plasma CCK levels and greater subjective sleepiness than those who had eaten low-fat/high-carbohydrate meals.[44] Geracioti and Liddle[52] found subnormal CCK levels postprandially in 14 women with bulimia nervosa, although fasting CCK plasma levels were similar in comparison with normal subjects. Bombesin, another gut-associated peptide released in response to feeding, has also shown sleep-promoting effects in rats.[53-55] The amino acid L-tryptophan, a precursor of serotonin, may have sleep-inducing effects, and bedtime snacks have been reported to have variable effects on sleep.[32] Some of these factors may contribute to sleepiness after eating binges in bulimia nervosa, although patients with anorexia nervosa typically maintain low-fat, low-carbohydrate, and low-protein diets and thus are unlikely to benefit from any direct sleep-inducing effects from their food.

Patients with anorexia nervosa, however, have alterations in several peptides with effects on feeding and sleep; they characteristically show reduced levels of leptin, a peptide produced by adipocytes that suppresses appetite, and increased levels of ghrelin, which increases appetite. Both ghrelin and leptin have been shown to increase SWS when administered intravenously to humans and rats, respectively.[56,57] In patients with anorexia nervosa, increased leptin levels were associated with increased amounts of SWS after refeeding.[58] As more is learned about the neuroendocrine factors and neural circuitry underlying feeding and satiety, it is likely that we will have a better idea of the mechanisms for sleep changes associated with primary eating disorders.

Treatment

The treatment of an eating disorder is based on a comprehensive assessment of the patient and the family. Treatment interventions vary and depend on the patient's age, premorbid functioning, duration of illness, severity of weight loss, the presence of coexisting psychiatric disorders or, in bulimia nervosa, the frequency of the binge eating/purging episodes.

Anorexia Nervosa

Hospitalization in specialty treatment programs is usually required for patients who have lost in excess of 25% IBW or who have a body mass index (weight in kilograms divided by height in meters squared) of less than 16, as well as for patients who refuse to drink fluids, or patients who have been unsuccessful in gaining weight in supervised outpatient treatment. No medications currently exist to treat the resistance to weight gain or the anxiety and guilt associated with eating and the fear of being overweight in anorexia nervosa; food is the only effective antidote. Depending on the comorbid diagnoses, antidepressant or antianxiety drugs may be indicated.

Sleeping medications may be helpful if insomnia is severe, although patients' sleep disturbances may improve with balanced nutrition sufficient for weight gain. Persistent sleep problems may also indicate a comorbid depressive illness or unresolved emotional conflicts. The patient's reasons for her strong investment in the weight loss process need to be explored in psychotherapy. Occasionally, the family's dysfunctional expectations and interaction pattern require attention through family treatment. Patients with restricting anorexia have been shown to share particular personality characteristics, including greater-than-normal tendencies toward perfectionism, self-control, inhibition, and conscientiousness, whereas those with bulimic anorexia nervosa tend to be more expressive and dramatic.[59] Treatment needs to take these personality differences into account. Treatment therefore occurs at several levels simultaneously: a supervised, clearly spelled-out nutritional regime; regular body weight measurements to ensure age- and height-adequate weight gain; treatment of dysfunctional personality characteristics to bring about changes in attitude, beliefs, and self-concept; treatment of psychiatric symptoms through individual, family, and peer group therapy; and occasionally pharmacotherapy. Although serotonin reuptake inhibitors are used frequently in these patients, there is little evidence that any currently available medications are particularly effective for eating disorders.[60] The goal is to help the patient relinquish her excessive reliance on body weight for improving her self-esteem and to use food again as nourishment so that she can gain control over herself and her life and proceed in growth and development through age-appropriate ways.

Bulimia Nervosa

Bulimia nervosa is largely treated on an outpatient basis, unless the bulimic behavior significantly disrupts work and psychosocial functioning or results in life-threatening medical symptoms or suicidality. Cognitive-behavioral methods and nutritional education are used first to assist the patient in organizing and controlling her eating behavior. In addition, antidepressant drugs,[61] including monoamine oxidase inhibitors (e.g., phenelzine)[62] and serotonin reuptake inhibitors (e.g., fluoxetine),[63] have been shown to reduce binging and purging behaviors. Recent studies have also suggested that the anticonvulsant and mood stabilizer topiramate may also be helpful in decreasing binging and purging.[64] Because emotional distress or uncontrollable feelings trigger eating binges in bulimia nervosa, individual, family, and group psychotherapy is usually necessary to explore dysfunctional interpersonal relationships or to treat a coexisting psychiatric disorder. Maturational issues germane to adolescence or young adulthood—such as lack of a sense of identity, a poor self-concept, and struggle with self-definition or separation–autonomy issues—are usually in the foreground. Thus, in bulimia nervosa, character and family issues need to be addressed so that eating can again serve a nutritional function instead of controlling emotions.

Sleep abnormalities usually resolve with return to more normal weight and eating behaviors. Persistent sleep disturbance may indicate the need for further assessment of possible psychiatric or medical causes of insomnia, including primary sleep disorders. Patients with bulimia nervosa have increased rates of alcoholism and substance abuse disorders, as well as depression, all of which can significantly affect sleep.[65,66]

SLEEP-RELATED EATING DISORDER

This sleeping and eating disorder (also called *nocturnal binge-eating disorder*) is classified as a Parasomnia in the newly revised International Classification of Sleep Disorders.[67] Its clinical and diagnostic features are presented here, along with its treatment.

Clinical Features

Sleep-related eating disorder (SRED) consists of recurrent episodes of involuntary eating and drinking during arousals from nocturnal sleep, with adverse consequences.[68-71] The episodes of eating always occur in an involuntary or "out-of-control" manner after an interval of sleep, and usually during partial arousals from sleep with subsequent partial recall. Some patients cannot be brought to full consciousness during an episode of eating, as with classic sleepwalking, and they may have no recall of having eaten during the night. On the other hand, some patients seemingly have considerable alertness during an episode and have substantial recall in the morning. High-calorie foods (fats, carbohydrates) are preferentially consumed, and healthful foods (fruits, vegetables) are rarely eaten. There can be consumption of odd types of food or of odd combinations of food, or even of inedible or toxic substances, such as frozen or uncooked foods, buttered cigarettes, animal food and salt sandwiches, coffee grounds and egg shells, and kitchen cleaning compounds. Simple foods or entire hot or cold meals can be prepared and consumed, often in a sloppy manner. External and internal injuries can occur during the food preparation and consumption process. Morning anorexia and abdominal distention are common complaints. Excessive weight gain commonly occurs.

Nightly frequency of eating, sometimes with multiple episodes of eating per night, is reported by most patients. The episodes of eating occur during any time in the sleep cycle. Hunger and thirst are notably absent during nocturnal binge eating.

Epidemiology and Risk Factors

The prevalence may exceed 4% in young adults, and may be as high as 8% to 17% in outpatient and inpatient eating disorders groups.[72] Women comprise approximated 75% of reported patients. Age of onset is most common during the third decade of life, but can begin in childhood and in midlife. Long-standing histories (more than 10 years) are often reported.

SRED can be idiopathic, but can also be associated with a primary sleep disorder, such as sleepwalking, restless legs syndrome, periodic limb movements during sleep, obstructive sleep apnea, and irregular sleep–wake cycling. Medication-induced sleep-related eating has been reported with zolpidem, triazolam, lithium, anticholinergics, and other agents.[69,73] Onset of SRED has also been reported with acute and chronic stress (usually involving major separation reactions), with cessation of cigarette smoking, with cessation of alcohol and substance abuse, after daytime dieting, and with the onset of narcolepsy, autoimmune hepatitis, encephalitis, and other conditions. Thus, SRED can be viewed as a "final common pathway disorder." A familial basis for SRED is not uncommon.

Various complications can occur on account of repeated, indiscriminate nocturnal binge eating: excessive weight gain/obesity; compromise in the control of type 1 or type 2 diabetes mellitus, or of hypercholesterolemia/hypertriglyceridemia; hypertension; risk of consuming foods to which one is allergic; and compromise of overnight fasting before next-day surgery; in addition, loss of dietary control during sleep may result in consumption of tyramine-rich foods followed by a hypertensive crisis in a patient being treated with a monoamine oxidase inhibitor. Furthermore, secondary depressive disorders may emerge from long-standing personal dejection and a sense of failure over the inability to control the nocturnal eating. There can also be interpersonal problems and marital discord related to various aspects of SRED, including disrupted sleep in the bed partner or roommate.

Diagnosis

Binge eating that is a direct nocturnal extension of daytime bulimia nervosa or binge-eating disorder must be excluded to diagnose SRED. Inappropriate compensatory behavior, such as self-induced vomiting, enemas, misuse of laxatives, diuretics, or other medications, or other purging activity, should not be present in SRED. However, a person with a daytime eating disorder can also have a coexisting SRED that is associated with confusional arousals, but not associated with purging behaviors during the night or on arising in the morning. These exclusion criteria should not apply to patients with long-standing SRED and excessive weight gain who may eventually restrict food intake during the daytime or engage in excessive exercise in a final effort to prevent progressive weight gain and obesity.

A history of excessive eating between the evening meal and sleep onset should not be present. Otherwise, the diagnosis would probably be night-eating syndrome (NES), also called *nocturnal eating syndrome*.[74-76] SRED must primarily be distinguished from NES, which is characterized by the following features that usually can distinguish it from SRED: overeating between the evening meal and nocturnal sleep onset; eating during complete awakenings from sleep with full subsequent recall; absence of bizarre food/substance choices and sloppy or bizarre eating behaviors; and absence of an associated primary sleep disorder. Nevertheless, SRED and NES share a considerable number of overlapping features and may exist along a common spectrum of pathophysiology. Thus, a complaint of abnormal nocturnal eating can be associated with either a parasomnia history or an insomnia history.

Treatment

Treatment is initially aimed at controlling any other sleep disorder that may be present, such as restless legs syndrome or obstructive sleep apnea, or at addressing major stress reactions with appropriate therapy. However, a focus on controlling the compulsive eating behavior may be the most effective approach in controlling SRED. Topiramate, 25 to 150 mg at bedtime (up to 300 to 400 mg) appears to be a promising agent,[77] and perhaps also zonisamide, 100 to 400 mg at bedtime. In cases when eating is controlled with these agents, but not recurrent arousals or awakenings, then the addition of low-dose clonazepam at bedtime can be effective. The treatment of restless legs syndrome with dopaminergics, opiates, or clonazepam is usually also effective in controlling SRED. Idiopathic SRED and SRED associated with sleepwalking or other conditions may also be controlled with bedtime dopaminergic (and opiate) therapy.[69,78,79]

PITFALLS AND CONTROVERSIES

Virtually all polysomnographic studies in eating disorders performed over the past several decades have focused on the question of whether sleep changes indicate the presence of a coexisting affective illness.[80,81] This question is difficult to answer, at best, in part because young patients, even if they are depressed, lack significant sleep abnormalities. Sleep-related eating disorders have been increasingly recognized over the past decade, and further work will be required to define these syndromes more clearly, as well as develop effective treatments for them.

The association of abnormal episodes of eating related to the sleep period, including NES and SRED, further suggests that systems involved in sleep and feeding are overlapping. It is not known whether these disorders are related to primary eating disorders, however, and few sleep electroencephalographic data are currently available for patients with SRED.

However, the study of sleep and eating disorders may yield important clues about the effects of various physiologic parameters on human sleep. Patients with anorexia nervosa can provide an opportunity to learn about the effects of chronic starvation, extreme weight loss, or undernutrition on sleep. In addition, the impact of hypercaloric intake on sleep in previously starving subjects, as well as the disturbed sleep patterns and sleep-related behaviors of patients with bulimia nervosa, require further study. Finally, basic research has begun on studying the effects of starvation and of weight restoration on the brain circuitry subserving sleep.[82] It is likely that more effective treatments for primary eating disorders as well as SRED and related disorders will be based on new pharmacologic agents that will be developed as we gain a better understanding of neural mechanisms involved in regulating appetite and sleep.

Clinical Pearl

Sleep and feeding, behaviors necessary for survival, are centrally regulated and, not surprisingly, interrelated. Sleep abnormalities may occur in patients with primary eating disorders and may require specific treatment. Sleep-related eating disorders often indicate the presence of a primary sleep disorder, but not necessarily a primary eating disorder.

REFERENCES

1. Casper RC, Kirschner B, Sandstead HH, et al: An evaluation of trace metals, vitamins, and taste function in anorexia nervosa. Am J Clin Nutr 1980;33:1801-1808.
2. Levy AB, Dixon KN, Stern SL: How are depression and bulimia related? Am J Psychiatry 1989;146:162-169.
3. Carroll BJ, Feinberg M, Greden JF, et al: A specific laboratory test for the diagnosis of melancholia: Standardization, validation, and clinical utility. Arch Gen Psychiatry 1981;38:15-22.
4. Byrne B, Nino-Murcia G, Gaddy JR, et al: Sleep patterns and dexamethasone suppression in nondepressed bulimics. Biol Psychiatry 1990;27:454-456.
5. Casper RC, Pandy GN, Jaspan JB, et al: Hormone and metabolite plasma levels after oral glucose in bulimia and healthy controls. Biol Psychiatry 1988;24.6:663-674.
6. Gwirtsman HE, Roy-Byrne P, Yager J, et al: Neuroendocrine abnormalities in bulimia. Am J Psychiatry 1983;140:559-563.

7. Hudson JI, Pope HG Jr, Jonas JM, et al: Hypothalamic-pituitary-adrenal-axis hyperactivity in bulimia. Psychiatry Res 1983;8:111-117.

8. Levy AB, Dixon KN: DST in bulimia without endogenous depression. Biol Psychiatry 1987;22:783-786.

9. Walsh BT, Katz JL, Levin J, et al: Adrenal activity in anorexia nervosa. Psychosom Med 1978;40:499-506.

10. Casper RC, Chatterton RT Jr, Davis JM: Alterations in serum cortisol and its binding characteristics in anorexia nervosa. J Clin Endocrinol Metab 1979;49:406-411.

11. Fichter MM, Pirke KM, Holsboer F: Weight loss causes neuroendocrine disturbances: Experimental study in healthy starving subjects. Psychiatry Res 1986;17:61-72.

12. Walsh BT, Stewart JW, Roose SP, et al: A double-blind trial of phenelzine in bulimia. J Psychiatr Res 1985;19:485-489.

13. Pope HG Jr, Hudson JI, Jonas JM, et al: Bulimia treated with imipramine: A placebo-controlled, double-blind study. Am J Psychiatry 1983;140:554-558.

14. Crisp AH, Stonehill E (eds): Sleep, Nutrition and Mood. London, John Wiley & Sons, 1971.

15. Guirguis WR: Sleepwalking as a symptom of bulimia. BMJ 1986;293:587-588.

16. Gupta MA: Sleep-related eating in bulimia nervosa-an underreported parasomnia disorder. Sleep Res 1991;20:182.

17. Hudson JI, Pope HG Jr, Jonas JM, et al: Sleep EEG in bulimia. Biol Psychiatry 1987;22:820-828.

18. Lauer CJ, Zulley J, Krieg J, et al: EEG sleep and the cholinergic REM induction test in anorexic and bulimic patients. Psychiatry Res 1988;26:171-181.

19. Levy AB, Dixon KN, Schmidt H: REM and delta sleep in anorexia nervosa and bulimia. Psychiatry Res 1987;20:189-197.

20. Levy AB, Dixon KN, Schmidt H: Sleep architecture in anorexia nervosa and bulimia. Biol Psychiatry 1988;23:99-101.

21. Walsh BT, Goetz RR, Roose SP, et al: EEG-monitored sleep in anorexia nervosa and bulimia. Biol Psychiatry 1985;20:947-956.

22. Neil JF, Merikangas JR, Foster FG, et al: Waking and all-night sleep EEG's in anorexia nervosa. Clin Electroencephalogr 1980;11:9-15.

23. Delvenne V, Kerkhofs M, Appelboom-Fondu J, et al: Sleep polygraphic variables in anorexia nervosa and depression: A comparative study in adolescents. J Affect Disord 1992;25:167-172.

24. Katz JL, Kuperberg A, Pollack CP, et al: Is there a relationship between eating disorder and affective disorder? New evidence from sleep recordings. Am J Psychiatry 1984;141:753-759.

25. Waller DA, Hardy BW, Pole R, et al: Sleep EEG in bulimic, depressed, and normal subjects. Biol Psychiatry 1989;25:661-664.

26. Lauer CJ, Krieg J-C, Riemann D, et al: A polysomnographic study in young psychiatric inpatients: Major depression, anorexia nervosa, bulimia nervosa. J Affect Disord 1990;18:235-245.

27. Benca RM, Obermeyer WH, Thisted RA, et al: Sleep and psychiatric disorders: A meta-analysis. Arch Gen Psychiatry 1992;49:651-668.

28. Sitaram N, Gillin JC, Bunney WEJ. Cholinergic and catecholaminergic receptor sensitivity in affective illness: Strategy and theory. In Post RM, Ballenger JC (eds): Neurobiology of Mood Disorders. Baltimore, Williams & Wilkins, 1984, pp 629-651.

29. Reynolds CF III, Kupfer DJ, Thase ME, et al: Sleep, gender and depression: An analysis of gender effects on the electroencephalographic sleep of 302 depressed outpatients. Biol Psychiatry 1990;28:673-684.

30. Jacobs BL, McGinty DJ: Effects of food deprivation on sleep and wakefulness in the rat. Exp Neurol 1971;30:212-222.

31. Treichler FR, Hall JF: The relationship between deprivation, weight loss and several measures of activity. J Compr Physiol Psychol 1962;55:348-349.

32. Evans FJ: Sleep, eating, and weight disorders. In Richard K (ed): Eating and Weight Disorders. New York, Springer, 1983, pp 147-178.

33. Crisp AH, Stonehill E, Fenton GW: The relationship between sleep, nutrition and mood: A study of patients with anorexia nervosa. Postgrad Med J 1971;47:207-213.

34. Lacey JH, Crisp AH, Kalucy RS, et al: Weight gain and the sleeping electroencephalogram: Study of 10 patients with anorexia nervosa. BMJ 1975;6:556-558.

35. MacFadyen UM, Oswald I, Lewis SA: Starvation and human slow-wave sleep. J Appl Physiol 1973;35:391-394.

36. Dewasmes G, Cohen-Adad F, Koubi H, et al: Sleep changes in long-term fasting geese in relation to lipid and protein metabolism. Am J Physiol 1984;247:R663-R671.

37. Dewasmes G, Buchet C, Geloen A, et al: Sleep changes in emperor penguins during fasting. Am J Physiol 1989;256:R476-R480.

38. Dewasmes G, Duchamp C, Minaire Y: Sleep changes in fasting rats. Physiol Behav 1989;46:179-184.

39. Karacan I, Rosenbloom AL, Londono JH, et al: The effect of acute fasting on sleep and the sleep-growth hormone response. Psychosomatics 1973;14:33-37.

40. Fara JW, Rubinstein EH, Sonnenschein RR: Visceral and behavioral responses to intraduodenal fat. Science 1969;166:110-111.

41. Zammit GK, Kolevzon A, Fauci M, et al: Postprandial sleep in healthy men. Sleep 1995;18:229-231.

42. Orr WC, Shadid G, Harnish MJ, et al: Meal composition and its effect on postprandial sleepiness. Physiol Behav 1997;62:709-712.

43. Wells AS, Read NW, Idzikowski C, et al: Effects of meals on objective and subjective measures of daytime sleepiness. J Appl Physiol 1998;84:507-515.

44. Wells AS, Read NW: Influences of fat, energy, and time of day on mood and performance. Physiol Behav 1996;59:1069-1076.

45. Antin J, Gibbs J, Holt J, et al: Cholecystokinin elicits the complete behavioral sequence of satiety in rats. J Comp Physiol Psychol 1975;89:784-790.

46. Kapas L, Obal FJ, Alföldi P, et al: Effects of nocturnal intraperitoneal administration of cholecystokinin in rats: Simultaneous increase in sleep, increase in EEG slow-wave activity, reduction of motor activity, suppression of eating, and decrease in brain temperature. Brain Res 1988;438:155-164.

47. Mansbach RS, Lorenz DN: Cholecystokinin (CCK-8) elicits prandial sleep in rats. Physiol Behav 1983;30:179-183.

48. Stacher G, Bauer H, Steinringer H: Cholecystokinin decreases appetite and activation evoked by stimuli arising from the preparation of a meal in man. Physiol Behav 1979;23:325-331.

49. Rojas-Ramirez JA, Crawley JN, Mendelson WB: Electroencephalographic analysis of the sleep-inducing actions of cholecystokinin. Neuropeptides 1982;3:129-138.

50. Riou F, Cespuglio R, Jouvet M: Endogenous peptides and sleep in the rat: I. Peptides decreasing paradoxical sleep. Neuropeptides 1982;2:243-254.

51. De Saint Hilaire-Kafi Z, Depoortere H, Nicolaidis S: Does cholecystokinin induce physiological satiety and sleep? Brain Res 1989;488:304-310.

52. Geracioti TD Jr, Liddle RA: Impaired cholecystokinin secretion in bulimia nervosa. N Engl J Med 1988;319:683-688.

53. Gibbs J, Fauser DJ, Rowe EA, et al: Bombesin suppresses feeding in rats. Nature 1979;282:208-210.

54. Gibbs J, Smith GP: Satiety: The roles of peptides from the stomach and the intestine. Fed Proc 1986;45:1391-1395.

55. De Saint Hilaire-Kafi Z, Gibbs J, Nicolaidis S: Satiety and sleep: The effects of bombesin. Brain Res 1989;478:152-155.

56. Weikel JC, Wichniak A, Ising M, et al: Ghrelin promotes slow-wave sleep in humans. Am J Physiol Endocrinol Metab 2003;284:E407-E415.

57. Sinton CM, Fitch TE, Gershenfeld HK: The effects of leptin on REM sleep and slow wave delta in rats are reversed by food deprivation. J Sleep Res 1999;8:197-203.

58. Lindberg N, Virkkunen M, Tani P, et al: Growth hormone-insulin-like growth factor-1 axis, leptin and sleep in anorexia nervosa patients. Neuropsychobiology 2003;47:78-85.

59. Casper RC, Hedeker D, McClough JF: Personality dimensions in eating disorders and their relevance for subtyping. J Am Acad Child Adolesc Psychiatry 1992;31:830-840.

60. Agras WS, Brandt HA, Bulik CM, et al: Report of the National Institutes of Health workshop on overcoming barriers to treatment research in anorexia nervosa. Int J Eat Disord 2004;35:509-521.

61. Bacaltchuk J, Hay P: Antidepressants versus placebo for people with bulimia nervosa. Cochrane Database Syst Rev 2003; 4:CD003391.

62. Walsh BT, Wilson GT, Loeb KL, et al: Medication and psychotherapy in the treatment of bulimia nervosa. Am J Psychiatry 1997;154:523-531.

63. Fluoxetine Bulimia Nervosa Collaborative Study Group: Fluoxetine in the treatment of bulimia nervosa: A multicenter, placebo-controlled, double-blind trial. Fluoxetine Bulimia Nervosa Collaborative Study Group. Arch Gen Psychiatry 1992;49:139-147.

64. Hoopes SP, Reimherr FW, Hedges DW, et al: Treatment of bulimia nervosa with topiramate in a randomized, double-blind, placebo-controlled trial: Part 1. Improvement in binge and purge measures. J Clin Psychiatry 2003;64:1335-1341.

65. Hatsukami D, Eckert E, Mitchell JE, et al: Affective disorder and substance abuse in women with bulimia. Psychol Med 1984;14:701-704.

66. Lacey JH, Moureli E: Bulimic alcoholics: Some features of a clinical sub-group. Br J Addict 1986;81:389-393.

67. American Academy of Sleep Medicine: International classification of sleep disorders: Diagnostic and coding manual, 2nd ed. Westchester, Ill: American Academy of Sleep Medicine, 2005.

68. Schenck CH, Hurwitz TD, Bundlie SR, et al: Sleep-related eating disorders: Polysomnographic correlates of a heterogeneous syndrome distinct from daytime eating disorders. Sleep 1991;14:419-431.

69. Schenck CH, Hurwitz TD, O'Connor KA, et al: Additional categories of sleep-related eating disorders and the current status of treatment. Sleep 1993;16:457-466.

70. Schenck CH, Mahowald MW: Review of nocturnal sleep-related eating disorders. Int J Eat Disord 1994;15:343-356.

71. Winkelman JW: Clinical and polysomnographic features of sleep-related eating disorder. J Clin Psychiatry 1998;59:14-19.

72. Winkelman JW, Herzog DB, Fava M: The prevalence of sleep-related eating disorder in psychiatric and non-psychiatric populations. Psychol Med 1999;29:1461-1466.

73. Morgenthaler TI, Silber MH: Amnestic sleep-related eating disorder associated with zolpidem. Sleep Med 2002;3:323-327.

74. Spaggiari MC, Granella F, Parrino L, et al: Nocturnal eating syndrome in adults. Sleep 1994;17:339-344.

75. Manni R, Ratti MT, Tartara A: Nocturnal eating: Prevalence and features in 120 insomniac referrals. Sleep 1997;20:734-738.

76. Birketvedt GS, Florholmen J, Sundsfjord J, et al: Behavioral and neuroendocrine characteristics of the night-eating syndrome. JAMA 1999;282:657-663.

77. Winkelman JW: Treatment of nocturnal eating syndrome and sleep-related eating disorder with topiramate. Sleep Med 2003;4:243-246.

78. Schenck CH, Mahowald MW: Combined bupropion-levodopa-trazodone therapy of sleep-related eating and sleep disruption in two adults with chemical dependency. Sleep 2000;23: 587-588.

79. Schenck CH: Dopaminergic and opiate therapy of nocturnal sleep-related eating disorder associated with sleepwalking or unassociated with another nocturnal disorder. Sleep 2002;25: A249-A250.

80. Strober M, Katz JL: Do eating disorders and affective disorders share a common etiology? A dissenting opinion. Int J Eat Disord 1987;6:171-180.

81. Casper RC: The dilemma of homonymous symptoms for evaluating comorbidity between affective disorders and eating disorders. In Maser JD, Cloninger CR (eds): Comorbidity of Mood and Anxiety Disorders. Washington, DC, American Psychiatric Press, 1990, pp 253-269.

82. Lauer CJ, Krieg JC: Sleep in eating disorders. Sleep Med Rev 2004;8:109-118.

115

Medication and Substance Abuse

J. Christian Gillin*

Sean P. A. Drummond

Camellia P. Clark

Polly Moore

ABSTRACT

Psychoactive substances are widely used in almost all cultures, and almost all of these substances have some impact on nocturnal sleep or daytime alertness. Furthermore, sleep is likely to be disturbed during acute and, typically, subacute withdrawal from almost any substance, legal or illegal. However, many of the effects of substances on sleep depend on the context. For example, is the use low-quantity social use, large quantities in the context of abuse or dependence, or secondary to a medical condition such as pain? Also, is the patient currently using or in withdrawal? In industrialized nations, the most commonly used substances that affect sleep are caffeine and alcohol. Caffeine use can lead to insomnia and shallow sleep for up to 10 hours, despite a half-life of approximately 3 to 7 hours. Alcohol results in lowered total sleep time, sleep efficiency, and slow wave sleep, particularly in the latter half of the night. Stimulants, on the other hand, may be used to self-medicate excessive daytime sleepiness secondary to a primary sleep disorder. In addition to directly disrupting sleep, some substances can exacerbate sleep disorders such as obstructive sleep apnea and periodic limb movements. The *Diagnostic and Statistical Manual of Mental Disorders*, 4th edition, allows for diagnosis of sleep disorders secondary to substance use, provided the sleep disorder occurs only during intoxication or withdrawal from the substance. Thus, the clinician should carefully screen patients for the presence of a primary sleep disorder before making a substance-related diagnosis. Similarly, clinicians should screen all patients with sleep disorders for the potential contribution of substance abuse or dependence to the patient's sleep disorder. In general, the choice of whether to treat the substance abuse or the sleep disorder depends on which is primary versus secondary. However, in some cases, it may be beneficial simultaneously to treat both, although insufficient research exists to allow for a formal recommendation for such.

Psychoactive substances are widely used in all cultures. Many of these substances are used according to social or medical norms, including alcohol, sedatives, hypnotics, anxiolytics, caffeine, tobacco, stimulants (e.g., prescription amphetamines for narcolepsy), and opioids (for medical analgesia). But psychoactive substances can also be abused or misused. In the United States, 18% of the population experiences a substance abuse disorder during their lifetime. Approximately 20% of the patients in general medical facilities and approximately 35% of patients in general psychiatric units present with substance abuse disorders.

Nearly all psychoactive substances affect the sleep–wake cycle, for better or worse. For this reason, sleep disorder clinicians should routinely assess substance use and abuse in their patients, including prescription and over-the-counter (OTC) drugs, recreational drugs, tobacco and caffeine, health foods, steroids or body-building aids, and botanical and natural substances (e.g., melatonin, valerian, or Saint John's wort). In this chapter, we focus primarily on substances of abuse and dependence.

The terms used to describe psychoactive substances are often misleading, controversial, or arbitrary. The terms *addiction* and *drug abuse*, for example, have been used extensively to condemn any drug with withdrawal symptoms; these drugs include methadone, amphetamine, sleeping pills, and anxiolytics. On the other hand, considerable scientific and clinical experience supports the value of these agents in the treatment of medical illnesses. For example, benzodiazepines may be helpful in the long-term clinical management of generalized anxiety disorder or chronic insomnia; amphetamines can be useful to treat attention-deficit/hyperactivity disorder (ADHD) or narcolepsy; and methadone is used in the management of heroin abuse. Box 115–1 defines some of the terms used to describe effects of psychoactive substances.

DIAGNOSIS OF SUBSTANCE ABUSE AND DEPENDENCE

Substance-related disorders are divided into two groups according to the *Diagnostic and Statistical Manual of Mental Disorders*, 4th edition (DSM-IV)[1]: substance use disorders (substance dependence, substance abuse), and substance-induced disorders (including substance-induced sleep disorders).

Substance abuse is defined as recurrent and significant adverse consequences related to repeated use of the substance (Box 115–2). These problems include failure to meet obligations, hazardous behaviors, legal problems, and other persistent problems.

Substance dependence is associated with repeated self-administered use of the substance despite significant substance-related problems (Box 115–3). It is usually characterized by drug craving, significant time spent in substance procurement, compulsive substance use, pharmacologic tolerance, and withdrawal symptoms on discontinuation. The DSM-IV diagnostic criteria for substance-induced sleep disorder are presented in Box 115–4. The diagnosis requires that the sleep disorder be sufficiently severe to warrant special attention and cause significant distress or impairment. Specific subtypes include

*Deceased.

Box 115–1.   Commonly Used Terms Related to Drugs of Abuse and Dependence

- *Intoxication:* A reversible substance-specific syndrome of maladaptive behavior or psychological changes associated with the recent exposure of a drug acting on the central nervous system. Significant changes may include belligerence, mood lability, cognitive impairment, and poor judgment (e.g., hallucinations associated with lysergic acid diethylamide [LSD] or drunkenness with alcohol).
- *Tolerance:* Following repeated exposure to a drug, a given dose of the drug produces a reduced effect or, conversely, higher doses are needed to induce the effects previously induced by the initial dose (e.g., increased doses of morphine may be needed to control severe pain over a period of time).
- *Cross-Tolerance and Cross-Dependence:* The ability of one drug to suppress manifestations of dependence produced by another drug and to maintain the physical dependence (e.g., between alcohol and barbiturates or benzodiazepines).
- *Withdrawal:* New physical and psychological manifestations following abrupt cessation of a dependence-producing drug (e.g., development of panic disorder during withdrawal from a benzodiazepine hypnotic in a patient without a history of panic disorder).
- *Relapse:* The recurrence of the original condition from which the patient suffered on discontinuing an effective medical treatment (e.g., reemergence of mania after cessation of a mood stabilizer).
- *Rebound:* The exaggerated expression of the original condition sometimes experienced by patients during immediate cessation of an effective treatment (e.g., emergence of insomnia that is worse than it was before treatment when discontinuing a short-acting benzodiazepine hypnotic).

Reprinted with permission from the American Psychiatric Association: Diagnostic and Statistical Manual of Mental Disorders, 4th ed. Washington, DC, American Psychiatric Press, 1994. Copyright 1994 American Psychiatric Association.

---

alcohol, amphetamines, caffeine, and opioids. The disorder can manifest as insomnia, hypersomnia, parasomnia, or mixed types of sleep disturbances. Of particular importance to sleep researchers and clinicians, sleep disorders are commonly associated with alcohol, stimulants (amphetamine, cocaine, methylphenidate), opioids, and sedative-hypnotics during both intoxication and withdrawal. In addition, caffeine can produce insomnia during intoxication, whereas nicotine is associated with insomnia typically during withdrawal.

SLEEP AND SPECIFIC SUBSTANCES

Alcohol and Alcoholism

Epidemiology and Risk Factors

In the United States, of those who drink alcohol, approximately 10% of men and 3% to 5% of women experience serious alcohol-related life problems. Twenty percent to 50% of men and 6% to 10% of women in general medical-psychiatric settings suffer from alcoholism. Nevertheless, only 20% to 50% of alcoholic patients are recognized and diagnosed in clinical practice. Most alcoholic people do not identify themselves as such. In addition to medical and psychiatric history and physical examination, the CAGE Questionnaire has been shown to increase the identification of alcohol abusers[2] (Box 115–5). A positive answer to two or more questions indicates that the patient is at risk. Laboratory tests also may help identify alcohol abusers. These tests measure blood and breath alcohol concentrations, liver enzymes (e.g., γ-glutamyltransferase, aspartate aminotransferase, alanine aminotransferase), high-density lipoprotein phospholipids, apolipoproteins, angiotensin I and angiotensin II, and mean corpuscular volume. Because genetic factors appear to predispose people to certain types of alcoholism, patients should be asked specifically about alcohol use and abuse in the family.

Pathogenesis

EFFECTS OF ALCOHOL ON SLEEP IN NONALCOHOLIC INDIVIDUALS

Alcohol may be mildly stimulating in some people,[3] but more commonly it has a transient sedative effect, especially in sleepy

---

Box 115–2.   DSM-IV Criteria for Substance Abuse

A. A maladaptive pattern of substance use, leading to clinically significant impairment or distress, as manifested by one (or more) of the following, occurring within a 12-month period:

1. Recurrent substance use resulting in a failure to fulfill major role obligations at work, school, or home (e.g., repeated absences or poor work performance related to substance use; substance-related absences, suspensions, or expulsions from school; neglect of children or household)
2. Recurrent substance use in situations in which it is physically hazardous (e.g., driving an automobile or operating a machine when impaired by the substance use)
3. Recurrent substance-related legal problems (e.g., arrests for substance-related disorderly conduct)
4. Continued substance use despite having persistent or recurrent social or interpersonal problems caused or exacerbated by the effects of the substance (e.g., arguments with spouse about consequences of intoxication, physical fights)

B. The symptoms have never met the criteria for Substance Dependence for this class of substance.

DSM-IV, Diagnostic and Statistical Manual of Mental Disorders, 4th edition.

Reprinted with permission from the American Psychiatric Association: Diagnostic and Statistical Manual of Mental Disorders, 4th ed. Washington, DC, American Psychiatric Press, 1994. Copyright 1994 American Psychiatric Association.

Box 115–3.   DSM-IV Criteria for Substance Dependence

A maladaptive pattern of substance use, leading to clinically significant impairment or distress, as manifested by three (or more) of the following, occurring at any time in the same 12-month period:

1. Tolerance, as defined by either of the following:
   a. A need for markedly increased amounts of the substance to achieve intoxication or desired effect
   b. Markedly diminished effect with continued use of the same amount of the substance
2. Withdrawal, as manifested by either of the following:
   a. The characteristic withdrawal syndrome for the substance
   b. The same (or a closely related) substance is taken to relieve or avoid withdrawal symptoms
3. The substance is often taken in larger amounts or over a longer period than was intended
4. There is a persistent desire or unsuccessful efforts to cut down or control substance use
5. A great deal of time is spent in activities necessary to obtain the substance (e.g., visiting multiple doctors or driving long distances), use the substance (e.g., chain-smoking), or recover from its effects
6. Important social, occupational, or recreational activities are given up or reduced because of substance use
7. The substance use is continued despite knowledge of having a persistent or recurrent physical or psychological problem that is likely to have been caused or exacerbated by the substance (e.g., current cocaine use despite recognition of cocaine-induced depression or continued drinking despite recognition that an ulcer was made worse by alcohol consumption)

Specify if:
- *With physiologic dependence:* Evidence of tolerance or withdrawal (i.e., either item 1 or 2 is present)
- *Without physiological dependence:* No evidence of tolerance or withdrawal (i.e., neither item 1 nor item 2 is present)

Course specifiers:
- Early Full Remission
- Early Partial Remission
- Sustained Full Remission
- Sustained Partial Remission
- On Agonist Therapy
- In a Controlled Environment

DSM-IV, Diagnostic and Statistical Manual of Mental Disorders, 4th edition.

Reprinted with permission from the American Psychiatric Association: Diagnostic and Statistical Manual of Mental Disorders, 4th ed. Washington, DC, American Psychiatric Press, 1994. Copyright 1994 American Psychiatric Association.

Box 115–4.   DSM-IV Diagnostic Criteria for Substance-Induced Sleep Disorder

A. A prominent disturbance in sleep that is sufficiently severe to warrant independent clinical attention.

B. There is evidence from the history, physical examination, or laboratory findings of either (1) or (2):
   1. The symptoms in criterion A developed during, or within a month of, substance intoxication or withdrawal
   2. Medication use is etiologically related to the sleep disturbance

C. The disturbance is not better accounted for by a sleep disorder that is not substance induced. Evidence that the symptoms are better accounted for by a sleep disorder that is not substance induced might include the following: the symptoms precede the onset of the substance abuse (or medication use), the symptoms persist for a substantial period of time (e.g., a month) after cessation of acute withdrawal or severe intoxication, or are substantially in excess of what would be expected given the type or amount of substance used or the duration of use; or there is other evidence that suggests the existence of an independent non–substance-induced sleep disorder (e.g., history of recurrent non–substance-related episodes).

D. The disturbance does not occur exclusively during the course of a delirium.

E. The sleep disturbance causes clinically significant distress or impairment in social, occupational, or other important areas of functioning.

Specify subtype: Alcohol, Amphetamine, Caffeine, Cocaine, Opioids, Sedative, Hypnotic, Anxiolytics, or Other
Specify type:
- *Insomnia type:* If the predominant sleep disturbance is Insomnia
- *Hypersomnia type:* If the predominant sleep disturbance is Hypersomnia
- *Parasomnia type:* If the predominant sleep disturbance is Parasomnia
- *Mixed type:* If more than one sleep disturbance is present and none predominates

Specify if:
- *With onset during intoxication*
- *With onset during withdrawal*

DSM-IV, Diagnostic and Statistical Manual of Mental Disorders, 4th edition.

Reprinted with permission from the American Psychiatric Association: Diagnostic and Statistical Manual of Mental Disorders, 4th ed. Washington, DC, American Psychiatric Press, 1994. Copyright 1994 American Psychiatric Association.

or anxious individuals. It is probably the most frequently used sleeping aid in the general population. In a survey of 18- to 45-year-olds in the general population, 13% reported using alcohol to help themselves sleep sometime during the previous year; of this 13%, 15%, or approximately 2% of the general population, had used it regularly for 1 month or more, and an additional 5% of the population used both alcohol and a hypnotic in order to sleep.[4]

When given to healthy control subjects shortly before bedtime, alcohol tends to shorten sleep latency, increase non–rapid eye movement (NREM) sleep, and reduce REM sleep in the first hours after ingestion,[5,6] which makes alcohol immediately rewarding as a hypnotic. Alcohol, however, is metabolized relatively rapidly, at the rate of approximately one glass of wine or one-half pint of beer per hour. Therefore, after four to five drinks in the hours before bedtime, alcohol concentrations in blood approach zero approximately halfway through the night.[7] As a consequence, withdrawal tends to occur in the last half of the night and produces shallow, disrupted sleep, increases REM sleep, increases dream or nightmare recall, and sympathetic arousal, including tachycardia and sweating. Sleep may also be interrupted by gastric irritation, headache, a full bladder, and a "rebound wakefulness." Thus, although alcohol decreases sleep latency and increases sleep at the beginning of the night, it decreases sleep at the end of the night, with a net result of overall diminished quality and quantity of sleep compared with not consuming alcohol. Alcohol also increases the risk of falls during the night. The effects of alcohol may be more pronounced in the elderly compared with younger individuals because a given dose produces higher blood and brain concentrations in older individuals. With nightly use of alcohol, some tolerance develops to the sedative and REM sleep–suppressing effects of alcohol.

Little is known about the effects of alcohol in infants, but some studies suggest that alcohol (or marijuana) in mother's milk helps infants go to sleep more easily but sleep less well overall than those infants who did not ingest alcohol.[8] Furthermore, Scher et al.[9] reported that infants whose mothers drank one drink per day during the first trimester of pregnancy showed more sleep disruptions than infants born to nondrinking women. The longer-term significance of these changes is unknown, however.

The adverse effects of alcohol may continue after blood alcohol concentrations are zero. Moderate drinking in the late afternoon—the so-called "happy hour"—may disrupt sleep during the last half of the night, long after alcohol has disappeared from the blood.[10] Likewise, when alcohol is administered in the morning, its sedative and detrimental effects continue on the Multiple Sleep Latency Test, a divided-attention task, and in simulated driving in the afternoon after the point when breath ethanol is undetectable.[11]

Interestingly, the sedative effects of alcohol in healthy subjects may reflect an "unmasking" of prior sleep loss.[12] Sleepiness potentiates the sedative effects of alcohol. For example, the risk of an automobile accident is probably greater after consumption of alcohol by a sleep-deprived individual than by a rested driver.

No systematic scientific data exist, to our knowledge, about the effects of alcohol taken at low doses at bedtime on sleep in nonalcoholic, chronic insomniac patients who regularly use alcohol to promote sleep at night. We do not know if tolerance has developed to the side effects or the soporific benefits of alcohol. In other words, it is not known whether a "nightcap" is helpful or harmful in individuals who imbibe every night. However, the information discussed previously would suggest that such a consumption pattern would not be beneficial.

ALCOHOL AND CLINICAL SLEEP DISORDERS

As mentioned earlier, the DSM-IV defines a substance-induced sleep disorder, alcohol subtype, which occurs in association with either intoxication or withdrawal, and which manifests itself as insomnia, hypersomnia, parasomnia, or mixed type (see Box 115–4). In contrast, the International Classification of Sleep Disorders (ICSD)[13] defines an alcohol-dependent sleep disorder in insomniac individuals without a diagnosis of alcoholism who have used alcohol as a bedtime sleep aid for over 30 days.

Alcohol-Related Sleep-Disordered Breathing and Periodic Limb Movements during Sleep

Alcohol increases the likelihood of snoring, inspiratory resistance, and apneic events in nonalcoholic individuals without a history of obstructive sleep apnea–hypopnea syndrome or snoring.[14] It apparently does this by potentiating upper airway atonia and inspiratory resistance,[15-17] although some studies report minimal effects of moderate alcohol on breathing or oxyhemoglobin saturation in patients with mild to severe apnea.[18] Nevertheless, sleep-disordered breathing (i.e., apneas, hypopneas, and desaturations) increases in an age-dependent manner in abstinent alcoholic patients,[19,20] particularly those older than 60 years of age. The risk of periodic limb movements during sleep (PLMS) was increased threefold with alcohol consumption in a general sleep disorders clinic sample,[21] but PLMS were not increased in another study of abstinent alcoholic patients.[19]

The effects of alcohol on both sleep-disordered breathing and PLMS may increase daytime sleepiness and fatigue. The risk of a fatigue-related automobile accident is increased fivefold in patients with obstructive sleep apnea who consume alcohol at the rate of two drinks or more per day compared with patients who drink little or not at all.[22] In addition, the combination of alcohol, obstructive sleep apnea, and snoring increases the risk of heart attacks, stroke, and sudden death.

Clinical Features: Sleep-Related Disturbances in Alcoholic Patients

Alcoholic patients commonly report insomnia, hypersomnia, circadian rhythm disturbances, and parasomnias.[23,24]

Nevertheless, the rate of insomnia in alcoholic people is not precisely known, although it was estimated at 36% to 67% in a recent review, compared with rates of 17% to 30% in the general population.[25] As alcohol dependence develops, patients often report difficulty sleeping without a drink.[26] Objective measures bear out the subjective complaints, with long sleep latencies, poor sleep efficiencies, and decrements in total sleep, slow wave sleep (SWS), and REM sleep.[27-29] The normal circadian patterns of sleep and wakefulness may become disrupted in alcoholic patients. In some patients, *polyphasic sleep–wake cycles* develop, for example during a binge, characterized by short periods of sleep induced by drinking, followed by short periods of wakefulness.

Finally, alcohol consumption at both the social and pathologic levels may lead to diurnal hypersomnolence. Hypersomnia may result from the direct hypnotic effects of alcohol after daytime consumption, especially in sleep-deprived individuals; the accumulative effects of alcohol and sleep deprivation may sometimes be followed by periods of hypersomnia or near coma; "terminal sleep," which can occur during withdrawal after delirium tremens, is a prolonged, deep sleep. Terminal sleep may be associated with a loss of delta and REM sleep, as well as with behavioral disturbances such as pavor nocturnus.[30] Finally, alcoholic individuals appear to be at greater risk for other primary sleep disorders such as apnea and PLMS.

Clinical Course and Prevention

SLEEP DURING RECOVERY AND ABSTINENCE IN ALCOHOLIC PATIENTS

Abnormal sleep patterns may persist for months to years during abstinence. At approximately the second or third week of abstinence, alcoholic patients show prolonged sleep latency; reduced total sleep time, especially NREM sleep and SWS; and increased *REM density* (a measure of ocular activity during REM sleep).[31,32] Patients with a history of secondary depression have shorter REM sleep latency and greater REM sleep percentage than patients without depression.[32] Even after 1 to 2 years of abstinence, sleep tends to be shortened, shallow, and fragmented. REM percentage is often elevated.[33-35] Figure 115–1 shows the slow recovery of total sleep time and lack of recovery in REM sleep in male veteran primary alcoholic patients over the course of 14 months of abstinence. Only a few abstinent, recovering alcoholic patients have been studied for 1 year or more, and they continued to show low levels of SWS and other subjective and objective sleep abnormalities.[33,35,36]

SLEEP MEASURES MAY PREDICT RELAPSE IN RECOVERING ALCOHOLIC PATIENTS

Does poor sleep contribute to relapse during subacute and long-term abstinence? Many patients rationalize drinking because they say it helps them sleep, at least at the beginning of the night during the first days of renewed drinking. In a recent study, alcoholic patients with insomnia admitted to an alcoholic treatment center were more likely to relapse at admission than patients without insomnia.[25] In an inpatient experimental ward, recovered alcoholic patients were given the opportunity to drink alcoholic beverages; those with subjective sleep complaints were more likely to drink than those without sleep problems.[37] Resumption of drinking appears to

ONE YEAR FOLLOW-UP IN SOBER ALCOHOLICS

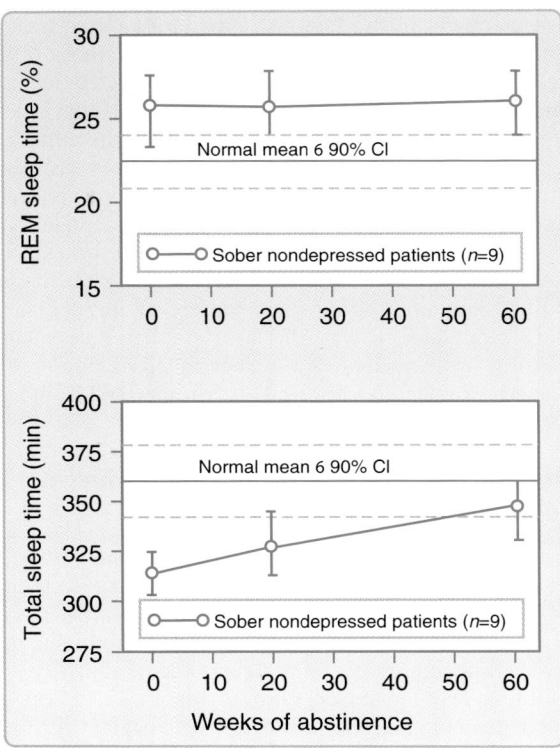

Figure 115–1. Polygraphic sleep recordings for rapid eye movement (REM) sleep percentage and total sleep time in nine male, sober, recovering, primary nondepressed, alcoholic patients for more than 1 year. Note that both measures differ from age-matched healthy control subjects for most of the recovery period. Values for the patients are mean ± standard error of the mean, and for healthy control subjects, mean ± 90% confidence interval (CI). (Data adapted from Drummond SPA, Gillin JC, Smith TL, Demodena A: The sleep of abstinent pure primary alcoholic patients: Natural course and relationship to relapse. Alcohol Clin Exp Res 1998;22:1796-1802.)

increase SWS and decrease wakefulness during the night, which may reinforce the impression that alcohol reduces complaints of sleep and daytime fatigue. Unfortunately, as drinking continues, both objective and subjective sleep patterns generally worsen.

Increasing evidence suggests that both objective and subjective measures of sleep during the acute and subacute abstinent recovery periods predict abstinence or relapse within 2 to 12 months. In the 1970s, Allen and Wagman and colleagues[38,39] suggested that low levels of SWS at baseline were associated with poor sobriety 2 months after discharge from an inpatient alcohol sleep research unit. More recently, studies have demonstrated that elevated REM sleep measures (short REM sleep latency, increased REM sleep percentage and REM density) at approximately 2 weeks of abstinence predicted relapse at 3 months after discharge in primary alcoholic patients with and without secondary depression.[40-43] Although age, duration and severity of alcoholism, marital status, employment, hepatic enzymes, cognitive performance, and depression ratings did not discriminate abstainers from relapsers, polygraphic sleep measures correctly classified approximately 75% to 80% of alcoholic patients; in the entire group of patients (both nondepressed and depressed alcoholic patients), elevated REM density during the first 1 to 2 weeks of abstinence was the best predictor of relapse at 3 months after discharge from the 1-month inpatient alcohol treatment program. In contrast, after approximately 5 months of abstinence, REM sleep measures no longer predicted relapse or abstinence at approximately 1 year; rather, long objective sleep latency and poor sleep efficiency (e.g., insomnia) were associated with relapse by the end of the first year.[35] In a longitudinal study of alcoholic patients who were initially evaluated at an average of 32 days of sobriety, patients who relapsed at an average of 5 months differed from those who remained sober on both subjective and objective sleep measures; after controlling for a variety of measures, polygraphic sleep latency was the best predictor of relapse.[34] Different sleep measures may reflect different phases of the protracted physical withdrawal syndrome associated with recovery from alcoholism.

Treatment: Alcoholism and Alcohol-Induced Sleep Disorders

Treatment of sleep disorders in alcoholic patients should be included as part of an overall treatment plan. Sleep disturbance is common during all phases of withdrawal, including sleep onset insomnia with significant loss of total sleep time and SWS, and increased REM sleep, fragmented sleep, and wakefulness. The potential chronic insomnia in long-term abstinent patients poses therapeutic challenges to the field of sleep disorders medicine. Many clinicians and alcoholic patients believe that successful alleviation of insomnia and other sleep complaints will improve long-term outcomes in the subacute and chronic abstinent phases. Unfortunately, the treatment of alcohol-related sleep problems has not been well studied. One question that often arises is whether sedative-hypnotics should be administered to abstinent alcoholic patients with insomnia. Except for management of acute symptoms of withdrawal, benzodiazepines or other sleeping pills usually are not recommended in managing abstinent alcoholic patients.[3] They are cross-tolerant with alcohol and can be abused or misused themselves. In a survey of addiction specialists, trazodone, sedating antidepressants, and antihistamines were used, but apparently reluctantly, by a minority of the respondents in abstinent, insomniac alcoholic patients.[43] These treatments have not been studied well enough to evaluate their benefits and risks, and they may be misused if the patient resumes drinking. Cognitive-behavioral approaches such as sleep hygiene instructions and stimulus-control should be included in any treatment plan, regardless of the use of pharmacotherapy.

Anxiolytics and Sedative-Hypnotics

Epidemiology and Risk Factors

Sedative hypnotics have been popular since antiquity, especially for the induction of sleep. Older drugs include alcohol, bromide, chloral hydrate, paraldehyde, and barbiturates. Approximately a century ago, chloral hydrate was a widely abused, addictive substance. For reasons poorly understood, it passed out of fashion as a drug of abuse even before the introduction of the newer sedative-hypnotics. Barbiturates were abused for many decades, but less so now because their use has declined dramatically since the introduction of the benzodiazepines.

At present, the major anxiolytics and sedative-hypnotic drugs include the benzodiazepines and atypical hypnotics (e.g., zolpidem and zaleplon). Other drugs that are infrequently used in clinical practice for the management of insomnia or anxiety include barbiturates, methyprylon, meprobamate, and others. All of these drugs probably increase the effects of gamma-aminobutyric acid (GABA), an inhibitory neurotransmitter in the brain. The sedative-hypnotics differ from one another to some degree in the exact mechanisms of action, but this common enhancement of GABA neurotransmission is probably responsible for the tendency for cross-tolerance between these drugs and alcohol.

Both clinical experience and laboratory studies in animals indicate that abuse and dependence can occur with the sedative-hypnotics. In general use, benzodiazepines are not usually strongly reinforcing or pleasurable for most individuals. Current alcohol use should always be evaluated carefully before prescribing a sedative-hypnotic to anyone, even if there is no known suggestion of substance abuse. Alcohol use increases the risk of cross-tolerance and withdrawal symptoms in benzodiazepine users, probably because both potentiate brain GABA neurotransmission. A strong family history of substance abuse should also be considered a risk factor because genetic factors play a role in the etiology of these disorders.

Many patients with mood disorders, anxiety and panic disorder, or severe insomnia may take benzodiazepines daily for long periods. Nevertheless, the risk of serious physical or behavioral dependency appears to be low. Epidemiologic surveys estimate that approximately 2.6% of the adult population in the United States has used a hypnotic agent within the past year. Approximately three fourths of hypnotic users take them for fewer than 2 weeks. Of the hypnotic users, approximately 10% to 11% (0.3% of the total sample) have taken the hypnotic more or less nightly for a year. Only approximately 35% of insomniac patients have actually taken sleeping pills; the reality is that many individuals with insomnia and other disorders are not using medications or other therapies that might be of benefit to them. The use of sleeping pills in the United States appears to be approximately average compared with other industrialized nations around the world.

Clinical Course

Concerns have been raised for decades about the benefits and risks of long-term treatment with benzodiazepines at more-or-less conventional doses. Nevertheless, there are few empirical data about the benefits and risks associated with long-term treatment of insomnia. If patients were randomly assigned in a double-blind fashion to hypnotic therapy or placebo for long periods (9 to 12 months), which group would fare better over time? We do not have the answer to that simple question at this time. We do know, however, from relatively short-term sleep laboratory studies (2 to 4 weeks), that the placebo group usually improves over time compared with the pretreatment baseline and that some pharmacologic tolerance develops to benzodiazepines. The benefits of the active drug compared with the placebo (the *effect size*) are usually statistically significant but small. Insomnia, even chronic insomnia, probably has a fluctuating course and is influenced by nonpharmacologic factors, such as the attention of the experimenters, the expectation of help, and the sleep hygiene schedules associated with sleep laboratory studies. A major study would be required to do justice to the question of long-term benefits and hazards of chronic hypnotic use.

Diagnosis

In evaluating the risks and benefits of sedative-hypnotic therapy in a patient, it is helpful to distinguish *drug-seeking behavior* from *therapy-seeking behavior*. The former involves drug use in a nontherapeutic context, at the expense of other activities, in excessive nontherapeutic amounts, with discriminable subjective effects, and on a chronic basis leading to tolerance and physical dependence. In contrast, with therapy-seeking behavior, the drug is taken for its therapeutic efficacy and is self-administered at a therapeutic dose for an appropriate period under medical supervision. Nevertheless, clinicians and patients should be cautious about long-term use of sedative-hypnotics.

In evaluating the clinical changes associated with discontinuation of drug therapy, it is useful to distinguish three groups of symptoms: (1) reemergence of the original symptoms for which the medication was ordered; (2) transient exacerbation of typical original symptoms, such as rebound insomnia for 1 to 2 nights after abrupt withdrawal from a short-acting benzodiazepine, such as triazolam; and (3) emergence of new symptoms. The ICSD defines a hypnotic-dependent sleep disorder, which is associated with withdrawal symptoms worse than the original complaint in individuals who used a hypnotic at night for at least 3 weeks.

Treatment of Withdrawal from Sedative-Hypnotics

If withdrawal from long-term use of sedative-hypnotics is desired, it should be done slowly and carefully. Patients should be cautioned about the potential withdrawal and rebound effects, especially insomnia and anxiety. Reemergence of the symptoms originally medicated may be a major risk factor for resumption of use. In fact, reemergence of some symptoms (e.g., panic attacks) may actually warrant resumption of sedative-hypnotic use, although insomnia does not usually fall into that category.

Caffeine

Epidemiology and Risk Factors

Caffeine and other methylxanthines are stimulants found not only in coffee but in tea, cola, chocolate, cocoa, and OTC analgesics, cold remedies, and stimulants.[44] A normal cup of brewed coffee contains approximately 100 to 150 mg of caffeine, and a cup of instant coffee approximately 85 to 100 mg of caffeine; tea contains approximately 60 to 75 mg per cup; cola contains approximately 40 to 75 mg per 12-oz drink; cocoa holds approximately 50 mg per cup; OTC cold preparations have approximately 15 to 60 mg per tablet; and OTC stimulants contain approximately 100 to 200 mg of caffeine.

Clinical Features

Whether caffeine is genuinely addictive has been debated for some time. Although in a sense a morning cup of coffee is apparently modestly "habit-forming," tolerance seems to develop to some of the subjective effects, and withdrawal

symptoms may develop after sudden cessation, caffeine is considered to be only a mildly reinforcing substance, with the possibility of physical dependence considered relatively low compared with other drugs of abuse.

Individuals differ in their response to caffeine, with some people becoming overstimulated with as little as 250 mg.[45,46] Others are less affected, especially chronic users who appear to develop some tolerance to the stimulating effect of caffeine. Caffeine intoxication is characterized by restlessness, nervousness, excitement, insomnia, flushed face, gastrointestinal disturbances, and other symptoms. Ingesting 500 mg of caffeine has the same altering effects as approximately 5 mg of amphetamine. For most people, doses of caffeine above 1 g may produce insomnia, dyspnea, delirium, and arrhythmias, and doses above 5 g can be fatal. Although the half-life of caffeine is approximately 3 to 7 hours, the effects may last as long as 8 to 14 hours. Therefore, caffeine may have significant effects on sleep at night even if it is consumed in the late afternoon or early evening. Six cups or more of coffee throughout the day are likely to cause insomnia at night, even if not taken shortly before bedtime. Under the circumstances, a vicious cycle can easily develop: although a few cups of coffee may reduce daytime sleepiness, this amount is sufficient to disrupt sleep at night and, therefore, exacerbate or perpetuate the daytime sleepiness. The effects of caffeine are prolonged in children and pregnant women, as well as the elderly and patients with hypothyroidism, who may become toxic at relatively low doses. In addition, caffeine may trigger panic attacks in some patients with panic disorder.

Caffeine has been used to produce experimental models of insomnia.[46] Many people, however, develop tolerance, and apparently sleep well, by subjective report. Caffeine has an important role in combating daytime fatigue and sleepiness in otherwise healthy people.[47-51] From the perspective of sleep–wake regulation, caffeine appears to promote wakefulness by blocking adenosine receptors in the brain. Adenosine may be an endogenous sleep-promoting substance.[52]

The combination of alcohol and caffeine can synergistically produce insomnia several hours later.[53] The two drugs are frequently consumed together, such as at dinner. The two substances initially have opposing effects when taken together: Alcohol is sedative and counteracts the stimulating effects of caffeine. The half-life of alcohol, however, is shorter than that of caffeine. Four to 6 hours after consumption, blood levels of alcohol have fallen to near zero. Therefore, the subject experiences the arousing withdrawal effects of alcohol at the same time that the blood levels of caffeine remain relatively high. Similar synergistic effects in coffee drinkers at bedtime may also occur in individuals who take a short-acting sleeping pill at bedtime and, perhaps, in cigarette smokers who go into withdrawal from nicotine at the end of the night.

Many patients and their physicians fail to recognize that caffeine may contribute to complaints of anxiety, insomnia, or other disorders. For patients with such symptoms who consume three or more cups of coffee per day (approximately 400 to 500 mg caffeine), gradual tapering off all caffeine may be helpful. Abrupt withdrawal, however, should be avoided because irritability, dysphoria, fatigue, sleepiness, headache, and flulike symptoms may ensue approximately 18 to 24 hours after the last dose.[54] These withdrawal symptoms suggest that heavy users of caffeine may develop dependence and may self-administer it to avoid the uncomfortable symptoms.

Sleep-related difficulties associated with caffeine can be classified under the DSM-IV criteria for a substance-induced sleep disorder, caffeine subtype. In addition, DSM-IV defines research criteria for caffeine withdrawal, which include marked fatigue or drowsiness after abrupt cessation of high amounts of caffeine daily.

Nicotine

Epidemiology and Risk Factors

Nicotine is addicting. Consistent with this characterization, most smokers report that they would like to quit, that they have tried unsuccessfully to quit, that they recognized that smoking is hazardous to their health, and that they often smoke to avoid the withdrawal symptoms that appear 1 to 2 hours after the last smoke, which matches the plasma half-life of nicotine. Approximately 20% of the adult population in the United States currently smokes cigarettes, 4% use pipes or cigars, and 3% use smokeless tobacco.[1] It is estimated that 20% to 50% of smokers meet diagnostic criteria for nicotine dependence. Nicotine dependence is approximately two to three times higher in patients with other psychiatric disorders than in the general population. Approximately half of people who smoke experience nicotine withdrawal. A rough but simple measure of nicotine dependence is to ask how long the smoker can go in the morning before the first cigarette: 30 minutes or less suggests that the smoker is strongly dependent on nicotine.

Clinical Features of Nicotine-Related Sleep Problems

The direct effects of nicotine on sleep in nonsmoking humans are not well characterized.[55,56] Some evidence suggests that it has sedating effects at low doses and alerting effects at high doses. In addition, nicotine appears to reduce total sleep time and REM sleep time in healthy control subjects.[55,56] Both polysomnography and questionnaire studies report increased sleep latency as well as increased arousals and difficulty staying asleep at night in active smokers versus nonsmokers.[55] Interestingly, nicotine may have novel effects in nonsmoking depressed patients compared with healthy control subjects, in that it increased rather than decreased REM sleep.[57,58] This same group later reported that the increase in REM sleep was correlated with next-day mood improvement.[59] Finally, some studies suggest that smoking is a risk factor for sleep-disordered breathing.[60]

Recently, a new withdrawal symptom has been described in active smokers and labeled *nocturnal sleep-disturbing nicotine craving*.[61] The prevalence of this symptom is approximately 20% and it is characterized by patients waking up one or more times in the middle of the night, unable to fall back to sleep without first smoking a cigarette. During acute withdrawal from nicotine (first several days of withdrawal), sleep tends to worsen in smokers, with increased arousals at night followed by sleepiness on the multiple sleep latency test the next day.[62] Oddly, despite the sleep-disturbing qualities of nicotine withdrawal both within a single night and across several nights, the nicotine patch, which is used as replacement therapy on smoking cessation, has been reported to have mixed results with regard to sleep complaints.[63,64] The patch also does not provide clinically significant improvements in

sleep-disordered breathing, although it may ameliorate other symptoms such as poor mood.

Stimulants

Epidemiology and Risk Factors

Prescription stimulants such as amphetamine, methylphenidate, fenfluramine, and pemoline may have important therapeutic effects, especially in narcolepsy and ADHD, and occasionally in patients with obesity or depression, negative-symptom schizophrenia, or other apathetic states. When taken in moderation for short periods, these stimulants counteract excessive daytime sleepiness and sleep loss and improve mood, performance, and endurance. Evidence suggests that stimulants may even improve nocturnal sleep disruption associated with ADHD.[65] Unfortunately, these prescription drugs can be abused, and there are increasing reports of methylphenidate misuse by adolescents and college students.[66,67] Other commonly abused stimulants include cocaine, methamphetamine, and ecstasy. Cocaine, amphetamine, methylphenidate, and many of the other stimulants apparently enhance neurotransmission of norepinephrine, dopamine, and serotonin, primarily by reuptake blockade or increased release of the neurotransmitter.

Modafinil is a promising new stimulant for the treatment of narcolepsy and sleepiness.[68] It appears to have a unique mode of action compared with other stimulants that may involve interaction with the histamine system, but the exact mechanism remains unclear.[69,70] Its utility for increasing alertness has also been investigated in shiftwork and sleep deprivation situations, in opiate-induced sedation, in sleepiness or fatigue in neurologic conditions, and in residual daytime somnolence associated with treated obstructive sleep apnea. At this time, it appears to be safer, less likely to be abused, and to have fewer side effects than other stimulants. Use of modafinil by graduate and professional students to facilitate increased productivity is a new and concerning trend, however.

Clinical Features: Sleep in Stimulant Use and Withdrawal

Relatively few studies have investigated sleep patterns during stimulant use or after withdrawal from stimulant dependence, and only a subset of these have used polysomnographic data to assess sleep. Amphetamine, methylphenidate, pemoline, and cocaine prolong sleep latency and REM sleep latency and reduce total sleep time and REM sleep time, presumably by stimulating dopaminergic arousal systems or, in the case of fenfluramine, releasing serotonin.[71-73] Tolerance may develop with long-term administration, not only in addicted patients but in patients with legitimate medical reasons for taking amphetamines or methylphenidate, such as narcolepsy or ADHD.[74] During bouts or runs of stimulant abuse, individuals may go for days without sleep, followed by periods of hypersomnia. With chronic use of stimulants at low to moderate doses, tolerance may develop to the sleep, anorectic, autonomic, and euphoric effects of stimulants, although activation of mood and behavior may persist. Stimulant abusers also use sedatives or alcohol to promote sleep and reduce anxiety.

The main subjective complaint during withdrawal is difficulty falling asleep, with one study reporting subjectively long sleep latencies for an entire 28-day study period.[75] The objective sleep data contain some inconsistencies, owing perhaps to the specific drugs abused by the subjects (e.g., diet pills versus methamphetamine), the quantity and frequency of use, and the age of the subjects studied. For example, although some studies reported greatly increased amounts of total sleep time compared with control or normative data during the first few days of withdrawal,[76] others reported no differences. The sleep abnormalities related to stimulant withdrawal include lowered sleep efficiency, increased nocturnal waking time, increased amounts of stage 1 sleep and REM sleep, and shortened REM sleep latency.[76] Sleep does not improve much during the first 2 weeks of abstinence, with the possible exception of a decrease in nocturnal waking time, stage 1 sleep, and REM density.[76] These measures were still abnormal compared with normative data in both studies, however.

Pathogenesis: Stimulants and Sleep Disorders

In the ICSD, a stimulant-dependent sleep disorder is "characterized by reduction of sleepiness or suppression of sleep by central stimulants, and resultant alterations in wakefulness following drug abstinence." This schema includes not only illicit stimulants but caffeine, theophylline, and thyroid hormones. In the Veterans Administration San Diego Healthcare System's Sleep Disorders Clinic, several stimulant-dependent patients have been diagnosed with sleep apnea who reported using stimulants as a self-medication for daytime hypersomnolence. Clinicians should screen patients who use excessive stimulants (e.g., caffeine) for sleep disorders, such as apnea, PLMS, or narcolepsy.

Before prescribing stimulants, sleep disorder specialists must objectively document the diagnosis and reasons for treatment. This concern reinforces the importance of establishing a diagnosis of narcolepsy by objective means. Objective diagnosis not only protects the physician against charges of malpractice, misdiagnosis, and "script writing," but also ultimately helps the narcoleptic patient obtain legitimate prescriptions in localities where family physicians and pharmacies are reluctant to supply stimulants. Likewise, patients who are prescribed stimulants need careful monitoring and education to ensure proper use; the first reported case of an amphetamine-induced psychosis occurred in a narcoleptic patient.

Opioids

Epidemiology and Risk Factors

When morphine was isolated from opium in 1803, it was named *morphine* after the Greek god responsible for dreams, Morpheus. Ironically, modern research has shown that short-term administration of morphine, heroin, and other opiates to healthy volunteers or abstinent addicts reduces REM sleep rather than increasing it, and also reduces total sleep time, sleep efficiency, and SWS.[77]

Today, the term *opioid* generally refers to natural, semisynthetic, and synthetic substances with opiate-like activity, including meperidine, methadone, and hydromorphone (Dilaudid); they are agonists at any of several endogenous opiate-like receptors, which are present in the brain, the gut, and elsewhere in the body. More than a dozen endogenous opioid peptides have been identified, falling into three different families: endorphins, enkephalins, and dynorphins. In addition, many different types of receptors have been characterized, including mu, kappa, epsilon, delta, and sigma receptors. Because of the complexity of these systems, it has been difficult to identify the normal physiologic roles of the endogenous opioid peptides and receptors. The effects of opioid drugs depend on the complex net agonist and antagonist action at a variety of receptor sites, as well as on the dose. The most commonly abused opioids include morphine, heroin, hydromorphone, and oxycodone (found in Percodan and Percocet). Heroin is metabolized in the body to morphine. The half-life of most narcotics is typically fairly short: 4 to 7 hours for codeine, morphine, hydromorphone, and propoxyphene; 3 to 5 hours for oxycodone and pentazocine; and 2 to 4 hours for meperidine. Nevertheless, the frequency with which these drugs are used by established substance abusers varies considerably: approximately every 2 to 3 hours with meperidine, hydromorphone, and codeine; approximately every 4 to 6 hours with heroin and morphine, and approximately every 8 to 12 hours with methadone. Methadone is occasionally but rarely abused. It generally lacks the euphoric effects of heroin, morphine, or commonly abused narcotics, and because of its relatively long half-life, it has been used to treat chronic opioid addicts.

Clinical Features

Opioids induce analgesia, sedation, apathy, poor concentration, mood changes, nausea, and vomiting. Rapid intravenous administration of an opioid causes a warm skin flushing and a "rush" that lasts approximately 45 seconds, associated with pleasure, relaxation, and satisfaction. Opioids also initially reduce secretion of gonadotropin-releasing hormone and corticotropin-releasing hormone. Constipation and pupillary constriction (miosis) are common. At high doses or overdose, respiratory depression is a danger, leading to death in some cases. Opioids are also absorbed subcutaneously and intramuscularly from the gut, nasal mucosa (as in snorting), and the lung (as in smoking opium). With repeated administration, tolerance to the pleasurable and neuroendocrine effects develops and dose escalation begins.

As mentioned earlier, the opioids tend to reduce total sleep time and REM sleep when first administered to a nontolerant, pain-free subject. For patients with pain, however, narcotics may increase sleep because of the reduction of pain. Opioids have also been used to treat restless legs syndrome with and without PLMS.[78] With chronic administration, tolerance develops to most of these effects. For example, the REM sleep–suppressing effects to morphine are lost within a week,[79] although the arousing effects may persist. Early studies indicated that methadone induces insomnia, and more recently it has been shown that chronic administration of methadone leads to increased central apneic events in addition to disrupted sleep architecture and increased arousals.[80] The mechanism by which morphine inhibits REM sleep may involve inhibition of acetylcholine in the pontine reticular formation[81] and direct agonist effects at specific mu receptors.

The signs and symptoms of opiate withdrawal vary with early, middle, and late phases of abstinence. During the early phase, yawning, lacrimation, rhinorrhea, and sweating are common. The middle phase is characterized by restless sleep, dilated pupils, anorexia, irritability, and gooseflesh. Finally, the late phase may be associated with increased severity of earlier symptoms, tachycardia, nausea, vomiting, diarrhea, abdominal cramps, depression, weakness, and pain. Death rarely, if ever, occurs with opioid withdrawal. Sleep is usually maximally disrupted or suppressed during early abstinence, and although this improves slightly over the next few weeks, sleep length usually remains below normal values indefinitely.

Insomnia is one of the most troublesome symptoms of withdrawal, particularly because it weakens the patient's resolve to remain drug free. Patients often cite sleep disturbance as the primary rationale for relapse. Flurazepam is reported to be well liked and tolerated by patients during withdrawal, but many of these patients have abused benzodiazepines in the past and therefore it should be used cautiously, if at all. Diphenhydramine and sedating antidepressants, such as amitriptyline, doxepin, and trazodone, have also been used.

Cannabis

A modest number of investigations have examined the effects of cannabis on objective measures of sleep. However, several methodologic problems limit their generalizability and make it difficult to compare them with one another. For example, most studies have examined experienced users. Only 17 subjects across four separate studies were cannabis-naive individuals (and 3 of those were psychiatric patients).[80-82] Other confounds include (1) baseline or placebo nights potentially including withdrawal effects,[83-88] (2) confounding the effects of chronic administration with those of escalating dosages,[86-88] and (3) use of either uncontrolled drug dosages or dosages much greater than those proposed for medicinal purposes (e.g., 70 to 120 mg tetrahydrocannabinol [THC]).[83,85-88] All of these issues result in a literature that is neither wholly consistent nor easy to interpret.

Despite these limitations, some general conclusions can be made regarding the effects of cannabis on sleep. First, acute administration (arbitrarily defined here as 7 days) of cannabis consistently decreases measures of REM sleep (e.g., REM as a percentage of total sleep time, minutes of REM sleep, or REM density), regardless of the dose administered. Second, acute administration often increases SWS. Third, with long-term administration (more than 7 days) some tolerance probably develops to the SWS effects, but not to the REM sleep effects. Finally, acute withdrawal seems to create a rebound in these measures (i.e., a decrease in SWS and an increase in REM sleep).

Only two of these reports have examined subjective sleep quality or quantity. The study with a lower cannabis dose found improvements in reported estimates of sleep latency and of sleep quality,[89] whereas the study with higher dosages reported the opposite[90]; the latter study used doses of cannabis high enough to produce significant anxiety, nausea, and other adverse consequences. Indirect evidence suggesting that cannabis may have subjectively beneficial effects on sleep comes from the fact that cannabis withdrawal is associated with sleep difficulties,[88-90] and patients in treatment for cannabis abuse reported reduced sleep quality during the first month of abstinence and cited self-treatment of sleep difficulties as a major reason for relapse.

Neuropharmacologic studies provide indirect evidence suggesting that THC may have persisting effects on sleep beyond the period of acute intoxication. Cannabinoid CB1 receptors are located in several brain regions known to play a role in the generation or maintenance of sleep, such as brainstem, pons, and the hypothalamus,[91,92] although brainstem

abundance of CB1 receptors has also been reported as minimal. CB1 receptors in the pons show both increased expression during the subjective sleep period and increased expression during recovery sleep after sleep deprivation.[93] It has been known for a number of years that the cannabinergic system plays a role in sleep, although the exact nature of this role is not fully understood. THC, cannabidiol, and anandamide (an endogenous cannabinoid that binds to the CB1 receptor) have all been shown to have soporific properties.[94-96] THC and cannabidiol also potentiate the hypnotic properties of ethanol, hexobarbital, and pentabaritone.[97,98] Moreover, the cannabinoids may interact with other systems to influence sleep. For example, it has been proposed that oleamide, a fatty acid amide with hypnotic properties, may act through the CB1 receptor to enhance the effects of 5-hydroxytryptamine (serotonin) and GABA,[99-101] both of which are involved in the initiation of NREM sleep.

Overall, additional well-controlled human studies need to be conducted in both healthy control subjects and patient populations to understand fully the impact of cannabis on sleep. This issue may become increasingly important if cannabis gains acceptance for its possible medicinal qualities. The Institute of Medicine and the National Institutes of Health have stimulated research into the medicinal properties of cannabis, with recent reports targeting specific diseases for study, including pain secondary to human immunodeficiency virus infection, chemotherapy, glaucoma, and multiple sclerosis.

Club Drugs

The term *club drugs* describes a set of recreational drugs increasingly used by adolescents and young adults in the United States and many other parts of the world. These "club drugs" are increasingly used at "raves" (crowded, all-night parties) or to facilitate sexual assault. Little is known about the effects of these drugs on sleep, but some information is provided here for the clinician because their use is likely to continue in the future.

MDMA

MDMA (3,4-methylenedioxymethamphetamine; "ecstasy"), a schedule I stimulant with hallucinogenic properties, is reputed to produce profound positive feelings (including elation, emotional closeness, sensory pleasure, and relaxation) and to increase sexual desire, satisfaction, and orgasmic intensity (despite its impairment of erectile function).[102] Its prolonged suppression of the desires to sleep, eat, and drink (permitting raves 2 to 3 days long) produces complications of electrolyte imbalances and exhaustion as well as the typical serious effects of amphetamine intoxication. The effects of overdose may include hypertension, uncontrolled hyperthermia, coma, seizures, and death. Physical dependence has been documented.[102] Considerable evidence (in humans as well as animals) demonstrates the serotonergic and dopaminergic toxicities and long-term sequelae of MDMA. Persistent use impairs total sleep time and NREM sleep time, particularly stage 2 sleep, with sleep disturbance reported well into abstinence.[103,104]

In addition to the psychotic features—especially paranoia—commonly seen with amphetamine misuse in general, chronic MDMA abuse has been linked to depressive syndromes, anxiety (including panic disorder), anorexia, anhedonia, and diminished sexual pleasure as well as difficulties with memory, concentration, impulse control, and executive function, with the severity of psychiatric sequelae in general increasing with increasing amounts of MDMA abuse.[104]

Ketamine

Ketamine ("special K," "K"), a general anesthetic used in veterinary medicine, has become less widely used in human therapeutics because of intense dysphoria and even psychotic phenomena occurring fairly frequently. A noncompetitive N-methyl-D-aspartate receptor antagonist,[105] ketamine produces symptoms of dissociation, psychosis, and memory disturbance in healthy volunteers, with psychotic and memory symptoms persisting up to 3 days in repeated users of ketamine.[106] Users describe the "trip" as qualitatively similar to, but better than, that with PCP (phencyclidine) or LSD (lysergic acid diethylamide) because its obvious hallucinogenic effects last only approximately an hour. Less obvious impairment of the senses, coordination, and judgment for up to 24 hours contributes to the morbidity of this drug. Ketamine dependence resembles cocaine dependence with its high tolerance and craving, although a physiologic withdrawal syndrome has not been reported.[107]

Gamma-Hydroxybutyrate

Gamma-hydroxybutyrate (GHB; "Georgia home boy," "grievous bodily harm"), marketed as Xyrem (sodium oxybate) for the treatment of cataplexy, has been frequently abused by body builders and connoisseurs of club drugs. Personal risks of misuse as well as widespread use of its intense amnestic properties to facilitate sexual assault have led to a tightly controlled system for its distribution for therapeutic purposes. The manufacturer and the U.S. Food and Drug Administration (FDA) have developed a carefully monitored patient and physician registry whereby GHB can be obtained only through a single pharmacy. (Unfortunately, it can be purchased through the Internet, where it is marketed as everything from bubble bath to furniture polish.) GHB is a schedule III drug for therapeutic purposes, but any illicit use is prosecuted under schedule I penalties.

Popular because of its production of euphoria, relaxation, and increased sexual pleasure,[108] GHB markedly increases brain dopamine and, to a lesser extent, dynorphin. Intoxication is similar to that of sedative-hypnotic agents, with coma, respiratory depression, seizures, and even death in overdose. Although withdrawal symptoms have not been reported in the context of therapeutic use, a withdrawal syndrome similar to that of benzodiazepines or alcohol is possible secondary to abuse.[109] More severe cases of GHB withdrawal may present with hallucinations, paranoia, delirium, and elevated heart rate and blood pressure. Barbiturates may be required for treatment because benzodiazepines are ineffective in the treatment of even lesser degrees of GHB withdrawal.[109,110-112]

Rohypnol

Rohypnol ("roofies"; flunitrazepam) is a benzodiazepine widely available in other countries for insomnia and use as a preoperative medication. Never approved by the FDA, flunitrazepam has sedative effects 7 to 10 times more intense than diazepam, with an onset of 15 to 20 minutes and a duration of 4 to 6 hours, and with some residual effects reported over 12 hours after administration. It is known mainly as a "date rape" drug in the United States.

PITFALLS AND CONTROVERSIES

One significant clinical controversy in the area of sleep and substance abuse is the use of sedative-hypnotics in abstinent alcoholic patients to treat sleeping difficulties, particularly insomnia. Many clinicians discourage the use of such medications in this population, other than to treat life-threatening withdrawal symptoms, because of the significant potential for cross-tolerance and abuse of these medications. This is particularly true for benzodiazapine-acting medications. Physicians often prefer to administer GABA-acting medications (e.g., gabapentin) or sedative antidepressants (e.g., trazodone) for insomnia in abstinent alcoholic, or other substance-dependent, patients. However, very little research has been done directly to examine the incident of abuse/dependence on benzodiazapine-acting medications in abstinent substance abusers, or to examine the efficacy of the other medications or cognitive-behavioral treatments for insomnia in this population. Furthermore, the findings that insomnia may confer an increased risk of relapse in abstinent alcoholic patients suggests that treating their insomnia should help them maintain abstinence, but this idea also requires further research.

Clinical Pearls

In assessing patients with sleep complaints, clinicians should always inquire about substance use, including types of substances and frequency, quantity, and timing of use. It is important to ask about specific substances, legal and illegal, rather than ask in general terms. Be sure to include alcohol, caffeine, nicotine, sleeping aids, stimulants, cannabis, and, in young adults, club drugs.

Many individuals believe that alcohol is beneficial for sleep because it decreases sleep latency and increases the depth of sleep (i.e., slow wave sleep) at the beginning of the night. However, alcohol can exacerbate sleep apnea, and it creates shallow, fragmented sleep in the latter half of the night, producing an overall night of lower total sleep time, poor sleep efficiency, and more wake and stage 1 sleep than would be the case without the use of alcohol.

Acknowledgments

The authors gratefully acknowledge the assistance of Sheila Neely and Carina Lopez. This research was supported by grants from the National Institutes of Mental Health NIMH 30914-24R, NIH R01 RR00827, MH18399, and MH01642. Support also was provided by the Veterans Affairs San Diego Healthcare System.

References

1. American Psychiatric Association: Diagnostic and Statistical Manual of Mental Disorders, 4th ed. Washington, DC, American Psychiatric Press, 1994.
2. Perdrix A, Decrey H, Pécoud A, et al: Detection of alcoholism in general practice: Applicability of the CAGE test by the general practitioner. Schweiz Med Wochenschr 1995;125:1772-1778.
3. Papineau KL, Roehrs TA, Petrucelli N, et al: Electrophysiological assessment (the multiple sleep latency test) of the biphasic effects of ethanol in humans. Alcohol Clin Exp Res 1998; 22:231-235.

4. Johnson EA, Roehrs T, Roth T, Breslau N: Epidemiology of alcohol and medication as aids to sleep in early adulthood. Sleep 1998;21:178-186.

5. Yules RB, Lippman ME, Freedman DX: Alcohol administration prior to sleep: The effect of EEG sleep stages. Arch Gen Psychiatry 1967;16:94-97.

6. Lobo LL, Tufik S: Effects of alcohol on sleep parameters of sleep-deprived healthy volunteers. Sleep 1997;20:52-59.

7. Madsen BW, Rossi L: Sleep and Michael-Menten elimination of ethanol. Clin Pharmacol Ther 1980;27:114-119.

8. Mennella JA, Gerrish CJ: Effects of exposure to alcohol in mother's milk on infant sleep. Pediatrics 1998;101:E2.

9. Scher MS, Richardson GA, Coble PA, et al: The effects of prenatal alcohol and marijuana exposure: Disturbances in neonatal sleep cycling and arousal. Pediatr Res 1988;24:101-105.

10. Landolt HP, Roth C, Dijk DJ, Borbely AA: Late-afternoon ethanol intake affects nocturnal sleep and the sleep EEG in middle-aged men. J Clin Psychopharmacol 1996;16:428-436.

11. Roehrs T, Beare D, Zorick F, Roth T: Sleepiness and ethanol effects on simulated driving. Alcohol Clin Exp Res 1994;18:154-158.

12. Zwyghuizen-Doorenbos A, Roehrs T, Timms V, Roth T: Individual differences in the sedating effects of alcohol. Alcohol Clin Exp Res 1990;14:400-404.

13. Diagnostic Classification Steering Committee: The International Classification of Sleep Disorders: Diagnostic and Coding Manual. Rochester, Minn, American Sleep Disorders Association, 1990.

14. Dawson A, Lehr P, Bigby BG, Mitler MM: Effect of bedtime ethanol on total inspiratory resistance and respiratory drive in normal non-snoring men. Alcohol Clin Exp Res 1993;17:256-262.

15. Krol RC, Knuth SL, Bartlett D Jr: Selective reduction of genioglossal muscle activity by alcohol in normal human subjects. Am Rev Respir Dis 1984;129:247-250.

16. Stradling JR, Crosby JH: Predictors and prevalence of obstructive sleep apnoea and snoring in 1001 middle aged men. Thorax 1991;46:85-90.

17. Dawson A, Bigby BG, Poceta JS, Mitler MM: Effect of bedtime alcohol on inspiratory resistance and respiratory drive in snoring and non-snoring men. Alcohol Clin Exp Res 1997;21:183-190.

18. Teschler H, Berthon-Jones M, Wessendorf T, et al: Influence of moderate alcohol consumption on obstructive sleep apnoea with and without AutoSet nasal CPAP therapy. Eur Respir J 1996;9:2371-2377.

19. Le Bon O, Verbanck P, Hoffmann G, et al: Sleep in detoxified alcoholics: Impairment of most standard sleep parameters and increased risk for sleep apnea, but not for myclonias—a controlled study. J Stud Alcohol 1997;58:30-36.

20. Aldrich MS, Shipley JE, Tandon R, et al: Sleep-disordered breathing in alcoholics: Association with age. Alcohol Clin Exp Res 1993;17:1179-1183.

21. Aldrich MS, Shipley JE: Alcohol use and periodic limb movements of sleep. Alcohol Clin Exp Res 1993;17:192-196.

22. Aldrich MS: Alcohol use, obstructive sleep apnea, and sleep-related motor vehicle accidents. Sleep Res 1997;26:308.

23. Gross MM, Hastey JM: Sleep disturbances in alcoholism. In Tarter RE, Sugarman A (eds): Alcoholism: Interdisciplinary Approaches to an Enduring Problem. Reading, Mass, Addison-Wesley, 1976, pp 257-309.

24. Zarcone V: Alcoholism and sleep. In Passonant P, Oswald I (eds): Pharmacology of the State of Alertness. Oxford, Pergamon Press, 1979, pp 9-38.

25. Brower KJ, Aldrich MS, Robinson EA, et al: Insomnia, self-medication, and relapse to alcoholism. Am J Psychiatry 2001;158:399-404.

26. Mello NK, Mendelson JH: Behavioral studies of sleep patterns in alcoholics during intoxication and withdrawal. J Pharmacol Exp Ther 1970;175:94-112.

27. Allen RP, Wagman A, Faillace LA, MacIntosh M: Electroencephalographic (EEG) sleep recovery following prolonged alcohol intoxication in alcoholics. J Nerv Ment Dis 1971;153:424-433.

28. Adamson J, Burdick JA: Sleep of dry alcoholics. Arch Gen Psychiatry 1973;28:146-149.

29. Benca RM, Obermeyer WH, Thisted RA, Gillin JC: Sleep and psychiatric disorders: A meta-analysis. Arch Gen Psychiatry 1992;49:651-668.

30. Kotorii T, Nakazawa Y, Yokoyama T: Terminal sleep following delirium tremens in chronic alcoholics: Polysomnographic and behavioral study. Drug Alcohol Depend 1982;10:125-134.

31. Gillin JC, Smith TL, Irwin M, et al: EEG sleep studies in "pure" primary alcoholism during subacute withdrawal: Relationships to normal controls, age, and other clinical variables. Biol Psychiatry 1990;27:447-488.

32. Gillin JC, Smith TL, Irwin M, et al: Short REM latency in primary alcoholics with secondary depression. Am J Psychiatry 1990;147:106-109.

33. Williams HL, Rundell OH: Altered sleep physiology in chronic alcoholics: Reversal with abstinence. Alcohol Clin Exp Res 1981;2:318-325.

34. Brower KJ, Aldrich MS, Hall JM: Polysomnographic and subjective sleep predictors of alcoholic relapse. Alcohol Clin Exp Res 1998;22:1864-1871.

35. Drummond SPA, Gillin JC, Smith TL, Demodena A: The sleep of abstinent pure primary alcoholic patients: Natural course and relationship to relapse. Alcohol Clin Exp Res 1998;22:1796-1802.

36. Skoloda TE, Alterman AI, Gottheil E: Sleep quality reported by drinking and non-drinking alcoholics. In: Gottheil EL (ed): Addiction Research and Treatment: Converging Trends. New York, Pergamon Press, 1979, pp 102-112.

37. Allen RP, Wagman AM: Do sleep patterns relate to the desire for alcohol? Adv Exp Med Biol 1975;59:495-508.

38. Allen RP, Wagman AM, Funderburk FR, Wells DT: Slow wave sleep: A predictor of individuals differences in response to drinking? Biol Psychiatry 1980;15:345-348.

39. Wagman AM, Allen RP, Funderburk F, Uprights D: EEG measures of functional tolerance to alcohol. Biol Psychiatry 1978;13:719-778.

40. Clark CP, Gillin JC, Golshan S, et al: Increased REM sleep density at admission predicts relapse by three months in primary alcoholics with a lifetime diagnosis of secondary depression. Biol Psychiatry 1998;43:601-607.

41. Gillin JC, Smith TL, Irwin M, et al: Increased pressure for rapid eye movement sleep at time of hospital admission predicts relapse in nondepressed patients with primary alcoholism at 3-month follow-up. Arch Gen Psychiatry 1994;51:189-197.

42. Clark CP, Gillin JC, Golshan S, et al: Polysomnography and depressive symptoms in primary alcoholics with and without a lifetime diagnosis of secondary depression and in patients with primary major depression. J Affect Disord 1999;52:177-185.

43. Bean-Bayog M: Alcoholics Anonymous. In Ciraulo DA, Shader RI (eds): Clinical Manual of Chemical Dependence. Washington, DC, American Psychiatric Press, 1991, pp 359-375.

44. James JE: Acute and chronic effects of caffeine on performance, mood, headache, and sleep. Neuropsychobiology 1998;38:32-41.

45. Bonnet MH, Arand DL: Caffeine use as a model of acute and chronic insomnia. Sleep 1992;15:526-536.

46. Johnson LC, Freeman CR, Spinweber CL, Gomez SA: Subjective and objective measures of sleepiness: Effect of benzodiazepine and caffeine on their relationship. Psychophysiology 1991;28:65-71.

47. Kelly TL, Mitler MM, Bonnet MH: Sleep latency measures of caffeine effects during sleep deprivation. Electroencephalogr Clin Neurophysiol 1997;102:397-400.

48. Rosenthal L, Roehrs T, Zwyghuizen-Doorenbos A, et al: Alerting effects of caffeine after normal and restricted sleep. Neuropsychopharmacology 1991;4:103-108.

49. Penetar D, McCann U, Thorne D, et al: Caffeine reversal of sleep deprivation effects on alertness and mood. Psychopharmacology (Berl) 1993;112:359-365.

50. Zwyghuizen-Doorenbos A, Roehrs T, Lipschutz L, et al: Effects of caffeine on alertness. Psychopharmacology (Berl) 1990; 100:36-39.

51. Portas CM, Thakkar M, Rainnie DG, et al: Role of adenosine in behavioral state modulation: A microdialysis study in the freely moving cat. Neuroscience 1997;79:225-235.

52. Stradling JR: Recreational drugs and sleep. BMJ 1993;306: 573-575.

53. Hughes JR, Higgins ST, Bickel WK, et al: Caffeine self administration, withdrawal, and adverse effects among coffee drinkers. Arch Gen Psychiatry 1991;48:611-617.

54. Ockene JKKJL: Tobacco. In Galanter M (ed): Textbook of Substance Abuse Treatment. Washington, DC, American Psychiatric Press, 1994, pp 157-177.

55. Salin-Pascual RJ, De La Fuente JR, Galicia-Polo L, Drucker-Colin R: Effects of transdermal nicotine on mood and sleep in nonsmoking major depressed patients. Psychopharmacology (Berl) 1995; 121:476-479.

56. Wetter DW, Young TB, Bidwell TR, et al: Smoking as a risk factor for sleep-disordered breathing. Arch Intern Med 1994;154: 2219-2224.

57. Salin-Pascual RJ, Drucker-Colin R: A novel effect of nicotine on mood and sleep in major depression. Neuroreport 1998;9:57-60.

58. Salin-Pascual RJ, Galicia-Polo L: REM sleep latency in major depressed patients predicts mood improvement after transdermal nicotine administration. Sleep Hypnosis 1999;1:32-34.

59. Prosise GL, Bonnet MH, Berry RB, Dickel MJ: Effects of abstinence from smoking on sleep and daytime sleepiness. Chest 1994;105:1136-1141.

60. Rieder A, Kunze U, Groman E, et al: Nocturnal sleep-disturbing nicotine craving: A newly described symptom of extreme nicotine dependence. Acta Med Austriaca 2001;28:21-22.

61. Wolter TD, Hauri PJ, Schroeder WJ, et al: Effects of 24-hour nicotine replacement on sleep and daytime activity during smoking cessation. Prev Med 1996;25:601-610.

62. Hughes JR, Higgins ST, Bickel WK: Nicotine withdrawal versus other drug withdrawal syndromes: Similarities and dissimilarities. Addiction 1994;89:1461-1470.

63. Hughes JR, Hatsukami D: Signs and symptoms of tobacco withdrawal. Arch Gen Psychiatry 1986;43:289-294.

64. Mitler MM: Evaluation of treatment with stimulants in narcolepsy. N Engl J Med 1995;17:103-106.

65. Teter CJ, McCabe SE, Boyd CJ, Guthrie SK: Illicit methylphenidate use in an undergraduate student sample: Prevalence and risk factors. Am Fam Physician 2003;23:609-617.

66. Klein-Schwartz W, McGrath J: Poison centers experience with methylphenidate abuse in pre-teens and adolescents. J Am Acad Child Adolesc Psychiatry 2003;42:288-294.

67. Goff DC, Ciraulo DA: Cocaine. In Ciraulo DA, Shader RI (eds): Clinical Manual of Chemical Dependence. Washington, DC, American Psychiatric Press, 1991, pp 233-259.

68. Touret M, Sallanon-Moulin M, Jouvet M: Awakening properties of modafinil without paradoxical sleep rebound: Comparative study with amphetamine in the rat. Neurosci Lett 1995;189: 43-46.

69. Engber TM, Dennis SA, Jones BE, et al: Brain regional substrates for the actions of the novel wake-promoting agent modafinil in the rat: comparison with amphetamine. Neuroscience 1998;87: 905-911.

70. Post RM, Gillin JC, Wyatt RJ, Goodwin FK: The effect of orally administered cocaine on sleep of depressed patients. Psychopharmacologia 1974;37:59-66.

71. Lewis SA: Comparative effects of some amphetamine derivatives on human sleep. In Costa E, Garattini S (eds): Amphetamines and Related Compounds. New York, Raven Press, 1970, pp 873-888.

72. Feinberg I, Hibi S, Cavness C, et al: Sleep amphetamine effects in MBDS and normal subjects. Arch Gen Psychiatry 1974; 31:723-731.

73. Weddington WW, Brown BS, Haertzen CA, et al: Changes in mood, craving, and sleep during short term abstinence reported by male cocaine addicts. Arch Gen Psychiatry 1990;47:861-868.

74. Watson R, Bakos L, Compton P, Gawin F: Cocaine use and withdrawal: The effect on sleep and mood. Am J Drug Alcohol Abuse 1992;18:21-28.

75. Watson R, Hartmann E, Schildkraut JJ: Amphetamine withdrawal: Affective state sleep patterns, and MHPG excretion. Am J Psychiatry 1972;129:39-45.

76. Thompson PM, Gillin JC, Golshan S, Irwin M: Polygraphic sleep measures differentiate alcoholics and stimulant abusers during short-term abstinence. Biol Psychiatry 1995;38:831-836.

77. Staedt J, Wassmuth F, Stoppe G, et al: Effects of chronic treatment with methadone and naltrexone on sleep in addicts. Eur Arch Psychiatry Clin Neurosci 1996;246:305-309.

78. Montplaisir J, Lapierre O, Warnes H, Pelletier G: The treatment of the restless leg syndrome with or without periodic leg movements in sleep. Sleep 1992;15:391-395.

79. Kay D: Human sleep and EEG through a cycle of methadone dependence. Electroencephalogr Clin Neurophysiol 1975; 38:35-43.

80. Teichtahl H, Prodromidis A, Miller B, et al: Sleep-disordered breathing in stable methadone programme patients: A pilot study. Addiction 2001;96:395-403.

81. Lydic R, Keifer JC, Baghdoyan HA, Becker L: Microdialysis of the pontine reticular formation reveals inhibition of acetylcholine release by morphine. Anesthesiology 1993;79:1003-1012.

82. Tassinari CA, Ambrosetto G, Peraita-Adrado MR, Gastaut H: The neuropsychiatric syndrome of delta-sup-9-tetrahydrocannabinol and cannabis intoxication in naive subjects: A clinical and polygraphic study during wakefulness and sleep. In Nahas GG, Sutin KM, Harvey DJ, Agurell S (eds): Marihuana Medicine. Totowa, Humana Press, Inc., 1999, pp 649-664.

83. Gillin JC, Kotin J, Post R, et al: Sleep during one week of administration of delta-9-tetrahydrocannabinol to psychiatric patients. Sleep Res 1972;1:44.

84. Karacan I, Fernandez-Salas A, Coggins WJ, et al: Sleep electroencephalographic-electrooculographic characteristics of chronic marijuana users: Part I. Ann N Y Acad Sci 1976;282: 348-374.

85. Barratt ES, Beaver W, White R: The effects of marijuana on human sleep patterns. Biol Psychiatry 1974;8:47-54.

86. Pranikoff K, Karacan I, Larson EA, et al: Effects of marijuana smoking on the sleep EEG: Preliminary studies. J Fla Med Assoc 1973;60:28-31.

87. Feinberg I, Jones R, Walker J, et al: Effects of marijuana extract and tetrahydrocannabinol on electroencephalographic sleep patterns. Clin Pharm Ther 1976;19:782-794.

88. Feinberg I, Jones R, Walker JM, et al: Effects of high dosage delta-9-tetrahydrocannabinol on sleep patterns in man. Clin Pharm Ther 1975;17:458-466.

89. Freemon FR: The effects of chronically administered delta-9-tetrahydrocannabinol upon polygraphically monitored sleep of normal volunteers. Drug Alcohol Depend 1982;10:345-353.

90. Haney M, Ward AS, Comer SD, et al: Abstinence symptoms following oral THC administration to humans. Pharmacology 1999;141:385-394.

91. Chait D: Subjective and behavioral effects of marijuana the morning after smoking. Psychopharmacology (Berl) 1990;100:328-333.

92. Budney AJ, Hughes JR, Moore BA, Novy PL: Marijuana abstinence effects in marijuana smokers maintained in their home environment. Arch Gen Psychiatry 2001;58:917-924.

93. Breivogel CS, Childers SR: The functional neuroanatomy of brain cannabinoid receptors. Neurobiol Dis 1998;5:417-431.

94. Martinez-Vargas M, Murillo-Rodriquez E, Gonzalez-Rivera R, et al: Cannabinoid receptor 1 increases with sleep rebound. Soc Neurosci Abstr 2001;27:1385.

95. Murillo-Rodriquez E, Cabeza R, Mendez-Diaz M, et al: Anandamide-induced sleep is blocked by SR141716A, a CB1 receptor antagonist and by U73122, a phospholipase C inhibitor. Neuroreport 2001;12:2131-2136.

96. Monti JM: Hypnoticlike effects of cannabidiol in the rat. Psychopharmacology (Berl) 1977;55:263-265.

97. Takahashi RN, Karniol IG: Pharmacological interaction between cannabinol and D9-tetrahydrocannabinol. Psychopharmacologia 1975;41:277-284.

98. McCoy DJ, Brown DJ, Forney RB: The effect of cannabinoid mixtures on induced sleep intervals and the disappearance of ethanol and hexobarbital. Res Commun Psychol Psychiatr Behav 1978;3:89-99.

99. Paton WD, Pertwee RG: Effects of cannabis and certain of its constituents on pentobarbitone sleeping time and phenazone metabolism. Br J Pharmacol 1972;44:250-261.

100. Mendelson WB, Basile AS: The hypnotic actions of the fatty acid amide, oleamide. Neuropsychopharmacology 2001;25:S36-S39.

101. Cheer JF, Cadogan AK, Marsden CA, et al: Modification of 5-HT2 receptor mediated behaviour in the rat by oleamide and the role of cannabinoid receptors. Neuropharmacology 1999;38:533-541.

102. Zemishlany Z, Aizenberg D, Weizman A: Subjective effects of MDMA ("ecstasy") on human sexual function. Eur Psychiatry 2001;16:127-130.

103. Jansen KL: Ecstasy (MDMA) dependence. Drug Alcohol Depend 1999;53:121-124.

104. Parrott AC: Human psychopharmacology of ecstasy (MDMA): A review of 15 years of empirical research. Hum Psychopharmacol 2001;16:557-577.

105. Allen RP, McCann UD, Ricaurte GA: Persistent effects of (±)3,4-methylenedioxymethamphetamine (MDMA, "ecstasy") on human sleep. Sleep 1993;16:560-564.

106. Parrott AC, Buchanan T, Scholey AB, et al: Ecstasy/MDMA attributed problems reported by novice, moderate and heavy recreational users. Hum Psychopharmacol 2002;17:309-312.

107. Curran HV, Monaghan L: In and out of the K-hole: A comparison of the acute and residual effects of ketamine in frequent and infrequent ketamine users. Addiction 2001;96:749-760.

108. Jansen KL, Darracot-Cankovic R: The nonmedical use of ketamine, part two: A review of problem use and dependence. J Psychoactive Drugs 2001;33:151-158.

109. Mamelak M: Gammahydroxybutyrate: An endogenous regulator of energy metabolism. Neurosci Biobehav Rev 1989;13:187-198.

110. Mason PE, Kerns WP: Gamma hydroxybutyric acid (GHB) intoxication. Acad Emerg Med 2002;9:730-739.

111. Mullins ME, Fitzmaurice SC: Lack of efficacy of benzodiazepines in treating gamma-hydroxybutyrate withdrawal. J Emerg Med 2001;20:418-420.

112. Sivilotti ML, Burns MJ, Aaron CK, Greenberg MJ: Pentobarbital for severe gamma-butyrolactone withdrawal. Ann Emerg Med 2001;38:660-665.

Monitoring and Staging Human Sleep

Mary A. Carskadon

Allan Rechtschaffen

ABSTRACT

Assessment of human sleep stages using electrophysiologic techniques—polysomnography (PSG)—is typically carried out in a sleep laboratory, although home-based PSG can also be performed. The scoring of sleep states and stages requires the acquisition of three core measures: the electroencephalogram (EEG), the electrooculogram (EOG), and the surface electromyogram (EMG). These basic PSG measures allow sleep staging according to conventions established in the 1960s to define two states of sleep—NREM and REM sleep—and four stages within NREM sleep. Stage 1 sleep is light sleep, occurring at sleep onset and transitions during the night; high levels indicate poor sleep. Stage 2 sleep is defined by sleep spindles and K-complexes in the EEG. Stages 3 and 4 sleep, collectively known as slow wave sleep, are characterized by high-voltage slow (two or fewer cycles per second) waves in the EEG, 20% to 50% for stage 3 and 50% or greater for stage 4. REM sleep is distinguished by a relatively low voltage mixed-frequency (desynchronized) EEG, bursts of rapid eye movements in the EOG, and suppression of EMG activity. The three core measures are usually supplemented by other measures, such as heart rate, breathing, limb movements, and so forth in the clinical setting. Sleep staging contributes to the definition of certain sleep disorders, can establish the severity of sleep disorders, and is useful for assessing the efficacy of therapeutic interventions.

The goal of this chapter is to summarize the procedures for monitoring and evaluating sleep in the laboratory setting. This material will not substitute for the standard manual; rather, it will be complementary. After recommended techniques and procedures are summarized, a few problematic areas are discussed briefly.

Although it is possible to monitor continuously and concurrently the activity of dozens of systems during sleep, just three systems need to be measured to assess sleep according to standard criteria.[1] This standard system of sleep recording and staging criteria is firmly rooted in the U.S. sleep research tradition, and although certain of its criteria have been challenged in recent years, it is the only system established by a consensus of experts. (A working group of the American Academy of Sleep Medicine is currently [2004] addressing the issue of preparing a new sleep staging manual.)

Among the earliest descriptions of electroencephalographic (EEG) activity during sleep were those from the laboratory of Loomis and colleagues.[2] These authors described five stages of sleep but failed to distinguish rapid eye movement (REM) sleep. Not until the landmark work of Kleitman's group at the University of Chicago was REM sleep described,[3] a description made possible by the addition of electrooculography (EOG) to the recording paradigm. The first comprehensive description of the nocturnal pattern of non–rapid eye movement (NREM) and REM sleep in humans[4] remains a foundation of modern human sleep research and represents one of the most outstanding scientific achievements of the 20th century. The standard sleep staging system[1] modified the EEG and EOG categorizations of Dement and Kleitman[4] primarily by adding electromyography (EMG). The addition of EMG to the criteria was based on the research of Berger[5] in humans and Jouvet and Michel[6] in cats, which linked muscle atonia with REM sleep. The EMG provided a more stable marker for REM sleep than the intermittent bursts of rapid eye movements.

PROCEDURES FOR MONITORING SLEEP

The EEG is the core measurement of polysomnography. The four stages of NREM sleep are distinguished from each other principally along this dimension.

Electroencephalogram

Application

The reliable recording of EEG begins with accurate measurement of the skull according to the international 10-20 system of electrode placement.[7] A skilled technologist can make the requisite measurements in 10 to 20 minutes. The "eyeball" or rule-of-thumb placement of EEG electrodes is not recommended because of the marked variability of electrode locations such practices engender, regardless of the technologist's skills.

Figure 116–1 illustrates the 10-20 placement system, by which a grid is marked on the skull and points of intersection denote electrode placement locations. The name of the system derives from measurements made at intervals of 10% or 20%

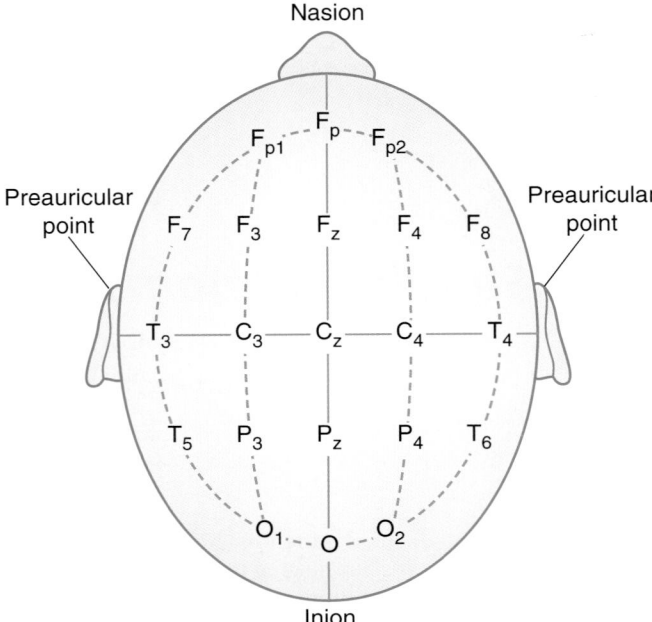

Figure 116–1. Schematic diagram showing measurements for the 10-20 electrode placement system. Measurements are made at 10% and 20% of the distances from inion to nasion, from left to right preauricular points, and around the circumference of the head. Intersecting points denote electrode placements. The most common placements for recording the electroencephalogram during sleep are C3 (left central), C4 (right central), O1 (left occipital), and O2 (right occipital). (Redrawn from Harner PF, Sannit T: A Review of the International Ten-Twenty System of Electrode Placement. Quincy, Mass, Grass Instrument Company, 1974.)

of the total distance between four landmarks: the nasion, the inion (external occipital protuberance), and the left and right preauricular points. Thus, the measurements are specific to each individual.

After measurements are made, the hair is separated and the scalp is cleaned in preparation for electrode application. In the past, technologists have used coarse-grained compounds to abrade the scalp, enabling better signal conduction. This practice has recently been discouraged in response to the increased risk of infection from blood-borne viruses.[8] Thorough cleansing and removal of dead skin layers by brisk rubbing with gauze are generally sufficient to ensure adequate conduction when the electrode is applied over a good conducting medium. One common method for overnight sleep studies is to attach EEG electrodes to the scalp using small patches of gauze soaked in collodion and dried with compressed air. The conducting medium may be added through a small hole in the electrode cup; if it is placed in the cup before application, an airtight seal prevents evaporation for at least 24 to 36 hours.

Derivations

The standard manual[1] recommends referential recording of one EEG lead, either C3 or C4, referenced to an indifferent, auricularly placed electrode on the contralateral mastoid or ear lobe: hence C3/A2 or C4/A1. The recommended sleep staging criteria, therefore, are intended to be used with this single, central EEG lead. The recommendations of the original committee acknowledged that use of a single EEG channel

was largely an economic issue for most laboratories, which at that time were limited to eight-channel recording systems on which two subjects were generally recorded simultaneously. Nevertheless, this economically dictated approach has proved to be a remarkably robust system.

Sleep stage scoring does not require measurement of focal EEG activity or regional comparisons, as might be performed in an EEG laboratory. Rather, all of the EEG waveforms used to distinguish sleep stages are well visualized at C3 or C4, particularly when signal amplitudes are optimized, with the relatively large interelectrode distance afforded by a contralateral reference. Thus, vertex sharp waves and K-complexes, which are maximal over the vertex, are clearly evident at C3 and C4; high-voltage slow waves characteristic of deep NREM sleep are seen maximally in frontal regions yet show clearly on central derivations; alpha rhythm, by contrast, is maximal over the occipital region but can be characterized centrally in most humans.[9,10]

Therefore, only C3/A2 or C4/A1 is used in the standard assessment of sleep stages.[1] Many laboratories, however, routinely record an occipital EEG (usually O1/A2 or O2/A1) as an adjunct to the central EEG, particularly for assessing sleep onset or arousals during sleep. Certain laboratories also routinely record from frontal placements. When the latter procedure is used for sleep staging, however, there is a tendency to observe a somewhat greater quantity of the deep NREM sleep stages (stages 3 and 4); therefore, such use should be documented in any published reports. Finally, clinical laboratories often record a more extensive EEG montage not used for sleep staging per se but for assessing potential regional or focal sleep-related EEG anomalies.

Electrooculogram

Eye movement activity is recorded during sleep for two primary reasons. The more obvious is to record the cardinal sign of REM sleep—the phasic bursts of rapid eye movements—which provide an essential sleep stage scoring criterion. In addition, the onset of sleep in most humans is heralded or accompanied by slow, rolling eye movements, which also occur with transitions to stage 1 during the night. Although these slow eye movements (SEMs) are not essential to sleep staging, they often provide very useful information.

The EOG recordings are based on the small electropotential difference from the front to the back of the eye. The cornea is positive with respect to the retina. Thus, the eyeball exists in the head as a potential field within a volume conductor. Because of this essentially constant potential difference, movement of the eyes can be measured from electrodes placed beside the eyes. An electrode nearest the cornea will register a positive potential; an electrode nearest the retina will register a negative potential. As the eye moves, the positions of the cornea and retina change relative to the fixed position of the electrode, and a potential change will register as a pen deflection at the polysomnograph.

Application

Standard EOG placements include the right outer canthus (ROC) and the left outer canthus (LOC). According to the standard manual,[1] the EOG electrodes should be offset from horizontal, one slightly above and one slightly below the horizontal plane. In this manner, the electrodes can detect horizontal and vertical eye movements. The EOG electrodes are usually applied with tape to a skin surface that has been thoroughly cleansed. An airtight seal over the electrode protects the conductivity of the electrode jelly for approximately 24 hours. The collodion electrode application technique is discouraged for EOG leads because of the risk of splashing collodion into the eyes.

Derivations

The standard manual[1] recommends continuous referential recording of two EOG leads: one outer canthus placement referred to the auricular reference on the opposite side and the other to the same auricular reference (e.g., ROC/A1 and LOC/A1). Certain laboratories[11] routinely use a contralateral reference for each outer canthus placement (ROC/A1 and LOC/A2). In the latter case, the contralateral references maximize the signal amplitude for both EOGs and equalize the amplitudes of pen deflections for conjugate eye movements. Either technique provides the capability to distinguish eye movements from electrode artifact. For example, in a montage recording ROC/A1 on one channel and LOC/A2 on another, conjugate eye movements will register as out-of-phase pen deflections, EEG activity reflected in the EOG channels (e.g., K-complexes) will be seen as in-phase deflections, and electrode artifacts will register in phase or in only one channel.

When a major goal of an experiment is to determine more precisely the direction of eye movements, the EOG may be simultaneously recorded from horizontal and vertical placements. Thus, in addition to placements on the outer canthi, electrodes would be placed supraorbitally and infraorbitally. For exact determination of eye position, direct current recordings are used.

Electromyogram

In a standard polysomnographic recording, the EMG from muscles beneath the chin is used as a criterion for staging REM sleep.[1] The EMG recordings from other muscle groups are sometimes used to assess certain sleep disorders. For example, the anterior tibialis EMG is useful to evaluate patients who have periodic leg movements during sleep. The intercostal EMG has been used to monitor respiratory effort in certain laboratories. Most EMG recordings during sleep require taping electrodes to the skin over the muscle group of interest.

Application

Three electrodes are placed beneath the chin, overlying the mentalis/submentalis muscles. These placements are typically used for the sake of convenience. The chin is very accessible, and the electrode wires can be drawn together with the others to form a bundle or "pony tail" at the back of the head. As in preparation for the EEG and EOG leads, the skin is thoroughly cleansed of oils and dead skin cells before applying the electrodes, which are generally secured with tape. Particularly in the case of a patient with a beard, the EMG electrodes may be affixed using a collodion-soaked gauze pad in the manner of the EEG leads.

Derivations

The chin EMG is recorded bipolarly. Any combination of the three placements can be used; the pair selected should produce the record of highest quality. The primary reason for using three electrodes (even though only two are recorded at any given time) is to ensure that there is always a backup electrode

in case of failure of one placement. Availability of a backup is important, especially if electrodes remain in place during the daytime when subjects are eating and talking. To monitor bruxism, EMG electrodes may be offset to a location over the masseter muscle.

General Considerations for Recording Sleep

A minimal four-channel montage for recording sleep is shown in Table 116–1. If channels are limited, it is possible to use a single EOG channel, although this practice is discouraged. If more channels can be devoted to the sleep portion of the recording, an occipital EEG will be the most helpful addition. In the rare cases when limited to four sleep channels, perhaps due to an extended clinical montage, some laboratories begin a night's recording with a central and an occipital EEG, a single EOG, and an EMG. After sleep onset, the occipital EEG is replaced with the second EOG.[11] Depending on the purpose of the recording, other selected parameters will be added to the montage to record respiration, heart rate, blood pressure, esophageal pH, penile circumference, or any of the many other available systems.

Most sleep laboratories use digital recording systems, often configured to appear as if recorded at a chart paper speed of 10 or 15 mm/sec. Thus, one screen displays about 30 seconds of data. More compressed views are discouraged because clear visualization of alpha rhythm and sleep spindles becomes extremely difficult. Less compressed displays may be useful for some clinical recording purposes; however, sleep staging that applies standard criteria is best accomplished with 30-second screen images. The display typically provides a sensitivity that gives a deflection of 7.5 or 10.0 mm for a 50-μV signal for the EEG and EOG channels. The chin EMG amplification is often adjusted to provide an acceptable EMG recording for distinguishing NREM and REM sleep (see later). A known calibration of the central EEG leads is *essential* because of the amplitude criterion for scoring NREM stage 3 and 4 sleep. A calibration of 50 μV/cm is common.

Electroencephalographic filtering should allow suitable visualization of a fairly wide range of signals, from slow waves (2 cycles per second [cps] or less) to sleep spindles (12 to 14 cps). A high-frequency filter setting in the range of 30 to 35 cps is common for visualizing a signal that passes through the essential waveforms while minimizing high-frequency (e.g., EMG) interference. A time constant of 0.3 second or slower (corresponding to a half-amplitude low-frequency filter setting of about 0.3 cps) ensures adequate visualization of slow wave activity.

Table 116–1. Montage for Monitoring Sleep States

Parameter	Derivation	Back-up or Option
EEG	C3/A2	C4/A1
EOG	ROC/A1 & LOC/A1	ROC/A1 & LOC/A2
EMG	Mentalis/submentalis	
If additional channels are available, add the following:		
EEG	O1/A2	O2/A1
EOG	Infraorbital/supraorbital	

The same settings are recommended for EOG channels to provide visualization of both the rapid eye movements essential to scoring REM sleep and the SEMs characteristic of sleep onset and transitional stage 1 sleep. A faster time constant has been used in certain laboratories to reduce the contamination of EOG by EEG signals. In slow wave (stages 3 and 4) sleep, however, the EEG activity seen in the EOG channels (with a slow time constant) tends to have fewer overriding fast components than the central leads and may therefore be helpful in distinguishing the slow EEG components. Thus, the slower time constant for EOGs may be doubly helpful.

The EMG is generally recorded with a much higher setting on both high- and low-pass filters. A low-pass setting of 70 or 75 cps is common (with notch filtering of alternating current interference—e.g., 60 Hz). High-pass filtering at 10 cps (time constant = 0.015 second) is useful to prevent slow signals from interfering with the EMG tracing. The standard manual recommends a time constant for EMG of 0.1 second or faster.[1] The absolute amplitude of EMG activity is not relevant to polysomnography; the emphasis, rather, is on relative changes in EMG amplitude. Thus, the EMG level is adjusted at the start of the record to provide an amplitude that permits such comparisons. An amplification of 20 μV/cm at the start of the recording will usually approximate a reasonable EMG level.

A number of special cases may require modification of the sensitivity, filter, and time constant settings just described. In most digital recording systems, such modifications can be achieved on line and during playback. In certain patients (especially older individuals), the amplitude of the EEG using the standard setting may be so small that the record is extremely difficult to evaluate and is more easily appreciated when a zoom function is used to provide, for example, a deflection of 15 mm for a 50-μV signal. By contrast, the amplitude of the EEG in some young children is very large and may require reduction of the amplification (or zoom out) to appreciate the recording—for example, a deflection of 5 mm for a 50-μV signal.

The EEG and EOG channels may also pick up a very low-frequency artifact related to sweat. In this instance, the low-frequency cutoff may be set at 1.0 cps (time constant = 0.1 second) during recording. Injudicious use of filtering holds some risk, however, of distorting the signals of interest. For example, a 5-cps low-frequency cutoff setting for an EEG will eliminate slow frequency signals important for assessing stages 3 and 4 NREM sleep.

A sleep recording requires vigilance during acquisition, and a key concern is that the technologist stay awake and alert. The recording must be observed frequently to ensure that proper electrode connections are maintained and that recording artifacts are minimized, as well as to monitor the safety and comfort of the patient and observe clinically relevant behaviors. This requirement for technologist vigilance makes the process of laboratory sleep recording a labor-intensive procedure; however, it also eliminates the necessity of retesting because of lost data.

PROCEDURES FOR STAGING SLEEP

General Considerations

The standard sleep staging manual[1] provides detailed guidelines and criteria for staging normal human sleep. The following material does not supersede the manual but is intended to be supplementary.

Several general concepts, referring primarily to the EEG, are helpful when approaching sleep stage scoring. It should first be noted that the sleep research community has adopted the EEG convention of "negative up," which simply means that a signal of negative polarity is shown as an upward pen deflection. Second, a number of the standard guidelines refer to the frequency of the EEG waves. Frequency is measured as cycles (each cycle is the complete series of potential changes before the series repeats) per second. A few common EEG frequency bands are as follows:

1. Alpha rhythm: 8 to 13 cps
2. Beta rhythm: more than 13 cps
3. Delta rhythm: less than 4 cps
4. Theta rhythm: 4 to 7 cps

The amplitude measures used in sleep staging are taken from trough to peak (or peak to trough) of the wave, rather than from baseline or zero crossing to peak or trough.

When a sleep recording is scored, it is customary to divide the recording into convenient segments and to assign a sleep stage value to each segment or epoch. The most common epoch length is 30 or 20 seconds, which corresponds to an analogue recording's single page of chart paper 300 mm wide recorded with a chart speed of 10 or 15 mm/sec. A 1-minute scoring epoch has also been used (see particularly Williams et al.[12]), although such a long epoch may overlook stage changes of relatively short duration.[13] A scoring epoch shorter than 20 seconds is considered too tedious by most groups, although epochs as short as 3 seconds have been used for specific research purposes.

Each epoch is assigned a score that most appropriately characterizes the predominant pattern occurring during that interval. Thus, the purpose of epoch staging is to determine the single descriptive factor that most fully characterizes the epoch. Any number of additional codes may be used to denote activities or events occurring within (or across) an epoch. Thus, for example, the standard manual describes "movement arousals," which are short-lived events occurring within an epoch but not descriptive of the majority of the epoch. With the increasing application of polysomnography to clinical assessments, the variety of possible events to be evaluated has grown markedly. Table 116–2 gives a partial listing of events that are coded by various laboratories. To date, these events have usually been defined within each laboratory because standard consensus descriptions are generally lacking. Laboratories typically select those events that are of local experimental or clinical relevance. Event coding is an extremely valuable adjunct to sleep staging, but it is not a substitute for sleep staging.

Sleep Staging in Normal Adult Humans

The following material summarizes the criteria described in the standard manual[1] for staging normal human sleep. Although these criteria apply most specifically to adults, they have also been used to characterize sleep in children and adolescents.[14,15] A separate set of criteria, however, is generally deemed necessary in newborns[16] and older infants.[17] The standard sleep staging criteria in adults, according to the three electrographic parameters, are outlined in Table 116–3 and described next.

Table 116–2. Partial Listing of Events That May Be Coded Within or Across Epochs

Body movement
Movement arousal
Transient arousal
Microsleep episodes
K-alpha complex
Esophageal pH abnormalities
Respiratory abnormalities
  Apnea
    Obstructive
    Central
    Mixed
  Hypopnea (usually ≥10 sec)
    Obstructive
    Central
    Mixed
  Paradoxical respiration
  Cheyne-Stokes respiration
  Periodic breathing
Periodic movements
  With arousal
  Without arousal

Penile tumescence
  T_{up}
  T_{max}
  T_{down}
Heart rate irregularities
  Asystole
  Premature ventricular contraction (PVC)
  Premature atrial contraction (PAC)
  Tachycardia
  Bradycardia
Oxygen saturation
  Below 90%
  Below 80%
REM sleep phasic events
  Twitches
  Rapid eye movements
  Middle ear muscle activity
  Periorbital integrated potentials

REM, rapid eye movement.

Relaxed Wakefulness

The majority of humans show an EEG of rhythmic alpha activity (in the range of 8 to 13 cps) when relaxed with the eyes closed (Fig. 116–2). This activity is maximal occipitally but also often occurs centrally. This rhythmic EEG pattern attenuates with attention, as well as when the eyes are open (Fig. 116–3), at which time the waking EEG pattern is best characterized as one of relatively low voltage and mixed frequency. In an excessively sleepy individual, rhythmic alpha activity may be present when the eyes are open and may attenuate with eye closure; in this case, alpha attenuation is related to the intrusion of stage 1 sleep.

When a person is awake, control of eye movements is voluntary. The waking EOG tracing generally consists of rapid eye movements and eye blinks when the eyes are open, and few or no eye movements with the eyes closed. Involuntary slow, rolling eye movements (with eyes closed) often characterize the EOG in the seconds to minutes preceding the EEG change to stage 1 sleep.

The EMG shows tonic activity of a relatively high level. Voluntary movements produce phasic increases of EMG amplitude. In very relaxed individuals, waking EMG tonus may be indistinguishable from NREM sleep.

NREM Sleep

The four NREM sleep stages are distinguished, as mentioned previously, principally by changes in EEG pattern. The EOG and EMG patterns contribute little to NREM sleep staging, except in the case of transitional stage 1 NREM sleep, in which both may be useful. Therefore, the discussion here will focus on EEG.

Stage 1

The transition from wakefulness to stage 1 sleep (Fig. 116–4) is most clearly visualized on the EEG when the waking pattern has well-defined rhythmic alpha activity. It is for this reason that an occipital derivation is frequently added to the sleep recording montage, because waking alpha activity is most prominent in this cortical region. The EEG pattern of stage 1 is described as relatively low-voltage, mixed-frequency activity. Especially during stage 1 sleep occurring at the beginning of the night, vertex sharp waves (Fig. 116–5) are common. In addition, the EEG activity with the highest relative amplitude during stage 1 sleep is generally in the theta (3 to 7 cps) range. Bursts of relatively high-voltage, very synchronous theta activity are common during the onset of stage 1 sleep in children and young adolescents (Fig. 116–6).

The SEMs commonly precede the EEG transition to stage 1 sleep from wakefulness. Although the onset of SEMs usually leads the EEG transition by only 1 or 2 minutes, the lead time may occasionally—particularly in daytime recordings—be as long as 15 minutes.[18] SEMs are very useful to distinguish stage 1 sleep transitions occurring during stage 2 NREM sleep or REM sleep.

Muscle tone is maintained during all NREM sleep stages and registers as low-amplitude EMG activity. There generally is no discrete change in EMG amplitude in the wake-to-sleep transition, although a gradual diminution of the EMG signal amplitude may occur within moments of the transition. During NREM sleep, the EMG is most helpful for distinguishing movement arousals, which is useful in certain stage change decisions. In addition, a rise in EMG activity is often the only discrete indicator of a transition to stage 1 sleep within a REM sleep episode (see Fig. 116–12).

Stage 2

The background EEG of stage 2 NREM sleep is a pattern of relatively low voltage, mixed-frequency activity. Stage 2 is distinguished from stage 1 on the basis of two specific EEG patterns that occur sporadically on this mixed-frequency background: the sleep spindle and the K-complex (Fig. 116–7).

Table 116–3.   Outline of Sleep Scoring Criteria According to Standard Manual

Stage/State	Electroencephalogram (EEG)	Electrooculogram (EOG)	Electromyogram (EMG)
Relaxed wakefulness	**Eyes closed:** rhythmic alpha (8-13 cps); prominent in occipital; attenuates with attention **Eyes open:** relatively low voltage mixed frequency	Voluntary control; REMs or none; blinks; slow eye movements (SEMs) when drowsy	Tonic activity, relatively high; voluntary movement
Non–rapid eye movement sleep (NREM)			
Stage 1	Relatively low voltage, mixed frequency May be theta (3-7 cps) activity with greater amplitude Vertex sharp waves Synchronous high-voltage theta bursts in children	SEMs	Tonic activity, may be slight decrease from waking
Stage 2	**Background:** relatively low voltage, mixed frequency **Sleep spindles:** waxing, waning, 12–14 cps (≥0.5 sec) **K-complex:** negative sharp wave followed immediately by slower positive component (≥0.5 sec); spindles may ride on Ks; Ks maximal in vertex; spontaneous or in response to sound	Occasionally SEMs near sleep onset	Tonic activity, low level
Stage 3	≥20%, ≤50% high amplitude (>75 μV), slow frequency (≤2 cps); maximal in frontal	None, picks up EEG	Tonic activity, low level
Stage 4	>50% high amplitude, slow frequency	None, picks up EEG	Tonic activity, low level
Rapid eye movement sleep (REM)	Relatively low voltage, mixed frequency Sawtooth waves Theta activity; slow alpha	Phasic REMs	Tonic suppression; phasic twitches
Movement time	Obscured	Obscured	Very high activity
Anomalous sleep*	Similar to REM	Phasic REMs	Tonic activity; phasic twitches

*Described in reference 44.

Modified from Rechtschaffen A, Kales A (eds): A Manual of Standardized Terminology: Techniques and Scoring System for Sleep Stages of Human Subjects. Los Angeles, Calif: UCLA Brain Information Service/Brain Research Institute; 1968.

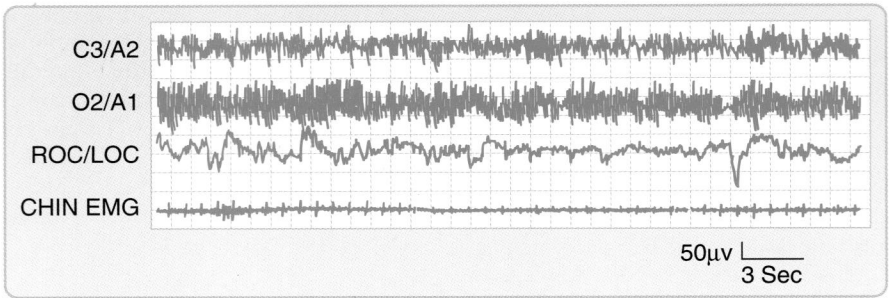

Figure 116–2. Rhythmic electroencephalographic (EEG) alpha activity is clearly evident in the C3/A2 and O2/A1 tracings of this young adult male volunteer who is awake with his eyes closed. Figures 116–2 to 116–7 and 116–9 to 116–13 are all taken from an overnight recording of this 19-year-old healthy man. All leads were recorded on a Grass Instruments Company Model 78 polygraph. The central and occipital EEGs and the electrooculograms (EOGs) used a low-frequency cutoff of 0.3 cps, a high-frequency cutoff of 30 cps, and a sensitivity of 50 μV/cm. The electromyogram (EMG) was recorded with a low-frequency cutoff of 10 cps, a high-frequency cutoff of 60 cps, and a sensitivity of 20 μV/cm. Paper speed was 10 mm/sec. In Figures 116–2 to 116–5, the EOG is monitored with a single lead (ROC/LOC). In Figures 116–9 to 116–13, the occipital tracing has been dropped, and the EOG is recorded from two leads, ROC/A1 and LOC/A2. (See text for comments on the latter procedure.)

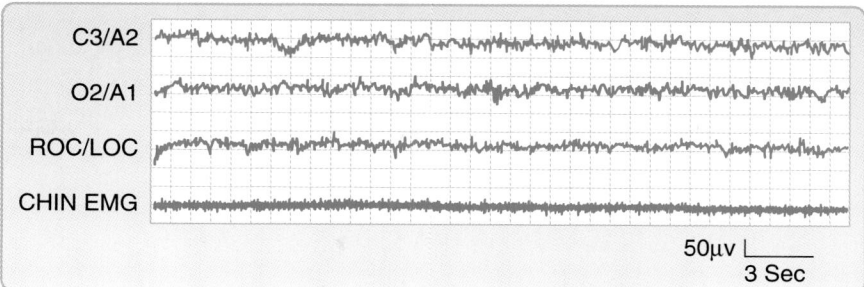

Figure 116–3. Attenuation of waking EEG alpha activity with eyes open is illustrated in this tracing. Note the characteristic "relatively low-voltage, mixed-frequency" EEG activity.

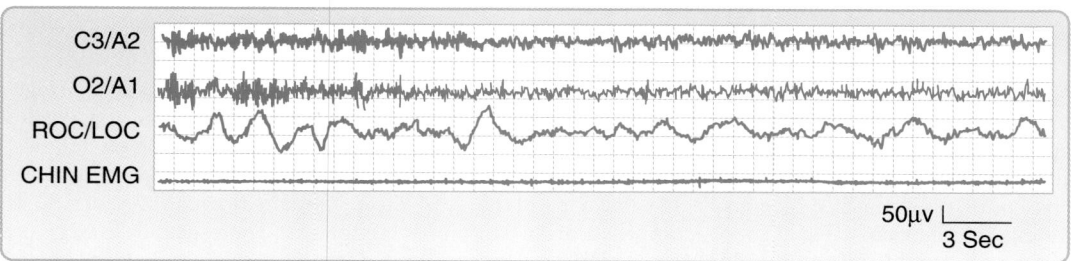

Figure 116–4. Transition from wakefulness to stage 1 sleep is illustrated, which clearly shows the attenuation of alpha that marks the onset of stage 1 sleep. As described in Figure 116–3 for an EEG of wakefulness with the eyes open, the EEG pattern of stage 1 sleep is one of "relatively low voltage, mixed frequency." Note, too, the presence of slow eye movements in the EOG tracing.

Figure 116–5. Vertex sharp waves are a common feature of the onset of stage 1 sleep. Few were seen in this volunteer, however, although one *(underlined)* is illustrated in this figure. Note that the vertex sharp wave is visible in the C3/A2 lead but not in the O2/A1 lead, emphasizing localization to the vertex region.

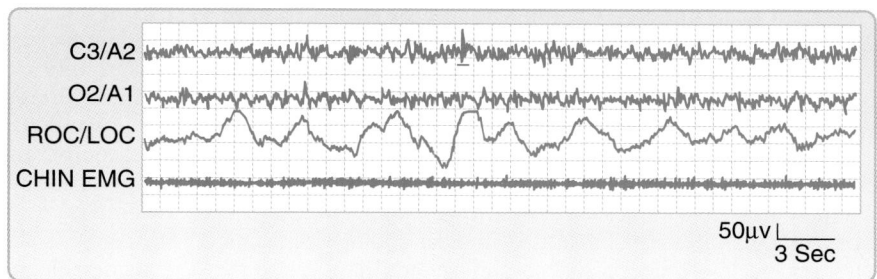

Figure 116–6. Very high voltage, highly synchronous theta activity *(underlined)* is common during sleep onset stage 1 in children and young adolescents. This phenomenon is illustrated here in a tracing from a 14-year-old male volunteer. (Recording parameters are as described in the legend for Figure 116–2, with the exception that EEGs were recorded with a low-frequency cutoff of 1.0 cps.)

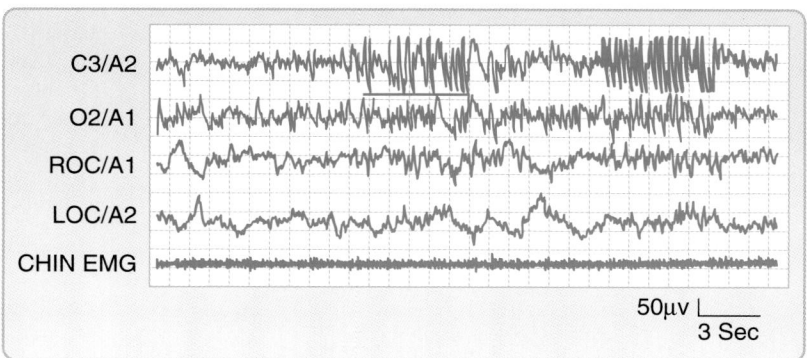

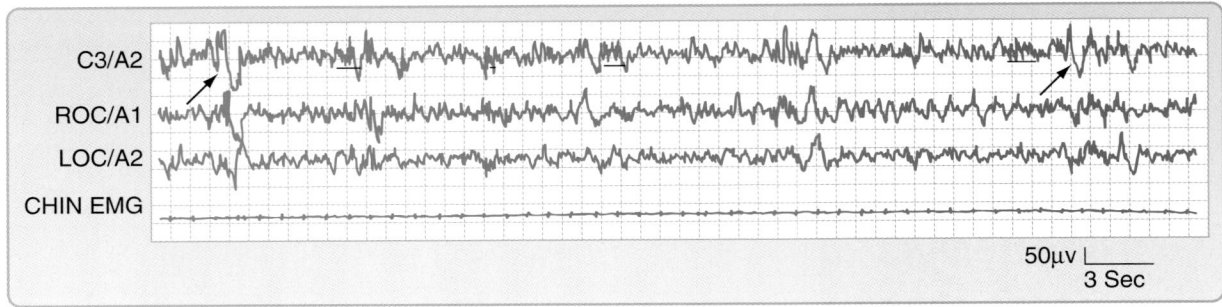

Figure 116–7. A stage 2 sleep pattern is illustrated. The *arrows* indicate K-complexes, and sleep spindles are *underlined*. Note that K-complexes are seen in the EOG tracings but are distinct from eye movements because the EOG tracings are in phase with one another. The last K-complex in this figure illustrates the coincidence of a sleep spindle and a K-complex, seen as relatively low voltage activity of spindle frequency (12 to 14 cps) on the trailing portion of the K-complex.

Because these stage 2–defining EEG patterns occur episodically, the standard staging criteria[1] provide for a default to stage 1 sleep if neither a sleep spindle nor a K-complex occurs within a 3-minute span when the EEG is of relatively low voltage and mixed frequency (the "3-min" rule).

In their most pure presentation, sleep spindles have a waxing and waning spindle shape (Fig. 116–8), composed of waves in the range of 12 to 14 cps, with a duration of about 0.5 to 1.5 seconds.[19] Sleep spindles are a common feature of mammalian sleep, and when recorded using identical techniques, they are indistinguishable—for example, between humans and cats.[20] Sleep spindle activity occurs during stage 2 sleep, with a frequency of about three to eight spindles per minute in normal adults[21] or insomniac adults,[22] and spindle rate appears to be a fairly stable individual characteristic.[21] "Incipient sleep spindles" may appear near the stage 1 to stage 2 transition early during sleep; however, "the presence of a spindle should not be defined unless it is of at least 0.5 sec duration, i.e., one should be able to count 6 or 7 distinct waves within the half-second period."[1]

From an ontogenetic perspective, sleep spindles in humans usually develop before age 3 months.[23,24] In infants with mental retardation, sleep spindles are slower to develop and occur less frequently than in normal infants.[25] In older adults, sleep spindles tend to lose their classic morphology and have a slightly slower frequency, lower amplitude, and shorter duration[26,27] than in the young adult. Benzodiazepine hypnotics tend to increase the density of sleep spindles in stage 2 sleep.[22,28]

Sleep spindles (the term will be used interchangeably with *K-complex* here) are absent in stage 1 NREM but may occur in REM sleep, particularly in subjects or patients whose sleep has been restricted or fragmented. If a single sleep spindle occurs in the middle of a REM sleep episode, it is not considered to be indicative of a stage change. If, however, two sleep spindles bracket half a scoring epoch or longer with no intervening REMs, the interval between spindles is considered a stage 2 sleep interruption of the REM episode.

The K-complex (see Fig. 116–7) is another sleep-specific EEG waveform that is characteristic of stage 2 sleep. This paroxysmal wave complex consists of a "well-delineated negative sharp wave which is immediately followed by a positive component. The total duration of the complex should exceed 0.5 sec."[1] The standard manual provides no amplitude criterion for K-complexes. There usually is very little difficulty in discerning K-complexes in stage 2 sleep. The following definition used by electroencephalographers for the term *complex* is very helpful when a K-complex distinction is in doubt, as may occur in stage 3 and 4 sleep, when it is sometimes difficult to differentiate K-complexes from high-voltage, slow wave activity. A complex is a "group of two or more waves, clearly distinguished from background activity and occurring with a well-recognized form or recurring with consistent form."[29] A key part of this definition is that the complex is distinct from the ongoing background activity, which makes the K-complex in stage 2 very clear, whereas the same morphology embedded within a series of high-voltage, slow wave activity during stage 3 or 4 would probably not stand out from the background.

K-complexes are maximal over the vertex. It is very common for spindle activity (12 to 14 cps) to ride over the K-complex. In young adults, the typical density of K-complexes in stage 2 is about 1 to 3 per minute,[21,30,31] although there is considerable individual variability. K-complexes occur spontaneously during stage 2 sleep and are also evoked in response to auditory stimuli.

At the beginning of the night, SEMs may infrequently and only very briefly persist after the appearance of sleep spindles and K-complexes. Because the EOG channels also register EEG activity, K-complexes can reflect on these channels (see Fig. 116–7). They are generally easily distinguished from rapid eye movements because the pens on the two channels deflect in phase and because the central EEG amplitude of a K-complex is usually much greater than any EEG activity related to eye movements. The EMG during stage 2 sleep is tonically active, generally at a low amplitude relative to wakefulness.

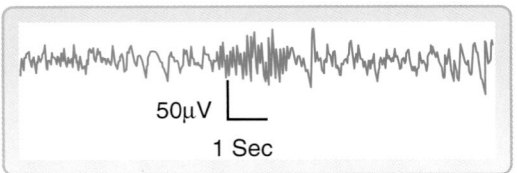

Figure 116–8. A sleep spindle from stage 2 sleep in a normal 16-year-old adolescent girl is illustrated. The activity is grossly spindle shaped, with waxing and waning amplitude. Older adult volunteers and many patients with sleep disorders no longer have spindles with this morphology. The "spindles" tend to be shorter and of lower amplitude in such individuals.

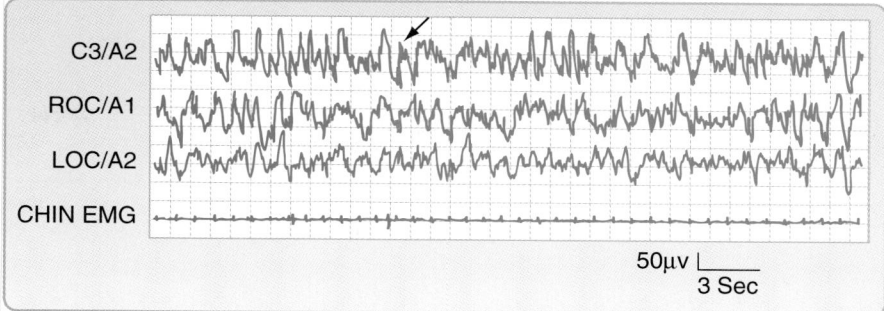

Figure 116–9. Stage 3 sleep is scored when the EEG pattern consists of high-voltage (≥75 μV), slow (≤2 cps) activity in 20% or more, but less than 50%, of a scoring epoch, as illustrated. Sleep spindles may occur in stage 3 sleep; the *arrow* indicates a spindle in this example of stage 3 sleep. Note that the EOG tracings pick up the high-voltage, slow wave activity, which can be seen in the ROC and LOC leads as in-phase deflections.

Stages 3 and 4

The EEG of stages 3 and 4 sleep is defined by the presence of high-voltage, slow wave activity (Figs. 116–9 and 116–10). In stage 3 sleep, "at least 20 per cent but not more than 50 per cent of the epoch consists of waves of 2 cps or slower which have amplitudes greater than 75 μV from peak to peak (the difference between the most negative and positive points of the wave)."[1] In stage 4 sleep, such waves predominate (more than 50% of the epoch). Sleep spindles can occur during stages 3 and 4, as can K-complexes; however, they are only infrequently distinct from the background EEG activity, particularly in stage 4 sleep. Eye movements do not occur during stage 3 and 4 sleep, although the EOG registers the high-voltage, slow wave activity. The EMG during stages 3 and 4 is tonically active, although the tracing may occasionally achieve very low levels, nearly indistinguishable from that of REM sleep.

REM Sleep

Staging REM sleep requires the coincidence of specific activities in all three electrographic measures: "activated" or desynchronized EEG, bursts of rapid eye movements, and suppression of EMG activity (Fig. 116–11). The REM sleep EEG pattern is characterized as one of "relatively low voltage, mixed frequency."[1] An EEG pattern called sawtooth waves—because of their notched morphology—is fairly common during REM sleep,[32] particularly in proximity to eye movements, but it is by no means a universal phenomenon. Thus, the presence of sawtooth activity is not required for staging REM sleep, although it may be very useful in equivocal instances. Sawtooth waves achieve the highest amplitude at the vertex[33] and, like much other REM sleep EEG activity, have a frequency in the theta range. Activity in the alpha range (usually 1 to 2 cps slower than waking alpha activity) may also be seen in the REM sleep EEG.[34]

Ponto-geniculo-occipital (PGO) spikes are a definitive feature of feline REM sleep,[35] and rhythmic hippocampal theta activity is a prominent REM feature in many primates, cats, dogs, and rodents.[36] In cats, PGO spikes occur singly in the transition to REM sleep and in bursts during REM sleep, usually leading other REM sleep phasic events. The scalp EEG routinely recorded in humans is not clearly related to these characteristic REM sleep patterns of other species. Hodes and Dement,[37] however, suggested that K-complexes in humans may be an analogue of the pre-REM PGO spikes because both pre-REM events are similarly associated with EMG and reflex suppression. Depth EEG recordings in humans have also suggested the presence of PGO spikes in REM sleep.[38]

The EOG reveals bursts of rapid eye movements at intervals during REM sleep (see Fig. 116–11). The acronym *REM* originated with these eye movements, of course, although the term is now used to denote the full constellation of physiologic events constituting this state. The density of rapid eye movement bursts within REM sleep varies with time of night; thus, earlier REM episodes contain fewer rapid eye movements than do later REM episodes.[39] The episodic nature of this sign of REM sleep often requires the sleep record scorer to scan the chart in advance of the epoch currently under scrutiny. The criteria of the standard manual[1] provide contingencies for such contextual decisions, as will be described later.

For an epoch to be considered REM sleep, in addition to the activated EEG and REM bursts, an EMG recorded in the manner described previously must obtain its lowest value. A universal feature of REM sleep in the intact organism is the tonic suppression of skeletal muscle tone and reflexes via a circuit that involves pontine activation of medullary inhibitory centers and culminates in postsynaptic hyperpolarization of brainstem and spinal motoneurons.[40] Superimposed on this background of tonic motor inhibition can be seen occasional twitches of distal muscles. In household pets, for example, paws, face, and

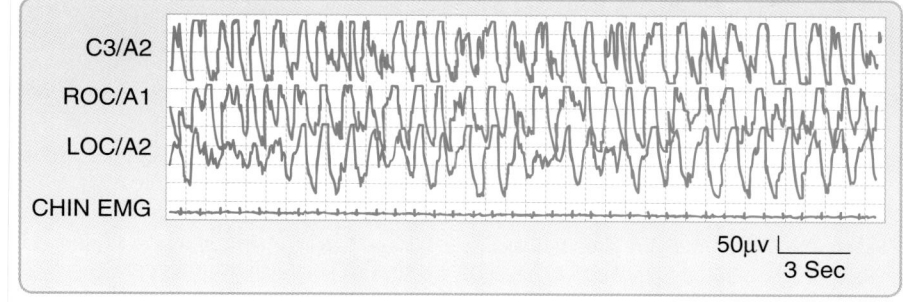

Figure 116–10. Stage 4 sleep is characterized by a predominance (less than 50%) of high-voltage slow waves in the EEG. In this sample tracing, the slow wave EEG amplitude is so great that the pen-swing limitation of the recorder is exceeded and pen "blocking" distorts the wave shapes.

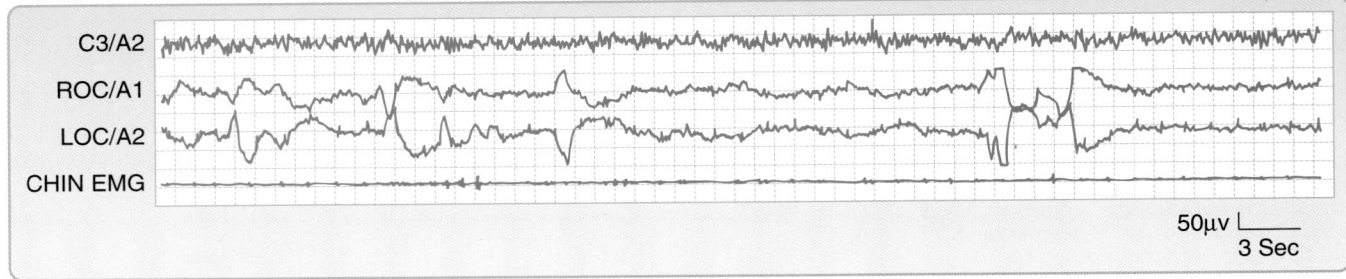

Figure 116–11. REM sleep is scored when the EEG pattern is one of relatively low voltage, mixed frequency; the EMG is tonically suppressed; and the EOG shows rapid eye movements. Each of these REM sleep components is present in this figure. The early and late portions of the figure, in which eye movement bursts occur along with EMG twitches in the earlier portion, might be characterized as phasic REM sleep, whereas the intervening segment containing no eye movements might be called tonic REM sleep. Note that eye movements appear as out-of-phase deflections in the ROC and LOC tracings.

whiskers show twitches in REM sleep. In human polysomnographic recordings, twitches appear as very short-lived EMG elevations, usually in proximity to eye movement bursts (see Fig. 116–11). Prolonged EMG elevation (15 seconds or longer) in REM sleep, even in the absence of an EEG change, requires a stage shift (Fig. 116–12). Brief EMG elevations associated with an alteration in EEG or EOG activity (i.e., movement arousal) may signal a stage change, depending on the relative size of this movement and duration of the EEG and EOG alterations.

Both REM sleep and NREM stage 2 sleep require the presence of episodic events: bursts of rapid eye movements in REM sleep and spindles or K-complexes in stage 2. In both, the background EEG is similar—that is, relatively low voltage, mixed frequency. Scoring the transitions from stage 2 to REM sleep (Fig. 116–13) and from REM level to stage 2, as well as stage 2 interruptions of REM sleep (Fig. 116–14), is therefore sometimes problematic. The following two fundamental guidelines from the standard manual[1] make it possible to deal with virtually every contingency:

1. Any section of record contiguous with stage REM sleep in which the EEG shows relatively low voltage and mixed frequency is scored stage REM sleep regardless of whether rapid eye movements are present, providing EMG is at the stage REM level and there are no intervening movement arousals.
2. An interval of relatively low-voltage, mixed-frequency EEG record between two sleep spindles or K-complexes is considered stage 2 regardless of EMG level, if there are no rapid eye movements or movement arousals during this interval and if the interval is less than 3 minutes long.

The manual provides a variety of specific examples that apply these guidelines, and the reader is urged to review them.

Movement Time

Gross postural readjustments are fairly common during sleep, often occurring in the vicinity of REM episodes.[4] When such movements arise from sleep or immediately precede sleep, and obscure the EEG activity (and usually the EOG as well) for at least one half of the scoring epoch, that epoch is designated "movement time." If this pattern is preceded or followed by wakefulness, it is scored as an awake pattern.

Considerations for Staging Sleep in Pathologies

The standard manual was developed to provide guidelines for staging sleep in normal adults, and its recommendations are suitable for many pathologic conditions as well. Nevertheless, full characterization of sleep in a number of sleep-related pathologies at times requires a departure from the standard procedures. The following material briefly reviews certain issues that may arise in specific disorders and suggests alternatives for addressing these issues.

Narcolepsy

The sleep of patients with narcolepsy is characterized by sleep onset REM episodes (the occurrence of rapid eye movements within 15 minutes of sleep onset), mixtures of stage 2 and REM sleep, and arousals that are more numerous than seen in healthy persons.[41] Each of these phenomena can be

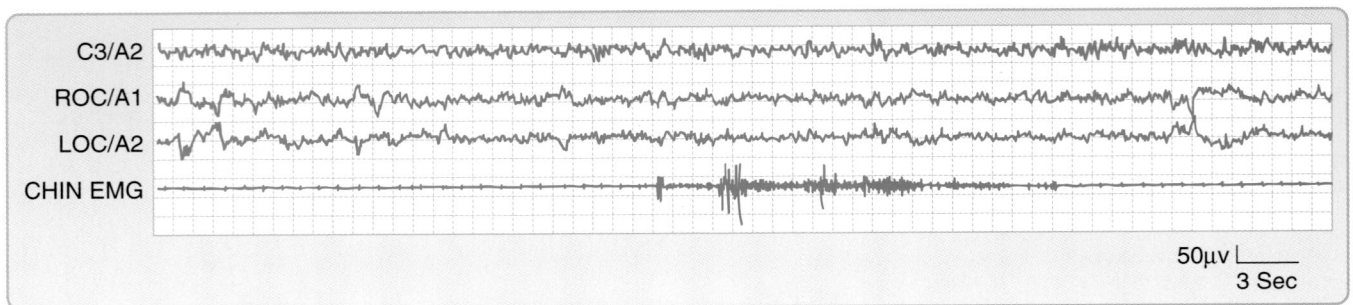

Figure 116–12. This figure shows an example of stage 1 sleep interrupting a REM episode. The interruption is seen as a tonic increase in EMG activity lasting longer than 50% of the scoring epoch. This change is scored even if the EEG pattern shows no discernible difference and even if no slow eye movements occur.

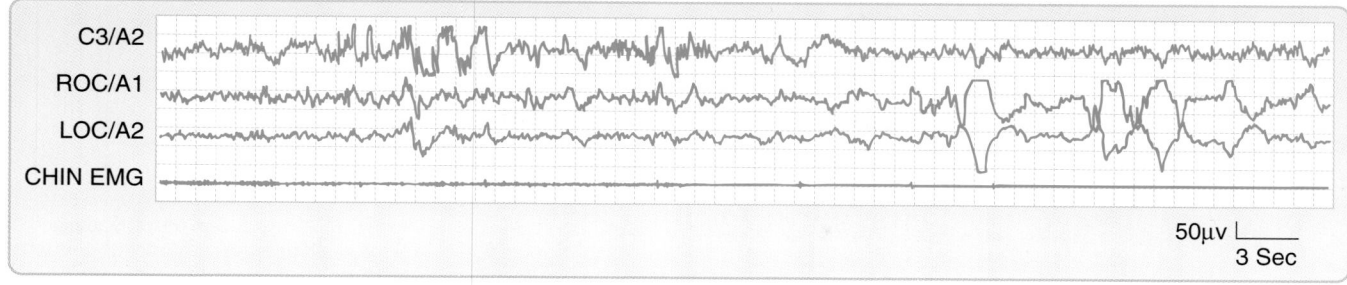

Figure 116–13. This figure illustrates a transition from stage 2 NREM sleep to REM sleep, in which the three markers of REM sleep occur in fairly close proximity. EMG suppression leads the EEG desynchronization by a few seconds, and bursts of rapid eye movements occur several seconds later. It is not uncommon for several minutes to elapse during such a transition.

characterized using the guidelines of the standard manual. Particular care is often required, however, and one may wish to use additional procedures, such as adding a vertical EOG, to assist in identifying a brief, early REM episode. An early REM episode may not last sufficiently long (e.g., longer than 15 seconds) to characterize a full epoch as REM sleep; its occurrence may nonetheless be diagnostically relevant and must be noted.

The most problematic area with narcolepsy generally involves patients whose medication regimen results in excessive motor activity during sleep, as characterized by an elevated EMG in the presence of an activated EEG and phasic rapid eye movements occurring with a periodicity similar to that of REM sleep.[42,43] (This pattern may also occur in nonnarcoleptic patients, such as those with Alzheimer's or Parkinson's disease.) This might be characterized as an anomalous state, as shown in Table 116–3. Thus, epochs of anomalous sleep may be accounted for outside the standard criteria and staged as neither REM nor NREM sleep.[44]

Sleep Apnea Syndromes

Patients with a sleep apnea syndrome experience a great increase in the frequency of arousals from sleep and in the number of body movements. Both types of activity have an impact on sleep staging. For example, a patient may be clearly asleep and apneic for 10 seconds, and movement associated with the termination of the apnea may obscure the remainder of the epoch (Fig. 116–15). Another common occurrence in patients with a sleep apnea syndrome is the appearance of K-complexes almost exclusively at the termination of the apneas. If scored exclusively using the standard guidelines

and a 30-second epoch, sleep might not be found in such patients or might appear as only stage 1 and movement time. The following suggestions (modified from Flagg and Coburn[45]) for scoring sleep in such patients attempt to account for these pathologic events:

1. Follow standard guidelines for entry into stage 1 from wakefulness and stage 2 from stage 1. (Coding "microsleep" episodes [less than half the epoch with stage 1 EEG] at the onset of sleep may be useful.)
2. Once stage 2 sleep is scored, continue stage 2 through any arousal that does not result in a transition to wakefulness (more than half the epoch with waking EEG). (Coding "transient arousals" [see later] may be useful.)
3. In REM sleep, ignore EMG elevations that are clearly associated with snoring.
4. In adults, stages 3 and 4 may be combined. (Some investigators[45] recommend combining stages 2, 3, and 4 in patients with sleep apnea. Such crude categorization may obscure clinically relevant information and is not recommended, particularly for children.)

Alpha-Delta Sleep

An EEG pattern of alpha intrusion into NREM sleep was first noted in patients with psychiatric disorders.[46] The pattern was described as "a mixture of 5-20 per cent delta waves (more than 75 μV, 0.5-2 cps) combined with relatively large amplitude, alpha-like rhythms (7-10 cps). These alpha rhythms are usually 1-2 cps slower than waking alpha." A similar pattern has been related to a complaint of nonrestorative sleep in patients with musculoskeletal pain or fibrositis.[47] This EEG

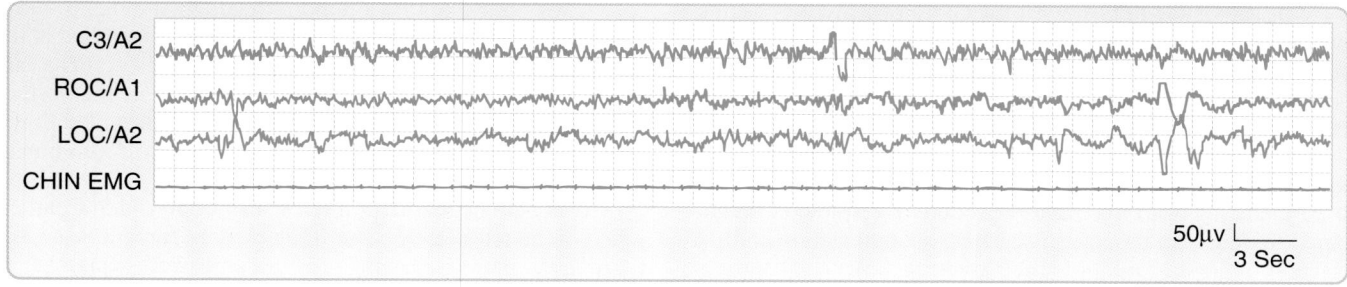

Figure 116–14. An isolated K-complex occurs in the midst of an REM episode. The episode is staged as REM sleep despite the K-complex (refer to the first guideline from the standard manual). Had a second K-complex or sleep spindle occurred, spanning more than 50% of the scoring epoch, the interval would be staged as stage 2 sleep, even if the background EEG resembled the REM pattern and the EMG were at the REM sleep level.

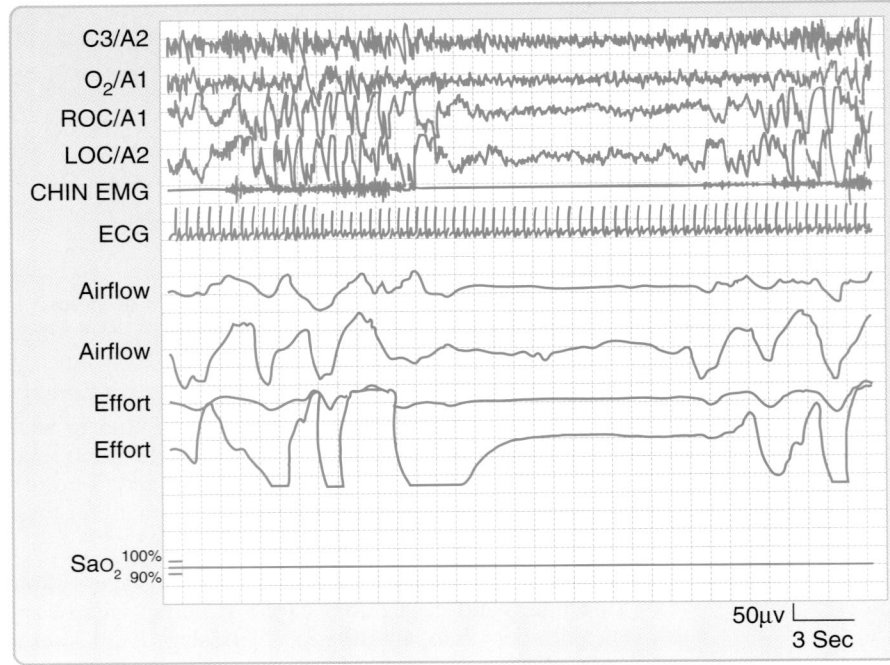

Figure 116–15. Sleep onset is aborted by a large movement associated with the termination of an episode of sleep apnea. Note that the "scorable" portion of this epoch contains only about 12 seconds of stage 1 sleep, which is insufficient to characterize the entire 30-second epoch. For this type of occurrence, the coding of a microsleep event might be useful, along with the coding of an apneic event.

pattern might legitimately be scored as NREM stage 1 or 2, but the clinical implications of this type of sleep require that it be noted and remarked on. Thus, one might define a separate sleep "stage" or use an event code to make this pattern accessible for separate analysis.

Transient Arousals

Many sleep disorders involve frequent, brief arousals that do not alter sleep stage scoring but that may be clinically relevant. Such arousals are a common feature of normal aging as well. Clinical implications of these brief arousals have been shown in several types of studies. For example, brief arousals induced experimentally into the sleep of normal volunteers resulted in daytime sleepiness, even though the total amount of sleep was unchanged.[48] In addition, spontaneously occurring transient arousals in older adults have been correlated with waking alertness level.[49] This type of arousal occurs frequently in patients with sleep apnea syndromes, periodic movements in sleep, and other sleep disorders. Therefore, cataloguing such events may be relevant in several clinical and nonclinical populations. The following definition has been proposed for transient arousals[49]: "Any clearly visible EEG arousal (usually alpha rhythm) lasting two seconds or longer, but not associated with any stage or state change in the epoch scoring. These brief arousals are sometimes, but not always, associated with a body movement or respiration event." To this definition we add the recommendation that transient arousals in REM sleep be coded only when EEG alpha activity is associated with another sign of arousal (e.g., increased heart rate, EMG elevation, or respiration irregularity), because alpha activity is a fairly common feature of REM sleep.[34] A task force of the American Sleep Disorders Association (ASDA) has defined a set of scoring rules and has provided examples for coding EEG arousals during sleep.[50]

The ASDA coding system has initiated a renewed interest in sleep-related arousals, an aspect of sleep staging that has beleaguered sleep researchers and clinicians for decades. For example, a 1999 task force of the American Academy of Sleep Medicine focused on the role of respiratory effort–related arousal events in helping define the severity of the obstructive sleep apnea–hypopnea syndrome (see Chapter 92).[51] Furthermore, as more investigators examine sleep in newly described sleep disorders and other medical disorders, this interest in sleep fragmentation strengthens. For example, the description of upper airway resistance syndrome[52] rekindled interest in EEG arousals because the respiratory signs of this syndrome are less obvious than those in frank obstructive sleep apnea syndrome and only subtle indicators may be available.[53] In addition, the ASDA arousal staging system and related research have stimulated an examination or a reexamination of arousals in other disorders such as allergic rhinitis,[54,55] juvenile rheumatoid arthritis,[56] and Parkinson's disease.[57]

Others have begun to examine variations of the ASDA arousal scoring schema, and still others suggest that non-EEG markers may be important and even more reliable signs of arousal than the EEG. Pitson and Stradling,[58] for example, note that transient changes in blood pressure may signify arousals more reliably than cortical EEG, although Lofaso and colleagues[59] indicate that autonomic changes are highly correlated with the extent of EEG arousals. Less well studied is the possibility that certain sleep-fragmenting phenomena are associated with subcortical events not visible in the cortical EEG signal. This may be the case in sleep studies of children who manifest few cortical arousals even with prominent obstructive sleep apnea syndrome.

A relatively new area of interest has established a pattern called cyclic alternating pattern, defined as "repetitive stereotyped EEG patterns lasting <60 seconds and separated by time-equivalent intervals of background activity."[60] A manual has been established for analyzing these patterns,[61] and clinical correlates are being identified. See Chapter 104 Appendix, "Technical Considerations and Scoring Criteria."

Automatic Sleep Stagers

Although many groups in the United States continue to analyze sleep data using human hand scoring of polysomnographic or digitally acquired tracings, several systems for automatically staging sleep have been proposed, and a number are commercially available.[62-67] Certain of these systems are based on the standard guidelines, although several approaches that confront the sleep staging issues more from the perspective of available technologies have also been used. Thus, instead of adapting digital computer technology to human eyeball scoring criteria, they use such techniques as frequency spectra analysis or multidimensional scaling,[62] adaptive segmentation and fuzzy subset theory,[63] or expert systems approaches.[64] No single automated stager has yet emerged as the ideal alternative to hand scoring, and space does not permit a review of available systems. The following questions are offered as a basis for evaluating automatic sleep staging systems:

1. Has the system been validated against another known assessment technique?
2. Is the system valid for the types of studies for which it will be used—for example, sleep only, sleep and breathing, sleep and movements, and so forth?
3. Is the system valid for the types of patients in whom it will be used—for example, patients with sleep apnea versus patients with narcolepsy, medicated versus nonmedicated patients, and so on?
4. Is the system valid for the age groups in which it will be used—children versus adults versus older adults?
5. Is the system compatible with available laboratory hardware?
6. Does the system require excessive operator input (e.g., knob turning, "tweaking," fine tuning) that takes as much time as hand scoring?
7. Does the system provide output verification? That is, can the raw data be reviewed?
8. If the system does not automatically assess relevant events, can hand-scored events be accurately correlated to the stager's output?
9. Is the system sufficiently flexible to support new foreseeable applications? Such applications might include changes in patient population, recording equipment, research orientation, and so forth.
10. Does the system reliably identify differences known to affect sleep staging, such as age, prior sleep history, and diagnosis?
11. Is the system supported by accessible consultants?

SUMMARIZING SLEEP STAGE DATA

After the sleep data are scored, they must be summarized into a comprehensible form. No consensus format has been achieved, and certain areas of controversy exist; however, a number of conventions are fairly common and include the following types of analysis. (Alternative calculation paradigms are sometimes used and have been noted where appropriate.) Figure 116–16 shows the output of one type of sleep data summary sheet.

Stages

A summary of the night of sleep will invariably include the time spent in each of the sleep stages, as well as the time awake and movement time. This type of summary is relatively straightforward and noncontroversial. Calculation of percentage distributions is not quite as clear cut, as various groups may calculate sleep stage percentages based on total recording time (dark time), on total sleep time (total NREM stages 1 to 4 plus REM), or on sleep period time (time from sleep onset to sleep offset, including intervening arousals). The example in Figure 116–16 uses all three alternatives.

Latencies

The topic of latencies is associated with a certain amount of controversy, particularly because the type of patient may affect the appropriateness of specific definitions. Thus, although sleep latency, defined as elapsed time from lights out until the first of three consecutive epochs of stage 1 or the first of any other stage, may be appropriate for normal, noncomplaining individuals or for hypersomnolent patients, it may not be appropriate for patients with sleep onset insomnia. One alternative to the this definition requires stage 2 sleep (spindle or K-complex) to define sleep onset.[68] To account for instances in which a patient may have 2 or 3 minutes of sleep followed by a lengthy awakening, definitions that require, for example, 5 consecutive minutes of sleep have been suggested by others.[69] The issue of the definition of sleep onset is not trivial because latencies to stage 4 or REM sleep are generally calculated from sleep onset. Certain analysis programs have the capability to provide several calculations of sleep onset, whereas others provide the flexibility to redefine the criterion for individual cases. In the absence of a comprehensive database, it is not possible to make a sweeping generalization. A safe alternative for most clinical studies is probably to choose the conservative 5-minute rule or even a 10-minute rule, although a briefer requirement might be more appropriate for patients with sleep syndromes in which frequent awakenings may preclude such a sleep onset entirely.

Once a definition of sleep onset is established, determining stage 3 or 4 or REM latency is fairly straightforward: elapsed time from the (start of) defined sleep onset to the first epoch of stage 3 (or 4) or REM sleep. Certain groups may apply a three-epoch rule to this definition—that is, three consecutive epochs of the target stage are required. One point of dispute regarding REM latency calculation concerns whether or not to include any waking intervals that may occur between sleep onset and REM onset.[70] No firm recommendation can be made; however, it is still generally assumed that waking is included in the calculation, unless otherwise noted. Such considerations are crucial when data are compared across groups, which is particularly relevant when norms from another laboratory are being used.

Cycles

A description of the NREM-REM cycle is a common feature of the night's sleep summary. Unfortunately, the defining characteristics for such a description are not standardized, and therefore, a number of idiosyncratic approaches have been used. One common way of defining cycles is as the elapsed time from the end of each REM episode to the end of the next REM episode, whereas another uses the time from the start of one REM episode to the start of the next. The consequences of choosing one alternative over the other have not been clearly established. Another difficulty for defining REM cycles arises

T.A.

Subject's name:	T.A.
Subject's gender:	M
Subject's age:	14.0000 years
Subject's date of birth:	1/11/73
Subject's tanner stage:	
Recording date:	1/11/87
Name of study:	T/A
Group:	
Recording condition:	Pretreatment
Recording technician:	Carskadon
Scoring technician:	Mancuso
Data entry technician:	Mancuso

Minimum epoch length: 0.4800 minutes (Epoch 478 of page 11)
Maximum epoch length: 0.5294 minutes (Epoch 965 of page 10)
Average epoch length: 0.4975 minutes

	Epochs	Minutes	%TDT	%SPT	%TST
TDT	1179	586.50	-	-	-
SPT	1067	530.95	90.53	-	-
TST	1031	513.00	87.47	96.62	-
WASO	38	18.93	3.23	3.56	3.69
WAFA	82	41.00	6.99	7.72	7.99
TS1	93	46.09	7.86	8.68	8.98
TS2	546	272.43	46.45	51.31	53.11
TS3	92	45.62	7.78	8.59	8.89
TS4	167	82.91	14.14	15.61	16.16
TNREM	898	447.05	76.22	84.20	87.14
TREM	115	56.98	9.71	10.73	11.11
TSW	259	128.53	21.91	24.21	25.05
TWT	148	73.50	12.53	13.84	14.33
TMT	18	8.97	1.53	1.69	1.75

REM summary:

	REM1	REM2	REM3	REM4	TOTAL	MEAN
TT	3.93	8.95	21.80	27.20	61.89	15.47
REMT	2.95	8.95	21.80	23.27	56.98	14.24
S1	0.00	0.00	0.00	2.95	2.95	0.74
S2	0.98	0.00	0.00	0.00	0.98	0.25
WT	0.00	0.00	0.00	0.98	0.98	0.25
MT	0.00	0.00	0.00	0.00	0.00	0.00
SEG	2	1	1	3	7	1.75
Cycles	192.77	111.64	104.66	111.89	520.95	130.24

End of last REM from end of night: 51:00

Analysis by fraction (1/3):

	1	2	3
Wake	0.00	6.98	12.20
SW	91.94	13.18	23.41
REM	0.00	11.90	45.08

T/A, Pretreatment

Milestones:

Lights out:	22:14:00 (Epoch 27 of page 1)
Sleep onset:	22:28:33 (Epoch 57 of page 1)
Last sleep epoch:	7:19:00 (Epoch 602 of page 13)
End of night:	8:00:30 (Epoch 685 of page 13)

	REM	NREM	WAKE
Body movement (1)	1	43	1
Transient arousal (2)	0	4	0
Slow eye movement(4)	0	4	4
Microsleep (5)	0	0	5
Central apnea/hypopnea (7)	2	6	0
Obstructive apnea/hypopnea (A)	0	83	0
Mixed apnea/hypopnea (B)	0	1	0
Sao$_2$<90% (C)	0	21	0
Sao$_2$<80% (D)	0	0	0

Latencies (minutes):

Lights out to S1	13.58
Lights out to S2	14.55
Lights out to S3	23.50
Lights out to S4	26.00
Lights out to sleep onset	13.58
LO to 10 minutes continuous sleep	14.55
Sleep onset to slow wave	8.95
Sleep onset to REM	188.83

Figure 116–16. A sleep stage summary sheet. This sample represents only one of many possible summary formats. The data are taken from a night of sleep recorded in a 14-year-old boy with enlarged tonsils and adenoids who had moderately disordered breathing during sleep. The 25-minute combining rule was used to define REM sleep periods. The following definitions were used to derive specific items presented in this summary: SPT, sleep period time (elapsed time from sleep onset to last epoch of sleep); TDT, total dark time (elapsed time from lights out to end of night); TMT, total amount of movement time; TNREM, total stages 1 + 2 + 3 + 4 sleep; TREM, total amount of REM sleep; TS1 to TS4, total amount of stage 1, 2, 3, and 4 sleep; TST, total sleep time; TSW, total amount of stages 3 + 4 sleep; TWT, total amount of wakefulness; WAFA, wake time after final awakening; WASO, wake time after sleep onset. Definitions in the REM summary are as follows: Cycles, elapsed time from sleep onset to end of first REM period, from end of first to end of second REM period, and so on; REMT, amount of REM sleep; S1, S2, WT, and MT, as defined for their total amounts; SEG, number of REM sleep segments within the REM period; TT, total time of the REM episode. All other items are self-explanatory.

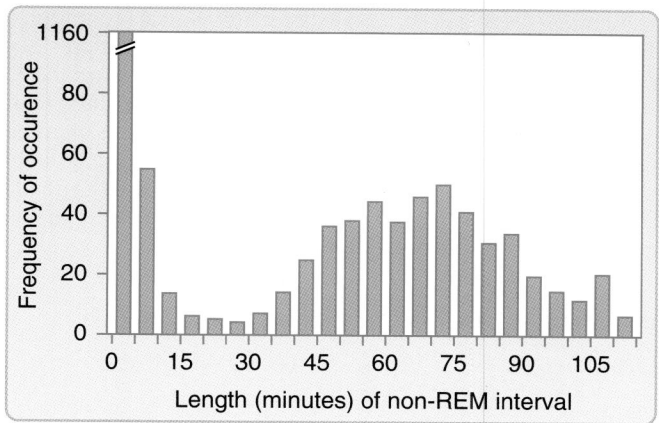

Figure 116–17. A frequency histogram illustrating the distribution of NREM (wakefulness, NREM sleep, and/or movement time) intervals of various duration during REM sleep episodes. Data are combined from the second laboratory night recorded from 82 adolescents, 18 young adults, and 26 older adults. Virtually no intervals of 15 to 30 minutes were recorded in these volunteers, suggesting that a combining rule in the range of 15 to 30 minutes will reflect the cyclic organization of REM sleep. (A 25-minute combining rule was used in the sleep stage summary sheet in Figure 116–16.)

from the fact that REM sleep episodes are noncontinuous—that is, as described earlier, REM sleep may be interrupted by stages 1 or 2, wakefulness, or movement time. Thus, one must choose a combining rule for defining REM episodes, which in turn defines the cycle. In the past, combining rules of 0, 5, 10, 15,

and 25 minutes have been used.[71] (This means that a new REM cycle is begun when the NREM interval exceeds the time designated by the combining rule.) When data are evaluated using a number of alternatives, a 15- to 25-minute rule is generally recommended.[71] Dement[72] originally recommended a 25-minute combining rule based on the frequency distribution of NREM intervals separating epochs of REM sleep. We replicated this finding, as illustrated in Figure 116–17, confirming Dement's results in adolescent, adult, and older adult volunteers. These data suggest that a combining rule of 15 to 30 minutes will provide the best description of REM sleep in humans.

Partitioning the Night

For many years, it has been a common practice to examine at least waking, slow wave (stages 3 plus 4) sleep, and REM sleep by thirds of the night. This practice, at least for REM sleep, seems to have originated in early studies of insomnia and sleeping pills.[73] Its usefulness derives primarily from normative studies in young adults, in which one sees a predominance of stage 3 and 4 NREM sleep in the first third of sleep and a predominance of REM sleep toward the last third of sleep. In patients with insomnia, preferential distribution of waking to a third of the night may provide insight regarding the type of sleep problem.[74] Although these specific comparisons are not always useful or appropriate, the thirds-of-night analysis remains a valuable thumbnail description of a night's sleep. Other variations of this partitioning technique may use halves or quarters of the night or even hour-by-hour assessment (Fig. 116–18).

Analysis by fraction (1/3):

	1	2	3
Wake	0.00	6.98	12.20
SW	91.94	13.18	23.41
REM	0.00	11.90	45.08

Analysis by fraction (1/4):

	1	2	3	4
Wake	0.00	1.00	8.45	9.72
SW	79.29	12.65	19.48	17.11
REM	0.00	2.95	20.09	33.93

Analysis by fraction (1/2):

	1	2
Wake	1.00	18.18
SW	91.94	36.59
REM	2.95	54.03

Analysis by interval (60 minutes):

	1	2	3	4	5	6	7	8	9
Wake	0.00	0.00	0.00	0.00	5.50	1.48	3.47	0.00	17.53
SW	43.82	22.67	25.45	0.00	0.00	17.50	1.98	13.19	3.91
REM	0.00	0.00	0.00	2.95	4.55	4.41	21.80	0.00	23.27

Figure 116–18. The sleep data summary may partition the night in one of several ways, depending on the purpose of the study or the questions being asked. The example in this figure, based on the night summarized in Figure 116-16, illustrates partitioning by thirds, quarters, and halves of the night, and hour by hour across the night.

Events

Events coded during sleep (see Table 116–2) are frequently tabulated according to whether they occurred in NREM or in REM sleep. Finer distinctions are rarely made. When the event (e.g., respiratory disturbance) spans more than one epoch, it is recommended that it be catalogued according to the stage in which it began.

Sleep Hypnogram

Another way to examine events is in correlation with the ongoing pattern of nocturnal sleep, as visualized using hypnogram plotting techniques. Figure 116–19 shows an example of such a plot. Sleep stages and transitions are illustrated in the upper portion of the plot and show the unfolding of sleep versus time. This type of graphic display has been used from the earliest modern sleep studies.[4] Events are usually plotted below the histogram, aligned temporally with their occurrence. This plotting technique provides a sometimes very helpful visual representation of the data, and many software packages that provide data reduction of sleep stages and events also have such plotting capabilities.

WHY STAGE SLEEP?

A number of investigators and clinicians coming to the field of sleep from other disciplines question the necessity for evaluating sleep stages, particularly in clinical conditions. Thus, for example, a pulmonary specialist may question sleep staging in a patient with apnea for whom the key issues to the specialist may be length of apnea, degree of desaturation, cardiac arrhythmias, and so forth. A urologist's focus may be penile circumference, which does not require distinctions of sleep staging. Thus, an argument can be and has been made for focusing on the pathologic event rather than sleep per se. A few counterarguments follow.

Regulatory Physiology Differs from Waking to NREM Sleep to REM Sleep

As increasing numbers of systems are evaluated during naturally occurring wakefulness and sleep, it has become quite clear that many regulatory mechanisms are affected by state.[75] For example, the ventilatory responses to oxygen and carbon dioxide (see Chapter 18) are somewhat damped in NREM sleep and may be absent in REM sleep.[76,77] Another dramatic example concerns thermoregulation. Thermoregulatory responses are only slightly altered in NREM sleep and almost totally lacking in REM sleep.[78] Such marked state-dependent alterations in regulatory physiology must be taken into account to assess fully the implications of observed sleep-related pathologies.

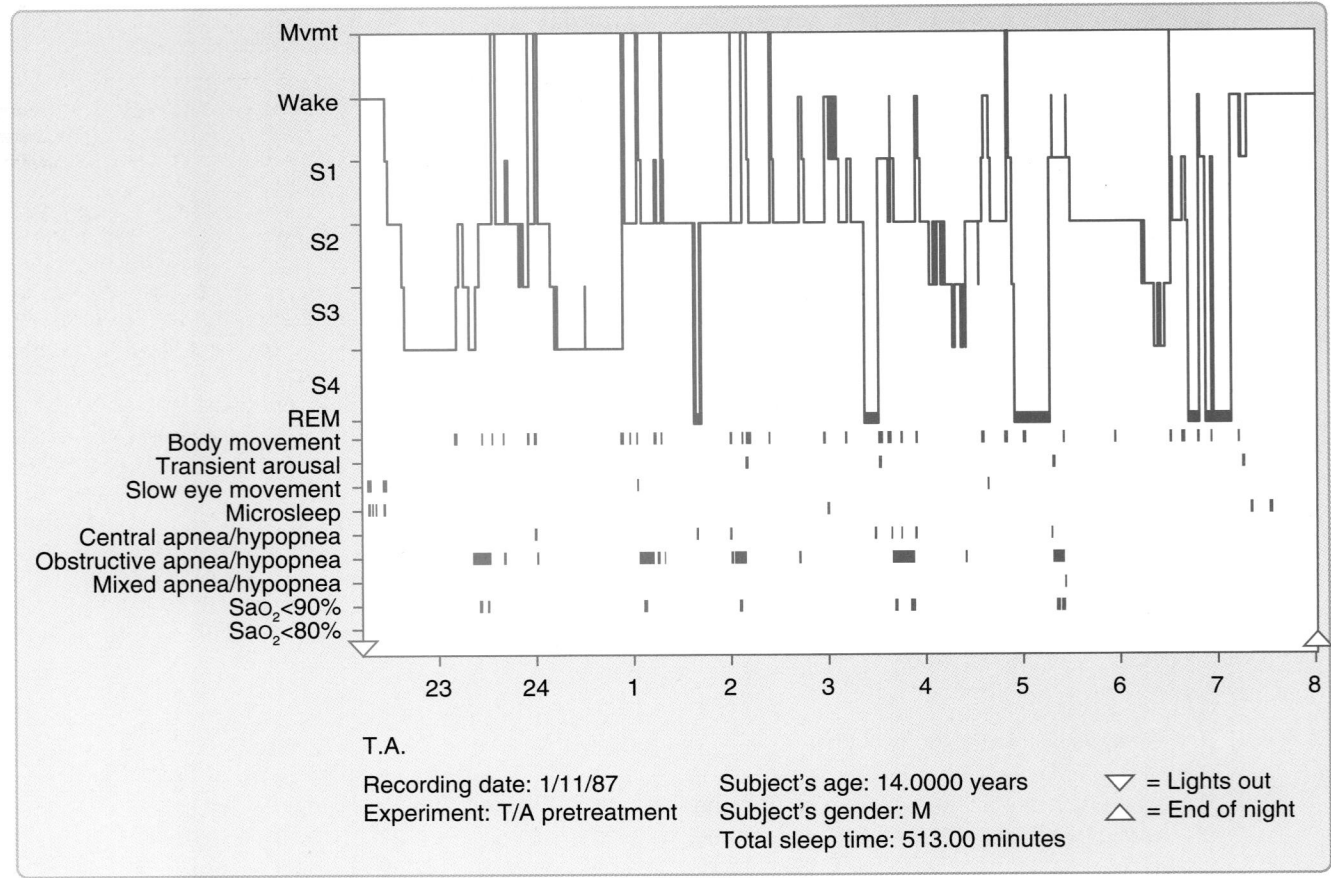

Figure 116–19. A sleep histogram of the same night of sleep summarized in Figure 116–16. The sleep histogram provides a graphic display of the night using an analogue plot of sleep–wake stages across time *(upper portion)*. Arrayed beneath this plot are event markers, which are temporally aligned.

Pathologic Events Disturb Sleep

Patients with sleep apnea syndromes, for example, have markedly disrupted sleep. In children, the disruption may preferentially reduce stage 3 and 4 sleep,[79] and sleep apnea may be associated with growth problems[80]; in adults, sleep apnea is more likely to occur during, and be disruptive of, REM sleep.[81] The possible clinical relevance of such a sleep disturbance in a child is obvious but cannot be appreciated if sleep states are not evaluated. Documentation of recovery sleep after treatment may also provide insights into therapeutic efficacy that may be unrelated to the pathologic events (i.e., the apneas) per se.

Arousals consequent to sleep pathologies are also clinically relevant and require assessment to fully characterize the pathology. Thus, as mentioned previously, arousals are clearly related to daytime sleepiness.[48,49] In the case of patients with sleep apnea syndromes, a given treatment may improve the apnea—as documented by the maintenance of arterial oxyhemoglobin saturation (SaO_2) at more than 85%, reduction in cardiac arrhythmias, and conversion of apneas to hypopneas—yet the patient may still suffer arousals from sleep sufficient to impair waking function or to be associated with a vulnerability to unintentional sleep episodes. Hence, it is relevant to evaluate sleep and arousals as well as the respiratory function in such patients. Arousals may be a relevant issue in the case of periodic movements during sleep as well. One study has documented clinical improvement of patients in whom periodic movements during sleep were treated with benzodiazepine hypnotics, although the number of movements was unchanged from pretreatment.[82] The number of associated arousals and the amount of transitional stage 1 sleep were reduced, however—a factor that would have been overlooked had sleep staging not been performed.

Sleep State May Affect Pathology

It has been known for many years that penile tumescence occurs in association with REM sleep in normal males of virtually all ages.[83] This phenomenon has been capitalized on to assess erectile dysfunction by recording REM sleep–related nocturnal penile tumescence (NPT).[84] Various clinicians, however, have attempted to perform studies of NPT in patients outside the sleep laboratory using such techniques as the "postage stamp" method.[85] Other methodologic considerations aside[86] (because the argument obtains even if appropriate NPT techniques are used without monitoring sleep stage), one cannot achieve a valid test of NPT if sleep is not assessed. This is true simply because an "abnormal" NPT can result if REM sleep is abnormal, disrupted, or absent. Sleep disorders themselves may have an impact on NPT as well.[87] Therefore, without evaluating sleep, it is not possible to determine whether tumescence did not occur because erectile function was impaired or because sleep was disturbed.

Another example again concerns sleep apnea syndromes. As mentioned previously, sleep apneas in a percentage of adult patients may occur preferentially in REM sleep.[81] It has been suggested that diagnostic assessment of sleep apneas can be performed by monitoring respiration during a daytime nap.[88] In this case, in particular, sleep monitoring is essential because REM sleep may not occur during a daytime nap (depending on the time of the nap[89]), and, therefore, the severity of sleep apnea may be very greatly underestimated. Without documentation

of sleep state, such important clinical judgments (including optimal continuous positive airway pressure) may not be possible.[90]

An Abnormal Sleep Architecture May Be a Marker of Pathology

Patients with narcolepsy often enter sleep through REM sleep rather than experiencing the normal transition from waking to NREM sleep.[41,91] Because the symptom presentation of narcolepsy is variable,[92] it is relevant to document the sleep onset transition in patients with complaints of hypersomnolence. Relatively short REM onset latencies are also thought to be a marker of endogenous depression.[93]

In summary, laboratory monitoring and staging of sleep remain important components in the assessment of patients with sleep disorders. The techniques derive directly from the earliest studies following the discovery of REM sleep in the 1950s, and some might criticize that the procedures have not kept pace with technologic advances. Because automated, ambulant systems that are inexpensive, validated, and reliable are marketed, it is likely that polysomnography has begun to advance accordingly.

The Newborn Infant

Because of rapid changes in the nervous system after birth, the well-defined *stages* seen in the adult are not present, and special criteria are used to define *states*. The standard scoring manual for neonates[16] defines sleep states using behaviors, respiration, eye movements, the EEG, and muscle tone. The following states were defined: active-REM sleep, quiet sleep, and indeterminate sleep. Criteria for defining these states with examples of sleep recordings in neonates are found in the standard scoring manual for neonates.[16]

Clinical Pearls

Although ancillary physiologic data collected during sleep are important for many diagnostic purposes, sleep staging and assessment of arousals remain crucial for a full evaluation of sleep and sleep-related processes. Sleep stage scoring in clinical settings may require certain modifications from the standard manual, such as combining stages 3 and 4 to slow wave sleep or collapsing across NREM stages. The appropriate definition of sleep onset latency may vary according to the nature of the clinical condition under study. Arousals during sleep are valuable to understanding the sleep-disrupting impact of clinical conditions that might otherwise be unappreciated.

Acknowledgments

We thank Joan Mancuso for assembling the figures and Sharon Keenan, Ph.D., REEGT, RPSGT, for her comments on the technical accuracy of versions of the manuscript.

REFERENCES

1. Rechtschaffen A, Kales A (eds): A Manual of Standardized Terminology: Techniques and Scoring System for Sleep Stages of Human Subjects. Los Angeles, UCLA Brain Information Service/Brain Research Institute, 1968.

2. Loomis AL, Harvey EN, Hobart GA: Electrical potentials of the human brain. J Exp Psychol 1936;19:249-279.

3. Aserinsky E, Kleitman N: Regularly occurring periods of eye motility, and concomitant phenomena, during sleep. Science 1953;118:273-274.

4. Dement WC, Kleitman N: Cyclic variations in EEG during sleep and their relation to eye movements, body motility, and dreaming. Electroencephalogr Clin Neurophysiol 1957;9:673-690.

5. Berger RJ: Tonus of extrinsic laryngeal muscles during sleep and dreaming. Science 1961;134:840.

6. Jouvet M, Michel M: Correlations electromyographiques du sommeil chez le chat décortiqué et mesencephalique chronique. CR Soc Biol (Paris) 1959;153:422-425.

7. Jasper HH (Committee Chairman): The ten twenty electrode system of the International Federation. Electroencephalogr Clin Neurophysiol 1958;10:371-375.

8. Grass ER: A Second AIDS Alert. Quincy, Mass: Grass Instrument Company Bulletin, September 1-2, 1985.

9. Blake H, Gerard RW, Kleitman N: Factors influencing brain potentials during sleep. J Neurophysiol 1939;2:48-60.

10. Brazier MAB: The electrical fields at the surface of the head during sleep. Electroencephalogr Clin Neurophysiol 1949;1:195-204.

11. Carskadon MA: Basics for polygraphic monitoring of sleep. In Guilleminault C (ed): Sleeping and Waking Disorders: Indications and Techniques. Menlo Park, Calif, Addison-Wesley, 1982, pp 1-16.

12. Williams RL, Karacan I, Hursch CJ: EEG of Human Sleep: Clinical Applications. New York, John Wiley & Sons, 1974.

13. Carskadon MA: The second decade. In Guilleminault C (ed): Sleeping and Waking Disorders: Indications and Techniques. Menlo Park, Calif, Addison-Wesley, 1982, pp 99-125.

14. Coble PA, Kupfer DJ, Taska LS, et al: EEG sleep of normal healthy children: Part I. Findings using standard measurement methods. Sleep 1984;7:289-303.

15. Carskadon MA, Orav EJ, Dement WC: Evolution of sleep and daytime sleepiness in adolescents. In Guilleminault C, Lugaresi E (eds): Sleep/Wake Disorders: Natural History, Epidemiology, and Long-Term Evolution. New York, Raven Press, 1983, pp 201-216.

16. Anders T, Emde R, Parmelee A (eds): A Manual of Standardized Terminology: Techniques and Criteria for Scoring of States of Sleep and Wakefulness in Newborn Infants. Los Angeles, UCLA Brain Information Service/Brain Research Institute, 1971.

17. Guilleminault C, Souquet M: Sleep states and related pathology. In Korobkin R, Guilleminault C (eds): Advances in Perinatal Neurology. New York, Spectrum, 1979, pp 225-247.

18. Carskadon MA: Determinants of daytime sleepiness: Adolescent development, extended and restricted nocturnal sleep (Dissertation). Stanford, Calif, Stanford University, 1979.

19. DiPerri R, Meduri M, DiRosa AE, et al: Sleep spindles in healthy people: I. Quantitative, automatic analysis in young-adult subjects. Boll Soc Ital Biol Sper 1977;53:983-989.

20. Dement WC: The nature and function of sleep. In Reynolds D, Sjoberg A (eds): Neuroelectric Research: Electroneuroprosthesis, Electroanesthesia, and Nonconvulsive Electrotherapy. Springfield, Ill, Charles C Thomas, 1970, pp 171-204.

21. Gaillard J-M, Blois R: Spindle density in sleep of normal subjects. Sleep 1981;4:385-391.

22. Johnson LC, Spinweber CL, Seidel WF, et al: Sleep spindle and delta changes during chronic use of a short-acting and a long-acting benzodiazepine hypnotic. Electroencephalogr Clin Neurophysiol 1983;55:662-667.

23. Crowell DH, Kapuniai LE, Boychuk RB, et al: Daytime sleep stage organization in three-month-old infants. Electroencephalogr Clin Neurophysiol 1982;53:36-47.

24. Ellingson RJ: Development of sleep spindle bursts during the first year of life. Sleep 1982;5:39-46.

25. Shibagaki M, Kiyono S, Watanabe K: Spindle evolution in normal and mentally retarded children: A review. Sleep 1982;5:47-57.

26. Prinz PN, Raskind M: Aging and sleep disorders. In Williams R, Karacan I (eds): Sleep Disorders: Diagnosis and Treatment. New York, John Wiley & Sons, 1978, pp 303-321.

27. Principe JC, Smith JR: Sleep spindle characteristics as a function of age. Sleep 1982;5:73-84.

28. Hirschkowitz M, Thornby JI, Karacan I: Sleep spindles: Pharmacologic effects in humans. Sleep 1982;5:85-94.

29. Van Leeuwen S (Chairman): Proposal for an EEG terminology by the Terminology Committee of the International Federation for Electroencephalography and Clinical Neurophysiology. Electroencephalogr Clin Neurophysiol 1966;20:293-304.

30. Johnson LC, Karpan WE: Autonomic correlates of the spontaneous K complex. Psychophysiology 1968;4:444-452.

31. Halász P, Pál I, Rajna P: K complex formation of the EEG in sleep: A survey and new examinations. Acta Physiol Acad Sci Hung 1985;65:3-35.

32. Berger RJ, Olley P, Oswald I: The EEG, eye movements and dreams of the blind. Q J Exp Psychol 1962;14:182-186.

33. Yasoshima A, Hayashi H, Iijima S, et al: Potential distribution of vertex sharp wave and saw-toothed wave on the scalp. Electroencephalogr Clin Neurophysiol 1984;58:73-76.

34. Johnson LC, Nute C, Austin MT, et al: Spectral analysis of the EEG during waking and sleeping. Electroencephalogr Clin Neurophysiol 1967;23:80.

35. Jouvet M: Neurophysiology of the states of sleep. Physiol Rev 1967;47:117-177.

36. Freemon FR: Sleep Research: A Critical Review. Springfield, Ill, Charles C Thomas, 1972.

37. Hodes R, Dement WC: Depression of electrically induced reflexes ("H-reflexes") in man during low voltage EEG "sleep." Electroencephalogr Clin Neurophysiol 1964;17:617-629.

38. Salzarulo P, Lairy GC, Bancaud J, et al: Direct depth recording of the striate cortex during REM sleep in man: Are there PGO potentials? Electroencephalogr Clin Neurophysiol 1975;38:192-202.

39. Aserinsky E: The maximal capacity for sleep: Rapid eye movement density as an index of sleep satiety. Biol Psychiatry 1969;1:147-159.

40. Chase MH: Synaptic mechanisms and circuitry involved in motoneuron control during sleep. Int Rev Neurobiol 1983;24:213-258.

41. Montplaisir J, Billiard M, Takahashi S, et al: Twenty-four-hour recording in REM-narcoleptics with special reference to nocturnal sleep disruption. Biol Psychiatry 1978;13:73-89.

42. Passouant P, Cadilhac J, Ribstein M: Les privations de sommeil avec mouvements oculaires par les antidépresseurs. Rev Neurol 1972;127:173-192.

43. Passouant P, Cadilhac J, Billiard M, et al: La suppression du sommeil paradoxal par la clomipramine. Thérapie 1973;28:379-392.

44. Raynal DM: Polygraphic aspects of narcolepsy. In Guilleminault C (ed): Narcolepsy. New York, Spectrum, 1976, pp 669-684.

45. Flagg WH, Coburn SC: Appendix 2: Polygraphic aspects of sleep apnea. In Guilleminault C, Dement WC (eds): Sleep Apnea Syndromes. New York, Alan R Liss, 1978, pp 357-363.

46. Hauri P, Hawkins DR: Alpha-delta sleep. Electroencephalogr Clin Neurophysiol 1973;34:233-237.

47. Moldofsky H, Scarisbrick P, England R, et al: Musculoskeletal symptoms and nonREM sleep disturbance in patients with "fibrositis syndrome" and healthy subjects. Psychosom Med 1975;37:341-351.

48. Stepanski E, Salava W, Lamphere J, et al: Experimental sleep fragmentation and sleepiness in normal subjects: A preliminary report. Sleep Res 1984;13:193.

49. Carskadon MA, Brown ED, Dement WC: Sleep fragmentation in the elderly: Relationship to daytime sleep tendency. Neurobiol Aging 1982;3:321-327.

50. Guilleminault C: EEG arousals: Scoring rules and examples. Sleep 1992;15:173-184.

51. American Academy of Sleep Medicine: Sleep related breathing disorders in adults: Recommendations for syndrome definition and measurement techniques in clinical research. Sleep 1999; 22:667-689.

52. Exar EN, Collop NA: The upper airway resistance syndrome. Chest 1999;115:1127-1139.

53. Hosselet JJ, Norman RG, Ayappa I, et al: Detection of flow limitation with a nasal cannula/pressure transducer system. Am J Respir Crit Care Med 1998;157:1461-1467.

54. Lavie P, Gertner R, Zomer J, et al: Breathing disorders in sleep associated with "microarousals" in patients with allergic rhinitis. Acta Otolaryngol 1981;92:529-533.

55. Craig TJ, Teets S, Lehman EB, et al: Nasal congestion secondary to allergic rhinitis as a cause of sleep disturbance and daytime fatigue and the response to topical nasal corticosteroids. J Allergy Clin Immunol 1998;101:633-637.

56. Zamir G, Press J, Tal A, et al: Sleep fragmentation in children with juvenile rheumatoid arthritis. J Rheumatol 1998;25: 1191-1197.

57. Stocchi F, Barbato L, Nordera G, et al: Sleep disorders in Parkinson's disease. J Neurol 1998;245:S15-S18.

58. Pitson DJ, Stradling JR: Autonomic markers of arousal during sleep in patients undergoing investigation for obstructive sleep apnoea, their relationship to EEG arousals, respiratory events and subjective sleepiness. J Sleep Res 1998;7:53-59.

59. Lofaso F, Goldenberg F, Dortho MP, et al: Arterial blood pressure response to transient arousals from NREM sleep in nonapneic snorers with sleep fragmentation. Chest 1998;113:985-991.

60. Terzano MG, Liborio P: Origin and significance of the cyclic alternating pattern (CAP). Sleep Med Rev 2000;4:101-123.

61. Terzano MG, Parrina L, Smerieri A, et al: Atlas, rules, and recording techniques for the scoring of cyclic alternating pattern (CAP) in human sleep. Sleep Med 2001;2:537-553.

62. Burger D, Cantani P, West J: Multidimensional analysis of sleep electrophysiological signals. Biol Cybern 1977;26:131-139.

63. Gath I, Bar-On E: Computerized method for scoring of polygraphic sleep recordings. Comput Prog Biomed 1980;11:217-223.

64. Ray SR, Lee WD, Morgan CD, et al: Computer sleep stage scoring—an expert system approach. Int J Biomed Comput 1986; 19:43-61.

65. Gaillard J-M, Tissot R: Principles of automatic analysis of sleep records with a hybrid system. Comput Biomed Res 1973;6:1-13.

66. Smith JR, Karacan I, Yang M: Automated analysis of human sleep EEG. Waking Sleep 1978;2:75-82.

67. Martens WLJ, Declerck AC, Kums DJT, et al: Considerations on a computerized analysis of long-term polygraphic recordings. In Stefan H, Burr W (eds): EEG Monitoring. Stuttgart, Germany, Gustav Fischer, 1982, pp 265-274.

68. Agnew HW, Webb WB: Measurement of sleep onset by EEG criteria. Am J EEG Technol 1972;12:127-134.

69. Webb WB: Recording methods and visual scoring criteria of sleep records: Comments and recommendations. Percept Mot Skills 1986;62:664-666.

70. Kupfer DJ, Targ E, Stack J: Electroencephalographic sleep in unipolar depressive subtypes: Support for a biological and familial classification. J Nerv Ment Dis 1982;170:494-498.

71. Webb WB, Dreblow LM: The REM cycle, combining rules and age. Sleep 1982;5:372-377.

72. Dement WC: Physiology of Dreaming (Dissertation). Chicago, University of Chicago, 1958.

73. Kales A, Allen C, Scharf M, et al: Hypnotic drugs and their effectiveness: All-night EEG studies of insomniac subjects. Arch Gen Psychiatry 1970;23:226-232.

74. Kales A, Bixler EO, Vela-Bueno A, et al: Biopsychobehavioral correlates of insomnia: III. Polygraphic findings of sleep difficulty and their relationship to psychopathology. Int J Neurosci 1984; 23:43-56.

75. Orem J, Barnes CD (eds): Physiology in Sleep. New York, Academic Press, 1980.

76. Phillipson EA, Sullivan CE, Read DJ, et al: Ventilatory and waking responses to hypoxia in sleeping dogs. J Appl Physiol 1978; 44:512-520.

77. Phillipson EA, Kozar LF, Rebuck AS, et al: Ventilatory and waking responses to CO_2 in sleeping dogs. Am Rev Respir Dis 1977; 115:251-259.

78. Parmeggiani PL: Temperature regulation during sleep: A study in homeostasis. In Orem J, Barnes CD (eds): Physiology in Sleep. New York, Academic Press, 1980, pp 98-145.

79. Guilleminault C, Eldridge FL, Simmons FB, et al: Sleep apnea in eight children. Pediatrics 1976;58:23-31.

80. Brouillette RT, Fernbach SK, Hunt CE: Obstructive sleep apnea in infants and children. J Pediatr 1982;100:31-40.

81. Sackner MA, Lauda J, Forrest T, et al: Periodic sleep apnea: Chronic sleep deprivation related to intermittent upper airway obstruction and central nervous system disturbance. Chest 1975;67:164-171.

82. Mitler MM, Browman CP, Menn SJ, et al: Nocturnal myoclonus: Treatment efficacy of clonazepam and temazepam. Sleep 1986;9:385-392.

83. Karacan I: The developmental aspect and the effect of certain clinical conditions upon penile erection during sleep. Excerpta Med 1966;150:2356-2359.

84. Karacan I: The clinical value of nocturnal erection in the prognosis and diagnosis of impotence. Hum Sex 1970;4:27-34.

85. Barry JM, Blank B, Bioleau M: Nocturnal penile tumescence monitoring with stamps. Urology 1980;15:171-172.

86. Karacan I, Aslan C, Williams RL: Reliability of stamp ring as indicator of penile rigidity in the diagnosis of impotence. Sleep Res 1982;11:202.

87. Pressman MR, DiPhillips MA, Kendrick JI, et al: Problems in the interpretation of nocturnal penile tumescence studies: Disruption of sleep by occult sleep disorders. J Urol 1986;136: 595-598.

88. Goode GB, Slyter HM: Daytime polysomnogram diagnosis of sleep apnea. Trans Am Neurol Assoc 1980;105:367-370.

89. Karacan I, Finley W, Williams R, et al: Changes in stage 1-REM and stage 4 sleep during naps. Biol Psychiatry 1970;2:261-265.

90. Oksenberg A, Silverberg DS, Arons E, et al: The sleep supine position has a major effect on optimal nasal continuous positive airway pressure: Relationship with rapid eye movements and non-rapid eye movements sleep, body mass index, respiratory disturbance index, and age. Chest 1999;116:1000-1006.

91. Vogel G: Studies in the psychophysiology of dreams: III. The dreams of narcolepsy. Arch Gen Psychiatry 1960;3:421-428.

92. Zarcone V: Narcolepsy: A review of the syndrome. N Engl J Med 1973;288:1156-1166.

93. Kupfer DJ: A psychobiologic marker for primary depressive disease. Biol Psychiatry 1976;11:159-174.

117

Monitoring Techniques for Evaluating Suspected Sleep-Disordered Breathing

Max Hirshkowitz

Meir H. Kryger

ABSTRACT

Sleep-disordered breathing is diagnosed in adults by objectively measuring specific pathophysiologies. Many methods are used to monitor breathing, to detect breathing abnormalities, and to evaluate physiologic alterations produced by abnormal breathing events in adults. Data acquisition systems, their operational paradigms, and the data collection setting (home versus laboratory) may vary a great deal. Some procedures are common to most laboratory settings and are based on expert opinion, consensus panels, and evidence-based recommendations. There is, however, some disagreement about what constitutes the most appropriate methodology, and experts do not always agree on what technique is best. Local medical resources vary. In fixed-resource environments, the clinician may have to make clinical management decisions with less-than-adequate diagnostic information. This, at times, may put the patient at risk.

OVERVIEW AND DEFINITIONS

Abnormal breathing during sleep goes by many names, including sleep apnea, sleep-disordered breathing, sleep-related breathing disorders, periodic breathing, Cheyne-Stokes respiration, and hypoventilation (Table 117–1). (Specific abnormal

Table 117–1. Definitions* for Some Sleep-Disordered Breathing Events and Parameters

Term	Definition
Apnea	The complete or near-complete cessation of breathing for 10 seconds, or more, in an adult
Hypopnea	A reduction in, but not cessation of, ventilation. A hypopnea is considered clinically significant if it is associated with an oxyhemoglobin desaturation event (see next), or with a CNS arousal characterized by alpha activity or EEG speeding. The CNS arousal is important because it represents a sleep continuity disturbance, and sleep fragmentation is correlated with daytime sleepiness.
Oxyhemoglobin desaturation event (ODE)	A decrease in blood oxygen saturation by 3% to 4%, or more
Desaturating hypopnea (DH)	Also know as a MediCare hypopnea, the DH is a hypopnea with a 4% or greater ODE.
Respiratory effort–related arousal (RERA) events	CNS arousals seen terminating obstructed events that do not meet the criteria for apnea or hypopnea (see reference 1)
Obstructive apnea or hypopnea episodes	Breathing events caused by obstruction of the upper airway
Central apnea or hypopnea episodes	Breathing events caused by absent or decreased respiratory effort (i.e., decreased output to the muscles of inspiration from the respiratory control system in the CNS)
Mixed apnea or hypopnea episodes	Breathing events with both obstructive and central features in the same event. Many laboratories consider mixed events to be essentially obstructive.
Sleep apnea	Sleep apnea (also known as sleep-disordered breathing or sleep-related breathing disorder) is any sleep-related respiratory abnormality diagnosed on the basis of apnea, hypopnea, and RERA events.
Periodic breathing	A regularly repeating pattern in which normal or increased ventilation alternates with and decreased or absent ventilation. Cheyne-Stokes respiration, which is found in heart failure, is an example.
Apnea index (AI)	The number of apnea episodes per hour of sleep
Apnea-hypopnea index (AHI)	The number of apnea and hypopnea episodes per hour of sleep
Oxygen desaturation index (ODI)	The number of oxyhemoglobin desaturation events per hour of sleep
Respiratory disturbance index (RDI)	The current definition for RDI is the number of apnea, hypopnea, and RERA events per hour of sleep. This term has been used differently over the years and is therefore the source of much confusion. It was first used for what is defined as ODI above; later it was used synonymously with AHI.

*Until recently, there was no official consensus on the definitions of these terms or how to document them.[1,12,72] This is the authors' interpretation of what most experts mean when they use these terms.

CNS, central nervous system; EEG, electroencephalographic.

Table 117–2. Severities of Obstructive Sleep Apnea Syndrome

Dimension	Mild	Moderate	Severe
Sleepiness or unintended sleep episodes	During activities requiring *little* attention (e.g., watching television)	During activities requiring *some* attention (e.g., business meeting)	During activities requiring *active* attention (e.g., driving a car)
Sleep-related obstructive breathing events per hour	5-15	15-30	>30

breathing patterns associated with neurologic lesions are described in Chapter 68.) Some terms distinguish between different types of sleep-related breathing impairments, but others are virtually synonymous. Sleep-disordered breathing events include apneas and hypopneas. Although apnea is defined fairly consistently, hypopnea definitions vary widely. Part of the difficulty is that hypopnea per se is not necessarily pathophysiologic—it is merely a shallow breath. When, however, a hypopnea is associated with abnormal or detrimental sequelae, it is deemed pathophysiologic. It is the abnormal consequence, be it an oxyhemoglobin desaturation or a central nervous system arousal, that makes a hypopnea relevant to sleep-disordered breathing. The second part of the difficulty stems from the widespread use of nonquantitative measures to index airflow. Thus, the airflow signal diminution and decreased tidal volume correlate poorly. Consequently, operational definitions for hypopnea based on percent flow decrease result in arbitrary cut-points. Apnea and hypopnea episodes are further categorized as obstructive, central, and mixed. This categorization reflects the presence or absence of respiratory effort during the event.

The severity of sleep-disordered breathing can be defined using a clinical dimension (e.g., sleepiness, as seen in Table 117–2) or it can based on pathophysiology (e.g., the apnea-hypopnea index [AHI] or the respiratory disturbance index). When the severity is defined by two measures (e.g., by the history and by laboratory assessment), the overall status of the patient should reflect the more severely affected dimension.[1]

There is no general agreement about assigning severity descriptors to indices of sleep-disordered breathing; however, two schemes are commonly used. In the first (the liberal) classification, an AHI between 5 and 15 is mild, between 15 and 30 is moderate, and greater than 30 is severe. In the second (the conservative) classification, an AHI between 10 and 20 is mild, between 20 and 50 is moderate, and greater than 50 is severe.[2] Finally, there is no consensus on how best to report the frequency of the physiologic changes in the upper airway resistance syndrome. A reasonable measure seems to be the number of *arousals per hour* related to obstructive breathing events (known as respiratory event–related arousals).[3]

METHODS TO DETECT AIRFLOW

Apnea in an adult is defined as cessation or near cessation of airflow for 10 seconds or more. Occasionally, unidirectional occlusion occurs, in which there is no airflow during attempted inspiration but tiny puffs in expiration. The airflow can be evaluated quantitatively using a pneumotachograph. Airflow can also be measured qualitatively or by detecting chemical or physical differences between expired air and ambient air.

Pneumotachography

Several types of pneumotachographs based on different physical principles are in use: differential pressure airflow transducers, ultrasonic flowmeters, and hot wire anemometers. This discussion focuses on the differential pressure flow transducer, which is the most widely used.

Airflow is directed through a cylinder. Before exiting the cylinder, the air passes through a small resistive field, usually small parallel tubes or a grill that promotes laminar flow. The pressure drop across this resistive field is measured by a differential manometer. When flow is laminar, there is a linear relationship between the pressure differences and flow. The pressure–flow relationship is altered by changes in gas density, viscosity, and temperature. Heating is required to prevent condensation on the resistive element, so calibration should be done when the pneumotachograph is heated. Correction factors can be used to minimize the error introduced by alterations in these physical factors. The flow signal can be integrated electronically or digitally to obtain volume.

In sleep research applications, the pneumotachograph is usually connected to a face mask. Although this combination of pneumotachograph and face mask is the most accurate means of assessing the volume of airflow, it is a relatively large, uncomfortable device, making it often unsuitable for many clinical respiratory studies during sleep. In awake patients, invasive devices alter breathing pattern; tidal volume increases, and breathing frequency is either decreased or unchanged. Some of the newer bilevel positive airway pressure and continuous positive airway pressure (CPAP) machines have pneumotachographs built in, so these devices can be used to monitor airflow and ventilation. Cardiogenic oscillations, which are markers of central apnea, can be detected with these systems.[4]

Nasal Airway Pressure

During inspiration, airway pressure is negative relative to atmosphere, and during expiration, airway pressure is positive relative to atmosphere. Some investigators have suggested that measurement of these pressure changes in the nasal airway may be used to estimate airflow.[5,6] It has been shown that such a pressure signal resembles that obtained with a pneumotachograph.[5] This measurement appears to be much more sensitive in detecting the type of flow limitation seen in the upper airway resistance syndrome than the thermistor (Fig. 117–1).[6] Airflow limitation is inferred when a plateau is present on the pressure trace during inspiration. It has been shown that such a system tracks changes in upper airway resistance and flow limitation in patients.[7] Such a system requires careful attention to signal conditioning. The optimal signal is obtained by using a direct current (DC) amplifier; if an alternating current (AC) amplifier is used, then a long

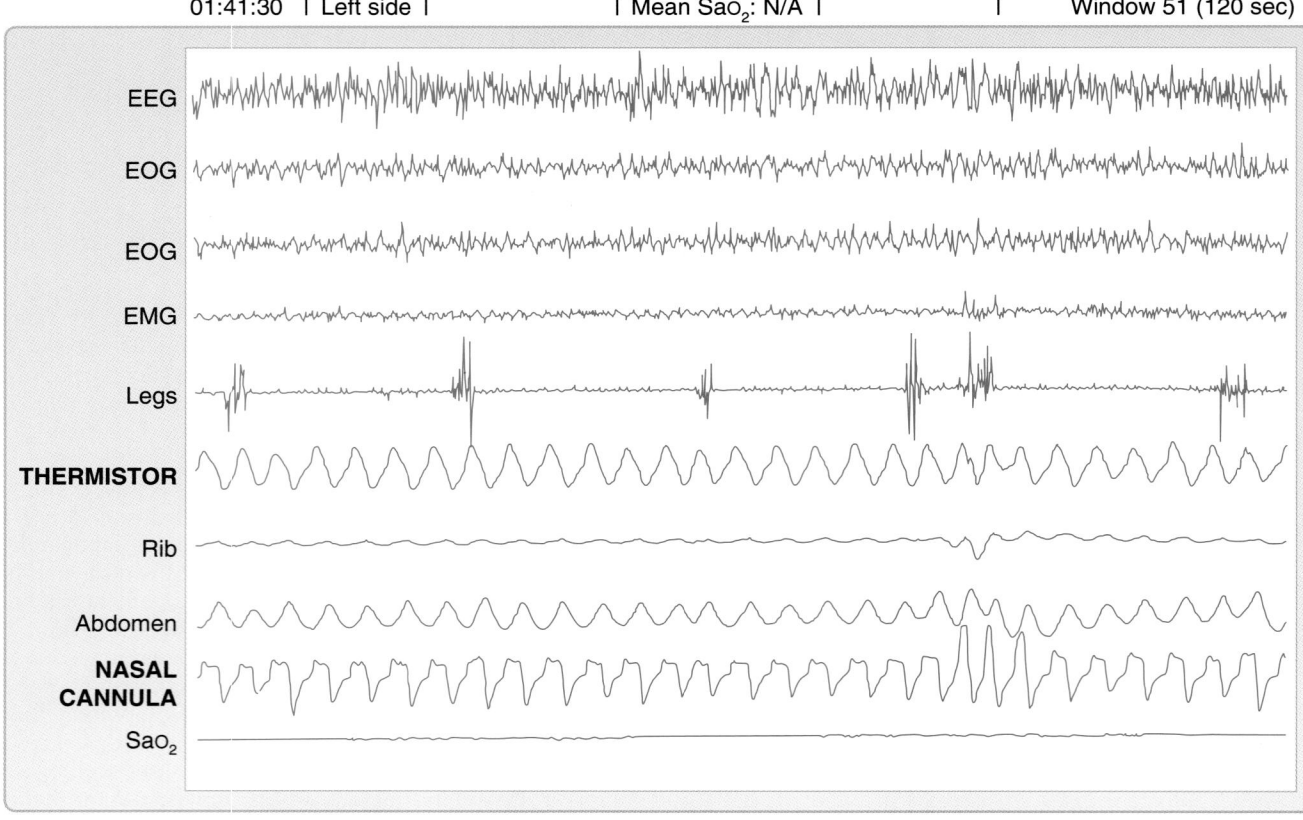

01:41:30 | Left side | | Mean Sao₂: N/A | | Window 51 (120 sec)

EEG

EOG

EOG

EMG

Legs

THERMISTOR

Rib

Abdomen

NASAL CANNULA

Sao₂

Figure 117–1. A 120-second section from a nocturnal polysomnogram in a subject undergoing simultaneous recording with a conventional thermistor and with a nasal cannula used for recording pressure. In this subject, there is nothing in the thermistor tracing to suggest a respiratory event, and there is only a suggestion of a movement in the rib and abdominal inductance plethysmographic tracings. However, in the nasal cannula tracing, the end of a hypopnea and the beginning of another are easily detected. Notice the plateaus (chopped off tops) of the pressure traces during hypopnea. EEG, electroencephalogram; EMG, electromyogram; EOG, electrooculogram; Sao₂, oxygen saturation in arterial blood. (Courtesy of Dr. David Rappaport.)

time-constant filter should be used. A short time-constant filter may result in artifacts (Fig. 117–2).[6] The role of this relatively new methodology is not entirely clear because some patients may not breathe via the nose. It does, however, seem more sensitive than the thermistor.

Thermistors and Thermocouples

During inspiration, air is rapidly heated so that air in the lungs reaches core body temperature. There is a large temperature difference between air coming out of the respiratory system (body temperature) and air going into the respiratory system. Therefore, simply measuring the temperature in front of the nose and mouth can be used to detect expiration.

A thermistor is a thermally sensitive resistor that is supplied with a constant but low current. The use of a low current reduces the tendency of the thermistor to heat itself. Thermistors are designed to maximize the sensing area while minimizing the size and mass of the sensor. This design results in the thermistor being more sensitive to changes in airflow. Small temperature changes should produce large resistance changes. Care must be taken to ensure that the operating temperature of the thermistor is below body temperature; otherwise, expiratory airflow may not always be detected. An unheated thermistor cannot accurately differentiate prolonged inspiratory activity

from a respiratory pause. A thermistor ceases being an airflow sensor if it touches the skin, because it will remain at body temperature.

A thermocouple likewise senses changes in temperature, but it uses a different approach. Essentially, it capitalizes on the fact that different metals have different coefficients of expansion and, when calibrated, a change can be transduced to voltage alterations displayable on polygraph systems. Thermistors or thermocouples are placed in the path of air flow from the nose and mouth. Expired airflow heats the sensor, increasing its resistance, and inspiratory airflow cools the sensor to ambient temperature, resulting in a relative decrease in the resistance that can then be recorded.

Expired Carbon Dioxide Sensing

Air leaving the lungs has a much higher concentration of CO_2 than ambient air. There is always a large CO_2 difference between air coming from the respiratory system and air going into the respiratory system. Thus, simply measuring CO_2 in front of the nose and mouth can detect expiration. An infrared analyzer is frequently used to measure the concentration of CO_2.

Measuring CO_2 pressure offers several advantages over measuring nasal pressure or using thermistors. First, in some patients, the end-of-breath concentration may yield an end-tidal P_{CO_2}.

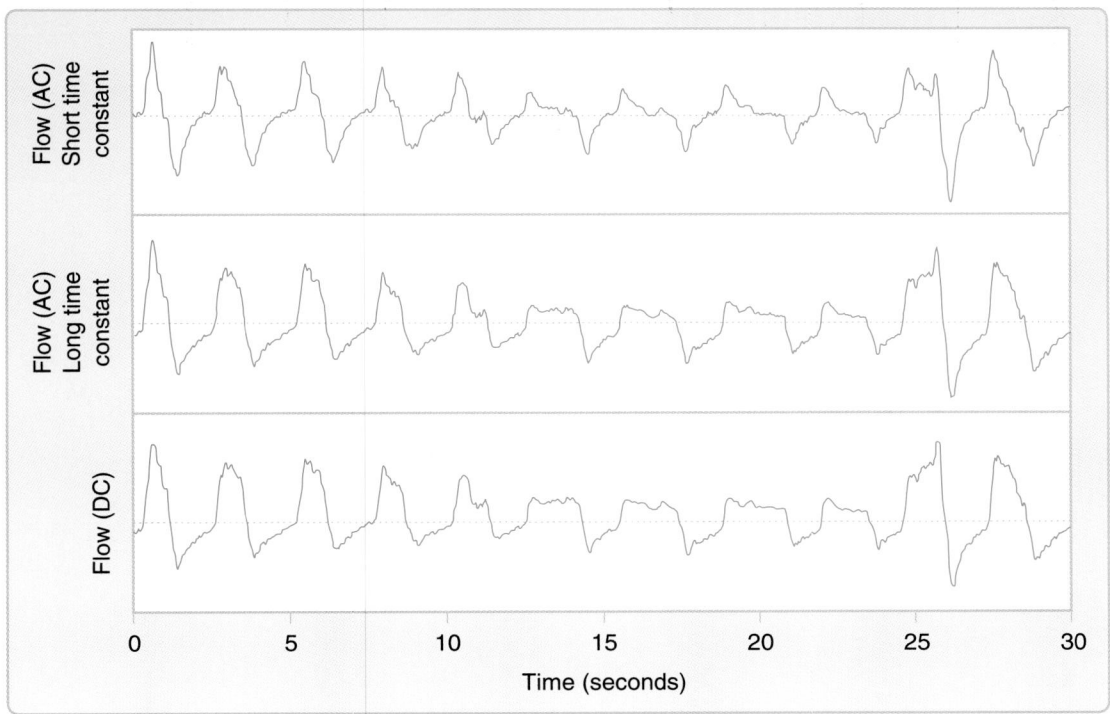

Figure 117–2. A. flow limitation event recorded from the nasal cannula measuring pressure simultaneously amplified by three different amplifiers. The *bottom* signal is from a direct current (DC) amplifier with no filtering. The top two signals are from alternating current (AC) amplifiers with low-frequency filters, with time constants of 1.6 *(top)* and 5.3 *(middle)*. The short time-constant filter *(top)* causes the flow signal to decay to baseline rapidly during a period of relatively constant flow (flow limitation plateau). The longer time-constant filter *(middle)* provides reasonably good reproduction of these constant flows.

Because the catheters sampling CO_2 may also entrain some room air, the CO_2 measured is likely to be lower than the end-tidal P_{CO_2}; thus, an elevated P_{CO_2} should be accepted as real, indicating that true P_{CO_2} is even higher. Therefore, this is the only noninvasive way to sample the air stream that can potentially confirm hypoventilation. Second, the shape of the expired curve may offer useful information. When a patient originally demonstrates an expired CO_2 curve with a clear-cut plateau, the loss of the plateau (or the curve becoming smaller or dome shaped) indicates a change in breathing pattern, usually a reduction in expiratory volume. Third, during central apnea, the CO_2 tracing may show cardiogenic oscillations. These oscillations are the result of small volume displacements caused by the beating heart. These oscillations are synchronized to the heartbeat, and they prove that the upper airway is wide open (Fig. 117–3). The catheter system should be of low volume and the analyzer set on its fastest response to detect these oscillations.

Infants and children with upper airway obstruction may develop severe hypoventilation during sleep without frank apnea; this can be detected by measuring expired CO_2, but it cannot be detected with a thermistor.[8]

Problems and Artifacts in Detecting Apnea

Thermistor and devices monitoring expired gases cannot reliably differentiate between a prolonged inspiration, central apnea, and obstructive apnea. Therefore, airflow is typically recorded in conjunction with measures of respiratory effort. The differential patterns of airflow and respiratory effort are commonly used to categorize apnea and hypopnea events as central, obstructive, or mixed. Nonetheless, extreme care must be taken when classifying respiratory activity on the basis of the relationship between detection of airflow and respiratory effort. In some cases, patients may have complete occlusion on inspiration but small puffs on expiration, detectable by thermistor or CO_2 analyzer. Such patients are erroneously categorized as having hypopneas, or even normal, unobstructed breathing. An example of this phenomenon is seen in Figure 117–4. Airflow is recorded simultaneously from a CO_2 analyzer and a pneumotachograph. During the obstructive apnea, periods of expiratory airflow occur (recorded by the pneumotachograph and the CO_2 analyzer) in the absence of inspiratory flow (obvious in the pneumotachograph recording, and unclear in the CO_2 recording). Without the information from the pneumotachograph, the recording from the CO_2 analyzer would be interpreted as evidence of uninterrupted inspiratory and expiratory airflow.

An additional useful finding when recording expired CO_2 is the occurrence of cardiogenic oscillations. When the typical CO_2 changes of expiration are absent, one cannot differentiate between a prolonged inspiration, obstructive apnea, and central apnea. In this setting, the presence of prolonged cardiogenic oscillations only is proof that the upper airway is patent and that central apnea is present.

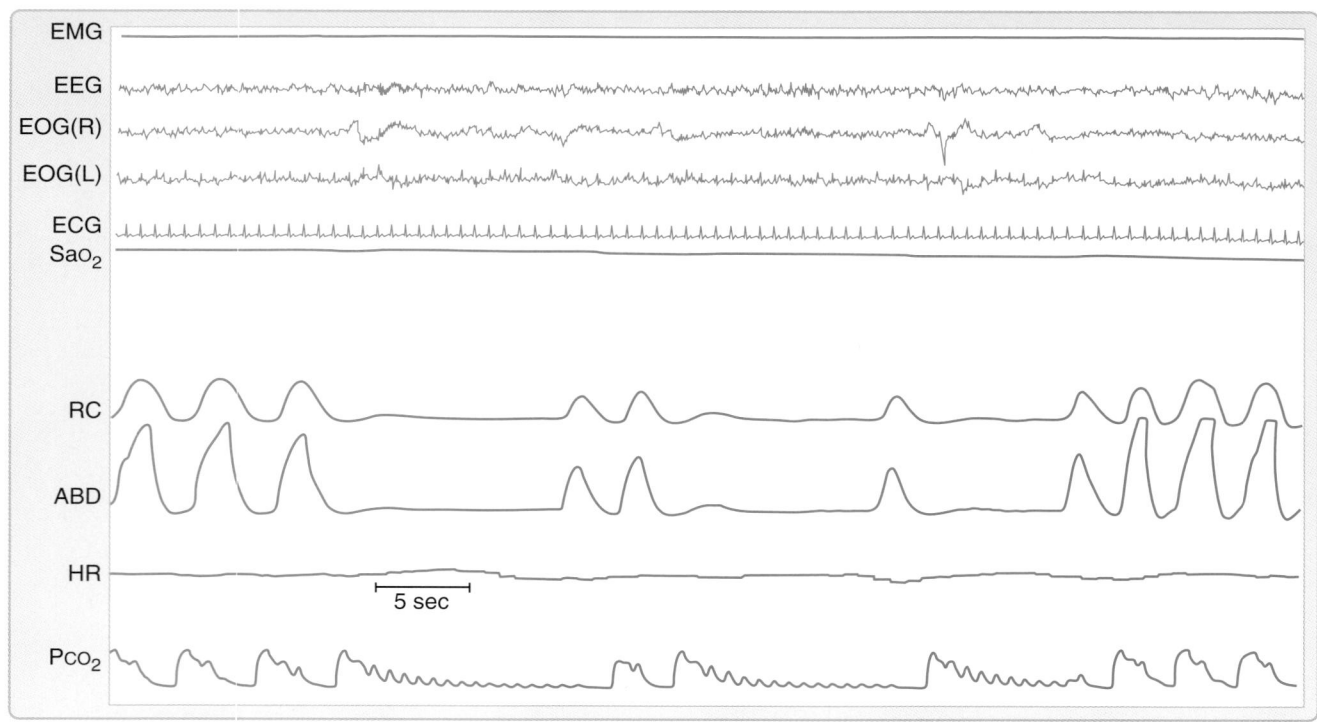

Figure 117–3. Cardiogenic oscillations in CO_2 are seen in the bottom channel in this example of central apnea. The presence of these oscillations, synchronous with the heartbeat, proves that the upper airway is patent. ABD, abdominal (movement); EEG, electroencephalogram; ECG, electrocardiogram; EMG, electromyogram; EOG, electrooculogram; HR, heart rate; RC, rib cage (movement); SaO_2, oxygen saturation in arterial blood.

ERROR IN DETECTING APNEA

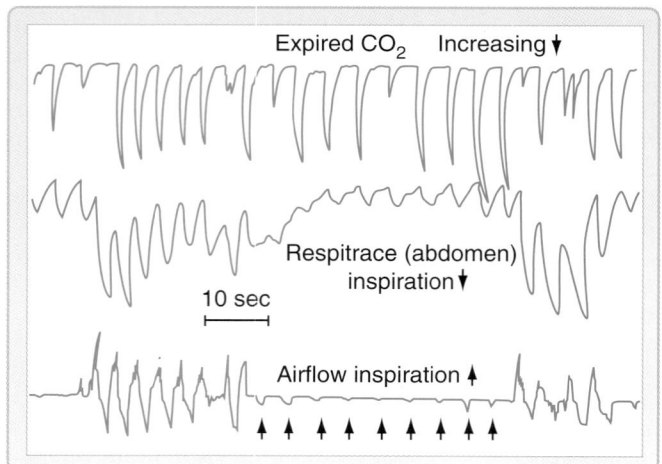

Figure 117–4. An example of the limitations of noninvasive airflow detection. *Top,* Airflow is detected with the CO_2 analyzer. *Middle,* Respiratory inductance plethysmograph (RIP). *Bottom,* Airflow measured with a pneumotachograph. With each apnea-related expiratory deflection documented by the pneumotachograph *(arrows, bottom),* there is a sustained shift in the baseline of the RIP. This suggests an incremental decrease in functional residual capacity resulting from absent inspirations with continued small expiratory puffs. If only the top two tracings were available, this pattern would have been mistakenly called hypoventilation or hypopnea, when it is clearly total occlusion on inspiration. (From West P, Kryger MH: Sleep and respiration: Terminology and methodology. Clin Chest Med 1985;6:706.)

Positive Airway Pressure as a Diagnostic Tool?

It was inevitable that positive airway pressure (PAP) systems with data collection capability would be developed. Although the information gathered focuses primarily on system utilization and adequacy of treatment, it was hardly a surprise that self-titrating machines (also called autoPAP) would be used as a de facto diagnostic system. With such systems, a patient is sent home for an empiric clinical trial with PAP, with or without a prior apnea diagnostic evaluation. The machine then monitors breathing according to flow curves, vibration, or pressure oscillation and adjusts pressure to maintain optimal breathing. A positive pressure is interpreted as indicating airway resistance or obstruction.

Several paradigms using this approach have been tried; however, results have not been well documented in a sample with a large number of patients.[9] In the first paradigm, a patient has an in-laboratory study for diagnosis followed by the use of self-adjusting PAP titration for one or more nights at home. A second option is for a patient to have level III study, followed by a home autoPAP titration study. A third paradigm is home trial with autoPAP based solely on clinical diagnosis; that is, autoPAP is initiated without any polysomnographic evaluation. The financial issues are quite complex, because reimbursement may not be available for some of this testing, and there might be expensive costs associated with such an approach if the patient or insurer has to pay for a CPAP mask, particularly in a patient who is found *not* to have sleep-disordered breathing.

There simply does not exist a scientific body of knowledge, or a consensus about the role of such types of evaluation, at this time.[10] As mentioned in Chapter 89, a clinical trial with CPAP is sometimes performed in complex cases when it is unclear whether snoring or mild sleep apnea is responsible for the symptom of daytime sleepiness in a patient with an equivocal level I study.

We frequently encounter clinical problems in patients who were initially evaluated by others using autoPAP. Sometimes patients had severe nasal obstructions that were not appreciated and consequently they could not tolerate the CPAP. Some patients slept with their mouths wide open while on nasal CPAP, and therefore the self-titrating process failed. Patients with severe respiratory disease (e.g., chronic obstructive pulmonary disease, kyphoscoliosis) may became intensely dyspneic on the self-titrating CPAP system and actually needed either bilevel positive airway pressure or home ventilation. AutoPAP titration failures include patients ultimately found to have central apnea and those with upper airway abnormalities that actually required a different modality of treatment (e.g., an oral appliance or surgical excision of tonsils and adenoids). These cases emphasize that a diagnostic system cannot rely solely on a self-titrating CPAP unit. Some patients with residual sleepiness notwithstanding treatment with CPAP turn out to have significant sleep-related movement disorder that remained untreated.

Thus, in our experience, using this mixed therapeutic–diagnostic mode as the sole "test" will result in significant problems in some subgroups of patients. We are aware of no outcome studies involving large numbers of patients that have examined the utility of such an approach. In the future, this situation will probably change as ventilatory devices are enhanced with more sophisticated diagnostic capabilities. However, it is unrealistic to expect computerized systems to deal with a claustrophobic patient panicking on CPAP, a patient complaining of a dry sore throat, a patient with severe nasal allergies, and the multitude of problems encountered in the clinic requiring troubleshooting of the mask (fit or leaks) or the CPAP machine.

METHODS TO DETECT RESPIRATORY EFFORT

Rib Cage and Abdominal Motion

Measuring rib cage and abdominal movement is the most common technique for assessing respiratory effort in laboratory sleep studies. During normal breathing, contraction of the major inspiratory muscle, the diaphragm, produces both rib cage expansion and a downward movement of the diaphragm. These movements cause the pressure around and in the lung to become negative relative to atmosphere. The pressure gradient between ambient air and the lung results in airflow into the lung. Thus, a change in lung volume is the sum of the volume changes of the structures surrounding the lungs, the rib cage and the abdomen.[11] Other respiratory muscles (intercostal, sternocleidomastoid, and so on) also play a role in stabilizing the thoracic cage. Some clinicians erroneously interpret the abdominal and rib cage motion changes as implying separate activities of abdominal and thoracic respiratory muscles, but this is not the case. Virtually all the changes in abdominal and rib cage volumes (including paradoxical motion) can be explained by changes in the respiratory muscles directly inserting onto the thoracic cage, as described later.

Normally, the enlargement of the thorax and the outward movement of the abdominal wall occur together, that is, they are *in phase*. For a given change in lung volume, one can thus quantify a change in rib cage volume and abdominal volume. For a given breath, the relative contributions of the rib cage and abdominal compartments also can be determined. If it is assumed that the fractional contributions of the abdomen and the rib cage are constant, then changes in lung volume can be measured by calibrating transducers sensitive to rib cage and abdominal displacement. The relative rib cage and abdominal contributions may change with posture and with the changes in muscle tone occurring in sleep; thus, the devices (mentioned later) can be calibrated, but their calibration may change markedly during the night.

Paradoxical motion of the rib cage and abdomen occurs with loss of tone of the diaphragm, with loss of tone of the other respiratory muscles, or with complete or partial upper airway obstruction. The mechanisms underlying this asynchronous motion of rib cage and abdomen are described in Table 117–3.

Respiratory Muscle Electromyography

One of the older techniques used to measure respiratory effort involved making electromyographic (EMG) recordings of intercostal muscle activity Figure 117–5. These uncalibrated recordings are made using standard surface electrodes placed in pairs in the intercostal space on the right anterior chest. Attaining an optimal signal requires practice and also trial and error; recordings are prone to artifact (especially artifact from the electrocardiogram [ECG]). These EMG recordings can be very helpful for classifying apnea and hypopnea episodes as central, obstructive, or mixed. Furthermore, although signals are not calibrated, cascading increases in respiratory effort are readily apparent from recordings.

Pleural Pressure

Some sleep centers use esophageal pressure to index inspiratory effort. In our experience, most patients undergoing all-night polysomnography find esophageal balloons unacceptable. However, the newer, thin, water-tip or catheter-tip piezoelectric transducers are better tolerated. Esophageal pressure measurements are especially helpful in two clinical applications: (1) to verify central apnea or hypopnea episodes with high certainty and (2) to diagnose upper airway resistance syndrome.

In upper airway resistance syndrome, the classic findings include pleural pressure that becomes progressively more negative until an arousal (sometimes associated with an audible snort) occurs (Fig. 117–6). After arousal, the pleural pressure swings temporarily decrease, to be followed by the next cycle of increased swings and arousal. At times, arousals may not fully meet the arousal scoring criteria of the American Sleep Disorders Association (ASDA, now the American Academy of Sleep Medicine [AASM]). However, these criteria included the 3-second rule to improve reliability for visually detecting spontaneous arousals. Electroencephalographic (EEG) changes of shorter duration are thought to represent central nervous system (CNS) arousals, as are spectral analysis indices of alpha power loading, even when it is difficult to see on the raw

Table 117–3. **Paradoxical Motion of the Rib Cage and Abdomen**

Cause	Mechanism
Loss of diaphragm tone	When the diaphragm ceases to contract and becomes flaccid, it merely reacts to pressure changes around it instead of generating pressure changes. In this situation, when the other respiratory muscles contract, the rib cage is enlarged, and pleural pressure becomes negative, sucking the diaphragm into the chest. This condition results in an increase in rib cage volume and a reduction in abdominal volume.
Loss of accessory respiratory muscles tone	When the accessory muscles lose tone, the rib cage, particularly the upper part of the rib cage, becomes unstable. When the diaphragm then contracts, the negative intrathoracic pressure causes the unstable part of the thorax to be sucked in during inspiration.
Partial upper airway obstruction	With partial upper airway obstruction, the diaphragm must generate very strong negative pressures for inspiration to occur. As the diaphragm contracts, it both pushes out the abdomen and creates great negative intrathoracic pressure. This highly negative intrathoracic pressure may overcome the mechanisms maintaining chest wall stability (accessory muscle tone and rigidity of the cage) and cause the least stable portions of the rib cage to move inward with inspiration. This inward movement of the rib cage is a problem mainly in the very young, who have a pliable rib cage.
Complete upper airway obstruction (obstructive apnea)	With complete upper airway obstruction, there is no movement of air into the lungs. Because the volume change is zero, the volume change of the abdomen (caused by diaphragmatic contraction) is equal and opposite in direction to the volume change of the rib cage. This volume change is a pathognomonic finding in obstructive sleep apnea.

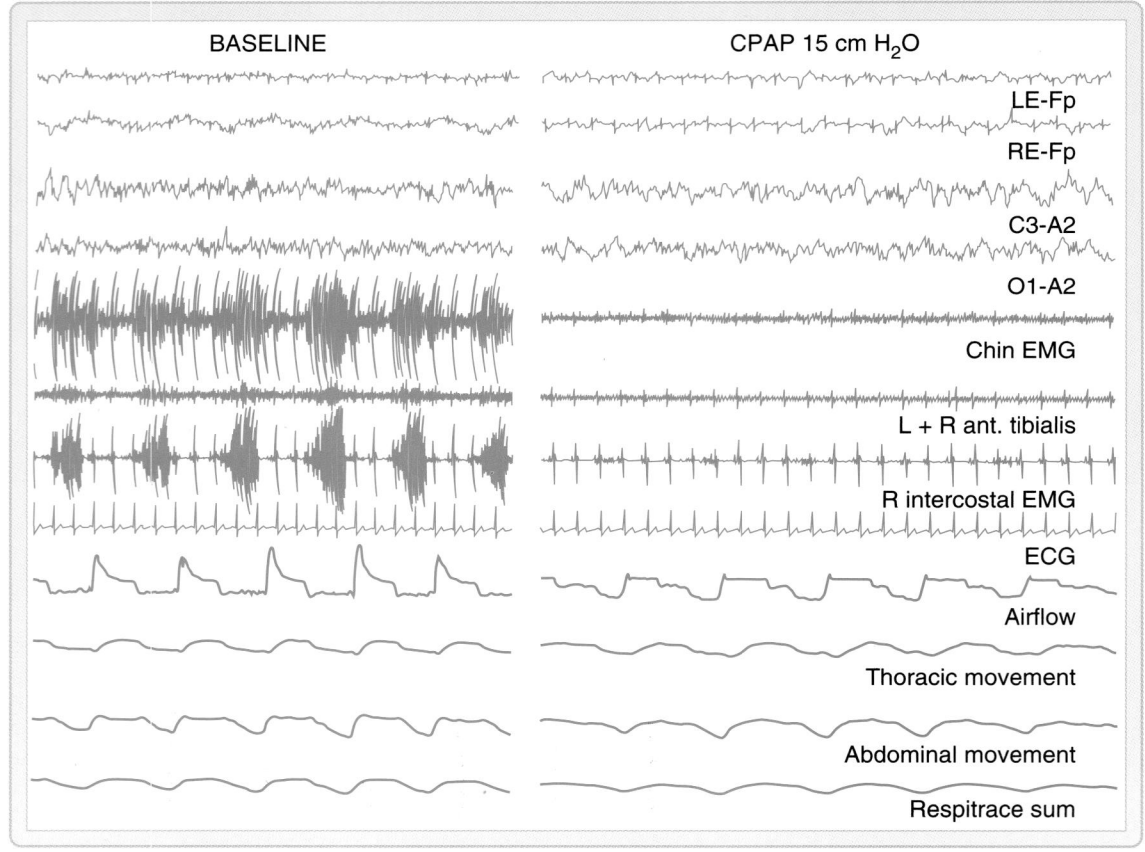

Figure 117–5. Surface respiratory (R intercostal) muscle EMG in sleep apnea. *Left,* The respiratory EMG is dramatically increased. *Right,* This signal is reduced on nasal continuous positive airway pressure (CPAP). ECG, electrocardiogram; EMG, electromyogram. (Courtesy of Dr. Catesby Ware.)

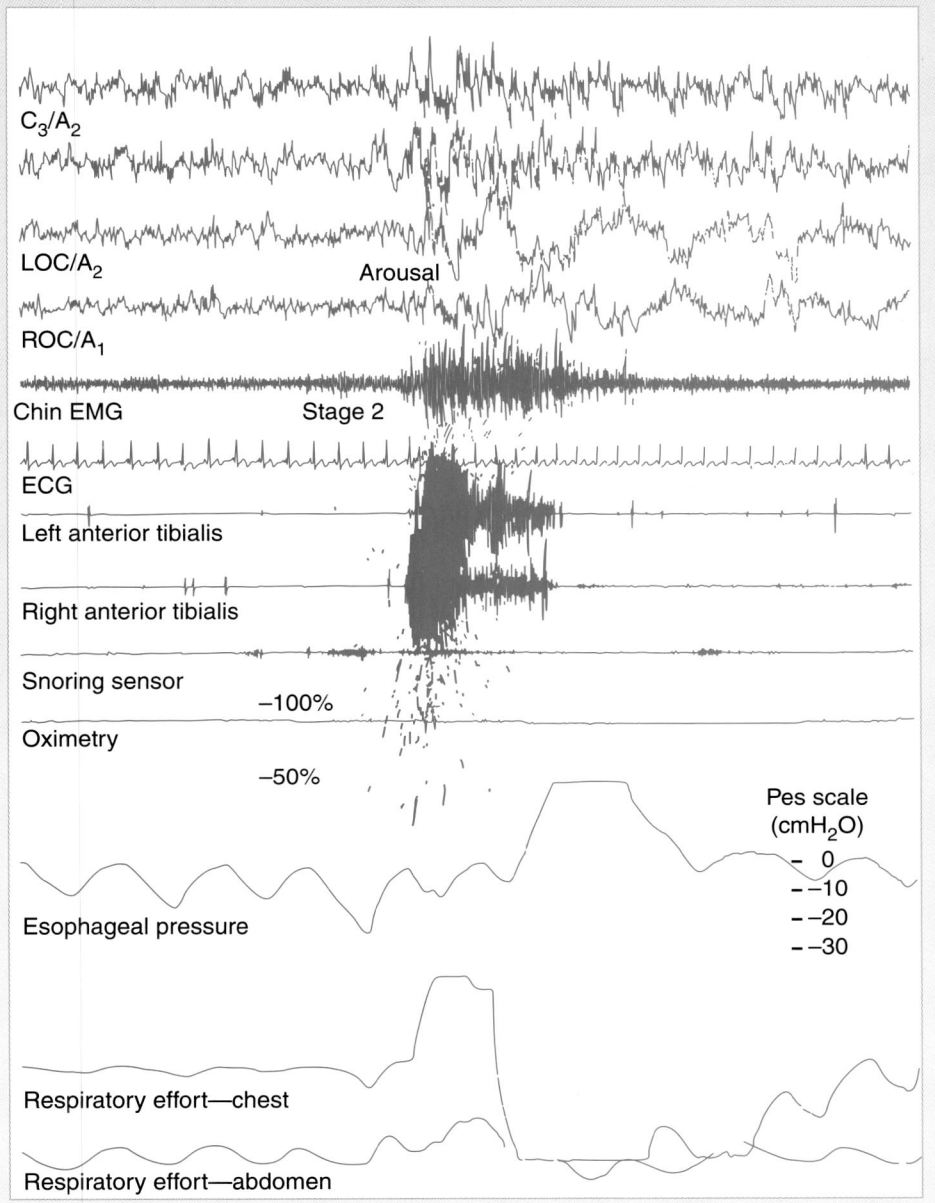

Figure 117–6. Esophageal pressure in the upper airway resistance syndrome. The esophageal pressure swing was greatest just before the arousal. ECG, electrocardiogram; EMG, electromyogram; LOC, left outer canthus; ROC, right outer canthus. (From Butkov N: Atlas of Clinical Polysomnography. Ashland, Ore, Synapse Media, 1996, p 224.)

data tracing. Sympathetic nervous system activation may be reflected by heart rate change.[12,13] Frequent (more than 10 per hour) negative pleural pressure swings with accompanying arousals in a sleepy patient who does not meet diagnostic criteria for sleep apnea is presumptive evidence of upper airway resistance syndrome.

Static Charge–Sensitive Bed

The static charge–sensitive bed technology has been evaluated in sleep disorders.[14] The transducer is part of a thin mattress that responds to the slightest movement. Output from the bed is exquisitely sensitive and can even detect heartbeat as a ballistocardiogram. Respiratory signal amplitude differs with body position changes; however, output is otherwise stable.

Digital Video

Although digital video recordings in some sleep laboratories are widely used in the evaluation of parasomnias and seizures, we believe that there may be an additional role for this technology in the evaluation of sleep breathing disorders.[15] When the digital video is perfectly synchronized with a digital polysomnogram, ambiguous or difficult-to-interpret polysomnographic events are frequently clarified. Digital video may be especially helpful for documenting upper airway resistance syndrome. For example, it is easy to recognize a small dip in arterial oxygen saturation (SaO_2) followed by oxygen resaturation as being significant when it corresponds to other events captured on video, such as an audible snort, a repetitive moving forward of the jaw or arching of the neck, or a closing of a gaping mouth, in an attempt to reestablish unobstructed breathing. The polysomnographic SaO_2 dip, without the other visual information, would quite likely be ignored or dismissed as artifact. We have found this approach to be particularly useful in thin individuals who may not have oxygen desaturation with their abnormal respiratory events. Furthermore, showing the sleep study video to patients so that they can see what they do during sleep can be a very effective tool to promote understanding of the problem and an appreciation of its severity.

METHODS TO DETECT CHANGES IN LUNG VOLUME

An assortment of techniques are available to not only measure respiratory movement but also to estimate tidal volume. These measures can provide semiquantitative information concerning presumed airflow while also documenting respiratory effort. When attempting to use these devices to gauge ventilation, calibration is crucial. Inaccuracies may be introduced by movements, changes in body position, and shifting in recording device placement. In sleep laboratories, strain gauges, inductance plethysmography, and impedance pneumography are most often used to measure volume changes. Other techniques include magnetometers, body plethysmography, canopy with neck seal, barometric method, and pneumotachography; however, these are seldom used in a clinical setting.[16-19]

Strain Gauges

A strain gauge consists of a sealed elastic tube filled with an electrical conductor, usually mercury, through which an electric current is passed.[20] When length is constant, current and resistance are constant. Stretching the strain gauge lengthens and narrows the cross-sectional area of the fixed-volume conductor. This produces a proportional increases in resistance. Current varies inversely to the length of the gauge, thereby becoming an index of gauge length. A Whetstone bridge amplifier transduces this change to voltage so it can be displayed as a tracing. These length-sensitive gauges can be used qualitatively to detect breathing abnormalities. If properly calibrated, the strain gauge can be used quantitatively to measure dynamic volume changes.[21] To properly quantify actual volume changes, the transducers must be calibrated against an independent volume-measuring system. The number and length of the gauges may vary, depending on the application. When it is not critical to measure exact volumes (as in most clinical sleep applications), a short strain gauge placed on the chest or abdominal wall will usually produce an adequate signal. When more exact volume measurements are required, two or more circumferential gauges are typically employed. Multiple linear regression techniques are then used to obtain calibration factors for each transducer.[21] In practice, two gauges—one for the rib cage and one for the abdomen—can give adequate precision for measuring changes in lung volume. The rib cage gauge is placed at the level of the axilla, and the abdominal gauge is placed just superior to the iliac crest. Once the gauges are calibrated, the sum of the rib cage and abdominal excursions will describe volume changes.

Differentiating central and obstructive breathing events is not possible solely on the basis of the summed rib cage and abdominal volume signals. Paradoxical rib cage and abdominal movement, which commonly occur during an obstructive apnea, results in zero summed net volume change. This results from the abdominal and rib cage volumes changing in equal but opposite directions. Similarly, central apnea (a cessation of all respiratory effort) is characterized by zero summed net volume change. To determine whether respiratory effort is present, an additional recording of either a rib cage or an abdominal transducer or of pleural pressure is required. If the gauge is being used solely as a relative index of respiratory movements, a single uncalibrated abdominal transducer will suffice.

The optimal working range of a mercury-filled strain gauge is narrow. An understretched gauge may not produce measurable resistance change as a function of its length. An overstretched gauge produces a high level of resistance. Most gauges have an optimal range where response is linear, and over- and understretching may shift output to a nonlinear range. Thus, these conditions preclude the gauge from correctly detecting changes in length. It is suggested that an unstretched gauge, if placed circumferentially, be at least 20% smaller than the circumference of the torso. Over time, there is deterioration in the function of the gauge due to the loss of tubing elasticity and the constant current through the conductor.

Piezoelectric transducers are also being used to monitor respiratory motion. These sensors are sensitive to changes in length; however, they are seldom calibrated in routine sleep laboratory applications.

Inductance Plethysmography

Changes in the cross-sectional area of the rib cage and abdominal compartments can be measured electronically by determining changes in inductance. Inductance is a property of electrical conductors characterized by the opposition to a change of current flow in the conductor.

Transducers are placed around the rib cage and abdomen—the physiologic equivalent of conductors. Each transducer consists of an insulated wire, sewn into the shape of a horizontally oriented sinusoid and onto an elasticized band. Changes in lung volumes alter the cross-sectional areas of the rib cage and abdomen, with a proportional change in the diameter of each transducer; this change directly affects the self-inductance of the transducer.[22] Considerations concerning transducer placement, volume calibration, and apnea identification are identical to those applied to strain gauges.

Additional factors must be considered in using these devices: there is sensitivity to artifact during changes in body position because the elasticized band may migrate from its original site, and the size of the band makes it deformable. These factors may adversely affect the accuracy and stability of the original volume calibration. As mentioned previously, the relative contributions of rib cage and abdomen may change with sleep and changes in posture, thereby causing the initial calibration to become less accurate.

Calibrated inductance plethysmography has been suggested as a method to infer the changes of upper airway resistance syndrome.[23] The following have been described: snoring may lead to rib cage–abdominal asynchrony with increased thoracic breathing and increased breathing cycle time taken up by inspiration; before arousal, one may detect evidence of flow limitation; and arousals may lead to increased variation of respiratory cycle time and increased tidal volume.

Impedance Pneumography

Impedance defines the combined effects of two previously discussed properties of an electrical conductor: *resistance* and *inductance*. In physical terms, when impedance pneumography is used, the conductor is the thorax. Impedance is measured by applying a small current across the thorax using a pair of electrodes placed at the site of maximal thoracic excursion. Changes in transthoracic impedance are related to variations in the amount of conductive materials (liquids, including interstitial fluid, blood and lymph, and tissue) and nonconductive material (air) between the electrodes. The conductive and nonconductive materials affect the total impedance differently. Increased air in the lung increases impedance, and increased fluid in the thorax decreases impedance. A recording of both the volume of air exchanged and the total of impedance changes may allow the differentiation of air-related and fluid-related changes in impedance. If total impedance is recorded in a single channel, both air volume–related and fluid-related changes are measured.

Changes in impedance in obstructive apnea are complex. During apnea, lung volume decreases, whereas the negative intrathoracic pressure most likely temporarily pools blood in the pulmonary circulation. For these reasons, a precise measurement of respiratory volume and pattern may not be possible.[24] Rate adapting cardiac pacemakers using transthoracic impedance to drive ventilation have been used for OSA screening.[24a]

METHODS TO DETECT PHYSIOLOGIC CONSEQUENCES

Blood Gas Changes

Oxyhemoglobin desaturation is a significant clinical consequence of sleep-disordered breathing. However, measuring blood oxygen content directly using an indwelling arterial catheter during sleep is highly invasive. Intermittent sampling fails to detect the incidence and severity of hypoxemia, which is now known to be highly variable in sleep.

Pulse Oximetry

Noninvasive technologies allow the continuous monitoring of SaO_2.[25-29] Pulse oximetry has become the standard approach for recording oxyhemoglobin desaturations during overnight sleep studies. Pulse oximeters determine SaO_2 using spectrophotoelectrical techniques via a two-wavelength light transmitter and a receiver placed on either side of a pulsating arterial vascular bed. Digit, ear, and nasal sites are recommended by the manufacturers. The amplitude of light detected by the receiver depends on the magnitude of the change in arterial pulse, the wavelengths transmitted through the arterial vascular bed, and the SaO_2 of the arterial hemoglobin. These devices are said to be sensitive only to tissues that pulsate; thus, venous blood, connective tissue, skin pigment, and bone theoretically do not interfere with SaO_2 measurement. A minimal pulse amplitude must be detected by the devices to prevent erroneous measurements. Dyshemoglobinemias, however, may cause problems.

The correct alignment of the light transmitter and receiver is critical to the proper operation of pulse oximeters. If the sensor is applied to a digit, that digit must be immobilized. Significant bending of the digit may restrict the ability of the devices to detect pulsatile flow, the absence of which precludes SaO_2 determination. Although all pulse oximeters are based on similar technology,[27] they have very different response characteristics, depending on the sensor location, the manufacturer, and the technology minimizing the effect of motion that can cause artifacts.[28,30] Indeed, the same model by the same manufacturer may have different software versions that may result in differing performance.[31,32] The difference in the response characteristics and dependence on sensor locations cannot be overemphasized (Fig. 117–7). Some oximeters may entirely miss episodes of hypoxemia easily detectable by other oximeters and thus may lead to an incorrect diagnosis and treatment (Fig. 117–8). The sensors are very lightweight and can be used in neonates.

In reflectance pulse oximetry, the light transmitter and receiver are on the same surface. The light transmitted into the vascular bed is scattered, absorbed, and reflected. Thus, only a small proportion of the light returns to the receiver. Reflectance devices deal with weaker pulse signals and therefore are more sensitive to changes in blood pressure and motion artifacts.

It is beyond the scope of this chapter to review the specific manufacturers and all their models.[31,33] However, generalizations about sensor location, instrument filters, and potential pitfalls are worth noting.

SENSOR LOCATIONS

In our experience, for most adults, the ear is the preferred location for the sensor. When perfusion is poor, we apply a trace amount of a vasodilator (nonylic acid vanillylamide and nicotinic acid, Finalgon ointment [Boehringer Ingelheim]). This is a powerful cutaneous vasodilator, and the technician must be careful to avoid its contact with eyes. We have used this ointment (which is not available in all countries) for more than 10 years without any problems. When the ear site is not usable, reflectance pulse oximeter sensors on the forehead or another well-perfused surface may be used. Recording from the ear also helps to reduce circulator delay. This becomes especially important for associating the respiratory and desaturation event when apnea episodes occur in rapid succession or the patient has congestive heart failure.

INSTRUMENT FILTERS AND SAMPLING RATE

Most pulse oximeters filter the SaO_2 signal. For some devices, the filter algorithms use the heart rate; thus, the degree of filtering becomes inversely related to rate, and at very low heart rates the signal is heavily filtered.[28] The greater the filtering, the less likely is the detection of brief, mild hypoxemic episodes.[34] It is recommended that the least filtering (i.e., the fastest response, or the highest sampling rate) be used so that transient changes are not missed.[35]

POTENTIAL PROBLEMS

Because pulse oximeters use two wavelengths of light in the process of estimating SaO_2, they are unable to distinguish three or more hemoglobin species. In the presence of carboxyhemoglobin, the SaO_2 will be overestimated in heavy smokers, whose carboxyhemoglobin level may reach 10% to 20%.[36] In the presence of a rising methemoglobin concentration, SaO_2 measured by oximetry will plateau toward 85%, regardless of whether the true SaO_2 is much higher or lower.[37] Because light is transmitted through tissue, pigment in the skin may

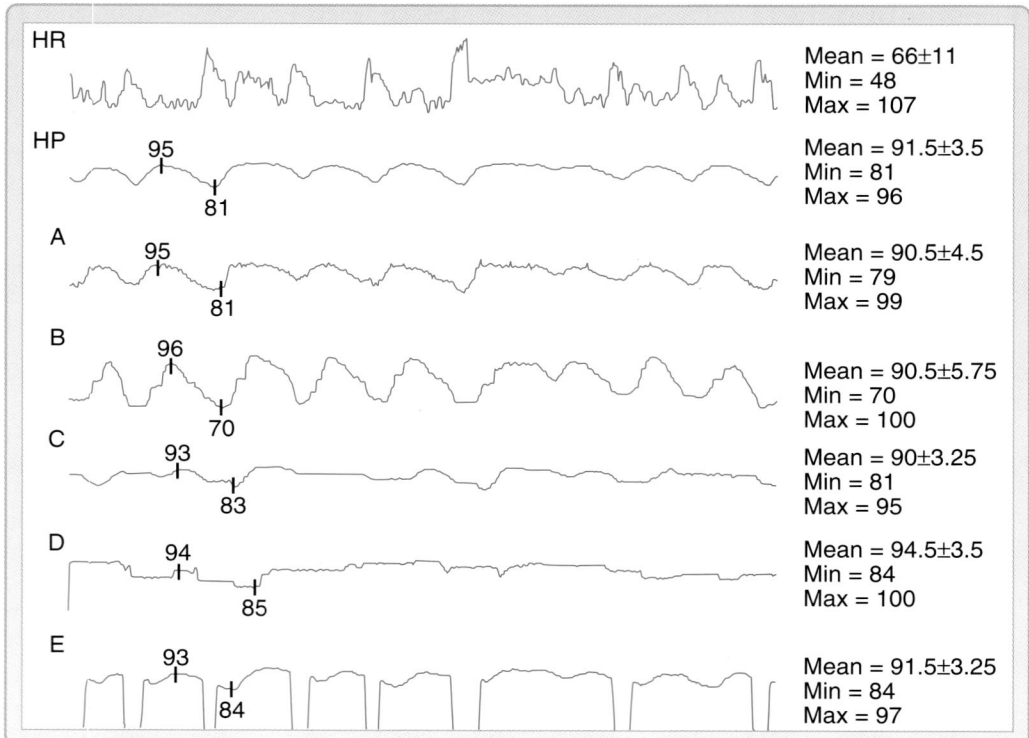

Figure 117–7. Heart rate (HR) and arterial oxygen saturation (Sao₂) during 5 minutes in a patient with sleep apnea. HP, Hewlett Packard oximeter; A to E, five different pulse oximeters. The scales for the six oximeters are identical. The numbers on the tracings represent the instantaneous Sao₂ measured during the peak and trough of an apneic episode. The numbers to the right of the figure are the mean, standard deviation, and minimum and maximum values for HR and Sao₂ for the six oximeters. Note that C and D do not track Sao₂, and that E has numerous artifacts.

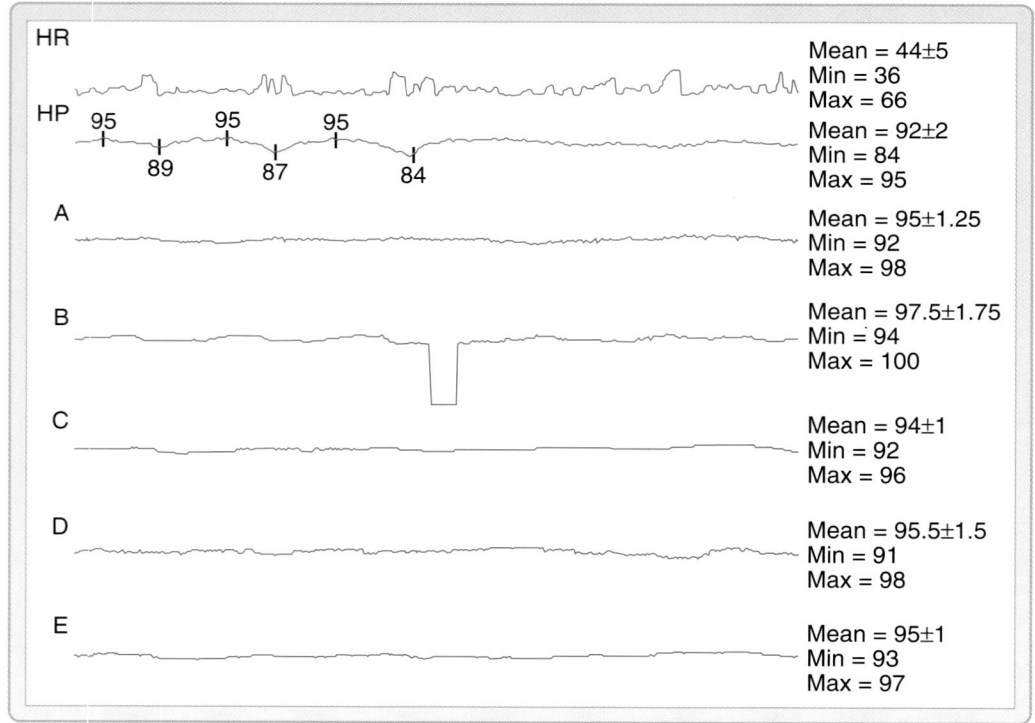

Figure 117–8. Heart rate (HR) and arterial oxygen saturation (Sao₂) during 5 minutes in a patient with sleep apnea and bradycardia. Tracings are taken from six oximeters, as described in Figure 117–7. In this example, three apneic episodes are missed entirely by all the pulse oximeters. This patient's problem would have been missed entirely by pulse oximetry screening.

degrade oximeter performance, with the device indicating a "probe off" or "perfusion low" message.[38] Although probe connectors from one manufacturer may fit perfectly into the unit of another, the wiring may be incompatible, and severe burns may result.[39] Pressure-related injuries to the digits have also been reported.[40]

Transcutaneous Oxygen and Carbon Dioxide

The estimation of partial pressure of arterial oxygen (PaO_2) from the surface of the skin is dependent on the oxygen flux through the skin, local oxygen consumption, and the diffusion barrier of the skin.[41] This measurement technique is most commonly used in neonates, whose skin is thin.

Accurate measurement of transcutaneous PO_2 ($tcPO_2$) requires maximal dilation of the local vasculature in the upper dermis, which is achieved by heating it to 43° C. Heating, however, shifts the oxyhemoglobin dissociation curve to the right, increases the resistance of the skin stratum corneum to oxygen permeation, increases the metabolic rate of the dermal tissue, and increases the rate of cutaneous blood flow. The shift in the oxyhemoglobin dissociation curve and the increase in metabolic rate effectively cancel each other out, leaving permeability and flow as the dependent factors in correlating $tcPO_2$ and PaO_2. An important advantage of heating is that the amount of blood present is maximal, and $tcPO_2$ will therefore be unaffected by small changes in blood supply to the tissue.

The $tcPO_2$ may be misinterpreted when the state of blood flow is unknown. When flow and PaO_2 are adequate, $tcPO_2$ reflects PaO_2. Under conditions of compromised flow and adequate PaO_2, $tcPO_2$ will change with flow. If SaO_2 and flow are compromised, $tcPO_2$ tracks oxygen delivery.

The accuracy of transcutaneous measurement also depends on correct sensor application. To convert $tcPO_2$ measurements to PaO_2 values precisely, a calibration curve for each subject is required; this is a prohibitive step in terms of time and labor. In practice, the $tcPO_2$ measurements are thus used to track, in relative terms, the status of arterial oxygen content. The responsiveness of the device is not adequate to rapidly track the blood gas changes of short apneas (less than 30 seconds), because oxygen diffuses slowly across the skin. The conditions that govern the transcutaneous measurement of PCO_2 are similar to those described for PaO_2. Transcutaneous blood gas determinations are of greatest value in neonates. Transcutaneous PCO_2 is used to assess hypoventilation and its treatment in adults[42] and in children.[12]

Central Nervous System Arousals and Awakenings

CNS arousals are derived from EEG recordings, preferably made from occipital sites. CNS arousals often take the form of bursts of alpha (7 to 13 cycles per second) activity, and the term *EEG speeding* is sometimes used to describe the event. A standard approach for visually scoring arousals was published by the ASDA in 1992. When scored visually, a 3- to 15-second burst of alpha activity in non–rapid eye movement sleep is considered an arousal. During rapid eye movement sleep, when alpha bursts can be an ongoing part of background activity, the alpha intrusion must be accompanied by increased muscle tone. In any sleep stage, bursts exceeding 15 seconds are scored as frank awakenings (the epoch is scored

as stage W). The reason the committee selected a lower limit of 3 seconds was not because they thought shorter bursts did not represent arousals but rather because bursts shorter than 3 seconds were not reliably identified across scorers when traces were reviewed visually. At the time the rule was developed, it was fully expected that computerized scoring would be able to identify shorter and more subtle events with adequate replicability.

The CNS arousal, as a clinically significant parameter of sleep, has both face and empirical validity. Face validity derives from the principle that disturbed or fragmented sleep is less restorative than undisturbed or consolidated sleep. Indeed, it can be empirically demonstrated that disrupted sleep is associated with tiredness, fatigue, and sleepiness. As a pathophysiologic consequence of obstructive sleep apnea, the arousal is thought to play a special role. Presumably resulting from respiratory effort, the arousal returns ventilation to voluntary control so that the airway can be dilated, and then breathing resumes. However, some controversy exists about resumption of breathing after an obstructive event without an arousal, and about the presence of arousals at the termination of central events. The role of the autonomic nervous system, especially sympathetic activation, is an area of active research.[43-45]

Blood Pressure Changes

Most sleep laboratories do not include the continuous measurement of blood pressure in routine clinical evaluations. The following techniques are currently practiced primarily in research settings.

Many pulse oximeters now include an output that tracks the pulse pressure, an index of the magnitude of the pulsation occurring at the site of the oximetry sensor. Pulse transit time (PTT) is the time taken for the pulse pressure wave to travel from the heart (R wave on the ECG) to the periphery. When pleural pressure is negative, there is a drop in blood pressure and thus a lengthening of the PTT. The progressive increase in pleural pressure during obstructive apnea is associated with a progressive rise in the amplitude of PTT oscillations. During central apnea, this does not occur. Thus, it has been suggested that the measurement of PTT may be a noninvasive estimate of inspiratory effort, which could be used to differentiate obstructive from central apnea.[46,47] It has also been suggested that the PTT might be useful to detect arousals in children, even when cortical arousals are not visible.[48]

Automatic self-inflating arm cuff sphygmomanometers are likely to be too "invasive" to be used routinely in the sleep laboratory, because the patient may arouse when the cuff inflates. A continuous measurement of blood pressure can be obtained using a device consisting of a miniature cuff that fits on the finger. The first generation of the device (Finapres, Datex-Ohmeda, Inc.) was validated in the anesthesia setting[49,50] and has been used in a sleep laboratory setting.[51] The current generation of this device (manufactured by Finapres Medical Systems, The Netherlands) can be used for prolonged periods because the measurements are obtained alternately from adjacent fingers, minimizing the risk of injury to the digits. In addition, there is automatic hydrostatic correction if the arm is moved. Measurements are sensitive to movement artifacts caused by flexion of the fingers, perhaps explaining the increased variability of the measurements. In general, this technique is acceptable for continuous measurement of mean blood pressure.[52,53]

Autonomic Nervous System Activation

Although autonomic nervous system (ANS) changes underlie heart rate and blood pressure changes, they can be difficult to measure. Direct measurement of sympathetic motor neurons during sleep is both difficult and invasive and is thus usually reserved for research.[54] In contrast, photoplethysmography is noninvasive and can be used to assess extremity blood flow. Vasoconstrictive responses can be detected; however, this technique is very prone to artifact. Recently, however, a tonometer that measures segmental pulsatile flow has become available.[55] This device, called Watch-PAT (Itimar Medical, Boston, MA), has an inflatable bladder inside a fingertip housing and a pulse volume sensor. Studies indicate sleep apnea and hypopnea episodes are associated with vasoconstriction detectable with this device. This autonomic activation is consistent with more global indicators of heightened sympathetic activation (e.g., norepinephrine turnover) in patients with sleep apnea. The device's sensitivity and specificity for detecting sleep-disordered breathing at an AHI of 20 were 90.9% and 84.2%, respectively. Thus, it appears to have some value as a screening device.[56]

SLEEP STUDY CLASSIFICATION

In addition to standard attended polysomnography, three levels of unattended overnight sleep recordings (portable polysomnography) were defined in 1992 by the ASDA. Table 117–4 summarizes the procedures performed at each level for sleep study classification. Selection of variables to be recorded is a matter of controversy. Most investigators recommend recording oximetry, effort to breathe, airflow, electrocardiography, and neurophysiologic variables (including EEG, electrooculography, submental EMG, and anterior tibialis EMG)[57,58]; others believe that monitoring oximetry (alone or

with video recording),[59] thoracoabdominal movement, and anterior tibialis EMG are sufficient to diagnose sleep apnea.[60] Surprisingly, nocturnal oximetry alone was found to be not cost effective because of poor diagnostic accuracy.[61,62] Level III recordings can be equivalent to the cardiorespiratory sleep studies by including channels for airflow, arterial oxygen saturation, respiratory effort, and ECG or heart rate. The bioparameters recorded by commercially available, self-contained, level II and III polysomnographic devices vary depending upon the manufacturer and user-defined protocols.

STANDARD OF PRACTICE

The AASM (formerly the ASDA) has published two position papers relevant to polysomnographic and cardiopulmonary testing to diagnose sleep apnea: "Practice Parameters for the Use of Portable Recording in the Assessment of Obstructive Sleep Apnea" in 1994, and "Practice Parameters for the Indications for Polysomnography and Related Procedures" in 1997. More recently, in a joint project involving the AASM, the American Thoracic Society, and the American College of Chest Physicians, an evidence-based medicine review of the literature concerning portable monitoring for diagnosing sleep-disordered breathing was compiled and published.[63] From this literature review, practice parameters were formulated.[64] It was concluded that there was not enough evidence to recommend the use of level II devices in either attended or unattended settings. Nonetheless, level III device application, when attended by a qualified technologist or the equivalent, can be used to determine if a patient has an AHI greater than 15 events per hour (of recording time). By contrast, evidence does not support using level III devices in unattended mode to rule out or rule in sleep-disordered breathing. Finally, level IV devices are not recommended for use in either attended or unattended mode.[64]

The older AASM guidelines provided some flexibility for using portable sleep studies under specific circumstances, such as (1) when the patient has severe symptoms, and

Table 117–4.   Recording Montages for Polysomnography (PSG) Levels

Parameter	Level I (Attended Standard PSG)	Level II (Comprehensive Portable PSG)	Level III (Modified Portable Sleep Apnea Testing)*	Level IV (Continuous Bioparameter Recording)†
Electroencephalogram (EEG)	+	+	—	—
Electrooculogram (EOG)	+	+	—	—
Electromyogram submentalis (chin) (EMG-SM)	+	+	—	—
Electrocardiogram (ECG)	+	+	+	—
Airflow	+	+	+	—
Respiratory effort	+	+	+	—
Arterial oxygen saturation (SaO₂)	+	+	+	+
Body position	+	Optional	Optional	—
Electromyogram anterior tibialis (EMG-AT)‡	+	+	—	—
Attended	+	—	—	—

*Typical montage, others exist.

†Single or dual; typical montage, others exist.

‡Recommended but optional for apnea studies.

standard polysomnography is not readily available, (2) when the patient cannot be studied in the sleep laboratory, and (3) when follow-up studies are needed after the original diagnosis was made with standard polysomnography and therapy was initiated.

Ultimately, the question is whether polysomnography is required for evaluating patients with suspected sleep-disordered breathing. In most cases, the answer is yes.[57] A single, brief clinical observation alone is an ineffective screening or diagnostic procedure for detecting the presence or severity of sleep apnea.[65] Thus, sleep recording is required and in most cases, all-night polysomnography is recommended. Many laboratories conduct split-night, diagnostic–pressure titration studies. In this paradigm, sleep-related breathing is evaluated during a baseline interval lasting 2 hours or more. If diagnostic criteria are met, positive airway pressure titration commences. This approach reportedly is acceptable for about 80% of patients.[66] Problems,[67] such as mask fit and leaks, difficulty sleeping, disorientation in the middle of the night when positive airway pressure is applied, and initial difficulty adjusting to the mask can make split-night studies less than optimal. If optimal pressure is not attained until the last hour of titration, the patient may not appreciate the full therapeutic benefit. By contrast, if optimal pressure is reached during the first 2 hours of a full-night titration, the remaining 5 or more hours may be judged as the best night of sleep the patient had in years. Consequently, perceived benefit will be high, which is the first step on the road to utilization.

Nap studies yield about 75% diagnostic sensitivity, at best, and tend to be inefficient.[68] Rapid eye movement (REM) sleep infrequently occurs on naps, and negative tests must be followed up with full polysomnography.

CONSIDERATIONS FOR USING NON–LEVEL I TECHNIQUES

In capitated health care systems, adequate funds for diagnostic sleep testing can be limited and this is a problem in several countries.[69] The clinician is forced to make difficult choices between providing the standard of care to fewer individual or lesser care to more individuals. Whether resources are available reflects not only medical issues but also the values of the health care system and how sleep disorders are viewed relative to other diseases.[70] In some cases, there is urgency for commencing treatment. Patient advocates argue that providing the standard of care ultimately serves the patient best. Providing substandard care creates a double standard that tends to perpetuate itself. Also, providing treatment other than the standard of practice may be construed as experimentation. If informed consent and institutional approval have not been granted, it could be an ethical violation of acceptable clinical practice.

Currently, to qualify for U.S. Medicare reimbursement, sleep studies must record the physiologic channels needed to score sleep stages.[71] Substituting total recording time for total sleep time in the denominator when calculating the AHI decreases overall magnitude and thereby diminishes sensitivity.

In a patient with severe sleep apnea, a level III test is likely to be positive. Consequently, the patient is scheduled for laboratory positive airway pressure titration. Thus, there will be one level III evaluation and one level I evaluation. However, if the patient's sleep-disordered breathing is severe, a split-night evaluation could have been conducted and the level III test would not have been needed. On the other hand, if a patient has mild sleep apnea, a level III test is likely to be negative. Consequently, the patient is scheduled for a laboratory full-night evaluation. Thus there will be one level III evaluation and one level I evaluation instead of only one level I evaluation. A savings (the difference in cost between a laboratory study and a level III study) is realized only when the disorder is not severe enough to have been split on a laboratory study (i.e., an AHI between 10 and 30) but severe enough to have been diagnosed with a level III device. To determine the savings afforded by using level III screening, first project from the database the number of patients falling in the AHI range of 10 to 30, and then multiply this by the cost difference between laboratory polysomnography and the level III test. Note this product as "screen savings." Next, determine the number of patients who (a) had split-night studies, (b) were appropriate for split-night study, and (c) had mild sleep apnea (AHI less than 10), and multiply this number by the cost of level III testing. Note this amount as "extra testing." The overall savings (or extra expense) is calculated by subtracting "extra testing" from "screen savings."

COMPUTERIZED SCORING

The central issue of the automatic scoring is accuracy. Automatic scoring may be unreliable in complicated OSAS patients.[72,73] Uncertainty about the accuracy of scoring can be framed in terms of confidence, or trust. Confidence can be increased by objective and appropriate system validation. Computerized polysomnographic systems differ between manufacturers and between different models or software updates produced by the same manufacturer. Additionally, because the system is a complex tool, it can also differ between users of identical systems. In other words, how a system performs in one laboratory may differ drastically from the way it performs elsewhere. Therefore, each laboratory should develop its own validation and normative data set. Specific focus should be on performance in different situations (e.g., with different patient groups, in the presence of various artifacts or suboptimal signals) and on whether there is systematic overestimation or underestimation of pathophysiologic events.

Clinical Pearl

At a minimum, measures of airflow and respiratory effort are needed to detect and classify apnea and hypopnea events as obstructive, central, or mixed. The laboratory diagnosis of upper airway resistance syndrome requires that an association be established between subtle respiratory events and sleep disruption. Although classically, diagnosing upper airway resistance syndrome required measurement of pleural pressure, surrogate measures for increased respiratory effort can be used.

REFERENCES

1. American Academy of Sleep Medicine: Sleep related breathing disorders in adults: Recommendations for syndrome definition and measurement techniques in clinical research. Sleep 1999;22:667-689.

2. Aldrich MS: Obstructive sleep apnea syndrome. In Aldrich MS (ed): Sleep Medicine. New York, Oxford University Press, 1999, pp 202-236.

3. Hirshkowitz M, Littner M, Kuna ST, et al: Sleep-Related Breathing Disorders: Sourcebook, 2nd ed. Milwaukee, Wisc, Healthcare Analysis and Information Group, 2003.

4. Ayappa I, Norman RG, Rapoport DM: Cardiogenic oscillations on the airflow signal during continuous positive airway pressure as a marker of central apnea. Chest 1999;116:660-666.

5. Montserrat JM, Farre R, Ballester E, et al: Evaluation of nasal prongs for estimating nasal flow. Am J Respir Crit Care Med 1997;155:211-215.

6. Norman RG, Ahmed MM, Walsleben JA, et al: Detection of respiratory events during NPSG: Nasal cannula/pressure sensor versus thermistor. Sleep 1997;20:1175-1184.

7. Hosselet J-J, Norman RG, Ayappa I, et al: Detection of flow limitation with a nasal cannula/pressure transducer system. Am J Respir Crit Care Med 1998;157(pt 1):1461-1467.

8. Morielli A, Desjardins D, Brouillette RT: To assess hypoventilation during pediatric polysomnography both transcutaneous and end-tidal CO_2 should be measured. Am Rev Respir Dis 1992;145:A180.

9. Berry RB, Parish JM, Hartse KM: The use of auto-titrating continuous positive airway pressure for treatment of adult obstructive sleep apnea: An American Academy of Sleep Medicine review. Sleep 2002;25:148-173.

10. Littner M, Hirshkowitz M, Davila D, et al: Practice parameters for the use of auto-titrating continuous positive airway pressure devices for titrating pressures and treating adult patients with obstructive sleep apnea syndrome: An American Academy of Sleep Medicine report. Sleep 2002;25:143-147.

11. Konno K, Mead J: Measurement of the separate volume changes of ribcage and abdomen during breathing. J Appl Physiol 1967;22:407-422.

12. Douglas NJ, Martin SE: Arousals and the sleep apnea/hypopnea syndrome. Sleep 1996;19(Suppl):S196-S197.

13. Martin SE, Wraith PK, Deary IJ, et al: The effect of nonvisible sleep fragmentation on daytime function. Am J Respir Crit Care Med 1997;155:1596-1601.

14. Svanborg E, Larsson H, Carlsson-Nordlander B, et al: A limited diagnostic investigation for obstructive sleep apnea syndrome. Chest 1990;98:1341-1345.

15. Banno K, Kryger MH: Use of polysomnography with synchronized digital video recording to diagnose pediatric sleep breathing disorders. CMAJ 2005;173:28-30.

16. Dubois A, Botelho SY, Bedell GN, et al: A new method for measuring airway resistance in man using a body plethysmograph: Values in normal subjects and in patients with respiratory disease. J Clin Invest 1956;35:327.

17. Epstein RA, Epstein MAF, Haddad GG, et al: Practical implementation of the barometric method for measurement of tidal volume. J Appl Physiol 1980;49:1107-1115.

18. Sharp JT, Druz WS, D'Souza V, et al: Use of the respiratory magnetometer in diagnosis and classification of sleep apnea. Chest 1980;3:350-353.

19. Sorkin B, Rapoport DM, Falk DB, et al: Canopy ventilation monitor for quantitative measurement of ventilation during sleep. J Appl Physiol 1980;48:724-730.

20. Shapiro A, Cohen HD: The use of mercury capillary length gauges for the measurement of the volume of thoracic and diaphragmatic components of human respiration: A theoretical analysis and a practical method. Trans N Y Acad Sci Ser II 1965;27:634-649.

21. Loveridge B, Perez-Padilla R, West P, et al: Comparison of the stability of the respiratory inductance plethysmograph versus mercury strain gauges in measuring ventilation. Am Rev Respir Dis 1984;129:A82.

22. Chadha TS, Watson H, Birch S, et al: Validation of respiratory inductive plethysmography using different calibration procedures. Am Rev Respir Dis 1982;125:644-649.

23. Bloch KE, Li Y, Sackner MA, et al: Breathing pattern during sleep disruptive snoring. Eur Respir J 1997;10:576-586.

24. Cohen KP, Ladd WM, Beams DM, et al: Comparison of impedance and inductance ventilation sensors on adults during breathing, motion, and simulated airway obstruction. IEEE Trans Biomed Eng 1997;44:555-566.

24a. Defaye P, Pepin JL, Poezevara Y, et al: Automatic recognition of abnormal respiratory events during sleep by a pacemaker transthoracic impedance sensor. J Cardiovasc Electrophysiol 2004;15:1034-1040.

25. Douglas NJ, Brash HM, Wraith PK, et al: Accuracy, sensitivity to carboxyhemoglobin, and speed of response of the Hewlett-Packard 47201A Ear Oximeter. Am Rev Respir Dis 1979;119: 311-313.

26. Rebuck AS, Chapman KR, D'Urzo A: The accuracy and response characteristics of a simplified ear oximeter. Chest 1983;83: 860-864.

27. Taylor MB, Whitwam JG: The accuracy of pulse oximeters: A comparative clinical evaluation of five pulse oximeters. Anaesthesia 1988;43:229-232.

28. West P, George CF, Kryger MH: Dynamic in-vivo response characteristics of three oximeters: Hewlett-Packard 47201A, Biox III, and Nellcor N-100. Sleep 1987;10:263-271.

29. Yelderman M, New W Jr: Evaluation of pulse oximetry. Anesthesiology 1983;59:349-352.

30. Trang H, Boureghda S, Leske V: Sleep desaturation: Comparison of two oximeters. Pediatr Pulmonol 2004;37:76-80.

31. Hannhart B, Haberer JP, Saulnir C, et al: Accuracy and precision of 14 pulse oximeters. Eur Respir J 1991;4:115-119.

32. Hannhart B, Michalski H, Delorme N, et al: Reliability of six pulse oximeters in chronic obstructive pulmonary disease. Chest 1991;99:842-846.

33. Severinghaus JW, Naifeh KH, Koh SO: Errors in 14 pulse oximeters during profound hypoxia. J Clin Monit 1989;5:72-81.

34. Farré R, Montserrat JM, Ballester E, et al: Importance of the pulse oximeter averaging time when measuring oxygen desaturation in sleep apnea. Sleep 1998;21:386-390.

35. Davila DG, Richards KC, Marshall BL, et al: Oximeter performance: The influence of acquisition parameters. Chest 2002;122: 1654-1660.

36. Barker SJ, Tremper KK, Hufstedler S: The effects of carbon monoxide inhalation on pulse oximetry and transcutaneous PO_2. Anesthesiology 1987;66:677-679.

37. Tremper KK, Barker SJ: Pulse oximetry. Anesthesiology 1989; 70:98-106.

38. Ries AL, Prewitt LM, Johnson JJ: Skin color and ear oximetry. Chest 1989;96:287-290.

39. Murphy KG, Secunda JA, Rockoff MA: Severe burns from a pulse oximeter. Anesthesiology 1990;73:350-352.

40. Meyer TJ, Eveloff J, Kline LR, et al: One negative polysomnography does not exclude OSA. Am Rev Respir Dis 1992;145:A724.

41. Lubbers DW: Theoretical basis of the transcutaneous blood gas measurements. Crit Care Med 1981;9:721-733.

42. Willson GN, Piper AJ, Norman M, et al: Nasal versus full face mask for noninvasive ventilation in chronic respiratory failure. Eur Respir J 2004;23:605-609.

43. Pillar G, Bar A, Betito M, et al: An automatic ambulatory device for detection of AASM defined arousals from sleep: The WP100. Sleep Med 2003;4:207-212.

44. Krieger J, Schroder C, Erhardt C: [Cortical arousal, autonomic arousal: Evaluation techniques and clinical importance]. Rev Neurol (Paris) 2003;159:6S107-112.

45. Levy P, Pepin J: Sleep fragmentation: Clinical usefulness of autonomic markers. Sleep Med 2003;4:489-491.

46. Pitson DJ, Stradling JR: Value of beat-to-beat blood pressure changes, detected by pulse transit time, in the management of the obstructive sleep apnoea syndrome. Eur Respir J 1998;12:685-692.

47. Argod J, Pepin JL, Levy P: Differentiating obstructive and central sleep respiratory events through pulse transit time. Am J Respir Crit Care Med 1998;158:1778-1783.

48. Katz ES, Lutz J, Black C, Marcus CL: Pulse transit time as a measure of arousal and respiratory effort in children with sleep-disordered breathing. Pediatr Res 2003;53:580-588.

49. Kurki T, Smith NT, Nead N, et al: Noninvasive continuous blood pressure measurement from the finger: Optimal measurement conditions and factors affecting reliability. J Clin Monit 1987;3:6-13.

50. Van Egmond J, Hasenbos M, Crul JF: Invasive v non-invasive measurement of arterial pressure. Br J Anaesthiol 1985;57:433-443.

51. Mateika JH, Slutsky AS, Hoffstein V: The effect of snoring on mean arterial blood pressure during non-REM sleep. Am Rev Respir Dis 1992;145:141-152.

52. Omboni S, Parati G, Castiglioni P, et al: Estimation of blood pressure variability from 24-hour ambulatory finger blood pressure. Hypertension 1998;32:52-68.

53. Voogel AJ, van Montfrans GA: Reproducibility of twenty-four-hour finger arterial blood pressure, variability and systemic hemodynamics. J Hypertens 1997;15:1761-1765.

54. Shamsuzzaman AS, Ackerman MJ, Kara T, et al: Sympathetic nerve activity in the congenital long-QT syndrome. Circulation 2003;107:1844-1847.

55. Bar A, Pillar G, Dvir I, et al: Evaluation of a portable device based on peripheral arterial tone for unattended home sleep studies. Chest 2003;123:695-703.

56. Ayas NT, Pittman S, MacDonald M, White DP: Assessment of a wrist-worn device in the detection of obstructive sleep apnea. Sleep Med 2003;4:435-442.

57. Phillipson EA, Remmers JE (Chairs): American Thoracic Society Consensus Conference on Indications and Standards for Cardiopulmonary Sleep Studies. Am Rev Respir Dis 1989; 139:559-568.

58. McAvoy RD: Guidelines for Respiratory Sleep Studies. Sydney, Australia, Thoracic Society of Australia and New Zealand, 1988.

59. British Thoracic Society: Facilities for the diagnosis and treatment of abnormal breathing during sleep including nocturnal ventilation. BTS News 1990;5:7-10.

60. Douglas NJ, Thomas JMA: Clinical value of polysomnography. Lancet 1992;339:347-350.

61. Epstein LJ, Dorlac GR: Cost-effectiveness analysis of nocturnal oximetry as a method of screening for sleep apnea-hypopnea syndrome. Chest 1998;113:97-103.

62. Hussain SF, Fleetham JA: Overnight home oximetry: Can it identify patients with obstructive sleep apnea-hypopnea who have minimal daytime sleepiness? Respir Med 2003;97:537-540.

63. Flemons WW, Littner MR, Rowley JA, et al: Home diagnosis of sleep apnea: A systematic review of the literature. Chest 2003;124:1543-1579.

64. Chesson AL, Berry RB, Pack A: Practice parameters for the use of portable monitoring devices in the investigation of suspected obstructive sleep apnea in adults. Sleep 2003;26:907-913.

65. Haponick EF, Smith PL, Meyers DA, et al: Evaluation of sleep-disordered breathing: Is polysomnography necessary? Am J Med 1984;77:671-677.

66. Iber C, O'Brien C, Schluter J, et al: Single night studies in obstructive sleep apnea. Sleep 1991;14:383-385.

67. Jamieson A: Split-night studies: A new standard? Forcing the examination of outcome. Sleep 1991;14:381-382.

68. Arias A, Antonio M, Dandamudi N, et al: Diagnostic yield of daytime nap polysomnography. Am Rev Respir Dis 1992;145:A724.

69. Flemons WW, Douglas NJ, Kuna ST, et al: Access to diagnosis and treatment of patients with suspected sleep apnea. Am J Respir Crit Care Med 2004;169:668-672.

70. Wittmann V, Rodenstein DO: Health care costs and the sleep apnea syndrome. Sleep Med Rev 2004;8:269-279.

71. Medicare Department of Health and Human Services: Coverage Issues Manual, Centers for Medicare and Medicaid Services (CMS), Transmittal 150: December 26, 2001 (Change request 1949).

72. George CF, Kryger MH: When is an apnea not an apnea? Am Rev Respir Dis 1985;131:485-486.

73. Cirlgnotta F, Mondini S, Gerardi R, et al: Unreliability of automatic scoring of MESAM 4 in assessing patients with complicated obstructive sleep apnea. Chest 2001;119:1387-1392.

118

Assessment of Sleep-Related Erections

J. Catesby Ware

Max Hirshkowitz

ABSTRACT

Sleep-related erections are involuntary, naturally occurring penile erections characteristically associated with rapid eye movement sleep. The historical background of this phenomenon's discovery and characterization is reviewed. Clinically, sleep-related erections are of interest because analyzing the pattern of these erections can provide information concerning the cause of erectile dysfunction. Specific clinical and laboratory procedures are reviewed and a quantitative approach is described. The techniques used to record, score, tabulate, classify, and summarize sleep-related erection information are discussed. Normative data, general guidelines, and specific questions helpful to guide interpretation are provided.

Penile erections normally occur in two situations: during sexual arousal and during rapid eye movement (REM) sleep. After German physiologists published the first scientific report on periodic sleep-related erections (SREs) in 1944,[1] Fisher and colleagues[2] and Karacan[3] determined that these erections occurred in association with REM sleep. (The physiology of SREs is reviewed in Chapter 25). SREs begin at age 3 to 6 months[4,5] and occur in healthy male human beings of all ages as well as in other mammals. In the flaccid penis, blood drawn from the corpora cavernosa has a PO_2 similar to that of venous blood (25 to 43 mm Hg).[6] Presumably, regular penile vasodilation during sleep provides the oxygenation, nutrition, and waste removal necessary to maintain erectile capability, thus adding a new meaning to the adage "use it or lose it."

SREs (also referred to as nocturnal penile tumescence [NPT]) are diagnostically useful in evaluating erectile dysfunction (ED). Because men with abnormal SREs are likely to have impairment in physiologic systems underlying normal erectile functioning, SREs are sensitive to organic factors that impair erectile functioning. Patients with abnormal SREs typically have abnormalities in vascular, neurologic, or hormonal systems necessary for normal sexual functioning. One study reported sensitivity to pathophysiology to be 90.6% and specificity to be 88.2% when compared with intracavernous injection, penile Doppler ultrasonography, and cavernosometry tests.[7]

Sleep appears to insulate SREs from psychological factors. For example, viewing a video before sleep, regardless of whether its content is neutral, dysphoric, or sexually explicit, does not affect subsequent erections in healthy subjects.[8] Nevertheless, the isolation of these sleep erections from psychiatric illnesses is not complete. Depression, a problem associated with altered sleep,[9] may cause an abnormal SRE pattern.[10] Furthermore, even after they are treated for depression, these patients have greater SRE variability than healthy subjects.[9] Any disorder that alters the basic sleep pattern, particularly REM sleep, may alter the SRE pattern.

Monitoring SRE provides an important objective measure of erectile capability that can be useful in assessing medications to treat ED; in evaluating legal cases, for example where the plaintiff claims that an injury resulted in ED[11]; in diagnosing problems in patients complaining of ED; in studying normal erectile physiology[12]; and in studying specific changes that occur from surgical trauma.[13]

PROCEDURES

This chapter focuses on the procedures that use SRE monitoring for the assessment of ED. There are a number of methods for monitoring erections during sleep. Minimum criteria for judging their validity should include the ability to assess erectile activity in conjunction with REM sleep, the presence of age-related normative data for that particular technique, and clinical trials demonstrating impairment in erections recorded from patient groups likely to have impairment in erectile capability. Here we describe details for measuring SREs using penile plethysmography with strain gauges and polysomnography. Examples of other techniques include use of the proprietary Snap Gauge and RigiScan (Timm Medical Technologies, New Albany, Ohio),[14,15] along with electrobioimpedance volumetric assessment.[16,17]

SRE data obtained in a vacuum are of limited utility, particularly when dealing with individual patients. To maximize the benefit of the data, the diagnostic assessment requires several steps. The process includes a history and physical examination, an explanation of the procedures to the patient, calibration and placement of correct-size strain gauges, measurement of penile rigidity, observation of the penis in its most erect state, and the determination of sleep stages, particularly REM sleep.

History, Physical Examination, and Other Procedures

In addition to the usual information obtained during the history, specific questions concerning the patient's sexual functioning are helpful. Some of these questions are included in Table 118–1. During the physical examination, palpate the penis for Peyronie's plaques. If there are other indications of hormonal abnormalities, an assay for testosterone and prolactin can be helpful. One study looking at 76 patients on renal replacement therapy, found that prognostic factors for ED were the number of cardiovascular events, the waist-to-hip ratio, body mass index, and acceleration time measured during penile pharmacologic duplex ultrasonography.[18] Penile duplex ultrasonography with papaverine injection can complement SRE testing and pinpoint specific vascular abnormalities, but

Table 118–1. **Examples of Potentially Helpful Questions When Taking Erectile Dysfunction History**

Question	Comment
What are the prior workups and treatments?	Most will have prior treatment attempts.
What is his best erection?	Usually asked with anchor points of 0 (floppy) to 50 (half hard) to 100 (completely firm).
What is the minimum percentage of a full erection necessary for penetration?	A full erection may not be needed for penetration.
How long can the patient maintain an erection?	Need to know in relation to ejaculation.
Is there penile pain or curvature during erection?	Pain or a bend may indicate an anatomical problem such as Peyronie's disease.
Is there any change in sensitivity or numbness?	Neuropathy or injury to penis?
Is there any change in level of sexual desire?	Loss of libido or erectile dysfunction?
Can the patient ejaculate, and can he ejaculate with a soft penis?	Most with ED report ability to ejaculate.
Does he have a regular sexual partner, and when was his last successful intercourse?	Lack of experience may be the issue.
How does the partner respond to his failures?	Lack of partner's empathy may increase performance anxiety.
Is the problem partner specific?	A "yes" does not necessarily indicate a psychogenic problem. Anatomy and experience may affect performance.
What are the patient's expectations?	Are they realistic?

duplex ultrasonography is normal in patients with neurogenic impotence, whereas SRE testing is likely to be abnormal.[19]

Assessment of Comorbidity Factors

Cardiovascular, endocrine, genitourinary, neurologic, and psychiatric conditions commonly exist in patients with ED. Disorders accompanying altered SREs include diabetes mellitus,[20-23] hypogonadism,[24] chronic obstructive pulmonary disease,[25] alcoholism,[26,27] spinal lesions,[28,29] end-stage renal disease,[30] hypercholesterolemia,[31] and hypertension.[32]

Although the SRE pattern usually continues to some degree in patients with these disorders, the changes from normal can be profound. For example, compared with potent subjects, SREs in patients with diabetes have smaller maximum circumference increases (often less than 10 mm) and greater variability in the circumference of each episode. Detumescence may be prolonged, penile rigidity is low (often less than 500 g), and SREs occur less frequently and have a shorter duration. SREs can be normal in some patient groups complaining of ED. For example, in patients with multiple sclerosis, less than 10% of those complaining of ED appear to have abnormal SRE.[33]

Endocrine functions can influence erectile arousal mechanisms. Decreased testosterone traditionally was thought to primarily reduce sexual drive. However, reduction in testosterone with gonadotropin-releasing hormone agonist decreases SREs in normal subjects without affecting REM sleep.[34] In addition, the withdrawal of androgen replacement therapy in hypogonadal men results in diminished SREs without changing the sleep patterns.[24]

Medication Review

Several classes of drugs adversely affect erectile function in men. Some medications reduce SREs by altering penile physiology; other agents suppress erections as a result of REM sleep disruption. Antihypertensives and medications that affect autonomic nervous system functioning may interfere with sexual function. Other medications associated with ED include antidepressants, antiandrogens, and antipsychotics. In addition, cimetidine, disulfiram, atropine, digoxin, and cancer chemotherapy agents may cause iatrogenic ED. Trazodone increases the duration of SREs in young healthy men.[35]

Four antidepressants appear not to reduce REM sleep: nefazodone,[36] bupropion,[37] trimipramine,[38] and mirtazapine.[39] Although well-controlled clinical trials are absent, these medications appear less likely to impair sexual functioning than antidepressants that suppress REM sleep. Conversely, medications such as phentolamine and sildenafil appear to improve SREs in healthy men[40] or in those complaining of ED.[41,42] Potentially, increasing oxygenation by increasing erectile activity during sleep over the long term may improve erectile functioning or help forestall the development of ED in at-risk patients such as those with diabetes mellitus.

Polysomnography

Recording

The polysomnographic study of SRE can help answer three practical questions: Can the patient attain a rigid erection? Is the erection anatomically normal? Can the patient maintain his erection (during REM sleep)?

A comprehensive evaluation requires a full polysomnographic study. In addition to the transducers used to assess sleep and respiratory function, strain gauges around the base of the penis (*base gauge*) and behind the glans at the coronal sulcus (*tip gauge*) monitor penile circumference changes. A strain gauge is a loop of mercury-filled Silastic tubing with a small wire inserted in each end; the tubes are sealed and tied together[43] so that a small electrical current can pass through the mercury. Penile expansion produces elongation and thinning of the gauge, so increased resistance reflects an increased circumference. The changes in circumference indicate the underlying dynamics of penile erections. The process involves initial vasodilation and filling of the corpora cavernosa, maintenance of the tumescence by mechanical occlusion of emissary veins, and detumescence associated with smooth muscle contraction and vasoconstriction. Table 118–2 summarizes SRE recording procedures and interpretations.

The measurement of penile circumference changes without measurement of rigidity provides limited information. Measurement of rigidity allows identification of patients who have normal penile circumference increases without rigidity increases. Our experience is that some patients may have typical 2-cm penile circumference increases with little increase in rigidity. Conversely, although less common, some patients have normal rigidity with little circumference increase (i.e., a maximum circumference increase [MCI] of less than 10 mm). Therefore, it is crucial to measure rigidity during the maximum circumference of a representative SRE.

For a clinical diagnosis, the few awakenings made to measure rigidity have little consequence on the overall sleep pattern, but for some research studies, these awakenings may require an additional study night. On the first night in the laboratory for normal subjects, the technician has only 6 minutes per episode (on average) to decide whether the patient has reached an MCI and to measure rigidity.[44] In patients with pathology, this window of opportunity is usually shorter; therefore, well before it is time to measure rigidity, the technician must prepare the force gauge, videotape, and camera.

Although the first episode of tumescence during the night may be unstable, it often indicates the minimum circumference increase and duration of subsequent episodes. The technician can skip measuring rigidity during the first erection and take a measurement during the second erection episode if the tip circumference reaches at least the circumference achieved during the first erection and stabilizes. Later, if the patient has a greater circumference increase than that accompanying the highest rigidity value, the technician takes additional measurements.

No device provides a continuous measure of the resistance of the penis to buckling; consequently, accuracy depends on the technician's skill at judging when to measure penile rigidity using a force gauge. After awakening the patient to measure penile rigidity, the technician reminds the patient of the procedure. (The patient also is given an explanation of the rigidity measurement procedure during the office intake, during the tour of the facilities after the office intake, and during the wiring in the evening before bed.)

To quickly measure rigidity, the technician pulls down the covers and the patient's pajamas, stabilizes the patient's penis at the base between the index finger and thumb, and applies the force gauge to the tip of the penis, parallel to the longitudinal axis. The technician increases the force gradually until either the penile shaft buckles or the meter reaches 1000 g. The technician then photographs the penis and instructs the patient to inspect and estimate the percentage of a full erection. The entire procedure takes less than 30 seconds. Generally, this is not sufficient time for detumescence to occur.

A normal healthy male is usually able to achieve an axial rigidity of 750 to 1200 g. Rigidities of 500 to 749 g are potentially functional. Rigidities of less than 500 g are abnormal and would rarely be adequate for penetration.

The patient estimates during rigidity measurement reveal a subgroup with normal SREs who perceive their erections as far below normal and judge them to be insufficient for intercourse. These patients may indicate that they have little or no erection notwithstanding the presence of a physiologically normal erection. Possibly, these patients also obtain full erections during sexual activity but have a distorted perception of their degree of erection. It is likely that men with *penis state misperception* require different treatment than patients with psychogenic ED arising from performance anxiety. This perceptual distortion is a possible variant of the body dysmorphic disorder described in the *Diagnostic and Statistical Manual of Mental Disorders, Fourth Edition*.[45]

Observation

The process of awakening the patient to measure rigidity allows detection of abnormalities that may not be obvious in the flaccid penis, such as a marked curve or bend in the penis caused by Peyronie's disease.

Consider the example of a 35-year-old, physically healthy man with diagnosed schizoid personality disorder and psychogenic ED. He presented with a 2-year history of an inability to obtain an erection sufficient for penetration. His tumescence pattern and rigidity were normal; however, he had a 75-degree upward bend in his penis. Examination of his penis during the office visit failed to detect a small plaque on the dorsal surface of his penis, and therefore the diagnosis of Peyronie's disease was missed. In addition, the patient failed to mention the bend during his history.

In some cases, photographic documentation of a normal SRE helps to persuade the patient of his ability to achieve a full erection. Photographing the erection is also helpful when considering surgical correction of Peyronie's disease. Documentation of the erect state, before and after surgery, is desirable. Finally, a photograph of the erection at the time of rigidity measurement provides independent evidence for cross-validating buckling (rigidity) values.

Number of Nights

An SRE evaluation usually requires two nights of polysomnography, although for some patients, a single night is sufficient to make a diagnosis. One study night usually suffices when a completely normal SRE pattern occurs. Many patients have reduced REM sleep during the first night sleeping in the laboratory.[46] Because REM sleep is a key ingredient for evaluating SREs, a second night is often required. Although the patient may obtain a full erection during the first night, shortened REM sleep episodes prevent accurate determination of his ability to maintain these erections. On the second night, the patient sleeps undisturbed to determine the duration of his erections. Short-duration SREs may accompany a complaint of inability to maintain erections. An extreme example occurs in some spinal cord–injured patients who obtain brief rigid erections (*reflex erections*) without the ability to sustain them.[28]

On the second night, if MCI exceeds that occurring during the first-night rigidity measurement and the maximal rigidity on the first night was less than 750 g, the patient must return for a third night so additional rigidity measurements can be collected. During the second night, if a full erection occurs near the patient's scheduled arising time, measuring rigidity may obviate the need for a third recording session.

Table 118–2.   Polysomnography Procedures for Evaluating Sleep-Related Erection

Procedure	Description or Purpose	Comment
Calibrate gauges	Gauges and amplifiers are calibrated on cylinders, typically 6-10 cm in circumference.	Gauge size must match calibration cylinder.
Gauge sizing and placement	Gauge circumference is approximately 0.5 cm less than flaccid penile circumference.	If gauge is too small, loss of linearity; if too large, loss of sensitivity.
Placement of strain gauges	Gauges are placed on penile base (base gauge) and behind the glans at the coronal sulcus (tip gauge) perpendicular to axis of penis.	Base and tip gauges may need to be different sizes.
Begin recording and adjust baseline	The record should indicate a circumference close to that of the calibration cylinder.	If the circumference is much greater, there is an incorrect gauge placement, gauge is too small, gauge is broken, or patient has an erection.
Detect artifact	Technician must recognize and correct artifact during study.	Common problems include a broken gauge or a tip gauge off the penis.
Rigidity measurement	Measure rigidity at maximum circumference.	Measuring at less than maximum circumference results in rigidity of less than normal and possibly a false positive study result.
Visual observation and photograph	Observe and photograph the erection when measuring rigidity. This can detect penile abnormalities such as Peyronie's disease.	The photograph helps if there is a discrepancy between rigidity reading and patient and technician estimate of fullness of erection. Should be repeated if less than normal rigidity
Poststudy calibration	This documents normally functioning gauges in the event of abnormal circumference changes during study.	Gauges may break during their removal in the morning if handled incorrectly.
Multinight recording	Testing usually requires two studies to determine rigidity and ability to maintain erections.	Poor sleep or a sleep disorder (e.g., sleep apnea) may necessitate additional recording nights.
Comparison to normal data	This is necessary to account for age-related changes.	Penile pathology or abnormal sleep can affect the results.

Scoring and Summarizing Data

SRE MEASURES

Parameters needed for diagnosis include SRE frequency, magnitude, and duration. In addition, indices of sleep continuity, integrity, and architecture complete the necessary quantitative picture of SREs. Four points—T_{up}, T_{max}, T_{down}, and T_{zero}—characterize an episode of penile tumescence; these are defined in Table 118–3 and illustrated in Figure 118–1.

SLEEP MEASURES

Because sleep, especially REM sleep, provides the essential physiologic milieu for SREs, polysomnography during assessment of sleep erection provides a number of benefits. Polysomnography prevents a false-positive test result—that is, an abnormal erection pattern due to abnormal sleep. If the duration of REM sleep is short, the erectile duration may be short as a result of sleep disturbance rather than erectile pathophysiology. This may occur during first-night evaluations conducted in a noisy hospital environment. It may also occur when a patient's medication suppresses REM sleep (e.g., medications with anticholinergic properties and many antidepressants). A false-positive test result increases the likelihood of misdiagnosis and nonoptimized treatment for patients with ED.

SLEEP DISORDERS

Because the elderly are particularly susceptible to sleep disturbances[47] and older men are more likely to complain of ED, assessment of sleep is an important part of the SRE evaluation in older men.

Sleep apnea is exceedingly common in men with erectile dysfunction.[48,49] In a group of 1025 patients complaining of ED, more than 25% had significant obstructive sleep apnea (apnea frequency of 10 or greater per hour of sleep).[50] In sleep apnea patients, neurogenic factors[51] and cardiovascular problems[52,53] may contribute to ED. In addition, hypoxia insults associated with apnea events and obesity-related hypoventilation may lower testosterone levels.

Table 118–3.   Sleep-Related Erection Scoring, Tabulation, and Summary Parameters

Parameter	Description
Maximum circumference increase (MCI)	The overall MCI above the flaccid state (baseline) that occurs during the recording period. The MCI also is determined for each tumescence episode.
T_{up} (tumescence up)	The beginning of tumescence. This is the point where there has been more than a 2-mm circumference increase above the baseline for 2 minutes. The term T_{up} also refers to the time between the points T_{up} and T_{max}.
T_{max} (tumescence maximum)	The point where penile circumference reaches 75% of the MCI for the entire night. T_{max} also refers to the time between the points T_{max} and T_{down}. If the MCI for a particular episode does not reach 75%, T_{max} for that episode begins and ends at the maximal point for that episode and T_{down} begins in the next minute.
T_{down} (tumescence down)	Begins where the circumference falls below the 75% T_{max} criterion and continues to T_{zero}. The term T_{down} also identifies the time between the points T_{down} and T_{zero}.
T_{zero} (tumescence zero)	The point where penile circumference reaches 2 mm or less above the baseline.
Tumescence episodes (TE)	Number of SREs during the sleep period. This closely parallels the number of REM periods. Episodes that overlap REM sleep by at least 1 minute (REM-related episodes) may be tabulated separately.
Total tumescence time (TTT)	Minutes during the recording in which penile circumference is more than 2 mm above the baseline. This is usually 125 ± 50 minutes.
Percentage total tumescence time (%TTT)	Percentage of the sleep period (interval from sleep onset to final awakening) during which there was a more than 2-mm increase in penile circumference above baseline.
Fluctuations (FLUC)	Transient decreases in circumference during T_{max}. The circumference drops below 75% of the MCI and may approach, but does not reach, baseline. Fluctuations may accompany anxiety-laden dreams and may occur to a greater degree in patients with vascular outflow problems. Because fluctuations allow for increased blood flow through the penis, they may be physiologically important during an erection.
TTT-to-REM sleep ratio (TTT/REM)	Ratio of total tumescence time to REM-sleep time facilitates comparisons between records with different durations of REM sleep.
T_{max}-to-REM sleep ratio (T_{max}/REM)	Ratio of the total duration of maximal tumescence (minutes between the points T_{max} and T_{down}) to REM sleep duration. This measures the erectile system's ability to maintain tumescence in the presence of an appropriate stimulus (i.e., REM sleep).
T_{up}–REM sleep onset differential (T_{up}–REM_{on})	Time between T_{up} and the beginning of REM sleep. In healthy subjects, T_{up} may precede an episode of REM sleep. In this situation, T_{up}–REM_{on} is a positive number. It is a negative number when tumescence onset follows the onset of REM.
REM sleep–T_{zero} offset differential (REM_{off}–T_{zero})	Time between the end of REM sleep and the end of tumescence. If tumescence ends before the end of REM sleep, the measure is a negative number. When tumescence ends after REM sleep, it is a positive number. In healthy subjects and patients free from vascular impotence, alpha-adrenergic receptor blocking will dramatically prolong REM_{off}–T_{zero}.[35]

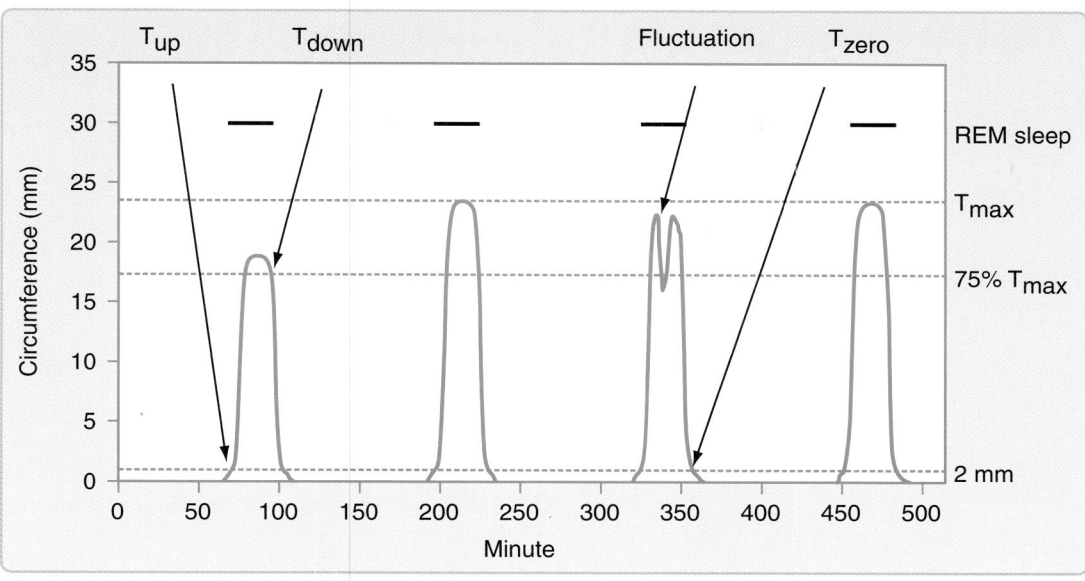

Figure 118–1. Normal sleep-related erection pattern illustrating T_{up}, T_{down}, T_{max}, a fluctuation, and T_{zero}. Note that the illustrated points actually occur on each of the four erections. The duration of T_{max} is measured from when circumference reaches more than 75% of the maximum circumference increase (T_{max}) to when it drops below the 75% line. Rapid eye movement (REM) sleep is indicated by the *dark bars* above the erections. Circumference is given in millimeters.

The treatment of obstructive sleep apnea does appear to increase testosterone levels and reverse a decrease in sexual function in some men.[54] Also, excessive daytime sleepiness, a prominent symptom of sleep apnea, can overwhelm the libido and result in falling asleep in bed rather than engaging in sexual activity. However, despite a number of possible reasons for ED to occur in sleep apnea patients, the available data do not yet confirm a cause-and-effect relationship between apnea and ED.[52]

Periodic limb movements in sleep also occur at a remarkably high rate in men with erectile dysfunction. Of 768 consecutively evaluated impotent men, 54% had 15 or more leg movements per hour of sleep.[55] Both apnea and periodic limb movements may reduce REM sleep, increase strain gauge artifact due to increased movement, correlate with an intervening factor, or directly contribute to ED.

INTERPRETING POLYSOMNOGRAPHY AND SRE RESULTS

Does the Patient Have Sustained REM Sleep Episodes?

During wakefulness, sexual stimulation initiates penile erections. During sleep, REM sleep provides an analogue to sexual stimulation. Interpretation of a polysomnographic SRE recording must be within the context of REM sleep. The amount of REM sleep required for a valid study depends on both the patient's complaint and the pattern of penile erections. Some patients complain of difficulty maintaining penile erections, and polysomnography reveals full but brief erections. Fragmented and short REM sleep episodes make it impossible to determine whether the short-duration erections reflect abnormal penile physiology or the REM sleep interruption. In other patients, brief REM sleep interruptions or short-duration REM periods do not substantially alter episodes of penile erections. Under these circumstances, the REM sleep fragmentation is irrelevant.

When the patient complains of an inability to attain a full erection, REM-sleep duration must be sufficient to obtain a stable maximum circumference for measuring rigidity. Although REM sleep totals approximately 100 minutes during a normal night, this duration may not be necessary. One sustained 20-minute REM episode may be sufficient to determine whether the patient can attain and maintain a normal erection. If a patient is taking medication, however, one normal erection at the end of the sleep period may not indicate that the patient can function normally during the day. It is possible that the medication suppresses erectile capability during wakefulness and the early part of the night. As the night progresses, blood levels may decline during sleep and allow a normal erection to occur toward the end of the night.

Does the Erection Progress Normally to the Maximum Circumference Increase?

The time between the onset of REM and the onset of SRE can be variable even in healthy subjects but decreases during the night.[56] In normal REM SREs, T_{up} is steep and steady. The development of an erection from onset to T_{max} takes approximately 10 minutes.

Does the Erection Continue throughout the REM Episode?

Once reached, the maximal erectile phase (T_{max}) should remain throughout most of the REM episode. Small oscillations (several millimeters) are common; however, an inability to sustain tumescence for more than 1 or 2 minutes during a normal REM sleep episode is unusual. Such a pattern suggests

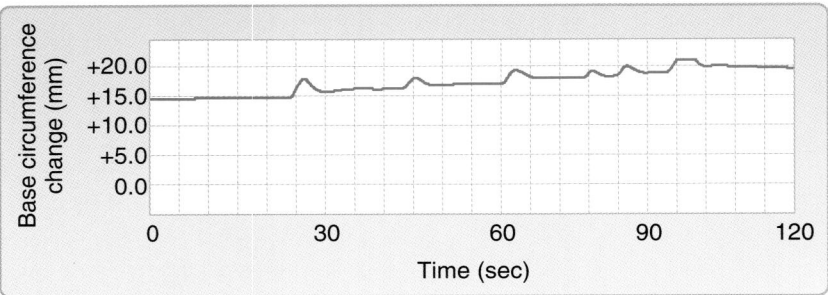

Figure 118–2. This tracing is from a strain gauge around the base of the patient's penis during a normal REM-sleep penile erection. The ordinate (y axis) indicates penile circumference increase from the flaccid baseline in millimeters. The abscissa (x axis) indicates time in 5-second blocks (*vertical lines*). The transient circumference increases are referred to as pulsations and are associated with bulbocavernosus and ischiocavernosus muscle activity.

venous leakage or some other penile pathophysiology. Detumescence typically starts just before the end of REM sleep and continues for 10 to 20 minutes (time from T_{down} to T_{zero}). The time from the end of REM sleep to T_{zero} ($REM_{off} - T_{zero}$) is typically 5 to 10 minutes.

Does Detumescence Proceed Quickly after the End of REM Sleep?

Detumescence is a physiologically active phase with increased sympathetic activity and vasoconstriction. Even to maintain the flaccid penis, some degree of sympathetic tone is necessary. The inability to proceed through detumescence rapidly (*fuzzy detumescence*) suggests an alteration in autonomic functioning. Blocking of the sympathetic nervous system pharmacologically with, for example, trazodone may cause tumescence to continue long after the end of REM sleep.[35]

Does Penile Buckling Force Indicate Functional Erectile Capacity?

Evidence suggests that 500 g is the minimal force required to achieve penetration under circumstances conducive to intercourse.[57] These data derive from direct measures during vaginal insertion, confidence ratings made by healthy subjects, and success-or-failure judgments made by patients. The presence of an erection with at least 750 g rigidity suggests adequate capacity for achieving penetration.

There are several exceptions. A patient complaining of difficulty maintaining an erection after achieving full tumescence may have completely rigid but short-lived tumescence episodes during sleep. Other instances in which rigidity values must be complemented by other measures are in assessment of men with spinal injuries, the pelvic steal syndrome,[58] and Peyronie's disease.

Are Penile Pulsations Present?

The resolution of the recording must be sufficient to detect penile pulsations. Pulsations are transient circumference increases that last approximately 1 second. Pulsations result from contractions of the bulbocavernosus and ischiocavernosus muscles. They normally occur during T_{up} and the first part of T_{max} at a frequency of several per minute (Fig. 118–2). They occur less frequently in patients with organic problems.[59] Absence of pulsations may indicate a problem of neurologic origin.

How Do SREs Compare with Age-Matched Normative Data?

Sleep-related erections change with age in normal subjects.[44] These changes occur not only as a result of changes in sleep pattern but also apparently as a result of erectile capability. Table 118–4 illustrates statistically reliable but modest changes with age. Importantly, these data indicate that sleep-related erections persist throughout life in healthy subjects. A comparison of the number and duration of erections in patients with age-matched normative values is helpful when interpreting nocturnal penile tumescence.

Does the Patient Have an Agenda?

Concurrent polysomnography during SRE testing safeguards against undetected intentional manipulation of data. Some patients strongly prefer one treatment to another. To fake an "organic pattern," a patient assessed without polysomnography need only remove the strain gauge or stay awake. A diagnosis of organic ED may increase the chance of obtaining a penile prosthesis, help obtain a more favorable judgment from a jury in an accident compensation case, or affect the ruling in a sexual assault trial.

Table 118–4.	Sleep-related Erection Parameters* by Age		
Age (Years)	Total Tumescence (Minutes)	REM Related Tumescence (Percentage)	Number of Episodes
20-29	100-200	20-30	2-5
30-49	65-165	19-29	2-5
40-49	60-160	14-24	2-4
50-59	60-160	13-23	2-4
60-69	40-140	12-22	1-3

*Approximate range for selected sleep-related erection (SRE) parameters at different ages. In the presence of a normal percentage of REM sleep, patient values less than the lower range suggest an abnormal SRE pattern.
REM, rapid eye movement.

SUMMARY

The measurement of SREs provides an objective assessment of erectile capability but must be combined with a clinical assessment. Performed correctly, a diagnostic evaluation of SREs consists of the following measures.

Measurement of sleep pattern is performed to prevent false-positive test results, to ease artifact detection, and to detect a subject's manipulation of data. An additional benefit is that the information obtained from sleep studies may be helpful in determining the presence of depression or sleep-related pathology.

Measurement of penile circumference patterns is performed to determine the number, magnitude, and duration of erections. An ability to attain and maintain an erection within REM sleep suggests an intact erectile physiology.

Measurement of penile rigidity is performed to determine erectile quality. The maximal circumference is not a guaranteed indicator of rigidity; thus, interpretation of the study requires rigidity measurements during MCIs.

Visual inspection of the penis during an erection is performed to determine penile anatomic problems that may not be obvious when the penis is flaccid. During an awakening when tumescence is present, asking the patient to estimate the degree of his erection allows identification of a penis-state misperception.

Accurate diagnostic methods become more essential as knowledge of the mechanisms controlling penile erections increases and as treatment techniques become more refined. When treatment options were limited to penile prosthesis, psychotherapy, or sex therapy, ED was classified as either organic or psychogenic. The degree of physical impairment and precise cause often made little difference. With improved surgical techniques and advancements in pharmacotherapy, detailed information concerning erectile function is more important to help match the treatment with the cause.

Sleep erection monitoring provides a wealth of objective information to facilitate understanding of ED and to guide therapeutic decisions. Because polysomnographic assessment of SREs is an unbiased, objective, noninvasive tool, it has the potential for furthering the advancement of the relatively understudied area of sexual dysfunction. The polysomnographic study of sexual dysfunction has the potential to advance the understanding of even central neuropathies that may contribute to impaired sexual performance when peripheral systems are intact.[60,61]

> *Clinical Pearl*
>
> *Sleep-related erections are naturally occurring and involuntary. They normally occur in close temporal association with REM sleep. They provide a unique opportunity to evaluate erectile physiology that is free from many sources of artifact and extraneous influences. Clinically, SRE pattern provides helpful etiologic information for assessment of erectile dysfunction.*

References

1. Ohlmeyer P, Brilmayer H, Hullstrung H: Periodische vorgange in schaf pflug. Arch Ges Physiol 1944;248:559-560.
2. Fisher C, Gross J, Zuch J: Cycle of penile erection synchronous with dreaming (REM) sleep: Preliminary report. Arch Gen Psychiatry 1965;12:29-45.
3. Karacan I: The effect of exciting presleep events on dream reporting and penile erections during sleep [dissertation]. Brooklyn, New York University, 1965.
4. Karacan I: The developmental aspect and the effect of certain clinical conditions upon penile erection during sleep. Proceedings of the Fourth World Congress of Psychiatry, Madrid, September 5-11, 1966. Excerpt Medical International Congress Series, vol 150, 1996, pp 2356-2359.
5. Korner A: REM organization in neonates. Arch Gen Psychiatry 1968;19:330-340.
6. Kim N, Vardi Y, Padma-Nathan H, et al: Oxygen tension regulates the nitric oxide pathway. Physiological role in penile erection. J Clin Invest 1993;91:437-442.
7. Basar MM, Atan A, Tekdogan UY: New concept parameters of RigiScan in differentiation of vascular erectile dysfunction: Is it a useful test? Int J Urol 2001;8:686-691.
8. Ware JC, Hirshkowitz M, Thornby J, et al: Sleep-related erections: Effects of presleep sexual arousal. J Psychosomat Res 1997;42:547-553.
9. Benca RM, Obermeyer WH, Thisted RA, et al: Sleep and psychiatric disorders: A meta-analysis. Arch Gen Psychiatry 1992;49:651-668.
10. Nofzinger EA, Thase ME, Reynolds CF, et al: Sexual function in depressed men: Assessment by self-report, behavioral, and nocturnal penile tumescence measures before and after treatment with cognitive behavior therapy. Arch Gen Psychiatry 1993;50:24-30.
11. Peled R, Pillar G, Berger Y, et al: Recording nocturnal erections following injuries and insurance claims: cost-effectiveness [Hebrew]. Harefuah 1999;136:432-434, 513, 514.
12. Lindsey I, Cunningham C, George BD, Mortensen NJ: Nocturnal penile tumescence is diminished but not ablated in postproctectomy impotence. Dis Colon Rectum 2003;46:14-19.
13. Schmidt MH, Valatx JL, Sakai K, et al: Role of the lateral preoptic area in sleep-related erectile mechanisms and sleep generation in the rat. J Neurosci 2000;20:6640-6647.
14. Chen J, Greenstein A, Sofer M, Matzkin H: RigiScan versus snap gauge band measurements: Is the extra cost justifiable? Int J Impot Res 1999;11:315-318; discussion 318.
15. Mizuno I, Fuse H, Fujiuchi Y: Snap-gauge band compared to RigiScan Plus in a nocturnal penile tumescence study for evaluation of erectile dysfunction. Urol Int 2003;71:96-99.
16. Knoll LD, Abrams JH: Application of nocturnal electrobioimpedance volumetric assessment: A feasibility study in men without erectile dysfunction. J Urol 1999;161:1137-1140.
17. Knoll LD, Abrams JH: Nocturnal electrobioimpedance volumetric assessment of patients with erectile dysfunction. Urology 1999;53:1200-1204.
18. Diemont WL, Hendriks JC, Lemmens WA, et al: Prognostic factors for the vascular components of erectile dysfunction in patients on renal replacement therapy. Int J Impot Res 2003;15:44-52.
19. Shabsigh R, Fishman IJ, Quesada ET, et al: Evaluation of vasculogenic erectile impotence using penile duplex ultrasonography. J Urol 1989;142:1469-1474.
20. Hirshkowitz M, Karacan I, Rando KC, et al: Diabetes, erectile dysfunction, and sleep-related erections. Sleep 1990;13:53-68.
21. Karacan I, Salis PJ, Ware JC, et al: Nocturnal penile tumescence and diagnosis in diabetic ED. Am J Psychiatry 1978;135:191-197.
22. Schiavi RC, Stimmel BB, Mandeli J, et al: Diabetes mellitus and male sexual function: A controlled study. Diabetologia 1993;36:745-751.
23. Zuckerman M, Neeb M, Ficher M, et al: Nocturnal penile tumescence and penile responses in the waking state in diabetic and nondiabetic sexual dysfunctionals. Arch Sex Behav 1985;14:109-129.
24. Cunningham GR, Hirshkowitz M, Korenman SG, et al: Testosterone replacement therapy and sleep-related erections in hypogonadal men. J Clin Endocrinol Metab 1990;70:792-797.

25. Fletcher EC, Martin RJ: Sexual dysfunction and erectile ED in chronic obstructive pulmonary disease. Chest 1982;81:413-421.

26. Karacan I, Moore CA: Sexual dysfunction in alcoholic men. In Wheatley D (ed): Psychopharmacology and Sexual Disorders. British Association for Psychopharmacology Monograph. Oxford, Oxford University, 1983, pp 113-122.

27. Snyder S, Karacan I: Effects of chronic alcoholism on nocturnal penile tumescence. Psychosomat Med 1981;43:423-429.

28. Halstead LS, Dimitrijevic M, Karacan I, et al: ED in spinal cord injury: Neurophysiological assessment of diminished tumescence and its relation to supraspinal influences. Curr Concepts Rehab Med 1984;1:8-14.

29. Suh DD, Yang CC, Clowers DE: Nocturnal penile tumescence and effects of complete spinal cord injury: Possible physiologic mechanisms. Urology 2003;61:184-189.

30. Karacan I, Dervent A, Cunningham G, et al: Assessment of nocturnal penile tumescence as an objective method for evaluating sexual functioning in ESRD patients. Dialysis Transplant 1978;7:872-876, 890.

31. Seftel AD, Strohl KP, Loye TL, et al: Erectile dysfunction and symptoms of sleep disorders. Sleep 2002;25:643-647.

32. Karacan I, Salis PJ, Hirshkowitz M, et al: Erectile dysfunction in hypertensive men: Sleep-related erections, penile blood flow, and musculovascular events. J Urol 1989;142:56-61.

33. Lottman PE, Jongen PJ, Rosier PF, Meuleman EJ: Sexual dysfunction in men with multiple sclerosis—a comprehensive pilot-study into etiology. Int J Impot Res 1998;10:233-237.

34. Hirshkowitz M, Moore CA, O'Connor S, et al: Androgen and sleep-related erections. J Psychosomat Res 1997;42:541-546.

35. Saenz de Tejada I, Ware JC, Blanco R, et al: Pathophysiology of prolonged penile erection associated with trazodone use. J Urol 1991;145:60-64.

36. Ware JC, Rose FV, McBrayer R: The acute effects of nefazodone, trazodone and buspirone on sleep and sleep-related penile tumescence in normal subjects. Sleep 1994;6:544-550.

37. Nofzinger EA, Reynolds CF 3rd, Thase ME, et al: REM sleep enhancement by bupropion in depressed men. Am J Psychiatry 1995;152:274-276.

38. Ware JC, Brown FW, Moorad PJ, et al: Effects on sleep: A double-blind study comparing trimipramine to imipramine in depressed insomniac patients. Sleep 1989;12:537-549.

39. Aslan S, Isik E, Cosar B: The effects of mirtazapine on sleep: A placebo controlled, double-blind study in young healthy volunteers. Sleep 2002;25:677-679.

40. Rochira V, Granata AR, Balestrieri A, et al: Effects of sildenafil on nocturnal penile tumescence and rigidity in normal men: Randomized, placebo-controlled, crossover study. J Androl 2002;23:566-571.

41. Hatzichristou DG, Apostolidis A, Tzortzis V, et al: Effects of oral phentolamine, taken before sleep, on nocturnal erectile activity: A double-blind, placebo-controlled, crossover study. Int J Impot Res 2001;13:303-308.

42. Montorsi F, Maga T, Strambi LF, et al: Sildenafil taken at bedtime significantly increases nocturnal erections: Results of a placebo-controlled study. Urology 2000;56:906-911.

43. Karacan I: A simple and inexpensive transducer for quantitative measurements of penile erection during sleep. Behav Res Methods Instrum 1969;1:251-252.

44. Ware JC, Hirshkowitz M: Characteristics of penile erections during sleep. J Clin Neurophysiol 1992;9:78-87.

45. American Psychiatric Association: Diagnostic and Statistical Manual of Mental Disorders, 4th ed. Washington, DC, American Psychiatric Association, 1994, pp 466-468.

46. Agnew HW, Webb WB, Williams RL: The first night effect: An EEG study of sleep. Psychophysiology 1966;2:263-266.

47. Avidan AY: Sleep changes and disorders in the elderly patient. Curr Neurol Neurosci Rep 2002;2:178-185.

48. Schmidt HS, Wise HA: Significance of impaired penile tumescence and associated polysomnographic abnormalities in the impotent patient. J Urol 1981;126:348-352.

49. Pressman MR, DiPhillipo MA, Kendrick JI, et al: Problems in the interpretation of nocturnal penile tumescence studies: Disruption of sleep by occult sleep disorders. J Urol 1986;136: 595-598.

50. Hirshkowitz M, Karacan I, Arcasoy MO, et al: Prevalence of sleep apnea in men with erectile dysfunction. Urology 1990;36: 232-234.

51. Fanfulla F, Malaguti S, Montagna T, et al: Erectile dysfunction in men with obstructive sleep apnea: An early sign of nerve involvement. Sleep 2000;23:775-781.

52. Arruda-Olson AM, Olson LJ, Nehra A, Somers VK: Sleep apnea and cardiovascular disease. Implications for understanding erectile dysfunction. Herz 2003;28:298-303.

53. Weiss JW, Remsburg S, Garpestad E, et al: Hemodynamic consequences of obstructive sleep apnea. Sleep 1996;19: 388-397.

54. Santamaria JD, Prior JC, Fleetham JA: Reversible reproductive dysfunction in men with obstructive sleep apnoea. Clin Endocrinol (Oxford) 1988;28:461-470.

55. Hirshkowitz M, Karacan I, Arcasoy MO, et al: The prevalence of periodic limb movements during sleep in men with erectile dysfunction. Biol Psychiatry 1989;26:541-544.

56. Mann K, Pankok J, Connemann B, Roschke J: Temporal relationship between nocturnal erections and rapid eye movement episodes in healthy men. Neuropsychobiology 2003;47: 109-114.

57. Karacan I, Moore CA, Sahmay S: Measurement of pressure necessary for vaginal penetration [abstract]. Sleep Res 1985;14:269.

58. Michal V, Kramar R, Pospichal J: External iliac "steal syndrome." J Cardiovasc Surg 1978;19:355-357.

59. Allen RP, Smolev JK: Bulbo-ischio-cavernosus muscle activity in determining etiology for organic ED. In Virag R, Virag H (eds): Proceedings of the First World Meeting on ED. Paris, CERI, 1984, pp 95-99.

60. Nofzinger EA: Sexual dysfunction in patients with diabetes mellitus: The role of a "central" neuropathy. Semin Clin Neuropsychiatry 1997;2:31-39.

61. Lavie P, Shlitner A, Nave R: Cardiac autonomic function during sleep in psychogenic and organic erectile dysfunction. J Sleep Res 1999;8:135-142.

PRECIPITATING/PERPETUATING FACTORS
CONTRIBUTING TO INSOMNIA OVER TIME

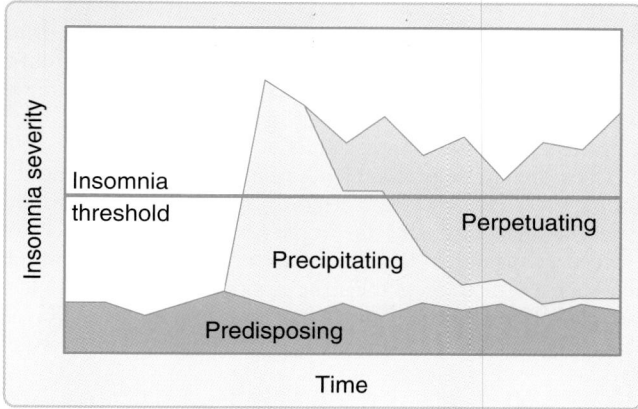

Figure 119–1. Conceptual model of the development of chronic insomnia and the changing factors that play a role over the course of the disorder. In this particular case, at the onset of the insomnia precipitating factors predominate. When the insomnia becomes chronic, perpetuating factors become the main feature contributing to the sleep disturbance (Adapted from Spielman AJ, Caruso L, Glovinsky PB: A behavioral perspective on insomnia. Psychiatr Clin North Am 1987;10:541-553.)

Loss of a job triggers a bout of insomnia. As our new insomniac begins to cope with unemployment, the precipitating factor's intensity is diminished. He speaks to colleagues, lines up interviews, and believes his prospects are good. However, he is determined to be at his best in this time of transition. He tries to get as much sleep as he can by going to bed early and oversleeping on weekends. He also drinks more coffee to maintain acuity and begins to worry about how his sleep

PREDISPOSING FACTORS CONTRIBUTING
TO INSOMNIA OVER TIME

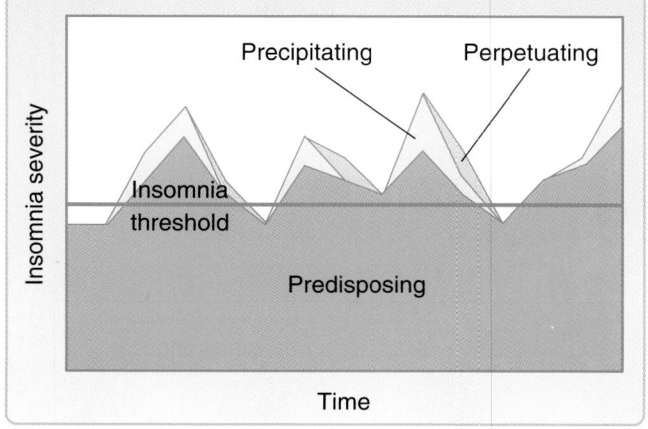

Figure 119–2. The conceptual model of insomnia applied to a case in which predisposing factors are prominent and are the single most important determinant of the insomnia. Precipitating factors episodically activate the predisposing factors. (Adapted from Spielman AJ, Caruso L, Glovinsky PB: A behavioral perspective on insomnia. Psychiatr Clin North Am 1987;10:541-553.)

problem will affect his performance at interviews. At the end of Figure 119–1 the intensity of the precipitating factor, the job loss, is barely present. Secondary perpetuating factors of sleep hygiene and worry about sleeplessness are now the main reasons the sleep problem persists.

In a second illustrative case (see Fig. 119–2) the person has a strong predisposition to insomnia. He is generally hyperaroused, overreactive to challenges, and a night owl. He often has trouble falling asleep and attaining an adequate amount of sleep. Although precipitating factors such as interpersonal conflicts, money problems, and health concerns trigger exacerbations of the sleep problem, the main ingredient producing the insomnia remains his underlying predisposition.

ASSESSMENT METHODS OF SLEEP DISORDERS CENTERS

To obtain a sense of evaluation procedures for insomnia, we conducted a quasi-random telephone survey of 40 sleep disorders centers for the first edition of this chapter. At the time, this sample represented more than 10% of the centers certified by the American Sleep Disorders Association.

We learned that a majority of centers used structured rating scales and questionnaires as adjuncts in the evaluation of patients complaining of insomnia. More than two thirds of the centers send questionnaires to the patient before the initial visit. Although virtually all centers use sleep logs, only about one third of patients fill out a sleep log before the sleep consultation. About three fourths of centers formally evaluate some of their patients for depression, whereas fewer than half evaluate their patients for anxiety. Although only a handful of centers use a separate instrument to assess beliefs and attitudes about sleep, this domain is often measured in sleep questionnaires. Two thirds of patients fill out a sleep and medical history questionnaire, and a similar percentage are evaluated by the clinician with the use of a semistructured interview. Half of the insomniacs have an evaluation by a psychologist or psychiatrist. After the initial consultation, a fourth of patients undergo nocturnal polysomnography. In the four centers that use actigraphy, only about 10% of patients receive this type of evaluation.

Unfortunately, most of the sleep logs, sleep history questionnaires, and semistructured interviews are custom made, unpublished, and unique to each center. Because of the absence of commonly accepted standard instruments, the lists that follow include published and unpublished methods even though they are not in common use. We refer to an instrument as *published* when the reference includes either a blank questionnaire or all the items, responses, and scoring necessary for use. Scales referred to as *available on request* can be purchased or obtained from the authors. The material in the tables is listed by date, except for Table 119–4 (assessment of specific causes), which groups according to categories. The following methods are arranged by the order in which clinicians typically proceed across the course of an evaluation.

Questionnaires, Diaries, and Logs

Some of the best methods for obtaining a balanced, comprehensive overview of a complaint of persistent insomnia involve having patients fill out retrospective questionnaires, inventories of current status, and prospective sleep diaries or logs.

Retrospective Instruments

A main benefit of adopting a guided retrospective approach to the assessment of insomnia is that it aids in forming an accurate picture of the sleep disturbance. Provided prompts to recognition memory as opposed to relying solely on recall, the patient is helped to gain a broader perspective on the problem. There is less need to focus only on those aspects that, in the judgment of the patient, would justify clinical attention.

SLEEP AND MEDICAL HISTORY QUESTIONNAIRES

Most useful if filled out by the patient before the first visit, sleep and medical history questionnaires can broach potentially sensitive topics for the patient's consideration in privacy, while also giving notice that the inquiry will necessarily be a broad one if the patient's complaint is to be adequately addressed. Questionnaires also have the benefit of introducing the long view and of moving the patient from the role of hapless victim of the vagaries of sleep into that of a coinvestigator.[22,24] Committing his or her experience to paper gives the patient the opportunity for reflection and revision common to all writing processes, which fosters a more considered and reliable assessment.

These methods do generate problems. The most obvious is that they often take a fair amount of the clinician's time to review. One such example is the venerable Cornell Medical Index, which contains 195 items, yielding a comprehensive survey.[33]

In addition to reviewing the patient's past medical history and current symptoms, it is essential to carefully consider the effects of all medications administered over the course of the insomnia disorder. This is partly accomplished with the sleep diary (see later), which asks the patient to list medication use. However, because the patient starts filling out the diary after the evaluation has begun, it does not yield information on the effect of drugs during the development of the insomnia. The clinical interview is the best way to weave together the features of medication use (e.g., type, amount, time of administration, frequency, side effects, withdrawal effects on discontinuation, and degree of drug tolerance) with other treatments and coping strategies in order to gauge the effects of these approaches on sleep.

There are two types of sleep history questionnaire. One assesses the adequacy and quality of sleep, and the other, more comprehensive type also includes a survey of potential etiologic factors (Tables 119–1 and 119–2). As noted above, we found that the overwhelming majority of clinicians use a sleep history questionnaire that is of their own design.

There are subtle problems associated with the use of questionnaires. They can create a false sense, on the part of both patient and clinician, that the inquiry has been comprehensive. There is a danger that in the interests of expediency, the clinician may choose "not to cover the same ground" as the questionnaire. Alternatively, due to the patient's positive response bias, the clinician may be obliged to follow up more intensively than would be otherwise necessary merely to rule out various diagnostic possibilities, and the interview will be prolonged. In other cases, patients simply are not capable of providing a faithful account by these means. However, even when a well-designed questionnaire is completed accurately, there is ample opportunity for confusion.

For these reasons, leaving the history taking to the form is tantamount to leaving out the history altogether. Rather than being misused in this way, questionnaires are properly used to structure the ensuing inquiry, to serve as an outline, and to guarantee that attention will be paid to all relevant areas as well as to the particular flags raised by the patient's responses.

PSYCHOPATHOLOGY AND PERSONALITY QUESTIONNAIRES

Although insomnia can result from a wide array of medical, environmental, and chronobiologic conditions, the high prevalence of psychopathology in patients with insomnia makes careful attention to this domain particularly important. Specific disorders such as depression, anxiety disorder, chaotic personality organizations, and psychoses may play a direct role in the genesis of insomnia. Even when overt psychopathology is not present, certain types of personality configuration may predispose toward insomnia. For example, a person who is prone to internalize conflict often experiences hyperarousal as a result.

Table 119–1. Sleep Quality Questionnaires*

Scale Name (Source)	No. of Items	Format
Published		
Post-sleep inventory[35] (p 989)	30	13-point bipolar scales
Leeds Sleep Evaluation Questionnaire[36] (pp 178-179)	10	Visual analogue scales Assessment of medication effects
St. Mary's Hospital Sleep Questionnaire[37] (pp 96-97)	14	Yes/no Frequency and severity ratings Fill in the blanks
Pittsburgh Sleep Quality Index[38] (pp 298-213)	24	Severity and frequency ratings Mainly symptom checklists Global score composed of a number of categories
Sleep Impairment Index[39] (pp 199-200)	15	Severity ratings Mainly symptom checklists
Available on Request		
Sleep questionnaire[40]	59	Mainly frequency ratings
Insomnia Symptom Questionnaire[41]	13	Visual analogue scales

*All scales assess the quality and adequacy of sleep. None survey etiologic factors.

Table 119–2.   Sleep History Questionnaires*

Scale Name (Source)	No. of Items	Format
Published		
Sleep Questionnaire and Assessment of Wakefulness[42] (pp 384-413)	863	Yes/no Symptom checklist Frequency and severity ratings Fill in the blanks
Sleep History Questionnaire[43] (pp 63-65)	48	Yes/no Fill in the blanks Links between particular questions and semistructured interview for follow-up
Sleep History Analysis[44] (p 24)	20	Yes/no Fill in the blanks
Available on Request		
Sleep Disorders Questionnaire[45]	176	Derived from Sleep Quality and Assessment of Wakefulness Frequency and severity ratings Not specific to insomnia
Brock Sleep and Insomnia Questionnaire[46]	103	Yes/no Severity and frequency ratings Fill in the blanks Separate sections on five diagnostic entities and a drug inventory

*All scales assess the quality and adequacy of sleep and survey etiologic factors.

Detail-oriented perfectionists may not allow themselves a respite from the day's challenges, instead bringing these into bed for further reflection. Persons with ruminative personalities may become caught in a cycle of misgivings or strategizing rather than settling into sleep.

Screening for psychopathology and personality typing are readily accomplished through the use of assessment instruments (Table 119–3). A large number of tests have been developed that permit valid inferences to be drawn about a patient's psychological makeup. Some cast a wide net and are useful in characterizing a broad range of pathology; others have a more specific focus. In any case, the use of psychological assessments does not relieve the clinician of responsibility for evaluating the patient's mental status. Often, clinical judgment is confirmed and treatment can proceed with greater assurance, whereas at other times, discrepancies between these forms of assessment may lead to fruitful new avenues of inquiry.

The Minnesota Multiphasic Personality Inventory (MMPI) is a widely used instrument that yields a personality profile and alerts the clinician to the possible existence of a broad range of psychopathology.[54] Extensive research has demonstrated that specific MMPI patterns are associated with insomnia.[6,7] If such personality configurations or psychopathologies are found, the clinician may bring specific remedies to bear on the sleep disturbance—for example, cognitive therapy or pharmacotherapy for depression may in turn relieve the symptom of early morning awakening. Instruction in self-hypnosis may give those who are prone to somaticizing a way to redirect their attention away from physical discomfort, thereby alleviating sleep-onset insomnia.

The MMPI has several drawbacks. Its comprehensive nature requires a lengthy administration. Although this is typically done before the initial visit, it can cause consternation in patients who feel they are being diverted back toward the general practice of psychology just when they thought they had reached a specialist who would focus on the complaint at hand. Depending on the type of scoring used, the turnaround time for results from the MMPI can also be long. Finally, the MMPI may be susceptible to some bias in the sleep disorders setting because questions regarding sleep disturbance contribute to the scoring of some clinical scales (such as the depression scale), and these items may receive more pronounced endorsement by the sleep clinic than they might otherwise have garnered.

Two instruments—the Beck Depression Inventory[55] and the Spielberger State-Trait Anxiety Scale[56]—deserve mention because they are in widespread use in sleep disorders centers, are relatively easy to administer and interpret, and target the most common types of psychopathology associated with insomnia: depression and anxiety. Because they offer a quick assessment of the intensity of depression or anxiety, these scales allow for rapid intervention in patients who may be at risk for serious psychological distress.

When choosing a scale, the clinician must become familiar with the content of the items that yield the scaled score, as different instruments may focus on different aspects of a disorder. For example, one depression scale may emphasize the biologic features of the disturbance, whereas another may focus on cognitive abnormalities. As there is no single scale appropriate to all circumstances, the clinician should be aware of the particular slant of the selected instrument. As with all questionnaires, these inventories are susceptible to response bias on the part of the patient. Some people tend to deny or minimize, others aim to give the clinician what he or she is thought to expect, others are careless in responding, and still others harbor some motivation to exaggerate their symptoms. The more comprehensive inventories, such as the MMPI, build in monitoring of various types of response bias, whereas shorter scales necessarily place greater, unchecked emphasis on relatively few endorsements.

Table 119–3.　**Assessment of Psychopathology and Personality**

Scale Name (Source)	No. of Items	Format	Scale Description
Published			
Hamilton Rating Scale of Depression[47] (pp 61-62)	21	Clinician rating of severity based on patient interview	Semistructured interview for depression Clinician needed for administration
Beck Depression Inventory[48] (pp 561-571)	21	Four levels of severity description	Assesses depressive state with a cognitive emphasis
Self Rating Depression Scale[49] (p 65)	20	Four-point frequency ratings	Depression survey
Beck Anxiety Inventory[50] (p 895)	21	Four-point severity ratings	Anxiety survey
Available on Request			
Symptom Checklist Revised[51]	90	Five-point frequency ratings	Psychiatric symptoms and descriptions Norms for different samples Nine primary symptom dimensions and three global indices Narrative interpretation may be obtained
Profile of Mood Scales[52]	65	Five-point severity ratings	Adjectives that describe mood states Norms published
State-Trait Anxiety Inventory[53]	40	Four-point severity ratings	Separate scales measure current and long-standing anxiety
Minnesota Multiphasic Personality Inventory 2[54]	567	True/false	Nine clinical subscales measure enduring personality and psychopathology Response bias correction Skilled interpretation necessary or narrative summary needs to be obtained

Current-Status Instruments

INVENTORIES OF COGNITIVE AND SOMATIC AROUSAL

Cognitive style will often determine whether a person is predisposed to develop insomnia. Although everyone must deal with some degree of stress in their lives, there is a great deal of variation in how this coping is accomplished. Some lucky souls can literally "sleep on it" when confronted with a problem, but many people dwell on issues, obsessing over them until they are too aroused to fall asleep. When the particular problem to be overcome is lack of sleep, the consequences can be especially pernicious. Several authors have described a vicious circle in which concern over the possibility of not sleeping will lead to hyperarousal as evening approaches, reaching such a peak that by bedtime, sleep is truly impossible. Past experiences of insomnia reinforce the belief that sleep will once more prove elusive, setting the stage for another evening of anxiety and failure to sleep.[3,24,57]

Many patients insist with bewilderment that there is nothing particularly upsetting that they are dealing with in their lives, yet their minds continue to race at night. Their thoughts range initially over all sorts of seemingly trivial issues, eventually gravitating to the fact that sleep is not occurring. It may in fact be that the contents of one's thoughts do not necessarily lead directly to arousal; rather, the problem may lie with the thought process itself: half-completed thoughts, racing, and the repetition of themes may represent operating characteristics of a mind that is temporarily incapable of sleep.

One reason hyperarousal so effectively forestalls sleep is that once it is triggered, baseline conditions of arousal are not reestablished for a long time. It has been noted that the response to a perceived threat is rapid, which makes sense from an evolutionary perspective, whereas the "fall time" to a level of calm that would be conducive to sleeping is prolonged.[58] According to the model we have discussed, hyperarousal may be a predisposing or perpetuating factor. Correct classification will help determine the appropriate treatment strategy.

Several inventories are available that help the clinician gauge the extent to which cognitively induced and somatic hyperarousal may be expected to interfere with sleep (Table 119–4). These scales have the benefit of targeting a factor that often perpetuates an insomniac condition regardless of whether other factors originally precipitated it. They can help to interrupt the vicious circle of insomnia by preventing the patient from catastrophizing the consequences of poor sleep and fostering instead a more detached, dispassionate attitude toward the disturbance. This in itself is often very beneficial to therapy. The clinician should be aware, however, of the potential for confrontation and harm to the therapeutic alliance that can occur by implying that a patient's beliefs are "faulty" and "unrealistic."

It is also important to try to assess the degree of physiologic activation that is fueling arousal. Muscle tension, psychomotor agitation, and heart pounding are reported by some insomniacs, and the role of treatments based on dearousal suggests that an assessment of this domain is relevant to a comprehensive evaluation of sleep disturbance.

ASSESSMENT OF SLEEP HYGIENE AND PREFERRED SLEEP PHASE

As noted earlier, the nature of the hours spent before bedtime often determines whether sleep will come easily. This guideline

Table 119–4. Assessment of Specific Causes

Scale Name (Source)	No. of Items	Format	Scale Description
Published			
Morningness-Eveningness[60] (pages 100-103)	19	Four-point severity ratings / Time of day ratings	Feeling and functioning best rhythm
Sleep Behavior Self Rating Scale[61] (pp 414-415)	20	Frequency ratings	Activities, practices, and circumstances of the day that affect sleep
Sleep Hygiene Awareness and Practice Scale[42] (pp 75-76)	31+	Frequency and effect on sleep ratings	Activities, practices, and circumstances of the day that affect sleep
Sleep Hygiene Questionnaire[43] (p 38)	10	Yes/no	Activities, practices, and circumstances of the day that affect sleep
Pres-Sleep Arousal Scale[62] (p 266)	16	Five-point severity ratings	Assesses cognitive and somatic arousal at bedtime
Arousability Predisposition Scale[63] (p 420)	12	Frequency ratings	Assesses cognitive and somatic arousal
Sleep Disturbance Questionnaire[65] (p 153)	12	Five-point severity ratings	Assesses sleep hygiene and cognitive and somatic arousal
Beliefs and Attitudes about Sleep Scale[39] (pp 201-204)	30	Visual analogue scale	Surveys dysfunctional sleep-related cognition

applies to the entire day, not just the evening hours. The amount of physical activity, bed rest, and light exposure obtained during the day affect one's propensity for sleep, the timing of that sleep, and its quality. Excessive caffeine, exposure to dreadful television news stories in the evening, extended periods of reading in bed, and other aspects of poor sleep hygiene will ultimately prove counterproductive, whereas regular bedtimes and an evening "buffer period" in which to wind down from the day's events will over time be beneficial. Several authors have developed scales that assess these factors (see Table 119–4).

The timing of the propensity for sleep and activity differs among individuals. This tendency toward greater activity in either the morning or evening hours may be constitutional. Disposition toward a morning lark or a night owl pattern is assessed by a number of circadian-typing scales; the best known is a questionnaire developed by Horne and Ostberg (see Table 119–4).[64]

Prospective Sleep Diaries (Sleep Logs)

Retrospective instruments such as those just described have the advantage of being able to quickly summarize events occurring over a long period of time, but along with this quick summary comes the distortion inevitably introduced when collapsing and distilling descriptions. Memories are often incomplete or selective. In the case of insomnia, there is a natural tendency to focus on the worst experiences and perhaps to amplify their importance. These pitfalls can be countered through the use of a prospective sleep diary or sleep log (Table 119–5). Sleep logs have an intuitive appeal, are user

Table 119–5. Sleep Diaries*

Scale Name (Source)	No. of Items	Format
Published		
Daily Sleep Diary[43] (p 71)	10	Severity ratings / Fill in the blanks
Sleep Log and Day Log[44] (pp 72-73)	11	Fill in the blanks / Severity ratings / Grid for daily activities
Sleep Diary[39] (p 210)	10	Five-point severity ratings / Fill in the blanks
Pittsburgh Sleep Diary[66] (pp 113-114)	24	Five-point frequency ratings / Visual analogue scales / Fill in the blanks
Sleep Log[67] (p 140)	9	Graphical depiction of sleep over time / Five-point severity ratings / Fill in the blanks
Available on Request		
Sleep Log[68]	12	Graphical depiction of sleep over time / Fill in the blanks

*All diaries assess sleep pattern and quality as well as presleep activities and practices.

friendly, and allow for repeated, accurate sampling of target behavior, whether lying in bed awake or consuming coffee, in a prospective manner that increases the reliability of the measure. Filling out a sleep log directs the patient's attention to aspects of behavior that might otherwise be overlooked. Some versions present the information in a graphical format that allows the clinician to quickly survey and appreciate patterns in large amounts of data. On the other hand, more precise information is obtained from fill-in-the-grid or question-type formats. Filling out a 2-week sleep log before the initial evaluation also provides a baseline against which treatment response may be measured.

Sleep logs have potential drawbacks as well. Some obsessive patients feel compelled to provide such accurate and complete information that the very act of logging clock times of various events interferes with sleep. Even in less-extreme cases, the act of logging information on a night-by-night basis often works against the therapeutic goal of instilling in the patient a longer view toward the sleep disturbance. This tendency may be countered by drawing attention to week-to-week changes shown on the logs, as opposed to focusing on nightly variations.

CASE ILLUSTRATIONS

The following cases illustrate the use of sleep logs in assessing and treating insomnia. They also demonstrate how application of the predisposing, precipitating, and perpetuating model of insomnia enhances understanding of the course of the disorder. These logs are based on actual cases but have been redrawn for clarity.

CASE 1

Figure 119–3 shows the key features of delayed sleep phase syndrome. Before the onset of her sleep problems, this 16-year-old was a late-night type, but she did not have trouble falling asleep by 11 PM and getting up early for school. During the summer she began to fight with her parents over staying out late; her bedtime drifted to 1 am and her rising time to 10 AM or later. When school resumed in the fall, she needed to get up at 6 AM to make her bus. In November she was still complaining of trouble falling asleep whenever she went to bed before 1 AM, and she had difficulty getting up in the morning. She was habitually late for school and slept in on the weekends. Groggy in the morning, she would become progressively more alert through the day, except for a dip in alertness around 4 PM. She got a "second wind" in the evening, and was not in the least bit sleepy at her former 11 PM bedtime.

CASE 2

The patient depicted in Figure 119–4 is depressed as a result of the miscarriage of her first pregnancy. She is spending too much time in bed, which is also contributing to her sleeping difficulties. In bed for 10 hours, she is achieving only 6 hours of fragmented sleep. Treatment required addressing both the insomnia's triggering event, her miscarriage, as well as the perpetuating factor, excess time in bed.

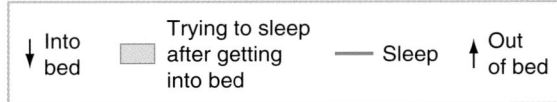
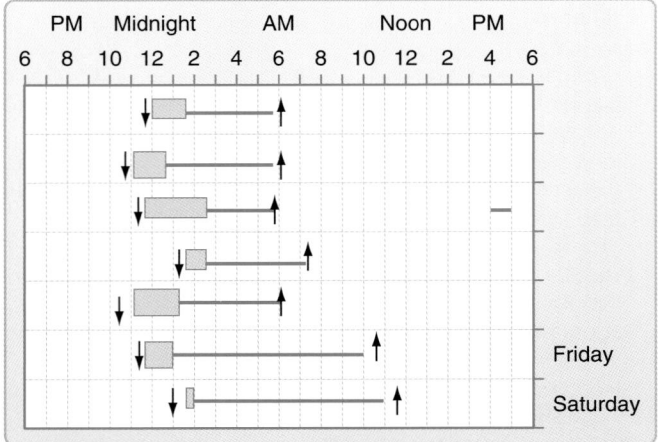

Figure 119–3. Delayed Sleep Phase Syndrome. Complaint: Very hard to fall asleep, easier to fall asleep if bedtime is later, hard to wake in the morning, late to school, sleeps late on weekends.
Predisposing factor: Late night type, rebellious adolescent
Precipitating factor: start of school in the fall with an early start time
Perpetuating factor: late wake-up time on weekends

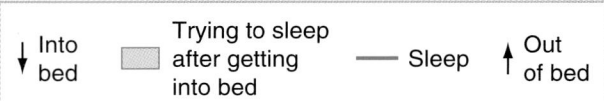
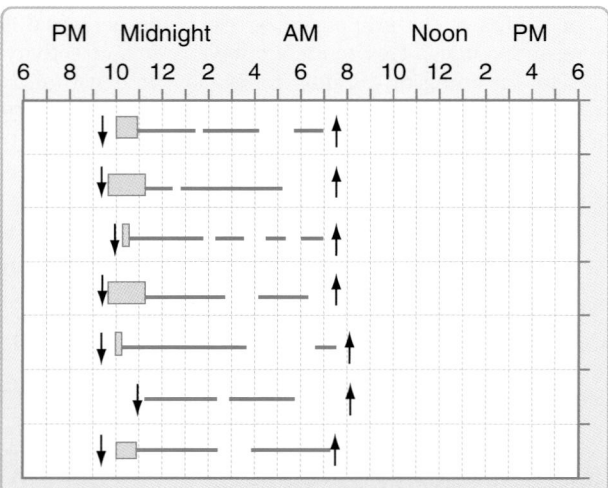

Figure 119–4. Depression and Inadequate Sleep Hygiene. Complaint: Trouble falling and staying asleep; onset after miscarriage.
Predisposing Factor: Unknown
Precipitating Factors: Post-pregnancy depression and hormonal changes
Perpetuating Factor: Too much time in bed

CASE 3

Bed was the hub of evening activity for the patient depicted in Figure 119–5. When she turned the lights off around 11 PM, she often had trouble falling asleep. Habitual association of the bed with waking activities conditioned her insomnia. The bed was no longer a clear signal for falling asleep, but instead it was perpetuating the sleep-onset problem.

CASE 4

Never a good sleeper, the patient portrayed in Figure 119–6 developed a medication strategy to prevent the development of drug tolerance. He used a different sleep medication each night at bedtime, and he usually took a second dose during the night. He felt desperate for sleep and unable to function if he did not get an adequate amount nightly. The onset of insomnia in early life often suggests a weak sleep-generating system. Hypnotic dependence was apparent in this patient's case, as was his preoccupation with sleep.

CASE 5

Figure 119–7 depicts a pattern of short sleep on weekdays and catch-up sleep on weekends. This somewhat agitated and overly stressed man was physiologically and cognitively hyperaroused. He was not able to wind down properly during weekday evenings. However, the discharge of his sleep debt on weekends was also perpetuating his poor weekday sleep pattern.

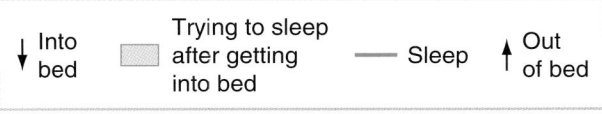

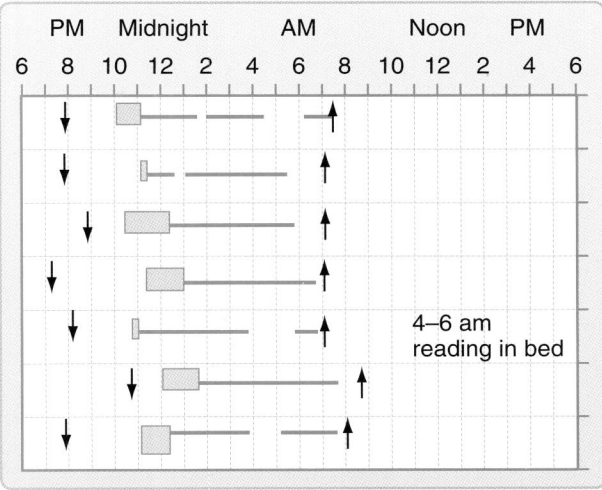

Figure 119–5. Psychophysiological Insomnia or Inadequate Sleep Hygiene. Complaint: Mainly trouble falling asleep; snacks, talks on phone, watches TV and reads in bed; stays in bed during awakenings. Predisposing Factor: Unknown
Precipitating Factor: Started to come home early after quitting second job in the evening
Perpetuating Factor: Engages in sleep-incompatible behaviors in bed

Figure 119–6. Insomnia associated with Hypnotic Dependence. Complaint: Light sleeper since childhood, can't sleep without medication; must sleep in order to function.
Predisposing Factor: Possible weak central nervous system sleep drive
Precipitating Factor: None
Perpetuating Factors: Hypnotic dependence, cognitive distortions, overly focused on sleep

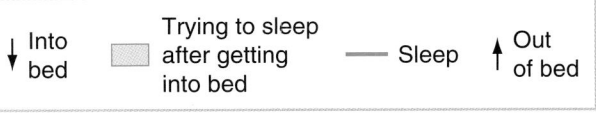

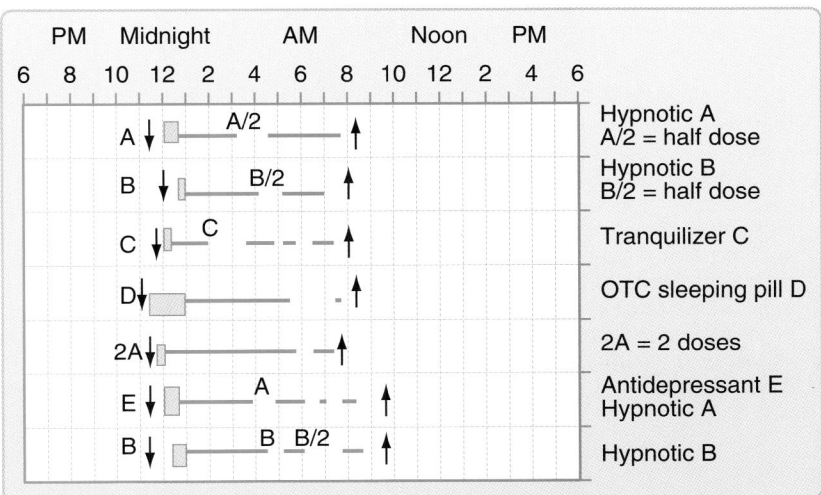

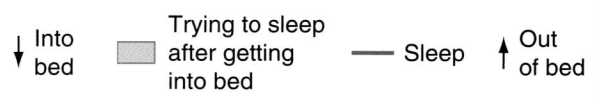

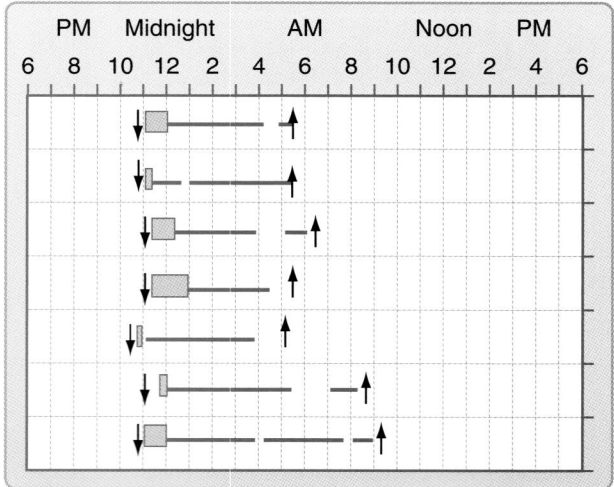

Figure 119–7. Inadequate Sleep Hygiene or Psychophysiological Insomnia. Complaint: Too little sleep; hard-driving businessman, catches up on sleep on weekends.
Predisposing Factor: Hyperarousal
Precipitating Factor: Unknown
Perpetuating Factors: Unequal distribution of sleep across seven days, irregular wake-up time

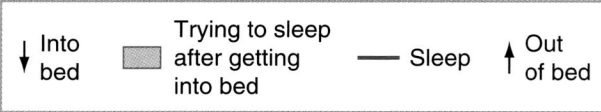

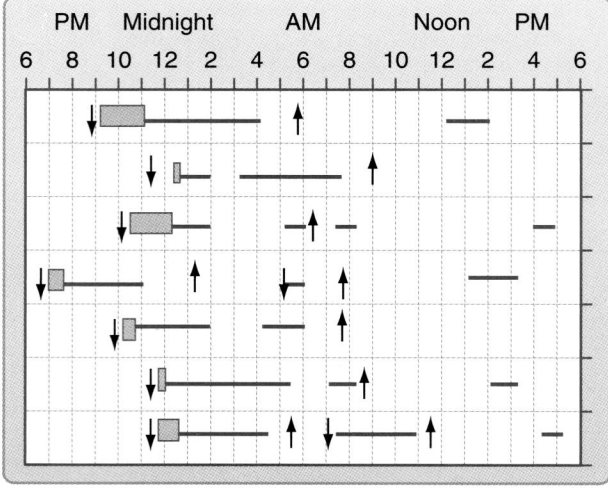

Figure 119–8. Irregular Sleep-Wake Schedule. Complaint: "I can't depend on my sleep, I wake up abruptly, I try to sleep whenever I can." Predisposing Factors: Robust autonomic arousal response, dependent personality
Precipitating Factor: Started freelance work, irregular work schedule
Perpetuating Factors: Irregular sleep-wake schedule, napping at different times of day for long periods of time, too much time in bed, over-concern about sleep

---

CASE 6

The patient with the variable sleep schedule depicted in Figure 119–8 was quite reactive physiologically. She had a robust startle response to loud noises, and her heart raced frequently during the day. She woke up abruptly in the middle of the night and had great difficulty going back to sleep. She felt she needed to seize sleep whenever she could get it and therefore avoided plans that might interfere with her sleep.

CASE 7

Figure 119–9 depicts a log of consistently solid sleep that was truncated after four hours. Wide awake in the middle of the night, the patient found that getting out of bed, working on his computer, and eating helped him get back to sleep for an hour or so in the morning. He did not use an alarm in the morning so that he could capture the last drop of sleep. This patient never required much sleep and was always an early riser. These traits predisposed him to early morning awakenings. Perpetuating factors included conditioned arousal secondary to working on the computer and eating in the middle of the night, variable arising time, and allowing too much time for sleep.

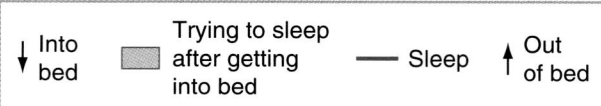

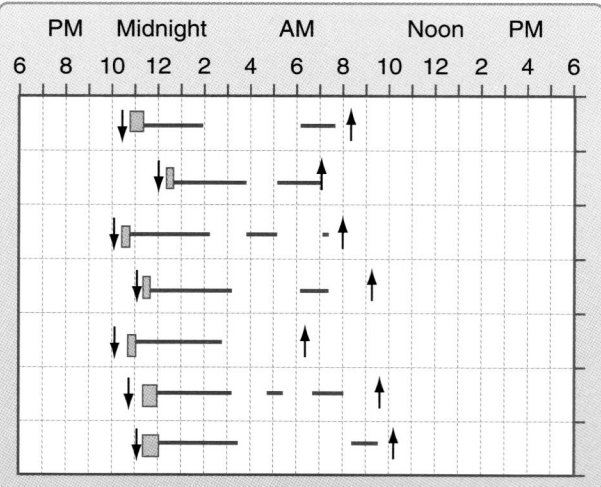

Figure 119–9. Psychophysiological Insomnia. Complaint: Trouble staying asleep, long awakening after 3-4 hours of solid sleep during which he works on the computer, gets refreshing sleep in the morning.
Predisposing Factor: Significant morning type, short sleeper
Precipitating Factor: Unknown
Perpetuating Factors: Variable morning rise time, too much time in bed, awakenings have become conditioned and associated with activating tasks

The Initial Consultation

Questionnaires and prospective logs certainly have their role in the assessment of insomnia, but it is in the face-to-face setting of the consultation that the clinician's skills and knowledge find full expression. Questionnaires do not ask follow-up questions. They cannot achieve the degree of nuance that is often necessary to decide, for example, whether episodes of awakening with gasping and palpitations likely represent a nocturnal anxiety attack or an apneic disturbance. They cannot probe for further examples or establish the context in which an event of interest occurs. It is up to the clinician, too, to recognize internal inconsistencies in a patient's history and to encourage the patient to be more exacting in his or her recollections in order to establish a more accurate reconstruction. Finally, within the course of interaction there may arise facets of the history that were not previously apparent to the patient and that would likely be wholly overlooked on a questionnaire.

A standard history-taking format usually serves well to elicit the essential features of an insomnia. However, an empirical study has shown that the non–sleep specialist clinician asks few pertinent questions of the insomnia patient.[69] The skilled clinician starts close to the patient's experience, allowing the patient the opportunity to expound the gist of the presenting problem with sufficient idiosyncratic detail to ensure that the experience does not fit too neatly and quickly into a preconceived diagnostic category—a potential pitfall for both patient and clinician. As these details emerge, the clinician develops hypotheses regarding the genesis of the insomnia and the factors that are maintaining it. These hypotheses are then tested via further questioning. For example, if it appears that a sleep-onset difficulty relates to concerns about performance at work, the clinician might ask about patterns in the severity of the disturbance and find that it is exacerbated on Sunday night, whereas the patient has experienced some asymptomatic periods during vacations.

After a working formulation has been established and a preliminary differential diagnosis is settled on, the clinician generally performs a systematic survey of the various domains that might have a bearing on the problem, such as the past medical history, family history, current psychosocial context,

and so on. Even when the clinician is fairly certain of the cause of a patient's insomnia and confident of an appropriate course of treatment, it still is important to piece together a comprehensive picture of the background conditions from which the disturbance evolved. There may be other ancillary or independent problems that also require attention.

The consultation interview is critical for establishing the trust and working alliance that will be necessary to carry the patient successfully through the treatment phase, especially when that treatment may involve changes in habits or lifestyle that are difficult to implement. The clinician must demonstrate caring, openness, and an ability to listen and understand, while bearing in mind that the patient is by definition in distress and likely to focus more on extreme experiences to garner aid.

Several semistructured interviews have been developed that help guide inquiry into a complaint of insomnia (Table 119–6). They have the advantage of cueing the clinician to cover relevant domains, and they include a survey of sleep hygiene practices. As with the use of any interview framework, the skilled clinician will be alert to instances where departures from the guide must be made to fully follow up on the patient's experience.

Testing and Referrals

Sleep specialists in almost all cases accumulate information from the broad categories just covered—retrospective questionnaires, prospective logs, and interviews. Referrals for testing or evaluation by another specialist are generally made more judiciously, based on the information gathered during the evaluation process. Sometimes the history will be sufficiently strong to warrant polysomnographic testing to confirm or rule out physiologic disturbance during sleep, such as sleep apnea or periodic limb movement disorder, before any treatments are applied. Similarly, further clinical evaluation may be indicated if the history is suggestive of psychiatric disturbance or specific disorders, such as hyperthyroidism or cardiac arrhythmia, that may be accompanied by insomnia. In other cases, testing or referral to a specialist takes place after a poor response to initial treatment is documented, to widen the base of potentially helpful information.

Table 119–6.   Semistructured Sleep Interviews*

Scale Name (Source)	No. of Items	Format
Published		
Structured Sleep History Interview[43] (pp 66-69)	53+	Open-ended questions
Insomnia Interview Schedule[39] (pp 195-198)	77	Open-ended questions Yes/no Severity ratings Fill in the blanks
CCNY Insomnia Interview[80] (pp 421-426)	41+	Open-ended questions Symptom checklists Severity ratings Rating of the degree to which factors covary with sleep disturbance Diagnostic entities linked to particular questions

*All interviews survey a wide range of symptoms and etiologic factors.

Nocturnal Polysomnogram

The nocturnal polysomnogram (NPSG) is the standard objective measure of sleep (see Chapter 116). Since the 1970s, a large body of research and clinical experience has accumulated regarding both normal sleep parameters and variants seen in disordered sleep. Evaluation with polysomnography allows the clinician to objectively compare the patient's sleep characteristics with normative data and with data gathered within various clinical populations to clarify the diagnosis. The NPSG is also helpful in uncovering covert disorders, such as periodic limb movement disorder, that might otherwise escape detection, especially if there is no bed partner available to observe sleep.

In addition to characterizing sleep, polysomnography affords the clinician several indices of arousal that may prove especially helpful in characterizing and addressing cases of insomnia. These include such measures as the percentage of non–rapid eye movement (NREM) stage 1 transitional sleep, the number of transient arousals, the number of stage changes across the record, and the intrusion of alpha wave activity into deeper sleep. Polysomnography also allows the clinician to compare objective parameters—such as total sleep time or the number of awakenings exceeding a specified duration—with the patient's subjective estimate of these same parameters. Sometimes, a large discrepancy between objective parameters and their corresponding subjective estimates characterizes the core of the presenting problem.[70,71]

The NPSG does have drawbacks. One is its expense, reflecting both its labor-intensive character and the investment in costly technology required. A consequence of this expense is that only one or two nights of data are typically obtained, resulting in a very limited sample of sleep. Given the increased night-to-night variability of sleep typically seen in insomnia, this may result in a biased estimate.

The effect of sleeping in a sleep laboratory can also result in an inaccurate representation of the patient's sleep, either exaggerating sleep difficulties—the classic "first night effect"[72]—or, paradoxically, resulting in better sleep than that typically obtained at home—the "reverse first night effect."[73] This latter effect can occur when associations have been established between the insomniac patient's bedroom environment and the experience of sleeping poorly that make continued insomnia more likely. These maladaptive cues are missing from the sleep laboratory, so sleep is improved there. Because of these drawbacks, NPSG is not indicated as a first-line diagnostic tool in the assessment of insomnia according to American Academy of Sleep Medicine guidelines.[74]

Actigraphy

Actigraphy is a relatively low cost method of estimating sleep parameters, such as total sleep time and the timing and duration of prolonged awakenings (see Chapter 124).[15,75-78] An actigraph is a device that records gross motor movements. Not much bigger than a wristwatch, it is attached to a limb and can be worn day or night without interfering with normal sleep or daily functioning. It can record motor activity (or in the case of sleep, the lack thereof) across many days and nights, employing various sampling rates. The collected data are usually downloaded to a computer for analysis.

The cost-effectiveness of actigraphy allows for multiple nights of sampling, avoiding the sampling error associated with the NPSG. However, it can overestimate the amount of sleep obtained in insomniac patients, who do not move much during the night even when they are awake. Furthermore, the various actigraphs available commercially have not been standardized. They have different sensitivities to the detection of movement and differing algorithms for converting raw data points into estimates of sleep and wakefulness.

Laboratory Urinalysis and Blood Work

Analyses of urine and blood samples routinely conducted by commercial laboratories at the behest of physicians in general medical practice may also prove helpful in the assessment of selected patients complaining of insomnia. Levels of thyroid-stimulating hormone and follicle-stimulating hormone and blood count profiles will help in evaluating whether hyperthyroidism, menopause, or infection is playing a role in the sleep disturbance.

A survey of the methods used to assess the numerous medical conditions associated with insomnia is beyond the scope of this chapter (see Section 14). We will comment on one test pertinent to the assessment of the conditions of restless legs syndrome (RLS) and periodic limb movement disorder (PLMD). Although the pathophysiology of these conditions is still under investigation, a subset of patients may have anemia, which can be assessed by obtaining ferritin levels.[79] Obtaining a set of blood panels on every insomnia patient is not recommended because of the low yield; however, when there is sufficient reason to suspect an underlying medical cause of insomnia, and testing proves negative, blood panels will allow behavioral interventions to be applied with more confidence and persistence.

Commonplace Technologies

Ubiquitous devices such as telephone answering machines or digital watches can be helpful in the assessment of insomnia. For example, patients complaining that they "get no sleep at all, or at best, just 1 or 2 hours" can be instructed to call on an hourly basis into a telephone answering machine equipped with a time stamp when they are unable to sleep. This provides an objective record of at least intermittent wakefulness across the night and may be useful in cases of sleep state misperception, also known as Paradoxical Insomnia. Digital watches that have an hourly chime function can be used to cue the patient to rate alertness or mood. Audiotape or videotape recordings can be useful as screening tools in those cases where sleep-maintenance difficulties are suspected of being secondary to a physiologic disturbance such as sleep apnea.

Trial Treatment As Assessment

There are times when a thorough evaluation yields only a probable cause underlying a patient's complaint of insomnia. In these cases, the most expeditious means of verifying that supposition may be through the application of a trial treatment. Of course, reasoning that a diagnostic impression is correct because improvement follows treatment is not necessarily valid; just because a cold improves after a few days of drinking chamomile tea does not mean that chamomile deficiency caused the cold in the first place. Similarly, good sleep hygiene practices are helpful for all sleepers, not just those whose sleep difficulties stem specifically from poor sleep hygiene. Therefore, if poor sleep hygiene is suspected as a causative factor, instruction in better practices can efficiently treat those who are correctly targeted, while not doing harm to those whose insomnia arises from other causes.

Another condition that deserves mention in this regard is sleep-maintenance insomnia due to suspected PLMD during sleep.[34] Very often, this condition responds to treatment with dopamine agonists or opioid drugs. These drugs are not of general benefit in other types of sleep-maintenance insomnia; therefore, if a case of suspected PLMD shows a positive response to these drugs, this response can usually be taken as indirect evidence that PLMD was the underlying culprit. Note that a positive response to one of the sedative-hypnotic medications, which can also be helpful in treating cases of insomnia due to PLMD, would not yield information regarding the presence of PLMD. This class of drug would be expected to benefit many different types of insomnia whether it is due to PLMD or not.

Other Reviews

For those interested in further reading on this topic, we recommend a chapter we have written[80] and two publications of the American Academy of Sleep Medicine that review the evaluation of chronic insomnia.[74,81]

SUMMARY

Very few medical or psychological disorders are associated with as diverse an array of diagnostic procedures as those summarized here in connection with the assessment of insomnia. This heterogeneity mirrors the multiple facets of the complaint, which range through physical discomfort, psychological distress, cognitive deficiencies, behavior impairment, and social disruption. Full evaluation of the complaint requires a multidimensional approach because those aspects of the sleep disorder that are most salient or distressing to the patient—and the facets where it might prove most amenable or recalcitrant to treatment—vary among individuals. The clinician who is prepared to meet a complaint of insomnia on its own terms, drawing from the range of diagnostic methods described in this chapter, will come to a more complete understanding of the problem and be better able to formulate effective recommendations for its treatment.

Clinical Pearls

The factors that increase risk for insomnia and those that trigger the onset of an episode are typically not the same as factors that maintain the disorder once it is established. Even if predisposing factors cannot be readily altered and precipitating factors are never positively identified, substantial relief from insomnia may be attained by addressing perpetuating factors.

Evaluation of insomnia is a multitiered process. It should virtually always make use of prospective sleep diaries and specialized questionnaires. A face-to-face clinical consultation is required to follow up responses on these instruments in order to articulate idiosyncratic features of the problem, establish a therapeutic alliance, and inform treatment decisions. While overnight polysomnography may be beneficial, especially in cases where covert sleep disorders are suspected, it is not considered a front-line diagnostic tool for insomnia.

REFERENCES

1. Kumar A, Vaidya AK: Anxiety as a personality dimension of short and long sleepers. J Clin Psychol 1984;40:197-198.
2. Mellinger GD, Balter MB, Uhlenhuth EH: Insomnia and its treatment: Prevalence and correlates. Arch Gen Psychiatry 1985;42:225-232.
3. Reynolds CF, Kupfer DJ: Sleep research in affective illness: State of the art. Sleep 1987;10:199-215.
4. Sweetwood HL, Kripke DF, Grant I, et al: Sleep disorder and psychobiological symptomatology. Psychosom Med 1976;38:373-378.
5. Vollrath M, Wicki W, Angst J: The Zurich Study, VIII: Insomnia: Association with depression, anxiety, somatic syndromes, and course of insomnia. Eur Arch Psychiatry Neurol Sci 1989;239:113-124.
6. Kales A, Caldwell AB, Preston TA, et al: Personality patterns in insomnia. Arch Gen Psychiatry 1976;33:1128-1134.
7. Kales A, Kales JD: Evaluation and Treatment of Insomnia. New York, Oxford University Press, 1984.
8. Espie CA, Lindsay WR: Paradoxical intention in the treatment of chronic insomnia: Six case studies illustrating variability in therapeutic response. Behav Res Ther 1985;23:703-709.
9. Killen JD, Coates TJ: The complaint of insomnia: What is it and how do we treat? Clin Behav Ther Rev 1979;1:1-15.
10. Lacks P: Behavioral Treatment for Persistent Insomnia. New York, Pergamon Press, 1987.
11. Carroll BJ, Feinberg M, Greden JF, et al: A specific laboratory test for the diagnosis of melancholia: Standardization, validation and clinical utility. Arch Gen Psychiatry 1981;38:15-22.
12. Czeisler CA, Moore-Ede MC, Regestein QR, et al: Episodic 24-hour cortisol secretory patterns in patients awaiting elective cardiac surgery. J Clin Endocrinol Metab 1976;42:273-283.
13. Sitaram N, Gillin JC: Development and use of pharmacological probes of the CNS in man: Evidence of cholinergic abnormality in primary affective illness. Biol Psychiatry 1980;15:925-955.
14. Bootzin RR, Rider SP: Behavioral techniques and biofeedback for insomnia. In Pressman MR, Orr WC (eds): Understanding Sleep: The Evaluation and Treatment of Sleep Disorders. Washington, DC, American Psychological Association, 1997, pp 315-338.
15. Sterman MD, Clemente CD, Wyricka W: Forebrain inhibitory mechanisms: Conditioning of basal forebrain induced EEG synchronization and sleep. Exp Neurol 1963;7:404-417.
16. Sterman MB, Szymusiask R, McGinty D: Quantitative analysis of basal forebrain stimulation effects: Sleep induction, sleep conditioning, and state distribution. Paper presented at the Fifth International Congress of Sleep Research, July 1987, Copenhagen, Denmark.
17. Bonnet MH, Arand DI: 24-Hour metabolic rate in insomniacs and matched normal sleepers. Sleep 1995;19:581-588.
18. Freedman R, Sattler HI: Physiological and psychological factors in sleep-onset insomnia. Abnorm Psychol 1982;91:380-389.
19. Johns MW, Gay MP, Masterton JP, et al: Relationship between sleep habits, adrenocortical activity and personality. Psychosomat Med 1971;3:499-508.
20. Kleitman N: Sleep and Wakefulness. Chicago, University of Chicago Press, 1939.
21. Hauri P: The Sleep Disorders, 2nd ed. Kalamazoo, Mich, Upjohn, 1982.
22. Hauri PJ: Consulting about insomnia: A method and some preliminary data. Sleep 1993;16:344-350.
23. Spielman AJ: Assessment of insomnia. Clin Psychol Rev 1986;6:11-26.
24. Espie CA: The Psychological Treatment of Insomnia. New York, Wiley, 1991.
25. Hauri P, Linde S: No More Sleepless Nights. New York, John Wiley, 1990.
26. Monroe LJ: Psychological and physiological differences between good and poor sleepers. J Abnorm Psychol 1967;72:255-264.

27. Torsvall L, Akerstedt T: Disturbed sleep while being on-call: An EEG study of ship's engineers. Sleep 1988;11:35-38.

28. Guilleminault C, Eldridge F, Dement WC: Insomnia, narcolepsy, and sleep apneas. Bull Physiopathol Respir 1972;8:1127-1138.

29. Symonds CP: Nocturnal myoclonus. J Neurol Neurosurg Psychiatry 1953;16:166-171.

30. Moore-Ede MC, Czeisler CA, Richardson GS: Circadian time-keeping in health and disease, I: Basic properties of circadian pacemakers. N Engl J Med 1983;309:469-476.

31. Moore-Ede MC, Czeisler CA, Richardson GS: Circadian time-keeping in health and disease, II: Clinical implications of circadian rhythmicity. N Engl J Med 1983;309:530-536.

32. Spielman AJ, Caruso L, Glovinsky PB: A behavioral perspective on insomnia. Psychiatr Clin North Am 1987;10:541-553.

33. Brodman K, Erdmann AJ Jr, Lorge I, et al: The Cornell Medical Index: An adjunct to medical interview. JAMA 1949;140:530-534.

34. American Sleep Disorders Association: International Classification of Sleep Disorders, Revised: Diagnostic and Coding Manual. Rochester, Minn, American Sleep Disorders Association, 1997.

35. Webb WB, Bonnet M, Blume G: A post-sleep inventory. Percept Motor Skills 1976;43:987-993.

36. Parrott AC, Hindmarch I: The Leeds Sleep Evaluation Questionnaire in psychopharmacological investigations—a review. Psychopharmacology 1980;71:173-179.

37. Ellis BW, Johns MW, Lancaster R, et al: The St. Mary's Hospital Sleep Questionnaire: A study of reliability. Sleep 1981;4:93-97.

38. Buysse DJ, Reynolds CF III, Monk TH, et al: The Pittsburgh Sleep Quality Index: A new instrument for psychiatric practice and research. Psychiatry Res 1989;28:193-213.

39. Morin CM: Insomnia: Psychological Assessment and Management. New York, Guilford Press, 1993.

40. Domino G, Blair G, Bridges A: Subjective assessment of sleep by sleep questionnaire. Percept Motor Skills 1985;59:163-170.

41. Spielman AJ, Saskin P, Thorpy MJ: Treatment of chronic insomnia by restriction of time in bed. Sleep 1987;10:45-56.

42. Miles I: Sleep Questionnaire and Assessment of Wakefulness (SQAW). In Guilleminault C (ed): Sleeping and Waking Disorders: Indications and Techniques. Menlo Park, Calif, Addison Wesley, 1982, pp 384-413.

43. Lacks P: Behavioral Treatment for Persistent Insomnia. New York, Pergamon Press, 1987.

44. Hauri P, Linde S: No More Sleepless Nights. New York, Wiley, 1990.

45. Douglass AB, Bornstein RF, Nino-Murcia G, et al: The Sleep Disorders Questionnaire, I: Creation and multivariate structure of SDQ. Sleep 1994;17:160-167.

46. Cote KA, Ogilvie RD: The Brock Sleep and Insomnia Questionnaire: Phase I. Sleep Res 1992;22:356.

47. Hamilton M: A rating scale for depression. J Neurol Neurosurg Psychiatry 1960;23:56-62.

48. Beck AT, Ward CH, Mendelson M, et al: An inventory for measuring depression. Arch Gen Psychiatry 1961;4:561-571.

49. Zung WWK: A self-rating depression scale. Arch Gen Psychiatry 1965;12:63-70.

50. Beck AT, Epstein N, Brown G, et al: An inventory for measuring clinical anxiety. J Consult Clin Psychol 1988;56:893-897.

51. Derogatis LR. SCL-90-R: Administration, Scoring, and Procedures Manual. Baltimore, Clinical Psychometrics Research, 1977.

52. McNair DM, Lorr M, Droppleman LF: EDITS manual for the Profile of Mood States. San Diego, Calif, Educational and Industrial Testing Service, 1981.

53. Spielberger CD, Gorsuch RL, Lushene R, et al: The State-Trait Anxiety Inventory for Adults. Palo Alto, Calif, Mind Garden, 1983.

54. Butcher JN, Dahlstrom WG, Graham JR, et al: MMPI-2: Minnesota Multiphasic Personality Inventory-2: Manual for Administration and Scoring. Minneapolis, University of Minnesota Press, 1989.

55. Beck AT, Ward CH, Mendelson M, et al: An inventory for measuring depression. Arch Gen Psychiatry 1961;4:561-571.

56. Spielberger CD, Gorsuch RL, Lushene R, et al: The State-Trait Anxiety Inventory for Adults. Palo Alto, Calif, Mind Garden, 1983.

57. Morin CM: Insomnia: Psychological Assessment and Management. New York, Guilford Press, 1993.

58. Hauri PJ: Personal communication, 1985.

59. Butcher JN, Dahlstrom WG, Graham JR, et al: MMPI-2: Minnesota Multiphasic Personality Inventory, 2. Manual for Administration and Scoring. Minneapolis, University of Minnesota Press, 1989.

60. Horne JA, Ostberg O: A self-assessment questionnaire to determine morningness-eveningness in human circadian rhythms. Int J Chronobiol 1976;4:97-110.

61. Kazarian SS, Howe MG, Csapo KG: Development of the Sleep Behavior Self-Rating Scale. Behav Ther 1979;10:412-417.

62. Nicassio PM, Mendlowitz DR, Fussell JJ, et al: The phenomenology of the pre-sleep state: the development of the pre-sleep arousal scale. Behav Res Ther 1985;23:263-271.

63. Coren S: Prediction of insomnia from arousability predisposition scores: scale development and cross-validation. Behav Res Ther 1988;26:415-420.

64. Horne JA, Ostberg O: A self-assessment questionnaire to determine morningness-eveningness in human circadian rhythms. Int J Chronobiol 1976;4:97-110.

65. Espie CA, Brooks DN, Lindsay WR: An evaluation of tailored psychological treatment of insomnia. J Behav Ther Exp Psychiatry 1989;20:143-153.

66. Monk TH, Reynolds CF III, Kupfer DJ, et al: The Pittsburgh Sleep Diary. J Sleep Res 1994;3:111-120.

67. Spielman AJ, Glovinsky PB: The diagnostic interview and differential diagnosis for complaints of insomnia. In Pressman MR, Orr WC (eds): Understanding Sleep: The Evaluation and Treatment of Sleep Disorders. Washington, DC, American Psychological Association, 1997,125-160.

68. Metrodesign Associates/Charles Pollak, MD, 90 Clinton Street, Homer, NY 13077, 1989.

69. Everitt DE, Avoran J: Clinical decision-making in the evaluation and treatment of insomnia. Am J Med 1990;89:357-362.

70. Frankel BL, Coursey RD, Buchbinder R, et al: Recorded and reported sleep in chronic primary insomnia. Arch Gen Psychiatry 1976;33:615-623.

71. McCall WV, Edinger JD: Subjective total insomnia: An example of sleep state misperception. Sleep 1992;15:71-73.

72. Agnew HW Jr, Webb WB, Williams RL: The first night effect: An EEG study of sleep. Psychophysiology 1966;2:263-266.

73. Hauri PJ, Olmstead EM: Reverse first night effect in insomnia. Sleep 1989;12:97-105.

74. Standards of Practice Committee of the American Academy of Sleep Medicine: Practice parameters for the evaluation of chronic insomnia. Sleep 2000;23:237-241.

75. Hauri PJ, Wisbey J: Wrist actigraphy in insomnia. Sleep 1992;15:293-301.

76. Jean-Louis G, von Gizycki H, Zizi F, et al: Determination of sleep and wakefulness with the actigraph data analysis software (ADAS). Sleep 1996;19:739-743.

77. Sadeh A, Hauri PJ, Kripke D, et al: The role of actigraphy in the evaluation of sleep disorders. Sleep 1995;18:288-302.

78. Standards of Practice Committee of the American Sleep Disorders Association: Practice parameters for the use of actigraphy in the clinical assessment of sleep disorders. Sleep 1995; 18:285-287.

79. Early C, Sun E, Chen C, et al: Iron relation to periodic leg movements and sleep disturbance in patients with the restless legs syndrome. Sleep 1998;21(suppl):142.

80. Spielman AJ, Anderson MW: The clinical interview and treatment planning as a guide to understanding the nature of insomnia: The CCNY insomnia interview. In Chokroverty S (ed): Sleep Disorders Medicine: Basic Science, Technical Considerations, and Clinical Aspects, 2nd ed. Boston, Butterworth-Heinemann, 1998, pp 385-426.

81. Sateia MJ, Doghramji K, Hauri PJ, et al: Evaluation of chronic insomnia. Sleep 2000;23:243-308.

120

Evaluating Sleepiness

Merrill M. Mitler

Mary A. Carskadon

Max Hirshkowitz

ABSTRACT

In this chapter, techniques for evaluating physiologic, manifest, and self-reported sleepiness are described. The technique and indications for using the Multiple Sleep Latency Test are reviewed in detail. Pupillography and electroencephalographic approaches are discussed. Manifest sleepiness, measured with the Maintenance of Wakefulness Test and vigilance testing, are contrasted with other approaches. The American Academy of Sleep Medicine practice parameters are summarized for using both the Multiple Sleep Latency Test and the Maintenance of Wakefulness Test in the clinical setting. Also, the limitations and advantages of self-reported sleepiness tests are compared. Finally, a few practical considerations and conclusions are discussed.

Excessive sleepiness during work activities is a serious, potentially life-threatening condition that affects not only sleepy individuals but also their families, coworkers, and society. Sleep regulation is currently conceptualized as involving two processes: circadian and homeostatic. The effect of these processes on self-reported, biologic, and behavioral measures of sleepiness is a topic of continuing research. With the growth and increasing interest in sleep disorders, tools are needed not only for conducting research but also for clinically assessing patients for sleepiness. It is helpful to remember that each tool has an optimal use and specific limitations. Although screws can be driven with a hammer, a screwdriver works better. Thus, the assessment goal should be considered when choosing a technique, the advantages and limitations should be considered, and specific evaluation protocols should be followed carefully.

The focus of this chapter is clinical assessment; therefore, special attention is directed to three specific measurement issues. The first issue relates to the difference between within-subject comparisons and between-subjects comparisons. For example, most valid and reliable tests of sleepiness can be used to assess the effects of sleep restriction in a before-and-after experimental design. However, examination of the data reveals instances in which the initial value for one person exceeds the final value for another. Consequently, this superb metric for assessing change in sleepiness may not be useful in determining whether a new patient in your office is sleepy.

The second issue concerns self-report. With increasing frequency, sleep specialists are being asked to make assessments for regulatory and judicial purposes. This makes parameters of testing more crucial. In such situations, an individual's self-assessment of sleepiness must be assumed to be colored by primary or secondary gain. Thus, some individuals are inclined to either exaggerate or minimize their own reports of sleepiness level.

The third issue is that clinical testing of sleepiness usually involves daytime testing. A large number of studies and normative data exist for physiologically based metrics of daytime sleepiness. When it is clinically necessary to assess sleepiness during the night, such as in shift workers, the choices of validated tools are more limited and mostly involve performance tests. Although physiologically based metrics can readily be used to detect nighttime drops in alertness in normal and sleep-deprived volunteers, the guidelines as to what degree of sleepiness is *pathologic* during the night have not been established; it is *normal* to be very sleepy at 4:00 AM.

One traditional conceptualization for characterizing sleepiness involved three factors: physiologic sleepiness, manifest sleepiness, and introspective sleepiness.[1] This model provides a useful organizational device for understanding sleepiness measurement, but different measurements may index quite different (although related) phenomena. Physiologic sleepiness can be thought of as the underlying biologic drive to sleep; consequently, the primary index is the speed with which an individual falls asleep. Manifest sleepiness can be considered from three perspectives: behavioral signs of sleepiness, inability to volitionally remain awake, and performance deficit on psychomotor or cognitive tasks. The common thread is the transformational effect of underlying sleepiness on outward behavior and abilities. Finally, introspective sleepiness concerns an individual's self-assessment of an internal state. Although the manifest and introspective measures may stem from the same underlying drive state, individual differences factor in and modify the measurable phenomena. Not only is it illogical to attempt to use these measures interchangeably but it misses the importance of the differences between them.

PHYSIOLOGIC SLEEPINESS

Multiple Sleep Latency Test

If sleepiness is considered a drive state, the rapidity with which an individual falls asleep can be used to evaluate the intensity of that drive. As such, sleep deprivation decreases latency to sleep on subsequent sleep opportunities. Homeostatic sleep drive builds across the normal waking day and is opposed in the evening by a circadian-dependent drive for alertness. Then as the circadian-dependent drive for alertness drops off with the homeostatic drive still increasing, sleep onset occurs. Sleepiness then rapidly rises to maximal levels as sleep deprivation and circadian factors combine in the nighttime hours.[2] During the normal nighttime hours, the physiologic drive to sleep quickly reaches maximum levels, and sleep onset becomes almost immediate when sleep opportunities are provided. It is standard practice to index physiologic sleepiness using the Multiple Sleep Latency Test (MSLT). The MSLT is a series of nap opportunities (four to six) presented at 2-hour intervals beginning approximately 2 hours after initial (morning) awakening (for details, see Carskadon et al.[3]). Individuals undergoing an MSLT are instructed to *allow themselves to fall asleep* or *to not to resist falling asleep*. Subjects are tested under standardized conditions in their street clothes and are not permitted to remain in bed between nap test sessions. Similarly, subjects should not engage in vigorous pretest activity because it will alter test outcome.[4] Standardization of testing conditions is necessary and critical to obtain reliable results.[5] Sleep rooms should be dark and quiet during testing. Electrophysiologic parameters needed to detect sleep onset and score sleep stages are recorded during nap opportunities. Recordings include central (required) and occipital (very strongly recommended) electroencephalograms (EEGs), left and right eye electrooculograms, and a submentalis electromyogram. MSLT guidelines also call for monitoring respiratory flow and sounds in patients known to snore (Table 120–1). In a series of elegant studies, the effects of age, partial sleep deprivation, and disorders of excessive somnolence were well characterized.[6-9] Key concepts concerning homeostatic influences on sleepiness derive directly from research with MSLT. MSLT demonstrations of the cumulative nature of sleep debt, the increased sleepiness during adolescence produced by sleep restriction, and reduction in sleepiness after sleep extension provide the foundation for understanding the interaction between sleep and wakefulness. Circadian influence can be seen in MSLT latencies on nap

Table 120–1.	**Multiple Sleep Latency Test: Recording Montage of Physiologic Activity**

Left or right central electroencephalogram (EEG) (C3 or C4)
Left or right occipital EEG (O1 or O2)
Left horizontal or oblique electrooculogram (EOG)
Right horizontal or oblique EOG
Vertical EOG
Submentalis (chin) electromyogram (EMG)
Electrocardiogram
Respiratory flow, as needed
Respiratory sounds, as needed

opportunities scheduled in the mid afternoon for subjects who were not already near maximal sleepiness or alertness.[10]

Two protocols exist for conducting the MSLT: clinical and research (Fig. 120–1). These two protocols differ with respect to the amount of allowable accumulated sleep if an individual falls asleep on a nap opportunity. In the research version, accumulated sleep is minimized by awakening the sleeper after sleep onset defined as (1) one epoch of unequivocal sleep or (2) three epochs of stage 1 sleep. Unequivocal sleep is an epoch of stage 2, 3, or 4, or of rapid eye movement (REM) sleep. The clinical version allows more sleep to occur because the test attempts to serve the dual role of indexing sleepiness and attempting to uncover abnormal REM sleep tendency (useful in the differential diagnosis of narcolepsy). Each test session is therefore allowed to continue for 15 minutes after sleep onset using these criteria (assuming sleep occurs) to determine whether a sleep-onset REM sleep episode will occur. If no sleep onset occurs, the nap opportunity is terminated in

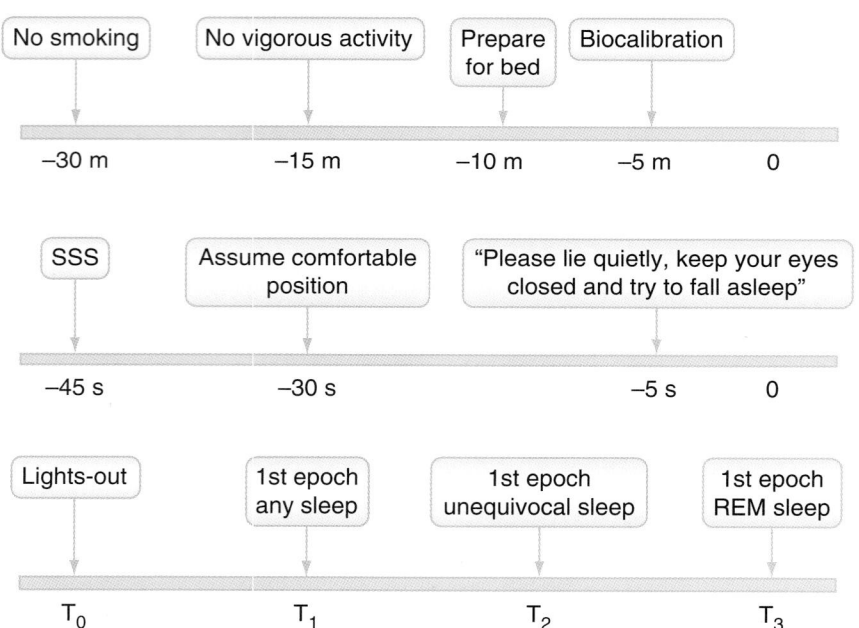

Figure 120–1. Timing of procedures for Multiple Sleep Latency Test nap opportunities.

Test session termination rules:
Experimental protocol: End at T_2
Clinical protocol: End at $T_1 + 15$ m
Either version, if no sleep occurs: $T_0 + 20$ m

both protocols after 20 minutes. Sleep latency is defined as the elapsed time from the start of the test to the first 30-second epoch scored as sleep. Sleep latency in normal adult control subjects ranges from 10 to 20 minutes. Pathologic sleepiness is defined as mean sleep latency of less than 5 or 6 minutes.[6] Latencies falling between the normal and the pathologic values are considered a diagnostic gray area. The clinical version of the MSLT reliably distinguishes patients with narcolepsy from control subjects with respect to both the number of episodes of REM sleep detected and sleep latency (Table 120–2).

The MSLT is useful for documenting treatment response.[11-13] It also can reveal residual sleepiness in patients who report no longer being sleepy after treatment.[14] The sensitivity of the MSLT to physiologic sleepiness makes it especially useful for detecting persistent sleepiness in the presumably well treated patient. Sleepiness may continue because of an occult comorbid sleep disorder, ineffective treatment, poor adherence to the treatment regimen, or concomitant soporific medication. Therefore, assessing sleep polysomnographically the night before MSLT testing and obtaining a careful history of drug use for the past month are essential. The MSLT should not be scheduled during drug withdrawal, while sedating medications are pharmacokinetically active, or after a night of profoundly disturbed sleep.

As a technique to demonstrate an individual's underlying sleepiness, the MSLT has several inherent advantages. The first is its direct, objective, quantitative approach. It is generally thought that individuals who are not sleepy cannot make themselves fall asleep. By contrast, one can succeed in remaining awake when sleepy if the sleepiness is not overwhelming. Thus, if a positive MSLT is one that indicates sleepiness, false-positive tests are theoretically minimal. A full polysomnogram, performed the night before MSLT testing, will assess prior sleep quality and quantity. If the prior night's sleep is significantly disrupted or disturbed, the MSLT can be rescheduled. Drug screening is also recommended to ensure that the physiologic sleepiness is not pharmacologically induced. The availability of normative values and test standardization made the MSLT the test of choice for assessing sleepiness for many years.

The American Academy of Sleep Medicine (AASM) Standards of Practice Committee has published new practice parameters for the clinical use of MSLT (Sleep, Nov 2004).[15] These parameters were developed on the basis of a comprehensive evidence-based medicine review process.[16] When data were insufficient, collective expert opinion was used to support recommendations. The Standard of Practice Committee recommendations were reviewed and approved by the board of directors. The conclusions can be summarized as follows:

1. The MSLT is indicated as part of the clinical evaluation for patients with suspected narcolepsy.
2. The MSLT may be helpful for clinical assessment of patients with suspected idiopathic hypersomnia.
3. The MSLT is not indicated for routine evaluation of obstructive sleep apnea.
4. The MSLT is not indicated for routine reevaluation of patients with sleep apnea treated with positive airway pressure therapy.
5. The MSLT is not indicated for routine clinical assessment of insomnia, circadian rhythm disorders, or dyssomnia associated with medical, psychiatric, or neurologic disorders (other than narcolepsy and idiopathic hypersomnia).

Other Measures of Physiologic Sleepiness

Pupillography

Pupil stability and size are affected by exposure to light and by an individual's arousal level. In a darkened room, a person's pupils dilate; however, if the person becomes sleepy and begins to fall asleep, the pupils constrict and become unstable. This change reflects autonomic nervous system changes and has been researched as a potential measure of sleep tendency.[17] Pupillometry was used in the clinical assessment of narcolepsy and its treatment for many years at the Mayo Clinic (Rochester, Minnesota),[18] and it continues to attract clinical interest.[19,20] Electronic pupillography is an objective method for monitoring the size of the pupil, but it is difficult to compare one subject with another and normative data are not available; consequently, the technique has not come into general use for clinically evaluating sleepiness.

Electroencephalography

Computerized quantitative analyses of EEG waveform features seem an obvious approach to the assessment of central nervous system arousal level. It has long been thought that EEG delta activity can be used to index sleepiness. Sleep-related EEG delta activity increases in response to experimental sleep deprivation.[21] Hasan et al.[22] reported EEG correlates of drowsiness using computerized analysis. In essence, the MSLT uses EEG markers (*macroarchitectural features*) of sleep onset to quantify sleepiness. It is reasonable to expect that subtle waveform patterns (*microarchitecture*) could provide a sensitive metric. Alpha EEG frequency decreases and amplitude increases occur just before sleep onset (marked by alpha EEG disappearance). Even further refinement using event-related potentials to directly index the neurologic reactivity to sensory stimuli has been explored as a way to assess sleepiness. Although these approaches hold promise, the lack of technique standardization and the absence of normative data limit their clinical usefulness. In addition, the high degree of between-subject variation makes it difficult to compare results between individuals.

Table 120–2.	Narcolepsy: Results of Multiple Sleep Latency Test	
Group	**Parameter**	**Value**
Patients with narcolepsy	n (men/women)	57 (33/24)
	Age (SD) in years	43.3 (12.3)
	Percent who slept	99.0
	Sleep latency, mean (SD)	3.0 (2.7)
	Minimum	0.6
	Maximum	14.1
	REM score	3.5
Controls	n (men/women)	17 (6/11)
	Age (SD) in years	33.4 (9.9)
	Percent who slept	63.5
	Sleep latency, mean (SD)	13.4 (4.0)
	Minimum	4.8
	Maximum	20
	REM score	0

REM, rapid eye movement; SD, standard deviation.

Finally, continuous EEG measures may not be as sensitive to episodes of sleepiness as continuous observation by a trained observer. Several investigators report that continuous EEG identified fewer episodes of sleepiness[23] and was less predictive of performance lapses than continuous video monitoring.[24]

MANIFEST SLEEPINESS

Maintenance of Wakefulness Test

The procedures used to conduct the Maintenance of Wakefulness Test (MWT) are similar to those used for the MSLT.[25] The major difference is the instruction given to the test subject. The person being tested is told *to attempt to remain awake*. In this manner, the MWT is used to assess an individual's capability to not be overwhelmed by sleepiness—that is, the functioning of the underlying wakefulness system is assessed. If the wakefulness system fails, sleepiness becomes manifest. This laboratory situation parallels circumstances in which sleep onset occurs inadvertently while a person is passive and sedentary in a nonstimulating environment. In the MWT, there is no task other than to remain awake. During the MWT, an individual is monitored for EEG sleep onset during four to six sessions, scheduled at 2-hour intervals beginning 2 hours after awakening from the previous night's sleep. In studies that compared MWT and MSLT sleep latencies, as expected, subjects were found to take longer to fall asleep when instructed to remain awake than when told not to resist sleep.

A major criticism of the MWT relates to the wide variety of protocols used. MWT session length has not been well standardized; 20-, 30-, and 40-minute tests have been used, with the longer tests devised to avoid ceiling effects. Also, a major drawback in the use of the MWT used to be the lack of normative data; however, this situation has changed.[26]

Remaining questions include the effect of acute sleep deprivation, age, time of testing, and drugs on MWT profiles. Nevertheless, the MWT has proved useful in evaluating treatment effects in patients with narcolepsy and sleep-related breathing disorders. Because the MWT poses the question of whether sleepiness is overwhelming, the test has attracted the attention of regulatory agencies. With growing interest in sleepiness and public safety, the demand for tests to assess sleepiness has increased. Indeed, the Federal Aviation Administration recognizes the MWT as a means to determine whether noncommercial pilots can be licensed after treatment for sleep apnea.[27] MWT measures often reveal improvement in treated patients who continue to be physiologically sleepy; thus, MWT is sometimes thought to be a way of extending the sensitivity range of MSLT.[28] It should be noted, however, that the MSLT and the MWT do not correlate well in patients complaining of excessive sleepiness.[29,30] Many patients who fall asleep rapidly when not resisting sleep can still retain the ability to remain awake if they desire. The underlying neurophysiologic mechanisms for maintaining alertness are quite distinct from those that regulate and coordinate sleep.

The AASM Standards of Practice Committee has developed practice parameters for clinical use of the MWT that are based on a critical review of the literature[16] and expert opinion (in cases where data were inadequate). MWT testing is indicated when assessing individuals whose inability to remain alert constitutes a safety hazard and in patients with narcolepsy (or idiopathic hypersomnia) to determine response to pharmacotherapy. Clinicians are warned that there is little evidence directly linking MWT sleep latency to real-world accidents and therefore assessment must integrate MWT findings with clinical history and treatment adherence. Specific recommendations include using a four-trial, 40-minute version of the MWT for assessing an individual's ability to remain awake when the issue is personal or public safety. Based on statistical analysis of normative data, a mean sleep latency of less than 8 minutes on the 40-minute MWT is abnormal. Scores between 8 and 40 (maximum value) are of uncertain significance. The mean sleep latency for presumed normal volunteer subjects was 30.4 minutes. The strongest evidence for an individual's ability to maintain wakefulness is provided by a capacity to remain awake throughout all trials of the 40-minute MWT (which is the upper limit of the 95% confidence interval). Clinical judgment is critical for assessing sleepiness, even when 40-minute MWT sleep latencies are collected, because completely normal values do not guarantee safety.

Performance and Vigilance Tests

Manifest sleepiness can be measured using a variety of performance tasks. Some of these tests attempt to measure cognitive slowing (e.g., the digit symbol substitution test), whereas others address alterations in attention. Arousal and attention have traditionally been difficult to tease apart; therefore, it is not surprising that long, experimenter-paced, monotonous tasks that tax the subject's endurance are sensitive to sleep loss. Such tests are called *vigilance tests*. These tests often attempt to mimic the tedious, palling situation of watching for blips on a radar screen or for ships on the horizon. Assessment of vigilance with nonstimulating tasks is clinically relevant in patients with disorders of sleep and arousal.

Regardless of the test used, several important measurement issues exist. The landmark studies, collectively labeled the Walter Reed experiments (named for the institute in which they were conducted), investigated, among other things, the effects of sleep deprivation on performance.[30,31] From these pioneering studies, it became clear that time-on-task, response slowing, and response lapsing were essential factors in *sustained attention* tasks (for an excellent review, see Dinges and Kribbs[32]).

A variety of performance, vigilance, and sustained attention tests are available.[33-35] One test in common use among sleep laboratories is the psychomotor vigilance test pioneered by David Dinges and colleagues at the University of Pennsylvania.[36,37] This metric employs trials with a duration of about 10 minutes in which a hand-held, computerized display-and-response unit quantifies response latency to multiple light emitting diode (LED) presentations of a stimulus. Data with this inexpensive method have been validated with the Stanford Sleepiness Scale (SSS) and the MSLT, and results have been reported for a wide variety of subject groups including normal control and sleep-deprived volunteers as well as patients with sleep apnea. The Oxford sleep resistance (OSLER) test[38,39] is another performance based metric used in the sleep laboratory setting that has been validated with the MWT. The OSLER test consists of four 40-minute-long trials during which there are multiple LED signal presentations. The subject is instructed to respond to each signal with a simple button press. Trials are ended after 40 minutes or after a failure to respond, which is considered to constitute a failure to maintain wakefulness.

The presentation modality, sensitivity, usefulness, and types of data available vary considerably among performance-based tests. With the exception of the psychomotor vigilance test, normative data are limited, and the meaningfulness of comparisons between individuals can be difficult to evaluate.

INTROSPECTIVE SLEEPINESS

Profile of Mood States

Although designed to assess mood, the Profile of Mood States (POMS) has often been used in sleep research.[40] The original test design included a dimension for sleepiness, but it was eliminated because it was found to overlap with other scales. Sleepiness loads several POMS scales, most notably, Vigor (negative), Confusion, and Fatigue. To a lesser extent, sleepiness is associated with increased scores on Depression and Anger scales. Interestingly, the Confusion scale may be differentially more responsive to severe sleepiness, and the Vigor scale may be differentially more responsive to partial sleep deprivation.[41] The *worn out syndrome* of oversleeping in the absence of marked sleep deficit described by Globus[36,42] is characterized in language comparable to the POMS Fatigue scale mood descriptors; however, fatigue can occur independent of sleepiness.

Stanford Sleepiness Scale

For many years, the SSS was the standard measure of introspective sleepiness.[43] Individuals taking the SSS choose one of seven statements to describe their self-assessed current state; the choices are shown in Table 120–3. The SSS is a momentary assessment scale and can therefore detect sleepiness as it waxes and wanes over the course of a day.

Advantages of SSS include its brevity and its ease of administration and the fact that it can be administered repeatedly. Experimentally induced sleep deprivation increases SSS scores; however, normative data do not exist. It is difficult to use the SSS to make clinical judgments and to compare introspective sleepiness between individuals.

Epworth Sleepiness Scale

The Epworth Sleepiness Scale (ESS) was developed by Murray Johns at the Epworth Hospital in Melbourne, Australia.[44] The ESS is a specialized, validated sleep questionnaire containing eight items that ask for self-reported disclosure of the expectation

Table 120–4. Epworth Sleepiness Scale

Question	Hypothetical Situation to Be Rated
1	Sitting and reading
2	Watching television
3	Sitting and inactive in a public place (e.g., a theater or a meeting)
4	As a passenger in a car for an hour without a break
5	Lying down to rest in the afternoon when circumstances permit
6	Sitting and talking to someone
7	Sitting quietly after a lunch without alcohol
8	In a car, while stopped for a few minutes in traffic

of "dozing" in a variety of situations. Dozing probability ratings are none (0), slight (1), moderate (2), or high (3) in the eight hypothetical situations shown in Table 120–4.

It is worth noting that in situations 1, 3, 6, and 7, the subject is explicitly sitting; in situations 2, 4, and 8, the subject is presumably sitting; and in situation 5, the subject is lying down. ESS also differs from other tests in that respondents are not being asked to interpret their internal state but rather to make a judgment about their behavior. Furthermore, in a sense, individuals completing the ESS are rating their *drive to sleep* in probability projections. This may explain why the ESS has a small but statistically significant correlation with the MSLT, an objective index of *sleep drive*. Johns[44,45] conducted reliability and validity studies on 54 patients with sleep-related breathing disorders (before and after treatment with continuous positive airway pressure) and 104 medical student control subjects. Student control subjects had a mean score of 7.6. Initially elevated scores (mean, 14.3) among patients with sleep-related breathing disorders declined to the normal range (mean, 7.4) after treatment. ESS scores increased as a function of increasing severity of their sleep-disordered breathing.[44,46] In another study, normative values were gathered from 942 patients waiting at outpatient clinics (e.g., dermatology, audiology, ophthalmology clinics) and 1120 healthy people attending health fairs or community health lectures. The mean ESS total score for these two groups were 8.1 and 5.2, respectively.[47] Considering an order of magnitude above the mean as profound sleepiness, we categorize ESS 0 to 8 as normal, 9 to 12 as mild, 13 to 16 as moderate, and greater than 16 as severe.

The popularity of ESS stems in part from its simplicity and brevity. This, in conjunction with the validation studies, has made it perhaps the most commonly administered self-report scale for daytime sleepiness. One disadvantage is the questionable usefulness of the test when readministered within a brief time interval; consequently, it is not useful for evaluating circadian rhythm influences on sleepiness. In addition, the sensitivity to age, acute sleep disturbance or deprivation, and drugs is not known.

PRACTICAL ISSUES AND CONCLUSIONS

Before sleepiness is assessed, a variety of questions should be considered, including whether the goal is to establish (1) the presence of sleepiness, (2) the absence of sleepiness, or

Table 120–3. Stanford Sleepiness Scale

Code	Scale Statements
1	Feeling active and vital, alert, wide awake
2	Functioning at a high level but not at peak; able to concentrate
3	Relaxed, awake, responsive, not at full alertness
4	A little foggy, not at peak; let down
5	Fogginess, beginning to lose interest in remaining awake; slowed down
6	Sleepiness, prefer to be lying down, fighting sleep, woozy
7	Almost in a reverie, sleep onset soon, lost struggle to remain awake

Table 120–5.   Comparison of Tests That Evaluate Sleepiness

Type of Sleepiness	Test Name	Normative Data Available	Possible to Fake Sleepiness?	Possible to Fake Alertness?
Physiologic	Multiple Sleep Latency Test*	Yes	No	Yes[†]
	Pupillography	No	No	Unknown
	Electroencephalography	No	No	Unknown
Manifest	Maintenance of Wakefulness Test*	Yes	Yes[‡]	No[‖]
	Vigilance and performance tests	No	Yes[§]	No
	Epworth Sleepiness Scale	Yes	Yes	Yes
Self-report	Stanford Sleepiness Scale	No	Yes	Yes
	Profile of Mood States	Yes	Yes	Yes

*Standard protocol described in an American Academy of Sleep Medicine Practice Parameter: Test involves four to six test sessions per day, at 2-hour intervals. Test sessions are sometimes scheduled at shorter intervals (e.g., for children), but we do not recommend practice.

[†]Assuming that an individual is not overwhelmingly sleepy, attempting to remain awake can undermine the test result.

[‡]Assuming that an individual is physiologically sleepy, not attempting to remain awake will make it appear that overwhelming sleepiness is present.

[§]Intentionally not attending or responding to the task can make an individual appear sleepy.

[‖]Assuming that the subject follows instructions and does not pinch him/herself or otherwise self inflict pain, engage in alerting action, or ingest wake-promoting substances.

(3) changes in sleepiness. Is testing being conducted for (4) clinical assessment, (5) research, or (6) legal purposes? Is there self-interest involved as part of a (7) primary or (8) secondary agenda? With increasing frequency, sleep specialists are being asked for opinions in legal cases involving accidents or disability claims and are often pressured to render opinions concerning "fitness for duty." In such cases, objective testing is critical because there are situational *demand characteristics*. Furthermore, a normal test result does not guarantee fitness for duty. Table 120–5 shows some characteristics of the tests described in this chapter. Ideally, physiologic, manifest, and introspective sleepiness should be assessed. In general, if an individual claims to be sleepy and the goal is to demonstrate sleepiness, the MSLT is the best confirmatory test. If an individual claims not to be sleepy and the goal is to demonstrate an ability to remain awake, the MWT has certain advantages.

For clinical purposes, self-reported measures combined with MSLT have long been the sine qua non for establishing sleepiness. Sometimes, however, in cases involving severe sleepiness, the MWT can demonstrate improved alertness after treatment, whereas the MSLT shows little or no change. Such individuals continue to be pathologically sleepy, but they are not overwhelmed by it during the brief testing interval. The relationship between this pattern of change and performance or behavior requires further study.

The dangers posed by excessive sleepiness are becoming increasingly apparent. The National Commission on Sleep Disorders Research[48] enumerated a substantial list of industrial and transportation accidents directly or indirectly related to sleepiness. Although it was originally thought that sleepiness stemmed from the accumulation of blood-borne neurotoxins, such substances have not been clearly identified. The search continues for sleep-inducing peptides (contemporary descendents of the hypothesized neurotoxins); however, a convenient and reliable blood test for sleepiness has yet to be developed. Nevertheless, evaluation techniques can assess not only the underlying physiologic drive to sleep but also its subjective, internalized consequences and its behavioral manifestations.

Clinical Pearl

Measuring sleepiness in a clinical setting is not a simple matter. Physiologic and manifest sleepiness testing has become standardized in the Multiple Sleep Latency Test and the Maintenance of Wakefulness Test. The MSLT is indicated for evaluating narcolepsy and idiopathic hypersomnia, whereas the MWT is indicated for testing a person's ability to remain awake when safety is at stake. Sleepiness testing must always be viewed within a larger context of an individual's clinical history and examination findings.

References

1. Carskadon MA, Dement WC: The multiple sleep latency test: What does it measure? Sleep 1982;5:S67-S72.
2. Carskadon MA, Acebo C, Labyak SE, et al: Circadian and homeostatic influences on sleep latency in adolescents. Paper presented at the sixth meeting of the Society for Research on Biological Rhythms. Amelia Island Plantation, Jacksonville, Fla, May 1998.
3. Carskadon MA, Dement WC, Mitler MM, et al: Guidelines for the multiple sleep latency test (MSLT): A standard measure of sleepiness. Sleep 1986;9:519-524.
4. Bonnet MH, Arand DL: Sleepiness as measured by modified multiple sleep latency testing varies as a function of preceding activity. Sleep 1998;21:477-483.
5. Roehrs TA, Carskadon MA: Standardization of method: essential to sleep science. Sleep 1998;21:445.
6. Carskadon MA, Dement WC: Cumulative effects of sleep restriction on daytime sleepiness. Psychophysiology 1981;18:107-113.
7. Carskadon MA, Dement WC: Daytime sleepiness: Quantification of behavioral state. Neurosci Biobehav Rev 1987;11:307-317.
8. Mitler MM, Nelson S, Hajdukovic R: Narcolepsy: Diagnosis, treatment, and management. Psychiatr Clin North Am 1987;10:593-606.
9. Carskadon MA, Harvey K, Duke P, et al: Pubertal changes in daytime sleepiness. Sleep 1980;2:453-460.
10. Richardson GS, Carskadon MA, Orav EJ, et al: Circadian variation in sleep tendency in elderly and young adult subjects. Sleep 1982;5:S82-S94.

11. Dement WC, Carskadon MA, Richardson GS: Excessive daytime sleepiness in the sleep apnea syndrome. In Guilleminault C, Dement WC (eds): Sleep Apnea Syndromes. Menlo Park, Calif, Alan R. Liss, 1978, pp 23-46.

12. Lamphere J, Roehrs T, Wittig R, et al: Recovery of alertness after CPAP in apnea. Chest 1989;96:1364-1367.

13. U.S. Modafinil in Narcolepsy Study Group (USMNSG): Randomized trial of modafinil for the treatment of pathological somnolence in narcolepsy. Ann Neurol 1998;43:88-97.

14. Zorick F, Roehrs T, Conway W, et al: Effects of uvulopalatopharyngoplasty on the daytime sleepiness associated with sleep apnea syndrome. Bull Eur Physiopathol Respir 1983;19:600-603.

15. Standards of Practice Committee of the American Academy of Sleep Medicine: Practice parameters for clinical use of the multiple sleep latency test and the maintenance of wakefulness test. Sleep 2005;28:113-121.

16. A Review by the MSLT and MWT Task Force of the Standards of Practice Committee of the American Academy of Sleep Medicine: The clinical use of the MSLT and MWT. Sleep 2005;28:123-144.

17. Schmidt HS, Fortin L: Electronic pupillography in disorders of arousal. In Guilleminault C (ed): Sleeping and Waking Disorders: Indications and Techniques. Menlo Park, Calif, Addison-Wesley, 1982, pp 127-143.

18. Yoss RE, Moyer NJ, Ogle KN: The pupillogram and narcolepsy: A method to measure decreased levels of wakefulness. Neurology 1969;19:921-928.

19. Morad Y, Lemberg H, Yofe N, Dagan Y: Pupillography as an objective indicator of fatigue. Curr Eye Res 2000;21:535-542.

20. Danker-Hopfe H, Kraemer S, Dorn H, et al: Time-of-day variations in different measures of sleepiness (MSLT, pupillography, and SSS) and their interrelations. Psychophysiology 2001;38:828-835.

21. Borbely AA, Baumann F, Brandeis D, et al: Sleep deprivation: Effect on sleep stages and EEG power density in man. Electroencephalogr Clin Neurophysiol 1981;51:483-493.

22. Hasan J, Hirvonen K, Varri A, et al: Validation of computer analyzed polygraphic patterns during drowsiness and sleep onset. Electroencephalogr Clin Neurophysiol 1993;87:117-127.

23. Mitler MM, Miller JC, Lipsitz JJ, et al: The sleep of long-haul truck drivers. N Engl J Med 1997;337:755-761.

24. Dinges DF, Mallis MM: Managing fatigue by drowsiness detection: Can technological promises be realized? Third International Conference on Fatigue in Transportation: Coping With the 24-Hour Society. Fremantle, Western Australia, February 9-13, 1998.

25. Mitler MM, Gujavarty KS, Browman CP: Maintenance of wakefulness test: A polysomnographic technique for evaluation of treatment efficacy in patients with excessive somnolence. Electroencephalogr Clin Neurophysiol 1982;53:658-661.

26. Doghramji K, Mitler MM, Sangal RB, et al: A normative study of the Maintenance of Wakefulness Test (MWT). Electroencephalogr Clin Neurophysiol 1997;103:554-562.

27. Federal Aviation Administration (FAA): Sleep Apnea Evaluation Specifications. Federal Aviation Administration specification letter dated October 6, 1992. U.S. Department of Transportation, 1992.

28. Mitler MM, Miller JC: Methods of testing for sleepiness. Behav Med 1996;21:171-183.

29. Sangal RB, Thomas L, Mitler MM: Disorders of excessive sleepiness: Treatment improves ability to stay awake but does not reduce sleepiness. Chest 1992;102:699-703.

30. Lubin A: Performance under sleep loss and fatigue. In Kety SS, Evarts EV, Williams HL (eds): Sleep and Altered States of Consciousness. Baltimore, Williams & Wilkins, 1967, pp 506-513.

31. Williams HL, Lubin A, Goodnow JJ: Impaired performance and acute sleep loss. Psychol Monogr 1959;73(pt 14):1-26.

32. Dinges DF, Kribbs NB: Performing while sleepy: Effects of experimentally induced sleepiness. In Monk TM (ed): Sleep, Sleepiness and Performance. Chichester, England, John Wiley & Sons, 1991, pp 97-128.

33. Wilkinson RT: Sleep deprivation: Performance tests for partial and selective sleep deprivation. In Abt LA, Reiss BF (eds): Progress in Clinical Psychology, vol 3. London, Grune & Stratton, 1968, pp 28-43.

34. Hirshkowitz M, De La Cueva L, Herman JH: The multiple vigilance test. Behav Res Meth Instrum Comput 1993;25:272-275.

35. Findley L, Unverzagt M, Guchu R, et al: Vigilance and automobile accidents in patients with sleep apnea or narcolepsy. Chest 1995;108:619-624.

36. Kribbs NB, Pack AI, Kline LR, et al: Effects of one night without nasal CPAP treatment on sleep and sleepiness in patients with obstructive sleep apnea. Am Rev Respir Dis 1993;147:1162-1168.

37. Doran SM, Van Dongen HP, Dinges DF: Sustained attention performance during sleep deprivation: Evidence of state instability. Arch Ital Biol 2001;139:253-267.

38. Bennett LS, Stradling JR, Davies RJ: A behavioural test to assess daytime sleepiness in obstructive sleep apnoea. J Sleep Res 1997;6:142-145.

39. Priest B, Brichard C, Aubert G, et al: Microsleep during a simplified maintenance of wakefulness test: A validation study of the OSLER test. Am J Respir Crit Care Med 2001;163:1619-1625.

40. McNair DM, Lorr M, Droppleman LF: Manual of the Profile of Mood States. San Diego, Calif, Educational and Industrial Testing Service, 1992.

41. Horne J: Dimensions to sleepiness. In Monk TM (ed): Sleep, Sleepiness and Performance. Chichester, England, John Wiley & Sons, 1991, pp 169-196.

42. Globus GG: A syndrome associated with sleeping late. Psychosomatic Med 1969;31:528-535.

43. Hoddes E, Zarcone V, Smythe H, et al: Quantification of sleepiness: A new approach. Psychophysiology 1973;10:431-436.

44. Johns MW: A new method for measuring daytime sleepiness: The Epworth Sleepiness Scale. Sleep 1991;14:540-545.

45. Johns MW: Reliability and factor analysis of the Epworth Sleepiness Scale. Sleep 1992;15:376-381.

46. Hirshkowitz M, Gokcebay N, Iqbal S, et al: Epworth Sleepiness Scale and sleep-disordered breathing: Replication and extension. Sleep Res 1995;24:249.

47. Sharafkhaneh A, Hirshkowitz M: Contextual factors and perceived self-reported sleepiness: A preliminary report. Sleep Med 2003;4:327-331.

48. National Commission on Sleep Disorders Research: Wake up America: A national sleep alert. Executive Summary and Executive Report, Report of the National Commission on Sleep Disorders Research. Washington, DC, National Institutes of Health, U.S. Government Printing Office, 1993;1:45.

121

Light Therapy

Michael Terman

Jiuan Su Terman

ABSTRACT

The susceptibility of the circadian system to selective phase shifting by timed light exposure has broad implications for the treatment of sleep-phase and depressive disorders. Light therapies have been devised that can normalize the patterns of delayed sleep phase syndrome (through circadian phase advances) and advanced sleep phase syndrome (through circadian phase delays). Doctors and patients need to become cognizant of the daily intervals when light exposure—and darkness—can facilitate or hamper adjustment. The primary intervals lie at the edges of the "subjective night," which coincide with the tails of the nocturnal melatonin cycle, but they can be inferred clinically through a chronotype questionnaire. The lighting schedule may have to be continually adjusted as the subjective night shifts gradually in the desired direction.

The treatment strategy for seasonal and nonseasonal depressive disorders is similar. In winter depression, the magnitude of phase advances correlates with the degree of mood improvement, and the optimum timing of light therapy must be specified relative to circadian rather than solar time. Apart from its use as a monotherapy, light therapy in both outpatient and inpatient trials indicates that light therapy accelerates remission of nonseasonal depression in conjunction with medication.

Exploratory applications for treatment of antepartum and premenstrual depression, bulimia nervosa, sleep disruption of senile dementia, and shift work and jet lag disturbance are considered. The chapter provides the clinician with guidelines for selecting lighting apparatus based on safety, efficacy, and comfort factors; summarizes adverse effects of light overdose; and offers a straightforward protocol for selecting treatment time of day.

Exposure of the eyes to light of appropriate intensity and duration, at an appropriate time of day, can have marked effects on the timing and duration of sleep and on the affective and physical symptoms of depressive illness. The most extensive clinical trials have focused on winter depression, or *seasonal affective disorder* (SAD).

Here, we review and evaluate the application of light therapy for circadian rhythm sleep disorders including delayed sleep phase syndrome (DSPS), advanced sleep phase syndrome (ASPS), non–24-hour sleep phase syndrome, and the displaced sleep of shift work and jet lag. Beyond SAD, we also cover light therapy for nonseasonal depressions (recurrent, chronic, premenstrual, and antepartum), including combination treatment with wake therapy and medication; bulimia nervosa; and the sleep-wake problems of senile dementia. We describe the critical features of light delivery systems; safety factors and potential adverse effects; and timing and dose optimization for light administration, including a set of clinical case studies. (For a review of the underlying circadian physiology, see Terman.[1])

LIGHT DELIVERY

Apparatus

Light Boxes

Many of the early research studies used a standard 60-cm by 120-cm (2-foot by 4-foot) fluorescent ceiling unit, with a plastic prismatic diffusion screen, placed vertically on a table about 1 meter (3 feet) from the user. A bank of fluorescent lamps—full spectrum or cool white—provided approximately 2500-lux illuminance. Smaller, more lightweight units have become commercially available; however, specific design features of marketed light boxes have most often not been clinically tested.

Factors include lamp type (output and spectrum), filter, ballast frequency (for fluorescent lamps), size and positioning of radiating surface, heat emission, and so on. One clinically tested model (Fig. 121–1) illustrates second-generation apparatus modifications, including smaller size, portability, raised and downward-tilted placement of the radiating surface, a smooth polycarbonate diffusion screen with complete ultraviolet (UV) filtering (see Resources), and high-output fluorescent lamps (nonglaring 4000 K color temperature) driven by high-frequency solid-state ballasts. The combination of elements in this configuration yields a maximum illuminance of approximately 10,000 lux with the patient seated in a position with the eyes about 30 cm (1 foot) from the screen.

With the direction of gaze downward toward the work surface, such a configuration provides pleasant illumination suitable for reading and, despite illuminance far higher than in normal home lighting, is generally well tolerated (see Side Effects of Exposure to Bright Light). The presentation of light from above eye level is supported by a study showing enhancement of melatonin suppression with directional illumination of the lower retina.[2] As the apparatus becomes miniaturized, however, the field of illumination narrows, and even small changes in head position can substantially reduce the intensity of light that reaches the eyes.

Although light boxes are simple in design, home construction of such an apparatus is discouraged because of the danger of excessive irradiation; some amateur assemblers have experienced corneal and eyelid burns. Because the critical design features have not been specified or regulated by the government or the profession, clinicians should seek documentation by the manufacturer of the safety and effectiveness of any apparatus under consideration.

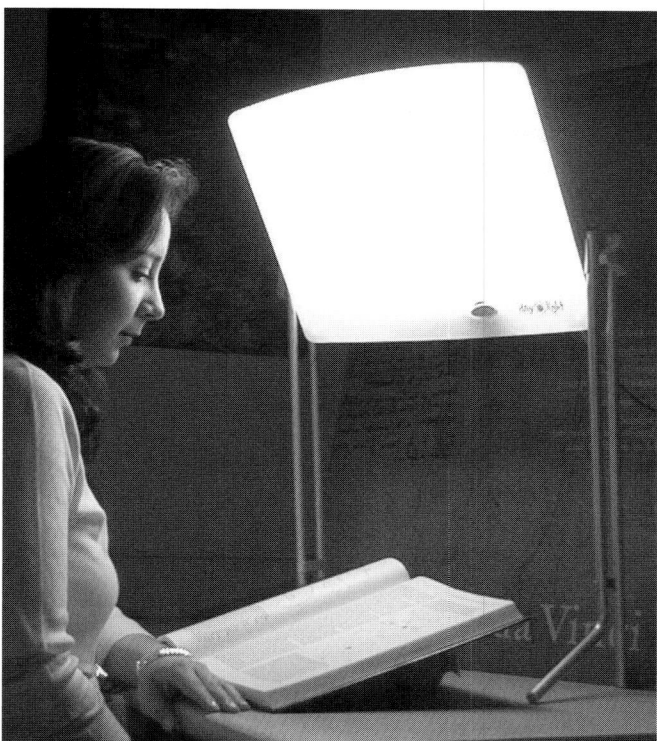

Figure 121–1. Table-mounted, tilted, 10,000-lux, UV-filtered 4000 Kelvin fluorescent light system. (Photograph courtesy of the Center for Environmental Therapeutics, www.cet.org.)

Claims for the specific efficacy of any particular lamp type or spectral distribution, although commonly given, are unsubstantiated. Unfortunately, systems are marketed that provide excessive visual glare, exposure of naked bulbs, direct intense illumination from below the eyes ("ski slope" effect), and intentionally augmented UV radiation. Claims that UV radiation is important for the therapeutic effect are unsubstantiated, and the risk of ocular and facial exposure must be avoided. Both the clinician and the consumer must be vigilant in the selection of an apparatus. Criteria are reviewed on the Suppliers website page of the nonprofit Center for Environmental Therapeutics, www.cet.org.

Light Visors

In an alternate configuration, head-mounted portable lighting units (in a visor configuration), which are intended to increase flexibility and convenience of use, have been marketed and are suited for novel applications such as in-flight treatment. However, despite a set of multicenter trials for SAD,[3-5] bright light exposure with this device has shown no advantage over dim light exposure (a putative placebo control), and there has been no convincing demonstration of clinical efficacy.[6] One visor study has demonstrated circadian phase shifting,[7] however, and pending design enhancements may yet show utility.

Dawn Simulators

Dawn simulation methodology provides a major contrast to bright light therapy. A computer-controlled lighting device delivers a mimic of gradual twilight transitions found outdoors in the spring or summer. The relatively dim, dynamically changing signals are presented to the patient while asleep, when eyes are adapted to the dark and the circadian system is most susceptible to phase advances (see Timing of Morning Light Exposure). As with bright light therapy, there is an antidepressant response and normalization of hypersomnic, phase-shifted, and fractionated sleep patterns.[8-10]

A laboratory study of healthy young adult subjects demonstrated that the addition of simulated, naturalistic dawn exposures blocks the delay drift of circadian rhythms under dim light-dark cycles.[11] A large, 6-week controlled clinical trial of log-linear light onset ramps (which differ from the curvilinear acceleration of naturalistic dawns) found signals rising to 250 lux between 4:30 and 6:00 AM significantly more antidepressant than dim red control signals rising to 0.5 lux.[12] Furthermore, the treatment was superior to postawakening bright light therapy administered between 6:00 and 6:30 AM.

The effectiveness of dawn simulation may depend on the presentation of diffuse, broad-field illumination that reaches the sleeper in varying postures. Such efficacy has not been demonstrated for inexpensive, commercial light "alarm clocks," which have small, directional fields.

Safety of Bright Light for the Eyes

Ophthalmologic evaluations of unmedicated patients with normal oculoretinal status have thus far shown no obvious acute light-induced pathology or long-term sequelae.[13] Although the intensity of bright light treatment falls well within the low outdoor daylight range, the exposure conditions differ from those outdoors, and prolonged use entails far greater cumulative light exposure than is normally experienced by urban dwellers and workers.[14,15]

Potentially damaging wavelengths above the UV range extend into the visible range up to 500 nm (blue light),[16-18] and one conservative proposal advocates screening out such low-wavelength light altogether.[19] On the other hand, recent data show that the blue wavelength range above 450 nm preferentially serves to suppress nocturnal melatonin production[20] and enhance circadian phase shifting.[21] Although selective therapeutic benefit of such light has yet to be ascertained, one already sees manufacturers rushing in with blue-light devices. A compromise solution may be assiduous filtering of wavelengths less than 450 nm—the blue-light hazard is magnified in that range.

At the opposite end of the light spectrum, ocular exposure to infrared illumination, which makes up about 90% of the output of incandescent lamps, poses risk of damage to the lens and cornea (as does UV) as well as the retina and pigment epithelium.[22] Thus, despite being marketed for light therapy, incandescent lamps are contraindicated.

Light box diffusion filters vary widely in short-wavelength transmission (for examples, see Remé et al.[19]). Transmission curves should be demanded of manufacturers and compared with published standards. Normal clouding of the lens and ocular media that begins in middle age, as well as cataract formation, serves to exacerbate perceptual glare, which can make high-intensity light exposure quite uncomfortable.[19]

Furthermore, both UV and short-wavelength blue light can interact with photosensitizing medications—including many standard antidepressant, antipsychotic, and antiarrhythmic agents, as well as common medications such as tetracycline—to promote or accelerate retinal pathology, whether acute or slow and cumulative.[22] In one reported case, a patient received combination treatment with clomipramine (an anticholinergic tricyclic antidepressant) and full-spectrum fluorescent light. After 5 days, the patient had reduced contrast sensitivity, foveal sensitivity and visual acuity, and central scotomas and lesions, fortunately with only minor residual aftereffects in contrast sensitivity and scotoma 1 year after discontinuation.[23]

Filtered wrap-around goggles are available (see Resources) that eliminate transmission of short-wavelength blue light while maximizing exposure above 500 nm, reducing glare, enhancing visual acuity and subjective brightness, and minimizing the risk of drug photosensitization.[24]

Although there are no definite contraindications for bright light treatment other than for the retinopathies, research studies have routinely excluded patients with glaucoma or cataract. Some of these patients have used light therapy effectively in open treatment; this should be done, however, only with ophthalmologic monitoring. A simple eye checkup is advised for all new patients, for which a structured examination chart has been designed (see Resources).[25] The examination has occasionally revealed preexisting ocular conditions that should be distinguished from potential consequences of bright light treatment.

Side Effects of Exposure to Bright Light

If evening light is timed too late, the patient may initially have insomnia and hyperactivity. If morning light is timed too early, the patient may awaken prematurely and be unable to resume sleep. These problems are responsive to timing and dose (duration and intensity) adjustments during treatment of both circadian sleep phase and mood disorders.

The emergence of side effects relates in part to the parameters of light exposure, including intensity, duration, spectral content, and method of exposure (diffuse, focused, direct, indirect, and angle of incidence relative to the eyes). Thus far, side effects have been assessed primarily in patients with seasonal and nonseasonal mood disorders, and information is lacking for sleep disorders without mood disturbance.

The earliest clinical trials of 2500-lux full-spectrum fluorescent light therapy for SAD noted infrequent side effects of hypomania, irritability, headache, and nausea.[26,27] Such symptoms often subside after several days of treatment. If persistent, they can be reduced or eliminated with dose decreases. Rarely have patients discontinued treatment due to side effects. Studies with portable head-mounted units containing incandescent bulbs near the eyes and providing illuminance of 60 to 3500 lux have also noted side effects of headache, eyestrain, and feeling "wired," but symptoms were not dose dependent.[28]

Two cases of induced manic episodes have been reported in drug-refractory nonseasonal unipolar depressives beginning after 4 to 5 days of light treatment.[29] A few cases of light-induced agitation and hypomania have been noted, also in nonseasonal depressives.[30] A patient with seasonally recurrent brief depressions developed rapid mood swings after light overexposure (far exceeding 30 minutes per day at 10,000 lux),[31] and a unipolar SAD patient with similar exposure showed his first manic episode[32]; both patients required discontinuation and medication. We had one bipolar patient with SAD who became manic after the use of light and was administered lithium as an effective countermeasure; others who have used mood stabilizers have responded to light therapy

without mania. Three cases of suicide attempt or ideation, also occurring in patients with SAD, were reported within 1 week of standard early-evening bright light treatment, and the patients required hospitalization.[33]

A 42-item side-effect inventory was administered to 30 patients with SAD after treatment with unfiltered full-spectrum fluorescent light at 2500 lux for 2 hours daily.[34] Other than for one case of hypomania, there were no clinically significant side effects. Patients given evening light (the timing relative to bedtime was unspecified) reported initial insomnia. Mild visual complaints included blurred vision, eyestrain, and photophobia.

Of specific interest is the side-effect profile for patients using a downward-tilted fluorescent light box protected by a smooth diffusion screen (see Fig. 121–1), with 30-minute daily exposures at 10,000 lux, because this method has had widespread application. A study of 83 patients with SAD who were evaluated for 88 potential side effects[35] identified a small number of emergent symptoms at a frequency of 6% to 16%, including nausea, headache, jumpiness or jitteriness, and eye irritation.[36] These results must be weighed against the improvement of other patients who showed similar symptoms at baseline but became asymptomatic after light treatment: All symptoms, except nausea, showed greater improvement than exacerbation, which forces attention to the risk-to-benefit ratio. Indeed, symptom emergence might reflect the natural course of depressive illness in nonresponders to light rather than a specific response to light exposure.

CASE MANAGEMENT, TIMING, AND DOSING

Patient Monitoring

Light treatment is typically self-administered at home on a schedule recommended by the clinician. To the extent that the timing of light exposure is important for obtaining a therapeutic effect, compliance is a sine qua non. When commencing treatment, therefore, it is helpful to ask the patient to call every few days or to fax log records of sleep, treatment times, and mood ratings; this will assist the clinician in managing timing and dose adjustments.

In contrast with structured research studies, the motivation and compliance of patients in open treatment can be problematic. Despite an agreement to awaken for light treatment at a specific hour, patients may ignore the alarm, considering additional sleep to be the priority of the moment, and may delay or skip treatment. Patients frequently attempt to test whether improvement can be achieved without rigid compliance, and they may quit if treatment is managed too rigidly. Indeed, the behavioral investment in a maintenance regimen of light treatment is considerable, far exceeding that of pharmacotherapy.

For hypersomnic patients who are unable to awaken when instructed, light exposure initially can be scheduled at the time of habitual awakening and then edged earlier across days toward the target interval. Some depressed patients compensate for earlier wake-up times with earlier bedtimes or napping (as do patients with DSPS), but others are comfortable with less sleep as the antidepressant effect sets in. Clinical experience suggests that most such patients could not sustain earlier awakening without the use of light.

Variability in the sleep pattern, if it occurs, may yield important information for determining the course of treatment. Online adjustments in scheduling, although labor intensive for the clinician, often succeed. Our strategy has been to encourage the adherence to a recommended light exposure schedule but to consider the obtained sleep pattern as a dependent measure that often reflects changes in mood state, sleep need, and circadian rhythm phase.

Timing of Morning Light Exposure

The thrust of recent clinical trials (see Seasonal Affective Disorder) leads to the recommendation that patients with SAD initially be given morning light shortly after awakening. A similar strategy applies to patients with DSPS. (In contrast, evening light is indicated for ASPS; see Case Example 6.) The dose of 10,000 lux for 30 minutes[37,38] appears to be most efficient. Although lower intensities also may be effective, they require exposure durations up to 2 hours,[39,40] and to accommodate such morning treatment, most patients would have to awaken far earlier than at baseline, with risk of a counterproductive circadian phase delay.

The advantage of morning light appears to lie in circadian rhythm phase advances, which can be measured as shifts in the time of nocturnal melatonin onset.[41] The magnitude of the antidepressant response varies with the magnitude of phase advances. In a protocol with 10,000-lux treatment for 30 minutes on habitual awakening, the magnitude of antidepressant response was negatively correlated with the interval between melatonin onset and treatment time ($r = -0.53$, a large effect size).[42] Indeed, light therapy given 7.5 to 9.5 hours after melatonin onset yields twice the remission rate (80% versus 38%) of light given 9.5 to 11.0 hours after melatonin onset.[43] The clock time of morning light administration is irrelevant, since baseline melatonin onset spans a 4-hour range or more. To maximize the likelihood of a treatment response, the clinician might therefore initiate morning light no later than 8.5 hours after a patient's melatonin onset.

Unfortunately, such diagnostic information is not readily available. A future solution may lie in the use of a salivary melatonin assay,[44] with home sampling and rapid turnaround by a commercial laboratory. An approximate solution, however, lies in the relation between melatonin onset and the Horne-Östberg Morningness-Eveningness Questionnaire (MEQ)[45] score, which for SAD patients are strongly correlated ($r = 0.80$, $N = 71$, $P < .001$).[46] One thus can schedule morning light exposure at individually specified circadian times by inferring the time of melatonin onset, a strategy that facilitates circadian rhythm phase advances as well as the antidepressant response.

A list of recommended light exposure times, derived from the regression of the MEQ score on melatonin onset, is shown in Table 121–1.

Sessions should begin within 10 minutes of scheduled wake-up time. In most cases, treatment will begin earlier than the baseline wake-up time—which is also highly correlated with melatonin onset and the MEQ score—depending on the patient's habitual sleep duration. For example, a short sleeper, whose bedtime is at midnight and who awakens at 6 AM, would start treatment on habitual awakening. In contrast, a long sleeper, with onset at 11:30 PM and awakening at 7:30 AM, would have to wake up 1 hour earlier, at 6:30 AM. For every half hour of sleep beyond 6 hours, awakening for light treatment

Table 121–1.	**Timing of Morning Light Therapy* Based on Morningness-Eveningness Score**
MEQ Score	**Start Time**
16-18	0845
19-22	0830
23-26	0815
27-30	0800
31-34	0745
35-38	0730
39-41	0715
42-45	0700
46-49	0645
50-53	0630
54-57	0615
58-61	0600
62-65	0545
66-68	0530
69-72	0515
73-76	0500
77-80	0445
81-84	0430
85-86	0415

*Start of 10,000-lux, 30-minute session, approximately 8.5 hours after estimated melatonin onset.

is 15 minutes earlier than habitual awakening at baseline—a maximum of 1.5 hours earlier if sleep duration extends to 9 hours. The algorithm should be considered a "best guess" strategy to determine the initial timing of light exposure, with a potential need for adjustment depending on early results. An online version of the MEQ,[47] at www.cet.org, automatically returns the recommended light exposure interval to the user. Although the algorithm is based on SAD data, it has been applied successfully to patients with nonseasonal depression[48] and delayed sleep phase.

LIGHT TREATMENT OF SPECIFIC DISORDERS

Circadian Sleep Phase Disorders

Delayed Sleep Phase Syndrome

Patients with DSPS have difficulty initiating sleep before 1 to 3 AM, and sometimes later, with commensurate difficulty awakening at an early hour (for a review and discussion of circadian rhythm correlates, see Terman et al.[49]). Once awake, most patients exhibit normal alertness and energy as long as they can maintain their displaced sleep schedule, but others report difficulties for several hours after awakening and spurts of energy after midnight. Not infrequently, patients with DSPS show comorbid mood and personality disorders.

Under delay chronotherapy,[50] the sleep episode is scheduled at successively later hours each night for about 1 week. Once the desired sleep phase is attained, the patient attempts to keep sleep-wake timing consistent. The original description of chronotherapy specified that sleep episodes occur in darkness. It follows that the timing of light exposure changes during and after the phase adjustment. An implication is that by the end of the procedure, the patient begins to receive a normalized pattern of daily light exposure that serves to maintain the target phase. Early morning artificial bright light exposure can forestall further drifting toward the original delayed sleep phase, which is always a risk.

Indeed, morning light treatment can often directly normalize the timing of the sleep episode without the need for progressive delays with chronotherapy. In one study, patients with DSPS were given 2 hours of early-morning light treatment at 2500 lux, along with light restriction after 4:00 pm.[51] The body temperature rhythm and daily cycle of sleep-onset latencies showed phase advances, and there was an increase in morning alertness within 1 week. These effects were not obtained with the use of a dim light control.

In open treatment, if morning light exposure fails to induce and maintain the desired phase advance, chronotherapy may be used to successively delay the sleep episode until the desired target phase is achieved. Light treatment can be used to facilitate chronotherapy with presleep exposures during the delay period, followed by postsleep exposures during maintenance.

These approaches require the clinician's active supervision, with continual adjustment in sleep and light exposure schedules in response to patient feedback and ability to comply. Bright light treatment is administered in the context of complex daily patterns of indoor and outdoor light exposure, including dark periods, all of which may influence treatment outcome. In fact, a procedure may require ensured dark exposure at certain times of day in coordination with light treatment at other times. The patient can accomplish this by using highly filtered goggles when going outdoors during daylight hours.[52]

An interesting novel therapeutic approach uses a sleep mask embedded with light emitting diodes that turn on gradually 4 hours before the end of sleep,[53] in the manner of dawn simulation.[8] A subgroup of delayed sleep phase subjects with relatively late melatonin cycles responded with earlier sleep onset accompanied by melatonin phase advances.

Mild Sleep Phase Delay (Subsyndromal Delayed Sleep Phase Syndrome)

The common problem of chronic but mild initial insomnia that falls short of DSPS, accompanied by difficulty arising and low morning alertness, is often readily treatable with postsleep light, leading to rapid adjustment. Many such insomniacs do not respond to hypnotic medication and are not depressed.

CASE EXAMPLE 1: Phase Advance with Postsleep Light

Patient T.W. (Fig. 121–2A) reported a lifelong history of DSPS with variable sleep onset averaging 5:00 AM and occasional hypersomnic episodes lasting 11 to 12 hours. Although not depressed while seeking help, he also reported experiencing subsyndromal symptoms of winter depression. The treatment consisted of gradually shifting light exposure earlier across days, beginning at 10:30 AM, a time of typical spontaneous awakening.

The patient monitored his level of sleepiness and time of awakening to determine the rate of shift. He was able to achieve successively earlier wake-up times over a period of 2 weeks while light-treatment sessions were advanced from 10:30 to 7:30 AM, but even at that point he could not fall asleep before 2:30 AM. However, when the treatment session was further advanced to 7 AM— an unprecedented time of awakening for this patient—sleep onset abruptly jumped approximately 2 hours earlier. The sleep episode stabilized at about 1:15 to 6:30 AM with light treatment on awakening.

After several months, the patient reported having increased light duration from 30 minutes (at 10,000 lux) to 45 or 60 minutes to enhance daytime energy. He also reported a relapse when he discontinued treatment twice within the next year. He managed his readjustments and reported the remission of depressed mood in the winter.

CASE EXAMPLE 2: Phase Delay with Chronotherapy Followed by Stabilization with Morning Light

Patient M.L. (see Fig. 121–2B) had chronic major depression and was referred for light therapy because of refractory response to drugs. She reported a long history of DSPS and daytime fatigue, often staying in bed all day. In addition, she reported occasionally sleeping at successively later hours until her delayed sleep phase was reestablished. She would not comply with most sleep scheduling requests, but when a free-run appeared to start spontaneously, she agreed to attempt to schedule successive delays of bedtime—in a loose application of chronotherapy—and aim to restabilize with midnight sleep onset and regular outdoor daylight exposure.

Sleep was often fragmented during the week of chronotherapy, and several days after reaching the target phase, sleep became restless throughout the night. The appearance of initial insomnia at that time suggested that there would be further delays over the next days, overshooting the target phase. At this point, the patient began 30-minute light sessions at 10,000 lux on awakening at 7:30 AM, with a second session in midafternoon. She became highly energized after the first day's exposure sessions and was unable to sleep at all the next night. Sleep onset continued to drift later, and she complained of sleep deprivation.

On one occasion when she skipped afternoon light, sleep onset occurred hours earlier than expected. Morning light treatment was then rescheduled about 1 hour later, and despite a few episodes of middle-to-late insomnia, she was able to fall asleep by 2 AM or earlier and to awaken by 8 AM. When monitored several months later, the pattern had stabilized, with sleep onsets occurring around 12:30 to 1:00 AM accompanied by uninterrupted sleep for 8 hours. Despite slightly improved daytime energy, however, her depression did not lift, and she remained dysfunctional.

T.W., ♂ 32 YR, BEG 16 JUL 88

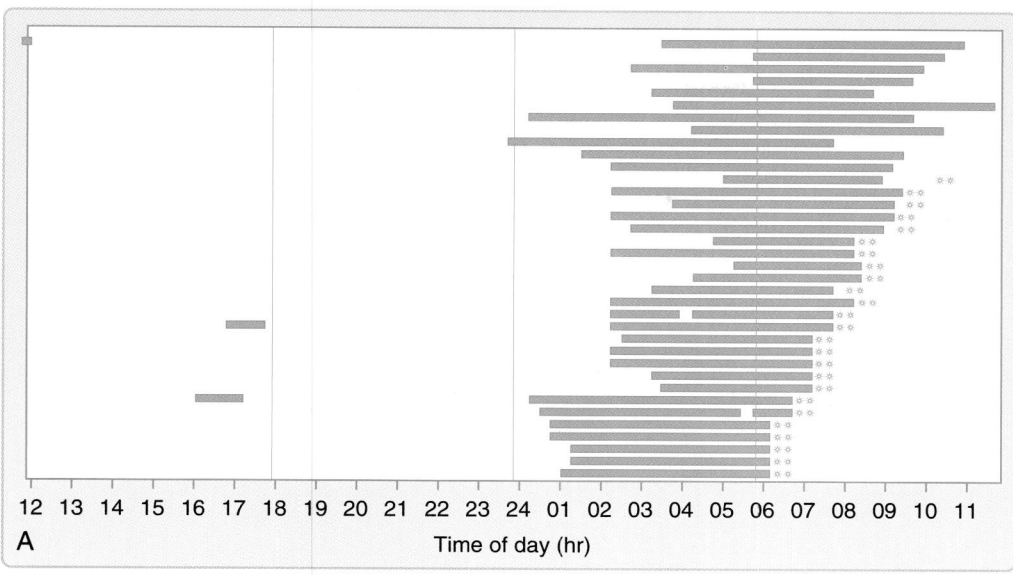

M.L., ♀ 25 YR, BEG 24 MAY 87

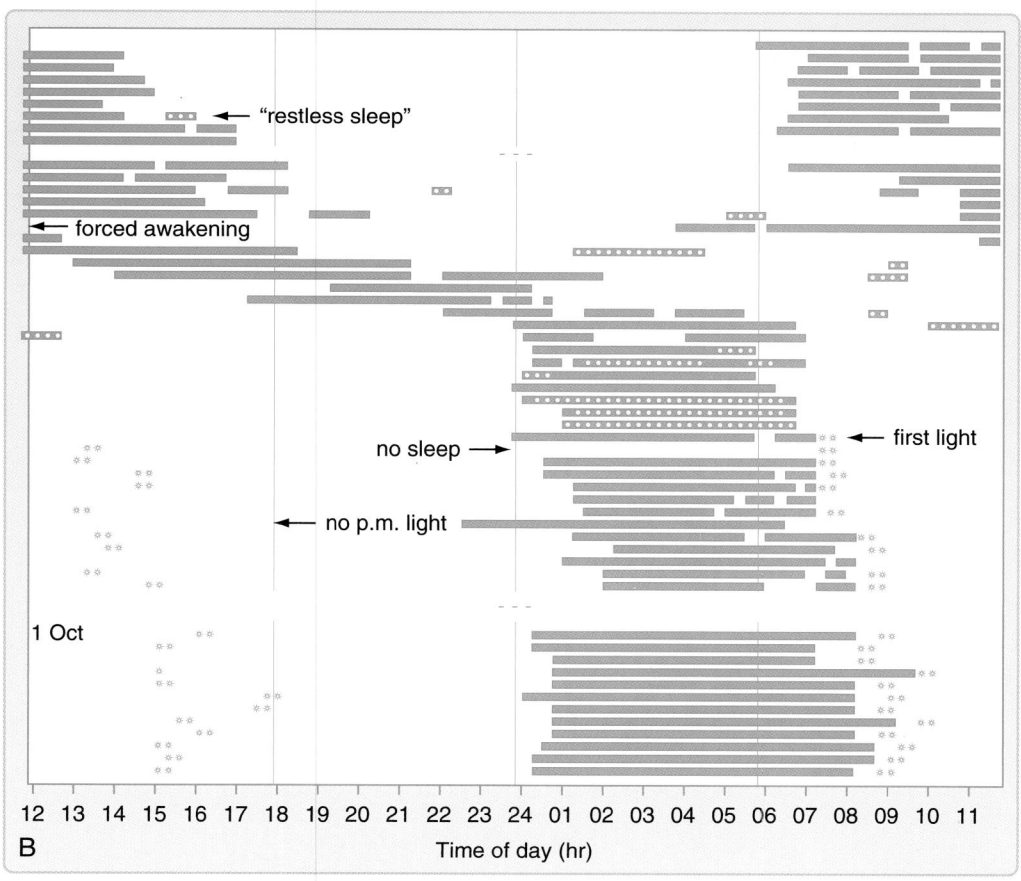

Figure 121–2. Self-report sleep records for five light-therapy patients with various sleep phase disturbances: **A-C**, delayed sleep phase syndrome (T.W., M.L., S.P.); **D**, mild sleep-phase delay (J.B.); **E**, non–24-h sleep-wake disorder (B.C.). Successive days are lined up, *top to bottom*, on the ordinate. *Bars* indicate intervals of sleep (including naps); *sun symbols* indicate 15-minute segments of bright light exposure; *ellipsis* indicates a gap in record. For patient M.L., *open circles* indicate "restless sleep." For patient S.P. (**C**), *B*, benzodiazepine hypnotic; *N*, waking due to noise. For patient B.C. (**E**), the duration of light exposure is indicated as the recommended average of 2.5 hours per day. In addition to morning light treatment, patients M.L. (**B**) and S.P. (**C**) used variations of chronotherapy to establish the desired sleep phase by successive delays of their sleep schedules.

Continued

CASE EXAMPLE 3: Phase Delay with Chronotherapy Followed by Stabilization with Morning Light

Patient S.P. (see Fig. 121–2C) showed a delayed sleep pattern similar to that of M.L. (Case Example 2), which was present since childhood. Although he was groggy on awakening, afternoon and evening energy levels were high, and he could work productively at those times. On nights when he used a benzodiazepine hypnotic, he could sometimes advance sleep onset by a few hours, which he considered trivial.

An attempt was then made to phase advance the sleep episode with the use of 10,000-lux, 30- to 45-minute light exposures on awakening. Despite intense effort over a 1-week trial, the patient could not be awakened before 12:30 PM, making successively earlier treatment sessions impossible. An alternative course of chronotherapy was then attempted.

The patient was instructed to delay successive sleep episodes by 2 hours, in conjunction with 1-hour light treatment sessions ending 2 hours before bedtime (a procedure intended to facilitate chronotherapy). However, he refused to enter bed until ready to fall asleep, resulting in successive daily delays that varied between 1 and 5 hours. After 6 days, the presleep light was discontinued, with instruction to substitute light exposure for 2 hours at 6 AM in an attempt to halt the delay drift. In the next weeks, the patient was able to maintain sleep onset between 11 PM and midnight and to awaken by 7:30 AM or earlier.

The resilience of the adjustment was tested on the occasion of two late-night parties after which the desired sleep pattern was easily recaptured. Subsequently, however, the patient discontinued treatment and resumed his former schedule, citing family stresses that he preferred to escape by sleeping during the day.

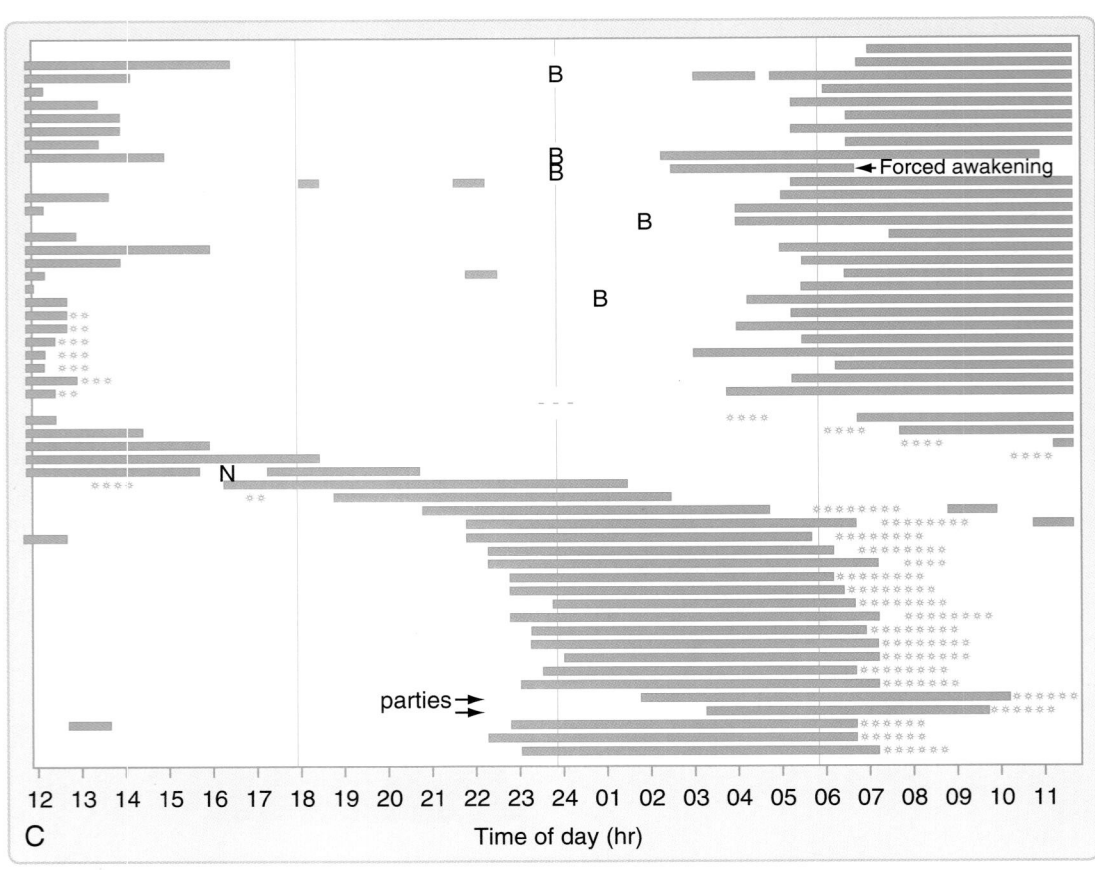

S.P., ♂ 47 YR, BEG 23 NOV 91

Figure 121–2. Cont'd.

Patient J.B. (see Fig. 121–2D) could rarely fall asleep before 1:30 AM or wake up in time for a normal work day. Although he was allowed to work from midmorning into the evening, he was handicapped by low alertness till midafternoon and headaches at a computer terminal during the late afternoon.

Light treatment began with 10,000-lux exposures at 8 AM for 30 minutes, with no effect for several days. When the session was advanced to 7:30 AM, sleep onset spontaneously advanced by about 1 hour. However, several days of late insomnia followed, with awakenings before 6 AM, signaling an overdose. Reducing the treatment duration to 15 minutes at 7:30 AM alleviated this problem, with sleep onset maintained around midnight. This regimen was continued, with effortless awakening accompanied by improved morning alertness and complete remission of the headache.

J.B., ♂ 34 YR, BEG 27 DEC 88

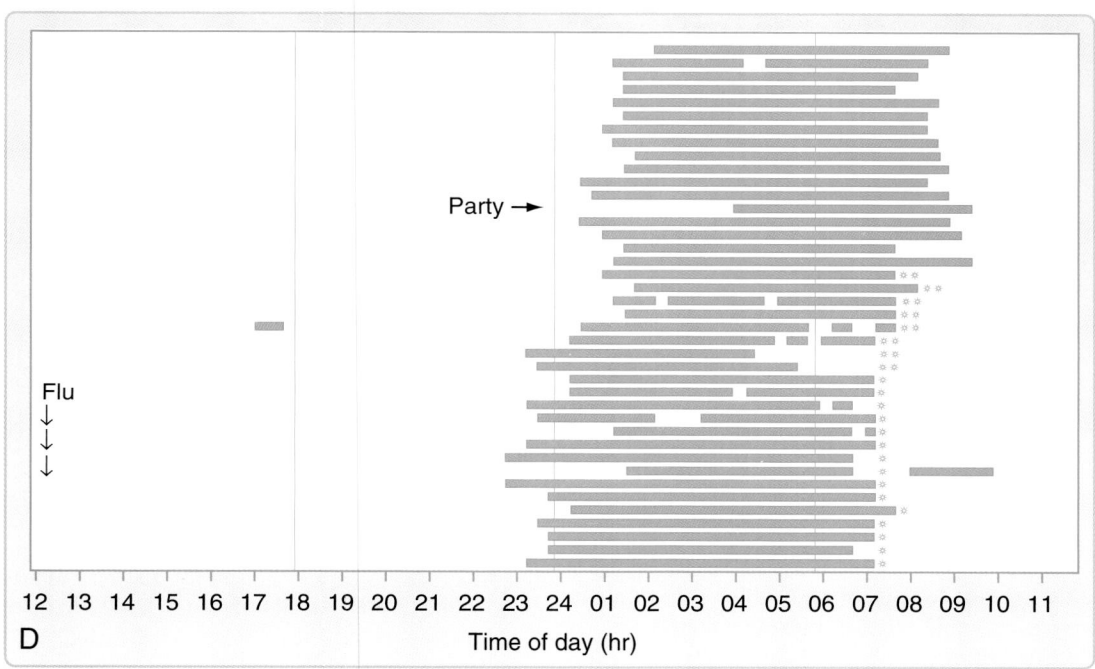

Figure 121–2. Cont'd.

Non–24-hour Sleep-Wake Syndrome

When sleep phase does not stabilize but continually shifts later relative to clock time, the pattern resembles the free-run seen in normal subjects under conditions of temporal isolation without day-night cues. However, in non–24-hour sleep-wake syndrome, despite the presence of such cues, a failure of entrainment is evidenced by a hypernychthemeral[54] sleep pattern. Some patients with DSPS break into transient hypernychthemeral patterns (e.g., patient M.L. in Fig. 121-2B and Case Example 2), which suggests that non–24-hour sleep-wake syndrome and DSPS are associated disorders of varying severity.[55] Light therapy aims to halt the delay drift by timing postsleep exposure to start when the subjective and objective nights coincide.

Patient B.C. (see Fig. 121–2E) showed a sleep-wake cycle length averaging 25 hours over approximately 13 years preceding treatment.[56] He was unemployed and socially withdrawn and refused to attempt to sleep when alert. Treatment began when sleep onset had drifted to midnight. The patient was exposed to light of 4000 to 8000 lux for 2 to 3 hours on awakening. The free-run immediately decelerated, and the sleep interval was maintained at approximately 1:30 to 8:15 AM for several weeks. In the long run, however, the sleep pattern continued to drift at a period of about 24.08 hours, a problem that might have been corrected with increased light dose.

B.C., ♂ 31 YR, ADAPTED FROM EASTMAN ET AL. (1988)

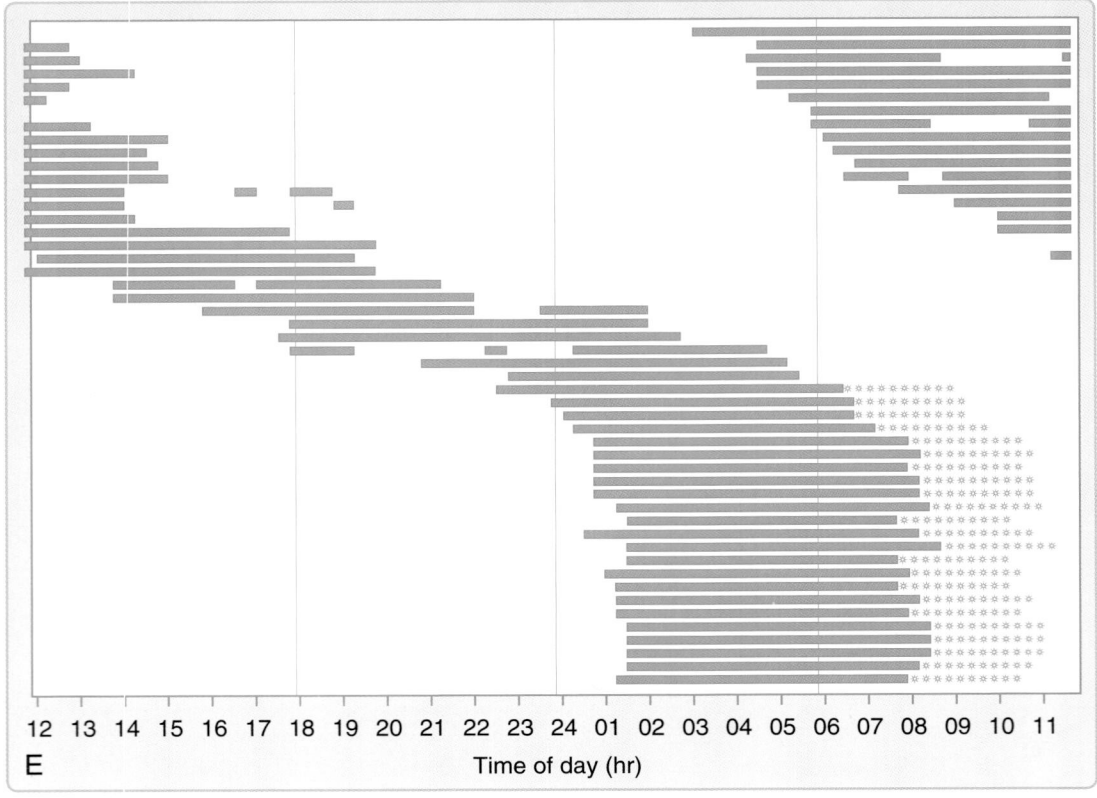

E   Time of day (hr)

Figure 121–2. Cont'd.

Advanced Sleep Phase Syndrome

ASPS, in which sleep onset occurs in the evening with awakening well before dawn, would seem to provide a counterpart to DSPS, treatable with late evening light,[57] but such treatment has not been extensively investigated. Light presented in the first part of the subjective night is known to elicit phase delays in the onset of nocturnal melatonin secretion[58] and the decline of body temperature,[59] which might induce later sleep onset. Although ASPS is not strictly age related, it is more prevalent among the elderly, whose early rise times are a common cause of concern.

> **CASE EXAMPLE 6: Phase Advance with Presleep Light**
>
> *The experience of a 38-year-old woman with lifetime history of ASPS[57] illustrates the potential use—and limitations—of evening light treatment. Patient K.W. was a mildly hypomanic high achiever, without seasonal pattern, who typically fell asleep at about 9:00 PM, and woke up between 2 and 4 AM, a pattern that led to marital stress. She could remain awake for occasional late-evening engagements, compensating with delayed time of arising at 5 to 6 AM. At baseline, she showed an early melatonin onset, at about 7:45 PM (Fig.121–3). Light exposure for up to 2 hours beginning at 8 PM hardly affected sleep phase or melatonin onset, whereas light exposure beginning at 9 PM succeeded in maintaining sleep onset at about 11 PM and wake-up between 4 and 5 AM, accompanied by a 1-hour delay in melatonin onset.*

Campbell et al.[60] compared the effects of evening bright light exposure (more than 4000 lux for 2 hours) with a dim red light control in elderly subjects with histories of sleep maintenance insomnia. The bright light group showed improved sleep efficiency; after 12 days of treatment, nighttime wakefulness decreased by about 1 hour. Despite this benefit, most subjects were reluctant to continue treatment given the long exposure sessions and glare discomfort.

These drawbacks might be corrected with shorter exposures to higher intensity light with the use of an apparatus that minimizes short-wavelength blue glare (see Apparatus), which is exacerbated in elderly people due to normal clouding of the lens and ocular media.

Seasonal Affective Disorder

Patients with SAD experience annually recurrent mood disturbance often accompanied by an increased appetite for carbohydrates, weight gain, daytime fatigue and loss of concentration, anxiety, and increased sleep duration. The appetitive and sleep symptoms are considered atypical, in contrast with the poor appetite, weight loss, and late insomnia seen in melancholic depression. For a set of diagnostic and clinical assessment instruments, see Resources and the discussion in Terman et al.[61]

Most light therapy studies have focused on parameters that influence treatment response, such as time of day, duration of exposure, intensity, and wavelength. The original regimen tested at the National Institute of Mental Health used 2500-lux

K.W., ♀ 38 YR, BEG 30 NOV 86 (C.M. Singer, pers. comm.)

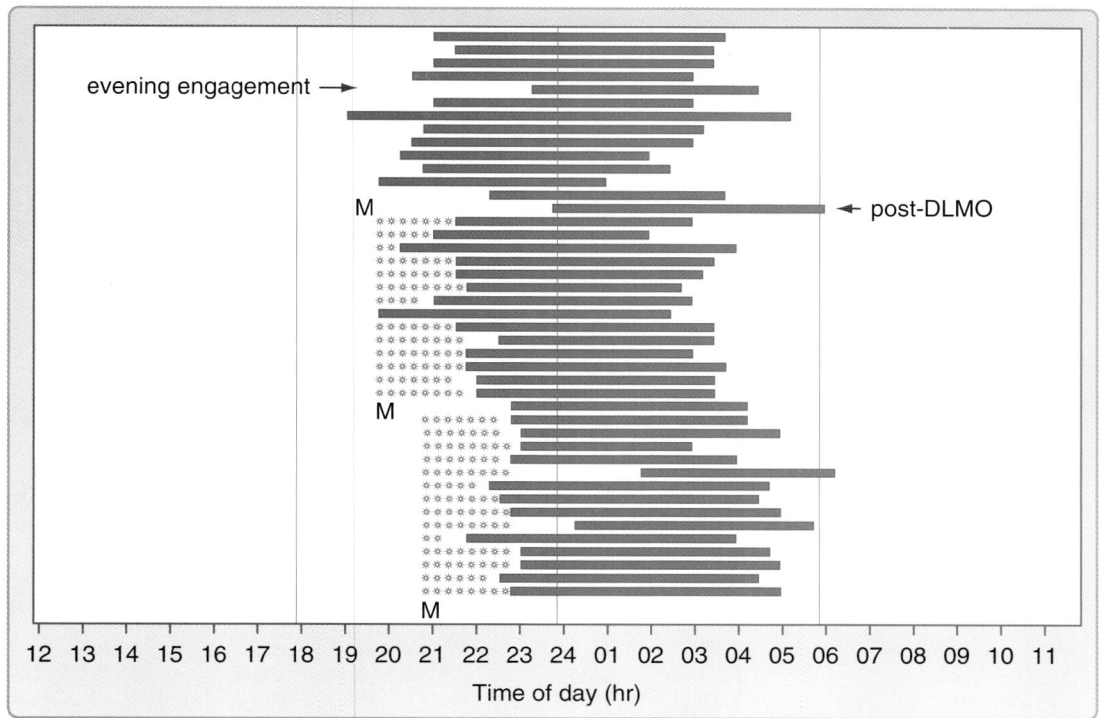

Figure 121–3. Self-report sleep record for a patient with advanced sleep phase disorder. *Bars* indicate intervals of sleep (including naps); *Sun symbols* indicate 15-minute segments of bright light exposure; M indicates the phase of dim light melatonin onset (DLMO), as determined on nights when treatment was omitted.

fluorescent illumination in 3-hour sessions in the morning and the evening.[26] A cross-center analysis of more than 25 studies that included 332 patients[62] summarized the results for dual daily sessions at 2500 lux for 2 hours; single morning, midday, and evening sessions; brief sessions (30 minutes); and lower light intensity (less than 500 lux). One week of morning bright light treatment produced a significantly higher remission rate (53%) than did evening (38%) or midday (32%) treatment. Dual daily sessions provided no benefit over morning light alone. All three bright light regimens were more effective than the dim light control; only morning (or morning plus evening) light was superior to the brief light control.

Two subsequent studies increased light intensity to 10,000 lux in 30- to 40-minute exposure sessions, with remission rates of approximately 75%, matching the most successful 2500-lux, 2-hour studies.[37,63] At these short durations, both dim light (400 lux) and lower-level bright light (3000 lux) were significantly less effective.

Until recently, individual studies of light therapy with standard fluorescent light boxes were limited by small sample sizes and did not consistently demonstrate time-of-day effects. The lack of convincing placebo controls led to controversy about whether improvement reflected the specific action of light. These problems have been successfully addressed in a set of three large clinical trials (for a summary, see Table 121–2).[38-40]

Eastman's group[39] administered light in the morning or evening, and an inert placebo (inactive negative ion generator), to parallel groups. Although all groups showed progressive

Table 121–2. Summary of Remission Rates in Controlled Clinical Trials of Bright Light Therapy for Seasonal Affective Disorder

	Remission Rate* (%/No. of Patients)		
Negative Ion Generator	**Morning Light**	**Evening Light**	**Placebo**
Terman et al.[38†]			
First treatment	54 (25/46)	33 (13/39)	11 (2/19)
Crossover	60 (28/47)	30 (14/47)	ND
Eastman et al.[39‡]			
First treatment	55 (18/33)	28 (9/32)	16 (5/31)
Lewy et al.[40§]			
First treatment	22 (6/27)	4 (1/24)	ND
Crossover	27 (14/51)	4 (2/51)	ND

From Wirz-Justice A. Beginning to see the light. Arch Gen Psychiatry 1998;55:861–862. Copyright 1998, American Medical Association.

*Baseline-to-posttreatment score reduction of ≥50%, with final score ≤8, on the Structured Interview for the Hamilton Depression Scale–Seasonal Affective Disorder Version (SIGH-SAD).

†6-year study; 10,000 lux for 0.5 h, 2 weeks.

‡6-year study; 6000 lux for 1.5 h, 4 weeks.

§4-year study; 2500 lux for 2 h, 2 weeks.

ND, not done

improvement over 4 weeks, patients administered morning light were most likely to show remissions, exceeding the placebo rate. Lewy's group[40] conducted a crossover study of morning and evening light. Although there was no placebo control, morning light proved to be more effective than evening light. Terman's group[38] performed both crossover and balanced parallel-group comparisons, which included nonphotic control groups that received negative air ions at a low or high concentration. Morning light produced a higher remission rate than evening light and the putative placebo, low-density ions. However, the response to evening light also exceeded that for placebo. Indeed, in the trials of both Lewy's group[40] and Terman's group,[38] a minority of patients responded preferentially to evening light.

Figure 121–4 presents sleep and light exposure logs for three patients who received 10,000-lux light treatment in 30-minute sessions. Treatment schedules were determined according to reported sleep habits and daytime commitments. The patients were urged to maintain consistent sleep times whether on or off treatment, waking up shortly before the time planned for morning treatment and keeping free a block of time for evening treatment at least 2 hours before bedtime. However, the patients often showed variations in sleep pattern that depended on the time of treatment (morning or evening), treatment response, and washout periods.

CASE EXAMPLE 7: Selective Antidepressant Response to Morning Light

Patient S.H. (see Fig. 121–4A) was depressed at baseline, showed middle insomnia, and overslept on weekends. During the course of evening light treatment, sleep onset was gradually delayed, with reduced insomnia, but she remained depressed. In contrast, under morning light treatment, sleep onset returned to the baseline pattern and sleep interruptions were largely eliminated, but sleep onset became earlier and duration became longer. Nevertheless, the depression remitted.

CASE EXAMPLE 8: Selective Antidepressant Response to Morning Light

Patient A.R. (see Fig. 121–4B), although depressed at baseline, showed fragmented sleep including napping, with highly variable total sleep duration. Under morning light, napping was eliminated, and although there was some late insomnia, the depression remitted. Under evening light—which failed clinically—sleep duration increased without a marked delay in sleep onset, and there were interruptions during the second half of sleep.

S.H., ♀ 37 YR, BEG 4 NOV 88

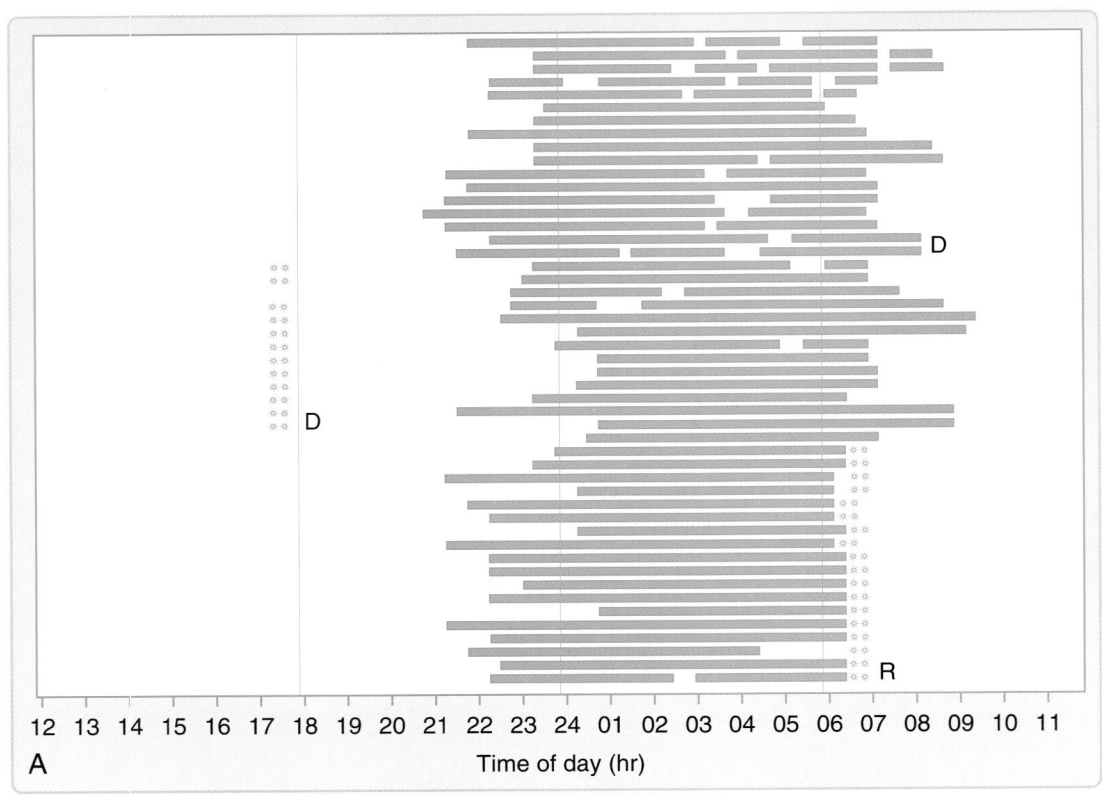

Figure 121–4. Self-report sleep records for three patients with winter depression, during baseline, light treatment, and withdrawal periods, for patients S.H. (**A**), A.R. (**B**), and D.F. (**C**). *Bars* indicate intervals of sleep (including naps); *sun symbols* indicate 15-min segments of bright light exposure. Clinical state is noted at the end of each period. *D*, depressed; *R*, responded (for quantitative criteria, see Terman et al.[58]).   *Continued*

A.R., ♀ 43 YR, BEG 2 FEB 89

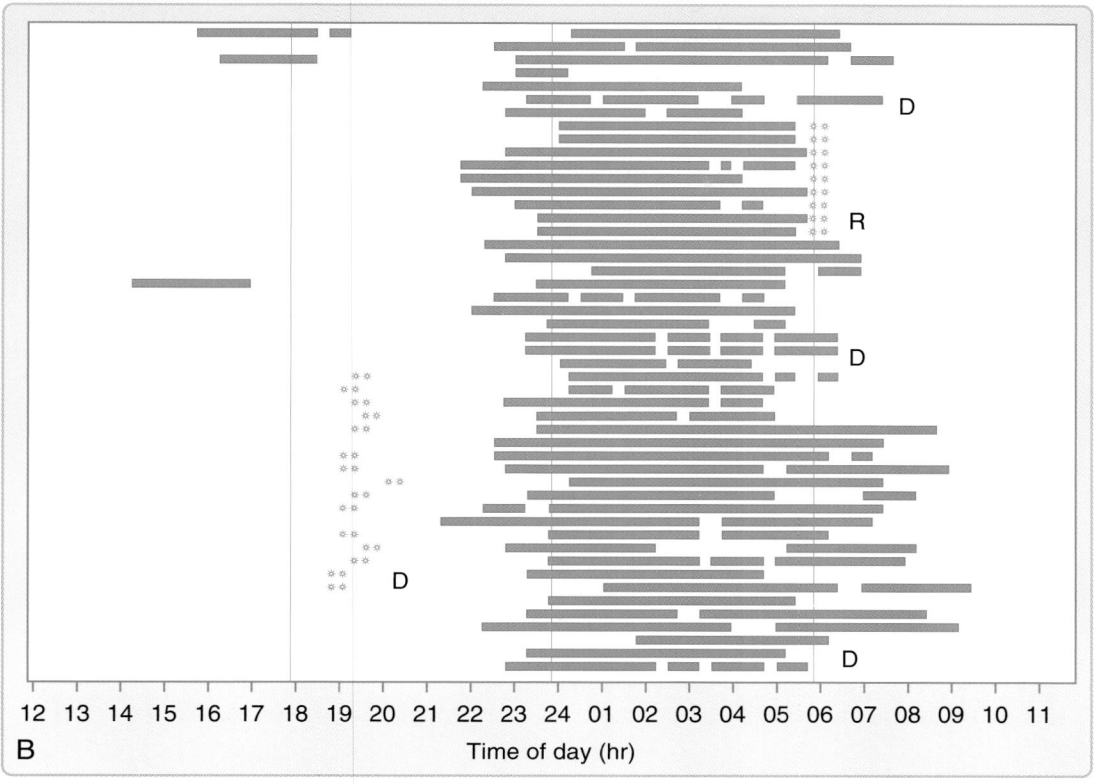

Figure 121–4. Cont'd.

CASE EXAMPLE 9: Nondifferential Antidepressant Response to Morning and Evening Light

Patient D.F. (see Fig. 121–4C) was monitored only briefly at baseline but reported consistent hypersomnia (subsequently also observed during washout phases) and agreed to attempt a 10:30 PM to 7:30 AM sleep schedule. Under evening light, tested twice, both sleep onset and time of arising were delayed relative to target, but sleep did not overshoot 9:30 AM. On both trials of evening light, the depression remitted. Over two washouts, sleep duration gradually increased, with relapse of depressive symptoms. Under morning light—which also was successful—the patient succeeded in advancing his wake-up time by several hours and was able to fall asleep, on target, at 10:30 PM, for modestly reduced sleep duration of 9 hours. Even though treatment was effective at both times of day, the patient preferred morning because of increased opportunity for activities given the earlier time of arising.

In summary, a lack of clinical response to evening light (patients S.H. and A.R.) appears to be correlated with delayed sleep onset, time of arising relative to baseline, or both. Morning light, which was uniformly effective, served to truncate morning sleep; in some cases, sleep onset also advanced,

conserving sleep duration, whereas in others, duration decreased only modestly. Although baseline patterns of interrupted sleep often disappeared under effective treatment, initial, middle, or late insomnia sometimes emerged during treatment. These symptoms may be signs of light overdose that can be eliminated by reducing light intensity or duration (see Side Effects of Exposure to Bright Light) or by scheduling evening sessions earlier or morning sessions later.

Subsyndromal Seasonal Affective Disorder

The phenomenology of subsyndromal SAD, or winter doldrums, is similar to that of SAD, although major depression is absent. However, the presence and severity of atypical neurovegetative symptoms (including food cravings and difficulty awakening) can be similar to those in SAD, as can fatigability (leading to characterization as a seasonal anergic syndrome).[64] Clinical trials have demonstrated significant improvement with bright light therapy,[65] as well as dawn simulation therapy,[66] for subsyndromal SAD. For bright light, optimum light scheduling and dose appear to be similar for subsyndromal SAD and SAD; in other words, the lower severity of depressed mood does not imply that a lower light dose will be sufficient to relieve symptoms.

D.F., ♂ 28 YR, BEG 2 FEB 90

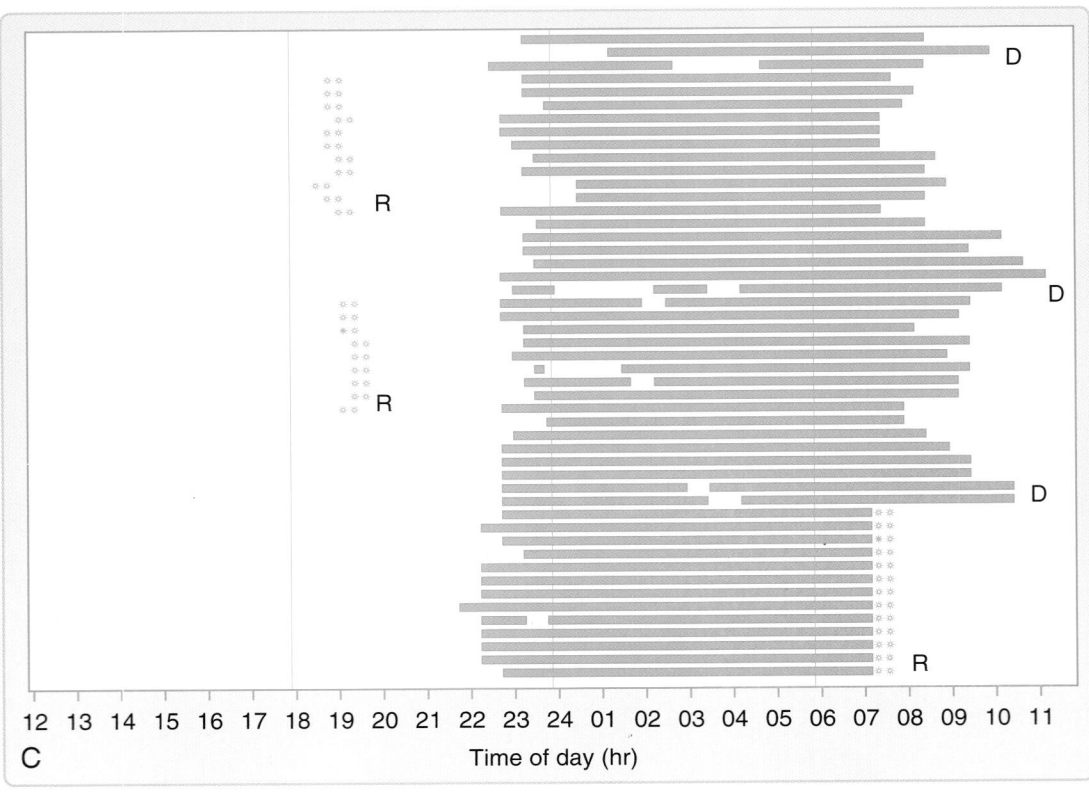

Figure 121–4. Cont'd.

FURTHER APPLICATIONS OF LIGHT THERAPY

Nonseasonal Depression

Beyond its established application for SAD, light therapy for nonseasonal depression appears both safe and effective. Kripke[67] compared several controlled trials in terms of the relative benefit of light versus placebo, and with light for as little as 1 week the results fell within the range of classic antidepressant drug studies of 4-16 weeks.

For example, a Japanese study of nonseasonal major depression gave 7 days of light therapy to 27 subjects, admitted as inpatients for the study, and obtained a benefit of 24% over a dim light placebo.[68] However, morning or evening exposure times showed no difference, nor did phase shifts of body temperature relate to clinical improvement. Goel and colleagues[69] gave 5 weeks of morning bright light therapy (10,000 lux, 60 minutes) to outpatients with chronic major depression lasting 2 years or longer. The study subjects experienced a remission rate of 50%; a control group given low-density negative air ionization showed only minor improvement. Using a ceiling-light installation at 3000-4000 lux, a 10-day open-label trial with 28 nonmedicated hospitalized patients in Switzerland resulted in depression rating scale improvement greater than 50% in 17 cases.[70]

Several investigators have combined light with drugs and found accelerated improvement relative to drugs alone (for an early review, see Kasper et al.[71]) and the method already has seen widespread use with European hospital patients.[71a] One such study demonstrated benefit among hospitalized patients with either unipolar or bipolar depression who were given 10,000-lux illumination in 30-minute morning sessions, with less improvement at 2500 lux.[72] In Denmark, a large-scale outpatient trial has combined 10,000-lux or 50-lux light therapy with standard sertraline medication.[73] Both remission rate and speed of improvement were greater under the active light condition.

Another study combined light with drugs and a single session of late-night sleep deprivation[74] ("wake therapy") at the start of treatment and achieved marked improvement in 1 day and benefit over a dim light control within 1 week.[75] In Italy, this model has been extended for general inpatient use, following treatment studies of nonseasonal major depression (in conjunction with citalopram medication)[48] and bipolar disorder (in conjunction with lithium)[76] that showed large benefits attributable to morning light exposure. Combined light and wake therapy can be feasibly self-administered at home. One controlled study yielded a remission rate of 43% in a group for whom standard antidepressants and psychotherapy had been deemed inadequate.[77] The recent successful completion of large-scale trials in Europe strongly supports the implementation of adjuvant light and wake therapy for treatment of major depression, with the prospect of reduced duration of hospitalization (F. Benedetti, personal communication).

Antepartum and Premenstrual Depression

Both open-label[78] and controlled[79] studies have successfully employed light therapy for major depression during pregnancy, which offers a safe somatic treatment alternative to antidepressant drugs whether or not the woman has a history of seasonality. Both efficacy and side effects have been shown to be dose-dependent.[79] For example, a nonresponder to 60 minutes of 7000-lux light administered upon awakening for 5 weeks showed full remission when session duration was increased to 75 minutes. A responder who developed irritable hypomania under the same initial treatment conditions became depressed when duration was reduced to 45 minutes but responded without hypomania when duration was increased to 50 minutes.

Although larger-scale, definitive trials are needed, morning light therapy is a viable option for open treatment of antepartum depression. Patients with both seasonal and nonseasonal premenstrual dysphoric disorder (PMDD) or milder premenstrual syndrome (PMS) have responded favorably to 1 week of bright light therapy (2500 lux for 2 hours) during the luteal phase, in a series of clinical trials by Parry and colleagues.[80] A placebo-controlled crossover study showed no difference between morning and evening exposures in 1-month trials, however.[81] Furthermore, bright and dim light had similar effects. By contrast, a 2-month study by Lam and coworkers[82] using 10,000-lux, 30-minute evening light during the luteal phase found significant improvement relative to a dim light control, with alleviation of both depressed mood and physical symptoms. Although larger controlled trials are needed and the relative advantage of morning light awaits investigation, Lam's method is a viable option for the open treatment of PMDD and PMS, especially for women who have not responded to medication.

Bulimia Nervosa

Lam and coworkers[83] became interested in this potential application of light therapy when a seasonal mood pattern was noted in many patients with bulimia; beyond the spectrum of SAD symptoms, this included binge eating and purging. In a 2-week crossover study, they showed a marked superiority of morning bright light therapy (30 minutes, 10,000 lux) over dim light, for both mood and bulimic symptoms. Furthermore, a 4-week open-treatment study yielded average reductions of 46% in binge eating and 36% in purging, along with 56% reduction in depression scale scores.[84]

In a placebo-controlled, parallel group study of morning light therapy during the winter months, Braun and colleagues[85] also obtained greater reductions in bingeing and purging under bright light than under a dim-light placebo. Interestingly, their patients did not have comorbid SAD, and mood improvement was unrelated to light intensity. The data thus augur well for the use of light therapy in seasonal bulimia with or without SAD.

Senile Dementia

Numerous small studies have found that symptoms of night wandering, sundowning, and daytime sleep are responsive to bright light therapy. Hospital trials in Japan indicated benefits of morning treatment over 1 month or longer,[86] and evening light exposure also succeeded in reducing disruptive nighttime activity.[87] A further trial of 27 patients ascertained significant increases in actigraphic sleep efficiency, with decreased number of awakenings and daytime napping; there was also a small improvement in cognitive state, although dementia ratings did not change.[88]

In another study, Dutch investigators installed diffuse indirect bright light tested for 2-week intervals in the hospital living quarters of demented patients.[89] Those without severe visual deficit showed significant reductions in day-to-day variability of the rest-activity rhythm (measured by actigraphy), whereas visually impaired patients showed no effect. For long-term management, such whole-room illumination may be more feasible than light boxes for patients with dementia, since light boxes require a stationary posture and direction of gaze. A further possibility is dusk-to-dawn simulation: When administered for 3 weeks at the bedside, it yielded trend improvements in sleep-onset latency, sleep duration, and nocturnal activity.[90]

In a crossover study of bright versus dim morning light therapy given for 4 weeks to patients with agitation, the active treatment selectively increased total nighttime sleep by nearly 2 hours, although agitation failed to improve.[91] Mishima et al.[92] distinguished patients with Alzheimer's-type from those with vascular dementia. After 2 weeks of morning bright light therapy, significant reduction in nocturnal activity was limited to the latter group, while neither group responded to dim light. A recent Norwegian 2-week open-label trial of 2-hour morning bright light exposure achieved the most dramatic improvement thus far.[93] Eleven patients with baseline actigraphic sleep efficiency averaging 73% improved to 86% within 2 weeks and nocturnal wake time reduced by 2 hours. Remarkably, post-treatment benefits lasted one month or longer.

All these very promising leads must be tempered by the results of the largest controlled trials to date, by Ancoli-Israel's group in San Diego. In one trial of 72 demented nursing home patients, separate groups received morning or evening bright light (2 hours, 2500 lux) or evening dim red light (<50 lux) for 10 days.[94] Actigraphic analyses found no improvement in nighttime sleep or daytime activity, even though morning light affected circadian rhythm parameters. A second trial of 92 patients with agitated behavior compared morning or evening bright light or morning dim red light (<300 lux).[95] Raters could not detect improvement in agitation under any condition, even though morning light phase-shifted the daily cycle of agitated behavior.

In summary, although we are impressed by the research activity in this very difficult area, the key to effective treatment has been elusive. Factors of diagnostic heterogeneity, stage and severity of disease, circadian system status, ocular status, optimal timing of light treatment, and exposure parameters and duration of treatment still need to be sorted out.[95a]

Shift Work Adjustment

Most research has focused on laboratory simulation studies in which sleep patterns and circadian measures can be closely monitored, work assignments can be kept simple and constant, and the interferences of family obligations and distractions can be minimized.[96] There have been few field tests, although bright light exposure regimens have been developed to phase shift circadian rhythms into synchrony with shift work schedules, either as a preparatory measure,[97] during the shift itself,[98] or both.[98a]

Eastman's group has pioneered simulation protocols that accelerate circadian phase delays by carefully timed light exposure in combination with light restriction, using filtered lenses during the morning commute home and when outdoors and fully darkened bedrooms during daytime sleep.[99] This combination of interventions, they have shown, specifically benefits subjects with relatively early baseline circadian phase, for whom the phase delay presents the greatest challenge.[100] The model has been successfully applied to night-shift nurses, who have shown increased alertness,[100a] and achieved virtually complete reentrainment given bright nighttime light exposure timed for phase delays.[101] However, performance benefits have not yet been demonstrated.

The feasibility of these approaches for industrial shift workers has been questioned. The attempted reentrainment can be incompatible with standard rapid rotation schedules, further exacerbating worker distress. Additionally, most shift workers choose to revert to a normal schedule on days off, which jeopardizes their workweek adjustment with incompatible patterns of light exposure. Potential adverse long-term consequences of repeated shifts under lighting protocols have not been evaluated.

Even with complete reentrainment, it has not been demonstrated that night-shift performance is significantly enhanced. After one early field test in which the lighting regimen succeeded in suppressing nocturnal melatonin, shifting rhythms, and increasing subjective alertness, most workers recommended against continuing the protocol.[102] A major complaint was difficulty readapting to their daytime routine. A North Sea oil platform trial successfully addressed this problem by using light to reentrain workers after they returned home; however, the treatment did not benefit initial adaptation to the night shift.[103]

A priority is to demonstrate that light-guided phase shifting does in fact enhance night shift performance. If it does, the procedure might be acceptably imposed on workers in critical occupations (hospital, military, power station), whether or not it is subjectively favored. An alternative approach would be to increase nighttime illumination only moderately, without imposing large circadian phase shifts.[96,104]

Jet Lag Adjustment

Although laboratory simulation paradigms for jet lag and shift work adjustment correspond closely, in the field, geographic relocation has the advantage of establishing a new, consistent light-dark cycle without competing day-night cues.[96] However, jet lag is also compounded by travel stresses (e.g., in-flight sleep disruption) beyond circadian phase displacement. Timing recommendations for natural and artificial bright light exposure (and light avoidance), which vary with direction and distance of travel, have been generated to accelerate circadian rhythm reentrainment based on properties of the phase response curve.[105,106] Although there have been anecdotal successes with such strategies, both laboratory and field trials have had equivocal success (for a review, see Samel and Wegmann[107]).

One positive lead comes from a polysomnographic study of four subjects before and after a Tokyo-to-San Francisco flight.[108] Two of them, who received 3 hours of bright light at 11 AM (3 AM Tokyo time) for 3 days after arrival, showed enhanced sleep efficiency compared with the other two, who received dim light.

In a Zurich-to-New York trial, Boulos and coworkers[7] provided 20 subjects with a bright or dim head-mounted unit on the first two evenings after arrival. The bright-light group showed significantly larger phase delays in melatonin onset, but behavioral indices of jet leg, including actigraphic sleep efficiency, showed little benefit. At this writing, Boulos's group is proceeding with a bidirectional trial, New York-to-Zurich-to-New York, using an enhanced head-mounted device for within-subject ascertainment of both eastward and westward jet lag adjustment.

OFFICIAL RECOMMENDATIONS AND GUIDELINES

Society for Light Treatment and Biological Rhythms

The Society for Light Treatment and Biological Rhythms (SLTBR) was the first organization to conduct a consensus-building process for clinical applications of light therapy and safety issues, with recommendations published in 1991.[109] Clinical trials completed by that time had already demonstrated efficacy for SAD and probable efficacy for subsyndromal SAD. Furthermore, the report cited "ample evidence that light can advance, delay, and entrain human circadian rhythms" (p. 47)[109] based on timing of exposure according to human phase-response curves. Basic safety standards for light-therapy devices were outlined, including control of thermal and short wavelength radiation (ultraviolet and blue) through appropriate choice of lamp and filtering and evaluation of patients' oculoretinal status.

U.S. Public Health Service Agency for Health Care Policy and Research

In 1990, the Depression Guidelines Panel of the U.S. Public Health Service Agency for Health Care Policy and Research (now, Agency for Health Care Research and Quality) commissioned a critical review of clinical trials of light therapy,[110] and in 1993 the panel issued guidelines for the treatment of SAD in primary care practice. The guidelines include the treatment for subsyndromal SAD: "Light therapy is a treatment consideration only for well-documented mild to moderate seasonal, nonpsychotic, winter depressive episodes in patients with recurrent depressive or bipolar II disorders or milder seasonal episodes" (p. 102).[111] The panel cautioned against unsupervised treatment: "It should be administered by a professional with experience and training in its use who deems it suitable for the particular patient" (p. 103).[111] The panel further noted that "light therapy can be useful to augment the response (if partial) to antidepressant medication and vice versa" (p. 103).[111]

American Psychiatric Association

In its 1993 clinical practice guidelines for major depressive disorder,[112] the American Psychiatric Association (APA) noted that "in some patients with [SAD], depressive manifestations respond to supplementation of environmental light by means of exposure to bright white artificial light" (p. 10). Possible side effects were listed, and the APA noted that "no adverse interactions between light therapy and pharmacotherapy have been identified" (but see Safety of Bright Light for the Eyes). In a 2003 meta-analysis of light therapy studies, the APA Committee on Research in Psychiatric Treatments concluded that "bright light treatment for SAD…and non-seasonal depression [appears] efficacious, with effect sizes equivalent to those found in most antidepressant trials."[113]

American Academy of Sleep Medicine

In 1993, the American Academy of Sleep Medicine (AASM; at that time, the American Sleep Disorders Association) and SLTBR jointly commissioned the Task Force on Light Treatment for Sleep Disorders. The task force published an extensive literature review and critique of the field in the Journal of Biological Rhythms[1] preparatory to review by the AASM Standards of Practice Committee. This committee conducted an evidence-based review of clinical trials of light therapy for the circadian sleep phase disorders, shift work and jet lag disturbances, dementia, and sleep complaints in the healthy elderly. (Guidelines for treatment of depression were deferred to the APA.) In 1999, the committee issued syndrome-specific guidelines, which concluded that "light therapy can be useful in treatment of DSPS and ASPS" (p. 641),[114] but they expressed less confidence in other applications. These guidelines have been incorporated by the National Guidelines Clearinghouse (www.guideline.gov), a collaboration of professional organizations, government agencies, and industry that includes the American Association of Health Plans.

Canadian Consensus Guidelines for the Understanding and Management of Seasonal Depression

Canadian specialists in SAD have published a thorough multicenter critical review (including evidence tables) of SAD diagnosis, epidemiology, pathophysiology, light treatment, medication management, and combination treatment.[115] Level 1 evidence from large, controlled trials was presented to justify recommending that the starting dose for light therapy with a fluorescent light box is 10,000 lux for 30 minutes a day; light boxes should use white, fluorescent light with the UV wavelengths filtered out; and light therapy should be started in the early morning, on awakening, to maximize treatment response.

Cochrane Collaboration

In a 2004 review of 49 randomized, controlled trials of light therapy for nonseasonal depression—most of which applied light as an adjuvant to drug treatment, wake therapy, or both—the reviewers concluded that light therapy "offers modest though promising antidepressive efficacy, especially when administered during the first week of treatment, in the morning, and as an adjunctive treatment to sleep deprivation responders. Hypomania as a potential adverse effect needs to be considered. Due to limited data and heterogeneity of studies these results need to be interpreted with caution" (p. 1).[116]

U.S. Food and Drug Administration

Despite the emerging professional consensus, the U.S. Food and Drug Administration (FDA) has not yet approved (or disapproved) light therapy for SAD or for other conditions, in part because the commercial community has yet to file applications for premarket approval. However, the agency intermittently continues to require that individual manufacturers of light therapy apparatuses cease sales and modify advertising copy that contains explicit or implicit medical claims.

The lack of FDA approval has discouraged third-party reimbursement, which, in turn, has limited the number of prospective patients and served to encourage self-treatment by consumers who obtain apparatuses on the open market. (In 1997, the Swiss Federal Department of the Interior mandated insurance reimbursement for light boxes used to treat SAD, although not for other therapeutic applications.[117])

Because regulatory standards have not been issued in the United States, there has been a proliferation of untested commercial products on the market. Some of these products explicitly violate consensus recommendations of the SLTBR, such as lack of lamp protection and UV shielding. There have been several unofficial attempts to promulgate safety standards and advise consumers and physicians (Consumer Reports on Health,[118] SLTBR,[109] and the Center for Environmental Therapeutics; see Resources), but these have had far less impact than marketing initiatives, some of which even have appeared under the guise of "medical education." The development of federal standards remains a priority.

RESOURCES

Tilted, 10,000-lux light boxes with polycarbonate UV filter diffusers are distributed by the nonprofit Center for Environmental Therapeutics (www.cet.org). Short-wavelength protective fit-over wrap-around lenses (product L-58, U-58, or S-58) are distributed by NoIR Medical Technologies, Inc. (www.noir-medical.com).

The *Columbia Eye Examination for Users of Light Treatment* (a structured chart for optometrists and ophthalmologists) and a set of questionnaires and structured interview guides for depressive disorders, written and tested by the Columbia group, is included in the Clinical Assessment Tools Packet distributed by the Center for Environmental Therapeutics. The website also includes an Ask the Doctor forum and on-line assessments of morningness-eveningness chronotype, depression, and seasonality, with individualized feedback.

The Society for Light Treatment and Biological Rhythms (www.sltbr.org) offers a continuing medical education course associated with its annual scientific meeting and hosts a lively listserv for members.

Clinical Pearl

Appropriately timed artificial light exposure can correct sleep-phase maladjustment and counteract seasonal and nonseasonal depression. The clinician's tasks are to determine the interval of the individual patient's "subjective night" and to schedule light at its end for phase advances or at its beginning for phase delays.

Acknowledgments

Preparation of this chapter and the authors' related research was supported in part by National Institute of Mental Health Grant MH42931.

REFERENCES

1. Terman M (ed): Task force report on light treatment for sleep disorders. J Biol Rhythms 1995;10:101-176.
2. Glickman G, Hanifin JP, Rollag MD, et al: Inferior retinal light exposure is more effective than superior retinal exposure in suppressing melatonin in humans. J Biol Rhythms 2003;18:71-79.
3. Joffe RT, Moul DE, Lam RW, et al: Light visor treatment for seasonal affective disorder: A multicenter study. Psychiatry Res 1993;46:29-39.
4. Rosenthal NE, Moul DE, Hellekson CJ, et al: A multicenter study of the light visor for seasonal affective disorder: No difference in efficacy found between two different intensities. Neuropsychopharmacology 1993;8:151-160.
5. Teicher MH, Glod CA, Oren DA, et al: The phototherapy light visor: More to it than meets the eye. Am J Psychiatry 1995; 152:1197-1202.
6. Terman M: Clinical efficacy of the light visor, and its broader implications. Light Treatment Biol Rhythms 1991;3:37-40.
7. Boulos Z, Macchi MM, Stürchler MP, et al: Light visor treatment for jet lag after westward travel across six time zones. Aviation Space Environ Med 2002;73:953-963.
8. Terman M, Schlager D, Fairhurst S, et al: Dawn and dusk simulation as a therapeutic intervention. Biol Psychiatry 1989;25:966-970.
9. Terman M, Schlager DS: Twilight therapeutics, winter depression, melatonin, and sleep. In Montplaisir J, Godbout R (eds): Sleep and Biological Rhythms. New York, Oxford University Press, 1990, pp 113-128.
10. Terman M: Light on sleep. In Schwartz WJ (ed): Sleep Science: Integrating Basic Research and Clinical Practice. Basel, Karger, 1997, pp 229-249.
11. Danilenko KV, Wirz-Justice A, Kräuchi K, et al: The human circadian pacemaker can see by the dawn's earlylight. J Biol Rhythms 2000;15:437-446.
12. Avery DH, Eder DN, Bolte MA, et al: Dawn simulation and bright light in the treatment of SAD: A controlled study. Biol Psychiatry 2001;50:205-216.
13. Gallin PF, Terman M, Remé CE, et al: Ophthalmologic examination of patients with seasonal affective disorder, before and after bright light therapy. Am J Ophthalmol 1995;119:202-210.
14. Okudaira N, Kripke DF, Webster JB: Naturalistic studies of human light exposure. Am J Physiol 1983;245:R613-R615.
15. Terman M: Research problems and prospects for the use of light as a therapeutic intervention. In Wetterberg L (ed): Biological Rhythms and Light in Man. Oxford, Pergamon Press, 1993, 421-436.
16. Remé CE, Williams TP, Rol P, et al: Blue-light damage revisited: Abundant retinal apoptosis after blue-light exposure, little after green. Invest Ophthalm Vis Sci 1998;39:S128.
17. Bynoe LA, Del Priore LV, Hornbeck R: Photosensitization of retinal pigment epithelium by protoporphyrin IX. Graefe's Arch Clin Exp Ophthalm 1998;236:230-233.
18. Remé CE, Wenzel A, Grimm C, et al: Mechanisms of blue-light induced retinal degeneration and the potential relevance for age-related macular degeneration and inherited retinal diseases. Chronobiol Int 2003;20:1186-1187.
19. Remé CE, Rol P, Grothmann K, et al: Bright light therapy in focus: Lamp emission spectra and ocular safety. Technol Health Care 1996;4:403-413.
20. Brainard GC, Hanifin JP, Greeson JM, et al: Action spectrum for melatonin regulation in humans: Evidence for a novel circadian photoreceptor. J Neurosci 2001;21:6405-6412.
21. Wright HR, Lack LC, Kennaway DJ: Differential effects of light wavelength in phase advancing the melatonin rhythm. J Pineal Res 2004;36:140-144.
22. Terman M, Remé CE, Rafferty B, et al: Bright light therapy for winter depression: Potential ocular effects and theoretical implications. Photochem Photobiol 1990;51:781-792.
23. Gallenga P, Lobefalo L, Mastropasqua L, et al: Photic maculopathy in a patient receiving bright light therapy. Am J Psychiatry 1997; 154:1319.
24. Zigman S: Vision enhancement using a short wavelength light-absorbing filter. Optom Vis Sci 1990;67:100-104.
25. Gallin PF, Terman M, Remé CE, et al: The Columbia Eye Examination for Users of Light Treatment. New York, New York State Psychiatric Institute, 1993.
26. Rosenthal NE, Sack DA, Gillin JC, et al: Seasonal affective disorder: A description of the syndrome and preliminary findings with light therapy. Arch Gen Psychiatry 1984;41:72-80.
27. Wirz-Justice A, Bucheli C, Graw P: Light treatment of seasonal affective disorder in Switzerland. Acta Psychiatr Scand 1986; 74:193-204.
28. Levitt AJ, Joffe RT, Moul DE, et al: Side effects of light therapy in seasonal affective disorder. Am J Psychiatry 1993;150: 650-652.
29. Schwitzer J, Neudorfer C, Blecha H-G, et al: Mania as a side effect of phototherapy. Biol Psychiatry 1990;28:532-534.
30. Kripke DF: Timing of phototherapy and occurrence of mania. Biol Psychiatry 1991;29:1156-1157.
31. Meesters Y, Van Houwelingen C: Rapid mood swings after unmonitored light exposure. Am J Psychiatry 1998;155:306.
32. Chan PK, Lam RW, Perry KF: Mania precipitated by light therapy for patients with SAD. J Clin Psychiatry 1994;55:454.
33. Praschak-Rider N, Neumeister A, Hesselmann B, et al: Suicidal tendencies as a complication of light therapy for seasonal affective disorder: A report of three cases. J Clin Psychiatry 1997; 58:389-392.
34. Labbate LA, Lafer B, Thibault A, et al: Side effects induced by bright light treatment for seasonal affective disorder. J Clin Psychiatry 1994;55:189-191.
35. National Institute of Mental Health: Systematic Assessment for Treatment Emergent Effects (SAFTEE). Rockville, Md, National Institute of Mental Health, 1986.
36. Terman M, Terman JS: Bright light therapy: Side effects and benefits across the symptom spectrum. J Clin Psychiatry 1999; 60:799-808.
37. Terman JS, Terman M, Schlager DS, et al: Efficacy of brief, intense light exposure for treatment of winter depression. Psychopharmacol Bull 1990;26:3-11.
38. Terman M, Terman JS, Ross DC: A controlled trial of timed bright light and negative air ionization for treatment of winter depression. Arch Gen Psychiatry 1998;55:875-882.
39. Eastman CI, Young MA, Fogg LF, et al: Bright light treatment for winter depression: A placebo-controlled trial. Arch Gen Psychiatry 1998;55:883-889.
40. Lewy AJ, Bauer VK, Cutler NL, et al: Morning vs evening light treatment of patients with winter depression. Arch Gen Psychiatry 1998;55:890-896.
41. Lewy AJ, Sack RL, Miller S, et al: Antidepressant and circadian phase-shifting effects of light. Science 1987;235:352-354.
42. Terman M: On the specific action and clinical domain of light treatment. In Lam RW (ed): Seasonal Affective Disorder and Beyond: Light Treatment for SAD and Non-SAD Conditions. Washington, DC, American Psychiatric Press, 1998, pp 91-115.
43. Terman JS, Terman M, Lo ES: Circadian time of morning light administration and therapeutic response in winter depression. Arch Gen Psychiatry 2001;58:69-75.
44. Weber JM, Schwander JC, Unger I, et al: A direct ultrasensitive RIA for the determination of melatonin in human saliva: Comparison with serum levels. Sleep Res 1997;26:757.
45. Horne JA, Östberg O: A self-assessment questionnaire to determine morningness-eveningness in human circadian rhythms. Int J Chronobiol 1976;4:97-110.
46. Terman M, Terman JS: Morningness-eveningness, circadian phase and the timing of sleep in patients with seasonal affective disorder. Soc Light Treatment Biol Rhythms Abst 2001;13:26.

47. Terman M, White TM, Jacobs J: Automated Morningness-Eveningness Questionnaire. New York, New York State Psychiatric Institute, 2002, www.cet.org/AutoMEQ.

48. Benedetti F, Colombo C, Pontiggia A, et al: Morning light treatment hastens the antidepressant effect of citalopram: A placebo-controlled trial. J Clin Psychiatry 2003;64:648-653.

49. Terman M, Lewy AJ, Dijk D-J, et al: Light treatment for sleep disorders: Consensus report, IV: Sleep phase and duration disturbances. J Biol Rhythms 1995;10:135-147.

50. Czeisler CA, Richardson GS, Coleman RM, et al: Chronotherapy: Resetting the circadian clocks of patients with delayed sleep phase insomnia. Sleep 1981;4:1-21.

51. Rosenthal NE, Joseph-Vanderpool JR, Levendosky AA, et al: Phase-shifting effects of bright morning light as treatment for delayed sleep phase syndrome. Sleep 1990;13:354-361.

52. Eastman CI, Stewart KT, Mahoney MP, et al: Dark goggles and bright light improve circadian rhythm adaptation to night-shift work. Sleep 1994;17:535-543.

53. Cole RJ, Smith JS, Alcalà YC, et al: Bright-light mask treatment of delayed sleep phase syndrome. J Biol Rhythms 2002;17:89-101.

54. Kokkoris CP, Weitzman ED, Pollak CP, et al: Long-term ambulatory temperature monitoring in a subject with a hypernychthemeral sleep-wake disturbance. Sleep 1978;1:177-190.

55. Weitzman ED, Czeisler CA, Coleman RM, et al: Delayed sleep phase syndrome: A chronobiological disorder with sleep-onset insomnia. Arch Gen Psychiatry 1981;38:737-746.

56. Eastman CI, Anagnopoulos CA, Cartwright RD: Can bright light entrain a free-runner? Sleep Res 1988;17:372.

57. Singer CM, Lewy AJ: Case report: Use of the dim light melatonin onset in the treatment of ASPS with bright light. Sleep Res 1989;18:445.

58. Terman M, Terman JS, Rafferty B: Experimental design and measures of success in the treatment of winter depression by bright light. Psychopharmacol Bull 1990;26:505-510.

59. Czeisler CA, Allan JS, Strogatz SH, et al: Bright light resets the human circadian pacemaker independent of the sleep-wake cycle. Science 1986;233:667-671.

60. Campbell SS, Dawson D, Anderson M: Alleviation of sleep maintenance insomnia with timed exposure to bright light. J Am Geriatr Soc 1993;41:829-836.

61. Terman M, Terman JS, Williams JBW: Seasonal affective disorder and treatments. J Prac Psychiatry Behav Health 1998;5:287-303.

62. Terman M, Terman JS, Quitkin FM, et al: Bright light therapy for winter depression: A review of efficacy. Neuropsychopharmacology 1989;2:1-22.

63. Magnússon A, Kristbjarnarson H: Treatment of seasonal affective disorder with high-intensity light. J Affect Disord 1991;21:141-147.

64. Wirz-Justice A, Graw P, Bucheli C, et al: Seasonal affective disorder in Switzerland: A clinical perspective. In Thompson C, Silverstone T (eds): Seasonal Affective Disorder. London, CNS Clinical Neuroscience, 1989, pp 69-76.

65. Kasper S, Rogers S, Yancey A, et al: Phototherapy in individuals with and without seasonal affective disorder. Arch Gen Psychiatry 1989;46:837-844.

66. Avery DH, Norden MJ: Dawn simulation and bright light therapy in subsyndromal seasonal affective disorder. In Lam RW (ed): Seasonal Affective Disorder and Beyond: Light Treatment for SAD and Non-SAD Conditions. Washington, DC, American Psychiatric Press, 1998, pp 143-157.

67. Kripke DF: Light treatment for nonseasonal depression: Speed, efficacy, and combined treatment. J Affect Disord 1998;49:109-117.

68. Yamada N, Martin-Iverson MT, Daimon K, et al: Clinical and chronobiological effects of light therapy on nonseasonal affective disorders. Biol Psychiatry 1995;37:866-873.

69. Goel N, Terman JS, Macchi MM, et al: A placebo-controlled trial of light and negative ion treatment for chronic depression: Preliminary results. Chronobiol Int 2003;20:1207-1209.

70. Wirz-Justice A, Graw P, Röösli H, et al: An open trial of light therapy in hospitalised major depression. J Aff Disord 1999;52:291-292.

71. Kasper S, Ruhrmann S, Schuchardt H-M: The effects of light therapy in treatment indications other than seasonal affective disorder (SAD). In Jung EG, Holick MF (eds): Biologic Effects of Light. Berlin, de Gruyter, 1994, pp 206-218.

71a. Kaper S, Ruhrmann S, Neumann S, et al: Use of light therapy in German psychiatric hospitals. Eur Psychiatry 1994;9:288-292.

72. Beauchemin KM, Hays P: Phototherapy is a useful adjunct in the treatment of depressed inpatients. Acta Psychiatr Scand 1997;95:424-427.

73. Martiny K: Adjunctive bright light in non-seasonal major depression. Acta Psychiatr Scand Suppl 2004; 425:7-28.

74. Wirz-Justice A, van den Hoofdakker RH: Sleep deprivation in depression: What do we know, where do we go? Biol Psychiatry 1999;46:445-453.

75. Neumeister A, Goessler R, Lucht M, et al: Bright light therapy stabilizes the antidepressant effect of partial sleep deprivation. Biol Psychiatry 1996;39:16-21.

76. Colombo C, Lucca A, Benedetti F, et al: Total sleep deprivation combined with lithium and light therapy in the treatment of bipolar depression: Replication of main effects and interaction. Psychiatry Res 2000;95:43-53.

77. Loving RT, Kripke DF, Shuchter SR: Bright light augments antidepressant effects of medication and wake therapy. Depress Anx 2002;16:1-3.

78. Oren DA, Wisner KL, Spinelli M, et al: An open trial of morning light therapy for treatment of antepartum depression. Am J Psychiatry 2002;159:666-669.

79. Epperson CN, Terman M, Terman JS: Randomized clinical trial of bright light therapy for antepartum depression: preliminary findings. J Clin Psychiatry 2004;65:421-425.

80. Parry BL: Light therapy of premenstrual depression. In Lam RW (ed): Seasonal Affective Disorder and Beyond: Light Treatment for SAD and Non-SAD Conditions. Washington, DC, American Psychiatric Press, 1998, pp 173-191.

81. Parry BL, Mahan AM, Mostofi N, et al: Light therapy of late luteal phase dysphoric disorder: An extended study. Am J Psychiatry 1993;150:1417-1419.

82. Lam RW, Carter D, Misri S, et al: A controlled study of light therapy in women with late luteal phase dysphoric disorder. Psychiatry Res 1999;86:185-192.

83. Lam RW, Goldner EM: Seasonality of bulimia nervosa and treatment with light therapy. In Lam RW (ed): Seasonal Affective Disorder and Beyond: Light Treatment for SAD and Non-SAD Conditions. Washington, DC, American Psychiatric Press, 1998, pp 193-220.

84. Lam RW, Lee SK, Tam EM, et al: An open trial of light therapy for women with seasonal affective disorder and comorbid bulimia nervosa. J Clin Psychiatry 2001;62:164-168.

85. Braun DL, Sunday SR, Fornari VM, et al: Bright light therapy decreases winter binge frequency in women with bulimia nervosa: A double-blind, placebo-controlled study. Comprehen Psychiatry 1999;40:442-448.

86. Mishima K, Okawa M, Hishikawa Y, et al: Morning bright light therapy for sleep and behavior disorders in elderly patients with dementia. Acta Psychiatrica Scand 1994;89:1-7.

87. Satlin A, Volicer L, Ross V, et al: Bright light treatment of behavioral and sleep disturbances in patients with Alzheimer's disease. Am J Psychiatry 1992;149:1028-1032.

88. Yamadera H, Ito T, Suzuki H, et al: Effects of bright light on cognitive and sleep-wake (circadian) rhythm disturbances in Alzheimer-type dementia. Psychiatry Clin Neurosci 2000;54:352-353.

89. Van Someren EJW, Kessler A, Mirmiran M, et al: Indirect bright light improves circadian rest-activity rhythm disturbances in demented patients. Biol Psychiatry 1997;41:955-963.

90. Fontana GP, Kräuchi K, Cajochen C, et al: Dawn-dusk simulation light therapy of disturbed circadian rest-activity cycles in demented elderly. Exp Gerontol 2003;38:207-216.

91. Lyketsos C, Veiel LL, Baker A, et al: A randomized, controlled trial of bright light therapy for agitated behaviors in dementia patients residing in long-term care. Int J Geriatr Psychiatry 1999;14:520-525.

92. Mishima K, Hishikawa Y, Okawa M: Randomized, dim light controlled, crossover test of morning bright light therapy for rest-activity rhythm disorders in patients with vascular dementia and dementia of Alzheimer's type. Chronobiol Int 1998; 15:647-654.

93. Fetveit A, Bjorvatn B: The effects of bright-light therapy on actigraphical measured sleep last for several weeks post-treatment: A study in a nursing home population; J Sleep Res 2004;13:153-158.

94. Ancoli-Israel S, Martin JL, Kripke DF, et al: Effect of light treatment on sleep and circadian rhythms in demented nursing home patients. J Am Geriatr Soc 2002;50:282-289.

95. Ancoli-Israel S, Martin JL, Gehrman P, et al: Effect of light on agitation in institutionalized patients with severe Alzheimer disease. Am J Geriatr Psychiatry 2003;11:194-203.

95a. Skjerve A, Bjorvatn B, Holsten F: Light therapy for behavioural and psychological symptoms of dementia. Int J Geriat Psychiatry 2004;19:516-522.

96. Boulos Z: Bright light treatment for jet lag and shift work. In Lam RW (ed): Seasonal Affective Disorder and Beyond: Light Treatment for SAD and Non-SAD Conditions. Washington, DC, American Psychiatric Press, 1998, pp 253-287.

97. Czeisler CA, Hiasera AJ, Duffy JF: Research on sleep, circadian rhythms and aging: Applications to manned spaceflight. Exp Gerontol 1991;26:217-232.

98. Czeisler CA, Johnson MP, Duffy JF, et al: Exposure to bright light and darkness to treat physiological maladaptation to night work. N Engl J Med 1990;322:1253-1259.

98a. Stewart KT, Hayes BC, Eastman CI: Light treatment for NASA shiftworkers. Chronobiol Int 1995;12:141-151.

99. Eastman CI, Martin SK: How to use light and dark to produce circadian adaptation to night shift work. Ann Med 1999; 31:87-98.

100. Crowley SJ, Lee C, Tseng CY, et al: Combinations of bright light, scheduled dark, sunglasses, and melatonin to facilitate circadian entrainment to night shift work. J Biol Rhythms 2003;18:513-523.

100a. Yoon YI, Jeong DU, Kwon KB, et al: Bright light exposure at night and light attenuation in the morning improve adaptation of night shift workers. Sleep 2002;25:351-356.

101. Boivin DB, James FO: Circadian adaptation to night-shift work by judicious light and dark exposure. J Biol Rhythms 2002;17: 556-567.

102. Budnick LD, Lerman SE, Nicolich MJ: An evaluation of scheduled bright light and darkness on rotating shiftworkers: Trial and limitations. Am J Industr Med 1995;27:771-782.

103. Bjorvatn B, Kecklund G, Åkerstedt T: Bright light treatment used for adaptation to night work and re-adaptation back to day life: A field study at an oil platform in the North Sea. J Sleep Res 1999;8:105-112.

104. Campbell SS, Dijk D-J, Boulos Z, et al: Light treatment for sleep disorders: Consensus report, III: Alerting and activating effects. J Biol Rhythms 1995;10:129-132.

105. Oren DA, Reich W, Rosenthal NE, et al: How to Beat Jet Lag: A Practical Guide for Air Travellers. New York, Henry Holt, 1993.

106. Houpt TA, Boulos Z, Moore-Ede MC: MidnightSun: software for determining light exposure and phase-shifting schedules during global travel. Physiol Behav 1996;59:561-568.

107. Samel A, Wegmann HM: Bright light: A countermeasure for jet lag? Chronobiol Int 1997;14:173-183.

108. Sasaki M, Kurosaki Y, Onda M, et al: Effects of bright light on circadian rhythmicity and sleep after transmeridian flight. Sleep Res 1989;18:442.

109. Society for Light Treatment and Biological Rhythms: Consensus statements on the safety and effectiveness of light therapy of depression and disorders of biological rhythms. Light Treatment Biol Rhythms 1991;3:45-50.

110. Terman M, Terman JS: Light Therapy for Winter Depression: Report to the Depression Guidelines Panel, USPHS Agency for Health Care Policy and Research. New York, New York State Psychiatric Institute, 1991.

111. Agency for Health Care Policy and Research: Depression in Primary Care: Treatment of Major Depression. Clinical Practice Guideline No. 5. Rockville, Md, US Department of Health and Human Services, 1993.

112. American Psychiatric Association: Practice guideline for major depressive disorder in adults. Am J Psychiatry 1993; 150(suppl):1-26.

113. Golden RN, Gaynes BN, Ekstrom RD, et al: The efficacy of phototherapy in the treatment of mood disorders: A review and meta-analysis of the evidence. Am J Psychiatry (in press).

114. Chesson AL, Littner M, Davila D, et al: Practice parameters for the use of light therapy in the treatment of sleep disorders. Sleep 1999;22:641-660.

115. Lam RW, Levitt AJ, eds: Canadian Consensus Guidelines for the Treatment of Seasonal Affective Disorder. Vancouver, British Columbia, Clinical and Academic Publishing, 1999.

116. Tuunainen A, Kripke DF, Endo T: Light therapy for non-seasonal depression (Cochrane review). In The Cochrane Library, Issue 2, Chichester, England, John Wiley, 2004.

117. Wirz-Justice A: Light therapy for SAD is now reimbursed by medical insurance in Switzerland. Light Treatment Biol Rhythms 1996;8:45.

118. Consumer Reports on Health: The winter of your discontent? 1993;February:15-16.

122

Neurologic Monitoring Techniques

Beth A. Malow

ABSTRACT

Patients with nocturnal spells present a unique challenge to the sleep specialist and the sleep laboratory. While standard polysomnography (PSG) provides valuable information about the stage of sleep from which spells emerge and the time of the spell relative to sleep onset, the characterization of these spells is enhanced by video and extended electroencephalogram (EEG). Addition of video and an extended (12 or more channels, and sometimes as many as 21 or more) EEG to the standard PSG is essential for precise definition of nocturnal spells, including epileptic seizures, rapid eye movement (REM) sleep behavior disorder, and arousal disorders. The video component provides information on the behavioral and motor manifestations of the nocturnal spell.

The EEG may show a rhythmic evolving discharge characteristic of an epileptic seizure, or it may show interictal epileptiform discharges that occur apart from epileptic seizures. Lack of an EEG change, however, does not exclude some types of epilepsy, particularly those of frontal lobe origin. The movement artifact frequently associated with nocturnal seizures may also obscure the EEG. A stereotyped series of movements on the video is highly suggestive of epileptic seizures, even in the absence of EEG changes.

Pitfalls in the interpretation of recorded events are common; the inexperienced interpreter may mistakenly identify an artifact as EEG activity characteristic of seizures or parasomnias. A clinician who is in doubt about an EEG-PSG pattern should consult a trained electroencephalographer. Apart from artifacts, many other normal physiologic variants may be mistaken for epileptic activity.

Sophisticated digital video and EEG-PSG computer systems facilitate the acquisition, review, and storage of large quantities of data, with synchronization of behavioral manifestations and the EEG-PSG. Depending on the clinical situation, a daytime EEG, an ambulatory EEG, daytime short-term monitoring, 1 to 2 nights of polysomnography, or long-term (several days and nights) monitoring may be indicated.

Nocturnal spells often present diagnostic problems in sleep medicine because the history alone may not provide sufficient information to differentiate among the various diagnostic possibilities. Standard polysomnography (PSG) is helpful in defining the state and stage of sleep from which such nocturnal spells emerge, but it has limitations in diagnosis because behavioral analysis often is not included and the number of channels devoted to electroencephalography (EEG) is limited. These shortcomings are especially pertinent to the evaluation of suspected nocturnal epileptic seizures, which are defined by behavioral and motor manifestations in addition to EEG criteria.[1] Both behavioral and EEG analyses are critical for characterizing epileptic seizures and for distinguishing them from parasomnias.

The behavioral and EEG manifestations of nocturnal spells caused by parasomnias, neurologic disorders, and psychiatric disorders can be characterized more precisely by combining standard PSG with video recordings and extensive (12 or more channels) EEG montages.[2] This chapter emphasizes the methodology and indications for video–EEG PSG (VPSG) in the diagnosis of nocturnal events. In addition, the methodology and roles of routine EEG, short-term continuous video-EEG monitoring (STM), long-term continuous video–EEG monitoring (LTM), and ambulatory monitoring are addressed.

METHODOLOGY

Technical Aspects of Electroencephalography

The EEG measures the difference in electrical potential between pairs of electrodes placed on the scalp. These signals, reflecting synchronous postsynaptic potentials in large groups of neurons, are amplified and filtered to produce an analog or digital recording.[3] The international 10-20 system of EEG electrode placement is customarily used, in which the 10-20 refers to 10% and 20% of the distances between standard cranial landmarks (Fig. 122–1).[4,5] Each electrode site is identified with

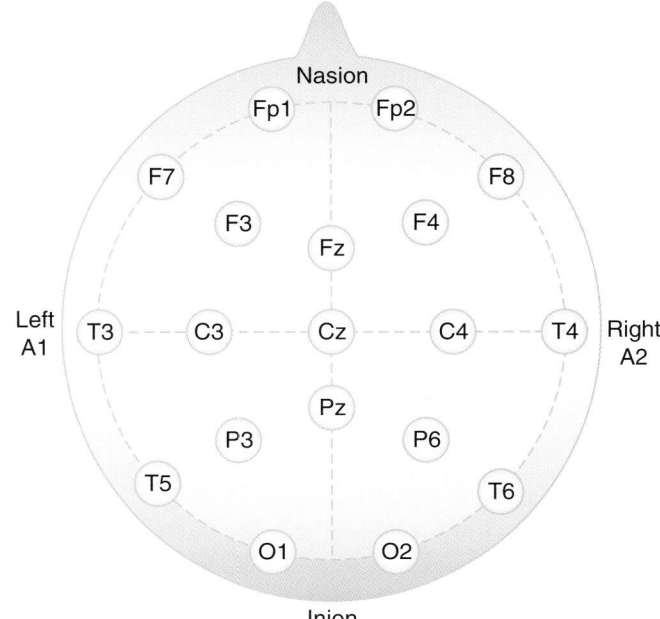

Figure 122–1. Standard international 10-20 electrode placement: Electrodes are placed at 10% or 20% of the distances between standard cranial landmarks. (From Keenan SA: Polysomnographic technique: an overview. In Chokroverty S [ed]: Sleep Disorders Medicine. Boston, Butterworth-Heinemann, 1994, p 84.)

Table 122–1.   Sample Attended Electroencephalographic Montages

Number of Available Channels	Montage
8	F7-T3, T3-T5, T5-O1, F8-T4, T4-T6, T6-O2, F3-C3, F4-C4
10	Fp1-F7, F7-T3, T3-T5, T5-O1, Fp2-F8, F8-T4, T4-T6, T6-O2, F3-C3, F4-C4
12	Fp1-F7, F7-T3, T3-T5, T5-O1, Fp2-F8, F8-T4, T4-T6, T6-O2, F3-C3, C3-P3, F4-C4, C4-P4
14	Fp1-F7, F7-T3, T3-T5, T5-O1, Fp2-F8, F8-T4, T4-T6, T6-O2, F3-C3, C3-P3, P3-O1, F4-C4, C4-P4, P4-O2
16	Fp1-F7, F7-T3, T3-T5, T5-O1, Fp2-F8, F8-T4, T4-T6, T6-O2, Fp1-F3, F3-C3, C3-P3, P3-O1, Fp2-F4, F4-C4, C4-P4, P4-O2
18	Fp1-F7, F7-T3, T3-T5, T5-O1, Fp2-F8, F8-T4, T4-T6, T6-O2, Fp1-F3, F3-C3, C3-P3, P3-O1, Fp2-F4, F4-C4, C4-P4, P4-O2, Fz-Cz, Cz-Pz
24	Fp1-F7, F7-T3, T3-T5, T5-O1, Fp2-F8, F8-T4, T4-T6, T6-O2, Fp1-F3, F3-C3, C3-P3, P3-O1, Fp2-F4, F4-C4, C4-P4, P4-O2, Fz-Cz, Cz-Pz, T1-T3, T3-C3, C3-Cz, Cz-C4, C4-T4, T4-T2

a letter representing the underlying region of the brain and with a number indicating a specific position above that region, with odd numbers indicating the left hemisphere and even numbers indicating the right hemisphere (e.g., T3 represents a left midtemporal electrode).

Each recording channel is derived from the signals from a pair of electrodes, and several pairs of electrodes, or derivations, are combined to form a montage. Montages may be either referential or bipolar. In referential montages, one of the electrodes in each pair is connected to a common electrode (e.g., channel 1: Fp1-A1; channel 2: F7-A1; channel 3: T3-A1; channel 4: T5-A1; channel 5: O1-A1). In bipolar montages, there is no common electrode. Bipolar montages are usually arranged in a chain with the same electrode in adjacent derivations (e.g., channel 1: Fp1-F7; channel 2: F7-T3; channel 3: T3-T5; channel 4: T5-O1).

The EEG montages used in a combined EEG-PSG study depend on the clinical indication and the number of channels available for recording (Table 122–1). Physicians and technicians involved in the use of EEG monitoring techniques require a solid knowledge of the principles of EEG recording and interpretation. Additional information regarding EEG methodology is available in a standard EEG text.[6]

Computerized digital EEG-PSG systems are an alternative to conventional analog EEG-PSG, and they are rapidly replacing the analog systems because of their numerous advantages.[7] These systems facilitate the review of large amounts of EEG-PSG data by displaying scoring and event information in a format that allows the user to, for example, click on the stage or event of interest and bring up the corresponding EEG-PSG.

The recording may be viewed at a variety of display settings that correspond to different paper speeds of conventional recordings. Filters, sensitivities, and montages may be adjusted to characterize events of interest and to help distinguish abnormalities from artifacts or normal variants. For example, certain montages may more easily identify and distinguish artifacts from *interictal epileptiform discharges* (IEDs),

defined as epileptic activity occurring between seizures. Digital EEG enhances the detection and review of IEDs by allowing for remontaging, changing the display settings that influence temporal resolution, and isolating specific channels for review (Fig. 122–2A and B). For example, by altering the display settings, synchronous delta or theta activity characteristic of non-rapid eye movement (NREM) arousal disorders may be more easily distinguished from spike-wave activity or an evolving ictal (seizure) pattern characteristic of an epileptic seizure disorder.

Several digital EEG-PSG systems share a common platform with epilepsy monitoring systems, allowing data obtained during a PSG to be analyzed by IED detection programs. Conversely, a study performed in the epilepsy-monitoring unit can be enhanced via the addition of electrooculogram (EOG) and chin electromyogram (EMG) electrodes to score sleep and determine the stage of sleep that precedes a particular event. This can be diagnostic in the case of distinguishing dissociative events, which rarely occur during sleep,[8] from epileptic seizures, which may occur during sleep or wakefulness.

Daytime Electroencephalography

Daytime EEG is used to look for IEDs, which support the diagnosis of a seizure disorder in many clinical settings.[6] In addition to the electrodes listed above, central (Fz, Cz, Pz) and ear (A1, A2) electrodes are included. Nasopharyngeal electrodes, although used in the past, are not recommended because they are uncomfortable and prone to artifact and rarely provide additional information.[9] The activating techniques of hyperventilation and intermittent photic stimulation are routinely performed and may bring out focal asymmetries or epileptiform activity.

Although seizures are not uniformly recorded during a routine EEG, focal IEDs or generalized spike-and-wave discharges may be observed and may assist in the classification of an epileptic syndrome as partial or generalized. The location of IEDs, which can be determined with the use of an extended

Figure 122–2. Use of different montages to enhance the review of interictal epileptiform discharges (IEDs). **A,** Left temporally dominant IEDs *(arrows)* on an extended electroencephalogram (EEG) montage that are not apparent in the central to ear channels *(asterisk).* **B,** Digital EEG allows the interpreter to select the relevant left temporal and parasagittal channels for review. The arrows highlight IEDs with phase reversals *(asterisks)* at T3 and F3, indicating maximal negativity at these electrodes, which defines the approximate location of the epileptic region. Both are 30-second epochs. Calibration symbol at bottom right, 100 μV.

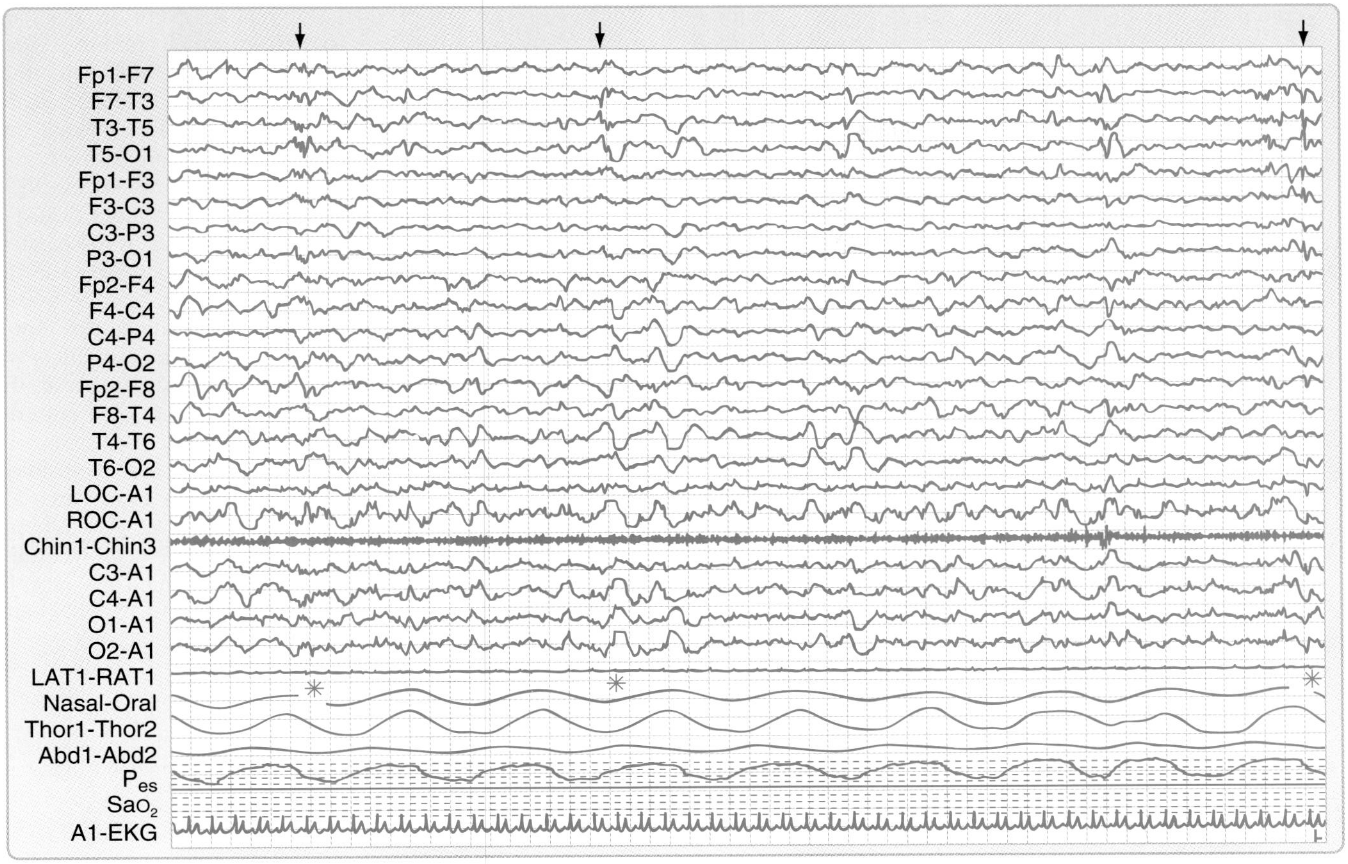

A

B

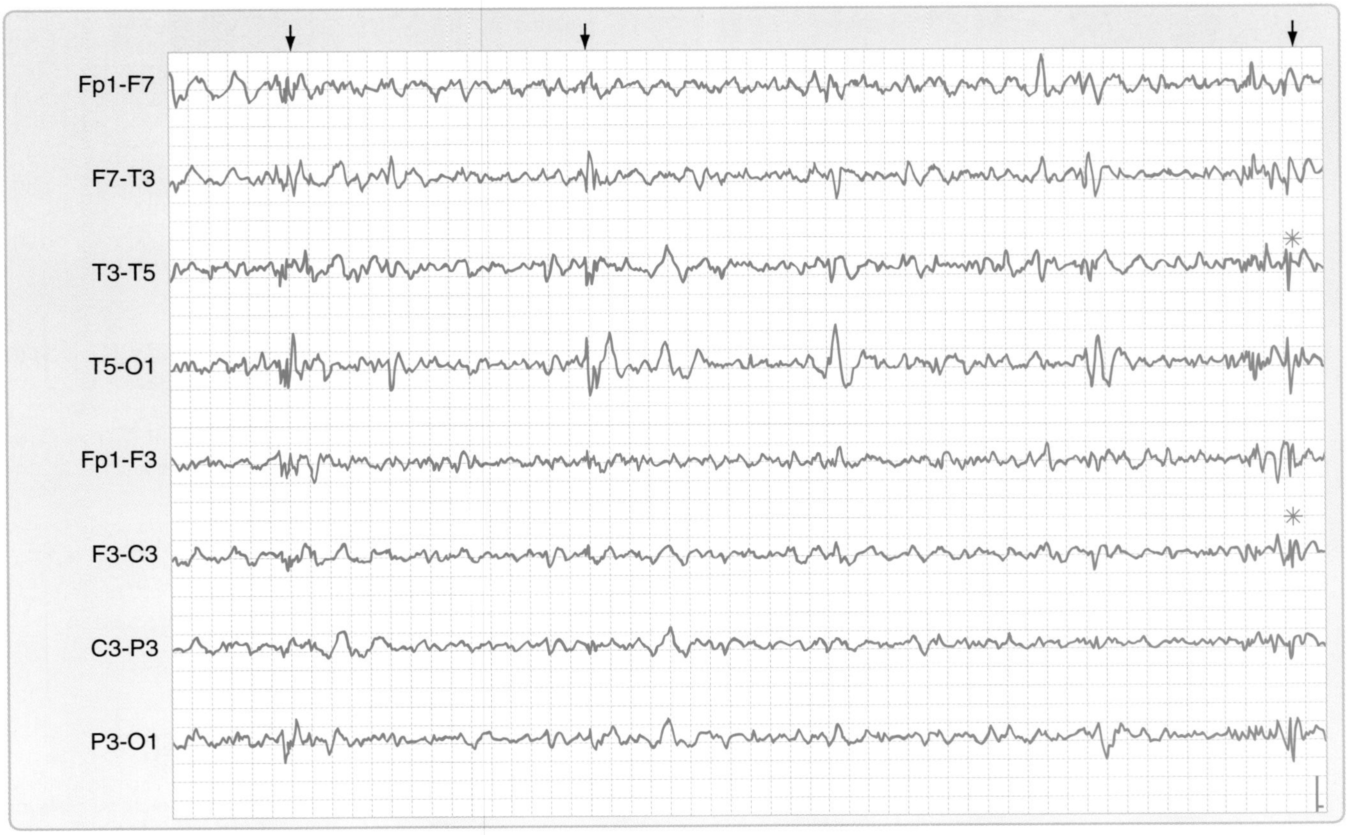

EEG montage, may clarify the nature of the epilepsy syndrome and its prognosis. For example, benign epilepsy of childhood with centrotemporal spikes has an excellent prognosis (Fig. 122–3). In contrast, some temporal lobe IEDs may be refractory to medical treatment and the patients may become candidates for epilepsy surgery.

Daytime studies performed while the patient is asleep for at least a portion of the recording increase the yield of finding abnormalities, because in many patients, IEDs are more common in drowsiness and NREM sleep. Stage 2 NREM sleep is usually, but not always, recorded on the routine EEG, whereas NREM stage 3 and 4 sleep and REM sleep are rarely recorded. When the routine EEG does not show IEDs and the physician has a high suspicion for seizures, a sleep-deprived EEG improves the yield of finding epileptiform activity, at least in part because sleep is more likely to be recorded. Analog EEG recordings use a variety of montages to display ongoing brain activity, whereas digital EEG recordings permit the viewing of a segment of EEG in a variety of montages and speeds, which can help distinguish an IED from an artifact.

Video–Electroencephalography Polysomnography

When the history does not allow the physician to diagnose nocturnal spells associated with complex movements and behavior, recording of the sleep-related event in question might allow definitive diagnosis. VPSG, which combines video recording with an extended EEG montage and with other standard PSG physiologic monitoring, is useful in characterizing unusual behavior and movements during sleep. Diagnostic considerations for patients with complex actions at night may include epileptic seizures, NREM arousal disorders, REM sleep behavior disorder (RBD), rhythmic movement disorder, or psychiatric disorders such as panic disorder or dissociative disorder. Episodes associated with these disorders have specific clinical features as discussed in Chapters 72 and 74-79. Events recorded with VPSG are reviewed to characterize the motor and behavioral manifestations of the event and the EEG-PSG features, including the stage of sleep preceding the event, the time of the event relative to sleep onset, and EEG patterns occurring during the event or between events.

Video recordings may be played back in real time or at slower speeds to define the event of interest. A slow tape (extended play) speed allows for continuous monitoring for 6 to 8 hours without changing tapes. Infrared cameras are useful for recording nighttime events. Movable cameras can be mounted in a patient's room and display close-ups or full-body views. Double cameras are useful for focusing on the face while simultaneously monitoring the body. During recorded events, the technologist should interact with the patient to test for level of consciousness and ability to perform commands.

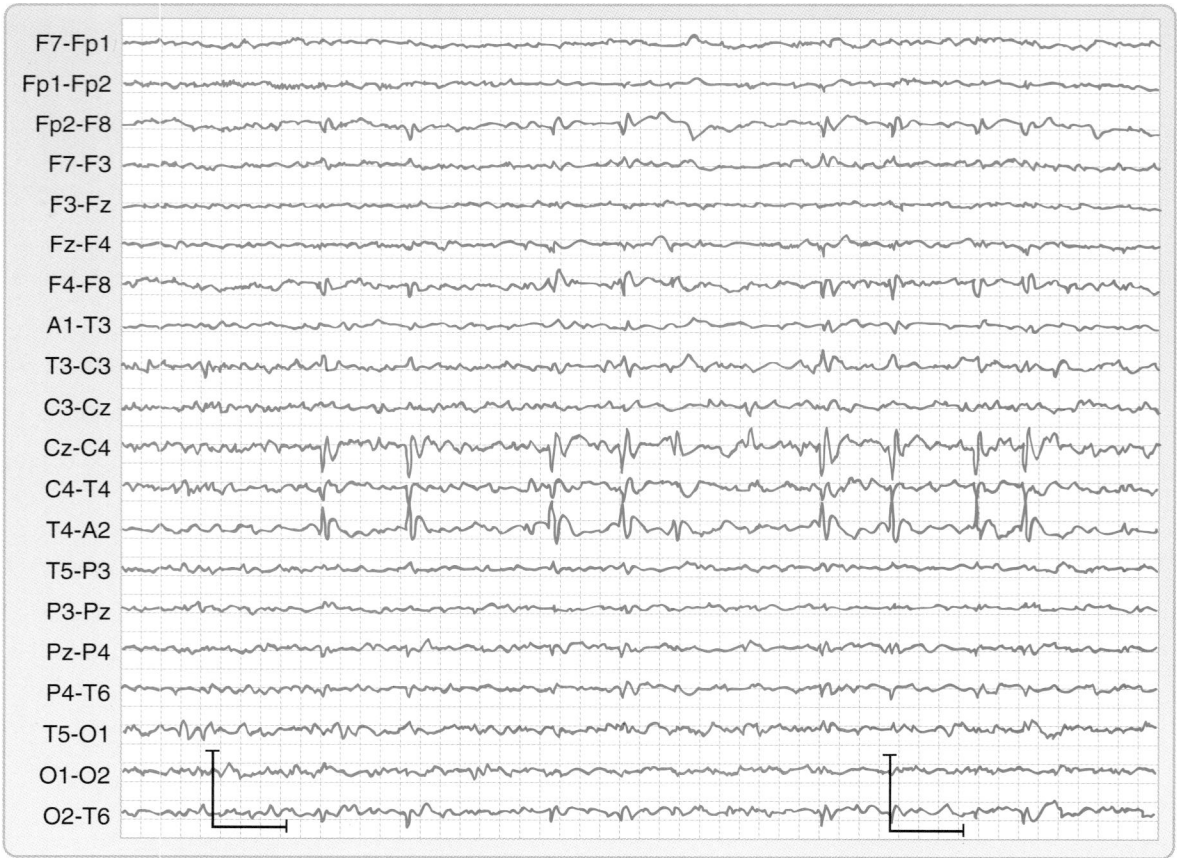

Figure 122–3. Runs of interictal epileptiform discharges with a centrotemporal dominance in benign epilepsy of childhood with centrotemporal spikes. The bipolar montage readily demonstrates peak negativity at the C4 and T4 electrodes. Such localization is not possible with electroencephalogram (EEG) montages commonly used with standard polysomnography (PSG). Calibration symbol, 500 μV, 1 sec. (From Malow BA: Sleep and epilepsy. Neurol Clin 1996;14:774.)

The EEG-PSG signal can be recorded as a multiplexed analog signal directly onto videotape and stored with the video signal, or it can be recorded digitally onto magnetic or optical media with a synchronizing signal to time-lock the actions to the PSG signals. For review, the video signal can be combined with EEG-PSG on a single "split" screen. Alternatively, the EEG-PSG signal and video signal can be synchronously replayed on two monitors. The EEG-PSG also can be played back onto paper at a variety of speeds to display sleep features or EEG features as indicated. Information regarding the date and time encoded onto the videotape and paper printout allows for synchronous review. Digital video recordings are rapidly replacing videotape recordings.

The stage of sleep from which the spells emerge and the time of the spell relative to sleep onset provide useful diagnostic information. For example, the actions accompanying the NREM arousal disorders arise from delta NREM sleep, usually in the first third of the sleep period (see Chapter 74), whereas those associated with RBD emerge from REM sleep, most commonly in the last third of the sleep period (see Chapter 75). Epileptic seizures are more common during NREM sleep than during REM sleep (see Chapter 72).[10] Rhythmic movements associated with rhythmic movement disorder usually occur during sleep-wake transitions, and dissociative episodes emerge from wakefulness. Nocturnal panic attacks occur from NREM sleep, usually at the transition from stage 2 to stage 3.[11]

Specific EEG patterns associated with nocturnal spells are discussed in "Relative Indications, Advantages, Disadvantages, and Limitations." If complex partial seizures are a diagnostic consideration, the EEG montage should emphasize the use of electrodes placed over the temporal lobes (e.g., F7, T1, T3, T5). If benign childhood epilepsy with centrotemporal spikes is a consideration, the montage should include the parasagittal region (e.g., C3, C4). The specific montage that is used depends on the number of channels available for EEG. Sample montages for 8, 10, 12, 14, 16, 19, and 24 channels are shown in Table 122–1.

The following montage of 16 electrodes in anterior-to-posterior chains provides excellent coverage for suspected seizures: left temporal: Fp1-F7, F7-T3, T3-T5, and T5-O1; left parasagittal: Fp1-F3, F3-C3, C3-P3, and P3-O1; right parasagittal: Fp2-F4, F4-C4, C4-P4, and P4-O2; and right temporal: Fp2-F8, F8-T4, T4-T6, and T6-O2. This montage allows for the evaluation of interictal and ictal activity during sleep. Two additional anterior temporal electrodes, T1 and T2, can be added because they are particularly useful for the detection of anterior temporal IEDs. In one study comparing abbreviated EEG montages with a standard 18-channel bipolar montage, seizures were more readily distinguished from arousal patterns using 7- and 18-EEG channel montages as compared with 4-channel EEG records.[12]

Short-Term and Long-Term Monitoring

When the history suggests frequent daytime spells or spells occurring during daytime naps, STM, a video-EEG recording typically performed in an EEG or sleep laboratory for 6 to 8 hours during the day, may be helpful. The value of such studies for the assessment of patients with strictly nocturnal spells, however, is limited. Occasionally, STM is useful if *sleep attacks*, spells of diminished responsiveness due to sleepiness, are included in the differential diagnosis of daytime spells.

Unfortunately, one or two nights of monitoring in the sleep laboratory is not always sufficient to capture and characterize spells. LTM, an extension of STM that allows for continuous recordings of up to several weeks, is used mainly for patients with known or suspected seizures.[13] For patients who are taking antiepileptic medications, these drugs may be tapered and discontinued during LTM; intermittent sleep deprivation also is commonly used to facilitate spells. Because frequent seizures or status epilepticus may occur in epileptic patients undergoing medication discontinuation, LTM is generally performed in a hospital setting, usually a specialized epilepsy-monitoring laboratory.

Eye movement leads and chin electromyographic leads may be added to the standard EEG electrodes to stage sleep. Semi-invasive sphenoidal electrodes, placed in the subtemporal fossa to record from the inferior temporal region and adjacent areas of the inferior frontal lobe, are usually reserved for patients with previously diagnosed epilepsy refractory to medication trials who are undergoing evaluation for epilepsy surgery. They are generally not required when the goal of monitoring is to identify EEG activity consistent with seizures or parasomnias rather than to precisely characterize an epileptic focus.

Even though sphenoidal electrodes may increase the number of IEDs recorded, the detection of IEDs from a sphenoidal electrode alone rarely occurs, particularly if ear, T1, and T2 electrodes are used.[14] In addition, although ictal patterns from sphenoidal electrodes may appear earlier and be better developed than those from surface electrodes, EEG seizure patterns are generally evident in both surface and sphenoidal electrodes.[15]

Even if additional electrodes are used, the lack of scalp or sphenoidal ictal activity during a clinical event does not exclude a seizure, particularly if awareness is preserved during the clinical event (e.g., a simple partial seizure) or if the event originates in the frontal lobe. Ictal activity may be apparent only with intracranial electrodes, such as depth electrodes that penetrate the brain parenchyma, subdural strips, and subdural grids.[16-18] These invasive electrodes, which are rarely used in the diagnosis of nocturnal spells because of the risks of infection and hemorrhage, are generally reserved for patients who require localization of epileptic foci before surgical resection and in whom scalp recordings are inconclusive. If an ictal pattern is not recorded but clinical seizures are highly suspected based on the history and stereotyped behavioral spells recorded on videotape, an empirical trial of an antiepileptic medication may be appropriate.

Ambulatory Monitoring

Ambulatory monitoring combines the extended recording time of VPSG with the convenience of recording in a patient's home. Several commercial products allow patients to go home with 12 or more channels of EEG electrodes and a recording device, which sometimes includes video monitoring. Ambulatory recording systems may use analog or digital recorders. Patients and their bed partners are instructed to keep an activity log to document events.

The indications for ambulatory monitoring in the differential diagnosis of nocturnal events are not established. This monitoring technique appears promising for the evaluation of interictal epileptiform activity during sleep. Depending on the sophistication of the video recordings, ambulatory monitoring may identify some cases of epileptic seizures, NREM arousal disorders, RBD, rhythmic movement disorder, panic disorder, and dissociative disorder.

ARTIFACTS AND PITFALLS

Artifacts, which are common during sleep-related spells recorded with any of these modalities, must be distinguished from interictal and ictal epileptiform activity and from EEG activity associated with parasomnias. Although artifacts may obscure the EEG and make diagnosis more difficult, they are sometimes helpful; for example, head or body rocking artifact may be diagnostic of rhythmic movement disorder, and rhythmic myogenic artifact may support bruxism (Fig. 122–4). Other examples of frequently encountered artifacts include those caused by head tremor, eye movements, and tongue movements (*glossokinetic artifact*). Associated rhythmic activities may resemble ictal EEG patterns.

Pitfalls in the interpretation of recorded events are common; the inexperienced interpreter may mistakenly identify an artifact as EEG activity characteristic of seizures or parasomnias. When the clinician is in doubt about an EEG-PSG pattern, a trained electroencephalographer should be consulted. Apart from artifacts, many other normal physiologic variants may be mistaken for epileptic activity; these include positive occipital sharp transients of sleep (see Fig. 122–4), frequent and sharply contoured vertex waves, particularly in young patients (Fig. 122–5), sawtooth waves, benign epileptiform transients of sleep, wicket spikes, and rhythmic temporal theta of drowsiness.[19]

RELATIVE INDICATIONS, ADVANTAGES, DISADVANTAGES, AND LIMITATIONS

Although VPSG and other neurologic monitoring techniques can be useful in diagnosing nocturnal events, the incremental cost of these techniques over standard PSG necessitates that specific indications be met. Unfortunately, no standards exist for determining when to choose a specific monitoring technique, and the reliability and validity of the monitoring techniques described here have not been formally studied. Consensus guidelines for interpretation have not been developed. In addition, the role of ambulatory EEG in monitoring parasomnias is not well defined. The indications, advantages, disadvantages, and limitations outlined here are based on the experiences of the authors and others.

Video–Electroencephalography Polysomnography

Indications for VPSG include suspected sleep-related epileptic seizures, suspected NREM arousal disorders, RBD, or suspected dissociative disorder.

Suspected Sleep-Related Epileptic Seizures

Although some epileptic seizures can be diagnosed on the basis of history (e.g., generalized tonic-clonic activity witnessed by a reliable observer), most events occurring frequently and

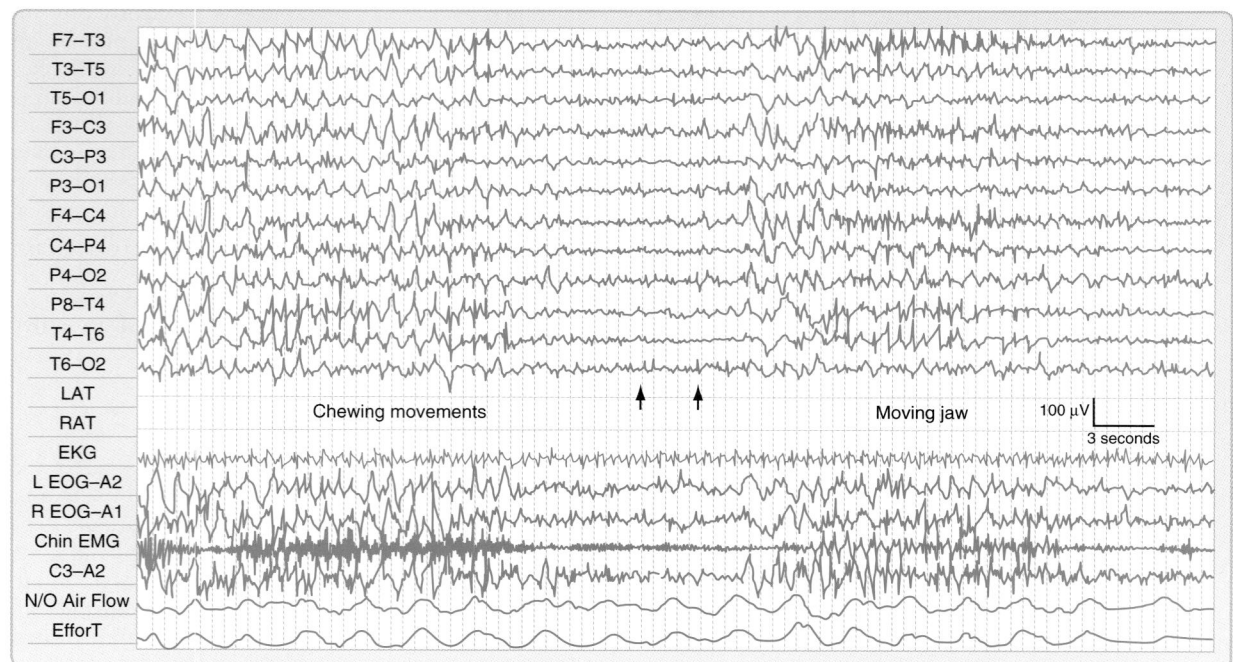

Figure 122–4. Artifacts resembling interictal epileptiform activity. Chewing movements produced by bruxism cause rhythmic activity with superimposed myogenic artifact in the electroencephalogram (EEG) channels, bearing a superficial resemblance to generalized spike-wave discharges. The arrows identify posterior occipital sharp transients of sleep (POSTS), normal features of non–rapid eye movement (NREM) stage 1 sleep that appear sharply contoured and may be mistaken for pathologic occipital sharp waves at the standard polysomnograph (PSG) paper speed of 10 mm/sec.

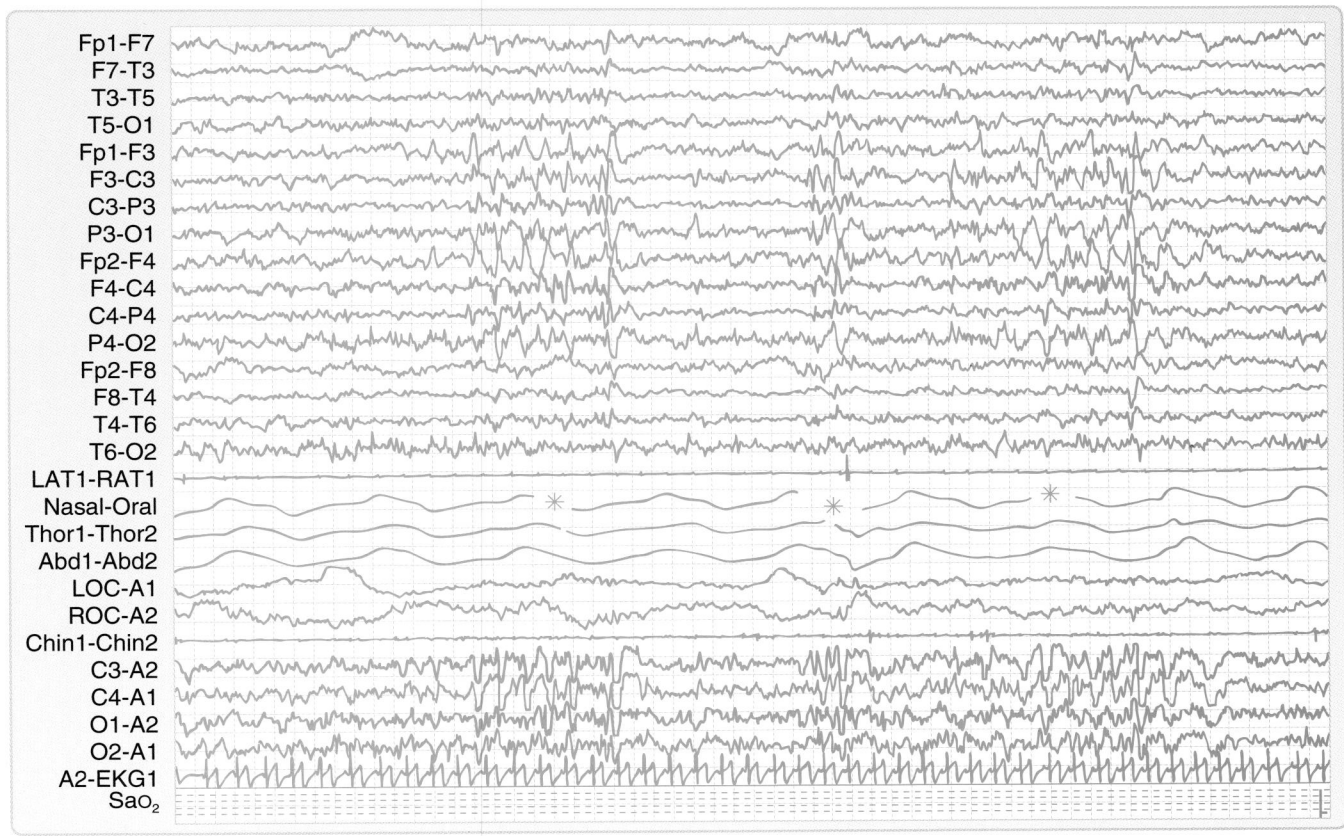

Figure 122–5. Sharply contoured vertex waves in a 6-year-old child. Although these physiologic waves resemble abnormal epileptiform activity, their morphology and distribution distinguish them from pathologic discharges. Compare with Figure 122–2. Thirty-second epoch. Calibration symbol at bottom right, 100 µV.

suspected to be complex partial seizures are best confirmed with VPSG monitoring, especially if they include the features of thrashing, kicking, hyperventilating, head rocking, screaming, or subtle arousals from sleep observed in parasomnias or dissociative disorders.

The advantage of VPSG over conventional PSG or EEG without video in suspected epileptic seizures is the ability to analyze stereotyped behaviors, characteristic of epileptic seizures, in association with ictal EEG activity. Figure 122–6A and B shows a recording with an extended EEG montage of an epileptic seizure, illustrating a clear evolution of activity. Apart from recording epileptic seizures, PSG with an expanded EEG montage allows for sampling of IEDs throughout the night. The IEDs associated with partial epilepsy are usually more prevalent in sleep, especially delta NREM sleep, than in wakefulness.[20,21] Therefore, occasionally, IEDs missed on a routine daytime EEG are detected on an overnight recording.[22]

CASE EXAMPLE 1

A 34-year-old woman with a remote history of daytime complex partial seizures presented with nightly nocturnal spells. Her husband reported that within 45 minutes of falling asleep she aroused, sat up, appeared frightened, breathed rapidly, looked around the room with a blank, wide-eyed stare, and then returned to sleep. These episodes were stereotyped and lasted less than 1 minute. She responded almost immediately and did not recall the episodes.

The differential diagnosis includes an NREM arousal disorder, dissociative episodes, or epileptic seizures. Nocturnal panic disorder is unlikely because she does not recall the episodes. RBD is possible, but it would be unusual in a young woman, usually does not cause stereotyped behavior, and rarely occurs soon after sleep onset.

Because the history was insufficient for diagnosis and because the spells were occurring nightly, VPSG was performed, during which the patient had several stereotyped spells occurring from all stages of NREM sleep. These spells were associated with ictal discharges beginning over the right temporal lobe consisting of rhythmic theta activity that increased in frequency and decreased in amplitude.

She was treated for complex partial seizures with carbamazepine, and the spells resolved. If this patient had been on antiepileptic medication chronically and had spells that were less frequent (e.g., once a week), an alternative approach would have been LTM with tapering of medications to promote seizure occurrence.

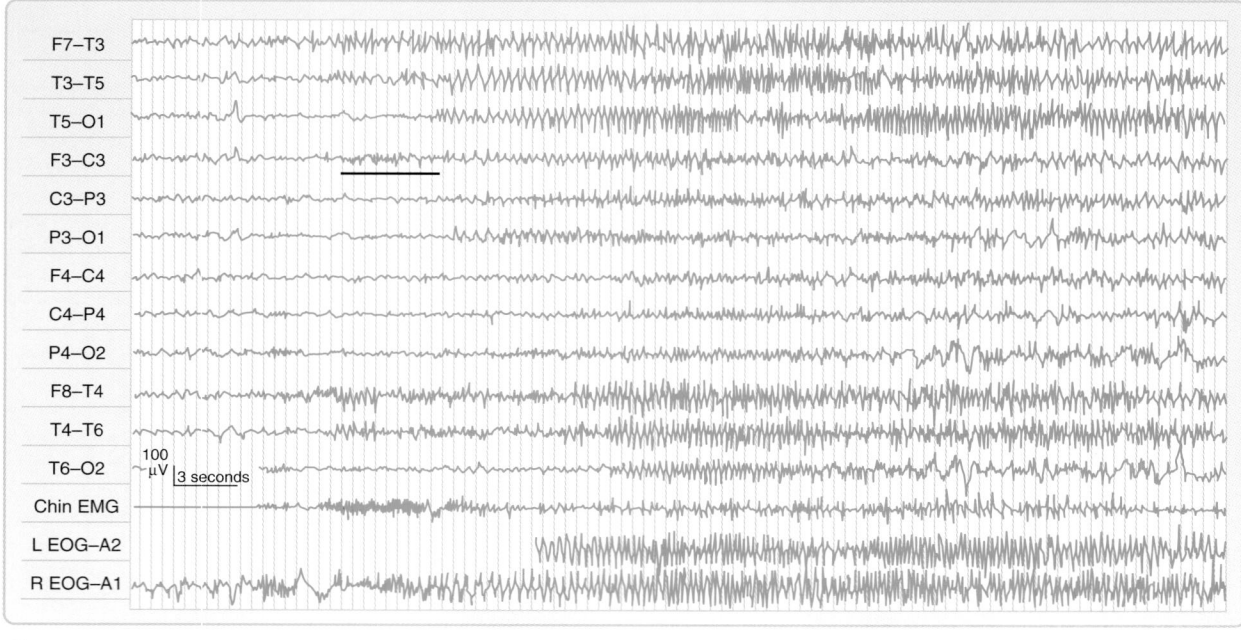

A

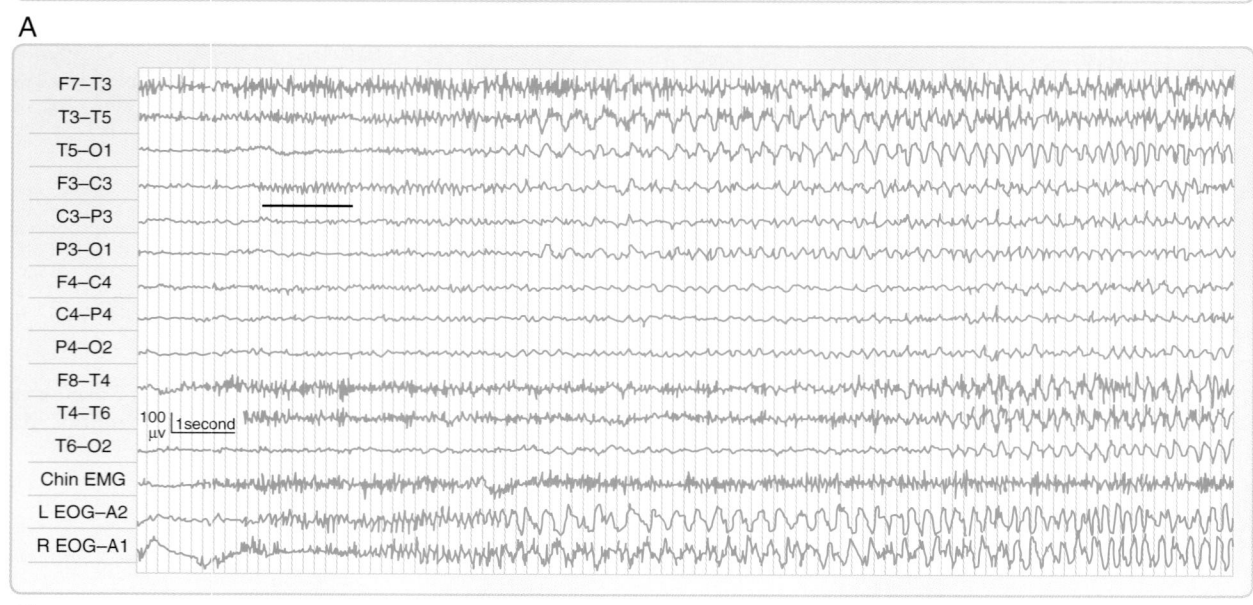

B

Figure 122–6. Partial seizure beginning during non–rapid eye movement (NREM) sleep. **A,** recorded at 10 mm/sec paper speed. Clinically, the seizure began with an abrupt arousal, followed by turning of head and eyes to the left and movements of the arms beneath the bedclothes. On electroencephalogram (EEG), an initial reduction in voltage is followed by a progressive increase in the amplitude of the ictal discharge over the left hemisphere, with spread to the right hemisphere derivations. The underlined activity from the F3-C3 derivation appears to be muscle artifact; however, in **B,** at 30 mm/sec paper speed, it is clear that the same underlined segment is the initial focal surface representation of the ictal discharge. Additional polysomnographic measures recorded on channels 16 to 21 are not shown. (Modified from Aldrich MS, Jahnke B: Diagnostic value of video-EEG polysomnography. Neurology 1991;41:1060-1066.)

Suspected NREM Arousal Disorders

Although confusional arousals, sleepwalking, and sleep terrors often can be diagnosed on the basis of history, VPSG is indicated if behavioral features are atypical or stereotyped, multiple nightly episodes occur, onset is in adulthood, or spells do not respond to a trial of medications. An advantage of VPSG in the diagnosis of NREM arousal disorders is the combination of video to characterize the event of interest,

sleep scoring channels to determine the stage of sleep involved, and an extended EEG montage to exclude ictal EEG activity characteristic of epileptic seizures.

The VPSG may capture a confusional arousal, night terror, or sleepwalking episode arising out of delta NREM (stage 3 or 4) sleep, accompanied by synchronous delta activity (Fig. 122–7). Alternatively, the VPSG recorded during an NREM arousal event may show asynchronous delta or theta activity, synchronous theta activity, a drowsy pattern, or nonreactive

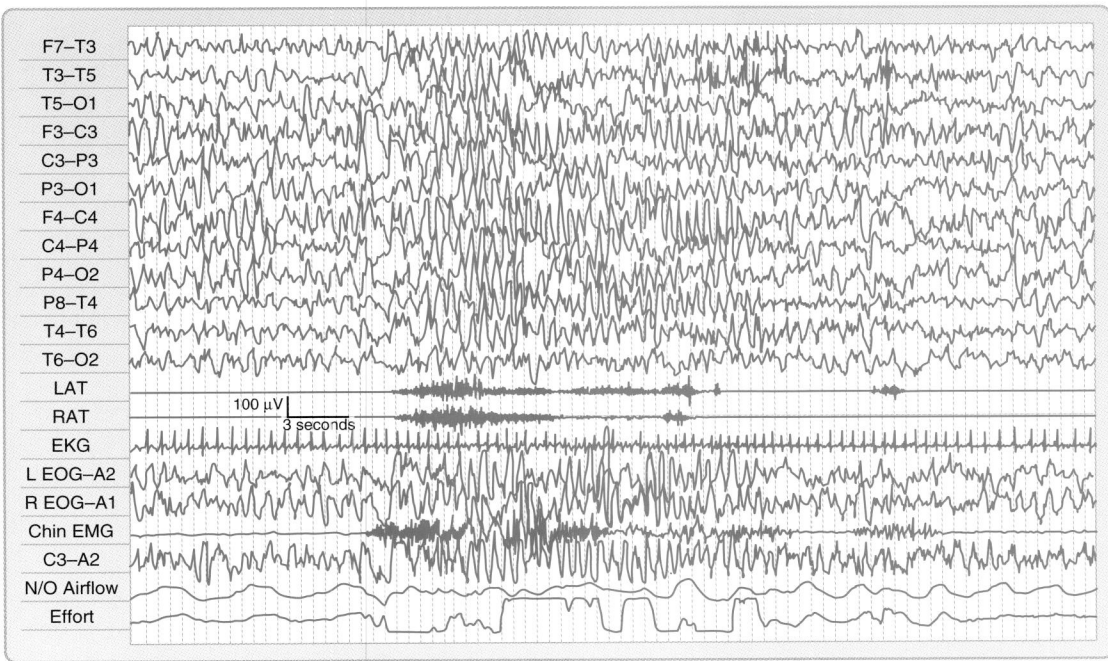

Figure 122–7. Arousal from delta non–rapid eye movement (NREM) sleep in a child with an NREM arousal disorder. Note synchronous delta activity during arousal from delta NREM sleep, associated with a tonic increase in chin electromyogram (EMG) and LAT and RAT electroencephalogram (EEG). In contrast to the EEG of an epileptic seizure, the delta activity does not evolve in amplitude or frequency.

CASE EXAMPLE 2

A 4-year-old girl had near-nightly episodes of screaming loudly about 1 hour after falling asleep. During these episodes, her parents found her agitated and inconsolable. On rare occasions, she got out of bed and wandered out of her room. She was amnestic for these spells. An older sibling had had similar spells.

Because the history is compelling for night terrors, evaluation with VPSG is not necessary. If any atypical features were present (e.g., automatisms or stereotyped behavior, multiple nightly episodes, or onset in adulthood) or if symptoms did not respond to treatment, a VPSG would be warranted.

---

alpha activity. Apart from clinical events, the EEG may show synchronous delta during arousals from stage 3 or 4 sleep, a nonspecific finding that is more common in patients with arousal disorders than in healthy subjects.[23]

Suspected REM Sleep Behavior Disorder

Although the definitive diagnosis of RBD may be suspected based on the history, definitive diagnosis requires capturing a behavioral event on a video recording or demonstrating abnormal muscle tone or excessive limb movements during REM sleep (Chapter 75). The advantage of VPSG is that video is combined with sleep staging to identify REM, and an extended EEG montage is used to exclude ictal EEG activity.

Suspected Dissociative Disorder

Dissociative episodes and other psychogenic spells occur during wakefulness, although the patient may appear asleep and

may believe that he or she is asleep.[8] Because the manifestations of dissociative episodes may be quite bizarre and include thrashing, screaming, or bicycling movements, it is often impossible to distinguish these spells from epileptic seizures or parasomnias based on the history alone. When nocturnal psychogenic episodes are suspected, VPSG is advantageous in documenting the behavior of the patient, the presence of waking background EEG preceding the onset of the spells, and the absence of ictal EEG activity.

CASE EXAMPLE 3

A 32-year-old man developed spells of unresponsiveness associated with asynchronous jerking movements of all four extremities for up to 30 minutes. These spells occurred nightly during sleep and rarely during the day. When they occurred during the day, he recalled portions of the spells and stated that he could hear people around him, but that he could not respond. His wife could shake him out of the spells, and then he would regain full alertness.

Based on the history of prolonged spells with bilateral extremity jerking and preserved consciousness, a dissociative episode was likely, although occasionally, epileptic seizures, especially of frontal lobe origin, manifest with bilateral jerking movements of the extremities and rapid return to full alertness. Depending on the relative frequency of the nocturnal and daytime spells, VPSG, STM, or LTM may be appropriate. In this case, because of the relative frequency of nocturnal spells, VPSG was performed. It documented an awake background preceding and during the spell, with an absence of ictal EEG activity, characteristic of a dissociative disorder. After psychiatric evaluation and treatment, the frequency of the spells decreased.

The major disadvantage of VPSG in the evaluation of suspected epileptic seizures, parasomnias, and dissociative disorders is the cost of the study. Additional technologist time is needed to place an extended EEG montage and to continuously observe patients throughout the study. In addition, physicians must review each spell to assess behavior and EEG patterns. Equipment must allow for review capabilities at EEG paper speed (30 mm/sec). These review capabilities are standard on most digital PSG equipment, although the additional channels require more space on storage media.

The VPSG also has limitations. The EEG recorded during a spell may not demonstrate an abnormality. Because epileptic seizures may lack surface EEG correlates, the absence of surface ictal EEG activity does not ensure that an epileptic seizure has not occurred. In addition, it can be difficult to differentiate an ictal EEG seizure pattern (which consists of rhythmic activity that evolves in frequency and amplitude) from the synchronous delta or theta activity or diffuse alpha activity occurring during an NREM arousal disorder. The most well-developed portion of the ictal EEG pattern may be rhythmic delta or theta without a clear evolution, seizures may have bilateral onsets, seizures may arise from delta NREM sleep, and muscle or movement artifact may obscure the EEG. Two consecutive nights of VPSG are often scheduled so if no events are captured on the first night, the second night is available for study.

Daytime Electroencephalography

The advantage of daytime EEG over VPSG, standard PSG, or any of the other monitoring techniques is its brief recording time and low cost. The disadvantage is that spells, particularly sleep-related spells, are rarely captured. When the history is highly suggestive of epileptic seizures, a routine EEG may demonstrate epileptic activity as supportive evidence of epilepsy. However, IEDs are not the equivalent of epileptic seizures and may be present in patients without epilepsy, such as occurs in relatives of patients with benign childhood epilepsy with centrotemporal spikes. Conversely, patients with epilepsy may not have IEDs during EEG recordings. In addition, patients with epilepsy may have coexisting parasomnias. Therefore, in the absence of a compelling history, the occurrence of abnormal interictal epileptiform activity should not be used by itself to definitively diagnose nocturnal spells as epileptic seizures.

Short-Term and Long-Term Monitoring

The advantages of STM and LTM over routine EEG are a longer recording time and simultaneous video monitoring. In patients with exclusively sleep-related spells, VPSG is preferred over STM because the recording is performed during sleep. In patients with a mixture of daytime and sleep-related spells, STM is sometimes appropriate.

LTM is an alternative in patients in whom antiepileptic medication taper or discontinuation is planned. Medication taper or discontinuation is especially useful in facilitating seizure activity in epileptic patients with infrequent spells (e.g., once a week or less). The disadvantages of LTM are the cost of inpatient hospitalization and the need for a specialized epilepsy-monitoring laboratory. The limitations of LTM are similar to those of PSG in that spells may lack EEG correlates or may not occur, despite many days of monitoring.

Ambulatory Monitoring

The advantage of ambulatory monitoring is the convenience of recording in a patient's home and the lack of need for continuous monitoring by a technologist. Cost varies, but it is usually lower than that of a recording in a sleep laboratory.

A major disadvantage of ambulatory monitoring relates to the fidelity of the recording in the absence of a technologist. If electrodes become detached, ground wires break, or conductive media become dry during the study, adjustments cannot be made. In addition, most systems use a reduced number of channels, thereby limiting the information provided, although technologic advances should increase the capability for expanded montages.

Furthermore, in contrast to the other monitoring techniques, the patient is not under constant observation and a technologist is not present. Consequently, interactions with the patient, which are critical for evaluation of the level of consciousness, are not possible, and the interpretation of rhythmic activities that resemble ictal discharges may be difficult in the absence of an assessment of behavior and consciousness. The addition of synchronized video recordings to ambulatory monitoring has potential for facilitating correlation between EEG activity and clinical events.

> *Clinical Pearl*
>
> *The clinician should consider performing video–EEG in suspected cases of nocturnal seizures and parasomnias such as REM sleep behavior disorder or NREM arousal disorders. The video may be as helpful as the EEG in documenting stereotyped behavior typical of epileptic seizures.*

References

1. Commission on Classification and Terminology of the International League Against Epilepsy: Proposal for revised clinical and electrographic classification of epileptic seizures. Epilepsia 1981;22:489-501.
2. Aldrich MS, Jahnke B: Diagnostic value of video-EEG polysomnography. Neurology 1991;41:1060-1066.
3. Epstein CM: Technical aspects of EEG: An overview. In Wyllie E (ed): The Treatment of Epilepsy: Principles and Practices. Philadelphia, Lea & Febiger, 1993, pp 202-210.
4. Jasper H: The 10-20 electrode system of the International Federation. Electroencephalogr Clin Neurophysiol 1958; 10:370-375.
5. Keenan SA: Polysomnographic technique: An overview. In Chokroverty S (ed): Sleep Disorders Medicine (2nd ed). Boston, Butterworth-Heinemann, 1999, pp 151-169.
6. Daly D, Pedley T: Current Practice of Clinical Electroencephalography. New York, Raven Press, 2002.
7. Lagerlund T, Cascino G, Cicora K, et al: Long-term electroencephalographic monitoring for diagnosis and management of seizures. Mayo Clin Proc 1996;71:1000-1006.
8. Thacker K, Devinsky O, Perrine K, et al: Nonepileptic seizures during apparent sleep. Ann Neurol 1993;33:414-418.
9. Kaplan PW, Lesser RP: Focal cortical resection evaluation: Noninvasive EEG. In Wyllie E (ed): The Treatment of Epilepsy: Principles and Practice. Philadelphia, Lea & Febiger, 1993, pp 1014-1022.
10. Malow B: Sleep and epilepsy. Neurol Clin 1996;14:765-789.
11. Mellman T, Uhde T: Electroencephalographic sleep in panic disorder. Arch Gen Psychiatry 1989;46:178-184

12. Foldvary N, Caruso AC, Mascha E, et al: Identifying montages that best detect electrographic seizure activity during polysomnography. Sleep 2000;23:211-229.

13. Kaplan P, Lesser R. Long-Term monitoring. In Daly D, Pedley T (eds): Current Practice of Clinical Electroencephalography. New York, Raven Press, 1990, pp 513-534.

14. Sperling MR, Engel J Jr: Sphenoidal electrodes. J Clin Neurophysiol 1986;3:67-73.

15. King DW, So EL, Marcus R, et al: Techniques and applications of sphenoidal recording. J Clin Neurophysiol 1986;3: 51-65.

16. So NK: Depth electrode studies in mesial temporal epilepsy. In Luders HO (ed): Epilepsy Surgery. New York, Raven Press, 1992, pp 371-384.

17. Wyler AR: Subdural strip electrodes in surgery of epilepsy. In Luders HO (ed): Epilepsy Surgery. New York, Raven Press, 1992, pp 395-398.

18. Lesser RP, Gordon B, Fisher R, et al: Subdural grid electrodes in surgery of epilepsy. In Luders HO (ed): Epilepsy Surgery. New York, Raven Press, 1992, pp 399-408.

19. Drury I: Epileptiform patterns of children. J Clin Neurophysiol 1989;6:1-39.

20. Sammaritano M, Gigli GL, Gotman J: Interictal spiking during wakefulness and sleep and the localization of foci in temporal lobe epilepsy. Neurology 1991;41:290-297.

21. Malow BA, Lin X, Kushwaha R, et al: Interictal spiking increases with sleep depth in temporal lobe epilepsy. Epilepsia 1998; 39:1309-1316.

22. Malow BA, Selwa LM, Ross DA, et al: Lateralizing value of interictal spikes on overnight sleep-EEG studies in temporal lobe epilepsy. Epilepsia 1999;40:1587-1592.

23. Blatt I, Peled R, Gadoth N, et al: The value of sleep recording in evaluating somnambulism in young adults. Electroencephalogr Clin Neurophysiol 1991;78:407-412.

123

Gastrointestinal Monitoring Techniques

William C. Orr

Chien Lin Chen

ABSTRACT

Symptoms suggestive of unexplained arousals from sleep resulting in complaints of insomnia or daytime sleepiness may well have nocturnal gastroesophageal reflux (GER) as an underlying contributing factor. In addition, nocturnal GER may be the cause of exacerbations from bronchial asthma and repeated pulmonary infections as a result of pulmonary aspiration of refluxed gastric contents. For most clinical circumstances, 24-hour ambulatory pH monitoring studies with careful documentation of the sleeping interval are suitable and allow a reasonable assessment of waking GER and sleep-related GER, as well as acid contact time during the total interval and the sleep interval. When patients present with unexplained extraesophageal symptoms, such as chronic cough, uncontrolled nocturnal wheezing, or repeated pulmonary aspiration, dual pH monitoring may provide unique data concerning the role of GER in the pathogenesis of these symptoms. In most instances, ambulatory studies provide adequate information for clinical management. In certain circumstances, however, more precise information may be needed concerning specific responses to reflux or infused acid, necessitating a complete polysomnographic evaluation.

Gastroesophageal reflux (GER) is a common problem associated with considerable morbidity.[1] Studies have shown the highest incidence of esophagitis, as well as the most severe complications (erosion and stricture), to be associated with recumbent reflux that occurs during sleep, a situation permitting prolonged acid–mucosal contact.[2,3] This is presumably the result not only of an incompetent lower esophageal sphincter (LES) but of an inability effectively to clear the refluxed material. Poor clearance of acid from the esophagus and subsequent acid neutralization have been documented to be impaired during sleep.[4,5]

GER may be viewed as consisting of two components:

1. The retrograde flow of gastric contents through the antireflux barrier at the esophagogastric junction
2. The return of the acid gastric juice to the stomach and subsequent neutralization of the distal esophagus to a pH of 4 (i.e., *esophageal acid clearing*)

The critical parameter in determining the extent of GER, and its potential damage to the esophageal mucosa, is the percentage of time the esophagus is exposed to a pH lower than 4. In view of the previous research documenting the importance of sleep-related GER in the pathogenesis of reflux esophagitis, it is important to determine the percentage of acid contact time (ACT) at night, as well as during the day.

Postprandial reflux has been shown to be "physiologic" and, when confined to the postprandial interval, it is considered benign.[6] In determining the clinical significance of GER, it is important to assess the 24-hour pattern (see Chapter 107). Twenty-four–hour patterns of GER can be evaluated with commercially available devices. Two types of pH studies are described here: (1) ambulatory pH studies in which sleep monitoring does not occur, and (2) in-laboratory pH studies that include simultaneous pH monitoring with polysomnography (PSG). More recent developments include techniques that allow the assessment of both acidic and nonacidic reflux by impedance measurement.

AMBULATORY pH MONITORING

Ambulatory esophageal pH monitoring can be accomplished by using commercially available pH probes and portable data acquisition devices. The techniques are similar to those in Holter monitoring; the patient is intubated with either a glass- or antimony-tipped pH electrode, the output of which is attached to a small box (3.5-inch width × 7.25-inch length × 1-inch depth) that the patient wears either at the waist with a belt or across the shoulder with a shoulder strap.

Our laboratory specifically conducted a validation study of one of these units, which included simultaneous monitoring of input to the computer system and polygraphic tracing of the pH. Although this was not an ambulatory study, because the patient had to be tethered to a recording device, there was excellent agreement between the computer-detected reflux events and those detected by visual inspection from the paper tracing.[7]

The decision to use antimony or glass electrodes depends on a variety of factors; each has advantages and disadvantages. The glass electrode is somewhat more accurate and linear across a large pH range, whereas the antimony electrode is somewhat more durable. From a clinical standpoint, there is little difference between the two with regard to the accuracy of the data collected. These commercially available devices have internal calibration techniques that should be performed before every intubation.

For the best readings, the pH probe is placed 5 cm above the proximal border of the manometrically determined LES. The LES must be determined manometrically, which can be somewhat inconvenient because it may require two separate intubations (the first to determine the LES location and the second to insert the pH probe). However, a pH probe has been developed that allows LES determination and pH probe placement with a single intubation. Data have shown that an approximation of the ideal site can be accomplished by using pH determinations only. This method requires placing the pH probe distally until a clearly acidic (approximately 1.5 to 2.5) pH is established (indicating that the pH probe is in the stomach) and then slowly withdrawing the probe until the pH rises to approximately 4. At that point, the pH probe is most likely out of the stomach and in the esophagogastric junction. The probe is then withdrawn 5 to 7 cm above this level and affixed at that point. Although not as accurate as the manometric method of determination, for clinical purposes this is an acceptable placement method. This method, however, has been shown to be most problematic with regard to accuracy in patients who actually have substantial GER and most accurate in healthy volunteers.[8] Thus, whenever feasible, the manometric method should be used to locate the LES for accurate pH probe placement.

With the increasing clinical interest in establishing GER as the cause of a variety of extraesophageal symptoms such as bronchial asthma, chronic cough, laryngopharyngitis, and pulmonary aspiration, dual pH probe monitoring has become substantially more popular. It entails monitoring at least two sites in the esophagus: one at the standard site in the distal esophagus (placed as described earlier) and one in the more proximal esophagus. The exact location in the more proximal esophagus varies from the mid-esophagus to the pharynx, and there is little in the way of currently accepted standards as to the proximal probe placement. Studies have shown that proximal esophageal and pharyngeal acid exposure effectively discriminates individuals with posterior laryngitis.[9] Another study by Jacob and colleagues[10] has shown that supine (primarily during sleep) proximal acid exposure best discriminates patients with laryngeal symptoms from those with reflux esophagitis and healthy individuals.[10] These data would suggest that some proximal acid exposure has clinically significant correlates.

Dual pH probe monitoring assumes additional clinical significance in reviewing data from Koufman, who has shown in an animal model that even minute amounts of acid exposure can create cancerous lesions in the larynx.[11] In addition, numerous studies have shown that patients with aerodigestive symptoms such as chronic cough and pulmonary aspiration have greater proximal esophageal and pharyngeal acid exposure.[10,12,13] Although much work needs to be done to assess the importance of, and specific parameters relating to, proximal esophageal acid exposure in the pathogenesis of extraesophageal symptoms of reflux, it is clear that the trend is moving increasingly toward the use of dual pH monitoring.

Once the intubation has been accomplished, the patient is instructed concerning the operation of the data acquisition system. Patients may be given special dietary instructions to avoid acidic foods; in general, my preference is *not* to have the patient adopt a special diet. GER and heartburn are both significantly affected by dietary intake, and, therefore, a more accurate clinical picture of the frequency and severity of GER can be obtained if patients eat their usual meals. The patient completes a log to document significant events. The patient is instructed to indicate the start and end time of meals, time of going to sleep and waking up, time of medication intake, and time of occurrence of clinical symptoms. The patient is instructed to return to the laboratory approximately 24 hours from the time of departure.

On returning to the laboratory, the patient is extubated and the data are downloaded into a computer system that analyzes a variety of reflux parameters over the total recording interval. These parameters include number of reflux episodes, average duration of the reflux episodes, longest reflux episode, percentage of ACT, and a summary of these events according to upright (primarily waking) and supine (primarily sleeping) postures.

The computer printout summarizes the timing of meals, sleep, and clinical symptoms as well. This information allows the clinician to determine the relationship of symptoms to episodes of GER.

A technique for monitoring pH by wireless telemetry is also now available. The Medtronic Bravo pH monitoring system was recently approved for use in the United States. This pH system involves the attachment of a radiotelemetry pH capsule to the mucosal wall of the esophagus using a prepackaged assembly, which incorporates both a delivery system and the pH capsule. The capsule is oblong in shape ($6 \times 5.5 \times 25$ mm) and contains a well (4-mm diameter, 3.5-mm in depth) for delivery, antimony pH electrode and reference electrode, and an internal battery and transmitter. The pH capsule sends a data signal to the external receiver by radiofrequency telemetry. Using endoscopic measurement, the pH probe is positioned 6 cm above the squamocolumnar junction, which approximates the placement method targeting a position 5 cm proximal to the upper margin of LES, as is typically used in conventional pH recordings.[14] The wireless pH monitoring system has demonstrated usefulness by successfully recording up to 2 days in 89% of all enrolled subjects.[15] The Bravo system has been shown to have minimal impact on daily acidity as well as diet. It is a viable option for patients who are unwilling or unable to undergo conventional pH studies using a transnasally placed pH electrode, and who will be undergoing endoscopy or part of an evaluation for gastroesophageal reflux disease (GERD).

The power of the wireless pH recording system in distinguishing patients with esophagitis from control subjects has been demonstrated to be comparable to that obtained using conventional pH monitoring system.[15-17] In fact, the discriminative power of the wireless pH study is comparable with that of the conventional pH monitoring system when data from the first 24-hour recording are used, but its sensitivity is improved if data from the worst day of the 48-hour recording are used. It takes advantage of the observation that esophageal acid exposure can exhibit day-to-day variability.[18] The comparable ability of the wireless pH system was also observed in discriminating endoscopy-negative GERD from control subjects. However, in this patient population, there was no significant improvement in sensitivity or specificity using data from the worst day of the 48-hour recording.[15] This is likely because excessive acid exposure is one of several pathophysiologic factors contributing to nonerosive GERD, in which hypersensitivity to acid reflux and symptoms may occur without pathologic acid reflux.[19] Although more work needs to be done on symptom analysis, the wireless pH monitoring system using 48-hour recording may be particularly beneficial in the diagnosis of nonerosive GERD by increasing the possibility of documenting an association between symptoms and reflux over a longer duration of recording.

Multichannel intraluminal impedance (MII) has been introduced as a new technique to study esophageal motility and the reflux of gastric contents (both acidic and nonacidic) based on differences in conductivity to alternating current of intraluminal contents.[20] Impedance is the average electric resistance between two adjacent electrodes and is measured using a specialized, 2.1-mm diameter catheter consisting of a series of cylindrical electrodes that make up measuring segments, each 2 cm in length, corresponding to one recording channel. The impedance between the two electrodes is inversely proportional to the electrical conductivity and the cross-sectional area of the material through which the current must travel. If a highly conductive bolus arrives at the measuring segment (i.e., saliva), impedance decreases, and the opposite occurs with a resistive bolus (i.e., air). In addition, increasing the luminal diameter (i.e., arrival of bolus into the measuring segment) results in an impedance drop, whereas a luminal narrowing (i.e., contraction wave) causes an impedance increase. Studies have indicated that MII can be used as a discriminative test of esophageal function for evaluating bolus transport.[21] It has been shown that combining MII with esophageal manometry (MII-EM) allows simultaneous measurement of intra-esophageal pressure and bolus movement.[22] These data would suggest that combined MII-EM is a more sensitive tool in assessing esophageal function compared with standard manometry because impedance can distinguish different bolus transit patterns.

The use of MII allows determination of the direction of bolus movement in the esophagus. Progression of impedance changes from distal to proximal is indicative of retrograde bolus movement, as found in GER. MII allows for prolonged monitoring and detection of bolus presence independent of the chemical (i.e., pH) composition, as well as detection of the proximal migration of the refluxate. In combined MII-pH monitoring, the pH sensor is used to define whether the refluxate is acid or nonacid based on predefined criteria. Combined MMI-EM-pH has been used to study the patterns of gas and liquid reflux in adults or patients with GERD.[23-25] Using this approach in subjects in the sitting position, Sifrim and colleagues have shown that patients with GERD had more acid reflux, less nonacid reflux, and higher proportions of pure liquid reflux compared with healthy subjects.[24,25]

MII is able to detect small volumes of liquid reflux of more neutral pH that are not detected by the traditional pH sensor. MII combined with pH monitoring allows the detection of most reflux episodes: very acid (pH below 4), moderately acid (pH 4 to 6), and nonacid (pH between 6 and 7). A pH drop below 4 is usually indicative of acidic GER. All other reflux events could be categorized as nonacidic reflux. The pathophysiologic relevance of nonacidic reflux in GERD is still unknown, but previous data suggest that it does not play a role in the development of esophageal mucosal damage because there is no difference in the patterns of nonacidic reflux between patients with GERD and healthy control subjects.[26] However, nonacidic reflux might be more important as a cause of persistent symptoms on acid-suppressant therapy[27] or in patients with endoscopy-negative GERD. Nonacidic reflux episodes in the most proximal impedance segment have been shown to be less frequent than traditional acid reflux episodes, both in patients with GERD and control subjects.[28]

POLYSOMNOGRAPHIC RECORDING

In certain circumstances, a PSG recording during pH monitoring may be desirable. For example, there may be specific interest in the possibility that a patient is having sleep-related reflux and pulmonary aspiration. In addition, nocturnal recordings of reflux or the clearance time of externally infused acid may identify individuals who are at high risk for pulmonary aspiration. Such individuals are specifically identified by prolonged clearance of spontaneous reflux or infused acid associated with poor arousal responses from sleep. Furthermore, it may be clinically useful to note whether reflux

itself is triggered by periodic arousal responses as a result of disturbed sleep. Such a relationship (i.e., sleep-related reflux preceded by a brief arousal response) has been reported.[29]

Electrode placement is as described for ambulatory studies. A reference lead is placed on the ventral surface of the forearm or the forehead. The reference lead and the pH probe should always be recorded through an electrical isolation box attached to the pH meter. Any commercially available pH meter is suitable, but it must have an external output to allow polygraphic recording. The output needs to be in a range of 0 to 1 V for most direct-current amplifiers. This measurement is made simultaneously with the standard polygraphic measurements for monitoring sleep (i.e., electroencephalogram, electrooculogram, electromyogram, electrocardiogram).

Reflux is defined by a drop in the pH of the distal esophagus below a level of 4. Clearance is arbitrarily defined by a return of the esophageal pH to 4. The time between the drop in the pH below 4 and its return to 4 is referred to as the *clearing duration* or *clearance interval*. A pH of 4 has been arbitrarily chosen as the criterion to determine a reflux event because the esophageal pH level is routinely between 5.5 and 6.5. Thus, in order for the pH to drop below 4, it is assumed that the electrode must be in contact with acid. Furthermore, there is little if any peptic activity associated with a pH of 4, although such activity increases logarithmically as the pH decreases below 4.

With regard to evaluating esophageal function during sleep, we have chosen to focus on the patient's ability to clear infused acid from the esophagus. This method has several advantages. First, spontaneous reflux during sleep—even in symptomatic patients with esophagitis—is relatively infrequent and unpredictable. Second, important parameters such as when the event occurs and the volume of the refluxate are uncontrolled with spontaneous reflux. Our method was designed to evaluate reflux by simulating an event using a controlled infusion of a specified volume at a specific point in time (i.e., waking versus a particular stage of sleep). Although this method does not allow the study of the effects of physiologic reflux, it does allow the control of the other critical factors. Although acidity per se does not necessarily produce mucosal damage, we assume that the arousal response from sleep is the result of the afferent stimulus caused by the low pH.

Volume is an important parameter in producing arousal responses, and it is therefore important to take this variable into consideration in evaluating reflux during sleep. For example, studies in our laboratory have shown that acid clearance and arousal responses are markedly altered by the volume infused into the esophagus.[30] Other obvious advantages of performing sleep studies relate to the determination of important responses to esophageal acidification such as polygraphic arousal responses and swallowing responses. These are important parameters with regard to acid clearance (assuming normal esophageal motor function) that cannot be assessed by 24-hour ambulatory studies.

The schematic diagram in Figure 123–1 illustrates the parameters that are obtained from a single infusion of a controlled volume of acid. The acid clearance time is determined as the interval of time elapsing between the drop in pH to 4 until the pH returns to 4 or 5. The arousal response latency is the elapsed time from a pH drop to 4 until polygraphic evidence of an arousal response. The latency to the first swallow is defined as the elapsed time from the drop in pH to 4 until the

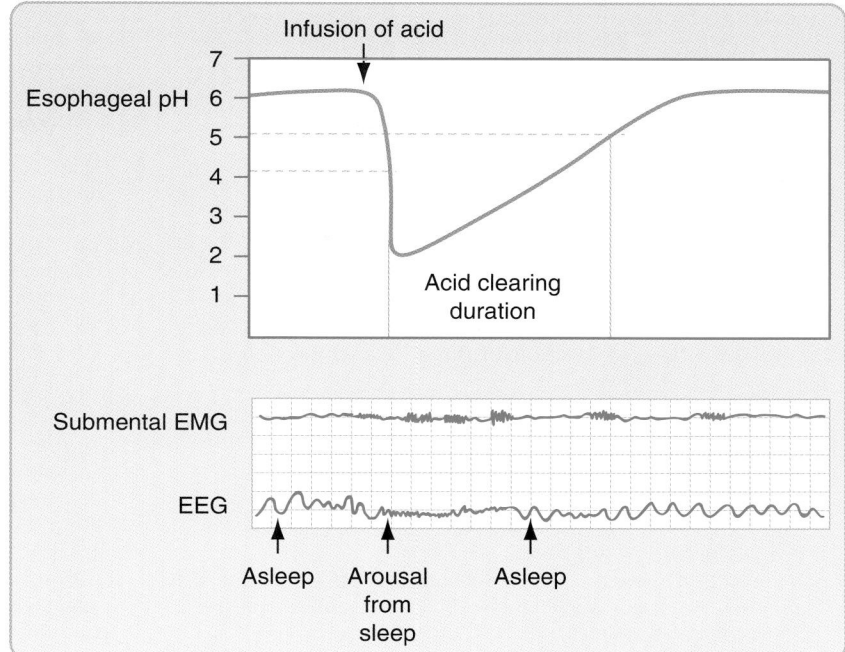

Figure 123–1. Schematic representation of the acid infusion paradigm. As with spontaneous gastroesophageal reflux, the duration of acid clearing is determined as the time from the drop in pH below 4 until the pH reaches 5 (in some studies the value is 4). EEG, electroencephalogram; EMG, electromyogram.

first swallow, defined as a transient burst of muscle activity from the submental electromyogram recording. Studies in our laboratory have determined normal parameters for these measures.[4,5]

CLINICAL INTERPRETATION

GERD is a complex, multifactorial disorder involving not only physiologic mechanisms that determine the retrograde flow of acid contents from the stomach into the esophagus but anatomic aspects of mucosal resistance.[1,31] Current diagnostic methodology confines itself only to evaluating GER and mucosal–esophageal ACT. Important aspects of the pathogenesis of esophagitis, such as hydrogen ion back-diffusion, constituents of the acid contents of the stomach (i.e., pepsin, bile salts, and pancreatic enzymes), and esophageal mucosal potential difference are not routinely available for evaluation in patients. As noted earlier, however, the 24-hour ambulatory pH study allows the clinician to assess a number of parameters thought to be important in the development of esophagitis.

Clinically, the most important parameters relate to the total percentage of ACT, percentage of ACT in the upright and supine positions, longest reflux episode, and number of reflux episodes longer than 5 minutes. The assessment of each of these parameters and the extent to which they occur in the waking state versus sleep are all clinically relevant. Normal parameters for reflux events have been published in a number of sources and have been reviewed by de Caestecker.[32]

Clinical interpretation of these studies is, to a large extent, subjective, but most experts agree that the most important parameter is ACT. For a normal individual, total ACT is usually between 4% and 6%. An ACT of 8% or more is considered a clinically significant elevation. If the majority of ACT occurs in the sleeping interval or if the sleeping ACT exceeds 4% to 5%, however, the clinical impact is considerably greater. This clinical difference occurs because patients who are susceptible to

sleep-related reflux have prolonged acid clearance associated with episodes of reflux during sleep, and such episodes are thought to be more damaging to the esophageal mucosa than short waking episodes, even if the latter are more numerous.[3,6]

With regard to pH studies conducted as part of a PSG evaluation, several variables are clinically important. First, the occurrence of spontaneous GER needs to be documented by identifying each time the esophageal pH drops below 4. The length of the subsequent arousal latency response is also significant. For example, an arousal response that is delayed beyond 2 to 3 minutes might indicate some alteration in arousal mechanisms. A prolongation of the arousal latency or the acid clearance time suggests that the individual may be at risk for pulmonary aspiration. Also of considerable clinical significance is the association of multiple short awakenings with repeated reflux events, which might suggest that fragmented sleep may be contributing to a complaint of daytime sleepiness.

As with the ambulatory studies, the percentage of time the esophageal pH is below 4 is relevant, as is the number of spontaneous episodes of reflux. Healthy individuals rarely have reflux during sleep; thus, the spontaneous occurrence of GER during sleep is an important clinical event. Having more than two to three episodes a night is clinically significant, particularly if any one of these events is associated with prolonged ACT (longer than 5 to 10 minutes). An acid exposure time exceeding 4% to 5% during sleep probably represents a clinically significant finding, and nocturnal acid suppression would be an appropriate approach to treatment.

There are minimal normative data with regard to proximal acid exposure. Because there is no standardization with regard to the placement of the proximal probe, it is impossible to describe normative values across a large population of patients. In general, this is done in each laboratory, where a standardized procedure is used. Most useful information with regard to normative data in the proximal esophagus is described in a review article by Richter.[33] In general, most studies in which control data have been collected describe proximal acid contact time in healthy individuals to be between 0% and 1%.[33]

> *Clinical Pearl*
>
> *Esophageal pH monitoring may be helpful in explaining symptoms suggestive of unexplained arousals from sleep resulting in complaints of insomnia or daytime sleepiness because nocturnal GER may be an underlying contributing factor. In addition, nocturnal GER may be the cause of exacerbations of bronchial asthma and repeated pulmonary infections as a result of pulmonary aspiration of refluxed gastric contents.*

REFERENCES

1. Richter JE, Bradley LA, Castell DO: Esophageal chest pain: Current controversies in pathogenesis, diagnosis and therapy. Ann Intern Med 1989;110:66-78.
2. Johnson LF, DeMeester TR: Twenty-four hour pH monitoring of the distal esophagus, a quantitative measure of gastroesophageal reflux. Am J Gastroenterol 1974;62:325-332.
3. Johnson LF, DeMeester TR, Haggitt RC: Esophageal epithelial response to gastroesophageal reflux, a quantitative study. Am J Dig Dis 1978;23:478-509.
4. Orr WC, Robinson MG, Johnson LF: Acid clearing during sleep in the pathogenesis of reflux esophagitis. Dig Dis Sci 1981;26:423.
5. Orr WC, Johnson LF, Robinson MC: The effect of sleep on swallowing, esophageal peristalsis, and acid clearance. Gastroenterology 1984;86:814-819.
6. DeMeester TR, Johnson LF, Guy JJ, et al: Patterns of gastroesophageal reflux in health and disease. Ann Surg 1976;184:459-470.
7. Allen M, Woodruff D, Robinson MG, et al: Validation of an ambulatory esophageal pH monitoring system. Am J Gastroenterol 1988;83:287-290.
8. Klauser AG, Schindlbeck NE, Muller-Lissner SA: Esophageal 24-pH monitoring: Is prior manometry necessary for correct positioning of the electrode? Am J Gastroenterol 1990;85:1463-1467.
9. Shaker R, Milbrath M, Ren J, et al: Esophagopharyngeal distribution of refluxed gastric acid in patients with reflux laryngitis. Gastroenterology 1995;109:1575-1582.
10. Jacob P, Kahrilas PJ, Herzon G: Proximal esophageal pH-metry in patients with "reflux laryngitis." Gastroenterology 1991;11:305-310.
11. Koufman JA: The otolaryngologic manifestations of gastroesophageal reflux disease (GERD): A clinical investigation of 225 patients using ambulatory 24-hour pH monitoring and an experimental investigation of the role of acid and pepsin in the development of laryngeal injury. Laryngoscope 1991;101:1-78.
12. Patti MG, Debas HT, Pellegrini CA: Esophageal manometry and 24-hour pH monitoring in the diagnosis of pulmonary aspiration secondary to gastroesophageal reflux. Am J Surg 1992; 163:401-406.
13. Paterson WG, Murat BW: Combined ambulatory esophageal manometry and dual-probe pH-metry in evaluation of patients with chronic unexplained cough. Dig Dis Sci 1994;39:1117-1125.
14. Kahrilas PJ, Lin S, Chen J, Manka M: The effect of hiatus hernia on gastro-oesophageal junction pressure. Gut 1999;44:476-482.
15. Pandolfino JE, Richter JE, Ours T, et al: Ambulatory esophageal pH monitoring using a wireless system. Am J Gastroenterol 2003;98:740-749.
16. Johnson F, Joelsson B, Isberg PE: Ambulatory 24-hour intra-esophageal pH-monitoring in the diagnosis of gastroesophageal reflux disease. Gut 1987;28:1145-1150.
17. Matioli S, Pilotti V, Spangaro M, et al: Reliability of 24-hour home esophageal pH monitoring in diagnosis of gastroesophageal reflux. Dig Dis Sci 1989;34:71-78.
18. Wiener GJ, Morgan TM, Copper JB, et al: Ambulatory 24-hour esophageal pH monitoring: Reproducibility and variability of pH parameters. Dig Dis Sci 1988;33:1127-1133.
19. Shi G, Bruley des Varannes S, Scarpignato C, et al: Reflux related symptoms in patients with normal oesophageal exposure to acid. Gut 1995;37:457-464.
20. Silay J: Intraluminal multiple electric impedance procedure for measurements of gastrointestinal motility. J Gastrointest Motil 1991;3:151-162.
21. Srinivasan R, Vela MF, Katz PO, et al: Esophageal function testing using multichannel intraluminal impedance. Am J Physiol 2001;289:G457-G462.
22. Tutuian R, Vela MF, Balaji NS, et al: Esophageal function testing with combined multichannel intraluminal impedance and manometry: Multicenter study in healthy volunteers. Clin Gastroenterol Hepatol 2003;1:174-182.
23. Sifrim D, Silny J, Holloway RH, Janssens JJ: Patterns of gas and liquid reflux during transient lower oesophageal sphincter relaxation: A study using intraluminal electrical impedance. Gut 1999; 44:47-54.
24. Sifrim D, Holloway R: Transient lower esophageal sphincter relaxations: How many or how harmful? Am J Gastroenterol 2001;96:2529-2532.
25. Sifrim D, Holloway R, Silny J, et al: Composition of the postprandial refluxate in patients with gastroesophageal reflux disease. Am J Gastroenterol 2001;98:647-655.
26. Sifrim D, Holloway R, Silny J, et al: Acid, non-acid, and gas reflux in patients with gastroesophageal reflux disease during ambulatory 24-hour pH impedance recordings. Gastroenterology 2001;120:1588-1598.
27. Vela MF, Camacho-Lobato L, Srinivasan R, et al: Simultaneous intraesophageal impedance and pH measurement of acid and non-acid gastroesophageal reflux: Effect of omeprazole. Gastroenterology 2001;120:1599-1606.
28. Sifrim D, Tack J, Lerut T, Janssens J: Transient lower esophageal sphincter relaxations and esophageal body muscular contractile response in reflux esophagitis. Dig Dis Sci 2000;45:1293-1300.
29. Dent J, Dodds WJ, Friedman RH, et al: Mechanism of gastroesophageal reflux in recumbent asymptomatic human subjects. J Clin Invest 1980;65:256-267.
30. Orr WC, Robinson MG, Johnson LF: The effect of esophageal acid volume on arousals from sleep and acid clearance. Chest 1991;99:351-354.
31. Johnson LF, Harmon JW: Experimental esophagitis in a rabbit model: clinical relevance. J Clin Gastroenterol 1986;8(Suppl 1):26-44.
32. de Caestecker JS: Twenty-four-hour oesophageal pH monitoring: Advances and controversies. Neth J Med 1989;34:S20-S39.
33. Richter JE: Ambulatory esophageal pH monitoring. Am J Med 1997;103:130S-134S.

124

Actigraphy

Sonia Ancoli-Israel

ABSTRACT

Wrist actigraphy is based on the fact that during sleep there is little movement activity, whereas during wake there is increased movement. Wrist actigraphy has the advantages of being cost efficient, of allowing the recording of sleep in the natural environment, of recording behavior that occurs both during the night and during the day, and of recording for long time periods. Although actigraphy is not a replacement for electroencephalography or polysomnography, there are times when it provides clear advantages for data collection. Actigraphy is particularly useful for studying individuals who cannot tolerate sleeping in the laboratory—for example, patients with the complaint of insomnia, small children, and older adults. It may provide a more accurate estimate of typical sleep durations by providing an opportunity for patients to adhere more closely to their customary sleep and wake times. Actigraphy is also becoming an important tool in follow-up studies and for examining efficacy in clinical outcome. It has some value in the assessment of sleep disorders, although it may not help in distinguishing between different sleep disorders.

The newer scoring algorithms have great accuracy in determining the variables that are most important in insomnia—that is, they have improved ability to detect wake versus sleep, sleep latency, awakenings during the night, and total sleep time. Actigraphy is superior to sleep logs particularly in detecting brief arousals during the night. It can also be used for the evaluation and clinical diagnosis of circadian rhythm disorders. The ability to detect movements holds promise in the identification of sleep disorders characterized by frequent movements, such as periodic limb movements during sleep, sleep apnea, or rapid eye movement sleep behavior disorders. The ability to measure for long time periods makes actigraphy particularly useful in situations where long-term changes in sleep are of interest. Actigraphy is (1) reliable and valid for detecting sleep in healthy populations, but less reliable for detecting disturbed sleep; (2) a useful adjunct to the routine evaluation of insomnia, circadian rhythm disorders, and excessive sleepiness, and helpful in the diagnosis of periodic limb movements during sleep and restless legs syndrome; and (3) useful in special populations such as children or older adults who are demented.

The gold standard for the evaluation of sleep is polysomnography (PSG) with a minimum of electroencephalogram (EEG), electrooculogram (EOG), and submentalis electromyogram (EMG) recordings. Other physiologic variables are added depending on the patient's sleep complaints (e.g., respiration, heart rate, tibialis muscle movement, oximetry). PSG thus allows the collection of detailed information. The EEG, EOG, and EMG records can be scored for stages of sleep (non–rapid eye movement [non-REM] stages 1 to 4, REM), total sleep time, total wake time, sleep onset latency, and percent time in REM as opposed to non-REM sleep.

This information is very important for certain types of evaluations; however, the PSG recording process may disturb a patient's sleep and is often very costly both to record and to score. In addition, PSG provides data about sleep episodes only during the time of recording, which often is 6 to 10 hours long. Because recordings are generally done during the major sleep period, little information is available about daytime (waking) or napping behavior. In some instances, it is not essential to know the specific stage of sleep or the status of other physiologic variables but only whether the person is awake or asleep.

Actigraphy is much less expensive than PSG, and records 24 hours of activity, from which wake and sleep can be scored. Actigraphs (or actimeters) record limb movement. Traditionally, the actigraphs are placed on a wrist, although sometimes activity from the leg is recorded. The data collected are displayed on a computer and are examined for activity/inactivity and analyzed for wake/sleep. This chapter will review the development of actigraphy, the major areas where it can be used, tips for its successful use, and its limitations.

BACKGROUND

Wrist activity technology is based on the fact that during sleep there is little movement, whereas during wake there is increased movement. Although activity monitors had been around for many years,[1] the laboratories of Kupfer, Colburn, and Kripke were among the first to use activity to differentiate wake from sleep. The initial models, developed in the early 1970s by Kupfer and colleagues, were self-contained activity counters with integrated circuits and memory that provided off-line data retrieval.[2,3] At about the same time, Colburn and colleagues developed a similar actigraph with different transducers and timing devices.[4] Kripke and his colleagues were among the first to publish reliability data on the use of wrist actigraphy for the assessment of sleep.[5-8] Several years later, other actigraphs were developed by Redmond and Hegge,[9] and by Borbély and colleagues.[10,11] The analogue actigraphs were small but used telemetry or needed to be attached to a Medilog recorder, and they were hand scored. The first digital actigraphs were about half the size of a chalkboard eraser, and computer algorithms were written for automatic scoring of sleep and wake.

Most contemporary actigraphs, coming after the advent of microprocessors and miniaturization, have a movement detector (such as an accelerometer) and sufficient memory to record for long periods. The only time the actigraph needs to be removed is during bathing or swimming, although many models now available are water resistant, thus allowing for nearly continuous 24-hour recordings for several days or weeks. Newer models are the size of a wristwatch and collect digitized data. Physical movement is generally sampled several times per second and stored in 1-minute epochs, although sampling and epoch rates can be set by the clinician or investigator. The digitized data are then translated into a numeric representation and stored until downloaded to a computer.

The way the analogue signal is digitized varies with the actigraph, and sometimes it can be chosen by the user. As described in a recent review by Ancoli-Israel et al., the three ways that signals can be digitized are time above threshold, zero crossing, and integration[12] (Fig. 124–1). Time above threshold counts the amount of time per epoch that the motion signal is above a given threshold, typically 0.1 to 0.2 g. However, neither the amplitude of the signal nor the acceleration of the movement is reflected in this strategy. The zero-crossing method counts the number of times per epoch that the signal crosses zero. In this strategy, once again neither the amplitude nor the acceleration is taken into account, and high-frequency artifact can potentially be counted as movement. Digital integration, on the other hand, samples the accelerometry output signal at a high rate and then, for each epoch, calculates the area under the curve. This reflects the amplitude and acceleration of the signal but does not reflect its duration or frequency. In studies comparing the three methodologies, digital integration was best for identifying movement amplitude, followed by time

TIME ABOVE THRESHOLD

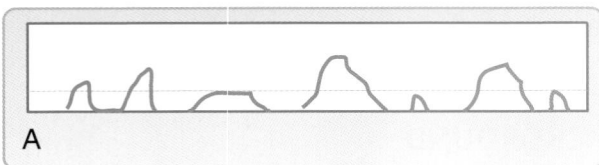

ZERO CROSSING

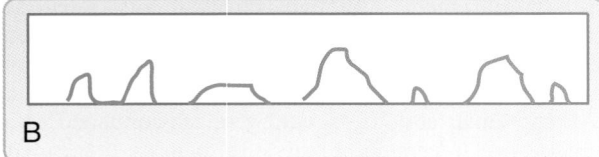

DIGITAL INTEGRATION

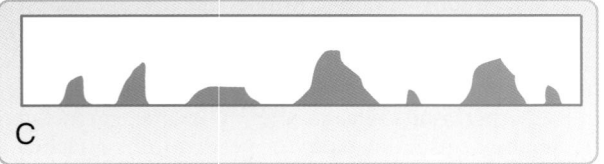

Figure 124–1. Three methods of deriving activity counts in actigraphy. **A,** Time above threshold derives the amount of time per epoch that the activity is above some defined threshold (represented by the *thin blue line*). **B,** Zero crossing counts the number of times the activity reaches zero (represented by the *solid baseline*). **C,** Digital integration calculates the area under the curves, represented by *dark blue shading.* (Reprinted with permission from Ancoli-Israel S, Cole R, Alessi C, et al: The role of actigraphy in the study of sleep and circadian rhythms. Sleep 2003;26:342-392.)

above threshold and zero crossing.[13] Some newer actigraphs utilize more than one method, thus decreasing the deficits of each method alone.

Once the data are digitized, computer algorithms are used to automatically score wake and sleep and provide the user with summary statistics. These computer algorithms generally supply information on total sleep time, percent of time spent asleep, total wake time, percent of time spent awake, number of awakenings, time between awakenings, and sleep onset latency.[7,12,14] The use of actigraphy in sleep disorders medicine has gained popularity. Research has compared the reliability of actigraphy and that of EEG for distinguishing wake from sleep. Results vary depending on the populations studied and on the actigraph and scoring software used. Most studies agree that actigraphy data correlate well with PSG data, particularly in normal sleep, where reliability coefficients have ranged from 0.89 to 0.98.[5,12,15,16] Correlations are somewhat lower for severely disturbed sleep. For example, in patients in sleep disorders clinics, reliability ranges from 0.78 to 0.88.[17-19] In infants and in children, the reliability ranges from 0.90 to 0.95.[20,21] Although total sleep time correlates well with EEG, the actigraphy data do not necessarily correlate well on a minute-by-minute basis, particularly if sleep is very disturbed.

Ancoli-Israel and colleagues[22] compared actigraphy to sleep and wake EEG in demented nursing home patients. Correlations with total sleep time were 0.91 for averaged activity (i.e., the average activity recorded per minute) and 0.81 for maximal activity (i.e., the maximal activity recorded per minute). Given the problems with obtaining EEG recordings in demented patients, the authors concluded that actigraphy is the more feasible approach for studying wake and sleep in this population.

Most studies are in agreement that, with correct use, the actigraph is reliable for certain populations. Actigraphs with different algorithms are now commercially available; therefore, reliability has become a major question. Each actigraph needs its own reliability studies, and results from one population may not generalize to other populations. Cole and colleagues[15] concluded, however, that even algorithms based on different mathematical principles had similar reliabilities. Sadeh and colleagues,[23] in a review of actigraphy, concluded that the validation studies for healthy subjects show greater than 90% agreement and are very promising. However, to date, there has been no head-to-head comparison between different actigraphs; therefore, no conclusion can be drawn about which method of collecting and scoring data is more valid than PSG.[12]

Wrist actigraphy can be used to record continuously for long periods, so behavior occurring both during the night and during the day can be studied in the patient's home environment. This is particularly useful when examining sleep of patients complaining of insomnia, because their sleep can vary from night to night and is easily disturbed by novel environments. The actigraph economically allows a pattern of difficulty sleeping to be seen. The resulting data are similar to those of a sleep diary, but the actigraphy data are continuous and objective rather than discrete and subjective.

Another advantage of collecting data over long periods is the ability to examine the circadian rhythms of the sleep or activity cycle, particularly in studies of patients with sleep–wake schedule disorders (e.g., jet lag, shift work, and advanced or delayed sleep phase). Cosinor analyses, including the computation of the mesor, the amplitude, and the acrophase, are possible. These analyses can be computed from 24 hours of data; however, a longer time period of data recording provides more accurate cosinor analyses.

The wrist actigraph is often valuable for studying individuals who would have difficulty sleeping in a sleep laboratory or with the wires associated with traditional PSG, such as insomniacs, children, and older adults who are demented. Furthermore, in the last group, it is difficult to distinguish wake from sleep with an EEG.[24] Actigraphy avoids both these problems, enabling the recording of sleep–wake activity in an easy, unobtrusive manner.

Some actigraphs record both activity and light exposure (for example, the Actillume by Ambulatory Monitoring, Inc., or the Actiwatch-L by Mini-Mitter Co., Inc.). Some devices also have the ability to record core body temperature, allowing both clinical and investigational studies of circadian rhythms in the home environment. Most actigraphs have event buttons that subjects can push when, for example, they turn out the lights.

The concurrent recording of light exposure enables the investigator to determine when the lights were turned off as well as when the sun begins to rise. This is helpful in studies of advanced and delayed sleep phase, when the amount and duration of light a person is normally exposed to needs to be determined. For example, several studies using activity monitors that also record light exposure have found that healthy older adults are exposed to only 58 minutes of bright light per day,[25] patients with Alzheimer's disease living at home are exposed to 30 minutes,[26] and patients in nursing homes are exposed to only 1.7 minutes.[27] These data are useful in understanding the changes that occur in sleep in these populations and can be used to devise treatment programs.

There are still many unknowns about how the environment affects activity recordings. Sadeh and coworkers[23] suggest that the bed surface (e.g., waterbed) and presence of a bed partner may affect the activity signal. Additional research is needed in these areas.

CLINICAL APPLICATIONS OF WRIST ACTIGRAPHY

Actigraphy has been used to help in the diagnosis of sleep disorders—for example, in large studies of sleep apnea, periodic limb movements during sleep (PLMS), and insomnia (as described later), and in case studies of fatal familial insomnia,[28] REM sleep behavior disorder,[29] non–24-hour sleep–wake syndrome,[30] and posttraumatic delayed sleep phase syndrome.[31] Because actigraphy is unobtrusive and can record for many days and nights, it is a useful tool in the evaluation of insomnia, the symptoms of which can vary from night to night. In addition, actigraphy eliminates laboratory effects, as patients can be recorded sleeping in their own beds in their own homes. However, the convenience of actigraphy must be weighed against the relative reliability and validity of PSG.[12]

The American Academy of Sleep Medicine has updated recommendations on the use of actigraphy in clinical assessment of sleep disorders.[32] They concluded that actigraphy is reliable and valid for detecting sleep in healthy populations but less reliable for assessing disturbed sleep. Actigraphy is a useful adjunct to the routine evaluation of insomnia, circadian rhythm disorders, and excessive sleepiness, and it helps in the diagnosis of PLMS and restless legs syndrome. They also concluded that actigraphy is useful in special populations such as children or older adults who are demented.

A complete description of studies using actigraphy can be found in Ancoli-Israel et al.[12] Here, the major issues involved with the use of actigraphy in sleep disorders medicine will be described. See Figures 66–2 to 66–5 for examples.

Insomnia

Several recent studies used actigraphy to evaluate sleep in the patient with insomnia, yet few of them validated the actigraphy findings with PSG. In an analysis of previously published data, Chambers[33] concluded that actigraphy is useful for assessing sleep variability and treatment effects. Although actigraphy cannot determine the etiology of insomnia, it can help evaluate the severity. In patients with insomnia, the most difficult distinctions for the actigraph to recognize are the transitions between sleep and wake and the ultrashort sleep–wake cycles. In patients with insomnia secondary to circadian rhythm disturbances, actigraphy can detect sleep phase alterations.

Sleep Apnea

Actigraphy cannot determine the presence or absence of breathing abnormalities. However, because patients with sleep apnea have more disrupted sleep and thus more body movements, several studies have been conducted on the efficacy of wrist activity in recognizing patients with sleep apnea, with some conflicting results. Aubert-Tulkens and coworkers[34] used wrist activity to obtain a movement index and a fragmentation index during sleep in patients with sleep apnea and in controls. Those with sleep apnea had significantly higher movement and fragmentation indices. Once treatment was begun, activity recordings showed decreased indices, indicating successful treatment. Sadeh et al.[20] also found that activity measures of sleep differentiated patients with sleep apnea from those with insomnia and from controls.

Middelkoop and colleagues[35] conducted an epidemiologic study of 116 subjects who reported snoring habitually, experienced excessive daytime sleepiness, or had a spousal report of respiratory cessations. Both wrist activity and respiration (oronasal thermistry) were recorded for 1 night in the subject's home. Results indicated that patients with an apnea index greater than 5 events per hour of sleep had higher movement and higher fragmentation indices than those with an apnea index less than 5.

In general, studies have concluded that actigraphy may be capable of distinguishing healthy subjects from those with moderate or severe sleep apnea, particularly because actigraphy is more sensitive than sleep logs in identifying brief awakenings, but that it is unlikely that a distinction could be made between different types of sleep disorders that cause brief arousals.[12] The real value of actigraphy in sleep apnea is in combination with stand-alone devices—that is, with recording equipment used to screen for sleep apnea without measures of wake or sleep. The addition of an actigraph to such a recording allows one to determine if all respiratory events actually occurred during sleep.

Periodic Limb Movements during Sleep

PLMS is generally evaluated by measuring the EMG at the tibialis muscle. Because leg movement is the primary characteristic of this disorder, actigraphy's ability to measure movement is thought to be an advantage. Kazenwasel and coworkers[36] found high reliability between tibialis EMG and actigraphy for the number of leg movements per hour of sleep. Because PLMS can vary greatly from night to night, actigraphy, which easily records for multiple nights, may give a better assessment. Actigraphy tends to underestimate the frequency of leg movements during sleep, however, which limits its diagnostic value.[12] Several studies have suggested that actigraphy is useful in the assessment of treatment efficacy.[37,38]

Treatment Effects

Actigraphy is particularly appropriate in the study of treatment effects, as it can identify changes over time. In a study of insomnia in older adults, Brooks and colleagues[18] used actigraphy to examine treatment effects of sleep restriction therapy and found the actigraph sufficiently sensitive to detect effects of therapy. The authors concluded that because actigraphy is less invasive and less expensive than PSG, it is a promising device for assessing treatment effects. Chambers,[33] in a critical evaluation, also concluded actigraphy, with its night-to-night reliability, is especially appropriate for assessing changes in sleep after treatment. Others have used actigraphy to measure the effects of drugs treatments on sleep.[39-44] These data suggest that, for some patients, actigraphy can be used as a screening device before the more expensive PSG is ordered. It also can be used for follow-up once treatment has begun or after the termination of treatment.

Circadian Rhythms

Actigraphy allows the study of rhythms occurring over many days, so it is well suited for the study of circadian rhythms. See Figure 58–2 for examples. Activity is a valid marker of entrained PSG sleep phase and correlates strongly with entrained endogenous circadian phase.[12] It is also useful in identifying sleep that has been disturbed by circadian rhythm changes.

Mormont et al.[45] used actigraphy to study circadian rhythms and sleep–wake cycles in patients with cancer, as a preliminary step toward the advancement of chronotherapy. Studies have also examined sleep schedules of adolescents,[46] shift workers,[47,48] flight crews,[49] and jet lag.[42]

A variety of methodologies can be used to analyze circadian parameters of activity,[50-54] but no studies have compared methodologies, and, to date, no standard methodology has been accepted.

Pediatrics

Increasing numbers of studies have been published that used actigraphy in children, particularly those with behavioral, psychiatric, or neurologic problems. Actigraphy has been used successfully to characterize the sleep of infants,[55] of developmental differences,[56] and of children with autism,[57] and to demonstrate differences in sleep between children with depression, abused children, and unaffected children.[58] Sadeh[59] used wrist activity to study treatment effects on the sleep patterns of 50 infants whose parents complained of sleep disturbances in their children. Objective activity recordings were compared with parental reports. The activity records showed that percent sleep increased and the number of awakenings during the night decreased with behavioral treatments. By examining data from each successive night, Sadeh determined that most changes occurred during the first night of intervention. In addition, parental subjective reports significantly differed from objective actigraphy on quality of sleep, with parents reporting fewer awakenings during the night. The objective measures allow an evaluation of activity during sleep that would be missed by observation alone.

Older Adults

At the other end of the age spectrum, actigraphy has been used to study sleep–wake patterns of older adults, who are particularly susceptible to sleep complaints secondary to circadian rhythm changes, sleep-disordered breathing, PLMS, medical illness, and medication use.[60] Although some of these complaints can be examined in the laboratory, older adults are often more comfortable in their customary surroundings, or they need to stay home to take care of a spouse.

Van Hilten and colleagues[61] examined the influence of age on nocturnal behavior in 100 healthy older adults who wore an activity monitor for 6 consecutive days and nights. The authors concluded that without illness, age itself has only marginal effects on nocturnal activity and immobility (i.e., sleep and wake). This type of study could not have been done in the laboratory without an isolation unit, and even then it is unlikely that 100 subjects could have been studied. The only way this large-scale study could have been accomplished was with the use of actigraphy.

In the same group of subjects, van Hilten et al.[62] also examined the night-to-night and intrasubject variability of actigraphy. Results indicated that the first-night effect, typical of laboratory sleep studies, did not occur (i.e., data from the first night did not differ from those of subsequent nights, and the data were rather stable from night to night). Similarly, Jean-Louis et al.[63] found no first-night effect with actigraphy in younger subjects. These results suggest that, unlike in traditional laboratory studies, subjects do not need time to adapt to the actigraphy monitor.

Using actigraphy, Ancoli-Israel and colleagues[64-66] have shown that sleep in patients in nursing homes is extremely fragmented, with most patients never sleeping for a full hour and never awake for a full hour throughout the 24-hour day. Actigraphy was then used to show that a trial of treatment with light consolidated sleep but did not improve agitation in this population.[52,53,67] Alessi et al., using actigraphy, found that a combined treatment of increased physical activity and improvements in the environment improved sleep.[68]

Schizophrenia

Ancoli-Israel and colleagues[69,70] studied the 24-hour sleep–wake patterns of 28 older patients with schizophrenia (mean age, 58 years). In general, these patients slept for only 67% of the night and napped for 9% of the day. Patients taking neuroleptic medications were significantly sleepier both at night and during the day. Wirz-Justice and colleagues[71] used actigraphy to examine the rest–activity cycle of a patient with schizophrenia. By recording wrist activity for 220 days, they were able to determine that under stable haloperidol treatment, the patient had an arrhythmic rest–activity cycle. When treatment was switched to clozapine, the circadian rhythmicity improved.

Other Medical Conditions

Actigraphy is increasingly used in clinical research in populations that it would be difficult to conduct PSG studies on. Actigraphy is used in sleep intervention trials to show evidence of beneficial treatment with multiple days and nights of recording. Studies on sleep in menopausal women have shown that they experience more sleep disturbance.[72] Studies on patients with cirrhosis suggest that they have decreased motor activity, more sleep fragmentation, and dampened rhythms.[73] Studies on patients with coronary artery disease suggest that the strength of the circadian rhythm, as measured by actigraphy, is related to recovery from surgery and length of hospital stay.[74] Studies of patients with cancer demonstrate that those with more robust rhythms have less fatigue.[45,75,76]

Epidemiologic Studies of Sleep

Actigraphy is useful for studying sleep in large populations, particularly when recording in the laboratory might be cost prohibitive and might jeopardize the compliance rate. Ancoli-Israel and Kripke, along with their colleagues,[77-79] used actigraphy to determine wake and sleep patterns in large samples of older (sample size of 426) and middle-aged adults (sample size of 355). Measurements were used to determine the prevalences of sleep apnea and PLMS (recorded with additional sensors). Many of these volunteers would have been less willing to participate if they had been required to sleep in the laboratory.

TRICKS OF THE TRADE

Actigraphs are traditionally placed on the wrist of the nondominant hand. However, two groups of investigators have shown that either wrist can be used. Sadeh et al.[21] compared data from both wrists and found that although activity levels were different between the two hands, agreement rates with PSG were essentially the same for data collected from either hand. Chung and coworkers[80] found similar results. In studies on babies, actigraphs have also been placed on the babys' legs.[81]

Most actigraphs come with bands similar to plastic watch bands. For individuals who might be sensitive to such bands, or who find it uncomfortable to wear them for long periods, bands of terrycloth and Velcro can be sewed. Figure 124–2 illustrates the type of band used in our laboratory for studying demented older adult patients in nursing homes. To discourage patients from removing the bands, the two Velcro straps were reversed, with one opening from right to left and the other from left to right. This has worked to keep even the most diligent patient from removing the band. This technique also works with young children.

Patients wearing actigraphs should be asked to keep an actigraph log. They should note information about daily time to bed, time out of bed, and any unusual activity or times when the device is removed (such as for showers or swimming). This information is extremely helpful for editing and analyzing data.

When data are collected in 1-minute epochs for more than 1 week, it is prudent to download data every week to minimize data loss. In units with batteries that need to be replaced, battery levels should be checked when initializing the device and again during downloading. Batteries with levels below 90% of the original battery voltage should be discarded because they are likely to fail. The battery life is approximately 30 days. In our laboratory, a battery log is kept of the battery number, the date the activity monitor was initialized, the date the data were downloaded, the total number of days the battery was used, and the starting and ending battery levels.

Figure 124–2. Diagram of a terrycloth band that can be sewn for use with the Actillume. This band is used by Ancoli-Israel's laboratory in the study of sleep in demented nursing home patients who have extremely fragile and delicate skin. Note that the straps are reversed to make removal more difficult.

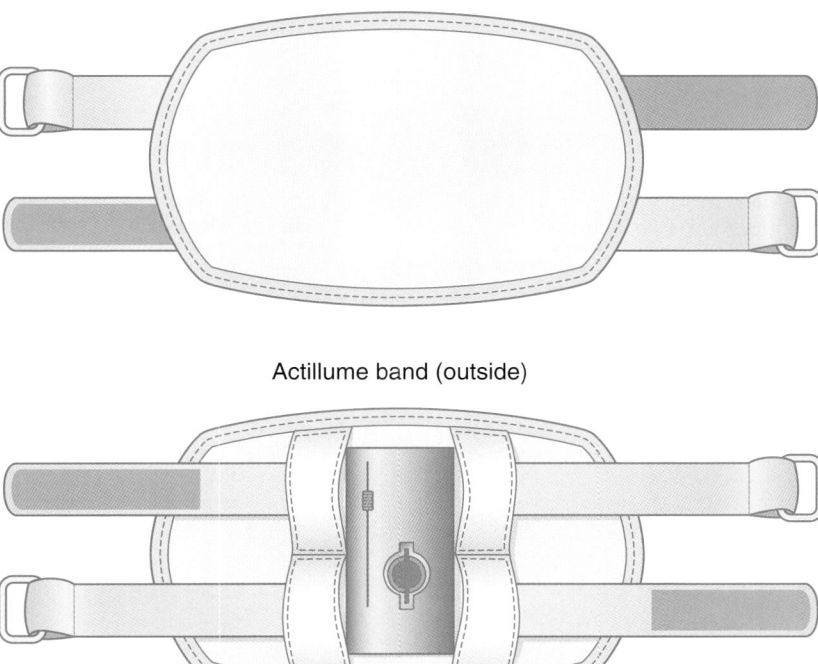

Actillume band (inside)

Actillume band (outside)

With devices that also record light, it is extremely important that the light sensor not be covered by the person's sleeve. The sleeve can be tucked under the actigraph or pinned up to ensure that it does not occlude the light sensor. Because the angle of the wrist differs from the angle of the eye, the lux reading from a light sensor may differ from ambient illumination. Figure 124–3 shows the lux level during a light treatment session. Although a photometer reading at the level of the eye confirmed a reading of 2500 lux, the lux reading at the level of the wrist was lower. Some devices have external light sensors in addition to the internal sensor, which can be clipped to a collar and might give more exact readings. All activity and light monitors should be checked on a regular basis to determine if calibration is needed.

In patients with sensitive skin, the bands can be removed for a few minutes each day to avoid pressure sores. The time the device is removed, the time it is replaced, and whether or not the person was awake for the few minutes it was removed should be noted on the log. This information is needed during the data editing process.

EDITING ACTIGRAPHY DATA

Different software packages are available for scoring the rest–activity data and inferring sleep–wake cycles. Because the experience of our laboratory is with the Actillume recorder and its accompanying software, Action3 (both by Ambulatory Monitoring, Inc., Ardsley, NY), editing and scoring techniques with this device will be reviewed.

Data are edited on a computer screen with the use of the daily sleep log. Time intervals that the device is removed are automatically scored as sleep by the Action3 software program, because there is no movement. Such time intervals can be manually changed to wake if the log indicates the person was involved in an activity where they were clearly awake (e.g., while bathing). If light exposure data is also being recorded, light data need not be edited when the Actillume is removed but left in the same room as the subject. Lack of movement that was scored as sleep because the device was removed for especially vigorous activity can also be manually changed to wake. For example, Israel and Ancoli-Israel[82] recorded activity in adolescents. Some subjects removed the Actillume during football or volleyball practice. No activity was recorded during that time period; however, it was clear that the subjects were awake. If there is no information on the log about the activity during the time the device was removed, that time period should be scored as missing data.

Channels of information can also be added to the data. For example, interval channels with information about time in bed and time out of bed can be added, as can times of treatment intervals. Figure 124–3 shows an example of two 24-hour periods with the activity data, sleep–wake scoring, and added interval channels.

LIMITATIONS

The actigraph user needs to be aware of the limitations of this device.[12] When compared to PSG, actigraphy is somewhat valid and reliable in healthy individuals. It is best at estimating total sleep time. As sleep becomes more disturbed, the actigraphy becomes less accurate. In general, actigraphy may overestimate sleep and underestimate wake, particularly during the day.

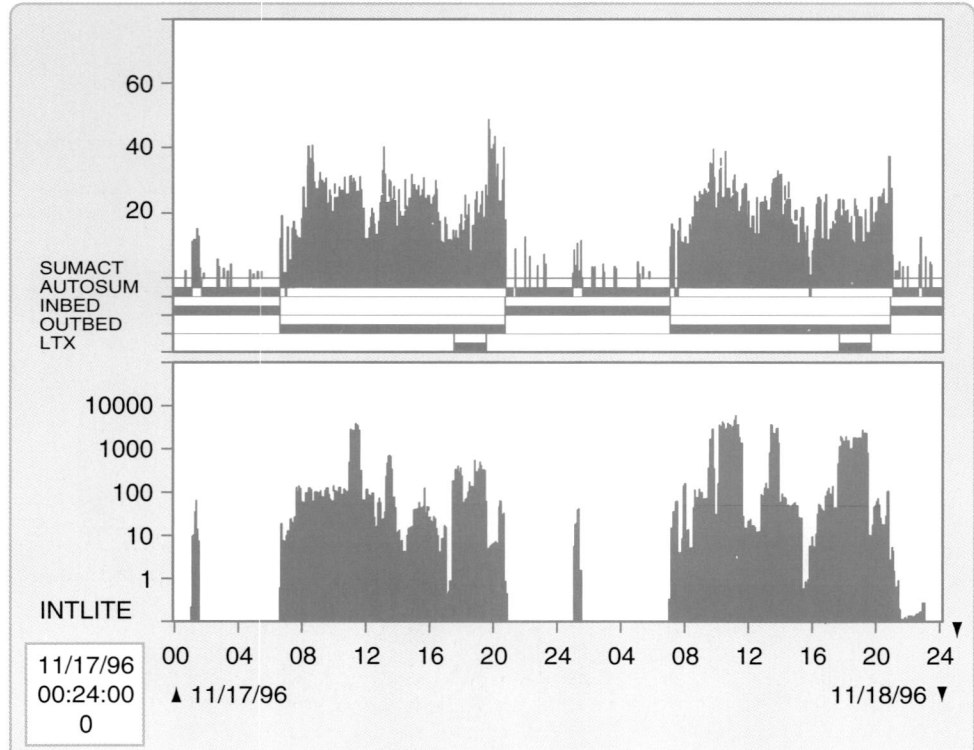

Figure 124–3. Action3 printout of an Actillume recording. Two 24-hour periods are shown with activity data (SUMACT); sleep/wake scoring (AUTOSUM); in-bed, out-of-bed, and treatment (LTX) intervals; and light exposure (INTLITE).

SUMMARY

Wrist activity has the advantages of being cost efficient, allowing the recording of sleep in the natural environment, recording behavior that occurs both during the night and during the day, and recording for long periods. Although it is not a replacement for EEG or PSG recordings, there are times when actigraphy provides clear advantages for data collection.

Actigraphy is particularly useful for studying individuals who cannot tolerate sleeping in the laboratory—for example, patients with insomnia, small children, and older adults. It may provide a more accurate estimate of typical sleep durations by providing an opportunity for patients to adhere more closely to their scheduled sleep and wake times. Actigraphy is also becoming an important tool in follow-up studies and for examining efficacy in clinical outcome.

The literature suggests that actigraphy has some value in the assessment of sleep disorders, although it may not be able to distinguish between different sleep disorders. The newer scoring algorithms have great accuracy in determining those variables that are most important in insomnia: they have improved ability to detect wake versus sleep, sleep latency, awakenings during the night, and total sleep time. Actigraphy is superior to sleep logs in detecting brief arousals during the night. It can also be used for the evaluation and clinical diagnosis of circadian rhythm disorders. The ability to detect movements holds promise in the identification of sleep disorders characterized by frequent movements, such as PLMS, sleep apnea, and REM sleep behavior disorders. The ability to measure for long periods makes actigraphy useful in situations where long-term changes in sleep are of interest.

As summarized in a recent review by Sadeh and Acebo,[14] the number of publications using actigraphy has sharply risen over the last 10 years. Over the next decade, additional improvements will be made that will allow the opportunities for using actigraphy in clinical settings and research to expand.

Clinical Pearl

Actigraphy is reliable and valid for detecting sleep in healthy populations, but less reliable for detecting disturbed sleep. It is a useful adjunct to the routine evaluation of insomnia, circadian rhythm disorders, and excessive sleepiness, and it is a help in the diagnosis of periodic limb movements during sleep and restless legs syndrome. It is also useful in special populations such as children or demented older adults.

Acknowledgment

This work is supported by NIA AG08415, NCI CA85264, NIA AG15301, NHLBI HL44915, the Sam and Rose Stein Institute for Research on Aging, the VA VISN-22 Mental Illness Research, Education and Clinical Center, and the Research Service of the Veterans Affairs San Diego Healthcare System.

REFERENCES

1. Tryon WW: Activity Measurement in Psychology and Medicine. New York, Plenum Press, 1991.
2. Kupfer DJ, Weiss BL, Foster FG, et al: Psychomotor activity in affective states. Arch Gen Psychiatry 1974;30:765-768.
3. McPartland RJ, Kupfer DJ, Foster FG: The movement-activated recording monitor: A third generation motor-activity monitoring system. Behav Res Meth Instr 1976;8:357-360.
4. Colburn TR, Smith BM, Guarini JJ, et al: An ambulatory activity monitor with solid state memory. ISA Transact 1976;15:149-154.
5. Kripke DF, Mullaney DJ, Messin S, et al: Wrist actigraphic measures of sleep and rhythms. Electroencephalogr Clin Neurophysiol 1978;44:674-676.
6. Mullaney DJ, Kripke DF, Messin S: Wrist-actigraphic estimation of sleep time. Sleep 1980;3:83-92.
7. Webster JB, Kripke DF, Messin S, et al: An activity-based sleep monitor system for ambulatory use. Sleep 1982;5:389-399.
8. Webster JB, Messin S, Mullaney DJ, et al: Transducer design and placement for activity recording. Med Biol Eng Comput 1982;20:741-744.
9. Redmond DP, Hegge FW: Observations on the design and specification of a wrist-worn human activity monitoring system. Behav Res Meth Instr Comp 1985;17:659-669.
10. Borbely AA: Long-term recording of the rest-activity cycle in man. In Zbinden G, Cuomo V, Racagni G, Wiess B (eds): Application of Behavioral Pharmacology in Toxicology. New York, Raven Press, 1983, pp 39-44.
11. Borbely AA: New techniques for the analysis of the human sleep-wake cycle. Brain Dev 1986;8:482-488.
12. Ancoli-Israel S, Cole R, Alessi CA, et al: The role of actigraphy in the study of sleep and circadian rhythms. Sleep 2003;26:342-392.
13. Gorny SW, Spiro JR: Comparing different methodologies used in wrist actigraphy. Sleep Rev 2001;Summer:40-42.
14. Sadeh A, Acebo C: The role of actigraphy in sleep medicine. Sleep Med Rev 2002;6:113-124.
15. Cole RJ, Kripke DF, Gruen W, et al: Automatic sleep/wake identification from wrist activity. Sleep 1992;15:461-469.
16. Jean-Louis G, von Gizycki H, Zizi F, et al: Determination of sleep and wakefulness with the actigraph data analysis software (ADAS). Sleep 1996;19:739-743.
17. Hauri PJ, Wisbey J: Wrist actigraphy in insomnia. Sleep 1992;15:293-301.
18. Brooks JO, Friedman L, Bliwise DL, et al: Use of the wrist actigraph to study insomnia in older adults. Sleep 1993;16:151-155.
19. Verbeek I, Arends J, Declerck G, et al: Wrist actigraphy in comparison with polysomnography and subjective evaluation in insomnia. In Coenen AML (ed): Sleep-Wake Research in The Netherlands. Leiden, Dutch Society for Sleep-Wake Research, 1994, pp 163-170.
20. Sadeh A, Alster J, Urbach D, et al: Actigraphically based automatic bedtime sleep-wake scoring: Validity and clinical applications. J Ambul Monit 1989;2:209-216.
21. Sadeh A, Sharkey KM, Carskadon MA: Activity-based sleep-wake identification: An empirical test of methodological issues. Sleep 1994;17:201-207.
22. Ancoli-Israel S, Clopton P, Klauber MR, et al: Use of wrist activity for monitoring sleep/wake in demented nursing home patients. Sleep 1997;20:24-27.
23. Sadeh A, Hauri PJ, Kripke DF, et al: The role of actigraphy in the evaluation of sleep disorders. Sleep 1995;18:288-302.
24. Bliwise DL: Review: Sleep in normal aging and dementia. Sleep 1993;16:40-81.
25. Espiritu RC, Kripke DF, Ancoli-Israel S, et al: Low illumination by San Diego adults: Association with atypical depressive symptoms. Biol Psychiatry 1994;35:403-407.
26. Campbell SS, Kripke DF, Gillin JC, et al: Exposure to light in healthy elderly subjects and Alzheimer's patients. Physiol Behav 1988;42:141-144.
27. Ancoli-Israel S, Kripke DF: Now I lay me down to sleep: The problem of sleep fragmentation in elderly and demented residents of nursing homes. Bull Clin Neurosci 1989;54:127-132.
28. Plazzi G, Schultz Y, Cortelli P, et al: Motor overactivity and loss of motor circadian rhythm in fatal familial insomnia: An actigraphic study. Sleep 1997;20:739-742.

29. Kunz D, Bes F: Melatonin effects in a patient with severe REM sleep behavior disorder: Case report and theoretical considerations. Neuropsychobiology 1997;34:211-214.

30. Shibui K, Uchiyama M, Iwama H, et al: Periodic fatigue symptoms due to desynchronization in a patient with non-24-h sleep-wake syndrome. Psychiatry 1998;52:477-481.

31. Quinto C, Gellido C, Chokroverty S, et al: Posttraumatic delayed sleep phase syndrome. Neurology 2000;54:250-252.

32. Littner M, Kushida CA, Anderson WM, et al: Practice parameters for the role of actigraphy in the study of sleep and circadian rhythms: An update for 2002. Sleep 2003;26:337-341.

33. Chambers MJ: Actigraphy and insomnia: A closer look—Part I. Sleep 1994;17:405-408.

34. Aubert-Tulkens G, Culee C, Rijckevorsel KH, et al: Ambulatory evaluation of sleep disturbance and therapeutic effects in sleep apnea syndrome by wrist activity monitoring. Am Rev Respir Dis 1987;136:851-856.

35. Middelkoop HA, Knuistingh NA, van Hilten JJ, et al: Wrist actigraphic assessment of sleep in 116 community based subjects suspected of obstructive sleep apnoea syndrome. Thorax 1995;50:284-289.

36. Kazenwadel J, Pollmacher T, Trenkwalder C, et al: New actigraphic assessment method for periodic leg movements (PLM). Sleep 1995;18:689-697.

37. Trenkwalder C, Stiasny K, Pollmacher T, et al: L-Dopa therapy of uremic and idiopathic restless legs syndrome: A double-blind, crossover trial. Sleep 1995;18:681-688.

38. Collado-Seidel V, Kazenwadel J, Wetter TC, et al: A controlled study of additional sr-L-dopa in L-dopa-responsive restless legs syndrome with late-night symptoms. Neurology 1999;52:285-290.

39. Wolter TD, Hauri PJ, Schroeder DR, et al: Effects of 24-hr nicotine replacement on sleep and daytime activity during smoking cessation. Prev Med 1996;25:601-610.

40. Garfinkel D, Laudon M, Nof D, et al: Improvement of sleep quality in elderly people by controlled-release melatonin. Lancet 1995; 346:541-544.

41. Friedman L, Benson K, Noda A, et al: An actigraphic comparison of sleep restriction and sleep hygiene treatments for insomnia in older adults. J Geriatr Psychiatry Neurol 2000;13:17-27.

42. Lavie P: Effects of midazolam on sleep disturbances associated with westward and eastward flights: evidence for directional effects. Psychopharmacology (Berlin) 1990;1012:250-254.

43. Tirosh E, Lavie P, Sadeh A, et al: Effects of methylphenidate on sleep in children with attention-deficit hyperactivity disorder. Am J Dis Child 1994;147:1313-1315.

44. Lavie P, Lorber M, Tzischinsky O, et al: Wrist actigraphic measurements in patients with rheumatoid arthritis: A novel method to assess drug efficacy. Drug Invest 1992;2(Suppl):15-21.

45. Mormont MC, De Prins J, Levi F: Assessment of activity rhythms by wrist actigraphy: preliminary results in 30 patients with colorectal cancer. Biol Rhythm Res 1995;6:423.

46. Carskadon MA, Acebo C, Richardson GS, et al: An approach to studying circadian rhythms of adolescent humans. J Biol Rhythms 1997;12:278-289.

47. Tzischinsky O, Epstein R, Lavie P: Sleep-wake cycles in rotating shift workers: Comparison between 3- and 5-day shift system. In Costa G, Geaana G, Cogi K, Wedderbrun A (eds): Shift Work: Health, Sleep and Performance. Frankfurt, Peter Lang, 1990, pp 651-656.

48. Lavie P, Tzischinsky O, Epstein R, et al: Sleep-wake cycles in rotating shift work: Effects of changing from phase advance to phase delay rotation. Isr J Med Sci 1992;28:636-644.

49. Buck A, Tobler I, Borbely AA: Wrist activity monitoring in air crew members: A method for analyzing sleep quality following transmeridian and North-South flights. J Biol Rhythms 1989; 4:93-105.

50. Middleton B, Arendt J, Stone BM: Complex effects of melatonin on human circadian rhythms in constant dim light. J Biol Rhythms 1997;12:467-477.

51. Martin J, Marler MR, Shochat T, Ancoli-Israel S: Circadian rhythms of agitation in institutionalized patients with Alzheimer's disease. Chronobiol Int 2000;17:405-418.

52. Ancoli-Israel S, Martin JL, Gehrman P, et al: Effect of light on agitation in institutionalized patients with severe Alzheimer's disease. Am J Geriatr Psychiatry 2003;11:194-203.

53. Ancoli-Israel S, Martin JL, Kripke DF, et al: Effect of light treatment on sleep and circadian rhythms in demented nursing home patients. J Am Geriatr Soc 2002;50:282-289.

54. van Someren E, Swaab DF, Colenda CC, et al: Bright light therapy: Improved sensitivity to its effects on rest-activity rhythms in Alzheimer's patients by application of nonparametric disorder. Chronobiol Int 1999;16:505-518.

55. Sadeh A, Dark I, Vohr BR: Newborns' sleep-wake patterns: The role of maternal, delivery and infant factors. Early Hum Dev 1996;44:113-126.

56. Sadeh A, Raviv A, Gruber R: Sleep patterns and sleep disruptions in school-age children. Dev Psychol 2000;36:291-301.

57. Hering E, Epstein R, Elroy S, et al: Sleep patterns in autistic children. J Autism Dev Disord 1999;29:143-147.

58. Glod CA, Teicher MH, Hartman CR, et al: Increased nocturnal activity and impaired sleep maintenance in abused children. J Am Acad Child Adolesc Psychiatry 1997;36:1236–1243.

59. Sadeh A: Assessment of intervention for infant night waking: Parental reports and activity-based home monitoring. J Consult Clin Psychol 1994;62:63-68.

60. Ancoli-Israel S: Sleep problems in older adults: Putting myths to bed. Geriatrics 1997;52:20-30.

61. van Hilten JJ, Middelkoop HA, Braat EA, et al: Nocturnal activity and immobility across aging (50-98 years) in healthy persons. J Am Geriatr Soc 1993;41:837-841.

62. van Hilten JJ, Braat EAM, van der Velde EA, et al: Ambulatory activity monitoring during sleep: An evaluation of internight and intrasubject variability in healthy persons aged 50-98 years. Sleep 1993;16:146-150.

63. Jean-Louis G, von Gizycki H, Zizi F, et al: The actigraph data analysis software: I. A novel approach to scoring and interpreting sleep-wake activity. Percept Mot Skills 1997;85:207-216.

64. Ancoli-Israel S, Jones DW, Hanger MA, et al: Sleep in the nursing home. In Kuna ST, Suratt PM, Remmers JE (eds): Sleep and Respiration in Aging Adults. New York, Elsevier Press, 1991, pp 77-84.

65. Pat-Horenczyk R, Klauber MR, Shochat T, Ancoli-Israel S: Hourly profiles of sleep and wakefulness in severely versus mild-moderately demented nursing home patients. Aging Clin Exp Res 1998;10:308-315.

66. Ancoli-Israel S, Parker L, Sinaee R, et al: Sleep fragmentation in patients from a nursing home. J Gerontol 1989;44:M18-M21.

67. Ancoli-Israel S, Gehrman PR, Martin JL, et al: Increased light exposure consolidates sleep and strengthens circadian rhythms in severe Alzheimer's disease patients. Behav Sleep Med 2003;1:22-36.

68. Alessi CA, Yoon EJ, Schnelle JF, et al: A randomized trial of a combined physical activity and environmental intervention in nursing home residents: Do sleep and agitation improve? J Am Geriatr Soc 1999;47:784-791.

69. Martin J, Jeste DV, Caligiuri M, et al: Actigraphic estimates of circadian rhythms and sleep/wake in older schizophrenia patients. Schizophr Res 2001;47:77-86.

70. Martin J, Jeste DV, Patterson T, Ancoli-Israel S: Light exposure and quality of life in older schizophrenia and schizoaffective disorder patients. In Holick MF, Jung EG (eds): Biologic Effects of Light. Hingham, Mass, Kluwer Academic, 1999, pp 471-473.

71. Wirz-Justice A, Cajochen C, Nussbaum P: A schizophrenic with an arrhythmic circadian rest-activity cycle. Psychiatry Res 1997; 73:83-90.

72. Baker A, Simpson A, Dawson D: Sleep disruption and mood changes associated with menopause. J Psychosom Res 1997;43:359-369.

73. Cordoba J, Cabrera J, Lataif L, et al: High prevalence of sleep disturbance in cirrhosis. Hepatology 1998;27:339-345.

74. Redeker NS, Wykpisz E: Effects of age on activity patterns after coronary artery bypass surgery. Heart Lung 1998;28:5-14.

75. Ancoli-Israel S, Moore P, Jones V: The relationship between fatigue and sleep in cancer patients: A review. Eur J Cancer Care 2001;10:245-255.

76. Berger AM: Patterns of fatigue and activity and rest during adjuvant breast cancer chemotherapy. Oncol Nurs Forum 1998;25:51-62.

77. Ancoli-Israel S, Kripke DF, Klauber MR, et al: Sleep disordered breathing in community-dwelling elderly. Sleep 1991;14:486-495.

78. Ancoli-Israel S, Kripke DF, Klauber MR, et al: Periodic limb movements in sleep in community-dwelling elderly. Sleep 1991;14:496-500.

79. Kripke DF, Ancoli-Israel S, Klauber MR, et al: Prevalence of sleep disordered-breathing in ages 40-64 years: A population-based survey. Sleep 1997;20:65-76.

80. Chung L, Kripke DF, Ancoli-Israel S, et al: Dominant versus non-dominant wrist movements during sleep. Sleep Res 1995; 24A:80.

81. Gershoni-Baruch R, Epstein R, Tzischinsky O, et al: Actigraphic home-monitoring of the sleep pattern of in vitro fertilization children and their matched controls. Dev Med Child Neurol 1994;36:639-645.

82. Israel SL, Ancoli-Israel S: Light exposure, sleep and delayed sleep phase in middle-school adolescents. Sleep Res 1997; 26:159.

125

Chronobiologic Monitoring Techniques

John H. Herman

ABSTRACT

This chapter serves as an introduction to fundamental methodologies in circadian rhythm research. Although methods can be described for molecular, genetic, cellular, organ, or in vivo exploration, this chapter concentrates exclusively on methodologies applicable to mammalian and, most specifically, human research. This chapter examines controversies and unresolved issues, and critically evaluates varying chronobiologic protocols.

The purpose of chronobiologic monitoring techniques in humans is to measure biologic and behavioral properties of circadian rhythms. Chronobiology research is based on the assumption that a given organism contains within it a core mechanism or clock for generating rhythmic expression of physiologic parameters. The fluctuations in any biologic or behavioral parameter that display an approximately 24-hour periodicity are assumed to be the direct or indirect consequence of an underlying pacemaker that has its own inherent and autonomous periodicity.

The internal clock has a variety of properties that are indirectly studied in circadian rhythm research by examining output variables. These include (1) amplitude, or the quantity of change in a parameter that occurs from apogee to nadir, in variables such as temperature, cortisol, or cognitive problem solving; (2) period length (or tau), or the temporal duration of one complete circadian cycle under free running conditions; (3) phase, or the relation of the internal clock to the environment, such as sunrise and morning awakening; (4) rate of change, or the rapidity with which a circadian parameter switches from its active to dormant or dormant to active modes; and (5) the duration of activity relative to the duration of sleep. Chronobiologic techniques have evolved to measure each of these variables, how they may be manipulated, and how they are interrelated.

The process by which the internal clock is kept in synchrony with the environment is called *entrainment*. Stimuli, such as light, that bring about entrainment are called *zeitgebers*. The circadian mechanism is always subject to the influences of "masking." Masking is the ability of an external variable, such as light, sound, or physical activity, to alter a behavioral or physiologic rhythm without affecting the core pacemaker. The distinction between entrainment and masking is not clearly defined. Exposure to daily sunlight, for example, entrains us to our local time zone and masks our internal clock from expressing its endogenous rhythm. In animals, masking influences may be removed by placing the animal in continuous light conditions. As simple and straightforward as it would seem to measure the period length of the human circadian rhythm, the field of circadian rhythms research has undergone continual

upheaval as methodologic errors have been repeatedly revealed and new paradigms designed to correct them. In humans, for example, there have been continued corrections of the period length of the circadian rhythm of activity, which is now estimated at slightly greater than 24 hours, 24.18 hours being the most recent value.[1]

In addition to a core pacemaker, each circadian system has input and output components. Input components are principally responsive to photic information but respond to a variety of stimuli, each of which is manipulated in circadian studies to examine the effect on output variables such as the sleep–wake cycle, temperature, or behaviors such as reaction time or problem-solving ability.

METHODOLOGIC QUESTIONS IN THE FIELD OF CIRCADIAN RHYTHMS

During the preceding three decades, various estimates have placed the human circadian period length at 13 to 65 hours, and the free-running circadian period of the human activity rhythm was believed to average slightly more than 25 hours.[2] Also, greater interindividual inconstancy in circadian variables in humans had been observed than that observed in other mammals. These findings showed a disparity between humans and nonhuman mammals, in which circadian rhythms are remarkably stable from day to day. In humans, there have been continued corrections of the period length of the circadian rhythm of activity, which has been most recently estimated at slightly greater than 24 hours.

Disagreements continue over which stimuli are capable of acting as zeitgebers to entrain or shift circadian rhythms. Initially, only bright light was considered to be capable of shifting the timing of circadian rhythms.[3] Subsequently, light of moderate intensity was described as being capable of shifting circadian rhythms,[4] and, most recently, studies now maintain that ordinary room light is capable of inducing a circadian shift.[5,6] Some authors have claimed that extraocular light is capable of influencing circadian rhythms. One study demonstrated that behind-the-knee (popliteal region) bright light is capable of inducing shifts in circadian timing,[7] but there have been multiple failures to replicate this finding.[8-11] As chronobiology research progressed, a series of modifications of experimental design successively eliminated some masking artifacts and external zeitgebers that previously introduced artifact.[1]

The field has also been inundated by controversy over what constitutes a zeitgeber, or a stimulus capable of entraining a circadian rhythm. There is evidence that nonphotic stimuli are capable of entraining individuals.[12] Exercise,[13,14] social activity,[15] feeding schedule,[16] ambient temperature,[17] napping in darkness,[18] administration of melatonin,[19] and knowledge of time of day or night[20] each might act as an entraining phenomenon. Some studies suggest a major role for such nonvisual zeitgebers,[12] whereas other studies imply a more modest role.[21] The extent to which melatonin is capable of shifting circadian rhythms remains controversial.[22]

Another area of research involves separating behavioral and biologic properties of circadian rhythms from other physiologic processes. Many behavioral and biologic phenomena are influenced by the sleep–wake cycle, or the duration of prior wakefulness. This is known as the *homeostatic model*, which describes an increasing "pressure" to sleep with increased duration of wakefulness and a decreased pressure to sleep with increased duration of sleep.[23] Circadian rhythm studies must separate variance in a biologic or behavioral parameter into homeostatic and circadian components; that is, they must identify what proportion of the parameter's variance is circadian and what proportion is homeostatic.[24,25] Neither the circadian nor the homeostatic models can explain in a compelling manner why humans are most wide awake in the hour or two preceding sleep and sleepiest in the hour after morning awakening.

An additional area of continued controversy is what biologic metric is best used to approximate the properties of the underlying core pacemaker, such as period length. Core body temperature[24] and melatonin[26] secretory profiles have been used in most studies. Some research uses dim-light melatonin onset as the marker of the beginning of a new circadian cycle, others use dim-light melatonin offset,[26] and many use the temperature nadir. However, there is no obvious point that can be identified as the minimum of temperature or the onset of melatonin secretion. Temperature fluctuates from moment to moment, and the minimum or maximum must be extracted mathematically. Melatonin rises gradually after sunset, and an arbitrary level must be selected to denote onset or offset. In addition, it must be emphasized that extracting circadian rhythm data relies on complex data analysis based on mathematical criteria and data analytic techniques selected in each experimental protocol.[1]

The amount of information uncovered in the past few decades in the field of circadian rhythm research has been truly astounding, and includes the identification of basic anatomy, novel photoreceptors, and genetic mechanisms. The field has not accepted specific definitions in the areas of contention listed previously, nor has it accepted a single chronobiologic monitoring technique as being the gold standard. Various studies using different experimental paradigms have contributed to the turbulence in this field. This chapter briefly reviews the various paradigms recently used in circadian rhythm research and discusses the strengths and weaknesses of each. This chapter does not present an in-depth description of the details of each model, but the reader is directed to a few key references in which a fuller exposition is offered.

PARADIGMS

Fixed Light–Dark Schedules, Double Plotted

The most common model for animal studies of circadian variables and activity schedule consists of placing the animal in a cage with a running wheel and subjecting the animal to a fixed schedule of light and dark (Fig. 125–1). The running wheel's turns are counted continuously. Typically, the animal's running behavior on the wheel is plotted as a vertical or horizontal line

per unit time, or wheel turns per unit time. These counts are plotted successively for 24 hours, yielding a visual representation of when and how much the animal ran that day. Successive days are stacked, enabling the reader visually to appreciate changes in the timing of activity that occurred during the experiment. The entire plot is duplicated side by side, called *double plotting*, because seeing the image next to itself enables the reader to appreciate what happened in the experiment more readily. For example, if the animal's principal expression of wheel-running activity "drifts" from before to after midnight, double plotting allows the reader to more easily follow the continuity of changed running wheel times. Drinking or feeding may be plotted in the same manner. Protocols are labeled as LL (constant light), LD (fixed light–dark schedule, most commonly 12 hours light/12 hours dark), or DD (constant darkness). Constant dim light is sometimes used in such protocols, of a low enough level of illumination to prevent influence on the rat's secretion of melatonin. In some studies the LD period length may be longer than or shorter than 24 hours, and as rapid as 1 hour in some studies.

The DD paradigm has been successful in demonstrating the remarkable consistency of a given species' free-running activity rhythm in constant darkness or dim light, successfully elucidating the period length of its biologic clock.[1] Frequently, the timing of light and dark are abruptly changed to measure the animal's reaction, which may take several days to adapt. Such paradigms are at the core of much genetic research, in which normal animals (+/+) are compared with partial (+/−) or complete (−/−) knockouts. Studies reveal genetic phenotypes (behavioral expression) because knockout animals display altered periodicity, diminished rhythmicity, or lack of any circadian rhythm in running, feeding, or drinking behavior. Such changes may occur only in LL or DD, but other knockouts remain arrhythmic in an LD paradigm.

The obvious strength of the fixed light–dark schedule with activity monitoring is its ability accurately and economically to measure an animal's rest–activity schedule. Alterations in activity schedules after genetic alterations have become the basis for a standard phenotype–genotype model. Weaknesses of this design include its inability to examine complex interactions that would occur in more natural circumstances that could have an impact on the circadian system. If only light, dark, or light versus dark are studied, then all effects appear to be a function of the animal's illumination schedule. The paradigm is subject to overly simple interpretation unless caution is used.

Entrained Twenty-Four–Hour Studies

In such studies, subjects live in laboratory conditions with constant bedtime, wakeup time, meal time, and timed activities. Subjects are aware of time of day and are not isolated from normal zeitgebers such as light from windows. This protocol is used to study biologic or behavioral parameters such as hormone secretory profiles or cognitive processes under constant conditions. Frequently, indwelling catheters with recurrent blood draws are used in such studies.

Phase-Shifting Protocols

One of the most experimentally robust findings in the area of circadian rhythm research is the capacity of zeitgebers such as bright light to change the time of day at which the circadian

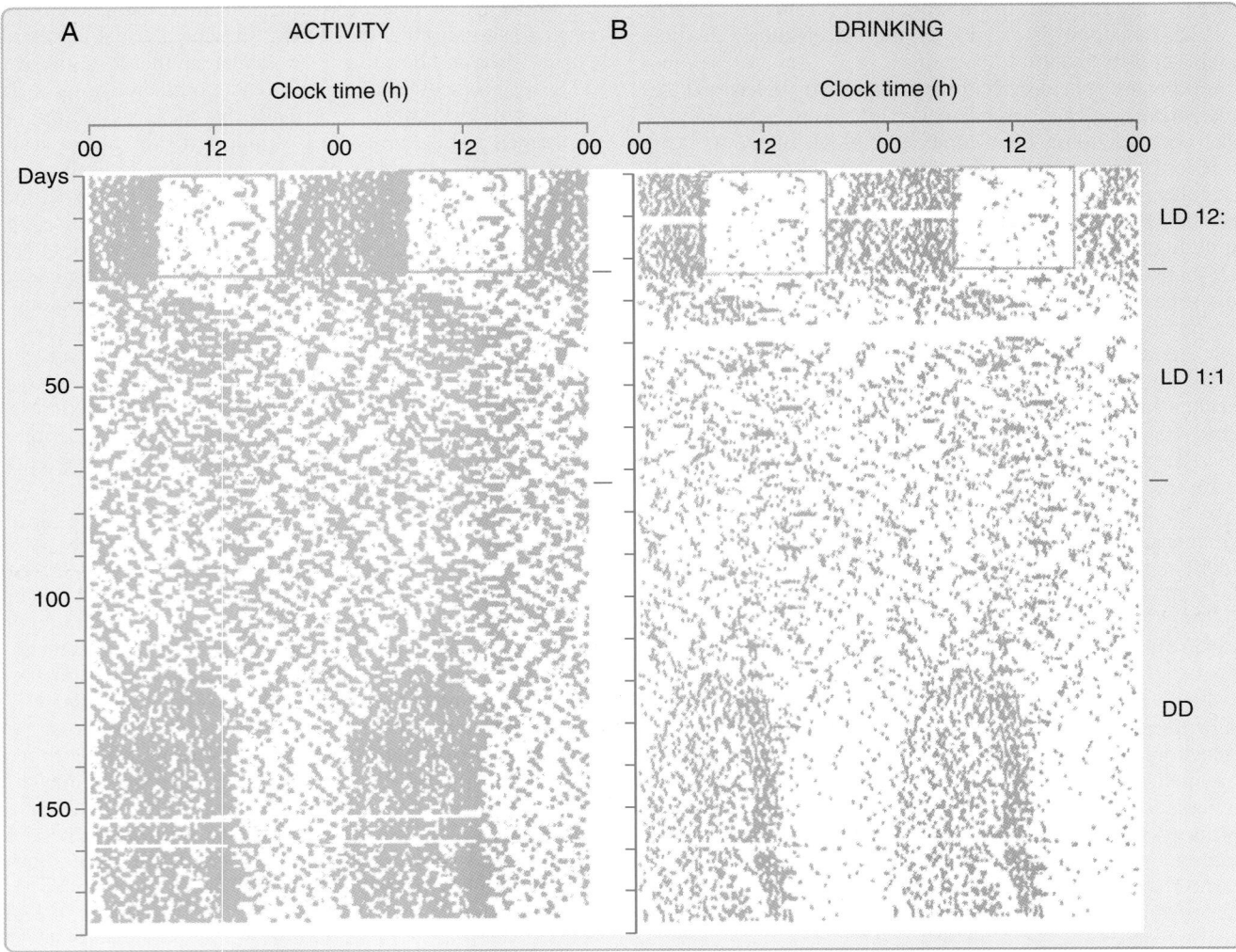

Figure 125–1. Typical double-plotted circadian rhythm study in a rodent. The double plot begins at midnight (00) and extends for 48 hours, or two complete dark and light cycles, through 6 hours of darkness (clock time 06:00) and three ensuing 12-hour periods of light and dark, and ends with 6 hours of darkness at midnight (00). This 180-day experiment shows double-plotted wheel-running behavior (*left*) and drinking behavior (*right*) under three consecutive experimental conditions.[42] The animal is in a light–dark (LD) 12:12 (light 12 hours, dark 12 hours) schedule for the first 24 days, followed by 50 days of LD 1:1 (light 1 hour, dark 1 hour), followed by constant darkness (DD) for 104 days. Note that during the first 24 days, the animal is active continually in the dark and does little wheel running in the light portion. When the animal is changed to an LD 1:1 schedule, it first shows a phase delay of approximately 1 hour per day and becomes almost completely arrhythmic after approximately 25 days in this LD schedule. Returning to DD gradually returns the animal to a 24-hour schedule of running activity, unlike the 25-hour schedule first induced by the LD 1:1 schedule, suggesting that the ultrashort LD schedule initially induced an activity rhythm distinct from the animal's endogenous rhythmicity. (From Usui S, Okazak T: Loss of circadian behavioural rhythms in rats kept in constant darkness. Psychiatry Clin Neurosci 2002;56:217.)

system switches from its active or "day" mode to its dormant or "night" mode. This is referred to as a *phase shift*. Many studies have examined the capacity of light of varying intensities and durations to alter the timing of sleep, melatonin secretion, or the temperature nadir. These studies share in common a baseline in which environmental light is controlled but typically is similar to the timing of natural environmental light. Frequently the baseline consists of dim light (more than 70 lux to as low as 1.5 lux). In the experimental condition, light is then delivered to the subject in what would normally be the dark or "night" portion of the circadian rhythm.[27] Light is delivered in the same manner during this experimental condition for 1 or several days. In some studies there is then a subsequent condition in which the subject is in constant dim light or in a constant routine (see later).

Circadian variables such as wheel running, the timing of sleep, or the timing of melatonin secretion are monitored during each condition.[1-3] The magnitude of the change in a circadian variable after the altered timing of light is measured. A "phase response curve" shows the effects of light exposure at different times throughout the circadian cycle in changing the timing of a circadian output variable.[28] Most studies show circadian rhythm shifts in response to light occurring only if the light is delivered at specific times, typically at or near normal hours of darkness, and indicate that mammals are not responsive to bright light administered during normal hours of daylight.[29] Other studies claim there is no "dead zone" and that bright light delivered at any hour, including normal daylight hours, will have a phase-shifting effect.[30]

Time-Isolation Protocols

Animals may be kept in total darkness or in light dim enough to have no effect on their circadian timing mechanism. Humans have typically been isolated in an environment free of time cues, such as an underground facility or an internal suite of rooms in an enclosed bunker. Great pains are taken not to give subjects any clues as to time, including double-door entry chambers and randomized schedules for technicians interacting with subjects. In such studies, subjects were permitted to turn off their room lights and retire when they wished and awaken when they wished. Subjects were instructed not to nap.

One of the more unexpected findings in circadian rhythm research is that the subjective sense of sleepiness, or the objective wish to sleep, is the least at the normal time of sleep initiation and greatest at the normal time of awakening.[31-35] This propensity to be alert at the normal hour of onset of sleep has bedeviled studies attempting to assess the period length of the human circadian clock using time-isolation protocols. Under conditions of time isolation, a variety of studies showed great variability in human sleep–wake cycle length, unlike studies in any other mammal. Studies showed sleep–wake cycles as long as 36 hours and great day-to-day variability in both sleep and wake duration.[36] Subjects who remained in time-isolation conditions for a sufficient interval developed desynchrony between their temperature rhythm and their sleep–wake cycle. Under normal conditions, the temperature minimum occurs near the middle of the sleep period, but in subjects in temporal isolation protocols, the interval from one temperature minimum to the next would have a cycle length of approximately 25 hours, whereas the interval between sleep initiation on successive nights would be of greater duration and show greater variability.[37]

Time-isolation protocols are no longer used because results from these studies are widely disparate from those of circadian rhythm studies of all other mammalian species. In disregarding this experimental approach, a basic attribute of human behavior is being ignored: Most individuals appear to prefer a sleep–wake schedule longer than 24 hours, when allowed. This perhaps unique human preference for longer wake and sleep episodes has been overlooked in the circadian rhythm field's fervor to produce human data as similar as possible to that from other mammals, invertebrates, and plants.

Forced Desynchrony Protocols

In forced desynchrony protocols, subjects are scheduled for rest–activity cycles anywhere from every 20 minutes to 28 hours. In such studies, core body temperature, melatonin, or both are monitored continuously. Subjects live in dim light during the active part of their rest–activity cycle and in darkness during scheduled sleep episodes. Dim light is defined as any level from 1 to 70 lux in various studies. Under such conditions, the endogenous circadian pacemaker, as measured by dim light melatonin onset or temperature rhythm, displays a stable period and is unable to follow the scheduled 28-hour (or 20-minute) sleep–wake cycle. The temperature rhythm then becomes desynchronized from the imposed sleep–wake schedule. The 20-minute sleep–wake cycle is referred to as the *ultrashort sleep schedule.*[38]

In forced desynchrony protocols, subjects are placed in a sound-attenuated and windowless room in which they have no access to any timepiece for the duration of the study. The contacts with staff members are limited and the staff is trained not to transmit any information about the time of day. In such studies, technicians have only brief contact with the subjects to announce the moments for rising, meals, showering, testing, and going to bed. Subjects watch videos, listen to music, or engage in their own preference of leisure activities. In some studies, subjects are allowed caffeine-containing beverages in the scheduled morning.

In forced desynchrony protocols, subjects spend two thirds of their time in active or waking conditions and one third of their time in dark or sleep conditions—for example, 60 minutes of activity and 30 minutes of scheduled sleep in a 90-minute day, and 18.66 hours of activity and 9.33 hours of scheduled sleep in a 28-hour day paradigm. Studies with day lengths of various durations share in common that the scheduled day length is outside the range of entrainment of the human circadian clock under dim light conditions whether the activity–sleep cycle duration is less than or greater than 24 hours (frequently 20 hours[39] or 28 hours). Under such conditions, the circadian clock becomes unmasked as it continues to oscillate at its near–24-hour intrinsic period despite sleep permitted only on the 28-hour schedule (Fig. 125–2).

Constant-Routine Protocols

This protocol requires the subjects to remain in a semirecumbent posture throughout the constant-routine experimental phase, typically 24 to 48 hours, sometimes continuously awake. During constant routine, the subject remains in temporal isolation in dim light. Subjects are fed their normal caloric and liquid intake in 24 equally divided portions. Food and beverages are at room temperature. In such studies, salivary melatonin samples may be acquired hourly, core body temperature may be monitored continuously, and psychometric testing may be administered at hourly intervals. Blood samples may be drawn at hourly intervals through an indwelling intravenous catheter. Constant-routine protocols eliminate the effects of activity, light–dark cycles, sleep, and meals on temperature, enabling a more accurate estimate of the circadian contribution to changes in amplitude of variables such as temperature or cognitive performance.[40]

Long Nights Protocol

In the long nights protocol, subjects have an enforced dark period longer than the permitted light period. Such studies have been used in adults and adolescents. This protocol reveals an aspect of the human circadian rhythm that is typically ignored: the capacity of humans to adapt to an extended dark period with enforced immobility. Historically, humans in temperate zones of both the northern and southern hemispheres obviously spent approximately half of the year with dark periods exceeding light periods. Society has used artificial light to impose permanent light conditions similar to the long days of summer, to which humans are capable of entraining. The long nights protocol reverses the circumstances, testing the ability of the human circadian system to adapt to short days (10 hours) and long nights (14 hours). Such studies have revealed increased total sleep time, increased duration of cortisol suppression, increased duration of melatonin secretion, increased duration of temperature suppression, and decreased daytime sleepiness under these conditions.[41] During long

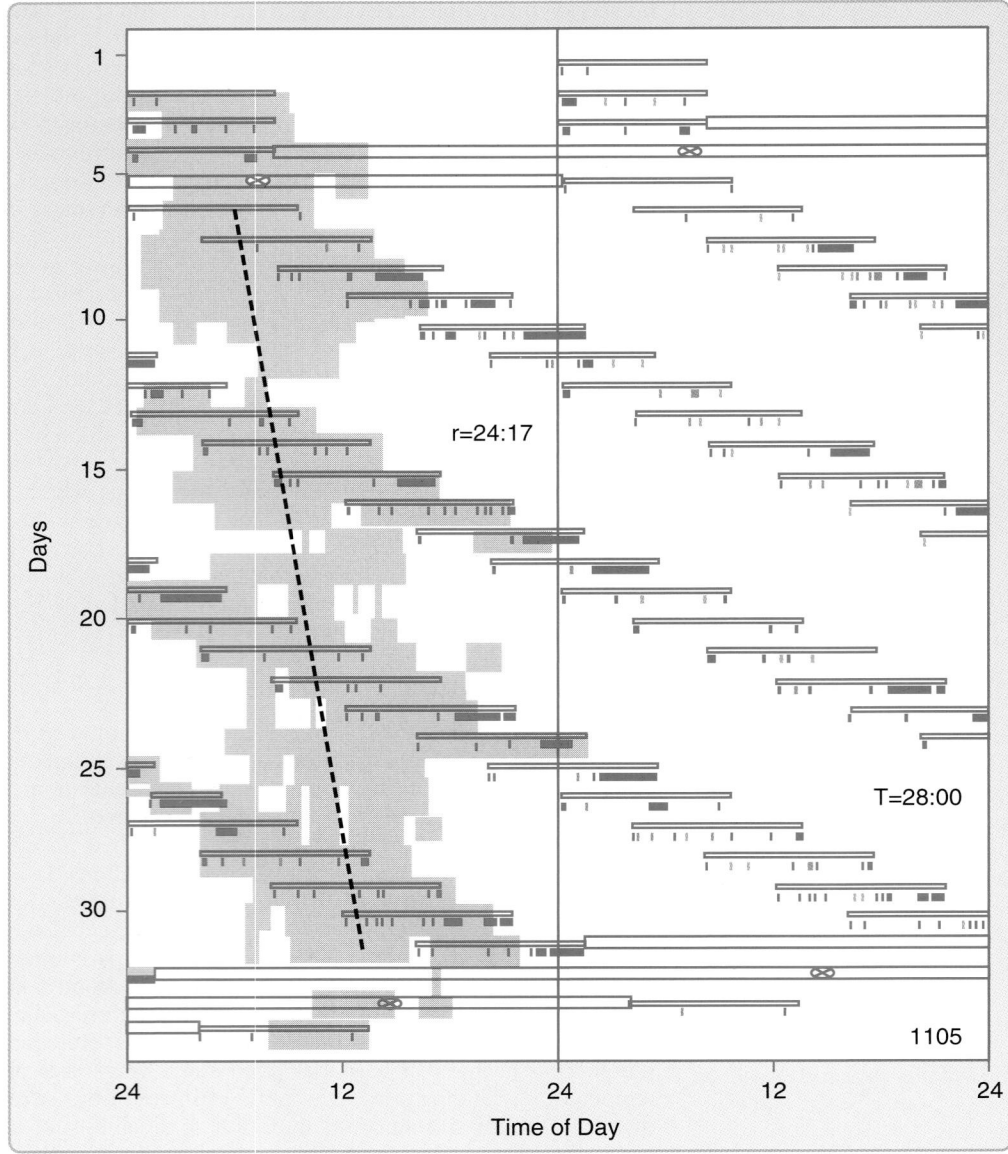

Figure 125–2. Double plot of forced desynchrony protocol using same display properties as Figure 125–1. Days 1 to 4 are baseline, followed by 40 hours of constant routine, followed by 26 days of forced desynchrony. Successive days are plotted both next to and beneath each other. Scheduled sleep episodes (*open narrow bars*), wakefulness within each sleep episode (*light and dark blue tick marks* below the narrow open bars), and intervals during which core body temperature was below the mean (*gray areas*) are indicated. An intrinsic temperature cycle period of 24.17 hours was statistically estimated by analysis of the core body temperature data during the forced desynchrony part of the protocol. The *dashed line* indicates the timing of the minimum of the circadian temperature rhythm. The minimum of the endogenous circadian rhythm—the minimum of core body temperature, as unmasked by a 40-hour constant-routine protocol—is indicated by the circled "x." (From Dijk DJ, Czeisler CA: Paradoxical timing of the circadian rhythm of sleep propensity serves to consolidate sleep and wakefulness in humans. Neurosci Lett 1994;166:63-68.)

nights, subjects spend some of this time awake, typically after rapid eye movement sleep periods.[42] In this manner, the ratio of the time spent below the circadian mean is increased and the time spent above the circadian mean is decreased. This demonstrates an aspect of adaptability in the human circadian system that is not revealed in other circadian protocols.

Indirectly Measuring Circadian Rhythms

A frequently employed technique in human circadian research is measurement of salivary melatonin. This non-invasive procedure permits a clinician or investigator to measure indirectly circulating melatonin levels, which may be consecutively plotted to estimate time of melatonin onset and offset, thereby determining a subject or patient's circadian phase.[43] Salivary melatonin correlates directly with sleep propensity and inversely with core body temperature.[44]

Saliva Collection

During the sampling period subjects typically avoid heavy exercise. Samples are taken under controlled light conditions to avoid light inhibition of melatonin: 250 to 300 lux for daytime and less than 50 lux for nighttime. Saliva is collected by placing a wool swab in the mouths of subjects and having them chew for 5 minutes. Saliva samples may be acquired once or multiple times over a 24-hour period. Samples are kept in refrigerated tubes at ± 4° C for up to one month. The tubes are then centrifuged for 15 min at 3000 g and are frozen at −20° C until assayed.[45]

Salivary Melatonin and Cortisol Assay

Melatonin in saliva is measured by a direct radioimmunoassay (RIA). Various kits are manufactured in North America and Europe and are specially made for the quantitative determination of melatonin in saliva. The cross-reactivity of the assay for closely related chemical structures is <1%. The sensitivity of the assay is approximately 1 ng/L. The intra- and inter-reliabilities are 11.3% and 12%, respectively.[45]

Statistics

To characterize the salivary melatonin profile for a given subject, the periodic function may be fitted to a set of data points using the baseline cosine mathematical function. The peak height (amplitude), acrophase, and duration of secretion are then calculated and may be subjected to further calculations or common statistical analysis.

FUTURE DIRECTIONS

Current methods for assessing circadian pacemaker properties are indirect. In the future, they will probably be viewed as clever but rudimentary. Temperature is an indirect output of the core pacemaker, and melatonin is also indirectly related to it. Genetic advances in chronobiologic technique could allow measurement of gene transcription or translation products that are direct outputs of the circadian pacemaker. Imaging studies with techniques such as functional magnetic resonance imaging could make it possible directly to monitor functional activity of neuronal assemblies with purported pacemaker activity, such as the suprachiasmatic nuclei.

DISCUSSION

Methodologies in circadian rhythm research are in a state of flux. Much has been learned about the circadian pacemaker in humans, its inputs and outputs, and the factors that affect circadian rhythms. Forced desynchrony protocols are probably the best current methodology for studying period length of circadian variables. Currently, constant-routine and forced desynchrony methodologies have gained wide acceptance in the field of circadian rhythm research. These protocols are continually being refined as additional controls are incorporated to eliminate unintended factors that could have masking effects. These protocols are complex and require sophisticated laboratories with extensive time-isolated floor space and equipment. Much of the data has been gathered from young male subjects, and little is yet known concerning sex effects.

Forced desynchrony studies must have a major impact in disrupting the emotional well-being of subjects, who live continuously in a timeless environment, have no contact with the outside world, are awakened at various times throughout the night and day, are permitted to sleep only at times when sleeping is unlikely, and have meals at times when one would not be hungry. In countries where physical torture is not permitted, circumstances similar to forced desynchrony are used to interrogate prisoners of war. It is possible that the results from forced desynchrony protocols are affected by the unusual and unsustainable nature of the experimental conditions.

The long nights protocol reveals great flexibility in the human capacity to adapt to long periods of darkness, both biologically and behaviorally. It reveals biologic changes, such as longer cortisol suppression and decreased daytime sleepiness, that could prove advantageous in certain populations, such as children, narcoleptic patients, or patients with affective disorders. Little is yet known about this chronobiologic approach.

Chronobiology research in humans appears to be searching for experimental protocols that minimize any differences between humans, other animals, and plants. Rodent studies have become the gold standard to which human circadian research aspires. Rodent studies maximize stability of period length and minimize variability. If gathering phenotypic information for genetic studies is the goal, it is understandable that maximal stability and minimal variance are sought. But something about what makes us human is lost when we abandon paradigms that show individual variance in preferred day length, and that some individuals prefer to remain awake and asleep for extended periods.

Clinical Pearl

Much of human biology and behavior fluctuates with a temporal period close to the 24-hour cycle of day and night, and these fluctuations are called circadian rhythms. *Defining the properties of human circadian rhythms requires complex experimental paradigms that are at the heart of chronobiologic research. Studies following these paradigms now show the endogenous circadian pacemaker to have a period length of 24.18 hours, similar to that of many mammals. Human circadian rhythms are flexible and can adapt, for example, to very long (14-hour) nights by suppressing cortisol longer, secreting melatonin longer, and dropping temperature for a more extended period.*

REFERENCES

1. Czeisler CA, Duffy JF, Shanahan TL, et al: Stability, precision, and near-24-hour period of the human circadian pacemaker. Science 1999;284:2177-2181.
2. Weitzman ED, Czeisler CA, Zimmerman JC, Ronda JM: Timing of REM and stages 3 + 4 sleep during temporal isolation in man. Sleep 1980;2:391-407.
3. Czeisler CA, Allan JS, Strogatz SH, et al: Bright light resets the human circadian pacemaker independent of the timing of the sleep-wake cycle. Science 1986;233:667-671.
4. Boivin DB, Duffy JF, Kronauer RE, Czeisler CA: Sensitivity of the human circadian pacemaker to moderately bright light. J Biol Rhythms 1994;9:315-331.
5. Boivin DB, Czeisler CA: Resetting of circadian melatonin and cortisol rhythms in humans by ordinary room light. Neuroreport 1998;9:779-782.
6. Waterhouse J, Minors D, Folkard S, et al: Light of domestic intensity produces phase shifts of the circadian oscillator in humans. Neurosci Lett 1998;245:97-100.
7. Campbell SS, Murphy PJ: Extraocular circadian phototransduction in humans. Science 1998;279:396-399.
8. Lushington K, Galka R, Sassi LN, et al: Extraocular light exposure does not phase shift saliva melatonin rhythms in sleeping subjects. J Biol Rhythms 2002;17:377-386.
9. Lindblom N, Hatonen T, Laakso M, et al: Bright light exposure of a large skin area does not affect melatonin or bilirubin levels in humans. Biol Psychiatry 2000;48:1098-1104.
10. Lindblom N, Heiskala H, Hatonen T, et al: No evidence for extraocular light induced phase shifting of human melatonin, cortisol and thyrotropin rhythms. Neuroreport 2000;11:713-717.
11. Hebert M, Martin SK, Eastman CI: Nocturnal melatonin secretion is not suppressed by light exposure behind the knee in humans. Neurosci Lett 1999;274:127-130.
12. Klerman EB, Rimmer DW, Dijk DJ, et al: Nonphotic entrainment of the human circadian pacemaker. Am J Physiol 1998;274:R991-R996.

13. Baehr EK, Fogg LF, Eastman CI: Intermittent bright light and exercise to entrain human circadian rhythms to night work. Am J Physiol 1999;277:R1598-R1604.
14. Redlin U, Mrosovsky N: Exercise and human circadian rhythms: what we know and what we need to know. Chronobiol Int 1997 Mar;14(2):221-9.
15. Duffy JF, Kronauer RE, Czeisler CA: Phase-shifting human circadian rhythms: Influence of sleep timing, social contact and light exposure. J Physiol (Lond) 1996;495:289-297.
16. Mistlberger RE: Circadian food anticipatory activity: Formal models and physiological mechanisms. Neurosci Biobehav Rev 1994;18:1-25.
17. Herzog ED, Huckfeldt RM: Circadian entrainment to temperature, but not light, in the isolated suprachiasmatic nucleus. J Neurophysiol 2003;90:763-770.
18. Buxton OM, L'Hermite-Baleriaux M, Turek FW, van Cauter E: Daytime naps in darkness phase shift the human circadian rhythms of melatonin and thyrotropin secretion. Am J Physiol 2000;278:R373-R382.
19. Lockley SW, Skene DJ, James K, et al: Melatonin administration can entrain the free-running circadian system of blind subjects. J Endocrinol 2000;164:R1-R6.
20. Mills JN: Circadian rhythms during and after three months in solitude underground. J Physiol (Lond) 1964;174:217.
21. Waterhouse J, Minors D, Folkard S, et al: Lack of evidence that feedback from lifestyle alters the amplitude of the circadian pacemaker in humans. Chronobiol Int 1999;16:93-107.
22. Arendt J: Complex effects of melatonin. Therapie 1998;53:479-488.
23. Borbely AA, Achermann P: Sleep homeostasis and models of sleep regulation. J Biol Rhythms 1999;14:557-568.
24. Akerstedt T, Hume K, Minors D, Waterhouse J: Experimental separation of time of day and homeostatic influences on sleep. Am J Physiol 1998;274:R1162-R1168.
25. Van Dongen HP, Dinges DF: Investigating the interaction between the homeostatic and circadian processes of sleep-wake regulation for the prediction of waking neurobehavioural performance. J Sleep Res 2003;12:181-187.
26. Lewy AJ, Cutler NL, Sack RL: The endogenous melatonin profile as a marker for circadian phase position. J Biol Rhythms 1999;14:227-236.
27. Reebs SG, Mrosovsky N: Large phase-shifts of circadian rhythms caused by induced running in a re-entrainment paradigm: the role of pulse duration and light. J Comp Physiol [A] 1989;165:819-825.
28. Rosenwasser AM, Dwyer SM: Circadian phase shifting: Relationships between photic and nonphotic phase response curves. Physiol Behav 2001;73:175-183.
29. Minors DS, Waterhouse JM, Wirz-Justice A: A human phase-response curve to light. Neurosci Lett 1991;133:36-40.
30. Jewett ME, Rimmer DW, Duffy JF, et al: Human circadian pacemaker is sensitive to light throughout subjective day without evidence of transients. Am J Physiol 1997;273:R1800-R1809.
31. Webb WB, Agnew HW: Sleep efficiency for sleep-wake cycles of varied length. Psychophysiology 1975;12:637-641.
32. Weitzman ED, Nogeire C, Perlow M, et al: Effects of a prolonged 3-hour sleep-wake cycle on sleep stages. plasma cortisol, growth hormone and body temperature in man. J Clin Endocrinol Metab 1974;38:1018-1030.
33. Carskadon MA, Dement WC: Sleep studies on a 90-minute day. Electroencephalogr Clin Neurophysiol 1975;39:145-155.
34. Carskadon MA, Dement WC: Distribution of REM sleep on a 90-minute sleep wake schedule. Sleep 1980;2:309-317.
35. Dijk D, Czeisler C: Paradoxical timing of the circadian rhythm of sleep propensity serves to consolidate sleep and wakefulness in humans. Neurosci Lett 1994;166:63-68.
36. Weitzman ED, Moline ML, Czeisler CA, Zimmerman JC: Chronobiology of aging: Temperature, sleep-wake rhythms and entrainment. Neurobiol Aging 1982;3:299.
37. Aschoff J, Wever R: Spontaneous period of human sleep without zeitgebers. Naturwissenschaften 1962;49:337-342.
38. Shochat T, Luboshitzky R, Lavie P: Nocturnal melatonin onset is phase locked to the primary sleep gate. Am J Physiol 1997;273:R364-R370.
39. Wyatt JK, Cecco AR, Czeisler CA, Dijk DJ: Circadian temperature and melatonin rhythms, sleep, and neurobehavioral function in humans living on a 20-h day. Am J Physiol 1999;277:R1152-R1163.
40. Dijk DJ, Duffy JF, Czeisler CA: Circadian and sleep/wake dependent aspects of subjective alertness and cognitive performance. J Sleep Res 1992;1:112-117.
41. Wehr TA, Aeschbach D, Duncan WC: Evidence for a biological dawn and dusk in the human circadian timing system. J Physiol (Lond) 2001;535:937-951.
42. Barbato G, Barker C, Bender C, Wehr TA: Spontaneous sleep interruptions during extended nights: Relationships with NREM and REM sleep phases and effects on REM sleep regulation. Clin Neurophysiol 2002;113:892-900.
43. Carskadon MA, Labyak SE, Acebo C, Seifer R: Intrinsic circadian period of adolescent humans measured in conditions of forced desynchrony. Neurosci Lett 1999;260:129-132.
44. Wehr TA, Aeschbach D, Duncan WC: Evidence for a biological dawn and dusk in the human circadian timing system. J Physiol 2001;535(Pt 3):937-951.
45. Fei GH, Liu RY, Zhang ZH, Zhou JN: Alterations in circadian rhythms of melatonin and cortisol in patients with bronchial asthma. Acta Pharmacol Sin 2004;25:651-656.

Index

Note: Page numbers followed by f refer to figures; page numbers followed by t refer to tables; page numbers followed by b refer to text in shaded boxes.

A

Abdominal movement. *See also* Rib cage movement.
  chest movement with, in central sleep apnea evaluation, 978
  during NREM sleep, 235
  during REM sleep, 238
The Abnormalities of Sleep in Man, 8
Abulia
  after stroke, 822
  fatigue vs., 1225
Accidents, sleep-related. *See also* Motor vehicle accidents, sleep-related; Transportation safety.
  among shift workers
    caffeine use and, 486
    due to sleep deprivation, 649
    on graveyard shift, 47
  insomnia-related, 706
  Maintenance of Wakefulness Test and, 1420
  modern societal changes and, 648-649
  peak hours of, 650
  with daytime sleepiness, 47
Accreditation Council for Graduate Medical Education (ACGME), regulation of medical resident hours by, 652
Acetazolamide
  for central sleep apnea, 979
    in heart failure, 1215
  for high altitude sleep disturbances, 251-252, 251f-252f
Acetylcholine
  in dreaming, 554
  in REM sleep atonia, 128, 129f
  in schizophrenia, 1331
  in waking, 137f, 142-143
Acetylcholine antagonist(s), brainstem-thalamic effects of, 111, 117
Acid clearance, esophageal, 1258-1259, 1456-1457, 1457f. *See also* Gastroesophageal reflux (GER).
Acromegaly
  etiology of, 1237
  narcolepsy associated with, 1239
  obstructive sleep apnea associated with, 640
  sleep apnea in
    disease activity and, 1238-1239
    epidemiology of, and risk factors for, 1237, 1238f
    growth hormone deficiency in, 1239
    morbidity and mortality in, 1239
    pathogenesis of, 1237-1238, 1238f
ACTH. *See* Adrenocorticotrophic hormone (ACTH).
Actigraphy, 1459-1465
  advantages of, 1460-1462
  background of, 1459-1461, 1460f
  bands for, 1463, 1463f
  editing of data from, 1464, 1464f
  for treatment effects assessment, 1462
  in advanced sleep phase syndrome, 694f-695f, 697
  in cancer-related sleep disruption, 1219
  in children, 1462
  in circadian rhythm studies, 1462

Actigraphy *(Continued)*
  in delayed sleep phase syndrome, 693, 694f-695f
  in epidemiologic studies, 1463
  in idiopathic hypersomnia, 795
  in insomnia assessment, 711, 1414, 1461
  in older adults, 1462
  in periodic limb movements during sleep, 1461-1462
  in schizophrenia, 1462
  in sleep apnea, 1461
  light sensing by, 1464
  limitations of, 1464
  logs for, 1463
  reliability and validation of, 1460, 1464
  signal digitization in, 1460, 1460f
  technique of, 1463-1464, 1463f-1464f
Action potentials, of motoneurons, 157f, 158, 158f
Activating system. *See* Brainstem reticular formation, ascending activating system of.
Activation-Deactivation Adjective Check List (AD-ACL), 435
Activation-input-modulation model, of dreaming, 554
Activation synthesis model, of dreaming, 554, 561, 905
Active sleep. *See* Rapid eye movement (REM) sleep.
Activity. *See* Exercise.
Adaptive nonresponding, in immobilization theory, 97
Adaptive pressure support servoventilation (APSSV)
  for central sleep apnea, in heart failure, 1214
  for stroke-related breathing disorders, 817
Adenosine
  aging effects on, 28
  in homeostatic sleep regulation, 42
  in nitric oxide synthase production, 261
  in slow wave sleep, 145
  sleep homeostasis hypothesis and, 300
  sleep-promoting role of, 178-179
Adenosine receptor(s), caffeine as antagonist of, 479
Adolescents
  breathing patterns of, during sleep, 240
  bruxism in, management of, 955b
  sleep deprivation effects in, 653
  sleep in, gender differences in, 1268-1269
Adrenergic uptake inhibition, effect on antidepressants, in narcolepsy with cataplexy, 763t, 763-764
Adrenocorticotrophic hormone (ACTH)
  plasma measures of, in hyperarousal, 715-716
  release of, suprachiasmatic nucleus regulation of, 345
  sex differences in, 1267t
Adults
  older. *See* Age/aging.
  sleep in, gender differences in, 1269-1270
  young
    pattern of sleep in, 17-19, 18f
    sleep deprivation effects in, 61, 62t, 653

Advanced sleep phase syndrome (ASPS), 696-698
  clinical features of, 693f, 696
  clock gene alleles in, 370
  depression and, 1317
  diagnosis of, 697
  epidemiology of, 696
  idiopathic hypersomnia vs., 797
  light therapy for, 697, 1432, 1433f
  pathogenesis of, 696-697
  treatment of, 697
Aerophagia, in noninvasive positive-pressure ventilation, 1151
Affect, aroused negative, reduction of, by normal dreaming, 567-571
African Americans
  genetics of obstructive sleep apnea in, 1016, 1017
    linkage analysis of, 1018-1019
  hot flash occurrence in, 1289
  insomnia risk in, 706
  narcolepsy and, HLA DQA1*0102 and DQB1*0602 genes in, 765, 766f, 766t-767t
  OSA-related hypertension in, 1195
Age/aging, 24-36
  accelerated, in Alzheimer's disease, 854
  as interindividual variable, in circadian rhythm, 438
  body temperature rhythms in, 299
  breathing effects of, during sleep, 240
  bruxism risk and, 947
  chronologic vs. physiologic age, 24
  circadian desynchronization due to, dream effects of, 545
  circadian rhythms and
    deterioration of, 331-332
    during menopause, 1288-1289
    melatonin in regulation of, 400
    misalignment of, 428
    physiologic changes in, 29-31, 30f
    sleep homeostasis interaction with, 428, 429f
    sleep-wake regulation and, 389, 389f
  corticotropin activity and, 269
  dementia and cognitive impairment in, 24
  dream content and, 527-528
  falls in, due to benzodiazepines, 754
  in pain-related sleep disturbance, 1247
  insomnia and. *See* Insomnia, in older adults.
  napping and sleepiness in, 35-36
  nightmare occurrence and, 928
  nocturnal cardiac risk associated with, 1167
  OSA-related hypertension and, 1195
  pain perception related to, 1249
  penile erectile dysfunction related to, 1398
  periodic limb movements and, 32
  restless legs syndrome and, 32, 840
  shift work and, 675-676
  sleep alterations in
    actigraphy in, 1461, 1462
    decline of sleep quality in, 1289
    endocrine function effects of, 277-279, 278f
    in eating disorders, 1339
    in mood disorders, 1316
  sleep architecture and, 25-28, 25t-26t, 26f-27f